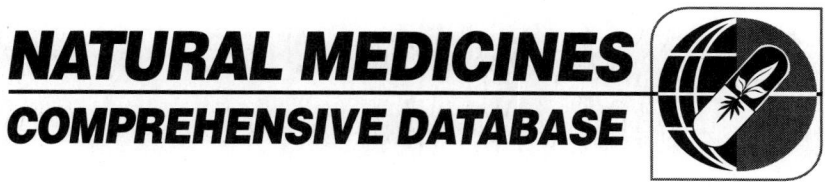

NATURAL MEDICINES
COMPREHENSIVE DATABASE

Fourth Edition

Published by: **Therapeutic Research Faculty**

3120 W. March Lane • P.O. Box 8190 • Stockton CA 95208
phone (209) 472-2244 • fax (209) 472-2249
Mail@NaturalDatabase.com • www.NaturalDatabase.com

Compiled by the Editors of:

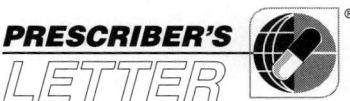 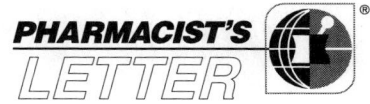

When referencing this *Database*, use the following format for the citation:

Jellin JM, Gregory PJ, Batz F, Hitchens, K, et al. *Pharmacist's Letter/ Prescriber's Letter Natural Medicines Comprehensive Database*. 4th ed. Stockton, CA: Therapeutic Research Faculty; 2002:pg xx-xx.

The authors have attempted to compile a comprehensive database of clinically important data on natural medicines. Errors, inaccuracies, or omissions are always possible in a work of this sort. The publisher assumes no responsibility for any patient care based on the application of the data contained in this database. Health professionals who use this database must rely on their own judgment before applying this data to any specific medical situation. People who are not health professionals should seek appropriate professional guidance on the use of any medicinal agent before using it.

For information on obtaining additional copies of this edition, or to receive a subscription to the printed version or the Web version of *Pharmacist's Letter/ Prescriber's Letter Natural Medicines Comprehensive Database*
see the last pages of this book, or contact:
Therapeutic Research Faculty, 3120 W. March Lane,
PO Box 8190, Stockton, CA 95208
TEL: 209-472-2244 • FAX: 209-472-2249
E-MAIL: mail@NaturalDatabase.com • WEBSITE: www.NaturalDatabase.com

Printed in the United States of America
ISBN #0-9676136-6-3

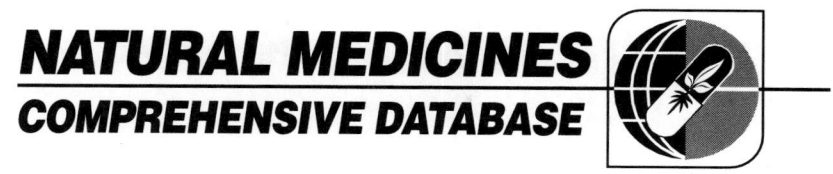

Table of Contents

Research and Writing Team 1

How to get data from this *Database* 4

Data on Natural Medicines 11

References 1385

Brand Names Index 1561

Chart: Herbs and Supplements with Therapeutic Efficacy 1821

Chart: Drug/Natural Medicines Interactions 1836

Chart: Natural Medicines/Drug Interactions 1853

Chart: Drug Influences on Nutrient Levels and Depletion 1869

General Index 1879

Natural Medicines Comprehensive Database Team

EDITOR
Jeff M. Jellin, Pharm.D.
  Editor, *Pharmacist's Letter*
  Editor, *Prescriber's Letter*

ASSOCIATE EDITOR
Philip J. Gregory, Pharm.D.
  Associate Editor, *Pharmacist's Letter*
  Associate Editor, *Prescriber's Letter*
  Director of Natural Medicines

CONTRIBUTING EDITORS
Forrest Batz, Pharm.D.
Robert Bonakdar, M.D.

RESEARCHERS & WRITERS
Gayle Nicholas Scott, Pharm.D., BCPS
Mary Birchfield, Pharm.D.
Judith Marshall, R.Ph.
Jennifer Obenrader, Pharm.D.
Kathy Hitchens, Pharm.D., MSBA
Jacintha Cauffield, Pharm.D., BCPS
Camene Wilson, Pharm.D.
Nicole Howard, Pharm.D.
Marie Mulligan, M.D.
Ben Mills, M.D., M.P.H.
James Ables, Pharm.D.
John Cathey, M.S., Pharm.
Gary Holt, R.Ph., Ph.D.
Paul Roberts, R.Ph.
Neeta O'Mara, Pharm.D., BCPS
Lynn Limon, Pharm.D.
John Morozumi, Pharm.D.
Loan Cat, Pharm.D.
Gary Choy, Pharm.D.
Tina Madej, R.Ph.
Sandra Downing, Pharm.D.
Lori Kolczak, R.Ph.

EDITORIAL REVIEW
Dan Perri, B.Sc.Phm, M.D.
  McMaster University
Barbara Miller, Pharm.D.
  Kaiser Permanente
Vivian Dickerson, M.D.
  Samueli Center for Complementary & Alternative Medicine
  University of California, Irvine
Cyndey McQueen, Pharm.D.
  Clinical Assistant Professor
  University of Missouri, Kansas City
Wadie Najm, M.D.
  Samueli Center for Complementary & Alternative Medicine
  University of California, Irvine
Shiraz Mishra, M.D., Ph.D.
  Samueli Center for Complementary & Alternative Medicine
  University of California, Irvine
Kevin Clausen, Pharm.D.
  Natural Products Research Fellow
  University of Missouri, Kansas City

Stephen McKernan, BS Pharm, N.D., D.O.
Ben Mills, M.D., M.P.H.
Mary Wilson, Ph.D., R.D.
Todd Reynolds, M.D.
Vincent Ferrari, BS Pharm.
Richard Filice, R.Ph.
John Weeks, M.D.
Joe Pepping, Pharm.D.
  Kaiser Permanente

SPECIAL CONSULTANTS
Karen Davidson, Pharm.D.
  Senior Associate Editor, *Pharmacist's Letter*
  Senior Associate Editor, *Prescriber's Letter*
Stephen C. Burson, R.Ph.
  Associate Editor, *Pharmacist's Letter*
  Associate Editor, *Prescriber's Letter*
  Director of Continuing Education
Kimberly Palacioz, Pharm.D.
  Assistant Editor, *Pharmacist's Letter*
  Assistant Editor, *Prescriber's Letter*
Kay A. Shaver, Pharm.D.
  Assistant Editor, *Pharmacist's Letter*
  Assistant Editor, *Prescriber's Letter*

DATABASE COORDINATORS
Linda Hneitina
Haydee Gobert

PROJECT MANAGEMENT
Timothy Swaim
  Editorial Project Manager
Shelby Butler
  Editorial Assistant

WEB SITE MANAGEMENT
Karen Wilson
  Web Editor
David Prothero
  Director of Information Technology
Mike Acosta
  Database Engineer
Jon Rombough
  Web Engineer
Russ Johnson
  Network Manager

STAFF
Dennis Himes, Director	Danae Harris
Daisy Plovnick, Director	Don Jacobsen
Lisa Shawhan, Manager	Connie Johnson
Georgene Albertini	Olga Oback
Myleen Arcangel	Gloria Rios
Rhonda Bigelow	Neng Vang
Jocosa Bottemiller	Patrice Verhines
Estella Freeman	Kathy Webb
Jan Garr	Tim Williams
Tillie Giovannetti	David Yanez

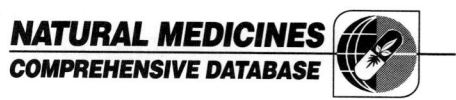

Dear Practitioner:

This 4th edition marks a milestone for the *Natural Medicines Comprehensive Database*.

The first edition was released in September 1999 when few reliable resources existed. There were high hopes for German Commission E, but clinicians found that it fell short of expectations...no references, questionable information, and outdated. Lots of new books were hitting the market. Biased authors or heavy reliance on German Commission E tainted most. *Natural Medicines Comprehensive Database* was a welcome newcomer ...comprehensive...up-to-date...evidence-based...totally unbiased. Plus it was created by the trusted editors of *Pharmacist's Letter* and *Prescriber's Letter*...seasoned drug information professionals with more than 18 years of experience.

Since that time, the *Natural Medicines Comprehensive Database* has grown not only in volume, but also in recognition. It is now recognized as the scientific gold standard for evidence-based information on this topic. Leaders in conventional medicine as well as complementary, alternative, and integrative medicine recognize the *Database* as the go-to resource for the most complete and practical information.

Some things have changed in this edition. The *Database* still provides all of the clinically relevant information in the same easy-to-use format, but we have added a lot of new info. Hundreds of monographs have been updated with tons of new references...more than 2000 since the last edition. We've also added lots of new practical data...new drug interactions...new safety concerns...and many Effectiveness Ratings have been raised or lowered based on new findings. We've also added more than 1500 new brand name listings.

This edition also contains expanded charts. A new chart provides a disease state index so that finding natural medicines with an Effectiveness Rating for a certain condition is a snap. We've also expanded the drug-herb and herb-drug interaction charts to be more comprehensive.

This 4th edition includes updates made to the Web version since the 3rd edition was printed. Our team updates the Web version literally every day. Research is now booming in this subject area. We continue to add huge amounts of new data...5-10 new studies every day of the week.

The Web version gives users the latest updated data along with easy-to-use and comprehensive search features. For the latest information go to www.NaturalDatabase.com.

We have also created a brand new database and web site specifically for patients. This gives patients reliable information in patient-friendly wording based on *Natural Medicines Comprehensive Database*. The content of the patient-oriented web site is integrated into the professional web site so health professionals who use www.NaturalDatabase.com can print the patient education info for a patient at any time.

If you are a new user of the *Natural Medicines Comprehensive Database*, please take a moment to read the following pages. They explain how each monograph is laid out and how you can use each section to answer your questions.

We hope you enjoy this new edition. If you have suggestions, comments, or inquiries, please don't hesitate to contact us: e-mail: mail@NaturalDatabase.com; phone: (209) 472-2244.

Sincerely,

Jeff M. Jellin

Jeff M. Jellin, PharmD
Editor

How to Get Data From
Natural Medicines Comprehensive Database

Monograph Name

Every one of the 1000+ monographs in the *Natural Medicines Comprehensive Database* is given a name based on the most widely used or most recognized name. These appear in ALL CAPS at the top of every monograph.

Also Known As

Most herbal and non-herbal natural medicines go by a variety of names. The most common name is chosen as the name of the monograph. Other colloquial, non-scientific names are included in this section and indexed at the end of the book. This makes finding a natural medicine by any of its names quick and easy.

In many cases, different natural medicines may have similar sounding names. For example, there are numerous varieties of ginseng: Siberian ginseng, American ginseng, Panax ginseng, and others. The *Database* has a separate monograph for each of these. This section will alert you when there are other monographs that have similar names.

Scientific Names

This section contains all botanical, chemical, or other scientific names. Often there is not just one botanical name for a plant. In these cases, we have provided as many botanical names as are known. We have also included any synonyms. For plants, a family name is also listed.

People Use This For

There are a wide variety of uses for most natural medicines. However, not all uses have been validated through clinical study. In this field, ALL known uses are listed without regard for effectiveness. A use listing in this section does NOT mean the product is effective for that use. Efficacy is discussed in the Effectiveness section (see below).

Safety

For each natural medicine in the *Database* you get an evidence-based safety rating.

These are PRACTICAL ratings that are STANDARDIZED throughout the *Natural Medicines Comprehensive Database*.

You will see that different uses of a product often get different safety ratings. For example, camphor is rated "LIKELY SAFE" when used topically, but it is rated "UNSAFE" when used orally.

Questions often come up about using products during pregnancy or lactation, or in children. If there are safety considerations that apply specifically to children, a special mention in the safety field will address the concern. Every listing includes a rating for safety in PREGNANCY and LACTATION.

Our team has been very meticulous in analyzing the medical literature to assign the safety ratings. Each rating is assigned according to specific criteria:

> **LIKELY SAFE** = The product has undergone a rigorous scientific evaluation equivalent to a review by the FDA, Health Canada, or other governmental authority and has been found to be safe when used appropriately. Or reputable references generally agree that the product is safe when used appropriately based on two or more randomized, controlled, clinical trials involving several hundred to several thousand patients and published in refereed journals; or based on large-scale post-marketing surveillance showing a low incidence of significant adverse effects.

POSSIBLY SAFE = Reputable references agree that the product might be safe when used appropriately, and there are human studies reporting no serious adverse effects.

POSSIBLY UNSAFE = There is some evidence suggesting that use of the product might be unsafe.

LIKELY UNSAFE = Reputable references agree that the product can be harmful, based on human studies or reliable case reports of significant adverse effects.

UNSAFE = The product has undergone a rigorous scientific evaluation or a review by a reliable regulatory agency and found to often cause clinically significant harm to humans. Or large-scale post-marketing surveillance shows a high incidence of significant adverse effects.

Effectiveness

For each natural medicine in the *Database* you get an evidence-based effectiveness rating.

These are PRACTICAL ratings that are STANDARDIZED throughout the *Natural Medicines Comprehensive Database.*

The "effectiveness" rating differs depending on the use, so you will often see more than one rating for a product.

Our team has been very meticulous in analyzing the medical literature to assign the efficacy ratings. Each product is rated by the following scale:

EFFECTIVE = The product has passed a rigorous scientific review equivalent to a review by the FDA, Health Canada, or other governmental authority and has been found to be effective for a specific indication as an OTC drug, orphan drug, or prescription drug product.

LIKELY EFFECTIVE = Reputable references generally agree that the product is effective for the given indication, based on two or more randomized, controlled, clinical trials involving several hundred to several thousand patients, giving positive results for clinically relevant end-points and published in established, refereed journals.

POSSIBLY EFFECTIVE = Reputable references suggest that the product might work for the given indication based on one or more clinical trials giving positive results for clinically relevant end-points.

POSSIBLY INEFFECTIVE = Reputable references suggest that the product might not work for the given indication based on one human study giving negative results for clinically relevant end-points.

LIKELY INEFFECTIVE = Reputable references generally agree that the product is not effective for the given indication, based on two or more randomized, controlled, clinical trials giving negative results for clinically relevant end-points and published in established, refereed journals.

INEFFECTIVE = Most reputable references agree that the product is not effective for the given indication, or multiple high-quality studies resulted in negative results; there are no equally reliable human studies offering convincing contradictory data.

When possible, we have included one very useful bit of information in this Effectiveness section...the SPECIFIC FORMULA OR EXTRACT that was used in studies that found the product to be effective or ineffective.

This information is not easily found elsewhere, but it is very important.

For example, a significant study was published in the *Journal of the American Medical Association* providing evidence that ginkgo has a positive role in delaying the progression of Alzheimer's disease. Its effects have been likened to *Aricept*. Many published works, and many ginkgo manufacturers have since stated ginkgo's effectiveness in this area.

But this information is not useful without knowing what formulation of ginkgo was shown to have a positive effect.

The *Natural Medicines Comprehensive Database* states that the formulations of ginkgo that contain Egb 761 (Tanakan) or LI 1370 (Lichtwer Pharma), consisting of 24-25% flavone glycosides and 6% terpene lactones, are the formulations in the prominent studies that were shown to have beneficial effect. It cannot be inferred from this that other formulations of ginkgo will also have the same effect.

Mechanism of Action and Active Ingredients

In this field you will find a description of the known constituents...and pharmacological actions that might be attributable to these constituents. Keep in mind that most of the natural products are used because people have observed, or think they observed, some benefit to using the product. In many cases there has been relatively little scientific inquiry into the active ingredients and the exact mechanism of action. Also recognize that most herbal medicines are combinations of many constituents. It is quite possible that herbal medicines work by the combined effects of multiple constituents, and the concept of identifying a single specific active ingredient is flawed. Even when a single, specific active ingredient is identified, it is possible that other active ingredients may be discovered later. For example, authorities used to think that St. John's wort exerted its effect due to hypericin content. More recent findings suggest that maybe hyperforin exerts significant activity.

Adverse Reactions

In this field you get information about all the known adverse reactions and side effects associated with the product. These are typically derived from the side effects reported in clinical trials and from reliable case reports regarding adverse effects.

In some cases, certain adverse reactions are suspected based on pharmacological properties of the product. Information about suspected adverse reactions and documented adverse reactions is clearly distinguished.

Known allergies are also listed. This can help you anticipate potential problems. For example, people who are allergic to one herb coming from the asteraceae family might also be allergic to other herbs in the same family.

Interactions

There are five separate fields listing different categories of possible interactions. For each product, this *Database* lists possible interactions with...

> Herbs and Other Dietary Supplements
> Drugs
> Foods
> Lab Tests
> Diseases and Conditions

This is a very important part of the *Database*. There are hundreds of potential interactions...and many practitioners are not on the look-out for them. The usual computerized checking systems do not have all this info in their systems...and patients do not recognize the potential problems like they do with regular drugs. To use the information in these interaction fields, it is important to understand the origin of the data. In some cases, it comes from documented reports. In other cases, the data are theoretical, based on the pharmacological profile of the natural medicine. For example, horse chestnut seed contains coumarin derivatives and theoretically increases bleeding time. At this point in time there are very few well-documented interactions. Much of the information regarding potential interactions is theoretical. A synopsis of documented reports and theoretical predictions appears in this field. We have also prepared a separate pair of charts in the back of the book to give you a listing of the potential interactions between drugs and natural medicines.

Nutrient Depletion

Some nutrients are thought to be depleted from the body by certain drugs. Data about nutrient depletion appear in this field. This is the only field in the *Database* that appears ONLY for those natural medicines that are involved in nutrient depletion interactions. Most of these include vitamins and minerals. The natural medicines listed in this *Database* are typically the substances that are being depleted, and are not the entities causing the depletion. For this reason, the editors have chosen to only list this field when there are important data to present.

Dosage and Administration

The dosages in this field are not necessarily recommended doses, safe doses, or efficacious doses. If clinical trials have been conducted, then the doses used in the studies are listed. Other doses listed are the common or traditional doses or those typically used in supplements. Many products included in this *Database* may not be safe or effective. This needs to be considered even when a typical dose is listed.

Comments

This field presents a potpourri of info. For example, the comments on Siberian ginseng point out that it is a completely different herb than American or Panax ginseng. American or Panax ginseng is considerably more expensive. It is said that the Soviet Union wanted to provide its athletes with any advantage offered by ginseng but wanted a less expensive version. Therefore, Siberian ginseng became popular, and this is why most studies on Siberian ginseng are written in Russian.

Scattered throughout the *Database* you will see statements like, "Insufficient reliable information available." This means that data do not exist, or the literature is too contradictory, or the studies are not of high enough quality. This information is valuable because it is important for practitioners to know what is NOT known. Many references state that certain products are effective or safe when data do not exist to support this conclusion. This *Database* states when there is insufficient information to meet the reliability standards of this *Database*.

References

This *Database* is thoroughly referenced with thousands of reference citations. In each monograph you will see numbers in parentheses appearing at the end of statements. These refer to reference citations that are listed in the back of the book in numerical order. The fact that so many references were used to create this *Database* allows this *Database* to be both a scientific consensus of clinical information and a comprehensive collection of data on natural medicines.

Brand Names Listing

There are really two separate databases of natural products within the *Natural Medicines Comprehensive Database*. There is a compilation of over 1000 monographs on natural medicines or ingredients. There is another database consisting of several thousand brand name products and their ingredients. Each brand name listing provides the name of the manufacturer and all of the ingredients. This information is towards the back of the book following the reference citations.

Within the Brand Name listing, you will sometimes find the term "**Editor's Comment.**" In these instances there will be some important commentary from the editors related to the particular brand name product. For example, the listing of all the ingredients in a brand name product may serve to answer some questions about the product, but the use of all these ingredients in COMBINATION form may require additional commentary. Or there may be some data related to this particular brand that the editors wish for you to know about. For example, some brand name products contain substances derived from animal organs. Since there is some theoretical risk of contamination with diseased animal tissue (e.g., mad cow disease), our editors have included an "Editor's Comment" about this risk.

Keep in mind that manufacturers can change the ingredients of their brand name products at any time. This has been creating problems for years. Remember when *Ex-Lax* contained phenolphthalein? Some people did not realize that it was changed to contain sennosides and docusate sodium. The same thing happens frequently with natural medicines.

"Tell The Editors" form

It is unrealistic to believe that all clinicians, researchers, and other experts will always agree with every statement in this *Database*. The Editors recognize that new information is surfacing all the time and new interpretations develop all the time. A team of researchers and editors work full-time to constantly update this *Database*. These editors respect intelligent differences of opinion, and in fact, invite and encourage any professional user of this *Database* to share new knowledge, or new interpretations with us. If you recommend a change to any statement in this *Database*, please use the form at the back of the book and send it to us. Please include the reference citation. The Editors review all suggestions. We thank you for helping to make this the best resource possible.

General Index

There are a couple different ways you can find data on a particular product in this *Database*. One way is to just flip to the listing…it's all in alphabetical order based on the most common name. If you don't see a listing for the product you want, you can use the index in the back of the book. The index is very complete. It allows you to search by scientific name, common names, and botanical name of every product in the *Database*. Keep in mind that the index does NOT include brand names. These are listed in the brand name section in alphabetical order.

Differences between the Book and Web versions of
Natural Medicines Comprehensive Database

Everything in this Book version of the *Database* is also contained in the Web site (www.NaturalDatabase.com). In addition, the Web version has added features and information.

Updates

The Web version of the *Database* is updated daily. Our team of editors and researchers work full-time to constantly add new, practical data. This allows users to quickly find answers to all the questions their patients are asking about the latest products and latest hype. The info on the Web version is periodically downloaded to create the Book version.

Searchability

Users of the Web version can quickly search the entire *Database* for whatever they are looking for. The advanced search helps you quickly answer questions about drug interactions, side effects, Effectiveness Ratings for specific diseases, precautions for certain conditions, etc.

Patient Education

The Web version provides a full set of patient education handouts covering all of the monographs in the book. For each of the 1000+ monographs written for professionals, there is a corresponding patient education handout. This allows you to provide patient-friendly information to all of your patients interested in these products. Patient information is updated right along with the professional monographs so your patients get the most up-to-date information.

Research Abstracts

The *Natural Medicines Comprehensive Database* is a great clinical tool. It's also an efficient research tool. The *Database* is completely referenced with several thousand reference citations. For each citation that is indexed on MEDLINE, the Web version of the *Database* links directly to the original abstract.

Colleagues Interact

Connect with your colleagues. *Colleagues Interact* is an online discussion group that allows users to post questions and discuss interesting cases. Our editors routinely monitor *Colleagues Interact* and frequently provide answers to subscribers' questions. Subscribers to the Web version have access.

Whether you get the Book version, the Web version, or both depends on your specific needs. The Book version allows you to quickly flip through a few pages to find the answers you need. Some practitioners like to keep a copy handy so they can go over the info face-to-face with their patients.

The Web version offers the same great content with some additional capabilities that can only be made available in the dynamic online format.

Many practitioners choose to get BOTH the Book and Web versions...the best of both worlds.

5-HTP

Also Known As
5HTP, 5-hydroxytryptophan, L-5 HTP, Oxitriptan.
CAUTION: See separate listing for L-tryptophan.

Scientific Names
5-hydroxytryptophan; L-5 hydroxytryptophan.

People Use This For
Orally, 5-HTP is used for sleep disorders, depression, anxiety (915), migraine and tension-type headaches (2204), fibromyalgia (913), binge eating associated with obesity (914), attention deficit disorder (ADD) (913), cerebellar ataxia (916), Ramsey-Hunt syndrome (917), Down syndrome (5050), and as adjunctive therapy in seizure disorder and Parkinson's disease.
In combination with carbidopa, 5-HTP is used for treating intention myoclonus (1403,1404) and as an orphan drug for treating post-anoxia myoclonus.

Safety
POSSIBLY UNSAFE ...when used orally. There is a lot of controversy about the safety of 5-HTP. There is some concern that 5-HTP might cause eosinophilia myalgia syndrome (EMS) (902,919,3575,7067). However, there is speculation that only certain contaminated 5-HTP products can cause this serious adverse effect. So far, there is not enough evidence to know if EMS is caused by 5-HTP, contaminants, or other unknown factors (919,7067). Until more is known, advise patients against using 5-HTP.
PREGNANCY AND LACTATION: POSSIBLY UNSAFE ...when used orally (919); avoid using.

Effectiveness
LIKELY EFFECTIVE ...when used orally for treating post-anoxic myoclonus. Post-anoxic myoclonus, also known as Land-Adams Syndrome, is a rare complication of successful cardiopulmonary resuscitation (14).
POSSIBLY EFFECTIVE ...when used orally for depression (903,904,912,2203). 5-HTP seems to significantly improve symptoms of depression (903), including in patients with treatment resistant depression (904). There is some evidence that 5-HTP might be comparable to the conventional antidepressants fluvoxamine (Luvox) and imipramine (Tofranil) (904,2203). ...when used orally for fibromyalgia (913). ...when used orally for obesity (914). ...when used orally for anxiety (915). ...when used orally for cerebellar ataxia (916). ...when used orally for Ramsey-Hunt syndrome (917).
POSSIBLY INEFFECTIVE ...when used orally for Alzheimer's disease (918).
There is insufficient reliable information available to rate the effectiveness of 5-HTP for its other uses. However, there is some preliminary evidence that 5-HTP might help reduce pain in patients with chronic tension-type headaches (2204). More evidence is needed to rate 5-HTP for this use.

Mechanism of Action
5-Hydroxytryptophan (5-HTP) is related to both L-tryptophan and serotonin. In the body L-tryptophan is converted to 5-HTP, which can then be converted to serotonin. 5-HTP readily crosses the blood-brain barrier and increases central nervous system (CNS) synthesis of serotonin. Serotonin can affect sleep, appetite, temperature, sexual behavior, and pain sensation. Serotonin also has a significant role in depression, anxiety, and aggression (901). Since 5-HTP can increase synthesis of serotonin, 5-HTP is tried for several disease states where serotonin plays a significant role including depression, insomnia, obesity, and numerous other conditions.

Adverse Reactions
Orally, 5-HTP can cause gastrointestinal side effects such as heartburn, stomach pain, belching and flatulence, nausea, vomiting, diarrhea, and anorexia (2203). There is also concern that 5-HTP, like L-tryptophan, can cause asymptomatic eosinophilia and eosinophilia myalgia syndrome (EMS) (902,919,3575,7067). There is speculation that many commercial 5-HTP products can contain a contaminant called peak X, an impurity that might cause EMS (919). However, the presence of peak X or other contaminant has not been verified in all cases of EMS. So far there is not enough evidence to determine if 5-HTP, a contaminant, or some other factor is responsible for EMS (902,919,7067). Until more is known, tell patients to avoid taking 5-HTP supplements.

Interactions with Herbs & Other Dietary Supplements
Insufficient reliable information available.

Interactions with Drugs
CARBIDOPA: Combining 5-HTP and carbidopa can increase the risk of serotonergic side effects. Carbidopa is sometimes used with 5-HTP to minimize peripheral 5-HTP metabolism and boost the amount that reaches the brain.

But using the combination can increase the risk of developing hypomania, restlessness, rapid speech, anxiety, insomnia, and aggressiveness (14). Combining carbidopa plus 5-HTP might also cause an eosinophilia myalgia (EMS)-like syndrome including scleroderma-like skin changes (1403,1404). It is suspected that decreased 5-HTP metabolism and an increase in either serotonin or a metabolite kynurenine are responsible for this adverse effect (1403,1404).

SEROTONIN AGONISTS: Combining other serotonergic drugs with 5-HTP might increase the risk of serotonergic side effects such as serotonin syndrome. Some serotonergic drugs include monoamine oxidase inhibitors (MAOIs), reserpine, selective serotonin reuptake inhibitors (SSRIs), tricyclic, and atypical antidepressants (14).

SEROTONIN ANTAGONISTS: There is some concern that 5-HTP might inhibit the effectiveness of serotonin antagonists. Some of these drugs include methysergide and cyproheptadine (14).

Interactions with Foods
No interactions are known to occur, and there is no known reason to expect a clinically significant interaction with 5-HTP.

Interactions with Lab Tests
No interactions are known to occur, and there is no known reason to expect a clinically significant interaction with 5-HTP.

Interactions with Diseases or Conditions
DOWN SYNDROME: 5-HTP is reported to cause seizures in some patients with Down syndrome. In one case series, 15% of patients receiving long-term 5-HTP treatment experienced seizures (5050).

PEPTIC ULCERS, PLATELET DISORDERS, AND RENAL DISEASE: Some experts caution against using 5-HTP in people with these conditions (14). These cautions appear to be based on indirect reasoning using various in vitro and animal data. Currently, there are no reported animal or human studies to support these cautions.

Dosage and Administration
ORAL: For depression, the typical dose of 5-HTP is 150-300 mg daily (903,2203). For post-anoxic myoclonus, 5-HTP has an orphan drug status. The sponsor of the orphan drug is Circa Pharmaceuticals (1-516-842-8383).

Comments
5-HTP is often produced commercially from the seeds of the African plant Griffonia simplicfolia.

7-KETO-DHEA

Also Known As
3-acetyl-7-oxo-dehydroepiandrosterone, 3beta-acetoxy-androst-5-ene-7,17-dione, 5-androsten-3-beta-17-one-DHEA, 7-Keto, 7-keto dehydroepiandrosterone, 7 KETO DHEA, 7-keto DHEA, 7-ketodehydroepiandrostenedione, 7-ODA, 7-oxo-dehydroepiandrosterone-3-acetate, 7-oxo-DHEA, 7-oxo-DHEA-acetate, 7keto DHEA.
CAUTION: See separate listing for DHEA.

Scientific Names
3-acetyl-7-oxo-dehydroepiandrosterone; 3beta-acetoxy-androst-5-ene-7,17-dione.

People Use This For
Orally, 7-keto-DHEA is used to increase metabolism and thermogenesis and promote weight loss, to improve lean body mass and build muscle, to increase activity of the thyroid gland and immune system, to boost memory, and to reduce aging (5834,5835,5836).

Safety
There is insufficient reliable information available about the safety of 7-keto-DHEA.
Pregnancy and Lactation: Insufficient reliable information available; avoid using.

Effectiveness
There is insufficient reliable information available to rate the effectiveness of 7-keto-DHEA. However, there is preliminary evidence that 7-keto-DHEA might significantly decrease body weight and fat composition in obese female patients (5842). More evidence is needed to rate 7-keto-DHEA for this use.

Mechanism of Action
7-keto-DHEA is a metabolite of dehydroepiandrosterone (DHEA) which is formed in the body (5837).
Unlike DHEA, 7-keto-DHEA is not converted to androgens and estrogens (5837,5840,5842). 7-keto-DHEA is thought

to be beneficial in weight loss by increasing metabolism and thermogenesis. Early evidence in animals suggests 7-keto-DHEA can increase thermogenesis, possibly by stimulation of thermogenic enzymes in the liver (5837); however this effect has not yet been reported in humans. Clinical evidence suggests 7-keto-DHEA might increase basal metabolism. One study in obese subjects showed significant increases in thyroid hormone triiodothyronine (T3) when 7-keto-DHEA was used over 4 weeks (5842). Other preliminary studies have shown other effects. In one study in rats, 7-keto-DHEA improved chemically-induced and age-related memory impairment (5839). In another study, 7-keto-DHEA was reported have immunomodulatory effects by stimulating interleukin-2 production by human lymphocytes in vitro (5841).

Adverse Reactions
None reported.

Interactions with Herbs & Other Dietary Supplements
Insufficient reliable information available.

Interactions with Drugs
No interactions are known to occur, and there is no known reason to expect a clinically significant interaction with 7-keto-DHEA.

Interactions with Foods
No interactions are known to occur, and there is no known reason to expect a clinically significant interaction with 7-keto-DHEA.

Interactions with Lab Tests
No interactions are known to occur, and there is no known reason to expect a clinically significant interaction with 7-keto-DHEA.

Interactions with Diseases or Conditions
No interactions are known to occur, and there is no known reason to expect a clinically significant interaction with 7-keto-DHEA.

Dosage and Administration
ORAL: For weight loss, 100 mg twice daily was used in one study (5842).

Comments
None.

ABSCESS ROOT

Also Known As
American Greek Valerian, Blue Bells, False Jacob's Ladder, Sweatroot.
CAUTION: See separate listing for Jacob's Ladder.

Scientific Names
Polemonium reptans.
Family: Polemoniaceae.

People Use This For
Orally, abscess root is used to reduce fevers. It has also been used orally to reduce inflammation, stimulate sweating, as an astringent, and expectorant (18).

Safety
There is insufficient reliable information available about the safety of abscess root.
Pregnancy and Lactation: Insufficient reliable information available; avoid using.

Effectiveness
There is insufficient reliable information available about the effectiveness of abscess root.

Mechanism of Action

Abscess root contains triterpene saponins. These substances are from colloidal solutions in water that foam when they are shaken. They are often irritating to mucous membranes and could cause symptoms such as sneezing and GI irritation (18,4077).

Adverse Reactions

Orally, abscess root can irritate the GI tract. It might cause sneezing and GI upset (18,4077).

Interactions with Herbs & Other Dietary Supplements

Insufficient reliable information available.

Interactions with Drugs

No interactions are known to occur, and there is no known reason to expect a clinically significant interaction with abscess root.

Interactions with Foods

No interactions are known to occur, and there is no known reason to expect a clinically significant interaction with abscess root.

Interactions with Lab Tests

No interactions are known to occur, and there is no known reason to expect a clinically significant interaction with abscess root.

Interactions with Diseases or Conditions

No interactions are known to occur, and there is no known reason to expect a clinically significant interaction with abscess root.

Dosage and Administration

ORAL: A tea is made from the ground root (18).

Comments

Abscess root is also called false Jacob's ladder because it has astringent activity similar to Jacob's ladder (see separate listing). These two plants are used in similar ways, but differ chemically. Be cautious with use, because one can be confused with the other (18).

ABUTA

Also Known As

Bejunco de Cerca, Butua, False Pareira, Pareira, Patacon, Velvetleaf.
CAUTION: See separate listing for Pareira.

Scientific Names

Cissampelos pareira.
Family: Menispermaceae.

People Use This For

Orally, abuta is used for acne, asthma, dog bites, snake bites, boils, bronchitis, burns, chills, cholera, colds, colic, convulsions, coughs, cystitis, delirium, diabetes, diarrhea, dropsy, dysentery, dyspepsia, erysipelas, fertility in women, fevers, hematuria, hemorrhage, hypertension, itching, jaundice, leukorrhea, malaria, menorrhagia, nephritis, palpitation, parturition, purgative, rabies, rheumatism, sores, stimulating menstrual flow, stomachache, veneral diseases, wounds, a diuretic, expectorant, stimulant, styptic, tonic (513), for eye infections, nervous children, toothaches, and as an aphrodisiac (3913).

Safety

There is insufficient reliable information available about the safety of abuta.
Pregnancy and Lactation: Insufficient reliable information available; avoid using.

Effectiveness

There is insufficient reliable information available about the effectiveness of abuta.

Mechanism of Action

The applicable part of abuta is the bark. There is insufficient reliable information available about the possible mechanism of action and active ingredients.

Adverse Reactions

None reported.

Interactions with Herbs & Other Dietary Supplements

Insufficient reliable information available.

Interactions with Drugs

No interactions are known to occur, and there is no known reason to expect a clinically significant interaction with abuta.

Interactions with Foods

No interactions are known to occur, and there is no known reason to expect a clinically significant interaction with abuta.

Interactions with Lab Tests

No interactions are known to occur, and there is no known reason to expect a clinically significant interaction with abuta.

Interactions with Diseases or Conditions

No interactions are known to occur, and there is no known reason to expect a clinically significant interaction with abuta.

Dosage and Administration

ORAL: People typically use 1 to 2 grams of powdered abuta bark in tablets or capsules twice daily. Abuta is also taken as a 4:1 tincture in a dose of 2 to 4 mL twice daily (5255).

Comments

Avoid confusion with Abuta grandifolia, which is also referred to as abuta and is a South American medicinal plant used for making arrow poison and other curaré preparations (518).

There is very little scientific information about this product. Our staff is continually analyzing the available information on natural medicines and will add data here as it becomes available.

ACACIA

Also Known As

Gomme Arabique, Gomme de Senegal, Gum Acacia, Gum Arabic, Gum Senegal, Gummae Mimosae, Kher.
CAUTION: See separate listing for Cassie Absolute.

Scientific Names

Acacia senegal.
Family: Leguminosae or Fabaceae.

People Use This For

Orally, acacia is used to reduce cholesterol levels.
In manufacturing, it is used as a pharmaceutical ingredient in making emulsions, troches, a demulcent for throat or stomach inflammation, a masking agent for acrid substances (e.g., capsicum), and as a film forming agent in peel-off skin masks (11).

Safety

POSSIBLY SAFE ...when used orally (11).
PREGNANCY AND LACTATION: Insufficient reliable information available; avoid using.

Effectiveness

POSSIBLY INEFFECTIVE ...when used orally for reducing cholesterol levels. It may actually elevate serum or tissue cholesterol levels (11).

Mechanism of Action

The applicable part of acacia is the gum. Acacia gum consists mostly of arabic acid which becomes arabinose, galactose, and arabinosic acid when hydrolyzed. It is almost completely soluble in twice its weight of water (16).

Adverse Reactions

Allergy to acacia dust manifests as skin lesions and severe asthmatic attacks (11).

Interactions with Herbs & Other Dietary Supplements

Insufficient reliable information available.

Interactions with Drugs

ORAL DRUGS: The fiber in acacia can impair absorption of oral drugs (19).
ALKALOIDS: If mixed with certain alkaloids, acacia gum causes partial destruction of them. These alkaloids include atropine, hyoscyamine, scopolamine, homatropine, morphine, apomorphine, cocaine, and physostigmine (11).
IRON: Acacia can be gelatinized by solutions of ferric iron salts (19).
ETHYL ALCOHOL: Mixing acacia with a substance containing greater than 50% concentration of ethyl alcohol can cause acacia to become insoluble (19).

Interactions with Foods

ALCOHOL: Acacia gum used with alcohol or alcoholic solutions can cause precipitation from suspensions (16).

Interactions with Lab Tests

SERUM CHOLESTEROL: Theoretically, acacia might increase serum cholesterol concentrations and test results (11).

Interactions with Diseases or Conditions

No interactions are known to occur, and there is no known reason to expect a clinically significant interaction with acacia.

Dosage and Administration

ORAL: Acacia is usually dissolved in water to make a mucilage. The usual dose is 1 to 4 teaspoons (5263).

Comments

Avoid confusion with sweet acacia (Acacia farnesiana).

ACEROLA

Also Known As

Barbados Cherry, Puerto Rican Cherry, West Indian Cherry.
CAUTION: See separate listings for Cherokee Rosehip, Rose Hip, and Vitamin C.

Scientific Names

Malpidnia glabra; Malpidnia punicifolia.
Family: Malpighiaceae.

People Use This For

Orally, acerola is used to treat or prevent scurvy, colds, heart disease, cancer, pressure sores, retinal hemorrhages, tooth decay, gum infections, atherosclerosis, depression, hay fever, for preventing blood clots, collagen disorders, and to enhance physical endurance.

Safety

POSSIBLY SAFE ...when used orally (6,15).
PREGNANCY AND LACTATION: Insufficient reliable information available; avoid using.

Effectiveness

POSSIBLY EFFECTIVE ...when used orally to prevent scurvy (6,15).
There is insufficient reliable information available about the effectiveness of acerola for its other uses.

Mechanism of Action

The applicable part of acerola is the fruit. Acerola contains 1000-2330 mg of vitamin C per 100 grams (6). Vitamin C is an essential coenzyme required for normal metabolic function. It is important for collagen formation and tissue repair.

Vitamin C is involved in tyrosine metabolism, folic acid conversion, carbohydrate metabolism, synthesis of lipids and proteins, iron metabolism, resistance to infections, and cellular respiration. Vitamin C also acts as an antioxidant (6,15). It regenerates and restores oxidized vitamin E (127,128). However, the dry acerola fruit and powder are unlikely to be a good source of vitamin C because much of the vitamin C is destroyed during the drying and processing (2,11). Acerola fruit also contains vitamin A, thiamine, riboflavin, and niacin (6).

Adverse Reactions
Orally, the vitamin C in acerola can cause nausea, abdominal cramps, fatigue, insomnia, and sleepiness. Doses greater than 1 gram might cause diarrhea (15).

Interactions with Herbs & Other Dietary Supplements
VITAMIN C SUPPLEMENTS: Concomitant use interacts with the vitamin C in acerola and increases total dose of vitamin C which might increase the risk of adverse effects.

Interactions with Drugs
WARFARIN (Coumadin): Concomitant use interacts with the vitamin C in acerola and can reduce anticoagulant activity (506).
IRON: Concomitant use interacts with the vitamin C in acerola and increases GI absorption of iron in foods (ferric) but not from supplements (ferrous) (15).
ESTROGEN: Concomitant use interacts with the vitamin C in acerola and might increase absorption and effects (129,130).
FLUPHENAZINE (Prolixin): Concomitant use interacts with the vitamin C in acerola and decreases blood levels (15).
ACIDIC or BASIC DRUGS: Concomitant use interacts with the vitamin C in acerola and might acidify urine affecting excretion (15).

Interactions with Foods
No interactions are known to occur, and there is no known reason to expect a clinically significant interaction with acerola.

Interactions with Lab Tests
URINE GLUCOSE TESTS: Doses of vitamin C greater than 500 mg can cause false-decreases with glucose oxidase tests (e.g. Clinistix). The vitamin C in acerola might also cause false increases with cupric sulfate tests (e.g. Clinitest) (15).
STOOL OCCULT BLOOD TESTS: The vitamin C in acerola can cause false-negative results if it is ingested 48-72 hours before amine-dependent tests (506).

Interactions with Diseases or Conditions
GOUT: The vitamin C in acerola might increase uric acid levels (15).
KIDNEY STONE FORMING TENDENCY: The vitamin C in acerola in large doses might cause precipitation of urate, cystine, or oxalate stones (15).

Dosage and Administration
No typical dosage.

Comments
None.

ACETYL-L-CARNITINE

Also Known As
Acetyl L-Carnitine, Acetyl-Carnitine, Acetyl-Levocarnitine, Acetylcarnitine, ALC, Alcar, ALCAR, Carnitine Acetyl Ester, Gamma-Trimethyl-Beta-Acetylbutyrobetaine, L-acetylcarnitine, Levacecarnine, N-Acetyl-Carnitine, N-Acetyl-L-Carnitine, ST-200, Vitamin B(t) Acetate.
CAUTION: See separate listings for L-Carnitine and Propionyl-L-Carnitine.

Scientific Names
2-(acetyloxy)-3-carboxy-N,N,N-trimethyl-1-propanaminium inner salt; (3-carboxy-2-hydroxy-propyl)trimethylammonium hydroxide inner salt acetate.

People Use This For

Orally, acetyl-L-carnitine is used for Alzheimer's disease (14,1584,1586,3082), age-related memory deficits, senile depression, Down syndrome (1586,1588), alcoholism-related cognitive deficits (1589), cerebrovascular insufficiency after stroke (14), peripheral neuropathies (14), diabetic neuropathy, neuropathy due to anti-viral drugs used in the treatment of AIDS (1585), and facial paralysis (1590).

In combination with L-carnitine, fructose, and citric acid (in ProXeed), acetyl-L-carnitine is used to improve sperm quality in male infertility.

Intravenously, acetyl-L-carnitine is used for dementia (14) and cerebral ischemia (1591,1592).

Intramuscularly, acetyl-L-carnitine is used for peripheral neuropathy with pain (1593).

Safety

POSSIBLY SAFE ...when used orally and appropriately. Due to the limited data available, periodic monitoring of blood cell counts and liver and renal function has been recommended during acetyl-L-carnitine therapy (14). ...when used parenterally and appropriately under medical supervision.

PREGNANCY AND LACTATION: Insufficient reliable information available; avoid using.

Effectiveness

POSSIBLY EFFECTIVE ...when used orally for improving memory and slowing the rate of decline in Alzheimer's disease. Acetyl-L-carnitine might slow the rate of disease progression and improve some measures of cognitive function and behavioral performance in people with Alzheimer's disease. It is most likely to be effective in those with early onset Alzheimer's disease who are less than 66 years of age and have a faster rate of disease progression and mental decline (1594,1595,1596,1597,1598,1599). Acetyl-L-carnitine may not be beneficial for patients with early onset Alzheimer's disease who do not have rapid disease progression and rapid rate of cognitive decline (6495). In some cases, acetyl-L-carnitine may need to be taken between 1-6 months before any improvement is seen (14). ...when used for improving some measures of cognitive function and memory in elderly people with age-related mental impairment (42,3600,3601). ...when used for decreasing symptoms of depression in elderly people (3602,3603,3604). ...when used for improving some measures of cognitive function in people recovering from strokes, vascular dementia, or other forms of cerebral insufficiency (14,43). ...when used intravenously for producing short-term improvements in cerebral blood flow in people with chronic cerebral ischemia after single doses (1591,1592). ...when used orally to improve memory and visuo-spatial capacity in 30 to 60 year-old non-drinking alcoholics with cognitive impairment (1589). There is insufficient reliable information about the effectiveness of acetyl-L-carnitine for its other uses.

Mechanism of Action

Acetyl-L-carnitine occurs naturally in the body, within the inner membrane of mitochondria (14). It is an ester of L-carnitine, and is converted to L-carnitine in the body by carnitine acetyltransferase (14). It is also structurally related to acetylcholine (14). It may act as a cholinergic-enhancing agent by serving as a mitochondrial precursor to acetyl coenzyme A (acetyl CoA), thus contributing acetyl moieties for acetylcholine (14). It is an intracellular carrier of acetyl groups across mitochondrial membranes and promotes acetylcholine release and increases choline acetyltransferase activity (44). These effects have lead to the study of acetyl-L-carnitine in Alzheimer's disease, in which there is substantial cholinergic neuronal loss and acetylcholine depletion (1594). Acetyl-L-carnitine also participates in cellular energy production by acting as a shuttle between the cytoplasm and mitochondria for long-chain fatty acids (1594). Other potentially beneficial actions of acetyl-L-carnitine include neuroprotective actions, enhancement of choline acetyltransferase activity, facilitatory actions on serotonergic pathways, enhancement of synaptic transmission, increased hippocampal binding of nerve growth factor, and reduction of age-dependent losses of hippocampal glucocorticoid receptors (14). An increase in cerebral blood flow has been reported following acetyl-L-carnitine administration to people with cerebrovascular disease (14). In asymptomatic people with AIDS, acetyl-L-carnitine has been reported to slow the loss of CD4 lymphocytes by reducing apoptosis and increasing the serum level of insulin-like growth factor 1 which is protective against apoptosis (3605). Plasma levels of acetyl-L-carnitine have also been reported to be lower in people who developed neuropathy while taking anti-HIV drugs than in those who did not develop neuropathy (3606). Acetyl-L-carnitine and L-carnitine are present in human sperm and seminal fluid (3607). Their levels increase in sperm during the maturation process in the epididymis and coincide with the acquisition of progressive motility (3608,3609). Levels of acetyl-L-carnitine, and the ratio of acetyl-L-carnitine to L-carnitine, have been reported to be lower in infertile semen and sperm samples with low motility (3610,3611), and an increase in sperm motility is seen in vitro when acetyl-L-carnitine or L-carnitine is added to the sample (3612).

Adverse Reactions

Orally, acetyl-l-carnitine may cause nausea and vomiting (14,1599) and agitation (restlessness and motor overactivity) (14,1596). Side effects reported in people with Alzheimer's disease include psychiatric disturbances, such as depression, mania, confusion and aggression, but it is not clear whether these are due to acetyl-L-carnitine or the disease itself (14).

Interactions with Herbs & Other Dietary Supplements
Insufficient reliable information available.

Interactions with Drugs
No interactions are known to occur, and there is no known reason to expect a clinically significant interaction with acetyl-L-carnitine.

Interactions with Foods
No interactions are known to occur, and there is no known reason to expect a clinically significant interaction with acetyl-L-carnitine.

Interactions with Lab Tests
No interactions are known to occur, and there is no known reason to expect a clinically significant interaction with acetyl-L-carnitine.

Interactions with Diseases or Conditions
HYPERSENSITIVITY: Contraindicated in people with known hypersensitivity to acetyl-L-carnitine or L-carnitine (14).

Dosage and Administration
ORAL: In Alzheimer's disease, 1500 to 4000 mg daily has been used, usually divided into two or three doses during the day (14,1584,1586,1594,1595,1599). In age-related memory impairment, 1500 to 2000 mg daily has been used (1586,3601). In people recovering from stroke, a dose of 1500 mg daily has been used (14). For depression in the elderly, 1500 to 3000 mg daily in divided doses has been used (1586,3602,3603). In Down syndrome 10 mg per pound of body weight has been recommended (1586). In some infertile men, 4000 mg daily has been used to improve sperm function (3607).
INTRAVENOUS: A dose of 20 mg/kg/day has been used in people with dementia (14). Single doses of 1500 mg have been used in people with chronic cerebral ischemia (1591,1592).
INTRAMUSCULAR: In people with peripheral neuropathy, 500 to 1000 mg daily has been used (1593).

Comments
None.

ACKEE

Also Known As
Akee, Aki, Arbre Fricasse, Seso Vegetal.

Scientific Names
Blighia sapida.
Family: Sapindaceae.

People Use This For
Orally, ackee is used as a treatment for colds, fever, edema, and epilepsy (6).
For food uses, the ripe fruit is eaten (6).

Safety
LIKELY SAFE ...when the ripe fruit is used in traditional Jamaican cooking (6).
UNSAFE ...when the unripe fruit and seeds are ingested. It can cause severe hypoglycemia, convulsions, and death (6).
CHILDREN: UNSAFE ...when the unripe fruit and seeds are ingested. Children are more sensitive to the toxic effects of ackee than adults (6). There is insufficient reliable information available about the safety of the ripe fruit for children.
PREGNANCY AND LACTATION: UNSAFE ...when the unripe fruit and seeds are ingested (6).
There is insufficient reliable information available about the safety of the ripe fruit during pregnancy and lactation.

Effectiveness
There is insufficient reliable information available about the effectiveness of ackee.

Mechanism of Action
The applicable parts of ackee are the seed and fruit. Unripe fruit and seeds contain liver toxins (hypoglycin A,

hypoglycin B). By inactivating flavoprotein acyl-CoA dehydrogenases and inhibiting the oxidation of long-chain fatty acids, the toxins inhibit gluconeogenesis and induce hypoglycemia (5609,5610).

Adverse Reactions

Orally, there are two forms of toxicity that can occur from ingestion of the unripe fruit and seeds of ackee. One form is referred to as "vomiting sickness". The symptoms include vomiting, remission for 8-10 hours, renewed vomiting, convulsions, and eventually coma. The second type of toxicity includes convulsions and coma at the onset. Both forms lead to severe hypoglycemia (6) known as toxic hypoglycemic syndrome (THS) (5602). Electrolyte and fluid disturbances may occur due to vomiting (6). Urticaria and anaphylaxis has been reported after ingestion of ackee (5610).

Interactions with Herbs & Other Dietary Supplements

Insufficient reliable information available.

Interactions with Drugs

DIABETES THERAPY: Monitor blood glucose level closely due to claims that ackee has hypoglycemic effects (19).

Interactions with Foods

No interactions are known to occur, and there is no known reason to expect a clinically significant interaction with ackee.

Interactions with Lab Tests

No interactions are known to occur, and there is no known reason to expect a clinically significant interaction with ackee.

Interactions with Diseases or Conditions

DIABETES: Monitor blood glucose level closely due to claims that ackee has hypoglycemic effects (19).

Dosage and Administration

No typical dosage.

Comments

Ackee was brought to Jamaica from West Africa during the end of the 18th century, and the ripe fruit has since become a common ingredient in traditional Jamaican cooking (6). Avoid use of unripe fruit and seeds or water in which unripe ackee has been cooked due to toxicity (5602). Ackee is also found in southern Florida, Central America, and Africa (5602,5609).

ACONITE

Also Known As

Aconiti Tuber, Autumn Monkshood, Blue Monkshood Root, Chuan-wu, Monkshood, Monkshood Tuber, Wolfsbane.

Scientific Names

Aconitum napellus; Aconitum species.
Family: Ranunculaceae.

People Use This For

Orally, aconite is used for pain, facial paralysis, joint pain, arthritis, gout, rheumatic complaints, inflammation, pleurisy, pericarditis sicca, fever, skin and mucosal diseases, disinfection, and wound treatment (2,11).
Topically, aconite is used as a counterirritant in liniment (11).
Historically, aconite has been used orally as a cardiac depressant and an agent to induce mild sweating. Aconite has been used topically for facial neuralgia, rheumatism, and sciatica (11).

Safety

UNSAFE ...when used orally or topically. Aconite root is a strong, fast-acting poison that affects the heart and CNS (11). All species of this herb are dangerous. Severe poisoning has been reported after ingestion of 0.2 mg of aconitine or 6 grams of processed and cured aconite (3490). Aconite can also be absorbed through the skin (11). Even when used in the therapeutic dose range, aconite can cause toxicity including nausea, vomiting, dizziness, muscle spasms, hypothermia, paralysis of respiratory system, and heart rhythm disorders (2,11).
PREGNANCY AND LACTATION: UNSAFE ...when used orally or topically (11,12); avoid using.

Effectiveness

There is insufficient reliable information available about the effectiveness of aconite.

Mechanism of Action

The applicable part of aconite is the root. Aconite contains alkaloids including aconitine, mesoconitine, and hypaconitine, which have widespread effects on cardiac, neural, and muscle tissue by activating sodium channels (559,3490). In the heart muscle, this activation enhances inward currents during the plateau phase of the cardiac action potential, prolonging repolarization, and inducing afterdepolarization, leading to tachyarrhythmias (2634). Aconitine, the principal alkaloid of aconite, is considered to be a fast-acting, lethal poison (2,11).

Adverse Reactions

Orally, aconite causes symptoms of intoxication including nausea, vomiting, weakness, sweating, restlessness, dizziness, numbness, paresthesias (beginning in the mouth and then spreading to the limbs), hypotension, palpitations, hypokalemia, metabolic and/or respiratory acidosis, cardiac toxicity (sustained ventricular tachycardia, ventricular fibrillation), reduced consciousness, and death (558,559,561,562,563,3490). Symptoms of intoxication usually begin 30 minutes after ingestion of aconite (559). Life-threatening symptoms and fatalities have been reported after aconite ingestion (3490,3491). No specific antidote is available. Cardioversion has been reported to be ineffective, but the use of antiarrhythmic agents such as amiodarone has been successful in some cases (2634,3490). Some Chinese medicine practitioners still commonly use aconite rootstocks in their preparations. They cure the rootstocks of aconite by soaking in water (with frequent changes to fresh water) and then boiling or steaming for prolonged periods of time. The process hydrolyzes the aconite alkaloids into less toxic derivatives, but toxicities and fatalities can also occur after ingestion of these cured and processed aconite roots (2634,3490). Aconite is also a common ingredient in numerous homeopathic products. Since most homeopathic products are so diluted that they contain virtually no active molecules, these products are not likely to have any pharmacological or toxic effects.

Interactions with Herbs & Other Dietary Supplements

Insufficient reliable information available.

Interactions with Drugs

No interactions are known to occur, and there is no known reason to expect a clinically significant interaction with aconite.

Interactions with Foods

No interactions are known to occur, and there is no known reason to expect a clinically significant interaction with aconite.

Interactions with Lab Tests

No interactions are known to occur, and there is no known reason to expect a clinically significant interaction with aconite.

Interactions with Diseases or Conditions

No interactions are known to occur, and there is no known reason to expect a clinically significant interaction with aconite.

Dosage and Administration

ORAL: People typically use a homeopathic preparation of aconite of 6c to 30c potency strength (5011). A 6c potency is made by diluting one part of aconite tincture to 99 parts of water or alcohol. One part of the resulting solution is taken and diluted again with 99 parts of water or alcohol. The process is repeated four additional times resulting in a 6c potency (5011).
TOPICAL: No typical dosage.

Comments

None.

ACTIVATED CHARCOAL

Also Known As
Animal Charcoal, Charcoal, Gas Black, Lamp Black, Medicinal Charcoal.
CAUTION: See separate listing for Coffee Charcoal.

Scientific Names
Carbon.

People Use This For
Orally, activated charcoal is used as an antiflatulent, for reducing blood lipid levels, acute management of poisonings (6), and cholestasis of pregnancy (126).

Safety
LIKELY SAFE ...when used orally short-term (6).
PREGNANCY AND LACTATION: POSSIBLY SAFE ...when used orally short-term (126).

Effectiveness
LIKELY EFFECTIVE ...when used orally as part of a standard treatment for some acute poisonings (15).
POSSIBLY EFFECTIVE ...when used orally for reducing serum cholesterol levels (6). ...when used orally for cholestasis of pregnancy (126). ...when used orally as an antiflatulent (15).

Mechanism of Action
Activated charcoal has a very large surface area which adsorbs chemicals and therefore prevents their systemic absorption. Activated charcoal may interrupt enterohepatic recirculation of drugs and other compounds that are excreted into the bile (6).

Adverse Reactions
Orally, activated charcoal can cause GI obstruction, pulmonary aspiration, hypernatremic dehydration, and prolonged GI transit time (6). Poisoning cases: Be cautious when using activated charcoal along with an emetic. There is a risk of pulmonary aspiration (6) (see Typical Dosage, Comments).

Interactions with Herbs & Other Dietary Supplements
MICRONUTRIENTS: Activated charcoal may cause reduced absorption of micronutrients (15).

Interactions with Drugs
SYRUP OF IPECAC: Activated charcoal adsorbs and inactivates syrup of ipecac; avoid co-administration (506).
ORAL DRUGS: Activated charcoal may reduce or prevent absorption of drugs including acetaminophen, barbiturates, carbamazepine, digitoxin, digoxin, furosemide, glutethimide, hydantoins, methotrexate, nizatidine, phenothiazines, phenylbutazones, propoxyphene, salicylates, sulfones, sulfonylureas, tetracyclines, theophyllines, tricyclic antidepressants, and valproic acid (506). Avoid co-administration.

Interactions with Foods
MICRONUTRIENTS: Activated charcoal can reduce absorption of micronutrients (15).
MILK, ICE CREAM OR SHERBET AND OTHER DAIRY PRODUCTS: Co-administration of these foods along with activated charcoal may decrease the adsorptive capacity of activated charcoal (506).

Interactions with Lab Tests
SERUM CHOLESTEROL: Activated charcoal can reduce serum total cholesterol and LDL cholesterol concentrations and test results (6).

Interactions with Diseases or Conditions
GI OBSTRUCTION: Avoid using activated charcoal in conditions of GI obstruction (see Adverse Reactions).

Dosage and Administration
ORAL: The usual antiflatulent dose is 520-975 mg after meals or at first sign of discomfort. Separate activated charcoal doses from other drugs by at least two hours to avoid interaction.

Comments
In case of POISONING, use caution if an emetic is given, due to the risk of pulmonary aspiration. Laxatives are often co-administered to reduce GI transit time and speed removal of poison from the body (6).

ADAM'S NEEDLE

Also Known As
Adams Needle.

Scientific Names
Yucca filamentosa.
Family: Liliaceae.

People Use This For
Orally, Adam's needle is used to treat liver and gallbladder disorders (18).

Safety
There is insufficient reliable information available about the safety of Adam's needle.
Pregnancy and Lactation: Insufficient reliable information available; avoid using.

Effectiveness
There is insufficient reliable information available about the effectiveness of Adam's needle.

Mechanism of Action
The applicable part of Adam's needle is the root of the nonflowering plant. Adam's needle contains saponins, including gitogenin and tigogenin. These substances are from colloidal solutions in water that foam when they are shaken. They are often irritating to mucous membranes and could cause symptoms such as sneezing and GI irritation (18,4077).

Adverse Reactions
Orally, Adam's needle might cause dyspepsia and related abdominal symptoms (18).

Interactions with Herbs & Other Dietary Supplements
Insufficient reliable information available.

Interactions with Drugs
No interactions are known to occur, and there is no known reason to expect a clinically significant interaction with Adam's needle.

Interactions with Foods
No interactions are known to occur, and there is no known reason to expect a clinically significant interaction with Adam's needle.

Interactions with Lab Tests
No interactions are known to occur, and there is no known reason to expect a clinically significant interaction with Adam's needle.

Interactions with Diseases or Conditions
No interactions are known to occur, and there is no known reason to expect a clinically significant interaction with Adam's needle.

Dosage and Administration
ORAL: The grounded root has been used and sometimes an extract is made from the root (18).

Comments
Adam's needle is a native to the southern states in the US, and is used as an ornamental plant in Europe (18). There is very little scientific information about this product. Our staff is continually analyzing the available information on natural medicines and will add data here as it becomes available.

ADRENAL EXTRACT

Also Known As
ACE, Adrenal, Adrenal Complex, Adrenal Concentrate, Adrenal Cortex Extract, Adrenal Factors, Adrenal Substance, Glandular, Whole Adrenal Extract.

Scientific Names
None.

People Use This For
Orally, adrenal extract is used for low adrenal function; fatigue; stress; impaired resistance to illness; and for treating severe allergies, asthma, eczema, psoriasis, rheumatoid arthritis, and other inflammatory conditions (6616).
Sublingually, adrenal extract is used for stress induced fatigue or exhaustion, poor stress tolerance, general fatigue, allergies, auto-immune disorders, depression, physical or emotional stress, inflammation, low blood pressure, hypoglycemia, drug and alcohol withdrawal, and discontinuing cortisone drugs (6618).
Intravenously, adrenal extract has been used for treating adrenal cortical insufficiency, hyperkalemia, ulcerative colitis, status thymicolymphaticus, and preventing spontaneous abortion (6619).

Safety
LIKELY UNSAFE …when used parenterally. Use of injectable adrenal extract has been associated with at least 50 cases of serious bacterial infections at injection sites (6620). Adrenal extracts are derived from animals so there is concern about contamination with diseased animal parts (see Adverse Reactions). So far, there are no reports of disease transmission to humans due to use of contaminated adrenal extracts.
There is insufficient reliable information available about the safety of adrenal extract for its other uses.
PREGNANCY AND LACTATION: Insufficient reliable information available; avoid using.

Effectiveness
There is insufficient reliable information available about the effectiveness of adrenal extract.

Mechanism of Action
Adrenal extracts are derived from raw cow, pig, or sheep adrenal glands gathered from slaughterhouses (6616,6620). There is no scientific evidence that adrenal extract constituents are or are not absorbed intact in the gastrointestinal tract. Some suggest that adrenal extract constituents are too large for absorption or are destroyed by digestion. Supporters of glandular therapy cite indirect evidence that adrenal extracts constituents can be absorbed (6616).
No human studies are reported regarding the absorption or efficacy of adrenal extracts.

Adverse Reactions
Orally, no adverse reactions have been reported; however, adrenal extracts are derived from raw cow, pig, or sheep adrenal glands gathered from slaughterhouses and possibly from sick or diseased animals (6616,6620). Products made from contaminated or diseased organs might present a human health hazard. There is also some concern that adrenal extracts produced from cows in countries where bovine spongiform encephalitis (BSE) has been reported might be contaminated with diseased tissue. Countries where BSE has been reported include Great Britain, France, The Netherlands, Portugal, Luxembourg, Ireland, Switzerland, Oman, and Belgium (1825); however, there have been no reports of BSE transfer to humans from contaminated adrenal extract products. Until more is known, tell patients to avoid these products unless country of origin can be determined. Patients should avoid products that are produced in countries where BSE has been found.
Intravenously, adrenal extract can cause infection and abscess at the site of injection (6620). In 1996, the FDA issued a nationwide alert regarding an injectable adrenal cortex extract after more than 50 cases of serious bacterial infections at injection sites were reported (6620).

Interactions with Herbs & Other Dietary Supplements
Insufficient reliable information available.

Interactions with Drugs
No interactions are known to occur, and there is no known reason to expect a clinically significant interaction with adrenal extract.

Interactions with Foods
No interactions are known to occur, and there is no known reason to expect a clinically significant interaction with adrenal extract.

Interactions with Lab Tests

No interactions are known to occur, and there is no known reason to expect a clinically significant interaction with adrenal extract.

Interactions with Diseases or Conditions

IMMUNOCOMPROMISED: Theoretically, adrenal extracts might increase the risk of infection. Adrenal extracts might harbor pathogens. Injectable adrenal extract reportedly caused more than 50 serious infections at injection sites (6620); avoid using.

Dosage and Administration

No typical dosage.

Comments

None.

ADRUE

Also Known As

Guinea Rush.

Scientific Names

Cyperus articulatus.
Family: Cyperaceae.

People Use This For

Orally, adrue is used as an anti-emetic and for digestive disorders including nausea, colic, and flatulence. It is also used orally as a sedative (18).

Safety

There is insufficient reliable information available about the safety of adrue.
Pregnancy and Lactation: Insufficient reliable information available; avoid using.

Effectiveness

There is insufficient reliable information about the effectiveness of adrue.

Mechanism of Action

The applicable part of adrue is the root. Adrue produces a volatile oil that contains sesquiterpene alcohols and sesquiterpene hydrocarbons, including cyperenone. At present, we don't know how these components relate to the uses of adrue (18).

Adverse Reactions

None reported.

Interactions with Herbs & Other Dietary Supplements

Insufficient reliable information available.

Interactions with Drugs

No interactions are known to occur, and there is no known reason to expect a clinically significant interaction with adrue.

Interactions with Foods

No interactions are known to occur, and there is no known reason to expect a clinically significant interaction with adrue.

Interactions with Lab Tests

No interactions are known to occur, and there is no known reason to expect a clinically significant interaction with adrue.

Interactions with Diseases or Conditions

No interactions are known to occur, and there is no known reason to expect a clinically significant interaction with adrue.

Dosage and Administration

ORAL: A liquid extract is obtained from the root (18).

Comments

Adrue is native to Turkey, Jamaica, and the Nile River region. It has a bitter taste and an aroma reminiscent of lavender (18).

There is very little scientific information about this product. Our staff is continually analyzing the available information on natural medicines and will add data here as it becomes available.

AFRICAN WILD POTATO

Also Known As

African Potato, Bantu Tulip, Hypoxis Plant, South African Star Grass, Sterretjie.
CAUTION: See separate listing for Potato.

Scientific Names

Hypoxis rooperi.

People Use This For

Orally, the African wild potato is used for bladder and urinary disorders including cystitis, prostate problems including prostatic hyperplasia (7,5943,5944) and prostate cancer (5945), lung disease (5944), and cancer (5943). It is also used in maintaining health in individuals who are HIV positive, for TB, "yuppie flu", arthritis, and psoriasis (5945). Topically, the African wild potato is used for wound healing (5944).

Safety

There is insufficient reliable information available about the safety of the African wild potato. Preliminary human trials indicate the African wild potato glucoside constituent is non-toxic (5943).
Pregnancy and Lactation: Insufficient reliable information available; avoid using.

Effectiveness

POSSIBLY EFFECTIVE ...when used orally to increase volume of urine excreted and improve urine flow in individuals with prostate problems (7).
There is insufficient reliable information available about the effectiveness of African wild potato for its other uses.

Mechanism of Action

The African wild potato tuber contains 3.5%-4.5% lignans, particularly norlignan glucoside (5944). It also contains beta-sitosterol and beta-sitosterolin (7). The activity of the African wild potato is attributed to the phytosterols that inhibit the production of prostaglandin synthase (5944). It is also believed to stimulate and regulate the immune system by activating the body's T-cells (5946).

Adverse Reactions

Orally, the African wild potato constituent beta-sitosterol has been associated with erectile dysfunction and loss of libido (5942).

Interactions with Herbs & Other Dietary Supplements

Insufficient reliable information available.

Interactions with Drugs

No interactions are known to occur, and there is no known reason to expect a clinically significant interaction with African wild potato.

Interactions with Foods

No interactions are known to occur, and there is no known reason to expect a clinically significant interaction with African wild potato.

Interactions with Lab Tests

No interactions are known to occur, and there is no known reason to expect a clinically significant interaction with African wild potato.

Interactions with Diseases or Conditions

No interactions are known to occur, and there is no known reason to expect a clinically significant interaction with African wild potato.

Dosage and Administration

ORAL: To boost the immune system, a typical dose is 15 drops in a glass of water three times daily before meals (5945).

Comments

The African wild potato was originally grown in South Africa (5944).

AGA

Also Known As

Fly Agaric, Soma.

Scientific Names

Amanita muscaria.
Family: Agariacaceae.

People Use This For

Orally, aga is used as a hallucinogen. It is also used orally in homeopathic dilutions for nerve pain, fever, anxiety, alcohol poisoning, and joint pains (18).

Safety

UNSAFE …when used orally (see Mechanism of Action) (18).
PREGNANCY AND LACTATION: UNSAFE …when used orally because of its toxicity (18); avoid using.

Effectiveness

There is insufficient reliable information available about the effectiveness of aga.

Mechanism of Action

The applicable parts of aga are the above ground mushroom parts. Aga is not a true hallucinogen. The illusions which occur with aga ingestion are primarily a misinterpretation of sensory stimuli. These mind altering effects are due to the isoxazoles ibotenic acid, muscimol, muscazone (14), and traces of muscarine (18). Ibotenic acid mimics the neurotransmitter glutamic acid in the brain. It is rapidly converted to muscimol, which imitates the action of the neurotransmitter GABA. Ibotenic acid also acts as a flavor enhancer and may produce an unusual aftertaste in people who use it orally. Toxicity also depends on the isoxazole content. It occurs with about 6 mg of mucsimol and 30-60 mg ibotenic acid. These can occur in a single aga mushroom. Isoxazole content can vary as much as 10 times higher depending on when it is collected. Mind-altering effects have occurred with ingestion of 2-4 mushrooms, and 20 large mushrooms have been ingested with survival. The toxic threshold for humans is approximately 6 mg for muscimol and 30-60 mg for ibotenic acid (14). Death due to aga ingestion is rare (less than 1%). Aga does not contain enough muscarine to produce cholinergic symptoms (14).

Adverse Reactions

Orally, people develop symptoms within 30-90 minutes of using aga. The effects peak at 2-3 hours. The initial symptom is drowsiness. This is quickly followed by confusion, ataxia, dizziness, euphoria, alcohol-like intoxication, and may proceed to hyperactivity, muscle jerks and spasms, and delirium. In the later stages, deep sleep or coma occurs and usually lasts from 4-8 hours. The whole episode lasts 8-10 hours. Severe vomiting is rare (14).

Interactions with Herbs & Other Dietary Supplements

Insufficient reliable information available.

Interactions with Drugs

No interactions are known to occur, and there is no known reason to expect a clinically significant interaction with aga.

Interactions with Foods

No interactions are known to occur, and there is no known reason to expect a clinically significant interaction with aga.

Interactions with Lab Tests

No interactions are known to occur, and there is no known reason to expect a clinically significant interaction with aga.

Interactions with Diseases or Conditions

No interactions are known to occur, and there is no known reason to expect a clinically significant interaction with aga.

Dosage and Administration

No typical dosage.

Comments

Aga is a mushroom with a red cap spotted with white. It is present in sandy, acid soils in the United States. Aga is also known as "fly agaric" because ibotenic acid and muscimol are toxic to the common housefly (14).

AGAR

Also Known As

Agar-Agar, Agarweed, Chinese Gelatin, Colle du Japon, Gelatin, Gelosa, Gelosae, Japanese Isinglas, Layor Carang, Vegetable Gelatin.

Scientific Names

Gelidiella acerosa; Gelidium amanasii; Gelidium cartilagineum; Gelidium crinale; Gelidium divaricatum; Gelidium pacificum; Gelidium vagum; Garacilaria confervoides.
Family: Sphaerococcaceae. Species of the genera Pterocladia; Ahnfeltia; Acanthopeltis; Suhria.

People Use This For

Orally, agar is used as a bulk laxative for chronic constipation.
In dentistry, agar is used to make dental impressions (11).
In manufacturing processes, agar is used as an ingredient in emulsions, suspensions, gels, and hydrophilic suppositories.

Safety

LIKELY SAFE ...when used orally with at least 250 mL of water (12).
PREGNANCY AND LACTATION: Insufficient reliable information available.

Effectiveness

POSSIBLY EFFECTIVE ...when used orally as a bulk laxative (11).

Mechanism of Action

Agar consists of two major polysaccharides, neutral agarose and charged agaropectin. Agarose is the gelling fraction (11).

Adverse Reactions

Potential to cause esophageal or bowel obstruction if taken with insufficient volume of water (12). Possibly can increase cholesterol levels (11).

Interactions with Herbs & Other Dietary Supplements

Insufficient reliable information available.

Interactions with Drugs

ORAL DRUGS: The fiber in agar can impair absorption of oral drugs (19).

Interactions with Foods

No interactions are known to occur, and there is no known reason to expect a clinically significant interaction with agar.

Interactions with Lab Tests

No interactions are known to occur, and there is no known reason to expect a clinically significant interaction with agar.

Interactions with Diseases or Conditions

BOWEL OBSTRUCTION OR DIFFICULTY SWALLOWING: Contraindicated (12).

Dosage and Administration

ORAL: A typical dose is 4-16 grams, one to two times daily (12). Take each dose with at least 250 mL of water (11) (see Safety).

Comments

OTC products must be labeled: "Warning, taking this product without adequate fluid may cause it to swell and block your throat or esophagus and may cause choking. Do not take this product if you have difficulty swallowing. If you experience chest pain, vomiting, or difficulty swallowing or breathing after using this product, seek immediate medical attention" (12).

AGRIMONY

Also Known As

Agromonia, Agrimoniae herba, Ackerkraut, Cocklebur, Fragrant Agrimony, Funffing, Funffingerkraut, Herba eupatoriae, Herbe d'Aigremoine, Herbe de Saint-Guillaume, Liverwort, Stickwort.
CAUTION: See separate listing for Potentilla.

Scientific Names

Agrimonia eupatoria; Agrimonia procera.
Family: Rosaceae.

People Use This For

Orally, agrimony is used for sore throat, upset stomach, and mild, nonspecific diarrhea.
Topically, agrimony is used as a mild astringent and for mild skin inflammation. The ethanolic extracts of agrimony are used for their antiviral properties (6).
Historically, agrimony has been used for gallbladder disorders, tuberculosis, bleeding, corns, warts, as a gargle, antitumor agent, cardiotonic, diuretic, sedative, and antihistamine.

Safety

LIKELY SAFE ...when the dried above ground parts are used orally and appropriately short-term (2,12). ...when used topically (2).
POSSIBLY UNSAFE ...when used orally or topically in excessive doses due to its high tannin content (12).
PREGNANCY AND LACTATION: POSSIBLY UNSAFE ...when used orally because of the possible effects on the menstrual cycle (4,12).

Effectiveness

There is insufficient reliable information available about the effectiveness of agrimony.

Mechanism of Action

The applicable parts of agrimony are the dried, above ground parts. The aerial plant parts contain 4-10% condensed tannins which can account for its astringent properties (6). Because of the tannin content and astringent properties of agrimony, it is thought to be helpful for gastrointestinal conditions such as diarrhea.

Adverse Reactions

The use of agrimony can cause photodermatitis and can affect blood pressure (6).

Interactions with Herbs & Other Dietary Supplements

Insufficient reliable information available.

Interactions with Drugs

ANTICOAGULANTS: Excessive doses of agrimony can potentiate anticoagulant therapy (4).

BLOOD PRESSURE ALTERING DRUGS: Excessive doses of agrimony might cause hypotension, interfering with therapy for hypertension or hypotension (4).

DIABETES THERAPY: Monitor blood glucose level closely due to claims that agrimony has hypoglycemic effects (19).

Interactions with Foods

No interactions are known to occur, and there is no known reason to expect a clinically significant interaction with agrimony.

Interactions with Lab Tests

No interactions are known to occur, and there is no known reason to expect a clinically significant interaction with agrimony.

Interactions with Diseases or Conditions

No interactions are known to occur, and there is no known reason to expect a clinically significant interaction with agrimony.

Dosage and Administration

ORAL: The typical dose of agrimony is 3 grams per day (2).

TOPICAL: A poultice is commonly applied several times daily using approximately 10% water extract, which is prepared by boiling the herb at low heat for 10-20 minutes (8).

Comments

None.

AGROPYRON

Also Known As

Couch Grass, Cutch, Dog Grass, Dog-grass, Doggrass, Durfa Grass, Graminis rhizoma, Quack Grass, Quackgrass, Quitch Grass, Scotch Quelch, Triticum, Twitchgrass, Witch Grass.

Scientific Names

Agropyron repens, synonyms Elytrigia repens, Triticum repens, Elymus repens.
Family: Gramineae or Poaceae.

People Use This For

Orally, agropyron is used for cystitis, urethritis, prostatitis, benign prostatic hypertrophy, renal calculus (kidney stones) (4), and "irrigation therapy" (use of a mild diuretic and copious fluid intake to increase urine flow) (2,11).

It is also used orally for common cold, cough and bronchitis, fever and colds, inflammation of mouth and pharynx, and tendency to infection (18).

In folk medicine, agropyron has been used as a diuretic, expectorant, for diabetes aid, gout, liver disorders, rheumatic pain, and chronic skin problems (11,18).

In foods and beverages, agropyron extracts are used as a flavoring component (11).

Safety

LIKELY SAFE ...when rhizome or root are used orally in food amounts. Agropyron has Generally Recognized as Safe (GRAS) status in the US. The maximum level used in foods is 0.003% (11).

POSSIBLY SAFE ...when used orally and appropriately for irrigation therapy for short periods of time (2,4).

There is insufficient reliable information available about the safety of agropyron for its other uses.

PREGNANCY AND LACTATION: Insufficient reliable information available; avoid using.

Effectiveness

POSSIBLY EFFECTIVE ...when used orally for irrigation therapy for inflammatory diseases of the urinary tract and prevention of urine stones (2,4,10).

There is insufficient reliable information available about the effectiveness of agropyron for its other uses.

Mechanism of Action

Agropyron is a plant that is rich in beta-carotene (19). Agropyrene and its oxidative product seem to have broad antibiotic activity (11). The essential oil has antimicrobial effects (2,6). Agropyron contains flavonoid constituents (4). Agropyron seems to produce diuretic and sedative activity (4,11).

Adverse Reactions

Orally, excessive or prolonged use of agropyron may cause hypokalemia (4).

Interactions with Herbs & Other Dietary Supplements

Insufficient reliable information available.

Interactions with Drugs

POTASSIUM DEPLETING DIURETICS: Theoretically, concomitant use may cause potassium depletion (4).

Interactions with Foods

No interactions are known to occur, and there is no known reason to expect a clinically significant interaction with agropyron.

Interactions with Lab Tests

No interactions are known to occur, and there is no known reason to expect a clinically significant interaction with agropyron.

Interactions with Diseases or Conditions

EDEMA: Irrigation therapy with agropyron is contraindicated in edema due to heart or kidney conditions (2).

Dosage and Administration

ORAL: The dried rhizome is commonly used as 4-8 grams three times daily, or as a tea (simmer 1-2 grams herb in 150 mL boiling water 5-10 minutes, strain) three times daily. The typical dosage of liquid extract (1:1 in 25% alcohol) is 4-8 mL three times daily. Tincture (1:5 in 40% alcohol) 5-15 mL three times daily has also been used (4). Use for "irrigation therapy" requires copious fluid intake (2).

Comments

None.

ALCHEMILLA

Also Known As

Feuilles d'Alchemille, Frauenmantelkraut, Lady's Mantle, Ladys Mantle, Leontopodium, Lion's Foot, Lions Foot, Marienmantel, Nine Hooks, Silerkraut, Stellaria.
CAUTION: See separate listing for Alpine Lady's Mantle.

Scientific Names

Alchemilla xanthochlora, synonym Alchemilla vulgaris.
Family: Rosaceae.

People Use This For

Orally, alchemilla is used for mild diarrhea (2,8), heavy menstrual flow (8), and diabetes (6).
Topically, alchemilla is used as an astringent for bleeding and to improve wound healing (8).
In folk medicine, alchemilla is used orally for menopausal complaints, painful menses, gastrointestinal disorders, as a relaxant for muscle spasms, an anti-inflammatory, a diuretic (6), and as a gargle for mouth and throat inflammation (18). Alchemilla is used topically in folk medicine for ulcers, eczema, skin rashes, and as a bath additive for treating lower-abdominal ailments (18).

Safety

POSSIBLY SAFE …when used orally and appropriately. Alchemilla has been used for many years without reports of significant toxicity (2,6,8,12).
There is insufficient reliable information available about the safety of the topical use of alchemilla.
PREGNANCY AND LACTATION: Insufficient reliable information available; avoid using.

Effectiveness
There is insufficient reliable information available about the effectiveness of alchemilla.

Mechanism of Action
The applicable parts of alchemilla are the above ground parts. Alchemilla contains 6-8% tannins (8), which might account for its perceived astringent activity (6). An aqueous extract of Alchemilla xanthochlora demonstrates lipid peroxidation and superoxide anion scavenging activity (6). Flavonoid extracts inhibit proteolytic enzymes, including elastase, trypsin, and alpha-chymotrypsin. This property suggests alchemilla might have a role in protecting conjunctive and elastic tissues (6).

Adverse Reactions
Rarely, alchemilla can cause liver damage (8).

Interactions with Herbs & Other Dietary Supplements
Insufficient reliable information available.

Interactions with Drugs
No interactions are known to occur, and there is no known reason to expect a clinically significant interaction with alchemilla.

Interactions with Foods
No interactions are known to occur, and there is no known reason to expect a clinically significant interaction with alchemilla.

Interactions with Lab Tests
No interactions are known to occur, and there is no known reason to expect a clinically significant interaction with alchemilla.

Interactions with Diseases or Conditions
No interactions are known to occur, and there is no known reason to expect a clinically significant interaction with alchemilla.

Dosage and Administration
ORAL: For diarrhea, one cup tea, prepared by steeping 1-4 grams above ground parts in boiling water for 10 minutes and then straining (8), used up to three times per day between meals. The average amount used per day is 5-10 grams. Equivalent preparations can also be used (2). Diarrhea persisting for more than 3-4 days should be medically evaluated (8).
TOPICAL: No typical dosage.

Comments
Although the German Standard License warns about possible liver damage, some experts consider the concern to be exaggerated (8).

ALDER BUCKTHORN

Also Known As
Alder Dogwood, Arrow Wood, Black Dogwood, Buckthorn, Buckthorn Bark, Dog Wood, Frangula, Frangula Bark, Frangulae Cortex, Glossy Buckthorn.
CAUTION: See separate listings for European Buckthorn, Sea Buckthorn, and Cascara.

Scientific Names
Rhamnus frangula, synonym Frangula alnus.
Family: Rhamnaceae.

People Use This For
Orally, alder buckthorn is used as a laxative (11).
Traditionally, alder buckthorn has been used as a tonic and a component in the Hoxsey cancer cure (11).

Safety

LIKELY SAFE ...when used orally and appropriately for no more than 8 to10 days (2,12). Only properly aged bark should be used, and the recommended dose should not be exceeded (12).
POSSIBLY UNSAFE ...when used orally for more than 8 to 10 days (2,12).
CHILDREN: LIKELY UNSAFE ...when used orally in children younger than 12 years of age (2,12); avoid using.
PREGNANCY AND LACTATION: LIKELY UNSAFE ...when used orally (2,12); avoid using.

Effectiveness

LIKELY EFFECTIVE ...when used orally as a laxative (3,4,7,12). Alder buckthorn is comparable to the gentle, laxative effects of cascara (3).
There is insufficient reliable information available about the effectiveness of alder buckthorn for its other uses.

Mechanism of Action

The applicable part of alder buckthorn is the bark. The anthraglycosides and particularly the diglycosides are cathartic in the large intestine (1,8,11). They can increase intestinal motility by inhibiting stationary contractions, stimulating propulsive contractions, stimulating active chloride secretion, and increasing water and electrolytes in the intestinal contents (2). The fresh bark contains free anthrone, which can cause severe vomiting and is destroyed by aging the bark naturally for one year or artificially with heat and aeration (2). Anthroid laxative use is not associated with an increased risk of developing colorectal ademoma or carcinoma (6138).

Adverse Reactions

Orally, alder buckthorn can cause cramp-like discomfort (2). Chronic use can cause pseudomelanosis coli (pigment spots in intestinal mucosa) which is harmless, usually reverses with discontinuation (2), and is not associated with an increased risk of developing colorectal ademoma or carcinoma (6138). Chronic use or abuse of the bark can lead to potassium depletion, albuminuria, and hematuria. Potassium depletion can lead to disturbed heart function and muscle weakness (2). The fresh or improperly aged bark can cause severe vomiting due to the presence of the free anthrone, an emetic constituent.

Interactions with Herbs & Other Dietary Supplements

LICORICE: Concomitant use of alder buckthorn with licorice can increase the risk of potassium depletion (2).
STIMULANT LAXATIVE HERBS: Theoretically, concomitant use of alder buckthorn with other stimulant laxative herbs can increase the risk of potassium depletion. Stimulant laxative herbs include aloe dried leaf sap, wild cucumber fruit (Ecballium elaterium), blue flag rhizome, butternut bark, cascara bark, castor oil, colocynth fruit pulp, gamboge bark exudate, jalap root, black root, manna bark exudate, podophyllum root, rhubarb root, senna leaves and pods, and yellow dock root (19).
POTASSIUM DEPLETING HERBS: Theoretically, concomitant use of alder buckthorn with horsetail plant or licorice rhizome increases the risk of potassium depletion.

Interactions with Drugs

CARDIAC GLYCOSIDES: Theoretically, overuse or abuse of alder buckthorn increases the risk of adverse effects from cardiac glycoside drugs, like digoxin (Lanoxin).
CORTICOSTEROIDS, POTASSIUM DEPLETING DIURETICS: Concomitant use with alder buckthorn can increase the risk of potassium depletion (2).
ORAL DRUGS: Theoretically, alder buckthorn can reduce absorption of some drugs due to reduced GI transit time (500).

Interactions with Foods

No interactions are known to occur, and there is no known reason to expect a clinically significant interaction with alder buckthorn.

Interactions with Lab Tests

COLORIMETRIC TESTS: Alder buckthorn can discolor urine (pink, red, purple, orange, rust), interfering with diagnostic tests that depend on a color change, due to its anthraquinone content (1,12,275).
POTASSIUM: Excessive use of alder buckthorn can cause potassium depletion, reducing serum potassium concentrations and test results (1,2,4,12,19).

Interactions with Diseases or Conditions

GI CONDITIONS: Alder buckthorn is contraindicated in individuals with intestinal obstruction; abdominal pain of unknown origin; and intestinal inflammation, including appendicitis, Crohn's disease, irritable bowel syndrome (IBS), and ulcerative colitis (12).

Dosage and Administration

ORAL: The typical dose of alder buckthorn is 0.5-2.5 grams of the dried bark (4) or as a tea, which is prepared by steeping 2 grams of the herb in 150 mL boiling water for 5-10 minutes and then straining (12). The average dose per day of the bark is 1 gram (3) or 20-30 mg of the hydoxyanthracene derivatives calculated as glycofrangulin A (2). The common dose of the liquid extract: (1:1 in 25% alcohol) is 2-5 mL three times daily (2). The individual dose of the bark is the minimum amount required to produce a soft stool (2). Limit its use to a maximum of seven to ten days. This preparation should be used only if no effect can be obtained through change of diet or the use of bulk-forming laxative products (2).

Comments

Avoid confusion with European buckthorn. The American Herbal Products Association (AHPA) recommends the following label statement: "Do not use this product if you have abdominal pain or diarrhea. Consult a health care provider prior to use if you are pregnant or nursing. Discontinue use in the event of diarrhea or watery stools. Do not exceed dose. Not for long-term use." (12). Today, alder buckthorn is primarily used as a dye.

ALETRIS

Also Known As

Ague Grass, Ague Root, Aloerot, Blazing Star, Colic Root, Crow Corn, Devil's-bit, Stargrass, Starwort, Unicorn Root, Whitetube Stargrass.

Scientific Names

Aletris farinosa.
Family: Liliaceae.

People Use This For

Orally, aletris is used for rheumatism (6,11), as a general tonic, a sedative, to relieve menstrual disorders, as a laxative, an antiflatulent, an antispasmodic (6), for colic, as an antidiarrheal, and a diuretic (11).

Safety

POSSIBLY SAFE ...when used orally and appropriately (6,12).
PREGNANCY AND LACTATION: POSSIBLY UNSAFE ...when used orally due to the possibility that aletris contains components that cause estrogenic activity (11) and oxytocin (Pitocin) antagonism (12); avoid using.

Effectiveness

POSSIBLY EFFECTIVE ...when used orally to treat menstrual disorders (11).
There is insufficient reliable information available about the effectiveness of aletris for its other uses.

Mechanism of Action

Some aletris constituents may have estrogenic activity (6).

Adverse Reactions

Orally, small doses of aletris may induce colic, stupefaction, and vertigo (6).

Interactions with Herbs & Other Dietary Supplements

Insufficient reliable information available.

Interactions with Drugs

ACID-INHIBITING DRUGS: Theoretically, due to claims that aletris increases stomach acid, it might interfere with antacids, sucralfate (Carafate), H-2 antagonists, or proton pump inhibitors (19).
PITOCIN: Aletris may antagonize activity of oxytocin (Pitocin) (12).

Interactions with Foods

No interactions are known to occur, and there is no known reason to expect a clinically significant interaction with aletris.

Interactions with Lab Tests

No interactions are known to occur, and there is no known reason to expect a clinically significant interaction with aletris.

Interactions with Diseases or Conditions

GASTROINTESTINAL DISEASES: Aletris can irritate gastrointestinal tract. It is contraindicated in individuals with infectious or inflammatory gastrointestinal conditions (19).

HORMONE SENSITIVE CANCERS/CONDITIONS: Aletris might have estrogenic effects (6). Women with hormone sensitive conditions should avoid aletris. Some of these conditions include breast, uterine, and ovarian cancer, and endometriosis and uterine fibroids.

Dosage and Administration

ORAL: Aletris is used as the powdered root, a liquid extract, and an infusion (18). One common dosage recommendation is 0.3 to 0.6 grams three times daily (18). The infusion is prepared by adding 1.5 grams of aletris to 100 mL of water, and the fluid extract (1:1) is commonly produced with 45% ethanol water (18).

Comments

None.

ALFALFA

Also Known As

Feuille De Luzerne, Lucerne, Medicago, Phytoestrogen, Purple Medick.

Scientific Names

Medicago sativa.
Family: Leguminosae or Fabaceae.

People Use This For

Orally, alfalfa is used as a diuretic, for kidney, bladder and prostate conditions, for asthma (6), arthritis, diabetes, indigestion (5,6), and thrombocytopenic purpura. (4). It is also used as a source of vitamins A, C, E, and K4; and minerals calcium, potassium, phosphorous, and iron (4).

Safety

LIKELY SAFE ...when the above ground parts are used orally in moderation (4,5,6,12).
LIKELY UNSAFE ...when large amounts of seeds are consumed. It is associated with pancytopenia (5,6).
PREGNANCY AND LACTATION: POSSIBLY SAFE ...when used in food amounts (4). Avoid amounts in excess of food because alfalfa contains constituents with possible estrogenic activity (11).

Effectiveness

POSSIBLY EFFECTIVE ...when used orally to lower cholesterol. ...when used for type II hyperlipoproteinemia (4). There is insufficient reliable information available about the effectiveness of alfalfa for its other uses.

Mechanism of Action

The applicable parts of alfalfa are the above ground parts. The alfalfa leaf contains saponins which appear to decrease plasma cholesterol without creating a change in HDL levels (4). Constituents of alfalfa seem to decrease cholesterol absorption, and increase excretion of neutral steroids and bile acids (4,6). Alfalfa contains manganese which might be responsible for hypoglycemic effects (4). Alfalfa contains medicagol which appears to have antifungal properties. Alfalfa also contains coumetrol, genistein, biochanin A, and daidzein which all seem to have estrogenic properties (11).

Adverse Reactions

Alfalfa might cause photosensitivity (605). Ingestion of ground alfalfa seeds is associated with a case of pancytopenia (381).

Interactions with Herbs & Other Dietary Supplements

VITAMIN E: Alfalfa contains saponins which interfere with the absorption or activity of vitamin E (11).
HERBS WITH CLOTTING POTENTIAL: Excessive use of herbs that contain vitamin K, an essential coagulation factor, can increase the risk of clotting in people using anticoagulants. These herbs include alfalfa, parsley, nettle, plantain, and others.

Interactions with Drugs

ANTICOAGULANTS: Excessive use of alfalfa may interfere with anticoagulant therapy (4).

ORAL CONTRACEPTIVES or HORMONE THERAPY: Excessive doses of alfalfa may interfere with hormone therapy (4).

CHLORPROMAZINE: Excessive doses of alfalfa may potentiate drug-induced photosensitivity (605).

Interactions with Foods

No interactions are known to occur, and there is no known reason to expect a clinically significant interaction with alfalfa.

Interactions with Lab Tests

CHOLESTEROL: Alfalfa seed might lower serum cholesterol concentrations and test results in individuals with type II hyperlipoproteinemia (4).

Interactions with Diseases or Conditions

SYSTEMIC LUPUS ERYTHEMATOSUS (SLE): Consumption of seeds (not stems/leaves) might reactivate latent disease (6,605).

DIABETES: Alfalfa might reduce blood sugar levels; monitor closely (4).

HORMONE SENSITIVE CANCERS/CONDITIONS: Because alfalfa seems to have estrogenic effects (11), women with hormone sensitive conditions should avoid alfalfa. Some of these conditions include breast, uterine, and ovarian cancer, and endometriosis and uterine fibroids.

Dosage and Administration

ORAL: A typical dosage is 5-10 grams, or as steeped strained tea, three times a day (4).
Liquid extract (1:1 in 25% alcohol) 5-10 mL three times a day has also been used (4).

Comments

There is some evidence to suggest that saponins from alfalfa stem and leaves might lower cholesterol. Stems and leaves are reportedly free of systemic lupus erythematosus (SLE) triggering substance(s) found in seeds (4). There is one case report of listeriosis traced to the consumption of alfalfa tablets from which Listeria monocytogenes was isolated (5600).

ALGIN

Also Known As

Alginates, Sodium Alginate.
CAUTION: See separate listings for Laminaria and Bladderwrack.

Scientific Names

Ascophyllum nodosum; Laminaria digitata; Macrocystis pyrifera.
Family: Lessoniaceae.

People Use This For

Orally, algin is used to lower serum cholesterol levels and to reduce absorption of strontium, barium, tin, cadmium, manganese, zinc, and mercury (11).

In folk medicine, algin has been used for the prevention and treatment of hypertension (11).

In foods, algin is used in candy, gelatins, puddings, condiments, relishes, processed vegetables, fish products, and imitation dairy products.

In manufacturing, algin is used as a binding and disintegrating agent in tablets, as binding and demulcent in lozenges, and as film in peel-off facial masks (11).

Safety

LIKELY SAFE ...when used orally in amounts typically found in foods. It is approved in the US for use in foods with a maximum use level of 1%.

PREGNANCY AND LACTATION: Insufficient reliable information available.

Effectiveness

POSSIBLY EFFECTIVE ...when used orally to reduce cholesterol and blood pressure. ...when used to reduce absorption of strontium (11).
There is insufficient reliable information available about the effectiveness of algin for its other uses.

Mechanism of Action

Algin is the purified carbohydrate product extracted from brown seaweeds by use of dilute alkali. Algin is comprised of the sodium salt of alginic acid, a linear polymer of L-guluronic and D-mannuronic acid. Although mannuronic acid is the major component, there is variation depending on the algal source (13). Cholesterol lowering effects may be related to viscosity of gel and inhibiting cholesterol absorption (11). Hypotensive effects may be due to laminine dioxalate (11). Algin is believed, but not confirmed, to be indigestible (11).

Adverse Reactions

None reported.

Interactions with Herbs & Other Dietary Supplements

Insufficient reliable information available.

Interactions with Drugs

ORAL DRUGS: The fiber in algin can impair absorption of oral drugs (19).

Interactions with Foods

No interactions are known to occur, and there is no known reason to expect a clinically significant interaction with algin.

Interactions with Lab Tests

CHOLESTEROL: Theoretically, algin might reduce serum cholesterol concentrations and test results (11).
BLOOD PRESSURE: Theoretically, algin might lower blood pressure and blood pressure readings (11).

Interactions with Diseases or Conditions

No interactions are known to occur, and there is no known reason to expect a clinically significant interaction with algin.

Dosage and Administration

No typical dosage.

Comments

Algin is isolated from a variety of brown algae (seaweeds, Class: Phaeophyceae), particularly from the genera Ascophyllum, Macrocystis, and Laminaria (11).

ALKANNA

Also Known As

Alkanet, Alkanna Radix, Anchusa, Dyer's Bugloss, Henna, Orchanet, Radix Anchusae.
CAUTION: See separate listing for Henna.

Scientific Names

Alkanna tinctoria.
Family: Boraginaceae.

People Use This For

Historically, alkanna was used topically by the ancient Greeks to heal skin wounds (18). It was also used as an astringent (6,8), for skin diseases, and diarrhea (6,8).

Safety

POSSIBLY UNSAFE …when the root preparations are used topically on broken or abraded skin (12) because they contain toxic unsaturated pyrrolizidine alkaloids (UPAs) that might be absorbed systemically.
LIKELY UNSAFE …when used orally. Repeated exposure to low concentrations of UPAs is linked to serious liver toxicity (4,12). UPAs are also thought to be carcinogenic and mutagenic (12).
There is insufficient reliable information available about the safety of alkanna used topically on unbroken skin.
PREGNANCY: POSSIBLY UNSAFE …when used topically (12). LIKELY UNSAFE …when used orally because it contains UPAs.
LACTATION: POSSIBLY UNSAFE …when used topically. LIKELY UNSAFE …when used orally. There is concern that UPAs could be excreted in breast milk (4,12,18).

Effectiveness
POSSIBLY EFFECTIVE …when used topically for enhancing wound healing of leg ulcers (6,18).
There is insufficient reliable information available about the effectiveness of alkanna for its other uses.

Mechanism of Action
The applicable part of alkanna is the root. Alkanna contains napthazarine esters, pyrrozolidine alkaloids, and tannins (18). Some pyrrolizidine alkaloids have shown carcinogenic and mutagenic properties, and there are reports of renal toxicity. However, the primary concern is veno-occlusive disease (12). Unsaturated pyrrolizidine alkaloids are known to be hepatotoxic (4). The color of alkanna comes from a mixture of 5-6% red pigments which consist mainly of fat-soluble naphthazarin (6).

Adverse Reactions
Chronic exposure to plants containing UPA constituents has been associated with veno-occlusive disease (4021). Symptoms of acute veno-occlusive disease are characterized by a dull, dragging ache in the right upper abdomen and marked distention of the abdomen. These symptoms are sometimes accompanied by reduced urine output. Subacute veno-occlusive disease is associated with vague symptoms and persistent liver enlargement (4021).

Interactions with Herbs & Other Dietary Supplements
EUCALYPTUS: Theoretically, concomitant use might increase the risk of unsaturated pyrrolizidine alkaloid toxicity due to enzyme induction by eucalyptus (19).
PYRROLIZIDINE ALKALOID-CONTAINING HERBS: Concomitant use is contraindicated due to the risk of additive toxicity. Herbs containing unsaturated pyrrolizidine alkaloids include alkanna (12), borage (271), gravel root (4), hemp agrimony (271), hound's tongue (19), petasites (19), comfrey (271), coltsfoot; and the Senecio species plants dusty miller (19), alpine ragwort (19), groundsel (271), golden ragwort (19), and tansy ragwort (271).

Interactions with Drugs
No interactions are known to occur, and there is no known reason to expect a clinically significant interaction with alkanna.

Interactions with Foods
No interactions are known to occur, and there is no known reason to expect a clinically significant interaction with alkanna.

Interactions with Lab Tests
No interactions are known to occur, and there is no known reason to expect a clinically significant interaction with alkanna.

Interactions with Diseases or Conditions
LIVER DISEASE: Alkanna is contraindicated due to hepatotoxic potential (19).

Dosage and Administration
No typical dosage.

Comments
Although alkanna is used as a reddish pigment in foods and cosmetics, many countries have banned its use in food (8).

ALLSPICE

Also Known As
Aqua Pimentae, Clove Pepper, Jamaica Pepper, Kiln-Dried Allspice, Pimenta, Pimento, Pimento Oil, Pimento Water, Spanish Pimienta, Water of Pimento.

Scientific Names
Pimenta dioica, synonyms Pimenta officinalis, Eugenia pimenta.
Family: Myrtaceae.

People Use This For
Topically, allspice is used for muscle pain, toothache, and as an antiseptic.
In dentistry, some dentists use eugenol, an active ingredient in allspice, as a local antiseptic and as an antiseptic for teeth and gums (7200).

In folk medicine, allspice is used to treat indigestion and flatulence (11), and as a purgative. It is also used for stomachache, menorrhagia, vomiting, diarrhea (6), fever, influenza, and colds.

For food uses, allspice is used as an aromatic spice. In manufacturing, it is used in toothpaste as a flavoring.

Safety

LIKELY SAFE ...when used orally in amounts found in foods (12). Allspice has Generally Recognized As Safe status (GRAS) for use in foods in the US (7112).

There is insufficient reliable information about the safety of allspice in amounts typically found in foods.

PREGNANCY AND LACTATION: LIKELY SAFE ...when used orally in amounts found in foods (7112).

There is insufficient reliable information available about the safety of allspice when used in greater amounts for women who are pregnant or breast-feeding.

Effectiveness

There is insufficient reliable information available about the effectiveness of allspice.

Mechanism of Action

The applicable parts of allspice are the unripe fruit and leaf. The eugenol in allspice may explain this product's effects on the digestive system and its pain relief properties. Eugenol seems to decrease intestinal pain by depressing the CNS and inhibiting prostaglandin activity in the human colon mucosa (11). It also increases the activity of some digestive enzymes, including trypsin (7200). Eugenol may be responsible for allspice's anesthetic effects when the crushed berries are applied topically.

Adverse Reactions

Orally, excessive doses of allspice may cause nausea, vomiting, CNS depression, and convulsions due to eugenol content (6).

Topically, allspice may irritate mucous membranes (6).

Interactions with Herbs & Other Dietary Supplements

Insufficient reliable information available.

Interactions with Drugs

ANTICOAGULANT and ANTIPLATELET DRUGS: Eugenol inhibits platelet activity. Individuals on anticoagulant or antiplatelet therapy who choose to use this product should use caution (4).

Interactions with Foods

No interactions are known to occur, and there is no known reason to expect a clinically significant interaction with allspice.

Interactions with Lab Tests

No interactions are known to occur, and there is no known reason to expect a clinically significant interaction with allspice.

Interactions with Diseases or Conditions

No interactions are known to occur, and there is no known reason to expect a clinically significant interaction with allspice.

Dosage and Administration

ORAL: Typical dose for flatulence is 0.05-0.2 mL allspice oil (11).
TOPICAL: No typical dosage.

Comments

The commercially available allspice powder consists of whole ground dried fruit (6).

ALOE dried juice from leaf, latex

Also Known As

Aloe Juice, Aloe Latex, Burn Plant, Elephant's Gall, Hsiang-Dan, Lily of the Desert, Lu-Hui, Miracle Plant, Plant of Immortality.
CAUTION: See separate listing for Aloe gel.

Scientific Names

Aloe africana; Aloe arborescens natalenis; Aloe barbadensis, synonym Aloe vera; Aloe ferox; Aloe perfoliata; Aloe perryi; Aloe spicata.
Family: Liliaceae.

People Use This For

Orally, aloe dried juice from leaf, latex is used as a laxative or cathartic (5). It is also used for seizures, asthma, colds, ulcers, bleeding, amenorrhea, colitis, depression, diabetes, glaucoma, multiple sclerosis, hemorrhoids, peptic ulcers, varicose veins, bursitis, arthritis, and vision problems.

Safety

POSSIBLY SAFE ...when used orally and appropriately short-term (2,12).
LIKELY UNSAFE ...when used orally long-term (8). Prolonged use can lead to tolerance (2,4). ...when used orally in high doses. Lethal dose: 1 gram per day for several days (8). ...when used orally during menstruation (8) or by women who have bleeding between periods, because it might increase blood to the uterus (19).
CHILDREN: LIKELY UNSAFE ...when used orally in children younger than 12 years (2,4).
PREGNANCY: LIKELY UNSAFE ...when used orally because it can induce abortions and stimulate menstruation (19).
LACTATION: LIKELY UNSAFE ...when used orally because genotoxic aloe-emodin might pass into milk (2,4,19).

Effectiveness

LIKELY EFFECTIVE ...when used orally as a stimulant laxative due to the cathartic effects of the anthraquinones in the aloe (2,4,5,8).
There is insufficient reliable information available about the effectiveness of aloe dried juice from leaf, latex for its other uses.

Mechanism of Action

It is likely that the anthracene derivatives are cleaved into aloe-emodin anthrone in the colon. Anthrones irritate mucous membranes, causing increased mucous secretion and peristalsis. Aloe increases motility of the colon and therefore, increases propulsion and reduces transit time. It also causes fluids and electrolytes to be secreted in the lumen. The effects of aloe cause a feeling of distention. These cathartic effects happen within about ten hours of taking the dose. Water and electrolyte reabsorption are inhibited (8). Aloe juice and latex causes loss of potassium, which paralyzes the intestinal muscles. With continued use, the dose must be increased to maintain a laxative effect (8). Anthroid laxative use is not associated with an increased risk of developing colorectal ademoma or carcinoma (6138).

Adverse Reactions

Orally, aloe dried juice from leaf, latex occasionally leads to abdominal pain and cramps (2,4). Long-term use or abuse of aloe can cause diarrhea, sometimes with blood and sometimes without blood; nephritis; potassium depletion; albuminuria; hematuria; muscle weakness; weight loss; pseudomelanosis coli; and heart disturbances (4). Pseudomelanosis coli (pigment spots in intestinal mucosa) is harmless, usually reverses with discontinuation (2), and is not associated with an increased risk of developing colorectal ademoma or carcinoma (6138).
Tolerance: Aloe dried juice from leaf and latex causes loss of potassium, which paralyzes the intestinal muscles. With continued use, the dose must be increased to maintain the laxative effect (8).

Interactions with Herbs & Other Dietary Supplements

CARDIAC GLYCOSIDE-CONTAINING HERBS: Theoretically, overuse of aloe can increase the risk of cardiac glycoside toxicity. Watch for possible interactions with herbs that contain cardiac glycosides such as black hellebore, Canadian hemp roots, digitalis leaf, hedge mustard, figwort, lily of the valley roots, motherwort, oleander leaf, pheasant's eye plant, pleurisy root, squill bulb leaf scales, and strophanthus seeds (2,18,19,500).
STIMULANT LAXATIVE HERBS: Theoretically, concomitant use of aloe with other stimulant laxative herbs may increase the risk of potassium depletion. Stimulant laxative herbs include wild cucumber fruit (Ecballium elaterium), blue flag rhizome, alder buckthorn, European buckthorn, butternut bark, cascara bark, castor oil, colocynth fruit pulp, gamboge bark exudate, jalap root, black root, manna bark exudate, podophyllum root, rhubarb root, senna leaves and pods, and yellow dock root (19).
LICORICE/HORSETAIL: Theoretically, concomitant use of aloe with horsetail plant or licorice rhizome increases the risk of potassium depletion (19).

Interactions with Drugs

CARDIAC GLYCOSIDES: Theoretically, overuse of aloe increases the risk of adverse effects from the cardiac glycoside drugs. Overuse of aloe along with drugs that contain cardiac glycosides, such as digoxin (Lanoxin) (19), can increase the risk of toxicity from increased cardiac glycoside effects.

ANTIARRHYTHMIC DRUGS: Overuse of aloe can increase the risk of drug toxicity (664).
DIURETICS: Overuse of aloe can compound potassium loss (2).
CORTICOSTEROIDS: Overuse of aloe can compound potassium loss (2).
ORAL DRUGS: Aloe can reduce drug absorption of some other drugs because aloe causes shorter GI transit time (500).

Interactions with Foods
No interactions are known to occur, and there is no known reason to expect a clinically significant interaction with aloe dried juice from leaf, latex.

Interactions with Lab Tests
BLOOD GLUCOSE: Small amounts of dried aloe juice might reduce blood glucose concentrations and test results (4).
COLORIMETRIC DIAGNOSTIC TESTS: Dried aloe juice discolors alkaline urine (red) and can interfere with diagnostic tests that depend on a color change (2,4).
SERUM POTASSIUM: Excessive use of dried aloe juice can cause potassium depletion, reducing serum potassium concentrations and test results (2,4,5,8,19).

Interactions with Diseases or Conditions
GI CONDITIONS: Contraindicated in individuals with intestinal obstruction, acute intestinal inflammation (Crohn's disease, ulcerative colitis, appendicitis), ulcers, abdominal pain of unknown origin, nausea, or vomiting (2,4) due to the irritating effect of anthranoid aloins (19).
HEMORRHOIDS: Contraindicated due to the possibility of causing stenosis, thrombosis or prolapse (19).
HEART CONDITIONS: Theoretically, overuse of aloe dried juice/latex might lead to potassium depletion (8).
KIDNEY DISORDERS: Contraindicated; theoretically, excessive doses can cause nephritis (19).

Dosage and Administration
ORAL: The common laxative dose is 100-200 mg aloe or 50 mg aloe extract taken in the evening (8). People also typically use 50-200 mg daily of the capsules (5011) that contain aloe leaf gel and/or latex, which is the residue resulting after the liquid from cut aloe evaporates (5012). Aloe juice product manufacturers suggest taking 1 to 8 ounces of the juice containing 99.7% of the whole leaf aloe vera juice daily (5015).

Comments
Aloe juice/latex is obtained from the cells beneath the plant's skin and contains cathartic laxative anthraquinones (101). Avoid confusion with aloe gel, which is obtained from the thin-walled mucilaginous cells of the inner central zone of the leaf. Aloe gel products sold for internal consumption might be contaminated with aloe juice/latex which can cause cathartic laxative effects (5). Aloe of the Bible is an unrelated fragrant wood used as incense (5).

ALOE gel

Also Known As
Aloe, Aloe Capensis, Aloe Leaf Gel, Aloe Vera, Salvia.
CAUTION: See separate listing for Aloe dried juice from leaf, latex.

Scientific Names
Aloe africana; Aloe arborescens natalenis; Aloe barbadensis, synonym Aloe vera; Aloe ferox; Aloe perfoliata; Aloe perryi; Aloe spicata.
Family: Liliaceae.

People Use This For
Orally, aloe gel is used for inflammation, arthritis, fever, anesthesia, itching, as a general tonic, antiseptic, and moisturizer (5). Aloe gel is also used orally for gastroduodenal ulcers, diabetes, and asthma.
Topically, aloe gel is used for burns and wound healing (5), inflammation, arthritis, and cold sores.

Safety
LIKELY SAFE ...when applied topically, although the maximum duration of treatment is not established (4).
POSSIBLY UNSAFE ...when used orally due to potential contamination with the anthraquinone constituents (4). Anthraquinones act as stimulant laxative.
PREGNANCY AND LACTATION: LIKELY SAFE ...when used topically (4). POSSIBLY UNSAFE ...when used orally; avoid using because of the potential for anthraquinone contamination (4).

Effectiveness
POSSIBLY EFFECTIVE ...when applied topically for reducing pain and inflammation; and enhancing the healing of burns, skin ulcerations, dermabrasion, psoriasis, and frostbite injury (4,5,6,101).
There is insufficient reliable information available about the effectiveness of aloe gel for its other uses.

Mechanism of Action
The carboxypeptidase and salicylate components of aloe gel can inhibit bradykinin, which is a pain-producing agent. The magnesium lactate component can inhibit histamine to reduce itching. Other components appear to slow the formation of thromboxane and thereby speed the healing of burns. Some evidence suggests aloe gel has antibacterial and antifungal properties (101).

Adverse Reactions
Orally, the potential exists for adverse reactions with aloe gel products that are contaminated with anthraquinones, which act as cathartic laxatives.

Interactions with Herbs & Other Dietary Supplements
Insufficient reliable information available.

Interactions with Drugs
GLYBURIDE: Concomitant use with glyburide (Diabeta, Micronase, Glynase) may increase hypoglycemic effects. Monitor blood glucose (19).
DIABETES THERAPY: Monitor blood glucose levels closely due to claims that aloe gel has hypoglycemic effects (19).
HYDROCORTISONE: Theoretically, concomitant topical use with hydrocortisone might increase anti-inflammatory effects (19).

Interactions with Foods
No interactions are known to occur, and there is no known reason to expect a clinically significant interaction with aloe gel.

Interactions with Lab Tests
No interactions are known to occur, and there is no known reason to expect a clinically significant interaction with aloe gel.

Interactions with Diseases or Conditions
GI OR KIDNEY CONDTIONS: Aloe gel could be contaminated with aloe latex and should be used cautiously or avoided by individuals with intestinal obstruction, Crohn's disease, ulcerative colitis, appendicitis, peptic ulcers, abdominal pain of unknown origin, nausea, vomiting, hemorrhoids (2,4), and kidney disease (2,4).
DIABETES: Monitor blood glucose levels closely due to claims that aloe gel has hypoglycemic effects (19).

Dosage and Administration
ORAL: People typically use 50-200 mg daily of the capsules that contain aloe leaf gel (5011,5012). Some people take 30 mL of aloe gel internally three times daily (5011) or 15-60 drops of an aloe tincture (1:10, 50% alcohol) as needed (5013). Many strengths of capsules are available, such as 75 mg, 100 mg and 200 mg (5008).
TOPICAL: People commonly apply aloe gel liberally as needed three to five times daily (5011). The aloe gel is available in 99.5%, 99.6%, 98% (5008), and 100% purity strengths (5014).

Comments
Aloe gel is the clear, jelly-like substance that is obtained from the thin-walled, sticky cells of the inner portion of the leaf. Avoid confusion with aloe juice or latex which is obtained from the cells beneath the plant's skin and contains the cathartic laxative anthraquinones (101). Aloe gel products sold for internal consumption can be contaminated with aloe juice or latex (5). Stabilized aloe gel is not always topically effective (5).

ALPHA HYDROXY ACIDS

Also Known As

AHA, Alpha-Hydroxy Acids, Alpha-hydroxyethanoic Acid, Apple Acid, Citric Acid, Dihydroxysuccinic Acid, Gluconolactone, Glycolic Acid, Hydroxyacetic Acid, Hydroxycaprylic Acid, Hydroxypropionic Acid, Hydroxysuccinic Acid, Lactic Acid, Malic Acid, Mixed Fruit Acid, Monohydroxysuccinic Acid, Tartaric Acid.

Scientific Names

Hydroxysuccinic acid; Monohydroxysuccinic acid (Malic acid); 2-hydroxypropionic acid (Lactic acid); Hydroxyacetic acid (Glycolic acid); Dihydroxysuccinic acid (Tartaric acid); Gluconolactone.

People Use This For

Orally, malic acid (an alpha hydroxy acid) is used with magnesium for treating pain and tenderness associated with fibromyalgia (3262).

Topically, alpha hydroxy acids are used for moisturizing and removing dead skin cells (6), for treating acne (947), improving the appearance of photo-aged skin (952,953,954), and for xerosis (pathologic dry skin) (949,955).

Safety

LIKELY SAFE ...when used topically and appropriately (947,949,952). Preparations containing concentrations of 10% or less can be safely used for self-treatment. However higher concentrations should only be used with the supervision of a cosmetologist or physician (6079).

POSSIBLY SAFE ...when malic acid (an alpha hydroxy acid) is used orally and appropriately. Malic acid has been safely used for up to 6 months (3262).

PREGNANCY AND LACTATION: LIKELY SAFE ...when used topically and appropriately (947,949,952). There is insufficient reliable information available about the safety of the oral use of malic acid during pregnancy and lactation; avoid using.

Effectiveness

LIKELY EFFECTIVE ...when used in a lotion or cream topically and daily for treating photo-damaged skin (952,953,954). ...when used in a lotion or cream topically for treating dry skin (949,955).

POSSIBLY EFFECTIVE ...when used topically for treating acne (947). ...when malic acid (an alpha hydroxy acid) is used orally with magnesium hydroxide (Super Malic tablets) for reducing pain and tenderness associated with fibromyalgia (3262).

LIKELY INEFFECTIVE ...when used topically in short-contact skin peels for treating photo-damaged skin (953).

Mechanism of Action

Alpha hydroxy acids are a group of natural fruit acids including citric, glycolic, lactic, and malic acids; and gluconolactone (6,6064). Hyperkeratinization is thought to contribute to acne, dry skin, and photo-aging. Alpha hydroxy acids work by exfoliating the top layers of dead skin cells (948,950,6064,6079). Alpha-hydroxy acids seem to improve the appearance of aging skin by increasing smoothness and reducing dark spots (6064). The degree of exfoliation is determined by the type, concentration, and pH of the alpha hydroxy acid; and other ingredients in the product. The lower the pH of the alpha hydroxy acid, the more rapidly it is absorbed into the skin (6079). Alpha-hydroxy acids can also enhance skin barrier function (951) and decrease cohesiveness of corneocytes by weakening intracellular bonding (6). The alpha-hydroxy acid, malic acid, plus magnesium hydroxide seems to decrease pain and tenderness in patients with fibromyalgia, but the mechanism is not known (3262).

Adverse Reactions

Orally, the alpha-hydroxy acid, malic acid, seems to be well tolerated. Some patients can experience gastrointestinal upset including diarrhea and nausea (3262).

Topically, alpha-hydroxy acids are generally well tolerated when used in concentrations below 10% (947,949,952). However, these products can increase sensitivity to the sun and ultraviolet (UV) light. This can increase damage to the skin, and after long-term use might increase the risk of skin cancer. Advise patients to protect themselves from the sun by using sunscreen and/or protective clothing. Also, tell patients to test the product on a small area of skin before applying it to a larger area. Adverse reactions can range from mild irritation and stinging to severe redness, swelling, itching, blistering, bleeding, rash, burns, and skin discoloration (6079,6080). Higher concentrations are more likely to cause severe skin irritation, burning, and sloughing (6).

Interactions with Herbs & Other Dietary Supplements
MAGNESIUM: Malic acid (an alpha hydroxy acid) is used with magnesium hydroxide for reducing pain and tenderness associated with fibromyalgia (3262).

Interactions with Drugs
MAGNESIUM: Malic acid (an alpha hydroxy acid) is used with magnesium for reducing pain and tenderness associated with fibromyalgia (3262).

Interactions with Foods
No interactions are known to occur, and there is no known reason to expect a clinically significant interaction with alpha hydroxy acids.

Interactions with Lab Tests
No interactions are known to occur, and there is no known reason to expect a clinically significant interaction with alpha hydroxy acids.

Interactions with Diseases or Conditions
INDIVIDUALS WITH SENSITIVE SKIN: Alpha hydroxy acids can worsen skin conditions by causing skin irritation and sloughing (6).

Dosage and Administration
ORAL: For reducing pain and tenderness associated with fibromyalgia, malic acid (an alpha hydroxy acid) 800-1200 mg per day orally with magnesium hydroxide 200-300 mg twice daily, equivalent to 4-6 Super Malic tablets twice daily, has been used (3262).
TOPICAL: For treating photo-aged skin alpha-hydroxy acid products are typically used in a concentration of 8% as lactic acid, tartaric acid, gluconolactone, or glycolic acid. They are usually applied to facial or other photo-aged skin twice daily (950,952). The alpha-hydroxy acid glucolactone has also been used in a 14% solution. A 12% lactic acid lotion has also been used (955).

Comments
Alpha-hydroxy acid-containing cosmetic products may lack concentration information on labeling. Try to use products that identify the concentration of active ingredients.

ALPHA-KETOGLUTARATE

Also Known As
A-Ketoglutaric Acid, Alpha Ketoglutarate, Alpha Ketoglutaric Acid, Alpha-Keto Glutarate, Alpha-Ketoglutarates, Alpha-Ketoglutaric Acid, Alpha KG, AKG.

Scientific Names
2-Oxopentanedoicic acid, 2-Oxoglutaric acid.

People Use This For
Orally, alpha-ketoglutarate is used for treating chronic kidney and gastrointestinal dysfunction, bacterial overgrowth, intestinal toxemia, liver dysfunction, and chronic candidiasis (5305). It is also used as an adjunct to diet and training for improving peak athletic performance (5307), and improving amino acid metabolism in hemodialysis patients (5311). Intravenously, alpha-ketoglutarate is used for preventing ischemic injury during heart surgery (5312,5313), improving renal blood flow after heart surgery (5308), and preventing muscle protein depletion after surgery or trauma (5309,5310).

Safety
POSSIBLY SAFE …when used orally and appropriately (5311). …when used intravenously and appropriately (5308,5309,5310,5311,5312,5313).
PREGNANCY AND LACTATION: Insufficient reliable information available; avoid using.

Effectiveness
POSSIBLY EFFECTIVE …when used intravenously for preventing ischemic injury during heart surgery (5312,5313). …when used for preventing muscle protein depletion after surgery or trauma (5309,5310).
There is insufficient reliable information available about the effectiveness of alpha-ketoglutarate for its other uses.

Mechanism of Action

Alpha-ketoglutarate, the carbon skeleton of glutamate and glutamine, is an intermediate compound in the Krebs cycle (5308). As a precursor of glutamate, alpha-ketoglutarate is taken up by fibroblasts involved in wound healing (5314). The availability of alpha-ketoglutarate determines the recovery of muscle protein synthesis after surgical trauma (5309). Some evidence suggests that rapidly growing cells use alpha-ketoglutarate when cellular glutamine uptake is limited (5314). Hemodialysis patients who take alpha-ketoglutarate with calcium carbonate have improved amino acid metabolism and reduced hyperphosphatemia (5311).

Adverse Reactions

None reported.

Interactions with Herbs & Other Dietary Supplements

Insufficient reliable information available.

Interactions with Drugs

No interactions are known to occur, and there is no known reason to expect a clinically significant interaction with alpha-ketoglutarate.

Interactions with Foods

No interactions are known to occur, and there is no known reason to expect a clinically significant interaction with alpha-ketoglutarate.

Interactions with Lab Tests

No interactions are known to occur, and there is no known reason to expect a clinically significant interaction with alpha-ketoglutarate.

Interactions with Diseases or Conditions

No interactions are known to occur, and there is no known reason to expect a clinically significant interaction with alpha-ketoglutarate.

Dosage and Administration

ORAL: A typical dose of alpha-ketoglutaric acid is 500 mg 10 to 30 minutes before a workout, then again with food 30 minutes after a workout (5307). To improve amino acid metabolism in hemodialysis patients, 1.187 grams are typically used three times daily (5311).
INTRAVENOUS: For cardiac surgery, a dose of 28 grams of alpha-ketoglutarate has been added to blood cardioplegia (5312,5313). For preventing muscle protein depletion after surgery or trauma, 280 mg/kg of body weight is added to parenteral nutrition (5310).

Comments

Suppliers of athletic nutritional supplements claim alpha-ketoglutaric acid may be an important adjunct to proper diet and training for the athlete desiring peak performance. They base this claim on studies that show excessive ammonia in the body can combine with alpha-ketoglutarate to reduce ammonia toxicity. So far, the only studies that show alpha-ketoglutarate can reduce ammonia toxicity have been performed in hemodialysis patients (5311).

ALPHA-LINOLENIC ACID

Also Known As

ALA, Alpha Linolenic Acid, Essential Fatty Acid, LNA, n-3 Fatty Acid, n-3 Polyunsaturated Fatty Acid, Omega-3 Fatty Acid, Omega-3 Polyunsaturated Fatty Acid.
CAUTION: See separate listings for Blue-Green Algae, Chasteberry, DHA, Emu Oil, English Walnut, EPA, Fish Oils, Flaxseed Oil, Gamma-Linolenic Acid, Lecithin, Safflower, Sea Buckthorn, and Sour Cherry.

Scientific Names

Alpha-Linolenic Acid.

People Use This For

Orally, alpha-linolenic acid is used to treat hypertension, rheumatoid arthritis, multiple sclerosis, lupus, diabetes, hypercholesterolemia, renal disease, ulcerative colitis, Crohn's disease, chronic obstructive pulmonary disease (COPD), migraine headache, skin cancer, depression, and allergic and inflammatory conditions such as psoriasis and eczema (7140,7148). Alpha-linolenic acid is also used to prevent cardiovascular disease and cancer (7140,7168).

Safety

LIKELY SAFE …when used orally in amounts typically found in foods (7141,7142,7144). There is insufficient reliable information available about the safety of alpha-linolenic acid when used in amounts exceeding those typically found in foods.

PREGNANCY AND LACTATION: LIKELY SAFE …when used orally in amounts typically found in foods (7141,7142,7145). There is insufficient reliable information available about the safety of alpha-linolenic acid during pregnancy and lactation when used in amounts exceeding those typically found in foods; avoid using.

Effectiveness

POSSIBLY EFFECTIVE …when used orally as a part of the diet for the primary prevention of coronary heart disease. There is some evidence that high dietary intake of alpha-linolenic acid over a period of 6 years can reduce the risk of myocardial infarction by as much as 59% in both men and women (7152). In women, a high dietary intake of alpha-linolenic acid over 10 years can reduce the risk of fatal ischemic heart disease by 65% (7153); however, it is not known if alpha-linolenic acid supplements have these same benefits. …when used orally as a part of the diet for secondary prevention of coronary heart disease. Starting a Mediterranean diet rich in alpha-linolenic acid and low in saturated fat and cholesterol after an initial myocardial infarction can significantly reduce the rate of occurrence of a second myocardial infarction and death rate. Over a 27 month period, patients using this diet seem to be 73% less likely to have a second myocardial infarction and 70% less likely to die from any cause, compared to the standard postinfarction diet (7150); however, it is not known if alpha-linolenic acid supplements have this same benefit. There is insufficient reliable information available about the effectiveness of alpha-linolenic acid for its other uses.

Mechanism of Action

Alpha-linolenic acid is an essential omega-3 fatty acid. Dietary alpha-linolenic acid is found in vegetable oils such as flaxseed (linseed) oil, canola (rapeseed) oil, and soybean oil. It is also found in margarines and salad dressings that contain vegetable oils (7141,7142). Walnuts and other edible nuts also contain significant amounts of alpha-linolenic acid. Alpha-linolenic acid is found in smaller amounts in green leafy vegetables, chocolate, and milk (7141). Alpha-linolenic acid is also a component of human milk, infant formulas, and intravenous fat emulsions (7143). The body converts some alpha-linolenic acid into longer and more unsaturated omega-3 fatty acids, such as eicosapentaenoic (EPA) and docosahexaenoic acids (DHA); however, the effects of EPA and DHA are not duplicated by alpha-linolenic acid, even at high doses (7141,7165). In some disease states, such as type 1 diabetes, chronic alcoholism, and schizophrenia, the amount of alpha-linolenic acid converted to longer chain fatty acids is reduced (7165); however, the reason for this is not known. Omega-6 fatty acids, such as linoleic acid, that are found in corn, safflower, sunflower, and peanut oils compete for enzyme systems that elongate alpha-linolenic acid into EPA and DHA (7142). The Western diet, including vegetarian diets, usually provides a disproportionate amount of omega-6 fatty acids. For example, the typical Western diet often includes an omega-6/omega-3 fatty acid ratio of 20-30:1 (7148,7149). There is some concern that a diet high in omega-6 fatty acids can lead to long-chain omega-3 fatty acid deficiency and produce a physiologic state that is favorable for platelet aggregation and clot formation and an increased risk of heart disease (7141,7142). The ideal omega-6/omega-3 fatty acid ratio in the diet should probably be no more than 4:1 (7141,7148). Some researchers theorize that adding omega-3 fatty acids, such as alpha-linolenic acid, can normalize this ratio and therefore decrease the risk of heart disease. Although alpha-linolenic acid itself does not appear to significantly affect coagulation, increased dietary alpha-linolenic acid can increase EPA levels and the omega-3 polyunsaturated fatty acid content of platelet phospholipids and plasma lipids (7149,7166). Accumulation of omega-3 fatty acids such as EPA and DHA in platelet phospholipids might inhibit platelet aggregation (2561). Although alpha-linolenic acid seems to have beneficial effects on the cardiovascular system and to reduce risk of heart disease it does not appear to have a significant effect on cholesterol or triglyceride levels (7146,7165). Alpha-linolenic acid does seem to increase arterial compliance and decrease cardiac workload (7165). There is also some evidence that alpha-linolenic acid has antiarrhythmic effects, but researchers are not sure if this is due to alpha-linolenic acid itself, or due to the longer-chain fatty acids EPA and DHA, to which alpha-linolenic acid is converted (7153,7156). Some researchers are interested in alpha-linolenic acid for prevention of breast cancer. There is some evidence that women with higher levels of alpha-linolenic acid in breast adipose tissue have a lower risk of breast cancer. Fatty acid composition of adipose tissue is thought to reflect past dietary intake, so researchers think high intake of alpha-linolenic acid might have a cancer protective effect (7168). However, there is some concern that high intake of alpha-linolenic acid might actually increase risk for prostate cancer (1334,1335,1336,2558,2559,7147,7167). Alpha-linolenic acid might increase free radical formation (2558); however, this mechanism has not been confirmed and the increased prostate cancer risk is probably more likely attributable to high animal fat intake and consumption of red meat and dairy products that contain alpha-linolenic acid rather than alpha-linolenic acid itself (1337,2558).

Adverse Reactions

Orally, alpha-linolenic acid from dietary sources is very well tolerated; however, alpha-linolenic acid is high in calories and may result in weight gain if consumed in excess. Patients should be advised that it's best to substitute alpha-linolenic acid in the diet for other sources of fat, such as saturated fats. Very high intake of alpha-linolenic acid from some dietary sources, such as margarine, which also contain high concentrations of linoleic and trans-fatty acids, can increase the risk of heart disease and myocardial infarction. This effect is probably attributable to trans-fatty acid content, and not alpha-linolenic acid (7155). There is also some concern that high intake of alpha-linolenic acid might increase risk for prostate cancer (1334,1335,1336,2558,2559,7147,7167); however, this risk may be attributable to high animal fat intake and consumption of red meat and dairy products that contain alpha-linolenic acid (1337,2558). Alpha-linolenic acid itself has not been shown to cause prostate cancer. Tell patients not to be concerned about moderate dietary intake of alpha-linolenic acid.

Interactions with Herbs & Other Dietary Supplements
Insufficient reliable information available.

Interactions with Drugs
No interactions are known to occur, and there is no known reason to expect a clinically significant interaction with alpha-linolenic acid.

Interactions with Foods
No interactions are known to occur, and there is no known reason to expect a clinically significant interaction with alpha-linolenic acid.

Interactions with Lab Tests
BLOOD PRESSURE: Alpha-linolenic acid might decrease diastolic blood pressure in patients with hypertension when consumed in place of dietary linoleic acid (7151).

Interactions with Diseases or Conditions
ALCOHOLISM: The synthesis of long-chain omega-3 fatty acids from alpha-linolenic acid may be reduced in chronic alcohol abuse (7165).
DIABETES: Diabetes may reduce the synthesis of long-chain omega-3 fatty acids from alpha-linolenic acid (7141,7165).
SCHIZOPHRENIA: The synthesis of long-chain omega-3 fatty acids from alpha-linolenic acid may be reduced in people with schizophrenia (7165).

Dosage and Administration
ORAL: For primary prevention of coronary heart disease, approximately 1.2-2 grams per day from dietary sources seems to be associated with the greatest benefit (7152,7153,7156). For secondary prevention of coronary heart disease, approximately 1.6 grams per day as part of a Mediterranean diet appears to be beneficial (7150). Fatty acid dosing is often done based on percentage of daily calories it provides. Some researchers suggest that alpha-linolenic acid should make up roughly 1% of daily calories. This comes to approximately 2 grams based on a 2000 kilocalorie diet (149,7165).

Comments
Use caution in extrapolating information about other omega-3 fatty acids, including EPA and DHA, to alpha-linolenic acid. Although some alpha-linolenic acid is converted to long-chain fatty acids, clinical effects may be different.

ALPHA-LIPOIC ACID

Also Known As
a-Lipoic Acid, Acetate Replacing Factor, ALA, Alpha Lipoic Acid, Alpha-Lipoic Acid Extract, Biletan, Lipoic Acid, Lipoicin, Thioctacid, Thioctan, Thioctic Acid.

Scientific Names
Alpha Lipoic Acid; 1,2-dithiolane-3-pentanoic acid; 1,2-dithiolane-3-valeric acid; 6,8-thioctic acid; 5-(1,2-dithiolan-3-yl) valeric acid; 6,8-dithiooctanoic acid.

People Use This For
Orally, alpha-lipoic acid is used as an antioxidant (1547). People with diabetes use alpha-lipoic acid to decrease blood glucose, treat and prevent peripheral neuropathy (1547,3540,3541,3557) and cardiac autonomic neuropathy (3543), and to improve insulin resistance in type 2 diabetes (3544,3545). Alpha-lipoic acid is used for preventing retinopathy (3543), cataracts (3546), and treating glaucoma (1551,1552). Alpha-lipoic acid is also used orally for treating HIV/AIDS, cancer, liver disease, Wilson's disease, cardiovascular disease, and lactic acidosis caused by inborn errors of metabolism (1554,1555,1556,1557,1570).
Intravenously, alpha-lipoic acid is used for improving insulin-resistance and glucose disposal in type 2 diabetes (3557,3874,3875), diabetic neuropathy (3540,3557), and Amanita mushroom poisoning (1547,1548,1549,3871).

Safety

POSSIBLY SAFE ...when used orally and appropriately. Oral alpha-lipoic acid has been used safely in clinical trials lasting from 4 months to 2 years (3540,3541,3542). ...when used intravenously and appropriately. Intravenous alpha-lipoic acid has been used safely in clinical trials lasting up to 3 weeks (3540,3557).

PREGNANCY AND LACTATION: Insufficient reliable information available; avoid using.

Effectiveness

POSSIBLY EFFECTIVE ...when used intravenously for improving symptoms of diabetic peripheral neuropathy (3540,3557). Clinical trials demonstrated significant improvement in Total Symptom Scores when diabetics with peripheral neuropathy were given alpha-lipoic acid 600 mg or 1200 mg intravenously daily. Improvement was seen after 5 days of treatment and continued until treatment was discontinued after 3 weeks (3540,3557). Lower doses have not shown to be effective (3869). ...when given orally or intravenously for improving insulin sensitivity and glucose disposal in type 2 diabetics (3545,3846,3874,3875,3876). Type 2 diabetics taking alpha-lipoic acid 600 to 1800 mg orally or 500 to 1000 mg intravenously daily had significant improvement in insulin resistance and glucose effectiveness after 4 weeks of oral treatment or after a single dose to 10 days of intravenous administration (3545,3846,3874,3875,3876).

POSSIBLY INEFFECTIVE ...when used orally for improving symptoms of diabetic peripheral neuropathy (3540,3541,3868). Placebo-controlled clinical trials demonstrated significant improvement in neuronal conduction measurements in diabetics with neuropathy who took alpha-lipoic acid orally, but this did not translate into significant symptom reduction (3540,3541,3868). ...when used orally for improving symptoms associated with cardiac autonomic neuropathy in diabetics (3542). A placebo-controlled clinical trial showed that autonomic nerve function indices measured by ECG improved in patients with cardiac autonomic neuropathy who took alpha-lipoic acid orally, but this did not translate into significantly improved symptoms (3541). ...when used orally for lowering glycosylated hemoglobin (HgbA1c) levels in patients with type 2 diabetes (3540). In one human study, alpha-lipoic acid failed to lower HgbA1c after 6 months of oral treatment in patients with type 2 diabetes (3540). ...when used orally for alcoholic liver disease (3880). People with alcohol-related liver disease taking alpha-lipoic acid 300 mg per day for 6 months did not demonstrate significant improvement compared to placebo (3880)...when used orally for HIV-related dementia (1556). Alpha-lipoic acid had no effect on HIV-associated cognitive impairment in a small trial comparing alpha-lipoic acid alone or in combination with selegiline (Deprenyl) and placebo (1556).

There is insufficient reliable information available about the effectiveness of alpha-lipoic acid for its other uses.

Mechanism of Action

Alpha-lipoic acid was identified as a vitamin when it was isolated 50 years ago, but was reclassified upon the finding that it is synthesized in humans and animals (3871). Endogenous alpha-lipoic acid is a coenzyme that, together with pyrophosphatase, is involved in carbohydrate metabolism and production of adenosine triphosphate (ATP) (6). Exogenous alpha-lipoic acid and the metabolite, dihydrolipoic acid (DHLA), have antioxidant activity and can scavenge free radicals both intra- and extra-cellularly (3871). Alpha-lipoic acid is both water and fat soluble and can regenerate endogenous antioxidants, such as vitamin E, vitamin C, and glutathione, and prevent oxidative damage (1547,1550,3546,3871). Alpha-lipoic acid is about 30% absorbed from dietary or supplemental sources, and is reduced to DHLA in many tissues (1561,3871,3872). Preliminary data suggests that these antioxidant effects might provide protection in cerebral ischemia, excitotoxic amino acid brain injury, mitochondrial dysfunction, diabetes, diabetic neuropathy, and other causes of damage to brain or neural tissue (1561,3546,3871). In experimental diabetic models, alpha-lipoic acid increases neuronal blood flow, improves neuronal glucose uptake, increases amounts of reduced glutathione in neurons, and improves neuronal conduction velocity (3873,3878). Preliminary evidence suggests that DHLA in combination with vitamin E might prevent oxidative stress in cardiac ischemia-reperfusion injury (3871,3877). The antioxidant effects of alpha-lipoic acid might be beneficial in liver diseases in which oxidative stress is a factor (3879). Alpha-lipoic acid has been used in combination with other treatments for Amanita mushroom poisoning (105,1548,1549,3871). Evidence of effectiveness in humans is anecdotal, and alpha-lipoic acid has been ineffective in laboratory models of Amanita poisoning, leading some groups to recommend eliminating it from treatment regimens for this condition (3871,3879). Alpha-lipoic acid has shown promise in experimental models to prevent aminoglycoside-induced cochlear damage, and metal (lead, arsenic, cadmium, mercury) and chemical (hexachlorobenzene, n-hexane) poisoning (3871,3879,3881,3882,3883,3884). Children treated with alpha-lipoic acid, alone or in combination with vitamin E, showed normalized organ function and lessened indices of oxidative damage following radiation exposure in the Chernobyl accident (3871). Case reports indicate that it may be helpful in various inborn errors of metabolism which result in lactic acidosis (1554,1555,1557). Preliminary data suggests that alpha-lipoic acid can inhibit replication of the human immunodeficiency virus (HIV) by inhibiting reverse transcriptase (1280,3871). Reactive oxygen species may act as intracellular messengers for HIV gene expression and transcription, and the antioxidant effects of alpha-lipoic acid could inhibit this process (1562,1563). Alpha-lipoic acid supplementation might improve blood antioxidant status and blood peroxidation products, and increase T-helper lymphocytes and T-helper to T-helper suppressor cell ratio, based on a small open trial in HIV positive patients (3885).

Adverse Reactions

Orally, skin rash has been reported after use of alpha-lipoic acid.

Intravenously, local allergic reactions have occurred at the injection site (14,1547). Paresthesias have been reported to worsen temporarily at the beginning of therapy. Rarely, platelet disorders and purpura have been observed after IV therapy (14). Alpha-lipoic acid can cause gastrointestinal upset, including nausea, vomiting, and headache. Adverse effects are more common in patients receiving higher intravenous doses (3557).

Preliminary evidence suggests that high doses of alpha-lipoic acid might cause thiamine deficiency. For people taking high doses of alpha-lipoic acid and who are at risk for thiamine deficiency (e.g., alcoholism), thiamine supplementation may be warranted (3871).

Interactions with Herbs & Other Dietary Supplements

HERBS WITH HYPOGLYCEMIC POTENTIAL: Theoretically, alpha-lipoic acid might have additive effects with herbs that decrease blood glucose levels. Herbs with hypoglycemic potential include devil's claw, fenugreek, garlic, guar gum, horse chestnut seed, Panax ginseng, psyllium, and Siberian ginseng.

HERBS WITH HYPERGLYCEMIC POTENTIAL: Theoretically, herbs that increase blood glucose levels might antagonize the antidiabetic effects of alpha-lipoic acid. Herbs with hyperglycemic potential include ephedra, ginger, gotu kola, and the above ground parts of the stinging nettle.

Interactions with Drugs

ANTI-DIABETES DRUGS: Theoretically, concomitant use might cause additive hypoglycemic effects (6,3545). Dosing adjustments for insulin or oral hypoglycemic agents may be necessary; however, in one study, co-administration of single doses of alpha-lipoic acid and glyburide or acarbose did not cause detectable drug interactions in healthy volunteers (3870).

CHEMOTHERAPEUTIC AGENTS: Theoretically, concomitant use might decrease the effectiveness of chemotherapy. Preliminary evidence from an unpublished study suggests antioxidants may decrease the effectiveness of chemotherapy (14,391).

ETHANOL: Concomitant use decreases the effects of alpha-lipoic acid (14).

Interactions with Foods

FOOD: Administration of alpha-lipoic acid with food decreases bioavailability (14). Alpha-lipoic acid should be taken on an empty stomach.

Interactions with Lab Tests

BLOOD GLUCOSE: Alpha-lipoic acid might decrease blood glucose levels and test results in patients with type 2 diabetes. Alpha-lipoic acid reduces insulin resistance and improves blood glucose disposal in patients with type 2 diabetes (3545); however, alpha-lipoic acid has no effect on glycosylated hemoglobin (HgbA1c) levels (3540,3557).

T HELPER/SUPPRESSOR LYMPHOCYTE RATIO: Alpha-lipoic acid might increase the T helper/suppressor ratio in patients infected with the human immunodeficiency virus (HIV) (6).

Interactions with Diseases or Conditions

BLOOD DYSCRASIAS: Intravenous alpha-lipoic acid has rarely been associated with platelet disorders and purpura (14). Theoretically, in these cases, alpha-lipoic acid may affect existing blood disorders.

DIABETES: Alpha-lipoic acid can decrease blood glucose levels (6,3545). Dosing adjustments for insulin or oral hypoglycemic agents may be necessary.

Dosage and Administration

ORAL: For treatment of diabetes and peripheral neuropathy, doses of 1200 mg daily or 600 mg three times daily have been used (3540,3541). For cardiac autonomic neuropathy in patients with type 2 diabetes, 800 mg daily has been used (3542). As a general antioxidant, people typically take 20 to 50 mg per day (3894).

INTRAVENOUS: For peripheral neuropathy in patients with type 2 diabetes, doses of 100 mg, 600 mg, or 1200 mg daily have been used (3540,3557); however, doses of 600 mg and 1200 mg daily appear to be more effective than 100 mg daily (3557).

Comments

High doses of alpha-lipoic acid are approved in Germany for the treatment of diabetic neuropathy. Clinical trials using alpha-lipoic acid in higher doses, which might be more effective, and of sufficient duration to show any long-term therapeutic effects are needed (3871). Good dietary sources of alpha-lipoic acid are yeast and liver; other sources include spinach, broccoli, potatoes, and kidney (6).

ALPINE CRANBERRY

Also Known As
Cowberry, Dry Ground Cranberry, Foxberry, Lingen, Lingenberry, Lingon, Lingonberry, Lowbush Cranberry, Moss Cranberry, Partridgeberry, Red Bilberry, Redberries, Red Whortleberry, Rock Cranberry, Shore Cranberry, Vine of Mount Ida.
CAUTION: See separate listings for Cranberry, Cramp Bark , and Uva Ursi.

Scientific Names
Vaccinium vitis-idaea.
Family: Ericaceae.

People Use This For
Orally, alpine cranberry is used for urinary tract irritation, gout, arthritis and kidney stones. It is also used orally as a urinary tract disinfectant, diuretic, and antiviral (18).

Safety
LIKELY UNSAFE …when the preparations of the leaves are used orally long-term because the arbutin constituent could be toxic (18).
There is insufficient reliable information available about the safety of the short-term oral use of alpine cranberry leaf.
CHILDREN: LIKELY UNSAFE …when used orally in children under 12 years of age because alpine cranberry might be hepatotoxic (18).
PREGNANCY AND LACTATION: LIKELY UNSAFE …when used orally because constituents have mutagenic effects (18); avoid using.

Effectiveness
There is insufficient reliable information available about the effectiveness of alpine cranberry.

Mechanism of Action
The applicable part of alpine cranberry is the leaf or berry. When ingested, alpine cranberry releases hydroquinones. In alkaline urine, the hydroquinones act as a disinfectant. Because hydroquinones can cause liver damage, long-term use is not recommended. There is also concern about long-term use because the constituents, arbutin and hydrochinon, are mutagenic and carcinogenic. (18).

Adverse Reactions
Orally, alpine cranberry may cause nausea and vomiting due to its high tannin content (18).

Interactions with Herbs & Other Dietary Supplements
Insufficient reliable information available.

Interactions with Drugs
ANTIGOUT AGENTS: Theoretically, medications that increase uric acid concentrations in the bladder may counteract effects (18).

Interactions with Foods
No interactions are known to occur, and there is no known reason to expect a clinically significant interaction with alpine cranberry.

Interactions with Lab Tests
No interactions are known to occur, and there is no known reason to expect a clinically significant interaction with alpine cranberry.

Interactions with Diseases or Conditions
LIVER DISEASE: Theoretically, the hydroquinones in alpine cranberry may worsen liver disease (18).

Dosage and Administration
ORAL: The typical daily dose is 2 grams of dried leaf or one cup of tea taken orally. The tea is prepared by steeping 2 grams dried leaf in 150 mL of boiling water for 10-15 minutes and straining (18).

Comments
Alpine cranberry leaves are sometimes used as a substitute for bearberry (uva ursi) leaves (18).

ALPINE LADY'S MANTLE

Also Known As
Alchemillae alpinae herba, Alpine Ladys Mantle.
CAUTION: See separate listing for Alchemilla (Lady's Mantle).

Scientific Names
Alchemilla alpina.
Family: Rosaceae.

People Use This For
Orally, alpine lady's mantle is used as a diuretic, antispasmodic, and cardioactive agent. It is also used for unspecific female complaints (2).

Safety
There is insufficient reliable information available about the safety of alpine lady's mantle.
Pregnancy and Lactation: Insufficient reliable information available; avoid using.

Effectiveness
There is insufficient reliable information available about the effectiveness of alpine lady's mantle.

Mechanism of Action
There is insufficient reliable information available about the possible mechanism of action and active ingredients.

Adverse Reactions
None reported.

Interactions with Herbs & Other Dietary Supplements
Insufficient reliable information available.

Interactions with Drugs
No interactions are known to occur, and there is no known reason to expect a clinically significant interaction with alpine lady's mantle.

Interactions with Foods
No interactions are known to occur, and there is no known reason to expect a clinically significant interaction with alpine lady's mantle.

Interactions with Lab Tests
No interactions are known to occur, and there is no known reason to expect a clinically significant interaction with alpine lady's mantle.

Interactions with Diseases or Conditions
No interactions are known to occur, and there is no known reason to expect a clinically significant interaction with alpine lady's mantle.

Dosage and Administration
No typical dosage.

Comments
Avoid confusion with alchemilla (lady's mantle).

ALPINE RAGWORT

Also Known As
Life Root, Liferoot, Senecio Herb, Squawweed, Squaw Weed.
CAUTION: See separate listing for Golden Ragwort (Senecio aureus).

Scientific Names
Senecio nemorensis.
Family: Asteraceae or Compositae.

People Use This For
Orally, alpine ragwort is used for diabetes mellitus, hemorrhage, high blood pressure, spasms, and as a uterine stimulant (2,18).
In folk medicine, it has been used to control bleeding after tooth extraction (18).

Safety
LIKELY UNSAFE ...when used orally, due to potential for liver toxicity and possible carcinogenicity and mutagenicity (4,12,18).
PREGNANCY AND LACTATION: LIKELY UNSAFE ...when used orally due to constituent hepatotoxic pyrrolizidine alkaloids contained in alpine ragwort (2). Pyrrolizidine alkaloids might also be excreted in milk (19).

Effectiveness
There is insufficient reliable information available about the effectiveness of alpine ragwort.

Mechanism of Action
The applicable parts of alpine ragwort are the above ground parts. Alpine ragwort contains the pyrrolizidines senecionine, fuschsisencionine, 7-angeloylretronecin, bulgarsenine, nemorensin, platyphyllin, and sarracin (18). Hepatotoxicity and carcinogenicity may result from the pyrrolizidine alkaloids and the unsaturated parent compounds (18). Some unsaturated pyrrolizidine alkaloids have shown carcinogenic and mutagenic properties, and there are reports of renal toxicity. However, the primary concern is veno-occlusive liver disease (12). Unsaturated pyrrolizidine alkaloids are known to be hepatotoxic in animals and humans (4).

Adverse Reactions
Chronic exposure to plants containing UPA constituents has been associated with veno-occlusive disease (4021). Symptoms of acute veno-occlusive disease are characterized by a dull, dragging ache in the right upper abdomen and marked distention of the abdomen. These symptoms are sometimes accompanied by reduced urine output. Subacute veno-occlusive disease is associated with vague symptoms and persistent liver enlargement (4021). Alpine ragwort can cause an allergic reaction in individuals sensitive to the Asteraceae/Compositae family. Members of this family include ragweed, chrysanthemums, marigolds, daisies, and many other herbs.

Interactions with Herbs & Other Dietary Supplements
EUCALYPTUS: Theoretically, concomitant use may increase the risk of unsaturated pyrrolizidine alkaloid toxicity due to enzyme induction by eucalyptus (19).
PYRROLIZIDINE ALKALOID-CONTAINING HERBS: Concomitant use is contraindicated due to the risk of additive toxicity. Herbs containing unsaturated pyrrolizidine alkaloids include alkanna (12), borage (271), gravel root (4), hemp agrimony (271), hound's tongue (19), petasites (19), comfrey (271), coltsfoot, and the Senecio species plants; dusty miller (19), alpine ragwort (19), groundsel (271), golden ragwort (19), and tansy ragwort (271).

Interactions with Drugs
No interactions are known to occur, and there is no known reason to expect a clinically significant interaction with alpine ragwort.

Interactions with Foods
No interactions are known to occur, and there is no known reason to expect a clinically significant interaction with alpine ragwort.

Interactions with Lab Tests
No interactions are known to occur, and there is no known reason to expect a clinically significant interaction with alpine ragwort.

Interactions with Diseases or Conditions
LIVER DISEASE: Contraindicated due to hepatotoxic potential (19).
CROSS-ALLERGENICITY: Can cause an allergic reaction in individuals sensitive to the Asteraceae/Compositae family. Members of this family include ragweed, chrysanthemums, marigolds, daisies, and many other herbs.

Dosage and Administration
No typical dosage.

Comments
Alpine ragwort is considered likely unsafe; avoid using. Avoid confusion with golden ragwort (Senecio aureus) also referred to as squaw weed.

ALPINIA

Also Known As
Catarrh Root, China Root, Chinese Ginger, Colic Root, East India Catarrh Root, East India Root, Galanga, Galangal, Gargaut, India Root, Rhizome Galangae.

Scientific Names
Alpinia officinarum.
Family: Zingiberaceae.

People Use This For
Orally, alpinia is used as an aromatic, stimulant, antiflatulent (6), antibacterial, antispasmodic, anti-inflammatory agent, and as a fever reducer (18).

Safety
LIKELY SAFE ...when used orally (6,12). There are no reports of health risks or side effects (18).
PREGNANCY AND LACTATION: Insufficient reliable information available; avoid using.

Effectiveness
POSSIBLY INEFFECTIVE ...when used orally for inflammation (6).
There is insufficient reliable information available about the effectiveness of alpinia for its other uses.

Mechanism of Action
The applicable part of alpinia is the rhizome. The gingerols and diaryheptanoids constituents are potent inhibitors of PG synthetase (prostaglandin biosynthesizing enzyme). Their structures indicate they can also be active against 5-lipoxygenase, an enzyme involved in leukotriene biosynthesis (6).

Adverse Reactions
None reported.

Interactions with Herbs & Other Dietary Supplements
Insufficient reliable information available.

Interactions with Drugs
ACID-INHIBITING DRUGS: Theoretically, due to claims that alpinia increases stomach acid, it might interfere with antacids, sucralfate (Carafate), H-2 antagonists (Zantac, Pepcid, Tagamet), or proton pump inhibitors (Prilosec, Prevacid) (19).

Interactions with Foods
No interactions are known to occur, and there is no known reason to expect a clinically significant interaction with alpinia.

Interactions with Lab Tests
No interactions are known to occur, and there is no known reason to expect a clinically significant interaction with alpinia.

Interactions with Diseases or Conditions

No interactions are known to occur, and there is no known reason to expect a clinically significant interaction with alpinia.

Dosage and Administration

ORAL: The typical dose of alpinia is 2-4 grams of the herb per day or one cup of the tea 30 minutes before meals (18). The tea is prepared by steeping 0.5-1 grams in 150 mL hot water for 10 minutes and then straining.

Comments

Alpinia is related to ginger in its botanical and pharmacological properties (6002). The uses of alpinia do not reflect its pharmacological properties. Some constituents possess antifungal activity while others inhibit prostaglandin biosynthesis and can inhibit leukotriene biosynthesis. The other Alpinia genus plants are also pharmacologically active (6).

AMARANTH

Also Known As

Lady Bleeding, Love-Lies-Bleeding, Lovely Bleeding, Pilewort, Prince's Feather, Red Cockscomb, Velvet Flower. CAUTION: See separate listings for Bulbous Buttercup and Lesser Celandine.

Scientific Names

Amaranthus hypochondriacus.

People Use This For

Orally, amaranth is used for ulcers, diarrhea, and inflammation of the mouth and throat (18).
In foods, amaranth is used similarly to wheat as a cereal grain (6189).

Safety

There is insufficient reliable information available about the safety of amaranth.
Pregnancy and Lactation: Insufficient reliable information available; avoid using.

Effectiveness

POSSIBLY INEFFECTIVE ...when used orally for lowering cholesterol in hypercholesterolemic adults (6188). Amaranth muffins added to a National Cholesterol Education Program (NCEP) step one low-fat diet failed to reduce cholesterol levels in a group of hypercholesterolemic adults beyond the reduction achieved by a group who ate only the low-fat diet (6188).
There is insufficient reliable information available about the effectiveness of amaranth for its other uses.

Mechanism of Action

The applicable part of amaranth is the whole plant. Amaranth is considered an astringent (18). The leaf contains a small amount of vitamin C (3833).

Adverse Reactions

None reported.

Interactions with Herbs & Other Dietary Supplements

Insufficient reliable information available.

Interactions with Drugs

No interactions are known to occur, and there is no known reason to expect a clinically significant interaction with amaranth.

Interactions with Foods

No interactions are known to occur, and there is no known reason to expect a clinically significant interaction with amaranth.

Interactions with Lab Tests

No interactions are known to occur, and there is no known reason to expect a clinically significant interaction with amaranth.

Interactions with Diseases or Conditions

No interactions are known to occur, and there is no known reason to expect a clinically significant interaction with amaranth.

Dosage and Administration

ORAL: People typically prepare amaranth as a tea, adding 1 teaspoon of leaves to 1 cup of cold water. The tea is taken cold, 1 to 2 cups a day. As a tincture amaranth is dosed up to 1 teaspoon (5263).

Comments

Avoid confusion with bulbous buttercup (Ranunculus bulbosus) or lesser celandine (Ranunculus ficaria), also known as pilewort.

AMBRETTE

Also Known As

Abelmosk, Ambretta, Egyptian Alcee, Muskmallow, Musk Seed, Okra, Target-Leaved Hibiscus.

Scientific Names

Abelmoschus moschatus, synonym Hibiscus abelmoschus.
Family: Malvaceae.

People Use This For

Orally, ambrette is used as a stimulant, antispasmodic (11), for snakebites, stomach and intestinal disorders with cramps, loss of appetite, and headaches (18).
In folk medicine, it is used for stomach cancer, hysteria, gonorrhea, and respiratory disorders (6).
For food uses, ambrette is an ingredient in vermouths, bitters, and other food products (11).
In manufacturing, ambrette is used in cosmetics such as perfumes, soaps, detergents, creams, and lotions (11).

Safety

POSSIBLY SAFE ...when the seeds or extracts are used orally. The extract has Generally Recognized as Safe (GRAS) status in the US. The maximum level is less than 0.001% (11). ...when the oil or absolute is used topically. The maximum use for the oil is 0.12% in perfumes (11).
There is insufficient reliable information available about the safety of larger amounts of ambrette used orally.
PREGNANCY: Insufficient reliable information available; avoid using.
LACTATION: POSSIBLY UNSAFE ...when used orally or topically because ambrette persists in mother's milk (6), but the effect is unknown.

Effectiveness

There is insufficient reliable information available about the effectiveness of ambrette.

Mechanism of Action

The applicable part of ambrette is the seed. The volatile oil is high in fatty acids, including palmitic and myristic acids (6). Ambrettolide and (Z)-5-tetradecen-14-olide are thought to be responsible for its characteristic musk-like odor (11).

Adverse Reactions

Topically, the use of ambrette can cause dermal irritation (6).

Interactions with Herbs & Other Dietary Supplements

Insufficient reliable information available.

Interactions with Drugs

No interactions are known to occur, and there is no known reason to expect a clinically significant interaction with ambrette.

Interactions with Foods

No interactions are known to occur, and there is no known reason to expect a clinically significant interaction with ambrette.

Interactions with Lab Tests

No interactions are known to occur, and there is no known reason to expect a clinically significant interaction with ambrette.

Interactions with Diseases or Conditions

No interactions are known to occur, and there is no known reason to expect a clinically significant interaction with ambrette.

Dosage and Administration

ORAL: Ambrette is typically used as a tea or tincture (18).

Comments

There is very little scientific information about this product. Our staff is continually analyzing the available information on natural medicines and will add data here as it becomes available.

AMERICAN ADDER'S TONGUE

Also Known As

American Adders Tongue, Dog's Tooth Violet, Dogs Tooth Voilet, Erythronium, Lamb's Tongue, Lambs Tongue, Rattlesnake Violet, Serpent's Tongue, Serpents Tongue, Snake Leaf, Yellow Snakeleaf, Yellow Snowdrop.
CAUTION: See separate listing for English Adder's Tongue.

Scientific Names

Erythronium americanum.
Family: Liliaceae.

People Use This For

Topically, American adder's tongue is used for ulcers (18).

Safety

There is insufficient reliable information available about the safety of American adder's tongue.
Pregnancy and Lactation: Insufficient reliable information available; avoid using.

Effectiveness

There is insufficient reliable information available about the effectiveness of American adder's tongue.

Mechanism of Action

The applicable parts of American adder's tongue are the leaves and tubers. The leaves can have emollient effects and treat skin ulcers when applied as a poultice. Used internally, they act as an emetic (18).

Adverse Reactions

Cross-sensitivity can occur with the use of American adder's tongue in individuals allergic to tulip, fritallaria, lily, alstroemeria, or Bomarea (18).

Interactions with Herbs & Other Dietary Supplements

Insufficient reliable information available.

Interactions with Drugs

No interactions are known to occur, and there is no known reason to expect a clinically significant interaction with American adder's tongue.

Interactions with Foods

No interactions are known to occur, and there is no known reason to expect a clinically significant interaction with American adder's tongue.

Interactions with Lab Tests

No interactions are known to occur, and there is no known reason to expect a clinically significant interaction with American adder's tongue.

Interactions with Diseases or Conditions

PLANT ALLERGIES: Cross-sensitivity can occur in individuals allergic to tulip, fritallaria, lily, alstroemeria, or Bomarea (18).

Dosage and Administration

TOPICAL: The fresh leaves of American adder's tongue are commonly applied as a poultice (18).

Comments

Avoid confusion with English adder's tongue.

AMERICAN BITTERSWEET

Also Known As

False Bittersweet, Waxwork.

Scientific Names

Celastrus scandens.
Family: Celastraceae.

People Use This For

Historically, American bittersweet was used orally for arthritis, menstrual disorders, and liver disorders. It was also used orally as a diuretic and to stimulate sweating (18).
American bittersweet is rarely used today.

Safety

There is insufficient reliable information available about the safety of American bittersweet.
Pregnancy and Lactation: Insufficient reliable information available; avoid using.

Effectiveness

There is insufficient reliable information available about the effectiveness of American bittersweet.

Mechanism of Action

The applicable parts of American bittersweet are the root and bark. American bittersweet contains tannins and a yellow quinoide nortriterpene called celastrol (18).

Adverse Reactions

None reported.

Interactions with Herbs & Other Dietary Supplements

Insufficient reliable information available.

Interactions with Drugs

No interactions are known to occur, and there is no known reason to expect a clinically significant interaction with American bittersweet.

Interactions with Foods

No interactions are known to occur, and there is no known reason to expect a clinically significant interaction with American bittersweet.

Interactions with Lab Tests

No interactions are known to occur, and there is no known reason to expect a clinically significant interaction with American bittersweet.

Interactions with Diseases or Conditions

No interactions are known to occur, and there is no known reason to expect a clinically significant interaction with American bittersweet.

Dosage and Administration

No typical dosage.

Comments

There is very little scientific information about this product. Our staff is continually analyzing the available information on natural medicines and will add data here as it becomes available.

AMERICAN CHESTNUT

Also Known As

None.
CAUTION: See separate listing for European Chestnut.

Scientific Names

Castanea dentata, synonym Castanea americana.
Family: Fagaceae.

People Use This For

Historically, American chestnut has been used orally for cough; pertussis; and respiratory ailments; and as an antirheumatic, sedative, tonic, and astringent agent (11). It has been used topically for pharyngitis (11).
In foods, an extract of American chestnut is used in beverages (11).

Safety

LIKELY SAFE ...when used orally in amounts found in beverages (11). American chestnut is approved for food use in the US (11).
There is insufficient reliable information available about the safety of the oral or topical use of American chestnut for medicinal purposes.
PREGNANCY AND LACTATION: Insufficient reliable information available; avoid using.

Effectiveness

There is insufficient reliable information available about the effectiveness of American chestnut.

Mechanism of Action

American chestnut contains 8-9% tannins (11), which could theoretically exert an astringent effect on the mucosal tissue. This effect dehydrates the tissue, reducing internal secretions and forming external cells into a protective layer (12).

Adverse Reactions

Orally, though no cases have been reported, adverse effects from the use of American chestnut are theoretically possible. Plants with at least 10% tannins may cause gastrointestinal disturbances, kidney damage, and necrotic conditions of the liver (12). Some animal experiments show that tannins may cause cancer; others show they may prevent it (12). Regular consumption of herbs with high tannin concentrations correlates with increased incidence of esophageal or nasal cancer (12).

Interactions with Herbs & Other Dietary Supplements

TANNIN-CONTAINING HERBS: Theoretically, herbs that contain high percentages of tannins (such as American chestnut) may cause precipitation of constituents of other herbs (19).

Interactions with Drugs

ORAL DRUGS: Theoretically, concomitant oral administration may cause precipitation of some drugs due to the high tannin content of American chestnut (19). Separate administration of oral drugs and tannin-containing herbs by the longest period of time practical (19).

Interactions with Foods

No interactions are known to occur, and there is no known reason to expect a clinically significant interaction with American chestnut.

Interactions with Lab Tests

No interactions are known to occur, and there is no known reason to expect a clinically significant interaction with American chestnut.

Interactions with Diseases or Conditions

No interactions are known to occur, and there is no known reason to expect a clinically significant interaction with American chestnut.

Dosage and Administration

ORAL: People typically prepare American chestnut as a tea with 1 teaspoon of leaves and bark boiled in a covered container with 2 cups of water for 30 minutes. The liquid is cooled slowly in the closed container and taken cold, 1 to 2 cups per day (5254).

Comments

Recently, American chestnut (Castanea dentata) has been devastated by fungal disease (11). Chestnut leaves used in commerce usually come from European chestnut (Castanea sativa) or other Castanea species (11).

AMERICAN DOGWOOD

Also Known As

Bitter Redberry, Box Tree, Boxwood, Budwood, Cornel, Cornelian Tree, Dog-Tree, Dogwood, False Box, Green Ozier, Osier, Rose Willow, Silky Cornel, Swamp Dogwood.
CAUTION: See separate listing for Jamaican Dogwood.

Scientific Names

Cornus florida.
Family: Cornaceae.

People Use This For

Orally, American dogwood is used for headaches and fatigue. It is also used orally to increase strength, for fever, chronic diarrhea and to stimulate appetite. It is also used orally as a tonic.
Topically, American dogwood is used as an astringent for boils and wounds (18).
Historically, American dogwood was used orally as a substitute for quinine.

Safety

There is insufficient reliable information available about the safety of American dogwood.
Pregnancy and Lactation: Insufficient reliable information available; avoid using.

Effectiveness

There is insufficient reliable information available about the effectiveness of American dogwood.

Mechanism of Action

The applicable part of American dogwood is the bark. American dogwood destroys the snails that carry the tropical human parasite species Schistosoma. A methanol extract has a dose-dependent inhibiting effect on heart activity, and stops the heartbeat at high doses. Animal data suggests the water-insoluble fraction of American dogwood has antimalarial effects comparable to quinine and sulfadiazine (18).

Adverse Reactions

None reported.

Interactions with Herbs & Other Dietary Supplements

Insufficient reliable information available.

Interactions with Drugs

No interactions are known to occur, and there is no known reason to expect a clinically significant interaction with American dogwood.

Interactions with Foods

No interactions are known to occur, and there is no known reason to expect a clinically significant interaction with American dogwood.

Interactions with Lab Tests

No interactions are known to occur, and there is no known reason to expect a clinically significant interaction with American dogwood.

Interactions with Diseases or Conditions

No interactions are known to occur, and there is no known reason to expect a clinically significant interaction with American dogwood.

Dosage and Administration

No typical dosage.

Comments

American dogwood is rarely used. Be careful not to confuse it with Jamaican dogwood (18).

AMERICAN ELDER

Also Known As

American Elderberry, Common Elderberry, Elder Flower, Elderberry, Sambucus, Sweet Elder.
CAUTION: See separate listings for Dwarf Elder, Elderberry, and Elderflower.

Scientific Names

Sambucus canadensis.
Family: Caprifoliaceae.

People Use This For

In folk medicine, American elder is used for asthma, bronchitis, bruises, cancer, flatulence, colds, edema associated with weak heart function, epilepsy, fever, gout, headache, neuralgia, psoriasis, rheumatism, to stimulate healing, for sore throat, sores, swelling, syphilis, toothache, as a cathartic laxative, to cause sweating, as a diuretic, emetic, eye wash, mouthwash, poultice, "purifier", and stimulant.
For food uses, American elder is cooked and eaten and used to make elderberry wine (6). American elder is also used as a flavor component in foods and beverages (11).
In manufacturing, extracts of American elder are used in perfumes (11).

Safety

LIKELY SAFE …when the fruit or flower is used in amounts found in foods. The flowers have Generally Recognized as Safe (GRAS) status in the US (11). The maximum use level of the flower is 0.049% (11). Cooked, ripe fruit has few if any adverse effects (6).
POSSIBLY SAFE …when flowers are used orally for medicinal purposes (12).
POSSIBLY UNSAFE …when leaves, stems, or unripe fruit are used. All contain cyanogenic glycosides (12). Limit juice consumption to avoid toxicity (6).
PREGNANCY AND LACTATION: POSSIBLY UNSAFE …when leaves, stems, or unripe fruit are used (6). There is insufficient reliable information available about the safety of the flower or cooked fruit; avoid using amounts greater than those found in foods.

Effectiveness

There is insufficient reliable information available about the effectiveness of American elder.

Mechanism of Action

The applicable parts of American elder are the flower and ripe fruit. Elder flowers are believed to have diuretic and laxative effects (6). They are a rich source of vitamin C (19). Elder leaves (6) and unripe berries (12) contain cyanogenic glycosides. If ingested, the leaves or unripe berries can cause cyanide poisoning (6). Sambucus species contain plant lectins with hemagglutinin characteristics that might be useful in blood typing and other blood testing (11).

Adverse Reactions

Orally, ingesting several glasses of elderberry juice can cause nausea, vomiting, weakness, dizziness, numbness and stupor (6).

Interactions with Herbs & Other Dietary Supplements

Insufficient reliable information available.

Interactions with Drugs

OTHER DRUGS: There is preliminary evidence that American elder can inhibit the cytochrome P450 (CYP450) 3A4 enzyme (6450). Theoretically, American elder might increase levels of drugs metabolized by CYP450 3A4; however, this interaction has not been reported in humans. Some drugs metabolized by CYP450 3A4 include lovastatin (Mevacor), ketoconazole (Nizoral), itraconazole (Sporanox), fexofenadine (Allegra), triazolam (Halcion), and numerous others. Use American elder cautiously or avoid in patients taking these drugs.

Interactions with Foods

No interactions are known to occur, and there is no known reason to expect a clinically significant interaction with American elder.

Interactions with Lab Tests

No interactions are known to occur, and there is no known reason to expect a clinically significant interaction with American elder.

Interactions with Diseases or Conditions

No interactions are known to occur, and there is no known reason to expect a clinically significant interaction with American elder.

Dosage and Administration

No typical dosage.

Comments

Though making a pea shooter from an American elder stem seems innocuous, it is not a good idea. The stem contains cyanogenic glycosides and has been reported to cause toxicity in children (6).

AMERICAN HELLEBORE

Also Known As

American Veratrum, American White Hellebore, Bugbane, Devil's Bite, Earth Gall, False Hellebore, Green Hellebore, Green Veratrum, Indian Poke, Itchweed, Tickleweed, Veratro Verde.
CAUTION: See separate listings for Black Hellebore, Pheasant's Eye, and White Hellebore.

Scientific Names

Veratrum viride.
Family: Liliaceae.

People Use This For

In folk medicine, American hellebore has been used orally as an antispasmodic, diuretic, sedative, and antipyretic (18). It has also been used for hypertension.
In manufacturing, American hellebore has been used as an insecticide (13).

Safety

LIKELY UNSAFE ...when used orally (18,1502) or topically. The alkaloids can be absorbed through unbroken skin and should be avoided (18).
UNSAFE ...when used orally in large amounts. American hellebore can cause death (18).
PREGNANCY AND LACTATION: LIKELY UNSAFE ...when used orally or topically; avoid using.

Effectiveness

There is insufficient reliable information available about the effectiveness of American hellebore.

Mechanism of Action

The applicable part of American hellebore is the rhizome and root. The principal active constituents are steroid ester alkaloids (13,18), which reduce blood pressure even in small doses (13,18,1502). At therapeutic dosages, they have cardiac depressant, bradycardic, and sedative effects (13,18). The alkaloids inhibit inactivation of sodium-ion channels in excitable cells, especially those regulating cardiac activity (18).

Adverse Reactions

Orally, American hellebore in therapeutic amounts can cause numerous adverse effects, including irritation of mucous membranes and cardiac depression (18). Large doses can cause sneezing, lacrimation, salivation, vomiting, diarrhea, burning sensations in the mouth and pharynx, dysphagia, paresthesias, vertigo, possible blindness, paralysis, mild convulsions, bradycardia, arrhythmias, hypotension, and death due to cardiac arrest or asphyxiation (17,18).

Interactions with Herbs & Other Dietary Supplements

Insufficient reliable information available.

Interactions with Drugs

No interactions are known to occur, and there is no known reason to expect a clinically significant interaction with American hellebore.

Interactions with Foods

No interactions are known to occur, and there is no known reason to expect a clinically significant interaction with American hellebore.

Interactions with Lab Tests

No interactions are known to occur, and there is no known reason to expect a clinically significant interaction with American hellebore.

Interactions with Diseases or Conditions

CARDIAC DISEASE: Theoretically, American hellebore can worsen cardiac disease by depressing cardiac activity or causing bradycardia. (13,18).

GI IRRITATION: American hellebore can irritate the gastrointestinal tract and is contraindicated in individuals with infectious or inflammatory gastrointestinal conditions (19).

Dosage and Administration

No typical dosage.

Comments

Avoid confusion with European hellebore and pheasant's eye.

AMERICAN IVY

Also Known As

American Woodbine, Creeper, False Grapes, Five Leaves, Ivy, Virginia Creeper, Wild Woodbine, Wild Woodvine, Woody Climber.
CAUTION: See separate listings for Gelsemium, Honeysuckle, and Woodbine.

Scientific Names

Parthenocissus quinquefolia.
Family: Vitaceae.

People Use This For

Orally, American ivy is used for digestive disorders. It is also used orally to stimulate sweating, as an astringent, and a tonic (18).

Safety

There is insufficient reliable information available about the safety of American ivy.
Pregnancy and Lactation: Insufficient reliable information available; avoid using.

Effectiveness

There is insufficient reliable information available about the effectiveness of American ivy.

Mechanism of Action

The applicable part of American ivy is the bark. There is insufficient reliable information available about the possible mechanism of action and active ingredients.

Adverse Reactions

Orally, ingestion of the berries, containing 2% oxalic acid, is considered poisonous. There is one case of a child's death following ingestion of the berries (18).

Interactions with Herbs & Other Dietary Supplements

Insufficient reliable information available.

Interactions with Drugs
No interactions are known to occur, and there is no known reason to expect a clinically significant interaction with American ivy.

Interactions with Foods
No interactions are known to occur, and there is no known reason to expect a clinically significant interaction with American ivy.

Interactions with Lab Tests
No interactions are known to occur, and there is no known reason to expect a clinically significant interaction with American ivy.

Interactions with Diseases or Conditions
No interactions are known to occur, and there is no known reason to expect a clinically significant interaction with American ivy.

Dosage and Administration
ORAL: People typically drink a tea made from the ground bark (18).

Comments
Avoid confusion with woodbine (Clematis virginiana). Also, avoid confusing American ivy with gelsemium or honeysuckle, which are also known as woodbine.

AMERICAN MISTLETOE

Also Known As
Mistletoe.
CAUTION: See separate listing for European Mistletoe.

Scientific Names
Phoradendron leucarpum, synonyms Phoradendron serontium, Phoradendron flavescens; Phoradendron macrophyllum, synonym Phoradendron tomentosum.
Family: Viscaceae.

People Use This For
Traditionally, American mistletoe has been used as a smooth muscle stimulant for increasing blood pressure, and uterine and intestinal contractions (515). It has also been used as an abortifacient (6).

Safety
LIKELY UNSAFE ...when the flower, fruit, leaf, or stem are taken orally (6,515). All American mistletoe plant parts are considered toxic (6).
PREGNANCY: LIKELY UNSAFE ...when used orally; contraindicated. American mistletoe is considered an abortifacient (19).
LACTATION: LIKELY UNSAFE ...when used orally; avoid using.

Effectiveness
There is insufficient reliable information available about the effectiveness of American mistletoe.

Mechanism of Action
The applicable parts of American mistletoe are the flower, fruit, leaf, and stem. Constituent phoratoxins produce dose-dependent hypertension or hypotension, bradycardia, and increased uterine and intestinal motility (6,14). Experimental exposure to phoratoxins causes depolarization of skeletal muscle, contraction of smooth muscle, vasoconstriction, and cardiac arrest (6,14), similar to the effects reported with cardiotoxins from cobra venom (6,14).

Adverse Reactions
Some people who have ingested American mistletoe have reported nausea, bradycardia, hypertension, delirium, hallucinations, vasoconstriction, and cardiac arrest (6). Diarrhea and vomiting from ingestion of this product can lead to serious dehydration, hypovolemic shock, and cardiovascular collapse (6,14). Double vision was noted after ingestion of a large amount of bee pollen containing Phoradendron (14). Mild cases of acute gastroenteritis have been observed with ingestion of a few berries (14). Deaths have been reported after ingestion of teas used as an abortifacient (mistletoe

species not identified) (6). However, no fatalities were reported in a review of 1754 accidental American mistletoe exposures extracted from the American Association of Poison Control Centers national data collection system from 1985-1992 (3706). The review concluded that the ingestion of one to three berries or one or two leaves of American mistletoe is unlikely to result in any significant toxicity (3706).

Interactions with Herbs & Other Dietary Supplements
Insufficient reliable information available.

Interactions with Drugs
No interactions are known to occur, and there is no known reason to expect a clinically significant interaction with American mistletoe.

Interactions with Foods
No interactions are known to occur, and there is no known reason to expect a clinically significant interaction with American mistletoe.

Interactions with Lab Tests
No interactions are known to occur, and there is no known reason to expect a clinically significant interaction with American mistletoe.

Interactions with Diseases or Conditions
HEART DISEASE: Avoid in individuals with heart disease; theoretically, may exacerbate.

Dosage and Administration
No typical dosage.

Comments
American mistletoe is considered likely unsafe; avoid using. Avoid confusion with European mistletoe, as well as mistletoe from Australia, Korea, New Zealand, and other areas. Mistletoe is a parasite. Some Australian mistletoe species are reported to extract toxic constituents from the host plant on which they grow (515), suggesting the importance of identifying the host plant before use of mistletoe is considered.

AMERICAN PAWPAW

Also Known As
Custard Apple.
CAUTION: See separate listings for Papaya and Papain.

Scientific Names
Asimina triloba.
Family: Annonaceae.

People Use This For
Orally, American pawpaw is used for treating fever, vomiting, and inflammation of the mouth and throat (18).

Safety
There is insufficient reliable information available about the safety of American pawpaw.
Pregnancy and Lactation: Insufficient reliable information available; avoid using.

Effectiveness
There is insufficient reliable information available about the effectiveness of American pawpaw.

Mechanism of Action
The applicable parts of American pawpaw are the bark, leaf, and seed. American pawpaw contains multiple acetogenin constituents; of these asimin, asiminacin and asininecin are reported to be highly cytotoxic (258). Based on preliminary animal studies and in vitro studies of human cancer lines, scientists report some acetogenins show activity against certain lung and breast cancers (256). An acetogenin mixture also demonstrates pesticide activity (257).

Adverse Reactions

Orally, American pawpaw can cause nausea and urticaria (18).
Topically, American pawpaw extract can cause contact dermatitis (1525).

Interactions with Herbs & Other Dietary Supplements

Insufficient reliable information available.

Interactions with Drugs

No interactions are known to occur, and there is no known reason to expect a clinically significant interaction with American pawpaw.

Interactions with Foods

No interactions are known to occur, and there is no known reason to expect a clinically significant interaction with American pawpaw.

Interactions with Lab Tests

No interactions are known to occur, and there is no known reason to expect a clinically significant interaction with American pawpaw.

Interactions with Diseases or Conditions

No interactions are known to occur, and there is no known reason to expect a clinically significant interaction with American pawpaw.

Dosage and Administration

No typical dosage.

Comments

There is very little scientific information about this product. Our staff is continually analyzing the available information on natural medicines and will add data here as it becomes available.

AMERICAN SPIKENARD

Also Known As

Indian Root, Life of Man, Life-of-Man, Old Man's Root, Pettymorell, Small Spikenard, Spikenard, Spignet.

Scientific Names

Aralia racemosa.
Family: Araliaceae.

People Use This For

Orally, American spikenard is used for colds, chronic coughs, asthma, and arthritis. It is also used orally as an expectorant, to stimulate tissue renewal, and to promote sweating.
Topically, American spikenard is used as an alternative to sarsaparilla for treating skin diseases (18).

Safety

There is insufficient reliable information available about the safety of American spikenard.
PREGNANCY: UNSAFE ...when used orally; avoid using (12).
LACTATION: Insufficient reliable information available; avoid using.

Effectiveness

There is insufficient reliable information available about the effectiveness of American spikenard.

Mechanism of Action

There is insufficient reliable information available about the possible mechanism of action and active ingredients.

Adverse Reactions

Topically, American spikenard could theoretically cause skin sensitization secondary to its polyyne content (18).

Interactions with Herbs & Other Dietary Supplements

Insufficient reliable information available.

Interactions with Drugs

No interactions are known to occur, and there is no known reason to expect a clinically significant interaction with spikenard.

Interactions with Foods

No interactions are known to occur, and there is no known reason to expect a clinically significant interaction with spikenard.

Interactions with Lab Tests

No interactions are known to occur, and there is no known reason to expect a clinically significant interaction with spikenard.

Interactions with Diseases or Conditions

No interactions are known to occur, and there is no known reason to expect a clinically significant interaction with spikenard.

Dosage and Administration

ORAL: People typically drink a tea prepared by steeping 15 grams root in 500 mL of boiling water for 10-15 minutes and straining. A liquid extract equivalent to 0.8-1.9 grams root has also been used (18).

Comments

There is very little scientific information about this product. Our staff is continually analyzing the available information on natural medicines and will add data here as it becomes available.

AMERICAN WHITE POND LILY

Also Known As

Cow Cabbage, Water Cabbage, Water Lily, Water Nymph.

Scientific Names

Nymphaea odorata.

People Use This For

Orally, American white pond lily is used to treat chronic diarrhea (18).
Topically, American white pond lily is used for vaginal conditions, diseases of the throat and mouth, and as a poultice for burns and furuncles (18).

Safety

There is insufficient reliable information available about the safety of American white pond lily.
Pregnancy and Lactation: Insufficient reliable information available; avoid using.

Effectiveness

There is insufficient reliable information available about the effectiveness of American white pond lily.

Mechanism of Action

The applicable part of American white pond lily is the rhizome and root. American white pond lilly contains tannins which are probably responsible for astringent and antiseptic activity (18).

Adverse Reactions

None reported.

Interactions with Herbs & Other Dietary Supplements

Insufficient reliable information available.

Interactions with Drugs

No interactions are known to occur, and there is no known reason to expect a clinically significant interaction with American white pond lily.

Interactions with Foods

No interactions are known to occur, and there is no known reason to expect a clinically significant interaction with American white pond lily.

Interactions with Lab Tests

No interactions are known to occur, and there is no known reason to expect a clinically significant interaction with American white pond lily.

Interactions with Diseases or Conditions

No interactions are known to occur, and there is no known reason to expect a clinically significant interaction with American white pond lily.

Dosage and Administration

ORAL: People typically use one cup of tea (steep 1-2 grams dried root in 150 mL boiling water 5-10 minutes, strain) (18). Liquid extract (1:1 in 25% ethanol), 1-4 mL has also been used (18).
TOPICAL: American white pond lily has been used as a douche, gargle, or hot poultice (18).

Comments

There is very little scientific information about this product. Our staff is continually analyzing information on natural medicines and will add data here as it becomes available.

ANDIROBA

Also Known As

Andiroba-Saruba, Bastard Mahogany, Brazilian Mahogany, Carapa, Cedro, Crabwood, Iandirova, Mahongany, Requia.

Scientific Names

Carapa guianensis.
Family: Meliaceae.

People Use This For

Orally, andiroba bark and leaf are used to treat fevers, herpes, as an anthelmintic, and as a tonic (517,518). Andiroba fruit oil is taken orally for coughs (517).
Topically, andiroba bark and leaf are used as a wash for dermatoses, sores, ulcers, and skin troubles (517,518). It is used topically for removing ticks from the head and for skin parasites (517). The seed oil is used topically to treat inflammation, arthritis (517), for rashes, muscle and joint aches and injuries, wounds, boils, and herpes ulcers (3918). Other uses of andiroba include use as a solvent for extracting plant colorants, as a lamp oil, and in soaps (as an insect repellent) (3918). Seed oil is also used for mummification of human heads (3918).

Safety

There is insufficient reliable information available about the safety of andiroba.
Pregnancy and Lactation: Insufficient reliable information available; avoid using.

Effectiveness

There is insufficient reliable information available about the effectiveness of andiroba.

Mechanism of Action

The applicable parts of andiroba are the bark, leaf, fruit oil, and seed oil. There is insufficient reliable information available about the possible mechanism of action and active ingredients.

Adverse Reactions

None reported.

Interactions with Herbs & Other Dietary Supplements

Insufficient reliable information available.

Interactions with Drugs

No interactions are known to occur, and there is no known reason to expect a clinically significant interaction with andiroba.

Interactions with Foods
No interactions are known to occur, and there is no known reason to expect a clinically significant interaction with andiroba.

Interactions with Lab Tests
No interactions are known to occur, and there is no known reason to expect a clinically significant interaction with andiroba.

Interactions with Diseases or Conditions
No interactions are known to occur, and there is no known reason to expect a clinically significant interaction with andiroba.

Dosage and Administration
ORAL: As a tea brewed from the bark and/or leaf (517,518).
TOPICAL: As a tea.

Comments
There is very little scientific information about this product. Our staff is continually analyzing the available information on natural medicines and will add data here as it becomes available.

ANDRACHNE

Also Known As
None.

Scientific Names
Andrachne aspera; Andrachne cordifolia; Andrachne phyllanthoides
Family: Euphorbiaceae.

People Use This For
In Yemen folklore, andrachne is used to treat eye inflammation (6).

Safety
There is insufficient reliable information available about the safety of andrachne.
Pregnancy and Lactation: Insufficient reliable information available.

Effectiveness
There is insufficient reliable information available about the effectiveness of andrachne.

Mechanism of Action
There is insufficient reliable information available about the possible mechanism of action and active ingredients.

Adverse Reactions
None reported.

Interactions with Herbs & Other Dietary Supplements
Insufficient reliable information available.

Interactions with Drugs
No interactions are known to occur, and there is no known reason to expect a clinically significant interaction with andrachne.

Interactions with Foods
No interactions are known to occur, and there is no known reason to expect a clinically significant interaction with andrachne.

Interactions with Lab Tests
No interactions are known to occur, and there is no known reason to expect a clinically significant interaction with andrachne.

Interactions with Diseases or Conditions

No interactions are known to occur, and there is no known reason to expect a clinically significant interaction with andrachne.

Dosage and Administration

No typical dosage.

Comments

There is very little scientific information about this product. Our staff is continually analyzing the available information on natural medicines and will add data here as it becomes available.

ANDROGRAPHIS

Also Known As

Andrographolide, Bidara, Carmantina, Chiretta, Chuan Xin Lian, Chuan Xin Lin, Creat, Fa Tha Lai Jone, Fa-Tha-Lai-Jone, Indian Echinacea, Kalmegh, Kariyat, King of Bitters, Kirta, Nabin Chanvandi, Sadilata, Sambilata, Takila, Vizra Ufar.

Scientific Names

Andrographis paniculata, synonym Justicia paniculata.
Family: Acanthaceae.

People Use This For

Orally, andrographis is used for preventing and treating the common cold, influenza, pharyngotonsillitis, allergies, and sinusitis (2744,2747,2748,5784). It has also been used orally to treat HIV/AIDS (6767).

In traditional medicine, andrographis is used for anorexia, atherosclerosis, snake and insect bites, bronchitis, cachexia, prevention of cardiovascular disease, cholera, colic, diabetes, diarrhea, flatulence, gastritis, gonorrhea, hemorrhoids, hepatomegaly, drug-induced hepatotoxicity, other hepatic disorders, myocardial ischemia, jaundice, leprosy, leptospirosis, malaria, pharyngitis, pneumonia, pruritus, pyelonephritis, rabies, skin wounds, unspecified skin diseases, syphilis, tuberculosis, tonsillitis, and ulcers (2743,2745,2746,2749). Andrographis is also used as an astringent, antiseptic, antidote, analgesic, antipyretic, anti-inflammatory, antithrombotic, expectorant, anthelmintic, laxative, and tonic (2743,2746,2758).

Safety

POSSIBLY SAFE …when used orally and appropriately, short-term (12). Andrographis extracts have been shown to be safe in one clinical trial using low doses lasting 3 months and in others using higher doses lasting 4-7 days (12,2744,2748,2772,2773,2774).

There is insufficient reliable information available about the safety of augmented andrographis preparations which contain elevated concentrations of the constituent andrographolide (see Comments).

PREGNANCY: LIKELY UNSAFE …when used orally due to abortifacient effects; avoid using (12).

LACTATION: Insufficient reliable information available; avoid using.

Effectiveness

POSSIBLY EFFECTIVE …when used orally for decreasing the severity of symptoms of the common cold. Andrographis seems to significantly improve symptoms of the common cold when started within 72 hours of symptom onset. Some symptoms can improve after 2 days of treatment (2744,2773), but it typically takes 4-5 days of treatment before there is maximal symptom relief (2744,2773,2774,5784). …when used orally for prevention of the common cold. There is some evidence that use of andrographis can decrease the relative risk of developing a cold by approximately 50%. However, this beneficial effect does not seem to occur until after at least 2 months of continuous treatment (2772). It is unclear how long this benefit lasts. So far, this benefit has only been assessed for up to 3 months of treatment. …when used orally for symptoms of pharyngotonsillitis. There is some evidence that high doses of andrographis are comparable to acetaminophen after 3 and 7 days of treatment for fever and sore throat associated with pharyngotonsillitis (2748).

Most clinical trials used Andrographis paniculata dried extract (Kan Jang, Swedish Herbal Institute), standardized to contain 4-5.6 mg of the constituent andrographolide per tablet (2744,2772,2773,2774,5784).

There is insufficient reliable information available about the effectiveness of andrographis for its other uses.

Mechanism of Action

The applicable parts of andrographis are the leaf and rhizome (12,2758,2767). Several active andrographis compounds have been identified, including andrographolide, deoxyandrographolide, and other diterpenes (2750,2760,2768,2771). Although andrographis is used for a wide variety of indications in Ayurvedic and herbal medicine, clinical evidence of effectiveness in humans is limited to the common cold. People use andrographis for the common cold because it is thought to have immunostimulant properties. There is some preliminary evidence that it might increase antibody activity and phagocytosis by macrophages (2766). Preliminary evidence also suggests that andrographis might also have mast cell-stabilizing and antiallergy activity (2750,2751). People try andrographis for HIV/AIDS because some of its constituents have been found to have anti-HIV in vitro (2765). High doses of the purified andrographolide constituent can also increase CD4+ cell counts in HIV patients. Andrographolide is thought to work through correction of T-lymphocyte function rather than by direct inhibition of viral replication (6767). Andrographis might also have leukemia cell differentiation-inducing activity (2766,2768). Possible analgesic, antipyretic, and anti-ulcerogenic effects of andrographis have been described (2753,2754). Andrographis has traditionally been used for infectious diseases. Antibacterial activity was not detected by one group of investigators, but preliminary evidence suggests potential use against bacteria in raw water, human roundworm (Ascaris lumbricoides), Toxoplasma gondii, malaria, and E. coli enterotoxin secretion (2752,2753,2764,2767,2777,2779,2780,2781). Andrographis might protect the liver against hepatotoxic drugs (e.g., acetaminophen) and chemicals possibly by increasing bile flow, bile salt, and bile acids (2761,2762,2763,2778). The andrographis constituent, andrographolide, is a more potent hepatoprotectant than silymarin, an active constituent of milk thistle (see separate listing) (2762,2778). Andrographis may be beneficial in cardiovascular disease. Early evidence suggests that andrographis might lower blood pressure, prevent arteriosclerosis, inhibit platelet aggregation, and reduce myocardial ischemia and reperfusion injury (2755,2756,2757,2758,2759,2760,2782,2783). Andrographis is reported to have abortifacient activity (12). The mechanism of abortifacient action is unknown (2771). Preliminary evidence suggests that andrographis might also have detrimental effects on male and female fertility. In animals, andrographis decreased fertility of both males and females (2769,2770,2776); however, this has not been demonstrated in humans.

Adverse Reactions

Orally, large doses of andrographis are reported to cause gastrointestinal distress, anorexia, and emesis (12,2743). Urticaria has also been reported (2743,2773). Preliminary evidence suggests that andrographis might inhibit male and female fertility (2769,2770,2776), but this has not been demonstrated in humans. High doses of the purified andrographolide constituent (5 mg/kg three times daily) have caused headache, fatigue, rash, abnormal taste, diarrhea, itching, lymphadenopathy, and anaphylactic reactions. The andrographolide constituent can also cause dose-related increases in liver enzymes such as ALT, which return to normal when andrographolide is discontinued (6767); however, these effects have not yet been reported.

Interactions with Herbs & Other Dietary Supplements

HERBS WITH ANTICOAGULANT/ANTIPLATELET POTENTIAL: Theoretically, concomitant use with herbs that have anticoagulant or antiplatelet activity might enhance therapeutic effects and increase the risk of bleeding (2758,2759). These include angelica, anise, arnica, asafoetida, bogbean, boldo, capsicum, celery, chamomile, clove, danshen, fenugreek, feverfew, garlic, ginger, ginkgo, Panax ginseng, horse chestnut, horseradish, licorice, meadowsweet, prickly ash, onion, papain, passionflower, poplar, quassia, red clover, turmeric, wild carrot, wild lettuce, willow, and others (4,19).

HERBS/SUPPLEMENTS WITH HYPOTENSIVE ACTIVITY: Theoretically, concurrent use might enhance therapeutic effects and increase the risk of hypotension (2755,2760). These include black cohosh, celery seed, Panax ginseng, and others (4).

Interactions with Drugs

ANTICOAGULANT/ANTIPLATELET DRUGS: Theoretically, concomitant use might enhance therapeutic effects and increase the risk of bleeding (2758,2759).

ANTIHYPERTENSIVE DRUGS: Theoretically, concomitant use might enhance therapeutic effects and increase the risk of hypotension (2755,2760).

IMMUNOSUPPRESSANTS: Theoretically, andrographis might interfere with immunosuppressive drugs because of its immunostimulant activity (2766). Immunosuppressant drugs include azathioprine (Imuran), basiliximab (Simulect), cyclosporine (Neoral, Sandimmune), daclizumab (Zenapax), muromonab-CD3 (OKT3, Orthoclone OKT3), mycophenolate (CellCept), tacrolimus (FK506, Prograf), sirolimus (Rapamune), prednisone (Deltasone, Orasone), and other corticosteroids (glucocorticoids).

Interactions with Foods

No interactions are known to occur, and there is no known reason to expect a clinically significant interaction with andrographis.

Interactions with Lab Tests

No interactions are known to occur, and there is no known reason to expect a clinically significant interaction with andrographis.

Interactions with Diseases or Conditions

BLEEDING DISORDERS: Theoretically, andrographis might have antiplatelet activity and increase the risk of bleeding in patients with bleeding disorders (2758,2759).

HYPOTENSION: Theoretically, andrographis might lower blood pressure and exacerbate hypotension (2755,2760).

INFERTILITY: Theoretically, andrographis might have detrimental effects on male and female fertility (2769,2770,2776). Avoid in couples with infertility.

Dosage and Administration

ORAL: Most clinical trials used andrographis dried extract (Kan Jang, Swedish Herbal Institute), standardized to contain 4-5.6 mg andrographolide. For decreasing symptoms of the common cold, doses of 400 mg three times daily have been used in clinical trials (2744,2773,2774,5784). For preventing the common cold, a dose of 200 mg daily for 5 days each week has been used in a clinical trial (2772). For relieving fever and sore throat in pharyngotonsillitis, doses of 3 grams and 6 grams daily were used (2748).

Comments

Andrographis is native to Asian countries such as India and Sri Lanka, and is cultivated and naturalized in other areas of the world (2775). Andrographis products have reportedly been used in Scandinavia for more than a decade (2772). One writer credits Andrographis with arresting the 1919 flu epidemic in India, although this has not been verified (2774). Some Internet vendors offer andrographis augmented to contain up to 30% andrographolide (2746). The safety and effectiveness of andrographis preparations with augmented andrographolide content is unknown.

ANDROSTENEDIOL

Also Known As

4-AD, 4-Androstenediol, 5-AD, 5-Androstenediol, Androdiol.

Scientific Names

4-androstene-3beta,17beta-diol; 5-androstene-3beta,17beta-diol.

People Use This For

Orally, androstenediol is used to increase endogenous testosterone production to increase energy, enhance recovery and growth from exercise, heighten sexual arousal and function, and to promote a greater sense of well being (8304).

Safety

There is insufficient reliable information available about the safety of androstenediol.
Pregnancy and Lactation: Insufficient reliable information available; avoid using.

Effectiveness

There is insufficient reliable information available about the effectiveness of androstenediol.

Mechanism of Action

There is some evidence that exogenous androstenediol is converted to testosterone in humans; but this is not yet scientifically established.

Adverse Reactions

Orally, androstenediol may cause masculinization and increased growth of facial hair in women.

Interactions with Herbs & Other Dietary Supplements

Insufficient reliable information available.

Interactions with Drugs

ANDROGENIC DRUGS: Theoretically, concomitant use with androstenediol may increase activity and risk of side effects.

ESTROGENIC DRUGS: Theoretically, concomitant use with androstenediol may reduce or inhibit activity (8304).

Interactions with Foods

No interactions are known to occur, and there is no known reason to expect a clinically significant interaction with androstenediol.

Interactions with Lab Tests

No interactions are known to occur, and there is no known reason to expect a clinically significant interaction with androstenediol.

Interactions with Diseases or Conditions

PROSTATE CONDITIONS: Androstenediol might aggravate prostate conditions due to its androgenic activity.
BREAST CANCER: Androstenediol might aggravate breast cancer due to its estrogenic activity (8304).

Dosage and Administration

No typical dosage.

Comments

There is some concern that the potency and purity of androstenediol products are not always the same as is labeled.

ANDROSTENEDIONE

Also Known As

Andro, Androstene.

Scientific Names

4-androstene-3,17-dione; Androst-4-ene-3,17-dione.

People Use This For

Orally, androstenedione is used to increase endogenous testosterone production to enhance athletic performance (674), increase energy, keep red blood cells healthy, enhance recovery and growth from exercise, and for heighten sexual arousal and function.

Safety

POSSIBLY UNSAFE ...when used orally. Androstenedione has been associated with significant side effects, including increased risk of breast, pancreatic, and prostate cancer (see Adverse Reactions) (672,3861,6000).
CHILDREN: LIKELY UNSAFE ...when used orally. Androstenedione could potentially cause premature closure of the bone growth plates (674).
PREGNANCY: LIKELY UNSAFE ...when used orally. Androstenedione might induce labor (673).
LACTATION: Insufficient reliable information available; avoid using.

Effectiveness

LIKELY INEFFECTIVE ...when used orally for improving muscle size or strength in weight trainers. Androstenedione in doses of 100-300 mg per day does not add any significant increase in muscle strength, muscle size, or lean body mass when used for 2-3 months in conjunction with weight training (1365,1905,6000,6795).

Mechanism of Action

Androstenedione is a steroid hormone produced by the adrenal glands, testes, and ovaries (3861). It is a direct precursor of testosterone and estrone in both men and women (674). Androstenedione production peaks in the mid-twenties and declines steadily after age 30 (1365). Androstenedione is a precursor to testosterone. A lot of people use it as an alternative to anabolic steroids to increase testosterone levels and to improve athletic performance and build muscle. Short-term use (less than 1 month) can sometimes increase testosterone levels (3861,1905); however, with continued use, testosterone levels return to normal (1365,1905,6000,6795,7236). When used for longer than one month, luteinizing hormone secretion seems to decline by about a third. This indicates that androstenedione might actually down-regulate testosterone synthesis (1905). Androstenedione also does not seem to have anabolic effects and does not significantly affect markers of muscle anabolism or growth; increase lean body mass or physical strength; or produce any perceived changes in mood, health, or libido (1365,1905,3862,7236). Furthermore, androstenedione consistently increases estrogen levels (1905,3861,3862,6000,7236). This might increase the risk of estrogenic side effects in both men and women using androstenedione (674,6000). Androstenedione also raises dehydroepiandrosterone (DHEA) concentrations, and lowers high-density lipoprotein (HDL) cholesterol (1905).

Adverse Reactions

Orally, side effects can be different for men and women.
In men, androstenedione might decrease endogenous testosterone production and increase estrogen. Theoretically, androstenedione might cause decreased spermatogenesis, acne, testicular atrophy, gynecomastia, behavioral changes, and potentially increase the risk of pancreatic and prostate cancer (672,674,6000). There is preliminary evidence that

androstenedione might stimulate prostate cancer cell growth (672). There is also some concern that androstenedione might increase risk of heart disease in men. Androstenedione decreases high-density lipoprotein (HDL) cholesterol (1905,6000). Some male patients might also be at risk for developing priapism. There is one case report of two episodes of priapism associated with androstenedione use in a 30-year-old man (5089).

In women, androstenedione theoretically might cause masculinization with the deepening of voice, hirsutism, acne, clitoral hypertrophy, menorrhea, male-pattern baldness, and coarsening of the skin (674). There is also some concern that androstenedione might cause or worsen depression in women. Some women with severe major depression seem to have increased endogenous androstenedione concentrations; however, it is not known if supplements can actually cause this adverse effect (6796).

In children, androstenedione might cause premature bone growth plate closure and decrease adult height (674). Androstenedione might cause early development of secondary sex characteristics in boys; and acne, oligomenorrhea or amenorrhea, hirsutism, and virilization in girls (217).

Testosterone derivatives similar to androstenedione have also been associated with hepatic toxicity (3861). Consider monitoring liver function tests (LFTs) in patients using androstenedione.

Interactions with Herbs & Other Dietary Supplements

Insufficient reliable information available.

Interactions with Drugs

ESTROGENS: There is some concern that taking androstenedione with estrogens might increase estrogenic effects and potential side effects. Androstenedione is a precursor to estrogen and seems to increase estrogen levels (674).

Interactions with Foods

No interactions are known to occur, and there is no known reason to expect a clinically significant interaction with androstenedione.

Interactions with Lab Tests

ESTRONE ASSAYS: Androstenedione is a precursor to estrone and might increase results of estrone assays (674,1905).
HIGH DENSITY LIPOPROTEIN (HDL) CHOLESTEROL: Androstenedione can lower HDL levels (7236).
NANDROLONE: Trace contamination of androstenedione with 19-norandrostenedione can result in positive urine test results for nandrolone use (1906).
TESTOSTERONE: Androstenedione is a precursor to testosterone and can increase results of total and free testosterone assays during the first month of androstenedione use. However, testosterone levels tend to normalize when androstenedione is used for longer than 1 month (674,1905).

Interactions with Diseases or Conditions

DEPRESSION: Theoretically, androstenedione supplementation might cause or worsen depression in women. There is evidence that some women with severe major depression have elevated endogenous androstenedione levels (6796). However, it is not known if taking androstenedione supplements causes this adverse effect.
HORMONE SENSITIVE CANCERS/CONDITIONS: Androstenedione is a precursor to testosterone and estrogen and seems to increase estrogen levels (674). Men and women with hormone sensitive conditions should avoid androstenedione. Some of these conditions include breast, uterine, ovarian and prostate cancer; endometriosis; and uterine fibroids.
LIVER DISEASE: There is some concern that androstenedione might adversely effect the liver. So far there are no cases of this adverse effect, but steroids similar to androstenedione have been associated with liver abnormalities. Androstenedione should be avoided by people with hepatic disease (3861). Consider checking liver function tests (LFTs) in patients taking androstenedione.
PROSTATE CANCER: There is some concern that androstenedione might increase the risk of developing prostate cancer. There is preliminary evidence that androstenedione can stimulate human prostate tumor cell growth (672). Avoid using in patients with prostate cancer.

Dosage and Administration

ORAL: For improving muscle strength and size in weight trainers, 50-150 mg twice daily has been used in studies. However, androstenedione does not seem to be effective for this use (1365,1905,3861,6000,6795).

Comments

Androstenedione gained popularity as the supplement used by home run-hitter Mark McGwire. Androstenedione is not prohibited by Major League Baseball, but is banned by the International Olympics Committee (IOC), the National Collegiate Athletic Association (NCAA), the National Basketball Association (NBA), the National Football League (NFL), and the World Natural Body Building Federation (217,5041). There are some concerns that the potency and purity of androstenedione products can differ from the product labeling.

ANGEL'S TRUMPET

Also Known As
Devil's Trumpet.
CAUTION: See separate listing for Jimson Weed (Datura stramonium).

Scientific Names
Datura sauveolens.
Family: Solanaceae.

People Use This For
Orally, Angel's trumpet is used to induce hallucinations and euphoria (5624,5625,5626,5627).
Historically, Angel's trumpet has been used to treat asthma (5625).

Safety
UNSAFE ...when used orally (5624,5625,5626,5627). All parts of the plant contain tropane alkaloids and are considered poisonous (5624,5625,5627); the foliage and seeds contain the highest concentration of toxic alkaloids (5627).
CHILDREN: UNSAFE ...when used orally (5624,5625,5626,5627). Severe toxicity has occurred in cases of accidental ingestion and in teenagers experimenting with Angel's trumpet for recreational use (5626).
PREGNANCY AND LACTATION: UNSAFE ...when used orally. The entire plant is considered poisonous (5624,5627); avoid using.

Effectiveness
There is insufficient reliable information available about the effectiveness of Angel's trumpet.

Mechanism of Action
The applicable parts of Angel's trumpet are the leaf and flower. Angel's trumpet contains tropane alkaloids, particularly atropine, hyoscyamine, and hyoscine (scopolamine), which are responsible for the anticholinergic effects and toxicity (5625,5627).

Adverse Reactions
Orally, Angel's trumpet can cause severe toxicity. Ingestion of Angel's trumpet can cause acute anticholinergic poisoning, which often requires medical attention (5624,5625,5626,5627). Oral use has been associated with delirium, dilated pupils, hyperactivity, disorientation, intense thirst, dry skin and mucous membranes, flushing, fever, widened pulse pressure, systolic hypertension, tachycardia (5624,5625), audio-visual disassociation (5627), hyperexcitability, visual hallucinations, anxiety, amnesia, combativeness, ataxia, clonus, muscular weakness, expressive aphasia, muscular paralysis, seizure, urinary retention (5624,5625), decreased GI motility (5627), alternating levels of consciousness, convulsions, and coma (5624,5625). Death may result from respiratory arrest (5624). Each flower contains approximately 0.20 mg of atropine and 0.65 mg of scopolamine. Reports suggest ingestion of tea made from 3-6 flowers can produce hallucinations, and 9 flowers can produce total paralysis (5624).

Interactions with Herbs & Other Dietary Supplements
Insufficient reliable information available.

Interactions with Drugs
ANTICHOLINERGIC DRUGS: Concomitant use may increase anticholinergic effects and adverse effects. Drugs include amantadine, atropine, belladonna alkaloids, phenothiazines, scopolamine, and tricyclic antidepressants (506).

Interactions with Foods
No interactions are known to occur, and there is no known reason to expect a clinically significant interaction with Angel's trumpet.

Interactions with Lab Tests
No interactions are known to occur, and there is no known reason to expect a clinically significant interaction with Angel's trumpet.

Interactions with Diseases or Conditions
CONGESTIVE HEART FAILURE (CHF): Angel's trumpet might cause tachycardia and exacerbate CHF due to its hyoscyamine (atropine) and scopolamine content (15).

CONSTIPATION: Angel's trumpet might cause constipation due to its hyoscyamine (atropine) and scopolamine content (15).

DOWN SYNDROME: Caution, patients with Down syndrome might be hypersensitive to the antimuscarinic effects (mydriasis, positive chronotropic heart effects, etc.) of hyoscyamine (atropine) and scopolamine contained in Angel's trumpet (15).

ESOPHAGEAL REFLUX: Angel's trumpet might delay gastric emptying and decrease lower esophageal pressure, promoting gastric retention and exacerbating reflux due to its hyoscyamine (atropine) and scopolamine content (15).

FEVER: Angel's trumpet might increase the risk of hyperthermia in patients with fever due to its hyoscyamine (atropine) and scopolamine content (15).

GASTRIC ULCER: Angel's trumpet might delay gastric emptying and exacerbate gastric ulcers due to its hyoscyamine (atropine) and scopolamine content (15).

GI INFECTIONS: Angel's trumpet might suppress GI motility causing retention of infecting organisms or toxins due to its hyoscyamine (atropine) and scopolamine content (15).

HIATAL HERNIA: Angel's trumpet might delay gastric emptying and decrease lower esophageal pressure, promoting gastric retention and exacerbating reflux due to its hyoscyamine (atropine) and scopolamine content (15).

TOXIC MEGACOLON: Contraindicated; Angel's trumpet might suppress intestinal motility, which might produce paralytic ileus and exacerbate toxic megacolon, due to its hyoscyamine (atropine) and scopolamine content (2,15).

NARROW-ANGLE GLAUCOMA: Angel's trumpet might increase ocular tension in patients with narrow-angle (angle-closure) glaucoma due to its hyoscyamine (atropine) and scopolamine content (2,15).

OBSTRUCTIVE GI TRACT DISEASE: Angel's trumpet might exacerbate obstructive GI tract diseases (including atony, paralytic ileus, and stenosis) due to its hyoscyamine (atropine) and scopolamine content (15).

TACHYARRHYTHMIAS: Angel's trumpet might cause tachycardia due to its hyoscyamine (atropine) and scopolamine content (2,15).

URINARY RETENTION: Angel's trumpet might increase urinary retention due to its hyoscyamine (atropine) and scopolamine content (2,15).

ULCERATIVE COLITIS: Angel's trumpet might suppress intestinal motility, which might produce paralytic ileus and precipitate toxic megacolon, due to its hyoscyamine (atropine) and scopolamine content (15).

Dosage and Administration
No typical dosage.

Comments
Angel's trumpet is usually cultivated as an ornamental plant in the southeastern United States (5625,5626) and may be confused with Jimson Weed which grows wild throughout the United States (5621,5622).

ANGELICA herb, seed

Also Known As
Angelicae, Angelicae Fructus, Angelicae Herba.
CAUTION: See separate listings for Angelica root and Dong Quai.

Scientific Names
Angelica archangelica.
Family: Apiaceae/Umbelliferae.

People Use This For
Historically, people used angelica herb and seed orally as a diuretic and as a diaphoretic (2).
In food use, angelica herb and seed is used in candied products to decorate cakes and pastries (5,6).

Safety
LIKELY UNSAFE ...when used orally due to the furocoumarins contained in the stem and other plant parts (2,12). Angelica contains a volatile oil. The furocoumarins are angelicin, bergapten, imperatorin, and xanthotoxin. These are photosensitizers and photocarcinogenic (5,8).
PREGNANCY AND LACTATION: UNSAFE ...when used orally because it seems to be a menstrual and uterine stimulant (12); avoid using.

Effectiveness
There is insufficient reliable information available about the effectiveness of angelica herb and seed.

Mechanism of Action

Angelica herb and seed contains a volatile oil. It contains furocoumarin which consists of angelicin, bergapten, imperatorin, and xanthotoxin which can make the skin more photosensitive (2).

Adverse Reactions

Orally, angelica herb and seed may cause photosensitivity (2,6,12).
Topically, photodermatitis is possible following contact with plant juice (18).

Interactions with Herbs & Other Dietary Supplements

HERBS WITH ANTICOAGULANT/ANTIPLATELET POTENTIAL: Concomitant use of herbs that have coumarin constituents or affect platelet aggregation could theoretically increase the risk of bleeding in some people. These herbs include anise, arnica, asafoetida, bogbean, boldo, capsicum, celery, chamomile, clove, danshen, fenugreek, feverfew, garlic, ginger, ginkgo, Panax ginseng, horse chestnut, horseradish, licorice, meadowsweet, prickly ash, onion, papain, passionflower, poplar, quassia, red clover, turmeric, wild carrot, wild lettuce, willow, and others (4,19).

Interactions with Drugs

ACID-INHIBITING DRUGS: Theoretically, due to claims that angelica increases stomach acid, it might interfere with antacids, sucralfate (Carafate), H-2 antagonists, or proton pump inhibitors (19).
ANTICOAGULANTS: Excessive doses of angelica herb and seed can potentiate effects and adverse effects of anticoagulants (4).
HEXOBARBITONE: Theoretically, hepatic metabolism of hexobarbitone might be inhibited by furanocoumarin constituents in angelica herb and seed (4).

Interactions with Foods

No interactions are known to occur, and there is no known reason to expect a clinically significant interaction with angelica herb and seed.

Interactions with Lab Tests

No interactions are known to occur, and there is no known reason to expect a clinically significant interaction with angelica herb and seed.

Interactions with Diseases or Conditions

No interactions are known to occur, and there is no known reason to expect a clinically significant interaction with angelica herb and seed.

Dosage and Administration

ORAL: People typically use 1 teaspoon of the powdered seeds or leaves in 1 cup boiling water and drink as a tea twice daily. As a tincture, angelica is dosed up to 1 teaspoon up to twice a day (5250).

Comments

There has been confusion in the past between angelica and water hemlock. Water hemlock is highly toxic (6).

ANGELICA root

Also Known As

Garden Angelica, European Angelica, Root of the Holy Ghost, Wild Angelica.
CAUTION: See separate listings for Angelica seed, herb, and Dong Quai.

Scientific Names

Angelica archangelica, synonym Archangelica officinalis; Angelica atropurpurea, Angelica sylvestris; Angelica curtisi; Angelica rosaefolia; Angelica pubescens.
Family: Apiaceae/Umbelliferae.

People Use This For

Orally, angelica root is used for loss of appetite, gastrointestinal spasms, feeling of fullness, and flatulence (2).
Topically, it is used to create warmth in neuralgia and rheumatism (6,8), and is used for skin disorders (6). It is also used as part of a multi-ingredient preparation for treating premature ejaculation (2537).
Historically, angelica root has been used to promote menstrual flow, as an abortifacient, antiseptic, expectorant, diuretic (5,8,11), and as a cure for the plague (6).

Safety

POSSIBLY SAFE …when the root is used as a medicinal tea or a steam-distilled oil. Although the root contains furanocoumarin constituents that can be phototoxic, photomutagenic, and carcinogenic when exposed to UV light, they are only slightly soluble in water (8), and they are absent in the steam-distilled oil (11). …when used in foods. Angelica has Generally Recognized as Safe (GRAS) status in the US but Canada does not allow archangelica as a nonmedicinal ingredient (12). …when used topically, short-term as part of a multi-ingredient preparation (SS Cream). This preparation was used safely for premature ejaculation in a clinical trial where the cream was applied and left on the glans penis for 1-hour (2537). Further evaluation is needed to determine its safety after prolonged, repetitive use.
POSSIBLY UNSAFE …when the root or root extracts are used orally in medicinal amounts (2) because they contain photosensitizing furanocoumarin constituents. …when applied topically in medicinal amounts. The International Fragrance Association recommends limiting angelica root to a maximum of 0.78% in products to be applied to the skin and exposed to the sun (4,8).
LIKELY UNSAFE …when used orally in large amounts angelica root preparations can cause poisoning (5). …when used topically in high concentrations.
PREGNANCY: LIKELY UNSAFE …when used orally. angelica root can have an abortifacient effect (4,12); contraindicated. POSSIBLY UNSAFE …when used topically; avoid using.
LACTATION: POSSIBLY UNSAFE …when used topically; avoid using. There is insufficient reliable information available about the safety of oral use during lactation; avoid using (4).

Effectiveness

POSSIBLY EFFECTIVE …when used topically as part of a multi-ingredient preparation for treating premature ejaculation. In one controlled clinical trial, a multi-ingredient cream preparation containing Panax ginseng root, Angelica root, Cistanches deserticola, Zanthoxyl species, Torlidis seed, clove flower, Asiasari root, cinnamon bark, and toad venom (SS Cream) was applied to the glans penis 1-hour prior to intercourse and washed off immediately before intercourse. Men suffering from premature ejaculation who were treated with the cream had significantly improved ejaculatory latency compared to placebo (2537).
There is insufficient reliable information available about the effectiveness of angelica root for its other uses.

Mechanism of Action

The constituent, alpha-angelica lactone, can have calcium antagonist effects (11). The coumarins in angelica are responsible for its phototoxicity (12). Volatile emissions from the angelica root can have fungistatic activity (6). The coumarin constituents of related Angelica species can inhibit human platelet aggregation in vitro (736). The related species, Angelica sinensis, can lower prothrombin time in rabbits when coadministered with warfarin (737). The multi-ingredient preparation containing Angelica root is thought to work in premature ejaculation by increasing the penile vibratory threshold and reducing the amplitude of penile somatosensory evoked potentials (2537).

Adverse Reactions

Angelica is a photosensitizer, and when used, prolonged exposure to sunlight should be avoided (2,12). Severe poisoning can occur from large doses (5). When the multi-ingredient cream preparation (SS Cream) has been applied topically to the glans penis, sporadic erectile dysfunction, excessively delayed ejaculation, mild pain, and local irritation and burning has occurred (2537).

Interactions with Herbs & Other Dietary Supplements

HERBS WITH ANTICOAGULANT/ANTIPLATELET POTENTIAL: Concomitant use of herbs that have coumarin constituents or affect platelet aggregation could theoretically increase the risk of bleeding in some people. These herbs include anise, arnica, asafoetida, bogbean, boldo, capsicum, celery, chamomile, clove, danshen, fenugreek, feverfew, garlic, ginger, ginkgo, Panax ginseng, horse chestnut, horseradish, licorice, meadowsweet, prickly ash, onion, papain, passionflower, poplar, quassia, red clover, turmeric, wild carrot, wild lettuce, willow, and others (4,19).

Interactions with Drugs

ACID-INHIBITING DRUGS: Theoretically, due to claims that angelica increases stomach acid, it might interfere with antacids, sucralfate (Carafate), H-2 antagonists, or proton pump inhibitors (19).
ANTICOAGULANTS: Concomitant use of the angelica root can potentiate the anticoagulant effects of these drugs due to its coumarin constituents (737).
ANTIPLATELET DRUGS: Concomitant use can potentiate the antiplatelet effects (736).
PHOTOSENSITIZING DRUGS: Theoretically, angelica can compound photosensitization and side effects, and concomitant use with these drugs should be avoided.

Interactions with Foods

No interactions are known to occur, and there is no known reason to expect a clinically significant interaction with angelica root.

Interactions with Lab Tests

No interactions are known to occur, and there is no known reason to expect a clinically significant interaction with angelica root.

Interactions with Diseases or Conditions

No interactions are known to occur, and there is no known reason to expect a clinically significant interaction with angelica root.

Dosage and Administration

ORAL: The typical dose of angelica is 4.5 grams per day of the crude root or equivalent preparations for appetite loss and digestive problems, including mild GI tract spasms and flatulence (2). The dose of the fluid extract (1:1) is commonly 1.5-3 grams per day (2). The tincture (1:5) is usually dosed as 1.5 grams per day (2). Do not store angelica root preparations in plastic, because plastic can react with the essential oil (8).

Comments

According to legend, humans began to use the angelica root after an angel explained to them that the plant was a cure for the plague (6). Angelica is often planted in herb gardens as a decorative border and to protect other herbs from the wind (6).

ANGOSTURA

Also Known As

Angustura, Carony Bark, Cusparia, Cusparia Bark, True Angostura.

Scientific Names

Galipea officinalis.
Family: Rutaceae.

People Use This For

Orally, angostura is used for preventing recurrence of malaria, as an antipyretic, antidiarrheal, and antispasmodic (11). Large doses of angostura can be cathartic and emetic (11).
In foods, angostura is used in alcoholic beverages (11).

Safety

LIKELY SAFE ...when used orally, in average food amounts. Average maximum use of extract in alcoholic beverages is 0.3% (11).
There is insufficient reliable information available about the safety of the use of angostura in amounts larger than typical food amounts.
PREGNANCY AND LACTATION: Insufficient reliable information available.

Effectiveness

There is insufficient reliable information available about the effectiveness of angostura.

Mechanism of Action

The applicable part of angostura is the bark. Contains angostura bitters 1 and 2, alkaloids, and a volatile oil. Researchers report the alkaloids, cusparine and galipine, have antispasmodic properties (11).

Adverse Reactions

Orally, large doses of angostura may cause nausea and vomiting (18).

Interactions with Herbs & Other Dietary Supplements

Insufficient reliable information available.

Interactions with Drugs

No interactions are known to occur, and there is no known reason to expect a clinically significant interaction with angostura.

Interactions with Foods

No interactions are known to occur, and there is no known reason to expect a clinically significant interaction with angostura.

Interactions with Lab Tests

No interactions are known to occur, and there is no known reason to expect a clinically significant interaction with angostura.

Interactions with Diseases or Conditions

No interactions are known to occur, and there is no known reason to expect a clinically significant interaction with angostura.

Dosage and Administration

ORAL: People typically use 300 to 1000 mg of the powdered bark. As a liquid extract, angostura is dosed 0.3 to 2 mL (5264).

Comments

"Angostura bitters" which is sometimes used in mixing alcoholic beverages, no longer contains angostura. It is now made from gentian and other bitters.

There is very little scientific information about this product. Our staff is continually analyzing the available information on natural medicines and we will add data here as it becomes available.

ANISE

Also Known As

Aniseed, Anisi Fructus, Phytoestrogen, Semen Anisi, Sweet Cumin.

Scientific Names

Pimpinella anisum.
Family: Apiaceae or Umbelliferae.

People Use This For

Orally, anise is used for dyspepsia (2) and as a pediatric antiflatulent and expectorant (6).
Topically, it is used for lice, scabies, and psoriasis treatment (6).
In folk medicine, anise is used to increase lactation, induce menstruation (8), facilitate birth, increase libido, and alleviate the symptoms of male climacteric, which is the period of life after reproduction functions stop (4).
For food uses, anise is used as a licorice flavor substitute (6). It is also used as a fragrance in food.
In manufacturing, anise is often used as a fragrance in soap, creams, and perfumes.

Safety

LIKELY SAFE ...when used orally in amounts typically found in food. Anise oil has Generally Recognized as Safe (GRAS) status in the US and is approved for food use (4).
POSSIBLY UNSAFE ...when used topically, because anise contains coumarin constituents that cause photosensitivity reactions when skin is exposed to UV light. The constituent bergapten is also believed to be carcinogenic (4).
LIKELY UNSAFE ...when the undiluted oil is used orally. Ingestion of 1-5 mL can cause nausea, vomiting, seizures, and pulmonary edema (4).
PREGNANCY: LIKELY SAFE ...when used in food amounts. POSSIBLY UNSAFE ...when used in larger amounts because it might have abortifacient activity (4,12).
LACTATION: LIKELY SAFE ...when used in amounts commonly found in foods (4). POSSIBLY UNSAFE: ...when used in larger amounts because anise contains anethole and estragole, which are structurally similar to safrole, a known hepatotoxin and carcinogen (4).

Effectiveness

LIKELY EFFECTIVE ...when used orally as an expectorant or mild antispasmodic (2,6,7,11).
There is insufficient reliable information available about the effectiveness of anise for its other uses.

Mechanism of Action

The applicable parts of anise are the dried fruit, seed, and oil. Anise is rich in calcium and iron (19). The trans-anethole, a major component of the anise oil, is responsible for its characteristic taste, smell, and medicinal properties. Anethole has a structure similar to catecholamines, such as adrenaline, noradrenaline, and dopamine (4); and to the hallucinogenic compound, myristicin (4). Estrogenic activity can be due to anethole and the anethole polymers, dianethole and photoanethole (4,11). The other constituents of anise include the coumarins umbelliferone, umbelliprenine, bergapten, and scopoletin (6).

Adverse Reactions

Allergic reactions to anise include reactions of the skin, respiratory, and GI tract, and photosensitivity (4). Excessive doses of anise can cause adverse neurological effects (4). The ingestion of 1-5 mL of the oil can cause nausea, vomiting, seizures, and pulmonary edema (4).

Interactions with Herbs & Other Dietary Supplements

HERBS WITH ANTICOAGULANT/ANTIPLATELET POTENTIAL: Concomitant use of herbs that have coumarin constituents or affect platelet aggregation could theoretically increase the risk of bleeding in some people. These herbs include angelica, arnica, asafoetida, bogbean, boldo, capsicum, celery, chamomile, clove, danshen, fenugreek, feverfew, garlic, ginger, ginkgo, Panax ginseng, horse chestnut, horseradish, licorice, meadowsweet, prickly ash, onion, papain, passionflower, poplar, quassia, red clover, turmeric, wild carrot, wild lettuce, willow, and others (4,19).

Interactions with Drugs

EXCESSIVE DOSES: Excessive doses of anise can interfere with anticoagulant therapy, monoamine oxidase inhibitors (MAOIs), and hormone therapy (4).

Interactions with Foods

No interactions are known to occur, and there is no known reason to expect a clinically significant interaction with anise.

Interactions with Lab Tests

BLOOD PRESSURE: Theoretically, anise might increase blood pressure and blood pressure readings, due to the catecholamine activity of the constituent anethole (4,11).
HEART RATE: Theoretically, anise might increase heart rate and pulse rate due to the catecholamine activity of the constituent anethole (4,11).
INTERNATIONAL NORMALIZED RATIO (INR), PROTHROMBIN TIME (PT): Theoretically, excessive use of anise might prolong coagulation, increasing PT/INR and test results, due to coumarins contained in anise (4).

Interactions with Diseases or Conditions

ANTICOAGULANT and CATECHOLAMINE-SENSITIVE: Anise should be used with caution in these conditions. Anise contains coumarin constituents with anticoagulant and catecholamine-like properties. Theoretically these could interact with diseases or conditions sensitive to such ingredients.
HORMONE SENSITIVE CANCERS/CONDITIONS: Because anise might have estrogenic effects (4,11), women with hormone sensitive conditions should avoid using it. Some of these conditions include breast, uterine, and ovarian cancer, and endometriosis and uterine fibroids.
SKIN REACTONS: Anise oil potentially can be irritating and photosensitizing. Avoid its use in cases of dermatitis and inflammatory or allergic skin reactions (4).

Dosage and Administration

ORAL: The typical dose of anise is 0.5-1 grams of the dried fruit, 50-200 mL of the essential oil, or as a tea, three times per day (4). The tea is prepared by steeping 1-2 teaspoons of the crushed seed for 10-15 minutes and then straining (4). As an expectorant, one cup of tea is commonly taken in the morning and/or at night. As an antiflatulent, 1 tablespoon of the tea is usually taken several times a day. For nursing babies and infants, the typical dose is one teaspoon of the tea (8).

Comments

Anise is not considered a primary irritant, but its use can be associated with skin and mouth irritation and sensitization. Bergapten, a constituent, can cause photosensitivity and could be carcinogenic (6). As a flavoring agent, anise has a sweet, aromatic taste similar to licorice. It is commonly used in alcohols and liqueurs, such as Ouzo, Benedictine, Boonekamp, and Danziger Goldwasser. It is also used in dairy products, gelatins, meats, candies, breath fresheners, perfumes, soaps, and sachets (8).

ANNATTO

Also Known As
Achiote, Achiotillo, Annotta, Arnotta.

Scientific Names
Bixa orellana.
Family: Bixaceae.

People Use This For
In foods, annatto is used as a coloring agent (11).

Safety
LIKELY SAFE ...when used in food amounts (12).

Effectiveness
There is insufficient reliable information available about the effectiveness of annatto.

Mechanism of Action
The applicable part of annatto is the seed. Researchers think the coloring principles are carotenoids, mostly bixin and norbixin (11), which do not have vitamin A activity (11).

Adverse Reactions
None reported.

Interactions with Herbs & Other Dietary Supplements
Insufficient reliable information available.

Interactions with Drugs
DIABETES THERAPY: Monitor blood glucose level closely due to claims that annatto has hyperglycemic effects (19).

Interactions with Foods
No interactions are known to occur, and there is no known reason to expect a clinically significant interaction with annatto.

Interactions with Lab Tests
No interactions are known to occur, and there is no known reason to expect a clinically significant interaction with annatto.

Interactions with Diseases or Conditions
No interactions are known to occur, and there is no known reason to expect a clinically significant interaction with annatto.

Dosage and Administration
ORAL: People typically use 1 to 2 grams of powdered leaf in tablets or capsules twice daily. Annatto is also used as a 4:1 tincture in a dose of 2 to 4 mL twice daily (5255).

Comments
This product is used commercially as a food coloring agent (11).

APPLE

Also Known As
Apples.

Scientific Names
Malus sylvestris
Family: Rosaceae.

People Use This For

Orally, apples are used to control diarrhea or constipation (6); and for the softening, passage, and collection of gallstones. Apples are also used for treating cancer, diabetes, dysentery, fever, heart ailments, scurvy, warts, and cleaning teeth.

Safety

LIKELY SAFE ...when used orally in food amounts. Tell patients to avoid eating apple seeds, which can be toxic (6).
PREGNANCY AND LACTATION: LIKELY SAFE ...when used orally in food amounts. Tell patients to avoid eating apple seeds, which can be toxic (6).

Effectiveness

POSSIBLY EFFECTIVE ...when used orally for diarrhea and constipation (6).
There is insufficient reliable information to rate the effectiveness of apple for its other uses. However, there is some preliminary evidence that increasing apple consumption might decrease the risk of developing lung cancer (3470). There is also some preliminary evidence apple juice used orally for seven days, with olive oil used on the seventh day before going to bed, might be effective for the softening, passage, and collection of gallstones in the stool (3472). More evidence is needed to rate apple for these uses.

Mechanism of Action

The applicable part of apple is the fruit. The pectin in apples probably accounts for their effect on diarrhea and constipation. Pectin absorbs water in the gastrointestinal (GI) tract and swells to a gummy mass. The mass provides bulk which tends to normalize bowel function (6). Apples also contain phloretin, which has antibacterial activity (6). There is some interest in using apples for improving lung function. There is some evidence that consuming 5 or more apples per week can improve lung function as measured by maximum forced expiration in one second (FEV1) (3469). The constituent quercetin is an antioxidant flavonoid found in high concentrations in apples. Quercetin is thought to be responsible for apples potential benefit in preventing lung cancer (3469,3470).

Adverse Reactions

No adverse reactions are generally known or predicted to occur with apple fruit. However, one death is attributed to ingestion of a large amount (a cupful) of apple seeds, which contain hydrogen cyanide (HCN) (6). Ingestion of large amounts of seeds may cause cyanide poisoning, leading to death. To release cyanide, seeds must be hydrolyzed in the stomach, and several hours may elapse before poisoning symptoms occur (6). Patients allergic to other fruits in the Rosaceae family can also be allergic to apples. Cross-reactivity among the apple fruit and other members of the Rosaceae family, including apricot, almond, plum, peach, pear, and strawberry, has been demonstrated (7129).

Interactions with Herbs & Other Dietary Supplements

Insufficient reliable information available.

Interactions with Drugs

FEXOFENADINE (Allegra): Apple juice can significantly decrease oral absorption and blood levels of fexofenadine when used together. Apple juice decreases bioavailability of fexofenadine by about 78%. Apple juice seems to inhibit organic anion transporting polypeptide (OATP), which is involved in drug uptake in the gut, liver, and kidney (7046). It's not yet known how long apple juice inhibits OATP. Separating administration times might not prevent this interaction. Tell patients it's best to take their medications with a plain glass of water.

Interactions with Foods

CROSS-ALLERGENICITY: Patients allergic to other fruits in the Rosaceae family can also be allergic to apples. Cross-reactivity among the apple fruit and other members of the Rosaceae family, including apricot, almond, plum, peach, pear, and strawberry, has been demonstrated (7129).

Interactions with Lab Tests

No interactions are known to occur, and there is no known reason to expect a clinically significant interaction with apple.

Interactions with Diseases or Conditions

CROSS-ALLERGENICITY: Patients allergic to other fruits in the Rosaceae family can also be allergic to apples. Cross-reactivity among the apple fruit and other members of the Rosaceae family, including apricot, almond, plum, peach, pear, and strawberry, has been demonstrated (7129).

Dosage and Administration

ORAL: People typically use 500 mg apple pectin capsules daily as a supplement. Dried apple peels are used to make a tea: 1 to 2 teaspoons with 1 cup simmering water. The usual dose is from 1 to 3 cups per day (5250,5263,6006). For the softening of gallstones, one liter of apple juice used daily for seven days with 1 cup of olive oil used on the seventh day before going to bed has been used (3472).

Comments

None.

APPLE CIDER VINEGAR

Also Known As

Cider Vinegar.
CAUTION: See separate listing for Apple.

Scientific Names

None.

People Use This For

Orally, apple cider vinegar is used alone or with honey for weight loss, leg cramps and pain, queasy stomach, sore throats, sinus problems, high blood pressure, arthritis, to help rid the body of toxins (5904,5906), stimulate thinking, slow the aging process (5906), regulate blood pressure, fight infection, and osteoporosis (5907).

In combination with grapefruit and kelp, apple cider vinegar is used orally for weight loss (5904). Apple cider vinegar combined with cayenne, ginger, bromelain, and citrin, is used orally to maintain healthy cholesterol levels and for weight reduction (5903). In combination with gotu kola, apple cider vinegar is used orally for curbing appetite; detoxifying the body; weight loss; boosting the immune system; treating arthritis; lowering cholesterol; improving circulation; supplying amino acids, minerals, and vitamins; and aiding in the effective metabolism of food (5905). Topically, apple cider vinegar is used for acne; as a skin toner; as an ingredient in hair rinse (5904,5910); to soothe sunburn, shingles, and bites; and to prevent dandruff, baldness and itchy scalp (5907). It is also used in the bath for vaginitis (5910).

In food, apple cider vinegar is used as a flavoring agent.

Safety

LIKELY SAFE ...when used orally as a food flavoring. ...when used topically, diluted.
POSSIBLY UNSAFE ...when used orally in amounts of 250 mL per day long-term. There is one report of an individual who developed hypokalemia, elevated renin levels, and osteoporosis after 6 years of ingesting 250 mL apple cider vinegar per day (5911).
There is insufficient reliable information available about the safety of apple cider vinegar for its other uses.
PREGNANCY AND LACTATION: LIKELY SAFE ...when used orally as a food flavoring. POSSIBLY UNSAFE ...when used in larger amounts; avoid using.

Effectiveness

There is insufficient reliable information available about the effectiveness of apple cider vinegar.

Mechanism of Action

Cider vinegar is fermented juice from crushed apples. Like apple juice, it probably contains some pectin; vitamins B1, B2, and B6; biotin; folic acid; niacin; pantothenic acid; and vitamin C. It also contains small amounts of the minerals sodium, phosphorous, potassium, calcium, iron, and magnesium (5912).

Adverse Reactions

Orally, there has been one published report of an individual who developed hypokalemia, high renin levels, and osteoporosis after ingesting 250 mL apple cider vinegar daily for 6 years.

Interactions with Herbs & Other Dietary Supplements

HERBS WITH CARDIAC ACTIVITY: Theoretically, the overuse of apple cider vinegar can increase the risk of cardiotoxicity due to potassium depletion. Cardioactive herbs include digitalis, lily-of-the-valley, pheasant's eye, and squill.
STIMULANT LAXATIVE HERBS: Theoretically, overuse of apple cider vinegar and stimulant laxative herbs can increase the risk of potassium depletion. Stimulant laxative herbs include aloe vera, alder buckthorn, European buckthorn, cascara sagrada, castor oil, rhubarb, and senna.

HORSETAIL/LICORICE: Theoretically, overuse of apple cider vinegar can increase the risk of potassium depletion from overuse of horsetail or licorice.

Interactions with Drugs
POTASSIUM DEPLETING DIURETICS: Theoretically, overuse of apple cider vinegar concomitantly with potassium-depleting diuretics might increase the risk of hypokalemia (5911)
INSULIN: Theoretically, overuse of apple cider vinegar concomitantly with insulin might cause hypokalemia (5911).
CARDIOVASCULAR DRUGS: Theoretically, overuse of apple cider vinegar could decrease potassium levels, increasing the risk of toxicity of cardiovascular drugs such as digoxin (Lanoxin).

Interactions with Foods
No interactions are known to occur, and there is no known reason to expect a clinically significant interaction with apple cider vinegar.

Interactions with Lab Tests
POTASSIUM LEVEL: Theoretically, long-term use or high doses can reduce serum potassium level and increase urine potassium level (5911).
URINARY ANION GAP: In one case report, long-term use of 250 mL apple cider vinegar per day was associated with high positive urinary anion gap (5911).

Interactions with Diseases or Conditions
DIABETES: Theoretically, long-term use or high doses of apple cider vinegar might increase potassium loss of individuals using insulin.
OSTEOPOROSIS: Theoretically, long-term use or high doses might cause osteoporosis (5911).

Dosage and Administration
ORAL: To aid digestion, a 285 mg tablet taken with each meal, has been used (5909). A typical dose for weight loss is 1 ounce apple cider vinegar, 1 teaspoon of honey in 1-4 ounces of warm water before each meal (5904). A dose for a cold is 2 tablespoons cider vinegar in 1 cup water three times daily (5904). A dose for arthritis is 2 teaspoons of apple cider vinegar and two teaspoon of honey in a glass of water daily (5905). A dose for high blood pressure is 2 teaspoons of apple cider vinegar mixed in water in the morning (5905).
TOPICAL: For vaginitis add 3 cups of apple cider vinegar to hot bath and soak, spreading legs to allow water into vagina (5910).

Comments
None.

APRICOT

Also Known As
Amygdaloside, Apricots, Armeniaca, Chinese Almond, Laetrile, Madelonitrile, Vitamin B17.

Scientific Names
Prunus armeniaca.
Family: Rosaceae.

People Use This For
In Chinese medicine very small amounts of toxic kernel constituent, hydrocyanic acid, a source of HCN is used for asthma, cough, and constipation (6).
In folk medicine, uses of apricot include hemorrhage, infertility, eye inflammation, spasm, and vaginal infections (6). Historically, laetrile, the semi-synthetic derivative of amygdalin constituent, has been fraudulently acclaimed as a cancer treatment (4).
In manufacturing, apricot oil is used in cosmetics or as a vehicle for pharmaceutical preparations (6).

Safety
POSSIBLY SAFE ...when apricot oil is used topically (6).
LIKELY UNSAFE ...when apricot kernels are used orally because they are a source of cyanide. Acute poisonings may progress to respiratory failure, coma and death within 15 minutes (4). The lethal dose is 50-60 kernels (12) but amount may vary (4). Chronic poisoning can also occur (4).

CHILDREN: POSSIBLY SAFE …when apricot oil is used topically (6). LIKELY UNSAFE …when apricot kernels are ingested. The lethal dose is 7-10 kernels (12) but amount may vary (4).
PREGNANCY AND LACTATION: POSSIBLY SAFE …when apricot oil is used topically (6). LIKELY UNSAFE …when apricot kernels are ingested (4,12).

Effectiveness

INEFFECTIVE …when used to treat cancer (4,5).
There is insufficient reliable information available about the effectiveness of apricot for its other uses.

Mechanism of Action

The applicable parts of apricot are the kernel and oil. Apricot contains fruit acids, a variety of sugars, vitamins C, K, beta-carotene, thiamine, niacin, and iron. The seed contains the glycoside amygdalin which yields laetrile and hydrocyanic acid (6). Related glucosides include prunasin, sambunigrin and prulaurasin (6673). Several popular theories that have now been disproved claimed preferential uptake and conversion of amygdalin to hydrogen cyanide in tumor cells. Actually, research shows that amygdalin is slowly hydrolyzed to HCN in the stomach, rapidly absorbed via the GI tract, and then diffused through the body (4).

Adverse Reactions

Apricot may cause acute poisoning, with symptoms including dizziness, headache, nausea, vomiting, drowsiness, dyspnea, palpitations, marked hypotension, convulsions, paralysis, coma, and death (4). Apricot may also cause chronic poisoning, with symptoms of increased blood thiocyanate, goiter, thyroid cancer, optic nerve lesions, blindness, ataxia, hypertonia, cretinism and mental retardation. Demyelinating lesions and neuromyopathies reportedly occur secondary to chronic exposure, including long-term therapy (4).

Interactions with Herbs & Other Dietary Supplements

Insufficient reliable information available.

Interactions with Drugs

No interactions are known to occur, and there is no known reason to expect a clinically significant interaction with apricot.

Interactions with Foods

No interactions are known to occur, and there is no known reason to expect a clinically significant interaction with apricot.

Interactions with Lab Tests

No interactions are known to occur, and there is no known reason to expect a clinically significant interaction with apricot.

Interactions with Diseases or Conditions

No interactions are known to occur, and there is no known reason to expect a clinically significant interaction with apricot.

Dosage and Administration

ORAL: People typically take from 3 to 9 grams of apricot seed (5268).

Comments

The apricot seed constituent, amygdalin, is the generic name for laetrile, which is also referred to as amygdaloside, madelonitrile, or vitamin B17 (6673). In 1984, amygdalin, was classified prescription-only to protect the general public (4). In 1987, laetrile was ruled to be an unapproved drug and its importation into the USA under an affidavit system created in 1977 ended (6672).
The FDA is seeking a permanent injunction against three corporations for unlawfully promoting and marketing laetrile (injectable and oral) and apricot seeds for treating cancer on their Internet websites (6669). The companies named in the action are Without Cancer, Inc. and The Health World International, Inc. both located in Florida, and Health Genesis Corporation located in Arizona.

ARECA

Also Known As

Areca Nut, Betel Nut, Betel Quid, Pinag, Pinlag.

Scientific Names
Areca catechu.
Family: Palmaceae.

People Use This For
Orally, areca is used as a recreational drug (18) because of its central nervous system (CNS) stimulating properties (18). It is also used orally for treatment of schizophrenia (6081), but is otherwise rarely used therapeutically. Historically, areca has been used for glaucoma and as a mild stimulant or digestive aid (6).
In veterinary medicine, an extract of areca is used for expelling tapeworms in cattle, dogs, and horses (6,18); as a cathartic; and for treating intestinal colic in horses (6).

Safety
LIKELY UNSAFE ...when used orally, long-term or in high doses. Constituents of areca have documented carcinogenic potential and have been commonly associated with precancerous lesions and squamous cell carcinoma in long-term users (6,17). Other constituents are poisonous. Ingesting 8-30 grams of areca nut can cause death (6). There is insufficient reliable information available about the safety of short-term use of areca.
PREGNANCY AND LACTATION: LIKELY UNSAFE ...when used orally. Areca has carcinogenic potential as well as central nervous system (CNS) stimulant and cholinergic properties and might adversely effect pregnancy and nursing infants (6,17); avoid using.

Effectiveness
There is insufficient reliable information available to rate the effectiveness of areca. However, there is some preliminary evidence that areca might be helpful for schizophrenia. Some patients with schizophrenia who chew areca nut seem to have less severe symptoms (6081). More evidence is needed to rate areca for this use.

Mechanism of Action
The applicable part of areca is the nut. Researchers think alkaloid components have cholinergic action similar to pilocarpine, but with greater central nervous system (CNS) action (6). The most abundant alkaloid is arecoline (6081). Arecoline's cholinergic effects are thought to be the reason for improvement in psychotic symptoms in patients with schizophrenia who chew areca nut (6081). Arecoline also has anthelmintic activity (6). The constituents, arecaidine, and arecoline have carcinogenic potential (6) and chewing areca nut has been associated with oral cancer (329). Areca was also historically tried for glaucoma due to its cholinergic effects.

Adverse Reactions
Orally, areca may cause pupil dilation, increased salivation, vomiting, diarrhea, gingivitis, and periodontitis (6). High doses can cause convulsions and death (6). Chewing areca nut results in red-stained mouth, lips, and feces (18). Chewing areca quids is likely to produce central nervous system (CNS) stimulation similar to caffeine and tobacco (6). Areca quid chewing can cause oral submucous fibrosis in susceptible individuals (327,328,329). Chronic use of areca has also been associated with cardiovascular disease, diabetes, asthma (326), and oral cancer (329).

Interactions with Herbs & Other Dietary Supplements
Insufficient reliable information available.

Interactions with Drugs
ANTI-CHOLINERGIC DRUGS: Theoretically, due to cholinergic effects (6) areca nut can interfere with anti-cholinergic drug therapy. Avoid concomitant use.
CHOLINERGIC DRUGS: Theoretically, due to cholinergic effects (6) areca nut can increase the effects and risk of side effects of cholinergic drugs. Avoid concomitant use.
PROCYCLIDINE: Concomitant use can reduce anticholinergic effects of procyclidine (Kemadrin) given to treat the extrapyramidal effects of fluphenazine (19).

Interactions with Foods
No interactions are known to occur, and there is no known reason to expect a clinically significant interaction with areca.

Interactions with Lab Tests
FECAL LAB TESTS: Chewing areca nuts stains feces red (18). This coloration may interfere with fecal lab tests.

Interactions with Diseases or Conditions
ASTHMA: Areca may aggravate asthma (6).

Dosage and Administration
ORAL: An average of approximately 11 whole nuts per day is commonly used (6081).

Comments
Areca nut is chewed alone or in the form of quids, a mixture of tobacco, powdered or sliced areca nut, and slaked lime wrapped in the leaf of "betel" vine (Piper betel) (6).

ARENARIA RUBRA

Also Known As
Common Sandspurry, Sabline Rouge, Sandwort.

Scientific Names
Spergularia rubra.
Family: Not available.

People Use This For
Orally, arenaria rubra is used to treat urinary tract disorders, cystitis, dysuria, and urinary calculi (18).

Safety
There is insufficient reliable information available about the safety of arenaria rubra.
Pregnancy and Lactation: Insufficient reliable information available; avoid using.

Effectiveness
There is insufficient reliable information available about the effectiveness of arenaria rubra.

Mechanism of Action
Arenaria rubra is stated to have diuretic effects (18).

Adverse Reactions
None reported.

Interactions with Herbs & Other Dietary Supplements
Insufficient reliable information available.

Interactions with Drugs
No interactions are known to occur, and there is no known reason to expect a clinically significant interaction with arenaria rubra.

Interactions with Foods
No interactions are known to occur, and there is no known reason to expect a clinically significant interaction with arenaria rubra.

Interactions with Lab Tests
No interactions are known to occur, and there is no known reason to expect a clinically significant interaction with arenaria rubra.

Interactions with Diseases or Conditions
No interactions are known to occur, and there is no known reason to expect a clinically significant interaction with arenaria rubra.

Dosage and Administration
ORAL: People typically prepare the herb as a liquid extract and take 2 to 4 mL (5264).

Comments
There is very little scientific information about this product. Our staff is continually analyzing the available information on natural medicines and will add data here as it becomes available.

ARISTOLOCHIA

Also Known As

Birthwort, Long Birthwort, Pelican Flower, Red River Snakeroot, Sangree Root, Sangrel, Serpentaria, Snakeroot, Snakeweed, Texas Snakeroot, Virginia Serpentary, Virginia Snakeroot.

Scientific Names

Aristolochia auricularia; Aristolochia clematitis; Aristolochia fangchi; Aristolochia heterophylla; Aristolochia kwangsiensis; Aristolochia moupinensis; Aristolochia reticulata; Aristolochia serpentaria; other Aristolochia species. Family: Aristolochiaceae.

People Use This For

Orally, aristolochia is used as an aphrodisiac, anticonvulsant, immune stimulant, and to promote menstruation [400]. It is also used orally to treat allergic gastrointestinal colic and gallbladder colic [18].

Safety

UNSAFE ...when used orally. Aristolochia contains aristolochic acid, which is nephrotoxic and carcinogenic [18,6073,6118,6119]. The FDA considers all products containing aristolochic acid to be unsafe and adulterated [6119].

PREGNANCY AND LACTATION: UNSAFE ...when used orally; avoid using [6118,6119].

Effectiveness

LIKELY INEFFECTIVE ...when used orally for any use [400].

Mechanism of Action

The applicable parts of aristolochia are the above ground parts and root. Aristolochia contains aristolochic acid which is nephrotoxic and carcinogenic. Aristolochic acid has been associated with cancers of the kidney, bladder, stomach, lung, and lymphoma in rodents and cancers of the bladder, ureter, and/or renal pelvis in people with aristolochic acid-associated nephropathy (see Adverse Reactions) [6118].

Adverse Reactions

Orally, use of aristolochia can cause vomiting, gastroenteritis, spasms, severe kidney damage, and death [18]. There have been more than 100 cases of nephropathy, referred to as "Chinese herb nephropathy," characterized by interstitial fibrosis and associated with tea believed adulterated with aristolochia. Of these cases, 43 progressed to end stage renal failure requiring dialysis or transplantation [564,6073,6142] and 18 developed urothelial carcinomas of the bladder, ureter, and/or renal pelvis [6073,6142]. The risk of developing urothelial carcinoma seems to be related to cumulative intake of the herb [6073].

Interactions with Herbs & Other Dietary Supplements

Insufficient reliable information available.

Interactions with Drugs

ACID-INHIBITING DRUGS: Theoretically, due to claims that aristolochia increases stomach acid, it might interfere with antacids, sucralfate (Carafate), H-2 antagonists, or proton pump inhibitors [19].

Interactions with Foods

No interactions are known to occur, and there is no known reason to expect a clinically significant interaction with aristolochia.

Interactions with Lab Tests

KIDNEY FUNCTION TESTS: Aristolochia can cause nephropathy and abnormal kidney function results [564].

Interactions with Diseases or Conditions

GI IRRITATION: Aristolochia can irritate gastrointestinal tract. It is contraindicated in individuals with infectious or inflammatory gastrointestinal conditions [19].

Dosage and Administration

ORAL: When the plant is in flower, the entire plant is used. The root alone is also used. A liquid preparation of aristolochia is prepared by adding 2 teaspoons of the fresh plant or root to 1 cup of water and boiling for 10 minutes. A cold extract is prepared by adding 2 teaspoons of the plant or root to 1 cup cold water, which is allowed to stand for 6 to 8 hours. Sources warn against the toxicity of aristolochia and suggest that a dosage should be obtained from a health care professional (5263).

Comments

The FDA considers all products containing aristolochic acid to be unsafe and adulterated (6119). The FDA intends to automatically detain, without physical examination, any product which contains plants known or suspected to contain aristolochic acid, or which might be adulterated with plants known to contain aristolochic acid. Each detained product will be released only after the responsible party provides direct analytical evidence that it is free of aristolochic acid (6119). Aristolochia is also banned in Germany, Austria, France, Great Britain, Belgium, and Japan (367). Health Canada, the Canadian health authority, removed five aristolochia-containing Chinese herbal medicine products from sale. The products include, Touku Natural Herbal Rheumatic Pills, two brands of Tri-Snakegall & Fritillary Powder, Tracheitis Pills, and Gastropathy Capsules (367).

ARNICA

Also Known As

Arnica Flos, Arnica Flower, Arnikablüten, Bergwohlverleih, Fleurs d'Arnica, Kraftwurz, Leopard's Bane, Mountain Tobacco, Wolf's Bane, Wundkraut.

Scientific Names

Arnica montana; Arnica fulgens; Arnica sororia; Arnica latifolia; Arnica cordifolia.
Family: Asteraceae or Compositae.

People Use This For

Topically, arnica is used for the inflammation and immune system stimulation associated with bruises, aches, and sprains (5,11), for mouth and throat inflammation (2), insect bites, and superficial phlebitis (2).
Historically, arnica has been used as an abortifacient (8).
For food uses, arnica is a flavor ingredient in alcoholic beverages, nonalcoholic beverages, frozen dairy desserts, candy, baked goods, gelatins, and puddings (11).
In manufacturing, arnica is used in hair tonics and anti-dandruff preparations. The oil is used in perfumes and other cosmetic preparations (11).

Safety

POSSIBLY SAFE ...when used as a flavoring in alcoholic beverages (12), although Canadian regulations do not allow its use as a nonmedicinal ingredient in oral products (12). Flavoring use is allowed in the US (12), but maximum use level is usually 0.03%. ...when used topically for short-term use on unbroken skin (12).
LIKELY UNSAFE ...when taken orally. Arnica is considered poisonous and has caused severe or fatal poisonings (5). It can be cardiotoxic and cause large increases in blood pressure (5,17). Arnica is irritating to mucous membranes and can cause gastroenteritis, muscle paralysis (voluntary and cardiac), an increase or decrease in pulse rate, heart palpitations, shortness of breath, and death (4,17).
PREGNANCY AND LACTATION: LIKELY UNSAFE when used orally or topically; avoid using (12).

Effectiveness

There is insufficient reliable information available about the effectiveness of arnica.

Mechanism of Action

The applicable part of arnica is the flowerhead. The sesquiterpenoid lactones of arnica are the active principles and produce anti-inflammatory and analgesic effects. They also can have some antibiotic activity (5). Two components of arnica, helenalin and 11 alpha,13-dihyrohelenalin, inhibit human platelet function (104).

Adverse Reactions

Arnica taken orally can cause irritation of mucous membranes, drowsiness, stomach pain, vomiting, diarrhea, tachycardia, shortness of breath, coma, and death (4,6,11). It can cause an allergic reaction in individuals sensitive to the Asteraceae/Compositae family. Members of this family include ragweed, chrysanthemums, marigolds, daisies, and many other herbs. Topically, arnica can cause contact dermatitis and mucous membrane irritation (6,11).

Interactions with Herbs & Other Dietary Supplements

HERBS WITH ANTICOAGULANT/ANTIPLATELET POTENTIAL: Concomitant use of herbs that have coumarin constituents or affect platelet aggregation could theoretically increase the risk of bleeding in some people. These herbs include angelica, anise, asafoetida, bogbean, boldo, capsicum, celery, chamomile, clove, danshen, fenugreek, feverfew, garlic, ginger, ginkgo, Panax ginseng, horse chestnut, horseradish, licorice, meadowsweet, prickly ash, onion, papain, passionflower, poplar, quassia, red clover, turmeric, wild carrot, wild lettuce, willow, and others (4,19).

Interactions with Drugs

ANTICOAGULANTS AND ANTIPLATELET DRUGS: There is some concern that arnica might potentiate the effects of anticoagulant and antiplatelet drugs and possibly increase the risk of bleeding. Constituents of arnica can decrease platelet aggregation in vitro (104). However, this effect has not yet been demonstrated in humans. Until more is known, use cautiously in patients taking anticoagulant or antiplatelet drugs. Some of these drugs include aspirin, clopidogrel (Plavix), dalteparin (Fragmin), enoxaparin (Lovenox), heparin, ticlopidine (Ticlid), warfarin (Coumadin), and others.

Interactions with Foods

No interactions are known to occur, and there is no known reason to expect a clinically significant interaction with arnica.

Interactions with Lab Tests

PLATELET FUNCTION: Theoretically, arnica might inhibit platelet function and test results (104).

Interactions with Diseases or Conditions

BROKEN SKIN: Avoid the use of arnica on broken or damaged skin (2,4).
CROSS-ALLERGENICITY: Arnica can cause reactions in individuals allergic to plants in the Asteraceae or Compositae family, which include ragweed, chrysanthemums, marigolds, daisies, and many other herbs (12,17).
GI IRRITATION: Can irritate gastrointestinal tract. Contraindicated in individuals with infectious or inflammatory gastrointestinal conditions (19).

Dosage and Administration

TOPICAL: The typical strength of arnica is 2 grams of the flowerheads in 100 mL water (8). For a poultice, the tincture of arnica is diluted three to ten times with water (8). For a mouthwash, the tincture is diluted ten times (8). The mouthwash should not be swallowed. Ointments commonly have a maximum of 20-25% of the tincture or 15% of the oil (8). The tincture is usually a 1:10 dilution (2), and the oil is usually made with 1 part herb extract to 5 parts vegetable fixed oil (2,8).

Comments

Avoid internal use of arnica because it can be poisonous and cardiotoxic.

ARRACH

Also Known As

Dog's Arrach, Goat's Arrach, Goosefoot, Netchweed, Oraches, Stinking Arrach, Stinking Goosefoot, Stinking Motherwort.

Scientific Names

Chenopodium vulvaria.

People Use This For

Orally, arrach is used to relieve cramps and induce menstruation (18).
Topically, arrach is used to relieve cramps (18).

Safety

There is insufficient reliable information available about the safety of arrach.
Pregnancy and Lactation: Insufficient reliable information available; avoid using.

Effectiveness

There is insufficient reliable information available about the effectiveness of arrach.

Mechanism of Action

The applicable part of arrach is the whole flowering plant. Chenopodium species are stated to be potentially photosensitizing (19).

Adverse Reactions

Orally, arrach can be potentially photosensitizing. Excessive periods in the sun should be avoided (19).

Interactions with Herbs & Other Dietary Supplements

Insufficient reliable information available.

Interactions with Drugs

PSORALENS: Theoretically, concomitant use of arrach can increase risk of adverse effects, as unspecified Chenopodium species are associated with photosensitivity (19).

Interactions with Foods

No interactions are known to occur, and there is no known reason to expect a clinically significant interaction with arrach.

Interactions with Lab Tests

No interactions are known to occur, and there is no known reason to expect a clinically significant interaction with arrach.

Interactions with Diseases or Conditions

No interactions are known to occur, and there is no known reason to expect a clinically significant interaction with arrach.

Dosage and Administration

ORAL: People typically use a liquid extract of arrach, 2 to 4 mL 3 or 4 times daily (5264).

Comments

There is very little scientific information about this product. Our staff is continually analyzing the available information on natural medicines and will add data here as it becomes available.

ARROWROOT

Also Known As

Maranta.

Scientific Names

Maranta arundinaceae.
Family: Marantaceae.

People Use This For

Orally, arrowroot is used as a nutritional food for infants and convalescents. Babies cut teeth on arrowroot cookies. It is also used as a dietary aid in gastrointestinal disorders and acute diarrhea.
Topically, arrowroot is used as a soothing agent for painful, irritated or inflamed mucous membranes (18).
In foods, arrowroot is used as an ingredient in cooking.

Safety

LIKELY SAFE ...when the starch from the root or rhizome are used orally in amounts found in foods (12).
POSSIBLY SAFE ...when used orally or topically in medicinal amounts (12).
PREGNANCY AND LACTATION: POSSIBLY SAFE ...when used in amounts found in foods. There is insufficient reliable information available about the safety of larger amounts used during pregnancy and lactation; avoid using.

Effectiveness

There is insufficient reliable information available about the effectiveness of arrowroot.

Mechanism of Action

The applicable part of arrowroot is the starch from the root and rhizome. Animal data suggests that arrowroot may reduce deposited cholesterol in the aorta and heart muscle. This may be due to an increase in the elimination of cholesterol in the form of bile acids (18).

Adverse Reactions

None reported.

Interactions with Herbs & Other Dietary Supplements

Insufficient reliable information available.

Interactions with Drugs

No interactions are known to occur, and there is no known reason to expect a clinically significant interaction with arrowroot.

Interactions with Foods

No interactions are known to occur, and there is no known reason to expect a clinically significant interaction with arrowroot.

Interactions with Lab Tests

No interactions are known to occur, and there is no known reason to expect a clinically significant interaction with arrowroot.

Interactions with Diseases or Conditions

No interactions are known to occur, and there is no known reason to expect a clinically significant interaction with arrowroot.

Dosage and Administration

ORAL: Arrowroot starch is extracted from the chopped root and rhizome by a specific process using water. The powdered starch is usually boiled with water and used orally (18).

Comments

Arrowroot is often replaced with cheaper starches, including potato, corn, wheat, or rice starch (18).

ARTICHOKE

Also Known As

Alcachofa, Alcaucil, Artichaut Commun, Artischocke, Cardo, Cardo de Comer, Cardon d'Espagne, Cardoon, Garden Artichoke, Gemuseartischocke, Globe Artichoke, Kardone, Tyosen-Azami.

Scientific Names

Cynara scolymus, synonym Cynara cardunculus.
Family: Asteraceae or Compositae.

People Use This For

Orally, artichoke is used for dyspepsia, hyperlipidemia, nausea (2056), and irritable bowel syndrome (IBS) (2562). It is also used orally as a diuretic and choleretic. Artichoke is also used orally for treating snakebites, renal insufficiency, anemia, edema, arthritis, cystitis, liver dysfunction (4), preventing gallstones, lowering blood pressure, as a hypoglycemic, stimulant, and a tonic (3272).

In foods, artichoke leaves and extracts are used as flavoring agents in beverages. The constituents, cynarin and chlorogenic acid, are sometimes used as sweeteners (11).

Safety

LIKELY SAFE ...when used orally in amounts found in food. Artichoke is approved for food use in the US in alcoholic beverages in concentrations up to 0.00016% (16 ppm) (4,11).

POSSIBLY SAFE ...when used orally and appropriately in therapeutic amounts (2,11,2056).

PREGNANCY AND LACTATION: LIKELY SAFE ...when used orally in amounts found in food (11). There is insufficient reliable information about the safety of therapeutic amounts of artichoke used during pregnancy or lactation; avoid using (4).

Effectiveness

POSSIBLY EFFECTIVE ...when used orally for dyspepsia (2056). Both artichoke leaf and artichoke leaf extract are used (7,2056). Artichoke leaf extract seems to significantly reduce symptoms such as nausea, vomiting, flatulence, and abdominal pain in idiopathic dyspepsia and dyspepsia associated with biliary disease. Improvement can take up to 2-6 weeks of treatment (2056). ...when used orally for irritable bowel syndrome (IBS). There is some evidence that artichoke extract can significantly reduce abdominal pain and cramping, bloating, flatulence, and constipation associated with IBS after 6 weeks of treatment (2562). ...when used orally for treating hyperlipidemia (6282). Artichoke extract seems to significantly reduce total and low-density lipoprotein (LDL) cholesterol, and the LDL/high-density lipoprotein (HDL) ratio over 6 weeks of treatment (6282).
There is insufficient reliable information available about the effectiveness of artichoke for its other uses.

Mechanism of Action

The applicable parts of artichoke are the leaf, stem, and root (4,11). The primary constituents include up to 2% phenolic acids, primarily chlorogenic acid, cynarin, and caffeic acid. Also, up to 4% sesquiterpene lactones and 1% flavonoids, including scolymoside, cynaroside, and luteolin (20,2056). Artichoke's therapeutic benefit in dyspepsia has centered around its choleretic effects, or ability to stimulate bile flow, which has been demonstrated in several studies (20,2056). Constituents responsible for this effect are thought to be cynarin, chlorogenic acid, and scolymoside (4,2056). Antiemetic, spasmolytic, and carminative effects of artichoke have also been described. These effects may be responsible for potential benefits in patients with irritable bowel syndrome (IBS) (2562). Cynarin and chlorogenic acid may also have cholesterol-lowering effects, although studies with cynarin for hyperlipidemia have produced mixed results (1423,1424). Cynaroside and its derivative, luteolin, might also indirectly inhibit HMG-CoA reductase (1425,1426,2056). Several constituents are reported to have antioxidant activity (1422). Preliminary research suggests that artichoke leaf extract might also protect liver cells from damage (1421,1422,2056,3269). A mixture of polyphenols and flavonoids, including caffeic acid, chlorogenic acid, cynarin, luteolin-7-O-glycoside (cynaroside), and luteolin might contribute to hepatoprotective activity (3269,2056).

Adverse Reactions

Orally, artichoke extract might increase flatulence in some patients (2562). Artichoke can cause an allergic reaction in some patients. Patients sensitive to the Asteraceae/Compositae family may be at greatest risk. Members of this family include ragweed, chrysanthemums, marigolds, daisies, and many other herbs.
Topically, allergic contact dermatitis can occur with the use of artichoke. This has been attributed to the constituent cynaropicrin (11).

Interactions with Herbs & Other Dietary Supplements

Insufficient reliable information available.

Interactions with Drugs

No interactions are known to occur, and there is no known reason to expect a clinically significant interaction with artichoke.

Interactions with Foods

No interactions are known to occur, and there is no known reason to expect a clinically significant interaction with artichoke.

Interactions with Lab Tests

No interactions are known to occur, and there is no known reason to expect a clinically significant interaction with artichoke.

Interactions with Diseases or Conditions

BILE DUCT OBSTRUCTION: Theoretically, artichoke might worsen bile duct obstruction by increasing bile flow (2,11,2056); avoid using.
GALLSTONES: Theoretically, artichoke might worsen gallstones by increasing bile flow (2,11,2056); use with caution.
CROSS-ALLERGENICITY: Artichoke might cause an allergic reaction in individuals sensitive to Asteraceae/Compositae family plants. Members of this family include ragweed, chrysanthemums, marigolds, daisies, and many other herbs (11,2056).

Dosage and Administration

ORAL: A typical dose using artichoke stem or root is 1-4 grams three times daily (4). The typical dose of the dried leaf is 2 grams three times daily (2). The typical dose of 12:1 dry leaf extract is 500 mg daily (20). For irritable bowel syndrome (IBS), 640 mg leaf extract three times daily has been used (2562). For lowering serum cholesterol, an artichoke extract 1800 mg per day has been used in one clinical study. The isolated constituent cynarin 60-1500 mg per day has also been used to lower cholesterol (1423,1424,2056). For extract preparations, appropriate dosing will vary depending on the specific extract being used.

Comments

Avoid confusion with Jerusalem artichoke (Helianthus tuberosus) (11).

ARUM

Also Known As

Adder's Root, Bobbins, Cocky Baby, Cuckoo Pint, Cypress Powder, Dragon Root, Friar's Cowl, Gaglee, Kings and Queens, Ladysmock, Lords and Ladies, Parson and Clerk, Portland Arrowroot, Quaker, Ramp, Starchwort, Wake Robin.

Scientific Names

Arum maculatum.
Family: Araceae.

People Use This For

Orally, arum is used for colds and inflammation of the throat. It is also used orally to stimulate sweating and as an expectorant (18).

Safety

UNSAFE ...when used orally for any medicinal use (see Mechanism of Action).
PREGNANCY AND LACTATION: UNSAFE ...whe used orally because of its toxicity (18); avoid using.

Effectiveness

There is insufficient reliable information available about the effectiveness of arum.

Mechanism of Action

The applicable part of arum is the root. Arum can cause severe mucous membrane irritation and bleeding. This is probably due to sharp oxalate crystals present in the root. These injure the mucous membranes, and may also introduce impurities into the wounds. Arum also contains cyanogenic glycosides, but the levels are probably too low to cause poisoning (18).

Adverse Reactions

Orally, arum can cause swelling of the tongue, bloody vomiting, and bloody diarrhea (18).

Interactions with Herbs & Other Dietary Supplements

CALCIUM, IRON, ZINC: Concurrent use might decrease mineral absorption. Arum contains oxalate (18), which can bind multivalent metal ions in the gastrointestinal tract and decrease mineral absorption.

Interactions with Drugs

No interactions are known to occur, and there is no known reason to expect a clinically significant interaction with arum.

Interactions with Foods

CALCIUM, IRON, ZINC: Concurrent use might decrease mineral absorption from foods. Arum contains oxalate (18), which can bind multivalent metal ions in the gastrointestinal tract and decrease mineral absorption.

Interactions with Lab Tests

No interactions are known to occur, and there is no known reason to expect a clinically significant interaction with arum.

Interactions with Diseases or Conditions

No interactions are known to occur, and there is no known reason to expect a clinically significant interaction with arum.

Dosage and Administration

No typical dosage.

Comments

None.

ASAFOETIDA

Also Known As

Asa Foetida, Asafetida, Assant, Devil's Dung, Food of the Gods, Fum, Giant Fennel, Heeng.

Scientific Names

Ferula assa-foetida; Ferula foetida; Ferula rubricaulis.
Family: Apiaceae/Umbelliferae.

People Use This For

Orally, asafoetida is used for chronic bronchitis [4], asthma [11], pertussis [4], hoarseness, hysteria, flatulent colic [4], chronic gastritis, dyspepsia, irritable colon [18], and convulsions [11].
Topically, asafoetida is used for corns and calluses [6].
In Chinese medicine, asafoetida is used as a nerve stimulant in treating neurasthenia [11].
In folk medicine, asafoetida has been used for amenorrhea, croup, insanity, and sarcomas [6].
In manufacturing, asafoetida is used as a fragrance or fixative in cosmetics [11], and it is used as a flavoring ingredient in foods and beverages [11].
Other uses for asafoetida include its use as a cat, dog, and wildlife repellent.

Safety

LIKELY SAFE ...when used orally in amounts typically found in foods. Asafoetida is approved for food use in the US. Its maximum safe use level is less than 0.004%.
POSSIBLY SAFE ...when used orally and appropriately. It is contraindicated in people with CNS conditions that could result in convulsions [12].
CHILDREN: UNSAFE ...when used orally in infants due to the possible risk of methemoglobinemia (see Adverse Reactions) [4].
PREGNANCY: UNSAFE ...when used orally in amounts greater than those typically found in foods, because it might cause abortion [4].
LACTATION: UNSAFE ...when used orally due to possible risk of methemoglobinemia in infants [4].

Effectiveness

There is insufficient reliable information available about the effectiveness of asafoetida.

Mechanism of Action

The applicable part of asafoetida is the root resin. Asafoetida may contain sulfur compounds in its volatile oil which may protect against fat-induced hyperlipidemia. Asafoetida may contain coumarin constituents with anticoagulant activity [4]. There is some evidence to suggest that its constituents treat irritable bowel syndrome (IBS) [4].

Adverse Reactions

Orally, 50-100 mg of asafoetida may cause convulsions in people with nervousness [12]. There is one report of methemoglobinemia in an infant [4]. Large amounts are reported to cause swelling of the lips, belching, flatulence, diarrhea, headache, or convulsions [18].
Topically, genital organ swelling was reported after external use of asafoetida on the abdomen [18].

Interactions with Herbs & Other Dietary Supplements

HERBS WITH ANTICOAGULANT/ANTIPLATELET POTENTIAL: Concomitant use of herbs that have coumarin constituents or affect platelet aggregation could theoretically increase the risk of bleeding in some people. These herbs include: angelica, anise, arnica, bogbean, boldo, capsicum, celery, chamomile, clove, danshen, fenugreek, feverfew, garlic, ginger, ginkgo, ginseng (Panax), horse chestnut, horseradish, licorice, meadowsweet, prickly ash, onion, papain, passionflower, poplar, quassia, red clover, turmeric, wild carrot, wild lettuce, willow, and others [4,19].

Interactions with Drugs

ANTICOAGULANT, ANTITHROMBOTIC DRUGS: Theoretically, asafoetida might increase the risk of bleeding (4).

ANTIHYPERTENSIVE, ANTIHYPOTENSIVE DRUGS: Theoretically, excessive doses might interfere with blood pressure control (4).

Interactions with Foods

No interactions are known to occur, and there is no known reason to expect a clinically significant interaction with asafoetida.

Interactions with Lab Tests

No interactions are known to occur, and there is no known reason to expect a clinically significant interaction with asafoetida.

Interactions with Diseases or Conditions

BLEEDING DISORDERS: Theoretically, asafoetida might increase the risk of bleeding (4).

HYPERTENSION, HYPOTENSION: Theoretically, asafoetida might interfere with blood pressure control (4).

GI IRRITATION: Asafoetida can irritate gastrointestinal tract. It is contraindicated in individuals with infectious or inflammatory gastrointestinal conditions (19).

Dosage and Administration

ORAL: A typical dose is 300-1000 mg powdered resin three times daily (4). Tincture of asafetida (concentration unspecified), 2-4 mL (4), or 20 drops as a single dose (18) have also been used.

TOPICAL: No typical dosage.

Comments

Asafoetida resin is produced by solidifying juice exuded from incisions in living roots of Ferula foetida and other Ferula species. Asafoetida is known to have putrid odor and tastes bitter. The acrid taste is the basis for its name, devil's dung (6). Various species of this plant have somewhat different constituents. The related species Ferula communis, contains toxic coumarin constituents. Other related species are Ferula galbaniflua and Ferula rubricaulis. These seem to cause contact dermatitis (4).

ASARABACCA

Also Known As

Asaroun, Asarum, Azarum, False Coltsfoot, Hazelwort, Public House Plant, Snakeroot, Wild Ginger, Wild Nard. CAUTION: See separate listings for Bitter Milkwort and Senega.

Scientific Names

Asarum europaeum.
Family: Aristolochiaceae.

People Use This For

Orally, asarabacca is used for acute and chronic bronchitis, bronchial spasms, and bronchial asthma (18).

In folk medicine, it has been used as an emetic, antitussive, menstrual stimulant, abortifacient, and to treat pneumonia, angina pectoris, migraines, liver disease and jaundice, and dehydration (18).

Safety

POSSIBLY SAFE ...when used orally and appropriately short-term (12).

POSSIBLY UNSAFE ...when used orally in large amounts or long-term (12). Large doses have been associated with significant side effects, including burning tongue, gastroenteritis, diarrhea, skin rashes, and partial paralysis (18).

...when the essential oil is taken orally. The essential oil contains a potential hepatocarcinogenic constituent, beta-asarone (12).

UNSAFE ...when aristolochic acid-contaminated asarabacca is used orally. Asarabacca is commonly contaminated with aristolochic acid, which is nephrotoxic and carcinogenic. The FDA considers all products containing aristolochic acid to be unsafe and adulterated. Only products analytically verified to be aristolochic acid-free should be used (6119).

PREGNANCY: LIKELY UNSAFE ...when used orally. Asarabacca might act as a menstrual or uterine stimulant (12); contraindicated.

LACTATION: Insufficient reliable information available; avoid using.

Effectiveness

There is insufficient reliable information available about the effectiveness of asarabacca.

Mechanism of Action

The applicable part of asarabacca is the rhizome. The constituent phenylpropanol may be responsible for the effects of asarabacca on bronchitis/bronchial asthma. Some products are standardized for content of this constituent (18). Researchers think emetic and spasmolytic effects may be due to the constituent trans-isoasarone (18). Local anesthetic effect demonstrated in humans may be due to constituents, trans-isoasarone and trans-isomethyleugenol (18).

Adverse Reactions

Asarabacca may cause nausea and vomiting (12). Severe poisoning has also been reported (553). Symptoms of poisoning include burning of tongue, gastroenteritis, diarrhea, skin rashes, and partial paralysis (18). Asarabacca is commonly contaminated with aristolochic acid, which is nephrotoxic and carcinogenic (6119).

Interactions with Herbs & Other Dietary Supplements

Insufficient reliable information available.

Interactions with Drugs

No interactions are known to occur, and there is no known reason to expect a clinically significant interaction with asarabacca.

Interactions with Foods

No interactions are known to occur, and there is no known reason to expect a clinically significant interaction with asarabacca.

Interactions with Lab Tests

No interactions are known to occur, and there is no known reason to expect a clinically significant interaction with asarabacca.

Interactions with Diseases or Conditions

GI IRRITATION: Asarabacca can irritate the gastrointestinal tract; contraindicated in individuals with infectious or inflammatory gastrointestinal conditions (19).

Dosage and Administration

ORAL: 30 mg dry extract is the average daily dose for adults and children over 13 years old (18).

Comments

Asarabacca has been reported as obsolete for medicinal use (18); safer alternatives are available. Avoid confusion with bitter milkwort (Polygala amara), or senega (Polygala senega) also known as snakeroot.

Asarabacca is frequently contaminated with aristolochic acid, which is nephrotoxic and carcinogenic. The FDA considers all products containing aristolochic acid to be unsafe and adulterated (6119). The FDA intends to automatically detain, without physical examination, any product which contains plants known or suspected to contain aristolochic acid, or which might be adulterated with plants known to contain aristolochic acid. Each detained product will be released only after the responsible party provides direct analytical evidence that it is free of aristolochic acid (6119).

ASH

Also Known As

Bird's Tongue, Common Ash, European Ash, Weeping Ash, White Ash.
CAUTION: See separate listings for Northern Prickly Ash and Southern Prickly Ash.

Scientific Names

Fraxinus americana; Fraxinus excelsior.
Family: Oleaceae.

People Use This For

Orally, ash is used for fever, arthritis, gout, bladder complaints, as a laxative, diuretic (2), and tonic (18).

Safety

There is insufficient reliable information available about the safety of ash.

Pregnancy and Lactation: Insufficient reliable information available; avoid using.

Effectiveness

There is insufficient reliable information available about the effectiveness of ash.

Mechanism of Action

The applicable parts of ash are the bark and leaf. There is insufficient reliable information available about the possible mechanism of action and active ingredients.

Adverse Reactions

None reported.

Interactions with Herbs & Other Dietary Supplements

Insufficient reliable information available.

Interactions with Drugs

No interactions are known to occur, and there is no known reason to expect a clinically significant interaction with ash.

Interactions with Foods

No interactions are known to occur, and there is no known reason to expect a clinically significant interaction with ash.

Interactions with Lab Tests

No interactions are known to occur, and there is no known reason to expect a clinically significant interaction with ash.

Interactions with Diseases or Conditions

No interactions are known to occur, and there is no known reason to expect a clinically significant interaction with ash.

Dosage and Administration

No typical dosage.

Comments

Avoid use due to lack of safety and effectiveness information. Avoid confusion with northern prickly ash, southern prickly ash. There is very little scientific information about this product. Our staff is continually analyzing the available information on natural medicines and will add data here as it becomes available.

ASHWAGANDHA

Also Known As

Ajagandha, Amangura, Amukkirag, Asan, Asgand, Asgandh, Asgandha, Ashagandha, Ashvagandha, Ashwaganda, Asoda, Asundha, Asvagandha, Aswagandha, Avarada, Ayurvedic Ginseng, Clustered Wintercherry, Ghoda Asoda, Indian Ginseng, Kanaje Hindi, Kuthmithi, Samm Al Ferakh, Turangi-Ghanda, Winter Cherry, Withania.
CAUTION: See separate listings for Blue Cohosh, Canaigre, Codonopsis, Ginseng American, Ginseng Panax, Ginseng Siberian, and Winter Cherry.

Scientific Names

Withania somnifera.
Family: Solanaceae.

People Use This For

Orally, ashwagandha is used for arthritis, anxiety, insomnia, tumors, tuberculosis, and chronic liver disease. Ashwagandha is also used as a so-called "adaptogen," for increasing resistance to environmental stress, and as a general tonic. It is also used orally for immunomodulatory effects, improving cognitive function, decreasing inflammation, and preventing the effects of aging. Ashwagandha is also used orally for emaciation, infertility in men and women, menstrual disorders, and hiccups. It is also used orally as an aphrodisiac, and emmenagogue; and for treating asthma, leukoderma, bronchitis, backache, and arthritis.
Topically, ashwagandha is used for treating ulcerations, backache, and hemiplegia.

Safety

POSSIBLY SAFE ...when used orally and appropriately (12,3710).

There is insufficient reliable information available about the safety of ashwagandha for its other uses.

PREGNANCY: **LIKELY UNSAFE** ...when used orally. Ashwagandha has abortifacient effects (12,19).

LACTATION: Insufficient reliable information available; avoid using.

Effectiveness

There is insufficient reliable information available about the effectiveness of ashwagandha.

Mechanism of Action

The applicable parts of ashwagandha are the root and berry. Ashwagandha contains several active constituents including withanolides (4116), the essential oil known as ipuranol, and withaniol (6). Ashwagandha does not contain nicotine as some researchers have reported (3710). Ashwagandha is thought to have a variety of pharmacological effects including analgesic, antipyretic, sedative, hypotensive, anti-inflammatory, and antioxidant effects (3710,3711,4113,4116). It might also stimulate respiratory function, cause smooth muscle relaxation, and stimulate thyroid synthesis and/or secretion (3710). Ashwagandha was once thought to act as a diuretic, but preliminary evidence shows it does not have this effect (6). Some researchers think ashwagandha has a so-called "antistressor" effect. There is preliminary evidence that ashwagandha might suppress stress-induced increases in dopamine receptors in the corpus striatum of the brain (3710). Ashwagandha might also have anxiolytic effects, possibly by acting as a gamma-aminobutyric acid (GABA) mimetic agent. It might also have anticonvulsant activity, by binding to the GABA receptor (3710). Ashwagandha and its constituents also seem to have immunomodulatory effects. The constituents withaferin-A and withanolide-D seem to cause immunosuppression (6), but other constituents seem to have immunostimulating and antitumor activity. It is unclear what net effect whole ashwagandha preparations have on the immune system (3710,3711); however, there is preliminary evidence that ashwagandha might reduce cyclophosphamide-induced immunosuppression and leukopenia (3711,4114). Ashwagandha also seems to increase bone marrow cell and white blood cell count in radiation-treated animals (3711).

Adverse Reactions

Orally, ashwagandha seems to be well tolerated at typical doses. Large doses may cause gastrointestinal upset, diarrhea, and vomiting secondary to irritation of the mucous and serous membranes (3710).

Interactions with Herbs & Other Dietary Supplements

HERBS/SUPPLEMENTS WITH SEDATIVE PROPERTIES: Theoretically, concomitant use with herbs that have sedative properties might enhance therapeutic and adverse effects. Some of these include 5-HTP, calamus, calendula, California poppy, catnip, capsicum, celery, couch grass, elecampane, Siberian ginseng, German chamomile, goldenseal, gotu kola, hops, Jamaican dogwood, kava, lemon balm, sage, St. John's wort, sassafras, scullcap, shepherd's purse, stinging nettle, valerian, wild carrot, wild lettuce, and yerba mansa (4,19).

Interactions with Drugs

AMPHETAMINE: Theoretically, concomitant use of ashwagandha extracts might increase the effects of amphetamine (6).

BARBITURATES, OTHER SEDATIVES AND ANXIOLYTICS: Theoretically, ashwagandha's sedative effect can potentiate the effects of barbiturates, other sedatives, and anxiolytics (19).

BENZODIAZEPINES: Theoretically, ashwagandha might increase the effects of benzodiazepines (3710). There is preliminary evidence that ashwagandha might have an additive effect with diazepam (Valium) and clonazepam (Klonopin) (3710). This can probably also occur with other benzodiazepines such as alprazolam (Xanax), flurazepam (Dalmane), lorazepam (Ativan), and midazolam (Versed).

IMMUNOSUPPRESSANTS: Theoretically, ashwagandha might decrease the effectiveness of immunosuppressant therapy because of its potential immunostimulating effects. There is preliminary evidence that ashwagandha might decrease immunosuppression caused by cyclophosphamide (3711,4114). It might also decrease the effectiveness of other immunosuppressant drugs such as azathioprine (Imuran), basiliximab (Simulect), cyclosporine (Neoral, Sandimmune), daclizumab (Zenapax), muromonab-CD3 (OKT3, Orthoclone OKT3), mycophenolate (CellCept), tacrolimus (FK506, Prograf), sirolimus (Rapamune), prednisone (Deltasone, Orasone), and other corticosteroids (glucocorticoids).

THYROID, LEVOTHYROXINE (Synthroid), LIOTHYRONINE (Cytomel): Theoretically, ashwagandha might have additive effects when used with thyroid supplements. There is preliminary evidence that ashwagandha might boost thyroid hormone synthesis and/or secretion (3710).

Interactions with Foods

No interactions are known to occur, and there is no known reason to expect a clinically significant interaction with ashwagandha.

Interactions with Lab Tests

THYROID FUNCTION TESTS: Theoretically, ashwagandha might suppress thyroid stimulating hormone (TSH) or increase triiodothyronine (T3) or thyroxine (T4) values. There is some evidence that ashwagandha might stimulate thyroid hormone synthesis or secretion (3710).

Interactions with Diseases or Conditions

PEPTIC ULCER DISEASE: Theoretically, ashwagandha should be avoided by people with peptic ulcer disease because of its irritant effect on the gastrointestinal tract (3710).

Dosage and Administration

ORAL: People typically use 1 to 6 grams daily of the whole herb in capsule or tea form (3710). The tea is prepared by boiling ashwagandha roots in water for 15 minutes and cooled. The usual dose is 3 cups daily. Tincture or fluid extracts are dosed 2 to 4 mL 3 times per day (6006).
TOPICAL: No typical dosage.

Comments

The name Ashwagandha is from the Sanskrit language and is a combination of the word ashva, meaning horse, and gandha, meaning smell. The root has a strong aroma that is described as "horse-like" (3710). In Ayurvedic, Indian, and Unani medicine, ashwagandha is described as "Indian ginseng" (6). Ashwagandha is sometimes substituted or adulterated with a similar plant, Withania coagulans (3710). Avoid confusing ashwagandha with Physalis alkekengi, also known as winter cherry.

ASPARAGUS

Also Known As

Asparagi Rhizoma Root, Asperge, Garden Asparagus, Sativari, Spargelkraut, Spargelwurzelstock, Sparrow Grass.

Scientific Names

Asparagus officinalis.
Family: Liliaceae.

People Use This For

Orally, asparagus is used along with copious fluid consumption as "irrigation therapy" to increase urine output. It is also used orally for treating urinary tract infections and other inflammatory conditions of the urinary tract, preventing kidney and bladder stones (2,18), rheumatic joint pain and swelling, female hormone imbalances, dryness in the lungs and throat, AIDS, and to prevent anemia due to folic acid deficiency (3900).
Topically, asparagus is used for cleaning the face, drying sores, and acne (6).
In Chinese medicine, it is used orally as a laxative, for neuritis, and for treating parasitic diseases and cancer (11).
For food uses, the newly-formed shoots, or spears, are eaten as a vegetable (11). The seed and root extracts of asparagus are used in alcoholic beverages (11).

Safety

LIKELY SAFE ...when consumed in amounts typically found in food (11).
POSSIBLY SAFE ...when used orally and appropriately for medicinal purposes (2,12).
There is insufficient reliable information available for the safety of the topical uses of asparagus.
PREGNANCY: LIKELY SAFE ...when consumed as food. POSSIBLY UNSAFE ...when used for medicinal purposes because the extracts have been used as a contraceptive (6); avoid using.
LACTATION: LIKELY SAFE ...when consumed as food. There is insufficient reliable information available about the safety of asparagus for its other uses.

Effectiveness

There is insufficient reliable information available about the effectiveness of asparagus.

Mechanism of Action

The applicable parts of asparagus are the rhizome and root. Asparagus is a vitamin E rich plant source (19). The asparagus root has diuretic effects in animal experiments (2). Asparagus also has hypotensive (11), antibacterial, and antiviral effects in vitro (3900). Fibers from the plant can have mutagen-adsorbing (cancer-preventing) activity (11). The saponin constituents can irritate mucous membranes and can be cytotoxic (6,3901). Asparagus can also cause urinary tract irritation (19).

Adverse Reactions

Orally, asparagus can cause mucous membrane irritation (3901).

Topically, asparagus can cause allergic skin reactions (2).

Interactions with Herbs & Other Dietary Supplements

Insufficient reliable information available.

Interactions with Drugs

No interactions are known to occur, and there is no known reason to expect a clinically significant interaction with asparagus.

Interactions with Foods

No interactions are known to occur, and there is no known reason to expect a clinically significant interaction with asparagus.

Interactions with Lab Tests

No interactions are known to occur, and there is no known reason to expect a clinically significant interaction with asparagus.

Interactions with Diseases or Conditions

KIDNEY DISEASE: Asparagus is contraindicated in individuals with inflammatory kidney disease because the mucosal irritant effect of asparagus can exacerbate this condition (2,6,12).

EDEMA: Irrigation therapy with asparagus is contraindicated in individuals with edema caused by heart or kidney disorders (2).

Dosage and Administration

ORAL: Typically, asparagus is used daily as a tea prepared by steeping 40-60 grams of the cut rhizome or root in 150 mL of boiling water for 5-10 minutes and then straining (2). Ensure ample fluid intake when used as "irrigation therapy" (2,18).

TOPICAL: No typical dosage.

Comments

Asparagus seeds are used medicinally in a few cultures. The consumption of asparagus spears produces a pungent odor in the urine of some people.

ASPARTATES

Also Known As

Aspartate Chelated Minerals, Aspartate Mineral Chelates, Mineral Aspartates.

CAUTION: See separate listing for Chelated Minerals.

Scientific Names

None.

People Use This For

Orally, aspartates are used to increase absorption of mineral supplements (5140) and enhance athletic performance (5133).

Safety

There is insufficient reliable information available about the safety of aspartates.

Pregnancy and Lactation: Insufficient reliable information available; avoid using.

Effectiveness

There is insufficient reliable information available about the effectiveness of aspartates.

Mechanism of Action

Aspartate is an amino acid that is metabolized in resting muscles (5141). People theorize that aspartate mineral salts of copper, iron, magnesium, manganese, potassium, or zinc have better absorption or improve athletic ability. There is no evidence to suggest that this is true (5133). Except in cases of mineral deficiency, such as iron-deficiency anemia, a well-balanced diet typically provides the RDA of minerals (5133).

Adverse Reactions
None reported.

Interactions with Herbs & Other Dietary Supplements
Insufficient reliable information available.

Interactions with Drugs
No interactions are known to occur, and there is no known reason to expect a clinically significant interaction with aspartates.

Interactions with Foods
No interactions are known to occur, and there is no known reason to expect a clinically significant interaction with aspartates.

Interactions with Lab Tests
No interactions are known to occur, and there is no known reason to expect a clinically significant interaction with aspartates.

Interactions with Diseases or Conditions
No interactions are known to occur, and there is no known reason to expect a clinically significant interaction with aspartates.

Dosage and Administration
ORAL: Aspartate mineral supplements typically contain the following, either as individual or combination products: copper aspartate 2 mg, iron aspartate 18 mg, magnesium aspartate 400 mg, manganese aspartate 7 mg, potassium aspartate 99 mg, and zinc aspartate 15 mg. The dose is usually once daily (5265).

Comments
None.

ASPEN

Also Known As
Populi cortex, Populi folium.

Scientific Names
Populus tremuloides; Populus tremula.
Family: Salicaceae.

People Use This For
Orally, aspen is used as a component in various medicinal herbal combinations for treating rheumatic disorders, prostate discomforts, sciatica, neuralgia, and bladder problems (2).

Safety
There is insufficient reliable information available about the safety of aspen.
Pregnancy and Lactation: Insufficient reliable information available; avoid using.

Effectiveness
There is insufficient reliable information available about the effectiveness of aspen or aspen-containing herb combinations.

Mechanism of Action
The applicable parts of aspen are the bark and leaf. Aspen contains salicin, a precursor to salicylate (3700), and therefore aspen may have anti-inflammatory activity (2,7).

Adverse Reactions
Topically, salicin is associated with skin rashes (4). Pollen sensitization and allergic contact dermatitis may occur following contact with the bud resin (2,14).

Interactions with Herbs & Other Dietary Supplements

SALICYLATE-CONTAINING HERBS: Theoretically, concomitant use with aspen may potentiate effects of other herbs that contain salicylates (19).

HERBS WITH ANTICOAGULANT/ANTIPLATELET POTENTIAL: Concomitant use of herbs that have coumarin constituents or effect platelet aggregation could theoretically increase the risk of bleeding in some people. These herbs include angelica, anise, arnica, asafoetida, bogbean, boldo, capsicum, celery, chamomile, clove, danshen, fenugreek, feverfew, garlic, ginger, ginkgo, Panax ginseng, horse chestnut, horseradish, licorice, meadowsweet, prickly ash, onion, papain, passionflower, poplar, quassia, red clover, turmeric, wild carrot, wild lettuce, willow, and others (4,19).

Interactions with Drugs

No interactions are known to occur, and there is no known reason to expect a clinically significant interaction with aspen.

Interactions with Foods

ALCOHOL: Theoretically, concomitant use with aspen increases the incidence, severity, and risk of salicylate-induced gastrointestinal bleeding (15).

Interactions with Lab Tests

Theoretically, salicylate-containing herbs may interfere with lab tests affected by salicylates, such as serum uric acid, urine glucose, vanillylmandelic acid (VMA), and 5-HIAA tests.

Interactions with Diseases or Conditions

SALICYLATE HYPERSENSITIVITY: Theoretically contraindicated, due to salicylate (salicin) content. Avoid or use aspen with caution in people with active peptic ulcer disease, diabetes, gout, hemophilia, hypoprothrombinemia, kidney, or liver disease (15).

Dosage and Administration

ORAL: People typically use 1 to 5 grams of powdered aspen bark. A liquid is prepared using 1 to 2 teaspoons of the bark simmered in a cup of water for 10 to 15 minutes. This is taken three times daily. The liquid extract is commonly dosed 1 to 5 mL (5253,5264).

Comments

None.

ASTRAGALUS

Also Known As

Astragali, Beg Kei, Bei Qi, Buck Qi, Huang Qi, Huang qi, Hwanggi, Membranous Milk Vetch, Milk Vetch, Mongolian Milk, Ogi.
CAUTION: See separate listing for Tragacanth.

Scientific Names

Astragalus membranaceus; Astragalus mongholicus.
Family: Leguminosae or Fabaceae.

People Use This For

Orally, astragalus is used for treating the common cold and upper respiratory infections; to strengthen and regulate the immune system; and to increase the production of blood cells particularly in individuals with chronic degenerative disease or in individuals with cancer undergoing chemotherapy or radiation therapy. It is also used orally for chronic nephritis and diabetes. Astragalus is also used orally as an antibacterial and antiviral; a tonic; liver protectant; anti-inflammatory; antioxidant; and as a diuretic, vasodilator, or hypotensive agent (11,303).
Topically, astragalus is used as a vasodilator and to speed healing (11).
In combination with Ligustrum lucidum (glossy privet), astragalus is used orally for treating breast, cervical, and lung cancers (303).

Safety

POSSIBLY SAFE ...when used orally and appropriately (12). Significant toxic reactions have not been reported (11,303); however, specific safety evaluations have not been performed. ...when used topically (12).
PREGNANCY AND LACTATION: Insufficient reliable information available.

Effectiveness

There is insufficient reliable information available to rate the effectiveness of astragalus; however, there is some preliminary evidence that astragalus might help for certain conditions. There is some evidence that long-term ingestion of astragalus can reduce the chance of developing the common cold. There is also some evidence that adjunctive use of astragalus in combination with glossy privet (Ligustrum lucidum) can increase survival rates in patients being treated conventionally for breast or lung cancer. There is also some preliminary evidence that intravenous use of astragalus can be beneficial for patients with chronic hepatitis (303). More evidence is needed to rate astragalus for these uses.

Mechanism of Action

The applicable part of astragalus is the root. Astragalus contains a variety of active constituents including more than 40 saponins such as astragaloside, several flavonoids, polysaccharides, multiple trace minerals, amino acids, and coumarins (11,303). Astragalus is an antioxidant. It inhibits free radical production, increases superoxide dismutase, and decreases lipid peroxidation (303). Astragalus is often promoted for its effects on the immune system, liver, and cardiovascular system. Astragalus does seem to affect the immune system. Astragalus is thought to improve the immune response by potentiating the effects of interferon. Astragalus also seems to increase antibody levels of IgA and IgG in nasal secretions (303). There is preliminary evidence that astragalus extracts can restore or improve immune function in cases of immune deficiency (423,3713). For example, astragalus seems to restore suppressed T-cell function in cancer patients (423). In animal models, an astragalus extract can reverse cyclophosphamide-induced immune deficiency (3713). Lower doses of astragalus appear to stimulate the immune system, but doses in excess of 28 grams might suppress immunity (303). When administered intravenously, some evidence suggests astragalus extract might increase proliferation and differentiation of bone marrow stem cells and progenitor cells (303). Astragalus also shows evidence of broad-spectrum antibiotic activity (303). In individuals with chronic hepatitis, astragalus seems to improve liver function as demonstrated by improvement in serum glutamate pyruvate transaminase (SGPT) levels (303). Astragalus is also thought to cause vasodilation and increase cardiac output which might be beneficial in angina, congestive heart failure, and post-myocardial infarction (11,303).

Adverse Reactions

Toxicity of astragalus root is reportedly "very low" (11). Although side effects have not been reported, doses greater than 28 grams might cause immunosuppression (303).

Interactions with Herbs & Other Dietary Supplements

Insufficient reliable information available.

Interactions with Drugs

CYLCLOPHOSPHAMIDE: Some evidence suggests astragalus might reduce immunosuppression caused by cyclophosphamide (Cytoxan, Neosar) (303,3713).
IMMUNOSUPPRESSANTS: Theoretically, concurrent use might interfere with immunosuppressive therapy (303); avoid concurrent use. Immunosuppressant drugs include azathioprine (Imuran), basiliximab (Simulect), cyclosporine (Neoral, Sandimmune), daclizumab (Zenapax), muromonab-CD3 (OKT3, Orthoclone OKT3), mycophenolate (CellCept), tacrolimus (FK506, Prograf), sirolimus (Rapamune), prednisone (Deltasone, Orasone), and other corticosteroids (glucocorticoids).

Interactions with Foods

No interactions are known to occur, and there is no known reason to expect a clinically significant interaction with astragalus.

Interactions with Lab Tests

No interactions are known to occur, and there is no known reason to expect a clinically significant interaction with astragalus.

Interactions with Diseases or Conditions

AUTO-IMMUNE DISORDERS: Astragalus might increase immune system activity and may not be appropriate for individuals with auto-immune disorders (303).
ORGAN TRANSPLANT RECIPIENTS: Astragalus might interfere with immunosuppressive therapy; avoid concurrent use (303).

Dosage and Administration

ORAL: Astragalus powder 1-30 grams per day is typically used (11,303). For enhancing immune function for prevention of the common cold, 4-7 grams per day is commonly used (303). In some cases, people have used astragalus powder 30-60 grams per day (303). However, this should be avoided because some research suggests that doses greater than 28 grams per day offers no additional benefit and might even cause immune suppression (303).

Astragalus decoction 0.5-1 L per day (maximum of 120 grams of whole root per liter of water) has been used (303). As a soup, mix 30 grams in 3.5 L of soup and simmer with other food ingredients (303).
TOPICAL: No typical dosage.

Comments
Astragalus is most commonly used in combination with other herbs (303).

AUTUMN CROCUS

Also Known As
Colchicum, Crocus, Fall Crocus, Meadow Saffran, Meadow Saffron, Mysteria, Naked Ladies, Upstart, Vellorita, Wonder Bulb.

Scientific Names
Colchicum autumnale; Colchicum speciosum; Colchicum vernum.
Family: Liliaceae.

People Use This For
Orally, autumn crocus is used for arthritis, gout, and familial Mediterranean fever (2,400).

Safety
UNSAFE ...when used orally for self-medication because it is a potential poison (6,500). Human intoxication can occur when corms, which are the underground bulb-like stems, are mistaken for onions and ingested (6).
PREGNANCY AND LACTATION: UNSAFE ...when used orally because autumn crocus is a potential mutagen and toxin (500); avoid using.

Effectiveness
POSSIBLY EFFECTIVE ...when used orally for acute gout attacks and familial Mediterranean fever; however, autumn crocus is unsafe for self-medication (8,400).

Mechanism of Action
The applicable parts of autumn crocus are the seed, tuber, and flower. The seeds of this plant contain at least 0.4% colchicine, which is the constituent responsible for its therapeutic benefit (2).

Adverse Reactions
Orally, autumn crocus can cause burning of the mouth and throat, thirst, nausea, vomiting, diarrhea, liver necrosis, hypovolemic shock, kidney impairment, multiorgan failure, and death (6,553). Long-term use of colchicine is associated with agranulocytosis, aplastic anemia, and peripheral neuritis (6). Human intoxication can occur when corms, which are the underground bulb-like stems, are mistaken for onions or when contaminated milk is ingested (6).
Topically, the handling of fresh corm slices can cause finger numbness (6).

Interactions with Herbs & Other Dietary Supplements
Insufficient reliable information available.

Interactions with Drugs
COLCHICINE: Avoid concomitant use of autumn crocus with colchicine because it can increase therapeutic and adverse effects (2).

Interactions with Foods
No interactions are known to occur, and there is no known reason to expect a clinically significant interaction with autumn crocus.

Interactions with Lab Tests
URIC ACID: Autumn crocus can lower serum uric acid concentrations and test results due to its colchicine content (8,400).

Interactions with Diseases or Conditions
No interactions are known to occur, and there is no known reason to expect a clinically significant interaction with autumn crocus.

Dosage and Administration

ORAL: Dosing is related to the colchicine content (2). Due to its toxic potential, use the standardized, FDA-approved colchicine. Gout and familial Mediterranean fever require diagnosis, treatment, and monitoring by a medical professional.

Comments

Colchicine is available by prescription and used to treat acute gout attacks and familial Mediterranean fever (506).

AVENS

Also Known As

Benedict's Herb, Bennet's Root, Colewort, Geum, Herb Bennet.

Scientific Names

Geum urbanum.
Family: Rosaceae.

People Use This For

Orally, avens is used to treat diarrhea, catarrhal colitis, uterine bleeding, intermittent fevers, and ulcerative colitis (4). In foods, avens is used as a source of food flavoring (4).

Safety

LIKELY SAFE ...when used in amounts typically found in foods. The Council of Europe allows avens as a natural source of food flavoring (4).
There is insufficient reliable information available about the safety of avens for its other uses.
PREGNANCY AND LACTATION: POSSIBLY UNSAFE ...when used orally because avens seems to have an affect on the menstrual cycle; avoid using (4).

Effectiveness

There is insufficient reliable information available about the effectiveness of avens.

Mechanism of Action

The applicable part of avens is the above ground parts. The tannin-type constituents of avens have an astringent action; this supports the traditional use of avens for treating diarrhea (4).

Adverse Reactions

None reported.

Interactions with Herbs & Other Dietary Supplements

Insufficient reliable information available.

Interactions with Drugs

No interactions are known to occur, and there is no known reason to expect a clinically significant interaction with avens.

Interactions with Foods

No interactions are known to occur, and there is no known reason to expect a clinically significant interaction with avens.

Interactions with Lab Tests

No interactions are known to occur, and there is no known reason to expect a clinically significant interaction with avens.

Interactions with Diseases or Conditions

No interactions are known to occur, and there is no known reason to expect a clinically significant interaction with avens.

Dosage and Administration

ORAL: People typically use 1-4 grams steeped in boiling water, strained, three times a day (4).
Liquid extract (1:1 in 25% alcohol) 1-4 mL three times a day has also been used (4).

Comments
Avens is very rarely used medicinally today (18).

AVOCADO

Also Known As
Ahuacate, Alligator Pear, Avocato.

Scientific Names
Laurus persea; Persea americana, synonym Persea gratissima.
Family: Lauraceae.

People Use This For
Orally, avocado fruit is used to reduce serum cholesterol levels (6).
Topically, avocado oil is applied to soothe and heal skin, treat sclerosis of the skin, pyorrhea, and arthritis (11).
The fruit pulp is used topically to promote hair growth and hasten wound healing (6).
In folk medicine, avocado fruit has been used as an aphrodisiac and to stimulate menstrual flow (11). The seeds, leaves and bark have been used for dysentery and diarrhea (6), and to relieve toothache (11).
For food uses, avocado fruit is edible.

Safety
LIKELY SAFE ...when the fruit is consumed in amounts commonly found in foods (11,18).
There is insufficient reliable information available about the safety of avocado for its other uses.
PREGNANCY AND LACTATION: LIKELY SAFE ...when consumed in food amounts. There is insufficient reliable information available about the safety of avocado for its other uses during pregnancy and lactation.

Effectiveness
LIKELY EFFECTIVE ...when used orally for reducing total serum cholesterol, LDL cholesterol, and apolipoprotein B; and increasing HDL cholesterol serum levels (668,669,670,671).
POSSIBLY EFFECTIVE ...when used topically as a skin emollient (6,18).
There is insufficient reliable information available about the effectiveness of avocado for its other uses.

Mechanism of Action
The applicable parts of avocado are the fruit, leaves, and seed. The cholesterol lowering and skin soothing/healing effects may be due to the high content of unsaturated fatty acids and other compounds (oleic acid, tocopherols, vitamin E, sterols, volatile oils) in avocado (6).

Adverse Reactions
Allergic cross-sensitivity may be seen in latex-sensitive individuals (676).

Interactions with Herbs & Other Dietary Supplements
Insufficient reliable information available.

Interactions with Drugs
WARFARIN (Coumadin): Avocado may antagonize the anticoagulant effects of warfarin, but there has been only one case report of this interaction (667).

Interactions with Foods
No interactions are known to occur, and there is no known reason to expect a clinically significant interaction with avocado.

Interactions with Lab Tests
CHOLESTEROL: Avocado can lower serum total cholesterol, LDL cholesterol and apolipoprotein B concentrations and test results. Avocado can increase serum HDL cholesterol concentrations and test results (668,669,670,671).

Interactions with Diseases or Conditions
Insufficient reliable information available.

Dosage and Administration
ORAL: Variable dosing used; related to dietary calorie content or fat intake (668,669,670,671,675).

Comments

Avocado oil is derived from the fruit pulp (6). The fruit pulp is a good source of potassium and vitamin D (6,11). The Mexican avocado, a variant available in the US, is reported to contain estragole and anethole (6) which are hepatotoxic in animals and structurally similar to safrole, a known carcinogen (4).

BA JI TIAN

Also Known As

Morinda, Morinda Root, Morindae officinalis, Morindae radix.
CAUTION: See separate listing for Morinda.

Scientific Names

Morinda officinalis.
Family: Rubiaceae.

People Use This For

Orally, ba ji tian is used for cancer, cholecystitis, debility, enuresis, polyuria, hernia, impotence and premature ejaculation, lumbago (mid- and lower-back pain), dorsalgia (upper back pain) (513), depression (3558), increasing white blood cell count, stimulating the endocrine system (445), improving kidney function, and strengthening the skeletal and nervous systems (446,447).

In traditional Chinese medicine, ba ji tian is used as a kidney tonic to strengthen the yang (449).

In some commercial preparations, Morinda officinalis (ba ji tian) is combined with Morinda citrifolia (see separate listing for Morinda).

Safety

LIKELY SAFE ...when used orally and appropriately (12).
PREGNANCY AND LACTATION: Insufficient reliable information available; avoid using.

Effectiveness

There is insufficient reliable information available about the effectiveness of ba ji tian.

Mechanism of Action

The applicable part of ba ji tian is the root. The root contains several potentially active constituents, including an iridoid lactone called morindolide, iridoid glucosides including morofficinaloside, anthraquinones, a monoterpene glycoside, sterols including beta-sitosterol, an ursane-type triterpene, a lactone compound, and 24-ethylcholesterol (448,451,452). However, the role of specific constituents for the purported uses has not been described. Constituents reported to have antidepressant activity have been isolated (succinic acid, nystose, 1F-fructofuranosylnystose, inulin-type hexasaccharide, and heptasaccharide) (449). Ba ji tian is thought to work in depression by increasing serotonergic effects (3558). A study in mice reported that ba ji tian had anti-fatigue properties, reversed radiation-induced leukopenia, and reduced excitability of the parasympathetic nervous system associated with hypothyroidism (453).

Adverse Reactions

None reported.

Interactions with Herbs & Other Dietary Supplements

Insufficient reliable information available.

Interactions with Drugs

No interactions are known to occur, and there is no known reason to expect a clinically significant interaction with ba ji tian.

Interactions with Foods

No interactions are known to occur, and there is no known reason to expect a clinically significant interaction with ba ji tian.

Interactions with Lab Tests

No interactions are known to occur, and there is no known reason to expect a clinically significant interaction with ba ji tian.

Interactions with Diseases or Conditions

DYSURIA: Theoretically, ba ji tian may exacerbate urinary difficulties. Ba ji tian is reported to stimulate the kidneys. Use with caution (12).

Dosage and Administration

No typical dosage.

Comments

None.

BAEL

Also Known As

Bel, Bengal Quince, Indian Bael.

Scientific Names

Aegle marmelos.
Family: Rutaceae.

People Use This For

Orally, bael is used for constipation and diarrhea (18).

Safety

There is insufficient reliable information available about the safety of bael.
Pregnancy and Lactation: Insufficient reliable information available; avoid using.

Effectiveness

There is insufficient reliable information available about the effectiveness of bael.

Mechanism of Action

The applicable parts of bael are the unripe fruit, root, leaf, and branch. Bael is stated to have digestive and astringent properties. Constituents include tannins and furocoumarins (18). In vitro, the essential oil isolated from the leaves exhibits variable antifungal activity and inhibits spore germination of fungi isolates (3832).

Adverse Reactions

Orally, consuming large amounts of bael may cause GI upset and constipation (18).

Interactions with Herbs & Other Dietary Supplements

Insufficient reliable information available.

Interactions with Drugs

No interactions are known to occur, and there is no known reason to expect a clinically significant interaction with bael.

Interactions with Foods

No interactions are known to occur, and there is no known reason to expect a clinically significant interaction with bael.

Interactions with Lab Tests

No interactions are known to occur, and there is no known reason to expect a clinically significant interaction with bael.

Interactions with Diseases or Conditions

No interactions are known to occur, and there is no known reason to expect a clinically significant interaction with bael.

Dosage and Administration

ORAL: People typically use 4 to 8 mL of the liquid extract (5264).

Comments

There is very little scientific information about this product. Our staff is continually analyzing the available information on natural medicines and will add data here as it becomes available.

BAIKAL SKULLCAP

Also Known As

Baikal Scullcap, Baikal Skullcap Root, Huang Qin, Huangquin, Hwanggum, Ogon, Skullcap, Scute, Wogon.
CAUTION: See separate listing for Scullcap.

Scientific Names

Scutellaria baicalensis.
Family: Lamiaceae or Labiatae.

People Use This For

In combination with seven other herbs, Baikal scullcap is used in PC-SPES to treat prostate cancer (5548). In combination with shung hua, the Baikal skullcap constituent baicalin is used to treat upper respiratory tract infections (5541). In combination with other herbs, Baikal skullcap is used to treat minimal brain dysfunction (5551). In Chinese medicine, the Baikal skullcap root is used orally to treat respiratory and gastrointestinal infections (5542), jaundice, viral hepatitis, nephritis, pelvitis, sores or swelling, and fever. It is also used for scarlet fever, headache, irritability, red eyes, flushed face, and a bitter taste in the mouth (5541,5544).

Safety

POSSIBLY SAFE ...when used orally and appropriately (12,5548,5549,5550,5551). ...when used orally and appropriately in a specific herbal combination (PC-SPES) (5548).
PREGNANCY AND LACTATION: Insufficient reliable information available; avoid using.

Effectiveness

POSSIBLY EFFECTIVE ...when used orally in a specific herbal combination for prostate cancer. Studies using Baikal skullcap in combination with seven other herbs (PC-SPES), found that it significantly decreases prostate-specific antigen (PSA) levels (3576,5122,5548,6284,6286), causes clinically significant reductions in serum testosterone (5548), improves quality of life, and reduces pain (6286) in patients with prostate cancer. In two reports, PSA levels fell significantly within one month of treatment (5122,5548).
There is insufficient reliable information available about the effectiveness of Baikal skullcap for its other uses.

Mechanism of Action

The applicable part of Baikal skullcap is the root (12). Most pharmacological activity has been attributed to flavonoid constituents, including baicalin, baicalein, wogonin, and scutellarein. These flavonoids all appear to bind to GABAA receptors with possibly benzodiazepine-like effects (6290,6291). The constituent baicalein has weak antipyretic properties and might also have antimutagenic (6294) alpha-glucosidase (6292) activity, according to preliminary evidence. Baicalin, a glycoside constituent, has potent anti-inflammatory and antitumor properties (5541). Some evidence suggests it can inhibit tumor growth and suppress carcinoma cell proliferation (5541). Baicalin also shows evidence that it might inhibit HIV-1 infection and replication by inhibiting HIV reverse transcriptase (5541). Baicalein and baicalin are reported to be more active free-radical scavengers than alpha-tocopherol (vitamin E) (5541,6293) Baikal skullcap also appears to have antibacterial and antiviral properties, as well as antifungal activity, particularly against Candida albicans (5541,6295). It also might have diuretic and antihypertensive properties (5541).

Adverse Reactions

Several case reports implicate the Baikal skullcap in hepatotoxicity (5542), although the use of Baikal skullcap has generally been considered relatively nontoxic (5541). Use of Baikal skullcap as an intramuscular injection can cause fever and a sudden drop in the leukocyte count (5541). Theoretically, Baikal skullcap could cause sedation (6290,6291).

Interactions with Herbs & Other Dietary Supplements

HERBS WITH SEDATIVE PROPERTIES: Theoretically, concomitant use with herbs that have sedative properties might enhance therapeutic and adverse effects. These include calamus, calendula, California poppy, catnip, capsicum, celery, couch grass, elecampane, Siberian ginseng, German chamomile, goldenseal, gotu kola, hops, Jamaican dogwood, kava, lemon balm, sage, St. John's wort, sassafras, scullcap, shepherd's purse, stinging nettle, wild carrot, wild lettuce, ashwaganda root, valerian and yerba mansa and others (6290,6291).

Interactions with Drugs

ALCOHOL: Theoretically, Baikal skullcap can potentiate the sedative effects of alcohol (6290,6291); use with caution.
ANTIDIABETES DRUGS: Theoretically, concomitant use might enhance blood glucose lowering effects due to alpha-glucosidase activity (6292). Monitor blood glucose levels closely.
BENZODIAZEPINES: Theoretically, concomitant use with benzodiazepines can cause additive therapeutic and adverse effects (6290,6291); use with caution.
OTHER DRUGS WITH SEDATIVE PROPERTIES: Theoretically, concomitant use of Baikal skullcap and drugs with sedative properties can cause additive therapeutic and adverse effects (6290,6291); use with caution.

Interactions with Foods

No interactions are known to occur, and there is no known reason to expect a clinically significant interaction with Baikal skullcap.

Interactions with Lab Tests

BLOOD GLUCOSE: Theoretically, Baikal skullcap might reduce postprandial blood glucose concentrations and test results due to alpha-glucosidase activity (6292).

Interactions with Diseases or Conditions

DIABETES: Theoretically, Baikal skullcap could have hypoglycemic activity (6292). Use in diabetics might increase the risk of hypoglycemic episodes; use with caution.
STOMACH DYSFUNCTION: Baikal skullcap should not be used by individuals with stomach or spleen dysfunction (5544).

Dosage and Administration

ORAL: A typical dose is 6-15 grams of Baikal skullcap, toasted to moderate the effect (5544). A typical dose of the Baikal skullcap constituent baicalin to treat viral hepatitis is 500 mg three times daily (5541). A typical dose to treat an upper respiratory tract infection is a tablet containing 50 mg of the Baikal skullcap constituent baicalin in combination with 100 mg of shung hua. Two to three tablets are taken four to six times per day (5541).

Comments

Common substitutions for Scutellaria baicalensis (Baikal scullcap) in Chinese medicine include Scutellaria viscidula, Scutellaria amonea, and Scutellaria ikoninikovii (5541).

BAMBOO

Also Known As

None.

Scientific Names

Arundinaria japonica.
Family: Poaceae.

People Use This For

In Chinese medicine, bamboo is used orally for asthma, coughs, and gallbladder disorders (18).

Safety

There is insufficient reliable information available about the safety of bamboo.
Pregnancy and Lactation: Insufficient reliable information available; avoid using.

Effectiveness

There is insufficient reliable information available about the effectiveness of bamboo.

Mechanism of Action

The applicable part of bamboo is the young shoot. There is insufficient reliable information available about the possible mechanism of action and active ingredients.

Adverse Reactions

None reported.

Interactions with Herbs & Other Dietary Supplements

Insufficient reliable information available.

Interactions with Drugs

No interactions are known to occur, and there is no known reason to expect a clinically significant interaction with bamboo.

Interactions with Foods

No interactions are known to occur, and there is no known reason to expect a clinically significant interaction with bamboo.

Interactions with Lab Tests

No interactions are known to occur, and there is no known reason to expect a clinically significant interaction with bamboo.

Interactions with Diseases or Conditions

No interactions are known to occur, and there is no known reason to expect a clinically significant interaction with bamboo.

Dosage and Administration

ORAL: Typically, juice from the young shoots hardened into bamboo sugar is used (18).

Comments

There is very little scientific information about this product. Our staff is continually analyzing the available information on natural medicines and will add data here as it becomes available.

BARLEY

Also Known As

Dietary Fiber, Hordeum, Mai Ya, Pearl Barley, Pot Barley, Scotch Barley.

Scientific Names

Hordeum distychum; Hordeum vulgare.
Family: Gramineae or Poaceae.

People Use This For

Orally, barley is used for bronchitis; cancer prevention; diarrhea; gastritis; inflammatory bowel conditions; lowering blood sugar, cholesterol, and lipid levels (6); and weight loss (5078).

Historically, barley has been used for boils, gastrointestinal inflammation, and increasing strength and stamina (6). For food uses, barley is utilized as a source of folic acid, riboflavin (vitamin B2), niacin (vitamin B3), pantothenic acid (vitamin B5), pyridoxine (vitamin B6), vitamin E, carbohydrates, proteins, and fatty oils (13,18).

In manufacturing, barley is used as a food grain, natural sweetener, and as an ingredient for brewing beer and making alcoholic beverages (6).

Safety

LIKELY SAFE ...when used orally (18).
PREGNANCY: LIKELY SAFE ...when used in moderate amounts as a food. POSSIBLY UNSAFE ...when used in the relatively high doses found in medicinal products. Excessive amounts of barley sprouts should not be consumed during pregnancy (12,19).
LACTATION: Insufficient reliable information available; avoid using.

Effectiveness

POSSIBLY EFFECTIVE ...when used orally for reducing blood cholesterol, lipid and sugar levels, and reducing the risk of colon cancer (6). A group of overweight adults who ate barley muffins rich in beta-glucan lost an average of 1/2 pound per week, reduced total cholesterol 11% and LDL cholesterol 12%, compared to a group who ate wheat muffins containing no beta-glucan and gained 1/2 pound per week. Each group followed the National Cholesterol Education Program's Step I diet supplemented with muffins for 4 weeks. The results of this unpublished study were presented at the Experimental Biology 2000 meeting (5078).
There is insufficient reliable information available about the effectiveness of barley for its other uses.

Mechanism of Action

The applicable part of barley is the grain. The fiber content of barley is responsible for the observed reduction of cholesterol levels in healthy and hypercholesterolemic people, the reduction of blood sugar and insulin levels in healthy people, and the reduction of the colon cancer risk in rats (6). Researchers think that the beta-glucan contained in barley helps control appetite by slowing stomach emptying, prolonging the feeling of fullness, and stabilizing blood sugar (5078). Hordenine, a sympathomimetic constituent of barley, stimulates peripheral blood circulation and bronchodilation (6). The enzyme, diastase, is responsible for barley's ability to ferment (216).

Adverse Reactions

Orally, beer made with barley can cause anaphylaxis in sensitive individuals (317). Occupational exposure to barley flour can cause asthma (1300).

Interactions with Herbs & Other Dietary Supplements

Insufficient reliable information available.

Interactions with Drugs

DRUGS IN GENERAL: Theoretically, fiber can reduce the absorption of some drugs by reducing the gastrointestinal transit time (6).
SYMPATHOMIMETICS: Theoretically, the use of barley with sympathomimetics can result in duplication of activity due to the hordenine component (6). Concurrent use of barley should be avoided.
DIABETES THERAPY: Monitor blood glucose level closely due to claims that barley has hypoglycemic effects (19).

Interactions with Foods

No interactions are known to occur, and there is no known reason to expect a clinically significant interaction with barley.

Interactions with Lab Tests

CHOLESTEROL: Barley might reduce serum total cholesterol and LDL cholesterol concentrations and test results (6).
GLUCOSE: Barley might reduce blood glucose concentrations and test results (6).
The barley constituent, hordenine, can yield false-positive test results with ELISA, RIA and TLC urine assays for a number of opiate drugs. Positive urine test results should be confirmed with the more sensitive GC/MS or HPLC assay (1302).

Interactions with Diseases or Conditions

CELIAC DISEASE: The gluten content in barley can exacerbate celiac disease (6); avoid using.
SYMPATHOMIMETICS: Barley can contain the sympathomimetic constituent, hordenine, and it should be avoided or used with CAUTION in conditions sensitive to this activity.

Dosage and Administration

ORAL: The malt extract is used in medicinal preparations and combination products (18).

Comments

Barley is a common grain that is used world-wide as a food and in the brewing processes of alcoholic beverages. Avoid confusion with malt extract products that do not contain the enzyme diastase and are intended for use as bulk laxatives (13).

BASIL

Also Known As
Basilici Herba, Common Basil, Garden Basil, Holy Basil, St. Josephwort, Sweet Basil.

Scientific Names
Ocimum basilicum.
Family: Labiatae or Lamiaceae.

People Use This For
In Chinese medicine, basil is used for stomach spasms, kidney conditions, before and after childbirth to promote blood circulation, and to treat snakebites and insect bites (11).
In folk medicine, the above ground parts of basil are used as an antiflatulent, diuretic, lactation stimulant, gargle and mouth astringent, and in maggot-infested nasal disease (8). Basil has traditionally been used to treat head colds and worms (11) and as an appetite stimulant and a cure for warts.
For food uses, basil is used as an oil or oleoresin at levels usually below 0.005%.

Safety
LIKELY SAFE ...when the above ground parts are used as a spice. It has Generally Recognized as Safe (GRAS) status in the US. Generally used at low levels, below 0.005% in foods (11).
POSSIBLY SAFE ...when the above ground parts are used orally and appropriately short-term (2,8,12).
POSSIBLY UNSAFE ...when the above ground parts of basil are used orally long-term. ...when the oil of basil is used orally (12). Both the above ground parts and the oil contain estragole which shows evidence that it might be hepatocarcinogenic (8) and mutagenic (2).
CHILDREN: LIKELY SAFE ...when the above ground parts are used as a spice. POSSIBLY UNSAFE ...when used in larger amounts due to the estragole constituents (2,8).
PREGNANCY AND LACTATION: LIKELY SAFE ...when the above ground parts are used as a spice. POSSIBLY UNSAFE ...when used in larger amounts due to the estragole constituent of the essential oil. Estragole might have mutagenic effects (2,12).

Effectiveness
There is insufficient reliable information available about the effectiveness of basil.

Mechanism of Action
The applicable parts of basil are the above ground plant parts. The basil plant is a rich source of vitamin C, calcium, magnesium, potassium, and iron (19). The basil constituents methyl cinnamate, methyl chavicol, ocimene, cineole, and linalool have insecticidal activities (11). The volatile oil of basil can have antagonistic activity on worms (11). The essential oil contains up to 85% estragole (2) (methyl chavicol), which can produce liver tumors in mice (11). The constituent, xanthomicrol, can have cytotoxic and antineoplastic activities (11).

Adverse Reactions
Basil is known to cause hypoglycemia (214). Due to the adverse effects of the constituents of basil, CAUTION should be used in long-term treatment, which may be unsafe (12).

Interactions with Herbs & Other Dietary Supplements
Insufficient reliable information available.

Interactions with Drugs
No interactions are known to occur, and there is no known reason to expect a clinically significant interaction with basil.

Interactions with Foods
No interactions are known to occur, and there is no known reason to expect a clinically significant interaction with basil.

Interactions with Lab Tests
No interactions are known to occur, and there is no known reason to expect a clinically significant interaction with basil.

Interactions with Diseases or Conditions
No interactions are known to occur, and there is no known reason to expect a clinically significant interaction with basil.

Dosage and Administration
ORAL: The typical dose of basil leaf for distention or flatulence is 1 cup of the fresh brewed tea 2-3 times a day between meals. The tea is prepared by steeping 2-4 grams in 150 mL boiling water for 10-15 minutes and straining (8). For chronic flatulence the usual oral dose is 1 cup 2-3 times daily between meals for 8 days, then stopped for 14 days, and resumed for another 8 days (8).

Comments
Due to the carcinogenic potential of basil oil; avoid using (18).

BAYBERRY

Also Known As
Candleberry, Myrica, Southern Bayberry, Southern Wax Myrtle, Tallow Shrub, Vegetable Tallow, Wax Myrtle, Waxberry.
CAUTION: See separate listing for Sweet Gale (Myrica gale) also known as Bayberry.

Scientific Names
Myrica cerifera; Myrica pensylvanica.
Family: Myricaceae.

People Use This For
Orally, bayberry is used for head colds (5), mucous colitis, diarrhea, as an antipyretic, a circulatory stimulant (4), and an emetic in large doses (5).
Topically, bayberry is used as a gargle for sore throat (4), as a douche for leukorrhea (vaginal discharge) (4), for indolent ulcers (5), and wound healing (6).
In folk medicine, bayberry is used to treat diarrhea (5).

Safety
POSSIBLY UNSAFE ...when used orally. The root bark and berries contain high amounts of tannins (6). Large doses may have mineralocorticoid activity (4). Root bark can also contain a carcinogen (5).
There is insufficient reliable information available about the safety of bayberry for its other uses.
PREGNANCY AND LACTATION: POSSIBLY UNSAFE ...when used orally or topically because of possible carcinogenic, or mineralocorticoid activities; avoid using (4,5).

Effectiveness
POSSIBLY EFFECTIVE ...when used topically as an astringent (5).
There is insufficient reliable information available about the effectiveness of bayberry for its other uses.

Mechanism of Action
The applicable parts of bayberry are the root bark and berry. The tannin constituents of bayberry are responsible for its astringent action (4).

Adverse Reactions
Orally, bayberry can cause gastrointestinal irritation, vomiting, liver damage (possibly due to tannin content), and can act as an irritant and sensitizer (6).

Interactions with Herbs & Other Dietary Supplements
Insufficient reliable information available.

Interactions with Drugs
Large amounts of tannin-containing herbs can interfere with hypertension, hypotension, or steroid therapy (4).

Interactions with Foods
No interactions are known to occur, and there is no known reason to expect a clinically significant interaction with bayberry.

Interactions with Lab Tests

No interactions are known to occur, and there is no known reason to expect a clinically significant interaction with bayberry.

Interactions with Diseases or Conditions

HYPERTENSION: Large amounts of tannin-containing herbs can interfere with this condition.
SODIUM AND WATER RETENTION: Avoid bayberry use due to the potential mineralocorticoid activity, which can influence salt metabolism (4).

Dosage and Administration

ORAL: The typical dose of bayberry is 0.6-2 grams powdered bark, steeped in boiling water and strained, used three times a day (4). The liquid extract of bayberry (1:1 in 45% alcohol) is typically used 0.6-2 mL three times a day (4).
TOPICAL: No typical dosage.

Comments

Bayberry is a shrub that is commonly found in Texas and the eastern US. The wax extract taken from the berries is used in fragrances and candles.

BEAN POD

Also Known As

Common Bean, Green Bean, Kidney Bean, Legume, Navy Bean, Phaseoli fructus, Pinto Bean, Seed-Free Bean Pods, Sine Semine, Snap Bean, String Bean, Wax Bean.

Scientific Names

Phaseolus vulgaris varieties.
Family: Leguminosae or Fabaceae.

People Use This For

Orally, bean pod is used for urinary tract infections, kidney or bladder stones, and the promotion of urine flow (2,18).
In herbal tea combinations, bean pod is used for kidney and bladder problems (7,18).
In folk medicine, bean pod is used as a diuretic and for diabetes (18).

Safety

POSSIBLY SAFE ...when the ripe, dried pods are used orally and appropriately in medicinal amounts (18).
POSSIBLY UNSAFE ...when large amounts of fresh bean husks are ingested. Raw bean husks contain lectins that can cause gastrointestinal upset. Cooking destroys lectins (18).
PREGNANCY AND LACTATION: Insufficient reliable information available; avoid using.

Effectiveness

POSSIBLY EFFECTIVE ...when used orally as a supportive treatment for the inability to urinate (2).
There is insufficient reliable information available about the effectiveness of bean pod for its other uses.

Mechanism of Action

The applicable part of bean pod is the pod without the seeds. Bean pods demonstrate a weak diuretic effect in animals and humans (18). The chromium salts found in bean pods play a role in its antidiabetic effect (18).

Adverse Reactions

Orally, large amounts of green bean husks, or raw green beans, can cause vomiting, diarrhea, and gastroenteritis due to the content of the plant protein lectin. Cooking usually destroys lectins (18).

Interactions with Herbs & Other Dietary Supplements

Insufficient reliable information available.

Interactions with Drugs

DIABETES THERAPY: Monitor blood glucose level closely due to claims that bean pod has hypoglycemic effects (19).

Interactions with Foods

No interactions are known to occur, and there is no known reason to expect a clinically significant interaction with bean pod.

Interactions with Lab Tests

No interactions are known to occur, and there is no known reason to expect a clinically significant interaction with bean pod.

Interactions with Diseases or Conditions

DIABETES: Monitor blood glucose level closely due to claims that bean pod has hypoglycemic effects (19).

Dosage and Administration

ORAL: The typical dose of bean pod is one cup of tea several times per day, prepared by simmering 2.5 grams bean pods in 150 mL boiling water for 10-15 minutes and straining (2,18). The amount of bean pod typically used is 5-15 grams of bean pods per day (2,18).

Comments

None.

BEAR'S GARLIC

Also Known As

Bears Garlic, Broad-leaved Garlic, Ramsons, Wild Garlic.

Scientific Names

Allium ursinum.

People Use This For

Orally, bear's garlic is used for GI complaints, indigestion accompanied by the fermentation of stomach contents, flatulence, high blood pressure, and arteriosclerosis (18).
Topically, bear's garlic is used for chronic rashes (18).

Safety

There is insufficient reliable information available about the safety of bear's garlic.
Pregnancy and Lactation: Insufficient reliable information available; avoid using.

Effectiveness

There is insufficient reliable information available about the effectiveness of bear's garlic.

Mechanism of Action

The applicable parts of bear's garlic are the herb and bulb. The bear's garlic constituents, glucopyranoside, kaempferol, and flavonoids, inhibit human platelet aggregation (3830). In vitro, bear's garlic exhibits cardioprotective properties. In vitro and in vivo, bear's garlic moderately inhibits the angiotensin converting enzyme (ACE), which could contribute to the suggested cardioprotective and blood pressure lowering action. (3831).

Adverse Reactions

None reported.

Interactions with Herbs & Other Dietary Supplements

Insufficient reliable information available.

Interactions with Drugs

No interactions are known to occur, and there is no known reason to expect a clinically significant interaction with bear's garlic.

Interactions with Foods

No interactions are known to occur, and there is no known reason to expect a clinically significant interaction with bear's garlic.

Interactions with Lab Tests

No interactions are known to occur, and there is no known reason to expect a clinically significant interaction with bear's garlic.

Interactions with Diseases or Conditions

No interactions are known to occur, and there is no known reason to expect a clinically significant interaction with bear's garlic.

Dosage and Administration

ORAL: People typically use 3 capsules of dried bear's garlic leaf daily. The quantity of garlic in each capsule, which varies from lot to lot, is determined by the potency of active principals. There are claims that bear's garlic must be used fresh, only the bulb may be dried and suggests using the fresh plant in unspecified quantities as an ingredient in soup, salad, or as a vegetable (5263,5266).
TOPICAL: No typical dosage.

Comments

There is very little scientific information about this product. Our staff is continually analyzing the available information on natural medicines and will add data here as it becomes available.

BEE POLLEN

Also Known As

Bee Pollen Extract, Buckwheat Pollen, Honeybee Pollen, Honey Bee Pollen, Maize Pollen, Pine Pollen, Pollen, Pollen D'Abeille.
CAUTION: See separate listings for Bee Venom, Honey, and Royal Jelly.

Scientific Names

None.

People Use This For

Orally, bee pollen is used for nutrition, as an appetite stimulant, to improve stamina and athletic performance, for premature aging, preventing hay fever or allergic rhinitis, mouth sores, rheumatism, painful urination, prostate conditions, and radiation sickness. It is also used for bleeding problems including coughing or vomiting blood, bloody diarrhea, nosebleed, cerebral hemorrhage, and menstrual problems. Bee pollen is also used for gastrointestinal problems including constipation, diarrhea, enteritis, and colitis, and as a general tonic (5,6,11).
Topically, bee pollen is used for skin care and in skin softening products (11).
In Chinese medicine, bee pollen is used orally as a diuretic, and for alcohol intoxication (11); and topically for eczema, pustular eruptions, and diaper rash (11).

Safety

POSSIBLY SAFE ...when used orally and appropriately (5,6,11,7062,7063).
POSSIBLY UNSAFE ...when used orally by individuals with pollen allergies. Bee pollen can cause allergic reactions including anaphylaxis (5,6,11).
PREGNANCY: POSSIBLY UNSAFE ...when used orally. There is some concern that bee pollen might have uterine stimulant effects (5,6,11); avoid using.
LACTATION: Insufficient reliable information available; avoid using.

Effectiveness

POSSIBLY INEFFECTIVE ...when taken orally for increasing athletic performance or stamina (7062,7063).
There is insufficient reliable information available about the effectiveness of bee pollen for its other uses.

Mechanism of Action

Bee pollen refers to the pollen from flowers that collects on the legs and bodies of worker bees. It can also include amounts of nectar and bee saliva. Bee pollen composition varies depending on plant source and geographic region. Up to 50% of bee pollen can be made up of polysaccharides. The other constituents include lipids, protein, simple sugars, vitamin C, and carotenoids (5). Proponents often claim that enzymes in bee pollen provide a variety of therapeutic benefits. However, any enzymes in bee pollen are likely to be digested in the gastrointestinal tract. There is no reliable evidence that bee pollen enzymes or other constituents in bee pollen offer any therapeutic benefit.

Adverse Reactions

Orally, bee pollen seems to be well tolerated in most patients. However, patients with pollen allergies are at risk for serious allergic reactions. Allergic reactions can include itching, swelling, shortness of breath, light headedness, and anaphylaxis. Chronic allergy symptoms due to bee pollen include gastrointestinal and neurologic symptoms and eosinophilia (5,6,11). There have also been two cases of acute hepatitis associated with bee pollen use. One case involved ingestion of two tablespoons of pure bee pollen daily for several months. Another case involved ingestion of 14 tablets per day of a combination herbal product containing bee pollen, chaparral, and 19 other herbs for 6 weeks (1351). In this case it is not known if bee pollen or another herb might have caused the adverse event.

Interactions with Herbs & Other Dietary Supplements

Insufficient reliable information available.

Interactions with Drugs

No interactions are known to occur, and there is no known reason to expect a clinically significant interaction with bee pollen.

Interactions with Foods

No interactions are known to occur, and there is no known reason to expect a clinically significant interaction with bee pollen.

Interactions with Lab Tests

LIVER FUNCTION TESTS: Bee pollen might increase alkaline phosphatase (Alk Phos), alanine aminotransferase (ALT), aspartate aminotransferase (AST), lactate dehydrogenase (LDH), total bilirubin, prothrombin time (PT), and test results. Bee pollen has been associated with two cases of acute hepatitis and abnormally high results for these tests (1351).

Interactions with Diseases or Conditions

LIVER DISEASE: Use of bee pollen has been associated with two cases of acute hepatitis (1351). Avoid using in patients with existing liver disease.
POLLEN ALLERGY: Patients with pollen allergies are at risk for serious allergic reactions. Allergic reactions can include itching, swelling, shortness of breath, light headedness, and anaphylaxis. (5,6).

Dosage and Administration

ORAL: People typically take 500 mg two to three times daily (6006).

Comments

Pollens come from various plants, including buckwheat, maize, pine (songhuafen), rape, and typha (puhuang) (11). Avoid confusion with bee venom, honey, and royal jelly.

BEE VENOM

Also Known As

Apis Venenum Purum, Apitoxin, Bald-Faced Hornet, Bee Sting Venom, Bumblebee Venom, Honeybee Venom, Mixed Vespids, Pure Bee Venom, Wasp Venom, White-Faced Hornet, Yellow Hornet, Yellow-Jacket Venom.
CAUTION: See separate listings for Bee Pollen, Honey, and Royal Jelly.

Scientific Names

Apis mellifera (Honeybee); Bombus terrestis (Bumblebee); Vespula maculata (Hornet, Wasp).
Family: Apidae; Vespidae.

People Use This For

Parenterally, bee venom is used for rheumatoid arthritis, neuralgias, multiple sclerosis, desensitization to bee stings (venom immunotherapy), tendonitis and tendosynovitis, and muscle conditions such as fibromyositis and enthesitis (6,507,2619,6041).

Safety

LIKELY SAFE ...when used by subcutaneous injection by a trained medical professional (2619,6070). Purified bee venom for subcutaneous injection is a FDA approved product (2619).
PREGNANCY AND LACTATION: POSSIBLY SAFE ...when used by subcutaneous injection by a trained medical professional. Significant adverse effects to fetus or mother have not been reported. However, some clinicians decrease

maintenance dose by half during pregnancy (2619). POSSIBLY UNSAFE ...when used by subcutaneous injection in high doses. High doses of bee venom can increase release of histamine, which can cause uterine contraction (2619); avoid using in high doses.

Effectiveness

LIKELY EFFECTIVE ...when used subcutaneously for bee sting desensitization in patients with severe allergy to bee stings. Bee venom immunotherapy provides 98-99% protection from systemic reactions to bee stings. Once immunotherapy is stopped, the risk of a systemic reaction over the next 5 to 10 years is about 5-15% (6075,6076). Bee venom is a FDA-approved subcutaneous injectable product for the treatment of severe allergies to bee stings (2619).
POSSIBLY EFFECTIVE ...when bumblebee venom is used for immunotherapy in patients with severe allergic reactions to bumblebee stings (6043).
POSSIBLY INEFFECTIVE ...when used by injection for the treatment of arthritis. Some early reports seemed to indicate a possible benefit of bee venom in the treatment of arthritis; however, results are conflicting and most clinical studies do not show a benefit (6045).
There is insufficient reliable information available about the effectiveness of bee venom for its other uses.

Mechanism of Action

Bee venom contains several physiologically active components. Two of the most toxic compounds are melittin and phospholipase A2 (PLA2). Melittin constitutes 30-50% of dry bee venom (6041,6045,6046), and PLA2 makes up about 10-12% of bee venom (6041). Mellitin is a potent hemolytic (6042,6045) that causes mast cell degranulation and activates PLA2 (6045). Other constituents in bee venom include hyaluronidase, apamin, mast cell degranulating peptide (MCD peptide), procamine, secapin, tertiapin, and other small peptides including adolapin (6). Some other components are histamine, dopamine, and noradrenaline (6041). In desensitization to bee stings, hymenoptera venom stimulates an allergenic response, decreases leukocyte sensitivity to the allergen, and increases the number of T-suppressor cells (2619). There were early suggestions that bee venom could be a useful treatment in patients with arthritis. This theory was largely due to purported anti-inflammatory effects of bee venom, and the observation that many beekeepers don't develop arthritis (6). While some components in bee venom have been shown to have anti-inflammatory effects, studies have also shown that some components of bee venom are pro-inflammatory. For example, activators of PLA2 such as melittin, are thought to cause an increase in the synthesis of cytokines (tumor necrosis factor and interleukin 1) and stimulate arachidonic acid release resulting in an immune or inflammatory response (6044,6071).
PLA2 is an enzyme which catalyzes the hydrolysis of phospholipid bonds, destroying the major component of cell membranes and leading to cell death (6041,6046). PLA2 causes smooth muscle contraction, blood pressure reduction, increased capillary permeability, and mast cell destruction. PLA2 also reduces blood coagulation, possibly by reducing the activity of coagulation factors II, V, and VIII (6046). Melittin might also be partially responsible for bee venom's anticoagulant effects (6046). Some components in bee venom seem to cause neutrophil degranulation and superoxide production (6,6044), but other actions of bee venom components seem to decrease superoxide production (6,6041,6045,6072). The formation of superoxide anions can be destructive to tissues. The melittin component of bee venom possesses antimicrobial activity, but due to its hemolytic effects, melittin is unsuitable as a treatment for infections (6042). Hyaluronidase is an enzyme which hydrolyzes hyaluronic acid. The adhesive properties of hyaluronic acid hold cells together, so once hydrolyzed, other venom components can penetrate into the cell. For this reason, hyaluronidase is termed a spreading factor (6041). Apamin is a neurotoxin (6045). It blocks many inhibitory effects, including alpha-adrenergic, cholinergic, and neurotensin-induced relaxation, by blocking calcium-dependent potassium channels (6041). MCD peptide is chemically similar to apamin. It causes mast cell degranulation and release of histamine at extremely low concentrations. Histamine causes dilation and increased permeability of capillaries (6041). The constituent adolapin inhibits inflammation and the prostaglandin-synthase system (6). In animals, whole bee venom, melittin, and apamin have also been shown to cause increases in cortisol levels (6039,6040). The mechanism of other peptides is not yet understood (6041).

Adverse Reactions

Parenterally, local erythema and swelling at the injection site are the most common reactions to bee venom treatment (1343). Less common adverse effects ranging from itching, urticaria, edema, malaise, and anxiety to anaphylaxis occur in about 20% of patients (1343). Adverse reactions most often occur during the dose increase phase of immunotherapy, particularly with rapid dose increases (1343,6077). Risk of adverse effects seems to be increased in people treated with honeybee venom (1343,6077). Women seem to have more severe and more frequent adverse effects (1343). Anaphylaxis is most likely to occur in extremely sensitive individuals or in the case of an overdose (2169,6074,6077). Other adverse reactions include chest tightness, palpitations, dizziness, nausea, vomiting, diarrhea, somnolence, respiratory distress, hypotension, confusion, fainting, and laryngeal edema or asthma (1343,2619,6070,6078). Uncommon reactions are abdominal pain, incontinence, chest pain, or visual disturbances (6078). Rarely, coagulation abnormalities can occur, and are usually associated with severe reactions to bee stings (6046).

Interactions with Herbs & Other Dietary Supplements
Insufficient reliable information available.

Interactions with Drugs
HYDROCORTISONE: Co-administration may enhance effects in arthritis (507).

Interactions with Foods
No interactions are known to occur, and there is no known reason to expect a clinically significant interaction with bee venom.

Interactions with Lab Tests
COAGULATION TESTS: Bee venom might increase the prothrombin time (PT) and partial thromboplastin time (PTT) (6046). The PLA2 component of bee venom seems to reduce the activity of clotting factors II, V, and VIII (6046).

Interactions with Diseases or Conditions
No interactions are known to occur, and there is no known reason to expect a clinically significant interaction with bee venom.

Dosage and Administration
PARENTERAL: Bee venom is used subcutaneously, intradermally, and intra-arterially for these uses. For arthritis, purified, sterile bee toxin (apitoxin 2 mg/mL) has been used starting with 0.05-0.1 mL. The dose is gradually increased to 0.25 mL, 0.5 mL, and 1 mL, with dose intervals usually from 5 to 7 days (507). For bee venom immunotherapy in people hypersensitive to bee stings, increased doses of venom are given at selected intervals, usually weekly (6078). There are many possible protocols for immunotherapy. Some start with 0.0001 or 0.001 mcg of venom extract (6077). This is continued until a maintenance dose is achieved, usually 100 micrograms per venom. Once the maintenance dose is achieved, therapy can continue for years. Patients have varying sensitivities to venom and tolerability to immunotherapy, so it is not possible to provide a general dosing schedule for all patients. Venom immunotherapy should only be done by physicians thoroughly familiar with the use of these products, including the treatment of anaphylactic and other adverse reactions. It is also advised to have injectable epinephrine and emergency facilities nearby in case an anaphylactic reaction occurs (507,2619,6074,6078). Alcohol and tincture of iodine rapidly destroy the activity of bee venom and should not be applied at the site of injection (507). In China, bee venom is also commonly administered by electrophoresis, ultrasonophoresis, and acupuncture.

Comments
Avoid confusion with bee pollen, honey, and royal jelly. Other venoms are derived from related members of the insect order, Hymenoptera (6).

BEER

Also Known As
None.
CAUTION: See separate listings for Barley, Hops, Wine, and Yeast.

Scientific Names
None.

People Use This For
Orally, beer is used for reducing the risk of cardiovascular disease, including coronary heart disease, atherosclerosis, and myocardial infarction, and for reducing the risk of ischemic stroke and type 2 diabetes. It is also used orally for preventing cognitive decline in later life, Alzheimer's disease, loss of bone mineral density, cancer, gallstones, and kidney stones. Beer is also used orally as an appetite and digestive stimulant.

Safety
LIKELY SAFE ...when used orally in moderation. Beer seems to be safe when 24 oz or less is consumed daily (14,2060).
POSSIBLY UNSAFE ...when consumed in large amounts. Greater than 24 oz per day can cause significant adverse effects (14,2060,6840).
PREGNANCY: LIKELY UNSAFE ...when used orally. Alcohol is a teratogen. Use during pregnancy, especially

during the first two months after conception, is associated with significant risk of spontaneous abortion, fetal alcohol syndrome, and developmental and behavioral dysfunction in infants and children exposed to alcohol in utero (4260); avoid using.

LACTATION: LIKELY UNSAFE ...when used orally. Alcohol is secreted in breast milk. It can cause abnormal psychomotor development, pseudo-Cushing syndrome, alcohol poisoning, and potentiate severe hypoprothrombic bleeding in infants (4260); avoid using.

Effectiveness

LIKELY EFFECTIVE ...when used orally for preventing cardiovascular disease, including coronary heart disease, atherosclerosis, and myocardial infarction. Consuming alcoholic drinks, including beer, in moderation, one to two drinks per day, seems to reduce risk of developing cardiovascular disease by 30-50% (2058,2060,2261,2267,2268,2270,2271,6835,6837,6840,6841,6888). Tell patients not to exceed two drinks per day. More than two drinks daily can increase the risk of cardiovascular and overall mortality (841,2060,2261,6173,6889,6890). Alcoholic beverage consumption does not seem to reduce morbidity and mortality in people with established cardiovascular disease (6173).

POSSIBLY EFFECTIVE ...when used orally for reducing the risk of all-cause mortality. There is some evidence that moderate consumption of alcoholic drinks, including beer, one to two drinks per day, can reduce the risk of all-cause mortality in people who are middle-aged or older (2261,6823,6835,6837,6843). Tell patients not to exceed more than two drinks per day. More than two drinks per day can increase the risk of all-cause mortality (841,2261). ...when used orally in moderation to reduce mortality in people with ischemic left ventricular (LV) dysfunction. Consumption of 1 to 14 alcoholic drinks, including beer, per week is associated with reduced all-cause mortality compared with non-drinkers in people with ischemic LV dysfunction. However, this association has not been found for those with non-ischemic LV dysfunction (6827). ...when used orally for reducing the risk of type 2 diabetes. Light to moderate alcohol consumption (from 2 drinks per week up to 3 or 4 drinks per day) is associated with a reduced risk of type 2 diabetes in healthy men (6172,6891). ...when used orally for preventing ischemic stroke. Moderate alcohol consumption (up to 2 drinks per day) appears to reduce the risk of having an ischemic stroke (841,2271,2279,6834,6842,6893). Tell patients to avoid heavy consumption of alcohol. Seven or more drinks per day seems to increase the risk of ischemic stroke (6842). There is also some evidence that any alcohol consumption can increase the risk of hemorrhagic stroke (841,2271). ...when used orally in moderation to maintain cognitive function in later life. Elderly men who have a history of consuming one alcoholic drink per day seem to maintain better general cognitive function during their late 70's and 80's compared to non-drinkers (6824,6829). However, consumption of more than 4 drinks per day during middle age seems to be associated with significantly poorer cognitive function later in life (6824).

POSSIBLY INEFFECTIVE ...when used orally for reducing morbidity and mortality in men with established coronary heart disease (CHD). Consumption of 1-14 alcoholic drinks per week, including beer, has no effect on CHD, cardiovascular disease, or all-cause mortality compared to drinking less than 1 drink per week. More than 3 drinks per day is associated with increased mortality in men with a history of heart attacks (6173). ...when used orally for decreasing the risk of mortality from cancer. Although wine consumption has been associated with some reductions in cancer mortality, beer consumption does not seem to have this effect (2058). In fact, there is some evidence that beer consumption might slightly increase cancer-related mortality (6823,6843). There is some evidence that consumption of one or more alcoholic drinks might increase mortality from breast cancer (6843).

There is insufficient reliable information available to rate the effectiveness of beer for its other uses. However, there is some evidence that 1-2 alcoholic drinks per day can reduce the risk of Alzheimer's disease in both men and women compared to non-drinkers (6603). There is also some preliminary evidence that moderate alcohol consumption in postmenopausal women is associated with increased bone mineral density in the trochanter and spine (6825,6836). There does not appear to be an effect on sites such as the femoral neck which are predominantly cortical bone (6825,6836), and women who drink may be at increased risk for hip fractures due to falls (6836). The effect of alcohol on anxiety is complex and may be affected by the psychological state of the user. It sometimes reduces anxiety, sometimes increases it, and sometimes has no effect (2266). More evidence is needed to rate the effectiveness of beer for these uses.

Mechanism of Action

Beers vary in ethanol content between 2-6%, with regular American beers averaging 4-5% ethanol by volume (17). Ethanol is a central nervous system depressant (2263).

Several mechanisms have been proposed for the protective effects of alcohol against coronary heart disease, including increased high-density lipoprotein (HDL) cholesterol levels, lowered low-density lipoprotein (LDL) cholesterol, lowered fibrinogen, increased prostacyclin/thromboxane ratio, and inhibitory effects on platelets and blood clotting (2060,2261,2268,2270,6838,6839,6840,6841). One to two alcoholic drinks per day increases HDL cholesterol by about 12% (6892). The increase in HDL cholesterol levels might account for about 50% of the cardioprotective effect of moderate alcohol consumption (2261,6838,6841). A further 18% of the effect has been attributed to a decrease in LDL cholesterol, but this is counterbalanced by a 17% increase in risk due to increases in blood pressure (6841). The explanation for the remainder of the protective effect is unknown but may include effects on clotting and thrombosis (6841). Effects of alcohol on blood clotting include a reduction in clotting potential and enhancement of clot breakdown (2261). Alcohol consumption decreases platelet aggregation, possibly via inhibition of prostaglandin synthesis (6892). Moderate alcohol consumption is also associated with an increase in plasma levels of tissue-type plasminogen activator, an indicator of fibrinolytic capacity (6894). Moderate alcohol consumption produces a reduction in coronary narrowing due to atherosclerosis (2261,6840). Beer also contains folate and vitamin B6 (pyridoxine) (6832). Vitamin B6 is involved in homocysteine breakdown, and its presence may explain why the increase in plasma homocysteine levels seen with other alcoholic beverages is not seen with beer (6832). Increased homocysteine levels are a risk factor for cardiovascular disease. Dark beers also contain flavonoids (6892). These polyphenolic compounds, which are found in higher concentrations in red wine, have antioxidant properties and may contribute to protection against CHD by reducing oxidation of LDL cholesterol (2268). The loss of any protective effect of alcohol against cardiovascular disease at higher intakes may be due to an increase in hypertension, fatal arrhythmias and direct damage to heart muscle (alcoholic cardiomyopathy) (2060,2261,2267,2270). Possible mechanisms by which alcohol could have a protective effect against ischemic stroke include increasing HDL and prostacyclin, decreasing fibrinogen, and inhibiting platelet aggregation (6842). Moderate alcohol intake may be protective against the development of type 2 diabetes due to an increase in insulin sensitivity (6891). Moderate alcohol consumption may be protective against postmenopausal bone loss due to an increase in estrogen levels, increased calcitonin secretion and reduced parathyroid hormone secretion (6825,6836). However, heavy and chronic alcohol consumption reduces bone mineral density, possibly due to increased calcium and magnesium excretion, increased cortisol secretion, and reduced osteoblast activity (6836). Chronic alcoholics also often have other risk factors for osteoporosis, including poor nutrition, smoking, sedentary lifestyle, and lower body weight (6825,6836). Preliminary studies suggest that substances in beer may have inhibitory effects on heterocyclic amines, which are carcinogenic substances formed during cooking of some foods (6833).

Adverse Reactions

Orally, beer can cause a variety of side effects, depending on the amount ingested. They can include flushing, confusion, emotional lability, perceptual and sensational disturbances, possible blackout spells, incoordination, trouble walking, central nervous system depression, seizures, drowsiness, respiratory depression, hypothermia, hypoglycemia, lactic or ketoacidosis, hypokalemia, anemia, thrombocytopenia, nausea, vomiting, diarrhea, abdominal pain and bleeding, and arrhythmias (14). The effects of chronic heavy ethanol ingestion (3 or more alcoholic drinks per day) vary with individuals, but include physical dependence, malnutrition, amnesia, dementia, somnolence, cardiac myopathy, hepatotoxicity, cirrhosis, pancreatitis, hypomagnesemia, acute and chronic skeletal myopathies, Wernicke's encephalopathy, Korsakoff's psychosis, chronic cerebellar syndrome (14), and cancers of the mouth, esophagus, pharynx, larynx, and liver (14,6843). Chronic intake of three or more drinks per day is associated with an increased risk of all-cause mortality, ischemic stroke, and hypertension (2261,6892). Consumption of any amount of alcohol can increase the risk of hemorrhagic stroke (841,2271). Consuming more than one alcoholic drink daily might increase mortality from breast cancer by as much as 30% higher in women (6843). Beer made with barley can cause anaphylaxis in sensitive individuals (317). There have been occasional reports of asthma triggered by beer consumption (6174).

Interactions with Herbs & Other Dietary Supplements

HERBS/SUPPLEMENTS WITH SEDATIVE PROPERTIES: Theoretically, concomitant use with herbs that have sedative properties might enhance adverse effects. These include 5-HTP, calamus, calendula, California poppy, catnip, capsicum, celery, couch grass, elecampane, Siberian ginseng, German chamomile, goldenseal, gotu kola, hops, Jamaican dogwood, kava, lemon balm, melatonin, sage, St. John's wort, sassafras, scullcap, shepherd's purse, stinging nettle, valerian, wild carrot, wild lettuce, ashwaganda root, yerba mansa, and others (2,4,19).

Interactions with Drugs

ASPIRIN/NSAIDs: Concomitant use of aspirin or nonsteroidal anti-inflammatory drugs with alcohol can increase the risk of gastrointestinal bleeding (2262).
BENZODIAZEPINES, BARBITURATES, NARCOTICS: Concomitant consumption of large amounts of alcohol may decrease metabolism of narcotics, barbiturates, and benzodiazepines (15,2262).
CISAPRIDE: Concomitant use of cisapride (Propulsid) might increase blood alcohol levels and effects (2262).
CNS DEPRESSANTS: Concomitant use of antihistamines, barbiturates, benzodiazepines, and tricyclic antidepressants with alcohol may increase sedative and other adverse effects (2262).
DRUGS THAT CAUSE DISULFIRAM-LIKE REACTIONS: Disulfiram-like reactions can occur when alcohol is used concomitantly with chlorpropamide (Diabinese) (506), disulfiram (Antabuse), tolbutamide (Orinase), metronidazole (Flagyl), sulfonamides, griseofulvin (Fulvicin), cefoperazone (Cefobid), and cefamandole (Mandol) (2262).
ERYTHROMYCIN: Concomitant use with alcohol can increase blood alcohol levels and effects (2262).
H2-RECEPTOR ANTAGONISTS: Concomitant use of cimetidine (Tagamet) and ranitidine (Zantac) with alcohol may increase blood alcohol levels and adverse effects (2262).
HEPATOTOXIC DRUGS: Concomitant use with acetaminophen, isoniazid, and phenylbutazone can increase the risk of hepatotoxicity (2262).
HYPOGLYCEMIC DRUGS: Alcohol may cause hypoglycemia secondary to decreased gluconeogenesis (2263).

Concomitant use may increase the risk of hypoglycemia with long-acting sulfonylureas such as chlorpropamide (Diabinese) (2262).

METFORMIN: Concomitant consumption of large amounts of alcohol may increase the risk of lactic acidosis with metformin (Glucophage) (2262).

PHENYTOIN: Concomitant consumption of large amounts of alcohol may induce metabolism, reducing therapeutic effectiveness of phenytoin (Dilantin) (15,2262).

WARFARIN: Acute alcohol intoxication can decrease metabolism and increase effects of warfarin (Coumadin) (15,2262). In contrast, chronic intoxication can induce metabolism of warfarin, reducing therapeutic effectiveness (15,2262).

Interactions with Foods

FOOD: Chronic use of alcohol might interfere with absorption of B vitamins and other nutrients (2263).

Interactions with Lab Tests

FOLATE: Chronic alcohol ingestion may decrease folate levels and test results (2263).

LIVER FUNCTION TESTS: Chronic alcohol ingestion can increase alkaline phosphatase (Alk phos), alanine aminotransferase (ALT), aspartate aminotransferase (AST), gamma-glutamyltransferase (GGT), and bilirubin test results (2263).

MEAN CORPUSCULAR VOLUME (MCV): Chronic alcohol ingestion can increase MCV (2263).

TRIGLYCERIDES: Chronic alcohol ingestion can increase triglycerides (2263).

Interactions with Diseases or Conditions

ASTHMA: There have been occasional reports of asthma triggered by beer consumption (6174).

GOUT: Alcohol use can exacerbate gout (2263).

HEART CONDITIONS: Alcohol use can exacerbate variant angina, congestive heart failure (2261,2263,6889), and idiopathic cardiomyopathy (6889).

HIGH BLOOD PRESSURE: Consuming three or more alcoholic drinks a day can increase blood pressure and exacerbate hypertension (2261).

HYPERTRIGLYCERIDEMIA: Alcohol ingestion can exacerbate hypertriglyceridemia (2261,2263,6892).

INSOMNIA: Alcohol use can exacerbate insomnia (2263).

LIVER DISEASE: Alcohol use can exacerbate liver disease (2261).

NEUROLOGICAL CONDITIONS: Alcohol use can exacerbate degenerative neurological conditions (6889).

PANCREATITIS: Alcohol use can exacerbate pancreatitis (2261).

PEPTIC ULCER DISEASE (PUD)/GASTROESOPHAGEAL REFLUX DISEASE (GERD): Alcohol use can exacerbate PUD and GERD (2261,2263).

PORPHYRIA: Alcohol use can exacerbate porphyria (2261).

PSYCHIATRIC DISORDERS: Consuming three or more drinks of alcohol a day can also exacerbate psychiatric disorders and increase cognitive impairment (2261).

Dosage and Administration

ORAL: For reducing the risk of cardiovascular disease, ischemic stroke, and all-cause mortality, 1 or 2 drinks (12 oz) per day has been used (2261,2271,6835,6837,6840,6841,6842,6888,6892,6893). Up to one drink per day has been associated with less cognitive decline in older men (6824,6829). Between 2 drinks per week and 3 or 4 drinks per day has been associated with reduced risk of type 2 diabetes in healthy men (6172,6891). Alcohol intake is often measured in number of "drinks". One drink is equivalent to a 4 oz (120 mL) glass of wine, 12 oz of beer, or 1 oz of spirits (14).

Comments

None.

BEESWAX

Also Known As

Bees Wax, Bleached Beeswax, White Beeswax, White Wax, Yellow Beeswax, Yellow Wax.

Scientific Names

Apis cerana; Apis mellifera.
Family: Apidae.

People Use This For

Orally, beeswax is used for lowering lipids (4051), as an anti-inflammatory (4052), and anti-ulcer agent (4053).

In Chinese medicine, it has been used orally for diarrhea, hiccups, and pain relief (11).
In foods and beverages, white beeswax and beeswax absolute are utilized as stiffening agents (11).
In manufacturing, yellow and white beeswax are used as thickeners, emulsifiers, and as stiffening agents in cosmetics (11). Beeswax absolute is used as a fragrance ingredient in soaps and perfumes (11). White beeswax and beeswax absolute are also used as tablet polishing components in pharmaceutical products (11,16).

Safety

LIKELY SAFE ...when consumed in amounts found in foods (11). Beeswax has Generally Recognized as Safe (GRAS) status in the US (11), and is listed in the United States Pharmacopoeia (10) as an inert ingredient (16).
...when used orally as a medicinal agent (11). ...when used topically (11).
PREGNANCY AND LACTATION: LIKELY SAFE ...when consumed in food amounts.

Effectiveness

There is insufficient reliable information available about the effectiveness of beeswax.

Mechanism of Action

A natural mixture of high molecular weight alcohols isolated and purified from beeswax, termed D-002, had mild anti-inflammatory effects in experimental animals (4052). In rats, injected D-002 partially inhibited experimentally-induced gastric damage (4053,4054).

Adverse Reactions

Orally, beeswax may cause allergic reactions (11).

Interactions with Herbs & Other Dietary Supplements

Insufficient reliable information available.

Interactions with Drugs

NONSTEROIDAL ANTI-INFLAMMATORY DRUGS (NSAIDs): Theoretically, concomitant use may protect against NSAID-induced ulcers (4053,4054).

Interactions with Foods

No interactions are known to occur, and there is no known reason to expect a clinically significant interaction with beeswax.

Interactions with Lab Tests

No interactions are known to occur, and there is no known reason to expect a clinically significant interaction with beeswax.

Interactions with Diseases or Conditions

No interactions are known to occur, and there is no known reason to expect a clinically significant interaction with beeswax.

Dosage and Administration

No typical dosage.

Comments

The three major beeswax products are yellow beeswax, white beeswax, and beeswax absolute. Yellow beeswax is the crude product obtained from the honeycomb. White beeswax is derived from yellow beeswax by bleaching, and beeswax absolute is derived from yellow beeswax by extraction with alcohol. Beeswax is obtained from the honeycomb of the honeybee (Apis mellifera) and other Apis species.

BEET

Also Known As

Beets, Fodder Beet, Garden Beet, Mangel, Mangold, Red Beet, Sugarbeet, Yellow Beet.

Scientific Names

Beta vulgaris.
Family: Chenopodiaceae.

People Use This For

Orally, beets are used as a supportive therapy in the treatment of liver diseases and fatty liver (18).

Safety

LIKELY SAFE …when consumed as a food or in amounts typically found in foods.

There is insufficient reliable information available about the safety of the oral medicinal use of beets.

PREGNANCY AND LACTATION: LIKELY SAFE …when consumed as a food or in amounts typically found in foods. Avoid using amounts greater than those typically found in foods (18).

Effectiveness

There is insufficient reliable information available about the effectiveness of beets.

Mechanism of Action

The applicable part of beet is the root. Animal data suggests that beets may be effective against fat deposition in the liver. A component called betaine may play a role (18).

Adverse Reactions

Orally, ingestion of large quantities of beets could lead to hypocalcemia and kidney damage because of the oxaluric acid content (18).

Interactions with Herbs & Other Dietary Supplements

Insufficient reliable information available.

Interactions with Drugs

No interactions are known to occur, and there is no known reason to expect a clinically significant interaction with beet.

Interactions with Foods

No interactions are known to occur, and there is no known reason to expect a clinically significant interaction with beet.

Interactions with Lab Tests

No interactions are known to occur, and there is no known reason to expect a clinically significant interaction with beet.

Interactions with Diseases or Conditions

KIDNEY DISEASE: Ingestion of large quantities of beets could worsen kidney disease (18).

Dosage and Administration

ORAL: Beet is used as a standardized granular powder (18).

Comments

None.

BELLADONNA

Also Known As

Deadly Nightshade, Devil's Cherries, Devil's Herb, Divale, Dwale, Dwayberry, Great Morel, Naughty Man's Cherries, Poison Black Cherries.

CAUTION: See separate listings for Bittersweet Nightshade and Henbane.

Scientific Names

Atropa belladonna; Atropa belladonna acuminata.

Family: Solanaceae.

People Use This For

Orally, belladonna is used as a sedative, an antispasmodic in bronchial asthma and whooping cough, cold and hay fever remedy, for Parkinson's disease, intestinal and biliary colic, and motion sickness (11).

Topically, belladonna is used in liniments for rheumatism, sciatica, and neuralgia (11).

Rectally, belladonna is used in hemorrhoid suppositories (11).

In Chinese medicine, belladonna is used as anesthetics (11).

In folk medicine, belladonna is used in topical medicinal plasters for treating psychiatric disorders, hyperkinesis, hyperhidrosis, and bronchial asthma (18).

Historically, belladonna berry juice has been used by Italian women to dilate their pupils giving them a striking appearance.

Safety

POSSIBLY SAFE ...when the standardized extract is used orally and appropriately under the supervision of a medical professional trained in the use of belladonna (2). Belladonna is available as a prescription drug in the US and has a narrow therapeutic index.

LIKELY UNSAFE ...when the standardized extract is used orally without medical supervision (12). ...when the leaf, root, or other preparation is used orally (12).

There is insufficient reliable information available about the safety of belladonna for its other uses.

CHILDREN: POSSIBLY SAFE ...when used orally in children older than 6 years old only under medical supervision. LIKELY UNSAFE ...when the leaf, root, or extract is used orally in children under 6 years old (12). There is insufficient reliable information available about the safety of the topical or rectal use of belladonna in children.

PREGNANCY: LIKELY UNSAFE ...when the leaf or root are used orally without medical supervision. There is insufficient reliable information about the safety of belladonna for its other uses during pregnancy.

LACTATION: LIKELY UNSAFE ...when the leaf, root, standardized extract, or other preparation are used orally. Use should be avoided because it can reduce milk production and is secreted into breast milk (15). There is insufficient reliable information available about the safety of belladonna for its other uses during lactation.

Effectiveness

LIKELY EFFECTIVE ...when used orally for spasms and colic-like pain in the GI tract and the bile ducts (2). There is insufficient reliable information available about the effectiveness of belladonna for its other uses.

Mechanism of Action

The applicable parts of belladonna are the leaf and root. Its anticholinergic activity is due to the 0.3%-0.5% tropane alkaloid constituents composed mainly of l-hyoscyamine and traces of l-scopolamine and atropine (dl-hyoscyamine) (11). On extraction, most of the l-hyoscyamine is racemized to atropine (11).

Adverse Reactions

Orally, belladonna can cause dry mouth, decreased perspiration, dilation of pupils, blurred vision, red dry skin, hyperthermia, tachycardia, difficulty urinating, hallucinations, spasms, acute psychosis, convulsions, and coma (2,11,553).

Interactions with Herbs & Other Dietary Supplements

Insufficient reliable information available.

Interactions with Drugs

ANTICHOLINERGIC DRUGS: Belladonna can increase the anticholinergic effects and adverse effects of amantadine, antihistamines, phenothiazines, procainamide, quinidine, tricyclic antidepressants, and others (2).

Interactions with Foods

No interactions are known to occur, and there is no known reason to expect a clinically significant interaction with belladonna.

Interactions with Lab Tests

No interactions are known to occur, and there is no known reason to expect a clinically significant interaction with belladonna.

Interactions with Diseases or Conditions

CONGESTIVE HEART FAILURE (CHF): Belladonna might cause tachycardia and exacerbate CHF due to its hyoscyamine (atropine) and scopolamine content (15).

CONSTIPATION: Belladonna might cause constipation due to its hyoscyamine (atropine) and scopolamine content (15).

DOWN SYNDROME: Caution, patients with Down syndrome might be hypersensitive to the antimuscarinic effects (mydriasis, positive chronotropic heart effects, etc.) of hyoscyamine (atropine) and scopolamine contained in belladonna (15).

ESOPHAGEAL REFLUX: Belladonna might delay gastric emptying and decrease lower esophageal pressure, promoting gastric retention and exacerbating reflux due to its hyoscyamine (atropine) and scopolamine content (15).

FEVER: Belladonna might increase the risk of hyperthermia in patients with fever due to its hyoscyamine (atropine) and scopolamine content (15).

GASTRIC ULCER: Belladonna might delay gastric emptying and exacerbate gastric ulcers due to its hyoscyamine (atropine) and scopolamine content (15).

GI INFECTIONS: Belladonna might suppress GI motility causing retention of infecting organisms or toxins due to its hyoscyamine (atropine) and scopolamine content (15).

HIATAL HERNIA: Belladonna might delay gastric emptying and decrease lower esophageal pressure, promoting gastric retention and exacerbating reflux due to its hyoscyamine (atropine) and scopolamine content (15).

TOXIC MEGACOLON: Belladonna might suppress intestinal motility, which might produce paralytic ileus and exacerbate toxic megacolon, due to its hyoscyamine (atropine) and scopolamine content (2,15).

NARROW-ANGLE GLAUCOMA: Belladonna might increase ocular tension in patients with narrow-angle (angle-closure) glaucoma due to its hyoscyamine (atropine) and scopolamine content (2,15).

OBSTRUCTIVE GI TRACT DISEASE: Belladonna might exacerbate obstructive GI tract diseases (including atony, paralytic ileus, and stenosis) due to its hyoscyamine (atropine) and scopolamine content (15).

TACHYARRHYTHMIAS: Belladonna might cause tachycardia due to its hyoscyamine (atropine) and scopolamine content (2,15).

URINARY RETENTION: Belladonna might increase urinary retention due to its hyoscyamine (atropine) and scopolamine content (2,15).

ULCERATIVE COLITIS: Belladonna might suppress intestinal motility, which might produce paralytic ileus and precipitate toxic megacolon, due to its hyoscyamine (atropine) and scopolamine content (15).

Dosage and Administration

ORAL: The belladonna leaf powder is typically an average single dose of 50-100 mg. The maximum single dose is 200 mg, which is equivalent to 0.6 mg total alkaloids, calculated as hyoscyamine. The maximum daily dose is 600 mg, which is equivalent to 1.8 mg total alkaloids, calculated as hyoscyamine. The root powder is commonly used in an average single dose of 50 mg. The maximum single dose is 100 mg, which is equivalent to 0.5 mg total alkaloids, calculated as hyoscyamine. The maximum daily dose of the root powder is 300 mg, equivalent to 1.5 mg total alkaloids calculated as hyoscyamine. The belladonna extract has an average single dose of 10 mg. The maximum single dose is 50 mg, equivalent to 0.73 mg total alkaloids calculated as hyoscyamine, and the maximum daily dosage is 150 mg, equivalent to 2.2 mg total alkaloids calculated as hyoscyamine (2).

TOPICAL: No typical dosage.

RECTAL: No typical dosage.

Comments

The name, belladonna, means beautiful lady. The belladonna berry juice has been used historically in Italy to dilate the pupils of women giving them a striking appearance (11). Avoid confusion with bittersweet nightshade (Solanum dulcamara) and henbane (nightshade).

BENZOIN

Also Known As

Benzoe, Gum Benjamin, Gum Benzoin, Sumatra Benzoin.

Scientific Names

Styrax benzoin; Styrax paralleloneurus.
Family: Styraceae.

People Use This For

Orally, benzoin is used for throat and bronchial inflammation.

Topically, benzoin is used as an antiseptic, astringent, skin protectant, and styptic on small cuts. Benzoin is also used topically for skin ulcers, bedsores, cracked nipples, and fissures of the lips and anus (11,13).

By inhalation, benzoin is used to treat laryngitis, croup, and other respiratory conditions.

In combination with other herbs, benzoin tincture (benzoin, aloe, storax, and tolu balsam) is used as a skin protectant.

In dentistry, benzoin is used for gum inflammation and oral herpes lesions.

In manufacturing, benzoin is used in making pharmaceutical preparations (11).

Safety

LIKELY SAFE ...when used as a food flavoring. It is approved for food use; the maximum level is 0.014% in candy and baked goods (11).

POSSIBLY SAFE ...when preparations of the gum resin are used orally for medicinal purposes (12). ...when used topically (11). Tincture of benzoin can cause contact dermatitis.
There is insufficient reliable information available about the safety of benzoin for its other uses.
PREGNANCY AND LACTATION: Insufficient reliable information available; avoid using.

Effectiveness
There is insufficient reliable information available about the effectiveness of benzoin.

Mechanism of Action
The applicable part of benzoin is the gum resin. Benzoin has antiseptic, stimulant, expectorant, astringent, diuretic, and skin protectant effects (11,13).

Adverse Reactions
Topically, the compound benzoin tincture (benzoin, aloe, storax, and tolu balsam) can cause contact dermatitis (11) and should be avoided in sensitive individuals.

Interactions with Herbs & Other Dietary Supplements
Insufficient reliable information available.

Interactions with Drugs
No interactions are known to occur, and there is no known reason to expect a clinically significant interaction with benzoin.

Interactions with Foods
No interactions are known to occur, and there is no known reason to expect a clinically significant interaction with benzoin.

Interactions with Lab Tests
No interactions are known to occur, and there is no known reason to expect a clinically significant interaction with benzoin.

Interactions with Diseases or Conditions
SENSITIVE INDIVIDUALS: Avoid contact with benzoin and the compound benzoin tincture due to contact dermatitis (11).

Dosage and Administration
ORAL: No typical dosage.
TOPICAL: People apply no more than a few drops of compound benzoin tincture (USP) every two hours (5008). Compound benzoin tincture contains 100 grams of benzoin powder, 20 grams of aloe powder, 80 grams of storax, and 40 grams of tolu balsam per 1000 mL of tincture (16).
INHALATION: People typically add 5 mL of a compound benzoin tincture (USP) to 473 mL of hot water or place the tincture directly on a handkerchief (5008).

Comments
Benzoin is the gum resin of Styrax species trees. Avoid confusion with Siam benzoin (Styrax tonikensis), which is used only in manufacturing and has no medicinal uses (11,13).

BERGAMOT OIL

Also Known As
Bergamot, Bergamot Orange, Bergamota, Bergamotier, Bergamoto, Bergamotte, Bergamotto Bigarade Orange, Oleum Bergamotte.
CAUTION: See separate listings for Bitter Orange flower, Bitter Orange peel, Oswego Tea, and Sweet Orange.

Scientific Names
Citrus bergamia, synonym Citrus aurantium bergamia.
Family: Rutaceae.

People Use This For

Topically, bergamot oil is used to treat psoriasis in conjunction with long-wave ultraviolet light (11). Bergamot oil is also used topically for vitiligo and mycosis fungoides (11).

Historically, it has been used as an insecticide to protect the body against lice and other vermin (215).

For food uses, bergamot oil is widely used as a citrus flavoring agent, up to 0.02% in gelatins and puddings (11).

In manufacturing of cosmetics, bergamot oil is used (up to 3% in perfumes and 0.25% in creams and lotions), in soaps (11), and suntan oils (9).

Safety

LIKELY SAFE ...when bergamot oil is used orally in food amounts (12).

POSSIBLY UNSAFE ...when used topically, because it can act as a photosensitizer and can induce malignant changes (6).

CHILDREN: POSSIBLY UNSAFE ...when large amounts are ingested. Bergamot oil can cause intestinal colic, convulsions, and death (12).

PREGNANCY AND LACTATION: POSSIBLY UNSAFE ...when used topically. There is insufficient reliable information available about the safety of bergamot oil in amounts greater than those found in foods.

Effectiveness

POSSIBLY EFFECTIVE ...when used with long-wave UV light for treating mycosis fungoides (11).

There is insufficient reliable information available about the effectiveness of bergamot oil for its other uses.

Mechanism of Action

The applicable part of bergamot oil is the peel. Bergamot oil is cold-expressed from the peel (11). Further distillation produces rectified (terpeneless) bergamot oil (11). The photosensitivity of bergamot oil is linked to the furocoumarin constituents, bergapten (5-methoxypsoralen) and xanthotoxin (8-methoxypsoralen) (6).

Adverse Reactions

Occupational Sensitization: Frequent contact with the peel or oil can cause erythema, blisters, pustules, dermatoses leading to scab formation, and pigment spots (18).

Topically, bergamot oil can cause photosensitivity, skin rash, and hyperpigmentation of the face and other areas. Photosensitivity reaches its peak two hours after topical application (6). Some skin changes can be malignant in nature (6).

Interactions with Herbs & Other Dietary Supplements

Insufficient reliable information available.

Interactions with Drugs

PHOTOSENSITIZING DRUGS: Theoretically, topical use of bergamot oil can compound the photosensitizing effects and increase the risk of side effects. Concomitant use should be avoided.

Interactions with Foods

No interactions are known to occur, and there is no known reason to expect a clinically significant interaction with bergamot oil.

Interactions with Lab Tests

No interactions are known to occur, and there is no known reason to expect a clinically significant interaction with bergamot oil.

Interactions with Diseases or Conditions

SUN SENSITIVE INDIVIDUALS: Avoid the topical use of bergamot oil due to its photosensitivity adverse effects.

Dosage and Administration

No typical dosage.

Comments

Avoid confusion with scarlet bergamot (oswego tea, mondara didyma) (6).

BETA-CAROTENE

Also Known As
A-Beta-Carotene, Beta Carotene, Betacarotene, Provitamin A.
CAUTION: See separate listing for Vitamin A.

Scientific Names
Beta-carotene.

People Use This For
Orally, beta-carotene is taken as a dietary source of vitamin A, for treating vitiligo, and reducing photosensitivities, including erythropoietic protoporphyria (EPP) and polymorphous light eruption. Beta-carotene is also used orally for decreasing exercise-induced asthma, and reducing the risk of some cancers, cardiovascular disease, cataracts, and age related macular degeneration.

Safety
LIKELY SAFE ...when used orally and appropriately (139,6393). Beta-carotene is safe for most people when used in doses up to 300 mg per day (14,15). However, higher doses are more likely to cause side effects such as yellowing of the skin (9).
POSSIBLY UNSAFE ...when used orally in people who smoke. Beta-carotene 20 mg daily for 5-8 years seems to increase the risk of lung and prostate cancer, intracerebral hemorrhage, and cardiovascular and total mortality in people who smoke cigarettes (1371,3359,3937,4257,5028,6393). Beta-carotene from foods does not seem to have this effect.
CHILDREN: LIKELY SAFE ...when used orally in amounts found in foods (6268). There is insufficient reliable information available about the safety of beta-carotene in children when larger amounts are used.
PREGNANCY: POSSIBLY SAFE ...when used orally in doses up to 30 mg daily (10). LIKELY UNSAFE ...when used orally in excessive amounts. Very high doses of beta-carotene can be toxic to the fetus (15).
LACTATION: LIKELY SAFE ...when used orally in amounts found in foods (9). There is insufficient reliable information available about the safety of beta-carotene in breast-feeding women when larger amounts are used.

Effectiveness
LIKELY EFFECTIVE ...when used orally for erythropoietic protoporphyria. Beta-carotene can reduce photosensitivity in patients with erythropoietic protoporphyria (15).
POSSIBLY EFFECTIVE ...when dietary beta-carotene is used to prevent breast cancer in premenopausal women. There is some evidence that a diet rich in beta-carotene may reduce the risk of breast cancer in premenopausal women at high risk due to family history or high alcohol intake (1444). ...when used orally from dietary sources for preventing age-related macular degeneration (ARMD). People consuming a diet high in beta-carotene seem to have a lower risk of developing ARMD (1470). ...when used orally in combination with antioxidant vitamins and zinc to slow progression age-related macular degeneration (ARMD). Taking beta-carotene 15 mg plus vitamin C 500 mg, vitamin E 400 IU, and elemental zinc 80 mg daily seems to provide a risk reduction of 27% for visual acuity loss and a risk reduction of 28% for progression to more advanced ARMD in patients with intermediate and advanced ARMD (7303). There isn't enough evidence to know if this combination is beneficial for people with less advanced disease or for preventing ARMD. Supplemental beta-carotene with antioxidants, but without zinc, doesn't seem to have any significant effect on ARMD (7303,7304). ...when dietary beta-carotene is used to prevent bronchitis and dyspnea in male smokers (2580). The prevalence of bronchitis and dyspnea in male smokers seems to be lower in those patients that consume a diet containing high amounts of beta-carotene (2580). ...when used orally to reduce the risk of prostate cancer in men who have plasma beta-carotene concentrations less than 153.25 ng/mL (1473). However, it doesn't seem to help prevent prostate cancer in men with plasma beta-carotene concentrations greater than 153.25 ng/mL (148,1470,1473,2406). ...when used orally to induce remission in patients with oral leukoplakia. There's also an increased risk of disease progression over 12 months if beta-carotene is stopped (1470,1472). ...when a mixture of beta-carotene isomers is taken orally to prevent exercise-induced asthma (1474). ...when used orally to prevent sunburn in individuals that are sensitivity to sun exposure. There is some evidence that 25 mg of mixed beta-carotene daily for 12 weeks reduces skin redness after exposure to UV light in sun-sensitive individuals (6134). However, beta-carotene doesn't seem to be helpful for people without sun sensitivity (15), and it doesn't seem to reduce the incidence of skin cancers associated with sun exposure (1297,2599). ...when used orally by malnourished women to reduce pregnancy-related maternal mortality. All-trans beta-carotene (synthetic beta-carotene) taken weekly before, during and after pregnancy by malnourished women seems to reduce pregnancy-related mortality by 49% (6153). ...when used orally by malnourished women to reduce the occurrence of pregnancy-related night blindness, and post-partum diarrhea and fever . All-trans beta-carotene (synthetic beta-carotene) taken weekly before, during and after pregnancy by malnourished women reduces, but does not eliminate, the occurrence of pregnancy-related night blindness, diarrhea and fever (2581,6154). ...when used orally to slow progression of osteoarthritis. Beta-carotene doesn't seem to prevent osteoarthritis, but might slow progression of the disease (5881). ...when used orally for preventing gastric cancer in high risk patients with premalignant gastric

lesions. Beta-carotene 30 mg daily seems to increase the rate of regression of premalignant gastric lesions in these high risk patients (2579). ...when used orally with other antioxidants for preventing gastric cancer in malnourished, high risk patients. There is some evidence that beta-carotene 15 mg daily plus vitamin E and selenium can decrease gastric cancer incidence by 21% in high-risk, malnourished Chinese population (2658).

POSSIBLY INEFFECTIVE ...when used orally to prevent stroke in male smokers. All-trans beta-carotene (synthetic beta-carotene) 20 mg/day for a median of 6 years has no effect on the overall incidence of stroke in male smokers (1371). There is some evidence that beta-carotene actually increases the risk of intracerebral hemorrhage by 62% in patients who also drink alcohol (1371,3359). ...when used orally to reduce symptoms of chronic obstructive pulmonary disease (COPD) in smokers. Beta-carotene 20 mg daily for 5 to 8 years doesn't reduce chronic cough, phlegm or dyspnea in male smokers with COPD (2580). ...when used orally by malnourished women to reduce fetal and early infant mortality. All-trans beta-carotene (synthetic beta-carotene) taken weekly before, during and after pregnancy by malnourished women do not reduce fetal and early infant mortality (6152). ...when used orally in combination with antioxidant vitamins ad zinc for cataracts. Taking elemental beta-carotene 15 mg plus vitamin C 500 mg, vitamin E 400 IU, and zinc 80 mg daily does not seem to have any effect on the development or progression of age-related lens opacities (cataracts) or the need for cataract surgery in well-nourished people (7304).

LIKELY INEFFECTIVE ...when used orally to reduce the risk of heart disease and cardiovascular mortality. In male and female patients with no history of cardiovascular disease, beta-carotene 50 mg daily or every other day has no effect on death rates from cardiovascular causes (1448,2646,2657). In people who smoke, beta-carotene 20 to 30 mg daily actually increases cardiovascular mortality by 12 to 26% (2642,3949). In men who smoke and have had a prior myocardial infarction, the risk of fatal coronary heart disease increases by as much as 43% with beta-carotene 20 mg daily (3937). These adverse effects do not seem to occur in people who eat foods high in beta-carotene content (1440,2657). ...when used orally to reduce cancer incidence and mortality in adults. Beta-carotene 20 to 50 mg daily, or 50 mg on alternate days, does not affect the incidence of a variety of cancers, including colon, rectal, uterine, ovarian, cervical, thyroid, bladder, brain, pancreatic, and blood (140,1448,2642,2646,2657,3949). ...when used orally to prevent lung cancer in smokers. Beta-carotene 20 to 30 mg daily actually seems to increase the risk of lung cancer by 18% to 28%, in people who smoke (especially those smoking more than 20 cigarettes per day), former smokers, people exposed to asbestos, and those who ingest significant amounts of alcohol (1 or more drinks per day) in addition to smoking (139,1471,2582,2642,3949). However, beta-carotene from food does not seem to have this adverse effect. ...when used orally to prevent non-melanoma skin cancer (NMSC) (1297,2599). Beta-carotene 30 mg daily or 50mg on alternate days, taken for several years, doesn't affect the incidence of NMSC, including basal cell carcinoma (BCC) and squamous cell carcinoma (SCC) (1297,2599).

Mechanism of Action

Beta-carotene belongs to a class of red, orange, and yellow pigments called carotenoids. There are hundreds of varieties of carotenoids, which are present in many fruits and vegetables. Carotenoid absorption is improved by dietary fat, and carotenoids are carried in the blood mainly in low-density lipoproteins (2628). Typical dietary intake of beta-carotene in American adults varies from 0.5 to 6.5 mg per day (2628). Absorption of beta-carotene from foods is only about 5% to 30% of that from synthetic supplements due to complex formation with proteins and fiber, although heating food may break down these complexes (2628). Beta-carotene is closely related to alpha-carotene and both are precursors for vitamin A. Some ingested beta-carotene is converted to vitamin A in the intestinal mucosa. The amount converted depends on the vitamin A status of the individual (2628). Although beta-carotene is partly metabolized to vitamin A, high intake of beta-carotene does not result in vitamin A toxicity because the proportion converted to vitamin A decreases as beta-carotene intake increases (9). Beta-carotene also has activity independent of its conversion to vitamin A (139,1470). Beta-carotene consists of a number of isomers. Synthetic beta-carotene, the form used in most clinical studies, is composed of the all-trans form. Natural beta-carotene sources contain 9-cis-, 13-cis-, and 15-cis-beta-carotene (1474). The 9-cis-beta-carotene isomer is poorly absorbed, and most is converted to all-trans-beta-carotene in the intestine (2628). The cis isomers account for less than 5% of the beta-carotene in plasma, but 10% to 25% of that stored in the tissues (2628). Little is known about the pharmacology of beta-carotene and the differences that might exist between the various isomers, and the natural and synthetic forms (2628). Beta-carotene does seem to have antioxidant activities and prevents lipid peroxidation (139). It has been proposed that the antioxidant effects may help prevent cancer by reducing free radical-induced DNA damage (2592,2599). There seems to be an inverse relationship between dietary carotenoid intake, or serum beta-carotene levels, and the incidence of various cancers, and in-vitro studies show that beta-carotene inhibits tumor cell growth (2592,2628). However, anticancer effects of beta-carotene supplementation have not been effectively demonstrated in humans. There is now also some concern that beta-carotene metabolites with pharmacological activity can accumulate and have carcinogenic effects (6377,6393). Components of cigarette smoke can degrade beta-carotene, and lower concentrations of beta-carotene have been reported in both active and passive smokers (2592,2593). Smoking might enhance production of carcinogenic beta-carotene oxidation metabolites which, if not neutralized by other antioxidants (such as tocopherol and ascorbate, which are often depleted in smokers), could lead to increased risk of lung cancer (2628,6377). In addition, beta-carotene metabolites might increase the binding of carcinogenic metabolites to DNA and inhibit gap-junction communication between normal cells and tumor cells. Beta-carotene itself might also increase the levels of certain cytochrome P450 dependent enzymes that can hydroxylate and activate certain compounds into highly carcinogenic forms (6393), as well as increase catabolism of retinoic acid, which controls lung epithelial cell proliferation and differentiation (2592).

Adverse Reactions

Orally, beta-carotene is typically well tolerated and safe when used in appropriate amounts. High doses can cause yellow or orange skin pigmentation called carotenoderma (9,15). This is generally considered harmless in the short-term, but has occasionally been associated with neutropenia and amenorrhea when it occurs long-term (9). Although beta-carotene is partly metabolized to vitamin A, high intake of beta-carotene does not result in vitamin A toxicity because the proportion converted to vitamin A decreases as beta-carotene intake increases (9). Advise smokers not to use beta-carotene supplements. Beta-carotene in doses of 20 mg per day for 5-8 years has been associated with an increased risk of lung and prostate cancer and increased total mortality in people who smoke cigarettes (4257,6393). In people who smoke, beta-carotene 20 to 30 mg daily also seems to increase cardiovascular mortality by 12 to 26% (2642,3949). In men who smoke and have had a prior myocardial infarction, the risk of fatal coronary heart disease increases by as much as 43% with beta-carotene 20 mg daily (3937). These adverse effects do not seem to occur in people who eat foods high in beta-carotene content (1440,2657).

Interactions with Herbs & Other Dietary Supplements

Insufficient reliable information available.

Interactions with Drugs

No interactions are known to occur, and there is no known reason to expect a clinically significant interaction with beta-carotene (see Drug Influences on Nutrient Levels and Depletion).

Drug Influences on Nutrient Levels and Depletion

SOME DRUGS CAN AFFECT BETA-CAROTENE LEVELS:

CHOLESTYRAMINE (Questran): Cholestyramine can reduce dietary beta-carotene absorption and serum levels (4457).

COLESTIPOL (Colestid): Colestipol can reduce dietary beta-carotene absorption and serum levels (4461).

MINERAL OIL: Concomitant administration can reduce supplemental beta-carotene absorption (4495,4496). Separate administration of mineral oil and beta-carotene by 2 hours to avoid this interaction.

ORLISTAT (Xenical): Concomitant administration can decrease supplemental beta-carotene absorption (6001). Separate administration of orlistat and beta-carotene by 2 hours to avoid this interaction.

PROTON PUMP INHIBITORS: Lansoprazole (Prevacid), Omeprazole (Prilosec, Losec), Rabeprazole (Aciphex), Pantoprazole (Protonix, Pantoloc). Loss of stomach acid interferes with the absorption of beta-carotene. Consider supplementation only if clinical judgment warrants it (31).

Interactions with Foods

OLESTRA: Concomitant use can decrease the absorption of beta-carotene.

Interactions with Lab Tests

No interactions are known to occur, and there is no known reason to expect a clinically significant interaction with beta-carotene.

Interactions with Diseases or Conditions

ANGIOPLASTY: There is some concern that when antioxidant vitamins, including beta-carotene, are used together they might have harmful effects in patients after angioplasty. A combination of beta-carotene 30,000 IU, vitamin C 500 mg, and vitamin E 700 IU daily started 30 days before angioplasty, and continued for 6 months thereafter, seems to prevent beneficial vascular remodeling in patients after angioplasty by promoting fibrosis at the site of angioplastic intervention (1317). Tell patients to avoid taking supplements of these vitamins immediately before and following angioplasty without the supervision of a health care professional.

SMOKERS: Supplemental beta-carotene in doses greater than 20 mg per day is associated with a significantly higher risk of lung and prostate cancer in smokers (139,3949,4257,6382,6393). Tell smokers to avoid taking beta-carotene supplements.

Dosage and Administration

ORAL: For erythropoietic protoporphyria, 30-300 mg daily for adults and 30-150 mg daily for children is typically used. The dose is adjusted to individual requirements and response and can be adjusted to maintain blood carotene levels at 4-6 mcg/mL (15). For decreasing the risk of prostate cancer in men with plasma beta-carotene concentrations less than 153.25 ng/mL, 50 mg every other day has been used (1473). For oral leukoplakia, 30 mg orally twice daily for a total of 6 months has been used (1472). For preventing sunburn in sun-sensitive people, beta-carotene 25 mg orally daily has been used (6134). For preventing gastric cancer in people at high risk, 15 to 30 mg daily has been used (2579,2658).

For treating age-related macular degeneration (ARMD), vitamin C 500 mg plus zinc oxide 80 mg, vitamin E 400 IU, and beta-carotene 15 mg has been given daily (7303).

The Institute of Medicine recently reviewed beta-carotene, but did not make recommendations for daily intake, citing lack of sufficient evidence (6268). Supplemental beta-carotene is similarly absorbed when taken with high-fat (36 grams) or low-fat (3 grams fat) meals (6133).

Comments

The American Heart Association recommends obtaining antioxidants, including beta-carotene, from a diet high in fruits, vegetables and whole grains rather than through supplements until more information is known from randomized clinical trials (1440). Similar statements have been released by the American Cancer Society, the World Cancer Research Institute in association with the American Institute for Cancer Research, and the World Health Organization's International Agency for Research on Cancer (1470).

BETA GLUCANS

Also Known As

Beta Glucan, Beta-Glucan, Beta-Glucans, Beta Glycans, Beta-Glycans, Gifolan (GRN), Lentinan, PGG Glucan, PGG-Glucan, Poly-[1-6]-Beta-D-Glucopyranosyl-[1-3]-Beta-D-Glucopyranose, Schizophyllan (SPG), SSG, Yeast-Derived Beta Glucan.

CAUTION: See separate listings for Barley, Brewer's Yeast, Brewer's Yeast (Hansen CBS 5926), Maitake Mushroom, Oat above ground parts, Oat Bran, Oats, Salep, and Shiitake Mushroom.

Scientific Names

1-3,1-6-beta-glucan; beta-1,3-D-glucan; beta-1-6,1,3-beta-glucan.

People Use This For

Orally, beta glucans are used for hypercholesterolemia, diabetes, cancer, and HIV/AIDS. Beta glucans are also used orally as an immunostimulant in people with conditions that may compromise their immune system such as chronic fatigue syndrome, physical and emotional stress, and patients receiving chemotherapy or radiation treatment. It is also used orally for colds (common cold), flu (influenza), allergies, hepatitis, Lyme disease, asthma, ear infections, aging, ulcerative colitis and Crohn's disease, fibromyalgia, rheumatoid arthritis, and multiple sclerosis.

Topically, beta glucans are used for dermatitis, eczema, wrinkles, bedsores, wounds, burns, diabetic ulcers, and radiation burns.

Intravenously and intramuscularly, beta glucans are used for treating cancer and as an immunostimulant in patients with HIV/AIDS and AIDS-related disorders. It is also used intravenously for preventing sepsis in trauma patients after undergoing exploratory laparotomy or thoracotomy and for preventing infection in surgical patients.

Subcutaneously, beta glucans are used for treating and reducing the size of subcutaneous tumors resulting from malignant metastatic disease.

In manufacturing, beta glucans are used as a food additive in products such as salad dressings, frozen desserts, sour cream, and cheese spreads.

Safety

LIKELY SAFE ...when used orally in amounts found in foods. Beta glucans derived from baker's yeast or brewer's yeast (Saccharomyces cerevisiae) have Generally Recognized as Safe (GRAS) status in the US (7273).

POSSIBLY SAFE ...when used orally and appropriately, short-term in medicinal amounts. There is some evidence that yeast-derived beta-glucans 15 grams per day can be used safely for up to 8 weeks (7272). ...when used intravenously or intramuscularly and appropriately. Both yeast and fungal beta-glucans seem to be safe when soluble forms are used (7261,7263,7264,7266,7267,7269,7270,7271). Particulate beta glucans may not be safe. There is preliminary evidence that intravenous beta glucans in the microparticulate form might cause serious side effects such as hepatosplenomegaly, granuloma formation, and microembolization (7241). Most studies evaluating parenteral use of beta glucans have used specific forms including PGG-glucan (Betafectin) from a proprietary strain of Saccharomyces cerevisiae (7269,7270,7271) and specific fungal-derived beta glucans lentinan and schizophyllan (SPG) (7261,7263,7264,7266, 7267). Lentinan and SPG have been safely used in studies lasting for up to 12 months (7263,7264,7267). PGG-glucan has been safely used in studies when given 24 hours prior to surgery and lasting up to 96 hours after surgery (7269,7270,7271).

There is insufficient reliable information available about the safety of beta glucans when used subcutaneously or topically.

PREGNANCY AND LACTATION: Insufficient reliable information available; avoid using.

Effectiveness

POSSIBLY EFFECTIVE ...when used orally for hypercholesterolemia. Yeast-derived beta glucan 7.5 grams twice daily appears to reduce serum total cholesterol concentrations by 6-8 % in patients with hypercholesterolemia after 7-8 weeks of treatment (7272). ...when used intravenously for immunostimulation in patients with HIV infection (7267). There is preliminary evidence that the specific beta glucan lentinan 2-10 mg once or twice weekly can increase levels of CD4 cells by 5.5-18 % and decrease p24 antigen levels (a marker of viral replication) by 11.5 % after 12-20 weeks of treatment in asymptomatic patients with HIV (7267). ...when used intravenously or intramuscularly to prolong survival in patients with cancer. Studies show that the specific fungal beta glucans lentinan and schizophyllan (SPG) can prolong survival time of cancer patients when given in addition to conventional cancer treatment regimens. Lentinan 1-2 mg once or twice weekly for at least 1 year increases survival time by 6-9 months in people with advanced (stage III or IV) unresectable cancers (7266). SPG 20-40 mg once or twice weekly for at least 1 year significantly improves 4-5 year survival rates in people with cervical and head and neck cancer (7261,7263,7264). ...when used intravenously to prevent sepsis in trauma patients following exploratory laparotomy or thoracotomy. There is some evidence that intravenous soluble yeast-derived beta glucans 50 mg/M2 daily for 7 days decreases the rate of septic morbidity by 39.5% in trauma patients following exploratory surgical procedures (7268). ...when used intravenously to prevent postoperative infection in surgical patients at high risk for infection. A proprietary beta glucan preparation from Saccharomyces cerevisiae called PGG-glucan given intravenously 12-24 hours before and 4-96 hours after surgery at 0.5-1 mg/kg per dose reduces the occurrence of postoperative infection by 10-16%, decreases the number of days of intravenous antibiotic use by 10 days, and shortens the length of stay in the intensive care unit (ICU) by 3 days (7269,7271).

There is insufficient reliable information available about the effectiveness of beta glucans for their other uses.

Mechanism of Action

Beta glucans are polysaccharides that consist of (1-3)-beta-D-linked polymers of glucose that are either non-branched or with 1-6-beta-branches (3394,7242). Beta glucans are primary components in cell walls of bacteria, fungi, yeasts, algae, lichens, plants such as oats and barley, or are excreted extracellularly by various fungi (3394,7242,7250). The beta glucans most extensively studied to date are yeast-derived beta glucans from Saccharomyces cerevisiae, the fungal-derived beta glucans such as lentinan from Lentinus edodes, gifolan (GRN) from Grifola frondosa, schizophyllan (SPG) from Schizophyllum commune, SSG from Sclerotinia sclerotiorum, and beta glucans from oats (7241,7248,7273). Mammals cannot digest and absorb beta glucans because they lack the enzyme beta-1-3-glucanase needed to break down large beta glucan molecules. Since beta glucans cannot be absorbed orally, clinical studies have usually administered beta glucans by the parenteral route (3393). Beta glucans seem to have antibacterial, antiviral, antifungal, antiparasitic, and antitumor activity, and have the ability to promote recovery from sepsis and immunosuppression associated with various disease states or conditions such as HIV infection or whole body radiation (7238,7243,7250). Laboratory findings suggest beta glucans specifically bind to monocyte and macrophage cell lines, increase the proliferation and activation of macrophages, and increase the production of cytokine interleukin-1 (IL-1) by macrophages which in turn promotes the release of IL-2 by T-cells (7243,7268,7248,7249,7250,7252). Beta glucans also seem to have anticancer effects. Beta glucans don't seem to have direct antitumor or antibacterial activity, but are thought to act as biological response modifiers (BRMs) that restore or enhance humoral and cell-mediated immune responses (3394,7237,7251). Beta glucans increase macrophage phagocytosis of tumor cells, increase the cytotoxicity of natural killer cells (NK), and stimulate the release of interleukin-1 (IL-1) and tumor necrosis factor (TNF) (7237,7238,7240,7265). Beta glucans bind to a beta glucan receptor on macrophages, neutrophils, and NK cells and activate a complement receptor on the cells which bind to tumor or bacterial cells that are opsonized with complement and antibodies (7237,7239,7248,7269,7270,7271). Many cells, including cancer cells and bacteria, can acquire mechanisms to resist the action of complement, but there is some evidence that beta glucans can override this mechanism and allow the phagocytosis to occur (7237). For wound healing after surgery, there is some evidence beta glucans can decrease inflammation and accelerate the repair of surgical wounds by stimulating macrophages and increasing macrophage infiltration, causing increased tissue granulation and enhanced re-epithelization of tissue (7246). For hypercholesterolemia, beta glucans are thought to lower cholesterol by forming a layer adjacent to the intestinal mucosa that prevents cholesterol absorption (7273). Beta glucans might also bind bile acids in the intestinal lumen (7272).

Adverse Reactions

Orally, yeast-derived beta glucans seem to be well-tolerated. No adverse effects have been reported (7272). Intravenously, beta glucans can cause chills and fever (7267,7271), redness, pain and swelling at the injection site, lymph node swelling (7261,7263), joint pain, lower back pain, headache, diarrhea, dizziness, flushing (7267), hypotension, hypertension, vasodilation, nausea, vomiting, leukocytosis (7270,7271), hives (7267), maculopapular rash (7270,7271), and excessive urination (7267).

Interactions with Herbs & Other Dietary Supplements

Insufficient reliable information available.

Interactions with Drugs

IMMUNOSUPPRESSANTS: Theoretically, beta glucans might decrease the effects of immunosuppressants because of its immunostimulant effects (7243,7268,7248,7249,7250,7252). Immunosuppressant drugs include azathioprine (Imuran), basiliximab (Simulect), cyclosporine (Neoral, Sandimmune), daclizumab (Zenapax), muromonab-CD3 (OKT3, Orthoclone OKT3), mycophenolate (CellCept), tacrolimus (FK506, Prograf), sirolimus (Rapamune), prednisone (Deltasone, Orasone), and other corticosteroids (glucocorticoids).

Interactions with Foods
No interactions are known to occur, and there is no known reason to expect a clinically significant interaction with beta glucans.

Interactions with Lab Tests
WHITE BLOOD CELL COUNT: Beta glucans can cause a transient increase in the number of white cells (leukocytosis) (7270).

Interactions with Diseases or Conditions
ACQUIRED IMMUNODEFICIENCY SYNDROME (AIDS) or AIDS-RELATED COMPLEX (ARC): Keratoderma of the palms and soles can develop in patients with AIDS/HIV or ARC who are receiving yeast beta glucans. The condition can begin during the first two weeks of therapy and resolves two to four weeks after discontinuation of beta glucans (7252).

Dosage and Administration
ORAL: For hypercholesterolemia, 7.5 grams twice daily of yeast-derived beta glucans fiber added to juice has been used (7272).
INTRAVENOUS: For HIV infection, 1-10 mg of the fungal beta glucan lentinan, administered over 10-30 minutes and given once to twice weekly has been used (7267). To prolong survival time in patients with cancer, 1-2 mg of the fungal beta glucan lentinan or 20-40 mg of the fungal beta glucan schizophyllan (SPG) administered once or twice weekly for at least one year has been used (3393,7261,7263,7264,7266). To prevent infection in trauma patients undergoing exploratory surgical procedures, 50 mg/M2 of soluble yeast-derived beta-glucan per day for 7 days has been used (7268). In surgical patients at high-risk for infection, 0.5-2 mg/kg of PGG-glucan given 1-6 hours before surgery and then repeated 4 hours, 48 hours, and 96 hours after surgery has been used (7270,7271).

Comments
There are several beta glucan supplement products that claim beta glucan taken orally can only be absorbed if the product is prepared by a special patented process that micronizes beta glucan particles to a size of 1 micron or less. However, there is no reliable evidence to support such a claim.

BETA-SITOSTEROL

Also Known As
24-ethyl-cholesterol, Angelicin, B-sitosterol 3-B-D-glucoside, B-sitosterolin, Beta sitosterin, Beta Sitosterol, Beta-sitosterol glucoside, Beta-sitosterol glycoside, Betasitosterol, Cinchol, Cupreol, Phytosterols, Plant sterols, Quebrachol, Rhamnol, Sitosterin, Sitosterol, Sitosterolins, Sitosterols, Sterinol, Sterolins.
CAUTION: See separate listing for Sitostanol.

Scientific Names
22,23-dihydrostigmasterol; 24-beta-ethyl-delta-5-cholesten-3beta-ol; 24-ethyl-cholesterol; 3-beta-stigmast-5-en-3-ol.

People Use This For
Orally, beta-sitosterol is used for coronary heart disease and hypercholesterolemia (9,14,3658,5330,5331,5332,5333,5334,5336), benign prostatic hyperplasia (BPH) and prostatitis (9,14,5327,5328,5329), and gallstones (14). It is also used orally for enhancing sexual activity (5323) and for preventing colon cancer (5322). Beta-sitosterol is also used orally for boosting the immune system, preventing immune suppression and inflammation following participation in a marathon (5335), common cold and flu (influenza), HIV/AIDS, rheumatoid arthritis, tuberculosis, psoriasis, allergies, cervical cancer (3654), fibromyalgia, systemic lupus erythematosus, asthma, alopecia, bronchitis, idiopathic thrombocytopenia purpura (ITP), migraine headache, chronic fatigue syndrome, and symptoms of menopause (3655).
In foods, beta-sitosterol is added to some margarines designed for use as part of a cholesterol-lowering diet and for preventing heart disease (6668).

Safety

LIKELY SAFE ...when used orally and appropriately. Beta-sitosterol has been safely used in studies lasting up to 18 months (9,14,5327,5328,5329,5330,5331,5332,5333,5334,5336) (5337,5338,5339,7198).

PREGNANCY AND LACTATION: Insufficient reliable information available; avoid using.

Effectiveness

LIKELY EFFECTIVE ...when used orally for symptoms of benign prostatic hyperplasia (BPH). Beta-sitosterol significantly improves urinary symptoms and increases maximum urinary flow and decreases postvoid residual urine volume; however, it does not affect prostate size (7,14,5327,5328,5329,7195,7198). ...when used orally for hypercholesterolemia. Beta-sitosterol significantly reduces total and low-density lipoprotein (LDL) cholesterol levels, but has little or no effect on high-density lipoprotein (HDL) cholesterol levels (14,5330,5331,5332,5333,5334,5336,6668,7195).

POSSIBLY INEFFECTIVE ...when used orally as adjunctive treatment for tuberculosis. There is some evidence that adding beta-sitosterol to conventional treatment for tuberculosis can increase lymphocyte counts; however, beta-sitosterol does not seem to decrease the time to cure based on negative sputum culture (14,5337).

LIKELY INEFFECTIVE ...when used orally for gallstones (14,5338,5339).

There is insufficient reliable information about the effectiveness of beta-sitosterol for its other uses.

Mechanism of Action

Beta-sitosterol is a plant sterol with a chemical structure similar to cholesterol with an ethyl group added at position 24 (14). Plant sterols, including beta-sitosterol and others such as stigmasterol, campesterol, and sitosterolins are widely distributed in fruits, vegetables, nuts, and seeds (3654,3655). Plant sterols are potentially atherogenic because they are so similar to cholesterol; however, atherogenesis does not occur with beta-sitosterol or other plant sterols because less than 5% is actually absorbed. About 175-200 mg of beta-sitosterol is consumed daily in the average diet (14). Beta-sitosterol is commonly added to margarines to be used as a cholesterol reducing aid. Fats are needed to solubilize plant sterols so margarines are an ideal vehicle. Capsules containing beta-sitosterol may not disperse properly in the gut, limiting their ability to reduce cholesterol absorption (5814). Beta-sitosterol actually inhibits intestinal absorption of cholesterol by competing for the limited space for cholesterol in mixed micelles. Cholesterol absorption is decreased by about 50% (5814). It also seems to accelerate the esterification rate of the lecithin-cholesterol acyltransferase (LCAT) enzyme, resulting in reduction of cholesterol-rich lipoprotein (14). Because there is decreased availability of cholesterol in the body, compensatory mechanisms kick in and can increase cholesterol synthesis in the liver (5814). This might explain why some patients do not respond to treatment with beta-sitosterol. In benign prostatic hyperplasia (BPH), beta-sitosterol binds to prostatic tissue, inhibits prostaglandin synthesis in the prostate, and has anti-inflammatory activity (7,14). There is some preliminary evidence that beta-sitosterol might also have anticancer and immune stimulant effects. Beta-sitosterol can inhibit the growth of human colon cancer cells in vitro (3667,3668). Mixtures of beta-sitosterol and its glycoside sitosterolin seem to also enhance proliferative responses of T-cells in vitro (3669,5342). Beta-sitosterol might also reduce the mild immune suppression and inflammation seen in marathon runners after a race (5335).

Adverse Reactions

Orally, beta-sitosterol is usually well tolerated. In some patients it can cause nausea, indigestion, gas, diarrhea, or constipation (14,5327,5328).

Interactions with Herbs & Other Dietary Supplements

CAROTENE, VITAMIN E: Beta-sitosterol may reduce absorption and blood levels of alpha- and beta-carotene and vitamin E (5814).

CHOLESTEROL LOWERING HERBS/SUPPLEMENTS: Beta-sitosterol might have additive effects with herbs and supplements that also lower cholesterol levels. Some of these herbs and supplements include chromium, flaxseed, garlic, guar gum, niacin, oat bran, psyllium, red yeast, and others.

Interactions with Drugs

ANTIHYPERLIPIDEMIC DRUGS: Theoretically, combining beta-sitosterol with cholesterol lowering drugs might have additive lowering effects on cholesterol levels. Some of these drugs include atorvastatin (Lipitor), cerivastatin (Baycol), cholestyramine (Questran), colestipol (Colestid), clofibrate (Atromid-S), fenofibrate (Tricor), fluvastatin (Lescol), gemfibrozil (Lopid), lovastatin (Mevacor), niacin, simvastatin (Zocor), and others.

PRAVASTATIN (Pravachol): There is some evidence that pravastatin can lower blood levels of beta-sitosterol (3672). Theoretically, this might occur with other HMG-CoA reductase inhibitors ("statins"); however, simvastatin (Zocor) does not seem to affect beta-sitosterol levels (3673). Other statin drugs include atorvastatin (Lipitor), cerivastatin (Baycol), fluvastatin (Lescol), and lovastatin (Mevacor).

Interactions with Foods
CAROTENE, VITAMIN E: Beta-sitosterol may reduce absorption and blood levels of alpha- and beta-carotene and vitamin E (5814).

Interactions with Lab Tests
CHOLESTEROL: Beta-sitosterol decreases total serum cholesterol and low-density lipoprotein (LDL) levels (5331,5336).

Interactions with Diseases or Conditions
SITOSTEROLEMIA: Taking beta-sitosterol can exacerbate sitosterolemia, a rare inherited lipid storage disease (14,5326). People with this disorder have increased absorption of cholesterol and beta-sitosterol from the diet, and decreased clearance of beta-sitosterol. Total body stores of beta-sitosterol are increased up to 17-fold. Elevated hepatic beta-sitosterol levels competitively inhibit cholesterol catabolism, contributing to hypercholesterolemia (3663). Patients with sitosterolemia are prone to premature coronary artery disease and xanthomas (3661,3662). Beta-sitosterol and its glycoside sitosterolin are contraindicated in patients with sitosterolemia.

Dosage and Administration
ORAL: For benign prostatic hyperplasia (BPH) and prostatitis, a typical dose is 60 to 130 mg of beta-sitosterol divided and given in 2-3 doses daily (9,14,5327,5328,5329). After symptoms improve, the dose is often reduced to 10 to 65 mg daily (9,14). For hypercholesterolemia, the usual dose is 800 mg to 6 grams per day divided and given before meals. Beta-sitosterol is typically given in conjunction with a low-fat diet (14,5327,5328,5329,5330,5331,5332,5333,5334,5336) (5337,5338,5339). In more severe hypercholesterolemia, doses of 10 to 15 grams per day have also been used (14). Doses should be taken at least 30 minutes, but not more than 90 minutes, before meals for maximum effect on cholesterol absorption (3658).

Comments
Beta-sitosterol is a supplement that is also found in the functional food product Take Control. The FDA authorized the use of labeling health claims for foods containing plant sterol esters, including beta-sitosterol, for reducing the risk of coronary heart disease (CHD) (6668). This rule is based on the FDA's conclusion that plant sterol esters may reduce the risk of CHD by lowering blood cholesterol levels. Although there is plenty of evidence that beta-sitosterol does lower cholesterol levels, there is no proof that long-term use actually lowers the risk of developing CHD. Avoid confusing beta-sitosterol with sitostanol, the saturated beta-sitosterol derivative contained in Benecol (5340,5341). Both sitostanol and beta-sitosterol are used for lowering cholesterol levels in people with hypercholesterolemia and appear to be equally effective (7196).

BETAINE ANHYDROUS

Also Known As
Betaine, Cystadane, Trimethyl Glycine, Trimethylglycine, TMG.
CAUTION: See separate listing for Betaine Hydrochloride.

Scientific Names
Trimethylglycine anhydrous.

People Use This For
Orally, betaine anhydrous is used for homocystinuria caused by cystathionine beta-synthase deficiency, 5,10-methylenetetrahydrofolate reductase deficiency, or cobalamin cofactor metabolism defect (15). It is also used orally for homocystinuria not responsive to pyridoxine (145). Betaine anhydrous is also used orally for hyperhomocysteinemia (6810).
Topically, betaine anhydrous is used as an ingredient in toothpastes to reduce the subjective symptoms of dry mouth (6812).

Safety
LIKELY SAFE ...when used orally and appropriately. Betaine anhydrous is a FDA-approved prescription product.
PREGNANCY AND LACTATION: Insufficient reliable information available; avoid using.

Effectiveness
EFFECTIVE ...when used orally for homocystinuria. Homocystinuria is commonly caused by cystathionine beta-synthase deficiency, 5,10-methylenetetrahydrofolate reductase deficiency, or cobalamin cofactor metabolism defect (14). In homocystinuria, betaine anhydrous reduces plasma homocysteine levels to 20-30% of the pretreatment levels (15). Betaine anhydrous is FDA-approved for this indication.

POSSIBLY EFFECTIVE ...when used topically as an ingredient of toothpastes to reduce the subjective symptoms of dry mouth (6812).

There is insufficient reliable information available about the effectiveness of betaine anhydrous for its other uses; however, there is some evidence that betaine supplementation for 3 weeks can produce a small (5.5 to 8%) decrease in plasma homocysteine levels in people with normal levels (<15 micromol/L). It is not clear whether this results in a decreased risk for cardiovascular disease (6810). More evidence is needed to rate betaine anhydrous for this use.

Mechanism of Action

Betaine anhydrous occurs naturally in the body. It is the major metabolite of choline and is present in small amounts in foods such as beets, spinach, cereals, seafood, and wine. It is a methyl group donor and facilitates the remethylation of homocysteine to methionine (14). Accumulation of homocysteine, leading to homocystinuria and hyperhomocysteinemia, can occur as a result of inborn errors of synthesis of the enzymes cystathionine beta-synthase, 5,10-methylenetetrahydrofolate reductase, or cobalamin cofactor. The resulting hyperhomocysteinemia can lead to thrombosis, osteoporosis, skeletal abnormalities, ocular lens dislocation, weakness, incoordination, peripheral neuropathies and paresthesias, memory impairment, and a high frequency of mental retardation (14). Elevated homocysteine levels can be reduced by two mechanisms: trans-sulfuration to cysteine using pyridoxine as a cofactor, or remethylation to methionine. This latter reaction uses either 5-methyltetrahydrofolate, derived from folic acid, as a methyl donor, with vitamin B12 as a cofactor, or betaine anhydrous (6810). In patients with homocystinuria, plasma total homocysteine concentrations are very high (>50 micromol/L) (6810), compared with levels in the normal population of 5 to 15 micromol/L (3047). Levels greater than 15 micromol/L are referred to as hyperhomocysteinemia and have been identified as a risk factor for cardiovascular disease (3047). The potential role of betaine anhydrous in lowering normal or slightly elevated homocysteine levels in order to reduce the risk of cardiovascular disease is not known. It has been suggested that the betaine content of wine may contribute to the lower incidence of cardiovascular disease in countries with a high wine consumption such as France, but it is not known whether the levels present (approximately 3 mg per glass) would have any signficant effect (6811). Preliminary studies in animals suggest that dietary supplementation with betaine can increase methionine and S-adenosylmethionine (SAM) biosynthesis from homocysteine in the liver when they have been inhibited by ethanol, and reduce ethanol-induced liver damage (6813).

Topically, betaine anhydrous has been reported to reduce irritant effects of sodium lauryl sulfate on the skin and oral mucosa, and may reduce subjective symptoms of dry mouth (6812).

Adverse Reactions

Orally, betaine anhydrous can cause nausea, GI distress, and diarrhea (698).

Interactions with Herbs & Other Dietary Supplements

Insufficient reliable information available.

Interactions with Drugs

No interactions are known to occur, and there is no known reason to expect a clinically significant interaction with betaine anhydrous.

Interactions with Foods

No interactions are known to occur, and there is no known reason to expect a clinically significant interaction with betaine anhydrous.

Interactions with Lab Tests

No interactions are known to occur, and there is no known reason to expect a clinically significant interaction with betaine anhydrous.

Interactions with Diseases or Conditions

No interactions are known to occur, and there is no known reason to expect a clinically significant interaction with betaine anhydrous.

Dosage and Administration

ORAL: For homocystinuria, a maintenance dose of 3 grams is typically taken twice daily in both adults and children. Dose titration is preferable in children. For children under three years old, the starting dose is 100 mg/kg per day, increased in weekly intervals in increments of 100 mg/kg daily. All patients can receive dose increases until plasma homocysteine concentrations are undetectable or very low, which can require doses up to 20 grams per day. Dissolve the powder in water immediately before administration (15). For reducing plasma homocysteine levels, 3 grams betaine anhydrous twice daily orally has been used (6810).

TOPICAL: Betaine has been added to toothpastes in a concentration of 4% for treatment of symptoms of dry mouth (6812).

Comments
Betaine anhydrous has Orphan Drug status in the US. Avoid confusion with betaine hydrochloride, a dietary supplement with variable purity and potency that has not been demonstrated safe or effective for treating homocystinuria.

BETAINE HYDROCHLORIDE

Also Known As
Betaine, Betaine HCl, Trimethyl Glycine, Trimethylglycine, TMG.
CAUTION: See separate listing for Betaine Anhydrous.

Scientific Names
Trimethylglycine hydrochloride.

People Use This For
Orally, betaine hydrochloride is used as a supplemental source of hydrochloric acid, to treat hypokalemia, and as a liver protectant (16,144).

Safety
There is insufficient reliable information available about the safety of betaine hydrochloride.
Pregnancy and Lactation: Insufficient reliable information available; avoid using.

Effectiveness
There is insufficient reliable information available about the effectiveness of betaine hydrochloride.

Mechanism of Action
Insufficient reliable information available.

Adverse Reactions
Orally, theoretically, betaine hydrochloride can irritate gastric or duodenal ulcers or impede ulcer healing by increasing gastric acid (9).

Interactions with Herbs & Other Dietary Supplements
Insufficient reliable information available.

Interactions with Drugs
No interactions are known to occur, and there is no known reason to expect a clinically significant interaction with betaine hydrochloride.

Interactions with Foods
No interactions are known to occur, and there is no known reason to expect a clinically significant interaction with betaine hydrochloride.

Interactions with Lab Tests
No interactions are known to occur, and there is no known reason to expect a clinically significant interaction with betaine hydrochloride.

Interactions with Diseases or Conditions
GASTRIC and DUODENAL ULCERS: Theoretically, betaine hydrochloride can irritate ulcers or impede healing by increasing gastric acid; avoid using in patients with gastric or duodenal ulcers (9).

Dosage and Administration
ORAL: People typically use 325 to 650 mg daily after a meal that contains protein. Do not take on an empty stomach (6006).

Comments
Avoid confusion with betaine anhydrous. Betaine is manufactured in various salt forms around the world, including betaine hydrochloride. The purity and potency of these dietary supplement products can vary. There are no data to support the effectiveness of betaine hydrochloride in any condition, including homocystinuria. Use only the FDA-approved betaine anhydrous for the treatment of homocystinuria (see separate listing for betaine anhydrous).

BETH ROOT

Also Known As
Birthroot, Coughroot, Ground Lily, Jew's Harp Plant, Indian Balm, Indian Shamrock, Lamb's Quarters, Milk Ipecac, Pariswort, Rattlesnake Root, Snakebite, Stinking Benjamin, Three–Leafed Nightshade, Wake-Robin.

Scientific Names
Trillium erectum.
Family: Liliaceae.

People Use This For
Orally, beth root is used for long, heavy menstruation and pain relief. It is also used orally as an astringent and expectorant.
Topically, beth root is used for varicose veins and ulcers, hematomas, and hemorrhoid bleeding (18).

Safety
POSSIBLY UNSAFE ...when used orally. Beth root is a gastrointestinal irritant (12).
There is insufficient reliable information available about the safety of beth root for its other uses.
PREGNANCY AND LACTATION: LIKELY UNSAFE ...when used orally; avoid using. Beth root might have menstrual or uterine stimulant activity (12,18).

Effectiveness
There is insufficient reliable information available about the effectiveness of beth root.

Mechanism of Action
The applicable parts of beth root are the rhizome, and dried root and leaf. There is insufficient reliable information about the possible mechanism of action or active ingredients.

Adverse Reactions
Orally, ingestion of large amounts of the plant or volatile oil might produce GI irritation severe enough to cause vomiting (12,18). In pregnant women, the drastic purgative effects can cause reflex uterine contractions.
Topically, beth root causes extreme irritation (18).

Interactions with Herbs & Other Dietary Supplements
Insufficient reliable information available.

Interactions with Drugs
No interactions are known to occur, and there is no known reason to expect a clinically significant interaction with beth root.

Interactions with Foods
No interactions are known to occur, and there is no known reason to expect a clinically significant interaction with beth root.

Interactions with Lab Tests
No interactions are known to occur, and there is no known reason to expect a clinically significant interaction with beth root.

Interactions with Diseases or Conditions
CARDIAC CONDITIONS: Due to potential cardiotoxicity from the convallamarin-like glycoside, patients with a cardiac condition should be cautioned against the use of this herb (214).

Dosage and Administration
ORAL: No typical dosage.
TOPICAL: The ground plant parts are used as a poultice (18).

Comments
None.

BETONY

Also Known As
Bishopswort, Bishop Wort, Hedge Nettles, Wood Betony.

Scientific Names
Stachys officinalis; Betonica officinalis.
Family: Labiatae.

People Use This For
Orally, betony is used to treat diarrhea, irritation of mucous membranes (5), stress and tension, headache, facial pain (6), coughs as an expectorant, bronchitis, and asthma (18).

In combination with other herbs, betony is used for treatment of neuralgia and anxiety (18).

In folk medicine, betony is considered a cure-all and thought effective in 47 different diseases (5), as an antidiarrheal, antiflatulent, and sedative. Betony is also used in folk medicine to treat inflammation of the nose, throat and lung air passages, heartburn, gout, nervousness, bladder and kidney stones, and bladder inflammation (18).

Safety
POSSIBLY SAFE ...when the dried above ground parts are used orally in medicinal amounts (5,6,12).
POSSIBLY UNSAFE ...when used in large amounts because it contains 15% tannins and these can cause gastrointestinal irritation (5,12).
PREGNANCY: POSSIBLY UNSAFE ...when used orally; avoid using (6).
LACTATION: Insufficient reliable information available; avoid using.

Effectiveness
POSSIBLY EFFECTIVE ...when taken orally in small doses for headache, nervous tension, facial pain, congestion, and diarrhea (5,6). ...when taken in large doses as a purgative or emetic (6). ...when used topically as a mouth rinse or gargle for gum, mouth, and throat irritations (5,6).
There is insufficient reliable information available about the effectiveness of betony for its other uses.

Mechanism of Action
The applicable parts of betony are the dried above ground parts. The high tannin content (15%) is responsible for its astringent properties (5). The glycoside mixture can have a hypotensive effect, possibly explaining its effectiveness in mild anxiety states and headache (5,6). One constituent, stachydrine, is a systolic depressant that is also active against rheumatism (6).

Adverse Reactions
Large doses can cause significant GI irritation due to the tannin component (5,6).

Interactions with Herbs & Other Dietary Supplements
Insufficient reliable information available.

Interactions with Drugs
DRUGS THAT ALTER BLOOD PRESSURE: Theoretically, betony can increase the blood pressure lowering effects of antihypertensive drugs and interfere with the activity of pressor drugs.

Interactions with Foods
No interactions are known to occur, and there is no known reason to expect a clinically significant interaction with betony.

Interactions with Lab Tests
No interactions are known to occur, and there is no known reason to expect a clinically significant interaction with betony.

Interactions with Diseases or Conditions
No interactions are known to occur, and there is no known reason to expect a clinically significant interaction with betony.

Dosage and Administration
ORAL: Betony is typically taken as a tea or an infusion (6002). Use small doses to avoid GI irritation.

Comments
None.

BIFIDOBACTERIA

Also Known As
B. bifidum, Bifido, Bifidobacteria bifidus, Bifidobacterium, Bifidum, Probiotics.
CAUTION: See separate listings for Brewer's Yeast (Hansen CBS 5926), Lactobacillus, Saccharomyces Boulardii, and Yogurt.

Scientific Names
Bifidobacterium adolescentis; Bifidobacterium bifidum; Bifidobacterium breve; Bifidobacterium infantis; Bifidobacterium lactis; Bifidobacterium longum.
Family: Actinomycetaceae.

People Use This For
Orally, bifidobacteria are used for preventing acute diarrhea in infants and children; preventing necrotizing entercolitis in neonates; treating atopic eczema in infants; preventing traveler's diarrhea; improving immune function; and replenishing intestinal normal flora depleted by diarrhea, radiation, chemotherapy, antibiotics, or other causes. Bifidobacteria are also used orally for candidiasis, the common cold and flu (influenza), hepatitis, hypercholesterolemia, lactose intolerance, mastitis, mumps, and cancer. They are also used orally to treat ulcerative colitis and pouchitis following surgery for ulcerative colitis.

Safety
POSSIBLY SAFE ...when used orally and appropriately. Bifodobacteria seem to be safe when used for up to 9 months (162,6087).
CHILDREN: POSSIBLY SAFE ...when used orally and appropriately. Bifodobacteria seem to be safe in children including those under two years of age and critically ill neonates when used for up to 8 months (161,3162,3169,3458).
PREGNANCY AND LACTATION: Insufficient reliable information available; avoid using.

Effectiveness
POSSIBLY EFFECTIVE ...when used orally to prevent acute rotaviral diarrhea in infants. Bifidobacterium bifidum combined with Streptococcus thermophilus or Bifidobacterium Bb12 strain appears to reduce the incidence of diarrhea and rotavirus shedding in infants (153,161,3169). ...when used orally to prevent necrotizing entercolitis (NEC) in neonates. Bifidobacterium infantis in combination with Lactobacillus acidophilus seems to reduce the incidence of NEC and NEC-assoicated mortality in critically ill neonates (3162). ...when used orally in infants to treat atopic eczema. Bifidobacterium lactis seems to reduce the severity of atopic eczema and the markers for allergic responses including soluble CD4 in serum and eosinophilic protein X in urine (3458). ...when used orally for preventing traveler's diarrhea. Bifidobacterium in combination with Lactobacillus acidophilus, Lactobacillus bulgaricus, or Streptococcus thermophilus seems to decrease the chance of developing traveler's diarrhea (155). ...when used orally to prevent antibiotic-induced gastrointestinal adverse effects. Ingestion of bifidobacterium longum can reduce stool frequency, abdominal discomfort, and stool clostridial spore count when used in patients concurrently taking erythromycin (1233). ...when used orally to maintain remission from ulcerative colitis. In patients intolerant to 5-aminosalicylic acid, bifidobacteria plus lactobacilli and Streptococcus thermophilus seem to prevent increases in pathogenic bacteria and relapse in some patients with ulcerative colitis (3261). ...when used orally for chronic pouchitis, a complication of surgery for ulcerative colitis. A combination of Bifidobacterium longum, Bifidobacterium breve, Lactobacillus species, and Streptococcus thermophilus seems to prevent chronic pouchitis flare-ups (6087). Daily consumption of bifidobacteria is usually required to maintain effectiveness, although effects may persist a week after discontinuation (154,1731).
There is insufficient reliable information available to rate the effectiveness of bifidobacterium for its other uses; however, there is preliminary evidence that antibiotic-resistant Bifidobacterium longum can help improve short-term survival in the treatment of radiation sickness. In combination with prophylactic antibioitics, bifidobacteria appear to inhibit colonization and overgrowth of intestinal opportunistic pathogens, preventing post-irradiation sepsis (3457). More evidence is needed to rate bifidobacteria for this use.

Mechanism of Action
Bifidobacteria are anaerobic, rod-shaped, Gram-positive bacteria that normally colonize the human colon (1060,1137).

Bifidobacteria belong to a group of bacteria called lactic acid bacteria. Lactic acid bacteria, which also include the lactobacilli species, are found in fermented foods like yogurt and cheese (1055,3589). Bifidobacteria are used therapeutically as so-called probiotics, the opposite of antibiotics. They are considered "friendly" bacteria and are used with the purpose of re-colonizing areas of the body where they normally would occur. The human body relies on the normal flora for several functions, including metabolizing foods, absorbing nutrients, and preventing colonization by pathogenic bacteria. Probiotics such as bifidobacteria are typically used in cases when a disease occurs or might occur due to depleted normal flora. Bifidobacteria, especially Bifidobacterium bifidum, are the predominant intestinal flora of breast-fed infants (161). Bifiodobacteria might contribute to the protection that breast-feeding provides against gastrointestinal infections in infants (1060). Bifidobacteria appear to produce antimicrobial substances that protect the intestine (1060). Bifidobacteria are also in the adult colon, but are less predominant (1060). When used orally, some species of bifidobacteria, such as Bifobacterium infantis, and some strains of Bifidobacterium breve and Bifidobacterium longum, pass through the gut and bind to the intestinal mucosa, preventing attachment of pathogenic coliform bacteria (1137,1735). Bifidobacteria disappear from the feces within 2 weeks of discontinuation of bifidobacteria, suggesting that there is no long-term colonization (1117,4363). For continued effect, bifidobacteria must be used regularly. In addition to acting as a barrier to pathogenic bacterial adhesion, some researchers think bifidobacteria and other probiotics might have immunomodulating effects (1137). Quantatitive differences in the compositon of intestinal microflora appear to affect immunological homeostasis (3458). Bifidobacteria seem to modulate non-specific cellular and humoral immunity possibly by stimulating lymphocyte and macrophage activity and cytokine production by mononuclear cells (6099). Due to these immunomodulating effects, some researchers think bifidobacteria and other probiotics might not only fight intestinal pathogens, but might also be helpful for conditions such as inflammatory bowel disease and pouchitis (6087). The addition of Bifidobacterium lactis to milk enhances cellular immunity in healthy middle-aged and elderly people, improving phagocyte function and natural killer cell activity, and increasing production of interferon-alpha (1055,1117). In infants, bacterial colonization appears to be essential in the development of oral tolerance instead of sensitization to dietary antigens (3458). There is also some preliminary evidence that bifidobacteria and other probiotics might help protect against cancer. Bifidobacteria decrease fecal enzymes such as beta-glucuronidase, beta-glucosidase, nitroreductase, and urease, which are involved in the metabolic activation of some mutagens and carcinogens (6099). Bifidobacteria might also fight cancer by alteration of colonic physiochemical conditions and production of antitumorigenic or antimutagenic compounds in the colon (1154). Most researchers agree that the effectiveness of bifidobacteria and other probiotics for all indications depends on their ability to colonize an area of tissue. To do this, bifidobacteria preparations must contain live and viable organisms. Products stored for long periods of time or stored improperly may contain few live and active organisms to start with. For oral preparations, bacteria must also remain viable after passing through the gut (3589). Bifidobacterium longum is particularly resistant to gastric acid (3589). They must also be able to latch on to the intestinal epithelium. Bifidobacteria strains might vary in their effectiveness due to differences in their ability to adhere to epithelial cells (1137). Complex sugars, such as fructo-oligosaccharides, inulin, and oligofructose, are selectively fermented by bifidobacteria in the colon, and increase indigenous bifidobacteria quantities (4363). The addition of oligosaccharides to bifidobacteria also seems to enhance the activity of bifidobacteria (1117). However, there are no trials confirming the clinical benefit of combining bifidobacteria with complex sugars.

Adverse Reactions

Orally, bifidobacteria seem to be well tolerated by most people. In children, bifidobacteria can cause diarrhea (3169). Adverse effects from ingestion of bifidobacteria have not been reported; however, with other probiotics, patients can sometimes experience gastrointestinal upset including bloating and flatulence. This effect is usually mild and typically subsides with continued use. Most bifidobacteria species are considered nonpathogenic and nontoxigenic; however, the Bifidobacterium dentium species, has been associated with dental caries (1137,1236). Sepsis with the Bifidobacterium longum species has occurred in one patient following acupuncture. This was likely due to needle contamination. This effect would not be expected to occur from taking oral bifidobacteria supplements in most healthy patients (1236).

Interactions with Herbs & Other Dietary Supplements

Insufficient reliable information available.

Interactions with Drugs

ANTIBIOTICS: There is some concern that concomitant administration of antibiotics might decrease the effectiveness of bifidobacteria. Since bifidobacteria preparations usually contain live and active organisms, simultaneously taking antibiotics might kill a significant number of the organisms (1740). Tell patients to separate administration of antibiotics and bifidobacteria preparations by at least 2 hours.

Interactions with Foods

No interactions are known to occur, and there is no known reason to expect a clinically significant interaction with bifidobacteria.

Interactions with Lab Tests

No interactions are known to occur, and there is no known reason to expect a clinically significant interaction with bifidobacteria.

Interactions with Diseases or Conditions

IMMUNOCOMPROMISE: There is some concern that bifidobacteria preparations might cause pathogenic colonization in patients who are immunocompromised. Although this has not occurred specifically with bifidobacteria, there have been rare cases involving other probiotic species such as lactobacillus. Pathogenic colonization seems to be more likely to occur in severely immunocompromised patients (4380,4391,4393,4398). Use with caution in these patients.

Dosage and Administration

ORAL: The strength of bifidobacteria preparations is usually quantified by the number of living organisms per capsule. People typically take 1 to 10 billion viable cells daily in 3 to 4 divided doses (5009).

Comments

None.

BILBERRY dried ripe fruit

Also Known As

Airelle, Black Whortles, Bleaberry, Blueberry, Burren Myrtle, Dwarf Bilberry, Dyeberry, Huckleberry, Hurtleberry, Myrtilli Fructus, Trackleberry, Whortleberry, Wineberry.
CAUTION: See separate listings for Bilberry leaf, Blueberry, and Bog Bilberry.

Scientific Names

Vaccinium myrtillus.
Family: Ericaceae.

People Use This For

Orally, bilberry dried, ripe fruit is used to treat non-specific, acute diarrhea, and to improve visual acuity (2,11), including night vision (6). The dried, ripe fruit extracts are used orally for angina, venous insufficiency of the lower limbs, varicose veins, atherosclerosis, and degenerative retinal conditions (11).
Topically, the dried, ripe fruit of bilberry is used for mild inflammation of the mouth and throat mucous membranes (2,11).

Safety

LIKELY SAFE ...when consumed in amounts typically found in foods (11).
There is insufficient reliable information available about the safety of the use of bilberry dried ripe fruit in medicinal amounts (2).
PREGNANCY AND LACTATION: LIKELY SAFE ...when consumed in amounts typically found in foods. There is insufficient reliable information available about the safety of the use of bilberry dried, ripe fruit in larger amounts.

Effectiveness

POSSIBLY EFFECTIVE ...when used orally to treat circulatory problems (6). ...when used orally for mild inflammation of the mouth and throat mucous membranes (2). ...when used orally to improve retinal lesions from diabetic or hypertensive retinopathy (39,40). Clinical studies of bilberry's effectiveness have used formulations containing 25% of the bioflavonoid complex anthocyanoside.
There is insufficient reliable information available about the effectiveness of bilberry dried ripe fruit for its other uses.

Mechanism of Action

Astringent tannin components of bilberry dried, ripe fruit are responsible for the observed benefits in diarrhea and irritation of the mouth and throat mucosa (6). Anthocyanoside (anthocyandin) constituents increase the synthesis of glycosaminoglycans, decrease vascular permeability, reduce basement membrane thickness, and aid in the redistribution of microvascular blood flow and the formation of interstitial fluid (6,41). An anthocyanadin pigment found in bilberry might have anti-ulcer and gastroprotective effects (6).

Adverse Reactions

None reported.

Interactions with Herbs & Other Dietary Supplements
Insufficient reliable information available.

Interactions with Drugs
No interactions are known to occur, and there is no known reason to expect a clinically significant interaction with bilberry dried ripe fruit.

Interactions with Foods
No interactions are known to occur, and there is no known reason to expect a clinically significant interaction with bilberry dried ripe fruit.

Interactions with Lab Tests
No interactions are known to occur, and there is no known reason to expect a clinically significant interaction with bilberry dried ripe fruit.

Interactions with Diseases or Conditions
No interactions are known to occur, and there is no known reason to expect a clinically significant interaction with bilberry dried ripe fruit.

Dosage and Administration
ORAL: The typical dose of the dried, ripe berries is 20-60 grams daily. People also drink a decoction of the berries, which is prepared by placing 5-10 grams (1-2 teaspoons) of mashed berries in cold water, bringing the water to a simmer for 10 minutes, and then straining the water. A dose of 160 mg of bilberry extract taken twice daily has been used in patients with retinopathy (39). Clinical studies of bilberry's effectiveness have used formulations containing 25% of the bioflavonoid complex anthocyanoside.
TOPICAL: The berries are usually applied as a 10% decoction, made by boiling the dried berries in water for 10 minutes and straining (2).

Comments
None.

BILBERRY leaf

Also Known As
Airelle, Black Whortles, Bleaberry, Blueberry, Burren Myrtle, Dwarf Bilberry, Dyeberry, Huckleberry, Hurtleberry, Myrtilli Fructus, Trackleberry, Whortleberry, Wineberry.
CAUTION: See separate listings for Bilberry dried ripe fruit, Blueberry, and Bog Bilberry.

Scientific Names
Vaccinium myrtillus.
Family: Ericaceae.

People Use This For
Orally, bilberry leaf is used for diabetes; arthritis; gout; dermatitis; hemorrhoids; poor circulation; functional heart problems; "stimulating metabolism"; "purifying the blood"; and prevention and treatment of gastrointestinal, kidney, and urinary tract symptoms and diseases (2,8).

Safety
POSSIBLY UNSAFE ...when used orally in high doses or with prolonged use. Death can occur with chronic dose of 1.5 g/kg/day (2).
PREGNANCY AND LACTATION: UNSAFE ...when used orally due to potential toxicity; avoid using.

Effectiveness
There is insufficient reliable information available about the effectiveness of bilberry leaf.

Mechanism of Action
Bilberry leaves contain polyphenols, tannins, flavonoids (1265) and a relatively high concentration of chromium (9.0 ppm) (8). Preliminary evidence suggests that a bilberry leaf extract might have blood glucose and triglyceride lowering effects (1264). The chromium in bilberry leaf is theorized to play a role in potential blood glucose lowering activity (8). Some researchers think that flavonoids in bilberry leaf might also be useful for diabetic circulatory disorders (8).

Adverse Reactions
None reported; however, chronic intoxication has been reported in animals. Symptoms include wasting, anemia, jaundice, acute excitatory states, disturbances of muscle contraction, and death (2).

Interactions with Herbs & Other Dietary Supplements
Insufficient reliable information is available.

Interactions with Drugs
ANTI-DIABETES DRUGS: Theoretically, concomitant use might require dosing adjustment of anti-diabetes drugs. Preliminary evidence suggests that a bilberry leaf extract might have blood glucose lowering activity (1264); monitor closely.
DISULFRAM: A disulfram reaction might occur with herbal products containing alcohol; avoid concurrent use (214).

Interactions with Foods
No interactions are known to occur, and there is no known reason to expect a clinically significant interaction with bilberry leaf.

Interactions with Lab Tests
BLOOD GLUCOSE: Theoretically, bilberry leaf might lower blood glucose and test results. Preliminary evidence suggests that a bilberry leaf extract might have blood glucose lowering activity (1264).
TRIGLYCERIDES: Theoretically, bilberry leaf might lower serum triglycerides and test results. Preliminary evidence suggests that a bilberry leaf extract might have triglyceride lowering activity (1264).

Interactions with Diseases or Conditions
DIABETES: Theoretically, bilberry leaf might lower blood glucose. Preliminary evidence suggests that a bilberry leaf extract might have blood glucose lowering activity (1264); monitor closely.

Dosage and Administration
ORAL: Bilberry leaf is commonly used as a tea [steep 1 gram (1-2 teaspoons) finely chopped dried leaf in 150 mL boiling water for 5-10 minutes, strain]; avoid prolonged use (8).

Comments
For short-term use only.

BIOTIN

Also Known As
Coenzyme R, D-Biotin, Vitamin H, W Factor.

Scientific Names
Cis-hexahydro-2-oxo-1H-thieno[3,4-d]-imidazole-4-valeric acid.

People Use This For
Orally, biotin is used for preventing and treating biotin deficiency associated with pregnancy, long-term parenteral nutrition, malnutrition, rapid weight loss, and multiple carboxylase deficiency. It is also used orally for hair loss, brittle nails, seborrheic dermatitis of infancy, and diabetes.

Safety
LIKELY SAFE ...when used orally and appropriately (9,1900).
CHILDREN: POSSIBLY SAFE ...when used orally and appropriately (173).
PREGNANCY AND LACTATION: POSSIBLY SAFE ...when used orally and appropriately (1901).

Effectiveness

LIKELY EFFECTIVE ...when used orally as a supplement to prevent or treat biotin deficiency (1901).
POSSIBLY EFFECTIVE ...when used orally for increasing the thickness of finger and toenails in individuals with brittle nails (171). ...when used orally for treating seborrheic dermatitis of infancy (173).
There is insufficient reliable information available about the effectiveness of biotin for its other uses.

Mechanism of Action

Biotin is a vitamin that is found in small amounts in numerous foods. In food, biotin is protein bound and is cleaved by the enzyme biotinidase. Biotin is also synthesized in animals by intestinal microflora. Researchers think biotin is stored in the mitochondria and that it acts as a coenzyme in bicarbonate-dependent carboxylation reactions (3915). Biotin-containing enzymes are involved in gluconeogenesis, fatty acid synthesis, propionate metabolism, and the catabolism of leucine in mammals. Biotin is recycled endogenously. This may be the reason why deficiency symptoms take a long time to develop and are rarely seen in humans (173). Biotin deficiency is most likely to occur in people with congenital biotinidase deficiency, malabsorption syndromes, such as short-gut syndrome, and in people receiving long-term parenteral nutrition. Symptoms of deficiency include thinning of the hair, frequently with loss of hair color, and red scaly rash around the eyes, nose, and mouth. Neurological symptoms, including depression, lethargy, hallucinations, and paresthesias of the extremities are also common in biotin deficiency (3915).

Adverse Reactions

Orally, biotin is well tolerated when used at recommended dosages (3915). There is one case of eosinophilic pleuropericardial effusion with biotin 10 mg per day in combination with pantothenic acid 300 mg for 2 months (3914).

Interactions with Herbs & Other Dietary Supplements

Insufficient reliable information available.

Interactions with Drugs

CARBAMAZEPINE AND PRIMIDONE: These drugs can reduce biotin absorption in vitro (172,176).
PHENYTOIN AND PHENOBARBITAL: These drugs can reduce biotin levels (175,176).

Interactions with Foods

EGG WHITES: Consumption of large amounts of egg whites can cause biotin deficiency (173,3915).

Interactions with Lab Tests

THYROID STIMULATING HORMONE (TSH): There is one report of a false-low TSH on the assay by the Boehringer Mannheim ES 700 analyzer due to high serum biotin levels in a neonate (170).
FREE THYROXINE (FT4): There is one report of a false-high FT4 on the assay by the Boehringer Mannheim ES 700 analyzer due to high serum biotin levels in a neonate (170).

Interactions with Diseases or Conditions

BIOTINIDASE DEFICIENCY: Biotin requirements may be higher in people with genetic biotinidase deficiency (3915).
RENAL DIALYSIS: Biotin requirements may be higher in people receiving hemodialysis or peritoneal dialysis (3915).

Dosage and Administration

ORAL: There is no recommended dietary allowance (RDA) established for biotin. The adequate intakes (AI) for biotin are 7 mcg for infants 0-12 months, 8 mcg for children 1-3 years, 12 mcg for children 4-8 years, 20 mcg for children 9-13 years, 25 mcg for adolescents 14-18 years, 30 mcg for adults over 18 years and pregnant women, and 35 mcg for lactating women (3915).

Comments

None.

BIRCH

Also Known As

Betula, Betulae folium, Downy Birch, Silver Birch, White Birch.

Scientific Names

Betula pendula, synonym Betula verrucosa; Betula pubescens.
Family: Betulaceae.

People Use This For
Orally, birch is used as a diuretic, for rheumatic ailments; "irrigation therapy" (use of a mild diuretic along with copious fluid intake to increase urine flow); and to treat pyelonephritis, ureteritis, cystitis, and urethritis (8).
In folk medicine, birch is used for arthritis, rheumatism, loss of hair, skin rashes, and in "spring cures" for "purifying the blood" (8).

Safety
LIKELY SAFE ...when used orally and appropriately as irrigation therapy (2,12).
PREGNANCY AND LACTATION: Insufficient reliable information available; avoid using.

Effectiveness
There is insufficient reliable information available about the effectiveness of birch.

Mechanism of Action
The applicable part of birch is the leaf. The aquaretic and possibly saluretic effects are due to the flavonoid constituents of the birch leaf. Aquaretics increase urine volume (water loss) but not sodium excretion (512). The high vitamin C content of the leaf can enhance the effect (8).

Adverse Reactions
None reported.

Interactions with Herbs & Other Dietary Supplements
Insufficient reliable information available.

Interactions with Drugs
DIURETICS: Theoretically, birch leaf might increase sodium retention and interfere with diuretic therapy (512).

Interactions with Foods
No interactions are known to occur, and there is no known reason to expect a clinically significant interaction with birch.

Interactions with Lab Tests
No interactions are known to occur, and there is no known reason to expect a clinically significant interaction with birch.

Interactions with Diseases or Conditions
EDEMA DUE TO HEART OR KIDNEY CONDITIONS: Irrigation therapy is contraindicated (2).
HYPERTENSION: Theoretically, birch leaf might increase sodium retention and worsen hypertension (512).
URINARY TRACT INFECTIONS: Herbal "irrigation therapy" can be insufficient and requires the addition of an antibacterial agent and close monitoring (8).

Dosage and Administration
ORAL: The typical dose of birch leaf is several times daily as a tea, which is prepared by steeping 2-3 grams of finely cut dried leaf in 150 mL boiling water for 10-15 minutes and straining (2,8). The tea should be taken with plenty of water (8).

Comments
None.

BISHOP'S WEED

Also Known As
Ajava Seeds, Ajowan, Ajowan Caraway, Ajowan Seed, Ajowanj, Bishop's Flower, Bishops Weed, Bullwort, Carum, Flowering Ammi, Omum, Yavani.
CAUTION: See separate listings for Goutweed and Khella.

Scientific Names
Ammi majus.
Family: Apiaceae/Umbelliferae.

People Use This For

Orally, bishop's weed is used for digestive disorders, asthma, angina, kidney stones, and as a diuretic (7161).
Topically, bishop's weed is used for psoriasis and vitiligo (9,7161).

Safety

There is insufficient reliable information available about the safety of bishop's weed.
PREGNANCY: LIKELY UNSAFE ...when used orally. The active constituent, khellin, has uterine stimulant
activity (19); avoid using.
LACTATION: Insufficient reliable information available; avoid using.

Effectiveness

There is insufficient reliable information available about the effectiveness of bishop's weed.

Mechanism of Action

The applicable parts of bishop's weed are the seeds (7161). Bishop's weed contains several active ingredients including
khellin, 8-methoxsalen, xanthotoxin, bergapten, and umbelliferone (1332,7162). The constituent, khellin, seems to have
calcium channel blocking effects. There is some evidence it might also increase high-density lipoprotein (HDL) levels
without affecting total cholesterol or triglyceride concentrations (2522,7162). The 8-methoxsalen (8-MOP,
methoxypsoralen) constituent is one of the first agents used along with ultraviolet-A (UVA) radiation to treat psoriasis.
It binds pyrimidine bases in DNA and suppresses cell division. This constituent also seems to contribute to the
phototoxicity caused by bishop's weed (15,2528). Another constituent, xanthotoxin, also seems to have antipsoriatic
activity (7162). The bergapten (5-methoxypsoralen) has antipsoriatic activity and antiplatelet activity (7162). Bergapten
also appears to inhibit the cytochrome P450 3A4 (CYP3A4) system, which might lead to numerous interactions with
drugs metabolized by this system (7163). The umbelliferone constituent is a hydroxycoumarin. Some researchers are
interested in coumarins such as umbelliferone from bishop's weed because of in vitro evidence that they can inhibit
reverse transcriptase in human immunodeficiency virus (HIV) replication (1332,1333). Further research is being done to
see if these constituents have this effect in humans. Although people use bishop's weed for kidney stones, animal
models show that it does not seem to decrease calcium oxalate deposition in the kidneys (2526).

Adverse Reactions

Orally, bishop's weed can cause nausea, vomiting, and headache (7161). Bishop's weed can also cause allergic reactions
including rhinitis and urticaria in sensitive patients (2520). There is some concern that bishop's weed might increase liver
enzymes. The isolated constituent khellin can increase transaminase levels (2522); however, so far this effect has not
been reported for bishop's weed. Bishop's weed might also cause photosensitivity due to the 8-MOP constituent. In
some patients bishop's weed can also cause contact dermatitis (2520,2521). There is also concern based on preliminary
evidence that bishop's weed might cause ophthalmic changes, such as pigmentary retinopathy (2527).
Topically, bishop's weed might cause skin malignancies in patients predisposed to cancer (214).

Interactions with Herbs & Other Dietary Supplements

HEPATOTOXIC HERBS: Theoretically, bishop's weed might have additive effects with herbs that cause
hepatotoxicity. The khellin constituent can cause elevated transaminase levels in some patients (2522). Other products
that might affect the liver include borage, chaparral, uva ursi, and others (2,2522).
HERBS WITH ANTICOAGULANT/ANTIPLATELET POTENTIAL: Concomitant use of herbs that affect
platelet aggregation might increase the risk of bleeding. These herbs include angelica, anise, arnica, asafoetida,
bogbean, boldo, capsicum, celery, chamomile, clove, fenugreek, feverfew, garlic, ginger, ginkgo, Panax ginseng, horse
chestnut, horseradish, licorice, meadowsweet, onion, prickly ash, papain, passionflower, poplar, quassia, red clover,
turmeric, wild carrot, wild lettuce, willow, and others (7162).
PHOTOSENSITIZING HERBS: Theoretically, bishop's weed might have an additive effect with products that
increase sun sensitivity, such as St. John's wort (2521,7162).

Interactions with Drugs

ANTICOAGULANT, ANTIPLATELET DRUGS: There is some concern that bishop's weed might have additive
effects with anticoagulant or antiplatelet drugs and possibly increase the risk of bleeding. The bergapten constituent of
bishop's weed has antiplatelet effects. Some anticoagulant or antiplatelet drugs include aspirin, clopidogrel (Plavix),
dalteparin (Fragmin), enoxaparin (Lovenox), heparin, ticlopidine (Ticlid), warfarin (Coumadin), and others (7162).
HEPATOTOXIC DRUGS: Theoretically, bishop's weed might have additive adverse effects on the liver
when used with hepatotoxic drugs. The khellin constituent of bishop's weed can increase liver transaminases (2,2522).
Some drugs that can adversely effect the liver include acetaminophen (Tylenol), amiodarone (Cordarone),
carbamazepine (Tegretol), isoniazid (INH), methotrexate (Rheumatrex), methyldopa (Aldomet), and many others.
PHOTOSENSITIZING DRUGS: Theoretically, concomitant use might result in increased photosensitivity. Bishop
weed constituents seem to cause photosensitivity (2521,7162). Some drugs that cause photosensitivity include

amitriptyline (Elavil), quinolones (Ciprofloxacin, others), sulfa drugs (Septra, Bactrim, others), and tetracycline.
OTHER DRUGS: Theoretically, bishop's weed might inhibit elimination and increase blood levels of drugs metabolized by the cytochrome P450 3A4 (CYP3A4) isoenzyme (7029). The bergapten constituent of bishop's weed is the same constituent as in bitter orange, which inhibits the CYP3A4 metabolism of drugs. Some drugs metabolized by CYP3A4 that might be affected include alprazolam (Xanax), amitriptyline (Elavil), amiodarone (Cordarone), buspirone (Buspar), cerivastatin (Baycol), citalopram (Celexa), felodipine (Plendil), fexofenadine (Allegra), itraconazole (Sporanox), ketoconazole (Nizoral), lansoprazole (Prevacid), losartan (Cozaar), lovastatin (Mevacor), ondansetron (Zofran), prednisone (Deltasone, Orasone), sertraline (Zoloft), sibutramine (Meridia), sildenafil (Viagra), simvastatin (Zocor), verapamil (Calan, Covera-HS, Isoptin), and many others.

Interactions with Foods
No interactions are known to occur, and there is no known reason to expect a clinically significant interaction with bishop's weed.

Interactions with Lab Tests
HIGH-DENSITY LIPOPROTEIN (HDL): Theoretically, bishop's weed might increase HDL levels. The isolated bishop's weed constituent, khellin, seems to increase in HDL levels without affecting total cholesterol or triglycerides (2522).
LIVER FUNCTION TESTS: There is some concern that bishop's weed might increase liver function tests in some patients. It is known that the isolated constituent khellin can increase aspartic acid transaminase (AST) and alanine aminotransferase (ALT, SGPT) (2522). However, this effect has not yet been reported specifically for bishop's weed.

Interactions with Diseases or Conditions
LIVER DISEASE: Theoretically, bishop's weed might exacerbate liver dysfunction in patients with liver disease. The isolated khellin constituent of bishop's weed is known to increase liver enzymes in some patients (2522).

Dosage and Administration
No typical dosage.

Comments
The prescription drug methoxsalen (Oxasoralen, Methoxypsoralen) was originally prepared from bishop's weed, but is now made synthetically (9,15). Bishop's weed is sometimes confused with its more used relative, khella (Ammi visnaga). The two species do have some common chemical constituents and pharmacological effects. Bishop's weed is more commonly used for dermatological conditions, and khella is usually used for cardiac and pulmonary conditions (7161). The isolated active constituent, khellin, is also used medicinally for angina pectoris, asthma, in conjunction with phototherapy for vitiligo, psoriasis, and alopecia areata (9,560,849,868).

BISTORT

Also Known As
Adderwort, Dragonwort, Easter Giant, Easter Mangiant, Oderwort, Osterick, Patience Dock, Red Legs, Snakeweed, Sweet Dock.

Scientific Names
Polygonum bistorta.
Family: Polygonaceae.

People Use This For
Orally, bistort is used for digestive disorders, particularly diarrhea.
Topically, bistort is used for mouth and throat infections, and for wounds (18).

Safety
There is insufficient reliable information available about the safety of bistort.
Pregnancy and Lactation: Insufficient reliable information available; avoid using.

Effectiveness
There is insufficient reliable information available about the effectiveness of bistort.

Mechanism of Action

The applicable parts of bistort are the rhizome and root. Bistort contains 15-21% tannins, which have astringent effects. Tannins work internally by dehydrating mucosal tissue, which reduces secretions. Externally, tannin astringent effects result in a protective layer of constricted, harder cells. Plants with at least 10% tannins can cause gastrointestinal upset, kidney damage, and liver damage. Animal data conflicts with respect to the carcinogenicity of tannins. They may be carcinogenic or may have anti-carcinogenic effects. An increased risk of esophageal or nasal cancer may be linked to people who regularly ingest herbs with high tannin concentrations (12).

Adverse Reactions

None reported.

Interactions with Herbs & Other Dietary Supplements

TANNIN-CONTAINING HERBS: Theoretically, herbs that contain high percentages of tannins, such as bistort, may cause precipitation of constituents of other herbs (19).

Interactions with Drugs

ORAL DRUGS: Theoretically, concomitant use may cause precipitation of some drugs due to the high tannin content of bistort (19). Separate administration of oral drugs and tannin-containing herbs by the longest period of time practical (19).

Interactions with Foods

No interactions are known to occur, and there is no known reason to expect a clinically significant interaction with bistort.

Interactions with Lab Tests

No interactions are known to occur, and there is no known reason to expect a clinically significant interaction with bistort.

Interactions with Diseases or Conditions

No interactions are known to occur, and there is no known reason to expect a clinically significant interaction with bistort.

Dosage and Administration

ORAL: The rhizome and root are powdered and used to make an infusion (18).
TOPICAL: The powdered root is used as an extract or ointment (18).

Comments

None.

BITTER ALMOND

Also Known As

Amygdala Amara, Bitter Almond Oil, Volatile Almond Oil.
CAUTION: See separate listing for Sweet Almond Oil.

Scientific Names

Prunus amygdalus amara, synonym Prunus dulcis amara.
Family: Rosaceae.

People Use This For

Orally, bitter almond is used as an antispasmodic, local anesthetic, and for its narcotic properties (11).
Historically, bitter almond has been used as a cough suppressant and antipruritic (11).

Safety

POSSIBLY SAFE ...when small amounts of HCN-free volatile oil are used orally HCN (hydrocyanic acid) is also known as FFPA (free form prussic acid). When the oil is HCN-free, it is nearly pure benzaldehyde, which has Generally Recognized as Safe (GRAS) status in the US (11).
LIKELY UNSAFE ...when the volatile oil containing HCN is used orally (11,12). ...when large amounts of HCN-free volatile oil are used orally. Ingesting 50-60 mL benzaldehyde can cause fatal CNS depression and respiratory failure (11).

PREGNANCY AND LACTATION: LIKELY UNSAFE ...when the volatile oil containing HCN is used orally (11). There is insufficient reliable information available about the safety of the oral of the HCN-free oil during pregnancy and breast-feeding; avoid using.

Effectiveness

There is insufficient reliable information available about the effectiveness of bitter almond.

Mechanism of Action

The applicable part of bitter almond is the volatile oil. The bitter almond kernel contains 3-4% amygdalin, which is hydrolyzed to poisonous hydrocyanic acid (HCN, prussic acid). The volatile oil contains 95% benzaldehyde and 2-4% HCN. For food and flavor use, HCN is removed. High doses of benzaldehyde can have narcotic properties and the potential for adverse reactions (11).

Adverse Reactions

Orally, 50-60 mL of benzaldehyde (sole constituent of HCN-free oil) can have high toxicity and be fatal due to CNS depression with respiratory failure (11). There is a report of one death of an adult after ingestion of 7.5 mL of the volatile oil (11).

Interactions with Herbs & Other Dietary Supplements

Insufficient reliable information available.

Interactions with Drugs

CNS DEPRESSANTS: Theoretically, bitter almond oil use with CNS depressants increases the risk of severe or fatal CNS and respiratory depression.

Interactions with Foods

No interactions are known to occur, and there is no known reason to expect a clinically significant interaction with bitter almond.

Interactions with Lab Tests

No interactions are known to occur, and there is no known reason to expect a clinically significant interaction with bitter almond.

Interactions with Diseases or Conditions

No interactions are known to occur, and there is no known reason to expect a clinically significant interaction with bitter almond.

Dosage and Administration

No typical dosage.

Comments

The volatile oil of bitter almond contains 95% benzaldehyde and 2-4% poisonous HCN. It is made by water maceration and steam distillation of partially defatted bitter almond (Prunus amygdalus amara), apricot (Prunus armeniaca), peach (Prunus persica), and plum (Prunus domestica) kernels. The fixed almond oil (sweet almond oil) is prepared by pressing the kernels of both sweet almond and bitter almond and contains no benzaldehyde or hydrocyanic acid (HCN). Sweet almond does not yield a volatile oil (11). Bitter almond volatile oil consists of distilled, partially defatted oil of the kernels of bitter almond (Prunus amygdalus amara) and kernels of other Prunus species.

BITTER MELON

Also Known As

African Cucumber, Balsam Pear, Balsam-Apple, Balsambirne, Balsamo, Bitter Apple, Bitter Cucumber, Bitter Gourd, Bittergurke, Carilla Gourd, Chinli-Chih, Cundeamor, Karela, Kuguazi, K'u-Kua, Lai Margose, Momordique, Pepino Montero, P'u-T'ao, Sorosi, Wild Cucumber.

Scientific Names

Momordica charantia, synonym Momordica murcata.
Family: Cucurbitaceae.

People Use This For

Orally, bitter melon is used to treat diabetes and psoriasis, and as supportive therapy for individuals with HIV (1900).

Safety

There is insufficient reliable information available about the safety of bitter melon.
PREGNANCY: LIKELY UNSAFE ...when used orally because the juice can stimulate menstruation and cause abortion (19).
LACTATION: Insufficient reliable information available; avoid using.

Effectiveness

POSSIBLY EFFECTIVE ...when used orally to improve glucose tolerance, and reduce blood sugar and glycosylated hemoglobin in type 2 diabetics (34,35,36).
There is insufficient reliable information available about the effectiveness of bitter melon for its other uses.

Mechanism of Action

The applicable parts of bitter melon are the fruit and seeds. The bitter melon fruit and fruit extracts exhibit hypoglycemic activity in normal and diabetic animal models (3762,3763,3764,3765). Bitter melon contains an insulin-like polypeptide called polypeptide P, plant insulin, or p-insulin. P-insulin has pharmacologic effects similar to bovine insulin with an onset of action between 30 and 60 minutes and a peak effect at about 4 hours. (6,37,38). The constituents alpha- and beta-momorcharin have immunosuppressive activity in vitro and in mice (3724). A protein constituent designated as MAP-30 exhibits antiviral and antitumor activity in human cells in vitro (3720,3721). Bitter melon extracts show antitumor and antileukemia activity in mice (3722,3723).

Adverse Reactions

None reported.

Interactions with Herbs & Other Dietary Supplements

STIMULANT LAXATIVE HERBS: Theoretically, concomitant use of bitter melon with other stimulant laxative herbs can increase the risk of potassium depletion. Stimulant laxative herbs include aloe dried leaf sap, wild cucumber fruit (Ecballium alterium), blue flag rhizome, alder buckthorn, European buckthorn, butternut bark, cascara bark, castor oil, colocynth fruit pulp, gamboge bark exudate, jalap root, black root, manna bark exudate, podophyllum root, rhubarb root, senna leaves and pods, and yellow dock root (19).
POTASSIUM DEPLETING HERBS: Theoretically, concomitant use of bitter melon with horsetail plant or licorice rhizome increases the risk of potassium depletion.
HYPOGLYCEMIC HERBS: Theoretically, concomitant use of bitter melon with other hypoglycemic herbs can have additive effects (19).

Interactions with Drugs

DIABETES THERAPY: Theoretically, concomitant use of bitter melon can enhance hypoglycemic drug effects and alter blood glucose control (19). Monitor blood glucose levels if bitter melon is used.
INSULIN: Insulin dosage adjustments might be necessary due to the hypoglycemic effects of bitter melon (19).
CHLORPROPAMIDE (Diabinese): Concomitant use of bitter melon can cause additive hypoglycemic effects (19).

Interactions with Foods

No interactions are known to occur, and there is no known reason to expect a clinically significant interaction with bitter melon.

Interactions with Lab Tests

BLOOD GLUCOSE: Theoretically, bitter melon can lower blood glucose and test results (19).

Interactions with Diseases or Conditions

DIABETES: Theoretically, bitter melon can alter blood glucose control (19), and blood glucose levels should be monitored with its use.

Dosage and Administration

ORAL: People typically use 1 to 2 grams of powdered leaf in tablets or capsules daily. Bitter melon is also taken as a 4:1 tincture in a dose of 1 to 3 mL twice daily (5255).

Comments

None.

BITTER MILKWORT

Also Known As
European Bitter Polygala, European Senega, Evergreen Snakeroot, Flowering Wintergreen, Little Pollom, Snakeroot. CAUTION: See separate listings for Asarabacca and Senega.

Scientific Names
Polygala amara.

People Use This For
Orally, bitter milkwort is used for upper and lower respiratory disorders, cough, and bronchitis (18).

Safety
There is insufficient reliable information available about the safety of bitter milkwort.
Pregnancy and Lactation: Insufficient reliable information available; avoid using.

Effectiveness
There is insufficient reliable information available about the effectiveness of bitter milkwort.

Mechanism of Action
The applicable parts of bitter milkwort are the flowering plant and root. Bitter milkwort can have mild expectorant properties (18). The active constituents are saponin (senegin), bitter substances, and methylestersalizylic acid (18).

Adverse Reactions
None reported.

Interactions with Herbs & Other Dietary Supplements
Insufficient reliable information available.

Interactions with Drugs
No interactions are known to occur, and there is no known reason to expect a clinically significant interaction with bitter milkwort.

Interactions with Foods
No interactions are known to occur, and there is no known reason to expect a clinically significant interaction with bitter milkwort.

Interactions with Lab Tests
No interactions are known to occur, and there is no known reason to expect a clinically significant interaction with bitter milkwort.

Interactions with Diseases or Conditions
No interactions are known to occur, and there is no known reason to expect a clinically significant interaction with bitter milkwort.

Dosage and Administration
ORAL: People typically prepare a tea, adding 1 teaspoon of the plant to 1 cup of boiling water. This is taken once daily. Four tablespoons of the leaves are also combined with water and boiled for an extended time. This liquid is taken at a dose of 1 tablespoon every 3 hours (5263).

Comments
Avoid confusion with asarabacca (Asarum europaeum) or senega (Polygala senega), also known as snakeroot. There is very little scientific information about this product. Our staff is continually analyzing the available information on natural medicines and will add data here as it becomes available.

BITTER ORANGE

Also Known As

Aurantii Pericarpium, Bitter Orange Flower, Bitter Orange Peel, Green Orange, Kijitsu, Neroli Oil, Seville Orange, Shangzhou Zhiqiao, Sour Orange, Zhi Qiao, Zhi Shi.
CAUTION: See separate listings for Bergamot Oil, Oswego Tea, and Sweet Orange.

Scientific Names

Citrus aurantium, synonyms Citrus aurantium amara, Citrus bergamia, Citrus bigaradia, Citrus vulgaris.
Family: Rutaceae.

People Use This For

Orally, bitter orange peel is used as an appetite stimulant and for dyspepsia (2). Bitter orange fruit and peel are also used orally for weight loss and nasal congestion (4800,6967,6970). The bitter orange flower and its oil are used orally for gastrointestinal (GI) disturbances, duodenal ulcers, constipation, regulating blood lipid levels, lowering blood sugar in diabetes, blood purification, functional disorders of liver and gallbladder, stimulation of the heart and circulation, frost bite, as a sedative for sleep disorders, for kidney and bladder diseases, general feebleness, anemia, imbalances of mineral metabolism, impurities of the skin, and hair loss (2,11,6977).

Topically, bitter orange peel is used for inflammation of the eye lid, conjunctiva, and retina; retinal hemorrhage; exhaustion accompanying colds; headaches; neuralgia; muscular pain; rheumatic discomfort; bruises; phlebitis; and bed sores (2).

In aromatherapy, the essential oil of bitter orange is used topically and by inhalation as an analgesic (7107).

In Chinese medicine, bitter orange peel is used for prolapsed uterus, prolapsed anus or rectum, diarrhea, and blood in the stools (11).

Traditionally, bitter orange peel is used as a tonic, antiflatulent, and for cancer (11).

For food use, the oil is approved as a flavoring agent by the FDA (11,6966).

In manufacturing, the oil is used in pharmaceuticals, cosmetics, and soaps (11).

Safety

LIKELY SAFE ...when used orally in the amounts found in foods (11). Bitter orange has Generally Recognized as Safe (GRAS) status in the US (11).

POSSIBLY SAFE ...when the bitter orange peel is used orally and appropriately for medicinal purposes (2). ...when the essential oil is used topically and by inhalation as aromatherapy (7107).

POSSIBLY UNSAFE ...when the fruit or peel are used orally in high doses. Bitter orange fruit and peel contain the stimulant synephrine. In high doses or when used recreationally in combination with other stimulants such as ephedra, it can cause cardiotoxicity (see Adverse Reactions) (6979,6980).

There is insufficient reliable information available about the safety of bitter orange flower and oil when used orally for medicinal purposes.

CHILDREN: POSSIBLY UNSAFE ...when used orally in high doses. High doses can cause intestinal colic, convulsions, and death (11).

PREGNANCY AND LACTATION: Insufficient reliable information available; avoid using.

Effectiveness

POSSIBLY EFFECTIVE ...when bitter orange oil is used topically for treating tinea corporis, cruris, or pedis (6972). There is insufficient reliable information available about the effectiveness of bitter orange for its other uses.

Mechanism of Action

The applicable parts of bitter orange are the peel, flower, leaf, and fruit. Bitter orange has numerous active constituents and pharmacological effects; however, the amount of each constituent can vary depending on the part of bitter orange plant used. For example, the flavonoid content is higher in the flowers than the leaves (6971). The fruit and peel of bitter orange contain synephrine, a sympathetic alpha-adrenergic agonist similar to phenylephrine (4800,6968). Commercially available bitter orange extracts usually contain from 1-6% synephrine. But some manufacturers boost synephrine content to as much as 30%. Bitter orange preparations are often promoted for weight loss due to purported thermogenic effects (4800). In animal models, synephrine causes weight loss, but also increases cardiovascular toxicity (6969). There is some evidence that bitter orange can cause vasoconstriction and increase mean arterial pressure (MAP), but reduce portal pressure (6975). Bitter orange plus a synthetic preparation of the active components synephrine and N-methyltyramine have been used successfully to treat infectious shock in preliminary research. N-methyltyramine seems to increase blood pressure by increasing norepinephrine release (6978). Bitter orange peel is also commonly used for dyspepsia due to spasmolytic effects. Bitter orange peel might also have anti-inflammatory activity, which might be due to the flavonoids naringin and nobiletin (11,1281). The pectin content of bitter orange might also lower cholesterol levels (11). Bitter orange preparations have a variety of antimicrobial properties. The oil of the bitter orange peel seems to have insecticidal activity (6973). Flavonoids and pectin from the bitter orange peel and from the oil of the flower have antifungal and antibacterial activities in vitro (11). Two active components of the bitter orange fruit, neohesperidin and hesperidin, also seem to have antiviral activity against rotavirus infection (6976). Early research indicates that compounds found in bitter orange, auraptene, marmin, tangeretin, nobiretin, and a psoralen compound, might have antitumor effects (6974). Furocoumarins found in bitter orange peel are thought responsible for photosensitivity (2,11,18). The furocoumarins bergamottin and dihydroxybergamottin in bitter orange fruit and juice can inhibit the cytochrome P450 3A4 (CYP3A4) isoenzyme. These are the same constituents found in grapefruit that are responsible for numerous drug interactions. However, grapefruit juice contains a significantly higher concentration of these constituents than bitter orange juice (7029). Although the bitter orange juice can inhibit CYP3A4, it's not known if commonly used bitter orange extracts contain enough of the furocoumarins to cause a clinically significant interaction.

Adverse Reactions
Case reports and laboratory evidence suggest that bitter orange fruit, which contains synephrine and N-methyltyramine, might cause hypertension and cardiovascular toxicity (6969,6979,6980). Photosensitivity can also occur, especially in fair-skinned people (2). Frequent contact with the peel or oil can cause erythema, blisters, pustules, dermatoses leading to scab formation, and pigment spots (18). The ingestion of large amounts of bitter orange peel in children can cause intestinal colic, convulsions, and death (11).

Interactions with Herbs & Other Dietary Supplements
STIMULANTS: Theoretically, herbs and supplements with stimulant properties, such as caffeine, coffee, cola nut, ephedra, guarana, and mate, might increase the risk of hypertension and adverse cardiovascular effects with bitter orange fruit or peel due to synephrine content (6979,6980).

Interactions with Drugs
ACID-INHIBITING DRUGS: Theoretically, due to reports that bitter orange peel increases stomach acid, it might interfere with antacids, sucralfate (Carafate), H2 antagonists, or proton pump inhibitors (19).
FELODIPINE (Plendil): Consumption of bitter orange juice 240 mL can significantly increase felodipine levels. Bitter orange juice inhibits cytochrome P450 3A4 (CYP3A4) metabolism of felodipine (7029).
MIDAZOLAM (Versed): Bitter orange juice can significantly inhibit cytochrome P450 3A4 (CYP3A4) metabolism of the midazolam, and potentially increase drug levels and adverse effects (7029).
MONOAMINE OXIDASE INHIBITORS (MAOIs): Concurrent use of MAOIs with synephrine containing bitter orange preparations might increase the blood pressure raising effects of synephrine and potentially cause hypertensive crisis. Tell patients taking MAOIs to avoid using synephrine containing bitter orange preparations. Some MAOIs include phenelzine (Nardil), tranylcypromine (Parnate), and others.
SAQUINAVIR (Fortovase, Invirase): Bitter orange juice can significantly inhibit cytochrome P450 3A4 (CYP3A4) metabolism of the protease inhibitor saquinavir, and potentially increase drug levels and adverse effects (7029). So far, this effect has only been shown for saquinavir, but other protease inhibitors are also likely to be affected. Patients taking these medications should avoid taking bitter orange juice. Other protease inhibitors include amprenavir (Agenerase), nelfinavir (Viracept), and ritonavir (Norvir).
STIMULANTS: Theoretically, drugs with CNS stimulant properties, such as phenylpropanolamine, pseudoephedrine, and caffeine might increase the risk of hypertension and adverse cardiovascular effects with bitter orange fruit or peel due to synephrine content (6979,6980).
OTHER DRUGS: Bitter orange juice can inhibit cytochrome P450 3A4 (CYP3A4) metabolism of drugs (7029), causing increased drug levels and potentially increasing the risk of adverse effects. Some of these drugs include calcium channel blockers (diltiazem, nicardipine, verapamil), chemotherapeutic agents (etoposide, paclitaxel, vinblastine, vincristine, vindesine), antifungals (ketoconazole, itraconazole), glucocorticoids, cisapride (Propulsid), losartan (Cozaar), fexofenadine (Allegra), NNRTI-type antiretroviral drugs including nevirapine (Viramune), delavirdine (Rescriptor), efavirenz (Sustiva), and numerous others.

Interactions with Foods
CAFFEINE: Theoretically, large amounts of caffeine-containing beverages might increase the risk of hypertension and adverse cardiovascular effects with bitter orange fruit or peel due to synephrine content (6979,6980).

Interactions with Lab Tests
No interactions are known to occur, and there is no known reason to expect a clinically significant interaction with bitter orange peel.

Interactions with Diseases or Conditions
HYPERTENSION: Theoretically, bitter orange fruit or peel might worsen hypertension due to synephrine content (6979,6980).

Dosage and Administration

ORAL: The typical dose of bitter orange peel is 4-6 grams per day of the dry peel, which is free of the white pulp layer (2). Bitter orange peel can be used as a tea, which is prepared by steeping 2 grams of the peel in 150 mL boiling water for 10-15 minutes and straining. A typical dose of the peel tincture is 2-3 grams per day. For the peel extract a typical dose is 1-2 grams per day (2). As a mild sedative, 1-2 grams of bitter orange flower is commonly used as a tea (8). For weight loss, people typically use bitter orange extract 100 to 200 mg daily in combination with other herbs and supplements (6967). Bitter orange extracts commonly contain from 1.5-6% synephrine (6967,6969).
TOPICAL: For treatment of fungal skin infections, pure oil of bitter orange has been applied once daily for 1 to 3 weeks (6972).

Comments

None.

BITTERSWEET NIGHTSHADE

Also Known As

Bitter Nightshade, Bittersweet, Blue Nightshade, Common Nightshade, Deadly Nightshade, Dulcarara, Fellen, Fellonwood, Felonwort, Fever Twig, Mortal, Scarlet Berry, Snake Berry, Staff Vine, Violet Bloom, Woody, Woody Nightshade.
CAUTION: See separate listings for Belladonna and Henbane.

Scientific Names

Solanum dulcamara.
Family: Solanaceae.

People Use This For

Orally, bittersweet nightshade is used for chronic eczema, itchy skin conditions, acne, furuncles, skin abrasions, and warts.
Topically, bittersweet nightshade is used for chronic eczema.
Historically, bittersweet nightshade has been used as an antirheumatic, diuretic, narcotic, sedative, and for nail bed inflammations (2,6,7,18).

Safety

POSSIBLY SAFE ...when used orally or topically and appropriately (2,18).
LIKELY UNSAFE ...when the leaves or berries are used orally. The plant contains the toxic compounds solanine, solanidine, and dulcamarin (6).
CHILDREN: LIKELY UNSAFE ...when used orally; unripe berries have caused poisonings. A lethal dose is estimated to be 200 berries (18). There is insufficient reliable information available about the safety of the stem used topically in children.
PREGNANCY: LIKELY UNSAFE ...when used orally. The stem, leaf, or berries are contraindicated. The alkaloids of the plant, solasodine, soladulcine, and related compounds have been linked to malformations in animals (6). Some of these constituents might be present in the stem (296). There is insufficient reliable information available about the safety of the topical use of the stem during pregnancy.
LACTATION: LIKELY UNSAFE ...when the leaves or berries are used orally; avoid using. There is insufficient reliable information available about the safety of the oral or topical use of the stem during lactation; avoid using.

Effectiveness

POSSIBLY EFFECTIVE ...when used topically as supportive therapy for chronic eczema (2). ...when used orally for treating itchy skin conditions (2,7).
There is insufficient reliable information available about the effectiveness of bittersweet nightshade for its other uses.

Mechanism of Action

The applicable part of bittersweet nightshade is the stem. It has astringent, antimicrobial, and mucous membrane-irritating actions (2). The steroidal alkaloid constituents of the stem can have anticholinergic effects (2). The component, solasodin, can prevent inflammation (2).

Adverse Reactions

Orally, the bittersweet nightshade plant can cause the symptoms of solanine poisoning, commonly associated with old potatoes. Symptoms include scratchy throat, headache, vertigo, dilated pupils, speech difficulties, subnormal temperature, vomiting, diarrhea, GI bleeding, cyanosis, convulsions, circulatory and respiratory depression, and

even death (6). The ingestion of unripe berries can cause poisoning in children (18).
Topically, there are no reports of adverse effects doe to the low alkaloid content.
In adults, toxicity associated with the stem (2,6,7,18) is uncommon due to the low alkaloid content. There are no reports of adverse effects relating to the topical use of the stem (2,6,7,18).

Interactions with Herbs & Other Dietary Supplements
Insufficient reliable information available.

Interactions with Drugs
No interactions are known to occur, and there is no known reason to expect a clinically significant interaction with bittersweet nightshade.

Interactions with Foods
No interactions are known to occur, and there is no known reason to expect a clinically significant interaction with bittersweet nightshade.

Interactions with Lab Tests
No interactions are known to occur, and there is no known reason to expect a clinically significant interaction with bittersweet nightshade.

Interactions with Diseases or Conditions
GI IRRITATION: Bittersweet nightshade can irritate the gastrointestinal tract. It is contraindicated in individuals with infectious or inflammatory gastrointestinal conditions (19).

Dosage and Administration
ORAL: The typical dose of the bittersweet nightshade stem is 1-3 grams of the dried herb per day, and can be taken as a tea, which is prepared by steeping the herb in 150 mL boiling water for 5-10 minutes and straining (2).
TOPICAL: The stem is used as a compress prepared by steeping 1-2 grams of the dried herb in 250 mL boiling water for 5-10 minutes and straining (2).

Comments
Bittersweet nightshade is a perennial vine-like plant that is found throughout the United States, Canada, and Eurasia and is a member of the same family that includes tomatoes and potatoes.

BLACK ALDER

Also Known As
Betula Alnus, Common Alder, English Alder, European Alder, European Black Alder, Owler.

Scientific Names
Alnus glutinosa.
Family: Betulaceae.

People Use This For
Orally, black alder is used for intestinal bleeding and pharyngitis.
Topically, black alder is used for streptococcal sore throat.

Safety
There is insufficient reliable information available about the safety of black alder.
Pregnancy and Lactation: Insufficient reliable information available; avoid using.

Effectiveness
There is insufficient reliable information about the effectiveness of black alder.

Mechanism of Action
The applicable part of black alder is the bark. There is insufficient reliable information available about the possible mechanism of action and active ingredients.

Adverse Reactions
None reported.

Interactions with Herbs & Other Dietary Supplements
Insufficient reliable information available.

Interactions with Drugs
No interactions are known to occur, and there is no known reason to expect a clinically significant interaction with black alder.

Interactions with Foods
No interactions are known to occur, and there is no known reason to expect a clinically significant interaction with black alder.

Interactions with Lab Tests
No interactions are known to occur, and there is no known reason to expect a clinically significant interaction with black alder.

Interactions with Diseases or Conditions
No interactions are known to occur, and there is no known reason to expect a clinically significant interaction with black alder.

Dosage and Administration
TOPICAL: The bark is prepared as a decoction and used as a gargle (18).

Comments
There is very little scientific information about this product. Our staff is continually analyzing the available information on natural medicines and will add data here as it becomes available.

BLACK BRYONY

Also Known As
Blackeye Root.

Scientific Names
Tamus communis.

People Use This For
Orally, black bryony is used for intestinal mucous membrane irritation and as an emetic (18).
Topically, black bryony is used for agitation and redness of the skin, bruises, strains, torn muscles, gout, rheumatic disorders, hair loss, and improving blood circulation to the scalp (18).

Safety
POSSIBLY UNSAFE ...when the fresh root is used topically. Skin contact can cause severe skin irritation (18).
UNSAFE ...when used orally. It can cause seizures, respiratory and kidney failure (18).
PREGNANCY AND LACTATION: POSSIBLY UNSAFE ...when used topically; avoid using (18). UNSAFE ...when used orally.

Effectiveness
There is insufficient reliable information available about the effectiveness of black bryony.

Mechanism of Action
The applicable part of black bryony is the root. It can stimulate external nerve endings. Applied topically, it acts as a mechanical irritant, penetrating the skin with tiny, needle-like crystals of calcium oxalate (3829). The rhizome contains histamine (3829), which can have a role in producing skin irritation (3829). In rats, an ethanolic extract of the root exhibited local anti-inflammatory activity (3828).

Adverse Reactions
Orally, black bryony can cause severe mouth, pharyngeal and GI irritation, as well as vomiting, diarrhea, spasms, colic, decreased kidney function, and respiratory depression (18).
Topically, the fresh root can cause reddening of skin (18). The fresh plant used topically can cause skin irritation, rash, swelling, pustules, wheals, and mucous membrane irritation (18).

Interactions with Herbs & Other Dietary Supplements
Insufficient reliable information available.

Interactions with Drugs
No interactions are known to occur, and there is no known reason to expect a clinically significant interaction with black bryony.

Interactions with Foods
No interactions are known to occur, and there is no known reason to expect a clinically significant interaction with black bryony.

Interactions with Lab Tests
No interactions are known to occur, and there is no known reason to expect a clinically significant interaction with black bryony.

Interactions with Diseases or Conditions
No interactions are known to occur, and there is no known reason to expect a clinically significant interaction with black bryony.

Dosage and Administration
ORAL: People typically use 1 to 5 drops of the tincture.
TOPICAL: The fresh root is scraped and the pulp rubbed into affected areas (5264,5267).

Comments
None.

BLACK COHOSH

Also Known As
Baneberry, Black Snakeroot, Bugbane, Bugwort, Cimicifuga, Cimicifuga racemosa, Phytoestrogen, Rattle Root, Rattle Snakeroot, Rattlesnake Root, Rattleweed, Squawroot.
CAUTION: See separate listings for Blue Cohosh and White Cohosh.

Scientific Names
Cimicifuga racemosa, Actaea racemosa, Actaea macrotys.
Family: Ranunculaceae.

People Use This For
Orally, black cohosh is used for symptoms of menopausal (3382,4614), inducing labor in pregnant women (1122), premenstrual syndrome (PMS), dysmenorrhea, nervous tension (3382), dyspepsia, rheumatism, fever, sore throat, cough, as an insect repellent, and as a mild sedative (3382,4611).
Topically, the fresh root is used for rattlesnake bites (4621).

Safety
LIKELY SAFE ...when used orally and appropriately. Black cohosh has been safely used in studies lasting up to 6 months (141,4614,4620,7054).
PREGNANCY: POSSIBLY SAFE ...when used orally in pregnant women at term. Midwives commonly use black cohosh for labor induction in pregnant women at term. This practice does not appear to adversely affect the mother or fetus (1122). However, black cohosh should not be used without the supervision of a health care professional.
LIKELY UNSAFE ...when used orally in pregnant women who are not at term. Black cohosh has menstrual and uterine stimulant effects, which can increase the risk of miscarriage (3382); contraindicated.
LACTATION: POSSIBLY UNSAFE ...when used orally. There is some concern that black cohosh, particularly in large doses, may adversely effect a nursing child (3382). Until more is known, tell nursing mothers to avoid taking black cohosh.

Effectiveness
POSSIBLY EFFECTIVE ...when taken orally for symptoms of menopause. Black cohosh seems to significantly reduce symptoms of menopause, such as hot flashes, in perimenopausal women. There is some evidence it can be as effective as estrogen replacement for some patients. Treatment for 4 weeks is usually required before there is significant improvement in symptoms (141,4611,4614,4620).

Most clinical studies on the effectiveness of black cohosh have used a specific black cohosh formulation standardized to contain 1 mg triterpene glycosides, calculated as 27-deoxyacetin (Remifemin, GlaxoSmithKline).
POSSIBLY INEFFECTIVE ...when used orally for hot flashes in women with a history of breast cancer. Taking black cohosh for 2 months does not seem to significantly reduce frequency or intensity of hot flashes in breast cancer survivors (7054).
There is insufficient reliable information available about the effectiveness of black cohosh for its other uses.

Mechanism of Action

The applicable parts of black cohosh are the rhizome and root. Black cohosh contains phytosterin; isoferulic acid; salicylic acid; sugars; tannins; long-chain fatty acids; and triterpene glycosides, including acetin, cimicifugoside, and 27-deoxyacetin (4611). The presence of an isoflavone, formononetin, is questionable (1122,4611,4616). Earlier reports of isoflavone content may have been a result of contamination with other similar plant species (4615). Laboratory evidence of estrogenic activity has been conflicting (4618,4619). A black cohosh extract competitively inhibits estradiol binding to estrogen receptors (6180). It also increases uterine weight and increases serum ceruloplasmin oxidase activity (a measure of estrogenic activity in the liver) in female rats with their ovaries removed (6180). The mechanism of action of black cohosh remains unknown. Some clinical evidence suggests that black cohosh suppresses LH secretion, while a more recent study showed no change in LH, FSH, sex hormone-binding globulin (SHBG) prolactin, and estradiol in postmenopausal women (512,4611,4614). Unidentified compounds acting synergistically may be responsible for the pharmacological effect of black cohosh (512). Whether black cohosh has an estrogen-like beneficial effect on osteoporosis and cardiovascular disease is unknown. Concomitant use with hormone replacement therapy has not been studied. Some authors have suggested that black cohosh can be safely used in women with a history of breast cancer, citing laboratory evidence that black cohosh does not stimulate the proliferation of estrogen receptor-positive breast cancer cells (4611,4616,4621). Large-scale epidemiological studies looking retrospectively at the association of black cohosh with breast cancer have not been performed.

Adverse Reactions

Orally, black cohosh can commonly cause gastrointestinal upset (3382,4615,4616). Other potential adverse effects include headache, dizziness, weight gain, feeling of heaviness in the legs, and cramping (3382,4621,7054). Some patients taking tamoxifen plus black cohosh have experienced endometrial hyperplasia and vaginal bleeding. However, these effects are more likely due to tamoxifen than black cohosh (7054). An overdose of black cohosh can cause nausea, vomiting, nervous system and visual disturbances, reduced heart rate (bradycardia), and perspiration (4). There is one case report of nocturnal seizures in a woman who used black cohosh, evening primrose oil, and chasteberry (588). There has been a case report of severe complications, including seizures, renal failure and respiratory distress, in an infant whose mother was given an unknown dose of black and blue cohosh at 42 weeks gestation to induce labor (1122). However, this adverse effect may have been attributable to blue cohosh. Studies on black cohosh mutagenicity, teratogenicity, and carcinogenicity have been negative (4611,4615).

Interactions with Herbs & Other Dietary Supplements

Insufficient reliable information.

Interactions with Drugs

No interactions are known to occur, and there is no known reason to expect a clinically significant interaction with black cohosh.

Interactions with Foods

No interactions are known to occur, and there is no known reason to expect a clinically significant interaction with black cohosh.

Interactions with Lab Tests

LUTEINIZING HORMONE (LH): Black cohosh might reduce serum LH concentrations and test results (1331).

Interactions with Diseases or Conditions

HORMONE SENSITIVE CANCERS/CONDITIONS: Because black cohosh seems to have estrogenic effects (6180), women with hormone sensitive conditions should avoid black cohosh. Some of these conditions include breast, uterine, and ovarian cancer; endometriosis; and uterine fibroids.

Dosage and Administration

ORAL: The usual dose of black cohosh is 300-2000 mg of the dried rhizome or root three times daily. A decoction can also be taken three times daily and is prepared by bringing the dried rhizome or root to a boil in water, simmering for 5-10 minutes, and straining (4). The typical dose of the liquid extract (1:1 in 90% alcohol) is 0.3-2.0 mL (4). Tincture of black cohosh (1:10 in 60% alcohol) is usually taken in a dose of 2-4 mL (4). For menopause and premenstrual syndrome (PMS), clinical studies have used a specific black cohosh extract (Remifemin, Enzymatic Therapy and Phytopharmica) standardized to contain 1 mg triterpene glycosides, calculated as 27-deoxyacetin, per 20 mg tablet. Most studies used doses of 40-80 mg twice daily, providing 4-8 mg triterpene glycosides. The manufacturer now claims that improvement in the extraction process permits using their currently recommended lower dose of 20 mg twice daily, providing 2 mg triterpene glycosides (4615).

Comments

Black cohosh was first used medicinally by native Americans who introduced it to European colonists (4611). It was introduced into Germany in the late 19th century (2). Remifemin, a branded black cohosh product, has been used in Germany since the mid-1950s to manage menopause (141). Black cohosh was also used as the main ingredient in Lydia Pinkham's Vegetable Compound (3382).

The genus name of black cohosh, cimicifuga, comes from the Latin words for "bedbug" and "repel". Although less fragrant than other species of the genus, black cohosh was used as an insect repellent, hence the common name "bugbane". Do not confuse black cohosh with two unrelated plants, blue cohosh and white cohosh.

BLACK CURRANT berry

Also Known As
Blackcurrant, Cassis.
CAUTION: See separate listing for Black Currant Seed Oil, and Black Currant leaf.

Scientific Names
Ribes nigrum.
Family: Grossulariaceae.

People Use This For
Orally, black currant berry is used for coughs.
For food uses, it is utilized as a flavor component in liqueurs and as a food (513).

Safety
LIKELY SAFE …when consumed as food or flavoring (513). …when used orally in medicinal amounts (12).
PREGNANCY AND LACTATION: LIKELY SAFE …when used orally (12).

Effectiveness
There is insufficient reliable information available about the effectiveness of black currant berry.

Mechanism of Action
Insufficient reliable information available.

Adverse Reactions
None reported.

Interactions with Herbs & Other Dietary Supplements
Insufficient reliable information available.

Interactions with Drugs
No interactions are known to occur, and there is no known reason to expect a clinically significant interaction with black currant berry.

Interactions with Foods
No interactions are known to occur, and there is no known reason to expect a clinically significant interaction with black currant berry.

Interactions with Lab Tests
No interactions are known to occur, and there is no known reason to expect a clinically significant interaction with black currant berry.

Interactions with Diseases or Conditions
No interactions are known to occur, and there is no known reason to expect a clinically significant interaction with black currant berry.

Dosage and Administration

No typical dosage.

Comments

There is very little scientific information about this product. Our staff is continually analyzing the available information on natural medicines and will add data here as it becomes available.

BLACK CURRANT dried leaf

Also Known As

Ribes nigri folium.
CAUTION: See separate listing for Black Currant Seed Oil and Black Currant berry.

Scientific Names

Ribes nigrum.
Family: Grossulariaceae.

People Use This For

Orally, black currant dried leaf is used for arthritis, gout, rheumatism, diarrhea, colic, hepatitis, liver ailments, convulsions, and inflammatory disorders of the mouth and throat (18). It is also used for coughs and colds, whooping cough (18), disinfecting the urine (7), promoting diuresis, treating bladder stones (7,18), and as a cleansing tea (18). Topically, black currant dried leaf is used for the treatment of wounds and insect bites (18).

Safety

There is insufficient reliable information available about the safety of black currant dried leaf.
Pregnancy and Lactation: Insufficient reliable information available; avoid using.

Effectiveness

There is insufficient reliable information available about the effectiveness of black currant dried leaf.

Mechanism of Action

Black currant leaves can have diuretic, hypotensive, and cooling effects (18). The leaves of black currant contain flavonoids, including astragalin, isoquercitrin, and rutin. The volatile oil contains trace amounts of ascorbic acid (18).

Adverse Reactions

None reported.

Interactions with Herbs & Other Dietary Supplements

Insufficient reliable information available.

Interactions with Drugs

No interactions are known to occur, and there is no known reason to expect a clinically significant interaction with black currant dried leaf.

Interactions with Foods

No interactions are known to occur, and there is no known reason to expect a clinically significant interaction with black currant dried leaf.

Interactions with Lab Tests

No interactions are known to occur, and there is no known reason to expect a clinically significant interaction with black currant dried leaf.

Interactions with Diseases or Conditions

CARDIAC DISORDERS: Avoid the use of black currant in individuals with edema associated with reduced cardiac function (18).
KIDNEY DISORDERS: Avoid its use in individuals with edema associated with reduced kidney function (18).

Dosage and Administration

ORAL: The typical dose of black currant is 3-4 cups of the tea daily. The tea is prepared by adding 1-2 teaspoons or 2-4 grams of the black currant leaves to 150 mL of boiling water for ten minutes and then straining (18).

TOPICAL: Black currant is commonly applied to wounds as a compress, which is made using the freshly grated leaves or leaves soaked in warm water and dried (18). The freshly grated leaves are also rubbed onto insect bites (18).

Comments
None.

BLACK CURRANT SEED OIL

Also Known As
European Black Currant, European Blackcurrant, Casis, Cassis, Ribes Nero.
CAUTION: See separate listings for Borage Seed Oil, Black Currant berry, Black Currant dried leaf, Evening Primrose Oil, Gamma Linolenic Acid, and Omega-6 Oils.

Scientific Names
Ribes nigrum.
Family: Grossulariaceae.

People Use This For
Orally, black currant seed oil is used for menopause symptoms, premenstrual syndrome, dysmenorrhea, mastodynia (512,515), and for boosting immunity (4016).

Safety
POSSIBLY SAFE ...when used orally to boost immunity in the elderly (4016).
There is insufficient reliable information available about the safety of black currant seed oil for its other uses.
PREGNANCY AND LACTATION: Insufficient reliable information available; avoid using.

Effectiveness
POSSIBLY EFFECTIVE ...when used orally for increasing immunity in the elderly (4016).
There is insufficient reliable information available about the effectiveness of black currant seed oil for its other uses.

Mechanism of Action
Black currant seed oil contains 6-19% gamma-linolenic acid (GLA) (512,515). Researchers think it may be beneficial in people unable to metabolize cis-linolenic acid to GLA and produce adequate prostaglandin E1 (PGE1). People with this condition have an imbalance in the ratio of inflammatory to noninflammatory prostaglandins. GLA is thought to improve this ratio (512,4016) and researchers think this is why black currant seed oil increases immune response in elderly people (4016).

Adverse Reactions
None reported.

Interactions with Herbs & Other Dietary Supplements
Insufficient reliable information available.

Interactions with Drugs
No interactions are known to occur, and there is no known reason to expect a clinically significant interaction with black currant seed oil.

Interactions with Foods
No interactions are known to occur, and there is no known reason to expect a clinically significant interaction with black currant seed oil.

Interactions with Lab Tests
No interactions are known to occur, and there is no known reason to expect a clinically significant interaction with black currant seed oil.

Interactions with Diseases or Conditions
No interactions are known to occur, and there is no known reason to expect a clinically significant interaction with black currant seed oil.

Dosage and Administration

ORAL: People typically use 500-1000 mg black currant oil daily. A 500 mg capsule is typically labeled to contain about 230 mg cis-linoleic acid, 85 mg cis-gamma-linoleic acid, 65 mg alpha-linoleic acid, and 15 mg stearidonic acid (6006). A dose of 4500 mg per day was used to boost immunity in the elderly in a clinical study (4016).

Comments

Black currant seed oil is the fixed oil obtained from seeds of the black currant (Ribes nigrum). Avoid confusion with black currant berry.

BLACK HAW

Also Known As

Blackhaw, Southern Black Haw, Stag Bush, Viburnum.

Scientific Names

Viburnum prunifolium; Viburnum prunifolium ferrugineum, synonym Viburnum rufidulum.
Family: Caprifoliaceae.

People Use This For

Orally, the root bark and extracts of black haw are used as a tonic, uterine sedative, antidiarrheal, diuretic, and antispasmodic (11).
Traditionally, black haw has been used for painful menses, preventing miscarriage, asthma, and as a postpartum antispasmodic (11).

Safety

LIKELY SAFE …when the stem bark is used orally in food amounts. It is approved for food use in the US. The maximum level used is 0.001% (11).
POSSIBLY SAFE …when the root bark is used orally and appropriately in medicinal amounts (12).
PREGNANCY: POSSIBLY UNSAFE …when used orally. Some evidence suggests black haw has uterine relaxant effects (11); avoid using.
LACTATION: Insufficient reliable information available.

Effectiveness

POSSIBLY EFFECTIVE …when used orally as an uterine antispasmodic (11,142).
There is insufficient reliable information available about the effectiveness of black haw for its other uses.

Mechanism of Action

The applicable parts of black haw are the root bark and stem bark. The root bark contains several active constituents, including scopoletin, tannins, oxalic acid, salicin and salicylic acid (11,296). Scopoletin is thought to be a uterine relaxant (11).

Adverse Reactions

None reported.

Interactions with Herbs & Other Dietary Supplements

CALCIUM, IRON, ZINC: Concurrent use might decrease mineral absorption. Black haw contains oxalic acid (oxalate) (11,296), which can bind multivalent metal ions in the gastrointestinal tract and decrease mineral absorption.

Interactions with Drugs

No interactions are known to occur, and there is no known reason to expect a clinically significant interaction with black haw.

Interactions with Foods

CALCIUM, IRON, ZINC: Concurrent use might decrease mineral absorption from foods. Black haw contains oxalic acid (oxalate) (11,296), which can bind multivalent metal ions in the gastrointestinal tract and decrease mineral absorption.

Interactions with Lab Tests

No interactions are known to occur, and there is no known reason to expect a clinically significant interaction with black haw.

Interactions with Diseases or Conditions

HISTORY OF KIDNEY STONES: Avoid the use of black haw because it contains oxalic acid and might increase stone formation in individuals with a history of kidney stones (11,12).

ASPIRIN ALLERGY: Theoretically, the salicylate constituents in black haw could trigger allergic reaction in individuals with aspirin allergy or asthma.

Dosage and Administration

ORAL: People typically use 2 teaspoons of the dried bark in 1 cup of water, boiled and simmered for 10 minutes. This is taken three times daily. In tincture form, black haw is taken 5 to 10 mL three times daily (5253).

Comments

Black haw is a shrub that has serrated oval leaves, clusters of white flowers, and blue-black berries. It is native to the woodlands of central and southern North America (4201).

BLACK HELLEBORE

Also Known As

Christe Herbe, Christmas Rose, Christmas Rose Plant, Melampode.
CAUTION: See separate listings for American Hellebore, Pheasant's Eye, and White Hellebore.

Scientific Names

Helleborus niger.
Family: Ranunculaceae.

People Use This For

In folk medicine, black hellebore is used for nausea, worm infestations, regulating menstruation, acute nephritis, head colds, as a laxative, and as an abortifacient (18).

Safety

LIKELY UNSAFE ...when used orally. Black hellebore contains cardiac glycosides with structure, activity, and adverse effects similar to digitalis (3).

PREGNANCY: LIKELY UNSAFE ...when used orally because it can have menstrual stimulant (19) or abortifacient effects (18); avoid using.

LACTATION: LIKELY UNSAFE ...when used orally; avoid using.

Effectiveness

There is insufficient reliable information available about the effectiveness of black hellebore.

Mechanism of Action

Black hellebore root contains cardioactive glycosides with digitalis-like effects (18). It also contains saponins that irritate mucous membranes and can cause toxicity (18). Black hellebore is a GI irritant (19), and the fresh plant has local irritant properties (19).

Adverse Reactions

Oral use of black hellebore can cause GI irritation (19). The symptoms of poisoning from black hellebore include scratchy throat or mouth, salivation, nausea, vomiting, diarrhea, dizziness, shortness of breath, spasm, and asphyxiation (18). Topically, the fresh plant may cause irritation or inflammation when handled (19).

Interactions with Herbs & Other Dietary Supplements

CARDIAC GLYCOSIDE-CONTAINING HERBS: Contraindicated; concomitant use can increase the risk of cardiac glycoside toxicity. Cardiac glycoside-containing herbs, including black hellebore, Canadian hemp roots, digitalis leaf, hedge mustard, figwort, lily of the valley roots, motherwort, oleander leaf, pheasant's eye plant, pleurisy root, squill bulb leaf scales, and strophanthus seeds (2,18,19,500).

OTHER CARDIOACTIVE HERBS: Avoid concomitant use with other cardioactive herbs due to unpredictability of effects and adverse effects. Other cardioactive herbs include: calamus, cereus, cola, coltsfoot, devil's claw, European mistletoe, fenugreek, fumitory, ginger, Panax ginseng, hawthorn, white horehound, mate, parsley, quassia, scotch broom flower, shepherd's purse, and wild carrot (4).

STIMULANT LAXATIVE HERBS: Theoretically, overuse or misuse of stimulant laxatives with cardiac glycoside-containing herbs increases the risk of cardiac toxicity due to potassium depletion. Stimulant laxative herbs include aloe dried leaf sap, blue flag rhizome, alder buckthorn, European buckthorn, butternut bark, cascara bark, castor oil, colocynth fruit pulp, gamboge bark exudate, jalap root, black root, manna bark exudate, podophyllum root, rhubarb root, senna leaves and pods, wild cucumber fruit (Ecballium elaterium), and yellow dock root (19).

LICORICE/HORSETAIL: Theoretically, overuse/misuse of licorice rhizome or horsetail plant with cardiac glycoside-containing herbs increases the risk of toxicity due to potassium depletion (19).

Interactions with Drugs

DIGOXIN: Contraindicated; therapeutic duplication increases risk of cardiac glycoside toxicity (2).

CARDIAC DRUGS: Theoretically, concomitant use can increase the risk of cardiac toxicity (152).

STIMULANT LAXATIVES: Theoretically, overuse/misuse can increase risk of cardiac glycoside toxicity due to potassium depletion (2,506).

POTASSIUM DEPLETING DIURETICS, QUININE: Can increase the risk of digitalis toxicity (2,506).

QUININE: Theoretically, concomitant use can increase risk of cardiac toxicity (2,506).

TETRACYCLINES and MACROLIDE ANTIBIOTICS (erythromycin-like drugs): Theoretically, concomitant use might increase risk of cardiac glycoside toxicity (152,17).

Interactions with Foods

No interactions are known to occur, and there is no known reason to expect a clinically significant interaction with black hellebore.

Interactions with Lab Tests

No interactions are known to occur, and there is no known reason to expect a clinically significant interaction with black hellebore.

Interactions with Diseases or Conditions

GI INFLAMMATION: Because black hellebore can aggravate GI inflammation, its use is contraindicated (19).

HEART DISEASE: Self-use contraindicated; requires diagnosis, treatment, and monitoring (515).

Dosage and Administration

No typical dosage.

Comments

Black hellebore is likely unsafe for self-use (3). Avoid confusion with white hellebore (Veratrum album). Black hellebore is an obsolete and dangerous natural product (18).

BLACK HOREHOUND

Also Known As

Ballota, Black Stinking Horehound.
CAUTION: See separate listing for White Horehound.

Scientific Names

Ballota nigra.
Family: Labiatae or Lamiaceae.

People Use This For

Orally, black horehound is used for nausea, vomiting, sedation in hysteria and hypochondria (4,18), increasing bile flow, whooping cough, and as an antispasmodic (18). It is used in France for symptomatic relief of nervous disorders in adults and children, especially mild sleep disorders, and for cough (18).

Topically, black horehound is used as a mild astringent (4) and for gout (18).

Traditionally, black horehound has been used for nervous dyspepsia (4,18).

Other uses include rectal enemas against ascaridae, or intestinal worms (18).

Safety

POSSIBLY SAFE ...when the above ground parts are used orally and appropriately in medicinal amounts (12). There is insufficient reliable information available about the safety of the topical use of black horehound.

PREGNANCY: LIKELY UNSAFE ...when used orally because it is believed to affect the menstrual cycle (4). There is insufficient reliable information available about the safety of black horehound used topically during pregnancy.

LACTATION: Insufficient reliable information available; avoid using.

Effectiveness
There is insufficient reliable information available about the effectiveness of black horehound.

Mechanism of Action
The applicable parts of black horehound are the above ground parts. Chemicals isolated from black horehound include flavonoids (apigenin-7-glucoside, vicenin-2, tangeretin), diterpenoids (ballotinone, ballonigrine, 7-alpha-acetoxymarrubiin, ballotenol, preleosibirin, 13-hydroxyballonigrinolide), and phenylpropanoids (caffeoyl-L-malic acid, verbascoside, forsythoside B, arenarioside, ballotetroside, alyssonoside, lavandulifolioside, angoroside A). In vitro studies indicate that caffeoyl-L-malic acid, verbascoside, forsythoside B, and arenarioside are able to bind to dopaminergic D2, benzodiazepine and morphine (mu) receptors. Verbascoside, forsythoside B, caffeoyl-L-malic acid, arenarioside, and ballotetroside (in order of decreasing potency) also have antioxidant properties, as demonstrated by scavenging of reactive oxygen species and reducing their release from polymorphonuclear neutrophils in vitro (5880). Black horehound also has antiemetic (4,18), sedative, mild astringent (4), antispasmodic, and stimulant effects (18). Preliminary evidence shows that the aqueous extracts of black horehound can reduce arterial blood pressure and heart rate and increase gallbladder secretions (18).

Adverse Reactions
None reported.

Interactions with Herbs & Other Dietary Supplements
Insufficient reliable information available.

Interactions with Drugs
DOPAMINE AGONISTS: Theoretically, black horehound might have additive effects when used with dopamine agonists. Some constituents of black horehound bind to dopamine D2 receptors in vitro (5880); however, this has not yet been reported in humans. Some dopamine agonists include bromocriptine (Parlodel), levodopa (Dopar, component of Sinemet), pramipexole (Mirapex), ropinirole (Requip), and others.

Interactions with Foods
No interactions are known to occur, and there is no known reason to expect a clinically significant interaction with black horehound.

Interactions with Lab Tests
No interactions are known to occur, and there is no known reason to expect a clinically significant interaction with black horehound.

Interactions with Diseases or Conditions
PARKINSON'S DISEASE: Theoretically, black horehound might affect therapy for Parkinson's disease. Some constituents of black horehound bind to dopamine D2 receptors in vitro (5880); however, this has not yet been reported in humans.
SCHIZOPHRENIA, PSYCHOTIC DISORDERS: Theoretically, black horehound might adversely effect people with schizophrenia and psychotic disorders. Some constituents of black horehound bind to dopamine D2 receptors in vitro (5880); however, this has not yet been reported in humans.

Dosage and Administration
ORAL: The typical dose of black horehound is 2-4 grams of its above ground parts or one cup of the tea three times daily (4). The tea is prepared by steeping 2-4 grams of the above ground parts in 150 mL boiling water for 10-15 minutes and then straining. The usual dose of the liquid extract (1:1 in 25% alcohol) is 1-3 mL three times daily (4). The common dose of the tincture (1:10 in 45% alcohol) is 1-2 mL three times daily (4).
TOPICAL: No typical dosage.

Comments
Avoid confusion with white horehound.

BLACK MULBERRY

Also Known As
Mulberry, Purple Mulberry, White Mulberry.

Scientific Names
Morus nigra.

People Use This For
Orally, black mulberry is taken as a laxative and for chronic rhinitis (18).

Safety
There is insufficient reliable information available about the safety of black mulberry.
Pregnancy and Lactation: Insufficient reliable information available; avoid using.

Effectiveness
There is insufficient reliable information available about the effectiveness of black mulberry.

Mechanism of Action
The applicable parts of black mulberry are the ripe berry and root bark. The fruit contains small amounts of vitamin C (0.17%), rutin, and pectin (18). The pectin may have laxative activity (7).

Adverse Reactions
None reported.

Interactions with Herbs & Other Dietary Supplements
Insufficient reliable information available.

Interactions with Drugs
DIABETES THERAPY: Monitor blood glucose level closely due to claims that some species of mulberry leaves have hypoglycemic effects (19).

Interactions with Foods
No interactions are known to occur, and there is no known reason to expect a clinically significant interaction with black mulberry.

Interactions with Lab Tests
No interactions are known to occur, and there is no known reason to expect a clinically significant interaction with black mulberry.

Interactions with Diseases or Conditions
No interactions are known to occur, and there is no known reason to expect a clinically significant interaction with black mulberry.

Dosage and Administration
ORAL: The average amount used daily is 2-4 mL of syrup (18).

Comments
None.

BLACK MUSTARD oil

Also Known As
Mustard Oil.
CAUTION: See separate listings for Black Mustard seed, Hedge Mustard, and White Mustard.

Scientific Names
Brassica nigra.
Family: Brassicaceae.

People Use This For
Topically, black mustard oil is used for symptoms of the common cold including pulmonary congestion (11), rheumatism and arthritis, as a counterirritant (3,272), and in footbaths for aching feet (6).
In foods and beverages, black mustard oil is used as a flavoiring agent.
In manufacturing, it is used as a lubricant and illuminant in soap and an ingredient in cat and dog repellents (11).

Safety

LIKELY SAFE ...when used orally in the amounts commonly found in foods (11,12). The average maximum level should not exceed 0.02% (11).

POSSIBLY SAFE ...when used topically in concentrations of 0.5-5% applied 3-4 times daily (3,272).

LIKELY UNSAFE ...when used orally, undiluted. Black mustard oil is an extremely powerful topical irritant and ingesting large amounts can cause irritant poisoning (12). ...when inhaled (11).

CHILDREN: LIKELY UNSAFE ...when used orally; contraindicated in children under 6 years of age (12,19). There is insufficient reliable information available about the safety of the topical use in children.

PREGNANCY: LIKELY UNSAFE ...when used orally. Black mustard oil is contraindicated because it might have abortifacient and menstrual stimulant effects (19). There is insufficient reliable information available about the safety of topical use during pregnancy; avoid using.

LACTATION: Insufficient reliable information available; avoid using.

Effectiveness

LIKELY EFFECTIVE ...when used topically as a counterirritant if applied in concentrations ranging from 0.5-5% (3,272).

There is insufficient reliable information available about the effectiveness of black mustard oil for its other uses.

Mechanism of Action

Black mustard oil consists mainly of allyl isothiocyanate, which is produced after the glucosinolate sinigrin is hydrolyzed and distilled (3,6,11). The allyl isothiocyanate of black mustard oil has strong antimicrobial (bacterial and fungi) properties (11), lacrimatory effects, and can act as a counterirritant when diluted (1:50) (6,11). Black mustard oil has powerful irritant properties that can cause pain and increased inflammation of the skin (6,11).

Adverse Reactions

Orally, large amounts of black mustard oil can lead to vomiting, stomach pain, diarrhea, somnolence, cardiac failure, breathing difficulties, coma, and possibly death (18). Rarely, black mustard oil exacerbates stomach and intestinal ulcers (18,19) and causes kidney irritation (19). The isothiocyanate constituents can cause endemic goiters (6,11). Topically, the oil can cause skin blistering and necroses (6,11), and can rarely cause contact allergies (18).

Interactions with Herbs & Other Dietary Supplements

Insufficient reliable information available.

Interactions with Drugs

ACID-INHIBITING DRUGS: Theoretically, due to claims that black mustard oil increases stomach acid, it might interfere with antacids, sucralfate (Carafate), H-2 antagonists, or proton pump inhibitors (19).

Interactions with Foods

No interactions are known to occur, and there is no known reason to expect a clinically significant interaction with black mustard oil.

Interactions with Lab Tests

No interactions are known to occur, and there is no known reason to expect a clinically significant interaction with black mustard oil.

Interactions with Diseases or Conditions

GASTROINTESTINAL ULCERS: Black mustard oil can exacerbate stomach and intestinal ulcers by irritating the mucus membranes (19).

Dosage and Administration

TOPICAL: As a counterirritant, black mustard oil is typically used in concentrations from 0.5-5% and as frequently as 3-4 times daily (3,272).

Comments

Avoid confusion with black mustard, hedge mustard, white mustard (Brassica alba or Sinapis alba), brown mustard (Brassica juncea), Indian mustard (Brassica juncea), and Chinese mustard (Sinapis juncea). Derivatives of mustard oil (allyl isothiocyanate) have formed the basis for toxic agents such as the "mustard gases" and antineoplastic agents (11). The volatile oil of mustard is prepared by steam distillation from brown or black mustard after expressing the fixed oil and macerating in water to allow hydrolysis of sinigrin by enzyme myrosin. The volatile oil mainly consists of allyl isothiocyanate.

BLACK MUSTARD seed

Also Known As
Mustard.
CAUTION: See separate listings for Black Mustard oil, Hedge Mustard, and White Mustard.

Scientific Names
Brassica nigra.
Family: Brassicaceae.

People Use This For
Topically, black mustard seed is used as a poultice for bronchial pneumonia, pleurisy (18), arthritis, lumbago, and aching feet (11). It is also used topically for rheumatism (11,18) and as a counterirritant (3).
Traditionally, black mustard seed has been used as an emetic, diuretic, and appetite stimulant (6,11).
For food uses, black mustard seed is a flavoring agent in condiments, foods, and beverages (6,11); and is a culinary spice (6).

Safety
LIKELY SAFE ...when used orally in the amounts commonly found in foods (11,12). Black mustard seed has Generally Recognized as Safe (GRAS) status in the US (3,11).
POSSIBLY SAFE ...when used topically and appropriately for less than 2 weeks (18).
LIKELY UNSAFE ...when used orally as an emetic. Black mustard seed is an irritant and when used as an emetic, it re-exposes the esophageal tissue to its corrosive effects (19). Ingesting a large amount can cause irritant poisoning (12). ...when pure mustard powder is applied topically for more than 15-30 minutes, it can cause severe burns (12). ...when it is used topically for more than 2 weeks (18).
CHILDREN: LIKELY UNSAFE ...when used orally; contraindicated for use in children under 6 years of age (12,19). There is insufficient reliable information available about the safety of the topical use of black mustard seed in children.
PREGNANCY: LIKELY UNSAFE ...when used orally because it might have abortifacient and menstrual stimulant effects (19). There is insufficient reliable information available about the safety of the topical use of black mustard seed during pregnancy; avoid using.
LACTATION: Insufficient reliable information available; avoid using.

Effectiveness
There is insufficient reliable information available about the effectiveness of black mustard seed.

Mechanism of Action
Black mustard powder contains the glucosinolate sinigrin, which produces allyl isothiocyanate when mixed with warm water (3,6,11,18). Allyl isothiocyanate has strong antimicrobial (bacterial and fungi) properties (11), lacrimatory effects, and can act as a counterirritant when diluted (1:50) (6,11). Mustard oil (produced from powder by hydrolysis) is absorbed through the skin and eliminated through the lungs. This could explain its inclusion in liniment preparations to treat lung congestion (11). Black mustard has powerful irritant properties that can cause pain and increased inflammation of the skin (6,11,18). Sinigrin can be toxic to certain insect larvae (11). The glucosinolate products can have protective effects against carcinogens (11).

Adverse Reactions
Orally, large amounts of black mustard seed can lead to vomiting, stomach pain, diarrhea, somnolence, cardiac failure, breathing difficulties, coma, and possibly death (18). The isothiocyanate constituents can cause endemic goiters (6,11). Topically, the allyl isothiocyanate found in black mustard seed can cause skin blistering and necroses (6,11,18) but rarely cause contact allergies (18).

Interactions with Herbs & Other Dietary Supplements
Insufficient reliable information available.

Interactions with Drugs
ACID-INHIBITING DRUGS: Theoretically, due to claims that black mustard seed increases stomach acid, it might interfere with antacids, sucralfate (Carafate), H-2 antagonists, or proton pump inhibitors (19).

Interactions with Foods
No interactions are known to occur, and there is no known reason to expect a clinically significant interaction with black mustard seed.

Interactions with Lab Tests
No interactions are known to occur, and there is no known reason to expect a clinically significant interaction with black mustard seed.

Interactions with Diseases or Conditions
ASTHMA: Coughing, sneezing, and possible asthma attacks can result from handling mustard flour (18).
GI IRRITATION: Can irritate gastrointestinal tract. Contraindicated in individuals with infectious or inflammatory gastrointestinal conditions (19).

Dosage and Administration
TOPICAL: To prepare a mustard plaster, typically 100 grams of mustard flour (ground mustard) is mixed with warm water to make a paste. The paste is packed in linen and applied to the affected area for 10 minutes (3-5 minutes for children over 6 years old) (18). Mustard plaster applied for longer than 15-30 minutes is associated with severe burns and skin necroses (12). Treatment should not exceed two weeks (19).

Comments
Avoid confusion with black mustard oil, hedge mustard, white mustard (Brassica alba or Sinapis alba), brown mustard (Brassica juncea), Indian mustard (Brassica juncea), and Chinese mustard (Sinapis juncea).

BLACK NIGHTSHADE

Also Known As
Garden Nightshade, Houndsberry, Petty Morel, Poisonberry.

Scientific Names
Solanum nigrum.
Family: Solanaceae.

People Use This For
Orally, black nightshade is used for gastric irritation and cramps.
Topically, black nightshade is used for psoriasis, hemorrhoids, and abscesses. The bruised, fresh leaves are used topically to treat inflammation, burns and ulcers.
In folk medicine, people used black nightshade orally as an antispasmodic, pain reliever, sedative, and narcotic (18).

Safety
LIKELY UNSAFE …when used orally (4009).
There is insufficient reliable information available about the safety of black nightshade for its other uses.
PREGNANCY AND LACTATION: LIKELY UNSAFE …when used orally because of concerns it could be teratogenic (4009); avoid using.

Effectiveness
There is insufficient reliable information available about the effectiveness of black nightshade.

Mechanism of Action
Most of the toxic effects of black nightshade can be attributed to the solanine constituent. The green fruits have higher solanine concentrations and are therefore more toxic than the other plant parts. However, among plant strains, toxicity varies widely (4009).

Adverse Reactions
Orally, ingestion of large quantities of the green berries or fresh foliage with high alkaloid content can result in overdose. Symptoms include nausea, vomiting, headache, and in rare cases, dilation of the pupils (18). At doses of 200-400 mg, solanine can cause gastroenteritis, tachycardia, dyspnea, vertigo, drowsiness, lethargy, twitches of the arms and legs, and cramping. Other symptoms of poisoning include diarrhea, panic, excitation, coma, hyperthermia. This is followed later by a dazed state, paralysis, and rarely, death due to respiratory arrest and hypothermia (4009).

Interactions with Herbs & Other Dietary Supplements
Insufficient reliable information available.

Interactions with Drugs

No interactions are known to occur, and there is no known reason to expect a clinically significant interaction with black nightshade.

Interactions with Foods

No interactions are known to occur, and there is no known reason to expect a clinically significant interaction with black nightshade.

Interactions with Lab Tests

No interactions are known to occur, and there is no known reason to expect a clinically significant interaction with black nightshade.

Interactions with Diseases or Conditions

No interactions are known to occur, and there is no known reason to expect a clinically significant interaction with black nightshade.

Dosage and Administration

ORAL: No typical dosage.
TOPICAL: A handful of herb is placed in boiling water for 10 minutes, and used as a compress or a rinse (18).

Comments

Black nightshade is sometimes referred to as petty morel. This name is a corruption of the original, petit morel. Originally, black nightshade was called petit morel to differentiate it from the more poisonous species, deadly nightshade that is known as great morel. Black nightshade has a musk-like fragrance when wilting. (18).

BLACK PEPPER AND WHITE PEPPER

Also Known As

Black Pepper, Blanc Poivre, Kosho, Pepe, Pepper, Pepper Extract, Pepper Plant, Peppercorn, Pfeffer, Pimenta, Pimienta, Piper, Poivre, Poivre Noir, White Pepper.

Scientific Names

Piper nigrum.
Family: Piperaceae.

People Use This For

Orally, black pepper is used for stomach upset, bronchitis, and cancer. White pepper is used orally for stomach upset, malaria, cholera, and cancer (11).
Topically, black pepper is used for treating neuralgia and scabies (18). Black and white pepper are also used topically as a counterirritant for pain (11,7107).
In foods and beverages, black pepper, white pepper, and pepper oil are used as flavoring agents (11).

Safety

LIKELY SAFE …when used orally in amounts found in foods. Black and white pepper have Generally Recognized as Safe (GRAS) status in the US (11).
POSSIBLY SAFE …when used orally and appropriately in medicinal amounts (12). …when black pepper oil is used topically. Black pepper oil is nonirritating and is typically well tolerated (11).
CHILDREN: LIKELY SAFE ...when used orally in amounts found in food (11). POSSIBLY UNSAFE ...when used orally in large amounts. Fatal cases of pepper aspiration have been reported in some patients (5619,5620). There is insufficient reliable information available about the safety of topical pepper oil when used in children.
PREGNANCY: LIKELY SAFE ...when used orally in amounts found in foods (11). LIKELY UNSAFE ...when used orally in large amounts. Black pepper might have abortifacient effects (11,19); contraindicated. There is insufficient reliable information available about the safety of topical pepper when used during pregnancy.
LACTATION: LIKELY SAFE ...when used orally in amounts found in foods (11). There is insufficient reliable information available about the safety of black and white pepper when used in medicinal amounts during breast-feeding.

Effectiveness
There is insufficient reliable information available about the effectiveness of black pepper and white pepper.

Mechanism of Action
The applicable part of black pepper and white pepper is the fruit. Piper nigrum is said to have antiflatulent and diuretic properties (11), antimicrobial and insecticidal effects (18). It is thought to influence liver and metabolic functions (11), stimulate thermal receptors, induce sweating, and stimulate taste buds causing a reflex increase in gastric secretions (18). It might also have lipolytic activity related to the outer layer of the fruit (11). Piper nigrum contains piperine which increases oral absorption of drugs and other substances, possibly by modulating intestinal membrane dynamics (3757). Some evidence suggests piper nigrum might protect against colon cancer (3761); however, other evidence suggests black pepper might induce hepatic enzymes (3760) or cause liver tumors (3759).

Adverse Reactions
Orally, pepper can cause a burning aftertaste.
Topically, eye contact with ground pepper can cause redness of eyes and swelling of eyelids (5619). Deaths due to aspiration of large amounts of pepper have been reported (5619,5620).

Interactions with Herbs & Other Dietary Supplements
SPARTEINE: Piperine increases the bioavailability of sparteine, a constituent of scotch broom (19).

Interactions with Drugs
PHENYTOIN: Concomitant administration speeds absorption and slows elimination of phenytoin (Dilantin) (537).
PROPRANOLOL: Concomitant administration speeds and increases absorption, and increases serum concentrations of propranolol (Inderal) (538).
THEOPHYLLINE: Concomitant administration increases absorption and serum concentrations of theophylline (Theo-dur) (538).

Interactions with Foods
No interactions are known to occur, and there is no known reason to expect a clinically significant interaction with black pepper and white pepper.

Interactions with Lab Tests
SERUM DRUG ASSAYS: Can increase phenytoin, propranolol, and theophylline serum concentrations and test results (537,538).

Interactions with Diseases or Conditions
No interactions are known to occur, and there is no known reason to expect a clinically significant interaction with black pepper and white pepper.

Dosage and Administration
ORAL: Typically, a single dose ranges from 300-600 mg (18) up to 1.5 grams per day (18).
TOPICAL: No typical dosage.

Comments
Black pepper is the dried, full grown but unripe fruit of Piper nigrum (11). White pepper is the dried ripe fruit of Piper nigrum with the outer covering that is known as a pericarp removed (11). Pepper oil is distilled from black pepper (11). Indian long pepper contains piperine. Red pepper and cayenne contain no piperine.

BLACK PSYLLIUM

Also Known As
Brown Psyllium, Dietary Fiber, Fleaseed, Fleawort, French Psyllium, Plantain, Psyllion, Psyllios, Psyllium Seed, Spanish Psyllium.
CAUTION: See separate listings for Blond Psyllium, Buckhorn Plantain, Great Plantain, and Water Plantain.

Scientific Names
Plantago psyllium, synonym Psyllium afra; Psyllium indica, synonym Psyllium arenaria.
Family: Plantaginaceae.

People Use This For
Orally, black psyllium is used for chronic constipation and for softening stools in conditions such as hemorrhoids, anal fissures, anorectal surgery, and pregnancy. It is also used for diarrhea, irritable bowel syndrome (IBS) (2,6,11,18), reducing elevated cholesterol (6,11,18), dysentery (6), and treating cancer (11).

Safety
LIKELY SAFE ...when used orally with appropriate fluid intake (4,12,272).
LIKELY UNSAFE ...when used orally without adequate fluid intake because it can cause esophageal obstruction (2,4,18). ...when the seeds of non-commercial preparations of black psyllium are chewed, crushed, or ground because they release a pigment that deposits in renal tubules (11) and can be nephrotoxic (6). This pigment has been removed from most commercial products (6).
PREGNANCY AND LACTATION: LIKELY SAFE ...when used orally with appropriate fluid intake (272).

Effectiveness
EFFECTIVE ...when used orally as a supplemental source of dietary fiber (272). ...when used as a bulk laxative (272).
POSSIBLY EFFECTIVE ...when used orally for reducing serum total and LDL cholesterol, and reducing the LDL:HDL ratio (6,11).
There is insufficient reliable information available about the effectiveness of black psyllium for its other uses.

Mechanism of Action
The applicable part of black psyllium is the seed. Its constituents are not absorbed and have no systemic effects (1). Black psyllium seed forms a mucilaginous mass when mixed with water and has a bulk laxative effect (1,4,6). In people with diarrhea, the mucilage absorbs water, provides mass, and prolongs gastrointestinal transit (1,6). In individuals with constipation, the mucilage absorbs water, swells, and stimulates peristalsis, reducing gastrointestinal transit time (1,4,6). Black psyllium can decrease abdominal pain in people with irritable bowel syndrome (IBS) by reducing rectosigmoidal pressure (405). Psyllium reduces peak blood glucose levels by slowing carbohydrate absorption (1,6) and can decrease cholesterol by absorbing dietary fats in the gastrointestinal tract, thereby preventing systemic absorption. It can also increase cholesterol elimination in the fecal bile acids (1,6,11,12). Chewing or crushing the seeds can release a pigment that deposits in renal tubules (11) and can be nephrotoxic (6). This pigment is removed from most commercial products (6).

Adverse Reactions
Orally, black psyllium can cause transient flatulence and abdominal distention (4). When consumed without water, it can cause esophageal (4) and bowel obstruction (4,604). Chewing or crushing the seeds can release a pigment that deposits in the renal tubules (11) and can be nephrotoxic (6). This pigment is removed from most commercial products (6). Allergic reactions to black psyllium include allergic rhinitis, conjunctivitis, urticaria, and asthma (18). Occupational exposure to black psyllium can cause sensitization, of which symptoms include sneezing, watery eyes, chest congestion, and anaphylactoid reaction (6).

Interactions with Herbs & Other Dietary Supplements
VITAMIN/MINERAL SUPPLEMENTS: The long-term use of black psyllium with vitamin or mineral supplements can reduce the absorption of calcium, iron, zinc, and vitamin B12 (1,12). Supplements should be taken one hour before or four hours after black psyllium to avoid this interaction (4,12).

Interactions with Drugs
CARBAMAZEPINE (Tegretol): Black psyllium can reduce carbamazepine absorption (539).
WARFARIN (Coumadin): Concomitant use might reduce warfarin absorption (1), requiring dose adjustment (12).
DIGOXIN (Lanoxin): Concomitant use might reduce digoxin absorption (1), requiring dose adjustment (12).
LITHIUM: Black psyllium use can reduce serum lithium levels (540).
INSULIN: Black psyllium use can reduce peak blood glucose levels decreasing insulin requirements in individuals with diabetes (1,18).
DIABETES THERAPY: Monitor blood glucose level closely due to claims that black psyllium has hypoglycemic effects (19).
ORAL DRUGS: Oral drugs should be administered one hour before or four hours after black psyllium to avoid decreased or delayed absorption (4,12).

Interactions with Foods
NUTRIENT ABSORPTION: The long-term use of black psyllium with meals can reduce nutrient absorption requiring vitamin or mineral supplementation (12).

Interactions with Lab Tests

BLOOD GLUCOSE: Theoretically, black psyllium might lower postprandial blood glucose levels and test results (1,6,1405).

SERUM CHOLESTEROL: Black psyllium can lower total cholesterol and LDL cholesterol levels, LDL:HDL ratio, and test results (1,6,1405).

Interactions with Diseases or Conditions

GI CONDITIONS: Black psyllium is contraindicated in people with fecal impaction, GI atony (1), GI tract narrowing, and obstruction or conditions that can lead to obstruction, such as spastic bowel (1,2,4,12,18).

DIABETES: Use with caution and monitor closely in patients with diabetes. Black psyllium might alter blood glucose levels by reducing carbohydrate absorption (1,2). In addition, commercially available psyllium products can contain sugar and other absorbable carbohydrates (272).

KIDNEY DYSFUNCTION: Chewing, crushing, or grinding the seeds releases a potentially nephrotoxic pigment (6). This pigment is removed from most commercial products (6).

SWALLOWING DIFFICULTIES: Contraindicated (12).

PSYLLIUM HYPERSENSITIVITY: Contraindicated.

PHENYLKETONURIA: Avoid products containing aspartame (Nutrasweet) (272).

Dosage and Administration

The amount of black psyllium seed required for an individual can vary. For best results, start with small amounts and increase to the desired response. Follow the package labeling when available.

ORAL: As a laxative, the typical dose of black psyllium seed is 10-30 grams per day (2,18), in divided amounts. Mix 10 grams seed in 100 mL water, to be followed by at least 200 mL water (18). Avoid chewing or crushing the seeds which can release a pigment that deposits in renal tubules (11). Adequate fluid intake is necessary and should be at least 150 mL water for each 5 grams of drug. The FDA labeling recommends at least 8 ounces (a full glass) of water or other fluid with each dose. Taking this product without enough liquid can cause choking (12). Black psyllium should be taken 30-60 minutes after a meal or the administration of other drugs (272).

Comments

Black psyllium is an aggressive-growing, perennial weed found throughout the world. The plant was spread with the colonization of the New World and was nicknamed "Englishman's foot" by the North American Indians.

The FDA requires that psyllium be labeled: "WARNING: Taking this product without adequate fluid may cause it to swell and block your throat or esophagus and may cause choking. Do not take this product if you have difficulty in swallowing. If you experience chest pain, vomiting, or difficulty in swallowing or breathing after taking this product, seek immediate medical attention" (12).

BLACK ROOT

Also Known As

Beaumont Root, Bowman's Root, Culveris Root, Culver's Physic, Culver's Root, Culvers, Hini, Oxadoddy, Physic Root, Purple Leptandra, Tall Speedwell, Tall Veronica, Veronica Virginica Root, Veronicastrum Virginicum, Whorlywort.

CAUTION: See separate listings for Brooklime (Veronica beccabungo), Veronica (Veronica officinalis), Indian Physic, and Comfrey.

Scientific Names

Leptandra virginica.
Family: Scrophulariaceae.

People Use This For

Orally, black root is used for chronic constipation and disorders of the liver and gallbladder (18). It has also been used as an emetic (214).

Historically, early American doctors used black root to treat bilious fever (6002).

Safety

POSSIBLY SAFE ...when the dried root is used orally (12). The dried root has a milder action than the fresh root (18).

POSSIBLY UNSAFE ...when the fresh root is used orally (12).

PREGNANCY: LIKELY UNSAFE ...when the fresh root is used orally because it has abortifacient and teratogenic effects (19). There is insufficient reliable information available about the safety of the dried root, avoid using.

LACTATION: Insufficient reliable information available; avoid using.

Effectiveness
There is insufficient reliable information available about the effectiveness of black root.

Mechanism of Action
The applicable parts of black root are the rhizome and root. Black root is stated to have antiflatulent, laxative, and bowel evacuant properties (18). It can stimulate bile flow into the duodenum and induce sweating. It contains tannic acid, which has astringent properties that act on the GI mucosa. Tannic acid can also form insoluble complexes with alkaloids, glycosides, and certain heavy metals (214).

Adverse Reactions
Orally, black root can cause abdominal pain or cramps, changes in stool color or odor, drowsiness, headache, nausea, and vomiting. Hepatotoxicity has been reported after ingestion of large amounts (214).

Interactions with Herbs & Other Dietary Supplements
STIMULANT LAXATIVE HERBS: Theoretically, concomitant use with other stimulant laxative herbs can increase the risk of potassium depletion. Stimulant laxative herbs include aloe dried leaf sap, wild cucumber fruit (Ecballium elaterium), blue flag rhizome, alder buckthorn, European buckthorn, butternut bark, cascara bark, castor oil, colocynth fruit pulp, gamboge bark exudate, jalap root, manna bark exudate, podophyllum root, rhubarb root, senna leaves and pods, and yellow dock root (19).
POTASSIUM DEPLETING HERBS: Theoretically, concomitant use with horsetail plant or the licorice rhizome can increase the risk of potassium depletion (19).

Interactions with Drugs
CARDIAC GLYCOSIDES: Theoretically, the overuse or abuse of black root can increase the risk of adverse effects of cardiac glycoside drugs, e.g., digoxin (Lanoxin). Black root chemically binds with the glycosides while in the gastrointestinal (GI) tract, which may reduce their effectiveness if used concomitantly (214).

Interactions with Foods
No interactions are known to occur, and there is no known reason to expect a clinically significant interaction with black root.

Interactions with Lab Tests
No interactions are known to occur, and there is no known reason to expect a clinically significant interaction with black root.

Interactions with Diseases or Conditions
GALLSTONES/BILE DUCT OBSTRUCTION: Black root is contraindicated, because it theoretically has bile stimulatory effects and could aggravate these conditions (19).
HEMORRHOIDS/ MENSTRUATION: Theoretically, black root is contraindicated due to its cathartic properties (19).
GI INFLAMMATION: Black root is contraindicated in individuals with inflammation of the GI tract due to the irritant, emetic, and stimulant laxative effects (19).

Dosage and Administration
ORAL: People typically use 1 teaspoon of dried black root in 1 cup boiling water, which is allowed to steep for 30 minutes, to make a tea. The suggested dose is 1/3 cup before each meal. A black root tincture is taken as 2 to 4 drops in water. The powdered root bark is taken in a dose of 1 to 4 grams. (5263,5264).

Comments
Black root grows in the United States and Canada and has a bitter and nauseous taste.

BLACK SEED

Also Known As
Ajenuz, Arañuel, Baraka, Black Cumin, Black Caraway, Charnuska, Cominho Negro, Cominho-Negro, Fennel Flower, Fennel-Flower, Fitch, Love in a Mist, Nigelle de Crète, Nutmeg Flower, Nutmeg-Flower, Roman-Coriander, Schwarzkümmel, Toute Épice.
CAUTION: See separate listings for Caraway, Coriander, Cumin, Fennel, and Nutmeg.

Scientific Names

Nigella sativa.
Family: Ranunculaceae.

People Use This For

Orally, black seed is used for treating gastrointestinal conditions including gas, colic, diarrhea, dysentery, constipation and hemorrhoids. It is also used orally for respiratory conditions, including asthma, allergies, cough, bronchitis, emphysema, flu and congestion. Additionally, it is used orally as an antihypertensive, immunoprotectant, anticancer agent, and vermifuge. It is used orally for women's health: including as a contraceptive, for stimulation of menstruation, and increasing milk flow (6).

Topically, black seed is used for inflammatory conditions including rheumatism, headache and skin conditions (6). Traditionally, black seed has been used for headache, toothache, nasal congestion, and intestinal worms. It has also been used for conjunctivitis, abscesses, and parasites (6).

In combination with cysteine, vitamin E, and saffron, black seed is used to decrease cisplatin-induced side effects (6).
In foods, black seed is used as a flavoring or spice (6).

Safety

LIKELY SAFE ...when used orally in amounts found in foods (6).
There is insufficient reliable information available about the safety of black seed for its other uses.
PREGNANCY: LIKELY UNSAFE ...when used orally in amounts exceeding those found in food. Black seed may decrease or inhibit uterine contractions (241) and may have contraceptive activity (242).
LACTATION: Insufficient reliable information available; avoid using.

Effectiveness

There is insufficient reliable information available about the effectiveness of black seed.

Mechanism of Action

The applicable part of black seed is the seed itself. In allergic conditions, black seed might have antihistamine effects. Although not yet demonstrated in humans, low concentration of the constituent nigellone has been shown to inhibit the release of histamine from mast cells in animals (233). Black seed is thought to have immunoprotectant effects. Preliminary evidence suggests it may help minimize chemotherapy-induced decreases in hemoglobin and leukocyte counts. It may also enhance the production of certain human interleukins and alter macrophages (234). Black seed is also used as an anticancer agent. According to preliminary studies, black seed may inhibit stomach tumors, carcinoma, and Ehrlich ascites carcinoma (236,239). The black seed constituents thymoquinone and dithymoquinone are actually cytotoxic toward human cells (238). Although some evidence suggests thymoquinone may offer protection against chemically induced hepatotoxicity (237,240), a study in rats indicates that black seed may actually be hepatotoxic. A fixed oil from black seed is reported to have anti-eicosanoid and antioxidant effects, which may support anti-inflammatory activity (235), but this effect has not been studied in humans. The essential oil may have antimicrobial and anthelmintic activity, particularly against staphylococcus as well as other gram-positive and gram-negative bacteria (243,1516). Black seed may have anti-oxytocic potential, and may inhibit spontaneous contractions (241). It may also have contraceptive activity (242).

Adverse Reactions

Topical use of black seed oil can cause allergic contact dermatitis (6). Black seed may be associated with hepatotoxicity based on preliminary animal research (245).

Interactions with Herbs & Other Dietary Supplements

Insufficient reliable information available.

Interactions with Drugs

No interactions are known to occur, and there is no known reason to expect a clinically significant interaction with black seed.

Interactions with Foods

No interactions are known to occur, and there is no known reason to expect a clinically significant interaction with black seed.

Interactions with Lab Tests

No interactions are known to occur, and there is no known reason to expect a clinically significant interaction with black seed.

Interactions with Diseases or Conditions

No interactions are known to occur, and there is no known reason to expect a clinically significant interaction with black seed.

Dosage and Administration

No typical dosage.

Comments

Black seed is reported to have been used for over 2000 years. Recordings mention it as far back as 1400 years. Black seed was found in the tomb of King Tutankhamen (6).

An issued patent covers the use of black seed to stimulate immune-competent cells in humans; however, this should not be taken as evidence for the safety and efficacy of black seed as an immunostimulant (246).

BLACK TEA

Also Known As

Black Leaf Tea, Chinese Tea, Tea.
CAUTION: See separate listings for Caffeine and Green Tea.

Scientific Names

Camellia sinensis, synonyms Camellia thea, Camellia theifera, Thea bohea, Thea sinensis, Thea viridis.
Family: Theaceae.

People Use This For

Orally, black tea is used for improving cognitive performance (4221,4224), headache (6,18), reducing the risk of cancer (4223), atherosclerosis (3450), myocardial infarction (4222), and preventing Parkinson's disease (6022). It is also used for stomach disorders, vomiting, diarrhea (6,18), preventing dental caries (4214), preventing kidney stones (4216), and as a diuretic (6,18).

In combination with various other products, black tea is used for weight loss (18).

For food use, black tea is consumed as a hot or cold beverage.

Safety

LIKELY SAFE ...when used orally in moderate amounts (12).

POSSIBLY UNSAFE ...when used orally in large amounts. Black tea contains a significant amount of caffeine. Consumption of more than 300 mg caffeine, which is equivalent to approximately 5 cups of black tea per day, has been associated with significant adverse effects (see Adverse Reactions) (18). These effects would not be expected to occur with the consumption of decaffeinated black tea.

CHILDREN: LIKELY UNSAFE ...when used orally by infants because it has been associated with impaired iron metabolism and microcytic anemia (6). This might be caused by tannins in black tea which bind and prevent iron absorption in the gastrointestinal tract (19). Children are also more susceptible to the adverse effects of caffeine present in black tea (15).

PREGNANCY: POSSIBLY SAFE ...when used orally in moderate amounts. Due to the caffeine content of black tea, mothers should closely monitor their intake to ensure moderate consumption. Fetal blood concentrations of caffeine approximate maternal concentrations (4260). Caffeine use in pregnancy is controversial; however, moderate consumption has not been associated with adverse fetal effects (6). Some sources suggest keeping caffeine consumption below 200 mg per day (2078). Black tea provides approximately 10-80 mg caffeine per cup (18,4218). POSSIBLY UNSAFE ...when used orally in large amounts. Caffeine in black tea crosses the placenta, producing fetal blood concentrations similar to maternal levels (4260). Although controversial, some evidence suggests that high doses of caffeine might be associated with premature delivery, low birth weight, and loss of the fetus (6). Excessive use of black tea in pregnancy should be avoided.

LACTATION: POSSIBLY SAFE ...when used in moderate amounts. Due to the caffeine content of black tea, mothers should closely monitor their intake to ensure moderate consumption. Breast milk concentrations of caffeine are thought to be approximately 50% of maternal serum concentrations. Moderate consumption of black tea would likely result in very small amounts of caffeine exposure to a nursing infant (6). POSSIBLY UNSAFE ...when used orally in large amounts. Consumption of black tea might cause irritability and increased bowel activity in nursing infants (6026). Large doses or excessive intake of black tea should be avoided during lactation.

Effectiveness

POSSIBLY EFFECTIVE ...when used orally to enhance cognitive performance (4221,4224). Consumption of black tea and other caffeinated beverages seems to prevent a decline in alertness and cognitive capacity when consumed throughout the day (4224). ...when used orally for reducing the risk of severe aortic atherosclerosis, especially in women (3450). Epidemiological evidence shows that black tea consumption seems to reduce the risk of severe aortic atherosclerosis (3450). ...when used orally for reducing the risk of myocardial infarction. There is some epidemiological evidence that black tea consumption is inversely associated with the risk of myocardial infarction (4222). ...when used orally for diarrhea and as a diuretic (7,18). ...when used orally for reducing the risk of kidney stones. Women consuming black tea seem to have an 8% decreased risk of developing kidney stones (4216). ...when used orally for preventing Parkinson's disease. There is some evidence from large-scale epidemiological studies that people who consume caffeinated beverages such as coffee, tea, and cola have a decreased risk of Parkinson's disease. For men, the effects seem to be dose related. For example, men consuming a total of 421-2716 mg of caffeine from any source daily, seem to have the greatest reduction in risk. However, there seems to be a significant reduction in risk even with consumption of as little as 124-208 mg caffeine per day (6022). In women, the effects do not seem to be dose related. Moderate consumption of caffeine (equivalent to 1-4 cups black tea daily), seems to provide the most reduction in risk (1238). There is insufficient reliable information available about the effectiveness of black tea for its other uses. However, there is some preliminary evidence that black tea might be beneficial for preventing osteoporosis by improving some measures of bone mineral density (6404). More evidence is needed to rate black tea for this use.

Mechanism of Action

The applicable parts of black tea are the leaf and stem. Flavonoids such as catechins, thearubigins, and theaflavins are abundant in black tea, and are thought to be responsible for many of its proposed benefits by acting as antioxidants (6032,6033). Black tea also contains 2-4% caffeine (519). It's not clear why black tea seems to be beneficial for preventing heart disease. Black tea may be beneficial in atherosclerosis due to flavonoid constituents which might reduce lipoprotein oxidation (6032,6033). There is also some preliminary evidence that black tea can increase blood vessel dilation. In people with heart disease, consumption of 4 cups of black tea seems to restore blood vessel dilation to near-normal. Constituents other than caffeine are thought to be responsible for this effect (1328). For osteoporosis, the mechanism is not known, but it is thought that isoflavonoids in black tea have weak estrogenic effects that might become beneficial in postmenopausal women with low endogenous estrogen levels (6404). The caffeine in black tea acts as a central nervous system stimulant (12,15,18) and is thought to be responsible for improving cognitive performance (4221,4224). Caffeine also increases blood pressure (1452,6663), heart rate and contractility (7,18), inhibits platelet aggregation (6,18), stimulates gastric acid secretion, causes diuresis (15,18), relaxes extracerebral vascular and bronchial smooth muscle, stimulates the release of catecholamines (18), and might indirectly inhibit histamine release (6130). The tannin constituents in black tea have antidiarrheal effects (7,18). In infants, the tannin constituents can bind and reduce iron absorption, causing microcytic anemia (631). For prevention of Parkinson's disease, caffeine in black tea may prevent adenosine's inhibition of dopaminergic transmission. This may result in a reduction in the clinical expression of Parkinsonism (6022).

Adverse Reactions

Orally, black tea can cause gastrointestinal upset (12) and constipation (7). High doses of black tea, due to the caffeine constituent, can cause headache, diuresis, anxiety, nervousness, insomnia, restlessness, agitation, tremor, irritability, tachyarrhythmias, palpitations, premature heartbeat, quickened respiration, tremor, heartburn, loss of appetite, nausea, vomiting, diarrhea, dizziness, ringing in the ears, elevated blood sugar, elevated cholesterol, hepatotoxicity, delirium, and convulsions (6,7,15,18,505). Although acute administration of black tea can cause increased blood pressure, regular consumption does not seem to increase either blood pressure or pulse, even in mildly hypertensive patients (1451,1452,6663). Chronic use of black tea that contains caffeine, especially in large amounts, can sometimes produce tolerance, habituation, and psychological dependence (15). The abrupt discontinuance of black tea that contains caffeine can sometimes result in physical withdrawal symptoms, including headaches, irritation, nervousness, anxiety, and dizziness (15). Some evidence shows caffeine is associated with fibrocystic breast disease in women; however, this is controversial and has been disputed (14,15). The adverse effects of caffeine found in black tea can be more severe in children than adults (15). In infants, black tea can cause microcytic anemia (631).

Interactions with Herbs & Other Dietary Supplements

CAFFEINE CONTAINING HERBS/SUPPLEMENTS: Concomitant use can increase therapeutic and adverse effects. Natural products that contain caffeine include coffee, tea (black or green), guarana, mate, and cola.
EPHEDRA (ma huang): Concomitant use interacts with the caffeine in black tea and can potentiate the stimulant effects and the risk of adverse effects (6).

Interactions with Drugs

ADENOSINE (Adenocard): The caffeine in black tea might interact with adenosine and inhibit the hemodynamic and anti-arrhythmic effects of adenosine (19).
ANTIPSYCHOTICS: Theoretically, the caffeine in black tea might decrease absorption of fluphenazine (Permitil, Prolixin) or haloperidol (Haldol) (626,627).

ASPIRIN, ACETAMINOPHEN: The caffeine in black tea might increase the action of these drugs by as much as 40% (3).

BARBITURATES: These drugs might decrease the effects of the caffeine in black tea (151).

BENZODIAZEPINES: The caffeine in black tea might decrease sedative effects of benzodiazepines (19).

BETA-ADRENERGIC AGONISTS: The caffeine in black tea can increase cardiac inotropic effects of these drugs (15). Beta-adrenergic agonists include albuterol (Proventil, Ventolin, Volmax), metaproterenol (Alupent), terbutaline (Bricanyl, Brethine), and isoproterenol (Isuprel).

BETA-BLOCKERS: Concomitant use of propranolol (Inderal) or metoprolol (Lopressor) can increase blood pressure by interacting with the caffeine in black tea (19).

CHLORPROMAZINE: Theoretically, the caffeine in black tea might inhibit the cataleptic effects of chlorpromazine (Thorazine) (19).

CIMETIDINE: Cimetidine (Tagamet) interacts with the caffeine in black tea and decreases caffeine clearance by 30-50% (14).

CLOZAPINE: The caffeine in black tea might interact with clozapine (Clozaril) and cause acute exacerbation of psychotic symptoms. Caffeine can increase effects and toxicity of clozapine (151). Caffeine doses of 400-1000 mg per day inhibit clozapine metabolism (5051).

CNS DEPRESSANTS: Concomitant use can increase the toxic effects of the caffeine in black tea (151).

DISULFIRAM (Antabuse): Concomitant use can decrease clearance and increase the half-life of caffeine, increasing effects and risk of adverse effects (15).

ERGOTAMINE: The caffeine in black tea can increase GI absorption of ergotamine (15).

LITHIUM: Abrupt withdrawal of the caffeine in black tea can increase serum lithium levels (609), worsening lithium tremor (610).

MAO INHIBITORS: The intake of large amounts of the caffeine in black tea can precipitate a hypertensive crisis (500).

ORAL CONTRACEPTIVES: Concomitant use of oral contraceptives interacts with the caffeine in black tea and can decrease caffeine clearance by 40-65%, increasing effects and risk of adverse effects (14).

PHENYLPROPANOLAMINE (Propagest, Rhindecon): Concomitant use can increase blood pressure and/or cause mania through interaction with the caffeine in black tea (19).

PHENYTOIN (Dilantin): Concomitant use can enhance metabolism and excretion of caffeine (19).

QUINOLONES: Concomitant use can decrease caffeine clearance and increase effects and risk of adverse effects (606,607,608). Quinolones include ciprofloxacin (Cipro), enoxacin (Penetrex), norfloxacin (Chibroxin, Noroxin), sparfloxacin (Zagam), trovafloxacin (Trovan), and grepafloxacin (Raxar).

THEOPHYLLINE: The caffeine in black tea can increase theophylline (Theo-Dur) levels (151).

TRICYCLICS: Theoretically, concomitant use might decrease absorption of amitriptyline (Elavil) or imipramine (Tofranil, Janimine) through interaction with the caffeine in black tea (626,627).

VERAPAMIL (Calan, Covera, Isoptin, Verelan): Concomitant use can increase plasma caffeine levels by 25%, increasing effects and risk of adverse effects (14).

Interactions with Foods

GRAPEFRUIT JUICE: Concomitant use can increase caffeine levels and the risk of adverse effects (504).

MILK: When taken together, milk might bind the antioxidants in black tea and reduce their beneficial effects (220); however, in one study this interaction did not occur (6032).

Interactions with Lab Tests

BLEEDING TIME: The caffeine in black tea can prolong bleeding time and increase the results of a bleeding time test (1701).

SERUM URATE (Bittner method): The caffeine in black tea can cause false-positive test results (15).

CREATINE: The caffeine in black tea can increase urine creatine levels (1701).

URINE CATECHOLAMINES, 5-HYDROXYINDOLEACETIC ACID, VANILLYLMANDELIC ACID (VMA): The caffeine in black tea can cause slight increases in these levels (15).

TESTS FOR PHEOCHROMOCYTOMA, NEUROBLASTOMA: High urine catecholamines or VMA can result in false-positive results. The caffeine in black tea should be avoided while testing for these diseases (15).

Interactions with Diseases or Conditions

GASTRIC, DUODENAL ULCERS: The caffeine in black tea can aggravate these conditions and should be avoided (14,16).

DEPRESSION, ANXIETY DISORDERS: The caffeine in black tea can aggravate these conditions (14).

HEART CONDITIONS: The caffeine in black tea can induce cardiac arrhythmias in sensitive individuals (14,16).

HORMONE SENSITIVE CANCERS/CONDITIONS: Because black tea might have weak estrogenic effects (6404), women with hormone sensitive conditions should avoid high doses of black tea. Some of these conditions include breast, uterine, and ovarian cancer, and endometriosis and uterine fibroids.

HYPERTENSION: The caffeine in black tea might increase blood pressure in people with high blood pressure (2272). However, this doesn't seem to occur in people who consume black tea or other caffeinated products regularly (1451,1452,6663).

KIDNEY DISEASE: The diuretic effect of caffeine in tea might aggravate certain kidney disorders (19).

Dosage and Administration

ORAL: A typical dose as a stimulant is several cups per day. A typical dose as an antidiarrheal is one cup 2-3 times daily. For reducing the risk of heart attack, kidney stones, and improving cognitive functioning, a dose of at least one cup per day has been used (4216,4222,4224). A current trial in women at high risk for breast cancer is using 4 cups of tea per day (4273). For preventing atherosclerosis, consumption of 125-500 mL (1-4 cups) of brewed black tea daily has been used (3450). For preventing Parkinson's disease, men consuming 421-2716 mg total caffeine (approximately 5-33 cups of black tea) daily have the lowest risk of developing Parkinson's disease. However, a significantly lower risk is also associated with consumption of as little as 124-208 mg of caffeine (approximately 1-3 cups of black tea) daily (6022). In women, more moderate caffeine consumption seems to be best; equivalent to approximately 1-4 cups of black tea per day (1238). To make tea pour boiling water over a teaspoon of tea, cover and allow to steep for 2 minutes, strain (8).

Comments

Green tea and black tea are derived from leaves of the same plant. Leaves used for green tea are prepared immediately after harvest, which limits enzymatic changes. Leaves used for black tea are fermented before preparation, promoting enzymatic changes. Consequently, green tea can have higher concentrations of the natural constituents than black teas (6,7).

BLACK WALNUT

Also Known As

Nogal Americano, Nogueira-preta, Noyer Noir, Schwarze Walnuss.
CAUTION: See separate listing for English Walnut hull and English Walnut leaf.

Scientific Names

Juglans nigra.
Family: Juglandaceae.

People Use This For

Orally, black walnut is used for diphtheria, leukemia, syphilis, and as an anthelmintic (513).
Topically, black walnut is used as a gargle, hair dye, insecticide, and for wounds (513).

Safety

POSSIBLY SAFE ...when used orally and appropriately, short-term (12).
POSSIBLY UNSAFE ...when used topically because it contains the constituent juglone (2). Daily use of the juglone-containing bark of a related species (English walnut) is associated with increased risk of tongue cancer and lip leukoplakia (2,12).
PREGNANCY AND LACTATION: POSSIBLY UNSAFE ...when used topically; avoid using (12).
There is insufficient reliable information about the safety of the oral use of black walnut during pregnancy or lactation; avoid using.

Effectiveness

There is insufficient reliable information available about the effectiveness of black walnut.

Mechanism of Action

The applicable part of black walnut is the hull. Black walnut hulls contain approximately 45% tannins (19) which exert an astringent effect on the mucosal tissue. Tannins work internally by dehydrating mucosal tissue, which reduces secretions. Externally, tannin astringent effects result in a protective layer of constricted, harder cells. Plants with at least 10% tannins can cause gastrointestinal upset, kidney damage, and liver damage. Animal data conflicts with respect to the carcinogenicity of tannins. They may be carcinogenic or may even have anti-carcinogenic effects. An increased risk of esophageal or nasal cancer may be linked with people who regularly ingest herbs with high tannin concentrations (12).

Adverse Reactions

None reported.

Interactions with Herbs & Other Dietary Supplements

TANNIN-CONTAINING HERBS: Theoretically, herbs such as black walnut contain high percentages of tannins, which might cause precipitation of constituents of other herbs (19).

Interactions with Drugs

ORAL DRUGS: Theoretically, concomitant oral administration might cause precipitation of some drugs due to the high tannin content of black walnut hulls (19). Separate administration of oral drugs and tannin-containing herbs by the longest period of time practical (19).

Interactions with Foods

No interactions are known to occur, and there is no known reason to expect a clinically significant interaction with black walnut.

Interactions with Lab Tests

No interactions are known to occur, and there is no known reason to expect a clinically significant interaction with black walnut.

Interactions with Diseases or Conditions

No interactions are known to occur, and there is no known reason to expect a clinically significant interaction with black walnut.

Dosage and Administration

ORAL: A typical oral dose of black walnut hull is 1000 mg three times daily with water (351), not to exceed 6 weeks (352).

Comments

None.

BLACKBERRY leaf

Also Known As

Black Berry, Bramble, Dewberry, Goutberry, Rubi Fruticosi Folium, Thimbleberry.
CAUTION: See separate listings for Blackberry root and Raspberry.

Scientific Names

Rubus fruticosus.
Family: Rosaceae.

People Use This For

Orally, blackberry leaf is used for non-specific, acute diarrhea.
Topically, blackberry leaf is used as a mouth rinse for mild inflammation of the mucosa of the oral cavity and throat (2,12).

Safety

LIKELY SAFE ...when used orally for short-term use (2,12).
There is insufficient reliable information available about the safety of long-term use of blackberry leaf.
PREGNANCY AND LACTATION: Insufficient reliable information available; avoid using.

Effectiveness

There is insufficient reliable information available about the effectiveness of blackberry leaf.

Mechanism of Action

The astringent property of the tannin constituents can relieve mucosal inflammation and diarrhea (2,12).

Adverse Reactions

None reported.

Interactions with Herbs & Other Dietary Supplements

Insufficient reliable information available.

Interactions with Drugs

No interactions are known to occur, and there is no known reason to expect a clinically significant interaction with blackberry leaf.

Interactions with Foods

No interactions are known to occur, and there is no known reason to expect a clinically significant interaction with blackberry leaf.

Interactions with Lab Tests

No interactions are known to occur, and there is no known reason to expect a clinically significant interaction with blackberry leaf.

Interactions with Diseases or Conditions

No interactions are known to occur, and there is no known reason to expect a clinically significant interaction with blackberry leaf.

Dosage and Administration

ORAL: The usual dose of the blackberry leaf is 2-5 grams per day taken as a tea, which is prepared by steeping 1-2 teaspoons (1.5 grams) dried herb in 150 mL boiling water for 5-10 minutes and then straining. For equivalent preparations, 2-5 grams per day of the leaf is also used (2,18).
TOPICAL: The blackberry leaf tea can be used as a mouth rinse.

Comments

Avoid confusion with blackberry root. The leaf extract of the related species, Rubus ellipticus, has shown uterotropic activity at 300 mg/kg and can potentiate estrogenic activity (11). The related species, Rubus odoratus, has shown antitumor activity against Walker 256 carcinosarcoma (11).

BLACKBERRY root

Also Known As

Black Berry, Bramble, Dewberry, Goutberry, Rubi Fruticosi Radix, Thimbleberry.
CAUTION: See separate listing for Blackberry leaf.

Scientific Names

Rubus fruticosus.
Family: Rosaceae.

People Use This For

Orally, blackberry root is used to prevent edema (2).

Safety

There is insufficient reliable information available about the safety of blackberry root.
Pregnancy and Lactation: Insufficient reliable information available; avoid using.

Effectiveness

There is insufficient reliable information available about the effectiveness of blackberry root.

Mechanism of Action

Insufficient reliable information available.

Adverse Reactions

None reported.

Interactions with Herbs & Other Dietary Supplements

Insufficient reliable information available.

Interactions with Drugs

No interactions are known to occur, and there is no known reason to expect a clinically significant interaction with blackberry root.

Interactions with Foods

No interactions are known to occur, and there is no known reason to expect a clinically significant interaction with blackberry root.

Interactions with Lab Tests

No interactions are known to occur, and there is no known reason to expect a clinically significant interaction with blackberry root.

Interactions with Diseases or Conditions

No interactions are known to occur, and there is no known reason to expect a clinically significant interaction with blackberry root.

Dosage and Administration

ORAL: People typically use 1 teaspoon of the root added to 1 cup water. The liquid is taken cold, 1 to 2 cups per day. The root in tincture form is taken 15 to 40 drops in water as needed (5263).

Comments

Avoid confusion with blackberry leaf. The related species, Rubus odoratus, has shown antitumor activity against Walker 256 carcinosarcoma (11). The leaf extract of the related species, Rubus ellipticus, has shown uterotropic activity at 300 mg/kg and can potentiate estrogenic activity (11).

BLACKTHORN berry

Also Known As

Blackthorn Fruit, Pruni Spinosae Fructus, Sloe, Sloe Berry.
CAUTION: See separate listing for Blackthorn flower.

Scientific Names

Prunus spinosa.
Family: Rosaceae.

People Use This For

Orally, blackthorn berry is used as a mouth rinse (gargle) for mild inflammation of the oral and pharyngeal mucosa (2). In folk medicine, the berry juice is utilized as the gargle for mouth, throat, and gum inflammation (18). The syrup and wine of the blackthorn berry is used for purging the bowels and as a diuretic (18). The berry marmalade is used for dyspepsia (18).

Safety

LIKELY SAFE ...when used orally and appropriately as a mouth rinse, short-term (2,12).
POSSIBLY UNSAFE ...when used orally; not recommended for long-term use (12).
PREGNANCY AND LACTATION: Insufficient reliable information available; avoid using.

Effectiveness

POSSIBLY EFFECTIVE ...when used as an oral mouth rinse for mild inflammation of the oral and pharyngeal mucosa (2).
There is insufficient reliable information available about the effectiveness of blackthorn berry for its other uses.

Mechanism of Action

The astringent properties of the tannin constituents can contribute to the reduction of mucous membrane inflammation (2,7).

Adverse Reactions

None reported.

Interactions with Herbs & Other Dietary Supplements

Insufficient reliable information available.

Interactions with Drugs

No interactions are known to occur, and there is no known reason to expect a clinically significant interaction with blackthorn berry.

Interactions with Foods

No interactions are known to occur, and there is no known reason to expect a clinically significant interaction with blackthorn berry.

Interactions with Lab Tests

No interactions are known to occur, and there is no known reason to expect a clinically significant interaction with blackthorn berry.

Interactions with Diseases or Conditions

No interactions are known to occur, and there is no known reason to expect a clinically significant interaction with blackthorn berry.

Dosage and Administration

ORAL: The blackthorn berry is typically used as a mouth rinse up to two times per day. The rinse is obtained from the tea, which is prepared by steeping 1-2 grams in 150 mL boiling water for 10-15 minutes and then straining (2,12). There is no typical dosage for the other uses of blackthorn berry.

Comments

None.

BLACKTHORN flower

Also Known As

Pruni Spinosae Llos, Sloe Flower, Wild Plum Flower.
CAUTION: See separate listing for Blackthorn berry.

Scientific Names

Prunus spinosa.
Family: Rosaceae.

People Use This For

Orally, blackthorn flower is used for common colds, ailments of the respiratory tract, bloating, general exhaustion, dyspepsia, kidney and bladder ailments, and to treat and prevent gastric spasms. The blackthorn flower is also used orally as a laxative, diuretic, diaphoretic, expectorant, and as a component in "blood cleansing" teas (2,18). Topically, blackthorn flower is used for rashes, skin impurities, and "blood purification" (2). In foods, blackthorn flower is utilized in herbal teas as a coloring agent (2).

Safety

POSSIBLY SAFE …when used as a coloring agent for oral herbal tea mixtures (2).
POSSIBLY UNSAFE …when used orally in medicinal amounts. Contains cyanogenic glycosides that could be toxic (12).
LIKELY UNSAFE …when used orally long-term or in excessive amounts (12).
There is insufficient reliable information available about the safety of blackthorn flower for its other uses.
PREGNANCY AND LACTATION: LIKELY UNSAFE …when used orally; avoid using. HCN can be teratogenic (12).

Effectiveness

There is insufficient reliable information available about the effectiveness of blackthorn flower.

Mechanism of Action

There is insufficient reliable information available about the possible mechanism of action and active ingredients of blackthorn flower.

Adverse Reactions

None reported.

Interactions with Herbs & Other Dietary Supplements

Insufficient reliable information available.

Interactions with Drugs

No interactions are known to occur, and there is no known reason to expect a clinically significant interaction with blackthorn flower.

Interactions with Foods

No interactions are known to occur, and there is no known reason to expect a clinically significant interaction with blackthorn flower.

Interactions with Lab Tests

No interactions are known to occur, and there is no known reason to expect a clinically significant interaction with blackthorn flower.

Interactions with Diseases or Conditions

No interactions are known to occur, and there is no known reason to expect a clinically significant interaction with blackthorn flower.

Dosage and Administration

ORAL: Blackthorn flower is usually taken as a tea, 1-2 cups during the day or 2 cups in the evening. The tea is prepared by steeping 1-2 heaping teaspoons (1-2 grams) in 150 mL boiling water for 5-10 minutes and then straining (18). Blackthorn is for short-term use only (12).

Comments

Blackthorn can be stored for up to one year away from light and moisture (18).

BLADDERWORT

Also Known As

None.
CAUTION: See separate listing for Bladderwrack.

Scientific Names

Utricularia vulgaris.
Family: Lentibulariaceae.

People Use This For

Orally, bladderwort is used for urinary tract disorders including kidney stones and urinary tract infections (UTIs). It is also used orally for weight loss, as a diuretic, antispasmodic, anti-inflammatory, and to stimulate gall bladder secretions.
Topically, bladderwort is used for burns and skin and mucous membrane inflammation.

Safety

There is insufficient reliable information available about the safety of bladderwort.
Pregnancy and Lactation: Insufficient reliable information available; avoid using.

Effectiveness

There is insufficient reliable information available about the effectiveness of bladderwort.

Mechanism of Action

There is insufficient reliable information available about the possible mechanism of action and active ingredients of bladderwort.

Adverse Reactions

None reported.

Interactions with Herbs & Other Dietary Supplements

Insufficient reliable information available.

Interactions with Drugs

No interactions are known to occur, and there is no known reason to expect a clinically significant interaction with bladderwort.

Interactions with Foods

No interactions are known to occur, and there is no known reason to expect a clinically significant interaction with bladderwort.

Interactions with Lab Tests

No interactions are known to occur, and there is no known reason to expect a clinically significant interaction with bladderwort.

Interactions with Diseases or Conditions

No interactions are known to occur, and there is no known reason to expect a clinically significant interaction with bladderwort.

Dosage and Administration

ORAL: As a diuretic, two cups are taken daily. The tea is prepared by steeping 2 grams dried leaf in 100 mL of boiling water for 10-15 minutes and then straining.
TOPICAL: As an anti-inflammatory, a tea is used in mouthwashes, cleansers, cosmetic, and medical packs. The tea is prepared by steeping 6 grams dried leaf in 100 mL of boiling water for 10-15 minutes and then straining (18).

Comments

Bladderwort use is nearly obsolete in Germany. It continues to be used in other countries (18).

BLADDERWRACK

Also Known As

Black Tang, Bladder Fucus, Bladder Wrack, Blasentang, Cutweed, Fucus, Kelp, Kelp-Ware, Kelpware, Knotted Wrack, Meereiche, Quercus Marina, Rockweed, Rockwrack, Schweintang, Seawrack, Tang, Varech.
CAUTION: See separate listings for Algin, Bladderwort, and Laminaria.

Scientific Names

Ascophyllum nodosum; Fucus vesiculosis; other Fucus species and other brown seaweed species.
Family: Fucaceae.

People Use This For

Orally, bladderwrack is used for thyroid disorders (2), iodine deficiency (9), lymphadenoid goiter (4), myxedema (4), obesity, arthritis, and rheumatism (4).
In folk medicine, bladderwrack is used for arteriosclerosis, digestive disorders, "blood cleansing" (2), constipation (9), bronchitis, emphysema, genitourinary disorders, decreased resistance to disease, anxiety, skin diseases, burns, and insect bites (5).

Safety

POSSIBLY UNSAFE ...when used orally because 1 gram of bladderwrack might contain as much as 600 mcg iodine (12). Ingesting more than 150 mcg iodine per day can cause hyperthyroidism or exacerbate existing hyperthyroidism (2). Heavy metal poisoning has also been reported (645).
CHILDREN: POSSIBLY UNSAFE ...when used orally; avoid using (14).
PREGNANCY AND LACTATION: LIKELY UNSAFE ...when used orally; avoid using (4,12).

Effectiveness

There is insufficient reliable information about the effectiveness of bladderwrack.

Mechanism of Action

Iodine, which is the essential substrate for the thyroid hormone, can have a concentration that varies from 0.03-1.0% (18). The constituent algin (sodium alginate) has bulk laxative and demulcent (soothing) effects (4,5). The isolated fraction, fucoidin, has 40-50% of the blood anticoagulant activity of heparin (4). Fucus can concentrate heavy metals (4). There is limited information available for Fucus vesiculosis, but the pharmacological activities are recognized for the individual constituents and other brown seaweed species.

Adverse Reactions

Bladderwrack can induce or exacerbate hyperthyroidism (2,12) and acne (4). Prolonged ingestion can reduce iron absorption (4). High sodium content can adversely affect individuals with restricted sodium intake (5). Iodine can cause idiosyncratic or allergic reactions (2,18). There is one case report of heavy metal poisoning where arsenic poisoning occurred with ingestions of a contaminated kelp product (645).

Interactions with Herbs & Other Dietary Supplements

IRON: Prolonged ingestion of bladderwrack can reduce iron absorption (4).

Interactions with Drugs

ANTICOAGULANTS: Theoretically, concomitant use might increase bleeding risk (4).
DIURETICS: Bladderwrack can decrease the effectiveness of diuretics due to high sodium content (5).
LITHIUM (ESKALITH, LITHOBID): Theoretically, concomitant use might enhance hypothyroid activity due to high iodine content in bladderwrack (19).
THYROID HORMONES: The high iodine content of bladderwrack might interfere with thyroid hormone replacement therapy (4).

Interactions with Foods

IRON: Prolonged ingestion of bladderwrack can reduce iron absorption (4).

Interactions with Lab Tests

ACTIVATED PARTIAL THROMBOPLASTIN TIME (aPTT): Theoretically, bladderwrack might increase aPTT test results due to the heparin-like activity of one of its constituents (4).
RADIOACTIVE IODINE UPTAKE: Theoretically, bladderwrack might interfere with the results of thyroid function tests using radioactive iodine uptake (15).
THYROID STIMULATING HORMONE (TSH): Theoretically, bladderwrack might increase serum TSH levels and test results (1701).
THYROXINE (T4): Theoretically, bladderwrack might increase serum T4 levels and test results (1701).

Interactions with Diseases or Conditions

CONDITIONS REQUIRING SODIUM RESTRICTION: The high sodium content can exacerbate these conditions (5).
HYPERTHYROIDISM, ACNE: Bladderwrack can exacerbate these conditions (2,4,12).
IODINE ALLERGY: Avoid bladderwrack use in those sensitive to iodine (2,18).
IRON DEFICIENCY: Bladderwrack can exacerbate this deficiency by reducing iron absorption (4).

Dosage and Administration

ORAL: The usual dose is 5-10 grams of the plant or as a tea three times a day. The tea is prepared by steeping the herb in 150 mL boiling water for 5-10 minutes and then straining (4). The typical dose of the liquid extract (1:1) is 4-8 mL three times a day. Bladderwrack can contain over 600 mcg iodine per gram seaweed (12).

Comments

Avoid confusion with bladderwort.

BLESSED THISTLE

Also Known As

Carbenia Benedicta, Cardo Santo, Carduus, Carduus Benedictus, Cnici Benedicti Herba, Cnicus, Holy Thistle, St. Benedict Thistle, Spotted Thistle.
CAUTION: See separate listing for Milk Thistle above ground parts and Milk Thistle fruit, seed.

Scientific Names

Cnicus benedictus.
Family: Asteraceae or Compositae.

People Use This For

Orally, blessed thistle is used for loss of appetite and indigestion (2), as an antidiarrheal, expectorant, antibiotic (4), and for promoting lactation (314).

Topically, blessed thistle is used as a poultice for boils, wounds, and ulcers (4,11).

In traditional medicine, blessed thistle has been used as a diuretic (11), and for treating colds and fever (11).

In manufacturing, it is used as a flavoring in alcoholic beverages (12).

Safety

LIKELY SAFE ...when used as flavoring, regulated in the US as an allowable flavoring for alcoholic beverages (12).

POSSIBLY SAFE ...when used orally and appropriately (12).

PREGNANCY: LIKELY UNSAFE ...when used orally; avoid using (4,12).

LACTATION: Insufficient reliable information available; avoid using (4).

Effectiveness

There is insufficient reliable information available about the effectiveness of blessed thistle.

Mechanism of Action

The applicable parts of blessed thistle are the flowering top, leaf, and upper stem. The bacteriostatic properties are due to the volatile oil of blessed thistle. The sesquiterpene lactone constituent, cnicin, can have antibacterial and antitumor activity (11). Metabolism of the constituents, arctiin and tracheoloside, following oral ingestion results in compounds that inhibit cyclic-AMP phosphodiesterase and histamine release from mast cells (11). Blessed thistle contains 8% tannins (4).

Adverse Reactions

Orally, blessed thistle used in high doses, greater than five grams per cup of tea, can cause stomach irritation and vomiting (12). It can cause an allergic reaction in individuals sensitive to the Asteraceae/Compositae family. Members of this family include ragweed, chrysanthemums, marigolds, daisies, and many other herbs.

Interactions with Herbs & Other Dietary Supplements

Insufficient reliable information available.

Interactions with Drugs

ACID-INHIBITING DRUGS: Theoretically, due to claims that blessed thistle increases stomach acid, it might interfere with antacids, sucralfate (Carafate), H-2 antagonists, or proton pump inhibitors (19).

Interactions with Foods

No interactions are known to occur, and there is no known reason to expect a clinically significant interaction with blessed thistle.

Interactions with Lab Tests

No interactions are known to occur, and there is no known reason to expect a clinically significant interaction with blessed thistle.

Interactions with Diseases or Conditions

CROSS-ALLERGENICITY: Can cause an allergic reaction in individuals sensitive to the Asteraceae/Compositae family. Members of this family include ragweed, chrysanthemums, marigolds, daisies, and many other herbs.

GI IRRITATION: Can irritate the gastrointestinal tract. Contraindicated in individuals with infectious or inflammatory gastrointestinal conditions (19).

Dosage and Administration

ORAL: The typical dose of the dried, flowering tops is 1.5-3 grams themselves or as a tea three times daily. The tea is prepared by steeping the dried, flowering tops in boiling water and then straining. The liquid extract (1:1 in 25% alcohol) is commonly taken as 1.5-3 mL three times daily (4).

TOPICAL: No typical dosage.

Comments

Blessed thistle was commonly used during the Middle Ages to treat the bubonic plague and as a tonic for monks. Avoid confusion with milk thistle (Silybum marianum).

BLOND PSYLLIUM

Also Known As
Blond Plantago, Blonde Psyllium, Dietary Fiber, Englishman's Foot, Indian Plantago, Ispaghula, Ispagol, Pale Psyllium, Plantaginis ovatae semen, Plantaginis ovatae testa, Psyllium, Sand Plantain, Spogel.
CAUTION: See separate listings for Black Psyllium seed, Buckhorn Plantain, Great Plantain, and Water Plantain.

Scientific Names
Plantago ovata, synonyms Plantago decumbens, Plantago isphagula.
Family: Plantaginaceae.

People Use This For
Orally, blond psyllium is used for constipation, softening stools in patients with hemorrhoids, anal fissures, post-anorectal surgery, and during pregnancy. It is also used for diarrhea, irritable bowel syndrome (IBS), hypercholesterolemia, hyperglycemia in patients with diabetes, dysentery, and cancer.
Topically, blond psyllium seed is used as a poultice for furunculosis (boils).
In food manufacturing, blond psyllium seed husk mucilage is used as a thickener or stabilizer in some frozen dairy desserts.

Safety
LIKELY SAFE ...when used orally and appropriately. Commercial blond psyllium preparations have been safely used in doses up to 20 grams per day for up to 6 months (12,272,1376). Tell patients not to use non-commercial preparations. The chewed or crushed seeds of these preparations can contain a dangerous pigment that can cause renal damage (11). Commercial preparations typically have this pigment removed and are safe.
PREGNANCY AND LACTATION: LIKELY SAFE ...when used orally and appropriately (1,4,272).

Effectiveness
EFFECTIVE ...when used orally as a bulk laxative for constipation or softening stools (272).
LIKELY EFFECTIVE ...when used orally for mild to moderate hypercholesterolemia. Blond psyllium seed husk in combination with a low-fat diet can significantly reduce total serum cholesterol, low-density lipoprotein (LDL) cholesterol, and the LDL:high-density lipoprotein (HDL) ratio in patients with high cholesterol (1376,6262,6263). Blond psyllium seed husk added to food or as a separate supplement in a dose of approximately 10 grams daily can reduce total cholesterol by 3-6% and LDL cholesterol by 5-9% after 6 months of treatment (1376,6261,6262,6263). Blond psyllium does not seem to significantly increase HDL levels in these patients (1376). Some clinical studies have used a specific blond psyllium powder preparation (Metamucil).
POSSIBLY EFFECTIVE ...when used orally for diarrhea. Psyllium seems to delay gastric emptying and slow colonic transit in patients with diarrhea (5246). ...when used orally for irritable bowel syndrome (IBS) (2). ...when used orally to prevent gastrointestinal (GI) side effects of orlistat (Xenical). Blond psyllium given with each dose of orlistat seems to relieve orlistat side effects such as flatulence, borborygmi, abdominal cramps, oily spotting, and fecal incontinence without decreasing the weight-reducing effect of orlistat (5245). ...when used orally for type 2 diabetes. There is some evidence that blond psyllium seed husk can significantly reduce postprandial glucose and serum total cholesterol and low-density lipoprotein (LDL) cholesterol levels in patients with type 2 diabetes and hypercholesterolemia (1405). There is insufficient reliable information available about the effectiveness of blond psyllium for its other uses.

Mechanism of Action
The applicable parts of blond psyllium are the seed and seed husk. The blond psyllium husk and intact seed are soluble fibers, are not digested in the small intestine, and are resistant to colonic bacterial degradation (5246). The husks of the psyllium seed form a mucilaginous mass when mixed with water. The mucilage tends to normalize bowel function (1,4,5246). In patients with constipation, the mucilage has a bulk laxative effect and stimulates peristalsis, which decreases gastrointestinal transit time (1,4,6). In patients with diarrhea, the mucilage increases meal viscosity which delays gastric emptying. It also prolongs gastrointestinal transit, possibly by delaying the production of gaseous fermentation products (5246). In patients with irritable bowel syndrome (IBS), blond psyllium is thought to normalize bowel function and relieve symptoms of abdominal pain by reducing rectosigmoidal pressure (405). In patients with high cholesterol, blond psyllium seems to decrease serum cholesterol levels by adsorbing dietary fats in the gastrointestinal tract and decreasing systemic absorption of the fat. Blond psyllium also seems to increase cholesterol elimination in fecal bile acids (1376). In diabetes patients, blond psyllium reduces postprandial blood glucose levels probably by slowing carbohydrate absorption (1405).

Adverse Reactions
Orally, blond psyllium can cause transient flatulence, abdominal pain, diarrhea, constipation, dyspepsia, and nausea (4,1376). Starting with a low dose and slowly titrating to the desired dose can often minimize gastrointestinal side

effects. There is some concern that blond psyllium can cause esophageal or bowel obstruction when consumed without water (604). Tell patients to consume plenty of water when taking blond psyllium. Suggest at least 240 mL of fluid 3.5-5 grams of seed husk or 7 grams of seed (12,272,1376). Occasionally, headache, backache, rhinitis, increased cough, and sinusitis have also been reported in patients taking psyllium (1376). Some patients can have an allergic response to blond psyllium. Allergy symptoms include allergic rhinitis, conjunctivitis, urticaria, and asthma (18). Occupational exposure to psyllium can cause sensitization, which can lead to symptoms include sneezing, watery eyes, chest congestion, and anaphylactoid reactions (6).

Steer patients away from using non-commercial blond psyllium preparations. Chewing, crushing, or grinding the seeds of these preparations can release a dangerous pigment which deposits in renal tubules and might cause renal damage (11). This pigment is typically removed from commercial preparations of blond psyllium.

Interactions with Herbs & Other Dietary Supplements

VITAMIN/MINERAL SUPPLEMENTS: Long-term use of psyllium with vitamin or mineral supplements can reduce nutrient absorption, including calcium, iron, zinc, and vitamin B12 (1,12). Take supplements one hour before or four hours after psyllium to avoid this interaction (4,12).

Interactions with Drugs

ANTIDIABETES DRUGS: Blond psyllium can reduce blood glucose levels in patients with type 2 diabetes (1405) and might have additive effects on glucose levels when used with antidiabetes drugs. Monitor blood glucose levels closely. Medication dose adjustments may be necessary. Some antidiabetes drugs include glimepiride (Amaryl), glyburide (Diabeta, Glynase PresTab, Micronase), insulin, pioglitazone (Actos), rosiglitazone (Avandia), and others.

CARBAMAZEPINE (Tegretol): Blond psyllium can reduce carbamazepine absorption and serum levels (539).

DIGOXIN (Lanoxin): Concomitant use with psyllium can require digoxin dosing adjustment (12) due to retarded drug absorption (1).

LITHIUM: There is one case report of reduced serum lithium levels associated with psyllium use and was reversed when psyllium stopped (540).

WARFARIN (Coumadin): Concomitant use with blond psyllium can require warfarin dosing adjustment (12) due to retarded drug absorption (1).

ORAL DRUGS: Blond psyllium may decrease absorption of drugs taken orally. Take oral drugs one hour before or four hours after blond psyllium to avoid decreased or delayed absorption (4,12).

Interactions with Foods

NUTRIENT ABSORPTION: Long-term use of psyllium with meals can reduce nutrient absorption (12) requiring vitamin or mineral supplementation. However, use of blond psyllium husk for up to six months did not clinically alter vitamin or mineral status in a review of eight human trials (1376).

Interactions with Lab Tests

GLUCOSE: Blond psyllium can reduce postprandial blood glucose levels and test results (1,6,1405).

CHOLESTEROL: Blond psyllium reduces serum total cholesterol and LDL cholesterol levels, LDL:HDL ratio, and test results (1,6,1405,1376).

Interactions with Diseases or Conditions

DIABETES: Blond psyllium can lower blood glucose levels in people with type 2 diabetes by retarding carbohydrate absorption (1,2,1405). Monitor blood glucose levels closely. Doses of conventional antidiabetes medications may require adjustment. Also, warn patients with diabetes that some commercial blond psyllium products can contain added sugars and other absorbable carbohydrates which might increase blood glucose levels.

GASTROINTESTINAL CONDITIONS: Blond psyllium is contraindicated in people with fecal impaction, GI atony (1), and GI tract narrowing, obstruction, or conditions that can lead to obstruction, such as spastic bowel (1,2,4,12,18).

HYPERSENSITIVITY: Some patients can have severe hypersensitivity reactions to blond psyllium This is more likely to occur in patients with previous occupation exposure to blond psyllium (1). Blond psyllium is contraindicated in these patients.

PHENYLKETONURIA: Some blond psyllium preparations are sweetened with aspartame (Nutrasweet) and should be avoided in patients with phenylketonuria (272).

SWALLOWING DISORDERS: Patients with swallowing disorders might be at greater risk for esophageal obstruction when using blond psyllium (12). Blond psyllium is contraindicated in these patients.

Dosage and Administration

ORAL: As a bulk laxative for constipation, blond psyllium seed 7-40 grams per day, in two to three divided doses is commonly used (1,2,18). For lowering serum cholesterol, blond psyllium seed husk 3.4 grams three times daily or 5.1 grams twice daily has been used (6261,6262,6264). However, doses up to 20.4 grams per day have been tried (1,1376).

For irritable bowel syndrome (IBS), blond psyllium husk 7 grams one to three times daily has been used (1).
For reducing the gastrointestinal (GI) side effects of orlistat, 6 grams three times daily with each orlistat dose has been used (5245). Tell patients to ensure adequate fluid intake. Inadequate fluid intake can lead to choking and esophageal or bowel obstruction. Suggest a minimum of 240 mL per 5.1 grams or less of blond psyllium husk or 7 grams of blond psyllium seed (1,12,272). To minimize some of the common gastrointestinal side effects, suggest that patients start with a low dose and titrate slowly to the desired dose.

Comments

There are some blond psyllium containing foods with labeling that claims these foods, when consumed as part of a low-fat diet, may reduce the risk of coronary heart disease (CHD) (6264). It is true that blond psyllium can help lower cholesterol levels; however, there is not yet proof that taking blond psyllium reduces the risk of developing heart disease.

BLOODROOT

Also Known As

Blood Root, Coon Root, Indian Plant, Indian Red Paint, Pauson, Red Indian Paint, Red Puccoon, Red Root, Sanguinaria, Sanguinaria canadensis, Snakebite, Sweet Slumber, Tetterwort.

Scientific Names

Sanguinaria canadensis.
Family: Papaveraceae.

People Use This For

Orally, bloodroot is used as an emetic, cathartic, antispasmodic, and expectorant (4).
Topically, bloodroot is used as an irritant and debriding agent (4).
In dentistry, bloodroot is used topically to reduce plaque (4,6).
In traditional medicine, bloodroot has been used for bronchitis, asthma, croup, laryngitis, pharyngitis, deficient capillary circulation, nasal polyps (4), rheumatism, warts, cancer (Fell technique), dental analgesic (6), fever, and as a general tonic (11).

Safety

POSSIBLY SAFE ...when used orally and appropriately short-term (4).
POSSIBLY UNSAFE ...when excessive doses are used orally because sanguinarine, although thought to be poorly absorbed, is a toxic alkaloid (6,12).
There is insufficient reliable information available about the safety of bloodroot for its other uses.
PREGNANCY: LIKELY UNSAFE ...when used orally; avoid using (12).
LACTATION: POSSIBLY UNSAFE ...when used orally; avoid using (4).

Effectiveness

POSSIBLY EFFECTIVE ...when used topically in dental products for reducing dental plaque (4,6). ...when used topically for treating carcinomas of the nose and ear (6).
There is insufficient reliable information available about the effectiveness of bloodroot for its other uses.

Mechanism of Action

The applicable part of bloodroot is the rhizome. The isoquinolone alkaloid constituents, primarily sanguinarine, have antimicrobial, anti-inflammatory, antihistamine, cardiotonic (exerts a favorable effect on the heart), and antiplaque activity (4). The negative ion of sanguinarine can bind to dental plaque (6).

Adverse Reactions

Orally, bloodroot can cause nausea, vomiting (12), slight CNS depression, and narcosis (6). High doses can cause hypotension, shock, coma, and glaucoma (6).
Topically, skin contact with fresh bloodroot can cause irritation or contact dermatitis (19).

Interactions with Herbs & Other Dietary Supplements

Insufficient reliable information available.

Interactions with Drugs

No interactions are known to occur, and there is no known reason to expect a clinically significant interaction with bloodroot.

Interactions with Foods
No interactions are known to occur, and there is no known reason to expect a clinically significant interaction with bloodroot.

Interactions with Lab Tests
No interactions are known to occur, and there is no known reason to expect a clinically significant interaction with bloodroot.

Interactions with Diseases or Conditions
GI IRRITATION: Bloodroot can irritate the gastrointestinal tract and is contraindicated in individuals with infectious or inflammatory gastrointestinal conditions (19).
GLAUCOMA: Bloodroot might affect glaucoma treatment. Do not exceed the recommended dose (12).

Dosage and Administration
ORAL: The dose of the bloodroot rhizome is typically 60-500 mg three times a day (4). The usual dose of the liquid extract (1:1 in 60% alcohol) is 0.06-0.3 mL three times a day (4). The common dose of the tincture (1:5 in 60% alcohol) is 0.3-2 mL three times a day (4). Avoid contact with the eyes and mucous membranes because of its irritant properties.
TOPICAL: No typical dosage.
EMETIC DOSE: As an emetic, 1-2 of the rhizome, 1-2 mL of the liquid extract (1:1 in 60% alcohol), or 2-8 mL of the tincture (1:5 in 60% alcohol) are commonly used (4).

Comments
During the mid-1800s, topical preparations of the bloodroot extracts were used in the Fell Technique for treatment of breast tumors (6).

BLUE COHOSH

Also Known As
Blue Ginseng, Caulophyllum, Papoose Root, Squaw Root, Yellow Ginseng.
CAUTION: See separate listings for Black Cohosh, White Cohosh, Ginseng American, Canaigre, Codonopsis, Ginseng Siberian, Ginseng Panax, and Ashwaganda.

Scientific Names
Caulophyllum thalictroides.
Family: Berberidaceae.

People Use This For
Orally, blue cohosh is used for stimulating the uterus and inducing labor (5,1122,3383), inducing menstruation (5), as an antispasmodic (5), for antirheumatic effects (4), and as a laxative (11).
Historically, blue cohosh has been used for colic, sore throat, cramps, hiccups, epilepsy, hysterics, inflammation of the uterus, and to facilitate childbirth (5,1122).
In food use, the roasted seeds of blue cohosh are often used as a coffee substitute (6).

Safety
LIKELY UNSAFE ...when used orally (4,12). Poisonings have occurred after ingestion of blue cohosh leaf or seeds (4).
CHILDREN: LIKELY UNSAFE ...when used orally. Blue cohosh can cause serious toxicity (4,102,1207).
PREGNANCY AND LACTATION: LIKELY UNSAFE ...when used orally. Blue cohosh is a uterine stimulant and can act as an abortifacient (12). Many midwives still use blue cohosh to facilitate delivery. However, there is evidence that this is a dangerous practice that should be avoided (5,1122,1207). Use of blue cohosh near term can cause life-threatening toxicity in the infant (see Adverse Reactions) (102,1207,7109). Blue cohosh also contains a constituent that might cause congenital malformations in newborns (1122).

Effectiveness
There is insufficient reliable information available about the effectiveness of blue cohosh.

Mechanism of Action
The applicable parts of blue cohosh are the rhizome and root. Blue cohosh has several pharmacological effects. However, most of these effects are undesirable. Blue cohosh constricts coronary arteries and seems to decrease the flow of oxygen to the heart (3383). Blue cohosh also contains several alkaloid constituents that are suspected teratogens. There is some evidence that the constituent anagyrine might cause birth defects in humans (7110). Another constituent,

N-methylcytosine also seems to be teratogenic (7110). N-methylcytosine seems to act similarly to nicotine, which can increase blood pressure, stimulate the small intestine, and produce hyperglycemia the developing fetus (4,11,7110). Blue cohosh also contains taspine, which is chemically related to morphine and its congeners (7110). Taspine seems to be cytotoxic and lethal to embryos even at very low concentrations (7110). Another constituent, caulosaponin, can have oxytocic effects (4) and possibly anti-fertility effects (4). There is preliminary evidence that blue cohosh might have estrogenic effects. A blue cohosh extract seems to enhance estradiol binding to estrogen receptors and increase estradiol-induced transcription activity in estrogen-responsive cells (6180). In animal models, it also decreases luteinizing hormone (LH) levels and increases serum ceruloplasmin oxidase activity, which is a measure of estrogenic activity in the liver (6180).

Adverse Reactions

Orally, blue cohosh can cause significant adverse effects including mucus membrane irritation, stomach upset including diarrhea and cramping, chest pain (angina), hypertension, and hyperglycemia (4,6002). Blue cohosh has been attributed to a case neonatal acute myocardial infarction (MI), congestive heart failure (CHF), and shock following maternal use of a blue cohosh combination product one month before delivery (566,3383). There is also some concern that use of blue cohosh in mothers might cause other cardiovascular adverse effects in infants. There are reports of stroke and aplastic anemia in infants following maternal use of blue cohosh containing products (7109).

Interactions with Herbs & Other Dietary Supplements

Insufficient reliable information available.

Interactions with Drugs

ANTIDIABETES DRUGS: There is some concern that blue cohosh might increase blood glucose levels (6002). Theoretically, it might decrease the effectiveness of medicines used for diabetes.

CARDIOVASCULAR DRUGS: There is some concern that blue cohosh might interfere with cardiovascular drug therapy (4). Constituents in blue cohosh contains might cause coronary vasoconstriction and possibly increase blood pressure (5,6002). Theoretically, it might decrease the effectiveness of drugs used for angina and high blood pressure.

NICOTINE: Blue cohosh can increase the effects of nicotine (6002).

Interactions with Foods

No interactions are known to occur, and there is no known reason to expect a clinically significant interaction with blue cohosh.

Interactions with Lab Tests

No interactions are known to occur, and there is no known reason to expect a clinically significant interaction with blue cohosh.

Interactions with Diseases or Conditions

CARDIOVASCULAR CONDITIONS: There is some concern that blue cohosh might worsen cardiovascular conditions such as angina and hypertension. There is evidence that blue cohosh can cause coronary vasoconstriction and decrease oxygen flow to the heart. It might also increase blood pressure (4,5,6002). Avoid using in these patients.

DIABETES: There is some concern that blue cohosh might worsen diabetes. It can increase blood glucose levels in some patients (6002).

DIARRHEA: Blue cohosh might worsen symptoms in patients with diarrhea (4). Blue cohosh seems to increase gastrointestinal motility (5).

HORMONE SENSITIVE CANCERS/CONDITIONS: Because blue cohosh might have estrogenic effects (6404), women with hormone sensitive conditions should avoid blue cohosh. Some of these conditions include breast, uterine, and ovarian cancer, and endometriosis and uterine fibroids.

Dosage and Administration

ORAL: The typical dose of the dried rhizome or root is 0.3-1 grams or as a tea three times daily. The tea is prepared by steeping the herb in 150 mL boiling water and then straining. The usual dose of the liquid extract (1:1 in 70% alcohol) is 0.5-1.0 mL three times daily (4).

Comments

Cohosh is from the Algonquin word "rough," referring to the appearance of the roots (7110). Blue cohosh was listed in the US Pharmacopoeia from 1882 to 1905 for inducing labor (7110).

BLUE FLAG

Also Known As
Iris, Sweet Flag.
CAUTION: See separate listing for Orris.

Scientific Names
Iris caroliniana; Iris versicolor; Iris virginica.
Family: Iridaceae.

People Use This For
Orally, blue flag is used as a laxative and diuretic and for dermatological, anti-inflammatory, and antiemetic uses. It is also used as a bile stimulant, for liver dysfunction, and specifically for skin eruptions (4).

Safety
LIKELY UNSAFE ...when used orally; contraindicated in all but small doses (4). The fresh root can cause nausea, vomiting, and mucosal irritation (4,12). The blue flag oil is a mucous membrane irritant (4).
PREGNANCY AND LACTATION: LIKELY UNSAFE ...when used orally; avoid using (4,12).

Effectiveness
There is insufficient reliable information available about the effectiveness of blue flag.

Mechanism of Action
The applicable part of blue flag is the rhizome. Little is known about blue flag's phytochemical, pharmacological, and toxicological properties, or those of its constituents. Some related species can be toxic (4).

Adverse Reactions
Blue flag can cause nausea and vomiting, and the fresh root can irritate mucosa or skin (4,19). The volatile oil constituent irritates mucous membranes and causes lacrimation, eye inflammation, irritation of the throat, or headache (4).

Interactions with Herbs & Other Dietary Supplements
POTASSIUM DEPLETING HERBS: Theoretically, concomitant use with horsetail plant or the licorice rhizome increases the risk of potassium depletion.
STIMULANT LAXATIVE HERBS: Theoretically, concomitant use of blue flag with other stimulant laxative herbs can increase the risk of potassium depletion. Stimulant laxative herbs include aloe dried leaf sap, wild cucumber fruit (Ecballium elaterium), alder buckthorn, European buckthorn, butternut bark, cascara bark, castor oil, colocynth fruit pulp, gamboge bark exudate, jalap root, black root, manna bark exudate, podophyllum root, rhubarb root, senna leaves and pods, and yellow dock root (19).

Interactions with Drugs
CARDIAC GLYCOSIDES: Theoretically, overuse or abuse of this product increases the risk of adverse effects from cardiac glycoside drugs, e.g. digoxin (Lanoxin).

Interactions with Foods
No interactions are known to occur, and there is no known reason to expect a clinically significant interaction with blue flag.

Interactions with Lab Tests
No interactions are known to occur, and there is no known reason to expect a clinically significant interaction with blue flag.

Interactions with Diseases or Conditions
GI IRRITATION: Blue flag can irritate the gastrointestinal tract and is contraindicated in individuals with infectious or inflammatory gastrointestinal conditions (19).

Dosage and Administration
No typical dosage.

Comments

Little is known about blue flag's phytochemical, pharmacological, or toxicological properties, or those of its constituents. Some related species can be toxic (4). Though orris root is sometimes used as a common name for blue flag, it is also used to describe the Iris species.

BLUE-GREEN ALGAE

Also Known As

AFA, BGA, Blue Green Algae, Cyanobacteria, Dihe, Klamath Blue/Green Algae, Blue-Green Micro-Algae, Spirulina, Tecuitlatl.

Scientific Names

Microcystis aeruginosa, Microcystis wesenbergii, and other Microcystis species; Spirulina maxima, Spirulina platensis, and other Spirulina species; Anabaena species; Lyngbya wollei; Aphanizomenon flos-aquae.

People Use This For

Orally, blue-green algae products are used as a source of dietary protein, B-vitamins, and iron (14). They are also used orally for weight loss, oral leukoplakia (6), obstetric and gynecological disorders (14), attention deficit hyperactivity disorder (ADHD), premenstrual syndrome, diabetes, stimulating the immune system, stress, fatigue, anxiety, depression, improving memory, increasing energy and metabolism, lowering cholesterol, decreasing cardiovascular disease, wound healing, and for promoting digestion and bowel health (3532,3533).

Safety

POSSIBLY SAFE ...when non-contaminated, non-microcystin containing Spirulina species of blue-green algae are consumed orally (6). Some manufacturers grow Spirulina species in controlled environments, perform analytical safety testing, and claim their products are uncontaminated and safe (3534).
POSSIBLY UNSAFE ...when contaminated Spirulina species of blue-green algae are used orally. Spirulina species can be contaminated with microbes, heavy metals (including mercury, cadmium, lead, or arsenic), and radioactive divalent and trivalent metal ions (6). Spirulina species grown in uncontrolled environments, including lakes and ponds, are more likely to be contaminated (3534). ...when Anabaena, Aphanizomenon, or Microcysitis species of blue-green algae are used orally. These types of blue-green algae often contain hepatotoxic microcystins (3534,3535,3536).
LIKELY UNSAFE ...when any microcystin-containing blue-green algae products are used orally; avoid using all untested blue-green algae products.
CHILDREN: LIKELY UNSAFE ...when any microcystin-containing blue-green algae products are used orally. Children are more sensitive to poisoning by microcystins produced by blue-green algae (3536).
PREGNANCY AND LACTATION: Insufficient reliable information available; avoid using.

Effectiveness

LIKELY EFFECTIVE ...when spirulina blue-green algae are used orally as a source of dietary protein and iron (6).
POSSIBLY EFFECTIVE ...when spirulina blue-green algae are taken orally for treating oral leukoplakia (6).
POSSIBLY INEFFECTIVE ...when spirulina blue-green algae are taken orally as a vitamin B12 supplement (6).
...when spirulina blue-green algae are taken orally for weight loss (6).
There is insufficient reliable information available about the effectiveness of non-spirulina blue-green algae.

Mechanism of Action

Spirulina blue-green algae consists of approximately 65% crude protein, high concentrations of B vitamins, phenylalanine, and iron and other minerals (6). The B vitamins are thought to be analogs of vitamin B12 and nutritionally insignificant (6). The phenylalanine content is promoted as being responsible for reducing appetite and causing weight loss (6). The FDA reviewed this claim and found no evidence to support using blue-green algae for weight loss (6). The iron in spirulina blue-green algae has been found to be highly bioavailable in humans (6). As much as 1.5–2 mg of iron can be absorbed from a dose of 10 grams of blue-green algae (6). Evidence suggests that spirulina blue-green algae might enhance antibody production, reduce serum lipids, liver triglycerides, and gastric secretions (6). It might also protect against the effects of gamma radiation, enhance the regression of oral carcinoma, and have antiviral effects (6). The blue-green algae Aphanizomenon flos-aquae (AFA) may stimulate the immune system by increasing T lymphocytes, and B lymphocytes (2534). AFA contains 1.9-2.9 times less of the polyunsaturated fatty acid (PUFA) alpha-linolenic acid (LNA), and 32-44 times less linoleic acid than soybean oil. However, an animal study indicates that AFA-supplementation in animals with a PUFA-deficient diet may increase linoleic acid plasma levels to 67-71% of those found in animals consuming a soybean oil-supplemented diet. Furthermore, preliminary evidence suggests that an AFA-supplemented diet may be more effective than the soybean oil-supplemented diet at lowering triglycerides and total cholesterol (2535).

Researchers at the National Cancer Institute have isolated an antiviral protein, cyanovirin-N (CV-N), which might prove useful in treating human immunodeficiency virus (HIV) infection. Isolated from the blue green algae Nostoc ellipsosporum, CV-N binds irreversibly to sites on the viral envelope, inactivating HIV and inhibiting its entry into cells. CV-N has unique temperature (heat and cold) stability which might allow for its use in applications not typical for proteins. The researchers hypothesize that, attached to a solid matrix, CV-N might be used to adsorb and remove HIV from infected blood products. This unpublished research was presented at the Microbicides 2000 International Conference (1375).

Adverse Reactions

Adverse effects have not been reported for non-contaminated, non-microcystin-containing Spirulina species blue-green algae products. Microcystin-containing blue-green algae products can cause hepatotoxicity, jaundice, abdominal pain and distention, nausea, vomiting, weakness, excessive thirst, rapid and weak pulse, shock, and death (3535). Symptoms of poisoning usually occur 30 minutes to 24 hours after ingestion (3535). Children are more sensitive to micorcystin poisoning than adults (3536).

Interactions with Herbs & Other Dietary Supplements

Insufficient reliable information available.

Interactions with Drugs

No interactions are known to occur, and there is no known reason to expect a clinically significant interaction with blue-green algae.

Interactions with Foods

No interactions are known to occur, and there is no known reason to expect a clinically significant interaction with blue-green algae.

Interactions with Lab Tests

No interactions are known to occur, and there is no known reason to expect a clinically significant interaction with blue-green algae.

Interactions with Diseases or Conditions

PHENYLKETONURIA: Theoretically, the phenylalanine content of Spirulina species blue-green algae products might exacerbate phenylketonuria (6); avoid Spirulina species blue-green algae products (6).

Dosage and Administration

ORAL: The typical dose of spirulina blue-green algae is 3-5 grams daily before meals (6002). Some people mix one or two teaspoons of 100% spirulina blue-green algae powder in fruit juice or smoothies (5022).
There is insufficient reliable information available for dosing non-spirulina blue-green algae.

Comments

Blue-green algae are commonly found in tropical or subtropical alkaline waters that have a high-salt content (6002). The natural color of these algae can give bodies of water a dark-green appearance (6). Blue-green algae (cyanophyta) comprises thousands of species, including Spirulina species blue-green algae and non-Spirulina species blue-green algae (3532,3534,3536). Most commercial products contain Aphanizomenon flos-aquae, Spirulina maxima, or Spirulina platensis. Commercial Spirulina species blue-green algae are usually grown under controlled conditions while some non-Spirulina blue-green algae (Klamath blue-green algae and others) are grown in natural setting (lakes, etc.) where contamination and microcystin production is more likely (3536). Select blue-green algae products that have been tested to avoid products contaminated with heavy metals, microbes, or microcystins (3532,3534,3536). A study by Canadian health authorities found all non-Spirulina species blue-green algae products tested were contaminated with hepatotoxic microcystins, while none of the Spirulina species blue-green algae products tested were contaminated (3536). While blue-green algae products are promoted as an excellent source of dietary protein, they are no better than meat or milk and are estimated to cost more than 30 times as much as beef on a per gram basis (6).

BLUEBERRY

Also Known As

Blueberries, Highbush Blueberry, Hillside Blueberry, Lowbush Blueberry, Rabbiteye Blueberry.
Caution: See separate listing for Bilberry (Vaccinium myrtillus).

Scientific Names

Vaccinium angustifolium, Vaccinium ashei, Vaccinium corymbosum, Vaccinium pallidum.
Family: Ericaceae.

People Use This For

Orally, blueberry fruit is used for preventing cataracts and glaucoma, ulcers, urinary tract infections (UTI), multiple sclerosis, fever, varicose veins, hemorrhoids, improving circulation, and as a laxative (503,804). The dried fruit and leaves are used for diarrhea (512). Tea made from the dried leaves is used for sore throat and other inflammations of the mouth or mucous membranes of the throat (814). Blueberry juice is also used as a contrast agent in magnetic resonance imaging.

In traditional medicine, blueberry has been used as a "blood purifier", for colic, labor pains, and as a tonic after miscarriage (519).

By inhalation, fumes of the burning dried flowers have been inhaled for treatment of insanity (519).

Safety

LIKELY SAFE …when used orally and appropriately (12).
PREGNANCY AND LACTATION: Insufficient reliable information available; avoid using.

Effectiveness

There is insufficient reliable information available about the effectiveness of blueberry for its uses.

Mechanism of Action

The applicable parts of the blueberry are the fruit and leaves (512). Blueberry fruit is high in fiber and vitamin C (833). Blueberries also contain anthocyanins and proanthocyanidins, which appear to have antioxidant activity (900,907,908). Preliminary research from animal models suggests that the antioxidant effects of blueberry extracts might have anticancer activity and potentially reduce normal oxidative cellular damage that occurs with aging (888,889,908). Blueberry, like its relative, the cranberry, also appears to prevent bacterial adhesion to the bladder and bacterial colonization (2813,6757); however, clinical studies have not yet been performed.

Adverse Reactions

None reported.

Interactions with Herbs & Other Dietary Supplements

Insufficient reliable information available.

Interactions with Drugs

ANTIDIABETES DRUGS: Theoretically, blueberry leaf might lower blood glucose (909); however, this effect has not yet been reported in humans. Until more is known, monitor blood glucose levels more closely in patients with diabetes who are taking blueberry. Dose adjustments may be necessary in patients taking diabetes medications.

Interactions with Foods

No interactions are known to occur, and there is no known reason to expect a clinically significant interaction.

Interactions with Lab Tests

BLOOD GLUCOSE: Theoretically, blueberry leaf might lower blood glucose and test results (909); however, this effect has not yet been reported in humans.
TRIGLYCERIDES: Theoretically, blueberry leaf, which is related to the bilberry, might lower serum triglycerides and test results (909); however, this effect has not yet been reported in humans.

Interactions with Diseases or Conditions

DIABETES: Theoretically, blueberry leaf might lower blood glucose (909); however, this effect has not yet been reported in humans. Until more is known, monitor blood glucose levels more closely in patients with diabetes who are taking blueberry. Dose adjustments may be necessary in patients taking diabetes medications.

Dosage and Administration

ORAL: For diarrhea, people typically chew 3 tablespoons of the dried berries or prepare a decoction of the crushed fruits (814). The leaves are also prepared as a tea using 1 to 2 teaspoons of chopped leaves per cup of cold water, taken up to 3 times daily (814).

Comments

Don't confuse blueberry with bilberry. Blueberry in the US refers to the species of Vaccinium listed in this monograph. However, elsewhere in the world, blueberry may refer to the European plant, Vaccinium myrtillus, which is called bilberry in the US [512].

BOG BILBERRY

Also Known As

None.
CAUTION: See separate listings for Bilberry fruit and Bilberry leaf.

Scientific Names

Vaccinium uliginosum.
Family: Ericaceae.

People Use This For

Orally, bog bilberry is used for mucous membrane inflammation of the gastric and intestinal tract, diarrhea, and bladder complaints [18].

Safety

POSSIBLY UNSAFE …when used orally in large amounts. Poisoning has been reported when individuals ingest fruit from fungus-infested plants [18].
There is insufficient reliable information available about the safety of dried bog bilberry fruit used in medicinal amounts.
PREGNANCY AND LACTATION: Insufficient reliable information available; avoid using.

Effectiveness

There is insufficient reliable information available about the effectiveness of bog bilberry.

Mechanism of Action

The applicable part of bog bilberry is the dried, ripe fruit. The active constituents of bog bilberry are tannins, anthocyanoside, and flavonoids [18].

Adverse Reactions

Orally, poisonings from the ingestion of large quantities of the bog bilberry fruit are rare and could have been due to contamination with a fungus, Sclerroyina megalospora [18]. The symptoms of poisoning include queasiness, vomiting, states of intoxication, feelings of weakness, and visual disorders [18].

Interactions with Herbs & Other Dietary Supplements

Insufficient reliable information available.

Interactions with Drugs

No interactions are known to occur, and there is no known reason to expect a clinically significant interaction with bog bilberry.

Interactions with Foods

No interactions are known to occur, and there is no known reason to expect a clinically significant interaction with bog bilberry.

Interactions with Lab Tests

No interactions are known to occur, and there is no known reason to expect a clinically significant interaction with bog bilberry.

Interactions with Diseases or Conditions

No interactions are known to occur, and there is no known reason to expect a clinically significant interaction with bog bilberry.

Dosage and Administration

ORAL: The usual dose of bog bilberry is one cup of the unsweetened tea once or twice daily [18]. The tea is prepared by steeping 2 heaping teaspoons of the dried, ripe fruit in 250 mL cold water for 10-12 hours and then straining.

Comments
Avoid confusion with bilberry fruit or bilberry leaf.

BOGBEAN

Also Known As
Buckbean, Marsh Trefoil, Menyanthes, Water Shamrock.

Scientific Names
Menyanthes trifoliata.
Family: Menyanthaceae.

People Use This For
Orally, bogbean is used for rheumatism, rheumatoid arthritis (4), loss of appetite, and dyspepsia (2).
In food manufacturing, bogbean is used as a flavoring agent (4).

Safety
LIKELY SAFE ...when used orally in amounts commonly found in foods. The Council of Europe lists bogbean as a natural food flavoring (4).
POSSIBLY SAFE ...when used orally in medicinal amounts (12).
POSSIBLY UNSAFE ...when used orally in excessive amounts. Bogbean leaf preparations can irritate the GI tract (4).
PREGNANCY AND LACTATION: POSSIBLY UNSAFE ...when used orally due to the lack of toxicity information and its possible purgative action (4); avoid using.

Effectiveness
POSSIBLY EFFECTIVE ...when used orally as an appetite stimulant (2).
There is insufficient reliable information available about the effectiveness of bogbean for its other uses.

Mechanism of Action
The applicable part of bogbean is the leaf. The bitter principles, or iridoids, can stimulate saliva and gastric juices (2,4). Bogbean can have purgative actions (4). An unidentified constituent has hemolytic activity (4).

Adverse Reactions
Orally, excessive doses of bogbean can irritate the GI tract, and cause diarrhea, pain, nausea, and vomiting. Theoretically, it can cause bleeding (4).

Interactions with Herbs & Other Dietary Supplements
HERBS WITH ANTICOAGULANT/ANTIPLATELET POTENTIAL: Concomitant use of herbs that have coumarin constituents or affect platelet aggregation could theoretically increase the risk of bleeding in some people. These herbs include: angelica, anise, arnica, asafoetida, boldo, capsicum, celery, chamomile, clove, danshen, fenugreek, feverfew, garlic, ginger, ginkgo, ginseng (Panax), horse chestnut, horseradish, licorice, meadowsweet, prickly ash, onion, papain, passionflower, poplar, quassia, red clover, turmeric, wild carrot, wild lettuce, willow, and others (4,19).

Interactions with Drugs
ANTICOAGULANT, ANTIPLATELET DRUGS: Theoretically, bogbean can increase the risk of bleeding.

Interactions with Foods
No interactions are known to occur, and there is no known reason to expect a clinically significant interaction with bogbean.

Interactions with Lab Tests
No interactions are known to occur, and there is no known reason to expect a clinically significant interaction with bogbean.

Interactions with Diseases or Conditions
DIARRHEA, DYSENTERY, COLITIS: Contraindicated (12).
PEOPLE AT RISK FOR BLEEDING: Theoretically, bogbean can increase bleeding risk.

Dosage and Administration

ORAL: The typical dose of bogbean is 1-3 grams of the dried leaf three times daily or as a tea three times daily. The tea is prepared by steeping 1-3 grams of the dried leaf in 150 mL boiling water for 5-10 minutes and then straining (2,4). The common dose of the liquid extract (1:1 in 25% alcohol) is 1-2 mL three times daily (4). The tincture (1:5 in 45% alcohol) is usually given as 1-3 mL three times daily (4).

Comments

The bogbean fruit resembles a small bean and is commonly found in swamps or bogs, which is the reason for its name (6002).

BOIS DE ROSE OIL

Also Known As

Cayenne Rosewood Oil, Distilled Oil from Aniba Rosaeodora Wood, Rosewood Oil.

Scientific Names

Aniba rosaeodora.
Family: Lauraceae.

People Use This For

No medicinal uses are reported (11).
For food use, bois de rose oil is a flavoring.
In manufacturing, bois de rose oil is used in cosmetics (maximum use level 1.2% in perfumes).

Safety

LIKELY SAFE ...when used orally in amounts contained in foods. It has Generally Recognized as Safe (GRAS) status in US (11). ...when used topically in cosmetics; reported to be nontoxic (11).
PREGNANCY AND LACTATION: Insufficient reliable information available.

Effectiveness

There is insufficient reliable information about the effectiveness of bois de rose oil.

Mechanism of Action

The major constituent, linalool, is reported to have anticonvulsant activity in mice and rats, spasmolytic activity on isolated guinea pig ileum, antimicrobial properties, and weak tumor promoting properties in mice (11).

Adverse Reactions

None reported.

Interactions with Herbs & Other Dietary Supplements

Insufficient reliable information available.

Interactions with Drugs

No interactions are known to occur, and there is no known reason to expect a clinically significant interaction with bois de rose oil.

Interactions with Foods

No interactions are known to occur, and there is no known reason to expect a clinically significant interaction with bois de rose oil.

Interactions with Lab Tests

No interactions are known to occur, and there is no known reason to expect a clinically significant interaction with bois de rose oil.

Interactions with Diseases or Conditions

No interactions are known to occur, and there is no known reason to expect a clinically significant interaction with bois de rose oil.

Dosage and Administration

No typical dosage.

Comments

There is very little scientific information about this product. Our staff is continually analyzing the available information on natural medicines and will add data here as it becomes available.

BOLDO

Also Known As

Boldine, Boldo Folium, Boldoak Boldea, Boldus, Boldus Boldus.

Scientific Names

Peumus boldus.
Family: Monimiaceae.

People Use This For

Orally, boldo is used for mild GI spasms, gallstones, rheumatism, cystitis, hepatic disease, and gonorrhea. It is also used as a diuretic, sedative, bile stimulant, and antiseptic.

Safety

LIKELY SAFE ...when consumed in the small amounts commonly found in food. Boldo is approved for use in alcoholic beverages with a maximum use level of 0.0002% (11).
LIKELY UNSAFE ...when used excessively for oral medicinal purposes, because of the presence of the volatile oil (2.5% in leaf), which contains ascaridole (4). If taken by mouth, ascaridole-free preparations should be used (2).
PREGNANCY AND LACTATION: UNSAFE ...when the volatile oil is used, due to ascaridole.

Effectiveness

POSSIBLY EFFECTIVE ...when used orally as a cathartic or diuretic (4) and used for mild GI spasms (2). There is insufficient reliable information available about the effectiveness of boldo for its other uses.

Mechanism of Action

The applicable part of boldo is the leaf. The alkaloidal constituents are responsible for actions that include stimulating bile and bile flow, stimulating stomach function, and diuresis (4). The diuretic and mild urinary antiseptic properties probably result from the irritant volatile oil (4). There's some evidence that the boldine constituent, can inhibit thromboxane A2 production, resulting in antiplatelet activity (5191).

Adverse Reactions

Orally, boldo can cause convulsions.
Topically, boldo can irritate the skin (4).

Interactions with Herbs & Other Dietary Supplements

HERBS WITH ANTICOAGULANT/ANTIPLATELET POTENTIAL: Concomitant use of herbs that have coumarin constituents or affect platelet aggregation could theoretically increase the risk of bleeding in some people. These herbs include: angelica, anise, arnica, asafoetida, bogbean, capsicum, celery, chamomile, clove, danshen, fenugreek, feverfew, garlic, ginger, ginkgo, ginseng (Panax), horse chestnut, horseradish, licorice, meadowsweet, prickly ash, onion, papain, passionflower, poplar, quassia, red clover, turmeric, wild carrot, wild lettuce, willow, and others (4,19).

Interactions with Drugs

ANTICOAGULANT/ANTIPLATELET DRUGS: There is some concern that boldo might have additive effects when used with anticoagulant or antiplatelet drugs and increase the risk of bruising and bleeding. Boldo constituents seem to have antiplatelet effects (5191). Some of these drugs include aspirin, clopidogrel (Plavix), nonsteroidal anti-inflammatory drugs (NSAIDs) such as diclofenac (Voltaren, Cataflam, others), ibuprofen (Advil, Motrin, others), naproxen (Anaprox, Naprosyn, others), dalteparin (Fragmin), enoxaparin (Lovenox), heparin, and others.
WARFARIN (Coumadin): Boldo can have additive effects with warfarin and increase the international normalized ratio (INR). Boldo constituents seem to have antiplatelet activity (5191).

Interactions with Foods

No interactions are known to occur, and there is no known reason to expect a clinically significant interaction with boldo.

Interactions with Lab Tests

No interactions are known to occur, and there is no known reason to expect a clinically significant interaction with boldo.

Interactions with Diseases or Conditions

KIDNEY DISORDERS: Avoid boldo products which are not certified as ascaridole-free (4).
LIVER DISEASE: Contraindicated (8,12).
BILE DUCT OBSTRUCTION: Contraindicated (12).
GALLSTONES: Boldo should not be used for self-medication of gallstones, which requires monitoring (12).

Dosage and Administration

ORAL: The typical dose of boldo is 60-200 mg of the dried leaf three times daily or as a tea three times a day. The tea is prepared by steeping 1 gram of the dried leaf in 150 mL boiling water for 5-10 minutes and then straining (2,4). The common dose of the liquid extract (1:1 in 45% alcohol) is 0.1-0.3 mL three times daily (4). The tincture (1:10 in 60% alcohol) is usually given as 0.5-2 mL three times daily (4). The average daily dose of the boldo leaf by infusion is 3 grams (2).

Comments

Fossilized boldo leaves that are over thirteen thousand years old have been found in Chile with the imprints of human teeth on them (6002).

BONESET

Also Known As

Agueweed, Crosswort, Feverwort, Indian Sage, Sweating Plant, Teasel, Thoroughwort, Vegetable Antimony.
CAUTION: See separate listings for Gravel Root and Sage.

Scientific Names

Eupatorium perfoliatum.
Family: Asteraceae or Compositae.

People Use This For

Orally, boneset is used as an antipyretic (5,6), diuretic, laxative, emesis, and cathartic (6).
Traditionally, boneset is used to treat influenza (especially with aching muscles) (4), acute bronchitis (4), nasal inflammation (4), rheumatism (6), edema (6), dengue fever (6), and pneumonia (6); and as a stimulant (11) and a diaphoretic (4,5,11).

Safety

POSSIBLY UNSAFE ...when used orally. Large doses are both cathartic and emetic. Though the alkaloids have not been characterized, hepatotoxic unsaturated pyrrolizidine alkaloids are common in this genus (12).
PREGNANCY AND LACTATION: POSSIBLY UNSAFE ...when used orally; avoid using.

Effectiveness

POSSIBLY EFFECTIVE ...when used orally as an immunostimulant and anti-inflammatory agent (4).
There is insufficient reliable information available about the effectiveness of boneset for its other uses.

Mechanism of Action

The applicable parts of boneset are the dried leaf and flowering parts. Researchers think the sesquiterpene lactones may have immunostimulant activity (4).

Adverse Reactions

Orally, boneset can cause an allergic reaction in individuals sensitive to the Asteraceae/Compositae family. Members of this family include ragweed, chrysanthemums, marigolds, daisies, and many other herbs.

Interactions with Herbs & Other Dietary Supplements

Insufficient reliable information available.

Interactions with Drugs

No interactions are known to occur, and there is no known reason to expect a clinically significant interaction with boneset.

Interactions with Foods

No interactions are known to occur, and there is no known reason to expect a clinically significant interaction with boneset.

Interactions with Lab Tests

No interactions are known to occur, and there is no known reason to expect a clinically significant interaction with boneset.

Interactions with Diseases or Conditions

CROSS-ALLERGENICITY: Boneset can cause an allergic reaction in individuals sensitive to the Asteraceae/Compositae family. Members of this family include ragweed, chrysanthemums, marigolds, daisies, and many other herbs.

Dosage and Administration

ORAL: Drink 1 cup tea (steep 1-2 grams herb in 150 mL boiling water 5-10 minutes, strain) three times daily (4). Liquid extract (1:1 in 25% alcohol) 1-2 mL three times daily (4) and tincture: (1:5 in 45% alcohol) 1-4 mL three times daily have also been used (4).

Comments

Avoid confusion with gravel root (Eupatorium purpureum) also known as boneset. Snakeroot is a common name used for poisonous Eupatorium species (4).

BORAGE flower, dried above ground parts

Also Known As

Bee plant, Beebread, Borago, Burrage, Common Borage, Common Bugloss, Cool Tankard, Ox's Tongue. CAUTION: See separate listing for Borage Seed Oil.

Scientific Names

Borago officinalis.
Family: Boraginaceae.

People Use This For

Orally, borage is used for fever, cough, depression, arthritis, pain relief, phlebitis, and menopausal disorders. It is also used as an agent to restore the adrenal cortex, for "blood purification" and diuresis, as a preventative for inflammation of lungs and peritoneum, an anti-inflammatory agent, cardiac tonic, sedative, to induce sweating, and increase circulatory capacity.
Topically, borage is used as a poultice and as an emollient.
Historically, borage was used to promote "happiness and courage", increase breast milk production, and to treat rheumatism, bronchitis, colds, and breast or facial cancers.
For food uses, borage is found in various products including preserved leaves, salads, and soups.
In manufacturing, borage is used in skin care products.

Safety

POSSIBLY SAFE ...when used orally in amounts found in foods (6).
LIKELY UNSAFE ...when used orally for medicinal uses. Borage flower and dried above ground parts contain hepatotoxic pyrrolizidine alkaloids (4,12). Excessive doses or long-term use increases risk of adverse effects (2,4,12).
PREGNANCY AND LACTATION: LIKELY UNSAFE ...when used orally (4,12); avoid using.

Effectiveness

There is insufficient reliable information available about the effectiveness of the oral or topical use of borage flower and dried above ground parts.

Mechanism of Action

Borage flower and dried above ground parts contain tannins which are thought to give it astringent properties. The mucilage may contribute to reported expectorant effect. Malic acid and potassium nitrate constituents may have a diuretic effect (6). Borage contains variable amounts of toxic pyrrolizidine alkaloids which are organotoxic, hepatotoxic, and carcinogenic in animal models (2). Unlike borage seed, the above ground parts of the plant do not contain gamma-linolenic acid (GLA) (7162).

Adverse Reactions

Orally, use of borage can cause constipation (5,6). The potential for hepatotoxicity (due to presence of pyrrolizidine alkaloids) increases with larger doses and longer periods of use (4,12).

Interactions with Herbs & Other Dietary Supplements

EUCALYPTUS: Theoretically, concomitant use might increase the risk of unsaturated pyrrolizidine alkaloid toxicity due to enzyme induction by eucalyptus (19).

PYRROLIZIDINE ALKALOID-CONTAINING HERBS: Concomitant use is contraindicated due to the risk of additive toxicity. Herbs containing unsaturated pyrrolizidine alkaloids include: alkanna (12), borage (271), gravel root (4), hemp agrimony (271), hound's tongue (19), petasites (19), comfrey (271), coltsfoot, and the Senecio species plants; dusty miller (19), alpine ragwort (19), groundsel (271), golden ragwort (19), and tansy ragwort (271).

Interactions with Drugs

HEPATOTOXIC DRUGS: Theoretically, borage flower and dried above ground parts could have additive toxicity with drugs with hepatotoxic potential (2). Some of these drugs are: amidarone (Codarone), fluconazole (Diflucan), itraconazole (Sporanox), carbamazepine (Tegretol), erythromycin (Erythrocin, Illosone, others), estrogens, isoniazid (INH), phenytoin (Dilantin), lovastatin (Mevacor), pravastatin (Pravachol), simvastatin (Zocor), and others.

Interactions with Foods

No interactions are known to occur, and there is no known reason to expect a clinically significant interaction with borage flower and dried above ground parts.

Interactions with Lab Tests

No interactions are known to occur, and there is no known reason to expect a clinically significant interaction with borage flower and dried above ground parts.

Interactions with Diseases or Conditions

HEPATIC DISEASE: Theoretically, borage flower and dried above ground parts could worsen hepatic disease. Borage flower and dried above ground parts contain hepatotoxic pyrrolizidine alkaloids (2).

Dosage and Administration

No typical dosage.

Comments

Avoid confusion with borage seed oil.

BORAGE SEED OIL

Also Known As

Borage Oil, Bugloss, Burage, Burrage, Huile De Bourrache, Starflower.
CAUTION: See separate listings for Borage flower, Black Currant Seed Oil, Evening Primrose Oil, Gamma Linolenic Acid, and Omega-6 Oils.

Scientific Names

Borago officinalis.
Family: Boraginaceae.

People Use This For

Orally, borage seed oil is used for rheumatoid arthritis, neurodermatitis, stress, atopic eczema, premenstrual syndrome (PMS), diabetes, alcoholism, inflammation, and for preventing heart disease and stroke.

Safety

POSSIBLY SAFE ...when used orally and appropriately. Only products that are labeled as unsaturated pyrrolizidine alkaloid (UPA) free should be used (3,214).

LIKELY UNSAFE ...when products containing UPAs are used orally, although borage seed oil is reported to contain only small amounts of UPAs (502). ...when therapeutic doses are used because UPA amounts may reach toxic levels (214). UPAs are associated with serious hepatic and possibly renal toxicity (3). The German Federal Health Agency limits consumption of toxic UPAs to not more than 1 mcg per day (3). Borage seed oil containing UPAs dosed at 1-2 grams per day might provide as much as 10 mcg of UPAs, which exceeds the German recommendation by 10 times (214).

PREGNANCY AND LACTATION: Insufficient reliable information available; avoid using.

Effectiveness

POSSIBLY EFFECTIVE ...when used orally in combination with analgesics or anti-inflammatory agents for improving symptoms of rheumatoid arthritis (1985). Two small-scale studies have suggested that borage seed oil might decrease symptoms of rheumatoid arthritis after 12-24 weeks of treatment in combination with conventional analgesics or anti-inflammatory agents (214). ...when used orally for reducing symptoms of atopic dermatitis (3900). There is insufficient reliable information available about the effectiveness of borage seed oil for its other uses.

Mechanism of Action

Borage seed oil is the fatty oil of the seeds of Borago officinalis. Borage oil contains 20-26% of the essential fatty acid gamma-linolenic acid (GLA) (3), making it useful as a supplemental source of fatty acid. For inflammatory conditions such as rheumatoid arthritis and atopic dermatitis, the GLA constituent is thought to act as an anti-inflammatory. In humans, GLA is rapidly metabolized to dihomogammalinolenic acid, which is a precursor to prostaglandin E1 (PGE1). PGE1 has potent anti-inflammatory properties (214). The mechanism of borage seed oil for reducing the cardiac response to stress is not known (4). The GLA constituent of borage seed oil also lowers plasma triglycerides, increases high-density lipoprotein (HDL) levels, and prolongs bleeding time (1979). It has been theorized that low arachidonic acid levels in breast milk of atopic mothers might increase the risk for development of atopy in infants and that maternal supplementation with borage seed oil might increase arachidonic acid levels in breast milk. However, oral borage seed oil supplements failed to increase breast milk arachidonic acid concentrations in lactating, atopic women (6106). Some borage seed oil preparations contain toxic constituents known as unsaturated pyrrolizidine alkaloids (UPAs). The UPA constituents, including amabiline, are hepatotoxic even in minute amounts (3) and there are some reports of renal toxicity (12). Some UPAs have shown carcinogenic and mutagenic properties; however, the primary concern is veno-occlusive disease (12). Borage seed oil preparations are available that are UPA-free (3).

Adverse Reactions

Gamma linolenic acid can prolong bleeding time (1979).

Interactions with Herbs & Other Dietary Supplements

HERBS WITH ANTICOAGULANT/ANTIPLATELET POTENTIAL: Concomitant use of herbs that have coumarin constituents or affect platelet aggregation could theoretically increase the risk of bleeding in some people. These herbs include: angelica, anise, arnica, asafoetida, bogbean, boldo, capsicum, celery, chamomile, clove, danshen, fenugreek, feverfew, garlic, ginger, ginkgo, ginseng (Panax), horse chestnut, horseradish, licorice, meadowsweet, prickly ash, onion, papain, passionflower, poplar, quassia, red clover, turmeric, wild carrot, wild lettuce, willow, and others (4,19).

EUCALYPTUS: Theoretically, unless the oil is certified pyrrolizidine-free, concomitant use with eucalyptus can increase the risk of unsaturated pyrrolizidine alkaloid toxicity due to enzyme induction by eucalyptus (19).

PYRROLIZIDINE ALKALOID-CONTAINING HERBS: Concomitant use is contraindicated due to the risk of additive toxicity. Herbs containing unsaturated pyrrolizidine alkaloids include: alkanna (12), borage (271), gravel root (4), hemp agrimony (271), hound's tongue (19), petasites (19), comfrey (271), coltsfoot, and the Senecio species plants; dusty miller (19), alpine ragwort (19), groundsel (271), golden ragwort (19), and tansy ragwort (271).

Interactions with Drugs

ANESTHESIA: Theoretically, concomitant use can increase the risk of seizures based on one case report of evening primrose oil (source of gamma linolenic acid) and possibly other drugs (613).

ANTICOAGULANT/ANTIPLATELET DRUGS: Borage seed oil, which contains gamma linolenic acid (GLA) could have anticoagulant effects (1979). Theoretically, taking borage seed oil with other anticoagulant or antiplatelet drugs might increase the risk of bruising and bleeding. Some of these drugs include aspirin, clopidogrel (Plavix), nonsteroidal anti-inflammatory drugs (NSAIDs) such as diclofenac (Voltaren, Cataflam, others), ibuprofen (Advil, Motrin, others), naproxen (Anaprox, Naprosyn, others), dalteparin (Fragmin), enoxaparin (Lovenox), heparin, warfarin (Coumadin), and others.

PHENOTHIAZINES: Theoretically, concomitant use of borage seed oil can increase the risk of seizures in people with schizophrenia treated with phenothiazines (4). This is based on reports involving evening primrose oil. Some phenothiazines are chlorpromazine (Thorazine), fluphenazine (Prolixin), promethazine (Phenergan), trifluoperazine (Stelazine), thioridazine (Mellaril), and others.

Interactions with Foods

No interactions are known to occur, and there is no known reason to expect a clinically significant interaction with borage seed oil.

Interactions with Lab Tests
BLEEDING TIME: Borage seed oil might prolong bleeding time. Borage seed oil contains gamma linolenic acid (GLA), which can inhibit platelet aggregation (1979).
LPID PROFILE: Borage seed oil might affect lipid levels. Borage seed oil contains gamma linolenic acid (GLA), which can lower plasma triglycerides and increase high-density lipoprotein (HDL) cholesterol (1979).

Interactions with Diseases or Conditions
BLEEDING DISORDERS: There is some concern that borage seed oil might prolong bleeding time and increase the risk of bruising and bleeding. Borage seed oil contains gamma linolenic acid (GLA), which can inhibit platelet aggregation (1979).
LIVER DISEASE: Borage seed oil might exacerbate liver disease. Borage seed oil can contain hepatotoxic pyrrolizidine alkaloids (19). Tell patients with liver disease to only use products certified to be pyrrolizidine alkaloid-free.
SCHIZOPHRENIA: Theoretically, concomitant use of phenothiazines and borage seed oil might increase the risk of seizures in people with schizophrenia (4). This is based on reports of evening primrose oil, another source of gamma linolenic acid.

Dosage and Administration
ORAL: For rheumatoid arthritis, studies have used either 1.1 or 1.4 grams borage seed oil daily (214,3900).

Comments
Some sources have suggested that borage seed oil could be used as an alternative to evening primrose oil because both are good sources of gamma-linolenic acid (GLA) (214).

BORON

Also Known As
Borate, Borates, Boric Acid, Boric Anhydride, Boric Tartate, Sodium Borate.

Scientific Names
Boron; B; atomic number 5.

People Use This For
Orally, boron is used for promoting bone health, treating osteoarthritis, as an aid for building muscle and increasing testosterone levels, and for enhancing cognitive function and fine motor skills.
Topically, boric acid, the most common form of boron, is used as an astringent, to prevent skin infection, and as an ophthalmological irrigant.

Safety
LIKELY SAFE ...when used orally and appropriately. Boron is safe in amounts that do not exceed 20 mg per day, the Tolerable Upper Intake Level (UL) (7135). ...when used topically and appropriately. Boric acid, the most common form of boron, can be safely applied to non-broken skin (6).
POSSIBLY UNSAFE ...when used orally in high doses. Tell patients to avoid exceeding the UL of 20 mg per day. Higher doses might theoretically cause adverse effects on the testes and male fertility (7135). Poisoning has occurred after ingestion of equivalent of 2.12 grams boron per day for 3-4 weeks (17).
CHILDREN: LIKELY SAFE ...when used orally and appropriately. Boron is safe in children in amounts that do not exceed the UL of 3 mg per day in children 1 to 3 years, 6 mg per day in children 4 to 8 years; 11 mg per day in children 9 to 13 years; 17 mg per day in adolescents 14 years or older (7135). The UL for infants has not been determined. (7135). POSSIBLY UNSAFE ...when used orally in high doses. Tell patients to avoid exceeding the UL of 3 mg per day in children 1 to 3 years, 6 mg per day in children 4 to 8 years, 11 mg per day in children 9 to 13 years, and 17 mg per day in adolescents 14 years or older (7135). Higher doses might theoretically cause adverse effects on the testes and male fertility (7135).
PREGNANCY AND LACTATION: LIKELY SAFE ...when used orally and appropriately. Boron is safe in amounts that do not exceed the 20 mg per day or 17 mg per day for pregnant women ages 14 to 18, the UL for pregnancy and lactation (7135). POSSIBLY UNSAFE ...when used orally in high doses. Tell patients to avoid exceeding the UL of 20 mg per day or 17 mg per day for pregnant women ages 14 to 18 (7135). Higher doses might theoretically cause adverse effects in the developing fetus (7135).

Effectiveness
LIKELY INEFFECTIVE ...when used orally for building muscle or increasing testosterone levels (944).

There is insufficient reliable information available about the effectiveness of boron for its other uses. However, early evidence suggests that boron might be useful for treating osteoarthritis (941). It might also improve cognitive function and fine motor skills in older people (943). More evidence is needed to rate boron for these uses.

Mechanism of Action

Boron is a trace mineral for which as a clear biological function for boron in humans has not been established. There is some evidence, though, that boron might be have a role in reproduction and development (945,7135). Boron is well absorbed from dietary beverages including prune and grape juice, wine, coffee, milk, and in some geographical locations, water (7135). Avocado, peanuts, pecans, apples, dried beans and potatoes also contain boron (7135). Boron is excreted unchanged in the urine, with a half-life of 21 hours (7135).

Boron seems to be important in mineral metabolism and membrane function (943). Diets higher in boron seem to increase serum 17-beta-estradiol levels in postmenopausal women using estrogen replacement therapy (945). Supplemental boron may increase serum estradiol levels in postmenopausal women (945) and healthy men (937). Boron together with exercise seems to result in lower serum magnesium levels (942) and modestly lower serum phosphorus concentrations. The lower serum phosphorus concentrations are diminished by exercise (940). Preliminary evidence suggests that boron may have a role in hand-eye coordination, attention, and short-term memory (7135).

Adverse Reactions

Orally, boron appears to have low toxicity (7135). Adverse reactions in doses below 10 mg per day (937) are unlikely. Chronic use of 1 gram daily of boric acid or 25 grams daily of boric tartate can cause dermatitis, alopecia, anorexia, and indigestion (7135). Boric acid/borate can be fatal when taken orally in doses of 300 mg/kg (6).

Large doses can result in acute poisoning. Children who have ingested 5 grams of more of borates can have persistent nausea, vomiting, and diarrhea leading to acute dehydration, shock, and coma. Adults who have ingested 15-20 grams of borate can exhibit nausea, vomiting, diarrhea, epigastric pain, hematemesis and blue-green discoloration of feces and vomit (17). Symptoms in adults and children may also include skin erythema, desquamation, exfoliation, hyperexcitability, irritability, tremors, convulsions, weakness, lethargy, headaches, and depression (17).

Interactions with Herbs & Other Dietary Supplements

Insufficient reliable information available.

Interactions with Drugs

ESTROGENIC DRUGS: Concomitant administration may increase serum estrogen levels (945) (see Mechanism of Action).

Interactions with Foods

No interactions are known to occur, and there is no known reason to expect a clinically significant interaction with boron.

Interactions with Lab Tests

BONE MINERAL DENSITY (BMD): Supplemental boron might increase BMD and BMD measurements in young athletic females (942).

PHOSPHORUS: Supplemental boron might reduce serum phosphorus concentrations and test results in some individuals (942).

Interactions with Diseases or Conditions

HORMONE SENSITIVE CANCERS/CONDITIONS: Because boron might have estrogenic effects (945), women with hormone sensitive conditions should avoid supplemental boron or high amounts of boron from foods. Some of these conditions include breast, uterine, and ovarian cancer, and endometriosis and uterine fibroids.

KIDNEY DISEASE, IMPAIRED KIDNEY FUNCTION: Theoretically, avoid supplements; boron appears largely excreted by kidneys (939).

Dosage and Administration

ORAL: There is no RDA for boron since an essential biological role for it has not been identified (7135). Dietary intake of boron varies. Diets considered to be high in boron provide approximately 3.25 mg boron per 2000 kcal/day is a diet. Diets considered to be low in boron provide 0.25 mg boron per 2000 kcal/day (943). The Tolerable Upper Intake Level (UL), the maximum dose at which no adverse effects would be expected, is 20 mg per day for adults and pregnant or lactating women over 19 years (7135). For adolescents 14 to 18 years and pregnant or lactating women 14 to 18 years, the UL is 17 mg per day (7135). For children 9 to 13 years, the UL is 11 mg per day; children 4 to 8 years, 6 mg per day; and children 1 to 3 years, 3 mg per day. A UL has not been established for infants (7135).

Comments

Boron was used as a food preservative between 1870 and 1920, and during World Wars I and II (945).

BOVINE CARTILAGE

Also Known As

Antitumor Angiogenesis Factor (anti-TAF), Bovine Tracheal Cartilage (BTC), Catrix, Catrix-S, Processed Bovine Cartilage, Psoriacin, Psoriacin-T, Rumalon.

Scientific Names

None.

People Use This For

Orally, bovine cartilage is used for rheumatoid arthritis (2016), osteoarthritis (2016,2017), ulcerative colitis (2009,2017), scleroderma (2017), psoriasis, allergic reactions caused by chemical toxins (2017), herpes infection (2017), glioblastoma multiforme, and cancer (2010).

Topically, bovine cartilage is used for non-healing ulcerated wounds (2009), moist lesions including pruritus ani, external hemorrhoids, acne, poison oak or poison ivy dermatitis (2009), mandibular alveolitis (dry socket) (2009), and psoriasis (2009).

Rectally, bovine cartilage is used for internal hemorrhoids and fissure-in-ano (2009).

Subcutaneously, bovine cartilage is used for osteoarthritis, rheumatoid arthritis, psoriasis, ulcerative colitis, regional enteritis, progressive systemic sclerosis (2009), glioblastoma multiforme (2010), inoperable squamous cancer of the nose (2010), and cancers of the pancreas, lung, ovary, rectum, prostate, cervix, and thyroid (2010).

Safety

POSSIBLY SAFE ...when used orally. Up to 20 kg total have been used without evidence of toxicity (2010). Up to 40 grams per week and 300 grams total have been injected subcutaneously without evidence of toxicity. However, since these preparations are derived from animals, there is concern about contamination with diseased animal parts (see Adverse Reactions) (1825). So far, there are no reports of disease transmission to humans due to use of contaminated bovine cartilage.

PREGNANCY AND LACTATION: Insufficient reliable information available; avoid using.

Effectiveness

POSSIBLY EFFECTIVE ...when used topically for pruritus ani, poison oak and poison ivy dermatitis, acne, mandibular alveolitis, and psoriasis (2009). ...when used rectally for hemorrhoids and fissure-in-ano (2009). ...when used subcutaneously for osteoarthritis, rheumatoid arthritis, and psoriasis (2009).

There is insufficient reliable information available about the effectiveness of bovine cartilage for its other uses.

Mechanism of Action

Researchers theorize that bovine cartilage provides the needed biochemical components to support resynthesis of cartilage in individuals with osteoarthritis (2009). Bovine cartilage is also thought to have anti-inflammatory, immunoregulatory, hygroscopic-drying, and wound-healing activity (2009). Churning symptoms (appearance of new papules as the original lesions fade) may occur for 3-6 weeks during psoriasis treatment. These are thought to result from release of "psoriagens" from present lesions. Eventually, "psoriagens" are excreted or metabolized, resulting in symptomatic improvement (2009).

Adverse Reactions

Orally, bovine cartilage can cause osmotic diarrhea (2009), nausea, and scrotal edema (2019). When used subcutaneously, bovine cartilage might initially cause local redness, swelling, and itching (2010); the appearance of new psoriatic papules (2009); or nephrotic syndrome (2011). It can cause local allergic reaction (2010). Bovine cartilage products made from contaminated or diseased animals might present a human health hazard. There is some concern that bovine cartilage from cows in countries where bovine spongiform encephalitis (BSE) has been reported might be contaminated with diseased tissue. Countries where BSE has been reported include Great Britain, France, The Netherlands, Portugal, Luxembourg, Ireland, Switzerland, Oman, and Belgium (1825). However, there have been no reports of BSE transfer to humans from contaminated bovine cartilage products. Until more is known, tell patients to avoid these products unless country of origin can be determined. Patients should avoid products that are produced in countries where BSE has been found.

Interactions with Herbs & Other Dietary Supplements

Insufficient reliable information available.

Interactions with Drugs

No interactions are known to occur, and there is no known reason to expect a clinically significant interaction with bovine cartilage.

Interactions with Foods

No interactions are known to occur, and there is no known reason to expect a clinically significant interaction with bovine cartilage.

Interactions with Lab Tests

No interactions are known to occur, and there is no known reason to expect a clinically significant interaction with bovine cartilage.

Interactions with Diseases or Conditions

No interactions are known to occur, and there is no known reason to expect a clinically significant interaction with bovine cartilage.

Dosage and Administration

ORAL: Ulcerative colitis, 3 grams four times daily (2009). Cancer- typical amount for maintenance following parenteral loading phase, 3 grams every 8 hours (or 9 grams per day in at least two divided amounts), up to 20 kg during a complete course of treatment (2010).
TOPICAL: Pruritus ani, 5% cream applied two or more times daily, with resolution expected in 3 days (2009). Poison ivy/oak dermatitis, 5% cream applied every two hours initially and less frequently as the itching is controlled, with resolution in 1-2 weeks (2009). Acne, 5% cream applied at least twice daily after washing (2009). Mandibular alveolitis, powdered bovine cartilage mixed with saline to form a paste, packed into the dry socket following tooth extraction (2009). Psoriasis, parenteral therapy followed by 5% ointment applied two to three times daily after bathing (2009); bovine cartilage ointment with 0.1% coal tar for elevated, dry, horny lesions or without coal tar for smooth and red skin after initial sloughing has been achieved (2009).
RECTAL: 2.2 grams in the form of a 2% suppository administered at least three times daily with dioctyl sodium sulfosuccinate (DSS) 100 mg twice daily orally as a stool softener (2009).
SUBCUTANEOUS (SC): Bovine cartilage solution (diluted 1:10 with 1% lidocaine to alleviate discomfort) is reportedly used in a concentration 50 mg/mL in humans (2009,2010). In general, 1.25-2.5 grams (25-50 mL) slowly injected per site with an 18-gauge needle for total of 5 grams per treatment, given weekly or biweekly, to a total of 25 grams for most uses; exceptions are osteoarthritis up to 40 grams, psoriasis up to 75 grams, and cancer 100-300 grams (2009,2010). Boosters of 2.5 grams (50 mL) are administered every 3-4 weeks as needed (2009,2010). Potential sites of administration include the flanks, anterior thorax, abdomen, or anterior thighs, where subcutaneous space is readily distensible (2009,2010). Initial local allergic reaction may be prevented by limiting the first treatment to 2.5 grams, and giving diphenhydramine 25 mg orally for the first four treatments (2010).

Comments

Catrix is a name which refers to activated acid-pepsin-digested bovine tracheal cartilage of calf origin (2009).

BOVINE COLOSTRUM

Also Known As

Bovine Immunoglobulin, Colostrum, Cow Milk Colostrum, Hyperimmune Bovine Colostrum.

Scientific Names

None.

People Use This For

Orally, bovine colostrum is used for stimulating the immune system, healing injuries, repairing nervous system damage, burning fat, building lean muscle, increasing stamina and vitality, elevating mood and sense of well being, slowing and reversing aging, and as an antibacterial and antifungal agent (4902). Oral hyperimmune bovine colostrum is also used in treating AIDS-related diarrhea (FDA Orphan Drug Status) (14), diarrhea associated with graft versus host disease following bone marrow transplant (4907), and rotavirus diarrhea in children (4903,4904,4909).

Safety

LIKELY SAFE ...when used orally and appropriately. There are no reports of significant toxicity in multiple human trials (4901,4903,4904,4905,4906,4907,4908,4909). Bovine colostrum seems to be safe, however, it is derived from animals, and there is some concern about contamination with diseased animal parts (see Adverse Reactions) (1825). So far, there are no reports of disease transmission to humans due to use of contaminated bovine colostrum.

PREGNANCY AND LACTATION: Insufficient reliable information available; avoid using.

Effectiveness

POSSIBLY EFFECTIVE ...when used orally for treating infectious diarrhea in people with HIV/AIDS (4905,4906,4907,4908). Hyperimmune bovine colostrum has FDA orphan status for AIDS-related diarrhea (14). ...when used orally for infectious diarrhea associated with graft versus host disease following bone marrow transplant (4907). ...when used orally for diarrhea associated with rotavirus in children (4903,4904,4909). ...when used orally for treating diarrhea due to enterotoxigenic Escherichia coli (2067,2068,2069) or Shigella flexneri (2070). Most clinical trials have used colostrum from pregnant cows which have been immunized against specific pathogens. The hyperimmune colostrum provides high antibody titers against organisms for which the cow has been immunized (4905).

There is insufficient reliable information available about the effectiveness of bovine colostrum for its other uses.

Mechanism of Action

Colostrum is the milky fluid produced by mammals within the first few days after giving birth. Most nutritional colostrum preparations come from cows (3567). Bovine colostrum contains proteins, carbohydrates, fat, vitamins, minerals, and immunoglobulin A (IgA) and immunoglobulin G (IgG) in concentrations approximately 100 times higher than dairy milk (4901). Because of the antibody content, bovine colostrum was thought to offer passive immunotherapy to people with enteric infections; however, bovine colostrum contains only low concentrations of antibodies against enteric pathogens and does not provide high enough titers to prevent disease. Hyperimmune bovine colostrum can be produced by immunizing pregnant cows against specific pathogens (e.g. cryptosporidium or rotavirus) resulting in increased specific colostrum antibody titers (4903). Hyperimmune bovine colostrum has been primarily used in clinical trials; however, the small amounts of antibodies that have been recovered from people who ingested hyperimmune colostrum were nonreactive (2072). Bovine colostrum also contains insulin-like growth factors (IGF), and increases serum insulin-like growth factor I (IGF-I) and insulin in athletes (4901). Bovine colostrum reduces indomethacin-induced gastrointestinal injury in rats and addition of colostrum to drinking water prevents experimental small intestinal injury in mice (4911). Bovine colostrum promotes small intestinal growth in newborn piglets (4901). The phosphatidylethanolamine in hyperimmune bovine colostrum may prevent Helicobacter pylori from binding to the gastric mucosa (2065). The effectiveness of hyperimmune bovine colostrum may decrease when it is taken with a meal (2070), possibly due to stomach acid and digestive enzymes (2071).

Adverse Reactions

Orally, bovine colostrum has caused nausea and vomiting in an individual with HIV-related cryptosporidiosis. Elevated liver function tests and decreased serum hematocrit have also been reported in HIV patients treated for infectious diarrhea (4905). It may cause allergic reaction in individuals allergic to bovine milk products. There is also some concern that bovine colostrum that is obtained from cows in countries where bovine spongiform encephalitis (BSE) has been reported might be unsafe, however, there is no research indicating that colostrum can be contaminated with the BSE-causing prion. Countries where BSE has been reported include Great Britain, France, The Netherlands, Portugal, Luxembourg, Ireland, Switzerland, Oman, and Belgium (1825). Until more is known, tell patients to avoid these products unless country of origin can be determined. Patients should avoid products that are produced in countries where BSE has been found.

Interactions with Herbs & Other Dietary Supplements

Insufficient reliable information available.

Interactions with Drugs

No interactions are known to occur, and there is no known reason to expect a clinically significant interaction with bovine colostrum.

Interactions with Foods

MEALS: Taking hyperimmune bovine colostrum with food may decrease antibody activity due to the increase in stomach acid and digestive enzyme secretion (2070,2071,2072).

Interactions with Lab Tests

No interactions are known to occur, and there is no known reason to expect a clinically significant interaction with bovine colostrum.

Interactions with Diseases or Conditions

BOVINE MILK ALLERGY: Avoid using.

Dosage and Administration

ORAL: For enhanced athletic training, 125 mL colostrum whey product twice daily has been used, however, this product is not available in the US (4901). For AIDS-related Cryptosporidium parvum diarrhea, 10 grams powder four times daily for 21 days has been used (4905). For AIDS-related cryptosporidial and other infectious diarrhea, 10-20 grams daily for 10 days has been used (4906). For graft versus host disease following bone marrow transplant, 10 grams per day for 10 days has been used (4907). For rotavirus diarrhea in children 10 grams, equivalent to 3.6 grams antirotavirus antibodies, per day for 4 days has been used (4903). 100 mL four times per day for 4 days has also been used (4904).

Comments

Bovine colostrum is the milk secreted by cows during the first few days after calving (4901). Hyperimmune bovine colostrum is produced by cows immunized against specific pathogens. Bovine colostrum is not on the banned drug list of the International Olympic Committee (4901). Unpublished information indicates that micro-organisms, such as Lyme disease spirochete and human immunodeficiency virus (HIV), can pass from mother to nursing baby via colostrum (4910). Whether micro-organisms can be passed to humans via pasteurized animal colostrum is unknown.

BOXWOOD

Also Known As

Boxwood Extract, Bush Tree, Buxus, Dudgeon, SPV 30, SPV-30, SPV30.

Scientific Names

Buxus sempervirens.
Family: Buxaceae.

People Use This For

Orally, boxwood is used to treat HIV/AIDS and to boost immunity. Boxwood is also used for arthritis and as a "blood detoxifying agent."

Safety

POSSIBLY SAFE …when the leaf extract is used orally and appropriately. There is some evidence that the boxwood leaf extract can be used safely for up to 16 months (5643).
LIKELY UNSAFE …when the whole leaf is used orally (12,18). The whole boxwood leaf can cause life threatening side effects including seizures, paralysis, and death by asphyxiation (18).
PREGNANCY AND LACTATION: LIKELY UNSAFE …when the whole leaf is used orally (12,18); avoid using. There is insufficient reliable information available about the safety of the boxwood leaf extract when used during pregnancy and lactation; avoid using.

Effectiveness

There is insufficient reliable information available to rate the effectiveness of boxwood for its uses; however, there is preliminary evidence that a specific boxwood leaf extract (SPV30) 990 mg per day might delay disease progression in HIV infected patients. It seems to delay decreases in CD4 cell counts, increases in viral load, and/or progression to AIDS in asymptomatic patients with CD4 counts greater than 350 cells per microliter and a relatively low viral load. A higher dose of 1980 mg per day does not seem to be effective possibly due to oxidative stress induced by flavonoids in the extract (5643). More evidence is needed to rate boxwood for this use.

Mechanism of Action

The applicable part of boxwood is the leaf. The mechanism of boxwood in HIV is not known. There is some speculation that flavonoids in the boxwood extract inhibit viral replication; however, there is not yet scientific evidence to support this.

Adverse Reactions

Orally, boxwood leaf extract can cause diarrhea and abdominal cramps (14). Ingestion of whole-leaf boxwood can cause serious side effects including vomiting, diarrhea, severe clonic spasms, paralysis and death secondary to asphyxiation (18). The extract, however, does not seem to have these effects (5643).
Topically, the fresh plant can also cause contact dermatitis (18).

Interactions with Herbs & Other Dietary Supplements

Insufficient reliable information available.

Interactions with Drugs
PHENOTHIAZINES AND ANALEPTICS: Contraindicated during overdoses with boxwood (18).

Interactions with Foods
No interactions are known to occur, and there is no known reason to expect a clinically significant interaction with boxwood.

Interactions with Lab Tests
No interactions are known to occur, and there is no known reason to expect a clinically significant interaction with boxwood.

Interactions with Diseases or Conditions
No interactions are known to occur, and there is no known reason to expect a clinically significant interaction with boxwood.

Dosage and Administration
ORAL: For HIV, a specific boxwood leaf extract (SPV30) 330 mg every 8 hours has been used (5643). Higher doses do not appear to be effective (5643).

Comments
Boxwood extract (SPV 30) is not usually found on store shelves. Most users get it through Internet sources or AIDS buyers' clubs.

BRAHMI

Also Known As
Jalanimba, Jalnaveri, Sambrani Chettu, Thyme-Leave Gratiola.

Scientific Names
Bacopa monnieri, synonym Bacopa monniera; Herpestis monniera; Moniera cuneifolia.
Family: Scrophulariaceae.

People Use This For
Orally, brahmi is used to aid learning (6).
Traditionally, brahmi has been used orally for treating asthma, backache, hoarseness, insanity, epilepsy, rheumatism, sexual dysfunction in both men and women, as a nerve tonic, cardiotonic, and a diuretic (6,2085).

Safety
There is insufficient reliable information available about the safety of brahmi.
Pregnancy and Lactation: Insufficient reliable information available; avoid using.

Effectiveness
There is insufficient reliable information available about the effectiveness of brahmi.

Mechanism of Action
Pharmacological activity is attributed to the saponin bacoside and bacopasaponin constituents (6). Some evidence suggests that an extract containing saponins has tranquilizing effects without interfering with coordination (6). Other evidence suggests that purified bacosides A and B may facilitate learning ability and cognitive performance in controlled settings (6). Bacosine may have analgesic effects by acting on the opioid pathway (6). Further evidence suggests that an ethanolic extract can relax smooth muscle in arteries, the trachea and the small intestine (6).

Adverse Reactions
None reported.

Interactions with Herbs & Other Dietary Supplements
Insufficient reliable information available.

Interactions with Drugs
PHENOTHIAZINES: Theoretically, concomitant use of brahmi may potentiate chlorpromazine's effects (6).

Interactions with Foods
No interactions are known to occur, and there is no known reason to expect a clinically significant interaction with brahmi.

Interactions with Lab Tests
No interactions are known to occur, and there is no known reason to expect a clinically significant interaction with brahmi.

Interactions with Diseases or Conditions
No interactions are known to occur, and there is no known reason to expect a clinically significant interaction with brahmi.

Dosage and Administration
No typical dosage.

Comments
Brahmi is a well-known herb in India and is frequently used in Ayurvedic herbal preparations. Centella asiatica (gotu kola) and Merremia gangetica have also been referred to by the name "bramhi", but most authorities associate brahmi with Bacopa monnieri (6).

BRANCHED-CHAIN AMINO ACIDS

Also Known As
BCAA, BCAAs, Branched Chain Amino Acids, Isoleucine, Leucine, L-Isoleucine, L-Leucine, L-Valine, Valine.

Scientific Names
2-amino-3-methylvaleric acid; 2-amino-4-methylvaleric acid; 2-amino-3-methylbutanoic acid.

People Use This For
Orally, branched-chain amino acids are used to enhance exercise performance, prevent fatigue, improve concentration, and reduce protein and muscle breakdown during intense exercise (76,692,694). They are also used for amyotrophic lateral sclerosis (ALS, Lou Gehrig's disease) (678), latent portosystemic encephalopathy (684,685), and chronic hepatic encephalopathy (690). Branched-chain amino acids have also been used orally to treat anorexia in cancer patients, tardive dyskinesia, McArdle's disease (a genetic glycogen metabolic disorder), spinocerebellar degeneration, and to attenuate muscle-wasting during bed rest (67,71,72,73,74).

Intravenously, branched-chain amino acids are used for acute hepatic encephalopathy (686) and in conditions of high metabolic stress due to severe trauma or sepsis (266).

Safety
LIKELY SAFE …when used intravenously and appropriately. Branched-chain amino acids are a FDA-approved injectable product (15).

POSSIBLY SAFE …when used orally and appropriately, short-term. Branched-chain amino acids have not been associated with significant adverse effects in studies lasting from 1-2 weeks (68,72,73,74).

PREGNANCY AND LACTATION: Insufficient reliable information available; avoid using.

Effectiveness
LIKELY EFFECTIVE …when used orally for long-term treatment of latent hepatic encephalopathy (684,685). In latent hepatic encephalopathy, oral branched-chain amino acid administration improves psychomotor function and driving ability (684,685).

POSSIBLY EFFECTIVE …when used orally or intravenously for chronic hepatic encephalopathy (68,69,82,690). Branched chain amino acids can improve liver function tests and nitrogen balance in people with chronic hepatic encephalopathy (68,69,82). Oral branched-chain amino acids are recommended for malnourished people with chronic hepatic encephalopathy who cannot tolerate protein supplementation (69,4274). When the enteral route is unavailable and in patients who cannot tolerate general purpose amino acid solutions, intravenous solutions with branched-chain amino acids can be used for nutritional support; however, most patients can tolerate standard amino acid mixtures (4274).
…when used orally for reducing muscle breakdown during exercise (694).

POSSIBLY INEFFECTIVE …when used orally for enhancing exercise or athletic performance (692).

LIKELY INEFFECTIVE …when used orally for amyotrophic lateral sclerosis (ALS, Lou Gehrig's disease). Early studies indicated that branched-chain amino acids are effective for ALS; however, more recent studies show no benefit and possibly, excess loss of pulmonary function and mortality among patients using branched-chain amino acids (678,679,680,681).

There is insufficient reliable information available to rate the effectiveness of branched chain amino acids for other uses; however, there's some evidence that intravenous branch-chain amino acids might be helpful for reversing coma in acute hepatic encephalopathy. But so far, findings are conflicting (66,81,686,687,688,689,4274). There's also some preliminary clinical evidence that shows oral branched-chain amino acids might help for anorexia in cancer patients, spinocerebellar degeneration, and tardive dyskinesia (71,72,73). More evidence is needed to rate branched-chain amino acids for these uses.

Mechanism of Action

Branched-chain amino acids are essential amino acids, including leucine, isoleucine, and valine (15,66). Branched-chain amino acids are found in dietary protein, such as meat, dairy products, and legumes (905). Skeletal muscle is the major site of branched-chain amino acid metabolism. The brain and kidneys are also involved, but to a lesser degree (78). The oral administration of branched-chain amino acids before exercise increases serum ammonia levels during exercise (693,694) and decreases muscle breakdown (694). Branched-chain amino acids appear to inhibit muscle glycogen degradation during exercise (77). Branched-chain amino acids compete with tryptophan, tyrosine, phenylalanine, and methionine for access to the neural amino acid transport system that allows amino acid entry into the brain (66,79,80,1289). This competitive inhibition is used therapeutically for amino acid imbalances that produce false neurotransmitters in pathologic conditions such as hepatic encephalopathy (66,1289). Branched-chain amino acids are also used in hepatic encephalopathy as an energy source to prevent endogenous catabolism of proteins and reduce ammonia detoxification in the brain by increasing ammonia metabolism in skeletal muscle (69).

Adverse Reactions

Orally, there has been one case report of hepatic encephalopathy in a chronic alcoholic. This resolved when dietary branched-chain amino acids were discontinued and recurred with rechallenge (691). Increased mortality was reported in one study using branched-chain amino acids in the treatment of amyotrophic lateral sclerosis (ALS) (679). Branched-chain amino acids can increase plasma ammonia levels (693,694), which can lead to fatigue and loss of motor coordination. Branched-chain amino acids should be used cautiously before or during activities where performance depends on motor coordination (75).

Interactions with Herbs & Other Dietary Supplements

Insufficient reliable information available.

Interactions with Drugs

LEVODOPA: Theoretically, branched-chain amino acids may compete with levodopa for transport systems in the intestine and brain and decrease the effectiveness of levodopa (66,1289).

Interactions with Foods

No interactions are known to occur, and there is no known reason to expect a clinically significant interaction with branched-chain amino acids.

Interactions with Lab Tests

No interactions are known to occur, and there is no known reason to expect a clinically significant interaction with branched-chain amino acids.

Interactions with Diseases or Conditions

AMYOTROPHIC LATERAL SCLEROSIS (ALS, Lou Gehrig's disease): The use of branched-chain amino acids has been associated with accelerated pulmonary failure and increased mortality when used in patients with ALS (679,681).

CHRONIC ALCOHOLISM: Dietary use of branched-chain amino acids in alcoholics has been associated with hepatic encephalopathy (691).

Dosage and Administration

ORAL: For latent or chronic hepatic encephalopathy, 240 mg/kg/day up to 25 grams branched-chain amino acids have been used (68,685,690).

INTRAVENOUS (IV): For all types of hepatic encephalopathy in patients who are intolerant standard amino acid solutions and cannot take oral therapy, a typical dose of commercially available branched-chain amino acid solution (e.g., Hepatamine) is 80-120 grams per day, which provides 28-43 grams of branched-chain amino acids per day (68,266,687,689).

Comments

None.

BREWER'S YEAST

Also Known As
Brewers Yeast, Faex Medicinalis, Levure De Biere, Medicinal Yeast.
CAUTION: See separate listing for Brewer's Yeast (Hansen CBS 5926).

Scientific Names
Saccharomyces cerevisiae.
Family: Saccharomycetaceae, Candida utilis, or Cryptococcaceae.

People Use This For
Orally, brewer's yeast is used for diarrhea, loss of appetite, chronic acne, furunculosis (2), and high chromium type diabetes (6003). It has also been used as a source of B vitamins and protein (215).

Safety
POSSIBLY SAFE ...when used orally and appropriately, short-term.
There is insufficient reliable information available about the safety of the long-term use of brewer's yeast (2).
CHILDREN: POSSIBLY SAFE ...when used orally and appropriately; however, diarrhea should be evaluated by a medical professional before using brewer's yeast (2).
PREGNANCY AND LACTATION: Insufficient reliable information available; avoid using.

Effectiveness
There is insufficient reliable information available about the effectiveness of brewer's yeast; however, there is one case report of the resolution of recurrent Clostridium difficile colitis with the use of brewer's yeast for 4 months in combination with a 30-day course of vancomycin. Before this treatment the patient experienced four relapses; after this treatment there were no further relapses (6432). It is not certain what benefit the yeast product provided in the treatment. More evidence is needed to rate the effectiveness of brewer's yeast for this use (6432).

Mechanism of Action
Brewer's yeast can have some action against C. difficile and enterotoxic E. coli. It reduces water and electrolyte influx into the intestines stimulated by the C. vibrio toxin. Brewer's yeast can increase the activity of intestinal disaccharidases, saccharidases, maltase, and lactase to alleviate diarrhea symptoms (2). It can also increase insulin releases (6004).

Adverse Reactions
Brewer's yeast can cause migraine-like headaches in sensitive individuals, intestinal discomfort, and flatulence (2). Allergic reactions to brewer's yeast can occur in hypersensitive individuals and include itching, urticaria, local or general exanthemas, and Quincke's edema (2).

Interactions with Herbs & Other Dietary Supplements
Insufficient reliable information available.

Interactions with Drugs
ANTIMYCOTIC DRUGS: These drugs can reduce yeast activity (2).
MONOAMINE OXIDASE INHIBITORS (MAOIs): Brewer's yeast is contraindicated, because concomitant use can increase blood pressure (2).

Interactions with Foods
No interactions are known to occur, and there is no known reason to expect a clinically significant interaction with brewer's yeast.

Interactions with Lab Tests
ANTIMICROBIAL TESTS: Brewer's yeast can confound results. Report the use of brewer's yeast to the lab (2).

Interactions with Diseases or Conditions
No interactions are known to occur, and there is no known reason to expect a clinically significant interaction with brewer's yeast.

Dosage and Administration
ORAL: The typical dose is 6 grams of brewer's yeast per day (2).

Comments

Brewer's yeast is obtained as a by-product from the brewing of beer made from an extract of grains and hops.
See separate listing for brewer's yeast (Hansen CBS 5926).

BREWER'S YEAST (HANSEN CBS 5926)

Also Known As

Brewers Yeast Hansen CBS 5926, Probiotics, Saccharomyces cerevisiae Hansen CBS 5926.
CAUTION: See separate listings for Bifidobacteria, Brewer's Yeast, Lactobacillus, Saccharomyces Boulardii, and Yogurt.

Scientific Names

Saccharomyces cerevisiae Hansen CBS 5926.
Family: Saccharomycetaceae.

People Use This For

Orally, brewer's yeast (Hansen CBS 5926) is used for prevention and treatment of acute diarrhea, traveler's diarrhea, diarrhea associated with tube feedings, and as an adjuvant treatment for chronic acne [2].

Safety

POSSIBLY SAFE ...when used orally and appropriately, short-term.
There is insufficient reliable information available about the safety of the long-term use of brewer's yeast (Hansen CBS 5926) [2].
CHILDREN: POSSIBLY SAFE ...when used orally and appropriately. However, diarrhea should be evaluated by a medical professional before using brewer's yeast [2].
PREGNANCY AND LACTATION: Insufficient reliable information available; avoid using.

Effectiveness

POSSIBLY EFFECTIVE ...when taken orally for symptomatic relief of acute diarrhea, prophylactic and symptomatic treatment of diarrhea during travel, diarrhea during tube feeding, and as an adjuvant treatment for chronic forms of acne [2].

Mechanism of Action

Brewer's yeast can have some action against Clostridium difficile and enterotoxic E. coli. It can reduce water and electrolyte influx into the intestines stimulated by the Vibrio cholera toxin. Brewer's yeast can increase the activity of intestinal disaccharidases, saccharidases, maltase, and lactase to alleviate diarrhea symptoms [2].

Adverse Reactions

Orally, brewer's yeast can cause flatulence. Symptoms of intolerance to brewer's yeast include itching, urticaria, local or general exanthemas (skin eruptions), and Quincke's edema [2].

Interactions with Herbs & Other Dietary Supplements

Insufficient reliable information available.

Interactions with Drugs

MONOAMINE OXIDASE INHIBITORS (MAOIs): Brewer's yeast is contraindicated, because concomitant use can cause increased blood pressure [2].
ANTIFUNGAL DRUGS: These drugs can reduce the activity of brewer's yeast [2].

Interactions with Foods

No interactions are known to occur, and there is no known reason to expect a clinically significant interaction with brewer's yeast (Hansen CBS 5926).

Interactions with Lab Tests

STOOL TESTS FOR MICROBES: Report the use of brewer's yeast to the lab, because it can confound antimicrobial tests on stool samples, resulting in false positive results [2].

Interactions with Diseases or Conditions

YEAST ALLERGY: Contraindicated [2].

Dosage and Administration

ORAL: For prevention of traveler's diarrhea in adults and children older than two years, the typical dose of brewer's yeast is 250-500 mg daily starting five days before the trip (2). For the treatment of diarrhea, the usual dose is 250-500 mg daily, continued for several days after the diarrhea has stopped (2). For diarrhea associated with tube feedings, add 500 mg of brewer's yeast to each liter of nutrient preparation (2). For acne, the typical dose is 750 mg per day (2).

Comments

Avoid confusion with brewer's yeast. Hansen CBS 5926 is a specifically standardized product.

BROMELAIN

Also Known As

Bromelains, Bromelainum, Bromelin, Plant Protease Concentrate.
CAUTION: See separate listing for Papain.

Scientific Names

Pineapple: Ananas comosus, synonym Ananas sativus.
Family: Bromeliaceae.

People Use This For

Orally, bromelain is used for acute postoperative and post-traumatic conditions of swelling (960), especially of the nasal and paranasal sinuses (2). It is also used orally for burn debridement, anti-inflammatory action, prevention of epinephrine-induced pulmonary edema, smooth muscle relaxation, stimulation of muscle contractions, inhibition of blood platelet aggregation, enhanced antibiotic absorption, cancer prevention, shortening of labor, and enhanced excretion of fat (11). Bromelain is also used for mild ulcerative colitis (6253).
In combination with trypsin and rutin, bromelain is used orally for osteoarthritis (6252).

Safety

LIKELY SAFE ...when used orally in appropriate amounts unless allergic to pineapple or bromelain (2).
PREGNANCY AND LACTATION: Insufficient reliable information available; avoid using.

Effectiveness

POSSIBLY EFFECTIVE ...when used orally for treating acute postoperative and post-traumatic conditions of swelling (960), especially of the nasal and paranasal sinuses (2). ...when used orally in combination with trypsin and rutin for treating osteoarthritis (6252). In a double-blind trial, 73 patients with painful osteoarthritis of the knee were randomly assigned the combination enzyme product (Phlogenzym) or diclofenac (Voltaren) 50 mg three times daily during the first week and then twice daily in weeks 2 and 3. The enzyme product was similar to diclofenac in relieving pain and improving knee function (6252).
POSSIBLY INEFFECTIVE ...when used orally for reducing swelling after oral surgery (957).
There is insufficient reliable information available about the effectiveness of bromelain for its other uses; however, two case reports indicate improvement of ulcerative colitis symptoms in people with persistent disease despite standard therapy (6253).

Mechanism of Action

The observed effects of bromelain are due to an enzyme constituent that causes the release of a kinin, which stimulates the production of prostaglandin E1-like compounds (11). A polyenzyme preparation containing bromelain can increase the release of reactive oxygen species by polymorphonuclear neutrophils in healthy people (962).

Adverse Reactions

Orally, bromelain can cause GI disturbances or diarrhea. Allergic reactions to bromelain can occur (2) and include a cross-allergenicity between wheat flour and bromelain (959).

Interactions with Herbs & Other Dietary Supplements

ZINC (an oxidizing agent): Concomitant use inhibits bromelain activity (11).
MAGNESIUM: Acts as a reducing agent and activates bromelain (11).
HERBS THAT AFFECT BLEEDING: Theoretically, bromelain can increase the risk of bleeding when used concomitantly with herbs that have anticoagulant or antiplatelet potential (2), including alfalfa, angelica, aniseed, arnica, asafoetida, celery, chamomile, clove, fenugreek, feverfew, fucus, garlic, ginger, horse chestnut, licorice, meadowsweet, poplar, northern and southern prickly ash, quassia, red clover, and willow (4).

Interactions with Drugs

ANTICOAGULANT/ANTIPLATELET DRUGS: Theoretically, concomitant use might cause additive anticoagulant/antiplatelet effects and increase the risk of bleeding (2).

TETRACYCLINES: Concomitant therapy increases plasma and urine tetracycline levels (2).

Interactions with Foods

POTATO PROTEIN AND SOYBEAN: These foods can inhibit bromelain activity (958,961).

Interactions with Lab Tests

No interactions are known to occur, and there is no known reason to expect a clinically significant interaction with bromelain.

Interactions with Diseases or Conditions

No interactions are known to occur, and there is no known reason to expect a clinically significant interaction with bromelain.

Dosage and Administration

ORAL: The typical dose of bromelain is 80-320 mg (200-800 FIP units) in two or three doses per day for eight to ten days (2). The administration of bromelain can be prolonged longer than ten days if needed (2). For osteoarthritis, a combination enzyme product (Phlogenzym), which contains rutin 100 mg, trypsin 48 mg, and bromelain 90 mg, was given 2 tablets 3 times daily (6252).

Comments

None.

BROOKLIME

Also Known As

Beccabunga, Mouth-Smart, Neckweed, Speedwell, Water Pimpernel, Water Purslane.
CAUTION: See separate listings for Black Root and Veronica.

Scientific Names

Veronica beccabunga.

People Use This For

Orally, brooklime is used for lessening the elimination of urine (2), constipation, liver complaints, dysentery, lung infection, and bleeding gums (18).

Safety

There is insufficient reliable information available about the safety of brooklime.
Pregnancy and Lactation: Insufficient reliable information available; avoid using.

Effectiveness

There is insufficient reliable information available about the effectiveness of brooklime.

Mechanism of Action

Brooklime appears to have a diuretic effect (18).

Adverse Reactions

None reported.

Interactions with Herbs & Other Dietary Supplements

Insufficient reliable information available.

Interactions with Drugs

No interactions are known to occur, and there is no known reason to expect a clinically significant interaction with brooklime.

Interactions with Foods

No interactions are known to occur, and there is no known reason to expect a clinically significant interaction with brooklime.

Interactions with Lab Tests

No interactions are known to occur, and there is no known reason to expect a clinically significant interaction with brooklime.

Interactions with Diseases or Conditions

No interactions are known to occur, and there is no known reason to expect a clinically significant interaction with brooklime.

Dosage and Administration

ORAL: People typically use from 1 teaspoon to 3 tablespoons of brooklime plant juice 3 times daily. The juice is sometimes mixed in milk (5263).

Comments

Avoid confusion with black root (Leptandra virginica) and veronica (Veronica officinalis), which are both known as speedwell.

There is very little scientific information about this product. Our staff is continually analyzing the available information on natural medicines and will add data here as it becomes available.

BROOM CORN

Also Known As

Darri, Durri, Guinea Corn, Sorghum.

Scientific Names

Sorghum vulgare.

People Use This For

Orally, broom corn is used for digestive disorders.
For food use, broom corn is used as a cereal grain (18).

Safety

LIKELY SAFE …when used in food amounts (18). Although the fruit contains cyanogenic glycosides, the concentrations are very low (18).

There is insufficient reliable information available about the safety of broom corn used in amounts larger than those found in foods.

PREGNANCY AND LACTATION: Insufficient reliable information available.

Effectiveness

There is insufficient reliable information available about the effectiveness of broom corn.

Mechanism of Action

The applicable part of broom corn is the seed. Broom corn contains a high percentage of starch and a small amount of protein and fatty oil. It also contains thiamine and riboflavin. Dhurrin, a cyanogenic glycoside, is present in a very low amount in the fruit, 0.005-5 mg per 100 grams. In contrast, the foliage contains a much higher level, 250-700 mg per 100 grams. Broom corn is thought to have a soothing effect on the alimentary tract (18).

Adverse Reactions

None reported.

Interactions with Herbs & Other Dietary Supplements

Insufficient reliable information available.

Interactions with Drugs

No interactions are known to occur, and there is no known reason to expect a clinically significant interaction with broom corn.

Interactions with Foods

No interactions are known to occur, and there is no known reason to expect a clinically significant interaction with broom corn.

Interactions with Lab Tests

No interactions are known to occur, and there is no known reason to expect a clinically significant interaction with broom corn.

Interactions with Diseases or Conditions

No interactions are known to occur, and there is no known reason to expect a clinically significant interaction with broom corn.

Dosage and Administration

No typical dosage.

Comments

None.

BRYONIA

Also Known As

Bryoniae Radix, Devil's Turnip, English Mandrake, Ladies' Seal, Tamus, Tetterberry, White Bryony, Wild Hops, Wild Nep, Wild Vine, Wood Vine.
CAUTION: See separate listings for European Mandrake and Podophyllum (American mandrake).

Scientific Names

Bryonia cretica; Bryonia alba.
Family: Cucurbitaceae.

People Use This For

Orally, bryonia is used as a laxative, emetic, diuretic, for gastrointestinal diseases, respiratory tract diseases, arthritis, liver disease, metabolic disorders, and for prophylaxis against infections (2).

Safety

LIKELY UNSAFE ...when bryonia root is used orally (2). ...when bryonia berries are ingested, 40 berries might be fatal (18).
CHILDREN: LIKELY UNSAFE ...when berries are ingested, 15 berries can be fatal (18). ...when the root is used orally (2).
PREGNANCY: UNSAFE ...when the root is used orally. Contraindicated because it can cause abortion (2). ...when berries are ingested (2).
LACTATION: LIKELY UNSAFE ...when the root is used orally (2). ...when berries are ingested (2).

Effectiveness

POSSIBLY EFFECTIVE ...when used as an emetic and laxative (2).
There is insufficient reliable information available about the effectiveness of bryonia for its other uses.

Mechanism of Action

The applicable part of bryonia is the root. The resin from bryonia has strong purgative effects (18). Some evidence suggests the aqueous extract might be effective against tumors (18). Other evidence suggests the methanol extract could have hypoglycemic effects (18).

Adverse Reactions

Bryonia can cause dizziness, vomiting, convulsions, colic, bloody diarrhea, abortion, nervous excitement, kidney damage (2). Large doses can cause anuria, collapse, spasms, paralysis, or death (2). Skin contact with fresh bryonia may cause irritation (19). Ingestion of 15 berries is likely to be fatal to a child. Ingestion of 40 berries is likely to be fatal for adult (18).

Interactions with Herbs & Other Dietary Supplements

Insufficient reliable information available.

Interactions with Drugs

No interactions are known to occur, and there is no known reason to expect a clinically significant interaction with bryonia.

Interactions with Foods

No interactions are known to occur, and there is no known reason to expect a clinically significant interaction with bryonia.

Interactions with Lab Tests

No interactions are known to occur, and there is no known reason to expect a clinically significant interaction with bryonia.

Interactions with Diseases or Conditions

GI IRRITATION: May irritate the gastrointestinal tract. Contraindicated in individuals with infectious or inflammatory gastrointestinal conditions (19).

Dosage and Administration

No typical dosage.

Comments

Bryonia is no longer used as an emetic or laxative due to safety concerns (2).

BUCHU

Also Known As

Barosmae Folium, Bookoo, Bucco, Bucku, Diosma, Round Buchu, Short Buchu.

Scientific Names

Agathosma betulina, synonym Barosma betulina; Barosma crenulata; B. serratifolia.
Family: Rutaceae.

People Use This For

Historically, buchu has been used as a urinary tract disinfectant in cystitis, urethritis, prostatitis, acute cystitis (4), kidney infections (2), and venereal disease (5).
In manufacturing, the oil from buchu is used to give a fruit flavor (often black current) to foods.

Safety

LIKELY SAFE ...when the leaf is used in amounts found in foods; approved for food use in the US. The maximum level used is 0.002% (4,11).
POSSIBLY SAFE ...when the leaf is used orally and appropriately in medicinal amounts (2,12).
POSSIBLY UNSAFE ...when large amounts of buchu leaf are taken orally or when the oil is ingested. Buchu contains pulegone, a known hepatotoxin (4). Pulegone is a major component of the oil.
PREGNANCY: POSSIBLY SAFE ...when used in food amounts. LIKELY UNSAFE ...when used in larger amounts because buchu is reported to be an abortifacient (4).
LACTATION: POSSIBLY SAFE ...when used in food amounts. There is insufficient reliable information available about the safety of using larger amounts; avoid using.

Effectiveness

There is insufficient reliable information available about the effectiveness of buchu (2,4).

Mechanism of Action

Buchu camphor (also known as diosphenol) is the principal constituent of the oil. Researchers believe this constituent may be responsible for buchu's reported diuretic and antiseptic effects (5).

Adverse Reactions

Buchu leaf can cause GI and kidney irritation (4,6), and increase menstrual flow (6). Buchu is also a reported abortifacient (4).

Interactions with Herbs & Other Dietary Supplements

Insufficient reliable information available.

Interactions with Drugs
ANTICOAGULANTS: May possibly enhance the effects of anticoagulants (7200).

Interactions with Foods
No interactions are known to occur, and there is no known reason to expect a clinically significant interaction with buchu.

Interactions with Lab Tests
No interactions are known to occur, and there is no known reason to expect a clinically significant interaction with buchu.

Interactions with Diseases or Conditions
KIDNEY INFECTION: Contraindicated (4,12).
URINARY TRACT INFLAMMATION: Contraindicated (4,12).

Dosage and Administration
ORAL: 1 cup of tea (steep 1 gram dry leaf in 150 mL boiling water 5-10 minutes, strain) several times per day (8).

Comments
Liver function should be monitored in people who use buchu because of its potential hepatotoxicity.

BUCKHORN PLANTAIN

Also Known As
Buckhorn, Chimney-Sweeps, English Plantain, Headsman, Hoary Plantain, Plantaginis lanceolatae herba, Plantain, Ribgrass, Ribwort, Ribwort Plantain, Ripplegrass, Soldier's Herb, Spitzwegerichkraut.
CAUTION: See separate listings for Great Plantain, Blond Psyllium, Black Psyllium, and Water Plantain.

Scientific Names
Plantago lanceolata.
Family: Plantaginaceae.

People Use This For
Orally, buckhorn plantain is used to treat inflammation of mucous membranes in the respiratory tract (2,3,7), for the common cold, cough, bronchitis, and fevers (18).
Topically, buckhorn plantain is used for pharyngeal mucous membrane inflammation, inflammation of the skin, and for wound healing (2,3).
In folk medicine, juice pressed from the plant is used to treat wounds, inflammation, and to arrest hemorrhages (18).

Safety
POSSIBLY SAFE ...when used orally in recommended doses. ...when used topically (2).
PREGNANCY AND LACTATION: LIKELY UNSAFE ...when used orally or topically. Some evidence suggests buckhorn plantain affects muscle tone of the uterus (4275).

Effectiveness
POSSIBLY EFFECTIVE ...when used orally for relieving respiratory tract mucous membrane inflammation (2).
...when used topically for relieving oral and pharyngeal mucous membrane inflammation and inflammation of the skin (2).
There is insufficient reliable information available about the effectiveness of buckhorn plantain for its other uses.

Mechanism of Action
The applicable parts of buckhorn plantain are the above ground parts. The tannin constituents have an astringent and antibacterial effect (18). Mucilage constituents are believed to be responsible for reducing local irritation and protecting mucous membranes from irritants (7).

Adverse Reactions
Buckhorn plantain is an allergen and a common problem in the early spring (3901).

Interactions with Herbs & Other Dietary Supplements
Insufficient reliable information available.

Interactions with Drugs

No interactions are known to occur, and there is no known reason to expect a clinically significant interaction with buckhorn plantain.

Interactions with Foods

No interactions are known to occur, and there is no known reason to expect a clinically significant interaction with buckhorn plantain.

Interactions with Lab Tests

No interactions are known to occur, and there is no known reason to expect a clinically significant interaction with buckhorn plantain.

Interactions with Diseases or Conditions

No interactions are known to occur, and there is no known reason to expect a clinically significant interaction with buckhorn plantain.

Dosage and Administration

ORAL: People typically use one cup tea (steep 2-3 grams chopped plant parts in 150 mL boiling water for 10 minutes, strain) several times daily (8,18); average amount is 3-6 grams per day (2).
TOPICAL: No typical dosage.

Comments

Avoid confusion with common plantain (Plantago major). CAUTION: Digitalis leaves resemble plantain leaves; adulteration of plantain with digitalis has been reported (3905). Be careful not to confuse buckhorn plantain with digitalis which is an unsafe product (2,12).

BUCKWHEAT

Also Known As

None.

Scientific Names

Fagopyrum esculentum.
Family: Polygonaceae.

People Use This For

Orally, buckwheat is used to improve venous and capillary tone, and prevent hardening of the arteries. It is also used orally to alleviate venous stasis and varicose veins (18).

Safety

There is insufficient reliable information available about the safety of buckwheat.
Pregnancy and Lactation: Insufficient reliable information available; avoid using.

Effectiveness

There is insufficient reliable information available about the effectiveness of buckwheat.

Mechanism of Action

The applicable part of buckwheat are the leaves and flowers. Buckwheat contains naphthadianthrones, which have photosensitizing effects. Phototoxicity has occurred in animals that ingest large quantities of buckwheat (18).

Adverse Reactions

None reported.

Interactions with Herbs & Other Dietary Supplements

Insufficient reliable information available.

Interactions with Drugs

No interactions are known to occur, and there is no known reason to expect a clinically significant interaction with buckwheat.

Interactions with Foods

No interactions are known to occur, and there is no known reason to expect a clinically significant interaction with buckwheat.

Interactions with Lab Tests

No interactions are known to occur, and there is no known reason to expect a clinically significant interaction with buckwheat.

Interactions with Diseases or Conditions

No interactions are known to occur, and there is no known reason to expect a clinically significant interaction with buckwheat.

Dosage and Administration

ORAL: Buckwheat is typically used as a tea, extract or tablet (18).

Comments

There is very little scientific information about this product. Our staff is continually analyzing the available information on natural medicines and will add data here as it becomes available.

BUGLE

Also Known As

Bugula, Carpenter's Herb, Middle Comfrey, Middle Confound, Sicklewort.

Scientific Names

Ajuga reptans.
Family: Labiatae.

People Use This For

Orally, bugle is used for gallbladder and stomach disorders.
Topically, bugle is used as an astringent for the inflammation of the mouth and pharynx. It is also used topically for wound treatment (18).

Safety

There is insufficient reliable information available about the safety of bugle.
Pregnancy and Lactation: Insufficient reliable information available; avoid using.

Effectiveness

There is insufficient reliable information available about the effectiveness of bugle.

Mechanism of Action

The applicable parts of bugle are the above ground parts. There is insufficient reliable information available about the possible mechanism of action and active ingredients.

Adverse Reactions

None reported.

Interactions with Herbs & Other Dietary Supplements

Insufficient reliable information available.

Interactions with Drugs

No interactions are known to occur, and there is no known reason to expect a clinically significant interaction with bugle.

Interactions with Foods

No interactions are known to occur, and there is no known reason to expect a clinically significant interaction with bugle.

Interactions with Lab Tests

No interactions are known to occur, and there is no known reason to expect a clinically significant interaction with bugle.

Interactions with Diseases or Conditions

No interactions are known to occur, and there is no known reason to expect a clinically significant interaction with bugle.

Dosage and Administration

No typical dosage.

Comments

Some people use bugle in alcoholic extracts, in teas, and as a water infusion [18]. There is very little scientific information about this product. Our staff is continually analyzing the available information on natural medicines and will add data here as it becomes available.

BUGLEWEED

Also Known As

Archangle, Ashangee, Bugle Weed, Green Wolf's Foot, Gypsy Weed, Gypsywort, Hoarhound, Lycopi Herba, Paul's Betony, Sweet Bugle, Virginia Water Horehound, Water Bugle, Water Hoarhound, Water Horehound, Wolfstrapp.

Scientific Names

Lycopus americanus; Lycopus europaeus; Lycopus virginicus.
Family: Lamiaceae.

People Use This For

Orally, bugleweed is used for mild hyperthyroidism, premenstrual syndrome, breast pain, nervousness, and insomnia [2,18].
Traditionally, bugleweed is used for bleeding, especially nosebleeds and heavy bleeding during menses [7].

Safety

POSSIBLY SAFE ...when used orally and appropriately [12].
PREGNANCY: LIKELY UNSAFE ...when used orally [12,19] because it has anti-gonadotropic and anti-thyrotropic activity [7,19]; avoid using.
LACTATION: LIKELY UNSAFE ...when used orally [12,19] because it might have anti-prolactin activity [7,19]; avoid using.

Effectiveness

There is insufficient reliable information available about the effectiveness of bugleweed.

Mechanism of Action

The applicable parts of bugleweed are the above ground parts. Bugleweed demonstrates anti-gonadotropic and anti-thyrotropic activity. It lowers serum prolactin levels [2,7] and inhibits peripheral deiodination of T4 [2]. Bugleweed can also have hypoglycemic activity [19].

Adverse Reactions

Orally, bugleweed rarely can cause thyroid enlargement during extended therapy or with large amounts [2,7]. The sudden discontinuation of bugleweed can result in a sudden increase in thyroid function [2] and prolactin secretion [7].

Interactions with Herbs & Other Dietary Supplements

THYROID-SUPPRESSING HERBS: Theoretically, concomitant use of bugleweed with other thyroid suppressing herbs can have additive therapeutic and adverse effects [19]. Herbs with thyroid-suppressing effects include balm leaf and the wild thyme plant [19].

Interactions with Drugs

DIABETES THERAPY: Theoretically, concomitant use of bugleweed can increase the risk of hypoglycemia [19]. Blood glucose levels should be monitored closely.
THYROID HORMONES: Concomitant use of bugleweed is contraindicated because bugleweed reduces the effects of thyroid hormones by blocking peripheral conversion of thyroxin to T3 [19].

Interactions with Foods
No interactions are known to occur, and there is no known reason to expect a clinically significant interaction with bugleweed.

Interactions with Lab Tests
RADIOACTIVE ISOTOPES: Bugleweed can interfere with diagnostic procedures using radioactive isotopes (2).
THYROID FUNCTION TESTS: Bugleweed might improve thyroid function and test results in mildly hyperthyroid patients (2).

Interactions with Diseases or Conditions
THYROID DISEASE: Bugleweed is contraindicated in thyroid enlargement, thyroid hypofunction (2,12,19), and during administration of other thyroid treatments (12).
DIABETES: Theoretically, bugleweed can interfere with blood glucose control and increase the risk of hypoglycemia (19). Blood glucose levels should be monitored closely while using bugleweed in diabetic patients.

Dosage and Administration
ORAL: The typical dose of bugleweed is 0.2-2 grams per day of the above ground parts or equivalent preparations (2,7). The dose must be carefully individualized, taking age and weight into consideration (2).

Comments
None.

BULBOUS BUTTERCUP

Also Known As
Crowfoot, Cuckoo Buds, Frogsfoot, Frogwort, Goldcup, King's Cup, Meadowbloom, Pilewort, St. Anthony's Turnip.
CAUTION: See separate listings for Buttercup and Poisonous Buttercup.

Scientific Names
Ranunculus bulbosus.
Family: Ranunculaceae.

People Use This For
Orally, bulbous buttercup is used for skin diseases, arthritis, gout, neuralgia, influenza, and meningitis (18).

Safety
LIKELY UNSAFE …when used orally or topically because it can cause severe local irritation (18).
PREGNANCY AND LACTATION: LIKELY UNSAFE …when used orally or topically; avoid using (18).

Effectiveness
There is insufficient reliable information available about the effectiveness of bulbous buttercup.

Mechanism of Action
The applicable parts of bulbous buttercup are the latex and the whole fresh flowering plant. When the fresh plant is crushed or cut into small pieces, the glycoside ranunculin is enzymatically changed into a severely irritating protoanemonin, which, in turn, rapidly degrades into the less toxic anemonin (18). Both protoanemonin and ranunculin are destroyed to an unknown extent during the drying process (2). The constituents ranunculin, protoanemonin, anemonin, and labenzym can cause drowsiness, fatigue and depressive moods. Protoanemonin present in the freshly harvested, bruised plant is severely irritating to skin and mucous membranes (18).

Adverse Reactions
Orally, ingestion of bulbous buttercup can cause severe irritation of the gastrointestinal tract, with colic and diarrhea. Topically, irritation of the urinary tract can also occur. Skin contact can cause blisters and burns which are difficult to heal (18).

Interactions with Herbs & Other Dietary Supplements
Insufficient reliable information available.

Interactions with Drugs

No interactions are known to occur, and there is no known reason to expect a clinically significant interaction with bulbous buttercup.

Interactions with Foods

No interactions are known to occur, and there is no known reason to expect a clinically significant interaction with bulbous buttercup.

Interactions with Lab Tests

No interactions are known to occur, and there is no known reason to expect a clinically significant interaction with bulbous buttercup.

Interactions with Diseases or Conditions

No interactions are known to occur, and there is no known reason to expect a clinically significant interaction with bulbous buttercup.

Dosage and Administration

No typical dosage.

Comments

This product is rarely used. Avoid confusing bulbous buttercup with lesser celandine and amaranth; these plants are also referred to as pilewort (18).

BUPLEURUM

Also Known As

Bei Chai Hu, Chi Hu, Chinese Thoroughwax, Hare's Ear Root, Sho-saiko-to, Shrubby Hare's-ear, Sickle-leaf Hare's-ear, Thoroughwax.

Scientific Names

Bupleurum chinense; Bupleurum exaltatum; Bupleurum falcatum; Bupleurum fruticosum; Bupleurum longifolium; Bupleurum multinerve; Bupleurum octoradiatum; Bupleurum rotundifolium; Bupleurum scorzonerifolium. Family: Apiaceae.

People Use This For

Orally, bupleurum is used for fevers, flu, the common cold, cough, fatigue, headache, tinnitus, liver disorders, premenstrual syndrome (PMS), dysmenorrhea, depression, anorexia, cancer, inflammation, lung congestion, malaria, angina, epilepsy, pain, muscle cramps, rheumatism, asthma, bronchitis, indigestion, ulcers, hemorrhoids, diarrhea, constipation, as a sedative, antioxidant, antiseptic, antifungal, antiviral, as an immune stimulant, and for reducing cholesterol and triglyceride levels (6,513,3145,3148,3149). It is also used for increasing sweating, as a protectant against kidney problems, a liver tonic, and a spleen and stomach toner (6).

In combination, bupleurum is used in many herbal formulas. It is included in a Chinese herbal formula used for treating thrombocytopenic purpura (3146) and in a Japanese herbal formula (Sho-saiko-to, TJ-9, Xiao-chai-hu-tang) used for various chronic liver diseases (3147). Bupleurum is used orally in combination with Panax ginseng and licorice to help stimulate adrenal gland function, particularly in patients with a history of long-term corticosteroid use (3234).

Safety

There is insufficient reliable information available about the safety of bupleurum.
Pregnancy and Lactation: Insufficient reliable information available; avoid using.

Effectiveness

There is insufficient reliable information available about the effectiveness of bupleurum.

Mechanism of Action

The applicable part of bupleurum is the root (12). Compounds isolated from Bupleurum species used in traditional Chinese medicine include saikosaponins, polysaccharides, and polyacetylenes. Saikosaponins are triterpenoid saponins, known as saikosides (6). While the saikosaponin content of some species is very similar (3151), that of other species varies considerably, as well as pharmacologic activity (3152). The saikosaponin content is highest in Bupleurum falcatum (2-8%) and Bupleurum chinense (1.7%). For infections, including the flu and the common cold, bupleurum is theorized to work by improving immune function. Bupleurum falcatum is reported to cause proliferation of B-lymphocytes and stimulate them to produce immunoglobulins in vitro. It is also reported to stimulate in vitro macrophage activity, possibly by increasing the number of antibody-binding sites on the cell surface (2598). The constituent saikosaponin-d has immunoregulatory actions on T-lymphocytes, including promotion of interleukin-2 (IL-2) production and IL-2 receptor expression (3160). It also increases macrophage activity, IL-1 production and antibody response (3161). Bupleurum also is reported to have antitussive properties (6). For peptic ulcers, bupleurum is thought to decrease gastric acid and pepsin secretion and have mucosal protecting effects (3154,3155). Bupleurum is also reported to have antitumor (3157), antibacterial (3170), anti-inflammatory (2597,3166,3167,3168), antispasmodic (3167), antioxidant (3154,3155,3156), antiplatelet (3159), and hepatoprotectant effects (3163,3164,3165); however these effects have not been demonstrated in humans.

Adverse Reactions

Orally, bupleurum can cause increased bowel movements, flatulence, and sedation (3148). The Japanese herbal formula, Sho-saiko-to, which contains bupleurum, has been associated with eosinophilic pneumonia (354), pulmonary edema (361), and multiple cases of pneumonitis (355,356,357). Sho-saiko-to, used in combination with interferon-alpha in people with chronic active hepatitis, has been associated with multiple cases of pneumonitis (358,359,360).

Interactions with Herbs & Other Dietary Supplements

Insufficient reliable information available.

Interactions with Drugs

No interactions are known to occur, and there is no known reason to expect a clinically significant interaction with bupleurum.

Interactions with Foods

No interactions are known to occur, and there is no known reason to expect a clinically significant interaction with bupleurum.

Interactions with Lab Tests

No interactions are known to occur, and there is no known reason to expect a clinically significant interaction with bupleurum.

Interactions with Diseases or Conditions

No interactions are known to occur, and there is no known reason to expect a clinically significant interaction with bupleurum.

Dosage and Administration

ORAL: A dose of 1.5 to 6 grams per day of bupleurum root has been used (3148). As a fluid extract (1:2), 1.5-3 mL daily, up to 25-60 mL per week has been used (3148).

Comments

The Japanese herbal formula, Sho-saiko-to, which contains bupleurum, enhances the anti-HIV-1 activity of lamivudine (Epivir, 3TC) in vitro (362).

BURDOCK

Also Known As

Arctium, Bardana, Bardanae Radix, Bardane, Beggar's Buttons, Burr Seed, Clotbur, Cocklebur, Cockle Buttons, Edible Burdock, Fox's Clote, Great Bur, Great Burdocks, Happy Major, Hardock, Harebur, Lappa, Love Leaves, Personata, Philanthropium, Thorny Burr.

Scientific Names

Arctium lappa; Arctium minus; Arctium tomentosum.
Family: Asteraceae or Compositae.

People Use This For

Orally, burdock is used as a diuretic, "blood purifier" (5), antimicrobial, antipyretic (11), and to treat anorexia nervosa (4), GI complaints (2), rheumatism, gout, cystitis (2,4), and chronic skin conditions including acne and psoriasis (5). Topically, burdock is used for dry skin (ichthyosis) and eczema (4,18).

In folk medicine, burdock has been used for treating colds, catarrh, cancers, and as an aphrodisiac (6). Historically, burdock has been used in the past in the treatment of gout and syphilitic disorders. As a food, burdock is consumed in Asia (11).

Safety

LIKELY SAFE ...when burdock root preparations are consumed in amounts commonly found in foods. Burdock is listed as a food flavoring by the Council of Europe (4).
POSSIBLY SAFE ...when used orally and appropriately in medicinal amounts (12).
PREGNANCY: LIKELY UNSAFE ...when used orally; contraindicated because it could cause uterine stimulation (4,19).
LACTATION: Insufficient reliable information available; avoid using (4).

Effectiveness

There is insufficient reliable information available about the effectiveness of burdock.

Mechanism of Action

The applicable part of burdock is the root. The leaf and flower have Gram-positive and Gram-negative antibacterial activity; the root is active against Gram-negative bacteria (4). Arctiopiricin (constituent) is active against Gram-positive bacteria (4). In vivo, burdock has uterine stimulant activity in animals (4). The plant may have some antimutagenic and antitumor activity (4).

Adverse Reactions

Orally, burdock can cause an allergic reaction in individuals sensitive to the Asteraceae/Compositae family. Members of this family include ragweed, chrysanthemums, marigolds, daisies, and many other herbs. Topically, sensitization may occur via skin contact (18).

Interactions with Herbs & Other Dietary Supplements

Insufficient reliable information available.

Interactions with Drugs

HYPOGLYCEMIC DRUGS: Theoretically, large amounts of burdock might cause hypoglycemia (4).
INSULIN: Concomitant use might require insulin dosage adjustment due to hypoglycemic effect (19).

Interactions with Foods

No interactions are known to occur, and there is no known reason to expect a clinically significant interaction with burdock.

Interactions with Lab Tests

No interactions are known to occur, and there is no known reason to expect a clinically significant interaction with burdock.

Interactions with Diseases or Conditions

DIABETES: Theoretically, large amounts may affect blood sugar control (4).
CROSS-ALLERGENICITY: Can cause an allergic reaction in individuals sensitive to the Asteraceae/Compositae family. Members of this family include ragweed, chrysanthemums, marigolds, daisies, and many other herbs.

Dosage and Administration

ORAL: 2-6 grams dried root three times daily, or drink 1 cup tea (steep 1-2 grams dried root in 150 mL boiling water 5-10 minutes, strain) three times daily (4). Liquid extract: (1:1 in 25% alcohol) 2-8 mL three times daily (4). Tincture (1:10 in 45% alcohol) 8-12 mL three times daily (4).

Comments

Burdock has been associated with atropine poisoning as a result of being adulterated with root of belladonna or deadly nightshade (4,5).

BURNING BUSH leaf

Also Known As

Adiptam, Dittany, Fraxinella, Gas Plant, Herba dictamni herba.
CAUTION: See separate listing for Burning Bush root.

Scientific Names

Dictamnus albus.
Family: Rutaceae.

People Use This For

Historically, burning bush leaf was used orally for cramps, stomach disorders, and worm infestations. In the Middle Ages, people used burning bush leaf orally for epilepsy, as an aid for urination, to promote menstruation and aid in the expulsion of the afterbirth. It was also used topically for curing or treating wounds and for rheumatism [18].
In Greece, burning bush is used orally as a stimulant and tonic.

Safety

POSSIBLY UNSAFE …when used topically because it can cause photosensitivity [18].
There is insufficient reliable information available about the safety of burning bush leaf for its other uses.
PREGNANCY AND LACTATION: POSSIBLY UNSAFE …when used topically. There is insufficient reliable information available about the safety of burning bush leaf used orally during pregnancy or lactation; avoid using.

Effectiveness

There is insufficient reliable information available about the effectiveness of burning bush.

Mechanism of Action

There is evidence to support the use of burning bush leaf in treating worm infestations. It decreases the ability of a tropical liver fluke called Clonorchis sinesis to lay eggs. This same liver fluke can occur in sushi if the fish has been imported from Asia. Burning bush leaf contains psoralen, xanthotoxin, auraptene, and bergapten. These furocoumarins can cause phototoxic reactions when they are applied topically [18].

Adverse Reactions

Topically, skin contact can cause phototoxicity [18].

Interactions with Herbs & Other Dietary Supplements

Insufficient reliable information available.

Interactions with Drugs

No interactions are known to occur, and there is no known reason to expect a clinically significant interaction with burning bush leaf.

Interactions with Foods

No interactions are known to occur, and there is no known reason to expect a clinically significant interaction with burning bush leaf.

Interactions with Lab Tests

No interactions are known to occur, and there is no known reason to expect a clinically significant interaction with burning bush leaf.

Interactions with Diseases or Conditions

No interactions are known to occur, and there is no known reason to expect a clinically significant interaction with burning bush leaf.

Dosage and Administration

ORAL: The typical dose is 1 cup of tea taken orally 3 times daily. One cup of tea is also taken after main meals twice daily. The tea is prepared by steeping 20 grams of dried leaf in 1 L of boiling water for 10-15 minutes and straining. Alternately, 1 gram of fresh or 2 grams of dried herb is added to 1 cup of water [18].
TOPICAL: No typical dosage.

Comments

The alternate burning bush name, herba dictamni herba, sounds similar to herba dictamni cretici (dittany of crete, Origanum dictamnus). Use caution to ensure the two are not confused. Avoid confusion with Euonymus, which has also been referred to as burning bush. Euonymus is the dried bark of the root of Euonymus atropurpureus (Fam. Celastracaea). It was used in the past as a diuretic and cathartic. Burning bush has a distinctive lemon or cinnamon scent. Its oil is easily flammable [18].

BURNING BUSH root

Also Known As
Adiptam, Dittany, Fraxinella, Gas Plant, Herba Dictamni Herba.
CAUTION: See separate listing for Burning Bush leaf.

Scientific Names
Dictamnus albus.
Family: Rutaceae.

People Use This For
Orally, burning bush root is used for digestive and urogenital disorders, and to promote hair growth.
Topically, burning bush root is used for eczema, impetigo, and scabies.
In Chinese medicine (China and Korea), the root is applied topically for arthritis, fever, hepatitis, skin inflammation, thread fungus, uterine hemorrhages, to calm children crying as a result of a nervous state, and as a sedative and tonic [18].
In folk medicine, burning bush root has been used as a diuretic and spasmolytic. In the Middle Ages, it was used for desiccation, epilepsy, hysteria, worm infestations, and to promote menstruation.
In India, burning bush root is used for amenorrhea and birth control.

Safety
POSSIBLY UNSAFE …when used topically [18].
There is insufficient reliable information available about the safety of burning bush root for its other uses.
PREGNANCY AND LACTATION: POSSIBLY UNSAFE …when used topically. There is insufficient reliable information available about the safety of burning bush root used orally during pregnancy or lactation; avoid using.

Effectiveness
There is insufficient reliable information available about the effectiveness of burning bush.

Mechanism of Action
There is insufficient reliable information available about the possible mechanism of action and active ingredients.

Adverse Reactions
Topically, skin contact can cause phototoxicity [18].

Interactions with Herbs & Other Dietary Supplements
Insufficient reliable information available.

Interactions with Drugs
No interactions are known to occur, and there is no known reason to expect a clinically significant interaction with burning bush root.

Interactions with Foods
No interactions are known to occur, and there is no known reason to expect a clinically significant interaction with burning bush root.

Interactions with Lab Tests
No interactions are known to occur, and there is no known reason to expect a clinically significant interaction with burning bush root.

Interactions with Diseases or Conditions
No interactions are known to occur, and there is no known reason to expect a clinically significant interaction with burning bush root.

Dosage and Administration
ORAL: Tea is taken over the course of one day. The tea is prepared by steeping 1 teaspoon dried root in 2 glasses of hot water for 10-15 minutes and straining . It is also occasionally used in tea mixtures and in Swedish herb mixtures [18].
TOPICAL: No typical dosage.

Comments

The alternate burning bush name, herba dictamni radix, sounds similar to herba dictamni cretici (dittany of crete, Origanum dictamnus). Use caution to ensure the two are not confused. In addition, previous sources report confusion with Carophyllaceen roots. Avoid confusion with Euonymus, which has also been referred to as burning bush. Euonymus is the dried bark of the root of Euonymus atropurpureus (Fam. Celastracaea). It was used in the past as a diuretic and cathartic. Burning bush has a distinctive lemon or cinnamon scent. Its oil is easily flammable. Its use is mostly obsolete [18].

BURR MARIGOLD

Also Known As

Water Agrimony.

Scientific Names

Bidens tripartitia.
Family: Compositae.

People Use This For

Orally, burr marigold is used for hair loss, colitis, and gout. It is also used orally as an astringent, diuretic, and to promote sweating [18].

Safety

There is insufficient reliable information available about the safety of burr marigold.
Pregnancy and Lactation: Insufficient reliable information available; avoid using.

Effectiveness

There is insufficient reliable information available about the effectiveness of burr marigold.

Mechanism of Action

The applicable parts of burr marigold are the above ground parts. There is insufficient reliable information available about the possible mechanism of action and active ingredients.

Adverse Reactions

Orally, burr marigold can cause an allergic reaction in individuals sensitive to the Asteraceae/Compositae family. Members of this family include ragweed, chrysanthemums, marigolds, daisies, and many other herbs.

Interactions with Herbs & Other Dietary Supplements

Insufficient reliable information available.

Interactions with Drugs

No interactions are known to occur, and there is no known reason to expect a clinically significant interaction with burr marigold.

Interactions with Foods

No interactions are known to occur, and there is no known reason to expect a clinically significant interaction with burr marigold.

Interactions with Lab Tests

No interactions are known to occur, and there is no known reason to expect a clinically significant interaction with burr marigold.

Interactions with Diseases or Conditions

CROSS-ALLERGENICITY: Burr marigold can cause an allergic reaction in individuals sensitive to the Asteraceae/Compositae family. Members of this family include ragweed, chrysanthemums, marigolds, daisies, and many other herbs.

Dosage and Administration

No typical dosage.

Comments

There is very little scientific information about this product. Our staff is continually analyzing the available information on natural medicines and will add data here as it becomes available.

BUTANEDIOL (BD)

Also Known As

1,4-BD, 1,4-butylene glycol, 1,4-dihydroxybutane, 1,4-tetramethylene glycol, 2(3H)-Furanone di-dihydro, BD, BDO, Butane-1,4-diol, Butylene glycol, Pine Needle Oil, Tetramethylene glycol, Tetramethylene-1,4-diol.
CAUTION: See separate listings for Gamma Hydroxybutyrate (GHB) and Gamma Butyrolactone (GBL).

Scientific Names

1,4-butanediol.

People Use This For

Orally, butanediol has been used to stimulate growth hormone production and muscle growth, for bodybuilding, weight loss, and insomnia (3677,3678).

Safety

UNSAFE ...when used orally. Butanediol, and the closely related products gamma hydroxybutyrate (GHB) and gamma butyrolactone (GBL) have been linked to at least 131 serious illnesses, including 5 deaths (1318,3678).
PREGNANCY AND LACTATION: UNSAFE ...when used orally (1318,3678).

Effectiveness

There is insufficient reliable information about the effectiveness of butanediol.

Mechanism of Action

Butanediol is converted to gamma hydroxybutyrate (GHB, see separate listing) in the body (14,3678,5813). It is a powerful hypnotic, producing potentially dangerous sedative effects (3679). GHB can be converted in the brain to the neurotransmitter gamma aminobutyric acid (GABA) (14,3699), and specific GHB uptake systems, transport systems, and receptors have also been identified (14,713,3699,5800,5801). Stimulation of GHB receptors reduces dopamine release in the brain (14,713,3699,5801), and GHB has also been reported to affect the endogenous opioid system, raising dynorphin levels (3682,5803). GHB produces general anesthesia (14); induces REM and non-REM sleep, hypothermia, abnormalities on the EEG similar to those seen in petit mal epilepsy (5800,5803); and it stimulates growth hormone secretion (5804).

Adverse Reactions

Orally, butanediol, like gamma butyrolactone (GBL), is metabolized to gamma hydroxybutyrate (GHB), and therefore causes similar toxic effects, including breathing problems, respiratory depression requiring intubation, coma, amnesia, combativeness, confusion, agitation, vomiting, seizures, bradycardia, and death (14,1318,3678,3679). Butanediol, GHB, and GBL have been linked to at least 131 serious illnesses, including 5 deaths (1318,3678). Non-fatal toxicity has been reported with doses of 1 to 14 grams. Death has occurred with doses of 5 to 20 grams (1318). Withdrawal symptoms, including insomnia, tremor, and anxiety; can occur in chronic users of GHB and probably also with butanediol (1430). GHB-like withdrawal has also occurred in a patient who presented with butanediol toxicity (1318).

Interactions with Herbs & Other Dietary Supplements

HERBS WITH SEDATIVE EFFECTS: Likely to cause additive sedation with butanediol, increasing the risk of serious adverse effects.

Interactions with Drugs

ALCOHOL: Concomitant use with butanediol and its metabolite GHB may increase the risk of serious CNS and respiratory depression (1430,3678).
BENZODIAZEPINES, NEUROLEPTICS: Concomitant use with GHB (a metabolite of butanediol) can potentiate the effects of GHB (14,3682).
CNS DEPRESSANTS: Additive sedative effects with butanediol may be dangerous (3679).
D-AMPHETAMINE, NALOXONE, HALOPERIDOL, DRUGS USED FOR ABSENCE SEIZURES: Concomitant use with GHB (a metabolite of butanediol) may antagonize the effects of GHB, but these agents have not been assessed as possible treatments for GHB or butanediol overdose (3682).
NARCOTIC ANALGESICS: Concomitant use with GHB (a metabolite of butanediol) can potentiate the therapeutic and adverse effects of narcotic analgesics (14).

SKELETAL MUSCLE RELAXANTS: Concomitant use with GHB (a metabolite of GBL) can potentiate the therapeutic and adverse effects of skeletal muscle relaxants (14,3682).

Interactions with Foods

ALCOHOL: Concomitant use with butanediol and its metabolite GHB may increase the risk of serious CNS and respiratory depression (1430,3678).

Interactions with Lab Tests

GAMMA BUTYROLACTONE (GBL) / GAMMA HYDROXYBUTYRIC ACID (GHB): The mass spectrometry assay for GHB (a metabolite of butanediol) used in either urine or serum studies is unable to differentiate between GHB and GBL (14).

Interactions with Diseases or Conditions

CARDIAC CONDUCTION DEFECTS: GHB, a metabolite of butanediol, should be avoided due to the risk of bradycardia (14).
EPILEPSY: GHB (a metabolite of butanediol) should be avoided due to its possible capacity to induce seizures (14).
HYPERTENSION OR BRADYCARDIA: GHB (a metabolite of butanediol) should be avoided since it may exacerbate these conditions (14).
RENAL IMPAIRMENT: GHB (a metabolite of butanediol) should be avoided due to possible accumulation (14).

Dosage and Administration

ORAL: Doses of 0.25 to 1 gram butanediol have been used for stimulating growth hormone release and muscle growth and treating insomnia (3677), but are considered unsafe (3678).

Comments

Butanediol is used industrially to make floor stripper, paint thinner, and other solvent products (3678). It is illegal to sell any product for human consumption containing butanediol (3678). Some manufacturers have substituted butanediol in products previously containing GHB or GBL, but the effects of butanediol are just as dangerous (3679). GBL, GHB, and BD are associated with at least 122 reports of serious adverse effects including dangerously low respiratory rates (intubation might be required), unconsciousness, coma, vomiting, seizures, slowed heart rate, and death (4259).

BUTCHER'S BROOM

Also Known As

Box Holly, Butchers Broom, Butcher's Broom, Butchers' Broom, Butcherbroom, Jew's Myrtle, Kneeholm, Knee Holly, Pettigree, Sweet Broom, Rusci Aculeati, Rusci Aculeati Rhizoma.
CAUTION: See separate listings for Scotch Broom flower, Scotch Broom herb, and Spanish Broom.

Scientific Names

Ruscus aculeatus.
Family: Liliaceae.

People Use This For

Orally, butcher's broom is used to relieve the burning and itching of hemorrhoids (18) and for symptoms of chronic venous insufficiency, including pain, heaviness, leg cramps, leg edema, varicose veins, peripheral vascular disease, itching, and swelling (2).
Traditionally, butcher's broom has been used as a laxative (5,6), diuretic (5), an anti-inflammatory (6), for atherosclerosis (6), and to facilitate the healing of fractures (5).
Historically, the rhizome shoots were eaten as food in some cultures in a manner similar to asparagus (6).

Safety

LIKELY SAFE ...when used orally and appropriately (12). The use of butcher's broom is not associated with any significant toxicity (6).
PREGNANCY AND LACTATION: Insufficient reliable information available; avoid using.

Effectiveness

POSSIBLY EFFECTIVE ...when used orally to relieve the burning and itching of hemorrhoids and for symptoms of chronic venous insufficiency, including pain, heaviness, leg cramps, itching, and swelling (2,5,6).
There is insufficient reliable information available about the effectiveness of butcher's broom for its other uses.

Mechanism of Action
The applicable parts of butcher's broom are the rhizome and root. The steroidal saponin constituents, ruscogenin and neoruscogenin, produce vasoconstrictive effects by direct activation of alpha-adrenergic receptors (5).

Adverse Reactions
Butcher's broom taken orally can cause GI disorders and rarely nausea (2).

Interactions with Herbs & Other Dietary Supplements
Insufficient reliable information available.

Interactions with Drugs
No interactions are known to occur, and there is no known reason to expect a clinically significant interaction with butcher's broom.

Interactions with Foods
No interactions are known to occur, and there is no known reason to expect a clinically significant interaction with butcher's broom.

Interactions with Lab Tests
No interactions are known to occur, and there is no known reason to expect a clinically significant interaction with butcher's broom.

Interactions with Diseases or Conditions
No interactions are known to occur, and there is no known reason to expect a clinically significant interaction with butcher's broom.

Dosage and Administration
ORAL: The typical dose of the raw extract is equivalent to 7-11 mg of total ruscogenin, which is determined as the sum of neoruscogenin and ruscogenin obtained after fermentation or acid hydrolysis (2). Butcher's broom is available in capsules, ointments, and suppositories (5).

Comments
European butchers historically have used the leaves and twigs of this plant to clean and scrub their chopping blocks, which had led to its name, butcher's broom (6002). Avoid confusion with scotch broom flower, scotch broom herb, and Spanish broom.

BUTTERBUR

Also Known As
Blatterdock, Bog Rhubarb, Bogshorns, Butter Bur, Butterburr, Butter-Dock, Butterfly Dock, Capdockin, Flapperdock, Langwort, Petasites, Petasites flower, Petasites leaf, Petasites rhizome, Petasites root, Petasitidis folium (flower), Petasitidis rhizoma (rhizome), Petasitidis hybridus, Umbrella Leaves.

Scientific Names
Petasites hybridus; Petasites officinalis.
Family: Asteraceae or Compositae.

People Use This For
Orally, butterbur is used for pain, stomach upset, gastric ulcers, headaches including migraine headaches, chronic cough, chills, anxiety, plague, fever, insomnia whooping cough, asthma, and for irritable bladder and urinary tract spasms. It is also used orally as an antispasmodic and appetite stimulant.
Topically, butterbur is used to improve wound healing.

Safety
POSSIBLY SAFE …when used orally and appropriately. Rhizome extracts that are free of unsaturated pyrrolizidine alkaloid (UPA) constituents seem to be safe when used for up to 12 weeks (7230). Tell patients not to use butterbur products that are not certified to be free of UPAs. Preparations containing UPAs are likely unsafe.
LIKELY UNSAFE …when products containing UPAs are used orally (2,19). Repeated exposure to low concentrations of UPAs can cause severe veno-occlusive disease (4,12). UPAs might also be carcinogenic and mutagenic (12). Tell patients not to use butterbur preparations that are not certified to be free of UPAs.

...when products containing UPAs are used topically on abraded or broken skin. Absorption of UPAs through broken skin can lead to systemic toxicities (12). Tell patients not to use topical butterbur preparations that are not certified to be free of UPAs.

There is insufficient reliable information available about the safety of butterbur preparations that are free of UPAs when used topically on unbroken skin.

PREGNANCY: LIKELY UNSAFE ...when used orally. Butterbur preparations containing UPAs might be teratogenic and hepatotoxic (2,19). There is insufficient reliable information available about the safety of butterbur preparations that are free of UPAs when used during pregnancy.

LACTATION: POSSIBLY UNSAFE ...when used orally. UPA constituents in butterbur might be excreted in milk (2,19). There is insufficient reliable information available about the safety of butterbur preparations that are free of UPAs when used during lactation.

Effectiveness

POSSIBLY EFFECTIVE ...when used orally to prevent migraine headache. There's some evidence that a specific butterbur rhizome extract standardized to 7.5 mg of the constituents petasin and isopetasin (Petadolex), free of unsaturated pyrrolizidine alkaloids (UPAs), can reduce the frequency, intensity, and duration of migraine headache (7230).

There is insufficient reliable information available about the effectiveness of butterbur for its other uses.

Mechanism of Action

The applicable parts of butterbur are the leaf, rhizome, and root. Butterbur is thought to have antispasmodic effects on smooth muscle and vascular walls, possibly due to sesquiterpene constituents, petasin and isopetasin (7,18,7229). These constituents might also exert anti-inflammatory effects by inhibiting leukotriene synthesis. Butterbur extracts are standardized to contain a minimum of 7.5 mg petasin and isopetasin (7229). Butterbur extracts also contain volatile oils, flavonoids, tannins, and pyrrolizidine alkaloids (7229). Pyrrolizidine alkaloids with an unsaturated pyrrolizidine alkaloid (UPA) nucleus can be hepatotoxic in animals and humans (4). Herbs containing UPAs have shown carcinogenic, mutagenic, and renal toxic effects. However, the primary concern is veno-occlusive disease (12). Methods to remove UPAs from butterbur extracts are available (7231). However, it is not clear if commercial products containing butterbur commonly remove UPAs.

Adverse Reactions

Orally, butterbur products have not been associated with side effects (7230). However, butterbur preparations can contain unsaturated pyrrolizidine alkaloids (UPAs). Chronic exposure to other plants containing UPA constituents has been associated with veno-occlusive disease (4021). Symptoms of acute veno-occlusive disease are characterized by a dull, dragging ache in the right upper abdomen and marked distention of the abdomen. These symptoms are sometimes accompanied by reduced urine output. Subacute veno-occlusive disease is associated with vague symptoms and persistent liver enlargement (4021). Butterbur can cause an allergic reaction in individuals sensitive to the Asteraceae/Compositae family. Members of this family include ragweed, chrysanthemums, marigolds, daisies, and many other herbs.

Interactions with Herbs & Other Dietary Supplements

PYRROLIZIDINE ALKALOID-CONTAINING HERBS: Concomitant use is contraindicated due to the risk of additive toxicity. Herbs containing unsaturated pyrrolizidine alkaloids include alkanna (12), borage (271), gravel root (4), hemp agrimony (271), hound's tongue (19), comfrey (271), coltsfoot, and the Senecio species plants; dusty miller (19), alpine ragwort (19), groundsel (271), golden ragwort (19), and tansy ragwort (271).

Interactions with Drugs

No interactions are known to occur, and there is no known reason to expect a clinically significant interaction with butterbur.

Interactions with Foods

No interactions are known to occur, and there is no known reason to expect a clinically significant interaction with butterbur.

Interactions with Lab Tests

No interactions are known to occur, and there is no known reason to expect a clinically significant interaction with butterbur.

Interactions with Diseases or Conditions

CROSS-ALLERGENICITY: Butterbur can cause an allergic reaction in individuals sensitive to the Asteraceae/Compositae family. Members of this family include ragweed, chrysanthemums, marigolds, daisies, and many other herbs.

LIVER DISEASE: Contraindicated due to hepatotoxic potential (19).

Dosage and Administration

ORAL: For migraine headache prophylaxis, a pyrrolizine-free butterbur rhizome extract standardized to 7.5 mg of the constituents petasin and isopetasin has been used in doses of 50 to 100 mg twice daily with meals (7230). Some researchers suggest taking the extract for 4 to 6 months, then tapering the dose until migraine incidence begins to increase (7229). For acute spastic pain of the urinary tract, the typical dose of butterbur is 4.5-7 grams per day of the root or equivalent preparation (2).

Comments

None.

BUTTERCUP

Also Known As

Acrid Crowfoot, Batchelor's Buttons, Blisterweed, Burrwort, Globe Amaranth, Gold Cup, Meadowbloom, Yellows, Yellowweed.

CAUTION: See separate listings for Poisonous Buttercup and Bulbous Buttercup.

Scientific Names

Ranunculus acris.
Family: Ranunculaceae.

People Use This For

Orally, buttercup is used for arthritis, blisters, bronchitis, chronic skin complaints, and nerve pain (18).

Safety

LIKELY UNSAFE …when used orally or topically because it can cause severe local irritation (18).

There is insufficient reliable information about the safety of the medicinal use of the dried, cut above ground parts of buttercup.

PREGNANCY AND LACTATION: LIKELY UNSAFE ...when used orally or topically. Buttercup might also stimulate uterine contractions (19). There is insufficient reliable information about the safety of the oral or topical use of the dried, cut above ground parts of buttercup during pregnancy and lactation.

Effectiveness

There is insufficient reliable information available about the effectiveness of buttercup.

Mechanism of Action

The applicable parts of buttercup are the fresh above ground parts. When the fresh plant is crushed or cut into small pieces, the glycoside ranunculin is enzymatically changed into a severely irritating protoanemonin, which, in turn, rapidly degrades into the less toxic anemonin (18). Both protoanemonin and ranunculin are destroyed to an unknown extent during the drying process (2).

Adverse Reactions

Orally, ingestion of buttercup can cause severe irritation of the gastrointestinal tract, with colic and diarrhea. Irritation of the urinary tract can also occur.

Topically, skin contact can cause blisters and burns which are difficult to heal (18). Buttercup can also cause phototoxic skin reactions (19).

Interactions with Herbs & Other Dietary Supplements

Insufficient reliable information available.

Interactions with Drugs

No interactions are known to occur, and there is no known reason to expect a clinically significant interaction with buttercup.

Interactions with Foods

No interactions are known to occur, and there is no known reason to expect a clinically significant interaction with buttercup.

Interactions with Lab Tests

No interactions are known to occur, and there is no known reason to expect a clinically significant interaction with buttercup.

Interactions with Diseases or Conditions

No interactions are known to occur, and there is no known reason to expect a clinically significant interaction with buttercup.

Dosage and Administration

No typical dosage.

Comments

None.

BUTTERNUT

Also Known As

Butternussbaum, Lemon Walnut, Nogal Ceniciento, Noyer Cerdré, Oil Nut, White Walnut.

Scientific Names

Juglans cinerea.
Family: Juglandaceae.

People Use This For

Orally, butternut is used for gallbladder disorders, hemorrhoids and skin diseases. It is also used orally as a stimulant laxative, antimicrobial, antineoplastic, antiparasitic, and tonic.

Safety

POSSIBLY SAFE …when used orally (12).
PREGNANCY AND LACTATION: LIKELY UNSAFE …when used orally in large amounts, it can be cathartic (12); avoid using.

Effectiveness

There is insufficient reliable information available about the effectiveness of butternut.

Mechanism of Action

The applicable part of butternut is the bark. It is reported to have cathartic properties (12,19).

Adverse Reactions

Orally, butternut bark can cause diarrhea and gastrointestinal irritation (19).

Interactions with Herbs & Other Dietary Supplements

CARDIAC GLYCOSIDE-CONTAINING HERBS: Stimulant laxative herbs such as butternut bark can cause potassium depletion increasing the risk of cardiac toxicity. Cardiac glycoside-containing herbs include: black hellebore, Canadian hemp roots, digitalis leaf, hedge mustard, figwort, lily of the valley roots, motherwort, oleander leaf, pheasant's eye plant, pleurisy root, squill bulb leaf scales, and strophanthus seeds (2,18,19).
STIMULANT LAXATIVE HERBS: Theoretically, concomitant use with other stimulant laxative herbs may increase the risk of potassium depletion. Stimulant laxative herbs include: aloe dried leaf sap, blue flag rhizome, alder buckthorn, European buckthorn, cascara bark, castor oil, colocynth fruit pulp, gamboge bark exudate, jalap root, black root, manna bark exudate, podophyllum root, rhubarb root, senna leaves and pods, wild cucumber fruit (Ecballium elaterium), and yellow dock root (19).
LICORICE/HORSETAIL: Theoretically, concomitant use with horsetail plant or licorice rhizome increases the risk of potassium depletion (19).

Interactions with Drugs

ANTIARRHYTHMIC DRUGS: Overuse of butternut bark might cause potassium depletion increasing risk of anti-arrhythmic drug toxicity (664).

CORTICOSTEROIDS: Overuse of butternut bark might compound corticosteroid-induced potassium loss (2).

CARDIAC GLYCOSIDES: Theoretically, overuse of butternut bark increases the risk of adverse effects of cardiac glycoside drugs, including digoxin (Lanoxin) and digitoxin (Crystodigin).

LAXATIVE DRUGS: Concomitant use might compound fluid and electrolyte loss.

POTASSIUM-DEPLETING DIURETICS: Overuse of butternut bark might compound diuretic-induced potassium loss (2).

ORAL DRUGS: Concomitant use with butternut bark might reduce absorption of drugs due to reduced GI transit time (19).

Interactions with Foods

No interactions are known to occur, and there is no known reason to expect a clinically significant interaction with butternut.

Interactions with Lab Tests

No interactions are known to occur, and there is no known reason to expect a clinically significant interaction with butternut.

Interactions with Diseases or Conditions

No interactions are known to occur, and there is no known reason to expect a clinically significant interaction with butternut.

Dosage and Administration

ORAL: Butternut extract 1.25 - 6 mL is typically used orally three times daily with a meal and plenty of water or juice (3537,3538). Dried bark 2 - 6 grams is typically used orally three times daily (3538).

Comments

None.

CABBAGE

Also Known As

Colewort.

Scientific Names

Brassica oleracea; va. Capitata.
Family: Cruciferae.

People Use This For

Orally, cabbage is used for gastritis, gastric and duodenal ulcers, gastric pain, gastric hyperacidity, and Roemheld syndrome. Cabbage is also used orally to treat asthma, morning sickness, and prevent osteoporosis. It is also used orally to prevent lung cancer, stomach cancer, colorectal cancer, breast cancer, and other cancers.

Topically, cabbage leaves and cabbage leaf extracts are used to relieve swelling and to reduce breast engorgement.

Safety

LIKELY SAFE ...when used orally in amounts found in foods. ...when used topically and appropriately, short-term. Significant side effects have not been reported in short-term studies (6781,6782,6783,6784).

POSSIBLY SAFE ...when used orally and appropriately in medicinal amounts (18).

PREGNANCY: LIKELY SAFE ...when used orally in amounts found in foods. There is insufficient reliable information available about using cabbage for medicinal purposes during pregnancy; avoid using.

LACTATION: LIKELY SAFE ...when used topically and appropriately, short-term. Significant adverse effects have not been reported in short-term studies (6781,6782,6783,6784). POSSIBLY UNSAFE ...when used orally in amounts found in foods. There is some evidence that exclusively breast-fed infants develop colic if mothers consume cabbage as little as once per week (6789).

Effectiveness

POSSIBLY EFFECTIVE ...when used topically for treating breast engorgement in lactating women (6781,6782,6784). Whole cabbage leaves seem to produce subjective relief similar to the standard practice of applying chilled gel-packs to the engorged breast (6781,6784). Both chilled and room temperature cabbage leaves seem to provide the same relief (6782). A cabbage leaf extract applied as a cream has also been tried. The cabbage leaf extract cream seems to provide subjective relief, but not significantly better than a placebo cream (6783).

There is insufficient reliable information available about the effectiveness of cabbage for its other uses; however, there is some evidence that people who consume large amounts of cabbage and other Brassica vegetables such as kale, broccoli, and cauliflower have a lower risk of developing some cancers, such as lung, stomach, and rectal cancer (6790,6792,6793). More evidence is needed to rate cabbage for this use.

Mechanism of Action

The applicable part of cabbage is the leaf. Cabbage contains modest amounts of calcium, vitamin C, vitamin A, vitamin E, and several B vitamins. Cabbage also contains other active constituents including chlorogenic acid, caffeic acid, and goitrin. These constituents seem to have antithyroid effects, possibly by inhibiting iodine uptake (7162). There is some interest in cabbage for breast cancer prevention because it contains constituents called glucosinolates such as indole-3 carbinol. Indole-3-carbinol is released from cabbage when it is chewed and is thought to change how estrogen is metabolized. Estrogen can be converted to either 16-alpha-hydroxyestrone or 2-alpha-hydroxyestrone. The 16-alpha-hydroxyestrone metabolite is thought to have a role in developing cancer. The 2-alpha-hydroxyestrone seems to protect against breast cancer. Indole-3-carbinol induces cytochrome P450 1A1 and 1A2 which shifts metabolism away from 16-alpha-hydroxyestrone in favor of 2-alpha-hydroxyestrone (7175,7176,7177,7179,7180,7181,7182,7187). This means that indole-3-carbinol might boost levels of a protective estrogen metabolite and decrease levels of a harmful one. Indole-3-carbinol and other glucosinolates, including S-methyl cysteine sulfoxide, might also have anticarcinogenic properties. These constituents seem to inhibit the enzymatic transformation of promutagens (6790). Cabbage also has antioxidant effects (5234,6791).

Adverse Reactions

None reported.

Interactions with Herbs & Other Dietary Supplements

Insufficient reliable information available.

Interactions with Drugs

ACETAMINOPHEN (TYLENOL, others): Cabbage can increase metabolism and decrease levels of acetaminophen. A diet that includes daily consumption of cabbage and Brussels sprouts decreases acetaminophen levels by as much as 16%. Cabbage seems to boost elimination through glucuronide conjugation (3952).

OXAZEPAM (SERAX): Cabbage can increase metabolism and decrease levels of oxazepam. A diet that includes daily consumption of cabbage and Brussels sprouts decreases oxazepam levels by as much as 17%. Cabbage seems to boost elimination through glucuronide conjugation (3952).

WARFARIN (Coumadin): Cabbage might decrease the anticoagulant effects of warfarin due to its high vitamin K content (19).

OTHER DRUGS: There is some concern that cabbage might decrease the effectiveness of numerous other drugs. Cabbage might increase drug metabolism and elimination by increasing glucuronide conjugation (3952) and by stimulating cytochrome P450 1A2 (CYP1A2) activity (7176,7187). Cabbage might lower levels of drugs that are metabolized through glucuronide conjugation including acetaminophen (Tylenol, others) and oxazepam (Serax), haloperidol (Haldol), lamotrigine (Lamictal), morphine (MS Contin, Roxanol), zidovudine (AZT, Retrovir), and others (3952). Cabbage might also lower levels of drugs that are substrates of CYP1A2 (7176,7187) including clozapine (Clozaril), cyclobenzaprine (Flexeril), fluvoxamine (Luvox), haloperidol (Haldol), imipramine (Tofranil), mexiletine (Mexitil), olanzapine (Zyprexa), pentazocine (Talwin), propranolol (Inderal), tacrine (Cognex), theophylline, zileuton (Zyflo), zolmitriptan (Zomig), and others.

Interactions with Foods

No interactions are known to occur, and there is no known reason to expect a clinically significant interaction with cabbage.

Interactions with Lab Tests

THYROID STIMULATING HORMONE (TSH): Ingesting large quantities of cabbage juice might elevate TSH test results (7162).

Interactions with Diseases or Conditions

HYPOTHYROIDISM: There is some concern that cabbage might worsen hypothyroidism. Cabbage constituents have antithyroid properties and there is some evidence that cabbage can boost TSH levels (7162); avoid using.

Dosage and Administration

ORAL: Cabbage is chopped and pressed for its juice. For augmenting the diet, 1 liter of juice has been consumed daily. For gastric pain and hyperacidity, people typically use 1 teaspoon of the juice 3 times daily before meals (18).
TOPICAL: For breast engorgement, cabbage leaves were prepared in clinical studies by stripping out the large vein of the cabbage leaf, cutting a hole for the nipple, and then rinsing and chilling the leaf. The chilled cabbage leaf is worn inside the bra or as a compress under a cool towel until the cabbage leaf reaches body temperature (approximately 20 minutes). This procedure is repeated 1-4 times daily for 1-2 days (6781,6784).

Comments

None.

CADE OIL

Also Known As

Alquitran de Enebro, Goudron de Cade, Juniper Tar, Juniper Tar Oil, Kadeol, Oil of Cade, Oil of Juniper Tar, Oleum Cadinum, Oleum Juniperi Empyreumaticum, Pix Cadi, Pix Juniper, Pix Oxycedri, Pyroleum Juniperi, Pyroleum Oxycedri, Wacholderteer.
CAUTION: See separate listing for Juniper.

Scientific Names

Juniperus oxycedrus.
Family: Cupressaceae or Pinaceae.

People Use This For

Topically, cade oil is used for itching, psoriasis, eczema and seborrhea (14), parasitic skin conditions, as an antiseptic in wound dressings, and in analgesic and antipruritic preparations (11).
Historically, cade oil has been used for treating various skin disorders, scalp conditions, hair loss, and cancers (11).
In manufacturing, cade oil is an ingredient in dermatologic creams and ointments, and in anti-dandruff shampoos (11).

Safety

POSSIBLY UNSAFE ...when used topically (14). Cade oil might lead to potentially carcinogenic DNA changes (14).
PREGNANCY AND LACTATION: POSSIBLY UNSAFE ...when used topically (14); avoid using.

Effectiveness

There is insufficient reliable information available about the effectiveness of cade oil.

Mechanism of Action

Cade oil contains a constituent called creosol. Creosol is a mild to moderate irritant (14). It has antipruritic and keratolytic activity, and antimicrobial activity in vitro (11).

Adverse Reactions

Topically, cade oil may cause eye irritation (14).

Interactions with Herbs & Other Dietary Supplements

Insufficient reliable information available.

Interactions with Drugs

No interactions are known to occur, and there is no known reason to expect a clinically significant interaction with cade oil.

Interactions with Foods

No interactions are known to occur, and there is no known reason to expect a clinically significant interaction with cade oil.

Interactions with Lab Tests

No interactions are known to occur, and there is no known reason to expect a clinically significant interaction with cade oil.

Interactions with Diseases or Conditions

No interactions are known to occur, and there is no known reason to expect a clinically significant interaction with cade oil.

Dosage and Administration

TOPICAL: Cade oil found in OTC ointments, shampoos, and scalp preparations in concentrations of 1-20%, and in Compound Resorcinol Ointment USP (14).

Comments

Avoid confusion with juniper berry (Juniperus communis). Cade oil is obtained by distilling the wood of the juniper tree (Juniperus oxycedrus).

CAFFEINE

Also Known As

Anhydrous Caffeine, Caffeine and Sodium Benzoate, Caffeine Citrate, Citrated Caffeine.
CAUTION: See separate listings for Black Tea, Green Tea, Coffee, Cola, Guarana, and Mate.

Scientific Names

1,3,7-trimethylxanthine.

People Use This For

Orally, caffeine is used in combination with analgesics and ergotamine for treating migraine headaches (3). It is used orally with analgesics for simple headaches and preventing and treating postoperative and postdural puncture headaches (15,2725,2726,2727,2728). It is also used orally for asthma, increasing blood pressure in hypotension (7), increasing mental alertness (15), enhancing athletic performance (7,6370), and for neonatal apnea (6023,6371).
In combination, caffeine is used with ephedrine or other stimulants and diuretics for weight loss (695,696,1704). Very high doses are used as euphoriants, often in combination with ephedrine as an alternative to illicit stimulants (7,2707).
Rectally, caffeine is used in combination with ergotamine for migraine headaches (15).
Topically, caffeine cream preparations have been used for reducing erythema and itching in dermatitis (14).
Parenterally, caffeine is used for postoperative and postdural puncture headache (15,6023), neonatal apnea (15,6023,6371), acute respiratory depression, and as a diuretic (13). It is also used for extending the length of seizure with electroconvulsive therapy (14).
In foods, caffeine is used as an ingredient in soft drinks and other beverages.

Safety

LIKELY SAFE ...when used orally, parenterally, or rectally and appropriately. Caffeine is a FDA-approved product and component of several over-the-counter and prescription products (14,15)
POSSIBLY UNSAFE ...when used orally long-term or in high doses. Chronic use, especially in large amounts, can produce tolerance, habituation, psychological dependence, and other significant adverse effects (15). Doses greater than 250-300 mg per day have been associated with significant adverse effects such as tachyarrhythmias and sleep disturbances (see Adverse Reactions) (14,18).
LIKELY UNSAFE ...when used orally in very high doses. Single doses of 3-10 grams have been associated with serious toxicity, including death (7).
CHILDREN: POSSIBLY SAFE ...when used orally or intravenously and appropriately in neonates (6371). POSSIBLY UNSAFE ...when used orally in amounts significantly greater than typical food amounts. Children are more susceptible to the adverse effects of caffeine (15).
PREGNANCY: POSSIBLY SAFE ...when used orally in small amounts or amounts found in food. Mothers should closely monitor their intake of caffeine. Use of caffeine in pregnancy is controversial (2708,2709,2710,2711); however, moderate consumption has not been associated with adverse fetal effects (6). Caffeine crosses the human placenta, but is not considered a teratogen. Fetal blood and tissue levels are similar to maternal concentrations (4260). Mothers should keep caffeine consumption below 200 mg per day. This is similar to the amount of caffeine found in 1-2 cups of coffee or tea (2708). POSSIBLY UNSAFE ...when used orally in large amounts. Caffeine crosses the placenta, producing fetal blood concentrations similar to maternal levels (4260). Mothers should avoid consuming more than 200 mg of caffeine daily or more than 1-2 cups of tea or coffee per day (2708). Maternal doses of greater than 200 mg per day throughout pregnancy has resulted in symptoms of caffeine withdrawal in newborn infants (14). High doses of caffeine have been

associated with spontaneous abortion, premature delivery, and low birth weight (6,2709,2711).

LACTATION: POSSIBLY SAFE …when used orally in small amounts or amounts found in food. Nursing mothers should closely monitor caffeine intake. Breast milk concentrations of caffeine are thought to be approximately 50% of maternal serum concentrations. Minimal consumption would likely result in limited exposure to a nursing infant (6). POSSIBLY UNSAFE …when used orally in large amounts. Caffeine is excreted slowly in infants and may accumulate. Caffeine can cause sleep disturbances, irritability, and increased bowel activity in breast-fed infants exposed to caffeine (18,2708,6026).

Effectiveness

LIKELY EFFECTIVE …when used orally for increasing mental alertness (14,15). Caffeine is FDA-approved as a stimulant for improving psychomotor performance (14). …when used orally in combination with analgesics for simple headache and analgesia (14,15,2718). Caffeine is a FDA-approved product for use with analgesics for improving pain relief (14). …when used orally in combination with acetaminophen and aspirin to treat migraine headache (2715,2716,2717). Caffeine is a FDA-approved product for use with analgesics for the treatment of migraine (14). …when used orally or intravenously to prevent postoperative headache (2725,2726). Caffeine is a FDA-approved product for preventing headache in postoperative patients who regularly consume caffeinated products.

POSSIBLY EFFECTIVE …when used orally for preventing or delaying onset of Parkinson's disease. There is some evidence from large-scale epidemiological studies that people who consume caffeinated beverages such as coffee, tea, and cola have a decreased risk of Parkinson's disease. For men, the effects seem to be dose related. For example, men consuming the greatest amount of caffeinated coffee, 3-4 cups (28 ounces) per day, or a total of 421-2716 mg of caffeine from any source daily, seem to have the greatest reduction in risk. However, there seems to be a significant reduction in risk even with consumption of as little as 124-208 mg caffeine per day (6022). In women, the effects do not seem to be dose related. Moderate consumption of caffeinated coffee, 1-3 cups daily, seems to provide the most reduction in risk (1238). …when used orally or intravenously to prevent postdural puncture headache (2727,2728). …when used orally for asthma (14). …when used orally for increasing blood pressure in hypotension (15). …when used orally in combination with ephedrine for weight loss (695,696,1704). …when used intravenously for respiratory depression secondary to CNS depressant overdose (14). …when used orally or intravenously for neonatal apnea of prematurity in infants 28-32 weeks postconception (14,6023,6371). Caffeine citrate seems to reduce the number of apnea episodes by at least 50% over 7-10 days of treatment (6371).

POSSIBLY INEFFECTIVE …when used orally for sustained, submaximal exercise endurance (14).

LIKELY INEFFECTIVE …when used orally for improving short-term, high-intensity performance and anaerobic capacity or power (14).

There is insufficient reliable information available about the effectiveness of caffeine for its other uses.

Mechanism of Action

Caffeine is a methylxanthine compound, structurally related to theophylline, theobromine, and uric acid (6372). It is 100% bioavailable after oral administration and is metabolized principally in the liver to paraxanthine, theophylline, and theobromine (6370). Caffeine stimulates the central nervous system (CNS), heart, muscles (15), and possibly the pressor centers that control blood pressure (7,15,2722). Possible mechanisms include adenosine receptor blockade and phosphodiesterase inhibition (2722). By blocking adenosine receptors, caffeine is thought to increase the release of neurotransmitters such as dopamine (6370). It has also been proposed that caffeine may decrease GABA and serotonin signaling (6370). Caffeine constricts cerebral vasculature (3) and stimulates gastric acid secretion (15). Caffeine can have positive inotropic and chronotropic effects on the heart with a duration of action from one to three hours (7). Caffeine can also acutely elevate both diastolic and systolic blood pressure, but might not have this effect in habitual users (6636). Caffeine exerts a diuretic effect, with water losses estimated at 1.17 mL per milligram of caffeine (15,2712). Tachyphylaxis to the diuretic effect develops rapidly, diminishing fluid losses associated with caffeine intake (3). Caffeine-containing beverages consumed during moderate endurance exercise do not appear to compromise bodily hydration status (2713). Caffeine's CNS stimulant effects are thought to improve vigilance and psychomotor performance (2720). For improving athletic performance, caffeine has been shown to decrease perceived levels of exertion, which enables the athlete to feel less tired and increase their performance (6370). Studies have also suggested caffeine possibly influences cardiovascular stress reactivity, either by potentiating the stress response itself or adding to the level reached during stress (6372). Caffeine may cause a slight decrease in heart rate after consumption and appears to raise blood pressure during psychological stress (6372). Large amounts of caffeine (>10 mg/kg/day) can also produce tachycardia and premature ventricular contractions (6372). Caffeine has been reported to cause increases and decreases in blood glucose (14). However, one study found that type 1 diabetics taking 200 mg of caffeine twice daily had increased frequency and intensity of warning signs of hypoglycemia (6024). This may be due to a reduction in blood flow to the brain and increase in glucose utilization by the brain (6024). For prevention of Parkinson's disease, caffeine may prevent adenosine's inhibition of dopaminergic transmission. This may result in a reduction in the clinical expression of Parkinsonism (6022). Evidence suggests tolerance to caffeine's neuroendocrine and cardiovascular effects may develop during consumption throughout the day, but tolerance appears to be lost during overnight abstinence of caffeine (6372). Preliminary evidence also suggests caffeine may increase plasma levels of cortisol and ACTH, decrease levels of extracellular potassium, and increase levels of intracellular calcium in skeletal muscle, but the mechanisms are poorly understood (6370).

Adverse Reactions

Caffeine can cause insomnia, nervousness, restlessness (7,15), gastric irritation (7), nausea and vomiting (15), tachycardia, quickened respiration, tremors, delirium, convulsions, and diuresis (15,505). Large doses can produce headache, anxiety, agitation, ringing in the ears, premature heartbeat, and arrhythmias (15). The adverse effects can be more severe in children than adults (15). Caffeine may cause feeding intolerance and gastrointestinal irritation in infants (6023). Some evidence shows caffeine is associated with fibrocystic breast disease in women; however, this is controversial and has been disputed (14,15). Past epidemiological studies on the relationship between caffeine use and the risk for osteoporosis have been conflicting. A recent study of 92 Caucasian, postmenopausal women does not support idea that caffeine use causes an increased risk for osteoporosis (6025). Chronic use of caffeine, especially in large amounts, can sometimes produce tolerance, habituation, and psychological dependence (15). The abrupt discontinuation of caffeine can sometimes result in physical withdrawal symptoms, including headaches, irritation, nervousness, anxiety, and dizziness (15); although some evidence suggests that clinically significant symptoms may be uncommon (2723).

Interactions with Herbs & Other Dietary Supplements

CAFFEINE CONTAINING HERBS/SUPPLEMENTS: Concomitant use can increase the therapeutic and adverse effects. Natural products that contain caffeine include coffee, black or green tea, guarana, mate, and cola.
CREATINE: There is one report of ischemic stroke in an athlete who consumed caffeine 400-600 mg, ephedra 40-60 mg, creatine monohydrate 6 grams, and a variety of other supplements daily for six weeks (1275). Caffeine can interfere with the ergogenic effects of creatine supplementation (2117).
EPHEDRA (Ma Huang): Concomitant use can increase the risk of adverse effects (7). One unpublished report associated jitteriness, hypertension, seizures, temporary loss of consciousness, and hospitalization requiring life support with the use of a combination ephedra and guarana (caffeine) product (1380). There is one report of ischemic stroke in an athlete who consumed caffeine 400-600 mg, ephedra 40-60 mg, creatine monohydrate 6 grams, and a variety of other supplements daily for six weeks (1275).

Interactions with Drugs

ACETAMINOPHEN (Tylenol): Concomitant use can increase the analgesic effect of acetaminophen by up to 40% (512).
ALCOHOL: Concomitant use of alcohol can increase caffeine serum concentrations and the risk of caffeine adverse effects. Alcohol reduces caffeine metabolism (6370).
ASPIRIN: Concomitant use can increase the analgesic effect of aspirin by up to 40% (512).
BENZODIAZEPINES: Concomitant use reduces the sedative and anxiolytic effects of benzodiazepines (14).
BETA-ADRENERGIC AGONISTS: Concomitant use can increase the positive inotropic effects of beta-agonists on the heart (15). Beta-adrenergic agonists include albuterol (Proventil, Ventolin), metaproterenol (Alupent), terbutaline (Brethine), and isoproterenol (Isuprel).
CIMETIDINE (Tagamet): Concomitant use can increase serum caffeine concentrations and the risk of caffeine adverse effects. Cimetidine decreases the rate of caffeine clearance by 30-50% (14).
CLOZAPINE (Clozaril): Co-administration can acutely exacerbate psychotic symptoms. Caffeine can also increase the effects and toxicity of clozapine (151). Caffeine doses of 400-1000 mg per day inhibit clozapine metabolism (5051).
CNS STIMULANTS: Concomitant use can increase the risk of adverse CNS effects (151,2719). Some CNS stimulants include nicotine, cocaine, sympathomimetic amines, and amphetamines.
DIABETES THERAPY: Theoretically, concomitant use of caffeine and diabetes drugs might interfere with blood glucose control. Some reports claim that caffeine might have hyperglycemic effects (19).
DISULFIRAM (Antabuse): Concomitant use can increase caffeine serum concentrations and the risk of adverse effects. Disulfiram decreases the rate of caffeine clearance (15).
EPHEDRINE: Concomitant use can increase the risk of stimulatory adverse effects of ephedrine and caffeine (7,19). An unpublished report associated jitteriness, hypertension, seizures, temporary loss of consciousness, and hospitalization requiring life support with the use of a combination ephedra (ephedrine) and caffeine-containing guarana product (1380).
ESTROGEN (Estrace): Concomitant use can increase serum caffeine concentrations and the risk of caffeine adverse effects. Estrogen inhibits caffeine metabolism (2714).
ERGOTAMINE: Concomitant use increases the gastrointestinal absorption of ergotamine (15).
FLUVOXAMINE (Luvox): Concomitant use can increase caffeine serum concentrations and the risk of caffeine adverse effects. Fluvoxamine reduces caffeine metabolism (6370).
LITHIUM (Eskalith, Lithobid): Abrupt caffeine withdrawal might increase serum lithium levels (609). There are two case reports of lithium tremor that worsened upon abrupt coffee withdrawal (610).
MEXILETINE (Mexitil): Concomitant use can increase serum caffeine concentrations and the risk of caffeine adverse effects. Mexiletine reduces caffeine metabolism (14).
MONOAMINE OXIDASE INHIBITORS (MAOIs): Concomitant intake of large amounts of caffeine

with MAOIs might precipitate a hypertensive crisis [19].

ORAL CONTRACEPTIVES (OCs): Concomitant use can increase serum caffeine concentrations and adverse effects. OCs decrease the rate of caffeine clearance by 40-65% [14].

PHENYLPROPANOLAMINE (Dexatrim, Propagest): Concomitant use can cause an additive increase in blood pressure. Phenylpropanolamine can also increase serum caffeine concentrations [14].

QUINOLONES: Concomitant use can increase serum caffeine concentrations and the risk of caffeine adverse effects. Quinolones decrease caffeine clearance [606,607,608]. Quinolones (fluoroquinolones) include ciprofloxacin (Cipro), enoxacin (Penetrex), gatifloxacin (Tequin), levofloxacin (Levaquin), lomefloxacin (Maxaquin), moxifloxacin (Avelox), norfloxacin (Noroxin), ofloxacin (Floxin), sparfloxacin (Zagam), and trovafloxacin (Trovan).

RILUZOLE (Rilutek): Concomitant use might increase serum concentrations and the risk of adverse effects of both caffeine and riluzole. Caffeine and riluzole are both metabolized by cytochrome P450 1A2, and concomitant use might reduce metabolism of one or both agents [14].

TERBINAFINE (Lamisil): Concomitant use can increase serum caffeine concentrations and the risk of caffeine adverse effects. Terbinafine decreases the clearance of intravenous caffeine by 19% [14].

THEOPHYLLINE (Theo-Dur): Large amounts of caffeine might inhibit theophylline metabolism, increase serum theophylline concentrations and the risk of adverse effects [14].

VERAPAMIL (Calan, Isoptin, Verelan): Concomitant use can increase plasma caffeine concentrations and the risk of caffeine adverse effects. Verapamil increases plasma caffeine concentrations by 25% [14].

Interactions with Foods

CAPSAICIN: Concomitant use of red-pepper extract capsaicin can increase caffeine levels and increase the risk of adverse effects [6370].

GRAPEFRUIT JUICE: Concomitant use can increase caffeine levels and increase the risk of adverse effects [504].

Interactions with Lab Tests

5-HYDROXYINDOLEACETIC ACID: Caffeine can cause slight increases in these levels and test results [15].

BLEEDING TIME: Caffeine can prolong bleeding time and increase the results of a bleeding time test [1701].

CREATINE: Caffeine can increase urine creatine levels [1701].

DIPYRIDAMOLE THALLIUM IMAGING: Caffeine attenuates the characteristic cardiovascular responses to dipyridamole and can alter test results [14].

SERUM URATE (Bittner method): Caffeine can cause false-positive test results [15].

TESTS FOR PHEOCHROMOCYTOMA, NEUROBLASTOMA: High urine catecholamines or VMA can result in false-positive results. Avoid caffeine while testing for these diseases [15].

URINE CATECHOLAMINES: Caffeine can cause slight increases in these levels and test results [15].

VANILLYLMANDELIC ACID (VMA): Caffeine can cause slight increases in these levels and test results [15].

Interactions with Diseases or Conditions

CARDIAC CONDITIONS: Caffeine can induce cardiac arrhythmias in sensitive individuals [14,16]; use with caution.

DEPRESSION, ANXIETY DISORDERS: Caffeine might aggravate these conditions [14]; use with caution.

DIABETES: Caffeine may enhance the frequency and intensity of hypoglycemic warning symptoms in type 1 diabetics. This may increase the ability of diabetics to detect and treat hypoglycemia early. However, it might also increase the frequency of hypoglycemic events [6024]; use with caution.

HYPERTENSION: Consuming caffeine might increase blood pressure in people with high blood pressure [2272,6663]. However, this effect, might be less in habitual caffeine users [6663].

KIDNEY DISEASE: The diuretic effect of caffeine might aggravate some kidney disorders [19].

PEPTIC ULCER DISEASE (PUD): Caffeine can aggravate PUD by increasing gastric acid secretion [14,16]; avoid using.

Dosage and Administration

ORAL: The typical dose of caffeine for headache or restoring mental alertness is up to 250 mg per day [14,15]. For fatigue, the common dose is 100-325 mg up to three times a day [13]. For increasing exercise performance, 2-10 mg/kg or more has been used [14]. However, doses in excess of 10 mg/kg can result in urine levels greater than the 12 mcg/mL allowed by the International Olympic Committee and the National Collegiate Athletic Association [14,6370]. For weight loss, the ephedrine and caffeine combination products are commonly dosed 20 mg/200 mg three times per day [695,696,1704]. For postdural puncture headache, 300 mg orally has been used [14]. For preventing Parkinson's disease, men consuming 3-4 cups (28 oz) of caffeinated coffee per day or 421-2716 mg total caffeine had the lowest risk of developing Parkinson's disease. However, a significantly lower risk was also associated with consumption of as little as 124-208 mg of caffeine [6022]. In women, more moderate caffeinated coffee consumption seems to be best; 1-3 cups per day [1238].

TOPICAL: For dermatitis, a 30% caffeine cream has been used [14].

INTRAVENOUS: For apnea in infants one study used an initial intravenous dose of caffeine benzoate of 10 mg/kg.

Some infants required a second dose of 5 mg/kg 18-24 hours later (6023). Another study used a 20 mg/kg loading dose of caffeine citrate intravenously followed by a daily dose of 2.5 mg/kg intravenously or orally for 10 days for maintenance (6371). For extended seizure in electroconvulsive therapy (ECT), 500 mg IV 5 minutes before the procedure has been used (14). For postdural puncture headache, 500 mg caffeine sodium benzoate in 1000 mL normal saline infused over 90 minutes following anesthesia has been used. The same dose has also been administered as a bolus dose and repeated in 8 hours as necessary (14).

Comments

People with voice disorders, singers, and other voice professionals are often advised against the use of caffeine; however, this recommendation has been based on anecdotal evidence. Now preliminary research seems to indicate that caffeine ingestion may actually adversely affect subjective voice quality. Further study is necessary to confirm these preliminary findings (2724). One cup of coffee, tea and cocoa contain approximately 75-200 mg, 50 mg, and 5 mg of caffeine respectively (6372). A 12 oz bottle of cola drink contains approximately 30-50 mg caffeine (6372).

CAJEPUT OIL

Also Known As

Cajuput, Cajeputi Aetheroleum, Paperbark Tree Oil, Punk Tree.
CAUTION: See separate listings for Niauli Oil and Tea Tree Oil.

Scientific Names

Melaleuca leucodendra, synonym Melaleuca leucodendron; Melaleuca quinquenervia.
Family: Myrtaceae.

People Use This For

Orally, cajeput oil is used as an expectorant (2) or tonic (11).
Topically, cajeput oil is used either alone or in combination with other ingredients in commercially available antiseptic liniments to treat rheumatic and neuralgic discomforts (2).
As an inhalant, it is used as an expectorant (2) and tonic (11).
In dentistry, cajeput oil is used to relieve dry socket discomfort (11).
Historically, cajeput oil has been used to treat colds, headaches, toothache, and indolent tumors (11). It has also been used topically for its anti-parasitic effect in scabies and tinea versicolor (215).
In food and beverages, it is used as a flavoring in very small amounts .

Safety

LIKELY SAFE ...when cajeput oil is used orally in food amounts. The maximum use is less than 0.001% (11).
POSSIBLY SAFE ...when used topically on unbroken skin (2,7).
POSSIBLY UNSAFE ...when inhaled. Inhalation can cause bronchospasm (7). ...when undiluted cajeput oil is used orally or topically (3527).
There is insufficient reliable information available about the safety of cajeput oil for its other uses or in amounts exceeding those found in food.
CHILDREN: LIKELY UNSAFE ...when used topically on facial areas, especially the nose (2,7) because it might cause bronchospasm.
PREGNANCY AND LACTATION: Insufficient reliable information available; avoid using.

Effectiveness

POSSIBLY EFFECTIVE ...when used orally as an expectorant (7). ...when used topically as counterirritant for arthritis and rheumatism (2). A counterirritant is an agent that causes mild inflammation of the skin for the purpose of relieving a deep-seated inflammatory process. (2).
There is insufficient reliable information available about the effectiveness of cajeput oil for its other uses.

Mechanism of Action

Cajeput oil contains 14-65% cineole (7,11), which is reported to have antispasmodic, antimicrobial and fungicidal properties (2,7). Cineole may act as a counterirritant (7). Cineole is identical to eucalyptol (215).

Adverse Reactions

Orally, use of cajeput oil can lead to dyspepsia (7).
Topically, use can produce hypersensitivity, allergic reactions and irritation of mucous membranes (7).
Inhalation can cause bronchospasm (7).

Interactions with Herbs & Other Dietary Supplements

Insufficient reliable information available.

Interactions with Drugs

No interactions are known to occur, and there is no known reason to expect a clinically significant interaction with cajeput oil.

Interactions with Foods

No interactions are known to occur, and there is no known reason to expect a clinically significant interaction with cajeput oil.

Interactions with Lab Tests

No interactions are known to occur, and there is no known reason to expect a clinically significant interaction with cajeput oil.

Interactions with Diseases or Conditions

ASTHMA: Inhalation of cajeput oil may provoke bronchospasm (7).

Dosage and Administration

No typical dosage.

Comments

Avoid confusion with tea tree oil (Maleleuca alternifolia) and niauli oil (Malaleuca viridiflora). Cajeput oil is produced by steam distillation of fresh leaves and twigs of Melaleuca leucodendra and Melaleuca quinquenervia.

CALABAR BEAN

Also Known As

Chop Nut, Esere Nut, Faba Calabarica, Legume, Ordeal Bean, Physotigma.

Scientific Names

Physostigma venenosum.
Family: Leguminosae or Fabaceae.

People Use This For

Orally, calabar bean is used for visual disorders, constipation, epilepsy, cholera, and tetanus. Calabar bean is a source of the prescription drug physostigmine (Isopto Eserine, Antilirium).

Safety

UNSAFE ...when used orally. The calabar bean is extremely toxic. Its active constituent, physostigmine, can cause death by impairing heart contractility and causing respiratory paralysis (6).
PREGNANCY AND LACTATION: UNSAFE ...when used orally (6); avoid using.

Effectiveness

There is insufficient reliable information available about the effectiveness of calabar bean.

Mechanism of Action

The applicable part of calabar bean is the dried, ripe seed. The major constituent, physostigmine, prolongs activity of neurotransmitter acetylcholine (6). It increases parasympathetic nervous system and striated muscle tone, stimulates glandular secretions, increases GI peristalsis, reduces heart rate, and causes pupil contraction leading to a reduction in intraocular pressure (18).

Adverse Reactions

Orally, overdose of physostigmine, the constituent of calabar bean, causes cholinergic crisis characterized by excessive salivation and sweating, constricted pupils of eye, nausea, vomiting, diarrhea, bradycardia or tachycardia, hypotension or hypertension, confusion, seizures, coma, severe muscle weakness, paralysis, and death (15).

Interactions with Herbs & Other Dietary Supplements

Insufficient reliable information available.

Interactions with Drugs

ANTICHOLINERGIC DRUGS: Physostigmine reverses the effect of belladonna and other drugs with anticholinergic action. These drugs include antihistamines, some emetics, some anti-Parkinson agents, and phenothiazines (15).

Interactions with Foods

No interactions are known to occur, and there is no known reason to expect a clinically significant interaction with calabar bean.

Interactions with Lab Tests

No interactions are known to occur, and there is no known reason to expect a clinically significant interaction with calabar bean.

Interactions with Diseases or Conditions

Avoid in patients with Parkinson's disease, bradycardia, asthma, gangrene, diabetes, cardiovascular disease, and mechanical obstruction of intestinal or urogenital tract.

Dosage and Administration

No typical dosage.

Comments

Historically, African tribes used calabar bean, the "ordeal bean," to identify witches and people possessed by evil spirits. They believed that people who regurgitated the bean and lived were innocent. Ritual uses continue in Africa despite being outlawed (6). Subjects of the "ordeal" can increase their chance of survival by not chewing the bean and swallowing it whole. Chewing releases the toxic constituents.

CALAMINT

Also Known As

Basil Thyme, Mill Mint, Mountain Balm, Mountain Mint.

Scientific Names

Calamintha ascendens.
Family: Labiatae or Lamiaceae.

People Use This For

Orally, calamint is used for respiratory illnesses and colds with fever. It is also used orally to promote sweating and as an expectorant (18).

Safety

There is insufficient reliable information available about the safety of calamint.
Pregnancy and Lactation: Insufficient reliable information available; avoid using.

Effectiveness

There is insufficient reliable information available about the effectiveness of calamint.

Mechanism of Action

The applicable parts of calamint are the above ground parts. There is insufficient reliable information available about the possible mechanisms of action or active ingredients.

Adverse Reactions

None reported.

Interactions with Herbs & Other Dietary Supplements

Insufficient reliable information available.

Interactions with Drugs

No interactions are known to occur, and there is no known reason to expect a clinically significant interaction with calamint.

Interactions with Foods

No interactions are known to occur, and there is no known reason to expect a clinically significant interaction with calamint.

Interactions with Lab Tests

No interactions are known to occur, and there is no known reason to expect a clinically significant interaction with calamint.

Interactions with Diseases or Conditions

No interactions are known to occur, and there is no known reason to expect a clinically significant interaction with calamint.

Dosage and Administration

No typical dosage.

Comments

There is very little scientific information about this product. Our staff is continually analyzing the available information on natural medicines and will add data here as it becomes available.

CALAMUS

Also Known As

Cinnamon Sedge, Gladdon, Grass Myrtle, Myrtle Flag, Myrtle Sedge, Sweet Cane, Sweet Cinnamon, Sweet Flag, Sweet Grass, Sweet Myrtle, Sweet Root, Sweet Rush, Sweet Sedge.

Scientific Names

Acorus calamus.
Family: Araceae.

People Use This For

Orally, calamus is used for digestive disorders including ulcers, gastritis (18), and flatulence (9), and to stimulate appetite and digestion. Some people use calamus to induce sweating (4). Others chew it to remove the smell of tobacco (6). Historically, calamus has been used orally as a sedative and for acute and chronic dyspepsia, gastritis, gastric ulcer, anorexia (4), rheumatoid arthritis, and strokes and topically for skin diseases (11). Native Americans of the Cree tribe chewed the root for its stimulant, euphoric, and hallucinogenic effects (214).
In food use, calamus is utilized in cooking as a spice (5).

Safety

LIKELY UNSAFE ...when used orally. FDA prohibits calamus use in food products (12) due to the presence of the carcinogenic constituent, beta-isoasarone (5) in three of the four distinct strains. However, the beta-isoasarone content varies widely among strains (from 0% to 96%) (6), so some products may be safer than others.
PREGNANCY AND LACTATION: LIKELY UNSAFE ...when used orally; avoid using (4,500).

Effectiveness

There is insufficient reliable information about the effectiveness of calamus.

Mechanism of Action

The applicable part of calamus is the rhizome. The constituent asarone, which is chemically related to reserpine, may explain calamus' sedative effects (6). It is not known exactly which constituent is responsible for calamus' ability to relieve smooth muscle spasms, though it is probably not isoasarone, because preparations without isoasarone have a measurable spasmolytic effect (6).

Adverse Reactions

Calamus oil may contain beta-isoasarone, a known carcinogen associated with kidney damage, tremors, and convulsions.

Interactions with Herbs & Other Dietary Supplements

HERBS WITH SEDATIVE PROPERTIES: Theoretically, concomitant use with herbs that have sedative properties might enhance therapeutic and adverse effects. These include calendula, California poppy, catnip, capsicum, celery, couch grass, elecampane, Siberian ginseng, German chamomile, goldenseal, gotu kola, hops, Jamaican dogwood, kava, lemon balm, sage, St. John's wort, sassafras, scullcap, shepherd's purse, stinging nettle, valerian, wild carrot, wild lettuce, ashwaganda root, and yerba mansa (4,19).

Interactions with Drugs
ACID-INHIBITING DRUGS: Theoretically, due to claims that calamus increases stomach acid, it might interfere with antacids, sucralfate (Carafate), H-2 antagonists, or proton pump inhibitors (19).
MAO INHIBITORS: Theoretically, calamus might potentiate the effects and adverse effects of monoamine oxidase inhibitor drugs (4).
CNS DEPRESSANTS: Theoretically, concomitant use with drugs with sedative properties can cause additive effects and side effects (4).

Interactions with Foods
No interactions are known to occur, and there is no known reason to expect a clinically significant interaction with calamus.

Interactions with Lab Tests
No interactions are known to occur, and there is no known reason to expect a clinically significant interaction with calamus.

Interactions with Diseases or Conditions
No interactions are known to occur, and there is no known reason to expect a clinically significant interaction with calamus.

Dosage and Administration
ORAL: 1-3 grams rhizome three times daily, or one cup tea (steep 1-3 grams rhizome in 150 mL boiling water 5-10 minutes, strain) three times daily (4). Liquid extract (1:1 in 60% alcohol) 1-3 mL three times daily (4). Tincture (1:5 in 60% alcohol) 2-4 mL three times daily (4).

Comments
Four different types of herbs/volatile oil exist, each in a different geographic region of the world. The North American variety is isoasarone free and the European form contains less than 10% isoasarone in the volatile oil. Others contain up to 96% carcinogenic beta-isoasarone in the volatile oil (5).

CALCIUM

Also Known As
Bone Meal, Calcium Acetate, Calcium Aspartate, Calcium Carbonate, Calcium Chelate, Calcium Chloride, Calcium Citrate, Calcium Citrate Malate, Calcium Gluconate, Calcium Lactate, Calcium Lactogluconate, Calcium Orotate, Calcium Phosphate, Di-calcium Phosphate, Dicalcium Phosphate, Heated Oyster Shell-Seaweed Calcium, Hydroxyapatite, Oyster Shell Calcium, Tricalcium Phosphate.
CAUTION: See separate listing for Dolomite.

Scientific Names
Calcium; Ca; atomic number 20.

People Use This For
Orally, calcium is used for treatment and prevention of hypocalcemia, osteoporosis, rickets, and latent tetany. It is also used orally for hypoparathyroidism, osteomalacia, premenstrual syndrome (PMS), leg cramps associated with pregnancy, and reducing the risk of colorectal cancer. Calcium is also used orally for diarrhea and rectal epithelial hyperproliferation following intestinal bypass, reducing excess fluoride levels in children, hypertension, and high low-density lipoprotein (LDL) levels. Calcium carbonate is used orally as an antacid. Calcium carbonate and calcium acetate are also used orally as phosphate binders in renal failure.
Intravenously, calcium gluconate, acetate, gluceptate or chloride are used for severe hypocalcemia and hypocalcemic tetany, and during cardiopulmonary resuscitation. Calcium gluconate and gluceptate are also given intramuscularly when intravenous administration is not possible.

Safety
LIKELY SAFE ...when used orally and appropriately. Routine dietary intake and supplementation in recommended doses are not associated with significant adverse effects (15). ...when used intravenously and appropriately (15).

POSSIBLY UNSAFE ...when used orally in excessive doses. Amounts exceeding 2.4 grams per day can cause kidney stones, which might result in renal damage (945,1816). ...when calcium chloride is used orally. Ingestion of calcium chloride has been reported to cause gastrointestinal hemorrhage (15).

PREGNANCY AND LACTATION: LIKELY SAFE ...when used orally and appropriately (945,3263,3264). There is insufficient reliable information available about the safety of the intravenous use of calcium during pregnancy and lactation.

Effectiveness

EFFECTIVE ...when used orally for treating and preventing hypocalcemia (15). ...when used orally for rickets (14). ...when calcium carbonate is used as an antacid (9). ...when calcium carbonate or calcium acetate are used orally as phosphate binders in renal failure (9). Calcium citrate is not recommended for this purpose because it increases aluminum absorption (14). ...when calcium gluconate, acetate, gluceptate, or chloride are used intravenously for severe hypocalcemia or hypocalcemic tetany, or during cardiopulmonary resuscitation (15).

LIKELY EFFECTIVE ...when used orally to prevent osteoporosis in postmenopausal women. Calcium supplementation has very little effect on bone loss in the 5 years immediately after menopause (2569,2570,2573,2575,2576). The rapid loss of estrogen causes a very high bone resorption rate, which increases serum calcium levels and inhibits intestinal absorption of calcium (2570). After this period, calcium supplementation has a significant benefit on bone loss. The typical rate of bone loss in postmenopausal women who are not taking calcium supplements is 2% per year (2572,2576). Calcium 1000 to 1600 mg per day (as the carbonate, citrate, lactate gluconate, or citrate malate) decreases this rate by 0.25-1% annually (977,979,981,2569,2571,2572,2573,2574,2575,2576,2578,6850). The greatest reductions (1% or more) are seen in the first 1 to 2 years of supplementation when bone remodeling foci are filled in (2569,2574,2576). After this period, the differences in rate of loss between supplemented and unsupplemented women are closer to 0.25% per year (2569,2574,2577). Despite the "first year effect" it is estimated that 30 years of continuous calcium supplementation after menopause might result in a 10% improvement in bone mineral density, and a 50% overall reduction in fracture rates, compared with women who do not take calcium supplements (2570). Most studies show that long-term calcium supplementation decreases fracture rates for specific bones by 30-35% for vertebral bone and 25% for hip bone (2576). Supplements must also be continued indefinitely since the effects of 2 years of calcium supplements on bone mineral density are largely lost within 2 years after discontinuing the supplements (981,2576,6853). Calcium has additive effects on bone density with other agents such as vitamin D, estrogens, or calcitonin. Whereas calcium alone generally reduces or prevents loss of bone density, combination with other agents can produce small increases in bone density (e.g., 0.3 to 3.3% depending on the combination and doses used) (978,980,1835,1836,2570,2571,2572,2576). A combination of calcium, vitamin D, and estrogen is likely the most efficacious for preventing bone loss in postmenopausal women (2573). ...when used orally in premenopausal women over 40 to prevent bone loss. Maximal bone growth occurs in the teenage years, then bone density remains relatively constant until age 30 to 40. After that, losses typically occur at rates of 0.5 to 1% per year, especially if dietary calcium intake is below the RDA, which is the case in for many Americans (2571,2578). This bone loss in premenopausal women over 40 can be reduced significantly by supplementing with 1000 mg calcium per day (2578). ...when used orally in combination with other agents for the treatment of osteoporosis in postmenopausal women. The full potential of osteoporosis treatments cannot be realized without adequate calcium intake (2569,2570,2571,2572,2573). Advise women taking agents such as estrogens, calcitonin, biphosphonates, or raloxifene (Evista) to ensure their daily calcium intake meets the RDA, using supplements if necessary. ...when used in mothers during pregnancy to improve fetal bone mineralization and density. Calcium supplements in pregnant women who have low dietary calcium intake (less than 562 mg elemental calcium per day), increase fetal bone mineralization. However, in women with adequate dietary intake, calcium supplementation won't offer any additional benefit (3263,3264). ...when used orally for reducing the symptoms of premenstrual syndrome (PMS) (1822,1823,1824,6847). There seems to be a link between low dietary calcium intake and symptoms of PMS (6847). Taking calcium 1-1.2 grams daily seems to significantly reduce depressed mood, water retention, and pain associated with PMS (1822,1823,1824). There is a high placebo response in PMS treatment trials, but calcium seems to decrease symptom scores by about 18 percentage points more than placebo (1822). ...when calcium carbonate is used orally for reducing secondary hyperparathyroidism in patients with chronic renal failure (1827,1828,1829).

POSSIBLY EFFECTIVE ...when used in combination with vitamin D as adjunctive therapy for reducing bone mineral density loss in people with conditions requiring long-term corticosteroid use (982,1046,1830,1831,1832,4462,4463,4464,4465,4466,4467). ...when used for reducing bone turnover during weight reduction in postmenopausal women (987). ...when used orally to reduce the risk of colorectal cancer (970,994,1047). ...when used orally for hypertension. Calcium supplementation produces a very modest reduction in blood pressure, usually around 2 mmHg. However, it may be more effective for certain subpopulations of patients, such as salt-sensitive people and African-American patients with low dietary calcium intake (945,972,974,976,984,1818,1819,1820,1821,6852). ...when used orally for reducing blood pressure in individuals with end-stage renal disease (975). ...when used orally for reducing pregnancy-related hypertension and pre-eclampsia in women with insufficient dietary calcium intake (973,1833,1834). Supplementation in women with adequate dietary intake does not seem to help (971). ...when used orally to reduce the incidence of pregnancy-related leg cramps (2567). There is some evidence that calcium 1 gram twice daily (as a mixture of salts) can reduce pregnancy-related leg cramping during the second half of pregnancy (2567). ...when used orally in

conjunction with a low-fat diet for mild to moderate hypercholesterolaemia. Calcium carbonate 400 mg three times daily produced a 4.4% reduction in low-density lipoprotein (LDL) cholesterol and a 4.1% increase in high-density lipoprotein (HDL) after 6 weeks of treatment when used in combination with a low-fat diet (American Heart Association step 1) starting 8 weeks prior to calcium carbonate (2557). ...when used orally for treating diarrhea and rectal epithelial hyperproliferation due to intestinal bypass (1826). ...when used in combination with ascorbic acid and vitamin D supplements for reducing excessive fluoride levels in children and improving symptoms of fluorosis (990). ...when used orally to prevent ischemic stroke. There is some evidence that increasing dietary calcium intake might decrease the relative risk of ischemic stroke in women (4822).
POSSIBLY INEFFECTIVE ...when used for preventing bone mineral density loss in lactating women (988). ...when used orally for preventing bone loss after bone marrow transplantation (1817). ...when used orally for preventing bone loss associated with renal transplantation (4823).

Mechanism of Action

The bones and teeth contain greater than 99% of calcium in the human body. It is also present in blood, extracellular fluid, and muscle and other tissues. It is essential for nerve transmission, muscle contraction, vascular contraction, vasodilation, glandular secretion, cell membrane and capillary permeability, enzyme reactions, respiration, renal function, and blood coagulation. It also plays a role in neurotransmitter and hormone release and storage, uptake and binding of amino acids, cyanocobalamin (vitamin B12) absorption, and gastrin secretion (15). Calcium in bone is present mainly as hydroxyapatite and also serves as a reserve source of calcium that can be mobilized to maintain extracellular calcium concentrations. About half of serum calcium is bound to plasma proteins. The free or ionized calcium is tightly regulated and a useful clinical indicator of calcium status (1834). In heart muscle and nerve terminals, calcium channels open when membranes are depolarized and stored calcium is released (945). The subsequent rise in cytosolic calcium concentration triggers contraction (945). Calcium balance is generally positive during growth, neutral in the mature adult, and negative in older adults (1834). Conditions associated with reduced levels of estrogens in women result in reduced calcium absorption and retention, increased bone turnover, and lower bone mass (15). Calcium is lost in varying amounts through the feces, urine, sweat, and sloughed skin cells (1834). Calcium absorption varies with age, environmental and dietary conditions, and race (1837). Asians and Africans absorb calcium more efficiently than Caucasians (1837). In healthy premenopausal women, the proportion of dietary calcium absorbed varies from 10 to 60%, and is positively correlated with body mass index, dietary fat, and serum vitamin D level (6851). It is inversely correlated with total dietary calcium, dietary fiber, alcohol intake, and physical activity (6851). There is a link between a low fat, high fiber diet and poor calcium absorption, possibly due to a faster rate of intestinal transit (6851). Calcium exhibits threshold absorption. Below the threshold, an increase in calcium intake results in improved response; above the threshold, increased calcium intake has no effect. The many variables of calcium absorption complicates interpretation of calcium absorption studies (1834). Some evidence suggests that calcium citrate and heated oyster shell-seaweed calcium are absorbed better than calcium carbonate, while other research indicates similar bioavailability (1838,1839,1840,1841,1842,1847). Contrary to laboratory evidence, lactose does not enhance calcium bioavailability in lactose tolerant people (4824). Dietary oxalate and phytate, which tend to be higher in vegetarian diets, reduce calcium bioavailability (15). Calcium taken orally can bind with phosphate in the gut, preventing its absorption and reducing the hyperphosphatemia associated with renal failure. Calcium carbonate or calcium acetate are used for this purpose, whereas calcium citrate is not recommended because it increases aluminum absorption (14). Calcium may help to lower serum cholesterol levels by forming insoluble complexes with saturated fatty acids in the gut, causing them to be excreted in the feces without being absorbed (2557). In women, calcium levels may be lower in the premenstrual period (due to effects of variations in estrogen levels on calcium absorption and metabolism), which may contribute to the mood changes and other symptoms associated with the premenstrual syndrome (PMS) (2639,6847).

Adverse Reactions

Orally, calcium can cause gastrointestinal irritation, belching, and flatulence (9,1843). Although constipation is frequently cited as an adverse effect of calcium, there is no scientific substantiation of this side effect (1843,1844,1845). Calcium chloride can cause gastrointestinal hemorrhage when taken orally (15). Extended use of calcium carbonate for gastric hyperacidity can cause acid rebound (9). Prolonged ingestion of large amounts of calcium carbonate (usually greater than 20 grams per day) can cause hypercalcemia, milk-alkali syndrome (1843,6123), nephrocalcinosis, and renal insufficiency (6122). In patients with impaired renal function, doses as low as 4 grams per day might cause hypercalcemia and milk-alkali syndrome (1843,6849). There is concern that calcium supplements, both oyster shell and refined calcium products, can be contaminated with lead (997,6459,6460). In one report, 8 of 23 nationally available calcium carbonate products contained small amounts of lead (6459). However, these findings are likely clinically insignificant. The amount of lead in these calcium supplements is substantially less than that found in common foods, such as green salads, grapes, and wine. Also, calcium significantly decreases lead absorption. Small amounts of lead in a calcium supplement would not likely be significantly absorbed or achieve clinically relevant levels in the body (6460). So far, there have not been reports of significant lead toxicity from appropriate use of calcium supplements (996). Epidemiological evidence suggests that a high intake of dietary calcium might increase the risk for prostate cancer (4825,4827).

Interactions with Herbs & Other Dietary Supplements

VITAMIN D: Concomitant administration with vitamin D increases active absorption of oral calcium (945).
IRON, ZINC, MAGNESIUM: Concomitant administration decreases gastrointestinal absorption of iron, zinc, and magnesium, but does not appear to have any clinically significant effect on the status of these minerals in the body (998,1848,1849,1850). Administration of calcium and other mineral supplements should be done at different times.

Interactions with Drugs

BISPHOSPHONATES (alendronate, etidronate, risedronate, etc.): Absorption is decreased by concomitant administration with calcium. Administer alendronate at least 30 minutes before calcium (14).
CAFFEINE: High doses of caffeine can increase urinary calcium excretion (2570).
ESTROGEN: Concomitant use of estrogen increases supplemental calcium absorption in postmenopausal women (995).
FLUOROQUINOLONES (ciprofloxacin, levofloxacin, ofloxacin, etc.): Concomitant administration decreases the absorption of these drugs and calcium (9). Administer these drugs at least two hours before or after calcium supplements.
LEVOTHYROXINE (Synthroid, Levothroid, Levoxyl): Concomitant administration reduces levothyroxine absorption (14). Calcium carbonate reduces levothyroxine absorption and effectiveness in hypothyroid patients on levothyroxine replacement therapy (5081,5082,6137). Separate the administration of levothyroxine and calcium by at least 4 hours (14). In some studies, long-term levothyroxine therapy has been associated with decreased bone density in the hip and spine in pre- and post-menopausal women. This is thought to be due to increased urinary loss of calcium. There is currently no evidence that calcium supplementation is either helpful or necessary (27,28,29).
TETRACYCLINES (demeclocycline, doxycycline, minocycline, etc.): Concomitant administration decreases the absorption of these drugs and calcium (9). Administer these drugs at least two hours before or after calcium supplements.
THIAZIDE AND THIAZIDE-LIKE DIURETICS (hydrochlorothiazide, indapamide, metolazone, etc.): Concomitant use of thiazide diuretics along with moderately large amounts of calcium carbonate increases the risk of milk-alkali syndrome (hypercalcemia, metabolic alkalosis, renal failure) (9,14). Reduce the calcium dose and monitor serum calcium level and/or parathyroid function (14).
VERAPAMIL (Calan, Isoptin, Verelan): Pretreatment with intravenous calcium gluconate can prevent or reduce hypotensive effects of intravenous verapamil without affecting the antiarrhythmic effects of verapamil (6124).

Drug Influences on Nutrient Levels and Depletion

SOME DRUGS CAN AFFECT CALCIUM LEVELS:
TETRACYCLINES: Tetracyclines can form complexes with dietary or supplemental calcium in the GI tract and reduce absorption of both tetracyclines and calcium. Tetracyclines should be dosed 2 hours before or after calcium-containing foods/products to avoid calcium malabsorption (4412).
LOOP DIURETICS and THIAZIDE DIURETICS: Use of loop diuretics and thiazide diuretics can increase urinary calcium excretion and possibly reduce serum levels. This is more likely with higher doses or when used in combination with diuretics of another class (4412).
ALUMINUM SALTS: Use of aluminum salts can indirectly lead to increased urinary calcium excretion. Avoid prolonged administration of large doses of aluminum-containing products which might lead to hypocalcemia (4400).
MAGNESIUM SALTS: Use of magnesium salts can indirectly lead to increased urinary calcium excretion. Avoid prolonged administration of large doses of magnesium-containing products which might lead to hypocalcemia (4400).
MINERAL OIL: Mineral oil can reduce dietary calcium absorption. Avoid long-term use of mineral oil (4495).
STIMULANT LAXATIVES: Stimulant laxatives can reduce dietary calcium absorption. Limit stimulant laxatives to short-term use (4425). Some stimulant laxatives include cascara (CitraMax Plus), senna (Senokot), bisacody (Dulcolax), and others.
CORTICOSTEROIDS: Use of corticosteroids can cause calcium depletion and osteoporosis with long-term administration. Calcium depletion creates a greater need for both supplemental calcium and vitamin D, which is necessary for calcium absorption. It may be prudent to supplement calcium and vitamin D (Calcitriol) before, during, and after long term and/or high dose corticosteroids (4462,4463,4464,4465,4466,4467).
THYROID HORMONES: In some studies, long-term levothyroxine therapy has been associated with decreased bone density in the hip and spine in pre- and post-menopausal women. This is thought to be due to increased urinary loss of calcium. There is not yet any proof that calcium supplementation is either helpful or necessary (27,28,29).

Interactions with Foods

CAFFEINE: High caffeine intake from foods and beverages increases urinary calcium excretion (2570).
DAIRY FOODS: Foods that are high in phosphorus, mainly dairy products, may reduce calcium absorption by forming insoluble complexes with calcium ions. Separate calcium supplements from dairy products and other high-phosphorus foods by two hours (14).
FIBER: Certain constituents of dietary fiber inhibit calcium absorption. These include phytic acid (found in wheat bran), oxalic acid (found in spinach and rhubarb), and uronic acid (a common plant fiber constituent) (14,945).

Separate administration of calcium supplements from these foods by two hours (14).
SODIUM: High sodium intake from foods increases urinary calcium excretion (1834,2570).
VITAMIN D: Ingestion of food high in vitamin D increases absorption of supplemental calcium (945).

Interactions with Lab Tests

GASTRIN: Calcium carbonate can increase serum gastrin concentrations and test results within 30-75 minutes after calcium carbonate ingestion (275).

GLUCOSE: Calcium gluconate can decrease serum glucose concentrations and test results. This interaction was reported in newborns (275).

11-HYDROXYCORTICOSTEROIDS: Calcium gluconate given intravenously can increase plasma 11-hydroxycorticosteroid concentrations and test results (275).

17-HYDROXYCORTICOSTEROIDS: Calcium gluconate can reduce urinary 17-hydroxycorticosteroid concentrations and test results. One case of this interaction is reported (275).

INSULIN: Calcium gluconate can increase plasma insulin concentrations and test results. This interaction was reported in newborns (275).

I-131 UPTAKE: Calcium gluconate can decrease serum uptake of I-131 (275).

LIPASE: Calcium ions can falsely decrease test results when measuring serum lipase concentrations greater than 5 mmol/L using the method of Teitz (275). Calcium ions do not affect test results when measuring serum lipase concentrations up to 5 mmol/L using the method of Teitz (275).

MAGNESIUM: Calcium gluconate can falsely decrease test results for serum magnesium measured by titan-yellow, but will not affect test results measured by the dihydroxyazobenzene method (275). Calcium gluconate can falsely decrease test results for urine magnesium measured by titan-yellow (275).

BONE MINERAL DENSITY (BMD): Supplemental calcium taken orally can prevent or reduce the rate of bone mineral loss as reflected in BMD measures (977,978,981).

Interactions with Diseases or Conditions

HYPERPARATHYROIDISM: Hyperparathyroid activity predisposes individuals to increased calcium absorption (945).

HYPERPHOSPHATEMIA: Use cautiously in indviduals with high serum phosphate levels. The product of serum phosphate and calcium levels should not exceed 60 to prevent precipitation of calcium phosphate and soft tissue calcification (6479).

HYPOTHYROIDISM: People taking levothyroxine (L-thyroxine, Levothroid, Synthroid) replacement therapy are cautioned to separate administration of levothyroxine and calcium carbonate by four hours for maximum levothyroxine effectiveness (14). Calcium carbonate reduces levothyroxine absorption and effectiveness in hypothyroid patients on levothyroxine replacement therapy (5081,5082,6137).

RENAL INSUFFICIENCY: Calcium carbonate supplementation increases the risk of hypercalcemia and alkalosis (9). Renal insufficiency predisposes individuals to reduced calcium absorption (945).

SARCOIDOSIS: This condition results in increased risk of excessive calcium absorption and hypercalcemia (945).

SMOKING: Cigarette smoking decreases intestinal calcium absorption (1846).

Dosage and Administration

ORAL: The typical adult dose for prevention of hypocalcemia is 1 gram elemental calcium daily (15).
Calcium replacement requirements in people with hypocalcemia can be estimated by clinical condition or serum calcium determinations, but a typical starting dose is 1 to 2 grams daily (15). The symptoms of rickets in children have been reversed with a dose of 1 gram calcium daily (14). The typical dose of calcium carbonate as an antacid is 0.5 to 1.5 grams when needed (14). To control hyperphosphatemia in adults with chronic renal failure, the initial dose of calcium acetate is 1.334 grams (338 mg elemental calcium) with each meal, increasing to 2 to 2.67 grams (500-680 mg elemental calcium) with each meal if necessary (15).

For prevention of osteoporosis in postmenopausal women, doses of 1 to 1.6 grams elemental calcium daily (as the carbonate, citrate, lactate gluconate, or citrate malate) have been used (977,979,981,2569,2571,2574,2575,2576,2578), and should be chosen to bring the total daily calcium intake from diet and supplements up to the relevant dietary reference intake (see below) (981,2569,2571,2575,2578). For prevention of bone loss in premenopausal women over 40 a dose of 1 gram daily has been used (2578). For pregnant women with low dietary calcium intake, the dose for increasing fetal bone density ranges from 300-1300 mg/day beginning at gestation week 20-22 (3263,3264). A dose of 1 to 1.2 grams calcium per day as calcium carbonate has reduced symptoms of premenstrual syndrome (PMS) (1822,1824). For treatment of secondary hyperparathyroidism in people with chronic renal failure, doses of 2 to 21 grams calcium carbonate daily have been used (14). To prevent bone loss associated with chronic corticosteroid therapy, a dose of 1.5 grams elemental calcium daily has been recommended (15). For reducing the risk of recurrence of colorectal adenomas, calcium carbonate 3 to 4 grams (1.2 to 1.6 grams calcium) daily has been used (14). As an adjunct to other treatments for hypertension, 1 to 1.5 grams calcium daily has been used (14). Typical doses used to reduce the risk of pre-eclampsia are 1 to 2 grams elemental calcium daily as calcium carbonate (14). For pregnancy-associated leg cramps, 1 gram calcium twice daily has been used (14). For treating diarrhea and rectal epithelial hyperproliferation due to intestinal bypass, a dose of 2.4 to 3.6 grams daily calcium as calcium carbonate has been used (1826). For hypercholesterolemia, 400 mg calcium (as calcium carbonate) three times daily has been used in conjunction with a low-fat diet (2557). High serum fluoride levels and symptoms of fluorosis in children have been reduced with calcium 125 mg twice daily, in combination with ascorbic acid and vitamin D (14).

Calcium carbonate and calcium citrate are the two most commonly used forms of calcium (945). Calcium carbonate contains 400 mg calcium/gram and calcium citrate contains 211 mg calcium/gram (15) (1000 mg elemental calcium = 2500 mg calcium carbonate = 4700 mg calcium citrate). Calcium carbonate and calcium phosphate should be taken with food (1816,1842). Other calcium salts may be taken without regard to meals and may be preferable in people with achlorhydria or on drugs that reduce gastric acidity (e.g., H2 antagonists, proton pump inhibitors) (1816). Calcium supplements are usually divided into three to four doses daily (9); absorption of calcium from supplements is greatest when taken with food in doses of 500 mg or less since the active transport system for calcium in the small bowel is easily saturated (15,2574,6122).

The daily Dietary Reference Intakes (DRI) for elemental calcium are: Age 1-3 years, 500 mg; 4-8 years, 800 mg; 9-18 years, 1300 mg; 19-50 years, 1000 mg; 51+ years, 1200 mg; Pregnant or Lactating (under 19 years), 1300 mg; Pregnant or Lactating (19-50 years), 1000 mg (998). The daily upper intake level (UL) for calcium is 2.5 grams for everyone over one year of age (3094).

INTRAVENOUS: Calcium injections are prescription products which must be administered slowly (maximum rate of 1.8 mEq/minute (15) and under medical supervision. The usual initial dose for severe hypocalcemia is 7 to 14 mEq elemental calcium (1 mEq = 20 mg elemental calcium) (15). Subsequent doses are given according to the patient's response and serum calcium levels. For hypocalcemic tetany, 4.5 to 16 mEq doses are given until a response occurs (15). Doses of calcium used in cardiopulmonary resuscitation are 0.027-0.054 mEq/kg calcium chloride, 4.5-6.3 mEq calcium gluceptate, or 2.3-3.7 mEq calcium gluconate (15).

Comments

To assure calcium needs are met, nutrition experts recommend consuming calcium throughout the day as a calcium-rich food or up to 500 mg supplemental calcium at each meal (307). Calcium-rich foods include milk and dairy products, kale and broccoli, as well as the calcium-enriched citrus juices, mineral water (6356), canned fish with bones, and tofu processed with calcium.

CALCIUM D-GLUCARATE

Also Known As
Calcium Glucarate, Calcium-D Glucarate, Calcium-D-Glucarate, D-Glucarate (GA).
CAUTION: See separate listing for Calcium.

Scientific Names
D-glucaro-1,4-lactone (1,4 GL).

People Use This For
Orally, calcium D-glucarate is used for preventing breast, prostate, and colon cancer; and for removing carcinogens, toxins, and steroid hormones from the body.

Safety
There is insufficient reliable information available about the safety of calcium D-glucarate.
Pregnancy and Lactation: Insufficient reliable information available; avoid using.

Effectiveness
There is insufficient reliable information available about the effectiveness of calcium D-glucarate.

Mechanism of Action
Glucaric acid is found in human tissues and body fluids. Glucaric acid is also found in foods such as fruits and vegetables including oranges, apples, Brussels sprouts, broccoli, and cabbage (772,3952). Dietary sources provide from 1.12-1.73 mg/100 grams (broccoli and potatoes) to a high of 4.53 mg/100 grams (oranges) (772). Glucaric acid is combined with calcium to form calcium D-glucarate, which is used in supplements. There is a lot of interest in using calcium D-glucarate for preventing estrogen-related cancer such as breast cancer and other hormone-related cancers. Calcium D-glucarate is thought to decrease estrogen levels by affecting estrogen's elimination. Estrogen is normally metabolized hepatically in phase II metabolism by combining with glucuronic acid. It's then excreted in the bile, but a bacterial enzyme in the intestine called beta-glucuronidase normally breaks the estrogen-glucuronide bond. Breaking the bond allows estrogen to be reabsorbed. Calcium D-glucarate works at this step by inhibiting beta-glucuronidase.

Blocking this enzyme is thought to decrease the amount of estrogen that is reabsorbed and lower circulating estrogen levels. There is some evidence that beta-glucuronidase activity might be increased in patients with hormone-dependent cancers like breast and prostate cancer (773,774). Dietary glucarate can inhibit beta-glucuronidase activity and inhibits animal models of mammary tumor development (775). In vitro, D-glucarate decreases tumor cell proliferation (776). Urinary excretion of D-glucaric acid may be an indicator of drug metabolizing enzyme activity in people with impaired renal function (778).

Adverse Reactions
None reported.

Interactions with Herbs & Other Dietary Supplements
Insufficient reliable information available.

Interactions with Drugs
ALCOHOL: Theoretically, concomitant use with alcohol might decrease calcium D-glucarate activity. There is some evidence that urinary excretion of D-glucarate is increased in people consuming alcohol (779).
GLUCURONIDATED DRUGS: Theoretically, calcium D-glucarate might increase the clearance of drugs that undergo glucuronidation, such as lorazepam (Ativan), lamotrigine (Lamictal), entacapone (Comtan), and others (772,3952).
KANAMYCIN: Theoretically, D-glucarate may increase the rate of kanamycin elimination and possibly reduce the risk of drug-induced renal impairment (777).

Interactions with Foods
ALCOHOL: Theoretically, concomitant use with alcohol might decrease calcium D-glucarate activity. There is some evidence that urinary excretion of D-glucarate is increased in people consuming alcohol (779).

Interactions with Lab Tests
No interactions are known to occur, and there is no known reason to expect a clinically significant interaction with calcium D-glucarate.

Interactions with Diseases or Conditions
No interactions are known to occur, and there is no known reason to expect a clinically significant interaction with calcium D-glucarate.

Dosage and Administration
No typical dosage.

Comments
None.

CALENDULA

Also Known As
Garden Marigold, Gold-Bloom, Holligold, Marigold, Marybud, Pot Marigold.

Scientific Names
Calendula officinalis.
Family: Asteraceae/Compositae.

People Use This For
Orally, calendula flower is used as an antispasmodic (3,4), to initiate menstrual periods (4), reduce fever, for treating cancer (6), and inflammation of oral and pharyngeal mucosa (2).
Topically, calendula is used as an anti-inflammatory and for poorly healing wounds and leg ulcers (2).
Traditionally, calendula has been taken orally for gastric and duodenal ulcers and dysmenorrhea. It has been used topically for nosebleeds, varicose veins, hemorrhoids, proctitis, and conjunctivitis (4).

Safety
LIKELY SAFE ...when the flower preparations are used orally and appropriately (4). ...when the flower preparations are used topically and appropriately (4).

PREGNANCY: LIKELY UNSAFE …when used orally; contraindicated because it has spermatocide, antiblastocyst, and abortifacient effects. There is insufficient reliable information available about the safety of the topical use of calendula during pregnancy (4).

LACTATION: Insufficient reliable information available; avoid using.

Effectiveness

There is insufficient reliable information available about the effectiveness of calendula.

Mechanism of Action

The applicable part of calendula is the flower. Some evidence suggests calendula is useful in wound healing. It has an anti-inflammatory effect and it also stimulates tissue granulation (2). The faradiol monoester is believed to play an important role in anti-inflammatory activity. Some evidence suggests the water-soluble flavonoids might be responsible for the wound-healing effects (515). Calendula also shows some evidence of antibacterial, antiviral, and antitumor activity (4).

Adverse Reactions

Calendula can cause an allergic reaction in individuals sensitive to the Asteraceae/Compositae family. Members of this family include ragweed, chrysanthemums, marigolds, daisies, and many other herbs. Despite the widespread use of calendula and the occurrence of allergies to other family members, there has been only one report of anaphylaxis (6).

Interactions with Herbs & Other Dietary Supplements

HERBS WITH SEDATIVE PROPERTIES: Theoretically, concomitant use with herbs that have sedative properties might enhance therapeutic and adverse effects. These include calamus, California poppy, catnip, capsicum, celery, couch grass, elecampane, Siberian ginseng, German chamomile, goldenseal, gotu kola, hops, Jamaican dogwood, kava, lemon balm, sage, St. John's wort, sassafras, scullcap, shepherd's purse, stinging nettle, valerian, wild carrot, wild lettuce, ashwaganda root, and yerba mansa (4,19).

Interactions with Drugs

BARBITURATES: Theoretically, concomitant use of calendula with barbiturates can cause additive therapeutic and adverse effects (19).

OTHER DRUGS WITH SEDATIVE PROPERTIES: Theoretically, concomitant use of calendula with drugs having sedative properties can cause additive therapeutic and adverse effects (19).

Interactions with Foods

No interactions are known to occur, and there is no known reason to expect a clinically significant interaction with calendula.

Interactions with Lab Tests

No interactions are known to occur, and there is no known reason to expect a clinically significant interaction with calendula.

Interactions with Diseases or Conditions

CROSS-ALLERGENICITY: Can cause an allergic reaction in individuals sensitive to the Asteraceae/Compositae family. Members of this family include ragweed, chrysanthemums, marigolds, daisies, and many other herbs.

Dosage and Administration

ORAL: One cup of the tea is commonly taken three times daily, and the tea is prepared by steeping 1-2 grams of the dried flowers in 150 mL boiling water for 5-10 minutes and then straining (2,4). The typical dose of the liquid extract (1:1 in 40% alcohol) is 0.5-1 mL three times daily (4). The tincture (1:5 in 90% alcohol) is usually given as 0.3-1.2 mL three times daily (4).

TOPICAL: The tea is commonly used as a gargle, mouthwash, or poured over an absorbent cloth and applied as a poultice to skin ailments (3). For topical use, 2-4 mL of the tincture is usually diluted into 0.25-0.5 L water. Ointments typically contain 2-5 grams of the herb in 100 grams ointment (2).

Comments

Avoid confusion with ornamental marigolds of the Tagets species, which are commonly grown in vegetable gardens (11).

CALIFORNIA POPPY

Also Known As
California Poppies, Poppy California.
CAUTION: See separate listing for Corn Poppy.

Scientific Names
Eschscholzia californica.
Family: Papaveraceae.

People Use This For
Orally, California poppy is used for insomnia, sedation, aches, nervous agitation, enuresis in children, and diseases of the bladder and liver (18).
In combination with other herbs, California poppy is used orally for depression, neurasthenia, neuropathy, various psychiatric conditions, foehn illness (sleep and mood disturbance associated with strong, warm wind in the Alps), vasomotor dysfunction, sensitivity to weather changes, and sedation (2).

Safety
POSSIBLY UNSAFE ...when used orally and appropriately. Although only the dried aerial parts are used medicinally, the freshly harvested plant contains cyanogenic glycosides that could potentially cause cyanide poisoning (18).
PREGNANCY AND LACTATION: POSSIBLY UNSAFE ...when used orally; avoid using (2).

Effectiveness
There is insufficient reliable information available about the effectiveness of California poppy.

Mechanism of Action
The applicable parts of California poppy are the dried, above ground parts. The active constituents are thought to be isoquinoline alkaloids (2,18). One alkaloid, cryptonine, may have uterine stimulating activity in guinea pigs (2). The tincture is reported to prolong pentobarbital-induced sleep in mice and to prevent chemically-induced spasms in rat jejunum (2).

Adverse Reactions
None reported.

Interactions with Herbs & Other Dietary Supplements
HERBS WITH SEDATIVE PROPERTIES: Theoretically, concomitant use with herbs that have sedative properties might enhance therapeutic and adverse effects. These include calamus, calendula, catnip, capsicum, celery, couch grass, elecampane, Siberian ginseng, German chamomile, goldenseal, gotu kola, hops, Jamaican dogwood, kava, lemon balm, sage, St. John's wort, sassafras, scullcap, shepherd's purse, stinging nettle, valerian, wild carrot, wild lettuce, ashwaganda root, and yerba mansa (4,19).

Interactions with Drugs
MONOAMINE OXIDASE INHIBITORS: California poppy may potentiate MAOI activity (12).
BARBITURATES: Theoretically, concomitant use of California poppy with barbiturates may cause additive effects and side effects (19).
OTHER DRUGS WITH SEDATIVE PROPERTIES: Theoretically, concomitant use of California poppy with drugs with sedative properties may cause additive effects and side effects (19).

Interactions with Foods
ALCOHOL: Theoretically, California poppy may increase the risk of drowsiness and impair motor skills; avoid concomitant use.

Interactions with Lab Tests
No interactions are known to occur, and there is no known reason to expect a clinically significant interaction with California poppy.

Interactions with Diseases or Conditions
No interactions are known to occur, and there is no known reason to expect a clinically significant interaction with California poppy.

Dosage and Administration

ORAL: People typically drink 1 cup tea (made by steeping 2 grams herb in 150 mL boiling water 10-15 minutes, strain) up to four times daily (12). Liquid extract, 1-2 mL per day (18).

Comments

Avoid use of the freshly harvested plant due to presence of cyanogenic glycosides. Avoid confusion with corn poppy (Papaver rhoeas). The California poppy (Eschscholzia californica) is sometimes confused with the opium poppy (Papaver somniferum). Both are members of the Papaveraceae family, but they are members of a different genera. They are distant relatives and the California poppy does not provide opium like the opium poppy.

CALOTROPIS

Also Known As

Mudar Bark, Muder Yercum.

Scientific Names

Calotropis procera.
Family: Asclepiadaceae.

People Use This For

Orally, calotropis is used for toothache, syphilis, digestive disorders, dysentery, and diarrhea (18).
In inhalation therapy, smoke from the bark is inhaled for coughs, asthma, and to induce sweating (18).
In folk medicine, calotropis is used orally for boils, ulcers, swellings, rheumatism epilepsy, hysteria, cramps, cancer, warts, leprosy, elephantiasis, worms, fever, gout, and snake bites (18). Historically, it has been used for fever, joint pain, muscular spasm, and constipation (3822).

Safety

LIKELY UNSAFE ...when used orally, especially in high doses. Calotropis contains cardiac glycosides. High doses can cause vomiting, diarrhea, bradycardia, convulsions, and death (18).
There is insufficient reliable information available about the safety of calotropis for its other uses.
PREGNANCY AND LACTATION: LIKELY UNSAFE ...when used orally; avoid using (18).

Effectiveness

There is insufficient reliable information available about the effectiveness of calotropis.

Mechanism of Action

Calotropis contains cardioactive glycosides (cardenolides) (13,18) that show some antitumor effects on human cells in vitro (18). Calotropis also has expectorant and diuretic properties (18). Animal studies of calotropis extract have shown anti-inflammatory (3823), antibacterial (3824), antipyretic, analgesic, and neuromuscular blocking activity (3822). In one animal study, the extract produced contractions that were blocked by atropine; this supports a use in constipation (3822). In another animal study, an extract of the root showed significant anti-ulcer activity against aspirin, indomethacin, ethanol, indomethacin + ethanol, or stress-induced ulcerations. This anti-ulcer activity may be attributable to the inhibition of 5-lipoxygenase (3825).

Adverse Reactions

Orally, high doses can cause vomiting, diarrhea, bradycardia, convulsions, and death (18).

Interactions with Herbs & Other Dietary Supplements

CARDIAC GLYCOSIDE-CONTAINING HERBS: Concomitant use can increase the risk of cardiac glycoside toxicity. Cardiac glycoside-containing herbs include black hellebore, Canadian hemp roots, digitalis leaf, hedge mustard, figwort, lily of the valley roots, motherwort, oleander leaf, pleurisy root, squill bulb leaf scales, strophanthus seeds, and uzara (2,18,19,500).
CARDIOACTIVE HERBS: Avoid concomitant use with cardioactive herbs due to unpredictability of effects and adverse effects. These include: calamus, cereus, cola, coltsfoot, devil's claw, European mistletoe, fenugreek, fumitory, ginger, ginseng Panax, hawthorn, white horehound, maté, parsley, quassia, scotch broom flower, shepherd's purse, and wild carrot (4).
LICORICE/HORSETAIL: Theoretically, the overuse or misuse of licorice rhizome or horsetail plant increases the risk of toxicity due to potassium depletion (19).
STIMULANT LAXATIVE HERBS: Theoretically, the overuse or misuse of stimulant laxatives increases the risk of cardiac toxicity due to potassium depletion. Stimulant laxative herbs include: aloe dried leaf sap, blue flag rhizome,

alder buckthorn, European buckthorn, butternut bark, cascara bark, castor oil, colocynth fruit pulp, gamboge bark exudate, jalap root, black root, manna bark exudate, podophyllum root, rhubarb root, senna leaves and pods, wild cucumber fruit (Ecballium elaterium), and yellow dock root (19).

Interactions with Drugs
DIGOXIN: Theoretically, concomitant use increases risk of cardiac glycoside toxicity.
POTASSIUM DEPLETING DIURETICS, STIMULANT LAXATIVES: Theoretically, concomitant use may increase risk of cardiac glycoside toxicity due to potassium loss.

Interactions with Foods
No interactions are known to occur, and there is no known reason to expect a clinically significant interaction with calotropis.

Interactions with Lab Tests
No interactions are known to occur, and there is no known reason to expect a clinically significant interaction with calotropis.

Interactions with Diseases or Conditions
No interactions are known to occur, and there is no known reason to expect a clinically significant interaction with calotropis.

Dosage and Administration
ORAL: As an expectorant or diuretic, 200 to 600 mg daily; as an emetic, 2-4 grams daily has been used (18). It is also smoked.
TOPICAL: It is used as a powder (18).

Comments
In India, calotropis has been used as a suicidal and infanticidal poison (215).

CAMPHOR

Also Known As
Camphora, Camphor Tree, Cemphire, Gum Camphor, Laurel Camphor.

Scientific Names
Cinnamomum camphora.
Family: Lauraceae.

People Use This For
Topically, camphor is used to relieve pain. It has been used specifically on warts, cold sores, and hemorrhoids. It has also been applied topically as an analgesic and an antipruritic. It has been used as a counterirritant, and to increase local blood flow (18). Camphor has frequently been used topically to treat respiratory tract diseases involving mucous membrane inflammation. It has sometimes been used topically to treat cardiac symptoms (2). Camphor is also used topically as an eardrop, and for treating minor burns.
In inhalation therapy, camphor is used as an antitussive (272).
Traditionally, camphor has been used orally as an expectorant (272), antiflatulent (16), and for treating respiratory tract diseases.

Safety
LIKELY SAFE ...when used topically in low concentrations short-term. Concentrations ranging from 0.1%-11% seem to be safe for short-term topical use on intact skin (12,272). ...when used by inhalation and appropriately (272).
LIKELY UNSAFE ...when used topically on broken or injured skin. Application of camphor to broken skin can result in systemic absorption and toxicity (272).
UNSAFE ...when used orally. Ingestion of camphor can cause significant toxicity including death (12). Oral preparations of camphor are no longer available in the US (17,159).
CHILDREN: POSSIBLY UNSAFE ...when used topically on young children (2,12). Young children might be might be more susceptible to adverse effects associated with even minor systemic absorption of camphor. UNSAFE ...when used orally. Ingestion of camphor can cause significant toxicity including death (17,159).

PREGNANCY AND LACTATION: UNSAFE …when used orally. Ingestion of camphor can cause serious toxicity including death (2,12,17,159). There is insufficient reliable information available about the safety of camphor when used topically during pregnancy and breast-feeding.

Effectiveness

POSSIBLY EFFECTIVE …when used topically for itching and irritation, cold sores (0.1%-3%), as a counterirritant (3%-11%), for treating minor burns (0.1%-3% or 3%-11% combined with light mineral oil), for hemorrhoids (0.1%-3%), as an antitussive (camphor ointment 4.7%-5.3%) (2,272).
LIKELY INEFFECTIVE …when used topically for treating warts (272).
There is insufficient reliable information available about the effectiveness of camphor for its other uses.

Mechanism of Action

The applicable part of camphor is the wood distillate. Camphor seems to exert its effect as a nasal decongestant because it induces local vasoconstriction (16). Camphor's vasoconstriction effects cause a counterirritant action which often improves local circulation, and therefore provides analgesic and antipruritic effects (16). Camphor also has weak expectorant effects.

Adverse Reactions

Orally, camphor can cause significant toxicity. Symptoms of camphor toxicity occur rapidly and start with nausea and vomiting, oral and intestinal burning, feeling of warmth, and headache. This can progress to confusion, vertigo, excitement, restlessness, delirium, hallucinations, muscular excitability, tremors, jerky movements, epileptiform convulsions, and depression. This is sometimes followed by central nervous system depression and coma. Death can occur from respiratory failure or status epilepticus (17). Other adverse effects that can occur after oral ingestion include tachycardia, mydriasis, visual disturbances, urinary retention, albuminuria, mild transient elevations of aspartate dehydrogenase and lactic dehydrogenase (LDH), and rarely, hepatic failure (17). While adults have recovered after ingesting as much as 42 grams of camphor, as little as 2 grams is usually enough to produce significant toxic effects. Much less is required to cause toxicity in children. In children, ingestion of as little as 700-1000 mg of camphor has been fatal. For example, 20 mL of a 5% camphor product can be lethal in a child (4814). In patients who survive camphor ingestion, recovery from toxicity is usually slow. Although topical application of camphor is not as likely to cause adverse effects, some camphor can be absorbed through intact skin. A considerable amount of camphor can also be absorbed when used by inhalation. Excessive use of camphor either topically or by inhalation can result in the development of symptoms of toxicity (17). Topical use of camphor has also been associated with contact eczema (2,12). There is also a report of increased liver enzymes in an infant who received a camphor-containing topical cold remedy. The liver enzymes normalized after stopping treatment (4608). Camphor products can contain safrole, which has been found to be a mild carcinogen in vitro (12,400); however, carcinogenic effects due to use of safrole containing camphor preparations have not yet been reported in humans (12). Due to the potential risk, camphor products should only be used short-term.

Interactions with Herbs & Other Dietary Supplements

Insufficient reliable information available.

Interactions with Drugs

No interactions are known to occur, and there is no known reason to expect a clinically significant interaction with camphor.

Interactions with Foods

No interactions are known to occur, and there is no known reason to expect a clinically significant interaction with camphor.

Interactions with Lab Tests

LIVER FUNCTION TESTS: Oral use of camphor can cause transient elevations of liver enzymes in both adults and children (17). There is also a report of increased liver enzymes in an infant who received a camphor-containing topical cold remedy. The enzymes affected included aspartate aminotransferase (AST), alanine aminotransferase (ALT), alkaline phosphatase, and lactate dehydrogenase (LDH). The liver enzymes normalized after stopping the topical cold formula (4608).

Interactions with Diseases or Conditions

GI IRRITATION: Might irritate gastrointestinal tract. Contraindicated in individuals with infectious or inflammatory gastrointestinal conditions (19).

Dosage and Administration

TOPICAL: Itching: 0.1%-3% three to four times daily (272). Cold sores: 0.1%-3% topically three to four times daily (272). Counterirritant: 3%-11% three to four times daily (272). Antitussive: (4.7%-5.3% camphor ointment) to throat and chest as a thick layer. Area may be covered with a warm, dry cloth or left uncovered (272). Hemorrhoids: 0.1%-3%. Any of these topical uses should be limited to 3-4 times daily (272).
INHALATION: 1 tablespoon of solution per quart of water is placed directly into a hot steam vaporizer, bowl, or washbasin. Sometimes 1.5 teaspoons of solution are added to a pint of water and boiled. The medicated vapors are breathed. This inhalation may be repeated up to three times a day (272).
ORAL: 30-300 mg per day (2,12).

Comments

Camphor is a well-established folk remedy and is commonly used. This presents problems because camphor can cause toxicity. The American Academy of Pediatrics says non-prescription camphor products should not exceed 11% strength. They also recommend that camphor not be used in treating children (272). Camphorated oil (20% camphor in cottonseed oil) has been removed from the US market due to toxicity (272).

CANADA BALSAM

Also Known As

Balm of Gilead, Balsam, Balsam Canada, Balsam Fir, Balsam Fir Canada, Balsam of Fir, Canada Turpentine, Canadian Balsam, Eastern Fir.
CAUTION: See separate listing for Oregon Fir Balsam.

Scientific Names

Abies balsamea.
Family: Pinaceae.

People Use This For

Topically, Canada balsam is used for hemorrhoids and as an antiseptic (11).
In dentistry, Canada balsam is used in root canal sealers and dentifrices (11).
Historically, Canada balsam has been used for burns, sores, cuts, tumors, heart and chest pains (11), cancer, mucous membrane inflammation, colds, coughs, warts, wounds, urogenital complaints, and as a pain-reliever.
In foods, Canada balsam is an ingredient in foods and beverages (11).
In manufacturing, Canada balsam is used in cosmetics as a fixative and fragrance (11) and in ointments and creams. It is also used as a cement for lenses and prepared microscope slides (11).

Safety

LIKELY SAFE ...when the appropriate parts of the plant are consumed in food; only needles, twigs (and their derivatives) of Canada balsam are approved for food use in the US (11).
POSSIBLY SAFE ...when used topically (11).
There is insufficient reliable information available about the safety of Canada balsam used orally in amounts greater than those found in foods.
PREGNANCY AND LACTATION: Insufficient reliable information available; avoid using.

Effectiveness

There is insufficient reliable information available about the effectiveness of Canada balsam.

Mechanism of Action

Insufficient reliable information available.

Adverse Reactions

None reported.

Interactions with Herbs & Other Dietary Supplements

Insufficient reliable information available.

Interactions with Drugs

No interactions are known to occur, and there is no known reason to expect a clinically significant interaction with Canada balsam.

Interactions with Foods
No interactions are known to occur, and there is no known reason to expect a clinically significant interaction with Canada balsam.

Interactions with Lab Tests
No interactions are known to occur, and there is no known reason to expect a clinically significant interaction with Canada balsam.

Interactions with Diseases or Conditions
No interactions are known to occur, and there is no known reason to expect a clinically significant interaction with Canada balsam.

Dosage and Administration
ORAL: People typically take 2 to 6 tablespoons of weak tea of Canada balsam. As a tincture (1:5 with 50% ethanol), Canada balsam is usually dosed 5 to 20 drops.
TOPICAL: A weak liquid is usually applied to affected areas (5276).

Comments
Avoid confusion with poplar (Populus tacamahacca, P. balsamifera, P. candicans) or spruce (Picea excelsa) also known as balm of Gilead. Oregon fir balsam (Pseudotsuga menziesii) has been detected as an adulterant in Canada balsam (Abies balsamea) (11). Canada balsam is an oleoresin (rather than a true balsam) collected from punctures in the bark of the Canadian balsam tree (Abies balsamea).

CANADIAN FLEABANE

Also Known As
Canadian Trailing Arbutus, Coltstail, Flea Wort, Horsewood, Prideweed.

Scientific Names
Erigeron canadensis.
Family: Compositae.

People Use This For
Orally, Canadian fleabane is used for bronchitis, diarrhea, dysentery, edema, uterine bleeding, and tumors. It is also used orally as an anthelmintic, mild hemostyptic, and to counteract or prevent inflammation and fever. In African folk medicine, Canadian fleabane is used for the treatment of granuloma annulare, sore throats, and urinary tract infections (18).

Safety
There is insufficient reliable information available about the safety of Canadian fleabane.
Pregnancy and Lactation: Insufficient reliable information available; avoid using.

Effectiveness
There is insufficient reliable information available about the effectiveness of Canadian fleabane.

Mechanism of Action
The applicable parts of Canadian fleabane are the above ground parts. There is insufficient reliable information available about the possible mechanism of action and active ingredients.

Adverse Reactions
Orally, Canadian fleabane can cause an allergic reaction in individuals sensitive to the Asteraceae/Compositae family. Members of this family include ragweed, chrysanthemums, marigolds, daisies, and many other herbs.

Interactions with Herbs & Other Dietary Supplements
Insufficient reliable information available.

Interactions with Drugs
No interactions are known to occur, and there is no known reason to expect a clinically significant interaction with Canadian fleabane.

Interactions with Foods

No interactions are known to occur, and there is no known reason to expect a clinically significant interaction with Canadian fleabane.

Interactions with Lab Tests

No interactions are known to occur, and there is no known reason to expect a clinically significant interaction with Canadian fleabane.

Interactions with Diseases or Conditions

CROSS-ALLERGENICITY: Canadain fleabane can cause an allergic reaction in individuals sensitive to the Asteraceae/Compositae family. Members of this family include ragweed, chrysanthemums, marigolds, daisies, and many other herbs.

Dosage and Administration

No typical dosage.

Comments

There is very little scientific information about this product. Our staff is continually analyzing the available information on natural medicines and will add data here as it becomes available.

CANADIAN HEMP

Also Known As

Bitterroot, Catchfly, Dogbane, Fly-Trap, Honeybloom, Indian Physic, Indian-Hemp, Milk Ipecac, Milkweed, Wallflower, Wild Cotton.
CAUTION: See separate listing for Indian Physic.

Scientific Names

Apocynum cannabinum.
Family: Apocynaceae.

People Use This For

Orally, Canadian hemp is used for arthritis, asthma, coughs, edema, and syphilis.
It is also used orally for valvular insufficiency, senile heart, and to strengthen weak heart muscles following pneumonia. Canadian hemp is also used orally as a diuretic (18).
Topically, the fresh juice of Canadian hemp is used for warts.

Safety

LIKELY UNSAFE …when used orally. Contains digitalis-like cardiac glycosides that can cause toxicity (18). There is insufficient reliable information available about the safety of Canadian hemp for its other uses.
PREGNANCY AND LACTATION: LIKELY UNSAFE …when used orally due to toxic potential of digitalis-like cardiac glycosides (18); avoid using.

Effectiveness

There is insufficient reliable information available about the effectiveness of Canadian hemp.

Mechanism of Action

The applicable part of Canadian hemp is the root. Canadian hemp contains cardenolide or digitalis-type glycosides, including cymine. These may cause bradycardia with low blood pressure, increased heart contractions, and reflex hypertension. It also may increase diuresis. It is more irritating to the intestinal mucosa than digitalis and strophanthus preparations. It has a lower therapeutic effect on atrial fibrillation than digitalis (18).

Adverse Reactions

Canadian hemp causes topical irritation of the gastrointestinal mucous membranes. This can cause nausea and vomiting more commonly than in other cardenolide glycoside containing plants (such as digitalis). It can also cause bradycardia with low blood pressure, increased heart contractions, and reflex hypertension (18).

Interactions with Herbs & Other Dietary Supplements

CARDIAC GLYCOSIDE-CONTAINING HERBS: Canadian hemp is contraindicated with these herbs, and concomitant use can increase the risk of cardiac glycoside toxicity. Cardiac glycoside containing herbs include black hellebore, digitalis leaf, hedge mustard, figwort, lily of the valley roots, motherwort, oleander leaf, pheasant's eye plant, pleurisy root, squill bulb leaf scales, strophanthus seeds, and uzara (2,18,19,500).

Interactions with Drugs
CARDIAC GLYCOSIDES: Concomitant use of Canadian hemp with digoxin (Lanoxin) or digitoxin (Crystodigin) might increase effects and adverse effects.

Interactions with Foods
No interactions are known to occur, and there is no known reason to expect a clinically significant interaction with Canadian hemp.

Interactions with Lab Tests
No interactions are known to occur, and there is no known reason to expect a clinically significant interaction with Canadian hemp.

Interactions with Diseases or Conditions
No interactions are known to occur, and there is no known reason to expect a clinically significant interaction with Canadian hemp.

Dosage and Administration
ORAL: Some people take 10 to 30 drops of the liquid extract three times daily or 0.3 to 0.6 mL of the tincture (1:10) (18).
TOPICAL: No typical dosage.

Comments
The tough, fibrous barks of both Canadian hemp and Indian hemp have been used as a substitute for hemp; hence, both are known as hemp (18).

CANAIGRE

Also Known As
Red American Ginseng, Wild Red American Ginseng, Wild Red Desert Ginseng.
CAUTION: See separate listings for Ashwaganda, Blue Cohosh, Codonopsis, Ginseng American, Ginseng Panax, and Ginseng Siberian.

Scientific Names
Rumex hymenosepalus.
Family: Polygonaceae.

People Use This For
Orally, canaigre, an inexpensive alternative to ginseng (6), is used for improving physical and athletic stamina, cognitive function and concentration, and work efficiency or athletic stamina; and as a general tonic to improve well-being. It is also used orally for soothing irritated or inflamed tissues, as a diuretic, and an antidepressant. Historically, canaigre has been used as an astringent (5) and for conditions ranging from lack of vitality to leprosy (515). In manufacturing, it is used for tanning leather and dying wool (5).

Safety
LIKELY SAFE ...when used orally (12). The petioles, or stems, are edible like rhubarb (6). Avoid excessive amounts. There is some speculation that high tannin contents (such as in canaigre) could be carcinogenic (5,6).
PREGNANCY AND LACTATION: Insufficient reliable information available; avoid using.

Effectiveness
There is insufficient reliable information available about the effectiveness of canaigre.

Mechanism of Action
The applicable part of canaigre is the root. High tannin content (25%) has astringent effect when applied topically. Leucoanthocyanin fraction may have antitumor activity (6).

Adverse Reactions
None reported.

Interactions with Herbs & Other Dietary Supplements
Insufficient reliable information available.

Interactions with Drugs
No interactions are known to occur, and there is no known reason to expect a clinically significant interaction with canaigre.

Interactions with Foods
No interactions are known to occur, and there is no known reason to expect a clinically significant interaction with canaigre.

Interactions with Lab Tests
No interactions are known to occur, and there is no known reason to expect a clinically significant interaction with canaigre.

Interactions with Diseases or Conditions
No interactions are known to occur, and there is no known reason to expect a clinically significant interaction with canaigre.

Dosage and Administration
No typical dosage.

Comments
Avoid confusion with Panax ginseng, Siberian ginseng, and red ginseng. Canaigre root is unrelated to ginseng. A 1976 Herb Trade Association policy states that "any herb products consisting of whole or part of Rumex hymenosepalus should not be labeled as containing 'ginseng' " (5).

CANANGA OIL

Also Known As
None.
CAUTION: See separate listing for Ylang Ylang Oil.

Scientific Names
Cangana odorata macrophylla, synonym Canagnium odoratum macrophylla.
Family: Annonaceae.

People Use This For
In foods, cananga oil is used as a flavoring agent in gelatins, puddings, and beverages.
In manufacturing, cananga oil is used to make fragrances in cosmetics and soaps.

Safety
LIKELY SAFE ...when used orally in amounts typically found in foods. It has Generally Recognized as Safe (GRAS) status in the US (11). The maximum use level is 0.003% (11).
POSSIBLY SAFE ...when used topically. The maximum level allowed is 0.8% in perfumes (11).
PREGNANCY AND LACTATION: LIKELY SAFE ...when used orally in amounts typically found in foods (11). There is insufficient reliable information available about the safety of using greater amounts during pregnancy and breast-feeding; avoid using.

Effectiveness
There is insufficient reliable information available about the effectiveness of cananga oil.

Mechanism of Action
Insufficient reliable information available.

Adverse Reactions
Cananga oil can cause allergic skin reactions in sensitive people (5244).

Interactions with Herbs & Other Dietary Supplements
Insufficient reliable information available.

Interactions with Drugs

No interactions are known to occur, and there is no known reason to expect a clinically significant interaction with cananga oil.

Interactions with Foods

No interactions are known to occur, and there is no known reason to expect a clinically significant interaction with cananga oil.

Interactions with Lab Tests

No interactions are known to occur, and there is no known reason to expect a clinically significant interaction with cananga oil.

Interactions with Diseases or Conditions

No interactions are known to occur, and there is no known reason to expect a clinically significant interaction with cananga oil.

Dosage and Administration

No typical dosage.

Comments

Cananga oil is used predominately as a food and cosmetic ingredient. Avoid confusion with ylang ylang oil (oil from Canangium odorata genuina).

CANELLA

Also Known As

White Cinnamon, White Wood, Wild Cinnamon.

Scientific Names

Canella alba.

People Use This For

For food uses, canella is used as a cooking spice (18).
There are no known medicinal uses.

Safety

There is insufficient reliable information available about the safety of canella.
Pregnancy and Lactation: Insufficient reliable information available; avoid using.

Effectiveness

There is insufficient reliable information available about the effectiveness of canella.

Mechanism of Action

The applicable part of canella is the bark. Canella bark is stated to have stimulant, tonic, and antimicrobial properties (18).

Adverse Reactions

None reported.

Interactions with Herbs & Other Dietary Supplements

Insufficient reliable information available.

Interactions with Drugs

No interactions are known to occur, and there is no known reason to expect a clinically significant interaction with canella.

Interactions with Foods

No interactions are known to occur, and there is no known reason to expect a clinically significant interaction with canella.

Interactions with Lab Tests

No interactions are known to occur, and there is no known reason to expect a clinically significant interaction with canella.

Interactions with Diseases or Conditions

No interactions are known to occur, and there is no known reason to expect a clinically significant interaction with canella.

Dosage and Administration

ORAL: People typically use 10 to 40 grains which is 650 to 2600 mg (5267).

Comments

There is very little scientific information about this product. Our staff is continually analyzing the available information on natural medicines and will add data here as it becomes available.

CANTHAXANTHIN

Also Known As

Canthaxanthine, Carophyll Red, CI Food Orange 8, Colour Index No. 40850, E161, Roxanthin Red 10. CAUTION: See separate listing for Beta-carotene.

Scientific Names

4,4-diketo-beta-carotene; Beta,beta-carotene-4,4-dione;Canthaxanthin.

People Use This For

Orally, canthaxanthin is used to reduce photosensitivity associated with erythropoietic protoporphyria (EPP) (14,5644,5645); and light-sensitive skin diseases including polymorphous light eruptions, drug-induced photosensitivity and solar urticaria (14). It is also used orally to color the skin and produce an artificial suntan (9,14).
In foods, canthaxanthin is used as a food coloring additive (9,14,5630) and added to animal feed to enhance the color of chicken skins, egg yolks (14), salmon, and trout (9).
In manufacturing, canthaxanthin has been used in cosmetics (9) and as a tablet excipient (14).

Safety

LIKELY SAFE ...when consumed in amounts commonly found in foods (14). Canthaxanthin is approved for use in human food. It has Generally Recognized as Safe (GRAS) status in the US (5637) but is not to exceed 30 mg per pint of liquid food or per pound of solid or semisolid food (5630).
POSSIBLY UNSAFE ...when used orally in doses to treat and reduce photosensitivities. Development of retinal changes has been reported in patients with erythropoietic protoporphyria (EPP) being treated with canthaxanthin to prevent photosensitization, including deposition of crystals around the macula of the retina (5644), slowing of dark-adaptation curves, and decreased amplitudes in electroretinograms (5632,5638,5645). Deposition of retinal crystals appears dose related (5638). Evidence suggests individuals taking a cumulative dose of 37 grams will have retinal changes 50% of the time, while those taking a total cumulative dose of 60 grams of canthaxanthin will demonstrate definite retinal changes upon examination (5636,5641).
LIKELY UNSAFE ...when used orally in large amounts to color and produce an artificial tan (5628,5629). Retinal changes have been reported in individuals ingesting large amounts of canthaxanthin chronically for tanning purposes (9,14,5636,5639,5641). Altered eye function, decreased visual acuity (5639), and aplastic anemia (5635) have also been reported.
PREGNANCY AND LACTATION: LIKELY SAFE ...when consumed in amounts found in foods (5630). POSSIBLY UNSAFE ...when consumed in doses to treat and reduce photosensitivities due to reported retinal changes with use (9,5632); avoid using. LIKELY UNSAFE ...when used orally in large amounts for artificial tanning purposes due to reported retinal changes with use (9,14); avoid using.

Effectiveness

LIKELY EFFECTIVE ...when used orally for reducing photosensitivity in erythropoietic protoporphyria (EPP) (rash, itching, or eczema) due to sunlight exposure (5644,5645).
There is insufficient reliable information available about the effectiveness of canthaxanthin for its other uses.

Mechanism of Action

Canthaxanthin is a carotenoid that is found naturally and produced synthetically (5637). It is not a precursor of vitamin A, has no vitamin A activity (9), is highly lipid soluble (5635), and accumulates in fatty tissue (5632). Oral canthaxanthin is thought to color the skin by accumulating in the epidermis and subcutaneous fat tissue (5635). Evidence suggests canthaxanthin and other carotenoids protect against photosensitization due to their antioxidant activity against reactive oxygen species by deactivating electronically excited molecules or acting as chain-breaking agents (5645,5649). In vitro and in vivo animal studies suggest canthaxanthin may inhibit the growth and transformation of tumor cells (5642,5647,5648) by inducing the gap junctional communication between cells (5649). Animal studies have not shown any toxic, carcinogenic, or mutagenic effects with canthaxanthin (14). Human studies are needed to determine whether canthaxanthin has a role in cancer prevention.

Adverse Reactions

Orally, large amounts of canthaxanthin can cause orange-brown coloration of the skin (5632), brick-red coloration of stools (5631), orange discoloration of plasma (5632), discolored body secretions (5634), diarrhea, nausea, stomach cramps (14), dry and itchy skin (5634), urticaria (5637), welts (9), gold and yellow crystalline deposits around the macula of the retina (5632,5635,5636,5638,5639,5640,5641), and hepatitis (14,5635). Decreased visual acuity (5639), diminished retinal sensitivity (5641), and aplastic anemia (5635) have been associated with large doses of canthaxanthin ingestion. A fatal case of aplastic anemia (5635) associated with the ingestion of canthaxanthin for tanning purposes has been reported. The patient refused treatment with human blood products due to religious beliefs and died (5635).

Interactions with Herbs & Other Dietary Supplements

Insufficient reliable information available.

Interactions with Drugs

No interactions are known to occur, and there is no known reason to expect a clinically significant interaction with canthaxanthin.

Interactions with Foods

No interactions are known to occur, and there is no known reason to expect a clinically significant interaction with canthaxanthin.

Interactions with Lab Tests

Canthaxanthin can interfere with carotene and vitamin A laboratory assays (14,5634).

Interactions with Diseases or Conditions

HYPERSENSITIVITY TO VITAMIN A AND CAROTENOIDS: Individuals with known hypersensitivities to vitamin A and carotenoids might also be hypersensitive to canthaxanthin (14).

Dosage and Administration

ORAL: The typical dose for reducing and treating photosensitivities associated with erythropoietic protoporphyria (EPP) is 60 to 90 mg daily on average for three to five months per year (5640). The typical dose for artificial tanning is 120 mg per day for several days (14,5633).

Comments

Orobronze (canthaxanthin) is sold in Canada as a nonprescription drug for artificial tanning purposes as 30 mg oral capsules (5631,5633). Oral tanning preparations containing canthaxanthin have been found to be readily available to consumers in the United States through mail order and tanning salons despite the FDA warning (5635,5638). A combination product containing beta-carotene and canthaxanthin (Phenoro: 10 mg beta-carotene and 15 mg canthaxanthin) is used in Europe for treatment of photosensitivities associated with EPP (5637). Other combination products containing beta-carotene and canthaxanthin are manufactured (Carotinoid-N, Apotrin), but are not available in the US (5628,5645).

CAPERS

Also Known As
Cappero.

Scientific Names
Capparis spinosa.
Family: Capparidaceae.

People Use This For

Topically, capers are used for skin disorders, improving the function of enlarged capillaries, and dry skin (6).
Capers are consumed as food, and used as a flavoring (6).

Safety

LIKELY SAFE ...when used orally. The pickled flower buds are commonly used without reports of adverse effects. There is insufficient reliable information available about the safety of the topical use of capers. Compresses soaked in fluid containing capers can cause contact dermatitis (6).
PREGNANCY AND LACTATION: LIKELY SAFE ...when used orally in amounts typically found in foods; avoid large amounts. There is insufficient reliable information available about the safety of the topical use of capers during pregnancy and lactation.

Effectiveness

There is insufficient reliable information available about the effectiveness of capers.

Mechanism of Action

The applicable part of capers is the unopened flower bud. Some evidence suggests that unknown constituents of caper extract may improve dry skin and functioning of enlarged capillaries (6).

Adverse Reactions

Topically, capers can cause contact dermatitis (6).

Interactions with Herbs & Other Dietary Supplements

Insufficient reliable information available.

Interactions with Drugs

No interactions are known to occur, and there is no known reason to expect a clinically significant interaction with capers.

Interactions with Foods

No interactions are known to occur, and there is no known reason to expect a clinically significant interaction with capers.

Interactions with Lab Tests

No interactions are known to occur, and there is no known reason to expect a clinically significant interaction with capers.

Interactions with Diseases or Conditions

PEOPLE WITH SENSITIVE SKIN: Capers may cause skin irritation (6); avoid topical use.

Dosage and Administration

No typical dosage.

Comments

CAUTION: Leaves of related species (Capparis fasicularis, Capparis tumentosa) are reported to be poisonous (6).

CAPSICUM

Also Known As

African Chillies, African Pepper, Bird Pepper, Capsaicin, Capsicum Fruit, Cayenne, Chili Pepper, Garden Pepper, Goat's Pod, Grains Of Paradise, Green Bell Pepper, Green Chili Pepper, Hot Pepper, Hungarian Pepper, Ici Fructus, Louisiana Long Pepper, Louisiana Sport Pepper, Mexican Chilies, Paprika, Pimento, Red Pepper, Sweet Pepper, Tabasco Pepper, Zanzibar Pepper.
CAUTION: See separate listing for Grains of Paradise.

Scientific Names

Capsicum frutescens; Capsicum annuum; Capsicum chinense; Capsicum baccatum; Capsicum pubscens; and other Capsicum species.
Family: Solanaceae.

People Use This For

Orally, capsicum is used to stimulate digestion (5), as an antiflatulent, for colic (4), diarrhea, cramps (11), toothache (11), to improve peripheral circulation (4), for reducing blood clotting tendencies (5), seasickness (18), alcoholism (18), malarial fever, yellow and other fevers (18), for reducing cholesterol (5), and preventing arteriosclerosis and heart disease (18). Topically, capsicum is used for the pain of shingles, and for post-herpetic, trigeminal, diabetic, post-mastectomy, and post-surgical neuralgias, HIV-associated peripheral neuropathy (6,3891), and fibromyalgia (6489). It is also used as a counterirritant to desensitize nerves and to create a feeling of warmth (7,11). Capsicum is also used to relieve muscle spasms (2), as a gargle for laryngitis (4), and as a deterrent to thumb-sucking or nail biting (11).

Capsicum has also been used as an inhalational provocation test to distinguish sensory hyperreactivity of the airways from asthma (5885).

In food, capsicum is used as a condiment (3).

In manufacturing, capsicum is the main ingredient used in many self-defense sprays, also referred to as pepper spray (6,1394).

Safety

LIKELY SAFE ...when used orally in amounts typically found in food. Capsicum has Generally Recognized as Safe (GRAS) status in the US. ...when used topically and appropriately. The active capsicum constituent capsaicin used in topical preparations is a FDA-approved over-the-counter product (272).

POSSIBLY SAFE ...when used orally and appropriately, short-term in medicinal amounts (4,12).

POSSIBLY UNSAFE ...when used orally, long-term or in high doses. Long-term use or use of excessive doses can sometimes cause hepatic or renal damage (4,12).

CHILDREN: POSSIBLY UNSAFE ...when used topically in children under 2 years old (272,506). There is insufficient reliable information available about the safety of oral use in children.

PREGNANCY: LIKELY SAFE ...when used orally in the amounts typically found in foods (4). ...when used topically and appropriately (272). There is insufficient reliable information available about the safety of capsicum during pregnancy when used orally in medicinal amounts.

LACTATION: LIKELY SAFE ...when used topically and appropriately (272). POSSIBLY UNSAFE ...when used orally. Dermatitis can sometimes occur in breast-fed infants when mothers ingest foods heavily spiced with capsicum peppers (739).

Effectiveness

EFFECTIVE ...when used topically for temporary relief of pain from rheumatoid arthritis, osteoarthritis, and neuralgias including shingles and diabetic neuropathy. The active capsicum constituent capsaicin used in topical preparations is FDA-approved for these uses (272,506).

POSSIBLY EFFECTIVE ...when used topically for fibromyalgia. There is some evidence that applying cream containing 0.025% of the active capsicum constituent capsaicin 4 times daily to tender points for 4 weeks can reduce tenderness in patients with fibromyalgia (7038).

POSSIBLY INEFFECTIVE ...when used topically for HIV-associated peripheral neuropathy (3891).

There is insufficient reliable information available about the effectiveness of capsicum for its other uses.

Mechanism of Action

The applicable part of capsicum is the fruit (4). Capsicum contains capsaicinoid constituents which stimulate digestion and therefore are said to aid in digestion (4). When used topically, the capsaicin constituent causes the release of substance P in the nerves. This initially causes pain, but after repeated applications, substance P is depleted. This reduces the ability of the nerves to transmit sensations and reduces pain (506). Capsaicin also stimulates the unmyelinated slow C-fibers of the sensory nervous system, which can induce cough, dyspnea, nasal congestion, and eye irritation after inhalation (5885). Some evidence shows the crude juice of fresh capsicum has antibacterial properties (11).

Adverse Reactions

Orally, capsicum can cause gastrointestinal (GI) irritation (4). Sweating and flushing of the head and neck, lacrimation, and rhinorrhea have also been reported (7005). Excessive amounts of capsicum can lead to gastroenteritis and hepatic or renal damage (4). There are also reports of dermatitis in breast-fed infants whose mothers' food is heavily spiced with capsicum (739). Capsicum can also decrease blood coagulation (7006).

Topically, capsicum can cause burning (6) and urticaria (2). Skin contact with fresh capsicum fruit can cause irritation or contact dermatitis (19). Inhalation of capsicum can cause cough, dyspnea, nasal congestion, eye irritation, and allergic alveolitis (4,5885). Capsicum can be extremely irritating to the eyes and mucous membranes.

Interactions with Herbs & Other Dietary Supplements

COCA: Theoretically, concomitant use of capsicum (including exposure to the capsicum in pepper spray) and coca might increase the effects and risk of adverse effects of the cocaine in coca (1394).

HERBS WITH SEDATIVE PROPERTIES: Theoretically, concomitant use with herbs that have sedative properties might enhance therapeutic and adverse effects. These include calamus, calendula, California poppy, catnip, celery, couch grass, elecampane, Siberian ginseng, German chamomile, goldenseal, gotu kola, hops, Jamaican dogwood, kava, lemon balm, sage, St. John's wort, sassafras, scullcap, shepherd's purse, stinging nettle, valerian, wild carrot, wild lettuce, ashwaganda root, and yerba mansa (4,19).

HERBS WITH ANTICOAGULANT/ANTIPLATELET POTENTIAL: Concomitant use of herbs that have coumarin constituents or affect platelet aggregation could theoretically increase the risk of bleeding in some people. These herbs include: angelica, anise, arnica, asafoetida, bogbean, boldo, celery, chamomile, clove, danshen, fenugreek, feverfew, garlic, ginger, ginkgo, Panax ginseng, horse chestnut, horseradish, licorice, meadowsweet, prickly ash, onion, papain, passionflower, poplar, quassia, red clover, turmeric, wild carrot, wild lettuce, willow, and others (4,19).

Interactions with Drugs

ACE INHIBITORS (ACEIs): Topically applied capsicum might contribute to the cough reflex in patients using ace inhibitors (7002).

ACID-INHIBITING DRUGS: Theoretically, capsicum might interfere with antacids, sucralfate (Carafate, Sulcrate in Canada), H-2 antagonists, or proton-pump inhibitors, due to claims that capsicum increases stomach acid (19).

ANTIHYPERTENSIVE DRUGS: Theoretically, capsicum might interfere with the activity of antihypertensive drugs by increasing catecholamine secretion (4).

ANTIPLATELET DRUGS: Theoretically, capsicum might increase the effects and adverse effects of antiplatelet drugs (19).

ASPIRIN: Chili powder, taken thirty minutes before aspirin, might reduce gastric mucosal damage (19).

BARBITURATES: Theoretically, concomitant use of capsicum with barbiturates might enhance sedative effects and the risk of adverse effects (19).

COCAINE: Theoretically, concomitant use of capsicum (including exposure to the capsicum in pepper spray) and cocaine might increase cocaine effects and the risk of adverse effects, including death (1394).

DRUGS WITH SEDATIVE PROPERTIES: Theoretically, concomitant use of capsicum and drugs with sedative activity might enhance sedative effects and the risk of adverse effects (19).

HEPATICALLY METABOLIZED DRUGS: Theoretically, capsicum might increase hepatic metabolism of drugs by increasing glucose-6-phosphate dehydrogenase and adipose lipase activity (4).

MONOAMINE OXIDASE INHIBITORS (MAOIs): Theoretically, capsicum might interfere with the activity of MAOIs by increasing catecholamine secretion (4).

THEOPHYLLINE (Theo-Dur): Theoretically, oral administration of capsicum before or at the same time as theophylline might enhance theophylline absorption (19).

Interactions with Foods

No interactions are known to occur, and there is no known reason to expect a clinically significant interaction with capsicum.

Interactions with Lab Tests

Capsicum has led to increased fibrinolytic activity and may lead to prolonged times in coagulation studies (7006).

Interactions with Diseases or Conditions

GI IRRITATION: Oral capsicum causes GI irritation but does not interfere with ulcer healing (4). Contraindicated in individuals with infectious or inflammatory gastrointestinal conditions (19).

DAMAGED SKIN: Capsicum is contraindicated in situations involving injured skin. Do not apply capsicum if the skin is open.

PEPPER ALLERGY: Avoid the use of capsicum (2). Contraindicated in individuals with infectious or inflammatory gastrointestinal conditions (19).

Dosage and Administration

ORAL: The capsicum fruit is usually used in doses of 30-120 mg three times daily (4). The tincture is usually given in doses of 0.0.6-2 mL (4). Capsicum is also sometimes administered as an oleoresin in doses of 0.6-2 mg (4).

TOPICAL: For pain syndromes, including rheumatoid and osteo-arthritis, neuropathy, and fibromyalgia, creams contain the active capsicum constituent capsaicin are typically applied 3-4 times daily. It can take up to 3 days for the full analgesic effect (4). Most creams contain 0.025% to 0.075% capsaicin concentrations. However, sometimes higher potency preparations are used for diabetic neuropathy. Tell patients to make sure they wash their hands after applying capsaicin cream (506). Tell patients they can use a diluted vinegar solution to remove capsicum cream. The active constituent, capsaicin is not water washable (5). Warn against using capsicum preparations near the eyes or on sensitive skin (5).

Comments

In nature, capsaicin occurs only as a trans stereoisomer. However, civamide, the cis isomer also has activity. Products labeled capsaicin sometimes include nonivamide which is an adulterant or pelargonic acid vanillylamide, referred to as "synthetic capsaicin" (7007). Capsaicin is being studied for use in treating urinary urgency as an intravesical injection (214). Capsicum powder has been reported to prevent radiation-induced damage to bacterial DNA and thereby protect certain bacteria (Escherichia coli, Bacillus megaterium, and Bacillus pumilus spores) from gamma irradiation used to preserve some foods (5886).

CARAMEL COLOR

Also Known As
Caramel.

Scientific Names
None.

People Use This For
In manufacturing, caramel color is used as a food color in medications, cosmetics and foods.
It does not have any known medicinal uses (11).

Safety
LIKELY SAFE ...when used in amounts found in foods and medications. It has Generally Recognized as Safe (GRAS) status in the US, and is official in both the FCC and the National Formulary (10,11). The highest average maximum level is 5.4% (11).
PREGNANCY AND LACTATION: POSSIBLY SAFE ...when used orally in food amounts. There is insufficient reliable information available for the safety of caramel color used in larger amounts during pregnancy and lactation.

Effectiveness
There is insufficient reliable information available about the effectiveness of caramel color.

Mechanism of Action
Caramel color is burnt sugar coloring and caramel. This is the color obtained by heating sugar with ammonia or ammonium salts under controlled temperature and pressure until the taste is eliminated and the desired color is achieved (11).

Adverse Reactions
Orally, some evidence from short-term and long-term studies suggest that large amounts of caramel might suppress immunity (11).

Interactions with Herbs & Other Dietary Supplements
Insufficient reliable information available.

Interactions with Drugs
No interactions are known to occur, and there is no known reason to expect a clinically significant interaction with caramel color.

Interactions with Foods
No interactions are known to occur, and there is no known reason to expect a clinically significant interaction with caramel color.

Interactions with Lab Tests
No interactions are known to occur, and there is no known reason to expect a clinically significant interaction with caramel color.

Interactions with Diseases or Conditions
No interactions are known to occur, and there is no known reason to expect a clinically significant interaction with caramel color.

Dosage and Administration
No typical dosage.

Comments
None.

CARAWAY dried fruit, seed

Also Known As
Anis des Vosges, Carvi Fructus, Cumin des Pres, Kummel, Kummich, Semen Cumini Pratensis, Semences de Carvi, Wiesen-Feldkummel.
CAUTION: See separate listing for Caraway Oil.

Scientific Names
Carum carvi, synonym Apium carvi.
Family: Apiaceae/Umbelliferae.

People Use This For
Orally, the dried fruit and seed of caraway is used for dyspepsia, distention, flatulence (2,8), and mild spastic conditions of the gastrointestinal tract (2). It is also used orally as an antibacterial (8), laxative, and digestive aid (11).
Traditionally, caraway has been used as an expectorant, to promote lactation, to relieve menstrual discomforts, for incontinence, and as a mouthwash (8,11).
In foods, caraway is used as a cooking spice (11).

Safety
LIKELY SAFE ...when consumed in amounts commonly found in foods. Caraway has Generally Recognized as Safe (GRAS) status in the US and is approved for food use with a maximum use level of 0.02% (11). ...when used orally for medicinal purposes in appropriate amounts (12).
There is insufficient reliable information available about the safety of caraway in large amounts.
PREGNANCY AND LACTATION: LIKELY SAFE ...when used orally in the amounts commonly found in food.

Effectiveness
POSSIBLY EFFECTIVE ...when used orally as an antiflatulent and for dyspeptic problems, such as mild, spastic conditions of the gastrointestinal tract, and fullness (2). ...when used orally for increasing gastric secretion and stimulating appetite (8).
There is insufficient reliable information available about the effectiveness of caraway for its other uses.

Mechanism of Action
Caraway produces a warm sensation and promotes postprandial gas elimination (7). The caraway fruits contain 2-7% volatile oil, consisting mainly of carvone and limonene (7). Carvone induces glutathione S-transferase (GST) in mouse tissues, which can inhibit carcinogenesis (11). There is some evidence that caraway oil has antispasmodic effects, but they are probably weak. There may also be some antihistaminic activity. It is possible that the antispasmodic effects are slightly more pronounced with the alcoholic extract, and less pronounced with the essential oil (7,11).

Adverse Reactions
Topically, caraway can cause contact dermatitis (19).

Interactions with Herbs & Other Dietary Supplements
Insufficient reliable information available.

Interactions with Drugs
No interactions are known to occur, and there is no known reason to expect a clinically significant interaction with caraway dried fruit and seed.

Interactions with Foods
No interactions are known to occur, and there is no known reason to expect a clinically significant interaction with caraway dried fruit and seed.

Interactions with Lab Tests

No interactions are known to occur, and there is no known reason to expect a clinically significant interaction with caraway dried fruit and seed.

Interactions with Diseases or Conditions

No interactions are known to occur, and there is no known reason to expect a clinically significant interaction with caraway dried fruit and seed.

Dosage and Administration

ORAL: The typical dose of caraway is 1.5-6 grams of the dried fruit per day or one cup of the freshly prepared tea two to four times daily between meals (8). The tea is prepared by steeping 1-2 teaspoons of the freshly crushed fruit in 150 mL boiling water for 5-10 minutes and then straining. The dose for infants and small children is usually one teaspoonful of the tea, and if necessary, given in a bottle (8).

Comments

Superstitions held that caraway had the power to prevent the theft of any object that contained the seed and to keep lovers from losing interest with one another (6002). Avoid confusion with caraway oil (distilled oil of caraway fruit/seed).

CARAWAY OIL

Also Known As

Roman Cumin, Wild Cumin.
CAUTION: See separate listing for Caraway dried fruit, seed.

Scientific Names

Carum carvi, synonym Apium carvi.
Family: Apiaceae or Umbelliferae.

People Use This For

Orally, caraway oil is used for digestive problems including mild gastrointestinal (GI) spasms, flatulence, fullness, and dyspepsia (2,6740,6741).

Traditionally, caraway oil has also been used to stimulate menstruation and relieve menstrual cramps, and to increase milk flow in nursing mothers (6747,6748). It has also been used as a component of mouthwashes (6) and topically in skin frictions to improve local blood flow (6).

In manufacturing, caraway oil is used as a flavoring agent in pharmaceutical compounding (11). It is a fragrance commonly utilized in the manufacturing of toothpaste, soap, and cosmetics (11).

Safety

LIKELY SAFE ...when used orally in amounts found in food (2). Caraway oil has Generally Regarded as Safe (GRAS) status in the US (6747).

POSSIBLY SAFE ...when used orally in medicinal amounts (2,6740,6741,6742).

PREGNANCY: LIKELY SAFE ...when used orally in amounts found in food (6747). POSSIBLY UNSAFE ...when used in medicinal amounts. (6746,6747). Caraway has been used to stimulate menstruation (6746,6748); avoid using.

LACTATION: LIKELY SAFE ...when used orally in amounts found in food.

There is insufficient reliable information available about the safety of caraway oil when used in medicinal amounts in breast-feeding women.

Effectiveness

POSSIBLY EFFECTIVE ...when used orally for digestive problems, including mild gastrointestinal (GI) spasms, and fullness (2). ...when used orally in combination with peppermint oil for non-ulcer dyspepsia (6740,6741). The combination of enteric-coated peppermint oil 90 mg and caraway oil 50 mg, which is not available in the US, appears to be superior to placebo and similar to cisapride for relieving dyspepsia (6740,6741).

There is insufficient reliable information available about the effectiveness of caraway oil for its other uses.

Mechanism of Action

Caraway oil is obtained from the distilled oil of caraway fruit and seed. Caraway oil has antibacterial, antifungal, and larvicidal activity in vitro (6,11). Some experts believe that caraway oil has antispasmodic effects, but this is controversial (7,11,512). There's preliminary evidence that peppermint oil in combination with caraway oil can reduce gastroduodenal motility when administered orally in enteric-coated capsules (6742). Preliminary evidence also indicates that the constituent carvone induces glutathione S-transferase (GST), which might inhibit carcinogenesis (11,911). Topically applied caraway oil has shown activity against skin tumors in early laboratory research (6745).

Adverse Reactions
Orally, when caraway oil was used in combination with peppermint oil only a few patients experienced substernal burning sensation, belching, and nausea (6741,6742). Nausea, vomiting, and CNS depression are manifestations of toxicity (17).
Topically, caraway oil can also cause contact dermatitis when used topically (19).

Interactions with Herbs & Other Dietary Supplements
Insufficient reliable information available.

Interactions with Drugs
No interactions are known to occur, and there is no known reason to expect a clinically significant interaction with caraway oil.

Interactions with Foods
No interactions are known to occur, and there is no known reason to expect a clinically significant interaction with caraway oil.

Interactions with Lab Tests
No interactions are known to occur, and there is no known reason to expect a clinically significant interaction with caraway oil.

Interactions with Diseases or Conditions
No interactions are known to occur, and there is no known reason to expect a clinically significant interaction with caraway oil.

Dosage and Administration
ORAL: The typical dose of the oil is 3-6 drops per day (2). For non-ulcer dyspepsia, caraway oil 50-100 mg per day has been used in combination with peppermint oil (6740,6741).

Comments
Caraway has been used as a love potion, because people superstitiously believed that it had a power of retention and could prevent lovers from losing interest in one another (6002).

CARDAMOM

Also Known As
Bai Dou Kou, Cardamon, Cardomomi Fructus.

Scientific Names
Elettaria cardamomum, synonym Amomum cardamomum.
Family: Zingiberaceae.

People Use This For
Orally, cardamom is used for dyspepsia (2), intestinal spasm, irritable bowel syndrome (IBS) (1504), common cold, cough, bronchitis, inflammation of the mouth and pharynx, liver and gallbladder complaints, loss of appetite, and tendency toward infection (18). It is also used as an antiflatulent and laxative (11).
In Chinese medicine, cardamom is used as a stimulant and for urinary problems (11).
For food uses, cardamom is consumed as a spice in many parts of the world (11).

Safety
LIKELY SAFE ...when used orally and appropriately (2).
PREGNANCY AND LACTATION: Insufficient reliable information available; avoid using amounts greater than those used in food.

Effectiveness
There is insufficient reliable information available about the effectiveness of cardamom.

Mechanism of Action

The applicable part of cardamom is the seed. The active principals of cardamom are thought to be volatile oils, including cineole (2,11). Volatile oils are believed to have antispasmodic (11), antiflatulent, virustatic (2,18), and motility-enhancing effects (18).

Adverse Reactions

None reported.

Interactions with Herbs & Other Dietary Supplements

Insufficient reliable information available.

Interactions with Drugs

No interactions are known to occur, and there is no known reason to expect a clinically significant interaction with cardamom.

Interactions with Foods

No interactions are known to occur, and there is no known reason to expect a clinically significant interaction with cardamom.

Interactions with Lab Tests

No interactions are known to occur, and there is no known reason to expect a clinically significant interaction with cardamom.

Interactions with Diseases or Conditions

GALLSTONES: The cardamom seed can trigger gallstone colic (spasmodic pain) (18) and is not recommended for self-medication in patients with gallstones (2).

Dosage and Administration

ORAL: The typical dose of cardamom is 1.5 grams of the ground seeds per day. The usual dose of the tincture is 1-2 grams per day (2).

Comments

None.

CARLINA

Also Known As

Carlinae Radix, Dwarf Carline, Eberwurz, Ground Thistle, Racine de Carline Acaule, Radix Cardopatiae, Radix Chamaeleontis Albae, Silberdistelwurz, Stemless Carlina Root, Southernwood Root.

Scientific Names

Carlina acaulis.
Family: Asteraceae or Compositae.

People Use This For

Orally, carlina is used for gallbladder disease, poor digestion, and alimentary tract spasms (18).
Topically, carlina is used for dermatosis, rinsing wounds and ulcers, and to alleviate cancer of the tongue (18).
Acetic extracts are used for herpes eruptions, skin pustules, and toothaches (8).
In combination herbal products, carlina is used for gallbladder disorders and gastrointestinal spasms (8).
In folk medicine, carlina is used as a diuretic, tonic, gargle, catarrh, and to induce sweat (8).

Safety

There is insufficient reliable information available about the safety of carlina.
Pregnancy and Lactation: Insufficient reliable information available; avoid using.

Effectiveness

There is insufficient reliable information available about the effectiveness of carlina.

Mechanism of Action

The applicable part of carlina is the root. Acetone extract and essential oil have antibacterial activity but aqueous extract does not (8).

Adverse Reactions

Orally, carlina can cause an allergic reaction in individuals sensitive to the Asteraceae/Compositae family. Members of this family include ragweed, chrysanthemums, marigolds, daisies, and many other herbs.

Interactions with Herbs & Other Dietary Supplements

Insufficient reliable information available.

Interactions with Drugs

No interactions are known to occur, and there is no known reason to expect a clinically significant interaction with carlina.

Interactions with Foods

No interactions are known to occur, and there is no known reason to expect a clinically significant interaction with carlina.

Interactions with Lab Tests

No interactions are known to occur, and there is no known reason to expect a clinically significant interaction with carlina.

Interactions with Diseases or Conditions

CROSS-ALLERGENICITY: Can cause an allergic reaction in individuals sensitive to the Asteraceae/Compositae family. Members of this family include ragweed, chrysanthemums, marigolds, daisies, and many other herbs.

Dosage and Administration

ORAL: Carlina has been used as one cup tea (steep 1.5-3 grams finely cut dried root in 150 mL boiling water 5-10 minutes, strain) three times daily between meals (8,18), or as a tincture (steep 20 grams chopped root in 80 grams of 60% ethanol) 40-50 drops, four to five times daily (18). It has also been used with wine, (steep 50 grams root in 1 L white wine minimum 12 days, strain) one small glass before mealtime (18).
TOPICAL: Tea (simmer 30 grams root in 1 L boiling water 5-10 minutes, strain) applied externally has been used(18).

Comments

Carlina is rarely used today (8).

CARNOSINE

Also Known As

B-alanyl-L-histidine, B-alanyl histidine, L-carnosine.
CAUTION: See separate listings for Carnitine, L-Carnitine.

Scientific Names

Beta-alanyl-L-histidine.

People Use This For

Orally, carnosine is used to prevent aging and for preventing or treating complications of diabetes such as neuropathy, cataracts, and renal dysfunction.

Safety

There is insufficient reliable information available about the safety of carnosine.
Pregnancy and Lactation: Insufficient reliable information available; avoid using.

Effectiveness

There is insufficient reliable information available about the effectiveness of carnosine.

Mechanism of Action

Carnosine is a naturally occurring di-peptide found in skeletal muscle, heart, brain and other innervated tissues. Carnosine is formed by a process involving the enzyme carnosine-synthetase, which bonds the amino acids beta-alanine and L-histidine. Enzymes called carnisinase, maintain carnosine equilibrium by inactivating carnosine in tissues or blood (3381,3391). Carnosine seems to be concentrated in actively contracting muscles. In patients with muscular dystrophies carnosine levels may be lower. The concentration of carnosine in muscles also appears to correlate with age. Older patients have lower muscle carnosine levels (3391). Carnosine is of interest as an anti-aging product because of its effects on so-called advance glycosylation end-products (AGEs). AGEs are abnormal, cross-linked, and oxidized proteins that might play a role in the aging process. Carnosine appears to block protein glycosylation and the formation of AGEs. Because carnosine appears to block protein glycosylation, there is also some interest in using carnosine for complications of diabetes such as cataracts, neuropathy, and kidney failure, which arise from glycosylation (3364). There is some evidence that carnosine might help prevent lipid peroxidation within the cell membranes. Carnosine may block malondialdehyde (MDA) production, which is a lipid peroxidation end-product. Theoretically, blocking MDA might decrease oxidative damage to lipids, enzymes, and DNA. This raises the question of whether carnosine might play a role in preventing atherosclerosis, joint inflammation, and cataract formation (3364,3381). Carnosine binds heavy metals, and may provide some protection from zinc and copper mediated neurotoxicity (7219). Preliminary information also suggests that carnosine may play a role in the regulation of intracellular calcium and contractility in cardiac tissue (3390).

Adverse Reactions
None reported.

Interactions with Herbs & Other Dietary Supplements
Insufficient reliable information available.

Interactions with Drugs
No interactions are known to occur, and there is no known reason to expect a clinically significant interaction with carnosine.

Interactions with Foods
No interactions are known to occur, and there is no known reason to expect a clinically significant interaction with carnosine.

Interactions with Lab Tests
No interactions are known to occur, and there is no known reason to expect a clinically significant interaction with carnosine.

Interactions with Diseases or Conditions
No interactions are known to occur, and there is no known reason to expect a clinically significant interaction with carnosine.

Dosage and Administration
No typical dosage.

Comments
There is very little scientific information about this product. Our staff is continually analyzing the available information on natural medicines and will add data here as it becomes available.

CAROB

Also Known As
Locust Bean, Locust Pods, St. John's Bread, Sugar Pods.

Scientific Names
Ceratonia siliqua.
Family: Leguminosae or Fabaceae.

People Use This For
Orally, carob is used for acute nutritional disorders, celiac disease, obesity, diarrhea, dyspepsia, entero-colitis, vomiting during pregnancy, and sprue. In infants, it is used for vomiting, retching cough (18), and diarrhea (11).
In foods and beverages, carob is used as a flavoring agent. It is used in health food products, including weight-loss formulations, "energy" bars, tea formulations, and as a chocolate substitute (11). Carob flour and extracts are used as ingredients in food.

Safety

LIKELY SAFE …when used orally in amounts found in foods. It has Generally Recognized as Safe (GRAS) status in the US (6). …when used orally in medicinal amounts (12).
PREGNANCY AND LACTATION: Insufficient reliable information available; avoid using.

Effectiveness

There is insufficient reliable information available about the effectiveness of carob.

Mechanism of Action

The applicable part of carob is the fruit. Tannins contained in carob strongly inhibit digestive enzymes. Animal data suggest that a 15% carob gum diet fed for 2-6 weeks may result in weight loss. Decreases in blood glucose levels, cholesterol plasma levels and insulin levels, and an increased glucose tolerance are also suggested (11).

Adverse Reactions

None reported.

Interactions with Herbs & Other Dietary Supplements

Insufficient reliable information available.

Interactions with Drugs

No interactions are known to occur, and there is no known reason to expect a clinically significant interaction with carob.

Interactions with Foods

No interactions are known to occur, and there is no known reason to expect a clinically significant interaction with carob.

Interactions with Lab Tests

No interactions are known to occur, and there is no known reason to expect a clinically significant interaction with carob.

Interactions with Diseases or Conditions

No interactions are known to occur, and there is no known reason to expect a clinically significant interaction with carob.

Dosage and Administration

ORAL: People typically use 20-30 grams carob added to water, tea, or milk and taken over one day.

Comments

Avoid confusing carob with carob tree, Jacaranda procera and Jacaranda caroba. The term "carat" evolved from the use of carob seeds as weight units for measuring gold (6).

CARRAGEENAN

Also Known As

Carrageenin, Carragheenan, Chondrus Extract, Irish Moss Extract, Mousse D'Irlande.

Scientific Names

Chondrus crispus; Euchema species; Gigartina mamillosa and other Gigartina species; related red algae.
Family: Gigartinaceae.

People Use This For

Orally, carrageenan is used to soothe mucous membranes irritated by coughs, bronchitis, tuberculosis, and intestinal problems. The French use a form that has been degraded by low pH and high temperatures to treat peptic ulcers (11), and as a bulk laxative (13); this degraded form has lost the gelling properties of the original product.
Topically, carrageenan is used for anorectal symptoms (14).
In manufacturing, carrageenan is used as a binder, emulsifier, thickening agent, and as a stabilizer in pharmaceuticals, foods, and toothpaste. Carrageenan is also an ingredient in weight loss products.

Safety

LIKELY SAFE ...when used orally and appropriately for medicinal use (11). ...when used in food amounts; it is approved for food use in the US (11).

LIKELY UNSAFE ...when used orally in degraded form. The degraded form was associated with lesions in animals (14).

CHILDREN: POSSIBLY UNSAFE ...when used orally in infants. UK Food Advisory Committee recommended against use in infant formulas because some evidence suggests carrageenan could have adverse effects on the immune system (14).

PREGNANCY AND LACTATION: LIKELY SAFE ...when used in food amounts. There is insufficient reliable information available about the safety of using larger amounts; avoid using.

Effectiveness

POSSIBLY EFFECTIVE ...when used orally for peptic ulcers (11).

There is insufficient reliable information available about the effectiveness of carrageenan for its other uses.

Mechanism of Action

In animals, carrageenan has been reported to lower blood cholesterol, reducing GI secretions and food absorption, increasing water content of the gut when large amounts are given. Parenterally it has shown anticoagulant, hypotensive, and immunosuppressive activities; it may also have anti-inflammatory properties (11).

Adverse Reactions

Orally, carrageenan can cause bleeding, cramping, diarrhea, hypotension, and can lead to infection. Theoretically, carrageenan may be a problem for infants. It can be absorbed by their immature gut and may affect their immune system adversely (14).

Interactions with Herbs & Other Dietary Supplements

Insufficient reliable information available.

Interactions with Drugs

Carrageenan may increase the risk of bleeding in patients taking anticoagulants, and may enhance hypotensive effects of antihypertensive agents. Additionally, it can impair GI absorption of other drugs (214).

Interactions with Foods

No interactions are known to occur, and there is no known reason to expect a clinically significant interaction with carrageenan.

Interactions with Lab Tests

No interactions are known to occur, and there is no known reason to expect a clinically significant interaction with carrageenan.

Interactions with Diseases or Conditions

No interactions are known to occur, and there is no known reason to expect a clinically significant interaction with carrageenan.

Dosage and Administration

ORAL: A one cup decoction of Irish moss is sometimes used two to three times daily. The decoction is prepared by adding 1 ounce of the dried plant in 1-1.5 pints boiling water, simmering, and then straining. The decoction can be sweetened with lemon, honey, or cinnamon (6002).

Comments

Carrageenan consists of hydrocolloids from various red algae or seaweeds.

CASCARA

Also Known As

Bitter Bark, Buckthorn, California Buckthorn, Cascara Sagrada, Chittem Bark, Dogwood Bark, Purshiana Bark, Rhamni Purshianae Cortex, Sacred Bark, Sagrada Bark, Yellow Bark.

Scientific Names

Rhamnus purshiana, synonym Frangula purshiana.
Family: Rhamnaceae.

People Use This For

Orally, cascara is used most commonly as a laxative (7,11). Cascara is also used for gallstones, liver ailments, cancer, and as a bitter tonic (11).
In foods and beverages, a bitterless extract of cascara is sometimes used as a flavoring agent (11).
In manufacturing, cascara is used in processing of some sunscreens (11).

Safety

LIKELY SAFE ...when the bark preparations are used orally and appropriately for short periods of time (2). Cascara has FDA approval for use as a nonprescription medication.
POSSIBLY UNSAFE ...when cascara is used orally for more than 1-2 weeks. Chronic use can lead to dependence and electrolyte loss, specifically low levels of potassium (6).
CHILDREN: POSSIBLY SAFE ...when used orally and appropriately in children more than 2 years old. Should be used cautiously, if at all, in children less than 2 years old (272).
PREGNANCY: Insufficient reliable information available; avoid using (4258).
LACTATION: POSSIBLY UNSAFE ...when used orally because it is excreted into breast milk and might cause diarrhea (272).

Effectiveness

EFFECTIVE ...when used as a laxative (2,4,272), and has been approved by the FDA.
There is insufficient reliable information available about the effectiveness of cascara for its other uses.

Mechanism of Action

The applicable part of cascara is the dried bark. The anthraglycoside constituents in cascara are cascarosides A and B. These stimulate peristalsis and evacuation leading to its stimulant laxative effect (6). Cascara exerts its effect on the large intestine and does not have much effect on the small intestine. Bacteria in the intestine are required to transform the anthraglycosides into stimulant laxatives. The fresh bark contains free anthrone which is an emetic compound that can cause severe vomiting. But the free anthrone is destroyed by aging the bark for at least one year, or by artificial aging with heat and aeration (2). Anthroid laxative use is not associated with an increased risk of developing colorectal ademoma or carcinoma (6138).

Adverse Reactions

Orally, cascara can commonly cause mild abdominal discomfort, colic, and cramps (4). Long-term use can lead to potassium depletion, albuminuria, hematuria, disturbed heart function, muscle weakness (2), finger clubbing, and cachexia (4). In some cases chronic use can also cause pseudomelanosis coli (pigment spots in intestinal mucosa) which is harmless, and usually resolves with discontinuation (6138). Fresh or improperly aged cascara bark can cause severe vomiting due to the presence of free anthrone constituents. There is also some concern about potential liver problems. In one case, cascara aged bark 425 mg (containing approximately 21 mg cascaroside) three times daily for three days resulted in cholestatic hepatitis, ascites, and portal hypertension. Symptoms resolved over about 3 months following discontinuation of cascara (6895). This adverse effect is suspected to be the result of a hypersensitivity reaction.

Interactions with Herbs & Other Dietary Supplements

LICORICE: Using cascara concomitantly with licorice can increase the risk of potassium depletion (2).
DIGITALIS, LILY OF THE VALLEY, SQUILL: Overuse of cascara can increase the risk of cardiac toxicity, because these herbs are also cardiac glycoside-containing herbs (2,500) and because of potassium loss (4).
STIMULANT LAXATIVE HERBS: Theoretically, cascara used concomitantly with other herbs that are stimulant laxatives can increase the risk of potassium depletion. Stimulant laxative herbs include: aloe, wild cucumber fruit (Ecballium elaterium), blue flag rhizome, alder buckthorn, European buckthorn, butternut bark, castor oil, colocynth fruit pulp, gamboge bark exudate, jalap root, black root, manna bark exudate, podophyllum root, rhubarb root, senna leaves and pods, and yellow dock root (19).
POTASSIUM DEPLETING HERBS: Theoretically, concomitant use of cascara along with horsetail plant or licorice rhizome can increase the risk of potassium depletion.

Interactions with Drugs

CARDIAC GLYCOSIDES: Theoretically, overuse of cascara increases the risk of adverse effects of cardiac glycoside drugs, such as digoxin (Lanoxin).
CORTICOSTEROIDS, POTASSIUM DEPLETING DIURETICS: Concomitant use of these drugs along with cascara can increase the risk of potassium depletion (2).
LAXATIVES: Concomitant use of cascara along with many laxatives can cause electrolyte and fluid depletion.
ORAL DRUGS: Theoretically, cascara can reduce the absorption of some drugs due to the reduced transit time through the GI tract (500).

Interactions with Foods

No interactions are known to occur, and there is no known reason to expect a clinically significant interaction with cascara.

Interactions with Lab Tests

COLORIMETRIC TESTS: Cascara can discolor urine (pink, red, purple, orange, rust), interfering with diagnostic tests that depend on a color change, due to its anthraquinone content (1,12,275).
POTASSIUM: Excessive use of cascara can cause potassium depletion, reducing serum potassium concentrations and test results (1,2,4,12,19).

Interactions with Diseases or Conditions

GI CONDITIONS: Cascara is contraindicated in people with intestinal obstruction, or acute intestinal inflammation. This includes people with Crohn's disease, ulcerative colitis, and appendicitis. It is also contraindicated for people who have ulcers, and abdominal pain of unknown origin (2,4,8).

Dosage and Administration

ORAL: 20-30 mg per day of the active ingredient, hyroxyanthracene derivatives. This is calculated as cascaroside A, from the cut bark, powder, or extracts (2). A typical dose includes 1 cup of tea which is made by steeping 2 grams of finely chopped bark in 150 mL of boiling water for 5-10 minutes, and then straining (18). The cascara liquid extract is given in a dose of 2-5 mL three times daily (4). The appropriate amount of cascara is the smallest dose that is necessary to maintain soft stools (2).

Comments

American Herbal Products Association (AHPA) recommends the following label statement: "Do not use this product if you have abdominal pain or diarrhea. Consult a health care provider prior to use if you are pregnant or nursing. Discontinue use in the event of diarrhea or watery stools. Do not exceed recommended dose. Not for long-term use." (12). Non-standardized anthraquinone-containing preparations should be avoided, as their effects are not predictable (4).

CASCARILLA

Also Known As

Bahama Cascarilla, Sweet Bark, Sweet Wood Bark.

Scientific Names

Croton eleuteria.
Family: Euphorbiaceae.

People Use This For

Orally, cascarilla is used for digestive disorders, diarrhea, and vomiting (18).

Safety

There is insufficient reliable information available about the safety of cascarilla.
Pregnancy and Lactation: Insufficient reliable information available; avoid using.

Effectiveness

There is insufficient reliable information available about the effectiveness of cascarilla.

Mechanism of Action

The applicable part of cascarilla is the bark. Constituents reported to have stimulant and tonic properties (18).

Adverse Reactions
None reported.

Interactions with Herbs & Other Dietary Supplements
Insufficient reliable information available.

Interactions with Drugs
No interactions are known to occur, and there is no known reason to expect a clinically significant interaction with cascarilla.

Interactions with Foods
No interactions are known to occur, and there is no known reason to expect a clinically significant interaction with cascarilla.

Interactions with Lab Tests
No interactions are known to occur, and there is no known reason to expect a clinically significant interaction with cascarilla.

Interactions with Diseases or Conditions
No interactions are known to occur, and there is no known reason to expect a clinically significant interaction with cascarilla.

Dosage and Administration
No typical dosage.

Comments
In the past, cascarilla was added to tobacco before smoking, due to its pleasant odor when burned. It also produced vertigo and intoxication during this process (215).

CASHEW

Also Known As
East Indian Almond.

Scientific Names
Anacardium occidentale.
Family: Anarcardiaceae.

People Use This For
Orally, cashew is used for gastrointestinal ailments.
Topically, cashew is used as a skin stimulant and cauterizing agent for ulcers, warts and corns (18).
Cashew is also consumed as a food.

Safety
LIKELY SAFE ...when consumed as a food (18).
There is insufficient reliable information available about the safety of cashew when used medicinally in amounts exceeding those found in foods.
PREGNANCY AND LACTATION: LIKELY SAFE ...when consumed as a food; avoid using amounts greater than typically found in foods.

Effectiveness
There is insufficient reliable information available about the effectiveness of cashew.

Mechanism of Action
The applicable part of cashew is the nut. A dried ethanolic extract is effective in vitro against gram-positive bacteria Bacillus subtilis and Staphylococcus aureus. Alkyl phenols contained in the cashew nut shell are strong skin irritants. Cashew contains alkyl phenols that are chemically related to constituents in poison ivy, poison oak, mango, and ginkgo. The adverse reactions resulting from cashew are related to the adverse reactions that sometimes occur with these other irritants. Roasted cashew nuts are free of the alkyl phenols (18).

Adverse Reactions
Topically, contact can lead to redness and nodule and blister formation.

Interactions with Herbs & Other Dietary Supplements
Insufficient reliable information available.

Interactions with Drugs
No interactions are known to occur, and there is no known reason to expect a clinically significant interaction with cashew.

Interactions with Foods
No interactions are known to occur, and there is no known reason to expect a clinically significant interaction with cashew.

Interactions with Lab Tests
No interactions are known to occur, and there is no known reason to expect a clinically significant interaction with cashew.

Interactions with Diseases or Conditions
No interactions are known to occur, and there is no known reason to expect a clinically significant interaction with cashew.

Dosage and Administration
No typical dosage.

Comments
Acajou oil, oleum anacardiae, and fatty oil are extracted from cashew nuts (18).

CASSIA

Also Known As
Bastard Cinnamon, Canton Cassia, Cassia Aromaticum, Cassia Bark, Cassia Cinnamon, Cassia Lignea, Chinese Cinnamon, Cinnamomi cassiae cortex, Cortex Cinnamomi, False Cinnamon, Nees, Rou Gui.
CAUTION: See separate listings for Cinnamon flower and Cinnamon bark.

Scientific Names
Cinnamomum aromaticum, synonym Cinnamomum cassia.
Family: Lauraceae.

People Use This For
Orally, cassia is used for gas (flatulence), muscle and GI spasms, preventing nausea and vomiting, diarrhea, infections, the common cold, and loss of appetite. It is also used for impotence, enuresis, rheumatic conditions, testicle hernia, menopausal symptoms, amenorrhea, and as an abortifacient. Cassia is also used for angina, kidney disorders, hypertension, cramps, and cancer.
Topically, cassia is used in suntan lotions, nasal sprays, mouthwashes, gargles, toothpaste, and as a counterirritant in liniments.
In food and beverages, cassia is used as a flavoring agent.

Safety
LIKELY SAFE ...when used orally in amounts found in foods. Cassia has Generally Recognized as Safe (GRAS) status in the US. The maximum use level is 0.047% (11).
POSSIBLY SAFE ...when used orally and appropriately for medicinal purposes (12).
LIKELY UNSAFE ...when used topically in concentrations greater than 0.2% (4).
PREGNANCY AND LACTATION: LIKELY SAFE ...when used orally in amounts found in foods (11). There is insufficient reliable information available about the safety of cassia when used in greater amounts during pregnancy and breast-feeding; avoid using.

Effectiveness
There is insufficient reliable information available about the effectiveness of cassia.

Mechanism of Action

The applicable part of cassia is the bark. Cinnamaldehyde, found in the volatile oil fraction of Cassia, causes CNS stimulation at a low dose, but sedation at a high dose. Cinnamaldehyde also has antibacterial and antifungal activity. It accelerates catecholamine release from adrenal glands, increases blood flow, reduces blood pressure and heart rate, and causes hyperglycemia (4).

Adverse Reactions

Topically, allergic skin reactions and dermal and membrane irritation have been reported (4).

Interactions with Herbs & Other Dietary Supplements

Insufficient reliable information available.

Interactions with Drugs

ANTIDIABETES DRUGS: There is some concern that cassia might increase blood glucose levels and possibly decrease the effectiveness of drugs used for diabetes (4).
ANTIHYPERTENSIVES: Cassia can lower blood pressure and might have additive effects in patients treated with antihypertensives; use with caution (4).

Interactions with Foods

No interactions are known to occur, and there is no known reason to expect a clinically significant interaction with cassia.

Interactions with Lab Tests

BLOOD GLUCOSE: Cassia might increase blood glucose levels in some patients (4).

Interactions with Diseases or Conditions

ALLERGY TO CINNAMON, PERU BALSAM: Contraindicated (2).
CARDIOVASCULAR CONDITIONS: There is concern that cassia might adversely effect patients with cardiovascular conditions such as high or low blood pressure, or congestive heart failure. Some constituents in cassia seem to slow heart rate and might lower blood pressure (4); however, the clinical significance of these effects in patients is not known. Until more is known, advise patients with cardiovascular conditions to avoid or use cassia preparations cautiously.
DIABETES: There is some concern that cassia might interfere with blood glucose control in patients with diabetes. Some cassia constituents seem to increase blood glucose levels (4). So far, the clinical significance of this effect in patients with diabetes is not known. Tell patients with diabetes to use cassia products cautiously. Suggest they monitor blood glucose levels more closely. Dose adjustments to diabetes medications might be necessary.
SENSITIVE INDIVIDUALS: Avoid contact, may cause contact dermatitis (12).

Dosage and Administration

ORAL: People use 0.5-1 grams of dried bark three times daily, or drink 1 cup tea (steep 0.5-1 grams of dry bark in 150 mL boiling water 5-10 minutes, strain) three times daily (2,4). Essential oil, 0.05-0.2 mL three times daily has also been used (2,4).

Comments

Reported to be inferior to true cinnamon in flavor (4,11).

CASSIE ABSOLUTE

Also Known As

Huisache, Popinac Absolute, Sweet Acacia.

Scientific Names

Acacia farnesiana; Mimosa farnesiana.
Family: Leguminosae or Fabaceae.

People Use This For

Orally, cassie absolute is used as an antispasmodic, antidiarrheal, stimulant, aphrodisiac, and to treat fever (11).
Topically, cassie absolute is used for dry skin and as an insecticide (11).
In Chinese medicine, cassie absolute is used for rheumatoid arthritis and pulmonary tuberculosis (11).
In other countries, various plant parts are used for medicinal purposes. In India, tea made from cassie absolute

leaves is used for gonorrhea (11), and the root is chewed for sore throat (11). In Venezuela, it is used for stomach cancer (11).

For food uses, cassie absolute is a flavor ingredient in foods and beverages (11).

In manufacturing, cassie absolute is used as a fragrance in perfumes (11).

Safety

LIKELY SAFE ...when used orally in amounts found in foods (maximum use level 0.002%); approved for food use in the US (11).

There is insufficient reliable information available about the safety of cassie absolute used in amounts greater than those found in foods.

PREGNANCY AND LACTATION: Insufficient reliable information available; avoid using.

Effectiveness

There is insufficient reliable information available about the effectiveness of cassie absolute.

Mechanism of Action

Cassie absolute is reported to have antispasmodic, aphrodisiac, astringent, demulcent, antidiarrheal, antipyretic, antirheumatic and stimulant properties (11). It contains glycosides which reportedly have anti-inflammatory and bronchodilator effects (1505).

Adverse Reactions

None reported.

Interactions with Herbs & Other Dietary Supplements

Insufficient reliable information available.

Interactions with Drugs

No interactions are known to occur, and there is no known reason to expect a clinically significant interaction with cassie absolute.

Interactions with Foods

No interactions are known to occur, and there is no known reason to expect a clinically significant interaction with cassie absolute.

Interactions with Lab Tests

No interactions are known to occur, and there is no known reason to expect a clinically significant interaction with cassie absolute.

Interactions with Diseases or Conditions

No interactions are known to occur, and there is no known reason to expect a clinically significant interaction with cassie absolute.

Dosage and Administration

No typical dosage.

Comments

Cassie absolute is an extract of Acacia farnesiana flowers. Limited pharmacologic and toxicologic information is available (11).

CASTOR OIL

Also Known As

African Coffee Tree, Bofareira, Castor, Castor Oil Plant, Mexico Weed, Palma Christi, Tangantangan Oil Plant, Wonder Tree.

CAUTION: See separate listing for Castor seed.

Scientific Names

Ricinus communis; Ricinus sanguines.

Family: Euphorbiaceae.

People Use This For

Orally, castor oil is used as a stimulant laxative (6) and to stimulate labor (1022).

Topically, castor oil is used as an emollient (11). It has also been used topically to dissolve cysts, growths, or warts, and to soften bunions and corns. Castor oil has been used in the eyes to soothe the irritated conjunctiva after the presence of foreign bodies there (214).

Historically, castor oil has been used alone or with quinine sulfate to induce labor at term, and applied topically as a cervical abortifacient and vaginal contraceptive (6). It has also been used orally to promote the flow of breast milk (1022).

Safety

LIKELY SAFE ...when used orally and appropriately, short-term (16).

POSSIBLY UNSAFE ...when used orally in high doses or for extended periods. Taking castor oil for greater than one week or exceeding the recommended dose of 15 to 60 mL per day can increase the risk of fluid and electrolyte disturbances (272).

CHILDREN: LIKELY SAFE ...when used orally and appropriately, short-term (14,16). POSSIBLY UNSAFE ...when used orally in high doses or for extended periods. Taking castor oil for greater than one week or exceeding the recommended dose of 1-15 mL, depending on age, can increase the risk of fluid and electrolyte disturbances (14,272).

PREGNANCY: POSSIBLY SAFE ...when used orally for inducing labor in pregnant women at term. Midwives routinely use castor oil for labor induction in pregnant women at term. This practice does not appear to adversely affect the mother or fetus (1122,7191). However, castor oil should not be used without the supervision of a clinician. LIKELY UNSAFE ...when used orally in pregnant women who are not at term. Castor oil might induce premature labor and induce miscarriage (12,18); avoid using.

LACTATION: Insufficient reliable information available; avoid using.

Effectiveness

EFFECTIVE ...when used orally, short-term as a stimulant laxative for constipation (6,14,272). ...when used orally for total colonic evacuation prior to surgery, or radiologic or intestinal examination procedures (14,15).

POSSIBLY EFFECTIVE ...when used orally to stimulate labor. A single 60 mL dose of castor oil appears to stimulate labor within 24 hours in at least 50% of women at term pregnancy with no prior signs of labor (7191). There is also some evidence that women at term pregnancy with premature membrane rupture who take castor oil have a higher incidence of labor onset and a lower incidence of cesarean section than women who take no medication (1122).

There is insufficient reliable information available about the effectiveness of castor oil for its other uses.

Mechanism of Action

Castor oil is produced by cold pressing ripe seeds of Ricinus communis. Unlike the seeds from this plant, castor oil does not contain the deadly poison risin (16,17). Castor oil is a glyceride that can be absorbed from the intestine and metabolized as a fatty acid (272). Castor oil is hydrolyzed in the duodenum by pancreatic lipase to release ricinoleic acid, which might have stimulant laxative effects (6,272). Although the exact mechanism of ricinoleic acid is unknown, the laxative effect appears to result from fluid secretion induced by cyclic adenosine monophosphate, rather than the increased peristalsis due to an irritant effect (272). Onset of bowel evacuant action is usually within 2 hours, but sometimes can take up to 6 hours (16). In pregnancy, castor oil is thought to induce labor by producing hyperemia in the intestinal tract, which causes reflex stimulation of the uterus (16). Castor oil might also increase prostaglandin production, which stimulates uterine activity (7191).

Adverse Reactions

Orally, castor oil, like all stimulant laxatives, can cause abdominal discomfort, cramping, nausea, and faintness (15,272). Nausea can also occur because of the unpleasant taste of castor oil (7191). Using flavored products might reduce this effect. Castor oil can also cause fluid and electrolyte loss, particularly potassium, which can result in hypokalemia. It can also cause malabsorption from intestinal hypermotility (15,272). Chronic ingestion over long periods of time can lead to cathartic colon (15,1060). There is some concern that castor oil might cause amniotic fluid embolism. There is one case of amniotic fluid embolism and cardiopulmonary arrest within one hour of ingestion of 30 mL of castor oil at full-term pregnancy (1219).

Interactions with Herbs & Other Dietary Supplements

CARDIAC GLYCOSIDE-CONTAINING HERBS: Theoretically, castor oil can increase the risk of cardiac glycoside toxicity (2,18,19,500).

LICORICE/HORSETAIL: Theoretically, concomitant use with horsetail plant or licorice rhizome increases the risk of potassium depletion (18).

MALE FERN: Concomitant use with oil-soluble anthelmintic herbs, such as the male fern, should be avoided due to enhanced absorption of castor oil (19).

STIMULANT LAXATIVE HERBS: Theoretically, concomitant use with other stimulant laxative herbs might increase the risk of potassium depletion (19).
WORMSEED: Concomitant use with wormseed oil might reduce both toxicity and efficacy of wormseed oil (19).

Interactions with Drugs
CARDIAC GLYCOSIDES: Theoretically, can increase the risk of adverse effects of cardiac glycoside drugs, e.g. digoxin (Lanoxin).
CORTICOSTEROIDS, POTASSIUM DEPLETING DIURETICS: Concomitant use may increase risk of potassium depletion (18).
LAXATIVES: Concomitant use may lead to electrolyte and fluid depletion.
ORAL DRUGS: Theoretically, may reduce absorption of drugs due to reduced transit time.

Interactions with Foods
No interactions are known to occur, and there is no known reason to expect a clinically significant interaction with castor oil.

Interactions with Lab Tests
No interactions are known to occur, and there is no known reason to expect a clinically significant interaction with castor oil.

Interactions with Diseases or Conditions
INTESTINAL DISORDERS: Contraindicated in intestinal obstruction (appendicitis, Crohn's disease, irritable bowel syndrome (IBS), ulcerative colitis), abdominal pain of unknown origin (18), abdominal pain of unknown origin (18), biliary tract obstruction and other biliary disorders (7).

Dosage and Administration
ORAL: For constipation, 15 mL is commonly used (15). For total colonic evacuation, such as before surgery, or radiologic or colonoscopic procedures, the dose for adults and children over 12 is 15-60 mL given 16 hours prior to surgery or colonic examination (15). For children age 2 to 11 years, 5-15 mL is typically used. In children younger than 2 years, 1-5 mL is commonly used. For induction of labor, a variety of dosage regimens have been used (1122). Single doses vary from 5-120 mL (1122). A one-time dose of 60 mL in fruit juice is a commonly used regimen (7191). Other regimens that have been used include 5 mL in peppermint tea every 2 hours, 15 mL three times daily, 30 mL every 2 hours, 30 mL every 6 hours, 30 mL every 3 hours for 3 doses, 60 ml daily, and 60 ml daily for 2 days (1122). Castor oil is most effective when taken on an empty stomach (7). Castor oil should not be given at bedtime because of its quick onset of action (2 to 6 hours) (1066).

Comments
Castor oil has been used medicinally for centuries and was mentioned in the Ebers Papyrus (16). The taste of castor oil is bland, followed by a slightly bitter and usually nauseating taste (16). Castor oil is sometimes flavored with cinnamon, peppermint, or other flavorings to mask the unpleasant taste (16).

CASTOR seed

Also Known As
African Coffee Tree, Bofareira, Castor Bean, Mexico Weed, Palma Christi, Tangantangan Oil Plant, Wonder Tree.
CAUTION: See separate listing for Castor Oil.

Scientific Names
Ricinus communis; Ricinus sanguines.
Family: Euphorbiaceae.

People Use This For
Orally, castor seeds are used as a birth control, a laxative, for leprosy, and syphilis (5611,7127,7128).
Topically, castor seed paste is used as a poultice for inflammatory skin disorders, boils, carbuncles, abscesses, inflammation of the middle ear, and migraines (18).

Safety
POSSIBLY SAFE ...when the hulled seed is used orally and appropriately, short-term. There is some evidence that a single dose of castor seed with the outer coat removed (hulled) can be used safely (7127,7128).

UNSAFE ...when the whole seed is used orally. Safety depends on whether or not the seed is chewed or if the outer coat is ruptured. Chewing as few as 1-6 whole seeds can be lethal in an adult. If the seed is swallowed intact, poisoning is less likely (6,5611); however, prompt medical attention should be sought after ingestion of any whole castor seed (5611). There is insufficient reliable information available about the safety of castor seed when applied topically.

CHILDREN: UNSAFE ...when the whole seed is used orally. The chewed or uncoated seeds can cause severe toxic effects (5611,5612) and death (5611). There is insufficient reliable information available about the safety of the hulled seed or topical use in children.

PREGNANCY AND LACTATION: UNSAFE ...when the whole seed is used orally. The chewed or uncoated seeds can cause severe toxic effects, including death (6,5611); avoid using. There is insufficient reliable information available about the safety of the hulled seed or topical use during pregnancy and lactation.

Effectiveness

POSSIBLY EFFECTIVE ...when the hulled seed is used orally as a contraceptive. There is some evidence that a single dose of seeds with the outer coat removed (hulled) can work as a contraceptive for up to 8-12 months (7127,7128). There is insufficient reliable information available about the effectiveness of castor seed for its other uses.

Mechanism of Action

Castor seeds are the seeds of the evergreen castor shrub (7122). The seeds are used to produce castor oil. Castor seeds are best known for their toxic effects. They contain the toxic glycoprotein ricin. Ricin can be fatal when ingested, inhaled, or given intravenously. Ricin is an N-glycosidase that affects an RNA subunit and interferes with protein synthesis, causing cell death (6,5611). Toxic effects typically occur 2-5 days after ingestion (5611). There is some preliminary evidence that ricin might also have analgesic effects and activity against leukemia (6). It is unclear how castor seeds work as a contraceptive; however, its effects do not seem to be hormonally mediated (7127,7128).

Adverse Reactions

Orally, castor seed can cause severe toxicity. Chewing whole seeds can cause nausea, vomiting, diarrhea, abdominal pain, dehydration, shock, hemolysis, severe fluid and electrolyte disturbances, peripheral vascular collapse, renal failure secondary to hypovolemia, and death. Cellular damage to liver, kidneys, and pancreas typically occurs 2-5 days after ingestion (5611,5612). As few as 1-6 seeds can be lethal in humans (6,5611). Rupture of the seed hull seems to be necessary to cause toxicity. Swallowing seeds whole, without chewing, is less likely to cause toxic effects; however, prompt medical attention should be received after ingestion of any whole seed. Serum chemistries should be monitored for at least 5 days after ingestion in symptomatic patients (5611). Hulled castor seeds, with the outer coat carefully removed, seem to be well-tolerated, and without toxic side effects (7127,7128); however, some patients taking hulled seeds can have transient anorexia and weight loss (1727).

Topically, the castor plant, crushed seeds, or seed dust can cause dermatitis in some patients (5611).

Castor seed is also an inhalant allergen in workers in the coffee industry (6). Anaphylaxis can occur in these patients after exposure to castor beans, plants, or dust (5611).

Interactions with Herbs & Other Dietary Supplements

Insufficient reliable information available.

Interactions with Drugs

No interactions are known to occur, and there is no known reason to expect a clinically significant interaction with castor seed.

Interactions with Foods

No interactions are known to occur, and there is no known reason to expect a clinically significant interaction with castor seed.

Interactions with Lab Tests

No interactions are known to occur, and there is no known reason to expect a clinically significant interaction with castor seed.

Interactions with Diseases or Conditions

No interactions are known to occur, and there is no known reason to expect a clinically significant interaction with castor seed.

Dosage and Administration

ORAL: No typical dosage.
TOPICAL: Paste made with ground seeds applied to affected skin twice daily has been used; treatment takes up to 15 days (18). For use on intact skin; avoid use on broken or damaged skin.

Comments

The plant is used mainly for ornamental purposes (6). Because of its toxic effects, the castor seed constituent, ricin, has been evaluated as a possible chemical warfare agent. (6).

CASTOREUM

Also Known As

Canadian Beaver, European Beaver, Siberian Beaver.

Scientific Names

Castor canadensis; Castor fiber.
Family: Castoridae.

People Use This For

In traditional medicine, castoreum is used for absence of menstrual periods, painful menses, hysteria, restless sleep, and as a calming and restorative agent (11).
In foods and beverages, castoreum extract is used as a flavoring agent.
In manufacturing, castoreum tincture is used as a fragrance or fixative in cosmetics and soaps (11).

Safety

LIKELY SAFE ...when used in amounts found in foods; the maximum use level is 0.009% (11). It has Generally Recognized as Safe (GRAS) status in the US (11). ...when used topically. Castoreum tincture is reported to be nontoxic in dermatological tests (11); the maximum use level is 0.4% in perfumes (11).
There is insufficient reliable information available about the safety of castoreum for its other uses.
PREGNANCY AND LACTATION: Insufficient reliable information available; avoid using.

Effectiveness

There is insufficient reliable information available about the effectiveness of castoreum.

Mechanism of Action

Castoreum is reported to have calming and sedating effects (11).

Adverse Reactions

None reported.

Interactions with Herbs & Other Dietary Supplements

Insufficient reliable information available.

Interactions with Drugs

No interactions are known to occur, and there is no known reason to expect a clinically significant interaction with castoreum.

Interactions with Foods

No interactions are known to occur, and there is no known reason to expect a clinically significant interaction with castoreum.

Interactions with Lab Tests

No interactions are known to occur, and there is no known reason to expect a clinically significant interaction with castoreum.

Interactions with Diseases or Conditions

No interactions are known to occur, and there is no known reason to expect a clinically significant interaction with castoreum.

Dosage and Administration

No typical dosage.

Comments

Castoreum is a secretion collected from scent glands of Canadian, European, and Siberian beavers. Castoreum from the Canadian beaver is considered superior in quality to that of the Siberian beaver (11).

CAT'S CLAW

Also Known As
Cats Claw, Griffe Du Chat, Life-Giving Vine of Peru, Samento, Uña De Gato.
CAUTION: See separate listing for Cat's Foot.

Scientific Names
Uncaria guianensis; Uncaria tomentosa.
Family: Rubiaceae.

People Use This For
Orally, cat's claw is used for diverticulitis, peptic ulcers, colitis, gastritis, hemorrhoids, parasites, and leaky bowel syndrome. Cat's claw is also used orally for viral infections including herpes zoster, herpes simplex, and human immunodeficiency virus (HIV). It is also used orally for wound healing, arthritis, asthma, cancer (especially urinary tract cancer), gonorrhea, dysentery, birth control, bone pains, and "cleansing" the kidneys.

Safety
POSSIBLY SAFE …when used orally, short-term. A specific freeze-dried aqueous extract seems to be safe when used for up to 4 weeks (7317).
PREGNANCY: POSSIBLY UNSAFE …when used orally. There is concern that cat's claw might be unsafe based on its use as a contraceptive (12); avoid using.
LACTATION: Insufficient reliable information available; avoid using.

Effectiveness
POSSIBLY EFFECTIVE …when used orally for treating osteoarthritis of the knee. A specific freeze-dried cat's claw extract (Uncaria guianensis) appears to relieve knee pain related to physical activity within one week of treatment, but it does not decrease pain at rest or decrease knee swelling (7317).

Mechanism of Action
The applicable part of cat's claw is the root and bark. The major alkaloid of cat's claw is rhynchophylline. There is some evidence that it might have cardiovascular effects including dilating peripheral blood vessels, lowering heart rate, and possibly lowering blood cholesterol. Rhynchophylline might also inhibit sympathetic nervous system activity (6). Cat's claw is thought to work for osteoarthritis due to anti-inflammatory effects. It seems to inhibit the production of prostaglandin E2 and tumor necrosis factor-alpha (TNF-alpha) (7317). There is also interest in cat's claw for cancer and viral infections because some of its constituents seem to have antioxidant, immunostimulant, and antiviral effects (7225,7317). These constituents include quinovic acid alkaloids and the alkaloids pteropodine and isopteropodine (7225). Extracts of cat's claw increase phagocytosis and might have antimutagenic activity (7224). There is also preliminary evidence that cat's claw extracts can induce tumor cell death (apoptosis) and inhibit proliferation of leukemia and lymphoma cells (7225), but cat's claw does not appear to be cytotoxic to normal cells (7227). Some cat's claw alkaloids may have a beneficial effect on memory in cases of amnesia caused by cholinergic dysfunction. These alkaloids seem to enhance central cholinergic transmission by increasing acetylcholine levels or by affecting dopaminergic systems that can enhance cholinergic function (7226). Another constituent, uncarine E, might also affect the glutameteric system, which might also play a critical role in memory and cognition (7226). The constituent mitraphylline seems to have diuretic activity (6). The hirsutine constituent seems to inhibit bladder contractions, cause local anesthesia at low doses, and have curare-like actions at high dose (6).

Adverse Reactions
Orally, cat's claw can cause headache, dizziness, and vomiting (7317).

Interactions with Herbs & Other Dietary Supplements
Insufficient reliable information available.

Interactions with Drugs
ANTI-HYPERTENSIVES: Since cat's claw may lower blood pressure, exercise caution if it is being used along with an antihypertensive.
IMMUNOSUPPRESSANTS: Theoretically, cat's claw may interfere with immunosuppressant therapy (7225) because of its immunostimulating activity. It stimulates phagocytosis and increases respiratory cellular activity and the mobility of leukocytes. Immunosuppressant drugs include azathioprine (Imuran), basiliximab (Simulect), cyclosporine (Neoral, Sandimmune), daclizumab (Zenapax), muromonab-CD3 (OKT3, Orthoclone OKT3), mycophenolate (CellCept), tacrolimus (FK506, Prograf), sirolimus (Rapamune), prednisone (Deltasone, Orasone),

and other corticosteroids (glucocorticoids).

OTHER DRUGS: There's preliminary evidence that cat's claw can inhibit the cytochrome P450 (CYP450) 3A4 enzyme (6450). Theoretically, cat's claw might increase levels of drugs metabolized by CYP450 3A4; however, so far, this interaction has not been reported in humans. Some drugs metabolized by CYP450 3A4 include lovastatin (Mevacor), ketoconazole (Nizoral), itraconazole (Sporanox), fexofenadine (Allegra), triazolam (Halcion), and numerous others. Use cat's claw cautiously or avoid in patients taking these drugs.

Interactions with Foods

No interactions are known to occur, and there is no known reason to expect a clinically significant interaction with cat's claw.

Interactions with Lab Tests

No interactions are known to occur, and there is no known reason to expect a clinically significant interaction with cat's claw.

Interactions with Diseases or Conditions

AUTOIMMUNE DISEASES: There is some concern that cat's claw might adversely affect patients autoimmune disorders because of its immune stimulating effects (7225). Avoid using in patients with multiple sclerosis, systemic lupus erythematosus (SLE), rheumatoid arthritis, or other autoimmune disorders.

HYPOTENSION: Cat's claw might reduce blood pressure and exacerbate hypotension (6).

Dosage and Administration

ORAL: For osteoarthritis of the knee, 100 mg daily of a specific freeze-dried aqueous cat's claw extract has been used (7317).

Comments

Cat's claw was ranked as the seventh most popular herb in US sales in 1997 (2). Two species of cat's claw are of primary interest for medicinal use: Uncaria tomentosa and Uncaria guianensis. Uncaria tomentosa is most commonly used in the US, and Uncaria guianensis is typically used in Europe (6).

CAT'S FOOT

Also Known As

Antennariase Dioicae Flos, Cats Ear Flower, Cat's Ear Flower, Cats Foot, Cudweed, Katsenpfotchenbluten, Life Everlasting, Mountain Everlasting.
CAUTION: See separate listings for Cudweed and Cat's Claw.

Scientific Names

Antennaria dioica.
Family: Asteraceae or Compositae.

People Use This For

Orally, cat's foot is used to treat intestinal disease (2).
In folk medicine, cat's foot is used as a diuretic (18).

Safety

There is insufficient reliable information available about the safety of cat's foot.
Pregnancy and Lactation: Insufficient reliable information available; avoid using.

Effectiveness

There is insufficient reliable information available about the effectiveness of cat's foot.

Mechanism of Action

The applicable part of cat's foot is the fresh or dried flowers. Mild spasmolytic and choleric effects have been reported in animals (18).

Adverse Reactions

Orally, cat's foot can cause an allergic reaction in individuals sensitive to the Asteraceae/Compositae family. Members of this family include ragweed, chrysanthemums, marigolds, daisies, and many other herbs.

Interactions with Herbs & Other Dietary Supplements
Insufficient reliable information available.

Interactions with Drugs
No interactions are known to occur, and there is no known reason to expect a clinically significant interaction with cat's foot.

Interactions with Foods
No interactions are known to occur, and there is no known reason to expect a clinically significant interaction with cat's foot.

Interactions with Lab Tests
No interactions are known to occur, and there is no known reason to expect a clinically significant interaction with cat's foot.

Interactions with Diseases or Conditions
CROSS-ALLERGENICITY: Can cause an allergic reaction in individuals sensitive to the Asteraceae/Compositae family. Members of this family include ragweed, chrysanthemums, marigolds, daisies, and many other herbs.

Dosage and Administration
ORAL: The fluid extract of cat's foot is sometimes taken as 14-28 grains three times daily (6002).

Comments
Avoid confusion with ground ivy, which is also sometimes referred to as cat's foot (214).

CATECHU

Also Known As
Black Catechu: Acacia Catechu Heartwood Extract, Black Cutch, Cachou, Cashou, Catechu nigrum, Cutch, Dark Catechu, Pegu Catechu.
Pale Catechu: Cube Gambir, Gambier, Gambir, Gambir Catechu, Terra Japonica, Uncaria Gambier Leaf/Twig Extract.

Scientific Names
Black catechu: Acacia catechu.
Family: Leguminosae or Fabaceae.
Pale catechu: Uncaria gambier.
Family: Rubiaceae.

People Use This For
Orally, catechu is used for diarrhea (6,9,11), chronic mucous membrane inflammation, dysentery, colitis, bleeding (18), and cancer (11). Catechu is used orally in some parts of the world as an anti-fertility drug (214).
Topically, catechu is used for skin diseases, hemorrhoids, traumatic injuries, to stop bleeding, and for dressing wounds.
Catechu is included in mouthwashes and gargles for gingivitis, stomatitis, pharyngitis, and oral ulcers (11,18).
In Chinese medicine, black catechu is used to treat indigestion in children (11).
In foods and beverages, catechu is used as a flavoring agent (11).
Catechu is used in some parts of the world as an anti-fertility drug (214).

Safety
LIKELY SAFE ...when used orally in amounts found in foods (maximum use level 0.016%); approved for use in foods in US (11).
POSSIBLY UNSAFE ...when used as a medicinal. Catechu contains tannins with possible carcinogenic and hepatotoxic properties (11). Another constituent, (+)-catechin (cianidanol), is associated with fatal hemolytic anemia (9). There is insufficient reliable information available about the safety of the topical use of catechu.
PREGNANCY AND LACTATION: POSSIBLY UNSAFE; avoid using.

Effectiveness
There is insufficient reliable information available about the effectiveness of catechu.

Mechanism of Action

Both black and pale catechu are applicable. Researchers think the astringent and antibacterial properties of catechu result from its high tannin content (11). Gambrine (in pale catechu) has hypotensive effects (11). D-catechin (in black and pale catechu) causes blood vessel constriction (11). Fisetin (in black catechu) and (+)-catechin (in black and pale catechu) and may protect against liver damage; (+)-catechin (cianidanol) is also thought to protect against experimentally-induced ulcers in animals (11); (+)-catechin (cianidanol) is associated with fatal hemolytic anemia (9).

Adverse Reactions

None reported.

Interactions with Herbs & Other Dietary Supplements

Insufficient reliable information available.

Interactions with Drugs

No interactions are known to occur, and there is no known reason to expect a clinically significant interaction with catechu.

Interactions with Foods

No interactions are known to occur, and there is no known reason to expect a clinically significant interaction with catechu.

Interactions with Lab Tests

No interactions are known to occur, and there is no known reason to expect a clinically significant interaction with catechu.

Interactions with Diseases or Conditions

No interactions are known to occur, and there is no known reason to expect a clinically significant interaction with catechu.

Dosage and Administration

ORAL: Typical dose ranges 0.3-2 grams three times daily, or a single 500 mg dose (18).
TOPICAL: Catechu tincture, 20 drops in a glass of lukewarm water (mouth rinse) or applied undiluted with a toothbrush has been used (18).

Comments

Though black catechu and pale catechu differ somewhat chemically, they are used for the same purposes at the same dose (11). Unstandardized products may contain high amounts of aflatoxin, a metabolite of Aspergillus, which is toxic and may lead to certain cancers.

CATNIP

Also Known As

Catmint, Catnep, Catswort, Field Balm.

Scientific Names

Nepeta cataria.
Family: Labiatae/Lamiaceae.

People Use This For

Orally, catnip is used for insomnia; migraine headaches; cold; flu; fever; hives; and gastrointestinal upset, including indigestion, colic, cramping, and flatulence (5,6). It has also been used orally for conditions associated with anxiety, diuresis, as a tonic (6), for upper respiratory tract infections, and headaches (6121).
Topically, catnip has been used for arthritis, hemorrhoids, and as a poultice to relieve swelling (6).
In folk medicine, catnip has also been used for lung and uterine congestion, eradicating worms, and for initiating menses in girls with delayed onset of menstruation (6). Catnip is smoked for respiratory conditions and recreationally for inducing a euphoric high (6).
Catnip has been used as a pesticide and insecticide (6).

Safety

POSSIBLY SAFE …when used orally and appropriately (6,12). Significant adverse effects have not been reported when catnip tea is used in cupful amounts (6).

POSSIBLY UNSAFE …when used orally in excessive doses. Higher doses may be associated with significant adverse effects (6). …when inhaled by smoking dried leaves. Smoking the dried leaves of catnip has been associated with a euphoric high (6), which might impair judgment; however, whether catnip can truly produce this effect in humans remains controversial (6).

There is insufficient reliable information available about the safety of topically applied catnip.

CHILDREN: POSSIBLY UNSAFE …when used orally. One child developed stomach pain and irritability followed by lethargy and hypnotic state after ingesting catnip leaves and tea (5,2596).

PREGNANCY: LIKELY UNSAFE …when used orally. Catnip tea has been reported to have uterine stimulant properties (12); contraindicated.

LACTATION: Insufficient reliable information available; avoid using.

Effectiveness

There is insufficient reliable information available about the effectiveness of catnip.

Mechanism of Action

The applicable part of catnip is the flowering tops. The pharmacological effect that catnip is famous for is the euphoric state it induces in cats. It is thought that the constituent cis-trans-nepetalcatone produces the characteristic stimulation in cats only when they smell it (5). Although humans have used catnip to induce a euphoric high, whether or not this effect actually occurs in humans is controversial. In humans, the constituent nepetalactone is thought to be responsible for catnip's calming effects in insomnia, anxiety, gastrointestinal conditions, and migraine headache. Nepetalactone is the major component (80-95%) of the volatile oil of catnip and is structurally related to the valepotriates found in valerian. Catnip provides approximately 0.2-1% volatile oil. Catnip reportedly also has antipyretic and diaphoretic effects, which have been attributed to its use for colds, flu, and fever. Other reported pharmacological effects, include diuretic and stimulation of gallbladder activity (6).

Adverse Reactions

Catnip abuse may result in headache and malaise. Large amounts of tea may cause vomiting (6). One case report exists of a nineteen-month-old child who developed a stomachache and irritability, followed by lethargy and a hypnotic state after ingesting raisins soaked in catnip tea and chewing on the tea bag (5,2596).

Interactions with Herbs & Other Dietary Supplements

HERBS WITH SEDATIVE PROPERTIES: Theoretically, concomitant use with herbs that have sedative properties might enhance therapeutic and adverse effects. These include calamus, calendula, California poppy, capsicum, celery, couch grass, elecampane, Siberian ginseng, German chamomile, goldenseal, gotu kola, hops, Jamaican dogwood, kava, lemon balm, sage, St. John's wort, sassafras, scullcap, shepherd's purse, stinging nettle, valerian, wild carrot, wild lettuce, ashwaganda root, and yerba mansa (4,19).

Interactions with Drugs

BARBITURATES: Theoretically, concomitant use with barbiturates may cause additive effects and side effects (19).
OTHER DRUGS WITH SEDATIVE PROPERTIES: Theoretically, concomitant use with drugs with sedative properties may cause additive effects and side effects (19).

Interactions with Foods

No interactions are known to occur, and there is no known reason to expect a clinically significant interaction with catnip.

Interactions with Lab Tests

No interactions are known to occur, and there is no known reason to expect a clinically significant interaction with catnip.

Interactions with Diseases or Conditions

PELVIC INFLAMMATORY DISEASE (PID) AND EXCESSIVE MENSTRUAL BLEEDING: Because catnip is also used to stimulate menstruation, theoretically it is contraindicated in pelvic inflammatory disease (PID) and excessive menstrual bleeding (12).

Dosage and Administration

ORAL: People typically use two 380 mg capsules three times daily at meals or prepared as a tea using 1 to 2 teaspoons in 6 ounces of boiling water (6006).

Comments
Today, in the US, catnip tea is still commonly used in Appalachia for many of the traditional uses (6).

CATUABA

Also Known As
Caramuru, Catuaba Casca, Chuchuhuasha, Golden Trumpet, Pau De Reposta, Piratancara, Tatuaba.

Scientific Names
Erythroxylum catuaba.
Family: Erythroxylaceae.

People Use This For
Orally, catuaba is used as an aphrodisiac, for male sexual impotency, agitation, exhaustion and fatigue, insomnia related to hypertension, nervousness, neurasthenia, poor memory or forgetfulness, as a tonic (3918), and for skin cancer (513).

Safety
There is insufficient reliable information available about the safety of catuaba.
Pregnancy and Lactation: Insufficient reliable information available; avoid using.

Effectiveness
There is insufficient reliable information available about the effectiveness of catuaba.

Mechanism of Action
The applicable part of catuaba is the bark. An alkaline catuaba extract shows antibacterial effects in mice. It also inhibits the human immunodeficiency virus (HIV) in vitro (3916).

Adverse Reactions
None reported.

Interactions with Herbs & Other Dietary Supplements
Insufficient reliable information available.

Interactions with Drugs
No interactions are known to occur, and there is no known reason to expect a clinically significant interaction with catuaba.

Interactions with Foods
No interactions are known to occur, and there is no known reason to expect a clinically significant interaction with catuaba.

Interactions with Lab Tests
No interactions are known to occur, and there is no known reason to expect a clinically significant interaction with catuaba.

Interactions with Diseases or Conditions
No interactions are known to occur, and there is no known reason to expect a clinically significant interaction with catuaba.

Dosage and Administration
ORAL: People typically use 450 mg daily (5262).

Comments
Some think that Juniperus brasiliensis is a synonym for Erythroxylum catuaba (Family: Erythroxylaceae) (3918); however, Juniperus genus plants are classified as members of the Cupressaceae plant family (513,815).
There is very little scientific information about this product. Our staff is continually analyzing the available information on natural medicines and will add data here as it becomes available.

CEDAR leaf

Also Known As
American Arborvitae, Arborvitae, Eastern Arborvitae, Eastern White Cedar, Hackmatack, Northern White Cedar, Swamp Cedar, Thuga, Thuja, Tree of Life, White Cedar.
CAUTION: See separate listings for Cedar Leaf Oil, Cedarwood Oil, and Cedarwood bark, berry, leaf, seed, twig.

Scientific Names
Thuja occidentalis.
Family: Cupressaceae.

People Use This For
Orally, cedar leaf is used to treat respiratory tract infections, in conjunction with antibiotics for bacterial skin infections and herpes simplex, for bronchitis, rheumatism, trigeminal neuralgia, and strep throat. It is also used as an abortifacient (18).
Topically, cedar leaf is used to manage joint pain, arthritis, and muscle rheumatism (18).

Safety
LIKELY SAFE ...when used orally in amounts found in foods; approved for use in foods in the US, if thujone-free (12).
POSSIBLY SAFE ...when used orally as a medicinal for occasional use in recommended amounts (12); not for long-term use.
There is insufficient reliable information available about the safety of cedar leaf for its other uses.
PREGNANCY: UNSAFE ...when used orally due to abortifacient activity (12); avoid using.
LACTATION: Insufficient reliable information available; avoid using.

Effectiveness
There is insufficient reliable information available about the effectiveness of cedar leaf.

Mechanism of Action
Cedar leaf is reported to be a urinary irritant (19), a uterine stimulant, and affect menstrual cycle (12). Thujone, a constituent, is a neurotoxin that can cause convulsions (1304). The glycoprotein and polysaccharide fractions have been used therapeutically (18). Some evidence suggests the polysaccharides might have antiviral and immunostimulating (1305) properties, and might inhibit HIV-1-specific antigens and reverse transcriptase activity (1306).

Adverse Reactions
Orally, symptoms of overdose include queasiness, vomiting, painful diarrhea, and mucous membrane hemorrhage. Deaths have been reported (18). Other side effects include asthma, CNS stimulation, and seizures (214).

Interactions with Herbs & Other Dietary Supplements
THUJONE CONTAINING HERBS: Avoid; concomitant use may increase the risk of thujone toxicity. Thujone-containing herbs include: oak moss (12), oriental arborvitae (12), sage (2,4,12), tansy (2,4,12), tree moss (12), and wormwood (2,12).

Interactions with Drugs
ANTI-CONVULSANTS: Cedar leaf may lower the seizure threshold in those individuals taking anti-convulsants (214).

Interactions with Foods
No interactions are known to occur, and there is no known reason to expect a clinically significant interaction with cedar leaf.

Interactions with Lab Tests
No interactions are known to occur, and there is no known reason to expect a clinically significant interaction with cedar leaf.

Interactions with Diseases or Conditions
GI CONDITIONS: Cedar leaf can irritate gastrointestinal tract. Contraindicated in individuals with infectious or inflammatory gastrointestinal conditions (19).

Dosage and Administration
ORAL: The typical dose of liquid extract (unspecified concentration) is 2-4 mL only for occasional use (12).
TOPICAL: No typical dosage.

Comments
CAUTION: Do not confuse with other Thuja species.

CEDAR LEAF OIL

Also Known As
American Arborvitae, Arborvitae, Eastern Arborvitae, Eastern White Cedar, Hackmatack, Northern White Cedar, Swamp Cedar, Thuja, Thuja Oil, Tree of Life, White Cedar.
CAUTION: See separate listings for Cedar Leaf, Cedarwood Oil, and Cedarwood.

Scientific Names
Thuja occidentalis.
Family: Cupressaceae.
CAUTION: Do not confuse with other Thuja species.

People Use This For
Orally, cedar leaf oil is used as an immune stimulant, expectorant, and diuretic (11).
Topically, cedar leaf oil is used to treat skin diseases, condyloma, cancers, as an insect repellent, and as a counterirritant to treat warts (11).
In foods and beverages, cedar leaf oil is used as a flavoring (11).
In manufacturing, cedar leaf oil is used as a fragrance in cosmetics and soaps (11).

Safety
LIKELY SAFE ...when used orally in amounts found in foods (maximum use level 0.002% in condiments and relishes); approved for food use in the US if thujone-free (11).
POSSIBLY SAFE ...when used topically. It is used in perfumes at concentrations of less than 0.4% (11).
UNSAFE ...when used orally for medicinal use (11). A constituent, thujone, is a neurotoxin (1304).
PREGNANCY: UNSAFE ...when used orally or topically due to toxicity and uterine stimulant activity (11); avoid using.
LACTATION: UNSAFE ...when used orally or topically due to toxicity (11); avoid using.

Effectiveness
There is insufficient reliable information available about the effectiveness of cedar leaf oil.

Mechanism of Action
Thujone, a constituent of cedar leaf oil, is a neurotoxin that can cause convulsions (1304). Polysaccharides have demonstrated in vitro antiviral, immunostimulating (1305), inhibition of HIV-1-specific antigens and reverse transcriptase activity (1306).

Adverse Reactions
Orally, use of cedar leaf oil can result in poisoning. Symptoms of thujone poisoning include hypotension, convulsion, and death (11). Other side effects include asthma, CNS stimulation, and seizures (214).

Interactions with Herbs & Other Dietary Supplements
THUJONE CONTAINING HERBS: Avoid; concomitant use may increase the risk of thujone toxicity.
Thujone-containing herbs include: oak moss (12), oriental arborvitae (12), sage (2,4,12), tansy (2,4,12), tree moss (12), and wormwood (2,12).

Interactions with Drugs
ANTI-CONVULSANTS: Cedar leaf oil may lower the threshold in those individuals taking anti-convulsants (214).

Interactions with Foods
No interactions are known to occur, and there is no known reason to expect a clinically significant interaction with cedar leaf oil.

Interactions with Lab Tests

No interactions are known to occur, and there is no known reason to expect a clinically significant interaction with cedar leaf oil.

Interactions with Diseases or Conditions

No interactions are known to occur, and there is no known reason to expect a clinically significant interaction with cedar leaf oil.

Dosage and Administration

ORAL: People typically use 2 to 4 mL of the liquid extract (5263).
TOPICAL: No typical dosage.

Comments

Avoid confusion with cedar leaf, cedarwood oil, cedarwood bark/berry/seed/stem, and other Thuja species. Cedar leaf oil is produced by steam distillation of Thuja occidentalis leaves and twigs (11).

CEDARWOOD bark, berry, leaf, seed, twig

Also Known As

Ashe Juniper, Cedar, Eastern Red Cedar, Red Cedarwood, Red Juniper, Texas Cedarwood, Virginia Cedarwood.
CAUTION: See separate listings for Cedar Leaf Oil, Cedar leaf, and Cedarwood Oil.

Scientific Names

Juniperus virginiana.
Family: Cupressaceae.

People Use This For

In traditional folk medicine, cedarwood has been used for cough, bronchitis, rheumatism, venereal warts, and skin rash (11).

Safety

POSSIBLY SAFE ...when the berry or leaf is used orally (12).
There is insufficient reliable information available about the safety of the oral or topical use of the bark, seed or twig.
PREGNANCY AND LACTATION: LIKELY UNSAFE ...when used orally. Virginia cedarwood berry or leaf is contraindicated in pregnancy (12). There is insufficient reliable information available about the safety of the oral or topical use of cedarwood bark, seed, or twig; avoid using.

Effectiveness

There is insufficient reliable information available about the effectiveness of cedarwood.

Mechanism of Action

Steam distillation of Virginia cedarwood produces an oil that contains alpha- and beta-cedrene, cedrol, and cedreol. It also contains the toxic constituent thujone (11).

Adverse Reactions

None reported.

Interactions with Herbs & Other Dietary Supplements

THUJONE CONTAINING HERBS: Avoid; concomitant use may increase the risk of thujone toxicity. Thujone-containing herbs include: oak moss (12), oriental arborvitae (12), sage (2,4,12), tansy (2,4,12), tree moss (12), and wormwood (2,12).

Interactions with Drugs

BARBITURATES: Theoretically, inhaling red cedar chip fragrance might reduce efficacy of hexobarbital or pentobarbital (19).
DICOUMAROL: Theoretically, inhaling red cedar chip fragrance might reduce efficacy of dicoumarol (19).

Interactions with Foods

No interactions are known to occur, and there is no known reason to expect a clinically significant interaction with cedarwood bark, berry, leaf, seed, and twig.

Interactions with Lab Tests

No interactions are known to occur, and there is no known reason to expect a clinically significant interaction with cedarwood bark, berry, leaf, seed, and twig.

Interactions with Diseases or Conditions

No interactions are known to occur, and there is no known reason to expect a clinically significant interaction with cedarwood bark, berry, leaf, seed, and twig.

Dosage and Administration

No typical dosage.

Comments

Avoid confusion with cedarwood oil.

CEDARWOOD OIL

Also Known As

None.
CAUTION: See separate listings for Cedar Leaf, Cedar Leaf Oil, and Cedarwood bark, berry, leaf, seed, twig.

Scientific Names

Juniperus mexicana (Cedarwood Oil Texas); Juniperus virginiana (Cedarwood Oil Virginia).
Family: Cupressaceae.
Cedrus atlantica (Cedarwood Oil Atlas).
Family: Pinaceae.

People Use This For

Topically, cedarwood oil is used for alopecia areata. It is also used topically as an insect repellent.
In manufacturing, cedarwood oils are used as fragrance or fixatives in cosmetics, soaps, and perfumes (11).

Safety

POSSIBLY SAFE ...when used topically and appropriately. Cedarwood oil has been used safely for up to 7 months (5177). The maximum use level in perfumes is 0.8%.
PREGNANCY AND LACTATION: Insufficient reliable information available; avoid using.

Effectiveness

POSSIBLY EFFECTIVE ...when used topically in combination with other essential oils for alopecia areata. Cedarwood oil in combination with the essential oils from thyme, lavender, and rosemary seem to improve hair growth by 44% after 7 months of treatment (5177).
There is insufficient reliable information available about the effectiveness of cedarwood oil for its other uses.

Mechanism of Action

Steam distillation of Virginia cedarwood produces an oil that contains alpha- and beta-cedrene, cedrol, and cedreol. It also contains the constituent thujone (11). It's not clear how cedarwood oil works in alopecia areata, but it may have a stimulatory effect on hair growth (5177). Dermatological studies have shown that all three cedarwood oils (Virginia, Texas, Atlas) are generally non-toxic (11); however, there is other evidence that cedarwood oil (probably Virginia) can produce tumors on mouse skin (11).

Adverse Reactions

There is some evidence that cedarwood oil (Virginia and/or Texas) is an allergenic and is a local irritant (11).

Interactions with Herbs & Other Dietary Supplements

THUJONE CONTAINING HERBS: Avoid; concomitant use may increase the risk of thujone toxicity. Thujone-containing herbs include: oak moss (12), oriental arborvitae (12), sage (2,4,12), tansy (2,4,12), tree moss (12), and wormwood (2,12).

Interactions with Drugs

No interactions are known to occur, and there is no known reason to expect a clinically significant interaction with cedarwood oil.

Interactions with Foods

No interactions are known to occur, and there is no known reason to expect a clinically significant interaction with cedarwood oil.

Interactions with Lab Tests

No interactions are known to occur, and there is no known reason to expect a clinically significant interaction with cedarwood oil.

Interactions with Diseases or Conditions

No interactions are known to occur, and there is no known reason to expect a clinically significant interaction with cedarwood oil.

Dosage and Administration

TOPICAL: For the treatment of alopecia areata, a combination of the essential oils including cedarwood 2 drops or 94 mg, rosemary 3 drops or 114 mg, thyme 2 drops or 88 mg, and lavender 3 drops or 108 mg, all mixed with 3 mL jojoba oil and 20 mL grapeseed oil has been used. Each night, the mixture is massaged into the scalp for 2 minutes with a warm towel placed around the head to increase absorption (5177).

Comments

There are several cedarwood oils with different physical and chemical properties, each produced by steam distillation of wood from various trees. The most common are: cedarwood oil Virginia (synonym cedar oil, red cedarwood oil), cedarwood oil Atlas (synonym cedarwood oil Moroccan), cedarwood oil Texas. Avoid confusion with cedar leaf, cedar leaf oil, cedarwood bark/berry/leaf/seed/twig.

CELERY

Also Known As

Ache des Marais, Apii Fructus, Celery Fruit, Celery Seed, Fruit de Celeri, Smallage, Selleriefruchte, Selleriesamen.

Scientific Names

Apium graveolens.
Family: Umbelliferae/Apiaceae.

People Use This For

Orally, celery is used to treat rheumatism, gout, hysteria, nervousness, headache, weight loss due to malnutrition, loss of appetite, and exhaustion (2). Celery is also used as a sedative (4), mild diuretic, urinary antiseptic (4,6), digestive aid, menstrual stimulant, antiflatulent, aphrodisiac, to reduce lactation (6), for regulating bowel movements, stimulating glands, and for blood purification.
In Oriental medicine, celery is used to treat headaches (6).

Safety

LIKELY SAFE ...when the oil or seeds are consumed in amounts found in foods. Celery seed has Generally Recognized as Safe (GRAS) status in the US. The maximum use of celery seed oil in food is 0.005% in condiments and relishes (11).
POSSIBLY SAFE ...when used orally and appropriately in medicinal amounts (12).
PREGNANCY: LIKELY SAFE ...when consumed in food amounts. LIKELY UNSAFE ...when the oil or seeds are used orally in larger amounts, because they might have uterine stimulant or abortifacient effects (4,19).
LACTATION: LIKELY SAFE ...when consumed in food amounts. There is insufficient reliable information available about the safety of larger amounts of celery during lactation.

Effectiveness

There is insufficient reliable information available about the effectiveness of celery.

Mechanism of Action

The applicable parts of celery are the fruit and seed. Sedative, diuretic, and antispasmodic effects of celery seed could be due to phthalide constituents (d-limonene, selinene, and related phthalides) (4,6). Plant extracts have hypotensive and hypoglycemic effects (4). In preliminary research, five of 23 celery-based preparations show antiarthritis effects, but no anti-inflammatory or antipyretic effects. The celery seed activity is thought to be dependent on processing at low temperatures (6131). Another constituent, apiogenin, shows evidence of antiplatelet activity. The essential oil can increase kidney inflammation by irritating epithelial tissue (8). Celery juice has been reported to show bile stimulating activity (4). Celery seed oil has shown bacteriostatic effects (4). Celery also contains the furocoumarins bergapten and celereodise, a dihydrofurocoumarin glycoside (isoquercitrin), and the coumarin glycoside apiumoside (6). Celery is a rich plant source of calcium, magnesium, and iron (19).

Adverse Reactions
Celery can cause contact dermatitis (19). Allergic and anaphylactic reactions have also been documented (4,6). Cross-allergenicity is possible between celery and pollen, carrots, dandelion, or wild carrot (4,6). Consuming large amounts of celery seed oil can induce CNS depression (6). Contact with celery stems could lead to photosensitivity (4).

Interactions with Herbs & Other Dietary Supplements
HERBS WITH SEDATIVE PROPERTIES: Theoretically, concomitant use with herbs that have sedative properties might enhance therapeutic and adverse effects. These include calamus, calendula, California poppy, catnip, capsicum, couch grass, elecampane, Siberian ginseng, German chamomile, goldenseal, gotu kola, hops, Jamaican dogwood, kava, lemon balm, sage, St. John's wort, sassafras, scullcap, shepherd's purse, stinging nettle, valerian, wild carrot, wild lettuce, ashwaganda root, and yerba mansa (4,19).
HERBS WITH ANTICOAGULANT/ANTIPLATELET POTENTIAL: Concomitant use of herbs that have coumarin constituents or affect platelet aggregation could theoretically increase the risk of bleeding in some people. These herbs include: angelica, anise, arnica, asafoetida, bogbean, boldo, capsicum, chamomile, clove, danshen, fenugreek, feverfew, garlic, ginger, ginkgo, Panax ginseng, horse chestnut, horseradish, licorice, meadowsweet, prickly ash, onion, papain, passionflower, poplar, quassia, red clover, turmeric, wild carrot, wild lettuce, willow, and others (4,19).

Interactions with Drugs
ANTICOAGULANTS AND ANTIPLATELET DRUGS: Theoretically, celery can potentiate the effects of these drugs.
DRUGS WITH SEDATIVE PROPERTIES: Theoretically, concomitant use with these drugs may cause additive effects (4).
PUVA: Theoretically, celery might increase the phototoxic response to PUVA therapy due to its psoralen content (6178). Drugs used in PUVA therapy include, methoxsalen (8-methoxypsoralen, 8-MOP, Oxsoralen) and Trioxsalen (Trisoralen).

Interactions with Foods
No interactions are known to occur, and there is no known reason to expect a clinically significant interaction with celery.

Interactions with Lab Tests
No interactions are known to occur, and there is no known reason to expect a clinically significant interaction with celery.

Interactions with Diseases or Conditions
KIDNEY CONDITIONS: Contraindicated in kidney disorders; celery might increase inflammation (8).

Dosage and Administration
ORAL: People typically use 0.5-2 grams of dried fruit three times daily, or one cup prepared tea (simmer 1 gram of fresh crushed dried fruit in 150 mL boiling water 5-10 minutes, strain) three times daily (4,8).
Liquid extract (1:1 in 60% alcohol) 0.3-1.2 mL three times daily has also been used (4).

Comments
Furocoumarin (a potential carcinogen) content increases 100-fold in injured or diseased celery (6). Celery is available in capsule form, containing 450 or 505 mg of the oil. The ancient Greeks used celery to make wine, which was served as an award at athletic games (214).

CENTAURY

Also Known As
Bitter Herb, Common Centaury, Drug Centaurium, Lesser Centauru, Minor Centaury.

Scientific Names
Centaurium erythraea, synonym Erythraea centaurium; Centaurium minus; Centaurium umbellatum.
Family: Gentianaceae.

People Use This For
Traditionally, centaury is used orally for anorexia and dyspepsia (4).
In beverages, it is used as a flavoring.

Safety
LIKELY SAFE ...when consumed in the very small amounts commonly found in food. Centaury is listed by the Council of Europe as a food flavoring. In the US, it is used in alcoholic and nonalcoholic beverages at maximum-permitted doses between 0.0002% and 0.0008% (4).
POSSIBLY SAFE ...when used orally for medicinal purposes in amounts greater than those found in food (12). There is no documented toxicity (4).
PREGNANCY AND LACTATION: Insufficient reliable information available; avoid the use of centaury in amounts greater than those commonly found in foods.

Effectiveness
POSSIBLY EFFECTIVE ...when used orally for peptic discomfort (2).
There is insufficient reliable information available about the effectiveness of centaury for its other uses.

Mechanism of Action
The applicable parts of centaury are the dried, above ground parts. The bitter constituents amarogentin, gentiopicroside, swertiamarin, and the related bitters (3,7) can act as an appetite stimulant, although with less activity than comparable bitter herbs (4). Its antipyretic activity can result from the phenolic acid constituents. The constituent, gentiopicrin, can have antimalarial properties. Animal evidence suggests that centaury has anti-inflammatory activity (4).

Adverse Reactions
None reported.

Interactions with Herbs & Other Dietary Supplements
Insufficient reliable information available.

Interactions with Drugs
No interactions are known to occur, and there is no known reason to expect a clinically significant interaction with centaury.

Interactions with Foods
No interactions are known to occur, and there is no known reason to expect a clinically significant interaction with centaury.

Interactions with Lab Tests
No interactions are known to occur, and there is no known reason to expect a clinically significant interaction with centaury.

Interactions with Diseases or Conditions
No interactions are known to occur, and there is no known reason to expect a clinically significant interaction with centaury.

Dosage and Administration
ORAL: The typical dose of centaury is 2-4 grams or as a tea three times daily. The tea is prepared by steeping 2-4 grams in 150 mL boiling water (4). The average daily dose of centaury is 6 grams (2). The usual dose of the liquid extract (1:1 in 25% alcohol) is 2-4 mL three times daily (4).

Comments
None.

CEREUS

Also Known As
Night Blooming Cereus, Sweet Scented Cactus.

Scientific Names
Selenicereus grandiflorus, synonyms Cereus grandiflorus, Cactus grandiflorus.
Family: Cactaceae.

People Use This For
Orally, cereus is used for angina pectoris (18), edema associated with weak heart function (4), and as a cardiac stimulant (sometimes instead of digitalis). Cereus is also used orally for urinary ailments (18).
In folk medicine, cereus is used orally for hemoptysis, menorrhagia, dysmenorrhea, hemorrhage, cystitis, and shortness of breath (18); and topically as a skin stimulant for rheumatism (18).

Safety
POSSIBLY SAFE ...when the flower or stem are used orally for non-cardiac conditions (12). Although it contains cactine, which may have a digitalis-like effect, there are no reports of human toxicity (12).
POSSIBLY UNSAFE ...when used orally to self-medicate cardiac conditions.
There is insufficient reliable information available about the safety of cereus for its other uses.
PREGNANCY AND LACTATION: Insufficient reliable information available; avoid using.

Effectiveness
There is insufficient reliable information available about the effectiveness of cereus.

Mechanism of Action
The applicable parts of cereus are the flower, stem, and young shoots. There is some evidence that cereus can stimulate the heart and dilate peripheral vessels (18), as well as stimulate spinal cord motor neurons (18). Researchers think tyramine, a cardiotonic amine, can strengthen heart muscle action (4). The reputed digitalis effect of cereus is claimed to be non-cumulative (12).

Adverse Reactions
Orally, fresh cereus juice may cause burning of the mouth, queasiness, nausea, vomiting, and diarrhea (4,18).
Topically, it may cause itching and skin pustules (18).

Interactions with Herbs & Other Dietary Supplements
Insufficient reliable information available.

Interactions with Drugs
MONOAMINE OXIDASE INHIBITORS (MAOIs): Theoretically, excessive doses of cereus may interact with MAOIs, because of the tyramine content (4).
CARDIAC GLYCOSIDES: Cereus may potentiate the actions of cardiac glycosides such as digoxin, and may enhance the effect of other cardiac drugs (214).

Interactions with Foods
No interactions are known to occur, and there is no known reason to expect a clinically significant interaction with cereus.

Interactions with Lab Tests
No interactions are known to occur, and there is no known reason to expect a clinically significant interaction with cereus.

Interactions with Diseases or Conditions
HEART CONDITIONS: Theoretically, cereus may affect individuals with existing heart conditions or interfere with therapy (4).

Dosage and Administration
ORAL: Typical doses are fluid extract (1:1) 0.6 mL one to ten times daily (4,18), tincture of cereus (1:10) 0.12-2 mL two to three times daily (4,18), or tincture in sweetened water (1:10) 10 drops three to five times daily (18). Should not be used as self-medication for cardiac conditions.

Comments
None.

CETYL MYRISTOLEATE

Also Known As
Cerasomal-cis-9-cetylmyristoleate, Cetylmyristoleate, CM, CMO.

Scientific Names
Cis-9-cetylmyristoleate.

People Use This For
Orally, cetyl myristoleate is used for rheumatoid arthritis, osteoarthritis, systemic lupus erythematosus, multiple sclerosis, ankylosing spondylitis, Reiter's syndrome, Behcet's syndrome, Sjogren's syndrome, psoriasis, fibromyalgia, emphysema, benign prostate hyperplasia (BPH), silicone breast disease, leukemia and other cancers, and relief of various types of back pain.

Safety
There is insufficient reliable information available about the safety of cetyl myristoleate.
Pregnancy and Lactation: Insufficient reliable information available; avoid using.

Effectiveness
There is insufficient reliable information available about the effectiveness of cetyl myristoleate.

Mechanism of Action
Cetyl myristoleate is a substance isolated from mice that are immune to chemically-induced arthritis (677). Researchers hypothesize that cetyl myristoleate has surfactant effects. They think cetyl myristoleate might cause lubrication of joints and muscles, softening of tissues, and increased pliability. They theorize that cetyl myristoleate might also be a modulator of the immune system and a mediator of inflammatory process. So far, the evidence to back these theories is sketchy.

Adverse Reactions
None reported.

Interactions with Herbs & Other Dietary Supplements
Insufficient reliable information available.

Interactions with Drugs
METHOTREXATE: Cetyl myristoleate may interfere with methotrexate absorption; avoid concomitant use.
STEROIDS: Cetyl myristoleate may interfere with steroid therapy; avoid concomitant use.
ALCOHOL: Alcohol may interact with cetyl myristoleate; avoid concomitant use.

Interactions with Foods
No interactions are known to occur, and there is no known reason to expect a clinically significant interaction with cetyl myristoleate.

Interactions with Lab Tests
No interactions are known to occur, and there is no known reason to expect a clinically significant interaction with cetyl myristoleate.

Interactions with Diseases or Conditions
No interactions are known to occur, and there is no known reason to expect a clinically significant interaction with cetyl myristoleate.

Dosage and Administration
No typical dosage.

Comments
There is very little scientific information about this product. Our staff is continually analyzing the available information on natural medicines and will add data here as it becomes available.

CHANCA PIEDRA

Also Known As

Chanca-Piedra Blanca, Chancapiedra, Child Pick-a-Back, Derriere Dos, Derrière-Dos, Des Dos, Dukong Anak, Feuilles la Fievre, Memeniran, Meniran, Niruri, Pitirishi, Quebra Pedra, Quebrapedra, Quinina Criolla, Quinine Créole, Rami Buah, Sacha Foster, Sasha Foster, Seed on the Leaf, Shatter Stone, Stone Breaker, Stonebreaker, Tamalaka, Turi Hutan.

Scientific Names

Phyllanthus niruri.
Family: Euphorbiaceae.

People Use This For

Orally, chanca piedra is used for urinary tract infections and inflammation (518,3918), kidney stones (517), urethral or vaginal mucous discharge (517,3919), as a diuretic (3913), an antiflatulent (517,3919), aperitif, appetite stimulant (517,3919), liver tonic, and blood purifier. It is also used orally for diabetes (3913), gallstones (517), colic (517,3919), stomachache (3913), dyspepsia (517,3919), intestinal infections (3923), constipation, dysentery, flu (3913), tenesmus (517,3918), jaundice (3913), hepatitis B (3923), abdominal tumors (3913), fever, pain, venereal problems (3913), syphilis, gonorrhea (517,3919), malaria, tumors (3913), caterpillar stings, cough, edema, itching, miscarriage, rectitis, tremors, typhoid, vaginitis, anemia, asthma, bronchitis, thirst, tuberculosis, and vertigo (3918).

Safety

There is insufficient reliable information available about the safety of chanca piedra.
Pregnancy and Lactation: Insufficient reliable information available; avoid using.

Effectiveness

POSSIBLY INEFFECTIVE ...when used orally for treating hepatitis B (3924,3925).
There is insufficient reliable information available about the effectiveness of chanca piedra for its other uses.

Mechanism of Action

Chanca piedra is thought to have multiple properties; antispasmodic, antiviral, bactericidal, antipyretic, and diuretic. It is also thought that chanca piedra reduces blood sugar and protects the liver (517); however, not all of these properties are supported by scientific evidence. In vitro, the constituent niuriside, inhibits specific HIV-protein binding activity, but does not protect cells from acute HIV infection (3927). In isolated animal tissue, an extract from the related plant, Phyllanthus sellowianus, has antispasmodic activity (3921). Preliminary studies in humans show the related species, Phyllanthus amarus, has diuretic, hypotensive and hypoglycemic effects (3928).

Adverse Reactions

None reported.

Interactions with Herbs & Other Dietary Supplements

Insufficient reliable information available.

Interactions with Drugs

DIABETES THERAPY: Monitor blood glucose level closely due to claims that chanca piedra has hypoglycemic effects (19).

Interactions with Foods

No interactions are known to occur, and there is no known reason to expect a clinically significant interaction with chanca piedra.

Interactions with Lab Tests

No interactions are known to occur, and there is no known reason to expect a clinically significant interaction with chanca piedra.

Interactions with Diseases or Conditions

No interactions are known to occur, and there is no known reason to expect a clinically significant interaction with chanca piedra.

Dosage and Administration

ORAL: People typically use 1 to 2 grams of powdered herb in tablets or capsules twice daily. Chanca piedra is also taken as a 4:1 tincture in a dose of 1 to 3 mL twice daily (5255).

Comments

Older studies published in India were reportedly conducted with Phyllanthus niruri, which is thought to be indigenous to the West Indies (514). A report from India mentions Phyllanthus niruri is a synonym for Phyllanthus amarus (3928); however, these appear to be different species (513,816).

CHAPARRAL

Also Known As

Creosote Bush, Greasewood, Hediondilla.

Scientific Names

Larrea divaricata; Larrea tridentata.
Family: Zygophyllaceae.

People Use This For

Orally, chaparral is used for arthritis, cancer, venereal disease, tuberculosis, bowel cramps, colds (4), and chronic cutaneous disorders (3497). It is also used orally for weight loss (3497).

Historically, chaparral has been used as a tonic, antiparasitic, antiflatulent, "blood purifier" for genitourinary and respiratory tract infections, and a treatment for musculoskeletal inflammation, skin diseases, GI conditions, CNS conditions (11), chickenpox and snakebite pain (3497).

Safety

LIKELY UNSAFE ...when used orally; avoid using. There are reports of serious poisoning, acute hepatitis, kidney and liver damage, and irreversible renohepatic failure (4).

PREGNANCY AND LACTATION: LIKELY UNSAFE ...when used orally due to demonstrated in vitro uteroactivity in addition to reported toxicity (4).

Effectiveness

There is insufficient reliable information available about the effectiveness of chaparral (4,6,11).

Mechanism of Action

Nordihydroguaiaretic acid (NDGA), a constituent of chaparral, may have antioxidant properties (4). Chaparral is thought to have analgesic, expectorant, emetic, diuretic, and anti-inflammatory properties (5). Reports of antimutagenic and anticarcinogenic activity are largely based on an observation in one patient (11). Theorized anticancer effects are thought to result from blocking of cellular respiration by NDGA (6).

Adverse Reactions

Orally, jaundice, fatigue, abdominal pain (right upper quadrant), dark urine, light stools, nausea, diarrhea, weight loss, fever, anorexia, increased serum liver enzyme levels (alkaline phosphatase, alanine aminotransferase, aspartate aminotransferase, total bilirubin, gamma-glutamyltransferase, lactate dehydrogenase), cirrhosis, cholestasis, cholangitis (3497), acute hepatitis, kidney and liver failure (4,3497) and mesenteric lymph node lesions have been reported (6). There are multiple reports of hepatotoxicity, including at least two requiring liver transplant (568,569,570,571,3497).

Topically, chaparral can cause contact dermatitis (4).

Interactions with Herbs & Other Dietary Supplements

Insufficient reliable information available.

Interactions with Drugs

MAO INHIBITORS: Theoretically, excessive amounts may interfere with MAO inhibitor therapy, due to documented amino acid constituents (4).

Interactions with Foods

No interactions are known to occur, and there is no known reason to expect a clinically significant interaction with chaparral.

Interactions with Lab Tests

No interactions are known to occur, and there is no known reason to expect a clinically significant interaction with chaparral.

Interactions with Diseases or Conditions

Theoretically, individuals with impaired liver function or renal function would have increased risk of adverse effects.

Dosage and Administration

No typical dosage.

Comments

Anecdotal reports of anticancer effects may justify further testing; however, use may stimulate growth of certain tumors (6). Herp-Eeze is a dietary supplement promoted for preventing and treating herpes infections. The manufacturer states that a patented manufacturing process renders the product nontoxic. However, toxicity information about this product is limited to the manufacturer's claims (267).

CHASTEBERRY

Also Known As

Agnolyt, Agnus Castus, Agnus-Castus, Chaste Berry, Chaste Tree, Chaste Tree Berry, Chastetree, Gattilier, Hemp Tree, Monk's Pepper, Vitex, Vitex Agnus Castus.

Scientific Names

Vitex agnus-castus.
Family: Verbenaceae.

People Use This For

Orally, chasteberry is used for menstrual irregularities including dysmenorrhea, secondary amenorrhea, metrorrhagia, oligomenorrhea, and polymenorrhea. Chasteberry is also used for symptoms of menopause and for symptoms of premenstrual syndrome (PMS) including mastalgia and other symptoms. It is also used orally for acne, female infertility, preventing miscarriage in patients with progesterone insufficiency, fibrocystic breasts, benign prostatic hyperplasia (BPH), reducing sexual desire, and controlling of postpartum bleeding and aiding expulsion of the placenta. Chasteberry is also used orally for increasing lactation, impotence and decreased libido, nervousness, dementia, rheumatic conditions, colds, and dyspepsia.

Safety

LIKELY SAFE ...when used orally and appropriately. Chasteberry has been used safely in studies lasting up to 1.5 years (6500,6557,7055,7076,7077,7078).
PREGNANCY: LIKELY UNSAFE ...when used orally. Chasteberry can have uterine stimulant properties and should be avoided during all stages of pregnancy (12,6557). Some clinicians use chasteberry during the first trimester of pregnancy to prevent miscarriage in patients with progesterone insufficiency (6500). However, because it is not known if chasteberry is helpful or safe in these patients, avoid using.
LACTATION: POSSIBLY UNSAFE ...when used orally. Chasteberry is thought to be a dopamine agonist and inhibit prolactin secretion. This might result in decreased breast milk production (6500). However, this is controversial. Some clinicians actually use low doses of chasteberry to increase milk production with some reports of benefit (6500,6557). Until more is known, avoid using chasteberry in breast-feeding mothers.

Effectiveness

POSSIBLY EFFECTIVE ...when used orally for symptoms of premenstrual syndrome (PMS). Chasteberry seems to decrease some symptoms of PMS, especially breast pain or tenderness (mastalgia), edema, constipation, irritability, depressed mood or mood alterations, anger, and headache (6500,6557,7055,7076,7078,7079). In some patients these symptoms can be decreased by as much as 50% (7055). Chasteberry may not be as effective for symptoms of bloating (7055) or in patients with a specific type of PMS with symptoms consisting mostly of craving sweets, sweating, palpitations, and dizziness (6500). Some evidence suggests that women who have PMS primarily due to low progesterone levels and higher estrogen levels are most likely to respond to treatment with chasteberry (6500,6557). Patients may not respond to therapy immediately. Treatment for 4-12 weeks can be required before there is significant improvement in symptoms (6557). ...when used orally for menstrual disorders. There is some evidence that chasteberry might normalize menstruation in patients with secondary amenorrhea, polymenorrhea (short cycle), oligomenorrhea (infrequent menstruation), and menorrhagia (prolonged menstruation). Chasteberry might be most effective in patients with low levels of progesterone (6500). Use for at least 8 weeks or more is often required before there is significant improvement (6557). ...when used for acne. There is some evidence that chasteberry can significantly improve acne in up to 70% of patients treated. Treatment for at least 6 months is usually required before there is significant improvement (6500). ...when used orally for infertility in women. There is some preliminary clinical evidence that chasteberry can increase the chance of getting pregnant in women who are infertile due to relative progesterone deficiency. But chasteberry does not seem to work quickly. Some researchers suggest it can take from 3-7 months of treatment to achieve pregnancy (6500,7012,7077).

Some clinical studies have used a specific extract of chasteberry (Agnolyt) standardized to contain 6% of the constituent agnoside. In the US, this formulation is found in the brand product Femaprin (Nature's Way).

There is insufficient reliable information available to rate the effectiveness of chasteberry for its other uses. However, there is some preliminary evidence that chasteberry might increase breast milk production in lactating women when used in low doses (6500,7012,7013). More evidence is needed to rate chasteberry for this use.

Mechanism of Action

The applicable part of the chasteberry tree is the fruit. The active constituents of chasteberries are the essential oils, iridoid glycosides, and flavonoids (7012,7013). The primary essential oils consist of limonene, cineol, pinene, and sabinene (7013). The primary flavonoids include casticin, kaempferol, quercetagetin, orientin, and isovitexin (6500,7013). The relevant iridoid glycosides are aucubin and agnoside (6500). Many chasteberry extracts are standardized to contain 6% agnoside. Although not generally considered key constituents, chasteberries also contain several essential fatty acids, including oleic acid, linolenic acid, palmitic acid, and stearic acid (7012). The therapeutic effects of chasteberry have primarily been attributed to its indirect effects on various hormones. Chasteberry's hormonal effects seem to be dose dependent. Lower doses of chasteberry extract of approximately 120 mg per day, are thought to diminish follicle stimulating hormone (FSH) release and increase luteinizing hormone (LH) release, resulting in decreased estrogen levels and increased progesterone and prolactin levels (6500,7013,7016). However, in higher doses of approximately 480 mg per day, chasteberry extract seems to result in decreased prolactin release (6500,7016). Chasteberry extracts contain multiple active constituents that seem to have agonistic effects at dopamine (D2) receptors when used in higher doses. This dopaminergic activity inhibits basal and thyrotropin-releasing hormone (TRH)-stimulated prolactin release (7014,7015), but higher doses of chasteberry do not seem to affect basal or luteinizing-hormone releasing hormone (LHRH)-stimulated gonadotropin release. FSH and LH do not seem to be affected by higher doses of chasteberry (6500,7015,7016). These dose-related effects explain why low dose chasteberry might be beneficial for increasing breast milk production in lactating women, while higher doses likely diminish breast milk production. Chasteberry's effects on prolactin and progesterone have led to its use for conditions in which there may be progesterone deficiencies and hyperprolactinemia such as menstrual irregularities, premenstrual syndrome (PMS), and infertility. Some sources suggest that chasteberry might also be beneficial for patients with acne due to some antiandrogenic effects (6500), but this has not been verified in studies. In fact, chasteberry appears to have no significant effect on testosterone (7016). In addition to hormonal effects, chasteberry also seems to have antibacterial and antifungal effects. Extracts of chasteberry have in vitro activity against Staphylococcus aureus, Streptococcus faecalis, Escherichia coli, Bacillus anthracoides, Candida species, Trichophyton mentagrophytes, Epidermophyton floccosum, Microsporum species, and Penicillium viridicatum (6500).

Adverse Reactions

Orally, chasteberry is usually well tolerated. However, some patients can experience gastrointestinal upset, headache, nausea, itching and urticaria, rash, acne, and intramenstrual bleeding (6500,7055,7076). Some patients have also had alopecia, headaches, tiredness, agitation, tachycardia, and dry mouth while taking chasteberry (6500). Side effects are relatively rare, occurring in approximately 2-5% of patients (6557). Changes in menstrual flow can also occur when chasteberry is first started (6557). Allergic reactions can occur in some patients, but typically resolve spontaneously when chasteberry is stopped.

Interactions with Herbs & Other Dietary Supplements

Insufficient reliable information available.

Interactions with Drugs

DOPAMINE ANTAGONISTS [Antipsychotics, Metoclopramide (Reglan)]: Theoretically, chasteberry might interfere with the action of dopamine antagonists due to dopaminergic effects of chasteberry (7014,7015).

ORAL CONTRACEPTIVES and HORMONE REPLACEMENT THERAPY: Theoretically, chasteberry can interfere with the efficacy of oral contraceptives and hormone replacement therapy because chasteberry seems to have hormone regulating activity (19).

Interactions with Foods

No interactions are known to occur, and there is no known reason to expect a clinically significant interaction with chasteberry.

Interactions with Lab Tests

No interactions are known to occur, and there is no known reason to expect a clinically significant interaction with chasteberry.

Interactions with Diseases or Conditions

HORMONE SENSITIVE CANCERS/CONDITIONS: Because chasteberry seems to have hormonal effects and might affect estrogen levels (6180), women with hormone sensitive conditions should avoid chasteberry. Some of these conditions include breast, uterine, and ovarian cancer, and endometriosis and uterine fibroids.

IN VITRO FERTILIZATION: There is some evidence that using chasteberry during in vitro fertilization procedures might prevent an ensuing pregnancy despite having a viable embryo. In one case, a woman undergoing in vitro fertilization began taking chasteberry. During her fourth in vitro fertilization treatment cycle she was found to have signs of ovarian hyperstimulation syndrome and a viable embryo did not result in pregnancy (6556).

Dosage and Administration

ORAL: For premenstrual syndrome (PMS) and other conditions doses vary considerably. The dosing regimen used depends on the formulation of chasteberry. In one study a specific chasteberry extract (Ze440) 20 mg per day has been used (7055). In a study using a different specific chasteberry extract (Agnolyt), 4 mg daily has been used (7076). Crude herb extracts are typically used in doses of 20-240 mg per day up to 1800 mg per day in 2-3 divided doses (6500,7055). Chasteberry fluid extract 40 drops daily has also been used (6500). Chasteberry fluid extract 40 drops daily has also been used (6500).

Some experts suggest that chasteberry should be taken on an empty stomach and in the morning for the most benefit (6500); however, potential benefits of this administration schedule have not been verified.

Comments

Historians say that monks chewed chaste tree parts to make it easier for them to maintain their celibacy. Progesterone, 17-alpha-hydroxyprogesterone, testosterone, and epitestosterone have been detected in chaste tree flower extract (11). Androstenedione has been detected in chaste tree leaf extract (11).

CHAULMOOGRA

Also Known As

Gynocardia Oil, Hydnocarp, Hydnocarpus, Oleum Chaulmoograe.

Scientific Names

Hydnocarpus species.

People Use This For

Topically, chaulmoogra is used for skin disorders, psoriasis, and eczema (18).
Parenterally, chaulmoogra is used for leprosy (18).

Safety

LIKELY UNSAFE ...when used orally. The seeds are considered very toxic due to their cyanogenic glycoside content (18).
There is insufficient reliable information available about the safety of the topical use of chaulmoogra.
PREGNANCY AND LACTATION: Insufficient reliable information available; avoid using.

Effectiveness

There is insufficient reliable information available about the effectiveness of chaulmoogra; however, chaulmoogra oil has demonstrated efficacy against Mycobacterium leprae in laboratory experiments and in case reports.

Mechanism of Action

The applicable part of chaulmoogra is the seed. Chaulmoogra is thought to have sedative, antipyretic, and skin effects (18). In mice, intraperitoneal and subcutaneous administration of chaulmoogra fatty acids demonstrated antimicrobial activity against Mycobacterium leprae (3826). The cyanogenic glycoside content of the seeds renders them extremely poisonous (18).

Adverse Reactions

Orally, ingestion of the seed can cause cough, dyspnea, laryngospasms, nephrotoxicity, visual disorders, head and muscle pain, and central paralysis (18).
Topically, use can cause skin irritation (18). No adverse effects are reported for parenteral use.

Interactions with Herbs & Other Dietary Supplements

Insufficient reliable information available.

Interactions with Drugs

No interactions are known to occur, and there is no known reason to expect a clinically significant interaction with chaulmoogra.

Interactions with Foods

No interactions are known to occur, and there is no known reason to expect a clinically significant interaction with chaulmoogra.

Interactions with Lab Tests

No interactions are known to occur, and there is no known reason to expect a clinically significant interaction with chaulmoogra.

Interactions with Diseases or Conditions

No interactions are known to occur, and there is no known reason to expect a clinically significant interaction with chaulmoogra.

Dosage and Administration

ORAL: No typical dosage.
TOPICAL: People typically use chaulmoogra as a powder, oil, emulsion, or in ointments.
PARENTERALLY: No typical dosage.

Comments

Chaulmoogra seeds provided the elemental materials for synthesizing the first antileprostatic agents (214).

CHEKEN

Also Known As

Arryan, Chekan, Myrtus.

Scientific Names

Eugenia chequen (dried leaf).

People Use This For

Orally, cheken leaf preparations are used as a tonic, diuretic, and expectorant (18). Preparations of the leaf oil are used orally for hyperlipoproteinemia (18).
In folk medicine, cheken has been used for diarrhea, fever, gout, and as a tonic, diuretic, antihypertensive, and digestive aid (18).

Safety

There is insufficient reliable information available about the safety of cheken.
Pregnancy and Lactation: Insufficient reliable information available; avoid using.

Effectiveness

There is insufficient reliable information available about the effectiveness of cheken.

Mechanism of Action

The applicable parts of cheken are the leaf and leaf oil. The essential oil of the leaf affects fat metabolism. The oil is used to counter hyperlipoproteinemia. It also has antibacterial and antimycotic properties (18).

Adverse Reactions

None reported.

Interactions with Herbs & Other Dietary Supplements

Insufficient reliable information available.

Interactions with Drugs

No interactions are known to occur, and there is no known reason to expect a clinically significant interaction with cheken.

Interactions with Foods

No interactions are known to occur, and there is no known reason to expect a clinically significant interaction with cheken.

Interactions with Lab Tests

No interactions are known to occur, and there is no known reason to expect a clinically significant interaction with cheken.

Interactions with Diseases or Conditions

No interactions are known to occur, and there is no known reason to expect a clinically significant interaction with cheken.

Dosage and Administration

ORAL: People typically use as a liquid extract or as tea (boil the leaves in water for 10-15 minutes; strain) (18).

Comments

There is very little scientific information about this product. Our staff is continually analyzing the available information on natural medicines and will add data here as it becomes available.

CHELATED MINERALS

Also Known As

Chelated Boron, Chelated Calcium, Chelated Chromium, Chelated Cobalt, Chelated Copper, Chelated Iron, Chelated Magnesium, Chelated Manganese, Chelated Molybdenum, Chelated Potassium, Chelated Selenium, Chelated Trace Minerals, Chelated Vanadium, Chelated Zinc.
CAUTION: See separate listings for Aspartates and individual minerals.

Scientific Names

Mineral-amino acid complex.

People Use This For

Orally, chelated minerals are used as dietary mineral supplements (marketed to be more bioavailable than non-chelated minerals) (1163,1164,1165,1166), for supporting normal growth, building strong muscles and bones, improving immune protection, healthy blood, and glowing skin (1163).

Safety

There is insufficient reliable information available about the safety of chelated minerals.
Pregnancy and Lactation: Insufficient reliable information available; avoid using.

Effectiveness

There is insufficient reliable information available about the effectiveness of chelated minerals.

Mechanism of Action

Chelated minerals are marketed to be better absorbed and utilized by the body than non-chelated minerals (1163,1164,1165,1166). However, no evidence supports these claims. Fatty liver-hemorrhagic syndrome is reported in commercial chickens which are fed diets containing chelated minerals (1162).

Adverse Reactions

None reported.

Interactions with Herbs & Other Dietary Supplements

Insufficient reliable information available.

Interactions with Drugs

No interactions are known to occur, and there is no known reason to expect a clinically significant interaction with chelated minerals.

Interactions with Foods

No interactions are known to occur, and there is no known reason to expect a clinically significant interaction with chelated minerals.

Interactions with Lab Tests

No interactions are known to occur, and there is no known reason to expect a clinically significant interaction with chelated minerals.

Interactions with Diseases or Conditions

No interactions are known to occur, and there is no known reason to expect a clinically significant interaction with chelated minerals.

Dosage and Administration

See separate listings for specific minerals.

Comments

The term, chelated mineral, refers to formation of a complex of a mineral and an amino acid.

CHENOPODIUM OIL

Also Known As

Epazote, Jesuit Tea, Mexican Tea.
CAUTION: See separate listings for Wormseed, Wormwood Oil, and Wormwood.

Scientific Names

Chenopodium ambrosioides; Chenopodium ambrosioides anthelminticum.
Family: Chenopodiaceae.

People Use This For

Historically, chenopodium oil has been used as an oral antiparasitic against roundworms and hookworms (11).

Safety

UNSAFE ...when used orally due to toxicity (11).
PREGNANCY AND LACTATION: UNSAFE ...when used orally due to toxicity (11).

Effectiveness

POSSIBLY EFFECTIVE ...when used orally as an anthelmintic (11,400) but toxicity precludes use.

Mechanism of Action

The constituent ascaridole is thought to paralyze roundworms, hookworms, and dwarf tapeworms (but not large tapeworms) within the intestines (11,400). Chenopodium oil may explode when heated or treated with acids due to high ascaridole content (11). Handle with caution!

Adverse Reactions

Ingestion of chenopodium oil can cause skin and mucous membrane irritation, vomiting, headache, vertigo/dizziness, kidney and liver damage, temporary deafness, convulsions, circulatory collapse, paralysis, and death (11,400).

Interactions with Herbs & Other Dietary Supplements

Insufficient reliable information available.

Interactions with Drugs

No interactions are known to occur, and there is no known reason to expect a clinically significant interaction with chenopodium oil.

Interactions with Foods

No interactions are known to occur, and there is no known reason to expect a clinically significant interaction with chenopodium oil.

Interactions with Lab Tests

No interactions are known to occur, and there is no known reason to expect a clinically significant interaction with chenopodium oil.

Interactions with Diseases or Conditions

No interactions are known to occur, and there is no known reason to expect a clinically significant interaction with chenopodium oil.

Dosage and Administration

No typical dosage.

Comments

Authorities disagree on whether chenopodium oil is the distilled oil of fresh above ground flowering and fruiting parts (11) or seed oil (18) of Chenopodium ambrosioides. Chenopodium oil may explode when heated or treated with acids (11). Handle with caution!

CHEROKEE ROSEHIP

Also Known As

Chinese Rosehip, Fructus Rosae Laevigatae, Jinyingzi.
CAUTION: See separate listings for Acerola, Vitamin C, and Rose Hip.

Scientific Names

Rosa laevigata, synonyms Rosa sinica, Rosa cherokensis, Rosa ternata, Rosa nivea, Rosa camellia.
Family: Rosaceae.

People Use This For

In Chinese medicine, Cherokee rosehip is used for male sexual dysfunction (nocturnal emission, spermatorrhea, neurasthenia), gynecologic problems (leukorrhea, uterine bleeding), night sweats, polyuria, enuresis, chronic diarrhea, chronic cough, hypertension, and enteritis (11,1506).

Safety

POSSIBLY SAFE ...when used orally and appropriately. It contains vitamin C as a major constituent (11).
POSSIBLY UNSAFE ...when used orally in large amounts. Hyperoxaluria, hyperuricosuria, hematuria, and crystalluria can occur in some people taking 1 gram of vitamin C (67 grams of Cherokee rosehip) or more per day (14,3042). Prolonged use of large amounts of vitamin C can increase its metabolism, and scurvy might occur when intake is reduced (15).
PREGNANCY: POSSIBLY UNSAFE ...when used orally in large doses because it is associated with newborn scurvy (14,15). There is insufficient reliable information available about the safety of smaller amounts.
LACTATION: Insufficient reliable information available.

Effectiveness

POSSIBLY EFFECTIVE ...when used for diarrhea and enteritis (1506).
There is insufficient reliable information available about the effectiveness of Cherokee rosehip for its other uses.

Mechanism of Action

Cherokee rosehip contains vitamin C (approximately 1.5%) (11). An antidiarrheal effect occurs in humans (11).

Adverse Reactions

Orally, the vitamin C in Cherokee rosehip may cause nausea, abdominal cramps, fatigue, insomnia, and sleepiness. Doses greater than 1 gram may cause diarrhea (15).

Interactions with Herbs & Other Dietary Supplements

VITAMIN CONTAINING HERBS: Due to the vitamin C content, concomitant use of Cherokee rosehip with other products containing vitamin C increases total dose of vitamin C and may increase risk of adverse effects.

Interactions with Drugs

ASPIRIN: Theoretically, the vitamin C in large amounts of Cherokee rosehip might decrease excretion of aspirin (15).
ESTROGEN: Theoretically, the vitamin C in large amounts of Cherokee rosehip might increase absorption and effects of estrogen (129,130).
FLUPHENAZINE: Theoretically, the vitamin C in large amounts of Cherokee rosehip might decrease blood levels of fluphenazine (15).
IRON: Theoretically, the vitamin C in large amounts of Cherokee rosehip might increase GI absorption of food iron (ferric) but not supplement iron (ferrous) due to vitamin C content (15).
WARFARIN (Coumadin): Theoretically, the vitamin C in large amounts of Cherokee rosehip might reduce anticoagulant activity (506).
OTHER DRUGS: Theoretically, the vitamin C in large amounts of Cherokee rosehip might acidify urine, affecting excretion of other drugs (15).

Interactions with Foods

No interactions are known to occur, and there is no known reason to expect a clinically significant interaction with Cherokee rosehip.

Interactions with Lab Tests

URINE GLUCOSE TESTS: Theoretically, large amounts of Cherokee rosehip (containing greater than 500 mg vitamin C) may cause false decreases with glucose oxidase tests (e.g. Clinistix) and may cause false increases with cupric sulfate tests (e.g. Clinitest) (15).
STOOL OCCULT BLOOD TESTS: Theoretically, large amounts of Cherokee rosehip may cause a false-negative result if ingested 48-72 hours before amine-dependent tests due to vitamin C content (506).

Interactions with Diseases or Conditions

GOUT: Theoretically, the vitamin C in large amounts of Cherokee rosehip might increase uric acid levels (15).
KIDNEY STONE FORMING TENDENCY: Theoretically, the vitamin C in large amounts of Cherokee rosehip might cause precipitation of urate, cystine, or oxalate stones (15).
DIABETES: Large amounts may affect blood sugar control because of the vitamin C content (15).

Dosage and Administration

ORAL: Typically, 6 to 18 grams has been used (5269).

Comments

Cherokee rosehip contains vitamin C (approximately 1.5%) (11).

CHERRY LAUREL WATER

Also Known As

Common Cherry Laurel, Laurocerasus Leaves.
CAUTION: See separate listing for Wild Cherry.

Scientific Names

Prunus laurocerasus, synonym Laurocerasus officinalis.
Family: Rosaceae.

People Use This For

Orally, cherry laurel water is used as a sedative, pain reliever, and antispasmodic (11,18).
Topically, cherry laurel water is used in eye lotions (11).
As an inhalant, cherry laurel water is used as an aromatic, and breathing stimulant (18).
In traditional medicine, the leaves of cherry laurel are used for treating cough, colds, insomnia, stomach and intestinal spasms, vomiting, and cancer (11).

Safety

POSSIBLY SAFE ...when used orally and appropriately (18).
LIKELY UNSAFE ...when use orally in high doses. Cherry laurel water contains 0.1% hydrocyanic acid (11). Overdose can be fatal (18).
PREGNANCY AND LACTATION: Insufficient reliable information available; avoid using.

Effectiveness

There is insufficient reliable information available about the effectiveness of cherry laurel water.

Mechanism of Action

Cherry laurel water contains prunasin, a cyanogenic glycoside (11,18).

Adverse Reactions

Orally, adverse effects have not been reported with typical doses. However, cherry laurel water contains 0.1% hydrocyanic acid (11) and overdoses can cause significant toxicity and death (18).

Interactions with Herbs & Other Dietary Supplements

Insufficient reliable information available.

Interactions with Drugs

No interactions are known to occur, and there is no known reason to expect a clinically significant interaction with cherry laurel water.

Interactions with Foods

No interactions are known to occur, and there is no known reason to expect a clinically significant interaction with cherry laurel water.

Interactions with Lab Tests

No interactions are known to occur, and there is no known reason to expect a clinically significant interaction with cherry laurel water.

Interactions with Diseases or Conditions

No interactions are known to occur, and there is no known reason to expect a clinically significant interaction with cherry laurel water.

Dosage and Administration

ORAL: People typically use a dose of 2 to 8 mL cherry laurel water (5264,5267).

Comments

Cherry laurel water is produced by water distillation of cherry laurel (Prunus laurocerasus) leaves.
Avoid confusion with wild cherry bark, sweet bay leaf (laurel).

CHERVIL

Also Known As

Garden Chervil, Salad Chervil.

Scientific Names

Anthriscus cerefolium, synonym Anthriscus longirostris.
Family: Apiaceae or Umbelliferae.

People Use This For

In folk medicine, chervil is used as a diuretic, expectorant, digestive aid, and an antihypertensive (11). Juice from fresh chervil is used for eczema, gout, and abscesses (11).
In foods and beverages, chervil is used as a flavoring agent (11).

Safety

LIKELY SAFE ...when the above ground parts are used orally in amounts found in foods. Chervil has Generally Recognized as Safe (GRAS) status in the US. The maximum level used is 0.114% in meat products (11).
There is insufficient reliable information available about the safety of the oral use of chervil in medicinal amounts.
PREGNANCY AND LACTATION: LIKELY SAFE ...when used orally in food amounts. LIKELY UNSAFE ...when used orally in amounts larger than those found in foods. Chervil contains estragole which might be mutagenic (12).

Effectiveness

There is insufficient reliable information available about the effectiveness of chervil.

Mechanism of Action

The applicable parts of chervil are the dried flowering parts and leaf. Chervil is a plant source rich in calcium and potassium (19). Estragole, the major constituent of the volatile oil, is reported to produce tumors in mice (11).

Adverse Reactions

None reported.

Interactions with Herbs & Other Dietary Supplements

Insufficient reliable information available.

Interactions with Drugs

No interactions are known to occur, and there is no known reason to expect a clinically significant interaction with chervil.

Interactions with Foods

No interactions are known to occur, and there is no known reason to expect a clinically significant interaction with chervil.

Interactions with Lab Tests

No interactions are known to occur, and there is no known reason to expect a clinically significant interaction with chervil.

Interactions with Diseases or Conditions

No interactions are known to occur, and there is no known reason to expect a clinically significant interaction with chervil.

Dosage and Administration

ORAL: Chervil is typically prepared by adding 1 teaspoon of fresh or dried herb to water. The dose is up to 1 cup a day, unsweetened, consumed a mouthful at a time (5263).

Comments

None.

CHICKEN COLLAGEN

Also Known As

Chicken Collagen Type II, Chicken Type II Collagen, Type II Collagen.

Scientific Names

Chicken collagen type II.

People Use This For

Orally, chicken collagen is used to treat pain syndromes associated with rheumatoid arthritis, osteoarthritis, gouty arthritis, juvenile rheumatoid arthritis, post-surgical joint pain, post-traumatic pain, fibrositis, back pain, and neck pain (3110,3112).

Safety

There is insufficient reliable information available about the safety of chicken collagen.
Pregnancy and Lactation: Insufficient reliable information available; avoid using.

Effectiveness

There is insufficient reliable information available about the effectiveness of chicken collagen.

Mechanism of Action

The rationale of using chicken collagen for pain syndromes is based on the theory of oral tolerance. This theory hypothesizes that oral administration of small quantities of antigens causes biological processes that suppress inflammation at the cellular level, suppress response to delayed-hypersensitivity antigens, and eliminate the cells that respond to antigens. Although evidence suggests this theory might be true in animals, it is unproven in humans (3126). Based on the theory of oral tolerance, when individuals with rheumatoid arthritis take oral collagen, the collagen should cause certain areas of the gut to generate T-cells that are absorbed by the body. Then, in the body, these

T-cells are activated by joint collagen and they secrete cytokines that suppress inflammation. Cytokines thought to be involved include interleukin 4, 10, and transforming growth factor beta (3111,3112,3125). Oral administration of collagen is also believed to decrease the expression of pro-inflammatory cytokines including interleukins 1, 2, 6, and 8; tumor necrosis factor alpha; and interferon gamma (3111). So far, the studies determining the efficacy of chicken collagen demonstrate conflicting results (3125,3112,3128), but these studies have used microgram doses. Not everyone agrees with the theory of oral tolerance. One supplement manufacturer recommends a dose of 2 grams of chicken collagen per day, attributing effectiveness to the 15% glucosamine sulfate and 15% chondroitin sulfate contained in collagen type II (3110).

Adverse Reactions

Although no significant adverse effects have been reported in the small trials of chicken collagen (3111,3112), allergic reactions to other collagen products have occurred, e.g., bovine collagen used in corneal shields, catgut suture for eye surgery, and dietary collagen in the form of gelatin (3127). If large doses are used, side effects associated with glucosamine sulfate or chondroitin might occur. These include nausea, heartburn, diarrhea and constipation, drowsiness, skin reactions, and headache (14,2608).

Interactions with Herbs & Other Dietary Supplements

Insufficient reliable information available.

Interactions with Drugs

No interactions are known to occur, and there is no known reason to expect a clinically significant interaction with chicken collagen.

Interactions with Foods

No interactions are known to occur, and there is no known reason to expect a clinically significant interaction with chicken collagen.

Interactions with Lab Tests

No interactions are known to occur, and there is no known reason to expect a clinically significant interaction with chicken collagen.

Interactions with Diseases or Conditions

ALLERIGES: Theoretically, individuals who are allergic to chicken or eggs should not use chicken collagen. Collagen products have been associated with allergic reactions (e.g., bovine collagen used in corneal shields, catgut suture for eye surgery, and dietary collagen in the form of gelatin) (3127).

Dosage and Administration

ORAL: For rheumatoid arthritis, doses of 20 to 2500 mcg per day of chicken collagen have been used. For juvenile arthritis, doses of 100 mcg per day for the first month then 500 mcg per day thereafter have been used (3111,3112). However, some supplement manufacturers recommend doses of 2 grams per day (3110).

Comments

The manufacturer of Colloral, an oral chicken collagen product, stopped product development because it failed to demonstrate efficacy in humans (3128). Bovine collagen products have also been used in the treatment of rheumatoid arthritis.

CHICKWEED

Also Known As

Star Chickweed, Starweed.

Scientific Names

Stellaria media.
Family: Caryophyllaceae.

People Use This For

Orally, chickweed is used for constipation, bronchial asthma, stomach and bowel problems, blood disorders, lung disease, obesity, scurvy (5), psoriasis (6), rabies (5), itching, and muscle and joint pain (11).
Topically, chickweed is used for skin problems including boils, abscesses, and ulcers (5).
For food uses, chickweed is eaten in salads or served as cooked greens (5).

Safety

LIKELY SAFE ...when used orally (12).

There is insufficient reliable information available about the safety of the topical use of chickweed.

PREGNANCY AND LACTATION: Insufficient reliable information available; avoid using in amounts greater than those found in food.

Effectiveness

LIKELY INEFFECTIVE ...for all uses (5,6).

Mechanism of Action

The applicable part of chickweed is the leaf. There is no indication that any of the constituents have therapeutic value (5,6). While chickweed does contain some vitamin C, the concentrations are too small to be effective (6).

Adverse Reactions

Orally, chickweed is generally well-tolerated (6). There are, however, some poorly documented human cases of paralysis from consumptions of large amounts of chickweed tea (6) . There is one case of alleged nitrate toxicity leading to paralysis, but the chickweed implicated in this case may have been contaminated (12).

Interactions with Herbs & Other Dietary Supplements

Insufficient reliable information available.

Interactions with Drugs

No interactions are known to occur, and there is no known reason to expect a clinically significant interaction with chickweed.

Interactions with Foods

No interactions are known to occur, and there is no known reason to expect a clinically significant interaction with chickweed.

Interactions with Lab Tests

No interactions are known to occur, and there is no known reason to expect a clinically significant interaction with chickweed.

Interactions with Diseases or Conditions

No interactions are known to occur, and there is no known reason to expect a clinically significant interaction with chickweed.

Dosage and Administration

ORAL: People typically use 1155 to 3450 mg per day in 2 to 3 divided doses. One chickweed supplier suggests three daily doses based on body weight: under 100 pounds, 385 mg per dose; 100 to 175 pounds, 770 mg; and over 175 pounds, 1155 mg. Chickweed is also prepared as a tea with 1 to 2 teaspoons in 6 ounces of boiling water. Chickweed is available as a tincture of unspecified concentration with a typical dose of 1 to 5 mL per day (6006).

TOPICAL: No typical dosage.

Comments

None.

CHICLE

Also Known As

Breiapfelbaum, Chicle, Chico Sapote, Kaugummibaum, Naseberry, Níspero, Sabojira, Sapodilla, Sapodillbaum, Sapote, Sapotier, Sapotillier, Zapote, Zapotillo.

Scientific Names

Manilkara zapota, synonyms Manilkara zapotilla, Manilkara achras, Sapota achras, Achras sapota, Achras zapotilla. Family: Zapotaceae.

People Use This For

In manufacturing, chicle is an ingredient in hair preparations (11), and a gum base in chewing gum (11).

Safety

LIKELY SAFE ...when used orally in amounts found in gum (20%) (11); approved for use in foods as a chewing gum base in the US (11).
PREGNANCY AND LACTATION: LIKELY SAFE ...when used orally in amounts found in chewing gum (11).

Effectiveness

There is insufficient reliable information available about the effectiveness of chicle.

Mechanism of Action

There is insufficient reliable information available about the possible mechanism of action and active ingredients.

Adverse Reactions

None reported.

Interactions with Herbs & Other Dietary Supplements

Insufficient reliable information available.

Interactions with Drugs

No interactions are known to occur, and there is no known reason to expect a clinically significant interaction with chicle.

Interactions with Foods

No interactions are known to occur, and there is no known reason to expect a clinically significant interaction with chicle.

Interactions with Lab Tests

No interactions are known to occur, and there is no known reason to expect a clinically significant interaction with chicle.

Interactions with Diseases or Conditions

No interactions are known to occur, and there is no known reason to expect a clinically significant interaction with chicle.

Dosage and Administration

No typical dosage.

Comments

Chicle is derived from the latex collected from the trunk of the chicle tree (Manilkara zapota). Refined chicle is not a true gum (11). It has characteristics similar to natural resins and rubber, it is soft and plastic when chewed and insoluble in saliva (11). Chewing gum consists of approximately 20% chicle, plus sugar, corn syrup, and flavorings (11).

CHICORY

Also Known As

Blue Sailors, Cichorii Herba, Cichorii Radix, Common Chicory Root, Hendibeh, Succory, Wild Chicory.

Scientific Names

Cichorium intybus.
Family: Asteraceae or Compositae.

People Use This For

Orally, chicory is used as a tonic, diuretic, laxative (5), liver protectant, to balance the stimulant effect of coffee (5), for loss of appetite, dyspepsia (2), liver and gallbladder disorders (11), and cancer.
Topically, chicory leaves are used as a poultice for swelling and inflammation (5).
In folk medicine, chicory is used for tachycardia (5) and as a laxative in children (18).
For food uses, chicory leaves are often eaten like celery, and the roots are boiled and eaten. Chicory is used as a culinary spice (6), and the leaf buds and roots are eaten as vegetables (6,11).
In food manufacturing, chicory is used as a flavoring component in foods and beverages (11). The roasted root is also ground and used in coffee mixes to enhance richness (11) and as a coffee substitute (6).

Safety

LIKELY SAFE ...when consumed in amounts commonly found in food (5). Chicory has Generally Recognized as Safe (GRAS) status for food use in the US (6).
POSSIBLY SAFE ...when used orally in medicinal amounts (2,12).
There is insufficient reliable information available about the safety of chicory for its other uses.
PREGNANCY: LIKELY UNSAFE ...when used orally due to concerns that chicory can induce menstruation or miscarriage (19).
LACTATION: Insufficient reliable information available; avoid using.

Effectiveness

POSSIBLY EFFECTIVE ...when used orally as an appetite stimulant (2).
There is insufficient reliable information available about the effectiveness of chicory for its other uses.

Mechanism of Action

The applicable parts of chicory are the root and dried, above ground parts. Chicory root has a mild laxative effect and stimulates bile production. It is also believed to slow heart rate (2,11), perhaps due to the presence of a digitalis-like compound (5). Chicory has a sedative effect that has been attributed to the constituent lactucopicrin (5) and other water-soluble components (6). The sedative effect antagonizes the stimulant effects of coffee and tea (6). The sesquiterpene alkaloid constituents show evidence of bacteriostatic properties (11). The extracts seem to have anti-inflammatory activity (11). Chicory is a rich source of beta-carotene (19).

Adverse Reactions

Topically, chicory can cause contact dermatitis (6,11). It can cause an allergic reaction in individuals sensitive to the Asterceae/Compositae family. Members of this family include ragweed, chrysanthemums, marigolds, daisies, and many other herbs.

Interactions with Herbs & Other Dietary Supplements

Insufficient reliable information available.

Interactions with Drugs

No interactions are known to occur, and there is no known reason to expect a clinically significant interaction with chicory.

Interactions with Foods

No interactions are known to occur, and there is no known reason to expect a clinically significant interaction with chicory.

Interactions with Lab Tests

No interactions are known to occur, and there is no known reason to expect a clinically significant interaction with chicory.

Interactions with Diseases or Conditions

CHICORY ALLERGY: Contraindicated (11).
GALLSTONES: Chicory should only be used with monitoring due to its bile stimulating effect (2,6,11).
CROSS-ALLERGENICITY: Can cause an allergic reaction in individuals sensitive to the Asteraceae/Compositae family. Members of this family include ragweed, chrysanthemums, marigolds, daisies, and many other herbs.

Dosage and Administration

ORAL: The typical dose of chicory is one cup of the tea, which is prepared by steeping 2-4 grams of the root in 150 mL boiling water for 10 minutes and then straining (18). The average amount of chicory is 3-5 grams of the root per day (18).
TOPICAL: No typical dosage.

Comments

Chicory can be contaminated with bacteria (6,3807) or foreign substances, including fungicides (6).

CHINESE CLUB MOSS

Also Known As
Huperazon, Qian Ceng Ta.
CAUTION: See separate listing for Huperzine A.

Scientific Names
Huperzia serrata.
Family: Lycopodiaceae.

People Use This For
Orally, Chinese club moss is used for Alzheimer's disease and other memory disorders (3150).
In Chinese medicine, Chinese club moss is used for fever, inflammation, blood loss, irregular menstruation, and as a diuretic (3130,3131).

Safety
There is insufficient reliable information available about the safety of Chinese club moss.
Pregnancy and Lactation: Insufficient reliable information available; avoid using.

Effectiveness
There is insufficient reliable information available about the effectiveness of Chinese club moss.

Mechanism of Action
Chinese club moss contains the alkaloid huperzine A, a reversible acetylcholinesterase (AChE) inhibitor which crosses the blood-brain barrier (3082).

Adverse Reactions
None reported with Chinese club moss.
Orally, huperzine A which is found in Chinese club moss can cause dizziness, nausea and sweating (3140,3143).

Interactions with Herbs & Other Dietary Supplements
Insufficient reliable information available.

Interactions with Drugs
ANTICHOLINERGIC DRUGS: Theoretically, concurrent use of anticholinergic drugs and Chinese club moss might decrease the effectiveness of Chinese club moss or the anticholinergic agent. In an animal model, huperzine A, an active constituent of Chinese club moss, reversed cognitive deficits induced by scopolamine (5537). Other anticholinergic drugs include atropine, benztropine (Cogentin), biperiden (Akineton), procyclidine (Kemadrin), and trihexyphenidyl (Artane) (15).
CHOLINERGIC DRUGS, ACETYLCHOLINESTERASE (AChE) INHIBITORS: Theoretically, concurrent use with Chinese club moss might have additive effects with drugs that promote acetylcholine activity because huperzine A has AChE inhibitor properties (14). AChE inhibitors and cholinergic drugs include bethanechol (Urecholine), donepezil (Aricept), echothiophate (Phospholine Iodide), edrophonium (Enoln, Reversol, Tensilon), neostigmine (Prostigmin), physostigmine (Antilirium), pyridostigmine (Mestinon, Regonol), succinylcholine (Anectine, Quelicin), and tacrine (Cognex) (14).

Interactions with Foods
No interactions are known to occur, and there is no known reason to expect a clinically significant interaction with Chinese club moss.

Interactions with Lab Tests
No interactions are known to occur, and there is no known reason to expect a clinically significant interaction with Chinese club moss.

Interactions with Diseases or Conditions
VARIOUS DISEASES: Acetylcholinesterase (AchE) inhibitors are used with caution or are contraindicated in people with asthma, chronic obstructive pulmonary disease, cardiovascular disease, obstruction of the intestinal or urogenital tracts, gastrointestinal ulcer disease, or seizures (14). Avoid using Chinese club moss in people with these conditions until more is known about its effects in humans.

Dosage and Administration

ORAL: Currently available products contain isolated huperzine A extracted from Chinese club moss (see separate listing for Huperzine A).

Comments

Don't let your patients confuse club moss and Chinese club moss. Only Chinese club moss contains huperzine A.

CHINESE CUCUMBER fruit

Also Known As

Chinese Snake Gourd, Compound Q, Gua Lou, Gua-Lou, Trichosanthes.
CAUTION: See separate listings for Chinese Cucumber root and Chinese Cucumber seed.

Scientific Names

Trichosanthes kirilowii.
Family: Curcurbitaceae.

People Use This For

Orally, Chinese cucumber fruit is used for coughing, reducing fever, swelling, tumors, and diabetes.
Intravaginally, Chinese cucumber fruit is used as an abortifacient (6).

Safety

POSSIBLY SAFE ...when used orally and appropriately (12).
There is insufficient reliable information available about the safety of the intravaginal use of Chinese cucumber fruit.
PREGNANCY: LIKELY UNSAFE ...when used orally because it might induce abortion (6).
LACTATION: Insufficient reliable information available; avoid using.

Effectiveness

There is insufficient reliable information available about the effectiveness of Chinese cucumber fruit.

Mechanism of Action

Some evidence suggests a 50% ethanolic extract might have protective effects against ulcers (4044). A sponge containing Chinese cucumber juice might induce abortions when inserted intravaginally (6).

Adverse Reactions

Orally, Chinese cucumber fruit may cause mild diarrhea and gastric discomfort (12).

Interactions with Herbs & Other Dietary Supplements

Insufficient reliable information available.

Interactions with Drugs

No interactions are known to occur, and there is no known reason to expect a clinically significant interaction with Chinese cucumber fruit.

Interactions with Foods

No interactions are known to occur, and there is no known reason to expect a clinically significant interaction with Chinese cucumber fruit.

Interactions with Lab Tests

No interactions are known to occur, and there is no known reason to expect a clinically significant interaction with Chinese cucumber fruit.

Interactions with Diseases or Conditions

Insufficient reliable information available.

Dosage and Administration

ORAL: People typically use 10 to 20 grams of the dried fruit (5269).

Comments

None.

CHINESE CUCUMBER root

Also Known As
Chinese Snake Gourd, Compound Q, Tian Hua Fen, Tian-Hua-Fen, Trichosanthes.
CAUTION: See separate entries for Chinese Cucumber fruit and Chinese Cucumber seed.

Scientific Names
Trichosanthes kirilowii.
Family: Curcurbitaceae.

People Use This For
Orally, Chinese cucumber root is used to treat HIV infection (6).
Intramuscularly, Chinese cucumber root is used to induce abortions (by intramuscular injection) (6).
In Chinese medicine, cucumber root is used orally to treat coughs, fever, swelling, tumors and diabetes (6). A starch extract is used for treating abscesses, amenorrhea, jaundice, frequent urination, and tumors (6).

Safety
LIKELY UNSAFE ...when used orally or by injection for self-medication; requires monitoring (6). Extracts of Chinese cucumber can be very toxic (6).
PREGNANCY: LIKELY UNSAFE ...when used orally or by injection due to abortifacient effects and possible teratogenicity (6,12).
LACTATION: LIKELY UNSAFE ...when used orally or by injection; avoid using (6).

Effectiveness
POSSIBLY EFFECTIVE ...when administered parenterally as an abortifacient (6).
There is insufficient reliable information available about the effectiveness of Chinese cucumber root for its other uses.

Mechanism of Action
Chinese cucumber root contains several constituents that demonstrate anti-HIV activity. Trichosanthin and protein "TAP 29" can block HIV replication and some evidence suggests they might selectively kill HIV infected cells in the immune system. Other constituents of the root, trichosanthin and momorcharin, can have abortifacient effects. Trichosanthin injected intramuscularly or extra-amniotically can induce first-trimester abortions. It has also been used to terminate ectopic pregnancies (6). Some evidence suggests trichosanthin and momorcharin might cause birth defects (12). Trichosanthin also shows antitumor activity. It has been used to treat invasive moles and certain types of liver tumors. Some evidence suggests that a water extract of the root might have hypoglycemic activity in individuals with normal blood glucose. Subsequent fractionation of the extract yielded five compounds. The activity of one of these suggests it might be useful in reducing blood sugars in individuals with diabetes (4045).

Adverse Reactions
Chinese cucumber root extracts are extremely toxic, particularly when they are injected. Trichosanthin injections can be fatal. They can also cause severe reactions including seizures, fever, lung and cerebral edema, cerebral hemorrhage, and heart damage. People receiving trichosanthin injections to cause abortion can develop a severe allergy. After a single exposure, the risk of anaphylaxis from a second exposure can persist for more than a decade (6).

Interactions with Herbs & Other Dietary Supplements
ANTIDIABETES HERBS: Theoretically, concomitant use may potentiate effects of other herbs with hypoglycemic effects (6,4045).

Interactions with Drugs
ANTIDIABETES DRUGS: Theoretically, concomitant use may have additive effects and adverse effects (6,4045). Monitor blood glucose closely, dose adjustment may be needed.

Interactions with Foods
No interactions are known to occur, and there is no known reason to expect a clinically significant interaction with Chinese cucumber root.

Interactions with Lab Tests
BLOOD GLUCOSE: Theoretically, may decrease blood glucose levels and test results (6,4045).

Interactions with Diseases or Conditions
DIABETES: Theoretically, use of Chinese cucumber root may alter blood glucose control (6,4045).

Dosage and Administration

ORAL: People typically use 9 to 15 grams of the root (5268).

Comments

Avoid confusion with Chinese cucumber fruit and Chinese cucumber seed.

CHINESE CUCUMBER seed

Also Known As

Chinese Snake Gourd, Compound Q, Gua Luo Ren, Gua-Luo-Ren, Trichosanthes.
CAUTION: See separate listings for Chinese Cucumber root and Chinese Cucumber fruit.

Scientific Names

Trichosanthes kirilowii.
Family: Curcurbitaceae.

People Use This For

Orally, Chinese cucumber seed is used for coughs, reducing fever, swelling, tumors and diabetes (6).

Safety

POSSIBLY SAFE ...when used orally (12).
PREGNANCY AND LACTATION: Insufficient reliable information available; avoid using.

Effectiveness

There is insufficient reliable information available about the effectiveness of Chinese cucumber seed.

Mechanism of Action

Some evidence suggests three triterpene compounds isolated from the seed might have anti-inflammatory effects (4042). Other information suggests that a 50% ethanolic seed extract might have anti-inflammatory and analgesic effects (4043).

Adverse Reactions

None reported.

Interactions with Herbs & Other Dietary Supplements

Insufficient reliable information available.

Interactions with Drugs

No interactions are known to occur, and there is no known reason to expect a clinically significant interaction with Chinese cucumber seed.

Interactions with Foods

No interactions are known to occur, and there is no known reason to expect a clinically significant interaction with Chinese cucumber seed.

Interactions with Lab Tests

No interactions are known to occur, and there is no known reason to expect a clinically significant interaction with Chinese cucumber seed.

Interactions with Diseases or Conditions

No interactions are known to occur, and there is no known reason to expect a clinically significant interaction with Chinese cucumber seed.

Dosage and Administration

ORAL: People typically use 9 to 15 grams of the seeds (5268).

Comments

None.

CHIRATA

Also Known As
Bitter Stick, Bitterstick, Chirayta, Chiretta, East Indian Balmony, Indian Bolonong, Indian Gentian.

Scientific Names
Swertia chirata.
Family: Gentianaceae.

People Use This For
In folk medicine, chirata is used as a bitter tonic, antipyretic, laxative, anthelmintic (11), for dyspepsia, loss of appetite, skin diseases, and cancer (11,18).
In India, it has been used as an anti-malarial, combined with the seeds of Guilandina Bonducella (215).
In manufacturing, chirata is used for alcoholic and non-alcoholic beverages (11).

Safety
LIKELY SAFE ...when used in amounts found in alcoholic (maximum use level 0.0016%) and non-alcoholic drinks (maximum use level 0.0008%) (11).
At higher levels, there is insufficient reliable information available about the safety of chirata for other uses; however, no adverse reactions reported (18).
PREGNANCY AND LACTATION: Insufficient reliable information available; avoid using.

Effectiveness
There is insufficient reliable information available about the effectiveness of chirata.

Mechanism of Action
The applicable parts of chirata are the above ground parts. The extract is reported to have anti-inflammatory activity in animals (11). Constituents and their reported activity include: chirata stimulates gastric juice secretion (18); swerchirin has antimalarial activity (in vivo) (11); amarogentin has hepatoprotective activity (in vitro) (11); xanthones claimed to have antituberculous activity (11).

Adverse Reactions
None reported.

Interactions with Herbs & Other Dietary Supplements
Insufficient reliable information available.

Interactions with Drugs
No interactions are known to occur, and there is no known reason to expect a clinically significant interaction with chirata.

Interactions with Foods
No interactions are known to occur, and there is no known reason to expect a clinically significant interaction with chirata.

Interactions with Lab Tests
No interactions are known to occur, and there is no known reason to expect a clinically significant interaction with chirata.

Interactions with Diseases or Conditions
DUODENAL ULCERS: Use of chirata may exacerbate (18); avoid using.

Dosage and Administration
ORAL: People typically use 0.5 to 2 grams of the powdered herb or 2 to 4 mL of the liquid extract (5264).

Comments
Adulteration reported with Andrographis paniculata, roots of Rubia cordifolia, and Swertia species, including Swertia angustifolia (11).

CHITOSAN

Also Known As

Chitosan Ascorbate, N-Carboxybutyl Chitosan, N,O-Sulfated Chitosan, O-Sulfated N-Acetylchitosan, Sulfated N-Carboxymethylchitosan, Sulfated O-Carboxymethylchitosan.

Scientific Names

Chitosan.

People Use This For

Orally, chitosan is used for weight loss (3243). It is also used orally by some people with renal failure on chronic hemodialysis for reducing high cholesterol, improving anemia, enhancing physical strength, appetite, and sleep (1942). Topically, chitosan is used for treating periodontitis (1945) and promoting donor site tissue regeneration in plastic surgery (1944).

In pharmaceutical manufacturing, chitosan is used as an excipient in tablets, as a disintegrant to improve drug dissolution, as a vehicle for parenteral drug delivery devices, and as a carrier in controlled release drug systems (1940,1941).

Safety

POSSIBLY SAFE ...when used orally (1942). ...when used topically (1944,1945,4269,4270).
PREGNANCY AND LACTATION: Insufficient reliable information available; avoid using.

Effectiveness

POSSIBLY EFFECTIVE ...when used orally by patients with renal failure on chronic hemodialysis for reducing high cholesterol, improving anemia, enhancing physical strength, appetite, and sleep (1942). ...when used topically for treating periodontitis (1945) and promoting donor site tissue regeneration in plastic surgery (1944).
LIKELY INEFFECTIVE ...when used orally for weight loss (3243,3244).
There is insufficient reliable information available about the effectiveness of chitosan for its other uses.

Mechanism of Action

Reported hemostatic activity is believed to be due to an interaction between erythrocyte cell membranes and chitosan; this appears to be independent of the classical coagulation cascade (1943). Chitosan ascorbate acts as a surgical cement in treatment of periodontitis, protecting periodontal pockets from oxygen and allowing for proliferation of periodontal tissues (1945). While it is theorized that chitosan might aid in weight reduction, clinical trials with chitosan show no effect on weight loss (3243,3244). The effect of chitosan on serum lipids is unclear. In one study, chitosan had no effects (3243), in a second study it was associated with a slight reduction in LDL and a slight increase in triglycerides (3244), and in a third study significantly reduced total serum cholesterol in patients with renal failure on chronic hemodialysis (1942).

Adverse Reactions

People with shellfish allergies should use caution when using chitosan (6).

Interactions with Herbs & Other Dietary Supplements

Insufficient reliable information available.

Interactions with Drugs

No interactions are known to occur, and there is no known reason to expect a clinically significant interaction with chitosan.

Interactions with Foods

No interactions are known to occur, and there is no known reason to expect a clinically significant interaction with chitosan.

Interactions with Lab Tests

CHOLESTEROL: May reduce serum cholesterol levels, and test results, in patients with renal failure on chronic hemodialysis (1942).
HEMOGLOBIN: May increase serum hemoglobin levels, and test results, in patients with renal failure on chronic hemodialysis (1942).
UREA/CREATININE: May reduce blood urea and creatinine levels, and test results, in patients with renal failure on chronic hemodialysis (1942).

Interactions with Diseases or Conditions

RENAL FAILURE: May reduce serum cholesterol, urea and creatinine levels, and increase hemoglobin levels in patients on chronic hemodialysis (1942).

Dosage and Administration

ORAL: Renal failure with chronic hemodialysis: 1.35 grams (30 x 45 mg tablets) three times daily (1942). No typical dosage for other uses and routes of administration.

Comments

Chitosan is a mucopolysaccharide component of crab, lobster, shrimp and other marine organism exoskeletons.

CHIVE

Also Known As

Chives, Cives.

Scientific Names

Allium schoenoprasum.
Family: Liliaceae.

People Use This For

Orally, chive is used to expel parasitic worms (18).
For food uses, chives are used commonly as a food flavoring agent.

Safety

LIKELY SAFE …when used in food amounts.
POSSIBLY SAFE …when used orally in amounts larger than those found in foods (12).
PREGNANCY AND LACTATION: LIKELY SAFE …when used in food amounts; avoid amounts larger than those found in foods.

Effectiveness

There is insufficient reliable information available about the effectiveness of chive.

Mechanism of Action

The applicable parts of chive are the above ground parts. There is insufficient reliable information available about the possible mechanism of action and active ingredients.

Adverse Reactions

Orally, intake of large quantities of chives can lead to dyspepsia (18).

Interactions with Herbs & Other Dietary Supplements

Insufficient reliable information available.

Interactions with Drugs

No interactions are known to occur, and there is no known reason to expect a clinically significant interaction with chive.

Interactions with Foods

No interactions are known to occur, and there is no known reason to expect a clinically significant interaction with chive.

Interactions with Lab Tests

No interactions are known to occur, and there is no known reason to expect a clinically significant interaction with chive.

Interactions with Diseases or Conditions

No interactions are known to occur, and there is no known reason to expect a clinically significant interaction with chive.

Dosage and Administration
ORAL: Chive is used fresh, dried, or powdered.

Comments
None.

CHLORELLA

Also Known As
None.

Scientific Names
Chlorella Vulgaris; Chlorella pyrenoidosa; other Chlorella species.

People Use This For
Orally, chlorella is used as a food supplement and source of nutrients, including protein, nucleic acids, fiber, vitamins, and minerals (5843,5846). Chlorella is also used orally for cancer prevention, stimulating the immune system (5843,5844), increasing white blood cell counts (e.g., in people with HIV infection or cancer) (5843), preventing colds (5843), to protect the body from the effects of radiation (e.g., during cancer therapy) (5843,5844), to protect the body from toxic metals such as lead and mercury (5844), and to slow aging (5843). It is also used orally to increase beneficial flora in the gastrointestinal tract in order to improve digestion (5843,5844), and to help treat ulcers, colitis, Crohn's disease, and diverticulosis (5843). It is also promoted for the prevention of stress-induced ulcers (5844); treatment of constipation, bad breath, and hypertension (5844); as an antioxidant (5844); to reduce serum cholesterol; to increase energy; to detoxify the body (5843); and as a source of magnesium to promote mental health, relieve premenstrual syndrome (PMS), and reduce asthma attacks (5843). It is also used orally for fibromyalgia (5890).

Topically, chlorella is used for treating ulcers, postirradiation dermatitis, vulval leukoplakias, and trichomoniasis (5851).

Safety
POSSIBLY SAFE ...when used as a food to supplement a normal diet (5846).
There is insufficient reliable information about the safety of chlorella for its other uses.
PREGNANCY AND LACTATION: Insufficient reliable information available; avoid using.

Effectiveness
POSSIBLY EFFECTIVE ...when used orally as a source of nutrients to supplement a normal diet (5846).
There is insufficient reliable information available about the effectiveness of chlorella for its other uses. However, preliminary clinical research shows subjective improvements in general symptom and pain scores in people with fibromyalgia who took chlorella tablets plus liquid extract containing malic acid daily for two months (5890). Early research also shows that chlorella tablets plus liquid extract might help people with brain tumors better tolerate chemotherapy and radiotherapy, possibly by improving immune system function; however, there appears to be no effect on tumor progression or survival (5890,6804). More evidence is needed to rate chlorella for these uses.

Mechanism of Action
Chlorella is a single-celled, freshwater green alga, also referred to as a seaweed (5846,5850). The whole plant is processed for medicinal use and is a rich source of chlorophyll (5846). The cell wall must be broken down before the organism can be digested by humans (5890). Chlorella contains significant amounts of protein, lipid, carbohydrates, fiber, nucleic acids, vitamins, and minerals (5846,5890). There is some evidence that consuming chlorella can increase serum vitamin B12 levels (5848). However, it has been suggested that the vitamin B12 found in chlorella might be in an inactive form which can raise serum levels without contributing biological activity (5849).

In vitro and animal studies indicate that substances in chlorella might have antitumor, immune system enhancing, and antiviral activities (5846,5850,5891,5892). Chlorella might stimulate the immune system by increasing the number and activity of macrophages and polymorphonuclear leukocytes. A polysaccharide from the cell wall of chlorella might also induce production of interferon (6804). However, these effects have not been verified in humans. The photosensitizing components in chlorella have been identified as pheophorbides (5846,5847).

Adverse Reactions
Orally, chlorella can cause diarrhea, abdominal cramping, flatus, and nausea, especially during the first week of treatment (5890,6804). Green discoloration of the feces has also been reported, presumably due to the chlorophyll content of chlorella (6804). Allergic reactions, including asthma and anaphylaxis, have been reported in people taking chlorella, and in those preparing chlorella tablets (5846,5847). Photosensitivity reactions have also occurred following ingestion of chlorella (5846,5852). There is a case report of human infection with chlorella, and several reports in animals (5853).

Interactions with Herbs & Other Dietary Supplements
Insufficient reliable information available.

Interactions with Drugs
ANTICOAGULANTS: Chlorella contains significant amounts of vitamin K, which may inhibit the anticoagulant activity of warfarin (Coumadin) and related drugs (5846).

Interactions with Foods
No interactions are known to occur, and there is no known reason to expect a clinically significant interaction with chlorella.

Interactions with Lab Tests
No interactions are known to occur, and there is no known reason to expect a clinically significant interaction with chlorella.

Interactions with Diseases or Conditions
ALLERGIES, INCLUDING IODINE SENSITIVITY: Chlorella has been associated with significant allergic reactions (5846,5847), and is also reported to contain iodine (5845).

Dosage and Administration
ORAL: As a general dietary supplement, a dose of 3 grams daily of chlorella tablets or 30 mL daily of a liquid extract (Wakasa Gold) has been used (5890). For fibromyalgia, doses of 10 gram tablets plus 100 mL liquid extract daily have been used (5890). For improving tolerability of chemotherapy and radiotherapy in people with brain tumors, chlorella tablets, up to 20 grams daily, plus 150 mL liquid extract daily have been used (6804).
TOPICAL: No typical dosage.

Comments
Commercial producers of chlorella report that it is a source of protein, including the amino acids: lysine, leucine, isoleucine, threonine, valine, methionine, phenylalanine, tryptophan, histidine, arginine, serine, proline, glycine, alanine, glutamic acid, and aspartic acid (5845). It is also reported to contain chlorophyll, saturated and unsaturated fatty acids, RNA, magnesium, potassium, calcium, iron, zinc, phosphorus, iodine, niacin, beta carotene, thiamine, riboflavin, pyridoxine, pantothenic acid, biotin, inositol, folic acid, vitamin B12, vitamin E, and vitamin C (5843,5844,5845).
Since chlorella is a naturally occurring organism, its content can vary with growing, harvesting, and processing conditions. By varying the cultivation conditions, it has been reported that a dried preparation of chlorella can contain from 7 to 88% protein, 6 to 38% carbohydrate, and 7 to 75% fat (5851). Most chlorella sold in the United States is cultivated in Japan or Taiwan (5846). Processing of the chlorella cultures includes destroying the cell walls, dehydration and sterilization (5851). Commercially available products include tablets and liquid extracts. The latter contain "chlorella growth factor", described as a water soluble extract of chlorella, containing amino acids, peptides, proteins, vitamins, sugars, and nucleic acids (5890).

CHLOROPHYLL

Also Known As
None.
CAUTION: See separate listing for Chlorophyllin.

Scientific Names
Chlorophyll a; Chlorophyll b; Chlorophyll c; Chlorophyll d.

People Use This For
Orally, chlorophyll is used for reducing colostomy odor (1322), bad breath, constipation, detoxification, and wound healing (1900).
Intravenously, chlorophyll is used for treating chronic relapsing pancreatitis (1324).

Safety
LIKELY SAFE ...when used orally (1324).
POSSIBLY SAFE ...when used intravenously (1324).
PREGNANCY AND LACTATION: POSSIBLY SAFE ...when used orally. There is insufficient reliable information available about the safety of the intravenous use of chlorophyll during pregnancy and lactation.

Effectiveness
POSSIBLY EFFECTIVE ...when used intravenously for chronic relapsing pancreatitis (1324).
POSSIBLY INEFFECTIVE ...when used orally for reducing colostomy odor (1322).

Mechanism of Action
Chlorophyll contains components that are activated by light. It appears that chlorophyll can cause a photosensitization when it is taken internally (1326). Derivatives of chlorophyll which have been extracted from silkworm droppings seem to have a cytotoxic effect on certain cancer cells (1314,1315). Certain carotenoids such as beta-carotene and canthaxanthin seem to prevent or lessen the photosensitivity that results from taking chlorophyll (1326).

Adverse Reactions
None reported.

Interactions with Herbs & Other Dietary Supplements
CAROTENOIDS (beta-carotene, canthaxanthin): Theoretically, may prevent or lessen chlorophyll-induced photosensitivity (1326).

Interactions with Drugs
PHOTOSENSITIZING DRUGS: Theoretically, use of chlorophyll may exacerbate effects (1326).

Interactions with Foods
No interactions are known to occur, and there is no known reason to expect a clinically significant interaction with chlorophyll.

Interactions with Lab Tests
No interactions are known to occur, and there is no known reason to expect a clinically significant interaction with chlorophyll.

Interactions with Diseases or Conditions
No interactions are known to occur, and there is no known reason to expect a clinically significant interaction with chlorophyll.

Dosage and Administration
ORAL: No typical dosage.
INTRAVENOUS: For pancreatitis; infusion of 5-20 mg water soluble chlorophyll-a per day for 1-2 weeks, followed by intermittent administration has been used (1324).

Comments
Avoid confusion with chlorophyllin, a semisynthetic derivative of chlorophyll. Commercial sources of chlorophyll include alfalfa (Medicago sativa) and silk worm droppings (11). Chlorophyll is a group of related green pigments found in photosynthetic organisms including: Chlorophyll a (found in higher plants, red and green algae), Chlorophyll b (found in higher plants), Chlorophyll c (found in brown algae, diatoms, flagellates), and Chlorophyll d (found in red algae).

CHLOROPHYLLIN

Also Known As
None.
CAUTION: See separate listing for Chlorophyll.

Scientific Names
Chlorophyllin.

People Use This For
Orally, chlorophyllin is used for controlling body, fecal, and urine odors, and for treating constipation and flatulence (1321,1323).

Safety
POSSIBLY SAFE ...when used orally (1321,1323).
PREGNANCY AND LACTATION: Insufficient reliable information available; avoid using.

Effectiveness

POSSIBLY EFFECTIVE ...when used orally for controlling body and fecal odors, and treating constipation and flatulence in geriatric patients (1321).
POSSIBLY INEFFECTIVE ...when used orally for controlling urinary odor in incontinent geriatric patients with indwelling catheters (1323).

Mechanism of Action

Chlorophyllin has antimutagenic activity in human lymphocytes (in vitro) (1312). Mechanisms may include reduced carcinogen DNA-binding (in fish) (1309), reduced chromosome damage (in vitro) (1311), and reduced carcinogen-induced cell transformation (in vitro) (1307). Bacteriologic studies failed to confirm reports of antibacterial properties for chlorophyllin (1321).

Adverse Reactions

None reported.

Interactions with Herbs & Other Dietary Supplements

Insufficient reliable information available.

Interactions with Drugs

No interactions are known to occur, and there is no known reason to expect a clinically significant interaction with chlorophyllin.

Interactions with Foods

No interactions are known to occur, and there is no known reason to expect a clinically significant interaction with chlorophyllin.

Interactions with Lab Tests

No interactions are known to occur, and there is no known reason to expect a clinically significant interaction with chlorophyllin.

Interactions with Diseases or Conditions

No interactions are known to occur, and there is no known reason to expect a clinically significant interaction with chlorophyllin.

Dosage and Administration

ORAL: Typically, 100 mg per day is used for controlling urinary odor in incontinent geriatric patients with indwelling catheters (1323).

Comments

Avoid confusion with Chlorophyll.

CHOLINE

Also Known As

Choline Bitartrate, Choline Chloride, Intrachol, Lipotropic Factor.
CAUTION: See separate listings for Lecithin and Phosphatidylcholine.

Scientific Names

Trimethylethanolamine; (beta-hydroxyethyl) trimethylammonium hydroxide.

People Use This For

Orally, choline is used for liver disease including chronic hepatitis and cirrhosis, hypercholesterolemia, depression, memory loss, Alzheimer's disease and dementia (5168,5169,5170), and schizophrenia (5171,5172). It is also used orally for body building (5160), delaying fatigue in endurance sports (5164), Huntington's chorea (5167), Tourette's disease, cerebellar ataxia (5161,5173), complex partial seizures (5162), asthma (5165,5166), and as a supplement in infant formulas (16,4921). Intravenously, choline has orphan drug status for TPN-associated hepatic steatosis (5163,5173,5174).

Safety

LIKELY SAFE ...when used orally and appropriately (3094,4921). ...when used intravenously and appropriately (5173,5174).

POSSIBLY UNSAFE ...when used orally in excessive doses. High doses can increase the risk of adverse effects. Tell patients not to exceed 3.5 grams per day for adults over age 18 (3094).

CHILDREN: LIKELY SAFE ...when used orally and appropriately (3094). POSSIBLY UNSAFE ...when used orally in excessive doses. High doses can increase the risk of adverse effects. Tell patients not to exceed 1 gram daily for children 1-8 years of age, 2 grams daily for children 9-13 years of age, and 3 grams daily for children 14-18 years of age (3094).

PREGNANCY AND LACTATION: LIKELY SAFE ...when used orally and appropriately. Doses up to 3 grams daily for women up to 18 years of age, and 3.5 grams daily for women 19 years and older are not likely to cause adverse effects (3094). There is insufficient reliable information about the safety when higher doses are used in pregnant or lactating patients.

Effectiveness

LIKELY EFFECTIVE ...when used intravenously to treat parenteral nutrition-associated hepatic dysfunction (5163,5173,5174). ...when used orally as a supplement in infant formulas (16,4921).

POSSIBLY EFFECTIVE ...when used orally for asthma. Choline supplements seem to decrease the severity of symptoms, number of symptomatic days (5165), and the need to use bronchodilators (5166) in patients with asthma. There is some evidence that higher doses of 3 grams daily might be more effective than lower doses of 1.5 grams daily (5165).

POSSIBLY INEFFECTIVE ...when used orally for treating cerebellar ataxia (5161,5173). ...when used orally for delaying fatigue in endurance sports (5164).

LIKELY INEFFECTIVE ...when used orally for treating memory loss, Alzheimer's disease, and dementia (9,5170). ...when used orally for treating schizophrenia (5171,5172).

There is insufficient reliable information available to rate the effectiveness of choline for its other uses. However, some case reports show that high doses of choline, 12-16 grams daily, might be helpful for some patients with complex partial seizures (5162). More evidence is needed to rate choline for this use.

Mechanism of Action

Choline has traditionally been considered a B vitamin. However, this is controversial because choline can be synthesized by the human body (4921,5139). Choline is produced in the liver via the methylation of phosphatidylethanolamine. S-adenosylmethionine is the methyl donor for this reaction (1949). Choline is also readily available in the typical diet (4921,5139). Foods that supply large amounts of choline are liver, muscle meats, fish, nuts, beans, peas, eggs, and others (16). A typical diet provides 200-600 mg daily (4921). Deficiency of choline is uncommon except in people receiving long-term total parenteral nutrition (TPN) (4921,5139,5174). Choline deficiency related to long-term TPN use can result in fatty liver and liver damage. Adding choline to the TPN solution usually resolves liver abnormalities (1949). This indicates that dietary choline is required in addition to the choline normally synthesized by the body (4921,5139,5174). Choline, or its metabolites, is needed for the synthesis of cell membrane phospholipids and is a methyl donor for the synthesis of other compounds (1949,4921). For example, the choline metabolite betaine is a methyl donor during the methylation of homocysteine to form methionine (1949). Choline is found in most living cells, but it concentrates in nervous tissue (4921). There is preliminary evidence that supplemental choline during pregnancy and lactation probably affects the birth, death, and migration of cells in the hippocampus during fetal brain development and possibly changes the distribution and morphology of neurons responsible for memory function in the brain (1949). Some researchers are interested in choline for Alzheimer's disease because it is a precursor to acetylcholine. However, there is evidence that oral choline does not affect concentrations of choline metabolites such as acetylcholine in the brain. This might be the reason oral choline does not seem to be effective for neurodegenerative disorders of cholinergic transmission (5175). In asthma, choline is thought to have anti-inflammatory effects by lowering lipophosphatidylcholine levels. Some researchers speculate that choline might also have a role in cancer prevention (5178,5179,5180). In animal models, long-term withdrawal of choline from the diet can cause hepatocarcinoma (5178,5180).

Adverse Reactions

Orally, adverse reactions can include sweating, a fishy body odor, gastrointestinal distress, and vomiting (4921,5160,5163). Large doses can cause diarrhea (4921).

Interactions with Herbs & Other Dietary Supplements

Insufficient reliable information available.

Interactions with Drugs

No interactions are known to occur, and there is no known reason to expect a clinically significant interaction with choline.

Interactions with Foods

No interactions are known to occur, and there is no known reason to expect a clinically significant interaction with choline.

Interactions with Lab Tests

No interactions are known to occur, and there is no known reason to expect a clinically significant interaction with choline.

Interactions with Diseases or Conditions

No interactions are known to occur, and there is no known reason to expect a clinically significant interaction with choline.

Dosage and Administration

ORAL: For asthma, 500-1000 mg three times daily has been used (5165,5166). An average diet supplies 200-600 mg of choline daily (4921). Adequate Intake (AI), as established by the Food and Nutrition Board of the National Institute of Medicine, for adults is 550 mg per day for males and lactating women; females, 425 mg per day; pregnant females, 450 mg per day (3094). For children 1-3 years the AI is 200 mg per day; 4-8 years, 250 mg per day; 9-13 years, 375 mg per day (3094); for infants less than 6 months, 125 mg per day; infants 7-12 months, 150 mg per day (3094). Daily Upper Intake Levels (UL, the highest level of intake that is likely to pose no risk of adverse effects) for choline are 1 gram daily for children 1-8 years, 2 grams for children 9-13 years, 3 grams for children 14-18 years, and 3.5 grams for adults over 18 years of age (3094).

Comments

Many people think choline, phosphatidylcholine, and lecithin are synonymous. Choline is a component of phosphatidylcholine, which is a component of lecithin (16). Although closely related, these terms are not synonymous. See separate listings for Phosphatidylcholine and Lecithin.

CHONDROITIN SULFATE

Also Known As

CDS, Chondroitin Sulfate A, Chondroitin Sulfates, Chondroitin Sulfate B, Chondroitin Sulfate C, Chondroitin Sulphate A Sodium, Condroitin, CSA, CSC, GAG, Galactosaminoglucuronoglycan Sulfate.

Scientific Names

Chondroitin 4-sulfate; chondroitin 4- and 6-sulfate.

People Use This For

Orally, chondroitin sulfate is used for osteoarthritis (14,1970,1971,1972). It is frequently used in combination with other products, including manganese ascorbate, glucosamine sulfate, glucosamine hydrochloride, or N-acetyl glucosamine for osteoarthritis (760,4237). Chondroitin sulfate is also used orally for ischemic heart disease, osteoporosis, and hyperlipidemia (9,1955). Chondroitin is also used in a complex with iron for treating iron-deficiency anemia (9). Intramuscularly, chondroitin sulfate is used for osteoarthritis (14,1970,1971,1972).

Topically, chondroitin sulfate is used for keratoconjunctivitis sicca (dry eyes) (14,1974), as a viscoelastic agent in cataract surgery (14), and as a medium for preservation of corneas used for transplantation (9). Chondroitin sulfate is also used topically in combination with other products for osteoarthritis (384).

Safety

LIKELY SAFE ...when used orally and appropriately. Chondroitin sulfate has been used safely in studies lasting from 2 months to 6 years (14,1342,1955,1970,1971,1972,2533). However, since chondroitin is often derived from bovine cartilage there is some concern about contamination with diseased animal parts (see Adverse Reactions) (1825). So far, there are no reports of disease transmission to humans due to use of contaminated chondroitin preparations. ...when used topically and appropriately as an ophthalmic product, which is a FDA-approved and prescription-only product that also contains sodium hyaluronate (Viscoat).
POSSIBLY SAFE ...when used intramuscularly (14).
PREGNANCY AND LACTATION: Insufficient reliable information available; avoid using.

Effectiveness

LIKELY EFFECTIVE ...when used orally in combination with analgesics or non-steroidal anti-inflammatory drugs (NSAIDs) for reducing the symptoms of osteoarthritis. Several studies have shown that chondroitin sulfate added to conventional analgesics or NSAIDs is significantly better than analgesics or NSAIDs alone for reducing pain and improving functionality indices in patients with osteoarthritis of the hip and knee (14,322,323,324,1342,1970,1971,1972,2533,4237). Several studies found that patients taking chondroitin sulfate could decrease their use or dose of analgesics and NSAIDs, but could not completely discontinue them. Treatment with chondroitin sulfate for 2-4 months may be required before significant improvement is experienced (1342). One clinical trial has evaluated the combination of chondroitin sulfate, glucosamine HCl, and manganese ascorbate (Cosamin-DS). The combination was superior to placebo, but was not compared to the individual components alone. It is unclear if the combination adds any benefit compared to chondroitin sulfate alone (4237). Although there have been several trials that have shown positive results, many of them have enrolled small numbers of patients and have been methodologically flawed. Two meta-analytical reviews of the literature have pooled and evaluated the data from these studies and found that chondroitin sulfate likely provides significant benefit in patients with hip and knee osteoarthritis (1342,2533). Additional large-scale, high quality studies are needed to clarify the potential role of chondroitin in treatment of osteoarthritis. ...when used in combination with sodium hyaluronate and applied topically to the eye as a surgical aid in cataract extraction or lens implantation. A combination product containing chondroitin sulfate and sodium hyaluronate (Viscoat) is a FDA-approved, prescription ophthalmic product (266).

POSSIBLY EFFECTIVE ...when used intramuscularly for reducing the symptoms of osteoarthritis (14). ...when used as an ophthalmic preparation for dry eyes (1974).

There is insufficient reliable information available about the effectiveness of chondroitin sulfate for its other uses. However, there is some preliminary evidence that oral chondroitin sulfate might reduce the occurrence of myocardial infarction in people who have previously had a myocardial infarction (MI) or who have unstable angina (1955). More evidence is needed to rate chondroitin sulfate for this use.

Mechanism of Action

Chondroitin sulfate belongs to a class of very large molecules called glucosaminoglycans (GAGs). Chondroitin is manufactured from natural sources, such as shark and bovine cartilage (6). People use chondroitin for osteoarthritis because it is endogenously found in cartilaginous tissues of most mammals and serves as a substrate for the formation of the joint matrix structure (1972,1973). Some researchers think chondroitin might have cardiovascular applications due to potential antiatherogenic properties (1955); however, this effect has not been verified. Since chondroitin is a minor component (~4%) of the low molecular weight heparinoid mixture, danaparoid (Orgaran), some concern has been expressed about possible anticoagulant activity of chondroitin sulfate. However, significant hematological changes have not been found in studies (760). Early evidence that chondroitin is not absorbed orally (4202) has been refuted by more recent studies. Studies show that people absorb 8-18% of orally administered chondroitin (760,3242,4203,4205,4237). Lower molecular weight derivatives of chondroitin formed in the gastrointestinal tract are more readily absorbed (3242) and might also contribute to the pharmacological activity of orally administered chondroitin.

Adverse Reactions

Orally, chondroitin sulfate is usually well-tolerated, but can cause epigastric pain and nausea in some patients (14). Diarrhea, constipation, eyelid edema, lower limb edema, alopecia, and extrasystoles have also been reported in clinical trials (1342). Some patients have also had allergic reactions (14). When used as an ophthalmic product, it can cause intraocular hypertension, discomfort, and corneal edema after cataract surgery (14). Concern has been expressed about possible anticoagulant activity of chondroitin sulfate. However, hematological changes have not occurred in patients taking chondroitin sulfate in clinical trials (760). Since chondroitin is usually produced from bovine cartilage, typically the trachea, there is some concern about the potential risk of contamination with diseased animals and transmission of bovine spongiform encephalopathy (BSE, mad cow disease) and other diseases. Although bovine trachea tissue does not seem to carry a high risk of BSE disease infectivity, in some cases manufacturing methods might lead to contamination with other diseased animal tissues. So far there are no reports of BSE or other disease transmission to humans from dietary supplements containing animal materials and the risk of potential disease transmission is thought to be low. Although many manufacturers 'guarantee' the safety of their chondroitin products, most manufacturers do not seem to take adequate measures to eliminate the risk of contamination.

Interactions with Herbs & Other Dietary Supplements

GLUCOSAMINE SULFATE: Although chondroitin sulfate and glucosamine sulfate are often administered together, no human studies have compared this combination to either product alone; there is no evidence that the combination has greater benefit than either product alone.

Interactions with Drugs

ANTIPLATELET/ANTICOAGULANT AGENTS: Theoretically, concurrent use of parenteral chondroitin sulfate with ardeparin (Normiflo), aspirin, NSAIDs, dalteparin (Fragmin), dextran, dipyridamole (Persantine), enoxaparin (Lovenox), or heparin, warfarin (Coumadin) (15) might increase the risk of bleeding.

HYALURONIC ACID: Concomitant use of chondroitin sulfate provides a beneficial synergistic effect in cataract surgery (14).

Interactions with Foods

No interactions are known to occur, and there is no known reason to expect a clinically significant interaction with chondroitin sulfate.

Interactions with Lab Tests

ANTI-FACTOR Xa: Theoretically, because it is a component of danaparoid, chondroitin sulfate administered by injection might increase the anti-factor Xa level and test results. No significant hematological changes were noted in a group of patients during six months of oral chondroitin therapy (760).

Interactions with Diseases or Conditions

COAGULATION DISORDERS: Theoretically, parenterally administered chondroitin sulfate might affect coagulation and increase the risk of bleeding when used in patients with clotting disorders; avoid use.

Dosage and Administration

ORAL: For osteoarthritis, the typical dose of chondroitin sulfate is 200-400 mg two to three times daily (14,1970,1971,1972,3278,4237) or 1200 mg as a single daily dose (1971). For prevention of recurrent myocardial infarction (MI), 10 grams daily in 3 divided doses for 3 months, followed by 1.5 grams in 3 divided doses as maintenance therapy has been used (1955).

INTRAMUSCULAR: For osteoarthritis, the most common dose is 50-100 mg per day in a single daily injection or divided into two daily injections (14). Parenteral chondroitin sulfate products are not available in the US.

Comments

Although chondroitin sulfate and glucosamine sulfate are frequently marketed together in combination products (760), there is no evidence that the combination has greater benefit than either product alone. The National Institutes of Health (NIH) is sponsoring a clinical trial of glucosamine sulfate and chondroitin sulfate. The 16-week, parallel group, double-blind RCT includes four separate treatment arms, in which patients will ingest: 1. placebo, 2. 500 mg of glucosamine sulfate 3 times per day, 3. 400 mg of chondroitin sulfate 3 times per day, or 4. a combination of glucosamine sulfate and chondroitin (3573). Tell patients to look out for chondroitin plus glucosamine combination products that also contain manganese (e.g., Cosamin DS). When taken according to the manufacturers' directions, these products can sometimes supply greater than the tolerable upper limit (UL) for manganese of 11 mg per day. Ingestion of more than 11 mg per day of manganese might cause significant central nervous system toxicity (7135) (See separate listing for Manganese).

CHROMIUM

Also Known As

Chromic Chloride, Chromium Acetate, Chromium Chloride, Chromium Nicotinate, Chromium Picolinate, Chromium Polynicotinate, Chromium Trichloride, Chromium Tripicolinate, Chromium III, Chromium III Picolinate, Chromium (III), Chromium 3, Chromium 3+, Chromium-3+, Cr III, Cr-III, Cr-3, Cr3+, Cr-3+, Glucose Tolerance Factor, Glucose Tolerance Factor-Cr, GTF, GTF-Cr, GTF Cr, Trivalent Chromium.

Scientific Names

Chromium; Cr; atomic number 24.

People Use This For

Orally, chromium is used for improving glycemic control in type 1 and 2 diabetes, corticosteroid-induced hyperglycemia, and reactive hypoglycemia; for hypercholesterolemia; and for increasing high-density lipoprotein (HDL) cholesterol levels in patients taking beta-blockers. It is also used orally for weight loss, to increase muscle mass and fat-free mass, and decrease body fat. Chromium is also used orally to enhance athletic performance, to increase energy and vigor, and to treat dysthymic disorder (a mild form of depression). Intravenously, chromium is used as a supplement in total parenteral nutrition (TPN).

Safety

LIKELY SAFE ...when used orally and appropriately. Chromium is safe in amounts found in foods or supplemental amounts not exceeding adequate intake (AI) levels. The AI for chromium is different based on gender and age. For men aged 14-50, the AI is 35 mcg per day. For men aged 51 and older, the AI is 30 mcg. For women aged 19-50 years, the AI is 25 mcg per day. For women aged 51 and older, the AI is 20 mcg (7135).

POSSIBLY SAFE ...when used orally and appropriately, short-term in amounts greater than adequate intake (AI) levels. Short-term, chromium picolinate has been safely used in doses up to 1000 mcg per day (1934,6867,7135,7137); however, there is insufficient information to establish safe and tolerable upper intake levels (7135). There is also some concern that long-term supplemental use may not be safe due to potential mutagenic effects (6863,6869). Until more is known, tell patients not to take chromium supplements long-term.

CHILDREN: LIKELY SAFE ...when used orally and appropriately. Chromium is safe in amounts not exceeding the adequate intake (AI) levels (7135). For infants 0 to 6 months, the AI is 0.2 mcg per day; 7 to 12 months, 5.5 mcg. For children 1 to 3 years, the AI is 11 mcg; 4 to 8 years, 15 mcg. For boys 9 to 13 years, the AI is 25 mcg. For girls 9 to 13 years, the AI is 21 mcg; 14 to 18 years, 24 mcg. There is insufficient reliable information available about the safety of chromium in higher amounts when used in children.

PREGNANCY: LIKELY SAFE ...when used orally and appropriately. Chromium is safe in amounts not exceeding adequate intake (AI) levels. The AI for pregnant women aged 14-18 years is 29 mcg per day. For pregnant women aged 19-50 years, it is 30 mcg per day (7135). POSSIBLY SAFE ...when used orally in amounts exceeding the adequate intake (AI) levels. There is some evidence that pregnant patients with gestational diabetes can safely use chromium in doses of 4-8 mcg per kilogram (1953); however, patients should not take chromium supplements during pregnancy without medical supervision.

LACTATION: LIKELY SAFE ...when used orally and appropriately. Chromium is safe in amounts not exceeding adequate intake (AI) levels. The AI for lactating women aged 14-18 years is 44 mcg per day. For lactating women aged 19-50 years it is 45 mcg per day (7135). Chromium supplements do not seem to increase normal chromium concentration in human breast milk (1937). There is insufficient reliable information available about the safety of chromium in higher amounts when used in breast-feeding women.

Effectiveness

POSSIBLY EFFECTIVE ...when used orally for type 2 diabetes. There is some evidence that certain patients can benefit by adding chromium picolinate to their conventional diabetes treatment regimen. Chromium seems to significantly decrease fasting blood glucose and insulin levels, and decrease glycosylated hemoglobin (HbA1c) (6862,6867,7137). Higher doses may be more effective and work more quickly. Doses of 500 mcg twice daily significantly decrease HbA1c after 2 months of treatment. Lower doses of 100 mcg twice daily can take up to 4 months. Higher doses of 200 mcg three times daily or 500 mcg twice daily also seem to significantly reduce triglyceride and total serum cholesterol levels after 2-4 months of treatment, indicating it might also be helpful for diabetic patients with metabolic syndrome (syndrome X) (1934,6867). There is some evidence that chromium picolinate might have the same benefits in patients with type 1 diabetes (1935). There is speculation that chromium supplements might only help certain patients with low chromium levels, since it only has a blood glucose-lowering effect in 40% to 80% of people with elevated blood glucose (6858). Chromium levels are often below normal in patients with diabetes (7058). There is not yet enough evidence to recommend chromium for all diabetes patients. Clinicians might consider trial use in interested patients to see if it helps. Stick with chromium picolinate preparations. Chromium chloride may not be as effective (7060). Remind patients that chromium is not an alternative to conventional medicines and should not be used in place of conventional treatments. ...when used orally for steroid-induced diabetes. There is some evidence chromium 200 mcg three times daily initially, followed by 200 mcg once daily for maintenance, can help improve blood glucose levels in patients taking corticosteroids (5039). ...when used orally for symptoms of reactive hypoglycemia. Treatment for 3 months with chromium chloride 200 mg daily seems to improve symptoms and increase blood glucose levels in patients with reactive hypoglycemia following an oral glucose load (6859). ...when used orally for low serum high-density lipoprotein (HDL) cholesterol in patients taking beta-blockers. There is some evidence that yeast-derived chromium 600 mcg daily for 2 months can increase HDL levels by 16% in men taking beta-blockers (5040).

POSSIBLY INEFFECTIVE ...when used orally for body building or to improve body composition. The use of chromium for this purpose is controversial. There is some evidence showing overall weight loss, body fat loss, and increased lean body mass in people taking chromium picolinate 200 to 400 mcg per day in conjunction with resistance training (6860,6861,6868). However, the results of these studies are unreliable due to questionable methods (6861). More reliable studies show that adding chromium picolinate or chloride 177-200 mcg daily to a weight-training program has no additional beneficial effect on body composition (6861,6862). ...when used orally for weight loss in obese patients. Using chromium picolinate 400 mcg alone or adding it to an aerobic exercise program does not seem to help increase weight loss or decrease body fat (6860).

There is insufficient reliable information available to rate the effectiveness of chromium for its other uses. However, there is some preliminary evidence that chromium might improve the response to antidepressants in people with dysthymic disorder. Chromium picolinate or chromium polynicotinate 200 mcg once or twice daily appears to improve mood in people who have only a partial response to antidepressants such as sertraline or nortriptyline (2659). More evidence is needed to rate chromium for this use.

Mechanism of Action

Chromium is an essential trace element. The activity of chromium depends on its valance state. Metallic chromium, or chromium 0, has no activity. The other two common forms, chromium III (Cr III) and chromium VI (Cr VI), have different activities. Cr VI is typically used in chemical and welding industries and is carcinogenic to humans. Cr III is the form found in foods and supplements. Chromium is sometimes referred to as glucose tolerance factor (GTF), but GTF is actually a complex of molecules found in the body that includes chromium bound to single molecules of glycine, cysteine, glutamic acid, and two molecules of nicotinic acid. Chromium is thought to be the active component of the complex. Some dietary sources of chromium include canned foods (due to chromium leaching from the can), meats and animal fats, fish, brown sugar, coffee, tea, some spices, calf liver, whole wheat bread, rye bread, and brewer's yeast (7061). Symptomatic chromium deficiency is rare. When it does occur it is most often due to malnutrition, pregnancy, stress, or long-term use of chromium deficient total parenteral nutrition (TPN) (6863). Other people might also be at risk for low chromium levels. Although not yet confirmed, some researchers suspect that tissue levels of chromium might decline with age (6863). Some athletes might also be at risk for low chromium levels since strenuous aerobic exercise seems to increase urinary excretion of chromium (6860,6861). However, exercise induced losses seem to be less in those who regularly exercise (6862). People doing strength training seem to have increased absorption of chromium (7136). It is difficult to measure chromium status to determine who might require supplementation. Blood chromium levels are not in equilibrium with chromium stores and therefore do not provide a good indicator of chromium status (6859). Similarly, levels in the urine and hair do not reflect overall chromium status (6867). There is no reliable method available to diagnose chromium deficiency, other than observing outcome following supplementation in patients suspected of being deficient (3859,6869). Symptoms of chromium deficiency can include impaired insulin function and glucose tolerance, increased serum cholesterol and triglycerides, and others (6863,6869). Discovery of the role of chromium in insulin function occurred when patients on long-term total parenteral nutrition (TPN), developed symptoms of diabetes that did not respond to insulin, but were reversed by chromium (6869). Because of the symptoms associated with chromium deficiency, researchers have speculated that chromium supplementation might be an effective treatment for diabetes and hypercholesterolemia. Chromium has a normal role in insulin function, so it might help patients with diabetes who are chromium deficient. There is some evidence that patients with diabetes might have lower than normal levels of chromium due to increased chromium excretion (6858). However, patients with diabetes also seem to have increased gastrointestinal absorption of chromium. It's also theorized that patients with diabetes may not be able to adequately convert chromium from the diet to a usable form in the body (6867). Chromium seems to be transported to insulin-sensitive cells by transferrin, in response to increases in plasma insulin levels (6869). It is suspected to potentiate insulin by increasing receptor numbers and affinity, and increasing insulin binding to cells (6859,6867). In the absence of chromium, insulin binding and the number of insulin receptors seems to decrease. In chromium-deficient tissue supplemental chromium potentiates glucose uptake by cells, oxidation of glucose, and incorporation of glucose into fatty acids and cholesterol (14). In animal models, a chromium-containing peptide called chromodulin has been identified, which potentiates the actions of insulin at its receptors, including activation of receptor tyrosine kinase activity (6869). In patients with diabetes, these actions seem to translate into decreased insulin resistance, improved glucose tolerance, and lower blood glucose levels (6862). Researchers are interested in chromium for treatment of obesity and metabolic syndrome (syndrome X) due to its potential effects on lipids and body composition. It is theorized that chromium might also sensitize insulin-sensitive glucoreceptors in the brain, resulting in appetite suppression, activation of the sympathetic nervous system and stimulation of thermogenesis, and down-regulation of insulin secretion (6170,6860). It is also theorized that chromium might enhance glucose utilization in the brain, stimulate norepinephrine release, and increase serotonin synthesis, which could lead to beneficial effects in dysthymic disorder (mild depression) (2659). Chromium is also hypothesized to increase muscle mass by increasing amino acid uptake into muscle cells via potentiation of insulin activity (6862). Chromium supplements come in several salt forms. The most common are chromium picolinate and chromium chloride. Chromium picolinate is a complex of chromium and picolinic acid, which is a naturally occurring metabolic derivative of tryptophan. Adding the picolinate salt increases absorption, retention and accumulation of chromium compared to inorganic salts such as chromium chloride (6861,6864). When ingested most chromium is excreted unabsorbed in the feces. The small percentage that is absorbed, typically 0.4 to 2.5%, is rapidly excreted in the urine (7135). Once absorbed, chromium concentrates in the kidney, heart, liver, brain, muscle, spleen, testes, epididymis, and lungs (6863). Excretion of chromium picolinate from tissue stores has a half-life of 3 years (14). Chromium picolinate seems to be handled differently in the body than dietary chromium (6869). There is some evidence that chromium picolinate can enter cells unchanged and then produce hydroxyl radicals when the chromium is released, which might cause DNA damage (1299,6869). The clinical significance of this potential harmful effect is not known.

Adverse Reactions

Orally, chromium in the trivalent form (Cr III) is typically well tolerated. However, some patients can experience cognitive, perceptual, and motor dysfunction at doses as low as 200-400 mcg per day of chromium picolinate. Chromium picolinate has also been associated with weight gain in young women who do not exercise and in those on a weight-lifting program (1938). Some patients can also experience headaches, insomnia, sleep disturbances, irritability, and mood changes (6860). Some of these side effects might be due to the picolinate salt form, which might affect dopamine, serotonin, and norepinephrine metabolism in the brain (217). There is some concern that chronic use of chromium picolinate in higher doses might cause significant adverse effects. In some cases, doses of 600-2400 mcg per day can cause anemia, thrombocytopenia, hemolysis, hepatic dysfunction, and renal failure in some patients (554); however, it is not clear if chromium is responsible for these effects. For example, chromium picolinate has been associated with chronic interstitial nephritis in two case reports, but contradictory laboratory evidence shows that chromium does not seem to cause kidney tissue damage even after long-term, high dose exposure (7135). Short-term use of chromium picolinate in a dose of 600 mcg daily for two days has also been associated with a case of rhabdomyolysis (14); however, it is unclear if chromium was the causative agent. Although there are reports of severe adverse events in people taking chromium supplements, in most instances it is unclear if chromium was actually responsible for the adverse event. Furthermore, there does not appear to be any dose-effect relationship for severe adverse effects.

Occupational inhalation of hexavalent chromium fumes can cause ulceration of the nasal mucosa (chrome ulcers) and perforation of the nasal septum (chrome holes) and has been associated with pneumoconiosis, allergic asthma, and increased susceptibility to respiratory tract carcinomas (14). Industrial hexavalent chromium is considered cytotoxic and genotoxic (6863). It penetrates the cells easily (unlike trivalent chromium) and appears to induce oxidative damage to DNA (7326).

Intravenously, chromium is associated with decreased glomerular filtration rate (GFR) in children who receive long-term chromium-containing total parenteral nutrition (TPN) (9).

Interactions with Herbs & Other Dietary Supplements

IRON: Chromium competes with iron for binding to the transport protein, transferrin, and could predispose people to iron deficiency. This effect is unlikely to be clinically significant at usual supplemental doses of chromium (6861,6865,6866).

VITAMIN C: Concomitant vitamin C use might increase chromium absorption (1900).

ZINC: Theoretically, co-administration might decrease absorption of both chromium and zinc (1950).

Interactions with Drugs

ANTACIDS: There is some evidence that antacids might decrease chromium levels by inhibiting absorption of chromium. Increasing gastric pH seems to decrease chromium absorption and retention (7135).

BETA-BLOCKERS: Concomitant use of chromium supplements and beta-blockers, including atenolol (Tenormin) or propranolol (Inderal), modestly increases serum high density lipoprotein (HDL) cholesterol concentrations (5040).

CORTICOSTEROIDS: Chromium might decrease corticosteroid-induced increases in blood sugar in patients with or without pre-existing diabetes. In two patients with type 2 diabetes, oral chromium supplements reversed increases in blood glucose associated with dexamethasone (Decadron) or prednisone (Deltasone). In a third case, chromium reduced the insulin dose required by a patient who experienced prednisone-induced diabetes after a kidney transplant (5039).

H2-BLOCKERS: There is some evidence that H2-blockers might decrease chromium levels by inhibiting absorption of chromium. Increasing gastric pH seems to decrease chromium absorption and retention (7135). Some of these drugs include cimetidine (Tagamet), rinitidine (Zantac), famotidine (Pepcid), and others.

INSULIN: Theoretically, concomitant use might increase the risk of hypoglycemia (1952).

NICOTINIC ACID: Combining chromium and nicotinic acid might have additive effects on improving glucose tolerance (1936).

NONSTEROIDAL ANTI-INFLAMMATORY DRUGS (NSAIDs): There is some evidence that NSAIDs might increase chromium levels by increasing chromium absorption and retention. Drugs that are prostaglandin inhibitors seem to increase chromium absorption and retention (7135). Some of these drugs include ibuprofen (Advil, Motrin, Nuprin, others), indomethacin (Indocin), naproxen (Aleve, Anaprox, Naprelan, Naprosyn), piroxicam (Feldene), aspirin, and others.

PROTON PUMP INHIBITORS (PPIs): There is some evidence that PPIs might decrease chromium levels by inhibiting chromium absorption. Increasing gastric pH might decrease chromium absorption and retention (7135). These drugs include lansoprazole (Prevacid), omeprazole (Prilosec), rabeprazole (Aciphex), and pantoprazole (Protonix, Pantoloc).

Drug Influences on Nutrient Levels and Depletion

SOME DRUGS CAN AFFECT CHROMIUM LEVELS:

CORTICOSTEROIDS: use of corticosteroids can increase urinary chromium excretion, which might lead to chromium deficiency and/or corticosteroid-induced hyperglycemia. Three cases are reported of oral chromium supplements reversing dexamethasone (Decadron) or prednisone (Deltasone) induced hyperglycemia in patients with or without pre-existing diabetes. Consider chromium supplements based on clinical judgment (5039).

Interactions with Foods

IRON: Chromium competes with iron for binding to the transport protein, transferrin, and could predispose people to iron deficiency. This effect is unlikely to be clinically significant at usual supplemental doses of chromium (6861,6865,6866).

SIMPLE SUGARS: Intake of high levels of simple sugars may increase chromium losses in urine (14).

Interactions with Lab Tests

GLUCOSE: Chromium might reduce blood glucose concentrations and test results in some patients' corticosteroid-induced hyperglycemia. Three cases are reported of oral chromium supplements reversing dexamethasone (Decadron) or prednisone (Deltasone) induced hyperglycemia in patients with or without pre-existing diabetes (5039).

CHOLESTEROL: Chromium can reduce fasting serum cholesterol concentrations and test results in patients with type 2 diabetes (14). Chromium can modestly increase serum HDL cholesterol concentrations and test results in men taking beta-blockers, including atenolol (Tenormin) and propranolol (Inderal) (5040).

GLYCOSYLATED HEMOGLOBIN (HbA1c): Chromium might improve blood glucose control and decrease HbA1c values in some patients with type 1, type 2, and gestational diabetes (14).

TRIGLYCERIDES: Chromium can reduce serum triglyceride concentrations and test results in patients with type 2 diabetes (14,1934).

Interactions with Diseases or Conditions

BEHAVIORAL AND PSYCHIATRIC DISORDERS: Theoretically, chromium picolinate preparations might affect behavioral and psychiatric conditions. Picolinic acid in chromium picolinate preparations can alter serotonin, dopamine, and norepinephrine metabolism in the central nervous system (1935).

CHROMATE/LEATHER CONTACT ALLERGY: Oral chromium supplements can cause allergic reactions in people with chromate or leather contact allergy, including dermatitis, erythema, and scaling on the extremities (6624).

DIABETES: Chromium might lower blood glucose levels (1939); monitor closely.

RENAL INSUFFICIENCY: Chromium supplements might exacerbate renal insufficiency (1951). Tell patients with renal dysfunction to avoid chromium supplements.

Dosage and Administration

ORAL: For lowering blood glucose and lipid levels in patients with type 2 diabetes, 200 to 1000 mcg daily in divided dose has been used (1934,6867). For increasing serum HDL cholesterol in men taking beta-blockers, 200 mcg three times daily has been used (5040). For corticosteroid-induced hyperglycemia or exacerbation of pre-existing diabetes, 400 mcg per day or 200 mcg three times daily has been used (5039). Chromium picolinate has been used in most studies. For preventing reactive hypoglycemia, 200 mcg daily of chromium chloride has been used (6859). For treating dysthymic disorder (mild depression) 200 mcg once or twice daily of chromium picolinate or polynicotinate has been used (2659). Daily adequate intake (AI) levels for chromium have been established: Infants 0 to 6 months, 0.2 mcg; 7 to 12 months, 5.5 mcg; children 1 to 3 years, 11 mcg; 4 to 8 years, 15 mcg; boys 9 to 13 years, 25 mcg; men 14 to 50 years, 35 mcg; men 51 and older, 30 mcg; girls 9 to 13 years, 21 mcg; 14 to 18 years, 24 mcg; women 19 to 50 years, 25 mcg; women 51 and older, 20 mcg; pregnant women 14 to 18 years, 29 mcg; 19 to 50 years, 30 mcg; lactating women 14 to 18 years, 44 mcg; 19 to 50 years, 45 mcg. Sometimes chromium amounts are listed in micromols. The conversion factor to micrograms is: 1.92 micromol Cr = 100 mcg (6867).

INTRAVENOUS: No typical dosage.

Comments

Chromium was discovered in France in the late 1790s, but it took until the 1960s before it was recognized as being an important trace element and important for insulin function (7058). Supplemental chromium is not required for short term total parenteral nutrition (TPN). Sufficient amounts of chromium (as contaminants) are contained in amino acid products used for TPN (9,14).

CHRYSANTHEMUM

Also Known As

Florist's Chrysanthemum, Ju Hua, Mum.

Scientific Names

Anthemis grandiflorum; Anthemis stipulacea; Chrysanthemum morifolium; Chrysanthemum sinense; Chrysanthemum stipulaceum; Dendranthema morifolium; Matricaria morifolia.
Family: Asteraceae or Compositae.

People Use This For

Orally, chrysanthemum is frequently used in herbal combinations. In one specific combination with seven other herbs (PC-SPES), the dried chrysanthemum flower is used to treat prostate cancer (5548). In combination with licorice (Glycyrrhiza uralensis) and Panax notoginseng, the dried chrysanthemum flower is used to treat precancerous lesions (5555).

In Chinese medicine, the dried chrysanthemum flower is commonly used orally to treat angina and hypertension (5545). The chrysanthemum product, jiangtangkang, is used to treat non-insulin dependent diabetes (5546).

In folk medicine, the dried chrysanthemum flower is widely used as an antipyretic, to clear the eye and the mind, and as an antitoxin. It is also used orally for colds, headache, dizziness, and swelling (5545).

In southern China, chrysanthemum is very popular as a summertime tea (5545).

Safety

POSSIBLY SAFE ...when used orally in a specific herbal combination (PC-SPES) (5548).

There is insufficient reliable information available about the safety of chrysanthemum for its other uses.

PREGNANCY AND LACTATION: Insufficient reliable information available; avoid using.

Effectiveness

POSSIBLY EFFECTIVE ...when used orally in a specific herbal combination for prostate cancer. Studies using chrysanthemum in combination with seven other herbs (PC-SPES), found that it significantly decreases prostate-specific antigen (PSA) levels (3576,5122,5548,6284,6286), causes clinically significant reductions in serum testosterone (5548), improves quality of life, and reduces pain (6286) in patients with prostate cancer. In two reports, PSA levels fell significantly within one month of treatment (5122,5548).

There is insufficient reliable information about the effectiveness of chrysanthemum for its other uses.

Mechanism of Action

The dried chrysanthemum flower contains the essential oil bornol, chrysantheonon, camphor, the alkaloid stachydrine and several glycosides. It also contains adenine, choline, B vitamins and substances similar to vitamin A. Some evidence suggests that chrysanthemum might increase coronary vasodilatation and blood flow without increasing coronary contractility or oxygen consumption. Chrysanthemum has antibacterial and antipyretic effects. It can also reduce the capillary permeability induced by histamine (5545). Preliminary information suggests the chrysanthemum product jiangtangkang used by individuals with non-insulin dependent diabetes might improve insulin sensitivity and decrease blood viscosity (5546). A preliminary trial suggests Hua-sheng-ping, a combination of chrysanthemum, licorice, and Panax notoginseng can reverse precancerous gastrointestinal lesions (5555). The chrysanthemum constituents chrysin and acetin-7-O-beta-D-galactopyranoside inhibit HIV replication (5545,5547).

Adverse Reactions

Chrysanthemum flowers can cause photosensitivity and contact dermatitis (5552,5553,5554,5556,5557). Chrysanthemum flowers can cause an allergic reaction in individuals sensitive to the Asteraceae/Compositae family. Members of this family include ragweed, chrysanthemums, marigolds, daisies and many other herbs.

Interactions with Herbs & Other Dietary Supplements

CARDIOACTIVE HERBS: Avoid concomitant use with other cardioactive herbs due to unpredictability of effects and adverse effects. Cardioactive herbs include: calamus, cereus, cola, coltsfoot, devil's claw, European mistletoe, fenugreek, fumitory, ginger, Panax ginseng, hawthorn, white horehound, mate, parsley, quassia, Scotch broom flower, shepherd's purse, and wild carrot (4). Cardiac glycoside containing herbs include black hellebore, Canadian hemp root, digitalis leaf, hedge mustard, figwort, lily of the valley root, motherwort, oleander leaf, pheasant's eye plant, pleurisy root, squill bulb leaf scales, and strophanthus seeds (2,18,19,500).

Interactions with Drugs

CARDIOACTIVE DRUGS: Theoretically, chrysanthemum could interfere with cardiovascular therapy; avoid using.

Interactions with Foods

No interactions are known to occur, and there is no known reason to expect a clinically significant interaction with chrysanthemum.

Interactions with Lab Tests

No interactions are known to occur, and there is no known reason to expect a clinically significant interaction with chrysanthemum.

Interactions with Diseases or Conditions

No interactions are known to occur, and there is no known reason to expect a clinically significant interaction with chrysanthemum.

Dosage and Administration

ORAL: To make the water extract, 300 mg of the dried chrysanthemum flower are condensed into 500 mL water. A typical dose is 25 mL three times daily or used as tea (5545).

Comments
The name chrysanthemum is from the Greek words for "gold" and "flower."

CHYMOTRYPSIN

Also Known As
Alpha-Chymotrypsin, Chymotrypsin A, Chymotrypsin B, Chymotrypsinum, Quimotripsina.

Scientific Names
Alpha-chymotrypsin; chymotrypsinum.

People Use This For
Orally, chymotrypsin is used for reducing inflammation and edema associated with abscesses, ulcers, surgery or traumatic injuries; as an expectorant in asthma, bronchitis, pulmonary diseases, and sinusitis (9). It is used in minimizing initial rise in serum liver enzymes in burn patients, reducing liver stress, and associated degradative changes during wound repair (716).
Topically, chymotrypsin is used for inflammatory and infectious disorders (509).
As an inhalant, chymotrypsin is used for inflammatory and infectious disorders (509).
Intramuscularly, chymotrypsin is used to reduce inflammation and edema associated with abscesses, ulcers, surgery or traumatic injuries (9), and as an expectorant in asthma, bronchitis, pulmonary diseases, and sinusitis (9), and for inflammatory and infectious disorders (509).
Ophthalmically, chymotrypsin is used as an adjunct in cataract surgery to reduce trauma to the eye (9,509).

Safety
LIKELY SAFE ...when used ophthalmically, as approved by the FDA.
POSSIBLY SAFE ...when used orally for inflammation due to surgery or trauma injuries (9,717,718). ...when used topically for treating burns (716).
There is insufficient reliable information available about the safety of chymotrypsin for its other uses.
PREGNANCY AND LACTATION: Insufficient reliable information available; avoid using.

Effectiveness
EFFECTIVE ...when used as an adjunct in cataract surgery according to FDA approved prescription product labeling (9,509).
POSSIBLY EFFECTIVE ...when used orally for reducing inflammation and edema associated with surgery or trauma injuries (9,717,718). ...when used for treating burns (716).
There is insufficient reliable information available about the effectiveness of chymotrypsin for its other uses.

Mechanism of Action
Chymotrypsin has ingredients that have proteolytic (9,509), anti-inflammatory (9,509,715), and antioxidant activities that reduce tissue destruction (715).

Adverse Reactions
Orally, anaphylactic reaction (rare) is characterized by dyspnea, urticaria, edema of the glottis or lip, shock and vascular collapse, loss of consciousness, and death (9,509). If hypersensitivity is suspected, a sensitivity test should be made before administration (9).
Opthamalmically, chymotrypsin leads to increased intraocular pressure (9,509), corneal edema, striation, moderate uveitis (9), iridoplegia, and filamentary keratitis (509).

Interactions with Herbs & Other Dietary Supplements
Insufficient reliable information available.

Interactions with Drugs
No interactions are known to occur, and there is no known reason to expect a clinically significant interaction with chymotrypsin.

Interactions with Foods
No interactions are known to occur, and there is no known reason to expect a clinically significant interaction with chymotrypsin.

Interactions with Lab Tests
No interactions are known to occur, and there is no known reason to expect a clinically significant interaction with chymotrypsin.

Interactions with Diseases or Conditions
OCULAR SURGERY: Contraindicated in ocular surgery cases involving congenital cataracts, high vitreous pressure and a gaping incisional wound, or if individual is 20 years of age or younger (9).

Dosage and Administration
ORAL: For inflammation, edema and respiratory secretions, 6:1 ratio (trypsin: chymotrypsin) in a combined amount of 100,000 units USP four times daily has been used (9,717,718). For burns, as 6:1 ratio (trypsin:chymotrypsin) in a combined amount of 200,000 units USP four times daily for 10 days has been used (716).
INTRAMUSCULAR: For inflammation, edema and respiratory secretions: 5000 USP units one to three times daily has been used (9).
OPHTHALMIC: As an adjunct in cataract surgery, 1:5000 or 1:10,000 solution of chymotrypsin in sterile sodium chloride injection (0.9%) injected to irrigate the posterior chamber has been used (9).
TOPICAL: No typical dosage.

Comments
None.

CIGUATERA

Also Known As
Ciguatera, Ciguatera Poisoning.

Scientific Names
Gambierdiscus toxicus.

People Use This For
There are no medicinal uses for this product, but it may be encountered inadvertently by eating tainted fish (6).

Safety
UNSAFE ...when ingested. Up to 20% mortality has been reported (6). A single bite of fish contaminated with this toxin will produce symptoms (6).
PREGNANCY: UNSAFE ...when ingested. There has been one report of a fetus being aborted during acute phase of maternal poisoning. However, no lasting adverse effects have been reported in liveborn infants (6).
LACTATION: UNSAFE ...when ingested. Ciguatera is excreted in breast milk; GI symptoms and itching reported in infants breast-fed by symptomatic mothers; infant symptoms resolved with discontinuation of breast-feeding (6).

Effectiveness
There is insufficient reliable information available about the effectiveness of ciguatera.

Mechanism of Action
The applicable part of ciguatera is the toxin. Ciguatoxin increases cell permeability to sodium, causing sustained depolarization (6). Action in humans is dependent on anti-cholinesterase activity and also to a transmitter-like cholinomimetic activity (6).

Adverse Reactions
Poisoning has many different manifestations. But in general, poisoning is characterized by abdominal cramps, nausea, vomiting, diarrhea within 1-6 hours of ingestion; itching, numbness of lips, tongue, throat, paresthesias, blurred vision, hypotension, bradycardia; reversal of hot and cold sensations, and coma (rarely). In severe cases, shock, muscular paralysis, and death are possible (6). GI symptoms usually resolve within 24 hours. Muscle weakness/numbness may last weeks to months (6). Tumultuous fetal movements and intermittent fetal shivering have been reported with maternal poisoning. There has been one case of a fetus aborted during the acute phase of maternal poisoning (6).

Interactions with Herbs & Other Dietary Supplements
Insufficient reliable information available.

Interactions with Drugs

No interactions are known to occur, and there is no known reason to expect a clinically significant interaction with ciguatera.

Interactions with Foods

No interactions are known to occur, and there is no known reason to expect a clinically significant interaction with ciguatera.

Interactions with Lab Tests

No interactions are known to occur, and there is no known reason to expect a clinically significant interaction with ciguatera.

Interactions with Diseases or Conditions

No interactions are known to occur, and there is no known reason to expect a clinically significant interaction with ciguatera.

Dosage and Administration

No typical dosage.

Comments

Ciguatera poisoning is caused by eating normally safe, bottom-feeding, coral-reef fish that have accumulated ciguatoxin via the marine food chain (6). The red snapper, barracuda, and grouper are most often involved. Florida and Hawaii have the greatest incidence of ciguatera poisoning. Avoid consumption of fish in areas of recently disturbed coral reefs (includes waterfront construction). Ciguatoxic fish appear normal, including smell and taste. Local "rules of thumb" for detection are unsubstantiated. Testing for ciguatoxin is available in some areas (6). Over 400 (normally safe) fish species may contain toxin, including red snapper, barracuda, parrotfish, jacks and grouper (6).

CINCHONA

Also Known As

Chinarinde, Ecorce de Quina, Fieberrinde, Jesuit's Bark, Peruvian Bark, Quinine, Red Cinchona Bark.

Scientific Names

Cinchona calisaya; Cinchona ledgeriana; Cinchona pubescens, synonym Cinchona succirubra.
Family: Rubiaceae.

People Use This For

Orally, cinchona is used for stimulating appetite, promoting GI secretions (8), bloating and fullness (2), hemorrhoids, varicose veins, colds, and leg cramps (11).
Topically, cinchona is used in eye lotions for astringent, bactericidal, and anesthetic effects (11). Cinchona extract is also used topically for hemorrhoids, stimulating hair growth, and managing varicose veins (8).
In folk medicine, cinchona is used for mild attacks of influenza (8), malaria, fever, cancer, mouth and throat diseases (6), enlarged spleen, muscle cramps, and gastric disorders (18).

Safety

POSSIBLY SAFE ...when used orally and appropriately (12).
LIKELY UNSAFE ...when excessive amounts are used orally. 2 to 8 grams of the quinine constituent (505) or 2.5-8 grams quinidine constituent (17) can cause serious toxicity including death (505); however, the amount of these constituents varies according to the cinchona species (13).
PREGNANCY: LIKELY UNSAFE ...when used orally; avoid using (12).
LACTATION: Insufficient reliable information available; avoid using.

Effectiveness

POSSIBLY EFFECTIVE ...when used orally for peptic discomforts, such as fullness (2).
There is insufficient reliable information available about the effectiveness of cinchona for its other uses.

Mechanism of Action

The applicable part of cinchona is the bark. The cinchona bark can stimulate saliva and gastric juice secretion (2). The antimalarial effects can be attributed to quinine, an alkaloid constituent. The constituents, quinidine and quinine, have cardiac depressant properties (11).

Adverse Reactions

Cinchona used orally can cause thrombocytopenia, bleeding, and hypersensitivity reactions, including hives and fever (2). Overdose or hypersensitivity to cinchona can cause cinchonism; symptoms include headache (505), nausea, diarrhea, vomiting, ringing in the ears (6), and vision disturbance (8,505). Topically, the cinchona bark can cause contact dermatitis (11).

Interactions with Herbs & Other Dietary Supplements

ANTICOAGULANT HERBS: Theoretically, the cinchona bark can potentiate the activity of herbs with anticoagulant or antiplatelet properties, including alfalfa, angelica, aniseed, arnica, asafoetida, celery, chamomile, clove, fenugreek, feverfew, fucus, garlic, ginger, Panax ginseng, horse chestnut, licorice, northern and southern prickly ash, quassia, and red clover (4).

Interactions with Drugs

ACID-INHIBITING DRUGS: Theoretically, due to claims that cinchona increases stomach acid, it might interfere with antacids, sucralfate (Carafate), H-2 antagonists, or proton pump inhibitors (19).
ANTICOAGULANTS: Cinchona can increase the drug effects and risk of bleeding due to its quinine content (2).
CARBAMAZEPINE, PHENOBARBITAL: Cinchona can increase serum drug levels of carbamazepine and phenobarbital due to its quinine content (540).
QUINIDINE, QUININE: Concomitant use of cinchona can increase the therapeutic and adverse effects of these drugs (505).

Interactions with Foods

No interactions are known to occur, and there is no known reason to expect a clinically significant interaction with cinchona.

Interactions with Lab Tests

No interactions are known to occur, and there is no known reason to expect a clinically significant interaction with cinchona.

Interactions with Diseases or Conditions

GASTRIC OR INTESTINAL ULCERS: Cinchona is contraindicated (8,12) in conditions with an increased risk of bleeding.

Dosage and Administration

ORAL: The typical dose of cinchona is one cup of the tea up to three times daily (18). The tea is prepared by steeping 500 mg of the dried bark in 150 mL boiling water for 5-10 minutes and then straining. The maximum amount of cinchona is 1-3 grams of the bark per day (18) or 0.05-0.2 grams of the essential oil per day (12). The usual dose of the cinchona liquid extract (4-5% total alkaloids) is 0.6-3 grams per day (18). The cinchona extract (15-20% total alkaloids) is commonly given as 0.15-0.6 grams per day (18).

Comments

Cinchona bark contains quinine and related alkaloids, including quinidine (a cardiac depressant) and cinchotannic acid (can cause constipation). While quinine is effective for preventing or suppressing malaria caused by susceptible organisms (15), people treated with cinchona bark are exposed to the risks of quinidine, cinchotannic acid, and other alkaloid constituents. It is recommended that only purified quinine, or other appropriate antimalarial agents, be used to prevent or suppress malaria (15). US drug regulations require products containing cinchona derivatives to contain the labeling, "Discontinue use if ringing in the ears, deafness, skin rash or visual disturbances occur" (12).

CINNAMON bark

Also Known As

Batavia Cassia, Batavia Cinnamon, Ceylon Cinnamon, Cinnamonum, Padang-Cassia, Panang Cinnamon, Saigon Cassia, Saigon Cinnamon.
CAUTION: See separate listings for Cassia and Cinnamon flower.

Scientific Names

Cinnamomum verum, synonym Cinnamomum zeylanicum, Laurus Cinnamomum.
Family: Lauraceae.

People Use This For

Orally, cinnamon bark is used as an antispasmodic, antiflatulent, appetite stimulant (2,4), antidiarrheal, antimicrobial, anthelmintic, and for treating the common cold and influenza (4).

Topically, cinnamon bark is used as part of a multi-ingredient preparation for treating premature ejaculation (2537).

Historically, cinnamon bark has been used for GI upset and dysmenorrhea (6).

For food uses, cinnamon is commonly consumed as a spice in food and a flavoring agent in beverages (11).

In manufacturing, the volatile oil is commonly used in small amounts in toothpaste, mouthwashes, gargles, lotions, liniments, soaps, detergents, and other pharmaceutical products and cosmetics.

Safety

LIKELY SAFE ...when consumed in amounts commonly found in foods (11). Cinnamon bark has Generally Recognized as Safe (GRAS) status in the US (11).

POSSIBLY SAFE ...when used orally and appropriately in amounts slightly greater than those found in foods (4,12). ...when used topically, short-term as part of a multi-ingredient preparation (SS Cream). This preparation was used safely in a clinical trial where the cream was applied and left on the glans penis for 1-hour (2537). Further evaluation is needed to determine its safety after prolonged, repetitive use.

POSSIBLY UNSAFE ...when used orally in large amounts or long-term (4,12). Consumption of up to 700 mcg per kilogram of the constituent, cinnamaldehyde, is considered the highest acceptable level (4).

PREGNANCY: LIKELY UNSAFE ...when used orally in amounts greater than those found in foods (4,12).

LACTATION: Insufficient reliable information available; avoid using amounts greater than found in foods.

Effectiveness

POSSIBLY EFFECTIVE ...when used orally as an antiflatulent, antispasmodic, and appetite stimulant (2,4). ...when used topically as part of a multi-ingredient preparation for treating premature ejaculation. In one controlled clinical trial, a multi-ingredient cream preparation (SS Cream) containing Panax ginseng root, Angelica root, Cistanches deserticola, Zanthoxyl species, Torlidis seed, clove flower, Asiasari root, cinnamon bark, and toad venom was applied to the glans penis one hour prior to intercourse and washed off immediately before intercourse. Men suffering from premature ejaculation who were treated with the cream had significantly improved ejaculatory latency compared to placebo (2537).

There is insufficient reliable information available about the effectiveness of cinnamon bark for its other uses.

Mechanism of Action

The volatile oils of cinnamon bark are thought to be responsible for the proposed antispasmodic, antiflatulent, and appetite stimulant effects (4). The constituent cinnamaldehyde makes up 60-80% of the volatile oil (4,4800). Cinnamaldehyde is thought to have central nervous system (CNS) stimulant effects at low doses and sedative effects at high doses. It is also thought to have hypothermic, antipyretic, antibacterial, and antifungal activity. Cinnamaldehyde might also increase peripheral blood flow, slow heart rate, reduce blood pressure, and increase blood sugar levels (4). However, these pharmacological effects are thought to be fairly weak. Furthermore, much of the active volatile oil in cinnamon is thought to evaporate away when the cinnamon is prepared as a tea (4). It is unclear to what extent the volatile oil contributes to any therapeutic activity. The tannin constituents in cinnamon bark have astringent properties and are thought to be responsible for an antidiarrheal effect (4). Cinnamon bark is also a urinary irritant (19). A multi-ingredient topical preparation containing cinnamon bark and several other herbs (SS Cream) is thought to work in premature ejaculation by increasing the penile vibratory threshold and reducing the amplitude of penile somatosensory evoked potentials (2537). There is some preliminary research that suggests the constituent, methylhydroxy chalcone polymer (MHCP), might improve insulin sensitivity (6657). However, this has not yet been demonstrated in humans.

Adverse Reactions

Orally, no adverse reactions tend to occur with the use of the cinnamon bark; however, the oil can irritate mucous membranes and is a skin irritant and sensitizer.

Topically, preparations in concentrations greater than 0.01% may cause allergic dermatitis in sensitive individuals (4). When the multi-ingredient cream preparation (SS Cream) has been applied topically to the glans penis, sporadic erectile dysfunction, excessively delayed ejaculation, mild pain, and local irritation and burning has occurred (2537).

Interactions with Herbs & Other Dietary Supplements

Insufficient reliable information available.

Interactions with Drugs

ACID-INHIBITING DRUGS: Theoretically, due to claims that cinnamon bark increases stomach acid, it might interfere with antacids, sucralfate (Carafate), H-2 antagonists, or proton pump inhibitors (19).

Interactions with Foods

No interactions are known to occur, and there is no known reason to expect a clinically significant interaction with cinnamon bark.

Interactions with Lab Tests

No interactions are known to occur, and there is no known reason to expect a clinically significant interaction with cinnamon bark.

Interactions with Diseases or Conditions

CARDIOVASCULAR CONDITIONS: There is concern that cinnamon bark might adversely effect patients with cardiovascular conditions such as high or low blood pressure or congestive heart failure. Some constituents in cinnamon bark seem to slow heart rate and might lower blood pressure (4). However, the clinical significance of these effects in patients is not known. Until more is known, advise patients with cardiovascular conditions to avoid or use cinnamon bark preparations cautiously.

CINNAMON OR PERU BALSAM ALLERGY: Contraindicated due to potential cross-allergenicity (2).

DIABETES: There is some concern that cinnamon bark might interfere with blood glucose control in patients with diabetes. Some cinnamon constituents seem to increase blood glucose levels (4) and others seem to lower blood glucose levels (6657). So far, the clinical significance of these effects in patients with diabetes is not known. Tell patients with diabetes to use cinnamon bark cautiously. Suggest they monitor blood glucose levels more closely. Dose adjustments to diabetes medications might be necessary.

GASTROINTESTINAL (GI) CONDITIONS: Cinnamon bark can irritate the GI tract. Cinnamon bark might worsen infectious or inflammatory GI conditions such as peptic ulcer disease (PUD) (19).

Dosage and Administration

ORAL: The typical dose of cinnamon bark is one cup of the tea three times daily (4). The tea is prepared by steeping 0.5-1 grams of the bark in 150 mL boiling water for 5-10 minutes and then straining. The maximum dose of cinnamon is 2-4 grams of the bark or 0.05-0.2 grams of the essential oil per day (12). The usual dose of the liquid extract (1:1 in 70% alcohol) is 0.51 mL three times daily (4).

TOPICAL: No typical dosage.

Comments

Avoid confusion with Chinese cinnamon (cassia). Cinnamon has been used as a recreational drug by youth (214).

CINNAMON flower

Also Known As

Cinnamon Flos, Cinnamonum, Zimbluten.
CAUTION: See separate listings for Cinnamon bark and Cassia.

Scientific Names

Cinnamomum aromaticum, synonym Cinnamomum cassia.
Family: Lauraceae.

People Use This For

Orally, cinnamon flower is used as a blood purifier.
Historically, cinnamon flower has been used to remove undesirable agents from the blood.
Cinnamon flower is also a flavoring agent (2).

Safety

LIKELY SAFE ...when consumed in amounts commonly found in food (2).
There is insufficient reliable information available about the safety of medicinal uses of cinnamon flower.
PREGNANCY AND LACTATION: Insufficient reliable information available; avoid amounts greater than those used in foods.

Effectiveness

There is insufficient reliable information available about the effectiveness of cinnamon flower.

Mechanism of Action

There is insufficient reliable information available about the possible mechanism of action and active ingredients.

Adverse Reactions

Cinnamon flower can cause allergic reactions with skin and mucous membrane contact in people who are sensitive to cinnamon (2).

Interactions with Herbs & Other Dietary Supplements

Insufficient reliable information available.

Interactions with Drugs

No interactions are known to occur, and there is no known reason to expect a clinically significant interaction with cinnamon flower.

Interactions with Foods

No interactions are known to occur, and there is no known reason to expect a clinically significant interaction with cinnamon flower.

Interactions with Lab Tests

No interactions are known to occur, and there is no known reason to expect a clinically significant interaction with cinnamon flower.

Interactions with Diseases or Conditions

No interactions are known to occur, and there is no known reason to expect a clinically significant interaction with cinnamon flower.

Dosage and Administration

No typical dosage.

Comments

None.

CITRONELLA OIL

Also Known As

None.
CAUTION: See separate listings for Lemongrass and Stone Root.

Scientific Names

Cymbopogon nardus, synonym Andropogon nardus; Cymbopogon winterianus.
Family: Graminaea or Poaceae.

People Use This For

Topically, citronella oil is used as an insect repellent for people and pets (11).
Historically, citronella oil has been used orally as a vermifuge, diuretic, antispasmodic (6), and digestive stimulant (11).
In foods and beverages, citronella oil is used as a flavoring agent (11).
In manufacturing, citronella oil is used as a fragrance in cosmetics and soaps (110).

Safety

LIKELY SAFE ...when used orally in amounts found in foods. It has Generally Recognized as Safe (GRAS) status in the US (11). The maximum use level is 0.005% (11).
LIKELY UNSAFE ...when used orally in large amounts (6,11). ...when inhaled. There have been reports of toxic alveolitis (2).
CHILDREN: LIKELY UNSAFE ...when used orally. There are reports of poisoning in children and one toddler died after ingesting insect repellent that contained citronella oil (2,6,17).
PREGNANCY AND LACTATION: Insufficient reliable information available; avoid using.

Effectiveness

There is insufficient reliable information available about the effectiveness of citronella oil (2).

Mechanism of Action

There is insufficient reliable information available about the possible mechanism of action and active ingredients.

Adverse Reactions

There has been at least one report of death following ingestion of insect repellent containing citronella oil (2). Topical use has caused contact dermatitis (6,11). Inhalation has caused toxic alveolitis (2).

Interactions with Herbs & Other Dietary Supplements

Insufficient reliable information available.

Interactions with Drugs

No interactions are known to occur, and there is no known reason to expect a clinically significant interaction with citronella oil.

Interactions with Foods

No interactions are known to occur, and there is no known reason to expect a clinically significant interaction with citronella oil.

Interactions with Lab Tests

No interactions are known to occur, and there is no known reason to expect a clinically significant interaction with citronella oil.

Interactions with Diseases or Conditions

No interactions are known to occur, and there is no known reason to expect a clinically significant interaction with citronella oil.

Dosage and Administration

No typical dosage.

Comments

Avoid confusion with lemongrass (Cymbopogon citratus). Citronella oil is the essential oil produced by steam distillation of lemongrass (Cymbopogon species), Ceylon or Lenabatu citronella oil (Cymbopogon nardus), Java or Maha Pengiri citronella oil (Cymbopogon winterianus).

CIVET

Also Known As

African Civet, Large Indian Civet, Zibeth.

Scientific Names

African Civet: Viverra civetta, synonym Civettictis civetta
Indian Civet: Viverra zibetha.
Family: Viverridae.

People Use This For

In Chinese medicine, civet is used for pain relief, and as a sedative (11).
In foods and beverages, civet is used as a flavoring agent (11).
In cosmetics, it is used as a fixative and fragrance component of perfumes, cosmetics, and soaps (11).

Safety

LIKELY SAFE ...when used in amounts found in foods (maximum use level less than 0.0014%) (11). It has Generally Recognized as Safe (GRAS) status in the US (11).
There is insufficient reliable information available about the safety of the use of civet in amounts larger than those found in foods.
PREGNANCY AND LACTATION: Insufficient reliable information available; avoid using.

Effectiveness

There is insufficient reliable information available about the effectiveness of civet.

Mechanism of Action

The applicable part of civet is the secretion. There is insufficient reliable information available about the possible mechanism of action and active ingredients.

Adverse Reactions
None reported.

Interactions with Herbs & Other Dietary Supplements
Insufficient reliable information available.

Interactions with Drugs
No interactions are known to occur, and there is no known reason to expect a clinically significant interaction with civet.

Interactions with Foods
No interactions are known to occur, and there is no known reason to expect a clinically significant interaction with civet.

Interactions with Lab Tests
No interactions are known to occur, and there is no known reason to expect a clinically significant interaction with civet.

Interactions with Diseases or Conditions
No interactions are known to occur, and there is no known reason to expect a clinically significant interaction with civet.

Dosage and Administration
No typical dosage.

Comments
Reportedly, crude civet is frequently adulterated (11).
There is very little scientific information about this product. Our staff is continually analyzing the available information on natural medicines and will add data here as it becomes available.

CLARY SAGE

Also Known As
Clary, Clary Wort, Clear Eye, Eyebright, Muscatel Sage, See Bright.
CAUTION: See separate listings for Sage and Eyebright.

Scientific Names
Salvia sclarea.
Family: Lamiaceae/Labiatae.

People Use This For
Orally, clary sage is used for upset stomach, digestive disorders, and kidney diseases (11,400).
Topically, clary sage mucilage is used to remove foreign objects from the eye, to remove thorns and splinters from the skin, and for treating tumors (11,400).
In foods and beverages, the oil from clary sage is used as a flavoring agent (11).
In manufacturing, the oil from clary sage is used as a fragrance in soaps and cosmetics (11).

Safety
LIKELY SAFE ...when used orally in amounts found in beverages and food products; maximal use level is 0.016% of oil in alcoholic beverages.
There is insufficient reliable information available about the safety of medicinal uses of clary sage.
PREGNANCY AND LACTATION: Insufficient reliable information available; avoid using.

Effectiveness
There is insufficient reliable information available about the effectiveness of clary sage.

Mechanism of Action
The applicable parts of clary sage are the flowering top and leaf. The oil has some anticonvulsant activity in animals (11), and it seems to potentiate the effects of hexobarbitone and chloral hydrate (11). The mucilaginous and sticky solution is thought to be able to pull objects from under the eyelid and from the skin (400).

Adverse Reactions
None reported.

Interactions with Herbs & Other Dietary Supplements
Insufficient reliable information available.

Interactions with Drugs
CHLORAL HYDRATE, HEXOBARBITONE: Reportedly potentiates narcotic effects (9,11).

Interactions with Foods
No interactions are known to occur, and there is no known reason to expect a clinically significant interaction with clary sage.

Interactions with Lab Tests
No interactions are known to occur, and there is no known reason to expect a clinically significant interaction with clary sage.

Interactions with Diseases or Conditions
No interactions are known to occur, and there is no known reason to expect a clinically significant interaction with clary sage.

Dosage and Administration
No typical dosage.

Comments
Avoid confusion with sage leaf (Salvia officinalis).

CLEMATIS

Also Known As
Upright Virgin's Bower.
CAUTION: See separate listings for Traveler's Joy and Woodbine.

Scientific Names
Clematis recta.
Family: Ranunculaceae.

People Use This For
Orally, clematis is used for treatment of rheumatic pains, headaches, and varicose veins (18).
Traditionally, clematis was used to treat syphilis, gout, rheumatism, bone disorders, chronic skin conditions, and used as a diuretic (18).
In folk medicine, it is used topically for blisters and as a poultice to treat purulent wounds and ulcers (18).

Safety
POSSIBLY UNSAFE ...when the fresh plant is used topically (18).
LIKELY UNSAFE ...when the fresh plant is used orally because it is severely irritating to mucous membranes and the gastrointestinal tract (18).
There is insufficient reliable information available about the safety of the oral or topical use of dried clematis (4226).
PREGNANCY AND LACTATION: LIKELY UNSAFE ...when the fresh plant is used orally. There is insufficient reliable information available for the safety of the dried plant; avoid using.

Effectiveness
There is insufficient reliable information available about the effectiveness of clematis.

Mechanism of Action
When the fresh plant is crushed or cut into small pieces, the glycoside ranunculin is enzymatically changed into a severely irritating protoanemonin, which, in turn, rapidly degrades into the non-toxic anemonin (18). Both protoanemonin and ranunculin are destroyed to an unknown extent during the drying process (2), and both have fungicidal activity (4). Since Clematis recta contains low levels of protoanemonin-forming agents, the adverse effects and toxicity may not be as severe as compared to other species of Ranunculaceae. Clematis also contains saponins (18).

Adverse Reactions

Orally, freshly harvested clematis can cause colic, diarrhea, and severe irritation to the gastrointestinal and urinary tracts (18). After prolonged skin contact, clematis can cause slow-healing blisters and burns(18).

Interactions with Herbs & Other Dietary Supplements

Insufficient reliable information available.

Interactions with Drugs

No interactions are known to occur, and there is no known reason to expect a clinically significant interaction with clematis.

Interactions with Foods

No interactions are known to occur, and there is no known reason to expect a clinically significant interaction with clematis.

Interactions with Lab Tests

No interactions are known to occur, and there is no known reason to expect a clinically significant interaction with clematis.

Interactions with Diseases or Conditions

No interactions are known to occur, and there is no known reason to expect a clinically significant interaction with clematis.

Dosage and Administration

ORAL: Clematis recta is available orally as drops, extracts, and tea (18). The tea is used for poultices (18).

Comments

Avoid confusion with other Clematis species (6). Clematis recta is considered a poisonous plant and is rarely used today (18). Plants that are grown in the sun have a higher ranunculin content than those grown in the shade, and therefore have stronger effects (18).

CLIVERS

Also Known As

Barweed, Bedstraw, Catchweed, Cleavers, Cleaverwort, Coachweed, Eriffe, Everlasting Friendship, Gallium, Goose Grass, Goose bill, Goosegrass, Gosling Weed, Grip Grass, Hayriffe, Hayruff, Hedge-Burs, Hedgeheriff, Love-Man, Mutton Chops, Robin-Run-in-the-Grass, Scratchweed, Stick-a-Back, Sweethearts.

Scientific Names

Galium aparine.
Family: Rubiaceae.

People Use This For

Orally, clivers is used as a diuretic, a mild astringent, for dysuria, lymphadenitis, psoriasis, and specifically for enlarged lymph nodes (4).
Topically, clivers is used for ulcers, festering glands, breast lumps, and skin rashes (18).

Safety

POSSIBLY SAFE ...when used orally and appropriately (12). There is no documented toxicity (4).
There is insufficient reliable information available about the safety of the topical use of clivers.
PREGNANCY AND LACTATION: Insufficient reliable information available; avoid using.

Effectiveness

There is insufficient reliable information available about the effectiveness of clivers.

Mechanism of Action

The applicable parts of clivers are the dried or fresh above ground parts. Clivers contain tannins, which are reported to have astringent properties (4).

Adverse Reactions
None reported.

Interactions with Herbs & Other Dietary Supplements
Insufficient reliable information available.

Interactions with Drugs
No interactions are known to occur, and there is no known reason to expect a clinically significant interaction with clivers.

Interactions with Foods
No interactions are known to occur, and there is no known reason to expect a clinically significant interaction with clivers.

Interactions with Lab Tests
No interactions are known to occur, and there is no known reason to expect a clinically significant interaction with clivers.

Interactions with Diseases or Conditions
DIABETES: Use expressed juice with caution (4).

Dosage and Administration
ORAL: 2-4 grams dried above ground parts three times daily, or one cup tea (steep 2-4 grams herb in 150 mL boiling water 5-10 minutes, strain) three times daily (4). Liquid extract (1:1 in 25% alcohol) 2-4 mL three times daily (4). Expressed juice, 3-15 mL three times daily (4).
TOPICAL: No typical dosage.

Comments
None.

CLOVE dried flowerbud, leaf, stem

Also Known As
Caryophylli, Caryophyllus, Clous de Girolfe, Cloves, Flores Caryophyllum, Gewurznelken Nagelein.
CAUTION: See separate listing for Clove Oil.

Scientific Names
Syzygium aromaticum, synonyms Caryophyllus aromaticus, Eugenia aromatica, Eugenia caryophyllata, Eugenia caryophyllus.
Family: Myrtaceae.

People Use This For
Orally, clove is used for gastrointestinal upset, including flatulence, nausea, and vomiting (4,11). It is also used orally as an expectorant (6).
Topically, clove is used for toothache, as a counterirritant for pain (4,7107), and for mouth and throat inflammation (2,8). It is also used topically as part of a multi-ingredient preparation for treating premature ejaculation (2537).
In manufacturing, clove is used as a flavoring in foods, beverages, and cigarettes (6,11).

Safety
LIKELY SAFE ...when consumed in amounts commonly found in foods (11). Clove has Generally Recognized as Safe (GRAS) status for food use in the US (11).
POSSIBLY SAFE ...when taken orally and appropriately for medicinal purposes (12). ...when used topically, short-term as part of a multi-ingredient preparation (SS Cream). This preparation was used safely for premature ejaculation in a clinical trial where the cream was applied and left on the glans penis for 1-hour (2537). Further evaluation is needed to determine its safety after prolonged, repetitive use.
LIKELY UNSAFE ...when inhaled due to its harmful effects. Smoking the clove cigarettes can cause respiratory injury (17). Clove cigarettes contain more tar, nicotine, and carbon monoxide than tobacco cigarettes (6,17).
There is insufficient reliable information available about the safety of cloves for its other uses.
PREGNANCY AND LACTATION: POSSIBLY SAFE ...when taken orally in the amounts found in foods. Avoid amounts that greatly exceed those in foods (4).

Effectiveness

POSSIBLY EFFECTIVE ...when used topically as part of a multi-ingredient preparation for treating premature ejaculation. In one controlled clinical trial, a multi-ingredient cream preparation containing Panax ginseng root, Angelica root, Cistanches deserticola, Zanthoxyl species, Torlidis seed, clove flower, Asiasari root, cinnamon bark, and toad venom (SS Cream) was applied to the glans penis 1-hour prior to intercourse and washed off immediately before intercourse. Men suffering from premature ejaculation who were treated with the cream had significantly improved ejaculatory latency compared to placebo (2537).

There is insufficient reliable information available about the effectiveness of cloves for its other uses.

Mechanism of Action

Cloves contain a volatile oil that can be up to 90% eugenol (11). The mild anesthetic and analgesic properties of clove are attributed to eugenol (4,512). Applied topically, eugenol depresses sensory receptors involved in pain perception by inhibiting prostaglandin biosynthesis (512). Eugenol inhibits platelet activity (4). Some evidence suggests the sesquiterpene constituents might have anticancer activity (838). Other evidence suggests whole cloves might have chemoprotective activity against liver and bone marrow toxicity (6). The multi-ingredient preparation containing clove flower is thought to work in premature ejaculation by increasing the penile vibratory threshold and reducing the amplitude of penile somatosensory evoked potentials (2537).

Adverse Reactions

The inhalation of cloves can cause respiratory injury including hemoptysis, bronchospasm, hemorrhagic and nonhemorrhagic pulmonary edema, pleural effusion, respiratory insufficiency, respiratory infection, and aspiration of foreign material. There have been two deaths associated with the smoking of the clove cigarettes (17). Used topically on the oral mucosa, it can cause oral tissue sensitivity, local tissue irritation, and damage to dental pulp or the supporting periodontium (214). When the multi-ingredient cream preparation containing clove flower (SS Cream) has been applied topically to the glans penis, sporadic erectile dysfunction, excessively delayed ejaculation, mild pain, and local irritation and burning has occurred (2537).

Interactions with Herbs & Other Dietary Supplements

HERBS WITH ANTICOAGULANT/ANTIPLATELET POTENTIAL: Concomitant use of herbs that have coumarin constituents or affect platelet aggregation could theoretically increase the risk of bleeding in some people. These herbs include: angelica, anise, arnica, asafoetida, bogbean, boldo, capsicum, celery, chamomile, danshen, fenugreek, feverfew, garlic, ginger, ginkgo, ginseng (Panax), horse chestnut, horseradish, licorice, meadowsweet, prickly ash, onion, papain, passionflower, poplar, quassia, red clover, turmeric, wild carrot, wild lettuce, willow, and others (4,19).

Interactions with Drugs

ANTICOAGULANTS AND ANTIPLATELET DRUGS: Theoretically, clove can potentiate the effects of these drugs.

Interactions with Foods

No interactions are known to occur, and there is no known reason to expect a clinically significant interaction with clove dried flowerbud, leaf, and stem.

Interactions with Lab Tests

No interactions are known to occur, and there is no known reason to expect a clinically significant interaction with clove dried flowerbud, leaf, and stem.

Interactions with Diseases or Conditions

No interactions are known to occur, and there is no known reason to expect a clinically significant interaction with clove dried flowerbud, leaf, and stem.

Dosage and Administration

ORAL: A typical dose of cloves is 120-300 mg (4). Limit clove ingestion to the equivalent of 3.6 mg/kg clove oil per day (4). The buds yield 15-18% volatile oil, The stems yield 4-6% (11).
TOPICAL: Clove is commonly used as a mouthwash, and products usually contain 1-5% clove essential oil (8). A 15% clove tincture can be effective in treating athletes foot (4).

Comments

Clove cigarettes, also called kreteks, generally contain 60% tobacco and 40% ground clove (6). Eugenol in clove cigarettes acts as a topical anesthetic to the posterior oropharynx. It reduces the noxious elements of smoking and can facilitate learning of smoking techniques (17).

CLOVE OIL

Also Known As
Caryophyllum, Caryophyllus, Clous de Girolfe, Flores Caryophylli, Gewurznelken Nagelein, Oil of Clove.
CAUTION: See separate listing for Clove.

Scientific Names
Syzygium aromaticum, synonyms Caryophyllus aromaticus, Eugenia aromatica, Eugenia caryophyllata, Eugenia caryophyllus.
Family: Myrtaceae.

People Use This For
Orally, clove oil is used as an antiemetic (11) and antiflatulent (4).
In Chinese medicine, clove oil is used to manage diarrhea, hernia, and halitosis (11).
In dentistry, clove oil is used topically for toothache (11), as a dental anesthetic (2), for treating postextraction alveolitis (dry socket) (11), and for mouth and throat inflammation (2,8). It is sometimes used as a counterirritant (272). It is also used a component in dental cements and fillings (11).
In foods and beverages, clove oil is used as a flavoring (11).
In manufacturing, clove oil is used for fragrance in toothpaste, soaps, cosmetics, and perfumes (11).

Safety
LIKELY SAFE ...when taken orally in amounts found in foods (11). It has Generally Recognized as Safe (GRAS) status in the US (11).
POSSIBLY SAFE ...when applied topically (272,512). Should not be used for self-medication, especially when undiluted. Repeated application can cause gingival damage, skin and mucous membrane irritation (4,272).
LIKELY UNSAFE ...when taken orally undiluted. 5-15 mL may induce high anion gap acidosis, seizures, coagulopathy, acute liver damage, behavorial changes, and coma (17).
PREGNANCY AND LACTATION: LIKELY UNSAFE ...when used orally and undiluted; avoid in amounts greater than those found in foods (4).

Effectiveness
POSSIBLY EFFECTIVE ...when applied topically as a dental analgesic (2,512), for mouth and throat mucosal inflammation, and for post-extraction alveolitis (dry socket) (6).
There is insufficient reliable information available about the effectiveness of clove oil for its other uses.

Mechanism of Action
Researchers attribute mild anesthetic and analgesic properties of clove to eugenol (3,4). On contact, eugenol acts to depress sensory receptors involved in pain perception by a profound inhibition of prostaglandin biosynthesis (3). It is also a powerful inhibitor of platelet activity (6). Clove bud oil contains 60-90% eugenol, clove leaf oil contains 82-88% eugenol, clove stem oil contains 90-95% eugenol (11). Clove oil has antihistaminic and antispasmodic properties, most likely due to eugenyl acetate (6). Clove oil inhibits gram-positive and gram-negative bacteria. It also has fungistatic action, anthelmintic and larvicidal properties. One report suggests it suppresses aflatoxin production (6). Another suggests eugenol from clove oil may counter some effects of environmental mutagens found in foods (6).

Adverse Reactions
Oral use of clove oil can cause nervous system depression, seizures, lactic acidosis, disseminated intravascular coagulation, hepatic dysfunction (17), and irritation to mucosal tissues (2,4,6,512). This is one report of disseminated intravascular coagulation and liver failure following clove ingestion by a two-year-old (6). There is one report of depression and electrolyte imbalance following accidental ingestion by a seven-month-old (6). Topical use of clove oil can be irritating to mucosal tissues and skin (2,4,6,512). There is one report of permanent local facial anesthesia and absence of sweating after clove spilled on an individual's face (6). Used topically to the oral mucosa, it can cause oral tissue sensitivity, local tissue irritation, and damage to dental pulp or the supporting periodontium (214).

Interactions with Herbs & Other Dietary Supplements
HERBS WITH ANTICOAGULANT/ANTIPLATELET POTENTIAL: Concomitant use of herbs that have coumarin constituents or affect platelet aggregation could theoretically increase the risk of bleeding in some people. These herbs include: angelica, anise, arnica, asafoetida, bogbean, boldo, capsicum, celery, chamomile, clove, danshen, fenugreek, feverfew, garlic, ginger, ginkgo, ginseng (Panax), horse chestnut, horseradish, licorice, meadowsweet, prickly ash, onion, papain, passionflower, poplar, quassia, red clover, turmeric, wild carrot, wild lettuce, willow, and others (4,19).

Interactions with Drugs

ANTICOAGULANT/ANTIPLATELET DRUGS: Theoretically, concomitant use may enhance antiplatelet or anticoagulant effects and adverse effects, due to eugenol content of clove oil (6).

Interactions with Foods

No interactions are known to occur, and there is no known reason to expect a clinically significant interaction with clove oil.

Interactions with Lab Tests

No interactions are known to occur, and there is no known reason to expect a clinically significant interaction with clove oil.

Interactions with Diseases or Conditions

PLATELET ABNORMALITIES: Theoretically, clove oil is contraindicated in people with reduced platelet counts or platelet function abnormalities (6).

Dosage and Administration

ORAL: Dosages for products containing clove oil vary. These dosages can be 5-30 drops of the fluid extract, 1-5 drops of the oil extract, and 1/2-1 ounce of a mouth rinse containing clove oil (6002).
TOPICAL: As mouthwash, products equivalent to 1-5% clove essential oil (8).

Comments

Undiluted clove oil is unsafe for self-use, requires application by a trained professional (512). Clove bud oil is considered more valuable than clove leaf and clove stem oils (11). Clove oil is obtained by distillation of the bud, leaf, or stem of the Clove Tree (Syzygium aromaticum).

CLOWN'S MUSTARD PLANT

Also Known As

Bitter Candy Tuft, Bitter Candytuft, Candytuft, Clowns Mustard Plant.
CAUTION: See separate listings for Black Mustard Oil, Black Mustard Seed, Hedge Mustard, and White Mustard.

Scientific Names

Iberis amara.
Family: Cruciferae.

People Use This For

Orally, clown's mustard plant is used for gastrointestinal conditions such as dyspepsia, irritable bowel syndrome (IBS), gastritis, and bloating. It is also used for gout, musculoskeletal aches and pains (rheumatism), tachycardia, asthma, bronchitis, and edema (dropsy).

Safety

POSSIBLY SAFE ...when used orally, short-term. There is some evidence that clown's mustard plant extract can be used safely for up to 7 days (7049).
PREGNANCY AND LACTATION: Insufficient reliable information available; avoid using.

Effectiveness

There is insufficient reliable information available about the effectiveness of clown's mustard plant. However, there is some preliminary evidence that a specific combination product containing clown's mustard plant extract as a primary ingredient (Ibergast, Phytopharmica) might be helpful for some patients with dyspepsia (7049). More evidence is needed to rate clown's mustard plant for this use.

Mechanism of Action

The applicable parts of clown's mustard plant are the leaves, stem, root, and seeds. The active ingredients and how it might work for gastrointestinal conditions are not known. Some people think it may contain glycosides or flavonoids that could be responsible for any pharmacological effect. However, this has not been verified by scientific studies. Clown's mustard plant does contain the constituent sinapic acid, which has antioxidant properties (7050).

Adverse Reactions

Orally, clown's mustard plant can cause nausea and diarrhea in some patients. Some patients might be hypersensitive to clown's mustard plant. There is one case of a facial rash following oral use (7051).

Interactions with Herbs & Other Dietary Supplements

Insufficient reliable information available.

Interactions with Drugs

No interactions are known to occur, and there is no known reason to expect a clinically significant interaction with clown's mustard plant.

Interactions with Foods

No interactions are known to occur, and there is no known reason to expect a clinically significant interaction with clown's mustard plant.

Interactions with Lab Tests

No interactions are known to occur, and there is no known reason to expect a clinically significant interaction with clown's mustard plant.

Interactions with Diseases or Conditions

No interactions are known to occur, and there is no known reason to expect a clinically significant interaction with clown's mustard plant.

Dosage and Administration

No typical dosage.

Comments

There is very little scientific information about this product. Our staff is continually analyzing the available information on natural medicines and will add data here as it becomes available.

CLUB MOSS

Also Known As

Lycopodium, Stags Horn, Vegetable Sulfur, Witch Meal, Wolfs Claw.
CAUTION: See separate listings for Chinese Club Moss and Huperzine A.

Scientific Names

Lycopodium clavatum.
Family: Lycopodiaceae.

People Use This For

In folk medicine, club moss is used orally for bladder and kidney disorders, and as a diuretic (18).

Safety

POSSIBLY UNSAFE ...when used orally. Club moss contains toxic alkaloids but no poisonings are reported (18).
PREGNANCY AND LACTATION: POSSIBLY UNSAFE ...when used orally; avoid using.

Effectiveness

There is insufficient reliable information available about the effectiveness of club moss.

Mechanism of Action

The applicable parts of club moss are the plant and spores. Club moss contains potentially toxic alkaloids, including lycopodine, dihydrolycopodine and traces of nicotine (18).

Adverse Reactions

None reported.

Interactions with Herbs & Other Dietary Supplements

Insufficient reliable information available.

Interactions with Drugs
No interactions are known to occur, and there is no known reason to expect a clinically significant interaction with club moss.

Interactions with Foods
No interactions are known to occur, and there is no known reason to expect a clinically significant interaction with club moss.

Interactions with Lab Tests
No interactions are known to occur, and there is no known reason to expect a clinically significant interaction with club moss.

Interactions with Diseases or Conditions
No interactions are known to occur, and there is no known reason to expect a clinically significant interaction with club moss.

Dosage and Administration
No typical dosage.

Comments
Avoid confusion with Chinese club moss. Only Chinese club moss contains huperzine A.

COCA

Also Known As
Bolivian Coca, Cocaine Plant, Huanuco Coca, Java Coca, Mate-de-Coca, Mate de Coca, Peruvian Coca, Spadic, Truxillo Coca.
CAUTION: See separate listing for Cocoa.

Scientific Names
Erythroxylum coca, synonym Erythroxylon coca; Erythroxylum novogranatense.
Family: Erythroxylaceae.

People Use This For
Topically, people use the prescription drug cocaine for corneal, nasal, throat mucosa anesthesia, severe ophthalmologic pain, and local vasoconstriction (11,15).
Coca is used as the source of cocaine. Cocaine is smoked and snorted for mind-altering effects (17).
Historically, coca has been chewed for relief of hunger and fatigue (11). Coca extracts have been used to stimulate stomach function, as a sedative, and for treating asthma, colds, and other ailments (11).
In manufacturing, decocainized coca extract is used to flavor cola drinks and food products (11).

Safety
LIKELY SAFE ...when decocainized coca extract is used in amounts found in foods (maximum use level 0.055%). It has Generally Recognized as Safe (GRAS) status in the US. ...when the constituent, cocaine, is used as a FDA-approved product for topical use.
LIKELY UNSAFE ...when the constituent, cocaine, is used as an oral medicinal (17).
UNSAFE ...when the constituent, cocaine, is ingested or inhaled as a recreational drug (17). 20 mg of cocaine can cause severe side effects and 1.2 grams can be fatal Cocaine is a Schedule II controlled substance in the US due to extremely high potential for addiction (17).
PREGNANCY: UNSAFE ...when inhaled or used orally. Coca, and the constituent cocaine, are contraindicated because they can have abortifacient and teratogenic effects (17,6187). ...when used during pregnancy because it is also associated with a high incidence of Sudden Infant Death Syndrome (SIDS) (17).
LACTATION: UNSAFE ...when inhaled. Coca and the constituent, cocaine, are contraindicated. Cocaine is excreted into breast milk and intoxication can occur in infants breast-fed by mothers recently exposed to cocaine (17,18).

Effectiveness

EFFECTIVE ...when the constituent, cocaine, is applied topically for ophthalmologic anesthesia, ophthalmologic pain, topical anesthesia and local vasoconstriction (15). It is an FDA-approved Schedule C-II drug.
LIKELY EFFECTIVE ...when the constituent, cocaine, is used orally as a stimulant (17). ...when the constituent, cocaine, is inhaled to cause altered consciousness. The risk of toxicity and potential for addiction are extremely high (17).

Mechanism of Action

The applicable part of coca is the leaf. Cocaine, the major alkaloid constituent, has local anesthetic, beta-1, beta-2 and alpha adrenergic stimulating properties (17).

Adverse Reactions

Adverse effects of coca generally pertain to the cocaine constituent. Initially, these effects can include euphoria, hyperactivity, and restlessness. Later tremors, hyperreflexia, and seizures can develop. Finally, coma, hyporeflexia, respiratory depression, cardiovascular depression, and death may occur. In the central nervous system (CNS), cocaine can also cause migraine headaches, stroke, and intracranial and intracerebral hemorrhage (17,5092). Unpublished research indicates that cocaine use is associated with an increased risk of hemorrhagic stroke and increased risk of death caused by stroke (5048,6375). There is also evidence that patients with a history of cocaine abuse have a 30% coronary aneurysm rate and angina, myocardial infarction, or other coronary events (378). The highest incidence of aneurysm previously reported was 5% in a study of patients undergoing coronary bypass surgery (378). Other cardiovascular adverse effects include extreme elevations of heart rate and blood pressure, vasoconstriction, myocardial ischemia, myocardial infarction, cardiac arrhythmias, cardiomyopathies, myocarditis, endocarditis, aortic rupture, and diffuse micro-aneurysms (17). There is also some evidence that cocaine use can cause platelet activation, platelet microaggregate formation and platelet alpha granule release, which might increase the risk of thrombosis and accelerate the development of atherosclerosis (6374). Gastrointestinal adverse effects include mesenteric ischemia and malnutrition. Cocaine can cause rhabdomyolysis-induced renal failure (17). Liver adverse effects include hepatic necrosis, and elevation of serum transaminase and serum creatinine phosphokinase (17). Metabolic adverse effects include lactic acidosis, hyperthermia, hypoglycemia, and hypoxia (17). Use during pregnancy might cause spontaneous abortion, abruptio placentae, and fetal malformation (17). Fetal exposure to cocaine, a constituent of coca, is associated with impaired auditory information processing in newborns (6187). Psychiatric adverse effects include paranoia, depression, and violence (17). Respiratory adverse effects include exacerbation of asthma, thermal airway injury, adult respiratory distress syndrome, pneumothorax, pneumomediastinum, pulmonary thrombosis, bronchiolitis obliterans, pulmonary edema, pulmonary infiltrates, pulmonary vascular disease, and pulmonary hemorrhage (17). Chronic intranasal cocaine abuse is associated with orbital wall (bone) destruction, acquired nasolacrimal duct obstruction, and orbital cellulitis (1258).

Interactions with Herbs & Other Dietary Supplements

CAPSICUM: Theoretically, concomitant use of coca and capsicum (including exposure to pepper spray which contains capsicum) might increase the effects and risk of adverse effects of the cocaine in coca (1394).
MARIJUANA: Concomitant use can have additive effects, including increased heart rate (17).

Interactions with Drugs

ALCOHOL: Concomitant use of alcohol and coca or the cocaine constituent may have additive negative effects on neurocognitive functioning in the brain (6373).
NIFEDIPINE: Nifedipine (Adalat, Procardia) use just prior to cocaine use increases the likelihood of seizures and death (17).
PSEUDOCHOLINESTERASE INHIBITORS: Ingesting organophosphate or carbamate insecticides, echothiophate eye drops (Phospholine Iodine), neostigmine (Prostigmin) or pyridostigmine (Mestinon, Regonol) can increase the risk of cardiovascular side effects, seizures, death (17).

Interactions with Foods

No interactions are known to occur, and there is no known reason to expect a clinically significant interaction with coca.

Interactions with Lab Tests

URINE DRUG TEST: Using coca preparations can cause a positive urine drug test for cocaine. Even some "decocainized" tea preparations can contain 5 mg of cocaine per bag.

Interactions with Diseases or Conditions

ASTHMA: Cocaine use is associated with more severe exacerbations in people with asthma. One study found exacerbations were more severe among cocaine users, compared to non-users, who presented to an emergency room during an asthma attack (6186).

CARDIOVASCULAR DISORDERS: People with cardiovascular disorders might be at increased risk for cocaine-induced cardiovascular side effects (17).

INTRACEREBRAL HEMORRHAGE: Cocaine use is associated with increased morbidity and mortality in patients who sustain intracerebral hemorrhage (5092).

PLASMA PSEUDOCHOLINESTERASE DEFICIENCY (PPD): People with PPD are at increased risk for cocaine-induced cardiovascular side effects, including seizures and death (17).

Dosage and Administration

No typical dosage.

Comments

Coca is considered unsafe and illegal for self-use. Avoid confusion with Cocoa Seed (Theobroma cacao).

COCILLANA

Also Known As

Grape Bark, Guapi, Trompillo, Upas.

Scientific Names

Guarea spiciflora; Guarea rusbyi, synonym Sycocarpus rusbyi; Guarea tricholoides; related Guarea species.
Family: Meliaceae.

People Use This For

Orally, cocillana is used as an ingredient in cough syrups (11).
Traditionally, cocillana was used orally as an expectorant (11). The root bark of Guarea spiciflora was used topically for skin indurations, and the leaf of Guarea trichiloides was used for skin tumors (11).

Safety

There is insufficient reliable information available about the safety of cocillana.
Pregnancy and Lactation: Insufficient reliable information available; avoid using.

Effectiveness

There is insufficient reliable information available about the effectiveness of cocillana.

Mechanism of Action

The applicable part of cocillana is the bark. Reported (in the late 1800s) to have expectorant and emetic properties; no recent pharmacological or toxicological data available (11).

Adverse Reactions

None reported.

Interactions with Herbs & Other Dietary Supplements

Insufficient reliable information available.

Interactions with Drugs

No interactions are known to occur, and there is no known reason to expect a clinically significant interaction with cocillana.

Interactions with Foods

No interactions are known to occur, and there is no known reason to expect a clinically significant interaction with cocillana.

Interactions with Lab Tests

No interactions are known to occur, and there is no known reason to expect a clinically significant interaction with cocillana.

Interactions with Diseases or Conditions

No interactions are known to occur, and there is no known reason to expect a clinically significant interaction with cocillana.

Dosage and Administration

ORAL: People typically use 0.5 to 1 gram of the powdered bark. In liquid extract form, the dose is 0.5 to 1 mL (5264).

Comments

None.

COCOA

Also Known As

Cacao, Chocola, Cocoa Bean, Cocoa Oleum, Cocoa Seed, Cocoa Semen, Cocoa Testae, Theobroma.
CAUTION: See separate listing for Coca.

Scientific Names

Theobroma cacao.
Family: Sterculiaceae or Byttneriaceae.

People Use This For

Orally, cocoa seed is used for infectious intestinal diseases and diarrhea (18), asthma, bronchitis, and as an expectorant for lung congestion (11). The seed coat is used for liver, bladder and kidney ailments, diabetes, as a tonic, and as a general remedy (18). Cocoa powder, enriched with flavonoid constituents, is used for prevention of cardiovascular disease (1329).
Topically, cocoa butter has been used to treat wrinkles on the skin and to prevent stretch marks during pregnancy (214).
In foods, cocoa seed is used as a flavoring agent (6). Chocolate is produced from cocoa powder (214).
In manufacturing, cocoa butter is used as a compounding base for various pharmaceutical preparations (6).

Safety

LIKELY SAFE ...when used orally in amounts found in foods (2,6,3900). ...when used orally in moderate amounts for medicinal purposes (2,6). ...when used topically. Cocoa butter is used extensively as a base for ointments and suppositories and is generally considered safe (11,3900).
POSSIBLY UNSAFE ...when used in large amounts. Due to the caffeine content, when used in excessive doses, significant adverse effects may occur, including tachyarrhythmias and sleep disturbances (18).
PREGNANCY: POSSIBLY SAFE ...when used in moderate amounts or in amounts found in foods. Due to the caffeine content of cocoa preparations, mothers should closely monitor their intake to ensure moderate consumption. Fetal blood concentrations of caffeine approximate maternal concentrations (4260). Caffeine use in pregnancy is controversial; however, moderate consumption has not been associated with adverse fetal effects (6). Some sources suggest keeping caffeine consumption below 200 mg per day (2078). Chocolate products provide 2-35 mg caffeine per serving (2078) and a cup of hot chocolate provides approximately 10 mg (3900). POSSIBLY UNSAFE ...when used orally in large amounts. Caffeine found in cocoa crosses the placenta producing fetal blood concentrations similar to maternal levels (4260). Although controversial, some evidence suggests that high doses of caffeine might be associated with premature delivery, low birth weight, and loss of the fetus (6). Some sources suggest keeping caffeine consumption below 200 mg per day (2078). Excessive use of cocoa in pregnancy should be avoided.
LACTATION: POSSIBLY SAFE ...when used in moderate amounts or amounts found in foods. Due to the caffeine content of cocoa preparations, mothers should closely monitor their intake to ensure moderate consumption. Breast milk concentrations of caffeine are thought to be approximately 50% of maternal serum concentrations. Moderate consumption of cocoa would likely result in very small amounts of caffeine exposure to a nursing infant (6). POSSIBLY UNSAFE ...when used orally in large amounts. Consumption of excess chocolate (16 oz per day) may can cause irritability and increased bowel activity in the infant (6026). Large doses or excessive intake of cocoa should be avoided during lactation.

Effectiveness

There is insufficient reliable information available about the effectiveness of cocoa.

Mechanism of Action

The applicable parts of cocoa are the seed, seed coat, cocoa powder, and butter. Cocoa seed contains oils, tannins, and alkaloids, including theobromine 1-4%, caffeine 0.07-0.36%, trigonelline, and others. Cocoa butter, also referred to as theobroma oil, is the fat obtained from roasted cocoa seeds. It contains oleic acid 37%, stearic acid 34%, palmitic acid 26%, and linoleic acid 2% (13). Cocoa also contains flavonoids, tyramine, phenylethylamine (PEA), magnesium, and possibly N-acylethanolamines (6018,6019). Cocoa has CNS stimulant, cardiac stimulant, coronary dilatory, and diuretic actions (6). Theobromine is the major methylxanthine found in cocoa and has only one-tenth of the cardiac activity of caffeine. In one study, consumption of 1.5 g/kg body weight of chocolate had no acute hemodynamic or physiologic effects on the hearts of healthy, young adults (1373). There has been recent analyses of the health effects of stearic acid, which is found in substantial amounts in cocoa. Unlike other saturated fatty acids, stearic acid does not increase total and low-density lipoprotein (LDL) cholesterol. However, it has been shown that stearic acid can lower high-density lipoprotein (HDL) levels and increase lipoprotein(a). Because of this, the stearic acid content in cocoa products is not thought to provide a reduction in the risk for coronary heart disease as was once proposed (6017,6027). However, preliminary research indicates that flavonoid constituents found in cocoa might be beneficial in cardiovascular disease, much like aspirin. In vitro data has shown that cocoa can stimulate the formation of nitric oxide and inhibit cyclo-oxygenase formation. In a human trial, patients receiving cocoa powder enriched with flavonoids had decreased epinephrine- or ADP-stimulated expression of fibrinogen-binding glycoprotein IIb-IIIa, indicating that it might inhibit platelet aggregation (1329,6085). Dark chocolate contains higher amounts of flavonoids than milk chocolate (6018). Preliminary evidence suggests a defatted-cocoa extract might also prevent arteries from constricting in the presence of cholesterol. This effect might be due to the flavonoids contained in cocoa which are eliminated in the chocolate manufacturing process (see Comments) (5057). It has been suggested that stearic acid might activate coagulation factor VII and impair fibrinolysis (6027). In contrast, one study concluded that diets high in stearic acid do not increase the tendency toward thrombosis (6020). PEA found in cocoa is structurally and pharmacologically similar to catecholamines and amphetamine. PEA may be a modulator of mood. N- acylethanolamines are pharmacologically related to anandamide, which activates cannabinoid receptors in the brain (6019).

Adverse Reactions

Orally, cocoa can cause allergic skin reactions (18), shakiness, increased urination, rapid pulse (2,6), constipation (2), and might trigger migraine headaches (18). The cocoa in chocolate can cause nausea, gastrointestinal discomfort, borborygmi, and flatus (1373). Topically, cocoa butter has occassionally caused a rash. In animals, it has been shown to be comedogenic; however, this has not been found in humans (11).

Interactions with Herbs & Other Dietary Supplements

CAFFEINE CONTAINING HERBS/SUPPLEMENTS: Concomitant use interacts with the caffeine in cocoa and may increase effects and risk of adverse effects. Natural products that contain caffeine include coffee, tea (black or green), guarana, mate, and cola.

EPHEDRA (ma huang): Concomitant use interacts with the caffeine in cocoa and may potentiate stimulant effects and risk of adverse effects (6).

Interactions with Drugs

ACETAMINOPHEN: Theoretically, concomitant use of large amounts of cocoa might increase acetaminophen effectiveness by up to 40%, due to cocoa's caffeine content (3).

ASPIRIN: Theoretically, concomitant use of large amounts of cocoa might increase aspirin effectiveness by up to 40%, due to cocoa's caffeine content (3).

BARBITURATES: Theoretically, concomitant use might decrease the effects of caffeine found in cocoa (151).

BETA-ADRENERGIC AGONISTS: Theoretically, concomitant use of large amounts of cocoa might increase cardiac inotropic effects of beta-agonists, due to cocoa's caffeine content (15). Beta-adrenergic agonists include albuterol (Ventolin, Proventil), metaproterenol (Alupent), terbutaline (Brethine, Bricanyl), and isoproterenol (Isuprel).

CIMETIDINE (Tagamet): Theoretically, concomitant use might increase the effects of caffeine found in cocoa. Cimetidine decreases caffeine clearance by 30-50% (14).

CLOZAPINE (Clozaril): Theoretically, co-administration of clozapine and large amounts of cocoa might acutely exacerbate psychotic symptoms, due to cocoa's caffeine content. Caffeine increases the effects and toxicity of clozapine (151). Caffeine doses of 400-1000 mg per day inhibit clozapine metabolism (5051).

DIABETES DRUGS: Concomitant use might interfere with blood glucose control. Cocoa is reported to have hyperglycemic effects (19).

DISULFIRAM (Antabuse): Theoretically, concomitant use of disulfiram and large amounts of cocoa might increase the effects of caffeine found in cocoa. Disulfiram reduces caffeine clearance (15).

ERGOTAMINE: Theoretically, concomitant use of ergotamine and large amounts of cocoa might increase the GI absorption of ergotamine, due to cocoa's caffeine content (15).

FLUCONAZOLE (Diflucan): Theoretically, concomitant use might increase the effects of caffeine found in cocoa. Fluconazole decreases caffeine metabolism (19).

LITHIUM: Theoretically, abrupt withdrawal of large amounts of cocoa might cause lithium toxicity, due to cocoa's caffeine content. Abrupt caffeine withdrawal reportedly increases serum lithium levels (609).

MONOAMINE OXIDASE INHIBITORS (MAOIs): Theoretically, concomitant use of MAOIs with large amounts of cocoa might precipitate a hypertensive crisis due to cocoa's tyramine content (19).

MEXILETINE (Mexitil): Theoretically, concomitant use might increase the effects of caffeine found in cocoa. Mexiletine reduces caffeine elimination by 30-50% (506).

ORAL CONTRACEPTIVES: Theoretically, concomitant use might increase the effects of caffeine found in cocoa. Oral contraceptives reduce caffeine clearance by 40-65% (14).

PHENYLPROPANOLAMINE (Propagest, Rhindecon): Theoretically, concomitant use might increase the effects of caffeine found in cocoa. Phenylpropanolamine might increase serum caffeine concentrations (506).

QUINOLONES: Theoretically, concomitant use might increase the effects of caffeine found in cocoa. Quinolones decrease caffeine clearance (606,607,608). Quinolones (fluoroquinolones) include ciprofloxacin (Cipro), enoxacin (Penetrex), norfloxacin (Chibroxin, Noroxin), sparfloxacin (Zagam), trovafloxacin (Trovan), and grepafloxacin (Raxar).

THEOPHYLLINE: Theoretically, concomitant use of theophylline and large amounts of cocoa might increase the risk of theophylline toxicity, due to cocoa's caffeine content. Caffeine decreases theophylline clearance 23-29% (506).

VERAPAMIL (Calan, Covera-HS, Isoptin, Verelan): Theoretically, concomitant use might increase the effects of caffeine found in cocoa. Verapamil can increase plasma caffeine levels by 25% (14).

Interactions with Foods

GRAPEFRUIT JUICE: Theoretically, concomitant use might increase the caffeine effects of cocoa. Grapefruit might decrease caffeine clearance (4300).

Interactions with Lab Tests

BLEEDING TIME: Theoretically, large amounts of cocoa might prolong bleeding time and increase test results, due to its caffeine content (1701).

BLOOD PRESSURE: Theoretically, large amounts of cocoa might increase blood pressure and blood pressure readings, due to its caffeine content (4).

URATE: Theoretically, large amounts of cocoa might falsely increase serum urate test results determined by the Bittner method, due to its caffeine content (15).

CATECHOLAMINES: Theoretically, large amounts of cocoa might increase urine catecholamine concentrations and test results, due to its caffeine content (15).

CREATINE: Theoretically, large amounts of cocoa might increase urine creatine concentrations and test results, due to its caffeine content (1701).

5-HYDROXYINDOLEACETIC ACID: Theoretically, large amounts of cocoa might increase urine 5-hydroxyindoleacetic acid concentrations and test results, due to its caffeine content. Caffeine can increase urine catecholamine concentrations (15).

VANILLYLMANDELIC ACID (VMA): Theoretically, large amounts of cocoa might increase urine VMA concentrations and test results, due to its caffeine content (15).

Interactions with Diseases or Conditions

ANXIETY: Theoretically, large amounts of cocoa might aggravate anxiety disorders, due to its caffeine content (506).

DEPRESSION: Theoretically, large amounts of cocoa might aggravate depression disorders, due to its caffeine content (506).

GASTRIC ULCERS, DUODENAL ULCERS: Theoretically, large amounts of cocoa might aggravate ulcers, due to its caffeine content (506).

GASTROESOPHAGEAL REFLUX DISEASE (GERD): Avoid cocoa which reduces lower esophageal sphincter pressure (1374).

HEART CONDITIONS: Theoretically, large amounts of cocoa might induce cardiac arrhythmias in sensitive individuals, due to its caffeine content (506). Limit amount ingested; avoid excessive amounts (2).

IRRITABLE BOWEL SYNDROME (IBS): Avoid cocoa-containing products including chocolate which might aggravate irritable bowel syndrome (6).

MIGRAINE HEADACHES: Theoretically, cocoa might trigger migraines in sensitive individuals (2).

Dosage and Administration

No typical dosage.

Comments

Avoid confusion with coca leaf (Erythroxylon coca). Bitter chocolate is produced by pressing roasted cocoa kernels between hot rollers. Cocoa powder is produced by expressing the cocoa butter from bitter chocolate and powdering the remaining residue. Sweet chocolate is produced by adding sugar and vanilla to bitter chocolate (13).

The candy company, Mars, Inc., plans to seek a health claim for chocolate from the Food and Drug Administration in the next few years based on preliminary research they sponsored regarding the potential role of cocoa flavonoids in cardiovascular health (1329).

COD LIVER OIL

Also Known As

Cod Oil, Fish oil, Liver Oil, n-3 Fatty Acids, Omega-3 Fatty Acids, Polyunsaturated Fatty Acids.
CAUTION: See separate listings for DHA (docosahexaenoic acid), EPA (eicosapentaenoic acid), Fish Oil, and Shark Liver Oil.

Scientific Names

None.

People Use This For

Orally, cod liver oil is used for hyperlipidemia, hypertriglyceridemia, hypertension, coronary heart disease, osteoarthritis, and systemic lupus erythematosus (SLE).
Topically, it is used to accelerate wound healing.

Safety

LIKELY SAFE ...when used orally and appropriately (3398,3399,4026).
POSSIBLY UNSAFE ...when used orally in excessive doses. Doses greater than 25 mL daily might decrease blood coagulation and increase the risk of bleeding (4025,4026). There is also some concern about vitamin A and vitamin D toxicity. On average 20 mL of cod liver oil provides 15,000 IU vitamin A and 1500 IU vitamin D (4003,4004).
There is insufficient reliable information available about the safety of cod liver oil when used topically.
PREGNANCY AND LACTATION: Insufficient reliable information available; avoid using.

Effectiveness

LIKELY EFFECTIVE ...when used orally for hypertriglyceridemia. Cod liver oil can reduce triglyceride levels by 20-50% (3399,4026,5705,5706).
POSSIBLY EFFECTIVE ...when used orally for mild hypertension. Cod liver oil seems to produce modest, but significant, reductions in systolic and diastolic blood pressure in patients with mild hypertension (1001,1020,3399).
POSSIBLY INEFFECTIVE ...when used orally for osteoarthritis. Cod liver oil in combination with non-steroidal anti-inflammatory drugs (NSAIDs) does not seem to decrease pain or inflammation when compared to NSAID treatment alone (3398).
There is insufficient reliable information available about the effectiveness of cod liver oil for its other uses.

Mechanism of Action

Cod liver oil contains high amounts of long-chain, polyunsaturated fats called omega-3 fatty acids. Cod liver oil is especially high in the omega-3 fatty acids docosahexaenoic acid (DHA) and eicosapentaenoic acid (EPA). Cod liver oil also contains a significant amount of vitamins A and D. On average, 20 mL of cod liver oil contains 1.8 grams EPA, 2.2 grams DHA, 15,000 IU vitamin A, and 1500 IU vitamin D (4003,4004,4026). Cod liver oil fatty acids compete with arachidonic acid for the cyclooxygenase and lipoxygenase pathways (4026). Cod liver oil's anti-inflammatory effects are likely due to inhibition of leukotriene synthesis (3392,4026). Because of this effect, there is interest in cod liver oil for heart disease prevention. Cod liver oil also has antithrombotic effects. It decreases blood viscosity and increases red blood cell deformability, increases prostacyclin synthesis and related vasodilation, reduces platelet adhesiveness, and reduces platelet count (3399,4005,4022,4025). The DHA and EPA fatty acids found in cod liver oil make up a third of all lipids in the brain's grey matter (425). DHA and EPA play a key role in the structural development of retinal, neural, and synaptic membranes and are thought to be important for normal neural function (424,425). Animals who are deficient in omega-3 fatty acids develop learning and vision disturbances (424). In hypertriglyceridemia, cod liver oil is thought to lower triglycerides by decreasing secretion of very low-density lipoproteins (VLDLs), increasing VLDL apolipoprotein B secretion, possibly by increasing VLDL clearance, decreasing VLDL size, and reducing triglyceride transport (3397,3399,4026).

Adverse Reactions

Orally, cod liver oil can have a fishy taste and might cause belching, nosebleeds, halitosis, and heartburn. High doses can cause nausea and loose stools. Some gastrointestinal side effects can be minimized if cod liver oil is taken with meals and if doses are started low and gradually increased (507). Doses greater than 25 mL might also decrease blood coagulation and potentially increase the risk of bleeding (1313,4025,4026). Long-term cod liver oil supplementation is associated with an increased risk of cutaneous malignant melanoma in women (3395). There is one case of lipoid pneumonia as a result of long-term cod liver oil use (3396). There is also some concern about vitamin A and vitamin D toxicity in people using cod liver oil long-term. On average, 20 mL of cod liver oil provides 15,000 IU vitamin A and 1500 IU vitamin D (4003,4004).

Interactions with Herbs & Other Dietary Supplements

HERBS & SUPPLEMENTS WITH ANTICOAGULANT/ANTIPLATELET POTENTIAL: Concomitant use of herbs that have coumarin constituents or affect platelet aggregation could theoretically increase the risk of bleeding in some people. These herbs include angelica, anise, arnica, asafoetida, bogbean, boldo, borage seed oil, capsicum, celery, chamomile, clove, danshen, evening primrose oil, fenugreek, feverfew, fish oils, garlic, ginger, ginkgo, Panax ginseng, horse chestnut, horseradish, licorice, meadowsweet, prickly ash, onion, papain, passionflower, poplar, quassia, red clover, turmeric, wild carrot, wild lettuce, willow, and others.

Interactions with Drugs

ANTICOAGULANTS/ANTIPLATELET DRUGS: Concomitant use with anticoagulant or antiplatelet drugs can increase the risk of bleeding (507). Some of these drugs include aspirin, clopidogrel (Plavix), dalteparin (Fragmin), dipyridamole (Persantine), enoxaparin (Lovenox), heparin, ticlopidine (Ticlid), warfarin (Coumadin), and others.
ANTIDIABETES DRUGS: There is some concern that cod liver oil might decrease the effectiveness of drugs used for diabetes. Omega-3 fatty acids in cod liver oil can increase blood glucose levels (3397); use with caution.
ANTIHYPERTENSIVE DRUGS: Cod liver oil can lower blood pressure and might have additive effects in patients treated with antihypertensives (1001,1020,3399); use with caution.

Interactions with Foods

No interactions are known to occur, and there is no known reason to expect a clinically significant interaction with cod liver oil.

Interactions with Lab Tests

BLOOD PRESSURE: Cod liver oil might moderately lower blood pressure and reduce blood pressure readings (1001,1020,3399,4026).
INTERNATIONAL NORMALIZED RATIO (INR), PROTHROMBIN TIME (PT): High doses of greater than 25 mL per day might decrease blood coagulation, increase INR and PT, and increase the risk of bleeding (1313,4025,4026).
TRIGLYCERIDES: Cod liver oil can reduce serum triglyceride concentrations and test results in patients with hypercholesterolemia (3399,4026,5705,5706).

Interactions with Diseases or Conditions

ASPIRIN-SENSITIVE INDIVIDUALS: Cod liver oil should be used with caution because omega-3 fatty acids in cod liver oil can decrease pulmonary function in aspirin-sensitive individuals (507).
DIABETES: Cod liver oil should be used with caution because omega-3 fatty acids in cod liver oil might increase blood glucose levels (3397). Monitor blood glucose levels closely. Dose adjustments may be necessary.
HYPERTENSION: Cod liver oil can lower blood pressure and might have additive effects in patients treated with antihypertensives (1001,1020,3399,4026); use with caution.

Dosage and Administration

ORAL: For lowering triglycerides, 20 mL of cod liver oil per day has been used (3399,4026). For lowering blood pressure, 20 mL of cod liver oil per day has been used (3399,4026).

Comments

None.

CODONOPSIS

Also Known As

Bastard Ginseng, Bellflower, Bonnet Bellflower, Dangshen, Radix Codonopsis.
CAUTION: See separate listings for Ashwaganda, Blue Cohosh, Canaigre, Ginseng American, Ginseng Panax, and Ginseng Siberian.

Scientific Names

Codonopsis pilosula; Codonopsis pilosula modesta; Codonopsis tangsheng; Codonopsis tubulosa; other Codonopsis species.
Family: Campanulaceae.

People Use This For

Orally, codonopsis is used to treat HIV infection (1510) and as a protective adjuvant to radiotherapy in cancer treatment (1509).

Codonopsis has been studied as a component of an herbal mixture for minimal brain dysfunction (1508).
In Chinese medicine, codonopsis is used as a substitute for ginseng; in tonic formulas; to stimulate the immune system and replenish qi (Chi, vital energy); and for weakness, anorexia, chronic diarrhea, dyspnea, palpitations, asthma, cough, thirst, diabetes, and spleen and blood deficiencies (11).

Safety

POSSIBLY SAFE ...when used orally and appropriately (12).
PREGNANCY AND LACTATION: Insufficient reliable information available; avoid using.

Effectiveness

There is insufficient reliable information available about the effectiveness of codonopsis.

Mechanism of Action

Codonopsis seems to be able to stimulate the central nervous system. It seems to promote weight gain, increase endurance, increase tolerance to anoxia, elevate temperature, increase macrophage activity, increase red and white blood cell counts, promote peripheral vasodilation (11). Codonopsis also has hypotensive, adrenergic blocking, radioprotective and ulcer-protective effects (11).

Adverse Reactions

None reported.

Interactions with Herbs & Other Dietary Supplements

Insufficient reliable information available.

Interactions with Drugs

No interactions are known to occur, and there is no known reason to expect a clinically significant interaction with codonopsis.

Interactions with Foods

No interactions are known to occur, and there is no known reason to expect a clinically significant interaction with codonopsis.

Interactions with Lab Tests

No interactions are known to occur, and there is no known reason to expect a clinically significant interaction with codonopsis.

Interactions with Diseases or Conditions

No interactions are known to occur, and there is no known reason to expect a clinically significant interaction with codonopsis.

Dosage and Administration

ORAL: People typically use 12 to 15 grams codonopsis added to 3 to 4 cups water and boiled until the volume is reduced by one-half. The cooled liquid is taken in 2 doses on an empty stomach (5251).

Comments

No ginseng saponins have been found in codonopsis (11).

COENZYME Q-10

Also Known As

Co-Enzyme Q10, Coenzyme Q10, Co-Enzyme Q-10, Co Enzyme Q 10, CoQ, CoQ10, Co Q 10, Co-Q-10, Co-Q10, CoQ-10, CO Q10, Q10.

Scientific Names

Ubiquinone; Ubidecarenone; Mitoquinone.

People Use This For

Orally, CoQ-10 is used for congestive heart failure (CHF), angina, diabetes, hypertension, preventing cardiotoxicity associated with doxorubicin (Adriamycin) chemotherapy, breast cancer, Huntington's disease, muscular dystrophy, increasing exercise tolerance, reducing symptoms of chronic fatigue syndrome, warfarin-induced alopecia, stimulating the immune system of people with HIV/AIDS, life extension, male infertility, and quinone-responsive mitochondrial encephalomyelopathy. CoQ-10 is also used for preventing "statin"-induced myopathy. A specific CoQ-10 formulation (UbiQGel) also has FDA Orphan Drug status for mitochondrial cytopathies, including MELAS syndrome, Kearns-Sayre syndrome, and MERRF.

Topically, CoQ-10 is used for treating periodontal disease.

Safety

LIKELY SAFE ...when used orally and appropriately. There have been no reports of significant toxicity associated with CoQ-10 in studies lasting up to a year (14,2134,6037,6038,6407). ...when used topically on the gums (2107).

POSSIBLY UNSAFE ...when used orally in high doses. Doses greater than 300 mg per day might adversely effect the liver (see Adverse Reactions) (14,2134,3370).

PREGNANCY AND LACTATION: Insufficient reliable information available; avoid using.

Effectiveness

POSSIBLY EFFECTIVE ...when used orally as adjunctive treatment for congestive heart failure (CHF). Adding Coenzyme Q-10 (CoQ-10) to conventional treatments seems to significantly improve quality of life (6408) and decrease hospitalization rates, pulmonary edema, cardiac asthma (6407), and other signs and symptoms of CHF such as dyspnea, peripheral edema, enlarged liver, insomnia, and others (6409) in patients with mild to severe (New York Heart Association Class II-IV) CHF. However, CoQ-10 does not seem to improve ejection fraction or exercise tolerance (5090,6037,6038,6408). ...when used orally for improving angina (2121). ...when used orally for hypertension (2122,3365). ...when used orally for reducing cardiotoxicity associated with doxorubicin (Adriamycin) chemotherapy (14). ...when used orally for improving immune function in people with HIV/AIDS (2123,2124). ...when used orally for treating muscular dystrophy (2127).

POSSIBLY INEFFECTIVE ...when used orally for treating Huntington's disease (1357). ...when used orally for improving blood sugar control in people with diabetes (456,492,2125,2126). CoQ-10 does not appear to improve glycemic control or reduce insulin requirement in patients with type 1 or type 2 diabetes (456,492,2126).

LIKELY INEFFECTIVE ...when used orally for improving exercise performance (2109,2110). ...when applied topically for treating periodontal disease (2107,2108).

There is insufficient reliable information available to rate the effectiveness of CoQ-10 for its other uses. However, there is some preliminary evidence that CoQ-10 might prevent progressive insulin secretory defect, exercise intolerance, and hearing loss in people with a rare form of diabetes called maternally inherited diabetes mellitus and deafness (MIDD) (2125). There's also preliminary evidence that CoQ-10 might be helpful in advanced breast cancer along with surgery and conventional therapy plus other antioxidants and omega-3 and omega-6 fatty acids (3993,3995). There is also some preliminary evidence that CoQ-10 might be helpful for warfarin-induced hair loss (455). More evidence is needed to rate CoQ-10 for these uses.

Mechanism of Action

Coenzyme Q-10 (CoQ-10) is a vitamin-like compound present endogenously in high concentrations in the heart, liver, kidney, and pancreas. Within the cell, 25-30% of total CoQ-10 is found in the nucleus, 40-50% in the mitochondria, 15-20% in the microsomes, and 5-10% in the cytosol. CoQ-10 is fat soluble and acts similar to a vitamin (2134). Its primary functions include activity as an antioxidant, a membrane stabilizer (2134,6037,6048), and as a cofactor in many metabolic pathways, particularly in the production of adenosine triphosphate (ATP) in oxidative respiration (2134,6037,6048,6410). The human body produces CoQ-10 naturally, but it is also ingested in small amounts from dietary sources, including meats and seafood. However, the amounts ingested in foods do not approach therapeutic doses (214). CoQ-10 formulated in soy bean oil appears to have superior bioavailability compared to other formulations (457). Peak levels of CoQ-10 after oral administration occur in 5-10 hours and the half-life is approximately 34 hours (2134). Many of the therapeutic benefits of coenzyme Q-10 are primarily attributed to its role in the generation of ATP and its antioxidant effects (214). In addition, many people with certain diseases for which CoQ-10 is thought to be helpful, have lower levels of CoQ-10, including congestive heart failure (CHF), hypertension, periodontal disease, certain muscular diseases, and AIDS (2134,6410). In the treatment of CHF, the mechanism is thought to involve prevention of oxidative damage. The greatest benefit seems to occur in people with the largest deficiency of CoQ-10 (2134). The effect in the treatment of angina may be due to increased ATP synthesis, reduction of free radicals, or membrane protection (2134). CoQ-10 has also been shown to help preserve myocardial sodium-potassium ATP-ase activity and stabilize myocardial calcium-dependent ion channels. CoQ-10 is metabolized to ubiquinol, which prolongs the antioxidant effect of vitamin E (6,14). CoQ-10 also seems to protect against doxorubicin (Adriamycin) cardiotoxicity, possibly through correction of CoQ-10 deficiencies and scavenging of free radicals (2134). Researchers are also interested in CoQ-10's possible anticancer effects related to its antioxidant properties. CoQ-10 might also have immunostimulatory activity (3993). There is also some evidence that CoQ-10 concentrations are lower in cancerous breast tissue than healthy tissue (4846,5158). Some researchers speculate that very low levels of CoQ-10 might be an indicator of a poor prognosis (4846).

Adverse Reactions

Orally, coenzyme Q-10 (CoQ-10) is generally well tolerated. In clinical studies, there have been no reports of significant adverse effects (2134,6037,6038,6047). CoQ-10 can cause mild side effects including gastric distress in 0.39% of patients, loss of appetite in 0.23% of patients, nausea in 0.16% of patients, and diarrhea in 0.12% of patients (6,14,2134,3370). Some of these adverse effects can be minimized if total daily doses exceeding 100 mg are divided and administered 2-3 times per day (3370). When taken in amounts exceeding 300 mg per day, CoQ-10 might cause asymptomatic elevations of liver function tests including LDH and mild elevations in SGOT. However, symptomatic liver disease has not been reported (14,2134,3370).

Interactions with Herbs & Other Dietary Supplements

RED YEAST: Theoretically, since red yeast has HMG-CoA reductase inhibitor ("statin") constituents (512), it might reduce CoQ-10 levels.

Interactions with Drugs

ANTIHYPERTENSIVE DRUGS: CoQ-10 might affect blood pressure and have additive effects with medications used for hypertension (2122); use with caution.

CHEMOTHERAPEUTIC AGENTS: There is some concern that taking antioxidants such as CoQ-10 might protect tumor cells from chemotherapeutic agents that work by inducing oxidative stress, such as the alkylating agents (eg, cyclophosphamide, Cytoxan) and radiation therapy (5158,5159). However, this potential interaction has not yet been verified. Tell cancer patients not to use Co-Q10 without the advice of their oncologist.

INSULIN: There is some concern that CoQ-10 might affect blood glucose and decrease the insulin requirement in patients with diabetes (3370). However, the majority of evidence shows that CoQ-10 does not have this effect in most patients (456,492,2126). Tell patients with diabetes that CoQ-10 probably won't decrease blood glucose levels or the amount of insulin they need.

WARFARIN (Coumadin): Concomitant use can reduce the anticoagulation effects of warfarin (2128,6048,6199). CoQ-10 is chemically similar to menaquinone and may have vitamin K-like procoagulant effects. Four cases of decreased warfarin efficacy thought to be due to CoQ-10 have been reported (2128,6048). Closely monitor patients taking warfarin and CoQ-10. Dose adjustment may be necessary.

Drug Influences on Nutrient Levels and Depletion

SOME DRUGS CAN AFFECT COENZYME Q-10 LEVELS:

BETA-BLOCKERS: Beta-blockers can reduce serum CoQ-10 levels (3368,3369,3370). Common beta-blockers include atenolol (Tenormin), metoprolol (Lopressor, Toprol), nadolol (Corgard), and propranolol (Inderal). The clinical significance is yet to be determined, and the need for supplementation has not been adequately studied.

HMG CoA REDUCTASE INHIBITORS (Statins): HMG CoA reductase inhibitors can reduce serum CoQ-10 levels (4404,4405,4406,4407,4408,4409,4410). One recent study has shown that although serum levels were reduced during short-term (4 weeks) simvastatin treatment, muscle tissue levels of CoQ-10 were not affected, and therefore cellular respiration was not negatively affected as suspected (3367). Further long-term studies are necessary to determine the clinical significance of these findings, and the need for supplementation has not been adequately studied. "Statin" drugs include cerivastatin (Baycol), lovastatin (Mevacor), simvastatin (Zocor), pravastatin (Pravachol), and fluvastatin (Lescol).

ORAL HYPOGLYCEMIC AGENTS: Some oral hypoglycemic agents can reduce serum CoQ-10 levels. These agents include glyburide (Micronase), acetohexamide (Dymelor), and tolazamide (Tolinase). The clinical significance is yet to be determined, and the need for supplementation has not been adequately studied. Consider CoQ-10 supplements based on clinical judgment (4479). Chlorpropamide (Diabinese), glipizide (Glucotrol), and tolbutamide (Orinase) do not seem to reduce CoQ-10 serum levels. There is no data concerning glimepiride (Amaryl).

Interactions with Foods

No interactions are known to occur, and there is no known reason to expect a clinically significant interaction with CoQ-10.

Interactions with Lab Tests

LIVER ENZYMES: CoQ-10 doses in excess of 300 mg per day can elevate SGOT and LDH concentrations (14,2134).
T4/T8 RATIO: CoQ-10 can increase the T4/T8 ratio in normal patients and some HIV-positive patients (2123).
BLOOD PRESSURE: CoQ-10 can lower blood pressure and reduce blood pressure readings in patients with essential hypertension (2122).

Interactions with Diseases or Conditions

BILIARY OBSTRUCTION, HEPATIC INSUFFICIENCY: CoQ-10 levels can increase when patients have either biliary obstruction or hepatic insufficiency (14).

HYPERTENSION: CoQ-10 might affect blood pressure and have additive effects with medications used for hypertension (2122); use with caution.

Dosage and Administration

ORAL: For heart failure, most studies have used 100 mg per day divided into 2 or 3 doses (14,6037,6038,6047). For angina, 50 mg three times per day has been used (2121). For treating cardiotoxicity associated with doxorubicin (Adriamycin) chemotherapy, 50 mg per day has been used (14). For HIV/AIDS, 200 mg per day has been used (2123,2124). For diabetes, 150 mg per day has been used (2125). For muscular dystrophy, 100 mg per day has been used (2127). For hypertension, 120 mg per day divided into 2 doses has been used (3365). For quinone-responsive mitochondrial encephalomyopathy, 5 mg/kg/day has been used (3366). To minimize adverse effects, divided daily doses of CoQ-10 are generally recommended when doses exceed 100 mg/day (3370).

TOPICAL: No typical dosage.

Comments

CoQ-10 was first identified in 1957. It is widely used in Japan. Millions of Japanese patients receive CoQ-10 as part of their treatment for cardiovascular disease. The Japanese government approved CoQ-10 for the treatment of congestive heart failure in 1974. CoQ-10 is also used extensively in Europe and Russia. Most of the CoQ-10 used in the US and Canada is supplied by Japanese companies. CoQ-10 is manufactured by beets fermenting and sugar cane with special strains of yeast (507). One unique formulation of CoQ-10 (UbiQGel) has received FDA Orphan Drug status for treating mitochondrial cytopathies (6608).

COFFEE

Also Known As

Cafe, Caffea, Espresso, Java, Mocha.
CAUTION: See separate listings for Caffeine and Coffee Charcoal.

Scientific Names

Coffea arabica; Coffea canephora, synonym Coffea robusta; Coffea liberica; other Coffea species.
Family: Rubiaceae.

People Use This For

Orally, coffee is used as a common beverage for short-term relief of mental and physical fatigue, to increase performance capabilities, to prevent Parkinson's disease, and to prevent Gallstone disease.
Rectally, coffee is used as an enema to treat cancer.

Safety

LIKELY SAFE ...when used orally and appropriately. Drinking decaffeinated coffee or coffee containing caffeine in low to moderate amounts is safe (14,15). Drinking up to 5 cups of caffeinated coffee (approximately 500 mg caffeine) daily can also be safe in regular users who have developed caffeine tolerance (18).

POSSIBLY UNSAFE ...when used orally in excessive amounts. Drinking caffeinated coffee in amounts greater than 5 cups per day short-term or long-term can cause caffeinism with symptoms of anxiety progressing to delirium and agitation (14). Chronic use of caffeine, especially in large amounts, can sometimes produce tolerance, habituation, and psychological dependence (15). Abrupt discontinuance of caffeine can cause physical withdrawal symptoms.

LIKELY UNSAFE ...when used rectally as an enema. Coffee enemas can cause severe electrolyte abnormalities and sometimes septicemia leading to severe side effects including death (3026,3349).

CHILDREN: POSSIBLY UNSAFE ...when coffee containing caffeine is taken orally in amounts significantly greater than typical beverage amounts. The adverse effects are usually more severe in children than adults (15).

PREGNANCY: POSSIBLY SAFE ...when used orally in small amounts. Three cups of coffee (approx. 300 mg caffeine) consumed throughout the day seems to be safe (15). Caffeine crosses the human placenta but is not considered a teratogen. Fetal blood and tissue levels are similar to maternal concentrations (4260). POSSIBLY UNSAFE ...when used orally in large amounts. More than 3 cups of coffee (300 mg caffeine) consumed daily may be harmful to the fetus (15,18,4260).

LACTATION: POSSIBLY UNSAFE ...when used orally. Caffeine from coffee can cause sleep disturbances in breast-fed infants (18); avoid using.

Effectiveness

EFFECTIVE ...when used orally for increasing mental alertness (14,15).

POSSIBLY EFFECTIVE ...when used orally for preventing or delaying onset of Parkinson's disease. There is evidence that people who consume caffeinated beverages such as coffee, tea, and cola have a decreased risk of Parkinson's disease. For men, the effects seem to be dose related. Men consuming the greatest amount of caffeinated coffee, 3-4 cups (28 ounces) per day, or a total of 421-2716 mg of caffeine from any source daily, seem to have the greatest reduction in risk. However, a significant reduction in risk exists even with consumption of as little as 124-208 mg caffeine per day (approximately 1-2 cups of coffee) (6022). In women, the effects do not seem to be dose related. Moderate consumption of caffeinated coffee, 1-3 cups daily, provides the most reduction in risk (1238). ...when used orally for preventing symptomatic gallstone disease in men. Men consuming caffeinated beverages including coffee that provide 400-800 mg caffeine per day (2-3 cups of coffee) have a significantly reduced risk of developing symptomatic gallstone disease. The effect seems to be dose-dependent. Men consuming 800 mg caffeine per day (4 or more cups of coffee) have the greatest reduction in risk (3345).

LIKELY INEFFECTIVE ...when used orally for improving short-term, high-intensity performance, anaerobic capacity, or power (14).

INEFFECTIVE ...when used orally for sustained, sub-maximal endurance exercise (14).

There is insufficient reliable information available about the effectiveness of coffee for its other uses.

Mechanism of Action

Coffee contains 1-2.6% caffeine (7,12,13) which is the primary active ingredient. Other active constituents include chlorogenic acid, caffeol, and diterpenes. Caffeine acts as a central nervous system stimulant (12,15), increases heart rate and contractility (7), increases blood pressure (6663), inhibits platelet aggregation (6), stimulates gastric acid secretion, causes diuresis (15), relaxes extracerebral vascular and bronchial smooth muscle, stimulates the release of catecholamines (18), and might indirectly inhibit histamine release (6130). The chlorogenic acid constituent is believed to increase gastric acid secretion (13). The diterpene constituents, cafestol and kahweol, increase serum cholesterol (1353). Green coffee beans contain high levels of antioxidant polyphenols, which are thought to be antitumorogenic. Most of these polyphenols are destroyed during the roasting process. Some researchers have reported that a new roasting process maintains higher levels of polyphenols without affecting the flavor. They theorize that such coffee might be healthier to drink (6601); however, this has not been demonstrated. For prevention of Parkinson's disease, caffeine may prevent adenosine's inhibition of dopaminergic transmission. This may result in a reduction in the clinical expression of Parkinsonism (6022). Coffee also seems to enhance gallbladder contractility, stimulate cholecystokinin (CCK) release, and may increase colonic motility, which are all factors related to the development of gallstone disease (3345). Proponents of caffeinated coffee enemas believe that caffeine is absorbed into the portal circulation, causing dilation of the bile ducts and stimulation of hepatocellular function to detoxify tumor cell metabolism products. However, these claims have not been substantiated (3026,3346,3347,6653).

Adverse Reactions

Orally, coffee containing caffeine can cause headache, increased intraocular pressure, diuresis (12), gastric distress, nervousness, vomiting, insomnia (7,18), anxiety, agitation, ringing in ears, and heart arrhythmias (15). Coffee consumption providing over 250 mg of caffeine can increase blood pressure, but this doesn't seem to occur in habitual coffee drinkers (6663). Adverse effects of caffeine are usually more severe in children (15). Chronic use of caffeine, especially in large amounts, can produce tolerance, habituation, and psychological dependence (15). Abrupt discontinuance of caffeine can sometimes cause physical withdrawal symptoms, including headaches, irritability, nervousness, anxiety, and dizziness (15). Unfiltered coffee can also adversely effect cholesterol levels. Drinking one liter of strong, unfiltered coffee daily for two weeks can raise serum cholesterol by 10% (1353). Tell patients to use coffee filters to decrease this adverse effect. Coffee can also adversely affect homocysteine levels. Higher homocysteine levels have been associated with cardiovascular disease. One liter of unfiltered coffee for 2 weeks can increase plasma homocysteine levels by 10% (1353). The same amount of filtered coffee can raise plasma homocysteine levels by 20% (3344). There is some evidence that coffee might increase the risk of pancreatic cancer (12). In women, coffee seems to be associated with increased risk of heart attack (12), breast cancer (in obese women), and ovarian cancer (12). Some evidence shows caffeine is associated with fibrocystic breast disease in women (14,15). However, these potential adverse effects are controversial. There is preliminary evidence that use of greater than 4 cups of coffee per day can increase the risk of rheumatoid factor positive rheumatoid arthritis, but this association has not been confirmed (6482). Combining ephedra with coffee can increase the risk of adverse effects, due to the caffeine contained in coffee (2729). Jitteriness, hypertension, seizures, temporary loss of consciousness, and hospitalization requiring life support has been associated with the combined use of ephedra and caffeine (1380). There is also a report of ischemic stroke in an athlete who consumed ephedra 40-60 mg, creatine monohydrate 6 grams, caffeine 400-600 mg, and a variety of other supplements daily for 6 weeks (1275). Rectally, coffee enemas have been associated with 3 deaths. Two of these deaths are related to severe electrolyte imbalance, and a third is associated with polymicrobial septicemia following use of coffee enema (3026,3347,3349,6652).

Interactions with Herbs & Other Dietary Supplements

CAFFEINE CONTAINING HERBS/SUPPLEMENTS: Concomitant use of coffee and caffeine-containing herbs/supplements constitutes therapeutic duplication (due to the caffeine contained in coffee) which increases the risk of caffeine-related adverse effects. Other natural products which contain caffeine include black tea, cocoa, cola nut, green tea, guarana, and mate.

CALCIUM: Coffee consumption can increase excretion of calcium (12).

EPHEDRA (Ma Huang): Concomitant use can increase the risk of stimulatory adverse effects, due to the caffeine contained in coffee (7). One unpublished report associated jitteriness, hypertension, seizures, temporary loss of consciousness, and hospitalization requiring life support with the use of a combination ephedra and guarana (caffeine) product (1380).

MAGNESIUM: Coffee consumption can increase excretion of magnesium (12).

ZINC: Separate coffee consumption and zinc administration by two hours. Concomitant administration reduces zinc absorption by up to 50% (14).

Interactions with Drugs

ACETAMINOPHEN (Tylenol): Theoretically, concomitant use might increase the pain-relieving activity of acetaminophen, due to the caffeine contained in coffee. Caffeine increases the pain-relieving activity of acetaminophen by up to 40% (512).

ACID-INHIBITING DRUGS: Theoretically, concomitant use might interfere with antacids, sucralfate (Carafate), H-2 antagonists, or proton pump inhibitors. This is based on the claim that coffee increases stomach acid (19).

ALENDRONATE (Fosamax): Separate coffee ingestion and alendronate administration by two hours. Coffee reduces alendronate bioavailability by 60% (14).

ASPIRIN: Theoretically, concomitant use might increase the pain-relieving activity of aspirin, due to the caffeine contained in coffee. Caffeine increases the pain-relieving activity of aspirin by up to 40% (512).

BENZODIAZEPINES: Theoretically, concomitant use might reduce the sedative and anxiolytic effects of benzodiazepines, due to the caffeine contained in coffee (14).

BETA-ADRENERGIC AGONISTS: Theoretically, concomitant use might increase the cardiac inotropic effects of beta agonists, due to the caffeine contained in coffee (15). Beta-adrenergic agonists include albuterol (Proventil, Ventolin), metaproterenol (Alupent), terbutaline (Brethine), and isoproterenol (Isuprel).

CIMETIDINE (Tagamet): Theoretically, concomitant use might increase serum caffeine concentrations and the risk of adverse effects, due to the caffeine contained in coffee. Cimetidine decreases the rate of caffeine clearance by 30-50% (14).

CLOZAPINE (Clozaril): Theoretically, co-administration might acutely exacerbate psychotic symptoms, due to the caffeine contained in coffee. Caffeine can increase the effects and toxicity of clozapine (151). Caffeine doses of 400-1000 mg per day inhibit clozapine metabolism (5051).

CNS STIMULANTS: Concomitant use might increase the risk of stimulant adverse effects, due to the caffeine contained in coffee (151,2719). CNS stimulants include nicotine, cocaine, sympathomimetic amines, and amphetamines.

DIABETES THERAPY: Theoretically, concomitant use of coffee and diabetes drugs might interfere with blood glucose control, due to the caffeine contained in coffee. This is based in the claim that caffeine might have hyperglycemic effects (19).

DISULFIRAM (Antabuse): Theoretically, concomitant use might increase serum caffeine concentrations and the risk of adverse effects, due to the caffeine contained in coffee. Disulfiram decreases the rate of caffeine clearance (15).

EPHEDRINE: Concomitant use might increase the risk of stimulatory adverse effects, due to the caffeine contained in coffee (7,19). An unpublished report associated jitteriness, hypertension, seizures, temporary loss of consciousness, and hospitalization requiring life support with the use of a combination ephedra (ephedrine) and guarana (caffeine) product (1380).

ESTROGEN (Estrace): Theoretically, concomitant use might increase serum caffeine concentrations and the risk of adverse effects, due to the caffeine contained in coffee. Estrogen inhibits caffeine metabolism (2714).

ERGOTAMINE: Theoretically, concomitant use might increase the GI absorption of ergotamine, due to the caffeine contained in coffee. Caffeine increases the GI absorption of ergotamine (15).

LITHIUM (Eskalith, Lithobid): Theoretically, abrupt coffee withdrawal might increase serum lithium levels, due to the caffeine contained in coffee. There are two case reports of lithium tremor that worsened upon abrupt coffee withdrawal (609,610).

MEXILETINE (Mexitil): Theoretically, concomitant use might increase serum caffeine concentrations and the risk of adverse effects, due to the caffeine contained in coffee. Mexiletine reduces caffeine metabolism (14).

MONOAMINE OXIDASE INHIBITORS (MAOIs): Theoretically, concomitant intake of large amounts of coffee with MAOIs might precipitate a hypertensive crisis, due to the caffeine contained in coffee. This is based on the claim that intake of large amounts of caffeine with MAOIs might precipitate a hypertensive crisis (19).

ORAL CONTRACEPTIVES (OCs): Theoretically, concomitant use might increase serum caffeine concentrations and the risk adverse effects, due to the caffeine contained in coffee. OCs decrease the rate of caffeine clearance by 40-65% (14).

PHENYLPROPANOLAMINE (Dexatrim, Propagest): Theoretically, concomitant use might cause an additive increase in blood pressure and serum caffeine concentrations, due to the caffeine contained in coffee [14]. Concomitant use of caffeine and phenylpropanolamine can cause an additive increase in blood pressure, and increase serum caffeine concentrations [14].

QUINOLONES: Theoretically, concomitant use might increase serum caffeine concentrations and the risk of adverse effects, due to the caffeine contained in coffee. Quinolones decrease caffeine clearance [606,607,608]. Quinolones (also referred to as fluoroquinolones) include ciprofloxacin (Cipro), enoxacin (Penetrex), gatifloxacin (Tequin), levofloxacin (Levaquin), lomefloxacin (Maxaquin), moxifloxacin (Avelox), norfloxacin (Noroxin), ofloxacin (Floxin), sparfloxacin (Zagam), and trovafloxacin (Trovan).

RILUZOLE (Rilutek): Theoretically, concomitant use might increase serum caffeine and riluzole concentrations and the risk of adverse effects of both caffeine and riluzole, due to the caffeine contained in coffee. Caffeine and riluzole are both metabolized by cytochrome P450 1A2 and concomitant use might reduce metabolism of one or both agents [14].

TERBINAFINE (Lamisil): Theoretically, concomitant use might increase serum caffeine concentrations and the risk of adverse effects, due to the caffeine contained in coffee. Terbinafine decreases the rate of caffeine clearance [14].

THEOPHYLLINE (Theo-Dur): Theoretically, concomitant use might increase serum theophylline concentrations and the risk of adverse effects, due to the caffeine contained in coffee. Large amounts of caffeine might inhibit theophylline metabolism [14].

VERAPAMIL (Calan, Isoptin, Verelan): Theoretically, concomitant use might increase plasma caffeine concentrations and the risk of adverse effects, due to the caffeine contained in coffee. Verapamil increases plasma caffeine concentrations by 25% [14].

Interactions with Foods
GRAPEFRUIT JUICE: Interacts with the caffeine in coffee and plasma caffeine concentrations can be elevated, increasing effects and risk of adverse effects [504].

Interactions with Lab Tests
BLEEDING TIME: Coffee might prolong bleeding time and increase test results, due to its caffeine content [1701].
BLOOD PRESSURE: Coffee might increase blood pressure and blood pressure readings, due to its caffeine content [4].
URATE: Coffee might falsely increase serum urate test results determined by the Bittner method, due to its caffeine content. Caffeine causes false elevations in serum urate test results determined by the Bittner method [15].
CATECHOLAMINES: Coffee might increase urine catecholamine concentrations and test results, due to its caffeine content. Caffeine can increase urine catecholamine concentrations [15].
CREATINE: Coffee might increase urine creatine concentrations and test results, due to its caffeine content [1701].
DIPYRIDAMOLE THALLIUM IMAGING: Coffee might interfere with dipyridamole thallium imaging studies, due to its caffeine content. Caffeine attenuates the characteristic cardiovascular responses to dipyridamole and has altered test results [14].
5-HYDROXYINDOLEACETIC ACID: Coffee might increase urine 5-hydroxyindoleacetic acid concentrations and test results, due to its caffeine content. Caffeine can increase urine catecholamine concentrations [15].
VANILLYLMANDELIC ACID (VMA): Coffee might increase urine VMA concentrations and test results, due to its caffeine content. Caffeine can increase urine VMA concentrations [15].
TESTS FOR NEUROBLASTOMA: Coffee (due to its caffeine content) might cause false-positive diagnosis of neuroblastoma, when diagnosis is based on tests of urine vanillylmandelic acid (VMA) or catecholamine concentrations. Caffeine can increase urine catecholamine and VMA concentrations [15].
TESTS FOR PHEOCHROMOCYTOMA: Coffee (due to its caffeine content) might cause false-positive diagnosis of pheochromocytoma, when diagnosis is based on tests of urine vanillylmandelic acid (VMA) or catecholamine concentrations. Caffeine can increase urine catecholamine and VMA concentrations [15].

Interactions with Diseases or Conditions
ANXIETY DISORDERS: The caffeine in coffee can aggravate anxiety disorders [14].
CARDIOVASCULAR DISEASE: Consumption of unfiltered coffee increases plasma homocysteine levels, which are associate with an increased risk of cardiovascular disease [1353].
CANCER: Coffee might increase the risk of pancreatic cancer, breast cancer (in obese women), and ovarian cancer [12].
DEPRESSION: The caffeine in coffee can aggravate depression [14].
GASTRIC, DUODENAL ULCERS: The caffeine in coffee can aggravate ulcers; avoid using [14,16].
HEART CONDITIONS: The caffeine in coffee can induce cardiac arrhythmias and tachycardia in sensitive individuals [14,16]. Theoretically, large amounts of caffeinated coffee might increase the risk of heart attacks [12].
HYPERCHOLESTEROLEMIA: Avoid unfiltered, fresh-brewed coffee which can increase serum cholesterol levels [7,12,18,1353,4200]. However, drinking filtered coffee does not increase serum cholesterol levels [18,4200].

HYPERTENSION: The caffeine in coffee might increase blood pressure in people with high blood pressure (2272,6663). However, this doesn't seem to occur in people who habitually drink coffee (6663).
HYPERTHYROID: Avoid use of coffee (18).
KIDNEY DISEASE: The diuretic effect of the caffeine in coffee might aggravate some kidney disorders (19).
OSTEOPOROSIS: Coffee can increase excretion of calcium and magnesium, and thus increase the risk of osteoporosis (12).
SEIZURE PREDISPOSITION: Avoid use of coffee (18).

Dosage and Administration

ORAL: For preventing Parkinson's disease, men consuming 3-4 cups (28 oz) of caffeinated coffee per day or 421-2716 mg total caffeine had the lowest risk of developing Parkinson's disease. However, a significantly lower risk was also associated with consumption of as little as 124-208 mg of caffeine (approximately 1-2 cups of coffee) (6022). In women, more moderate caffeinated coffee consumption seems to be best; 1-3 cups per day (1238). For preventing symptomatic gallstone disease, men consuming 400-800 mg caffeine per day (2-3 cups of coffee) have a significant risk reduction. However, men consuming at least 800 mg caffeine per day (4 or more cups of coffee) seem to have the greatest reduction in risk (3345). Use filtered coffee to avoid some adverse effects. Choice of coffee, grind, ratio of coffee to water, and other factors determine flavor and strength of beverage. Caffeine content of coffee (per average cup): percolated, 100-150 mg caffeine; instant, 85-100 mg caffeine; and decaffeinated, approximately 8 mg caffeine (13). Darker roasts contain less caffeine due to sublimation during roasting (13).

Comments

Coffee enemas are used as a part of the "Gerson Therapy." Cancer patients are treated with caffeinated coffee, in the form of four-hourly enemas on a daily basis. The enemas are combined with a diet of liver, vegetables, and a variety of oral medications, including potassium, pepsin, Lugol's solution, niacin, pancreatin, and thyroid extracts (3348,6653). The Gerson Therapy is considered an unacceptable medical practice in the United States, but continues to be used at The Hospital of the Baja California in Tijuana, Mexico, one mile from the USA (3346,3347,3348,6652,6653).

COFFEE CHARCOAL

Also Known As
None.
CAUTION: See separate listings for Activated Charcoal and Coffee.

Scientific Names
Coffea arabica; Coffea canephora; Coffea liberica.
Family: Rubiaceae.

People Use This For
Orally, coffee charcoal is used for nonspecific, acute diarrhea (2).
Topically, coffee charcoal is used for inflammation of the oral and pharyngeal mucosa (2).
In folk medicine, coffee charcoal has been used as a topical treatment for festering wounds (18).

Safety
POSSIBLY SAFE ...when used orally or topically (2).
PREGNANCY AND LACTATION: Insufficient reliable information available; avoid using.

Effectiveness
POSSIBLY EFFECTIVE ...when used topically for mild inflammation of the oral and pharyngeal mucosa (2). There is insufficient reliable information about the effectiveness of coffee charcoal for its other uses.

Mechanism of Action
Coffee charcoal can have adsorbent and astringent properties (2).

Adverse Reactions
None reported.

Interactions with Herbs & Other Dietary Supplements
Insufficient reliable information available.

Interactions with Drugs
ORAL DRUGS: Coffee charcoal can reduce the absorption of orally administered drugs (2) and should be separated from oral drug administration by at least two hours.

Interactions with Foods
No interactions are known to occur, and there is no known reason to expect a clinically significant interaction with coffee charcoal.

Interactions with Lab Tests
No interactions are known to occur, and there is no known reason to expect a clinically significant interaction with coffee charcoal.

Interactions with Diseases or Conditions
No interactions are known to occur, and there is no known reason to expect a clinically significant interaction with coffee charcoal.

Dosage and Administration
ORAL: The average single dose of coffee charcoal is 3 grams (18), and the total daily dose is 9 grams per day (2). Store coffee charcoal in a well-sealed container (18). Diarrhea persisting beyond 3 to 4 days should be evaluated by a health care professional (2).
TOPICAL: No typical dosage.

Comments
Coffee charcoal is produced by roasting the outer portion of the coffee beans until blackened or charred. Avoid confusion with coffee seed or activated charcoal.

COLA NUT

Also Known As
Bissy Nut, Cola Seed, Guru Nut, Kola Nut.
CAUTION: See separate listings for Caffeine and Gotu Kola.

Scientific Names
Cola acuminata, synonym Sterculia acuminata; Cola nitida; and related species.
Family: Sterculiaceae.

People Use This For
Orally, cola nut is used for short-term relief of mental and physical fatigue (2) and depressive states, especially those associated with general muscle weakness. It is also used orally for melancholy, atony, exhaustion, dysentery, atonic diarrhea, anorexia, and migraines (4).
In foods and beverages, cola nut is used as a flavoring ingredient (11).

Safety
LIKELY SAFE ...when consumed in amounts commonly found in foods and beverages. The cola nut has Generally Recognized as Safe (GRAS) status in the US (11).
POSSIBLY SAFE ...when used orally and appropriately (12,18).
POSSIBLY UNSAFE ...when used in excessive amounts or long-term due to its caffeine content (12). Chronic use of caffeine, especially in large amounts, can sometimes produce tolerance, habituation, and psychological dependence (15). The abrupt discontinuance can result in physical withdrawal symptoms (15).
CHILDREN: POSSIBLY UNSAFE ...when used orally in amounts significantly greater than typical food amounts. The adverse effects of caffeine can be more severe in children than adults (15).
PREGNANCY: Insufficient reliable information available. Although the caffeine content of a typical dose should not cause concern, other constituents could be unsafe.
LACTATION: POSSIBLY UNSAFE ...when used orally; avoid using. It can cause sleep disturbances in breast-fed infants (18).

Effectiveness
POSSIBLY EFFECTIVE ...when used orally for mental and physical fatigue (2).
There is insufficient reliable information available about the effectiveness of cola nut for its other uses.

Mechanism of Action
Cola nut has central nervous system (CNS) stimulant, antidepressant, diuretic, and antidiarrheal effects (4). Cola nut contains 1-3.5% caffeine (13) which acts as a CNS stimulant (12,15,18), increases heart rate and contractility (7,18), increases blood pressure (6663), inhibits platelet aggregation (6,18), stimulates gastric acid secretion, causes diuresis (15,18), relaxes extracerebral vascular and bronchial smooth muscle, stimulates the release of catecholamines (18), and might indirectly inhibit histamine release (6130).

Adverse Reactions
Cola nut can cause sleeplessness, anxiety, tremor, palpitations (4), over-excitability, nervous restlessness, and gastric irritation (2). The caffeine constituent can cause a fast heartbeat, quickened respiration, tremors, delirium, vomiting, convulsions, diuresis (15,505), agitation, ringing in the ears, premature heartbeat, and arrhythmias (15). High doses of cola nut providing 250 mg of caffeine can also increase blood pressure. This doesn't seem to occur in people who habitually consume caffeine products (6663). The adverse effects of caffeine are usually more severe in children (15). Some evidence shows caffeine is associated with fibrocystic breast disease in women; other evidence disputes this (14,15). Chronic use of caffeine, especially in large amounts, can sometimes produce tolerance, habituation, and psychological dependence (15). The abrupt discontinuance can sometimes result in physical withdrawal symptoms, including headaches, irritation, nervousness, anxiety, and dizziness (15). The chewing of cola nuts can cause staining of the oral mucosa to a bright yellow. The chewing of these nuts can also increase the risk of oral carcinoma in smokers (214). Combining ephedra with cola nut increases the risk of adverse effects, due to the caffeine contained in cola nut (2729). One unpublished report associated jitteriness, hypertension, seizures, temporary loss of consciousness, and hospitalization requiring life support with the use of a combination ephedra and guarana (caffeine) product (1380). There is one report of ischemic stroke in an athlete who consumed ephedra 40-60 mg, creatine monohydrate 6 grams, caffeine 400-600 mg, and a variety of other supplements daily for six weeks (1275).

Interactions with Herbs & Other Dietary Supplements
CAFFEINE CONTAINING HERBS/SUPPLEMENTS: Concomitant use of cola nut and caffeine-containing herbs/supplements constitutes therapeutic duplication (due to the caffeine contained in cola nut) which increases the risk of caffeine-related adverse effects. Other natural products which contain caffeine include black tea, cocoa, coffee, green tea, guarana, and mate.
EPHEDRA (Ma Huang): Concomitant use can increase the risk of stimulatory adverse effects, due to the caffeine contained in cola nut (7). One unpublished report associated jitteriness, hypertension, seizures, temporary loss of consciousness, and hospitalization requiring life support with the use of a combination ephedra and guarana (caffeine) product (1380).

Interactions with Drugs
ACETAMINOPHEN (Tylenol): Theoretically, concomitant use might increase the pain-relieving activity of acetaminophen, due to the caffeine contained in cola nut. Caffeine increases the pain-relieving activity of acetaminophen by up to 40% (512).
ASPIRIN: Theoretically, concomitant use might increase the pain-relieving activity of aspirin, due to the caffeine contained in cola nut. Caffeine increases the pain-relieving activity of aspirin by up to 40% (512).
BENZODIAZEPINES: Theoretically, concomitant use might reduce the sedative and anxiolytic effects of benzodiazepines, due to the caffeine contained in cola nut (14).
BETA-ADRENERGIC AGONISTS: Theoretically, concomitant use might increase the cardiac inotropic effects of beta agonists, due to the caffeine contained in cola nut (15). Beta-adrenergic agonists include albuterol (Proventil, Ventolin), metaproterenol (Alupent), terbutaline (Brethine), and isoproterenol (Isuprel).
CIMETIDINE (Tagamet): Theoretically, concomitant use might increase serum caffeine concentrations and the risk of adverse effects, due to the caffeine contained in cola nut. Cimetidine decreases the rate of caffeine clearance by 30-50% (14).
CLOZAPINE (Clozaril): Theoretically, co-administration might acutely exacerbate psychotic symptoms, due to the caffeine contained in cola nut. Caffeine can increase the effects and toxicity of clozapine (151). Caffeine doses of 400-1000 mg per day inhibit clozapine metabolism (5051).
CNS STIMULANTS: Concomitant use might increase the risk of stimulant adverse effects, due to the caffeine contained in cola nut (151,2719). CNS stimulants include nicotine, cocaine, sympathomimetic amines, and amphetamines.
DIABETES THERAPY: Theoretically, concomitant use of coffee and diabetes drugs might interfere with blood glucose control, due to the caffeine contained in cola nut. This is based in the claim that caffeine might have hyperglycemic effects (19).
DISULFIRAM (Antabuse): Theoretically, concomitant use might increase serum caffeine concentrations and the risk of adverse effects, due to the caffeine contained in cola nut. Disulfiram decreases the rate of caffeine clearance (15).
EPHEDRINE: Concomitant use might increase the risk of stimulatory adverse effects, due to the caffeine contained in cola nut (7,19). An unpublished report associated jitteriness, hypertension, seizures, temporary loss of consciousness,

and hospitalization requiring life support with the use of a combination ephedra (ephedrine) and guarana (caffeine) product (1380).

ESTROGEN (Estrace): Theoretically, concomitant use might increase serum caffeine concentrations and the risk of adverse effects, due to the caffeine contained in cola nut. Estrogen inhibits caffeine metabolism (2714).

ERGOTAMINE: Theoretically, concomitant use might increase the GI absorption of ergotamine, due to the caffeine contained in cola nut (15).

LITHIUM (Eskalith, Lithobid): Theoretically, abrupt cola nut withdrawal might increase serum lithium levels, due to the caffeine contained in cola nut. There are two case reports of lithium tremor that worsened upon abrupt coffee withdrawal (609,610).

MONOAMINE OXIDASE INHIBITORS (MAOIs): Theoretically, concomitant intake of large amounts of cola nut with MAOIs might precipitate a hypertensive crisis, due to the caffeine contained in cola nut. This is based on the claim that intake of large amounts of caffeine with MAOIs might precipitate a hypertensive crisis (19).

MEXILETINE (Mexitil): Theoretically, concomitant use might increase serum caffeine concentrations and the risk of adverse effects, due to the caffeine contained in cola nut. Mexiletine reduces caffeine metabolism (14).

ORAL CONTRACEPTIVES (OCs): Theoretically, concomitant use might increase serum caffeine concentrations and the risk of adverse effects, due to the caffeine contained in cola nut. OCs decrease the rate of caffeine clearance by 40-65% (14).

PHENYLPROPANOLAMINE (Dexatrim, Propagest): Theoretically, concomitant use might cause an additive increase in blood pressure and serum caffeine concentrations, due to the caffeine contained in cola nut (14).

QUINOLONES: Theoretically, concomitant use might increase serum caffeine concentrations and the risk of adverse effects, due to the caffeine contained in cola nut. Quinolones decrease caffeine clearance (606,607,608). Quinolones (also referred to as fluoroquinolones) include ciprofloxacin (Cipro), enoxacin (Penetrex), gatifloxacin (Tequin), levofloxacin (Levaquin), lomefloxacin (Maxaquin), moxifloxacin (Avelox), norfloxacin (Noroxin), ofloxacin (Floxin), sparfloxacin (Zagam), and trovafloxacin (Trovan).

RILUZOLE (Rilutek): Theoretically, concomitant use might increase serum caffeine and riluzole concentrations and the risk of adverse effects of both caffeine and riluzole, due to the caffeine contained in cola nut. Caffeine and riluzole are both metabolized by cytochrome P450 1A2 and concomitant use might reduce metabolism of one or both agents (14).

TERBINAFINE (Lamisil): Theoretically, concomitant use might increase serum caffeine concentrations and the risk of adverse effects, due to the caffeine contained in cola nut. Terbinafine decreases the rate of caffeine clearance (14).

THEOPHYLLINE (Theo-Dur): Theoretically, concomitant use might increase serum theophylline concentrations and the risk of adverse effects, due to the caffeine contained in cola nut. Large amounts of caffeine might inhibit theophylline metabolism (14).

VERAPAMIL (Calan, Isoptin, Verelan): Theoretically, concomitant use might increase plasma caffeine concentrations and the risk of adverse effects, due to the caffeine contained in cola nut. Verapamil increases plasma caffeine concentrations by 25% (14).

Interactions with Foods

CAFFEINE-CONTAINING BEVERAGES: Concomitant use can have additive therapeutic and adverse effects due to the caffeine content.

GRAPEFRUIT JUICE: Grapefruit juice interacts with the caffeine in cola nut and can increase caffeine levels, its activity, and the risk of adverse effects (504).

Interactions with Lab Tests

BLEEDING TIME: Cola nut might prolong bleeding time and increase test results, due to its caffeine content (1701).

BLOOD PRESSURE: Cola nut might increase blood pressure and blood pressure readings, due to its caffeine content (4).

URATE: Cola nut might falsely increase serum urate test results determined by the Bittner method, due to its caffeine content. Caffeine causes false elevations in serum urate test results determined by the Bittner method (15).

CATECHOLAMINES: Cola nut might increase urine catecholamine concentrations and test results, due to its caffeine content.

CREATINE: Cola nut might increase urine creatine concentrations and test results, due to its caffeine content (1701).

DIPYRIDAMOLE THALLIUM IMAGING: Cola nut might interfere with dipyridamole thallium imaging studies, due to its caffeine content. Caffeine attenuates the characteristic cardiovascular responses to dipyridamole and has altered test results (14).

5-HYDROXYINDOLEACETIC ACID: Cola nut might increase urine 5-hydroxyindoleacetic acid concentrations and test results, due to its caffeine content. Caffeine can increase urine catecholamine concentrations (15).

VANILLYLMANDELIC ACID (VMA): Cola nut might increase urine VMA concentrations and test results, due to its caffeine content.

TESTS FOR NEUROBLASTOMA: Cola nut (due to its caffeine content) might cause false-positive diagnosis of neuroblastoma, when diagnosis is based on tests of urine vanillylmandelic acid (VMA) or catecholamine concentrations. Caffeine can increase urine catecholamine and VMA concentrations (15).

TESTS FOR PHEOCHROMOCYTOMA: Cola nut (due to its caffeine content) might cause false-positive diagnosis of pheochromocytoma, when diagnosis is based on tests of urine vanillylmandelic acid (VMA) or catecholamine concentrations. Caffeine can increase urine catecholamine and VMA concentrations (15).

Interactions with Diseases or Conditions

DEPRESSION, ANXIETY DISORDERS: The caffeine in cola nut can aggravate these conditions (14).

GASTRIC, DUODENAL ULCERS: The caffeine in cola nut can aggravate these conditions and should be avoided (14,16).

HEART CONDITIONS: The caffeine in cola nut can induce cardiac arrhythmias in sensitive individuals (14,16).

HYPERTENSION: The caffeine in cola nut might increase blood pressure in people with high blood pressure (2272). Consumption of 250 mg caffeine can increase blood pressure in healthy people; however, this doesn't seem to occur in people who habitually consume caffeine products (6663).

KIDNEY DISEASE: The diuretic effect of caffeine in cola nut might aggravate some kidney disorders (19).

Dosage and Administration

ORAL: The typical dose of cola nut is 1-2 grams of the powdered nut or one cup of the tea three times daily (2,4). The tea is prepared by simmering 1-2 grams of the powdered nut in 150 mL boiling water for 5-10 minutes and then straining. The usual dose of the liquid extract of cola nut (1:1 in 60% alcohol) is 0.6-1.2 mL (4). The common dose of the tincture of cola nut (1:5 in 60% alcohol) is 1-4 mL (4).

Comments

Avoid confusion with gotu kola.

COLLOIDAL MINERALS

Also Known As

Bioelectrical Minerals, Clay Suspension Products, Colloidal Trace Minerals, Humic Shale, Plant-Derived Liquid Minerals.

Scientific Names

Anhydrous aluminum silicates.

People Use This For

Orally, colloidal minerals are used as a supplemental source of trace minerals, a dietary supplement to increase energy, for improving blood sugar levels in diabetes, arthritis symptoms, reducing blood cell clumping, reversing early cataracts, turning gray hair dark again, flushing poisonous heavy metals from the body, improving general well being, reducing aches and pains (1157).

Safety

POSSIBLY UNSAFE ...when used orally. These products contain varying amounts of aluminum, arsenic, lead, barium, nickel and titanium (1157). Some products contain as much as 1800-4400 ppm aluminum and 20 ppm arsenic (1159); generally, foods do not contain more than 10 ppm of aluminum (1159). While no cases of toxicity have been reported, there are concerns about colloidal mineral supplements containing unsafe levels of radioactive metals (1161).

PREGNANCY AND LACTATION: POSSIBLY UNSAFE ...when used orally; avoid using.

Effectiveness

There is insufficient reliable information about the effectiveness of colloidal minerals.

Mechanism of Action

Commercial colloidal mineral products are derived from clay or humic shale deposits (1159). Clay minerals are layer type aluminosilicates that figure in terrestrial biogeochemical cycles, in the buffering capacity of the oceans, and in the containment of toxic waste materials (1160). Humic shale is a common source of plant-derived colloidal minerals (1157). When mixed with water, the surfaces of clay particles become negatively charged. This allows the particles to bind with ionic minerals, such as magnesium, sodium, calcium, and potassium (1159). The content of trace minerals in individual products depends upon the rock source used (1159). Proponents claim that, due to mineral depletion of soil, many people do not take in the dietary trace minerals once plentiful in the human diet (1158). However, there is no evidence that there is increased bioavailability of ingested minerals in this form (1159).

Adverse Reactions
None reported.

Interactions with Herbs & Other Dietary Supplements
Insufficient reliable information available.

Interactions with Drugs
No interactions are known to occur, and there is no known reason to expect a clinically significant interaction with colloidal minerals.

Interactions with Foods
No interactions are known to occur, and there is no known reason to expect a clinically significant interaction with colloidal minerals.

Interactions with Lab Tests
No interactions are known to occur, and there is no known reason to expect a clinically significant interaction with colloidal minerals.

Interactions with Diseases or Conditions
HEMOCHROMATOSIS, WILSON'S DISEASE: Theoretically, colloidal minerals could exacerbate conditions in which metal accumulation is a problem.

Dosage and Administration
No typical dosage.

Comments
The medicinal use of clay-based products in modern days was first encouraged by a southern Utah rancher. Historically, some Native American tribes used clay medicinally (1157). There is a tremendous amount of promotional claims for colloidal mineral products. There is no reliable medical evidence to support using these products. Commercial colloidal mineral products are derived from clay or humic shale deposits (1159).

COLLOIDAL SILVER

Also Known As
Colloidal Silver Protein, Silver Protein.

Scientific Names
Silver in suspending agent.

People Use This For
Orally, colloidal silver is used to treat ear infections, emphysema (5519), bronchitis (5523), fungal infections, Lyme disease, Rosacea, sinus infections, stomach ulcers, yeast infections (5519), chronic fatigue syndrome (5521), AIDS (5522), and tuberculosis (5523). It is used orally for antibacterial properties (5519), for food poisoning (5523), to promote rapid healing and subdue inflammation (5519), and to treat gum disease (5521). It is used to improve digestion, and to prevent flu and colds (5519,5521). Colloidal silver is used during pregnancy to aid the baby's growth and health as well as the mother's delivery and recovery. (5522).

Topically, colloidal silver is used for acne, burns, eye infections, fungal infections, throat infections, skin infections, and Staphylococcus infections (5519).

Traditionally, colloidal silver has been used for allergies; appendicitis; arthritis; blood parasites; bubonic plague; cancer; cholera; colitis; cystitis; conjunctivitis; atopic dermatitis (cradle cap); diabetes; dysentery; eczema; gastritis; gonorrhea; impetigo; hay fever; herpes; leprosy; leukemia; lupus; lymphangitis; malaria; meningitis; parasitic infections; pneumonia; pneumococci; psoriasis; prostatitis; rhinitis; ringworm; scarlet fever; septic conditions of the eyes, ears, mouth, and throat; Salmonella; septicemia; shingles; skin cancer; syphilis; tonsillitis; toxemia; trench foot; viruses; warts; and yeast infections (5520).

Safety
POSSIBLY SAFE ...when colloidal silver is used orally in amounts that do not exceed a total intake (including food and water) of 14 mcg/kg/day of silver (350 microgram/day/70kg person). 2L of water meeting EPA standards could contain up to 200 mcg, plus a regular diet could contain 90 mcg (5525) for a total of 290 mcg without any additional oral or topical silver use.

POSSIBLY UNSAFE ...when colloidal silver is used orally or topically for medicinal use. According to the FDA final rule, no over the counter products containing colloidal silver are generally recognized as safe (5524).

LIKELY UNSAFE ...when colloidal silver is used orally or topically in large amounts or long-term. Silver accumulates in the body causing an irreversible bluish skin discoloration known as argyria. Neurological deficits, diffuse silver deposition in visceral organs, renal damage, and metal flume fever can occur (5526).

PREGNANCY AND LACTATION: POSSIBLY UNSAFE ...when used orally. Epidemiological evidence links increased silver levels to babies born with developmental anomalies of the ear, face, and neck (5525).

Effectiveness
There is insufficient reliable information available about the effectiveness of colloidal silver.

Mechanism of Action
Compounds that contain inorganic silver are germicidal. Silver binds to the reactive groups of proteins, causing denaturation and precipitation. Silver can also inactivate enzymes by binding to sulfhydryl, amino, carboxyl, phosphate, and imidazole groups. When absorbed, silver is most concentrated in the skin, liver, spleen, and adrenals with lesser amounts in the muscle and brain. The half-life depends on the silver salt used. Half-life can range from days to months. Silver deposited in the skin has a much longer half-life. Silver primarily leaves the body via fecal elimination with active biliary excretion (5525).

Adverse Reactions
Oral or topical use of colloidal silver can lead to argyria, an irreversible bluish skin discoloration. Argyria first appears in the gingiva with a slate-blue silver line. Colloidal silver can also stimulate melanin production in skin. Areas exposed to the sun will become increasingly discolored. Colloidal silver can also cause neurological deficits, diffuse silver deposition in visceral organs, renal damage, and metal flume fever (5525).

Interactions with Herbs & Other Dietary Supplements
Insufficient reliable information available.

Interactions with Drugs
DRUGS THAT COMPLEX WITH IRON: Theoretically, drugs such as tetracycline, ciprofloxacin (Cipro), methyldopa (Aldomet), norfloxacin (Noroxin), ofloxacin (Floxin), penicillamine (Cupramine), and thyroxine replacement therapy might have reduced absorption if given with colloidal silver.

Interactions with Foods
No interactions are known to occur, and there is no known reason to expect a clinically significant interaction with colloidal silver.

Interactions with Lab Tests
No interactions are known to occur, and there is no known reason to expect a clinically significant interaction with colloidal silver.

Interactions with Diseases or Conditions
No interactions are known to occur, and there is no known reason to expect a clinically significant interaction with colloidal silver.

Dosage and Administration
ORAL: A typical dose is 1 teaspoon of a 5 ppm colloid (25 mcg silver) (5520). A typical antibiotic dose is 1-3 teaspoons of 5 ppm colloid up to three times daily (5527), (75-225 mcg silver) which could exceed the total amount/day considered possibly safe for a 70 kg adult.

Comments
Interestingly, there are many internet ads for the components of a generator to produce colloidal silver at home. Those who produce colloidal silver at home will likely have no means to assay the product to assure any standard potency. There are many products that are far safer and more effective than colloidal silver.

COLOCYNTH

Also Known As
Bitter Apple, Bitter Cucumber, Colocynth Pulp, Colocynthidis Fructus, Koloquinthen.

Scientific Names
Citrullus colocynthis.
Family: Cucurbitaceae.

People Use This For
Orally, colocynth is used in combination products for acute and chronic constipation (including during pregnancy), and for liver and gallbladder ailments (2).

Safety
UNSAFE ...when used orally. Colocynth was banned by the FDA in 1991, due to toxicity (17).
PREGNANCY AND LACTATION: UNSAFE ...when used orally; avoid using.

Effectiveness
LIKELY EFFECTIVE ...when used orally for constipation, but risks preclude use.
There is insufficient reliable information available about the effectiveness of colocynth for its other uses.

Mechanism of Action
The applicable part of colocynth is the ripe fruit. It contains up to 3% cucurbitacin, a poisonous constituent that irritates mucous membranes, including GI mucosa (2) .

Adverse Reactions
Orally, ingestion of 0.6-1 grams of colocynth can cause severe irritation of the gastric mucosa, bloody diarrhea, kidney damage, hemorrhagic cystitis, and diuresis leading to anuria (2,18). Doses of 2 grams or more can cause convulsions, paralysis, and if untreated, death from circulatory collapse (18).

Interactions with Herbs & Other Dietary Supplements
STIMULANT LAXATIVE HERBS: Theoretically, concomitant use with other stimulant laxative herbs may increase the risk of potassium depletion. Stimulant laxative herbs include: aloe dried leaf sap, wild cucumber fruit (Ecballium elaterium), blue flag rhizome, alder buckthorn, European buckthorn, butternut bark, cascara bark, castor oil, gamboge bark exudate, jalap root, black root, manna bark exudate, podophyllum root, rhubarb root, senna leaves and pods, and yellow dock root (19).
POTASSIUM DEPLETING HERBS: Theoretically, concomitant use with horsetail plant or licorice rhizome increases the risk of potassium depletion.

Interactions with Drugs
CARDIAC GLYCOSIDES: Theoretically, overuse/abuse of this product increases the risk of adverse effects of cardiac glycoside drugs, such as digoxin (Lanoxin).

Interactions with Foods
No interactions are known to occur, and there is no known reason to expect a clinically significant interaction with colocynth.

Interactions with Lab Tests
POTASSIUM: Excessive use of colocynth might cause potassium depletion, reducing serum potassium concentrations and test results (19).
URINE OUTPUT: Excessive use of colocynth might lead to cessation of urine output (anuria) (18).

Interactions with Diseases or Conditions
GI CONDITIONS: Colocynth can irritate gastrointestinal tract. It is contraindicated in individuals with infectious or inflammatory gastrointestinal conditions (19).

Dosage and Administration
No typical dosage.

Comments
Colocynth is considered unsafe; avoid using. The use of colocynth is not justified due to significant risks (2). Death has resulted from the consumption of as little as 1 1/2 teaspoons of the powder. In the management of poisoning, a dilute tannic acid solution should be taken, followed by large quantities of albuminous drinks (215).

COLOMBO

Also Known As
Calomba Root, Calumba, Calumbo Root.

Scientific Names
Jateorhiza palmata, synonym Wateorhiza palmata.
Family: Menispermaceae.

People Use This For
Orally, colombo is used to treat gastritis, dyspepsia, chronic enterocolitis (18), and diarrhea (18,7).

Safety
There is insufficient reliable information available about the safety of colombo.
Pregnancy and Lactation: Insufficient reliable information; avoid using.

Effectiveness
There is insufficient reliable information available about the effectiveness of colombo.

Mechanism of Action
The applicable part of colombo is the root. Colombo contains alkaloids that have narcotic properties (18,7) and side effects (7) similar to morphine. Both increase the resting tone of smooth muscle in the intestinal tract (18,7). In frogs, the alkaloids appear to act as a central nervous system (CNS) paralyzing agent (18). Palmatine, the main alkaloid component, has a similar effect in mammals (18). Colombo's use as a digestive aid is empirically based upon the bitter principle content, which is believed to increase stomach acid secretion via vagal nerve stimulation (19).

Adverse Reactions
Orally, large doses of colombo may cause vomiting and epigastric pain (18). Overdose can lead to paralysis and unconsciousness (18).

Interactions with Herbs & Other Dietary Supplements
Insufficient reliable information available.

Interactions with Drugs
ANTACIDS, H-2 ANTAGONISTS: Antacids and H-2 antagonists decrease stomach acid secretion, which is contradictory to Colombo's theoretical action (19). H-2 antagonists include cimetidine, famotidine, nizatidine, and ranitidine.

Interactions with Foods
No interactions are known to occur, and there is no known reason to expect a clinically significant interaction with colombo.

Interactions with Lab Tests
No interactions are known to occur, and there is no known reason to expect a clinically significant interaction with colombo.

Interactions with Diseases or Conditions
No interactions are known to occur, and there is no known reason to expect a clinically significant interaction with colombo.

Dosage and Administration
ORAL: A typical dose is 2 teaspoons of the boiled root as tea taken every hour (18). For single use, 20 drops of the extract or 2.5 grams of the tincture has been used (18). The root should be stored in a dry area (18).

Comments
Colombo is no longer used as a digestive aid and is rarely used as an antidiarrheal agent because of its morphine-like effects (18).

COLTSFOOT

Also Known As
Ass's Foot, Brandlattich, British Tobacco, Bullsfoot, Colts Foot, Coughwort, Farfarae Folium leaf, Fieldhove, Filuis Ante Patrem, Flower Velure, Foal's Foot, Foalswort, Guflatich, Hallfoot, Horsefoot, Horsehoof, Kuandong Hua, Pas Diane, Pas d'Ane, Pferdefut, Tussilage.

Scientific Names
Tussilago farfara.
Family: Asteraceae or Compositae.

People Use This For
Historically, coltsfoot leaf has been used orally for bronchitis, asthma, laryngitis, pertussis (4), acute respiratory tract mucous membrane inflammation with cough and hoarseness, acute or mild inflammation of the oral and pharyngeal mucosa (2), and sore throat (6). Coltsfoot has also been used as an inhalant for coughs and wheezing (6).

Safety
UNSAFE ...when used orally (2,7,12,515). All parts of coltsfoot contain unsaturated pyrrolizidine alkaloids (UPAs) in varying amounts (2,7). The unsaturated pyrrolizidine alkaloids are considered to be hepatotoxic and hepatocarcinogenic (7,515) UPAs are released into teas when prepared from coltsfoot leaves (7). Repeated exposure to low concentrations of UPAs is linked to veno-occlusive disease (4,12,515). UPAs are considered to be also possibly mutagenic (12). Dietary supplement products sold in the United States are not required to include the amount of UPAs they may contain; therefore, all preparations used orally containing coltsfoot should be considered potentially unsafe (3484).
PREGNANCY AND LACTATION: UNSAFE ...when used orally; contraindicated due to its potential to be abortifacient (4,19) and hepatotoxic (4,12,575). Hepatotoxic pyrrolizidine alkaloids may be excreted in breast milk (4,12,18).

Effectiveness
There is insufficient reliable information available about the effectiveness of coltsfoot.

Mechanism of Action
The applicable part of coltsfoot is the leaf. Coltsfoot has been documented to have expectorant, antitussive, demulcent, and anti-inflammatory effects on mucous membranes (4). The mucilage content of coltsfoot has a soothing effect on the throat (6,515). Coltsfoot contains the unsaturated pyrrolizidine alkaloids senkirkirine and senecionine (4,7,515). Unsaturated pyrrolizidine alkaloids are known to be hepatotoxic in animals and humans (4,7,515). UPAs destroy and damage centrilobular hepatocytes of the liver and also destroy small branches of the hepatic vein (7). Animals fed various amounts of coltsfoot have been reported to develop cancerous tumors in the liver (515,3484). In animals, coltsfoot has anti-inflammatory and antibacterial activity against gram negative bacteria (4). It also contains an inhibitor of the platelet activating factor (PAF). PAF is known to play a key role in the inflammatory cascade. The presence of a PAF inhibitor in coltsfoot can account for the effect of coltsfoot in asthma (4). The constituent tusilagone has respiratory stimulant and cardiovascular (including pressor) activities (4). Cardiovascular effects are thought to be mediated by peripheral mechanisms and the respiratory effects by central mechanisms (4). An isolated coltsfoot constituent interacts with the cardiac calcium channel blocker receptor complex (dihydropyridine receptor), but it also has calcium channel blocking activity (4). In animals, coltsfoot is reported to have a pressor effect similar to dopamine but without tachyphylaxis and to be phototoxic (4).

Adverse Reactions
Nonspecific symptoms such as anorexia, lethargy and abdominal pain can result after chronic use of coltsfoot (7). Further use can lead to hepatotoxicity (4,7). There is one case report of fatal hepatic veno-occlusive disease in a neonate associated with regular maternal consumption during pregnancy of an herb tea containing several pyrrolizidine alkaloid herbs, including coltsfoot (575). It can cause an allergic reaction in individuals sensitive to the Asteraceae/Compositae family. Members of this family include ragweed, chrysanthemums, marigolds, daisies, and many other herbs.

Interactions with Herbs & Other Dietary Supplements
EUCALYPTUS: Theoretically, concomitant use can increase the toxicity of coltsfoot due to enzyme induction by eucalyptus (19).
PYRROLIZIDINE ALKALOID-CONTAINING HERBS: Concomitant use is contraindicated due to the risk of additive toxicity. Herbs containing unsaturated pyrrolizidine alkaloids include: alkanna (12), borage (271), gravel root (4), hemp agrimony (271), hound's tongue (19), petasites (19), comfrey (271), coltsfoot, and the Senecio species plants; dusty miller (19), alpine ragwort (19), groundsel (271), golden ragwort (19), and tansy ragwort (271).

Interactions with Drugs

ANTIHYPERTENSIVE and CARDIOVASCULAR DRUGS: Theoretically, excessive doses of coltsfoot can interfere with antihypertensive or cardiovascular therapy (4).

Interactions with Foods

No interactions are known to occur, and there is no known reason to expect a clinically significant interaction with coltsfoot.

Interactions with Lab Tests

No interactions are known to occur, and there is no known reason to expect a clinically significant interaction with coltsfoot.

Interactions with Diseases or Conditions

HYPERTENSION, CARDIOVASCULAR DISEASE: Excessive amounts of coltsfoot can interfere with therapy for hypertension or cardiovascular disease (4).
LIVER DISEASE: Coltsfoot is contraindicated due to its hepatotoxic potential (19).
CROSS-ALLERGENICITY: Can cause an allergic reaction in individuals sensitive to the Asteraceae/Compositae family. Members of this family include ragweed, chrysanthemums, marigolds, daisies, and many other herbs.

Dosage and Administration

No typical dosage.

Comments

None.

COLUMBINE

Also Known As

Culverwort.

Scientific Names

Aquilegia vulgaris.
Family: Ranunculaceae.

People Use This For

Orally, columbine is used for general gastrointestinal disorders, to stimulate bile flow, and to regulate gallbladder contraction. It is also used for scurvy, jaundice and as a tranquilizer in patients with agitation (18).

Safety

There is insufficient reliable information available about the safety of columbine.
Pregnancy and Lactation: Insufficient reliable information available; avoid using.

Effectiveness

There is insufficient reliable information available about the effectiveness of columbine.

Mechanism of Action

The applicable parts of columbine are the above ground parts. There is insufficient reliable information available about the possible mechanism of action and active ingredients.

Adverse Reactions

None reported.

Interactions with Herbs & Other Dietary Supplements

Insufficient reliable information available.

Interactions with Drugs

No interactions are known to occur, and there is no known reason to expect a clinically significant interaction with columbine.

Interactions with Foods

No interactions are known to occur, and there is no known reason to expect a clinically significant interaction with columbine.

Interactions with Lab Tests

No interactions are known to occur, and there is no known reason to expect a clinically significant interaction with columbine.

Interactions with Diseases or Conditions

No interactions are known to occur, and there is no known reason to expect a clinically significant interaction with columbine.

Dosage and Administration

No typical dosage.

Comments

There is very little scientific information about this product. Our staff is continually analyzing the available information on natural medicines and will add data here as it becomes available.

COMFREY

Also Known As

Ass Ear, Black Root, Blackwort, Bruisewort, Common Comfrey, Consolidae Radix, Consound, Gum Plant, Healing Herb, Knitback, Knitbone, Salsify, Slippery Root, Symphytum Radix, Wallwort.

Scientific Names

Symphytum officinale.
Family: Boraginaceae.

People Use This For

Topically, comfrey is used for ulcers, wounds, and fractures (4,5). The above ground parts of comfrey are used for bruises and sprains (2).

Traditionally, comfrey has been used as a tea for ulcers, excessive menstrual flow, diarrhea, bloody urine, persistent cough, rheumatism, pleuritis, bronchitis, cancer, angina, as a gargle for gum disease, and pharyngitis (11,18,214).

Safety

POSSIBLY SAFE ...when the above ground parts are used topically on unbroken skin for less than 10 days (4). ...when the above ground parts are used topically for a maximum of 4-6 weeks per year in amounts at or below a daily dosage of 100 mcg of the hepatotoxic unsaturated pyrrolizidine alkaloids (UPAs) (2).

UNSAFE ...when the root or above ground parts are used orally because of its potential for acute or chronic liver toxicity (2,4,5) . Teas made from comfrey leaf contain lesser levels of alkaloids (4), but regular consumption can lead to toxicity (17,515). Dietary supplement products sold in the United States are not required to include the amount of UPAs they may contain; therefore, all preparations used orally containing comfrey should be considered potentially unsafe (3484).

PREGNANCY AND LACTATION: UNSAFE ...when the above ground parts or root are used orally (4,12). There is insufficient reliable information available about the safety of the topical use of comfrey during pregnancy or lactation; avoid using.

Effectiveness

POSSIBLY EFFECTIVE ...when used topically as an anti-inflammatory agent and for treating and sprains (2,9). Comfrey should be used only on unbroken skin (2).

There is insufficient reliable information available about the effectiveness of comfrey for its other uses.

Mechanism of Action

The applicable parts of comfrey are the leaf, rhizome, and root. Comfrey contains unsaturated pyrrolizidine alkaloids (UPAs) which are considered to be hepatotoxic and hepatocarcinogenic (4,7,515). UPAs destroy and damage centrilobular hepatocytes of the liver and also destroy small branches of the hepatic vein (7). The pyrrolizidine alkaloid content of the roots is ten times that of the leaves (5). Sarracind and platyphylline, non-hepatotoxic pyrrolizidine alkaloid constituents, have been used for treating gastrointestinal hypermotility and peptic ulcers (4). The healing activity of comfrey is due to its constituent, allantoin (9). The constituent, rosmarinic acid, shows evidence of anti-inflammatory activity (4) and that it can inhibit microvascular pulmonary injury (3).

Adverse Reactions
Chronic exposure to plants containing UPA constituents has been associated with veno-occlusive disease (4021). Symptoms of acute veno-occlusive disease are characterized by anorexia, lethargy (7) and a dull, dragging ache in the right upper abdomen with marked distention of the abdomen. These symptoms are sometimes accompanied by reduced urine output. Subacute veno-occlusive disease is associated with vague symptoms and persistent liver enlargement (4021).

Interactions with Herbs & Other Dietary Supplements
EUCALYPTUS: Theoretically, concomitant use might increase the risk of unsaturated pyrrolizidine alkaloid toxicity due to enzyme induction by eucalyptus (19).
PYRROLIZIDINE ALKALOID-CONTAINING HERBS: Concomitant use is contraindicated due to the risk of additive toxicity. Herbs containing unsaturated pyrrolizidine alkaloids include: alkanna (12), borage (271), gravel root (4), hemp agrimony (271), hound's tongue (19), petasites (19), comfrey (271), coltsfoot, and the Senecio species plants: dusty miller (19), alpine ragwort (19), groundsel (271), golden ragwort (19), and tansy ragwort (271).

Interactions with Drugs
No interactions are known to occur, and there is no known reason to expect a clinically significant interaction with comfrey.

Interactions with Foods
No interactions are known to occur, and there is no known reason to expect a clinically significant interaction with comfrey.

Interactions with Lab Tests
No interactions are known to occur, and there is no known reason to expect a clinically significant interaction with comfrey.

Interactions with Diseases or Conditions
BROKEN, DAMAGED SKIN: Contraindicated. Apply only to unbroken skin (2,4).

Dosage and Administration
TOPICAL: Ointments and other external preparations are commonly made with 5-20% of comfrey. The daily use of comfrey should not exceed 100 mcg of the pyrrolizidine alkaloids. Comfrey should not be used for more than ten days (4,5), and the maximum use is four to six weeks per year (2). It only should be applied externally on unbroken skin (4,12).

Comments
Prickly comfrey is more toxic than common comfrey, but either might be labeled comfrey. Some products labeled common comfrey or Symphytum officinale instead contain the more toxic prickly comfrey (3,515). The American Herbal Products Association recommends all products with toxic pyrrolizidine alkaloids be labeled with the statement, "For external use only. Do not apply to broken or abraded skin. Do not use while nursing" (12).

COMMON STONECROP

Also Known As
Bird Bread, Creeping Tom, Gold Chain, Golden Moss, Jack-of-the-Buttery, Mousetail, Prick Madam, Wall Ginger, Wallpepper.

Scientific Names
Sedum acre.

People Use This For
Orally, common stonecrop is used for coughs and hypertension.
Topically, common stonecrop is used for wounds, burns, hemorrhoids, warts, eczema, and mouth ulcers (18).

Safety

There is insufficient reliable information available about the safety of common stonecrop.

Pregnancy and Lactation: Insufficient reliable information available; avoid using.

Effectiveness

There is insufficient reliable information available about the effectiveness of common stonecrop.

Mechanism of Action

There is insufficient reliable information available about the possible mechanism of action and active ingredients.

Adverse Reactions

Orally, common stonecrop can cause vomiting and diarrhea if consumed in greater then medicinal amounts (18).

Interactions with Herbs & Other Dietary Supplements

Insufficient reliable information available.

Interactions with Drugs

No interactions are known to occur, and there is no known reason to expect a clinically significant interaction with common stonecrop.

Interactions with Foods

No interactions are known to occur, and there is no known reason to expect a clinically significant interaction with common stonecrop.

Interactions with Lab Tests

No interactions are known to occur, and there is no known reason to expect a clinically significant interaction with common stonecrop.

Interactions with Diseases or Conditions

GI AND LOWER URINARY TRACT INFLAMMATION: Contraindicated (18).

Dosage and Administration

ORAL: Typically, one cup tea (simmer 1 teaspoon or 1.5 grams in 150 mL boiling water for 10-15 minutes, strain) twice daily (18).
TOPICAL: Crush fresh plant and place on eczematous skin or warts.

Comments

None.

CONDURANGO

Also Known As

Condurango Cortex, Eagle-Vine Bark.

Scientific Names

Marsdenia condurango; Gonolobus condurango.
Family: Asclepiadaceae.

People Use This For

Orally, condurango is used as an appetite stimulant and for dyspeptic complaints (2,18).
In folk medicine, condurango has been used for stomach cancer (8,18).

Safety

LIKELY SAFE ...when used orally and appropriately (2).
PREGNANCY AND LACTATION: Insufficient reliable information available; avoid using.

Effectiveness

POSSIBLY EFFECTIVE ...when used orally as an appetite stimulant (2).
There is insufficient reliable information available about the effectiveness of condurango for its other uses.

Mechanism of Action

The applicable part of condurango is the bark. The condurango alkaloid constituents, which as a group are referred to as condurangin, stimulate salivation and the secretion of gastric juices (8).

Adverse Reactions

Orally, anaphylaxis can occur with the use of condurango bark (1501).

Interactions with Herbs & Other Dietary Supplements

Insufficient reliable information available.

Interactions with Drugs

No interactions are known to occur, and there is no known reason to expect a clinically significant interaction with condurango.

Interactions with Foods

No interactions are known to occur, and there is no known reason to expect a clinically significant interaction with condurango.

Interactions with Lab Tests

No interactions are known to occur, and there is no known reason to expect a clinically significant interaction with condurango.

Interactions with Diseases or Conditions

LATEX ALLERGY: Cross-sensitivity to condurango can occur in individuals allergic to natural rubber latex (1500), including anaphylaxis (1501). Avoid the use of condurango in these individuals.

Dosage and Administration

ORAL: The typical dose of the bark is 2-4 grams per day (2). The usual dose of the water extract is 200-500 mg per day (2). The common dose of the liquid extract is 2-4 grams per day (2), and the tincture is usually given as 2-5 grams per day (2).

Comments

None.

CONJUGATED LINOLEIC ACID

Also Known As

CLA, Linoleic.

Scientific Names

cis-9,trans-11 conjugated linoleic acid; trans-10,cis-12 conjugated linoleic acid.

People Use This For

Orally, conjugated linoleic acid (CLA) is used for cancer, obesity, cachexia, bodybuilding, for limiting food allergy reactions, and for atherosclerosis.

Safety

LIKELY SAFE ...when used orally in amounts found in foods. Conjugated linoleic acid occurs naturally in milk fat, beef, and meat of other ruminant animals (5924,5925,5932,5933).
POSSIBLY SAFE ...when used orally and appropriately in medicinal amounts (3153).
PREGNANCY AND LACTATION: LIKELY SAFE ...when used orally in amounts found in foods (5924,5932,5933). There is insufficient reliable information available about the safety of conjugated linoleic acid when used in medicinal amounts during pregnancy or lactation; avoid using.

Effectiveness

There is insufficient reliable information available to rate the effectiveness of conjugated linoleic acid (CLA). However, there is preliminary evidence that CLA might help obese people lose weight or lose body fat mass when 3.4 grams per day is taken over a period of 12 weeks (3153). More evidence is needed to rate CLA for this use.

Mechanism of Action

Conjugated linoleic acid (CLA) refers to a group of conjugated dienoic isomers of linoleic acid, including cis-9, trans-11 linoleic acid and trans-10, cis-12 linoleic acid. Different isomeric forms might have different physiological effects (3158). Dairy products and beef are the major dietary sources. These primarily contain the cis-9, trans-11 isomer. Plant oils contain only small amounts of CLA. However, plant oils are good sources of linoleic acid, but in humans linoleic acid does not seem to be converted to CLA in significant amounts (5933). CLA can also be produced synthetically by exposing oils rich in linoleic acid, such as safflower and soybean, to base and heat. This CLA product is high in both the cis-9, trans-11 and the trans-10, cis-12 isomers (3001). There's a lot of interest in using CLA for weight loss in obesity. Researchers think that CLA might reduce body fat deposits by promoting apoptosis in adipose tissue (3070,5928). There is some evidence that only the trans-10, cis-12 isomer has an effect on body fat mass (3001). There is also interest in using CLA for cancer prevention. There is some evidence it can enhance immune function, and inhibiting cyclooxygenase and lipoxygenase pathways in tumor cells (5926,5934). CLA might also modulate cellular response to tumor necrosis factor-alpha (TNF-alpha) (5924). CLA may have a variety of other pharmacological properties, including hypoglycemic and antiplatelet effects (5934,5936).

Adverse Reactions

Orally, the most common adverse effect of conjugated linoleic acid is gastrointestinal upset and in some cases, fatigue (3153).

Interactions with Herbs & Other Dietary Supplements

VITAMIN A: Some evidence suggests conjugated linoleic acid might increase vitamin A (retinol) storage in the liver and breast (5931).

Interactions with Drugs

No interactions are known to occur, and there is no known reason to expect a clinically significant interaction with conjugated linoleic acid.

Interactions with Foods

No interactions are known to occur, and there is no known reason to expect a clinically significant interaction with conjugated linoleic acid.

Interactions with Lab Tests

CHOLESTEROL: Conjugated linoleic acid appears to reduce total, low-density lipoprotein (LDL), and high-density lipoprotein (HDL) cholesterol levels (3153).

Interactions with Diseases or Conditions

No interactions are known to occur, and there is no known reason to expect a clinically significant interaction with conjugated linoleic acid.

Dosage and Administration

ORAL: For weight loss in obese patients, 2-7 grams per day has been used. However, doses greater than 3.4 grams per day do not seem to offer any additional benefit (3153).

Comments

None.

CONTRAYERVA

Also Known As

None.

Scientific Names

Dorstenia contrayerva.

People Use This For

Orally, contrayerva is used to increase stamina and as a snakebite antidote (18).

Safety

POSSIBLY UNSAFE …when root preparations are used orally. Contrayerva contains cardenolides that are cardioactive steroids and could affect the heart (18).
PREGNANCY AND LACTATION: POSSIBLY UNSAFE …when used orally; avoid using.

Effectiveness

There is insufficient reliable information available about the effectiveness of contrayerva.

Mechanism of Action

The applicable part of contrayerva is the root. Contrayerva is believed to act as a stimulant and induce sweating (18).

Adverse Reactions

Topically, skin contact with plant can increase sensitivity to ultraviolet light (18).

Interactions with Herbs & Other Dietary Supplements

Insufficient reliable information available.

Interactions with Drugs

No interactions are known to occur, and there is no known reason to expect a clinically significant interaction with contrayerva.

Interactions with Foods

No interactions are known to occur, and there is no known reason to expect a clinically significant interaction with contrayerva.

Interactions with Lab Tests

No interactions are known to occur, and there is no known reason to expect a clinically significant interaction with contrayerva.

Interactions with Diseases or Conditions

No interactions are known to occur, and there is no known reason to expect a clinically significant interaction with contrayerva.

Dosage and Administration

ORAL: People typically use 1/2 teaspoon of the powdered root. Contrayerva is also prepared as a tea with 1 ounce added to 2 cups boiling water (5267).

Comments

There is very little scientific information about this product. Our staff is continually analyzing the available information on natural medicines and will add data here as it becomes available.

COOLWORT

Also Known As

Foam Flower, Mitrewort.

Scientific Names

Tiarella cordifolia.

People Use This For

Orally, coolwort is used for urinary tract and digestive disorders (18), as a tonic, diuretic, for bladder diseases and stones, indigestion, and dyspepsia (3821).

Safety

There is insufficient reliable information available about the safety of coolwort.
Pregnancy and Lactation: Insufficient reliable information available; avoid using.

Effectiveness

There is insufficient reliable information available about the effectiveness of coolwort.

Mechanism of Action
Coolwort is thought to have diuretic and tonic properties (18).

Adverse Reactions
None reported.

Interactions with Herbs & Other Dietary Supplements
Insufficient reliable information available.

Interactions with Drugs
No interactions are known to occur, and there is no known reason to expect a clinically significant interaction with coolwort.

Interactions with Foods
No interactions are known to occur, and there is no known reason to expect a clinically significant interaction with coolwort.

Interactions with Lab Tests
No interactions are known to occur, and there is no known reason to expect a clinically significant interaction with coolwort.

Interactions with Diseases or Conditions
No interactions are known to occur, and there is no known reason to expect a clinically significant interaction with coolwort.

Dosage and Administration
ORAL: Coolwort is used as a tea (18).

Comments
There is very little scientific information about this product. Our staff is continually analyzing the available information on natural medicines and will add data here as it becomes available.

COPAIBA BALSAM

Also Known As
Balsam, Copaiba, Copaiba Oleoresin, Copaiva, Jesuit's Balsam.

Scientific Names
Copaifera officinalis; Copaifera langsdorfii; Copaifera reticulata; and other Copaifera species.
Family: Leguminosae or Fabaceae.

People Use This For
Traditionally, copaiba balsam has been used for chronic bronchitis, hemorrhoids, chronic diarrhea, chronic cystitis (11), urinary tract infections, as a stimulant, and a laxative (18).
In foods and beverages, copaiba balsam oleoresin is used as an ingredient (11).
In manufacturing, copaiba balsam oleoresin and oil are used in soaps, cosmetics, and perfumes (11).
In pharmaceutical preparations, both the oleoresin and oil are used in cough medicines and diuretics (11).

Safety
POSSIBLY SAFE …when used orally in food amounts. Maximum use level is usually less than 0.002%. Both the oleoresin and oil have been approved for food use. …when used topically in cosmetics. Maximum use level in perfumes is 0.8%.
POSSIBLY UNSAFE …when used orally for medicinal purposes. Copaiba balsam can irritate mucous membranes. Ingesting 5 grams can cause stomach pains (18).
PREGNANCY AND LACTATION: POSSIBLY UNSAFE …when used orally for medicinal purposes; avoid using.

Effectiveness
There is insufficient reliable information available about the effectiveness of copaiba balsam.

Mechanism of Action

Copaiba balsam contains a volatile oil consisting of alpha and beta-caryophyllene, L-cadinenes, and copene. It also has resins, including diterpenoid oleoresins. Some evidence suggests copaiba balsam might have bacteriostatic (18), diuretic, expectorant, disinfectant, and stimulant activity (11). In addition to these properties, the oil exhibits antibacterial activity (11). Some evidence suggests the oleoresin of the Brazilian Copaifera species might have anti-inflammatory effects (11).

Adverse Reactions

Orally, ingesting 5 grams of copaiba balsam orally can cause stomach pains (18); repeated doses can cause shivers, tremor, groin pain, and insomnia (18). Large amounts may cause vomiting, diarrhea, and measles-like rash (11). Topically, copaiba balsam can cause contact dermatitis with erythema, papular or vesicular rash, urticaria, petechiae, and the rash may leave brown spots after healing (18).

Interactions with Herbs & Other Dietary Supplements

Insufficient reliable information available.

Interactions with Drugs

No interactions are known to occur, and there is no known reason to expect a clinically significant interaction with copaiba balsam.

Interactions with Foods

No interactions are known to occur, and there is no known reason to expect a clinically significant interaction with copaiba balsam.

Interactions with Lab Tests

No interactions are known to occur, and there is no known reason to expect a clinically significant interaction with copaiba balsam.

Interactions with Diseases or Conditions

No interactions are known to occur, and there is no known reason to expect a clinically significant interaction with copaiba balsam.

Dosage and Administration

No typical dosage.

Comments

Copaiba balsam is an oleoresin rather than a true balsam collected from the trunk of Copaifera species trees (11). Copaiba oil is distilled from the oleoresin (11). Copaiba balsam is considered obsolete for medicinal purposes (18).

COPPER

Also Known As

Cuivre, Elemental Copper.

Scientific Names

Copper; Cu; atomic number 29.

People Use This For

Orally, copper is used for treating copper deficiency and anemia due to copper deficiency, zinc-induced copper deficiency, improving wound healing, osteoarthritis, and osteoporosis.

Safety

LIKELY SAFE ...when used orally and appropriately. Copper is safe in amounts that do not exceed 10 mg per day, the Tolerable Upper Intake Level (UL) (7135).
POSSIBLY UNSAFE ...when used orally in high doses. Tell patients to avoid exceeding the UL of 10 mg per day. Higher intake can cause liver damage (7135). Renal failure and death can occur with ingestion of as little as 1 gram of copper sulfate (17).
CHILDREN: LIKELY SAFE ...when used orally and appropriately. Copper is safe in amounts that do not exceed the UL of 1 mg per day for children 1 to 3 years, 3 mg per day for children 4 to 8 years, 5 mg per day for children 9 to 13 years, and 8 mg per day for adolescents (7135). POSSIBLY UNSAFE ...when used orally in high doses.

Tell patients to avoid exceeding the UL of 1 mg per day for children 1 to 3 years, 3 mg per day for children 4 to 8 years, 5 mg per day for children 9 to 13 years, and 8 mg per day for adolescents (7135). Higher intake can cause liver damage (7135).

PREGNANCY: LIKELY SAFE …when used orally and appropriately. Copper is safe in amounts that do not exceed the UL of 8 mg per day (7135). POSSIBLY UNSAFE …when used orally in high doses. Tell patients to avoid exceeding the UL of 8 mg per day. Higher intake can cause liver damage (7135).

LACTATION: LIKELY SAFE …when used orally and appropriately. Copper is safe in amounts that do not exceed the UL of 10 mg per day or 8 mg per day for breast-feeding women ages 14 to 18 years (7135). POSSIBLY UNSAFE …when used orally in high doses. Tell patients to avoid exceeding the UL of 10 mg per day or 8 mg per day for breast-feeding women ages 14 to 18 years. Higher intake can cause liver damage (7135).

Effectiveness

LIKELY EFFECTIVE …when taken orally or intravenously for treating copper deficiency and anemia due to copper deficiency (505). Copper deficiency is rare. It is seen most commonly in people receiving prolonged parenteral nutrition (7135).

There is insufficient reliable information available about the effectiveness of copper for its other uses.

Mechanism of Action

Copper is an essential trace mineral. It is widely distributed in foods, particularly organ meats, seafood, nuts, seeds, wheat bran cereals, grain products, and cocoa products (7135). Absorption occurs primarily in the small intestine with lesser absorption in the stomach (7135). The majority of body copper is in the skeleton and muscles, with the liver maintaining plasma copper concentrations. Excretion of copper into the gastrointestinal tract regulates copper homeostasis, with greater excretion the result of increased absorption (7135). Biochemically, copper acts as a catalytic agent via a many copper metalloenzymes which act as oxidases (7135). Amine oxidases are important in a variety of processes including allergic reactions, serotonin and catacholamine degredation, and connective tissue development. Ferroxidases, copper enzymes in the plasma, are required for ferrous iron oxidation and binding of iron to transferrin. The main copper protein in plasma Ferroxidase I, also called ceruloplasmin, might have antioxidant functions. Another copper enzyme, cytochrome c oxidase is a mitochondrial enzyme that catalyzes the reduction of oxygen to water to fuel ATP synthesis. Cytochrome c oxidase is most abundant in highly metabolic tissues, including the heart, brain, and liver. Other copper enzymes are responsible for precursors of dopa and melatonin formation, conversion of dopamine to norepinephrine, production of amides, and protection from free radical damage (7135). The activity of copper enzymes decreases with copper depletion (7135). Copper deficiency in humans is rare, but has been associated with excessive zinc intake (505,706,707,708), intestinal bypass surgery, parenteral nutrition, and malnourished infants (505). Copper deficiency is manifested by normocytic hypochromic anemia, leukopenia, and neutropenia (7135). In infants and children, osteoporosis may been seen (7135). No single lab test is available to determine copper deficiency. Diagnosis of copper deficiency is made by several indicators, including serum or plasma copper concentration, ceruloplasmin concentration, and erythrocyte superoxide dismutase activity (7135).

Adverse Reactions

Orally, copper is most commonly associated with gastrointestinal side effects including abdominal pain, cramps, nausea, diarrhea and vomiting. Copper toxicity is rare in humans, except in those people with a heredity defect in copper homeostasis.

Acute hepatic failure has been reported in a patient taking 30 to 60 mg of copper daily for more than 2 years (7135). Renal failure and death can occur with ingestion of as little as 1 gram of copper sulfate (17). Symptoms of acute copper poisoning include nausea, vomiting, bloody diarrhea, hypotension, hemolytic anemia, uremia, and cardiovascular collapse (159). Chronic exposure symptoms include sporadic fever, vomiting, epigastric pain, diarrhea, and jaundice (159).

Interactions with Herbs & Other Dietary Supplements

IRON: In infants, high iron intake may interfere with copper absorption (7135).
VITAMIN C (ascorbic acid): 1500 mg of Vitamin C taken daily may decrease copper-dependent enzyme (ceruloplasmin) activity significantly (710).
ZINC: Large amounts of zinc can inhibit copper absorption (707,708) and cause copper deficiency (706).

Interactions with Drugs

PENICILLAMINE: Copper inhibits penicillamine (Cuprimine, Depen) activity; avoid concomitant use (15).

Drug Influences on Nutrient Levels and Depletion

SOME DRUGS CAN AFFECT COPPER LEVELS:

PENICILLAMINE (Cuprimine, Depen): Penicillamine chelates copper in the gastrointestinal tract and decreases absorption. Separate administration by at least 2 hours. The need for supplementation has not been adequately studied (4453,4531,4534,4535).

Interactions with Foods

No interactions are known to occur, and there is no known reason to expect a clinically significant interaction with copper.

Interactions with Lab Tests

No interactions are known to occur, and there is no known reason to expect a clinically significant interaction with copper.

Interactions with Diseases or Conditions

IDIOPATHIC COPPER TOXICOSIS: Copper supplementation can worsen this genetic condition (7135).
INDIAN CHILDHOOD CIRRHOSIS: Copper supplementation can worse this genetic condition (7135).
WILSON'S DISEASE: Copper supplementation can worsen this condition or interfere with penicillamine therapy (15,505).

Dosage and Administration

ORAL: For copper deficiency, doses up to 0.1 mg/kg cupric sulfate per day have been used (505). The National Institute of Medicine has determined Adequate Intake (AI) of copper for infants: 0 to 6 months, 200 mcg (30 mcg/kg/day); 7 to 12 months, 220 mcg (24 mcg/kg/day). For children, a Recommended Dietary Allowance (RDA) has been set: 1 to 3 years, 340 mcg/day; 4 to 8 years, 440 mcg/day; 9 to 13, 700 mcg/day; 14 to 18 years, 890 mcg/day. For men and women age 19 years and older, the RDA is 900 mcg/day. For pregnancy, the RDA is 1000 mcg/day, and lactation 1300 mcg/day for women of all ages (7135). The average dietary intake of copper by US women is 1.0 to 1.1 mg/day, men consume 1.2 to 1.6 mg/day (7135). Tolerable Upper Intake Levels (UL) have been established for children and adults. All copper intake by infants should be from food or formula, unless under medical supervision (7135). The Uls for copper are: children 1 to 3 years, 1 mg/day; 4 to 8 years, 3 mg/day; 9 to 13 years, 5 mg/day; 14 to 18 years (including pregnancy and lactation) 8 mg/day; adults age 19 and older (including lactation), 10 mg/day; pregnancy age 19 and older, 8 mg/day (7135).

INTRAVENOUS: For copper deficiency, 1 to 2 mg per day is added to the parenteral nutrition solution (505).

Comments

There is no evidence that copper supplementation is needed or beneficial for people eating a normal diet, including athletes (505,703,704,705,709).

CORAL

Also Known As

Calcium Carbonate Matrix, Sea Coral.
CAUTION: See separate listing for Coral Root.

Scientific Names

Goniopora species; Porites species.

People Use This For

Orthopedically, coral is used as a substrate for growing new bone in areas damaged by trauma, maxillofacial reconstruction, cosmetic facial surgery, and damaged weight-bearing bones (6).

Safety

LIKELY SAFE ...when used in orthopedic surgery. Coral may reduce adverse effects inherent in bone graft surgery (6).
PREGNANCY AND LACTATION: Insufficient reliable information available; avoid using.

Effectiveness

LIKELY EFFECTIVE ...when used in orthopedic surgery as substrate for growing new bone in maxillofacial reconstruction (6).
There is insufficient reliable information available about the effectiveness of coral for its other uses.

Mechanism of Action

Coral (calcium carbonate matrix) is harvested and treated with heat, pressure, and chemicals to convert it to hydroxyapatite (6). Researchers think it provides a long-lasting matrix that is very similar to natural bone (6).

Adverse Reactions

None reported.

Interactions with Herbs & Other Dietary Supplements

Insufficient reliable information available.

Interactions with Drugs

No interactions are known to occur, and there is no known reason to expect a clinically significant interaction with coral.

Interactions with Foods

No interactions are known to occur, and there is no known reason to expect a clinically significant interaction with coral.

Interactions with Lab Tests

No interactions are known to occur, and there is no known reason to expect a clinically significant interaction with coral.

Interactions with Diseases or Conditions

No interactions are known to occur, and there is no known reason to expect a clinically significant interaction with coral.

Dosage and Administration

No typical dosage.

Comments

Avoid confusion with coral root (Corallorhiza odontorhiza).

CORAL ROOT

Also Known As

Chicken Toe, Crawley, Crawley Root, Fever Root, Scaley Dragon's Claw, Turkey Claw.
CAUTION: See separate listing for Coral.

Scientific Names

Corallorhiza odontorihiza.
Family: Orchidaceae.

People Use This For

Orally, coral root is used for colds and inducing perspiration (18).

Safety

There is insufficient reliable information available about the safety of coral root.
Pregnancy and Lactation: Insufficient reliable information available; avoid using.

Effectiveness

There is insufficient reliable information available about the effectiveness of coral root.

Mechanism of Action

The applicable part of coral root is the rhizome and root. Reported to have diaphoretic, antipyretic, and sedative effects (18).

Adverse Reactions

None reported.

Interactions with Herbs & Other Dietary Supplements
Insufficient reliable information available.

Interactions with Drugs
No interactions are known to occur, and there is no known reason to expect a clinically significant interaction with coral root.

Interactions with Foods
No interactions are known to occur, and there is no known reason to expect a clinically significant interaction with coral root.

Interactions with Lab Tests
No interactions are known to occur, and there is no known reason to expect a clinically significant interaction with coral root.

Interactions with Diseases or Conditions
No interactions are known to occur, and there is no known reason to expect a clinically significant interaction with coral root.

Dosage and Administration
ORAL: People typically prepare coral root as a tea, adding 1 teaspoon of root to 1 cup of water. The tea is taken hot or cold, 1 to 2 cups per day. In tincture form, the coral root dose is 10 to 20 drops (5263).

Comments
Avoid confusion with coral. Scarcity of this plant limits use (18).

CORDYCEPS

Also Known As
Caterpillar Fungus, Cs-4, Dong Chong Xia Cao, Dong Chong Zia Cao, Hsia Ts'Ao Tung Ch'Ung, Vegetable Caterpillar.

Scientific Names
Cordyceps sinensis.
Family: Ascomycetes or Clavicipitaceae.

People Use This For
Orally, cordyceps is used for strengthening the immune system, for reducing the effects of aging (321), promoting longevity, treating lethargy (512), and improving liver function in people with hepatitis B. It is also used to treat coughs, chronic bronchitis, respiratory disorders, kidney disorders (512), frequent nocturia (3408), male sexual dysfunction (512), anemia, heart arrhythmias, high cholesterol, liver disorders (321), dizziness, weakness, tinnitus (3408), wasting, and opium addiction. It is also used as a stimulant, a tonic, and an adaptogen which is used to increase energy, enhance stamina, and reduce fatigue (512).

Safety
POSSIBLY SAFE ...when used orally and appropriately (12). There are no reports of cordyceps toxicity in humans.
PREGNANCY AND LACTATION: Insufficient reliable information available; avoid using.

Effectiveness
POSSIBLY EFFECTIVE ...when used orally following cancer chemotherapy for improving quality of life and cellular immunity (3417). ...when used orally by patients with hepatitis B for improving liver function (3435).
There is insufficient reliable information available about the effectiveness of cordyceps for its other uses.

Mechanism of Action
Cordyceps sinensis has beneficial effects on the immune, endocrine, cardiovascular, respiratory, renal, sexual, hepatic, immunologic, and nervous systems (3403,3404). Preliminary studies suggest cordyceps might stimulate immune function by increasing the number of T helper cells (3431); increasing the natural killer cell activity (3425,3427); stimulating the blood mononuclear cells (3414); increasing the levels of interferon-gamma, tumor necrosis factor-alpha, and interleukin-1 (3414); and prolonging the survival of lymphocytes (3432). Studies in animals with cancer suggest cordyceps improves immune response, reduces tumor size (3409,3431,3434), and lengthens survival time (3434,3437).

Some evidence suggests cordyceps might be cytotoxic to cancer cells (3410,3416,3420), particularly lung carcinoma (3407) and melanoma (3427). Other evidence suggests that cordyceps might reduce the risk of renal toxicity from cyclosporine or aminoglycoside drugs (3411,3418,3419), and prove beneficial in chronic renal failure (3428). Cordyceps shows evidence that it can inhibit platelet aggregation and thrombus formation (3429). Other information suggests it might counteract or prevent arrhythmias, while decreasing heart rate and contractility (3436). Cordyceps polysaccharides show evidence that they might increase corticosterone production (3412). Other studies suggest they might reduce blood glucose (3415) without reducing plasma insulin levels (3415,3421), as well as reduce plasma triglycerides and cholesterol (3415). Preliminary animal studies suggest cordyceps could possibly be beneficial in treating systemic lupus erythematosus (3424). Limited human evidence suggests cordyceps can improve liver function in patients with chronic hepatitis B (3435).

Adverse Reactions
None reported.

Interactions with Herbs & Other Dietary Supplements
Insufficient reliable information available.

Interactions with Drugs
CYCLOSPORINE: Concomitant administration can reduce nephrotoxicity in kidney-transplant recipients (3418).
AMINOGLYCOSIDES: Concomitant administration can reduce amikacin-induced nephrotoxicity in older people (3419).
CYCLOPHOSPHAMIDE: Theoretically, concomitant use might protect helper T-cells and natural killer cells from immunosuppressive drug effects (3427,3431).
PREDNISOLONE: Theoretically, concomitant use might protect helper T-cells from immunosuppressive drug effects (3431,3437).

Interactions with Foods
No interactions are known to occur, and there is no known reason to expect a clinically significant interaction with cordyceps.

Interactions with Lab Tests
LIVER FUNCTION TESTS: Cordyceps might improve liver function and test results in people with chronic hepatitis B (3435).

Interactions with Diseases or Conditions
HEPATITIS B: Based on limited human evidence, cordyceps might improve liver function and provide other benefits for people with chronic hepatitis B (3435).

Dosage and Administration
ORAL: A typical dosage of fermented Cordyceps sinensis is 3 grams per day (3403,3404).

Comments
Cordyceps sinensis is a fungus parasite that lives on caterpillars in high mountain regions of China (512). For commercial purposes, the cordyceps cells (Cs-4 strain) can be artificially propagated in the laboratory (512). Jinshuibao capsules are the commercially available form of fermented Cordyceps sinensis Cs-4 (3403).

CORIANDER

Also Known As
Chinese Parsley, Cilantro, Coriandri Fructus, Koriander.

Scientific Names
Coriandrum sativum.
Family: Apiaceae or Umbelliferae.

People Use This For
Orally, coriander is used for dyspepsia, loss of appetite (2), as a stomach function stimulant, spasmolytic, antiflatulent, bactericide, fungicide, and for diarrhea (8).
In Chinese medicine, coriander is used to treat measles, dysentery, hemorrhoids, and toothaches (11). The whole plant is used for stomachache, nausea, measles, and painful hernia (11).

In folk medicine, coriander is used for worms, rheumatism, and joint pain (8).

For food uses, coriander is used as a culinary spice (11).

In manufacturing, coriander is used as a flavoring agent in pharmaceutical preparations, as a fragrance component in cosmetics and soaps, and for flavoring tobacco (11).

Safety

LIKELY SAFE ...when consumed in amounts commonly found in foods. Coriander has Generally Recognized as Safe (GRAS) status for food use in the US and has a maximum use level of 0.52% (11).

POSSIBLY SAFE ...when used orally and appropriately for medicinal purposes (12).

PREGNANCY AND LACTATION: Insufficient reliable information available; avoid amounts in excess of those found in foods.

Effectiveness

There is insufficient reliable information available about the effectiveness of coriander.

Mechanism of Action

The applicable part of coriander is the seed/fruit. Coriander is a rich source of vitamin C, calcium, magnesium, potassium, and iron (19). The odor and taste of coriander are due to the volatile oil, which consists mainly of linalool (60-70%) (7). In animals, coriander has shown hypoglycemic activity (11). Coriander oil can possess larvicidal properties (11).

Adverse Reactions

Powdered coriander and especially the oil can cause allergic reactions and photosensitivity (8). Like other members of the carrot family, coriander can cause contact dermatitis (19).

Interactions with Herbs & Other Dietary Supplements

Insufficient reliable information available.

Interactions with Drugs

No interactions are known to occur, and there is no known reason to expect a clinically significant interaction with coriander.

Interactions with Foods

No interactions are known to occur, and there is no known reason to expect a clinically significant interaction with coriander.

Interactions with Lab Tests

No interactions are known to occur, and there is no known reason to expect a clinically significant interaction with coriander.

Interactions with Diseases or Conditions

No interactions are known to occur, and there is no known reason to expect a clinically significant interaction with coriander.

Dosage and Administration

ORAL: The typical dose of coriander is 3 grams per day of the dried fruit/seed or one cup of the tea between meals, up to three times daily (2,8,18). The tea is prepared by steeping 1 gram of the crushed seed or fruit in 150 mL boiling water for 5-10 minutes. The usual dose of the tincture is 10-20 drops after meals (18).

Comments

None.

CORIOLUS MUSHROOM

Also Known As

Boletus Versicolor, Coriolus, Kawaratake, Krestin, Polyporus Versicolor, Polysaccharide Peptide, Polysaccharide-K, Polystictus Versicolor, PSK, PSP, Turkey Tail, Yun-Zhi (cloud mushroom).

Scientific Names

Coriolus versicolor, synonym Trametes versicolor.
Family: Polyporaceae.

People Use This For

Orally, coriolus mushroom or its derivatives are used for stimulating the immune system; treating herpes, chronic fatigue syndrome, hepatitis (5495,5496), treating pulmonary disorders; reducing phlegm; improving body building; increasing energy; curing ringworm and impetigo; treating upper respiratory, urinary, and digestive tract infections; curing liver disorders including hepatitis (5497), ameliorating the toxic effects and pain of chemotherapy and radiation therapy; promoting curative effect of chemotherapy; prolonging life and raising the quality of life; increasing appetite (5498), and improving the effectiveness of cancer chemotherapy (1640,1641,1648,1649,1650,1651,1652,1653,1654,1655,1656) (1657,1658,1659,1660,1661,1662).

Safety

POSSIBLY SAFE ...when coriolus mushroom is used orally and appropriately (5477). ...when isolated PSK and PSP are used orally and appropriately (1635,1636,1640,1641,1648,1649,1650,1651,1652,1653,1654) (1655,1656,1657,1658,1659,1660,1661,1662).
PREGNANCY AND LACTATION: Insufficient reliable information available; avoid using.

Effectiveness

POSSIBLY EFFECTIVE ...when isolated PSP and PSK which are found in coriolus are used orally as adjuncts in cancer chemotherapy regimens (1640,1641,1648,1649,1650,1651,1652,1653,1654,1655,1656) (1657,1658,1659,1660,1661,1662). There is insufficient reliable information available about the effectiveness of coriolus for its other uses.

Mechanism of Action

The applicable parts of coriolus mushroom are the fruiting body and mycelium (5494,5496). Coriolus mushrooms have a long history in folk medicine, but researchers are just beginning to isolate and identify substances in coriolus that have pharmacological activity (5477,1635). Coriolus contains several polysaccharides, including polysaccharide peptide (PSP) and polysaccharide-K (PSK, krestin), shown to have antitumor and immunomodulating effects (5484,5494,5499,1600,1635,1636,1637,1638,1639,1640,1641) (1642,1648,1649,1650). PSK has been used in Japan as a biological response modifier in cancer chemotherapy regimens with varying results (1640,1641,1651,1652,1653,1654,1655,1656,1657,1658,1659) (1660,1661,1662). Coriolus might have activity against the human immunodeficiency virus (HIV) (1643,1644). Preliminary evidence suggests that coriolus might have analgesic activity and protect against acetaminophen-induced hepatotoxicity (1645,1646,1647).

Adverse Reactions

None reported with coriolus (1635,1636). Patients receiving PSK as an adjunct to chemotherapy experienced nausea, leukopenia, and liver function impairment (1651); however, this may have been due to the chemotherapy.

Interactions with Herbs & Other Dietary Supplements

Insufficient reliable information available.

Interactions with Drugs

ACETAMINOPHEN: Theoretically, coriolus might protect against acetaminophen-induced hepatotoxicity.

Interactions with Foods

No interactions are known to occur, and there is no known reason to expect a clinically significant interaction with coriolus mushroom.

Interactions with Lab Tests

No interactions are known to occur, and there is no known reason to expect a clinically significant interaction with coriolus mushroom.

Interactions with Diseases or Conditions

No interactions are known to occur, and there is no known reason to expect a clinically significant interaction with coriolus mushroom.

Dosage and Administration

ORAL: People drink a tea prepared with 20 grams of dried coriolus fruiting bodies three times daily, or take capsules containing up to 5 grams per day of the dried fruiting bodies. As an adjuvant to cancer chemotherapy, 3 grams of PSK is taken daily (1650,1654,1656,1658). A typical dose of PSP is 1 gram 3 times daily (5497,5498).

Comments

None.

CORKWOOD TREE

Also Known As

Pituri.

Scientific Names

Duboisia myoporoides.
Family: Solanaceae.

People Use This For

Orally, corkwood quids (cured and rolled leaves) are chewed to ward off hunger, pain, and tiredness (6).
Alkaloids derived from the plant are used as a therapeutic substitute for atropine (6).

Safety

LIKELY UNSAFE ...when used orally. Corkwood tree leaves contain tropane alkaloids that are potent anticholinergics (6). Large doses of scopolamine and related alkaloids can be fatal (6).
PREGNANCY AND LACTATION: LIKELY UNSAFE ...when used orally; avoid using.

Effectiveness

POSSIBLY EFFECTIVE ...when chewed for conditions which would be treated with hyoscyamine and hyoscine, scopolamine, and atropine (6).
There is insufficient reliable information available about the effectiveness of corkwood tree for its other uses.

Mechanism of Action

The applicable part of corkwood tree is the leaf. Researchers document tropane alkaloids (atropine, scopolamine, etc.) as constituents (6). Stimulant and hallucinogenic properties are due to anticholinergic effects (6).

Adverse Reactions

Orally, corkwood tree can cause central nervous system disturbances (6).

Interactions with Herbs & Other Dietary Supplements

Insufficient reliable information available.

Interactions with Drugs

No interactions are known to occur, and there is no known reason to expect a clinically significant interaction with corkwood tree.

Interactions with Foods

No interactions are known to occur, and there is no known reason to expect a clinically significant interaction with corkwood tree.

Interactions with Lab Tests

No interactions are known to occur, and there is no known reason to expect a clinically significant interaction with corkwood tree.

Interactions with Diseases or Conditions

No interactions are known to occur, and there is no known reason to expect a clinically significant interaction with corkwood tree.

Dosage and Administration

ORAL: Leaves are cured and rolled into a quid which Australian natives chew (6).

Comments

Although at one time used as a source of scopolamine, other sources are more commercially viable (6).

CORN COCKLE

Also Known As

Cockle, Corn Campion, Corn Rose, Crown-of-the-Field, Purple Cockle.

Scientific Names

Agrostemma githago.
Family: Caryophyllaceae.

People Use This For

Historically, corn cockle seeds were used for treating cancers, hard tumors, warts, hard swelling of the uterus, and to induce inflammation of the conjunctiva and cornea (6). The root was used historically for exanthemata (acute skin eruptions signifying a viral or coccal infection) and hemorrhoids (6). Various plant parts have also been used as a diuretic, expectorant, menstrual stimulant, poison, vermifuge, and for jaundice (6).

Safety

LIKELY UNSAFE ...when used orally, due to toxicity (6).
There is insufficient reliable information available about the safety of the topical use of corn cockle.
PREGNANCY AND LACTATION: **LIKELY UNSAFE** ...when used orally; avoid using (6).

Effectiveness

There is insufficient reliable information available about the effectiveness of corn cockle.

Mechanism of Action

The applicable parts of corn cockle are the root and seed. Poisonous constituents, githagin and agrostemmic acid, are reportedly absorbed from the GI tract causing GI irritation, severe muscle pain and twitching, depression, and coma (6).

Adverse Reactions

Oral use can cause GI irritation, severe muscle pain and twitching, depression, and coma (6). Acute poisoning symptoms include: diarrhea, salivation, vertigo, vomiting, paralysis, and respiratory depression (6). Repeated poisoning by small doses is referred to as "githagism" (6).

Interactions with Herbs & Other Dietary Supplements

Insufficient reliable information available.

Interactions with Drugs

No interactions are known to occur, and there is no known reason to expect a clinically significant interaction with corn cockle.

Interactions with Foods

No interactions are known to occur, and there is no known reason to expect a clinically significant interaction with corn cockle.

Interactions with Lab Tests

No interactions are known to occur, and there is no known reason to expect a clinically significant interaction with corn cockle.

Interactions with Diseases or Conditions

No interactions are known to occur, and there is no known reason to expect a clinically significant interaction with corn cockle.

Dosage and Administration

No typical dosage.

Comments

None.

CORN POPPY

Also Known As
Copperose, Corn Rose, Cup-Puppy, Headache, Headwark, Red Poppy, Rhoeados Flos.
CAUTION: See separate listing for California Poppy.

Scientific Names
Papaver rhoeas.
Family: Papaveraceae.

People Use This For
Orally, corn poppy is used for respiratory tract diseases and discomforts, disturbed sleep, and pain relief (2).
Historically, corn poppy has been used in children's cough syrup (18).
For food uses, corn poppy is an ingredient in some "metabolic" teas (18). In other teas, it is used as a brightening agent.

Safety
POSSIBLY SAFE ...when the dried corn poppy flower petals are used orally and appropriately in medicinal amounts (2,18).
CHILDREN: POSSIBLY UNSAFE ...when the fresh leaves or blossoms are eaten because this can cause poisoning (18). There is insufficient reliable information available for the safety of dried corn poppy flower petals used in children.
PREGNANCY AND LACTATION: Insufficient reliable information available; avoid using.

Effectiveness
There is insufficient reliable information available about the effectiveness of corn poppy.

Mechanism of Action
The applicable part of corn poppy is the flower. There is insufficient reliable information available about the possible mechanism of action and active ingredients.

Adverse Reactions
No adverse effects in adults have been reported (2). However, poisonings have been reported in children who consumed the fresh leaves and blossoms. Symptoms include vomiting and stomach pain (18).

Interactions with Herbs & Other Dietary Supplements
Insufficient reliable information available.

Interactions with Drugs
No interactions are known to occur, and there is no known reason to expect a clinically significant interaction with corn poppy.

Interactions with Foods
No interactions are known to occur, and there is no known reason to expect a clinically significant interaction with corn poppy.

Interactions with Lab Tests
No interactions are known to occur, and there is no known reason to expect a clinically significant interaction with corn poppy.

Interactions with Diseases or Conditions
No interactions are known to occur, and there is no known reason to expect a clinically significant interaction with corn poppy.

Dosage and Administration
ORAL: For bronchial irritation, one cup tea (steep 2 teaspoons dried petals in boiling water 5-10 minutes, strain) 2 to 3 times daily (may be sweetened with honey) has been used (18).

Comments
None.

CORN SILK

Also Known As
Cornsilk, Indian Corn, Maidis Stigma, Maize Silk, Stigma Maydis, Zea.

Scientific Names
Zea mays.
Family: Gramineae.

People Use This For
Orally, corn silk is used for cystitis, urethritis, nocturnal enuresis, prostatitis, and acute chronic inflammation of the urinary system (4).
In Chinese medicine, corn silk is used as a diuretic for congestive heart failure, to treat diabetes, and hypertension. Corn silk is decocted with watermelon peel and bananas (11).

Safety
LIKELY SAFE ...when consumed in amounts found in foods (maximum use level 0.002%) (11); Corn silk has Generally Recognized as Safe (GRAS) status in the US (11).
POSSIBLY SAFE ...when used orally and appropriately in medicinal amounts (12).
PREGNANCY: POSSIBLY SAFE ...when consumed in food. LIKELY UNSAFE ...when used orally in larger amounts because it might have uterine stimulant effects (4).
LACTATION: Insufficient reliable information available.

Effectiveness
There is insufficient reliable information available about the effectiveness of corn silk.

Mechanism of Action
Corn silk contains tannins, which are astringents, and Cryptoxanthin, which has vitamin A activity (4).

Adverse Reactions
Orally, prolonged use may cause hypokalemia (4).
Topically, allergy to cornsilk, corn pollen, or cornstarch may result in contact dermatitis or urticaria (4).

Interactions with Herbs & Other Dietary Supplements
Insufficient reliable information available.

Interactions with Drugs
ANTICOAGULANTS: Corn silk contains vitamin K. Individuals using anticoagulant drug therapy should consume a consistent daily amount to maintain anticoagulation levels (19).
DIABETES THERAPY: Theoretically, because some evidence suggests corn silk can reduce blood glucose level, excessive amounts might interfere with diabetes therapy (4).
BLOOD PRESSURE TREATMENT: Theoretically, excessive doses might cause hypotension and interfere with drugs used to treat hypertension or hypotension (4).
POTASSIUM-DEPLETING DRUGS: Theoretically, prolonged use might have additive effects with drugs that deplete potassium, including diuretics (4).

Interactions with Foods
No interactions are known to occur, and there is no known reason to expect a clinically significant interaction with corn silk.

Interactions with Lab Tests
No interactions are known to occur, and there is no known reason to expect a clinically significant interaction with corn silk.

Interactions with Diseases or Conditions
DIABETES: Theoretically, excessive doses might reduce blood glucose level (4), interfering with control.
HYPERTENSION, HYPOTENSION: Theoretically, excessive doses might interfere with control of these conditions (4).
POTASSIUM DEPLETION: Theoretically, excessive doses might exacerbate this condition (4).

Dosage and Administration

ORAL: 4-8 grams dried style/stigma three times daily, or one cup tea (steep 0.5 grams dried corn silk in 150 mL boiling water 5-10 minutes, strain) several times daily (4,8). Liquid extract of maize stigmas, 4-8 mL (4). Tincture (1:5 in 25% alcohol), 5-15 mL three times daily (4). Syrup of maize stigmas, 8-15 mL (4).

Comments

Corn silk is the so-called "silk" of an ear of ordinary Indian corn or maize.

CORNFLOWER

Also Known As

Batchelor's Buttons, Blue Cap, Blue Centaury, Bluebonnet, Bluebottle, Bluebow, Corn Flower, Cyani Blossoms, Cyani Flos, Cyani Flower, Cyani Petals, Hurtsickle.

Scientific Names

Centaurea cyanus.
Family: Asteraceae or Compositae.

People Use This For

Orally, cornflower is used for fever, menstrual disorders, vaginal candidiasis, as a laxative, diuretic, expectorant, tonic, bitter, and liver and gallbladder stimulant (2).
Topically, cornflower is used for eye irritation or discomfort (1502).
For food uses, cornflower is utilized in herbal teas as a coloring agent (2).

Safety

LIKELY SAFE ...when used as a coloring agent in herbal teas (2).
There is insufficient reliable information available about the safety of the other oral or topical uses of cornflower.
PREGNANCY AND LACTATION: Insufficient reliable information available; avoid using.

Effectiveness

There is insufficient reliable information available about the effectiveness of cornflower.

Mechanism of Action

The applicable part of cornflower is the dried flower. The color is due to anthocyanin constituents (1502).

Adverse Reactions

Cornflower can cause an allergic reaction in individuals sensitive to the Asteraceae/Compositae family. Members of this family include ragweed, chrysanthemums, marigolds, daisies, and many other herbs.

Interactions with Herbs & Other Dietary Supplements

Insufficient reliable information available.

Interactions with Drugs

No interactions are known to occur, and there is no known reason to expect a clinically significant interaction with cornflower.

Interactions with Foods

No interactions are known to occur, and there is no known reason to expect a clinically significant interaction with cornflower.

Interactions with Lab Tests

No interactions are known to occur, and there is no known reason to expect a clinically significant interaction with cornflower.

Interactions with Diseases or Conditions

CROSS-ALLERGENICITY: Can cause an allergic reaction in individuals sensitive to the Asteraceae/Compositae family. Members of this family include ragweed, chrysanthemums, marigolds, daisies, and many other herbs.

Dosage and Administration
ORAL: People typically use the crushed dried flowers to make a tea, adding 1 gram of cornflower per cup of water (5252).

Comments
None.

CORYDALIS

Also Known As
Early Fumitory, Squirrel Corn, Turkey Corn.
CAUTION: See separate listing for Turkey Corn.

Scientific Names
Corydalis cava.
Family: Fumariaceae.

People Use This For
Orally, corydalis is used for mild depression, neuroses, emotional disturbances, severe nerve damage, and limb tremors. It is also used orally as a mild sedative and tranquilizer, hallucinogen, to lower blood pressure, and to relax small intestine peristalsis (18).

Safety
There is insufficient reliable information available about the safety of corydalis.
PREGNANCY: LIKELY UNSAFE ...when used orally because corydalis might promote menstrual flow and stimulate uterine contractions (12).
LACTATION: Insufficient reliable information available; avoid using.

Effectiveness
There is insufficient reliable information available about the effectiveness of corydalis.

Mechanism of Action
The applicable part of corydalis is the tuber and root. There is insufficient reliable information available about the possible mechanism of action and active ingredients.

Adverse Reactions
Orally, clonic spasms and muscle tremors may occur with overdoses of corydalis (18).

Interactions with Herbs & Other Dietary Supplements
Insufficient reliable information available.

Interactions with Drugs
No interactions are known to occur, and there is no known reason to expect a clinically significant interaction with corydalis.

Interactions with Foods
No interactions are known to occur, and there is no known reason to expect a clinically significant interaction with corydalis.

Interactions with Lab Tests
No interactions are known to occur, and there is no known reason to expect a clinically significant interaction with corydalis.

Interactions with Diseases or Conditions
No interactions are known to occur, and there is no known reason to expect a clinically significant interaction with corydalis.

Dosage and Administration
ORAL: Corydalis has been taken as an extract (18).

Comments

There is very little scientific information about this product. Our staff is continually analyzing the available information on natural medicines and will add data here as it becomes available.

COSTUS OIL

Also Known As

Auckland Costus, Mokko, Mu Xiang.
CAUTION: See separate listing for Costus root.

Scientific Names

Saussurea lappa, synonym Aucklandia costus.
Family: Asteraceae or Compositae.

People Use This For

In Chinese and Indian medicine, costus oil is used as a tonic; gastric stimulant; antiflatulent; and for treating asthma, cough, dysentery, and cholera.
In foods and beverages, costus oil is used as a flavoring component (11).
In manufacturing, costus oil is used as a fixative and fragrance in cosmetics (11).

Safety

LIKELY SAFE ...when used in amounts found in foods. Costus oil is approved for food use in the US (11).
UNSAFE ...when aristolochic acid-contaminated costus oil is used orally. Costus oil is commonly contaminated with aristolochic acid, which is nephrotoxic and carcinogenic. The FDA considers all products containing aristolochic acid to be unsafe and adulterated. Only products analytically verified to be aristolochic acid-free should be used (6118,6119). There is insufficient reliable information available about the safety of costus oil when used for medicinal purposes.
PREGNANCY AND LACTATION: Insufficient reliable information available; avoid using.

Effectiveness

There is insufficient reliable information available about the effectiveness of costus oil.

Mechanism of Action

Costus oil is reported to inhibit bronchospasm and lower blood pressure in animals (11).

Adverse Reactions

Orally, costus oil might cause allergic reactions, including contact dermatitis (11). Costus oil can cause an allergic reaction in individuals sensitive to the Asteraceae/Compositae family. Members of this family include ragweed, chrysanthemums, marigolds, daisies, and many other herbs. Costus oil is commonly contaminated with aristolochic acid, which is nephrotoxic and carcinogenic (6119).

Interactions with Herbs & Other Dietary Supplements

Insufficient reliable information available.

Interactions with Drugs

No interactions are known to occur, and there is no known reason to expect a clinically significant interaction with costus oil.

Interactions with Foods

No interactions are known to occur, and there is no known reason to expect a clinically significant interaction with costus oil.

Interactions with Lab Tests

No interactions are known to occur, and there is no known reason to expect a clinically significant interaction with costus oil.

Interactions with Diseases or Conditions

CROSS-ALLERGENICITY: Costus oil can cause an allergic reaction in individuals sensitive to the Asteraceae/Compositae family. Members of this family include ragweed, chrysanthemums, marigolds, daisies, and many other herbs.

Dosage and Administration

No typical dosage.

Comments

Costus oil is distilled, extracted oil from the root of Saussurea lappa. Avoid confusion with costus root.
Costus oil is frequently contaminated with aristolochic acid, which is nephrotoxic and carcinogenic. The FDA considers all products containing aristolochic acid to be unsafe and adulterated (6119). The FDA intends to automatically detain, without physical examination, any product which contains plants known or suspected to contain aristolochic acid, or which might be adulterated with plants known to contain aristolochic acid. Each detained product will be released only after the responsible party provides direct analytical evidence that it is free of aristolochic acid (6118,6119).

COSTUS root

Also Known As

Auckland Costus, Mokko, Mokkou, Mu Xiang.
CAUTION: See separate listing for Costus Oil.

Scientific Names

Saussurea lappa, synonym Aucklandia costus.
Family: Asteraceae or Compositae.

People Use This For

Orally, costus root is used as an antinematode therapy (1516).

Safety

POSSIBLY SAFE ...when used orally and appropriately (12).
UNSAFE ...when aristolochic acid-contaminated costus root is used orally. Costus root is commonly contaminated with aristolochic acid, which is nephrotoxic and carcinogenic. The FDA considers all products containing aristolochic acid to be unsafe and adulterated. Only products analytically verified to be aristolochic acid-free should be used (6118,6119).
PREGNANCY AND LACTATION: Insufficient reliable information available; avoid using.

Effectiveness

POSSIBLY EFFECTIVE ...when used orally against nematodes when the root or methanol extract of root is taken (1516).

Mechanism of Action

In children, costus reduces the number of fecal eggs per gram similarly to treatment with pyrantel pamoate (1516).

Adverse Reactions

Orally, costus root can cause an allergic reaction in individuals sensitive to the Asteraceae/Compositae family. Members of this family include ragweed, chrysanthemums, marigolds, daisies, and many other herbs. Costus root is commonly contaminated with aristolochic acid which is nephrotoxic and carcinogenic (6119).

Interactions with Herbs & Other Dietary Supplements

Insufficient reliable information available.

Interactions with Drugs

No interactions are known to occur, and there is no known reason to expect a clinically significant interaction with costus root.

Interactions with Foods

No interactions are known to occur, and there is no known reason to expect a clinically significant interaction with costus root.

Interactions with Lab Tests

No interactions are known to occur, and there is no known reason to expect a clinically significant interaction with costus root.

Interactions with Diseases or Conditions

CROSS-ALLERGENICITY: Costus root can cause an allergic reaction in individuals sensitive to the Asteraceae/Compositae family. Members of this family include ragweed, chrysanthemums, marigolds, daisies, and many other herbs.

Dosage and Administration

ORAL: As an antinematodal, 50 mg/kg root (or equivalent amount of methanol extract of root) as a single dose has been used (1516).

Comments

Avoid confusion with costus oil.

Costus root is frequently contaminated with aristolochic acid, which is nephrotoxic and carcinogenic. The FDA considers all products containing aristolochic acid to be unsafe and adulterated (6119). The FDA intends to automatically detain, without physical examination, any product which contains plants known or suspected to contain aristolochic acid, or which might be adulterated with plants known to contain aristolochic acid. Each detained product will be released only after the responsible party provides direct analytical evidence that it is free of aristolochic acid (6118,6119).

COTTON

Also Known As

Cotton Root.
CAUTION: See separate listing for Gossypol.

Scientific Names

Gossypium herbaceum; Gossypium hirsutum; other Gossypium species.
Family: Malvaceae.

People Use This For

Orally, cotton is used for amenorrhea; dysmenorrhea; irregular, painful, or profuse menstrual bleeding; climacteric complaints; poor lactation; nausea; fever; headache; diarrhea; dysentery; urethritis; nerve inflammation; hemorrhage; as an oxytocic; and to expel afterbirth (18).

Cotton has been used as an anti-fertility drug in males, as well as in topical, vaginal contraceptive preparations (214).

Safety

POSSIBLY SAFE ...when used orally in medicinal amounts (12). ...when preparations of the root bark are used in amounts found in foods. Canadian regulations limit use to less than 450 ppm of free gossypol (including cotton seed meal and oil) (12).

PREGNANCY: LIKELY UNSAFE ...when used orally because it is a possible abortifacient and uterine stimulant (12).

LACTATION: Insufficient reliable information available; avoid using.

Effectiveness

There is insufficient reliable information available about the effectiveness of cotton.

Mechanism of Action

The applicable part of cotton is the root bark. It is believed to stimulate menstrual flow, act as an oxytocic, and male contraceptive (18). Some evidence suggests cotton root can cause histamine release (18). The constituent, gossypol that is extracted from cotton seed is used as a male contraceptive (6).

Adverse Reactions

There is insufficient reliable information available for oral uses; no adverse reactions reported (18). However, in animals, long-term feeding with cotton seed cakes has been linked to poisonings and deaths (18).

Interactions with Herbs & Other Dietary Supplements

Insufficient reliable information available.

Interactions with Drugs

No interactions are known to occur, and there is no known reason to expect a clinically significant interaction with cotton.

Interactions with Foods

No interactions are known to occur, and there is no known reason to expect a clinically significant interaction with cotton.

Interactions with Lab Tests

No interactions are known to occur, and there is no known reason to expect a clinically significant interaction with cotton.

Interactions with Diseases or Conditions

UROGENITAL IRRITATION OR SENSITIVITY: Contraindicated (12).

Dosage and Administration

ORAL: People typically prepare cotton root bark using one teaspoon boiled in a covered container with 3 cups of water for 30 minutes. The liquid is cooled slowly in the closed container and taken cold, 1 to 2 cups per day (5254).

Comments

Avoid confusion with gossypol (cotton seed extract).

Cotton's use as a male contraceptive agent is in question because it may potentially cause irreversible sterility (214).

COUCH GRASS

Also Known As

Couchgrass, Cutch, Dog Grass, Dog-Grass, Doggrass, Durfa Grass, Quack Grass, Quackgrass, Scotch Quelch.
CAUTION: See separate listings for German Sarsaparilla, Sarsaparilla, and Tormentil.

Scientific Names

Agropyron repens, synonyms Elytrigia repens, Triticum repens; Elymus repens.
Family: Gramineae or Poaceae.

People Use This For

Orally, couch grass is used for cystitis, specifically with irritation or inflammation of the urinary tract (4). It is also used orally for urethritis, prostatitis, benign prostatic hypertrophy (BPH), renal calculus, and "irrigation therapy," to increase urine flow for inflammatory diseases of the urinary tract and the prevention of urine stones (2,11). Couch grass is used to treat the common cold, cough and bronchitis, fever and colds, inflammation of the mouth and pharynx, and a tendency toward infection (18).

In folk medicine, couch grass has been used as a diuretic and expectorant and for diabetes, gout, liver disorders, rheumatic pain, and chronic skin problems (11,18).

In foods and beverages, couch grass extracts are used as flavor components (11).

Safety

LIKELY SAFE ...when used orally and appropriately for medicinal purposes for short periods of time (2,4). ...when consumed in amounts commonly found in foods. Couch grass is Generally Recognized as Safe (GRAS) in the US for food use (11).

PREGNANCY AND LACTATION: Insufficient reliable information available; avoid amounts greater than those used in foods.

Effectiveness

POSSIBLY EFFECTIVE ...when used orally for "irrigation therapy," where it is used as a mild diuretic along with copious fluid intake to increase urine flow to treat inflammatory diseases of the urinary tract and for prevention of urine stones (2,4,10).

There is insufficient reliable information available about the effectiveness of couch grass for its other uses.

Mechanism of Action

The applicable parts of couch grass are the root and rhizome. Couch grass is a rich source of beta-carotene (19). Couch grass can have diuretic and sedative activities in animals (4,11). The constituent agropyrene and its oxidative product can have broad antibiotic activity (11). The essential oil of couch grass has antimicrobial effects (2,6).

Adverse Reactions

Excessive or prolonged use of couch grass can cause hypokalemia (4).

Interactions with Herbs & Other Dietary Supplements

HERBS WITH SEDATIVE PROPERTIES: Theoretically, concomitant use with herbs that have sedative properties might enhance therapeutic and adverse effects. These include calamus, calendula, California poppy, catnip, capsicum, celery, elecampane, Siberian ginseng, German chamomile, goldenseal, gotu kola, hops, Jamaican dogwood, kava, lemon balm, sage, St. John's wort, sassafras, scullcap, shepherd's purse, stinging nettle, valerian, wild carrot, wild lettuce, ashwaganda root, and yerba mansa (4,19).

Interactions with Drugs

POTASSIUM-DEPLETING DIURETICS: Theoretically, concomitant use of couch grass with these diuretics can enhance potassium loss (4).

DRUGS WITH SEDATIVE PROPERTIES: Theoretically, concomitant use with drugs having sedative properties can cause additive therapeutic and adverse effects (4).

Interactions with Foods

No interactions are known to occur, and there is no known reason to expect a clinically significant interaction with couch grass.

Interactions with Lab Tests

No interactions are known to occur, and there is no known reason to expect a clinically significant interaction with couch grass.

Interactions with Diseases or Conditions

EDEMA: "Irrigation therapy," or the use of a mild diuretic and copious fluid intake to increase urine flow, is contraindicated in edema due to heart or kidney disease (2).

Dosage and Administration

ORAL: The typical dose of couch grass is 4-8 grams of the dried rhizome or one cup of the tea three times daily (4). The tea is prepared by simmering 1-2 grams of the herb in 150 mL boiling water for 5-10 minutes and then straining. The usual dose of the liquid extract (1:1 in 25% alcohol) is 4-8 mL three times daily (4). The tincture (1:5 in 40% alcohol) is commonly given as 5-15 mL three times daily (4). When used for "irrigation therapy," couch grass requires copious fluid intake (2).

Comments

Avoid confusion with German sarsaparilla, also known as red couch grass.

COUNTRY MALLOW

Also Known As

Bala, Bariar, Heartleaf, Khareti.
CAUTION: See separate listings for Mallow flower, Mallow leaf, and Marshmallow.

Scientific Names

Sida cordifolia.
Family: Malvaceae.

People Use This For

In herbal combinations country mallow is used orally for weight loss (4307,4309,4316,4318,4320,4323,4324), to burn fat (4319), to increase energy (4308), for impotence (4312,4315), sinus (4305), allergy (4306), throat diseases (4312), asthma and bronchitis (4313), and to promote a strong skeletal system (4317). In combination with ginger, country mallow root is used orally for intermittent fever. In combination with milk and sugar, country mallow root is used for urinary urgency and leukorrhea (4310).

Traditionally, country mallow is used orally to treat bronchial asthma, colds, flu, chills, lack of perspiration, headaches, nasal congestion, cough and wheezing, urinary infections, and edema. It is also traditionally used orally for heart disease, facial paralysis, healing chronic tissue inflammation, sciatica, insanity, neuralgia, nerve inflammation, chronic rheumatism, and emaciation. Country mallow is also traditionally used orally as a stimulant, analgesic, diuretic, tonic, aphrodisiac, and before and after cancer chemotherapy to aid recovery. Country mallow is traditionally used topically for numbness, nerve pain, muscle cramps, skin disorders, tumors, joint diseases, wounds, ulcers, and as a massage oil.

Safety

LIKELY UNSAFE ...when the seeds are used orally for self-medication. Country mallow contains ephedrine and it is most concentrated in the seeds. ...when the country mallow constituent ephedrine is used orally in combination with caffeine. The FDA has proposed banning caffeine in combination with ephedrine alkaloids (2729).
There is insufficient reliable information available about the safety of country mallow aerial parts or root.
PREGNANCY: LIKELY UNSAFE ...when used orally; avoid using. The country mallow ephedrine constituent can stimulate uterine contractions (12).
LACTATION: Insufficient reliable information available; avoid using.

Effectiveness

There is insufficient reliable information available about the effectiveness of country mallow.

Mechanism of Action

The applicable parts of country mallow are the root, leaves, and seeds. Country mallow contains 0.8%-1.2% ephedrine (4304,4310), but ephedrine is most concentrated in the seeds (4314). Some evidence suggests country mallow has anticonvulsant, antipyretic, antibacterial, antifungal, and antiviral activity (4310). Other information suggests the extracts of the aerial and root parts have analgesic, anti-inflammatory, and hypoglycemic properties (4299). An aqueous extract shows evidence that it limits the virulence of dental bacteria, reducing the rate of plaque formation (4303).

Adverse Reactions

Orally, the country mallow ephedrine constituent can cause dizziness, motor restlessness, irritability, insomnia, headache, anorexia, nausea, vomiting, flushing, tingling, difficulty urinating, tachycardia, and heart palpitations (2,6,7,13). Use of botanical sources of ephedrine such as country mallow have been associated with muscle conditions including myalgia, cardiomyopathy, rhabdomyolysis, eosinophilia myalgia syndrome (1270), and hypersensitivity myocarditis (1271). Botanical sources of ephedrine such as country mallow have also been associated with kidney stones (1272), acute hepatitis, (1273), psychosis (1276), and sudden death (1274). The country mallow constituent ephedrine can also cause a drastic increase in blood pressure, cardiac arrhythmias (2), heart failure, asphyxia, and hyperthermia (18).

Interactions with Herbs & Other Dietary Supplements

CAFFEINE: Concomitant use with the country mallow constituent ephedrine can cause increased stimulatory adverse effects (7).
COFFEE, GUARANA, TEA: Theoretically, concomitant use with the country mallow constituent ephedrine can cause additive stimulatory adverse effects (7).
DIGITALIS: Theoretically, using digitalis with the country mallow constituent ephedrine can cause cardiac arrhythmias (2).
SECALE ALKALOID DERIVATIVES (Ergot): Concomitant use with the country mallow constituent ephedrine can cause hypertension (2).

Interactions with Drugs

METHYLXANTHINES (Caffeine/Theophylline): Concomitant use with the country mallow constituent ephedrine can cause increased stimulatory adverse effects (7,19), and can enhance thermogenesis and weight loss (19).
DIGITALIS: Theoretically, concomitant use with the country mallow constituent ephedrine might cause cardiac arrhythmias (2).
SECALE ALKALOID DERIVATIVES (Ergot): Concomitant use with the country mallow constituent ephedrine might cause hypertension (2).
OXYTOCIN: Concomitant use with the country mallow constituent ephedrine can cause hypertension (2).
DIABETES THERAPY: The country mallow constituent ephedrine can raise blood glucose levels, but country mallow extract shows evidence it might reduce blood glucose. Monitor closely (19).
DEXAMETHASONE: The country mallow constituent ephedrine can increase the clearance and reduce the effectiveness of dexamethasone (19).
URINARY ACIDIFIERS: Concomitant use can increase the excretion of the country mallow ephedrine constituent due to reabsorption effects on kidney tubules (19).
URINARY ALKALINIZERS: Concomitant use can slow the excretion of the country mallow ephedrine constituent due to reabsorption effects on kidney tubules (19).
AMITRIPTYLINE (Elavil): Concomitant use can block the hypertensive effects caused by the country mallow ephedrine constituent (19).
RESERPINE: Concomitant use with the country mallow constituent ephedrine can antagonize the sympathomimetic effects of the resperine (19).
MONOAMINE OXIDASE INHIBITORS (MAOIs): Contraindicated; concomitant use of the country mallow ephedrine constituent with MAOIs might increase the risk of hypertension (15).

Interactions with Foods

COFFEE, TEA: Theoretically, concomitant use of the country mallow constituent ephedrine and large amounts of caffeinated coffee or tea might increase the stimulatory effects and adverse effects of caffeine and ephedrine.

Interactions with Lab Tests

URINE: The country mallow ephedrine constituent can cause positive urine tests for ephedrine, a substance banned by many athletic organizations.
BLOOD GLUCOSE: The country mallow ephedrine constituent might increase blood glucose levels (19), or other constituents of country mallow might reduce blood glucose levels (4299).

Interactions with Diseases or Conditions

ANGINA: Contraindicated; the country mallow ephedrine constituent might induce or exacerbate angina due to its cardiac stimulant effects (15,512).
ANOREXIA: Contraindicated; the country mallow ephedrine constituent might suppress the appetite (12,19).
ANXIETY: Large doses of the country mallow ephedrine constituent might cause or exacerbate anxiety due to its CNS stimulant effects (2,12,15,512).
BULIMIA: Contraindicated; bulimic patients might be at increased risk for the adverse effects of the country mallow ephedrine constituent due to inadequate nutritional status (12,19).
BENIGN PROSTATIC HYPERTROPHY (BPH): The country mallow ephedrine constituent might exacerbate urinary retention in patients with BPH due to its effects on the detrusor muscle (15,512).
CEREBRAL INSUFFICIENCY: Contraindicated; the country mallow ephedrine constituent might further decrease cerebral blood flow because it has vasoconstrictive effects (2,12,512).
DIABETES: The country mallow ephedrine constituent might interfere with blood sugar control, and exacerbate high blood pressure and circulatory problems in people with diabetes (15,19,512). However, extract of country mallow shows evidence of hypoglycemic effect (4299). Monitor closely.
ESSENTIAL TREMOR: The country mallow ephedrine constituent could exacerbate tremor (1715).
NARROW-ANGLE GLAUCOMA: The country mallow ephedrine constituent might exacerbate narrow-angle (angle-closure) glaucoma by causing mydriasis (2,12,15,512).
HEART DISEASE: Contraindicated; the country mallow ephedrine constituent might cause tachycardia, arrhythmias, or induce angina in patients with heart disease due to its cardiac stimulant effects (15,512).
HYPERTHYROID, THYROTOXICOSIS: Contraindicated; the country mallow ephedrine constituent might stimulate the thyroid and exacerbate hyperthyroid symptoms (2,12,15,512).
HYPERTENSION: The country mallow ephedrine constituent might exacerbate hypertension (2,12,15,512); contraindicated in uncontrolled hypertension.
KIDNEY STONES: The country mallow ephedrine constituent can cause kidney stones (1272).
MYASTHENIA GRAVIS: Large doses of the country mallow ephedrine constituent might increase muscle strength in patients with myasthenia gravis (15).
PHEOCHROMOCYTOMA: Contraindicated; the country mallow ephedrine constituent might exacerbate the symptoms of pheochromocytoma (2).
URINARY RETENTION: Large doses of the country mallow ephedrine constituent might exacerbate urinary retention due to its effects on the detrusor muscle (2,12,15,512).

Dosage and Administration

ORAL: A typical dose of powder (root, leaves, seeds) is 0.5 -1 gram twice daily. A typical dose of the fresh juice is 15-30 mL twice daily (4310).
TOPICAL: No typical dosage.

Comments

Country mallow is used extensively in Ayurvedic medicine because it is reported to simultaneously balance the three laws of physiology (Vata, Pitta, Kapha) (4321).

COWHAGE

Also Known As

Atmagupta, Couhage, Cowitch, Feijao macaco, HP 200, HP-200, Kaunch, Kawanch, Kiwach, Mucuna, Mucuna prurient, Pica Pica, Pica-Pica, Velvet Bean.

Scientific Names

Mucuna pruriens, synonym Stizolobium pruriens.
Family: Leguminosae or Fabaceae.

People Use This For

Orally, cowhage is used for Parkinson's disease, anxiety, arthritis, hyperprolactinemia, and for parasitic infections. It's also used as an analgesic for pain, for fever, to induce vomiting, and as an aphrodisiac. Cowhage is also used prophylactically as snakebite remedy.

Topically, cowhage is used as a rubefacient or counterirritant for rheumatic conditions, myalgias, to stimulate cutaneous blood flow in paralytic conditions, and to treat scorpion stings.

Safety

POSSIBLY SAFE …when used orally and appropriately. Powdered formulations of cowhage seed have been used safely for up to 20 weeks (6899,7020,7203).

POSSIBLY UNSAFE …when the hair of the cowhage bean pod is used orally or topically. The bean pod hairs are strong irritants and can cause severe itching, burning, and inflammation (18).

PREGNANCY AND LACTATION: POSSIBLY UNSAFE …when the hair of the cowhage bean pod is used orally or topically. The bean pod hairs are strong irritants and can cause severe itching, burning, and lasting inflammation (18). There is insufficient reliable information available about the safety of cowhage bean when used orally during pregnancy or in breast-feeding mothers; avoid using.

Effectiveness

There is insufficient reliable information available to rate the effectiveness of cowhage. However, there is preliminary evidence that some cowhage preparations might help improve symptoms of Parkinson's disease when used in combination with conventional drugs such as amantadine, selegiline, and anticholinergic agents. Cowhage contains 3-6% levodopa (L-dopa). Specific cowhage extracts standardized to 3.3% L-dopa (HP-200) and other powdered formulations providing 75 to 220 mg per day of L-dopa are being used for patients with Parkinson's (6899,7020,7203). There is also some evidence that cowhage might be useful for chlorpromazine-induced hyperprolactinemia in men (7207), but it does not appear to be effective for hyperprolactinemia of unknown cause in women (7206). More evidence is needed to rate cowhage for these uses.

Mechanism of Action

The applicable parts of cowhage are the bean or seed and the hair on the bean pod. Cowhage is thought to work for Parkinson's disease because it contains a significant amount of levodopa (L-dopa). The whole cowhage bean contains about 3-6% L-dopa (7020,7021). The inner layer (endocarp) of the pericarp, which has also been studied in patients with Parkinson's disease, usually contains the highest amount of L-dopa, about 5.3% (7020). Symptoms of Parkinson's disease occur in patients due to a depletion of the neurotransmitter dopamine. L-dopa is a precursor to dopamine. To be effective for Parkinson's disease, L-dopa must cross the blood-brain barrier where it is then decarboxylated to dopamine. However, the majority of L-dopa is metabolized peripherally and probably less than 1% actually reaches the brain (15). Some powdered cowhage seed preparations containing L-dopa seem to lessen symptoms of Parkinson's disease at a relatively low dose, compared to conventional L-dopa products. So there is some speculation that constituents other than levodopa might have antiparkinson activity (7203).

Cowhage also contains prurieninin, which might slow heart rate, decrease blood pressure, and stimulate intestinal peristalsis (18). Cowhage has also been reported to have anthelmintic, antiflatulent, and cholesterol lowering properties (18), but these effects have not been verified in humans.

Animal studies show that cowhage might lower blood glucose levels (7221) and possibly slow the development of diabetic nephropathy (7220). Cowhage contains significant amounts of minerals, including calcium, mangesium, phosphorus, iron, manganese, zinc, and copper. Some researchers speculate that cowhage might exert its hypoglycemic effect due to trace element stimulation of insulin or possibly because of orally active insulin-like compounds in cowhage (7221).

There is interest in using cowhage for snakebite. Cowhage extract seems to have a procoagulant effect against the venom of the saw scaled viper (Echis carinatus), when given at least 24 hours prior to laboratory exposure to the venom (7222).

Cowhage also possesses counterirritant and rubefacient properties (18). The hairs (spicules) of the bean pod or seed cause severe itching, burning, and inflammation when they penetrate the epidermis (18,6898). Serotonin and protein constituents such as mucunain are released into the skin, causing blood vessel dilation, redness, and inflammation (18,6898). Repeated boiling of the bean is sometimes used to eliminate the pharmacologically and toxicologically active principles so that the bean can be consumed as food (7021,7205).

Adverse Reactions

Orally, cowhage seems to be fairly well tolerated when a standardized powdered formulation, known as HP-200, made from the inner portion (endocarp) of the bean wall (pericarp) is used. The most common side effects reported are nausea and a sensation of abdominal distention. Other side effects less frequently reported are vomiting, dyskinesias, and insomnia (7020). Adverse effects reported with other cowhage bean preparations include headache; palpitations; sweating; flatulence; diarrhea; dry mouth; rash and pruritus; changes in urine color; and symptoms of psychosis including confusion, giddiness, agitation, hallucinations, and paranoid delusions (7203,7021). Cowhage-induced psychosis has been successfully treated with intravenous chlorpromazine (Thorazine) (7021). Theoretically, due to the levodopa (L-dopa) constituent, cowhage is likely to cause the same adverse effects that have been attributed to the purified L-dopa prescription drug. Some of these side effects include elevated liver enzymes, respiratory disturbances, urinary rentention, darkening of bodily fluids, muscle cramps, headache, and priapism (15). However, these effects have not yet been reported for cowhage. Ingestion of hairs from the bean pod or seed can result in significant mucosal irritation and should be avoided.

Topically, hairs from the cowhage bean pod or seed can cause severe itching, burning, inflammation, and erythematous macular rashes (18,6898). Symptoms resolve spontaneously within several hours, but may also be relieved with antihistamines (6898). The hairs can be removed from the skin by washing, but the hairs can also be retained, and transferred to other people, in fabrics and carpets. Clothing and other materials that come in contact with the cowhage hairs should also be thoroughly washed (6898).

Interactions with Herbs & Other Dietary Supplements

HERBS AND SUPPLEMENTS WITH HYPOGLYCEMIC EFFECTS: There is some evidence that cowhage might have hypoglycemic effects (7221). Theoretically, concomitant use with other herbs and supplements that decrease blood glucose levels might increase the risk of hypoglycemia. Some of these products include bitter melon, ginger, goat's rue, fenugreek, kudzu, willow bark, and others.

KAVA: Theoretically, kava might reduce the effectiveness of cowhage. There is some evidence that kava might have antidopaminergic effects and possibly decrease the effects of levodopa (L-dopa) in cowhage (19).

VITAMIN B6 (Pyridoxine): Vitamin B6 can decrease the effectiveness of the cowhage constituent levodopa (L-dopa) in patients with Parkinson's disease. Vitamin B6 increases peripheral decarboxylation of L-dopa to dopamine (15). Tell patients taking cowhage for Parkinson's disease to avoid taking vitamin B6 supplements.

Interactions with Drugs

ANESTHESIA: Concomitant use of some anesthetics and the cowhage constituent, levodopa (L-dopa) has resulted in cardiac arrhythmia. This effect has only been associated with cyclopropane and the halogenated hydrocarbons. Other anesthetics have not been implicated (15). Use other anesthetics in patients taking cowhage or tell patients to stop taking cowhage at least 2 weeks before surgery.

ANTIDIABETES DRUGS: There is some evidence that cowhage might have hypoglycemic effects (7221). Theoretically, concomitant use with drugs that decrease blood glucose levels might increase the risk of hypoglycemia. Dosing adjustments for insulin or oral hypoglycemic agents may be necessary. Oral hypoglycemic drugs include glimepiride (Amaryl), glipizide (Glucotrol), glyburide (Diabeta, Micronase), tolazamide (Tolinase), tolbutamide (Orinase), and others.

ANTIPSYCHOTIC AGENTS: Due to the antidopaminergic effects of antipsychotic medications, concomitant use of cowhage and these drugs might decrease the effectiveness of cowhage for Parkinson's disease (15). Some of these drugs include chlorpromazine (Thorazine), clozapine (Clozaril), fluphenazine (Prolixin), haloperidol (Haldol), olanzapine (Zyprexa), perphenazine (Trilafon), prochlorperazine (Compazine), quetiapine (Seroquel), risperidone (Risperdal), thioridazine (Mellaril), and thiothixene (Navane).

GUANETHIDINE (Ismelin): Cowhage might have additive hypotensive effects when used concomitantly with guanethidine (15); avoid using.

METHYLDOPA (Aldomet): Cowhage might have additive hypotensive effects when used concomitantly with methyldopa. Furthermore, methyldopa can inhibit peripheral decarboxylation of the cowhage constituent levodopa (L-dopa). This could increase the amount of L-dopa reaching the central nervous system and potentially lead to toxicity (15).

MONOAMINE OXIDASE INHIBITORS (MAOIs): Due to the levodopa (L-dopa) content of cowhage, it should not be given with non-selective MAOIs such as phenelzine (Nardil) and tranylcypromine (Parnate). Concomitant use can cause hypertensive crisis. However, cowhage can be used concurrently with the MAO-B selective inhibitor selegiline (Deprenyl) (15).

TRICYCLIC ANTIDEPRESSANTS (TCAs): There is some concern that TCAs might decrease absorption of the active cowhage constituent, levodopa (L-dopa). TCAs can slow gastric emptying which can prevent L-dopa from being fully absorbed. There have also been rare reports of hypertension and dyskinesias in some patients taking both TCAs and L-dopa (15). Concomitant use of cowhage and TCAs should be done cautiously or avoided. Some TCAs include amitriptyline (Elavil), clomipramine (Anafranil), desipramine (Norpramin), doxepin (Sinequan), imipramine (Tofranil), nortriptyline (Pamelor), and Protriptyline (Vivactil).

Interactions with Foods

No interactions are known to occur, and there is no known reason to expect a clinically significant interaction with cowhage.

Interactions with Lab Tests

GLUCOSE: Due to the levodopa (L-dopa) content, cowhage might cause false-positive urine glucose tests when cupric sulfate reagents, such as Benedict's reagent or Clinitest tablets, are used. Cowhage might cause false-negatives when glucose oxidase tests such as Clinistix and Tes-Tape are used (15).

KETONES: Due to the levodopa (L-dopa) content, cowhage might cause a false positive urine ketones reaction when sodium nitroprusside reagents such as Acetest, Ketostix, and Labstix are used (15).

LIVER FUNCTION TESTS: Due to the levodopa content, cowhage might cause elevated liver function tests. L-dopa has caused transiently increased liver function tests including alkaline phosphatase, aspartate aminotransferase (AST or SGOT), alanine aminotransferase (ALT or SGPT), lactate dehydrogenase (LDH), and bilirubin (15). However, this effect has not yet been reported for cowhage.

URIC ACID: Due to the levodopa (L-dopa) content of cowhage, serum and urine uric acid levels might appear elevated when colorimetric tests are used. However, cowhage does not effect tests using uricase (15).

Interactions with Diseases or Conditions

CARDIOVASCULAR DISEASE: Due to the levodopa (L-dopa) content of cowhage, it should be avoided or used cautiously in patients with cardiovascular disease. L-dopa can frequently cause orthostatic hypotension, dizziness, and syncope. Much less frequently, L-dopa can also cause palpitations and cardiac arrhythmias (15).

DIABETES: There is some evidence that cowhage can lower blood glucose levels and might cause hypoglycemia (7221). Advise patients to increase blood glucose monitoring. Dosing adjustments to diabetes medications may be necessary.

HEPATIC DISEASE: Due to the levodopa (L-dopa) content of cowhage, use cautiously in patients with liver disease. L-dopa has been reported to cause increased liver function tests (15).

HYPOGLYCEMIA: There is some evidence that cowhage can lower blood glucose levels and might exacerbate hypoglycemia (7221).

MELANOMA: Since levodopa (L-dopa) in cowhage is a precursor to the skin pigment melanin, there is some concern that it might worsen melanoma (15). Tell patients with malignant melanoma, history of melanoma or a suspicious undiagnosed skin lesions to avoid cowhage.

PEPTIC ULCER DISEASE (PUD): Since cowhage contains levodopa (L-dopa), there is some concern that it might induce gastrointestinal bleeding in patients with peptic ulcer disease. L-dopa has been reported to cause gastrointestinal bleeding in patients with PUD (15). However, this has not yet been reported with cowhage.

PSYCHIATRIC DISEASE: Due to the levodopa (L-dopa) content, cowhage might worsen psychiatric disease in patients with an existing condition (15). Furthermore, patients with a history of mental illness might be more likely to experience a cowhage-induced psychiatric disturbance.

Dosage and Administration

ORAL: For Parkinson's disease, a powdered cowhage extract known as HP-200, standardized to contain 3.3% levodopa (L-dopa) has been used. Dosages ranged from 22.5 to 67.5 grams divided into 2 to 5 doses per day (7020). Nonstandardized ground cowhage preparations have also been used. These contain 4.5% to 5.5% levodopa (L-dopa) and have been taken in doses of 40 to 60 grams per day in 4 divided doses (7203).

Comments

Cowhage is a legume that grows wild in the tropics, including India and the Bahamas, and its range may extend to southern Florida (6898). It has been used since ancient times in Ayurvedic medicine for the treatment of Parkinson's disease (7223). Prior to commercial synthesis of levodopa from vanillin, cowhage was investigated as a potential source of the drug with efforts to increase the yield of levodopa from the seeds and leaves (7203,7204). The barbed spicules detach easily from the fruiting pods and have been sold commercially as itching powder (6898).

COWSLIP

Also Known As

Arthritica, Buckels, Butter Rose, Crewel, English Cowslip, Fairy Caps, Herb Perter, Key Flower, Key of Heaven, Mayflower, Our Lady's Keys, Paigle, Paigle Peggle, Palsywort, Password, Peagle, Peagles, Petty Mulleins, Plumrocks, Primrose, Primula.

Scientific Names

Primula veris, synonym Primula officinalis; Primula elatier.
Family: Primulaceae.

People Use This For
Orally, cowslip flower is used for respiratory tract mucous membrane inflammation (2), cough, bronchitis, insomnia, nervous excitability, headache, hysteria, neuralgia, tremors, hydroticum, as a diuretic, antispasmodic, and as a heart tonic for sensations of dizziness and cardiac insufficiency (4,18).

Orally, cowslip root is used for respiratory tract mucous membrane inflammation (2), cough, bronchitis, whooping cough, asthma, gout, and neurologic complaints (18).

In combination with gentian root, European elder flower, verbena, and sorrel, cowslip is used orally for maintaining healthy sinuses (373) and treating sinusitis (7,374,379).

Safety
POSSIBLY SAFE ...when used orally in appropriate amounts (2,12). ...when used orally with gentian root, European elder flower, verbena, and sorrel (Quanterra Sinus Defense, Sinupret) (7,374,379).

PREGNANCY AND LACTATION: Insufficient reliable information available; avoid using.

Effectiveness
POSSIBLY EFFECTIVE ...when used orally for treating respiratory tract mucous membrane inflammation (2). ...when used orally with gentian root, European elder flower, verbena, and sorrel (Quanterra Sinus Defense, Sinupret) for treating acute or chronic sinusitis (7,374,379). ...when the root is used orally for treating respiratory tract mucous membrane inflammation (2).

There is insufficient reliable information available about the effectiveness of cowslip for its other uses.

Mechanism of Action
The applicable parts of cowslip are the flower and root. Cowslip is a rich source of beta-carotene and vitamin C (19). Cowslip is reported to have antispasmodic, diuretic, expectorant, hypnotic, laxative, secretion-reducing, and sedative activities (2,4). Evidence suggests the saponin fraction might initially cause hypotension followed by long-lasting hypertension (4). Flavonoid constituents might have anti-inflammatory and antispasmodic effects. The tannin constituents have astringent effects (4).

Adverse Reactions
Orally, cowslip can cause gastric discomfort and nausea (2,4,12). It may cause an allergic reaction in sensitive individuals (4). Toxicity, when it occurs, seems to be associated with saponin constituents of the underground parts of the plant (4).

Interactions with Herbs & Other Dietary Supplements
Insufficient reliable information available.

Interactions with Drugs
HYPERTENSIVE, HYPOTENSIVE DRUGS: Theoretically, excessive amounts of cowslip flower might interfere with the actions of these drugs (4).

DIURETICS: Cowslip may potentiate effects of diuretics (214).

SEDATIVES: Cowslip may potentiate effects of sedatives (214).

Interactions with Foods
No interactions are known to occur, and there is no known reason to expect a clinically significant interaction with cowslip.

Interactions with Lab Tests
No interactions are known to occur, and there is no known reason to expect a clinically significant interaction with cowslip.

Interactions with Diseases or Conditions
HYPERTENSION, HYPOTENSION: Theoretically, excessive doses may interfere with control of these conditions (4).

Dosage and Administration
ORAL (flower): One cup tea (1-2 grams dried flowers steeped in 150 mL of boiling water 5-10 minutes, strain) three times daily (4). Liquid extract (1:1 in 25% alcohol), 1-2 mL three times daily (4). Tincture, 2.5-7.5 grams per day (2). For acute or chronic sinusitis, two Sinupret tablets three times daily for up to two weeks has been used in clinical trials (7,374,379), equivalent to gentian root 12 mg, European elder flower 36 mg, verbena 36 mg, cowslip flower 36 mg, and sorrel 36 mg three times daily. For maintaining healthy sinuses, a typical dose is one tablet of Quanterra Sinus Defense three times daily with water, equivalent to gentian root 9 mg, European elder flower 29 mg, verbena 29 mg,

cowslip flower 29 mg, and sorrel 29 mg three times daily (373). Each tablet of Quanterra Sinus Defense contains 125 mg of the herbal combination found in Sinupret (373).

ORAL (root): 0.5-1.5 grams dried root per day, or as prepared tea. Tincture, 1.5-3 grams per day (2).

Comments

None.

CRAMP BARK

Also Known As

Common Guelder-Rose, Crampbark, European Cranberry-Bush, Guelder Rose, Guelder-Rose, High-Bush Cranberry, Snowball Bush.

CAUTION: See separate listings for Alpine Cranberry, Black Haw, Cranberry, and Uva Ursi.

Scientific Names

Viburnum opulus.
Family: Caprifoliaceae.

People Use This For

In folk medicine, cramp bark or root bark has been used for relieving cramps, muscle spasms, menstrual cramps, cramps during pregnancy, as a kidney stimulant in painful or spasmodic urinary conditions (862), cancer, hysteria, infection, nervous disorders, scurvy, and uteritis. It has also been used as a diuretic, emetic, purgative, and sedative.

Safety

POSSIBLY SAFE …when used orally (12).
PREGNANCY AND LACTATION: Insufficient reliable information available; avoid using.

Effectiveness

There is insufficient reliable information available about the effectiveness of cramp bark.

Mechanism of Action

The applicable parts of cramp bark are the bark and root bark. There is insufficient reliable information available about the possible mechanism of action and active ingredients.

Adverse Reactions

None reported.

Interactions with Herbs & Other Dietary Supplements

Insufficient reliable information available.

Interactions with Drugs

No interactions are known to occur, and there is no known reason to expect a clinically significant interaction with cramp bark.

Interactions with Foods

No interactions are known to occur, and there is no known reason to expect a clinically significant interaction with cramp bark.

Interactions with Lab Tests

No interactions are known to occur, and there is no known reason to expect a clinically significant interaction with cramp bark.

Interactions with Diseases or Conditions

No interactions are known to occur, and there is no known reason to expect a clinically significant interaction with cramp bark.

Dosage and Administration

ORAL: A common dose is 2-4 grams of the dried bark, 2-4 mL of a liquid extract (1:1 in 25% alcohol), or 5-10 mL of a tincture (1:5 in 45% alcohol), three times daily (2822).

Comments

Canadian regulations prohibit cramp bark as a non-medicinal ingredient for oral use products (12). Avoid confusion with black haw (Vibernum prunifolium), which is sometimes referred to as cramp bark (214).

CRANBERRY

Also Known As

American Cranberry, Arandano Americano, Arandano Trepador, Cranberries, European Cranberry, Grosse Moosbeere, Kranbeere, Large Cranberry, Moosebeere, Mossberry, Ronce d'Amerique, Small Cranberry, Trailing Swamp Cranberry, Tsuru-kokemomo.
CAUTION: See separate listings for Alpine Cranberry, Cramp Bark (European Cranberry-Bush), and Uva Ursi (Mountain Cranberry).

Scientific Names

Vaccinium macrocarpon, synonym Oxycoccus macrocarpos; Vaccinium oxycoccos, synonyms Oxycoccus hagerupii, Oxycoccus microcarpus, Oxycoccus palustris, Oxycoccus quadripetalus, Vaccinium hagerupii, Vaccinium microcarpum, Vaccinium palustre.
Family: Ericaceae.

People Use This For

Orally, cranberry is used for prevention and treatment of urinary tract infections (UTIs) (3333), as a urinary deodorizer for people with incontinence (3333), prevention of urinary catheters blockage, and to heal skin around urostomy stomas (3333). Cranberry is also used for scurvy (2810), pleurisy (6084), as a diuretic, antiseptic, antipyretic, and for cancer (2810).
In foods, cranberry fruit is used in fruit juice, jelly, and sauce (11).

Safety

LIKELY SAFE ...when used orally and appropriately (515,6756,6758,6761,7008).
CHILDREN: LIKELY SAFE ...when used orally and appropriately (2811,6759).
PREGNANCY AND LACTATION: LIKELY SAFE ...when used orally in food amounts (5). There is insufficient reliable information about the safety of cranberry when used therapeutically during pregnancy or lactation; avoid using.

Effectiveness

POSSIBLY EFFECTIVE ...when used orally for preventing urinary tract infections (UTIs). There is some evidence that daily consumption of cranberry juice 10 oz (300 mL) can prevent recurrent UTIs in some young and elderly women (6756,6758,6761,7008). A combination product containing cranberry juice plus alpine cranberry also seems to be helpful for prevention (6761). But tell patients not to try cranberry juice for treating UTIs. There's not enough evidence it works. Some patients are trying encapsulated forms of concentrated cranberry. So far, there is little reliable evidence that these preparations offer the same benefits as the juice (6760). For now, tell patients interested in trying cranberry for prevention to stick with the juice. ...when used orally as a urinary deodorizer for incontinent individuals (3333,3334).
POSSIBLY INEFFECTIVE ...when used orally for reducing the frequency of UTIs in children with neurogenic bladder and intermittent catheterization (2811,6759).
There is insufficient reliable information available about the effectiveness of cranberry for its other uses.

Mechanism of Action

The applicable part of the cranberry plant is the fruit. The cranberry is acidic, but does not acidify the urine, as was previously thought. Cranberries contain proanthocyanidin, also known as condensed tannins, and a high-molecular weight compound that has not yet been identified. These constituents seem to interfere with bacterial adherence to the urinary tract epithelial cells (3,2812,2813,2814,3335,3337,3339,6753,6755,6757). For example, proanthocyanidins seem to be capable of "wrapping" around Escherichia coli (E. coli), which causes most urinary tract infections (UTIs), and preventing it from adhering to the urinary tract wall (3333,3338,6690). It probably also has this effect against other urinary tract pathogens (2815). Laboratory evidence suggests that fructose in cranberries might also contribute to the anti-infective activity (3,2813,3333,6757). Cranberry juice has shown antibacterial activity in culture medium against E. coli, Staphylococcus aureus, Klebsiella pneumoniae, Pseudomonas aeruginosa, and Proteus mirabilis (3333,3338,6753). Whether urinary concentrations of the active constituents reach bacteriocidal levels is currently a topic of research (6753). Preliminary data suggest that a high molecular weight cranberry constituent might also prevent adhesion of plaque bacteria that cause periodontal disease (2816,6690). There is also some evidence that cranberry compounds might prevent adhesion of Helicobacter pylori (H. pylori) in the stomach. There is some interest in cranberry for use in cancer. There is some early evidence that cranberry juice might increase the antioxidant capacity of plasma (6754). There is also preliminary evidence that the proanthocyanidin fraction of cranberry might have anticarcinogenic activity (7009).

Cranberry juice and cranberry products can reduce the number of breast cancer tumors, delay tumor development, and reduce the spread of tumors to the lungs and lymph nodes in an animal model of cancer. Additionally, cranberry juice seems to have antioxidant activity and inhibits low-density lipoprotein (LDL) cholesterol oxidation in vitro (5058).

Adverse Reactions

Orally, cranberry is usually well-tolerated (6756,6758,6761,7008). However, in very large doses, for example 3-4 L per day of cranberry juice, patients can experience gastrointestinal upset like diarrhea. Consuming more than 1 L per day over a prolonged period of time might also increase the risk of uric acid kidney stone formation (3334).

Interactions with Herbs & Other Dietary Supplements

Insufficient reliable information available.

Interactions with Drugs

PROTON PUMP INHIBITORS: Cranberry juice might increase absorption of dietary vitamin B-12 in people taking proton pump inhibitors, due to its acidity (2817). Proton pump inhibitors include lansoprazole (Prevacid), omperazole (Prilosec), and Rabeprazole (Aciphex).

Interactions with Foods

No interactions are known to occur, and there is no known reason to expect a clinically significant interaction with cranberry.

Interactions with Lab Tests

No interactions are known to occur, and there is no known reason to expect a clinically significant interaction with cranberry.

Interactions with Diseases or Conditions

ATROPHIC GASTRITIS: Cranberry juice might increase absorption of dietary vitamin B12 in people with atrophic gastritis due to its acidity (2817).
DIABETES: Caution patients with diabetes to avoid cranberry juice cocktail products sweetened with sugar and instead to use cranberry juice cocktail products sweetened with artificial sweeteners.
HYPOCHLORHYDRIA: Cranberry juice might increase absorption of dietary vitamin B12 in people with hypochlorhydria due to its acidity (2817).
KIDNEY STONES (Nephrolithiasis): There is some concern that cranberry juice and cranberry extracts might increase the risk of kidney stones because of its high oxalate content. Drinking cranberry juice 30 mL typically provides approximately 1.9 mg of oxalate. Concentrated cranberry extracts might contain higher amounts of oxalate. There is some evidence that some cranberry extracts tablets can boost urinary oxalate concentration by as much as 43% (7074). Tell patients with a history of kidney stones to avoid cranberry extract products or excessive consumption of cranberry juice.

Dosage and Administration

ORAL: For preventing urinary tract infections (UTIs), cranberry juice 1-10 oz per day has been used (6756,6758,7008). However, the ideal dose has not yet been determined. Some people drink up to 10-32 oz per day of cranberry juice for treating UTIs (515). Some sources suggest that six capsules of dried cranberry powder are equivalent to 3 oz cranberry juice cocktail (515). But this has not been verified. Encapsulated formulations are often taken in doses of 300-400 mg twice daily (7010). Fresh or frozen cranberries may also be used, 1.5 oz is equivalent to 3 oz cranberry juice cocktail (3). Approximately 1500 grams of fresh fruit produce 1 L of juice. Cranberry juice cocktail is approximately 26%-33% pure cranberry juice, sweetened with fructose or artificial sweetener (515,3335).

Comments

Avoid confusing cranberry fruit with high-brush cranberry (Viburnum opulus), which is also known as cramp bark (6,11). The American cranberry (Vaccinium macrocarpon) is native to the northeastern and north central US and eastern Canada, and the fruit is cultivated commercially for food use and as a beverage base (2818). Cranberries, along with blueberries and Concord grapes, are the only fruits native to North America (2821). The Pilgrims called the cranberry "crane berry" because the stem and flower resembled the neck, head, and beak of the crane, and the name was shortened to the word used today (2821).
The European cranberry (Vaccinium oxycoccos) is native to the same areas of North America as its American cousin, as well as central and northern Europe and temperate areas of Asia (2819). The fruit of European cranberry is commercially important in Russia (2820). Approximately 1500 grams of fresh cranberries produce 1 L of pure cranberry juice.

CREATINE

Also Known As
Cr, Creatine Monohydrate.

Scientific Names
N-amidinosarcosine; N-(aminoiminomethyl)-N methyl glycine.

People Use This For
Orally, creatine is used for improving exercise performance and increasing muscle mass in athletes and older adults. Creatine is also used orally for congestive heart failure (CHF), neuromuscular disease, mitochondrial cytopathies, gyrate atrophy of the choroid and retina, and hyperlipidemia. It is also used orally for slowing the progression of amyotrophic lateral sclerosis (ALS, Lou Gehrig's disease), rheumatoid arthritis, McArdle disease, and for various muscular dystrophies. Intravenously, creatine is used in cardiac surgery and for congestive heart failure.

Safety
POSSIBLY SAFE ...when used orally and appropriately. Creatine supplementation appears generally to be safe when used in appropriate doses in healthy adults (1367,2100,2101,2103,3996,4569,6052,6117). Creatine has been safely used daily for up to 5 years (3996,6117).
POSSIBLY UNSAFE ...when used orally in high doses. There is some concern that very high doses of creatine might adversely effect renal, hepatic, or cardiac function and have other adverse effects, such as hypertension (1367,6052); however, a clear association between high dose creatine and significant adverse effects has not yet been established.
PREGNANCY AND LACTATION: Insufficient reliable information available; avoid using.

Effectiveness
POSSIBLY EFFECTIVE ...when used orally for enhancing muscle performance during repeated bouts of brief, high-intensity exercise. Numerous studies have shown creatine to be beneficial for certain types of high-intensity exercises (2100,2101,2102,4591,4592,4593,4594,4601,4602,4604) (4605,6015); however, for other exercises, creatine appears to offer no benefit (4582,4595,4596,4597,4606,6117,6183). Creatine seems to be more effective for increasing muscular power in healthy young adults during repeated, short, maximal energy bursts than for single event performances (4593,4598,4599,4600,6052). It might also be beneficial for exercise of longer-duration with the intensity alternating between anaerobic and aerobic metabolism (6926). Many variables seem to determine the effect of creatine on performance, including the subject's training status, the type of sport being tested, diet, age of the subject, and the dose regimen of creatine. Creatine does not seem to improve performance in aerobic exercises. It also does not seem to be beneficial in older individuals. It is possible that the benefit in certain sports is offset by weight gain from creatine supplementation (2106,4576,4601,4604,4605,6015,6052). Acute creatine loading may also be more effective than chronic continuous use (4603). Most studies have used 20 grams daily for 5 days for creatine loading; however, various other regimens have been studied. One study used 9 grams daily for 5 days and was beneficial in weight lifters, while another study used 20 grams daily for 3 days and was not beneficial for single sprints in cyclists (4576,4599,6015). Due to the variety of study methodologies and some conflicting findings, it has yet to be determined exactly who can benefit from creatine supplementation and what dosing schedule might be most effective. All studies have been limited by small sample size; all have involved less than 40 subjects and most less than 25. ...when used orally or intravenously for congestive heart failure (CHF). Oral creatine seems to improve exercise tolerance, but does not affect ejection fraction (4562,4563). Intravenous creatine improves cardiac function, including ejection fraction, even in the presence of conventional pharmacologic therapy. Following an infusion of 6 grams of IV creatine, improvements in ejection fraction persist for l more than 12 hours (1369). ...when used orally to treat gyrate atrophy of the choroid and retina (4577,4578). Creatine supplementation seems to slow visual deterioration in patients with gyrate atrophy (4577,4578). ...when used orally to treat McArdle disease. There is some preliminary clinical evidence that daily high-dose creatine supplementation can increase exercise capacity and decreases exercise-induced muscle pain in some patients with McArdle disease (70). ...when used orally short-term to improve muscle strength and daily-life activity in adults and children with various muscular dystrophies (6182). Creatine monohydrate daily for eight weeks seems to mildly improve muscle strength and daily-life activity in children and adults with facioscapulohumeral dystrophy, Becker dystrophy, Duchenne dystrophy, or sarcoglycan-deficient limb girdle muscular dystrophy (6182).
POSSIBLY INEFFECTIVE ...when used orally for rheumatoid arthritis. Creatine supplementation can increase muscle creatine content and muscle strength, but has no significant effect on physical functional ability or disease activity (6929).
LIKELY INEFFECTIVE ...when used for increasing endurance or for improving performance in highly trained athletes (2103,2105,2106,4607). ...when used to improve isometric strength and body composition in adults over age 60 (4570,4571,4572). In three well-designed studies, creatine dosed at 20 grams per day for 5 days followed by

lower maintenance doses had no beneficial effect on exercise except reducing muscle fatigue (4570,4571,4572). In one study it had no effect on quadriceps fatigue after repeated sets of explosive work (6183).
There is insufficient reliable information available about the effectiveness of creatine for its other uses.

Mechanism of Action

Creatine is found primarily in skeletal muscle (95%), but also in heart, brain, testes, retina, and other tissues (3997,3998). The body synthesizes 1 to 2 grams of creatine a day, primarily in the liver, kidneys, and pancreas (3997). Dietary sources, such as fish and meats, supply an additional 1 to 2 grams (3977). For example, one pound of fresh uncooked steak contains about 2 grams of creatine (4575). Intestinal absorption of creatine is nearly 100% (6052). Creatine is irreversibly converted to creatinine and excreted by the kidneys (3997). Creatine in skeletal muscles exists in dynamic equilibrium with phosphocreatine (3997). Body stores of phosphocreatine in skeletal muscle serve as a precursor to the energy molecule, adenosine triphosphate (ATP). Higher levels of creatine are thought to enhance the ability to renew ATP for short 10-20 second energy bursts and improve resynthesis of phosphocreatine during recovery from intense exercise. However, there is debate about whether increased phosphocreatine resynthesis actually occurs (2103,3997,4576,4580,6925,6927). Supplementation does seem to increase total creatine (4574,4583). People who have lower initial total creatine, such as vegetarians, are more likely to respond to supplemental creatine, while people with higher initial levels may not respond (4574). Skeletal muscle has a saturation point at which additional supplemental creatine will not increase intracellular creatine levels. This occurs within the first few days of loading (3999,6052). Excess supplementation increases urinary creatine and creatinine (4576). Exogenous creatine supplementation also appears to reduce endogenous creatine production; whether this has any clinically significant negative effect on metabolic regulation within the liver is unknown (6052). After discontinuing supplementation, endogenous creatine production and creatine levels typically return to baseline within 28 days (2101,4582,6052). Although some laboratory evidence identifies creatine as a potential muscle builder, most clinical evidence supports increased water retention as the primary cause of creatine-induced weight gain (4569,4575,4576,4579,4588,6061). The muscle enlargement due to increased water retention is short term. This is compared to the muscle enlargement from strength training, which results in an increase in contractile and structural muscle proteins (6052). Creatine may allow athletes to train harder due to increased phosphocreatine resynthesis and subsequent energy production (6061). Creatine might also reduce lactate production (4604); however, this has not been consistently found in studies (4592). In patients with congestive heart failure (CHF), the cardiac creatine phosphate/adenosine triphosphate is lower than in people with normal cardiac function and correlates with the severity of heart failure (1369). Creatine phosphate appears to improve CHF by preserving intracellular high-energy phosphates in the myocardium, stabilizing the sarcolemma, preventing peroxidative damage, and improving microcirculation (1369). In patients with gyrate atrophy, an inherited metabolic disease in which phosphocreatine is depleted, supplemental creatine increased myofibrillar protein synthesis resulting in muscle accretion (4576,4587). In myophosphorylase deficiency, known as McArdle disease, a rare genetic metabolic disease in which ATP cannot be formed from glycogen in skeletal muscle, supplemental creatine is thought to serve as a source of energy (70). Creatine appears to also effect lipid metabolism. There is some preliminary evidence that it can modestly reduce total cholesterol and very low-density lipoprotein (VLDL) cholesterol (4573). Early laboratory evidence also suggests that creatine might be useful in diseases such as amyotrophic lateral sclerosis, Huntington's disease, and Parkinson's disease, possibly due to neuroprotective effects (4566,4567,4568). There is conflicting evidence on creatine and cancer. Some research suggests that creatine and its analogs, such as cyclocreatine, inhibit tumor growth (1393,1406,1432,1481). Creatine might alter energy production by the creatine kinase system, which appears to play a role in controlling some types of tumors such as breast tumors and neuroblastomas (1393,1406). Other research suggests that creatine or its metabolites can form mutagenic substances when combined at room temperature with sugars or heated (1486,1487), but this has not been verified.

Adverse Reactions

Orally, creatine use can cause gastrointestinal pain, nausea, and diarrhea (2103,4576,6052). Although not reported in clinical studies (6930), 25% of male collegiate athletes taking creatine have reported muscle cramping (4584). A theoretical increase in risk of dehydration due to intracellular fluid shifts has led most creatine manufacturers to caution about adequate hydration with creatine supplementation (217,4576). Tell people who are controlling weight and engaging in strenuous exercise and/or exercising in hot environments to avoid creatine supplementation (6052). Creatine typically causes a weight gain of 0.5 to 1.6 kg (see Mechanism of Action) that increases with prolonged supplementation (3997). This fat-free weight gain, most likely due to water retention, has been thought to also increase the risk for high blood pressure. However, a recent study showed no effect of 20 grams daily of creatine for 5 days on blood pressure (4569). Creatine might also cause renal dysfunction (184,2118), but this appears to be rare in people with healthy kidneys (1368,2120,3996). Most studies have not found alterations in renal function in people taking 5-20 grams of creatine daily for up to 5 years (3996,4569,6117). However, there is one report of acute interstitial nephritis and focal tubular injury after four weeks of creatine at 5 grams four times daily (184). In another case, supplemental creatine, loaded at 15 grams per day for one week, then 2 grams per day, caused a significant decline in creatinine clearance in a man receiving cyclosporine for steroid-resistant focal segmental glomerulosclerosis (2118). Medical supervision is suggested for people with kidney disease or a high risk of kidney disease who use creatine (4569,6052). There is one report of ischemic stroke in an athlete who consumed creatine monohydrate 6 grams, caffeine 400-600 mg, ephedra 40-60 mg, and a variety of other supplements daily for six weeks (1275). The FDA has received a total of 32 complaints of adverse effects linked to creatine, including seizures, cardiomyopathy, arrhythmias, rhabdomyolysis, and cardiac arrest, although causality has not been proven (4585).

Interactions with Herbs & Other Dietary Supplements

EPHEDRA: There is some concern that combining ephedra, caffeine, and creatine might increase the risk of serious adverse effects. There is a report of ischemic stroke in an athlete who consumed creatine monohydrate 6 grams, caffeine 400-600 mg, ephedra 40-60 mg, and a variety of other supplements daily for 6 weeks (1275).

CAFFEINE: There is some concern that combining caffeine, ephedra, and creatine might increase the risk of serious adverse effects. There is a report of ischemic stroke in an athlete who consumed creatine monohydrate 6 grams, caffeine 400-600 mg, ephedra 40-60 mg, and a variety of other supplements daily for 6 weeks (1275). Caffeine might also decrease creatine's beneficial effects on athletic performance. Some researchers think caffeine can inhibit phosphocreatine resynthesis (2117,4575).

Interactions with Drugs

NEPHROTOXIC DRUGS: There is some concern about using creatine with drugs that can be nephrotoxic. Since high doses of creatine might adversely effect renal function (6052), combining creatine with potentially nephrotoxic drugs might have additive harmful effects on kidney function. However, this effect has not yet been reported. Some potentially nephrotoxic drugs include cyclosporine (Neoral, Sandimmune); aminoglycosides including amikacin (Amakin), gentamicin (Garamycin, Gentak, others), and tobramycin (Nebcin, others); nonsteroidal anti-inflammatory drugs (NSAIDs) including ibuprofen (Advil, Motrin, Nuprin, others), indomethacin (Indocin), naproxen (Aleve, Anaprox, Naprelan, Naprosyn), piroxicam (Feldene); and numerous others.

Interactions with Foods

No interactions are known to occur, and there is no known reason to expect a clinically significant interaction with creatine.

Interactions with Lab Tests

SERUM CREATININE (SCr): Creatine is metabolized to creatinine. Higher than normal serum creatinine levels can result in patients taking creatine, despite normal renal function (2100,2103).

Interactions with Diseases or Conditions

KIDNEY DYSFUNCTION: Creatine should be avoided by people with pre-existing renal disease or by people with diseases such as diabetes that increase the risk for renal dysfunction (4576). There is some concern that creatine might exacerbate renal dysfunction in these patients.

Dosage and Administration

ORAL: For improving physical performance, several dosing regimens have been tried. Creatine is typically acutely loaded with 20 grams per day (or 0.3 grams per kg) for 5 days followed by a maintenance dose of 2 or more grams (0.03 grams per kg) daily (4576). Although 5 day loading is typical, 2 days of loading has also been used (4576). A loading dose of 9 grams per day for 6 days has also been used (6015). Some sources suggest that, instead of acutely loading, similar results can be obtained with 3 grams per day for 28 days (2104). During creatine supplementation, the water intake should be 64 ounces per day (2103,2104). For heart failure, 20 grams per day for 5-10 days has been used in clinical trials (4562,4563). For gyrate atrophy, 1.5 grams per day has been used (4577,4578). For McArdle disease, 150mg/kg daily for 5 days followed by 60 mg/kg per day has been used (70). For muscular dystrophies, 10 grams per day has been used by adults and 5 grams per day has been used by children (6182).

Comments

Creatine is allowed by the International Olympic Committee, National Collegiate Athletic Association (NCAA), and professional sports (3998,4575,4576). However, the NCAA no longer allows colleges and universities to supply creatine to their students with school funds. Students are permitted to buy creatine on their own and the NCAA has no plans to ban creatine unless sufficient medical evidence indicates that it is harmful (6140). With current testing methods, detection of supplemental creatine use would not be possible (4575). Creatine use is widespread among professional and amateur athletes and has been acknowledged by well-known athletes such as Mark McGuire, Sammy Sosa, and John Elway (3998). Following the finding that carbohydrate solution further increased muscle creatine levels more than creatine alone, creatine sports drinks have become popular (4576,4589). Annual consumption of creatine in the US is estimated to exceed 4 million kg (3998).

CROTON SEEDS

Also Known As
Croton, Tiglium, Tiglium Seeds.

Scientific Names
Croton tiglium.
Family: Euphorbiaceae.

People Use This For
Orally, croton is used as a purgative (3800).
In Chinese medicine, croton is used orally to treat gallbladder colic, bowel obstruction, and malaria (18); and topically for rheumatism, gout, neuralgia, and bronchitis (3819).

Safety
LIKELY UNSAFE ...when used orally. One drop of the oil can be toxic, and one mL (20 drops) of oil is considered lethal (18). Also, the phorbol esters in the oil are co-carcinogens (18). ...when used topically; avoid using (18).
PREGNANCY: UNSAFE ...when used orally due to abortifacient properties (19); avoid using.
LACTATION: UNSAFE ...when used orally; avoid using.

Effectiveness
POSSIBLY EFFECTIVE ...when used orally as a purgative (3800,3819), but risk precludes use.
There is insufficient reliable information available about the effectiveness of croton seed oil for its other uses.

Mechanism of Action
The applicable part of croton seeds is the oil from the seed. Croton seeds possess powerful, irritant, cathartic properties due to phorbol esters (3800). The diterpene, TPA, is carcinogenic, affecting prostaglandin metabolism (18).

Adverse Reactions
Orally, croton seeds can cause burning of mouth, vomiting, dizziness, stupor, painful bowel movements, and collapse (18).
Topically, croton seeds can cause itching, burning and blistering of skin (18).

Interactions with Herbs & Other Dietary Supplements
Insufficient reliable information available.

Interactions with Drugs
No interactions are known to occur, and there is no known reason to expect a clinically significant interaction with croton seeds.

Interactions with Foods
No interactions are known to occur, and there is no known reason to expect a clinically significant interaction with croton seeds.

Interactions with Lab Tests
No interactions are known to occur, and there is no known reason to expect a clinically significant interaction with croton seeds.

Interactions with Diseases or Conditions
No interactions are known to occur, and there is no known reason to expect a clinically significant interaction with croton seeds.

Dosage and Administration
No typical dosage.

Comments
None.

CUBEBS

Also Known As
Cubeb, Cubeb Berries, Cubeba, Java Pepper, Tailed Chubebs, Tailed Pepper.

Scientific Names
Cubeba officinaliz; Piper cubeba.
Family: Piperaceae.

People Use This For
Orally, cubebs is used as a diuretic, urinary antiseptic, and for amoebic dysentery (11).
Traditionally, cubebs was used as an antiflatulent, stimulating expectorant, for gonorrhea, and cancer (11).
For food uses, cubebs oil is used as a flavoring ingredient (11).

Safety
LIKELY SAFE ...when used in amounts found in foods (maximum use level for oil is 0.004%); approved for use in foods in the US (11).
POSSIBLY SAFE ...when used orally and appropriately for medicinal purposes (12).
PREGNANCY AND LACTATION: Insufficient reliable information available; avoid using.

Effectiveness
There is insufficient reliable information available about the effectiveness of cubebs.

Mechanism of Action
The applicable part of cubebs is the dried, fully grown but unripe fruit. Researchers think that the constituent cubebic acid is responsible for the stimulant effect on urinary and respiratory tract (11).

Adverse Reactions
None reported.

Interactions with Herbs & Other Dietary Supplements
Insufficient reliable information available.

Interactions with Drugs
ACID-INHIBITING DRUGS: Theoretically, due to claims that cubebs increases stomach acid, it might interfere with antacids, sucralfate (Carafate), H-2 antagonists, or proton pump inhibitors (19).

Interactions with Foods
No interactions are known to occur, and there is no known reason to expect a clinically significant interaction with cubebs.

Interactions with Lab Tests
No interactions are known to occur, and there is no known reason to expect a clinically significant interaction with cubebs.

Interactions with Diseases or Conditions
GI CONDITIONS: Can irritate gastrointestinal tract. Contraindicated in individuals with infectious or inflammatory gastrointestinal conditions (19).
NEPHRITIS: Contraindicated in individuals with nephritis (12).

Dosage and Administration
ORAL: People typically use 2 to 4 grams of the powdered fruit or 2 to 4 mL of the liquid extract (5264).

Comments
None.

CUDWEED

Also Known As
Cotton Dawes, Cotton Weed, Dysentery Weed, Everlasting, Mouse Ear, Wartwort.
CAUTION: See separate listings for Cat's Foot and Mouse Ear.

Scientific Names
Gnaphalium uliginosum.
Family: Asteraceae or Compositae.

People Use This For
Topically, cudweed is used as a gargle or rinse for diseases of the mouth or throat (18).

Safety
There is insufficient reliable information available about the safety of cudweed.
Pregnancy and Lactation: Insufficient reliable information available; avoid using.

Effectiveness
There is insufficient reliable information available about the effectiveness of cudweed.

Mechanism of Action
The applicable parts of cudweed are the above ground parts. Cudweed has astringent effects, and promotes and improves appetite (18). Unsubstantiated sources report it has antidepressant, aphrodisiac, and hypotensive effects (18).

Adverse Reactions
Topically, cudweed can cause an allergic reaction in individuals sensitive to the Asteraceae/Compositae family. Members of this family include ragweed, chrysanthemums, marigolds, daisies, and many other herbs.

Interactions with Herbs & Other Dietary Supplements
Insufficient reliable information available.

Interactions with Drugs
No interactions are known to occur, and there is no known reason to expect a clinically significant interaction with cudweed.

Interactions with Foods
No interactions are known to occur, and there is no known reason to expect a clinically significant interaction with cudweed.

Interactions with Lab Tests
No interactions are known to occur, and there is no known reason to expect a clinically significant interaction with cudweed.

Interactions with Diseases or Conditions
CROSS-ALLERGENICITY: Can cause an allergic reaction in individuals sensitive to the Asteraceae/Compositae family. Members of this family include ragweed, chrysanthemums, marigolds, daisies, and many other herbs.

Dosage and Administration
ORAL: People typically use 2 to 4 mL of the liquid extract (5264).

Comments
Avoid confusion with cat's foot (Antennaria dioica), which is also referred to as cudweed. Avoid confusion with Pilosella officinarum, also known as mouse ear.

CUMIN

Also Known As
Cummin.

Scientific Names
Cuminum cyminum; Cuminum odorum.
Family: Apiaceae/Umbelliferae.

People Use This For
Orally, cumin is used as an antiflatulent (11).
Traditionally, cumin was used as a stimulant, antispasmodic, diuretic, aphrodisiac, for stimulating menstrual flow (11), treating diarrhea, colic, and flatulence (18).
In spices, foods, and beverages, cumin is used as a flavoring component (11).
In other manufacturing processes, cumin oil is used as a fragrance component in cosmetics (maximum use level 0.4% in perfumes).

Safety
LIKELY SAFE ...when used in amounts used as spice (cumin maximum use level 0.4%). ...when used in amounts found in foods (cumin oil maximum use level 0.025%); Generally Recognized as Safe (GRAS) status in the US.
POSSIBLY SAFE ...when used orally and appropriately for medicinal purposes (12).
PREGNANCY AND LACTATION: Insufficient reliable information available; avoid in excess of food amounts.

Effectiveness
There is insufficient reliable information available about the effectiveness of cumin.

Mechanism of Action
The applicable part of cumin is the fruit/seed. Cumin is a rich source of iron (19). Cumin oil and constituent, cuminaldehyde, have been reported to exhibit strong larvicidal and antibacterial activity (6). Demonstrated phototoxic effects are reportedly not due to cuminaldehyde (11). Some evidence suggests the dried extract might inhibit platelet aggregation (18) and prolong phenobarbiturate hypnosis in mice; however, a higher dose shortened phenobarbiturate hypnosis (18).

Adverse Reactions
Orally, cumin oil has phototoxic effects (6).

Interactions with Herbs & Other Dietary Supplements
Insufficient reliable information available.

Interactions with Drugs
DIABETES THERAPY: Monitor blood glucose levels closely due to claims that cumin has hypoglycemic effects (19).
BARBITURATES: Theoretically, might increase or decrease activity of barbiturates (18).

Interactions with Foods
No interactions are known to occur, and there is no known reason to expect a clinically significant interaction with cumin.

Interactions with Lab Tests
No interactions are known to occur, and there is no known reason to expect a clinically significant interaction with cumin.

Interactions with Diseases or Conditions
No interactions are known to occur, and there is no known reason to expect a clinically significant interaction with cumin.

Dosage and Administration
ORAL: Average single amount used, 5-10 fruits (18).

Comments
Fine grinding of seed can cause loss of 50% of volatile oil, most within 1 hour (6).

CUP PLANT

Also Known As
Indian Gum, Pilot Plant, Polar Plant, Prairie Dock, Ragged Cup, Rosinweed, Turpentine Weed.
CAUTION: See separate listing for Rosinweed.

Scientific Names
Silphium perfoliatum.

People Use This For
Orally, cup plant is used for digestive disorders (18).

Safety
There is insufficient reliable information available about the safety of cup plant.
Pregnancy and Lactation: Insufficient reliable information available; avoid using.

Effectiveness
There is insufficient reliable information available about the effectiveness of cup plant.

Mechanism of Action
The applicable part of cup plant is the root. Cup plant is stated to have tonic and diaphoretic effects (18).

Adverse Reactions
None reported.

Interactions with Herbs & Other Dietary Supplements
Insufficient reliable information available.

Interactions with Drugs
No interactions are known to occur, and there is no known reason to expect a clinically significant interaction with cup plant.

Interactions with Foods
No interactions are known to occur, and there is no known reason to expect a clinically significant interaction with cup plant.

Interactions with Lab Tests
No interactions are known to occur, and there is no known reason to expect a clinically significant interaction with cup plant.

Interactions with Diseases or Conditions
No interactions are known to occur, and there is no known reason to expect a clinically significant interaction with cup plant.

Dosage and Administration
ORAL: Cup plant is used to make a tea; typically 1 teaspoon of cup plant root is added to 1 cup of water. The usual dose is 1 cup daily. The powdered root dose is 20 grains which is 1300 mg, and tincture 5 to 20 drops (5263).

Comments
Avoid confusion with Silphium laciniatum, also known as rosinweed.
There is very little scientific information about this product. Our staff is continually analyzing the available information on natural medicines and will add data here as it becomes available.

CUPMOSS

Also Known As
Chin Cups.

Scientific Names
Cladonia pyxidata.

People Use This For
Orally, cupmoss is used for coughs, bronchitis, and whooping cough (18).

Safety
There is insufficient reliable information available about the safety of cupmoss.
Pregnancy and Lactation: Insufficient reliable information available; avoid using.

Effectiveness
There is insufficient reliable information available about the effectiveness of cupmoss.

Mechanism of Action
Cupmoss is stated to have expectorant and antitussive effects (18).

Adverse Reactions
None reported.

Interactions with Herbs & Other Dietary Supplements
Insufficient reliable information available.

Interactions with Drugs
No interactions are known to occur, and there is no known reason to expect a clinically significant interaction with cupmoss.

Interactions with Foods
No interactions are known to occur, and there is no known reason to expect a clinically significant interaction with cupmoss.

Interactions with Lab Tests
No interactions are known to occur, and there is no known reason to expect a clinically significant interaction with cupmoss.

Interactions with Diseases or Conditions
No interactions are known to occur, and there is no known reason to expect a clinically significant interaction with cupmoss.

Dosage and Administration
ORAL: A suggested dose is 2 ounces of liquid, prepared by adding cupmoss to water, mixed with honey as needed for cough (5267,5264).

Comments
There is very little scientific information about this product. Our staff is continually analyzing the available information on natural medicines and will add data here as it becomes available.

CYCLAMEN

Also Known As
Cyclamen europaeum, Groundbread, Ivy-Leafed Cyclamen, Sowbread, Swinebread.

Scientific Names
Cyclamen europaeum.
Family: Primulaceae

People Use This For
Orally, cyclamen is used for menstrual complaints, "nervous emotional states," and digestive problems (18).

Safety
LIKELY UNSAFE ...when used orally. Doses as low as 300 mg can cause poisoning (18).
PREGNANCY AND LACTATION: LIKELY UNSAFE ...when used orally; avoid using.

Effectiveness
There is insufficient reliable information available about the effectiveness of cyclamen.

Mechanism of Action
The applicable parts of cyclamen are the rhizome and root. There is insufficient reliable information available about the possible mechanism of action and active ingredients.

Adverse Reactions
Orally, poisoning has been reported with doses as low as 300 mg; symptoms include stomach pain, nausea, vomiting, and diarrhea (18). High doses can cause severe poisoning; symptoms include spasm and asphyxiation (18,553).

Interactions with Herbs & Other Dietary Supplements
Insufficient reliable information available.

Interactions with Drugs
No interactions are known to occur, and there is no known reason to expect a clinically significant interaction with cyclamen.

Interactions with Foods
No interactions are known to occur, and there is no known reason to expect a clinically significant interaction with cyclamen.

Interactions with Lab Tests
No interactions are known to occur, and there is no known reason to expect a clinically significant interaction with cyclamen.

Interactions with Diseases or Conditions
No interactions are known to occur, and there is no known reason to expect a clinically significant interaction with cyclamen.

Dosage and Administration
ORAL: People typically use 20 to 40 grains (1300 to 2600 mg) of powdered cyclamen root (5267). One source specifies that cyclamen should not be used without medical supervision (5263).

Comments
None.

CYPRESS

Also Known As
None.

Scientific Names
Cupressus sempervirens.
Family: Coniferae.

People Use This For
Topically, cypress is used for head colds, cough, bronchitis, and as an expectorant (18).

Safety
There is insufficient reliable information available about the safety of cypress.
Pregnancy and Lactation: Insufficient reliable information available; avoid using.

Effectiveness
There is insufficient reliable information available about the effectiveness of cypress.

Mechanism of Action
The applicable parts of cypress are the branch, cone, and oil. There is insufficient reliable information available about the possible mechanism of action and active ingredients.

Adverse Reactions
Orally, cypress may cause kidney irritation (18).

Interactions with Herbs & Other Dietary Supplements
Insufficient reliable information available.

Interactions with Drugs
No interactions are known to occur, and there is no known reason to expect a clinically significant interaction with cypress.

Interactions with Foods
No interactions are known to occur, and there is no known reason to expect a clinically significant interaction with cypress.

Interactions with Lab Tests
No interactions are known to occur, and there is no known reason to expect a clinically significant interaction with cypress.

Interactions with Diseases or Conditions
No interactions are known to occur, and there is no known reason to expect a clinically significant interaction with cypress.

Dosage and Administration
TOPICAL: Cypress is used as an ointment (18).

Comments
There is very little scientific information about this product. Our staff is continually analyzing the available information on natural medicines and will add data here as it becomes available.

CYPRESS SPURGE

Also Known As
None.

Scientific Names
Euphorbia cyparissias.

People Use This For
Orally, cypress spurge is used for diseases of the respiratory organs, diarrhea, and skin diseases (18).

Safety
UNSAFE ...when used orally. The plant contains poisonous white latex (milky liquid) and cocarcinogenic agents (18). Both the fresh and dried latex are toxic (18).
PREGNANCY AND LACTATION: UNSAFE ...when used orally due to toxicity (18); avoid using.

Effectiveness
There is insufficient reliable information available about the effectiveness of cypress spurge.

Mechanism of Action
The applicable parts of cypress spurge are the flowering plant and root. Cypress spurge contains varied diterpenes and triterpenes. The ingenan esters are potent inflammatory and cocarcinogenic agents (18). Euphorbia species have topical irritant, GI irritant, emetic, and purgative effects (19).

Adverse Reactions
Orally, cypress spurge, which is part of the Euphorbia species, may cause GI irritation, nausea, vomiting, and diarrhea (19). Ingestion of the latex can cause burning of the mouth, vomiting, mydriasis, dizziness, painful bowel

movements, stupor, cardiac arrhythmias, and collapse (18).

Topically, Euphorbia species may cause contact dermatitis (19). Skin contact with the latex causes reddening, itching, burning, and blisters (18). Eye contact can cause eyelid swelling, conjunctival inflammation, and corneal defects (18).

Interactions with Herbs & Other Dietary Supplements
Insufficient reliable information available.

Interactions with Drugs
No interactions are known to occur, and there is no known reason to expect a clinically significant interaction with cypress spurge.

Interactions with Foods
No interactions are known to occur, and there is no known reason to expect a clinically significant interaction with cypress spurge.

Interactions with Lab Tests
No interactions are known to occur, and there is no known reason to expect a clinically significant interaction with cypress spurge.

Interactions with Diseases or Conditions
DIARRHEA: Avoid using; Euphorbia species have purgative effects (19).
GI IRRITATION, INFLAMMATION: Avoid using; Euphorbia species have GI irritant effects (19).
NAUSEA, VOMITING: Avoid using; Euphorbia species have emetic effects (19).

Dosage and Administration
No typical dosage.

Comments
None.

DA QING YE

Also Known As
Quing Dai.

Scientific Names
Isatis indigota.
Family: Brassicaceae.

People Use This For
In Chinese medicine, da qing ye is used to treat acute parotitis, upper respiratory infection, encephalitis, hepatitis, lung abscess, dysentery, acute gastroenteritis, and HIV (5541).
In combination with seven other herbs (PC-SPES), da qing ye is used to treat prostate cancer (5548).

Safety
POSSIBLY SAFE ...when used orally in a specific herbal combination (PC-SPES) (5548).
There is insufficient reliable information available about the safety of da qing ye when used in other preparations.
PREGNANCY AND LACTATION: LIKELY UNSAFE ...when used orally. It is reported to cause uterine contractions (5541); avoid using.

Effectiveness
POSSIBLY EFFECTIVE ...when used orally in a specific herbal combination for prostate cancer. Studies using da qing ye in combination with seven other herbs (PC-SPES), found that it significantly decreases prostate-specific antigen (PSA) levels (3576,5122,5548,6284,6286), causes clinically significant reductions in serum testosterone (5548), improves quality of life, and reduces pain (6286) in patients with prostate cancer. In two reports, PSA levels fell significantly within one month of treatment (5122,5548).
There is insufficient reliable information available about the effectiveness of da qing ye for its other uses.

Mechanism of Action

The applicable part of da qing ye is the dried leaf. The dried leaf appears to have antibacterial and antiviral activity and can increase the phagocytic activity of leukocytes. It also shows evidence of antipyretic, anti-inflammatory, and biliary stimulant properties. Da qing ye seems to relax smooth muscles but contracts the uterine muscle. The dried leaf of da qing ye contains the glycosides indican and isatin B. Of the ingested dose of da qing ye, 90% is excreted in the urine (5541).

Adverse Reactions

Orally, da qing ye can cause nausea and vomiting (5541).
Intramuscularly, it can cause blood in the urine (5541).

Interactions with Herbs & Other Dietary Supplements

Insufficient reliable information available.

Interactions with Drugs

No interactions are known to occur, and there is no known reason to expect a clinically significant interaction with da qing ye.

Interactions with Foods

No interactions are known to occur, and there is no known reason to expect a clinically significant interaction with da qing ye.

Interactions with Lab Tests

No interactions are known to occur, and there is no known reason to expect a clinically significant interaction with da qing ye.

Interactions with Diseases or Conditions

No interactions are known to occur, and there is no known reason to expect a clinically significant interaction with da qing ye.

Dosage and Administration

No typical dosage.

Comments

Other herbs considered to be da qing ye include Isatis tinctoria, Baphicacanthus cusia, Clerodendron cyrtophyllum, and Polyconum tinctorium (5541).

DAFFODIL

Also Known As

Lent Lily.

Scientific Names

Narcissus pseudonarcissus.
Family: Amaryllidaceae.

People Use This For

Orally, daffodil is used to soothe mucous membrane irritation resulting from whooping cough, colds, asthma, bronchial catarrh (18), and as an emetic (7200).
Historically, a plaster made from daffodil bulbs was used topically for wounds, burns, strains, and joint pain (7200).

Safety

POSSIBLY UNSAFE ...when used topically. Severe cases of dermatitis have been reported (5004).
LIKELY UNSAFE ...when used orally (19). Merely chewing on the stem may be enough to cause a chill, shivering, and fainting. The constituent lycorine can cause salivation, vomiting, diarrhea at low doses, and paralysis and collapse at higher doses (514).
PREGNANCY AND LACTATION: LIKELY UNSAFE when used orally or topically; avoid using.

Effectiveness

There is insufficient reliable information available about the effectiveness of daffodil.

Mechanism of Action

The applicable parts of daffodil are the bulb, leaf, and flower. Daffodil contains numerous active constituents including alkaloids (lycorine and galanthamine) and chelidonic acid (18). In small amounts, lycorine causes salivation, vomiting, and diarrhea. At higher doses, it causes paralysis and collapse. Galanthamine is a cholinesterase inhibitor and analgesic (514), and it is being investigated for use in the treatment of Alzheimer's disease (5007). Lycorine, narciclasine, and other constituents are cytotoxic (514). The mucus and sap of daffodil plants and bulbs contain calcium oxalate crystals, which are most likely responsible for the skin irritation (5004). "Micro trauma" to the skin from the oxylate crystals allows penetration of other irritants and worsens dermatitis (5004).

Adverse Reactions

Orally, daffodil can cause irritation and swelling of the mouth, tongue, and throat (19), as well as vomiting, salivation, diarrhea, central nervous disorders, and respiratory or CV collapse and subsequent death (18). This is due to the lycorine component (214). Topical use can cause dermatitis (5004,5005) . People who simply handle daffodil plants or bulbs can get "Lily rash" or "daffodil itch" (18,5004).

Interactions with Herbs & Other Dietary Supplements

CALCIUM, IRON, ZINC: Concurrent use might decrease mineral absorption. Daffodil contains oxalate (5004), which can bind multivalent metal ions in the gastrointestinal tract and decrease mineral absorption.

Interactions with Drugs

No interactions are known to occur, and there is no known reason to expect a clinically significant interaction with daffodil.

Interactions with Foods

CALCIUM, IRON, ZINC: Concurrent use might decrease mineral absorption from foods. Daffodil contains oxalate (5004), which can bind multivalent metal ions in the gastrointestinal tract and decrease mineral absorption.

Interactions with Lab Tests

No interactions are known to occur, and there is no known reason to expect a clinically significant interaction with daffodil.

Interactions with Diseases or Conditions

No interactions are known to occur, and there is no known reason to expect a clinically significant interaction with daffodil.

Dosage and Administration

ORAL: Used as a powder and an extract (amount unspecified) (18).

Comments

None.

DAMIANA

Also Known As

Damiana Herb, Damiana Leaf, Herba de la Pastora, Mexican Damiana, Mizibcoc, Old Woman's Broom, Rosemary, Turnerae diffusae folium, Turnerae diffusae herba.

Scientific Names

Turnera diffusa, synonyms Damiana aphrodisiaca, Turnera aphrodisiaca, Turnera microphylla.
Family: Bignoniaceae/Turneraceae.

People Use This For

Orally, damiana is used to treat headache, bedwetting (6), depression, nervous dyspepsia, atonic constipation (4), for prophylaxis and treatment of sexual disturbances, strengthening and stimulation during exertion (overwork), boosting and maintaining mental and physical capacity, and as an aphrodisiac (2). It is also used orally as a tea.
By inhalation, damiana is used for a subtle "high" (5).

Safety

LIKELY SAFE ...when used orally in amounts found in foods (maximum use level 0.125%.); Damiana is approved for food use in the US (11).

POSSIBLY SAFE ...when used orally and appropriately for medicinal purposes (12).
PREGNANCY AND LACTATION: Insufficient reliable information available; avoid using (4).

Effectiveness
There is insufficient reliable information available about the effectiveness of damiana.

Mechanism of Action
The applicable parts of damiana are the leaf and stem. Ethanolic extracts are reported to exhibit CNS depressant activity (4). The quinone arbutin may be responsible for antibacterial properties (4).

Adverse Reactions
Orally, 200 grams of damiana extract has caused tetanus-like convulsions and paroxysms resulting in symptoms similar to rabies or strychnine poisoning (4).

Interactions with Herbs & Other Dietary Supplements
Insufficient reliable information available.

Interactions with Drugs
HYPOGLYCEMIC DRUGS: Theoretically, damiana may interfere with hypoglycemic therapy (4).

Interactions with Foods
No interactions are known to occur, and there is no known reason to expect a clinically significant interaction with damiana.

Interactions with Lab Tests
No interactions are known to occur, and there is no known reason to expect a clinically significant interaction with damiana.

Interactions with Diseases or Conditions
DIABETES: Theoretically, may interfere with blood glucose control (4).

Dosage and Administration
ORAL: 2-4 grams dried leaf three times daily, or one cup tea (steep 2-4 grams dried leaf in 150 mL boiling water 5-10 minutes, strain) three times a day has been used (4). Liquid extract of damiana, 2-4 mL has also been used (4).

Comments
None.

DANDELION above ground parts

Also Known As
Blowball, Cankerwort, Common Dandelion, Dandelion Herb, Lion's Tooth, Pissenlit, Priest's Crown, Swine Snout, Taraxaci herba, Taraxacum, Wild Endive.
CAUTION: See separate listing for Dandelion entire plant.

Scientific Names
Taraxacum officinale, synonyms, Taraxacum vulgare, Leontodon taracum.
Family: Asteraceae/Compositae.

People Use This For
Orally, dandelion above ground parts are used for loss of appetite and dyspepsia, flatulence, and feelings of fullness (2). It is also used as a laxative, promoter of healthy circulation, skin toner, blood vessel cleanser and strengthener (5), for rheumatism, arthritic joints, and as a tonic (5).
For food uses, dandelion above ground parts are used in salad greens, soups, and wine (6).

Safety
LIKELY SAFE ...when used orally and appropriately for medicinal purposes (12). ...when used in amounts found in foods (12).
PREGNANCY AND LACTATION: Insufficient reliable information available; avoid using amounts greater than those in foods.

Effectiveness

There is insufficient reliable information available about the effectiveness of dandelion above ground parts.

Mechanism of Action

The sesquiterpene lactones are responsible for the diuretic effects and can contribute to dandelion's mild anti-inflammatory activity. Dandelion also contains an appetite-stimulating bitter identified as eudesmanolides, which was previously called taraxacin (6). Dandelion can have a slight laxative effect (5).

Adverse Reactions

Dandelion can cause contact dermatitis in sensitive individuals (6). Dandelion can cause an allergic reaction in individuals sensitive to the Asteraceae/Compositae family. Members of this family include ragweed, chrysanthemums, marigolds, daisies, and many other herbs.

Interactions with Herbs & Other Dietary Supplements

Insufficient reliable information available.

Interactions with Drugs

No interactions are known to occur, and there is no known reason to expect a clinically significant interaction with dandelion above ground parts.

Interactions with Foods

No interactions are known to occur, and there is no known reason to expect a clinically significant interaction with dandelion above ground parts.

Interactions with Lab Tests

No interactions are known to occur, and there is no known reason to expect a clinically significant interaction with dandelion above ground parts.

Interactions with Diseases or Conditions

OBSTRUCTION: The use of dandelion is contraindicated in patients with obstruction of bile ducts or the gallbladder. If gallstones are present, physician consultation is necessary before the use of dandelion (2).
OTHER: Dandelion is contraindicated in patients with puss in the pleural cavity or obstruction of the bowels (2).
CROSS-ALLERGENICITY: Can cause an allergic reaction in individuals sensitive to the Asteraceae/Compositae family. Members of this family include ragweed, chrysanthemums, marigolds, daisies, and many other herbs.

Dosage and Administration

ORAL: The typical dose of dandelion is 4-10 grams of the dried above ground parts three times daily. The common dose of the liquid extract (1:1 in 25% alcohol) is 4-10 mL three times daily (2).

Comments

Dandelions contain more vitamin A than carrots (6002). Avoid confusion with dandelion as a whole plant.

DANDELION entire plant

Also Known As

Blowball, Cankerwort, Common Dandelion, Lion's Tooth, Pissenlit, Priest's Crown, Swine Snout, Taraxacum, Wild Endive.
CAUTION: See separate listing for Dandelion above ground parts.

Scientific Names

Taraxacum officinale, synonyms Leontodon taraxacum, Taraxacum vulgare.
Family: Asteraceae or Compositae.

People Use This For

Orally, dandelion plant is used for gallstones, bile stimulation, muscle aches, low urine output, indigestion (4), constipation (4,9,11), flatulence, as a tonic (11), and in anti-smoking preparations (11).
In Chinese medicine, dandelion plant is used for treating breast cancer (6,11).
Traditionally, dandelion plant has been used for diabetes, rheumatic conditions, heartburn, bruises, gout, stiff joints, eczema, and cancer (11).

For food uses, dandelion leaves are added to salads. The roasted root and extract are used as coffee substitutes (11). In food manufacturing, dandelion plant is a flavoring component for foods as well as beverages (11).

Safety
LIKELY SAFE ...when consumed in amounts commonly found in foods. Dandelion has Generally Recognized Safe (GRAS) status in the US for food use with a maximum level of 0.014% for the fluid extract and 0.003% for the solid extract (11).
POSSIBLY SAFE ...when used orally and appropriately for medicinal purposes (12).
PREGNANCY: POSSIBLY SAFE ...when used in food amounts; avoid amounts greater than those found in foods (4).
LACTATION: Insufficient reliable information available; avoid using.

Effectiveness
POSSIBLY EFFECTIVE ...when used orally for disturbances in bile flow (2). ...when used orally for stimulating diuresis (2). ...when used orally in combination with uva ursi to prevent recurrent urinary tract infections (UTIs) (1932). A specific combination of dandelion root and uva ursi leaf extracts seems to help reduce the recurrence rate of UTIs in women (1932). In this combination uva ursi is used for its antibacterial properties and dandelion is used to increase urination. However, this combination should not be used long-term against recurrent UTI because uva ursi is not thought to be safe for extended use.
There is insufficient reliable information available about the effectiveness of dandelion for its other uses.

Mechanism of Action
The dandelion constituent taraxacin favorably effects digestion. The bitter constituents in dandelion root are responsible for increasing bile flow (7). The extracts demonstrate diuretic effects in animals and antitumor activity in vitro (4). The root extract has anti-inflammatory activity in animals (4). Hypoglycemic activity can also occur with the use of dandelion in animals (4). The sesquiterpene lactone constituents can be responsible for allergic reactions (4).

Adverse Reactions
The dandelion plant taken orally can cause gastric hyperacidity (2). Topically, the plant can cause contact dermatitis (4). It can cause an allergic reaction in individuals sensitive to the Asteraceae/Compositae family. Members of this family include ragweed, chrysanthemums, marigolds, daisies, and many other herbs.

Interactions with Herbs & Other Dietary Supplements
DIURETIC HERBS: Theoretically, dandelion can have additive effects with herbs having diuretic properties. Herbs thought to have diuretic properties include agrimony, artichoke, broom, buchu, burdock, celery, cornsilk, couch grass, elder, guaiacum, juniper, pokeroot, shepherd's purse, squill, uva ursi, and yarrow.
HYPOGLYCEMIC HERBS: Theoretically, dandelion can have additive effects with herbs having hypoglycemic effects.

Interactions with Drugs
DIURETICS, HYPOGLYCEMIC DRUGS: Theoretically, concomitant use of the dandelion plant can interfere with drug therapy (4).
LITHIUM (Eskalith, Lithobid): Theoretically, concomitant use can cause lithium toxicity due to sodium loss brought about by dandelion (19).
ACID-INHIBITING DRUGS: Theoretically, due to claims that dandelion increases stomach acid, it may interfere with antacids, sucralfate (Carafate), H-2 antagonists (Zantac, Pepcid, etc.), or proton-pump inhibitors (Prilosec, Prevacid) (19).
DIABETES THERAPY: Monitor blood glucose levels closely because dandelion can exhibit hypoglycemic effects (19).

Interactions with Foods
No interactions are known to occur, and there is no known reason to expect a clinically significant interaction with dandelion entire plant.

Interactions with Lab Tests
No interactions are known to occur, and there is no known reason to expect a clinically significant interaction with dandelion entire plant.

Interactions with Diseases or Conditions
Contraindicated in cases of acute gallbladder inflammation, bile duct obstruction, and intestinal blockage (2).
DIABETES: Monitor blood glucose levels closely because dandelion can exhibit hypoglycemic effects (19).
GALLSTONES: Professional evaluation is needed before the use of the dandelion plant in individuals

with gallstones (2).

CROSS-ALLERGENICITY: Can cause an allergic reaction in individuals sensitive to the Asteraceae/Compositae family. Members of this family include ragweed, chrysanthemums, marigolds, daisies, and many other herbs.

Dosage and Administration

ORAL: The typical dose of the dandelion leaf is 4-10 grams of the dried leaf or one cup of the tea three times daily (4). The tea is prepared by steeping 4-10 grams of the dried leaf in 150 mL boiling water for 5-10 minutes and then straining. The usual dose of the liquid leaf extract (1:1 in 25% alcohol) is 4-10 mL three times a day (4). The typical dose of the dandelion root is 2-8 grams of the dried root or one cup of the tea three times daily (4). The tea is prepared by steeping 3-8 grams of the dried root in 150 mL boiling water for 5-10 minutes and then straining (4). The usual dose of the root tincture (1:5 in 45% alcohol) is 5-10 mL three times daily (4). The common dose of the whole plant is as a tea, which is prepared by steeping 3-4 grams of the powdered whole plant in 150 mL boiling water for 5-10 minutes and then straining (2). The dose of the liquid extract of taraxacum is typically 2-8 mL (4). The juice of taraxacum is given as 4-8 mL (4).

Comments

The dandelion plant contains more vitamin A than carrots (6002). Avoid confusion with the above ground parts of dandelion.

DANSHEN

Also Known As

Ch'ih Shen, Dan Shen, Dan-Shen, Huang Ken, Pin-Ma Ts'ao, Red Rooted Sage, Red Sage, Salvia Root, Shu-Wei Ts'ao, Tan-Shen, Tzu Tan-Ken.
CAUTION: See separate listing for Sage.

Scientific Names

Salvia bowelyana; Salvia miltiorrhiza; Salvia przewalskii; Salvia przewalskii mandarinorum; Salvia yunnanensis. Family: Labiatae/Lamiaceae.

People Use This For

Orally, danshen is used for circulation problems, ischemic stroke, angina pectoris, and other cardiovascular diseases. It is also used orally for menstrual problems, chronic hepatitis, abdominal masses, insomnia due to palpitations and tight chest, acne, psoriasis, eczema, and other skin conditions. Danshen is also used orally to relieve bruising and to aid in wound healing.

Safety

POSSIBLY SAFE ...when used orally and appropriately (12).
PREGNANCY AND LACTATION: Insufficient reliable information available; avoid using.

Effectiveness

There is insufficient reliable information available about the effectiveness of danshen.

Mechanism of Action

The applicable part of danshen is the root. The constituents protocatechualdehyde and 3,4-dihydroxyphenyl-lactic acid may play a role in vasoactivity (6048). Other constituents in danshen, including salvianolic acid and tanshinone derivatives, seem to have anticoagulant properties (7162). Danshen appears to interfere with hemostasis by inhibiting platelet aggregation, interfering with extrinsic blood coagulation, mimicking the activity of antithrombin III, and promoting fibrinolytic activity (2237). Danshen and digoxin have some structural and pharmacological similarities. The tanshinone constituents of danshen have an aglycon ring that contains a common phenanthrene ring structure like digoxin and other cardiac glycosides (7311). Danshen is thought to work for cardiovascular diseases by dilating coronary arteries and affecting cardiac function. It appears to produce dose-dependent hypotensive effects, positive inotropic effects, and negative chronotropic effects (5884,6048,7311).

Adverse Reactions

Orally, danshen can cause pruritus, upset stomach, and reduced appetite (12).

Interactions with Herbs & Other Dietary Supplements

CARDIAC GLYCOSIDE-CONTAINING HERBS: Theoretically, using danshen with herbs containing cardiac glycosides might increase the risk cardiovascular effects and side effects such as arrhythmia. Danshen has structural and pharmacological similarities to cardiac glycosides (5884,6048,7311). Cardiac glycoside containing herbs include black hellebore, Canadian hemp roots, digitalis leaf, hedge mustard, figwort, lily of the valley roots, motherwort, oleander leaf, pheasant's eye plant, pleurisy root, squill bulb leaf scales, and strophanthus seeds.

HERBS WITH ANTICOAGULANT/ANTIPLATELET POTENTIAL: Taking danshen with herbs that affect platelet aggregation could theoretically increase the risk of bleeding in some people (7162). These herbs include angelica, anise, arnica, asafoetida, bogbean, boldo, capsicum, celery, chamomile, clove, fenugreek, feverfew, garlic, ginger, ginkgo, ginseng Panax, horse chestnut, horseradish, licorice, meadowsweet, prickly ash, onion, papain, passionflower, poplar, quassia, red clover, turmeric, wild carrot, wild lettuce, willow, and others.

METHYL SALICYLATE OIL: There is one case report of increased international normalized ratio (INR) with concomitant use of topical methyl salicylate oil, oral danshen, and warfarin (612).

Interactions with Drugs

ANTICOAGULANT, ANTIPLATELET DRUGS: Concomitant use might increase the risk of bleeding due to decreased platelet aggregation. Danshen has been reported to have antithrombotic effects (6048); avoid concomitant use. Some of these drugs include aspirin, clopidogrel (Plavix), dalteparin (Fragmin), enoxaparin (Lovenox), heparin, ticlopidine (Ticlid), warfarin (Coumadin), and others.

DIGOXIN (Lanoxin): Theoretically, using danshen with digoxin might increase cardiovascular effects and side effects such as arrhythmia. Danshen has structural and pharmacological similarities to cardiac glycosides (5884,6048,7311).

WARFARIN (Coumadin): Concomitant use increases the anticoagulant effects of warfarin and the risk of bleeding (611,612). There have been several case reports of increased international normalized ratio (INR) after concomitant use of danshen and warfarin (611,612,2237,5883,5884). Elevations in INR have occurred as early as 3-5 days after start of danshen. Danshen might increase the rate of absorption and decrease the elimination rate of warfarin (5884,6048). Avoid concomitant use.

Interactions with Foods

No interactions are known to occur, and there is no known reason to expect a clinically significant interaction with danshen.

Interactions with Lab Tests

DIGOXIN: Danshen can interfere with serum digoxin measurements. It falsely elevates serum digoxin concentrations when fluorescence polarization immunoassay (FPIA) is used. It falsely lowers digoxin concentrations when microparticle enzyme immunoassay (MEIA) is used. This interference is likely related to the structural similarity of danshen to digoxin. Danshen interference can be eliminated by monitoring the free digoxin concentration. This assay takes advantage of the stronger plasma protein binding of danshen than digoxin (7311).

Interactions with Diseases or Conditions

BLEEDING DISORDERS: Avoid using; theoretically, danshen may increase the risk of bleeding (2237).

Dosage and Administration

No typical dosage.

Comments

None.

DATE PALM

Also Known As

None.

Scientific Names

Phoenix dactylifera.
Family: Palmae.

People Use This For

In folk medicine, date palm is used for coughs and other respiratory symptoms (18).

Safety

There is insufficient reliable information available about the safety of the oral use of date palm fruit in amounts exceeding those found in foods.

Pregnancy and Lactation: Avoid using in amounts greater than those typically found in foods.

Effectiveness

There is insufficient reliable information available about the effectiveness of date palm.

Mechanism of Action

The applicable part of date palm is the fruit. There is insufficient reliable information available about the possible mechanism of action and active ingredients.

Adverse Reactions

None reported.

Interactions with Herbs & Other Dietary Supplements

Insufficient reliable information available.

Interactions with Drugs

No interactions are known to occur, and there is no known reason to expect a clinically significant interaction with date palm.

Interactions with Foods

No interactions are known to occur, and there is no known reason to expect a clinically significant interaction with date palm.

Interactions with Lab Tests

No interactions are known to occur, and there is no known reason to expect a clinically significant interaction with date palm.

Interactions with Diseases or Conditions

No interactions are known to occur, and there is no known reason to expect a clinically significant interaction with date palm.

Dosage and Administration

ORAL: Juice from the fruits is sun-dried to a "honey" and used orally [18].

Comments

There is very little scientific information about this product. Our staff is continually analyzing the available information on natural medicines and will add data here as it becomes available.

DEANOL

Also Known As

2-Dimethyl Aminoethanol, Deanol aceglumate, Deanol acetamidobenzoate, Deanol benzilate, Deanol bisorcate, Deanol cyclohexylpropionate, Deanol hemisuccinate, Deanol pidolate, Deanol tartrate, Dimethylaminoethanol, Dimethylethanolamine, DMAE.

Scientific Names

2-Dimethylaminoethanol.

People Use This For

Orally, deanol is used for treating attention deficit disorder (ADD) [1664,1669,1677,1678,1679], enhancing memory and mood, boosting cognitive function [1664], treating Alzheimer's disease [1665,1680,1681], increasing intelligence and physical energy, improving athletic performance [1666], preventing aging or liver spots, improving red blood cell function, improving muscle reflexes and increasing oxygen efficiency, extending life span [1667,1671], treating autism [1670], and treating tardive dyskinesia [1665,1672,1673,1674,1675,1676,1803].

Safety

POSSIBLY SAFE ...when used orally and appropriately [1668,1669,1671,1672,1673,1674,1675,1676,1677,1678] [1679,1680,1681,2706].
PREGNANCY AND LACTATION: Insufficient reliable information available; avoid using.

Effectiveness

POSSIBLY EFFECTIVE ...when used orally in combination with ginseng, vitamins, and minerals for improving exercise performance [1671]. The combination increases total work load and maximal oxygen consumption during exercise (1671).

LIKELY INEFFECTIVE ...when used orally for treating Alzheimer's disease (1680,1681). ...when used orally for treating tardive dyskinesia (1665,1672,1673,1674,1675,1676,1803,1804).

Clinical studies using deanol for treating attention deficit disorder have produced inconclusive results (1669,1677,1679). There is insufficient reliable information available about deanol for its other uses.

Mechanism of Action

Deanol is a precursor to choline and might enhance central acetylcholine formation (9,1669). Deanol has been formulated in a variety of salts and esters, including deanol aceglumate, deanol acetamidobenzoate, deanol bisorcate, deanol cyclohexylpropionate (cyprodenate, cyprodemanol), deanol hemisuccinate, deanol pidolate, and deanol tartrate (9). The hydrochloride salt of deanol benzilate (deanol diphenylglycoate, benzacine) has been included in antispasmodic preparations (9). Preliminary research with deanol has demonstrated no effect on life span (1682,1683).

Adverse Reactions

Orally, deanol can cause constipation, urticaria, headache, drowsiness, insomnia, overstimulation, vivid dreams, confusion, depression, blood pressure elevation, hypomania, an increase in schizophrenia symptoms, and orofacial and respiratory tardive dyskinesia (1674,1680,1684,1685,1686,2706).

Interactions with Herbs & Other Dietary Supplements

Insufficient reliable information available.

Interactions with Drugs

ANTICHOLINERGIC DRUGS: Theoretically, concomitant use might decrease the effect of drugs with anticholinergic activity, due to the potential cholinergic activity of deanol.

Interactions with Foods

No interactions are known to occur, and there is no known reason to expect a clinically significant interaction with deanol.

Interactions with Lab Tests

No interactions are known to occur, and there is no known reason to expect a clinically significant interaction with deanol.

Interactions with Diseases or Conditions

SCHIZOPHRENIA: Deanol can worsen schizophrenia symptoms (1674); avoid using in patients with schizophrenia.
DEPRESSION: Deanol might worsen depression. It is reported to cause depression as an adverse effect (1685).
CLONIC-TONIC SEIZURES: Deanol is relatively contraindicated in people with clonic-tonic seizure disorders (2706).

Dosage and Administration

ORAL: People typically begin with 100 mg per day and gradually increase to 500 mg per day (1664). Doses have ranged from 300 to 2000 mg per day in clinical studies (1669,1672,1673).

Comments

Deanol was previously marketed as the prescription drug, Deaner, by Riker Laboratories for the management of children with behavior problems and learning difficulties (1669,2706). According to 3M (Riker), Deaner was removed from the US market in 1983 because of insufficient evidence of efficacy (1895). Deanol is not an approved food additive in the US, nor is it an orphan drug, as some supplement advertising suggests (1805).

DEER VELVET

Also Known As

Cornu Cervi Parvum, Deer Antler, Deer Antler Velvet, Horns of Gold, Lu Rong, Nokyong, Rokujo, Velvet Antler, Velvet of Young Deer Horn.

Scientific Names

Cervus nippon; Cervus elaphus.

People Use This For

Orally, deer velvet is used to boost strength and endurance, for muscle aches and pains, to promote youthfulness, increase mental clarity, as an aphrodisiac, to treat sexual dysfunction (5507,5509), to boost estrogen and testosterone levels (5516), to counter the effects of stress, to improve immune system functioning, and to promote rapid recovery from illness (5508). It is used to improve fertility, for menstrual and menopause problems, to reduce hormone replacement therapy dose, to reduce cholesterol and high blood pressure, for liver and kidney disorders, to protect the liver from toxins, for migraines, asthma, indigestion, osteoporosis, and acne (5510,5511,5516). It is also used for its anticancer and anti-inflammatory properties, as a source of growth factors IGR-1 & IGF-2 (5508), to stimulate production and circulation of blood (5513), to increase blood count, and lower the level of free radicals (5516).

In herbal combinations, deer velvet is used to improve athletic performance, for an anti-aging effect, arthritis and osteoporosis, anemia, gonadotropic disorders, gynecological disorders, skin conditions, tissue and bone rejuvenation (5506). It is also used to increase mental capacity and performance, increase blood circulation to the brain, reduce early stages of muscular degeneration, to improve eyesight and hearing, to help PMS, impotence, and reduce stress (5506,5515).

In Chinese medicine, deer velvet is used to treat symptoms of impotence; cold extremities; soreness and weakness in the lower back and knees; leukorrhea; uterine bleeding; chronic skin ulcers; and frequent, copious, clear urination. It has also been used as a tonic for children with failure to thrive, mental retardation, learning disabilities, insufficient growth, or skeletal deformities including rickets (5501).

In Korean medicine, deer velvet is used at the onset of winter to ward off infections (5512).

Safety

There is insufficient reliable information available about the safety of deer velvet.

Pregnancy and Lactation: Insufficient reliable information available; avoid using.

Effectiveness

There is insufficient reliable information available about the effectiveness of deer velvet.

Mechanism of Action

By weight, deer velvet is approximately 50% amino acids (5502). Chondroitin sulfate is a major glycosaminoglycan (5517). Deer velvet also contains vitamin A, estrone and estradiol, sphingomyelin, ganglioside, some prostaglandins (5502), and epidermal growth factor (5518). The sex hormones estrone and estradiol can stimulate sexual function in females (5502). Gangliosides and sphingomyelins are thought to be involved with cell metabolism and growth (5514). Deer velvet is believed to stimulate the growth of body tissues, particularly the reticuloendothelial cells and leukocytes. It also appears to stimulate wound healing. Deer velvet seems to reduce fatigue by improving sleep and stimulating appetite. It is believed to improve health, especially in children and the elderly (5502). Preliminary evidence suggests that athletes taking deer velvet experience increased muscular strength and endurance in training. They also seem to recover faster from muscle tissue damage that results from exercise (5505). Other evidence suggests deer velvet extract might counteract certain effects of repeated doses of morphine, such as the development of tolerance (5503).

Adverse Reactions

None reported.

Interactions with Herbs & Other Dietary Supplements

Insufficient reliable information available.

Interactions with Drugs

MORPHINE: Some evidence suggests use of deer velvet might inhibit the development of tolerance to repeated doses of morphine (5503).

Interactions with Foods

No interactions are known to occur, and there is no known reason to expect a clinically significant interaction with deer velvet.

Interactions with Lab Tests

No interactions are known to occur, and there is no known reason to expect a clinically significant interaction with deer velvet.

Interactions with Diseases or Conditions

ESTROGEN-SENSITIVE CONDITIONS: Theoretically, women with conditions sensitive to estrogen, i.e. history of breast or cervical cancer, should avoid using deer velvet.

Dosage and Administration

ORAL: A typical dose of deer velvet powder for a protective effect is 400-600 mg (5512). A typical dose for treatment is 0.9-2.4 grams. Double-boiled, 3-4.5 grams are used. Alternately, it can be soaked in wine (5501) or prepared as a 20% tincture in wine (5502).

Comments

Deer velvet is the epidermis that covers the inner structure of the growing bone and cartilage that will become deer antlers (5504). The velvet is removed either by a veterinarian or a producer who has been accredited by a veterinarian. Tourniquets of rubber or plastic are placed around the pedicles to prevent bleeding (5514).

DEERTONGUE

Also Known As

Carolina Vanilla, Deer's Tongue, Hound's Tongue, Liatris, Vanilla Leaf, Vanilla Plant, Vanilla Trilisa, Wild Vanilla. CAUTION: See separate listing for Hound's Tongue (Cyonglossum officinale).

Scientific Names

Trilisa odoratissima, synonyms Carphephorus odoratissimus, Liatris odoratis.
Family: Asteraceae or Compositae.

People Use This For

Orally, deertongue is used for malaria (11).
In manufacturing, deertongue extracts are used to flavor tobacco, as a fragrance in cosmetics and soaps, and as a fixative in some products (11).

Safety

LIKELY UNSAFE ...when used orally for medicinal purposes. ...when used in amounts found in foods. The use of deertongue is not permitted in foods in the US (11).
PREGNANCY AND LACTATION: LIKELY UNSAFE ...when used orally due to potential effects of coumarin constituents; avoid using.

Effectiveness

There is insufficient reliable information available about the effectiveness of deertongue.

Mechanism of Action

The applicable part of deertongue is the dried leaf. Coumarin constituents are reported to cause liver injury and hemorrhage (11).

Adverse Reactions

Liver injury and hemorrhage are possible due to coumarin content (11). It can cause an allergic reaction in individuals sensitive to the Asteraceae/Compositae family. Members of this family include ragweed, chrysanthemums, marigolds, daisies, and many other herbs.

Interactions with Herbs & Other Dietary Supplements

HERBS THAT AFFECT BLOOD CLOTTING: Theoretically, may enhance effects of other herbs which affect blood clotting, including alfalfa, angelica, aniseed, arnica, asafoetida, celery, chamomile, clove, fenugreek, feverfew, fucus, garlic, ginger, Panax ginseng, horse chestnut, licorice, northern and southern prickly ash, quassia, and red clover (4).

Interactions with Drugs

ANTICOAGULANTS, ANTITHROMBOTICS: Theoretically, concomitant use may increase risk of bleeding.

Interactions with Foods

No interactions are known to occur, and there is no known reason to expect a clinically significant interaction with deertongue.

Interactions with Lab Tests

No interactions are known to occur, and there is no known reason to expect a clinically significant interaction with deertongue.

Interactions with Diseases or Conditions

BLOOD CLOTTING DISORDERS: Theoretically, may increase the risk of bleeding in these condition.
CROSS-ALLERGENICITY: Can cause an allergic reaction in individuals sensitive to the Asteraceae/Compositae family. Members of this family include ragweed, chrysanthemums, marigolds, daisies, and many other herbs.

Dosage and Administration

No typical dosage.

Comments

None.

DELPHINIUM

Also Known As

Delphinii Flos, Knight's Spur, Lark Heel, Lark's Claw, Lark's Toe, Larkspur, Ritterspornblüten, Staggerweed.

Scientific Names

Delphinium consolida.
Family: Ranunculaceae.

People Use This For

Orally, delphinium is used as an anthelmintic, diuretic, sedative, and appetite stimulant.
In herbal teas, delphinium is used as a brightening agent.

Safety

POSSIBLY SAFE ...when used in tea mixtures (less than 1%) (2).
LIKELY UNSAFE ...when used orally except in very low doses because it is toxic to the heart and respiratory systems (2,17).
PREGNANCY AND LACTATION: LIKELY UNSAFE ...when used orally; avoid using (2,17).

Effectiveness

There is insufficient reliable information available about the effectiveness of delphinium.

Mechanism of Action

The applicable part of delphinium is the flower. The alkaloid constituents are cardiotoxic and seem to be responsible for the curare-like, central paralysis of the respiratory system (2).

Adverse Reactions

Orally, delphinium can cause bradycardia, hypotension, cardiac arrest, and respiratory failure (2). Animal deaths from poisoning are common (18).

Interactions with Herbs & Other Dietary Supplements

Insufficient reliable information available.

Interactions with Drugs

No interactions are known to occur, and there is no known reason to expect a clinically significant interaction with delphinium.

Interactions with Foods

No interactions are known to occur, and there is no known reason to expect a clinically significant interaction with delphinium.

Interactions with Lab Tests

No interactions are known to occur, and there is no known reason to expect a clinically significant interaction with delphinium.

Interactions with Diseases or Conditions

No interactions are known to occur, and there is no known reason to expect a clinically significant interaction with delphinium.

Dosage and Administration

No typical dosage.

Comments

None.

DEVIL'S CLAW

Also Known As

Devils Claw, Devil's Claw Root, Grapple Plant, Griffe Du Diable, Harpagophyti Radix, Harpagophytum, Wood Spider.

Scientific Names

Harpagophytum procumbens.
Family: Pedaliaceae.

People Use This For

Orally, devil's claw is used for arteriosclerosis (5), osteoarthritis (4,5,6472), gout, myalgia, fibrositis, lumbago, pleuritic chest pain, rheumatic disease (4), gastrointestinal (GI) upset or dyspepsia (2,5), loss of appetite (2,11), and degenerative disorders of the locomotor system (2).
Topically, devil's claw is used for skin injuries and disorders (18).
Traditionally, devil's claw has also been used for kidney and bladder disease, and menstrual problems (5).

Safety

POSSIBLY SAFE ...when used orally and appropriately, short-term (4,5,8,12,6472). Devil's claw seems to be well tolerated when used daily for up to 16 weeks (6472).
There is insufficient reliable information available about the safety of topical or long-term oral use of devil's claw.
PREGNANCY: LIKELY UNSAFE ...when used orally. Devil's claw seems to have oxytocic effects (4); contraindicated.
LACTATION: Insufficient reliable information available; avoid using.

Effectiveness

POSSIBLY EFFECTIVE ...when used orally for osteoarthritis in conjunction with non-steroidal anti-inflammatory drugs (NSAIDs) (2,6472). Devil's claw seems to be comparable to diacerhein (a slow-acting drug for osteoarthritis; not available in the US) for improving pain in osteoarthritis of the hip and knee after 16 weeks of treatment. Patients taking devil's claw also seem to be able to decrease use of NSAIDs for pain relief (6472). This study used a specific powdered devil's claw root product (Harpadol) containing 2% of the constituent harpagoside (9.5 mg per capsule) and 3% total iridoid glycosides (14.5 mg per capsule) (6472).
There is insufficient reliable information available about the effectiveness of devil's claw for its other uses.

Mechanism of Action

The applicable part of devil's claw is the tuber. Devil's claw contains iridoid glycoside constituents, primarily harpagoside. People try devil's claw for osteoarthritis and other inflammatory conditions because iridoid glycoside constituents seem to have an anti-inflammatory effect (4,6472). There is also some evidence that devil's claw products might be cardioactive due to an harpagide constituent. Low doses seem to slow the heart rate and increase the strength of contraction. High doses seem to weaken heart contraction and coronary blood flow. Devil's claw extracts also seem to have hypoglycemic effects (4), stimulate production of stomach acid, increase bile production (19), and have weak antifungal activity (4).

Adverse Reactions

Orally, devil's claw is generally well tolerated. The most common adverse effect is diarrhea, occurring in approximately 8% of patients in one study (6472). There is also a report of throbbing frontal headache, tinnitus, anorexia, and loss of taste associated with devil's claw (4).

Interactions with Herbs & Other Dietary Supplements

Insufficient reliable information available.

Interactions with Drugs

ACID-INHIBITING DRUGS: Theoretically, due to claims that devil's claw increases stomach acid, it might interfere with antacids, H2 antagonists [cimetidine (Tagamet), famotidine (Pepcid), nizatidine (Axid), ranitidine (Zantac)], or proton pump inhibitors [lansoprazole (Prevacid), omeprazole (Prilosec), Pantoprazole (Pantoloc, Protonix),

Rabeprazole (Aciphex)] (19).

BLOOD PRESSURE THERAPY: Since devil's claw can affect blood pressure (4), it might adversely effect drug therapy for blood pressure; use cautiously.

CARDIAC DRUGS: Since devil's claw can affect heart rate and contractility of the heart (4), it might interfere with drug therapy for heart conditions such as congestive heart failure or cardiac arrhythmia; use cautiously.

DIABETES THERAPY: Devil's claw might decrease blood glucose levels (4) and have additive effects with medications used for diabetes. Monitor blood glucose levels closely. Dose adjustments may be necessary.

WARFARIN (Coumadin): Purpurea has occurred in a patient taking warfarin and devil's claw concurrently, suggesting over-anticoagulation (613). Devil's claw should be avoided or used cautiously in patients taking warfarin. Warfarin dose adjustments may be necessary.

Interactions with Foods

No interactions are known to occur, and there is no known reason to expect a clinically significant interaction with devil's claw.

Interactions with Lab Tests

No interactions are known to occur, and there is no known reason to expect a clinically significant interaction with devil's claw.

Interactions with Diseases or Conditions

PEPTIC ULCER DISEASE (PUD): Since devil's claw might increase gastric acid secretion (2,19), it might adversely effect people with gastric or duodenal ulcer; avoid using.

GALLSTONES: Devil's claw might increase bile production and adversely affect people with gallstones (2,8); avoid using.

DIABETES: Devil's claw might decrease blood glucose levels (4) and have additive effects with medications used for diabetes. Monitor blood glucose levels closely. Dose adjustments may be necessary.

CARDIAC DISORDERS, HYPERTENSION, HYPOTENSION: Since devil's claw can affect heart rate, contractility of the heart, and blood pressure (4), it might adversely effect people with cardiovascular conditions; use cautiously.

Dosage and Administration

ORAL: For stimulating appetite, the typical dose of devil's claw is 1.5 grams of the root per day (2). For osteoarthritis, one clinical study used a specific powdered devil's claw root product (Harpadol) dosed at 2.6 grams per day. This dose provided a total of 57 mg of the harpagoside constituent and 87 mg of total iridoid glycosides daily. Each 435 mg capsule contained 2% harpagoside (9.5 mg per capsule) and 3% total iridoid glycosides (14.5 mg per capsule) (6472). For other uses, the usual dose is from 1-4.5 grams of the root per day (2,6472). It is also used as a tea, consumed in three portions. The tea is prepared by steeping 4.5 grams of the root in 300 mL boiled water for 8 hours at room temperature and then straining (2).

Comments

The name for this plant is derived from the appearance of its fruit, which is covered with hooks meant to attach onto animals in order to spread the seeds (6002).

DEVIL'S CLUB

Also Known As

Cukilanarpak, Devils Club, Fatsia.

Scientific Names

Oplopanax horridus; Panax horridum; Echiopanax horridum.
Family: Araliaceae.

People Use This For

Orally, devil's club is used for arthritis, as a purgative, an emetic, for wound healing, fever, tuberculosis, stomach trouble, coughs, colds, and pneumonia (6).

Topically, it is used as a treatment for swollen glands, boils, sores, and skin infections. The ashes have been used to treat burns (4215).

Safety

POSSIBLY SAFE ...when used orally (12).

There is insufficient reliable information available about the safety of devil's club for its other uses.

PREGNANCY AND LACTATION: Insufficient reliable information available; avoid using.

Effectiveness

There is insufficient reliable information available about the effectiveness of devil's club.

Mechanism of Action

The applicable part of devil's club is the root bark. Several animal studies found no evidence of activity (6).

Adverse Reactions

Orally, devil's club may have a hypoglycemic effect (6).

Interactions with Herbs & Other Dietary Supplements

Insufficient reliable information available.

Interactions with Drugs

DIABETES THERAPY: Monitor blood glucose levels closely due to claims that devil's club has hypoglycemic effects (19).

Interactions with Foods

No interactions are known to occur, and there is no known reason to expect a clinically significant interaction with devil's club.

Interactions with Lab Tests

No interactions are known to occur, and there is no known reason to expect a clinically significant interaction with devil's club.

Interactions with Diseases or Conditions

DIABETES: Might reduce blood sugar levels. There are repeated anecdotal reports of hypoglycemic activity in individuals with diabetes (6).

Dosage and Administration

ORAL: People typically use 15 to 30 drops of the extract mixed in warm water three times daily between meals. The alcohol content is 55 to 65% (6006).

TOPICAL: The inner bark is baked slowly until it is very dry, then rubbed between the hands until broken and soft. The pulp is placed on the affected area to draw out infection (4215).

Comments

Devil's club is a common plant in southeastern Alaska. It is considered the most important medicinal and magical plant of the Yakutat Tlingit. Both the shaman and the layman chew the stem bark (with the thorns removed) for its effects as an emetic, a purgative, and a general cure all (4215).

DHA (DOCOSAHEXAENOIC ACID)

Also Known As

DHA, Docosahexaenoic, Fish Oil Fatty Acid, N-3 Fatty Acid, Neuromins, Omega 3 Fatty Acid, Omega Fatty Acid, Omega-3 Fatty Acid, W-3 Fatty Acid.

CAUTION: See separate listings for Cod Liver Oil, EPA (eicosapentaenoic acid), and Fish Oils.

Scientific Names

Docosahexaenoic acid.

People Use This For

Orally, docosahexanoic acid (DHA) is used as a supplement for preterm infants (1045), as an ingredient in infant formula (5941), during the first four months of life to enhance mental development of infants (5941), for reducing aggressive behavior in stressed individuals (1043), for preventing depression, reducing symptoms of dementia, and enhancing vision (1048).

In combination with eicosapentaenoic acid (EPA), DHA is used for a variety of conditions, including the prevention and reversal of heart disease, decreasing ectopic ventricular beats, asthma, cancer, painful menses, hay fever, lung diseases, lupus erythematosus, lupus nephritis, and IgA nephropathy (507). EPA and DHA are also used in combination for migraine headache prophylaxis in adolescents (5097), atopic dermatitis, Behcet's syndrome, hyperlipidemia, hypertension, psoriasis, Raynaud's syndrome, rheumatoid arthritis, bipolar disorder, and ulcerative colitis (9). DHA is also used in combination with arachidonic acid during the first four to six months of life to enhance mental development of infants (424,5941).

Safety

LIKELY SAFE ...when used orally and appropriately (9,945,1016).
POSSIBLY UNSAFE ...when used orally in high doses. Doses greater than 3 grams daily might decrease blood coagulation and increase the risk of bleeding (1313).
CHILDREN: POSSIBLY SAFE ...when used orally and appropriately as a supplement to infant formula (5941). ...when used orally and appropriately in combination with arachidonic acid as a supplement to infant formula (424,5941).
PREGNANCY AND LACTATION: Insufficient reliable information available; avoid using.

Effectiveness

POSSIBLY EFFECTIVE ...when used orally for reducing aggressive behavior in stressed individuals (1043). ...when given orally to preterm infants for improving visual attention later in childhood (1045). ...when used orally to improve night vision in children with dyslexia. Dyslexic children who received fish oils rich in DHA developed significantly better dark adaptation when compared with controls (5708). ...when used orally in combination with evening primrose oil, thyme oil, and vitamin E (Efalex) to improve movement disorders in children with dyspraxia. One small clinical trial has shown that this combination significantly decreases movement disorders as determined by objective measures (5708).
POSSIBLY INEFFECTIVE ...when used as a supplement in infant formula for improving cognitive and mental development or growth up to 18 months of age (424).
There is insufficient reliable information available about the effectiveness of DHA for its other uses.

Mechanism of Action

DHA is a long chain n-3 polyunsaturated fatty acid that competes with arachidonic acid for inclusion in cyclo-oxygenase and lipoxygenase pathways (9). Long-chain polyunsaturated fatty acids make up a third of all lipids in the brain's grey matter (425). DHA decreases blood viscosity and increases red blood cell deformability (9). DHA can be converted into EPA (eicosapentaenoic acid) in humans (1044). Pure DHA reduces serum triglycerides in adults (1014,6143), and increases serum HDL2 cholesterol, LDL cholesterol, LDL particle size and fasting insulin, but has no effect on total cholesterol or fasting glucose in mildly hypercholesterolemic men (6143). DHA plays a key role in the structural development of retinal, neural and synaptic membranes, and is thought to be important for normal neural function (424,425). DHA is present in human breast milk but not in standard infant formulas. Formula-fed infants have lower plasma and cerebral cortex DHA levels than breast milk-fed infants; the clinical significance of this, if any, is unknown. Animals who are deficient in n-3 fatty acids (such as DHA) develop learning and vision disturbances. These disturbances do not occur when the parent fatty acid, linolenic acid, is adequately supplied (424).

Adverse Reactions

Adverse reactions have not been reported for DHA alone. However, for fish oils containing EPA and DHA, side effects can include fishy taste, belching (507), nosebleeds (9), nausea, and loose stools (9). Three people with pre-existing familial adenomatous polyposis were diagnosed with malignant lesions during the course of long-term fish oil use (999). High doses of fish oils might also decrease blood coagulation and increase the risk of bleeding (1313).

Interactions with Herbs & Other Dietary Supplements

HERBS WITH ANTICOAGULANT/ANTIPLATELET POTENTIAL: Concomitant use of herbs that have coumarin constituents or affect platelet aggregation could theoretically increase the risk of bleeding in some people. These herbs include: angelica, anise, arnica, asafoetida, bogbean, boldo, capsicum, celery, chamomile, clove, danshen, fenugreek, feverfew, garlic, ginger, ginkgo, Panax ginseng, horse chestnut, horseradish, licorice, meadowsweet, prickly ash, onion, papain, passionflower, poplar, quassia, red clover, turmeric, wild carrot, wild lettuce, willow, and others (4,19).

Interactions with Drugs

ANTICOAGULANTS/ANTIPLATELET DRUGS: Theoretically, concomitant use of DHA with anticoagulant or antiplatelet drugs, including aspirin, can increase risk of bleeding (9,507).

Interactions with Foods

No interactions are known to occur, and there is no known reason to expect a clinically significant interaction with DHA.

Interactions with Lab Tests

CHOLESTEROL: DHA can increase serum HDL2 cholesterol concentrations, LDL cholesterol concentrations and LDL particle size and test results in mildly hypercholesterolemic patients (6143).
INSULIN: DHA can increase fasting insulin concentrations and test results in mildly hypercholesterolemic patients (6143).
INTERNATIONAL NORMALIZED RATIO (INR), PROTHROMBIN TIME (PT): Doses greater than 3 grams per day might decrease blood coagulation, increase INR and PT, and increase the risk of bleeding (1313).
PULMONARY FUNCTION TESTS: DHA might cause a decline in pulmonary function tests in aspirin-sensitive individuals (507).
TRIGLYCERIDES: DHA can reduce serum triglyceride concentrations and test results in patients with hypercholesterolemic (6143).

Interactions with Diseases or Conditions

ASPIRIN-SENSITIVE INDIVIDUALS: Fish oils and other omega-3 fatty acids can lower pulmonary function tests in some aspirin sensitive patients (507).
DIABETES: Fish oils containing EPA and DHA can interfere with blood glucose control (9). Monitor blood glucose levels closely. Dose adjustments may be necessary.
HYPERTENSION: Fish oils including DHA can lower blood pressure and might have additive effects in patients with high blood pressure who are treated with antihypertensives (1001,1020,1030,1033).

Dosage and Administration

ORAL: DHA is usually administered with EPA (eicosapentaenoic acid) in fish oil. A wide range of doses have been used. The typical amount is 5 grams of fish oil containing 169-563 mg of EPA and 72-312 mg of DHA per day (9,507). As a supplement in infant formula, 0.32% DHA has been used (424). For improving dark adaptation of vision in dyslexic individuals, a daily oral fish oil dose containing 480 mg DHA has been used (5708). For improving movement disorders in children with dyspraxia, a daily oral tuna fish oil dose containing 480 mg DHA, combined with 35 mg arachidonic acid, 96 mg gamma-alpha linoleic acid from evening primrose oil, 24 mg thyme oil, and 80 mg vitamin E (Efalex) has been used (5708).

Comments

Preliminary evidence suggests that DHA might prevent or reverse some of the effects of cystic fibrosis. In mice with cystic fibrosis, the lungs, pancreas and intestine show high levels of arachidonic acid. This means the organs are at risk for inflammation and mucus secretion. DHA, which regulates the arachidonic acid and the cellular fluid balance, is significantly reduced. When researchers restored a more normal balance of DHA and arachidonic acid, they were able to prevent lung and intestine abnormalities. It's too soon to know if this might work in humans, but it looks promising and trials are planned (309). Avoid confusing DHA with EPA (eicosapentaenoic acid).

DHEA

Also Known As

Dehydroepiandrosterone, GL701, Prasterone.
CAUTION: See separate listing for 7-Keto-DHEA.

Scientific Names

Dehydroepiandrosterone; Prasterone.

People Use This For

Orally, DHEA is used for slowing or reversing aging; promoting weight loss; stimulating immunity; treating systemic lupus erythematosus (SLE); treating multiple sclerosis; and increasing strength, energy, and muscle mass. It is also used orally for improving cognitive function; slowing the progression of Parkinson's disease and Alzheimer's disease; treating erectile dysfunction; depression; and preventing heart disease, breast cancer, and diabetes. For people with HIV disease, DHEA is used to improve depressed mood and fatigue. It is also used orally by women who have adrenal insufficiency to improve well-being and sexuality.
Vaginally, DHEA is used in postmenopausal women for vaginal atrophy and increasing bone mineral density.
Intravenously, DHEA is being investigated for improving skin graft-site healing.

Safety

POSSIBLY SAFE ...when used orally and appropriately. DHEA has been used safely in men and women in several studies. Most studies have been small and lasted from a few weeks to 6 months (793,2133,3231,4249,4251,4252,4253,4254,4255). Three studies have used oral DHEA safely for up to 12 months (1295,2113,6446). ...when used intravaginally and

appropriately. DHEA has been safely used intravaginally by postmenopausal women in a study lasting 12 months (4242).
POSSIBLY UNSAFE ...when used orally long-term or in high doses. There is concern that long-term use or use of amounts that cause higher than normal physiological DHEA levels might increase the risk of prostate cancer (2111,2116), breast cancer or other hormone-sensitive cancers (4256,6445). In some cases, 50-100 mg daily can produce slightly higher than normal physiological DHEA levels (4249,4251).
PREGNANCY AND LACTATION: POSSIBLY UNSAFE ...when used orally. DHEA can cause higher than normal androgen levels (2133,4249,4251,4253) which might adversely effect pregnancy or a nursing infant.

Effectiveness

POSSIBLY EFFECTIVE ...when taken orally for depression and dysthymia (3270,3892,4233). ...when taken orally for sexual dysfunction in men. Men with erectile dysfunction treated for 24 weeks have improved erectile function, orgasmic function, sexual desire, and overall sexual satisfaction (793). ...when taken orally as replacement therapy by women with adrenal insufficiency to improve well-being and sexuality (3231). ...when taken orally as an adjunctive treatment for systemic lupus erythematosus (SLE). Use of DHEA in conjunction with conventional treatment helps reduce disease activity, frequency of flare-ups, and decreases corticosteroid doses needed (1295,2113,2114,2136,6447,6068). DHEA also seems to improve bone mineral density in SLE patients being treated with high dose corticosteroids (6068,6097,6447). ...when used orally for improving skin in elderly men and women. DHEA seems to increase epidermal thickness, sebum production, skin hydration, and decrease facial skin pigmentation in elderly men and women (6446). ...when used vaginally to treat vaginal atrophy and increase bone density in postmenopausal women (4242).
POSSIBLY INEFFECTIVE ...when taken orally to improve cognitive function (3892,3893).
There is insufficient reliable information available about the effectiveness of DHEA for its other uses. However, researchers report that DHEA might be beneficial for autologous skin grafting. Intravenously administered DHEA might improve the rate of re-epithelialization patients undergoing autologous skin grafting for burn wound closure (1399). More evidence is needed to rate DHEA for this use.

Mechanism of Action

DHEA is endogenously produced in the adrenal glands and liver of humans. DHEA and its sulfate ester, dehydroepiandrosterone sulfate (DHEA-S), are interconvertible. DHEA is initially converted to DHEA-S, which is considered the storage form of DHEA (5874). Peripheral tissues and target organs convert DHEA-S back to DHEA, which is then metabolized to androstenedione, the major human precursor to androgens and estrogens (3232,6098). DHEA and DHEA-S levels are higher in men than in women, and naturally decline with age in both sexes (4248,6013,6014). Because of this decline, some suggest that replacing DHEA with supplementation might prevent some of the diseases and conditions associated with aging (6446).

DHEA supplementation seems to change the circulating androgen/estrogen ratio in a gender-specific manner. That is, there appears to be significant increases in the levels of estrogens, but not as much increase in the amount of androgens, in the blood of men given DHEA. Conversely, women given DHEA develop significant increases in the levels of androgens, but not as much increase in estrogen levels (6010,6011). For example, in elderly men, administration of DHEA 50 mg daily for 12 months, increases DHEA-S to levels comparable with young adults. Testosterone levels don't significantly increase, but estradiol levels do significantly increase. In elderly women, administration of the same dose initially increases DHEA-S levels above those of young adults, but after 12 months of use, levels fall back to the young adult range. Testosterone levels increase to levels comparable with young adults and estradiol increases, but not as high as levels in young adults (6446). In both men and women, extended use seems to result in increased elimination of DHEA-S. After continuous oral administration of DHEA, DHEA-S levels seem to significantly increase after 6 months of use, but after 12 months of use, DHEA-S levels fall back some; however, DHEA-S levels remain higher than before supplementation began (6446). This suggests that the human body might have an adaptive mechanism, which limits the accumulation of DHEA-S and androgenic compounds (6446). The androgen-like or estrogen-like effects might be responsible for some of the benefits of DHEA (2115).

Some researchers speculate that DHEA might have similar therapeutic benefits as estrogen-progestin hormone replacement therapy (HRT). Some of DHEA's effects in postmenopausal women are similar to HRT including increasing estradiol, estrone, osteocalcin, growth hormone, and insulin-like growth factor 1 (IGF-1) (7327); however, unlike HRT, DHEA also increases androstenedione and testosterone.

Although DHEA and DHEA-S declines with age, there does not appear to be an association between prematurely low DHEA-S levels and increased risk for diseases commonly seen with old age (6013,6014). It has also not been possible to demonstrate any correlation between DHEA-S levels and cognitive status or cognitive decline in elderly men (5874); however, endogenous DHEA levels are affected by certain activities and disease states. For example, exercising at maximal and submaximal levels and consuming food naturally increase the endogenous DHEA level.

DHEA is decreased in cases of anorexia nervosa, depression, end-stage renal disease, type 2 diabetes mellitus, schizophrenia, and patients with systemic lupus erythematosus (SLE) (4248,5872). Because decreased serum DHEA-S levels have been reported in men under age 60 with erectile dysfunction (5868), DHEA supplements are being tried for erectile dysfunction. DHEA-S levels are also decreased in men with congestive heart failure, in proportion to its severity, possibly due to effects of oxidative stress on electron transport required for DHEA synthesis (5871). DHEA is tried for SLE because endogenous DHEA levels are decreased in SLE patients. It is thought that a high-estrogen, low-androgen state may contribute to the presence or activity of SLE, and that an increase in the level of androgens could help patients with this disease. DHEA has also been reported to correct defective interleukin-2 production in T-lymphocytes from people with SLE (5872,6098). The effects of DHEA on stimulation of bone formation in SLE patients has been attributed to the androgenic properties of DHEA (6447); however, a reduction in corticosteroid dose that DHEA permits might also be responsible for this effect.

In addition to the adrenals, DHEA is also produced in the central nervous system and is concentrated in the limbic regions, and may function as an excitatory neuroregulator, antagonizing gamma-aminobutyric acid transmission (5870). DHEA has been used for HIV disease because of some reports of modest antiviral effects of DHEA, possible immunomodulating effects, and the finding that DHEA decreases with declining CD4 lymphocyte counts (3865,3866,3867); however, DHEA does not affect CD4 counts, even at doses as high as 2.25 grams per day (3865).

Endogenous DHEA is increased in some individuals taking diltiazem and alprazolam. Danazol, insulin, and morphine decrease DHEA (4248). Exogenous glucocorticoids also seem to suppress DHEA production. In vivo, glucocorticoids and DHEA are secreted concomitantly. Some researchers speculate that concurrent administration of DHEA with exogenous glucocorticoids might help combat the adverse effects of glucocorticoids (7328).

Male sex hormones appear to have a harmful effect on organ function after trauma hemorrhage. DHEA attenuates depressed cardiac and hepatic function secondary to trauma hemorrhage in male rats, possibly due to estrogenic activity (6101). Estrogenic activity, together with nitric oxide release, may also be responsible for an antiatherosclerotic effect of DHEA observed in animal models (5869).

Adverse Reactions

Orally, DHEA can cause acne, hair loss, hirsutism, voice deepening, insulin resistance, decreased HDL cholesterol, changes in menstrual pattern, hepatic dysfunction, abdominal pain, and hypertension (2111,2116,6098). When used in very high doses it can cause mild insomnia (4248). In individuals with HIV, it is associated with nasal congestion, fatigue, and headache (4248). Doses up to 2.25 grams taken for four months were well tolerated with no serious adverse effects in people with mild HIV (3865). There are three cases of mania in men taking DHEA (5870,6102,7023). This has occurred in people with no history of psychiatric disease (6102) and in those with a history of mania (5870) and bipolar disorder (7023). Mania can occur with doses ranging from 50-300 mg per day. However, mania may not occur for 2-6 months after starting DHEA (6102,7023).

Interactions with Herbs & Other Dietary Supplements

SOY: Theoretically, soy might decrease the effects of DHEA. Soy consumption seems to decrease serum DHEA-S levels in premenopausal women (6445).

Interactions with Drugs

GLUCOCORTICOIDS: Glucocorticoid drugs can suppress endogenous DHEA production (7328). Some glucocorticoid drugs include dexamethasone (Decadron), hydrocortisone (Cortef), methylprednisolone (Medrol), and prednisone (Deltasone).

TRIAZOLAM (Halcion): DHEA can increase plasma triazolam concentrations. Administration of DHEA 200 mg/day for two weeks was shown to inhibit cytochrome P450 3A (CYP3A) metabolism of triazolam and is due to DHEA-S, rather than DHEA (1389).

OTHER DRUGS: DHEA may potentially increase levels of drugs metabolized through cytochrome P450 3A (CYP 3A) due to enzyme inhibition (1389); however, the clinical significance of these potential interactions is not known. Drugs that are substrates of CYP3A include alfentanil (Alfenta), alprazolam (Xanax), amitriptyline (Elavil), amiodarone (Cordarone), buspirone (Buspar), cerivastatin (Baycol), citalopram (Celexa), felodipine (Plendil), fexofenadine (Allegra), itraconazole (Sporanox), ketoconazole (Nizoral), lansoprazole (Prevacid), losartan (Cozaar), lovastatin (Mevacor), midazolam (Versed), ondansetron (Zofran), prednisone (Deltasone, Orasone), sertraline (Zoloft), sibutramine (Meridia), sildenafil (Viagra), simvastatin (Zocor), verapamil (Calan, Covera-HS, Isoptin), and many others.

Interactions with Foods

VEGETARIAN DIET: Pure vegetarians and lactovegetarians have higher serum DHEA levels than non-vegetarians. However, this difference is not apparent in postmenopausal vegetarians (6445). The clinical significance of these findings is not known.

Interactions with Lab Tests

TRIAZOLAM: DHEA can increase plasma triazolam concentrations and test results. DHEA-S, the activated form of DHEA, inhibits triazolam metabolism (1389).

Interactions with Diseases or Conditions

DIABETES: DHEA can increase insulin resistance or sensitivity. Monitor blood glucose level closely (2112,4249,4250).
HORMONE SENSITIVE CANCERS/CONDITIONS: Because DHEA has estrogenic effects (6445), there is some concern that it might increase the risk of breast cancer and other hormone sensitive conditions. DHEA should be avoided in patients with hormone sensitive conditions such as breast, uterine, and ovarian cancer, and endometriosis and uterine fibroids.
LIVER DYSFUNCTION: DHEA can exacerbate liver dysfunction (2111,2116).
MOOD DISORDERS: There is some concern that patients with a history of depression and bipolar disorder might be at an increased risk of psychiatric adverse events associated with DHEA. DHEA has been found to cause hypomania, mania, irritability, sexual inappropriateness and psychosis in some patients with suspected mood disorders (4233,5870,7023).

Dosage and Administration

ORAL: In postmenopausal women and in men, doses of 25-50 mg daily have commonly been used (4249,4251,4252,4254,4255). For depression, clinical trials have used doses of 30-90 mg daily either alone or in combination with conventional antidepressant therapy (3270,4233). For replacement therapy in individuals with adrenal suppression, clinical trials have used 50 mg, either given daily or as a single dose (2133,3231,4253,6012). For systemic lupus erythematosus (SLE), the typical dose is 200 mg per day as an adjunct to conventional medical treatment (2113,2114), but doses up to 600 mg per day have been used (5872). For erectile dysfunction, 50 mg per day has been used (793).
VAGINAL: A 10% cream applied daily has been used (4242).

Comments

DHEA is manufactured from constituents of wild yam extract. The wild yam constituents, such as diosgenin, are converted in the laboratory to DHEA. However, diosgenin from ingested wild yam cannot be converted to DHEA in the human body, as has been reported. So, taking wild yam extract will not increase DHEA levels in humans (2112). People interested in taking DHEA should avoid wild yam products labeled as "natural DHEA."
DHEA is banned by the National Basketball Association (NBA) (5041).

DIBENCOZIDE

Also Known As

Adenosylcobalamin, Cobalamin Enzyme, Cobamamide, Co-enzyme B-12, Coenzyme B-12.
CAUTION: See separate listing for Vitamin B12.

Scientific Names

None.

People Use This For

Orally or sublingually, dibencozide is used as a preparation to stimulate protein metabolism (5132); increase muscle mass and strength (5133); increase mental concentration (5135), and to treat depression, anxiety, and panic attacks (5134).

Safety

LIKELY SAFE …when used orally. There are no reports of toxicity from excessive amounts of cobalamins (4921,5133). When tissue binding sites are saturated, excessive dibencozide is excreted in urine and bile (5133).
PREGNANCY AND LACTATION: Insufficient reliable information available; avoid using.

Effectiveness

LIKELY INEFFECTIVE …when used orally or sublingually for uses in individuals without vitamin B12 deficiency (5133,5137).
There is insufficient reliable information available about the effectiveness of dibencozide for its other uses.

Mechanism of Action

The term vitamin B12 refers to all cobalamins that are active as coenzymes in humans, including dibencozide (adenosylcobalamin), methylcobalamin, and hydroxocobalamin (5133,4921). Cyanocobalamin, the most stable of the cobalamins, is metabolized in the body to an active coenzyme (4921,5133). Vitamin B12 is involved in fat, protein, and carbohydrate metabolism. It is active in all cells, particularly in the bone marrow, CNS, and GI tract (4921). Produced almost exclusively by microorganisms, vitamin B12 is found in animal protein and in some legumes in small amounts (4921). Adults who eat meat in their diet usually ingest more than the RDA of 2.4 mcg (5138). Vitamin B12 is conserved by enterohepatic circulation. Deficiency takes about three years to develop in people with normal absorption (4921). No benefit has been shown from taking large quantities of cobalamins unless an individual is deficient (4921).

Adverse Reactions
None reported.

Interactions with Herbs & Other Dietary Supplements
ALCOHOL: Excessive alcohol intake lasting longer than two weeks can decrease vitamin B12 absorption from the gastrointestinal tract (14,15).

Interactions with Drugs
AMINOGLYCOSIDES: Aminoglycoside antibiotics can decrease vitamin B12 absorption from the gastrointestinal tract (14,15).
CHLORAMPHENICOL: May impair hematopoietic response to vitamin B12 (15).
COLCHICINE: Colchicine can decrease vitamin B12 absorption from the gastrointestinal tract (14,15).
ACID INHIBITING DRUGS : Cimetidine (Tagamet), ranitidine (Zantac), omeprazole (Prilosec) can decrease vitamin B12 absorption from the gastrointestinal tract (14,15).
POTASSIUM: Extended-release potassium preparations can decrease vitamin B12 absorption from the gastrointestinal tract (14,15).
AMINOSALICYLIC ACID: Aminosalicylic acid and its salts can decrease vitamin B12 absorption from the gastrointestinal tract (14,15).
ANTICONVULSANTS: Phenytoin (Dilantin), phenobarbital, and primidone (Mysoline) can decrease vitamin B12 absorption from the gastrointestinal tract (14,15).
VITAMIN C: Large amounts of vitamin C can destroy vitamin B12 and should not be taken within an hour of oral vitamin B12 (15).

Interactions with Foods
No interactions are known to occur, and there is no known reason to expect a clinically significant interaction with dibencozide.

Interactions with Lab Tests
No interactions are known to occur, and there is no known reason to expect a clinically significant interaction with dibencozide.

Interactions with Diseases or Conditions
GI CONDITIONS: Ileal disease or resection, intrinsic factor deficiency can cause vitamin B12 malabsorption (4921).

Dosage and Administration
No typical dosage.

Comments
Cyanocobalamin and hydroxocobalamin are the only forms of vitamin B12 stable for storage (5139).

DIGITALIS

Also Known As
Dead Man's Bells, Digitalis purpurea, Fairy Cap, Fairy Finger, Foxglove, Lady's Thimble, Lion's Mouth, Purple Foxglove, Scotch Mercury, Throatwort, Witch's Bells, Wolly Foxglove.

Scientific Names
Digitalis purpurea; Digitalis lanata.
Family: Scrophulariaceae.

People Use This For
Orally, digitalis is used for congestive heart failure and atrial fibrillation or flutter.
Historically, digitalis has been used for diureses in edema, asthma, as an emetic, for epilepsy, tuberculosis, constipation, headache, spasm, and wound and burn healing (6,7,400).

Safety
UNSAFE ...when used orally for self-medication. Use requires monitoring by a medical professional (12). Can cause heart arrhythmias and death (17). All parts of the plant are toxic (501). US regulations require labeling to inform consumers that digitalis is inappropriate for use as an anti-obesity agent (12). Canadian regulations prohibit digitalis in foods (12). Deaths have occurred when digitalis was mistaken for comfrey (501).

CHILDREN: LIKELY UNSAFE ...sucking on the flowers, ingesting seeds, or parts of the leaves has caused children to become ill (6).
PREGNANCY AND LACTATION: UNSAFE ...when used orally for self-medication; avoid using (12).

Effectiveness

LIKELY EFFECTIVE ...when used orally for atrial fibrillation or flutter, congestive heart failure, and removal of edema associated with heart failure (6).
There is insufficient reliable information available about the effectiveness of digitalis for its other uses.

Mechanism of Action

The applicable part of digitalis is the leaf. Digitalis contains varied glycosides, primarily glycoside A and glycoside B, which are precursors to digitoxin and gitoxin, respectively. Digitalis lanata contains lanatosides A,B,C,D, and E that yield digitoxin, gitoxin, digoxin, digitalin, and gitaloxin, respectively (6). Cardiac glycosides increase cardiac contractility, decrease heart rate and reduce AV node conduction, stabilize the heart rate, increase cardiac output, and relieve pulmonary congestion and peripheral edema (6).

Adverse Reactions

Chronic use of digitalis can lead to intoxication symptoms including visual halos, yellow-green vision, and GI upset (6). Acute poisoning of digitalis includes GI upset, contracted pupils, blurred vision, strong slow pulse, nausea, vomiting, dizziness, excessive urination, fatigue, muscle weakness and tremors, stupor, confusion, convulsions, atrial arrhythmias, AV block, and death (6,159,501).

Interactions with Herbs & Other Dietary Supplements

CARDIAC GLYCOSIDE-CONTAINING HERBS: Contraindicated; concomitant use can increase the risk of cardiac glycoside toxicity. Cardiac glycoside containing herbs, including black hellebore, Canadian hemp roots, digitalis leaf, hedge mustard, figwort, lily of the valley roots, motherwort, oleander leaf, pheasant's eye plant, pleurisy root, squill bulb leaf scales, and strophanthus seeds (2,18,19,500).
OTHER CARDIOACTIVE HERBS: Avoid concomitant use with other cardioactive herbs due to unpredictability of effects and adverse effects. Other cardioactive herbs include: calamus, cereus, cola, coltsfoot, devil's claw, European mistletoe, fenugreek, fumitory, ginger, Panax ginseng, hawthorn, white horehound, mate, parsley, quassia, scotch broom flower, shepherd's purse, and wild carrot (4).
STIMULANT LAXATIVE HERBS: Theoretically, overuse/misuse of stimulant laxatives with cardiac glycoside-containing herbs increases the risk of cardiac toxicity due to potassium depletion. Stimulant laxative herbs include: aloe dried leaf sap, blue flag rhizome, alder buckthorn, European buckthorn, butternut bark, cascara bark, castor oil, colocynth fruit pulp, gamboge bark exudate, jalap root, black root, manna bark exudate, podophyllum root, rhubarb root, senna leaves and pods, wild cucumber fruit (Ecballium elaterium), and yellow dock root (19).
LICORICE/HORSETAIL: Theoretically, overuse/misuse of licorice rhizome or horsetail plant with cardiac glycoside-containing herbs increases the risk of toxicity due to potassium depletion (19).

Interactions with Drugs

DIGOXIN (Lanoxin): Contraindicated; therapeutic duplication increases risk of cardiac glycoside toxicity (2).
CARDIOACTIVE DRUGS: Theoretically, concomitant use can increase the risk of cardiac toxicity (152).
STIMULANT LAXATIVES: Theoretically, overuse/misuse can increase risk of cardiac glycoside toxicity due to potassium depletion (2,506).
POTASSIUM DEPLETING DIURETICS, QUININE: Can increase the risk of digitalis toxicity (2,506).
TETRACYCLINES and MACROLIDE ANTIBIOTICS (erythromycin-like drugs): Theoretically, concomitant use might increase risk of cardiac glycoside toxicity (152,17).

Interactions with Foods

No interactions are known to occur, and there is no known reason to expect a clinically significant interaction with digitalis.

Interactions with Lab Tests

ELECTROCARDIOGRAM (ECG): Digitalis can normalize arrhythmias, and ECG readings, associated with atrial fibrillation or flutter in patients with congestive heart failure (15).

Interactions with Diseases or Conditions

HEART DISEASE: Self-use contraindicated; requires diagnosis, treatment, and monitoring (515,150).
RENAL DISEASE: May reduce excretion of digitalis, increasing the potential for toxicity (150).

Dosage and Administration
No typical dosage.

Comments
Digitalis is unsafe for self-medication. Digitalis lanata is the major source of digoxin in the US (6).

DILL above ground parts

Also Known As
American Dill, Anethi herba, Dill Herb, Dill Weed, Dillweed, Dilly, European Dill.
CAUTION: See separate listing for Dill seed.

Scientific Names
Anetheum graveolens.
Family: Apiaceae or Umbelliferae.

People Use This For
Orally, dill above ground parts are used for diseases and disorders of the gastrointestinal tract, kidney, and urinary tract. Dill is also used for spasms (2), flatulence, and sleep disorders (11).
In foods, dill and dill oil are used as flavoring agents (11).
In manufacturing, dill oil is used as a fragrance component in cosmetics, soaps, and perfumes (11).

Safety
LIKELY SAFE ...when consumed in amounts commonly found in foods. It has Generally Recognized as Safe (GRAS) status for food use in the US (11).
POSSIBLY SAFE ...when used orally and appropriately for medicinal purposes (12).
PREGNANCY AND LACTATION: Insufficient reliable information available; avoid using amounts greater than those found in foods.

Effectiveness
There is insufficient reliable information available about the effectiveness of dill above ground parts.

Mechanism of Action
An aqueous dill extract administered intravenously lowers blood pressure, dilates blood vessels, stimulates respiration, and slows heart rate in animals (11). The dill leaf is reported to be a rich source of beta carotene, iron, and potassium (19).

Adverse Reactions
Topically, photodermatosis is possible after contact with juice from the freshly harvested plants (18,19). Dill can also cause contact dermatitis (19).

Interactions with Herbs & Other Dietary Supplements
Insufficient reliable information available.

Interactions with Drugs
No interactions are known to occur, and there is no known reason to expect a clinically significant interaction with dill above ground parts.

Interactions with Foods
No interactions are known to occur, and there is no known reason to expect a clinically significant interaction with dill above ground parts.

Interactions with Lab Tests
No interactions are known to occur, and there is no known reason to expect a clinically significant interaction with dill above ground parts.

Interactions with Diseases or Conditions
CROSS REACTIVITY: The use of dill above ground parts can cause allergic reactions in people with allergies to the carrot family plants, which include asafoetida, caraway, celery, coriander, and fennel (19).

Dosage and Administration

ORAL: The common dose of the dried fruits is 1 to 4 grams three times daily (6002). The usual dose of the dill oil is 0.05-2 mL three times daily (6002).

Comments

Dill oil (dillweed oil, dill herb oil) is distilled from freshly harvested dill (Anetheum graveolens). During the Middle Ages, people sometimes used dill as a charm against witchcraft and enchantments (6002). Avoid confusion with dill seed.

DILL seed

Also Known As

American Dill, Anethi fructus, Dilly, European Dill.
CAUTION: See separate listing for Dill above ground parts.

Scientific Names

Anetheum graveolens.
Family: Umbelliferae/Apiaceae.

People Use This For

Orally, dill seed is used for loss of appetite, fever and colds, cough, bronchitis, tendency towards infection, liver and gallbladder complaints (18), and as a digestive aid (11).
Topically, dill seed is used for mouth and throat inflammation (18).
Historically, dill seed has been used for flatulence, hemorrhoids, bronchial asthma, neuralgias, renal colic, dysuria, genital ulcers, and dysmenorrhea (11).
In foods, dill seed is used as a culinary spice (11).

Safety

LIKELY SAFE ...when dill seed is used orally in amounts found in foods. It has Generally Recognized as Safe (GRAS) status in the US (11).
POSSIBLY SAFE ...when used orally and appropriately for medicinal purposes (12).
PREGNANCY: LIKELY SAFE ...when used in food amounts. LIKELY UNSAFE ...when used in amounts greater than those found in foods because dill seed might stimulate menstrual flow (19).
LACTATION: Insufficient reliable information available; avoid amounts greater than those found in foods.

Effectiveness

There is insufficient reliable information available about the effectiveness of dill seed.

Mechanism of Action

Dill seed contains an essential oil rich in carvone (2). Dill seed has antibacterial, antispasmodic, sedative, and diuretic effects. They also think it stimulates lactation (2,11) and is a urinary irritant (19). Dill seed oil has spasmolytic effects on smooth muscle (11). Some evidence suggests an intravenous emulsion might increase respiratory volume and lower blood pressure (2,11).

Adverse Reactions

Topically, photodermatosis is possible after contact with juice from freshly harvested plants (18,19).

Interactions with Herbs & Other Dietary Supplements

Insufficient reliable information available.

Interactions with Drugs

No interactions are known to occur, and there is no known reason to expect a clinically significant interaction with dill seed.

Interactions with Foods

No interactions are known to occur, and there is no known reason to expect a clinically significant interaction with dill seed.

Interactions with Lab Tests

No interactions are known to occur, and there is no known reason to expect a clinically significant interaction with dill seed.

Interactions with Diseases or Conditions

URINARY TRACT INFLAMMATION: Avoid due to claims that dill seed is a urinary irritant (19).

Dosage and Administration

ORAL: People typically use 3 grams of dill seed daily. People also add 2 teaspoons bruised seeds to a cup of boiling water and drink up to 3 cups per day. As a tincture, dill is taken up to 1 teaspoon up to 3 times daily. As a breath freshener, up to 1 teaspoon is chewed. Oil of dill is taken 100 to 300 mg (2 to 6 drops) daily (5250,5252).

Comments

Avoid confusion with dill above ground parts. Dill seed oil is distilled from the crushed, dried fruit (seed) of the dill plant (Anetheum graveolens).

DIMETHYLGLYCINE

Also Known As

Dimethyl Glycine, (Dimethylamino)acetic Acid, DMG, N,N-dimethylaminoacetic Acid, N-methylsarcosine. CAUTION: Dimethylglycine is one of the compounds found in pangamic acid formulations. See separate listing for Pangamic Acid.

Scientific Names

N,N-dimethylglycine.

People Use This For

Orally, dimethylglycine is used to improve speech and behavior in autism (5817); for attention deficit disorder (ADD) (5818); to treat epilepsy; to reduce physical and environmental stress; to improve oxygen utilization; to enhance liver function; to optimize athletic performance; to improve neurological function; for anti-inflammatory and anti-aging effects; to improve immune response and enhance anti-viral, anti-bacterial and anti-tumor defenses; and to treat tumors, chronic fatigue syndrome, allergies, respiratory disorders, alcoholism, and drug addiction (5816). It is also used orally to lower blood cholesterol and triglycerides, and to help normalize blood pressure and blood glucose (5815).

Safety

POSSIBLY UNSAFE ...when used orally. Dimethylglycine may react with nitrites in the gastrointestinal tract to form the potent carcinogen, dimethylnitrosamine (5,5827), although this has been questioned (5830).
PREGNANCY AND LACTATION: POSSIBLY UNSAFE ...when used orally; avoid using.

Effectiveness

POSSIBLY EFFECTIVE ...when used orally for enhancing humoral and cell mediated immune responses (14).
LIKELY INEFFECTIVE ...when used orally for improving athletic performance (14).
POSSIBLY INEFFECTIVE ...when used orally for treatment of epilepsy (14,5823) and autism (5819).
There is insufficient reliable information about the effectiveness of dimethylglycine for its other uses.

Mechanism of Action

Dimethylglycine is the dimethylated form of the amino acid glycine, but it only exists in the body for seconds at a time, and in very small quantities (14,5827). It is formed from betaine during methylation of homocysteine (5828). The effects of supplemental doses in excess of naturally occurring amounts are unknown (14).
Preliminary evidence suggests that dimethylglycine enhances humoral and cell-mediated immune responses in humans and some, but not all, animals (5820,5822,5825). Dimethylglycine has been reported to have anticonvulsant effects in animals (5828), including antagonizing strychnine- and penicillin-induced seizures (5824,5829). A single case report described a dramatic improvement in a person with mixed complex partial and grand mal seizures (5826), but a small study in people with generalized or akinetic/myoclonic seizures found no benefit with dimethylglycine 300 to 600 mg per day (5823). Several small studies in athletes have not found any benefit of dimethylglycine on athletic performance (5821), including maximal treadmill performance, as measured by maximal and recovery heart rates, treadmill time, and pre-test and post-test blood glucose and lactate levels (2645). A small study using low-dose dimethylglycine did not find any benefit in children with autism (5819).

Adverse Reactions

Dimethylglycine may react with nitrites in the gastrointestinal tract to form carcinogenic substances (5,5827).

Interactions with Herbs & Other Dietary Supplements

Insufficient reliable information available.

Interactions with Drugs

No interactions are known to occur, and there is no known reason to expect a clinically significant interaction with dimethylglycine.

Interactions with Foods

No interactions are known to occur, and there is no known reason to expect a clinically significant interaction with dimethylglycine.

Interactions with Lab Tests

No interactions are known to occur, and there is no known reason to expect a clinically significant interaction with dimethylglycine.

Interactions with Diseases or Conditions

No interactions are known to occur, and there is no known reason to expect a clinically significant interaction with dimethylglycine.

Dosage and Administration

ORAL: As a dietary supplement, divided doses of 125 to 1000 mg per day sublingual dimethylglycine have been recommended (5816).

Comments

Dimethylglycine is found in low levels in such foods as cereal grains, beans, and liver (5816). In the 1980s, a federal court in Chicago forbade interstate sale of a brand of dimethylglycine stating that it was an unsafe food additive (5827).

DIOSMIN

Also Known As

Citrus Bioflavonoid, Citrus Bioflavonoids, Diosmetin.
CAUTION: See separate listings for Quercetin, Rue, and Rutin.

Scientific Names

Diosmetin, Diosmin.

People Use This For

Orally, diosmin is used for treating acute internal hemorrhoids (4861,4898,4900), preventing relapse of acute internal hemorrhoids (4861), treating varicose veins, venous stasis (4861,4898), subconjunctival and retinal hemorrhage, and gingival bleeding (4898). Diosmin has also been used to protect against liver toxicity (4954).

Safety

POSSIBLY SAFE ...when used orally and appropriately, short-term. Diosmin seems to be safe when used for up to 3 months (4861,4898).
There is insufficient reliable information available about the safety of diosmin when used for greater than 3 months.
PREGNANCY AND LACTATION: Insufficient reliable information available; avoid using.

Effectiveness

POSSIBLY EFFECTIVE ...when used orally in combination with hesperidin for internal hemorrhoids. The combination of diosmin 1350 mg plus hesperidin 150 mg twice daily for 4 days followed by diosmin 900 mg and hesperidin 100 mg twice daily for 3 days seems to significantly improve signs and symptoms of internal hemorrhoids. The combination can stop acute bleeding in up to 92% of patients after 4 days of treatment. It can also reduce symptoms such as anal discomfort, pain, discharge, and local lesions. Subjective symptoms can be relieved within 2 days of treatment. The combination also seems to reduce the duration and intensity of hemorrhoidal flare-ups (4861,4900). Some clinicians use diosmin in lower doses and in combination with bulk laxatives instead of hesperidin. Diosmin 600 mg three times daily for 4 days, then 300 mg twice daily for 10 more days plus the bulk laxative psyllium 11 grams daily does seem to slightly help after 4 days of treatment (4898). But this combination does not seem to be as effective as the higher dose of diosmin plus hesperidin combination. ...when used orally in combination with hesperidin to prevent relapse in patients with internal hemorrhoids. Maintenance use of diosmin 450 mg plus hesperidin 50 mg twice daily for 3 months in patients following acute treatment for hemorrhoids seems to significantly decrease the relapse rate (4861).

Clinical trials have used specific brand name formulations of diosmin (Daflon 500 and Daflon, Les Laboratoires Servier, France). Each tablet of Daflon 500 contains a micronized formulation of diosmin 450 mg and hesperidin 50 mg extracted from rutaceae species. Each tablet of Daflon contains only diosmin 150 mg.

There is insufficient reliable information available about the effectiveness of diosmin for its other uses.

Mechanism of Action

Diosmin is one of over 4,000 flavonoids found in plants (4919,4959,5006). Diosmin is in a class of flavonoids primarily derived from citrus fruits and is known as a citrus bioflavonoid. It is closely related to other citrus bioflavonoids such as quercetin, rutin, and hesperidin. Diosmin alone, or in combination with other citrus bioflavonoids, is most often used for vascular conditions such as hemorrhoids and varicose veins. Diosmin seems to work by improving venous tone, reducing stasis, restoring normal capillary permeability, and improving lymphatic drainage. Diosmin might improve venous tone and reduce stasis by improving vasculature response to adrenergic stimulation. Diosmin's anti-inflammatory effects seem to help restore normal capillary permeability. Diosmin inhibits phosphodiesterase and increases intracellular cyclic adenosine monophosphate (cAMP), which causes decreased production of inflammatory prostaglandins E2 and F2 and thromboxane B2. Diosmin can also reduce the generation of free radicals (4861,4898,4900,4954). Some diosmin preparations use a micronized formulation. The smaller particle size seems to help increase absorption (4900). There is preliminary evidence that a diosmin metabolite, diosmetin, might also be hepatoprotective. Diosmetin might have direct antioxidant effects, increase glutathione (GSH) levels, and decrease lipid peroxidation (4954).

Adverse Reactions

Orally, diosmin can cause gastrointestinal side effects, including abdominal pain, diarrhea, and gastritis. Headache can also occur in some patients (4861,4898,4900).

Interactions with Herbs & Other Dietary Supplements

Insufficient reliable information available.

Interactions with Drugs

No interactions are known to occur, and there is no known reason to expect a clinically significant interaction with diosmin.

Interactions with Foods

No interactions are known to occur, and there is no known reason to expect a clinically significant interaction with diosmin.

Interactions with Lab Tests

No interactions are known to occur, and there is no known reason to expect a clinically significant interaction with diosmin.

Interactions with Diseases or Conditions

No interactions are known to occur, and there is no known reason to expect a clinically significant interaction with diosmin.

Dosage and Administration

ORAL: For the treatment of internal hemorrhoids, diosmin 1350 mg plus hesperidin 150 mg twice daily for 4 days followed by diosmin 900 mg and hesperidin 100 mg twice daily for 3 days has been used (4861,4900). Some clinicians also try diosmin 600 mg three times daily for 4 days, followed by 300 mg twice daily for 10 days, in combination with psyllium 11 grams daily (4898). However, this lower diosmin dose does not seem to be as effective. For prevention of relapse internal hemorrhoids diosmin 450 mg plus hesperidin 50 mg twice daily for 3 months of therapy has been used (4861).

Comments

None.

DIVI-DIVI

Also Known As
Divi Divi, Nichol Seeds, Nikkar Nuts.

Scientific Names
Caesalpinia bonducella.
Family: Leguminosae or Fabaceae.

People Use This For
Orally, divi-divi is used for fever and diabetes (18).

Safety
There is insufficient reliable information available about the safety of divi-divi.
Pregnancy and Lactation: Insufficient reliable information available; avoid using.

Effectiveness
There is insufficient reliable information available about the effectiveness of divi-divi.

Mechanism of Action
The applicable part of divi-divi is the seed. Divi-divi is stated to have antipyretic effects (18). In normal rats, ethanolic and aqueous seed extracts exhibited hypoglycemic effects, with the aqueous extract showing a longer duration of action (3834). In rats with experimentally-induced diabetes, both extracts produced antihyperglycemic effects. However, only the aqueous extract demonstrated an effect in reducing cholesterol and triglyceride levels (3834).

Adverse Reactions
None reported.

Interactions with Herbs & Other Dietary Supplements
Insufficient reliable information available.

Interactions with Drugs
No interactions are known to occur, and there is no known reason to expect a clinically significant interaction with divi-divi.

Interactions with Foods
No interactions are known to occur, and there is no known reason to expect a clinically significant interaction with divi-divi.

Interactions with Lab Tests
No interactions are known to occur, and there is no known reason to expect a clinically significant interaction with divi-divi.

Interactions with Diseases or Conditions
No interactions are known to occur, and there is no known reason to expect a clinically significant interaction with divi-divi.

Dosage and Administration
No typical dosage.

Comments
The seed is ground or roasted (18). There is very little scientific information about this product. Our staff is continually analyzing the available information on natural medicines and will add data here as it becomes available.

DIVINER'S SAGE

Also Known As

Divine Mexican Mint, Diviner's Mint, Diviners Sage, Divinorin, Divinorin A, Herb-of-the-Virgin, Herba de María, Hierba de la Virgen, Hojas de la Pastora, La Hembra, Leaves of the Virgin Shepherdess, Mexican Sage, Mexican Sage Incense, Pipiltzintzintli, Sadi, Salvia, Salvinorin, Salvinorin A, Sage of the Seers, Ska Maria, Ska Maria Pastora, Yerba de Maria.
CAUTION: See separate listings for Boneset, Clary Sage, Danshen, German Sarsaparilla, Purple Loosestrife, Sage, Spearmint, and Wood Sage.

Scientific Names

Salvia divinorum.
Family: Labiatae or Lamiaceae.

People Use This For

Orally and by inhalation, diviner's sage is used as a hallucinogen.
Orally, diviner's sage is used for diarrhea, headache, rheumatism, abdominal distension, and as a tonic and end-of-life remedy. It is also used orally to regulate urination and defecation.

Safety

There is insufficient reliable information available about the safety of diviner's sage.

Effectiveness

There is insufficient reliable information available about the effectiveness of diviner's sage.

Mechanism of Action

The applicable part of diviner's sage is the leaf. The leaves are chewed and swallowed, made into an infusion (tea), or smoked for hallucinogenic effects. Unlike other hallucinogens, the active constituent of diviner's sage is not an alkaloid. It contains the diterpene salvinorin A, which is also called divinorin A (7350,7351,7352). Salvinorin A is the most potent hallucinogen known. It causes hallucinations in doses of 200 to 500 mcg when vaporized and inhaled (7351). Salvinorin A is absorbed by the oral mucosa when chewed, but is inactivated by the gastrointestinal system when swallowed. It also seems to be absorbed and produce pharmacological activity when inhaled (7352). The onset of hallucinogenic activity occurs within 5 to 10 minutes when chewed and within 30 seconds when inhaled. The effects last about an hour when chewed and 20 to 30 minutes via inhalation (7352). However, the duration of effect appears to be dose-dependent (7351). It's not clear how diviner's sage constituents cause hallucinations. Diviner's sage does not appear to affect receptor sites such as serotonin, dopamine, or monoamine oxidase that are often affected by other hallucinogens (7352).

Adverse Reactions

Orally, diviner's sage can cause nausea, dizziness, and slurred speech. It can also cause confusion and hallucinations (7350,7351).

Interactions with Herbs & Other Dietary Supplements

Insufficient reliable information available.

Interactions with Drugs

No interactions are known to occur, and there is no known reason to expect a clinically significant interaction with diviner's sage.

Interactions with Foods

No interactions are known to occur, and there is no known reason to expect a clinically significant interaction with diviner's sage.

Interactions with Lab Tests

No interactions are known to occur, and there is no known reason to expect a clinically significant interaction with diviner's sage.

Interactions with Diseases or Conditions

No interactions are known to occur, and there is no known reason to expect a clinically significant interaction with diviner's sage.

Dosage and Administration
No typical dosage.

Comments
Diviner's sage has been used for centuries in religious ceremonies by the Mazatec Indians, a native people who live in Oaxaca, Mexico. The Mazatecs believe it is an incarnation of the Virgin Mary (7350). Diviner's sage is widely available on the Internet. Its possession and use is legal in the US, but the Drug Enforcement Agency (DEA) is reviewing it for possible controlled substance regulation (7349).

DMSO (DIMETHYLSULFOXIDE)

Also Known As
Dimethyl Sulfoxide, Dimethyl Sulphoxide, Dimethylis sulfoxidum, Methyl sulphoxide, NSC-763, SQ-9453, Sulphinybismethane.

Scientific Names
Dimethylsulfoxide.

People Use This For
Orally, DMSO is used for the management of amyloidosis and related symptoms (14,6304).

Topically, DMSO is used to decrease pain and speed the healing of wounds and burns (6322). DMSO is also used topically to treat headache, tic doloreaux, cataracts, glaucoma, retinal degeneration, bunions, calluses, fungus toenails, asthma, to flatten raised keloid scars (6322), and for cancer (6327). It is also used topically to prevent tissue necrosis after extravasation with antineoplastic agents (14,5698,5699), to treat symptoms associated with acute musculoskeletal injuries and inflammation (14,6304,6305,6322), osteoarthritis (6304), rheumatoid arthritis (6304,6313), scleroderma (6304,6313,6314), and amyloidosis (14). It is also used topically for reducing skin flap ischemia following surgery (14,6307), complex regional pain syndromes (6317), as a vehicle in combination with idoxuridine to decrease the development of inflammatory reactions and lesions associated with herpes zoster infection (14,6308,6309,6311,6312), and decrease the pain associated with postherpetic neuralgia (14,6310,6311,6312).

Intravenously, DMSO is used to manage symptoms associated with secondary amyloidosis (6304) and to lower intracranial hypertension (6300,6301). DMSO is administered by intravesical instillation to treat symptoms of interstitial cystitis such as urinary frequency, urgency, nocturia and suprapubic pain (14,5692,5694). It is also used by intravesical instillation to treat symptoms associated with chronic inflammatory bladder disease (5695,5696,5697). DMSO is infused alternatively with methyl-tert-butyl ether and a buffer solution of EDTA and sodium deoxycholate through a nasobiliary catheter for the dissolution of bile duct stones (6315,6316). DMSO is used for the cryopreservation of hematopoietic stem cells to be infused and transplanted at a later date (6318,6319).

In manufacturing, DMSO is used as an industrial solvent for herbicides, fungicides, antibiotics, and plant hormones (6326).

Safety
LIKELY SAFE ... when used by intravesical instillation (14,5692,5694,5695,5696,5697). An aqueous 50% solution of DMSO is FDA approved for intravesical use in the treatment of interstitial cystitis (14,5692,5694).

POSSIBLY UNSAFE ...when used topically (14). It has been reported that industrial grade DMSO is being used topically for self-treatment of several disease conditions. Industrial grade DMSO is not of the same quality of that used for drug research purposes since it may contain impurities. DMSO readily penetrates the skin and enhances the absorption of impurities and other substances, which may be hazardous to health (14,5691,6326).

PREGNANCY AND LACTATION: Insufficient reliable information available; avoid using.

Effectiveness
EFFECTIVE ...when used by intravesical instillation for treatment of intersitial cystitis (14,5692,5694). This is the only indication for DMSO in humans that has been approved by the FDA (14,5691).

POSSIBLY EFFECTIVE ...when used topically for the prevention of tissue necrosis after extravasation with antineoplastic agents (5698,5699). ...when used topically for symptoms associated with osteoarthritis (6303,6304). ...when used topically for symptoms associated with rheumatoid arthritis (14,6303,6304). ...when used topically for the treatment of amyloidosis (14,6304,6306). ...when used topically to reduce skin flap ischemia after surgery (14,6307). ...when used topically as a vehicle in combination with idoxuridine (40% idoxuridine in DMSO) to reduce the number lesions and decrease the inflammatory reaction associated with herpes zoster infection (14,6308,6309,6311,6312). ...when used topically as a vehicle in combination with idoxuridine (40% idoxuridine in DMSO) to decrease the pain associated with postherpetic neuralgia (6310,6311,6312). Trigeminal herpes zoster seems most responsive (14,6312). ...when used intravenously to lower intracranial pressure (6300,6301) ...when used by intravesical instillation for treatment of symptoms associated with chronic inflammatory bladder disease (5695,5696,5697). ...when infused alternatively with methyl-tert-butyl ether and a buffer solution of EDTA and sodium deoxycholate through a nasobiliary catheter for the dissolution of bile duct stones (6315,6316).

POSSIBLY INEFFECTIVE ...when used topically to treat symptoms of scleroderma such as open ulcers (14,6313). Neither 2% DMSO or 70% DMSO have been found to be better than placebo (6313). There have been conflicting open studies with DMSO (6304,6313,6314).

LIKELY INEFFECTIVE ...when used topically to treat patients with cancer (6327).

There is insufficient reliable information available about the effectiveness of DMSO for its other uses.

Mechanism of Action

DMSO is a highly polar substance and is used in industry as a solvent for many organic and inorganic substances (14). It also interacts with other substances such as proteins, carbohydrates, lipids, water and ethanol (6331). DMSO easily penetrates the skin (6326), is widely distributed in body fluids and tissues after administration and is metabolized to dimethyl sulfone and dimethyl sulfide (14). Dimethyl sulfide is thought to cause the distinctive body odor commonly associated with DMSO use (14). Concentrations of DMSO of 80-100% penetrate more effectively than concentrations less than 70%. This is thought to be due to DMSOs ability to exchange and interchange water in cell membranes (6326) and its interference with and conformational changes of cell membrane phospholipids (6331,6330). DMSO facilitates topical penetration of many medications (6326,6330) depending on the medication used (14). It has been used to aid the penetration and enhance the effects of idoxuridine (9). The exact mechanism is unknown (6330). Most of the effects of DMSO have been demonstrated in laboratory studies (6326,6330). DMSO has been found to decrease skin adhesions by possibly dissolving only collagen fibers and not elastic fibers (14,6330). DMSO also stabilizes lysosomal membranes (14) and causes vasodilation (6330). DMSO has free hydroxyl radical scavenging properties (6326,6330) that are thought to be responsible for DMSOs anti-inflammatory, cryopreservative, cryoprotective, anti-ischemic properties and possible radioprotective activity (6326). DMSO also demonstrates antimicrobial activity (6326,6330) which is possibly due to a loss of the RNA conformational structure that is necessary for protein synthesis (6330). Cardiovascular and vasoactive effects of DMSO such as lowered vagal threshold and increased response to nerve and muscle stimulation on skeletal, smooth, and cardiac muscle are thought to be due to its inhibition of anticholinesterase activity (6326,6330). In vitro, DMSO appears to protect against ischemic injury by increasing levels of prostaglandin-E1 (PGE1) which in turn increases cyclic-AMP levels and reduces platelet aggregation. DMSO also appears to protect against ischemic injury by decreasing the secretion of vasoactive substances such as fibrinogen and thromboxane A2 from platelets that can cause vasoconstriction, vasospasm or obstruction of a vessel (6302,6330). There is evidence DMSO can decrease cerebral edema (14) and antagonizes the release of calcium from cells and platelets to possibly prevent arteriolar-wall muscle spasms (6302,6330). Evidence also suggests DMSO slows the conduction of C-type nerve fibers which may be responsible for its analgesic effect (6329). DMSO causes histamine release from mast cells which is thought to be responsible for the eosinophilia (6524) and the hypersensitivity reactions associated with its use (14). Evidence suggests DMSO affects sensory nerves during bladder instillations by stimulating bladder afferent pathways, causing release of nitrogen oxide from afferent neurons (9,5693). Nitrogen oxide is thought to act as a peripheral neurotransmitter to control lower urinary tract function (5693). Other data suggests DMSO could help antineoplastic agents cross the blood-brain barrier (6327) but results show DMSO does not significantly increase uptake of any compounds (6330). There is evidence DMSO may induce differentiation of tumor cells present in frozen cryopreserved marrow (6328). Preliminary evidence suggests DMSO may be effective in treating duodenal ulceration in patients infected with Helicobacter pylori (6321).

Adverse Reactions

Topically, DMSO can cause sedation, headache, dizziness, drowsiness, nausea, vomiting, diarrhea, constipation, anorexia, and eosinophilia (14). Topical DMSO can also cause erythema, pruritus, burning, blistering, drying and scaling skin, dry or sore throat, cough, dry nasal passages, dyspnea, worsening of bronchial asthma, and an influenza-like syndrome (14). Intravenously, DMSO can cause facial flushing, fluid overload, hypernatremia, electrolyte disturbances, diuresis (14), increased serum osmolality (14,6325), eosinophilia, hemolysis, hematuria, weakness, confusion, lethargy, disorientation, agitation, dysarthria, hypoactive reflexes, decreased consciousness, jaundice, vasodilation, hypotension, chest pains, sinus tachycardia, increased liver enzymes, increased serum bilirubin, increased serum creatinine, and encephalopathy (14).

Intravesical instillation of DMSO may cause a chemical cystitis (14), and bladder discomfort and spasm (9). Infusion of hematopoietic stem cells cryopreserved with DMSO can cause pyrexia, rigors (14), nausea, vomiting (14,6318), hypertension with tachycardia, bradycardia, chest tightness, fever, chills, abdominal cramps, ventricular extrasystoles (6320), electrolyte disturbances, and decreased hemoglobin (14). Garlic-like taste, breath and garlic-onion-oyster body odor may be experienced with all routes of administration (14). Hypersensitivity reactions may be experienced by all routes of administration, rarely causing anaphylaxis (14). Transient photophobia and color vision disturbances have been reported (14). DMSO is absorbed via all routes of administration (14) and theoretically could cause any of the above adverse effects regardless of route. Headache and transient eye, nose, and throat irritations have been reported by individuals caring for patients with DMSO body odor (6323).

Interactions with Herbs & Other Dietary Supplements

Insufficient reliable information available.

Interactions with Drugs

SULINDAC (Clinoril): Peripheral neuropathy has been reported with the combined use of oral sulindac and topical DMSO (14). In vitro and animal studies have shown DMSO inhibits enzyme reduction activity of sulindac (14).
ALL MEDICATIONS: DMSO may potentiate the effects of other medications given concomitantly (14). Evidence from animal studies suggest DMSO may potentiate the action of numerous medications (6330).

Interactions with Foods

No interactions are known to occur, and there is not known reason to expect a clinically significant interaction with DMSO.

Interactions with Lab Tests

No interactions are known to occur, and there is not known reason to expect a clinically significant interaction with DMSO.

Interactions with Diseases or Conditions

ASTHMA: DMSO can potentially worsen symptoms associated with asthma (14).
CARDIAC CONDITIONS: DMSO causes vasodilation, diuresis and can also cause fluid overload, hypernatremia, electrolyte disturbances, chest pains and sinus tachycardia (14). Theoretically, DMSO may worsen existing cardiac diseases and conditions.
DIABETES: Topical administration of DMSO has been reported to potentiate the effects of insulin (6326); use with caution. Increased monitoring of blood glucose and insulin dosing adjustments may be necessary.
HEMATOLOGIC CONDITIONS: A complete blood count is recommended every 6 months (14). Eosinophilia with topical use and dose-related hemolysis with intravenous use has been reported (14); use with caution.
INTRACRANIAL PRESSURE: Fluid overload, electrolyte disturbances (14) and extreme serum hyperosmolality have been reported in patients with elevated intracranial pressure who were treated with DMSO (6325).
LIVER CONDITIONS: Liver function tests are recommended every 6 months (14). Hepatotoxicity with infusion of DMSO has been reported (14); use with caution.
NEUROLOGIC CONDITIONS: Sedation, headache, dizziness, agitation, confusion and decreased consciousness has been reported with use (14). Theoretically, DMSO might worsen existing neurologic diseases or conditions; use with caution.
OCULAR CONDITIONS: Full eye examinations are recommended before and during treatment. Toxicological animal studies suggest lens opacities and changes in refractive index may occur with high concentrations or chronic use of DMSO. There have been no case reports of similar ocular effects in humans (14).
RENAL CONDITIONS: Renal function tests are recommended every 6 months (14). Increases in serum creatinine have been reported (14); use with caution.
URINARY TRACT MALIGNANCIES: Caution is advised when used in patients with urinary tract malignancies since DMSO induces vasodilation (14).

Dosage and Administration

ORAL: For symptoms of amyloidosis, 7-15 grams of DMSO daily has been used (14,6304).
TOPICAL: For prevention of tissue necrosis after extravasation with antineoplastic agents, 77-90% DMSO is typically applied every 3-8 hours for 10-14 days. For acute musculoskeletal injuries and inflammation, 60-90% DMSO solution or gel is typically applied to the affected area 1-3 times daily for 1-3 weeks (14,6304). For osteoarthritis, 60-90% DMSO is typically applied to the affected area daily (6304). For rheumatoid arthritis, 60-90% DMSO solution is typically applied to the affected area 2-4 times daily (6304,6313). For scleroderma, 50-90% DMSO solution is typically applied to the affected area or the affected area is immersed in solution twice daily (6304). For amyloidosis, 50-100% DMSO solution is typically applied twice weekly to the affected area (14). For amyloid-produced itching, 50-100% DMSO solution has been applied to the affected area daily (14). For surgical flaps, 60% DMSO has been applied to the flaps every 4 hours for 10 days (6307). For herpes zoster, 5-40% idoxuridine in DMSO has been started within 48 hours after the appearance of a rash and applied every 4 hours for 4 days (14,6508). For neuropathic pain, 50% DMSO solution has been used 4 times daily for up to 3 weeks (6517).
INTRAVENOUS: For intracranial hypertension, a 10% solution of DMSO has been infused rapidly at a dose of 1 g/kg or a 20% DMSO solution is infused and titrated against the intracranial pressure (6300). A 28% solution of DMSO has also been used by infusing rapidly at a dose of 1.12 g/kg (6301).
INTRAVESICAL INSTILLATION: For interstitial cystitis, typically 50 ml of aqueous 50% DMSO solution is instilled into the bladder, the catheter is removed and the patient is instructed to hold the medication in the bladder for 15-20 minutes before voiding (14,5692). Treatment is usually repeated every 2 weeks until symptoms decrease or patient is symptom free (14). 100 mg of hydrocortisone has been added to the solution before instillation for

added anti-inflammatory action in patients who do not respond favorably (5694). For chronic inflammatory bladder disease, 50 ml of aqueous 50% DMSO solution is typically instilled every 2 weeks for 3 treatments and then once every 4 weeks until symptoms decrease or patient is symptom free. Patient is usually instructed to hold medication for 30 minutes after instillation before voiding (5695).

NASOBILIARY CATHETER: For dissolution of bile duct stones, a mixture of 70/30 DMSO/methyl tert-butyl ether and a mixture of 26 mM ethylene diamine tetraacetic acid with 40 mM sodium deoxycholate and 30% DMSO has been infused alternatively and continuously for 2 hours via a nasobiliary catheter in the common bile duct until disappearance of stones (6315,6316).

Comments

DMSO has been self-prescribed by individuals as a remedy for acute musculoskeletal injuries and inflammation (14,6322) and for arthritis (14). Many of the DMSO products for sale are not for human use and are for veterinary or industrial purposes only (14). The FDA is concerned of the widespread use of DMSO for various conditions and there are studies under way to determine DMSOs effectiveness for many conditions (14). DMSO for bladder instillation is available as a 50% solution (14). 100% DMSO is also available (14). A 70% solution of DMSO for treating scleroderma is available in Canada (14).

DODDER

Also Known As

Beggarweed, Cuscutae, Devil's Guts, Dodder Of Thyme, Hellweed, Lesser Dodder, Scaldweed, Strangle Tare, Tu Si Zi, Tu Sizi.

Scientific Names

Cuscuta epithymum; Cuscuta chinensis.
Family: Convolvulaceae.

People Use This For

Orally, dodder is used for urinary tract, spleen, and hepatic disorders (18).

Safety

There is insufficient reliable information available about the safety of dodder.
Pregnancy and Lactation: Insufficient reliable information available; avoid using.

Effectiveness

There is insufficient reliable information available about the effectiveness of dodder.

Mechanism of Action

The applicable parts of dodder are the above ground parts. Dodder is reported to have hepatic and laxative effects (18).

Adverse Reactions

Orally, dodder may cause intestinal colic (18).

Interactions with Herbs & Other Dietary Supplements

Insufficient reliable information available.

Interactions with Drugs

No interactions are known to occur, and there is no known reason to expect a clinically significant interaction with dodder.

Interactions with Foods

No interactions are known to occur, and there is no known reason to expect a clinically significant interaction with dodder.

Interactions with Lab Tests

No interactions are known to occur, and there is no known reason to expect a clinically significant interaction with dodder.

Interactions with Diseases or Conditions

No interactions are known to occur, and there is no known reason to expect a clinically significant interaction with dodder.

Dosage and Administration

ORAL: People typically use 7 to 12 grams of dodder added to 3 to 4 cups of water and boiled until the volume is reduced by one-half. The cooled liquid is taken in 2 doses on an empty stomach (5251).

Comments

There is very little scientific information about this product. Our staff is continually analyzing the available information on natural medicines and will add data here as it becomes available.

DOLOMITE

Also Known As

Dolomitic Limestone.
CAUTION: See separate listings for Calcium and Magnesium.

Scientific Names

None.

People Use This For

Orally, dolomite is used as a mineral supplement of calcium and magnesium (6).

Safety

LIKELY SAFE ...when used orally and appropriately.
CHILDREN: POSSIBLY UNSAFE ...when used orally long-term due to the presence of lead in some products. Children are more sensitive to lead than adults (152).
PREGNANCY AND LACTATION: Insufficient reliable information available; avoid using unless certain of purity (6).

Effectiveness

LIKELY EFFECTIVE ...when used as a source of calcium and magnesium supplementation (6).

Mechanism of Action

Dolomite is a type of limestone. It is rich in magnesium and calcium carbonate, with smaller amounts of several other minerals. Some evidence suggests that the minerals in dolomite are well-absorbed (6).

Adverse Reactions

Orally, some dolomite products are contaminated with heavy metals including aluminum, arsenic, lead, mercury, nickel, and others that may cause heavy metal poisoning (6). Contaminated products have induced seizure activity in otherwise well-controlled patients who have seizure disorders (6). Calcium used orally can cause gastrointestinal irritation and constipation (9). Calcium carbonate can cause acid rebound (9). Large amounts of calcium carbonate can cause hypercalcemia and alkalosis (9). Magnesium can cause gastrointestinal irritation, nausea, vomiting, and diarrhea (9,14,15). Larger amounts may cause hypermagnesemia (9) with symptoms including thirst, hypotension, drowsiness, confusion, loss of tendon reflexes, muscle weakness, respiratory depression, cardiac arrhythmias, coma, cardiac arrest, and death (9).

Interactions with Herbs & Other Dietary Supplements

BORON: Can increase serum magnesium levels (940).
MAGNESIUM: Theoretically, concomitant use with other magnesium containing supplements can cause diarrhea.
CALCIUM: Theoretically, concomitant use with other calcium containing supplements can cause constipation.

Interactions with Drugs

EXCRETION-ENHANCING DRUGS: Magnesium levels can be reduced by concomitant use of drugs that increase renal excretion. These drugs include amphotericin B, cisplatin, aminoglycoside antibiotics, cyclosporine, thiazide and loop diuretics, mannitol, and intravenous glucose (945).
EXCRETION-REDUCING DRUGS: Magnesium levels can be increased by concomitant use of drugs that decrease renal excretion. These drugs include calcitonin, glucagon, and potassium-sparing diuretics (945).
ESTROGEN: Concomitant use of estrogen increases calcium absorption in postmenopausal women (995).

GLUCOCORTICOIDS: Concomitant use can decrease calcium absorption (15).
REDUCED-ABSORPTION DRUGS: Concomitant use of calcium decreases absorption of fluoride, fluoroquinolones, and tetracyclines (9). Separate administration by at least 2 hours.
THIAZIDE DIURETICS: Concomitant use with moderately large amounts of calcium carbonate increases the risk of milk-alkali syndrome (9).

Interactions with Foods
FOOD: Concomitant ingestion with food, and food high in vitamin D, increases absorption of supplemental calcium (945).
DIETARY FIBER: Certain constituents of dietary fiber inhibit calcium absorption, including phytic acid that is found in wheat bran and uronic acid, a common plant fiber constituent (945).
IRON: Calcium carbonate taken with iron supplements and food might decrease supplemental iron absorption. Calcium carbonate taken with iron supplements on an empty stomach appears to have little effect on supplemental iron absorption (945).
VITAMIN D: Concomitant use can increase active absorption of oral calcium (945).

Interactions with Lab Tests
ALKALINE PHOSPHATASE: The magnesium component might cause a false increase in serum alkaline phosphatase test results due to enzyme activation (275).
ANGIOTENSIN-CONVERTING ENZYME: The magnesium component might decrease serum ACE levels and test results (275).
CALCIUM: The magnesium component might cause a false increase in serum calcium test results in some procedures using edetate disodium (EDTA) (275).
DIAGNEX BLUE: The magnesium component might increase urine diagnex blue excretion due to heavy metal displacement of diagnex blue (275).
GASTRIN: The calcium component might cause a physiological increase in serum levels 30-75 minutes after using (275).
LIPASE: The calcium component might cause an analytical decrease in serum concentrations above 5 mmol/L on method of Tietz (275).

Interactions with Diseases or Conditions
HEART BLOCK: Magnesium is contraindicated in people with heart block (9).
HYPERPARATHYROIDISM: Primary hyperparathyroidism predisposes individuals to increased calcium absorption (945).
HYPOPARATHYROIDISM: Predisposes individuals to reduced calcium absorption (945).
RENAL INSUFFICIENCY: Magnesium is contraindicated in people with severe renal disease. Use cautiously in individuals with reduced kidney function due to increased risk of hypermagnesemia (9). Calcium supplementation increases the risk of hypercalcemia and alkalosis in people with renal disease (9). Renal insufficiency predisposes individuals to reduced calcium absorption (945).
SARCOIDOSIS: Increases the risk of excessive calcium absorption and hypercalcemia (945).

Dosage and Administration
ORAL: The recommended amount of elemental magnesium as a dietary supplement for adults is 54-483 mg daily in divided doses (14). The daily Dietary Reference Intakes of elemental calcium for adults is 1000 mg to age 50, 1200 mg thereafter (998).

Comments
None.

DONG QUAI

Also Known As
Chinese Angelica, Dang Gui, Danggui, Dong Qua, Ligustilides, Phytoestrogen, Tan Kue Bai Zhi, Tang Kuei.
CAUTION: See separate listings for Angelica root and Angelica seed.

Scientific Names
Angelica sinensis, synonym Angelica polymorpha sinensis.
Family: Apiaceae or Umbelliferae.

People Use This For

Orally, dong quai is used for gynecological ailments including menstrual cramps, irregularity, retarded flow, weakness during the menstrual period, and symptoms of menopause (515). It is also used orally as a "blood purifier"; to manage hypertension, rheumatism, ulcers, anemia, and constipation; and in the prevention and treatment of allergic attacks (6,515). Dong quai is also used orally is used for the treatment of skin depigmentation and psoriasis (6). In Chinese medicine, dong quai is generally used in combination with other ingredients (515).

Safety

POSSIBLY SAFE ...when using orally and appropriately (12).
POSSIBLY UNSAFE ...when using orally in large amounts. Large amounts can cause severe photodermatitis (6,515). Dong quai constituents can be carcinogenic, mutagenic, and photocarcinogenic even without light exposure (6). However, the phototoxic constituents are not found in the steam-distilled oils of the root and seed (12).
PREGNANCY: UNSAFE ...when used orally due to uterine stimulant and relaxant effects (12,19,515).
LACTATION: Insufficient reliable information available; avoid using.

Effectiveness

POSSIBLY INEFFECTIVE ...when used orally for treating menopausal symptoms (738). One well designed study found dong quai (as a single agent) had no effect on endometrial wall thickness or menopausal symptoms (738). Human studies are needed to determine the effect(s) of dong quai in combination with other herbs for treating menopausal symptoms.
There is insufficient reliable information available about the effectiveness of dong quai for its other uses.

Mechanism of Action

The applicable part of dong quai is the root. Dong quai has several coumarin constituents including osthol, psoralen, and bergapten. Some coumarins can act as vasodilators and antispasmodics. Osthol has central nervous system stimulant effects (5). Psoralen and bergapten are photosensitizing and can cause severe photodermatitis (6). Psoralens are photocarcinogenic and mutagenic (6). Safrole, a constituent of the dong quai essential oil, is carcinogenic (6). A dong quai extract competitively inhibits estradiol binding to estrogen receptors and induces transcription activity in estrogen-responsive cells (6180). It also increases uterine weight, decreases LH (luteinizing hormone) levels, and increases serum ceruloplasmin oxidase activity (a measure of liver estrogenic activity) in female rats that have had their ovaries removed (6180). Dong quai can improve abnormal protein metabolism in people with chronic hepatitis or hepatic cirrhosis (4). An injected aqueous extract can show efficacy in treating acute ischemic cerebrovascular disease (11). In animals, dong quai speeds neurocyte growth and prevents the decline of process branches in vitro, which suggests it can have some activity in humans for promoting nerve growth and delaying atrophy (6). The related species, Angelica dahurica, can have anti-inflammatory, analgesic, and antipyretic activity (6). Another related Angelica species inhibits human platelet aggregation (736).

Adverse Reactions

The use of dong quai can cause photosensitivity and photodermatitis and is potentially carcinogenic and mutagenic (6).

Interactions with Herbs & Other Dietary Supplements

HERBS WITH ANTICOAGULANT/ANTIPLATELET POTENTIAL: Concomitant use of herbs that have coumarin constituents or affect platelet aggregation could theoretically increase the risk of bleeding in some people. These herbs include: angelica, anise, arnica, asafoetida, bogbean, boldo, capsicum, celery, chamomile, clove, danshen, fenugreek, feverfew, garlic, ginger, ginkgo, ginseng (Panax), horse chestnut, horseradish, licorice, meadowsweet, prickly ash, onion, papain, passionflower, poplar, quassia, red clover, turmeric, wild carrot, wild lettuce, willow, and others (4,19).

Interactions with Drugs

ANTICOAGULANT, ANTIPLATELET DRUGS: Theoretically, dong quai might potentiate the therapeutic and adverse effects of these drugs. Dong quai has been reported to inhibit platelet aggregation (6048).
WARFARIN (Coumadin): Concomitant use increases the anticoagulant effects of warfarin and the risk of bleeding (3526,6048). In one case, after 4 weeks of dong quai 565 mg once or twice daily, INR increased to 4.9. INR normalized 4 weeks after discontinuation of dong quai. Dong quai is thought to inhibit platelet activation and aggregation (6048).

Interactions with Foods

No interactions are known to occur, and there is no known reason to expect a clinically significant interaction with dong quai.

Interactions with Lab Tests
PROTHROMBIN TIME (PT), INTERNATIONAL NORMALIZATION RATIO (INR): Dong quai can enhance the effects of warfarin, resulting in increased PT and INR test results (3526).

Interactions with Diseases or Conditions
HORMONE SENSITIVE CANCERS/CONDITIONS: Dong quai seems to have estrogenic effects (6180). Women with hormone sensitive conditions including breast, uterine, and ovarian cancer, and endometriosis and uterine fibroids, should avoid using dong quai.

Dosage and Administration
ORAL: Women typically use 3 to 4 grams per day in divided doses with meals. One dong quai supplier suggests three daily doses based on body weight: under 100 pounds, 520 mg per dose; 100 to 175 pounds, 1040 mg; over 175 pounds, 1560 mg. Dong quai is sometimes prepared as a tea. An extract of dong quai is used in a dose of 1 mL (20 to 40 drops) three times daily. The extract contains alcohol and glycerin, but the concentration is not specified (6006).

Comments
Dong quai is an aromatic herb that is commonly used throughout the Orient (6). Some references classify Angelica atropurpurea and Angelica dahurica as dong quai (Chinese angelica) (6), while others do not (5,11,12).

DRAGON'S BLOOD

Also Known As
Draconis Resina, Dracorubin, Dragons Blood, Dragon's-Blood Palm, Sanguis Draconis, Xue Jie.
CAUTION: See separate listings for Herb Robert and Sangre de Grado.

Scientific Names
Daemonorops draco, synonym Calamus draco.
Family: Arecaceae or Palmae.

People Use This For
Orally, dragon's blood is used for diarrhea, digestive disorders and as a coloring agent.
Topically, dragon's blood is used as an astringent (18).

Safety
POSSIBLY SAFE …when used orally (12). There is insufficient reliable information available about the safety of the topical use of dragon's blood.
PREGNANCY AND LACTATION: Insufficient reliable information available; avoid using.

Effectiveness
There is insufficient reliable information available about the effectiveness of dragon's blood.

Mechanism of Action
The applicable part of dragon's blood is the fruit. There is insufficient reliable information available about the possible mechanism of action and active ingredients.

Adverse Reactions
None reported.

Interactions with Herbs & Other Dietary Supplements
Insufficient reliable information available.

Interactions with Drugs
No interactions are known to occur, and there is no known reason to expect a clinically significant interaction with dragon's blood.

Interactions with Foods
No interactions are known to occur, and there is no known reason to expect a clinically significant interaction with dragon's blood.

Interactions with Lab Tests
No interactions are known to occur, and there is no known reason to expect a clinically significant interaction with dragon's blood.

Interactions with Diseases or Conditions
No interactions are known to occur, and there is no known reason to expect a clinically significant interaction with dragon's blood.

Dosage and Administration
ORAL: Dragon's blood has been used as a powder (18).
TOPICAL: No typical dosage.

Comments
Dragon's blood is the red resin extracted from the fruit of Daemonorops draco (18).

DUCKWEED

Also Known As
None.

Scientific Names
Lemna minor.
Family: Lemnaceae.

People Use This For
Orally, duckweed is used for inflammation of the upper respiratory tract, jaundice, and arthritis (18).

Safety
There is insufficient reliable information available about the safety of duckweed.
Pregnancy and Lactation: Insufficient reliable information available; avoid using.

Effectiveness
There is insufficient reliable information available about the effectiveness of duckweed.

Mechanism of Action
There is insufficient reliable information available about the possible mechanism of action and active ingredients.

Adverse Reactions
None reported.

Interactions with Herbs & Other Dietary Supplements
Insufficient reliable information available.

Interactions with Drugs
No interactions are known to occur, and there is no known reason to expect a clinically significant interaction with duckweed.

Interactions with Foods
No interactions are known to occur, and there is no known reason to expect a clinically significant interaction with duckweed.

Interactions with Lab Tests
No interactions are known to occur, and there is no known reason to expect a clinically significant interaction with duckweed.

Interactions with Diseases or Conditions
No interactions are known to occur, and there is no known reason to expect a clinically significant interaction with duckweed.

Dosage and Administration
ORAL: Duckweed is used as a powder or an extract (18).

Comments
There is very little scientific information about this product. Our staff is continually analyzing the available information on natural medicines and will add data here as it becomes available.

DUSTY MILLER

Also Known As
None.

Scientific Names
Senecio cineraria, synonym Cineraria maritima.
Family: Compositae.

People Use This For
Orally, dusty miller is used in preparations for eyesight problems (spots before the eyes), migraine, and to promote menstrual flow (18).

Safety
LIKELY UNSAFE ...when any parts of the plant are used orally. Dusty miller contains hepatotoxic unsaturated pyrrolizidine alkaloids (UPAs) (18,19). Repeated exposure to low concentrations of UPAs are linked to veno-occlusive disease (4,12). UPAs may also be carcinogenic and mutagenic (12). ...when used topically on abraded or broken skin because it might be absorbed systemically (12,19).
PREGNANCY AND LACTATION: LIKELY UNSAFE ...when used orally because it contains UPA constituents (12). There is insufficient reliable information available about the safety of the topical use of dusty miller during pregnancy and lactation; avoid using.

Effectiveness
There is insufficient reliable information available about the effectiveness of dusty miller.

Mechanism of Action
Some pyrrolizidine alkaloids have shown carcinogenic and mutagenic properties, and there are reports of renal toxicity. However, the primary concern is veno-occlusive disease (12). Unsaturated pyrrolizidine alkaloids are known to be hepatotoxic in animals and humans (4).

Adverse Reactions
Orally, dusty miller may cause acute toxicity which may result in hepatic necrosis; chronic toxicity may cause veno-occlusive liver disease. The potential for hepatotoxicity (due to presence of pyrrolizidine alkaloids) increases with larger doses and longer periods of use (4,12). It can cause an allergic reaction in individuals sensitive to the Asteraceae/Compositae family. Members of this family include ragweed, chrysanthemums, marigolds, daisies, and many other herbs.

Interactions with Herbs & Other Dietary Supplements
EUCALYPTUS: Theoretically, concomitant use with dusty miller might increase the risk of unsaturated pyrrolizidine alkaloid toxicity due to enzyme induction by eucalyptus (19).
PYRROLIZIDINE ALKALOID-CONTAINING HERBS: Concomitant use with dusty miller is contraindicated due to the risk of additive toxicity. Herbs containing unsaturated pyrrolizidine alkaloids include: alkanna (12), borage (271), gravel root (4), hemp agrimony (271), hound's tongue (19), petasites (19), comfrey (271), coltsfoot, and the Senecio species plants; dusty miller (19), alpine ragwort (19), groundsel (271), golden ragwort (19), and tansy ragwort (271).

Interactions with Drugs
No interactions are known to occur, and there is no known reason to expect a clinically significant interaction with dusty miller.

Interactions with Foods
No interactions are known to occur, and there is no known reason to expect a clinically significant interaction with dusty miller.

Interactions with Lab Tests

No interactions are known to occur, and there is no known reason to expect a clinically significant interaction with dusty miller.

Interactions with Diseases or Conditions

LIVER DISEASE: Contraindicated.
CROSS-ALLERGENICITY: Can cause an allergic reaction in individuals sensitive to the Asteraceae/Compositae family. Members of this family include ragweed, chrysanthemums, marigolds, daisies, and many other herbs.

Dosage and Administration

No typical dosage.

Comments

American Herbal Products Association recommends labeling all botanical products that contain toxic pyrrolizidine alkaloids "For external use only. Do not apply to broken or abraded skin; do not use when nursing" (12).

DWARF ELDER

Also Known As

Blood Elder, Blood Hilder, Danewort, Walewort.
CAUTION: See separate listings for American Elder, Elderberry, Elderflower.

Scientific Names

Sambucus ebulus.
Family: Caprifoliaceae.

People Use This For

Orally, dwarf elder is used for arthritis, weight reduction, and as a diuretic (18).

Safety

LIKELY UNSAFE …when large quantities of any part of the plant are used orally. It can cause loss of consciousness and death (18).
There is insufficient reliable information available about the safety of the oral use of dwarf elder in small amounts.
PREGNANCY AND LACTATION: LIKELY UNSAFE …when used orally in large quantities (18).

Effectiveness

There is insufficient reliable information available about the effectiveness of dwarf elder.

Mechanism of Action

Dwarf elder contains iridoide monoterpene glycosides. The constituents that cause nausea or purgative effects have not been identified (18).

Adverse Reactions

Orally, ingestion of large quantities of any plant part of dwarf elder may cause vomiting, bloody diarrhea, cyanosis, dizziness, headache and unconsciousness. Death has been reported (18). Cyanide poisoning can be caused by any plant part of dwarf elder. Sambunigrine, a cyanogenic glycoside, is present in the plant.

Interactions with Herbs & Other Dietary Supplements

Insufficient reliable information available.

Interactions with Drugs

No interactions are known to occur, and there is no known reason to expect a clinically significant interaction with dwarf elder.

Interactions with Foods

No interactions are known to occur, and there is no known reason to expect a clinically significant interaction with dwarf elder.

Interactions with Lab Tests
No interactions are known to occur, and there is no known reason to expect a clinically significant interaction with dwarf elder.

Interactions with Diseases or Conditions
No interactions are known to occur, and there is no known reason to expect a clinically significant interaction with dwarf elder.

Dosage and Administration
No typical dosage.

Comments
Dwarf elder is considered unsafe; avoid using. Dwarf elder is considered obsolete as a medicinal herb in many countries (18). Avoid confusion with Elderberry and American Elder, which are the berries of other members of the Sambucus genus (214).

DWARF PINE NEEDLE

Also Known As
None.
CAUTION: See separate listings for Fir, Fir Needle Oil, Pine, Poplar, and Scotch Pine Needle Oil.

Scientific Names
Pinus mugo, synonym Pinus montana; Pinus pumilio, synonym Pinus mugo pumilio.
Family: Pinaceae.

People Use This For
There are no known medicinal uses of dwarf pine needle (11).
In foods and beverages, dwarf pine needle is used as a flavoring agent (11).
In other manufacturing processes, dwarf pine needle is used as a flavoring and fragrance component in pharmaceutical preparations (cough and cold medicines, vaporizer fluids, nasal decongestants, analgesic ointments), and as a fragrance ingredient in soaps and cosmetics (maximum use level 1.2% in perfumes) (11).

Safety
LIKELY SAFE ...when used in amounts found in foods. The maximum use level is 0.001% (11); approved for food use in the US (11).
POSSIBLY SAFE ...when used topically. There is possible human skin irritation and demonstrated sensitizing in some individuals (11).
PREGNANCY AND LACTATION: Insufficient reliable information available; avoid using.

Effectiveness
There is insufficient reliable information available about the effectiveness of dwarf pine needle.

Mechanism of Action
The applicable part of dwarf pine needle is the oil. Constituents bornyl acetate, dipentene, and limonene are believed to have antibacterial and antiviral properties (11).

Adverse Reactions
Topically, dwarf pine needle can cause skin irritation (11). It also may be sensitizing in some individuals (11).

Interactions with Herbs & Other Dietary Supplements
Insufficient reliable information available.

Interactions with Drugs
No interactions are known to occur, and there is no known reason to expect a clinically significant interaction with dwarf pine needle.

Interactions with Foods
No interactions are known to occur, and there is no known reason to expect a clinically significant interaction with dwarf pine needle.

Interactions with Lab Tests

No interactions are known to occur, and there is no known reason to expect a clinically significant interaction with dwarf pine needle.

Interactions with Diseases or Conditions

ALLERGY: Avoid dwarf pine needle if allergic or sensitive to pine oil.

Dosage and Administration

No typical dosage.

Comments

Dwarf pine needle oil is produced by distillation of dwarf pine (Pinus mugo) needles and twigs. Avoid confusion with fir needle oil and scotch pine needle oil.

DYER'S BROOM

Also Known As

Broom Flower, Dyers Broom, Dyer's Greenwood, Dyer's Weed, Dyer's Whin, Furze, Green Broom, Greenweed, Wood Waxen.

Scientific Names

Genista tinctoria.
Family: Leguminosae or Fabaceae.

People Use This For

Orally, dyer's broom is used for digestive disorders, gout, as an emetic or purgative, and to remove bladder stones. It is also used orally to "detoxify" blood, to increase heart rate, strengthen blood vessels, stimulate blood flow to the kidneys, and to alter metabolism. It has been used to deepen breathing and alleviate pain in the lower back and pelvis (18).

Safety

POSSIBLY UNSAFE …when above ground parts are used orally (12).
PREGNANCY: LIKELY UNSAFE …when used orally because it could have uterine-stimulant activity (12).
LACTATION: POSSIBLY UNSAFE …when used orally; avoid using.

Effectiveness

There is insufficient reliable information available about the effectiveness of dyer's broom.

Mechanism of Action

Dyer's broom contains quinolizidine alkaloids, including methylcytisine, anagyrine, isopsarteine, lupanine, tinctorin, and cysisine. It also contains flavonoids (including luteolin glycosides), isoflavonoids (including genistein and genistin), and lectins (18).

Adverse Reactions

Orally, dyer's broom may cause nausea and vomiting. Overuse of dyer's broom can lead to diarrhea (18).

Interactions with Herbs & Other Dietary Supplements

Insufficient reliable information available.

Interactions with Drugs

No interactions are known to occur, and there is no known reason to expect a clinically significant interaction with dyer's broom.

Interactions with Foods

No interactions are known to occur, and there is no known reason to expect a clinically significant interaction with dyer's broom.

Interactions with Lab Tests

No interactions are known to occur, and there is no known reason to expect a clinically significant interaction with dyer's broom.

Interactions with Diseases or Conditions

No interactions are known to occur, and there is no known reason to expect a clinically significant interaction with dyer's broom.

Dosage and Administration

No typical dosage.

Comments

None.

ECHINACEA

Also Known As

American Cone Flower, Black Sampson, Black Susans, Brauneria Angustifolia, Brauneria Pallida, Comb Flower, Coneflower, Echinaceawurzel, Hedgehog, Igelkopfwurzel, Indian Head, Kansas Snakeroot, Narrow-leaved Purple Cone Flower, Pale Coneflower, Purple Cone Flower, Purpursonnenhutkraut, Purpursonnenhutwurzel, Racine d'echininacea, Red Sunflower, Rock-Up-Hat, Roter Sonnenhut, Schmallblaettrige Kegelblumenwurzel, Schmallblaettriger Sonnenhut, Scurvy Root, Snakeroot, Sonnenhutwurzel.

Scientific Names

Echinacea angustifolia; Echinacea pallida; Echinacea purpurea.
Family: Asteraceae or Compositae.

People Use This For

Orally, echinacea is used for treating and preventing the common cold and other upper respiratory infections. Echinacea is also used orally as an immunostimulant for fighting a variety of other infections, including urinary tract infections (UTIs), vaginal candidiasis (yeast infections), genital herpes (HSV Type 1 and 2). Echinacea is also used orally for septicemia, nasopharyngeal catarrh, pyorrhea, tonsillitis, rheumatism, migraines, streptococcus infections, dyspepsia, pain, dizziness, rattlesnake bites, syphilis, typhoid, malaria, and diphtheria.
Topically, echinacea is used for boils, abscesses, skin wounds and ulcers, eczema, psoriasis, herpes simplex, bee stings, and hemorrhoids.
Intravenously, echinacea has been used for recurrent vaginal candidiasis (yeast infections), and urinary tract infections (UTI).
Intravenously and intramuscularly, echinacea is used to prolong survival time in patients with advanced hepatocellular carcinoma and colorectal cancer.

Safety

LIKELY SAFE ...when used orally and appropriately, short-term. Echinacea has been used safely in trials lasting up to 12 weeks (1412,3279,3280,3281,3282,6417). ...when used topically and appropriately (12).
There is insufficient reliable information available about the safety of echinacea when used long-term.
PREGNANCY: POSSIBLY SAFE ...when used orally, short-term. There is some evidence that mothers can safely use echinacea for 5-7 days during the first trimester of pregnancy without adversely effecting the fetus (7056). However, this evidence is preliminary. Tell pregnant patients not to use echinacea without the supervision of their health care provider.
LACTATION: Insufficient reliable information available; avoid using.

Effectiveness

POSSIBLY EFFECTIVE ...when used orally for treating influenza-like upper respiratory infections such as the common cold and flu. Echinacea preparations seem to decrease the severity and duration of symptoms associated with influenza-like upper respiratory infections if started when symptoms are first noticed and used for 7-10 days (1412,3279,3280,3281,6206,6384,6385); however, the formulation and species that might offer the most benefit is unclear. Most studies have used Echinacea purpurea species, but several preparations have been used including extracts of Echinacea purpurea herb; combination root and herb extracts; and root extracts of Echinacea pallida, Echinacea angustifolia, and Echinacea purpurea (1412,3280,3281,6206,6417). Studies have also used echinacea compound herbal teas (6384) and fixed combination herbal preparations containing echinacea (3281,6392). ...when used orally in combination with a topical antifungal cream for preventing recurrence of vaginal yeast infection. Herb juice of Echinacea purpurea in combination with topical econazole (Spectazole) lowers recurrence rate to 16.7% compared to 60.5% with econazole alone (4800).
POSSIBLY INEFFECTIVE ...when used orally for preventing the common cold or influenza-like respiratory infections. Echinacea angustifolia, Echinacea purpurea, and Echinacea pallida herb extract or root extract preparations

are ineffective when used prophylactically for 8-12 weeks for reducing the rate of respiratory infections (3280,3281,3282,6417,6386). Some researchers suggest that when used greater than 8 weeks, the immunostimulatory effects might decline, making it less effective (6417,6418). To prevent this decline in activity, it is often recommended that a 1-week drug holiday be taken after each 8-week treatment period (6418). However, there is no reliable evidence to support either of these claims. ...when used orally for recurrent genital herpes. A specific Echinacea purpurea extract (Echinaforce) 800 mg twice daily for 6 months does not seem to prevent or reduce frequency or duration of recurrent genital herpes in patients with herpes simplex virus (HSV) type 1 or 2 (7087). Clinical studies have used a wide variety of specific extracts and dosage forms of echinacea. Some of these include a Echinacea purpurea 95% herb and 5% root extract (Echinaforce, Bioforce), a fixed combination of Echinacea purpurea plus cedar and wild indigo extracts (Esberitox N, Enzymatic Therapy), and a tea containing a blend of Echinacea purpurea and Echinacea augustifolia leaves, stems, and flowers plus a dry extract of Echinacea purpurea root (Echinacea Plus, Traditional Medicinals).

There is insufficient reliable information available about the effectiveness of echinacea for its other uses.

Mechanism of Action

The applicable parts of echinacea are the roots and the above ground parts. Echinacea is used for the upper respiratory tract infections such as the common cold and influenza infections because it is reported to have antiviral and immune system stimulatory effects (11,3279). Echinacea seems to have indirect antiviral activity, possibly by stimulating interferon-like effects (11). Echinacea increases phagocytosis and increases lymphocyte activity, possibly by promoting release of tumor necrosis factor (TNF), interleukin-1 (IL-1), and interferon (3,4,14,3279,6388,6389). Several constituents of echinacea seem to be involved in stimulating this non-specific immune response. Some of these include high-molecular weight polysaccharides, such as heteroxylan and arabinogalactan; and lower molecular weight compounds, including alkylamides and cafeoyl conjugates such as chicoric acid and echinacosides (3279). Heteroxylan might activate phagocytosis (3279), and arabinogalactan seems to induce macrophages to produce the cytokines TNF, IL-1, and interferon beta-2. Macrophages activated by arabinogalactan have been found to be cytotoxic against tumor cells and micro-organisms (6,14,6388). The constituents chicoric and echinacosides are thought to also play a role in enhancing phagocytosis (3279). Polysaccharides in echinacea also seem to have moderate effects on B-lymphocytes, but no apparent activity on T-lymphocytes (4,6389). Echinacea is also reported to have antifungal properties, so people try it for yeast infections (vaginal candidiasis). Polyacetylenic compounds in echinacea, including ketoalkenes and ketoalkynes, seem to have antifungal activity, including activity against yeasts such as candida (6390). For wound healing, echinacea seems to promote the formation of mesenchymal mucopolysaccharides, stimulate histogenic and hematogenic phagocytes, promote differentiation of fibrocytes from fibroblasts, and stimulate of the anterior pituitary-adrenal cortex (11). Several conjugates isolated from echinacea have also been reported to inhibit tissue and bacterial hyaluronidase and have anti-inflammatory activity (6,11,3279). The constituent echinacin has also been found to promote tissue granulation (3279). Preliminary research suggests that high concentrations of Echinacea purpurea might reduce sperm and ova fertility (4239,4240). However, this has not yet been demonstrated in humans. Animal research shows that very high doses of Echinacea do not seem to have genotoxic or carcinogenic effects (1413).

Adverse Reactions

Orally, echinacea is usually very well tolerated (1412,3279,3280,3282,6387); however, some patients may experience allergic reactions, fever, nausea, vomiting (2), unpleasant taste, abdominal pain, diarrhea, sore throat (6), and dizziness (14). Allergic reactions can include urticaria, erythema nodosum (7057), acute asthma and dyspnea, anaphylaxis, and angioedema (638,1358). Allergic reactions seem to be relatively uncommon, but some people are more likely to be sensitive. For example, atopic individuals are at increased risk for allergic reactions to echinacea (1358). Individuals sensitive to the Asteraceae/Compositae plant family might also be more likely to experience an allergic reaction to echinacea. Members of this family include ragweed, chrysanthemums, marigolds, daisies, and many other herbs. There is some preliminary evidence that high doses of echinacea might reduce male and female fertility (4239,4240). However, this effect has not yet been demonstrated in humans.

Topically, echinacea can cause erythema, exanthema, and pruritus (14).

Parenterally, echinacea has been associated with shivering, muscle weakness (6), and slight reddening with transient pain at the injection site (6387).

Interactions with Herbs & Other Dietary Supplements

Insufficient reliable information available.

Interactions with Drugs

IMMUNOSUPPRESSANTS: Theoretically, echinacea may interfere with immunosuppressant therapy (4) because of its immunostimulating activity. Echinacea stimulates phagocytosis and increases respiratory cellular activity and the mobility of leukocytes. Immunosuppressant drugs include azathioprine (Imuran), basiliximab (Simulect), cyclosporine (Neoral, Sandimmune), daclizumab (Zenapax), muromonab-CD3 (OKT3, Orthoclone OKT3), mycophenolate (CellCept), tacrolimus (FK506, Prograf), sirolimus (Rapamune), prednisone (Deltasone, Orasone), and other corticosteroids (glucocorticoids).

ECONAZOLE NITRATE (Spectazole): Concomitant use of echinacea and topical econazole can decrease the recurrence rate of vaginal candida infections (19).

OTHER DRUGS: There's preliminary evidence that echinacea can inhibit the cytochrome P450 (CYP450) 3A4 enzyme (6450). Theoretically, echinacea might increase levels of drugs metabolized by CYP450 3A4. However, so far, this interaction has not been reported in humans. Some drugs metabolized by CYP450 3A4 include lovastatin (Mevacor), ketoconazole (Nizoral), itraconazole (Sporanox), fexofenadine (Allegra), triazolam (Halcion), and numerous others. Use echinacea cautiously or avoid in patients taking these drugs.

Interactions with Foods

No interactions are known to occur, and there is no known reason to expect a clinically significant interaction with echinacea.

Interactions with Lab Tests

No interactions are known to occur, and there is no known reason to expect a clinically significant interaction with echinacea.

Interactions with Diseases or Conditions

ATOPY: Individuals with atopy (a genetic tendency toward allergic conditions) may be more likely to experience an allergic reaction when taking echinacea. Unpublished case reports, presented at the American Academy of Allergy, Asthma and Immunology (AAAAI) 2000 annual meeting, describe 23 cases of allergic reactions to echinacea consistent with IgE mediated hypersensitivity. Thirty-four percent of the reactions were in patients with atopy. In a related study, 20% of 100 atopic patients tested who had never taken echinacea had positive skin test reactions to echinacea, indicating hypersensitivity without previous exposure (1358).

AUTOIMMUNE AND PROGRESSIVE SYSTEMIC DISEASES: There is some concern that echinacea might exacerbate autoimmune and related disorders due to its immunostimulant effects. Some of these conditions include leukosis, collagenosis, multiple sclerosis, collagen disorders, rheumatoid arthritis, systemic lupus erythematosus (SLE) and others (2,7,8). Some experts also warn against using echinacea in patients with HIV/AIDs. However, the rational for this is not known and there is no reliable evidence to support this warning.

DIABETES: Parenteral administration might worsen metabolic control (8).

CROSS-ALLERGENICITY: Individuals sensitive to the Asteraceae/Compositae plant family may be more likely to experience an allergic reaction to echinacea. Members of this family include ragweed, chrysanthemums, marigolds, daisies, and many other herbs.

INFERTILITY: Preliminary evidence suggests that echinacea might inhibit oocyte fertilization and alter sperm DNA (4239,4240). This effect has not yet been demonstrated in humans; however, until more is known, use with caution in couples attempting to conceive and avoid use in couples having difficulty conceiving.

Dosage and Administration

ORAL: For treatment of upper respiratory infections including the common cold and influenza, a wide variety of doses have been used depending on the formulation. A tablet containing 6.78 mg of Echinacea purpurea crude extract based on 95% herb and 5% root (Echinaforce, Bioforce AG) is dosed as two tablets given 3 times daily (1412). Echinacea purpurea herb juice has been used in a daily dose of 6-9 mL for up to a maximum of 8 weeks (3282). Echinacea purpurea herb juice has also been used in a dose of 20 drops every 2 hours for the first day followed by 20 drops three times daily until symptoms resolve. An echinacea pallida root tincture, equivalent to 900 mg herb daily, has also been used (3281). An echinacea herbal compound tea (Echinacea Plus, Traditional Medicinals) consisting of leaves, flowers, and stems of Echinacea purpurea and Echinacea angustifolia plus dried extract of Echinacea purpurea root, has been used by drinking 5-6 cups of tea on the first day of symptoms and titrating down to 1 cup per day over the next 5 days (6384). The tea is prepared by pouring 8 ounces of boiling water over one tea bag and steeping, covered, for 10-15 minutes (6384). For urinary tract infections, a daily dose of 6-9 mL Echinacea purpurea fresh herb juice for a maximum of 8 weeks has been used (2).

TOPICAL: A semi-solid preparation containing at least 15% pressed juice of Echinacea purpurea herb for a maximum of 8 weeks has been used (2).

INTRAVENOUS: No typical dosage.

Comments

There are three Echinacea species of medicinal interest: Echinacea angustifolia, Echinacea pallida, and Echinacea purpurea. Echinacea species are native to North America and were used as traditional herbal remedies by the Great Plains Indian tribes, and were adopted for medicinal use by settlers (3279). Echinacea angustifolia and Echinacea pallida were official in the US National Formulary from 1916 to 1950 (11). Conventional use of echinacea fell out of favor in the United States with the discovery of antibiotics and due to the lack of scientific data supporting its use, but it continued to be widely used in Europe (3279). The development of antibiotic resistance has contributed to renewed interest in echinacea. Echinacea products have been commonly adulterated. The results from clinical studies performed prior to 1991 might be unreliable unless the plant material used was positively confirmed (11,3279,1414). Now presence of Echinacea purpurea is now confirmable with HPLC analysis (11,1414). Although some echinacea extract products are standardized for their echinacoside content, echinacoside is not a specific marker for Echinacea purpurea, Echinacea angustifolia or Echinacea pallida (11). It has been suggested Echinacea preparations could be standardized according to their alkamide content as levels of alkamides have been found to vary significantly between parts of Echinacea purpurea plants and between different commercial Echinacea purpurea products (6391).

EDTA

Also Known As

Calcium Disodium Edathamil, Calcium Disodium Edetate, Calcium Disodium EDTA, Calcium Disodium Versenate, Calcium Edetate, Calcium EDTA, Disodium Edathamil, Disodium Edetate, Disodium EDTA, Disodium Tetraacetate, Iron EDTA, Sodium Edetate.

Scientific Names

Ethylenediamine tetraacetic acid; Disodium ethylenediamine tetraacetic acid; Trisodium ethylenediamine tetraacetic acid.

People Use This For

Topically, EDTA has been used as an ointment for skin irritations produced by metals such as chromium, nickel and copper (5729).

Intravenously and intramuscularly, EDTA is used for acute and chronic lead poisoning and lead encephalopathy (15,5730,5731,5732,5733,5734,5735,5736). Intravenous EDTA is also used in the calcium EDTA mobilization test which is used to evaluate a patient's response to chelation therapy for suspected lead poisoning (15,5733). EDTA is also used intravenously to treat poisonings by radioactive products such as plutonium, thorium, uranium, yttrium (15), and strontium (5728). It is also used intravenously for removing copper in patients with Wilson's disease (5728), hypercalcemia (9,15,5729,5763), cardiac glycoside-induced arrhythmias (9,15,5761,5762), atherosclerotic vascular disease (5737,5738,5739,5740,5741,5742,5743), scleroderma (15,5757,5758,5759,5760), porphyria, hypercholesterolemia, and in the diagnosis of hypoparathyroidism (15). EDTA has also been used intravenously to treat essential hypertension, Raynaud's syndrome, intermittent claudication, gangrene (5726), cancer (5727), rheumatoid arthritis, osteoarthritis (5738), decreased vision due to macular degeneration, diabetes, Alzheimer's disease, multiple sclerosis (5739), Parkinson's disease, psoriasis, and angina (5749).

Ophthalmically, EDTA is used for corneal calcium deposits in the eye (15).

In foods, EDTA is used as iron EDTA to fortify grain-based products such as breakfast cereals and cereal bars (5728). EDTA is also used as calcium disodium EDTA and disodium EDTA as an additive to preserve food (5725,5767); and to promote the color, texture, and flavor of food (5767).

In manufacturing, EDTA is used as disodium EDTA and trisodium EDTA to improve stability in pharmaceutical preparations (15,5725), detergents, liquid soaps, shampoos, agricultural chemical sprays, oil emulsion devices (5725), contact lens cleaners and cosmetics (9). It is also used in manufactured clinical laboratory evacuated blood collection tubes to anticoagulate blood specimens (9,5725).

Safety

LIKELY SAFE ...when used intravenously or intramuscularly and appropriately, short-term. Parenteral EDTA in the disodium and calcium disodium forms are FDA-approved prescription products (15).

POSSIBLY SAFE ...when used ophthalmically and appropriately (15,5774). Solutions of 0.35-1.85% EDTA in the disodium form seem to be safe (5774).

LIKELY UNSAFE ...when used intravenously or intramuscularly in excessive doses or long-term. Doses exceeding 50 mg/kg/day or greater than 3 grams per day, or used longer than 5-7 days per treatment course are associated with severe toxicity including nephrotoxicity (15,5733). ...when used intravenously and infused at an excessive rate. Infusion of the disodium form of EDTA over less than 3 hours can cause severe, life-threatening adverse effects including hypocalcemia and death (9,15,5737).

PREGNANCY AND LACTATION: Insufficient reliable information available; avoid using.

Effectiveness

EFFECTIVE ...when used intravenously and intramuscularly to treat acute and chronic lead poisoning and lead encephalopathy (15,5730,5731,5734,5735,5736). The calcium disodium form of EDTA is FDA approved for these uses (15). Calcium disodium EDTA is used when blood lead concentrations are 45 ug/dl or greater or when patients are symptomatic. Treatment of 3-5 days is usually required to lower blood lead levels below 40 ug/dl (15,5730,5733). A second treatment course can be required if blood lead concentrations rebound to 45 ug/dl or greater within 5-7 days after the initial treatment (15). Treatment with calcium disodium EDTA improves symptoms of lead poisoning such as abdominal pain, fatigue, constipation, and anorexia (5730). It also seems slow progression of renal dysfunction in patients who have had chronic lead poisoning (5732). Calcium disodium EDTA is preferred to disodium EDTA for lead poisoning because unlike calcium disodium EDTA, disodium EDTA can significantly lower serum calcium levels and cause hypocalcemia when used in doses necessary to treat lead poisoning (15).

LIKELY EFFECTIVE ...when used intravenously for emergency treatment of hypercalcemia. The disodium form of EDTA is approved by the FDA for this use (15). Disodium EDTA can temporarily lower serum calcium to safe levels (15). However, clinicians generally prefer other methods of treatment such as forced diuresis with saline or use of pamidronate (Aredia), calcitonin (Miacalcin, others), or glucocorticoids (5775). These treatments more effectively lower serum calcium concentrations over longer periods of time than would be achieved with disodium EDTA and are less likely to cause renal side effects (15). ...when used intravenously for emergency treatment of cardiac glycoside-induced ventricular arrhythmias. The disodium form of EDTA is approved by the FDA for this use. Disodium EDTA works rapidly to control ventricular arrhythmias, but it is very short acting (15,5761,5762). Clinicians do not consider it the preferred treatment (15). Other agents such as lidocaine or phenytoin (Dilantin) (3078) are typically used because they are safer and more effective (15).

POSSIBLY EFFECTIVE ...when used ophthalmically to treat corneal calcium deposits. A single application of the disodium form of EDTA can clear corneal calcium deposits (5773,5774) and improve eyesight (5774). However, debridement of the corneal epithelium prior to application of EDTA is required (5773,5774).

POSSIBLY INEFFECTIVE ...when used intravenously or intramuscularly in the diagnosis of suspected lead poisoning. Some clinicians use this diagnostic test, known as the calcium EDTA mobilization test. However, many experts consider the test obsolete due to technical inconsistencies in administering and interpreting the test (15,5733). Treatment of lead poisoning should not be delayed for performance of this test if blood lead levels are 45 mcg/dl or greater (15). ...when used intravenously to treat localized and systemic scleroderma. Although there have been some anecdotal reports showing benefit (5757,5760), clinical studies show no significant changes or improvements in the skin or joints of scleroderma patients treated with disodium EDTA (5757,5758,5759,5760).

LIKELY INEFFECTIVE ...when used intravenously to treat coronary heart disease (CHD) or peripheral arterial occlusive disease. The effectiveness of EDTA as chelation therapy is highly debated (5738,5739). Proponents often cite anecdotal reports or poorly controlled studies as evidence to support EDTA chelation therapy (5737,5738,5739,5740,5742,5743,5751,5770), but well-designed research shows that EDTA offers no significant benefit for these conditions (5737,5740,5742,5750,5752,5753,5754).

There is insufficient reliable information available about the effectiveness of EDTA for it other uses.

Mechanism of Action

Ethylenediaminetetraacetic acid (EDTA) is known as a chelating agent. It is a complex molecule with a claw-like structure, which binds and seizes divalent and trivalent metal ions such as calcium and aluminum to form a stable ring structure (5729,5749). EDTA binds and chelates metal ions in the following decreasing order: chromium, iron (ferric ion), mercury, copper, aluminum, nickel, zinc, calcium, cobalt, iron (ferrous ion), manganese, calcium, and magnesium (5737). After intravenous administration, accessible metal ions are chelated forming stable soluble complexes, which are then excreted in the urine (3078). EDTA is not metabolized, but elimination is decreased with renal dysfunction (5737). Calcium disodium EDTA and disodium EDTA are the two forms of EDTA available for clinical use (15). Calcium disodium EDTA is the form of EDTA used primarily for lead poisoning (9,15,5730,5731,5732,5733,5734,5735,5736). The calcium in calcium disodium EDTA is displaced by metal ions such as lead to form a soluble complex that is then excreted in the urine (15). Unlike disodium EDTA, calcium disodium EDTA can be administered in large quantities without causing substantial changes in serum or total body calcium concentrations (15). Radioactive isotopes such as uranium and plutonium can also be chelated to a limited extent by calcium disodium EDTA (15). Disodium EDTA antagonizes the ventricular inotropic and chronotropic effects of cardiac glycosides on the heart (15) by decreasing the amount of extracellular calcium in the blood (5761,5762). Some researchers think that decreased extracellular calcium can increase potassium re-entry into myocardial cells which then counteracts with the intracellular potassium depletion caused by cardiac glycosides (5762). Ophthalmically, disodium EDTA is used to dissolve corneal calcium deposits by binding with calcium in the eye (15,5774). EDTA can also disorganize the outer membrane of gram-negative bacteria, inhibit the coaggregation between pairs of microorganisms and is possibly an effective inhibitor of bacterial adhesins (5764). Chelation therapy using disodium EDTA has been purported by many as being efficacious in the treatment of many disease conditions, including atherosclerosis (5738,5739,5743,5751,5768). Many biochemical mechanisms have been proposed to justify the use of disodium EDTA in the treatment of atherosclerotic vascular disease (5738,5741,5743). Mechanisms claimed include that EDTA chelation therapy can extract calcium out of atherosclerotic plaques and clear atherosclerotic arteries (5742,5749) or that calcium removed by chelation is replaced by calcium from the bone, causing secretion of parathryoid hormone (PTH) which then promotes a transfer of calcium from hardened arterial tissue and plaque to bone (5749). Other mechanisms claimed also include that EDTA blocks production of free radicals involved in reactions causing atherosclerosis by reducing iron loads (5738), binds toxic metals released when blood clots in occluded arteries (5749), or that disodium EDTA prevents damage and mutation of arterial cells caused by free radicals (5749).

None of these proposed mechanisms have been scientifically proven (5749,5756), and controlled scientific clinical studies have been unable to confirm that EDTA can reverse peripheral arterial occlusive disease (5740,5742) or atherosclerotic vascular disease (5746,5750,5752,5753,5754,5769). Severe nephrotoxicity is the major toxicity that can result when disodium EDTA and calcium disodium EDTA is used in excessively large doses (15). The degeneration of proximal tubular cells that results is felt to be possibly due to an interaction between EDTA and endogenous metals in the tubular cells (3078). EDTA can also chelate and cause increased urinary excretion of magnesium (15), which may also result in decreased serum concentrations and increased excretion of potassium (15). Sudden decreases in calcium can occur if disodium EDTA is administered too rapidly resulting in tetany, cardiac arrythmias and respiratory arrest (15, 5763).

Adverse Reactions

Intravenously, EDTA can commonly cause abdominal cramps (14), anorexia, nausea, vomiting, diarrhea, headache (15), hypotension (14,15,5737), exfoliative dermatitis (15), and a burning sensation and pain at the site of infusion (15,5744). EDTA can also sometimes cause fever, chills, fatigue, malaise, thirst, sneezing and nasal congestion (15), arrhythmias (5771,5772), thrombophlebitis (14,15), anemia (15), prolonged prothrombin time (PT) (14,15,5737), transient bone marrow depression (15,5737,5772), and urinary urgency and frequency (14,15,5772). The calcium disodium form of EDTA can also cause zinc deficiency (15,5771,5772), hypercalcemia (5771,5772), mild elevations of serum alanine aminotransferase (ALT) and aspartate aminotransferase (AST) and decreased alkaline phosphatase levels (15). The disodium form of EDTA can occasionally cause muscle cramps, back pains, muscle weakness, tremors, tingling, myalgias, paresthesias (15), decreased magnesium and potassium serum concentrations (15,5771,5772), and rarely cause histamine-like reactions and insulin shock (5737). The most serious adverse effect of both forms of EDTA is nephrotoxicity (15,5772), which is dose dependent (15) and usually occurs only with doses greater than 3 grams per day (14). Both forms of EDTA can cause nocturia, hyperuricemia, polyuria, dysuria, oliguria, proteinuria, glycosuria, hematuria and distal tubule and glomeruli changes (15). Both forms of EDTA can also cause acute renal tubular necrosis, and renal insufficiency and failure (15,5772). Rapid infusion of disodium EDTA or when given in too concentrated a solution can cause hypocalcemia, tetany, convulsions, severe cardiac arrhythmias, respiratory arrest, (9,15) and death (15). When used ophthalmically, disodium EDTA can cause transient chemosis and stromal edema (15). Inhalation of disodium EDTA contained in nebulizer solutions has been reported to cause dose-related bronchoconstriction (9,5765).

Interactions with Herbs & Other Dietary Supplements

MAGNESIUM: EDTA can bind to and cause increased urinary excretion of magnesium (15).
TRACE METALS (copper, iron, zinc, etc.): EDTA can bind to and cause increased urinary excretion of trace metals (15,5733).

Interactions with Drugs

DIURETICS: EDTA can decrease serum potassium levels and increase excretion of potassium (15). There is some concern that people receiving EDTA along with potassium depleting diuretics might be at an increased risk for hypokalemia. Initiation of potassium supplementation or an increase in potassium supplement dose may be necessary for some patients. Some diuretics that can deplete potassium include chlorothiazide (Diuril), furosemide (Lasix), and hydrochlorothiazide (HCTZ, Hydrodiuril, Microzide).
INSULIN: Concomitant use of disodium EDTA with insulin can cause severe decreases in blood glucose concentrations (15,5737,5771). EDTA chelates zinc in insulin products (15) and might interfere with the designed onset and duration of activity of various insulin preparations.
WARFARIN (Coumadin): There is some concern that disodium EDTA can increase the anticoagulant effects of warfarin and potentially increase risk of bleeding. Disodium EDTA seems to increase in prothrombin time (PT) (5737).

Interactions with Foods

No interactions are known to occur, and there is no known reason to expect a clinically significant interaction with EDTA.

Interactions with Lab Tests

ALKALINE PHOSPHATASE: Disodium EDTA can decrease serum alkaline phosphatase concentrations (15,3314). Disodium EDTA can cause low magnesium serum concentrations, which decreases the activity of alkaline phosphatase (15).
ALANINE AMINOTRANSFERASE (ALT, SGPT): Calcium disodium EDTA can cause mild increases in serum ALT (15).
ASPARTATE AMINOTRANSFERASE (AST, SGOT): Calcium disodium EDTA can cause mild increases in AST (15).
CALCIUM: Calcium serum concentrations cannot be determined by colorimetric methods in patients receiving

disodium EDTA due to chelation of a calcium disodium complex. Oxalate and other precipitation methods may also give falsely decreased levels when disodium EDTA is present (15).

PROTHROMBIN TIME (PT): Disodium EDTA can increase prothrombin time (PT) in some patients (5737).

Interactions with Diseases or Conditions

ASTHMA: Nebulizer solutions containing disodium EDTA as a preservative can produce dose-related bronchoconstriction in some asthmatics (9,5765).

CARDIAC RHYTHM IRREGULARITIES: Calcium disodium EDTA can cause ECG changes such as T wave inversions (15). Disodium EDTA can have negative inotropic effects on the heart (15). Use with caution in patients with pre-existing cardiac rhythm irregularity conditions.

DIABETICS: Use of disodium EDTA may result in poor control of glucose levels in diabetic patients due to disodium EDTA's interactions with insulin preparations and serum glucose lowering effect (15).

HYPOCALCEMIA: Disodium EDTA can decrease serum calcium levels. Disodium EDTA may exacerbate hypocalcemia in patients with existing low calcium levels (15); avoid using.

HYPOKALEMIA: EDTA can increase urinary excretion of potassium and reduce serum potassium concentrations (15). EDTA might exacerbate hypokalemia in patients with existing potassium deficiency; avoid using.

HYPOMAGNESEMIA: EDTA can chelate and cause increased urinary excretion of magnesium resulting in depletion of serum magnesium concentrations (15). EDTA might exacerbate hypomagnesemia in patients with existing magnesium depletion; avoid using.

LIVER DYSFUNCTION AND HEPATITIS: Calcium disodium EDTA can cause mild increases in serum ALT (SGPT) and AST (SGOT) (15). Theoretically, EDTA might exacerbate liver dysfunction in patients with liver dysfunction or hepatitis; avoid using.

RENAL DYSFUNCTION: EDTA is nephrotoxic and might exacerbate existing renal disease. Avoid using in patients with severe renal disease and renal failure. EDTA doses should be reduced in patients with renal insufficiency (15).

SEIZURE DISORDERS: There is some concern that disodium EDTA might increase the risk of seizure in people with epilepsy or those prone to seizure (15). Disodium can cause severe decreases in serum calcium which can induce seizure (15).

TUBERCULOSIS: Use of disodium EDTA is contraindicated in people with active tuberculosis or healed calcified tubercular lesions (15). Theoretically, use of EDTA may cause the chelation of calcium from calcified tubercular lesions, resulting in possible reactivation of the tuberculosis disease process.

Dosage and Administration

TOPICAL: For corneal calcium deposits, a 0.35% to 1.85% solution is prepared with sterile 0.9% sodium chloride and commercially available disodium EDTA preparations for injection (15). Debridement of the corneal epithelium must be done before application of the solution since EDTA does not penetrate the epithelium (5773,5774). The solution is applied as a corneal bath one time for 15-20 minutes (15) followed by debridement of the calcium (5774). Or a cellulose sponge is soaked in disodium EDTA solution and wiped over the deposits until the calcium is removed (5774). The eye should be irrigated with 0.9% sodium chloride following application of disodium EDTA solution (15).

INTRAVENOUS: For acute and chronic lead poisoning and lead encephalopathy, a dose of calcium disodium EDTA 50 mg per kilogram body weight to a maximum daily dose of 3 grams (9,15) is diluted with 5% dextrose or 9% sodium chloride to a concentration of 2-4 mg/mL and given as a single infusion over 8-24 hours for up to 5 days (15). A minimal 2-day waiting period is suggested before starting a second 5-day course of chelation therapy to further minimize development of nephrotoxicity (15). For blood lead levels greater than 70 mcg/dl, it is recommended that dimercaprol (BAL, British Anti-Lewisite) be used in conjunction with calcium disodium EDTA (15,5731). For people exposed long-term to low levels of lead and with decreased renal function, 1 gram of calcium disodium EDTA has been used and mixed with 200 mL of 5% dextrose and infused over 2 hours once weekly for 2 months (5732). For hypercalcemia, a dose of disodium EDTA 50 mg/kg body weight up to a maximum daily dosage of 3 grams is diluted with 5% dextrose or 0.9 % sodium chloride to a concentration of 2-4 mg/ml and infused over 3 hours or more (15). For cardiac glycoside-induced ventricular arrhythmias, disodium EDTA is given in a dose of 15 mg/kg per hour to a maximum of 60 mg/kg infused in 5% dextrose (15). For the treatment of atherosclerotic vascular disease, people have used disodium EDTA in a dose of 50 mg/kg up to a maximum of 5 grams diluted in 500-1000 mL of a 150-osmolar carrier (5737). Heparin, sodium ascorbate, elemental magnesium, lidocaine, pyridoxine, and sodium bicarbonate is often added to the infusion with optional additives of adrenal cortex extract, cyanocobalamin, niacin, pantothenic acid, and vitamin-B complex (5737). People usually eat before treatment and bring snacks to eat during a 3-hour infusion (5738).

INTRAMUSCULAR: For acute and chronic lead poisoning and lead encephalopathy, the dosage of calcium disodium EDTA is the same as intravenous administration in divided doses every 8-12 hours (15). When given in conjunction with dimercaprol, the daily dosage is given in equally divided doses every 4 hours. To decrease pain at the injection site, 1 mL of 1% lidocaine HCl or 1 mL of 1% procaine HCl is added to each mL of calcium disodium EDTA to obtain a final lidocaine or procaine HCl concentration of 5 mg/mL (15).

Comments

The American College for Advancement of Medicine (ACAM) strongly supports using EDTA chelation therapy for cardiovascular conditions. ACAM has a standard chelation therapy protocol and has trained more than 6000 practitioners to administer chelation treatments for various conditions (5768). However, the majority of the medical community does not support chelation therapy due to the lack of supporting evidence (5747,5749,5756). An iron-EDTA chelate is also used for iron fortification of grain-based foods. The established acceptable daily intake (ADI) for iron EDTA is 2.5 mg/kg/day. Iron EDTA has Generally Recognized as Safe (GRAS) status in the US (5728).

ELDERBERRY

Also Known As

Baccae, Baises De Sureau, Black-Berried Alder, Black Elder, Black Elderberry, Boor Tree, Bountry, Elder, Ellanwood, Ellhorn, European Alder, European Elder Fruit, European Elderberry, Holunderbeeren, Sambuci Sambucus.
CAUTION: See separate listings for Elderflower, Dwarf Elder, and American Elder.

Scientific Names

Sambucus nigra.
Family: Caprifoliaceae.

People Use This For

Orally, elderberry juice-containing syrup is used for treating the flu (5260).
Historically, elderberry fruit has been used as a laxative, diuretic, to induce sweating, for catarrhal complaints, sciatica, neuralgia (8), and cancer (11).
In manufacturing, elderberry fruit is used for making wine (6) and as a food flavoring (4).

Safety

POSSIBLY SAFE ...when the cooked fruit is used orally (4,6,12).
POSSIBLY UNSAFE ...when the fruit is not cooked sufficiently because it can cause nausea and vomiting (8,12).
PREGNANCY AND LACTATION: Insufficient reliable information available; avoid using.

Effectiveness

POSSIBLY EFFECTIVE ...when used orally for reducing symptoms and duration of the influenza infection. Most patients taking an elderberry juice-containing syrup had significant symptom relief and clinical cure after 2-3 days. This clinical study used a specific elderberry juice preparation (Sambucol, JB Harris) (5260).
There is insufficient reliable information available about the effectiveness of elderberry fruit for its other uses.

Mechanism of Action

Elderberries contain the flavonoids rutin, isoquertin, and hyperoside (4,8). They also contain 3% tannins, as well as anthocyan glycosides, an essential oil, cyanogenic glycosides including sambunigrin (4,8,12), and a lectin (4151). Elderberry extract inhibits hemagglutinin activity and replication of several strains of influenza viruses A and B (5260). In one clinical trial, Elderberry juice-containing syrup (Sambucol, see Dosage) reduced the symptoms and duration of influenza in adults and children (5260).

Adverse Reactions

Raw and unripe fruit might cause nausea, vomiting, or severe diarrhea (4,12). Weakness, dizziness, numbness and stupor are reported following ingestion of elderberry juice (6). No adverse effects were reported in a clinical trial of elderberry syrup in children and adults (5260).

Interactions with Herbs & Other Dietary Supplements

Insufficient reliable information available.

Interactions with Drugs

No interactions are known to occur, and there is no known reason to expect a clinically significant interaction with elderberry.

Interactions with Foods

No interactions are known to occur, and there is no known reason to expect a clinically significant interaction with elderberry.

Interactions with Lab Tests

No interactions are known to occur, and there is no known reason to expect a clinically significant interaction with elderberry.

Interactions with Diseases or Conditions

No interactions are known to occur, and there is no known reason to expect a clinically significant interaction with elderberry.

Dosage and Administration

ORAL: Influenza, an adult dose of four tablespoons of elderberry juice-containing syrup (Sambucol) daily for three days has been used (5260); a dose of two tablespoons of Sambucol daily for three days has been used in children (5260).

Comments

Avoid confusion with American elder (Sambucus canadensis).

ELDERFLOWER

Also Known As

Black-Berried Alder, Black Elder, Boor Tree, Bountry, Common Elder, Ellanwood, Ellhorn, European Alder, European Elder Flower, Sambucus, Sweet Elder.
CAUTION: See separate listings for American Elder, Dwarf Elder, and Elderberry.

Scientific Names

Sambucus nigra.
Family: Caprifoliaceae.

People Use This For

Orally, elderflower is used as a diuretic, laxative, and to induce sweating (2,11,18). It is also used orally to treat colds (2,11,18), flu (11), cough, and bronchitis (18).
Topically, elderflower preparations are used as a gargle and mouthwash for coughs, headcolds, laryngitis, flu, and shortness of breath (18). It is used on the skin as an astringent for rheumatism (11), swelling, and inflammation (4,18).
In combination with gentian root, verbena, cowslip flower, and sorrel, elderflower is used orally for maintaining healthy sinuses (373) and treating sinusitis (7,374,379).
In foods and beverages, elderflowers are used as a flavoring component (11).
In manufacturing, elderflower extracts are used in perfumes (11). Elderflower water is used as a vehicle in eye and skin lotions.

Safety

LIKELY SAFE ...when consumed in amounts used in foods. It has Generally Recognized as Safe (GRAS) status in the US (11). ...when used orally and appropriately (2,4,12) in therapeutic amounts; no adverse effects have been reported (2,4,6,12).
POSSIBLY SAFE ...when used orally with gentian root, verbena, cowslip flower, and sorrel (Quanterra Sinus Defense, Sinupret) (7,374,379).
There is insufficient reliable information available about the safety of the topical use of elderflower.
PREGNANCY AND LACTATION: Insufficient reliable information available; avoid using.

Effectiveness

POSSIBLY EFFECTIVE ...when used orally with gentian root, verbena, cowslip flower, and sorrel (Quanterra Sinus Defense, Sinupret) for treating acute or chronic sinusitis (7,374,379).
There is insufficient reliable information available about the effectiveness of elderflower for its other uses.

Mechanism of Action

Elderflower may have sweat-inducing, diuretic, and laxative effects. It also soothes mucous membranes and stimulates bronchial secretions (2,4,11). Compounds responsible for diuretic and laxative properties have not yet been isolated. Elderflower has demonstrated anti-inflammatory, antiviral, and diuretic effects in animals (4). Constituents of a related species, Sambucus formosana, appear to have a hepatoprotective activity against liver damage (6).

Adverse Reactions

None reported.

Interactions with Herbs & Other Dietary Supplements
Insufficient reliable information available.

Interactions with Drugs
No interactions are known to occur, and there is no known reason to expect a clinically significant interaction with elderflower.

Interactions with Foods
No interactions are known to occur, and there is no known reason to expect a clinically significant interaction with elderflower.

Interactions with Lab Tests
No interactions are known to occur, and there is no known reason to expect a clinically significant interaction with elderflower.

Interactions with Diseases or Conditions
No interactions are known to occur, and there is no known reason to expect a clinically significant interaction with elderflower.

Dosage and Administration
ORAL: People typically use one cup tea (steep 2-4 grams dried flowers in 250 mL boiling water 10-15 minutes, strain) three times daily (4); average daily dose 10-15 grams dried flowers (2). Liquid extract (1:1 in 25% alcohol), 2-4 mL three times daily has also been used (4). For acute or chronic sinusitis, two Sinupret tablets three times daily for up to two weeks has been used in clinical trials (7,374,379), equivalent to gentian root 12 mg, elderflower 36 mg, verbena 36 mg, cowslip flower 36 mg, and sorrel 36 mg three times daily. For maintaining healthy sinuses, a typical dose is one tablet of Quanterra Sinus Defense three times daily with water, equivalent to gentian root 9 mg, elderflower 29 mg, verbena 29 mg, cowslip flower 29 mg, and sorrel 29 mg three times daily (373).
Each tablet of Quanterra Sinus Defense contains 125 mg of the herbal combination found in Sinupret (373).
TOPICAL: No typical dosage.

Comments
Avoid confusion with American elder (Sambucus canadensis). American elder (sambucus candadensis) and European elder (sambucus nigra), are discussed together despite the fact most of the information available pertains to elder (11).

ELECAMPANE

Also Known As
Alant, Elfdock, Elfwort, Horse-Elder, Horseheal, Inula, Scabwort, Velvet Dock, Wild Sunflower, Yellow Starwort.

Scientific Names
Inula helenium, synonyms Helenium grandiflorum, Aster officinalis, Aster helenium.
Family: Asteraceae or Compositae.

People Use This For
Orally, elecampane is used as an expectorant, antitussive, and diaphoretic (4), for diseases of the respiratory tract (2), as an anthelmintic, for improving stomach function, and as a diuretic (11).
In folk medicine, elecampane has been used for asthma, bronchitis, whooping cough (11), cough associated with tuberculosis (4), nausea, and diarrhea (11).
In foods and beverages, elecampane is used as a flavoring ingredient (11).
In other manufacturing processes, elecampane is used as a fragrance component in cosmetics and soaps (11).

Safety
LIKELY SAFE ...when consumed in amounts found in alcoholic beverages (11).
POSSIBLY SAFE ...when the root and rhizome preparations are used appropriately as an oral medicinal agent (12).
POSSIBLY UNSAFE ...when used orally in large amounts. Elecampane can cause gastrointestinal upset and symptoms of paralysis (12).
PREGNANCY AND LACTATION: LIKELY UNSAFE ...when used orally (12).

Effectiveness

POSSIBLY EFFECTIVE ...when used orally for treating hookworm, roundworm, threadworm and whipworm infections (4,11); alantolactone is used as an anthelmintic in Europe and the UK (11).
There is insufficient reliable information available about the effectiveness of elecampane for its other uses.

Mechanism of Action

The applicable parts of elecampane are the rhizome/root. Alantolactone and isoalantolactone, sesquiterpene alkaloids found in elecampane, show antibacterial and antifungal (11) activity in vitro and anthelmintic activity in humans (11).

Adverse Reactions

Large doses taken orally may cause vomiting, diarrhea, spasms, and symptoms of paralysis (12). Topically, elecampane may cause allergic contact dermatitis (4). It can cause an allergic reaction in individuals sensitive to the Asteraceae/Compositae family. Members of this family include ragweed, chrysanthemums, marigolds, daisies, and many other herbs.

Interactions with Herbs & Other Dietary Supplements

HERBS WITH SEDATIVE PROPERTIES: Theoretically, concomitant use with herbs that have sedative properties might enhance therapeutic and adverse effects. These include calamus, calendula, California poppy, catnip, capsicum, celery, couch grass, Siberian ginseng, German chamomile, goldenseal, gotu kola, hops, Jamaican dogwood, kava, lemon balm, sage, St. John's wort, sassafras, scullcap, shepherd's purse, stinging nettle, valerian, wild carrot, wild lettuce, ashwaganda root, and yerba mansa (4,19).

Interactions with Drugs

HYPOGLYCEMIC DRUGS: Theoretically, concomitant use may interfere with drug activity and blood glucose control (4).
ANTIHYPERTENSIVE, ANTIHYPOTENSIVE DRUGS: Theoretically, concomitant use may interfere with drug therapy and blood pressure control (4).
DRUGS WITH SEDATIVE PROPERTIES: Theoretically, concomitant use with drugs with sedative properties may cause additive effects (4).

Interactions with Foods

No interactions are known to occur, and there is no known reason to expect a clinically significant interaction with elecampane.

Interactions with Lab Tests

No interactions are known to occur, and there is no known reason to expect a clinically significant interaction with elecampane.

Interactions with Diseases or Conditions

DIABETES: Theoretically, elecampane may interfere with blood glucose control (4).
HYPERTENSION, HYPOTENSION: Theoretically, elecampane may interfere with blood pressure control (4).
CROSS-ALLERGENICITY: Can cause an allergic reaction in individuals sensitive to the Asteraceae/Compositae family. Members of this family include ragweed, chrysanthemums, marigolds, daisies, and many other herbs.

Dosage and Administration

ORAL: Typically, 1.5-4 grams of rhizome/root three times daily, or one cup tea (simmer 1.5-4 grams of rhizome/root in 150 mL boiling water 5-10 minutes, strain) three times daily is used (4). Liquid extract (1:1 in 25% alcohol) 1.5-4 mL three times daily is also used (4). As an anthelmintic for adults, alantolactone 300 mg daily for 2 courses of 5 days, with an interval of 10 days, is used. For children, alantolactone 50-200 mg daily is used (4).

Comments

None.

ELEMI

Also Known As
Elemi Oleoresin, Elemi Resin, Manila Elemi.

Scientific Names
Canarium commune; Canarium luzonicum.
Family: Burseraceae.

People Use This For
In folk medicine, elemi is used for improving stomach function, and as an expectorant and local stimulant.
In foods and beverages, elemi is used as a flavoring agent (11).
In other manufacturing processes, elemi is used as a fixative and fragrance in cosmetics and soaps (11).

Safety
LIKELY SAFE ...when used in amounts found in foods; approved for food use in the US (11).
There is insufficient reliable information available about the safety of the oral use of elemi in amounts greater than those found in foods.
PREGNANCY AND LACTATION: Insufficient reliable information available; avoid using.

Effectiveness
There is insufficient reliable information available about the effectiveness of elemi.

Mechanism of Action
The applicable parts of elemi are the gum and oil. There is insufficient reliable information available about the possible mechanism of action and active ingredients.

Adverse Reactions
None reported.

Interactions with Herbs & Other Dietary Supplements
Insufficient reliable information available.

Interactions with Drugs
No interactions are known to occur, and there is no known reason to expect a clinically significant interaction with elemi.

Interactions with Foods
No interactions are known to occur, and there is no known reason to expect a clinically significant interaction with elemi.

Interactions with Lab Tests
No interactions are known to occur, and there is no known reason to expect a clinically significant interaction with elemi.

Interactions with Diseases or Conditions
No interactions are known to occur, and there is no known reason to expect a clinically significant interaction with elemi.

Dosage and Administration
No typical dosage.

Comments
Elemi gum is resin exuded by the elemi tree (Canarium commune). Elemi oil is produced by distillation of elemi gum resin.

ELM BARK

Also Known As
Smooth-Leaved Elm.

Scientific Names
Ulmus minor.
Family: Ulmaceae.

People Use This For
Orally, elm bark is used for digestive disorders and severe diarrhea. Sometimes it is used as a diuretic and astringent. Topically, elm bark is used for cleaning open and/or festering wounds (18).

Safety
There is insufficient reliable information available about the safety of elm bark.
Pregnancy and Lactation: Insufficient reliable information available; avoid using.

Effectiveness
There is insufficient reliable information available about the effectiveness of elm bark.

Mechanism of Action
There is insufficient reliable information available about the possible mechanism of action and active ingredients.

Adverse Reactions
None reported.

Interactions with Herbs & Other Dietary Supplements
Insufficient reliable information available.

Interactions with Drugs
No interactions are known to occur, and there is no known reason to expect a clinically significant interaction with elm bark.

Interactions with Foods
No interactions are known to occur, and there is no known reason to expect a clinically significant interaction with elm bark.

Interactions with Lab Tests
No interactions are known to occur, and there is no known reason to expect a clinically significant interaction with elm bark.

Interactions with Diseases or Conditions
No interactions are known to occur, and there is no known reason to expect a clinically significant interaction with elm bark.

Dosage and Administration
ORAL: People have used one cup of tea orally 2-3 times daily. The tea is prepared by simmering 2 teaspoons of bark in 150 mL of boiling water for 10-15 minutes and straining. Alternately, 2-5 grams of powdered root daily has been used (18).
TOPICAL: A 20% tea diluted 1:1 with water has been used (18).

Comments
There is very little scientific information about this product. Our staff is continually analyzing the available information on natural medicines and will add data here as it becomes available.

EMU OIL

Also Known As
Emu.

Scientific Names

Dromiceius nova-hollandiae.

People Use This For

Orally, emu oil is used for improving cholesterol levels, as a source of polyunsaturated and monounsaturated fatty acids (5914), for weight loss (5920), and as a cough syrup for colds and flu (5914).

Topically, emu oil is used for relief from sore muscles; aching joints, pain or inflammation (5914); carpal tunnel syndrome; sciatica, shin splints (5918); and gout (5921). It is also used topically to improve healing of wounds and incisions, burns from radiation therapy, to reduce bruises and stretch marks (5914), to reduce scarring and keloids, to heal the donor site of skin grafting (5916), to diminish acne inflammation, soften dry cuticles and promote healthy nails (5914), for skin cancers (5916), athlete's foot, diaper rash, canker sores, chapped lips, circulation (5918), dry skin, eczema, psoriasis, wrinkles or age spots, dry or damaged hair (5914), dandruff (5918), in massage therapy (5914), for its anti-aging properties (5915), to protect skin from sun damage (5917), and to promote skin rejuvenation (5916). Emu oil is also used topically to reduce pain and irritation from shingles, bed sores, hemorrhoids, diabetic neuropathy (5914), insect bites (5917), earaches, eye irritation (5918), "growing pains" (5916), and frostbite (5918). It is used for rashes, razor burn and nicks, rosacea, and roseola (5918).

Intranasally, emu oil is used to treat colds and flu (5914).

In combination, emu oil (7%) is used with glycolic acid (10%) for lowering cholesterol, triglycerides, and low density lipoprotein; preventing and treating allergies; preventing scarring; treating headaches, especially migraines; preventing nosebleeds; treating and preventing cold and flu symptoms; and relieving discomfort associated with menstruation (5916).

In veterinary practice, emu oil is used to reduce swelling in joints, prevent cracked or peeling paws, calm "hot spots", and reduce irritation of flea bites (5914).

In manufacturing, emu oil is used to sharpen and oil industrial machinery, for polishing timber and leather, and for conditioning and waterproofing (5916).

Safety

POSSIBLY SAFE ...when used orally and appropriately. ...when used topically. There are no reports of adverse affects and the Australian government classifies emu meat as fit for human consumption (5916).
PREGNANCY AND LACTATION: Insufficient reliable information available; avoid using.

Effectiveness

There is insufficient reliable information available about the effectiveness of emu oil.

Mechanism of Action

Though not standardized, emu oil typically contains myristic, palmitic, palmitoleic, stearic, oleic, linoleic, and linolenic fatty acids (5919). Linoleic acid is believed to ease muscle ache and joint pain; oleic acid is considered to have a local anti-inflammatory effect (5922). Emu oil appears to have the ability to penetrate the skin, perhaps in part because it does not contain phospholipids (5922). Some animal evidence suggests emu oil is more effective in acute inflammation than in chronic inflammation (5923). A combination of 7% emu oil and 10% glycolic acid is patented for therapeutic use in methods for lowering cholesterol, triglycerides, and low density lipoprotein; preventing and treating allergies; preventing scarring; treating headaches; preventing nosebleeds; treating and preventing cold and flu symptoms; relieving discomfort associated with menstruation (5916). However, no studies have been published in refereed journals.

Adverse Reactions

None reported.

Interactions with Herbs & Other Dietary Supplements

HERBS WITH ANTICOAGULANT/ANTIPLATELET POTENTIAL: Concomitant use of herbs that have coumarin constituents or affect platelet aggregation could theoretically increase the risk of bleeding in some people. These herbs include: angelica, anise, arnica, asafoetida, bogbean, boldo, capsicum, celery, chamomile, clove, danshen, fenugreek, feverfew, garlic, ginger, ginkgo, ginseng Panax, horse chestnut, horseradish, licorice, meadowsweet, prickly ash, onion, papain, passionflower, poplar, quassia, red clover, turmeric, wild carrot, wild lettuce, willow, and others (4,19).

Interactions with Drugs

ASPIRIN AND ANTICOAGULANTS: Some information suggests the concomitant use of the emu oil constituent linolenic acid might increase risk of bleeding (5914).

Interactions with Foods

No interactions are known to occur, and there is no known reason to expect a clinically significant interaction with emu oil.

Interactions with Lab Tests

LIPID LEVELS: Some evidence suggests that emu oil might reduce lipid levels (5916).

Interactions with Diseases or Conditions

No interactions are known to occur, and there is no known reason to expect a clinically significant interaction with emu oil.

Dosage and Administration

ORAL: Emu oil 7% in combination with 10% glycolic acid, the preferable adult dose is 1 teaspoon daily (5916).
TOPICAL: For sore muscles, aching joints, pain or inflammation, apply emu oil to affected area three times daily for at least three days (5914).

Comments

The emu has been a sacred bird to the Australian Aborigines for thousands of years. The emu provided the Aborigines with clothing, food, and oil believed to have special healing properties (5914). The therapeutic uses of emu oil were patented in 1995 by Elf Resources, Inc., New Rochelle, NY (5916).

ENGLISH ADDER'S TONGUE

Also Known As

Christs Spear, Christ's Spear, English Adders Tongue, Green Oil of Charity, Serpents Tongue, Serpent's Tongue.
CAUTION: See separate listing for American Adder's Tongue.

Scientific Names

Ophioglossum vulgatum.

People Use This For

Topically, English adder's tongue is used to treat ulcers (18).

Safety

There is insufficient reliable information available about the safety of English adder's tongue.
Pregnancy and Lactation: Insufficient reliable information available; avoid using.

Effectiveness

There is insufficient reliable information available about the effectiveness of English adder's tongue.

Mechanism of Action

The applicable parts of English adder's tongue are the root and leaf. English adder's tongue is stated to have emollient properties when applied. When used orally, it is has emetic properties (18).

Adverse Reactions

None reported.

Interactions with Herbs & Other Dietary Supplements

Insufficient reliable information available.

Interactions with Drugs

No interactions are known to occur, and there is no known reason to expect a clinically significant interaction with English adder's tongue.

Interactions with Foods

No interactions are known to occur, and there is no known reason to expect a clinically significant interaction with English adder's tongue.

Interactions with Lab Tests

No interactions are known to occur, and there is no known reason to expect a clinically significant interaction with English adder's tongue.

Interactions with Diseases or Conditions

No interactions are known to occur, and there is no known reason to expect a clinically significant interaction with English adder's tongue.

Dosage and Administration

TOPICAL: Fresh English adder's tongue leaves are applied as a poultice.

Comments

Avoid confusion with American adder's tongue (Erythronium americanum).

ENGLISH HORSEMINT

Also Known As

None.

Scientific Names

Mentha longifolia.
Family: Labitae or Lamiceae.

People Use This For

Orally, English horsemint is used for digestive disorders, particularly flatulence.
Historically, English horsemint was used for pain in general, and specifically for headaches [18].

Safety

There is insufficient reliable information available about the safety of English horsemint.
Pregnancy and Lactation: Insufficient reliable information available; avoid using.

Effectiveness

There is insufficient reliable information available about the effectiveness of English horsemint.

Mechanism of Action

The applicable parts of English horsemint are the above ground parts. There is insufficient reliable information available about the possible mechanism of action and active ingredients.

Adverse Reactions

None reported.

Interactions with Herbs & Other Dietary Supplements

Insufficient reliable information available.

Interactions with Drugs

No interactions are known to occur, and there is no known reason to expect a clinically significant interaction with English horsemint.

Interactions with Foods

No interactions are known to occur, and there is no known reason to expect a clinically significant interaction with English horsemint.

Interactions with Lab Tests

No interactions are known to occur, and there is no known reason to expect a clinically significant interaction with English horsemint.

Interactions with Diseases or Conditions

No interactions are known to occur, and there is no known reason to expect a clinically significant interaction with English horsemint.

Dosage and Administration
ORAL: English horsemint is used as a tea (18).
TOPICAL: English horsemint is used as a bath additive (18).

Comments
There is very little scientific information about this product. Our staff is continually analyzing the available information on natural medicines and will add data here as it becomes available.

ENGLISH IVY

Also Known As
Gum Ivy, Hederae helicis folium, Ivy, True Ivy, Woodbind.

Scientific Names
Hedera helix.
Family: Araliaceae.

People Use This For
Orally, English ivy is used for inflammation of mucous membranes in respiratory passages, symptomatic treatment of chronic inflammatory bronchial conditions (2), as an expectorant (3), as an antispasmodic (18), and improvement of lung function in children with chronic obstructive bronchitis (3471).
Topically, English ivy is used for burn wounds, calluses, cellulitis, inflammations, neuralgia, parasitic disorders, ulcers, rheumatic complaints, and for phlebitis (18).
In folk medicine, English ivy is used orally for liver, spleen, and gallbladder disorders; gout; rheumatism; and scrofulosis (18).

Safety
POSSIBLY SAFE ...when used orally and appropriately (2).
There is insufficient reliable information available about the safety of English ivy for its other uses.
PREGNANCY AND LACTATION: Insufficient reliable information available; avoid using.

Effectiveness
POSSIBLY EFFECTIVE ...when used orally for inflammation of respiratory passage mucous membranes, symptomatic treatment of chronic inflammatory bronchial conditions (2), and improvement of lung function in children with chronic obstructive bronchitis (3471).
There is insufficient reliable information available about the effectiveness of English ivy for its other uses.

Mechanism of Action
The applicable part of English ivy is the leaf. English ivy has expectorant and antispasmodic actions. It irritates skin and mucosa (2). Researchers think the ivy leaf acts on the gastric mucosa to cause stimulation of mucous glands in the bronchi via parasympathetic sensory pathways (7). Fresh leaves contain the contact allergen falcarinol (7). Preliminary evidence suggests ivy leaf dried extract may improve lung function (measured as forced expiratory volume in one second) in children with chronic obstructive bronchitis due to its secretolytic and spasmolytic effects (3471). Human studies are needed to determine whether ivy leaf dried extract is as effective or beneficial as conventional agents used prophylactically to improve and maintain lung function such as bronchodilators and corticosteroids.

Adverse Reactions
Orally, fresh English ivy leaves can cause skin irritation (7). Saponin constituents, hederacosides, and hederin monodesmosides have acrid and/or bitter taste (7).

Interactions with Herbs & Other Dietary Supplements
Insufficient reliable information available.

Interactions with Drugs
No interactions are known to occur, and there is no known reason to expect a clinically significant interaction with English ivy.

Interactions with Foods
No interactions are known to occur, and there is no known reason to expect a clinically significant interaction with English ivy.

Interactions with Lab Tests

No interactions are known to occur, and there is no known reason to expect a clinically significant interaction with English ivy.

Interactions with Diseases or Conditions

No interactions are known to occur, and there is no known reason to expect a clinically significant interaction with English ivy.

Dosage and Administration

ORAL: People have used 300-800 mg dried leaf per day (2,18), or one cup tea, steep 1 heaping teaspoon of dried leaf in 1/4 cup boiling water 10 minutes, strain, up to three times daily (18). For chronic obstructive bronchitis in children, 35 mg dried leaf extract three times a day or 14 mg dried leaf alcohol-based extract three times a day has been used (3471).
TOPICAL: Fresh leaves placed on festering wounds and burns have been used (18). For rheumatism, prepare tea, simmer 200 grams of fresh leaves in 1 L boiling water 5-10 minutes, strain (18).

Comments

English ivy is most often used in the form of an extract and seldom used as a prepared tea (7).

ENGLISH WALNUT

Also Known As

Fructus Cortex, Juglans, Juglandis, Juglandis Folium, Walnussblätter, Walnussfrüchtschalen, Walnut, Walnut Fruit, Walnut Hull, Walnut Leaf.
CAUTION: See separate listing for Black Walnut.

Scientific Names

Juglans regia.
Family: Juglandaceae.

People Use This For

Orally, the English walnut fruit is used as a part of the diet for lowering cholesterol. The hull of English walnut is used to treat gastrointestinal mucous membrane inflammation (2,805,4800). The leaf is used orally for treating diarrhea. Topically, the hull is used for skin diseases, abscesses, and eye lid inflammation (2,805). The leaf is used topically for superficial inflammation of the skin; excessive hand and/or foot perspiration (2,4800); and for skin conditions such as acne, eczema, scrophula, pyodermia, and ulcers (8).
In combination with other herbs, English walnut hull is used to treat diabetes mellitus, gastritis, and anemia (2,4800). Traditionally, English walnut hull has been used to treat "blood poisoning" and as a "blood purifier" to remove undesirable agents from the blood (2,4800). The leaf is used traditionally for gastrointestinal mucous membrane inflammation, as an anthelmintic, and "blood-purifying" agent (8).
In foods, English walnut is commonly consumed, usually as a snack, in baking, and in salads.

Safety

LIKELY SAFE ...when the fruit is eaten in amounts normally found in foods.
POSSIBLY SAFE ...when the leaf is used topically and appropriately, short-term (2,18,4800).
POSSIBLY UNSAFE ...when the hull is used topically. English walnut hulls might contain the carcinogenic constituent juglone; however, the amount of juglone contained in hulls is not clear. Daily topical use of walnut preparations known to contain juglone has been associated with skin discoloration and increased risk of cancer of the tongue and lip leukoplakia (2,4800).
There is insufficient reliable information available about the safety of the oral use of English walnut for medicinal purposes.
PREGNANCY AND LACTATION: POSSIBLY UNSAFE ...when the hull is used topically. English walnut hulls might contain the carcinogenic constituent juglone (2,4800); avoid using. There is insufficient reliable information available about the safety of the oral use of English walnut leaf during pregnancy and lactation; avoid using.

Effectiveness

POSSIBLY EFFECTIVE ...when the fruit is used as part of a special diet for lowering cholesterol. One trial found that a diet with walnuts composing 35% of daily fat intake lowered total and low-density lipoprotein (LDL) cholesterol by 9% and 11.2% compared to 5% and 5.6%, respectively, with a Mediterranean diet (6431). ...when the leaf is used topically for mild, superficial inflammation of the skin, and excessive perspiration of the hands and feet (2,4800).

There is insufficient reliable information available about the effectiveness of English walnut hull or leaf for its other uses.

Mechanism of Action

The applicable parts of English walnut are the fruit, hull, and leaf. English walnut hull contains the tannins, galloylglucose and ellagitannins; naphthalene derivatives including juglone; and flavonoids including hyperoside and quercitrin (8,18). The leaf of the English walnut also contains tannins (2,4800). The astringent properties of English walnut hull and leaf can be attributed to the tannins (2,8,18,4800). Juglone and the essential juglone oil from the leaves have antifungal effects. The juglone component of the leaves may quickly break down when leaves are handled or dried (8,18). The fruit of English walnut is high in alpha-linolenic acid, a polyunsaturated fatty acid, which may be responsible for benefits in hyperlipidemia (6431).

Adverse Reactions

No adverse reactions with english walnut leaf have been reported. However, applying walnut preparations containing the juglone constituent to skin and mucous membranes leads to yellow or brown discoloration (2). Daily use of juglone-containing preparations is associated with tongue cancer and lip leukoplakia (2). Juglone is reported to have mutagenic effects in animals (12). English walnut hull is thought to contain juglone, but it is not clear what concentration of juglone it contains (2) and the extent of the risk. The fruit of English walnut has been reported to cause softening of stools, and mild bloating (6431).

Interactions with Herbs & Other Dietary Supplements

Insufficient reliable information available.

Interactions with Drugs

No interactions are known to occur, and there is no known reason to expect a clinically significant interaction with English walnut.

Interactions with Foods

No interactions are known to occur, and there is no known reason to expect a clinically significant interaction with English walnut.

Interactions with Lab Tests

No interactions are known to occur, and there is no known reason to expect a clinically significant interaction with English walnut.

Interactions with Diseases or Conditions

No interactions are known to occur, and there is no known reason to expect a clinically significant interaction with English walnut.

Dosage and Administration

ORAL: For lowering cholesterol, the fruit of approximately 8-11 English walnuts were consumed per day with the diet in one study (6431). For English walnut leaf, as an adjuvant for skin conditions, one cup tea (simmer 1.5 grams of finely chopped dried leaf in 150 mL boiling water 3-5 minutes, steep) one to three times daily (8).
TOPICAL: For dressing, lotion, poultice or hip bath, simmer 2-3 grams of finely chopped dried English walnut leaf per 100 mL boiling water (2,8). Average daily amount is 3-6 grams of dried leaf (18).

Comments

None.

EPA (EICOSAPENTAENOIC ACID)

Also Known As

EPA, Eicosapentaenoic, Eicosapentaenoic Acid, Fish Oil Fatty Acid, N-3 Fatty Acid, Omega Fatty Acid, Omega 3 Fatty Acid, Omega-3 Fatty Acid, W-3 Fatty Acid.
CAUTION: See separate listings for Cod Liver Oil, DHA (docosahexaenoic acid), and Fish Oils.

Scientific Names

Eicosapentaenoic acid.

People Use This For

Orally, eicosapentaenoic acid (EPA) is used for treating the symptoms of cystic fibrosis, reducing the risk of intrauterine growth retardation, and treating pregnancy induced hypertension in high-risk pregnancies (1027). In combination, EPA is used with docosahexanoic acid (DHA) in fish oil preparations for a variety of conditions, including preventing and reversing heart disease, decreasing ectopic ventricular beats, asthma, cancer, dysmenorrhea, hay fever, lung diseases, lupus erythematosus, lupus nephritis, and IgA nephropathy (507). They are also used in combination for migraine headache prophylaxis in adolescents (5097), atopic dermatitis, Behcet's syndrome, hyperlipidemia, hypertension, psoriasis, Raynaud's syndrome, rheumatoid arthritis, Crohn's disease, and ulcerative colitis (9).

Safety

LIKELY SAFE ...when used orally and appropriately (9,945,1016).
POSSIBLY UNSAFE ...when used orally in high doses. Doses greater than 3 grams daily might decrease blood coagulation and increase the risk of bleeding (1313).
PREGNANCY AND LACTATION: Insufficient reliable information available; avoid using.

Effectiveness

POSSIBLY EFFECTIVE ...when used orally as an adjunct to standard therapy for schizophrenia. One clinical study has shown EPA to be superior to both docosahexanoic acid (DHA) and linoleic acid (5073).
POSSIBLY INEFFECTIVE ...when taken orally as a single agent for treating symptoms of cystic fibrosis (1006,1027). ...when used orally for reducing the risk of intrauterine growth retardation (1027). ...when used orally for pregnancy-induced hypertension in women with high-risk pregnancies (1027). ...when taken orally to treat asthma. A clinical trial has shown that EPA has no effects on asthma symptoms when given for 4 weeks (1023). ...when taken orally to treat hayfever. A clinical trial has shown that EPA is no more effective than placebo for relieving hayfever symptoms, including wheezing, cough and nasal symptoms (1036).
There is insufficient reliable information available about the effectiveness of EPA for its other uses.

Mechanism of Action

EPA is a long chain n-3 polyunsaturated fatty acid that competes with arachidonic acid for inclusion in cyclo-oxygenase and lipoxygenase pathways (9). EPA decreases blood viscosity and increases red blood cell deformability (9). Pure EPA reduces serum triglyceride concentrations, increases fasting insulin concentrations, and has no effect on total, LDL, or HDL-cholesterol or fasting glucose concentrations in mildly hypercholesterolemic men (6143).

Adverse Reactions

Adverse reactions have not been reported for EPA alone. However, for fish oils containing EPA and DHA, side effects can include fishy taste, belching (507), nosebleeds (9), nausea, and loose stools (9). Three people with pre-existing familial adenomatous polyposis were diagnosed with malignant lesions during the course of long-term fish oil use (999). High doses of fish oils might also decrease blood coagulation and increase the risk of bleeding (1313).

Interactions with Herbs & Other Dietary Supplements

HERBS WITH ANTICOAGULANT/ANTIPLATELET POTENTIAL: Concomitant use of herbs that have coumarin constituents or affect platelet aggregation could theoretically increase the risk of bleeding in some people. These herbs include: angelica, anise, arnica, asafoetida, bogbean, boldo, capsicum, celery, chamomile, clove, danshen, fenugreek, feverfew, garlic, ginger, ginkgo, ginseng (Panax), horse chestnut, horseradish, licorice, meadowsweet, prickly ash, onion, papain, passionflower, poplar, quassia, red clover, turmeric, wild carrot, wild lettuce, willow, and others (4,19).

Interactions with Drugs

ANTICOAGULANTS/ANTIPLATELET DRUGS: Theoretically, concomitant use of EPA with anticoagulant or antiplatelet drugs, including aspirin can increase the risk of bleeding (9,507).
ETRETINATE: Concomitant use can have additive effects for treating psoriasis (1000). Fish oils containing EPA and DHA can attenuate cyclosporine-induced hypertension in people with kidney or heart transplants (507,1012,1021).

Interactions with Foods

No interactions are known to occur, and there is no known reason to expect a clinically significant interaction with EPA.

Interactions with Lab Tests

INSULIN: EPA can increase fasting insulin concentrations and test results in mildly hypercholesterolemic patients (6143).

INTERNATIONAL NORMALIZED RATIO (INR), PROTHROMBIN TIME (PT): High doses of greater than 3 grams per day might decrease blood coagulation, increase INR and PT, and increase the risk of bleeding (1313).
PULMONARY FUNCTION TESTS: EPA might cause a decline in pulmonary function tests in aspirin-sensitive individuals (507).
TRIGLYCERIDES: EPA can reduce serum triglyceride concentrations and test results in patients with hypercholesterolemia (6143).

Interactions with Diseases or Conditions

ASPIRIN-SENSITIVE INDIVIDUALS: Fish oils and other omega-3 fatty acids can lower pulmonary function tests in some aspirin sensitive patients (507).
DIABETES: Fish oils containing EPA and DHA can interfere with blood glucose control (9). Monitor blood glucose levels closely. Dose adjustments may be necessary.
HYPERTENSION: Fish oils including EPA can lower blood pressure and might have additive effects in patients with high blood pressure who are treated with antihypertensives (1001,1020,1030,1033).

Dosage and Administration

ORAL: EPA is usually administered with DHA (docosahexaenoic acid) as fish oil. A wide range of doses have been used. The usual amount is 5 grams of fish oil containing 169-563 mg of EPA and 72-312 grams of DHA (9,507). As an adjunct to standard therapy for schizophrenia, an oral EPA daily dose of 2 grams has been used (5703). Many fish oil preparations also contain small amounts of vitamin E as an antioxidant (9).

Comments

Avoid confusion with DHA (docosahexaenoic acid) and fish oils, which contain EPA and DHA. Most available data involving EPA are from research and clinical experience with fish oil products containing variable combinations of EPA and DHA. For more information, see the separate listing for Fish Oils. Researchers are investigating oils containing stearidonic acid (SDA) from genetically modified plants as an alternative source of omega-3 fatty acids. SDA is metabolized to EPA and DHA in animals. However, further research is needed on the effects of SDA in humans (6129).

EPHEDRA

Also Known As

Cao Mahuang, Desert Herb, Ephedrae herba, Ephedra sinensis, Herbal Ecstasy, Joint Fir, Ma Huang, Ma-Huang, Mahuang, Mahuanggen (ma huang root), Muzei Mahuang, Popotillo, Sea Grape, Teamster's Tea, Yellow Astringent, Yellow Horse, Zhong Mahuang.
CAUTION: See separate listing for Mormon Tea.

Scientific Names

Ephedra distachya; Ephedra equisetina; Ephedra gerardiana; Ephedra intermedia; Ephedra shennungiana; Ephedra sinica; and other Ephedra species.
Family: Ephedraceae.

People Use This For

Orally, ephedra is used for weight loss and obesity and to enhance athletic performance. It is also used for allergies and allergic rhinitis; nasal congestion; and respiratory tract conditions such as bronchospasm, asthma, and bronchitis (18). Ephedra is also used for colds, flu, fever, chills, headache, edema, anhydrosis, joint and bone pain, and as a diuretic for edema.

Safety

POSSIBLY UNSAFE ...when used orally. There is concern that use of ephedra can cause severe life-threatening or disabling adverse effects in some people. Several case reports have linked ephedra use to hypertension, myocardial infarction, seizure, stroke, and other significant adverse effects. Some suggest that ephedra is only harmful when used inappropriately in excessive doses. However, in several cases significant adverse events occurred with short-term use of relatively low doses ranging from 20-60 mg of ephedra alkaloids (2729,6486). Based on case reports, it is not possible to determine the incidence of these serious adverse effects or to determine who is at the greatest risk. However, people with existing conditions such as cardiovascular disease or those using ephedra products in combination with other stimulants such as caffeine, might be at increased risk. Until more is known, advise patients to avoid ephedra products. Tell them that any potential benefits of ephedra do not outweigh the potential risks.
LIKELY UNSAFE ...when used orally in high doses or long-term. Prolonged use or use of high doses can increase the risk of serious adverse effects (2729). Chronic use can also cause rapid development of tolerance and dependence (2,12).

CHILDREN: LIKELY UNSAFE ...when used orally. Children can be more susceptible to the adverse effects of ephedra (2,12).

PREGNANCY: LIKELY UNSAFE ...when used orally. Ephedra can stimulate uterine contraction (12); contraindicated.

LACTATION: Insufficient reliable information available; avoid using.

Effectiveness

POSSIBLY EFFECTIVE ...when used orally, short-term for obesity. There is preliminary evidence that a specific combination product containing ephedra, guarana, and 17 other vitamins, minerals, and supplements (Metabolife-356) might help reduce weight by approximately 2.7 kg over 8 weeks when used with a low-fat diet and exercise (3719). However, there are serious concerns about the safety of this product since it combines significant amounts of the stimulants ephedra and caffeine (See Adverse Reactions). Tell patients to avoid using this product. ...when taken orally for short-term treatment of respiratory conditions, including asthma, bronchitis, and bronchospasm (2,3,6,7). However, doses recommended for these indications often exceed the safe limit (2729) and better treatment alternatives are available.

There is insufficient reliable information available about the effectiveness of ephedra for its other uses.

Mechanism of Action

The applicable part of ephedra is primarily the dried, young branch. Less commonly, the root or whole plant is used (11,13,18). Ephedra in dietary supplements is usually either a formulation of powdered stems and aerial portions or a dried extract (6488). Dried extracts contain more ephedra alkaloids per unit weight of material, due to the extraction process. The principle alkaloid constituents are ephedrine, pseudoephedrine, and sometimes small amounts of phenylpropanolamine. Ephedrine is absorbed faster if it is consumed as the powdered extract. However, onset of action and extent of absorption does not differ greatly between the powdered extract and the powdered herb (6008,6009). Some sources claim ephedra is safer than pure ephedrine and pseudoephedrine because ephedrine from ephedra is absorbed more slowly. However, pharmacokinetic studies have found no differences in the pharmacokinetics of ephedrine from ephedra versus the purified form (6488). Ephedrine and pseudoephedrine are both non-selective alpha- and beta-receptor agonists. The ephedrine and pseudoephedrine constituents can directly and indirectly stimulate the sympathetic nervous system (2,3,6,7,9). They can increase systolic and diastolic blood pressure (3,6,11,18) and heart rate (3,6,11), cause peripheral vasoconstriction, bronchodilation (3,6,7,11), and central nervous system stimulation (2,3,7,11). Ephedra alkaloids have been linked to myocarditis and myocardial infarction. This has been attributed to coronary artery vasoconstriction and possibly vasospasm caused by ephedra. Ephedra might also cause cardiac arrhythmia due to adrenergic effects that shorten the cardiac refractory period, causing re-entrant arrhythmias. Cerebral hemorrhage associated with ephedra has been attributed primarily to hypertensive effects and possibly due to cerebral vasculitis, which has been reported with other adrenergic drugs. Ischemic stroke has been attributed to ephedra's vasoconstrictive effects on cerebral vasculature and possibly platelet aggregation effects due to adrenergic stimulation (6486). Ephedrine also seems to have antitussive (2,7), bacteriostatic (2), and anti-inflammatory (6,11) activity. Ephedrine can have diuretic effects, but can also exacerbate urinary retention (512). Ephedra can have either hypoglycemic or hyperglycemic effects. It can also stimulate uterine contraction, and theoretically can be catabolized to mutagenic nitrosamines (6,11). Ephedrine causes relaxation of the smooth muscle in the gastrointestinal tract, urinary retention by relaxing the detrusor muscle, and diminishes contraction of the bladder sphincter (11,15). Above ground parts of ephedra seem to cause sweating, but the root seems to inhibit sweating (11).

Adverse Reactions

Orally, ephedra most commonly causes dizziness, restlessness, anxiety, irritability, personality changes, insomnia, headache, dry mouth, anorexia, nausea, vomiting, flushing, tingling, difficulty urinating, tachycardia, heart palpitations, hyperthermia, and increased blood pressure (1276,3719,6008,6486). Long-term use or use in high doses has also been associated with dependence and tolerance (12,1381). There are also several reports of serious life-threatening or debilitating adverse effects with ephedra products. Psychosis, sometimes prolonged for several months after discontinuation, has been reported (1276,6998). There are reports of myopathies, including myalgia, cardiomyopathy, rhabdomyolysis, eosinophilia-myalgia syndrome (1270), and hypersensitivity myocarditis (1271,6487). Nephrolithiasis (1272) and acute hepatitis (1273) have also been reported. However, the single case of hepatitis is more likely the result of product contamination than due to ephedra itself (1273). Other reported events include chest tightness, myocardial infarction (6486), cardiac arrest and sudden death (1274,6486), stroke, transient ischemic attack, cerebral hemorrhage, seizure, and loss of consciousness (1275,1380,1381,2729,6486). Because most of these events have been described in case reports, it is impossible to determine the overall incidence of these adverse effects. It is also difficult to determine which patient groups might be most likely to experience an adverse event. Patients with a history of cardiovascular disease would be expected to be at a higher risk. However, there have been several reports of serious events in patients with no known pre-existing medical condition. In many cases, ephedra has been used in combination with another stimulant such as caffeine. However, there are also reports of serious adverse effects when ephedra has been used alone. The safety of ephedra is controversial and highly debated. Some claim that ephedra is only unsafe when it is used inappropriately in excessive doses. The supplement industry maintains that ephedra is safe when taken in doses recommended on labeling. However, there are several cases where severe life-threatening or debilitating effects occurred with short-term use of relatively low doses ranging from 20-60 mg ephedra alkaloids per day (6486). Until more is known, warn patients that the potential risks of using ephedra outweigh any potential benefit. Advise patients against using products containing ephedra, especially in combination with other stimulants such as caffeine or if they have a pre-existing condition such as cardiovascular disease.

Interactions with Herbs & Other Dietary Supplements

HERBS & SUPPLEMENTS WITH STIMULANT PROPERTIES: Use of ephedra and other stimulant herbs such as those containing caffeine can increase the risk of common side effects such as insomnia, jitteriness, tremulousness, dizziness, etc (7). Using ephedra with other stimulants might also increase the risk of more serious adverse effects such as hypertension, myocardial infarction, stroke, and death. There are several reports of serious life-threatening or debilitating adverse events in patients taking ephedra in combination with caffeine and other stimulants (1380,6486). Some herbs and supplements with significant caffeine content include black tea, coffee, cola nut, green tea, guarana, mate, and others.

DIGITALIS: Theoretically, use of ephedra with digitalis might cause cardiac arrhythmias (2).

SECALE ALKALOID DERIVATIVES (Ergot): Theoretically, concomitant use might cause hypertension (2).

Interactions with Drugs

AMITRIPTYLINE (Elavil): Theoretically, concomitant use might reduce the hypertensive effects of the ephedrine contained in ephedra. Amitriptyline blocks the hypertensive effects of ephedrine (19).

CAFFEINE: Use of ephedra with caffeine can increase the risk of stimulatory adverse effects of ephedra and caffeine (7,19), and possibly enhance thermogenesis and weight loss (19). There is also some evidence that using ephedra with caffeine might increase the risk of serious life-threatening or debilitating adverse effects such as hypertension, myocardial infarction, stroke, and death (1380,6486). Tell patients to avoid taking ephedra with caffeine and other stimulants.

DEXAMETHASONE (Decadron): Theoretically, concomitant use might reduce the effectiveness of dexamethasone, due to the ephedrine contained in ephedra. Ephedrine increases the clearance rate of dexamethasone (19).

DIABETES DRUGS: Ephedra can raise blood glucose levels and interfere with diabetes drug therapy. Monitor blood glucose concentrations closely (19).

DIGOXIN (Lanoxin): Theoretically, concomitant use might cause cardiac arrhythmias (2).

ERGOTAMINE (Migranol, D.H.E. 45, Ergomar): Theoretically, concomitant use of ephedra and ergot alkaloids might cause hypertension, due to the ephedrine contained in ephedra (2).

MONOAMINE OXIDASE INHIBITORS (MAOIs): Contraindicated; concomitant use of ephedra with MAOIs might increase the risk of hypertension (15). A hypertensive crisis and subarachnoid hemorrhage were reported after a patient took a 50 mg dose of ephedrine and an MAOI drug (15).

OXYTOCIN: Theoretically, concomitant use might cause hypertension (2).

RESERPINE: Theoretically, concomitant use might antagonize the indirect sympathomimetic effects of the ephedrine contained in ephedra (19).

THEOPHYLLINE: Theoretically, concomitant use might increase the risk of stimulatory adverse effects of theophylline and ephedrine (contained in ephedra) (7,19).

URINARY ACIDIFIERS: Theoretically, concomitant use of ephedra and urinary acidifying drugs might reduce the ephedrine-related effects of ephedra. Urinary acidifying drugs increase ephedrine excretion (19).

URINARY ALKALINIZERS: Theoretically, concomitant use of ephedra and urinary alkalinizing drugs might increase the ephedrine-related effects of ephedra. Urinary alkalinizing drugs reduce ephedrine excretion (19).

Interactions with Foods

COFFEE, TEA: Theoretically, concomitant use of large amounts of caffeinated coffee or tea might increase the stimulatory effects and adverse effects of caffeine and the ephedrine contained in ephedra.

Interactions with Lab Tests

AMPHETAMINE, METHAMPHETAMINE: Ephedra might cause false-positive urine amphetamine or methamphetamine test results. One unpublished case involved a false-positive urine methamphetamine assay in a woman who experienced life-threatening adverse effects associated with the use of an ephedra/guarana product (1381).

EPHEDRINE: Ephedra can cause a positive urine ephedrine test due to its ephedrine content. A case of an athlete whose urine tested positive for norpseudoephedrine was attributed to the use of an herbal supplement labeled to contain ephedra. However, the product might also have contained added norpseudoephedrine as an unlabeled ingredient (1259).

GLUCOSE: Ephedra might increase blood glucose levels and test results (19).

Interactions with Diseases or Conditions

ANGINA: Contraindicated; ephedra might induce or exacerbate angina due its cardiac stimulant effects (15,512).

ANOREXIA: Contraindicated due to the purported appetite suppressant effects of ephedra. Anorexic patients might be at increased risk for the adverse effects of ephedra due to inadequate nutritional status (12,19).

ANXIETY: Large doses of ephedra might cause or exacerbate anxiety due to its CNS stimulant effects (2,12,15,512).

BENIGN PROSTATIC HYPERTROPHY (BPH): Ephedra might exacerbate urinary retention in patients with BPH due to its effects on the detrusor muscle (15,512).

BULIMIA: Contraindicated; bulimic patients might be at increased risk for the adverse effects of ephedra due to inadequate nutritional status (12,19).

CEREBRAL INSUFFICIENCY: Contraindicated; ephedra might further decrease cerebral blood flow due to its vasoconstrictive effects (2,12,512).

DIABETES: Ephedra might interfere with blood sugar control, and exacerbate high blood pressure and circulatory problems in people with diabetes (15,19,512).

ESSENTIAL TREMOR: Ephedra might exacerbate essential tremor (1715).

HEART DISEASE: Contraindicated; ephedra might cause tachycardia, arrhythmias, or induce angina in patients with heart disease due to its cardiac stimulant effects (15,512).

HYPERTHYROID, THYROTOXICOSIS: Contraindicated; ephedra might stimulate the thyroid and exacerbate hyperthyroid symptoms (2,12,15,512).

HYPERTENSION: Ephedra might exacerbate hypertension (2,12,15,512); contraindicated in uncontrolled hypertension.

KIDNEY STONES: Ephedra and ephedrine can cause kidney stones (1272).

NARROW-ANGLE GLAUCOMA: Ephedra might exacerbate narrow-angle (angle-closure) glaucoma by causing mydriasis (2,12,15,512).

PHEOCHROMOCYTOMA: Contraindicated; ephedra might exacerbate the symptoms of pheochromocytoma (2).

URINARY RETENTION: Large doses of ephedra might exacerbate urinary retention due its effects on the detrusor muscle (2,12,15,512).

Dosage and Administration

ORAL: For reducing weight in obese patients, ephedra 12 mg in combination with guarana 40 mg three times daily plus 17 other vitamins, minerals, and supplements (Metabolife 356) has been used (3719). The typical dose of ephedra is 15-20 mg of the ephedra alkaloids calculated as ephedrine taken up to 3 times daily (2,7,12,6486). Doses up to 300 mg per day have been used (2,7,12). However, doses as low as 12-36 mg per day have been associated with severe adverse effects (see Adverse Reactions). One cup of ephedra tea is also commonly taken 3 times per day. The tea is prepared by steeping 1-4 grams in 150 mL boiling water for 5-10 minutes and then straining (18). The tincture (1:1) is usually given as 5 grams per dose (18). Another tincture (1:4) is given 6-8 mL three times per day (18). The typical dose of the extract is 1-3 mL three times per day (18). For children over the age of 6 years, some sources suggest a dose of 0.5 mg/kg up to a maximum of 2 mg/kg per day (2,7,12), but due to safety concerns, ephedra should not be used in children.

Comments

Mormon tea and ephedra are often confused. Mormon tea or American ephedra comes from Ephedra nevadensis and ephedra or ma huang comes primarily from Ephedra sinica. Mormon tea is alkaloid-free and lacks both the therapeutic effects and the toxicity of ephedrine (3,12).

There has been a lot of debate about the safety of ephedra. In June of 1997, the FDA proposed restrictions on the ephedrine content of dietary supplements, new warning labels for ephedra alkaloid-containing products, and a prohibition on combination products containing ephedra and other natural stimulants, such as guarana and cola nut, both of which contain significant amounts of caffeine (2729). These proposals were dropped after the link between ephedra use and serious adverse effects was challenged by the General Accounting Office (GAO) and the dietary supplement industry (1381). The FDA is currently reviewing numerous adverse event reports involving ephedra alkaloid-containing products, with 140 of the reports receiving in-depth clinical review by FDA and outside experts (1381,5047,6486). Findings from experts outside the FDA support the FDA's initial finding that ephedra is likely the cause of many of the 140 reports receiving in-depth clinical review (6486). Restrictions on ephedra products have not yet been implemented by the FDA. However, 28 states have independently implemented varying restrictions on ephedra use (6487).

Ephedra is now being marketed as a recreational drug "herbal ecstasy." The FDA has announced that ephedra products marketed as recreational drugs are unapproved and misbranded drugs subject to seizure and injunction (5047).

EPIMEDIUM

Also Known As

Barrenwort, Herba Epimedii, Horny Goat Weed, Japanese Epimedium, Xian Ling Pi, Yin Yang Huo.

Scientific Names

Epimedium acuminatum; Epimedium brevicornum; Epimedium grandiflorum; Epimedium koreanum; Epimedium pubescens; Epimedium sagittatum; Epimedium wushanese; and other Epimedium species.
Family: Berberidaceae.

People Use This For

Orally, epimedium is used for impotence, involuntary ejaculation, weak back and knees, arthralgia, mental and physical fatigue, memory loss, hypertension, coronary heart disease, bronchitis, chronic hepatitis, polio, chronic leukopenia (11), viral myocarditis (1513), and as a tonic and aphrodisiac (11).
Epimedium is included in some personal care products for its antimicrobial effects (11).

Safety

POSSIBLY SAFE ...when preparations of the leaf are taken orally, short-term (12).
POSSIBLY UNSAFE ...when used orally, long-term (12).
LIKELY UNSAFE ...when large amounts are used orally. Some species can cause respiratory arrest (12).
PREGNANCY AND LACTATION: Insufficient reliable information available; avoid using.

Effectiveness

There is insufficient reliable information available about the effectiveness of epimedium.

Mechanism of Action

The applicable part of epimedium is the leaf. Researchers think flavonoids, icariin, and polysaccharides are the active constituents. Some evidence suggests epimedium might cause peripheral vasodilation, increase coronary blood flow, increase platelet aggregation, and improve male sexual function (11). Epimedium also seems to inhibit catecholamine effects. It seems to have some hypotensive, immunomodulating, antimicrobial, anti-inflammatory, antitussive and expectorant effects (11). Evidence suggests epimedium might have activity against HIV (1512).

Adverse Reactions

Orally, extended use of Japanese epimedium may result in dizziness, vomiting, dry mouth, thirst, and nosebleed (12). Large doses of Japanese epimedium may cause respiratory arrest and exaggeration of tendon reflexes to the point of spasm (12). There is insufficient reliable information available for other Epimedium species.

Interactions with Herbs & Other Dietary Supplements

Insufficient reliable information available.

Interactions with Drugs

No interactions are known to occur, and there is no known reason to expect a clinically significant interaction with epimedium.

Interactions with Foods

No interactions are known to occur, and there is no known reason to expect a clinically significant interaction with epimedium.

Interactions with Lab Tests

No interactions are known to occur, and there is no known reason to expect a clinically significant interaction with epimedium.

Interactions with Diseases or Conditions

No interactions are known to occur, and there is no known reason to expect a clinically significant interaction with epimedium.

Dosage and Administration

No typical dosage.

Comments

The leaf of Japanese epimedium (Epimedium grandiflora) is generally used (12). Leaf, petiole, and stem of other Epimedium species are also sometimes used (11). As many as 15 Epimedium species are interchangeable as "yin yang huo" (11).

ERGOT

Also Known As
Cockspur Rye, Hornseed, Mother of Rye, Secale cornutum, Smut Rye, Spurred Rye.

Scientific Names
Plant host: Claviceps purpurea.
Family: Claviciptaceae.

People Use This For
Orally, ergot is used for obstetric and gynecologic conditions, including hemorrhage, climacteric hemorrhage, menorrhagia, metrorrhagia (before and after miscarriage), expulsion of placenta, shortening of afterbirth period, and atonia of the uterus (2,18).

Safety
UNSAFE ...when used orally due to poisoning risk and interactions with many disease states (2).
PREGNANCY AND LACTATION: UNSAFE ...when used orally due to high level of risk (2,400); avoid using.

Effectiveness
POSSIBLY EFFECTIVE ...when taken orally for hemorrhage, climacteric hemorrhage, menorrhagia, metrorrhagia (before and after miscarriage), expulsion of placenta, shortening of afterbirth period, and atonia of the uterus (2,17). However, high level of risk and availability of safer alternatives preclude use (2).

Mechanism of Action
Ergot is dried fungal growth that occurs on rye (Claviceps purpurea). Ergot alkaloids produce vasoconstriction, myometrial stimulation and alpha-adrenergic blockade (17).

Adverse Reactions
Orally, ergot can cause nausea, vomiting, leg weakness, myalgia, numbness of fingers, angina, tachycardia, bradycardia, localized edema, and itching (18). Overdose or long-term use can cause thrombosis, damage to blood vessels in the retina, optic atrophy, gangrene of extremities, convulsions, and hemiplegia (18). The symptoms of acute poisoning are queasiness, vomiting, diarrhea, thirst, skin coolness, itching of skin, rapid weak pulse, paresthesia, extremity numbness, confusion, and unconsciousness (18). The symptoms of chronic poisoning are ergotismus gangrenosus (painful blood flow disorders of the extremities with dry gangrene, angina, aphasia, visual field loss) (18) and ergotismus convulsivus (muscle twitching, followed by clonic spasms, tonic spasms, hemiplegia, loss of consciousness, death) (18).

Interactions with Herbs & Other Dietary Supplements
Insufficient reliable information available.

Interactions with Drugs
ERGOT ALKALOIDS: Co-administration increases risk of adverse effects.
SYMPATHOMIMETICS: Co-administration may increase risk of adverse effects (17).

Interactions with Foods
No interactions are known to occur, and there is no known reason to expect a clinically significant interaction with ergot.

Interactions with Lab Tests
No interactions are known to occur, and there is no known reason to expect a clinically significant interaction with ergot.

Interactions with Diseases or Conditions
CONTRAINDICATIONS: Raynaud's disease, thromboangitis obliterans, severe arteriosclerotic vascular changes, liver function disorders, coronary insufficiency, kidney disease, infectious disease, sepsis, hypotonia, and hypertonia (18).

Dosage and Administration
No typical dosage.

Comments
Alternatives include FDA-approved ergot alkaloid drug products (standardized potency and purity). These prescription drugs show far less toxicity and the same or higher specific effectiveness (2).

ERYNGO above ground parts

Also Known As
Eringo, Eryngii Herba, Sea Holly, Sea Holme, Sea Hulver.
CAUTION: See separate listing for Eryngo root.

Scientific Names
Eryngium campestre, synonyms Eryngium maritinum, Eyrnigium planum, Eryngium yuccifolium.
Family: Apiaceae.

People Use This For
Orally, people use eryngo above ground parts for urinary tract infections, inflammation of the urinary tract, prostatitis, and mucous membrane inflammation of the bronchi (18).

Safety
There is insufficient reliable information available about the safety of eryngo above ground parts.
Pregnancy and Lactation: Insufficient reliable information available; avoid using.

Effectiveness
There is insufficient reliable information about the effectiveness of eryngo above ground parts.

Mechanism of Action
Eryngo above ground parts are stated to have a diuretic effect (18).

Adverse Reactions
None reported.

Interactions with Herbs & Other Dietary Supplements
Insufficient reliable information available.

Interactions with Drugs
No interactions are known to occur, and there is no known reason to expect a clinically significant interaction with eryngo above ground parts.

Interactions with Foods
No interactions are known to occur, and there is no known reason to expect a clinically significant interaction with eryngo above ground parts.

Interactions with Lab Tests
No interactions are known to occur, and there is no known reason to expect a clinically significant interaction with eryngo above ground parts.

Interactions with Diseases or Conditions
No interactions are known to occur, and there is no known reason to expect a clinically significant interaction with eryngo above ground parts.

Dosage and Administration
ORAL: Eryngo above ground parts are typically administered as an extract (amount used unspecified) (18).

Comments
None.

ERYNGO root

Also Known As
Eringo, Eryngii Radix, Sea Holly, Sea Holme, Sea Hulver.
CAUTION: See separate listing for Eryngo above ground parts.

Scientific Names
Eryngium campestre, synonyms Eryngium maritimum, Eyrnigium planum, Eryngium yuccifolium.
Family: Apiaceae.

People Use This For
Orally, eryngo root is used for kidney and bladder stones, renal colic, kidney and urinary tract inflammation, urinary retention, edema, coughs, bronchitis, and skin and respiratory disorders (18).

Safety
POSSIBLY SAFE ...when used orally and appropriately (12).
PREGNANCY AND LACTATION: Insufficient reliable information available; avoid using.

Effectiveness
There is insufficient reliable information about the effectiveness of eryngo root.

Mechanism of Action
Eryngo root is reported to have mild expectorant and antispasmodic properties (18).

Adverse Reactions
None reported.

Interactions with Herbs & Other Dietary Supplements
Insufficient reliable information available.

Interactions with Drugs
No interactions are known to occur, and there is no known reason to expect a clinically significant interaction with eryngo root.

Interactions with Foods
No interactions are known to occur, and there is no known reason to expect a clinically significant interaction with eryngo root.

Interactions with Lab Tests
No interactions are known to occur, and there is no known reason to expect a clinically significant interaction with eryngo root.

Interactions with Diseases or Conditions
No interactions are known to occur, and there is no known reason to expect a clinically significant interaction with eryngo root.

Dosage and Administration
ORAL: Typical dose is 3 to 4 cups of tea (steep 1 teaspoon ground root in 150 mL of boiling water until cold; strain) daily (18). Alternatively, 2-3 cups decoction (boil 4 teaspoons of ground root in 1 L water for 10 minutes, steep for 15 minutes, strain) daily (18); or 50-60 drops tincture (soak 20 grams powdered root in 80 grams of 60% alcohol for 10 days) divided into 3 or 4 doses daily have been used.

Comments
None.

EUCALYPTUS dried leaf

Also Known As
Blue Gum, Eucalypti Folium, Eucalyptusblatter, Fever Tree, Fevertree, Fieberbaumblatter, Gum Tree, Red Gum, Stringy Bark Tree, Tasmanian Blue Gum.
CAUTION: See separate listing for Eucalyptus Oil.

Scientific Names
Eucalyptus globulus; Eucalyptus smithii; Eucalyptus fructicetorum, synonym Eucalyptus polybractea.
Family: Myrtaceae.

People Use This For
Orally, dried eucalyptus leaf is used as an antiseptic, antipyretic, expectorant [4], stimulant in respiratory ailments [11], and for treating respiratory tract mucous membrane inflammation [2].
In Chinese medicine, the leaf has been used for aching joints, bacterial dysentery, ringworms, and pulmonary tuberculosis [11].
In folk medicine, eucalyptus dried leaf has been used for asthma, acne, bleeding gums, bladder diseases, diabetes, fever, flu, gonorrhea, liver and gallbladder complaints, loss of appetite, neuralgia, poorly healing ulcers, rheumatism, stomatitis, whooping cough, wounds, as a gastrointestinal remedy [18], for burns, and cancer [11].
In foods, eucalyptus dried leaf is used as a flavoring agent [4,11].

Safety
POSSIBLY SAFE ...when the dried leaf is used orally and appropriately [12]. ...when preparations of the dried leaf are used topically.
CHILDREN: LIKELY UNSAFE ...when applied topically to the face or in the nose of infants and young children [2,12]. It can cause bronchospasm. There is insufficient reliable information available about the safety of oral use in young children; avoid using.
PREGNANCY AND LACTATION: Insufficient reliable information available; avoid using.

Effectiveness
POSSIBLY EFFECTIVE ...when used orally for respiratory tract mucous membrane inflammation [2]. ...when used as an expectorant, and depending on the species, the product must contain 70-85% eucalyptol or cineole [3].
There is insufficient reliable information available about the effectiveness of dried eucalyptus leaf for its other uses.

Mechanism of Action
The leaf can have secretion-stimulating, expectorant, antiseptic, and weakly antispasmodic properties [2,4]. The antiseptic and expectorant properties of the leaf are due to its volatile oils, particularly eucalyptol [4]. Other evidence suggests eucalyptus can be a urinary irritant [19].

Adverse Reactions
Orally, eucalyptus dried leaf rarely can cause nausea, vomiting, and diarrhea [2]. Signs of eucalyptus poisoning include epigastric burning, nausea, vomiting, diarrhea, dizziness, muscular weakness, miosis, feeling of suffocation, cyanosis, delirium, convulsions, and death [4]. The ingestion of 3.5 mL of the eucalyptus oil can be fatal [11].

Interactions with Herbs & Other Dietary Supplements
Insufficient reliable information available.

Interactions with Drugs
HYPOGLYCEMIC DRUGS: Eucalyptus can interfere with blood sugar control [4].
HEPATICALLY METABOLIZED DRUGS: Eucalyptus oil induces liver enzymes which can reduce the activity of drugs metabolized by the liver [2].

Interactions with Foods
No interactions are known to occur, and there is no known reason to expect a clinically significant interaction with eucalyptus dried leaf.

Interactions with Lab Tests
No interactions are known to occur, and there is no known reason to expect a clinically significant interaction with eucalyptus dried leaf.

Interactions with Diseases or Conditions

DIABETES: Theoretically, eucalyptus can interfere with blood glucose control (4).
OTHER CONDITIONS: Contraindicated in cases of GI tract and bile duct inflammation, liver disease (2), hypotension, and kidney inflammation (500).

Dosage and Administration

ORAL: The typical dose of the eucalyptus leaf is one cup of the freshly prepared tea 3 times daily (3). The tea is made by steeping 2 grams of the dried leaf in 150 mL boiling water and then straining. Limit the daily intake to 4-6 grams per day of the dried leaf or equivalent preparations (2). The usual dose of the tincture is 3-9 grams per day (2), and the fluid extract is dosed 2-4 grams per day (4).

Comments

None.

EUCALYPTUS OIL

Also Known As

None.
CAUTION: See separate listing for Eucalyptus dried leaf.

Scientific Names

Eucalyptus fructicetorum, synonym Eucalyptus polybractea; Eucalyptus globulus; Eucalyptus smithii.
Family: Myrtaceae.

People Use This For

Orally, eucalyptus oil is used for inflammation of respiratory tract mucous membranes (2), for suppressing coughs (3), as an expectorant (11).
Topically, eucalyptus oil is used for inflammation of respiratory tract mucous membranes, rheumatic complaints (2), and nasal stuffiness (7).
Traditionally, eucalyptus oil has been used as an antiseptic and antipyretic, for wounds, burns, ulcers, cancer, and in vaporizer fluids (11).
In dentistry, eucalyptus oil is a component of sealers and solvents for root canal fillings (11).
In manufacturing, eucalyptus oil is utilized as a flavoring and a fragrance component in perfumes (11). It is also used as a mouthwash (11), antiseptic, liniments, ointments, and in toothpaste (11), cough drops, and gum lozenges (7).

Safety

LIKELY SAFE ...when consumed in amounts commonly found in foods. Eucalyptus oil is approved for food use in the US (11). Eucalyptol is listed as a synthetic flavoring agent. The maximum level used in food is 0.002% (11).
POSSIBLY SAFE ...when used orally and appropriately for medicinal purposes (2,12). It must be used in very small amounts or diluted (2,12).
POSSIBLY UNSAFE ...when the undiluted oil is used topically (4).
LIKELY UNSAFE ...when undiluted oil is ingested orally. Ingesting 3.5 mL of undiluted oil can be fatal (4).
CHILDREN: LIKELY UNSAFE ...when used topically on the face, especially the nose, of infants and young children (2) because it can cause bronchospasm. ...when the oil is used orally (4).
PREGNANCY: LIKELY SAFE ...when used orally in food amounts. LIKELY UNSAFE ...when used orally in larger amounts; contraindicated (4).
LACTATION: Insufficient reliable information available; avoid using in amounts greater than found in foods (4).

Effectiveness

POSSIBLY EFFECTIVE ...when used orally for inflammation of respiratory tract mucous membranes (2). ...when applied topically for inflammation of respiratory tract mucous membranes (2) and rheumatic complaints (2).
There is insufficient reliable information available about the effectiveness of eucalyptus oil for its other uses.

Mechanism of Action

Eucalyptus oil contains 70-85% eucalyptol (1,8-cineole) that stimulates production and secretion of saliva (11). This, in turn, activates the swallowing reflex. Voluntary swallowing can suppress an impending cough (7). Taken by mouth, eucalyptus oil aids in expectorating secretions (2,4), has mild antibacterial action (4), and is mildly antispasmodic (2). In vitro, it has antibacterial and fungicidal effects. Topically, it acts as a mild counterirritant (2) and inhibits prostaglandin biosynthesis (18). The crude eucalyptus leaf extract has demonstrated hypoglycemic activity in rabbits (4). Eucalyptus can be a urinary irritant (19).

Adverse Reactions

Orally, eucalyptus oil can cause nausea, vomiting, and diarrhea (2). Signs of eucalyptus oil poisoning include epigastric burning, nausea, vomiting, dizziness, muscular weakness, constricted pupils of eyes, feeling of suffocation, cyanosis, delirium, and convulsions. The ingestion of 3.5 mL of the oil can be fatal (4).

Interactions with Herbs & Other Dietary Supplements

PYRROLIZIDINE ALKALOID CONTAINING PLANTS: Eucalyptus oil can potentiate the toxicity of borage, coltsfoot, comfrey, hound's tooth, and Senecio species (500).

Interactions with Drugs

DIABETES DRUGS: Theoretically, concomitant use of eucalyptus oil can interfere with blood sugar control (4).
HEPATICALLY METABOLIZED DRUGS: Eucalyptus oil induces liver enzymes and, theoretically, can alter the effects of drugs metabolized by the liver (2).

Interactions with Foods

No interactions are known to occur, and there is no known reason to expect a clinically significant interaction with eucalyptus oil.

Interactions with Lab Tests

No interactions are known to occur, and there is no known reason to expect a clinically significant interaction with eucalyptus oil.

Interactions with Diseases or Conditions

DIABETES: Theoretically, eucalyptus oil can interfere with blood sugar control (4).
OTHER CONDITIONS: Eucalyptus oil is contraindicated in cases of GI tract and bile duct inflammation, severe liver disease (2), hypotension, kidney inflammation, or low blood pressure (500).

Dosage and Administration

ORAL: The typical dose is 300-600 mg of the eucalyptus oil per day (2), and about 0.05-0.2 mL per dose (4).
TOPICAL: Semi-solid or vegetable oil preparations usually contain 5%-20% eucalyptus oil (2,4), and aqueous-alcoholic preparations contain 5%-10% eucalyptus oil (2). The oil is also typically used for local application by diluting 30 mL oil to 500 mL lukewarm water (4). Avoid the use of the undiluted essential oil. The essential oil diluted in vegetable oil is preferred for applications on the skin (4). Avoid use on areas of the face, especially the nose, of infants and young children (2).

Comments

Eucalyptus oil is the steam distilled volatile oil from fresh leaves and branch tops of various species of Eucalyptus.

EUPHORBIA

Also Known As

Pillbearing Spurge, Snakeweed.

Scientific Names

Euphorbia hirta, synonym Euphorbia capitata; Euphorbia pilulifera.
Family: Euphorbiaceae.

People Use This For

Orally, euphorbia is used for respiratory disorders including asthma, bronchitis, catarrh, laryngeal spasm (4), hay fever, and tumors (11), and as an expectorant and an emetic (12). It is also used orally for treating worms, dysentery, gonorrhea, and digestive problems in India (11).

Safety

There is insufficient reliable information available about the safety of euphorbia.
PREGNANCY AND LACTATION: POSSIBLY UNSAFE ...when used orally; avoid using. Euphorbia is reported to cause smooth muscle contraction and relaxation (4).

Effectiveness

There is insufficient reliable information available about the effectiveness of euphorbia.

Mechanism of Action

The applicable parts of euphorbia are the above ground parts. It is reported to have antispasmodic, histamine potentiator, antitumor, and antibacterial activity against gram positive and gram negative organisms in animals(4). The constituent choline is reported to produce contraction of isolated pig ileum. The constituent shikimic acid produces relaxation (11).

Adverse Reactions

Orally, euphorbia may cause nausea and vomiting (12). Skin contact with fresh euphorbia can cause irritation or contact dermatitis (19).

Interactions with Herbs & Other Dietary Supplements

Insufficient reliable information available.

Interactions with Drugs

No interactions are known to occur, and there is no known reason to expect a clinically significant interaction with euphorbia.

Interactions with Foods

No interactions are known to occur, and there is no known reason to expect a clinically significant interaction with euphorbia.

Interactions with Lab Tests

No interactions are known to occur, and there is no known reason to expect a clinically significant interaction with euphorbia.

Interactions with Diseases or Conditions

GI CONDITIONS: Euphorbia can irritate the gastrointestinal tract. Contraindicated in individuals with infectious or inflammatory gastrointestinal conditions (19).

Dosage and Administration

ORAL: Typical dose is one cup tea prepared by steeping 120-300 mg above ground parts in 150 mL boiling water 5-10 minutes and then straining (4). Liquid extract, concentration unspecified, 0.12-0.3 mL, and tincture, concentration unspecified, 0.6-2 mL have also been used (4). As and expectorant, 2 grams above ground parts has been used; emetic dose may be similar.

Comments

None.

EUROPEAN BARBERRY

Also Known As

Agracejo, Berberidis cortex, Berberidis fructus, Berberidis radicis cortex, Berberidis radix, Berberitze, Berberry, Berbis, Common Barberry, Épine-Vinette, Espino Cambrón, Jaundice Berry, Mountain Grape, Oregon Grape, Pipperidge, Piprage, Sauerdorn, Sow Berry, Vinettier.
CAUTION: See separate listing for Oregon Grape.

Scientific Names

Berberis vulgaris.
Family: Berberidaceae.

People Use This For

Orally, the fruit of European barberry is used for kidney, urinary tract, and gastrointestinal tract discomforts such as heartburn, stomach cramps, constipation, lack of appetite, liver and spleen disease, for bronchial and lung discomforts, spasms, as a stimulant for circulation, for people susceptible to infection, and as a supplemental source of vitamin C (2,18). The bark, root, and root bark of European barberry are also used orally for ailments and complaints of the GI tract, liver, gallbladder, kidney and urinary tract, respiratory tract, heart and circulatory system, as an antipyretic, "blood purifier" (2), and for narcotic withdrawal (18).
In folk medicine, European barberry root bark has been used for liver dysfunction, gallbladder disease, jaundice, splenopathy, diarrhea, indigestion, hemorrhoids, renal and urinary tract diseases, gout, rheumatism, arthritis, mid and low back pain, malaria, and leishmaniasis (18).

European barberry fruit is used in making jam, jellies, and wine (18).
In manufacturing, the fruit syrup is used for masking tastes in pharmaceutical preparations (18).

Safety
LIKELY SAFE …when the fruit is consumed in food amounts. The fruit is considered to contain only trace amounts of berberine (2,12,18).
POSSIBLY SAFE …when the fruit, root, bark, or root bark are used orally and appropriately for medicinal uses. Amounts of less than 500 mg of berberine are usually considered safe (2,12,18).
LIKELY UNSAFE …when more than 500 mg of berberine is consumed. Berberine is considered moderately toxic (12). The LD50 in humans is reported to be 27.5 mg/kg (12).
PREGNANCY: LIKELY UNSAFE ...when used orally; contraindicated because it can have uterine stimulant properties (11,12).
LACTATION: Insufficient reliable information is available; avoid using.

Effectiveness
There is insufficient reliable information available about the effectiveness of European barberry.

Mechanism of Action
The applicable parts of European barberry are the bark, fruit, root, and root bark. European barberry fruit contains vitamin C (18). Researchers think it has mild diuretic activity due to the acid content (18). The bark, root, and root bark of European barberry contain isoquinolone alkaloid constituents, including berberine, berbamine, columbamine, jatorrhizine, palmatine, and oxyacanthine (11,19). The constituents berberine, columbamine, and oxyacanthine show evidence of antibacterial activity (11). Berberine has anticonvulsant, sedative, hypotensive, antifibrillatory, and bile-stimulating effects. In low doses, it is a cardiac and respiratory stimulant. In high doses it is a depressant (11,12,515). Some evidence suggests berberine sulfate might be amebicidal and trypanocidal (11). Other information suggests the constituent berbamine might have antiarrhythmic, hypotensive, spasmolytic, and immunostimulating activity (11,515).

Adverse Reactions
Orally, ingestion of greater than 500 mg berberine, which is found in European barberry, can cause lethargy, nose bleed, skin and eye irritation, nephritis and kidney irritation (2). It might also cause dyspnea, hypotension, cardiac damage (12), nausea, vomiting, diarrhea, hemorrhagic nephritis, respiratory spasms and arrest, and death (2).

Interactions with Herbs & Other Dietary Supplements
BERBERINE-CONTAINING HERBS: Concomitant use can increase the risk of berberine toxicity. Berberine-containing herbs include: bloodroot, goldenseal, celandine, Chinese goldthread, goldthread, Oregon grape (Mahonia species), amur cork tree, and Chinese corktree (12).

Interactions with Drugs
No interactions are known to occur, and there is no known reason to expect a clinically significant interaction with European barberry.

Interactions with Foods
No interactions are known to occur, and there is no known reason to expect a clinically significant interaction with European barberry.

Interactions with Lab Tests
No interactions are known to occur, and there is no known reason to expect a clinically significant interaction with European barberry.

Interactions with Diseases or Conditions
KIDNEY DISEASE: Berberine, which is found in European barberry, can cause kidney irritation and nephritis (2).
GI IRRITATION: European barberry can irritate gastrointestinal tract. It is contraindicated in individuals with infectious or inflammatory gastrointestinal conditions (19).

Dosage and Administration
ORAL :A typical dose is one cup tea. To make tea, steep 1-2 teaspoons of whole or squashed berries in 150 mL boiling water 10-15 minutes and strain (18) or steep 2 grams of root bark in 250 mL boiling water 5-10 minutes and strain (18). Root bark is typically used as a tincture (1:10), 20-40 drops per day (18). Root tea is not recommended (2,18).

Comments
None.

EUROPEAN BUCKTHORN

Also Known As
Buckthorn, Buckthorn Berry, Hartshorn, Highwaythorn, Kreuzdornbeeren, Ramsthorn, Rhamni cathartica fructus, Waythorn.
CAUTION: See separate listings for Alder Buckthorn, Sea Buckthorn, and Cascara (California Buckthorn).

Scientific Names
Rhamnus catharticus.
Family: Rhamnaceae.

People Use This For
Orally, European buckthorn is used for constipation (2,18).

Safety
POSSIBLY SAFE ...when the standardized preparations of the berry are used orally and appropriately for less than eight to ten days (12). It is important not to exceed recommended amounts (12).
POSSIBLY UNSAFE ...when standardized preparations are used more than ten days (12).
LIKELY UNSAFE ...when nonstandardized preparations are used orally (2,12).
CHILDREN: LIKELY UNSAFE ...when used orally in children younger than 12 years of age (2,12).
PREGNANCY AND LACTATION: LIKELY UNSAFE ...when used orally (2,12); avoid using.

Effectiveness
LIKELY EFFECTIVE ...when taken orally as a stimulant laxative for constipation (2,3,4,7,12) and is comparable to the gentle, laxative effects of cascara (3).

Mechanism of Action
The applicable part of European buckthorn is the berry. The anthraquinones in the European buckthorn berry can increase intestinal GI motility by inhibiting stationary contractions and stimulating propulsive contractions (2). Stimulation of active chloride secretion increases the water and electrolytes in intestinal contents, increasing the risk of electrolyte loss with overuse or misuse of the berry (2). Anthroid laxative use is not associated with an increased risk of developing colorectal adenoma or carcinoma (6138).

Adverse Reactions
Orally, European buckthorn can cause abdominal pain, cramps, or watery diarrhea (12). Chronic use or abuse of the berry can lead to potassium depletion, albuminuria, and hematuria. Potassium depletion can lead to disturbed heart function and muscle weakness (2). Chronic use can cause pseudomelanosis coli (pigment spots in intestinal mucosa) which is harmless, usually reverses with discontinuation (2), and is not associated with an increased risk of developing colorectal ademoma or carcinoma (6138).

Interactions with Herbs & Other Dietary Supplements
STIMULANT LAXATIVE HERBS: Theoretically, concomitant use of European buckthorn with other stimulant laxative herbs can increase the risk of potassium depletion. Stimulant laxative herbs include aloe dried leaf sap, wild cucumber fruit (Ecballium elaterium), blue flag rhizome, alder buckthorn, butternut bark, cascara bark, castor oil, colocynth fruit pulp, gamboge bark exudate, jalap root, black root, manna bark exudate, podophyllum root, rhubarb root, senna leaves and pods, and yellow dock root (19).
HORSETAIL/LICORICE: Theoretically, concomitant use of European buckthorn berry with horsetail plant or licorice rhizome increases the risk of potassium depletion (19).
CARDIAC GLYCOSIDE-CONTAINING HERBS: Theoretically, overuse or abuse of European buckthorn can increase the risk of cardiac glycoside toxicity. Cardiac glycoside containing herbs include black hellebore, Canadian hemp roots, digitalis leaf, hedge mustard, figwort, lily of the valley root, motherwort, oleander leaf, pheasant's eye plant, pleurisy root, squill bulb leaf scales, and strophanthus seeds (2,18,19,500).

Interactions with Drugs
ORAL DRUGS: European buckthorn can decrease bowel transit time, reducing absorption of oral drugs (19).
CARDIAC GLYCOSIDE DRUGS: Theoretically, the overuse or abuse of European buckthorn increases the risk of adverse effects from cardiac glycoside drugs, like digoxin (Lanoxin).
DIURETICS: Concomitant use with potassium-depleting diuretics might result in hypokalemia (19).

Interactions with Foods

No interactions are known to occur, and there is no known reason to expect a clinically significant interaction with European buckthorn.

Interactions with Lab Tests

COLORIMETRIC TESTS: Due to its anthraquinone content, European buckthorn can discolor urine (pink, red, purple, orange, rust), interfering with diagnostic tests that depend on a color change.(12,275).
POTASSIUM: Excessive use of European buckthorn can cause potassium depletion, reducing serum potassium concentrations and test results (2,12,19).

Interactions with Diseases or Conditions

GI CONDITIONS: European buckthorn is contraindicated in individuals with intestinal obstruction; abdominal pain of unknown origin; and intestinal inflammation, including appendicitis, Crohn's disease, irritable bowel syndrome (IBS), and ulcerative colitis (2,12).

Dosage and Administration

ORAL: The typical dose of European buckthorn berry is 20-30 mg of the hydroxyanthracene derivative per day calculated as glucofrangulin A (2). One cup of the tea is commonly taken in the evening, and if needed, in the morning and afternoon (8,12). The tea is prepared by steeping 2-4 grams of the fruit in 150 mL boiling water for 10-15 minutes and then straining (8,12). Use the smallest amount necessary to achieve a soft stool (2) and discontinue in the event of diarrhea or watery stools (12). Limit the use of European buckthorn to a maximum of 8 to 10 days (12). This preparation should be used only if no effect can be obtained through a change of diet or use of bulk-forming laxative products (2).

Comments

Avoid confusion with alder buckthorn (Rhamus frangula). The American Herbal Products Association (AHPA) recommends the following label statement: "Do not use this product if you have abdominal pain or diarrhea. Consult a health care provider prior to use if you are pregnant or nursing. Discontinue use in the event of diarrhea or watery stools. Do not exceed dose. Not for long-term use." (12). Today, European buckthorn is primarily used as a dye.

EUROPEAN CHESTNUT

Also Known As

Castaneae Folium, Husked Nut, Jupiter's Nut, Kastanienblaetter, Sardian Nut, Spanish Chestnut, Sweet Chestnut.
CAUTION: See separate listing for American Chestnut leaf.

Scientific Names

Castanea sativa, synonyms Castanea vesca, Castanea vulgaris.
Family: Fagaceae.

People Use This For

Orally, European chestnut is used for respiratory tract complaints including bronchitis and whooping cough, disorders affecting the legs and circulation (2), diarrhea (18), fever, the passage of bloody stools, hydrocele, infection, inflammation, kidney disorders, myalgias, nausea, paroxysm, sclerosis, inflammation of the lymph nodes due to tuberculosis infection, and stomach disorders.
Topically, European chestnut is used as a gargle for sore throat (18) and for wounds.

Safety

POSSIBLY SAFE ...when used orally and appropriately (12).
There is insufficient reliable information available about the safety of European chestnut for its other uses.
PREGNANCY AND LACTATION: Insufficient reliable information available; avoid using.

Effectiveness

There is insufficient reliable information available about the effectiveness of European chestnut.

Mechanism of Action

The applicable part of European chestnut is the leaf. European chestnut contains 9% tannins, which exert an astringent effect on the mucosal tissue. This effect causes localized dehydration that turns the external cells into a protective layer (12). Plants with 10% tannins or more may cause gastrointestinal disturbances, kidney damage, and necrotic conditions of the liver (12). Some animal experiments show that tannins may cause cancer; others show that they may prevent it (12). Regular consumption of herbs with high tannin concentrations correlates with increased incidence of esophageal or nasal cancer (12).

Adverse Reactions
None reported.

Interactions with Herbs & Other Dietary Supplements
TANNIN-CONTAINING HERBS: Theoretically, herbs that contain high percentages of tannins (such as European chestnut) may cause precipitation of constituents of other herbs.

Interactions with Drugs
ORAL DRUGS: Theoretically, concomitant oral administration may cause precipitation of some drugs due to the high tannin content of European chestnut (19). Separate administration of oral drugs and tannin-containing herbs by the longest period of time practical (19).

Interactions with Foods
No interactions are known to occur, and there is no known reason to expect a clinically significant interaction with European chestnut.

Interactions with Lab Tests
No interactions are known to occur, and there is no known reason to expect a clinically significant interaction with European chestnut.

Interactions with Diseases or Conditions
No interactions are known to occur, and there is no known reason to expect a clinically significant interaction with European chestnut.

Dosage and Administration
ORAL: People typically prepare European chestnut as a tea with 1 teaspoon of leaves and bark boiled in a covered container with 2 cups of water for 30 minutes. The liquid is cooled slowly in the closed container and taken cold, 1 to 2 cups per day (5254).

Comments
None.

EUROPEAN FIVE-FINGER GRASS

Also Known As
Cinquefoil, European Five Finger Grass, Five-Finger Blossom, Five Fingers, Sunkfield, Synkfoyle.

Scientific Names
Potentilla reptans.
Family: Rosaceae.

People Use This For
Orally, European five-finger grass is used for diarrhea and fever.
Topically, European five-finger grass is used for inflammation of the mucous membranes of the mouth and gums, toothache, and heartburn. It is also used for an astringent and to treat open wounds (18).

Safety
There is insufficient reliable information available about the safety of European five-finger grass.
Pregnancy and Lactation: Insufficient reliable information available; avoid using.

Effectiveness
There is insufficient reliable information available about the effectiveness of European five-finger grass.

Mechanism of Action
The astringent effects of European five-finger grass are most likely secondary to tannin content (18).

Adverse Reactions
None reported.

Interactions with Herbs & Other Dietary Supplements
Insufficient reliable information available.

Interactions with Drugs
No interactions are known to occur, and there is no known reason to expect a clinically significant interaction with European five-finger grass.

Interactions with Foods
No interactions are known to occur, and there is no known reason to expect a clinically significant interaction with European five-finger grass.

Interactions with Lab Tests
No interactions are known to occur, and there is no known reason to expect a clinically significant interaction with European five-finger grass.

Interactions with Diseases or Conditions
No interactions are known to occur, and there is no known reason to expect a clinically significant interaction with European five-finger grass.

Dosage and Administration
ORAL: Typically, one cup of tea is taken 2-3 times daily. The tea is prepared by simmering 3 grams of dried plant in 100 mL of boiling water for 10-15 minutes and straining.
TOPICAL: A tea is made by simmering 6 grams of dried plant in 100 mL of boiling water for 10-15 minutes and strained before use. It is also used in baths as one handful of dried plant to a bathful of water (18).

Comments
European five-finger grass is easily confused with Potentilla canadensis (18).

EUROPEAN MANDRAKE

Also Known As
Alraunwurzel, Mandragora, Mandragore, Mandrake, Satan's Apple.
CAUTION: See separate listings for Bryonia (English Mandrake) and Podophyllum (American Mandrake).

Scientific Names
Mandragora officinarum, synonym Mandragora vernalis.
Family: Solanaceae.

People Use This For
In folk medicine, European mandrake root has been used orally as an emetic, purgative, sedative, anesthetic, pain killer and aphrodisiac; and for treating stomach ulcers, colic, asthma, hay fever, convulsions, rheumatism, and whooping cough (14,18,3144).
In folk medicine, European mandrake fresh leaves and leaf extracts have been used topically for treating ulcers (3144).

Safety
POSSIBLY UNSAFE …when used orally. European mandrake contains several anticholinergic alkaloids, which can cause significant side effects when used in therapeutic doses (12,14).
LIKELY UNSAFE …when used orally in large doses. European mandrake contains several anticholinergic alkaloids (14). Large doses of anticholinergic alkaloids can cause respiratory and cardiac arrest and death (15,17). There is insufficient reliable information available about the safety of European mandrake when used topically.
CHILDREN: LIKELY UNSAFE …when used orally. Children can be more susceptible to the adverse effects of anticholinergic alkaloid constituents of European mandrake (15); avoid using.
PREGNANCY AND LACTATION: LIKELY UNSAFE …when used orally. European mandrake contains anticholinergic alkaloids that can cross the placenta and adversely effect the fetus. There is also some evidence that these anticholinergic constituents might pass into breast milk (14); avoid using.

Effectiveness

There is insufficient reliable information available about the effectiveness of European mandrake.

Mechanism of Action

The applicable parts of European mandrake are the root and leaf. European mandrake contains atropine, belladonnine, hyoscyamine, mandragorine, scopolamine, and scopoletin (513,816). The root contains 0.4% tropane alkaloids, principally hyoscyamine (18). All plant parts contain tropane alkaloids, principally hyoscyamine and scopolamine (17). The tropane alkaloids have anticholinergic effects, inhibiting the actions of acetylcholine principally at muscarinic receptors (15). They reduce saliva and gastric acid production, inhibit gastrointestinal motility, decrease the tone and amplitude of contractions of the ureters and bladder, reduce bronchial secretions, produce bronchodilation, inhibit sweat gland secretions reducing the volume of perspiration, reduce the movement disorders associated with Parkinsonism, prevent motion-induced nausea and vomiting, and block the responses of the sphincter muscle of the iris and the ciliary muscle of the lens, producing mydriasis and cycloplegia (15). In large doses tropane alkaloids cause tachycardia (15).

Adverse Reactions

Orally, European mandrake most commonly causes anticholinergic side effects including confusion, drowsiness, dry mouth, tachycardia, mydriasis, blurred vision, photophobia, decreased urination, decreased sweating and overheating, and flushing (15,17,18). Although some adverse reactions can occur even with low doses, adverse effects are dose related. Large doses can cause severe adverse reactions include somnolence, central excitation (restlessness, hallucinations, delirium, manic episodes), exhaustion, respiratory and cardiac arrest, and death (17,18). All components of the European mandrake plant including root, leaves, and fruit contain anticholinergic alkaloids and can cause these effects (17). Elderly patients and children can be more susceptible to the adverse effects of anticholinergic constituents of European mandrake (15).

There is some evidence that subcutaneous injection can cause anaphylactic shock including swelling of lips and eyelids, nausea, tingling in palms and scalp, abdominal cramping, stool incontinence, and loss of consciousness. This reaction has occurred with a very low dose of 2 mL of a 3 mcg/mL solution of European mandrake extract. Although IgE antibodies to European mandrake may not be detected, in vitro evaluation may find strong T lymphocyte proliferation. Skin patch tests with European mandrake root powder in sensitive individuals is likely to produce a delayed-type reaction with erythema resembling acute dermatitis (7022). Skin patch tests should be performed to rule-out hypersensitivity before administration of subcutaneous European mandrake.

Interactions with Herbs & Other Dietary Supplements

HERBS WITH ANTICHOLINERGIC EFFECTS: Theoretically, concurrent use might have additive effects and adverse effects. Anticholinergic herbs include belladonna, henbane, scopolia, and bittersweet nightshade (2).

Interactions with Drugs

ORAL DRUGS: Theoretically, concurrent use might increase absorption of some drugs because of inhibited GI motility caused by European mandrake (15).
ANTICHOLINERGIC DRUGS: Concurrent use can cause additive anticholinergic effects and adverse effects. Anticholinergic drugs include conventional medications containing tropane alkaloids such as atropine, as well as phenothiazines, amantadine, some antiparkinson drugs, glutethimide, meperidine, tricyclic antidepressants, antiarrhythmic agents, and antihistamines (15).

Interactions with Foods

No interactions are known to occur, and there is no known reason to expect a clinically significant interaction with European mandrake.

Interactions with Lab Tests

No interactions are known to occur, and there is no known reason to expect a clinically significant interaction with European mandrake.

Interactions with Diseases or Conditions

NARROW/CLOSED-ANGLE GLAUCOMA: Contraindicated due to the anticholinergic effects of European mandrake (14).
REFLUX ESOPHAGITIS: Contraindicated due to the anticholinergic effects of European mandrake (14).
OBSTRUCTIVE GASTROINTESTINAL DISEASE: Contraindicated due to the anticholinergic effects of European mandrake (14).
ULCERATIVE COLITIS OR TOXIC MEGACOLON: Contraindicated due to the anticholinergic effects of European mandrake (14).
OBSTRUCTIVE UROPATHY: Contraindicated due to the anticholinergic effects of European mandrake (14).

UNSTABLE CARDIOVASCULAR STATUS IN ACUTE HEMORRHAGE OR THYROTOXICOSIS: Contraindicated due to the anticholinergic effects of European mandrake (14).

PARALYTIC ILEUS or INTESTINAL ATONY: Contraindicated due to the anticholinergic effects of European mandrake (14).

MYASTHENIA GRAVIS: Contraindicated due to the anticholinergic effects of European mandrake (14).

HEPATIC OR RENAL DYSFUNCTION: Avoid using European mandrake due to anticholinergic effects (14,15).

HYPERTHYROIDISM: Avoid using European mandrake due to anticholinergic effects (14,15).

CONGESTIVE HEART FAILURE: Avoid using European mandrake due to anticholinergic effects (14,15).

CORONARY ARTERY DISEASE: Avoid using European mandrake due to anticholinergic effects (14,15).

TACHYARRHYTHMIAS: Avoid using European mandrake due to anticholinergic effects (14,15).

PROSTATIC HYPERTROPHY: Avoid using European mandrake due to anticholinergic effects (14,15).

HYPERTENSION: Avoid using European mandrake due to anticholinergic effects (14,15).

GASTRIC ULCER: Avoid using European mandrake due to anticholinergic effects (14,15).

HIATAL HERNIA: Avoid using European mandrake due to anticholinergic effects (14,15).

GI INFECTIONS: Avoid using European mandrake due to anticholinergic effects (14,15).

DOWN SYNDROME: Avoid using European mandrake in people with Down syndrome. They may be hypersensitive to antimuscarinic effects of anticholinergics (15).

SPASTIC PARALYSIS/BRAIN DAMAGE: Avoid using European mandrake in children with spastic paralysis or brain damage. They may be hypersensitive to antimuscarinic effects of anticholinergics (15).

Dosage and Administration

No typical dosage.

Comments

European mandrake has had many superstitions associated with it and has been claimed to have magical properties (3144). It is now considered obsolete as a therapeutic agent (18). The FDA has issued a ban on the sale of mandrake-containing products as aphrodisiacs, due to lack of evidence of their safety or efficacy (14).

EUROPEAN MISTLETOE

Also Known As

All-Heal, Birdlime Mistletoe, Devil's Fuge, Drudenfuss, Eurixor, Helixor, Hexenbesen, Iscador, Isorel, Leimmistel, Mistlekraut, Mistletein, Mistletoe, Mystyldene, Visci, Visci albi folia, Visci albi fructus, Visci albi herba, Visci albi stipites, Vogelmistel, Vysorel.
CAUTION: See separate listing for American Mistletoe.

Scientific Names

Viscum album.
Family: Viscaceae.

People Use This For

Orally, European mistletoe is used for cancer, reducing side effects of chemotherapy and radiation therapy, cardiovascular conditions including high blood pressure, internal bleeding, hemorrhoids, epilepsy and infantile convulsions, arteriosclerosis, gout, psychiatric conditions such as depression, sleep disorders, headache, amenorrhea, symptoms of menopause, and for "blood purifying" (18). It is also used orally for treating mental and physical exhaustion, as a tranquilizer, for whooping cough, asthma, vertigo, diarrhea, chorea, and liver and gallbladder conditions (18).

Subcutaneously, European mistletoe injections are used for cancer and for degenerative joint disease (2,18).

Safety

POSSIBLY SAFE ...when used orally or subcutaneously and appropriately. There is some evidence that European mistletoe extracts can be used safely (4,12,7039). However, these have a narrow therapeutic range. High doses are not safe. Tell patients not to consume more than 3 mistletoe berries or 2 leaves (4,12). Advise patients not to use European mistletoe for self-medication.

LIKELY UNSAFE ...when used orally in high doses. Ingestion of high doses of mistletoe berry or leaf can cause serious adverse reactions. More than 3 berries or 2 leaves can cause seizures, slow heart rate, low blood pressure, and death in some patients (4,7039).

PREGNANCY: LIKELY UNSAFE ...when used orally or subcutaneously. European mistletoe might have uterine stimulant and abortifacient activity (4,19).

LACTATION: Insufficient reliable information available; avoid using.

Effectiveness

POSSIBLY INEFFECTIVE ...when used subcutaneously for pancreatic cancer. European mistletoe extract does not seem to improve rates of partial or complete remission in patients with stage IV pancreatic cancer (3707,7039). ...when used subcutaneously for kidney cancer. European mistletoe does not seem to improve survival in patients with stage IV kidney cancer (7039). ...when used subcutaneously for bronchial carcinoma (7). ...when used subcutaneously for glioma. Combining European mistletoe extract plus surgery or radiation for glioma does not improve overall survival or disease-free survival (7039). ...when used subcutaneously as adjuvant therapy for melanoma. European mistletoe extract does not seem to improve overall survival or disease-free survival in patients with stage I or stage IIB melanoma (7039). There is insufficient reliable information available about the effectiveness of European mistletoe for its other uses. However, some studies seem to indicate European mistletoe extracts can improve survival in patients with solid tumors of the breast, colon, and stomach (7039,7044,7045). However, most studies have been poorly designed and have produced inconsistent results. So far, there is no convincing evidence European mistletoe extract can improve survival in patients with any form of cancer. Discourage patients from relying on European mistletoe for treating cancer.

Mechanism of Action

The applicable parts of European mistletoe are the berries, leaf, and stem. European mistletoe is a parasitic plant that grows on several different trees, including pine, oak, apple, maple, and numerous others. So, the chemical composition of mistletoe preparations can vary depending on the species of tree it grows on, the time of harvest, and other factors (7039,7106). European mistletoe has several active constituents, including the glycoprotein lectins and viscotoxins and alkaloids. European mistletoe is best known as a potential anticancer agent. Researchers think it might work as a biological response modifier that both stimulates the immune system and has cytotoxic effects (7039). There is good evidence that European mistletoe can stimulate the immune system in both animal models and humans. It seems to cause leukocytosis and increase white blood cell (WBC) secretion of cytokines interleukin-1 (IL-1), IL-6, and tumor necrosis factor-alpha (TNF-alpha) (7,7039). There is also some evidence that European mistletoe can be cytotoxic to tumor cells in vitro and in animals. Some researchers think it might induce apoptosis in tumor cells. So far, evidence for cytotoxic or antitumor effects has been conflicting. The mistletoe lectin known as ML-I seems to be responsible for many of these effects. However, there is some evidence that viscotoxins and alkaloids might also have immune stimulating and cytotoxic effects (4,7039). Although European mistletoe does seem to affect the immune system in humans and possibly has cytotoxic effects, the clinical benefits in humans are unproven. Clinical studies show that European mistletoe does not improve survival in patients with a variety of cancers. Researchers theorize that it might not work in humans for several reasons. Mistletoe lectins may not be able to bind to certain humans cells. Human plasma proteins might interfere or break down active components of mistletoe; or humans may produce antibodies that destroy active constituents of mistletoe (7039). In addition to potential anticancer effects, European mistletoe might also have hypotensive, cardiac depressant, anti-inflammatory, and sedative effects (4,11).

Adverse Reactions

Orally, European mistletoe can be well tolerated when used in small amounts. Consumption of 3 berries or 2 leaves or less does not seem to cause significant adverse effects. However, potential toxicity is dose related. Higher doses can cause significant toxicity. Oral use can cause vomiting, diarrhea, intestinal cramps, hepatitis (14), hypotension, contraction of the pupil, uncontrollable movement of the eyeball, seizures, coma, and death (2,4,6,18). European mistletoe was once associated with hepatitis in a patient taking a combination herbal product (3932). However, it is unlikely that mistletoe actually caused this adverse effect. It was most likely attributable to another ingredient, scullcap, or product contamination. There have never been additional reports of hepatitis from European mistletoe.

Subcutaneously, European mistletoe can cause pain at the injection site, chills, high fever, headaches, angina, orthostatic circulatory disturbances, eosinophilia, and allergic reaction (2). Intraperitoneal injection and injection directly into a tumor can cause pain at the injection site, nausea, and eosinophilia (7106). Necrosis can also occur at the site of injection (2,8).

Interactions with Herbs & Other Dietary Supplements

HAWTHORN: There is some evidence that European mistletoe might have cardiotoxic and negative inotropic effects (4). Theoretically, European mistletoe might decrease the effectiveness of positive inotropic agents such as hawthorn.

Interactions with Drugs

ANTIHYPERTENSIVE DRUGS: There is some evidence that European mistletoe can cause hypotension (4). Theoretically, it might have additive blood pressure lowering effects and increase the risk of hypotension; use cautiously.

CARDIOVASCULAR THERAPY: There is some evidence that European mistletoe might have cardiotoxic and negative inotropic effects. Theoretically, European mistletoe might decrease the effectiveness of positive inotropic drugs or have additive effects with negative inotropic drugs (4). Use cautiously in patients taking digoxin (Lanoxin), amrinone (Inocor), milrinone (Primacor), bepridil (Vascor), diltiazem (Cardizem, Dilacor),

verapamil (Calan, Isoptin, Veralan), and others.
IMMUNOSUPPRESSANTS: There is some concern that European mistletoe might decrease the effectiveness of immunosuppressants (4). European mistletoe has immunostimulant effects and might counteract the effects of immunosuppressants. Immunosuppressant drugs include azathioprine (Imuran), basiliximab (Simulect), cyclosporine (Neoral, Sandimmune), daclizumab (Zenapax), muromonab-CD3 (OKT3, Orthoclone OKT3), mycophenolate (CellCept), tacrolimus (FK506, Prograf), sirolimus (Rapamune), prednisone (Deltasone, Orasone), and other corticosteroids (glucocorticoids).

Interactions with Foods
No interactions are known to occur, and there is no known reason to expect a clinically significant interaction with European mistletoe.

Interactions with Lab Tests
EOSINOPHILIA: Subcutaneous, intraperitoneal, and intratumoral administration has been associated with eosinophilia. Intratumoral administration has caused hypereosinophilia, up to 43% of the white blood cell count (7106).

Interactions with Diseases or Conditions
CARDIOVASCULAR DISEASE: There is some evidence European mistletoe can have cardiotoxic and negative inotropic effects and might worsen cardiovascular conditions (4).
ORGAN TRANSPLANT: There is some concern that European mistletoe might decrease the effectiveness of immunosuppressants in organ transplant patients (4). European mistletoe has immunostimulant effects and might potentially contribute to transplant rejection.

Dosage and Administration
No typical dosage.

Comments
Interest in mistletoe for cancer is growing in North America. A lot of patients are asking about it since Suzanne Somers announced on Larry King Live that she is using it to treat her breast cancer. European mistletoe has been used for treating cancer since the 1920s, especially in Europe. Several brand name mistletoe extracts are available there: Iscador, Eurixor, Helixor, Isorel, Vysorel, and ABNOBAviscum (7,7039). So far these products are not readily available in North America. There is no proof they work for breast or other cancers. Advise patients to avoid these and stick with proven cancer treatments.

EVENING PRIMROSE OIL

Also Known As
EPO, Evening Primrose, Fever Plant, Huile D'Onagre, King's Cureall, Night Willow-Herb, Primrose, Scabish, Sun Drop.
CAUTION: See separate listings for Black Currant Seed Oil, Borage Seed Oil, Gamma Linolenic Acid, and Omega-6 Fatty Acids.

Scientific Names
Oenothera biennis and other Oenothera species.
Family: Onagraceae.

People Use This For
Orally, evening primrose oil is used for premenstrual syndrome (PMS), cyclic and non-cyclic mastalgia, endometriosis, and symptoms of menopause such as hot flashes. It is also used orally for atopic eczema, psoriasis, acne, rheumatoid arthritis, Raynaud's syndrome, multiple sclerosis, and Sjogren's syndrome. Evening primrose oil is also used orally for cancer, hypercholesterolemia and coronary heart disease, intermittent claudication, alcoholism, Alzheimer's disease, and schizophrenia. It is also used orally for post-viral fatigue syndrome, asthma, diabetic neuropathy, neurodermatitis, hyperactivity in children and attention deficit hyperactivity disorder (ADHD), obesity and weight loss, whooping cough, and gastrointestinal disorders, including ulcerative colitis, irritable bowel syndrome, and peptic ulcer disease. Evening primrose oil has also been used orally in pregnancy for preventing preeclampsia, shortening the duration of labor, stimulating labor, and preventing postdate deliveries.
In foods, evening primrose oil is used as a dietary source of essential fatty acids.
In manufacturing, evening primrose oil is used in soaps and cosmetics.

Safety

LIKELY SAFE ...when used orally and appropriately. Evening primrose oil is generally considered safe and has been used in several studies without reports of significant side effects (1106,6034,6035,6036).

PREGNANCY: POSSIBLY UNSAFE ...when used orally. Evening primrose oil might increase the risk for pregnancy complications, including delayed rupture of membranes, oxytocin augmentation, arrest of descent, and vacuum extraction (1411); avoid using.

LACTATION: POSSIBLY SAFE ...when used orally. Nursing mothers who supplement their diets with evening primrose oil secrete high levels of the constituent gamma linolenic acid into breast milk (1982); however, the gamma linolenic acid constituent of evening primrose oil is normally present in significant proportions in breast milk (4).

Effectiveness

POSSIBLY EFFECTIVE ...when taken orally for mastalgia (6034,6406). There is some evidence that evening primrose oil can relieve cyclic mastalgia in 45% of patients and non-cyclic mastalgia in 27% of patients. Evening primrose oil seems to be less effective than danazol, but similarly effective as bromocriptine (6406). ...when taken orally for improving symptoms of rheumatoid arthritis. In one study, patients experienced a significant reduction in symptoms of arthritis after 6 months of treatment (6036). ...when taken orally for irritable bowel syndrome exacerbated by premenstrual syndrome (PMS) (6034). Some clinical studies on the effectiveness of evening primrose oil have used evening primrose formulations standardized to 9% gamma linolenic acid. This formulation is similar to Efamol's Pure Evening Primrose Oil.

POSSIBLY INEFFECTIVE ...when taken orally for relief of symptoms associated with premenstrual syndrome (PMS) (1105,1106,6034,6035). Multiple small-scale studies have not demonstrated significant benefit when compared to placebo (1105,1106). ...when used orally for attention deficit hyperactivity disorder (ADHD) in children. Evening primrose oil is comparable to placebo for most measures of improvement (6443,6462).

LIKELY INEFFECTIVE ...when taken orally for preventing pre-eclampsia (1409). ...when taken orally for shortening duration of labor (1409,1411). ...when taken orally for preventing post-date deliveries in pregnant women (1411). ...when taken orally for treating menopausal hot flashes (274).

There is insufficient reliable information available about the effectiveness of evening primrose oil for its other uses.

Mechanism of Action

Evening primrose oil is obtained from the plant seed. It contains 2-16% gamma-linolenic acid (GLA), 65-80% linoleic acid, and vitamin E (6036,3908). GLA is metabolized to dihomogammalinolenic acid (DGLA). Both GLA and DGLA are precursors of prostaglandin E2 (PGE2) and the prostaglandin E1 (PGE1). Taking supplemental GLA increases the concentration of DGLA, which is converted to 15-hydroxy-DGLA, which may competitively inhibit the production of the certain inflammatory prostaglandins and leukotrienes from arachidonic acid (6036). Taking GLA from evening primrose oil is thought to decrease inflammation in conditions such as rheumatoid arthritis by improving the inflammatory and noninflammatory ratio of prostaglandins and leukotrienes (6036). There is also interest in using evening primrose oil for conditions that might result from metabolic deficiencies. For example, patients with premenstrual syndrome (PMS) are thought to have lower levels of GLA, possibly due to a defect in the conversion of linoleic acid to GLA (6034). Some children with attention deficit hyperactivity disorder (ADHD) might also have deficiencies in certain essential fatty acids, including DGLA (6462). Evening primrose oil might have other pharmacological effects related to its GLA content, including lowering elevated plasma lipids and inhibiting platelet aggregation (1979). There is also preliminary evidence from animal models that evening primrose oil can prevent diabetic neuropathy possibly by improving neuronal blood supply (3909).

Adverse Reactions

Orally, evening primrose oil can cause indigestion, nausea, soft stools, and headache in some people (4). Large doses of evening primrose oil can lead to loose stools and abdominal pain (4). There is one case report of nocturnal seizures associated with the use of evening primrose oil, black cohosh, and chasteberry (588). Evening primrose oil might increase the risk for pregnancy complications, including prolonged rupture of membranes, oxytocin augmentation, arrest of descent, and vacuum extraction (1411).

Interactions with Herbs & Other Dietary Supplements

HERBS WITH ANTICOAGULANT/ANTIPLATELET POTENTIAL: Concomitant use of herbs that have coumarin constituents or affect platelet aggregation could theoretically increase the risk of bleeding in some people. These herbs include angelica, anise, arnica, asafoetida, bogbean, boldo, capsicum, celery, chamomile, clove, danshen, fenugreek, feverfew, garlic, ginger, ginkgo, ginseng (Panax), horse chestnut, horseradish, licorice, meadowsweet, prickly ash, onion, papain, passionflower, poplar, quassia, red clover, turmeric, wild carrot, wild lettuce, willow, and others (4,19).

Interactions with Drugs

ANESTHESIA: There is a case report of seizures associated with concomitant use of evening primrose oil and anesthesia; however, other drugs were also involved (613).

ANTICOAGULANT/ANTIPLATELET DRUGS: Evening primrose oil, which contains gamma-linolenic acid (GLA), could have anticoagulant effects (1979). Theoretically, taking evening primrose oil with other anticoagulant or antiplatelet drugs might increase the risk of bruising and bleeding. Some of these drugs include aspirin, clopidogrel (Plavix), nonsteroidal anti-inflammatory drugs (NSAIDs) such as diclofenac (Voltaren, Cataflam, others), ibuprofen (Advil, Motrin, others), naproxen (Anaprox, Naprosyn, others), dalteparin (Fragmin), enoxaparin (Lovenox), heparin, warfarin (Coumadin), and others.

PHENOTHIAZINES: Seizures have been reported in people with schizophrenia treated concomitantly with phenothiazine drugs and evening primrose oil (614); use with caution.

Interactions with Foods
No interactions are known to occur, and there is no known reason to expect a clinically significant interaction with evening primrose oil.

Interactions with Lab Tests
BLEEDING TIME: There is some concern that evening primrose oil might prolong bleeding time. Evening primrose oil contains gamma linolenic acid (GLA), which can inhibit platelet aggregation (1979).

LIPID PROFILE: Evening primrose oil might affect cholesterol levels. Evening primrose oil contains gamma-linolenic acid (GLA), which can lower plasma triglycerides and increase high-density lipoprotein (HDL) cholesterol (1979).

Interactions with Diseases or Conditions
BLEEDING DISORDERS: There is some concern that evening primrose oil might prolong bleeding time and increase the risk of bruising and bleeding. Evening primrose oil contains gamma-linolenic acid (GLA), which can inhibit platelet aggregation (1979).

EPILEPSY/SEIZURE DISORDER: There is concern that evening primrose oil might lower the seizure threshold or unmask undiagnosed temporal lobe epilepsy. However, current reports have only identified seizure in association with phenothiazine (4,614).

SCHIZOPHRENIA: Seizures have been reported in people with schizophrenia treated concomitantly with phenothiazine drugs and evening primrose oil (614); use with caution.

Dosage and Administration
ORAL: For mastalgia 3-4 grams daily has been used (6034,6406). For premenstrual syndrome (PMS), 2-4 grams daily has been used (6034). For rheumatoid arthritis, doses ranging from 540 mg daily to 2.8 grams daily have been used (6036). For atopic eczema, 6-8 grams daily has been used (4). Children take about 2-4 grams daily (4).

Comments
Evening primrose oil is approved in the United Kingdom as a "Prescription Only Medicine" for treating atopic eczema and is approved in Canada as a dietary supplement for increasing essential fatty acid intake (11).

EYEBRIGHT

Also Known As
Augentrostkraut, Euphraisia Eye Bright, Euphrasiae herba, Eye Bright, Herbed' Euphraise.
CAUTION: See separate listing for Clary Sage.

Scientific Names
Eurphrasia rostkoviana; Euphrasia officinalis.
Family: Scrophulariaceae.

People Use This For
Orally, eyebright is used to treat nasal mucous membrane inflammation and sinusitis (4).

Topically, eyebright is used as an ophthalmic in the form of a lotion, poultice, or eyebath. The eye conditions eyebright is used for include: conjunctivitis (4,6), blepharitis (6), eye fatigue (6), inflammation of the blood vessels, eyelids and conjunctiva, and for "glued" and inflamed eyes. Eyebright is also used topically to prevent mucous and mucous membrane inflammation of the eyes (2).

Historically, eyebright has been used in British Herbal Tobacco, which was smoked for chronic bronchial conditions and colds (6). It was also used historically for allergies, cancers, coughs, conjunctivitis, earaches, epilepsy, headaches, hoarseness, inflammation, jaundice, ophthalmia, rhinitis, skin ailments, sore throats (6), and as a poultice for styes (8,11). In foods, eyebright is used as a flavoring ingredient (4).

Safety
POSSIBLY SAFE ...when used orally and appropriately (12). ...when used orally in amounts found in foods. Eyebright is listed by the Council of Europe as a natural source of food flavoring (4).
POSSIBLY UNSAFE ...when used as an ophthalmic; avoid using due to hygienic concerns. Eye products may be subject to contamination (8,11).
PREGNANCY AND LACTATION: Insufficient reliable information available; avoid using.

Effectiveness
There is insufficient reliable information available about the effectiveness of eyebright.

Mechanism of Action
Tannin constituents may be responsible for astringent properties (4). The constituent caffeic acid has bacteriostatic activity (4). Constituents, aucubin and iridoid glycosides, have purgative activity (4).

Adverse Reactions
10-60 drops eyebright tincture (unspecified route of administration) may induce mental confusion, headache, increased eye pressure with lacrimation, itching, redness, swelling of eyelid margins, dim vision, photophobia, weakness, sneezing, nausea, toothache, constipation, cough, dyspnea, insomnia, polyuria, and sweating (4).

Interactions with Herbs & Other Dietary Supplements
Insufficient reliable information available.

Interactions with Drugs
No interactions are known to occur, and there is no known reason to expect a clinically significant interaction with eyebright.

Interactions with Foods
No interactions are known to occur, and there is no known reason to expect a clinically significant interaction with eyebright.

Interactions with Lab Tests
No interactions are known to occur, and there is no known reason to expect a clinically significant interaction with eyebright.

Interactions with Diseases or Conditions
No interactions are known to occur, and there is no known reason to expect a clinically significant interaction with eyebright.

Dosage and Administration
ORAL: 2-4 grams dried above ground parts three times daily (4), or one cup tea (steep 2-4 grams dried above ground parts in 150 mL boiling water 5-10 minutes, strain) three times daily (4). Liquid extract (1:1 in 25% alcohol), 2-4 mL three times daily (4). Tincture (1:5 in 45% alcohol), 2-6 mL three times daily (4).
TOPICAL: No typical dosage.

Comments
Avoid use of nonsterile solutions (including homemade products) in the eye(s), due to high risk of infection. Ophthalmic application of eyebright is not recommended (5).

FALSE UNICORN

Also Known As
Blazing Star, Fairywand, Helonias, Starwort.

Scientific Names
Chamaelirium luteum, synonyms Chamaelirium carolianum, Helonias dioica, Helonias lutea, Veratrum luteum. Family: Liliaceae.

People Use This For
Orally, false unicorn is used for ovarian cysts, menstrual problems, menopause (4201), threatened miscarriage (4), vomiting from pregnancy (4), digestive problems (4201), and to normalize hormones after oral contraceptive use. It is also used as a diuretic and to rid the intestines of worms.

Safety
POSSIBLY SAFE ...when the root preparations are used orally and appropriately (12).
PREGNANCY: LIKELY UNSAFE ...when used orally because it is a potential uterine stimulant (12,18).
LACTATION: Insufficient reliable information available; avoid using.

Effectiveness
There is insufficient reliable information available about the effectiveness of false unicorn.

Mechanism of Action
The applicable parts of false unicorn are the rhizome and root. False unicorn reportedly has anthelmintic, diuretic (18), uterine stimulant, and menstruation stimulant activity (12).

Adverse Reactions
Orally, large doses of false unicorn may cause nausea and vomiting (4).

Interactions with Herbs & Other Dietary Supplements
Insufficient reliable information available.

Interactions with Drugs
No interactions are known to occur, and there is no known reason to expect a clinically significant interaction with false unicorn.

Interactions with Foods
No interactions are known to occur, and there is no known reason to expect a clinically significant interaction with false unicorn.

Interactions with Lab Tests
No interactions are known to occur, and there is no known reason to expect a clinically significant interaction with false unicorn.

Interactions with Diseases or Conditions
GI CONDITIONS: Can irritate the gastrointestinal tract. Contraindicated in individuals with infectious or inflammatory gastrointestinal conditions (19).

Dosage and Administration
ORAL: 1-2 grams dried root 3 times per day, or, one cup tea (steep 1-2 grams dried root in 150 mL boiling water 5-10 minutes, strain) 3 times daily (4). Liquid extract (1:1 in 45% alcohol), 1-2 mL 3 times daily (4). Tincture (1:5 in 45% alcohol), 2-5 mL 3 times daily (4).

Comments
None.

FENNEL fruit, seed

Also Known As
Bitter Fennel, Carosella, Common Fennel, Finnochio, Florence Fennel, Garden Fennel, Large Fennel, Phytoestrogen, Sweet Fennel, Wild Fennel.
CAUTION: See separate listing for Fennel Oil.

Scientific Names
Foeniculum vulgare, synonyms Foeniculum officinale, Foeniculum capillaceum, Anethum foeniculum.
Family: Apiaceae or Umbilliferae.

People Use This For

Orally, fennel is used to enhance lactation, promote menstruation, facilitate birth, increase libido (6), treat indigestion, upper respiratory tract mucous membrane inflammation (2), cough, bronchitis (18), loss of appetite, visual problems, and colic in infants (6135).

In Chinese medicine, fennel has been used orally in combination formulas for cholera, backache, and bedwetting (11). Fennel powder has been used topically in Chinese medicine as a poultice for hard-to-heal snake bites (11).

Safety

LIKELY SAFE ...when the seed is used orally in food amounts (11,12).

POSSIBLY SAFE ...when used orally and appropriately for short periods of time (2,12).

POSSIBLY UNSAFE ...when used orally in medicinal amounts for prolonged periods of time. The constituent, estragole, is a procarcinogen (12).

PREGNANCY: LIKELY UNSAFE ...when used orally; avoid using (2).

LACTATION: Insufficient reliable information available; avoid using.

Effectiveness

There is insufficient reliable information available about the effectiveness of fennel fruit or seed.

Mechanism of Action

Fennel is a rich source of beta-carotene and vitamin C (19). The seed contains a volatile oil composed largely of trans-anethole, with lesser amounts of fenchone, estragole, and other constituents. It also contains significant amounts of calcium, magnesium, and iron, and lesser amounts of other metal cations (6135). Fennel seed can promote GI motility, and in higher concentrations, it can act as an antispasmodic (2). The constituents, anethole and fenchone, reduce upper respiratory tract secretions (11). Some evidence suggests the aqueous fennel extract might also increase mucociliary activity (11). The constituent anethole appears to be allergenic, insecticidal, and toxic. Polymers of anethole have estrogenic activity (11). The constituent estragole is a procarcinogen but the carcinogenic risk is minimal. It is not directly hepatotoxic or hepatocarcinogenic but requires activation by liver enzymes to reach full toxicity. In the liver, other enzymes inactivate the carcinogenic metabolites, limiting possible damage to the liver (12).

Adverse Reactions

Orally, fennel can cause allergic reactions affecting the skin and respiratory system (2). It can also cause photodermatitis. Avoid excessive sunlight or ultraviolet light exposure while using this product (19). Allergic cross-sensitivity is possible in people with allergies to carrot, celery, mugwort, or other Apiaceae family plants (6,18).

Interactions with Herbs & Other Dietary Supplements

Insufficient reliable information available.

Interactions with Drugs

CIPROFLOXACIN (Cipro): Concomitant administration might reduce the effectiveness of ciprofloxacin therapy. Preliminary evidence suggests that fennel reduces ciprofloxacin bioavailability by nearly 50%, possibly due to interaction with the metal cations contained in fennel. Evidence also suggests that fennel increases tissue distribution and slows elimination of ciprofloxacin (6135).

Interactions with Foods

No interactions are known to occur, and there is no known reason to expect a clinically significant interaction with fennel fruit or seed.

Interactions with Lab Tests

No interactions are known to occur, and there is no known reason to expect a clinically significant interaction with fennel fruit or seed.

Interactions with Diseases or Conditions

CELERY, CARROT, MUGWORT ALLERGY: Allergic cross-sensitivity to fennel possible (6,18).

HORMONE SENSITIVE CANCERS/CONDITIONS: Because fennel oil might have estrogenic effects (11), women with hormone sensitive conditions should avoid fennel oil. Some of these conditions include breast, uterine, and ovarian cancer, and endometriosis and uterine fibroids.

Dosage and Administration

ORAL: The typical dose of fennel is 5-7 grams of the dried fruit or seed per day or one cup of the tea three times daily (2,18). The tea is prepared by steeping 1-2 grams of the crushed or ground fruit or seed in 150 mL boiling water for 5-10 minutes and then straining. The common dose of the tincture compound is 5-7.5 grams per day (2). Fennel should be used on a short-term basis (2).

Comments

None.

FENNEL OIL

Also Known As

Foeniculi antheroleum, Phytoestrogen.
CAUTION: See separate listing for Fennel fruit, seed.

Scientific Names

Foeniculum vulgare, synonyms Foeniculum officinale, Foeniculum capillaceum, Anethum foeniculum.
Family: Apiaceae or Umbilliferae.

People Use This For

Orally, fennel oil is used for mild spastic disorders of the GI tract, feeling of fullness, flatulence, upper respiratory tract mucous membrane inflammation (2), cough, and bronchitis (18). Fennel honey syrup is used for upper respiratory tract mucous membrane inflammation in children (2).
Traditionally, fennel oil has been used for improving appetite, digestion, and other stomach complaints (11).
In foods and beverages, fennel oil is used as a flavoring agent (11).
In other manufacturing processes, fennel oil is used as a flavoring agent in some laxatives (11), and as a fragrance component in soaps and cosmetics (11).

Safety

LIKELY SAFE ...when consumed in amounts commonly found in foods. Fennel oil has Generally Recognized as Safe (GRAS) status for food use in the US. A maximum level of 0.119% is used in meat products (11).
POSSIBLY SAFE ...when used orally in medicinal amounts for less than 2 weeks (2,18).
POSSIBLY UNSAFE ...when used orally, long-term.
CHILDREN: LIKELY UNSAFE ...when used orally. Contraindicated for oral use in infants and toddlers (2).
PREGNANCY: LIKELY SAFE ...when used in food amounts. LIKELY UNSAFE ...when used orally in larger amounts (2).
LACTATION: Insufficient reliable information available; avoid using amounts larger than those found in foods.

Effectiveness

POSSIBLY EFFECTIVE ...when used orally for mild spastic disorders of the GI tract, feeling of fullness, and upper respiratory tract mucous membrane inflammation (including the use of the honey syrup in children) (2).
There is insufficient reliable information available about the effectiveness of fennel oil for its other uses.

Mechanism of Action

Fennel oil is composed largely of trans-anethole, with lesser amounts of fenchone, estragole, and other constituents. The oil can promote GI motility, and in higher concentrations, it can act as an antispasmodic (2). The constituents, anethole and fenchone, reduce upper respiratory tract secretions (11). The constituent anethole appears to be allergenic, insecticidal, and toxic. Polymers of anethole have estrogenic activity (11). The constituent estragole is a procarcinogen but the carcinogenic risk is minimal. It is not directly hepatotoxic or hepatocarcinogenic but requires activation by liver enzymes to reach full toxicity. In the liver other enzymes inactivate the carcinogenic metabolites, limiting possible damage to the liver (12).

Adverse Reactions

Allergic cross-sensitivity is possible in people with allergies to carrot, celery, mugwort, or other Apiaceae family plants (6,18). Allergic reactions that affect the skin and respiratory system are rare (2).

Interactions with Herbs & Other Dietary Supplements

Insufficient reliable information available.

Interactions with Drugs
No interactions are known to occur, and there is no known reason to expect a clinically significant interaction with fennel oil.

Interactions with Foods
No interactions are known to occur, and there is no known reason to expect a clinically significant interaction with fennel oil.

Interactions with Lab Tests
No interactions are known to occur, and there is no known reason to expect a clinically significant interaction with fennel oil.

Interactions with Diseases or Conditions
CELERY, CARROT, MUGWORT ALLERGY: Allergic cross sensitivity to fennel is possible (6,18).
DIABETES: Use caution with the fennel honey syrup in diabetics due to its carbohydrate content (2).
HORMONE SENSITIVE CANCERS/CONDITIONS: Because fennel oil might have estrogenic effects (11), women with hormone sensitive conditions should avoid fennel oil. Some of these conditions include breast, uterine, and ovarian cancer; endometriosis; and uterine fibroids.

Dosage and Administration
ORAL: The typical daily dose of fennel oil is 0.1-0.6 mL, which is equivalent to 100-600 mg of the dried fruit or seed. It should only be used up to two weeks without professional evaluation (2). The fennel honey syrup, which contains 500 mg fennel oil/kg, is usually dosed 10-20 grams per day (2).

Comments
Fennel oil is the distilled essential oil of the fennel (Foeniculum vulgare) fruit or seed.

FENUGREEK

Also Known As
Bird's Foot, Bockshornsame, Foenugraeci Semen, Foenugreek, Greek Hay, Greek Hay Seed, Hu Lu Ba, Methi, Trigonella.

Scientific Names
Trigonella foenum-graecum.
Family: Leguminosae or Fabaceae.

People Use This For
Orally, fenugreek seed is used for loss of appetite (2,4), for treating dyspepsia, gastritis (4), for lowering blood glucose in people with diabetes (220,622), constipation, atherosclerosis, high serum cholesterol and triglycerides (1900), and for promoting lactation (314).
Topically, fenugreek is used as a poultice for local inflammation (2), myalgia, lymphadenitis, gout, wounds, leg ulcers (6), and eczema (18).
In Chinese medicine, fenugreek is used for nutrition, kidney ailments, beriberi, hernia, impotence, and other male problems (11).
Traditionally, fenugreek has been taken to reduce fever, promote lactation, and treat mouth ulcers, boils, bronchitis, cellulitis, tuberculosis, chronic coughs, chapped lips, and cancer. It is also used as a cure for baldness (6,11).
For food use, fenugreek is included as an ingredient in spice blends. It is also used as a flavoring agent in imitation maple syrup, foods, beverages, and tobacco (11).
In other manufacturing processes, fenugreek extracts are used in soaps and cosmetics (11).

Safety
LIKELY SAFE ...when seed preparations are used in the amounts commonly found in foods, (maximum use level is 0.05% in meat). It has Generally Recognized as Safe (GRAS) status in the US (11).
POSSIBLY SAFE ...when used orally in medicinal amounts (2,4).
POSSIBLY UNSAFE ...when used topically, the repeated use of fenugreek can result in skin sensitization (2,18).
PREGNANCY: LIKELY UNSAFE ...contraindicated for oral use in amounts greater than those found in foods because of its potential oxytocic and uterine stimulant activity (4).
LACTATION: Insufficient reliable information available; avoid using.

Effectiveness

POSSIBLY EFFECTIVE ...when used orally for lowering blood sugar in people with diabetes (4,6). ...when used topically as a poultice for local inflammation (2).
There is insufficient reliable information available about the effectiveness of fenugreek for its other uses.

Mechanism of Action

The applicable part of fenugreek is the seed. Fenugreek affects gastrointestinal transit, slowing glucose absorption (163). The constituent, 4-isoleucine, appears to directly stimulate insulin (164). In healthy individuals, whole seed extracts, gum isolate, extracted seeds, cooked seeds, and the constituent, trigonelline, show evidence of a hypoglycemic effect (4). In people with noninsulin-dependent diabetes, the ingestion of the extracted seeds can improve plasma glucose and insulin response (4). In people with insulin-dependent diabetes, the ingestion of the seed powder can reduce plasma glucose, glycosuria, and the daily insulin requirement (4). Some studies suggest the seed powder can reduce serum cholesterol in people with diabetes (4). Other evidence suggests the seed consumption might decrease calcium oxalate deposition in the kidneys (720). The fenugreekine constituent shows evidence of cardiotonic, hypoglycemic, diuretic, anti-inflammatory, antihypertensive and antiviral properties (4).

Adverse Reactions

Orally, fenugreek can cause diarrhea and flatulence (622). With large doses, hypoglycemia is possible (6,164). Occupational exposure to fenugreek can cause asthma (6), and after inhalation of the seed powder, it can cause allergic symptoms, such as runny nose, wheezing, and fainting. The paste of fenugreek applied to the scalp can cause allergic symptoms, including head numbness, facial swelling, and wheezing (719).

Interactions with Herbs & Other Dietary Supplements

HERBS WITH ANTICOAGULANT/ANTIPLATELET POTENTIAL: Concomitant use of herbs that have coumarin constituents or affect platelet aggregation could theoretically increase the risk of bleeding in some people. These herbs include: angelica, anise, arnica, asafoetida, bogbean, boldo, capsicum, celery, chamomile, clove, danshen, feverfew, garlic, ginger, ginkgo, ginseng (Panax), horse chestnut, horseradish, licorice, meadowsweet, prickly ash, onion, papain, passionflower, poplar, quassia, red clover, turmeric, wild carrot, wild lettuce, willow, and others (4,19).

Interactions with Drugs

ANTICOAGULANT: Theoretically, fenugreek can enhance anticoagulant drug activity and increase the risk of bleeding (4).
CORTICOSTEROID: Theoretically, fenugreek can inhibit corticosteroid drug activity (4).
HORMONE THERAPY: Fenugreek theoretically can interfere with hormone therapy (4).
HYPOGLYCEMIC DRUGS: Fenugreek can alter blood glucose control (4), and when used, blood glucose levels should be monitored closely.
INSULIN: Insulin dosage might need to be adjusted due to the hypoglycemic effect of fenugreek (19).
MONOAMINE OXIDASE INHIBITORS (MAOIs): Theoretically, fenugreek can potentiate their drug activity (4).
ORAL DRUGS: Theoretically, the high mucilage content of fenugreek can decrease or delay the absorption of oral drugs (4,19).

Interactions with Foods

No interactions are known to occur, and there is no known reason to expect a clinically significant interaction with fenugreek.

Interactions with Lab Tests

URINE ODOR: Fenugreek can cause a maple syrup odor in urine (6). Avoid confusion with "maple syrup urine" disease (6).
BLOOD GLUCOSE: Fenugreek can lower blood glucose and test results (4,6).

Interactions with Diseases or Conditions

FENUGREEK ALLERGY: Contraindicated.
KIDNEY STONES: Theoretically, it can decrease calcium oxalate deposition and stone formation (720).
DIABETES: Fenugreek can alter blood sugar control in people with diabetes (4,6), and blood glucose levels should be monitored closely.

Dosage and Administration

ORAL: The typical dose is 1-2 grams of the seed or equivalent three times daily (2,4) or one cup of the tea several times a day. The tea is prepared by steeping 500 mg seed in 150 mL cold water for three hours and the straining. The maximum amount of fenugreek is 6 grams of the seed per day (2).
TOPICAL: It is typically used as a poultice, which is prepared by mixing 50 grams of the powdered seed in 0.25-1 L of hot water to form a paste (2,18).

Comments

The taste and odor of fenugreek resembles maple syrup, and it has been used to mask the taste of medicines (6).

FEVER BARK

Also Known As

Alstonia Bark, Australian Febrifuge, Australian Fever Bush, Australian Quinine, Devil's Bit, Devil Tree, Dita Bark, Pale Mara, Pali-Mara.

Scientific Names

Alstonia constricta.
Family: Apocynaceae.

People Use This For

Orally, fever bark is used for treating fever, hypertension, diarrhea, and malaria. It is also used as a stimulant and a uterine stimulant (18).
Historically, fever bark was used to treat rheumatism (18).

Safety

POSSIBLY UNSAFE ...when used orally and appropriately. Fever bark contains reserpine and yohimbine constituents (18) that can cause severe adverse effects including depression, psychosis, and acute renal failure (2,5,6,11,17,18,19).
PREGNANCY AND LACTATION: Insufficient reliable information available; avoid using.

Effectiveness

There is insufficient reliable information available about the effectiveness of fever bark.

Mechanism of Action

Fever bark contains various alkaloids including yohimbe. The constituents reserpine and deserpidine are likely responsible for its antihypertensive effects. Fever bark might also have antipyretic and antispasmodic properties (18).

Adverse Reactions

Orally, the reserpine constituent of fever bark can cause lethargy, nasal congestion, or depression (17). The yohimbine constituent of fever bark can cause salivation, irritability, fluid retention, skin eruptions, eye dilation, allergy, acute renal failure, and lupus-like syndrome (2,5,6,11,18,19). Yohimbine is reported to trigger psychosis in people predisposed to it (2,5,6,11,18). Symptoms of yohimbine toxicity include paralysis, severe hypotension, cardiac conduction disorders, cardiac failure, and death (6,18).

Interactions with Herbs & Other Dietary Supplements

ST. JOHN'S WORT: Theoretically, concomitant use of St. John's wort extract might antagonize effects of reserpine, a constituent of fever bark (19).
TURMERIC: Theoretically, concomitant use of tumeric might reduce the frequency of gastric and duodenal ulcers associated with reserpine, a constituent of fever bark (19).
YOHIMBE: Theoretically, concomitant use of fever bark with yohimbe can cause additive effects or adverse effects.
INDIAN SNAKEROOT: Theoretically, concomitant use of Indian snakeroot with fever root can cause additive effects and side effects due to reserpine and deserpidine content of both herbs.

Interactions with Drugs

GENERAL ANESTHETICS: Reserpine can increase the risk of cardiovascular instability in individuals receiving general anesthetics (151).
SYMPATHOMIMETICS: Reserpine might increase or decrease effects of sympathomimetics (151).

PHENOTHIAZINES: Theoretically, phenothiazines might increase the toxicity of yohimbine due to alpha-two adrenoreceptor antagonism (19).

NALOXONE: Concomitant use of yohimbine and naloxone can cause synergistic effects and adverse reactions (19).

Interactions with Foods

No interactions are known to occur, and there is no known reason to expect a clinically significant interaction with fever bark.

Interactions with Lab Tests

FFA: Reserpine can increase serum free fatty acids (275).

GUAIACOLA SPOT TEST: Reserpine can cause a false reading with urine screening test of Rogers (275).

HOMOVANILLIC ACID: Reserpine can increase urine levels of homovanillic acid; maximum on second day (275).

HYDROCHLORIC ACID: Reserpine can increase gastric hydrochloric acid levels (275).

17-HYDROXYCORTICOSTEROIDS: Reserpine can decrease urine levels (275).

5-HYDROXYINDOLEACETIC ACID (5-HIAA): Reserpine can increase test results (275).

NOREPINEPHRINE: Reserpine can decrease urine levels of norepinephrine (275). Yohimbine can increase plasma and cerebrospinal fluid norepinephrine levels and test results (275).

PEPSIN: Reserpine can increase gastric pepsin levels and test results (275).

PLATELETS: Reserpine can decrease blood platelet levels and test results (275).

PROLACTIN: Reserpine can increase plasma prolactin levels and test results (275).

PROTHROMBIN TIME: Reserpine can decrease plasma prothrombin time (275).

SEROTONIN: Reserpine can decrease plasma 5-HT and test results (275).

T-4: Reserpine can decrease thyroxine (T-4) serum levels and test results (275).

TYRAMINE: Reserpine can cause a false positive response to tyramine test (275).

VANILLYMANDELIC ACID: Reserpine can decrease urine levels and test results (275).

Interactions with Diseases or Conditions

MENTAL DEPRESSION: Theoretically, contraindicated in individuals with a history of mental depression due to reserpine constituent (17,18).

PEPTIC ULCER: Theoretically, contraindicated in individuals with active peptic ulcer due to reserpine constituent (17).

SCHIZOPHRENIA: Theoretically, contraindicated in individuals with schizophrenia because yohimbine constituent might induce psychotic episodes (19).

Dosage and Administration

ORAL: A typical dose is 15 to 20 mL of tea daily. Tea can be made by steeping one part ground bark to 20 parts boiling water for 10-15 minutes, strain. Alternatively, 2-4 mL tincture (1:8 or 1:10) daily; or 4-8 mL of liquid extract (1:1) daily has also been used (18).

Comments

Most of the information available for fever bark concerns its constituents.

FEVERFEW

Also Known As

Altamisa, Bachelor's Button, Featerfoiul, Featherfew, Featherfoil, Fever Few, Flirtwort Midsummer Daisy, Santa Maria, Tanaceti parthenii.

Scientific Names

Tanacetum parthenium, synonyms Chrysanthemum parthenium, Leucanthemum parthenium, Pyrethrum parthenium. Family: Asteraceae or Compositae.

People Use This For

Orally, feverfew is used for fever, headache, prevention of migraine, and menstrual irregularities (5,11,18). It is also used for arthritis (6933), psoriasis (6934), allergies (5121), asthma (214), tinnitus and vertigo (4), and nausea and vomiting (6121). Feverfew is also used for infertility, anemia, cancer, common cold, earache, liver disease, prevention of miscarriage, muscular tension and orthopedic disorders, swollen feet, diarrhea, and dyspepsia including indigestion and flatulence (6963).

Topically, feverfew is used for toothaches and as an antiseptic and insecticide (4,18). It is also used as a general stimulant and tonic and for intestinal parasites (4,11,18).

Safety

LIKELY SAFE ...when used orally and appropriately, short-term (12). Feverfew has been used safely in studies lasting up to 4 months (6959,6960,6961).

There is insufficient reliable information available about the safety of the long-term use of feverfew. Although no significant adverse effects have been reported with long-term use (12,6711,6959), long-term safety has not been sufficiently evaluated (6711).

PREGNANCY: LIKELY UNSAFE ...when used orally. Feverfew might cause uterine contractions and abortion (4); avoid using.

LACTATION: Insufficient reliable information available; avoid using.

Effectiveness

POSSIBLY EFFECTIVE ...when used orally for preventing migraine headaches. Taken prophylactically, feverfew can significantly reduce the frequency of migraine headaches. Migraine headaches that do occur tend to have less severe symptoms of pain, nausea, vomiting, and sensitivity to light and noise (6959,6960,6961,6965,6711). The US Headache Consortium 2000 guidelines for preventing migraine headaches suggest feverfew as a second-line preventive treatment (5080). Although most studies have used feverfew products standardized to contain 0.2-0.35% of the parthenolide constituent, this standardization does not seem necessary for effectiveness (726,6935,6938).

POSSIBLY INEFFECTIVE ...when used orally to treat or abort acute migraine headache (6940). ...when used orally to reduce the symptoms of rheumatoid arthritis (6933). ...when used orally for non-migraine headache (6940).

There is insufficient reliable information available about the effectiveness of feverfew for its other uses.

Mechanism of Action

The applicable part of feverfew is the leaf. At least 39 constituents of feverfew have been identified (724). However, there has been controversy about which constituents were responsible for feverfew's pharmacological effects. It used to be widely believed that the sesquiterpene lactone, parthenolide, was the active constituent (3,6935). It was suggested that at least 0.2% of parthenolide was required for efficacy (21,6935,6937,6940). However, a study using an alcoholic extract of feverfew standardized to 0.35% parthenolide was found ineffective for preventing migraine (6938), suggesting that parthenolide may not be the active ingredient and that other constituents are necessary for benefit in the prevention of migraine (49,512,6935,6938). It's not yet clear how feverfew works in the prevention of migraine. Laboratory evidence suggests that feverfew extracts might inhibit platelet aggregation and inhibit serotonin release from platelets and leucocytes (6935,6936,6942,6943,6944,6945); however, platelet studies in people have not found this effect (6951). Feverfew might also inhibit serum proteases and leukotrienes (6939,6946). Feverfew also appears to block prostaglandin synthesis by inhibiting phospholipase, which prevents the release of arachidonic acid (6943,6953,6954). Preliminary research shows that extracts of fresh feverfew leaves and parthenolide might cause irreversible inhibition of vascular muscle contraction (6948,5949,6950). Chrysanthenyl acetate, an essential oil of feverfew, has been suggested as one active component (6938). Chrysanthenyl acetate inhibits prostaglandin synthetase and might have analgesic properties (6711,6713). Feverfew also contains melatonin which might contribute to its pharmacological effect (50). Fresh or dried leaves contained significantly more melatonin than commercially prepared standardized feverfew tablets (50). Migraine attacks have been associated with decreased melatonin excretion (6712). Other pharmacological effects of feverfew include cytostatic effect on tumor cell growth (6957), inhibition of inflammation and pain transmission (6947), and anti-inflammatory effects (6941).

Adverse Reactions

Orally, feverfew can cause abdominal pain, indigestion, diarrhea, flatulence, nausea, and vomiting (1). The traditional method of feverfew administration, chewing fresh feverfew leaves, can result in mouth ulceration, inflamed oral mucosa and tongue, swelling of the lips, and occasionally, loss of taste (6935,6959). Mouth ulceration might result from direct contact with feverfew leaves during chewing, possibly attributable to the sesquiterpene lactone constituent (6959). Some researchers suggest that mouth ulceration is a systemic effect, but one study using dried feverfew capsules reported a higher incidence of mouth ulcers in subjects taking placebo than feverfew (6935,6959,6960). "Post-feverfew syndrome," including anxiety, headaches, insomnia, and muscle and joint stiffness, has been described in people who have taken feverfew over long periods of time (6959). Allergic contact dermatitis can occur with topical use of feverfew (1,6958). Overall, feverfew might be better tolerated than some conventional migraine drugs used for prophylaxis. For example, in clinical trials, feverfew did not affect blood pressure, heart rate, body weight, blood chemistry, or cytology, like some conventional drugs do, such as ergot derivatives, serotonin agonists ("triptans"), beta-blockers, valproic acid, and analgesics (6959,6960,6961,6965,6711). Feverfew could cause an allergic reaction in individuals sensitive to the Asteraceae/Compositae family. Members of this family include ragweed, chrysanthemums, marigolds, daisies, and many other herbs.

Interactions with Herbs & Other Dietary Supplements

HERBS WITH ANTICOAGULANT/ANTIPLATELET POTENTIAL: Some evidence suggests that feverfew can inhibit platelet aggregation. However, this has not been demonstrated in humans (6935,6936,6942,6943,6944,6945,6951).

Theoretically, concomitant use of feverfew and herbs that affect platelet aggregation could increase the risk of bleeding in some people. Some of these herbs include angelica, anise, arnica, asafoetida, bogbean, boldo, capsicum, celery, chamomile, clove, danshen, fenugreek, garlic, ginger, ginkgo, Panax ginseng, horse chestnut, horseradish, licorice, meadowsweet, prickly ash, onion, papain, passionflower, poplar, quassia, red clover, turmeric, wild carrot, wild lettuce, willow, and others [4,19].

Interactions with Drugs

ANTICOAGULANT, ANTIPLATELET DRUGS: Some evidence suggests that feverfew can inhibit platelet aggregation. However, this has not been demonstrated in humans [6935,6936,6942,6943,6944,6945,6951]. Theoretically, feverfew might have additive effects and increase the risk of bleeding when used with these drugs.
NONSTEROIDAL ANTI-INFLAMMATORY DRUGS (NSAIDs): Theoretically, NSAIDs might decrease the effectiveness of feverfew [6]. This potential interaction might be mediated through NSAIDs' effects on prostaglandins [21].

Interactions with Foods

No interactions are known to occur, and there is no known reason to expect a clinically significant interaction with feverfew.

Interactions with Lab Tests

No interactions are known to occur, and there is no known reason to expect a clinically significant interaction with feverfew.

Interactions with Diseases or Conditions

CROSS-ALLERGENICITY: Feverfew can cause an allergic reaction in individuals sensitive to the Asteraceae/Compositae family. Members of this family include ragweed, chrysanthemums, marigolds, daisies, and many other herbs.

Dosage and Administration

ORAL: For migraine headache prophylaxis, clinical studies have used 50 to 100 mg of feverfew extract daily. Although most extracts used in clinical studies were standardized to 0.2-0.35% parthenolide content, this standardization does not appear to be necessary for effectiveness [6935,6938,6959,6960,6961]. The typical dose of the fresh leaf is 2.5 leaves daily with or after food [4]. The freeze-dried leaf is taken at 50-125 mg per day with or after food [4,6,724,725].
TOPICAL: No typical dosage.

Comments

Some feverfew tablet products can contain little or no feverfew [5]. The Therapeutic Products Directorate of the Health Products and Food Branch of Health Canada issued a Drug Identification Number (DIN) to a feverfew leaf (capsules) product standardized to 0.2% parthenolide, with the labeling claim "used as a prophylactic against migraines" [724].

FICIN

Also Known As

Doctor Oje, Leche de Higueron, Leche de Oje, Oje.

Scientific Names

Ficus insipida, synonyms Ficin anthelmintica, Ficin glabrata, and Ficin laurfolia.
Family: Moraceae.

People Use This For

Orally, ficin is used as a digestive aid [11].
In medical procedures, ficin is used to clean and prepare intestinal submucosa for the production of sutures, to clean and prepare animal arteries for human implantation, and in serologic testing (e.g., for Rh factor determination) [11]. Historically, ficin has been used as an anthelmintic in South America [11,3766].
In manufacturing, ficin is used in European anti-inflammatory preparations [11], cheese manufacturing, chillproofing beer [11], preparation of protein hydrolysates, edible collagen films, and sausage casings [11]. Ficin is sometimes included in meat tenderizers, usually in combination with papain and/or bromelain [11].

Safety
LIKELY UNSAFE ...when used topically. Crude ficin is corrosive to skin and prolonged contact can cause bleeding (11).

There is insufficient reliable information available about the safety of the oral use of ficin.

PREGNANCY AND LACTATION: LIKELY UNSAFE ...when used topically (11). There is insufficient reliable information available about the safety of ficin for oral use during pregnancy or lactation; avoid using.

Effectiveness
There is insufficient reliable information available about the effectiveness of ficin.

Mechanism of Action
Ficin is a sulfhydryl proteinase and can hydrolyze proteins, amides, esters, and small peptides (11). Some evidence suggests ficin might be useful in treating helminthiasis (11,3766). Other evidence suggests ficin has anti-inflammatory activity (11).

Adverse Reactions
Orally, large amounts can cause catharsis (11).

Topically, crude ficin is corrosive to skin and can cause bleeding with prolonged contact (11). Ficin can also cause contact allergies (11).

Interactions with Herbs & Other Dietary Supplements
Insufficient reliable information available.

Interactions with Drugs
No interactions are known to occur, and there is no known reason to expect a clinically significant interaction with ficin.

Interactions with Foods
No interactions are known to occur, and there is no known reason to expect a clinically significant interaction with ficin.

Interactions with Lab Tests
No interactions are known to occur, and there is no known reason to expect a clinically significant interaction with ficin.

Interactions with Diseases or Conditions
No interactions are known to occur, and there is no known reason to expect a clinically significant interaction with ficin.

Dosage and Administration
ORAL: As an anthelmintic, 1.0 cc of prepared latex/kg per day for 3 days to be repeated every 3 months has been used (3766).

Comments
Ficin is the latex harvested from the trunk of felled Ficus insipida trees. Crude ficin consists of the latex combined with acetic acid to prevent coagulation and sodium benzoate as a preservative (11). Purified ficin is not pure ficin. Rather, it is a mixture of several proteases and small amounts of other enzymes and other constituents (11).

FIELD SCABIOUS

Also Known As
None.

Scientific Names
Knautia arvensis.

People Use This For
Orally, field scabious is used for cough and throat complaints (18).

Topically, field scabious is used for chronic skin conditions; eczema; anal fissures; anal itching; urticaria; scabies; favus (roundworm); and cleansing and healing ulcers, bruises and inflammation (18).

Safety

There is insufficient reliable information available about the safety of field scabious.

Pregnancy and Lactation: Insufficient reliable information available; avoid using.

Effectiveness

There is insufficient reliable information available about the effectiveness of field scabious.

Mechanism of Action

The applicable parts of field scabious are the above ground parts. Field scabious contains triterpene saponins including knatioside, knautioside A and B, iridoide monoterpenes including dipsacan, flavonoids, and tannins. It is reported to have astringent, antiseptic, expectorant, and purgative properties [18].

Adverse Reactions

None reported.

Interactions with Herbs & Other Dietary Supplements

Insufficient reliable information available.

Interactions with Drugs

No interactions are known to occur, and there is no known reason to expect a clinically significant interaction with field scabious.

Interactions with Foods

No interactions are known to occur, and there is no known reason to expect a clinically significant interaction with field scabious.

Interactions with Lab Tests

No interactions are known to occur, and there is no known reason to expect a clinically significant interaction with field scabious.

Interactions with Diseases or Conditions

No interactions are known to occur, and there is no known reason to expect a clinically significant interaction with field scabious.

Dosage and Administration

ORAL: For chronic eczema, people typically drink 2 glasses tea (add 4 teaspoons to 240 mL boiling water, steep for 10 minutes and strain) throughout day [18]. Product is used both orally and topically as an alcoholic extract and tea.

Comments

None.

FIG

Also Known As

Caricae Fructus, Feigen.

Scientific Names

Ficus carica.
Family: Moraceae.

People Use This For

Orally, fig is used as a laxative [2].

Safety

LIKELY SAFE ...when used orally in food amounts as fresh or dried fruit.
PREGNANCY AND LACTATION: LIKELY SAFE ...when used orally in food amounts as fresh or dried fruit.

Effectiveness

There is insufficient reliable information available about the effectiveness of fig.

Mechanism of Action

The applicable parts of fig are the fruit and leaf. However, very little is known about pharmacological effects of fig. An aqueous leaf extract can cause hypoglycemic activity in animals (6625).

Adverse Reactions

Orally, fig use can cause photodermatitis. Avoid excessive sunlight or ultraviolet light exposure while using this product (19).

Interactions with Herbs & Other Dietary Supplements

Insufficient reliable information available.

Interactions with Drugs

No interactions are known to occur, and there is no known reason to expect a clinically significant interaction with fig.

Interactions with Foods

No interactions are known to occur, and there is no known reason to expect a clinically significant interaction with fig.

Interactions with Lab Tests

No interactions are known to occur, and there is no known reason to expect a clinically significant interaction with fig.

Interactions with Diseases or Conditions

No interactions are known to occur, and there is no known reason to expect a clinically significant interaction with fig.

Dosage and Administration

No typical dosage.

Comments

None.

FIGWORT

Also Known As

Carpenter's Square, Common Figwort, Heal-all, Rosenoble, Scrophula Plant, Scrophularia, Throatwort.

Scientific Names

Scrophularia mailandica; Scrophularia nodosa (Scrophylariaceae).

People Use This For

Orally, figwort is used as a diuretic (4).
Topically, figwort is used for chronic skin diseases such as eczema, itching, and psoriasis (4), and hemorrhoids, swelling, and eruptions (201).

Safety

There is insufficient reliable information available about the safety of figwort.
Pregnancy and Lactation: Insufficient reliable information available; avoid using.

Effectiveness

There is insufficient reliable information available about the effectiveness of figwort.

Mechanism of Action

The applicable parts of figwort are the above ground parts and root. It is reported to have diuretic and laxative effects (18). Constituents, aucubin and catalpol, exert purgative action in mice; harpagide may have cardioactive and anti-inflammatory activity (4).

Adverse Reactions

None reported.

Interactions with Herbs & Other Dietary Supplements

CARDIAC GLYCOSIDE-CONTAINING HERBS: Contraindicated, and concomitant use can increase the risk of cardiac glycoside toxicity. Cardiac glycoside-containing herbs include black hellebore, Canadian hemp roots, digitalis leaf, hedge mustard, lily of the valley roots, motherwort, oleander leaf, pheasant's eye plant, pleurisy root, squill bulb leaf scales, strophanthus seeds, and uzara (2,18,19,500).

Interactions with Drugs
No interactions are known to occur, and there is no known reason to expect a clinically significant interaction with figwort.

Interactions with Foods
No interactions are known to occur, and there is no known reason to expect a clinically significant interaction with figwort.

Interactions with Lab Tests
No interactions are known to occur, and there is no known reason to expect a clinically significant interaction with figwort.

Interactions with Diseases or Conditions
DIABETES: Theoretically, may alter blood glucose control (4); monitor closely.
VENTRICULAR TACHYCARDIA: Contraindicated (4,12).

Dosage and Administration
ORAL: As a tea, use 2-8 grams dried above ground parts in 150 mL boiling water 5-10 minutes, steep (4). As a liquid extract (1:1 in 25% alcohol), 2-8 mL has been used (4). As a tincture (1:10 in 45% alcohol), 2-4 mL has been used (4).
TOPICAL: No typical dosage.

Comments
Figwort is stated to be a suitable substitute for devil's claw (due to similar chemical composition) (4).

FIR

Also Known As
Fir Tree, Norway Spruce, Piceae turiones recentes, Spruce, Spruce Fir.
CAUTION: See separate listings for Dwarf Pine Needle, Fir Needle Oil, Pine Needle Oil, Pine, Poplar, and Scotch Pine Needle.

Scientific Names
Abies alba, synonym Abies pectinata; Picea abies, synonym Picea excelsa.
Family: Pinaceae.

People Use This For
Orally, fir is used for respiratory tract inflammation (2), colds, cough, bronchitis, fever, inflammation of the mouth and pharynx, muscle and nerve pain, and tendency toward infection (18).
Topically, fir is used for mild myalgia, neuralgia, and rheumatic pain (2,18).
In folk medicine, fir has been used orally for tuberculosis (18) and applied externally as a bath additive for mental illness (18).

Safety
POSSIBLY SAFE ...when used orally and topically in appropriate amounts (2).
PREGNANCY AND LACTATION: Insufficient reliable information available; avoid using.

Effectiveness
There is insufficient reliable information available about the effectiveness of fir.

Mechanism of Action
The applicable part of fir is the shoot. Fir shoot can reduce secretions, enhance local circulation, and act as a mild antiseptic (2). The essential oil can have secretory and antibacterial effects on bronchial mucous membranes (18). The essential oil also acts as a rubefacient (counterirritant) and improves circulation when applied externally (18).

Adverse Reactions
None reported.

Interactions with Herbs & Other Dietary Supplements
Insufficient reliable information available.

Interactions with Drugs
No interactions are known to occur, and there is no known reason to expect a clinically significant interaction with fir.

Interactions with Foods
No interactions are known to occur, and there is no known reason to expect a clinically significant interaction with fir.

Interactions with Lab Tests
No interactions are known to occur, and there is no known reason to expect a clinically significant interaction with fir.

Interactions with Diseases or Conditions
ASTHMA, PERTUSSIS (whooping cough): The fir shoot can exacerbate these conditions [18].
Contraindicated for use as a bath additive for individuals with extensive skin injuries, acute skin diseases, feverish or infectious diseases, cardiac insufficiency, or hypertonia [18].

Dosage and Administration
ORAL: The typical dose is 5-6 grams of the fresh fir shoots per day [2,18]. The essential oil is usually given as 4 drops in water or on a sugar lump three times daily [18].
TOPICAL: Boil 200-300 grams of the shoots in 1 L water, steep for 5 minutes, strain, and add to a full bath [2,18].
INHALATION: Inhale the vapor of 2 grams of the essential oil in hot water several times per day [18].

Comments
Avoid confusion with fir needle oil.

FIR NEEDLE OIL

Also Known As
Fichtennadelöl, Piceae aetheroleum, White Spruce Oil.
CAUTION: See separate listing for Dwarf Pine Needle, Scotch Pine Needle Oil, Poplar, Fir, and Pine.

Scientific Names
Picea abies, synonym Picea excelsa; Piceae aetheroleum; Abies alba; Abies sachalinensis; Abies sibirica.
Family: Pinaceae.

People Use This For
Orally, fir needle oil is used for upper and lower respiratory tract infections and conditions [2].
Topically, fir needle oil is used for upper and lower respiratory tract infections and conditions [2]. It is also used topically for rheumatic, neuralgic, and muscle pains [2]. Fir needle oil is commonly used as a liniment in alcoholic solutions, ointments, gels, emulsions, and oils. It is also used topically as a bath additive [2].
Fir needle oil is also used as an inhalant [2].

Safety
POSSIBLY SAFE ...when used orally or applied topically [2].
PREGNANCY AND LACTATION: Insufficient reliable information available; avoid using.

Effectiveness
There is insufficient reliable information available about the effectiveness of fir needle oil.

Mechanism of Action
Fir needle oil is made from the tips of branches or twigs. Fir needle oil has mild antiseptic and counterirritant properties. It also breaks up respiratory secretions [2].

Adverse Reactions
Orally, the oil can increase bronchospasms [2].
Topically, fir needle oil increases skin and mucous membrane irritation [2].

Interactions with Herbs & Other Dietary Supplements
Insufficient reliable information available.

Interactions with Drugs

No interactions are known to occur, and there is no known reason to expect a clinically significant interaction with fir needle oil.

Interactions with Foods

No interactions are known to occur, and there is no known reason to expect a clinically significant interaction with fir needle oil.

Interactions with Lab Tests

No interactions are known to occur, and there is no known reason to expect a clinically significant interaction with fir needle oil.

Interactions with Diseases or Conditions

ASTHMA, PERTUSSIS (whooping cough): Fir needle oil is contraindicated in individuals with these conditions because it can increase bronchospasms (2).

Dosage and Administration

Dosage is individualized according to the type and intensity of the illness, the special areas of use, and the mode of administration (2).

Comments

None.

FIREWEED

Also Known As

Blood Vine, Blooming Sally, Flowering Willow, French Willow, French-Willow, Great Willowherb, Persian Willow, Purple Rocket, Rose Bay Willow, Rosebay Willow, Tame Withy, Wickup, Wicopy, Willow Herb, Willowherb.

Scientific Names

Epilobium angustifolium.
Family: Onagraceae.

People Use This For

In folk medicine, fireweed has been used for inflammation, fevers, tumors, wounds, as an astringent, and as a tonic.

Safety

POSSIBLY SAFE …when used orally (12).
PREGNANCY AND LACTATION: Insufficient reliable information available; avoid using.

Effectiveness

There is insufficient reliable information available about the effectiveness of fireweed.

Mechanism of Action

The applicable parts of fireweed are the above ground parts. Some evidence suggests that aqueous extracts of fireweed might affect reproduction (858). Other evidence suggests that extracts could have anti-inflammatory effects (859,860).

Adverse Reactions

None reported.

Interactions with Herbs & Other Dietary Supplements

Insufficient reliable information available.

Interactions with Drugs

No interactions are known to occur, and there is no known reason to expect a clinically significant interaction with fireweed.

Interactions with Foods

No interactions are known to occur, and there is no known reason to expect a clinically significant interaction with fireweed.

Interactions with Lab Tests

No interactions are known to occur, and there is no known reason to expect a clinically significant interaction with fireweed.

Interactions with Diseases or Conditions

No interactions are known to occur, and there is no known reason to expect a clinically significant interaction with fireweed.

Dosage and Administration

No typical dosage.

Comments

Other Epilobium species are also referred to as willow herb (18).

FISH OILS

Also Known As

Cod Liver Oil, Fish Oil Fatty Acids, Fish Body Oil, Fish Oil, Fish Liver Oil, Fish Liver Oils, Marine Oils, Menhaden Oil, N-3 Fatty Acids, N3-polyunsaturated Fatty Acids, Omega Fatty Acids, Omega 3 Fatty Acids, Omega-3 Fatty Acids, PUFA, W-3 Fatty Acids.
CAUTION: See separate listings for Cod Liver Oil, DHA, EPA, and Shark Liver Oil.

Scientific Names

None.

People Use This For

Orally, fish oils are used for hyperlipidemia, hypertriglyceridemia, coronary heart disease, hypertension, stroke, bipolar disorder, rheumatoid arthritis, psoriasis, atopic dermatitis, ulcerative colitis, Behcet's syndrome, and Raynaud's syndrome. Fish oils are also used orally for weight loss, asthma, cancer, painful menses, lung diseases, hay fever, Crohn's disease, chronic fatigue syndrome, albuminuria associated with diabetic neuropathy, restenosis after angioplasty, miscarriage, preeclampsia, preterm labor, and intrauterine growth retardation. Fish oils are used for systemic lupus erythematosus, cystic fibrosis, gingivitis, renal impairment associated with cirrhosis, hyperglycemia associated with type 2 diabetes and claudication. Fish oils are also used to treat attention deficit hyperactivity disorder (ADHD), dyslexia, and dyspraxia.
In combination with linoleic and gamma-linoleic acid, fish oils are used orally for treating post-viral fatigue syndrome. Fish oils are also used orally in combination with garlic to treat hypercholesterolemia.
Intravenously, fish oils are used to treat psoriasis.

Safety

LIKELY SAFE ...when used orally and appropriately. Doses of 3 grams per day and less can be safely used by most people. Fish oils have Generally Recognized as Safe (GRAS) status in the US (5703,7376).
POSSIBLY UNSAFE ...when used orally in high doses. Doses greater than 3 grams per day can inhibit blood coagulation and potentially increase the risk of bleeding. Doses greater than 3 grams per day might also suppress immune response (1313,7376,7383,7384).
CHILDREN: POSSIBLY SAFE ...when used orally and appropriately (5708,5711).
PREGNANCY AND LACTATION: LIKELY SAFE ...when used orally in amounts found in foods (5703). There is insufficient reliable information available about the safety of fish oils when used in amounts greater than those found in foods during pregnancy and breast-feeding.

Effectiveness

LIKELY EFFECTIVE ...when used orally for hypertriglyceridemia. Fish oils from supplements or from dietary sources can reduce triglyceride levels by 20-50% (1024,2299,2300,2301,2302,2315,2317,5702,5705) (5706,6394,6399,7368,7369,7380). This effect appears to be dose-dependent (5706,7380). However, fish oil supplements in doses of 4 grams per day do not seem to be as effective as gemfibrozil (Lopid) 1200 mg per day (7377).
POSSIBLY EFFECTIVE ...when used orally from dietary sources to reduce the risk of death from coronary heart disease. Epidemiological research suggests that long-term consumption of a diet that regularly includes fish reduces the risk of death from death from coronary heart disease, possibly by decreasing ventricular ectopic beats (7360). Consumption of one to two servings per week of fish oils from dietary sources appears to reduce the risk of coronary heart disease death by 25% (2309). ...when used orally to reduce cardiovascular events and mortality after myocardial infarction (MI). Fish oils 1 gram daily starting within 3 months after MI and continued for at least a year appears to

reduce the risk of total cardiac events, non-fatal MI, and total cardiac mortality by 15% (1007,2307). There is also some evidence that consuming dietary fish oil from 2 to 3 servings of fish each week seems to reduce the risk of death after myocardial infarction (7359). Fish oil supplements do not seem to reduce the risk of post-MI cardiovascular events in people whose diet already includes fish (7361). ...when used orally to reduce the risk of stroke. Consuming fish oils from dietary sources at least once a week seems to reduce the risk of ischemic stroke by 27% (7373). Higher serum levels of fish oils are also associated with decreased risk of stroke (7372). Dietary fish oils don't seem to further reduce stroke risk in people who already take aspirin (7373). It's not known if fish oil supplements have any effect on stroke risk. ..when used orally for mild hypertension. Fish oil seems to produce modest, but significant reductions in systolic and diastolic blood pressure in patients with mild hypertension with or without type 2 diabetes (1001,1020,2301). ...when used orally to decrease the incidence of vein graft occlusion following coronary artery bypass grafting. Supplemental fish oil appears to reduce the frequency of vein graft occlusions after coronary artery surgery (2314). ...when used orally for rheumatoid arthritis. Fish oils alone or in combination with naproxen (Naprosyn) seem to significantly decrease the duration of morning stiffness in patients with rheumatoid arthritis (1017,1039,1041). Use of fish oils might also allow reduction of non-steroidal anti-inflammatory drug (NSAID) requirements when used concomitantly (1031). ...when taken orally in combination with conventional therapy for bipolar disorder. Using fish oils with conventional therapies seems to improved symptoms of depression and increase length of remission (7202). However, fish oil does not seem to have beneficial effects on manic symptoms in bipolar patients (5713,7202). ...when used orally in combination with garlic for hypercholesterolemia. Combining fish oil 12 grams plus garlic 900 mg daily seems to lower total cholesterol, triglycerides and the ratios of total cholesterol to high-density lipoprotein (HDL) and low-density lipoprotein (LDL) to HDL in patients with hypercholesterolemia (2318,2319). The addition of garlic appears to prevent the typical rise in LDL normally seen when fish oil is used alone (2318). ...when used orally to prevent cyclosporine-induced hypertension following cardiac transplant. There is some evidence that fish oils can maintain pre-cyclosporine blood pressures in patients taking cyclosporine (507,1012). ...when used for preventing cyclosporine-induced nephrotoxicity. There is some evidence that fish oil can significantly improve glomerular filtration rate (GFR) and renal blood flow in individuals taking cyclosporine (1021). ...when used orally to prevent recurrent miscarriage in patients with antiphospholipid syndrome. There is some evidence that fish oils can increase live birth rate in pregnant women with a history of recurrent miscarriage associated with antiphospholipid syndrome (1032). ...when used orally in combination with linoleic and gamma-linoleic acid to treat symptoms of postviral fatigue syndrome. There is some evidence that fish oil plus linoleic acid can significantly improve overall symptoms, including degree of fatigue, myalgias, dizziness, and concentration (1019). ...when used orally to reduce albuminuria in individuals with diabetic nephropathy (1025). ...when used orally to improve appetite and increase lean body mass in patients with advanced pancreatic cancer (5701). ...when used orally to improve night vision in children with dyslexia. Dyslexic children who take fish oils seem to develop significantly better dark adaptation (5708). ...when used orally in combination with evening primrose oil, thyme oil, and vitamin E to improve movement disorders in children with dyspraxia (5708). ...when used orally with simvastatin to decrease postprandial hemostatic risk factors in hyperlipidemia (5704). ...when used orally for migraine headache prophylaxis in adolescents. There is some preliminary clinical evidence that fish oil preparations containing eicosapentaenoic acid (EPA) 756 mg and docosahexanoic acid (DHA) 498 mg daily for 2 months can significantly reduce frequency of migraine headaches. When migraine headaches do occur, duration and severity seems to less in patients taking fish oil (5097). ...when used orally from dietary sources for weight loss. There is some evidence that ingestion of fish oils from dietary fish sources can improve weight loss and decrease blood glucose and insulin concentrations in overweight and hypertensive patients (2049). ...when used orally from dietary sources to reduce the risk of age-related maculopathy. There is some evidence that people who ingest fish oils from dietary fish sources more than once per week have a reduced risk of developing age-related maculopathy (6260). ...when used orally from dietary sources to reduce the risk of prostate cancer. Population studies indicate that prostate cancer risk is 2 to 3 times lower in men who regularly include fish oils in the diet (7378). Men who have higher serum levels of eicosapentaenoic acid (EPA) and docosahexaenoic acid (DHA), fatty acids that are in fish, seem to have a lower risk of developing prostate cancer (6395). ...when used intravenously for certain types of acute and chronic psoriasis. There is some evidence that giving intravenous fish oils can decrease severity of symptoms in patients with acute, extended guttate psoriasis and chronic plaque psoriasis. Fish oils seem to be superior to omega-6 fatty acids for this use (1004,1034). However, fish oil taken orally does not seem to have this benefit (1035).

POSSIBLY INEFFECTIVE ...when taken orally to reverse progression of atherosclerosis. Long-term use of fish oils appears to have no effect on decreasing plaque size or increasing the luminal diameter of coronary arteries in patients with coronary atherosclerosis (1022,2311). ...when taken orally for systemic lupus erythematosus (SLE) and lupus nephritis (507). ...when taken orally for atopic dermatitis (507). ...when taken orally for gingivitis (1005). ...when taken orally for renal impairment associated with advanced cirrhosis (1013). ...when taken orally for stable claudication. Fish oils appear to have no effect on walking distance in patients with claudication (1002).

LIKELY INEFFECTIVE ...when taken orally in combination with evening primrose oil for preventing pre-eclampsia, preterm labor, and intrauterine growth retardation (1026,1027,1042). ...when taken orally to prevent restenosis after percutaneous transluminal coronary angioplasty (PTCA) (1028,1038,2320). ...when taken orally for type 2 diabetes. Fish oil appears to have no effect on fasting plasma glucose levels or serum hemoglobin A1c levels at doses less than 6 grams per day (2299,2300,2302,7368,7369). Several clinical studies have used fish oil products containing specific proportions of the fatty acids eicosapentaenoic acid (EPA) and docosahexanoic acid (DHA). Most commonly products have contained 35% EPA and 25% DHA. There is insufficient reliable information available to rate the effectiveness of fish oils for other uses. However, there is some evidence fish oils might be helpful for inflammatory bowel disease (IBD), but evidence is conflicting (1037,1040,5709,6257,6258,6259). More evidence is needed to rate fish oil for this use.

Mechanism of Action

Fish such as herring, kipper, mackerel, menhaden, pilchard, salmon, sardine, and trout contain oils with high amounts of long-chain, polyunsaturated fats called omega-3 fatty acids. These fish oils are especially high in the omega-3 fatty acids eicosapentaenoic acid (EPA) and docosahexanoic acid (DHA) (See separate listings for EPA and DHA). Omega-3 fatty acids from fish oil have anti-inflammatory effects because they compete with arachidonic acid in the cyclooxygenase and lipoxygenase pathways and inhibit leukotriene synthesis. Fish oils can also suppress mediators of immune function by reducing the production of cytokines such as interleukin-1(IL-1), interleukin-2 (IL-2), and tumor necrosis factor (TNF). Fish oils also suppress T- and B-cell proliferation and decrease delayed-type hypersensitivity skin response (DTH). They also decrease antibody production and increase free radical activity (7376,7383,7384).

Due to fish oil's anti-inflammatory effects, they are tried for a variety of inflammatory conditions, including psoriasis, systemic lupus erythematosus (SLE), inflammatory bowel disease, and others.

Fish oils seem to be beneficial in rheumatoid arthritis due to anti-inflammatory effects and epidemiological data that suggests EPA levels are decreased in total plasma fatty acids and synovial fluid, and DHA is decreased in the synovial fluid of patients with rheumatoid arthritis (5710).

Fish oils are also used for cardiovascular conditions, including stroke and heart disease, due anti-inflammatory and antithrombotic effects. Fish oils decrease blood viscosity and increase red blood cell deformability. The antithrombotic activity of fish oils results from increased prostacyclin synthesis and vasodilation, reduction of platelet adhesiveness, and reduced platelet count. Fish oils also seem to have an antiarrhythmic effect. Fish oils might regulate calcium movement through calcium channels in the heart and suppress intracellular calcium activity, which has been associated with arrhythmias. There's also some evidence that it might affect sodium channels and inhibit ischemia-induced arrhythmias (7360,7362,7363).

In hypertriglyceridemia, fish oils are thought to lower triglycerides by decreasing secretion of very low-density lipoproteins (VLDLs), increasing VLDL apolipoprotein B secretion, possibly by increasing VLDL clearance, decreasing VLDL size, and reducing triglyceride transport (5707). In addition, fish oils appear to decrease synthesis of VLDL by inhibiting 1,2-diacylglycerol-sterol o-acyltransferase or phosphatidate phosphatase (6394). Fish oils also seem to decrease chylomicron concentrations. More lipoprotein lipase becomes available due to decreased VLDL levels, which causes increased hydrolysis of chylomicrons (6394). Fish oils also increase fatty acid oxidation by peroxisomal and mitochondrial routes, reduce fatty acid synthesis, divert fatty acids into phospholipid synthesis, increase hepatic uptake of triglycerides, and down regulate fatty acid esterifying enzymes (5707). Fish oils also seem to decrease cholesterol absorption from the gut and decrease cholesterol synthesis (5707). Fish oils also might increase high-density lipoproteins (HDL) (2318,5707) and improve flow-mediated arterial dilation (5702). Fish oils also seem to increase low density lipoprotein (LDL) concentrations but the mechanism is unknown (2299,2318). It is thought that fish oils may cause a more buoyant LDL to be formed, which might be less atherogenic (2299).

Unlike some other kinds of dietary fat, omega-3 fatty acids from fish oils do not seem to impair endothelial function, which is thought to be a precursor to atherogenesis (5702,7382). In some patients fish oils actually seem to improve arterial compliance (1029,5707).

Omega-3 fatty acids compete metabolically with omega-6 fatty acids, which are found in vegetable oils. Omega-6 fatty acids seem to inhibit the incorporation of omega-3 fatty acids into tissue lipids. Omega-3 fatty acids inhibit the conversion of the major omega-6 fatty acid in vegetable oils, linoleic acid, into arachidonic acid. There is some concern that dietary vegetable oils in the diet might negate the beneficial cardiovascular effects of fish oils, but omega-3 fatty acids from fish oil seem to reduce cardiovascular risk factors despite concurrent omega-6 fatty acid ingestion. The total dose of omega-3 fatty acids, rather than the ratio of omega-6 fatty acids to omega-3 fatty acids seems to determine efficacy (7381).

Fish oils have been proposed as a treatment for attention deficit hyperactivity disorder (ADHD) due to epidemiological data that suggests symptoms of ADHD might be inversely related to the omega 3-fatty acid phospholipid content (5711). In individuals with bipolar disorder, the fatty acids in fish oils are thought to have an effect similar to lithium or valproate, slowing nerve signaling (7202).

Some researchers think fish oils might also help prevent some forms of cancer. People with high EPA and DHA levels in their erythrocytes seem to have decreased rates of prostate cancer (6395). EPA and DHA might compete with arachidonic acid as substrates for cyclooxygenases that produce prostaglandins that can enhance tumor growth (6385,7378). There is also preliminary evidence that high levels of EPA and DHA can be beneficial for prolonging cancer remission. Fish oils might decrease production of lactic acid by tumor cells. Lactic acidosis is a marker of unfavorable metabolic conditions associated with many cancers (6398). There is also some evidence that fish oils might be cytotoxic to some cancer cells (1008).

Adverse Reactions

Orally, fish oils are generally well-tolerated at doses of 3 grams or less per day. Fish oils sometimes have a fishy taste and can cause belching, halitosis, and heartburn (507,6258). High doses can cause nausea and loose stools. Some gastrointestinal side effects can be minimized if fish oils are taken with meals and if doses are started low and gradually increased.

At doses greater than 3 grams per day, fish oils can inhibit platelet aggregation and could cause bleeding and potentially increase the risk for hemorrhagic stroke (7376).

There's also some evidence that fish oils in doses greater than 3 grams per day might adversely affect immune function. Fish oils appear to suppress T- and B-cell function and to reduce the production of cytokines, which might be detrimental to elderly people and people with suppressed immune function such as patients with human immunodeficiency virus (HIV) infection (7376,7383,7384).

In some patients fish oils can increase low-density cholesterol (LDL) (7376). There is also some concern that polyunsaturated fatty acids, such as omega-3 fatty acids, might increase the oxidation of low-density lipoprotein (LDL), which could increase the risk of atherosclerosis (1011,2322,2323,7366). Although thiobarbituric acid reacting substances (TBARS) rise during fish oil supplementation, TBARS is now thought to inaccurately reflect LDL oxidation. More specific indicators of lipid peroxidation, such as F2-isoprostanes and malondialdehyde (MDA), suggest that fish oil is unlikely to have a negative effect on LDL and the risk for atherosclerosis (2323).

Some fish oil preparations (e.g., cod liver oil) contain large amounts of vitamin A and vitamin D. If these preparations are used long-term or in large doses, there is a risk of vitamin A and D toxicity (See separate listing for Cod Liver Oil) (6872,6874).

There is some concern that fish oil products might be contaminated with toxins or pesticides if the fish were caught in contaminated waters (6873,6875). Heavy metals, especially mercury, are a particular concern (259). However, laboratory analysis of some fish oil supplements found no detectable levels of mercury in the 20 products tested. Fish typically contain 10 to 1000 parts per billion of mercury. Mercury accumulates in fish meat much more so than fish oil, which might explain the lack of detectable mercury in fish oil supplements (7379).

Fish oils also contribute to caloric intake and may cause weight gain if used long-term. One gram of fat or oil provides 9 kcal (6871,6872). Fish oil capsules containing 500 mg omega-3 fatty acids in 1 gram of oil would supply about 13.5 kcal per capsule (6871,6874). Fish oil supplements also contain cholesterol in amounts from 1 to 6 mg per gram of fish oil (3022,6871).

Interactions with Herbs & Other Dietary Supplements

VITAMIN E: Fish oils can reduce vitamin E levels. The mechanism is unknown, but might result from reduced vitamin E absorption or increased vitamin E utilization by other tissues to block free radicals and prevent peroxidative damage (7384).

HERBS WITH ANTICOAGULANT/ANTIPLATELET POTENTIAL: Concomitant use of herbs that have coumarin constituents or affect platelet aggregation could theoretically increase the risk of bleeding in some people. These herbs include angelica, anise, arnica, asafoetida, bogbean, boldo, capsicum, celery, chamomile, clove, danshen, fenugreek, feverfew, garlic, ginger, ginkgo, Panax ginseng, horse chestnut, horseradish, licorice, meadowsweet, prickly ash, onion, papain, passionflower, poplar, quassia, red clover, turmeric, wild carrot, wild lettuce, willow, and others (4,19).

Interactions with Drugs

ANTICOAGULANTS/ANTIPLATELET DRUGS: Concomitant use with anticoagulant or antiplatelet drugs can increase the risk of bleeding (9,507). Some of these drugs include aspirin, clopidogrel (Plavix), dalteparin (Fragmin), dipyridamole (Persantine), enoxaparin (Lovenox), heparin, ticlopidine (Ticlid), warfarin (Coumadin), and others.

ANTIDIABETES DRUGS: Theoretically, concomitant use of fish oil at doses greater than 6 grams per day might interfere with blood glucose control. However, lower doses do not seem to affect blood glucose. (7368,7369).

ANTIHYPERTENSIVE DRUGS: Fish oils can lower blood pressure and might have additive effects in patients treated antihypertensives (1001,1020,1030,1033); use with caution.

CYCLOSPORINE: Fish oils can reduce cyclosporine-induced hypertension in individuals after heart transplants, and may help protect against cyclosporine-induced nephrotoxicity (507,1012,1021).

ETRETINATE: Concomitant use of etretinate with eicosapentaenoic (EPA) can enhance the effects in psoriasis treatment (1000).

Interactions with Foods

No interactions are known to occur, and there is no known reason to expect a clinically significant interaction with fish oils.

Interactions with Lab Tests

BLOOD PRESSURE: Fish oils can moderately lower blood pressure and reduce blood pressure readings in patients with hypertension (1001,1020,1030,1033).

ELECTROCARDIOGRAM (ECG): Fish oils might normalize ECG readings in some patients with ventricular ectopic beats. Fish oils might decrease ventricular ectopic beats (507).

INTERNATIONAL NORMALIZED RATIO (INR), PROTHROMBIN TIME (PT): High doses of fish oils, greater than 3 grams per day, might decrease blood coagulation, increase INR and PT, and increase the risk of bleeding (1313).

TRIGLYCERIDES: Fish oils can reduce serum triglyceride concentrations and test results by 20% to 50% in patients with elevated triglycerides (1003,1009,1014,1024).

Interactions with Diseases or Conditions

ASPIRIN-SENSITIVE INDIVIDUALS: Fish oils should be used with caution because omega-3 fatty acids can decrease pulmonary function in aspirin-sensitive individuals (507).

BIPOLAR DISORDER AND DEPRESSION: Symptoms of hypomania can develop in patients taking fish oils who have bipolar (5713,7202) or major depressive disorders (6396).

CIRRHOSIS: Theoretically, use of fish oils may lower mean arterial pressure (MAP) to hypotensive levels, and may increase risk of bleeding (1013); use with caution.

DIABETES: Fish oils in doses greater than 6 grams per day can increase blood glucose levels. However, lower doses don't seem to effect blood glucose. Tell patients with diabetes to avoid exceeding a dose of 3 grams per day (7368,7369).

FAMILIAL ADENOMATOUS POLYPOSIS: Fish oils might further increase the risk of cancer in people with familial adenomatous polyposis. Three people, who had pre-existing familial adenomatous polyposis, were diagnosed with malignant lesions during the course of long-term use of fish oils (999).

HYPERTENSION: Fish oils can lower blood pressure and might have additive effects in patients treated with antihypertensives (1001,1020,1030,1033).

IMMUNODEFICIENCY: Higher doses of fish oils might cause suppression of immune and inflammatory response (7376,7383,7384). Tell immunocompromised patients (e.g., patients with HIV/AIDS) to avoid exceeding a dose of 3 grams per day.

Dosage and Administration

ORAL: For lowering triglycerides, studies have used 1-4 grams of fish oils per day (5707,6394,6399). For lowering blood pressure, studies have used either 4 grams of fish oils or fish oils providing EPA 2.04 grams and DHA 1.4 grams daily (1001,1020). For hypertension secondary to cyclosporine in heart transplant patients, 4 grams per day has been used (1012). For cyclosporine nephrotoxicity, 12 grams per day containing 2.2 grams EPA and 1.4 grams DHA has been used (1021). For reducing mortality after a myocardial infarction, a daily oral dose of fish oils providing EPA 850 mg-1.08 grams with or without 882 mg DHA or a daily serving of 1.25 ounces or more of fish has been used (1007,2307). For improving endothelial function in individuals with hypercholesterolemia, 4 grams per day has been used (5702). For decreasing duration of morning stiffness secondary to rheumatoid arthritis, fish oils providing EPA 3.8 grams and DHA 2 grams per day have been used (1039). For preventing miscarriage in women with antiphospholipid antibody syndrome and a history of recurrent miscarriage, 5.1 grams fish oils with a 1.5 EPA:DHA ratio has been used (1032). As an adjunct to standard therapy for bipolar disorder, fish oils providing EPA 6.2 grams and DHA 3.4 grams daily have been used (7202). For weight loss, a daily serving of 2-7 ounces of fish containing approximately 3.65 grams omega-3 fatty acids (0.66 gram from EPA and 0.60 gram from DHA) has been used (2049). For improving appetite in individuals with pancreatic cancer fish oils providing EPA 2.2 grams and DHA 1.4 grams daily have been used (5701). For improving dark vision adaptation in dyslexic individuals, fish oils providing DHA 480 mg daily have been used (5708). For improving movement disorders in children with dyspraxia, fish oils providing DHA 480 mg combined with 35 mg arachidonic acid and 96 mg gamma-alpha linoleic acid from evening primrose oil, 24 mg thyme oil, and 80 mg vitamin E (Efalex) have been used (5708). For decreasing the frequency of vein graft occlusion after coronary bypass grafting, 4 grams of fish oil per day containing EPA 2.04 grams and DHA 1.3 grams has been used (2314). For combined hypertriglyceridemia and hypercholesterolemia, fish oil providing EPA 1800-2160 mg and DHA 1200-1440 mg combined with garlic powder 900-1200 mg daily has been used to lower total cholesterol, LDL, triglycerides, and the ratios of total cholesterol to HDL and LDL to HDL (2318,2319). Fish oil supplements often contain small amounts of vitamin E as an antioxidant to prevent spoilage. They might also be combined with calcium, iron, or vitamins A, B1, B2, B3, C, or D (507). Fish that are good sources of omega-3 fatty acids, including mackerel, tuna, salmon, sturgeon, mullet, bluefish, anchovy, sardines, herring, trout, and menhaden, provide about 1 gram of omega-3 fatty acids per 3.5 ounces of fish.

INTRAVENOUS: For chronic plaque psoriasis, a daily 200 mL intravenous dose of parenteral fish oil-based lipid emulsion (Omegavenous), containing 4.2 grams EPA and 4.2 grams DHA, has been used for 14 days (1004). For acute, extended guttate psoriasis, a daily intravenous dose of a parenteral fish oil product, containing 2.1 grams EPA and 21 grams DHA, has been used for 10 days (1034).

Comments

Fish oils come from a variety of marine life including mackerel, herring, tuna, halibut, salmon (945), cod liver, whale blubber, and seal blubber (1048). Products that are commercially available contain varying amounts and ratios of docosahexaenoic acid (DHA) and eicosapentaenoic acid (EPA) (507). Researchers are investigating oils containing stearidonic acid (SDA) from genetically modified plants as an alternative to fish oil as a source of omega-3 fatty acids. SDA is metabolized to DHA and EPA in animals. However, further research is needed on the effects of SDA in humans (6129).

FLAXSEED

Also Known As

Flax Seed, Graine De Lin, Leinsamen, Lini Semen, Linseed, Lint Bells, Linum, Phytoestrogen, Winterlien. CAUTION: See separate listings for Alpha Linolenic Acid, Conjugated Linoleic Acid (CLA), Decosahexaenoic Acid (DHA), Eicosapentaenoic Acid (EPA), Fish Oils, and Flaxseed Oil.

Scientific Names

Linum usitatissimum.
Family: Linaceae.

People Use This For

Orally, flaxseed is used for chronic constipation, colon damage due to laxative abuse, diverticulitis, irritable bowel syndrome (IBS) or irritable colon, gastritis, enteritis (2), bladder inflammation (18), hypercholesterolemia, atherosclerosis (6,6800,6808), protection against cancer (5893,6801), and improving renal function in people with systemic lupus erythematosus (SLE) nephritis (6802).
Topically, flaxseed is used as a poultice for skin inflammation (2).
Ophthalmically, flaxseed is used for the removal of foreign bodies from the eye (18).

Safety

LIKELY SAFE ...when taken orally in appropriate amounts with sufficient fluid intake, which is in a ratio of 1:10 (seed:liquid) (2,12). ...when applied topically (2), although the regular handling of flaxseed can cause sensitization (6).
PREGNANCY AND LACTATION: POSSIBLY SAFE ...but should be used with caution (2,12).

Effectiveness

LIKELY EFFECTIVE ...when taken orally for reducing serum cholesterol. Various flaxseed preparations, including raw, ground, partially defatted, and flaxseed bread and muffins seem to significantly reduce total cholesterol and low-density lipoprotein (LDL) cholesterol in healthy people (5899,6803) and people with hypercholesterolemia (6800,6808). Preparations providing flaxseed 50 grams per day seem to reduce total cholesterol by 5-9% and LDL cholesterol by 8-18% (5899,6800,6803,6808). However, flaxseed does not affect high-density lipoprotein (HDL) cholesterol. Most flaxseed preparations also do not affect triglyceride levels. But partially defatted flaxseed (flaxseed without as much alpha-linolenic acid content) can increase triglycerides by approximately 10% (6808). ...when taken orally as a bulk forming laxative for constipation (2,6803).
POSSIBLY EFFECTIVE ...when used orally to improve renal function in people with systemic lupus erythematosus (SLE) nephritis (6802).
There is insufficient reliable information available about the effectiveness of flaxseed for its other uses.

Mechanism of Action

Flaxseed is a bulk-forming fibrous product which stimulates intestinal peristalsis, producing a laxative effect (18). The soluble fiber in flaxseed is found primarily in the seed coat gum, which is a mixture of polysaccharides including glucuronic acids, rhamnose, arabinose, xylose, and galactose (6808). Ten grams of flaxseed typically provides approximately 44 kilocalories energy, 2 grams protein, 4 grams fat and 4 grams dietary fiber (6801). Flaxseed is a rich source of alpha-linolenic acid and long-chain n-3 polyunsaturated fatty acids. Supplementation with flaxseed significantly increases n-3 polyunsaturated fatty acids in plasma and erythrocytes (5899,6803). Flaxseed is used for atherosclerosis because it can reduce platelet aggregation and serum cholesterol and thereby might lower atherogenic risks (6,6808). In animal models, flaxseed supplementation seems to significantly reduce the risk of developing aortic atherosclerosis (6806,6807). The fiber content of flaxseed is thought to be important for flaxseed's lipid lowering effects. High fiber diets increase fecal elimination of bile acids which increases primary bile acid synthesis (6800,6808). The alpha-linolenic acid content of flaxseed might also help lower serum cholesterol (6800). However, because partially defatted flaxseed also seems to lower cholesterol, other mechanisms are likely involved (6807,6808). Alpha-linolenic acid may also be involved in the beneficial effects on platelets (6800). Flaxseed might also have hypoglycemic effects. The postprandial glucose response to a 50 gram carbohydrate load given as flaxseed bread is 27% lower compared with regular white bread (5899). Flaxseed is also an indirect source of lignans. Secoisolariciresinol diglycoside is found in high concentrations in flaxseed and is converted by bacteria in the colon to the lignans enterolactone and enterodiol. The lignan precursor content of flaxseed can vary significantly depending on growing location and harvest year (5897). Urinary excretion of these lignans increases in variable amounts in people taking flaxseed, showing that they are absorbed from the colon (5894,6801,6803). Lignans might have some beneficial effects. Lignans have platelet activating factor (PAF) receptor antagonist effects and antioxidant effects (6802,6806). Lignans might also stimulate production of sex-hormone binding globulin in the liver (6801). Lignans have weak estrogenic effects and possibly antiestrogenic effects. They seem to compete with endogenous steroids for various enzymes and receptors. This competition might reduce endogenous estrogen binding to estrogen receptors, resulting in an antiestrogen effect. These effects may inhibit growth of hormone-dependent cancer cells (6801). Supplementation with flaxseed increases urinary excretion of certain estrogen metabolites, which has been hypothesized to confer protective effects against breast cancer in postmenopausal women (5893). Lignans may also inhibit angiogenesis (6803). Inhibition of mammary and colon tumor growth by the lignans enterolactone and enterodiol has also been reported in vitro (5895). Flaxseed and the constituent secoisolariciresinol diglycoside have also been reported to be protective against chemical-induced carcinogenesis in animal models (5897). In animals, secoisolariciresinol diglycoside seems to be most effective against new tumor development, and flaxseed and its alpha-linolenic acid rich oil component, being more effective for reducing growth of established tumors (6805). Although both alpha-linolenic acid and lignans constituents have been reported to have antioxidant effects (6806), there is some evidence that partially defatted flaxseed might actually have pro-oxidant activity (6808). For systemic lupus erythematosus (SLE) flaxseed is thought to improve renal function by decreasing blood viscosity, reducing serum cholesterol, and reducing inflammatory response (6802). Both alpha-linolenic acid and lignans seem to have beneficial platelet effects. Alpha-linolenic acid also suppresses the production of interleukin-1 (IL-1), tumor necrosis factor (TNF) and leukotriene B4, and production of oxygen free radicals by polymorphonuclear (PMN) leukocytes and monocytes (6806).

Flaxseed also contains cyanogenic glycosides (linustatin, neolinustatin, and linamarin), which can increase blood levels and urinary excretion of thiocyanate in humans consuming raw flaxseed, and can cause toxicity in grazing animals (6,5899); however, these glycosides have not been detected after flaxseed is baked in muffins (5899).

Adverse Reactions

Oral consumption of flaxseed can significantly increase the number of bowel movements (6803). High doses, greater than 45 grams per day, may not be tolerated for this reason (6802). Consumption of flaxseed with inadequate liquid can cause intestinal blockage (18). Occasionally, allergic and anaphylactic reactions have been reported after ingestion of flaxseed and flaxseed oil. Workers processing flax products might be more likely to be hypersensitive (6,6809).

Interactions with Herbs & Other Dietary Supplements

Insufficient reliable information available.

Interactions with Drugs

ORAL DRUGS: The fiber in flaxseed can impair absorption of oral drugs (19).

ANTICOAGULANT/ANTIPLATELET AGENTS: There is some evidence that flaxseed oil can decrease platelet aggregation and increase bleeding time (5898). Theoretically, using flaxseed oil in combination with anticoagulant or antiplatelet drugs might have additive effects and increase the risk of bleeding. Some of these drugs include aspirin, clopidogrel (Plavix), dalteparin (Fragmin), enoxaparin (Lovenox), heparin, ticlopidine (Ticlid), warfarin (Coumadin), and others.

Interactions with Foods

No interactions are known to occur, and there is no known reason to expect a clinically significant interaction with flaxseed.

Interactions with Lab Tests

CHOLESTEROL: Flaxseed can lower total serum cholesterol and low-density lipoprotein cholesterol levels, and test results (6,5899,6800,6803).

TRIGLYCERIDES: Partially defatted flaxseed (flaxseed without as much alpha-linolenic acid content) can increase triglyceride levels, and test results (6808).

Interactions with Diseases or Conditions

BLEEDING DISORDERS: There is some evidence that flaxseed can decrease platelet aggregation and increase bleeding time (5898). Theoretically, flaxseed might increase the risk of severe bleeding in patients with bleeding disorders; use with caution.

GASTROINTESTINAL OBSTRUCTION: People with bowel obstruction, esophageal stricture, and acute intestinal inflammation should avoid flaxseed. Flaxseed is a bulk forming laxative and might further contribute to obstruction (2,12).

HORMONE SENSITIVE CANCERS/CONDITIONS: Because flaxseed might have estrogenic effects (6), women with hormone sensitive conditions should avoid flaxseed. Some of these conditions include breast, uterine, and ovarian cancer, and endometriosis and uterine fibroids.
HYPERTRIGLYCERIDEMIA: Partially defatted flaxseed (flaxseed with less alpha linolenic acid content) might increase triglyceride levels (6808) and should be avoided in patients with hypertriglyceridemia.

Dosage and Administration

ORAL: The typical dose of flaxseed is 1 tablespoon of the whole or bruised seed (not ground) with 6 oz (150 mL) of liquid 2-3 times daily (2,12). Sufficient liquid with each dose is important to prevent possible intestinal blockage.
TOPICAL: 30-50 grams of flaxseed flour is commonly used for a moist and hot poultice or compress (2).
OPHTHALMIC: A single flaxseed is moistened and placed under the eyelid until the foreign body sticks to the mucus secretion (18).

Comments

Flaxseed has been used for more than ten thousand years as a fiber for weaving and clothing (6).

FLAXSEED OIL

Also Known As

Flax Oil, Flax Seed Oil, Graine De Lin, Linoleic Acid, Linseed Oil.
CAUTION: See separate listings for Alpha Linolenic Acid, Conjugated Linoleic Acid (CLA), Decosahexaenoic Acid (DHA), Eicosapentaenoic Acid (EPA), Fish Oils, and Flaxseed.

Scientific Names

Linum usitatissimum.
Family: Linaceae.

People Use This For

Orally, flaxseed oil is used as a laxative for constipation (844,6809), for arthritis, cancer (843), anxiety (294), benign prostatic hyperplasia (BPH), vaginitis (844), weight loss (293), hypertriglyceridemia, hypercholesterolemia, and to prevent heart attacks (843). Flaxseed oil is also used as a supplemental source of dietary alpha-linolenic acid (843).
Topically, flaxseed oil is used for its demulcent and emollient properties (6).
In foods, flaxseed oil is used as a cooking oil and in margarines (6809).
In manufacturing, flaxseed oil is used as a component in paints, varnishes, linoleum, and soap; and as a waterproofing agent (6,6809).

Safety

LIKELY SAFE ...when used orally in amounts found in foods.
POSSIBLY SAFE ...when used orally and appropriately for medicinal purposes, short-term. Flaxseed oil has been used safely in studies lasting up to 3 months (845,3912,5898).
There is insufficient reliable information available about the safety of topical use of flaxseed oil.
PREGNANCY: LIKELY SAFE ...when used orally in amounts found in foods. LIKELY UNSAFE ...when used orally in medicinal amounts. Flaxseed oil might affect menstruation (19); contraindicated.
LACTATION: LIKELY SAFE ...when used orally in amounts found in foods. There is insufficient reliable information available about the safety of flaxseed oil in breast-feeding women when used in medicinal amounts; avoid using.

Effectiveness

POSSIBLY INEFFECTIVE ...when used orally for rheumatoid arthritis. Flaxseed oil taken daily for 3 months does not seem to improve symptoms of pain and stiffness, and has no effect on laboratory measures of rheumatoid arthritis, such as C-reactive protein and erythrocyte sedimentation rate (ESR) (5898).
There is insufficient reliable information available about the effectiveness of flaxseed oil for its other uses.

Mechanism of Action

Flaxseed oil contains linolenic, linoleic, and oleic acids (6). It is among the best sources of alpha-linolenic acid (6). Linoleic acid and alpha-linolenic acid are required for the structural integrity of all cell membranes. Alpha-linolenic acid raises serum omega-3 polyunsaturated fatty acids, including eicosapentaenoic acid (EPA) and docosahexaenoic acid (DHA) (845,6803). There is some evidence that flaxseed oil can lower triglyceride levels (3911). Flaxseed oil seems to have other potentially beneficial cardiovascular effects. There is also some preliminary evidence that a low fat diet plus the flaxseed oil can increase systemic arterial elasticity, which might improve circulatory function (5896). Some researchers think flaxseed oil can also decrease platelet aggregation (845,6806), and increase the bleeding time (5898), but data are conflicting (3912). Flaxseed oil is used for rheumatoid arthritis because it might have anti-inflammatory effects. Alpha-linolenic acid contained in flaxseed oil is a precursor of eicosapentaenoic acid (EPA) and docosahexaenoic acid (DHA) which are converted to non- or anti-inflammatory prostaglandins and leukotrienes in the body. Supplementation with flaxseed oil or alpha-linolenic acid increases the ratio of EPA and DHA to the pro-inflammatory arachidonic acid (5898). Alpha-linolenic acid has also been reported to suppress the production of interleukin-1 (IL-1), tumor necrosis factor (TNF), leukotriene B4, and oxygen free radicals by polymorphonuclear (PMN) leukocytes and monocytes (6806). There is some evidence that alpha-linolenic acid from flaxseed oil might have anti-tumor effects, possibly by increasing peroxidation of fatty acids in tumor cell membranes, or by altering the balance of prostaglandin production away from tumor promoting prostaglandins of the E2 series (6805). Flaxseed oil seems to reduce the volume of chemically-induced mammary tumors in animal models (6805).

Adverse Reactions
Orally, flaxseed oil is typically well-tolerated. However, doses of flaxseed oil of 30 grams per day and higher have been associated with loose stools and diarrhea (5898). Allergic and anaphylactic reactions have been reported with flaxseed oil ingestion and also in workers processing flaxseed products (6809).

Interactions with Herbs & Other Dietary Supplements
Insufficient reliable information available.

Interactions with Drugs
ANTICOAGULANT/ANTIPLATELET AGENTS: There is some evidence that flaxseed oil can decrease platelet aggregation and increase bleeding time (5898). Theoretically, using flaxseed oil in combination with anticoagulant or antiplatelet drugs might have additive effects and increase the risk of bleeding. Some of these drugs include aspirin, clopidogrel (Plavix), dalteparin (Fragmin), enoxaparin (Lovenox), heparin, ticlopidine (Ticlid), warfarin (Coumadin), and others.

Interactions with Foods
No interactions are known to occur, and there is no known reason to expect a clinically significant interaction with flaxseed oil.

Interactions with Lab Tests
PROTHROMBIN TIME (PT): Flaxseed oil may affect platelet aggregation and prolong bleeding time and test results (5898).
TRIGLYCERIDES: Flaxseed oil might decrease serum triglyceride concentrations and test results in some patients with hyperlipoproteinemia (3911).

Interactions with Diseases or Conditions
BLEEDING DISORDERS: There is some evidence that flaxseed oil can decrease platelet aggregation and increase bleeding time (5898). Theoretically, flaxseed oil might increase the risk of severe bleeding in patients with bleeding disorders; use with caution.

Dosage and Administration
ORAL: A typical dose is 15-30 mL daily (3912).
TOPICAL: No typical dosage.

Comments
Specific deficiencies from inadequate intakes of essential fatty acids are rare except in individuals with severe, untreated fat malabsorption or those suffering from famine. Symptoms include dry, cracked, scaly and bleeding skin, excessive water loss from the skin, and impaired liver function resulting from the accumulation of lipid in the liver (i.e. fatty liver) (298).

FO-TI

Also Known As
Chinese Cornbind, Chinese Knotweed, Climbing Knotweed, Flowery Knotweed, Fo Ti, Fo-Ti-Tient, Foti, He Shou Wu, He-Shou-Wu, Heshouwu, Ho Shou Wu, Ho-Shou-Wu, Hoshouwu, Multiflora Preparata, Polygonum, Radix Polygoni Multiflori, Shen Min, Radix Polygoni Shen Min, Shou Wu, Shou-Wu, Shouwu, Zhihe Shou Wu, Zhihe-Shou-Wu, Zhiheshouwu, Zi Shou Wu, Zi-Shou-Wu, Zishouwu.

Scientific Names

Polygonum multiflorum.
Family: Polygonaceae.

People Use This For

Orally, fo-ti is used for treating lymph node tuberculosis, cancer, and constipation. It is also used orally as a liver and kidney tonic; blood and vital essence toner; and to fortify muscles, tendons, and bones. Fo-ti is also used orally for hyperlipidemia, insomnia, limb numbness, lower back and knee soreness or weakness, premature graying, and dizziness with tinnitus.

Topically, fo-ti is used for sores, carbuncles, skin eruptions, and itching.

In manufacturing, fo-ti extract is used as an ingredient in hair and skin care products.

Safety

POSSIBLY SAFE ...when used orally and appropriately (5,12).

There is insufficient reliable information available about the topical use of fo-ti.

PREGNANCY: POSSIBLY UNSAFE ...when used orally. Fo-ti contains anthraquinone constituents, which can exert a stimulant laxative effect. Bulk-forming or emollient laxatives are preferred in pregnancy (272). There is insufficient reliable information available about the topical use of fo-ti during pregnancy.

LACTATION: POSSIBLY UNSAFE ...when used orally. Anthraquinone constituents can cross into breast milk and might cause loose stools in some breast-fed infants (272). There is insufficient reliable information available about the topical use of fo-ti while nursing.

Effectiveness

POSSIBLY EFFECTIVE ...when used orally as a laxative. Raw fo-ti contains a higher concentration of the stimulant laxative anthraquinone constituents than cured products (5).

There is insufficient reliable information available about the effectiveness of fo-ti for its other oral or topical uses.

Mechanism of Action

The applicable part of fo-ti is the rhizome. Fo-ti is either used raw (uncured) or processed (cured) by repeated steaming and sun drying. Raw fo-ti root contains the anthraquinone derivatives, chrysophanol and emodin, along with a small amount of rhein. These constituents have stimulant laxative effects, which probably accounts for fo-ti's use in constipation. Curing fo-ti reduces these constituents by 42-96% (5). Fo-ti reportedly has hypoglycemic effects (5,19). Some evidence suggests that isolated stilbene glycoside constituents in the raw fo-ti root might have liver protectant effects, including inhibition of alanine aminotransferase (ALT, formerly SGOT) and aspartate aminotransferase (AST) (11). Cured fo-ti shows evidence it might increase the levels of superoxide dismutase (SOD), serotonin, norepinephrine, dopamine, and decrease levels of monoamine oxidase-B (MAO-B), lipid peroxide, malonyl dialdehyde (MDA) (11); these are believed to be markers for anti-aging effects. Some evidence suggests fo-ti might also increase serum ceruloplasmin levels, reduce thymus gland atrophy, and inhibit atrophy of adrenal glands; enhancing nonspecific and cellular immunity, and antagonizing the immunosuppressive effects of prednisolone or hydrocortisone (11). Other evidence suggests the alcoholic extract might increase high-density lipoprotein (HDL) cholesterol, reduce total cholesterol, free cholesterol, triglycerides, and retard atherosclerosis (11). The aqueous extract appears to inhibit the replication of hepatitis B (11).

Adverse Reactions

Orally, fo-ti, particularly the raw root, may cause catharsis, diarrhea, abdominal pain, nausea, and vomiting (12).

Interactions with Herbs & Other Dietary Supplements

Insufficient reliable information available.

Interactions with Drugs

DIABETES THERAPY: Theoretically, concomitant use of fo-ti with antidiabetic agents might increase the risk of hypoglycemia. Fo-ti reportedly has hypoglycemic effects (5,19). Dosing adjustments for insulin or oral hypoglycemic agents may be necessary. Oral hypoglycemic drugs include glimepiride (Amaryl), glipizide (Glucotrol), glyburide (Diabeta, Micronase), tolazamide (Tolinase), tolbutamide (Orinase), and others. Monitor blood glucose levels closely.

DIGOXIN: Theoretically, overuse of anthraquinone laxatives (e.g., fo-ti) might increase the risk of hypokalemia and digoxin cardiotoxicity (151,272).

DIURETICS: Theoretically, concomitant use of potassium-depleting diuretics and fo-ti can increase risk of hypokalemia (151,272).

STIMULANT LAXATIVES: Theoretically, concomitant use of fo-ti with other laxatives can increase the risk of fluid and electrolyte depletion (151,272).

Interactions with Foods
No interactions are known to occur, and there is no known reason to expect a clinically significant interaction with fo-ti.

Interactions with Lab Tests
CHOLESTEROL: Theoretically, cured fo-ti might reduce serum total cholesterol concentrations and test results (11).
COLORIMETRIC TESTS: Fo-ti might discolor urine (pink, red, purple, orange, rust), interfering with diagnostic tests that depend on a color change, due to its anthraquinone content (11,275).
GLUCOSE: Theoretically, fo-ti might decrease blood glucose concentrations and test results (5,6,19).
POTASSIUM: Excessive use of fo-ti might cause hypokalemia, reducing serum potassium concentrations and test results due to its anthraquinone content (11).
TRIGLYCERIDES: Theoretically, cured fo-ti might reduce serum triglyceride concentrations and test results (11).

Interactions with Diseases or Conditions
GASTROINTESTINAL DISEASE: Fo-ti exerts a stimulant effect on the intestinal tract (5). Avoid its use in diarrhea, intestinal obstruction, acute intestinal inflammation (Crohn's disease, ulcerative colitis, appendicitis), ulcer, abdominal pain of unknown origin, nausea, and vomiting.
HEART CONDITIONS: Theoretically, the laxative effect of fo-ti might cause hypokalemia with overuse/misuse, potentially decreasing cardiac function (15).

Dosage and Administration
No typical dosage.

Comments
Avoid confusion with the commercial product Fo-ti-Teng which contains no fo-ti (6).

FOLIC ACID

Also Known As
B Complex Vitamin, B-Complex Vitamin, Folacin, Folate, Vitamin B9.

Scientific Names
Pteroylglutamic acid; Pteroylmonoglutamic acid; Pteroylpolyglutamate.

People Use This For
Orally, folic acid is used for preventing and treating folate deficiency. It is also used for megaloblastic anemia resulting from folate or vitamin B12 deficiency, megaloblastic anemia in sickle cell disease, and for folate deficiency in intestinal malabsorption or sprue (14). Folic acid is also used orally in conditions commonly associated with folate deficiency, including ulcerative colitis; liver disease; alcoholism; renal dialysis; and drug-induced deficiency related to phenytoin, primidone, barbiturates, oral contraceptives, and nitrofurantoin. Folic acid is also used orally for preventing neural tube defects, reducing the risk of colon cancer, preventing pregnancy loss, hyperhomocystinemia, fragile-X syndrome, gingival hyperplasia, memory deficit, vitiligo, osteoporosis, restless leg syndrome, insomnia, depression, peripheral neuropathy, myelopathy, and AIDS. It is also used for reducing lometrexol and methotrexate toxicity; and for preventing signs of aging, heart attack, and stroke (14,15,16,412,2165,2251,3323,3324,6667).
Topically, folic acid is used for treating gingival hyperplasia (14) and gingivitis (2152).
Parenterally, folic acid is used intramuscularly, subcutaneously, or intravenously for treating folate deficiency, particularly in patients with malabsorption or those who cannot take oral treatment (15). Folic acid has also been used parenterally to treat chronic fatigue syndrome (6082).

Safety
LIKELY SAFE ...when used orally or parenterally and appropriately. Folic acid is generally safe when used in doses less than 1000 mcg per day (14,15,6241). In certain malabsorption disorders, such as sprue, larger doses can also be safely used (6241).
POSSIBLY UNSAFE ...when used orally in large doses. Doses above 1000 mcg per day should be avoided to prevent precipitation or exacerbation of neuropathy related to vitamin B12 deficiency (6241,6242,6245). Very high doses of 15 mg per day can also cause significant central nervous system (CNS) and gastrointestinal side effects (14,15,16,505).
PREGNANCY AND LACTATION: LIKELY SAFE ...when used orally and appropriately. Folic acid is commonly used during pregnancy for prevention of neural tube defects (14,3094).

Effectiveness

EFFECTIVE ...when used orally or parenterally for treating folic acid deficiency (14,15,16,505).

LIKELY EFFECTIVE ...when used orally for reducing the risk of neural tube birth defects (14,15,3325). ...when used orally for treating hyperhomocysteinemia. Although there have been conflicting findings reported (1179), the majority of evidence shows that folic acid 400-1000 mcg can significantly lower homocysteine levels in people with elevated homocysteine levels (412,2146,2147,2148,2149,3323,3324,3886,6883,6884). At least 400 mcg per day of folate seems to be necessary to simultaneously normalize or maintain serum folate levels and decrease plasma total homocysteine concentrations (6366). Folic acid supplements and folic acid-fortified cereals appear to be more effective than folate-rich foods for reducing plasma total homocysteine concentrations (6367). Although folic acid lowers homocysteine levels, it's not clear if this results in decreased cardiovascular morbidity and mortality. However there is some preliminary evidence that high dose folic acid might lower blood pressure and homocysteine levels in people who have previously had a myocardial infarction or stroke (6667). ...when used orally for reducing methotrexate toxicity in the treatment of rheumatoid arthritis (14,2162,2163,2164).

POSSIBLY EFFECTIVE ...when used orally for reducing methotrexate-related gastrointestinal side effects in the treatment of psoriasis (768). ...when used orally for reducing the risk of colon cancer (505,2140,2141,2142,2143,2144,2145,2250). ...when used orally for treating vitiligo (14,2153,2154). ...when used topically for treating gingival hyperplasia secondary to phenytoin therapy (2151). ...when used topically for treating gingivitis in pregnancy (2152).

POSSIBLY INEFFECTIVE ...when used orally for treating gingival hyperplasia secondary to phenytoin therapy (14,2150,2151,2152). ...when used orally for reducing lometrexol toxicity (14,2161).

LIKELY INEFFECTIVE ...when used orally for treating fragile-X syndrome (14,2155,2156,2157,2158,2159,2160).

There is insufficient reliable information available about the effectiveness of folic acid for its other uses. However, early evidence suggests folic acid might prevent the progression of subclinical atherosclerosis to symptomatic disease in at-risk patients (3886,3887). Further evidence is needed to rate folic acid for this use.

Mechanism of Action

Folate is the general term that refers to a variety of chemical forms of the vitamin (6241). Folic acid, or pteroylmonoglutamic acid, is the form used in vitamin supplements and fortified foods (6241). Folate in food is pteroylpolyglutamate, which has a polyglutamate side chain with peptide linkages (6241). Folate in food is about 40% less bioavailable than synthetic folic acid, which is almost 100% bioavailable (6241). Before folate from food can be absorbed, the polyglutamate side chain must be cleaved to form the absorbable monoglutamate form (6241). After folic acid is absorbed, it is converted to tetrahydrofolate. In humans, tetrahydrofolate-based coenzymes play a major role in intracellular metabolism. Tetrahydrofolate plays an indirect role in the rate-limiting step in DNA synthesis. Abnormalities in this process that occur with folic acid deficiency cause megaloblastic anemia. Folic acid supplementation can correct this problem (14). Folic acid can also reduce damage to DNA and prevent replication errors (2139,2144). Tetrahydrofolate-based coenzymes are also involved in the conversion of homocysteine to methionine (14). Supplementation with folic acid increases conversion of homocysteine to methionine, lowering homocysteine levels and making it useful for hyperhomocystinemia (412,2146,2147,2148,2149,3886). Hyperhomocystinemia has been linked to cardiovascular disease, and low folic acid levels have been associated with elevated homocysteine levels and increased risk of acute coronary events, including myocardial infarction (1899,3323,3324). Although still poorly understood, it has been proposed that hyperhomocystinemia may alter anticoagulant properties of endothelial cells, cause dysfunction of vascular endothelium, or enhance lipid peroxidation. Folic acid supplementation might decrease the risk of cardiovascular disease through reducing plasma homocysteine levels (3323,6367). Folic acid might also be beneficial for reducing coronary events. There is some evidence people with low serum folate are at an increased risk for coronary events (3323). Early evidence suggests that folic acid alone or in combination with other B vitamins can reduce arterial endothelial dysfunction in people with elevated homocysteine levels (412,6235,6236). Folic acid also seems to play an important role in pregnancy. Low folate levels have been associated with recurrent spontaneous pregnancy loss (6237). Folic acid supplementation also prevents neural tube defects in the fetus. But the exact role of folic acid in this process is not completely understood (15). Folic acid might play a role in Alzheimer's disease. Preliminary evidence indicates that low folate concentrations might be related to atrophy of the cerebral cortex, particularly in people with neocortical lesions related to Alzheimer's disease (6234). Low serum folate levels are strongly correlated to cerebral atrophy on autopsy (6234). Functional and mental deterioration is also sometimes associated with low folate levels in elderly people (6238). Folate deficiency has also been attributed to melancholic depression and poor response to antidepressants (6239,3657). Some patients with chronic fatigue syndrome also have decreased folic acid levels (6082,6083), so some people try folic acid supplements for chronic fatigue. Crohn's disease has also been associated with decreased folate levels (6269). Low red blood cell folate levels have been associated with the development of dysplasia and cancer in ulcerative colitis (6270). Preliminary clinical evidence suggests folate supplementation might protect against cancer in people with ulcerative colitis (6271).

Adverse Reactions

Orally, high doses of folic acid can cause altered sleep patterns, vivid dreaming, irritability, excitability, overactivity, confusion, impaired judgment, exacerbation of seizure frequency and psychotic behavior, nausea, abdominal distention, flatulence, bitter taste in the mouth, allergic skin reactions, and zinc depletion (14,15). In one study, these effects were observed after administration of 15 mg per day for 30 days. Large doses of folic acid can also precipitate or exacerbate neuropathy in people deficient in vitamin B12 (6243). Allergic reactions have occurred rarely. Symptoms have included rash, erythema, itching, malaise, and bronchospasm. An anaphylactic reaction has been reported in one patient receiving intravenous folic acid. Use of folic acid for undiagnosed anemia has masked the symptoms of pernicious anemia, resulting in lack of treatment and eventual neurological damage (15). Patients should be warned to not self-treat suspected anemia.

Interactions with Herbs & Other Dietary Supplements

ZINC: Chronic administration of folic acid can decrease zinc levels (14,15).
VITAMIN B12: Long-term use of folic acid can deplete levels of vitamin B12 (15).

Interactions with Drugs

CHLORAMPHENICOL: Concomitant use can reduce the effectiveness of folic acid in the treatment of anemias (15).
CHOLESTYRAMINE (Questran): Concomitant use can decrease bioavailability of supplemental folic acid (4455).
COLESTIPOL (Colestid): Concomitant administration can decrease bioavailability of supplemental folic acid (14,4461).
PANCREATIC ENZYMES (Pancreatin): Concomitant use can interfere with folic acid absorption (14).
METHOTREXATE (MTX, Rheumatrex): Theoretically, concomitant use might interfere with the effectiveness of methotrexate cancer therapy (15). However, when methotrexate is used in rheumatoid arthritis and psoriasis therapy, large amounts of folic acid can reduce methotrexate side effects without interfering with effectiveness (767,768,2162,4492,4493,4494,4546).
PHENYTOIN (Dilantin), FOSPHENYTOIN (Cerebyx), PRIMIDONE (Mysoline), PHENOBARBITAL: Folic acid can increase metabolism and reduce the serum levels of these drugs (14,15,505). These drugs can also affect folic acid (see Drug Influences on Nutrient Levels and Depletion).
PYRIMETHAMINE (Daraprim): Concomitant use can decrease the effectiveness of pyrimethamine (14).
SULFASALAZINE (Azulfidine): Concomitant use can decrease folic acid absorption (14).

Drug Influences on Nutrient Levels and Depletion

SOME DRUGS CAN AFFECT FOLIC ACID LEVELS:
ANTIBIOTICS: Destruction of normal gastrointestinal flora by antibiotics can cause decreased production of B vitamins. The clinical significance of this decreased production is not known. Consider supplementation only if clinical judgment warrants it (4434,4435,4436,4437,4438,4439,4440,4441,4442,4443).
CARBAMAZEPINE (Tegretol): Treatment with carbamazepine is associated with decreased folic acid levels. However, the necessity for folic acid supplementation to prevent peripheral neuropathies or red cell dyscrasias has not been adequately studied (4426,4427,4428,4429).
CYCLOSERINE (Seromycin Pulvules): Use of cycloserine can impair dietary folic acid absorption and reduce serum folic acid levels. The need for supplementation has not been adequately studied (4531).
FUROSEMIDE (Lasix): Use of furosemide might increase the excretion of folic acid (1898). Long-term furosemide therapy (1894) in people with hypertension has been associated with decreased folic acid levels and increased homocysteine levels (1898). Elevated homocysteine levels are associated with atherosclerotic vascular disease, arterial and venous thromboembolism, coronary, cerebral, and peripheral arterial occlusive diseases, and increased risk of myocardial infarction in smokers (1891,1892,1893,1899). However, the need for folic acid supplementation during furosemide therapy has not been adequately studied.
METFORMIN (Glucophage): Metformin may reduce serum folic acid and vitamin B12 levels (32,4490). A multivitamin preparation may be valuable in some patients.
METHOTREXATE: Methotrexate binds to dihydrofolate reductase and prevents the conversion of folate to folic acid (1716,1719,4493,4494). Consider folic acid supplements for prolonged methotrexate therapy.
ORAL CONTRACEPTIVES: Use of oral contraceptives can impair dietary folic acid absorption and reduce serum folic acid levels. The need for folic acid supplementation has not been adequately studied (4459,4498).
p-AMINOSALICYLIC ACID (PAS, Aminosalicylic acid): Concomitant use can decrease folic acid absorption in the gastrointestinal tract. The need for supplementation has not been adequately studied. Consider supplementation only if clinical judgment warrants it (4557,4558,4559,4560).
PENTAMIDINE (NebuPent): Treatment with pentamidine can impair dietary folic acid absorption and reduce serum folic acid levels. The need for folic acid supplementation during pentamidine therapy has not been adequately studied (4351).
PHENOBARBITAL (Luminal), PRIMIDONE (Mysoline): These drugs can impair dietary folic acid absorption and reduce serum folic acid levels. The need for folic acid supplementation has not been adequately studied (4453,4530,4531).
PHENYTOIN (Dilantin), FOSPHENYTOIN (Cerebyx): These drugs can reduce serum folic acid levels. Clinical evidence suggests that giving supplemental folic acid with the initial dose of phenytoin might prevent folic acid deficiency (4471,4472,4473,4474,4477,4531).

PYRIMETHAMINE (Daraprim): Treatment with pyrimethamine can reduce serum folic acid levels. At lower pyrimethamine doses, the need for folic acid supplementation has not been adequately studied. However, with larger pyrimethamine doses (those required to treat toxoplasmosis), if signs of folic acid deficiency develop, administer folinic acid (Leucovorin) 5-15 mg/day (orally, IV, or IM) until normal hematopoiesis is restored (4425,4532).

SULFASALAZINE (Azulfidine): Sulfasalazine-induced blood dyscrasias might involve folic acid depletion. Foods high in folic acid rather than folic acid supplements have been recommended (4515,4516,4517).

THIAZIDE DIURETICS: These drugs might increase the excretion of folic acid. Long-term thiazide diuretic therapy (1894) in people with hypertension has been associated with decreased folic acid levels and increased homocysteine levels (1898). Elevated homocysteine levels are associated with atherosclerotic vascular disease, arterial and venous thromboembolism, coronary, cerebral, and peripheral arterial occlusive diseases, and increased risk of myocardial infarction in smokers (1891,1892,1893,1899). The need for folic acid supplementation during thiazide diuretic therapy has not been adequately studied.

TRIMETHOPRIM (Trimpex): Trimethoprim, including trimethoprim contained in the combination antibiotic trimethoprim/sulfamethoxazole (TMP/SMX, Septra) can interfere with folic acid metabolism, reduce serum folic acid levels, and cause mild folic acid deficiency in patients on long-term or high-dose therapy (4468,4531).

TRIAMTERENE (Dyrenium): Use of triamterene can decrease the utilization of dietary folic acid and reduce serum folic acid levels. The need for folic acid supplementation has not been adequately studied (14,4425,4536,4537).

Interactions with Foods

FOODS: Taking folic acid with food slightly decreases the absorption of folic acid (6241). With food, the bioavailability is estimated at 85% compared to nearly 100% when taken without food (6241).

Interactions with Lab Tests

MEAN CORPUSCULAR VOLUME (MCV): Folic acid supplementation can normalize megaloblastic anemia in cases of folic acid and vitamin B12 deficiencies. In cases of vitamin B12 deficiency or pernicious anemia, treatment with folic acid will normalize hematological findings, but will not prevent neurological damage (14).

Interactions with Diseases or Conditions

PERNICIOUS ANEMIA: Folic acid can mask pernicious anemia by decreasing megaloblastic anemia. This can prevent appropriate treatment with vitamin B12 and result in neurological damage (14,15,16,505). Patients should be warned to avoid treating undiagnosed anemia with folic acid.

SEIZURE DISORDERS: Supplemental folic acid can exacerbate seizures in people with seizure disorders. This was reported in a study using 800 mcg folic acid per day in pregnant women with seizure disorders (14).

SCHIZOPHRENIA: Folic acid supplementation might exacerbate psychotic behavior in schizophrenic patients, despite have normal folic acid blood levels initially (14).

Dosage and Administration

ORAL: For folate deficiency, the typical dose is 250-1000 mcg per day (14,15). For preventing neural tube defects, 400 mcg folic acid per day from supplements or fortified food should be taken by women capable of becoming pregnant and continued through the first month of pregnancy (3325,6241,6243). Women with a history of previous pregnancy complicated by such neural tube defects usually take 4 mg per day beginning one month before and continuing for three months after conception (14,15). For reducing colon cancer risk, 400 mcg per day has been used (2250). For hyperhomocystinemia and reducing atherogenesis, 400-1000 mcg per day has been used (412,2146,2147,2148,2149,6366). For decreasing blood pressure and homocysteine levels in patients with a history of stroke or myocardial infarction, 5 mg daily has been used (6667). For vitiligo, 5 mg is typically taken twice daily (14,2153). For the reduction of methotrexate toxicity, 5 mg a week or 1 mg daily is used (14,2162,2163,2164). For enhancing response to antidepressants, 500 mcg daily has been used (3657). The adequate intakes (AI) for infants are 65 mcg for infants 0-6 months and 80 mcg for infants 7-12 months of age (3094). The recommended dietary allowances (RDAs) for folate in DFE, including both food folate and folic acid from fortified foods and supplements are: Children 1-3 years, 150 mcg; Children 4-8 years, 200 mcg; Children 9-13 years, 300 mcg; Adults over 13 years, 400 mcg; Pregnant women 600 mcg; and Lactating women, 500 mcg (3094,6243). The maximum daily levels of folate not likely to pose a risk for adverse effects are 300 mcg for children 1-3 years of age, 400 mcg for children 4-8 years, 600 mcg for children 9-13 years, 800 mcg for adolescents 14-18 years, and 1000 mcg for everyone over 18 years of age (3094).

TOPICAL: For gingival hyperplasia secondary to phenytoin therapy, a 0.1% folate mouthwash is used twice daily (2166). For gingivitis in pregnancy, a folate mouthwash is used twice daily (2152). Dietary folate equivalents (DFE) are used to account for the differences in absorption of folate from food and synthetic folic acid, either from supplements or fortified food (6241,6243). The Institute of Medicine established these equivalencies: 1 mcg DFE equals 1 mcg food folate, equals 0.6 mcg folic-acid-fortified food, equals 0.5 mcg supplemental folic acid taken on an empty stomach (6243). Thus 1 mcg supplemental folic acid taken on an empty stomach equals 2 mcg DFE (6241).

Comments

Beginning in 1998, the US government required folic acid fortification of all cold cereals and baking flour, which extends to breads, pastas, bakery items, cookies, crackers, etc. (6241). Foods that are naturally high in folate content include spinach, okra, asparagus, legumes, beef liver, and orange and tomato juice (6241).

Folic acid is frequently used in combination with other B vitamins in vitamin B complex formulations. Vitamin B complex generally includes vitamin B1 (thiamine), vitamin B2 (riboflavin), vitamin B3 (niacin/niacinamide), vitamin B5 (pantothenic acid), vitamin B6 (pyridoxine), vitamin B12 (cyanocobalamin), and folic acid. However, some products do not contain all of these ingredients and some may include others, such as biotin, para-aminobenzoic acid (PABA), choline bitartrate, and inositol (3022,3060,3061).

FOOL'S PARSLEY

Also Known As

Dog Parsley, Dog Poison, Fool's-Cicely, Fools Parsley, Lesser Hemlock, Small Hemlock.
CAUTION: See separate listings for Parsley leaf, root; Parsley seed; and Parsley Piert.

Scientific Names

Aethusa cynapium.
Family: Apiaceae or Umbelliferae.

People Use This For

Orally, fool's parsley is used for gastrointestinal complaints in children, infantile cholera, Summer diarrhea, and convulsions (18).

Safety

LIKELY UNSAFE ...when used orally; avoid using. Plant parts are considered poisonous and are associated with serious, potentially life-threatening poisonings (18).
PREGNANCY AND LACTATION: UNSAFE ...when used orally; contraindicated, due to potential for poisoning (18).

Effectiveness

There is insufficient reliable information available about the effectiveness of fool's parsley.

Mechanism of Action

Fool's parsley contains varied flavone glycosides (rutoside, narcissine, camphor oil-3-glucorhamnoside). Freshly harvested leaves (only) contain polyenes aethusin, aethusanol A, and asthusanol B (18).

Adverse Reactions

Orally, there are reports that fool's parsley caused deaths when it was mistaken for garden parsley; however, there is some evidence that the botanical to blame was actually spotted hemlock (18). Nevertheless, caution is warranted.

Interactions with Herbs & Other Dietary Supplements

Insufficient reliable information available.

Interactions with Drugs

No interactions are known to occur, and there is no known reason to expect a clinically significant interaction with fool's parsley.

Interactions with Foods

No interactions are known to occur, and there is no known reason to expect a clinically significant interaction with fool's parsley.

Interactions with Lab Tests

No interactions are known to occur, and there is no known reason to expect a clinically significant interaction with fool's parsley.

Interactions with Diseases or Conditions

No interactions are known to occur, and there is no known reason to expect a clinically significant interaction with fool's parsley.

Dosage and Administration
No typical dosage.

Comments
Fool's parsley is considered unsafe; avoid using. Fool's parsley looks a lot like young garden parsley; hence its name. Be careful not to confuse the two, since fool's parsley is poisonous (18).

FORGET-ME-NOT

Also Known As
Forget Me Not.

Scientific Names
Myosotis arvensis.
Family: Borraginaceae.

People Use This For
Orally, forget-me-not is used for respiratory disorders and nose bleeds (18).

Safety
LIKELY UNSAFE ...when used orally. The flowering plant preparations contain hepatotoxic unsaturated pyrrolizidine alkaloids (UPAs) (18). Repeated exposure to low concentrations of UPAs is linked to serious liver toxicity. UPAs are also thought to be carcinogenic and mutagenic (12).
PREGNANCY AND LACTATION: LIKELY UNSAFE ...when used orally. It contains toxic UPAs (12,19).

Effectiveness
There is insufficient reliable information available about the effectiveness of forget-me-not.

Mechanism of Action
The applicable part of forget-me-not is the whole flowering plant. Forget-me-not contains unsaturated pyrrolizidine alkaloids that can cause toxicity (18).

Adverse Reactions
Orally, acute toxicity may result in hepatic necrosis; chronic toxicity may cause veno-occlusive liver disease. The potential for hepatotoxicity increases with larger doses and longer periods of use (4,12).

Interactions with Herbs & Other Dietary Supplements
Insufficient reliable information available.

Interactions with Drugs
No interactions are known to occur, and there is no known reason to expect a clinically significant interaction with forget-me-not.

Interactions with Foods
No interactions are known to occur, and there is no known reason to expect a clinically significant interaction with forget-me-not.

Interactions with Lab Tests
No interactions are known to occur, and there is no known reason to expect a clinically significant interaction with forget-me-not.

Interactions with Diseases or Conditions
No interactions are known to occur, and there is no known reason to expect a clinically significant interaction with forget-me-not.

Dosage and Administration
No typical dosage.

Comments
None.

FORSKOLIN

Also Known As

Borforsin, Colecus forskohlii, Coleus forskolii, Coleus forskohlii, Colforsin, Colius forskolii, Forscolin, Forskolin, HL-362, L-75-1362B.

Scientific Names

17beta-acetoxy-8,13-epoxy-1alpha,6beta,9alpha-trihydroxylabd-14-en-11-one.

People Use This For

Orally, forskolin is used for asthma, allergies, eczema, psoriasis, obesity, dysmenorrhea, irritable bowel syndrome (IBS), urinary tract infections (UTI) and bladder infections, hypertension, angina, metastatic cancer, thrombosis, impotence, insomnia, and convulsions.

Intravenously, forskolin is used for idiopathic congestive cardiomyopathy and congestive heart failure (CHF).

By inhalation, forskolin is used for asthma and bronchospasm.

Ophthalmologically, forskolin is used for glaucoma.

Safety

POSSIBLY SAFE …when used intravenously and appropriately, short term. Intravenous forskolin seems to be safe and well tolerated when given at an appropriate rate of 0.5 mcg/kg/minute and increased at 15 minute intervals to 1.0, 2.0, and 3.0 mcg/kg/minute up to 1 hour. (7278,7279). …when used by inhalation and appropriately. Single-dose inhalation of forskolin powder (10mg) from a Spinhaler inhalator seems to be safe and well tolerated (7281). …when used ophthamically and appropriately. Forskolin suspension eye drops (1%) seem and well-tolerated (7282,7283,7284,7402,7403,7405).

PREGNANCY AND LACTATION: Insufficient reliable information available; avoid using.

Effectiveness

POSSIBLY EFFECTIVE …when used intravenously for idiopathic congestive cardiomyopathy. There is some evidence that intravenous forskolin, starting at 0.5 mcg/kg/minute, increasing at 15 minute intervals to 1.0, 2.0 and 3.0 mcg/kg/minute, is effective in improving cardiac output and pulmonary vascular pressures in patients with idiopathic congestive cardiomyopathy (7278). …when used by inhalation for asthma. There is some evidence that a single-dose inhalation of forskolin powder 10 mg from a Spinhaler inhaler can significantly increase forced expiratory volume in 1 second (FEV1) in patients with asthma (7281).

There is insufficient reliable information available to rate forskolin for its other uses. However, there is some preliminary evidence that forskolin suspension eye drops (1%) can significantly decrease intraocular pressure in healthy people without eye disease (7282,7283,7284,7402,7403,7405). Forskolin has not yet been tested in patients with glaucoma. More evidence is need to rate forskolin for this use.

Mechanism of Action

Forskolin is a diterpene and the major active constituent found in the roots of the plant Coleus forskolii (7277). Forskolin stimulates and activates the enzyme adenylate cyclase in the heart and smooth muscle. This causes increased production of cyclic AMP (cAMP), which causes calcium channels to open and intracellular calcium concentrations to increase, resulting in increased contractility of heart muscle and relaxation of smooth muscle (7277,7406,7407,7408,7409). Researchers speculate that forskolin might also activate adenylate cyclase in other cells of the body such as platelet cells and cells in the thyroid, pancreas, adrenal or pituitary glands (7277). There is preliminary evidence that forskolin prevents platelet aggregation and adhesion (7410,7411) and may also block tumor cell-induced human platelet aggregation, prevent tumor cell growth, and prevent cancer metastasis (7412,7413).

Adverse Reactions

Intravenously, forskolin can cause flushing and hypotension (7279).

Inhalation of forskolin can cause throat and upper respiratory tract irritation, mild to moderate cough, tremor, and restlessness (7281).

Ophthamically, forskolin can cause stinging of the eyes and conjunctival hyperemia (7283).

Interactions with Herbs & Other Dietary Supplements

CARDIOACTIVE HERBS: Theoretically, concomitant use of forskolin and cardioactive herbs could potentiate the cardiac effects and adverse effects (7278,7279). Some cardioactive herbs include calamus, cereus, cola, coltsfoot, devil's claw, European mistletoe, fenugreek, fumitory, ginger, Panax ginseng, white horehound, mate, parsley, quassia, scotch broom flower, shepherd's purse, wild carrot, and some cardiac glycoside-containing herbs such as digitalis leaf or lily-of-the-valley roots.

HERBS WITH ANTICOAGULANT/ANTIPLATELET POTENTIAL: Theoretically, concomitant use of forskolin with herbs that affect platelet aggregation could potentially increase the risk of bruising and bleeding. Some of these herbs include angelica, anise, arnica, asafetida, bogbean, boldo, capsicum, celery, chamomile, clove, danshen, fenugreek, feverfew, garlic, ginger, ginkgo, Panax ginseng, horseradish, licorice, meadowsweet, prickly ash, onion, papain, passionflower, poplar, quassia, red clover, turmeric, wild carrot, wild lettuce, willow, and others.

Interactions with Drugs

ANTICOAGULANTS AND ANTIPLATELET DRUGS: Theoretically, concomitant use of forskolin and anticoagulant or antiplatelet agents might increase the risk of bruising and bleeding. There is some evidence forskolin can inhibit platelet aggregation and adhesion (7410,7411). Some anticoagulant and antiplatelet drugs include abciximab (Reopro), anagrelide (agrylin), antithrombin III (Thrombate III), ardeparin (Normiflo), cilostazol (Pletal), clopidogrel (Plavix), dalteparin (Fragmin), danaparoid (Orgaran), dicumarol, dipyridamole (Persantine), enoxaparin (Lovenox), eptifibitide (Integrilin), heparin, lepirudin (Refludan), (tirofiban (Aggrastat), and warfarin (Coumadin).
CORONARY VASODILATORS: Theoretically, using forskolin with theophylline, caffeine, papaverine, sodium nitrate, adenosine, epinephrine, and other coronary vasodilators might cause additive vasodilatory effects. Forskolin can cause vasodilation and significantly lower blood pressure (7278,7279).

Interactions with Foods

No interactions are known to occur, and there is no known reason to expect a clinically significant interaction with forskolin.

Interactions with Lab Tests

BLEEDING TIME: Theoretically, forskolin might increase measures of bleeding time and increase tests results for prothrombin time (PT) and international normalized ratio (INR). There is evidence forskolin inhibits platelet aggregation and adhesion (7410,7411).

Interactions with Diseases or Conditions

CARDIOVASCULAR DISEASE: There is some concern that forskolin might interfere with treatment for cardiovascular disease and potentially worsen cardiovascular conditions. Forskolin can cause vasodilation and significantly lower blood pressure (7278,7279). Use forskolin with caution in patients with cardiovascular conditions.
BLEEDING DISORDERS: Theoretically, forskolin increase the risk of bleeding. There is evidence forskolin inhibits platelet aggregation and adhesion (7278,7279).

Dosage and Administration

INTRAVENOUS: For idiopathic congestive cardiomyopathy, intravenous forskolin has been infused at 0.5 mcg/kg/min and increased at 15 minute intervals as tolerated up to 1.0, 2.0 and 3.0 mcg/kg/minutefor up to 1 hour (7278,7279).
INHALATION: For asthma, 10 mg of forskolin powder, using a Spinhaler inhalator, has been used (7281).
OPHTHALMIC: For lowering intraocular pressure, 50 microliters of forskolin suspension eye drops (1%), applied topically to the cornea, has been used in health people (7282,7283,7284,7402,7403,7405). An appropriate dose for patients with glaucoma is not known.
ORAL: No typical dosage.

Comments

Forskolin comes from Coleus forskolii, an herb that has been used since ancient times to treat heart and respiratory disorders. Herbal product manufacturers are now producing Coleus forskolii extracts with elevated levels of the constituent forskolin. These preparations are being promoted for the same conditions that forskolin has been used for. However, there is no reliable scientific information that shows Coleus forskolii extracts offer any therapeutic benefit.

FRANKINCENSE

Also Known As

Bible Frankincense, Olibanum.
CAUTION: See separate listing for Indian Frankincense.

Scientific Names

Boswellia carteri.
Family: Burseraceae.

People Use This For
Orally, frankincense is used for colic and flatulence.

Topically, frankincense is used in hand cream (18). The essential oil of frankincense is used topically and by inhalation as an analgesic (7107).

Safety
POSSIBLY SAFE ...when used orally (12). ...when the frankincense essential oil is used topically and by inhalation (7107).

PREGNANCY AND LACTATION: Insufficient reliable information available; avoid using.

Effectiveness
There is insufficient reliable information available about the effectiveness of frankincense.

Mechanism of Action
The applicable part of frankincense is the resin. There is insufficient reliable information available about the possible mechanism of action and active ingredients.

Adverse Reactions
Topically, frankincense can cause mild irritation (18).

Interactions with Herbs & Other Dietary Supplements
Insufficient reliable information available.

Interactions with Drugs
No interactions are known to occur, and there is no known reason to expect a clinically significant interaction with frankincense.

Interactions with Foods
No interactions are known to occur, and there is no known reason to expect a clinically significant interaction with frankincense.

Interactions with Lab Tests
No interactions are known to occur, and there is no known reason to expect a clinically significant interaction with frankincense.

Interactions with Diseases or Conditions
No interactions are known to occur, and there is no known reason to expect a clinically significant interaction with frankincense.

Dosage and Administration
No typical dosage.

Comments
Frankincense is the hardened gum resin extruded from incisions made in the trunk of Boswellia carteri. Olibanum is a term which refers to the oleogum resin exuded from incisions in the bark of several Boswellia species, including Boswellia serrata (Indian frankincense), Boswellia carterii (Bible frankincense), Boswellia frereana (African elemi), and Boswellia bhau-dajiana (11). The black kohl used by Egyptian women to paint their eyelids is an ingredient from charred frankincense. Frankincense is considered obsolete as a medicinal herb (18).

FRINGETREE

Also Known As
Chionanthus, Fringe Tree, Gray Beard Tree, Old Man's Beard, Poison Ash, Snowdrop Tree, Snowflower, White Fringe.

Scientific Names
Chionanthus virginicus.
Family: Oleaceae.

People Use This For

Orally, fringetree is used for the treatment of liver and gallbladder disorders, including gallstones. It is also used orally to stimulate bile flow, as a diuretic, and as a tonic (18).

Safety

There is insufficient reliable information available about the safety of fringetree.
Pregnancy and Lactation: Insufficient reliable information available; avoid using.

Effectiveness

There is insufficient reliable information available about the effectiveness of fringetree.

Mechanism of Action

There is insufficient reliable information available about the possible mechanism of action and active ingredients.

Adverse Reactions

None reported.

Interactions with Herbs & Other Dietary Supplements

Insufficient reliable information available.

Interactions with Drugs

No interactions are known to occur, and there is no known reason to expect a clinically significant interaction with fringetree.

Interactions with Foods

No interactions are known to occur, and there is no known reason to expect a clinically significant interaction with fringetree.

Interactions with Lab Tests

No interactions are known to occur, and there is no known reason to expect a clinically significant interaction with fringetree.

Interactions with Diseases or Conditions

No interactions are known to occur, and there is no known reason to expect a clinically significant interaction with fringetree.

Dosage and Administration

ORAL: Fringetree has been used as a liquid extract (18).

Comments

Fringetree is almost odorless and very bitter to taste (18).
There is very little scientific information about this product. Our staff is continually analyzing the available information on natural medicines and will add data here as it becomes available.

FROSTWORT

Also Known As

Frost Plant, Frostweed, Rock-Rose, Sun Rose.

Scientific Names

Helianthemum canadense.

People Use This For

Orally, frostwort is used for digestive disorders (18).
Topically, frostwort is used for ulcers (18).

Safety

There is insufficient reliable information available about the safety of frostwort.
Pregnancy and Lactation: Insufficient reliable information available; avoid using.

Effectiveness

There is insufficient reliable information available about the effectiveness of frostwort.

Mechanism of Action

The applicable parts of frostwort are the above ground parts. Frostwort contains tannins and the glycoside helianthinin. It appears to have astringent and tonic effects (18).

Adverse Reactions

None reported.

Interactions with Herbs & Other Dietary Supplements

Insufficient reliable information available.

Interactions with Drugs

No interactions are known to occur, and there is no known reason to expect a clinically significant interaction with frostwort.

Interactions with Foods

No interactions are known to occur, and there is no known reason to expect a clinically significant interaction with frostwort.

Interactions with Lab Tests

No interactions are known to occur, and there is no known reason to expect a clinically significant interaction with frostwort.

Interactions with Diseases or Conditions

No interactions are known to occur, and there is no known reason to expect a clinically significant interaction with frostwort.

Dosage and Administration

ORAL: Frostwort has been used as an extract (18).

Comments

There is very little scientific information about this product. Our staff is continually analyzing the available information on natural medicines and will add data here as it becomes available.

FRUCTO-OLIGOSACCHARIDES

Also Known As

FOS, Fructo Oligo Saccharides, Fructooligosaccharides, Oligofructose.

Scientific Names

Beta-D-fructofuranosidase.

People Use This For

Orally, fructo-oligosaccharides are used for prebiotic activity, specifically for bifidobacteria in the GI tract (742). Prebiotic refers to the use of a substance to promote the growth of GI flora. Fructo-oligosaccharides are also used orally for reducing serum cholesterol (743) and increasing fecal mass (744).
In foods, fructo-oligosaccharides are used as a sweetener (740,741).

Safety

POSSIBLY SAFE ...when used orally in amounts less than 30 grams per day (741,745).
PREGNANCY AND LACTATION: Insufficient reliable information available; avoid using.

Effectiveness

There is insufficient reliable information available about the effectiveness of fructo-oligosaccharides.

Mechanism of Action

Fructo-oligosaccharides (FOS) pass undigested through the small intestine and are fermented in the colon. In the colon, they specifically promote the growth of some species of the indigenous microflora, especially bifidobacteria. FOS are not hydrolyzed by human digestive enzymes (746), yet they are not recoverable in the feces suggesting complete colonic metabolism (747). Colonic fermentation leads to increased fecal biomass, decreased ceco-colonic pH, and production of short chain fatty acids. The short chain fatty acids exert systemic effects on lipid metabolism similarly to dietary fiber (744). FOS can counteract advanced stages of colon carcinogenesis in mice (748).

Adverse Reactions
Orally, the use of FOS can cause flatulence in amounts exceeding 10 grams (740), excessive flatus at 30 grams per day, GI sounds and bloating at 40 grams per day, and abdominal cramps and diarrhea at 50 grams per day (745).

Interactions with Herbs & Other Dietary Supplements
BIFIDOBACTERIUM BIFIDUM: Concomitant use of FOS can promote the growth of supplemental bifidobacteria.

Interactions with Drugs
No interactions are known to occur, and there is no known reason to expect a clinically significant interaction with fructo-oligosaccharides.

Interactions with Foods
No interactions are known to occur, and there is no known reason to expect a clinically significant interaction with fructo-oligosaccharides.

Interactions with Lab Tests
No interactions are known to occur, and there is no known reason to expect a clinically significant interaction with fructo-oligosaccharides.

Interactions with Diseases or Conditions
No interactions are known to occur, and there is no known reason to expect a clinically significant interaction with fructo-oligosaccharides.

Dosage and Administration
ORAL: For prebiotic effect (to increase fecal bifidobacteria), the typical dose is 4 to 10 grams per day (749,750).

Comments
Fructo-oligosaccharides are non-digestible plant sugars derived from asparagus, Jerusalem artichokes, and soybeans.

FUMITORY

Also Known As
Beggary, Earth Smoke, Fumiterry, Fumus, Hedge Fumitory, Herba fumariae, Vapor, Wax Dolls.

Scientific Names
Fumaria officinalis.
Family: Fumariaceae.

People Use This For
Orally, fumitory is used for GI spasms (2) and as a bile flow stimulant (4).
Historically, fumitory has been used for skin eruptions (4), eczema (6), conjunctivitis (4), and cardiovascular disorders (6), and as a diuretic and laxative (4,6).

Safety
POSSIBLY SAFE ...when above ground parts are used orally and appropriately. No significant toxicity usually occurs in standard doses (4,6).
POSSIBLY UNSAFE ...when used orally in large amounts because it contains the alkaloid protopine. Other Fumariaceae species that contain alkaloids including protopine can cause convulsions and death when large amounts are ingested (6). ...when homemade, non-sterile products are used for ophthalmic use (4).
PREGNANCY AND LACTATION: Insufficient reliable information available; avoid using (4).

Effectiveness
POSSIBLY EFFECTIVE ...when used orally for biliary disorders (4,6,280).
There is insufficient reliable information available about the effectiveness of fumitory for its other uses.

Mechanism of Action

The applicable parts of fumitory are the above ground parts. Fumitory can have weak antispasmodic effects on the smooth muscle of the bile duct and upper GI tract (2,4,18). The major alkaloid constituent, protopine, has antihistamine, hypotensive, bradycardic, and sedative activity in small doses, and it causes excitation and convulsions in large doses (4). Fumitory can exhibit bactericidal activity against gram-positive organisms, including Bacillus anthracis and Staphylococcus (4).

Adverse Reactions

Orally, adverse reactions to fumitory are not common; however, large quantities of alkaloids in other members of this family (Fumariaceae) have caused trembling, convulsions, and death (2).

Interactions with Herbs & Other Dietary Supplements

Insufficient reliable information available.

Interactions with Drugs

No interactions are known to occur, and there is no known reason to expect a clinically significant interaction with fumitory.

Interactions with Foods

No interactions are known to occur, and there is no known reason to expect a clinically significant interaction with fumitory.

Interactions with Lab Tests

No interactions are known to occur, and there is no known reason to expect a clinically significant interaction with fumitory.

Interactions with Diseases or Conditions

No interactions are known to occur, and there is no known reason to expect a clinically significant interaction with fumitory.

Dosage and Administration

ORAL: The typical dose of fumitory is 2-4 grams of the above ground parts per day or as a tea 3 times daily (4). The tea is prepared by steeping the herb in 150 mL boiling water for 5-10 minutes and then straining. The usual dose of the liquid extract (1:1 in 25% alcohol) is 2-4 mL 3 times daily, and the tincture (1:5 in 45% alcohol) is commonly dosed 1-4 mL 3 times daily (4).
INHALATION: Nebulizers have been used to administer the extract; no typical dosage. (6).

Comments

The fumitory plant is a low shrub with gray pointed leaves, and from a distance the plant can have the wispy appearance of smoke, because of this it received the name "earth smoke" (6).

GABA (GAMMA-AMINOBUTYRIC ACID)

Also Known As

GABA, Gamma Amino Butyric Acid, Gamma Amino-Butyric Acid, Gamma Aminobutyric Acid.

Scientific Names

Gamma-aminobutyric acid.

People Use This For

Orally, GABA is used for relieving anxiety, elevating mood, relieving premenstrual syndrome (PMS), promoting lean muscle growth, burning fat, stabilizing blood pressure, and relieving pain (5111,5112).
Sublingually, GABA is used for increasing feeling of well being, relieving injuries, improving exercise tolerance, decreasing body fat, and increasing lean body weight (5471).

Safety

There is insufficient reliable information available about the safety of GABA.
Pregnancy and Lactation: Insufficient reliable information available; avoid using.

Effectiveness

There is insufficient reliable information available about the effectiveness of GABA.

Mechanism of Action

In the central nervous system, GABA is the primary inhibitory neurotransmitter. It is synthesized in the brain by decarboxylation of glutamate (5109,5110). GABA exerts anticonvulsant, sedative, and anxiolytic effects at the cellular level (5109,5110). Single, oral doses of GABA given to people with photo-convulsant epilepsy had no effect (5113). Single, oral doses of 5 or 10 grams of GABA caused a rise in C-peptide, insulin, and glucagon but not serum glucose in healthy people (5114). GABA given intravenously can cause dysphoria and dose-related increases in blood pressure and pulse (5116). In healthy volunteers, a single 5 gram dose of GABA increased growth hormone, but chronic four-day administration of 18 grams of GABA decreased growth hormone and increased serum prolactin (5115).

Adverse Reactions

None reported.

Interactions with Herbs & Other Dietary Supplements

Insufficient reliable information available.

Interactions with Drugs

No interactions are known to occur, and there is no known reason to expect a clinically significant interaction with GABA.

Interactions with Foods

No interactions are known to occur, and there is no known reason to expect a clinically significant interaction with GABA.

Interactions with Lab Tests

No interactions are known to occur, and there is no known reason to expect a clinically significant interaction with GABA.

Interactions with Diseases or Conditions

No interactions are known to occur, and there is no known reason to expect a clinically significant interaction with GABA.

Dosage and Administration

ORAL: People typically use 500 to 2250 mg daily, although some products suggest doses ranging from 250 mg to 5000 mg daily (5117,5118,6006). Some products recommend bedtime dosing (6006).
SUBLINGUAL: People typically use 3 to 5 grams 1 to 2 times daily (5471).

Comments

Although GABA is promoted as an alternative to the benzodiazepines (5111,5112), no clinical trials support these uses.

GALBANUM

Also Known As

Galbanum Gum, Galbanum Gum Resin, Galbanum Oleogum Resin, Galbanum Oleoresin, Galbanum Resin.

Scientific Names

Ferula gummosa.
Family: Umbelliferae.

People Use This For

Orally, galbanum is used for digestive disorders and flatulence. It is used orally as an appetite stimulant, expectorant (18), and antispasmodic (11).
Topically, galbanum is used for wound treatment (18).
In food and beverages, galbanum oil and resin are used as flavor components.
In manufacturing, galbanum oil and resin are used as fragrance components in cosmetics. Galbanum is rarely used in pharmaceuticals (11).

Safety

LIKELY SAFE …when used orally in amounts typically found in foods (11). It is approved for food use in the US.
POSSIBLY SAFE …when used topically (11).
There is insufficient reliable information available about the safety of the oral use of galbanum in amounts greater than those typically found in foods.
PREGNANCY AND LACTATION: LIKELY SAFE …when used orally in amounts typically found in foods (11). Avoid using in amounts greater than those typically found in foods. There is insufficient reliable information available about the safety of the oral use of galbanum in amounts greater than those typically found in foods during pregnancy.

Effectiveness

There is insufficient reliable information available about the effectiveness of galbanum.

Mechanism of Action

The applicable part of galbanum is the gum resin from the roots and trunk. In vitro data suggest antimicrobial activity, particularly against Staphylococcus aureus. Galbanum may also be effective as an emulsion preservative. Emulsions containing galbanum were stable for up to 6 months (11).

Adverse Reactions

None reported.

Interactions with Herbs & Other Dietary Supplements

Insufficient reliable information available.

Interactions with Drugs

No interactions are known to occur, and there is no known reason to expect a clinically significant interaction with galbanum.

Interactions with Foods

No interactions are known to occur, and there is no known reason to expect a clinically significant interaction with galbanum.

Interactions with Lab Tests

No interactions are known to occur, and there is no known reason to expect a clinically significant interaction with galbanum.

Interactions with Diseases or Conditions

No interactions are known to occur, and there is no known reason to expect a clinically significant interaction with galbanum.

Dosage and Administration

No typical dosage.

Comments

None.

GAMBOGE

Also Known As

Camboge, Gambodia, Gummigutta, Gutta Cambodia, Gutta Gamba, Tom Rong.
CAUTION: See separate listing for Garcinia.

Scientific Names

Garcinia hanburyi.
Family: Clusiaceae.

People Use This For

Orally, gamboge is used for constipation, generally in combination with other laxatives (18).
Historically, gamboge has been used for the evacuation of intestinal worms (215).

Safety
POSSIBLY UNSAFE ...when used orally. Deaths have been reported with ingestion of 4 grams (18).
PREGNANCY AND LACTATION: POSSIBLY UNSAFE ...when used orally; avoid using.

Effectiveness
There is insufficient reliable information available about the effectiveness of gamboge.

Mechanism of Action
The applicable part of gamboge is the resin. It contains resins (benzophenones and xanthones) and mucilages. Gamboge reportedly has strong laxative effect (18).

Adverse Reactions
Orally, abdominal pain and vomiting has been reported with as little as 200 mg; deaths were reported with ingestion of 4 grams (18).

Interactions with Herbs & Other Dietary Supplements
DIGITALIS: Theoretically, overuse/misuse may cause potassium depletion and increase risk of cardiotoxicity.
STIMULANT LAXATIVE HERBS: Theoretically, concomitant use with other stimulant laxative herbs may increase the risk of potassium depletion. Stimulant laxative herbs include: aloe dried leaf sap, wild cucumber fruit (Ecballium elaterium), blue flag rhizome, alder buckthorn, European buckthorn, butternut bark, cascara bark, castor oil, colocynth fruit pulp, jalap root, black root, manna bark exudate, podophyllum root, rhubarb root, senna leaves and pods, and yellow dock root (19).
POTASSIUM DEPLETING HERBS: Theoretically, concomitant use with horsetail plant or licorice rhizome increases the risk of potassium depletion.

Interactions with Drugs
DIGOXIN: Theoretically, overuse/misuse may cause potassium depletion and increase risk of cardiotoxicity.
LAXATIVES: Theoretically, concomitant use may increase risk of fluid and electrolyte loss.
POTASSIUM DEPLETING DRUGS: Theoretically, concomitant use may increase risk of potassium depletion.
CARDIAC GLYCOSIDES: Theoretically, overuse/abuse of this product increases the risk of adverse effects of cardiac glycoside drugs, e.g., digoxin (Lanoxin).

Interactions with Foods
No interactions are known to occur, and there is no known reason to expect a clinically significant interaction with gamboge.

Interactions with Lab Tests
No interactions are known to occur, and there is no known reason to expect a clinically significant interaction with gamboge.

Interactions with Diseases or Conditions
HEART CONDITIONS: Theoretically, overuse/misuse may cause potassium depletion and exacerbate condition. Gamboge is contraindicated in intestinal obstruction, acute intestinal inflammation (Crohn's disease, ulcerative colitis, appendicitis), ulcer, abdominal pain of unknown origin, nausea, and vomiting.

Dosage and Administration
ORAL: People typically use 2 to 5 grains (130 to 325 mg) (5269). Some use a maximum dose of 10 mg (5264).

Comments
The resin is extracted from Garcinia hanburyi. Avoid confusion with garcinia (Garcinia cambogia).
Gamboge may be adulterated with rice and wheat starches, sand, and vegetable fragments. These adulterated products are usually coarser and hard (215).

GAMMA BUTYROLACTONE (GBL)

Also Known As
1,2-Butanolide, 2(3H)-Furanone Dihydro, 3-Hydroxybutyric Acid Lactone, 4-Butanolide, 4-Butyrolactone, 4-Hydroxybutanoic Acid Lactone, Butyrolactone, Butyrolactone Gamma, Dihydro-2(3H)-Furanone, Gamma Butyrolactone, Gamma Hydroxybutyric Acid Lactone, GBL, Tetrahydro-2-Furanone.
CAUTION: See seprate listings for Gamma Hydroxybutyrate (GHB) and Butanediol (BD).

Scientific Names

2,3 dihydro furanone; synonyms 2(3H) furanone dihydro, butyrolactone gamma, 2(3H)-furanone dihydro, butyrolactone, 4-butyrolactone, dihydro-2(3H)-furanone, 4-butanolide, tetrahydro-2-furanone.

People Use This For

Orally, gamma butyrolactone is used for relaxation, calming, increased mental clarity, fat loss, as a body or muscle "builder", recreational drug, for releasing growth hormone, improving athletic performance, inducing and improving sleep, relieving depression and stress, prolonging life, and improving sexual performance and pleasure (682,1430,1432).

Safety

UNSAFE ...when used orally. The use of GBL or the closely related substances gamma hydroxybutyrate (GHB) and butanediol (BD) has been linked to at least 3 deaths and 122 serious adverse effects (3678,3679). GBL can cause dangerously low respiratory rates and heart rates, seizures, and coma (4259).
PREGNANCY AND LACTATION: UNSAFE ...when used orally; avoid using.

Effectiveness

There is insufficient reliable information available about the effectiveness of gamma butyrolactone (GBL).

Mechanism of Action

Gamma butyrolactone (GBL) is metabolized in the body to gamma hydroxybutyrate (GHB) (see separate listing) (1430). However, it is more rapidly absorbed than GHB, has greater lipid solubility, and may avoid first-pass metabolism due to its lactone structure (5813). This can lead to higher serum concentrations and more marked hypnotic activity than with similar doses of GHB (5813). GHB can be converted in the brain to the neurotransmitter gamma aminobutyric acid (GABA) (14,3699), and specific GHB uptake systems, transport systems and receptors have also been identified (14,713,3699,5800,5801). Stimulation of GHB receptors reduces dopamine release in the brain (14,713,3699,5801), which may be the mechanism for GBL-induced reductions in dopamine neuronal impulse flow (5811). GBL has been reported to inhibit stereotyped behavior induced by dopamine agonists (5810,5811). The indirect dopamine agonist amphetamine has been reported to partially reverse effects of GBL (5810). GBL may also have some direct GABA agonist activity (5802), although the GABA antagonist bicuculline only partially reverses GBL-induced inhibition of apomorphine activity (5810). GBL, possibly through conversion to GHB, also affects the endogenous opioid system, and the opiate antagonists naloxone and naltrexone attenuate or abolish the electrical seizure activity, behavioral abnormalities, and increased striatal dopamine content produced by GBL (5812). GHB produces general anesthesia (14), induces REM and non-REM sleep, hypothermia, abnormalities on the EEG similar to those seen in petit mal epilepsy (5800,5803), and it stimulates growth hormone secretion (5804).

Adverse Reactions

GBL is converted to gamma hydroxybutyrate (GHB) (see separate listing) in the body and can therefore be associated with the same life-threatening adverse effects (14). Oral ingestion of GBL has been associated with at least 55 cases of adverse effects (at least five cases involving children), including involuntary muscle movements, fainting and seizures, bowel incontinence, vomiting, slow breathing, respiratory depression, apnea, slow heart rate, mental changes, severe central nervous system depression, agitation, combativeness and amnesia. One death, two cases of respiratory arrest, and one case of cardiac arrest have been reported. Nineteen of the 55 cases involved unconsciousness or coma, and in some cases intubation was required for assisted breathing (665,666,682,1430). Withdrawal symptoms, including insomnia, tremor and anxiety, can occur in chronic users of gamma hydroxybutyrate (GHB), and are predicted to occur in chronic GBL users (1430).

Interactions with Herbs & Other Dietary Supplements

PRODUCTS WITH SEDATIVE EFFECTS: Concomitant use is likely to cause additive sedation with GBL, increasing the risk of serious adverse effects.

Interactions with Drugs

ALCOHOL: GHB (a metabolite of GBL) acts synergistically with alcohol to produce CNS and respiratory depression (1430).
NARCOTIC ANALGESICS: Concomitant use with GHB (a metabolite of GBL) can potentiate the therapeutic and adverse effects of narcotic analgesics (14).
D-AMPHETAMINE: Theoretically, concomitant use might antagonize the effects of amphetamine (14), and amphetamine has been reported to partially reverse the effects of GBL (5810).
BENZODIAZEPINES, NEUROLEPTICS: Concomitant use with GHB (a metabolite of GBL) can potentiate the effects of GHB (14,3682).
DRUGS WITH SEDATIVE EFFECTS: Any sedative drug could theoretically increase the risk of serious adverse effects with GBL.

D-AMPHETAMINE, NALOXONE, HALOPERIDOL, DRUGS USED FOR ABSENCE SEIZURES: Concomitant use with GHB (a metabolite of GBL) may antagonize the effects of GHB, but these agents have not been assessed as possible treatments for GHB or GBL overdose (3682).

RITONAVIR (Norvir), SAQUINAVIR (Fortovase, Invirase): Concomitant use of the protease inhibitor-type antiretroviral drugs ritonavir and saquinavir with GHB (a metabolite of GBL) reportedly caused a near-fatal reaction, probalby due to inhibition of GHB metabolism (1431).

SKELETAL MUSCLE RELAXANTS: Concomitant use with GHB (a metabolite of GBL) can potentiate the therapeutic and adverse effects of skeletal muscle relaxants (14,3682).

Interactions with Foods

ALCOHOL: GHB (a metabolite of GBL) acts synergistically with alcohol to produce CNS and respiratory depression (1430).

Interactions with Lab Tests

GAMMA HYDROXYBUTYRATE (GHB): The mass spectrometry assay for GHB used in either urine or serum studies is unable to differentiate between GHB and GBL (14).

Interactions with Diseases or Conditions

HYPERTENSION OR BRADYCARDIA: GHB and GBL should be avoided since they may exacerbate these conditions (14).

CARDIAC CONDUCTION DEFECTS: GHB and GBL should be avoided due to the risk of bradycardia (14).

EPILEPSY: GHB and GBL should be avoided due to their possible capacity to induce seizures (14).

RENAL IMPAIRMENT: GHB and GBL should be avoided due to possible accumulation (14).

Dosage and Administration

No typical dosage.

Comments

FDA WARNING: Avoid all gamma butyrolactone containing products due to safety concerns (682). GBL has been marketed as an alternative to gamma hydroxybutyrate (GHB), but it is illegal to manufacture or market GBL or the related products GHB and butanediol (BD) (3678). Publication of a Federal Register notice on 3/13/00 brought into effect the Hillory J. Farias and Samantha Reid Date-Rape Drug Prohibition Act of 2000, which effected changes to the Controlled Substances Act, making GHB a schedule 1 controlled substance (like heroin), and GBL a list 1 chemical (3681). GBL, GHB and BD are associated with at least 122 reports of serious adverse effects including dangerously low respiratory rates (intubation might be required), unconsciousness/coma, vomiting, seizures, slowed heart rate, and death (4259).

GAMMA-HYDROXYBUTYRATE (GHB)

Also Known As

4-Hydroxy Butyrate, Gamma Hydrate, Gamma Hydroxybutyrate Sodium, Gamma Hydroxybutyric Acid, Gamma-OH, GHB, Sodium gamma-hydroxybutyrate, Sodium Oxybate, Sodium Oxybutyrate.
CAUTION: See separate listings for Gamma Butyrolactone (GBL) and Butanediol (BD).

Scientific Names

Gamma hydroxybutyrate; 4-hydroxybutyric acid; Sodium 4-hydroxybutyrate.

People Use This For

Orally, gamma hydroxybutyrate (GHB) is used for reducing weight, enhancing muscle growth, as an aphrodisiac (712,714), as an hypnotic (3693), for management of opiate withdrawal and alcohol dependence and withdrawal (3684,3686,3694,3695,3696), and for posthypoxic cerebral edema (3682). It is also used for improving pain, fatigue, and the alpha sleep anomaly in patients with fibromyalgia (711).

Traditionally, it has been used as a sedative alternative to the dietary supplement L-tryptophan (3682,3687).

As an investigational orphan drug, it has been designated by the FDA for treatment of narcolepsy (improving nighttime sleep, and the auxiliary symptoms of cataplexy, sleep paralysis, hypnagogic hallucinations, and automatic behavior) (14).

Intravenously, GHB has been used as part of an anesthetic regimen (14), and to reduce intracranial pressure associated with trauma (3685).

Safety

POSSIBLY SAFE ...when used orally and appropriately. GHB has FDA orphan drug status (4261).

UNSAFE ...Tell patients not to use GHB without medical supervision. It can cause serious side effects including dangerously low respiratory rates, tonic-clonic seizure, coma and death if used inappropriately (see Adverse Reactions) (3678,3679,3680,3688,4259).

There is insufficient reliable information available about the safety of intravenous GHB as a component of general anesthesia.

PREGNANCY AND LACTATION: UNSAFE ...when used orally. GHB has been associated with life-threatening toxicities (3678,3679,3680,3688,4259); contraindicated.

Effectiveness

POSSIBLY EFFECTIVE ...when used orally for improving overnight sleep quality and reducing cataplexy in people with narcolepsy (3683,3689,3690,3691,3692). GHB has FDA investigational orphan drug status for treatment of narcolepsy and associated symptoms (4261). ...when used orally as a hypnotic (3693). ...when used orally for fibromyalgia-associated pain, fatigue and alpha sleep anomaly (711). ...when used orally for management of opiate withdrawal and alcohol dependence and withdrawal (3684,3686,3694,3695,3696).

There is insufficient reliable information available about the effectiveness of GHB for its other uses. However, limited evidence suggests that low doses of GHB given intravenously might be effective as a part of an anesthetic regimen (3697,3698). Further evidence is needed to rate the effectiveness of GHB for this use.

Mechanism of Action

GHB occurs naturally in several areas of the brain, with the highest concentrations found in the basal ganglia (14), and is also found in peripheral tissues including kidneys, heart, skeletal muscle and brown fat (3682). In the brain, it is formed as a metabolite of the neurotransmitter gamma aminobutyric acid (GABA), and can also be converted back to GABA during metabolism (14,3699). Specific uptake and transport systems have been identified for GHB in the brain (3699,5800), and specific GHB receptors have been identified (14,713,5801). Stimulation of GHB receptors results in a reduction in dopamine release in the basal ganglia (14,713,5801), and it also influences dopamine release in the substantia nigra (3699). Some authors suggest that GHB interacts with GABA(B) receptors (14,713), but others report that GABA formed from GHB is likely involved and that GHB itself is not a GABA agonist (5801,5802). Another GHB metabolite, gamma butyrolactone (GBL) may have some GABA agonist activity (5802). GHB has also been reported to affect the endogenous opioid system, raising dynorphin levels (3682,5803).

GHB produces general anesthesia, possibly by a general suppressant action on the entire cerebrospinal axis, and muscle relaxation by an action on the spinal cord (14). It also induces REM and non-REM sleep, hypothermia, and abnormalities on the EEG similar to those seen in petit mal epilepsy (5800,5803). It stimulates growth hormone secretion which occurs during slow wave sleep (5804), and this has led to claims of anabolic effects (3688). It is also involved in preventing the production of, and scavenging oxygen-derived free radicals in the brain (3682,5805). It decreases brain glucose utilization (3683), lowers cerebral energy requirements and it may play a neuroprotective role, protecting against the effects of anoxia or excessive metabolic demand (3682,5800,5803). It has been suggested that the natural function of GHB may be to induce and maintain physiological states such as sleep and hibernation in which energy utilization is depressed (5803). Some of the effects of GHB are antagonized by the opiate antagonist, naloxone and anticonvulsant drugs (5800), but the stimulation of growth hormone release is antagonized by flumazenil (a benzodiazepine antagonist) and metergoline (a serotonin receptor antagonist) (5806).

The effects of GHB on sleep have been used to improve nighttime sleep quality, sleep continuity, stage 3 and 4 sleep, and cataplexy in people with narcolepsy, with some studies also reporting a reduction in the number of daytime sleep attacks (3689,3690,3691,3692).

Studies in rats indicate that a cross-tolerance can develop between GHB and ethanol with chronic exposure, leading to investigations of GHB for management of ethanol dependence and withdrawal (14,3686). Efficacy has also been reported in the management of opiate withdrawal (3694,3695), although a fatality occurred when GHB and heroin were taken concurrently (5807).

Adverse Reactions

Orally, GHB can cause headaches, hallucinations, dizziness, confusion, nausea, vomiting, drowsiness, agitation, and diarrhea. It can also cause sexual arousal, numbing of legs, loss of peripheral vision, tightness of chest, slowed heart rate, depressed respiration, nystagmus, ataxia, eosinophilia-myalgia syndrome, and seizure-like activity (14,6016). The symptoms usually occur within 15 to 60 minutes and subside within 2 to 96 hours, although dizziness can continue for up to 14 days. Doses of GHB greater than 10 mg/kg can cause amnesia and reduced muscle tone (14,6016). Doses between 20-30 mg/kg can cause somnolence (14), and doses greater than 50 mg/kg can cause abrupt unconsciousness and coma (14). GHB and the chemically-related products, gamma butyrolactone (GBL) and 1,4 butanediol, have been associated with at least 122 reports of serious adverse reactions including dangerously low respiratory rates, some requiring intubation; unconsciousness and coma; vomiting, seizures; bradycardia; and multiple deaths (3680,4259). At least two deaths involved the use of GHB and alcohol. Death occurred in less than 24 hours after ingestion and was due to circulatory and respiratory collapse. The amount of GHB consumed in these two cases is not known; however, the GHB levels in blood and urine were significantly elevated (6016). GHB can cause dependence requiring in-patient detoxification (6612,6613). Withdrawal symptoms have included insomnia, diarrhea, panic, terror, anxiety, and tremor (6612,6613).

Interactions with Herbs & Other Dietary Supplements

HERBS/SUPPLEMENTS WITH SEDATIVE PROPERTIES: Theoretically, concomitant use with herbs that have sedative properties might enhance therapeutic and adverse effects. These include calamus, calendula, California poppy, catnip, capsicum, celery, couch grass, elecampane, Siberian ginseng, German chamomile, goldenseal, gotu kola, hops, Jamaican dogwood, kava, lemon balm, Melatonin, sage, sassafras, scullcap, shepherd's purse, St. John's wort, stinging nettle, valerian, wild carrot, wild lettuce, ashwaganda root, and yerba mansa (4,19).

Interactions with Drugs

ALCOHOL: Concomitant use with GHB can potentiate the CNS and respiratory depression effects of alcohol and GHB (3682).
NARCOTIC ANALGESICS: Concomitant use with GHB can potentiate the therapeutic and adverse effects of narcotic analgesics (14); a fatality has been reported with concurrent use of GHB and heroin (5807).
BENZODIAZEPINES, NEUROLEPTICS: Concomitant use with GHB can potentiate the effects of GHB (14,3682).
DRUGS WITH SEDATIVE EFFECTS: Any sedative drug could theoretically increase the risk of serious adverse effects with GHB.
D-AMPHETAMINE, NALOXONE, HALOPERIDOL, DRUGS USED FOR ABSENCE SEIZURES: Concomitant use with GHB may antagonize the effects of GHB, but these agents have not been assessed as possible treatments for GHB overdose (3682).
SKELETAL MUSCLE RELAXANTS: Concomitant use with GHB can potentiate the therapeutic and adverse effects of skeletal muscle relaxants (14,3682).
RITONAVIR (Norvir), SAQUINAVIR (Fortovase, Invirase): Concomitant use of the protease inhibitor-type antiretroviral drugs ritonavir and saquinavir with GHB reportedly caused a near-fatal reaction, probably due to inhibition of GHB metabolism (1431).

Interactions with Foods

ALCOHOL: Concomitant use with GHB can potentiate the CNS and respiratory depression effects of alcohol and GHB (3682).

Interactions with Lab Tests

GAMMA BUTYROLACTONE (GBL): The mass spectrometry assay for GHB used in either urine or serum studies is unable to differentiate between GHB and GBL (14).

Interactions with Diseases or Conditions

HYPERTENSION OR BRADYCARDIA: GHB should be avoided since it may exacerbate these conditions (14).
CARDIAC CONDUCTION DEFECTS: GHB should be avoided due to the risk of bradycardia (14).
EPILEPSY: GHB should be avoided due to its possible capacity to induce seizures (14).
RENAL IMPAIRMENT: GHB should be avoided due to possible accumulation (14).

Dosage and Administration

ORAL: For narcolepsy and associate symptoms, a dose of 25 mg/kg at bedtime, repeated 3-hours later has been used (3689,3690). For treating alcohol dependence, 50 to 150 mg/kg divided into 3 to 6 doses per day has been used (3684,3696). As a hypnotic, 75-100 mg/kg has been used (3693).

Comments

Gamma butyrolactone (GBL) and butanediol (BD) (see separate listings) are closely related to GHB and produce similar adverse effects (3678,3679). Due to reports of serious adverse effects, the FDA removed GHB from the market in 1990, but clandestine manufacture continued, with the drug being widely available on the Internet, and being implicated as a date rape agent (3687). Publication of a Federal Register notice on 3/13/00 brought into effect the Hillory J. Farias and Samantha Reid Date-Rape Drug Prohibition Act of 2000, which effected changes to the Controlled Substances Act, making GHB a schedule 1 controlled substance (like heroin), which it is illegal to produce, sell or possess (3680,3681). Orphan Medical is expected to submit a new drug application to the FDA during 2001 for GHB under the generic name sodium oxybate and trade name Xyrem, for the treatment of cataplexy associated with narcolepsy (3680). If approved, the drug would be in Schedule 3 of the Controlled Substances Act for this indication (3680,3681). To access information on sodium oxybate (Xyrem) for narcolepsy contact: Orphan Medical (1-888-867-7426).

GAMMA LINOLENIC ACID

Also Known As
Gamma-Linolenic Acid, Gamolenic Acid, GLA.
CAUTION: See separate listings for Black Currant Seed Oil, Borage Seed Oil, Evening Primrose Oil, and Omega-6 Oils.

Scientific Names
(Z,Z,Z)-Octadeca-6,9,12-trienoic acid.

People Use This For
Orally, gamma linolenic acid (GLA) is used for rheumatoid arthritis, oral mucoceles (mucous polyps), hyperlipidemia, systemic sclerosis, diabetic neuropathy, and to hasten the response to tamoxifen in people with breast cancer.

Safety
LIKELY SAFE ...when used orally (1983).
PREGNANCY AND LACTATION: Insufficient reliable information available; avoid using.

Effectiveness
POSSIBLY EFFECTIVE ...when used orally for rheumatoid arthritis (14). ...when used orally for diabetic neuropathy (1980,1981,1984). ...when used orally to hasten the response to tamoxifen in patients with breast cancer (5902).
POSSIBLY INEFFECTIVE ...when used orally for systemic sclerosis (1977).
There is insufficient reliable information available about the effectiveness of gamma linolenic acid for its other uses.

Mechanism of Action
Gamma linolenic acid (GLA) can be converted to compounds that have anti-inflammatory and antiproliferative properties (1975), including prostaglandins with vasoactive properties. Preliminary evidence suggests GLA can hasten the response to tamoxifen in individuals with primary breast cancer that is estrogen-sensitive (5902). GLA is believed to benefit individuals who have ischemic lesions associated with systemic sclerosis (1977) and individuals with diabetic neuropathy (1980,1981). Some evidence suggests that gamma linolenic acid might lower plasma triglycerides, increase HDL cholesterol, and prolong bleeding time (1979).

Adverse Reactions
Orally, GLA might prolong bleeding time (1979).

Interactions with Herbs & Other Dietary Supplements
HERBS WITH ANTICOAGULANT/ANTIPLATELET POTENTIAL: Concomitant use of herbs that have coumarin constituents or affect platelet aggregation could theoretically increase the risk of bleeding in some people. These herbs include angelica, anise, arnica, asafoetida, bogbean, boldo, capsicum, celery, chamomile, clove, danshen, fenugreek, feverfew, garlic, ginger, ginkgo, ginseng (Panax), horse chestnut, horseradish, licorice, meadowsweet, prickly ash, onion, papain, passionflower, poplar, quassia, red clover, turmeric, wild carrot, wild lettuce, willow, and others (4,19).

Interactions with Drugs
ANTICOAGULANT/ANTIPLATELET DRUGS: Gamma-linolenic acid (GLA) appears to have anticoagulant effects (1979). Theoretically, taking GLA with other anticoagulant or antiplatelet drugs might increase the risk of bruising and bleeding. Some of these drugs include aspirin, clopidogrel (Plavix), nonsteroidal anti-inflammatory drugs (NSAIDs) such as diclofenac (Voltaren, Cataflam, others), ibuprofen (Advil, Motrin, others), naproxen (Anaprox, Naprosyn, others), dalteparin (Fragmin), enoxaparin (Lovenox), heparin, warfarin (Coumadin), and others.

Interactions with Foods
No interactions are known to occur, and there is no known reason to expect a clinically significant interaction with GLA.

Interactions with Lab Tests
BLEEDING TIME: Gamma linolenic acid inhibit platelet aggregation and prolong bleeding time and lab assay results (1979).
LIPID PROFILE: Gamma linolenic acid might lower plasma triglycerides and increase high-density lipoprotein (HDL) cholesterol (1979).

Interactions with Diseases or Conditions

BLEEDING DISORDERS: There is some concern that gamma linolenic acid (GLA) might prolong bleeding time and increase the risk of bruising and bleeding. GLA has platelet inhibiting effects (1979).

Dosage and Administration

ORAL: For rheumatoid arthritis, gamma linolenic acid (GLA) 1.1 grams per day has been used (1985). For diabetic neuropathy, 360 mg per day has been used (1984). For hyperlipidemia, 1.5-6 grams per day has been used (1976,1979).

Comments

Borage oil and evening primrose oil are often used as a source of gamma linolenic acid.

GAMMA ORYZANOL

Also Known As

Gamma-Oryzanol, Gamma-OZ, Oryzanol.

Scientific Names

Gamma oryzanol.

People Use This For

Orally, gamma oryzanol is used for hypercholesterolemia and dyslipidemia (752,754), increasing testosterone and human growth hormone levels (755), improving strength during resistance exercise training (751), and for treating symptoms associated with menopause and aging (757).

Safety

POSSIBLY SAFE ...when used orally and appropriately (751,752,753,754,755).
PREGNANCY AND LACTATION: Insufficient reliable information available; avoid using.

Effectiveness

POSSIBLY EFFECTIVE ...when used orally for lowering cholesterol in patients with dyslipidemia. There is some preliminary clinical evidence that gamma oryzanol can significantly decrease total cholesterol, low-density lipoprotein (LDL) cholesterol, and triglyceride levels. Effects on high-density lipoprotein (HDL) cholesterol levels are conflicting (752,757).
There is insufficient reliable information available about the effectiveness of gamma oryzanol for its other uses.

Mechanism of Action

Gamma oryzanol is a group of constituents derived primarily from rice bran oil. It is also found in wheat bran and some fruits and vegetables. Gamma oryzanol itself is poorly absorbed from the gut (755). Researchers think it might help lower cholesterol by decreasing cholesterol absorption from the gut (756). Gamma oryzanol is also often promoted for treating menopause, but it is unclear how it would work for this use. Some researchers suspect it might be helpful due to effects on luteinizing hormone (LH) (755). However, this effect has not been verified in humans. Some people use gamma oryzanol for increasing testosterone and growth hormone levels. However, gamma oryzanol appears to have no effect on these hormone levels (751). Animal studies using parenteral administration actually show gamma oryzanol can be anti-anabolic by suppressing the release of LH and increasing the release of catecholamines, dopamine, and norepinephrine in the brain (755). If this occurs in humans, gamma oryzanol might actually reduce testosterone production (755). There is some evidence gamma oryzanol can reduce elevated serum TSH levels in hypothyroid patients. Some researchers think gamma-oryzanol inhibits serum TSH levels by a direct action at the hypothalamus rather than the pituitary (753).

Adverse Reactions

None reported.

Interactions with Herbs & Other Dietary Supplements

Insufficient reliable information available.

Interactions with Drugs

No interactions are known to occur, and there is no known reason to expect a clinically significant interaction with gamma oryzanol.

Interactions with Foods

No interactions are known to occur, and there is no known reason to expect a clinically significant interaction with gamma oryzanol.

Interactions with Lab Tests

THYROID STIMULATING HORMONE (TSH): Gamma oryzanol can reduce serum TSH concentrations in patients with hypothyroidism (753).
CHOLESTEROL: Gamma oryzanol can reduce serum total cholesterol (752,757) and low-density lipoprotein (LDL) cholesterol (752) concentrations and test results. Gamma oryzanol might also increase serum high-density lipoprotein (HDL) cholesterol concentrations in some patients (757).
TRIGLYCERIDES: Gamma oryzanol can reduce serum triglyceride concentrations and test results (757).

Interactions with Diseases or Conditions

PRIMARY HYPOTHYROIDISM: Gamma oryzanol can decrease TSH serum levels (753).

Dosage and Administration

ORAL: For reducing serum cholesterol, the usual dose of gamma oryzanol is 300 mg daily (752,757). In one study, 100 mg three times daily was used (752).

Comments

Gamma oryzanol is an extraction product from rice bran oil.

GARCINIA

Also Known As

Brindal Berry, Brindall Berry, Brindle Berry, Garcinia Cambogi, Garcinia Cambogia, Gorikapuli, HCA, Hydroxycitrate, Hydroxycitric Acid, Malabar Tamarind.
CAUTION: See separate listings for Gamboge, Malabar Nut, and Tamarind.

Scientific Names

Garcinia cambogia.
Family: Clusiaceae.

People Use This For

Orally, garcinia is used for weight loss (728).
In folk medicine, garcinia is used for dysentery, as a purgative, and for treating worms and parasites (729).
For food uses, garcinia is used as a condiment in Thai and Indian cuisine (730).

Safety

POSSIBLY SAFE ...when used orally and appropriately for 12 weeks or less (728).
There is insufficient reliable information available about the safety of the long-term use of garcinia.
PREGNANCY AND LACTATION: Insufficient reliable information available; avoid using.

Effectiveness

POSSIBLY INEFFECTIVE ...when fruit rind extract is used orally for weight loss (728).
There is insufficient reliable information available about the effectiveness of garcinia for its other uses.

Mechanism of Action

The applicable parts of garcinia are the fruit and rind. Garcinia fruit rind extract reported to contain 50% hydroxycitric acid; theorized to interfere with lipogenesis (728).

Adverse Reactions

None reported.

Interactions with Herbs & Other Dietary Supplements

Insufficient reliable information available.

Interactions with Drugs

No interactions are known to occur, and there is no known reason to expect a clinically significant interaction with garcinia.

Interactions with Foods
No interactions are known to occur, and there is no known reason to expect a clinically significant interaction with garcinia.

Interactions with Lab Tests
No interactions are known to occur, and there is no known reason to expect a clinically significant interaction with garcinia.

Interactions with Diseases or Conditions
No interactions are known to occur, and there is no known reason to expect a clinically significant interaction with garcinia.

Dosage and Administration
ORAL: An extract containing 50% hydroxycitric acid has been used. Dosage of 1,000 mg three times daily was used in a study that found garcinia ineffective for weight loss (728).

Comments
Avoid confusion with gamboge resin (Garcinia hanburyi).

GARDEN CRESS

Also Known As
None.

Scientific Names
Lepidium sativum.
Family: Cruciferae.

People Use This For
Orally, garden cress is used for coughs and vitamin C deficiency.
In folk medicine, garden cress is used orally for constipation, poor immunity, and as a diuretic (18).

Safety
There is insufficient reliable information available about the safety of garden cress.
Pregnancy and Lactation: Insufficient reliable information available; avoid using.

Effectiveness
There is insufficient reliable information available about the effectiveness of garden cress.

Mechanism of Action
The applicable parts of garden cress are the above ground parts. Garden cress may have in vitro antibacterial activity, but the activity appears to be dependent on the age of the plant at harvest. It also appears to have antiviral activity against the encephalitis virus Columbia SH (animal data) (18).

Adverse Reactions
Orally, ingesting large amounts of garden cress may cause gastrointestinal irritation (18).

Interactions with Herbs & Other Dietary Supplements
Insufficient reliable information available.

Interactions with Drugs
No interactions are known to occur, and there is no known reason to expect a clinically significant interaction with garden cress.

Interactions with Foods
No interactions are known to occur, and there is no known reason to expect a clinically significant interaction with garden cress.

Interactions with Lab Tests

No interactions are known to occur, and there is no known reason to expect a clinically significant interaction with garden cress.

Interactions with Diseases or Conditions

No interactions are known to occur, and there is no known reason to expect a clinically significant interaction with garden cress.

Dosage and Administration

ORAL: Garden cress is used as a fresh use herb in oral preparations (18).

Comments

Garden cress is rarely adulterated because it is usually cultivated rather than harvested (18).

GARDEN VIOLET

Also Known As

None.
CAUTION: See separate listing for Sweet Violet.

Scientific Names

Viola odorata.
Family: Violaceae.

People Use This For

Orally, garden violet is used for acute and chronic bronchitis, bronchial asthma, acute and chronic inflammation of the respiratory tract, and cold symptoms.
Topically, garden violet is used in skin lavages for treating various skin diseases (18).
In folk medicine, garden violet is used orally for coughs, hoarseness, tuberculosis, as an expectorant for throat inflammation and bronchitis accompanied by fixed mucous, nervous strain, insomnia, and hysteria.

Safety

There is insufficient reliable information available about the safety of garden violet.
Pregnancy and Lactation: Insufficient reliable information available; avoid using.

Effectiveness

There is insufficient reliable information available about the effectiveness of garden violet.

Mechanism of Action

The applicable parts of garden violet are the whole plant and the essential oil from the leaves. There is insufficient reliable information available about the possible mechanism of action and active ingredients.

Adverse Reactions

None reported.

Interactions with Herbs & Other Dietary Supplements

Insufficient reliable information available.

Interactions with Drugs

No interactions are known to occur, and there is no known reason to expect a clinically significant interaction with garden violet.

Interactions with Foods

No interactions are known to occur, and there is no known reason to expect a clinically significant interaction with garden violet.

Interactions with Lab Tests

No interactions are known to occur, and there is no known reason to expect a clinically significant interaction with garden violet.

Interactions with Diseases or Conditions

No interactions are known to occur, and there is no known reason to expect a clinically significant interaction with garden violet.

Dosage and Administration

ORAL: Typically, one cup tea is taken 2-3 times daily. The tea is prepared by steeping 2 teaspoons of dried herb in 250 mL of boiling water for 10-15 minutes and straining [18].
TOPICAL: No typical dosage.

Comments

There is very little scientific information about this product. Our staff is continually analyzing the available information on natural medicines and will add data here as it becomes available.

GARLIC

Also Known As

Aged Garlic Extract, Ail, Ajo, Allii Sativi Bulbus, Allium, Camphor of the Poor, Clove Garlic, Garlic Clove, Nectar of the Gods, Poor Man's Treacle, Rust Treacle, Stinking Rose.

Scientific Names

Allium sativum.
Family: Amaryllidaceae or Liliaceae.

People Use This For

Orally, garlic is used for hypertension, hyperlipidemia and preventing coronary heart disease, preventing age-related vascular changes and atherosclerosis [2,4,3315,3319,3321], reducing reinfarction and mortality rate post-myocardial infarction [4], earaches, and menstrual disorders [6121]. Garlic is also used orally for HIV-drug induced lipid disorders, treatment of Helicobacter pylori infection, and cancer prevention [14,3316,3319,3320,3321,3322]. Other uses include immune system stimulation; treatment of diabetes, arthritis, allergies, traveler's diarrhea, colds and flu; prevention of tick bites; and prevention and treatment of bacterial and fungal infections [3318,3319,3321,4760]. An aged garlic extract has been used orally for enhancing circulation, fighting stress and fatigue, and maintaining healthy liver function [1872].
Topically, garlic oil is used for tinea pedis [14,5121], tinea corporis, tinea cruris [4766,4767,5121], and onychomycosis [5121]. Intravaginally, garlic is used alone or in combination with yogurt for vaginitis [5121].
In traditional Chinese medicine, garlic is used for diarrhea, amoebic and bacterial dysentery, tuberculosis, bloody urine, diphtheria, whooping cough, scalp ringworm, hypersensitive teeth, and vaginal trichomoniasis [11,3321]. Garlic has also been traditionally used to treat colds, flu symptoms, fever, coughs, headache, stomachache, sinus congestion, athlete's foot, gout, rheumatism, hemorrhoids, asthma, bronchitis, shortness of breath, arteriosclerosis, low blood pressure, hypoglycemia, hyperglycemia, cancer, old ulcers, snakebites, and as an aphrodisiac [5,11,3321]. It has also been used as a diuretic, stimulant, and cathartic [6084].
In foods and beverages, fresh garlic, garlic powder, and garlic oil are used as flavor components [11,3321].

Safety

LIKELY SAFE ...when ingested in amounts commonly found in foods. Garlic oil, extract, and oleoresin have Generally Recognized as Safe (GRAS) status in the US [11].
POSSIBLY SAFE ...when used orally and appropriately for medicinal purposes. Garlic has been used in clinical studies lasting up to 4 years without reports of significant toxicity [2,4,3321,4797,4798].
POSSIBLY UNSAFE ...when used orally in large amounts [4]. ...when used topically in large amounts [585].
CHILDREN: POSSIBLY SAFE ...when used orally and appropriately, short-term. In one study, garlic extract 300 mg three times daily had side effects comparable to placebo when used in children ages 8-18 years for 8 weeks [4796]. POSSIBLY UNSAFE ...when used orally in large amounts. Some sources suggest that high doses of garlic could be dangerous or even fatal to children [12]; however, the reason for this warning is not known. There are no case reports available of significant adverse events or mortality in children associated with ingestion of garlic. There is insufficient reliable information available about the safety of topical garlic use in children.
PREGNANCY: LIKELY SAFE ...when used orally in amounts typically found in foods [12,3319]. POSSIBLY UNSAFE ...when used orally in large amounts [4]. Theoretically, large amounts of garlic might act as an abortifacient, enable onset of menstruation, and cause uterine contractions [4,19]. One study also suggests that garlic constituents are distributed to the amniotic fluid after a single dose of garlic [4828]. However, there are no published reports of garlic adversely affecting pregnancy. There is insufficient reliable information available about the safety of topical garlic use during pregnancy.

LACTATION: LIKELY SAFE …when used orally in amounts typically found in foods (12). POSSIBLY UNSAFE …when used orally in amounts greater than those found in foods (2,12). Some authors suggest that use of garlic should be avoided during lactation (4,12); however, the reason for this warning is not known. There are no published reports of adverse effects in nursing infants whose mothers ingested garlic. Several small studies suggest that garlic constituents are secreted in breast milk, and that nursing infants of mothers consuming garlic are prone to extended nursing and an altered flavor in breast milk (3319,4829,4830). There is insufficient reliable information available about the safety of topical garlic use during lactation.

Effectiveness

POSSIBLY EFFECTIVE …when used orally for hyperlipidemia. There is some controversy about the clinical benefits of garlic for hyperlipidemia. Some studies show no significant benefit (731,732,4792,4793,4794,4795,4807). But the majority of evidence shows that garlic does modestly improve total cholesterol, low-density lipoprotein (LDL) cholesterol, and triglyceride levels (279,3321,4782,4783,4784,4785,4786,4787,4788,4789,4790) (4791,6457,6465,6897). When used for 4-25 weeks garlic usually lowers total cholesterol levels by about 4-12% (3321,4786,4788,6457). As a comparison, conventional "statin" drugs typically decrease cholesterol levels by 17-32% (6457). Garlic does not seem to affect high-density lipoprotein (HDL) cholesterol (6897). Because of the relatively minor cholesterol level reductions possible with garlic, some clinicians are questioning its value in reducing cardiovascular disease. There is also some concern that garlic may not produce long-term benefits. Some studies show no significant benefit when used for 6 months or longer (6465,6897). Tell patients garlic can offer modest benefits for lowering cholesterol. But garlic alone is probably not appropriate for patients that require significant reductions in cholesterol levels. Direct patients to garlic powder preparations standardized based on the active alliin constituent. Most studies have used this kind of preparation. Consider aged garlic extracts as an alternative. There is some evidence that these preparations might also be beneficial (1873,1875,1876). …when taken orally for hypertension. There is some evidence that garlic can modestly reduce blood pressure by 2-7% after 4 weeks of treatment (277,278,279,1873,3321,6897). …when taken orally for preventing age-related vascular changes and atherosclerosis. Lower doses of garlic powder, 300 mg per day, seem to lessen age related decreases in aortic elasticity. Higher doses of 900 mg per day seem to slow development of atherosclerosis in both aortic and femoral arteries when used over a 4 year period (3315,4797,4798). …when used orally for preventing colon cancer. Several population studies show that increased garlic consumption from the diet can decrease risk of developing colorectal cancer (3320,4770,4771,4772). However, garlic supplements do not seem to offer this benefit (4773). …when used orally for preventing stomach cancer. There is some evidence from population studies that increasing garlic consumption in the diet can decrease risk of developing stomach (gastric) cancer (3320,4775,4776). It's not known if garlic supplements have this same benefit. …when used orally for preventing prostate cancer. There is preliminary evidence from a population study that increasing garlic consumption in the diet or with supplements can decrease the risk of developing prostate cancer (4777). …when taken orally as a tick repellant. People consuming high doses of garlic (1200 mg daily) over a 20 week period seem to have a significant reduction in tick bites (3318). …when the garlic constituent, ajoene, is used topically for tinea infections (4766,4767). Ajoene 0.4% cream seems to be effective for tinea pedis in as many as 79% of patients when used for 7 days (4766). The ajoene 0.6% gel seems to be as effective as terbinafine 1% cream for tinea cruris and tinea corporis (4766,4767).

POSSIBLY INEFFECTIVE …when taken orally to treat Helicobacter pylori infection. The use of garlic for H. pylori infection used to look promising due to laboratory and epidemiological evidence showing potential activity against H. pylori. But when garlic cloves, powder, or oil is used in humans it doesn't seem to have any beneficial effect for treating patients infected with H. pylori (3316,3322,4761,4762,4763,4764,4765,4774). …when taken orally for peripheral arterial occlusive disease. After 12 weeks of treatment garlic does not seem to improve walking distance in patients with stage II peripheral arterial occlusive disease (4801,4809). …when used orally for diabetes (6465,6897). …when taken orally for hypercholesterolemia in children. In children with familial hyperlipidemia garlic powder extract standardized based on alliin content does not seem to significantly improve total serum cholesterol, low-density lipoprotein (LDL) or high-density-lipoprotein (HDL) cholesterol levels, triglycerides, lipoprotein (a), apolipoprotein B-100, homocysteine, fibrinogen, or blood pressure (4796). …when used orally for preventing breast cancer (4779). …when used orally for preventing lung cancer (4778).

Most clinical studies have used the brand name product Kwai (Lichtwer Pharma), a dried garlic powder preparation standardized to contain 1.3% alliin. Some studies have used the brand name product Kyolic (Wakunaga of America), an aged garlic extract.

There is insufficient reliable information available about the effectiveness of garlic for its other uses.

Mechanism of Action

The applicable parts of garlic are the bulb and clove. Garlic is mostly used for its antihyperlipidemic, antihypertensive, and antifungal effects. However, it is also reported to have antibacterial, anthelmintic, antiviral, antispasmodic, diaphoretic, expectorant, immunostimulant, and antithrombotic effects (2,4). Many of the pharmacological effects of garlic have been attributed to the constituents allicin and ajoene. However, when doses of fresh garlic clove 4 grams per day are used, only allicin appears to have clinically significant activity (4800). The effectiveness of garlic products seems to be determined by their ability to yield allicin which in turn triggers production of other active principles (13).

Intact garlic cells contain the odorless amino acid, alliin. When intact cells are broken, alliin comes into contact with the enzyme allinase, producing allicin, an unstable, odiferous compound (5,4768). Fresh garlic contains approximately 1% alliin. One milligram of alliin is converted to 0.458 mg allicin (4800). Further conversion yields ajoene (13). Garlic is aged to reduce the content of sulfur compounds and the odor commonly associated with garlic. This process can significantly decrease alliin content. Odorless aged garlic extract reduces the alliin content to only 3% of what is typically contained in fresh garlic (4800). Boiling garlic also causes allicin to denature and can decrease activity (3321). To improve effectiveness dried garlic preparations should also have enteric coating to protect the active constituents from degeneration by stomach acid (13). In patients with hyperlipidemia, garlic might lower cholesterol levels by acting as a HMG-CoA reductase inhibitor (statin) (4810,4811). For hypertension, garlic is thought to reduce blood pressure by causing smooth muscle relaxation and vasodilation by activating production of endothelium-derived relaxation factor (EDRF, Nitric oxide) (4812). For age-related vascular changes and atherosclerosis, garlic is thought to be beneficial by reducing oxidative stress and low-density lipoprotein (LDL) oxidation and through antithrombotic effects (1880,3321,4813). Garlic appears to prevent endothelial cell depletion of glutathione, which may be responsible for its antioxidant effects (1880). Garlic has been found to have antithrombotic properties and can increase fibrinolytic activity, decrease platelet aggregation, and increase prothrombin time (PT) (2,3321). Garlic powder and aged garlic preparations have been shown to have antiplatelet properties in both patients with cardiovascular disease and in healthy volunteers (1874,4802,4803). Garlic oil does not appear to effect platelet aggregation (4805). Raw garlic seems to have more potent antiplatelet properties than cooked garlic (4799,4804). Garlic also seems to have immunostimulant activity. Garlic might stimulate both humoral and cellular immunity, causing T-cell proliferation, restoring suppressed antibody responses, and stimulating macrophage cytotoxicity on tumor cells (3321). Several other constituents of garlic and derivatives of alliin seem to have pharmacological activity. The constituents, allylpropyl disulfide and S-allyl cysteine, can reduce blood sugar by stimulation of insulin secretion in the pancreas (4,3321). Fresh garlic, but not aged garlic, has shown activity against Escherichia coli, methicillin-resistant Staph aureus, salmonella enteritidis, and Candida albicans in the laboratory, and has been suggested as a food additive to prevent food poisoning (4808). Preliminary evidence suggests that garlic compounds might have activity against viruses such as herpes simplex virus type 1, herpes simplex virus type 2, parainfluenza virus type 3, vaccinia virus, vesicular stomatitis virus, and human rhinovirus type 2 (4769). S-allyl cysteine and S-allyl mercaptocysteine, garlic derivatives, might protect the liver against acetaminophen and carbon tetrachloride, according to laboratory studies (14). Other preliminary evidence suggests S-allyl cysteine might ameliorate doxorubicin-induced cardiac and hepatic toxicity (4780). An active component of aged garlic, s-allylcysteine, shows effectiveness in preventing experimental physiological aging, age-related immunodeficiency, and atherosclerosis. Another constituent, S-allylmercaptocysteine, has shown activity against erythroleukemic, breast, and prostate cancer cells (1871,1877,1878,1879,1880,1881,1882). Additionally, garlic might enhance selenium absorption with possible protection against tumorigenesis (4815). Preliminary reports regarding a possible hepatoprotective effect of aged garlic extract have been conflicting (1883,1884). Early evidence suggests a possible protective effect of aged garlic on methotrexate-induced intestinal toxicity (1885). There is some evidence that garlic might effect the cytochrome P450 enzyme system. Some findings indicate that garlic might mildly inhibit cytochrome P450 2D6 (CYP2D6) activity by about 9% in humans (1303). This limited inhibition is not likely to produce clinically meaningful increases in drugs that are metabolized by the CYP2D6 isoenzyme. However, researchers suspect that garlic induces the cytochrome P450 3A4 (CYP450) isoenzyme and can produce clinical significant decreases in levels of drugs metabolized by this enzyme (7027).

Adverse Reactions

Orally, garlic has dose-related adverse effects, which most commonly include breath and body odor, mouth and gastrointestinal burning or irritation, heartburn, flatulence, nausea, vomiting, and diarrhea. These effects can be more pronounced with consumption of raw garlic or in patients unaccustomed to eating garlic (3319,4783,4800). The oral use of garlic can also cause changes to the intestinal flora (3319,4800), which might result in gastrointestinal upset. Garlic is well known to affect platelet function and possibly increase the risk of bleeding. Excessive consumption of dietary garlic has caused spinal epidural hematoma and platelet dysfunction in one case (586) and postoperative bleeding and prolonged bleeding time in another case (587). Asthma in people working with garlic has been reported (4816). Other allergic reactions associated with garlic include rhinitis, conjunctivitis, urticaria, anaphylaxis, and angioedema (6897). True IgE-mediated garlic allergy seems to be relatively rare, but can occur more often in young people with pollen allergy (4816).

Topically, application of fresh garlic has caused dermatitis (4833). Allergic contact dermatitis and eczema have been reported following occupational exposure to garlic (3317,4832). One child developed blisters and subsequently scars on both wrists after several hours of contact with crushed garlic cloves (585).

Interactions with Herbs & Other Dietary Supplements

EICOSAPENTAENOIC ACID (EPA, Fish Oils): Concomitant use of garlic can enhance antithrombotic effects (4).
HERBS WITH ANTICOAGULANT/ANTIPLATELET POTENTIAL: Concomitant use of herbs that have coumarin constituents or affect platelet aggregation could theoretically increase the risk of bleeding in some people. These herbs include: angelica, anise, arnica, asafoetida, bogbean, boldo, capsicum, celery, chamomile, clove, danshen,

fenugreek, feverfew, garlic, ginger, ginkgo, ginseng (Panax), horse chestnut, horseradish, licorice, meadowsweet, prickly ash, onion, papain, passionflower, poplar, quassia, red clover, turmeric, vitamin E, wild carrot, wild lettuce, willow, and others (4,19).

Interactions with Drugs

ANTICOAGULANT/ANTIPLATELET AGENTS: Garlic can enhance the effects of warfarin (Coumadin) as measured by the INR (616). Monitor patients using this combination closely. Dose adjustment may be necessary. Theoretically, garlic might also enhance the effects and adverse effects of other anticoagulant and antiplatelet drugs, including aspirin, clopidogrel (Plavix), enoxaparin (Lovenox), and others (4).

ANTIDIABETES DRUGS/INSULIN: Theoretically, concomitant use might increase effects and adverse effects of hypoglycemic drugs and insulin (4,19). Dose adjustments may be necessary when used concomitantly (19).

CYCLOSPORINE (Neoral, Sandimmune): There is some concern that garlic supplements might decrease the effectiveness of cyclosporine. Researchers suspect that garlic can induce metabolism and decrease levels of drugs such as cyclosporine that are substrates of the cytochrome P450 3A4 (CYP3A4) isoenzyme (7027). Garlic might decrease cyclosporine to subtherapeutic levels and potentially cause transplant rejection. Advise patients taking cyclosporine to avoid garlic supplements.

NONNUCLEOSIDE REVERSE TRANSCRIPTASE INHIBITORS (NNRTIs): Concomitant use might decrease serum levels of NNRTIs. Garlic can substantially decrease plasma concentrations of the protease inhibitor saquinavir (Fortovase, Invirase) (7027). Since NNRTIs and protease inhibitors are metabolized through similar routes, NNRTIs might also be affected. Patients taking these medications should avoid using garlic. NNRTI-type antiretroviral drugs include nevirapine (Viramune), delavirdine (Rescriptor), and efavirenz (Sustiva).

ORAL CONTRACEPTIVES: There is some concern that taking garlic supplements might decrease the effectiveness of oral contraceptives. Researchers suspect that garlic can induce metabolism and decrease levels of drugs such as estrogen that are substrates of the cytochrome P450 3A4 (CYP3A4) isoenzyme (7027). Advise women taking garlic supplements and oral contraceptives concurrently to use an additional or alternative form of birth control.

SAQUINAVIR (Fortovase, Invirase): Concomitant use of garlic can significantly decrease serum concentrations of saquinavir. Garlic 600 mg twice daily (equivalent to 3600 mcg allicin content per capsule) can reduce saquinavir area under the curve (AUC) by 51%. Garlic can decrease peak levels of saquinavir by 54% and mean trough levels by 49% (7027). These subtherapeutic concentrations might cause therapeutic failure, increase development of viral resistance, and development of drug class resistance. Researchers suspect garlic induces cytochrome P450 3A4 (CYP3A4) metabolism of saquinavir. Prolonged use (e.g., 10 days) of garlic supplements seems to be necessary for significant enzyme induction. Therefore, even occasional moderate to high consumption of garlic from dietary sources is not expected to cause a significant interaction. So far, this interaction has only been shown for saquinavir, but other protease inhibitors are also likely to be affected. Patients taking these medications should avoid taking garlic. Other protease inhibitors include amprenavir (Agenerase), nelfinavir (Viracept), and ritonavir (Norvir).

OTHER DRUGS: Based on garlic's potential effects on cytochrome P450 3A4 (CYP450) isoenzyme, use caution when considering concomitant use of garlic and other drugs affected by this system. Drugs that might be affected include some calcium channel blockers (diltiazem, nicardipine, verapamil), chemotherapeutic agents (etoposide, paclitaxel, vinblastine, vincristine, vindesine), antifungals (ketoconazole, itraconazole), glucocorticoids, alfentanil (Alfenta), cisapride (Propulsid), fentanyl (Sublimaze), lidocaine (Xylocaine), losartan (Cozaar), fexofenadine (Allegra), midazolam (Versed), and others.

Interactions with Foods

No interactions are known to occur, and there is no known reason to expect a clinically significant interaction with garlic.

Interactions with Lab Tests

GLUCOSE: Garlic can lower blood glucose concentrations and test results (4).
INSULIN: Garlic can increase blood insulin concentrations and test results (4).
INTERNATIONAL NORMALIZED RATIO (INR), PROTHROMBIN TIME (PT): Garlic can increase INR in patients anticoagulated with warfarin (Coumadin). There are two case reports of increased INR associated with concomitant use of garlic products and warfarin (616).
CHOLESTEROL: Garlic can lower serum cholesterol concentrations and test results (2,4,277,278,279).
BLOOD PRESSURE: Garlic can lower blood pressure and blood pressure readings (2,4,277,278,279).

Interactions with Diseases or Conditions

BLEEDING DISORDERS: Theoretically, garlic might increase the risk of bleeding (4); contraindicated.
DIABETES: Theoretically, garlic might reduce blood sugar levels and interfere with control (4); use with caution.
GASTROINTESTINAL IRRITATION: Garlic can irritate the gastrointestinal tract; use with caution in individuals with infectious or inflammatory gastrointestinal conditions (19).

SURGERY: Garlic can prolong bleeding time and should be discontinued one to two weeks prior to scheduled surgery (587,4800).

Dosage and Administration

ORAL: For hyperlipidemia and hypertension, garlic extract 600-1200 mg divided and given three times daily has been used in clinical trials. Most clinical studies have used a standardized garlic powder extract containing 1.3% alliin content (279,3321,4782,4783,4784,4785,4786,4787,4788,4789,4790) (4791,6457,6465,6897). Aged garlic extract 600 mg to 7.2 grams per day has also been used. Aged garlic typically contains only 0.03% alliin (1874,1875,3319,3321). Fresh garlic 4 grams (approximately one clove) once daily has also been used. Fresh garlic typically contains 1% alliin (3319,4800). For prevention of colorectal and stomach cancer, fresh or cooked garlic 3.5-29 grams weekly has been used (3320). Garlic preparations are sometimes dosed based on the allicin constituent. For every milligram of alliin, 0.458 mg of allicin is typically generated. Therefore, a dose of garlic extract 600 mg that contains 1.3% alliin typically produces 3600 mcg allicin. A dose of fresh garlic 4 grams containing 1% alliin typically produces approximately 18300 mcg of allicin. **TOPICAL**: For tinea infections, clinical studies have used the garlic constituent ajoene as a 0.4% cream and 0.6% gel (4766,4767). For onychomycosis and other fungal infections, including tinea infections, some sources suggest applying liquified raw garlic or garlic extract to the affected area three times daily (5121).

Comments

There is some concern than marketed garlic preparations may not generate an adequate amount of the active ingredient allicin to be effective. In one report only 25% of the garlic products commercially available generated an amount of allicin equivalent to one clove of fresh garlic (13). Also, some odorless garlic preparations may not contain active compounds at all (4,1877).

GELSEMIUM

Also Known As

Caroline Jasmine, Evening Trumpet Flower, False Jasmin, Gelsemii Rhizoma, Gelsemin, Gelsemium sempervirens, Gelsemiumwurzelstock Jessamine, Trumpet Flower, Woodbine, Yellow Jasmine, Yellow Jessamine Root.
CAUTION: See separate listings for Jasmine, American Ivy, Honeysuckle, and Woodbine.

Scientific Names

Gelsemium sempervirens, synonyms Gelsemium nitidum, Bignonia sempervirens.
Family: Loganiaceae or Spigeliaceae.

People Use This For

Orally, gelsemium is used as an analgesic for trigeminal neuralgia and migraine headaches (9).
Historically, gelsemium has been used for asthma and in respiratory remedies (6).

Safety

UNSAFE ...when the rhizome or root are used orally. All parts of the plant contain toxic alkaloids (14). The adult lethal dose is 2-3 grams or 4 mL of the fluid extract (18).
CHILDREN: UNSAFE ...when used orally. The lethal dose is 500 mg (18).
PREGNANCY AND LACTATION: UNSAFE ...when used orally due to toxicity (6).

Effectiveness

There is insufficient reliable information available about the effectiveness of gelsemium.

Mechanism of Action

The applicable parts of gelsemium are the rhizome and root. Researchers think the active components in gelsemium are gelsamine alkaloids and related compounds (gelsemine, gelsemicine, gelsedine) (6). Gelsemium and the principal alkaloid, gelsemine, are reported to have CNS stimulant (6), CNS depressant (9) and analgesic effects (6).

Adverse Reactions

Orally, the use of gelsemium can be deadly. Toxicity symptoms include: headache, dilated pupils, drooping of the eyelid, double vision, difficulty in swallowing, dizziness, muscle weakness/rigidity, seizures (rare), shortness of breath and bradycardia. Death due to failure of respiratory muscles can occur (14).
Topically, the whole plant can cause contact dermatitis when used topically (14).

Interactions with Herbs & Other Dietary Supplements

Insufficient reliable information available.

Interactions with Drugs

ASPIRIN, PHENACETIN: May potentiate drug effects (6).

Interactions with Foods

No interactions are known to occur, and there is no known reason to expect a clinically significant interaction with gelsemium.

Interactions with Lab Tests

No interactions are known to occur, and there is no known reason to expect a clinically significant interaction with gelsemium.

Interactions with Diseases or Conditions

HEART DISEASE/WEAKNESS: Contraindicated (18).

Dosage and Administration

ORAL: People typically use 0.3 to 1 mL gelsemium tincture (5264).

Comments

There is a very narrow safety margin and medicinal preparations are considered obsolete (18). Avoid confusion with jasmine or woodbine (Clematis virginiana). Also, avoid confusing gelsemium with American ivy or honeysuckle, which are also known as woodbine.

GENTIAN

Also Known As

Bitter Root, Bitterwort, Gall Weed, Gentiana, Gentianae radix, Pale Gentian, Stemless Gentian, Yellow Gentian, Wild Gentian.

Scientific Names

Gentiana lutea; Gentiana acaulis.
Family: Gentianaceae.

People Use This For

Orally, gentian is used for digestive disorders, such as loss of appetite, fullness, and flatulence. (2). It is used orally for fever, for hysteria, to stimulate menstrual flow, as an anthelmintic, and antiseptic (5).
Topically, gentian is used for treating wounds and cancer (11).
In combination with European elder flower, verbena, cowslip flower, and sorrel, gentian is used orally for maintaining healthy sinuses (373) and treating sinusitis (7,374,379). It is used in combination with other products for malaria (5).
In traditional medicine, gentian has been used orally for diarrhea, gastritis, heartburn, and vomiting (11).
In foods and beverages, gentian is used as an ingredient (11).
In manufacturing, gentian is used in cosmetics (11).

Safety

LIKELY SAFE ...when the root preparations are consumed in amounts commonly found in foods.
Gentian root is approved for food use in the US. The maximum level of gentian extract used is 0.02%; for stemless gentian, 0.001% (11).
POSSIBLY SAFE ...when used orally in therapeutic amounts (2). ...when gentian root is used orally with European elder flower, verbena, cowslip flower, and sorrel (Quanterra Sinus Defense, Sinupret) (7,374,379).
There is insufficient reliable information available about the safety of the topical use of gentian.
PREGNANCY: LIKELY UNSAFE ...when used orally because gentian is a potential mutagen with effects on the menstrual cycle (4).
LACTATION: Insufficient reliable information available; avoid using.

Effectiveness

POSSIBLY EFFECTIVE ...when gentian is used orally with European elder flower, verbena, cowslip flower, and sorrel (Quanterra Sinus Defense, Sinupret) for treating acute or chronic sinusitis (7,374,379).
There is insufficient reliable information available about the effectiveness of gentian for its other uses.

Mechanism of Action

The applicable part of gentian is the root. The bitter constituents, gentiamarin, gentiopicrin, amarogentin, and swertiamarin, show evidence that they can increase saliva and digestive juice secretion (2,4). Some evidence suggests the constituent gentianine has anti-inflammatory activity (11). The constituents, gentisin and isogentisin, are both mutagenic (4). The constituent gentiopicrin is lethal to mosquito larvae (11).

Adverse Reactions

Orally, gentian root can cause GI irritation, nausea, and vomiting (6). It can also cause headaches in individuals sensitive to bitter substances (12).

Interactions with Herbs & Other Dietary Supplements

Insufficient reliable information available.

Interactions with Drugs

ACID-INHIBITING DRUGS: Theoretically, due to claims that gentian increases stomach acid, it might interfere with antacids, sucralfate (Carafate), H-2 antagonists, or proton pump inhibitors (19).
DOXYCYCLINE (Vibramycin): Concurrent use of gentian root, European elder flower, verbena, cowslip flower, and sorrel (Quanterra Sinus Defense, Sinupret) with doxycycline and a topical decongestant might improve the outcome of conventional (antibiotic/decongestant) therapy for acute bacterial sinusitis (374).

Interactions with Foods

No interactions are known to occur, and there is no known reason to expect a clinically significant interaction with gentian.

Interactions with Lab Tests

No interactions are known to occur, and there is no known reason to expect a clinically significant interaction with gentian.

Interactions with Diseases or Conditions

DUODENAL AND GASTRIC ULCERS: Contraindicated (2).
GASTRIC IRRITATION OR INFLAMMATION: Contraindicated (12).
HYPERTENSION: The gentian root may not be well-tolerated in hypertensive individuals (5).

Dosage and Administration

ORAL: The typical dose of gentian is 0.6-2 grams of the dried root three times daily with a maximum of 4 grams per day. One cup of the tea is also taken three times daily (2,4,18). The tea is prepared by steeping 0.6-2 grams of the dried root in 150 mL boiling water for 5-10 minutes and then straining (2,4,18). The tea can be sweetened with honey. The common dose of the tincture (1:5 in 45% alcohol) is 1-3 grams daily (2) or 1-4 mL three times daily (4). The usual dose of the fluid extract is 2-4 grams daily (2). The irritating qualities of the gentian root are minimized in the tea and maximized in the tincture form (12).
For acute or chronic sinusitis, two Sinupret tablets three times daily for up to two weeks has been used in clinical trials (7,374,379), equivalent to gentian root 12 mg, European elder flower 36 mg, verbena 36 mg, cowslip flower 36 mg, and sorrel 36 mg three times daily. For maintaining healthy sinuses, a typical dose is one tablet of Quanterra Sinus Defense three times daily with water, equivalent to gentian root 9 mg, European elder flower 29 mg, verbena 29 mg, cowslip flower 29 mg, and sorrel 29 mg three times daily (373). Each tablet of Quanterra Sinus Defense contains 125 mg of the herbal combination found in Sinupret (373).
TOPICAL: No typical dosage.

Comments

CAUTION: The highly toxic white hellebore (Veratrum album) can grow in proximity to gentian and has caused accidental poisoning when used in home-made preparations (11). A related Gentiana species is used in Chinese medicine for treating jaundice, headache, sores, inflammation, and rheumatoid arthritis (11). The gentian root is unrelated to the gentian violet dye.

GERMAN CHAMOMILE

Also Known As

Camomilla, Camomille Allemande, Chamomilla, Chamomile, Echte Kamille, Feldkamille, Fleur de Camomile, Hungarian Chamomile, Kamillen, Kleine Kamille, Manzanilla, Matricaire, Matricariae Flos, Pin Heads, Sweet False Chamomile, True Chamomile, Wild Chamomile.

Scientific Names

Matricaria recutita, synonyms Chamomilla recutita, Matricaria chamomilla.
Family: Asteraceae or Compositae.

People Use This For

Orally, German chamomile is used for flatulence, travel sickness, nasal mucous membrane inflammation, nervous diarrhea, restlessness and insomnia (4), gastrointestinal (GI) spasms, inflammatory diseases of the gastrointestinal (GI) tract (2,4), gastrointestinal (GI) ulcers associated with non-steroidal anti-inflammatory drugs (NSAIDs) and alcohol consumption (19), and as an antispasmodic for menstrual cramps (5).

Topically, German chamomile is used for hemorrhoids; mastitis; leg ulcers (4); skin, anogenital, and mucous membrane inflammation; and bacterial skin diseases, including those of the mouth and gums (2). It is also used topically for treating or preventing chemotherapy- or radiation-induced oral mucositis (6655).

As an inhalant, German chamomile is used to treat inflammation and irritation of the respiratory tract (2).

In foods and beverages, the essential oil and extracts are used as flavor components (11).

In manufacturing, German chamomile is used in cosmetics, soaps, and mouthwashes (11).

Safety

LIKELY SAFE ...when used in amounts commonly found in foods. It has Generally Recognized as Safe (GRAS) status for food use in the US (11).

POSSIBLY SAFE ...when preparations of the flower are used orally in medicinal amounts short-term (2,12). ...when used topically; avoid applying it near the eyes (8).

POSSIBLY UNSAFE ...when used as highly concentrated tea German chamomile can cause vomiting (12).

PREGNANCY: LIKELY UNSAFE ...when used orally because it is believed to be a teratogen, affect the menstrual cycle and have uterine stimulant effects (4).

LACTATION: Insufficient reliable information available; avoid using.

Effectiveness

POSSIBLY EFFECTIVE ...when used topically for treating or preventing mucositis induced by radiation therapy and some types of chemotherapy (6655). German chamomile oral rinse seems to prevent or treat mucositis secondary to radiation therapy and some types of chemotherapy including asparaginase (Elspar), cisplatin (CDDP, Platinol-AQ), cyclophosphamide (Cytoxan, Neosar), daunorubicin (DaunoXome), doxorubicin (Adriamycin, Rubex), etoposide (VP-16, Etopophos, VePesid, Toposar), hydroxyurea (Hydrea), mercaptopurine (6-MP, Purinethol), methotrexate (MTX, Rheumatrex), procarbazine (MIH, Mutlane), and vincristine (VCR, Oncovin, Vincasar) (6655). However, the rinse doesn't seem to be better than placebo for preventing fluorouracil (5-FU)-induced oral mucositis (6656). Some clinical studies have used German chamomile extracts and flowers standardized to 1.2% apigenin.

There is insufficient reliable information available about the effectiveness of German chamomile for its other uses.

Mechanism of Action

The applicable part of German chamomile is the flowerhead. German chamomile possesses multiple actions, including anti-allergic, antiflatulent, antispasmodic, mild sedative, anti-inflammatory, and antiseptic actions. It also soothes mucous membranes (4). Chamomile's anti-allergic and anti-inflammatory actions result from the azulene constituents which inhibit histamine release (4). The sesquiterpene bisabolol constituents are also pharmacologically active and they possess anti-inflammatory and anti-ulcer properties (3,4). The coumarin constituents can have antibacterial properties (4). German chamomile can affect the menstrual cycle and is known to cause animal teratogenicity (4).

Adverse Reactions

The highly concentrated tea can cause vomiting (12). Chamomile can cause allergic reactions including contact dermatitis, severe hypersensitivity reactions, and anaphylaxis (6,567). If used near the eyes, it can be irritating (19). It can cause an allergic reaction in individuals sensitive to the Asteraceae/Compositae family. Members of this family include ragweed, chrysanthemums, marigolds, daisies, and many other herbs.

Interactions with Herbs & Other Dietary Supplements

HERBS WITH SEDATIVE PROPERTIES: Theoretically, concomitant use with herbs that have sedative properties might enhance therapeutic and adverse effects. These include calamus, calendula, California poppy, catnip, capsicum, celery, couch grass, elecampane, Siberian ginseng, goldenseal, gotu kola, hops, Jamaican dogwood, kava, lemon balm, sage, St. John's wort, sassafras, scullcap, shepherd's purse, stinging nettle, valerian, wild carrot, wild lettuce, ashwaganda root, and yerba mansa (4,19).

HERBS WITH ANTICOAGULANT/ANTIPLATELET POTENTIAL: Concomitant use of herbs that have coumarin constituents or affect platelet aggregation could theoretically increase the risk of bleeding in some people. These herbs include: angelica, anise, arnica, asafoetida, bogbean, boldo, capsicum, celery, clove, danshen, fenugreek, feverfew, garlic, ginger, ginkgo, Panax ginseng, horse chestnut, horseradish, licorice, meadowsweet, prickly ash, onion, papain, passionflower, poplar, quassia, red clover, turmeric, wild carrot, wild lettuce, willow, and others (4,19).

Interactions with Drugs

ANTICOAGULANT, ANTIPLATELET DRUGS: Theoretically, concomitant use of large amounts of chamomile might increase anticoagulation effects and increase the risk of bleeding (4); however, this effect has not yet been reported in humans. Some anticoagulant and antiplatelet drugs include aspirin, clopidogrel (Plavix) dalteparin (Fragmin), enoxaparin (Lovenox), heparin, ticlopidine (Ticlid), warfarin (Coumadin), and others.

BENZODIAZEPINES: Theoretically, concomitant use with benzodiazepines might cause additive effects and side effects (19).

DRUGS WITH SEDATIVE PROPERTIES: Theoretically, concomitant use with drugs with sedative properties can cause additive effects and side effects (19).

OTHER DRUGS: There's preliminary evidence that German chamomile can inhibit the cytochrome P450 (CYP450) 3A4 enzyme (6450). Theoretically, German chamomile might increase levels of drugs metabolized by CYP450 3A4. However, so far, this interaction has not been reported in humans. Some drugs metabolized by CYP450 3A4 include lovastatin (Mevacor), ketoconazole (Nizoral), itraconazole (Sporanox), fexofenadine (Allegra), triazolam (Halcion), and numerous others. Use German chamomile cautiously or avoid in patients taking these drugs.

Interactions with Foods

No interactions are known to occur, and there is no known reason to expect a clinically significant interaction with German chamomile.

Interactions with Lab Tests

No interactions are known to occur, and there is no known reason to expect a clinically significant interaction with German chamomile.

Interactions with Diseases or Conditions

ASTHMA: Chamomile can exacerbate this condition (4).

CROSS-ALLERGENICITY: Can cause an allergic reaction in individuals sensitive to the Asteraceae/Compositae family. Members of this family include ragweed, chrysanthemums, marigolds, daisies, and many other herbs.

Dosage and Administration

ORAL: The typical dose of German chamomile is 2-8 grams of the dried flower heads three times daily (4) or one cup of the tea three to four times daily. The tea is prepared by steeping 3 grams of the dried flower heads in 150 mL boiling water for 5-10 minutes and then straining (2). The liquid extract (1:1 in 45% alcohol) is commonly dosed as 1-4 mL three times daily (4). Clinical studies on the effectiveness of German chamomile have used extracts and flowers standardized to 1.2% apigenin.

TOPICAL: German chamomile is used as poultices and rinses. The prepared tea is commonly used (steep 4 teaspoons of the dried flower heads in 1.5 cups boiling water for 15 minutes and then strain) (18). The 3-10% ointments and gels are for external use only (18). Avoid topical use near the eyes (12). For inflammation of mucous membranes of the mouth and throat, the freshly prepared tea is commonly used as a mouthwash or gargle (2). For chemotherapy- or radiation-induced oral mucositis, an oral rinse made with 10-15 drops of German chamomile liquid extract in 100 ml warm water has been used three times daily (6655).

INHALATION: No typical dosage.

Comments

Avoid confusion with Roman chamomile. Although ointments, creams, and lotions containing the volatile oil of chamomile are intended for the treatment of various skin conditions and are used in Europe, they have not been approved in the US (3).

GERMAN IPECAC

Also Known As
None.

Scientific Names
Cynanchum vincetoxicum.
Family: Asclepiadaceae.

People Use This For
Orally, German ipecac is used for digestive and kidney disorders, and dysmenorrhea.
Topically, German ipecac is used in poultices for healing swelling and bruising.
In folk medicine, German ipecac is used orally for edema. It was also used for kidney disorders, the plague, snake bite, and dysmenorrhea, as a diuretic, emetic, and to promote sweating [18].

Safety
POSSIBLY UNSAFE ...when used orally [18].
There is insufficient reliable information available about the safety of German ipecac for its other uses.
PREGNANCY AND LACTATION: POSSIBLY UNSAFE ...when used orally [18]; avoid using.

Effectiveness
There is insufficient reliable information available about the effectiveness of German ipecac.

Mechanism of Action
The applicable parts of German ipecac are the leaf and root/rhizome. There is insufficient reliable information available about the possible mechanism of action and active ingredients.

Adverse Reactions
Orally, high doses of German ipecac may cause vomiting, apnea, and cardiac arrest. Seed extracts may cause advancing paralysis of the central nervous system [18].

Interactions with Herbs & Other Dietary Supplements
Insufficient reliable information available.

Interactions with Drugs
No interactions are known to occur, and there is no known reason to expect a clinically significant interaction with German ipecac.

Interactions with Foods
No interactions are known to occur, and there is no known reason to expect a clinically significant interaction with German ipecac.

Interactions with Lab Tests
No interactions are known to occur, and there is no known reason to expect a clinically significant interaction with German ipecac.

Interactions with Diseases or Conditions
No interactions are known to occur, and there is no known reason to expect a clinically significant interaction with German ipecac.

Dosage and Administration
No typical dosage.

Comments
None.

GERMAN SARSAPARILLA

Also Known As
Caricis rhizoma, Red Couchgrass, Red Sage, Sandriedgraswurzelstock, Sand Sedge, Sea Sedge.
CAUTION: See separate listings for Couch Grass, Sarsaparilla, Sage, and Tormentil.

Scientific Names
Carex arenaria.
Family: Cyperaceae.

People Use This For
Orally, German sarsaparilla is used for preventing gout, inducing sweating, arthritis, skin ailments, and as a diuretic (2). It is also used orally for venereal disease, flatulence, colic, liver disorders, diabetes, edema, pulmonary tuberculosis, and amenorrhea (18).

Safety
There is insufficient reliable information available about the safety of German sarsaparilla.
Pregnancy and Lactation: Insufficient reliable information available; avoid using.

Effectiveness
There is insufficient reliable information available about the effectiveness of German sarsaparilla.

Mechanism of Action
The applicable part of German sarsaparilla is the underground stem. German sarsaparilla contains saponins, a volatile oil containing methyl salicylate and cineole, flavonoids, and tannins (18).

Adverse Reactions
Orally, the saponins contained in German sarasaparilla may cause local irritation (2).

Interactions with Herbs & Other Dietary Supplements
Insufficient reliable information available.

Interactions with Drugs
No interactions are known to occur, and there is no known reason to expect a clinically significant interaction with German sarsaparilla.

Interactions with Foods
No interactions are known to occur, and there is no known reason to expect a clinically significant interaction with German sarsaparilla.

Interactions with Lab Tests
There are no reports of lab interactions with German sarsaparilla. However, because it contains salicylate(s), use caution in interpreting test results known to be affected by salicylates.

Interactions with Diseases or Conditions
ASPIRIN ALLERGY/ASTHMA: Avoid or use cautiously in individuals who are allergic to aspirin or have asthma; contains salicylates.

Dosage and Administration
ORAL: German sarsaparilla is typically prepared as a liquid. For a tea, 3 grams is added to 1 cup boiling water; 1 cup is taken daily. A cold solution is prepared with 2 teaspoons sarsaparilla added to a cup of water; a cup is taken 2 to 3 times daily (5252).

Comments
There is very little scientific information about this product. Our staff is continually analyzing the available information on natural medicines and will add data here as it becomes available.

GERMANDER

Also Known As
Wall Germander, Wild Germander.

Scientific Names
Teucrium chamaedrys.
Family: Lamiaceae.

People Use This For
Topically, germander is used as a mouthwash for oral hygiene (514).

Traditionally, germander is used orally for treating gallbladder conditions, fever, stomachaches (14), mild diarrhea, as a digestive aid (18), an adjunct for weight loss (18), an antiseptic (14), and as "a rinse for gout" (18).

In manufacturing, germander is used as a flavoring agent in alcoholic beverages (14).

Safety
LIKELY UNSAFE ...when used orally. Germander is associated with multiple cases of hepatitis and death (17,18,514,3741,3742,3743,3744). France has banned its sale (17). Canada does not allow germander to be included in oral products as a non-medicinal ingredient (12,14). However, the US still allows germander to be used in small amounts as a flavoring agent in alcoholic beverages (12,14).

PREGNANCY AND LACTATION: LIKELY UNSAFE ...when used orally (17,18,514,3741,3742,3743,3744).

Effectiveness
There is insufficient reliable information available about the effectiveness of germander.

Mechanism of Action
The applicable parts of germander are the above ground parts. Germander contains teucrin A, a diterpene, which causes hepatic necrosis in mice (3740).

Adverse Reactions
Orally, germander has been associated with hepatitis, liver cell necrosis, and death (18,514,3741,3742,3743,3744).

Interactions with Herbs & Other Dietary Supplements
Insufficient reliable information available.

Interactions with Drugs
No interactions are known to occur, and there is no known reason to expect a clinically significant interaction with germander.

Interactions with Foods
No interactions are known to occur, and there is no known reason to expect a clinically significant interaction with germander.

Interactions with Lab Tests
No interactions are known to occur, and there is no known reason to expect a clinically significant interaction with germander.

Interactions with Diseases or Conditions
No interactions are known to occur, and there is no known reason to expect a clinically significant interaction with germander.

Dosage and Administration
No typical dosage.

Comments
None.

GERMANIUM

Also Known As
Bis-Carboxyethyl Germanium Sesquioxide, Carboxyethylgermanium Sesquioxide, Ge-132, GE-132, Ge-Oxy 132, Germanium Lactate Citrate, Inorganic Germanium, Organic Germanium.

Scientific Names
Germanium; Ge; atomic number 32; Bis-carboxyethyl germanium sesquioxide; Germanium lactate citrate.

People Use This For
Orally, germanium is used for osteoarthritis, pain relief, osteoporosis, low energy, AIDS, cancer, high blood pressure, high cholesterol, heart disease, glaucoma, and cataracts. It is used orally for rheumatoid arthritis, depression, hepatitis, cirrhosis, food allergies, candidiasis, chronic viral infections, and heavy metal poisoning (including mercury, cadmium). Germanium is also used orally for increasing circulation of blood to the brain, supporting the immune system, and as an antioxidant (2356,2357,2358,2359).

Safety
LIKELY UNSAFE ...when used orally; avoid using. There have been 31 reports of renal failure or death caused by ingestion of 15-300 grams over 2 to 36 months (2360).
PREGNANCY AND LACTATION: LIKELY UNSAFE ...when used orally due to reported toxicity (2360); avoid using.

Effectiveness
There is insufficient reliable information available about the effectiveness of germanium.

Mechanism of Action
There is insufficient reliable information available about the possible mechanism of action and active ingredients.

Adverse Reactions
Ingestion of germanium can cause renal tubular degeneration, anemia, muscle weakness, peripheral neuropathy, renal failure, and death (2360).

Interactions with Herbs & Other Dietary Supplements
Insufficient reliable information available.

Interactions with Drugs
FUROSEMIDE: One case report of furosemide resistance associated with a ginseng product containing germanium (770).

Interactions with Foods
No interactions are known to occur, and there is no known reason to expect a clinically significant interaction with germanium.

Interactions with Lab Tests
No interactions are known to occur, and there is no known reason to expect a clinically significant interaction with germanium.

Interactions with Diseases or Conditions
No interactions are known to occur, and there is no known reason to expect a clinically significant interaction with germanium.

Dosage and Administration
ORAL: People typically use 150 mg 1 to 5 times daily between meals or with meals (directions vary).
Available in capsule and tablet form. The tablet form may also be dissolved under the tongue (6006).

Comments
None.

GINGER

Also Known As
African Ginger, Black Ginger, Cochin Ginger, Gingembre, Ginger Root, Jamaica Ginger, Race Ginger, Zingiberis rhizoma.

Scientific Names
Zingiber officinale.
Family: Zingiberaceae.

People Use This For
Orally, ginger is used for motion sickness, morning sickness, colic, dyspepsia, flatulence, chemotherapy-induced nausea, rheumatoid arthritis, osteoarthritis, loss of appetite, post-surgical nausea and vomiting, and for discontinuing selective serotonin reuptake inhibitor (SSRI) drug therapy. It is also used orally for anorexia, upper respiratory tract infections, cough, and bronchitis.

Topically, the fresh juice of ginger is used for treating thermal burns. The essential oil of ginger is used topically as an analgesic.

In Chinese medicine, ginger is used as a diaphoretic, diuretic, and stimulant. Ginger is also used in Chinese medicine for treating stomachache, diarrhea, nausea, cholera, and bleeding. Fresh ginger is used orally for treating acute bacterial dysentery, baldness, malaria, orchitis, poisonous snake bites, rheumatism, and toothaches.

In foods and beverages, ginger is used as a flavoring agent.

In manufacturing, ginger is used as a fragrance component in soaps and cosmetics. The oleoresin of ginger is also used as an ingredient in digestive, laxative, antitussive, antiflatulent, and antacid preparations.

Safety
LIKELY SAFE ...when used orally in amounts found in foods. It has Generally Recognized as Safe (GRAS) status in the US. The maximum use level of ginger in food is 0.023% (11). ...when used topically (4,11).

POSSIBLY SAFE ...when used orally and appropriately for medicinal purposes (721,722,723,5343,7048,7400).

PREGNANCY: LIKELY SAFE ...when used orally in amounts found in foods (11). POSSIBLY UNSAFE ...when used orally for medicinal purposes. The use of ginger during pregnancy is controversial (1921,7083). So far, there is no conclusive evidence that ginger is harmful during pregnancy. Some pregnant patients have used ginger for morning sickness without noticeable harm (5343). However, there is a case report of spontaneous abortion during the twelfth week of pregnancy in a patient using ginger for morning sickness. It is unclear if ginger was responsible for this outcome (721). There is also some evidence that a high dose of the ginger constituent, 6-gingerol, can be mutagenic. It's not clear if the whole ginger preparation has this effect. Mutagenicity has not yet been confirmed in humans. Until more is known, avoid medicinal use of ginger during pregnancy.

LACTATION: Insufficient reliable information available: avoid using amounts greater than those found in foods.

Effectiveness
POSSIBLY EFFECTIVE ...when used orally for preventing motion sickness. Taking ginger up to 4 hours prior to travel seems to prevent some symptoms such as cold-sweating and vomiting. It might also decrease the severity of dizziness (vertigo) (7400). ...when used orally for morning sickness. Ginger seems to reduce feelings of nausea in some pregnant patients with morning sickness (721,1922,5343). However, since the safety of ginger during pregnancy is not clearly established, ginger should be avoided for this use (1919,1921). ...when used orally for preventing postoperative nausea and vomiting in the absence of narcotic anesthesia or analgesia (722,723,1919). There is some evidence that ginger might be as effective as metoclopramide (Reglan) for reducing postsurgical nausea and vomiting in patients not concurrently receiving anesthesia or narcotic analgesia (722,723,1919). However, ginger does not seem to help patients that do receive anesthesia or narcotic analgesics (3452,3453). ...when used orally to prevent chemotherapy-induced nausea. There is some evidence that ginger might help prevent chemotherapy-induced nausea when given following administration of intravenous (IV) prochlorperazine (Compazine) (1919).

LIKELY INEFFECTIVE ...when used orally for preventing postoperative nausea and vomiting in the presence of narcotic anesthesia or analgesia. Although ginger seems to help patients not receiving anesthesia or narcotic analgesia (722,723,1919), patients that do receive these medications don't seem to benefit from ginger (3452,3453).

There is insufficient reliable information available to rate the effectiveness of ginger for its other uses. However, there is preliminary evidence that ginger might offer very modest benefits in osteoarthritis. Two studies have evaluated a specific ginger extract (Eurovita Extract 33; EV ext-33) 170 mg three times daily or 255 mg twice daily (510 mg total daily dose) for 3-6 weeks (7048,7084). Ginger might modestly improve pain after standing or walking and joint stiffness in some patients, but it does not seem to significantly improve functionality, quality of life, or use of relief analgesics (7084,7085). Ginger does reduce pain as well as ibuprofen 400 mg three times daily (7048). There is some preliminary evidence that ginger might be helpful for decreasing joint pain in patients with rheumatoid arthritis (7401). More evidence is needed to rate ginger for these uses.

Mechanism of Action

The applicable parts of ginger are the rhizome and root. Ginger contains active constituents known as gingerols. These constituents seem to have a variety of pharmacological properties including antipyretic, analgesic, antitussive, cardiac inotropic, and sedative properties (5). However, all of these pharmacological effects may not occur when whole ginger preparations are used. For example, whole ginger-containing products do not seem to have antipyretic effects (6131). Ginger might work for reducing nausea and vomiting by increasing gastrointestinal motility and transport (1923), possibly due to the 6-gingerol constituent (1924). Other ginger constituents such as 6-shogaol and galanolactone also seem to act on serotonin receptors (5-HT receptors) (1924). Galanolactone seems to act primarily on 5-HT3 receptors in the ileum, which are the same receptors affected by some prescription antiemetics such as ondansetron (Zofran). There is some evidence that ginger constituents may also have central antiemetic activity (1924). Ginger is sometimes used for inflammatory conditions such as rheumatoid arthritis. Some researchers speculate that certain constituents of ginger might inhibit cyclooxygenase and lipoxygenase pathways (7401). The ginger constituent 6-gingerol (4), does seem to have anti-inflammatory effects, but the whole ginger preparation may not (6131). There is some preliminary evidence that ginger may also have hypoglycemic, hypotensive or hypertensive, hypocholesterolemic, anthelmintic, gastroprotective, and antiplatelet effects (4,11). There is preliminary evidence that some extracts and constituents of ginger might have mutagenic properties. However, these constituents may only be mutagenic when in the presence of other mutagens. Other ginger constituents such as zingerone have the opposite effect and are antimutagenic. Whole ginger preparations may not have mutagenic effects (4).

Adverse Reactions

Orally, ginger is usually well tolerated. However, some patients taking ginger can have some side effects including abdominal discomfort, heartburn, diarrhea, and a pepper-like irritant effect in the mouth and throat (5343,7400). Ginger can cause dermatitis in sensitive individuals (4). Large overdoses can cause central nervous system depression and cardiac arrhythmias (5).

Interactions with Herbs & Other Dietary Supplements

HERBS WITH ANTICOAGULANT/ANTIPLATELET POTENTIAL: Concomitant use of herbs that have coumarin constituents or affect platelet aggregation could theoretically increase the risk of bleeding in some people. These herbs include: angelica, anise, arnica, asafoetida, bogbean, boldo, capsicum, celery, chamomile, clove, danshen, fenugreek, feverfew, garlic, ginkgo, ginseng (Panax), horse chestnut, horseradish, licorice, meadowsweet, prickly ash, onion, papain, passionflower, poplar, quassia, red clover, turmeric, wild carrot, wild lettuce, willow, and others (4,19).

Interactions with Drugs

ACID-INHIBITING DRUGS: Theoretically, due to claims that ginger rhizome increases stomach acid, it might interfere with antacids, sucralfate (Carafate), H-2 antagonists, or proton pump inhibitors (19).
ANTICOAGULANT, ANTIPLATELET DRUGS: Theoretically, excessive amounts of ginger might increase the risk of bleeding. Ginger is thought to inhibit thromboxane synthetase and decrease in platelet aggregation (4,6048).
BARBITURATES: Theoretically, ginger might enhance barbiturate effects (6).
BLOOD PRESSURE THERAPY: Theoretically, due to hypertensive or hypotensive effects, ginger might interfere with blood pressure drug therapy (4).
CARDIAC DRUGS: Theoretically, ginger might interfere with cardiac drug therapy due to inotropic effects (2,4).
DIABETES DRUGS: Theoretically, ginger might interfere with diabetes therapy due to hypoglycemic effects (2,4).

Interactions with Foods

No interactions are known to occur, and there is no known reason to expect a clinically significant interaction with ginger.

Interactions with Lab Tests

No interactions are known to occur, and there is no known reason to expect a clinically significant interaction with ginger.

Interactions with Diseases or Conditions

GALLSTONES: Individuals with gallstones should not use ginger except after medical evaluation determines ginger will not worsen gallstone symptoms (12).
BLEEDING CONDITIONS: Theoretically, excessive doses of ginger can interfere with increase risk of bleeding (4).
DIABETES: Theoretically, excessive doses of ginger can cause hypoglycemia, necessitating change in dose of diabetes medication (4).
HEART CONDITIONS: Theoretically, excessive doses of ginger might have cardiotonic activity that can interfere with the therapy for heart conditions (4).
HIGH BLOOD PRESSURE, LOW BLOOD PRESSURE: Theoretically, excessive doses of ginger might increase or reduce blood pressure, interfering with blood pressure control (4).

Dosage and Administration

ORAL: For morning sickness, 250 mg ginger 4 times daily has been used in studies (721,5343). For motion sickness, 1 gram of dried powdered ginger root 30 minutes to 4 hours before travel has been used (1919,7400). For osteoarthritis, a specific ginger extract (Eurovita Extract 33; EV ext-33), 170 mg three times daily or 255 mg twice daily has been used (7048,7084). For nausea and disequilibrium resulting from selective serotonin reuptake inhibitor (SSRI) discontinuation or tapering, 550-1100 mg ginger 3 times daily has been used (3451). For preventing postoperative nausea and vomiting 1 gram powdered ginger root 1 hour before induction of anesthesia has been used (722,723). For chemotherapy-induced nausea, powdered ginger 2-4 grams daily has been used (1920). A ginger tea has also been used and is typically prepared and taken on the day of chemotherapy and continued for as long as needed (1920). As a general anti-emetic, powdered root 2 grams daily is typically used (1920). It is generally recommended that doses not exceed 4 grams per day (1920). Ginger tea is prepared by steeping 0.5-1 gram dried root in 150 mL boiling water for 5-10 minutes and then straining (4,18). Tinctures are typically taken in doses of 0.25–3 mL (4). **TOPICAL**: No typical dosage.

Comments

Ginger is commonly found in the warmer climates, including India, Jamaica, and China. Its flowers are similar to orchids. The rhizome is used as the source for the dried, powder spice.

GINKGO leaf (GINKGO leaf extract)

Also Known As

Adiantifolia, Bai Guo Ye, Fossil Tree, Gingko, Gingko Biloba, Ginkgo Biloba, Ginkgo Folium, Ginkgo leaf, Ginkgo leaf extract, Ginko Biloba, Ginkyo, Japanese Silver Apricot, Kew Tree, Maidenhair Tree, Salisburia, Salisburia Adiantifolia, Yinhsing.
CAUTION: See separate listing for Ginkgo seed.

Scientific Names

Ginkgo biloba.
Family: Ginkgoaceae.

People Use This For

Orally, ginkgo leaf is used for dementia, including Alzheimer's, vascular, and mixed dementia. Ginkgo leaf is also used orally for conditions associated with cerebral vascular insufficiency, especially in the elderly; including memory loss, headache, tinnitus, vertigo, dizziness, difficulty concentrating, mood disturbances, and hearing disorders. It is also used orally for relief of walking pain associated with intermittent claudication, particularly in patients with Fontaine's stage IIa or IIb peripheral arterial occlusive disease. Ginkgo leaf is also used orally to treat sexual dysfunction and to reverse sexual dysfunction caused by SSRI antidepressants. It is also used orally for cognitive disorders secondary to depression; eye problems, including macular degeneration and glaucoma; attention deficit hyperactivity disorder (ADHD); thrombosis; heart disease; arteriosclerosis; angina pectoris; hypercholesterolemia; cardiac reperfusion injury; premenstrual syndrome (PMS); dysentery and filariasis; and diabetic retinopathy. Ginkgo leaf is also used orally to improve cognitive behavior and sleep patterns in patients with depression. Ginkgo leaf has also been used orally to prevent acute mountain sickness. It is also used orally to treat asthma, allergies, bronchitis, and for various disorders of the central nervous system. Ginkgo leaf is also used for preventing aging, regulating gastric acidity, improving liver and gallbladder function, regulating bacterial flora, and controlling blood pressure.
Topically, ginkgo leaf is used to wash chilblains, which are lesions on the fingers, toes, heels, ears, and nose caused by exposure to extreme cold. It is also used topically in wound dressings to improve circulation in the skin.
Intravenously, ginkgo leaf is used to increase cerebral blood flow, improve cognition, and for psychiatric conditions in the elderly.
In manufacturing, ginkgo leaf extract has been used in cosmetics.

Safety

LIKELY SAFE ...when used orally and appropriately. Standardized ginkgo leaf extracts have been used safely in trials lasting from several weeks to a year (1514,1515,3461,5717,5718,6211,6212,6213,6214,6215) (6216,6222,6223,6224,6225,6490). Tell patients to avoid crude ginkgo plant parts, which can exceed concentrations of 5 ppm of the toxic ginkgolic acid constituents and can cause severe allergic reactions (2,17,5714).
LIKELY UNSAFE ...when used intravenously. The intravenous ginkgo product once available in Germany has been withdrawn from the market due to severe adverse reactions (6).
There is insufficient reliable information available about the safety of ginkgo leaf when used topically.
PREGNANCY AND LACTATION: Insufficient reliable information available; avoid using.

Effectiveness

POSSIBLY EFFECTIVE ...when used orally for Alzheimer's, vascular, or mixed dementias. Studies lasting from 3 months to a year show that ginkgo leaf extract can stabilize or improve some measures of cognitive function and social functioning in patients with multiple types of dementia (1514,1515,2665,2666,6222,6223,6225). Although there is one report with conflicting findings (5720), the majority of evidence indicates that ginkgo leaf extract can be modestly helpful. Some researchers suggest that the improvement with ginkgo leaf extract is roughly equivalent to a 6-month delay in disease progression (1514). However, outcome studies have not yet verified ginkgo's effects on disease progression. Doses ranging from 120 mg to 240 mg daily have been beneficial after 6-8 weeks of treatment. Ginkgo leaf extract has not been directly compared to conventional medicines for dementia, but improvement appears to be similar to that found with the prescription drugs donepezil (Aricept), tacrine (Cognex) (1514,1515,6224,6490), and possibly other cholinesterase inhibitors (6224). German practitioners consider ginkgo leaf extract the treatment of choice for dementia (6491). ...when used orally for improving cognitive function in elderly people with mild to moderate age-related memory impairment. Although there have been some conflicting findings (5720), the majority of evidence shows that ginkgo leaf extract can modestly improve some measures of cognitive function, particularly short-term visual memory and possibly speed of cognitive processing, in non-demented patients with age-related memory impairment (5717,5718,6216). ...when used orally to improve cognitive function in healthy young people. There is preliminary evidence that ginkgo leaf extract can modestly improve cognitive function, including memory and speed of cognitive processing, in people aged 30-59 with no complaints of memory impairment (6214,6215). Tell patients not to take high doses to get a greater effect. Lower doses of 120 mg per day seem to be as effective or more effective than higher doses up to 600 mg per day. There is also some evidence that older patients in this group, aged 50-59, might experience the most benefit (6214). A specific combination of ginkgo leaf extract 60 mg and Panax ginseng 100 mg twice daily also seems to improve memory in otherwise healthy people ages 38 to 66 years (1903). ...when used orally for increasing pain-free walking distance in patients with intermittent claudication (3461,6211,6212,6213). Ginkgo leaf extract seems to significantly improve pain-free walking distance in patients with Fontaine's IIb peripheral arterial occlusive disease (3461,6212). Although significant benefit has been found with doses as low as 120-160 mg per day (6211), there is some evidence that a higher dose of 240 mg per day might be more beneficial in some patients (3461,6212). ...when used orally for vertigo and equilibrium disorders (6208,6220,6221). There is evidence from two clinical studies that ginkgo leaf extract is significantly more effective than placebo (6220) and possibly as effective as betahistine for improving vertigo and dizziness caused by vascular vestibular disorders and vestibular disorders of unknown origin (6220,6221). ...when used orally for symptoms of premenstrual syndrome (PMS) (6229). There is some evidence that ginkgo leaf extract can produce significant relief in breast tenderness and neuropsychological symptoms associated with premenstrual syndrome (PMS) when started during the 16th day of the menstrual cycle and continued until the 5th day of the following cycle (6229). ...when used orally to prevent acute altitude sickness (6230). In mountain climbers, ginkgo leaf extract 80 mg twice daily seems to significantly reduce the occurrence of symptoms of altitude sickness, including headache, fatigue, dyspnea, nausea, and vomiting. Ginkgo leaf extract also seems to improve cold tolerance by approximately 23% (6230). ...when used orally for age-related macular degeneration (6227,6228). There is limited evidence that ginkgo leaf extract might significantly improve distance vision in patients with macular degeneration (6227). ...when used orally for improving color vision in diabetic retinopathy. There is some evidence that treatment with ginkgo leaf extract for six months can significantly improve measures of color vision in patients with early diabetic retinopathy (6175).

POSSIBLY INEFFECTIVE ...when used orally for tinnitus. The use of ginkgo leaf extract for tinnitus is controversial. Some studies have shown benefit, but the majority of evidence indicates that ginkgo leaf extract is not consistently effective for patients with tinnitus (221,910,6208,6218,6208,6219).

Most clinical studies on the effectiveness of ginkgo leaf have used the standardized extracts EGb 761 (Tanakan) and LI 1370 (Lichtwer Pharma). These two extracts are similar and prepared to contain approximately 24-25% flavone glycosides and 6% terpene lactones. Products with similar ingredients include Ginkai (Lichtwer Pharma), Ginkgo 5 (Pharmline), Ginkgold and Ginkgo (Nature's Way), and Quanterra Mental Sharpness (Warner-Lambert). There is insufficient reliable information available to rate the effectiveness of ginkgo leaf for its other uses. However, there is preliminary evidence that ginkgo biloba might be helpful for antidepressant-induced sexual dysfunction (599,3965,3967,3968), but not all findings have been positive (207,3966,3969). More evidence is needed to rate the effectiveness of ginkgo leaf for this use.

Mechanism of Action

Gingko leaf and its extracts contain several active constituents including flavonoids, terpenoids, and organic acids. Many ginkgo leaf extracts are standardized to contain 24-25% of the flavonoid glycosides and 6% of the terpenoids. The major flavonoids are primarily derived from rutin and include isorhamnetine, quercetin, kaempferol, and proanthocyanidins. The primary terpenoids are ginkgolides A, B, C, M, and J, and bilobalide (1515). Although many of ginkgo's constituents have intrinsic pharmacological effects individually, there is some evidence that the constituents work synergistically to produce more potent pharmacological effects than any individual constituent (1514,6494). Although the mechanism of action of ginkgo leaf is only partially understood, there are several theories about how it might work for various disease states. One theory is that ginkgo leaf might work by protecting tissues from oxidative damage. Gingko leaf flavonoids have antioxidant and free radical scavenging properties (2660,5715,5717,5719). These flavonoids seem to prevent or reduce cell membrane lipid peroxidation (1515), decrease oxidative damage to erythrocytes (5717), and protect neurons and retinal tissue from oxidative stress (1515,5719) and injury following ischemic episodes (1515,2660,5077). Protecting neurons and other tissues from oxidative damage might prevent progression of tissue degeneration in patients with dementia and other conditions. Central nervous system (CNS) disorders such as dementia and other conditions such as peripheral arterial disease, hypersensitivity disorders, allergies, asthma, bronchitis, etc. might also benefit from ginkgo's anti-inflammatory effects. Ginkgolides from the ginkgo leaf competitively inhibit platelet activating factor (PAF) binding at membrane receptors of numerous cells (5719). PAF inhibition decreases platelet aggregation (5717), decreases phagocyte chemotaxis, decreases smooth muscle contraction (1515), prevents degranulation of neutrophils, decreases free radical production (5716,5717), decreases damaging glycine production after brain injury, and reduces excitatory amino acid receptor function (2660). Ginkgo leaf's inhibition of PAF might also increase cardiac contractility and coronary blood flow. Ginkgo leaf products might also benefit CNS and vascular conditions by improving circulation. Ginkgo leaf seems to improve blood flow to capillaries throughout the body, including the CNS, eyes, ears, extremities, and other tissues. Ginkgo leaf likely improves circulation by both decreasing blood viscosity and affecting vascular smooth muscle. Ginkgo leaf seems to restore the balance between prostacyclin and thromboxane A2, resulting in improved vasoregulation. Therefore, ginkgo leaf relaxes spasmodic contracting vasculature and contracts abnormally dilated vessels. It is not clear exactly how ginkgo causes vascular contraction and improves venous tone, but these effects might be due to phosphodiesterase inhibition, resulting in increased cAMP levels and release of catecholamines (6492). Some ginkgo constituents may also have a potent relaxing effect on vascular smooth muscle (213). Overall, ginkgo leaf seems to increase cerebral and peripheral blood flow microcirculation, and reduce vascular permeability (5721,6492). Ginkgo is also thought to be helpful for erectile dysfunction due to relaxing effects on vascular smooth muscle and improvement in blood flow to the corpus cavernosum (213). In addition to antioxidant, anti-inflammatory, and circulatory effects, ginkgo leaf products have several other pharmacological effects. Ginkgo leaf extract might also be helpful for Alzheimer's disease due to effects on beta-amyloid proteins. There is preliminary evidence that ginkgo leaf extract can inhibit toxicity and cell death induced by beta-amyloid peptides (6494). However, this has not yet been demonstrated in vivo. Ginkgo might also influence certain neurotransmitter systems, such as the cholinergic system (6490), and seems to produce EEG changes similar to the acetylcholinesterase inhibitor tacrine (Cognex) (6067). There has been some speculation that ginkgo leaf inhibits monoamine oxidase A and B (5721), but so far studies have found conflicting results (6231,6232,6233). It is also suggested that ginkgo leaf inhibits catechol-O-methyl transferase (COMT, an enzyme which breaks down adrenergic transmitters) and increases the number of alpha-adrenoreceptors in the brain, which would help reverse the decline in brain alpha-adrenoceptor activity which occurs with aging (2660). There is some evidence that ginkgo flavonoids have GABA-ergic effects and might directly effect benzodiazepine receptors (6423). However, the clinical significance of this effect is not known. The ginkgolides A and B seem to decrease glucocorticoid biosynthesis, which might also play a role in gingko's proposed antistress and neuroprotective effects (5722,5723,5724). Ginkgo leaf might also have some antimicrobial activity, including activity against Pneumocystis carinii and possibly some gram-positive bacteria and yeast (6069). There is some preliminary evidence that ginkgo might have a role in fighting syndrome X. In healthy volunteers, gingko leaf extract can increase pancreatic beta-cell function in response to glucose loading and also seems to reduce blood pressure. Some researchers think it might decrease development of hyperinsulinemia associated with hypertension, which often precedes development of type 2 diabetes and atherosclerotic cardiovascular disease (5719). Some crude extracts from gingko leaves also contain the constituent ginkgolic acid. This constituent can have strong allergenic properties and might also have possible mutagenic and carcinogenic properties. Standardized gingko leaf extracts such as EGb 761 contain no greater than 5 ppm in concentration of ginkgolic acids (5714). There is some preliminary evidence that ginkgo leaf extract can inhibit cytochrome P450 1A2 activity by approximately 13% and 2D6 by approximately 9%. Ginkgo leaf extract seems to inhibit 2D6 more in males than females (1303). The effects of ginkgo leaf extract on cytochrome P450 3A4 are unclear. There is some in vitro evidence that ginkgo leaf extract might inhibit cytochrome P450 3A4 (6450). In vivo, ginkgo leaf extract does not seem to inhibit 3A4 activity (1303). However, there is anecdotal evidence that suggest ginkgo leaf extract might actually induce cytochrome P450 3A4 activity (6423). This effect has not yet been verified.

Adverse Reactions

Orally, ginkgo leaf extract in typical doses can cause mild gastrointestinal upset (4,12,17), headache (5719), dizziness (9), palpitations, constipation (5719), and allergic skin reactions (17). Large doses can cause restlessness, diarrhea, nausea, vomiting (5), lack of muscle tone, and weakness (2). Excessive spontaneous bleeding is one of the most concerning potential side effects. There are two case reports of subdural hematoma associated with ginkgo use (577,578), one report of a subarachnoid hemorrhage (4207), one report of a parietal hemorrhage (244), and one case report of a bleeding iris (spontaneous hyphema) associated with ginkgo use (579). Excessive postoperative bleeding requiring transfusion has also occurred following laparoscopic surgery in a patient who had been taking ginkgo leaf extract (887). Ginkgo leaf extract might cause serious allergic skin reactions in certain patients. There is one case of Stevens-Johnson syndrome following a second administration of a preparation containing ginkgo leaf extract, choline, vitamins B6, and vitamin B12 (208). There is some concern based on anecdotal reports that ginkgo might be associated with seizures in some patients. However, there is not yet enough evidence to prove that ginkgo can actually cause seizure (3575,7030). The ingestion of the crude plant is associated with severe allergic reactions (17). Skin contact with fresh ginkgo leaves can cause contact dermatitis (19). There is some in vitro evidence that suggests high concentrations of ginkgo might reduce male and female fertility (4239,4240); however, this has not been demonstrated in humans. Intravenously, ginkgo leaf extract can cause skin allergy, circulatory disturbances, and phlebitis (6). The German intravenous product has been withdrawn from the market due to safety concerns (6).

Interactions with Herbs & Other Dietary Supplements

HERBS WITH ANTICOAGULANT/ANTIPLATELET POTENTIAL: Concomitant use of herbs that affect platelet aggregation could theoretically increase the risk of bleeding in some people. These herbs include: angelica, anise, arnica, asafoetida, bogbean, boldo, capsicum, celery, chamomile, clove, danshen, fenugreek, feverfew, garlic, ginger, ginseng (Panax), horse chestnut, horseradish, licorice, meadowsweet, prickly ash, onion, papain, passionflower, poplar, quassia, red clover, turmeric, wild carrot, wild lettuce, willow, and others (4,19).

Interactions with Drugs

ANTICOAGULANT, ANTIPLATELET DRUGS: Concomitant administration can increase the risk of bleeding (5,18). Ginkgo leaf has been shown to decrease platelet aggregation. It is thought that the ginkgo constituent, ginkgolide B, displaces platelet-activating factor from its binding sites, decreasing blood coagulation (6048). Some of these drugs include aspirin, dalteparin (Fragmin), enoxaparin (Lovenox), heparin, indomethacin (Indocin), ticlopidine (Ticlid), warfarin (Coumadin), and others.

INSULIN: Gingko leaf extract can alter insulin secretion and metabolism and might affect blood glucose levels (5719). People taking insulin should monitor glucose levels closely. Insulin dose adjustments might be necessary.

MONOAMINE OXIDASE INHIBITORS (MAOIs): Theoretically, ginkgo might potentiate the activity of monoamine oxidase inhibitors (6,12). However, this effect has not been demonstrated in humans.

THIAZIDE DIURETICS: Ginkgo leaf can increase blood pressure when used concomitantly with thiazide diuretics (613).

TRAZODONE (Desyrel): Use of ginkgo leaf extract with trazodone has been associated with coma. In one case, an Alzheimer's patient taking trazodone 20 mg twice daily and ginkgo leaf extract 80 mg twice daily for 4 doses became comatose. The coma was reversed by administration of flumazenil (Romazicon). Coma might have been induced by excessive GABA-ergic activity. Ginkgo flavonoids are thought to have GABA-ergic activity and directly act on benzodiazepine receptors. Ginkgo might also increase metabolism of trazodone to active GABA-ergic metabolites, possibly by inducing cytochrome P450 3A4 metabolism (6423).

WARFARIN (Coumadin): Ginkgo leaf can increase the anticoagulant effects of warfarin and risk of bleeding (576). Monitor patients using this combination closely. Warfarin dose adjustment may be necessary.

OTHER DRUGS: There is preliminary evidence that ginkgo leaf extract can affect cytochrome P450 (CYP450) enzymes including 1A2, 2D6, and 3A4 (1303,6423,6450). Ginkgo leaf extract seems to mildly inhibit CYP1A2 and CYP2D6. Since ginkgo leaf extract seems to only mildly effect these enzymes, it is not likely to produce clinically significant interactions; however, it might slightly increase levels of some drugs metabolized by those enzymes. Ginkgo leaf extract might also affect CYP3A4. However, there is conflicting evidence about whether it induces or inhibits the enzyme (1303,6423,6450). Until more is known, use ginkgo cautiously in patients taking drugs metabolized by these enzymes. Some drugs metabolized by CYP1A2 include acetaminophen (Tylenol), amitriptyline (Elavil), clopidogrel (Plavix), clozapine (Clozaril), diazepam (Valium), estradiol, olanzapine (Zyprexa), ondansetron (Zofran), propranolol (Inderal), ropinirole (Requip), tacrine (Cognex), theophylline, verapamil (Calan, Covera-HS, Isoptin, Verelan), warfarin (Coumadin), and others. Some drugs metabolized by CYP2D6 include amitriptyline (Elavil), clozapine (Clozaril), codeine, desipramine (Norpramin), donepezil (Aricept), fentanyl (Duragesic), flecainide (Tambocor), fluoxetine (Prozac), meperidine (Demerol), methadone (Dolophine), metoprolol (Lopressor, Toprol XL), olanzapine (Zyprexa), ondansetron (Zofran), tramadol (Ultram), trazodone (Desyrel), and others. Some drugs metabolized by CYP450 3A4 include lovastatin (Mevacor), ketoconazole (Nizoral), itraconazole (Sporanox), fexofenadine (Allegra), triazolam (Halcion), and others.

Interactions with Foods

No interactions are known to occur, and there is no known reason to expect a clinically significant interaction with ginkgo leaf.

Interactions with Lab Tests

No interactions are known to occur, and there is no known reason to expect a clinically significant interaction with ginkgo leaf.

Interactions with Diseases or Conditions

BLEEDING DISORDERS: Ginkgo leaf can decrease platelet aggregation by inhibiting platelet-activation factor (PAF) and may exacerbate bleeding disorders (6); use with caution.

DIABETES: Theoretically, ginkgo may interfere with the management of diabetes. Ginkgo has been reported to increase pancreatic beta-cell function in response to glucose and may also increase the metabolic clearance of insulin (5719). Monitor blood glucose levels closely. Diabetes medications might require dose adjustment.

EPILEPSY: There is some concern that ginkgo might be associated with seizure. There are several anecdotal reports of seizure occurring in patients taking combination products containing ginkgo and single ingredient ginkgo products. However, there is not yet enough evidence to prove that ginkgo can actually cause seizure in certain patients (3575,7030). Until more is known, use cautiously or avoid in epileptic patients or patients prone to seizure.

INFERTILITY: Some evidence suggests that ginkgo biloba might inhibit oocyte fertilization and should be avoided in couples attempting to conceive (4239,4240). This effect has not yet been demonstrated in humans; however, until more is known, use with caution in couples attempting to conceive and avoid use in couples having difficulty conceiving.

SURGERY: Ginkgo leaf extract has antiplatelet effects and can cause excessive bleeding if used prior to surgery (887). Tell patients to discontinue ginkgo at least 2 weeks before elective surgical procedures.

Dosage and Administration

ORAL: For dementia syndromes a dosage of 120-240 mg per day of gingko leaf extract, divided in two or three doses has been used (2,1514,1515). To relieve walking pain in patients with intermittent claudication, a dosage of 120-240 mg per day of gingko leaf extract, divided into two or three doses has been used; however, the higher dose may be more effective (2,3461). For reversing sexual dysfunction due to SSRIs, the typical starting dose is 60 mg twice daily of gingko leaf extract. This dose can be titrated up to 240 mg twice daily (212). For vertigo or tinnitus dosages of 120-160 mg per day of gingko leaf extract, divided into two or three doses have been used (2). For prevention of altitude sickness, 80 mg of gingko leaf extract twice daily was used (6230). For premenstrual syndrome (PMS), 80 mg twice daily starting on the sixteenth day of the menstrual cycle until the fifth day of the next cycle has been used (6229). For all indications, start at a lower dose of not more 120 mg per day to avoid adverse gastrointestinal effect. Titrate to higher doses as needed. Most trials used specific standardized Ginkgo biloba leaf extracts. Dosing may vary depending on the specific formulation used. Some people take 0.5 mL of a standard 1:5 tincture of the crude ginkgo leaf three times daily (5011).

Comments

When people talk about Ginkgo biloba, they usually mean ginkgo leaf extract. However, traditionally Ginkgo biloba fruit was used. Ginkgo biloba comes from the Chinese Yin-Kuo, meaning "silver apricot" and biloba, describes its two-lobed, fan shaped leaves (6208). Ginkgo biloba is the oldest living tree species in the world. Ginkgo trees can live as long as a thousand years (6). Ginkgo use for asthma and bronchitis was described in the first pharmacopoeia, Chen Noung Pen T'sao, dating to 2600 BC (6208). Ginkgo is the most frequently prescribed herbal medicine in Germany (6208) and is the preferred treatment for dementia (6491). The National Center for Complementary and Alternative Medicine (NCCAM) is beginning a 5-year study of 3000 people aged 75 and older (the largest study ever of dementia) to determine if ginkgo 240 mg daily prevents dementia or Alzheimer's disease (6226).

GINKGO seed

Also Known As

Baiguo, Fossil Tree, Gingko, Ginkyo, Japanese Silver Apricot, Kew Tree, Maidenhair Tree, Yinhsing.
CAUTION: See separate listings for Ginkgo leaf and Ginkgo leaf extract. Ginkgo leaf extract (Ginkgo biloba) is the most commonly used form of Ginkgo.

Scientific Names

Ginkgo biloba.
Family: Ginkgoaceae.

People Use This For

Orally, ginkgo seed is used as an antitussive and expectorant, for asthma, bronchitis, genitourinary complaints, to aid digestion, and prevent drunkenness.
Topically, ginkgo seed is used for scabies and skin sores.
For food uses, roasted ginkgo seed, which has the pulp removed, is an edible delicacy in Japan and China.

Safety

POSSIBLY SAFE ...when the roasted seed is consumed as food. Limit consumption to a maximum of 8-10 per day (11).
POSSIBLY UNSAFE ...when the roasted seed is used orally for medicinal purposes, especially with long-term use (6,12).
UNSAFE ...when the fresh seed is used orally. Fresh seeds are toxic and potentially deadly (11).

There is insufficient reliable information available about the safety of the topical use of ginkgo seed.
PREGNANCY AND LACTATION: POSSIBLY SAFE ...when the roasted seed is eaten as food.
POSSIBLY UNSAFE ...when used orally for medicinal purposes; avoid using (4).

Effectiveness
There is insufficient reliable information available about the effectiveness of the ginkgo seed.

Mechanism of Action
The seeds contain cyanogenic glycosides (4), which are reported to have antibacterial and antifungal effects (6). The seeds also contain ginkgotoxin, a compound believed responsible for causing seizures, loss of consciousness, and death (4,11).

Adverse Reactions
Orally, fresh seeds can cause stomachache, nausea, diarrhea, restlessness, difficulty breathing, weak pulse, seizures, loss of consciousness, and shock (4,11). The fresh seeds have caused death in children (11). Ginkgo fruit and pulp is a potent contact allergen. Ingestion of even small amounts of pulp can cause redness around the mouth, rectal burning, and painful anal sphincter spasms (6).
Topically, ginkgo fruit and pulp can cause severe allergic skin reactions, irritation of mucous membranes and the gastrointestinal tract (4,12,17). Cross-reactivity is possible with ginkgo fruit in individuals allergic to poison ivy, poison oak, poison sumac, mango rind, and cashew shell oil (6,380).

Interactions with Herbs & Other Dietary Supplements
Insufficient reliable information available.

Interactions with Drugs
ANTICONVULSANTS: Theoretically, the use of ginkgo seed might interfere with the effectiveness of anticonvulsant drugs. Consumption of raw ginkgo seeds reportedly causes seizures, due to the presence of ginkgotoxin (4,11).

Interactions with Foods
No interactions are known to occur, and there is no known reason to expect a clinically significant interaction with ginkgo seed.

Interactions with Lab Tests
No interactions are known to occur, and there is no known reason to expect a clinically significant interaction with ginkgo seed.

Interactions with Diseases or Conditions
GINKGO ALLERGY: Contraindicated (2).
SEIZURE DISORDERS: Consumption of raw ginkgo seeds reportedly causes seizures, due to the presence of ginkgotoxin (4,11); contraindicated.

Dosage and Administration
ORAL: People typically use 120-240 mg ginkgo tablets or capsules daily in two or three divided doses (5008).

Comments
When people talk about ginkgo, they usually mean ginkgo leaf. Fossils of the ginkgo tree have been found to be over two hundred million years old, making the tree the oldest living species in the world, and the tree itself can live as long as one thousand years (6).

GINSENG, AMERICAN

Also Known As
American Ginseng, Anchi Ginseng, Canadian Ginseng, Ginseng, North American Ginseng, Ontario Ginseng, Red Berry, Ren Shen, Sang, Tienchi Ginseng, Wisconsin Ginseng.
CAUTION: See separate listings for Blue Cohosh, Canaigre, Codonopsis, Ginseng Siberian, Ginseng Panax, Panax Pseudoginseng, and Ashwaganda.

Scientific Names
Panax quinquefolius.
Family: Araliaceae.

People Use This For

Orally, American ginseng is used as an adaptogen, for increasing resistance to environmental stress, a general tonic, stimulant, diuretic, and digestive aid. It is also used for anemia, diabetes, insomnia, neurasthenia, gastritis, impotence, fever, hangover symptoms, stimulating immune function, and for eradicating Pseudomonas infection in cystic fibrosis (4,11,13).

In folk medicine, American ginseng has been used for improving stress resistance, preventing the effects of aging, improving stamina (4,6,13), blood and bleeding disorders, atherosclerosis, loss of appetite, vomiting, colitis, dysentery, cancer, insomnia, neuralgia, rheumatism, memory loss, dizziness, headaches, convulsions, and disorders of pregnancy and childbirth (4,6,11,13).

In food manufacturing, American ginseng is used in soft drinks (11).

In other manufacturing processes, American ginseng oil and extracts are used in soaps and cosmetics (11).

Safety

POSSIBLY SAFE ...when used orally and appropriately, short-term (12).

PREGNANCY AND LACTATION: Insufficient reliable information available; avoid using.

Effectiveness

POSSIBLY EFFECTIVE ...when used orally for reducing post-prandial blood glucose levels in type 2 diabetics. Administration of American ginseng 3 grams up to 2 hours before a meal can significantly reduce post-prandial glucose levels (1018,6461). However, doses greater than 3 grams do not seem to offer any addition benefit (6461).

Mechanism of Action

The applicable part of American ginseng is the root. The principle constituents of American ginseng are known as ginsenosides or as panaxosides (8,11). American ginseng contains primarily ginsenoside Rb-1, which reportedly lowers blood pressure (8,11); has antihemolytic, antipyretic, antipsychotic (11), CNS depressant (8,11), and ulcer protective activity; increases GI motility (11); and decreases islet insulin concentrations (4). Most research has focused on the related species, Panax ginseng, which contains ginsenosides Rb-1, Rc, and Rg-1 (4) (see separate listing for ginseng, Panax). An American ginseng extract decreases LH (luteinizing hormone) levels and increases serum ceruloplasmin oxidase activity (a measure of estrogenic activity in the liver) in female rats with their ovaries removed (6180). However, estrogenic effects in humans has been disputed (515). Preliminary research suggests that American ginseng extract might reduce breast cancer cell growth and that the extract combined with anti-breast cancer drugs might have a synergistic effect (389).

Adverse Reactions

No adverse reactions have been reported specifically with use of American ginseng. Adverse reactions reported for the related species Panax ginseng include insomnia (589), mastalgia (590), vaginal bleeding (591,592), tachycardia (7), mania (594), cerebral arteritis (595), Stevens Johnson syndrome (596), cholestatic hepatitis (associated with a panax-containing, multi-ingredient product, Prostata) (598), amenorrhea, decreased appetite, edema, hyperpyrexia, pruritus, rose spots, hypotension, palpitations, headache, vertigo, euphoria, and neonatal death (4,12). Diarrhea or allergic skin reactions can occur, especially with large amounts or prolonged use (4,9,515). Allergic reactions to ginseng include palpitations, insomnia, and itching (4). There are reports of ginseng abuse syndrome that includes hypertension, nervousness, insomnia, and increased libido (7); however, this is controversial (515) and has not been verified by other reports.

Interactions with Herbs & Other Dietary Supplements

CAFFEINE, COFFEE, GUARANA, MATE, TEA: Concomitant use of American ginseng can potentiate the stimulant effects of these drugs (4,12).

Interactions with Drugs

ANTIPSYCHOTIC DRUGS: Theoretically, American ginseng can interfere with antipsychotic drugs (4).

ANTIDIABETES DRUGS: American ginseng can lower blood glucose (1018,6461). Theoretically, concomitant use with antidiabetes drugs might enhance blood glucose lowering effects and possibly cause hypoglycemia. Monitor blood glucose levels closely. Some antidiabetes drugs include glimepiride (Amaryl), glyburide (Diabeta, Glynase PresTab, Micronase), insulin, pioglitazone (Actos), rosiglitazone (Avandia), and others.

HORMONES: Theoretically, American ginseng can interfere with hormone therapy (4).

MONOAMINE OXIDASE INHIBITORS (MAOIs): Theoretically, American ginseng can interfere with monoamine oxidase inhibitor therapy. There is one case report of insomnia, headache, and tremors with concomitant phenylzine (Nardil) and unspecified ginseng use (617). There is also one case report of hypomania with concomitant phenelzine (Nardil) and unspecified ginseng use (618).

STIMULANT DRUGS: Theoretically, concomitant use of American ginseng can potentiate the activity of stimulant drugs (4,12).

WARFARIN (Coumadin): Theoretically, concomitant use of American ginseng can interfere with warfarin therapy. There is one case report of a decreased international normalization ratio (INR) associated with the addition of a Panax ginseng product to warfarin therapy (619).

Interactions with Foods

COFFEE, TEA: Theoretically, concomitant use of ginseng can potentiate the stimulant effects of coffee or tea (4,12).

Interactions with Lab Tests

COAGULATION TESTS: Theoretically, American ginseng can prolong thrombin time (TT) and activated partial thromboplastin time (aPTT), which is based on in vitro studies with the related species, Panax ginseng (1522).
BLOOD GLUCOSE: American ginseng decrease postprandial blood glucose levels and test results (1018,6461).

Interactions with Diseases or Conditions

BLEEDING CONDITIONS: American ginseng has been reported to decrease blood coagulation (4); contraindicated in cases of hemorrhage or thrombosis.
CARDIAC CONDITIONS: American ginseng is reported to have negative inotropic and chronotropic activity and hypotensive effects. Ginseng might adversely effect patients with cardiac disorders (4); use with caution.
DIABETES: American ginseng has hypoglycemic activity (4,1018,6461). Use in diabetics might increase the risk of hypoglycemic episodes; use with caution.
HORMONE SENSITIVE CANCERS/CONDITIONS: Because American ginseng might have estrogenic effects (6180), women with hormone sensitive conditions should avoid American ginseng. Some of these conditions include breast, uterine, and ovarian cancer, and endometriosis and uterine fibroids.
INSOMNIA: High doses of American ginseng have been associated with insomnia (597). Theoretically, use in patients with insomnia might worsen the condition; use with caution.
SCHIZOPHRENIA: High doses of American ginseng have been associated with insomnia and agitation in schizophrenic patients (597); use with caution.

Dosage and Administration

ORAL: For young and healthy people, the typical dose of American ginseng is 0.25-0.5 grams of the root two times daily (4). For the elderly and debilitated people, 0.4-0.8 grams of the root is usually taken daily and can be used on a continuous basis (4). For reducing postprandial glucose levels in type 2 diabetics, 3-9 grams up to 2 hours before a meal has been used (1018,6461). However, there is no added benefit to taking more than 3 grams (6461). American ginseng should be taken within 2 hours of a meal to avoid potential hypoglycemia (4,1018,6461). Some sources recommend taking American ginseng for a course of 15-20 days with a ginseng-free period of two weeks between consecutive courses (4). But the reason for this recommendation is not clear.

Comments

Avoid confusion with eleutherococcus senticosus, also referred to as Siberian ginseng, and Panax ginseng, also referred to as Asian ginseng. Wild American ginseng is so extensively sought that it has been declared an endangered species in the US (515).

GINSENG, PANAX

Also Known As

Asian Ginseng, Asiatic Ginseng, Chinese Ginseng, Ginseng, Ginseng Asiatique, Ginseng Radix, Ginseng Root, Japanese Ginseng, Jintsam, Korean Ginseng, Korean Panax Ginseng Korean Red, Korean Red Ginseng, Ninjin, Oriental Ginseng, Panax Ginseng, Red Ginseng, Ren Shen, Sang, Seng.
CAUTION: See separate listings for Ginseng American, Blue Cohosh, Canaigre, Codonopsis, Ginseng Siberian, Panax Pseudoginseng, and Ashwaganda.

Scientific Names

Panax ginseng, synonym Panax schinseng.
Family: Araliaceae.

People Use This For

Orally, Panax ginseng is used as a so-called "adaptogen" for increasing resistance to environmental stress and as a general tonic for improving well-being. It is also used for stimulating immune function; improving physical and athletic stamina; and improving cognitive function, concentration, memory, and work efficiency. It is also used orally for depression, anxiety, Pseudomonas infection in cystic fibrosis, irritated or inflamed tissues, and as a diuretic. Panax ginseng is also used orally for anemia, diabetes, gastritis, neurasthenia, impotence and male fertility, fever, hangover, and asthma. It is also used orally for bleeding disorders, loss of appetite, vomiting, colitis, dysentery, cancer, insomnia, neuralgia, rheumatism, dizziness, headache, convulsions, disorders of pregnancy and childbirth, hot flashes due to menopause, and to slow the aging process.

Topically, Panax ginseng is used as part of a multi-ingredient preparation for treating premature ejaculation.

In manufacturing, Panax ginseng is used to make soaps, cosmetics, and as a flavoring in beverages.

Safety

POSSIBLY SAFE ...when used orally and appropriately, short-term. Panax ginseng seems to be safe when used for less than 3 months (12). ...when used topically, short-term as part of a multi-ingredient preparation (SS Cream). This preparation seems to be safe when applied and left on the glans penis for one hour (2537). Further evaluation is needed to determine its safety after prolonged, repetitive topical use.

POSSIBLY UNSAFE ...when used orally, long-term. There is some concern about the long-term safety due to potential hormone-like effects, which might be cause adverse effects with prolonged use (7). Tell patients to limit continuous use to less than 3 months.

CHILDREN: LIKELY UNSAFE ...when used orally in infants. Use of Panax ginseng in newborns is associated with intoxication that can lead to death (12). There is insufficient reliable information about use in older children; avoid using.

PREGNANCY AND LACTATION: Insufficient reliable information available; avoid using.

Effectiveness

POSSIBLY EFFECTIVE ...when used orally for improving cognitive function. There is preliminary evidence that Panax ginseng can improve abstract thinking, mental arithmetic skills, and reaction times in healthy, middle-aged people (2064). Panax ginseng alone does not seem to improve memory (2064), but there is some evidence that a combination of Panax ginseng 100 mg and ginkgo leaf extract 60 mg twice daily can improve memory in otherwise healthy people ages 38 to 66 years (1903). ...when used orally for type 2 diabetes. There is some evidence that Panax ginseng 200 mg daily can decrease fasting blood glucose levels and hemoglobin A1c (HbA1c) in patients with type 2 diabetes (4225). ...when used orally for improving resistance to stress. Panax ginseng in combination with multivitamins and minerals are more effective than multivitamins and minerals alone for improving quality of life in people exposed to stress (6254). ...when used orally in combination with influenza vaccination for preventing the common cold and flu (589,1427). When started 4 weeks prior to influenza vaccination and continued for 8 more weeks, Panax ginseng seems to significantly reduce the risk of contracting both the common cold and flu (589). ...when red ginseng, which is produced by steam-curing Panax ginseng prior to drying, is used orally for improving hemodynamics in patients with congestive heart failure (4243). ...when used orally for preventing cancer. Epidemiological data suggests that ginseng consumption, particularly fresh ginseng extract, might decrease the incidence of cancer in general and specifically for stomach, lung, liver, ovary, and skin cancers (2063,3122). ...when used topically as part of a multi-ingredient preparation for treating premature ejaculation. A multi-ingredient cream preparation containing Panax ginseng, angelica root, Cistanches deserticola, Zanthoxyl species, torlidis seed, clove flower, asiasari root, cinnamon bark, and toad venom (SS Cream) applied to the glans penis 1 hour prior to intercourse and washed off immediately before intercourse improves ejaculatory latency in men with premature ejaculation (2537).

POSSIBLY INEFFECTIVE ...when used orally for enhancing athletic performance in healthy, young adults (1427,4230,4231,4236,4244).

There is insufficient reliable information available about the effectiveness of Panax ginseng for its other uses.

Mechanism of Action

The applicable part of Panax ginseng is the root. Panax ginseng contains several active constituents. The constituents thought to be of most importance are triterpenoid saponins referred to as ginsenosides or panaxosides. Ginsenosides is the term developed by Asian researchers, and the term panaxosides was developed by early Russian researchers. Numerous subtypes of ginsenosides have been identified. Other constituents include pectin, B vitamins, and various flavonoids (8,11). The ginsenosides have a wide range of pharmacological activity. In some cases, these constituents seem to counteract each other's activity. For example, ginsenoside Rg1, raises blood pressure and acts as a central nervous system (CNS) stimulant. Ginsenoside Rb1 lowers blood pressure and acts as a CNS depressant (8,11). Ginseng is widely used as a general tonic or "adaptogen" for fighting stress. There is some evidence that it might work against stress by affecting the hypothalamic-pituitary-adrenal (HPA) axis. Panax ginseng saponins seem to increase serum cortisol concentrations (3256,3257) and stimulate adrenal function (6,13). Panax ginseng might also increase dehydroepiandrosterone sulfate (DHEA-S) levels in women (3863). There is some evidence that Panax ginseng can affect immune function and might have anticancer effects. Panax ginseng appears to stimulate natural-killer cell activity and possibly other immune-system activity. It might also have some antitumor activity (4,6,7,8,3122). Extracts of Panax ginseng decrease the production of tumor necrosis factor, diminish DNA strand breakage, and inhibit the formation of induced skin tumors (1956). Panax ginseng also increases antioxidant plasma levels and antioxidant activity (1956,4227). Ginsenosides have been shown to inhibit tumor cell invasion and suppress sister chromatid exchanges in human lymphoctes (1956). Panax ginseng also contains water insoluble polyacetylenic constituents such as panaxynol, panaxydol, and panaxytriol. Panaxydol seems to have antiproliferative effects on various types of cancer cells by inhibiting cancer cell growth at the cell cycle G1 to S transition phase (1955). In peptic ulceration, Panax ginseng has shown inhibitory activity on Helicobacter pylori-induced hemagglutination (3121). Ginseng might improve hemodynamics in patients with congestive heart failure and might work synergistically with digoxin (4243). Ginsenosides have a variety of other pharmacological effects. They seem to interfere with platelet aggregation and coagulation (4,1522). They also have papaverine-like effects on smooth muscle (6), and analgesic and anti-inflammatory effects (4,6). There is evidence that ginsenosides can relax human bronchial smooth muscle by stimulating the release of nitrous oxide from airway epithelium which may account for the potential anti-asthmatic effect of Panax ginseng (1957). Ginsenosides also potentiate nerve growth factor (11) and might confer neuroprotection through nicotinic activity (3109). Panax ginseng also seems to promote growth of normal intestinal flora while inhibiting Clostridial species (7). Panax ginseng may also lower serum cholesterol and triglycerides (6). Panax ginseng extract has been shown to increase serum ceruloplasmin oxidase activity (a measure of estrogenic activity in the liver) in animal models when ovaries are removed (6180). A multi-ingredient cream preparation containing Panax ginseng is thought to work in premature ejaculation by increasing the penile vibratory threshold and reducing the amplitude of penile somatosensory evoked potentials (2537). Some people try ginseng for cystic fibrosis because there is preliminary evidence that it has activity against Pseudomonas aeruginosa lung infections, but this effect has not yet been demonstrated in humans (3095,3096,6108). There is some evidence that a Panax ginseng root extract can mildly inhibit cytochrome P450 2D6 activity by approximately 6% in humans. However, it appears to have no effect on 3A4 activity (1303).

Adverse Reactions

Orally, Panax ginseng is usually well tolerated, but some patients can experience sides effects. The most common side effect is insomnia (589). Less commonly patients can experience mastalgia (590), vaginal bleeding (591,592,3354), amenorrhea, tachycardia and palpitations (7), hypertension, hypotension, edema, decreased appetite, diarrhea hyperpyrexia, pruritus, rose spots, headache, vertigo, euphoria, and mania (4,5,9,594). Uncommon side effects can include cerebral arteritis (595), Stevens-Johnson syndrome (596) cholestatic hepatitis (associated with a Panax ginseng-containing, multi-ingredient product, Prostata) (598), and neonatal death (4,12). Some patients can have allergic skin reactions, especially with use of large amounts or prolonged use (4,5,9). When the multi-ingredient cream preparation (SS Cream) has been applied topically to the glans penis, sporadic erectile dysfunction, excessively delayed ejaculation, mild pain, and local irritation and burning has occurred (2537).

There is a lot of controversy about the existence of a "ginseng abuse syndrome." In the late 1970s one author reported the existence of this syndrome that occurred after long-term use of ginseng. Symptoms included one or more of either hypertension, nervousness, insomnia, increased libido (7,3353), estrogenic effects (5,6), skin eruptions, edema, and diarrhea (3353). Experts now agree there is not a ginseng abuse syndrome (7,515). However, many of these individual side effects can occur in some patients, even after short-term use of Panax ginseng.

Interactions with Herbs & Other Dietary Supplements

COFFEE, GUARANA, TEA: Concomitant use may potentiate effects due to caffeine content of coffee, guarana or tea (4,12).

HERBS WITH ANTICOAGULANT/ANTIPLATELET POTENTIAL: Theoretically, concomitant use of ginseng with herbs that affect platelet aggregation may increase the risk of bleeding. Ginsenosides in ginseng are reported to inhibit platelet aggregation in vitro (4). This effect has not been demonstrated in humans. In two case reports, ginseng has actually been reported to decrease the effectiveness of the prescription drug warfarin (19,619,1288). Herbs with anticoagulant or antiplatelet properties include: angelica, anise, arnica, asafoetida, bogbean, boldo, capsicum, celery, chamomile, clove, danshen, fenugreek, feverfew, garlic, ginger, ginkgo, horse chestnut, horseradish, licorice, meadowsweet, prickly ash, onion, papain, passionflower, poplar, quassia, red clover, turmeric, wild carrot, wild lettuce, willow, and others (4,19).

Interactions with Drugs

ANTICOAGULANT/ANTIPLATELET AGENTS: There is some evidence from one case that Panax ginseng can decrease the effectiveness of warfarin (Coumadin) (619,1288). However, there is in vitro evidence that ginsenoside constituents in Panax ginseng might actually decrease platelet aggregation (4). Theoretically, concomitant use of ginseng and antiplatelet agents might increase the risk of bleeding. However, this effect has not been reported in humans. Use with caution in patients concurrently taking anticoagulant or antiplatelet agents. Some antiplatelet and anticoagulant drugs include aspirin, cilostazol (Pletal), clopidogrel (Plavix), dalteparin (Fragmin), enoxaparin (Lovenox), heparin, ticlopidine (Ticlid), and others.

ANTIDIABETES DRUGS: Theoretically, concomitant use might enhance blood glucose lowering effects (4225). Monitor blood glucose levels closely. Some antidiabetes drugs include glimepiride (Amaryl), glyburide (Diabeta, Glynase PresTabs, Micronase), insulin, pioglitazone (Actos), rosiglitazone (Avandia), and others.

ANTIPSYCHOTIC DRUGS: Theoretically, Panax ginseng might interfere with antipsychotic drugs by interfering with neurotransmitters (4).

CAFFEINE: There is some concern that long-term use of 3 grams of Panax ginseng daily in combination with caffeine might lead to hypertension in some patients (19).

FUROSEMIDE: There is some concern that Panax ginseng might contribute to diuretic resistance. There is one case of resistance to furosemide diuresis in a patient taking a germanium-containing ginseng product (770).

IMMUNOSUPPRESSANTS: Theoretically, concurrent use might interfere with immunosuppressive therapy. Panax ginseng might have immune system stimulating properties (4,6,7,8,3122). Immunosuppressant drugs include azathioprine (Imuran), basiliximab (Simulect), cyclosporine (Neoral, Sandimmune), daclizumab (Zenapax), muromonab-CD3 (OKT3, Orthoclone OKT3), mycophenolate (CellCept), tacrolimus (FK506, Prograf), sirolimus (Rapamune), prednisone (Deltasone, Orasone), and other corticosteroids (glucocorticoids).

INSULIN: There is some concern that Panax ginseng might have additive hypoglycemic effects when used with insulin. Insulin dose adjustments might be necessary in patients taking Panax ginseng (19); use with caution.

MAO INHIBITORS: Theoretically, Panax ginseng can interfere with monoamine oxidase inhibitor therapy. Concomitant use with phenelzine (Nardil) is associated with insomnia, headache, tremors (617), and hypomania (618).

STIMULANT DRUGS: Panax ginseng can potentiate stimulant drug effects (12).

WARFARIN (Coumadin): There is some evidence from one case that Panax ginseng can decrease the effectiveness of warfarin (619,1288); however, it's not clear how ginseng causes this interaction (2531). Monitor patients using this combination closely. Dose adjustments may be necessary.

OTHER DRUGS: There is some evidence that Panax ginseng can inhibit the cytochrome P450 2D6 (CYP2D6) enzyme by approximately 6% (1303). Although this effect is unlikely to produce clinically significant interactions, it might cause slightly elevated levels of drugs metabolized by the CYP2D6 enzyme. Some of these drugs include amitriptyline (Elavil), clozapine (Clozaril), codeine, desipramine (Norpramin), donepezil (Aricept), fentanyl (Duragesic), flecainide (Tambocor), fluoxetine (Prozac), meperidine (Demerol), methadone (Dolophine), metoprolol (Lopressor, Toprol XL), olanzapine (Zyprexa), ondansetron (Zofran), tramadol (Ultram), trazodone (Desyrel), and others.

Interactions with Foods

COFFEE, TEA: Concomitant use may potentiate effects due to caffeine content of coffee or tea (4,12).

Interactions with Lab Tests

ACTIVATED PARTIAL THROMBOPLASTIN TIME (aPTT), THROMBIN TIME (TT): Theoretically, Panax ginseng might prolong aPTT, TT, and increase test results (1522).

INTERNATIONAL NORMALIZED RATIO (INR), PROTHROMBIN TIME (PT): Panax ginseng can reduce PT/INR and test results in patients treated with warfarin (Coumadin) (619,1288).

GLUCOSE: Panax ginseng might reduce fasting blood glucose concentrations and test results (4225).

GLYCOSYLATED HEMOGLOBIN (HbA1c): Panax ginseng might improve glucose control and reduce HbA1c values in patients with type 2 diabetes (4225).

Interactions with Diseases or Conditions

BLEEDING CONDITIONS: Ginseng has been reported to decrease blood coagulation (4); contraindicated in cases of hemorrhage or thrombosis.

CARDIAC CONDITIONS: Ginseng is reported to have negative inotropic and chronotropic activity and hypotensive effects. Ginseng might adversely affect patients with cardiac disorders (4); use with caution.

DIABETES: Ginseng is reported to have hypoglycemic activity (4). Use in diabetics might increase the risk of hypoglycemic episodes; use with caution.

HORMONE SENSITIVE CANCERS/CONDITIONS: Because ginseng seems to have estrogenic effects (6180), women with hormone sensitive conditions should avoid ginseng. Some of these conditions include breast, uterine, and ovarian cancer, and endometriosis and uterine fibroids.

INSOMNIA: High doses of ginseng have been associated with insomnia (597). Theoretically, use in patients with insomnia might worsen the condition; use with caution.

ORGAN TRANSPLANT RECIPIENTS: Theoretically, concurrent use might interfere with immunosuppressive therapy. Panax ginseng might have immune system stimulating properties (4,6,7,8,3122); avoid concurrent use.

SCHIZOPHRENIA: High doses of ginseng have been associated with insomnia and agitation in schizophrenic patients (597); use with caution.

Dosage and Administration

ORAL: Root powder is commonly available in 1 ounce and 4 ounce containers. Cut or powdered root is commonly taken orally 0.6-3 grams 1-3 times per day (8,12), or one cup tea (Panax ginseng tea bags usually have 1500 mg of ginseng root. The tea is made by steeping 3 grams of root in 150 mL of boiling water for 10-15 minutes, and then straining). People consume this tea 1-3 times per day for 3-4 weeks (8). An extract is made using 2 ounces of root extract in an alcohol base. Capsules come in 100 mg, 250 mg, and 500 mg. People typically take from 200-600 mg per day (7). For reducing the risk of getting the common cold or flu, one study has used Panax ginseng 100 mg daily starting 4 weeks prior to influenza vaccination and continued for 8 weeks thereafter (589). Panax ginseng can also be taken in an extract form or as an oil. People usually take panax ginseng from 3 weeks to 3 months (2,4,12). Sometimes it is taken continuously. A panax-free period of two weeks is recommended between consecutive courses (2,4).

Comments

Ginseng has been used for medicinal purposes for over two thousand years. Approximately six million Americans use it regularly. Some consider the age of the ginseng roots important. In 1976, a four hundred year old root of Manchurian ginseng from the mountains of China reportedly sold for $10,000 per ounce. The contents of commercial preparations labeled as containing Panax ginseng can vary greatly; many contain little or no Panax ginseng (5,6,13). Sometimes you will hear people refer to ginseng as red or white ginseng. This distinguishes how some ginseng roots are prepared. For example, red ginseng is produced by steam-curing Panax. Heat treatment of ginseng at a temperature and pressure higher than what is conventionally used to prepare red ginseng has been found to cause increased production of the ginsenosides Rg3, Rg5, Rg6, Rh2, Rh3, Rh4, and Rs3 which are usually absent or present in only small amounts in preparations of white or red ginseng (1956).

GINSENG, SIBERIAN

Also Known As

Ci Wu Jia, Ciwujia, Devil's Bush, Devil's Shrub, Eleuthera, Eleuthero, Eleuthero Ginseng, Eleutherococ, Eleutherococci radix, Eleutherococcus, Ginseng, Phytoestrogen, Shigoka, Siberian Ginseng, Thorny Bearer of Free Berries, Touch-Me-Not, Untouchable, Wild Pepper, Wu Jia Pi, Wu-jia, Ussuri, Ussurian Thorny Pepperbrush. CAUTION: See separate listings for American Ginseng, Ashwaganda, Blue Cohosh, Canaigre, Codonopsis, Ginseng Panax, and Panax Pseudoginseng.

Scientific Names

Eleutherococcus senticosus, synonym Acanthopanax senticosus.
Family: Araliaceae.

People Use This For

Orally, people use Siberian ginseng as an adaptogen, for increasing resistance to environmental stress. It is also used orally for normalizing high or low blood pressure, atherosclerosis, pyelonephritis, craniocerebral trauma, rheumatic heart disease, neuroses, increasing work capacity (6,11), Alzheimer's disease, attention deficit disorder, chronic fatigue syndrome, diabetes, fibromyalgia, influenza, chronic bronchitis, tuberculosis, improving athletic performance, reducing toxicity of chemotherapy, symptomatic treatment of herpes simplex type II infections, and as an immune system stimulant (1427,1900).

In traditional Chinese medicine, Siberian ginseng is used as a stimulant, tonic, and diuretic; for insomnia, lower back or kidney pain, lack of appetite, rheumatoid arthritis; enhancing overall resistance to disease; and for stress (11).

In manufacturing, Siberian ginseng is added to skin care products (11).

Safety

LIKELY SAFE ...when used orally and appropriately, short-term. Studies have safely used Siberian ginseng in multiple course treatment regimens. Patients received daily treatment for 35-60 consecutive days followed by a 2-3 week ginseng-free period. Up to 8 treatment courses have been used, each separated by a ginseng-free period (4,12).
PREGNANCY AND LACTATION: Insufficient reliable information available; avoid using (4).

Effectiveness

POSSIBLY EFFECTIVE ...when used orally by healthy individuals for increasing speed, quality, and capacity for physical work (2,4) . ...when used orally as an adaptogen in people exposed to high temperatures, hypoxemia, and conditions that cause motion sickness (4). ...when used orally for preventing atherosclerosis (4). ...when used orally for normalizing blood pressure in people with hypertension or hypotension (4). ...when used orally for treating acute pyelonephritis (4). ...when used orally for treating diabetes (4). ...when used orally for treating acute craniocerebral trauma (4). ...when used orally for treating people with various types of neuroses (4). ...when used orally for treating rheumatic heart disease by reducing blood coagulation (4). ...when used orally for treating chronic bronchitis (4). ...when used orally for treating children with abating forms of pulmonary tuberculosis (4). ...when used orally as a tonic for invigoration during times of fatigue and debility and for building strength during convalescence (2). ...when used orally for reducing frequency, severity and duration of herpes simplex type II infections. Studies for management of herpes simplex have used Siberian ginseng extract standardized to contain eleutheroside 0.3%. This extract is found in the product Elagen (1427).

Mechanism of Action

The applicable part of Siberian ginseng is the root. It contains active compounds referred to as eleutherosides A through M (515,1954). The eleutherosides include a variety of diverse compounds including saponins (daucosterol, beta-sitosterol, hederasaponin B), coumarins (isofraxidin), lignans (sesamin, syringoresinol), phenylpropanoids (syringin, caffeic acid, sinapyl alcohol, coniferyl aldehyde), betulinic acid, vitamins (vitamin E), and provitamins (beta-carotene) (515,1954). Siberian ginseng and its lignan constituents, sesamin and syringin, seem to have immunostimulatory effects (7,11,1954). Several constituents are also thought to have antioxidant and possible anticancer effects including syringin, syringoresinol, sesamin, beta sitosterol, caffeic acid, and coniferyl aldehyde (1954). In addition, there is some evidence the constituent coniferyl aldehyde protects DNA against breakage caused by ultraviolet light (1954). There is also some evidence that Siberian ginseng can boost immune function in humans. Siberian ginseng increases lymphocyte counts and phagocyte activity (6206). Siberian ginseng constituents have a variety of other pharmacological effects. The dihydroxybenzoic acid constituent seems to inhibit platelet aggregation (4). Other constituents are also thought to have anti-inflammatory, diuretic, gonadotropic, and estrogenic activity (11). Siberian ginseng might also have protein-anabolic activity (11) and stimulate the pituitary-adrenocortical system (3,4,6).

Adverse Reactions

Orally, Siberian ginseng can sometimes cause slight drowsiness, anxiety, irritability, and melancholy (4,6). Mastalgia can also occur (4). These adverse effects are more likely with higher than normal doses. Siberian ginseng should be used cautiously in patients with cardiovascular disorders (e.g. atherosclerotic or rheumatic heart disease), because it can cause palpitations, tachycardia, and hypertension (4,6,6500). Headache and pericardial pain can also occur in patients with rheumatic heart disease (4,6). Long term use of Siberian ginseng is associated with inflamed nerves, often the sciatic nerve, which can then cause muscle spasms (4). There is one case report of neonatal androgenization following maternal use of Siberian ginseng (593,6500). However, it was later discovered that the androgenization was not due to Siberian ginseng, but due to silk vine (Periploca sepium) bark contamination (850,6500).

Interactions with Herbs & Other Dietary Supplements

HERBS WITH SEDATIVE PROPERTIES: Theoretically, concomitant use with herbs that have sedative properties might enhance therapeutic and adverse effects. These include calamus, calendula, California poppy, catnip, capsicum, celery, couch grass, elecampane, German chamomile, goldenseal, gotu kola, hops, Jamaican dogwood, kava, lemon balm, sage, St. John's wort, sassafras, scullcap, shepherd's purse, stinging nettle, valerian, wild carrot, wild lettuce, ashwaganda root, and yerba mansa (4,19).
COFFEE: Avoid concomitant use (4).
VITAMINS: Concomitant use with vitamins B1, B2 and C may increase the excretion of these vitamins (4).

Interactions with Drugs

ALCOHOL: Avoid concomitant use of Eleutherococcus (4).
ANTICOAGULANT/ANTIPLATELET DRUGS: Theoretically, concomitant use might increase effects or adverse of anticoagulant or antiplatelet drugs (4).
ANTIPSYCHOTIC DRUGS, HORMONES: Avoid concomitant use (4).
BARBITURATES: Theoretically, concomitant use with barbiturates may cause additive effects and side effects (19).
OTHER DRUGS WITH SEDATIVE PROPERTIES: Theoretically, concomitant use with drugs with sedative properties may cause additive effects and side effects (19).
DIABETES THERAPY: Monitor blood glucose levels closely due to claims that Eleutherococcus has hypoglycemic effects (19).
DIGOXIN: One case report of a product stated to contain Siberian ginseng associated with elevated serum digoxin levels, without symptoms of toxicity (543). However, it is not clear if this is due to an interaction or whether the product ingested in this case actually contained cardiac glycoside-like constituents. The product was found to be free of digoxin and digitoxin (543), but was not tested for the presence of eleutherosides (797). It is unclear whether the product actually contained Eleutherococcus. It has been postulated that it may have contained silk vine (Periploca sepium) which is reported to contain cardiac glycosides and silk vine is a common substitute for Eleutherococcus senticosus (797).
KANAMYCIN (Kantrex): Concomitant use might increase antibiotic efficacy, possibly due to increased T-lymphocyte activity (19).
HORMONES: Avoid concomitant use. Reason not specified (4).
INSULIN: Theoretically, the hypoglycemic effects of Siberian ginseng might cause a need for insulin dose adjustment (19).

Interactions with Foods

ALCOHOL, SPICY FOODS, BITTER SUBSTANCES: Avoid concomitant use (4).

Interactions with Lab Tests

No interactions are known to occur, and there is no known reason to expect a clinically significant interaction with Siberian ginseng.

Interactions with Diseases or Conditions

CARDIOVASCULAR CONDITIONS: Siberian ginseng can cause palpitations, tachycardia, and hypertension and should be used cautiously in patients with cardiovascular disorders (e.g. atherosclerotic or rheumatic heart disease) (4,6,6500). It can also cause headache and pericardial pain in patients with rheumatic heart disease (4,6).

HORMONE SENSITIVE CANCERS/CONDITIONS: Because Siberian ginseng might have estrogenic effects (6180), women with hormone sensitive conditions should avoid Siberian ginseng. Some of these conditions include breast, uterine, and ovarian cancer, and endometriosis and uterine fibroids.

HYPERTENSION: Siberian ginseng is contraindicated in individuals with blood pressures exceeding 180/90. Siberian ginseng can potentially exacerbate hypertension (4,12).

MYOCARDIAL INFARCTION: Theoretically, Siberian ginseng may exacerbate myocardial infarction (4); use with caution.

PSYCHIATRIC CONDITIONS: Theoretically, Siberian ginseng may exacerbate some psychiatric conditions, including hysteria, mania, and schizophrenia (4); use with caution.

OTHER CONDITIONS: Theoretically, Siberian ginseng might exacerbate numerous other conditions; however, documentation for these effects is lacking. Some authors suggest Siberian ginseng should be avoided in patients with hypertonic crisis, conditions with fever (6), and in individuals who are highly energetic, nervous, or tense (4).

Dosage and Administration

ORAL: The dry root, 0.6-3 grams daily for up to one month has been used (4). In healthy people, 2-16 mL of an ethanolic extract is taken one to three times daily up to 60 consecutive days. In unhealthy patients, 0.5-6 mL of an ethanolic extract is taken one to three times daily for up to 35 consecutive days. Studies have used a 2-3 week ginseng-free period after every 30-60 days of treatment with Siberian ginseng (4). For herpes type II infections, studies have used Siberian ginseng extract standardized to contain eleutheroside E 0.3%. Doses used were 400 mg per day (1427).

Comments

Adaptogen is a non-medical term used to suggest that a substance can act to strengthen the body and increase general resistance (1954). The chemical content and potency of various Siberian ginseng products varies. This variance depends, in part, on the time of year the product is harvested. The herb seems to have the highest content of the active ingredients if it is harvested in October, and lesser concentration if harvested in July (6). Siberian ginseng is often misidentified or adulterated (3). Siberian ginseng is a completely different herb than American or Panax ginseng. American or Panax ginseng is considerably more expensive. It is said that the Soviet Union wanted to provide its athletes with the advantage offered by ginseng but wanted a less expensive version. Therefore Siberian ginseng became popular, and this is why most studies on Siberian ginseng have been done in Russia. Exercise caution in differentiating ginseng products. Silk vine is a common substitute for Siberian ginseng (797).

GLOBE FLOWER

Also Known As
Globe Crowfoot, Globe Ranunculus, Globe Trollius.

Scientific Names
Trollius europaeus.
Family: Ranunculaceae.

People Use This For
Orally, globe flower is used for scurvy (18).

Safety
LIKELY UNSAFE ...when any part of the fresh plant is used orally or topically because it can cause severe local irritation (18).
There is insufficient reliable information available about the safety of the dried, cut globe flower plant.
PREGNANCY AND LACTATION: LIKELY UNSAFE ...when any part of the fresh plant is used orally or topically (18). There is insufficient reliable information available about the safety of the dried, cut globe flower plant during pregnancy and lactation.

Effectiveness
There is insufficient reliable information available about the effectiveness of globe flower.

Mechanism of Action
The applicable part is the whole fresh plant. When the fresh plant is crushed or cut into small pieces, the glycoside

ranunculin is enzymatically changed into a severely irritating protoanemonin, which, in turn, rapidly degrades into the less toxic anemonin (18). Both protoanemonin and ranunculin are destroyed to an unknown extent during the drying process (2).

Adverse Reactions
Orally, ingestion of globe flower can cause severe irritation of the gastrointestinal tract, with colic and diarrhea. Irritation of the urinary tract can also occur.
Topically, skin contact can cause blisters and burns that are difficult to heal (18).

Interactions with Herbs & Other Dietary Supplements
Insufficient reliable information available.

Interactions with Drugs
No interactions are known to occur, and there is no known reason to expect a clinically significant interaction with globe flower.

Interactions with Foods
No interactions are known to occur, and there is no known reason to expect a clinically significant interaction with globe flower.

Interactions with Lab Tests
No interactions are known to occur, and there is no known reason to expect a clinically significant interaction with globe flower.

Interactions with Diseases or Conditions
No interactions are known to occur, and there is no known reason to expect a clinically significant interaction with globe flower.

Dosage and Administration
No typical dosage.

Comments
None.

GLOSSY PRIVET

Also Known As
Chinese Privet, Dongqingzi, Ligustro, Ligustrum, Ligustrum Fruit, Nu Zhen, Nu Zhen Zi, Nuzhenzi, Privet, To-Nezumimochi, Troène De Chine, Trueno, White Waxtree.

Scientific Names
Ligustrum lucidum.
Family: Oleaceae.

People Use This For
Orally, glossy privet is used for promoting growth and darkening of hair, reducing facial dark spots (11), palpitations, rheumatism, swelling, tumors, vertigo, common cold, congestion, constipation, deafness, debility, fever, headache, hepatitis, insomnia, rejuvenation and longevity. It is also used as a diaphoretic and tonic (513), for improving immune function, and reducing the side effects of chemotherapy (415).
In traditional Chinese medicine, glossy privet is used for blurred vision, invigorating the liver and kidney, for dizziness, tinnitus, and for sore back and knees (11).

Safety
POSSIBLY SAFE ...when glossy privet is used orally and appropriately (12).
CHILDREN: UNSAFE ...when used orally. Glossy privet berries and leaves are considered toxic to children (414).
PREGNANCY AND LACTATION: Insufficient reliable information available; avoid using.

Effectiveness
There is insufficient reliable information available about the effectiveness of glossy privet.

Mechanism of Action

The applicable part of glossy privet is the ripe fruit (11). It contains triterpenoids, including oleanolic acid (ligustrin), acetyloleanolic acid, and ursolic acid; glycosides (including ligustroside, oleuropein, 4-hydroxy-beta-phenylethyl-beta-D-glucoside); mannitol; fatty oil, consisting mainly of linoleic, linolenic, oleic and palmitic acids; and a volatile oil consisting primarily of esters, alcohols, thioketones and hydrocarbons (11). Ligustrum is used clinically in China for treating leukopenia (11), although data involving experimentally-induced leukopenia did not show any effect (418). Ligustrum might also have immunomodulatory and antitumor effects (11). Preliminary evidence suggests that glossy privet fruit might inhibit growth of renal cell carcinoma, possibly via augmentation of phagocyte and lymphokine-activated killer cell activity (419). Glossy privet extracts inhibit mutagenicity in bacteria (420), stimulate T-cell function in cancer tissue (423), and reverse tumor-induced macrophage suppression (421). Preliminary evidence suggests that glossy privet fruit, and the ingredient ligustrin, might have anti-inflammatory, anti-allergic, mild cardiotonic, diuretic, sedative, lipid-lowering, blood flow enhancing, blood glucose lowering, and liver protectant effects (11).

Adverse Reactions

None reported. However, respiratory allergies (allergic rhinitis, asthma) and cross-allergenicity have been reported with the pollen of other Oleaceae species including common privet (Ligustrum vulgare), olive, ash and lilac (416,417).

Interactions with Herbs & Other Dietary Supplements

Insufficient reliable information available.

Interactions with Drugs

No interactions are known to occur, and there is no known reason to expect a clinically significant interaction with glossy privet.

Interactions with Foods

No interactions are known to occur, and there is no known reason to expect a clinically significant interaction with glossy privet.

Interactions with Lab Tests

No interactions are known to occur, and there is no known reason to expect a clinically significant interaction with glossy privet.

Interactions with Diseases or Conditions

No interactions are known to occur, and there is no known reason to expect a clinically significant interaction with glossy privet.

Dosage and Administration

ORAL: A common dose is 5-15 grams of powdered, encapsulated berries per day. Some people drink a tea prepared by steeping 2-5 grams of powdered berries in 250 mL (1 cup) of boiling water for ten to fifteen minutes, up to three times per day. As a tincture, 3-5 mL is taken three times per day (415).

Comments

Avoid confusion with other species of privet such as Japanese privet (Ligustrum japonicum), border privet (Ligustrum obtusifolium), Chinese privet (Ligustrum sinense), privet (Ligustrum tschonoskii), common privet (Ligustrum vulgare), and golden privet (Ligustrum x vicaryi) (413). The fruits of glossy privet (Ligustrum lucidum) and Ilex chinensis are both referred to by the Chinese name dongqingzi (11).

GLUCOMANNAN

Also Known As

Konjac, Konjac Mannan.

Scientific Names

Amorphophallus konjac.
Family: Araceae.

People Use This For

Orally, glucomannan is used for moderate constipation (6,9), weight loss in adults and children (6,180,181,182,183), blood glucose control, and reducing serum cholesterol (6).
For food uses, glucomannan is edible (6).

Safety

POSSIBLY SAFE ...when used orally in powder or encapsulated form is used (6,180,182).

LIKELY UNSAFE ...when used orally in tablet form. There have been numerous reports of esophageal and gastrointestinal obstruction (6,9). Oral tablets have been banned in Australia since 1985 (6,9).

PREGNANCY AND LACTATION: Insufficient reliable information available; avoid using.

Effectiveness

POSSIBLY EFFECTIVE ...when used orally for weight loss in obese adults (6,181,182,183), reducing serum cholesterol in obese adults and adults with diabetes (6,181,182,183), reducing blood glucose and triglycerides in obese adults (181,182), and reducing insulin or hypoglycemic drug requirements for people with diabetes (6).

There is insufficient reliable information available about the effectiveness of glucomannan for its other uses.

Mechanism of Action

Glucomannan is a polysaccharide derived from underground stems (tubors) of konjac (Amorphophallus konjac). Glucomannan relieves moderate constipation in 1-2 days. The effect is believed due to water absorption, increasing intestinal bulk (6). Glucomannan delays glucose absorption and reduces insulin or hypoglycemic agent requirements in people with diabetes (6). It aids in weight loss, improves lipid profile and glucose tolerance in obese adults (6,181,182,183). In obese children, there has been one report of weight loss, reduced triglycerides and cholesterol (180), but there is another report of no weight loss and increased triglycerides (179). Glucomannan reduces total serum cholesterol in healthy men (178), overweight adults and adults with diabetes; activity reportedly due to inhibited active transport of cholesterol in the jejunum and absorption of bile acids in the ileum (animal data) (6). In mice, glucomannan protects against chemically induced lung cancer (6).

Adverse Reactions

Orally, esophageal or gastrointestinal obstruction has been reported with tablet form (6,9).

Interactions with Herbs & Other Dietary Supplements

Insufficient reliable information available.

Interactions with Drugs

HYPOGLYCEMIC DRUGS, INSULIN: Glucomannan might reduce fasting blood glucose and postprandial blood glucose levels, interfering with blood sugar control in people with diabetes (6), monitor closely.

ORAL DRUGS: The fiber in glucomannan can impair absorption of oral drugs (19).

Interactions with Foods

No interactions are known to occur, and there is no known reason to expect a clinically significant interaction with glucomannan.

Interactions with Lab Tests

CHOLESTEROL: Glucomannan might reduce serum total cholesterol, LDL cholesterol, and test results in obese adults (6,181,182,183).

GLUCOSE: Glucomannan might reduce fasting and postprandial blood glucose concentrations and test results in patients with type 2 diabetes (6).

TRIGLYCERIDES: Glucomannan might reduce serum triglycerides and test results in obese adults (181,182).

Interactions with Diseases or Conditions

DIABETES: Glucomannan may interfere with blood sugar control (6), monitor closely.

Dosage and Administration

ORAL: Typical dose for adult weight loss, 1 gram three times daily (1 hour before each meal) (182), or 1.5 grams twice daily (6). Child weight loss, 2-3 grams per day (180). Diabetes, 3.6-7.2 grams per day (6), monitor blood glucose carefully. Reducing high cholesterol 3.9 grams per day (6). If glucomannan is used for treatment of diabetes or hyperlipidemia, therapy should be in conjunction with physician evaluation and effectiveness should be monitored.

Comments

None.

GLUCOSAMINE HYDROCHLORIDE

Also Known As
2-amino-2-deoxy-beta-D-glucopyranose, Glucosamine, Glucosamine HCL.
CAUTION: See separate listings for Glucosamine Sulfate and N-Acetyl Glucosamine.

Scientific Names
2-amino-2-deoxyglucose hydrochloride.

People Use This For
Orally, glucosamine hydrochloride is used for osteoarthritis (2608).
In combination with other products, glucosamine hydrochloride, chondroitin sulfate, and manganese ascorbate are used orally for osteoarthritis (4237).

Safety
POSSIBLY SAFE …when used orally and appropriately, short-term. Glucosamine hydrochloride has been used safely in studies lasting up to 16 weeks (1520,4237).
There is insufficient reliable information available about the safety of long-term use of glucosamine hydrochloride.
PREGNANCY AND LACTATION: Insufficient reliable information available; avoid using.

Effectiveness
POSSIBLY EFFECTIVE …when used orally for symptoms of osteoarthritis. There is some evidence that glucosamine hydrochloride alone can reduce subjective pain levels in some patients with osteoarthritis of the knee. However, it may not improve more objective measures of pain (1520). So far, the majority of evidence supporting glucosamine hydrochloride involves a specific combination product, which contains glucosamine hydrochloride, chondroitin sulfate, and manganese ascorbate (Cosamin DS). There is more evidence to support the combination than glucosamine hydrochloride alone. This combination seems to improve both objective and subjective measures of pain in patients with osteoarthritis of the knee (4237,7169). It is unknown if this effect is due to glucosamine hydrochloride or the other ingredients. Although evidence for glucosamine hydrochloride, including the combination product, looks promising, there is significantly more evidence supporting the glucosamine sulfate formulation (see separate listing for Glucosamine Sulfate) for osteoarthritis. Until more is known about the effectiveness of glucosamine hydrochloride, encourage patients interested in trying glucosamine to use the glucosamine sulfate formulation.

Mechanism of Action
Glucosamine hydrochloride is one salt form of the glycoprotein, glucosamine. Other salt forms are also available including glucosamine sulfate and N-acetyl glucosamine. Glucosamine is usually derived from marine exoskeletons or produced synthetically (6). Glucosamine is required for the synthesis of glycoproteins, glycolipids, and glycosaminoglycans, also known as mucopolysaccharides, which comprise the body's tendons, ligaments, cartilage, synovial fluid, mucus membranes, and structures in the eye, blood vessels, and heart valves. Glucosamine stimulates metabolism of chondrocytes in the articular cartilage and of synoviocytes in the synovial tissues. Preliminary evidence suggests glucosamine decreases glucose-induced insulin secretion by inhibiting pancreatic glucokinase in the beta cells of the islet of Langerhans (371,372,3406). Evidence also suggests glucosamine impairs insulin-mediated glucose uptake and metabolism in skeletal muscle. It is hypothesized that glucosamine desensitizes cell membranes to the effects of insulin (372,3406). Evidence also suggests that type 2 diabetes and glucosamine induce insulin resistance by acting on a common pathway (3405) and glucosamine-induced insulin resistance might be dose-dependent (3406).

Adverse Reactions
Orally, glucosamine hydrochloride can cause mild gastrointestinal symptoms such as gas, abdominal bloating, and cramps (1520). There is also concern that glucosamine hydrochloride products derived from marine exoskeletons might cause allergic reactions in people allergic to shellfish, although no reactions have been reported. Until more is known, and because the source of glucosamine hydrochloride products is not listed on product labels, use glucosamine hydrochloride cautiously in patients with shellfish allergy.

Interactions with Herbs & Other Dietary Supplements
Insufficient reliable information available.

Interactions with Drugs
ANTIDIABETES DRUGS: Theoretically, glucosamine hydrochloride might decrease the hypoglycemic effects of insulin and oral antidiabetes agents by increasing insulin resistance and/or decreasing insulin production.

Interactions with Foods

No interactions are known to occur, and there is no known reason to expect a clinically significant interaction with glucosamine hydrochloride.

Interactions with Lab Tests

BLOOD GLUCOSE: Theoretically, glucosamine hydrochloride might increase blood glucose levels and test results, by increasing insulin resistance and/or decreasing insulin production. There are also anecdotal reports of poorer control in people with diabetes who take glucosamine (22,1203,1204,3405,3406).

Interactions with Diseases or Conditions

DIABETES: Theoretically, glucosamine hydrochloride might exacerbate diabetes by increasing insulin resistance and/or decreasing insulin production.

SHELLFISH ALLERGY: There is concern that glucosamine hydrochloride products derived from marine exoskeletons might cause reactions in people allergic to shellfish, although no reactions have been reported. Until more is known, and because the source of glucosamine hydrochloride products is not listed on product labels, use glucosamine hydrochloride with caution in people with shellfish allergy.

Dosage and Administration

ORAL: People typically use 1 to 2 grams of glucosamine hydrochloride daily as a single dose or in divided doses (5261,6006). For osteoarthritis, one study used glucosamine hydrochloride 500 mg three times daily (1520). A combination of glucosamine hydrochloride (1500 mg/day), chondroitin sulfate (1200 mg/day), and manganese ascorbate (228 mg/day) (Cosamin-DS, Nutramax Laboratories) has also been used (4237).

Comments

Read glucosamine product labels carefully for content. Avoid confusion with glucosamine sulfate and N-acetyl glucosamine. These products may not be interchangeable. Glucosamine sulfate is the best studied form of glucosamine for osteoarthritis (see separate listing for Glucosamine Sulfate). However, there is no clinical evidence to support the use of N-acetyl glucosamine for osteoarthritis (see separate listing for N-Acetyl Glucosamine). Tell patients to look out for glucosamine plus chondroitin combination products that also contain manganese (e.g., Cosamin DS). When used according to the manufacturers' directions, these products can sometimes supply greater than the tolerable upper limit (UL) for manganese of 11 mg per day. Ingestion of more than 11 mg per day of manganese might cause significant central nervous system toxicity (see separate listing for Manganese).

GLUCOSAMINE SULFATE

Also Known As

D-Glucosamine, Glucosamine, Glucosamine Sulphate, Mono-Sulfated Saccharide, Sulfated Saccharide.
CAUTION: See separate listings for Glucosamine Hydrochloride and N-Acetyl Glucosamine.

Scientific Names

2-amino-2-deoxyglucose sulfate.

People Use This For

Orally, glucosamine sulfate is used for osteoarthritis and temporomandibular joint (TMJ) arthritis. Glucosamine sulfate is also used frequently in combination with other products, including chondroitin sulfate, glucosamine hydrochloride, or N-acetyl glucosamine.
Topically, glucosamine sulfate is used in combination with other products for osteoarthritis.
Parenterally, glucosamine sulfate is used short-term for reducing the symptoms of osteoarthritis.

Safety

LIKELY SAFE ...when used orally and appropriately. Glucosamine has been used safely in multiple clinical trials lasting from 4 weeks to 3 years (2533,2600,2602,2603,2604,2606,7026).
POSSIBLY SAFE ...when used intramuscularly and appropriately, short-term. Intramuscular glucosamine seems to be well tolerated when given twice weekly for up to 6 weeks (2605).
PREGNANCY AND LACTATION: Insufficient reliable information available; avoid using.

Effectiveness

LIKELY EFFECTIVE ...when used orally for osteoarthritis. Glucosamine sulfate can significantly improve symptoms of pain and functionality indices in patients with osteoarthritis of the knee compared to placebo. These benefits have been consistently demonstrated in studies lasting from a few weeks to 3 years (2533,2600,2602,2603,2604,2606,3377,7026). There is some evidence that glucosamine sulfate can be comparable to the non-steroidal anti-inflammatory drugs (NSAIDs) ibuprofen (2602,2604) and piroxicam (Feldene) for symptom relief (2606); however, NSAIDs appear to relieve symptoms within 2 weeks compared to 4 weeks with glucosamine sulfate (2602,2604,2606). In one study, ibuprofen provided superior symptom relief compared to glucosamine sulfate after 2 weeks of treatment, but after 8 weeks, glucosamine sulfate was significantly better than ibuprofen (2602). Unlike NSAIDs and analgesics, glucosamine might actually slow joint degeneration in patients with osteoarthritis. There is evidence that patients taking glucosamine for up to 3 years have significantly less knee joint degeneration, less joint space narrowing, and significant symptom improvement when compared to placebo (3377,7026). So far, most studies have only evaluated glucosamine sulfate for osteoarthritis of the knee. However, there is some preliminary clinical evidence that glucosamine sulfate might also help for osteoarthritis of the lumbar spine (1316). Some clinical trials used a specific patented oral formulation of glucosamine sulfate (Dona, Viartril-S, Rottapharm, Italy).

POSSIBLY EFFECTIVE ...when used orally for temporomandibular joint (TMJ) arthritis. Glucosamine sulfate appears to be at least as effective as analgesic doses of ibuprofen for relieving pain and improving temporomandibular joint function such as chewing, yawning, talking, and laughing. In some patients pain relief persists for up to 90 days after glucosamine sulfate is discontinued (3714). ...when used intramuscularly, short-term for reducing the symptoms of osteoarthritis. In one placebo-controlled clinical trial, intramuscular glucosamine sulfate given twice per week for six weeks significantly reduced the severity of symptoms of knee osteoarthritis in patients with mild to moderately severe disease (radiological stage I-III) compared to placebo. Improvement was significant after five weeks of treatment and symptom relief continued for two weeks after discontinuation of treatment (2605).

POSSIBLY INEFFECTIVE ...when used orally for reducing pain in severe, long-standing osteoarthritis. In one study, glucosamine sulfate added to an existing analgesic regimen failed to improve symptoms of osteoarthritis compared to placebo after two months of treatment. Patients in this study were generally older, heavier, and had more severe and a longer-duration of osteoarthritis than patients in previous studies with positive findings (1330).

Mechanism of Action

Glucosamine is a glycoprotein derived from marine exoskeletons or produced synthetically. It is required for the synthesis of glycoproteins, glycolipids, and glycosaminoglycans, also known as mucopolysaccharides, which comprise the body's tendons, ligaments, cartilage, synovial fluid, mucus membranes, and structures in the eye, blood vessels, and heart valves. Glucosamine stimulates metabolism of chondrocytes in articular cartilage and synoviocytes in synovial tissue. There is some evidence that glucosamine might stop or slow progression of osteoarthritis (7026). Glucosamine sulfate is 90% absorbed after oral administration. The bioavailability is approximately 26% after first pass metabolism (2608). Glucosamine is incorporated into plasma proteins during first-pass metabolism, and unbound glucosamine is concentrated in the articular cartilage (2608). Free glucosamine is undetectable in the plasma (2607). Some glucosamine preparations are provided as topical creams. It is not known if glucosamine is absorbed transdermally. Oral glucosamine might be better tolerated than the non-steroidal anti-inflammatory drugs (NSAIDs) because its mode of action seems to target the pathogenic mechanisms of osteoarthritis rather than affecting cyclooxygenase, which is responsible for anti-inflammatory, analgesic, and adverse gastrointestinal effects of NSAIDs (2604). Preliminary evidence suggests glucosamine decreases glucose-induced insulin secretion by inhibiting pancreatic glucokinase in the beta cells of the islet of Langerhans (371,372,3406). Evidence also suggests glucosamine impairs insulin-mediated glucose uptake and metabolism in skeletal muscle. It is hypothesized that glucosamine desensitizes cell membranes to the effects of insulin (372,3406). Evidence suggests that type 2 diabetes and glucosamine induce insulin resistance through a common pathway (3405) and glucosamine-induced insulin resistance might be dose-dependent (3406). In a recent unpublished study, announced at the Experimental Biology 2000 conference, non-diabetic subjects taking glucosamine sulfate 1500 mg per day for 12 weeks had significantly increased insulin levels compared to placebo (5059). Additional research is needed to determine the effects of glucosamine in people with diabetes.

Adverse Reactions

Orally, glucosamine sulfate can commonly cause mild gastrointestinal problems, including nausea, heartburn, diarrhea, and constipation. Drowsiness, skin reactions, headache have also been reported (2608). However, adverse effects in clinical studies have generally been comparable to placebo (7026). Glucosamine sulfate 1500 mg per day appears to be better tolerated than the non-steroidal anti-inflammatory drugs (NSAIDs) ibuprofen in doses of 1200 mg per day and piroxicam (Feldene) 20 mg per day (2604,2606). However, in one study there was no significant difference in adverse effects between glucosamine sulfate 1500 mg per day and ibuprofen 1200 mg per day (2602).

Elevated blood glucose levels in patients with diabetes have also been reported (22). There is preliminary evidence that glucosamine sulfate 1500 mg per day for 12 weeks in non-diabetic subjects can significantly increase insulin levels, possibly indicating insulin resistance (5059). Due to glucosamine sulfate's potential effects on insulin, there is also some concern that it might increase the risk of metabolic disturbances resulting in increased cholesterol levels and blood pressure. Increased insulin (hyperinsulinemia) is associated with elevated triglycerides, cholesterol, and blood pressure. So far there is not enough evidence to know if these adverse effects actually occur in patients taking glucosamine sulfate or if they are clinically significant (7075). Until more is known, tell patients at risk for diabetes, hyperlipidemia, or hypertension to use glucosamine sulfate cautiously. Blood glucose, serum lipids, and blood pressure monitoring should be done routinely in these patients.

There is concern that glucosamine sulfate products derived from marine exoskeletons might cause reactions in people allergic to shellfish, although no reactions have been reported. Some manufacturers claim that their glucosamine sulfate products are so purified, shellfish allergies should not be a concern. However, since preparation methods and quality standards can vary significantly, use glucosamine sulfate with caution or avoid using in patients with shellfish allergy.

Interactions with Herbs & Other Dietary Supplements

Insufficient reliable information available.

Interactions with Drugs

ANTIDIABETES DRUGS: Theoretically, glucosamine sulfate might decrease the hypoglycemic effects of insulin and oral antidiabetes agents by increasing insulin resistance and/or decreasing insulin production.

Interactions with Foods

No interactions are known to occur, and there is no known reason to expect a clinically significant interaction with glucosamine sulfate.

Interactions with Lab Tests

BLOOD GLUCOSE: Theoretically, glucosamine sulfate might increase blood glucose levels by increasing insulin resistance and/or decreasing glucose-induced insulin production. There are also anecdotal reports of poorer blood glucose control in people with diabetes who take glucosamine (22,1203,1204,3405,3406).

INSULIN: Glucosamine might increase blood insulin levels. An unpublished study found that glucosamine sulfate 1500 mg per day for 12 weeks increased blood insulin levels in a group of non-diabetic patients (5059). Additional research is needed to determine the effects of glucosamine in people with diabetes.

Interactions with Diseases or Conditions

DIABETES: Glucosamine sulfate might exacerbate diabetes by increasing insulin resistance and/or decreasing insulin production, resulting in elevated blood glucose levels. There have been anecdotal reports of poorer blood glucose control in people with diabetes who take glucosamine sulfate (22,1203,1204,3405,3406). Glucosamine sulfate 1500 mg per day also seems to significantly increase insulin levels compared to placebo, suggesting that glucosamine sulfate increases tissue insulin resistance (5059). Patients with diabetes should avoid glucosamine sulfate or use cautiously under the supervision of a health care provider.

HYPERLIPIDEMIA: There is some concern that glucosamine sulfate might increase cholesterol and triglyceride levels. There is preliminary evidence that glucosamine sulfate can increase insulin levels. Hyperinsulinemia is associated with elevated triglycerides and cholesterol (7075). Tell patients with hyperlipidemia to use glucosamine sulfate cautiously. Serum lipid levels should be monitored closely in patients with hyperlipidemia that take glucosamine sulfate.

HYPERTENSION: There is some concern that glucosamine sulfate might increase blood pressure. There is preliminary evidence that glucosamine sulfate can increase insulin levels. Hyperinsulinemia is associated with increased blood pressure levels (7075). Tell patients with hypertension to use glucosamine sulfate cautiously. Blood pressure should be monitored closely in patients with hypertension that take glucosamine sulfate.

SHELLFISH ALLERGY: Glucosamine sulfate products derived from marine exoskeletons might cause reactions in people allergic to shellfish, although no reactions have been reported. Some manufacturers claim that their glucosamine sulfate products are so purified, shellfish allergies should not be a concern. However, since preparation methods and quality standards can vary significantly, use glucosamine sulfate with caution or avoid using in patients with shellfish allergy.

Dosage and Administration

ORAL: For osteoarthritis and temporomandibular joint (TMJ) osteoarthritis, the typical dose is 500 mg three times daily (2600,2602,2603,2606,3714). However, 1500 mg once daily has also been used (3377,7026).

PARENTERAL: In other countries, intravenous, intramuscular, and intra-articular products are used (2601); however, these products are not available in the US. In one trial, glucosamine sulfate 400 mg intramuscularly twice per week was used (2605).

Comments

Although chondroitin sulfate and glucosamine sulfate are frequently marketed together in combination products (760), there is no evidence that the combination has greater benefit than either product alone. The National Institutes of Health (NIH) is sponsoring its first clinical trial of glucosamine sulfate in combination with chondroitin sulfate. The 16 week, parallel group, double-blind RCT includes four separate treatment arms, in which patients will ingest: 1. placebo, 2. glucosamine sulfate 500 mg three times per day, 3. chondroitin 400 mg three times per day, or 4. a combination of glucosamine sulfate and chondroitin (3573).

GLUTAMINE

Also Known As

GLN, Glutamate, Glutamic Acid, Glutaminate, Levoglutamide, Levoglutamine, L-Glutamic Acid, L-Glutamic Acid 5-Amide, l-Glutamine, L-Glutamine, Q.

Scientific Names

L-(+)-2-Aminoglutaramic acid.

People Use This For

Orally, glutamine is used for depression, moodiness, irritability, anxiety, insomnia, short bowel syndrome, Crohn's disease, and enhanced exercise performance. Glutamine is also used orally for HIV wasting, abnormal intestinal permeability in people with HIV, chemotherapy-induced mucositis, chemotherapy-induced diarrhea, chemotherapy-induced neuropathy, protection of immune and gut barrier function in people with esophageal cancer undergoing radiochemotherapy, cystinuria, peptic ulcer, ulcerative colitis, sickle cell anemia, improving recovery after bone marrow transplant, and for alcohol withdrawal support. It is also used orally as enteral nutrition, for preventing morbidity in trauma patients, preventing infectious complications in critically ill patients, and for paclitaxel-induced myalgia and arthralgia.< chemotherapy-induced preventing and transplant, marrow bone after surgery recovery improving for administered is glutamine>

Safety

POSSIBLY SAFE ...when used orally and appropriately. Glutamine seems to be safe in doses up to 40 grams per day (2334,2337,2338,2364,2365,5029,5462,7233,7288,7293). ...when used intravenously. Glutamine seems to be safe in doses up to 570 mg/kg/day when incorporated into parenteral nutrition (2363,2366,5448,5452,5453,5454,5458,7293).
PREGNANCY AND LACTATION: Insufficient reliable information available; avoid using.

Effectiveness

POSSIBLY EFFECTIVE ...when used orally for chemotherapy-induced mucositis (stomatitis). Glutamine appears to decrease the incidence, severity, and duration of mouth pain in some patients undergoing cancer chemotherapy or bone marrow transplant (2336,2364,2368,2704,5029), but glutamine is not effective for all patients (2365,5451,5462,7296). It's not clear yet which patients are most likely to benefit. However, some researchers speculate that those cancer patients with glutamine deficiency may benefit most (2368). Upcoming clinical trials will help clarify the best way to use glutamine and which patients are most likely to benefit (7288). ...when taken orally for HIV/AIDS-related wasting (2337,2702,5461,7310). Glutamine seems to decrease intestinal permeability and enhance intestinal absorption of nutrients and help HIV/AIDS patients gain weight. Doses of 40 grams per day seems to produce the best effect (2337,2702,5461). Lower doses (14 grams per day) might also be effective when used in combination with arginine and beta-hydroxy-beta-methylbutyrate (a leucine metabolite) (7310). ...when taken orally to prevent decreasing lymphocyte counts and attenuate gut permeability in people with esophageal cancer during radiochemotherapy (2705). ...when administered enterally for preventing morbidity in trauma patients and infectious complications in critically ill patients. Glutamine-fortified enteral nutrition formulas seem to improve nutritional and immunologic status and to reduce complications in critically ill medical (5450) and multiple trauma patients (5449,7309). ...when given intravenously for improving recovery after bone marrow transplant. Most patients receiving glutamine-supplemented parenteral nutrition after bone marrow transplantation seem to have improved nitrogen balance, a diminished incidence of clinical infection, lower rates of microbial colonization, and shortened hospital stay compared with patients receiving standard parenteral nutrition (2366,5454). It also seems to preserve hepatic function and promote lymphocyte recovery (5452,5453). However, not all patients seem to benefit (5451). It's not yet clear which patients glutamine might be most beneficial for. ...when taken orally in combination with growth hormone for treating short bowel syndrome. Glutamine plus growth hormone seems to decrease dependence on parenteral nutrition in some patients (2334,2361,2362,2701,2703). Glutamine has orphan drug status for this use (2701). ...when given intravenously to improve recovery following abdominal surgery. Glutamine-fortified parenteral nutrition appears to preserve intestinal mucosal structure and intestinal permeability (7299,7300). Glutamine seems to improve nitrogen balance, improve immune function, and shorten hospital stay in patients recovering from major abdominal surgery and other major surgeries (2363,5448,7299,7300).

POSSIBLY INEFFECTIVE ...when taken orally for treating cystinuria (2339). ...when taken orally for Crohn's disease (2338,6256). Neither supplemental glutamine 7 grams three times daily nor a glutamine-enriched diet has any benefit in patients with Crohn's disease (2338,6256,7297). ...when used orally in rehydration solution for acute diarrhea in infants. Glutamine administered in the standard World Health Organization (WHO) glucose-electrolyte solution doesn't seem to have any effect on diarrheal stool output, duration of diarrhea, or volume of rehydration solution required to achieve and maintain hydration (7298). ...when taken orally for enhancing exercise performance (2341,2342,5455,5456,5464,5465,5466). ...when administered in parenteral nutrition solution to prevent complications of cancer chemotherapy. Glutamine 26 grams per day appears to be similar to standard parenteral nutrition in outcomes such as neutropenia, fever, or antibiotic use (7295).

There is insufficient reliable information available to rate the effectiveness of glutamine for its other uses. However, there is early evidence that glutamine might also help to reduce paclitaxel-induced myalgia and arthralgia (6433). There is also preliminary evidence that glutamine might reduce the occurrence of chemotherapy-induced diarrhea (7235,7285). But so far research findings have been inconsistent (7233). More evidence is needed to rate glutamine for these uses.

Mechanism of Action

Glutamine is an amino acid produced primarily in skeletal muscle. It acts as an inter-organ nitrogen and carbon transporter (5467). Although traditionally classified as a non-essential amino acid, glutamine is essential for maintaining intestinal function, immune response, and amino acid homeostasis during times of severe stress (5468). Glutamine is also important for providing metabolic fuel to lymphocytes, macrophages, fibroblasts, and small intestine enterocytes (5468,5469). Glutamine also functions as a precursor of other amino acids, glucose, purines and pyrimidines, glutathione, and glutamate, an excitatory neurotransmitter (5468,5469,5470,7292). Glutamine promotes carbohydrate storage after exhaustive exercise (5457). The gastrointestinal tract is one of the largest utilizers of glutamine in the body (5469). Depletion of glutamine can result in atrophy, ulceration and necrosis of intestinal epithelium. Some cancer patients are thought to have reduced levels of glutamine (2368). Since gastrointestinal cells are rapidly dividing, they are highly susceptible to the cytotoxic effects of chemotherapy. Glutamine treatment is thought to help prevent chemotherapy and radiation induced gastrointestinal toxicity by maintaining viability of gastrointestinal tissues (2368).

Adverse Reactions

Orally and intravenously glutamine seems to be well tolerated (7293). Significant side effects have not been reported in clinical studies (2336,2364,2365,2368,2704,5029,5451,5462) (7233,7235,7285,7288). However, glutamine is metabolized to glutamate and ammonia, both of which might have neurological effects in people with neurological and psychiatric diseases (7293). Mania has been reported in people with bipolar disorder and supplementation with glutamine (7291).

There is also some concern that glutamine might be used by rapidly growing tumors and possibly stimulate tumor growth. Although tumors may utilize glutamine and other amino acids, preliminary research shows that glutamine supplementation does not increase tumor growth (5469,7233). In fact, there is preliminary evidence that glutamine might actually reduce tumor growth (5469).

Interactions with Herbs & Other Dietary Supplements

Insufficient reliable information available.

Interactions with Drugs

ANTIEPILEPTIC DRUGS: Theoretically, glutamine, which is metabolized to the excitatory neurotransmitter glutamate, might antagonize the anticonvulsant effects of medications taken for epilepsy (7292,7293,7294). Some antiepileptic drugs include phenobarbital, primidone (Mysoline), valproic acid (Depakene), gabapentin (Neurontin), carbamazepine (Tegretol), phenytoin (Dilantin), and others.

LACTULOSE: Theoretically, glutamine might antagonize the antiammonia effects of lactulose. Glutamine is metabolized to ammonia (7293).

Interactions with Foods

No interactions are known to occur, and there is no known reason to expect a clinically significant interaction with glutamine.

Interactions with Lab Tests

No interactions are known to occur, and there is no known reason to expect a clinically significant interaction with glutamine.

Interactions with Diseases or Conditions

HEPATIC ENCEPHALOPATHY: Theoretically, glutamine, which is metabolized to ammonia, might worsen hepatic encephalopathy (7293).

MONOSODIUM GLUTAMATE (MSG) HYPERSENSITIVITY: People who are sensitive to MSG, also known as "Chinese Restaurant Syndrome" might be sensitive to glutamine. Glutamine is metabolized to glutamate in the body (5469,7291).

MANIA, HYPOMANIA: Glutamine might cause affective changes in people with mania or hypomania (7291). Glutamine is a precursor of the excitatory neurotransmitter glutamate (7292).

SEIZURE DISORDERS: Theoretically excess amounts of glutamine, and its metabolite, glutamate, might lower the seizure threshold (7292,7293).

Dosage and Administration

ORAL: For reducing chemotherapy-induced mucositis (stomatitis), a variety of dosage regimens have been used. Most often glutamine suspension 4 grams swish and swallow every four hours around the clock starting with the first dose of chemotherapy and continued until discharge or resolution of symptoms has been used (5029). In some cases, 4 grams swish and swallow twice daily from day 1 of chemotherapy for 28 days or for 4 days past the resolution of symptoms has been used (2364). Other successful regimens include 2 grams per meter squared swish and swallow twice daily (2336) or 1 gram per meter squared swish and swallow 4 times daily (2368) on days of chemotherapy administration and for at least 14 additional days, or 500 mg/kg per day (2704). For chemotherapy-induced diarrhea, 6 grams mixed in water 3 times daily beginning 5 days before chemotherapy for 15 consecutive days has been used (7285). For short bowel syndrome, 630 mg/kg per day has been used (2334). For HIV wasting, 8-40 grams per day has been used. However, 40 grams daily may be the most beneficial (2335,2702,5461). For preventing drops in lymphocyte counts and attenuating gut permeability in people with esophageal cancer during radiochemotherapy, 30 grams per day has been used (2705). For Crohn's disease, 7 grams three times daily has been used (2338). For treating paclitaxel-induced myalgia and arthralgia, 10 grams three times daily starting 24 hours after paclitaxel infusion has been used (6433).

INTRAVENOUS: For improving recovery after bone marrow transplantation, 570 mg/kg/day has been used (2366). For improving recovery after major surgery, doses of 20 grams and 300 mg/kg/day have been added to parenteral nutrition (2363,5448).

Comments

Glutamine powder can be ordered through most wholesale drug suppliers.

GLUTATHIONE

Also Known As

gamma-Glutamylcysteinylglycine, gamma-L-Glutamyl-L-cysteinylglycine, L-Glutathione, GSH.

Scientific Names

N-(N-L-gamma-Glutamyl-L-cysteinyl)glycine.

People Use This For

Orally, glutathione is used for treating cataracts (5355,5356), glaucoma (5356), preventing aging (5356), treating or preventing alcoholism, asthma, cancer, heart disease (atherosclerosis and hypercholesterolemia), hepatitis (5356), liver disease (5355), immunosuppression (including AIDS and chronic fatigue syndrome) (5356), maintaining immune function (5365,5366), memory loss, Alzheimer's disease, osteoarthritis, Parkinson's disease, and detoxifying metal and drugs (5356).

Inhaled, glutathione is used for treating lung diseases (9), including idiopathic pulmonary fibrosis (5369), cystic fibrosis (5367), and lung disease in individuals with HIV disease (5368).

Intramuscularly, glutathione is used for preventing toxicity of chemotherapy (5374,5375) and for treating male infertility (5384).

Intravenously, glutathione is used for preventing anemia in patients undergoing hemodialysis (5359), preventing renal dysfunction after coronary bypass surgery (5360), treating Parkinson's disease (5344, 5354), improving blood flow and decreasing clotting in individuals with atherosclerosis (5385), treating diabetes (5357,5358), and preventing toxicity of chemotherapy (5373,5374,5375,5376,5377,5378,5379,5380,5381,5382,5383).

Safety

POSSIBLY SAFE …when used orally (5361,5362), by inhalation (9,5367,5368,5369), or by intramuscular (5374,5375,5384) or intravenous injection (5344,5354,5357,5358,5359,5360,5373,5374,5375,5376,5377) (5378,5379,5380,5381,5382,5383).

PREGNANCY AND LACTATION: Insufficient reliable information available; avoid using.

Effectiveness

POSSIBLY EFFECTIVE …when used by intravenous injection for preventing chemotherapy toxicity (5373,5374,5375,5376,5377,5378,5379,5380,5381,5382,5383).

LIKELY INEFFECTIVE …when used orally because it is not absorbed (5362).

There is insufficient reliable information available about the effectiveness of glutathione for its other uses.

Mechanism of Action

Glutathione is primarily synthesized in the liver (5387,5388). It is involved in DNA synthesis and repair, protein and prostaglandin synthesis, amino acid transport, metabolism of toxins and carcinogens, immune system function, prevention of oxidative cell damage, and enzyme activation (5344,5386). Cellular glutathione levels increase during exercise (5398,5386). Glutathione deficiency is associated with aging, age-related macular degeneration, diabetes, lung and gastrointestinal disease, pre-eclampsia, Parkinson's disease, and other neurodegenerative disorders, and a poor prognosis in AIDS (5344,5346,5347,5348,5349,5350,5351,5352,5353,5354,5393) (5394,5395,5396,5397). Although glutathione is present in fruits, vegetables, and meats, the levels in the body do not seem to correlate to dietary intake. This suggests that oral glutathione might be inactivated by peptidases in the gut (5344,5890,5891). Despite evidence that suggests that glutathione is bioavailable in rodents (5363,5364), oral doses of 3 grams cause negligible increases in human plasma levels (5362). Preliminary evidence suggests glutathione intake from fruits and vegetables might be associated with a reduced risk of pharyngeal cancer (5345). In individuals with cirrhosis, oral glutathione has no effect on liver function tests (5361). Researchers report that glutathione inhibits the activity of enzymes that help the flu virus colonize cells lining the mouth and throat. They also report that flu-infected mice fed glutathione-enriched drinking water had lower tissue virus levels than untreated mice. The researchers caution that human studies are needed to determine the effects of glutathione on humans with the flu. The results of these unpublished studies were presented at the Experimental Biology 2000 conference (5061).

Adverse Reactions
None reported.

Interactions with Herbs & Other Dietary Supplements
Insufficient reliable information available.

Interactions with Drugs
CISPLATIN: Concurrent use can prevent or reduce the severity of cisplatin-induced nephrotoxicity and neurotoxicity without altering the effectiveness of cisplatin (5373,5374,5378,5379,5380,5381).
GLUTATHIONE-DEPLETING DRUGS: Drugs that deplete glutathione (acetaminophen, alcohol, and others) might decrease the therapeutic effects of glutathione (5394).

Interactions with Foods
No interactions are known to occur, and there is no known reason to expect a clinically significant interaction with glutathione.

Interactions with Lab Tests
No interactions are known to occur, and there is no known reason to expect a clinically significant interaction with glutathione.

Interactions with Diseases or Conditions
ASTHMA: Inhaled (nebulized) glutathione can cause bronchospasm in individuals with asthma (5372).

Dosage and Administration
ORAL: Supplemental doses range from 50–600 mg per day, with a typical dose of 250 mg daily (5355,5356,5365,5366); however, orally administered glutathione is probably not bioavailable (5362).
INHALATION: A common dose is 600 mg, aerosolized twice daily (5367,5368,5369).
INTRAMUSCULAR: For infertility, 600 mg every other day for 2 months has been used (5384). As a chemotherapy adjunct, 600 mg on days 2 through 5 of chemotherapy has been used (5374,5375).
INTRAVENOUS: As a chemotherapy adjunct, 2.5 grams or 1.5 grams/meter squared immediately prior to chemotherapy has been used (5373,5374,5375,5376,5377,5378,5379,5380,5381,5382,5383).

Comments
The role of glutathione is being studied in the wasting of AIDS, heavy metal poisoning, sepsis, myocardial ischemia, renal dysfunction and nephrotoxicity, liver disorders, corneal disorders, and eczema (9,14,5355,5344,5345). Currently, researchers are investigating whether administering glutathione precursors, such as glutamine and n-acetylcysteine might increase glutathione levels (5344,5389,5392).

GLYCEROL

Also Known As
Glicerol, Glucerite, Glycerin, Glycerolum, Glyceryl Alcohol.

Scientific Names
Glycerol; 1,2,3-propanetriol.

People Use This For
Orally, glycerol is used for weight loss, enhancing exercise performance, improving rehydration during acute gastrointestinal disease, and reducing intraocular pressure (15,2479,2485). Glycerol is also used by athletes as an aid to hydration (217).

Intravenously, glycerol is used for reducing intra-cranial pressure in various conditions including stroke, meningitis, encephalitis, Reye's syndrome, pseudotumor cerebri, central nervous system (CNS) trauma, and CNS tumors or space-occupying lesions; for reducing brain volume for neurosurgical procedures; and for postural syncope (15,2477).

Ophthalmically, glycerol is an ingredient for reducing corneal edema to facilitate ophthalmic exams (15).

Rectally, glycerol is used as a laxative (15).

Safety
LIKELY SAFE ...when used rectally and appropriately (15). ...when used orally for reducing intraocular pressure; glycerol is a FDA-approved prescription product for this purpose.

POSSIBLY UNSAFE ...when used intravenously. In one study, hemolysis was reported in 98% of people treated for acute ischemic stroke (2482).

There is insufficient reliable information available about the safety of glycerol for its other uses.

PREGNANCY AND LACTATION: Insufficient reliable information available; avoid using.

Effectiveness
LIKELY EFFECTIVE ...when used rectally for constipation (15).

POSSIBLY INEFFECTIVE ...when used orally for weight loss (2485).

LIKELY INEFFECTIVE ...when used orally for enhancing exercise performance (2474,2475). ...when used intravenously for treating acute stroke (2480,2481,2482,2484,2486).

There is insufficient reliable information available about the effectiveness of glycerol for its other uses.

Mechanism of Action
Supplemental glycerol increases serum osmolality (2477). It also has hyperosmotic laxative activity (15). Glycerol consumption failed to enhance human exercise performance (2476,2492) or reduce water loss in underwater divers (2478). However, one study reported that following glycerol ingestion, participants had improved exercise tolerance and reduced heart rate during stationary cycling (2479). Intravenous glycerol failed to improve acute ischemic stroke survival in several clinical trials (2480,2481,2482,2484,2486). However, one study of elderly people with acute ischemic stroke found glycerol improved initial survival (2483).

Adverse Reactions
Orally, the use of glycerol can cause mild headache, dizziness, bloating, nausea, vomiting, thirst, and diarrhea (15,2475). Intravenously, the use of glycerol has caused hemolysis in people treated for acute ischemic stroke (2480,2482).

Interactions with Herbs & Other Dietary Supplements
Insufficient reliable information available.

Interactions with Drugs
No interactions are known to occur, and there is no known reason to expect a clinically significant interaction with glycerol.

Interactions with Foods
No interactions are known to occur, and there is no known reason to expect a clinically significant interaction with glycerol.

Interactions with Lab Tests
No interactions are known to occur, and there is no known reason to expect a clinically significant interaction with glycerol.

Interactions with Diseases or Conditions
No interactions are known to occur, and there is no known reason to expect a clinically significant interaction with glycerol.

Dosage and Administration
ORAL: For enhancing exercise performance, the usual dose of glycerol is 1 gram/kg with 1.5 L fluid 60-120 minutes

before competition (2475). For weight loss, 7.5 grams in a 25% solution is typically taken before meals (2485).

RECTAL: As an adult laxative, the common dose is a 2-3 grams suppository or a 5-15 mL enema (15). For children younger than six years old, the dose is a 1-1.7 grams suppository or a 2-5 mL enema (15).

OPHTHALMIC: Glycerol is a FDA-approved prescription product for reducing intraocular pressure.

INTRAVENOUS: No typical dosage.

Comments

None.

GOA POWDER

Also Known As

Araoba, Bahia Powder, Brazil Powder, Chrysatobine, Crude Chrysarobin, Ringworm Powder.

Scientific Names

Andira araroba.

People Use This For

Topically, goa powder is used for psoriasis and fungal infections of the skin (18).

Safety

POSSIBLY UNSAFE ...when used topically. Goa powder is severely irritating to skin and mucous membranes. It can also be absorbed through the skin with adverse effects. As little as 10 mg absorbed is associated with vomiting, diarrhea, and kidney inflammation (18).

PREGNANCY AND LACTATION: Insufficient reliable information available; avoid using.

Effectiveness

There is insufficient reliable information available about the effectiveness of goa powder.

Mechanism of Action

The applicable part of goa powder is the latex. Goa powder contains anthrone derivatives including chrysophanolanthrone. The powder is a strong reducing agent and inhibits glucose-6-phosphated-dehydrogenization in psoriatic skin conditions. It is considered a potent irritant to skin and mucous membranes and is easily absorbed through the skin (18).

Adverse Reactions

Orally, vomiting, diarrhea, and kidney inflammation can follow if ingested (18).

Topically, application of goa powder can cause redness, swelling, pustules, and conjunctivitis.

Interactions with Herbs & Other Dietary Supplements

Insufficient reliable information available.

Interactions with Drugs

No interactions are known to occur, and there is no known reason to expect a clinically significant interaction with goa powder.

Interactions with Foods

No interactions are known to occur, and there is no known reason to expect a clinically significant interaction with goa powder.

Interactions with Lab Tests

No interactions are known to occur, and there is no known reason to expect a clinically significant interaction with goa powder.

Interactions with Diseases or Conditions

No interactions are known to occur, and there is no known reason to expect a clinically significant interaction with goa powder.

Dosage and Administration

TOPICAL: People typically use a 2% goa powder ointment.

Comments

Goa powder has been replaced by synthetic anthranol (18). Goa should not be used internally (5264,5269).

GOAT'S RUE

Also Known As

French Honeysuckle, French Lilac, Galegae officinalis herba, Geissrautenkraut, Goats Rue, Goat's Rue Herb, Italian Fitch.
CAUTION: See separate listing for Rue.

Scientific Names

Galega officinalis.
Family: Leguminosae or Fabaceae.

People Use This For

Orally, goat's rue is used as supportive therapy for diabetes and as a diuretic (18).
In combination with other herbs, goat's rue is used for adrenal gland and pancreas stimulation, for glandular disturbances, blood purification, purifying the mesenchyma, digestive fluid secretion disturbances, fermentative dyspepsia, Roemheld syndrome, diarrhea, abnormal colonic bacterial flora, status lymphaticus and exudative diathesis, for stimulating lactation, as a tonic, and as a liver-protectant (2).

Safety

There is insufficient reliable information available about the safety of goat's rue.
Pregnancy and Lactation: Insufficient reliable information available; avoid using.

Effectiveness

There is insufficient reliable information available about the effectiveness of goat's rue.

Mechanism of Action

The applicable parts of goat's rue are the above ground parts. In vitro, the constituent galegine has hypoglycemic effects (2,18,4006), but these effects have not been demonstrated with goat's rue (2,18). In experimental rats, an intravenously administered aqueous extract suppresses platelet aggregation (4007). Fatal poisonings have been reported in grazing animals. Toxicity may involve galegine (4008).

Adverse Reactions

None reported in humans. However, fatal poisonings have been reported in grazing animals following ingestion of large amounts of goat's rue (2,18); poisoning symptoms in sheep, include salivation, spasms, paralysis, and asphyxiation (2,18).

Interactions with Herbs & Other Dietary Supplements

HYPOGLYCEMIC HERBS: Theoretically, concomitant use could potentiate effects of other herbs that cause hypoglycemia (2,4006).

Interactions with Drugs

ANTIDIABETES DRUGS: Theoretically, concomitant use could potentiate hypoglycemic drug effects. Monitor closely (2,4006).

Interactions with Foods

No interactions are known to occur, and there is no known reason to expect a clinically significant interaction with goat's rue.

Interactions with Lab Tests

BLOOD GLUCOSE: Theoretically, could cause a true decrease in blood glucose levels and test results (2,4006).

Interactions with Diseases or Conditions

DIABETES: Goat's rue may interfere with effective diabetes treatment; avoid using.

Dosage and Administration

ORAL: As prepared tea (steep 2 grams finely cut above ground parts in 150 mL boiling water 5-10 minutes, strain); frequency of use not specified (18).

Comments

Avoid confusion with rue (Ruta graveolens). Goat's rue is not recommended for diabetes mellitus therapy because its effectiveness is uncertain.

GOLDEN RAGWORT

Also Known As

Cocash Weed, Coughweed, False Valerian, Female Regulator, Golden Groundsel, Golden Senecio, Grundy Swallow, Life Root, Liferoot, Ragwort, Squaw Weed, Squawweed.
CAUTION: See separate listings for Alpine Ragwort and Tansy Ragwort.

Scientific Names

Senecio aureus.
Family: Asteraceae/Compositae.

People Use This For

Orally, golden ragwort is used for diabetes mellitus, high blood pressure, spasms, as a uterine stimulant, and to minimize bleeding. It is also used orally as a diuretic and mild expectorant (4).

In folk medicine, golden ragwort has been used orally for treating conditions involving the female reproductive tract, including functional amenorrhea, menopausal neurosis, dysmenorrhea, pain associated with childbirth, and for inducing uterine contractions (6,18).

In folk medicine, golden ragwort has been used topically for the treatment of bleeding after tooth extraction and as a douche for leukorrhea (18).

Safety

LIKELY UNSAFE ...when used orally. Golden ragwort contains hepatotoxic unsaturated pyrrolizidine alkaloids (UPAs) (12,19). Repeated exposure to low concentrations of UPAs linked to veno-occlusive disease, a serious condition (4,12). UPAs may also be carcinogenic and mutagenic (12). ...when used topically on abraded or broken skin, it might be unsafe due to the potential for systemic absorption (12,19).

PREGNANCY: UNSAFE ...when used orally due to the possibility it might stimulate menstruation, oxytocic activity, or cause teratogenic effects (19).

LACTATION: UNSAFE ...when used orally due to pyrrolizidine alkaloid content (19).

Effectiveness

There is insufficient reliable information available about the effectiveness of golden ragwort.

Mechanism of Action

Some pyrrolizidine alkaloids have shown carcinogenic and mutagenic properties, and there are reports of renal toxicity. However, the primary concern is veno-occlusive disease (12). Unsaturated pyrrolizidine alkaloids are known to be hepatotoxic in animals and humans (4).

Adverse Reactions

Orally, acute toxicity may result in hepatic necrosis; chronic toxicity may cause veno-occlusive liver disease. The potential for hepatotoxicity (due to presence of pyrrolizidine alkaloids) increases with larger doses and longer periods of use (4,12). It can cause an allergic reaction in individuals sensitive to the Asteraceae/Compositae family. Members of this family include ragweed, chrysanthemums, marigolds, daisies, and many other herbs.

Interactions with Herbs & Other Dietary Supplements

EUCALYPTUS: Theoretically, concomitant use might increase the risk of unsaturated pyrrolizidine alkaloid toxicity due to enzyme induction by eucalyptus (19).

PYRROLIZIDINE ALKALOID-CONTAINING HERBS: Concomitant use is contraindicated due to the risk of additive toxicity. Herbs containing unsaturated pyrrolizidine alkaloids include: alkanna (12), borage (271), gravel root (4), hemp agrimony (271), hound's tongue (19), petasites (19), comfrey (271), coltsfoot, and the Senecio species plants; dusty miller (19), alpine ragwort (19), groundsel (271), golden ragwort (19), and tansy ragwort (271).

Interactions with Drugs

No interactions are known to occur, and there is no known reason to expect a clinically significant interaction with golden ragwort.

Interactions with Foods
No interactions are known to occur, and there is no known reason to expect a clinically significant interaction with golden ragwort.

Interactions with Lab Tests
No interactions are known to occur, and there is no known reason to expect a clinically significant interaction with golden ragwort.

Interactions with Diseases or Conditions
LIVER DISEASE: Golden ragwort is hepatotoxic and may exacerbate liver conditions; contraindicated (6).
CROSS-ALLERGENICITY: Golden ragwort can cause an allergic reaction in individuals sensitive to the Asteraceae/Compositae family. Members of this family include ragweed, chrysanthemums, marigolds, daisies, and many other herbs.

Dosage and Administration
No typical dosage.

Comments
Even though golden ragwort is considered unsafe for oral use (12,18), it is still included in some herbal preparations designed to treat irregular menses and other gynecological disorders. Golden ragwort is sometimes confused with other plants credited with broad healing powers, such as mandrake and ginseng (6).

GOLDENROD

Also Known As
Aaron's Rod, European Goldenrod, Golden Rod, Woundwort.
CAUTION: See separate listing for Mullein.

Scientific Names
Solidago virgaurea (European goldenrod); Solidago canadensis (Canadian goldenrod); Solidago serotina, synonyms Solidago gigantea (Early goldenrod).
Family: Asteraceae or Compositae.

People Use This For
Orally, goldenrod is used as a diuretic, anti-inflammatory, and antispasmodic (3). It is also used as "irrigation therapy" where it is taken with copious fluids to increase urine flow to treat inflammatory diseases of the lower urinary tract, urinary calculi, and kidney gravel. As "irrigation therapy," it is also used as prophylaxis for urinary calculi and kidney gravel (2).
Topically, goldenrod is used as a mouth rinse for inflammation of the mouth and throat and externally for poorly healing wounds (8,18).
In folk medicine, goldenrod has been taken orally as a "blood purifying" agent in gout, rheumatism, arthritis, eczema, and other skin conditions (8). It has been used for acute exacerbations of pulmonary tuberculosis, diabetes, enlargement of the liver, hemorrhoids, internal bleeding, nervous bronchial asthma, and prostatic hypertrophy (18).

Safety
LIKELY SAFE ...when above ground parts are used orally and appropriately for "irrigation therapy" (as a mild diuretic along with copious fluid intake) (2).
There is insufficient reliable information available about the safety of the topical use of goldenrod.
PREGNANCY AND LACTATION: Insufficient reliable information available; avoid using.

Effectiveness
POSSIBLY EFFECTIVE ...when taken orally for "irrigation therapy" where goldenrod is used with copious fluid intake to increase urine flow for inflammatory diseases of the lower urinary tract and kidney gravel, and as prophylaxis for kidney gravel (2).
There is insufficient reliable information available about the effectiveness of goldenrod for its other uses.

Mechanism of Action
The applicable parts of goldenrod are the above ground parts. Goldenrod is classified as an aquaretic, a compound that increases urine volume (water loss) but not sodium excretion (512). The anti-inflammatory and aquaretic effects of goldenrod are due to the saponin and flavonoid constituents (8,512). Goldenrod also has bacteriostatic activity (512).

Adverse Reactions

Goldenrod can cause an allergic reaction in individuals sensitive to the Asteraceae/Compositae family. Members of this family include ragweed, chrysanthemums, marigolds, daisies, and many other herbs.

Interactions with Herbs & Other Dietary Supplements

Insufficient reliable information available.

Interactions with Drugs

DIURETICS: Theoretically, goldenrod might increase sodium retention and interfere with diuretic therapy (512).

Interactions with Foods

No interactions are known to occur, and there is no known reason to expect a clinically significant interaction with goldenrod.

Interactions with Lab Tests

No interactions are known to occur, and there is no known reason to expect a clinically significant interaction with goldenrod.

Interactions with Diseases or Conditions

EDEMA DUE TO HEART OR KIDNEY CONDITIONS: "Irrigation therapy," where goldenrod is taken with copious fluid intake to increase urine flow, is contraindicated in these conditions with edema (2).
HYPERTENSION: Theoretically, goldenrod might increase sodium retention and worsen hypertension (512).
URINARY TRACT INFECTIONS: Herbal "irrigation therapy" can be insufficient and require the addition of antibacterial agent. "Irrigation therapy" should be monitored closely (8).
CROSS-ALLERGENICITY: Can cause an allergic reaction in individuals sensitive to the Asteraceae/Compositae family. Members of this family include ragweed, chrysanthemums, marigolds, daisies, and many other herbs.

Dosage and Administration

ORAL: The typical dose of goldenrod is one cup of the tea two to four times daily between meals (18). The tea is prepared by steeping 1-2 teaspoons (3-5 grams) of the dried herb in 150 mL boiling water for 5-10 minutes and then straining. The usual dose ranges from 6-12 grams of the herb per day (2). The common dose of the liquid extract (1:1 in 25% ethanol) is 0.5-2 mL two to three times daily (18). The usual dose of the tincture (1:5 in 45% ethanol) is 0.5-1 mL two to three times daily (18). Drink plenty of water, at least 2 liters per day, with the use of goldenrod (18).
CAUTION: In cases of chronic kidney disorders, professional evaluation is needed (12).

Comments

Avoid confusion with mullein (Verbascum densiflorum; also referred to as goldenrod). Early goldenrod, European goldenrod, and Canadian goldenrod are used interchangeably.

GOLDENSEAL

Also Known As

Eye Balm, Eye Root, Golden Seal, Goldenroot, Goldsiegel, Ground Raspberry, Hydrastis, Hydrastis Canadensis, Indian Dye, Indian Plant, Indian Tumeric, Jaundice Root, Orange Root, Sceau D'Or, Turmeric Root, Warnera, Wild Curcuma, Yellow Indian Paint, Yellow Paint, Yellow Puccoon, Yellow Root.
CAUTION: See separate listings for Barberry, Goldthread, Javanese Turmeric, Oregon Grape, Ox-Eye Daisy, and Turmeric.

Scientific Names

Hydrastis canadensis.
Family: Ranunculaceae.

People Use This For

Orally, goldenseal is used for the common cold and other upper respiratory tract infections, nasal congestion, gastritis, peptic ulcers, colitis, diarrhea, constipation, flatulence, inflammation of vaginal and uretal mucous membranes, urinary tract infections (UTIs), menorrhagia, dysmenorrhea, hemorrhoids, anal fissures, internal hemorrhage, liver disorders, cancer, to mask urine tests for illicit drugs, jaundice, gonorrhea, child birth, post-partum hemorrhage, fever, pneumonia, malaria, whooping cough, and anorexia.
Topically, goldenseal is used as a mouthwash for sore gums and mouth. It is also used topically for skin rashes,

skin ulcers, wound infections, itching, eczema, acne, dandruff, ringworm, herpes blisters, and herpes labialis. Ophthalmically, goldenseal is used as an eyewash for eye inflammation and conjunctivitis.
Otologically, goldenseal is used for ringing of the ears, earache, and catarrhal deafness.

Safety

POSSIBLY SAFE ...when used orally and appropriately, short-term (12).

LIKELY UNSAFE ...when used orally in high doses or long-term. Doses providing more than 500 mg of the constituent, berberine, can cause significant toxicity. This may correspond to 8-100 grams of dry root, depending on the concentration of berberine (12). Overdoses of goldenseal can cause cardiac damage, spasms, and death (4). The LD50 of the berberine constituent in humans is thought to be 27.5 mg/kg (12). Prolonged use has also been associated with significant side effects, including digestive disorders and hallucinations (see Adverse Reactions) (18). Prolonged use has also been associated with significant side effects, including digestive disorders and hallucinations (see Adverse Reactions) (18).

CHILDREN: LIKELY UNSAFE ...when used orally in newborns. The berberine constituent of goldenseal can cause kernicterus in newborns, particularly preterm neonates with hyperbilirubinemia (2589).

PREGNANCY: LIKELY UNSAFE ...when used orally. Goldenseal is thought to affect menstruation and have oxytocic effects (4,12). Berberine and other constituents are also thought to cross the placenta and may cause harm to the fetus. Kernicteris has developed in newborn infants exposed to goldenseal (2589).

LACTATION: LIKELY UNSAFE ...when used orally. Berberine and other harmful constituents can be transferred to the infant through breast milk (2589).

Effectiveness

POSSIBLY INEFFECTIVE ...when used orally to cause a false negative immunoassay (EMIT and TDx) for marijuana and cocaine urine tests (260). ...when used orally to cause false negative results for Microgenics CEDIA DAU assay for amphetamines, barbiturates, benzodiazepines, cocaine, opiates, phencyclidine, and tetrahydrocannabinol. Drinking one gallon of water with goldenseal did not increase the number of false negatives over water alone (261). ...when used orally to cause false positives for the fluorescent polarization immunoassay (FPIA) or thin-layer chromatography (TLC) assays for amphetamines, opiates, cocaine metabolites, methadone, or their metabolites (2590). There is insufficient reliable information available about the effectiveness of goldenseal for its other uses.

Mechanism of Action

The applicable parts of goldenseal are the dried rhizome and root. The alkaloids hydrastine and berberine are the principle active constituents in goldenseal (7265). However, these alkaloids are poorly absorbed when given orally (2591). Berberine and hydrastine from goldenseal might not reach adequate concentrations to have significant pharmacological activity in humans.

The isolated constituents have a variety of pharmacological effects. The berberine constituent has antimicrobial effects including antibacterial, antifungal, and some antimycobacterial and antiprotozoal activity (7258,7259). Berberine has activity against Staphylococcus aureus, Streptococcus pyogenes, Eschericha coli, Shigella boydii, Vibrio cholerae, Mycobacterium tuberculosis, Candida albicans, Candida tropicalis, Trichophyton mentagrophytes, Microsporum gypseum, Cryptococcus neoformans, Sporotrichum schenkii, Entamoeba histolytica and Giardia lamblia (2530,2587,2588,7258,7259). These effects have not been demonstrated specifically for goldenseal. Due to the poor oral absorption of berberine, goldenseal preparations might not be capable of achieving berberine serum concentrations high enough to be effective in humans. However, berberine from goldenseal is thought to concentrate in the bladder. Theoretically, goldenseal could potentially have activity against the binding of urinary tract pathogens, such as Escherichia coli, to bladder walls (2583,6411).

There is also preliminary evidence that the berberine constituent might have antitumor properties (7260).

Isolated berberine and hydrastine seem to have cardiovascular effects. Berberine seems to increase coronary blood flow and stimulates the heart; although higher doses or long-term use are thought to inhibit cardiac activity (4,12). Berberine has antimuscarinic and antihistaminic activity (4). Hydrastine, in low doses, has hypotensive effects (4); however, at higher doses, hydrastine constricts peripheral blood vessels, potentially leading to hypertensive effects (4).

There is preliminary evidence goldenseal might stimulate IgM antibody production (2530).

Adverse Reactions

Orally, prolonged use of goldenseal can cause digestive disorders, constipation, excitatory states, hallucinations, and occasionally delirium (18). Overdoses can cause stomach upset, nausea, vomiting, nervousness, depression, dyspnea, bradycardia, cardiac damage, hypotension, seizures, paralysis, spasms, and death (4,6). High doses of the constituent hydrastine can cause exaggerated reflexes, convulsions, paralysis, and death from respiratory failure (4). The fresh plant can cause mucosal irritation (12). Using goldenseal vaginally as a douche can cause ulceration (4). Use of goldenseal during pregnancy, lactation or in newborn infants can cause kernicteris, and several resulting fatalities have been reported (2589). The LD50 of the berberine constituent in humans is reported to be 27.5 mg/kg (12).

Interactions with Herbs & Other Dietary Supplements

B VITAMINS: Theoretically, prolonged use of goldenseal can decrease B vitamin absorption (4).

HERBS WITH SEDATIVE PROPERTIES: Theoretically, concomitant use with herbs that have sedative properties might enhance therapeutic and adverse effects. These include calamus, calendula, California poppy, catnip, capsicum, celery, couch grass, elecampane, Siberian ginseng, German chamomile, gotu kola, hops, Jamaican dogwood, kava, lemon balm, sage, St. John's wort, sassafras, scullcap, shepherd's purse, stinging nettle, valerian, wild carrot, wild lettuce, ashwaganda root, and yerba mansa (4,19).

Interactions with Drugs

ACID-INHIBITING DRUGS: Theoretically, due to claims that goldenseal increases stomach acid, it might interfere with antacids, sucralfate (Carafate), H-2 antagonists, and proton pump inhibitors (19).

ANTIHYPERTENSIVE AGENTS: Theoretically, large amounts of goldenseal might interfere with blood pressure control due to vasoconstrictive action of constituent hydrastine (4).

BARBITURATES: Theoretically, goldenseal might potentiate barbiturate-induced sleep time (4).

HEPARIN: Theoretically, goldenseal can inhibit anticoagulant effects due to the constituent, berberine (4).

HIGHLY PROTEIN BOUND DRUGS: Theoretically, the berberine in goldenseal can displace highly protein bound drugs, such as phenylbutazone and papaverine (2589).

SEDATIVE DRUGS: Theoretically, concomitant use with drugs with sedative properties might cause additive effects and side effects (4).

OTHER DRUGS: There's preliminary evidence that goldenseal can inhibit the cytochrome P450 (CYP450) 3A4 enzyme (6450). Theoretically, goldenseal might increase levels of drugs metabolized by CYP450 3A4. However, so far, this interaction has not been reported in humans. Some drugs metabolized by CYP450 3A4 include lovastatin (Mevacor), ketoconazole (Nizoral), itraconazole (Sporanox), fexofenadine (Allegra), triazolam (Halcion), and numerous others. Use goldenseal cautiously or avoid in patients taking these drugs.

Interactions with Foods

No interactions are known to occur, and there is no known reason to expect a clinically significant interaction with goldenseal.

Interactions with Lab Tests

BILIRUBIN: Theoretically, goldenseal might increase bilirubin levels. This has been demonstrated with isolated berberine constituent, but not specifically with goldenseal. Berberine can cause a true increase in total and unbound bilirubin concentrations because it displaces bilirubin from albumin (2589).

Interactions with Diseases or Conditions

CARDIOVASCULAR DISEASE: Theoretically, low doses can increase coronary blood flow and stimulate the heart, while large doses can inhibit cardiac function (4).

GASTROINTESTINAL IRRITATION: Might irritate gastrointestinal tract. Contraindicated in individuals with infectious or inflammatory gastrointestinal conditions (19).

HYPERBILIRUBINEMIA: The berberine in goldenseal can cause kernicterus in newborns, particularly preterm neonates with hyperbilirubinemia (2589); contraindicated in newborns.

HYPERTENSION: Vasoconstrictive action of the constituent hydrastine might interfere with blood pressure control (4); use with caution.

Dosage and Administration

ORAL: Doses of 0.5 -1 gram three times daily of the dried root or rhizome or as a tea have been used. The tea is prepared by simmering 0.5-1 gram dried root or rhizome in 150 mL of boiling water for 5-10 minutes and then straining (4, 12). The liquid extract (1:1, 60% ethanol) is usually taken as 0.3-1.0 mL three times daily (12). The tincture (1:10, 60% ethanol) is dosed 2-4 mL three times daily (12).

TOPICAL: Goldenseal is used as a mouthwash 3-4 times daily. The mouthwash is prepared by steeping 2 teaspoons (6 grams) of dried herb in 150 mL boiling water for 5-10 minutes, straining, and allowing to cool (3).

Comments

Goldenseal is commonly found in the deep woods from Vermont to Arkansas and received its name from the golden-yellow scars on the base of the stem. When the stem is broken, the scar resembles a gold wax letter seal. In the 1900s, goldenseal was immensely popular and has become endangered due to over-harvesting (13). In 1997, goldenseal became listed under Appendix II of the Convention on International Trade in Endangered Species of Wild Flora and Fauna (CITIES), which controls export of the root to other countries. Goldenseal is now being cultivated in Washington state, and is considered a cash crop (6). Because it is so expensive, it is often adulterated. Common adulterants include Coptis and Xanthorrhiza (6). The concept of using goldenseal as an adulterant in drug screens came from the novel Stringtown on the Pike by the pharmacist John Uri Lloyd, but goldenseal caused a false positive for strychnine poisoning in this fictional situation (6).

GOLDTHREAD

Also Known As
Cankerroot, Chinese Goldthread, Coptide, Coptis, Coptis Chinesis, Gold Thread, Goldenthread, Huang Lian, Mouth Root, Yellowroot.

Scientific Names
Coptis chinensis; Coptis deltoidea; Coptis teetoides; Coptis trifolia, synonym Coptis groenlandica.
Family: Ranunculaceae.

People Use This For
Orally, goldthread is used for digestive disorders (18).

Safety
POSSIBLY UNSAFE ...when used orally in low doses. The constituent berberine is considered moderately toxic. Its LD50 in humans is 27.5 mg/kg (12).
PREGNANCY: LIKELY UNSAFE ...when used orally; avoid using. Goldthread may induce menstruation and uterine contractions (12,19).
LACTATION: Insufficient reliable information available; avoid using.

Effectiveness
There is insufficient reliable information available about the effectiveness of goldthread.

Mechanism of Action
The applicable part of goldthread is the rhizome. Goldthread contains the bitter berberine, which stimulates bile secretion (12). Berberine also has antimicrobial, diuretic, smooth muscle relaxant, and cardiac depressant activities (12). Small doses stimulate the cardiac and respiratory systems and decrease intestinal peristalsis (12). High doses stimulate smooth muscle in the intestines and uterus, and depress respiration and cardiac function (12). In animal studies, berberine depresses cardiac function by dilating blood vessels and stimulating the vagal nerve (12).

Adverse Reactions
Orally, purified berberine can cause lethargy, nosebleed, dyspnea, skin and eye irritation, kidney irritation, nephritis, nausea, vomiting, and diarrhea (2).

Interactions with Herbs & Other Dietary Supplements
Insufficient reliable information available.

Interactions with Drugs
ACID-INHIBITING DRUGS: Theoretically, due to claims that goldthread increases stomach acid, it might interfere with antacids, sucralfate (Carafate), H-2 antagonists, or proton pump inhibitors (19).

Interactions with Foods
No interactions are known to occur, and there is no known reason to expect a clinically significant interaction with goldthread.

Interactions with Lab Tests
No interactions are known to occur, and there is no known reason to expect a clinically significant interaction with goldthread.

Interactions with Diseases or Conditions
PEPTIC ULCER DISEASE: Contraindicated. Goldthread might increase stomach acid (19).

Dosage and Administration

ORAL: People typically use 0.5 to 1.2 grams of the powdered rhizome (5264). As a liquid, 1 teaspoon is boiled with 1 cup water, and dosed 1 tablespoon 3 to 6 times daily. The liquid is sometimes used as a mouthwash or gargle. The tincture is taken 5 to 10 drops at a time (5263).

Comments

None.

GOSSYPOL

Also Known As

Cottonseed Oil.
CAUTION: See separate listing for Cotton.

Scientific Names

Gossypium hirsutum; Gossypium herbaceum; other Gossypium species.
Family: Malvaceae.

People Use This For

Orally, gossypol is used as a male contraceptive (6,9,17).
Topically, gossypol is used as a spermicidal cream or gel (6).
Gossypol is being investigated for possible uses in treating uterine myoma, endometriosis, dysfunctional uterine bleeding, metastatic carcinoma of the endometrium or ovary, and HIV disease (6).

Safety

POSSIBLY UNSAFE ...when the cotton seed extract of gossypol is used orally (6,10). Inhibitory effects on spermatogenesis are not predictably reversible, although sperm counts usually return to normal within 3 months to 2 years after discontinuation (6). Chronic use might cause sterility (12). Gossypol might also be cytotoxic to endometrial cells (6).
There is insufficient reliable information available about the safety of the topical use of gossypol.
PREGNANCY: LIKELY UNSAFE ...when used orally because it possibly has abortifacient and uterine stimulant effects (6,12).
LACTATION: POSSIBLY UNSAFE ...when used orally; avoid using.

Effectiveness

EFFECTIVE ...when used orally for male contraception (6); adverse effects limit use.
POSSIBLY EFFECTIVE ...when applied topically as a spermicide (6).

Mechanism of Action

The applicable part of gossypol is the cotton seed extract. The contraceptive action of gossypol results from inhibition of an enzyme, lactate dehydrogenase X, that is crucial to energy metabolism in sperm and spermatogenic cells (6). Gossypol does not have estrogenic or androgenic activity, but it potentiates the androgenicity of methyltestosterone (6). Gossypol may act as an antifertility agent by inhibiting prostaglandin synthesis (17); it inhibits platelet activating factor and leukotrienes (6). Gossypol has shown activity against HIV and herpes simplex type 2 viruses (6); early evidence suggests possible inhibition of ovarian function and possible endometrial cell cytotoxicity (6).

Adverse Reactions

Orally, gossypol can cause fatigue (6,9,17), changes in appetite (6,9), loss of libido, persistent oligospermia (9), and hyperkalemia (17). Gossypol can cause hypokalemia resistant to potassium supplementation and potassium-sparing diuretics (9). GI effects associated with gossypol include mucosal sloughing, mucosal necrosis, ileus, and intestinal hemorrhage (21). The inhibitory effects on spermatogenesis are not predictably reversible, although sperm counts usually return to normal within 3 months to 2 years after discontinuation (6). Chronic use may cause sterility (12). High doses (100 to 700 times the contraceptive dose) may cause diarrhea, hair discoloration, malnutrition, circulatory problems, and heart failure (6). Gossypol might inhibit ovarian function (6).
Topically, it might cause a burning sensation on the face and hands (9,17).

Interactions with Herbs & Other Dietary Supplements

CARDIAC GLYCOSIDE-CONTAINING HERBS: Theoretically, concomitant use might increase the risk of cardiac glycoside toxicity due to the potassium depleting effects of gossypol. Cardiac glycoside containing herbs, including black hellebore, Canadian hemp roots, digitalis leaf, hedge mustard, figwort, lily of the valley roots, motherwort, oleander leaf, pheasant's eye plant, pleurisy root, squill bulb leaf scales, and strophanthus seeds (2,18,19,500).

STIMULANT LAXATIVE HERBS: Theoretically, overuse or misuse of stimulant laxatives with gossypol might increase the risk of potassium depletion. Stimulant laxative herbs include: aloe dried leaf sap, blue flag rhizome, alder buckthorn, European buckthorn, butternut bark, cascara bark, castor oil, colocynth fruit pulp, gamboge bark exudate, jalap root, black root, manna bark exudate, podophyllum root, rhubarb root, senna leaves and pods, wild cucumber fruit (Ecballium elaterium), and yellow dock root (19).

LICORICE/HORSETAIL: Theoretically, overuse/misuse of licorice rhizome or horsetail plant with gossypol might increase the risk of potassium depletion (19).

Interactions with Drugs
DIGOXIN: Theoretically, concomitant use might increase the risk of digoxin toxicity due to the potassium-depleting effects of gossypol (9).
NONSTEROIDAL ANTI-INFLAMMATORY DRUGS (NSAIDs): Concomitant use might increase the risk of gastrointestinal side effects (21).
POTASSIUM DEPLETING DIURETICS: Concomitant use increases the risk of potassium depletion and hypokalemia (9).
STIMULANT LAXATIVES: Theoretically, overuse or misuse of stimulant laxatives with gossypol might increase the risk of potassium depletion.

Interactions with Foods
No interactions are known to occur, and there is no known reason to expect a clinically significant interaction with gossypol.

Interactions with Lab Tests
No interactions are known to occur, and there is no known reason to expect a clinically significant interaction with gossypol.

Interactions with Diseases or Conditions
UROGENITAL IRRITATION OR SENSITIVITY: Contraindicated (12).
HYPOKALEMIA: Contraindicated; may induce or exacerbate hypokalemia (6).

Dosage and Administration
ORAL: Male contraception, 20 mg daily for 2.5 to 4 months followed by weekly maintenance dose of 50-60 mg (9,17); one reference mentions maintenance dose of 75-100 mg taken two times per month (6).
TOPICAL: No typical dosage.

Comments
Gossypol is considered unsafe for self-medication due to toxic potential; requires monitoring. Gossypol is found in cotton root, root bark, seed and stem, but is commercially extracted from cotton seed (6).

GOTU KOLA

Also Known As
Brahma-Buti, Brahma-Manduki, Centella, Centellase, Gota Kola, Gotu Cola, Gotu-Kola, Hydrocotyle, Hydrocotyle Asiatique, Indischer Wassernabel, Idrocotyle, Indian Pennywort, Indian Water Navelwort, Luei Gong Gen, Madecassol, Marsh Penny, Talepetrako, Thick-Leaved Pennywort, Tsubo-kusa, Tungchian, White Rot.
CAUTION: See separate listing for Cola Nut.

Scientific Names
Centella asiatica, synonym Hydrocotyle asiatica; Centella coriacea.
Family: Apiaceae or Umbelliferae.

People Use This For
Orally, gotu kola is used for reducing fatigue, improving memory and intelligence, venous insufficiency including varicose veins (6,18), wound healing, and increasing longevity (4,11,3901). It is also used for the common cold and influenza (flu), sunstroke, tonsillitis, pleurisy, urinary tract infection (UTI), hepatitis, jaundice (11,6887), abdominal pain, diarrhea, indigestion, gastritis, peptic ulcer disease (6887), dysentery, trauma, shingles (11), leprosy, cholera, syphilis, psychiatric disorders, epilepsy, asthma, anemia, diabetes, and hypertension (4,5,6,11,6887). Gotu kola is also used for amenorrhea, elephantiasis, systemic lupus erythematosus (SLE), tuberculosis, memory loss (11), and as an aphrodisiac (5,6).

Topically, gotu kola is used for skin conditions, including scabies, ulcers, psoriasis, and fungal infections (4,5,6,11,18), varicose veins, striae gravidarum, cellulitis (6887), keloids and hypertrophic scarring, and in poultices for snakebite (11). Parenterally, gotu kola is used for bladder lesions of schistosomiasis (6), post-phlebitis ulcers, and scleroderma (11). In manufacturing, gotu kola leaf extracts are used in cosmetics (11).

Safety
POSSIBLY SAFE ...when used orally or topically and appropriately (4,6,12,6887).
PREGNANCY: POSSIBLY UNSAFE ...when used orally. Gotu kola might be an abortifacient (4); avoid using.
LACTATION: Insufficient reliable information available; avoid using.

Effectiveness
POSSIBLY EFFECTIVE ...when used orally for chronic venous insufficiency (5,6,11,18,6887). ...when applied topically for improving wound healing (4,6,6887). ...when used topically for prevention of keloids and hypertrophic scarring (4). ...when used topically for psoriasis (4,6,6887). ...when given parenterally for bladder lesions of schistosomiasis (bilharzial infections) (6).
There is insufficient reliable information available about the effectiveness of gotu kola for its other uses.

Mechanism of Action
The applicable parts of gotu kola are the above ground parts. The pharmacological effects are thought to be due primarily to the 1 to 8% of saponin-containing triterpene acids and their sugar esters, including asiatic acid, madecassic acid, asiaticoside, asiaticoside A (madecassoside), and asiaticoside B. Gotu kola also contains essential oils, flavonoids, flavone derivatives including quercetin and kaempferol, sesquiterpenes, stigmasterol, and sitosterol (6887). The triterpenoid saponins (e.g., asiaticoside, madecassoside) seem to be involved in wound healing and decreasing venous pressure in venous insufficiency (4,5,6,11,18); asiaticoside and madecassoside have anti-inflammatory activity (4,5,6,11). There is also some evidence that asiaticosides might promote wound healing by stimulating collagen and glycosaminoglycan synthesis (1890,2700). Topical application of gotu kola extracts increase collagen synthesis, intracellular fibronectin content, and mitotic activity in the germ layer, and enlarges kerato-hyaline granules in scar tissue. There's preliminary evidence from animal models that asiaticosides might also have preventive and therapeutic effects on gastrointestinal ulcers (6887). The asiaticosides have several other pharmacological effects, including elevating blood glucose, triglycerides and cholesterol levels. They also seem to decrease blood urea nitrogen (BUN) and acid phosphatase levels. Some researchers think the asiaticoside derivatives, asiatic acid, asiaticoside 6, and SM2, might have a role in Alzheimer's disease. There is some early evidence that they might protect neurons from beta-amyloid toxicity (1889). There is preliminary evidence that gotu kola extracts might have sedative, anticonvulsant, and analgesic effects, possibly mediated in part via increased levels of the inhibitory transmitter, GABA (6887). The terpenoid constituents brahmoside and brahminoside might be responsible for sedative effects (4). Gotu kola extracts also seem to have antibacterial activity in vitro against Pseudomonas pyocyaneus, Trichoderma mentagrophytes, and Entamoeba histolytica, and antiviral activity against Herpes simplex type II (6887).

Adverse Reactions
Orally, gotu kola is usually well tolerated when used in typical doses. However, in some patients it can cause gastrointestinal upset and nausea (6887), widespread pruritus and photosensitivity (4). Caution patients using gotu kola to use sunscreen and wear adequate clothing to prevent sunburn. Large doses of gotu kola might increase blood pressure, glucose, and cholesterol levels (4). There is also some concern that large doses of gotu kola might cause sedation and drowsiness (4).
Topically, gotu kola can cause allergic contact dermatitis (6,6887) and burning sensation in some patients (4). Subcutaneous injection of gotu kola can cause pain and discoloration at injection site (6). This can be prevented by using intramuscular injections (6).

Interactions with Herbs & Other Dietary Supplements
HERBS WITH SEDATIVE PROPERTIES: Theoretically, concomitant use with herbs that have sedative properties might enhance therapeutic and adverse effects. These include calamus, calendula, California poppy, catnip, capsicum, celery, couch grass, elecampane, Siberian ginseng, German chamomile, goldenseal, hops, Jamaican dogwood, kava, lemon balm, sage, St. John's wort, sassafras, scullcap, shepherd's purse, stinging nettle, valerian, wild carrot, wild lettuce, ashwaganda, and yerba mansa (4,19).

Interactions with Drugs
CHOLESTEROL-REDUCING DRUGS: Theoretically, large doses can increase serum cholesterol, interfering with cholesterol-lowering drug therapy (4).
DIABETES DRUGS: Theoretically, large doses might increase blood glucose levels interfering with hypoglycemic drug therapy (4).

DRUGS WITH SEDATIVE PROPERTIES: Theoretically, concomitant use with drugs with sedative properties might cause additive effects and side effects (4).

Interactions with Foods
No interactions are known to occur, and there is no known reason to expect a clinically significant interaction with gotu kola.

Interactions with Lab Tests
No interactions are known to occur, and there is no known reason to expect a clinically significant interaction with gotu kola.

Interactions with Diseases or Conditions
DIABETES: Gotu kola can elevate blood glucose levels (4).
HYPERLIPIDEMIAS: Gotu kola can elevate triglyceride and cholesterol levels (4).

Dosage and Administration
ORAL: 600 mg dried leaves three times per day (18), or, one cup tea (steep 600 mg dried leaves in 150 mL boiling water 5-10 minutes, strain) three times per day (18). Clinical trials for venous insufficiency used 60-120 mg titrated extract per day for two months (780).
TOPICAL: No typical dosage.
INJECTION: No typical dosage.

Comments
Avoid confusion with cola nut.

GOUTWEED

Also Known As
Achweed, Ashweed, Bishop's Elder, Bishopsweed, Bishopswort, Eltroot, English Goatweed, Gout Herb, Goutwort, Ground Elder, Herb Gerard, Jack-Jump-About, Masterwort, Pigweed, Weyl Ash, White Ash.
CAUTION: See separate listings for Bishop's Weed and Masterwort.

Scientific Names
Aegopodium podagraria.

People Use This For
Orally, goutweed is used for gout and rheumatic disease. It is also used for hemorrhoids, kidney, bladder, and intestinal disorders (18).

Safety
There is insufficient reliable information available about the safety of goutweed.
Pregnancy and Lactation: Insufficient reliable information available.

Effectiveness
There is insufficient reliable information available about the effectiveness of goutweed.

Mechanism of Action
The applicable parts of goutweed are the above ground parts. Goutweed contains a volatile oil, flavonol glycosides (hyperoside, isoquercitrin), and caffeic acid derivatives including chlorogenic acid (18).

Adverse Reactions
None reported.

Interactions with Herbs & Other Dietary Supplements
Insufficient reliable information available.

Interactions with Drugs
No interactions are known to occur, and there is no known reason to expect a clinically significant interaction with goutweed.

Interactions with Foods

No interactions are known to occur, and there is no known reason to expect a clinically significant interaction with goutweed.

Interactions with Lab Tests

No interactions are known to occur, and there is no known reason to expect a clinically significant interaction with goutweed.

Interactions with Diseases or Conditions

No interactions are known to occur, and there is no known reason to expect a clinically significant interaction with goutweed.

Dosage and Administration

ORAL: People typically use 2 to 4 mL of liquid goutweed extract (5264).
TOPICAL: The fresh herb is squeezed or softened by soaking in water for poultices (18).

Comments

Avoid confusion with bishop's weed (Ammi visnagae) and masterwort (Heracleum sphondylium and Heracleum lanatum).

GRAINS OF PARADISE

Also Known As

Guinea Grains, Mallaguetta Pepper, Melegueta Pepper.
CAUTION: See separate listing for Capsicum.

Scientific Names

Aframomum melegueta, synonym Amomum melegueta.
Family: Zingiberaceae.

People Use This For

Orally, grains of paradise fruit and seeds are used as a stimulant (18).

Safety

POSSIBLY SAFE ...when used orally and appropriately (12).
PREGNANCY AND LACTATION: Insufficient reliable information available; avoid using.

Effectiveness

There is insufficient reliable information available about the effectiveness of grains of paradise.

Mechanism of Action

The applicable parts of grains of paradise are the fruit and seed. Grains of paradise contains a volatile oil and the constituents hydroxyphenylalkanones and hydroxyphenylalkanoles. The seed is said to be a stimulant (18).

Adverse Reactions

Theoretically, may cause GI and lower urinary tract irritation when taken orally (18).

Interactions with Herbs & Other Dietary Supplements

Insufficient reliable information available.

Interactions with Drugs

No interactions are known to occur, and there is no known reason to expect a clinically significant interaction with grains of paradise.

Interactions with Foods

No interactions are known to occur, and there is no known reason to expect a clinically significant interaction with grains of paradise.

Interactions with Lab Tests

No interactions are known to occur, and there is no known reason to expect a clinically significant interaction with grains of paradise.

Interactions with Diseases or Conditions

No interactions are known to occur, and there is no known reason to expect a clinically significant interaction with grains of paradise.

Dosage and Administration

ORAL: People typically use 4 to 6 grams added to 3 to 4 cups of water and boiled until the volume is reduced by one-half. The cooled liquid is taken in 3 doses on an empty stomach (5251).

Comments

Avoid confusion with capsicum (Capsicum annuum), also known as grains of paradise.

GRAPE fruit, skin

Also Known As

Black Grape Raisins, Cabernet Franc, Cabernet Sauvignon, Calzin, Chardonnay, Emperor, Enocianina, Flame Seedless, Grape, Grapes, Grape Fruit, Grape Fruit Skin, Grape Juice, Grape Skin, Grape Skin Extract, Merlot, Petite Sirah, Raisins, Red Globe, Red Malaga, Sauvignon Blanc, Sultanas, Table Grapes, Thompson Seedless, Wine Grapes. CAUTION: See separate listings for Grape leaf, Grape seed, Grapefruit, Resveratrol, and Wine.

Scientific Names

Vitis vinifera.
Family: Vitaceae.

People Use This For

Orally, grapes and grape preparations, including grape skin and grape juice are used to prevent coronary heart disease (3579). They are also used as a dietary source of antioxidants (3579). Grapes have also been used for varicose veins, hemorrhoids, capillary fragility, and as a mild laxative for constipation. Grape fasts have been used for "detoxification." Dried grapes, raisins or sultanas, have been used as an expectorant for cough (4201).
In beverages and drink mixes, including wine, grape skin extract is used as a coloring agent (11).

Safety

LIKELY SAFE …when used orally in amounts found in foods (11,18). Grape skin extracts have been approved for beverage use only (11).
There is insufficient reliable information available about the safety of grape fruit or skin for its other uses.
PREGNANCY AND LACTATION: LIKELY SAFE …when used orally in amounts found in foods (11,18). There is insufficient reliable information available about the safety of grape fruit or skin for its other uses.

Effectiveness

There is insufficient reliable information available about the effectiveness of grape fruit or skin.

Mechanism of Action

Grapes and grape preparations provide a variety of constituents that are thought to be pharmacologically active. Various types of phenolic compounds, including anthocyanins, cinnamates, and flavan-3-ols, are thought to provide benefit in the prevention of heart disease. These phenolic compounds are thought to have antioxidant properties and play a role in prevention of low-density lipoprotein (LDL) oxidation. In an in vitro study, a variety of grapes were tested for phenol content and ability to prevent LDL oxidation. Inhibition of oxidation ranged from 22% to 91% at higher concentrations. Red grape varieties tended to produce more oxidation protection than white or blush grape varieties. A similar trend has been seen with red versus white wines. There was a significant correlation between total phenol content and anthocyanin content and antioxidant activity. Phenol content in red grapes is primarily from anthocyanins, which are responsible producing the color in red grapes (3579). Grapes are also reported to have laxative and expectorant properties (4201). Black grape raisins are thought to have similar antioxidant potential as red wine (2540). Grape skin extract also contains anthocyanin pigments (11). Some evidence suggests that anthocyanins might strengthen capillaries and have antifungal and antibacterial activity (11). The anthocyanidins delphinidin and delphinidin/cyanidin dimer show some evidence that they might induce chromosomal damage (4074).

Adverse Reactions

Excessive consumption of grapes, dried grapes, raisins, or sultanas, might cause diarrhea due to laxative effects (4201). There is one report of an anaphylactic reaction to grape skin extract, which included urticaria and angioedema (4073).

Interactions with Herbs & Other Dietary Supplements

LACTOBACILLUS ACIDOPHILUS: Grape anthocyanins can inhibit the growth of Lactobacillus acidophilus. Concurrent administration might prevent Lactobacillus acidophilus colonization of the gastrointestinal tract (11); avoid concurrent use.

Interactions with Drugs

PHENACETIN: Grape juice decreases phenactin, but not acetaminophen plasma levels. It may decrease levels by inducing cytochrome P450 1A2 (CYP 1A2) metabolism (2539).
OTHERS: Grape juice is thought to induce cytochrome P450 1A2 (CYP 1A2) metabolism and may decrease plasma levels of substrates of CYP 1A2. Drugs metabolized by CYP 1A2 include amitriptyline (Elavil), caffeine, chlordiazepoxide (Librium), clomipramine (Anafranil), clopidogrel (Plavix), clozapine (Clozaril), cyclobenzaprine (Flexaril), desipramine (Norpramin), diazepam (Valium), estradiol (Estrace, others), flutamide (Eulexin), fluvoxamine (Luvox), grepafloxacin (Raxar), haloperidol (Haldol), imipramine (Tofranil), mexiletine (Mexitil), mirtazapine (Remeron), naproxen (Naprosyn), nortriptyline (Pamelor), olanzapine (Zyprexa), ondansetron (Zofran), propafenone (Rythmol), propranolol (Inderal), riluzole (Rilutek), ropinirole (Requip), ropivacaine (Naropin), tacrine (Cognex), theophylline (Theo-Dur, others), verapamil (Calan, Covera-HS, others), warfarin (Coumadin), and zileuton (Zyflo).

Interactions with Foods

No interactions are known to occur, and there is no known reason to expect a clinically significant interaction with grape fruit or skin.

Interactions with Lab Tests

No interactions are known to occur, and there is no known reason to expect a clinically significant interaction with grape fruit or skin.

Interactions with Diseases or Conditions

No interactions are known to occur, and there is no known reason to expect a clinically significant interaction with grape fruit or skin.

Dosage and Administration

No typical dosage.

Comments

None.

GRAPE leaf

Also Known As

Folia Vitis Viniferae, Grape Leaf Extract, Red Vine Leaf Extract, Red Vine Leaf AS 195.
CAUTION: See separate listings for Grape seed; Grape fruit, skin; Resveratrol; and Grapefruit.

Scientific Names

Vitis vinifera.
Family: Vitaceae.

People Use This For

Orally, grape leaf is used for vascular or circulatory disorders, especially venous diseases (18) such as chronic venous insufficiency (2538), varicose veins, and edema (4201). It is also used for attention deficit hyperactivity disorder (ADHD) (3578), diarrhea, heavy menstrual bleeding, uterine hemorrhage, hemorrhoids, and canker sores (4201). Intravaginally, grape leaf infusions are used as a douche (4201).
Grape leaf is used as a food, particularly in Greek cooking.

Safety

LIKELY SAFE ...when used orally in amounts found in foods (18).
POSSIBLY SAFE ...when used orally and appropriately for medicinal purposes. Significant adverse effects

have not been reported (18). In one study using a grape leaf extract, no significant adverse events were reported during 12 weeks of treatment (2538).

PREGNANCY AND LACTATION: Insufficient reliable information available; avoid using.

Effectiveness

POSSIBLY EFFECTIVE ...when used orally for mild to moderate chronic venous insufficiency. In one clinical trial, a specific grape leaf extract, known as red vine leaf extract AS 195 (Antistax, Boehringer Ingelheim), was given to 260 patients with stage I and stage II chronic venous insufficiency for 12 weeks. Leg edema significantly decreased after 6 weeks of treatment compared to placebo. Doses of 360 mg and 720 mg daily were both effective, but the higher dose produced a slightly greater effect. Patients also reported significant decreases in subjective complaints such as tired or heavy legs, tension, and tingling and pain after 12 weeks of treatment (2538).

There is insufficient reliable information available about the effectiveness of grape leaf for its other uses.

Mechanism of Action

Grape leaf preparations contain flavonoids that are thought to be responsible for its pharmacological effects (18). The red vine grape extract AS 195 (Antistax, Boehringer Ingelheim) used in one clinical trial primarily contains the flavonoids quercetin-3-O-beta-glucuronide and isoquercitrin (2538). However, its mechanism of action in chronic venous insufficiency is not clearly understood. Grape leaf is reported to have anti-inflammatory and astringent properties (18,4201). These properties are reported to be greatest in the red leaves (4201).

Adverse Reactions

In one study, the most common adverse effects were gastrointestinal and included abdominal discomfort, diarrhea, dyspepsia, dry mouth, and retching. Other adverse effects included infections, headache and musculoskeletal disorders. One case of leg hematoma following a minor trauma was also reported in a person using grape leaf extract (2538).

Interactions with Herbs & Other Dietary Supplements

Insufficient reliable information available.

Interactions with Drugs

No interactions are known to occur, and there is no known reason to expect a clinically significant interaction with grape leaf.

Interactions with Foods

No interactions are known to occur, and there is no known reason to expect a clinically significant interaction with grape leaf.

Interactions with Lab Tests

No interactions are known to occur, and there is no known reason to expect a clinically significant interaction with grape leaf.

Interactions with Diseases or Conditions

No interactions are known to occur, and there is no known reason to expect a clinically significant interaction with grape leaf.

Dosage and Administration

ORAL: For chronic venous insufficiency, one clinical trial used a standardized red vine grape extract AS 195 (Antistax, Boehringer Ingelheim). The dose used was 360 mg or 720 mg once daily (2538).

Comments

None.

GRAPE seed

Also Known As

Activin, Extrait De Pepins De Raisin, Grape Seed Extract, Grape Seed Oil, Grapeseed, Leucoanthocyanin, Muskat, Oligomeric Proanthocyanidins, Oligomeric Procyanidins, OPC, OPCs, PCO, PCOs, Proanthodyn, Procyanidolic Oligomers.

CAUTION: See separate listings for Grape leaf; Grape fruit, skin; Grapefruit Seed Extract; Pycnogenol; and Resveratrol.

Scientific Names

Vitis vinifera; Vitis coignetiae.
Family: Vitaceae.

People Use This For

Orally, grape seed is used for treating and preventing vascular or circulatory disorders including venous insufficiency, varicose veins, atherosclerosis, peripheral vascular disease, edema associated with injury or surgery, and myocardial or cerebral infarction (402,3900,3580). Grape seed is also used orally for hemorrhoids (3580), strengthening blood vessels, inflammation, diabetic complications such as neuropathy or retinopathy (3580,3900), improving wound healing, preventing dental caries (6,3900), cancer prevention, macular degeneration, poor night vision, liver cirrhosis, allergies, and prevention of collagen breakdown associated with collagen diseases and aging (3580,3900). Grape seed oil is used orally as a supplemental dietary source of essential fatty acids and tocopherols (6).

Safety

LIKELY SAFE ...when used orally in the amounts commonly found in foods (6,402).
POSSIBLY SAFE ...when used orally and appropriately for medicinal purposes (6,402).
PREGNANCY AND LACTATION: Insufficient reliable information available; avoid using amounts greater than those found in foods.

Effectiveness

POSSIBLY EFFECTIVE ...when used orally as a supplemental dietary source of essential fatty acids and tocopherols. Ground grape seeds produce an oil that is rich in essential fatty acids and tocopherols (6). ...when used orally for treating chronic venous insufficiency. Multiple small European clinical trials have shown grape seed extract or its procyanidin constituents to be superior to placebo for reducing subjective symptoms and improving venous tone (2541). ...when used orally for decreasing ocular stress from glare (2541). Multiple small European clinical trials have shown grape seed extract containing procyanidin constituents to be superior to placebo (2541).
There is insufficient reliable information available to rate the effectiveness of grape seed for its other uses. However, preliminary research suggests it might also be beneficial for improving night vision. In one 6-week unblinded study, healthy volunteers had improved night vision after using grape seed extract containing procyanidins (3580). Further research is needed to rate the effectiveness of grape seed for this use.

Mechanism of Action

Grape seeds are typically obtained as a by-product of the manufacturing of wine (6). Constituents called oligomeric proanthocyanidins (OPCs) or procyanidins are thought to be responsible for grape seed's pharmacological effects. OPCs from grape seed are theorized to be beneficial to prevent and treat cardiovascular and circulatory conditions due to antioxidant and potential antilipoperoxidant activity (6,3900). OPCs are also thought to inhibit the proteolytic enzymes collagenase, elastase, hyaluronidase, and beta glucuronidase, which are involved in the breakdown of structural components of the vasculature and skin (6,3900). For prevention of dental caries, grape seed is thought to work by inhibiting the growth of Streptococcus mutans and preventing glucan formation from sucrose (6). These pharmacological effects have not yet been clearly demonstrated in humans. Ground grape seeds also produce an oil that is rich in essential fatty acids, such as linoleic acid, and tocopherol (6,6870). The oil usually also contains traces of the oligomeric proanthocyanidins (OPCs) (6870).

Adverse Reactions

None reported.

Interactions with Herbs & Other Dietary Supplements

Insufficient reliable information available.

Interactions with Drugs

WARFARIN (Coumadin): Theoretically, due to the tocopherol content of grape seed oil, concomitant use with warfarin might increase warfarin's effects and the risk of bleeding (402); use with caution.

Interactions with Foods

No interactions are known to occur, and there is no known reason to expect a clinically significant interaction with grape seed.

Interactions with Lab Tests

No interactions are known to occur, and there is no known reason to expect a clinically significant interaction with grape seed.

Interactions with Diseases or Conditions

No interactions are known to occur, and there is no known reason to expect a clinically significant interaction with grape seed.

Dosage and Administration

ORAL: Grape seed extract as tablets or capsules dosed at 75-300 mg daily for three weeks followed by a maintenance dose of 40-80 mg daily has been suggested by some sources (402,3900). For chronic venous insufficiency, grape seed extract procyanidin doses of 150-300 mg per day have been used (2541). For reducing ocular stress due to glare, grape seed extract procyanidin doses of 200-300 mg per day have been used (2541).

Comments

Pycnogenol (pinebark extract) is similar to the grape seed extract in active ingredients and medicinal uses (7,402). Both pycnogenol and grape seed contain oligomeric proanthocyanidins (OPCs). Several other natural medicines contain constituents that are similar to the OPCs, including wine, cranberries, bilberries, green and black teas, black currant, onions, legumes, parsley, and hawthorn (3580).

GRAPEFRUIT

Also Known As

Paradisapfel, Pomelo, Toronja.
CAUTION: See separate listings for Grapefruit Seed Extract and Grapefruit Oil.

Scientific Names

Citrus paradisi.
Family: Rutaceae.

People Use This For

Orally, grapefruit is used for reducing cholesterol and reversing atherosclerosis; as a supplemental source of potassium, vitamin C, and fiber; for reducing hematocrit; as an anti-cancer agent; and as an aid in weight reduction (6).
In combination with cyclosporine, grapefruit is used for treating psoriasis (6).
For food uses, grapefruit is consumed as fruit and juice (6).

Safety

LIKELY SAFE ...when used orally in food amounts.
There is insufficient reliable information available about the safety of very large amounts of grapefruit.
PREGNANCY AND LACTATION: LIKELY SAFE ...when used in food amounts; avoid excessive amounts.

Effectiveness

There is insufficient reliable information available about the effectiveness of grapefruit. However, there's some evidence that consumption of vitamin C-rich citrus fruits, including grapefruit and others, might improve lung function in people with asthma. Intake of citrus fruits 1-2 times per week has produced this benefit in some studies (6049,6055,6056). However, other studies have not found this benefit (6057,6058). More evidence is needed to rate the effectiveness of grapefruit for this use.

Mechanism of Action

The applicable parts of grapefruit are the fruit and juice. Whole grapefruit is high in water and fiber. It is a good dietary source of potassium, vitamin C, pectin, and other nutrients (6). The potential benefits of grapefruit in asthma might be due to antioxidant properties of vitamin C or other fruit constituents (6049,6054,6055). Grapefruit pectin, which is found in whole fruit but not juice, can reduce cholesterol and promote regression of atherosclerosis (6). Studies suggest grapefruit can affect blood components. Some evidence suggests the constituent, naringin, might induce red cell aggregation. Consuming one half to one grapefruit per day can reduce an individual's hematocrit level (6). An analysis of grapefruit's anti-cancer effects suggests that consumption might reduce the risk of pancreatic cancer (6). Grapefruit juice contains furanocoumarins, including bergamottin and dihydroxybergamottin, which inhibit cytochrome P450 3A4 (CYP3A4) (3769,5070,5071). In addition, bergamottin inhibits CYPs 1A2, 2A6, 2C9, 2C19, 2D6, and 2E1 (5072). Grapefruit juice also contains naringin, naringenin, limonin, and obacunone which are known to inhibit human hepatic microsomes (6). Grapefruit juice inhibits hepatic and gut wall CYP3A4 and increases bioavailability and plasma concentrations of numerous drugs (see Interactions with Drugs) (1386). Human research indicates that blended grapefruit segments, and an extract of grapefruit core and peel, also inhibit CYP3A4 activity (1388). Evidence suggests that grapefruit juice inhibits p-glycoprotein counter-transport activity. P-glycoprotein is thought to reduce the absorption of some drugs by pumping them back into the gut (1390). However, the clinical effect of grapefruit juice on drugs affected by p-glycoprotein activity requires further investigation. It may be necessary to withhold grapefruit juice for 3 days to avoid interactions with felodipine and nisoldipine (5068,5069).

Adverse Reactions

Grapefruit has few reported adverse reactions. One study shows it can reduce hematocrit (531). One case report associates grapefruit juice with hypotension (6).

Interactions with Herbs & Other Dietary Supplements

RED YEAST (Cholestin): Concomitant use of grapefruit with red yeast increases the serum levels of lovastatin, a constituent of red yeast (527).

Interactions with Drugs

ARTEMETHER (Artenam, Paluther): Grapefruit juice increases the oral bioavailability of artemether in healthy men by 90-250% (5065,5066).

BENZODIAZEPINES: Some studies suggest that grapefruit juice increases the maximum blood levels and duration of effect of midazolam (Versed) and triazolam (Halcion); other studies suggest there is no effect (4300). Grapefruit juice increases the maximum blood levels and duration of effect of diazepam (Valium), but the clinical significance of this is not known (3228).

BUSPIRONE (Buspar): Grapefruit juice increases absorption and plasma concentrations of buspirone (3771).

CAFFEINE: Some studies suggest grapefruit juice decreases caffeine clearance, possibly increasing the effects or adverse effects; others disagree (4300).

CALCIUM CHANNEL BLOCKERS: Grapefruit juice increases absorption and plasma concentrations of amlodipine (Norvasc) (523), nifedipine (Procardia, Adalat) (528), nisoldipine (Sular) (529), felodipine (Plendil), nimodipine (Nimotop), nicardipine (Cardene), diltiazem (Cardizem) (524,528,1388,4300), and verapamil (Calan, Isoptin, Verelan) (3229). Some references dispute the clinical relevance of the interactions with amlodipine, diltiazem, and verapamil (3230,4300). In healthy older adults, the hemodynamic response to felodipine (Plendil) plus grapefruit juice might be influenced by altered autonomic regulation. In older healthy adults, a single dose of grapefruit juice and felodipine enhanced the blood pressure lowering effects of felodipine. However, after a week of grapefruit juice and felodipine (steady state), the hypotensive activity was reduced, possibly due to compensatory tachycardia (1392). Research indicates it is necessary to withhold grapefruit juice for 3 days to avoid interactions with felodipine and nisoldipine (5068,5069,6453).

CARBAMAZEPINE (Tegretol): Grapefruit juice increases absorption and plasma concentrations of carbamazepine (524).

CARVEDILOL (Coreg): Grapefruit juice is reported to increase the bioavailability of a single dose of carvedilol by 16% (5071).

CISAPRIDE (Propulsid): Grapefruit juice increases absorption and plasma concentrations of cisapride (1383,3226).

CLOMIPRAMINE (Anafranil): Grapefruit juice increases blood levels of clomipramine. Two cases are reported in which trough clomipramine blood levels increased significantly after adding grapefruit juice to the therapeutic regimen (5064).

CYCLOSPORINE (Neoral, Sandimmune): Grapefruit juice increases absorption and plasma concentrations of cyclosporine (522).

ESTROGENS: Grapefruit juice increases absorption and plasma concentrations of 17-beta-estradiol (526) and ethinyl-estradiol (525).

FEXOFENADINE (Allegra): Grapefruit juice can significantly decrease oral absorption and blood levels of fexofenadine when taken together. Quarter-strength grapefruit juice decreases bioavailability of fexofenadine by about 24% and full strength by 67%. Grapefruit juice seems to inhibit organic anion transporting polypeptide (OATP), which is a drug transporter in the gut, liver, and kidney (7046). It's not yet known how long grapefruit juice inhibits OATP. Separating administration times might not prevent this interaction. Tell patients it's best to take their medications with a plain glass of water.

HMG-CO A REDUCTASE INHIBITORS: Grapefruit juice increases absorption and plasma concentrations of lovastatin (Mevacor) (527), simvastatin (Zocor) (3774), and atorvastatin (Lipitor) (3227). It does not affect pravastatin (3227).

ITRACONAZOLE (Sporanox): Grapefruit juice impairs itraconazole absorption (310).

LOSARTAN (Cozaar): Concomitant use of grapefruit juice and losartan might reduce losartan effectiveness, but this requires further study. Losartan is an inactive prodrug which must be metabolized to its active form, E-3174, to be effective. In one human study, grapefruit juice reduced losartan metabolism, increased losartan AUC, and reduced the AUC of the major active losartan metabolite, E-3174 (1391).

METHYLPREDNISOLONE (Adlone, A-Methapred, depMedalone, Depoject, Medrol, Solu-Medrol): Grapefruit juice can increase plasma concentration of orally administered methylprednisolone. Grapefruit juice 200 mL 3 times daily given with methylprednisolone 16 mg increased methylprednisolone half-life by 35%, peak plasma concentration by 27%, and total area under the curve by 75% (3123). In some patients, consumption of large amounts of grapefruit juice with methylprednisolone might increase the risk of adverse effects; use cautiously.

QUINIDINE: Grapefruit juice decreases quinidine clearance and prolongs the half-life by about 20% (5067).

The clinical effect of this interaction is unknown.

SAQUINAVIR (Fortovase, Invirase): Grapefruit juice increases absorption and plasma concentrations of the protease inhibitor (PI)-type antiretroviral drug saquinavir (3773).

TERFENADINE (Seldane): Grapefruit juice increases absorption and plasma concentrations of terfenadine (530).

WARFARIN (Coumadin): Grapefruit juice might increase warfarin effects. One case is reported of significantly increased international normalized ratio (INR) associated with consumption of 50 ounces of grapefruit juice daily; no evidence of bleeding was reported. In a small clinical trial, consumption of 24 ounces of grapefruit juice daily for one week had no effect on INR in a group of men anticoagulated with warfarin.

Interactions with Foods

No interactions are known to occur, and there is no known reason to expect a clinically significant interaction with grapefruit.

Interactions with Lab Tests

DRUG ASSAYS: Grapefruit juice decreases metabolism, increasing plasma concentrations and test results of amlodipine (Norvasc) (523), nifedipine (Procardia, Adalat) (528), nisoldipine (Sular) (529), felodipine (Plendil), nimodipine (Nimotop), nicardipine (Cardene), diltiazem (Cardizem, Dilacor XR, Tiazac) (524,528,1388,4300), verapamil (Calan, Isoptin, Verelan) (3229), buspirone (BuSpar) (3771), midazolam (Versed) and triazolam (Halcion) (4300), diazepam (Valium) (3228), carbamazepine (Tegretol) (524), cisapride (Propulsid) (3226), cyclosporine (Sandimmune, Neoral) (522), 17-beta-estradiol (526), ethinyl-estradiol (525), lovastatin (Mevacor) (527), saquinavir (Fortovase, Invirase) (3773), simvastatin (Zocor) (3774), atorvastatin (Lipitor) (3227), and terfenadine (530).

LOSARTAN (Cozaaar): Grapefruit juice might increase plasma losartan concentrations, reduce plasma E-3174 concentrations, and test results. Losartan is an inactive prodrug which must be metabolized to its active form, E-3174, to be effective. In one human study, grapefruit juice reduced losartan metabolism, increased losartan AUC, and reduced the AUC of the major active losartan metabolite, E-3174 (1391).

Interactions with Diseases or Conditions

No interactions are known to occur, and there is no known reason to expect a clinically significant interaction with grapefruit.

Dosage and Administration

ORAL: The pharmacologic effects of grapefruit juice seem to be most pronounced when people consume over four glasses of the juice per day. When using grapefruit juice to increase effect and decrease dose of cyclosporine, it is important to avoid fluctuations in grapefruit juice intake, brand used if a commercial product used, variety of grapefruit if juice is freshly made, and the means of processing used to extract juice (6). However, grapefruit juice should not be used to lower the dose of cyclosporine because it is too unpredictable.

Comments

Drug interactions with grapefruit juice are well documented. The chemistry of the grapefruit varies by the species, the growing conditions, and the process used to extract the juice. Because grapefruit juice is not standardized, use as an adjunct to drug therapy is not recommended (3775).

GRAPEFRUIT OIL

Also Known As

Cold-Pressed Grapefruit Oil, Expressed Grapefruit Oil, Shaddock Oil.
CAUTION: See separate listings for Grapefruit and Grapefruit Seed Extract.

Scientific Names

Citrus X paradisi, synonyms Citrus racemosa, Citrus decumana, Citrus maxima.
Family: Rutaceae.

People Use This For

Topically, grapefruit oil is used to relieve muscle fatigue, to promote hair growth, for toning the skin, and for reducing acne and oily skin. It is also used to aid with the common cold and flu.

Inhaled, the vapors are used to help the body retain water and to relieve headache and stress. The aroma is used to relieve depression.

In food and beverages, grapefruit oil is used as a flavoring component (11).

In manufacturing, grapefruit oil is used as a fragrance component in soaps and cosmetics.

Safety

LIKELY SAFE ...when used in amounts found in foods. It has Generally Recognized as Safe (GRAS) status in the US. The highest concentrations of grapefruit oil in foods is 0.108% (11). ...when used in amounts found in perfumes and cosmetics. The highest concentrations of grapefruit oil in these products is 1.0% (11).

There is insufficient reliable information available about the safety grapefruit oil for its other uses.

PREGNANCY AND LACTATION: LIKELY SAFE ...when used in food amounts. There is insufficient reliable information available about the safety of larger amounts used during pregnancy and lactation; avoid using.

Effectiveness

There is insufficient reliable information available about the effectiveness of grapefruit oil.

Mechanism of Action

Grapefruit oil is obtained by cold expression from the fruit peel of the Citrus X paradisi tree (11). Antibacterial activity has been suggested. Grapefruit oil contains furocoumarins, including bergaptens, which are photosensitizing, phototoxic, and mutagenic (2). They are responsible for adverse dermatological reactions in other plants that contain them (see separate listings for Angelica and Rue) (11,515). Animal data suggests that 9,10-dimethyl-1,2-benzanthracene, the primary carcinogen, promoted tumor formation when grapefruit oil was applied directly to the skin. Dermatological studies have suggested that grapefruit oil is nonirritating, nonsensitizing, and nonphototoxic to human skin (11).

Adverse Reactions

Contact dermatitis and phototoxic reactions, including skin blisters, have occurred with other furocoumarin-containing herbs following topical exposure and exposure to sunlight (11).

Interactions with Herbs & Other Dietary Supplements

Insufficient reliable information available.

Interactions with Drugs

No interactions are known to occur, and there is no known reason to expect a clinically significant interaction with grapefruit oil.

Interactions with Foods

No interactions are known to occur, and there is no known reason to expect a clinically significant interaction with grapefruit oil.

Interactions with Lab Tests

No interactions are known to occur, and there is no known reason to expect a clinically significant interaction with grapefruit oil.

Interactions with Diseases or Conditions

No interactions are known to occur, and there is no known reason to expect a clinically significant interaction with grapefruit oil.

Dosage and Administration

No typical dosage.

Comments

None.

GRAPEFRUIT SEED EXTRACT

Also Known As

Bioflavonoid Concentrate, Citrus Grandis Extract, Citrus Seed Extract, CSE, Grapefruit Extract, Grapefruit Seed Glycerate, GSE, Standardized Extract of Grapefruit.

Caution: See separate listings for Grapefruit; Grapefruit Oil; Grape fruit, seed; and Grape Seed.

Scientific Names

Citrus paradisi.
Family: Rutaceae.

People Use This For

Orally, grapefruit seed extract is used for preventing and treating infections due to bacteria, viruses, fungi, and parasites (5858,5859). It is particularly promoted for yeast infections, and intestinal parasites such as Giardia lamblia and Entamoeba histolytica, including intestinal infections associated with travel (5858).

Topically, grapefruit seed extract is used as a facial cleanser, first-aid treatment, and treatment for mild skin irritations (5858). It is also used as an ear or nasal rinse for prevention and treatment of infections, a throat gargle for sore throat, a dental rinse to prevent gingivitis and to promote healthy gums and fresh breath, and a vaginal douche for candidiasis (5858). It has also been nebulized for the treatment of lung infections (5858).

In manufacturing, grapefruit seed extract is used in soaps and cosmetics; and as a household cleaner for fruits, vegetables, meats, kitchen surfaces, dishes, etc. (5858).

In agriculture, it is used as a bactericide and fungicide, a mold inhibitor and antiparasitic for animal feeds, a food preservative and antioxidant, and a water disinfectant (5858).

Safety

POSSIBLY SAFE ...when preservative-free products are used orally as a food additive. Unpreserved natural extracts of grapefruit seed have Generally Recognized as Safe (GRAS) status in the US (5860).

POSSIBLY UNSAFE ...when products with preservatives are used orally. The preservative benzethonium chloride has been detected in some commercial grapefruit seed extracts. This substance is restricted to use in rinse-off cosmetics and is not permitted for use in drugs or foods in Germany (5867). It can cause vomiting, collapse, convulsions and coma when ingested (3082).

There is insufficient reliable information about the safety of grapefruit seed extract for its other uses.

PREGNANCY AND LACTATION: Insufficient reliable information available; avoid using.

Effectiveness

There is insufficient reliable information available about the effectiveness of grapefruit seed extract. However, in one study, a citrus seed extract (ParaMycrocidin) used orally, produced improvements in complaints of constipation, flatulence and abdominal discomfort, possibly due to changes in intestinal microflora, in people with atopic eczema (5866). More evidence is needed to rate grapefruit seed extract for these uses.

Mechanism of Action

Grapefruit seeds contain numerous constituents including naringin, nomilin, deacetyl-nomilin, nomilinic-acid-17-O-beta-D-glucoside, deacetyl-nomilinic-acid-17-O-beta-D-glucoside, limonol, deoxy-limonol, 7-obacunol, obacunone, epi-iso-obacunoic-acid-17-O-beta-D-glucoside, iso-obacunoic-acid-17-O-beta-D-glucoside, and trans-obacunoic-acid-17-O-beta-D-glucoside (513). However, the role these play in any potential therapeutic actions of grapefruit seed extract is unknown. Naringin has been reported to induce red blood cell aggregation in vitro (6). Naringin and obacunone have been reported to have inhibitory effects on liver enzymes (6).

A commercial citrus seed extract used at a concentration of 0.5% has been reported to inhibit the in vitro growth of some bacteria, yeasts and molds (Streptococcus species, Staph. aureus, enterococci, Enterobacter, E. coli, Candida, Geotrichum, Aspergillus and Penicillium species) (5866). Grapefruit seed extracts have been reported to reduce counts of Salmonella Typhimurium when sprayed on chicken skins (5862), but to have no effect in controlling fungal growth on unshelled peanuts (5864,5865).

When examined by HPLC, a commercial grapefruit seed extract was found to contain significant amounts of the preservatives methyl-p-hydroxybenzoate and triclosan, which were not present in an ethanol extract of grapefruit seeds (5863). In another study, five of six commercial grapefruit seed extracts tested contained significant amounts of the preservative benzethonium chloride, and three of these also contained triclosan and methyl-p-hydroxybenzoate. These five extracts had significant antibacterial activity, as measured by in vitro tests, but a sixth commercial extract which was preservative-free had no in vitro antibacterial activity (5867). It has therefore been hypothesized that the reported antimicrobial activity of grapefruit seed extract products is due to the preservative content (5867).

Adverse Reactions

When used in the eyes, severe irritation may occur, and irritation of other mucous membranes may also occur (5858,5861). When preservative-containing products are used vomiting, collapse, convulsions and coma can occur (3082).

Interactions with Herbs & Other Dietary Supplements

RED YEAST (Cholestin): Theoretically, concomitant use of grapefruit seed extract with red yeast can increase the serum levels of lovastatin, a constituent of red yeast (527). Grapefruit seed extract products can contain grapefruit pulp and the naringin constituent, which can inhibit cytochrome P450 metabolism of lovastatin (6,5858).

Interactions with Drugs

ARTEMETHER (Artenam, Paluther): Theoretically, grapefruit seed extract can increase the oral bioavailability of artemether (5065,5066). Grapefruit seed extract contains grapefruit pulp and the constituent naringin, which can inhibit cytochrome P450 metabolism of this and other drugs (6,5858).

BENZODIAZEPINES: Theoretically, grapefruit seed extract might increase blood levels of some benzodiazepines, such as diazepam (Valium), midazolam (Versed), and triazolam (Halcion) (3228,4300). Grapefruit seed extract contains grapefruit pulp and the constituent naringin, which can inhibit cytochrome P450 metabolism of these and other drugs (6,5858).

BUSPIRONE (Buspar): Theoretically, grapefruit seed extract can plasma concentrations of buspirone (3771). Grapefruit seed extract contains grapefruit pulp and the constituent naringin, which can inhibit cytochrome P450 metabolism of this and other drugs (6,5858).

CAFFEINE: Theoretically, grapefruit seed extract can increase caffeine levels and adverse effects (4300). Grapefruit seed extract contains grapefruit pulp and the constituent naringin, which can inhibit cytochrome P450 metabolism of this and other drugs (6,5858).

CALCIUM CHANNEL BLOCKERS: Theoretically, grapefruit seed extract can increase plasma concentrations of amlodipine (Norvasc) (523), nifedipine (Procardia, Adalat) (528), nisoldipine (Sular) (529), felodipine (Plendil), nimodipine (Nimotop), nicardipine (Cardene), diltiazem (Cardizem) (524,528,1388,4300), and verapamil (Calan, Isoptin, Verelan) (3229). Grapefruit seed extract contains grapefruit pulp and the constituent naringin, which can inhibit cytochrome P450 metabolism of these and other drugs (6,5858).

CARBAMAZEPINE (Tegretol): Theoretically, grapefruit seed extract can increase plasma concentrations of carbamazepine (524). Grapefruit seed extract contains grapefruit pulp and the constituent naringin, which can inhibit cytochrome P450 metabolism of this and other drugs (6,5858).

CARVEDILOL (Coreg): Theoretically, grapefruit seed extract might increase plasma concentration of carvedilol (5071). Grapefruit seed extract contains grapefruit pulp and the constituent naringin, which can inhibit cytochrome P450 metabolism of this and other drugs (6,5858).

CISAPRIDE (Propulsid): Theoretically, grapefruit seed extract can increase plasma concentrations of cisapride (1383,3226). Grapefruit seed extract contains grapefruit pulp and the constituent naringin, which can inhibit cytochrome P450 metabolism of this and other drugs (6,5858).

CLOMIPRAMINE (Anafranil): Theoretically, grapefruit seed extract can increase blood levels of clomipramine (5064). Grapefruit seed extract contains grapefruit pulp and the constituent naringin, which can inhibit cytochrome P450 metabolism of this and other drugs (6,5858).

CYCLOSPORINE (Neoral, Sandimmune): Theoretically, grapefruit seed extract can increase plasma concentrations of cyclosporine (522). Grapefruit seed extract contains grapefruit pulp and the constituent naringin, which can inhibit cytochrome P450 metabolism of this and other drugs (6,5858).

ESTROGENS: Theoretically, grapefruit seed extract can increase plasma concentrations of 17-beta-estradiol (526) and ethinyl-estradiol (525). Grapefruit seed extract contains grapefruit pulp and the constituent naringin, which can inhibit cytochrome P450 metabolism of this and other drugs (6,5858).

HMG-CoA REDUCTASE INHIBITORS: Theoretically, grapefruit seed extract can increase plasma concentrations of lovastatin (Mevacor) (527), simvastatin (Zocor) (3774), and atorvastatin (Lipitor) (3227). Grapefruit seed extract contains grapefruit pulp and the constituent naringin, which can inhibit cytochrome P450 metabolism of these and other drugs (6,5858).

QUINIDINE: Theoretically, grapefruit seed extract can increase plasma levels (5067). Grapefruit seed extract contains grapefruit pulp and the constituent naringin, which can inhibit cytochrome P450 metabolism of this and other drugs (6,5858).

SAQUINAVIR (Fortovase, Invirase): Grapefruit juice increases absorption and plasma concentrations of the protease inhibitor (PI)-type antiretroviral drug saquinavir (3773).

TERFENADINE (Seldane): Theoretically, grapefruit seed extract can increase plasma concentrations of terfenadine (530). Grapefruit seed extract contains grapefruit pulp and the constituent naringin, which can inhibit cytochrome P450 metabolism of this and other drugs (6,5858).

WARFARIN (Coumadin): Theoretically, grapefruit seed extract might increase warfarin effects. Grapefruit seed extract contains grapefruit pulp and the constituent naringin, which can inhibit cytochrome P450 metabolism of this and other drugs (6,5858).

Interactions with Foods
No interactions are known to occur, and there is no known reason to expect a clinically significant interaction with grapefruit seed extract.

Interactions with Lab Tests
No interactions are known to occur, and there is no known reason to expect a clinically significant interaction with grapefruit seed extract.

Interactions with Diseases or Conditions
No interactions are known to occur, and there is no known reason to expect a clinically significant interaction with grapefruit seed extract.

Dosage and Administration

No typical dosage.

Comments

Grapefruit seed extract is processed from grapefruit seeds and pulp obtained as a byproduct from grapefruit juice production. Processing involves the use of ammonium chloride, ascorbic acid, hydrochloric acid, enzymes, and heat processes. Vegetable glycerin is added to the final product to reduce acidity and bitterness (5858).

GRAVEL ROOT

Also Known As

Joe Pye, Joe-Pye Weed, Kidney Root, Kydney Root, Purple Boneset, Queen of the Meadow, Roter Wasserhanf, Trumpet Weed.
CAUTION: See separate listing for Boneset.

Scientific Names

Eupatorium purpureum.
Family: Asteraceae or Compositae.

People Use This For

Orally, gravel root is used for urinary calculus, renal or vesicular calculi, cystitis, painful urination, urethritis, prostatitis, rheumatism, and gout (4). It is also used orally for fever from malaria, dengue virus, fever, typhus, as an antacid, aperitif, diuretic, emetic, stimulant, tonic, and for inducing sweating.

Safety

UNSAFE ...when used orally. Gravel root contains hepatotoxic unsaturated pyrrolizidine alkaloids (UPAs) (12,19). Repeated exposure to low concentrations of UPAs is linked to veno-occlusive disease, a serious condition (4,12). UPAs may also be carcinogenic and mutagenic (12). Topical use on abraded or broken skin might be unsafe due to potential for systemic absorption (12,19).
PREGNANCY: UNSAFE ...when used orally (12,19). Animal data suggests gravel root might be an abortifacient (19).
LACTATION: UNSAFE ...when used orally due to concern that UPAs might be excreted into breast milk (4,12,18,19).

Effectiveness

There is insufficient reliable information available about the effectiveness of gravel root.

Mechanism of Action

The applicable parts of gravel root are the above ground parts and rhizome/root. Although people think gravel root has antilithic, diuretic, and antirheumatic properties (4), this has not been studied. Some evidence suggests an ethanolic extract might have anti-inflammatory activity (4020). The above ground parts of gravel root contain echinatine, an unsaturated pyrrolizidine alkaloid (UPA) (4). Pyrrolizidine alkaloids with an unsaturated pyrrolizidine nucleus can be hepatotoxic in animals and humans (4). Herbs containing UPAs have shown carcinogenic, mutagenic, and renal toxic effects. However, the primary concern is veno-occlusive disease (12).

Adverse Reactions

Although no adverse effects are reported for gravel root/rhizome, chronic exposure to other plants containing UPA constituents has been associated with veno-occlusive disease (4021). Symptoms of acute veno-occlusive disease are characterized by a dull, dragging ache in the right upper abdomen and marked distention of the abdomen. These symptoms are sometimes accompanied by reduced urine output. Subacute veno-occlusive disease is associated with vague symptoms and persistent liver enlargement (4021). Gravel root can cause an allergic reaction in individuals sensitive to the Asteraceae/Compositae family. Members of this family include ragweed, chrysanthemums, marigolds, daisies, and many other herbs.

Interactions with Herbs & Other Dietary Supplements

EUCALYPTUS: Theoretically, concomitant use might increase the risk of unsaturated pyrrolizidine alkaloid toxicity due to enzyme induction by eucalyptus (19).
PYRROLIZIDINE ALKALOID-CONTAINING HERBS: Concomitant use is contraindicated due to the risk of additive toxicity. Herbs containing unsaturated pyrrolizidine alkaloids include: alkanna (12), borage (271), gravel root (4), hemp agrimony (271), hound's tongue (19), petasites (19), comfrey (271), coltsfoot, and the Senecio species plants; dusty miller (19), alpine ragwort (19), groundsel (271), golden ragwort (19), and tansy ragwort (271).

Interactions with Drugs
No interactions are known to occur, and there is no known reason to expect a clinically significant interaction with gravel root.

Interactions with Foods
No interactions are known to occur, and there is no known reason to expect a clinically significant interaction with gravel root.

Interactions with Lab Tests
No interactions are known to occur, and there is no known reason to expect a clinically significant interaction with gravel root.

Interactions with Diseases or Conditions
LIVER DISEASE: Contraindicated due to hepatotoxic potential (19).
CROSS-ALLERGENICITY: Can cause an allergic reaction in individuals sensitive to the Asteraceae/Compositae family. Members of this family include ragweed, chrysanthemums, marigolds, daisies, and many other herbs.

Dosage and Administration
No typical dosage.

Comments
None.

GREAT PLANTAIN

Also Known As
Common Plantain, General Plantain, Greater Plantain.
CAUTION: See separate listings for Buckhorn Plantain, Blond Psyllium, Black Psyllium, and Water Plantain.

Scientific Names
Plantago major.
Family: Plantaginaceae.

People Use This For
Historically, great plantain has been used for cystitis with hematuria, bronchitis, colds, irritated or bleeding hemorrhoids (4), dermatological conditions, and eye irritation or discomfort (514).

Safety
POSSIBLY SAFE ...when the leaf is used orally and appropriately (12).
POSSIBLY UNSAFE ...when used topically. Great plantain can cause allergic contact dermatitis (4).
PREGNANCY: LIKELY UNSAFE ...when used orally because it can increase uterine tone (4).
LACTATION: Insufficient reliable information available; avoid using.

Effectiveness
POSSIBLY EFFECTIVE ...when used orally for treating spastic and nonspastic chronic bronchitis, and for treating symptoms of the common cold (4).
There is insufficient reliable information available about the effectiveness of great plantain for its other uses.

Mechanism of Action
The applicable part of great plantain is the leaf. Great plantain contains low levels of tannins (4), and relatively high concentrations of vitamin K, beta-carotene, and calcium (19). It also contains a variety of acids, amino acids, carbohydrates, and iridoids (4). The anti-inflammatory and wound-healing effects demonstrated in animal studies are attributed to the constituents chlorogenic acid and neochlorogenic acid (4). Studies in humans show great plantain is beneficial in treating chronic bronchitis and the common cold (4). In guinea pigs, an aqueous extract had bronchodilator effects; however, effects were less and had shorter duration than salbutamol or atropine (4). In animals, great plantain extract also lowers blood pressure, and decreases total plasma lipids, cholesterol, and triglycerides (4). In vitro, an aqueous extract increases animal uterine tissue tone (4), and fresh juice has antibacterial activity (4). Great plantain inhibits carcinogenesis and mammary tumor formation in experimental animals (6).

Adverse Reactions

Orally, excessive amounts taken orally may have laxative and hypotensive effects (4).
Topically, application can cause allergic contact dermatitis (4).

Interactions with Herbs & Other Dietary Supplements

HERBS WITH CLOTTING POTENTIAL: Excessive use of herbs that contain vitamin K, an essential coagulation factor, can increase the risk of clotting in people using anticoagulants. These herbs include: alfalfa, parsley, nettle, plantain, and others.

Interactions with Drugs

WARFARIN (Coumadin): Theoretically, consumption of large amounts of great plantain may antagonize drug effects due to vitamin K content. Individuals using anticoagulants should consume a consistent daily amount to maintain effect of anticoagulation therapy (19).

Interactions with Foods

No interactions are known to occur, and there is no known reason to expect a clinically significant interaction with great plantain.

Interactions with Lab Tests

BLOOD CLOTTING TESTS: Theoretically, consumption of large amounts of great plantain may reduce clotting time and test results due to vitamin K content (19).

Interactions with Diseases or Conditions

PLANTAIN HYPERSENSITIVITY: Contraindicated.
MELON ALLERGY: Plantago species pollen may cause cross-reactivity in people allergic to melon (4075).

Dosage and Administration

ORAL: People typically used 2-4 grams dried leaf three times daily, or one cup tea (steep 2-4 grams dried leaf in 150 mL boiling water 5-10 minutes, strain) three times daily (4). Liquid extract (1:1 in 25% in ethanol) 2-4 mL three times daily. Tincture (1:5 in 45% in ethanol) 2-4 mL three times daily (4).

Comments

Avoid confusion with Buckhorn plantain (Plantago lanceolata), Blond psyllium (Plantago ovata), and Black psyllium (Plantago psyllium).

GREATER BINDWEED

Also Known As

Bearbind, Bear's-Bind, Devil's Vine, Hedge Bindweed, Hedge Convolvulus, Hedge Lily, Lady's Nightcap, Old Man's Night Cap, Rutland Beauty.

Scientific Names

Calystegia sepium.
Family: Convolvulaceae.

People Use This For

Orally, greater bindweed is used for fever, urinary tract diseases, as a purgative for constipation, and for increasing bile production (18).

Safety

POSSIBLY UNSAFE ...when the whole plant is used orally because it has strong contact cathartic effects (514).
PREGNANCY AND LACTATION: POSSIBLY UNSAFE ...when used orally; avoid using.

Effectiveness

There is insufficient reliable information available about the effectiveness of greater bindweed.

Mechanism of Action

Greater bindweed is said to be a potent smooth muscle stimulant and to increase bile production (18). Constituent gluco-resins (glycoretins) are contact cathartics which cause an increase in water elimination and peristalsis (514).

Adverse Reactions

Theoretically, large amounts may cause intestinal and stomach pain (18).

Interactions with Herbs & Other Dietary Supplements

STIMULANT LAXATIVE HERBS: Theoretically, concomitant use with other stimulant laxative herbs may increase the risk of potassium depletion. Stimulant laxative herbs include: aloe dried leaf sap, blue flag rhizome, alder buckthorn, European buckthorn, butternut bark, cascara bark, castor oil, colocynth fruit pulp, gamboge bark exudate, jalap root, black root, manna bark exudate, podophyllum root, rhubarb root, senna leaves and pods, wild cucumber fruit (Ecballium elaterium), and yellow dock root (19).

CARDIAC GLYCOSIDE-CONTAINING HERBS: Concomitant use may increase the risk of cardiac glycoside toxicity. Cardiac glycoside-containing herbs include: black hellebore, Canadian hemp roots, digitalis leaf, hedge mustard, figwort, lily-of-the-valley roots, motherwort, oleander leaf, pheasant's eye plant, pleurisy root, squill bulb leaf scales, and strophanthus seeds (2,18,19,500).

LICORICE/HORSETAIL: Theoretically, overuse/misuse of licorice rhizome or horsetail plant with cardiac glycoside-containing herbs increases the risk of cardiac toxicity due to potassium depletion. (19).

Interactions with Drugs

CARDIAC GLYCOSIDE DRUGS: Theoretically, overuse/abuse of this product increases the risk of adverse effects of cardiac glycoside drugs, e.g., digoxin (Lanoxin).

Interactions with Foods

No interactions are known to occur, and there is no known reason to expect a clinically significant interaction with greater bindweed.

Interactions with Lab Tests

No interactions are known to occur, and there is no known reason to expect a clinically significant interaction with greater bindweed.

Interactions with Diseases or Conditions

GI CONDITIONS: Contraindicated in individuals with intestinal obstruction, abdominal pain of unknown origin, or any inflammatory condition of intestines including appendicitis, colitis, Crohn's disease, irritable bowel syndrome (IBS), and others (12).

Dosage and Administration

ORAL: People typically use one level teaspoon of the powdered root once or twice daily. A liquid is prepared by boiling 1 teaspoon of the flowering plant in 1 cup of water. This is taken 1 tablespoon at a time, as needed.

Comments

None.

GREATER BURNET

Also Known As

Garden Burnet, Sanguisorba.

Scientific Names

Sanguisorba officinalis.
Family: Rosaceae.

People Use This For

Orally, greater burnet is used for heavy menstrual flow during menopause, hot flashes, irregular menstrual flow, ulcerative colitis, diarrhea, dysentery, enteritis, bladder restraint, hemorrhoids, phlebitis, and varicose veins (4,18). Topically, greater burnet is used in a plaster for wounds and boils (18).

Safety

There is insufficient reliable information available about the safety of greater burnet.
Pregnancy and Lactation: Insufficient reliable information available; avoid using.

Effectiveness

There is insufficient reliable information available about the effectiveness of greater burnet.

Mechanism of Action
The applicable parts of greater burnet are the flowering above ground parts. Greater burnet appears to have antihemorrhagic, antihemorrhoidal, astringent, and styptic properties (4).

Adverse Reactions
None reported.

Interactions with Herbs & Other Dietary Supplements
Insufficient reliable information available.

Interactions with Drugs
No interactions are known to occur, and there is no known reason to expect a clinically significant interaction with greater burnet.

Interactions with Foods
No interactions are known to occur, and there is no known reason to expect a clinically significant interaction with greater burnet.

Interactions with Lab Tests
No interactions are known to occur, and there is no known reason to expect a clinically significant interaction with greater burnet.

Interactions with Diseases or Conditions
No interactions are known to occur, and there is no known reason to expect a clinically significant interaction with greater burnet.

Dosage and Administration
ORAL: People typically use 2-6 grams dried above ground parts three times daily (4), or one cup tea (steep 2-6 grams herb in 150 mL boiling water 5-10 minutes, strain) three times daily (4). Liquid extract (1:1 in 25% alcohol) 2-6 mL three times daily (4). Tincture (1:5 in 45% alcohol) 2-8 mL three times daily (4).
TOPICAL: Used as plasters, no additional dosing or administration available (18).

Comments
None.

GREATER CELANDINE dried above ground parts

Also Known As
Bai Qu Cai, Celandine, Celandine Herb, Chelidonii, Chelidonii Herba, Schollkraut, Tetterwort.
CAUTION: See separate listings for Greater Celandine root, Jewelweed, and Lesser Celandine.

Scientific Names
Chelidonium majus.
Family: Papaveraceae.

People Use This For
Orally, greater celandine dried above ground parts are used for spastic discomfort of bile ducts and the gastrointestinal tract (2).
Topically, they are used for warts, blister rashes, scabies, tooth pain, and to ease tooth extraction (8,18).
In Chinese medicine, greater celandine dried above ground parts are used as an analgesic, antitussive, anti-inflammatory, and detoxicant (8).
In folk medicine, they are used orally for liver and gallbladder complaints, loss of appetite, gastroenteritis, stomach cancer, cramps, intestinal polyps, breast lumps, angina, edema, arteriosclerosis, hypertension, asthma, gout, and arthritis (8).

Safety
POSSIBLY UNSAFE ...when used orally. The above ground parts of greater celandine are considered safe when used orally and appropriately (2,7,12); however, they have been strongly implicated in at least ten cases of hepatitis involving five different brand products manufactured in Germany (363). Until more is known, avoid using products containing greater celandine dried above ground parts.

There is insufficient reliable information available about the safety of the topical use of greater celandine dried above ground parts.

CHILDREN: UNSAFE ...when used orally (12); avoid using.

PREGNANCY: UNSAFE ...when used orally because the berberine content might stimulate uterine contractions (12).

LACTATION: Insufficient reliable information available; avoid using.

Effectiveness

POSSIBLY EFFECTIVE ...when used orally for spastic discomfort of the bile ducts and gastrointestinal tract (2). There is insufficient reliable information available about the effectiveness of greater celandine dried above ground parts for its other uses.

Mechanism of Action

Greater celandine dried above ground parts contain 0.1-1% isoquinoline alkaloids (7,12), including chelidonine, which reportedly acts as an antispasmodic and weak central analgesic (7,8). This product is thought to have a papaverine-like effect on the upper gastrointestinal tract (2). In animal studies, an alcoholic extract increased bile flow (7), caused non-specific immune stimulation (2), and acted as a hepatoprotectant (8). The above ground parts of greater celandine also contain small amounts of berberine, which is a uterine stimulant and in large amounts can depress cardiac function (12).

Adverse Reactions

Orally, greater celandine dried above ground parts have been strongly implicated in at least ten cases of hepatitis (363). Large amounts can cause stomach pain, intestinal colic, urinary urgency, and hematuria accompanied by dizziness and stupor (7).

Interactions with Herbs & Other Dietary Supplements

Insufficient reliable information available.

Interactions with Drugs

DRUGS FOR GLAUCOMA: Use of greater celandine dried above ground parts may affect treatment (12).

Interactions with Foods

No interactions are known to occur, and there is no known reason to expect a clinically significant interaction with greater celandine dried above ground parts.

Interactions with Lab Tests

LIVER FUNCTION TESTS: Greater celandine-induced hepatitis can increase liver enzyme serum levels and results of liver function tests (363).

Interactions with Diseases or Conditions

BILE TRACT OBSTRUCTION: Use of greater celandine dried above ground parts may exacerbate condition (2).

GLAUCOMA: Use of greater celandine dried above ground parts may affect treatment (12).

HEPATITIS/LIVER DISEASE: Greater celandine taken orally has been strongly implicated in causing hepatitis (363); avoid using in people with liver disease.

Dosage and Administration

ORAL: Dried herb or herb powder 2-5 grams per day (equivalent to 12-30 mg total alkaloids calculated as chelidonine) has been used (2). Fluid extract: 1-2 mL three times daily has also been used (18). Do not use in children. Greater celandine tea preparations are difficult to dose properly and are not recommended (7).

TOPICAL: No typical dosage.

Comments

Recently, greater celandine dried above ground parts have been strongly implicated in at least ten cases of hepatitis involving five different brand products manufactured in Germany (363). Until more is known, avoid using products containing greater celandine dried above ground parts. Avoid confusion with greater celandine rhizome, root and lesser celandine (Family: Ranunculus ficaria).

GREATER CELANDINE rhizome, root

Also Known As

Celandine Root.

CAUTION: See separate listings for Greater Celandine dried above ground parts, Jewelweed, and Lesser Celandine.

Scientific Names

Chelidonium majus.
Family: Papaveraceae.

People Use This For

In Chinese medicine, greater celandine is used orally for irregular menses (18). The powdered root is applied topically to ease tooth extraction, and the fresh root is chewed to relieve toothache (18).

Safety

There is insufficient reliable information available about the safety of greater celandine rhizome, root.
Pregnancy and Lactation: Insufficient reliable information available; avoid using.

Effectiveness

There is insufficient reliable information available about the effectiveness of greater celandine rhizome, root.

Mechanism of Action

There is insufficient reliable information available about the possible mechanism of action and active ingredients.

Adverse Reactions

Orally, greater celandine rhizome/root can cause burning in the mouth, nausea, vomiting, bloody diarrhea, hematuria, and stupor (18).

Interactions with Herbs & Other Dietary Supplements

Insufficient reliable information available.

Interactions with Drugs

No interactions are known to occur, and there is no known reason to expect a clinically significant interaction with greater celandine rhizome/root.

Interactions with Foods

No interactions are known to occur, and there is no known reason to expect a clinically significant interaction with greater celandine rhizome/root.

Interactions with Lab Tests

No interactions are known to occur, and there is no known reason to expect a clinically significant interaction with greater celandine rhizome/root.

Interactions with Diseases or Conditions

No interactions are known to occur, and there is no known reason to expect a clinically significant interaction with greater celandine rhizome/root.

Dosage and Administration

ORAL: Standard dose is 500 mg (18). Store carefully (18).

Comments

There is very little scientific information about this product. Our staff is continually analyzing the available information on natural medicines and will add data here as it becomes available.

GREEK SAGE

Also Known As

None.

Scientific Names

Salvia triloba.
Family: Labiatae or Lamiaceae.

People Use This For

Orally, Greek sage is used for inflammation of the mouth and throat (8).

Safety

There is insufficient reliable information available about the safety of Greek sage.

Pregnancy and Lactation: Insufficient reliable information available; avoid using.

Effectiveness

There is insufficient reliable information available about the effectiveness of Greek sage.

Mechanism of Action

Greek sage contains 2-3% volatile oil. Of the volatile oil, 60% is cineole, 5% is thujone (8). Greek sage can inhibit smooth-muscle contractions induced by acetylcholine, histamine, serotonin and BaCl2 (4152). Constituents of the leaf can prolong hexobarbital sleep (4152). Some evidence suggests an aqueous extract of Greek sage might have a blood pressure-lowering effect (4152).

Adverse Reactions

None reported.

Interactions with Herbs & Other Dietary Supplements

Insufficient reliable information available.

Interactions with Drugs

HEXOBARBITAL: Greek sage can prolong the effects of hexobarbital (4152).

Interactions with Foods

No interactions are known to occur, and there is no known reason to expect a clinically significant interaction with Greek sage.

Interactions with Lab Tests

No interactions are known to occur, and there is no known reason to expect a clinically significant interaction with Greek sage.

Interactions with Diseases or Conditions

No interactions are known to occur, and there is no known reason to expect a clinically significant interaction with Greek sage.

Dosage and Administration

ORAL: Greek sage is used as a tea. The tea is prepared by pouring boiling water over 3 grams of finely chopped leaf. After 10 minutes, strain (8).

Comments

Greek sage is very rare but sometimes it is found as an adulterant of Salvia officinalis (4,5).

GREEN TEA

Also Known As

Chinese Tea, Tea, TeaGreen, Tea Green.

CAUTION: See separate listings for Black Tea and Caffeine.

Scientific Names

Camellia sinensis, synonyms Camellia thea, Camellia theifera, Thea sinensis, Thea bohea, Thea viridis.

Family: Theaceae.

People Use This For

Orally, green tea is used to improve cognitive performance (4221), treat stomach disorders, vomiting, diarrhea, and headaches. It is used as a diuretic and in combination products for weight loss (6,18). Green tea is also used to maintain remission in people with Crohn's disease (4209); to reduce the risk of prostate cancer (4210), colon cancer (4211), and gastric cancer (7033); to prevent Parkinson's disease (6022); and to protect against heart disease (4219), dental caries (4214), and kidney stones (4216). Green tea is also used to prevent skin damage and cancer related to ultraviolet (UV) radiation (e.g., sunburn) and other environmental causes (6065).

Topically, green tea bags are used as a wash to soothe sunburn, as a poultice for bags under the eyes, as a compress for headache or tired eyes, and to stop the bleeding of tooth sockets (11). Green tea is also used topically to prevent skin damage and cancer related to ultraviolet (UV) radiation (e.g., sunburn) and other environmental causes (6065). For food use, green tea is consumed as a beverage (11).

Safety

LIKELY SAFE ...when used orally in moderate amounts (18,733,6031). Green tea is often consumed daily in Asian cultures and has not been associated with significant adverse effects (6031).

POSSIBLY UNSAFE ...when used orally in large amounts. Green tea contains a significant amount of caffeine. Consumption of more than 300 mg caffeine, which is equivalent to approximately 5 cups of green tea, per day has been associated with significant adverse effects (see Adverse Reactions) (18). These effects would not be expected to occur with the consumption of decaffeinated green tea.

CHILDREN: LIKELY UNSAFE ...when taken orally by infants because it has been associated with impaired iron metabolism and microcytic anemia (6). This might be caused by tannins in green tea which bind and prevent iron absorption in the gastrointestinal tract (19). Children are also more susceptible to the adverse effects of caffeine present in green tea (15).

PREGNANCY: POSSIBLY SAFE ...when used in moderate amounts. Due to the caffeine content of green tea, mothers should closely monitor their intake to ensure moderate consumption. Fetal blood concentrations of caffeine approximate maternal concentrations (4260). Caffeine use in pregnancy is controversial; however, moderate consumption has not been associated with adverse fetal effects (6). Some sources suggest keeping caffeine consumption below 200 mg per day (2078). Green tea provides approximately 10-80 mg caffeine per cup (18,4218). POSSIBLY UNSAFE ...when used orally in large amounts. Caffeine found in green tea crosses the placenta, producing fetal blood concentrations similar to maternal levels (4260). Although controversial, some evidence suggests that high doses of caffeine might be associated with premature delivery, low birth weight, and loss of the fetus (6). Some sources suggest keeping caffeine consumption below 200 mg per day (2078). Green tea provides approximately 10-80 mg caffeine per cup (18,4218). Excessive use of green tea in pregnancy should be avoided.

LACTATION: POSSIBLY SAFE ...when used in moderate amounts. Due to the caffeine content of green tea, mothers should closely monitor their intake to ensure moderate consumption. Breast milk concentrations of caffeine are thought to be approximately 50% of maternal serum concentrations. Moderate consumption of green tea would likely result in very small amounts of caffeine exposure to a nursing infant (6). POSSIBLY UNSAFE ...when used orally in large amounts. Consumption of green tea might cause irritability and increased bowel activity in nursing infants (6026). Large doses or excessive intake of green tea should be avoided during lactation.

Effectiveness

POSSIBLY EFFECTIVE ...when used orally for improving cognitive performance (4221). ...when used orally to lower cholesterol and triglycerides. There is some epidemiological evidence that higher consumption of green tea is associated with significantly lowered serum total cholesterol, triglycerides, low-density lipoprotein (LDL), and increased high-density lipoprotein (HDL) levels (6403). ...when used orally for treatment of oral leukoplakia (4213). ...when used orally for prevention of bladder, esophageal, and pancreatic cancers. There is some evidence that people who consume green tea might have a lower risk of developing certain specific cancers (4218), including bladder (1457,1458,1459), esophageal, and pancreatic (733,6031). ...when used orally for treating diarrhea (7,18). ...when used orally for preventing or delaying onset of Parkinson's disease. There is some evidence from large-scale epidemiological studies that people who consume caffeinated beverages such as coffee, tea, and cola have a decreased risk of Parkinson's disease. For men, the effects seem to be dose related. For example, men consuming a total of 421-2716 mg of caffeine (approximately 5-33 cups of tea) from any source daily, seem to have the greatest reduction in risk. However, there seems to be a significant reduction in risk even with consumption of as little as 124-208 mg caffeine per day (approximately 1-3 cups tea) (6022). In women, the effects do not seem to be dose related. Moderate consumption of approximately 1-4 cups daily, seems to provide the most reduction in risk (1238).

POSSIBLY INEFFECTIVE ...when used orally for preventing gastric cancer. Consumption of green tea up to 5 or more cups per day does not seem to reduce the risk of developing gastric (stomach) cancer compared to people who drink less than one cup per day (7033).

There is insufficient reliable information available about green tea for its other uses.

Mechanism of Action

The applicable parts of green tea are the leaf, leaf bud, and stem. Green tea is different than black and oolong teas because it is not fermented. Green tea is produced by steaming fresh leaves at high temperatures. This process inactivates certain oxidizing enzymes, but does not adversely affect polyphenols (7034). Polyphenols such as gallic acid and catechins are abundant in green tea, and are thought to be responsible for many of its proposed benefits (6031). One cup of brewed green tea contains up to 200 mg of the catechin, epigallocatechin-3-gallate (EGCG) (6886). Green tea typically contains 2-4% caffeine or 10-80 mg per cup (512,519,4218). The caffeine in green tea acts as a central nervous system (CNS) stimulant (6031); increases blood pressure (1452,6663), heart rate, and contractility; inhibits platelet aggregation (733); stimulates gastric acid secretion; causes diuresis; relaxes extracerebral vascular and bronchial smooth muscle; stimulates the release of catecholamines; and might indirectly inhibit histamine release (6130). Caffeine content is thought to be responsible for green tea's use for improving cognitive performance (4221). Antioxidant catechins in green tea are thought to possibly have a protective effect against atherosclerosis and heart disease (1453,1463). They may lower total and low-density lipoprotein (LDL) cholesterol, and increase high-density lipoprotein (HDL) cholesterol (6882). Some preliminary studies show that flavonoids found in green tea might also reduce lipoprotein oxidation (6032,6033); however, benefits have not yet been described in humans. It is unclear exactly how green tea might reduce the risk of some cancers, but preliminary research suggests that green tea catechins, particularly EGCG, might prevent new blood vessel growth in tumors (1454,1455,1456). EGCG might also inhibit specific phases of cell division in breast epithelial cells stimulated by epidermal growth factor (6880), to inhibit cellular signal transduction pathways in cancer cells, and to induce apoptosis (programmed cell death) in various types of cancer cells in vitro (6886). Another catechin, epigallocatechin (ECC), might prevent radiation-induced increases of liver lipid peroxide. Green tea may also reduce oxidative DNA damage, lipid peroxidation, and free radical generation (4212); and might reduce mutagenic activity in smokers (4217). There is also evidence from in vitro studies that green tea polyphenols can inhibit the excessive release of nitric oxide from cells which has been implicated in tissue damage and inflammation (6881). Green tea is thought to be beneficial for preventing skin damage and cancer from ultraviolet (UV) radiation due to the antioxidant effects of polyphenols in green tea. It can reduce oxidative skin damage, skin inflammation, and epidermal hyperplasia due to UV radiation and other causes in animal models. Green tea might also prevent UV radiation induced immunosuppression and protect against development of skin tumors (6065). Green tea has also been used for weight loss. Early evidence indicates that a green tea extract rich in ECG can increase calorie and fat metabolism. Caffeine might also contribute to these effects (1453). In animals, EGCG causes a reduction in food intake and short-term weight loss, but tolerance develops to these effects (6882). In vitro studies show that EGCG inhibits fat cell functions and may affect cell proliferation and differentiation in fat tissues (6882). The impact of ECG and green tea on weight loss in obese humans remains to be determined. For diarrhea, tannins in green tea can produce antidiarrheal effects (7). For prevention of Parkinson's disease, caffeine in green tea may prevent adenosine's inhibition of dopaminergic transmission. This may result in a reduction in the clinical expression of Parkinsonism (6022).

Adverse Reactions

Orally, green tea can cause gastrointestinal upset and constipation (7,12). There is one report of liver dysfunction with the excessive use of green tea (65 grams of tea leaves daily for five years) (7). High doses of the caffeine constituent of green tea can cause headache, diuresis, anxiety, nervousness, insomnia, restlessness, agitation, tremor, irritability, tachyarrhythmias, palpitations, premature heartbeat, quickened respiration, heartburn, loss of appetite, nausea, vomiting, diarrhea, dizziness, ringing in the ears, elevated blood sugar, elevated cholesterol, hepatotoxicity, delirium, and convulsions (6,7,15,18,505). Although acute administration of green tea can cause increased blood pressure, regular consumption does not seem to increase either blood pressure or pulse when consumed on a regular basis, even in mildly hypertensive patients (1451,1452). The chronic use of caffeine, especially in large amounts, can sometimes produce tolerance, habituation, and psychological dependence (15). The abrupt discontinuation of caffeine can result in physical withdrawal symptoms, including headaches, irritation, nervousness, anxiety, and dizziness (15). Some evidence shows caffeine is associated with fibrocystic breast disease in women; however, this is controversial and has been disputed (14,15). The adverse effects of caffeine from green tea can be more severe in children than adults (15). In infants, green tea ingestion has been associated with impaired iron metabolism and microcytic anemia (6).

Interactions with Herbs & Other Dietary Supplements

CAFFEINE-CONTAINING HERBS/SUPPLEMENTS: Concomitant use interacts with the caffeine in green tea and can increase the effects and risk of adverse effects. Natural products that contain caffeine include coffee, black tea, guarana, mate, and cola.

EPHEDRA (ma huang): Concomitant use interacts with the caffeine in green tea and can potentiate the stimulant effects and risk of adverse effects (6).

IRON: The concomitant use of iron and green tea can impair iron metabolism in infants and children, resulting in a high incidence of microcytic anemia (6). However, a study in the elderly suggests concomitant use does not affect iron absorption (185).

Interactions with Drugs

ADENOSINE (Adenocard): Theoretically, concomitant use might inhibit the hemodynamic effects of adenosine (19).

ANTICOAGULANT, ANTIPLATELET AGENTS: Theoretically, green tea might increase the risk of bleeding when used concomitantly with these agents. Green tea is reported to have antiplatelet activity (733); however, this interaction has not been reported in humans. Antiplatelet agents include aspirin, clopidogrel (Plavix), dipyridamole (Persantine), ticlopidine (Ticlid), and others.

ASPIRIN, ACETAMINOPHEN (Tylenol): Concomitant administration can increase the effectiveness of these drugs by as much as 40%, due to the caffeine in green tea (3).

ANTIPSYCHOTIC DRUGS: Theoretically, green tea might cause precipitation of fluphenazine (Permitil, Prolixin), chlorpromazine (Thorazine), haloperidol (Haldol), prochlorperazine (Compazine), thioridazine (Mellaril), and trifluoperazine (Stelazine) (626,627).

BARBITURATES: Concomitant administration can decrease the effects of the caffeine in green tea (151).

BETA-ADRENERGIC AGONISTS: Concomitant use can increase the cardiac inotropic effect of beta-adrenergic agonist drugs due to the caffeine in green tea (15). Beta-adrenergic agonists include albuterol (Proventil, Ventolin), metaproterenol (Alupent), terbutaline (Brethine), and isoproterenol (Isuprel).

BENZODIAZEPINES: Concomitant use might reduce the sedative effects of benzodiazepines due to the caffeine in green tea (19).

CHLORPROMAZINE (Thorazine): Theoretically, concomitant use might inhibit the cataleptic effects of chlorpromazine due to precipitation with compounds in green tea (19).

CIMETIDINE (Tagamet): Concomitant use might increase the effects and adverse effects of caffeine in green tea. Cimetidine can reduce caffeine clearance by 30-50% (14).

CLOZAPINE (Clozaril): Theoretically, concomitant administration might cause acute exacerbation of psychotic symptoms due to the caffeine in green tea. Caffeine can increase the effects and toxicity of clozapine (19,151). Caffeine doses of 400-1000 mg per day inhibit clozapine metabolism (5051).

DISULFIRAM (Antabuse): Concomitant use might increase the risk of adverse effects of caffeine in green tea. Disulfiram decreases the clearance and increases the half-life of caffeine (15).

EPHEDRINE: Concomitant use might increase the risk of agitation, tremors, and insomnia due to the caffeine in green tea (19).

ERGOTAMINE (Ergomar): Concomitant administration might increase the GI absorption of ergotamine due to the caffeine in green tea (15).

LITHIUM (Eskalith, Lithobid): Abrupt caffeine withdrawal can increase serum lithium levels (609). Two case of lithium tremor which worsened with abrupt coffee withdrawal have been reported (610).

MAO INHIBITORS (MAOIs): Concomitant intake with large amounts of green tea might precipitate a hypertensive crisis due to the caffeine in green tea (19).

MEXILETINE (Mexitil): Concomitant use might increase the effects and adverse effects of caffeine in green tea. Mexiletine can decrease caffeine elimination by 50% (1260).

ORAL CONTRACEPTIVES: Concomitant use might increase the effects and adverse effects of caffeine in green tea. Oral contraceptives can decrease caffeine clearance by 40-65% (14).

PHENYTOIN (Dilantin): Concomitant use might reduce the effects of caffeine in green tea. Phenytoin enhances metabolism and excretion of caffeine (19).

PHENYLPROPANOLAMINE (Propagest, Rhindecon): Concomitant use might increase blood pressure and/or cause mania, due to the caffeine in green tea (19).

QUINOLONES: Concomitant use might increase the effects and risk of adverse effects of caffeine in green tea. Quinolones decrease caffeine clearance (606,607,608). Quinolones include ciprofloxacin (Cipro), enoxacin (Penetrex), norfloxacin (Chibroxin, Noroxin), sparfloxacin (Zagam), trovafloxacin (Trovan), and grepafloxacin (Raxar).

THEOPHYLLINE (Theo-Dur): Concomitant use might increase the effects and adverse effects of theophylline due to the caffeine in green tea. Caffeine can reduce theophylline clearance, increase elimination half-life, and increase serum levels (151).

VERAPAMIL (Calan, Isoptin): Concomitant use might increase the effects and adverse effects of caffeine in green tea. Verapamil can increase plasma caffeine levels by 25% (14).

WARFARIN (Coumadin): Consumption of large amounts of green tea is reported to antagonize the effects of warfarin. This has been attributed to the vitamin K1 in green tea (4211). However, there is so little vitamin K1 in green tea (0.03 +/- 0.1 mcg/mL) that the interaction is more likely due to other constituents (1460,1461,1462,1463).

Interactions with Foods

GRAPEFRUIT JUICE: Concomitant use can increase caffeine levels and the risk of adverse effects (504).

MILK: When taken together, milk might bind the antioxidants in tea and reduce their beneficial effects (220); however, in one study this interaction did not occur (6032).

Interactions with Lab Tests

BLEEDING TIME: The caffeine in green tea can prolong bleeding time and increase the results of a bleeding time test (1701).

SERUM URATE (Bittner method): The caffeine in green tea can cause false-positive test results (15).

CREATINE: The caffeine in green tea can increase urine creatine levels (1701).

URINE CATECHOLAMINES, 5-HYDROXYINDOLEACETIC ACID, VANILLYLMANDELIC ACID (VMA): The caffeine in green tea can cause a slight increase in these levels and test results (15).

TESTS FOR PHEOCHROMOCYTOMA, NEUROBLASTOMA: High urine catecholamines or VMA can result in false-positive results. Avoid caffeine while testing for these diseases (15).

Interactions with Diseases or Conditions

DEPRESSION, ANXIETY DISORDERS: Theoretically, the caffeine in green tea might aggravate depression or anxiety disorders (14).

DIABETES: Theoretically, the caffeine in green tea might have hyperglycemic effects (19); monitor blood sugar.

GASTRIC, DUODENAL ULCERS: Theoretically, the caffeine in green tea might aggravate these conditions by increasing acid secretion (14,16,19).

HEART CONDITIONS: Theoretically, the caffeine in green tea might induce cardiac arrhythmias in sensitive individuals (14,16).

HYPERTENSION: The caffeine in green tea might increase blood pressure in people with high blood pressure (2272). However, this doesn't seem to occur in people who regularly consume green tea or other caffeinated products (1451,1452,6663).

KIDNEY DISEASE: Theoretically, the diuretic effect of caffeine in green tea might aggravate some kidney disorders (19).

Dosage and Administration

ORAL: Doses of green tea vary significantly, but usually range between 1-10 cups daily (6002). The commonly used dose of green tea is based on the amount typically consumed in Asian countries, which is about 3 cups per day providing 240-320 mg of polyphenols. For improving cognitive performance, tea providing 60 mg of caffeine, or approximately 1 cup, has been used (4221). For reducing cholesterol, only 10 or greater cups per day has been associated with decreased cholesterol levels (6403). For preventing Parkinson's disease, men consuming 421-2716 mg total caffeine (approximately 5-33 cups of green tea) daily have the lowest risk of developing Parkinson's disease. However, a significantly lower risk is also associated with consumption of as little as 124-208 mg of caffeine (approximately 1-3 cups of green tea) daily (6022). In women, more moderate caffeine consumption seems to be best; equivalent to approximately 1-4 cups of green tea per day (1238). To make tea, people typically use 1 teaspoon of tea leaves in 8 ounces boiling water. Tablets and capsules containing standardized extracts of green tea polyphenols, particularly epigallocatechin, are available. Some provide up to 97% polyphenols, equivalent to drinking four cups of brewed green tea (6006). However, no studies have used evaluated tablet formulations and they cannot be considered equivalent to tea preparations.

TOPICAL: No typical dosage.

Comments

Camellia sinensis leaves and stems are used to manufacture green tea (non-fermented), oolong tea (partially fermented), and black tea (fermented) (4218). Leaves used for green tea are prepared immediately after harvest with limited enzymatic changes. Consequently, green teas can have a higher concentration of the natural constituents than oolong teas or black teas (6,7,4218).

GROUND IVY

Also Known As

Alehoof, Catsfoot, Cat's-Paw, Creeping Charlie, Gill-Go-By-The-Hedge, Gill-Go-Over-The-Ground, Haymaids, Hedgemaids, Lizzy-Run-Up-The-Hedge, Robin-Run-In-The-Hedge, Tun-Hoof, Turnhoof.

Scientific Names

Nepeta hederacea, synonym Glechoma hederacea.
Family: Labiatae.

People Use This For

Orally, ground ivy is used for mild upper respiratory complaints, coughs, arthritis, rheumatism, and as a diuretic in individuals with bladder and kidney stones (4,18).

Topically ground ivy is used for poorly healing wounds, ulcers, and other skin conditions (18).

In Chinese medicine, ground ivy is used for menstrual irregularities (18).

Historically, ground ivy has been used for bronchitis, chronic bronchial inflammation, tinnitus, diarrhea, intestinal inflammation, hemorrhoids, cystitis, and gastritis (4,18).

In food manufacturing, ground ivy is used as a flavoring agent (4).

Safety

POSSIBLY SAFE ...when preparations of the above ground parts are consumed in amounts found in foods; listed by the Council of Europe as natural source of food flavoring (4). ...when used orally in medicinal amounts (4,18).

PREGNANCY: LIKELY UNSAFE ...when used orally because of abortifacient activity (4).

LACTATION: Insufficient reliable information available; avoid using (4).

Effectiveness

There is insufficient reliable information available about the effectiveness of ground ivy.

Mechanism of Action

Contains rosmarinic acid, which may be an astringent (4). Contains the volatile oil pulegone, which has hepatotoxic, abortifacient, and irritant properties. The concentration of pulegone in ground ivy is low (4). Fatal poisonings have occurred in animals (18).

Adverse Reactions

Orally, ground ivy in excessive doses may irritate the GI mucosa and kidneys (4).

Interactions with Herbs & Other Dietary Supplements

PENNYROYAL: Avoid concomitant use, both herbs contain potentially hepatotoxic constituent, pulegone (4).

Interactions with Drugs

No interactions are known to occur, and there is no known reason to expect a clinically significant interaction with ground ivy.

Interactions with Foods

No interactions are known to occur, and there is no known reason to expect a clinically significant interaction with ground ivy.

Interactions with Lab Tests

No interactions are known to occur, and there is no known reason to expect a clinically significant interaction with ground ivy.

Interactions with Diseases or Conditions

KIDNEY DISEASE: The volatile oil is contraindicated due to potential for kidney irritation (4).
LIVER DISEASE: Contraindicated, due to presence of hepatotoxic pulegone (4).
SEIZURE DISORDERS: Contraindicated (4).

Dosage and Administration

ORAL: 2-4 grams dried plant three times daily (4), or, one cup tea (steep 2-4 grams dried plant in 150 mL boiling water 5-10 minutes, strain) three times daily (4). Liquid extract (1:1 in 25% alcohol), 2-4 mL three times daily (4).
TOPICAL: Apply crushed leaves to affected area(s) (18).

Comments

Ground ivy is a rich plant source of potassium and iron (19).

GROUND PINE

Also Known As

Bugle, Yellow Bugle.

Scientific Names

Ajuga chamaepitys.
Family: Lamiaceae.

People Use This For

Orally, the above ground parts of ground pine are used for stimulating menstrual flow, for gout, rheumatism, gynecological complaints (18), edema, malaria, and sclerosis. They are also used as a stimulant and diuretic (18), for inducing sweating, and as a tonic.
Topically, ground pine is used for wound healing.

Safety

There is insufficient reliable information available about the safety of ground pine.
Pregnancy and Lactation: Insufficient reliable information is available; avoid using.

Effectiveness

There is insufficient reliable information available about the effectiveness of ground pine.

Mechanism of Action

The applicable parts of ground pine are the above ground parts. There is insufficient reliable information available about the possible mechanism of action and active ingredients.

Adverse Reactions

None reported.

Interactions with Herbs & Other Dietary Supplements

Insufficient reliable information available.

Interactions with Drugs

No interactions are known to occur, and there is no known reason to expect a clinically significant interaction with ground pine.

Interactions with Foods

No interactions are known to occur, and there is no known reason to expect a clinically significant interaction with ground pine.

Interactions with Lab Tests

No interactions are known to occur, and there is no known reason to expect a clinically significant interaction with ground pine.

Interactions with Diseases or Conditions

No interactions are known to occur, and there is no known reason to expect a clinically significant interaction with ground pine.

Dosage and Administration

No typical dosage.

Comments

There is very little scientific information about this product. Our staff is continually analyzing the available information on natural medicines and will add data here as it becomes available.

GROUNDSEL

Also Known As

Common Groundsel, Ground Glutton, Grundy Swallow, Simson.

Scientific Names

Senecio vulgaris.
Family: Compositae.

People Use This For

Orally, groundsel is used for worm infestations and colic. The pressed juice is used orally in the treatment of dysmenorrhea and epilepsy (18).
Topically, groundsel pressed juice is used as a dental styptic (18).

Safety

UNSAFE …when taken orally (2,18). Excessive doses or long-term use increases risk of adverse effects due to unsaturated pyrrolizidine alkaloids (UPAs) (4,12). UPAs are linked to veno-occlusive disease (4,12) and are considered to be hepatotoxic and hepatocarcinogenic (7,515). They might also be mutagenic (12). Dietary supplements sold in the United States are not required to include the amount of UPAs they contain (3484); therefore, all preparations used orally containing groundsel should be considered potentially unsafe.
PREGNANCY AND LACTATION: UNSAFE …when used orally due to pyrrolizidine alkaloid content (12).

Effectiveness

There is insufficient reliable information available about the effectiveness of groundsel.

Mechanism of Action

The applicable part of groundsel is the whole flowering plant. Some pyrrolizidine alkaloids have shown carcinogenic and mutagenic properties, and there are reports of renal toxicity. However, the primary concern is veno-occlusive disease (12). Unsaturated pyrrolizidine alkaloids are known to be hepatotoxic and hepatocarcinogenic in animals and humans (4,7). UPAs destroy and damage centrilobular hepatocytes of the liver and also destroy small branches of the hepatic vein (7).

Adverse Reactions
Chronic exposure to other plants containing UPA constituents has been associated with veno-occlusive disease (4021). Symptoms of acute veno-occlusive disease are characterized by nausea, vomiting (5606), anorexia, lethargy (7), a dull, dragging ache in the right upper abdomen and marked distention of the abdomen (4021). These symptoms are sometimes accompanied by reduced urine output. Subacute veno-occlusive disease is associated with vague symptoms and persistent liver enlargement (4021). There is one case report of fatal hepatic veno-occlusive disease in an infant resulting from groundsel tea consumption (5606). It can cause an allergic reaction in individuals sensitive to the Asteraceae/Compositae family. Members of this family include ragweed, chrysanthemums, marigolds, daisies, and many other herbs.

Interactions with Herbs & Other Dietary Supplements
EUCALYPTUS: Theoretically, concomitant use might increase the risk of unsaturated pyrrolizidine alkaloid toxicity due to enzyme induction by eucalyptus (19).
PYRROLIZIDINE ALKALOID-CONTAINING HERBS: Concomitant use is contraindicated due to the risk of additive toxicity. Herbs containing unsaturated pyrrolizidine alkaloids include: alkanna (12), borage (271), gravel root (4), hemp agrimony (271), hound's tongue (19), petasites (19), comfrey (271), coltsfoot, and the Senecio species plants; dusty miller (19), alpine ragwort (19), groundsel (271), golden ragwort (19), and tansy ragwort (271).

Interactions with Drugs
No interactions are known to occur, and there is no known reason to expect a clinically significant interaction with groundsel.

Interactions with Foods
No interactions are known to occur, and there is no known reason to expect a clinically significant interaction with groundsel.

Interactions with Lab Tests
No interactions are known to occur, and there is no known reason to expect a clinically significant interaction with groundsel.

Interactions with Diseases or Conditions
LIVER DISEASE: Contraindicated.
CROSS-ALLERGENICITY: Can cause an allergic reaction in individuals sensitive to the Asteraceae/Compositae family. Members of this family include ragweed, chrysanthemums, marigolds, daisies, and many other herbs.

Dosage and Administration
No typical dosage.

Comments
Groundsel is considered unsafe for oral use; avoid using (18).

GUAIAC WOOD OIL

Also Known As
Champaca Wood Oil.
CAUTION: See separate listing for Guaiac Wood resin, wood.

Scientific Names
Bulnesia sarmienti.
Family: Zygophyllaceae.

People Use This For
There are no known medicinal uses for guaiac wood oil.
In foods and beverages, guaiac wood oil is used as a flavoring agent.
In other manufacturing processes, guaiac wood oil is used as a fixative, modifier, or fragrance in soaps and cosmetics.

Safety

POSSIBLY SAFE ...when consumed in amounts found in foods (maximum use level 0.002% in meat products); approved for food use in the US (11).
PREGNANCY AND LACTATION: Insufficient reliable information available.

Effectiveness

There is insufficient reliable information available about the effectiveness of guaiac wood oil.

Mechanism of Action

There is insufficient reliable information available about the possible mechanism of action and active ingredients.

Adverse Reactions

None reported.

Interactions with Herbs & Other Dietary Supplements

Insufficient reliable information available.

Interactions with Drugs

No interactions are known to occur, and there is no known reason to expect a clinically significant interaction with guaiac wood oil.

Interactions with Foods

No interactions are known to occur, and there is no known reason to expect a clinically significant interaction with guaiac wood oil.

Interactions with Lab Tests

No interactions are known to occur, and there is no known reason to expect a clinically significant interaction with guaiac wood oil.

Interactions with Diseases or Conditions

No interactions are known to occur, and there is no known reason to expect a clinically significant interaction with guaiac wood oil.

Dosage and Administration

No typical dosage.

Comments

The distilled oil is obtained from the wood of Bulnesia sarmienti.

GUAIAC WOOD resin, wood

Also Known As

Guaiac, Guaiac Heartwood, Guaiacum, Guajaci Lignum, Lingum Vitae, Pockwood.
CAUTION: See separate listing for Guaiac Wood Oil.

Scientific Names

Guaiacum officinale; Guaiacum sanctum.
Family: Zygophyllaceae.

People Use This For

Orally, guaiac wood is used for subacute and chronic rheumatism, chronic rheumatoid arthritis, and preventing gout (2,4,11).
Topically, guaiac wood is used as a bacteriostatic agent in mouthwashes (18).
In lab tests, guaiac resin is used as a diagnostic reagent in tests for occult blood (11).
In folk medicine, guaiac wood has been used for respiratory complaints, skin disorders, and syphilis (18).
As a flavoring agent, guaiac wood is used in foods and in edible oils and fats (4,11).

Safety

POSSIBLY SAFE ...when consumed in amounts commonly found in foods. Guaiac wood has Generally Recognized as Safe (GRAS) status for food use in the US (11). ...when taken orally for medicinal purposes in appropriate amounts.

The resin can have low toxicity (4).

There is insufficient reliable information available about the safety of guaiac wood/resin for its other uses.

PREGNANCY AND LACTATION: Insufficient reliable information available; avoid using.

Effectiveness

POSSIBLY EFFECTIVE ...when taken orally as supportive therapy for rheumatic complaints (2).

There is insufficient reliable information available about the effectiveness of guaiac wood/resin for its other uses.

Mechanism of Action

Guaiac wood can have antirheumatic, anti-inflammatory, diuretic, mild laxative, diaphoretic, and fungistatic activity (4,18).

Adverse Reactions

Orally, guaiac wood can cause skin rashes (18). High doses can cause diarrhea, gastroenteritis, or intestinal colic (18).

Interactions with Herbs & Other Dietary Supplements

Insufficient reliable information available.

Interactions with Drugs

No interactions are known to occur, and there is no known reason to expect a clinically significant interaction with guaiac wood/resin.

Interactions with Foods

No interactions are known to occur, and there is no known reason to expect a clinically significant interaction with guaiac wood/resin.

Interactions with Lab Tests

No interactions are known to occur, and there is no known reason to expect a clinically significant interaction with guaiac wood/resin.

Interactions with Diseases or Conditions

ACUTE INFLAMMATORY CONDITONS: Contraindicated in acute inflammatory conditions and individuals allergic or hypersensitive to the product (4).

Dosage and Administration

ORAL: The typical dose of guaiac wood is one cup of the tea three times daily (2,4,18). The tea is prepared by simmering 1.5 grams of the wood or resin in 150 mL boiling water for 5-10 minutes and then straining. The usual dose of the liquid extract (1:1 in 80% alcohol) is 1-2 mL per dose. The common dose of the tincture of is 1-4 mL, which is about 20-40 drops (4,18).

TOPICAL: No typical dosage.

Comments

Avoid confusion with guaiac wood oil.

GUAR GUM

Also Known As

Dietary Fiber, Guar Flour, Indian Cluster Bean, Indian Guar Plant, Jaguar Gum.

CAUTION: See separate listing for Guarana.

Scientific Names

Cyamopsis tetragonolobus, synonym Cyamopsis psoralioides.

Family: Leguminosae or Fabaceae.

People Use This For

Orally, guar gum is used as a bulk laxative, for reducing serum cholesterol, preventing atherosclerosis, for diabetes, and weight loss and obesity.

In foods and beverages, guar gum is used as a thickening, stabilizing, suspending and binding agent.

In manufacturing, guar gum is used as a binding and disintegrating agent in tablets, and as a thickening agent in lotions and creams.

Safety
LIKELY SAFE ...when used oral and appropriately (12,8305).
PREGNANCY: POSSIBLY SAFE ...when used orally (6).
LACTATION: Insufficient reliable information available; avoid using.

Effectiveness
LIKELY EFFECTIVE ...when used orally as a bulk laxative (7). ...when taken orally for hypercholesterolemia. Guar gum can reduce total cholesterol (6,7) and low-density lipoprotein (LDL) cholesterol (6).
POSSIBLY EFFECTIVE ...when taken orally for hypertriglyceridemia (7). ...when used orally for diabetes. Guar gum seems to lower post-prandial glucose levels when taken with meals (6).
LIKELY INEFFECTIVE ...when taken orally for weight loss or obesity (8305).
There is insufficient reliable information available about the effectiveness of guar gum for its other uses.

Mechanism of Action
Guar gum is a soluble dietary fiber produced from the seed of the guar plant. It works as a bulk laxative. When ingested, it swells 10-20 fold in the presence of water and tends to normalize bowel function. Like other fibers, it adsorbs glucose and lipids in the gut and decreases their absorption. The bulk forming properties may also cause a sense of fullness and cause decreased appetite (6).

Adverse Reactions
Orally, guar gum can cause flatulence, diarrhea, nausea, gastrointestinal discomfort (6,12). Gastrointestinal side effects can be minimized by starting with small doses and titrating up. When guar gum is consumed with inadequate amounts of fluids, it can also cause severe esophageal and small bowel obstruction (602). Tell patients to take guar gum with at least 8 ounces (250 mL) of water (12).
Topically, asthma may result from occupational exposure (600,601).

Interactions with Herbs & Other Dietary Supplements
VITAMIN/MINERAL SUPPLEMENTS: Guar gum can reduce vitamin and mineral absorption (12). Tell patients to take supplements one hour before or several hours after guar gum.

Interactions with Drugs
DIABETES THERAPY: There is some concern that guar gum can decrease glucose levels and might have additive effects with insulin and other diabetes medications (6,19). Monitor blood glucose levels closely. Dose adjustments may be necessary.
ORAL DRUGS: Guar gum can decrease absorption of orally administered drugs (6,12), including aspirin, anticoagulants, digoxin, metformin, penicillin, and numerous others (12,532,533). Tell patients to take drugs one hour before or several hours after guar gum.

Interactions with Foods
NUTRIENT ABSORPTION: Long term use with meals may reduce nutrient absorption (12) requiring vitamin/mineral supplementation.

Interactions with Lab Tests
CHOLESTEROL: Guar gum can reduce serum total cholesterol and low-density lipoprotein (LDL) cholesterol levels and test results (6,7).
GLUCOSE: Guar gum can reduce postprandial serum glucose concentrations and test results (6).
TRIGLYCERIDES: Guar gum might reduce triglyceride concentrations and test results (6,7).

Interactions with Diseases or Conditions
GASTROINTESTINAL OBSTRUCTION: Guar gum is contraindicated in cases of gastrointestinal obstruction or narrowing, anatomical predisposition to luminal obstruction (6,12).

Dosage and Administration
ORAL: Typically, 5 grams three times per day just before or with meals is used. Tell patients to take each dose with at least 8 ounces (250 mL) of fluid to prevent esophageal obstruction (7,12). Recommend starting with a small dose of 3 grams per day and titrating to reduce occurrence of gastrointestinal side effects.

Comments
None.

GUARANA

Also Known As
Brazilian Cocoa, Guarana Bread, Guarana Gum, Guarana Seed Paste, Paullinia, Zoom.
CAUTION: See separate listings for Caffeine and Guar Gum.

Scientific Names
Paullinia cupana, synonym Paullinia sorbilis.
Family: Sapindaceae.

People Use This For
Orally, guarana is used for weight loss (6,11), to enhance athletic performance, and to reduce fatigue (1900).
In folk medicine, guarana has been used as a stimulant (11,18), tonic (11,18), aphrodisiac (6), diuretic, and astringent (11).
It has also been used to prevent malaria and dysentery (6), and for chronic diarrhea, fever, heart problems, headache, rheumatism, lumbago, and heat stress (11).
In food manufacturing, guarana has been used as a flavoring ingredient in beverages and candy (11).

Safety
LIKELY SAFE ...when used in the amounts that are typically found in foods. Guarana's usage in foods is approved in the US (11).
POSSIBLY SAFE ...when used orally and appropriately short-term (12).
POSSIBLY UNSAFE ...when large amounts are used. Chronic use of caffeine, contained in guarana, can sometimes produce tolerance, habituation, and psychological dependence (15). The abrupt discontinuation of caffeine can sometimes cause physical withdrawal symptoms (15).
CHILDREN: POSSIBLY UNSAFE ...when taken orally in amounts significantly greater than typical food amounts. The adverse effects due to the caffeine content are usually more severe in children than adults (15).
PREGNANCY: Insufficient reliable information available. Although the caffeine content of a typical dose should not cause concern, other constituents could be unsafe.
LACTATION: POSSIBLY UNSAFE; avoid using. Caffeine can cause sleep disturbances in breast-fed infants (18).

Effectiveness
LIKELY EFFECTIVE ...when taken orally as a central nervous system stimulant (12,15,18).
POSSIBLY EFFECTIVE ...when taken orally as a diuretic (15,18), for headache, increasing blood pressure in hypotension (15), and weight loss (695,696,1704).
POSSIBLY INEFFECTIVE ...when taken orally for sustained, sub-maximal exercise endurance (14).
LIKELY INEFFECTIVE ...when taken orally for improving short-term, high-intensity performance, anaerobic capacity or power (14).
There is insufficient reliable information available about the effectiveness of guarana for its other uses.

Mechanism of Action
The applicable part of guarana is the seed. Guarana contains 2.5-7% caffeine (compared to 1-2% in coffee) (5,6,11,12,18) which acts as a central nervous system stimulant (12,15,18), increases heart rate and contractility (7,18), increases blood pressure (6663), inhibits platelet aggregation (6,18), stimulates gastric acid secretion, causes diuresis (15,18), relaxes extracerebral vascular and bronchial smooth muscle, stimulates the release of catecholamines (18), and might indirectly inhibit histamine release (6130). An unpublished study found that consumption of 250 mg caffeine acutely increases systolic and diastolic pressure in healthy people (6663). A second unpublished study found that 250 mg caffeine increases systolic blood pressure and muscle sympathetic nervous activity in healthy, non-habitual coffee drinkers, but not in habitual coffee drinkers (6663). Guarana also contains theophylline and theobromine, which have actions similar to caffeine (6,18). Guarana contains tannins with possible carcinogenic and hepatotoxic properties (6,11,12,18). It also contains trace amounts of timbonine, which is used as a fish poison (6).

Adverse Reactions
Overdose of guarana can cause painful urination, abdominal spasms, and vomiting (18). Caffeine constituents can cause insomnia, nervousness, restlessness, agitation (7,15), gastric irritation (7), nausea, vomiting, diuresis (15), fast heartbeat, arrhythmias, increased respiratory rate, muscle spasms, tinnitus, headache, delirium, and convulsions (15,505). High doses of guarana providing 250 mg of caffeine can also increase blood pressure. This doesn't seem to occur in people who habitually consume caffeine products (6663). The adverse effects of caffeine can be more severe in children (15). Some evidence shows caffeine is associated with fibrocystic breast disease in women; other evidence disputes this (14,15). The chronic use of caffeine, especially in large amounts, can sometimes produce tolerance, habituation, and psychological dependence (15). The abrupt discontinuation can sometimes result in physical withdrawal symptoms, including irritability, anxiety, headaches, and dizziness (15).

Combining ephedra with guarana increases the risk of adverse effects, due the caffeine contained in guarana (2729). One unpublished report associated jitteriness, hypertension, seizures, temporary loss of consciousness, and hospitalization requiring life support with the use of a combination ephedra and guarana (caffeine) product (1380). There is one report of ischemic stroke in an athlete who consumed ephedra 40-60 mg, creatine monohydrate 6 grams, caffeine 400-600 mg, and a variety of other supplements daily for six weeks (1275).

Interactions with Herbs & Other Dietary Supplements

CAFFEINE CONTAINING HERBS/SUPPLEMENTS: Concomitant use of guarana and caffeine-containing herbs/supplements constitutes therapeutic duplication (due to the caffeine contained in guarana) which increases the risk of caffeine-related adverse effects. Other natural products which contain caffeine include black tea, cocoa, coffee, cola nut, green tea, and mate.

EPHEDRA (Ma Huang): Concomitant use can increase the risk of stimulatory adverse effects, due to the caffeine contained in guarana (7). One unpublished report associated jitteriness, hypertension, seizures, temporary loss of consciousness, and hospitalization requiring life support with the use of a combination ephedra and guarana (caffeine) product (1380).

Interactions with Drugs

ACETAMINOPHEN (Tylenol): Theoretically, concomitant use might increase the pain-relieving activity of acetaminophen, due to the caffeine contained in guarana. Caffeine increases the pain-relieving activity of acetaminophen by up to 40% (512).

ASPIRIN: Theoretically, concomitant use might increase the pain-relieving activity of aspirin, due to the caffeine contained in guarana. Caffeine increases the pain-relieving activity of aspirin by up to 40% (512).

BENZODIAZEPINES: Theoretically, concomitant use might reduce the sedative and anxiolytic effects of benzodiazepines, due to the caffeine contained in guarana (14).

BETA-ADRENERGIC AGONISTS: Theoretically, concomitant use might increase the cardiac inotropic effects of beta agonists, due to the caffeine contained in guarana (15). Beta-adrenergic agonists include albuterol (Proventil, Ventolin), metaproterenol (Alupent), terbutaline (Brethine), and isoproterenol (Isuprel).

CIMETIDINE (Tagamet): Theoretically, concomitant use might increase serum caffeine concentrations and the risk of adverse effects, due to the caffeine contained in guarana. Cimetidine decreases the rate of caffeine clearance by 30-50% (14).

CLOZAPINE (Clozaril): Theoretically, co-administration might acutely exacerbate psychotic symptoms, due to the caffeine contained in guarana. Caffeine can increase the effects and toxicity of clozapine (151). Caffeine doses of 400-1000 mg per day inhibit clozapine metabolism (5051).

CNS STIMULANTS: Concomitant use might increase the risk of stimulant adverse effects, due to the caffeine contained in guarana (151,2719). CNS stimulants include nicotine, cocaine, sympathomimetic amines, and amphetamines.

DIABETES THERAPY: Theoretically, concomitant use of coffee and diabetes drugs might interfere with blood glucose control, due to the caffeine contained in guarana. This is based in the claim that caffeine might have hyperglycemic effects (19).

DISULFIRAM (Antabuse): Theoretically, concomitant use might increase serum caffeine concentrations and the risk of adverse effects, due to the caffeine contained in guarana. Disulfiram decreases the rate of caffeine clearance (15).

EPHEDRINE: Concomitant use might increase the risk of stimulatory adverse effects, due to the caffeine contained in guarana (7,19). An unpublished report associated jitteriness, hypertension, seizures, temporary loss of consciousness, and hospitalization requiring life support with the use of a combination ephedra (ephedrine) and guarana (caffeine) product (1380).

ESTROGEN (Estrace): Theoretically, concomitant use might increase serum caffeine concentrations and the risk of adverse effects, due to the caffeine contained in guarana. Estrogen inhibits caffeine metabolism (2714).

ERGOTAMINE: Theoretically, concomitant use might increase the GI absorption of ergotamine, due to the caffeine contained in guarana. Caffeine increases the GI absorption of ergotamine (15).

LITHIUM (Eskalith, Lithobid): Theoretically, abrupt guarana withdrawal might increase serum lithium levels, due to the caffeine contained in guarana. There are two case reports of lithium tremor that worsened upon abrupt coffee withdrawal (609,610).

MEXILETINE (Mexitil): Theoretically, concomitant use might increase serum caffeine concentrations and the risk of adverse effects, due to the caffeine contained in guarana. Mexiletine reduces caffeine metabolism (14).

MONOAMINE OXIDASE INHIBITORS (MAOIs): Theoretically, concomitant intake of large amounts of guarana with MAOIs might precipitate a hypertensive crisis, due to the caffeine contained in guarana. This is based on the claim that intake of large amounts of caffeine with MAOIs might precipitate a hypertensive crisis (19).

ORAL CONTRACEPTIVES (OCs): Theoretically, concomitant use might increase serum caffeine concentrations and the risk adverse effects, due to the caffeine contained in guarana. OCs decrease the rate of caffeine clearance by 40-65% (14).

PHENYLPROPANOLAMINE (Dexatrim, Propagest): Theoretically, concomitant use might cause an additive increase in blood pressure and serum caffeine concentrations, due to the caffeine contained in guarana (14).

Concomitant use of caffeine and phenylpropanolamine can cause an additive increase in blood pressure, and increase serum caffeine concentrations (14).

QUINOLONES: Theoretically, concomitant use might increase serum caffeine concentrations and the risk of adverse effects, due to the caffeine contained in guarana. Quinolones decrease caffeine clearance (606,607,608). Quinolones (also referred to as fluoroquinolones) include ciprofloxacin (Cipro), enoxacin (Penetrex), gatifloxacin (Tequin), levofloxacin (Levaquin), lomefloxacin (Maxaquin), moxifloxacin (Avelox), norfloxacin (Noroxin), ofloxacin (Floxin), sparfloxacin (Zagam), and trovafloxacin (Trovan).

RILUZOLE (Rilutek): Theoretically, concomitant use might increase serum caffeine and riluzole concentrations and the risk of adverse effects of both caffeine and riluzole, due to the caffeine contained in guarana. Caffeine and riluzole are both metabolized by cytochrome P450 1A2 and concomitant use might reduce metabolism of one or both agents (14).

TERBINAFINE (Lamisil): Theoretically, concomitant use might increase serum caffeine concentrations and the risk of adverse effects, due to the caffeine contained in guarana. Terbinafine decreases the rate of caffeine clearance (14).

THEOPHYLLINE (Theo-Dur): Theoretically, concomitant use might increase serum theophylline concentrations and the risk of adverse effects, due to the caffeine contained in guarana. Large amounts of caffeine might inhibit theophylline metabolism (14).

VERAPAMIL (Calan, Isoptin, Verelan): Theoretically, concomitant use might increase plasma caffeine concentrations and the risk of adverse effects, due to the caffeine contained in guarana. Verapamil increases plasma caffeine concentrations by 25% (14).

Interactions with Foods

GRAPEFRUIT JUICE: Interacts with the caffeine in guarana and can increase caffeine levels, and the effects and the risk of adverse effects (504).

Interactions with Lab Tests

BLEEDING TIME: Guarana might prolong bleeding time and increase test results, due to its caffeine content (1701).

BLOOD PRESSURE: Guarana might increase blood pressure and blood pressure readings, due to its caffeine content (4).

URATE: Guarana might falsely increase serum urate test results determined by the Bittner method, due to its caffeine content. Caffeine causes false elevations in serum urate test results determined by the Bittner method (15).

CATECHOLAMINES: Guarana might increase urine catecholamine concentrations and test results, due to its caffeine content. Caffeine can increase urine catecholamine concentrations (15).

CREATINE: Guarana might increase urine creatine concentrations and test results, due to its caffeine content (1701).

DIPYRIDAMOLE THALLIUM IMAGING: Guarana might interfere with dipyridamole thallium imaging studies, due to its caffeine content. Caffeine attenuates the characteristic cardiovascular responses to dipyridamole and has altered test results (14).

5-HYDROXYINDOLEACETIC ACID: Guarana might increase urine 5-hydroxyindoleacetic acid concentrations and test results, due to its caffeine content. Caffeine can increase urine catecholamine concentrations (15).

VANILLYLMANDELIC ACID (VMA): Guarana might increase urine VMA concentrations and test results, due to its caffeine content. Caffeine can increase urine VMA concentrations (15).

TESTS FOR NEUROBLASTOMA: Guarana (due to its caffeine content) might cause false-positive diagnosis of neuroblastoma, when diagnosis is based on tests of urine vanillylmandelic acid (VMA) or catecholamine concentrations. Caffeine can increase urine catecholamine and VMA concentrations (15).

TESTS FOR PHEOCHROMOCYTOMA: Guarana (due to its caffeine content) might cause false-positive diagnosis of pheochromocytoma, when diagnosis is based on tests of urine vanillylmandelic acid (VMA) or catecholamine concentrations. Caffeine can increase urine catecholamine and VMA concentrations (15).

Interactions with Diseases or Conditions

DEPRESSION, ANXIETY DISORDERS: The caffeine in guarana can aggravate these conditions (14).

GASTRIC, DUODENAL ULCERS: The caffeine in guarana can aggravate these conditions; avoid using (14,16).

HEART CONDITIONS: The caffeine in guarana can induce cardiac arrhythmias in sensitive individuals (14,16).

HYPERTENSION: The caffeine in guarana might increase blood pressure in people with high blood pressure (2272). Consumption of 250 mg caffeine can increase blood pressure in healthy people. But this doesn't seem to occur in people who habitually consume caffeine products (6663).

KIDNEY DISEASE: The diuretic effect of caffeine in guarana might aggravate some kidney disorders (19).

Dosage and Administration

ORAL: Guarana is often used along with other ingredients in weight loss products. People use 1-2 capsules or tablets containing 200-800 mg guarana extract (1:4) before breakfast or lunch (5018), not to exceed 3 grams daily (5008).

Comments

None.

GUAYULE

Also Known As

None.

Scientific Names

Parthenium argentatum.
Family: Asteraceae or Compositae.

People Use This For

Guayule is a source of natural rubber (6). There are no reported medicinal uses.

Safety

LIKELY UNSAFE ...when used orally or topically. Guayule is a potent contact allergen (6).
PREGNANCY AND LACTATION: LIKELY UNSAFE ...when used orally or topically. Guayule is a potent contact allergen (6).

Effectiveness

There is insufficient reliable information available about the effectiveness of guayule.

Mechanism of Action

Contact allergenicity may be caused by guayulin A, which is reported equal in potency to poison ivy (6).

Adverse Reactions

Guayule is a potent contact allergen (equivalent to poison ivy) and induces strong erythema at very low concentrations (0.003%); avoid contact (6). Guayule can cause an allergic reaction in individuals sensitive to the Asteraceae/Compositae family. Members of this family include ragweed, chrysandthemums, marigolds, daisies, and many other herbs.

Interactions with Herbs & Other Dietary Supplements

Insufficient reliable information available.

Interactions with Drugs

No interactions are known to occur, and there is no known reason to expect a clinically significant interaction with guayule.

Interactions with Foods

No interactions are known to occur, and there is no known reason to expect a clinically significant interaction with guayule.

Interactions with Lab Tests

No interactions are known to occur, and there is no known reason to expect a clinically significant interaction with guayule.

Interactions with Diseases or Conditions

CROSS-ALLERGENICITY: Can cause an allergic reaction in individuals sensitive to the Asteraceae/Compositae family. Members of this family include ragweed, chrysanthemums, marigolds, daisies, and many other herbs.

Dosage and Administration

No typical dosage.

Comments

None.

GUGGUL

Also Known As
Guggal, Guggulu, Gum Guggal, Gum Guggulu, Indian Bdellium-Tree.
CAUTION: See separate listing for Indian Frankincense.

Scientific Names
Commiphora mukul.
Family: Burseracaea.

People Use This For
Orally, guggul gum resin is used for arthritis, lowering high cholesterol (6,3267), nodulocystic acne (3268), and weight loss (6).

Safety
POSSIBLY SAFE ...when the prepared gum resin is used orally and appropriately (12). No significant adverse effects reported in clinical trials (6).
PREGNANCY: LIKELY UNSAFE ...when used orally. Guggul gum resin appears to stimulate menstrual flow and the uterus (12).
LACTATION: Insufficient reliable information available; avoid using.

Effectiveness
POSSIBLY EFFECTIVE ...when gugulipid preparations are used orally for lowering serum cholesterol and triglycerides in people with hyperlipidemia (366,3267). ...when used orally for treating nodulocystic acne (3268). There is insufficient reliable information available about the effectiveness of guggul for its other uses.

Mechanism of Action
The applicable part of guggul is the gum resin. Guggul extracts contain guggulsterone and gugulipid. Studies indicate that extracts containing these constituents can lower serum total cholesterol, LDL cholesterol, and triglycerides (366,3267). However, the effects on HDL cholesterol are unclear. In one study, guggul increased HDL cholesterol concentrations (366) while in another study it had no effect on HDL levels (3267). The constituent, guggulsterone has thyroid-stimulating activity (6). It also shows protective effects against drug-induced myocardial necrosis (6). Some evidence suggests guggul extracts might have anti-inflammatory activity (6). Guggul was comparable to oral tetracycline in the treatment of nodulocystic acne (3268). Both treatments decreased inflammation and the number of relapses (3268). Co-administration of gugulipid reduces bioavailability of single doses of propranolol and diltiazem in healthy people (383).

Adverse Reactions
Orally, guggul can cause gastrointestinal upset (366), headache, mild nausea, belching, and hiccups (3267).

Interactions with Herbs & Other Dietary Supplements
Insufficient reliable information available.

Interactions with Drugs
PROPRANOLOL (Inderal): Concomitant oral administration can reduce propranolol bioavailability and might reduce therapeutic effects (383).
DILTIAZEM (Cardizem): Concomitant oral administration can reduce diltiazem bioavailability and might reduce therapeutic effects (383).
THYROID DRUGS: Theoretically, concomitant use might interfere with therapy to normalize thyroid function; monitor.

Interactions with Foods
No interactions are known to occur, and there is no known reason to expect a clinically significant interaction with guggul.

Interactions with Lab Tests
SERUM CHOLESTROL: Guggul can reduce serum total cholesterol and LDL cholesterol concentrations and test results (366,3267). It is unclear what effect, if any, guggul has on serum HDL cholesterol concentrations or test results (366,3267).
SERUM TRIGLYCERIDES: Guggul can reduce serum triglycerides and test results (366,3267).

Interactions with Diseases or Conditions

THYROID DISORDERS: Theoretically, concomitant use might interfere with therapy for hyperthyroid or hypothyroid conditions; monitor use.

Dosage and Administration

ORAL: For hypercholesterolemia, doses of 100-500 mg gugulipid per day have been used (366,3267). For nodulocystic acne, a dose of gugulipid equivalent to 25 mg guggulsterone per day has been used (3268).

Comments

Guggul is of the same genus as Commiphora myrrha, the myrrh of the bible. The plant has been used in Ayurvedic medicine for centuries to treat a variety of disorders, particularly arthritis, and to aid weight loss (6).

GUMWEED

Also Known As

August Flower, Grindelia, Grindeliae herba, Gum Weed, Gumweed Herb, Rosin Weed, Tar Weed.

Scientific Names

Grindelia robusta; Grindelia squarrosa.
Family: Asteraceae or Compositae.

People Use This For

Orally, gumweed is used for cough, bronchitis, and inflammation of the upper respiratory tract mucous membrane (2,18).

Safety

POSSIBLY SAFE ...when used orally and appropriately (2,12).
PREGNANCY AND LACTATION: Insufficient reliable information; avoid using.

Effectiveness

POSSIBLY EFFECTIVE ...when taken orally for treating upper respiratory tract mucous membrane inflammation (2). There is insufficient reliable information available about the effectiveness of gumweed for its other uses.

Mechanism of Action

The applicable parts of gumweed are the dried top and leaf. Gumweed can have antibacterial effects in vitro (2).

Adverse Reactions

Orally, gumweed can cause gastric mucosa irritation (2,12), diarrhea (18), and kidney irritation (12). Gumweed can cause an allergic reaction in individuals sensitive to the Asteraceae/Compositae family. Members of this family include ragweed, chrysanthemums, marigolds, daisies, and many other herbs.

Interactions with Herbs & Other Dietary Supplements

Insufficient reliable information available.

Interactions with Drugs

No interactions are known to occur, and there is no known reason to expect a clinically significant interaction with gumweed.

Interactions with Foods

No interactions are known to occur, and there is no known reason to expect a clinically significant interaction with gumweed.

Interactions with Lab Tests

No interactions are known to occur, and there is no known reason to expect a clinically significant interaction with gumweed.

Interactions with Diseases or Conditions

CROSS-ALLERGENICITY: Can cause an allergic reaction in individuals sensitive to the Asteraceae/Compositae family. Members of this family include ragweed, chrysanthemums, marigolds, daisies, and many other herbs.

Dosage and Administration

ORAL: The typical dose of gumweed is 4-6 grams of the dried top or leaf per day (2). The usual dose of the fluid extract is 3-6 grams per day (2). The common dose of the 1:10 tincture (60-80% ethanol) is 1.5-3 mL per day, and the usual dose of the 1:5 tincture (60-80% ethanol) is 1.5-3 mL per day (2).

Comments

None.

GYMNEMA

Also Known As

Gur-Mar, Gurmar, Gurmarbooti, Merasingi, Meshashringi.

Scientific Names

Gymnema sylvestre; Asclepias geminate; Gemnema melicida; Periploca sylvestris.
Family: Asclepiadaceae.

People Use This For

Orally, gymnema leaf is used to treat diabetes (6).
In combination with other products, gymnema is used for metabolic control (6).
In Ayurvedic medicine, gymnema is a component in the Tribang shila compound, which contains tin, lead, zinc, gymnema leaves, neem leaves, jambul seeds, and Enicostemma littorale (6).
Traditionally, gymnema has been used as an antimalarial, digestive stimulant, laxative, and diuretic. It has also been used traditionally for coughs and as a snake bite antidote (14).

Safety

There is insufficient reliable information available about the safety of gymnema.
Pregnancy and Lactation : Insufficient reliable information available; avoid using.

Effectiveness

POSSIBLY EFFECTIVE ...when taken orally by patients with type 1 or 2 diabetes on insulin or oral hypoglycemics for further reductions in blood glucose and glycosylated hemoglobin (45,46). ...when taken orally for reducing total cholesterol and triglycerides in type 1 diabetics (45). Studies have used the GS4 extract.
There is insufficient reliable information available about the effectiveness of gymnema for its other uses.

Mechanism of Action

The applicable part of gymnema is the leaf. Gymnema lowers blood sugar (6), serum triglycerides, total cholesterol, and VLDL and LDL cholesterol in animals (14). The constituent, gymnemic acid, inhibits the ability to taste bitter (quinine) or sweet (sugar) without affecting the ability to taste sour, astringent, or pungent flavors (6). Gymnemic acids can reduce intestinal absorption of glucose and may stimulate pancreatic beta cell growth (47,48). Gymnema can increase serum C-peptide levels, suggesting an increase in endogenous insulin secretion (45).

Adverse Reactions

None reported.

Interactions with Herbs & Other Dietary Supplements

Insufficient reliable information available.

Interactions with Drugs

DIABETES DRUGS/INSULIN: Gymnema can enhance the blood glucose lowering effects of insulin and hypoglycemic drugs (45,46); blood glucose levels should be monitored closely.
IRON: Some gymnema preparations can decrease absorption of iron. However, the GS4 extract, which has been used in clinical studies, is thought to be free of constituents that can reduce iron absorption (6420).

Interactions with Foods

No interactions are known to occur, and there is no known reason to expect a clinically significant interaction with gymnema.

Interactions with Lab Tests

BLOOD GLUCOSE: Gymnema can lower blood sugar resulting in lower blood glucose test results.

Interactions with Diseases or Conditions

DIABETES: Gymnema can affect blood sugar control, and blood glucose levels should be monitored closely.

Dosage and Administration

ORAL: For lowering blood sugar, the typical dose of the extract GS4 is 400 mg daily.

Comments

The gymnema leaf is commonly found in Africa and India but is readily distributed worldwide (6).

HARONGA

Also Known As

Harongabládder leaf, Harongarinde bark, Harunganae madagascariensis cortex bark, Harunganae madagascariensis folium leaf.

Scientific Names

Haronga madagascariensis.
Family: Hypericaceae.

People Use This For

Orally, haronga is used for dyspepsia, mild exocrine pancreatic insufficiency, liver and gallbladder complaints, and loss of appetite (2,18).

Safety

POSSIBLY SAFE ...when used orally and appropriately (2). The recommended maximum safe duration of use is two months (2).
PREGNANCY AND LACTATION: Insufficient reliable information available; avoid using.

Effectiveness

POSSIBLY EFFECTIVE ...when taken orally for mild exocrine pancreatic insufficiency (2).
There is insufficient reliable information available about the effectiveness of haronga for its other uses.

Mechanism of Action

The applicable parts of haronga are the bark and leaf. Haronga can have gallbladder stimulating (2), liver protectant, pancreas stimulating, gastric juice secretion stimulating, and antimicrobial effects (18). It can also have possible anti-amoebic activity (1519).

Adverse Reactions

Photosensitivity is possible with the use of haronga, especially in fair-skinned people (2). Phototoxicity is theoretically possible with large doses (18).

Interactions with Herbs & Other Dietary Supplements

Insufficient reliable information available.

Interactions with Drugs

No interactions are known to occur, and there is no known reason to expect a clinically significant interaction with haronga.

Interactions with Foods

No interactions are known to occur, and there is no known reason to expect a clinically significant interaction with haronga.

Interactions with Lab Tests

No interactions are known to occur, and there is no known reason to expect a clinically significant interaction with haronga.

Interactions with Diseases or Conditions

CONTRAINDICATIONS: The use of haronga is contraindicated in acute pancreatitis and exacerbations of chronic pancreatitis, severe liver dysfunction, gallstones, biliary obstruction, gallbladder empyema, or obstruction of the bowels (2,18).

FAIR-SKINNED INDIVIDUALS: Haronga can cause photosensitivity in fair-skinned individuals (2).

Dosage and Administration

ORAL: The typical dose of the haronga dry extract is 7.5-15 mg per day, which corresponds to 25-50 mg of the herb (2,18). The recommended maximum safe duration of use is two months (2).

Comments

None.

HARTSTONGUE

Also Known As

Buttonhole, God's-Hair, Hind's Tongue, Horse Tongue.

Scientific Names

Scolopendrium vulgare.

People Use This For

Orally, hartstongue is used to treat digestive disorders and urinary tract diseases (18).

Safety

There is insufficient reliable information available about the safety of hartstongue.
Pregnancy and Lactation: Insufficient reliable information available; avoid using.

Effectiveness

There is insufficient reliable information available about the effectiveness of hartstongue.

Mechanism of Action

The applicable parts of hartstongue are the above ground parts. Hartstongue contains tannins, mucilage, flavonoids (kaempferol-7-rhamnoside-3 coffeoyl-7-diglucoside), thiaminase, and sugars (sucrose and invert sugar) (18). These constituents seem to produce diuretic and mild laxative and purgative actions.

Adverse Reactions

None reported.

Interactions with Herbs & Other Dietary Supplements

Insufficient reliable information available.

Interactions with Drugs

No interactions are known to occur, and there is no known reason to expect a clinically significant interaction with hartstongue.

Interactions with Foods

No interactions are known to occur, and there is no known reason to expect a clinically significant interaction with hartstongue.

Interactions with Lab Tests

No interactions are known to occur, and there is no known reason to expect a clinically significant interaction with hartstongue.

Interactions with Diseases or Conditions

No interactions are known to occur, and there is no known reason to expect a clinically significant interaction with hartstongue.

Dosage and Administration

ORAL: People typically use 2 to 4 grams of the dried hartstongue leaves 3 times daily. This is also made into a tea. A liquid extract in a 1:1 concentration with 25% ethanol is dosed 2 to 4 mL three times daily. A liquid extract in a 1:5 concentration with 55% ethanol is dosed 2 to 6 mL three times daily (5269).

Comments

There is very little scientific information about this product. Our staff is continually analyzing the available information on natural medicines and will add data here as it becomes available.

HAWAIIAN BABY WOODROSE

Also Known As

Baby Hawaiian Woodrose, Baby Wood-rose, Elephant-Climber, Elephant Creeper, Silver-Morning-Glory, Wood-Rose, Woolly Morning Glory, Woolly-Morning-Glory.

Scientific Names

Argyreia nervosa, synonyms, Argyreia speciosa, Convolvulus nervosus, Convolvulus speciosus, Lettsomia nervosa. Family: Convolvulaceae.

People Use This For

Orally, Hawaiian baby woodrose seeds are used for pain relief, promoting sweating (5299), for sacramental rituals (5300), and as a hallucinogen (5301,5304).

Safety

LIKELY UNSAFE ...when used orally (17,5301). The seeds of Hawaiian baby woodrose have effects similar to the hallucinogen lysergic acid diethylamide (LSD), including flashbacks (5301).
PREGNANCY AND LACTATION: LIKELY UNSAFE ...when used orally; avoid using (17,5301).

Effectiveness

There is insufficient reliable information about the effectiveness of Hawaiian baby woodrose.

Mechanism of Action

The applicable part of Hawaiian baby woodrose is the seeds. Hawaiian baby woodrose, an ornamental plant, has seeds that contain hallucinogens including ergonovine, isoergine (isolysergic acid amide), and ergine (lysergic acid amide) (17,5300,5301,5304). Four to eight seeds are equivalent to 10 to 100 mcg of lysergic acid diethylamide (LSD) (5301), a potent 5-HT1A agonist (17). The hallucinatory effects of Hawaiian baby woodrose are similar to alcohol intoxication with psychedelic visual effects such as enhanced colors. The effects last 6-8 hours (5301,5304).

Adverse Reactions

Orally, ingestion can cause nausea and vomiting, dizziness, auditory hallucinations, blurred vision, dilated pupils, involuntary, rapid, rhythmic movement of eyeballs, sweating, fast heart rate, and hypertension (5301).

Interactions with Herbs & Other Dietary Supplements

ST. JOHN'S WORT: Theoretically, Hawaiian baby woodrose might increase the effects and adverse effects of products that increase serotonin levels, including St. John's wort (14,17).

Interactions with Drugs

SELECTIVE SEROTONIN REUPTAKE INHIBITORS (SSRIs): Theoretically, because Hawaiian baby woodrose contains chemicals related to LSD, it might interact with drugs that increase serotonin including sertraline (Zoloft), paroxetine (Paxil), fluoxetine (Prozac) and other antidepressants. Seizures have occurred in people taking the related compound, LSD, with fluoxetine (Prozac) (14,17). Individuals who have previously used LSD have developed flashbacks and hallucinations when treated with serotonin reuptake inhibitors (17).
5-HT2 ANTAGONISTS: Theoretically, because selective 5-HT2 receptor antagonists antagonize the effect of LSD, they might also decrease the effect of Hawaiian baby woodrose. 5-HT2 antagonists include cyproheptadine (Periactin), clozapine (Clozaril), and risperidone (Risperidone) (17).

Interactions with Foods

No interactions are known to occur, and there is no known reason to expect a clinically significant interaction with Hawaiian baby woodrose.

Interactions with Lab Tests

No interactions are known to occur, and there is no known reason to expect a clinically significant interaction with Hawaiian baby woodrose.

Interactions with Diseases or Conditions

PYSCHOSIS: Theoretically, because Hawaiian baby woodrose has effects similar to LSD, individuals with psychotic tendencies might experience prolonged psychotic reactions (17).

Dosage and Administration

No typical dosage.

Comments

Hawaiian baby woodrose is likely unsafe for oral use; avoid using. Hawaiian baby woodrose, a relative of the morning glory, grows in Florida, California, and Hawaii (17). Touted as a "natural LSD" in Internet advertising (5302), the seeds are legal (5301) and easily purchased from Internet sources.

HAWTHORN

Also Known As

Aubepine, Bianco spino, Crataegi Flos, Crataegi Folium, Crataegi Folium Cum Flore, Crataegi Fructus, English Hawthorn, Épine Blanche, Épine de Mai, Haagdorn, Hagedorn, Harthorne, Haw, Hawthorn Extract, Hawthorn Flower, Hawthorn Fruit, Hawthorn Leaf, Hawthorne, Hedgethorn, LI 132, LI132, May, Maybush, Maythorn, Mehlbeebaum, Meidorn, Nan Shanzha, Oneseed Hawthorn, Shanzha, Weissdorn, Whitehorn, WS 1442, WS1442.

Scientific Names

Crataegus laevigata, synonym Crataegus cuneata; Crataegus oxyacantha; Crataegus monogyna; Crataegus pinnatifida. Family: Rosaceae.

People Use This For

Orally, hawthorn is used for cardiovascular conditions such as congestive heart failure (CHF), coronary circulation problems, and arrhythmias. It is also used to increase cardiac output reduced by hypertension or pulmonary disease, to treat both hypotension and hypertension, atherosclerosis, hyperlipidemia, and Buerger's disease. Hawthorn is also used as a sedative, antispasmotic, astringent, and diuretic. It is also used for gastrointestinal conditions such as indigestion, enteritis, epigastric distension, diarrhea, and abdominal pain. Hawthorn fruit is also used orally to treat tapeworm infections, acute bacillary dysentery, and amenorrhea.

Topically, hawthorn leaf is used as a poultice for boils, sores, and ulcers. Hawthorn fruit preparations are used as a wash for sores, itching, and frost bite.

In manufacturing, hawthorn fruit is used for making candied fruit slices, jam, jelly, and wine.

Safety

POSSIBLY SAFE …when used orally and appropriately, short-term. Hawthorn preparations seem to be safe when used for up to approximately 60 days (2,12,406). Although hawthorn might be safe for long-term use, current studies have not extended past 60 days.

There is insufficient reliable information about the safety of topical use of hawthorn.

PREGNANCY: UNSAFE …when used orally. Hawthorn has potential uterine activity (4).

LACTATION: Insufficient reliable information available; avoid using.

Effectiveness

LIKELY EFFECTIVE …when used orally for congestive heart failure (CHF). Specific standardized leaf with flower extracts LI132 or WS 1442 can improve ejection fraction, exercise tolerance, and reduce subjective symptoms associated with New York Heart Association stage II heart failure (4,7,406). The greatest benefit is usually seen after 6-8 weeks of therapy (7,406).

There is insufficient reliable information available about the effectiveness of other uses of hawthorn.

Mechanism of Action

The applicable parts of hawthorn are the leaf, fruit, and flower. Extracts of the leaf and flower, are most commonly used therapeutically. The constituents responsible for the pharmacological effects of hawthorn preparations include flavonoids and procyanidins. Other active compounds are vitexin, rutin, and hyperoside (406). Hawthorn preparations act on the myocardium by increasing force of contraction (4,6,7,11,406), lengthening the refractory period (7,406), reducing peripheral vascular resistance (18,406), reducing oxygen consumption (406), and increasing nerve conductivity (406).

Researchers think the constituent flavonoids and oligomeric procyanidins increase coronary blood flow due to vasodilation (18). They attribute hawthorn's cardiotrophic properties to increased membrane permeability for calcium and phosphodiesterase inhibition that increases intracellular cAMP. Increased cAMP leads to increased coronary blood flow, vasodilation, and positive inotropic effects (150). Hawthorn has also been reported to decrease uterine tone and motility and reduce lipid levels. It also has antibacterial, spasmolytic, and analgesic effects (11).

Adverse Reactions

Orally, hawthorn preparations can cause nausea, gastrointestinal complaints (4,406), fatigue, sweating, rash on hands (4), palpitations, headache, dizziness, sleeplessness, agitation, and circulatory disturbances (406) when used in therapeutic doses. Some German clinicians prefer hawthorn over digoxin in mild heart failure because hawthorn is thought to have a wider therapeutic range, lower risk in cases of dosage errors, less arrhythmogenic potential, safer for use in renal impairment (7). However, these potential advantages have not been verified.

Interactions with Herbs & Other Dietary Supplements

CARDIAC GLYCOSIDE-CONTAINING HERBS: Contraindicated; concomitant use may increase the risk of cardiac glycoside toxicity. Cardiac glycoside-containing herbs include black hellebore, Canadian hemp roots, digitalis leaf, hedge mustard, figwort, lily of the valley roots, motherwort, oleander leaf, pheasant's eye plant, pleurisy root, squill bulb leaf scales, and strophanthus seeds (2,18,19,500).

OTHER CARDIOACTIVE HERBS: Avoid concomitant use with other cardioactive herbs due to unpredictability of effects and adverse effects. Other cardioactive herbs include calamus, cereus, cola, coltsfoot, devil's claw, European mistletoe, fenugreek, fumitory, ginger, Panax ginseng, white horehound, mate, parsley, quassia, scotch broom flower, shepherd's purse, and wild carrot (4). See individual product listings.

Interactions with Drugs

CARDIOVASCULAR DRUGS: Hawthorn might potentiate or interfere with conventional drug therapy for heart failure, hypertension, angina, and arrhythmias (4,12).

CNS DEPRESSANTS: Concomitant use of hawthorn and CNS depressants might have additive CNS depressant effects (4,406).

CORONARY VASODILATORS: Using hawthorn with theophylline, caffeine, papaverine, sodium nitrate, adenosine, epinephrine, and other coronary vasodilators might cause additive vasodilatory effects (406).

DIGOXIN: Concomitant use of hawthorn and digoxin might potentiate digoxin effects requiring digoxin dose reduction (12,406).

Interactions with Foods

No interactions are known to occur, and there is no known reason to expect a clinically significant interaction with hawthorn.

Interactions with Lab Tests

No interactions are known to occur, and there is no known reason to expect a clinically significant interaction with hawthorn.

Interactions with Diseases or Conditions

CARDIOVASCULAR CONDITIONS: Concomitant use of hawthorn with conventional cardiovascular drug therapy might potentiate or interfere with the treatment of these conditions (4,12).

Dosage and Administration

ORAL: Dried hawthorn fruit powder 300-1000 mg is taken orally three times daily or as a prepared tea after meals (4,406). To make tea, pour hot water over a teaspoon of hawthorn leaves and flowers, steep for 20 minutes, and strain (8). Hawthorn fruit liquid extract (1:1 in 25% alcohol) 0.5-1 mL is taken three times daily (4,406). Hawthorn fruit tincture (1:5 in 45% alcohol) 1-2 mL is taken three times daily (4,406). Hawthorn fruit syrup is taken as 1 teaspoon two to three times daily (406). A hawthorn fruit solid extract is used in doses of 1/4 to 1/2 teaspoon (1.7-3.3 mL) daily (406). Hawthorn leaf is used as a water extract, a water-alcohol extract, wine tea, and fresh juice (2). A powder of the leaf and flower 200-500 mg is taken three times daily (406). Twenty drops of the leaf and flower tincture is given 2-3 times daily. Hawthorn leaf with flower extract 160-900 mg (3.5-19.8 mg of total flavonoids calculated as hyperoside or 30-160 mg of procyanidins) is divided and taken 2-3 times daily (2,406).

Comments

None.

HAY FLOWER

Also Known As

Cat's Tails, Common Couch, Foxtails, Graminis Flos, Grass Flower, Hay Sack, Hayflower, Kniepp Hay Sack, Lop Grass, Meadow Fescue, Perennial Rye-Grass, Rock's-Foot, Sweet Vernal Grass, Timothy.
CAUTION: See separate listing for Sweet Clover.

Scientific Names

Elymus repens; Anthoxantum odoratum; Lolium perenne; Bromus hordeaceus; Festuca pratensis; Phleum species; Alopecurus species; Dactylis species.
Family: Poaceae.

People Use This For

Topically, hay flower is used as heat therapy for degenerative disorders, including arthritis (2). It is used as a bath additive for musculoskeletal and joint disorders (9).
In folk medicine, hay flower has been used as a bath additive for rheumatic conditions, lumbago, chilblains, and neurasthenia. It has also been used as an inhalant for inflammatory conditions of the respiratory tract (8).

Safety

POSSIBLY SAFE ...when used topically (2).
PREGNANCY AND LACTATION: Insufficient reliable information available; avoid using.

Effectiveness

POSSIBLY EFFECTIVE ...when used topically as heat therapy for degenerative diseases such as arthritis (2).
There is insufficient reliable information available about the effectiveness of hay flower for its other uses.

Mechanism of Action

The applicable parts of hay flower are the fruit, flower, and above ground parts. Applied topically as a heat pack, hay flower produces moist heat (1517) and promotes local blood flow (2). It can also influence internal organs through cuti-visceral reflexes (2). Hay flower contains coumarins and furanocoumarins, which are thought to have a mild sedative effect when inhaled (8,1518).

Adverse Reactions

Topically, rare skin reactions and hay fever have occurred with the use of hay flower (2,8).
CAUTION: Avoid overheating the topical preparations in order to prevent burns.

Interactions with Herbs & Other Dietary Supplements

Insufficient reliable information available.

Interactions with Drugs

No interactions are known to occur, and there is no known reason to expect a clinically significant interaction with hay flower.

Interactions with Foods

No interactions are known to occur, and there is no known reason to expect a clinically significant interaction with hay flower.

Interactions with Lab Tests

No interactions are known to occur, and there is no known reason to expect a clinically significant interaction with hay flower.

Interactions with Diseases or Conditions

No interactions are known to occur, and there is no known reason to expect a clinically significant interaction with hay flower.

Dosage and Administration

TOPICAL: For use as a flower bag, one hay flower bag is commonly heated to 42 degrees C (108 degrees F) and applied directly to the affected area once or twice per day for 40-50 minutes (2). Avoid overheating the flower bag in order to prevent burns. As a bath additive, 500 grams of hay flower is typically boiled in 3-4 L, or about one gallon, of water for 1 minute, steeped for 30 minutes, strained, and then added to one normal bath. The individual usually bathes in the water for a maximum of 15 minutes followed by one hour bed rest (8).

INHALATION: The vapors from 5-10 grams of hay flower (1 teaspoon is approximately 2.3 grams) in one liter of boiling water is commonly inhaled (8). Remove from heat before inhaling and handle with care to prevent burns.

Comments
Hay flower includes parts of various plants sieved from cut hay grasses, and its composition varies widely (8).

HAZELNUT

Also Known As
Aveleira, Avelinier, Avellano, Cobnut, Coudrier, European Filbert, European Hazel, Haselnuss, Haselstrauch, Hazel, Hazel Nut, Noisetier.

Scientific Names
Corylus avellana; Corylus heterophylla
FAMILY: Betulaceae; Corylaceae.

People Use This For
Orally, hazelnut oil is used to reduce cholesterol and as an antioxidant (5992).
Hazelnuts are commonly consumed as food.

Safety
LIKELY SAFE ...when ingested in food amounts.
PREGNANCY AND LACTATION: LIKELY SAFE ...when used in amounts commonly found in foods. There is insufficient reliable information available about the safety of the use of hazelnut in larger amounts; avoid using.

Effectiveness
There is insufficient reliable information available about the effectiveness of hazelnut.

Mechanism of Action
Hazelnuts contain 54.6-63.2% oil, 14.3-18.2% protein, and 9.8%-13.2% fiber (5995). Preliminary information suggests hazelnut oil and beta-carotene together might increase aminopyrine-N-dimethylase activity in the cytochrome P-450 system (5599).

Adverse Reactions
Orally, hazelnut can cause an allergic reaction in sensitive individuals (5991). When ingested orally, hazelnut has been associated with exercise-induced anaphylactic reaction (5998) and one outbreak of botulism from contaminated yogurt (5999).

Interactions with Herbs & Other Dietary Supplements
Insufficient reliable information available.

Interactions with Drugs
No interactions are known to occur, and there is no known reason to expect a clinically significant interaction with hazelnut.

Interactions with Foods
No interactions are known to occur, and there is no known reason to expect a clinically significant interaction with hazelnut.

Interactions with Lab Tests
No interactions are known to occur, and there is no known reason to expect a clinically significant interaction with hazelnut.

Interactions with Diseases or Conditions
Hazelnut is believed to be cross reactive with peanuts (5991), mugwort pollen (5993), brazil nut (5994), birch pollen (5996), and macadamia nut (5997).

Dosage and Administration

No typical dosage.

Comments

None.

HEART'S EASE

Also Known As

European Wild Pansy, Field Pansy, Hearts Ease, Heartsease, Johnny-Jump-Up, Ladies' Delight, Pansy, Pensee Sauvage, Viola, Violae Tricoloris Herba, Wild Pansy.

Scientific Names

Viola tricolor.
Family: Violaceae.

People Use This For

Orally, heart's ease is used for promoting metabolism, as a demulcent for respiratory disorders such as throat inflammation and whooping cough, and as a laxative (18,400).

Topically, heart's ease is used for mild seborrheic skin disorders, milk scall (seborrhea of the scalp) in children, warts, mild skin inflammation, acne, exanthema (skin eruption), eczema, impetigo, and itching of the female external genitalia (2,400).

Safety

POSSIBLY SAFE ...when appropriately used for oral or topical medicinal purposes (2,12).
PREGNANCY AND LACTATION: Insufficient reliable information; avoid using.

Effectiveness

There is insufficient reliable information available about the effectiveness of heart's ease.

Mechanism of Action

The applicable parts of heart's ease are the above ground parts. Heart's ease can have anti-inflammatory and antioxidant properties (18).

Adverse Reactions

None reported.

Interactions with Herbs & Other Dietary Supplements

Insufficient reliable information available.

Interactions with Drugs

No interactions are known to occur, and there is no known reason to expect a clinically significant interaction with heart's ease.

Interactions with Foods

No interactions are known to occur, and there is no known reason to expect a clinically significant interaction with heart's ease.

Interactions with Lab Tests

No interactions are known to occur, and there is no known reason to expect a clinically significant interaction with heart's ease.

Interactions with Diseases or Conditions

No interactions are known to occur, and there is no known reason to expect a clinically significant interaction with heart's ease.

Dosage and Administration

ORAL: The typical dose of heart's ease is one cup of the tea three times per day (18). The tea is prepared by steeping 1.5 grams of the above ground parts in 150 mL boiling water for 5-10 minutes and then straining.
TOPICAL: Heart's ease is commonly applied externally three times per day as a poultice or the prepared tea (18).

Comments

Store heart's ease in a well-sealed container and away from light (18).

HEATHER

Also Known As

Callunae vulgaris herba, Calluna vulgaris flos, Ling, Scotch Heather.

Scientific Names

Calluna vulgaris.
Family: Ericaceae.

People Use This For

Orally, heather is taken for ailments of the kidney and lower urinary tract, prostate enlargement, diuresis, gastrointestinal ailments and diseases, diarrhea, gastrointestinal spasm, colic, disease of the liver and gallbladder, gout, arthritis, sleep disorders, respiratory disorders, cough, colds, and diaphoresis (2,18).
Topically, heather is used for wounds and inflamed eyes (2).
In combination with other herbs, heather is used for diabetes, menstrual discomfort, menopause, stimulation of digestion, nervous exhaustion, and regulation of the circulatory system (2).

Safety

POSSIBLY SAFE ...when used orally or topically and appropriately (12).
PREGNANCY AND LACTATION: Insufficient reliable information available; avoid using.

Effectiveness

There is insufficient reliable information available about the effectiveness of heather.

Mechanism of Action

The applicable parts of heather are the flower, leaf, and plant top. There is insufficient reliable information available about the possible mechanism of action and active ingredients.

Adverse Reactions

None reported.

Interactions with Herbs & Other Dietary Supplements

Insufficient reliable information available.

Interactions with Drugs

No interactions are known to occur, and there is no known reason to expect a clinically significant interaction with heather.

Interactions with Foods

No interactions are known to occur, and there is no known reason to expect a clinically significant interaction with heather.

Interactions with Lab Tests

No interactions are known to occur, and there is no known reason to expect a clinically significant interaction with heather.

Interactions with Diseases or Conditions

No interactions are known to occur, and there is no known reason to expect a clinically significant interaction with heather.

Dosage and Administration

ORAL: One cup of tea (simmer 1.5 grams of flower/leaf/plant top in 250 mL boiling water 3 minutes, strain) three times daily between meals (18).
TOPICAL: As a bath, 500 grams of flower/leaf/plant top in a few liters of water, strain and add to full bath (18).

Comments

None.

HEDGE MUSTARD

Also Known As
English Watercress, Erysimum, Singer's Plant, St. Barbara's Hedge Mustard, Thalictroc.
CAUTION: See separate listings for White Mustard, Black Mustard seed, and Black Mustard Oil.

Scientific Names
Sisymbrium officinale, synonym Erysimum officinale.
Family: Brassicaceae.

People Use This For
Orally, hedge mustard is taken to treat urinary tract diseases, coughs, chronic bronchitis, and inflammation of the gallbladder [18].
Topically, it is used as a gargle or mouthwash [18].

Safety
LIKELY UNSAFE ...when the flowering above ground parts are taken orally since they contain cardioactive glycosides [18].
There is insufficient reliable information available about the safety of hedge mustard for its other uses.
PREGNANCY AND LACTATION: LIKELY UNSAFE ...when used orally; avoid using.

Effectiveness
There is insufficient reliable information available about the effectiveness of hedge mustard.

Mechanism of Action
The applicable parts of hedge mustard are the above ground parts. The foliage contains vitamin C and 0.05% cardenolides (cardioactive glycosides) including sinigrin and gluconapin. Hedge mustard also contains the volatile mustard oil allyl isothiocyanate and 3-butenylisothiocyanate [18].

Adverse Reactions
Theoretically, digitalis-like effects are possible (vomiting, diarrhea, headache, and cardiac rhythm disorders) [18].

Interactions with Herbs & Other Dietary Supplements
CARDIAC GLYCOSIDE-CONTAINING HERBS: Contraindicated, and concomitant use can increase the risk of cardiac glycoside toxicity. Cardiac glycoside-containing herbs include black hellebore, Canadian hemp root, digitalis leaf, figwort, lily of the valley root, motherwort, oleander leaf, pheasant's eye plant, pleurisy root, squill bulb leaf scale, strophanthus seed, and uzara [2,18,19,500].
OTHER CARDIOACTIVE HERBS: Avoid concomitant use with other cardioactive herbs due to unpredictability of effects [4].
STIMULANT LAXATIVE HERBS: Theoretically, overuse or misuse of stimulant laxatives with cardiac glycoside-containing herbs increases the risk of cardiac toxicity due to potassium depletion [19].
LICORICE/HORSETAIL: Theoretically, overuse/misuse of licorice rhizome or horsetail plant with cardiac glycoside-containing herbs increases the risk of cardiac toxicity due to potassium depletion [19].

Interactions with Drugs
DIGOXIN: Contraindicated; concomitant use increases risk of cardiac glycoside toxicity [2].
CARDIAC DRUGS: Theoretically, concomitant may increase risk of cardiac toxicity [152].
STIMULANT LAXATIVES: Theoretically, overuse/misuse may increase risk of cardiac glycoside toxicity due to potassium depletion [2].
POTASSIUM-DEPLETING DIURETICS: Theoretically, concomitant use may increase risk of cardiac glycoside toxicity due to potassium depletion [2,506].
QUININE: Theoretically, concomitant use may increase risk of cardiac toxicity [2,506].
TETRACYCLINES AND MACROLIDE ANTIBIOTICS: Theoretically, concomitant use may increase risk of cardiac glycoside toxicity [152,17].

Interactions with Foods
No interactions are known to occur, and there is no known reason to expect a clinically significant interaction with hedge mustard.

Interactions with Lab Tests

No interactions are known to occur, and there is no known reason to expect a clinically significant interaction with hedge mustard.

Interactions with Diseases or Conditions

HEART DISEASE: Contraindicated; theoretically, cardiac glycosides contained in hedge mustard may exacerbate condition or interfere with existing drug therapy.

Dosage and Administration

ORAL: One cup tea (preparation unspecified) 3-4 times daily (18); average amount is 0.5-1 grams above ground parts per day (18).
TOPICAL: Tea is used as a mouthwash or gargle, several times daily (18).

Comments

Avoid confusion with black mustard (Brassica nigra), brown mustard (Brassica juncea), white mustard (Brassica alba or Sinapis alba), Indian mustard (Brassica juncea), and Chinese mustard (Sinapis juncea).

HEDGE-HYSSOP

Also Known As

Gratiola, Hedge Hyssop.

Scientific Names

Gratiola officinalis.
Family: Scrophulariaceae.

People Use This For

In folk medicine, people used hedge-hyssop orally for treating the liver, as an emetic, and to induce bowel evacuation. It has also been used in the elimination of intestinal parasites, and to increase urination (18).

Safety

UNSAFE ...when taken orally (18).
PREGNANCY AND LACTATION: UNSAFE ...when used orally due to toxic potential (18).

Effectiveness

There is insufficient reliable information available about the effectiveness of hedge-hyssop.

Mechanism of Action

The applicable parts of hedge-hyssop are the above ground parts. Hedge-hyssop contains cucurbitacin glycosides which are released in aqueous environments and are extremely irritating to mucous membranes (18).

Adverse Reactions

Orally, taken in toxic doses, hedge-hyssop may cause vomiting, bloody diarrhea, colic, and kidney irritation characterized by initial diuresis followed by anuria. When people ingest very large amounts, spasms, paralysis, and circulatory collapse occur. Death occurs rarely (18).

Interactions with Herbs & Other Dietary Supplements

Insufficient reliable information available.

Interactions with Drugs

No interactions are known to occur, and there is no known reason to expect a clinically significant interaction with hedge-hyssop.

Interactions with Foods

No interactions are known to occur, and there is no known reason to expect a clinically significant interaction with hedge-hyssop.

Interactions with Lab Tests

No interactions are known to occur, and there is no known reason to expect a clinically significant interaction with hedge-hyssop.

Interactions with Diseases or Conditions
No interactions are known to occur, and there is no known reason to expect a clinically significant interaction with hedge-hyssop.

Dosage and Administration
No typical dosage.

Comments
None.

HEMLOCK

Also Known As
California Fern, Carrot Weed, Conium, Conium maculata, Nebraska Fern, Poison Fool's Parsley, Poison-Hemlock, Spotted Hemlock, Wild Carrot.
CAUTION: See separate listings for Water Hemlock and Hemlock Water Dropwort.

Scientific Names
Conium maculatum.
Family: Umbelliferae.

People Use This For
Orally, hemlock is used as a sedative, antispasmodic (33,6342), and paralyzer (6342). It is also used orally for nervous motor excitability, teething in children, cramps, spasms of the larnyx and gullet, acute mania, bronchitis, whooping cough, asthma, and as an antidote to strychnine poisoning (6342).
Historically, hemlock has been used for the bite of a mad dog, indolent tumors, swollen joints, painful joints, skin infections (6342), epilepsy, Parkinson's disease, Sydenham's chorea, and acute cystitis (33).

Safety
UNSAFE ...when taken orally (6338). All parts of hemlock including seeds, flowers, and fruits are considered poisonous (6338,6339). Death has resulted after ingestion of hemlock (6340). Prompt medical attention is advised after ingestion of hemlock (6341).
CHILDREN: UNSAFE ...when taken orally (6340). Acute, sometimes lethal poisoning has resulted after ingestion of leaf material (6340) or when hollow stems are used as peashooters, flutes or whistles (6338).
PREGNANCY AND LACTATION: UNSAFE ...when taken orally (6338). Ingestion can be lethal; avoid using (6338).

Effectiveness
There is insufficient reliable information available about the effectiveness of hemlock.

Mechanism of Action
All plant parts of hemlock can cause toxicity. Coniceine and coniine are the alkaloids in hemlock which account for its toxicity (6338,6340,6341). The amount of poisonous alkaloids in hemlock increase as the plant and fruit ripens and is also dependent on the amount of solar exposure and soil moisture (6338). It is most toxic during early stages of growth in the spring (6338,6339). Green fruit contains larger amounts of toxic alkaloids than mature fruit and seeds. The amount of toxic alkaloids in hemlock decreases as the plant reaches maturity (6338). Coniine predominates in the plant during sunny dry weather. During cloudy and rainy weather, coniine and coniceine are produced in equal amounts in hemlock (6339). Coniceine predominates during early growth periods of hemlock and coniine predominates in mature hemlock plants and seeds (6339). The alkaloid's effects occur at the neuromuscular junction of the autonomic ganglia (6341), stimulating and then paralyzing nicotinic receptors (6340). Larger doses of the alkaloids produce narcotic-like depressant activity (6340). Death usually occurs by respiratory failure (6341).

Adverse Reactions
Orally, hemlock can cause salivation; burning of the mouth, throat and abdomen (6341); drowsiness (6340); mydriasis (6341); muscle pain; rapid swelling and stiffening of muscles (6340); tachycardia followed by bradycardia; loss of speech; paralysis; rhabdomyolysis (6341); unconsciousness; cardiovascular collapse; and death (6340).

Interactions with Herbs & Other Dietary Supplements
Insufficient reliable information available.

Interactions with Drugs

No interactions are known to occur, and there is no known reason to expect a clinically significant interaction with hemlock.

Interactions with Foods

No interactions are known to occur, and there is no known reason to expect a clinically significant interaction with hemlock.

Interactions with Lab Tests

No interactions are known to occur, and there is no known reason to expect a clinically significant interaction with hemlock.

Interactions with Diseases or Conditions

No interactions are known to occur, and there is no known reason to expect a clinically significant interaction with hemlock.

Dosage and Administration

No typical dosage.

Comments

Hemlock is native to Europe and western Asia and was introduced into North America as an ornamental plant (6338,6339,6341). It is frequently found in the United States and southern Canada (6338). Hemlock is found along fences, in modified soils, roadsides, ditches, abandoned construction sites, pastures, crops, and fields (6338,6341). Hemlock can remain in a vegetative state throughout the winter (6338,6339) and accidental ingestion occurs after mistaking the root for parsnip, leaves for parsley, and seeds for anise (6338,6344). Poisoning and death have been reported after human consumption of migratory wild birds that have eaten hemlock seeds. (6338,6340).

HEMLOCK SPRUCE

Also Known As

Balm of Gilead Fir, Balsam Fir, Canada Balsam, Fir Tree, Norway Pine, Norway Spruce, Picea aetheroleum, Picea turiones recentes, Spruce, Spruce Fir.

Scientific Names

Picea excelsa, synonym Picea abies; Abies excelsa.
Family: Coniferae.

People Use This For

Orally, hemlock spruce is used for coughs, the common cold, bronchitis, fever, inflammation of the mouth and pharynx, muscular and nerve pain, arthritis, and as an antibacterial.
Topically, it is used for inflammation of the respiratory tract, arthritis pain, nerve pain, and for feelings of tension. Hemlock spruce is also used externally as a counterirritant and to improve circulation.
In folk medicine, it was used orally for tuberculosis and topically as a bath additive for individuals who were mentally ill (18).

Safety

There is insufficient reliable information available about the safety of hemlock spruce.
Pregnancy and Lactation: Insufficient reliable information available; avoid using.

Effectiveness

There is insufficient reliable information available about the effectiveness of hemlock spruce.

Mechanism of Action

The applicable part of hemlock spruce is the oil obtained by steam distillation from the needles, branch tips or branches and the fresh fir shoots of Picea excelsa (18). There is insufficient reliable information available about the possible mechanism of action and active ingredients.

Adverse Reactions

None reported.

Interactions with Herbs & Other Dietary Supplements
Insufficient reliable information available.

Interactions with Drugs
No interactions are known to occur, and there is no known reason to expect a clinically significant interaction with hemlock spruce.

Interactions with Foods
No interactions are known to occur, and there is no known reason to expect a clinically significant interaction with hemlock spruce.

Interactions with Lab Tests
No interactions are known to occur, and there is no known reason to expect a clinically significant interaction with hemlock spruce.

Interactions with Diseases or Conditions
ASTHMA AND WHOOPING COUGH: Hemlock spruce may theoretically worsen asthma and whooping cough (18).
EXTENSIVE SKIN INJURIES, ACUTE SKIN DISEASES: Hemlock spruce should not be applied to broken skin (18).
CARDIAC INSUFFICIENCY: Avoid using of hemlock spruce (18).

Dosage and Administration
ORAL: The typical daily dose is 4 drops of oil on a lump of sugar taken three times daily. Alternately, 2 grams of oil can be added to hot water and inhaled several times daily (18).
TOPICAL: Hemlock spruce is used as a 10-50% semi-solid preparation. Several drops of this oil are rubbed into the affected area (18).

Comments
Hemlock spruce is very similar sounding to water hemlock and European water hemlock, which are entirely different plants. Be careful not to confuse hemlock spruce with either form of water hemlock, because the water hemlocks are very toxic (see separate listings) (18).

HEMLOCK WATER DROPWORT

Also Known As
Dead Tongue, Five-Fingered Root, Horsebane, Yellow Water Dropwort.
CAUTION: See separate listings for Water Hemlock and Hemlock.

Scientific Names
Oenanthe crocata.
Family: Umbelliferae.

People Use This For
Topically, hemlock water dropwort is used as a poultice for skin eruptions (6333).

Safety
UNSAFE ...when used orally (6334). Ingestion of very small amounts of root may be fatal (6335,6337). Accidental ingestion requires prompt medical attention (6334).
There is insufficient reliable information available about the safety of hemlock water dropwort when used topically.
CHILDREN: UNSAFE ...when used orally (6334). Poisoning has occurred after accidental ingestion of roots or tubers (6334).
PREGNANCY AND LACTATION: UNSAFE ...when used orally (6334). Ingestion can be lethal; avoid using (6334).

Effectiveness
There is insufficient reliable information available about the effectiveness of hemlock water dropwort.

Mechanism of Action
The applicable part of hemlock water dropwort is the root. Oenanthetoxin, a highly unsaturated alcohol (6334), is the active principle toxin found in hemlock water dropwort (6332). The roots of hemlock water dropwort are considered to

be the most poisonous part of the plant and the toxin is contained in a yellowish staining juice of the root (6334). The toxin is unstable when exposed to air and is chemically similar to cicutoxin found in water hemlock (Cicuta virosa) (6334). The exact mechanism of action of the toxin is unknown, but animal studies suggest that oenanthetoxin has an antagonizing effect on nerve impulses in the brain stem (6334).

Adverse Reactions

Orally, hemlock water dropwort can cause nausea, dizziness, (6334), abdominal pain (6335), vomiting, sweating (6332), salivation, weakness, confusion, slurred speech, muscle spasms, tonic-clonic movements, glycosuria, hematuria, hyperventilation, cyanosis, exhaustion (6334), seizures, metabolic acidosis (6335), generalized convulsions (6332), unconsciousness (6334), dilated pupils, and death (6332).

Interactions with Herbs & Other Dietary Supplements

Insufficient reliable information available.

Interactions with Drugs

No interactions are known to occur, and there is no known reason to expect a clinically significant interaction with hemlock water dropwort.

Interactions with Foods

No interactions are known to occur, and there is no known reason to expect a clinically significant interaction with hemlock water dropwort.

Interactions with Lab Tests

No interactions are known to occur, and there is no known reason to expect a clinically significant interaction with hemlock water dropwort.

Interactions with Diseases or Conditions

No interactions are known to occur, and there is no known reason to expect a clinically significant interaction with hemlock water dropwort.

Dosage and Administration

No typical dosage.

Comments

Hemlock water dropwort is commonly found in ditches, watering places (6333), marshy areas and banks (6334) in southwest England (6333,6337) and western France (6337). It is considered to be the most poisonous plant in the British Isles (6334). Hemlock water dropwort has been accidentally ingested after mistaking the tuber for wild parsnip, sweet flag or pignut (6334,6337).

HEMP AGRIMONY

Also Known As

Alpenkraut, Chanvrin, Donnerkraut, Dostenkraut, Drachenkraut, Dutch Agrimony, Dutch Eupatoire Commune, Eupatorium, Gemeiner Wasswedost, Herbe de Sainte Cunegonde, Hirshklee, Holy Rope, Kunigundendraut, Leberkraut, Origan De Marais, St. John's Herb, Sweet Mandulin, Sweet-Smelling Trefoil, Thoroughwort, Wasshanf, Waterhemp, Water Maudlin.

Scientific Names

Eupatorium cannabinum.
Family: Compositae.

People Use This For

Orally, hemp agrimony is used for liver and gallbladder disorders, colds, and fever (18).

Safety

LIKELY UNSAFE ...when used orally. Hemp agrimony contains hepatotoxic unsaturated pyrrolizidine alkaloids (UPAs) (12,19). Repeated exposure to low concentrations of UPAs are linked to veno-occlusive disease, a serious condition (4,12). UPAs may also be carcinogenic and mutagenic (12). ...when used topically on abraded or broken skin due to potential for systemic absorption (12,19).

PREGNANCY: UNSAFE ...when used orally; contraindicated due to possible menstrual stimulant and abortifacient activities (19).
LACTATION: LIKELY UNSAFE ...when used orally due to concern that UPAs might be excreted into breast milk (19).

Effectiveness
There is insufficient reliable information available about the effectiveness of hemp agrimony.

Mechanism of Action
The applicable part of hemp agrimony is the flowering herb. Some pyrrolizidine alkaloids have shown carcinogenic and mutagenic properties, and there are reports of renal toxicity. However, the primary concern is veno-occlusive disease (12). Unsaturated pyrrolizidine alkaloids are known to be hepatotoxic in animals and humans (4).

Adverse Reactions
When used orally, acute toxicity may result in hepatic necrosis; chronic toxicity may cause veno-occlusive liver disease. The potential for hepatotoxicity (due to presence of pyrrolizidine alkaloids) increases with larger doses and longer periods of use (4,12). It can cause an allergic reaction in individuals sensitive to the Asteraceae/Compositae family. Members of this family include ragweed, chrysanthemums, marigolds, daisies, and many other herbs.

Interactions with Herbs & Other Dietary Supplements
EUCALYPTUS: Theoretically, concomitant use might increase the risk of unsaturated pyrrolizidine alkaloid toxicity due to enzyme induction by eucalyptus (19).
PYRROLIZIDINE ALKALOID-CONTAINING HERBS: Concomitant use is contraindicated due to the risk of additive toxicity. Herbs containing unsaturated pyrrolizidine alkaloids include: alkanna (12), borage (271), gravel root (4), hemp agrimony (271), hound's tongue (19), petasites (19), comfrey (271), coltsfoot, and the Senecio species plants; dusty miller (19), alpine ragwort (19), groundsel (271), golden ragwort (19), and tansy ragwort (271).

Interactions with Drugs
No interactions are known to occur, and there is no known reason to expect a clinically significant interaction with hemp agrimony.

Interactions with Foods
No interactions are known to occur, and there is no known reason to expect a clinically significant interaction with hemp agrimony.

Interactions with Lab Tests
No interactions are known to occur, and there is no known reason to expect a clinically significant interaction with hemp agrimony.

Interactions with Diseases or Conditions
CROSS-ALLERGENICITY: Can cause an allergic reaction in individuals sensitive to the Asteraceae/Compositae family. Members of this family include ragweed, chrysanthemums, marigolds, daisies, and many other herbs.

Dosage and Administration
No typical dosage.

Comments
None.

HEMPNETTLE

Also Known As
Galeopsidis Herba.

Scientific Names
Galeopsis segetum, synonym Galeopsis ochroleuca.
Family: Lamiaceae.

People Use This For
Orally, hempnettle is used for mild respiratory tract inflammation (2), cough, and bronchitis (18). Traditionally, it has been used for pulmonary afflictions and as a diuretic (18).

Safety
POSSIBLY SAFE ...when used orally and appropriately (2).
PREGNANCY AND LACTATION: Insufficient reliable information available; avoid using.

Effectiveness
POSSIBLY EFFECTIVE ...when used orally for mild respiratory tract inflammation (2). There is insufficient reliable information available about the effectiveness of hempnettle for its other uses.

Mechanism of Action
The applicable parts of hempnettle are the above ground parts. Hempnettle can have astringent and expectorant effects (18).

Adverse Reactions
None reported.

Interactions with Herbs & Other Dietary Supplements
Insufficient reliable information available.

Interactions with Drugs
No interactions are known to occur, and there is no known reason to expect a clinically significant interaction with hempnettle.

Interactions with Foods
No interactions are known to occur, and there is no known reason to expect a clinically significant interaction with hempnettle.

Interactions with Lab Tests
No interactions are known to occur, and there is no known reason to expect a clinically significant interaction with hempnettle.

Interactions with Diseases or Conditions
No interactions are known to occur, and there is no known reason to expect a clinically significant interaction with hempnettle.

Dosage and Administration
ORAL: The typical dose of hempnettle is 6 grams of the above ground parts per day or one cup of the tea up to three times daily. The tea is prepared by steeping 2 grams of the above ground parts in 150 mL boiling water for 5-10 minutes and then straining (18). The use of hempnettle in children requires a dosing adjustment; however, no additional information is available on the exact dosing adjustments (510).

Comments
None.

HENBANE

Also Known As
Devil's Eye, Fetid Nightshade, Hen Bell, Hog Bean, Hyoscyami Folium, Jupiter's Bean, Poison Tobacco, Stinking Nightshade.
CAUTION: See separate listings for Belladonna and Bittersweet Nightshade.

Scientific Names
Hyoscyamus niger.
Family: Solanaceae.

People Use This For
Orally, henbane leaf is used for spasms of the gastrointestinal tract (2).
Topically, the leaf oil is used for treating scar tissue (18).

Safety
POSSIBLY SAFE ...when the leaf is used orally and appropriately short-term under medical supervision (2). Contains hyoscyamine and scopolamine alkaloids (2).
LIKELY UNSAFE ...when used orally for self-medication. Hyoscyamine and scopolamine have a narrow range of safe use. Excessive doses can cause poisoning and death (18).
There is insufficient reliable information available about the safety of henbane for its other uses.
PREGNANCY AND LACTATION: LIKELY UNSAFE ...contraindicated for oral use because of its risk of poisoning (18).

Effectiveness
POSSIBLY EFFECTIVE ...when taken orally for spasms of the GI tract (2).
There is insufficient reliable information available about the effectiveness of henbane for its other uses.

Mechanism of Action
The applicable part of henbane is the leaf. The alkaloid constituents, which include hyoscyamine and scopolamine, competitively inhibit acetylcholine, causing anticholinergic and parasympathetic effects (18). With storage, hyoscyamine converts to atropine. The inhibition of acetylcholine affects the muscarinic action but not the nicotinic effects of acetylcholine on ganglia and motor endplates. Henbane causes smooth muscle relaxation particularly in the GI tract, relieves muscle tremors of CNS origin, and has a sedative effect (2).

Adverse Reactions
Orally, henbane can cause dry mouth, red skin, constipation, overheating, reduced sweating, vision disturbances, tachycardia, and difficulty with urinating (2,18). Overdose poisoning symptoms include somnolence followed by CNS stimulation described as restlessness, hallucinations, delirium, and manic episodes followed by exhaustion and sleep. Henbane can cause death by asphyxiation (18).

Interactions with Herbs & Other Dietary Supplements
ANTICHOLINERGIC CONTAINING HERBS: Theoretically, concomitant use of henbane with other anticholinergic alkaloid-containing herbs, including belladonna, deadly nightshade, and jimson weed, can have additive therapeutic and adverse effects.

Interactions with Drugs
ANTICHOLINERGIC DRUGS: Concomitant use of henbane can have additive anticholinergic effects and adverse effects with amantadine, antihistamines, atropine, belladonna alkaloids, hyoscyamine, phenothiazines, procainamide, scopolamine, and tricyclic antidepressants (2).

Interactions with Foods
No interactions are known to occur, and there is no known reason to expect a clinically significant interaction with henbane.

Interactions with Lab Tests
No interactions are known to occur, and there is no known reason to expect a clinically significant interaction with henbane.

Interactions with Diseases or Conditions
CONGESTIVE HEART FAILURE (CHF): Contraindicated; henbane might cause tachycardia and exacerbate CHF due to its hyoscyamine (atropine) and scopolamine content (15).
CONSTIPATION: Contraindicated; henbane might cause constipation due to its hyoscyamine (atropine) and scopolamine content (15).
DOWN SYNDROME: Caution, patients with Down syndrome might be hypersensitive to the antimuscarinic effects (mydriasis, positive chronotropic heart effects, etc.) of hyoscyamine (atropine) and scopolamine contained in henbane (15).
ESOPHAGEAL REFLUX: Contraindicated; henbane might delay gastric emptying and decrease lower esophageal pressure, promoting gastric retention and exacerbating reflux due to its hyoscyamine (atropine) and scopolamine content (15).
FEVER: Contraindicated; henbane might increase the risk of hyperthermia in patients with fever due to its hyoscyamine (atropine) and scopolamine content (15).

GASTRIC ULCER: Contraindicated; henbane might delay gastric emptying and exacerbate gastric ulcers due to its hyoscyamine (atropine) and scopolamine content (15).

GI INFECTIONS: Contraindicated; henbane might suppress GI motility causing retention of infecting organisms or toxins due to its hyoscyamine (atropine) and scopolamine content (15).

HIATAL HERNIA: Contraindicated; henbane might delay gastric emptying and decrease lower esophageal pressure, promoting gastric retention and exacerbating hiatal hernia due to its hyoscyamine (atropine) and scopolamine content (15).

TOXIC MEGACOLON: Contraindicated; henbane might suppress intestinal motility, which might produce paralytic ileus and exacerbate toxic megacolon, due to its hyoscyamine (atropine) and scopolamine content (2,15).

NARROW-ANGLE GLAUCOMA: Contraindicated; henbane might increase ocular tension in patients with narrow-angle (angle-closure) glaucoma due to its hyoscyamine (atropine) and scopolamine content (2,15).

OBSTRUCTIVE GI TRACT DISEASE: Contraindicated; henbane might exacerbate obstructive GI tract diseases (including atony, paralytic ileus, and stenosis) due to its hyoscyamine (atropine) and scopolamine content (15).

TACHYARRHYTHMIAS: Contraindicated; henbane might cause tachycardia due to its hyoscyamine (atropine) and scopolamine content (2,15).

URINARY RETENTION: Contraindicated; henbane might increase urinary retention due to its hyoscyamine (atropine) and scopolamine content (2,15).

ULCERATIVE COLITIS: Contraindicated; henbane might suppress intestinal motility, which might produce paralytic ileus and precipitate toxic megacolon, due to its hyoscyamine (atropine) and scopolamine content (15).

Dosage and Administration

ORAL: The average single dose of the standardized henbane powder is 500 mg, which corresponds to 250-350 mg of the total alkaloid (2). The maximum single dose of henbane is 1 gram, which corresponds to 500-700 mg of the total alkaloid (2). The maximum daily dosage is 3 grams, which corresponds to 1.5-2.1 grams of the total alkaloid calculated as hyoscyamine (2).

TOPICAL: No typical dosage.

Comments

Avoid confusion with bittersweet nightshade (Solanum dulcamara) and belladonna (deadly nightshade). The flowering branches, dried seeds, and whole, fresh flowering plant of henbane may have medicinal uses (18).

HENNA

Also Known As

Alcanna, Egyptian Privet, Hennae folium, Henne, Jamaica Mignonette, Mehndi, Mendee, Mignonette Tree, Reseda, Smooth Lawsonia.

CAUTION: See separate listing for Alkanna (Alkanna tinctoria).

Scientific Names

Lawsonia inermis, synonym Lawsonia alba.
Family: Lythraceae.

People Use This For

Orally, henna leaf is used for gastrointestinal ulcers (18).

Topically, it is used for dandruff, eczema, scabies, fungal infections, and ulcers (18). Henna is also used topically for applying decorative henna "tattoos".

Traditionally, henna leaf has been used for amebic dysentery (11,18), cancer, enlarged spleen, headache, jaundice, and skin conditions (11).

In manufacturing, henna is used in cosmetics (18); hair dyes and hair care products (11); and as a dye for nails, hands and clothing (11). Lawsone, a constituent, can be used as an indicator for titration of strong acids with weak bases (11).

Safety

LIKELY SAFE ...when the leaf is used topically. It is approved for topical use as a color additive in hair cosmetics in the US (11). However, contact dermatitis and hypersensitivity reactions have been reported with topical use (1370,4146,4148,6144,6145,6146,6147,6148,6149,6150,6151).

UNSAFE ...when used orally (12).

CHILDREN: POSSIBLY UNSAFE ...when used topically on children, and especially on infants (4147,6144,6149,6150). Use is associated with hemolysis in infants deficient in glucose-6-phosphate dehydrogenase (G6PD) (4147). UNSAFE ...when used orally (12).

PREGNANCY: UNSAFE ...when used orally. Henna is believed to have abortifacient properties (12,19).
LACTATION: UNSAFE ...when used orally (12).

Effectiveness

There is insufficient reliable information available about the effectiveness of henna.

Mechanism of Action

The applicable part of henna is the leaf. Henna leaf contains lawsone, gallic acid and 5-10% tannin (11). It is thought to have astringent and diuretic properties (18). Some evidence suggests henna might have activity against Mycobacterium tuberculosis (4150). In female rats, henna leaves inhibit fertility (11). The constituents, lawsone and gallic acid, have antibacterial properties (11). Studies suggest that lawsone might also have antifungal, antitumor, antispasmodic and weak vitamin K activity (11). Evidence shows it might be able to decrease the formation of sickled cells in individuals with sickle cell anemia (4149). An ethanol extract containing luteolin, beta-sitosterol, and lawsone was claimed to have anti-inflammatory, antihyaluronidase, and analgesic activity (11).

Adverse Reactions

Orally, henna can cause an upset stomach, possibly due to tannin content (18).
Topically, henna can cause contact dermatitis, including redness, itching, burning, swelling, scaling, fissuring, papules, blisters, and scarring (1370,4146,6144,6145,6146,6147,6148,6149,6150). There are two reports of occupational exposure associated with immediate-type hypersensitivity involving urticaria, rhinitis, wheezing, and bronchial asthma (4148,6151). In infants with glucose 6-phosphate dehydrogenase (G6PD) deficiency, topical henna use has been associated with hemolysis, anemia, reticulocytosis, and indirect hyperbilirubinemia (4147). Prolonged use on hair may turn the hair orange-red, unless mixed with other dyes to get different shades (11).

Interactions with Herbs & Other Dietary Supplements

Insufficient reliable information available.

Interactions with Drugs

No interactions are known to occur, and there is no known reason to expect a clinically significant interaction with henna.

Interactions with Foods

No interactions are known to occur, and there is no known reason to expect a clinically significant interaction with henna.

Interactions with Lab Tests

No interactions are known to occur, and there is no known reason to expect a clinically significant interaction with henna.

Interactions with Diseases or Conditions

G6PD DEFICIENCY: There are reports of hemolysis in infants with glucose-6-phosphate dehydrogenase deficiency after topical exposure to henna (4147).
HENNA HYPERSENSITIVITY: Avoid topical exposure by individuals with henna hypersensitivity.

Dosage and Administration

No typical dosage.

Comments

Henna should not be confused with henna root (Alkanna tinctoria), also referred to as alkanna root (6).

HERB PARIS

Also Known As
Einbeere, Herb-Paris, One Berry, Oneberry, Tilki Uzumu, Uva De Raposa, Wang Sun.

Scientific Names
Paris quadrifolia.
Family: Trilliaceae.

People Use This For
Traditionally, Herb Paris has been used for headache; longevity; neuralgia; rheumatism; genital tumors; palpitation; spasms; and as an emetic, narcotic, poison, and purgative.

Safety
LIKELY UNSAFE ...when used orally. The plant and berry are poisonous (18).
PREGNANCY AND LACTATION: UNSAFE ...when used orally (18).

Effectiveness
There is insufficient reliable information available about the effectiveness of Herb Paris.

Mechanism of Action
The applicable part of Herb Paris is the whole plant with ripe fruit. Herb Paris contains triterpene saponins (pennogenintetra glycosides), also referred to as parissaponins, which cause local irritation, increasing absorption of the toxic constituent, paristyphnin (18). Paristyphnin causes miosis and respiratory paralysis (18).

Adverse Reactions
Herb Paris can cause nausea, vomiting, diarrhea, headache, miosis, and respiratory paralysis (18).

Interactions with Herbs & Other Dietary Supplements
Insufficient reliable information available.

Interactions with Drugs
No interactions are known to occur, and there is no known reason to expect a clinically significant interaction with Herb Paris.

Interactions with Foods
No interactions are known to occur, and there is no known reason to expect a clinically significant interaction with Herb Paris.

Interactions with Lab Tests
No interactions are known to occur, and there is no known reason to expect a clinically significant interaction with Herb Paris.

Interactions with Diseases or Conditions
No interactions are known to occur, and there is no known reason to expect a clinically significant interaction with Herb Paris.

Dosage and Administration
No typical dosage.

Comments
None.

HERB ROBERT

Also Known As
Dragon's Blood, Storkbill, Wild Crane's-Bill.
CAUTION: See separate listings for Dragon's Blood (Daemonorops draco) and Sangre de Grado.

Scientific Names
Geranium robertianum.
Family: Geraniaceae.

People Use This For
Orally, Herb Robert is used for diarrhea; to improve functioning of the liver and gallbladder; to reduce inflammation of the kidney, bladder, and gallbladder; and to prevent the formation of calculi (18).
Topically, Herb Robert is used as a mouthwash or gargle and the fresh leaves chewed to relieve inflammation of the mouth and throat (18).

Safety
There is insufficient reliable information available about the safety of Herb Robert.
Pregnancy and Lactation: Insufficient reliable information is available; avoid using.

Effectiveness
There is insufficient reliable information available about the effectiveness of Herb Robert.

Mechanism of Action
The applicable parts of Herb Robert are the above ground parts. Herb Robert contains several flavonoids including rutin. Some evidence suggests an ethanolic extract can inhibit the growth of E. coli, P. aeruginosa, and S. aureus. Other evidence indicates the extract of the fresh herb, including the root, has a mild antiviral effect against the vesicular stomatitis virus (18). Although general reviews report Herb Robert has hypotensive effects, no specific information is available (18). Some data show a crystalline fraction can protect the tobacco plant from pathogenic viruses (18).

Adverse Reactions
None reported.

Interactions with Herbs & Other Dietary Supplements
Insufficient reliable information available.

Interactions with Drugs
No interactions are known to occur, and there is no known reason to expect a clinically significant interaction with Herb Robert.

Interactions with Foods
No interactions are known to occur, and there is no known reason to expect a clinically significant interaction with Herb Robert.

Interactions with Lab Tests
No interactions are known to occur, and there is no known reason to expect a clinically significant interaction with Herb Robert.

Interactions with Diseases or Conditions
No interactions are known to occur, and there is no known reason to expect a clinically significant interaction with Herb Robert.

Dosage and Administration
ORAL: Herb Robert is used as tea, 2 to 3 cups daily between meals (18). To make tea, 1 teaspoon of herb is added to 500 mL of cold water, brought to a boil, allowed to draw, and strained.
TOPICAL: Prepared tea is used as mouthwash or gargle (18). Fresh leaves are chewed to relieve mouth or throat inflammation (18).

Comments
Herb Robert is characterized by an unpleasant smell of goats or bugs (18).

HESPERIDIN

Also Known As
Citrus Bioflavonoid, Citrus Bioflavonoids.
CAUTION: See separate listings for Diosmin, Quercetin, Rue, and Rutin.

Scientific Names
Hesperidin.

People Use This For
Orally, hesperidin is used for treating acute internal hemorrhoids (4861,4900), preventing relapse of acute internal hemorrhoids (4861), and treating varicose veins and venous stasis (4861).

Safety
POSSIBLY SAFE ...when used orally and appropriately, short-term. Hesperidin seems to be safe when used for up to 3 months (4861).
There is insufficient reliable information available about the safety of hesperidin when used for longer than 3 months.
PREGNANCY AND LACTATION: Insufficient reliable information available; avoid using.

Effectiveness
POSSIBLY EFFECTIVE ...when used orally in combination with diosmin for internal hemorrhoids. The combination of hesperidin 150 mg plus diosmin 1350 mg twice daily for 4 days followed by hesperidin 100 mg and diosmin 900 mg twice daily for 3 days seems to significantly improve signs and symptoms of internal hemorrhoids. The combination can stop acute bleeding in up to 92% of patients after 4 days of treatment. It can also reduce symptoms such as anal discomfort, pain, discharge, and local lesions. Subjective symptoms can be relieved within 2 days of treatment. The combination also seems to reduce the duration and intensity of hemorrhoidal flare-ups (4861,4900). ...when used orally in combination with diosmin to prevent relapse in patients with internal hemorrhoids. Maintenance use of hesperidin 50 mg plus diosmin 450 mg twice daily for 3 months in patients following acute treatment for hemorrhoids seems to significantly decrease the relapse rate (4861). Clinical trials have used specific brand name formulations of hesperidin (Daflon 500, Les Laboratoires Servier, France). Each tablet of Daflon 500 contains hesperidin 50 mg and a micronized formulation of diosmin 450 mg extracted from rutaceae species.
There is insufficient reliable information available about the effectiveness of hesperidin for its other uses.

Mechanism of Action
Hesperidin is one of over 4,000 flavonoids found in plants (4919,4959,5006). Hesperidin is in a class of flavonoids primarily derived from citrus fruits and is known as a citrus bioflavonoid. It is closely related to other citrus bioflavonoids such as quercetin, rutin, and diosmin. Hesperidin alone, or in combination with other citrus bioflavonoids, is most often used for vascular conditions such as hemorrhoids and varicose veins. Hesperidin seems to work by improving venous tone, reducing stasis, restoring normal capillary permeability, and improving lymphatic drainage. Hesperidin might improve venous tone and reduce stasis by improving vasculature response to adrenergic stimulation. Hesperidin's anti-inflammatory effects seem to help restore normal capillary permeability. Hesperidin inhibits phosphodiesterase and increases intracellular cyclic adenosine monophosphate (cAMP), which causes decreased production of inflammatory prostaglandins E2 and F2 and thromboxane B2. Hesperidin's analgesic effect seems to work through peripheral rather than central mechanisms. Hesperidin can also reduce the generation of free radicals and inhibit tumor growth (4861,4900,4919,4956).

Adverse Reactions
Orally, hesperidin can cause gastrointestinal side effects, including abdominal pain, diarrhea, and gastritis. Headache can also occur in some patients (4861,4900).

Interactions with Herbs & Other Dietary Supplements
Insufficient reliable information available.

Interactions with Drugs
No interactions are known to occur, and there is no known reason to expect a clinically significant interaction with hesperidin.

Interactions with Foods
No interactions are known to occur, and there is no known reason to expect a clinically significant interaction with hesperidin.

Interactions with Lab Tests

No interactions are known to occur, and there is no known reason to expect a clinically significant interaction with hesperidin.

Interactions with Diseases or Conditions

No interactions are known to occur, and there is no known reason to expect a clinically significant interaction with hesperidin.

Dosage and Administration

ORAL: For the treatment of internal hemorrhoids, hesperidin 150 mg plus diosmin 1350 mg twice daily for 4 days followed by hesperidin 100 mg and diosmin 900 mg twice daily for 3 days has been used (4861,4900). For prevention of relapse internal hemorrhoids hesperidin 50 mg plus diosmin 450 mg twice daily for 3 months of therapy has been used (4861).

Comments

None.

HIBISCUS

Also Known As

Guinea Sorrel, Jamaica Sorrel, Karkade, Red Tea, Roselle, Sudanese Tea.

Scientific Names

Hibiscus sabdariffa.
Family: Malvaceae.

People Use This For

Orally, hibiscus is used for loss of appetite, colds, upper respiratory tract and stomach mucous membrane inflammation, disorders of circulation, for dissolving phlegm, and as a gentle laxative and diuretic (2). Historically, hibiscus was used for treating heart and nerve diseases (11). In foods and beverages, hibiscus is used as a flavoring (11). It is also used to improve the odor, flavor, or appearance of tea mixtures (7).

Safety

LIKELY SAFE ...when used orally in amounts found in beverages (maximum use level 0.02%); approved for use in alcoholic beverages in the US (12).
POSSIBLY SAFE ...when used orally in medicinal amounts (2,12); there are no known risks (2).
PREGNANCY: LIKELY UNSAFE ...when used orally. Hibiscus is thought to be a menstrual stimulant, and might have abortifacient effects (19).
LACTATION: Insufficient reliable information available; avoid using.

Effectiveness

There is insufficient reliable information available about the effectiveness of hibiscus.

Mechanism of Action

The applicable part of hibiscus is the flower. People think the laxative effects of hibiscus are due to high content of poorly absorbable fruit acids (18). Extracts have intestinal and uterine muscle antispasmodic activity (11,18), hypotensive effects (11,18), anthelmintic properties (11), and in vitro antibacterial activity (11).

Adverse Reactions

None reported.

Interactions with Herbs & Other Dietary Supplements

Insufficient reliable information available.

Interactions with Drugs

No interactions are known to occur, and there is no known reason to expect a clinically significant interaction with hibiscus.

Interactions with Foods

No interactions are known to occur, and there is no known reason to expect a clinically significant interaction with hibiscus.

Interactions with Lab Tests

No interactions are known to occur, and there is no known reason to expect a clinically significant interaction with hibiscus.

Interactions with Diseases or Conditions

No interactions are known to occur, and there is no known reason to expect a clinically significant interaction with hibiscus.

Dosage and Administration

ORAL: To prepare tea, steep 1.5 grams of flowers in 150 mL boiling water 5-10 minutes, strain (18).

Comments

None.

HISTIDINE

Also Known As

Levo-Histidine, L-Histidine.

Scientific Names

L-2-Amino-3-(1H-imidazol-4-yl) propionic acid; alpha-amino-4-imidazole propanoic acid.

People Use This For

Orally, histidine is used for rheumatoid arthritis, allergic diseases, ulcers, and anemia (2344,2345,2346).

Safety

POSSIBLY SAFE ...when used orally and appropriately. Clinical studies note the absence of side effects at doses up to 4 grams per day (2347,2353).
PREGNANCY AND LACTATION: Insufficient reliable information available; avoid using.

Effectiveness

POSSIBLY INEFFECTIVE ...when taken orally for treating rheumatoid arthritis (2350,2351), anemia of uremia (2352), or anemia associated with chronic dialysis (2352,2353).
There is insufficient reliable information available about the effectiveness of histidine for its other uses.

Mechanism of Action

Histidine is an essential amino acid involved in a wide range of metabolic processes (2354).

Adverse Reactions

None reported.

Interactions with Herbs & Other Dietary Supplements

Insufficient reliable information available.

Interactions with Drugs

No interactions are known to occur, and there is no known reason to expect a clinically significant interaction with histidine.

Interactions with Foods

No interactions are known to occur, and there is no known reason to expect a clinically significant interaction with histidine.

Interactions with Lab Tests

URINE FORMIMINOGLUTAMIC ACID (FIGLU): Use of histidine in people with folic acid deficiency can cause accumulation of the metabolite formiminoglutamic (2355).

Interactions with Diseases or Conditions

FOLIC ACID DEFICIENCY: Use of histidine in individuals with folic acid deficiency can cause accumulation of the metabolite formiminoglutamic acid (FIGLU) (2355).

Dosage and Administration

ORAL: For rheumatoid arthritis, the usual dose of histidine is 3.7-4.5 grams daily (2347,2350,2351). For anemia of uremia or anemia associated with maintenance dialysis, the typical dose is 1-4 grams daily (2352,2353).

Comments

None.

HOLLY

Also Known As

Christ's Thorn, Holm, Holme Chase, Holy Tree, Hulm, Hulver Bush, Hulver Tree.

Scientific Names

Ilex aquifolium; Ilex opaca; Ilex vomitoria.
Family: Aquifoliaceae.

People Use This For

Orally, preparations of holly leaf are used as a diuretic, for coughs, digestive disorders, and jaundice (18). In Chinese medicine, Ilex aquifolium leaves are used for treating intermittent fevers and rheumatism, as an antipyretic, astringent, diuretic, and expectorant (6). Llex opaca leaves are used as a diuretic, tonic, purgative, and cardiac stimulant (6). Other Ilex species are used for treating coronary heart disease, dizziness, and hypertension (6). Historically, Ilex opaca fruit tea was used as a cardiac stimulant by American Indians (6). Ilex vomitoria was used as an emetic (6), and Youpon tea (mixed leaves of Ilex cassine, Ilex vomitoria, and Ilex dahoon) was used as a ceremonial "cleanser" in South America (6).

Safety

UNSAFE ...when the berries are ingested, poisoning can be fatal (18).
There is insufficient reliable information available about the safety of holly leaves.
CHILDREN: UNSAFE …when the berries are ingested. Eating berries can be fatal (6).
PREGNANCY AND LACTATION: UNSAFE ...when berries are ingested (6). There is insufficient reliable information available about the safety of holly leaves; avoid using.

Effectiveness

There is insufficient reliable information available about the effectiveness of holly.

Mechanism of Action

The applicable parts of holly are the leaf and berry. The constituent saponins are thought to cause GI irritation and emetic effects (6). Holly also contains a cyanogenic glycoside (4).

Adverse Reactions

Orally, ingestion of the leaf can cause GI irritation, diarrhea, nausea, and vomiting (6,18). Leaf spines may tear or puncture skin or mucous membranes (6). Ingestion of as few as 2 berries can cause vomiting and diarrhea in small children (6). Ingestion of more than 5 berries can cause nausea, vomiting, diarrhea, and stupor (6,18). Ingestion of 20-30 berries can cause death (18).

Interactions with Herbs & Other Dietary Supplements

Insufficient reliable information available.

Interactions with Drugs

No interactions are known to occur, and there is no known reason to expect a clinically significant interaction with holly.

Interactions with Foods

No interactions are known to occur, and there is no known reason to expect a clinically significant interaction with holly.

Interactions with Lab Tests

No interactions are known to occur, and there is no known reason to expect a clinically significant interaction with holly.

Interactions with Diseases or Conditions

DEHYDRATION: In addition to toxic effects, berry ingestion may cause or exacerbate dehydration by inducing vomiting and diarrhea (6).
ELECTROLYTE IMBALANCE: Berry ingestion may cause or exacerbate electrolyte imbalance by inducing vomiting and diarrhea (6).

Dosage and Administration

ORAL: People typically use 3.9 grams of powdered leaves in a tea, taken to reduce the effects of intermittent fevers (5254).

Comments

Many other Ilex species are referred to as holly. English holly, Oregon holly, American holly are used as ornamental Christmas holly (6). Yaupon, Appalachian tea, cassena, deer berry, Indian holly and Indian black drink may be included in discussions of holly (6). Leaf spines may tear or puncture skin or mucous membranes (6).

HOLLYHOCK

Also Known As

Althea Rose, Hollyhock Flower, Malvae arboreae flos, Malva, Malva Flower, Rose Mallow.

Scientific Names

Alcea rosea, synonym Althaea rosea.
Family: Malvaceae.

People Use This For

Orally, the mucilage of hollyhock flower is used for prevention and treatment of diseases and discomforts of the respiratory and gastrointestinal tracts (2).
Topically, it is used for ulcers and inflammation (2).
In herbal teas, hollyhock is used as a brightening agent (2).

Safety

POSSIBLY SAFE ...when used orally. No health hazards are known in conjunction with appropriate use (18). There are no reported safety concerns about the use of hollyhock as a brightening agent in herbal tea mixtures (2).
PREGNANCY AND LACTATION: Insufficient reliable information available; avoid using.

Effectiveness

There is insufficient reliable information available about the effectiveness of hollyhock.

Mechanism of Action

The applicable part of hollyhock is the flower. There is insufficient reliable information available about the possible mechanism of action and active ingredients.

Adverse Reactions

None reported.

Interactions with Herbs & Other Dietary Supplements

Insufficient reliable information available.

Interactions with Drugs

No interactions are known to occur, and there is no known reason to expect a clinically significant interaction with hollyhock.

Interactions with Foods

No interactions are known to occur, and there is no known reason to expect a clinically significant interaction with hollyhock.

Interactions with Lab Tests

No interactions are known to occur, and there is no known reason to expect a clinically significant interaction with hollyhock.

Interactions with Diseases or Conditions

No interactions are known to occur, and there is no known reason to expect a clinically significant interaction with hollyhock.

Dosage and Administration

ORAL: People typically use hollyhock flower as a tea (5263).

Comments

There is very little scientific information about this product. Our staff is continually analyzing the available information on natural medicines and will add data here as it becomes available.

HONEY

Also Known As

Clarified Honey, Honig, Mel, Miel Blanc, Purified Honey, Strained Honey.
CAUTION: See separate listings for Bee Pollen, Bee Venom, and Royal Jelly.

Scientific Names

Apis mellifera (honey bee).
Family: Apidae.

People Use This For

Orally, honey is used for cough, asthma, and as an expectorant. It is also used orally for diarrhea and gastric ulcer associated with Helicobacter pylori (6). Honey is also used orally for recuperation after exercise (6197).
Topically, honey is used to speed healing in mild sores, wounds, skin ulcerations, and burns; and for treating cataracts and postherpetic corneal opacities (6).
In foods, honey is used as a sweetening agent (11).
In manufacturing, honey is used as a fragrance and a moisturizer in soaps and cosmetics (11).

Safety

LIKELY SAFE ...when used orally in amounts typically found in foods. Honey has Generally Recognized as Safe (GRAS) status in the US (11).
POSSIBLY SAFE ...when used topically (395,396,397,398,399).
CHILDREN: POSSIBLY UNSAFE ...when used orally. Ingestion of honey contaminated with Clostridium botulinum spores may cause botulism poisoning in infants (6,11). This is not a danger for older children or adults.
PREGNANCY AND LACTATION: LIKELY SAFE ...when used orally in amounts typically found in foods.

Effectiveness

POSSIBLY EFFECTIVE ...when used topically for improving healing of mild sores, wounds, burns and skin ulcerations (6,395,396,397,398,399).
There is insufficient reliable information available about the effectiveness of honey for its other uses.

Mechanism of Action

Honey is produced by bees (Apis mellifera) from the nectar of several varieties of plants. Pharmacological activity can vary depending on the type of plant from which the nectar is obtained. For example, honey produced from poisonous plants can be poisonous (6). Honey has been reported to have an expectorant effect and to be useful for cough and asthma. Honey has antibacterial and antifungal activity (6), which might offer benefit in preventing wound infection and Helicobacter pylori infection in peptic ulcer disease (6). Antibacterial peptides (apidaecins and abaecin) have been isolated in honeybees (6). Researchers think that release of hydrogen peroxide contained in honey, high sugar content of honey, and/or phytochemicals contained in honey might play a role in the antimicrobial activity (1261,1428). Honey and solutions with similar sugar content (15% w/v) demonstrate similar effectiveness at inhibiting Helicobacter pylori (1428) and 2-4% v/v dilutions of various types of honey inhibit the growth of coagulase positive Staphylococcus aureus isolated from infected wounds (1261). Honey is thought to be useful after vigorous exercise to normalize blood glucose. Researchers report that eating protein supplemented with honey after intense weight training achieved more desirable blood sugar levels within the following two hours than protein supplemented with sugar or maltodextrin.

Honey consumption was also associated with hormone levels favorable to muscle recuperation in this unpublished research presented at the National Strength and Conditioning Association 2000 annual conference (6197).

Adverse Reactions

Orally, honey can cause allergic reactions. Some honey is contaminated with Clostridium botulinum spores, which pose a risk to infants, but not older children or adults (6,11). Botulinum spores can proliferate in the intestines of infants causing botulism poisoning (6,11).

Interactions with Herbs & Other Dietary Supplements

Insufficient reliable information available.

Interactions with Drugs

No interactions are known to occur, and there is no known reason to expect a clinically significant interaction with honey.

Interactions with Foods

No interactions are known to occur, and there is no known reason to expect a clinically significant interaction with honey.

Interactions with Lab Tests

No interactions are known to occur, and there is no known reason to expect a clinically significant interaction with honey.

Interactions with Diseases or Conditions

POLLEN ALLERGIES: Honey may cause allergic reactions (6).

Dosage and Administration

ORAL: Liberal amounts are used orally.
TOPICAL: Liberal amounts are applied topically.

Comments

Avoid confusion with bee pollen, bee venom, and royal jelly.

HONEYSUCKLE

Also Known As

Goat's Leaf, Honey Suckle, Jinyinhua, Lonicera, Woodbine.
CAUTION: See separate listings for American Ivy, Gelsemium, and Woodbine.

Scientific Names

Lonicera caprifolium; Lonicera japonica; and other Lonicera sp.
Family: Caprifoliaceae.

People Use This For

Orally, honeysuckle is used for digestive disorders, malignant tumors, and to promote sweating. It is also used orally as a laxative (18).
Topically, it is used for inflammation, itching, and as an astringent and antimicrobial (11).
In traditional Chinese medicine, honeysuckle is used orally for colds, fever, inflammation, swelling, boils, sores, and viral and bacterial infections.

Safety

There is insufficient reliable information available about the safety of honeysuckle.
Pregnancy and Lactation: Insufficient reliable information available; avoid using.

Effectiveness

There is insufficient reliable information available about the effectiveness of honeysuckle.

Mechanism of Action

The applicable parts of honeysuckle are the flower, seed, and leaf. In vitro data suggests antimicrobial activity against Staphylococcus aureus, Salmonella typhi, Mycobacterium tuberculosis, and bacilli which cause dysentery. It may also have antiviral activity against HIV and influenza virus. It is active, but less so, against dermatophytes. Animal data suggest anti-inflammatory effects, with possible increased resistance to infection, inhibited tumor formation, and decreased intestinal cholesterol absorption. Animal data also suggest that honeysuckle has stimulant effects at about one-sixth the activity of caffeine. Some of these biological activities are attributed to the saponin and chlorogenic acid content of honeysuckle. The LD50 of honeysuckle is low, approximately 53 g/kg when given subcutaneously to mice [11].

Adverse Reactions
Orally, honeysuckle may cause irritation of the gastrointestinal tract, kidneys, and urinary tract [18].

Interactions with Herbs & Other Dietary Supplements
Insufficient reliable information available.

Interactions with Drugs
No interactions are known to occur, and there is no known reason to expect a clinically significant interaction with honeysuckle.

Interactions with Foods
No interactions are known to occur, and there is no known reason to expect a clinically significant interaction with honeysuckle.

Interactions with Lab Tests
No interactions are known to occur, and there is no known reason to expect a clinically significant interaction with honeysuckle.

Interactions with Diseases or Conditions
No interactions are known to occur, and there is no known reason to expect a clinically significant interaction with honeysuckle.

Dosage and Administration
No typical dosage.

Comments
Avoid confusion with woodbine (Clematis virginiana). Also, avoid confusing honeysuckle with American ivy or gelsemium, which are also known as woodbine.

HOPS

Also Known As
Common Hops, European Hops, Hop Strobile, Hop Strobiles, Hopfenzapfen, Houblon, Lupuli Strobulus.

Scientific Names
Humulus lupulus.
Family: Cannabinaceae or Moraceae.

People Use This For
Orally, hops are used for restlessness, anxiety, sleep disorders, tension, excitability [1,2,3], nervousness, and irritability [6121]. They are also used orally as an appetite stimulant [1], a bitter tonic, and for indigestion [6121]. Topically, hops are used as an anti-bacterial [4].
In Chinese medicine, hops are used for tuberculosis and cystitis [11].
Traditionally, hops are used orally as a diuretic [11], for intestinal cramps, mucous colitis, neuralgia, and priapism [4,11]. Topically, they are used for leg ulcers.
In foods and beverages, the extracts and oil are used as flavor components [11]. The strobile is often used for brewing beer [11].
In manufacturing, the extract is used in skin creams and lotions [11].

Safety
LIKELY SAFE ...when consumed in amounts commonly found in foods and beverages. Hops have Generally Recognized as Safe (GRAS) status for food use in the US with a maximum level of 0.072% [11].

POSSIBLY SAFE ...when used orally and appropriately for medicinal purposes (12).
PREGNANCY AND LACTATION: Insufficient reliable information available; avoid using.

Effectiveness
POSSIBLY EFFECTIVE ...when used orally for tenseness and restlessness (1,2).
There is insufficient reliable information available about the effectiveness of hops for its other uses.

Mechanism of Action
The applicable part of hops is the dried, fruiting part. Hops can have sedative, hypnotic, anticonvulsant, antimicrobial, and pain- and fever-reducing properties (1,4,11). Its antimicrobial properties are due to the bitter acid constituents, lupulone and humulone (11). The constituent 2-methyl-3-butene-2-ol can have sedative effects in rats (11). The alcoholic extracts have been used to treat acute bacterial dysentery, leprosy, and pulmonary tuberculosis in humans with varying success (11). An extract of hops competitively inhibits estradiol binding to estrogen receptors and induces transcription activity in estrogen-responsive cells (6180). It also decreases LH (luteinizing hormone) levels in female rats that have had their ovaries removed (6180).

Adverse Reactions
Topically, allergic reactions are possible through contact with the fresh plant and plant dust. Contact dermatitis is attributed to the pollen (4).

Interactions with Herbs & Other Dietary Supplements
HERBS WITH SEDATIVE PROPERTIES: Theoretically, concomitant use with herbs that have sedative properties might enhance therapeutic and adverse effects. These include calamus, calendula, California poppy, catnip, capsicum, celery, couch grass, elecampane, Siberian ginseng, German chamomile, goldenseal, gotu kola, Jamaican dogwood, kava, lemon balm, sage, St. John's wort, sassafras, scullcap, shepherd's purse, stinging nettle, valerian, wild carrot, wild lettuce, ashwaganda root, and yerba mansa (4,19).

Interactions with Drugs
ALCOHOL, SEDATIVE DRUGS: Concomitant use of hops can potentiate the sedative effects of these drugs (4).
BARBITURATES: Theoretically, concomitant use of hops with barbiturates can cause additive therapeutic and adverse effects (19).
OTHER DRUGS WITH SEDATIVE PROPERTIES: Theoretically, concomitant use with drugs having sedative properties can cause additive therapeutic and adverse effects (19).

Interactions with Foods
ALCOHOL: Concomitant use of hops with alcohol can potentiate the sedative effects (4).

Interactions with Lab Tests
No interactions are known to occur, and there is no known reason to expect a clinically significant interaction with hops.

Interactions with Diseases or Conditions
DEPRESSION: Hops may contribute to depression (12).

Dosage and Administration
ORAL: The typical dose of hops is 0.5-1 grams of the strobile as a single dose (4) or one cup of the tea (4). The tea is prepared by steeping 0.5-1 grams of the strobile in 150 mL boiling water for 5-10 minutes and then straining (4). The usual dose of the liquid extract (1:1, 45% alcohol) is 0.5-2 mL (4). The common dose of the tincture (1:5, 60% alcohol) is 1-2 mL (4). For sleep, 1-2 grams of the strobile are typically used (4), and combination of hops with other plant sedatives can be beneficial (1,2).
TOPICAL: No typical dosage.

Comments
The hops themselves are not reported to interfere with the ability to drive and operate machines (1).

HORSE CHESTNUT branch bark

Also Known As
Buckeye, Hippocastani Cortex, Hippocastani Semen, Marron Europeen, Spanish Chestnut.
CAUTION: See separate listings for Horse Chestnut flower, Horse Chestnut leaf, and Horse Chestnut seed.

Scientific Names
Aesculus hippocastanum.
Family: Hippocastanaceae.

People Use This For
Orally, horse chestnut branch bark is used for malaria and dysentery (11).
Topically, horse chestnut branch bark is used for lupus and skin ulcers (11).
In combination with other herbs, horse chestnut branch bark together with the flower is used for treating varicose veins, strengthening veins, promoting and supporting cardiac function, treating hemorrhoids and rectal problems, prevention of embolism, improving circulation, ringing in the ears, low and high blood pressure, dizziness, stimulant effect, tendency towards uric acid disturbances, kidney or bladder disease, edema associated with weak heart function, dropsy, liver congestion, bile flow disturbances, and pancreatitis (2).

Safety
There is insufficient reliable information available about the safety of horse chestnut branch bark.
CHILDREN: LIKELY UNSAFE ...when used orally. Poisoning has been reported from children drinking tea made with twigs (6).
PREGNANCY AND LACTATION: Insufficient reliable information available; avoid using.

Effectiveness
There is insufficient reliable information available about the effectiveness of horse chestnut branch bark.

Mechanism of Action
Horse chestnut branch bark contains aescin (11). This is a mixture of triterpene saponins. Aescin seems to have a weak diuretic activity (6). In some countries, intravenous aescin is used after surgery (6). Horse chestnut branchbark also contains sterols, stigmasterol, alpha-spinasterol, and beta-sitosterol (11). These constituents seem to have anti-inflammatory activity (6). Horse chestnut bark and twigs contain the toxic glycoside aesculin (6). Aesculin is a hydroxycoumarin with potential antithrombin activity (19).

Adverse Reactions
Orally, there is the possibility of severe bleeding or bruising due to the antithrombotic activity of horse chestnut branch bark (19). Children have been poisoned by drinking tea made from horse chestnut leaves and twigs (6).

Interactions with Herbs & Other Dietary Supplements
HERBS WITH ANTICOAGULANT/ANTIPLATELET POTENTIAL: Concomitant use of herbs that have coumarin constituents or affect platelet aggregation could theoretically increase the risk of bleeding in some people. These herbs include: angelica, anise, arnica, asafoetida, bogbean, boldo, capsicum, celery, chamomile, clove, danshen, fenugreek, feverfew, garlic, ginger, ginkgo, Panax ginseng, horseradish, licorice, meadowsweet, prickly ash, onion, papain, passionflower, poplar, quassia, red clover, turmeric, wild carrot, wild lettuce, willow, and others (4,19).

Interactions with Drugs
ANTICOAGULANTS: Theoretically, the aesculin constituent in horse chestnut branch bark might increase the effect or adverse effects of anticoagulant drugs (19).
ASPIRIN: Theoretically, concomitant use should be avoided due to the antithrombin effects of aesculin (19).
DIABETES THERAPY: Monitor blood glucose level closely due to claims that horse chestnut branch bark has hypoglycemic effects (19).

Interactions with Foods
No interactions are known to occur, and there is no known reason to expect a clinically significant interaction with horse chestnut branch bark.

Interactions with Lab Tests
No interactions are known to occur, and there is no known reason to expect a clinically significant interaction with horse chestnut branch bark.

Interactions with Diseases or Conditions
BLEEDING DISORDERS: The antithrombin activity of aesculin can theoretically increase bleeding time (19).
GI CONDITIONS: Can irritate gastrointestinal tract. Contraindicated in individuals with infectious or inflammatory gastrointestinal conditions (19).

Dosage and Administration

ORAL: Tincture (1:5, 50% alcohol), 3-10 drops, use with care (886).

Comments

Sometimes buckeye is referred to as horse chestnut bark. Do not confuse horse chestnut bark with buckeye.

HORSE CHESTNUT flower

Also Known As

Buckeye, Hippocastani Flos, Marron Europeen, Spanish Chestnut.
CAUTION: See separate listings for Horse Chestnut branch bark, Horse Chestnut leaf, and Horse Chestnut seed.

Scientific Names

Aesculus hippocastanum.
Family: Hippocastanaceae.

People Use This For

Orally, horse chestnut flower, in various combinations with horse chestnut bark and other herbs, is used for hemorrhoids and rectal problems, prevention of embolism, improving circulation, strengthening veins, promoting and supporting cardiac function, ringing in the ears, low and high blood pressure, dizziness, stimulant, uric acid diathesis, kidney or bladder disease, edema due to weak heart function, dropsy, liver congestion, bile flow disturbances, and pancreatitis (2).

Safety

LIKELY UNSAFE ...when used orally (2,11).
There is insufficient reliable information available about the safety of the topical use of horse chestnut flower.
PREGNANCY AND LACTATION: LIKELY UNSAFE ...when used orally; avoid using (11).

Effectiveness

There is insufficient reliable information available about the effectiveness of horse chestnut flower.

Mechanism of Action

Horse chestnut flower contains aescin (11). This is a mixture of triperpene saponins. Horse chestnut flower also contains sterols, stigmasterol, alpha-spinasterol, and beta-sitosterol. These constituents seem to have anti-inflammatory activity (6). Aescin is a hydroxycoumarin and can lead to increased bleeding. In some countries, an intravenous mixture containing horse chestnut flower is used after surgery. It seems to have a weak diuretic activity.

Adverse Reactions

Orally, symptoms of horse chestnut flower poisoning include nervous muscle twitching, weakness, dilated pupils, vomiting, diarrhea, depression, paralysis, and stupor (11).

Interactions with Herbs & Other Dietary Supplements

HERBS WITH ANTICOAGULANT/ANTIPLATELET POTENTIAL: Concomitant use of herbs that have coumarin constituents or affect platelet aggregation could theoretically increase the risk of bleeding in some people. These herbs include: angelica, anise, arnica, asafoetida, bogbean, boldo, capsicum, celery, chamomile, clove, danshen, fenugreek, feverfew, garlic, ginger, ginkgo, Panax ginseng, horseradish, licorice, meadowsweet, prickly ash, onion, papain, passionflower, poplar, quassia, red clover, turmeric, wild carrot, wild lettuce, willow, and others (4,19).

Interactions with Drugs

No interactions are known to occur, and there is no known reason to expect a clinically significant interaction with horse chestnut flower.

Interactions with Foods

No interactions are known to occur, and there is no known reason to expect a clinically significant interaction with horse chestnut flower.

Interactions with Lab Tests

No interactions are known to occur, and there is no known reason to expect a clinically significant interaction with horse chestnut flower.

Interactions with Diseases or Conditions
No interactions are known to occur, and there is no known reason to expect a clinically significant interaction with horse chestnut flower.

Dosage and Administration
No typical dosage.

Comments
The horse chestnut flower can be toxic and should not be used. Avoid confusion with horse chestnut branch bark, leaf, and seed. Sometimes buckeye is referred to as horse chestnut. Do not confuse horse chestnut with buckeye. Horse chestnut seed is used to manufacture Venastat which is being shown to be likely effective against varicose veins.

HORSE CHESTNUT leaf

Also Known As
Buckeye, Hippocastani folium, Marron Europeen, Spanish Chestnut.
CAUTION: See separate listings for Horse Chestnut bark, Horse Chestnut flower, and Horse Chestnut seed.

Scientific Names
Aesculus hippocastanum.
Family: Hippocastanaceae.

People Use This For
Orally, the horse chestnut leaf is used for eczema, varicose veins, discomfort due to varicose veins, supportive treatment of varicose ulcers, treating phlebitis, thrombophlebitis, hemorrhoids, menstrual spastic pain, soft tissue swelling from bone fracture and sprains, and complaints after concussion (2,11).
In combination with other herbs, the horse chestnut leaf is used for discomfort due to hemorrhoids, anal fissures, and rhagades (linear cracks or fissures in the skin occurring especially at the angles of the mouth or about the anus). Also, the horse chestnut leaf is used in herbal combination products for follow-up treatment of hemorrhoid surgery, for colon stasis, preventing vein weakness, strengthening vein walls, maintaining normal blood supply in tissues, strengthening venous blood circulation, preventing leg and foot fatigue, and for severe disorders of the venous system. Combination products also use horse chestnut for preventing thromboembolism, arteriosclerosis, arthrosis deformans, arthritis, sciatica, rheumatism, lumbago, neuralgia, hematoma, bruises, brachialgia, and as a diuretic and purifying remedy (2).
In folk medicine, it has been used as a cough remedy and for arthritis and rheumatism (18).

Safety
LIKELY UNSAFE ...when taken orally.
There is insufficient reliable information available about the safety of horse chestnut leaf for its other uses.
CHILDREN: UNSAFE ...when used orally. The horse chestnut leaf is toxic (11) and should not be used in children due to the potential for poisoning (6).
PREGNANCY AND LACTATION:UNSAFE ...when used orally because the horse chestnut leaf can be toxic (11).

Effectiveness
There is insufficient reliable information available about the effectiveness of the horse chestnut leaf for its other uses.

Mechanism of Action
The horse chestnut leaf contains the toxic glycoside aesculin (esculin) (6). Aesculin is a hydroxycoumarin with potential antithrombin activity (19).

Adverse Reactions
Orally, symptoms of horse chestnut leaf poisoning include nervous muscle twitching, weakness, dilated pupils, vomiting, diarrhea, depression, paralysis, and stupor (11). There is also the possibility of severe bleeding or bruising due to the antithrombotic activity of aesculin contained in horse chestnut leaf (19). Children have been poisoned by drinking the tea made from horse chestnut leaves and twigs (6).
There is one case report of cholestatic liver damage associated with intramuscular injection of a horse chestnut leaf extract (2).

Interactions with Herbs & Other Dietary Supplements
HERBS WITH ANTICOAGULANT/ANTIPLATELET POTENTIAL: Concomitant use of herbs that have coumarin constituents or affect platelet aggregation could theoretically increase the risk of bleeding in some people.

These herbs include: angelica, anise, arnica, asafoetida, bogbean, boldo, capsicum, celery, chamomile, clove, danshen, fenugreek, feverfew, garlic, ginger, ginkgo, Panax ginseng, horseradish, licorice, meadowsweet, prickly ash, onion, papain, passionflower, poplar, quassia, red clover, turmeric, wild carrot, wild lettuce, willow, and others (4,19).

Interactions with Drugs
ANTICOAGULANTS AND ASPIRIN: Theoretically, the aesculin component in horse chestnut leaf might increase the effect or adverse effects of anticoagulant drugs or aspirin (19).

Interactions with Foods
No interactions are known to occur, and there is no known reason to expect a clinically significant interaction with horse chestnut leaf.

Interactions with Lab Tests
No interactions are known to occur, and there is no known reason to expect a clinically significant interaction with horse chestnut leaf.

Interactions with Diseases or Conditions
No interactions are known to occur, and there is no known reason to expect a clinically significant interaction with horse chestnut leaf.

Dosage and Administration
No typical dosage.

Comments
The horse chestnut leaf can be toxic and should not be used. Avoid confusion with the horse chestnut bark, flower, and seed. Sometimes buckeye is referred to as horse chestnut. Do not confuse horse chestnut with buckeye.

HORSE CHESTNUT seed

Also Known As
Chestnut, Escine, Hippocastani Semen, Horse Chestnut, Marron Europeen, Venastat, Venostat, Venostasin Retard.
CAUTION: See separate listings for Horse Chestnut leaf, Horse Chestnut flower, and Horse Chestnut branch bark.

Scientific Names
Aesculus hippocastanum.
Family: Hippocastanaceae.

People Use This For
Orally, horse chestnut seed has been used for the treatment of varicose veins, hemorrhoids, phlebitis, diarrhea, fever, and enlarged prostate (4). Standardized horse chestnut seed extract products are taken orally for the treatment of chronic venous insufficiency (2,7). A specially prepared product made from horse chestnut seed is taken orally for the treatment of varicose veins, hemorrhoids, phlebitis, diarrhea, fever, and enlarged prostate (4).

Safety
POSSIBLY SAFE ...when used orally as the standardized extract product. European preparations of horse chestnut extracts have removed the primary toxic constituent, esculin, and are generally considered safe (2,11,6420).
UNSAFE ...when used orally as the raw seed. Raw horse chestnut seed preparations contain significant amounts of the toxin esculin and can be lethal (6).
PREGNANCY AND LACTATION: UNSAFE ...when used orally as the raw seed. Raw horse chestnut preparations can be lethal (6); contraindicated. There is insufficient reliable information available about the safety of horse chestnut seed extract when used during pregnancy and lactation; avoid using.

Effectiveness
LIKELY EFFECTIVE ...when used orally for symptomatic treatment of chronic venous insufficiency, such as varicose veins, and relieving pain, tiredness, tension, swelling in the legs, itching, and edema (281,282,283,284,285). Clinical studies showing the effectiveness of horse chestnut seed have used extracts standardized to 16-20% aescin.
There is insufficient reliable information available about the effectiveness of horse chestnut seed for its other uses.

Mechanism of Action

Horse chestnut seed contains triterpene saponins referred to as aescin (escin) and the toxic glycoside aesculin (esculin) (11). Aesculin is a hydroxycoumarin which may increase bleeding time due to antithrombin activity (19). Aescin decreases the permeability of venous capillaries. In vitro, aescin, constricts veins and reduces the capillary permeability induced by histamine or serotonin (6). These properties of the saponin components are the basis for the cosmetic applications of horse chestnut seed extract (4). In some countries, an intravenous mixture containing aescin is used after surgery (6). It seems to have a weak diuretic activity (6). Aescin binds to plasma proteins (4).

Adverse Reactions

Orally, horse chestnut can cause GI irritation and toxic nephropathy (4). The symptoms of chestnut poisoning include muscle twitching, weakness, loss of coordination, dilated pupils, vomiting, diarrhea, depression, paralysis, and stupor (6). Horse chestnut seed extract taken orally can cause itching and gastric complaints (2). Isolated cases of kidney and liver toxicity have occurred after intravenous administration (512).

Intravenously, administration of aescin can cause anaphylaxis (18).

Interactions with Herbs & Other Dietary Supplements

HERBS WITH ANTICOAGULANT/ANTIPLATELET POTENTIAL: Concomitant use of herbs that have coumarin constituents or affect platelet aggregation could theoretically increase the risk of bleeding in some people. These herbs include: angelica, anise, arnica, asafoetida, bogbean, boldo, capsicum, celery, chamomile, clove, danshen, fenugreek, feverfew, garlic, ginger, ginkgo, Panax ginseng, horseradish, licorice, meadowsweet, prickly ash, onion, papain, passionflower, poplar, quassia, red clover, turmeric, wild carrot, wild lettuce, willow, and others (4,19).

HERBS WITH HYPOGLYCEMIC ACTIVITY: Theoretically, concomitant use with herbs having hypoglycemic activity could have additive effects and adverse effects (19).

Interactions with Drugs

ANTICOAGULANTS: Theoretically, horse chestnut can have additive effects and adverse effects with anticoagulants (4).

PROTEIN-BINDING DRUGS: Theoretically, the saponin constituent of horse chestnut seed or extract, aescin, might interfere with the binding of protein binding of drugs (4).

DIABETES THERAPY: Monitor blood glucose level closely due to claims that horse chestnut seeds can have hypoglycemic effects (19).

Interactions with Foods

No interactions are known to occur, and there is no known reason to expect a clinically significant interaction with horse chestnut seed.

Interactions with Lab Tests

No interactions are known to occur, and there is no known reason to expect a clinically significant interaction with horse chestnut seed.

Interactions with Diseases or Conditions

GI IRRITATION: Can irritate gastrointestinal tract; contraindicated in individuals with infectious or inflammatory gastrointestinal conditions (19).

RENAL IMPAIRMENT: Toxic nephropathy has been reported as an adverse effect (4); avoid using.

HEPATIC IMPAIRMENT: A report of liver injury associated with horse chestnut (4); avoid using.

DIABETES: Monitor blood glucose level closely due to claims that horse chestnut seeds can have hypoglycemic effects (19).

Dosage and Administration

ORAL: Typical preparations of horse chestnut capsules contain about 250 mg horse chestnut extract. The usual dose is 1 to 3 capsules daily in divided doses. Some preparations are labeled for aescin content (usually 16 to 21%). Some sources recommend taking an initial dose of 90 – 150 mg of aescin (about 450 to 750 mg horse chestnut extract), and decreasing the maintenance dose to 35 to 70 mg aescin (about 175 to 350 mg extract). A tincture formulation of horse chestnut extract is used in a dose of 1 to 4 mL three times per day (5261,6006).

Comments

Do not confuse the horse chestnut seed with the related species, Aesculus californica and Aesculus glabra, known respectively as the California and Ohio buckeye. Sometimes buckeye is referred to as horse chestnut. Do not confuse horse chestnut with buckeye.

HORSEMINT

Also Known As
Monarda Lutea, Spotted Monarda, Wild Bergamot.

Scientific Names
Monarda punctata.
Family: Labitae or Lamiaceae.

People Use This For
Orally, horsemint is used for digestive disorders, flatulence, and dysmenorrhea. It is also used orally to promote menstruation and as a stimulant (18).

Safety
There is insufficient reliable information available about the safety of horsemint.
PREGNANCY: UNSAFE …when used orally due to menstruation promoting and uterine stimulant effects (12).
LACTATION: Insufficient reliable information available; avoid using.

Effectiveness
There is insufficient reliable information available about the effectiveness of horsemint.

Mechanism of Action
There is insufficient reliable information available about the possible mechanism of action and active ingredients of horsemint.

Adverse Reactions
None reported.

Interactions with Herbs & Other Dietary Supplements
Insufficient reliable information available.

Interactions with Drugs
No interactions are known to occur, and there is no known reason to expect a clinically significant interaction with horsemint.

Interactions with Foods
No interactions are known to occur, and there is no known reason to expect a clinically significant interaction with horsemint.

Interactions with Lab Tests
No interactions are known to occur, and there is no known reason to expect a clinically significant interaction with horsemint.

Interactions with Diseases or Conditions
No interactions are known to occur, and there is no known reason to expect a clinically significant interaction with horsemint.

Dosage and Administration
ORAL: The average daily dose is 2-4 mL of syrup prepared from the herb (18).

Comments
Horsemint has a pungent, bitter taste, and has a scent reminiscent of thyme (18).

HORSERADISH

Also Known As
Amoraciae Rusticanae Radix, Great Raifort, Meerrettich, Mountain Radish, Pepperrot, Red Cole.

Scientific Names

Armoracia rusticana, synonym Armoracia lopathifolia; Cochlearia armoracia; Nasturtium armoracia; Roripa armoracia. Family: Brassicaceae/Cruciferae.

People Use This For

Orally, horseradish is used for urinary tract infection, urinary stones, edematous conditions, cough, and bronchitis (2,4,18).

Topically, it is used for inflamed joints or tissues and minor muscle aches (2,4).

Traditionally, horseradish has been used for expelling afterbirth, treating gout, rheumatism, gallbladder disorders, sciatica pain, relief of colic, increasing urination, and intestinal worms in children (6,18).

In foods, it is used as a flavoring agent (4).

Safety

LIKELY SAFE ...when the root is used orally in food amounts. It has Generally Recognized as Safe (GRAS) status in the US (4).

POSSIBLY SAFE ...when used orally and appropriately in larger amounts (2,4,6,12,18). ...when topical preparations containing 2% mustard oil, or less are used (2). Mustard oil is a constituent of horseradish.

CHILDREN: POSSIBLY SAFE ...when used as a spice. LIKELY UNSAFE ...when used orally in children less than 4 years of age because it can cause gastrointestinal problems (2,12,19).

PREGNANCY AND LACTATION: LIKELY SAFE ...when used orally in food amounts. LIKELY UNSAFE ...when used orally in larger amounts because horseradish contains toxic and irritating mustard oil constituents (4). ...when the tincture is taken regularly and in large amounts, it is considered an abortifacient (19).

Effectiveness

There is insufficient reliable information available about the effectiveness of horseradish.

Mechanism of Action

The applicable part of horseradish is the root. Researchers state horseradish has antimicrobial efficacy against gram negative and gram positive bacteria. It also has antispasmodic properties. Horseradish shows evidence that it can stimulate local blood flow; it might also be carcinostatic (2,18). The toxic mustard oil constituents of horseradish are extremely irritating to mucous membranes (2,4) and the urinary tract (19).

Adverse Reactions

Orally, consuming large amounts of horseradish can cause gastrointestinal upset, bloody vomiting and diarrhea (2,6), and irritation of mucous membranes (2,4) and the urinary tract (19). Horseradish, and other members of the cabbage and mustard family are associated with depressed thyroid function (4).

Topically, skin contact with fresh horseradish can cause irritation (4,19) or allergic reaction (4).

Interactions with Herbs & Other Dietary Supplements

HERBS WITH ANTICOAGULANT/ANTIPLATELET POTENTIAL: Concomitant use of herbs that have coumarin constituents or affect platelet aggregation could theoretically increase the risk of bleeding in some people. These herbs include: angelica, anise, arnica, asafoetida, bogbean, boldo, capsicum, celery, chamomile, clove, danshen, fenugreek, feverfew, garlic, ginger, ginkgo, Panax ginseng, horse chestnut, licorice, meadowsweet, prickly ash, onion, papain, passionflower, poplar, quassia, red clover, turmeric, wild carrot, wild lettuce, willow, and others (4,19).

Interactions with Drugs

LEVOTHYROXINE: Theoretically, concomitant use of horseradish can interfere with levothyroxine or hypothyroid therapy (4).

Interactions with Foods

No interactions are known to occur, and there is no known reason to expect a clinically significant interaction with horseradish.

Interactions with Lab Tests

No interactions are known to occur, and there is no known reason to expect a clinically significant interaction with horseradish.

Interactions with Diseases or Conditions

KIDNEY DISORDERS: Theoretically, because it has a strong diuretic effect (19), horseradish is contraindicated in individuals with kidney inflammation (2,18,19).

HYPOTHYROIDISM: Theoretically, horseradish might exacerbate hypothyroidism or interfere with therapy (19).
GI CONDITIONS: Horseradish can irritate gastrointestinal tract. Contraindicated in individuals with infectious or inflammatory gastrointestinal conditions, or stomach or intestinal ulcers (19).

Dosage and Administration
ORAL: The typical dose of horseradish is 6-20 grams per day of the root or equivalent preparations (4,6,18).
TOPICAL: Ointments with a maximum of 2% mustard oil content are commonly used (6,18).

Comments
Horseradish has been cultivated for more than two thousand years (6) and is sometimes added to toxic substances as a taste repellent for animals (6002).

HORSETAIL

Also Known As
Bottle Brush, Corn Horsetail, Dutch Rushes, Equisetum, Field Horsetail, Horse Tail, Horse Willow, Horsetail Grass, Horsetail Rush, Paddock-Pipes, Pewterwort, Prele, Scouring Rush, Souring Rush, Shave Grass, Shavegrass, Toadpipe.

Scientific Names
Equisetum arvense; Equisetum telmateia.
Family: Equisetaceae.

People Use This For
Orally, horsetail is used for diuresis, edema, kidney and bladder stones, urinary tract infections, and general disturbances of the kidney and bladder (2,6,7,18).
Topically, it is used for supportive treatment of wounds and burns (2,6,18).
In folk medicine, horsetail is used for alopecia; tuberculosis; brittle fingernails; nasal, pulmonary, and gastric hemorrhage; rheumatic diseases; gout; frostbite; and to halt profuse menstruation (18).

Safety
POSSIBLY UNSAFE ...when used orally and appropriately short-term (2,6,12).
LIKELY UNSAFE ...when used orally long-term. It can cause thiamine deficiency. The inorganic silica content can cause toxicity similar to nicotine poisoning.
CHILDREN: LIKELY UNSAFE ...when used orally. Horsetail contains inorganic silica and the powdered herb can cause toxicity similar to nicotine poisonings. Poisoning has been reported in children who chewed on the stem (12).
PREGNANCY AND LACTATION: Insufficient reliable information available; avoid using.

Effectiveness
There is insufficient reliable information available about the effectiveness of horsetail.

Mechanism of Action
Evidence suggests horsetail has a mild diuretic action (18), which is likely due to the constituents, equisetonin and flavone glycosides (6). It also contains minute amounts of nicotine (6).

Adverse Reactions
Orally, horsetail may lead to thiamine deficiency, and Canadian products are required to be certified as free from thiaminase-like effect (12). Toxicity has occurred in children who chewed the stems and is similar to nicotine poisoning (12).
Topically, horsetail can cause seborrheic dermatitis (6).

Interactions with Herbs & Other Dietary Supplements
CARDIAC GLYCOSIDE-CONTAINING HERBS: Concomitant use may increase the risk of cardiac glycoside toxicity. Cardiac glycoside-containing herbs, include black hellebore, Canadian hemp roots, digitalis leaf, hedge mustard, figwort, lily of the valley roots, motherwort, oleander leaf, pheasant's eye plant, pleurisy root, squill bulb leaf scales, and strophanthus seeds (2,18,19,500).
STIMULANT LAXATIVE HERBS: Theoretically, concomitant use increases the risk of potassium depletion. Stimulant laxative herbs include: aloe dried leaf sap, blue flag rhizome, alder buckthorn, European buckthorn, butternut bark, cascara bark, castor oil, colocynth fruit pulp, gamboge bark exudate, jalap root, black root, manna bark exudate, podophyllum root, rhubarb root, senna leaves and pods, wild cucumber fruit (Ecballium elaterium), and yellow dock root (19).

LICORICE: Theoretically, overuse/misuse of licorice rhizome with horsetail increases the risk of cardiac toxicity due to potassium depletion. (19).

Interactions with Drugs
DIGITALIS GLYCOSIDE: Increased digitalis toxicity might occur due to the loss of potassium associated with the diuretic effect of horsetail (19).
POTASSIUM-DEPLETING DRUGS: Theoretically, concomitant use with potassium-depleting diuretics or corticosteroids with mineral corticoid activity increases the risk of reduced potassium levels or hypokalemia (4,13).

Interactions with Foods
REGULAR DIET: Horsetail can breakdown thiamine and theoretically increases the risk of thiamine deficiency (19).

Interactions with Lab Tests
No interactions are known to occur, and there is no known reason to expect a clinically significant interaction with horsetail.

Interactions with Diseases or Conditions
THIAMINE DEFICIENCY: Theoretically, the horsetail stem can cause or exacerbate thiamine deficiency (12).
IMPAIRED HEART OR KIDNEY FUNCTION: The diuretic effect of horsetail can cause an increased excretion of potassium (19); avoid using.

Dosage and Administration
ORAL: The typical dose of horsetail is 6 grams of the dried stem per day with ample fluid intake (2,18). One cup of the tea is commonly taken several times per day between meals. The tea is prepared by steeping 1.5 grams of the dried stem in 150 mL boiling water for 10-15 minutes and then straining (18). The powdered stem should be used only on a short-term basis in adults. Avoid the use of the powdered stem in children due to its inorganic silica content (12). The usual dose of the liquid extract (1:1 in 25% alcohol) is 1-4 mL three times per day (18). Do not exceed 2 grams of the powdered extract per day (12).
TOPICAL: Horsetail is commonly used as a compress containing 10 grams of the dried stem per L of water (2,18).

Comments
Adulteration with Equisetum palustre, which contains the toxic alkaloid palustrine, has occurred. Palustrine can be toxic in cattle, but toxicity in humans has not yet been established (12).

HOUND'S TONGUE

Also Known As
Cynoglossi herba, Cynoglossi radix, Dog-Bur, Dog's Tongue, Dogs Tongue, Gypsy Flower, Hounds Tongue, Sheep-Lice, Woolmat.
CAUTION: See separate listing for Deertongue (Trilisa odoratissima).

Scientific Names
Cynoglossum officinale.
Family: Boraginaceae.

People Use This For
Orally, hound's tongue is used for diarrhea and other GI tract complaints, infections, skin diseases, and bronchitis. It is also used as an analgesic, expectorant, and cough sedative (2,18,400).
Topically, hound's tongue is used for painful discomfort of extremities, myalgia, neuralgia, trauma, nervous diseases, wound healing, and for care of scar tissue (2,18).

Safety
LIKELY UNSAFE ...when taken orally; contraindicated (2,18,400), due to significant amounts of unsaturated pyrrolizidine alkaloids (UPAs) (2,19). Repeated exposure to low concentrations of UPAs has been linked to serious liver toxicity (4,12). UPAs may also be carcinogenic and mutagenic (12).
There is insufficient reliable information available about the safety of hound's tongue for topical use; avoid using.
PREGNANCY AND LACTATION: LIKELY UNSAFE ...when used orally due to UPA content (2,18).

Effectiveness
There is insufficient reliable information available about the effectiveness of hound's tongue.

Mechanism of Action

Researchers think the constituent cynoglossin paralyzes peripheral nerve endings (18). Hound's tongue contains significant amounts of hepatotoxic and hepatocarcinogenic pyrrolizidine alkaloids (2,18). Unsaturated pyrrolizidine alkaloids are known to be hepatotoxic in animals and humans (4).

Adverse Reactions

Chronic exposure to plants containing UPA constituents has been associated with veno-occlusive disease (4021). Symptoms of acute veno-occlusive disease are characterized by a dull, dragging ache in the right upper abdomen and marked distention of the abdomen. These symptoms are sometimes accompanied by reduced urine output. Subacute veno-occlusive disease is associated with vague symptoms and persistent liver enlargement (4021).

Interactions with Herbs & Other Dietary Supplements

EUCALYPTUS: Theoretically, concomitant use may increase the risk of unsaturated pyrrolizidine alkaloid toxicity due to enzyme induction by eucalyptus (19).
PYRROLIZIDINE ALKALOID-CONTAINING HERBS: Concomitant use is contraindicated due to the risk of additive toxicity. Herbs containing unsaturated pyrrolizidine alkaloids include: alkanna (12), borage (271), gravel root (4), hemp agrimony (271), hound's tongue (19), petasites (19), comfrey (271), coltsfoot, and the Senecio species plants; dusty miller (19), alpine ragwort (19), groundsel (271), golden ragwort (19), and tansy ragwort (271).

Interactions with Drugs

No interactions are known to occur, and there is no known reason to expect a clinically significant interaction with hound's tongue.

Interactions with Foods

No interactions are known to occur, and there is no known reason to expect a clinically significant interaction with hound's tongue.

Interactions with Lab Tests

No interactions are known to occur, and there is no known reason to expect a clinically significant interaction with hound's tongue.

Interactions with Diseases or Conditions

LIVER DISEASE: Contraindicated due to hepatotoxic potential (19).

Dosage and Administration

No typical dosage.

Comments

Avoid oral or topical use of hound's tongue. It is without documented effectiveness and is likely to be unsafe.

HOUSELEEK

Also Known As

Aaron's Rod, Ayegreen, Ayron, Bullock's Eye, Hens and Chickens, Jupiter's Beard, Jupiter's Eye, Liveforever, Sengreen, Thor's Beard, Thunder Plant.

Scientific Names

Sempervivum tectorum.
Family: Crassulaceae.

People Use This For

Orally, houseleek is used for severe diarrhea.
Topically, houseleek is used for burns, ulcers, warts, and itchy, burning skin and swelling associated with insect bites. The diluted juice is used as a gargle for stomatitis (18).

Safety

There is insufficient reliable information available about safety of houseleek.
Pregnancy and Lactation: Insufficient reliable information available; avoid using.

Effectiveness
There is insufficient reliable information available about the effectiveness of houseleek.

Mechanism of Action
The applicable part of houseleek is the leaf of the nonflowering plant. There is insufficient reliable information available about the possible mechanism of action and active ingredients.

Adverse Reactions
None reported.

Interactions with Herbs & Other Dietary Supplements
Insufficient reliable information available.

Interactions with Drugs
No interactions are known to occur, and there is no known reason to expect a clinically significant interaction with houseleek.

Interactions with Foods
No interactions are known to occur, and there is no known reason to expect a clinically significant interaction with houseleek.

Interactions with Lab Tests
No interactions are known to occur, and there is no known reason to expect a clinically significant interaction with houseleek.

Interactions with Diseases or Conditions
No interactions are known to occur, and there is no known reason to expect a clinically significant interaction with houseleek.

Dosage and Administration
ORAL: Houseleek is used as a tea (18).
TOPICAL: Houseleek is used as freshly pressed leaves and juice (18).

Comments
None.

HUPERZINE A

Also Known As
HupA, Huperzine, Huperzine-A, Selagine.
CAUTION: See separate listing for Chinese Club Moss.

Scientific Names
Huperzine A.

People Use This For
Orally, huperzine A is used for Alzheimer's disease (3138,3140,3171,4624), memory and learning enhancement (4626), age-related memory impairment (3561), increasing alertness and energy (3130), protection from neurotoxic agents including organophosphate nerve gases (3137,3139,3561), glutamate toxicity (3561), and for treating myasthenia gravis (3140,3561).

Safety
POSSIBLY SAFE ...when used orally and appropriately, short-term. Huperzine A has been used safely in clinical trials lasting from 1-3 months (3138,3140,3171,3561,4624,4626).
PREGNANCY AND LACTATION: Insufficient reliable information available; avoid using.

Effectiveness
POSSIBLY EFFECTIVE ...when used orally for improving memory, cognitive function, and behavioral function in Alzheimer's, multi-infarct, and senile dementia (3138,3140,3171,4624). In one clinical trial, patients with Alzheimer's disease treated with huperzine A had significant improvement in memory, cognitive, and behavioral function scales compared to placebo after 8 weeks of treatment (3138). In a small-scale, placebo-controlled trial, multi-infarct and senile dementia

patients treated with huperzine A had significant improvement in memory function after 2-4 weeks of treatment (3140). Long-term, large scale trials are necessary to confirm these findings and determine huperzine A's potential role in dementia. ...when used intramuscularly for preventing muscle weakness in patients with myasthenia gravis. In a short-term, small-scale open-label trial, stabilized patients with myasthenia gravis given huperzine A intramuscularly for 10 days maintained muscle strength as well as patients treated with intramuscular neostigmine alternating with intramuscular huperzine A. Huperzine A was reported to have a 7 hour duration of effect compared to 4 hours for neostigmine (3561). Well-controlled, large-scale trials are necessary to confirm huperzine A's potential benefit in myasthenia gravis. ...when used orally in healthy adolescents for improving memory function. In a small-scale, placebo controlled trial, Chinese middle school children complaining of poor memory had significant improvement in memory quotient scores after taking huperzine A for 4 weeks compared to placebo (4626).

There is insufficient reliable information available about the effectiveness of huperzine A for its other uses.

Mechanism of Action

Huperzine A is an alkaloid isolated from Chinese club moss, Huperzia serrata and from Lycopodium selago (3082,3130). It is an optically active stereoisomer. Only the levorotatory-isomer is pharmacologically active (3561). Huperzine A is thought to be beneficial in dementia, memory impairment, and myasthenia gravis due to its effects on acetylcholine levels (3133,3134,3135,3136,3172). It is a reversible inhibitor of acetylcholinesterase (AChE) and crosses the blood-brain barrier (3082). Huperzine A inhibits AChE activity in the brain for up to three hours. It produces a variable degree of acetylcholine elevation in different areas of the brain, with maximal values in the frontal and parietal cortex (125% and 105% respectively), and 22-65% in other brain regions (3141). It might be more specific for AChE and have a longer duration of action than AChE inhibitors such as tacrine (Cognex) or donepezil (Aricept), which are marketed as prescription drugs for Alzheimer's disease (3131,3132). In animal studies, huperzine A was found to be 64 times more potent than tacrine. It also is more bioavailable and penetrates the blood-brain barrier better than tacrine (3561). Huperzine A protects neurons against toxic levels of glutamate by blocking glutamate-induce neuronal calcium influx and cell death (3131,3561). Although it has low affinity, huperzine A is also a cerebral cortex N-methyl-D-aspartate (NMDA) receptor antagonist (3129,3137). It might also protect against seizures and neuropathological changes caused by exposure to organophosphate nerve agents such as soman, by protecting peripheral and central stores of acetylcholine (3137,3139).

Adverse Reactions

Orally, huperzine A can cause nausea, sweating, blurred vision, hyperactivity, anorexia, decreased heart rate, and fasciculations (3140,3143,3172,3561,4625). It has been suggested that huperzine A might have fewer cholinergic side effects than tacrine (Cognex) and donepezil (Aricept), but this has not been confirmed in human trials (3131). Adverse effects that have been reported with other AChE inhibitors, and theoretically might occur with huperzine A, include vomiting, diarrhea, cramping, hypersalivation, increased urination/incontinence, and bradycardia (14).

Interactions with Herbs & Other Dietary Supplements

Insufficient reliable information available.

Interactions with Drugs

ANTICHOLINERGIC DRUGS: Theoretically, concurrent use of anticholinergic drugs and huperzine A might decrease the effectiveness of huperzine A or the anticholinergic agent. In an animal model, huperzine A reversed cognitive deficits induced by scopolamine (5537). Other anticholinergic drugs include atropine, benztropine (Cogentin), biperiden (Akineton), procyclidine (Kemadrin), and trihexyphenidyl (Artane) (15).

CHOLINERGIC DRUGS, ACETYLCHOLINESTERASE (AChE) INHIBITORS: Theoretically, concurrent use might have additive effects with drugs that promote acetylcholine activity because huperzine A has AChE inhibitor properties (14). AChE inhibitors and cholinergic drugs include bethanechol (Urecholine), donepezil (Aricept), echothiophate (Phospholine Iodide), edrophonium (Enoln, Reversol, Tensilon), neostigmine (Prostigmin), physostigmine (Antilirium), pyridostigmine (Mestinon, Regonol), succinylcholine (Anectine, Quelicin), and tacrine (Cognex) (14).

Interactions with Foods

No interactions are known to occur, and there is no known reason to expect a clinically significant interaction with huperzine A.

Interactions with Lab Tests

No interactions are known to occur, and there is no known reason to expect a clinically significant interaction with huperzine A.

Interactions with Diseases or Conditions

BRADYCARDIA/CARDIOVASCULAR DISEASE: Huperzine A can cause decreased heart rate and might

exacerbate bradycardia and other cardiac conditions sensitive to decreased heart rate (3561); use with caution.
EPILEPSY: Theoretically, huperzine A might exacerbate seizure disorders (14); use with caution.
GASTROINTESTINAL TRACT OBSTRUCTION: Theoretically, huperzine A might exacerbate gastrointestinal obstruction due to its pro-secretory effects (14); use with caution.
PEPTIC ULCER DISEASE: Theoretically, huperzine A might exacerbate peptic ulcer disease due to its pro-secretory effects (14); use with caution.
PULMONARY CONDITIONS: Theoretically, huperzine A might exacerbate pulmonary conditions such as asthma and chronic obstructive pulmonary disease due to its pro-secretory effects (14); use with caution.
UROGENITAL TRACT OBSTRUCTION: Theoretically, huperzine A might exacerbate urogenital tract obstruction due to its pro-secretory effects (14); use with caution.

Dosage and Administration
ORAL: For Alzheimer's disease and multi-infarct dementia, doses of 50-200 mcg twice daily have been used (3138,3140,4625). For senile or presenile dementia, doses of 30 mcg twice daily have been used (3140). For improving memory in adolescents, doses of 100 mcg twice daily have been used (4626).
INTRAMUSCULAR: For prevention of muscle weakness in myasthenia gravis, doses of 400 mcg daily have been used (3561).

Comments
The Cerebra brand name used for huperzine A has been confused with the prescription drugs Celebrex, Celexa, and Cerebyx (3142). Huperzine A is also referred to as selagine. Avoid confusion with the prescription drug selegiline (Eldepryl). Huperzine A is a drug that stretches the guidelines of the Dietary Supplement Health and Education Act (DSHEA). Although derived from a plant, huperzine A is a laboratory-manipulated, highly purified drug, unlike herbs which typically contain hundreds of constituents. Caution people that the moss from which huperzine A is derived is an expensive, rare Chinese herb (3143). To date, most clinical studies have been published in the Chinese literature. Synthetic derivatives of huperzine A are now being studied for Alzheimer's disease (3143). Chemical hybrids of huperzine A plus tacrine and huperzine A plus donepezil are being investigated (3143,4625). The hybrid of huperzine A plus donepezil has been referred to as huprine X (4625). Laboratory studies indicate that these hybrids have substantially greater affinity for AChE than tacrine or donepezil and show potential for enhanced efficacy at lower doses, with fewer side effects (3143,4625).

HYDRANGEA

Also Known As
Mountain Hydrangea, Seven Barks, Smooth Hydrangea, Wild Hydrangea.

Scientific Names
Hydrangea arborescens.
Family: Hydrangeaceae or Saxifragaceae.

People Use This For
Orally, hydrangea is used for conditions of the urinary tract, such as cystitis, urethritis, prostatitis, enlarged prostate, and urinary calculi (4,5,18).

Safety
POSSIBLY SAFE ...when used orally and appropriately, short-term (12).
LIKELY UNSAFE ...when used orally in excessive amounts (over 2 grams of dried rhizome/root per dose) (4,12).
...when used orally long-term (4,12).
PREGNANCY AND LACTATION: Insufficient reliable information available; avoid using.

Effectiveness
There is insufficient reliable information available about the effectiveness of hydrangea.

Mechanism of Action
The applicable parts of hydrangea are the rhizome and root. Researchers think hydrangea possesses mild diuretic activity and properties which prevent the formation of stones or calculus (4). The cyanogenic glycoside constituent, hydrangin, may be responsible for some of the potential adverse effects (12).

Adverse Reactions

Orally, hydrangea can cause gastroenteritis (4). Overdose symptoms include vertigo and a feeling of tightness in the chest (4). There is one case report of cholestatic hepatitis associated with Prostata, a multi-ingredient product containing hydrangea (598).

Interactions with Herbs & Other Dietary Supplements

Insufficient reliable information available

Interactions with Drugs

No interactions are known to occur, and there is no known reason to expect a clinically significant interaction with hydrangea.

Interactions with Foods

No interactions are known to occur, and there is no known reason to expect a clinically significant interaction with hydrangea.

Interactions with Lab Tests

No interactions are known to occur, and there is no known reason to expect a clinically significant interaction with hydrangea.

Interactions with Diseases or Conditions

No interactions are known to occur, and there is no known reason to expect a clinically significant interaction with hydrangea.

Dosage and Administration

ORAL: A typical dose is 2-4 grams dried rhizome and root three times daily or one cup tea (steep 2-4 grams dried rhizome and root in 150 mL boiling water 5-10 minutes, strain) three times daily (4,12). Liquid extract (1:1 in 25% alcohol), 2-4 mL three times daily has been used (4,12). Tincture (1:5 in 45% alcohol), 2-10 mL three times daily is commonly used (4). One reference states not to exceed 2 grams dried rhizome and root per dose (12).

Comments

None.

HYDRAZINE SULFATE

Also Known As

Hydrazine, Sehydrin.

Scientific Names

Hydrazine sulfate.

People Use This For

Orally, hydrazine sulfate is used for treating cancer and the general weight loss and wasting associated with it (14,8000).

Safety

POSSIBLY SAFE ...when used orally and appropriately (8004,8005).
UNSAFE ...when used topically or by inhalation; avoid using (14).
PREGNANCY: UNSAFE ...when used orally, topically, or by inhalation. Some evidence suggests hydrazine is embryotoxic, fetotoxic, genotoxic, and carcinogenic (14).
LACTATION: Insufficient reliable information available; avoid using.

Effectiveness

POSSIBLY INEFFECTIVE ...when used as a single agent for treating metastatic colorectal cancer (8002).
LIKELY INEFFECTIVE ...when used as an adjunct to chemotherapy for treating non-small cell lung cancer (8001,8003).
There is insufficient reliable information available about the effectiveness of hydrazine sulfate for its other uses.

Mechanism of Action

Hydrazine sulfate is an organic compound used in various industrial processes (14). Hydrazine, itself, can be inhaled or absorbed through the skin causing toxicity (14). As a sulfate salt, hydrazine inhibits phosphoenolpyruvate kinase (8000), an enzyme involved in gluconeogenesis. Scientists theorize that excessive gluconeogenesis might be partially responsible for the cachexia that occurs in people with cancer (8000,8005). By blocking gluconeogenesis, hydrazine sulfate might reduce cachexia (8000). Use of hydrazine sulfate has been associated with increased body weight in people with diverse cancers treated with varied chemotherapy regimens (8004). However, when compared to placebo, hydrazine sulfate failed to improve survival or anorexia, it was associated with greater sensory and motor neuropathy, and a poorer quality of life in people with non-small cell lung cancer treated with cisplatin and vinblastine (8003).

Adverse Reactions

Orally, hydrazine sulfate can cause nausea, vomiting, dizziness, drowsiness, peripheral neuropathies (8005), weakness, and irregular breathing, confusion, hypoglycemia or hyperglycemia, lethargy, violent behavior, restlessness, seizures, coma, renal toxicity, and hepatotoxicity (14).

Topically or inhaled, hydrazine comes in contact with the skin, eyes, or mucous membranes, it can cause irritation, burns, permanent damage to the eyes, bronchial mucus destruction, pulmonary edema, and death (14). Hydrazine is a sensitizer and can cause an allergic reaction (14).

Interactions with Herbs & Other Dietary Supplements

Insufficient reliable information available.

Interactions with Drugs

CNS DEPRESSANTS: Concomitant use with alcohol, barbiturates, or benzodiazepines can increase the toxicity and decrease the effectiveness of hydrazine (8005).

MAOIs: Theoretically, concomitant use might increase the effects and adverse effects associated with monoamine oxidase inhibitors (8005).

Interactions with Foods

TYRAMINE-CONTAINING FOODS: Avoid concomitant use, hydrazine sulfate may have monoamine oxidase inhibiting activity (8005). Tyramine-containing foods, include avocado, banana, brewer's yeast, broad beans, caviar, aged cheese, aged red wine, herring, liver, and pickled meats (151).

Interactions with Lab Tests

ALANINE AMINOTRANSFERASE (ALT): Can increase serum levels and test results secondary to hepatotoxicity (275).

ALKALINE PHOSPHATASE (Alk Phos): Can increase serum levels and test results secondary to hepatotoxicity (275).

ASPARTATE AMINOTRANSFERASE: Can increase serum levels and test results secondary to hepatotoxicity (275).

BILE: Can increase urine levels and test results secondary to hepatotoxicity (275).

BILIRUBIN: Can increase serum levels and test results secondary to hepatotoxicity (275).

BSP RETENTION: Can increase serum levels and test results secondary to hepatotoxicity (275).

ERYTHROCYTE SEDIMENTATION RATE (sed rate): Can increase sed rate results secondary to an SLE-type syndrome (275).

GLUCOSE: Can decrease serum glucose and test results by potentiating insulin effects (275).

5-HYDROXYINDOLACETIC ADIC (5-HIAA): Can decrease urine levels and test results (275).

LE CELLS: Can cause a positive blood test result by activating lupus erythematosus (275).

LYMPHOCYTES: Can decrease blood levels and test results with megadose supplementation (275).

METANEPHRINES (total): Can increase urine levels and test results (275).

NORMETANEPHRINE: Can increase urine levels and test results (275).

VANILLYLMANDELIC ACID: Can increase urine levels and test results (275).

Interactions with Diseases or Conditions

DIABETES: Might interfere with blood glucose control due to effects on gluconeogenesis (14,8000).

KIDNEY DISORDERS: Theoretically, might worsen kidney disorders (14).

LIVER DISORDERS: Theoretically, might worsen liver disorders (14).

PSYCHOSIS: Theoretically, might worsen psychoses (14).

SEIZURE DISORDERS: Can increase incidence of seizures (14).

Dosage and Administration

ORAL: A typical dose used for cachexia in people with cancer on a chemotherapy regimen is 60 mg three times daily for a cycle of 30-45 days followed by a rest period of 2-6 weeks (8004,8005).

Comments

Although some information shows hydrazine sulfate might be useful in the general weight loss and wasting associated with cancer, information is very limited and inconclusive.

HYDROXYMETHYLBUTYRATE (HMB)

Also Known As

B-Hydroxy B-Methylbutyrate Monohydrate, Beta-Hydroxy-Beta-Methylbutyric Acid, Beta-Hydroxy Beta-Methylbutyric Acid, HMB, Hydroxymethyl Butyrate.

Scientific Names

Beta-hydroxy-beta-methylbutyrate.

People Use This For

Orally, HMB is used for increasing the benefits from weight training and exercise, cardiovascular disease, hypercholesterolemia, and hypertension (2167,2168,3374). In combination with arginine and glutamine, HMB is also used orally for treating weight loss in people with AIDS (1909).

Safety

POSSIBLY SAFE ...when used orally and appropriately, short-term. Doses of 3 grams per day or less for up to 8 weeks seem to be safe (1909,2168,3374).
PREGNANCY AND LACTATION: Insufficient reliable information available; avoid using.

Effectiveness

POSSIBLY EFFECTIVE ...when used orally for increasing the benefits from weight training (1929,2168). There is some evidence that using HMB in combination with a weight training exercise program may be more effective than exercise alone for increasing upper body muscular strength (1929,2168). ...when used orally for mild hypertension. There is some evidence that HMB can lower systolic blood pressure by approximately 4-9 mmHg in some patients with high blood pressure (3374). ...when taken orally for hypercholesterolemia. HMB seems to decrease total cholesterol by 11-13 mg/dL in some patients with high cholesterol (3374). ...when used orally in combination with amino acids to prevent wasting in patients with AIDS (1909). HMB in combination with arginine and glutamine seems to increase body weight and lean body mass, and possibly improve immune function when used over 8 weeks (1909).
There is insufficient reliable information available about the effectiveness of HMB for its other uses.

Mechanism of Action

Hydroxymethylbutyrate (HMB) is a byproduct of metabolism of the amino acid leucine (2168). HMB is also a precursor to cholesterol. HMB found in the cytosol of liver and muscle cells is converted to beta-hydroxy-beta-methylglutarate-Co-A (HMG-CoA). HMG-CoA is used for the cellular synthesis of cholesterol, and might also promote muscle growth by reducing the catabolism of muscle protein (2168,3374). There is also some evidence that HMB lowers levels of creatine phosphokine (CK) and lactate dehydrogenase (LDH), and decreases the excretion of 3-methylhistidine (3-MH). This suggests that HMB might also prevent or decrease muscle membrane inflammation or injury, and prevent increased proteolysis that is often associated with intense exercise (1929,2168).

Adverse Reactions

Orally, HMB seems to be well tolerated (2168,3374). Use in doses less than 3 grams per day for 3-8 weeks seems to be safe. Adverse effects have not been reported (1909,3374).

Interactions with Herbs & Other Dietary Supplements

Insufficient reliable information available.

Interactions with Drugs

No interactions are known to occur, and there is no known reason to expect a clinically significant interaction with HMB.

Interactions with Foods

No interactions are known to occur, and there is no known reason to expect a clinically significant interaction with HMB.

Interactions with Lab Tests

No interactions are known to occur, and there is no known reason to expect a clinically significant interaction with HMB.

Interactions with Diseases or Conditions

No interactions are known to occur, and there is no known reason to expect a clinically significant interaction with HMB.

Dosage and Administration

ORAL: For muscle building and increasing body strength during weight training, doses of 1 gram three times daily (1929) or 1.5 grams once or twice daily has been used (3374). For lowering cholesterol and blood pressure, 3 grams daily has been used (3374). For treatment of AIDS-related wasting, 3 grams HMB in combination with 14 grams each of arginine and glutamine administered in two divided doses daily has been used (1909).

Comments

None.

HYSSOP

Also Known As

None.

Scientific Names

Hyssopus officinalis.
Family: Labiatae or Lamiaceae.

People Use This For

Orally, hyssop is used for liver and gallbladder complaints, intestinal inflammation (2,18), colds, respiratory and chest ailments (2,6,18), sore throats, asthma, urinary tract inflammation, gas and colic, to stimulate appetite and circulation (2,18), and as an expectorant (6).
Topically, hyssop is used as a gargle; in baths to induce sweating; and for treating skin irritations, burns, bruises, and frostbite (11).
Historically, hyssop was used for coughs, colds, breast and lung problems, menstrual complaints (11), and digestive and intestinal problems (11,18).
In foods, hyssop oil and extract are used as a flavoring (11).
In manufacturing, hyssop oil is used as a fragrance in soaps and cosmetics (11).

Safety

LIKELY SAFE ...when used orally in amounts found in foods (11). It has Generally Recognized as Safe (GRAS) status in the US (11). The maximum level of hyssop herb is 0.06% in alcoholic beverages. The maximum for the extract is 0.03%. The maximum for hyssop oil is 0.004% in alcoholic beverages (11).
POSSIBLY SAFE ...when used orally and appropriately for medicinal purposes (12).
POSSIBLY UNSAFE ...when used orally for medicinal purposes. There are reports that associate ingestion of the oil with tonic-clonic convulsions (2,18).
There is insufficient reliable information available about the safety of hyssop for its other uses.
CHILDREN: LIKELY UNSAFE ...when used orally because of a report that 2-3 drops over several days caused tonic-clonic convulsions (2,18); avoid using.
PREGNANCY: LIKELY UNSAFE ...when used orally because it might cause uterine stimulant and menstrual stimulant effects (12).
LACTATION: Insufficient reliable information available; avoid using.

Effectiveness

There is insufficient reliable information available about the effectiveness of hyssop.

Mechanism of Action

The applicable parts of hyssop are the above ground parts. Constituent marrubiin (11) has cardioactive effects and stimulates bronchial secretions (4). Caffeic acid and tannins may be responsible for the effect of extracts of dried leaves. Extracts show antiviral activity against herpes simplex virus and HIV in vitro (6,11). Hyssop oil causes convulsions (of CNS origin) and death in experimental rats (6), thought due to constituents pincamphone and isopincamphone (6). Hyssop oil is associated with tonic-clonic convulsions in adults and children (2,18).

Adverse Reactions
Orally, hyssop was associated with tonic-clonic convulsions in two adults (10-30 drops) and in one child (2-3 drops for several days) (2,18).

Interactions with Herbs & Other Dietary Supplements
Insufficient reliable information available.

Interactions with Drugs
No interactions are known to occur, and there is no known reason to expect a clinically significant interaction with hyssop.

Interactions with Foods
No interactions are known to occur, and there is no known reason to expect a clinically significant interaction with hyssop.

Interactions with Lab Tests
No interactions are known to occur, and there is no known reason to expect a clinically significant interaction with hyssop.

Interactions with Diseases or Conditions
SEIZURE DISORDERS: Theoretically, hyssop oil may exacerbate seizure disorders.

Dosage and Administration
ORAL: Typically people take two 445 mg capsules containing the hyssop herb three times daily (5019). Some people take 10-15 drops of the hyssop extract (12-14% by volume) in water two to three times daily (5023). People also consume or gargle the hyssop tea three times daily (5008). The tea is prepared by steeping 1-2 teaspoons of the dried hyssop flower tops in 150 mL boiling water for 10-15 minutes and then straining. Avoid internal use of hyssop oil due to possible neurotoxicity.
TOPICAL: No typical dosage.

Comments
None.

IBOGA

Also Known As
None.

Scientific Names
Tabernanthe iboga.
Family: Apocyanaceae.

People Use This For
Orally, iboga is used as an aperitif, aphrodisiac, tonic, for convalescence, debility, fever, flu, hypertension, neurasthenia (3919), and preventing fatigue and drowsiness (514).

Safety
There is insufficient reliable information available about the safety of iboga.
Pregnancy and Lactation: Insufficient reliable information available; avoid using.

Effectiveness
There is insufficient reliable information available about the effectiveness of iboga.

Mechanism of Action
The applicable part of iboga is the root. The hallucinogenic properties of iboga are due to the indole alkaloids, ibogaine, ibogamone, iboluteine, and tabernanthine (6,514). Ibogaine inhibits cholinesterase, leading to synaptic acetylcholine accumulation (6). The associated dose-dependent CNS stimulation ranges from mild excitation and euphoria to visual and auditory hallucinations (6,514). Ibogaine has kappa agonist effects; it is serotonergic; and it exhibits nicotinic and N-methyl-D-aspartate (NMDA) antagonism (813). Animal experiments suggest these effects may

have value in treating human addictions to alcohol, nicotine, opioids, cocaine, and other stimulants (812,813). The constituent tabernanthine demonstrates cardiac conduction effects similar to those of calcium channel antagonists (6).

Adverse Reactions
Iboga taken orally may cause bradycardia, hypotension, convulsions, paralysis, and respiratory arrest (6). Amounts large enough to induce hallucinations may also cause anxiety, apprehension, and death (6).

Interactions with Herbs & Other Dietary Supplements
Insufficient reliable information available.

Interactions with Drugs
ANTICHOLINERGIC DRUGS: Theoretically, concomitant use can antagonize anticholinergic effects.
CHOLINERGIC DRUGS: Theoretically, concomitant use may enhance effects and adverse effects.

Interactions with Foods
No interactions are known to occur, and there is no known reason to expect a clinically significant interaction with iboga.

Interactions with Lab Tests
No interactions are known to occur, and there is no known reason to expect a clinically significant interaction with iboga.

Interactions with Diseases or Conditions
No interactions are known to occur, and there is no known reason to expect a clinically significant interaction with iboga.

Dosage and Administration
ORAL: Dry root bark powder or root is chewed (6).

Comments
Iboga is used for ritual and ceremonial purposes in some African cultures (6,514,812).

ICELAND MOSS

Also Known As
Centraria, Eryngo-leaved Liverwort, Iceland Lichen, Lichen Islandicus.

Scientific Names
Cetraria islandica.
Family: Parmeliaceae.

People Use This For
Orally, Iceland moss is used for irritation of the oral and pharyngeal mucous membranes and associated dry cough, for loss of appetite (2), common cold, cough and bronchitis, dyspeptic complaints, fevers, and the tendency toward infection (18).
In folk medicine, Iceland moss has been used orally for lung disease, kidney and bladder complaints, and topically for poorly healing wounds (18).
For food uses, Iceland moss is utilized as an emergency food source in Iceland (3).
In manufacturing, Iceland moss is utilized as a flavoring agent in alcoholic beverages (12).

Safety
POSSIBLY SAFE ...when the dried plant is used orally, short-term for medicinal use (3,12). The dried plant can be contaminated with lead (3).
POSSIBLY UNSAFE ...when used in larger amounts as a food source because lead contamination can occur in amounts of up to 30 mg/kg of its dry weight (3). It is regulated in the US and allowable only as a flavoring agent in alcoholic beverages (12).
PREGNANCY AND LACTATION: POSSIBLY UNSAFE ...when used orally; avoid Iceland moss due to the potential for lead contamination (3).

Effectiveness

POSSIBLY EFFECTIVE ...when taken orally for irritation or inflammation of oral and pharyngeal mucous membranes (2).
There is insufficient reliable information available about the effectiveness of Iceland moss for its other uses.

Mechanism of Action

The applicable part of Iceland moss is the dried plant body. Iceland moss has soothing and mild antimicrobial action (2). The mucilage constituents, lichenin and isolichenin, and the bitter principles can be responsible for its effects (2,3). The bitter organic acid constituents can be responsible for an antibiotic effect (18).

Adverse Reactions

Orally, Iceland moss can cause GI irritation (12). Sensitization to Iceland moss is rare (18). It can be contaminated with lead up to 30 mg/kg of its dry weight (3).

Interactions with Herbs & Other Dietary Supplements

Insufficient reliable information available.

Interactions with Drugs

ORAL DRUGS: The fiber in Iceland moss can impair absorption of oral drugs (19).

Interactions with Foods

No interactions are known to occur, and there is no known reason to expect a clinically significant interaction with Iceland moss.

Interactions with Lab Tests

No interactions are known to occur, and there is no known reason to expect a clinically significant interaction with Iceland moss.

Interactions with Diseases or Conditions

GASTRODUODENAL ULCERS: The alcohol extract and powder of Iceland moss is contraindicated due to the potential for mucosal irritation (12).

Dosage and Administration

ORAL: The typical dose of Iceland moss is one cup of tea several times daily. The tea is prepared by steeping or simmering 1.5-3 grams of the dried plant in 150 mL boiling water for 5-10 minutes and then straining (3,7). The maximum dose of the moss is 4-6 grams per day of the dried plant or equivalent preparations (2).

Comments

Iceland moss is a lichen, or an algae and a fungus growing together in a symbiotic relationship (3). Iceland is one the least polluted countries in the world, which is important for lichens. Lichens derive their nutrients from the environment and are easily contaminated with radioactive or heavy metals. Most of the lichens in Europe were contaminated by the fallout from the Chernobyl accident, but Iceland only received negligible radioactive levels (6002).

IGNATIUS BEAN

Also Known As

None.

Scientific Names

Strychnos ignatii.
Family: Loganiaceae.

People Use This For

Orally, ignatius bean is used for faintness; as a bitter or tonic; and as an agent to invigorate, refresh, or restore body function (18).

Safety

UNSAFE ...when used orally due to its strychnine content (18). The FDA banned strychnine from nonprescription drug products in 1989 (14).
PREGNANCY AND LACTATION: UNSAFE ...when used orally due to toxic effects (18).

Effectiveness
LIKELY INEFFECTIVE ...when used orally for any medicinal use (14).

Mechanism of Action
Ignatius bean contains the centrally-acting neurotoxins strychnine and brucine (18). Strychnine competitively antagonizes post-synaptic binding of the inhibitory transmitter glycine, leading to heightened reflex excitability of muscles. External irritations or centrally-acting stimulants can trigger convulsions (2,14,505). Strychnine can selectively inhibit the spinal cord in subconvulsive amounts (2). However, strychnine accumulates with extended administration, particularly in individuals with liver damage. Chronic use of subconvulsive amounts can cause death after a period of weeks (18).

Adverse Reactions
Orally, 30-50 mg ignatius bean (5 mg strychnine) can cause restlessness, feelings of anxiety, heightening of sense perception, enhanced reflexes, equilibrium disorders, painful neck and back stiffness, followed later by twitching, tonic spasms of jaw and neck muscles, painful convulsions of the entire body triggered by visual or tactile stimulation with possible opisthotonos, muscle hypertonicity, and agitation. Dyspnea may follow spasm of respiratory muscles (14,18). Seizures occur within 15 minutes of ingestion (or 5 minutes of inhalation) and may result in hyperthermia, metabolic and respiratory acidosis, rhabdomyolysis, and myoglobinuric renal failure (14,17). 1-2 grams ignatius bean (50 mg strychnine) can be fatal (18); most deaths occur 3-6 hours post-ingestion from respiratory and subsequent cardiac arrest, anoxic brain damage, or multiple organ failure secondary to hyperthermia (14,18,505). Strychnine accumulates with extended administration, particularly in individuals with liver damage. Chronic use of subconvulsive amounts can cause death after a period of weeks (18).

Interactions with Herbs & Other Dietary Supplements
Insufficient reliable information available.

Interactions with Drugs
ANALEPTICS, PHENOTHIAZINES: Contraindicated in individuals with symptoms of poisoning (18).

Interactions with Foods
No interactions are known to occur, and there is no known reason to expect a clinically significant interaction with ignatius bean.

Interactions with Lab Tests
No interactions are known to occur, and there is no known reason to expect a clinically significant interaction with ignatius bean.

Interactions with Diseases or Conditions
LIVER DISEASE: Contraindicated; strychnine accumulates in individuals with liver damage. Also, strychnine accumulation can cause liver damage (18).

Dosage and Administration
ORAL: TOXIC, avoid using (18).

Comments
Strychnine may be detected by thin-layer chromatography (qualitative analysis) and high performance liquid chromatography (quantitative analysis). Urine and gastric aspirate are most useful in confirming poisoning (17). Strychnine pills are no longer marketed (14). Strychnos ianata and strychnos multiflora seeds were once treated in the same way as ignatius beans (18).

IMMORTELLE

Also Known As
Common Shrubby Everlasting, Eternal Flower, Goldilocks, Yellow Chaste Weed.
CAUTION: See separate listing for Sandy Everlasting.

Scientific Names
Helichrysum arenarium.
Family: Compositae/Asteraceae.

People Use This For
Orally, immortelle is used for liver and gallbladder disorders, including chronic gallstones with accompanying cramps. It is also used orally for dyspepsia, loss of appetite, to stimulate bile flow, and as an antimicrobial. In folk medicine, it is used orally as a diuretic [18].

Safety
There is insufficient reliable information available about the safety of immortelle.
Pregnancy and Lactation: Insufficient reliable information available; avoid using.

Effectiveness
There is insufficient reliable information available about the effectiveness of immortelle.

Mechanism of Action
The applicable part of immortelle is the dried flower. There is insufficient reliable information available about the possible mechanism of action and active ingredients.

Adverse Reactions
When immortelle is used in people with gallstones, it may cause colic [18]. Immortelle can cause an allergic reaction in individuals sensitive to the Asteraceae/Compositae family. Members of this family include ragweed, chrysanthemums, marigolds, daisies, and many other herbs.

Interactions with Herbs & Other Dietary Supplements
Insufficient reliable information available.

Interactions with Drugs
No interactions are known to occur, and there is no known reason to expect a clinically significant interaction with immortelle.

Interactions with Foods
No interactions are known to occur, and there is no known reason to expect a clinically significant interaction with immortelle.

Interactions with Lab Tests
No interactions are known to occur, and there is no known reason to expect a clinically significant interaction with immortelle.

Interactions with Diseases or Conditions
BILIARY OBSTRUCTION: Immortelle is contraindicated during biliary obstruction secondary to its possible stimulation of biliary flow.
CROSS-ALLERGENICITY: Can cause an allergic reaction in individuals sensitive to the Asteraceae/Compositae family. Members of this family include ragweed, chrysanthemums, marigolds, daisies, and many other herbs.

Dosage and Administration
ORAL: One cup of tea daily. The tea is prepared by steeping 3-4 grams dried flower in 150 mL of boiling water for 10 minutes and straining. The tea is sometimes drunk throughout the day, but must be made fresh each time. The average daily dose is 3 grams of immortelle [18].

Comments
Immortelle is a protected species. It can easily be confused with sandy everlasting (Helichrysum augustifolium, synonym Helichrysum italicum), or Helichrysum stoechas [18]. Avoid confusion with immortal (Asclepias asperula) [11].

INDIAN FRANKINCENSE

Also Known As

Boswellia, Boswellin, Boswellin Serrata Resin, Indian Olibanum, Salai Guggal.
CAUTION: See separate listings for Frankincense and Guggul.

Scientific Names

Boswellia serrata.
Family: Burseraceae.

People Use This For

Orally, Indian frankincense is used for arthritis, as an anti-inflammatory agent (11), and for ulcerative colitis (6).
Historically, it has been used for rheumatism, syphilis, painful menstruation, pimples, sores, tumors, cancers, asthma, sore throat, abdominal pain, stomach troubles, nervous problems, as a stimulant, respiratory antiseptic, diuretic, and for stimulating menstrual flow (11).
In manufacturing, the resin oil and extracts are used in soaps, cosmetics, foods, and beverages (11).

Safety

LIKELY SAFE ...when consumed in amounts found in foods (maximum use level 0.001% in meat products) (11); approved for food use in the US (11).
POSSIBLY SAFE ...when used orally and appropriately as a medicinal agent (6,12).
There is insufficient reliable information available about the safety of Indian frankincense for its other uses.
PREGNANCY AND LACTATION: Insufficient reliable information available.

Effectiveness

POSSIBLY EFFECTIVE ...when used orally for arthritis (11), and ulcerative colitis symptoms (6).
There is insufficient reliable information available about the effectiveness of Indian frankincense for its other uses.

Mechanism of Action

The applicable part of Indian frankincense is the resin. The principle constituents of Indian frankincense are boswellic acid and alpha-boswellic acid, which have anti-inflammatory properties (6,11,1706). In preliminary research, Indian frankincense extracts show anti-inflammatory and antiarthritis effects, but various Indian frankincense-containing products fail to show antiarthritis, anti-inflammatory, or antipyretic effects (6131). However, an Indian frankincense resin-containing herb/mineral combination product reduces pain and disability in people with arthritis symptoms (6). Indian frankincense resin might improve ulcerative colitis (1708), bronchial asthma symptoms, and indices of respiratory function (1709).

Adverse Reactions

None reported.

Interactions with Herbs & Other Dietary Supplements

Insufficient reliable information available.

Interactions with Drugs

No interactions are known to occur, and there is no known reason to expect a clinically significant interaction with Indian frankincense.

Interactions with Foods

No interactions are known to occur, and there is no known reason to expect a clinically significant interaction with Indian frankincense.

Interactions with Lab Tests

No interactions are known to occur, and there is no known reason to expect a clinically significant interaction with Indian frankincense.

Interactions with Diseases or Conditions

No interactions are known to occur, and there is no known reason to expect a clinically significant interaction with Indian frankincense.

Dosage and Administration

ORAL (gum resin preparation): Ulcerative colitis, 350 mg three times daily, reported in one clinical trial (1708). Bronchial asthma, 300 mg three times daily, reported in one clinical trial (1709).

Comments

Olibanum is a term which refers to the oleogum resin exuded from incisions in the bark of several Boswellia species, including Boswellia serrata (Indian frankincense), Boswellia carterii (Bible frankincense), Boswellia frereana (African elemi), and Boswellia bhau-dajiana (11).

INDIAN GOOSEBERRY

Also Known As

Aamalaki, Amalaki, Amblabaum, Amla, Aonla, Emblic, Emblic Myrobalan, Emblica, Groseillier de Ceylan, Indian-Gooseberry, Mirobalano, Myrobalan Emblic, Neli.

Scientific Names

Emblica officinalis, synonyms Mirobalanus embilica, Phyllanthus emblica.
Family: Euphorbiaceae.

People Use This For

Orally, Indian gooseberry is used for lowering cholesterol, treating atherosclerosis, cancer, dyspepsia, eye problems, joint pain, diarrhea, dysentery, "organ restoration", and as an anti-inflammatory and antimicrobial (6). It is also used orally for obesity (2075).
In Ayurvedic medicine, Indian gooseberry is used orally for treating diabetes and pancreatitis (6).
In India, Indian gooseberry is consumed as part of the diet (6).

Safety

LIKELY SAFE ...when consumed in amounts found in foods (6,2076).
There is insufficient reliable information available about the safety of Indian gooseberry when used in amounts greater than those found in foods.
PREGNANCY AND LACTATION: Insufficient reliable information available; avoid using.

Effectiveness

There is insufficient reliable information available about the effectiveness of Indian gooseberry.

Mechanism of Action

The applicable part of Indian gooseberry is primarily the fruit (2075), but extracts from the leaves have also been used (6,2078,2079). Indian gooseberry fruit and juice have been shown to lower total serum cholesterol, low-density lipoprotein (LDL), triglycerides, and phospholipids and to have positive effects on atherosclerosis in animals (6). Preliminary evidence suggests Indian gooseberry might also lower total serum cholesterol levels in humans, without affecting high-density lipoprotein (HDL) levels (2077). Indian gooseberry fruit juice also has antimicrobial, antimutagenic and antioxidant activity in animals (6,2080,2081). Indian gooseberry leaf extract has been shown to have anti-inflammatory activity (6,2078,2079).

Adverse Reactions

None reported.

Interactions with Herbs & Other Dietary Supplements

Insufficient reliable information available.

Interactions with Drugs

No interactions are known to occur, and there is no known reason to expect a clinically significant interaction with Indian gooseberry.

Interactions with Foods

No interactions are known to occur, and there is no known reason to expect a clinically significant interaction with Indian gooseberry.

Interactions with Lab Tests
No interactions are known to occur, and there is no known reason to expect a clinically significant interaction with Indian gooseberry.

Interactions with Diseases or Conditions
No interactions are known to occur, and there is no known reason to expect a clinically significant interaction with Indian gooseberry.

Dosage and Administration
No typical dosage.

Comments
Indian gooseberry is a native deciduous tree in India and the Middle East (6). Indian gooseberry has been used in Ayurvedic medicine for thousands of years. Reference to Indian gooseberry appeared in an Ayurvedic medicine text in the seventh century (3563).

INDIAN LONG PEPPER

Also Known As
Jaborandi Pepper, Langer Pfeffer, Long Pepper, Pimenta-Longa, Poivre Long.

Scientific Names
Piper longum.
Family: Piperaceae.

People Use This For
In folk medicine, Indian long pepper is used orally to treat headache, toothache, asthma, beri-beri, bronchitis, mucous membrane inflammation, cholera, coma, cough, diarrhea, dysentery, epilepsy, fever, frigidity, stomachache, stroke, heartburn, indigestion, insomnia, leprosy, lethargy, enlarged spleen, muscle pain, nasal discharge, painful menses, paralysis, psoriasis, sterility in women, snake bites, tetanus, thirst, tuberculosis, and tumors. It is also used during childbirth, and during the 3-6 weeks following childbirth while the uterus returns to normal size. Indian long pepper fruit is also used in folk medicine to stimulate menstrual flow, appetite, and bile flow; to improve digestion; induce sweating; and as an abortifacient, analgesic, antiflatulent, aphrodisiac, astringent, bactericide, diuretic, larvicide, sedative, stimulant, tonic, and vermifuge.

In Ayurvedic medicine, Indian long pepper fruit is used in combination herbal preparations (3755).

For food uses, Indian long pepper fruit has a role in cooking, both as an ingredient and a spice. It is used in fresh or dried form.

Safety
LIKELY SAFE ...when used orally in amounts found in foods.
There is insufficient reliable information available about the safety of Indian long pepper for its other uses.
PREGNANCY AND LACTATION: Insufficient reliable information is available; avoid amounts greater than found in foods.

Effectiveness
There is insufficient reliable information available about the effectiveness of Indian long pepper.

Mechanism of Action
The applicable part of Indian long pepper is the fruit. Piper longum contains piperine which can increase oral absorption of drugs and other substances, possibly by modulating intestinal membrane dynamics (3757). Some evidence suggests an ethanolic extract and isolated piperine might have amoebicidal activity (3758). An Ayurvedic herbal preparation containing piper longum (Pippali rasayana) shows evidence that it is useful for managing giardiasis (3754,3755). In mice, an ethanolic extract of piper longum administered chronically increased weights of lung, spleen, and reproductive organs. It also increased sperm count and motility without demonstrating acute or chronic toxicity (3756).

Adverse Reactions
None reported.

Interactions with Herbs & Other Dietary Supplements
SCOTCH BROOM: Piperine increases the bioavailability of sparteine, a constituent of scotch broom (19).

Interactions with Drugs
PHENYTOIN: Concomitant administration speeds absorption and slows elimination of phenytoin (Dilantin) (537).
PROPRANOLOL: Concomitant administration speeds and increases absorption, and increases serum concentrations of propranolol (Inderal) (538).
THEOPHYLLINE: Concomitant administration increases absorption and serum concentrations of theophylline (Theo-Dur) (538).

Interactions with Foods
No interactions are known to occur, and there is no known reason to expect a clinically significant interaction with Indian long pepper.

Interactions with Lab Tests
SERUM DRUG ASSAYS: Can increase phenytoin, propranolol, and theophylline serum concentrations and test results (537,538).

Interactions with Diseases or Conditions
No interactions are known to occur, and there is no known reason to expect a clinically significant interaction with Indian long pepper.

Dosage and Administration
No typical dosage.

Comments
Piper nigrum, the source of black pepper and white pepper, also contains the constituent piperine. However, red pepper and cayenne do not.

INDIAN PHYSIC

Also Known As
American Ipecacuanha, Bowman's Root, Gillenia, Indian Hippo.
CAUTION: See separate listings for Black Root and Canadian Hemp.

Scientific Names
Gillenia trifoliata.

People Use This For
Orally, Indian physic is used for digestive disorders and as an emetic (18).

Safety
There is insufficient reliable information available about the safety of Indian physic.
Pregnancy and Lactation: Insufficient reliable information available; avoid using.

Effectiveness
There is insufficient reliable information about the effectiveness of Indian physic.

Mechanism of Action
The applicable parts of Indian physic are the dried root and root bark. Indian physic is stated to have expectorant, emetic, and "blood purification" properties (18).

Adverse Reactions
None reported.

Interactions with Herbs & Other Dietary Supplements
Insufficient reliable information available.

Interactions with Drugs

No interactions are known to occur, and there is no known reason to expect a clinically significant interaction with Indian physic.

Interactions with Foods

No interactions are known to occur, and there is no known reason to expect a clinically significant interaction with Indian physic.

Interactions with Lab Tests

No interactions are known to occur, and there is no known reason to expect a clinically significant interaction with Indian physic.

Interactions with Diseases or Conditions

No interactions are known to occur, and there is no known reason to expect a clinically significant interaction with Indian physic.

Dosage and Administration

ORAL: Used as a powder in tea or tonic (18).

Comments

Avoid confusion with Canadian hemp (Apocynum cannabinum), also known as Indian physic (12). Avoid confusion with black root (Leptandra virginica), also known as bowman's root.

INDIAN SNAKEROOT

Also Known As

Chandrika, Chota-Chand, Covanamilpori, Dhanburua, Pagla-Ka-Dawa, Patalagandhi, Rauwolfae radix, Rauwolfia, Rauwolfia Serpentina, Rauwolfiawurzel, Sarpagandha.

Scientific Names

Rauvolfia serpentina.
Family: Apocynaceae.

People Use This For

Orally, Indian snakeroot is used for mild essential hypertension (2,18), symptomatic relief in individuals with agitated psychosis unable to tolerate other agents (13), for nervousness, and insomnia (18). As a prescription product, it is used to treat mild to moderate hypertension (15), schizophrenia, and vasospastic attacks due to peripheral vascular disorders (15). Traditionally, Indian snakeroot has been used for snake and reptile bites, insanity, fever, constipation, feverish intestinal diseases, liver ailments, rheumatism, dropsy (edema), as a tonic for general debilities (18), for mental illness, and epilepsy (514).

Safety

POSSIBLY SAFE ...when the prescription product is used orally (15). ...when the standardized extract is used orally under the supervision of a medical professional trained in the use of Indian snakeroot (18).
POSSIBLY UNSAFE ...when used orally for self-medication. Appropriate use of Indian snakeroot requires medical diagnosis and treatment. Large amounts or overdose can lead to CNS depression, convulsions, extrapyramidal effects, and coma (15). ...when used by individuals operating motor vehicles or machinery. Indian snakeroot can alter reaction time (2,15).
PREGNANCY: LIKELY UNSAFE ...when used orally (2,18) because the reserpine alkaloid constituents cross the placenta and can be potentially teratogenic (15,4260).
LACTATION: POSSIBLY UNSAFE ...when used orally because the reserpine alkaloids are excreted in breast milk although there are no reports of toxicity (4260); avoid using.

Effectiveness

There is insufficient reliable information available about the effectiveness of Indian snakeroot. However, early evidence indicates that Indian snakeroot in a specific combination with two other herbs might offer some benefit for insomnia (6051). More evidence is needed to rate the effectiveness for this use.

Mechanism of Action

The applicable part of Indian snakeroot is the root. The properties of the whole root of rauwolfia serpentina differ from those of reserpine. The whole root contains over 50 alkaloids (13). Rauwolfia serpentina demonstrates hypotensive, sedative, and tranquilizing effects (15). It also reduces heart rate (13), has anti-arrhythmic effects (18), and causes a general sense of euphoria (13). The principle constituents of the whole root include the rauwolfia alkaloids, reserpine, rescinnamine, and deserpidine (11-desmethoxyreseroine) (13). Hypotensive effects are believed to be due to the depletion of both catecholamine and serotonin stores and to the prevention of reabsorption (13,18). The greater the proportion of alkaloids present, the greater the hypotensive activity (13). The sedative effects of Indian snakeroot can result from the depletion of amine stores in the central nervous system (13).

Adverse Reactions

Orally, low amounts of Indian snakeroot can have adverse reactions including nasal congestion, abdominal cramps, diarrhea, nausea, vomiting, anorexia, increased gastric acid secretion, drowsiness, fatigue, lethargy, slowed reflexes, sexual dysfunction, and bradycardia (15). Cardiac and vascular effects begin with tachycardia and hypertension, and usually within 24 hours progress to bradycardia and hypotension (14). In larger amounts, mental depression can slowly develop. After discontinuation of Indian snakeroot, mental depression can persist for several months (15). In extremely large amounts, Parkinson-like symptoms, extrapyramidal reactions, and convulsions can occur (15). Allergic reactions from the use of Indian snakeroot are rare (15), and it can precipitate asthma (15).

Interactions with Herbs & Other Dietary Supplements

EPHEDRA: Theoretically, concomitant use of Indian snakeroot can decrease ephedrine effects (15).
CARDIOACTIVE GLYCOSIDE-CONTAINING HERBS: Theoretically, concomitant use can increase the risk of bradycardia (2,18), angina-like symptoms, and arrhythmias (15). Cardioactive glycoside containing herbs include black hellebore, digitalis, lily of the valley, oleander leaf, pheasant's eye, and squill (19).

Interactions with Drugs

ALCOHOL (Ethanol): Use Indian snakeroot with caution, because concomitant use increases the risk of additive CNS-depressant effects (15).
ANTIHYPERTENSIVE, DIURETICS: Concomitant use with Indian snakeroot can potentiate the hypotensive effects of rauwolfia alkaloids (15).
BARBITURATES: Concomitant use with Indian snakeroot can potentiate the effects of these drugs and the rauwolfia alkaloids (2,18).
DIGOXIN (Lanoxin): Concomitant use with Indian snakeroot can cause bradycardia (2,18), angina-like symptoms, and arrhythmias (15). Avoid large amounts of the rauwolfia alkaloids together with digitalis glycosides (15).
EPHEDRINE: Concomitant use with Indian snakeroot can reduce indirect-sympathomimetic drug activity (15).
LEVODOPA: Avoid the use of Indian snakeroot (15) because concomitant use can reduce drug effectiveness and increase extrapyramidal motor symptoms (2,18,15).
MONOAMINE OXIDASE INHIBITORS (MAOIs): Avoid concomitant or overlapping use of Indian snakeroot within several days, which can increase the risk of excitation and hypertension (15).
NEUROLEPTICS: Concomitant use with Indian snakeroot can potentiate the effects of these drugs and the rauwolfia alkaloids (2,18).
PROPRANOLOL (Inderal): Concomitant use with Indian snakeroot can enhance beta-blockade due to the rauwolfia alkaloid Catecholamine-depleting effects (15).
SYMPATHOMIMETIC DRUGS: Concomitant use with Indian snakeroot can cause an initial increase in blood pressure and enhance or prolong the pressor effects (2,18,15).
TRICYCLIC ANTIDEPRESSANTS: Concomitant use with Indian snakeroot can decrease the effectiveness of rauwolfia alkaloids (15).

Interactions with Foods

ALCOHOL (Ethanol): Indian snakeroot should be used with caution, because concomitant use with alcohol increases the risk of additive CNS-depressant effects (15).

Interactions with Lab Tests

BLOOD PRESSURE: Indian snakeroot might lower blood pressure and blood pressure readings in patients with mild to moderate hypertension, due to its rauwolfia alkaloid content (2,15).
BILIRUBIN: Theoretically, large doses of Indian snakeroot might cause falsely high serum bilirubin test results, due to its reserpine content. Reserpine concentrations greater than 61 mg/L can cause falsely high serum bilirubin test results when measured by the Jendrassik and Grof method (275).
CATECHOLAMINES: Overdose of Indian snakeroot might initially increase urinary catecholamine excretion and test results. Rauwolfia alkaloids (contained in Indian snakeroot) release stored norepinephrine, resulting in increased urinary catecholamine excretion. Chronic use of Indian snakeroot might decrease urinary catecholamine excretion, due

to its rauwolfia alkaloid content. Chronic use of rauwolfia alkaloids decreases urinary catecholamine excretion (15,275).

GLUCOSE: Theoretically, Indian snakeroot might increase blood glucose concentrations and test results, due to its reserpine content. Reserpine might increase blood glucose concentrations following administration (275).

GUAIACOLS SPOT TEST: Theoretically, Indian snakeroot might cause false-positive urine guaiacols spot test results, due to its reserpine content. Reserpine can cause a false-positive reaction for urinary guaiacols with the screening test of Rogers (275).

17-HYDROXYCORTICOSTEROIDS: Indian snakeroot might reduce urinary 17-hydroxycorticosteroid concentrations and test results, possibly due to suppression of central 17-hydroxycorticosteroid synthesis by its rauwolfia alkaloid content. Indian snakeroot might interfere with colorimetric assays of urinary 17-hydroxycorticosteroid concentrations by the Glenn-Nelson technique, due to its rauwolfia alkaloid content. Theoretically, Indian snakeroot might interfere with colorimetric assays of urinary 17-hydroxycorticosteroid concentrations which rely on the Porter-Silber reaction, due to its reserpine content (15,275).

5-HYDROXYINDOLEACETIC ACID (5-HIAA): Large doses of Indian snakeroot might increase urinary 5-HIAA excretion and test results. Large doses of rauwolfia alkaloids, which are contained in Indian snakeroot, can release serotonin (5-HT) from brain tissues, resulting in increased urinary 5-HIAA excretion (15,275).

4-HYDROXY-3-METHOXY PHENYLETHYLENE GLYCOL (HMPG): Theoretically, Indian snakeroot might increase or decrease urinary HMPG concentrations and test results, due to its reserpine content. Reserpine can increase urinary HMPG concentrations by causing release of stored norepinephrine. Long-term reserpine administration can decrease urinary HMPG concentrations (275).

17-KETOSTEROIDS: Indian snakeroot might interfere with colorimetric assays of urinary 17-ketosteroids by the Holtorff Koch modification of the Zimmerman reaction, due to its rauwolfia alkaloid content (15).

LUPUS ERYTHEMATOSUS (LE) CELLS: Theoretically, Indian snakeroot might trigger the presence of LE cells in the blood and positive LE cell test results, due to its reserpine content. Reserpine might cause systemic lupus erythematosus (SLE) and the presence of LE cells in the blood; however, this usually normalizes when reserpine is discontinued (275).

NOREPINEPHRINE: Theoretically, Indian snakeroot might decrease urinary norepinephrine concentrations, due to its reserpine content.

OCCULT BLOOD: Theoretically, Indian snakeroot might activate peptic ulcers, resulting in bleeding and positive fecal occult blood tests, due to its reserpine content. Reserpine might activate peptic ulcers, resulting in bleeding and occult blood (275).

PLATELETS: Theoretically, Indian snakeroot might cause thrombocytopenia, decreasing blood platelets and platelet counts. Reserpine might cause thrombocytopenia (275).

PROLACTIN: Theoretically, large doses of Indian snakeroot might increase plasma prolactin levels and test results in patients with hypertension, due to its reserpine content. Reserpine, in daily doses greater than 0.25 mg, can increase plasma prolactin levels in patients with hypertension (275).

THYROXINE (T4): Theoretically, Indian snakeroot might decrease serum T4 concentrations and test results, due to its reserpine content. Reserpine can decrease serum T4 concentrations by increasing hepatic T4 metabolism (275).

TYRAMINE: Theoretically, Indian snakeroot might cause false-negative tyramine test results, due to its reserpine content. Reserpine can inhibit patient responsiveness to tyramine tests (275).

VANILLYLMANDELIC ACID (VMA): Overdose of Indian snakeroot might initially increase urinary VMA excretion and test results. Rauwolfia alkaloids (contained in Indian snakeroot) release stored norepinephrine, resulting in increased urinary VMA excretion. Chronic use of Indian snakeroot might decrease urinary VMA excretion, due to its rauwolfia alkaloid content. Chronic use of rauwolfia alkaloids decreases urinary VMA excretion (15,275).

Interactions with Diseases or Conditions

GI CONDITIONS: Indian snakeroot is contraindicated in individuals with active peptic ulcer disease or ulcerative colitis (15). Use cautiously in individuals with a history of these diseases.

GALLBLADDER DISEASE: Use cautiously in individuals with a history of gallstones, because Indian snakeroot could precipitate biliary colic (15).

ELECTROCONVULSIVE THERAPY (ECT): Indian snakeroot is contraindicated during ECT (15), and one week should elapse between cessation of rauwolfia alkaloids and initiation of ECT (15).

HYPERSENSITIVITY: Contraindicated in individuals hypersensitive to rauwolfia alkaloids (15).

MENTAL DEPRESSION: Indian snakeroot is contraindicated, especially in individuals with a past history of depression or suicidal tendencies (15).

PHEOCHROMOCYTOMA: Contraindicated (18).

Dosage and Administration

ORAL: The average daily amount of Indian snakeroot is 600 mg of the powdered whole root, which is equivalent to 6 mg total alkaloids (2,18). Rauwolfia serpentina, deserpidine, and reserpine are available as FDA approved prescription drugs (15).

Comments

Reserpine is commercially obtained from Rauvolfia serpentina and the related species, Rauvolfia micrantha, Rauvolfia tetraphylla, and Rauvolfia vomitoria (13). Spelling note: The genus, Rauvolfia, is correctly spelled with a "v", while Rauwolfia or Rauwolfia serpentina (names for the dried root of Rauvolfia serpentina) are correctly spelled with a "w" (2,13).

INDOLE-3-CARBINOL

Also Known As

I3C, 3-Hydroxymethyl Indole, 3 Hydroxymethyl Indole, Indole 3 Carbinol, 3-(hydroxymethyl), 3 (hydroxymethyl) Indole, 3-Indolylcarbinol, 3 Indolylcarbinol, 3-Indolylmethanol, 3 Indolylmethanol, Indole, Indole 3 Carbinol, Indole-3 Carbinol, Indole 3-Carbinol.

Scientific Names

Indole-3-methanol.

People Use This For

Orally, indole-3-carbinol is used for prevention of breast cancer, colon cancer, and other types of cancer. Indole-3-carbinol is also used orally for fibromyalgia, laryngeal papillomatosis, cervical dysplasia, and systemic lupus erythematosus (SLE). It is also used to balance hormone levels, detoxify the intestines and liver, and to support the immune system (7170).

Safety

LIKELY SAFE …when used orally in amounts typically found in the diet. Dietary consumption of indole-3-carbinol is typically 20-120 mg per day (7170,7176).
POSSIBLY SAFE …when used orally and appropriately in medicinal amounts. Doses of 200-400 mg per day seem to be safe and well tolerated when used for up to 3 months (7173,7174,7175). There is also some evidence that lower doses of 100-200 mg per day can be used safely for up to 15 months (7172).
CHILDREN: LIKELY SAFE …when used orally in amounts typically found in the diet (7170,7176). POSSIBLY SAFE …when used orally and appropriately in medicinal amounts. There is some evidence that indole-3-carbinol can be safely used in children ages 2 to 12 years. Doses of 100-200 mg, based on body weight, seem to be safe and well tolerated when used for up to 15 months (7172).
PREGNANCY AND LACTATION: LIKELY SAFE …when used in amounts typically consumed in foods (7170). There is insufficient reliable information available about the safety of indole-3-carbinol when used in amounts greater than those found in the diet during pregnancy and lactation; avoid using.

Effectiveness

POSSIBLY EFFECTIVE …when used orally for cervical dysplasia (cervical intraepithelial neoplasia, CIN) (7173). Treatment with indole-3-carbinol for 12 weeks seems to cause complete regression of CIN in 45-50% of patients with stage II-III CIN. Lower doses of 200 mg per day seem to be just as effective as higher doses of 400 mg per day (7173). There is insufficient reliable information available about the effectiveness of indole-3-carbinol for its other uses. However, there is some preliminary clinical evidence that long-term use of indole-3-carbinol might reduce papilloma growth in patients with recurrent respiratory papillomatosis (7172). More evidence is needed to rate indole-3-carbinol for this use.

Mechanism of Action

Indole-3-carbinol is a constituent of cruciferous vegetables of the Brassica genus. Some of these vegetables include broccoli, Brussels sprouts, cabbage, collards, cauliflower, kale, kohlrabi, mustard greens, rapeseed, and root vegetables such as turnips and rutabagas (7170,7176). One head of cabbage contains approximately 1200 mg of indole-3-carbinol (7173). Daily dietary intake of indole-3-carbinol is typically 20-120 mg (7170,7176). In plant cells, indole-3-carbinol exists in the form of 3-indolylmethyl glucosinolate, which is then converted to indole-3-carbinol when the plant is cut or chewed (7170). However, indole-3-carbinol is also produced synthetically (7170). Indole-3-carbinol itself is not active. When indole-3-carbinol comes in contact with stomach acid it is converted to active metabolites, diindoylmethane and indolylcarbazole. Therefore, parenterally administered indole-3-carbinol does not produce active metabolites (7188). Researchers are interested in indole-3-carbinol for cancer prevention, particularly breast, cervical and endometrial, and colorectal cancer. Their reason is that diets with higher amounts of fruit and vegetable consumption are associated with a decreased risk of developing cancer. Researchers suspect indole-3-carbinol is one of several vegetable components that might be cancer protective (7174,7180,7181,7182,7187). However, researchers are finding that indole-3-carbinol has a variety of effects on liver metabolism of toxins. Some effects on metabolism seem to be cancer protective while others might potentially increase cancer risk. Some researchers think indole-3-carbinol might be particularly helpful against hormone-dependent cancers such as breast cancer. Indole-3-carbinol induces cytochrome P450 1A1 (CYP1A1) and 1A2 (CYP1A2), which alters estrogen metabolism. Estradiol is normally metabolized to both 16-alpha-hydroxyestrone and 2-alpha-hydroxyestrone. The 16-alpha-hydroxysestrone metabolite has both genotoxic and tumorigenic effects and is thought to increase the risk of breast and cervical cancers. Indole-3-carbinol shifts metabolism of estradiol from 16-alpha-hydroxyestrone to the weaker estrogen and more benign 2-alpha-hydroxyestrone metabolite, possibly producing a protective effect against hormone-mediated cancers (7175,7177,7179,7180,7181,7182). Indole-3-carbinol also induces cytochrome P450 2B1, 2B2, 3A1, and 3A2, as well as phase II enzymes including glutathione S-transferase (GST), quinone reductase, and uridine diphosphate glucuronide transferase (7176,7187). The phase II enzyme induction seems to have a detoxifying effect by increasing water solubility and increasing excretion of carcinogenic toxins (7176). There is some evidence that indole-3-carbinol might have other protective effects including antioxidant properties (7178,7188) and might also cause cancer cell apoptosis and cell cycle arrest (7176,7188). The majority of evidence seems to indicate that indole-3-carbinol has a protective effect against cancer. However, there is some concern that it might enhance carcinogenicity in some cases (7170,7171,7184,7185,7186). Some of the effects of indole-3-carbinol on metabolism actually seem to increase carcinogenicity of certain toxins. Since indole-3-carbinol induces CYP1A1 metabolism, it can also increase conversion of procarcinogens to their active carcinogenic form (7170). Ultimately, whether indole-3-carbinol has a cancer preventive effect or increases cancer risk in humans probably depends on several factors, including dietary factors, and duration and timing of exposure to indole-3-carbinol. For example, in animal models, there is some evidence that indole-3-carbinol has a protective role if administered before or in conjunction with a carcinogenic agent. If indole-3-carbinol is given after carcinogen exposure during the initiation phase of tumor induction, it might act as a tumor promoting agent and increase the risk of developing a tumor (7184,7185,7186). However, there is some conflicting evidence (7189). Indole-3-carbinol seems be active against diseases that are related to the human papilloma virus, including cervical cancer and laryngeal papillomatosis (7172,7173,7183). Indole-3-carbinol also seems to have immune modulating effects. In animal models, high doses of indole-3-carbinol seem to depress natural killer cell activity, but enhance delayed-type hypersensitivity in laboratory models (7190). Whether these immune system effects contribute to the effects of indole-3-carbinol on carcinogenicity is unknown (7190).

Adverse Reactions
Orally, indole-3-carbinol is usually well tolerated. However, some patients can experience skin rash and small increases in the liver enzyme alanine aminotransferase (ALT, SGPT) (7170,7174). However, this seems to rarely occur. In very high doses, greater than 400 mg per day, dysequilibrium symptoms, tremor, and nausea can occur (7172). There is some concern that certain patients might be at risk for tumor promoting effects of indole-3-carbinol. There is some preliminary evidence that indole-3-carbinol might promote tumorigenesis in patients who are in the initiation phase of tumor induction due to carcinogen exposure (7171). However, this potential risk is controversial and has never been documented in humans. Until more is known, it is not possible to determine if there is a real risk to humans or who might be susceptible to this risk.

Interactions with Herbs & Other Dietary Supplements
Insufficient reliable information available.

Interactions with Drugs
SUBSTRATES OF CYTOCHROME P450 1A2 (CYP1A2): There is some evidence that indole-3-carbinol induces the CYP1A2 isozyme (7197). Theoretically, indole-3-carbinol might increase the metabolism of CYP1A2 substrates and lower serum concentrations. Some substrates of CYP1A2 include clozapine (Clozaril), cyclobenzaprine (Flexeril), fluvoxamine (Luvox), haloperidol (Haldol), imipramine (Tofranil), mexiletine (Mexitil), olanzapine (Zyprexa), pentazocine (Talwin), propranolol (Inderal), tacrine (Cognex), theophylline, zileuton (Zyflo), zolmitriptan (Zomig), and others.

Interactions with Foods
No interactions are known to occur, and there is no known reason to expect a clinically significant interaction with indole-3-carbinol.

Interactions with Lab Tests
ALANINE AMINOTRANSFERASE (ALT, SGPT): A mild increase in ALT can occur in some patients taking indole-3-carbinol (7174). However, this effect seems to rarely occur. Routine liver function tests are probably not necessary.

Interactions with Diseases or Conditions
No interactions are known to occur, and there is no known reason to expect a clinically significant interaction with indole-3-carbinol.

Dosage and Administration

ORAL: For cervical dysplasia, 200-400 mg per day has been used. However, 200 mg seems to be as effective as the higher dose (7173). For breast cancer prevention, 300 mg per day has been used (7174). For adults with recurrent respiratory papillomatosis, 200 mg twice daily has been used (7172). For children with respiratory papillomatosis, dosing is weight based. For children weighing 6-10 kg, 50 mg twice daily has been used. For children weighing 11-19 kg, 75 mg twice daily has been used. For children weighing 20-29 kg, 100 mg twice daily has been used, etc. Children 60 kg and above have used the adult dose of 200 mg twice daily (7172).

Comments

Indole-3-carbinol is becoming a very popular dietary supplement. Usage of indole-3-carbinol is expected to grow by 3000% between the year 2000 and 2002 (7170,7176). The National Institutes of Health (NIH) has reviewed indole-3-carbinol as a possible cancer preventive agent and is now sponsoring clinical research for breast cancer prevention (7170).

INOSINE

Also Known As

Hypoxanthine Riboside, Hypoxanthosine.

Scientific Names

2,3-Diphosphoglycerate; 6,9-Dihydro-9-B-D-ribofuranosyl-1H-puin-6-one; 9-B-D-ribofuranosylhypoxanthine.

People Use This For

Orally, inosine is used for enhancing athletic performance (1900).

Safety

There is insufficient reliable information available about the safety of inosine.
Pregnancy And Lactation: Insufficient reliable information available; avoid using.

Effectiveness

LIKELY INEFFECTIVE ...when taken orally for improving athletic performance (2369,2370).

Mechanism of Action

Preliminary evidence suggests inosine might stimulate axon growth from uninjured nerve cells to injured nerve cells of the central nervous system. Further studies in humans are needed to establish whether this finding has significance in restoring function after spinal cord injuries (370).

Adverse Reactions

None reported.

Interactions with Herbs & Other Dietary Supplements

Insufficient reliable information available.

Interactions with Drugs

PROBENECID, ALLOPURINOL: Because inosine can make gout worse, concomitant use is not recommended. There is not a direct interaction between these drugs and inosine (217).

Interactions with Foods

No interactions are known to occur, and there is no known reason to expect a clinically significant interaction with inosine.

Interactions with Lab Tests

No interactions are known to occur, and there is no known reason to expect a clinically significant interaction with inosine.

Interactions with Diseases or Conditions

GOUT: Inosine can aggravate gout (217).

Dosage and Administration
ORAL: 5 to 6 grams per day used in clinical studies of effects on athletic performance (2369,2370).

Comments
None.

INOSITOL

Also Known As
Antialopecia Factor, Cyclohexitol, D-chiro-inositol, Dambrose, Inose, Inosite, Inositol Monophosphate, Liposital, Meso-inositol, Mouse Antialopecia Factor, Myo-inositol, Vitamin B8.
CAUTION: See separate listings for Inositol Nicotinate and IP-6.

Scientific Names
Hexahydroxycyclohexane, synonyms 1,2,3,4,5,6-Cyclohexanehexol, cis-1,2,3,5-trans-4,6-Cyclohexanehexol; D-chiro-inositol, synonym (+)-chiroinositol, 1,2,5/3,4,6-inositol, (1S)-inositol, (1S)-1,2,4/3,5,6-inositol.

People Use This For
Orally, inositol is used for diabetic neuropathy, conditions associated with disorders of fat transport and metabolism (14,2138), panic disorder, high cholesterol, insomnia (2180), cancer (2181), depression (2183), schizophrenia, Alzheimer's disease, attention deficit disorder, autism (2187), treating lithium-induced side effects (2027), and promoting hair growth (2182). Inositol is also used orally for treating conditions associated with polycystic ovary syndrome, including anovulation, hypertension, hypertriglyceridemia, and elevated serum concentrations of testosterone (2028). Parenterally, inositol is used for treating respiratory distress syndrome in premature infants (14).

Safety
POSSIBLY SAFE ...when used orally and appropriately. Inositol has been used in amounts up to 12 grams per day for up to 4 weeks with no significant adverse effects (2184,2185,2187).
CHILDREN: POSSIBLY SAFE ...when used parenterally and appropriately for treating respiratory distress syndrome in premature infants (2191,2192).
PREGNANCY: Insufficient reliable information available; avoid using.
LACTATION: Insufficient reliable information available; avoid using. Breast milk is rich in endogenous inositol (14,16,2138); however, the effects of exogenously administered inositol are not known.

Effectiveness
POSSIBLY EFFECTIVE ...when used orally for treating panic disorder with or without agoraphobia. In one small-scale, placebo-controlled trial, inositol significantly reduced the severity and rate of panic attacks and severity of agoraphobia compared to placebo over 4 weeks of treatment (2184). Large scale, long-term trials are needed to confirm inositol's potential benefit in panic disorders. ...when used orally for treating depression. In one small-scale, placebo-controlled trial, depressed patients receiving inositol for 4 weeks had significant improvement, based on Hamilton Depression Rating Scale scores, compared to placebo (2185). In a follow-up study, patients initially responding to inositol rapidly relapsed upon discontinuation of treatment (2026). Large scale, long-term trials are necessary to confirm inositol's potential benefit in depression. ...when used orally for treating obsessive-compulsive disorder (OCD). In one small-scale, placebo-controlled trial, OCD patients receiving inositol for 6 weeks had significant improvement, based on Yale-Brown Obsessive Compulsive Scale scores, compared to placebo (2186). ...when used parenterally as a nutritional supplement for improving survival and symptoms in premature infants with respiratory distress syndrome. Clinical trials have shown that inositol significantly lowered inspiratory oxygen requirements, mean airway pressure, and the incidence of bronchopulmonary dysplasia in premature infants not receiving surfactant compared to placebo and glucose (2191,2192). ...when used orally for treating symptoms associated with polycystic ovary syndrome. In one clinical trial, the inositol isomer D-chiro-inositol significantly decreased serum triglyceride and testosterone levels, modestly decreased blood pressure, and induced ovulation in obese women with polycystic ovary syndrome (2028).
POSSIBLY INEFFECTIVE ...when used orally for treating schizophrenia (2188). ...when used orally for treating Alzheimer's disease. Inositol was no more effective than placebo for improving symptoms of Alzheimer's disease in one clinical trial (2189). ...when used orally for treating autism. One clinical trial has shown inositol to be no better than placebo (2190). ...when used orally for treating attention deficit disorder. One clinical trial has shown inositol to be no better than placebo (2187). ...when used orally for enhancing the antidepressant effects of selective serotonin reuptake inhibitors (SSRIs). One small-scale clinical trial showed inositol to be no better than placebo when combined with an SSRI as measured by the Hamilton Depression Rating Scale after 4 weeks of combination therapy (2025). ...when used orally for reducing lithium-induced side effects. One uncontrolled trial has shown that inositol has no effect on the occurrence of lithium-induced adverse effects, including tremor, thirst, and thyroid and adrenal function (2027).

LIKELY INEFFECTIVE ...when used orally for reducing symptoms of diabetic neuropathy. Clinical trials suggest that inositol is incapable of significantly improving the symptoms of diabetic neuropathy (2193,2194,2195). There is insufficient reliable information available about the effectiveness of inositol for its other uses.

Mechanism of Action

Endogenous inositol is an essential component of cell membrane phospholipids. It has weak lipotropic activity, and can move fat out of liver and intestine cells (2187). Inositol has a variety of stereoisomers, including myo-inositol and D-chiro-inositol. Myo-inositol is the most abundant form in the central nervous system (CNS). Biological function varies among the isomers (2047,2048). Inositol might reverse desensitization of serotonin receptors (2187). Limited clinical evidence suggests exogenous inositol may have similar benefits as the selective-serotonin-reuptake inhibitors (SSRIs) in conditions such as panic disorder, depression, and obsessive-compulsive disorder. Limited evidence suggests that inositol might reverse desensitization of serotonin receptors (2187). Researchers think that D-chiro-inositol isomer induces ovulation in women with polycystic ovary syndrome by improving insulin sensitivity. Reduced insulin resistance is also thought responsible for improving other symptoms associated with polycystic ovary syndrome, including hypertension, hyperlipidemia, type 2 diabetes, obesity, and increased serum testosterone concentrations (2028). Previous research suggests that patients with insulin resistance, including those with impaired glucose intolerance and type 2 diabetes, might have D-chiro-inositol deficiency (2028).

Adverse Reactions

None reported.

Interactions with Herbs & Other Dietary Supplements

Insufficient reliable information available.

Interactions with Drugs

No interactions are known to occur, and there is no known reason to expect a clinically significant interaction with inositol.

Interactions with Foods

MINERALS: Phytic acid, the form of inositol found in foods, may interfere with absorption of minerals, especially calcium, zinc and iron (16).

Interactions with Lab Tests

No interactions are known to occur, and there is no known reason to expect a clinically significant interaction with inositol.

Interactions with Diseases or Conditions

No interactions are known to occur, and there is no known reason to expect a clinically significant interaction with inositol.`

Dosage and Administration

ORAL: For panic disorder and depression, inositol 12 grams per day has been used (2184,2185). For obsessive-compulsive disorder, inositol 18 grams per day has been used (2186). For treating symptoms associated with polycystic ovary syndrome, D-chiro-inositol 12 grams per day has been used (2028).
PARENTERAL: For respiratory distress syndrome in premature infants, inositol 80 mg/kg parenterally per day has been used (2191).

Comments

None.

INOSITOL NICOTINATE

Also Known As

Hexanicotinoyl Inositol, Inositol Hexaniacinate, Inositol Hexanicotinate, Inositol Niacinate, Meso-Inositol Hexanicotinate, No-Flush Niacin.
CAUTION: See separate listings for Inositol and Niacin and Niacinamide (Vitamin B3).

Scientific Names

Hexanicotinyl cis-1,2,3-5-trans-4,6-cyclohexane; Myo-inositol hexa-3-pyridine-carboxylate.

People Use This For

Orally, inositol nicotinate is used for improving circulation (491) and for treating peripheral vascular disease, cerebral vascular disease (9), intermittent claudication, stasis dermatitis, and Raynaud's disease (493,495,496). It is also used for hypercholesterolemia (9), atherosclerosis-related migraines, scleroderma (496), supporting nervous system and brain function, improving sleep, lowering blood pressure, calming effects (491), restless leg syndrome, acne, dermatitis herpetiformis, exfoliative glossitis, psoriasis (496), and schizophrenia and other mental illnesses (494).

Safety

POSSIBLY SAFE ...when used orally and appropriately (496).
PREGNANCY AND LACTATION: Insufficient reliable information available; avoid using.

Effectiveness

POSSIBLY EFFECTIVE ...when used orally for improving symptoms of peripheral vascular disorders, including intermittent claudication and Raynaud's disease (496,498,1544,1545). Several weeks of treatment may be necessary before the full beneficial effects are seen (1544,1545). ...when used orally for treating hyperlipidemia, especially in combination with clofibrate (496,499,1546).
There is insufficient reliable information available about inositol nicotinate for its other uses.

Mechanism of Action

Inositol nicotinate consists of six molecules of niacin (nicotinic acid) chemically linked to an inositol molecule. It is hydrolyzed in the body to free niacin and inositol, although this occurs slowly, with peak serum levels not occurring until approximately 10 hours after ingestion (496). It is theoretically possible that this slow conversion might reduce peak plasma levels and thereby reduce the incidence of side effects that have been associated with niacin such as flushing. Inositol nicotinate is reported to have vasodilatory, lipid lowering, and fibrinolytic actions (9,496). The mechanism of action of inositol nicotinate is believed to be the same as that of niacin (496). Several weeks of treatment may be necessary before the full beneficial effects of inositol nicotinate are seen in peripheral vascular disorders such as Raynaud's disease, suggesting that fibrinolysis, lipid lowering, and vasodilatory action contribute to its beneficial effects (1544,1545).

Adverse Reactions

Adverse effects from the use of inositol nicotinate in usual doses appear to be rare (496). However, inositol nicotinate is metabolized to niacin which is associated with numerous side effects including flushing, pruritus, GI complaints, hepatotoxicity, hyperuricemia, and impaired glucose tolerance (496).

Interactions with Herbs & Other Dietary Supplements

Insufficient reliable information available.

Interactions with Drugs

ANTICOAGULANTS/FIBRINOLYTIC AGENTS: Theoretically, concomitant use might increase the risk of bleeding, due to the fibrinolytic effects of inositol nicotinate (496).
ANTIDIABETES DRUGS: Theoretically, concomitant use might interfere with blood glucose control, requiring drug dosing adjustment. Niacin can interfere with blood glucose control (15). Inositol nicotinate is metabolized to niacin in the body (496). More frequent blood glucose monitoring may be necessary, particularly early in the course of treatment (15).
GANGLIONIC BLOCKING DRUGS: Theoretically, concomitant use might potentiate the hypotensive effects of ganglionic blocking drugs (15). Niacin can potentiate the hypotensive effects of these drugs (15). Inositol nicotinate is metabolized to niacin in the body (496).
HMG-CoA REDUCTASE INHIBITORS: Concomitant use of niacin and HMG-CoA reductase inhibitors increase the risk of myopathy (14,15). Inositol nicotinate is metabolized to niacin in the body (496). HMG-CoA reductase inhibitors include cerivastatin (Baycol), atorvastatin (Lipitor), lovastatin (Mevacor), pravastatin (Pravachol), and simvastatin (Zocor).
TRANSDERMAL NICOTINE (Nicoderm, Nicotrol): Concomitant use of niacin and transdermal nicotine increases the risk of flushing and dizziness (14). Inositol nicotinate is metabolized to niacin in the body (496).

Interactions with Foods

ETHANOL: Theoretically, inositol nicotinate should be used with caution in heavy ethanol drinkers. Both niacin and ethanol can increase the risk of hepatotoxicity. Niacin-induced flushing can be magnified by concomitant ingestion of ethanol. Inositol nicotinate is metabolized to niacin (14,15,1289).
HOT DRINKS: Niacin-induced flushing can be magnified by concomitant ingestion of hot drinks. Inositol nicotinate is metabolized to niacin (14,15,1289).

Interactions with Lab Tests

LIVER FUNCTION TESTS: Inositol nicotinate may increase levels of liver enzymes. Liver function should be monitored periodically when using doses of 2000 mg per day or more (496).

URINARY CATECHOLAMINES: Niacin, a metabolite of inositol nicotinate, can produce fluorescent substances in the urine, which cause false elevations in some fluorometric tests of urinary catecholamines (15).

URINE GLUCOSE: Niacin, a metabolite of inositol nicotinate, can give false-positive reactions with cupric sulfate solution (Benedict's reagent) for urine glucose tests (15).

Interactions with Diseases or Conditions

ALLERGIES: Niacin, a metabolite of inositol nicotinate, might exacerbate allergies by causing histamine release (14,15,496).

ARTERIAL HEMORRHAGE: Contraindicated; niacin, a metabolite of inositol nicotinate, can cause hypotension and might exacerbate hypotension associated with arterial hemorrhage (15,496).

CORONARY ARTERY DISEASE/UNSTABLE ANGINA: Large amounts of niacin, a metabolite of inositol nicotinate, can increase the risk of cardiac arrhythmias (15,496). One study showed an increased incidence of cardiac arrhythmias when niacin was used in patients with coronary artery disease (15); use with caution.

DIABETES: Niacin, a metabolite of inositol nicotinate, can interfere with blood glucose control requiring dosing adjustment of antidiabetic agents (15,496). Niacin and niacinamide can cause hyperglycemia, abnormal glucose tolerance, and glycosuria. Increased blood glucose monitoring might be necessary, particularly early in the course of treatment (15).

GALLBLADDER DISEASE: Niacin, a metabolite of inositol nicotinate, might exacerbate gallbladder disease (14,15,496); use with caution.

GOUT: Caution, large amounts of niacin might precipitate gout. Niacin can cause hyperuricemia. Inositol nicotinate is metabolized to niacin (14,15,496).

SEVERE HYPOTENSION: Contraindicated; niacin, a metabolite of inositol nicotinate, can cause hypotension (15,496).

KIDNEY DISEASE: Niacin, a metabolite of inositol nicotinate, is excreted unchanged in the urine and might accumulate in patients with kidney disease (14,15,496); use with caution.

LIVER DISEASE: Inositol nicotinate should be avoided in people with liver disease. Niacin has been associated with liver damage, and inositol nicotinate is metabolized to niacin (15,496).

NIACIN HYPERSENSITIVITY: Contraindicated; inositol nicotinate is metabolized to niacin (15,496).

PEPTIC ULCER DISEASE: Contraindicated in patients with active peptic ulcer disease. Large amounts of niacin, a metabolite of inositol nicotinate, might activate peptic ulcer disease (14,15,496).

Dosage and Administration

ORAL: For hyperlipoproteinemia, the typical dosing range is 1500-4000 mg daily given in 2-4 divided doses (496,497). For peripheral vascular disorders, the typical dosing range is 1500-4000 mg daily given in 2-4 divided doses (496,497).

Comments

Inositol nicotinate has been used in conventional medical practice in Great Britain for improving symptoms of peripheral vascular disorders and treating hyperlipidemia for many years, although it is not considered an agent of first choice (9,497).

IODINE

Also Known As

Potassium Iodide, Povidone Iodine.

Scientific Names

Iodine; I; atomic number 53.

People Use This For

Orally, iodine is used as an expectorant, for treating endemic goiter, thyroid storm, hyperthyroidism, treating radiation emergency associated with radioactive iodides, cutaneous sporotrichosis, and fibrocystic breast disease. Topically it is used as an antiseptic, for preventing mucositis from chemotherapy, and treating diabetic ulcers. Iodine is also used for water purification.

Safety

LIKELY SAFE ...when used orally and appropriately. Iodine is safe in amounts that do not exceed 1100 mcg per day, the Tolerable Upper Intake Level (UL) (7135). Higher doses can be safely used therapeutically with appropriate medical monitoring (2197,7080). Advise patients not to use doses greater than the UL without medical supervision.

...when used topically as a 2% solution (15). Iodine is a FDA-approved prescription product.

POSSIBLY UNSAFE ...when used orally in high doses. Tell patients to avoid prolonged use of doses exceeding the UL of 1100 mcg per day without proper medical supervision. Higher intake can increase the risk of side effects such as thyroid dysfunction (7135).

CHILDREN: LIKELY SAFE ...when used orally and appropriately (7135). Iodine is safe in amounts that do not exceed the UL of 200 mcg per day for children 1 to 3 years, 300 mcg per day for children 4 to 8 years, 600 mcg per day for children 9 to 13 years, and 900 mcg per day for adolescents (7135). ...when used topically as a 2% solution (15). Iodine is a FDA-approved prescription product. POSSIBLY UNSAFE ...when used orally in high doses. Tell patients to avoid prolonged use of doses exceeding the UL of 200 mcg per day for children 1 to 3 years, 300 mcg per day for children 4 to 8 years, 600 mcg per day for children 9 to 13 years, and 900 mcg per day for adolescents (7135). Higher intake can cause thyroid dysfunction (7135).

PREGNANCY AND LACTATION: LIKELY SAFE ... when used orally and appropriately. Iodine is safe in amounts that do not exceed the UL of 1100 mcg per day (7135). ...when used topically as a 2% solution (15). Iodine is a FDA-approved prescription product. POSSIBLY UNSAFE ...when used orally in high doses. Tell patients to avoid exceeding the UL of 1100 mcg per day or 900 mcg per day for pregnant women ages 14 to 18. Higher intake can cause thyroid dysfunction (7135).

Effectiveness

EFFECTIVE ...when used orally for treating thyroid storm (15). ...when used orally for radiation emergency associated with radioactive iodides (15,7080). ...when used orally for cutaneous sporotrichosis (15). ...when used orally for hyperthyroidism and endemic goiter (15). ...when used topically as an antiseptic (15). ...when used for water purification (14,15,16).

POSSIBLY EFFECTIVE ...when used orally for treating fibrocystic breast disease (2197). ...when used topically for preventing mucositis from chemotherapy (2198,2199). ...when used topically for treating diabetic foot ulcers (2200). There is insufficient reliable information available about the effectiveness of iodine for its other uses.

Mechanism of Action

Iodine is an essential nutrient in humans. About 90% of iodine, which is ingested in a variety of chemical forms, is absorbed (7135). The iodine content of most foods is low and is affected by agricultural factors such as soil quality and climate. Marine animals concentrate iodine from seawater and have a higher content than most other foods (7135). Processed foods may add to dietary iodine due to the addition of iodate to salt.

The thyroid gland in humans concentrates iodine for thyroid synthesis. Lesser amounts of iodine are found in the salivary glands, breast, choroid plexus, and gastric mucosa. Iodine is excreted by the kidney (7135). Iodine comprises 65% of thyroxine (T4) and 59% of triiodothyronine (T3). These iodine-rich thyroid hormones control many biochemical reactions, particularly protein synthesis and enzymatic processes. In people with hyperthyroidism, iodine inhibits the release and synthesis of thyroid hormone (15). Iodine deficiency is most devastating on the developing brain (7135). Thyroid hormone is responsible for myelination of the developing central nervous sytem. Iodine deficiency is associated with mental retardation, and in extreme cases, cretinism (7135). Most developed countries, including the US and Canada, screen for hypothryoidsm at birth (7135). The earliest clinical symptom of iodine deficiency is thryoid enlargement (goiter) (7135). Iodide salts, such as potassium iodide, might increase respiratory tract secretions and thereby decrease mucus viscosity, but there is limited supporting evidence for this effect (15). When used topically, iodine oxidizes organic substrates, killing microorganisms (15).

Adverse Reactions

Orally, iodine can cause marked sensitivity. Symptoms of iodine hypersensitivity are angioedema, cutaneous and mucosal hemorrhage, fever, arthralgia, lymph node enlargement, eosinophilia, urticaria, thrombotic thrombocytopenic purpura, and fatal periarteritis (15). Large amounts or chronic use of iodine can cause metallic taste, soreness in teeth and gums, burning in mouth and throat, increased salivation, coryza, sneezing, eye irritation and eyelid swelling, headache, cough, pulmonary edema, swelling of parotid and submaxillary glands, inflammation of the pharynx, larynx and tonsils; acneform skin lesions, gastric upset, diarrhea, anorexia, and depression (14,15,2138). Prolonged use of iodides can cause thyroid gland hyperplasia, thyroid adenoma, goiter, and severe hypothyroidism (15).

Topically, iodine may stain skin, irritate tissues, and cause sensitization in some individuals (15). Iodine burns are associated with application of 7% hydroalcoholic solution (15).

Interactions with Herbs & Other Dietary Supplements

Insufficient reliable information available.

Interactions with Drugs

AMIODARONE (Cordarone): Amiodarone contains 37.3% iodine. Plasma iodide levels may be increased and additive with iodine supplements (15,7135). Monitor thyroid function.

ANTITHYROID DRUGS: Concomitant use may result in additive hypothyroid activity, may cause hypothyroidism (2138).
LITHIUM: Concomitant use may have additive or synergistic hypothyroid effects (15).
POTASSIUM IODIDE: Concomitant use with potassium-containing products, potassium-sparing diuretics, or ACE inhibitors may cause hyperkalemia (15).

Interactions with Foods

No interactions are known to occur, and there is no known reason to expect a clinically significant interaction with iodine.

Interactions with Lab Tests

THYROID VOLUME: The di-iodotyrosine form of iodine can reduce thyroid volume in patients with goiter due to iodine deficiency (14).
THYROID HORMONES: Excess iodine intake can result in elevated thyroid stimulating hormone (TSH) levels. (7135). Short-term use of potassium iodide can reduce serum thyroid hormone concentrations and test results (14,15).

Interactions with Diseases or Conditions

AUTOIMMUNE THYROID DISEASE (AITD): People with AITD may have increased sensitivity to adverse effects of iodine (7135).
THYROID DYSFUNCTION: Prolonged use or excessive amounts of iodides may cause or exacerbate thyroid gland hyperplasia, thyroid adenoma, goiter, and hypothyroidism (14,15).

Dosage and Administration

ORAL: For fibrocystic breast disease, 80 mcg/kg molecular iodine has been used (2197). The National Institute of Medicine has set Adequate Intake (AI) of iodine for infants: 0 to 6 months, 110 mcg/day; 7 to 12 months, 130 mcg/day (7135). For children and adults, Recommended Dietary Amounts (RDA) have been set: children 1 to 8 years, 90 mcg/day; 9 to 13 years, 120 mcg/day; people age 14 and older, 150 mcg/day (7135). For pregnant women, the RDA is 209 mcg/day, and breast-feeding women, 290 mcg/day (7135). Tolerable Upper Intake Levels (UL) for iodine intake have been set: children 1 to 3 years, 200 mcg/day; 4 to 8 years, 300 mcg/day; 9 to 13 years, 600 mcg/day; 14 to 18 years (including pregnancy and lactation), 900 mcg/day. For adults older than age 19 including pregnant and breast-feeding women, the UL is 1100 mcg/day (7135).
TOPICAL: Antiseptic, 2% aqueous solution applied to affected skin areas (15). Preventing mucositis from chemotherapy, rinse mouth with povidone iodine solution 4 times daily (2198,2199). Treating diabetic foot ulcers, 0.9% iodine ointment (2200). CAUTION: Avoid occluding skin areas treated with iodine to reduce risk of iodine burn (15).
OTHER: Water purification, 3-10 drops tincture of iodine added to water (14).

Comments

Iodine deficiency is a common world health problem (7135). Early in the twentieth century, iodine deficiency was common in the US and Canada, but the addition of iodine to salt has improved public health. The addition of potassium iodide at 100 ppm, or 76 mg of iodine per kg of salt, is mandatory in Canada, and iodized salt is used optionally by half of the US population (7135).

IP-6

Also Known As

Fytic Acid, Inositol Hexaphosphate, IP6, Phytic Acid.
Caution: See separate listings for Inositol, Inositol Nicotinate, and Vitamin B3.

Scientific Names

Inositol hexaphosphate.

People Use This For

Orally, IP-6 is used to treat and prevent cancer, increase white blood cell production, prevent heart attacks, prevent and treat kidney stones, enhance the immune system, and as an antioxidant (1851,1852,1853).

Safety

LIKELY SAFE ...when used in amounts contained in foods (1854).
There is insufficient reliable information available about the safety of IP-6 when used in supplemental doses in amounts greater than those found in foods.
PREGNANCY AND LACTATION: LIKELY SAFE ...when used in amounts contained in foods (1854). There is insufficient reliable information available about the safety of IP-6 when used in amounts greater than those found in foods; avoid using.

Effectiveness

There is insufficient reliable information available about the effectiveness of IP-6.

Mechanism of Action

Inositol hexaphosphate (IP-6), the hexaphosphate ester of inositol, is the major phosphorus storage compound of plants, comprising about 1 to 7% of the dry weight of most cereals, nuts, and legumes (1855,1858). Inositol hexaphosphate and its less phosphorylated forms (e.g., inositol triphosphate) are also endogenous to most mammalian cells in much smaller amounts (1857). Cellular functions include signal transduction and cellular proliferation and differentiation (1857). Inositol hexaphosphate chelates multivalent metal ions (particularly zinc, calcium, and iron) forming insoluble salts in the gastrointestinal tract and decreasing mineral bioavailability (1858,1869,1870). Preliminary evidence suggests that the ability of inositol hexaphosphate to chelate minerals might decrease iron-mediated colon cancer risk, and lower serum cholesterol and triglycerides (1858). As a natural antioxidant, inositol hexaphosphate added to food reduces lipid peroxidation and retards spoilage (1855,1858). In preliminary research, inositol hexaphosphate inhibits cancer cell proliferation and increases cancer cell differentiation, sometimes resulting in reversion to a normal phenotype (1859). Inositol hexaphosphate has shown anticancer activity in breast, colon, liver, and prostate cells and experimental tumors (1860,1861,1862,1863,1864,1865). Inositol hexaphosphate might also inhibit platelet aggregation and lower serum cholesterol and triglycerides, according to preliminary studies (1867,1868).

Adverse Reactions

None reported.

Interactions with Herbs & Other Dietary Supplements

CALCIUM, IRON, ZINC: Concurrent use can decrease mineral absorption. IP-6 can chelate multivalent metal ions in the gastrointestinal tract, forming insoluble salts and decreasing mineral absorption (1858).
HERBS WITH ANTICOAGULANT/ANTIPLATELET POTENTIAL: Theoretically, concomitant use of IP-6 with herbs that affect platelet aggregation might increase the risk of bleeding. In vitro IP-6 can inhibit platelet aggregation (1867). This effect has not been demonstrated in humans. Herbs with anticoagulant or antiplatelet properties include: angelica, anise, arnica, asafoetida, bogbean, boldo, capsicum, celery, chamomile, clove, danshen, fenugreek, feverfew, garlic, ginger, ginkgo, Panax ginseng, horse chestnut, horseradish, licorice, meadowsweet, prickly ash, onion, papain, passionflower, poplar, quassia, red clover, turmeric, wild carrot, wild lettuce, willow, and others (4,19).

Interactions with Drugs

ANTICOAGULANT/ANTIPLATELET AGENTS: Theoretically, concomitant use of IP-6 with drugs that affect platelet aggregation may increase the risk of bleeding. In vitro IP-6 can inhibit platelet aggregation (1867). This effect has not been demonstrated in humans.

Interactions with Foods

No interactions are known to occur, and there is no known reason to expect a clinically significant interaction with IP-6.

Interactions with Lab Tests

CHOLESTEROL/TRIGLYCERIDES: Theoretically, may reduce serum cholesterol and triglyceride levels. Preliminary research suggests that IP-6 can lower cholesterol and triglyceride levels (1868). This effect has not been demonstrated in humans.

Interactions with Diseases or Conditions

IRON-DEFICIENCY ANEMIA: IP-6 might decrease dietary and supplemental iron absorption. IP-6 chelates multivalent metal ions in the gastrointestinal tract, preventing absorption (1858).
OSTEOPOROSIS/OSTEOPENIA (Paget's Disease): IP-6 may decrease dietary and supplemental calcium absorption. IP-6 chelates multivalent metal ions in the gastrointestinal tract, preventing absorption (1858).
CLOTTING DISORDERS: Theoretically, may increase risk of bleeding (1867). In vitro, IP-6 can inhibit platelet aggregation (1867). This effect has not been demonstrated in humans.

Dosage and Administration

ORAL: For cancer and cardiovascular disease prevention 500 mg to 2 grams twice daily has been used (1852). For those with existing cancer, 5 to 8 grams per day has been used (1852).

Comments

Preliminary studies of inositol hexaphosphate in cancer have been ongoing since 1988; however, to date, no studies in humans with cancer have been performed (1866). "IP-6, Nature's Revolutionary Cancer-Fighter," a book by prominent inositol hexaphosphate researcher, Abulkalam M. Shamsuddin, MD, PhD, has popularized inositol hexaphosphate (1851,1852,1853,1854).

IPECAC

Also Known As

Brazilian Ipecac, Brazil Root, Cartagena Ipecac, Ipecacuanha, Matto Grosso Ipecac, Nicaragua Ipecac, Panama Ipecac, Rio Ipecac.

Scientific Names

Cephaelis ipecacuanha, synonyms Uragoga ipecacuanha, Psychotria ipecacuanha; Cephaelis acuminata, synonym Uragoga granatensis.
Family: Rubiaceae.

People Use This For

Orally, ipecac is used as an expectorant and emetic (12,13), and for croupous bronchitis in children (18).
Intravenously, it is used for amebic abscesses and hepatitis (6).
Historically, ipecac has been used for amebic dysentery, as an appetite stimulant (small doses), and for treating cancer (11).

Safety

POSSIBLY SAFE ...when the rhizome or syrup of ipecac is used orally and appropriately short-term (12).
POSSIBLY UNSAFE ...when used orally long-term. Theoretically, prolonged use might blunt the emetic reflex (19). ...when in contact with skin or when inhaled. The constituent, emetine is a skin irritant. Ipecac powder is a respiratory irritant (6,18).
LIKELY UNSAFE ...when used orally in large amounts. Misuse can lead to serious toxicity or death (6,12). ...when a total dose of more than 1 gram is injected, it can cause nervous system symptoms, blood in the urine, and circulatory collapse (6).
CHILDREN: LIKELY SAFE ...when used orally and appropriately to treat poisoning (272). LIKELY UNSAFE ...for other uses. Contraindicated in infants under 1 year old (12,19). Children are more sensitive to large doses and effects on the nervous system than adults (19).
PREGNANCY: LIKELY UNSAFE ...when used orally because it is a potential uterine stimulant (12,19).
LACTATION: Insufficient reliable information available; avoid using.

Effectiveness

EFFECTIVE ...when used as an emetic (15). Ipecac is a FDA-approved prescription product.
There is insufficient reliable information available about the effectiveness of ipecac for its other uses.

Mechanism of Action

Ipecac contains the alkaloids, emetine and cephaeline (13). Ipecac produces emesis by irritating the GI mucosa and by stimulating the chemoreceptor trigger zone in the brain (6,13).

Adverse Reactions

Orally, ipecac causes nausea, vomiting (3,6,13,15,18), GI irritation, dizziness, hypotension, dyspnea, and tachycardia (11). Chronic use is associated with myopathies and death (6,18). Overdose is associated with erosion of GI tract mucous membranes, cardiac arrhythmias, disorders of respiratory function, convulsions, shock, and coma (18).
Topically, emetine is a skin irritant (6). Ipecac powder is a respiratory irritant.
Intravenously, emetine may cause inflammation of the muscle tissue at the injection site with chronic administration. In total doses over 1 gram, it can lead to gastrointestinal and nervous system symptoms, hematuria and circulatory collapse (6).

Interactions with Herbs & Other Dietary Supplements

PODOPHYLLUM: Ipecac reduces the intensity of the cathartic effect of podophyllum (19).

Interactions with Drugs
ORAL DRUGS: Emetics such as ipecac can prevent the absorption of drugs taken orally.

Interactions with Foods
No interactions are known to occur, and there is no known reason to expect a clinically significant interaction with ipecac.

Interactions with Lab Tests
No interactions are known to occur, and there is no known reason to expect a clinically significant interaction with ipecac.

Interactions with Diseases or Conditions
HEART DISEASES: Contraindicated (12), due to cardiotoxic potential of emetine (6), and its depressive effect on the heart (19).
UNCONSCIOUSNESS: Contraindicated (12).
GI CONDITIONS: Can irritate gastrointestinal tract. Contraindicated in individuals with infectious or inflammatory gastrointestinal conditions (19).
POISONINGS: Contraindicated in individuals poisoned with corrosives (risks re-exposure of esophageal tissue), petroleum distillates (risks aspiration pneumonia), strychnine (risk of convulsions) (12,19).

Dosage and Administration
ORAL: Expectorant (adults), 0.4-1.4 mL ipecac syrup (USP) (12). Emetic, 15 mL ipecac syrup (USP) followed by 1-2 glasses of water (12); may repeat once in 20 minutes if no results (12,13). Before using ipecac syrup to treat poisoning, call poison control for recommendation. Ipecac syrup is available both as a nonprescription product and as a FDA-approved prescription product.

Comments
None.

IPORURU

Also Known As
Iporoni, Iporuro, Ipurosa, Ipururo, Macochihua, Niando.

Scientific Names
Alchornea castaneifolia.
Family: Euphorbiaceae.

People Use This For
Orally, iporuru is used for coughs; rheumatism (517); impotence; lowering blood sugar levels in individuals with diabetes (3918); diarrhea (517); headache; toothache; snakebite; bronchitis; chancre; chills; conjunctivitis; dysentery; dysmenorrhea; gonorrhea; hemorrhoids; jaundice; leprosy; malaria; ophthalmia; ringworm; stimulating digestion; thrush; urethritis, and as a cathartic, diuretic, emetic (513), and aphrodisiac (517).
Topically, iporuru is used for arthritis, colds, muscle pain, rheumatism (517), and for stingray wounds (3918).

Safety
There is insufficient reliable information available about the safety of iporuru.
Pregnancy and Lactation: Insufficient reliable information available; avoid using.

Effectiveness
There is insufficient reliable information available about the effectiveness of iporuru.

Mechanism of Action
The applicable parts of iporuru are the bark, leaf, and root. There is insufficient reliable information available about the possible mechanism of action and active ingredients.

Adverse Reactions
None reported.

Interactions with Herbs & Other Dietary Supplements
Insufficient reliable information available.

Interactions with Drugs
No interactions are known to occur, and there is no known reason to expect a clinically significant interaction with iporuru.

Interactions with Foods
No interactions are known to occur, and there is no known reason to expect a clinically significant interaction with iporuru.

Interactions with Lab Tests
No interactions are known to occur, and there is no known reason to expect a clinically significant interaction with iporuru.

Interactions with Diseases or Conditions
No interactions are known to occur, and there is no known reason to expect a clinically significant interaction with iporuru.

Dosage and Administration
ORAL: Iporuru is typically prepared as a tea with 1 teaspoon of dried leaf added to 4 ounces of boiling water and taken 1 to 3 times daily. A 4:1 tincture is taken in a dose of 2 to 3 mL twice daily (5255).

Comments
None.

IPRIFLAVONE

Also Known As
7-Isopropoxy-Isoflavone, 7-Isopropoxy Isoflavone, FL-113, TC-80.
CAUTION: See separate listings for Red Clover and Soy.

Scientific Names
7-isopropoxyisoflavone.

People Use This For
Orally, ipriflavone is used for preventing and treating postmenopausal and senile osteoporosis, preventing drug-induced osteoporosis (4746), relieving osteoporotic pain, treating Paget's disease and renal osteodystrophy (14), and for reducing bone loss in hemiplegic stroke patients (429). Ipriflavone is also used by bodybuilders as an anabolic agent (4745).

Safety
LIKELY SAFE ...when used orally and appropriately. Ipriflavone seems to be safe when used for up to 3 years (427,428,430,431,432,433,1196,2169,2170,2171,2172,2173,2174,2175,4749). However, there is concern that ipriflavone can cause subclinical (asymptomatic) lymphocytopenia in some patients taking it for greater than 6 months (see Adverse Reactions) (1196). Monitor white blood cell (WBC) count in patients taking ipriflavone long-term. Tell patients not to take ipriflavone without proper medical supervision and monitoring.
PREGNANCY AND LACTATION: Insufficient reliable information available; avoid using.

Effectiveness
LIKELY EFFECTIVE ...when used orally for treating osteoporosis or low bone mass in postmenopausal women. Ipriflavone plus calcium 1000 mg daily can prevent further loss of bone mineral density (BMD) in postmenopausal women with osteoporosis or low bone mass (430,432,433,2169,2170,2175). There is some evidence it can actually increase BMD in some patients (428,2173,2175,4756). Concurrent use of calcium in doses of at least 1000 mg per day seems to be necessary for greatest benefit. One study using ipriflavone with only 500 mg per day of calcium found no effect on BMD (1196). Ipriflavone can also significantly reduce osteoporotic pain and seems to be as effective as inhaled calcitonin (432,2175,4756,4757). ...when used orally for preventing osteoporosis in postmenopausal women. There is evidence that ipriflavone plus calcium or vitamin D can maintain or possibly improve bone mineral density (BMD) in some postmenopausal women (2171,2174). However, using ipriflavone in combination with low-dose estrogen seems to be more beneficial. Ipriflavone plus conjugated estrogen 0.3 mg per day and

calcium 500-1000 mg daily seems to consistently increase BMD in postmenopausal women (427,2171,2172).
POSSIBLY EFFECTIVE ...when used orally in combination with estrogen for preventing osteoporosis in oophorectomized women. There is some evidence that combining ipriflavone with conjugated estrogen 0.625 mg per day decreases loss of bone mineral density (BMD) better than estrogen of ipriflavone alone (4749). ...when used orally to prevent drug-induced osteoporosis. There is some evidence that ipriflavone plus calcium can prevent loss of bone mineral density (BMD) induced by the gonadotropin hormone-releasing hormone agonist, leuprolide (Lupron) (4746). ...when used orally for Paget's disease. There is some evidence that ipriflavone 600 mg or 1200 mg given for 30 days can reduce serum alkaline phosphatase and hydroxyproline/creatinine excretion and decrease bone pain in patients with Paget's disease (2176). ...when used orally for renal osteodystrophy (2177). ...when used orally to prevent bone loss in hemiplegic stroke patients (429). In combination with vitamin D, ipriflavone seems to prevent bone mineral density (BMD) loss and significantly better than vitamin D alone (429).
There is insufficient reliable information available about the effectiveness of ipriflavone for its other uses.

Mechanism of Action

Ipriflavone is a semisynthetic isoflavone manufactured in the laboratory from daidzein, a compound derived from soy (431). Ipriflavone enhances osteoblast function and inhibits bone resorption, mainly by inhibiting recruitment of osteoclasts (14,2173,2176,2179). Preliminary evidence suggests that ipriflavone prevents bone density loss without suppressing the rate of bone formation (unlike 17-beta-estradiol which suppresses the rate of bone formation) (426). Ipriflavone has no direct estrogenic activity in postmenopausal women, but might potentiate the effects of estrogen on bone, increase uterotropic activity of estrogen, and stimulate estrogen-induced calcitonin secretion (14,434,2179). Clinical evidence suggests that using ipriflavone in combination with conjugated estrogens for postmenopausal osteoporosis might allow for use of a lower estrogen dose (427,2171,2172). Ipriflavone is metabolized extensively by the liver; some metabolites appear to possess pharmacologic activity (14). Ipriflavone, or its metabolite 7-hydroxy-isoflavone, might inhibit cytochrome P450 enzymes CYP1A2 and CYP2C9 (14,2178). Laboratory evidence suggests that isoflavones can inhibit oxidative and conjugative metabolism (4736). Isoflavones might also affect drug absorption and biliary excretion by interacting with drug transporters such as P-glycoprotein and the canalicular multispecific organic anion transporter (4736). Whether ipriflavone has similar activity is unknown.

Adverse Reactions

Orally, ipriflavone is usually well-tolerated. However, some patients taking ipriflavone can experience epigastric pain, diarrhea, and dizziness (432). There is some concern about ipriflavone causing lymphocytopenia. In one study, subclinical (asymptomatic) lymphocytopenia occurred in about 13% of patients. Decreased lymphocytes (less than 500/microliter) seems to be most likely to occur after 6 months of treatment, but may not occur until much later (1196). The clinical significance of this effect on lymphocytes is not known. Monitor white blood cell (WBC) counts in patients taking ipriflavone long-term. Consider discontinuing ipriflavone if lymphocytes drop below 1000 per microliter. Lymphocyte counts seem to normalize in most patients within 12 months after discontinuing ipriflavone (1196). Tell patients not to take ipriflavone without proper medical supervision and monitoring.

Interactions with Herbs & Other Dietary Supplements

VITAMIN D: Concomitant use may enhance effects in preventing osteoporosis (2174).
CALCIUM: Concomitant use may enhance effects in preventing osteoporosis (14,2169,2170,2171,2173,2175).

Interactions with Drugs

CALCITONIN: Theoretically, ipriflavone might enhance effects of calcitonin on relieving bone pain in patients with osteoporosis (432,2175,4756,4757).
ESTROGEN: Ipriflavone seems to have additive effects on bone mineral density (BMD) and bone resorption when used in combination with estrogen. Low dose estrogen plus ipriflavone seem to maintain or increase BMD in postmenopausal women better than either agent alone (427,2171,2172,4749).
IMMUNOSUPPRESSANTS: Theoretically, concurrent use of ipriflavone and immunosuppressant drugs might have additive inhibiting effects on immune function. Some patients taking ipriflavone experience subclinical (asymptomatic) lymphocytopenia (1196); avoid concurrent use. Immunosuppressant drugs include azathioprine (Imuran), basiliximab (Simulect), cyclosporine (Neoral, Sandimmune), daclizumab (Zenapax), muromonab-CD3 (OKT3, Orthoclone OKT3), mycophenolate (CellCept), tacrolimus (FK506, Prograf), sirolimus (Rapamune), prednisone (Deltasone, Orasone), and other corticosteroids (glucocorticoids).
THEOPHYLLINE: Concomitant use can increase serum theophylline levels. Increased theophylline levels have occurred in two cases after patients started taking ipriflavone (2178,6604). Ipriflavone is thought to decrease theophylline metabolism through competitive inhibition of the cytochrome P450 1A2 (CYP 1A2) enzyme (2178,6604).
OTHER DRUGS: Ipriflavone is thought to competitively inhibit cytochrome P450 1A2 and 2C9 (2178). Theoretically, concurrent use of ipriflavone and drugs metabolized by these enzymes might result in decreased drug elimination, increased serum levels, and potential toxicity. Some drugs metabolized by these enzymes include amitriptyline (Elavil), clopidogrel (Plavix), clozapine (Clozaril), diazepam (Valium), estradiol (Estrace), grepafloxacin (Raxar),

mirtazapine (Remeron), ondansetron (Zofran), tacrine (Cognex), verapamil (Calan), warfarin (Coumadin), zileuton (Zyflo), and others.

Interactions with Foods
FOOD: Increases ipriflavone bioavailability (14).

Interactions with Lab Tests
LYMPHOCYTES: Ipriflavone can decrease lymphocytes in some patients. Lymphocytes can often decrease by about 27% in patients after 6 months of use and then they stabilize. However, in a smaller number of patients, about 13% in one study, subclinical (asymptomatic) lymphocytopenia (less than 500/microliter) can occur (1196). White blood cell (WBC) count should be monitored in patients using ipriflavone long-term. Consider discontinuing ipriflavone if lymphocytes drop below 1000 per microliter. Lymphocyte counts seem to normalize in most patients within 12 months after discontinuing ipriflavone (1196).

Interactions with Diseases or Conditions
IMMUNOSUPPRESSION: Theoretically, ipriflavone might have additive immunosuppressive effects in patients with a compromised immune system. Ipriflavone can cause lymphocytopenia in some patients (1196); use with caution.
LIVER DYSFUNCTION: Ipriflavone is extensively metabolized in the liver (14) and might accumulate in people with liver dysfunction; use with caution.
LYMPHOCYTOPENIA: Since ipriflavone has been reported to cause lymphocytopenia in some patients (1196), it might further decrease lymphocyte counts when used in patients with pre-existing lymphocytopenia; use with caution.
RENAL INSUFFICIENCY: Ipriflavone is eliminated renally and might accumulate in patients with renal impairment (e.g., creatinine clearance less than 40 ml/minute) (14); use with caution.

Dosage and Administration
ORAL: The typical dose for postmenopausal osteoporosis is 200 mg three times daily (14,2169,2170,2171,2172,2173,2175). Senile osteoporosis, 600 mg daily (14). Paget's disease, 600-1200 mg daily (14,2176). Renal osteodystrophy, 400-600 mg daily (14). These conditions should not be self-medicated.

Comments
Ipriflavone is used in Italy and Japan for the treatment of osteoporosis (9).

IRON

Also Known As
Elemental Iron, Fer, Ferrous Carbonate Anhydrous, Ferrous Fumarate, Ferrous Gluconate, Ferrous Pyrophosphate, Ferrous Sulfate.

Scientific Names
Iron; Fe; atomic number 26.

People Use This For
Orally, iron salts are used for preventing and treating iron deficiency and iron deficiency anemia, for attention deficit disorder, improving athletic performance, treating oral canker sores, Crohn's disease, depression, female infertility, and menorrhagia.

Safety
LIKELY SAFE ...when used orally and appropriately (15). Iron is safe for people with adequate iron stores when used in doses below the tolerable upper intake level (UL) of 45 mg per day of elemental iron (7135). For people with iron deficiency, 300 mg per day can be safely taken by most people (15).
LIKELY UNSAFE ...when used orally in excessive doses. Doses greater than the UL of 45 mg frequently cause gastrointestinal side effects such as constipation and nausea (7135). Doses of 30 mg/kg are associated with acute toxicity. Long-term use of high doses of iron can cause hemosiderosis and multiple organ damage. The estimated lethal dose of iron is 180-300 mg/kg; however, doses as low as 60 mg/kg have also been lethal (15).
CHILDREN: LIKELY SAFE ...when used orally and appropriately (15). LIKELY UNSAFE ...when used orally in excessive amounts. Tell patients who are not iron-deficient not to use doses above the tolerable upper intake level (UL) of 40 mg per day of elemental iron for infants and children. Higher doses frequently cause gastrointestinal side effects such as constipation and nausea (7135). Iron is the most common cause of pediatric poisoning deaths. Doses as low as 60 mg/kg can be fatal (15).
PREGNANCY AND LACTATION: LIKELY SAFE ...when used orally and appropriately (15). Iron is safe for

pregnant and breast-feeding women with adequate iron stores when used in doses below the tolerable upper intake level (UL) of 45 mg per day of elemental iron (7135). LIKELY UNSAFE ...when used orally in high doses (15). Tell patients who are not iron deficient to avoid exceeding the tolerable upper intake level (UL) of 45 mg per day of elemental iron. Higher doses frequently cause gastrointestinal side effects such as nausea and vomiting. High hemoglobin concentrations at the time of delivery are associated with adverse pregnancy outcomes (7135).

Effectiveness

EFFECTIVE ...when used orally for treating iron deficiency anemia (9,945).
POSSIBLY EFFECTIVE ...when used orally for preventing iron deficiency in menstruating women with previous Roux-en-Y gastric bypass. Iron therapy begun one month after gastric bypass seems to reduce the incidence of iron deficiency in menstruating women (1089). ...when used orally for improving cognitive function in iron-deficient children and adolescents. Supplemental iron seems to improve verbal learning and memory in non-anemic iron-deficient adolescent girls (1095). It might also reverse developmental and learning deficits in iron-deficient children (1104). ...when given orally before surgery for reducing a postoperative decrease in hemoglobin. Supplemental iron given 1 month prior to joint replacement surgery seems to protect against a fall in hemoglobin during the immediate post-operative period (1092). ...when given orally to inhibit cough associated with angiotensin converting enzyme (ACE) inhibitors. Ferrous sulfate 256 mg daily might reduce or eliminate cough associated with ACE inhibitors such as captopril (Capoten), enalapril (Vasotec), Lisinopril (Prinivil, Zestril), and others (7307). There is insufficient reliable information available about the effectiveness of iron for its other uses.

Mechanism of Action

Iron is a trace mineral found in two forms in the body. It exists in a reduced state as ferrous iron and an oxidized state as ferric iron. Most iron in the body is found in hemoglobin in red blood cells and myoglobin in muscle cells where it is required for oxygen and carbon dioxide transport (403,1093). Iron also functions in the electron transport chain as an electron carrier in cytochromes. It is also found in the functional groups of most enzymes in the Krebs cycle (945) and plays a role in regulating dopamine activity (1093). Signs and symptoms of deficiency include microcytic, hypochromic anemia, lethargy, cognitive impairment, developmental delay, amenorrhea, hair loss, enlarged liver, and others (403,7135). Iron deficiency in pregnancy has been associated with adverse pregnancy outcomes and increased perinatal maternal mortality (7135). The rate of iron absorption from food and supplements is variable. Absorption of iron from foods depends on the source. Meats, such as red meat, poultry, and fish provide iron in heme and non-heme forms. Meats contain about 40% heme iron and 60% non-heme iron. Heme iron is absorbed at a rate of 23% compared to 2-20% for non-heme iron. Iron from plant sources is only in the non-heme form. Iron bioavailability from a vegetarian diet is estimated to be 5 to 10%. Meats and fish seem to enhance the absorption of non-heme iron (7135). Boiling, steaming or stir-frying appears to enhance the bioavailability of iron contained in many vegetables, including asparagus, broccoli, cabbage, red and green peppers, and tomatoes, but cold storage of cooked vegetables might greatly reduce the increases in iron bioavailability gained from cooking (5044). Overall, dietary iron absorption is only 10-15%. However, this varies significantly depending on the person and the iron demand of the body (403). Vegetarians and people who engage in intense physical exercise, particularly female athletes, may have increased iron requirements (7135). Blood loss and rapid growth also increase gastrointestinal absorption (403,1101). Iron is stored as ferritin or hemosiderin (7135). Body iron is highly conserved. In the absence of bleeding (including menstruation) or pregnancy, the body loses only a small quantity of iron each day, mostly through the feces (7135). Iron also seems to reduce nitric oxide production. This effect might be clinically useful in the suppression of cough associated angiotensin converting enzyme (ACE) inhibitors. Iron might reduce the generation of nitric oxide, which is thought to be increased by ACE inhibitors (7303).

Adverse Reactions

Orally, iron can cause gastrointestinal irritation, abdominal pain, constipation or diarrhea, nausea, and vomiting. At doses below the tolerable upper intake level (UL) of 45 mg per day of elemental iron in adults with normal iron stores, gastrointestinal adverse effects are uncommon (7135). Higher doses can be taken safely in adults with iron deficiency, but gastrointestinal side effects may occur. Taking iron supplements with food seems to reduce gastrointestinal side effects (7135). Liquid oral preparations can blacken teeth (9). Long-term use of high doses of iron can cause hemosiderosis that clinically resembles hemochromatosis (15). Acute overdosage (60 mg/kg and more) can cause vomiting and diarrhea, followed by cardiovascular or metabolic toxicity, and death (9). There is a lot of debate about the potential association between high levels or iron stores and cancer. So far, data are conflicting and inconclusive (1098,1099,1100,1102). There has also been a lot of debate about a potential link between coronary heart disease and high levels of iron stores, particularly from heme iron (1492). Some reports suggest there might be an association between high ferritin levels and coronary heart disease (1239,7135), but the majority of research has found no association. At present, there isn't convincing support for a causal relationship between the level of dietary iron intake and coronary heart disease (1097,1099).

Interactions with Herbs & Other Dietary Supplements

ACACIA: Combining the ferric salt of iron with acacia can cause acacia to precipitate out of an aqueous solution (16,19).

ANTACIDS: Concomitant administration with aluminum or calcium-containing antacids may decrease iron absorption (15). Separate dose administration times by at least 2 hours.

CALCIUM: Calcium inhibits the absorption of iron. People at risk for iron deficiency should avoid taking calcium supplements with meals to avoid inhibiting dietary iron absorption (7135,7308). Theoretically calcium supplements might reduce the absorption of iron supplements. Separate dose administration times by at least 2 hours.

OAK BARK: Theoretically, concomitant administration may precipitate iron salts due to the tannin content of oak bark (19).

SOY: Soy protein isolate reduces the absorption of non-heme iron from foods (5053). Non-heme iron is found in plant-based foods.

VITAMIN C (ASCORBIC ACID): Concomitant administration of more than 200 mg of ascorbic acid increases iron supplement absorption (15).

Interactions with Drugs

ANTACIDS (Maalox, Mylanta, others): Concomitant administration may decrease iron absorption; separate these agents by as much time as possible (15).

ASCORBIC ACID (VITAMIN C): Concomitant use can increase absorption of iron (15).

CHLORAMPHENICOL (Chloromycetin): Concomitant use can delay response to iron therapy (15).

ERYTHROPOIETIN (EPO, Epoetin): Concomitant use with oral iron can enhance effect in increasing hemoglobin (1087,1091).

FLUOROQUINOLONES (ciprofloxacin (Cipro), levofloxacin (Levaquin), ofloxacin (Floxin), and others): Concomitant use can decrease the absorption of fluoroquinolone antibiotics (15): Concomitant use can decrease the absorption of fluoroquinolone antibiotics (15). Administer fluoroquinolones at least two hours before or after iron-containing supplements.

LEVOTHYROXINE (Levoxyl, Synthroid): Concomitant use can decrease absorption of levothyroxine (15). Administer levothyroxine at least two hours before or after iron-containing supplements.

METHYLDOPA (Aldomet): Concomitant use can decrease absorption of methyldopa. Iron might also alter the metabolism of methyldopa, resulting in increased blood pressure (15). Administer methyldopa at least two hours before or after iron-containing supplements.

PENICILLAMINE (Cuprimine, Depen): Concomitant use can decrease absorption of penicillamine (15). Administer penicillamine at least two hours before or after iron-containing supplements.

TETRACYCLINES: Concomitant use can decrease absorption of tetracyclines (15). Some of these drugs include doxycycline (Vibramycin), minocycline (Minocin), tetracycline (Achromycin), and others. Administer tetracyclines at least two hours before or after iron-containing supplements.

Drug Influences on Nutrient Levels and Depletion

SOME DRUGS CAN AFFECT IRON LEVELS:

H2-BLOCKERS: Long-term use of high-dose H2-blockers may lead to iron malabsorption (4539,4540,4541). The mechanism of this is thought to be through inhibition of gastric acid secretion necessary for absorption of iron. Monitor for signs or symptoms of anemia. Some of these drugs include cimetidine (Tagamet), ranitidine (Zantac), famotidine (Pepcid), and others.

PROTON PUMP INHIBITORS: Concomitant use can decrease absorption of iron in gastrointestinal tract due to elevated pH. The need for supplementation has not been adequately studied. Consider supplementation only if clinical judgment warrants it (31,4483,4484,4485,4486,4539,4540,4541). Some of these drugs include lansoprazole (Prevacid), omeprazole (Prilosec), rabeprazole (Aciphex), pantoprazole (Protonix, Pantoloc), and others.

Interactions with Foods

COFFEE: Coffee inhibits absorption of iron and might lead to iron-deficiency anemia (19).

SOY: Soy protein isolate reduces the absorption of non-heme iron from foods (5053). Non-heme iron is found in plant-based foods.

Interactions with Lab Tests

GUAIAC TEST: Iron may cause a false-positive reading for occult fecal blood. However, the benzidine test for occult fecal blood is not likely to be affected (15).

Interactions with Diseases or Conditions

ACHLORHYDRIA: Decreased stomach acidity may impair iron absorption (7135).

CHRONIC UNDERNUTRITION, MICRONUTRIENT DEFICIENCY: Supplemental iron can normalize serum ferritin, but may not raise low hemoglobin in chronic undernutrition and multiple micronutrient deficiency (6923).

HEMODIALYSIS: Supplemental iron absorption is decreased in people requiring chronic hemodialysis (1088,1090).
HEMOGLOBIN DISEASES: Iron overload is likely to occur in people with hemoglobinopathies or other refractory anemias erroneously diagnosed as iron deficiency anemia (15).
IRON DEFICIENCY: Iron absorption is increased (945).
MALABSORPTION SYNDROMES: Oral iron therapy may be ineffective in individuals with diarrhea, post-gastrectomy, or other malabsorption syndromes (945).
PEPTIC ULCER DISEASE, REGIONAL ENTERITIS, ULCERATIVE COLITIS: Iron can exacerbate these conditions (15); contraindicated.
PREMATURE INFANTS: Use of oral iron preparations in premature infants with low serum vitamin E levels may cause hemolysis and hemolytic anemia (15); vitamin E deficiency should be corrected before administering supplemental iron (15).

Dosage and Administration

ORAL: For treating iron deficiency anemia in adults, 50-100 mg elemental iron is given three times daily. For children with iron deficiency anemia, the dose is 4-6 mg/kg per day divided into three doses (15). Treatment is usually continued 6 months to replenish iron stores (15). Two to three months of treatment may reverse anemia without replenishing iron stores (945). Iron deficiency due to chronic, uncontrolled bleeding requires continuous iron therapy (945). For preventing iron deficiency in menstruating women who have undergone gastric bypass surgery, 320 mg twice daily has been used (1089). For improving cognitive function in iron-deficient adolescents, 650 mg ferrous sulfate twice daily has been used (1095). For reducing angiotensin converting enzyme (ACE) inhibitor cough, 256 mg ferrous sulfate has been given daily (7307). The adequate intake (AI) of iron for infants 6 months of age and less is 0.27 mg/day (7135). For older infants and children, the recommended daily allowances (RDAs) for iron are: Infants 7 to 12 months, 11 mg/day; children 1 to 3 years, 7mg/day; 4 to 8 years, 10 mg/day; 9 to 13 years, 8 mg/day; boys 14 to 18 years, 11 mg/day; girls 14 to 18 years, 15 mg/day. For adults, the RDA for iron is 8 mg/day for men ages 19 and older, and women ages 51 and older. For women 19 to 50 years, the RDA is 18 mg/day. For pregnant women, the RDA is 27 mg/day. For lactating women, the RDA is 10 mg/day for ages 14 to 18 years, and 9 mg/day for ages 19 to 50 (7135). Tolerable upper intake levels (UL) for iron are: infants and children birth to age 13, 40 mg/day; people age 14 and older (including pregnancy and lactation), 45 mg/day (7135). UL recommendations do not apply to people under medical supervision for iron deficiency (7135). All forms of iron are not equivalent; 1 gram of ferrous gluconate =120 mg elemental iron (12% iron); 1 gram of ferrous sulfate =200 mg elemental iron (20% iron); 1 gram of ferrous fumarate =330 mg elemental iron (33% iron) (15).

Comments

Plants rich in iron include anise seed, basil leaves, celery seed, coriander, cumin seed, dill leaves, flax seed, lungwort leaves, marjoram leaves, parsley leaves, laminaria, thyme leaves, tumeric root, and yellow dock root and leaves (19).

JABORANDI

Also Known As

Arruda Bravam, Arruda Do Mato, Jamguarandi, Juarandi, Maranhao Jaborandi.

Scientific Names

Pilocarpus microphyllus.
Family: Rutaceae.

People Use This For

Topically, jaborandi is used for glaucoma.
In folk medicine, jaborandi is used orally for diarrhea and to promote sweating (18).

Safety

UNSAFE ...when the leaf is used orally or topically, because it contains pilocarpine. The lethal dose of jaborandi is estimated to be 5-10 grams of leaf (18).
PREGNANCY: UNSAFE ...when used orally or topically because it has teratogenic and uterine stimulant effects (19).
LACTATION: UNSAFE...when used orally or topically (18).

Effectiveness

EFFECTIVE ...when jaborandi component pilocarpine is used for the treatment of glaucoma. Pilocarpine is FDA approved for this indication (15).
There is insufficient reliable information available about the effectiveness of jaborandi for its other uses.

Mechanism of Action

The applicable part of jaborandi is the leaf. Jaborandi contains the parasympathetic system stimulant pilocarpine. Among its cholinergic effects are the stimulation of saliva secretion, sweat, and smooth muscle contraction in the gastrointestinal tract (18). It also causes ocular miosis (15).

Adverse Reactions

The lethal oral dose of the pilocarpine constituent in jaborandi is approximately 60 mg, corresponding to approximately 5-10 grams of jaborandi leaf. Symptoms of poisoning include bradycardia, bronchospasm, colic, cardiac collapse and possible arrest, convulsions, hypotension, dyspnea, nausea, severe salivation, strong secretion of sweat, and vomiting (18).

Interactions with Herbs & Other Dietary Supplements

Insufficient reliable information available.

Interactions with Drugs

No interactions are known to occur, and there is no known reason to expect a clinically significant interaction with jaborandi.

Interactions with Foods

No interactions are known to occur, and there is no known reason to expect a clinically significant interaction with jaborandi.

Interactions with Lab Tests

INTRAOCULAR PRESSURE: Jaborandi might reduce intraocular pressure due to its pilocarpine content (15,18).

Interactions with Diseases or Conditions

No interactions are known to occur, and there is no known reason to expect a clinically significant interaction with jaborandi.

Dosage and Administration

TOPICAL: Pharmaceutical pilocarpine eye drops are a prescription only medication (15,18).

Comments

Jaborandi is considered unsafe for oral use; avoid using. Jaborandi itself is obsolete as a medicinal herb, but it is used in the production of pilocarpine (18). Avoid confusing jaborandi with Pilocarpus jaborandi (Pernambuco jaborandi) (19) and Pilocarpus pennatifolius (Paraguay jaborandi).

JACOB'S LADDER

Also Known As

Charity, English Green Valerian, Jacobs Ladder.
CAUTION: See separate listings for Abscess Root and Lily-of-the-Valley.

Scientific Names

Polemonium coeruleum.
Family: Polemoniaceae.

People Use This For

Orally, Jacob's ladder is used for fever and inflammation. It is also used orally as an astringent, hemolytic, and to promote sweating (18).

Safety

There is insufficient reliable information available about the safety of Jacob's ladder.
Pregnancy and Lactation: Insufficient reliable information available; avoid using.

Effectiveness

There is insufficient reliable information available about the effectiveness of Jacob's ladder.

Mechanism of Action

The applicable parts of Jacob's ladder are the above ground parts. There is insufficient reliable information available about the possible mechanism of action and active ingredients.

Adverse Reactions

None reported.

Interactions with Herbs & Other Dietary Supplements

Insufficient reliable information available.

Interactions with Drugs

No interactions are known to occur, and there is no known reason to expect a clinically significant interaction with Jacob's ladder.

Interactions with Foods

No interactions are known to occur, and there is no known reason to expect a clinically significant interaction with Jacob's ladder.

Interactions with Lab Tests

No interactions are known to occur, and there is no known reason to expect a clinically significant interaction with Jacob's ladder.

Interactions with Diseases or Conditions

No interactions are known to occur, and there is no known reason to expect a clinically significant interaction with Jacob's ladder.

Dosage and Administration

ORAL: Jacob's ladder is used as a tea (18).

Comments

There is very little scientific information about this product. Our staff is continually analyzing the available information on natural medicines and will add data here as it becomes available.

JALAP

Also Known As

Jalapa, Jalape, Mechoacán.
CAUTION: See separate listings for Pokeweed berry, Pokeweed root, and Mexican Scammony Root.

Scientific Names

Ipomoea purga, synonym Exogonium purga; Convolvulus purga.
Family: Convolvulaceae.

People Use This For

Traditionally, jalap has been used as a cathartic, purgative, and diuretic.

Safety

UNSAFE ...when used orally. Jalap has potent purgative effects (12).
PREGNANCY AND LACTATION: UNSAFE ...when used orally. Jalap can be a menstrual stimulant (19); avoid using.

Effectiveness

There is insufficient reliable information available about the effectiveness of jalap.

Mechanism of Action

The applicable part of jalap is the root. The roots of the jalap (ipomoea purga) plant contain gluco-resins that act as a cathartic. They increase water elimination and cause peristalsis (514).

Adverse Reactions

Orally, jalap has potent purgative effects (12).

Interactions with Herbs & Other Dietary Supplements

STIMULANT LAXATIVE HERBS: Theoretically, concomitant use with other stimulant laxative herbs may increase the risk of potassium depletion. Stimulant laxative herbs include: aloe dried leaf sap, blue flag rhizome, alder buckthorn, European buckthorn, butternut bark, cascara bark, castor oil, colocynth fruit pulp, gamboge bark exudate, black root, manna bark exudate, podophyllum root, rhubarb root, senna leaves and pods, wild cucumber fruit (Ecballium elaterium), and yellow dock root (19).

HORSETAIL/LICORICE: Theoretically, concomitant use with horsetail plant or licorice rhizome increases the risk of potassium depletion (19).

CARDIAC GLYCOSIDE-CONTAINING HERBS: Overuse/abuse of jalap may increase the risk of cardiac glycoside toxicity. Cardiac glycoside-containing herbs include black hellebore, Canadian hemp roots, digitalis leaf, hedge mustard, figwort, lily of the valley roots, motherwort, oleander leaf, pheasant's eye plant, pleurisy root, squill bulb leaf scales, and strophanthus seeds (2,18,19,500). Jalap may increase risk of cardioglycoside toxicity due to increase risk of potassium loss.

Interactions with Drugs

CARDIAC GLYCOSIDE DRUGS: Theoretically, overuse/abuse of this product increases the risk of adverse effects of cardiac glycoside drugs, e.g., digoxin (Lanoxin). Increases risk of adverse effects of cardiac glycosides due to possible potassium loss.

Interactions with Foods

No interactions are known to occur, and there is no known reason to expect a clinically significant interaction with jalap.

Interactions with Lab Tests

No interactions are known to occur, and there is no known reason to expect a clinically significant interaction with jalap.

Interactions with Diseases or Conditions

GI CONDITIONS: Contraindicated; may have GI irritant effects (19). Contraindicated in individuals with infectious or inflammatory gastrointestinal conditions (19). Stimulant laxatives are contraindicated in individuals with symptoms of appendicitis (abdominal pain, nausea, and vomiting) (272).

Dosage and Administration

ORAL: Jalap is prepared as a liquid, using 1 teaspoon root to 1 cup of water. The dose is 1 cup daily, a mouthful at a time (5263). The usual dose of the powdered root is 3 to 20 grains (195 to 1300 mg) (5267). The resin from the root is dosed 60 to 300 mg, and the tincture is taken 2 to 4 mL (5264).

Comments

Avoid confusion with pokeweed (Phytolacca americana) or Mexican scammony root (Ipomoea orizabensis), also known as jalap.

JAMAICAN DOGWOOD

Also Known As

Fishfudle, Fish Poison Bark, Fish-Poison Tree, Jamaica Dogwood, West Indian Dogwood.
CAUTION: See separate listing for American Dogwood.

Scientific Names

Piscidia piscipula, synonym Piscidia communis; Piscidia erythrina; Ichthyomethia piscipula.
Family: Leguminosae or Fabaceae.

People Use This For

Orally, Jamaican dogwood is used for anxiety and fear, and as a daytime sedative (18).
Historically, it has been used for neuralgia, migraine, insomnia (especially sleeplessness due to nervous tension), and dysmenorrhea (4).

Safety

LIKELY UNSAFE ...when the root bark is used orally for self-medication because it is considered toxic (4). The elderly are particularly sensitive to potent neuro-muscular depressant effects (19).
CHILDREN: LIKELY UNSAFE ..when used orally; avoid using. Children are particularly sensitive to potent,

neuro-muscular depressant effects (19).
PREGNANCY: LIKELY UNSAFE ...when used orally; contraindicated due to possible uterine depressant effects (4).
LACTATION: LIKELY UNSAFE ...when used orally (4); avoid using.

Effectiveness
There is insufficient reliable information available about the effectiveness of Jamaican dogwood.

Mechanism of Action
The applicable part of Jamaican dogwood is the root bark. Animal studies have shown that an extract of Jamaican dogwood has sedative effects, marked antitussive and antipyretic activities, and also anti-inflammatory and antispasmodic action on smooth muscles (4,11). In some in vitro tests, the extract's antispasmodic effects have been at least as strong as papaverine's (4). The constituent rotenone has shown some anticancer activity towards lymphocytic leukemia and human epidermoid carcinoma of the nasopharynx; yet, paradoxically, rotenone is also documented to be carcinogenic (4). Rotenone is toxic to fish and insects, and to animals when administered parenterally, but non-toxic when administered orally (4). Another constituent, ichtynone, is toxic to fish (4).

Adverse Reactions
Jamaican dogwood is an irritant and toxic to humans (4). Overdose symptoms include numbness, tremors, salivation, and sweating (4).

Interactions with Herbs & Other Dietary Supplements
HERBS WITH SEDATIVE PROPERTIES: Theoretically, concomitant use with herbs that have sedative properties might enhance therapeutic and adverse effects. These include calamus, calendula, California poppy, catnip, capsicum, celery, couch grass, elecampane, Siberian ginseng, German chamomile, goldenseal, gotu kola, hops, kava, lemon balm, sage, St. John's wort, sassafras, scullcap, shepherd's purse, stinging nettle, valerian, wild carrot, wild lettuce, ashwaganda root, and yerba mansa (4,19).

Interactions with Drugs
DRUGS WITH SEDATIVE ACTION: Jamaican dogwood may potentiate sedative effects (4).

Interactions with Foods
No interactions are known to occur, and there is no known reason to expect a clinically significant interaction with Jamaican dogwood.

Interactions with Lab Tests
No interactions are known to occur, and there is no known reason to expect a clinically significant interaction with Jamaican dogwood.

Interactions with Diseases or Conditions
No interactions are known to occur, and there is no known reason to expect a clinically significant interaction with Jamaican dogwood.

Dosage and Administration
No typical dosage.

Comments
Jamaican dogwood is likely unsafe and without any documented effectiveness; avoid using. Root bark and liquid extract are reportedly no longer used (18). Avoid confusion with American dogwood (Cornus florida).

JAMBOLAN bark

Also Known As
Jambul, Jamum, Java Plum, Jumbul, Rose Apple, Syxygii cumini cortex.
CAUTION: See separate listing for Jambolan seed.

Scientific Names
Syzygium cumini, synonym Syzygium jambolana.
Family: Mytraceae.

People Use This For

Orally, jambolan bark is used for nonspecific, acute diarrhea (2).

Topically, it is used for mild inflammation of the oral-pharyngeal mucosa (2) and of the skin (2).

In folk medicine, jambolan has been used orally for bronchitis, asthma, and dysentery, and topically for ulcers (18).

Safety

POSSIBLY SAFE ...when used orally and appropriately for medicinal purposes (2,12).

PREGNANCY AND LACTATION: Insufficient reliable information available; avoid using.

Effectiveness

POSSIBLY EFFECTIVE ...when applied topically for mild inflammation of the oral-pharyngeal mucosa, or mild, superficial inflammation of the skin.

There is insufficient reliable information available about the effectiveness of jambolan bark for its other uses.

Mechanism of Action

The astringent effects of jambolan bark can result from the tannin constituents (2). Jambolan bark also possesses antibacterial, hypoglycemic, and CNS-depressant activities (4).

Adverse Reactions

None reported.

Interactions with Herbs & Other Dietary Supplements

Insufficient reliable information available.

Interactions with Drugs

No interactions are known to occur, and there is no known reason to expect a clinically significant interaction with jambolan bark.

Interactions with Foods

No interactions are known to occur, and there is no known reason to expect a clinically significant interaction with jambolan bark.

Interactions with Lab Tests

No interactions are known to occur, and there is no known reason to expect a clinically significant interaction with jambolan bark.

Interactions with Diseases or Conditions

No interactions are known to occur, and there is no known reason to expect a clinically significant interaction with jambolan bark.

Dosage and Administration

ORAL: The typical dose of jambolan is 3-6 grams of the dried bark per day (2,18). It can also be taken as a tea, which is prepared by simmering 1-2 teaspoons of the dried bark in 150 mL boiling water for 5-10 minutes and then straining (18).

TOPICAL: Jambolan bark is commonly used as a compress made from the tea (18).

Comments

Avoid confusion with jambolan seed.

JAMBOLAN seed

Also Known As

Jambul, Jamum, Java Plum, Jumbul, Rose Apple, Syxygii cumini semen.

CAUTION: See separate listing for Jambolan bark.

Scientific Names

Syzygium cumini, synonym Syzygium cumini jambolana.

Family: Myrtaceae.

People Use This For

Orally, jambolan seed is used for diabetes (2), flatulence, antispasmodic, stimulating stomach function, as an aphrodisiac, and tonic (2).

In herbal combinations, it is used for atonic and spastic constipation, diseases of the pancreas, gastric and pancreatic complaints, nervous disorders, depression, and exhaustion (2).

Safety

There is insufficient reliable information available about the safety of jambolan seed.

Pregnancy and Lactation: Insufficient reliable information available; avoid using.

Effectiveness

There is insufficient reliable information available about the effectiveness of jambolan seed.

Mechanism of Action

There is insufficient reliable information available about the possible mechanism of action and active ingredients.

Adverse Reactions

None reported.

Interactions with Herbs & Other Dietary Supplements

Insufficient reliable information available.

Interactions with Drugs

No interactions are known to occur, and there is no known reason to expect a clinically significant interaction with jambolan seed.

Interactions with Foods

No interactions are known to occur, and there is no known reason to expect a clinically significant interaction with jambolan seed.

Interactions with Lab Tests

No interactions are known to occur, and there is no known reason to expect a clinically significant interaction with jambolan seed.

Interactions with Diseases or Conditions

DIABETES THERAPY: Monitor blood glucose levels closely due to claims that jambolan seed has hypoglycemic effects (19).

Dosage and Administration

ORAL: People typically use 0.3 to 2 grams of the powdered seeds. As a liquid extract, the dose is 4 to 8 mL (5264).

Comments

Avoid confusion with jambolan bark. There is very little scientific information about this product. Our staff is continually analyzing the available information on natural medicines and will add data here as it becomes available.

JAPANESE MINT

Also Known As

Brook Mint, Chinese Mint Oil, Cornmint Oil, Field Mint Oil, Mentha arvensis aetheroleum, Mint Oil, Minzol, Poleo.

Scientific Names

Mentha arvensis var. piperascens, synonym Mentha canadensis.
Family: Lamiaceae.

People Use This For

Orally, Japanese mint oil is used for flatulence, improving gastrointestinal and gallbladder function (2), for gallstones, and irritable bowel syndrome (IBS) (11).

Topically, it is used for myalgia, neuralgic ailments (2), pruritus, urticaria, oral mucosal inflammation, and rheumatic conditions (11).

When inhaled, Japanese mint oil is used for mucous membrane inflammation of the upper respiratory tract (11).

In Chinese medicine, Japanese mint oil is used for the common cold, cough, bronchitis, fever, mouth and pharynx inflammation, pain, liver and gallbladder complaints, tendency to infection (18), for improving appetite and digestion, indigestion, nausea, sore throat, diarrhea, headaches, toothaches, cramps, earache, tumors, sores, cancer, as an aromatic, a stimulant, an antiseptic, a local anesthetic, and an antispasmodic (11).

In folk medicine, Japanese mint oil has been used for functional cardiac complaints, breathing difficulties, and sensitivity to weather changes (18).

In manufacturing, Japanese mint oil is also used as a fragrance in toothpaste, mouthwash, gargles, soaps, detergents, creams, lotions, and perfumes. Commercially it is used as a source of menthol (11).

Safety

POSSIBLY SAFE ...when the oil is used orally and appropriately (2). ...when used topically and appropriately (2). There is insufficient reliable information available about the safety of Japanese mint for its other uses.

CHILDREN: LIKELY UNSAFE ...when mint oil is used topically on the faces of infants and children, particularly in the nasal area, it can trigger glottal or bronchial spasm, asthma-like attacks, or even respiratory failure (2). There is insufficient reliable information about Japanese mint oil used for medicinal purposes; avoid using.

PREGNANCY AND LACTATION: Insufficient reliable information available; avoid using.

Effectiveness

POSSIBLY EFFECTIVE ...when used orally to improve gastrointestinal and gall bladder function (2). ...when used as an inhalation for upper respiratory tract mucous membrane inflammation (2). ...when used topically for myalgia and neuralgic ailments (2).

There is insufficient reliable information available about the effectiveness of Japanese mint oil for its other uses.

Mechanism of Action

Japanese mint oil is thought to have antiflatulent and cooling effects (2). It might also stimulate bile flow (2). Some evidence demonstrates that Japanese mint oil has cytotoxic properties. Other evidence suggests it might have antimicrobial activity (11). Japanese mint oil contains up to 95% menthol (11). Used topically it has the potential to cause sensitization (18). Processing removes some of the menthol in the Japanese mint oil that is commercially available (2,11).

Adverse Reactions

Japanese mint oil can cause stomach upset when taken orally (2). Contact dermatitis can result from topical use (11). In children, topical use on the face can trigger glottal or bronchial spasm, asthma-like attacks, or even respiratory failure (18). If inhaled, the menthol content of Japanese mint oil can worsen bronchial asthma spasms (18). Menthol can also cause allergic reactions including flushing or headache (11).

Interactions with Herbs & Other Dietary Supplements

Insufficient reliable information available.

Interactions with Drugs

No interactions are known to occur, and there is no known reason to expect a clinically significant interaction with Japanese mint.

Interactions with Foods

No interactions are known to occur, and there is no known reason to expect a clinically significant interaction with Japanese mint.

Interactions with Lab Tests

No interactions are known to occur, and there is no known reason to expect a clinically significant interaction with Japanese mint.

Interactions with Diseases or Conditions

GALLBLADDER CONDITIONS: Contraindicated in individuals with bile duct obstruction or gallbladder inflammation (2). Individuals with gallstones may experience pain and spasms (18).

LIVER DISEASE: Contraindicated in individuals with severe liver damage (2).

BRONCHIAL SPASMS: Theoretically, menthol content of Japanese mint oil might worsen bronchial asthma spasms (18).

Dosage and Administration

ORAL: A typical dose is 3-6 drops of oil daily (2).
TOPICAL: Rub several drops of oil or equivalent preparations into affected areas of skin (2). Japanese mint oil is also available as 5-20% oil and semi-solid preparations, in hydroalcoholic preparations of 5-10%, and as 1-5% essential oil in nasal ointments (2).
INHALATION: A typical dose is 3-4 drops of oil in hot water (2).

Comments

Japanese mint oil is the partially dementholated, distilled oil of the above ground parts of Japanese mint (Mentha arvensis var. piperascens) (2,11). There are 20 different species of Mentha with as many as 2300 named variations. Of these half are true names and half are synonyms. Commercial varieties of mint oil can be distinguished by their relative contents of menthol and carvone (11).

JASMINE

Also Known As

Catalonina Jasmine, Common Jasmine, Italian Jasmine, Poet's Jessamine, Royal Jasmine, Spanish Jasmine.
CAUTION: See separate listing for Gelsemium.

Scientific Names

Jasminium grandiflorum, synonym Jasminium officinale.
Family: Oleaceae.

People Use This For

Historically, jasmine has been used for pepatitis, hepatic pain due to cirrhosis, and abdominal pain due to dysentery (11). Many Jasminum species have been used as a sedative, aphrodisiac, or in cancer treatment (11).
For food uses, jasmine is utilized to flavor beverages, frozen dairy desserts, candy, baked goods, gelatins, and puddings (11).
In manufacturing, jasmine is used to add fragrance to creams, lotions, and perfumes (11).

Safety

LIKELY SAFE ...when used orally in the amount found in food (12). It has Generally Recognized as Safe (GRAS) status in the US (11). Maximum use level 0.001% (11).
There is insufficient reliable information available about the safety of the oral medicinal use of jasmine.
PREGNANCY AND LACTATION: Insufficient reliable information available; avoid using in amounts greater than those found in food.

Effectiveness

There is insufficient reliable information available about the effectiveness of jasmine.

Mechanism of Action

The applicable part of jasmine is the flower. There is insufficient reliable information available about the possible mechanism of action and active ingredients.

Adverse Reactions

Jasmine may possibly cause hypersensitivity (11).

Interactions with Herbs & Other Dietary Supplements

Insufficient reliable information available.

Interactions with Drugs

No interactions are known to occur, and there is no known reason to expect a clinically significant interaction with jasmine.

Interactions with Foods

No interactions are known to occur, and there is no known reason to expect a clinically significant interaction with jasmine.

Interactions with Lab Tests

No interactions are known to occur, and there is no known reason to expect a clinically significant interaction with jasmine.

Interactions with Diseases or Conditions

No interactions are known to occur, and there is no known reason to expect a clinically significant interaction with jasmine.

Dosage and Administration

ORAL: People typically prepare jasmine as a tea, adding 1 to 2 teaspoons of jasmine flowers to 1 cup of water. The dose is 1 cup daily (5263).

Comments

Concrétes are the fat-soluble abstracts of the flower. Absolutes, the alcoholic extracts of concrétes, are more commonly used as a fragrance (11).

JAVA TEA

Also Known As

Orthosiphon, Orthosiphonis folium.

Scientific Names

Orthosiphon spicatus, synonym Orthosiphon stamineus.
Family: Lamiaceae.

People Use This For

Orally, java tea is taken as "irrigation therapy" (where it is used as a mild diuretic along with copious fluid intake to increase urine flow), for bacterial and inflammatory diseases of the lower urinary tract, renal gravel (2), and liver and gallbladder complaints (18).
In folk medicine, java tea is used for bladder and kidney disorders, gallstones, gout, and rheumatism (18).

Safety

POSSIBLY SAFE ...when used orally and appropriately (2).
PREGNANCY AND LACTATION: Insufficient reliable information available; avoid using.

Effectiveness

There is insufficient reliable information available about the effectiveness of java tea.

Mechanism of Action

The applicable parts of java tea are the leaf and stem tip. Java tea is stated to have diuretic, weak antispasmodic, and antimicrobial effects (2,18).

Adverse Reactions

None reported.

Interactions with Herbs & Other Dietary Supplements

Insufficient reliable information available.

Interactions with Drugs

No interactions are known to occur, and there is no known reason to expect a clinically significant interaction with java tea.

Interactions with Foods

No interactions are known to occur, and there is no known reason to expect a clinically significant interaction with java tea.

Interactions with Lab Tests

No interactions are known to occur, and there is no known reason to expect a clinically significant interaction with java tea.

Interactions with Diseases or Conditions

EDEMA: Java tea is contraindicated for use as "irrigation therapy" in cases of edema due to limited heart or kidney function (2).

Dosage and Administration

ORAL: The typical dose of java tea is 6-12 grams of the dried leaf or stem tips per day or equivalent preparations, including the prepared tea (2,18). Adequate fluid intake is essential, at least 2 L per day (18).

Comments

None.

JAVANESE TURMERIC

Also Known As

Curcuma, Curcumae xanthorrhizae rhizoma, Temu Lawak, Temu Lawas, Tewon Lawa.
CAUTION: See separate listings for Goldenseal, Zedoary, and Turmeric.

Scientific Names

Curcuma xanthorrhiza.
Family: Zingiberaceae.

People Use This For

Orally, Javanese turmeric is used for indigestion, feelings of fullness, bloating after meals (18), flatulence (8), peptic disorders (2), and for improving appetite and digestion (8).
In folk medicine, Javanese turmeric is used for liver and gallbladder complaints (18).

Safety

POSSIBLY SAFE …when the dried rhizome is used orally and appropriately for short periods of time (2,8).
POSSIBLY UNSAFE …when used in large amounts or for prolonged use. It can cause gastric irritation and nausea (2,8).
PREGNANCY AND LACTATION: Insufficient reliable information available; avoid using.

Effectiveness

POSSIBLY EFFECTIVE …when taken orally for "peptic disorders" (2).
There is insufficient reliable information available about the effectiveness of Javanese turmeric for its other uses.

Mechanism of Action

The applicable part of Javanese turmeric is the root. Javanese turmeric root contains a volatile oil with the chief components of alpha-curcumene, xanthorrhizole, beta-curcumene, germacrene, furanodien, and furanodienone. The root also contains curcumin, demethoxycurcumin, and non-phenolic diarylheptanoids (18). Javanese turmeric is thought to stimulate bile production (2). It might also have antitumor effects (18).

Adverse Reactions

Orally, use of large amounts or for prolonged periods of time can cause gastric irritation and nausea (2,8).

Interactions with Herbs & Other Dietary Supplements

Insufficient reliable information available.

Interactions with Drugs

No interactions are known to occur, and there is no known reason to expect a clinically significant interaction with Javanese turmeric.

Interactions with Foods

No interactions are known to occur, and there is no known reason to expect a clinically significant interaction with Javanese turmeric.

Interactions with Lab Tests

No interactions are known to occur, and there is no known reason to expect a clinically significant interaction with Javanese turmeric.

Interactions with Diseases or Conditions

LIVER OR GALLBLADDER DISEASE: Contraindicated in people with acute bile duct inflammation, biliary tree inflammation (8), bile duct obstruction (2,8), or jaundice (8) due to bile stimulating effects (2). Individuals with gallstones should have medical evaluation before using (2).

Dosage and Administration

ORAL: To stimulate bile production, a typical oral dose is one cup tea several times daily between meals. To make tea, steep 0.5-1 grams coarsely powdered root in 150 mL boiling water for 5-10 minutes, and strain. The average daily amount used is 2 grams root or equivalent preparations (2). For improving appetite, digestion, or for flatulence, a typical dose is one cup tea before or during meals. To make tea, steep 0.5-1 grams coarsely powdered root in 150 mL boiling water for 5-10 minutes, and strain (8). The average daily amount used is 2 grams root or equivalent preparations (2).

Comments

Javanese turmeric is indigenous to the forests of Indonesia and the Malaysian peninsula (18).

JEWELWEED

Also Known As

Balsam-Weed, Garden Balsam, Jewel Balsam Weed, Jewel Weed, Quick-In-The-Hand, Silverweed, Slipper Weed, Speckled Jewels, Spotted Touch-Me-Not, Touch-Me-Not, Wild Balsam, Wild Celandine, Wild Lady's Slipper. CAUTION: See separate listings for Potentilla, Greater Celandine above ground parts, Greater Celandine rhizome/root, and Lesser Celandine.

Scientific Names

Impatiens biflora; Impatiens pallida; Impatiens balsamina; Impatiens capensis.
Family: Balsaminaceae.

People Use This For

Orally, jewelweed is used for mild digestive disorders (18).
Orally and topically, jewelweed is used for poison ivy dermatitis (3).

Safety

POSSIBLY SAFE ...when used orally. ...when used topically. There are no published reports of significant toxicity for either route of administration (18).
PREGNANCY AND LACTATION: Insufficient reliable information available; avoid using.

Effectiveness

There is insufficient reliable information available about the effectiveness of jewelweed.

Mechanism of Action

The applicable parts of jewelweed are the above ground parts. Impatiens balsamina has digestive and diuretic effects (18). One constituent, 2-methoxynaphthoquinone, has antifungal activity (6).

Adverse Reactions

None reported.

Interactions with Herbs & Other Dietary Supplements

Insufficient reliable information available.

Interactions with Drugs

No interactions are known to occur, and there is no known reason to expect a clinically significant interaction with jewelweed.

Interactions with Foods

No interactions are known to occur, and there is no known reason to expect a clinically significant interaction with jewelweed.

Interactions with Lab Tests

No interactions are known to occur, and there is no known reason to expect a clinically significant interaction with jewelweed.

Interactions with Diseases or Conditions

No interactions are known to occur, and there is no known reason to expect a clinically significant interaction with jewelweed.

Dosage and Administration

No typical dosage.

Comments

Avoid confusion with potentilla (Potentillae anserinae), also known as silverweed.

JIAOGULAN

Also Known As

Adaptogen, Amachazuru, Dungkulcha, Fairy Herb, Immortality Herb, Miracle Grass, Penta Tea, Southern Ginseng, Xianxao.
CAUTION: See separate listing for Panax Ginseng.

Scientific Names

Gynostemma pentaphyllum, synonym Gynostemma pedatum; Vitis pentaphylla.
Family: Cucurbitaceae.

People Use This For

Orally, jiaogulan is used for hyperlipidemia, hypertension, strengthening immune function, and increasing stamina and endurance. It is also used orally for appetite stimulation, chronic bronchitis, chronic gastritis, ulcers, constipation, gallstones, obesity, cancer, diabetes, insomnia, backache, and pain. Jiaogulan is also used orally for improving memory, improving coronary and cardiovascular functions, stress, preventing hair loss, and as an anti-aging agent. It is also used orally as an anti-inflammatory agent, antioxidant, detoxifying agent, decongestant and cough suppressant, and as an "adaptogen" for increasing resistance to environmental stress.

Safety

POSSIBLY SAFE ...when used orally and appropriately, short-term. There is preliminary evidence that jiaogulan can be safely used for up to 30 days [7069,7070].
PREGNANCY AND LACTATION: Insufficient reliable information available; avoid using.

Effectiveness

POSSIBLY EFFECTIVE ...when used orally for hypercholesterolemia. There is some evidence that jiaogulan can decrease total cholesterol and increase the high-density lipoprotein (HDL)/total cholesterol ratio in patients with high cholesterol levels [7069,7070].
There is insufficient reliable information available about the effectiveness of jiaogulan for its other uses.

Mechanism of Action

The applicable part of jiaogulan is the leaf. The leaves of jiaogulan contain a large number of triterpene saponins referred to as gypenosides. Many of the gypenosides are identical to the ginsenosides found in Panax ginseng. For example, gypenoside 3 is identical to ginsenoside Rb1, gypenoside 4 is the same as ginsenoside Rb3, and gypenoside 8 is the same as ginsenoside Rd [6]. The amount of saponins in the leaves of jiaogulan is similar to the amount found in ginseng roots. Due to the similar chemical make up between jiaogulan and ginseng, jiaogulan is often assumed to have the same effects as ginseng. However, most of the evidence about the pharmacological effects of jiaogulan comes from preliminary animal or in vitro research. There is some evidence that jiaogulan has antioxidant activity. In animal models it seems to increase tolerance to fatigue and lack of oxygen. There is also some evidence that the gypenoside constituents have several cardiovascular effects. In animal research it seems to lower blood pressure, heart rate, blood vessel resistance, increase coronary blood flow, inhibition of platelet aggregation, and possibly protect against cerebral ischemic damage [6,7071]. There is also evidence from human studies that jiaogulan has cholesterol lowering effects [7069,7070]. There is also preliminary evidence that jiaogulan has immunostimulatory effects and possible anti-cancer activity [6].

Adverse Reactions

Orally, use of jiaogulan might cause severe nausea and increased bowel movements [6].

Interactions with Herbs & Other Dietary Supplements

HERBS WITH ANTICOAGULANT/ANTIPLATELET POTENTIAL: Concomitant use of jiaogulan with herbs that inhibit platelet aggregation might increase the risk of bleeding in some people (7071). Some of these herbs include angelica, anise, arnica, asafoetida, bogbean, boldo, capsicum, celery, chamomile, clove, danshen, fenugreek, feverfew, garlic, ginger, ginkgo, ginseng (Panax), horse chestnut, horseradish, licorice, meadowsweet, prickly ash, onion, papain, passionflower, poplar, quassia, red clover, turmeric, vitamin E, wild carrot, wild lettuce, willow, and others.

Interactions with Drugs

ANTICOAGULANT/ANTIPLATELET AGENTS: Theoretically, using jiaogulan with drugs that have anticoagulant or antiplatelet effects might increase the risk of bruising and bleeding. Jiaogulan also seems to have antiplatelet effects (7071). Some of these drugs with anticoagulant or antiplatelet effects include aspirin, dalteparin (Fragmin), enoxaparin (Lovenox), heparin, indomethacin (Indocin), ticlopidine (Ticlid), warfarin (Coumadin), and others.
BARBITURATES: Theoretically, concomitant use might potentiate the effects and adverse effects of barbiturates (6).
IMMUNOSUPPRESSANTS: Theoretically, concurrent use might interfere with immunosuppressive therapy (6); avoid concurrent use. Immunosuppressant drugs include azathioprine (Imuran), basiliximab (Simulect), cyclosporine (Neoral, Sandimmune), daclizumab (Zenapax), muromonab-CD3 (OKT3, Orthoclone OKT3), mycophenolate (CellCept), tacrolimus (FK506, Prograf), sirolimus (Rapamune), prednisone (Deltasone, Orasone), and other corticosteroids (glucocorticoids).

Interactions with Foods

No interactions are known to occur, and there is no reason to expect a clinically significant interaction with jiaogulan.

Interactions with Lab Tests

BLEEDING TIME: Theoretically, jiaogulan might increase measures of bleeding time such as prothrombin time (PT) or international normalize ratio (INR) (7071).
BLOOD PRESSURE: Theoretically, jiaogulan might reduce blood pressure and blood pressure readings (6).
CHOLESTEROL: Jiaogulan might reduce serum total cholesterol concentrations and test results (6).

Interactions with Diseases or Conditions

BLEEDING DISORDERS: Theoretically, jiaogulan might increase the risk of bleeding due to its antiplatelet effects (7071).

Dosage and Administration

ORAL: For hypercholesterolemia, jiaogulan extract 10 mg three times daily has been used (7069).

Comments

Jiaogulan grows wild in China. It is sometimes referred to as Southern Ginseng because it grows in south central China and is used in similar ways as ginseng. Jiaogulan is a newcomer to traditional Chinese medicine. Jiaogulan has reportedly been adulterated with Cayratia japonica.

JIMSON WEED

Also Known As

Angel Tulip, Datura, Devil's Apple, Devil's Trumpet, Jamestown Weed, Locoweed, Mad-apple, Nightshade, Peru-apple, Stinkweed, Stinkwort, Stramonium, Thorn-apple.

Scientific Names

Datura stramonium.
Family: Solanaceae.

People Use This For

Orally, jimson weed is used to treat asthma, spastic or convulsive cough, pertussis during bronchitis and influenza, and as basic therapy for diseases of the autonomic nervous system (2,18). It is also used orally to induce hallucinations and euphoria (5622,5623).

Safety

UNSAFE ...when the leaf or seed are used orally, inhaled (2,13), or prepared as a tea (5622). Although all parts of the plant contain belladonna alkaloids and are poisonous, the seeds contain the most (5623). Ingestion of jimson weed can cause acute anticholinergic poisoning (17,5621,5622) and death (2,5622). The lethal dose for adults is 15-100 grams of leaf or 15-25 grams of the seeds (equivalent to 100 mg atropine) (18).

CHILDREN: UNSAFE ...when the seed or leaf are used orally or inhaled. Children are more sensitive to the effects than adults, and the lethal dose is less (18).

PREGNANCY AND LACTATION: UNSAFE ...when used orally (2); avoid using.

Effectiveness
There is insufficient reliable information available about the effectiveness of jimson weed.

Mechanism of Action
The applicable parts of jimson weed are the leaf and seed. Jimson weed contains 0.1-0.6% alkaloids including atropine, l-hyoscyamine and l-scopolamine which are responsible for anticholinergic action and toxicity (2).

Adverse Reactions
Orally, ingestion of jimson weed can cause dilated pupils, dry mouth, dry skin, extreme thirst (13,18), dry mucous membranes, tachycardia, blurred vision, nausea and vomiting, decreased bowel sounds, difficulty swallowing and speaking, auditory and visual hallucinations, hyperthermia, hypertension, seizure (5623), loss of consciousness (13,18) and coma (5623). Potential adverse effects also include confusion, emotional lability, reduced coordination, and headache (636). Death may result from central nervous system depression, circulatory collapse, and hypotension (18). Edema of the lungs and pectichial hemorrhages of the endocardium have been reported at autopsy (5622).

Interactions with Herbs & Other Dietary Supplements
Insufficient reliable information available.

Interactions with Drugs
ANTICHOLINERGIC DRUGS: Avoid using; concomitant use may increase anticholinergic effects and adverse effects; drugs include: amantadine, atropine, belladonna alkaloids, phenothiazines, scopolamine, tricyclic antidepressants (506).

Interactions with Foods
No interactions are known to occur, and there is no known reason to expect a clinically significant interaction with jimson weed.

Interactions with Lab Tests
No interactions are known to occur, and there is no known reason to expect a clinically significant interaction with jimson weed.

Interactions with Diseases or Conditions
CONGESTIVE HEART FAILURE (CHF): Contraindicated; jimson weed might cause tachycardia and exacerbate CHF due to its hyoscyamine (atropine) and scopolamine content (15).

CONSTIPATION: Contraindicated; jimson weed might cause constipation due to its hyoscyamine (atropine) and scopolamine content (15).

DOWN SYNDROME: Caution, patients with Down syndrome might be hypersensitive to the antimuscarinic effects (mydriasis, positive chronotropic heart effects, etc.) of hyoscyamine (atropine) and scopolamine contained in jimson weed (15).

ESOPHAGEAL REFLUX: Contraindicated; jimson weed might delay gastric emptying and decrease lower esophageal pressure, promoting gastric retention and exacerbating reflux due to its hyoscyamine (atropine) and scopolamine content (15).

FEVER: Contraindicated; jimson weed might increase the risk of hyperthermia in patients with fever due to its hyoscyamine (atropine) and scopolamine content (15).

GASTRIC ULCER: Contraindicated; jimson weed might delay gastric emptying and exacerbate gastric ulcers due to its hyoscyamine (atropine) and scopolamine content (15).

GI INFECTIONS: Contraindicated; jimson weed might suppress GI motility causing retention of infecting organisms or toxins due to its hyoscyamine (atropine) and scopolamine content (15).

HIATAL HERNIA: Contraindicated; jimson weed might delay gastric emptying and decrease lower esophageal pressure, promoting gastric retention and exacerbating reflux due to its hyoscyamine (atropine) and scopolamine content (15).

TOXIC MEGACOLON: Contraindicated; jimson weed might suppress intestinal motility, which might produce paralytic ileus and exacerbate toxic megacolon, due to its hyoscyamine (atropine) and scopolamine content (2,15).

NARROW-ANGLE GLAUCOMA: Contraindicated; jimson weed might increase ocular tension in patients with narrow-angle (angle-closure) glaucoma due to its hyoscyamine (atropine) and scopolamine content (2,15).

OBSTRUCTIVE GI TRACT DISEASE: Contraindicated; jimson weed might exacerbate obstructive GI tract diseases (including atony, paralytic ileus, and stenosis) due to its hyoscyamine (atropine) and scopolamine content (15).

TACHYARRHYTHMIAS: Contraindicated; jimson weed might cause tachycardia due to its hyoscyamine (atropine) and scopolamine content (2,15).

URINARY RETENTION: Contraindicated; jimson weed might increase urinary retention due to its hyoscyamine (atropine) and scopolamine content (2,15).

ULCERATIVE COLITIS: Contraindicated; jimson weed might suppress intestinal motility, which might produce paralytic ileus and precipitate toxic megacolon, due to its hyoscyamine (atropine) and scopolamine content (15).

Dosage and Administration
No typical dosage.

Comments
None.

JOJOBA

Also Known As
Deernut, Goatnut, Pignut.

Scientific Names
Simmondsia chinensis, synonym Buxus chinensis.
Family: Simmondsiaceae or Buxaceae.

People Use This For
Topically, jojoba is used for acne, psoriasis, sunburn, and chapped skin (11). It is also used topically as a hair restorer (11).

In manufacturing, jojoba is used as a component in shampoo; lipstick; makeup; cleansing products; and in face, hand, and body lotions (11).

For food uses, roasted jojoba seeds are used as a coffee substitute (11).

Safety
LIKELY SAFE ...when used topically (6).

LIKELY UNSAFE ...when used orally because it contains 14% erucic acid, which can cause myocardial fibrosis (6); avoid using.

PREGNANCY AND LACTATION: LIKELY SAFE ...when used topically for hygienic uses (6). LIKELY UNSAFE ...when used orally (6).

Effectiveness
There is insufficient reliable information available about the effectiveness of jojoba.

Mechanism of Action
The applicable parts of jojoba are the oil and wax. Jojoba seeds yield a colorless, odorless oil that is an emollient (11). Jojoba oil penetrates skin and skin oils easily, unclogging hair follicles and preventing sebum build up, which could lead to hair loss (6). Taken by mouth, jojoba wax passes through the body without being digested, but is stored in intestinal cells and the liver (18).

Adverse Reactions
Topically, contact dermatitis occurs with use of shampoos and hair conditioners containing jojoba oil (6). Hypoallergenic sensitivity to jojoba wax may occur (6).

Interactions with Herbs & Other Dietary Supplements
Insufficient reliable information available.

Interactions with Drugs
No interactions are known to occur, and there is no known reason to expect a clinically significant interaction with jojoba.

Interactions with Foods
No interactions are known to occur, and there is no known reason to expect a clinically significant interaction with jojoba.

Interactions with Lab Tests

No interactions are known to occur, and there is no known reason to expect a clinically significant interaction with jojoba.

Interactions with Diseases or Conditions

No interactions are known to occur, and there is no known reason to expect a clinically significant interaction with jojoba.

Dosage and Administration

TOPICAL: Jojoba oil ingredient levels vary. In skin care products 5-10%; shampoos and conditioners 1-2%; bar soaps 0.5-3% (6).

Comments

Jojoba oil and wax are produced from the seeds of jojoba, a shrub native to arid regions of northern Mexico and the southwestern US. (3901). Jojoba wax is unsuitable for food use (18).

JUJUBE

Also Known As

Black Date, Chinese Jujube, Da Zao, Hei Zao, Hong Zao, Jujube Plum, Jujubi, Red Date, Zao, Zizyphus.

Scientific Names

Zyzyphus jujube.
Family: Rhamnaceae.

People Use This For

Orally, jujube is used for improving muscular strength and to prophylax against liver diseases and stress ulcers. It is also used as a sedative (18).
In Chinese medicine, it is used for dry, itchy skin; neutralizing drug toxicities; lack of appetite; fatigue; diarrhea; hysteria; anemia; hypertension; purpura; and as a sedative.
In Arabic medicine, jujube is used orally for fever wounds, ulcers, inflammation, asthma, and eye diseases (11). Jujube is eaten as a food.
In manufacturing, jujube extracts are used in skin care products for anti-inflammatory, antiwrinkle, moisturizing, and relief from sunburn.

Safety

There is insufficient reliable information available about the safety of jujube.
Pregnancy and Lactation: Insufficient reliable information available; avoid using.

Effectiveness

There is insufficient reliable information available about the effectiveness of jujube.

Mechanism of Action

The applicable part of jujube is the fruit. Animal data suggests that jujube increases body weight, increases swimming endurance and protects against carbon tetrachloride-induced liver damage. Animal data also suggests anti-inflammatory effects and growth inhibition of Bacillus subtilis with an ethanolic extract. A methanolic extract containing oleanolic acid and ursolic acid inhibits the in vitro dental cavity-producing activity of Streptococcus mutans (11).

Adverse Reactions

None reported.

Interactions with Herbs & Other Dietary Supplements

Insufficient reliable information available.

Interactions with Drugs

No interactions are known to occur, and there is no known reason to expect a clinically significant interaction with jujube.

Interactions with Foods

No interactions are known to occur, and there is no known reason to expect a clinically significant interaction with jujube.

Interactions with Lab Tests

No interactions are known to occur, and there is no known reason to expect a clinically significant interaction with jujube.

Interactions with Diseases or Conditions

No interactions are known to occur, and there is no known reason to expect a clinically significant interaction with jujube.

Dosage and Administration

No typical dosage.

Comments

Jujube is no longer used medicinally (18).

JUNIPER

Also Known As

Common Juniper Berry, Enebro, Geniévre, Ginepro, Juniperi fructus, Wacholderbeeren, Zimbro.
CAUTION: See separate listing for Cade Oil.

Scientific Names

Juniperus communis.
Family: Cupressaceae or Pinaceae.

People Use This For

Orally, juniper is used for dyspepsia, flatulence, heartburn, bloating, loss of appetite, urinary tract infections (UTIs), kidney and bladder stones, snakebite, intestinal worms, gastrointestinal infections, and cancer.
Topically, juniper is used for rheumatic pains in joints and muscles, inflammatory diseases, and wounds.
As an inhalant, the essential oil of juniper is used as an analgesic for pain and for bronchitis as an inhaled vapor.
In foods, the juniper berry is often used as a culinary condiment, a flavor component in gin and bitter preparations, and the extract and oil are used as a flavoring agent in foods and beverages.
In manufacturing, the juniper oil is used as a fragrance component in soaps and cosmetics.

Safety

LIKELY SAFE ...when used orally in amounts commonly found in foods and beverages. The juniper berry has Generally Recognized as Safe (GRAS) status in the US. The maximum level used in food is 0.006% for the oil and 0.01% for the extracts (11).
POSSIBLY SAFE ...when used orally and appropriately short-term (12). ...when used topically on limited areas of skin (12,18). ...when the oil is used by inhalation and appropriately as aromatherapy (7107).
LIKELY UNSAFE ...when used orally in excessive amounts, long-term. Prolonged use of high doses can increase the potential for severe side effects such as convulsions or kidney damage (8,19). ...when used topically on large skin wounds or in individuals with acute skin conditions (18).
PREGNANCY: UNSAFE ...when used orally. Juniper can increase uterine tone, interfere with fertility and implantation, and cause abortion (4,19).
LACTATION: Insufficient reliable information available; avoid using.

Effectiveness

There is insufficient reliable information available about the effectiveness of juniper.

Mechanism of Action

The applicable part of juniper is the berry. Juniper berry has aquaretic, antiseptic, antiflatulent, and antirheumatic effects. It also stimulates stomach function (4,512). Aquaretics increase urine volume (water loss) but not sodium excretion (512). The constituent terpinen-4-ol increases the glomerular filtration rate, but it can also irritate the kidneys (4). In vitro, juniper berry exhibits antiviral activity against the herpes simplex virus and has antifungal activity (4). In experimental animals, the juniper berry extract shows abortifacient, antifertility, anti-inflammatory, anti-implantation, hypotensive, hypertensive, and hypoglycemic effects (4). The juniper berry oil stimulates uterine activity (4). It has diuretic, GI antiseptic, and irritant effects (11). The oil prevents antispasmodic effects in smooth muscle (11).

Adverse Reactions

Orally, excessive amounts of the juniper berry oil can cause kidney irritation (4). Overdose symptoms include kidney pain, diuresis, albuminuria, hematuria, purplish urine, tachycardia, hypertension, convulsions, metrorrhagia, and abortion (4).

Topically, juniper can cause skin irritation (4). Signs of topical poisoning include burning, erythema, inflammation with blisters, and edema (4). Repeated exposure to the juniper pollen can cause occupational allergies that affect the skin and respiratory tract (6).

Interactions with Herbs & Other Dietary Supplements

Insufficient reliable information available.

Interactions with Drugs

DIURETICS: Theoretically, juniper berry might interfere with diuretic therapy (4,512).
DIABETES: Theoretically, juniper berry might potentiate diabetes therapy (4).

Interactions with Foods

No interactions are known to occur, and there is no known reason to expect a clinically significant interaction with juniper.

Interactions with Lab Tests

URINE TESTS: The juniper berry can interfere with urine assays, and large amounts can cause purplish urine (4).

Interactions with Diseases or Conditions

DIABETES: Monitor blood glucose level closely due to claims that juniper has hypoglycemic effects (4,19).
HYPERTENSION, HYPOTENSION: Theoretically, juniper berry might interfere with blood pressure control (4,512).
KIDNEY DISEASE: Contraindicated (4,12).
SEIZURE DISORDERS: Theoretically, the juniper berry might exacerbate these conditions.
GI CONDITIONS: Juniper berry can irritate the gastrointestinal tract (19). It is contraindicated in individuals with infectious or inflammatory gastrointestinal conditions (19).
OTHER: Individuals with cardiac insufficiency, hypertonia, fever, acute skin disease, or large skin wounds should not use juniper berry (18).

Dosage and Administration

ORAL: The typical dose of juniper is 1-2 grams of the berry three times daily (4) or one cup of the tea three to four times daily (8). The tea is prepared by steeping 1 teaspoon of the crushed juniper berry, about 2-3 grams, in 150 mL boiling water for 10 minutes and then straining. Juniper should be used up to a maximum of 10 grams of the dried berry per day, corresponding to 20-100 mg of the essential oil (2). This dose should not be used longer than four weeks without physician consultation (8). The usual dose of the liquid extract (1:1 in 25% alcohol) is 2-4 mL three times daily (4). The common dose of the tincture (1:5 in 45% alcohol) is 1-2 mL three times daily (4). The berry oil (1:5 in 45% alcohol) is typically taken as 0.03-0.2 mL three times daily (4). CAUTION: The juniper berry oil should only be used under supervision (4).
TOPICAL: The juniper berry is commonly used in bath salts for treating rheumatism (18).

Comments

Avoid confusion with cade oil, which is distilled from juniper wood (Juniperus oxycedrus). Turpentine oil has been used to adulterate juniper berry oil (512).

KAMALA

Also Known As
Kamcela, Kameela, Rottlera Tinctoria, Spoonwood.

Scientific Names
Mallotus philippinensis.

People Use This For
Orally, kamala is used for treating tape worm infestation (18).

Safety
There is insufficient reliable information available about the safety of kamala.
Pregnancy and Lactation: Insufficient reliable information available; avoid using.

Effectiveness
There is insufficient reliable information available about the effectiveness of kamala.

Mechanism of Action
The applicable parts of kamala are the gland and hair of the fruit. Kamala contains berginin and tannins. It is reported to have anthelmintic and purgative effects (18).

Adverse Reactions
None reported.

Interactions with Herbs & Other Dietary Supplements
STIMULANT LAXATIVE HERBS: Theoretically, concomitant use with other stimulant laxative herbs may increase effects and adverse effects. Stimulant laxative herbs include: aloe dried leaf sap, blue flag rhizome, alder buckthorn, European buckthorn, butternut bark, cascara bark, castor oil, colocynth fruit pulp, gamboge bark exudate, jalap root, black root, manna bark exudate, podophyllum root, rhubarb root, senna leaves and pods, wild cucumber fruit (Ecballium elaterium), and yellow dock root (19).

Interactions with Drugs
No interactions are known to occur, and there is no known reason to expect a clinically significant interaction with kamala.

Interactions with Foods
No interactions are known to occur, and there is no known reason to expect a clinically significant interaction with kamala.

Interactions with Lab Tests
No interactions are known to occur, and there is no known reason to expect a clinically significant interaction with kamala.

Interactions with Diseases or Conditions
GI CONDITIONS: Stimulant laxatives are contraindicated in individuals with symptoms of appendicitis (abdominal pain, nausea and vomiting) (272).

Dosage and Administration
ORAL: People typically use 2 to 10 grams of kamala powder and 8 to 14 mL of the liquid extract (5264).

Comments
There is very little scientific information about this product. Our staff is continually analyzing the available information on natural medicines and will add data here as it becomes available.

KAOLIN

Also Known As
Argilla, Bolus Alba, China Clay, Heavy Kaolin, Light Kaolin, Porcelain Clay, White Bole.

Scientific Names
Hydrated aluminum silicate.

People Use This For
Orally, kaolin is used for mild to moderate acute diarrhea, cholera, enteritis, and dysentery (6).
Topically, it is used as a poultice, dusting powder, drying agent, and emollient (6,9,16,188,189).
In combination products, kaolin is used for symptomatic diarrhea control (6,9,14,16), in relief of radiation-induced mucositis (14,186,187), in the treatment of chronic ulcerative colitis (16), and to treat spontaneous pneumothorax (9).
Diagnostic uses include, as a contrast media agent (C,D), (6,16), automated testing for activated coagulation time (ACT) (6,192), serodiagnosis of tuberculosis (193), and the kaolin agglutination test (KAT) (254).
In manufacturing, kaolin is used as a diluent in tablet preparation (6,194), and a filtering or decolorizing agent (6,16).
It is also a food additive (9).

Safety
LIKELY SAFE ...when used orally in appropriate amounts (6,14). Kaolin is not absorbed systemically and is generally nontoxic (6). ...when used topically with appropriate use of sterile products (9,16). Kaolin is a FDA-approved prescription product.
PREGNANCY AND LACTATION: POSSIBLY UNSAFE ...when used orally in large amounts because of iron deficiency anemia and hypokalemia secondary to clay ingestion (14).

Effectiveness
POSSIBLY EFFECTIVE ...when taken alone or in combination with pectin and other drugs for the symptomatic control of mild to moderate acute diarrhea (excluding pseudomembranous enterocolitis) (14,15). Kaolin is a FDA-approved prescription product. ...when taken orally in combination with other drugs for relief of pain and to decrease the severity of radiation-induced mucositis (14,186,187). ...when used topically as a drying agent in dusting powder (6,9,16,188).
There is insufficient reliable information available about the effectiveness of kaolin for its other uses.

Mechanism of Action
Kaolin may absorb bacteria and toxins in the GI tract, increase fecal bulk and restore stool consistency (6,9,14,15,16). In radiation-induced mucositis, kaolin may act as a protective coating to decrease the severity of pain (14,186). Topically, kaolin acts as a drying agent adsorbing a wide variety of substances (6,9,16).

Adverse Reactions
Orally, kaolin can cause constipation, particularly in children and the elderly (14).
Occupational kalinosis (pulmonary disease) is reported in miners following inhalation (6,195,196,197).

Interactions with Herbs & Other Dietary Supplements
Insufficient reliable information available.

Interactions with Drugs
NUMEROUS DRUGS: Kaolin actively adsorbs a wide variety of substances (6,9). Concomitant use of kaolin or kaolin/pectin could decrease systemic absorption of digoxin, quinidine, lincomycin, clindamycin, phenothiazines, chloroquine, and trimethoprim (6,14,198,199,250,251,252,253). Separate doses of chloroquine and kaolin by at least four hours (14).

Interactions with Foods
No interactions are known to occur, and there is no known reason to expect a clinically significant interaction with kaolin.

Interactions with Lab Tests
No interactions are known to occur, and there is no known reason to expect a clinically significant interaction with kaolin.

Interactions with Diseases or Conditions
PSEUDOMEMBRANOUS ENTEROCOLITIS: Kaolin/pectin combination is contraindicated in the treatment of diarrhea from pseudomembranous enterocolitis or toxigenic bacteria (14).

Dosage and Administration
ORAL: For diarrhea the dose varies ranging between 15-60 grams (6,9) and 50-100 grams at three hour intervals (16). Kaolin is usually taken at first sign of diarrhea and after each loose bowel movement (14). Doses of 15-60 grams (6,9)

and doses of 50-100 grams at 3 hours intervals reported (16). For relief of radiation-induced mucositis, 15 ml (50% kaolin/pectin, 50% diphenhydramine) solution, rinse four times a day (14,186). Kaolin is a FDA-approved prescription product.

Comments

Kaolin is hydrated aluminum silicate (16) purified for pharmaceutical use by treatment with hydrochloric acid or sulfuric acid, or both, then washed with water (6,9,16). Heavy kaolin (Kaolinum ponderosum) is the purified natural form of variable composition (9,16), and light kaolin is prepared from heavy kaolin by elutriation (separation of finer from coarser particles by suspension in water) (9,16).

KARAYA GUM

Also Known As

Bassora Tragacanth, Indian Tragacanth, Kadaya, Kadira, Karaya, Katila, Kullo, Mucara, Sterculia Gum.

Scientific Names

Sterculia urens; Sterculia villosa; Sterculia tragacanth; other Sterculia species.
Family: Sterculiaceae.

People Use This For

Orally, karaya gum is used as a bulk laxative (6).
Historically, it has been used as an aphrodisiac (11).
In manufacturing, karaya gum is used as a thickener in pharmaceuticals and cosmetics (6,11); denture and ostomy adhesives (6,400); and a binder and stabilizer in foods and beverages (6,11).

Safety

LIKELY SAFE ...when used in amounts found in foods (maximum use level 0.805% in candy) (11); it has Generally Recognized as Safe (GRAS) status in the US (11). ...when used orally for medicinal purposes (6).
PREGNANCY AND LACTATION: Insufficient reliable information available.

Effectiveness

POSSIBLY EFFECTIVE ...when used as a bulk forming laxative (6,11).
There is insufficient reliable information available about the effectiveness of karaya gum for its other uses.

Mechanism of Action

Karaya gum is not digested or absorbed but swells in the presence of water, forming a viscous colloidal solution that stimulates peristalsis in the GI tract (6,11).

Adverse Reactions

None reported.

Interactions with Herbs & Other Dietary Supplements

Insufficient reliable information available.

Interactions with Drugs

ORAL DRUGS: Co-administration of oral drugs with bulk forming laxatives may decrease the absorption of the drugs (12).

Interactions with Foods

No interactions are known to occur, and there is no known reason to expect a clinically significant interaction with karaya gum.

Interactions with Lab Tests

No interactions are known to occur, and there is no known reason to expect a clinically significant interaction with karaya gum.

Interactions with Diseases or Conditions

BOWEL OBSTRUCTION: In general, bulk laxatives are contraindicated in individuals with bowel obstruction (12).

Dosage and Administration
No typical dosage.

Comments
Karaya gum is exuded from Sterculia species trees, that are native to India, when charred or scarred (6,3901).
Adequate fluid intake is important with bulk forming laxatives.

KAVA

Also Known As
Ava, Ava Pepper, Awa, Intoxicating Pepper, Kava Kava, Kava Pepper, Kava Root, Kava-kava, Kawa, Kawa Kawa, Kawa-Kawa, Kew, Rauschpfeffer, Sakau, Tonga, Wurzelstock, Yagona.

Scientific Names
Piper methysticum.
Family: Piperaceae.

People Use This For
Orally, kava is used to treat anxiety disorders, stress, insomnia, and restlessness. It is also used orally for epilepsy, psychosis, depression, headaches including migraines, common cold and other respiratory tract infections, tuberculosis, and musculoskeletal pain. Kava is also used orally for urinary tract infections (UTIs), uterine inflammation, venereal disease, menstrual discomfort, vaginal prolapse, and as an aphrodisiac.
Topically, kava is used for skin diseases including leprosy and to promote wound healing. It is also used topically as a poultice for otitis and abscesses.
Ceremonially, Kava is used as a beverage to induce relaxation.

Safety
POSSIBLY UNSAFE ...when used orally. There is concern that kava preparations can induce hepatotoxicity and liver failure in patients taking relatively normal doses, short-term. Kava extracts have been safely used under medical supervision in some studies lasting for up to 6 months (2092,2093,2094,2095,7325). However, there are at least 30 documented cases of liver toxicity following kava use. In some cases, use of kava for as little as 1-3 months has resulted in the need for liver transplants, and even death (7024,7068,7086). Based on these reports, kava has been banned from the market in Switzerland. German regulators are considering similar action. Some patients may be more at risk than others. There is speculation that "poor metabolizers" might be at greatest risk, but this has not been verified (7068). Until more is known, tell patients to avoid kava. Recommend routine liver function tests for those patients that continue to use kava.
PREGNANCY: POSSIBLY UNSAFE ...when used orally. There is some concern that pyrone constituents in kava can cause loss of uterine tone (12,19); avoid using.
LACTATION: POSSIBLY UNSAFE ...when used orally. There is concern that the toxic pyrone constituents of kava can pass into breast milk (19); avoid using.

Effectiveness
LIKELY EFFECTIVE ...when used orally for short-term treatment of anxiety disorders. Kava extracts standardized to 70% kava-lactones are superior to placebo (2093,2094,2095,7325), and possibly comparable to low-dose benzodiazepines (2092) for short-term treatment of anxiety. Treatment for 1-8 weeks may be necessary for significant improvement (2094,2095).
Most clinical studies on the effectiveness of kava for anxiety disorders have used the standardized extract WS 1490 (W. Schwabe). This extract is standardized to contain 70% kava-lactones (also known as kavapyrones). This extract is more than twice as concentrated as most products that are commercially available.
POSSIBLY EFFECTIVE ...when used orally for reducing symptoms of anxiety related to climacteric in menopausal women. Two small trials have shown that kava standardized to 15% or 70% kava-lactones is superior to placebo for short-term treatment of neurovegetative and anxiety symptoms related to climacteric. Significant improvement occurred after 1 week of treatment (7,2096). ...when used orally to prevent benzodiazepine withdrawal. There is some evidence that upwardly titrating kava over one week while tapering the benzodiazepine over 2 weeks can prevent withdrawal symptoms in some people with non-psychotic anxiety (7325).
There is insufficient reliable information available about the effectiveness of kava for its other uses.

Mechanism of Action
The applicable part of kava is the rhizome and root. Pharmacological activity has largely been attributed to the kava-lactones (also known as kavapyrones), kawain, dihydrokawain, methysticin, dihydromethysticin, and others. The dried herb typically provides 3.5% kava-lactones (7), but kava extracts commercially available are generally formulated to

provide from 30-70% kava-lactones. Kava has been found to have a variety of central nervous system effects, including anxiolytic, sedative, anticonvulsant, local anesthetic, spasmolytic, and analgesic activities; however, the exact mechanism for these effects is not known. Kava is not thought to affect benzodiazepine or GABA receptors (6401). Analgesia is not believed to occur by the opiate pathway because naloxone will not reverse it (6). Furthermore, kava is thought to produce motor sedation without affecting respiratory processes (2095). Some evidence suggests kava may affect the limbic system (214). When chewed kava root reportedly numbs the mouth similar to cocaine (1740). People consuming kava have reported feeling more sociable, tranquil, and generally happy (1740). The kavapyrones desmethoxyyangonin and methysticin can competitively inhibit monoamine oxidase B (MAO-B) (2500). Kava compounds can also be potent strychnine antagonists (6). The kavapyrone (+)-kawain can have antithrombic action on platelets, probably due to inhibition of cyclo-oxygenase and decreased thromboxane 2 (TXA2) production (2501).

Adverse Reactions

Orally, kava can cause gastrointestinal upset; headache; dizziness; enlarged pupils and disturbances of oculomotor equilibrium and accommodation; and rarely, allergic skin reactions (2,7). Unlike benzodiazepines, kava is not thought to be associated with impaired cognitive function (2097,2098); however, it does cause drowsiness and seems to affect motor reflexes (19).

Use of normal doses of kava may affect the ability to drive or operate machinery. Driving under the influence (DUI) citations have been issued to individuals observed driving erratically after drinking large amounts of kava tea (535,5079). Chewing kava can cause mouth numbness (6). There is also concern that kava might adversely effect the liver. Liver toxicity is primarily associated with prolonged use of very high doses (6401); however, kava can exacerbate hepatitis in patients with a history of recurrent hepatitis. Symptoms seem to resolve spontaneously after discontinuation of kava (390). There is also some concern that even short-term use of kava in typical doses might cause acute hepatitis in some patients. There are 24 documented cases of hepatotoxicity following use of kava (7024,7068,7086). In some cases, death or liver transplant has been required after as little as 1-3 months of kava use (7024,7068,7086). In one case, kava use resulted in acute hepatitis with severe hepatocellular necrosis, which required a liver transplant (7024). In another case, kava alone was used for three weeks. Then, following a single occasion of alcohol consumption, symptoms of liver toxicity occurred (7068). In susceptible patients, symptoms can show up after as little as 3-4 weeks of kava use, including yellowed skin (jaundice), fatigue, and dark urine (7024,7068). Liver function tests can be elevated after 3-8 weeks of use, possibly followed by hepatomegaly and onset of encephalopathy (7024). These cases have resulted in kava supplements being banned in Switzerland. German regulators are also considering removing kava from the market (7086). Most patients taking kava have not experienced such severe adverse effects. It is unclear which patients might be susceptible to adverse liver effects. There is some speculation that so-called "poor metabolizers" or those patients with deficiency in the cytochrome P450 2D6 (CYP2D6) isozyme may be at increased risk for hepatotoxic effects of kava. Until more is known, tell patients to avoid kava. Advise patients that continue to use to routinely monitor liver function. In patients who develop symptoms, discontinue kava and monitor liver function tests. Liver function tests may normalize within 8 weeks following discontinuation (7068). Long-term use of very large amounts of kava is also associated with overall poor health including symptoms of low body weight, reduced protein levels, puffy face, scaly rash, hematuria, increased red blood cell volume, decreased platelets and lymphocytes, and possibly pulmonary hypertension (6402). There is also a case of generalized abnormal movements of the body associated with high-dose, chronic kava consumption (534). Chronic use of high doses of kava has been associated with kava dermopathy, a pellagra-like syndrome that is unresponsive to niacinamide treatment (7,6240). The cause is unknown but may relate to interference with cholesterol metabolism (6240). Some experts speculate that kava's adverse effects on the liver function might contribute to the disorder. This syndrome consists of dry, flaky skin; reddened eyes; and temporary yellow discoloration of the skin, hair, and nails (7,6401). It usually occurs within 3 months to 1 year of kava use and resolves when the kava dose is decreased or discontinued (6401). Kava dose should be decreased or discontinued if kava dermopathy occurs (7,6401).

Interactions with Herbs & Other Dietary Supplements

HEPATOTOXIC HERBS AND SUPPLEMENTS: There is some concern that kava can adversely effect the liver (7024,7068). Theoretically, concomitant use with other potentially hepatotoxic products might increase the risk of developing liver damage. Some of these products include androstenedione, chaparral, coenzyme Q10 (only in high doses), comfrey, DHEA, germander, niacin, pennyroyal oil, red yeast, scullcap, valerian, and others.

HERBS AND SUPPLEMENTS WITH SEDATIVE PROPERTIES: Theoretically, concomitant use with herbs and supplements that have sedative properties might increase the risk of excessive drowsiness. Some of these include 5-HTP, calamus, calendula, California poppy, catnip, capsicum, celery, couch grass, elecampane, German chamomile, goldenseal, gotu kola, hops, Jamaican dogwood, lemon balm, melatonin, sage, St. John's wort, sassafras, scullcap, shepherd's purse, Siberian ginseng, stinging nettle, valerian, wild carrot, wild lettuce, ashwaganda root, and yerba mansa (4,19).

Interactions with Drugs

ALPRAZOLAM: There is one report of an individual who was hospitalized due to lethargy and disorientation that

---

occurred when alprazolam and kava were used concomitantly (536).

CNS DEPRESSANTS: Concomitant use of kava and alcohol, barbiturates, benzodiazepines, and other CNS depressants can increase the risk of drowsiness and motor reflex depression (2,6).

HEPATOTOXIC DRUGS: There is some concern that kava can adversely effect the liver (7024,7068). Theoretically, concomitant use with other potentially hepatotoxic drugs might increase the risk of developing liver damage. Some of these drugs include acarbose (Precose), amiodarone (Cordarone), atorvastatin (Lipitor), azathioprine (Imuran), carbamazepine (Tegretol), cerivastatin (Baycol), diclofenac (Voltaren), felbamate (Felbatol), fenofibrate (Tricor), fluvastatin (Lescol), gemfibrozil (Lopid), isoniazid, itraconazole, (Sporanox), ketoconazole (Nizoral), leflunomide (Arava), lovastatin (Mevacor), methotrexate (Rheumatrex), nevirapine (Viramune), niacin, nitrofurantoin (Macrodantin), pioglitazone (Actos), pravastatin (Pravachol), pyrazinamide, rifampin (Rifadin), ritonavir (Norvir), rosiglitazone (Avandia), simvastatin (Zocor), tacrine (Cognex), tamoxifen, terbinafine (Lamisil), valproic acid, and zileuton (Zyflo).

LEVODOPA (Larodopa, Dopar): There is some concern that kava might decrease the effectiveness of levodopa. In one case, kava seemed to reduce efficacy of levodopa. This effect might be due to dopamine antagonism by kava (19).

Interactions with Foods

ALCOHOL: Concomitant use with alcohol can increase the risk of kava side effects such as drowsiness and motor reflex depression (2,6,19). There is also some concern that concomitant use of kava and alcohol can increase the risk of developing hepatotoxicity (7068).

Interactions with Lab Tests

LIVER FUNCTION TESTS: There is some concern that kava can cause liver damage and increase liver function tests (LFTs) in some patients. Liver toxicity is primarily associated with prolonged use of high doses (6401). However, in some patients, short-term use (3-8 weeks) of typical doses might result in liver damage and increase liver function tests (390,7024,7068). Liver function tests affected include aspartate aminotransferase (AST), alanine aminotransferase (ALT), alkaline phosphatase, gamma-glutamyltransferase, lactate dehydrogenase (LDH), and total and conjugated bilirubin (7024,7068). Consider monitoring liver function tests in patients taking kava for more than one month or in patients symptoms of liver problems such as fatigue, yellowing of the skin (jaundice), or dark urine.

Interactions with Diseases or Conditions

DEPRESSION: There is some concern about using kava in depressed patients. Kava seems to have CNS depressant effects and theoretically might exacerbate depression in some patients (2,12,19); use with caution.

HEPATITIS: Kava might adversely effect the liver, especially when taken for prolonged periods or in high doses. Even when used short-term in typical doses, kava might exacerbate hepatitis in patients with a history of recurrent hepatitis (390). Tell patients with active hepatitis or a history of hepatitis to avoid kava.

Dosage and Administration

ORAL: For anxiety disorders, most clinical trials have used kava extract standardized to 70% kava-lactone content. Doses of the kava extract were most commonly 100 mg (70 mg kava-lactones) three times daily (7,2092,2093,2094,2095,2096). For preventing benzodiazepine withdrawal, the 70% kava-lactone standardized extract has been used in doses increasing from 50 mg to 300 mg per day over one week, while the benzodiazepine is tapered over 2 weeks (7325). For nervous anxiety, stress, and restlessness, a dose of 60-120 mg kava-lactones daily has been used (2). Kava is also taken as 1 cup of the tea up to 3 times per day. The tea is prepared by simmering 2-4 grams of the root in 150 mL boiling water for 5-10 minutes and then straining (12). Because kava-lactone content varies substantially among products, appropriate dosing will also vary.

TOPICAL: No typical dosage.

Comments

Kava was discovered by Captain Cook who named the plant, "intoxicating pepper" (6240). In the South Pacific, kava is a popular social drink, similar to alcohol in Western societies (6). Kava is also prepared in a defined ritual manner and used for ceremonial purposes and has been used for thousands of years by Pacific Islanders (782,6240). Commercially available kava extracts are prepared from the dried root of Piper methysticum with an ethanol-water mixture (for extracts containing 30% kavapyrones) and with an acetone-water mixture (for extracts containing 70% kavapyrones; one extract is designated WS 1490) (7).

KHAT

Also Known As

Abyssinian Tea, Chaat, Gat, Kat, Kus es Salahin, Qut, Tchaad, Tohai, Tohat, Tschut.

Scientific Names
Catha edulis.
Family: Celastraceae.

People Use This For
Orally, khat leaf is used for depression, fatigue, obesity, and gastric ulcers (6). The leaf and stem are chewed by people in East Africa and the Arabian countries as a euphoriant (6).

Safety
POSSIBLY UNSAFE ...when used orally. Khat leaf is not physically addicting but is associated with psychological dependence (6).
PREGNANCY: POSSIBLY UNSAFE ...when used orally. Khat may reduce infant birth weight (6).
LACTATION: POSSIBLY UNSAFE ...when used orally. Khat contains norpseudoephedrine, which passes into mother's milk (6); avoid using.

Effectiveness
There is insufficient reliable information available about the effectiveness of khat.

Mechanism of Action
The applicable parts of khat are the leaf and stem. Contains cathine, which has 1/10 the stimulant effect of d-amphetamine, and cathinone, a more powerful stimulant than cathine. Both decrease food intake and increase locomotor activity (6).

Adverse Reactions
Orally, consumption of Khat results in central stimulation including euphoria, increased alertness, excessive talkativeness, hyperactivity, excitement, aggressiveness, anxiety, elevated blood pressure, and manic behavior. Insomnia, malaise, and lack of concentration usually follow. True psychotic reactions occur much less often than with amphetamines. Cardiovascular effects include tachycardia, palpitations, and increased blood pressure. Other effects include increased respiratory rate, hyperthermia, sweating, pupil dilation and decreased intraocular pressure, stomatitis, esophagitis, gastritis, periodontal disease, temporomandibular joint dysfunction and keratosis of buccal mucosa, and constipation (6). Chronic use in young people is linked to hypertension. Severe adverse effects include migraine, cerebral hemorrhage, myocardial infarction, pulmonary edema, hepatic cirrhosis, initial increase in men's libido followed by loss of sexual drive, spermatorrhea, and impotence (6). Females report increased sexual desire and improved performance (6). There are also cases of infection with Fasciola hepatica following chewing khat leaves. Fasciola hepatica contamination might be most likely with freshly picked, damp leaves. Signs of Fasciola hepatica infection can include pain below the ribs, leukocytosis with eosinophilia, and large liver mass on CT examination (6464).

Interactions with Herbs & Other Dietary Supplements
Insufficient reliable information available.

Interactions with Drugs
No interactions are known to occur, and there is no known reason to expect a clinically significant interaction with khat.

Interactions with Foods
No interactions are known to occur, and there is no known reason to expect a clinically significant interaction with khat.

Interactions with Lab Tests
No interactions are known to occur, and there is no known reason to expect a clinically significant interaction with khat.

Interactions with Diseases or Conditions
DIABETES: Khat use suppresses appetite, causing people to skip meals, decrease adherence to dietary advice, and increase consumption of sweetened beverages aggravating hyperglycemia (6).

Dosage and Administration
No typical dosage.

Comments
None.

KHELLA

Also Known As

Ammi, Bischofskrautfruchte, Bishop's Weed, Bishop's Weed Fruit, Bishops Weed, Fruits De Khella, Khella Fruit, Khellin, Toothpick Ammi, Toothpick Plant, Visnaga, Visnagae, Visnagafruchte, Visnaga Fruit, Visnagin.
CAUTION: See separate listings for Goutweed and Bishop's Weed.

Scientific Names

Ammi visnaga, synonyms Ammi daucoides, Daucus visagna.
Family: Apiaceae/Umbelliferae.

People Use This For

Orally, khella is used for colic and abdominal cramps, kidney stones, menstrual pain, and premenstrual syndrome (PMS). Khella is also used for respiratory conditions including asthma, bronchitis, cough, and whooping cough. It is also used for cardiovascular disorders including hypertension, cardiac arrhythmias, congestive heart failure (CHF), angina, atherosclerosis, and hypercholesterolemia. It is also used for liver and gall bladder disorders, diabetes, and as a diuretic (7159,7160,7161).
Topically, khella is used for vitiligo, psoriasis, wound healing, inflammation conditions, and poisonous bites (7159,7160).

Safety

POSSIBLY UNSAFE ...when used orally in high doses. High doses of khella can cause increases in liver enzymes and possible liver damage (2).
PREGNANCY: LIKELY UNSAFE ...when used orally. The active constituent, khellin, has uterine stimulant activity (19); contraindicated.
LACTATION: Insufficient reliable information available; avoid using.

Effectiveness

There is insufficient reliable information available about the effectiveness of khella.

Mechanism of Action

The applicable parts of khella are the dried, ripe fruits (7161). Khella has several constituents with known pharmacological activity, including visnadin, visnagin, and khellin. All of these constituents seem to have cardiovascular effects due to calcium channel blocking actions (8,2525). Visnadin is the most active. It can inhibit vascular smooth muscle contraction and seems to dilate peripheral and coronary vessels and increase coronary circulation (8,9,2523,2524). Visnagin also has negative chronotropic and inotropic effects and reduces peripheral vascular resistance (869). The khellin constituent also acts as a vasodilator and has bronchodilatory activity (9). There is some preliminary evidence that khellin might also increase high-density lipoprotein (HDL) levels without affecting total cholesterol or triglyceride concentrations (2522). A khella extract seems to have some antimicrobial activity. This might be attributable to both the khellin and visnagin constituents, which both seem to have antifungal, antibacterial, and antiviral activity (1907). Researchers are interested in khella for use in psoriasis. The khellin constituent is structurally similar to the psoralen nucleus and might be useful as a photosensitizer in patients with psoriasis (1908).

Adverse Reactions

Orally, prolonged use or use of high doses of khella can cause nausea, dizziness, constipation, lack of appetite, headache, itching, and insomnia. In some patients, khella can cause elevated liver transaminase and gamma-glutamyltransferase (GGT) levels (2), probably due to the khellin constituent, which is known to affect liver enzymes (6,2522). Liver dysfunction and jaundice is typically reversible when khella is discontinued (2). There is also some concern that khella might cause photosensitivity because of the constituents khellin and furocoumarin (2,7162).

Interactions with Herbs & Other Dietary Supplements

DIGITALIS: Theoretically, khella might decrease the effectiveness of digitalis. The visnagin constituent of khella has negative inotropic effects, which might counter the effects of digitalis (869).
HEPATOTOXIC HERBS: Khella might have additive effects with herbs that cause hepatotoxicity. Khella can cause increase liver enzymes and liver dysfunction in some patients. Other products that might affect the liver include borage, chaparral, uva ursi, and others (2,2522).
PHOTOSENSITIZING HERBS: Theoretically, khella might have an additive effects with products that increase sun sensitivity, such as St. John's wort (7162).

Interactions with Drugs

DIGITOXIN (Crystodigin), DIGOXIN (Lanoxin): Theoretically, khella might decrease the effectiveness of cardiac glycosides like digoxin and digitoxin. The khella constituent visnadin has negative inotropic effects that might counter the effects of cardiac glycosides (19,869).

HEPATOTOXIC DRUGS: Theoretically, khella might have additive adverse effects on the liver when used with hepatotoxic drugs. Khella can increase liver transaminases (2,2522). Some drugs that can adversely effect the liver include acetaminophen (Tylenol), amiodarone (Cordarone), carbamazepine (Tegretol), isoniazid (INH), methotrexate (Rheumatrex), methyldopa (Aldomet) and many others.

PHOTOSENSITIZING DRUGS: Theoretically, concomitant use might result in increased photosensitivity. Khella constituents can cause photosensitivity (2521,7162). Some drugs that cause photosensitivity include amitriptyline (Elavil), quinolones (Ciprofloxacin, others), sulfa drugs (Septra, Bactrim, others), and tetracycline.

Interactions with Foods

No interactions are known to occur, and there is no known reason to expect a clinically significant interaction with khella.

Interactions with Lab Tests

HIGH-DENSITY LIPOPROTEIN (HDL): Theoretically, khella might increase HDL levels. The isolated khella constituent khellin seems to increase in HDL levels without affecting total cholesterol or triglycerides (2522).

LIVER FUNCTION TESTS: In some patients, khella can cause elevated liver transaminase and gamma-glutamyltransferase (GGT) levels (2), probably due to the khellin constituent, which is known to affect liver enzymes (6,2522). Liver dysfunction is typically reversible when khella is discontinued (2).

Interactions with Diseases or Conditions

LIVER DISEASE: Khella might exacerbate liver dysfunction in patients with liver disease. Khella can increase liver enzymes in some patients, probably due to the khellin constituent (2,2522).

Dosage and Administration

ORAL: Khella is typically given as an extract standardized based on khellin content. Extracts are usually standardized to 12% khellin (214). A typical dose of khella is an amount that provides 20 mg of the khellin constituent per day (8). For angina, khella in an amount providing doses of 30-300 mg of the khellin constituent has also been used (214). Khella is sometimes used as a tea. The tea is usually prepared by pouring boiling water over powdered fruit, steeping 10-15 minutes, and straining (8).

Comments

Several conventional drugs including amiodarone, nifedipine, and cromolyn, have been developed from khella (9,7161,7164). Khella is sometimes confused with its less used relative, bishop's weed (Ammi majus). The two species have some common chemical constituents and pharmacological effects, but khella is more commonly used for cardiac and pulmonary conditions, and bishop's weed is more commonly used for dermatological conditions (7161). Isolated khellin, a constituent of khella and bishop's weed, is used for angina pectoris; asthma; and in conjunction with phototherapy for vitiligo, psoriasis, and alopecia areata (9,560,849,868).

KINETIN

Also Known As

Kinerase, Kinetase.

Scientific Names

N-(2-furanylmethyl)-1H-purin-6-amine; N(6)furfuryladenine; 6-furfurylaminopurine.

People Use This For

Topically, kinetin is used to reduce the effects of skin aging; to reduce skin roughness; fine wrinkles; telangiectasias; and mottled, excessive pigmentation (4276).

In combination, kinetin is also used topically with retinol palmitate to treat signs of aging (4286).

Safety

POSSIBLY SAFE ...when kinetin is used topically and appropriately (4276).

There is insufficient reliable information about the safety of kinetin and retinol palmitate used in combination.

PREGNANCY AND LACTATION: Insufficient reliable information available; avoid using.

Effectiveness

There is insufficient reliable information available about the effectiveness of kinetin.

Mechanism of Action

Kinetin is a cytokinin, a potent plant growth factor (4277,4279). Kinetin prevents the aging of leaves; a green leaf dipped in kinetin will not turn brown. Some evidence suggests kinetin might also prevent age-related changes in human skin (4277). Although kinetin's mechanism of action is unknown, limited information suggests it acts as an antioxidant protecting DNA from oxidative damage (4278). Other evidence suggests that it also decreases skin water loss across the epidermis (4276). Unlike other growth agents, kinetin does not increase the maximum lifespan or ability of human skin cells to multiply in culture, suggesting it does not promote skin cancer (4277).

Adverse Reactions

Topically, kinetin 0.1% sometimes initially causes dry skin (4285).

Interactions with Herbs & Other Dietary Supplements

Insufficient reliable information available.

Interactions with Drugs

No interactions are known to occur, and there is no known reason to expect a clinically significant interaction with kinetin.

Interactions with Foods

No interactions are known to occur, and there is no known reason to expect a clinically significant interaction with kinetin.

Interactions with Lab Tests

No interactions are known to occur, and there is no known reason to expect a clinically significant interaction with kinetin.

Interactions with Diseases or Conditions

No interactions are known to occur, and there is no known reason to expect a clinically significant interaction with kinetin.

Dosage and Administration

TOPICAL: A typical dose is 0.05% cream or lotion or 0.1% cream or lotion applied twice daily (4280,4284). Although kinetin does not cause photosensitivity, using a sunscreen with SPF 15 is recommended as the basis of any skin care program (4285).

Comments

To date, no controlled trials in humans have been published in peer-reviewed journals. A study financed by a manufacturer evaluated 64 subjects who used 0.005% kinetin lotion or cream or placebo along with a mild facial cleanser and sunscreen (SPF 15). All study participants showed global improvement, 33-36% using kinetin showed good to excellent improvement compared to 12-21% in the placebo group (4276).

KIWI

Also Known As

China Gooseberry, Chinese Gooseberry, Kiwi Fruit.

Scientific Names

Actinidia chinensis.
Family: Actinidiaceae.

People Use This For

For food use, kiwi is eaten as a food, used as a meat tenderizer, and is a component in some sports drinks (6).

Safety

LIKELY SAFE ...when used in food amounts (6).
PREGNANCY AND LACTATION: LIKELY SAFE ...when used in food amounts (6).

Effectiveness

There is insufficient reliable information available to rate the effectiveness of kiwi. However, there's some evidence that consumption of vitamin C-rich citrus fruits, including kiwi and others, might improve lung function in people with asthma. Intake of citrus fruits 1-2 times per week has produced this benefit in some studies (6049,6055,6056). However, other studies have not found this benefit (6057,6058). More evidence is needed to rate the effectiveness of kiwi for this use.

Mechanism of Action
The applicable part of kiwi is the fruit. Kiwi fruit contains high concentrations of vitamin C and serotonin (6). The potential benefits of kiwi in asthma might be due to antioxidant properties of vitamin C or other fruit constituents (6049,6054,6055). The constituent, actinidin, is an enzyme with proteolytic activity similar to papain (6). Enzymatic components may be responsible for adverse effects (6).

Adverse Reactions
Orally, eating kiwi fruit or drinking the juice can lead to hypersensitivity reactions of the mouth, including dysphagia, urticaria, and vomiting immediately following ingestion (6).
Topically, use can cause contact urticaria (6).

Interactions with Herbs & Other Dietary Supplements
Insufficient reliable information available.

Interactions with Drugs
No interactions are known to occur, and there is no known reason to expect a clinically significant interaction with kiwi.

Interactions with Foods
No interactions are known to occur, and there is no known reason to expect a clinically significant interaction with kiwi.

Interactions with Lab Tests
URINE TESTS: Kiwi may elevate urine levels of 5-hydroxyindoleacetic acid and interfere with lab tests for this serotonin metabolite (6).

Interactions with Diseases or Conditions
No interactions are known to occur, and there is no known reason to expect a clinically significant interaction with kiwi.

Dosage and Administration
No typical dosage.

Comments
None.

KNOTWEED HERB

Also Known As
Allseed Nine-Joints, Armstrong, Beggarweed, Bird's Tongue, Birdweed, Centinode, Cow Grass, Crawlgrass, Doorweed, Hogweed, Knot Grass, Knotgrass, Knotweed, Ninety-Knot, Pigrush, Pigweed, Polygoni Avicularis Herba, Red Robin, Sparrow Tongue, Swine's Grass, Swynel Grass, Vogelknoeterichkraut.

Scientific Names
Polygonum aviculare.
Family: Polygonaceae.

People Use This For
Orally, knotweed herb is used for bronchitis, cough, and inflammation of the mouth and pharynx.
In folk medicine, knotweed herb is used orally for supportive treatment of pulmonary diseases, skin disorders, to suppress perspiration associated with tuberculosis, as a diuretic, and as a hemostatic in cases of hemorrhage (18).

Safety
POSSIBLY SAFE ...when used orally or topically (2,18).
PREGNANCY AND LACTATION: Insufficient reliable information available; avoid using.

Effectiveness
POSSIBLY EFFECTIVE ...when used orally to treat inflammation of the mouth or pharynx (2).
There is insufficient reliable information available about the effectiveness of knotweed herb for its other uses.

Mechanism of Action
The applicable part of knotweed herb is the whole flowering plant. Knotweed is suggested to have astringent and anticholinergic activity (2,18). There is insufficient reliable information about the possible mechanism of action or active ingredients.

Adverse Reactions
None reported.

Interactions with Herbs & Other Dietary Supplements
Insufficient reliable information available.

Interactions with Drugs
No interactions are known to occur, and there is no known reason to expect a clinically significant interaction with knotweed herb.

Interactions with Foods
No interactions are known to occur, and there is no known reason to expect a clinically significant interaction with knotweed herb.

Interactions with Lab Tests
No interactions are known to occur, and there is no known reason to expect a clinically significant interaction with knotweed herb.

Interactions with Diseases or Conditions
No interactions are known to occur, and there is no known reason to expect a clinically significant interaction with knotweed herb.

Dosage and Administration
ORAL: One cup of tea (simmer 1.4 grams dried ground herb in 150 mL of boiling water for 10-15 minutes, strain) is taken orally 3 to 5 times daily. The daily oral dose is 4-6 grams dried ground herb (2,18).

Comments
None.

KOMBUCHA TEA

Also Known As
Champagne Of Life, Combucha Tea, Dr. Sklenar's Kombucha Mushroom Infusion, Fungus Japonicus, Kargasok Tea, Kombucha Mushroom Tea, Kwassan, Manchurian Fungus, Manchurian Mushroom Tea, Spumonto, T'Chai from the Sea, Tschambucco.

Scientific Names
None.

People Use This For
Orally, kombucha tea is used for memory loss, premenstrual syndrome, rheumatism, aging, anorexia (6), AIDS, cancer (2650), hypertension, increasing T-cell counts (2652), strengthening the immune system and metabolism (2653), constipation, arthritis (2654), and hair regrowth (2655).
Topically, it is used for analgesia (2651).

Safety
POSSIBLY UNSAFE ...when taken orally because non-sterile home preparations have a high risk of contamination (2650,2651,2652,2653).
LIKELY UNSAFE ...when used orally by individuals with compromised immunity, including HIV/AIDS, due to the risk of transmission of opportunistic pathogens (2652,2653), including Aspergillus (2652,2653) and anthrax (Bacillus anthracis) (2651). ...when kombucha tea prepared in a lead-glazed ceramic container is used orally. Lead poisoning was

reported in two people who consumed kombucha tea prepared in a lead-glazed ceramic pot for six months (1366).
PREGNANCY AND LACTATION: POSSIBLY UNSAFE …when used orally; avoid using.

Effectiveness
There is insufficient reliable information available about the effectiveness of kombucha tea.

Mechanism of Action
Kombucha tea can contain up to 1.5% alcohol, vinegar (acetic acid), and a variety of other metabolites (2655). The product contains high levels of B vitamins (2653). No clinically relevant pharmacology has been defined for the kombucha symbiot or its products (6). Caffeine (black tea) and sugar are theorized to account for the increased energy claimed by some tea users (2654). Kombucha tea has the potential to incubate pathogenic organisms, including Aspergillus and anthrax, during its preparation, which is commonly ten days of fermentation at room temperature (2651,2652,2653). Due to the vinegar and ethanol content, it also has the potential to leach lead and other toxic chemicals from the walls of the preparation and storage containers (2650).

Adverse Reactions
Orally, kombucha tea can cause stomach problems, yeast infections (2652), allergic reactions, jaundice, nausea, vomiting, head and neck pain (2656), anthrax (2651), and possibly death (2655). Symptomatic lead poisoning requiring chelation decontamination therapy was reported in two people who consumed kombucha tea prepared in a lead-glazed ceramic pot for six months (1366).

Interactions with Herbs & Other Dietary Supplements
Insufficient reliable information available.

Interactions with Drugs
ACID-SENSITIVE DRUGS: Theoretically, concomitant use of kombucha tea with acid-sensitive oral drugs can interfere with drug therapy due to the acidity of kombucha tea.
DISULFIRAM (Antabuse): Theoretically, concomitant use can cause a disulfiram reaction due to the alcohol contained in the fermented tea (2650).

Interactions with Foods
No interactions are known to occur, and there is no known reason to expect a clinically significant interaction with kombucha tea.

Interactions with Lab Tests
LIVER FUNCTION TESTS: There is one report of increased liver function tests after three weeks of consumption of kombucha tea (6).

Interactions with Diseases or Conditions
ALCOHOLISM: Kombucha tea is contraindicated in people with stabilized or therapeutically-controlled alcoholism, because the alcohol content of the tea can aggravate this condition (2650).
COMPROMISED IMMUNITY: Contraindicated because kombucha tea can harbor or culture organisms that cause opportunistic infections (2652,2653).

Dosage and Administration
No typical dosage.

Comments
The kombucha "mushroom" is a yeast or bacteria fungal symbiot and not an actual mushroom. It is derived from the fermentation of yeasts and bacteria with black tea, sugar, and other ingredients (6,2650). The resulting liquid is called kombucha tea. Although advocates of kombucha tea have attributed many therapeutic effects to the drink in the popular press, there is no scientific evidence to support any therapeutic claims (6,2650,2652,2654,2655). An outbreak of anthrax in twenty people in Iran confirmed the tea is a good culture medium for Bacillus anthracis (2651).

KOUSSO

Also Known As
Cossoo, Kooso, Kosso.

Scientific Names

Brayera anthelmintica; Hagenia abyssinica.
Family: Rosaceae.

People Use This For

Historically, kousso was used orally for tapeworm infestations (18).

Safety

LIKELY UNSAFE ...when used orally (18).
PREGNANCY: UNSAFE ...when used orally; contraindicated due to abortifacient activity (19).
LACTATION: UNSAFE ...when used orally due to its potential for toxicity (18).

Effectiveness

There is insufficient reliable information available about the effectiveness of kousso.

Mechanism of Action

There is insufficient reliable information available about the possible mechanism of action or active ingredients.

Adverse Reactions

The side effects of kousso include gastrointestinal irritation, with accompanying salivation, headache, and general weakness. With overdose, people experience syncope and vision disorders. It can also cause colic, spasms, acidosis, and shock (18).

Interactions with Herbs & Other Dietary Supplements

Insufficient reliable information available.

Interactions with Drugs

No interactions are known to occur, and there is no known reason to expect a clinically significant interaction with kousso.

Interactions with Foods

No interactions are known to occur, and there is no known reason to expect a clinically significant interaction with kousso.

Interactions with Lab Tests

No interactions are known to occur, and there is no known reason to expect a clinically significant interaction with kousso.

Interactions with Diseases or Conditions

GI CONDITIONS: Can irritate the gastrointestinal tract. Contraindicated in individuals with infectious or inflammatory gastrointestinal conditions (19).

Dosage and Administration

No typical dosage.

Comments

None.

KUDZU

Also Known As

Daidzein, Fen Ke, Fenge, Gange, Ge Gen, Gegen, Isoflavone, Isoflavones, Japanese Arrowroot, Kudsu, Kudzu Vine, Kwaao Khruea, Mealy Kudzu, Pueraria, Pueraria Root, Radix Peurariae, Yege.

Scientific Names

Pueraria montana var. lobata, synonyms Pueraria lobata, Pueraria thunbergiana, Pueraria pseudohirsuta, Dolichos lobatus; Pueraria montana var. thomsonii, synonym Pueraria thomsonii; Pueraria mirifica; Pueraria tuberosa.
Family: Leguminosae or Fabaceae.

People Use This For

Orally, kudzu is used alone or in combination with other products for symptoms of alcohol hangover, such as headache, upset stomach, dizziness, and vomiting (11,766).

In traditional Chinese medicine, kudzu has been used for managing alcoholism and drunkenness, myalgia, measles (6,11), dysentery, gastritis (6), fever, diarrhea, thirst, cold, flu, neck stiffness, and as a diaphoretic (11). In recent years, kudzu has been used for hypertension, angina pectoris, arrhythmia, migraine (6,11), deafness, diabetes, traumatic injuries, sinusitis, urticaria, pruritus, and psoriasis (11).

Kudzu root is also consumed as food (11).

Safety

POSSIBLY SAFE ...when used orally and appropriately (11,12). Daily doses of 50-100 grams kudzu root does not produce adverse effects in humans (11).

PREGNANCY AND LACTATION: Insufficient reliable information available; avoid using.

Effectiveness

There is insufficient reliable information available about the effectiveness of kudzu.

Mechanism of Action

The applicable parts of kudzu are the root and flower. Isoflavone constituents (daidzin, daidzein, and puerarin) and their derivatives are thought to be reversible inhibitors of alcohol and aldehyde dehydrogenase (6). However, recent studies dispute this finding (1523,1524). Kudzu extract, daidzein, and daidzin decrease alcohol consumption and peak blood alcohol levels, and shorten alcohol-induced sleep in alcohol-craving animals (6,1523). Decreased peak blood alcohol levels might be due to delayed gastric emptying (1523). Preliminary evidence suggests that puerarin might decrease heart rate, plasma renin activity, capillary permeability, platelet aggregation (11). Puerarin demonstrates hypoglycemic, hypocholesterolemic, antiarrhythmic, antipyretic, and antioxidant activity (11). Kudzu root extracts dilate coronary and cerebral blood vessels and increase myocardial and cerebral blood flow, decrease vascular resistance, myocardial oxygen demand, and lactic acid production in anaerobic myocardial tissues; and increase the blood oxygen supply (11). Studies are needed to investigate the effect(s) of kudzu in humans.

Adverse Reactions

None reported.

Interactions with Herbs & Other Dietary Supplements

Insufficient reliable information available.

Interactions with Drugs

ANTICOAGULANTS: Theoretically, kudzu might potentiate the effects of anticoagulants. A constituent of kudzu inhibits platelet activating factor (11).

ASPIRIN: Theoretically, concomitant use might increase the potential for hypoglycemic effects with kudzu. Aspirin increases the hypoglycemic effects of a kudzu constituent in diabetic mice (11).

HYPOGLYCEMIC AGENTS: Theoretically, concomitant use might have additive hypoglycemic effects. A constituent of kudzu has hypoglycemic activity in animals (11).

CARDIOVASCULAR AGENTS: Theoretically, kudzu might interfere with cardiovascular therapies. Kudzu extracts decrease heart rate and have vasodilatory and antiarrhythmic effects in animals (11).

Interactions with Foods

No interactions are known to occur, and there is no known reason to expect a clinically significant interaction with kudzu.

Interactions with Lab Tests

BLOOD GLUCOSE: Theoretically, kudzu might decrease blood glucose levels and test results. A constituent of kudzu has hypoglycemic activity in animals (11).

SERUM CHOLESTEROL: Theoretically, kudzu might decrease serum cholesterol levels and test results. A constituent of kudzu reduces serum cholesterol levels in animals (11).

Interactions with Diseases or Conditions

DIABETES: Theoretically, kudzu might interfere with blood glucose control requiring dosing adjustment of diabetes drug therapy. A constituent of kudzu has hypoglycemic activity in animals (11).

CARDIOVASCULAR CONDITIONS: Theoretically, kudzu might interfere with cardiovascular treatments. Kudzu extracts decrease heart rate and have vasodilatory and antiarrhythmic effects in animals (11).

CLOTTING DISORDERS: Theoretically, kudzu might interfere with anticoagulant therapies. A constituent of kudzu inhibits platelet activating factor (11).

Dosage and Administration

ORAL: People take kudzu root extract 150-300 mg three times daily (5019). Kudzu root extract 300 mg once daily has also been used (3539). In China, people take kudzu root 9-15 grams daily (5011). Kudzu root tablets 30-120 mg (each 10 mg is equivalent to 1.5 grams of crude kudzu root) have also been used (5011).

Comments

Some commercial kudzu products are standardized for daidzin content (3538) (see Mechanism of Action).

L-ARGININE

Also Known As

Arg, Arginine, Arginine HCl, Arginine Hydrochloride, L Arginine, L-Arginine HCl, L-Arginine-HCl, L-Arginine Hydrochloride.

Scientific Names

2-Amino-5-guanidinopentanoic acid.

People Use This For

L-Arginine is used for cardiovascular conditions, including congestive heart failure (CHF), angina pectoris, and coronary artery disease (3330,3332,3593,3594,6028). L-arginine is also used for intermittent claudication (3592), erectile dysfunction (222), male infertility, prevention of the common cold, (3330,3592), interstitial cystitis (107,114,3330,3460), cyclosporine nephrotoxicity (112), and improving athletic performance (217). It is also used in combination with ibuprofen for migraine headaches (109), and as an adjunct to chemotherapy in breast cancer (3330,3331). In combination with hydroxymethylbutyrate (HMB) and glutamine, L-arginine is used orally for treating weight loss in people with AIDS (1909).

Topically, L-arginine is used as an aid in wound healing, for treating cold hands and feet, and for male and female sexual dysfunction (3259,3260,3591).

Intravenously, L-arginine is used for intermittent claudication (3330,3465), for detecting growth hormone deficiency, nutritional supplementation for the critically ill (111,113,115), metabolic acidosis (15), and persistent pulmonary hypertension in newborns (120).

Safety

LIKELY SAFE ...when used orally and appropriately. L-arginine is generally considered safe and has only been associated with minor side effects in clinical studies lasting a few days to 6 months (114,3330,3331,3460,3593,3595,3596,6028). ...when used intravenously and appropriately. Parenteral L-arginine is a FDA-approved prescription product (15). There is insufficient reliable information available about the safety of the topical use of L-arginine.

PREGNANCY AND LACTATION: Insufficient reliable information available; avoid using.

Effectiveness

POSSIBLY EFFECTIVE ...when used orally in combination with conventional treatment for congestive heart failure (CHF). There is some evidence from small-scale studies that L-arginine can significantly improve quality of life and exercise tolerance as measured by walking distance (3595,6028). There is also some preliminary evidence that L-arginine can improve renal function in patients with CHF. It seems to significantly improve glomerular filtration rate (GFR), creatinine clearance, and sodium and water elimination after saline loading (3596). ...when used orally for intractable angina pectoris associated with coronary artery disease. There is some evidence from a small-scale study that patients with class IV angina and frequent attacks at rest, despite treatment with standard antianginal agents, can have significant relief by adding L-arginine. Some patients can improve from class IV to class II. However, after discontinuation of L-arginine, patients seem to rapidly return to class IV angina (3593). ...when taken orally for erectile dysfunction (222). In one study, oral L-arginine improved subjective assessment of sexual function in men with organic erectile dysfunction (222). ...when taken orally for improving renal vasodilation and sodium excretion in renal transplant patients treated with cyclosporine (112). ...when used orally for symptoms (especially pain) associated with interstitial cystitis (107,114,3460). ...when used orally in combination with ibuprofen for migraine headache (109). ...when used intravenously for improving clinical symptoms of intermittent claudication associated with peripheral arterial occlusive disease (3465). ...when used orally for interstitial cystitis. Evidence suggests that patients with interstitial cystitis having a bladder capacity greater than 800 mL and/or a history of recurrent genitourinary infections might respond more favorably to L-arginine than patients with bladder capacity less than 800 mL and/or no history of recurrent genitourinary infections. Three months of treatment may be necessary before significant improvement occurs (3460).

...when used orally in combination with hydroxymethylbutyrate (HMB) and glutamine for wasting in people with HIV/AIDS. There is some evidence that when used over a period of 8 weeks, L-arginine plus HMB and glutamine can increase body weight, particularly lean body mass, and positively affect immune status (1909).

POSSIBLY INEFFECTIVE ...when used orally for preventing coronary heart disease (CHD)-related mortality. Population studies show that intake of L-arginine does not seem to have any overall effect on mortality (3332,6896). There is insufficient reliable information available about the effectiveness of L-arginine for its other uses.

Mechanism of Action

L-arginine is an essential amino acid necessary for protein synthesis. It is found naturally in foods such as red meat, poultry, fish, and dairy products (3330,3592). L-arginine has numerous physiological effects including stimulating release of growth hormone (GH), prolactin, glucagon, and insulin. It also increases gastrin concentrations, and inhibits tubular reabsorption of protein. However, L-arginine is best known for its effects on the vascular system. L-arginine is a substrate for the enzyme nitric oxide synthase. Nitric oxide synthase in vascular endothelial cells converts L-arginine to nitric oxide, also known as endothelium-derived relaxation factor (EDRF), which causes vasodilation (3331,3460). L-arginine can significantly improve peripheral vasodilation, peripheral blood flow, and arterial compliance (3595,6028). The vasodilatory effects of L-arginine are thought to be useful in cardiovascular conditions, including congestive heart failure (CHF), coronary heart disease (CHD) and angina, and erectile dysfunction. L-arginine can also improve coronary endothelial function and brachial artery endothelium-dependent dilation, and reduce monocyte/endothelial cell adhesion in patients with coronary artery disease or hypercholesterolemia (110,116,1362,1363,3330). However, it may not have these effects in healthy people (1361). Nitric oxide also increases the relaxation of urinary tract smooth muscle (3259,3460) and is involved in erectile function. Although L-arginine appears to be helpful for erectile dysfunction, L-arginine may not effect the hemodynamics of the corpus cavernosum (222). When used topically for sexual dysfunction in females, L-arginine is purported to increase blood flow to the clitoris and increase sensitivity (3591); however, this effect has not been demonstrated in humans. Nitric oxide might also be involved in host inflammatory and microbial killing responses (3460). L-arginine is a precursor for collagen synthesis and together with fibroblast nitric oxide production might be important for wound healing (3259,3260). There is interest in L-arginine for adjunctive use in treating breast cancer. There is some evidence that L-arginine modifies immune system function and might potentiate tumor cell response to anti-cancer drugs and possibly reduce the immunosuppressive effects of chemotherapy agents. L-arginine seems to increase lymphocyte reactivity to polyclonal mitogenic agents and might also enhance natural cytotoxicity (3331).

L-arginine has an oral bioavailability of 68% and an elimination half-life of approximately 80 minutes (108).

Adverse Reactions

L-arginine can cause abdominal pain and bloating (15); diarrhea; gout (3331,3595); decreased platelet count; elevations of blood-urea-nitrogen (BUN), serum creatine and creatinine (15); allergic response or airway inflammation (15,117); and exacerbation of airway inflammation in asthma (121). Allergic reactions, including macular rash with hand and facial swelling and redness, nasal obstruction, increased pulse, sweating, and choking, have occurred. Excessively rapid infusion of L-arginine has caused flushing, nausea and vomiting, local venous irritation, numbness, and headache. Extravasation has caused necrosis and superficial phlebitis (15,3330).

Interactions with Herbs & Other Dietary Supplements

Insufficient reliable information available.

Interactions with Drugs

ANTIHYPERTENSIVES: Theoretically, concomitant use might cause additive hypotensive effects; use with caution.

CYCLOSPORINE: L-arginine can counteract the anti-natriuretic effect of cyclosporine (112).

ESTROGENS AND ORAL CONTRACEPTIVES: Concomitant use can increase the growth hormone response to arginine, and reduce the glucagon and insulin response to L-arginine (15).

MEDROXYPROGESTERONE/NORETHINDRONE: Concomitant use can reduce the L-arginine-induced growth hormone response (15).

NITRATES: Theoretically, concomitant use might cause additive vasodilation and have a hypotensive effect; use with caution.

POTASSIUM INCREASING DRUGS (ACE inhibitors, potassium-sparing diuretics): These drugs can increase the risk of L-arginine-induced hyperkalemia (15).

SILDENAFIL (Viagra): There is some concern that concurrent use of sildenafil and L-arginine might result in additive vasodilation and cause hypotension. However, this interaction has not been reported. Until more is known, use with caution or avoid using in combination.

XYLITOL, AMINOPHYLLINE: Concomitant use can reduce the glucagon response to L-arginine (15).

Interactions with Foods
No interactions are known to occur, and there is no known reason to expect a clinically significant interaction with L-arginine.

Interactions with Lab Tests
BLOOD UREA NITROGEN (BUN): L-arginine has been reported to increase BUN (15).
PLATELET COUNT: In one case, L-arginine has been reported to decrease platelet count (15).
SERUM CREATINE/CREATININE: L-arginine has been reported to increase serum creatine and creatinine (15).

Interactions with Diseases or Conditions
ACROCYANOSIS: L-arginine can exacerbate this condition (15).
ALLERGIC TENDENCIES/ASTHMA: L-arginine can cause an allergic response or aggravate airway inflammation (15,117), and inhaled L-arginine can amplify the inflammatory airway response in people with asthma (121); use with caution.
CIRRHOSIS OF THE LIVER: L-arginine-containing infusions can lead to a hyperdynamic circulatory state related to an elevation of the plasma level of nitrous oxide by L-arginine (122); use with caution.
HERPES VIRUS: Theoretically, L-arginine might exacerbate this condition. Preliminary evidence suggests that L-arginine may be necessary for viral replication (118,119).
HYPERCHLOREMIC ACIDOSIS: The injection of L-arginine can affect the intracellular or extracellular potassium balance (15); avoid using.
RENAL FAILURE: Intravenous administration of L-arginine has been associated with life-threatening hyperkalemia and a high nitrogen load (15); contraindicated.
SICKLE CELL ANEMIA: L-arginine might exacerbate this condition (15); use with caution.

Dosage and Administration
ORAL: For congestive heart failure, doses ranging from 2-5 grams three times per day have been used in clinical studies (3595,3596,6028). For angina pectoris associated with coronary artery disease, 3 grams three times per day has been used (110,3593). For interstitial cystitis, 500 mg-1.5 grams per day has been used (114,3330,3460). For organic erectile dysfunction, 5 grams per day has been used (222). For stimulation of host defenses in breast cancer patients undergoing chemotherapy, an oral dose of 10 grams three times per day for 3 days has been used (3331).
INTRAVENOUS: For intermittent claudication associated with peripheral arterial occlusive disease, 8 grams two times a day for 3 weeks has been used (3465).

Comments
Arginine butyrate has orphan drug status for beta-hemoglobinopathy, beta-thalassemia, and sickle cell disease (10).

L-CARNITINE

Also Known As
B(t) Factor, Carnitine, Carnitor, D-Carnitine, DL-Carnitine, Levocarnitine, Vitacarn, Vitamin B(t).
CAUTION: See separate listings for Acetyl-L-Carnitine and Propionyl-L-Carnitine.

Scientific Names
3-carboxy-2-hydroxy-N,N,N-trimethyl-1-propanaminium inner salt; (3-carboxy2-hydroxypropyl)trimethylammonium hydroxide inner salt; B-hydroxy-N-trimethyl aminobutyric acid; beta-hydroxy-gamma-trimethylammonium butyrate; L-3-hydroxy-4-(trimethylammonium)-butyrate; (R)-(3-carboxy-2-hydroxypropyl) trimethylammonium hydroxide; (R)-3-hydroxy-4-trimethylammonio-butyrate; 3-hydroxy-4-N-trimethylaminobutyrate.

People Use This For
Orally, L-carnitine is used for treating primary L-carnitine deficiency, secondary L-carnitine deficiency due to inborn errors of metabolism, and L-carnitine deficiency in people requiring hemodialysis. It is also used orally for treating drug-induced L-carnitine deficiency and for treating valproate-induced toxicity. L-carnitine is also used orally for myopathies associated with zidovudine and isotretinoin; and myocarditis associated with diphtheria, Rett Syndrome, chronic stable angina pectoris, congestive heart failure (CHF), and myocardial infarction. It is also used orally as a supplement in low birthweight and preterm infants, in strict vegetarians or vegans, and in dieters. L-carnitine is also used for anorexia, chronic fatigue syndrome, diabetes, hyperlipidemia, peripheral vascular disease and intermittent claudication, leg ulcers, and to enhance athletic performance and endurance.
Intravenously, L-carnitine is used to treat secondary L-carnitine deficiencies in people with inborn errors of metabolism, who require hemodialysis and to treat severe valproic acid-induced hepatotoxicity, especially in patients treated for overdose or accidental ingestion of valproic acid. It is also used intravenously for increasing CD4 cell

counts in people with HIV/AIDS, acute myocardial infarction, and as a supplement in people receiving total parenteral nutrition.

Safety

LIKELY SAFE ...when L-carnitine is used orally and appropriately. ...when L-carnitine injection is used as a FDA-approved prescription medicine. Avoid using D-carnitine and DL-carnitine, because they can act as competitive inhibitors of L-carnitine and cause symptoms of L-carnitine deficiency (9,1946).
There is insufficient reliable information available about the safety of l-carnitine for its other uses.
PREGNANCY: Insufficient reliable information available; avoid using.
LACTATION: POSSIBLY SAFE ...when used orally. Supplemental doses of L-carnitine have been given to infants in breast milk and formula with no reported adverse effects (9). The effects of large doses used while nursing are unknown, but L-carnitine is secreted in the breast milk (3616).

Effectiveness

EFFECTIVE ...when used orally or intravenously for acute or chronic treatment of primary L-carnitine deficiency or secondary L-carnitine deficiency due to inborn errors of metabolism. This is a FDA-approved indication for L-carnitine (3616). ...when used intravenously for prevention and treatment of L-carnitine deficiency in people with end-stage renal disease who are undergoing hemodialysis. This is a FDA-approved indication for L-carnitine (3616).
POSSIBLY EFFECTIVE ...when used orally or intravenously to improve fat utilization in preterm infants on total parenteral nutrition (3633,3634,3635,3636,3637). ...when used orally for L-carnitine deficiency secondary to valproic acid. L-carnitine supplementation can increase total and unbound carnitine plasma concentrations in patients taking valproic acid with laboratory evidence of L-carnitine deficiency; however, improvement of nonspecific symptoms of L-carnitine deficiency such as fatigue, nausea and vomiting, or reduced appetite may not occur (4523,4528,5798). ...when used orally or intravenously for valproic acid-induced toxicities. There is some evidence that patients taking valproic acid who have neurologic or hepatic deterioration or hyperammonemia can have neurologic and hepatic function restored and plasma ammonia levels lowered to within normal limits when L-carnitine is supplemented (1438,1914,1915,1916,1917,4523,5798,5799). Valproic acid toxicities are often associated with L-carnitine deficiency. There is also some evidence that intravenous L-carnitine can prevent the development of severe valproic acid-induced hepatotoxicity when given to patients being treated for overdose and accidental ingestion of valproic acid (1438, 4528,5798,5799), especially if treatment is initiated early (4528). ...when used orally to improve exercise tolerance in people with chronic stable angina (9,3623,3624), to improve symptoms in people with congestive heart failure (3625,3626), or after myocardial infarction to reduce complications and mortality (9,3627,3628,3629). ...when used orally for reducing the morbidity and mortality of myocarditis associated with diphtheria (3620,3621).
LIKELY INEFFECTIVE ...when used orally for enhancing athletic performance or endurance (1947,3639).
There is insufficient reliable information available about the effectiveness of L-carnitine for its other uses.

Mechanism of Action

L-carnitine is found in all mammalian tissue, especially striated muscle and is synthesized in the liver, kidneys and brain from the amino acids lysine and methionine (14). Approximately 98% of L-carnitine in the body is found in cardiac and skeletal muscle, with the remaining 2% being stored in the brain, kidney, and liver (14). It plays an important role in the transport of free fatty acids across the mitochondrial membrane for energy production, in the beta oxidation of fatty acids, and in maintaining an adequate ratio of fatty acyl-CoA compounds to free CoA inside the mitochondria (14). Primary tissue deficiency of L-carnitine may arise from failure of hepatic synthesis, failure of membrane transport, or disorders of reabsorption by the kidney (9,14). It is characterized by low concentrations of L-carnitine in plasma, red blood cells and/or tissues (3616). It may be present with hypoglycemia, encephalopathy, skeletal myopathy, cardiomyopathy, hepatotoxicity, and multiple organ dysfunction (9,14). L-carnitine deficiency can also occur secondary to other disorders, such as inborn errors of metabolism, cirrhosis, and hypopituitarism (9,14). Muscle L-carnitine deficiency has been reported in children with Duchenne muscular dystrophy (3640), and in people with myopathies due to zidovudine (3618) or isotretinoin (3619). Increased urinary losses of L-carnitine have been reported with ifosfamide and cisplatin therapy (3641,3642). Low serum L-carnitine levels have been reported in people receiving valproic acid therapy (1910,1911,1912,1913,4528,4526), in pregnant women (14,3643), in people with chronic fatigue syndrome (3630), and in people with HIV infection (3617). However, the relationship between serum and tissue L-carnitine levels is not fully understood and it is not known whether low serum levels necessarily lead to symptomatic deficiency (4528,4529,5798). Symptomatic deficiency is unlikely to arise from insufficient dietary intake since the body is usually able to synthesize adequate quantities (9). However, preterm neonates have a reduced capacity to synthesize L-carnitine and they may become deficient, especially if receiving total parenteral nutrition without L-carnitine supplements (3633). Breast milk and some formulas contain L-carnitine; those that do not, generally do not induce symptomatic deficiencies in healthy, full-term infants unless a metabolic disorder is also present, although utilization of fats may be impaired (3644). Hemodialysis is associated with significant losses of L-carnitine (3616,3645), which may contribute to malaise, muscle weakness, cardiomyopathy, and cardiac arrhythmias (3616). L-carnitine supplements, usually given intravenously after dialysis, may improve exercise performance, reduce muscle cramps and hypotension, improve erythrocyte survival time, and decrease dose requirements for erythropoietin used to treat anemia (3645,3646,3647). In people with angina, a reduction in tissue L-carnitine levels has been observed during myocardial ischemia (14), and L-carnitine supplementation may improve exercise performance, reduce angina attacks, and reduce ST segment depression (9,3623,3624). In congestive heart failure, L-carnitine supplementation may improve symptoms and chance of survival (3625,3626). When used for one to twelve months after a myocardial infarction, L-carnitine has been reported to decrease infarct size, left ventricular dilation, angina attacks, heart failure, arrhythmias, and cardiac deaths (9,3627,3628,3629). Preliminary evidence suggests that L-carnitine may improve walking distances in people with peripheral vascular disease (9,3631). Maximal exercise in trained athletes has been associated with a fall in plasma L-carnitine levels (3648). Although increases in maximum oxygen uptake and power output have been reported with L-carnitine supplements in some studies (3649,3650), there is no evidence that L-carnitine supplementation will improve exercise performance in normal individuals or trained athletes (1947,3639). Preliminary studies have reported that daily infusions of L-carnitine may improve CD4 cell counts in people with HIV infection and reduce the percentage of CD4 and CD8 cells undergoing apoptosis (798,3632). Preliminary studies also suggest that intravenous infusions of L-carnitine may produce short-term improvements in insulin sensitivity in people with type 2 diabetes (3651,3652). Some experts think that L-carnitine supplementation improves some of the symptoms of Rett syndrome (1433). Recent evidence indicates that L-carnitine improves well-being and motor skills, but more studies are needed (1433,3622). L-carnitine and acetyl-L-carnitine are present in human sperm and seminal fluid (3607). Their levels increase in sperm during the maturation process in the epididymis and coincide with the acquisition of progressive motility (3608,3609). An increase in sperm motility is seen in vitro when L-carnitine or acetyl-L-carnitine is added to the semen sample (3612).

Adverse Reactions

L-Carnitine used orally or intravenously has been associated with nausea, vomiting, abdominal cramps, heartburn, gastritis, diarrhea, body odor, and seizures (9,14,3616).
DL-carnitine, but not L-carnitine, has been associated with myasthenia syndrome with severe weakness, muscle wasting, and discolored urine possibly due to myoglobinuria (9,14). This may be due to competitive inhibition of L-carnitine by D-carnitine, leading to symptoms of L-carnitine deficiency (14,1946).

Interactions with Herbs & Other Dietary Supplements

COENZYME Q10: Coenzyme Q10 and L-carnitine may have synergistic effects (3653).
D-CARNITINE: Taking D-carnitine may cause symptoms of L-carnitine deficiency (1946); avoid using.

Interactions with Drugs

ACENOCOUMAROL: L-carnitine may potentiate the anticoagulant effects of acenocoumarol (14).
HEPARIN: When used as an anticoagulant for whole plasma, heparin interferes with free and total L-carnitine radioenzyme assays, leading to inaccurate results (14).
VALPROIC ACID: L-carnitine deficiency may cause or potentiate valproic acid toxicity (4528,4529,5798).

Drug Influences on Nutrient Levels and Depletion

SOME DRUGS CAN AFFECT L-CARNITINE LEVELS:
VALPROIC ACID (Depakene, Depakote, VPA): Valproic acid induces L-carnitine deficiency by affecting carnitine metabolism in the mitochondria of cells, resulting in the formation of a valproylcarnitine ester that is excreted in the urine. This also interferes with the tubular reabsorption of free carnitine (4528,4529,5798). Oral L-carnitine supplementation is strongly suggested for symptomatic VPA-associated hyperammonemia, patients with multiple risk factors for VPA-associated hepatotoxicity, and infants and young children taking VPA, especially children younger than 2 years of age who are taking multiple anticonvulsant agents (4523,4524,4525,4526,4527,4528,4529,5798).

Interactions with Foods

No interactions are known to occur, and there is no known reason to expect a clinically significant interaction with L-carnitine.

Interactions with Lab Tests

CD4/CD8 COUNTS: L-carnitine infusions can increase CD4 and CD8 lymphocyte counts in some individuals with HIV-1 infection who have not been treated with antiretroviral therapy (798).
CHOLESTEROL: Intravenous L-carnitine supplementation can increase serum HDL cholesterol concentrations and test results in children on hemodialysis with type IV hyperlipoproteinemia (275).
L-CARNITINE RADIOENZYME ASSAY: Heparin, when used as an anticoagulant for whole plasma, interferes with free and total L-carnitine assays, leading to inaccurate results (14).
TRIGLYCERIDES: Intravenous L-carnitine supplementation can decrease serum triglyceride concentrations and test results in children on hemodialysis with type IV hyperlipoproteinemia (275).

Interactions with Diseases or Conditions

HEMODIALYSIS/ANURIA/UREMIA: Avoid DL-carnitine; reported to cause myasthenia-like symptoms when administered by IV after dialysis (L-carnitine not reported to have this effect) (9,14).

CHRONIC LIVER DISEASE: Avoid due to impaired L-carnitine metabolism or increased L-carnitine biosynthesis, and potential for intrinsically high L-carnitine levels (1931,1948).

SEIZURES: An increase in seizure frequency or severity has been reported in people with a history of seizures who have used L-carnitine orally or intravenously (3616).

Dosage and Administration

ORAL: For primary or secondary L-carnitine deficiencies in adults, 990 mg two to three times per day in tablets or oral solution is used (3616). For valproate-induced toxicities often associated with L-carnitine deficiency, 50 to 100 mg/kg/day in three or four divided doses, to a maximum of 3 grams/day is used (3616,4528,5798). For chronic stable angina and congestive heart failure (CHF), 1 gram twice daily has been used (3623,3624,3625,3626). Following myocardial infarction, 2 to 6 grams daily have been used (3627,3628,3629). For peripheral vascular disease, 2 grams L-carnitine twice daily has been used (14). People on hemodialysis have used 2 to 4 grams per day in divided doses (1933). For Rett syndrome, 100 mg/kg/day L-carnitine in three divided doses has been used (1433). For myocarditis associated with diphtheria, DL-carnitine 100 mg/kg/day for 4 days has been used (3620,3621).

INTRAVENOUS: For inborn error of metabolism resulting in secondary L-carnitine deficiency, 50 mg/kg given as a slow (2 to 3 minute) bolus injection or by infusion followed by 50 mg/kg administered in divided doses every 3 to 4 hours over the next 24 hours is used. Subsequent daily maintenance doses are usually in the range of 50 mg/kg (3616). For people with L-carnitine deficiency secondary to hemodialysis, 10 to 20 mg/kg adjusted according to plasma L-carnitine levels is used (3616). For treating and preventing valproic acid-induced hepatotoxicity in patients being treated for accidental ingestion or overdose of valproic acid, 150-500 mg/kg/day up to 3 grams/day is used (4528,5798). A dose of 10 mg/kg has been used to improve fat utilization in premature infants on total parenteral nutrition (3637), and 1 to 8 grams per day has been used as a supplement in adults on total parenteral nutrition (14). After acute myocardial infarction, doses of 100 mg/kg every 12 hours for 36 hours have been used (14).

Comments

L-carnitine is found in the diet in meat and dairy products (3613). It is FDA-approved for primary or secondary L-carnitine deficiencies (14). Only FDA approved, prescription L-carnitine should be used for these indications. Avoid D-carnitine and DL-carnitine which are often present in over-the-counter preparations and dietary supplements. Low serum L-carnitine levels are reported to be less than 20 micromoles/L in term infants and less than 40 to 50 micromoles/L in adults on dialysis (3616).

L-TRYPTOPHAN

Also Known As

L-trypt, Tryptophan.
CAUTION: See separate listing for 5-HTP.

Scientific Names

L-2-amino-3-(indole-3-yl) propionic acid.

People Use This For

Orally, L-tryptophan is used for insomnia, depression, myofascial pain, premenstrual syndrome (PMS), smoking cessation, bruxism, grinding teeth during sleep, attention deficit hyperactivity disorder (ADHD), Tourette's syndrome, and to improve athletic performance (512).

Safety

UNSAFE ...when used orally due to the risk of eosinophilia myalgia syndrome and death (9,512). The FDA recalled all over-the-counter L-tryptophan in 1990 (512).

PREGNANCY: UNSAFE ...when used orally because it can cause respiratory depression in utero (14,1142); avoid using.

LACTATION: UNSAFE ...when used orally (14); avoid using.

Effectiveness

POSSIBLY EFFECTIVE ...when used orally for treating sleep disorders (512,1144,1146). ...when used orally for depression (9,512,6245). In a double-blind, placebo-controlled study of 24 depressed patients receiving clomipramine, supplementation with L-tryptophan resulted in more rapid response to treatment (6245). ...when used orally for premenstrual syndrome (6246). In a randomized controlled, 37 patients with premenstrual dysphoric disorder treated with L-tryptophan 6 g per day had greater symptomatic improvement of dysphoria, mood swings, tension and irritability than 34 women receiving placebo (6246). ...when used orally as an adjunct treatment for smoking cessation (1138).

POSSIBLY INEFFECTIVE ...when used orally for treating bruxism (1139), myofascial pain (1140,1145), and improving athletic performance (1135).

Mechanism of Action

L-tryptophan is an essential amino acid present in concentrations of 1-2% in many plant and animal proteins (5). L-tryptophan is a precursor of serotonin and is also converted to nicotinic acid and nicotinamide (9). L-tryptophan has sedative effects in humans (1143). Dietary tryptophan depletion has been associated with bulimia relapse (1133) and deterioration of schizophrenia symptoms (1134), but it does not seem to worsen symptoms in people with untreated depression (1136). Preliminary clinical evidence suggests L-tryptophan might be helpful in seasonal affective disorder (6247).

Adverse Reactions

Orally, L-tryptophan can cause nausea, headache, lightheadedness, and drowsiness (9). Occasionally, sexual disinhibition, reversible dyskinesias, and reversible Parkinsonian-like rigidity can occur in people taking L-tryptophan with or after phenothiazines or benzodiazepines (9). Euphoria can happen with doses of 30-90 mg per kg body weight (14). Symptoms of eosinophilia myalgia syndrome include eosinophilia, fatigue, myalgias, multisystem organ involvement, and inflammatory disorders affecting the joints, skin, connective tissue, lungs, heart, and liver (9). More than 1500 cases of eosinophilia-myalgia syndrome and 37 deaths were associated with L-tryptophan use in the US (9,512), which led to the FDA recall of L-tryptophan in 1990 (512). All L-tryptophan-containing products that were suspected of causing EMS were traced to a single manufacturer in Japan (9). Seventeen contaminants, including 1,1'-ethylidenebis(L-tryptophan) and 3-(phenylamino)-L-alanine, were identified in a batch of L-tryptophan implicated in cases of eosinophilia myalgia syndrome; however, no causative agent was confirmed. Up to 5% of the cases were not linked to contaminated batches of L-tryptophan, suggesting that L-tryptophan can also cause eosinophilia myalgia syndrome (512).

Interactions with Herbs & Other Dietary Supplements

HERBS WITH SEDATIVE PROPERTIES: Theoretically, concomitant use with herbs that have sedative properties might enhance therapeutic and adverse effects. These include calamus, calendula, California poppy, catnip, capsicum, celery, couch grass, elecampane, Siberian ginseng , German chamomile, goldenseal, gotu kola, hops, Jamaican dogwood, kava, lemon balm, sage, St. John's wort, sassafras, scullcap, shepherd's purse, stinging nettle, valerian, wild carrot, wild lettuce, ashwaganda root, and yerba mansa (4,19).

SEDATIVE SUPPLEMENTS: Theoretically, it can cause additive effects when used with supplements having sedative activity, including melatonin.

Interactions with Drugs

SELECTIVE SEROTONIN REUPTAKE INHIBITORS (SSRIs): Concomitant use of L-tryptophan can result in serotonin syndrome (1141).

TRAZODONE, MONOAMINE OXIDASE INHIBITORS (MAOIs): Concomitant use of L-tryptophan can exacerbate conditions of psychosis or hypomania (14).

BENZODIAZEPINES, PHENOTHIAZINES: Concomitant use can cause sexual disinhibition, reversible dyskinesias, and reversible Parkinsonian-like rigidity (9).

SEDATIVE DRUGS: Theoretically, it can have additive effects when taken with sedative drugs.

Interactions with Foods

No interactions are known to occur, and there is no known reason to expect a clinically significant interaction with L-tryptophan.

Interactions with Lab Tests

EOSINOPHIL COUNT: In cases of eosinophilia myalgia syndrome, L-tryptophan can increase serum eosinophil counts and test results (9).

LIVER FUNCTION TESTS: In cases of eosinophilia myalgia syndrome, L-tryptophan can increase serum liver enzyme levels and test results (14).

Interactions with Diseases or Conditions

EOSINOPHILIA: L-tryptophan is contraindicated because it can exacerbate this condition.

KIDNEY OR LIVER DYSFUNCTION: Lower amounts of L-tryptophan can be required (9).

Dosage and Administration

ORAL: Clinical studies for sleep disorders have used doses from 1 to 2.5 grams (1144,1146). For depression, 300 mg daily in combination with antidepressants has been used (6245). For premenstrual syndrome, 6 grams daily was used in one study (6246). High dose L-tryptophan (50 mg/kg/day) has been used as adjunct therapy for smoking cessation (1138).

Comments

L-tryptophan is not available as a dietary supplement in the US (14). It is unclear whether supplement manufacturers are able to produce contaminant-free, pure L-tryptophan products (512). While L-tryptophan continues to be unavailable in the US, it was reintroduced in 1994 in the UK for restricted use under carefully monitored conditions (9). Older people may require lower amounts (9).

LABDANUM

Also Known As
Ambreine, Ciste, Cyste, Rockrose.

Scientific Names
Cistus ladanifer, synonym Cistus ladaniferus; Cistus incanus, synonym Cistus villosus; Cistus polymorphus; and other Cistus species.
Family: Cistaceae.

People Use This For
Orally, labdanum is used for inflammation of the respiratory tract mucous membrane (11), bronchitis, diarrhea (11), edema, hernia, tumors, leprosy, and spleen sclerosis. Labdanum is also used orally for its expectorant, stimulant, purgative, and cleansing properties (11).
Topically, labdanum is used for its astringent and hemostatic properties.
In foods and beverages, the absolute, oleoresin, and oil are used as flavoring agents (11).
In cosmetics, labdanum absolute and oil are used as fixative and fragrance components (11).
In addition, people use labdanum as a fumigant (11) and insecticide.

Safety
LIKELY SAFE …when used orally in amounts found in foods (11). Approved for food use in the US, the oil is used at a level less than 0.001%, the absolute is used at a level less than 0.002% (11). …when used topically in small amounts. In cosmetics, the maximum level used is 0.8% for the oil and 0.04% for the absolute (11).
POSSIBLY SAFE …when used topically for medicinal purposes. It is nontoxic and nonirritating to human skin (11). There is insufficient reliable information available about the safety of labdanum for its other uses.
PREGNANCY AND LACTATION: Insufficient reliable information available; avoid using.

Effectiveness
There is insufficient reliable information available about the effectiveness of labdanum.

Mechanism of Action
The applicable parts of labdanum are the above ground parts. Beta-pinene, eugenol, eucalyptol (cineole), and benzaldehyde are thought to be the most active constituents of labdanum (11). Some evidence suggests the essential oil of labdanum and resin might have antibacterial and antifungal activity (11). Other evidence indicates an aqueous extract of Cistus incanus might protect against gastric lesions (4050). One study in experimental animals found that a non-alkaloid substance extracted by alcohol but not water caused liver changes (11), which might indicate some safety risks.

Adverse Reactions
None reported.

Interactions with Herbs & Other Dietary Supplements
Insufficient reliable information available.

Interactions with Drugs
No interactions are known to occur, and there is no known reason to expect a clinically significant interaction with labdanum.

Interactions with Foods
No interactions are known to occur, and there is no known reason to expect a clinically significant interaction with labdanum.

Interactions with Lab Tests

No interactions are known to occur, and there is no known reason to expect a clinically significant interaction with labdanum.

Interactions with Diseases or Conditions

No interactions are known to occur, and there is no known reason to expect a clinically significant interaction with labdanum.

Dosage and Administration

No typical dosage.

Comments

Labdanum oleoresin (gum, gum cistus) is obtained by boiling the above ground parts of labdanum (Cistus ladanifer) in water and separating the resin layer (11). Labdanum oil is distilled from the above ground parts of labdanum (Cistus ladanifer). Labdanum absolute (cyste absolute) is obtained by evaporation of the alcohol extract of fat soluble portions of labdanum (Cistus ladanifer) after removal of alcohol insoluble substances (11).

LABRADOR TEA

Also Known As

Continental Tea, Marsh Rosemary, Marsh Tea, St. James's Tea, Wild Rosemary.
CAUTION: See separate listing for Marsh Tea.

Scientific Names

Ledum groenlandicum; Ledum latifolium; Ledum palustre.
Family: Ericaceae or Laminaceae.

People Use This For

Orally, labrador tea is used as an expectorant (18).
In folk medicine, it has been used orally as an abortifacient (18), for "female disorders," sore throat, cough, pulmonary infections and other chest ailments, dysentery, diarrhea, kidney problems, rheumatism, headache, and cancer (6).
Topically or in a bath, it has been used for skin problems (6,18).
As a beverage, it was used as a substitute for more traditional tea. Some people even added the leaves to beer to make it more intoxicating (6).

Safety

POSSIBLY SAFE ...when the leaves or flowering shoots are used orally as weak tea or in small amounts (6).
LIKELY UNSAFE ...when used orally in concentrated solutions or in large amounts. It can cause delirium, paralysis, and death (6).
PREGNANCY: UNSAFE ...when used orally because it might induce abortion (18).
LACTATION: Insufficient reliable information available; avoid using.

Effectiveness

There is insufficient reliable information available about the effectiveness of labrador tea.

Mechanism of Action

The applicable parts of labrador tea are the leaf and flowering shoot. Labrador tea has expectorant activity (18) and narcotic properties (6). The constituent ledol (ledum camphor) can cause gastrointestinal irritation (vomiting, gastroenteritis, diarrhea), central nervous system excitation, spasms, and paralysis (18). The constituent grayanotoxin (andromedotoxin), can cause bradycardia, hypotension, loss of coordination, convulsions, paralysis, and death (6).

Adverse Reactions

Orally, labrador tea can cause gastrointestinal irritation (vomiting, gastroenteritis, diarrhea), central nervous system excitation, spasms, paralysis, and death (6,18).

Interactions with Herbs & Other Dietary Supplements

Insufficient reliable information available.

Interactions with Drugs

No interactions are known to occur, and there is no known reason to expect a clinically significant interaction with labrador tea.

Interactions with Foods

No interactions are known to occur, and there is no known reason to expect a clinically significant interaction with labrador tea.

Interactions with Lab Tests

No interactions are known to occur, and there is no known reason to expect a clinically significant interaction with labrador tea.

Interactions with Diseases or Conditions

No interactions are known to occur, and there is no known reason to expect a clinically significant interaction with labrador tea.

Dosage and Administration

No typical dosage.

Comments

Medicinal uses of Labrador tea are now largely obsolete (18).

LABURNUM

Also Known As

Bean Trifoil, Golden Chain, Legume, Pea Tree.

Scientific Names

Cytisus laburnum.
Family: Leguminosae or Fabaceae.

People Use This For

Laburnum is used as a pesticide. (18).

Safety

UNSAFE ...when used orally (18).
PREGNANCY AND LACTATION: UNSAFE ...when used orally (18).

Effectiveness

There is insufficient reliable information available about the effectiveness of laburnum.

Mechanism of Action

The applicable part of laburnum is the seed. There is insufficient reliable information available about the possible mechanism of action and active ingredients.

Adverse Reactions

The fatal adult dose of laburnum is 20 seeds or 3-4 unripe berries. Symptoms of laburnum poisoning include nausea, dizziness, salivation, and pain in the mouth, throat and stomach. This is accompanied by sweating, headaches, and extended, severe, and occasionally bloody vomiting. The centrally-stimulating effects of laburnum lead to tonic-clonic spasms followed by paralysis. Some patients experience anuria or uremia. Death occurs by asphyxiation (18).

Interactions with Herbs & Other Dietary Supplements

Insufficient reliable information available.

Interactions with Drugs

No interactions are known to occur, and there is no known reason to expect a clinically significant interaction with laburnum.

Interactions with Foods
No interactions are known to occur, and there is no known reason to expect a clinically significant interaction with laburnum.

Interactions with Lab Tests
No interactions are known to occur, and there is no known reason to expect a clinically significant interaction with laburnum.

Interactions with Diseases or Conditions
No interactions are known to occur, and there is no known reason to expect a clinically significant interaction with laburnum.

Dosage and Administration
No typical dosage.

Comments
Laburnum is spelled very similarly to labdanum, but they are very different plants. The similar spelling could cause confusion.

LACTASE

Also Known As
None.

Scientific Names
Beta-galactosidase.

People Use This For
Orally, lactase is used for preventing symptoms of lactose intolerance, of which symptoms include cramps, diarrhea, and gas (1900).

Safety
LIKELY SAFE ...when used orally in appropriate amounts. There is an absence of adverse effects up to 9,900 IU of lactase (2371,2372,2373). It is a FDA-approved, nonprescription product available in the US.
PREGNANCY AND LACTATION: Insufficient reliable information available; avoid using.

Effectiveness
LIKELY EFFECTIVE ...when taken orally in lactose-intolerant people for reducing GI symptoms and when used before the consumption of lactose or when added to milk prior to consumption (2371,2372,2373).

Mechanism of Action
Lactase is a sugar-splitting enzyme that hydrolyzes lactose, a milk sugar, to produce glucose and galactose (9,511).

Adverse Reactions
None reported.

Interactions with Herbs & Other Dietary Supplements
Insufficient reliable information available.

Interactions with Drugs
No interactions are known to occur, and there is no known reason to expect a clinically significant interaction with lactase.

Interactions with Foods
No interactions are known to occur, and there is no known reason to expect a clinically significant interaction with lactase.

Interactions with Lab Tests
No interactions are known to occur, and there is no known reason to expect a clinically significant interaction with lactase.

Interactions with Diseases or Conditions

No interactions are known to occur, and there is no known reason to expect a clinically significant interaction with lactase.

Dosage and Administration

ORAL: The typical dose of lactase is 6,000-9,000 IU tablets chewed and swallowed at the start of a lactose-containing meal (2374) or 2000 IU of the solution added to 500 mL of milk immediately before consumption (2375).

Comments

Lactase deficiency can be one of several factors that predispose an individual to the development of osteoporosis, possibly through diminished calcium intake (2376,2377).

LACTOBACILLUS

Also Known As

Acidophilus, L. Acidophilus, L. johnsonii LC-1, Lacto Bacillus, Lactobacilli, Lactobacillus casei, Lactobacillus GG, Lactobacillus johnsonii, Lactobacillus rhamnosus GG, LC-1 L. johnsonii, Probiotics.
CAUTION: See separate listings for Bifidobacteria, Brewer's Yeast (Hansen CBS 5926), Saccharomyces Boulardii, and Yogurt.

Scientific Names

Lactobacillus acidophilus; Lactobacillus brevis; Lactobacillus bulgaricus; Lactobacillus casei sp. rhamnosus; Lactobacillus delbrueckii; Lactobacillus fermentum; Lactobacillus plantarum; Lactobacillus rhamnosus.
Family: Lactobacillaceae.

People Use This For

Orally, lactobacillus is used for treating and preventing diarrhea, including infectious types such as rotaviral diarrhea in children and traveler's diarrhea. It is also used orally to prevent and treat antibiotic-associated diarrhea. Lactobacillus is also used orally for general digestion problems, irritable bowel syndrome (IBS), inflammatory bowel syndrome (IBD, Crohn's disease, ulcerative colitis), relapsing Clostridium difficile colitis, and bacterial overgrowth in short bowel syndrome. It is also used orally for lactose intolerance, urinary tract infections, vaginal and Candida-related (yeast) infections, high cholesterol levels, hives, fever blisters, canker sores, and adolescent acne. Lactobacillus is also used orally to prevent cancer or the formation of carcinogens, to stimulate the immune system, and as a vaccine adjuvant. Intravaginally, lactobacillus is used to treat vaginitis and urinary tract infections.

Safety

LIKELY SAFE ...when used orally and appropriately. Several species of lactobacillus, including Lactobacillus acidophilus, Lactobacillus bulgaricus, Lactobacillus casei, Lactobacillus delbrueckii, Lactobacillus rhamnosus, and Lactobacillus plantarum have been safely used in studies lasting up to 9 months (4367,4380,6087).
POSSIBLY SAFE ...when used intravaginally and appropriately. Several species of lactobacillus including Lactobacillus casei sp. rhamnosus and Lactobacillus fermentum have been used safely in studies lasting from 10 weeks to 6 months (4397,6094,6095).
CHILDREN: LIKELY SAFE ...when used orally and appropriately. Lactobacillus GG, a specific strain of Lactobacillus rhamnosus, has been used safely in studies lasting from 7 days to 15 months (4369,4372,4373,4377,4383). The safety of other Lactobacillus species in children is not known.
PREGNANCY AND LACTATION: Insufficient reliable information available; avoid using.

Effectiveness

LIKELY EFFECTIVE ...when used orally for rotaviral diarrhea in children. Lactobacillus GG, a specific strain of Lactobacillus rhamnosus, can reduce the duration of the diarrheal phase of rotavirus infection by 1-3 days in infants and young children (4369,4377).
POSSIBLY EFFECTIVE ...when used orally to prevent antibiotic-associated diarrhea in children. Concurrent treatment with Lactobacillus GG, a specific strain of Lactobacillus rhamnosus, and antibiotics significantly decreases stool frequency and improves stool consistency compared to treatment with antibiotics alone in children (4371). Lactobacillus GG seems to reduce the rate of antibiotic-associated diarrhea by approximately 11% (4372). However, Lactobacillus GG does not seem to reduce the occurrence of antibiotic-associated diarrhea in hospitalized adults (7306). ...when used to prevent diarrhea in undernourished children. Lactobacillus GG, a specific strain of Lactobacillus rhamnosus, can significantly reduce the occurrence of diarrhea from all causes in undernourished children (4373,4383). ...when used orally to prevent traveler's diarrhea. Lactobacillus GG, a specific strain of Lactobacillus rhamnosus, seems to significantly reduce the occurrence of diarrhea in travelers (4374). ...when used orally with antibiotics or

following antibiotic therapy for recurrent Clostridium difficile diarrhea. Patients treated with metronidazole and vancomycin for Clostridium difficile diarrhea have a 20% chance for developing a secondary or recurring Clostridium difficile infection when antibiotic therapy is stopped. Adding Lactobacillus GG, a specific strain of Lactobacillus rhamnosus, during conventional antibiotic therapy seems to reduce the recurrence rate of Clostridium difficile diarrhea after antibiotics are stopped. Adding Lactobacillus GG during antibiotic treatment also seems to improve some symptoms of an active Clostridium difficile infection, including cramping and diarrhea (4392,4394). ...when used for atopic eczema in infants with food allergies. There is some evidence that Lactobacillus GG, a specific strain of Lactobacillus rhamnosus, can reduce symptoms of atopic eczema in infants allergic to cow's milk. Lactobacillus GG also seems to decrease markers of inflammation such as tumor necrosis factor and alpha 1-antitrypsin (4369). ...when used orally to prevent relapse in patients with chronic pouchitis. There is some evidence that continuous treatment for 9 months with a specific concentrated formulation of Lactobacillus, Bifidobacterium, and Streptococcus can maintain remission in 85% of patients (6087).

POSSIBLY INEFFECTIVE ...when used orally for irritable bowel syndrome (IBS). Substitution of Lactobacillus acidophilus milk for regular cow's milk seems to have no effect on symptoms of IBS (123). ...when used orally for lactose intolerance. Use of Lactobacillus acidophilus milk seems to produce similar symptoms of intolerance as regular cow's milk (123). ...when used orally for preventing antibiotic-associated diarrhea in adults. Lactobacillus GG, a specific strain of Lactobacillus rhamnosus, 20 billion live colony–forming units per day given at the initiation of antibiotic therapy appears to be ineffective for reducing the rate of occurrence of diarrhea in hospitalized adults (7306). ...when used intravaginally for reducing recurrence of bacterial vaginosis. A Lactobacillus acidophilus fermented milk product seems to be ineffective for bacterial vaginosis (6).

There is insufficient reliable information available to rate the effectiveness of Lactobacillus for its other uses. However, there is some preliminary evidence that intravaginal use of some Lactobacillus species might be helpful for preventing urinary tract infections (UTIs), but there have been some conflicting findings in studies (4581,6094,6095). More evidence is needed to rate Lactobacillus for this use.

Mechanism of Action

Lactobacillus refers to a group of lactic acid producing bacteria that make up some of the normal flora in the human gastrointestinal and genitourinary tracts (6,6089,6094,6096). They are also found in some fermented food products such as yogurt as well as in capsule form (6099). Some of the specific lactobacillus species include Lactobacillus acidophilus, Lactobacillus bulgaricus, Lactobacillus casei sp. rhamnosus, Lactobacillus delbrueckii, Lactobacillus fermentum, Lactobacillus rhamnosus, and Lactobacillus plantarum. Lactobacilli are used therapeutically as so-called probiotics, the opposite of antibiotics. They are considered "friendly" bacteria and are taken with the purpose of re-colonizing areas of the body where they normally would occur. The human body relies on the normal flora for several functions, including metabolizing foods, absorbing nutrients, and preventing colonization by pathogenic bacteria. Probiotics such as lactobacillus are typically used in cases when a disease occurs or might occur due to depleted normal flora. For example, treatment with antibiotics can kill off pathogenic bacteria and also the normal flora of the gastrointestinal and genitourinary tracts. Altering the normal flora allows for potential colonization by pathogenic organisms (6088) which can result in side effects such as diarrhea, cramping, and less commonly pseudomembranous colitis caused by Clostridium difficile. The theory is that taking lactobacillus probiotics can prevent or minimize normal flora depletion and prevent subsequent pathogenic bacteria colonization. There is some evidence to support this theory. When taken orally, lactobacilli pass through the gut and attach to the intestinal mucosa where they can persist for at least one week (5500). When probiotic lactobacilli latch on to and colonize the intestinal and urogenital mucosa, it seems to prevent epithelial attachment by pathogenic bacteria (4369,4378,6086,6089,6091,6092). Lactobacilli seem to have this effect by increasing epithelial mucus production (4388), competing with pathogens for mucosal binding sites, and possibly through steric hindrance (6086,6089,6091,6092). Lactobacilli also inhibit bacterial pathogens by producing lactic acid, and many lactobacilli also produce hydrogen peroxide (6,6089,6090,6096). In the vagina, lactic acid from lactobacilli lowers vaginal pH, which can prevent pathogen growth. Lactobacilli might also produce bacteriocin-like substances that can inhibit growth of some bacteria and fungi, and biosurfactants that can prevent some bacteria from adhering to the epithelium (6089,6090,6091,6096).

In addition to acting as a barrier to pathogen adhesion, some researchers think lactobacilli and other probiotics might have immunomodulating effects (4368,4369). Lactobacilli seem to modulate non-specific cellular and humoral immunity possibly by stimulating lymphocyte and macrophage activity (6089) and decreasing cytokine production by mononuclear cells (4379). However, the way lactobacilli affect immune function might be different depending on the health status of the patient. In people with a condition of immune system hypersensitivity, lactobacilli seem to down-regulate immune function. In healthy people without immune system hypersensitivity, lactobacilli seem to stimulate the immune system (4399). Due to these immunomodulating effects, some researchers think lactobacillus and other probiotics might not only fight intestinal and urogenital pathogens, but also be helpful for conditions such as inflammatory bowel disease, pouchitis, food allergy, and for use as an adjuvant to vaccination (4368,4379,4393,4399).

There is also some preliminary evidence that lactobacilli and other probiotics might help protect against cancer. In animal models, lactobacillus has been shown to bind dietary carcinogens (4376) and decrease development of tumors in the colon after carcinogen challenge (4382,4387). Most researchers agree that the effectiveness of lactobacilli and other probiotics for all indications depends on their ability to colonize an area of tissue. To do this, lactobacillus preparations must contain live and viable organisms. Products stored for long periods of time or stored improperly may contain few live and active organisms to start with. For oral preparations, bacteria must also remain viable after passing through the gut and then they must be able to latch on to the intestinal epithelium. Lactobacilli strains might vary in their effectiveness due to differences in their ability to adhere to epithelial cells (4373,6091,6094). Some strains might also have differing activity against specific pathogens (6094). Host factors such as hormone levels can also influence adherence and effectiveness. The ability of lactobacilli to attach to epithelial cells can change during a woman's menstrual cycle in response to changing hormone levels. In post-menopausal women, correcting low estrogen levels can help restore lactobacillus colonization without supplementation (6094,6089).

There is some evidence that Lactobacillus GG, a strain of Lactobacillus rhamnosus, appears to attach to intestinal epithelial cells better than Lactobacillus acidophilus (4373). Lactobacillus casei may adhere better to urogenital cells than other lactobacillus species (6091). Probiotic strains may differ in specific metabolic activities and that not all lactobacilli species inhibit a wide range of pathogenic bacteria (6093). Therefore, some researchers theorize that probiotic preparations containing several species might offer more benefit than a single species (6087,6094). However, this theory has not yet been evaluated in studies.

Adverse Reactions

Oral and intravaginal administration of lactobacillus species is usually well tolerated (15,6087,6094). With oral administration, the most common side effect is flatulence; however; it is usually mild and subsides as therapy continues (15). Since lactobacillus preparations contain live and active microorganisms, there is some concern that they might cause pathological infection in some patients. Lactobacillus bacteremia has been reported in severely ill or immunocompromised patients (4380). However, bacteremia has not been associated with taking lactobacilli supplements. There are also no reports of pathogenic colonization in relatively healthy patients with intact immune systems (4380,4389,4390,4391,4393,4398).

Interactions with Herbs & Other Dietary Supplements

Insufficient reliable information available.

Interactions with Drugs

ANTIBIOTICS: There is some concern that concomitant administration of antibiotics might decrease the effectiveness of lactobacillus. Since lactobacillus preparations usually contain live and active organisms, simultaneously taking antibiotics might kill a significant number of the organisms (1740). Tell patients to separate administration of antibiotics and lactobacillus preparations by at least 2 hours.

Interactions with Foods

No interactions are known to occur, and there is no known reason to expect a clinically significant interaction with lactobacillus.

Interactions with Lab Tests

No interactions are known to occur, and there is no known reason to expect a clinically significant interaction with lactobacillus.

Interactions with Diseases or Conditions

IMMUNOCOMPROMISE: There is some concern that lactobacillus preparations might cause pathogenic colonization, especially in patients who are immunocompromised. Although lactobacilli have caused bacteremia and other pathogenic infections, it rarely occurs. Pathogenic colonization is more likely to occur in severely immunocompromised patients (4380,4391,4393,4398).

Dosage and Administration

ORAL: The strength of lactobacillus preparations is usually quantified by the number of living organisms per capsule. Typical doses usually range from 1 to 10 billion viable organisms daily taken in 3-4 divided doses (5008). For children with diarrhea, 5-10 billion live Lactobacillus GG in a rehydrating solution has been used (4369,4370). For preventing antibiotic-associated diarrhea in children, 20 billion live Lactobacillus GG daily were used throughout the conventional antimicrobial treatment period (4372). For recurrent Clostridium difficile, 1.25 billion live Lactobacillus GG in two divided doses for 2 weeks has been used (4394). For milk hypersensitivity, 2600 million Lactobacillus GG daily has been used (4399). For chronic pouchitis, 3 grams twice daily of a specific concentrated formula containing 300 billion viable bacteria per gram of several strains of Lactobacillus, Bifidobacterium, and Streptococcus has been used (6087).
INTRAVAGINAL: For bacterial vaginitis, vaginal suppositories containing 1 billion live Lactobacillus GG twice daily for 7 days have been used (4397). For reducing the risk of recurrent urinary tract infection (UTI), lactobacillus suppositories containing 0.5 gram (1.6 billion organisms) of L. casei var rhamnosus and L. fermentum have been used

twice weekly for two weeks, then once a month for two months (6095). A vaginal solution containing 100 billion viable bacteria/mL in a dose of 1 mL twice weekly has also been used (6094).

Comments
Some products labeled to contain Lactobacillus acidophilus have been found to actually contain little or no Lactobacillus acidophilus. Products may also contain other strains of lactobacillus, including Lactobacillus bulgaricus. Some products have been found to also contain contaminants, including Enterococcus faecium, Clostridium sporogenes, and Pseudomonas species (6).

LACTOFERRIN

Also Known As
Bovine lactoferrin, lactoferrins.

Scientific Names
Lactoferrin.

People Use This For
Orally, lactoferrin is used for stimulating the immune system; preventing tissue damage related to aging; promoting healthy intestinal flora; regulating iron metabolism; and as an antioxidant, antibacterial, and antiviral agent (2489).

Safety
There is insufficient reliable information available about the safety of lactoferrin.
Pregnancy and Lactation: Insufficient reliable information available; avoid using.

Effectiveness
There is insufficient reliable information available about the effectiveness of lactoferrin.

Mechanism of Action
Lactoferrin is an iron binding protein (a transferrin) found in the milk of several mammalian species, including humans (511). In experimental animals, it appears to offer protection from bacterial infection (2490). Preliminary evidence in healthy males suggests supplementation may increase the phagocytic activity of polymorphonuclear leukocytes and the proportion of natural killer cells in the host defense system (2490). In vitro, lactoferrin B, a peptide derived from lactoferrin, has antibacterial activity against a wide range of gram positive and gram negative bacteria (2491).

Adverse Reactions
None reported.

Interactions with Herbs & Other Dietary Supplements
Insufficient reliable information available.

Interactions with Drugs
No interactions are known to occur, and there is no known reason to expect a clinically significant interaction with lactoferrin.

Interactions with Foods
No interactions are known to occur, and there is no known reason to expect a clinically significant interaction with lactoferrin.

Interactions with Lab Tests
No interactions are known to occur, and there is no known reason to expect a clinically significant interaction with lactoferrin.

Interactions with Diseases or Conditions
No interactions are known to occur, and there is no known reason to expect a clinically significant interaction with lactoferrin.

Dosage and Administration
ORAL: People typically take 250 mg daily (5272).

Comments

There is very little scientific information about this product. Our staff is continually analyzing the available information on natural medicines and will add data here as it becomes available.

LADY FERN

Also Known As

Brake Root, Common Polypod, Oak Fern, Rock Brake, Rock of Polypody.

Scientific Names

Athyrium filix-femina.
Family: Dryopteridaceae.

People Use This For

Orally, lady fern is used for respiratory and gastrointestinal illnesses, and as an expectorant [18].

Safety

There is insufficient reliable information available about the safety of lady fern.
Pregnancy and Lactation: Insufficient reliable information available; avoid using.

Effectiveness

There is insufficient reliable information available about the effectiveness of lady fern.

Mechanism of Action

The applicable part of lady fern is the root/rhizome. There is insufficient reliable information available about the possible mechanism of action and active ingredients.

Adverse Reactions

None reported.

Interactions with Herbs & Other Dietary Supplements

Insufficient reliable information available.

Interactions with Drugs

No interactions are known to occur, and there is no known reason to expect a clinically significant interaction with lady fern.

Interactions with Foods

No interactions are known to occur, and there is no known reason to expect a clinically significant interaction with lady fern.

Interactions with Lab Tests

No interactions are known to occur, and there is no known reason to expect a clinically significant interaction with lady fern.

Interactions with Diseases or Conditions

No interactions are known to occur, and there is no known reason to expect a clinically significant interaction with lady fern.

Dosage and Administration

ORAL: 1-2 tablets or 10-20 drops of a liquid preparation are taken 3 times daily when it is used for functional gastrointestinal illnesses or as a digestive [18].

Comments

There is very little scientific information about this product. Our staff is continually analyzing the available information on natural medicines and will add data here as it becomes available.

LADY'S BEDSTRAW

Also Known As
Cheese Rennet, Cheese Renning, Curdwort, Ladys Bedstraw, Maid's Hair, Petty Mugget, Yellow Cleavers, Yellow Galium.

Scientific Names
Galium verum.
Family: Rubiaceae.

People Use This For
In folk medicine, lady's bedstraw has been used orally for treating swollen ankles, as a diuretic for bladder and kidney mucous discharge (18), for cancer, epilepsy, hysteria, spasms, tumors, and for relief of chest and lung ailments. It is also used orally to induce sweating; as a tonic; to stimulate appetite; as an aphrodisiac; and for astringent, cleansing, and purgative effects. Lady's bedstraw has been used topically for poorly healing wounds (18) and to stop bleeding.

Safety
There is insufficient reliable information available about the safety of lady's bedstraw.
Pregnancy and Lactation: Insufficient reliable information available; avoid using.

Effectiveness
There is insufficient reliable information available about the effectiveness of lady's bedstraw.

Mechanism of Action
The applicable parts of lady's bedstraw are the above ground parts. There is insufficient reliable information available about the possible mechanism of action and active ingredients.

Adverse Reactions
None reported.

Interactions with Herbs & Other Dietary Supplements
Insufficient reliable information available.

Interactions with Drugs
No interactions are known to occur, and there is no known reason to expect a clinically significant interaction with lady's bedstraw.

Interactions with Foods
No interactions are known to occur, and there is no known reason to expect a clinically significant interaction with lady's bedstraw.

Interactions with Lab Tests
No interactions are known to occur, and there is no known reason to expect a clinically significant interaction with lady's bedstraw.

Interactions with Diseases or Conditions
No interactions are known to occur, and there is no known reason to expect a clinically significant interaction with lady's bedstraw.

Dosage and Administration
ORAL: Typically, lady's bedstraw is used as a tea (18).
TOPICAL: Lady's bedstraw is used as a poultice. To prepare, pour 250 mL cold water over 2 heaping teaspoons of above ground parts, bring to simmer, and allow to steep (18).

Comments
None.

LAMINARIA

Also Known As
Brown Algae, Horsetail, Kelp, Kombu, Makombu Thallus, Sea Girdles, Seagirdle Thallus.
CAUTION: See separate listings for Algin and Bladderwrack.

Scientific Names
Laminaria digitata; Laminaria japonica.
Family: Laminariaceae.

People Use This For
Orally, laminaria is used for weight loss, preventing cancer, hypertension, as a bulk laxative for constipation, and for treating radioactive intoxication (6).

Topically, it is used as a "tent" placed into the cervix to cause cervical dilation prior to D & C, for removal of intrauterine devices, diagnostic procedures, for relief of cervical stenosis, and to facilitate uterine placement of therapeutic radium (6). Laminaria tents are also used in pregnancy for near-term or term cervical ripening particularly for a first pregnancy, to facilitate labor, alone or as adjunct to prostaglandins, and for inducing first-trimester abortions (6).

Sodium alginate, a derivative of laminaria, is used orally as a bulk laxative and in combination with antacids for gastroesophageal reflux (272).

In folk medicine, laminaria has been used orally as a hypotensive agent (6).

Safety
POSSIBLY SAFE ...when the derivative, sodium alginate, is used as a bulk laxative or in combination with an antacid for gastro-esophageal reflux (272).

There is insufficient reliable information available about the safety of laminaria for its other uses.

PREGNANCY: POSSIBLY UNSAFE ...when used topically for cervical ripening because there is an increased risk of infection and the cervical wall could rupture (6). LIKELY UNSAFE ...when used topically to induce labor because use is associated with maternal endometriosis, neonatal sepsis, fetal hypoxia, and intrauterine death (6). UNSAFE ...when used orally because of potential hormonal effects (19); avoid using.

LACTATION: LIKELY UNSAFE ...when used orally because of potential toxicity (19).

Effectiveness
POSSIBLY EFFECTIVE ...when the derivative, sodium alginate, is used as a bulk laxative (6,11,272). ...when laminaria is used orally for absorption of strontium (11). ...when laminaria is used topically for cervical ripening (6).

There is insufficient reliable information available about the effectiveness of laminaria for its other uses.

Mechanism of Action
Laminaria contains iodine, and is considered to be a rich source of iron and potassium (19). The constituents of laminaria include alginate, lamine, and laminarin (6). Much of the utility of laminaria relates to its ability to form a viscous colloidal solution of gel in water. This allows laminaria to function as a bulk laxative (6). It also allows laminaria to be used to dilate the cervix for procedures or to ripen the cervix and hasten the onset of labor. For these uses, laminaria "tents" are inserted cervically. They absorb ambient moisture, gradually swelling to a diameter of 1/2 inch over 4-6 hours. This swelling causes cervical dilation that can induce labor (6). The mechanism of cervical "ripening" might be similar to that of a foreign body that disrupts the normal chorioamniotic balance and initiates prostaglandin synthesis. That, in turn, causes myometrial contractions and cervical ripening. An alternative theory is that laminaria causes ripening because it contains high levels of the prostaglandin precursor, arachidonic acid. Still another theory is that laminaria causes partial detachment of the placenta and induces cervical dilation (6). Although laminaria can reduce the duration of labor induction, it is associated with an increased risk for maternal endometritis and neonatal sepsis (6). Some laminaria constituents might also have medical uses. The polysaccharide constituent of laminaria, laminarin, has antilipemic activity when partially sulfated and anticoagulant activity similar to heparin when more extensively sulfated (6). The basal portion of laminaria blades are used as a hypotensive agent; the constituents histamine and lamine may be responsible for hypotensive effects (6). Alginate-containing kelp reduces absorption of radioactive strontium in animals and humans (6) and it has been used for managing radioactive intoxication (6). However, the risk of adverse effects resulting from laminaria's iodide content may outweigh the benefits of its use as a routine preventative measure (515).

Adverse Reactions
Topically, use for cervical ripening is associated with neonatal and maternal infection (6); however, in a small study of "tent" use (see People Use This For) with manufacturer recommended procedures, no infection occurred. Manufacturer recommendation included prior swabbing of the cervical canal with a suitable lubricant and antibacterial

agent, then packing the canal with antibacterial gel (6). Uterine contractions associated with laminaria use have been implicated in fetal hypoxia and subsequent intrauterine death (6). Tent use is also associated with possible rupture of the cervical wall and subsequent infection (6).

Interactions with Herbs & Other Dietary Supplements
POTASSIUM SUPPLEMENTS: Theoretically, concomitant use can increase the risk of hypokalemia (19).

Interactions with Drugs
POTASSIUM SUPPLEMENTS: Theoretically, concomitant use can increase the risk of hypokalemia (19).
POTASSIUM-SPARING DIURETICS: Contraindicated. Theoretically concomitant use may cause hyperkalemia (19).
ACE INHIBITORS: Use of angiotensin converting enzyme inhibitors is contraindicated. Theoretically, concomitant use might increase the risk of hyperkalemia (19).
DIGOXIN: Caution; theoretically, laminaria may cause hyperkalemia in susceptible individuals, potentiating digoxin effects and adverse effects (19). Use with caution.

Interactions with Foods
No interactions are known to occur, and there is no known reason to expect a clinically significant interaction with laminaria.

Interactions with Lab Tests
POTASSIUM: Theoretically, may increase serum levels and test results (19).

Interactions with Diseases or Conditions
RENAL INSUFFICIENCY: Theoretically, laminaria may induce hyperkalemia in people with renal insufficiency on a potassium restricted diet (19). Use with caution.

Dosage and Administration
ORAL: People typically use capsules or tablets containing 500 to 650 mg of ground laminaria once daily (5008).
TOPICAL: No typical dosage.

Comments
None.

LARCH ARABINOGALACTAN

Also Known As
AG, Ara-6, Arabinogalactan, Dietary Fiber, Larch, Larch Gum, Larix, Mongolian Larch, Mongolian Larchwood, Stractan, Western Larch, Wood Gum, Wood Sugar.
CAUTION: See separate listing for Larch Turpentine.

Scientific Names
Larix dahurica; Larix occidentalis.
Family: Pinaceae.

People Use This For
Orally, larch arabinogalactan is used for the common cold, flu, metastatic liver disease, pediatric otitis media, HIV/AIDS, adjunctive therapy during cancer chemotherapy, as a dietary fiber supplement, immunostimulant, anti-inflammatory agent, and for hepatic encephalopathy (6,3529,3530,3531).
In foods, Larch arabinogalactan is used as a stabilizer, emulsifier, binder, and sweetener (3529).

Safety
LIKELY SAFE ...when used in amounts found in foods. Larch arabinogalactan is approved by the FDA for use in foods (3529).
POSSIBLY SAFE ...when used orally, appropriately, and short-term in therapeutic amounts (6,3529,3530).
There is insufficient reliable information available about the safety of the long-term use of larch arabinogalactan.
PREGNANCY AND LACTATION: Insufficient reliable information available; avoid using.

Effectiveness
There is insufficient reliable information available about the effectiveness of larch arabinogalactan.

Mechanism of Action

Larch arabinogalactan is a polysaccharide produced from the bark of the Larch tree. Arabinogalactans are found throughout nature and are found in other plants with immunostimulatory activity, including echinacea. Larch arabinogalactan is thought to have immunostimulatory effects by increasing release of interferon gamma, tumor necrosis fact alpha, interleukin-1 and interleukin-6 and stimulating phagocytosis and natural killer cell activity. Larch arabinogalactan is a fibrous product which ferments in the gut. It increases gut microflora, e.g., Lactobacillus, increases short-chain fatty acid production, and minimizes ammonia production and absorption. These effects suggest it may be beneficial as a dietary fiber supplement for improving gastrointestinal health and as an adjunct for treating hepatic encephalopathy. Larch arabinogalactan has been shown to concentrate in the liver. Some people think it might block hepatic receptors for metastatic cells and decrease liver metastases (3529,3530).

Adverse Reactions

Orally, bloating and flatulence have been reported (3530).

Interactions with Herbs & Other Dietary Supplements

Insufficient reliable information available.

Interactions with Drugs

ORAL DRUGS: Theoretically, concurrent administration might decrease the absorption of some oral drugs due to the fibrous nature of larch arabinogalactan.

IMMUNOSUPPRESSANTS: Theoretically, larch arabinogalactan might interfere with immunosuppression therapy due its immunostimulatory activity (3529,3530). Immunosuppressant drugs include azathioprine (Imuran), basiliximab (Simulect), cyclosporine (Neoral, Sandimmune), daclizumab (Zenapax), muromonab-CD3 (OKT3, Orthoclone OKT3), mycophenolate (CellCept), tacrolimus (FK506, Prograf), sirolimus (Rapamune), prednisone (Deltasone, Orasone), and other corticosteroids (glucocorticoids).

Interactions with Foods

No interactions are known to occur, and there is no known reason to expect a clinically significant interaction with larch arabinogalactan.

Interactions with Lab Tests

No interactions are known to occur, and there is no known reason to expect a clinically significant interaction with larch arabinogalactan.

Interactions with Diseases or Conditions

TRANSPLANT RECIPIENTS: Theoretically, larch arabinogalactan might interfere with immunosuppression therapy.

Dosage and Administration

ORAL: For colds and the flu, one teaspoon of larch arabinogalactan powder in juice or water is usually taken 2-3 times daily until symptoms are relieved. (3531).

Comments

Larch arabinogalactan specifically concentrates in hepatocytes and might have future application as a diagnostic tool or as a vehicle for delivering drugs to the liver (3529,3530).

LARCH TURPENTINE

Also Known As

Terebinthina Laricina, Terebinthina Veneta, Venetian Turpentine.
CAUTION: See separate listing for Larch Arabinogalactan.

Scientific Names

Larix decidua.
Family: Pinaceae.

People Use This For

Topically, larch turpentine is used for treating neuralgia, rheumatic discomfort, furuncles (2), fevers, colds, cough, bronchitis, tendency toward infection, blood pressure problems, and inflammation of the mouth and pharynx (18).

Safety
POSSIBLY SAFE ...when larch turpentine preparations are used topically and appropriately on intact skin (2).
POSSIBLY UNSAFE ...when larch turpentine is used orally (18). ...when larch turpentine is used topically on damaged skin, particularly if used on large areas (18). Skin damage allows systemic absorption, which can cause kidney and central nervous system toxicity (18). ...when larch turpentine is inhaled, because it can cause acute airway inflammation (18).
PREGNANCY AND LACTATION: Insufficient reliable information available; avoid using.

Effectiveness
There is insufficient reliable information available about the effectiveness of larch turpentine.

Mechanism of Action
Larch turpentine is an oily exudate obtained by drilling into the trunks of Larix decidua trees. It contains up to 20% volatile oil (2). When topically applied, it increases local blood flow and can have an antiseptic effect (2).

Adverse Reactions
Topically, larch turpentine can cause allergic skin reactions (2).
When taken orally or applied to large areas of skin or damaged skin, it can cause kidney and central nervous system damage (18).
Inhalation can cause acute respiratory tract inflammation (18).

Interactions with Herbs & Other Dietary Supplements
Insufficient reliable information available.

Interactions with Drugs
No interactions are known to occur, and there is no known reason to expect a clinically significant interaction with larch turpentine.

Interactions with Foods
No interactions are known to occur, and there is no known reason to expect a clinically significant interaction with larch turpentine.

Interactions with Lab Tests
No interactions are known to occur, and there is no known reason to expect a clinically significant interaction with larch turpentine.

Interactions with Diseases or Conditions
BRONCHITIS: Inhalation of larch turpentine is contraindicated; may worsen respiratory tract inflammation (2).

Dosage and Administration
TOPICAL: The ointments, gels, emulsions, and oils commonly contain 10 to 20 percent larch turpentine as liniments for external application (2).

Comments
None.

LARKSPUR

Also Known As
Knight's Spur, Lark Heel, Lark's Claw, Lark's Toe, Staggerweed.

Scientific Names
Delphinium consolida.
Family: Ranunculaceae.

People Use This For
Orally, larkspur is used as an anthelmintic, diuretic, sedative, and appetite stimulant (18).

Safety

There is insufficient reliable information available about the safety of larkspur.
Pregnancy and Lactation: Insufficient reliable information available; avoid using.

Effectiveness

There is insufficient reliable information available about the effectiveness of larkspur.

Mechanism of Action

The applicable part of larkspur is the flower. Animal data suggests that larkspur may have a paralyzing effect on peripheral and motor nerve endings and the central nervous system. Fatal animal poisonings due to asphyxiation have been reported with larkspur [18].

Adverse Reactions

None reported.

Interactions with Herbs & Other Dietary Supplements

Insufficient reliable information available.

Interactions with Drugs

No interactions are known to occur, and there is no known reason to expect a clinically significant interaction with larkspur.

Interactions with Foods

No interactions are known to occur, and there is no known reason to expect a clinically significant interaction with larkspur.

Interactions with Lab Tests

No interactions are known to occur, and there is no known reason to expect a clinically significant interaction with larkspur.

Interactions with Diseases or Conditions

No interactions are known to occur, and there is no known reason to expect a clinically significant interaction with larkspur.

Dosage and Administration

No typical dosage.

Comments

Use of larkspur should probably be avoided [18]. Avoid confusing larkspur with Delphinium orientale [18].

LATHYRUS

Also Known As

Caley Pea, Chickling Vetch, Chick-Pea, Everlasting Pea, Flat-Podded Vetch, Singletary Pea, Spanish Vetchling, Sweet Pea, Wild Pea.

Scientific Names

Lathyrus cicera; Lathyrus clymenu; Lathyrus hirsutus; Lathyrus incanus; Lathyrus odoratus; Lathyrus pusillus; Lathyrus sativus; Lathyrus sylvestris.
Family: Leguminosae or Fabaceae.

People Use This For

In foods, Lathyrus sativus is used in unleavened Indian bread [6]. Lathyrus seeds are eaten as food and used as animal fodder throughout the world [6].
The flowers of sweet pea (Lathyrus odoratus) are cultivated for their color and fragrance [6].

Safety

LIKELY UNSAFE ...when used orally. The seeds of Lathyrus sativus, Lathyrus cicera, and Lathyrus clymenum can be neurotoxic [6].
PREGNANCY AND LACTATION: LIKELY UNSAFE; avoid using.

Effectiveness
There is insufficient reliable information available about the effectiveness of lathyrus.

Mechanism of Action
Lathyrus seeds contain multiple constituents including phytates, divicine, and a mixture of alkaloids (6). The toxicity of lathyrus results from several compounds. The neurotoxic effects are linked to constituent beta-N-oxalyl-L-alpha, beta-diaminopropionic acid (ODAP). Constituent beta-aminopropionitrile (BAPN) causes skeletal abnormalities and damage to blood vessels (6).

Adverse Reactions
Orally, lathyrus can cause neurotoxic manifestations including muscular rigidity, spasticity, weakness, paralysis of leg muscles, weak pulse, shallow breathing, convulsions, or death (6). Prolonged neurotoxicity is characterized by poor central motor coordination and reduced nerve conduction in the lower limbs (6).

Interactions with Herbs & Other Dietary Supplements
Insufficient reliable information available.

Interactions with Drugs
No interactions are known to occur, and there is no known reason to expect a clinically significant interaction with lathyrus.

Interactions with Foods
No interactions are known to occur, and there is no known reason to expect a clinically significant interaction with lathyrus.

Interactions with Lab Tests
No interactions are known to occur, and there is no known reason to expect a clinically significant interaction with lathyrus.

Interactions with Diseases or Conditions
No interactions are known to occur, and there is no known reason to expect a clinically significant interaction with lathyrus.

Dosage and Administration
No typical dosage.

Comments
Neurolathyrism and its complications are rare in western countries, yet they have been documented for more than a century in Europe, Africa, and Asia. Despite the attempt to ban the sale of Lathyrus sativus in several states of India, distribution continues. To deactivate the toxin, several methods have been tried. Typically they involve soaking the seeds in water followed by steaming or sun drying. Roasting the seeds at high temperatures for twenty minutes also helps to destroy the neurotoxic constituent. However, these methods are only 80-85% effective (6).

LAURELWOOD

Also Known As
Alexandrian-laurel, Alexandrinischer Lorbeer, Borneo-mahogany, Calanolide, Caulophyllum Tree, Indian-laurel, Kamani Punna, Mahogany, Palo de Santa Maria, Palo Maria, Punnanga, Undi.

Scientific Names
Calophyllum inophyllum.
Family: Clusiaceae, Guttiferae.

People Use This For
Orally, the laurelwood constituent (+)-calanolide A is used for HIV infection (4290).
Topically, tamanu oil from the nut of the laurelwood is used for skin ailments including sunburn, rashes, burns, psoriasis, dermatitis, scratches, skin blemishes, acne, skin allergies, bedsores, rosacea, and hemorrhoids; and for infant skin care.
In folk medicine, laurelwood is used for leprosy, piles, scabies, gonorrhea, vaginitis, and chicken pox.

Safety

POSSIBLY SAFE ...when the laurelwood constituent (+)-calanolide A is used orally by HIV-negative individuals (4290).

There is insufficient reliable information available about the safety of laurelwood for its other uses.

PREGNANCY AND LACTATION: Insufficient reliable information available; avoid using.

Effectiveness

There is insufficient reliable information about the effectiveness of laurelwood.

Mechanism of Action

Laurelwood is one of many species of Calophyllum. Each species contains somewhat different constituents but many species including Calophyllum cordato-oblongum, Calophyllum lanigerum, Calophyllum teysmannii (synonym Calophyllum miqueli), and Calophyllum cerasiferum as well as the laurelwood contain constituents that seem to have activity against the HIV virus. Recent interest has centered on the calanolide compounds, particularly (+)-calanolide A. This constituent, now in phase I testing, appears to be a unique and specific non-nucleoside inhibitor of the reverse transcriptase of the HIV-1 virus (4292,4293). It does not appear to have activity against HIV-2 (4295). Some evidence suggests calanolide A might have synergistic effects with zidovudine (Retrovir), lamivudine (Epivir), nelfinavir (Viracept) (4290), and nevirapine (Viramune) (4294). At least two isomers of calanolide A known as costatolide and dihydrocostatolide possess similar properties (4291,4292). Calanolide A also shows evidence of antituberculosis effects (4290).

Adverse Reactions

Orally, the use of the laurelwood constituent, (+)- calanolide A, by healthy individuals can cause dizziness, oily aftertaste, headache, and nausea (4290).

Topically, there are no reported adverse reactions when tamanu oil from the nut of laurelwood is used.

Interactions with Herbs & Other Dietary Supplements

Insufficient reliable information available.

Interactions with Drugs

No interactions are known to occur, and there is no known reason to expect a clinically significant interaction with laurelwood.

Interactions with Foods

No interactions are known to occur, and there is no known reason to expect a clinically significant interaction with laurelwood.

Interactions with Lab Tests

No interactions are known to occur, and there is no known reason to expect a clinically significant interaction with laurelwood.

Interactions with Diseases or Conditions

No interactions are known to occur, and there is no known reason to expect a clinically significant interaction with laurelwood.

Dosage and Administration

No typical dosage.

Comments

The laurelwood constituent (+)-canolide A is in Phase IB testing as an anti-HIV agent. The purpose of the current study is to determine its safety and its effect on development of resistance, CD4 count and viral load (4289). Phase IA testing in 94 healthy HIV-negative individuals showed it was well tolerated (4290). Sarawak MediChem Pharmaceuticals Inc. (Lemont, Illinois) is the agency supporting testing (4289). Avoid confusing laurelwood (Caulophyllum inophyllum) with blue cohosh (Caulophyllum thalictroides).

LAVENDER

Also Known As
Alhucema, Common Lavender, English Lavender, French Lavender, Garden Lavender, Spanish Lavender, Spike Lavender, True Lavender.
CAUTION: See separate listing for Lavender Cotton.

Scientific Names
Lavandula angustifolia, synonyms Lavandula officinalis, Lavandula vera, Lavandula spica; Lavandula dentata; Lavandula latifolia; Lavandula pubescens; Lavandula stoechas.
Family: Lamiaceae.

People Use This For
Orally, lavender is used for restlessness, insomnia, nervousness, meteorism (abdominal swelling from gas in the intestinal or peritoneal cavity), and loss of appetite. Lavender is also used orally for flatulence, upset stomach, giddiness, migraine headaches, toothaches, sprains, neuralgia, rheumatism, acne, sores, nausea, and vomiting. Lavender is also used orally to promote menstruation and treat cancer.
Topically, lavender is used for alopecia areata, pain, and in baths for circulation disorders.
By inhalation, lavender is used as aromatherapy for insomnia and pain.
In foods and beverages, lavender products are used as flavor components.
In manufacturing, lavender products are utilized in pharmaceutical products and as fragrance ingredients in soaps and cosmetics. Lavender is also used as an insect repellent.

Safety
LIKELY SAFE ...when consumed in amounts commonly found in foods and beverages (11). Lavender has Generally Recognized as Safe (GRAS) status for food use in the US (11).
POSSIBLY SAFE ...when used orally and appropriately (2,12). ...when used topically and appropriately (2,12,5177). Lavender oil has been used safely for up to 7 months (5177). ...when the essential oil is inhaled as a part of aromatherapy (7107).
PREGNANCY AND LACTATION: Insufficient reliable information available; avoid using.

Effectiveness
POSSIBLY EFFECTIVE ...when used topically in combination with other essential oils for alopecia areata. There is some evidence that lavender oil in combination with the essential oils from thyme, rosemary, and cedarwood might improve hair growth by as much as 44% after 7 months of treatment (5177). ...when used as aromatherapy for insomnia (6).
There is insufficient reliable information available about the effectiveness of lavender for its other uses.

Mechanism of Action
The applicable parts of lavender are the flower and oil. Lavender preparations and constituents seem to have several pharmacological effects in vitro and in animals. But effects in humans are less well known. Lavender seems to induce relaxation and sedation. Lavender decreases EEG potentials and decreases alertness in humans (7). Lavender might also have stimulant effects on hair growth (5177); however, the mechanism of this effect is not known. There is some evidence that lavender has spasmolytic effects on smooth muscle (6) and might have analgesic effects (7107). There is some interest in lavender as an anticancer agent. The constituent perillyl alcohol seems to have some anticancer activity in vitro and in animal models (6). There is also some evidence from animal models that lavender might have anticonvulsant effects and possibly potentiate chloral hydrate and pentobarbital effects (6,7).

Adverse Reactions
Topically, use of lavender rarely can cause contact dermatitis (6).

Interactions with Herbs & Other Dietary Supplements
HERBS WITH SEDATIVE OR ANTIFLATULENT EFFECTS: The use of combination products with other sedative and/or antiflatulent herbs can be beneficial (2).

Interactions with Drugs
BARBITURATES, CHLORAL HYDRATE: Theoretically, lavender can potentiate the effects of these drugs (6,7).
CNS DEPRESSANTS: Theoretically, lavender can enhance the therapeutic and adverse effects of CNS depressants.
HMG-CoA REDUCTASE INHIBITORS: Theoretically, lavender can potentiate the effects of these drugs due to the perillyl alcohol content (6).

Interactions with Foods
No interactions are known to occur, and there is no known reason to expect a clinically significant interaction with lavender.

Interactions with Lab Tests
SERUM CHOLESTEROL: Theoretically, lavender can decrease serum cholesterol levels and test results (6).

Interactions with Diseases or Conditions
No interactions are known to occur, and there is no known reason to expect a clinically significant interaction with lavender.

Dosage and Administration
ORAL: The typical dose of lavender is 1 cup of tea several times a day, especially before bedtime (8). The tea is prepared by steeping 1.5 grams of the flowers in 150 mL boiling water for 5-10 minutes and then straining. The usual dose of lavender oil is 1-4 drops (20-80 mg) on a sugar cube (2).
TOPICAL: For alopecia areata, one study used a combination of essential oils including lavender 3 drops (108 mg), rosemary 3 drops (114 mg), thyme 2 drops (88 mg), and cedarwood 2 drops (94 mg), all mixed with 3 mL jojoba oil and 20 mL grapeseed. Each night, the mixture is massaged into the scalp for 2 minutes with a warm towel placed around the head to increase absorption (5177). For bath therapy, 20-100 grams of the lavender flowers are commonly steeped in 2 L boiling water, strained, and then added to bath water (2,18).

Comments
Lavender is a popular component for perfumes, potpourri, and decorations (6002). Lavender is commonly adulterated with related species, including Lavandula hybrida, which is a cross between Lavandula angustifolia and Lavandula latifolia, from which lavandin oil is obtained (8).

LAVENDER COTTON

Also Known As
Santolina.
CAUTION: See separate listing for Lavender.

Scientific Names
Santolina chamaecyparissias.
Family: Asteraceae.

People Use This For
Orally, lavender cotton is used for digestive disorders, premenstrual syndrome, worm infestations, jaundice, and as a spasmolytic. It is also used as an anti-inflammatory (18).
Topically, lavender cotton is used as an insect repellent.

Safety
There is insufficient reliable information available about the safety of lavender cotton.
Pregnancy and Lactation: Insufficient reliable information available; avoid using.

Effectiveness
There is insufficient reliable information available about the effectiveness of lavender cotton.

Mechanism of Action
The applicable parts of lavender cotton are the above ground parts. There is insufficient reliable information available about the possible mechanism of action and active ingredients.

Adverse Reactions
Lavender cotton can cause an allergic reaction in individuals sensitive to the Asteraceae/Compositae family. Members of this family include ragweed, chrysanthemums, marigolds, daisies, and many other herbs.

Interactions with Herbs & Other Dietary Supplements
Insufficient reliable information available.

Interactions with Drugs

No interactions are known to occur, and there is no known reason to expect a clinically significant interaction with lavender cotton.

Interactions with Foods

No interactions are known to occur, and there is no known reason to expect a clinically significant interaction with lavender cotton.

Interactions with Lab Tests

No interactions are known to occur, and there is no known reason to expect a clinically significant interaction with lavender cotton.

Interactions with Diseases or Conditions

CROSS-ALLERGENICITY: Can cause an allergic reaction in individuals sensitive to the Asteraceae/Compositae family. Members of this family include ragweed, chrysanthemums, marigolds, daisies, and many other herbs.

Dosage and Administration

ORAL: People typically prepare lavender cotton root bark using one teaspoon boiled in a covered container with 3 cups of water for 30 minutes. The liquid is cooled slowly in the closed container and taken cold, 1 to 2 cups per day (5254).

Comments

The whole lavender cotton plant is used externally as a moth and insect repellent due to its strong smell (18). Lavender cotton is unrelated to lavender and its scent is distinctly different from that of lavender (513).

LECITHIN

Also Known As

Egg Lecithin, Ovolecithin, Soybean Lecithin, Vegilecithin, Vitellin.
CAUTION: See separate listings for Choline, Phosphatidylcholine, Phosphatidylserine, and Soy.

Scientific Names

None.

People Use This For

Orally, lecithin is used for treating dementia and Alzheimer's disease (5135,5136,5137,5149,5150,5151,5152), for extrapyramidal disorders (5138,5139), reducing hepatic steatosis (fat accumulation) in long-term parenteral nutrition patients (5140), treating gallbladder disease (5141,5142,5155), aiding ultrafiltration in peritoneal dialysis (5143), treating liver disease (5144), treating manic-depressive illness (5145), improving memory (5146), treating hypercholesterolemia (5147,5148), for anxiety (5154), and eczema (5154). It is also used as a source of choline, inositol, phosphorus, and linoleic and linolenic acids (5153).
Topically, lecithin is used as a moisturizing agent for dermatitis and dry skin (4921).
As a pharmaceutical and food additive, lecithin is used for emulsifying and stabilizing water-based products, (9), and as an antioxidant in foods and pharmaceutical preparations (16). In the manufacture of preparations for intravenous and subcutaneous use, lecithin is used both as an emulsifying agent and a stabilizing agent (15,19).

Safety

LIKELY SAFE ...when used orally in amounts found in foods. It has Generally Recognized as Safe (GRAS) status in the US (4912). ...when used orally and appropriately for medicinal purposes (2619,4914).
...when used topically (4914). ...when used intravenously or subcutaneously and appropriately (16,4914).
PREGNANCY AND LACTATION: Insufficient reliable information available; avoid using in amounts greater than found in foods.

Effectiveness

LIKELY EFFECTIVE ...when used intravenously for reducing hepatic steatosis in long-term parenteral nutrition patients (14,5140). ...when used topically for dermatitis and dry skin (4921).
POSSIBLY INEFFECTIVE ...when used orally for treating gallbladder disease (5141,5142,5155).
...when used orally for treating hypercholesterolemia (5147,5148).
LIKELY INEFFECTIVE ...when used orally for dementia and Alzheimer's disease (5135,5136,5149,5150,5151,5152).

...when used orally for extrapyramidal disorders (5138,5139).
There is insufficient reliable information available about the effectiveness of lecithin for its other uses.

Mechanism of Action

Lecithin is a phospholipid composed of phosphatidyl esters (phosphatides), chiefly consisting of phosphatidylcholine, phosphatidylethanolamine, phosphatidylserine and phosphatidylinositol, and varying amounts of other substances such as triglycerides, fatty acids, and carbohydrates, depending on source (9). For example, egg lecithin contains 69% phosphatidylcholine and 24% phosphatidylethanolamine, while soybean lecithin contains 24% phosphatidylcholine, 22% phosphatidylethanolamine, and 19% phosphatidylinositol. Lecithin is a precursor to acetylcholine (5156).

Adverse Reactions

Orally, lecithin can cause diarrhea, nausea, abdominal pain, or fullness (5136,5138,5140).

Interactions with Herbs & Other Dietary Supplements

Insufficient reliable information available.

Interactions with Drugs

No interactions are known to occur, and there is no known reason to expect a clinically significant interaction with lecithin.

Interactions with Foods

No interactions are known to occur, and there is no known reason to expect a clinically significant interaction with lecithin.

Interactions with Lab Tests

No interactions are known to occur, and there is no known reason to expect a clinically significant interaction with lecithin.

Interactions with Diseases or Conditions

No interactions are known to occur, and there is no known reason to expect a clinically significant interaction with lecithin.

Dosage and Administration

ORAL: A typical oral dose is 1.2–2.4 grams/day (5153). for reducing cholesterol 20-30 grams daily has been used in studies (5147,5148). For improving memory and Alzheimer's disease, 20-45 grams daily has been tried (5146,5149,5151,5152).

Comments

Unlike choline, lecithin does not cause unpleasant body and breath odor (5153). Lecithin contains phosphatidylcholine, which contains choline (16). Although closely related, these terms are not synonymous.

LEECH

Also Known As

Fresh Water Leech, Leeches, Medicinal Leech.

Scientific Names

Hirudo medicinalis.

People Use This For

Topically, leeches are used for stimulating blood flow and relieving venous congestion at postoperative surgical flap sites (2971,2972,2974,2978,2979,2989,2990,2991) and at sites of surgical reattachment, such as fingers, toes, or ears (2971,2978,2990). They are also used for hematoma drainage (2985); varicose veins (2973); purpura fulminans (2975); macroglossia (2976); bladder extrophy (2977); infectious myocarditis (2992); and ear diseases including tinnitus, otitis media, and acute external otitis (2981).

Safety

LIKELY SAFE ...when used topically to aid in blood flow and for venous congestion in post-surgical wound management of flaps and after surgical reattachment (6). Leeches should not be used for self-treatment.
PREGNANCY AND LACTATION: Insufficient reliable information available; avoid using.

Effectiveness

POSSIBLY EFFECTIVE ...when used topically for stimulating blood flow and treating venous congestion at postoperative surgical flap sites (2971,2972,2974,2978,2979,2989,2990,2991) and after surgical reattachment (2971,2978,2990). There is insufficient reliable information available about the effectiveness of leeches for other uses.

Mechanism of Action

In vitro, leech saliva inhibits platelet aggregation induced by thrombin, collagen, adenosine diphosphate (ADP), epinephrine, platelet activating factor, and arachidonic acid (2993,2994). No effects on coagulation time or prothrombin time were noted in one study (2962). Leech saliva contains a variety of substances including hirudin, which has anticoagulant properties (see Comments) (6). Hirudin inhibits thrombin when it is bound to a fibrin clot (2995). Other constituents of leech saliva include a vasodilator, a hyaluronidase that aids in the spread of the anticoagulant through the tissue, a collagenase, two fibrinases, callin, and a platelet adhesion inhibitor (6,2963,2996). There is conflicting evidence whether a constituent with anesthetic activity is present (2997,2998).

Adverse Reactions

The use of leeches can cause infections, including those caused by Aeromonas (2964,2965,2968,2970), and Vibrio (2966). Excessive blood loss, anemia (2967,2963), contact dermatitis (2969), allergic reactions (2969), loss of leeches in body orifices (2967), and adverse psychological responses can also occur (2967). In addition, the topical use of leeches can cause epistaxis (2980,2986), tracheal obstruction (2982), hematemesis (2984), and bleeding (2987,2988) due to unrecognized nasal, throat, and vaginal leech infestation.

Interactions with Herbs & Other Dietary Supplements

Insufficient reliable information available.

Interactions with Drugs

ASPIRIN, WARFARIN (Coumadin), NONSTEROIDAL ANTI-INFLAMMATORY DRUGS (NSAIDs): Theoretically, leeches can increase the risk of bleeding in people using these drugs.

Interactions with Foods

No interactions are known to occur, and there is no known reason to expect a clinically significant interaction with leeches.

Interactions with Lab Tests

HEMOGLOBIN, HEMATOCRIT: Leeches can decrease hemoglobin, hematocrit, and test results.

Interactions with Diseases or Conditions

ARTERIAL INSUFFICIENCY: Leeches are contraindicated due to an increased risk of infection (2983).
IMMUNOCOMPROMISED PATIENTS: Theoretically, there can be a risk of overwhelming sepsis with the use of leeches in these patients (2963).
CLOTTING ABNORMALITIES: Theoretically, leeches can increase the risk of excessive bleeding.

Dosage and Administration

TOPICAL: One leech is typically applied two to four times a day for up to one week (6). Leeches are for one-time use and never to be reused (2989). Dispose of used leeches properly per facility guidelines.

Comments

Leeches are unsafe for self-medication. Lepirudin (rDNA), a recombinant hirudin analog, is an FDA-approved prescription drug with specific, direct thrombin-inhibiting activity. Lepirudin is available as an injectable product.

LEMON

Also Known As

Limon.

Scientific Names

Citrus limon.
Family: Rutaceae.

People Use This For

Orally, lemon is used as a source of vitamin C in the treatment of scurvy, low resistance, and colds. It is also used as an anti-inflammatory, diuretic, and to improve vascular permeability.

In foods, lemon is used as a food and flavoring agent (18).

Safety

LIKELY SAFE …when used in amounts found in foods (12).

POSSIBLY SAFE …when used orally for medicinal purposes in amounts similar to those found in foods (12).

PREGNANCY AND LACTATION: Avoid using in amounts greater than those typically found in foods.

Effectiveness

There is insufficient reliable information available about the effectiveness of lemon.

Mechanism of Action

The applicable parts of lemon are the fruit and peel. There is insufficient reliable information about the possible mechanism of action or active ingredients. It does contain vitamin C (18).

Adverse Reactions

None reported.

Interactions with Herbs & Other Dietary Supplements

Insufficient reliable information available.

Interactions with Drugs

No interactions are known to occur, and there is no known reason to expect a clinically significant interaction with lemon.

Interactions with Foods

No interactions are known to occur, and there is no known reason to expect a clinically significant interaction with lemon.

Interactions with Lab Tests

No interactions are known to occur, and there is no known reason to expect a clinically significant interaction with lemon.

Interactions with Diseases or Conditions

No interactions are known to occur, and there is no known reason to expect a clinically significant interaction with lemon.

Dosage and Administration

ORAL: Lemon is taken as an oil, tincture, or fresh fruit (18).

Comments

None.

LEMON BALM

Also Known As

Balm, Cure-All, Dropsy Plant, Honey Plant, Melissa, Melissae folium, Melissenblatt, Sweet Balm, Sweet Mary.

Scientific Names

Melissa officinalis.
Family: Lamiaceae or Labiatae.

People Use This For

Orally, lemon balm is used for promoting digestion, as a mild tranquilizer, for stimulating appetite (11), as an antispasmodic, for Graves' disease (6), and for functional gastrointestinal disorders with distention and gas (2,18). Topically, it is used for cold sores (herpes labialis) (1,6).

Traditionally, lemon balm has been used for promoting sweating, promoting menstrual flow, for female discomforts, nervous problems, insomnia, cramps, headache, toothache, sores, tumors, insect bites (11), nervous stomach, hysteria and melancholia, chronic bronchial mucous membrane inflammation, nervous palpitations, vomiting, and high blood pressure (18).

In foods and beverages, the extract and oil are utilized (11).

Safety

LIKELY SAFE ...when consumed in amounts found in foods (11). It has Generally Recognized as Safe (GRAS) status in the US for food use with a maximum level of 0.5% in baked goods (11).

POSSIBLY SAFE ...when used appropriately for oral or topical medicinal purposes on a short-term basis (1,2). The maximum length of use is 14 days (1).

PREGNANCY AND LACTATION: Insufficient reliable information available; avoid using.

Effectiveness

POSSIBLY EFFECTIVE ...when used orally for nervous sleeping disorders and functional gastrointestinal complaints (2). ...when used topically for treating herpes labialis (cold sores) (1,790).

There is insufficient reliable information available about the effectiveness of lemon balm for its other uses.

Mechanism of Action

The applicable part of lemon balm is the leaf. Lemon balm has sedative, antiflatulent, spasmolytic, antibacterial, and antiviral activities (2). These activities were formerly attributed to volatile oil; however, a volatile oil-free hydroalcoholic extract shows sedative activity in mice (6). Hot water extracts have antiviral effects in egg and cell cultures against herpes simplex virus (6,11) mumps, vaccinia, Newcastle disease (11), and HIV-1 (6). Lemon balm's antiviral activity is due to the tannin and polyphenol constituents (6,11). Freeze-dried extracts containing the constituents, rosmarinic acid and lithospermic acid, bind thyrotropin and block activation of thyrotropin receptor sites (6).

Adverse Reactions

Hypersensitivity reactions have been reported (9).

Topically, there is one report of irritation and one report of exacerbation of herpes symptoms when lemon balm was applied (790).

Interactions with Herbs & Other Dietary Supplements

HERBS WITH SEDATIVE PROPERTIES: Theoretically, concomitant use with herbs that have sedative properties might enhance therapeutic and adverse effects. These include calamus, calendula, California poppy, catnip, capsicum, celery, couch grass, elecampane, Siberian ginseng, German chamomile, goldenseal, gotu kola, hops, Jamaican dogwood, kava, sage, St. John's wort, sassafras, scullcap, shepherd's purse, stinging nettle, valerian, wild carrot, wild lettuce, ashwaganda root, and yerba mansa (4,19).

Interactions with Drugs

THYROID HORMONE: Theoretically, may interfere with replacement therapy (6).

BARBITURATES: Theoretically, concomitant use with barbiturates may cause additive effects and side effects (19).

OTHER DRUGS WITH SEDATIVE PROPERTIES: Theoretically, concomitant use with drugs with sedative properties may cause additive effects and side effects (19).

Interactions with Foods

No interactions are known to occur, and there is no known reason to expect a clinically significant interaction with lemon balm.

Interactions with Lab Tests

No interactions are known to occur, and there is no known reason to expect a clinically significant interaction with lemon balm.

Interactions with Diseases or Conditions

HYPOTHYROID CONDITIONS: Contraindicated because lemon balm can exacerbate or interfere with treatment (500).

Dosage and Administration

ORAL: The typical dose of lemon balm is one cup of tea several times daily as needed (2,18). The tea is prepared by steeping 1.5-4.5 grams of the leaf in 150 mL boiling water for 10 minutes and then straining. The average amount of lemon balm is 8-10 grams of the leaves per day (18). Used as a combination product with other sedative or antiflatulent herbs can be beneficial (2). The common dose of the tincture (1:5 in 45% alcohol) is 2-6 mL three times daily (1).

TOPICAL: For herpes labialis (cold sores), the cream or ointment containing 1% of a 70:1 lyophilized aqueous extract is usually applied two to four times daily from first sign of prodrome to a few days after the lesions have healed (1). The maximum length of use is 14 days (1). Alternatively, a tea is applied to the lesions with a saturated cotton ball several times daily (3). The tea is prepared by steeping 2-3 teaspoons (2-3 grams) of the finely cut leaf in 150 mL boiling water for 5-10 minutes and then straining.

Comments
None.

LEMON VERBENA

Also Known As
Herb Louisa, Lemon-Scented Verbena, Louisa.
CAUTION: See separate listing for Verbena.

Scientific Names
Aloysia triphylla, synonyms Aloysia citriodora, Lippia citriodora, Verbena citriodora, Verbena triphylla.
Family: Verbenaceae.

People Use This For
Orally, lemon verbena is used for digestive disorders, agitation, and insomnia (18).
Historically, it has been used for asthma, cold, fever, flatulence, colic, diarrhea, indigestion (4), febrile hemorrhoids, varicose veins, skin conditions, chills, and constipation (18).
In foods and manufacturing, lemon verbena is used as an ingredient in herbal teas (4), as a fragrance component in perfumes (6), and also as an ingredient in alcoholic beverages (4).

Safety
LIKELY SAFE ...when consumed in amounts found in alcoholic beverages. It has Generally Recognized as Safe (GRAS) status in the US for human consumption in alcoholic beverages (4).
POSSIBLY SAFE ...when used in appropriate amounts as an oral medicinal agent (12).
There is insufficient reliable information available about the safety of the topical use of lemon verbena.
PREGNANCY AND LACTATION: Insufficient reliable information available; avoid excessive amounts (4).

Effectiveness
There is insufficient reliable information available about the effectiveness of lemon verbena.

Mechanism of Action
The applicable parts of lemon verbena are the leaf and flower top. Oil of verbena (the essential oil distilled from lemon verbena leaf) may be acaricidal and bactericidal (6). Terpene-rich volatile oils in the plant are considered irritants (4).

Adverse Reactions
During excretion, volatile oils may irritate the kidneys (4).
Topically, contact dermatitis is possible (6).

Interactions with Herbs & Other Dietary Supplements
Insufficient reliable information available.

Interactions with Drugs
No interactions are known to occur, and there is no known reason to expect a clinically significant interaction with lemon verbena.

Interactions with Foods
No interactions are known to occur, and there is no known reason to expect a clinically significant interaction with lemon verbena.

Interactions with Lab Tests
No interactions are known to occur, and there is no known reason to expect a clinically significant interaction with lemon verbena.

Interactions with Diseases or Conditions
KIDNEY DISEASE: Avoid excessive amounts due to possible kidney irritation (4).

Dosage and Administration

ORAL: One cup tea (steep 5-29 grams leaf in 1 L boiling water 10-15 minutes, strain) two to five times daily (18).
TOPICAL: No typical dosage.

Comments

None.

LEMONGRASS

Also Known As

British Indian Lemongrass, Capim-Cidrao, Ceylon Citronella Grass, Citronella, Cochin Lemongrass, East Indian Lemongrass, Fever Grass, Guatemala Lemongrass, Lemon Grass, Madagascar Lemongrass, West Indian Lemongrass. CAUTION: See separate listings for Citronella Oil and Stone Root.

Scientific Names

Cymbopogon citratus, synonym Andropogon citratus; Cymbopogon flexuosus; Cymbopogon nardis. Family: Gramineae or Poaceae.

People Use This For

Orally, lemongrass is used for treating gastrointestinal spasms, stomachache, hypertension, convulsions, pain and neuralgia, vomiting, cough, rheumatism, fever, common cold, and exhaustion. It is also used orally as an antiseptic and as a mild astringent.

Topically, lemon grass and its essential oil are used for headache, stomachache, abdominal pain, and musculoskeletal pain.

By inhalation, the essential oil of lemongrass is used as aromatherapy for musculoskeletal pain (7107).

In food and beverages, lemongrass is used as a flavoring (6,11).

In manufacturing, lemongrass is used as a fragrance in soaps and cosmetics. Lemongrass is also used in synthesizing vitamin A and natural citral (11).

Safety

LIKELY SAFE ...when used orally in amounts found in foods. It has Generally Recognized as Safe (GRAS) status in the US. The maximum use level is 0.004% in baked goods (11).

POSSIBLY SAFE ...when used orally or topically, short-term for medicinal purposes. Lemongrass has been safely used in studies lasting up to 2 weeks (6,12,2612,7107). ...when the essential oil of lemongrass is used by inhalation as a component of aromatherapy (7107).

PREGNANCY: LIKELY UNSAFE ...when used orally. Lemongrass seems to have uterine and menstrual flow stimulating effects (12); avoid using.

LACTATION: Insufficient reliable information available; avoid using.

Effectiveness

There is insufficient reliable information available about the effectiveness of lemongrass.

Mechanism of Action

The applicable part of lemongrass is the leaf and oil. The lemongrass leaves are commonly used as "lemon" flavoring in herbal teas. The essential oil from lemongrass contains geraniol, limonene, alpha-pinene, and alpha-terpineole, which have antimicrobial properties (2130,7162). The oil has in vitro antimicrobial activity against a variety of common gram positive and gram negative organisms, including Acinetobacter calcoacetica, Enterococcus faecalis, Escherichia coli, Klebsiella pneumoniae, Pseudomonas aeruginosa, Salmonella species, Serratia marcescens, Staphylococcus aureus, and the yeast Candida albicans (2131). Lemongrass oil also contains citral, 65-85%. Although citral is a central nervous system (CNS) depressant (11,7162), lemongrass does not seem to have significant CNS effects (2612). Lemongrass is also thought to have analgesic, antipyretic, and antioxidant properties (11), as well as uterine and menstrual flow stimulating effects (12).

Adverse Reactions

Topically, rare allergic reactions have occurred following use (2,18).
By inhalation, there have been two cases of toxic alveolitis associated with an unknown quantity of lemongrass oil (2).
Orally, there is a single report of fatal poisoning after a child ingested a lemongrass oil-based insect repellent (2).

Interactions with Herbs & Other Dietary Supplements

Insufficient reliable information available.

Interactions with Drugs

No interactions are known to occur, and there is no known reason to expect a clinically significant interaction with lemongrass.

Interactions with Foods

No interactions are known to occur, and there is no known reason to expect a clinically significant interaction with lemongrass.

Interactions with Lab Tests

AMYLASE, BILIRUBIN: Lemongrass may cause elevations in serum bilirubin (direct) and amylase levels (2612).

Interactions with Diseases or Conditions

No interactions are known to occur, and there is no known reason to expect a clinically significant interaction with lemongrass.

Dosage and Administration

ORAL: People typically use 1 to 2 teaspoons of lemongrass in 6 oz boiling water as a tea (6006).
TOPICAL: No typical dosage.

Comments

Avoid confusion with citronella oil.

LENTINAN

Also Known As

None.
CAUTION: See separate listing for Shiitake Mushroom.

Scientific Names

Polysaccharide derived from Lentinus edodes, synonyms Lenticus edodes, Lentinan edodes, Lentinula edodes, Tricholomopsis edodes.
Family: Polyporaceae.

People Use This For

Lentinan is given by intravenous, intramuscular, and intraperitoneal injection as an adjunctive treatment for cancer (6) and HIV infection (1107).

Safety

There is insufficient reliable information available about the safety of lentinan.
Pregnancy and Lactation: Insufficient reliable information available; avoid using.

Effectiveness

POSSIBLY EFFECTIVE ...when given by injection as adjunctive treatment for breast, gastric, and prostate cancer (6,1108,1109,1112,1113) and as adjunctive treatment with didanosine (ddI) in HIV infection (1107).

Mechanism of Action

Lentinan is not directly cytotoxic, but may augment natural killer cell activity, activate macrophages and may enhance T-helper cell function (6). It may enhance the anti-HIV effects of zidovudine (6).

Adverse Reactions

Mild thrombocytopenia (6); minor adverse effects (unspecified) were reported in clinical trials (one case report) (6). Rapid intravenous infusion of lentinan is reported to cause "oppression" of the anterior chest and dryness of the throat; these symptoms disappeared with slow drip infusion (1111).

Interactions with Herbs & Other Dietary Supplements

Insufficient reliable information available.

Interactions with Drugs

DIDANOSINE (ddI, Videx): Concomitant use of the nucleoside reverse transcriptase inhibitor (NRTI)-type antiretroviral drug didanosine with lentinan might enhance drug-induced increases in CD4 levels in HIV+ patients (1107).

Interactions with Foods

No interactions are known to occur, and there is no known reason to expect a clinically significant interaction with lentinan.

Interactions with Lab Tests

CD4 COUNTS: Intravenously administered lentinan, combined with didanosine (ddI, Videx), might enhance drug-induced increases in CD4 concentrations and test results in some HIV+ patients with low CD4 counts (1107).

Interactions with Diseases or Conditions

MALNUTRITION: In one clinical trial, gastric cancer patients with low serum protein levels (consistent with poor nutritional status) did not respond to lentinan therapy, while patients with normal serum protein levels (consistent with adequate nutritional status) had favorable responses to lentinan (1110).

Dosage and Administration

ORAL: No typical dosage.
INJECTION: 1-4 mg per week have been used in clinical trials (6,1108,1111).

Comments

Lentinan is a polysaccharide derived from shiitake mushroom (Lenticus edode).

LESSER CELANDINE

Also Known As

Ficaria, Figwort, Pilewort, Ranunculus, Smallwort.
CAUTION: See separate listings for Greater Celandine, Amaranth, Bulbous Buttercup, and Jewelweed.

Scientific Names

Ranunculus ficaria.
Family: Ranunculaceae.

People Use This For

Orally, lesser celandine is used for scurvy (18).
Topically, it is used for bleeding wounds and gums, swollen joints, warts, scratches (18), and hemorrhoids (internal or prolapsed piles, with or without hemorrhage) (4,18).
For food uses, fresh leaf sheaths are sometimes used in salads (18).

Safety

POSSIBLY SAFE ...when small amounts of fresh leaf sheaths are eaten (18).
POSSIBLY UNSAFE ...when used topically (4,18). Extended contact with the fresh, bruised plant can cause blisters (18).
LIKELY UNSAFE ...when used orally (4,18); avoid using.
PREGNANCY AND LACTATION: LIKELY UNSAFE ... when used orally (4); avoid using.

Effectiveness

There is insufficient reliable information available about the effectiveness of lesser celandine.

Mechanism of Action

The applicable parts of lesser celandine are the above ground parts. Lesser celandine contains large amounts of vitamin C (18). It also has astringent and demulcent effects (4). Protoanemonin, a constituent, is believed to be an acrid skin irritant (4). However, when the above ground parts are dried or prepared, protoanemonin changes into a pungent, volatile intermediate that quickly dimerizes to a form that does not irritate the mucous membrane (18). Some studies suggest the constituents, anemonin and protoanemonin, might have antibacterial and antifungal activity (4). The saponin constituents show some evidence of antihemorrhoidal activity (4). Large amounts of protoanemonin-forming plants have caused death of experimental animals by asphyxiation (18).

Adverse Reactions

Orally, use is associated with severe GI irritation, colic, diarrhea, and irritation of the urinary tract (18). One report associates the use of lesser celandine with a case of recurrent, acute hepatitis (390).

Topically, use can cause mucous membrane and skin irritation (18). Extended contact with fresh, bruised plant can cause blisters (18). Some Ranunculus species also cause photodermatitis (19).

Interactions with Herbs & Other Dietary Supplements

Insufficient reliable information available.

Interactions with Drugs

No interactions are known to occur, and there is no known reason to expect a clinically significant interaction with lesser celandine.

Interactions with Foods

No interactions are known to occur, and there is no known reason to expect a clinically significant interaction with lesser celandine.

Interactions with Lab Tests

No interactions are known to occur, and there is no known reason to expect a clinically significant interaction with lesser celandine.

Interactions with Diseases or Conditions

GI CONDITIONS: Can irritate gastrointestinal tract. Contraindicated in individuals with infectious or inflammatory gastrointestinal conditions (19).

Dosage and Administration

ORAL: No typical dosage.

TOPICAL: Liquid extract (1:1 in 25% alcohol), 2-5 mL 3 times daily (4). Ointment (3%) or Pilewort Ointment (30% fresh herb in benzoinated lard) (4). Liquid extract can be added to baths for hemorrhoids, warts, or scratches (18).

Comments

Avoid confusion with greater celandine (Chelidonium majus). Scrophularia nodosa (Family: Scrophulariaceae) is also referred to as figwort (4). Amaranth and bulbous buttercup are also referred to as pilewort.

LEVANT BERRY

Also Known As

Cocculus, Cocculus Indicus, Coculus Fructus, Fish Berries, Fish Killer, Hockle Elderberry, Indian Berry, Levant Nut, Louseberry, Poisonberry.

CAUTION: See seperate listings for Chenopodium Oil, Mugwort, Wormseed, Wormwood, and Wormwood Oil.

Scientific Names

Anamirta cocculus, synonyms Anamirta paniculata, Menispermum cocculus, Menispermum Lacunosum; Cocculus suberosus; Cocculus lacunosus.

Family: Menispermaceae.

People Use This For

Orally, levant berry is used for peripheral and vestibular nystagmus and peripherally-based dizziness (18).

Topically, it is used as a powder to treat scabies (6).

Historically, the constituent, picrotoxin, was used for treating epilepsy, night sweats, and as a stimulant for barbituric acid poisoning (6,18).

In India, the leaves are inhaled as snuff to relieve malaria (6); whole fruits are used for paralyzing fish and killing birds or dogs (6); picrotoxin is applied to arrow tips for hunting by jungle tribes (6), and was formerly used to paralyze fish in the fishing industry (18); extracts are applied topically for lice (6).

Safety

POSSIBLY UNSAFE …when used topically; avoid application to broken skin (6).

LIKELY UNSAFE …when used orally; avoid due to toxic potential (6). Picrotoxin 30 mg/kg or 2-3 cocculus kernels can cause death (6,18).

PREGNANCY AND LACTATION: LIKELY UNSAFE …when used orally or topically (6); avoid using.

Effectiveness

There is insufficient reliable information available about the effectiveness of levant berry.

Mechanism of Action

The applicable parts of levant berry are the dried fruit and seed. The seed contains highly toxic picrotoxin (6,18), which stimulates the central nervous system via parasympathetic nerves, is a GI irritant, stimulates the medulla oblongata resulting in changes in respiration rate, slows heart rate due to vagal nerve stimulation, and increases blood pressure (6,18).

Adverse Reactions

Picrotoxin is a GI irritant and central nervous system stimulant (6). Mild poisoning can lead to headache, dizziness, nausea, coordination disturbances, depression, and spasms or twitching (18). Larger amounts can cause salivation, vomiting, purging, rapid shallow breathing, drowsiness, palpitations or bradycardia, tonic-clonic spasms, stupor, loss of consciousness, and death (6). The lethal dose is stated to be 30 mg/kg (6) or 2-3 Cocculus kernels (seeds) (18).

Interactions with Herbs & Other Dietary Supplements

Insufficient reliable information available.

Interactions with Drugs

No interactions are known to occur, and there is no known reason to expect a clinically significant interaction with levant berry.

Interactions with Foods

No interactions are known to occur, and there is no known reason to expect a clinically significant interaction with levant berry.

Interactions with Lab Tests

No interactions are known to occur, and there is no known reason to expect a clinically significant interaction with levant berry.

Interactions with Diseases or Conditions

No interactions are known to occur, and there is no known reason to expect a clinically significant interaction with levant berry.

Dosage and Administration

Avoid using.

Comments

Although picrotoxin is used experimentally, medicinal use has been abandoned in the US and Europe (6).

LICORICE

Also Known As

Alcacuz, Alcazuz, Chinese Licorice, Gan Cao, Gan Zao, Glycyrrhiza, Isoflavone, Isoflavones, Lakritze, Licorice Root, Liquiritiae radix, Liquirizia, Liquorice, Orozuz, Phytoestrogen, Reglisse, Regliz, Russian Licorice, Spanish Licorice, Subholz, Sweet Root.

Scientific Names

Glycyrrhiza glabra; Glycyrrhiza glabra glandulifera; Glycyrrhiza glabra typica; Glycyrrhiza glabra violacea; Glycyrrhiza uralensis, Reglisse.
Family: Leguminosae or Fabaceae.

People Use This For

Orally, licorice is used for inflammation of the upper respiratory tract mucous membranes, gastric and duodenal ulcers (2), bronchitis, chronic gastritis, colic, primary adrenocortical insufficiency (4), dry cough, arthritis, lupus, and as an antibacterial and antiviral agent (4). It is also used to treat cholestatic liver disorders, hypokalemia, and hypertonia (6121).
Topically, licorice is used as a shampoo to reduce sebum secretion (6).
Intravenously, licorice components are used for treating hepatitis B and C (3247,3248,3249,3250,3251).
In combination with Panax ginseng and Bupleurum falcatum, licorice is used orally to help stimulate adrenal gland

function, particularly in patients with a history of long-term corticosteroid use (3234). As a component of the herbal formula, Shakuyaku-Kanzo-To, licorice is used to increase fertility in women with polycystic ovary syndrome (3245). In combination with seven other herbs, licorice is used in PC-SPES to treat prostate cancer (5548).

In Chinese medicine, licorice is used for sore throats, abdominal pain, infectious hepatitis, malaria, tuberculosis, sores, abscesses, food poisoning, diabetes insipidus, and contact dermatitis (11).

Licorice is used as a flavoring in foods, beverages (4,11), and tobacco (4,6).

Safety

LIKELY SAFE ...when used orally in amounts commonly found in foods. Foods generally contain less than 0.25% licorice and 0.01% of the constituent ammoniated glycyrrhizin (11). The maximum safe daily intake of licorice is equivalent to 100 mg glycyrrhizin (2). Licorice, glycyrrhiza, and ammoniated glycyrrhizin are Generally Recognized as Safe (GRAS) for food use in the US (11).

POSSIBLY SAFE ...when used orally and appropriately, short-term, for medicinal purposes. Prolonged use of licorice longer than four to six weeks or in large amounts should be supervised (2,12). ...when used orally in a specific herbal combination (PC-SPES) (5548).

PREGNANCY: UNSAFE ...when used orally. Licorice can have abortifacient, estrogenic, and steroid effects and can cause uterine stimulation (4); avoid using.

LACTATION: Insufficient reliable information available; avoid using.

Effectiveness

POSSIBLY EFFECTIVE ...when used orally in a specific herbal combination for prostate cancer. Studies using licorice in combination with seven other herbs (PC-SPES) in prostate cancer patients, found that it significantly decreases prostate-specific antigen (PSA) levels (5548,5122), causes tumor cell death, and causes clinically significant reductions in testosterone (5548). In two reports, PSA levels fell significantly within 1 month of treatment (5548,5122). There is insufficient reliable information available about the effectiveness of licorice for its other uses.

Mechanism of Action

The applicable part of licorice is the root. Licorice has antispasmodic, anti-inflammatory, expectorant, laxative, and soothing properties (4). The constituents, glycyrrhizin and glycyrrhetinic acid, inhibit 11-beta-hydroxysteroid dehydrogenase (4). This inhibition blocks metabolism of prostaglandins E and F2 alpha and may be responsible for peptic ulcer healing observed with these products (3). Glycyrrhizin may contribute to licorice-associated mineralocorticoid side effects including hypertension and hypokalemia both by binding directly to mineralocorticoid receptors and by decreasing the conversion of active cortisol to inactive cortisone (3252,3253,6600). Panax ginseng appears to compliment licorice by increasing serum cortisol concentrations (3257). Licorice decreases testosterone production, which might account for the decreased serum testosterone concentrations in young healthy men who eat licorice (3246). The glycyrrhizin constituent acts as an expectorant by increasing the bronchial secretion and transport of mucus by a reflex pathway, which originates in the stomach (3). Glycyrrhizin has antitussive activity, perhaps due to its sweetness, which is fifty times sweeter than sugar (3,7). Licorice has both anti-estrogenic and estrogenic action. The anti-estrogenic action, attributed to isoflavone constituents, occurs at relatively high concentrations and is associated with the blocking of estrogen receptors. Licorice also affects estrogen metabolism by decreasing the metabolism when estrogen concentrations are high and potentiating metabolism when concentrations are low (4). A licorice root extract enhances estradiol binding to estrogen receptors, induces transcription activity in estrogen-responsive cells, and enhances estradiol-induced transcription activity in estrogen-responsive cells in vitro (6180). It also increases serum ceruloplasmin oxidase activity (a measure of estrogenic activity in the liver) in female rats with their ovaries removed (6180). In vitro, a coumarin constituent of licorice has antiplatelet activity. Isoliquiritigenin, a constituent, reportedly inhibits aldose reductase and the resultant sorbitol accumulation (4). Liquiritigenin and isoliquiritigenin have MAO-inhibitory activities (11). Glycyrrhetinic acid exhibits anti-inflammatory action against UV erythema and is known to inhibit the Epstein-Barr virus activation by tumor promotors. The isoflavonoid constituents, glabridin, glabrol, and derivatives, show antimicrobial activity against S. aureus, M. smegmatis, and C. albicans. Glycyrrhetinic acid has shown antiviral activity against vaccinia, herpes simplex 1, Newcastle disease, and vesicular stomatitis viruses (4). Glycyrrhizin- and glycyrrhizic acid-containing intravenous preparations (Stronger Neominophagen C and Remefa S) show activity against hepatitis B and C in humans, but the trials are too small to draw any definitive conclusions (3247,3250,3251). In vitro data suggests that glycyrrhizin suppresses the production and expression of hepatitis B surface antigen (HbS-Ag) (3248,3249). Glycyrrhizic acid and the aglycone of glycyrrhizic acid can exert anti-inflammatory and anti-allergenic properties (3). In controlled, clinical trials, they accelerated the healing of gastric ulcers (2,4). Licorice reduces body fat but accompanying fluid retention offsets any change in body weight (6196). When seven healthy adults consumed 3.5 grams of licorice candy (7.6% glycyrrhizic acid) per day for two months, body fat as a percent of total body weight decreased, extracellular water as a percent of body weight increased, the renin aldosterone system was suppressed, and there was no change in body mass index. The results of this unpublished study were presented at the Endocrine society's 82nd annual meeting (6196).

Adverse Reactions

The use of licorice can cause amenorrhea. Consumption of 50 grams of licorice per day, or chronic use longer than six weeks, can cause pseudoaldosteronism with symptoms including hypertension, lethargy, headache, sodium and water retention, and edema. Pseudoaldosteronism can lead to increased blood pressure, hypokalemia, hypokalemic myopathy, rhabdomyolysis, myoglobinuria, severe congestive heart failure with pulmonary edema, lower extremity weakness, hypertensive encephalopathy, and quadriplegia (2,3,4,6,6600). The chronic consumption of large amounts of licorice candy has caused hypermineralocorticoidism (781). Because licorice can decrease serum testosterone and increase 17-hydroxyprogesterone it might cause decreased libido and sexual dysfunction in men (3246). Chewing tobacco flavored with licorice has also been associated with toxicity (6).

Interactions with Herbs & Other Dietary Supplements

HERBS WITH CARDIAC ACTIVITY: Theoretically, the overuse or misuse of licorice can increase the risk of cardiotoxicity due to potassium depletion. Cardioactive herbs include digitalis, lily-of-the-valley, pheasant's eye, and squill.
STIMULANT LAXATIVE HERBS: Theoretically, concomitant overuse or misuse of licorice can increase the risk of potassium depletion. Stimulant laxative herbs include aloe vera, alder buckthorn, European buckthorn, cascara sagrada, castor oil, rhubarb, and senna.
HERBS WITH ANTICOAGULANT/ANTIPLATELET POTENTIAL: Concomitant use of herbs that have coumarin constituents or affect platelet aggregation could theoretically increase the risk of bleeding in some people. These herbs include: angelica, anise, arnica, asafoetida, bogbean, boldo, capsicum, celery, chamomile, clove, danshen, fenugreek, feverfew, garlic, ginger, ginkgo, ginseng Panax, horse chestnut, horseradish, meadowsweet, prickly ash, onion, papain, passionflower, poplar, quassia, red clover, turmeric, wild carrot, wild lettuce, willow, and others (4,19).

Interactions with Drugs

ANTIHYPERTENSIVE DRUGS: Theoretically, licorice might reduce the effect of antihypertensive drug therapy. Large amounts of licorice can cause sodium and water retention, and hypertension (4,515).
ASPIRIN: Theoretically, concomitant use might protect against aspirin-induced damage to the gastrointestinal mucosa (19).
CORTICOSTEROIDS: Theoretically, concomitant use might potentiate the duration of activity of corticosteroids, e.g., hydrocortisone (19).
CARDIAC GLYCOSIDES: Overuse or misuse of licorice with cardiac glycoside therapy, e.g., digoxin (Lanoxin), might increase the risk of cardiac toxicity due to potassium loss (2).
CIMETIDINE (Tagamet): Theoretically, concomitant use might provide additive protection from gastrointestinal ulcers (19).
FUROSEMIDE (Lasix), ETHACRYNIC ACID (Edecrin): Theoretically, furosemide and ethacrynic acid might enhance the mineralocorticoid effects of licorice by inhibiting the enzyme that converts cortisol to cortisone; however, bumetanide (Bumex) does not appear to have this effect (3255).
HORMONES: Theoretically, licorice might interfere with estrogen or anti-estrogen therapy due to estrogenic and anti-estrogenic effects (4).
INSULIN: Theoretically, concomitant use might cause hypokalemia and sodium retention (19).
INTERFERON: The licorice component glycyrrhizin, as part of the Japanese intravenous preparation Stronger Neominophagen C (SNMC), might enhance the effectiveness of interferon for treating hepatitis C (3247).
MONOAMINE OXIDASE INHIBITORS (MAOIs): Theoretically, concomitant use might increase the effects of MAOI drugs due to the MAO-inhibiting effects of some licorice constituents (11).
NONSTEROIDAL ANTI-INFLAMMATORY DRUGS (NSAIDs): Theoretically, concomitant use can compound NSAID sodium and water retention (504), and protect against NSAID-induced damage to the gastrointestinal mucosa (19).
OTHER DRUGS: There's preliminary evidence that licorice can inhibit the cytochrome P450 (CYP450) 3A4 enzyme (6450). Theoretically, licorice might increase levels of drugs metabolized by CYP450 3A4; however, as of yet, this interaction has not been reported in humans. Some drugs metabolized by CYP450 3A4 include lovastatin (Mevacor), ketoconazole (Nizoral), itraconazole (Sporanox), fexofenadine (Allegra), triazolam (Halcion), and numerous others. Use licorice cautiously or avoid in patients taking these drugs.
POTASSIUM-DEPLETING DRUGS: Concomitant use of licorice and potassium-depleting drugs might increase potassium loss and the risk of potassium depletion. Overuse or misuse of licorice can cause potassium depletion (2,12).

Interactions with Foods

GRAPEFRUIT JUICE: Theoretically, grapefruit juice and its component naringenin might enhance the mineralocorticoid activities of licorice, by blocking the conversion of cortisol to cortisone (3254,3255).

Interactions with Lab Tests

BLOOD PRESSURE: Excessive use of licorice can increase blood pressure and blood pressure readings. Excessive licorice intake can cause hypertension (1372).

17-HYDROXYPROGESTERONE: Licorice can increase serum 17-hydroxyprogesterone concentrations and test results (3246).

POTASSIUM: Excessive use of licorice can cause hypokalemia, reducing serum potassium levels and test results (4).

TESTOSTERONE: Licorice can decrease serum testosterone concentrations and test results (3246).

Interactions with Diseases or Conditions

DIABETES: Contraindicated; licorice can interfere with blood glucose control (4,12).

HEART DISEASE: Licorice is contraindicated in congestive heart disease (4).

HORMONE SENSITIVE CANCERS/CONDITIONS: Licorice might have estrogenic effects (6180). Women with hormone sensitive conditions should avoid using licorice. Some of these conditions include breast, uterine, and ovarian cancer; and endometriosis and uterine fibroids.

HYPERTENSION: Contraindicated; licorice can cause hypertension (1372).

HYPERTONIA: Contraindicated in individuals with hypertonia (2).

HYPOKALEMIA: Contraindicated; licorice use can cause hypokalemia (2).

KIDNEY INSUFFICIENCY: Contraindicated in patients with severe renal insufficiency (2).

LICORICE HYPERSENSITIVITY: Contraindicated in individuals hypersensitive to licorice (14).

LIVER DISEASE: Licorice is contraindicated in cholestatic liver disorders and liver cirrhosis (2). Patients with liver disease might be more sensitive to the mineralocorticoid effects of licorice (4).

SEXUAL DYSFUNCTION: Theoretically, licorice might decrease libido and worsen erectile dysfunction by decreasing testosterone and increasing 17-hydroxyprogesterone serum concentrations (3246).

Dosage and Administration

ORAL: The typical dose of licorice is 1-4 grams of the powdered root or one cup of the tea three times daily (4). The tea is prepared by simmering 1-4 grams of the powdered root in 150 mL boiling water for 5-10 minutes and then straining. The usual dose of Succus liquiritiae is 0.5-1 gram for upper respiratory tract mucous membrane inflammation and 1.5-3 grams for gastric and duodenal ulcers.

TOPICAL: No typical dosage.

INTRAVENOUS: Nop typical dosage.

Comments

Deglycyrrizinated licorice (DGL) is usually free of adverse effects (12). Studies using DGL for ulcer treatment have been inconclusive (6). Carbenoxolone is a semisynthetic derivative of the licorice constituent, glycyrrhetic acid, which is used outside the US for treating gastric and duodenal disease (6). Many "licorice" products manufactured in the US actually contain no licorice, and instead, they contain anise oil that smells and tastes like licorice (3). Authentic licorice is more commonly used in products manufactured in Europe (5).

LILY-OF-THE-VALLEY

Also Known As

Constancy, Convallaria, Convallaria herba, Convall-Lily, Jacob's Ladder, Ladder-To-Heaven, Lily, Lily of the Valley, May Bells, May Lily, Muguet, Our Lady's Tears.
CAUTION: See separate listings for Abscess Root and Jacob's Ladder.

Scientific Names

Convallaria majalis.
Family: Liliaceae or Convallariaceae.

People Use This For

Orally, lily-of-the-valley is used for mild cardiac insufficiency, heart insufficiency due to old age, chronic cor pulmonale (2,18), arrhythmias, urinary tract infections, and kidney stones (18).
In folk medicine, it is used for weak contractions in labor, epilepsy, edema, strokes and ensuing paralysis, conjunctivitis, and leprosy.

Safety

POSSIBLY SAFE ...when the standardized extract is used orally under supervision (2,12). Poor oral absorption of its cardiac glycosides can reduce the risk of poisoning (18), but the number of glycosides and their varied properties makes controlled use difficult (7).

LIKELY UNSAFE ...when the standardized extract is used orally for self-medication (12).

PREGNANCY AND LACTATION: UNSAFE ...when used orally for self-medication.

Effectiveness
There is insufficient reliable information available about the effectiveness of lily-of-the-valley.

Mechanism of Action
The applicable parts of lily-of-the-valley are the root, rhizome, and dried flower tips. Lily-of-the-valley contains over 40 cardioactive glycosides, principally convallatoxin, and other minor glycosides, including canvallatoxol and convalloside (13). The cardiac glycosides exert positive inotropic, negative chronotropic, negative dromotropic (conduction), and positive bathmotropic (excitability) effects (7). They can lower the elevated left-ventricular diastolic pressure as well as the pathologically elevated venous pressure (2). Diuretic, natriuretic, and dose-dependent vasoconstrictive effects have been observed in experimental animals (18).

Adverse Reactions
Orally, lily-of-the-valley can cause nausea, vomiting, cardiac arrhythmias (2), headache, and stupor (18). Visual color disturbances can also occur (18).

Interactions with Herbs & Other Dietary Supplements
CARDIAC GLYCOSIDE-CONTAINING HERBS: Contraindicated. Concomitant use can increase the risk of cardiac glycoside toxicity. Cardiac glycoside-containing herbs include black hellebore, Canadian hemp root, digitalis leaf, hedge mustard, figwort, motherwort, oleander leaf, pheasant's eye plant, pleurisy root, squill bulb leaf scales, strophanthus seeds, and uzara (2,18,19,500).
OTHER CARDIOACTIVE HERBS: Avoid concomitant use with other cardioactive herbs due to the unpredictability of therapeutic and adverse effects. Other cardioactive herbs include calamus, cereus, cola, coltsfoot, devil's claw, European mistletoe, fenugreek, fumitory, ginger, ginseng panax, hawthorn, white horehound, mate, parsley, quassia, scotch broom flower, shepherd's purse, and wild carrot (4).
STIMULANT LAXATIVE HERBS: Theoretically, the overuse or misuse of stimulant laxatives with cardiac glycoside-containing herbs increases the risk of cardiac toxicity due to potassium depletion. Stimulant laxative herbs include aloe dried leaf sap, blue flag rhizome, alder buckthorn, European buckthorn, butternut bark, cascara bark, castor oil, colocynth fruit pulp, gamboge bark exudate, jalap root, black root, manna bark exudate, podophyllum root, rhubarb root, senna leaves and pods, wild cucumber fruit (Ecballium elaterium), and yellow dock root (19).
LICORICE/HORSETAIL: Theoretically, the overuse or misuse of licorice rhizomes or horsetail plant with cardiac glycoside-containing herbs increases the risk of cardiac toxicity due to potassium depletion (19).

Interactions with Drugs
CALCIUM: Calcium salts can enhance the therapeutic and adverse effects of lily-of-the-valley (18).
CARDIAC DRUGS: Theoretically, concomitant use can increase the risk of cardiac toxicity (152).
DIGOXIN: Contraindicated because therapeutic duplication increases the risk of cardiac glycoside toxicity (2).
GLUCOCORTICOIDS: Theoretically, concomitant, long-term glucocorticoid use can increase the risk of cardiac glycoside toxicity due to potassium depletion (2).
POTASSIUM-DEPLETING DIURETICS: Theoretically, concomitant use can increase the risk of cardiac glycoside toxicity due to potassium depletion (2,506).
QUININE: Theoretically, concomitant use can increase the risk of cardiac toxicity (2,506).
STIMULANT LAXATIVES: Theoretically, the overuse or misuse of stimulant laxatives can increase the risk of cardiac glycoside toxicity due to potassium depletion (2).
TETRACYCLINES and MACROLIDE ANTIBIOTICS (erythromycin-like drugs): Theoretically, concomitant use can increase the risk of cardiac glycoside toxicity (17,152).

Interactions with Foods
No interactions are known to occur, and there is no known reason to expect a clinically significant interaction with lily-of-the-valley.

Interactions with Lab Tests
No interactions are known to occur, and there is no known reason to expect a clinically significant interaction with lily-of-the-valley.

Interactions with Diseases or Conditions
HEART DISEASE: Self-medication of lily-of-the-valley is contraindicated; requires diagnosis, treatment, and monitoring (515).
POTASSIUM DEFICIENCY: Contraindicated (2).

Dosage and Administration

ORAL: The average daily amount is 600 mg of the standardized lily-of-the-valley powder (0.2-0.3% cardioactive glycosides) or equivalent preparations (2).

Comments

It is unsafe for self-use. The large number of cardiac glycosides in lily-of-the-valley makes monitoring and therapeutic control more difficult than digitalis or digoxin therapy (7). Lily-of-the-valley has a short duration of action. This correlates with lower absorption rates and makes treatment more difficult to control than with isolated cardiac glycosides, especially due to the narrow therapeutic range of these constituents (7). When indicated, digoxin of standard potency and purity is a safer alternative than nonstandardized lily-of-the-valley (7). Store lily-of-the-valley in well-sealed containers and protect from light (18).

LIME fruit, peel

Also Known As

Adam's Apple, Italian Limetta, Limette.
CAUTION: See separate listing for Lime oil.

Scientific Names

Citrus aurantifolia.
Family: Rutaceae.

People Use This For

Orally, lime is used as a source of vitamin C for treating scurvy and low resistance (18).

Safety

LIKELY SAFE …when used in food amounts (12).
POSSIBLY SAFE …when used orally in medicinal amounts (12).
PREGNANCY AND LACTATION: Avoid using in amounts greater than those typically found in foods.

Effectiveness

There is insufficient reliable information available about the effectiveness of lime.

Mechanism of Action

There is insufficient reliable information available about the possible mechanism of action and active ingredients.

Adverse Reactions

None reported.

Interactions with Herbs & Other Dietary Supplements

Insufficient reliable information available.

Interactions with Drugs

No interactions are known to occur, and there is no known reason to expect a clinically significant interaction with lime.

Interactions with Foods

No interactions are known to occur, and there is no known reason to expect a clinically significant interaction with lime.

Interactions with Lab Tests

No interactions are known to occur, and there is no known reason to expect a clinically significant interaction with lime.

Interactions with Diseases or Conditions

No interactions are known to occur, and there is no known reason to expect a clinically significant interaction with lime.

Dosage and Administration

ORAL: Lime is taken as a liquid extract or as the fresh fruit (18).

Comments

Lime flower is obtained from a species distinct from lime.

LIME oil

Also Known As

Adam's Apple, Italian Limetta, Key Lime, Limette.
CAUTION: See separate listing for Lime fruit, peel.

Scientific Names

Citrus aurantifolia, synonym Citrus medica var. acida.
Family: Rutaceae.

People Use This For

In cosmetics, expressed lime oil is used as a fragrance component. Distilled lime oil is used as a fixative in cosmetics (11).
In foods, lime oil is used as flavor component in foods and beverages (11).

Safety

LIKELY SAFE …when lime oil is used orally in amounts found in foods. It has Generally Recognized as Safe (GRAS) status in the US. The maximum level used is 0.078% (11).
POSSIBLY SAFE …when used topically in amounts found in cosmetics. Maximum use level for expressed and distilled oils is 1.5%.
POSSIBLY UNSAFE ...when used topically in larger amounts than those found in cosmetics. Lime oil can be associated with phototoxic skin reactions (11,19) and should not be used during periods of excessive exposure to sunlight.
PREGNANCY AND LACTATION: LIKELY SAFE ...when used orally in food amounts. There is insufficient reliable information available about the safety of the topical use of lime oil; avoid using.

Effectiveness

There is insufficient reliable information available about the effectiveness of lime oil.

Mechanism of Action

Expressed lime oil contains phototoxic furocoumarins, including bergapten (11). Some evidence suggests expressed and distilled lime oils might promote tumors in the presence of carcinogenic chemicals (11).

Adverse Reactions

Topically, use is associated with hypersensitivity (4058). Although distilled lime oil is reported to be nonirritating, non-sensitizing, and non-phototoxic to human skin (11), expressed lime oil and lime peel can cause phototoxic skin reactions (11,19).

Interactions with Herbs & Other Dietary Supplements

PHOTOSENSITIZING HERBS: Theoretically, concomitant use with other photosensitizing herbs may increase the risk of phototoxicity (19).

Interactions with Drugs

PSORALENS: Theoretically, concomitant use might potentiate effects and adverse effects (19); contraindicated.

Interactions with Foods

No interactions are known to occur, and there is no known reason to expect a clinically significant interaction with lime oil.

Interactions with Lab Tests

No interactions are known to occur, and there is no known reason to expect a clinically significant interaction with lime oil.

Interactions with Diseases or Conditions

No interactions are known to occur, and there is no known reason to expect a clinically significant interaction with lime oil.

Dosage and Administration

No typical dosage.

Comments

Distilled lime oil is the distilled essential oil of the whole crushed fruit of the lime tree. Expressed lime oil is obtained from unripe lime peel. Expressed lime oil is not as important economically as distilled lime oil (11).

LINDEN CHARCOAL

Also Known As

Basswood, European Linden, Lime Tree, Tiliae carbo.
CAUTION: See separate listings for Linden dried flower, Linden dried leaf, Linden dried sapwood, and Silver Linden.

Scientific Names

Tilia cordata; Tilia platyphyllos.
Family: Tiliaceae.

People Use This For

Orally, linden charcoal is used for intestinal disorders (2,18).
Topically, linden charcoal is used for lower leg abscesses (ulcus cruris) (2,18).

Safety

There is insufficient reliable information available about the safety of linden charcoal.
Pregnancy and Lactation: Insufficient reliable information available; avoid using.

Effectiveness

There is insufficient reliable information available about the effectiveness of linden charcoal.

Mechanism of Action

Linden charcoal is described as an extremely absorbent charcoal (18).

Adverse Reactions

None reported.

Interactions with Herbs & Other Dietary Supplements

Insufficient reliable information available.

Interactions with Drugs

No interactions are known to occur, and there is no known reason to expect a clinically significant interaction with linden charcoal.

Interactions with Foods

No interactions are known to occur, and there is no known reason to expect a clinically significant interaction with linden charcoal.

Interactions with Lab Tests

No interactions are known to occur, and there is no known reason to expect a clinically significant interaction with linden charcoal.

Interactions with Diseases or Conditions

No interactions are known to occur, and there is no known reason to expect a clinically significant interaction with linden charcoal.

Dosage and Administration

No typical dosage.

Comments

Linden charcoal is the charcoal obtained from the wood of the linden tree (Tilia cordata and Tilia platyphyllos). There is very little scientific information about this product. Our staff is continually analyzing the available information on natural medicines and will add data here as it becomes available.

LINDEN dried flower

Also Known As

Basswood, European Linden, Lime Blossom, Lime Flower, Lime Tree, Linden Tree, Tiliae flos.
CAUTION: See separate listings for Linden Charcoal, Linden dried leaf, Linden dried sapwood, and Silver Linden.

Scientific Names

Tilia cordata; Tilia platyphyllos.
Family: Tiliaceae.

People Use This For

Orally, linden dried flower is used for coughs, colds (2), nasal congestion, throat irritation, nervous palpitations, hypertension, headaches, insomnia, sinus headache, migraines, incontinence, and hemorrhage (6).
Topically, linden dried flower is used for itchy skin and rheumatism (6).
Traditionally, linden dried flower has been used for migraines, hysteria, arteriosclerotic hypertension, feverish colds, nervous tension (4), and as a diuretic (6).

Safety

POSSIBLY SAFE ...when used orally and appropriately (12).
PREGNANCY AND LACTATION: Insufficient reliable information available; avoid using.

Effectiveness

There is insufficient reliable information available about the effectiveness of linden dried flower.

Mechanism of Action

The linden dried flower has antispasmodic, diaphoretic, diuretic, sedative, and mild astringent properties (4), and antifungal activity (6). In vitro, its antispasmodic activity is attributed to p-coumaric acid and the flavonoid constituents (4). Diaphoretic effects can be due to kaempferol, p-coumaric acid, and quercetin (6), or perhaps due to the heat of the liquid as a tea combined with warm bed rest (7). The volatile oils, including citral, citronellal, citronellol, eugenol, and limonene, exert sedative and antispasmodic effects (4,6). A diuretic effect can be due to the irritant action of terpenoid on the kidneys (4).

Adverse Reactions

Orally, frequent use of the linden dried flower tea is associated with cardiac damage, but this is rare (6).
Topically, linden dried flower can cause contact urticaria (6).

Interactions with Herbs & Other Dietary Supplements

Insufficient reliable information available.

Interactions with Drugs

No interactions are known to occur, and there is no known reason to expect a clinically significant interaction with linden dried flower.

Interactions with Foods

No interactions are known to occur, and there is no known reason to expect a clinically significant interaction with linden dried flower.

Interactions with Lab Tests

No interactions are known to occur, and there is no known reason to expect a clinically significant interaction with linden dried flower.

Interactions with Diseases or Conditions

HEART DISEASE: Frequent use of linden dried flower tea is associated with cardiac damage and should be used with caution in individuals with heart disease (6).

Dosage and Administration

ORAL: The typical dose of linden dried flower is one to two cups of the tea used as hot as possible (8). The tea is prepared by steeping 2 grams of the flowers in 150 mL boiling water for 5-10 minutes and then straining. The linden dried flower should only be used up to 2-4 grams daily (2). The usual dose of the tincture (1:5 in 45% alcohol) is 2-4 mL (4). The common dose of the liquid extract (1:1 in 25% alcohol) is 1-2 mL (4).

Comments
Tilia sylvestris, a related species, has been reported to possess anti-inflammatory and wound healing effects (6).

LINDEN dried leaf

Also Known As
Basswood, European Linden, Lime Tree, Tiliae folium.
CAUTION: See separate listings for Linden Charcoal, Linden dried flower, Linden dried sapwood, and Silver Linden.

Scientific Names
Tilia cordata; Tilia platyphyllos.
Family: Tiliaceae.

People Use This For
Orally, linden dried leaf is used as a diaphoretic (2,18).

Safety
There is insufficient reliable information available about the safety of linden dried leaf.
Pregnancy and Lactation: Insufficient reliable information available; avoid using.

Effectiveness
There is insufficient reliable information available about the effectiveness of linden dried leaf.

Mechanism of Action
There is insufficient reliable information available about the possible mechanism of action and active ingredients.

Adverse Reactions
None reported.

Interactions with Herbs & Other Dietary Supplements
Insufficient reliable information available.

Interactions with Drugs
No interactions are known to occur, and there is no known reason to expect a clinically significant interaction with linden dried leaf.

Interactions with Foods
No interactions are known to occur, and there is no known reason to expect a clinically significant interaction with linden dried leaf.

Interactions with Lab Tests
No interactions are known to occur, and there is no known reason to expect a clinically significant interaction with linden dried leaf.

Interactions with Diseases or Conditions
No interactions are known to occur, and there is no known reason to expect a clinically significant interaction with linden dried leaf.

Dosage and Administration
No typical dosage.

Comments
There is very little scientific information about this product. Our staff is continually analyzing the available information on natural medicines and will add data here as it becomes available.

LINDEN dried sapwood

Also Known As
Basswood, European Linden, Lime Tree, Linden Wood, Tiliae lignum.
CAUTION: See separate listings for Linden Charcoal, Linden dried flower, Linden dried leaf, and Silver Linden.

Scientific Names
Tilia cordata; Tilia platyphyllos.
Family: Tiliaceae.

People Use This For
Orally, linden dried sapwood is used for liver disease, gallbladder disease, and cellulitis (2,18).

Safety
There is insufficient reliable information available about the safety of linden dried sapwood.
Pregnancy and Lactation: Insufficient reliable information available; avoid using.

Effectiveness
There is insufficient reliable information available about the effectiveness of linden dried sapwood.

Mechanism of Action
There is insufficient reliable information available about the possible mechanism of action and active ingredients.

Adverse Reactions
None reported.

Interactions with Herbs & Other Dietary Supplements
Insufficient reliable information available.

Interactions with Drugs
No interactions are known to occur, and there is no known reason to expect a clinically significant interaction with linden dried sapwood.

Interactions with Foods
No interactions are known to occur, and there is no known reason to expect a clinically significant interaction with linden dried sapwood.

Interactions with Lab Tests
No interactions are known to occur, and there is no known reason to expect a clinically significant interaction with linden dried sapwood.

Interactions with Diseases or Conditions
No interactions are known to occur, and there is no known reason to expect a clinically significant interaction with linden dried sapwood.

Dosage and Administration
No typical dosage.

Comments
There is very little scientific information about this product. Our staff is continually analyzing the available information on natural medicines and will add data here as it becomes available.

LIPASE

Also Known As
None.

Scientific Names
Triacylglycerol lipase.

People Use This For
Orally, lipase is used for indigestion, heartburn, celiac disease, Crohn's disease, and cystic fibrosis (2378).

Safety
LIKELY SAFE ...when used orally (15).
PREGNANCY AND LACTATION: Insufficient reliable information available; avoid using.

Effectiveness
There is insufficient reliable information available about the effectiveness of lipase.

Mechanism of Action
Lipase aids in fat digestion by hydrolyzing fat to yield fatty acids and glycerol (9).

Adverse Reactions
Taking large amounts of lipase orally can cause nausea, cramping, and/or diarrhea. Extremely large amounts of exogenous pancreatic enzymes (containing lipase) may be associated with hyperuricosuria and hyperuricemia (14).

Interactions with Herbs & Other Dietary Supplements
Insufficient reliable information available.

Interactions with Drugs
No interactions are known to occur, and there is no known reason to expect a clinically significant interaction with lipase.

Interactions with Foods
No interactions are known to occur, and there is no known reason to expect a clinically significant interaction with lipase.

Interactions with Lab Tests
No interactions are known to occur, and there is no known reason to expect a clinically significant interaction with lipase.

Interactions with Diseases or Conditions
GOUT: Excessive ingestion of lipase may exacerbate gout (14).
CYSTIC FIBROSIS: High doses of lipase appear to increase the risk of fibrosing colonopathy and colonic strictures in individuals with cystic fibrosis (2379,2380,2381,2382).

Dosage and Administration
No typical dosage.

Comments
Lipase is a digestive enzyme that is widely distributed in the plant world, in milk, milk products, bacteria, molds, and animal tissues (2383). Castor beans and dehulled oats are also plant sources of acid-stable lipases (2383). Lipase is included in many prescription and OTC combination pancreatic enzyme products. Most clinical studies use combination pancreatic enzyme products, rather than lipase-only products, although pancreatic enzyme dosing is often expressed in units of lipase (2384).

LIVER EXTRACT

Also Known As
Aqueous Liver Extract, Hydrolyzed Liver Extract, Liquid Liver Extract, Liver, Liver Concentrate, Liver Factors, Liver Fractions, Liver Hydrolysate, Liver Substance, Raw Liver.
CAUTION: See separate listing for Shark Liver Oil.

Scientific Names
None.

People Use This For
Orally, liver extract is used for improving liver function, treating chronic liver diseases (6614), preventing liver damage, and regenerating liver tissue (6650). It is also used for allergies; enhancing muscle development in bodybuilders;

improving stamina, strength, and physical endurance; enhancing detoxification; and as an aid to recovery from chemical addiction or poisoning (6648).

Safety
There is insufficient reliable information available to rate the safety of liver extract. However, since some preparations are derived from animals, there is concern about contamination with diseased animal parts (see Adverse Reactions) (1825). So far, there are no reports of disease transmission to humans due to use of contaminated liver extract.
PREGNANCY AND LACTATION: Insufficient reliable information available; avoid using.

Effectiveness
There is insufficient reliable information available about the effectiveness of liver extract.

Mechanism of Action
Liver extract is a concentrated product derived from animal liver, most commonly from cattle (6647). It contains vitamin B12, folic acid, and up to 3-4 mg of heme iron per gram of product (6614). Liver extract increases liver weight and shows evidence of stimulating liver cell proliferation in experimental animals after partial hepatectomy (6650). However, information about pharmacological effects in humans is not available.

Adverse Reactions
Adverse reactions have not been reported. However, there is some concern about the possibility of contamination. Liver extract is derived from raw animal liver gathered from slaughterhouses, possibly from sick or diseased animals (6616). Products made from contaminated or diseased organs might present a human health hazard. There is also concern that liver extracts produced from cows in countries where bovine spongiform encephalitis (BSE) has been reported might be contaminated with diseased tissue. Countries where BSE has been reported include Great Britain, France, The Netherlands, Portugal, Luxembourg, Ireland, Switzerland, Oman, and Belgium (1825). However, there have been no reports of BSE transfer to humans from contaminated liver extract products. Until more is known, tell patients to avoid these products unless the country of origin can be determined. Patients should avoid products that are produced in countries where BSE has been found.

Interactions with Herbs & Other Dietary Supplements
IRON: Concomitant use might increase the risk of iron overload. Liver extract can contain 3-4 mg heme iron per gram of product (6614).

Interactions with Drugs
IRON: Concomitant use might increase the risk of iron overload. Liver extract can contain 3-4 mg heme iron per gram of product (6614).

Interactions with Foods
No interactions are known to occur, and there is no known reason to expect a clinically significant interaction with liver extract.

Interactions with Lab Tests
IRON: Liver extract might increase iron concentrations and test results due to its iron content (6614).
HEMOGLOBIN: Liver extract might increase hemoglobin concentrations and test results due to its iron content (6614).

Interactions with Diseases or Conditions
IRON METABOLISM DISORDERS: Liver extract contains 3-4 mg of heme iron and might adversely effect people with iron metabolism disorders, including hemochromatosis (6614); contraindicated.

Dosage and Administration
No typical dosage.

Comments
None.

LIVERWORT

Also Known As

American Liverleaf, Anémone à Lobes Aigus, Anémone d'Amérique, Hepatici noblis herba, Hépatique à Lobes Aigus, Hépatique d'Amérique, Herb Trinity, Kidney Wort, Leberbluemchenkraut, Liverleaf, Liverweed, Liverwort-Leaf, Round-Leaved Hepatica, Round-Lobe Hepatica, Sharp-Lobe Hepatica, Trefoil.

Scientific Names

Anemone acutiloba, synonym Hepatica nobilis var. acuta; Anemone americana, synomym Hepatica nobilis var. obtusa; Anemone hepatica.
Family: Ranunculaceae.

People Use This For

Orally, liverwort is used for liver diseases, jaundice, liver enlargement, congestion, portal vein problems, hepatitis, and liver cirrhosis. It is also used orally for gastric and digestive discomfort, stimulating appetite, relieving sensation of fullness, for treating gallstones and gravel, for regulating bowel function, stimulating pancreatic function, regulating blood lipid levels, for varicose veins, stimulating systemic and cardiac circulation, increasing myocardium blood supply, strengthening nerves, "purifying" blood, stimulating metabolism, relief of menopausal symptoms, and as a general tonic or sedative (2).
Topically, liverwort is used for hemorrhoids (2) or as an external rinse (18).

Safety

LIKELY UNSAFE ...when the fresh above ground parts are used orally or topically (2).
There is insufficient reliable information available about the safety of dried liverwort.
PREGNANCY: LIKELY UNSAFE ...when used orally or topically (2).
LACTATION: LIKELY UNSAFE ...when the fresh above ground parts are used orally or topically (2). There is insufficient reliable information available about the safety of dried liverwort; avoid using.

Effectiveness

There is insufficient reliable information available about the effectiveness of liverwort.

Mechanism of Action

The applicable parts of liverwort are the fresh or dried above ground parts (2). Liverwort contains ranunculin (18), which hydrolyzes to toxic, unstable protoanemonin, which readily dimerizes to nontoxic anemonin (4). Some evidence suggests anemonin might be cytotoxic (4). Other evidence indicates anemonin and protoanemonin might have sedative and antipyretic activity (4). Protoanemonin has antimicrobial activity (2). It causes central nervous system stimulation, then paralysis in experimental animals (2). Kidney and urinary tract irritation might be due to the alkylating action of protoanemonin (2).

Adverse Reactions

Orally, fresh liverwort can cause colic, diarrhea, gastrointestinal irritation (18), and kidney and urinary tract irritation (2).
Topically, skin contact with fresh liverwort can cause irritation, mucous membrane irritation, itching, and pustule formation known a ranunculus dermatitis (2).
Inhalation of protoanemonin-containing volatile oil can cause nasal mucosal and conjunctival irritation (4).

Interactions with Herbs & Other Dietary Supplements

Insufficient reliable information available.

Interactions with Drugs

No interactions are known to occur, and there is no known reason to expect a clinically significant interaction with liverwort.

Interactions with Foods

No interactions are known to occur, and there is no known reason to expect a clinically significant interaction with liverwort.

Interactions with Lab Tests

No interactions are known to occur, and there is no known reason to expect a clinically significant interaction with liverwort.

Interactions with Diseases or Conditions

No interactions are known to occur, and there is no known reason to expect a clinically significant interaction with liverwort.

Dosage and Administration

No typical dosage.

Comments

None.

LOBELIA

Also Known As

Asthma Weed, Bladderpod, Emetic Herb, Gagroot, Indian Tobacco, Pukeweed, Vomit Wort, Wild Tobacco.

Scientific Names

Lobelia inflata.
Family: Lobeliaceae or Campanulaceae.

People Use This For

Orally, lobelia is used for asthma and bronchitis (4).

Topically, it is used for muscle inflammation, rheumatic nodules (4), bruises, sprains, insect bites, poison ivy, and ringworm (11).

Historically, lobelia has been used orally for whooping cough, inducing sweating, and as a sedative (4,11). Lobelia was also used as an ingredient in smoking cessation products (11,514) and for treating apnea in newborn infants (514).

In manufacturing, lobelia is used in cough preparations and counterirritant products (11).

Safety

LIKELY UNSAFE ...when used orally (3,11). 0.6-1 gram of the leaf is said to be toxic and 4 grams may be fatal (18). There is insufficient reliable information available about the safety of the topical use of lobelia.

PREGNANCY AND LACTATION: LIKELY UNSAFE ...when used orally because it has emetic effects (4,12). There is insufficient reliable information available about the safety of lobelia for topical use during pregnancy and lactation.

Effectiveness

LIKELY INEFFECTIVE ...when lobeline, a constituent of lobelia, is used orally for smoking cessation (13). There is insufficient reliable information available about the effectiveness of lobelia for its other uses.

Mechanism of Action

The applicable parts of lobelia are the above ground parts. Lobelia has some anti-asthmatic, antispasmodic, emetic, expectorant, and respiratory stimulant effects (4,13). The primary constituent, (-)-lobeline, is known as alpha lobeline, to distinguish it from the mixture of lobelia alkaloids formerly called lobeline. Like nicotine but weaker, alpha lobeline exhibits effects on the peripheral circulation, neuromuscular system and central nervous system (CNS) (4,13). Small amounts of lobeline stimulate respiration and have expectorant activity (11,18). Larger amounts have emetic, purgative, and diuretic effects (11). Lobeline first causes CNS stimulation then CNS and respiratory depression (505).

Adverse Reactions

Orally, lobelia can cause nausea, vomiting, diarrhea, coughing, dizziness, and tremors (4). Overdose may cause sweating, tachycardia, convulsions, hypothermia, hypotension, coma, and possibly death (4,11).

Interactions with Herbs & Other Dietary Supplements

TOBACCO: Concomitant use with lobelia may enhance nicotine effects and adverse effects (505).

Interactions with Drugs

No interactions are known to occur, and there is no known reason to expect a clinically significant interaction with lobelia.

Interactions with Foods

No interactions are known to occur, and there is no known reason to expect a clinically significant interaction with lobelia.

Interactions with Lab Tests
No interactions are known to occur, and there is no known reason to expect a clinically significant interaction with lobelia.

Interactions with Diseases or Conditions
HEART DISEASE: CAUTION, dose-dependent cardiac activity is reported with lobelia (12).
GI CONDITIONS: Lobelia can irritate the gastrointestinal tract. It is contraindicated in individuals with infectious or inflammatory gastrointestinal conditions (19).

Dosage and Administration
ORAL: A typical dose as an expectorant is 100 mg of leaf, 0.6-2.0 mL of the tincture (12). The dosage of specific products varies widely from 375 mg once daily to 820 mg three times daily. One supplier warns not to exceed 50 mg of the dried lobelia. An extract of lobelia is used in a dose of 2 to 5 drops three to four times daily. The extract contains alcohol (6006).

Comments
Clinical research was unable to demonstrate lobeline efficacy greater than placebo in smoking cessation (13) and it was disallowed as an ingredient in anti-smoking products in the US in 1993 (11).

LOGWOOD

Also Known As
Bloodwood, Peachwood.

Scientific Names
Haematoxylon campechianum; Haematoxylon lignum.
Family: Leguminosae or Fabaceae.

People Use This For
Orally, logwood is used for diarrhea, hemorrhage, and as an astringent.

Safety
There is insufficient reliable information available about the safety of logwood.
Pregnancy and Lactation: Insufficient reliable information available; avoid using.

Effectiveness
There is insufficient reliable information available about the effectiveness of logwood.

Mechanism of Action
There is insufficient reliable information available about the possible mechanism of action and active ingredients.

Adverse Reactions
None reported.

Interactions with Herbs & Other Dietary Supplements
Insufficient reliable information available.

Interactions with Drugs
No interactions are known to occur, and there is no known reason to expect a clinically significant interaction with logwood.

Interactions with Foods
No interactions are known to occur, and there is no known reason to expect a clinically significant interaction with logwood.

Interactions with Lab Tests
No interactions are known to occur, and there is no known reason to expect a clinically significant interaction with logwood.

Interactions with Diseases or Conditions
No interactions are known to occur, and there is no known reason to expect a clinically significant interaction with logwood.

Dosage and Administration
ORAL: Logwood is used as a tea or liquid extract (18).

Comments
There is very little scientific information about this product. Our staff is continually analyzing the available information on natural medicines and will add data here as it becomes available.

LOOSESTRIFE

Also Known As
Yellow Willowherb.
CAUTION: See separate listing for Purple Loosestrife.

Scientific Names
Lysimachia vulgaris.
Family: Primulaceae.

People Use This For
Orally, loosestrife is used for scurvy, diarrhea, dysentery, and as an astringent. It is also used for hemorrhages, including nose bleeds and heavy menstrual flow.
Topically, loosestrife is used for wounds (18).

Safety
There is insufficient reliable information available about the safety of loosestrife.
Pregnancy and Lactation: Insufficient reliable information available; avoid using.

Effectiveness
There is insufficient reliable information available about the effectiveness of loosestrife.

Mechanism of Action
There is insufficient reliable information available about the possible mechanism of action and active ingredients.

Adverse Reactions
None reported.

Interactions with Herbs & Other Dietary Supplements
Insufficient reliable information available.

Interactions with Drugs
No interactions are known to occur, and there is no known reason to expect a clinically significant interaction with loosestrife.

Interactions with Foods
No interactions are known to occur, and there is no known reason to expect a clinically significant interaction with loosestrife.

Interactions with Lab Tests
No interactions are known to occur, and there is no known reason to expect a clinically significant interaction with loosestrife.

Interactions with Diseases or Conditions
No interactions are known to occur, and there is no known reason to expect a clinically significant interaction with loosestrife.

Dosage and Administration
ORAL: No typical dosage.
TOPICAL: Loosestrife is used as a powder (18).

Comments
Both purple loosestrife (Lythrum salicaria) and Lysimachia vulgaris are known as loosestrife and can be confused for each other.
There is very little scientific information about this product. Our staff is continually analyzing the available information on natural medicines and will add data here as it becomes available.

LORENZO'S OIL

Also Known As
Lorenzos Oil, Glycerol Trierucate Oil, Glycerol Trioleate Oil.

Scientific Names
13-Docosenoic acid (erucic acid); cis-9-Octadecenoic acid (oleic acid).

People Use This For
Orally, Lorenzo's oil is used as a treatment for two related genetic neurological syndromes: adrenoleukodystrophy, which occurs in children, and adrenomyeloneuropathy, which occurs in adults (6).

Safety
There is insufficient reliable information available about the safety of Lorenzo's oil.
Pregnancy and Lactation: Insufficient reliable information available; avoid using.

Effectiveness
POSSIBLY EFFECTIVE ...when taken orally in slightly slowing clinical progression of adrenoleukodystrophy when given to asymptomatic patients (928).
LIKELY INEFFECTIVE ...when taken orally for treating adrenoleukodystrophy and adrenomyeloneuropathy (920,921,922,923,924,930). There was one case report of modest clinical benefit in a child with symptomatic adrenoleukodystrophy (929).

Mechanism of Action
Adrenoleukodystrophy and adrenomyeloneuropathy are rare genetic disorders that result in an impaired ability to oxidize saturated, very-long chain fatty acids. Buildup of these acids is thought to cause neurologic symptoms associated with the disorder (6). Monounsaturated fatty acids have been shown to inhibit production of very-long-chain fatty acids (6). However, when Lorenzo's oil is given to patients with adrenoleukodystrophy, eruric acid does not enter the brain in a significant quantity, which may be a factor in the negative results (931).

Adverse Reactions
Asymptomatic thrombocytopenia (924,927), asymptomatic neutropenia (6). One case report of purpura, petechia, and bleeding (926). May cause decrease in plasma docosahexanoic acid levels without essential fatty acid deficiency (individuals studied were also taking supplemental safflower and fish oils) (6).

Interactions with Herbs & Other Dietary Supplements
ESSENTIAL FATTY ACIDS: Supplemental essential fatty acids taken concomitantly may not prevent decreased plasma levels of docosahexaenoic acid (6).

Interactions with Drugs
No interactions are known to occur, and there is no known reason to expect a clinically significant interaction with Lorenzo's oil.

Interactions with Foods
No interactions are known to occur, and there is no known reason to expect a clinically significant interaction with Lorenzo's oil.

Interactions with Lab Tests
PLATELET COUNTS: May cause false low platelet counts (927). High monounsaturated fat diets may cause true thrombocytopenia (925,927). A hand-count of platelets is recommended in individuals taking Lorenzo's oil (927).

Interactions with Diseases or Conditions
THROMBOCYTOPENIA OR NEUTROPENIA: Lorenzo's oil may worsen existing thrombocytopenia or neutropenia.

Dosage and Administration
ORAL: People typically use a mixture of approximately 20% erucic acid and 80% oleic acid (5278). One clinical study used 0.3 gram per kg per day of erucic acid and 1.7 grams per kg of oleic acid per day (5277).

Comments
Lorenzo's oil is a combination of erucic acid and oleic acid in a 1:4 ratio.

LOTUS flower

Also Known As
Lian Fang, Lian Xu.
CAUTION: See separate listing for Lotus seed.

Scientific Names
Nelumbo nucifera.
Family: Nymphaeaceae.

People Use This For
Orally, lotus flowers are used as an astringent for bleeding (18).

Safety
There is insufficient reliable information available about the safety of lotus flower.
Pregnancy and Lactation: Insufficient reliable information available; avoid using.

Effectiveness
There is insufficient reliable information available about the effectiveness of lotus flower.

Mechanism of Action
There is insufficient reliable information available about the possible mechanism of action and active ingredients.

Adverse Reactions
None reported.

Interactions with Herbs & Other Dietary Supplements
Insufficient reliable information available.

Interactions with Drugs
No interactions are known to occur, and there is no known reason to expect a clinically significant interaction with lotus flower.

Interactions with Foods
No interactions are known to occur, and there is no known reason to expect a clinically significant interaction with lotus flower.

Interactions with Lab Tests
No interactions are known to occur, and there is no known reason to expect a clinically significant interaction with lotus flower.

Interactions with Diseases or Conditions
No interactions are known to occur, and there is no known reason to expect a clinically significant interaction with lotus flower.

Dosage and Administration
ORAL: Lotus flower is used as a powder or liquid extract (18).

Comments

There is very little scientific information about this product. Our staff is continually analyzing the available information on natural medicines and will add data here as it becomes available.

LOTUS seed

Also Known As

Lian Zi.
CAUTION: See separate listing for Lotus flower.

Scientific Names

Nelumbo nucifera.
Family: Nymphaeaceae.

People Use This For

Orally, lotus seed is used for digestive disorders and diarrhea (18).

Safety

POSSIBLY SAFE ...when used orally (12).
PREGNANCY AND LACTATION: Insufficient reliable information available; avoid using.

Effectiveness

There is insufficient reliable information available about the effectiveness of lotus seed.

Mechanism of Action

There is insufficient reliable information available about the possible mechanism of action and active ingredients.

Adverse Reactions

None reported.

Interactions with Herbs & Other Dietary Supplements

Insufficient reliable information available.

Interactions with Drugs

No interactions are known to occur, and there is no known reason to expect a clinically significant interaction with lotus seed.

Interactions with Foods

No interactions are known to occur, and there is no known reason to expect a clinically significant interaction with lotus seed.

Interactions with Lab Tests

No interactions are known to occur, and there is no known reason to expect a clinically significant interaction with lotus seed.

Interactions with Diseases or Conditions

GASTROINTESTINAL DISORDERS: Lotus seed is contraindicated in patients with constipation and stomach distention (12).

Dosage and Administration

ORAL: Lotus seed is used as a powder or liquid extract (18).

Comments

There is very little scientific information about this product. Our staff is continually analyzing the available information on natural medicines and will add data here as it becomes available.

LOVAGE

Also Known As
Lavose, Levistici radix, Love Parsley, Maggi Plant, Sea Parsley, Smallage, Smellage.

Scientific Names
Levisticum officinale, synonyms Angelica levisticum, Hipposelinum levisticum, Ligusticum levisticum.
Family: Apiaceae or Umbelliferae.

People Use This For
Orally, lovage is used as "irrigation therapy" for inflammation of the lower urinary tract, for prevention of kidney gravel (2,5,7,18), and as a diuretic for urinary tract infections (18) or pedal edema (6,8).
In folk medicine, lovage is used orally for indigestion, heartburn, stomach distention, and flatulence (5,6,8,11,18).
It is also used orally as an expectorant (11), to loosen secretions in respiratory conditions (6,8,18), for menstrual irregularities (5,8,11,12,18), sore throat (5,6), boils (5,6), jaundice, malaria, pleurisy, gout, rheumatism, and migraines (5).
In foods and beverages, lovage is used as a flavor component (11).
In manufacturing, lovage is used as a fragrance component in soaps and cosmetics (11).

Safety
LIKELY SAFE ...when used orally in amounts commonly found in food (11). Lovage is approved for food use in the US (11).
POSSIBLY SAFE ...when used orally and appropriately (2,12).
PREGNANCY: LIKELY UNSAFE ...when used orally because of possibile uterine or menstrual stimulation (12).
LACTATION: Insufficient reliable information available; avoid using.

Effectiveness
POSSIBLY EFFECTIVE ...when orally as "irrigation therapy" for inflammation of the lower urinary tract and prevention of kidney gravel (2,5,6,8,11). In "irrigation therapy," it is used as a mild diuretic along with copious fluid intake to increase urine flow.
There is insufficient reliable information available about the effectiveness of lovage for its other uses.

Mechanism of Action
The applicable parts of lovage are the rhizome and root. Lovage contains 0.2-2% volatile oil (5,6,8,11,18).
Its principal constituents are lactone derivatives known as phthalides. Of these, ligustilide has sedative (6,8,11,18), antispasmodic (2,6,8,11,18), and aquaretic (5,6,8,11,18,512) effects in experimental animals. Aquaretics increase urine volume (water loss) but not sodium excretion (512). It can also have varied actions including cholinergic and antimicrobial activity (18), increased uterine tone (12), and increased gastrointestinal blood flow (6). The bitter taste and aroma of lovage can increase the production of saliva and gastric juices (6,8,18). Theoretically, the coumarin constituents can cause phototoxic reactions including photosensitivity dermatitis (2,5,6,8,11,12).

Adverse Reactions
Orally, long term use may result in an increased risk of phototoxic reactions, including photosensitivity dermatitis (2,5,6,8,11,12). Avoid excessive exposure to the sun or UV light if using lovage (2,12).

Interactions with Herbs & Other Dietary Supplements
Insufficient reliable information available.

Interactions with Drugs
DIURETICS: Theoretically, lovage root might increase sodium retention and interfere with diuretic therapy (512).

Interactions with Foods
No interactions are known to occur, and there is no known reason to expect a clinically significant interaction with lovage.

Interactions with Lab Tests
No interactions are known to occur, and there is no known reason to expect a clinically significant interaction with lovage.

Interactions with Diseases or Conditions
HYPERTENSION: Theoretically, lovage root might increase sodium retention and worsen hypertension (512).
EDEMA: "Irrigation therapy," which is the use of a mild diuretic and copious fluid intake to increase urine flow, is

contraindicated in cases of edema that are due to limited heart or kidney function (2).

RENAL DISEASE: Lovage is contraindicated in acute kidney inflammation (2,8,12) or impaired kidney function (2,12).

Dosage and Administration

ORAL: The typical dose of lovage is one cup of the tea two to three times per day (8). The tea is prepared by steeping 1.5-3 grams of the dried root in 150 mL boiling water for 10-15 minutes and then straining. Lovage should only be used up to 4-8 grams of the dried root per day (2,7). Ample fluid intake is essential when used for "irrigation therapy" (18). For stomach complaints, one cup of the tea is commonly taken 30 minutes before meals (8). Avoid excessive sun or UV light exposure with prolonged use of lovage due to its phototoxic adverse effects.

Comments

None.

LUFFA

Also Known As

Angled Loofah, Dishcloth Sponge, Loofa, Loofah, Luffaschwamm, Sigualuo, Silky Loofah, Smooth Loofah, Sponge Cucumber, Vegetable Sponge, Water Gourd.

Scientific Names

Luffa aegyptiaca; Luffa acutangula; Luffa cylindrica.
Family: Cucurbitaceae.

People Use This For

Orally, luffa is used for treating and preventing colds, nasal inflammation, sinusitis, and suppuration of the sinuses (2,18).

Topically, luffa sponge is used to remove dead skin and stimulate the skin. Luffa charcoal is used topically for shingles in the face and eye region.

In Chinese medicine, luffa is used orally for arthritis and associated pain, muscle pain, chest pain, amenorrhea, and to promote lactation.

For food uses, young luffa fruits are eaten as vegetables (11).

In cosmetics, powdered luffa is used in skin care products as an anti-inflammatory and detoxicant.

Safety

LIKELY SAFE ...when used topically as a sponge for exfoliation (11).

POSSIBLY SAFE ...when used orally in amounts found in foods (11).

There is insufficient reliable information available about the safety of luffa for its other uses.

PREGNANCY AND LACTATION: POSSIBLY SAFE ...when used orally in amounts found in foods (11).

POSSIBLY UNSAFE ...when used orally in amounts greater than those typically found in foods.

Effectiveness

There is insufficient reliable information available about the effectiveness of luffa.

Mechanism of Action

The applicable part of luffa is the dried fiber structure from the ripe fruit. The toxicity of luffa is low.

Adverse Reactions

None reported.

Interactions with Herbs & Other Dietary Supplements

Insufficient reliable information available.

Interactions with Drugs

No interactions are known to occur, and there is no known reason to expect a clinically significant interaction with luffa.

Interactions with Foods

No interactions are known to occur, and there is no known reason to expect a clinically significant interaction with luffa.

Interactions with Lab Tests

No interactions are known to occur, and there is no known reason to expect a clinically significant interaction with luffa.

Interactions with Diseases or Conditions

No interactions are known to occur, and there is no known reason to expect a clinically significant interaction with luffa.

Dosage and Administration

ORAL: No typical dosage.
TOPICAL: Luffa is powdered and used in skin care products. The intact sponge is also used to remove dead skin (11).

Comments

None.

LUNGMOSS

Also Known As

Lungwort, Oak Lungs.
CAUTION: See separate listing for Lungwort.

Scientific Names

Lobaria pulmonaria.
Family: Lobariaceae.

People Use This For

Orally, lungmoss is used for bronchitis, asthma, and coughs, including irritable cough and smoker's cough. It is also used orally as an expectorant, anti-inflammatory, antimicrobial and to promote sweating (18).

Safety

There is insufficient reliable information available about the safety of lungmoss.
Pregnancy and Lactation: Insufficient reliable information available; avoid using.

Effectiveness

There is insufficient reliable information available about the effectiveness of lungmoss.

Mechanism of Action

There is insufficient reliable information available about the possible mechanism of action and active ingredients.

Adverse Reactions

None reported.

Interactions with Herbs & Other Dietary Supplements

Insufficient reliable information available.

Interactions with Drugs

No interactions are known to occur, and there is no known reason to expect a clinically significant interaction with lungmoss.

Interactions with Foods

No interactions are known to occur, and there is no known reason to expect a clinically significant interaction with lungmoss.

Interactions with Lab Tests

No interactions are known to occur, and there is no known reason to expect a clinically significant interaction with lungmoss.

Interactions with Diseases or Conditions

No interactions are known to occur, and there is no known reason to expect a clinically significant interaction with lungmoss.

Dosage and Administration

ORAL: Lungmoss is used as a powder or a liquid extract (18).

Comments

Lungmoss and Pulmonaria officinalis are both known as lungwort, but are physically distinct. Lungmoss is a lichen; Pulmonaria officinalis is a plant (18).

There is very little scientific information about this product. Our staff is continually analyzing the available information on natural medicines and will add data here as it becomes available.

LUNGWORT

Also Known As

Dage of Jerusalem, Lungenkraut, Pulmonariae herba.
CAUTION: See separate listing for Lungmoss.

Scientific Names

Pulmonaria officinalis.
Family: Boraginaceae.

People Use This For

Orally, lungwort is used for the treatment of conditions of the respiratory tract, gastrointestinal tract, the kidney and urinary tract.

Topically, it is used as an astringent and for wound treatment (2).

In folk medicine, it is used orally in irritant-relieving cough medicine, as a diuretic, and to treat lung diseases such as tuberculosis (18).

Safety

There is insufficient reliable information available about the safety of lungwort.
Pregnancy and Lactation: Insufficient reliable information available; avoid using.

Effectiveness

There is insufficient reliable information available about the effectiveness of lungwort.

Mechanism of Action

The applicable parts of lungwort are the above ground parts. Lungwort was thought to contain hepatotoxic pyrrolizidine alkaloids, but gas chromatography analysis of multiple samples failed to detect these compounds (12).

Adverse Reactions

None reported.

Interactions with Herbs & Other Dietary Supplements

Insufficient reliable information available.

Interactions with Drugs

No interactions are known to occur, and there is no known reason to expect a clinically significant interaction with lungwort.

Interactions with Foods

No interactions are known to occur, and there is no known reason to expect a clinically significant interaction with lungwort.

Interactions with Lab Tests

No interactions are known to occur, and there is no known reason to expect a clinically significant interaction with lungwort.

Interactions with Diseases or Conditions

No interactions are known to occur, and there is no known reason to expect a clinically significant interaction with lungwort.

Dosage and Administration

ORAL: One cup of tea taken as sips repeatedly with honey throughout the day. The tea is prepared by heating or scalding 1.5 grams dried herb rapidly in 150 mL of boiling water, then straining for 5-10 minutes (18).

Comments

The taste of lungwort is described as dry and slimy. Pulmonaria officinalis and lungmoss are both known as lungwort. However, they are physically distinct because Pulmonaria officinalis is a plant and lungmoss is a lichen (see separate listing). In addition, lungwort can easily be mistaken for other Pulmoniaria species, particularly Pulmonaria mollis (18).

LUTEIN

Also Known As

Xanthophyll, Zeaxanthin.

Scientific Names

Beta, Epsilon-Carotene-3, 31-diol.

People Use This For

Orally, lutein is used for preventing age-related macular degeneration (2394), cataracts (2386,2394), and colon cancer (3962).

Safety

LIKELY SAFE ...when used orally (219,3219,3220).
PREGNANCY AND LACTATION: LIKELY SAFE ...when used orally (219,3219,3220).

Effectiveness

POSSIBLY EFFECTIVE ...when dietary lutein is consumed to reduce the risk of age-related macular degeneration (219,2394). There is some evidence from epidemiological studies that shows reduced risk of developing age-related macular degeneration in people consuming higher amounts of lutein in their diet (219,2394). It is not known if supplemental lutein offers the same benefit. ...when dietary lutein is consumed for reducing the risk of developing cataracts severe enough to require surgical removal (2395,3219,3220). There is some evidence from epidemiological studies that shows reduced risk of developing severe cataracts in people consuming higher amounts of lutein in their diet (2395,3129,3220). It is not known if supplemental lutein offers the same benefit. ...when dietary lutein is consumed for reducing the risk of developing colon cancer (3962). There is some epidemiological evidence that shows reduced risk of developing colon cancer in people consuming higher amounts of lutein in their diet. It is not known if supplemental lutein offers the same benefit.

Mechanism of Action

Lutein is a carotenoid that is typically found in combination with its stereoisomer, zeaxanthin. They are the two major carotenoids found as a pigment in the human macula and retina (2388,3225). They are thought to function as antioxidants and as a blue light filter protecting underlying ocular tissues from photodamage. Epidemiological evidence associates high dietary lutein intake with reduced risk of developing age-related macular degeneration and cataracts (2394,2395,3219,3220). Increasing dietary lutein intake increases serum lutein levels and macular pigment density (2389). Low dietary lutein intake is associated with males, smokers, and people who drink alcohol (more than 2 drinks per week), while higher dietary lutein intake is associated with females, increasing age, and people with hypertension (2398). Foods containing high concentrations of lutein such as broccoli, spinach, and kale, are associated with the greatest eye health benefits (3219,3220). Other carotenoids and antioxidants such as vitamin A, lycopene, alpha- or beta-carotene, vitamin C, and vitamin E have not been associated with this benefit (3219,3220,3221,3222,3223). Epidemiologic studies have shown that carotenoids might be inversely associated with cancer (3963,3964). Supplemental esterified lutein is better absorbed when taken with high fat (36 grams fat) meals compared to low-fat (3 grams fat) meals (6133).

Adverse Reactions

None reported.

Interactions with Herbs & Other Dietary Supplements

BETA-CAROTENE: Concomitant administration may reduce bioavailability of lutein and may reduce or increase bioavailability of beta-carotene (2390,2391).

Interactions with Drugs
No interactions are known to occur, and there is no known reason to expect a clinically significant interaction with lutein.

Interactions with Foods
OLESTRA: Theoretically, may interfere with supplemental lutein activity. Olestra (fat substitute) lowers serum lutein concentrations in healthy people (2392).

Interactions with Lab Tests
No interactions are known to occur, and there is no known reason to expect a clinically significant interaction with lutein.

Interactions with Diseases or Conditions
No interactions are known to occur, and there is no known reason to expect a clinically significant interaction with lutein.

Dosage and Administration
ORAL: For reducing the risk of cataracts and macular degeneration, 6 mg of lutein per day, either through diet or supplementation has been suggested. People consuming 6.9-11.7 mg of lutein per day through diet had the lowest risk of developing age-related macular degeneration and cataracts (3219,3220). There is 44 mg of lutein per cup of cooked kale, 26 mg/cup of cooked spinach, and 3 mg/cup of broccoli (219,3219,3220). Commercial products containing 6 mg or 20 mg of lutein are available (5020). Supplemental esterified lutein is better absorbed when taken with high fat (36 grams fat) meals compared to low-fat (3 grams fat) meals (6133).

Comments
Centrum and Centrum Silver now contain lutein 0.25 mg per tablet, but probably not enough to provide much benefit (219,3219,3220). Avoid confusion with lutein extract (dried powdered hog corpora lutea) formerly used as a source of progesterone (511). Although dark green leafy vegetables contain 15-47% lutein, they have a very low zeaxanthin content (0-3%). Corn is richest in lutein (60% of total carotenoids), and orange pepper is richest in zeaxanthin (37% of total). Substantial amounts of lutein and zeaxanthin (30-50%) are also present in kiwi fruit, grapes, spinach, orange juice, zucchini, and different kinds of squash (3224).

LYCIUM

Also Known As
Chinese Wolfberry, Di Gu Pi, Digupi, Fructus Lycii, Fructus Lycii Berry, Gou Qi Zi, Gouqizi, Lycii Berries, Matrimony Vine, Wolfberry.

Scientific Names
Lycium chinense, Synonym Lycium barbarum.
Family: Solanaceae.

People Use This For
Orally, lycium is used for diabetes, hypertension, fever, malaria, and cancer. It's also used for improving circulation, erectile dysfunction, dizziness, and tinnitus. It is used as an eye tonic for blurred vision, macular degeneration, and other ophthalmic disorders. Lycium is also used orally to strengthen muscles and bone, and as a blood, liver, and kidney tonic. It is used orally in to reduce fever, sweating, irritability, thirst, nosebleeds, hemoptysis, cough and wheezing.
In foods, the berries are eaten raw and used in cooking.

Safety
POSSIBLY SAFE …when used orally and appropriately (12,7126).
PREGNANCY AND LACTATION: LIKELY UNSAFE …when used orally. Lycium contains betaine, which is an emmenagogue and abortifacient (12,7123); avoid using.

Effectiveness
There is insufficient reliable information available about the effectiveness of lycium.

Mechanism of Action
The applicable parts of lycium are the dried berries and root bark. Both the root bark and berries contain

pharmacologically active constituents. Both contain beta-sitosterol (see separate listing for Beta-Sitosterol) which can reduce cholesterol levels by preventing cholesterol absorption in the gastrointestinal tract (5814,7123,7126). The root bark also contains the constituent kukoamine, which might also have cholesterol lowering effects and antihypertensive effects (7123,7126). Lycium root bark also seems to have hypoglycemic effects. Peak blood glucose lowering effects are thought to occur after 3-4 hours and last for 7-8 hours. Lycium root bark is also thought to have antibacterial, antipyretic, and antihypersensitivity properties (7126). Both the root bark and berry contain betaine, which has uterine stimulant properties (7123,7126). The berries also contain beta-carotene, niacin, pyridoxine, and ascorbic acid (7123). There is some preliminary evidence that a cerebroside constituent found in lycium berry might also have hepatoprotective properties (7125).

Adverse Reactions
Orally, the dried root bark has been associated with nausea and vomiting (7126).

Interactions with Herbs & Other Dietary Supplements
HERBS WITH ANTICOAGULANT/ANTIPLATELET POTENTIAL: Concomitant use of herbs that affect platelet aggregation could theoretically increase the risk of bleeding in some people. Some of these herbs include angelica, anise, arnica, asafoetida, bogbean, boldo, capsicum, celery, chamomile, clove, danshen, fenugreek, feverfew, garlic, ginger, ginkgo, Panax ginseng, horse chestnut, horseradish, licorice, meadowsweet, prickly ash, onion, papain, passionflower, poplar, quassia, red clover, turmeric, wild carrot, wild lettuce, willow, and others (4,19).
HERBS AND SUPPLEMENTS WITH HYPOTENSIVE EFFECTS: Lycium root bark might have antihypertensive effects (7126). Theoretically, concurrent use of lycium root bark with other herbs and supplements that decrease blood pressure might increase risk of hypotension. Some of these products include danshen, ginger, Panax ginseng, turmeric, valerian, and others.
HERBS AND SUPPLEMENTS WITH HYPOGLYCEMIC EFFECTS: Lycium root bark might have hypoglycemic effects (7126). Theoretically, concomitant use with other herbs and supplements that decrease blood glucose levels might increase the risk of hypoglycemia. Some of these products include bitter melon, ginger, goat's rue, fenugreek, kudzu, willow bark, and others.

Interactions with Drugs
ANTIHYPERTENSIVE DRUGS: Lycium root bark might have hypotensive effects (7126). Theoretically, concomitant use with antihypertensives might have additive effects on blood pressure and increase the risk of hypotension.
ANTIDIABETES DRUGS: Lycium root bark might have hypoglycemic effects (7126). Theoretically, concomitant use with drugs used for diabetes might enhance blood glucose lowering effects and increase the risk of hypoglycemia. Monitor blood glucose levels closely. Some antidiabetes drugs include glimepiride (Amaryl), glyburide (Diabeta, Glynase PresTab, Micronase), insulin, pioglitazone (Actos), rosiglitazone (Avandia), and others.
WARFARIN (Coumadin): There is some evidence that lycium can increase the effects of warfarin and possibly increase the risk of bleeding. International normalized ratio (INR) can increase in patients stabilized on warfarin who begin taking lycium. Researchers think that lycium inhibits cytochrome P450 2C9 metabolism of warfarin and increases warfarin levels (7158). Use with caution. Warfarin dose adjustments may be necessary.

Interactions with Foods
No interactions are known to occur, and there is no known reason to expect a clinically significant interaction with lycium.

Interactions with Lab Tests
WHITE BLOOD CELL COUNT (WBC): Lycium berries might increase leukocyte and lymphocyte counts in some patients (7126).
BLOOD GLUCOSE: Lycium root bark might lower blood glucose levels in some patients (7126).

Interactions with Diseases or Conditions
DIABETES: Lycium root bark might have hypoglycemic effects (7126). Theoretically, use in patients treated with antidiabetes medications might enhance blood glucose lowering effects and increase the risk of hypoglycemia. Monitor blood glucose levels closely (7126).
HYPERTENSION: Lycium root bark might have hypotensive effects (7126). Theoretically, concomitant use in patients treated with antihypertensives might have additive effects on blood pressure and potentially increase the risk of hypotension.
HYPOTENSION: Lycium root bark might have hypotensive effects (7126). Theoretically, use in people with existing low blood pressure might exacerbate hypotension and possibly lead to syncope.

Dosage and Administration
ORAL: Lycium is usually taken as a tea. A typical dose is one or more cups of tea daily; however, the strength of the

tea can vary depending on the condition being treated. Typically the tea is made by boiling 20 grams of berries or root bark in 3 cups of water and simmered until the volume is reduced to 2 cups. For fever, one cup daily of this preparation is commonly used (7122). For diabetes, 6 to 12 grams is commonly boiled and consumed as a tea. For hypertension, 30 grams of the root bark boiled in 100 mL is commonly used. For treating malaria, 30 grams of the root bark is commonly boiled and consumed as a tea (7126).

Comments

Lycium is a native Chinese deciduous shrub with bright red berries. The use of lycium was first described in the first century AD in Chinese literature. Traditionally, lycium has been used to promote longevity. Legend reports that one herbalist who used lycium in combination with other tonic herbs lived 252 years (7122).

LYCOPENE

Also Known As
All-Trans Lycopene, Psi-Psi-Carotene.

Scientific Names
All-Trans-Lycopene, Lycopene, Psi-Psi-Carotene.

People Use This For
Orally, lycopene is used for preventing atherosclerosis and cancer.

Safety
LIKELY SAFE …when consumed in amounts found in foods.
There is insufficient reliable information available about the safety of lycopene supplements.
PREGNANCY AND LACTATION: LIKELY SAFE …when consumed in amounts found in foods. There is insufficient reliable information available about the safety of lycopene supplements; avoid using in amounts greater than those typically found in foods.

Effectiveness
POSSIBLY EFFECTIVE ...when dietary lycopene is used to prevent prostate cancer. There is epidemiological evidence that consumption of lycopene 6 mg per day or more from foods such as tomatoes and tomato products can significantly reduce the risk of prostate cancer (2406). ...when dietary lycopene and other carotenoids are used to prevent lung cancer. There is epidemiological evidence that consumption of lycopene from foods (12 mg per day or more for men, and 6.5 mg per day or more for women) decreases the risk of lung cancer in non-smoking men aged 40 to 75, and non-smoking women aged 30 to 55 (2595).
POSSIBLY INEFFECTIVE ...when dietary lycopene is used for reducing the risk of bladder cancer. Epidemiological studies find no association between dietary lycopene intake or serum lycopene levels and the risk of bladder cancer (2407).
There is insufficient reliable information available to rate the effectiveness of lycopene for its other uses. Epidemiological studies of serum lycopene concentrations and the risk of cancers of the breast, cervix, esophagus, larynx, ovaries, and pancreas are inconclusive (1444,2407). Epidemiological studies of dietary lycopene intake and prevention of atherosclerosis are also inconclusive (1446,1449).

Mechanism of Action
Lycopene is the pigment that gives fruits and vegetables such as tomatoes their red color (1928,2401). It is also found in watermelons, pink-grapefruits, apricots, and pink-guavas. In North America, 85% of dietary lycopene comes from tomato-derived products such as tomato juice or paste. One cup (240 mL) of tomato juice provides about 23 mg of lycopene (1499). Lycopene is considered a carotenoid, but it has no vitamin A activity (1928). Lycopene exists naturally in fresh fruits and vegetables in the trans-configuration, which is poorly absorbed (1928). Heat processing of foods such as tomatoes into products such as tomato paste, juice, ketchup, and others induces the isomerization of lycopene from the trans to the cis-configuration. The cis isomer has better bioavailability (1928,1497). Lycopene supplements seem to be similarly bioavailable as foods containing the cis-isomer since lycopene supplements can provide similar serum lycopene levels as tomato juice when ingested in equivalent amounts (1498). Lycopene is highly lipophilic and is commonly found within cellular membranes. Lycopene has antioxidant activity and can scavenge free radicals and quench singlet oxygen (2401). So some researchers are interested in lycopene for prevention of cancer, atherosclerosis, and other conditions. In vitro, lycopene does seem to inhibit the oxidation of low density lipoproteins (LDL) (1928). In cultures, lycopene also inhibits the proliferation of breast, lung, and prostate cancer cells (1928). There is also some evidence that decreased serum or tissue lycopene concentrations might increase the risk of developing prostate cancer (1447,1496,2405,2406,2407).

Adverse Reactions

None reported.

Interactions with Herbs & Other Dietary Supplements

BETA-CAROTENE: Concomitant ingestion may increase lycopene absorption (2403).

Interactions with Drugs

No interactions are known to occur, and there is no known reason to expect a clinically significant interaction with lycopene.

Interactions with Foods

No interactions are known to occur, and there is no known reason to expect a clinically significant interaction with lycopene.

Interactions with Lab Tests

No interactions are known to occur, and there is no known reason to expect a clinically significant interaction with lycopene.

Interactions with Diseases or Conditions

No interactions are known to occur, and there is no known reason to expect a clinically significant interaction with lycopene.

Dosage and Administration

ORAL: For reducing the risk of prostate cancer, at least 6 mg of lycopene per day from foods is needed (2406). For reducing the risk of lung cancer in non-smoking men, at least 12 mg of lycopene per day from foods is needed (2595). For reducing the risk of lung cancer in non-smoking women, at least 6.5 mg of lycopene per day from foods is needed (2595).

Comments

None.

LYSINE

Also Known As

L-Lysine, Lys, Lysine Hydrochloride, Lysine Monohydrochloride.

Scientific Names

L-2,6-diaminohexanoic acid.

People Use This For

Orally, lysine is used for preventing and treating clinical symptoms of recurrent herpes simplex labialis (1114). It is also used as an aid to improving athletic performance (217).
Lysine monohydrochloride is used to treat metabolic alkalosis (14).

Safety

POSSIBLY SAFE ...when used orally and appropriately for up to one year (1114,1120).
PREGNANCY AND LACTATION: Insufficient reliable information available; avoid using.

Effectiveness

POSSIBLY EFFECTIVE ...when used orally for reducing recurrences of herpes simplex labialis infections (1114,1115,1116,1118,1120) and for reducing severity and healing time of herpes simplex labialis infections (1119,1120). ...when lysine monohydrochloride is used for treating metabolic alkalosis (14).

Mechanism of Action

Lysine is required for collagen synthesis and it may be important to bone health (1124,1130). Lysine antagonizes herpes simplex virus (HSV) growth in vitro and this effect may be important clinically (119).

Adverse Reactions

Orally, diarrhea and abdominal pain occur with use of 10 grams per day for five days (14). There is one case report of supplemental lysine use associated with tubulointerstitial nephritis progressing to chronic renal failure (1121).

Interactions with Herbs & Other Dietary Supplements

CALCIUM SUPPLEMENTS: Concomitant use may increase supplemental calcium absorption and decrease urine calcium loss (1131).

Interactions with Drugs

CALCIUM: Concomitant use may increase supplemental calcium absorption and decrease urine calcium loss (1131).

Interactions with Foods

No interactions are known to occur, and there is no known reason to expect a clinically significant interaction with lysine.

Interactions with Lab Tests

No interactions are known to occur, and there is no known reason to expect a clinically significant interaction with lysine.

Interactions with Diseases or Conditions

KIDNEY DISEASES: There is one case report of supplemental lysine associated with tubulointerstitial nephritis progressing to chronic renal failure (1121).
OSTEOPOROSIS: Concomitant use of lysine and calcium supplements may increase supplemental calcium absorption and decrease urine calcium loss (1131).

Dosage and Administration

ORAL: Recurrent herpes simplex labialis infections, 1000 mg daily for twelve months and 1000 mg three times daily for six months reported in clinical trials (1114,1120). Metabolic alkalosis, 10 grams per day in divided doses for up to five days (14).

Comments

None.

MACA

Also Known As

Ayak Chichira, Ayuk Willku, Maca Maca, Maino, Maka, Peruvian Ginseng.

Scientific Names

Lepidium meyenii.
Family: Brassicaceae.

People Use This For

Orally, maca is used for anemia; chronic fatigue syndrome; enhancing energy, stamina, athletic performance and memory; female hormone imbalance, menstrual irregularities; enhancing fertility; menopause symptoms; stomach cancer; tuberculosis; as an aphrodisiac; for impotence; and as an immunostimulant (3918).
For food uses, maca is eaten baked or roasted, prepared as a porridge, and used for making a fermented drink (3918).

Safety

LIKELY SAFE ...when maca is consumed in food amounts (6).
There is insufficient reliable information available about the safety of maca when used orally in therapeutic amounts.
PREGNANCY AND LACTATION: LIKELY SAFE ...when consumed in food amounts (6). There is insufficient reliable information available about the safety of maca in amounts greater than used as food; avoid using amounts greater than found in food.

Effectiveness

There is insufficient reliable information available about the effectiveness of maca.

Mechanism of Action

The applicable part of maca is the root which contains fatty acids and essential amino acids (6).

Adverse Reactions

None reported.

Interactions with Herbs & Other Dietary Supplements

Insufficient reliable information available.

Interactions with Drugs

No interactions are known to occur, and there is no known reason to expect a clinically significant interaction with maca.

Interactions with Foods

No interactions are known to occur, and there is no known reason to expect a clinically significant interaction with maca.

Interactions with Lab Tests

No interactions are known to occur, and there is no known reason to expect a clinically significant interaction with maca.

Interactions with Diseases or Conditions

No interactions are known to occur, and there is no known reason to expect a clinically significant interaction with maca.

Dosage and Administration

ORAL: People typically use 1500 to 6000 mg or more per day in three divided doses. A teaspoon of root powder, containing 2800 mg of maca root, is used in 8 ounces of water three times daily.

Comments

Maca root has been cultivated as a vegetable crop in the Andes Mountains of Peru for at least 2000 years [6].

MADAGASCAR PERIWINKLE

Also Known As

Cape Periwinkle, Catharanthus, Church-Flower, Magdalena, Myrtle, Old Maid, Periwinkle, Ram-Goat Rose, Red Periwinkle.
CAUTION: See separate listing for Periwinkle.

Scientific Names

Catharanthus roseus, synonym Vinca rosea; Lochnera rosea, synonym Ammocallis rosea.
Family: Apocynaceae.

People Use This For

Orally, Madagascar periwinkle is used for diabetes, cancer [6], as a cough remedy, for easing lung congestion, throat inflammation, and as a diuretic [3820].
Topically, it is used as a hemostatic [3820], for insect bites [6], wasp stings, eye irritation, infection [3820], and inflammation [6].

Safety

LIKELY UNSAFE ...when the plant or root are used orally. Madagascar periwinkle contains vinca alkaloids which can cause death [6,3820].
There is insufficient reliable information available about the safety of the topical use of Madagascar periwinkle.
PREGNANCY: LIKELY UNSAFE ...when used orally because it has abortifacient and teratogenic properties [19].
LACTATION: LIKELY UNSAFE ...when used orally [6,3820]; avoid using.

Effectiveness

There is insufficient reliable information about the effectiveness of Madagascar periwinkle.

Mechanism of Action

The applicable parts of Madagascar periwinkle are the above ground parts. The constituent vinca alkaloids, vincristine and vinblastine, block cell mitosis, have immunosuppressive effects, and in high concentrations, exert effects on nucleic acid and protein synthesis [6,15]. The constituent, catharanthine, demonstrates diuretic properties [6]. Hypotensive constituents, reserpine and alstonine, have been isolated from Madagascar periwinkle root [6]. The constituent, ajmalicine, may improve cerebral blood flow, and has been combined with rauwolfia alkaloids for treating high blood pressure (6). Concentrated extracts are reported to lower blood glucose (6), but studies by one pharmaceutical company found the plant had no effect on blood glucose levels (6).

Adverse Reactions
Taken orally, the plant is an hallucinogen, and has caused seizures, GI upset, hepatotoxicity, and alopecia (17). Adverse effects of Vinca alkaloids include nausea, vomiting, alopecia, dizziness, nystagmus, vertigo, hearing impairment, leukopenia, thrombocytopenia, bleeding, hyperuricemia, neurotoxicity, (15), and possibly death (6).

Interactions with Herbs & Other Dietary Supplements
Insufficient reliable information available.

Interactions with Drugs
ANTIDIABETES DRUGS: Madagascar periwinkle may cause hypoglycemia (6,19); monitor blood glucose control closely.

Interactions with Foods
No interactions are known to occur, and there is no known reason to expect a clinically significant interaction with Madagascar periwinkle.

Interactions with Lab Tests
BLOOD GLUCOSE: Conflicting information about possible hypoglycemic activity (6,19); may lower blood glucose.

Interactions with Diseases or Conditions
DIABETES: May cause hypoglycemia (6,19).

Dosage and Administration
No typical dosage.

Comments
Madagascar periwinkle is considered likely unsafe; avoid, due to presence of toxic vinca alkaloids. The vinca alkaloids, vinblastine and vincristine, isolated from Madagascar periwinkle, are FDA approved for use as chemotherapeutic agents to treat cancers, including Hodgkin's disease, leukemia, Kaposi's sarcoma, malignant lymphomas, mycosis fungoides neuroblastoma, and Wilm's tumor (6).

MADDER

Also Known As
Dyer's Madder, Farberrote, Garance, Robbia, Rubia, Rubiae tinctorum radix.

Scientific Names
Rubia tinctorum.
Family: Rubiaceae.

People Use This For
Orally, madder is used for preventing kidney stones and for disintegrating kidney stones (2,18).
Historically, madder has been used for menstrual and urinary disorders (18).

Safety
LIKELY UNSAFE ...when used orally. It is potentially carcinogenic and mutagenic (2,18,19).
PREGNANCY: UNSAFE ...when used orally because it may be a potential menstrual stimulant and a genotoxin (2,19).
LACTATION: UNSAFE ...when used orally because it is a potential genotoxin (2,19). It also can cause red-colored breast milk (2).

Effectiveness
There is insufficient reliable information available about the effectiveness of madder.

Mechanism of Action
The applicable part of madder is the root. Madder contains lucidin, which is an anthracene derivative. The Ames test shows that anthracene has genotoxic activity, and causes dose-dependent increases in benign and malignant liver and

kidney tumors in experimental rats (3718). Madder also seems to decrease calcium oxalate crystallization in the kidney, which potentially could induce kidney or bladder stones (2).

Adverse Reactions
Orally, madder can cause red colored urine, saliva, perspiration, and breast milk (2). There is some concern that madder can stain contact lenses. Advise patients to be cautious (7003).

Interactions with Herbs & Other Dietary Supplements
Insufficient reliable information available.

Interactions with Drugs
No interactions are known to occur, and there is no known reason to expect a clinically significant interaction with madder.

Interactions with Foods
No interactions are known to occur, and there is no known reason to expect a clinically significant interaction with madder.

Interactions with Lab Tests
COLORIMETRIC TESTS: Theoretically, madder might interfere with colorimetric tests involving urine, saliva, perspiration, and breast milk due to red coloring of these body fluids (2).

Interactions with Diseases or Conditions
No interactions are known to occur, and there is no known reason to expect a clinically significant interaction with madder.

Dosage and Administration
ORAL: People typically prepare madder bark using one teaspoon boiled in a covered container with 3 cups of water for 30 minutes. The liquid is cooled slowly in the closed container and taken cold, 1 to 2 cups per day (5254).

Comments
None.

MAGGOTS

Also Known As
Botfly Maggot, Fly Larva, Grub, Living Antiseptic, Surgical Maggot, Viable Antiseptic.

Scientific Names
Lucilia sericata; Phormia regina; and other Calliphoridae family of flies.
Family: Calliphoridae.

People Use This For
Topically, maggots are used for treating infected or necrotic skin wounds including pressure ulcers (14,4946,4949,4994,4995,4996,4997), diabetic foot ulcers (14,4948), venous stasis ulcers (14,4994,4945,4996,4997), abscesses (14,4946,4947,4996,4997,4998), osteomyelitis (14,4989,4990,4991,4992,4993,4994,4995,4996,4997,4998), mastoiditis (4996,4999), empyema (4996), carbuncles (4995,4997), soft tissue wounds (4995,4996,4997,4998), burns (4996), and otitis media (14).

Safety
LIKELY SAFE ...when used topically and when sterile, laboratory-produced larvae are used (14,4951,4986).
LIKELY UNSAFE ...when used topically for self-treatment.
PREGNANCY AND LACTATION: Insufficient reliable information available; avoid using.

Effectiveness
POSSIBLY EFFECTIVE ...when used topically for treating infected or necrotic skin wounds including pressure ulcers (14,4946,4949,4994,4995,4996,4997), diabetic foot ulcers (14,4948), venous stasis ulcers (14,4994,4945,4996,4997), abscesses (14,4946,4947,4996,4997,4998), osteomyelitis (14,4989,4990,4991,4992,4993,4994,4995,4996,4997,4998), mastoiditis (4996,4999), empyema (4996), carbuncles (4995,4997), soft tissue wounds (4995,4996,4997,4998), burns (4996), and otitis media (14).

Mechanism of Action

Maggots can improve wound-healing by various mechanisms. They can kill bacteria by producing natural antibiotic-like substances, by raising wound pH, and by ingesting and destroying bacteria through normal feeding behavior (14,4946,4948,4950,5100). They can promote regrowth of healthy granulation tissue by secreting proteolytic enzymes that liquefy necrotic tissue, such as collagenase. They consume necrotic tissue as food. Maggots are irritating to the wound, which can induce serous exudate to mechanically wash out the bacteria. Substances with healing actions such as allantoin, urea, calcium carbonate, and ammonium bicarbonate can be secreted by maggots. The larvae also excrete growth-stimulating factors. In addition, the continuous crawling of the larvae mechanically stimulates viable tissue (14,4946,4948,4950,5101,5102). Maggots do not attack healthy tissue (4946) and cannot multiply within the wound, and the mature breeding insect cannot develop in the wound (4946).

Adverse Reactions

Topically, maggots can cause pain and intense local pruritus, which can require analgesics or sedation (14,4946,4948,4950,4986). If non-sterile larvae are used, wounds can become contaminated with pathogenic organisms, although bacteria cultured from leprous ulcers infected with maggots did not differ from uninfected ulcers (4946,4952). Rarely, a large number of larvae in a granulating wound have caused bleeding, possibly as a result of proteolytic enzymes produced by larvae (4946). Although allergic reactions have not been reported, theoretically they are possible due to the foreign protein of the larvae (4946).

Interactions with Herbs & Other Dietary Supplements

Insufficient reliable information available.

Interactions with Drugs

No interactions are known to occur, and there is no known reason to expect a clinically significant interaction with maggots.

Interactions with Foods

No interactions are known to occur, and there is no known reason to expect a clinically significant interaction with maggots.

Interactions with Lab Tests

No interactions are known to occur, and there is no known reason to expect a clinically significant interaction with maggots.

Interactions with Diseases or Conditions

No interactions are known to occur, and there is no known reason to expect a clinically significant interaction with maggots.

Dosage and Administration

TOPICAL: Depending on the size and depth of the wound, between 50 to 1000 maggots are typically applied to the skin two to five times weekly and left in place usually for 72 hours (14,4946,4948). No more than 10 larvae per square cm should be placed in a wound, and fewer should be used if the wound contains a limited amount of necrotic tissue (4986). About 200 to 600 maggots will consume 10 to 15 grams of necrotic tissue per day (4946). After 72 hours, the larvae will be about one-half inch long, readily visible, and actively crawling (4946). At this time, they should be removed with forceps and a saline lavage (14,4946,4986) and then destroyed (4946,4986). Repeat treatments might be required (4948,4946). Specialized dressings have been developed to prevent larval escape and to absorb exudate or liquefied necrotic tissue (4953,4986).

Comments

Maggots are the larvae of flies. For therapeutic purposes, the most commonly used are the larvae of the green bottle fly or green blow fly (Lucilia sericata) (14,4986) and the black blow fly or black bottle blow fly (Phormia regina) (14,4999). Maggots were commonly used by surgeons to treat skin and bone infections in the US and Europe during the 1930s and early 1940s (4945,4948). Lucilia sericata larva were produced commercially by Lederle (4988). With the advent of antibiotics and surgical debridement, the use of maggots was largely abandoned until the late 1980s (4948). Prior to therapy, patients should be counseled about efficacy and the possible adverse reactions. They should be reassured that maggots do not attack healthy tissue, do not multiply within the wound, and will be removed and killed before the larvae develop into mature insects (4986). Maggot treatment is also called biosurgery (4986).

MAGNESIUM

Also Known As

Magnesia, Chelated Magnesium, Magnesium Aspartate, Magnesium Carbonate, Magnesium Chloride, Magnesium Citrate, Magnesium Gluconate, Magnesium Hydroxide, Magnesium Lactate, Magnesium Orotate, Magnesium Oxide, Magnesium Sulfate, Magnesium Trisilicate, Epsom salts, Milk of Magnesia.
CAUTION: See separate listings for Chelated Minerals and Dolomite.

Scientific Names

Magnesium; Mg; atomic number 12.

People Use This For

Orally, magnesium is used for treating and preventing hypomagnesemia. It is also used orally as a laxative for constipation and preparation of the bowel for surgical or diagnostic procedures. Magnesium is also used orally for treating symptoms of asthma; for cardiovascular diseases including angina, arrhythmias, hypertension, coronary heart disease and hyperlipidemia, low high-density lipoprotein (HDL) levels, mitral valve prolapse, and myocardial infarction; and as an antacid for symptoms of gastric hyperacidity. It is also used orally for treating attention deficit hyperactivity disorder (ADHD), pregnancy-induced leg cramps, diabetes, kidney stones, migraine, osteoporosis, premenstrual syndrome, altitude sickness, urinary incontinence, kidney stones, and for preventing hearing loss. Magnesium is also used orally by athletes to increase energy and endurance.
Topically, magnesium is used for treating infected skin ulcers, boils, and carbuncles; and for speeding wound healing. It is also used topically as a cold compress in the treatment of erysipelas and as a hot compress for deep-seated skin infections.
Parenterally, magnesium is used for acute hypomagnesemia occurring in conditions such as pancreatitis, malabsorption disorders, and cirrhosis, and for treating preeclampsia and eclampsia. It is used as an additive to total parenteral nutrition (TPN) for prevention of hypomagnesemia.
Intravenously, magnesium is used for controlling seizures associated with epilepsy, glomerulonephritis, or hypothyroidism when low serum magnesium levels are present. It is also used intravenously for treatment of atrial and ventricular arrhythmias, including torsades de pointes, preventing arrhythmias after myocardial infarction, and for cardiac arrest. Magnesium is also used intravenously for treating acute exacerbations of asthma and chronic obstructive pulmonary disease (COPD), for migraine, neuropathic pain and postoperative pain, as an osmotic agent for cerebral edema, and for tetanus.
In combination with malic acid, magnesium is used orally for fibromyalgia.

Safety

LIKELY SAFE ...when used orally and appropriately (9,15,3566). ...when used parenterally and appropriately. Parenteral magnesium sulfate is a FDA-approved prescription product (15).
POSSIBLY SAFE ...when used orally and appropriately in combination with malic acid. In one study, magnesium hydroxide and malic acid were used safely in a trial lasting 6 months (3262).
POSSIBLY UNSAFE ...when used orally in high doses. High doses can cause loose stool and diarrhea. Although symptomatic hypermagnesemia, including hypotension, nausea, vomiting, and bradycardia, is rare in patients with normal renal function, it has occurred in patients ingesting magnesium sulfate 30 grams every 4 hours for 3 doses (14). Safe upper limit doses for magnesium have not been established (3566). ...when magnesium sulfate is used topically for prolonged periods or repeatedly, since it may damage the skin (9).
CHILDREN: LIKELY SAFE ...when used orally or parenterally and appropriately (15). LIKELY UNSAFE ...when used orally in large doses or for an extended period of time. There is one report of fatal hypermagnesemia in a 28-month old boy treated for constipation with oral magnesium oxide 800 mg per day, then 2400 mg per day for several days (see Adverse Reactions) (1360).
PREGNANCY AND LACTATION: LIKELY SAFE ...when used orally in amounts not exceeding the recommended dietary allowance (RDA) (15). POSSIBLY SAFE ...when given intramuscularly prior to delivery. Intramuscular magnesium sulfate is not thought to cause hypermagnesemia in the neonate when administered to toxemic mothers (15). LIKELY UNSAFE ...when used intravenously less than two hours before delivery. Intravenous infusions of magnesium sulfate can cause neonatal respiratory depression when given to toxemic mothers (14,15). There is insufficient reliable information available about the safety of the oral use of magnesium in pregnancy and lactation when doses exceed the recommended daily allowance (RDA); avoid using.

Effectiveness

EFFECTIVE ...when used orally or parenterally for treating and preventing hypomagnesemia (15). Magnesium deficiency typically only occurs in certain disease states such as alcoholism/cirrhosis of the liver, severe or prolonged diarrhea or vomiting, kidney dysfunction, inflammatory bowel disease, pancreatitis, and various other malabsorption syndromes (14,403,6280,6281). There is some controversy regarding whether parenteral or oral magnesium replacement is better. Because higher oral doses of magnesium might result in diarrhea, some suggest parenteral administration is better. However, oral magnesium can be used carefully in adequate doses for replacement without causing diarrhea. Magnesium gluconate or chloride is preferred for oral replacement because they do not cause as much diarrhea (14,6430). Magnesium oxide should be avoided due to greater risk for diarrhea. Magnesium carbonate may not be soluble enough to adequately replace magnesium levels and should also be avoided (14). ...when used orally as a laxative for constipation and for preparation of the bowel for surgical or diagnostic procedures (15). Magnesium citrate, sulfate, and hydroxide salts are typically used for this indication (14). The magnesium sulfate salt is the most potent (6430). ...when used orally as an antacid for reducing symptoms of gastric hyperacidity or gastroesophageal reflux disease (GERD). Typically, magnesium carbonate, hydroxide, oxide, or trisilicate salts are used (15). Magnesium hydroxide has the fastest onset of action. Magnesium carbonate is slower due to its crystal structure. Magnesium trisilicate has the slowest onset and longest duration due to its poor solubility (6844).

LIKELY EFFECTIVE ...when used parenterally for preventing and managing pre-eclampsia and eclampsia (9,15). Intravenous or intramuscular magnesium sulfate is considered the agent of choice for pre-eclampsia and eclampsia (15). ... when used intravenously for treatment of torsade de pointes. Magnesium sulfate is first line therapy for torsade de pointes (14,6844).

POSSIBLY EFFECTIVE ...when used orally for preventing migraine (6844), and premenstrual migraine (1186,6847). ...when used orally for relieving symptoms of premenstrual syndrome (PMS). There is some evidence that magnesium supplementation can improve symptoms, including mood changes and fluid retention, in some patients with PMS (1187,1188,6847). ...when used orally to increase bone density in osteoporosis associated with gluten-sensitive enteropathy (celiac disease). Magnesium seems to significantly improve bone density after 2 years of supplementation (14). ...when used orally to improve urinary incontinence in women with detrusor instability or sensory urgency (14). ...when used orally for attention deficit hyperactivity disorder (ADHD). There's some evidence magnesium can decrease activity level in ADHD patients with magnesium deficiency (1189). However, there's no proof magnesium works for ADHD in kids without magnesium deficiency. ...when used orally for treating pregnancy-induced leg cramps (1194). ...when used orally for reducing symptoms of mitral valve prolapse in people with low serum magnesium levels (14,1191). ...when used orally for reducing anginal attacks in people with coronary artery disease (1181). ...when used orally for treating mild to moderate hypertension. There is some evidence that doses of 600-1000 mg can produce additional small decreases in blood pressure in patients also taking antihypertensive medications (14,1192,1199). However, significantly lower doses do not seem to have this effect (1180,1195,1197). ...when used orally for hypercholesterolemia. There is some evidence that magnesium chloride and magnesium oxide can produce small decreases in low-density lipoprotein (LDL) and total cholesterol levels and small increases in high-density lipoprotein levels (14). However, magnesium does not seem to improve lipoprotein (a) levels (1193). ...when used orally for preventing recurrence of kidney stones. There is some evidence that prophylactic treatment with magnesium might decrease the recurrence rate of calcium stone formation (2007). Magnesium in combination with pyridoxine (vitamin B6) also seems to decrease urinary oxalate levels in people with hyperoxaluria who have previously had kidney stones (1201). However, it's unclear if this effect on urinary oxalate levels translates into a reduced incidence of kidney stones. ...when used orally for preventing hearing loss in individuals exposed to loud noise (1205). ...when used topically for treating skin ulcers and inflammatory conditions including boils and carbuncles (9). ...when used topically for speeding wound healing (14). ...when used intravenously for acute prevention of uterine contractions in preterm labor (tocolysis) (9,15). The use of magnesium for tocolysis is controversial. Not all experts agree it is beneficial (6844); however, most clinicians consider magnesium and beta-adrenergic agonists first-line therapy when tocolysis is indicated. Intravenous magnesium sulfate seems to be effective for delaying delivery for 24 to 48 hours (9,15). Oral magnesium therapy is not effective because it cannot achieve sufficiently high magnesium plasma levels (14,15). ...when used intravenously for cluster headaches (1184,1185). ...when used intravenously for acute migraine. (14,6844). Although some patients with normal magnesium levels can respond to intravenous magnesium, most patients who benefit from magnesium seem to have low magnesium levels (14,6844). ...when used intravenously in the management of seizures associated with low serum magnesium levels (14). ...when used intravenously in combination with conventional therapies for tetanus (14). ...when used intravenously for neuropathic pain associated with cancer. Single 500 mg to 1 gram doses of magnesium sulfate seem to relieve neuropathic pain for up to 4 hours (6846). ...when used intravenously for pain control after hysterectomy. There is some evidence that a high magnesium dose of 3 grams followed by a 500 mg per hour infusion can reduce discomfort and analgesic requirements in patients post-hysterectomy. However, lower doses of 200 mg followed by an infusion of 200 mg per hour is not effective and might actually increase pain in some patients (14,6846). ...when used intravenously to reduce arrhythmias and mortality after an acute myocardial infarction (MI). When given within 6 hours after symptom onset, intravenous magnesium sulfate seems to significantly reduce the rate of ventricular arrhythmias and slightly decrease mortality rate. Magnesium levels should be maintained above 2 mEq/L (14,15,6844). Administration beyond 6 hours cut off point might not provide this benefit (14,15). Oral magnesium supplementation seems to be ineffective for this use (1198,6844). ...when used intravenously for treating atrial tachycardia, ventricular fibrillation and tachycardia, and supraventricular tachycardia. There is some evidence that intravenous magnesium can be effective for various life-threatening arrhythmias in some patients who have not responded to standard antiarrhythmic drugs (14). ...when used intravenously for treating acute exacerbation of chronic obstructive pulmonary disease (1208). ...when used intravenously in moderate to severe asthmatics to treat acute attacks that have not responded to standard therapy (14,6844). ...when used in combination with malic acid for fibromyalgia. Magnesium hydroxide plus malic acid (Super Malic tablets) seems to decrease fibromyalgia-related pain and tenderness in some patients (3262). **POSSIBLY INEFFECTIVE** ...when used orally for asthma. Magnesium supplementation does not seem to improve FEV1 or reduce the need for bronchodilator use in patients with asthma (1173). ...when used orally for improving glycemic control in type 2 diabetes (14,1171,1172). ...when used intravenously for improving successful resuscitation in people with cardiac arrest (1190). ...when used to increase energy and endurance in athletic activity (2742,2825,2826,2827,2828,2829,2830).

Mechanism of Action

Magnesium is the second most plentiful cation in the intracellular fluid and the most plentiful cation in the body. Up to 50% of the magnesium in the body is present in bone. Magnesium is important to the normal bone structure (272) and it plays an essential role in more than 300 fundamental cellular reactions (945). Magnesium is required for the formation of cyclic AMP (cAMP) and is involved in ion movements across cell membranes (945). It is involved in protein synthesis and carbohydrate metabolism (272). Extracellular magnesium is critical to both maintaining nerve and muscle electrical potentials and transmitting impulses across neuromuscular junctions (272). Symptoms of deficiency include convulsions, confusion, muscle weakness, abnormal muscle movements, and others (403). As antacids, magnesium salts work by reacting with gastric acid to form magnesium chloride. Magnesium hydroxide has the fastest onset of action, magnesium carbonate is slower due to its crystal structure, and magnesium trisilicate has the slowest onset and longest duration due to its poor solubility (6844). The laxative effects and diarrhea produced by magnesium salts are due to the osmotic effects of unabsorbed salts in the intestine and colon, and stimulation of gastric motility due to the release of gastrin and cholecystokinin (6844). The inhibitory effect of magnesium on preterm labor contractions (tocolysis) is attributed to antagonism of calcium-mediated myometrial contractions (6844). Anticonvulsant actions of magnesium in eclampsia may be due to depression of neuromuscular transmission, a direct depressant effect on smooth muscle, and CNS depression (6844). There is also some evidence that magnesium is important in regulating blood pressure (1170,1182). Effects of magnesium on serum lipids may be due to decreased lipolysis and increased lipoprotein lipase activity (14). There is some evidence that low magnesium levels play a role in diabetes and migraine headaches (1168,1183,6844). Magnesium blood levels might play a role in insulin resistance (1168,6844). There is also some evidence that low dietary intake of magnesium increases the risk of developing type 2 diabetes (6845). Intracellular levels of magnesium, measured in erythrocytes and leukocytes, have been found to be lower in women with premenstrual syndrome (PMS), leading to the use of magnesium supplements for PMS (6847). Magnesium is also reported to be an antagonist at N-methyl-D-aspartate (NMDA) receptors which are involved in the potentiation of pain. This may also contribute to possible effects of magnesium in migraine, post-operative pain, neuropathic pain, and other pain syndromes (6846,6848). There is some evidence that magnesium metabolism is a factor in renal stone formation and prevention (2006,2007). In asthma, intravenous administration of magnesium might cause bronchodilation (2003).

Adverse Reactions

Orally, magnesium can cause gastrointestinal irritation, nausea, vomiting, and diarrhea (9,14,15). Although rare, larger amounts may cause hypermagnesemia (9) with symptoms including thirst, hypotension, drowsiness, confusion, loss of tendon reflexes, muscle weakness, respiratory depression, cardiac arrhythmias, coma, cardiac arrest, and death (9). Magnesium sulfate 30 grams every 4 hours for 3 doses has been associated with severe hypermagnesemia (14). A tolerable upper limit has not yet been determined (14). There is one report of fatal hypermagnesemia (serum magnesium 20.3 mg/dL) involving a child treated with oral magnesium oxide, calcium carbonate, multivitamins, essential fatty acids, lactobacillus, and bifidobacterium. The 28-month-old boy, with a history of severe mental retardation, spastic quadriplegia, and seizure disorder, was treated for constipation with 800 mg magnesium oxide per day, then 2400 mg magnesium oxide for several days before hospital admission (1360).
Topically, prolonged use of magnesium sulfate in the treatment of boils and carbuncles can cause damage to surrounding skin (9).
Intravenously (IV), Urticaria has been reported (9). Chronic use of magnesium-containing antacids, especially those that do not contain aluminum, can cause diarrhea leading to fluid and electrolyte imbalances (15).

Interactions with Herbs & Other Dietary Supplements

BORON: Can increase serum magnesium levels (940).
CALCIUM: Concomitant administration decreases gastrointestinal absorption of magnesium, but does not appear to have a clinically significant effect on magnesium status (998). Magnesium and calcium administration should be separated.
MALIC ACID: Malic acid is used with magnesium hydroxide for reducing pain and tenderness associated with fibromyalgia (3262).

Interactions with Drugs

EXCRETION-ENHANCING DRUGS: Concomitant use can reduce the effects of supplemental magnesium. Urinary excretion-enhancing drugs include amphotericin B, cisplatin, aminoglycoside antibiotics, cyclosporine, thiazide and loop diuretics, mannitol, and intravenous glucose (945).

EXCRETION-REDUCING DRUGS: Concomitant use can increase the effects of supplemental magnesium and magnesium serum levels. Urinary excretion-reducing drugs include calcitonin, glucagon, and potassium-sparing diuretics (945).

FLUOROQUINOLONES (ciprofloxacin, levofloxacin, ofloxacin, etc.): Concomitant administration decreases the absorption of the fluoroquinolone (15). Administer fluoroquinolones at least two hours before or four hours after magnesium-containing supplements or antacids.

NIFEDIPINE: Profound hypotension or neuromuscular blockade can occur in individuals using oral nifedipine concomitantly with intravenous magnesium sulfate (9).

SKELETAL MUSCLE RELAXANTS: Parenteral magnesium might potentiate the effects of skeletal muscle relaxants, e.g., tubocurarine chloride (9).

Drug Influences on Nutrient Levels and Depletion

SOME DRUGS CAN AFFECT MAGNESIUM LEVELS:

DIGOXIN (Lanoxin, Lanoxicaps): Digoxin can decrease renal tubule reabsorption and increase excretion of magnesium. The need for supplementation has not been adequately studied. Consider supplementation only if clinical judgment warrants it (4556).

LOOP DIURETICS and THIAZIDE DIURETICS: Use of loop diuretics and thiazide diuretics can increase urinary magnesium loss and reduce serum levels. This is more likely with higher doses or when used in combination with diuretics of another class (4412).

ESTROGENS and ESTROGEN-CONTAINING ORAL CONTRACEPTIVES: Use of estrogens and estrogen-containing oral contraceptives might shift magnesium from the serum to storage in other tissues, decreasing serum magnesium levels. The need for supplementation has not been adequately studied (4470).

PENICILLAMINE (Cuprimine): Penicillamine can reduce serum magnesium levels (4534).

Interactions with Foods

No interactions are known to occur, and there is no known reason to expect a clinically significant interaction with magnesium.

Interactions with Lab Tests

ALKALINE PHOSPHATASE (ALK PHOS): Magnesium salts can cause a false increase in serum alkaline phosphatase test results due to the activation of enzymes used in lab procedures (275).

ANGIOTENSIN-CONVERTING ENZYME (ACE): Magnesium sulfate can reduce serum ACE concentrations and test results (275).

BLOOD PRESSURE: Orally, magnesium can lower blood pressure and reduce blood pressure readings in patients with mild to moderate hypertension (1192,1199).

CALCIUM: Magnesium salts can cause a false increase in serum calcium test results in some procedures using edetate disodium (EDTA) (275).

CORTISOL: Intravenous magnesium sulfate can decrease plasma cortisol concentrations and test results (275).

DIAGNEX BLUE: Magnesium salts can increase urine diagnex blue concentrations and test results by heavy metal displacement of diagnex blue (275).

ELECTROCARDIOGRAM (ECG): Orally, magnesium can normalize arrhythmias and ECG readings in some patients with angina (1181). Intravenous magnesium can normalize arrhythmias and ECG readings in some people with atrial fibrillation or ventricular tachydysrhythmias (1202,3314).

PARATHYROID HORMONE: Intravenous magnesium sulfate can reduce plasma parathyroid hormone concentrations and test results (275).

TESTOSTERONE: Intravenous magnesium sulfate can reduce serum testosterone concentrations and test results (275).

Interactions with Diseases or Conditions

ELDERLY: The elderly have an increased risk for hypomagnesemia. Elderly are more prone to decreased magnesium absorption and increased urinary loss and disease states associated with abnormal magnesium status (1167).

HEART BLOCK: Contraindicated in people with heart block (9).

MALABSORPTION SYNDROMES: Intestinal magnesium absorption can be decreased in bile insufficiency states, gastrointestinal infections, gluten enteropathy, immune diseases with villous atrophy, inflammatory bowel disease, intestinal fistulas, lymphectasia, primary idiopathic hypomagnesemia, radiation enteritis, and sprue (945,6280,6281).

RENAL DISEASE: Use cautiously in individuals with reduced kidney function due to increased risk of hypermagnesemia (9).

Dosage and Administration

ORAL: Magnesium gluconate or chloride is preferred for oral use because they are highly soluble and less likely to cause diarrhea (14,6430). The initial dose used in hypomagnesemia is empirical; however, for mild deficiency, doses of 20-130 mg elemental magnesium daily to twice daily have been used. For chronic deficiency, 12-24 mg/kg given in divided doses has been used (6430). The dose is then adjusted to maintain normal serum levels (15). Normal serum levels of magnesium are 1.5-2.5 mEq/L (14,15). A typical dose used as a laxative in an adult is magnesium citrate 11-25 grams, or magnesium hydroxide 1.2-4.8 grams or 15-60 mL of milk of magnesia, or magnesium sulfate 10-30 grams (14,15). Magnesium used as a laxative should be used as single doses at infrequent intervals (15). A typical adult dose used as an antacid is magnesium hydroxide 400-1300 mg up to four times daily, or magnesium oxide 400-840 mg per day in divided doses (14). For prophylaxis of migraine headache, 600 mg daily of trimagnesium dicitrate has been used (not available in the US) (4891,4895). Doses of 200 to 360 mg magnesium daily have been used to reduce the symptoms of premenstrual syndrome (14). For improving bone density in osteoporosis, 504 to 576 mg/day has been used (14). In women with urinary incontinence associated with detrusor instability or sensory urgency, 350 to 700 mg daily of magnesium hydroxide has been used (14). For treatment of attention deficit hyperactivity disorder (ADHD) in children with magnesium deficiency 200 mg daily has been used (1189). For reducing the symptoms of altitude sickness, gradually increasing doses of magnesium citrate of 450 to 1200 mg/day have been used (14). For mild to moderate hypertension, 200-1000 mg elemental magnesium per day has been used (14,1192,1199). Beneficial effects on serum lipids have been seen with magnesium chloride doses averaging 432 mg/day or magnesium oxide 362 mg/day (14). For reducing pain and tenderness associated with fibromyalgia, magnesium hydroxide 200-300 mg is used orally with malic acid 800-1200 mg twice daily, equivalent to 4-6 Super Malic tablets twice daily (3262). For preventing kidney stones, magnesium hydroxide 200 mg/day or magnesium 300 mg daily plus pyridoxine (vitamin B6) 10 mg daily has been used (24,1201). To improve glycemic control in type 2 diabetes, 1000 mg elemental magnesium per day has been used (14,1172). For preventing recurrence of calcium-based kidney stones, 500 mg per day has been used (2007). The recommended amount of elemental magnesium as a dietary supplement is 54-483 mg daily in divided doses (14). The Adequate Intakes (AI) of magnesium for infants are: 0-6 months, 30 mg; and 7-12 months, 75 mg (3094). The RDAs for magnesium are: Children 1-3 years, 80 mg; Children 4-8 years, 130 mg; Children 9-13 years, 240 mg; Males 14-18 years, 410 mg; Males 19-30 years, 400 mg; Men 31 years and older, 420 mg; Females 14-18 years, 360 mg; Females 19-30 years, 310 mg; Women 31 years and older, 320 mg; Pregnant women up to 18 years, 400 mg; Pregnant women 19-30 years, 350 mg; Pregnant women over 30 years, 360 mg; Lactating women up to 18 years, 360 mg; Lactating women 19-30 years, 310 mg; and Lactating women over 30 years, 320 mg (3094). The maximum daily amount not likely to pose a risk of adverse effects from magnesium is 65 mg for children ages 1-3 years, 110 mg for children ages 4-8 years, and 350 mg for everyone over 8 years of age (3094).

PARENTERAL: For treatment of hypomagnesemia doses must be individualized according to serum magnesium levels, but a typical starting dose for mild deficiency is 1 gram intramuscularly (IM) every 6 hours for 4 doses. For more severe deficiency, 5 grams may be given in a 1 liter intravenous (IV) infusion over 3 hours (15). As part of total parenteral nutrition (TPN), adults typically receive 500 mg to 3 grams magnesium sulfate daily (15). For treatment of severe preeclampsia or eclampsia, a typical initial dose is 4 grams by IV infusion, followed by 4 to 5 grams IM every 4 hours, or 1 to 3 grams per hour by constant IV infusion. Doses should be adjusted according to serum levels and urinary excretion, and should not exceed 30 to 40 grams daily (15). As a tocolytic in preterm labor, an initial dose of 4 to 6 grams infused IV over 20 minutes has been used, followed by a maintenance infusion of 2 to 4 grams per hour, adjusted according to the response (15). For treatment of life-threatening ventricular arrhythmias such as torsades de pointes, 1 to 6 grams is given IV over several minutes, followed by an IV infusion, and for atrial tachycardia, 3 to 4 grams is given over 30 seconds. These IV push doses should be given with extreme caution (15). For reducing cardiovascular morbidity and mortality after a myocardial infarction, magnesium is started within 6 hours of symptoms. A dose of 2 grams IV over 5 to 15 minutes has been used, followed by an IV infusion of 18 grams over 24 hours (15). In the treatment of neuropathic pain associated with cancer, single 500 mg or 1 gram doses have been used (6846). In the management of cluster headaches and acute migraine 1 gram IV doses have been used (6844). As an adjunct to analgesics for pain after hysterectomy, a 3 gram bolus dose followed by an infusion of 0.5 grams/hour has been used (6848). As an adjunctive treatment in the management of acute asthmatic attacks, doses of 1 to 2 grams infused IV over 15 to 30 minutes have been used (14,6844). Acute exacerbations of COPD have also been treated with 1.2 grams magnesium sulfate IV (6844).

Comments

None.

MAGNOLIA bark

Also Known As
Beaver Tree, Holly Bay, Hou Po, Indian Bark, Red Bay, Swamp Laurel, Swamp Sassafras, Sweet Bay, White Bay, White Laurel.
CAUTION: See separate listing for Magnolia flower bud.

Scientific Names
Magnolia biondii, synonym Magnolia fargesii; Magnolia denudata, synonym Magnolia heptaperta; Magnolia glauca; Magnolia officinalis; Magnolia sprengeri; Magnolia sargentiana, synonym Magnolia emargenata; Magnolia wilsonii; Magnolia salicifolia; other Magnolia species.
Family: Magnoliaceae.

People Use This For
Orally, magnolia bark is used for digestive disorders, as an anti-inflammatory, a stimulant, and to promote sweating. It is also used orally as a tonic, which is an agent used to invigorate, refresh or restore body function [18].

Safety
There is insufficient reliable information available about the safety of magnolia bark.
Pregnancy and Lactation: Insufficient reliable information available; avoid using.

Effectiveness
There is insufficient reliable information available about the effectiveness of magnolia bark.

Mechanism of Action
There is insufficient reliable information available about the possible mechanism of action and active ingredients.

Adverse Reactions
None reported.

Interactions with Herbs & Other Dietary Supplements
Insufficient reliable information available.

Interactions with Drugs
No interactions are known to occur, and there is no known reason to expect a clinically significant interaction with magnolia bark.

Interactions with Foods
No interactions are known to occur, and there is no known reason to expect a clinically significant interaction with magnolia bark.

Interactions with Lab Tests
No interactions are known to occur, and there is no known reason to expect a clinically significant interaction with magnolia bark.

Interactions with Diseases or Conditions
No interactions are known to occur, and there is no known reason to expect a clinically significant interaction with magnolia bark.

Dosage and Administration
ORAL: Magnolia bark is used as a powder or liquid extract [18].

Comments
There is very little scientific information about this product. Our staff is continually analyzing the available information on natural medicines and will add data here as it becomes available.

MAGNOLIA flower bud

Also Known As
Flos Magnoliae, Hou Po, Magnolia Flower Bud.
CAUTION: See separate listing for Magnolia bark.

Scientific Names
Magnolia biondii, synonym Magnolia fargesii; Magnolia denudata, synonym Magnolia heptaperta; Magnolia glauca; Magnolia officinalis; Magnolia sprengeri; Magnolia sargentiana, synonym Magnolia emargenata; Magnolia wilsonii; Magnolia salicifolia; other Magnolia species.
Family: Magnoliaceae.

People Use This For
In Chinese medicine, magnolia flower bud is used both orally and topically for nasal congestion, runny nose, common cold, headache, and facial dark spots. It is also used topically for toothaches.
In skin care products, magnolia flower bud extract is used topically as a skin whitener and to minimize or counteract irritant effects of other ingredients (11).

Safety
There is insufficient reliable information available about safety of magnolia flower bud. Its regulatory status in the US has not been determined (11).
PREGNANCY: UNSAFE ...when used orally; contraindicated due to empiric uterine stimulating activity (11).
LACTATION: Insufficient reliable information available; avoid using.

Effectiveness
There is insufficient reliable information available about the effectiveness of magnolia flower bud.

Mechanism of Action
Magnolia flower bud has antihistaminic activity and protective activity against asthma in animals. In vitro animal data also suggests anti-inflammatory, hypotensive, uterine stimulating, antifungal, antibacterial, and antiviral effects. It may also have skeletal muscle blocking and muscle relaxant properties. Magnolia flower bud may have activity against allergic and chronic rhinitis as well as some forms of sinusitis (11).

Adverse Reactions
None reported.

Interactions with Herbs & Other Dietary Supplements
Insufficient reliable information available.

Interactions with Drugs
No interactions are known to occur, and there is no known reason to expect a clinically significant interaction with magnolia flower bud.

Interactions with Foods
No interactions are known to occur, and there is no known reason to expect a clinically significant interaction with magnolia flower bud.

Interactions with Lab Tests
No interactions are known to occur, and there is no known reason to expect a clinically significant interaction with magnolia flower bud.

Interactions with Diseases or Conditions
No interactions are known to occur, and there is no known reason to expect a clinically significant interaction with magnolia flower bud.

Dosage and Administration
ORAL: Magnolia flower bud is used as a powder or liquid extract (18).

Comments
Magnolia flower bud emits a strong eucalyptus scent when crushed (11).

MAIDENHAIR FERN

Also Known As
Five-Finger Fern, Hair of Venus, Maiden Fern, Rock Fern, Venus Hair.

Scientific Names
Adiantum pedatum, synonym Adiantum capillus-veneris.
Family: Adiantiaceae.

People Use This For
Orally, maidenhair fern is used for bronchitis, coughs, whooping cough, and painful and excessive menstruation. It is also used orally as an expectorant and demulcent.

Historically, it was used orally for various respiratory tract illnesses and severe coughs. It was also used topically for hair loss and to promote dark hair color (18).

Safety
POSSIBLY SAFE ...when used orally in amounts found in foods.
There is insufficient reliable information available about the safety of maidenhair fern for its other uses.
PREGNANCY: UNSAFE ...when used orally; contraindicated, most likely due to its emetic effects at higher doses (12).
LACTATION: Insufficient reliable information available; avoid using.

Effectiveness
There is insufficient reliable information available about the effectiveness of maidenhair fern.

Mechanism of Action
There is insufficient reliable information available about the possible mechanism of action and active ingredients.

Adverse Reactions
Orally, people using large amounts may experience emesis (12).

Interactions with Herbs & Other Dietary Supplements
Insufficient reliable information available.

Interactions with Drugs
No interactions are known to occur, and there is no known reason to expect a clinically significant interaction with maidenhair fern.

Interactions with Foods
No interactions are known to occur, and there is no known reason to expect a clinically significant interaction with maidenhair fern.

Interactions with Lab Tests
No interactions are known to occur, and there is no known reason to expect a clinically significant interaction with maidenhair fern.

Interactions with Diseases or Conditions
No interactions are known to occur, and there is no known reason to expect a clinically significant interaction with maidenhair fern.

Dosage and Administration
ORAL: Maidenhair fern is taken as a tea. A single dose is equivalent to 1.5 grams ground or powdered herb. The tea is prepared by steeping 1.5 grams dried herb in 150 mL of boiling water for 10-15 minutes and straining (18).

Comments
Maidenhair tree is another name for Ginkgo biloba, and is distinct from maidenhair fern (18).

MAITAKE MUSHROOM

Also Known As
Dancing Mushroom, Grifola, Hen Of The Woods, King Of Mushrooms, Maitake, Monkey's Bench, Shelf Fungi.

Scientific Names
Grifola frondosa.
Family: Polyporaceae.

People Use This For
Orally, maitake mushroom is used for cancer, HIV/AIDS, chronic fatigue syndrome (CFS), hepatitis, hay fever, diabetes, high blood pressure, hyperlipidemia, weight loss or control, and chemotherapy support (1900).
For food uses, maitake mushroom is edible (1210) and has been consumed in Asia for thousands of years (6).

Safety
POSSIBLY SAFE ...when used orally and appropriately (12).
PREGNANCY AND LACTATION: Insufficient reliable information available; avoid using.

Effectiveness
There is insufficient reliable information available about the effectiveness of maitake mushroom.

Mechanism of Action
The applicable parts of maitake mushroom are the fruiting body and mycelium. Maitake mushroom contains beta-glucan, which has been shown to possess antitumor activity. The "D-fraction" of betaglucan appears to be the most active and potent form (6). Maitake mushroom has immunostimulant effects and activates natural killer cells, cytotoxic T-cells, interleukin-1, and superoxide anions (6). Experiments have shown varied effects. In hypertensive rats, it lowers blood pressure (1213,1214), and it improves the lipid profile in hyperlipidemic rats (1209,1211). In genetically-induced diabetic mice, it lowers blood glucose (1212), and in overweight rats, it reduces weight (6). Maitake mushroom might improve the quality of life of people with cancer by improving cancer symptoms and reducing pain, and it can aid in weight loss in overweight people (6). However, controlled studies are needed to confirm these effects (6).

Adverse Reactions
None reported.

Interactions with Herbs & Other Dietary Supplements
Insufficient reliable information available.

Interactions with Drugs
DIABETES THERAPY: Monitor blood glucose levels closely due to claims that maitake mushroom has hypoglycemic effects (19).

Interactions with Foods
No interactions are known to occur, and there is no known reason to expect a clinically significant interaction with maitake mushroom.

Interactions with Lab Tests
No interactions are known to occur, and there is no known reason to expect a clinically significant interaction with maitake mushroom.

Interactions with Diseases or Conditions
No interactions are known to occur, and there is no known reason to expect a clinically significant interaction with maitake mushroom.

Dosage and Administration
ORAL: People typically take 500 to 1000 mg of maitake mushroom with water 2 or 3 times daily between meals. Maitake "D fraction" is typically dosed 6 mg twice daily between meals. The "D fraction" is also available as a liquid, approximately 1 mg/mL. For general use as a dietary supplement, the dose is 5 to 6 drops 3 times daily between meals. Health care professionals are directed to prescribe 0.5 to 1 mg/kg of body weight. If maitake mushroom causes stomach upset, the supplement is taken with food. Sometimes the dose is doubled or tripled (5273).

Comments

The potential for toxicity exists when other mushrooms are mistaken for maitake mushroom (6).

MALABAR NUT

Also Known As

Adulsa, Arusa.
CAUTION: See separate listing for Garcinia.

Scientific Names

Justicia Adhatoda.
Family: Acanthaceae.

People Use This For

In Indian medicine, malabar nut is used orally as an expectorant and secretory agent. It is also used as a bronchodilatory agent and mild spasmolytic (18).

Safety

There is insufficient reliable information available about the safety of malabar nut.
PREGNANCY: UNSAFE ...when used orally; contraindicated (18).
LACTATION: Insufficient reliable information available; avoid using.

Effectiveness

There is insufficient reliable information available about the effectiveness of malabar nut.

Mechanism of Action

The applicable part of malabar nut is the leaf. The quinazoline alkaloid vasicine has excitatory activity when taken in large amounts (18).

Adverse Reactions

None reported.

Interactions with Herbs & Other Dietary Supplements

Insufficient reliable information available.

Interactions with Drugs

No interactions are known to occur, and there is no known reason to expect a clinically significant interaction with malabar nut.

Interactions with Foods

No interactions are known to occur, and there is no known reason to expect a clinically significant interaction with malabar nut.

Interactions with Lab Tests

No interactions are known to occur, and there is no known reason to expect a clinically significant interaction with malabar nut.

Interactions with Diseases or Conditions

No interactions are known to occur, and there is no known reason to expect a clinically significant interaction with malabar nut.

Dosage and Administration

No typical dosage.

Comments

Vasicine was formerly used as the starting substance for production of mucolytics Bromhexin and Ambroxol. Neither of these products are available in the United States (18).

MALE FERN

Also Known As
American Aspidium, Bear's Paw, European Aspidium, Knotty Brake, Marginal Fern, Shield Fern.

Scientific Names
Dryopteris Filix-Mas.
Family: Aspleniaceae or Polypodiaceae.

People Use This For
In Chinese medicine, male fern has been used to treat recurrent nose bleeds, heavy menstrual bleeding, and wounds (6).
In veterinary medicine, male fern is used as an anthelmintic to treat worms (6).
Historically, male fern has been used orally for tumors and as an anthelmintic for treating worms (6).

Safety
LIKELY UNSAFE ...when used orally. Male fern can be a violent poison if absorbed (2,11). For this reason, it should no longer be used internally (2). Canada requires that it be labeled "For external use only" (12).
There is insufficient reliable information available about the safety of male fern for its other uses.
PREGNANCY AND LACTATION: LIKELY UNSAFE ...when used orally; contraindicated (12). There is insufficient reliable information available about the safety of male fern used topically; avoid using.

Effectiveness
POSSIBLY EFFECTIVE ...when used orally for treating tapeworm infestation (2,6).
POSSIBLY INEFFECTIVE ...when used orally for rheumatism and sleep disorders (2).
There is insufficient reliable information available about the effectiveness of male fern for its other uses.

Mechanism of Action
The applicable parts of male fern are the above ground parts, leaf and rhizome. Male fern contains filicin and filmarone. These are active anthelmintics and act as a vermifuge to kill worms. Active constituents are soluble derivatives of phloroglucinol. These constituents are inactivated in an alkaline environment. Male fern also contains volatile oils, tannin, albaspidin, and desaspidin. All of these compounds together are called filicin, and work together to kill tapeworms. It is important to remember that once the tapeworm has been killed, a simultaneously administered saline laxative is used expel the worm (6).

Adverse Reactions
Orally, male fern may cause headaches, dyspnea, nausea, diarrhea, vertigo, tremors, convulsions, cardiac and respiratory failure, and optic neuritis (6). Death has occurred with severe poisoning. Symptoms of toxicity include muscular weakness, coma, temporary or permanent blindness (11).

Interactions with Herbs & Other Dietary Supplements
Insufficient reliable information available.

Interactions with Drugs
CASTOR OIL: Enhances absorption and toxic potential of the male fern (6).

Interactions with Foods
FATS, OILS AND ALCOHOL: Increases absorption and side effects (2).

Interactions with Lab Tests
No interactions are known to occur, and there is no known reason to expect a clinically significant interaction with male fern.

Interactions with Diseases or Conditions
Theoretically, in damaged GI mucosa or conditions which prolong GI transit, absorption and risk of side effects may be increased.

Dosage and Administration
ORAL: Adults in a fasting state usually receive 3-6 mL orally. Children up to age two receive up to 2 mL in divided doses. Children over age two are given 0.25-0.5 mL per year of age up to a total of 4 mL in divided doses. The dose is typically given with a purgative (saline laxative) to aid expulsion of tapeworms (6,11).

Comments

High toxic potential precludes use (2,6). Treatment of overdose consists of giving saline cathartic followed by demulcent fluids. It is important to avoid fats and oils. If seizures occur, benzodiazepines may be used, and assisting respiration may be required. Since there are other products available that are effective and safer than male fern, it should not be used (7003).

MALLOW flower

Also Known As

Blue Mallow Flower, Cheeseflower, High Mallow, Malvae flos, Mauls.
CAUTION: See separate listings for Mallow leaf, Country Mallow, and Marshmallow.

Scientific Names

Malva sylvestris.
Family: Malvaceae.

People Use This For

Orally, mallow flower is used for irritation of the mucosa of the mouth and throat and the associated dry cough (2,8,18).
Topically, mallow flower has been used as a poultice or bath additive for wounds (8,18).
In folk medicine, it has been used for bronchitis (18), as a mild astringent for gastroenteritis, and for bladder complaints (8,18).
In foods, it is used as a food-coloring agent (8).

Safety

POSSIBLY SAFE ...when used orally and appropriately (2,12).
PREGNANCY AND LACTATION: Insufficient reliable information available; avoid using.

Effectiveness

POSSIBLY EFFECTIVE ...when taken orally for irritation of the mouth and throat (2).
There is insufficient reliable information available about the effectiveness of mallow flower for its other uses.

Mechanism of Action

Mallow flower contains mucilage, which protects and soothes mucous membranes (2,18). The anthocyanins constituents are a source of color (8).

Adverse Reactions

None reported.

Interactions with Herbs & Other Dietary Supplements

Insufficient reliable information available.

Interactions with Drugs

No interactions are known to occur, and there is no known reason to expect a clinically significant interaction with mallow flower.

Interactions with Foods

No interactions are known to occur, and there is no known reason to expect a clinically significant interaction with mallow flower.

Interactions with Lab Tests

No interactions are known to occur, and there is no known reason to expect a clinically significant interaction with mallow flower.

Interactions with Diseases or Conditions

No interactions are known to occur, and there is no known reason to expect a clinically significant interaction with mallow flower.

Dosage and Administration

ORAL: The typical dose of mallow flower is one cup of the tea several times daily (6,18). The tea is prepared by steeping 1.5-2 grams of the dried flowers in 150 mL boiling water for 10 minutes and then straining. Up to 5 grams of the dried flowers should be ingested per day (2,8,18).

Comments

Avoid confusion with mallow leaf, other malvae varieties, and marshmallow (Althaea officinalis).

MALLOW leaf

Also Known As

Blue Mallow, Dwarf Mallow, High Mallow, Malvae folium.
CAUTION: See separate listings for Mallow flower, Country Mallow, and Marshmallow.

Scientific Names

Malva sylvestris; Malva neglecta.
Family: Malvaceae.

People Use This For

Orally, mallow leaf is used for irritation of the mucosa of the mouth and throat and the associated dry cough (2,8).
In folk medicine, mallow leaf has been used for colds and upper respiratory mucous membrane inflammation (8), as a mild astringent for gastroenteritis (8), and topically as a poultice for wounds (8).

Safety

POSSIBLY SAFE ...when used orally and appropriately (2).
PREGNANCY AND LACTATION: Insufficient reliable information available; avoid using.

Effectiveness

POSSIBLY EFFECTIVE ...when taken orally for irritation of the mouth and throat (2).
There is insufficient reliable information available about the effectiveness of mallow leaf for its other uses.

Mechanism of Action

Mallow leaf contains mucilage which protects and soothes mucous membranes (2,18). The mucilage has been shown in vitro to inactivate the serum complement, which is a component in the host defense system (1526).

Adverse Reactions

None reported.

Interactions with Herbs & Other Dietary Supplements

Insufficient reliable information available.

Interactions with Drugs

No interactions are known to occur, and there is no known reason to expect a clinically significant interaction with mallow leaf.

Interactions with Foods

No interactions are known to occur, and there is no known reason to expect a clinically significant interaction with mallow leaf.

Interactions with Lab Tests

No interactions are known to occur, and there is no known reason to expect a clinically significant interaction with mallow leaf.

Interactions with Diseases or Conditions

No interactions are known to occur, and there is no known reason to expect a clinically significant interaction with mallow leaf.

Dosage and Administration

ORAL: The typical dose of mallow leaf is one cup of the tea several times per day and in the evening before going to sleep (6). It can be sweetened with honey (6). The tea is prepared by steeping 3-5 grams of the dried leaves in 150 mL boiling water for 10-15 minutes and then straining (6). The maximum use of mallow is 5 grams of the dried leaves per day (2).

Comments
Mallow leaf is a rich plant source of vitamin C (19).

MANACA

Also Known As
Pohl, Vegetable Mercury.

Scientific Names
Brunfelsia hopeana.
Family: Solanaceae.

People Use This For
Orally, manaca is used for arthritis, and as a diuretic (18).

Safety
There is insufficient reliable information available about the safety of manaca.
Pregnancy and Lactation: Insufficient reliable information available; avoid using.

Effectiveness
There is insufficient reliable information available about the effectiveness of manaca.

Mechanism of Action
The applicable part of manaca is the root. Animal data suggests that manaca may cause symptoms of anxiety, restlessness, increases in heart and respiratory rates, increased salivation, vomiting, muscle tremors, and may result in death (18).

Adverse Reactions
None reported.

Interactions with Herbs & Other Dietary Supplements
Insufficient reliable information available.

Interactions with Drugs
No interactions are known to occur, and there is no known reason to expect a clinically significant interaction with manaca.

Interactions with Foods
No interactions are known to occur, and there is no known reason to expect a clinically significant interaction with manaca.

Interactions with Lab Tests
No interactions are known to occur, and there is no known reason to expect a clinically significant interaction with manaca.

Interactions with Diseases or Conditions
No interactions are known to occur, and there is no known reason to expect a clinically significant interaction with manaca.

Dosage and Administration
ORAL: Manaca is taken as a liquid extract (18).

Comments
There is very little scientific information about this product. Our staff is continually analyzing the available information on natural medicines and will add data here as it becomes available.

MANGANESE

Also Known As
Manganese Amino Acid Chelate, Manganese Aminoate, Manganese Ascorbate, Manganese Aspartate Complex, Manganese Chloride, Manganese Chloridetetrahydrate, Manganese Dioxide, Manganese Gluconate, Manganese Sulfate, Manganese Sulfate Monohydrate, Manganese Sulfate Tetrahydrate, Manganum.

Scientific Names
Manganese; Mn; atomic number 25.

People Use This For
Orally, manganese is used for prevention and treatment of manganese deficiency, osteoporosis (1993), microcytic anemia (9), and symptoms of premenstrual syndrome (PMS) (2004).
In combination, Manganese is used with chondroitin sulfate and glucosamine hydrochloride for osteoarthritis (4237).
Intravenously, manganese is used as a trace element in total parenteral nutrition (TPN) preparations (9,14).

Safety
LIKELY SAFE ...when used orally and appropriately. Manganese is usually safe in doses up to 11 mg per day (7135). ...when used intravenously and appropriately as a component of total parenteral nutrition (TPN) (14).
POSSIBLY UNSAFE ...when used orally in high doses. Doses exceeding 11 mg per day can cause significant adverse effects (7135).
CHILDREN: LIKELY SAFE ...when used orally and appropriately. Manganese is usually safe in children when used in daily doses less than 2 mg in children 1 to 3 years, 3 mg in children 4 to 8 years, 6 mg in children 9 to 13 years, 9 mg in children 14 to 18 years (7135). POSSIBILY UNSAFE ...when used orally in high doses. Daily doses greater than 2 mg in children 1 to 3 years, 3 mg in children 4 to 8 years, 6 mg in children 9 to 13 years, 9 mg in children 14 to 18 years, are associated with a greater risk of toxicity (7135).
PREGNANCY AND LACTATION: LIKELY SAFE ...when used orally and appropriately. Manganese is usually safe in pregnant or lactating adult women aged 19 or older when used in doses of less than 11 mg per day. However, pregnant and lactating women under age 19 should limit doses to less than 9 mg per day (7135). POSSIBLY UNSAFE ...when used orally in high doses. Doses over 11 mg per day are associated with a greater risk of toxicity (7135).

Effectiveness
EFFECTIVE ...when used orally or intravenously for preventing or treating manganese deficiency (14).
POSSIBLY EFFECTIVE ...when used orally in combination with calcium, zinc, and copper for osteoporosis (1994). ...when used orally in combination with calcium for symptoms of premenstrual syndrome (PMS). There is some evidence that supplementing manganese with calcium can help improve symptoms of crying, loneliness, anxiety, restlessness, irritability, mood swings, depression, and tension (2004).
There is insufficient reliable information available about the effectiveness of manganese for its other uses.

Mechanism of Action
Manganese is an essential nutrient that acts as a cofactor in several metabolic and enzymatic reactions (14,2003,7135). Manganese is found in several foods including nuts, legumes, seeds, tea, whole grains, and leafy green vegetables (2005,2008,7135). However, typically less than 5% of dietary manganese is absorbed. It's not known if absorption of manganese from supplements is better or worse than manganese from dietary sources. Men seem to absorb less manganese than women. The reason for this is not known, but it might be due to higher serum ferritin concentrations in men. Ferritin is associated with decreased manganese absorption (7135). Manganese is involved in amino acid, cholesterol, and carbohydrate metabolism (7135). Manganese metalloenzymes include arginase, glutamine synthetase, phosphoenolpyruvate decarboxylase, and manganese superoxide (7135). Researchers think manganese might have a role in osteoporosis. Decreased plasma manganese concentrations have been linked to osteoporosis, and bone mineral density seems to improve when trace minerals including manganese are added to calcium supplementation (7135). Manganese may work by enhancing bone turnover (1993). Manganese might also have a role in the treatment of anemia. There is some evidence it can increase the hematinic action of iron (9). In patients with premenstrual syndrome (PMS), low dietary manganese has been associated with altered mood and increased pain (7135). Some researchers think that supplementing manganese in women with PMS might improve symptoms. Manganese is cleared hepatically and chronic liver disease can cause manganese accumulation and toxicity (1992). Manganese accumulation plays a role in Parkinsonian symptoms and encephalopathy associated with chronic liver disease (1992). Manganese is transported by transferrin. The globus pallidus and substantia nigra, areas of the brain associated with the extrapyramidal system, are high in transferrin receptor density, which may result in concentration of manganese (7135).

Adverse Reactions

Orally, manganese is usually well tolerated when used in doses below 11 mg per day (7135). There is some concern that higher doses might increase risk of neurotoxicity, including Parkinsonian-like extrapyramidal symptoms (7135). People with impaired manganese excretion can also experience these effects even with very low manganese intake. Manganese accumulation due to chronic liver disease seems to cause Parkinsonian-like extrapyramidal symptoms, encephalopathy, and psychosis (9,1992,7135). Chronic occupational exposure to manganese dust or fumes can also cause extrapyramidal reactions, orthostatic hypotension, decreased heart rate, mood disturbance, and dementia (1990,7135).

Interactions with Herbs & Other Dietary Supplements

CALCIUM: Concomitant administration can decrease manganese absorption (2000).
IP-6 (Phytic Acid): IP-6 found in foods, such as cereals, nuts, and beans, and in supplements can decrease manganese absorption (7135). IP-6 chelates multivalent metal ions in the gastrointestinal tract and prevents absorption (1858). Suggest that patients separate intake of manganese and IP-6 by at least two hours.
IRON: Concomitant administration can decrease manganese absorption (2004).
ZINC: Concomitant administration can increase manganese absorption and plasma levels (2000).

Interactions with Drugs

FLUOROQUINOLONES: Theoretically, manganese might reduce the absorption of fluoroquinolones. Interactions occur with other multivalent cations, such as calcium and iron (488). Fluoroquinolones include ciprofloxacin (Cipro), levofloxacin (Levaquin), gatifloxicin (Tequin), sparfloxacin (Zagam), and others.
TETRACYCLINES: Theoretically, manganese might reduce the absorption of tetracyclines. Interactions occur with other multivalent cations, such as calcium and iron (488). Tetracyclines include demeclocycline (Declomycin), minocycline (Minocin), and tetracycline (Achromycin).

Interactions with Foods

No interactions are known to occur, and there is no known reason to expect a clinically significant interaction with manganese.

Interactions with Lab Tests

ALKALINE PHOSPHATASE: Magnesium salts can cause a false increase in serum alkaline phosphatase test results due to enzyme activation in the laboratory procedure (275).
BONE MINERAL DENSITY (BMD): Manganese (in combination with calcium, zinc, and copper) might improve BMD and BMD test results in patients with osteoporosis (1994).
STOOL COLOR: Manganese dioxide might cause stool to turn dark brown to black (275).

Interactions with Diseases or Conditions

CHRONIC LIVER DISEASE: Use manganese cautiously. Chronic liver disease can lead to manganese accumulation and toxicity (9,14,1992,2001).
IRON-DEFICIENCY ANEMIA: Individuals with iron-deficiency anemia might have enhanced manganese absorption (2002).

Dosage and Administration

ORAL: For osteoporosis, 5 mg per day combined with 1000 mg elemental calcium, 15 mg zinc, and 2.5 mg copper has been used (1994).
No recommended dietary allowances (RDA) for manganese have been established. The daily Adequate Intake (AI) levels for manganese are: infants birth to 6 months, 3 mcg; 7 to 12 months, 600 mcg; children 1 to 3 years, 1.2 mg; 4 to 8 years 1.5 mg; boys 9 to 13 years, 1.9 mg; 14 to 18 years, 2.2 mg; girls 9 to 18 years, 1.6 mg; men age 19 and older 2.3 mg; women 19 and older 1.8 mg; pregnancy age 14 to 50, 2 mg; lactation 2.6 mg (7135). Tolerable Upper Intake Levels (UL) for manganese have been established (7135). The daily ULs for manganese are: children 1 to 3 years, 2 mg; 4 to 8 years, 3 mg; 9 to 13 years, 6 mg; 14 to 18 years (including pregnancy and lactation) 9 mg; for adults 19 years and older (including pregnancy and lactation), 11 mg (7135).
INTRAVENOUS: In parenteral nutrition, manganese is administered in doses of 150 to 800 mcg per day for adults and 2 to 10 mcg/kg per day for children (157).

Comments

Tell patients to look out for excessive manganese hidden in some supplements. Certain supplements, including those commonly used for osteoarthritis (e.g., Cosamin and Cosamin DS) provide more than the tolerable upper limit (UL) of 11 mg per day when used according to manufacturer's labeled directions.

MANNA

Also Known As
Flake Manna, Flowering Ash, Manna Ash.

Scientific Names
Fraxinus ornus.
Family: Oleaceae.

People Use This For
Orally, the dried sap of manna is used as a laxative for constipation (2,9,18) and a stool softener for anal fissure, hemorrhoids, and after anorectal surgery (2,18).

Safety
POSSIBLY SAFE ...when used orally and appropriately on a short-term basis (2); avoid extended use of manna (2,18).
PREGNANCY AND LACTATION: Insufficient reliable information available; avoid using.

Effectiveness
POSSIBLY EFFECTIVE ...when taken orally for constipation, and as a stool softener for anal fissure and after anorectal surgery (2).

Mechanism of Action
Manna consists of the dried sap collected from the splits in branches and trunk of Fraxinus ornus. The manna bark contains coumarins which can inactivate the serum complement, a component in the host defense system (1527). Manna contains 40-90% mannitol (9,18), which acts as an osmotic laxative (2,18).

Adverse Reactions
Manna can cause nausea or flatulence (2,18).

Interactions with Herbs & Other Dietary Supplements
STIMULANT LAXATIVE HERBS: Theoretically, concomitant use of manna with other stimulant laxative herbs can increase the risk of potassium depletion. Stimulant laxative herbs include aloe dried leaf sap, wild cucumber fruit (Ecballium elaterium), blue flag rhizome, alder buckthorn, European buckthorn, butternut bark, cascara bark, castor oil, colocynth fruit pulp, gamboge bark exudate, jalap root, black root, podophyllum root, rhubarb root, senna leaves and pods, and yellow dock root (19).
POTASSIUM DEPLETING HERBS: Theoretically, concomitant use of manna with horsetail plant or the licorice rhizome increases the risk of potassium depletion.

Interactions with Drugs
CARDIAC GLYCOSIDES: Theoretically, the overuse or abuse of this product increases the risk of adverse effects of cardiac glycoside drugs, e.g., digoxin (Lanoxin).

Interactions with Foods
No interactions are known to occur, and there is no known reason to expect a clinically significant interaction with manna.

Interactions with Lab Tests
No interactions are known to occur, and there is no known reason to expect a clinically significant interaction with manna.

Interactions with Diseases or Conditions
OBSTRUCTION: Manna is contraindicated in cases of bowel obstruction or ileus (2,18).

Dosage and Administration
ORAL: For adults, the typical dose of manna is 20-30 grams per day or equivalent preparations (2,18).
For children, the common dose is 2-16 grams per day (2,18). Manna should not be taken for prolonged use (2,18).

Comments
None.

MARIJUANA

Also Known As

Anashca, Banji, Bhang, Cannabis, Charas, Esrar, Gaga, Ganga, Grass, Hash, Hashish, Hemp, Kif, Mariguana, Marihuana, Pot, Sawi, Sinsemilla, Weed.

Scientific Names

Cannabis sativa.
Family: Cannabaceae.

People Use This For

Orally, marijuana is used recreationally as a euphoriant (18). A cannabinoid from marijuana is used in the prescription-only product dronabinol (Marinol) for the treatment of anorexia or appetite loss associated with AIDS and for cancer chemotherapy induced nausea and vomiting unresponsive to traditional medications (14). Cannabinoid constituents from marijuana have also been used orally to treat tremor and spasticity associated with multiple sclerosis (MS) (14).

As an inhalant, marijuana is smoked for treating nausea, reducing intraocular pressure in glaucoma, stimulation of appetite, and recreationally for altering senses (psychoactivity) and euphoria (18). Marijuana is also smoked for mucous membrane inflammation, leprosy, fever, dandruff, hemorrhoids, obesity, asthma, urinary tract infections, cough (6), anorexia associated with weight loss in AIDS patients (2619), chronic pain (5887), multiple sclerosis (14,5889), and for producing immunosuppression after renal transplantation (14).

Safety

LIKELY SAFE ...when the cannabinoid constituent dronabinol is used orally and appropriately. Dronabinol (Marinol) is a FDA-approved prescription product (6,14).

POSSIBLY UNSAFE ...when marijuana is used orally or inhaled (6).

PREGNANCY: UNSAFE ...when used orally or inhaled; marijuana passes through the placenta and can reduce fetal growth. Marijuana use during pregnancy is also associated with childhood leukemia (4260).

LACTATION: LIKELY UNSAFE ...when used orally or inhaled because dronabinol (THC) is concentrated and excreted in breast milk (6,2619,2620).

Effectiveness

EFFECTIVE ...when the cannabinoid constituent dronabinol is used orally for prevention and treatment of chemotherapy-induced nausea and vomiting, which is unresponsive to other drugs; and treatment of anorexia and weight loss in patients with AIDS. Dronabinol (Marinol) is FDA-approved for these uses (6,14,6606).

LIKELY EFFECTIVE ...when used orally or smoked as an euphoriant (6,13,18).

POSSIBLY EFFECTIVE ...when smoked as an antiemetic (2621,2622). ...when smoked as an appetite stimulant in AIDS patients (6,13,18). Marijuana cigarettes can increase caloric intake and weight gain in HIV positive patients also taking indinavir (Crixivan) or nelfinavir (Viracept) without affecting viral load (6606). ...when marijuana is smoked, or cannabinoids are taken orally for the treatment of spasticity and tremor associated with multiple sclerosis (14). ...when smoked for reducing intraocular pressure in patients with glaucoma (1268). There is some evidence marijuana can decrease intraocular pressure, but it also seems to decrease blood flow to the optic nerve. So far, it is not known if it can improve visual function (6,14,1268).

There is insufficient reliable information available about the effectiveness of marijuana for its other uses.

Mechanism of Action

The applicable parts of marijuana are the flower and leaf. Marijuana contains cannabinoids, including tetrahydrocannabinol (THC, dronabinol), that act on the central nervous system (CNS) (6,13). The THC concentration is highest in the flowers and leaves and lowest in the stems, roots, and seeds (6). THC can interact with cell-wall lipids or affect prostaglandin biosynthesis (18). It can act via cannabinoid receptors in neural tissues (2619) or opiate receptors in the forebrain, leading to indirect inhibition of the emetic center in the medulla oblongata (13). Two types of cannabinoid receptors have been identified in animals: CB1, which is found predominantly in the CNS and is thought to be responsible for the psychoactive effects, and CB2 which is found in high levels on immune system cells including leukocytes, and to a lesser extent in the brain (5887,5888,5889). Endogenous substances which bind to these receptors have been identified (5887,5888). Tetrahydrocannabinol is a partial CB1 receptor agonist and has limited CB2 agonist activity (5889). Marijuana suppresses the immune system in experimental animals (18). While short-term inhalation increases bronchodilation and reduces bronchospasm, long-term use impairs lung function, which can result in constrictive lung disease. The cannabinoids in marijuana are allergenic in animal models (6). THC is absorbed orally or by inhalation, is rapidly distributed throughout the body, and has a high affinity for fat tissues (6). The metabolites appear in the urine for ten days or more after a single exposure and for several weeks after chronic exposure (6). In an animal model of multiple sclerosis, tetrahydrocannabinol has been reported to reduce tremor and spasticity, possibly through its activity at CB1 receptors in the brain (5889). Cannabinoids have been reported to inhibit human breast cancer cell proliferation in vitro, and tetrahydrocannabinol produced tumor eradication or improvements in survival in a significant proportion of animals with experimentally induced malignant gliomas (a type of brain tumor) (5887). In these animal studies it was also found that tetrahydrocannabinol was inducing tumor cell apoptosis via CB1 and CB2 receptors expressed on the glioma cells (5887).

Adverse Reactions

The use of marijuana can cause xerostomia (dry mouth), nausea, vomiting, and a characteristic reddening of the conjunctiva (6,14). Cardiovascular effects include tachycardia, hypotension or hypertension, syncope, palpitations, and vasodilation (6,14). Intoxicating doses of marijuana impair reaction time, motor coordination, and visual perceptions, and can also produce panic reactions, hallucinations, flashbacks, depression and other emotional disturbances (6,14). An individual's driving ability can be impaired up to 8 hours (18). The chronic use of marijuana can cause laryngitis, bronchitis, apathy, psychic decline, sexual dysfunction, and abnormal menstruation (6,18), and has been associated with several cases of an unusual pattern of bullous emphysema (1395). Signs of acute poisoning from marijuana include nausea, vomiting, lacrimation, hacking cough, disturbed cardiac function, and limb numbness (18). Marijuana has a high abuse potential (6). Regular smoking of 3-4 marijuana cigarettes per day is reported to produce as many symptoms as an average of 22 tobacco cigarettes per day, and comparable airway histological effects as 20 tobacco cigarettes per day (1395).

Regular use of marijuana in middle-aged persons has been associated with an increased risk of myocardial infarction. Unpublished evidence indicates that there is a 4.8 fold increase in relative risk of myocardial infarction within the first hour following smoking marijuana. Regular marijuana smoking was defined as smoking marijuana less than once a month to daily (1356).

Interactions with Herbs & Other Dietary Supplements

Theoretically, marijuana can have additive or synergistic effects when used with herbs that possess CNS depressant or stimulant effects.

Interactions with Drugs

BARBITURATES: Marijuana can decrease barbiturate clearance rate (2619).
FLUOXETINE, DISULFIRAM: Concomitant use of marijuana can cause transient hypomanic episodes (2619).
THEOPHYLLINE: Concomitant use can increase theophylline metabolism (2619).
OTHER DRUGS: Use of dronabinol can have additive or synergistic effects with amphetamines, anticholinergics, antihistamines, cocaine, hypnotics, psychomimetics, sedatives, and sympathomimetics (2619).

Interactions with Foods

ALCOHOL: Concomitant use of alcohol with dronabinol can have additive or synergistic CNS effects (2619).

Interactions with Lab Tests

INTRAOCULAR PRESSURE: Marijuana smoking reduces intraocular pressure and test results in some patients with glaucoma (1268).

Interactions with Diseases or Conditions

CARDIOVASCULAR DISEASES: Avoid; marijuana has the potential to cause tachycardia and transient hypertension (6).
COMPROMISED IMMUNE FUNCTION: Theoretically, inhalation of marijuana smoke containing Aspergillus spores increases the risk of fungal infections and sensitization in individuals with compromised immune function (6).
RESPIRATORY DISEASES: Long-term use of marijuana can exacerbate respiratory conditions (6). Chronic marijuana use has been associated with several cases of an unusual pattern of bullous emphysema (1395).
SEIZURE DISORDERS: Marijuana might exacerbate, or help control, seizure disorders in some individuals (6).

Dosage and Administration

ORAL: People typically use 5 to 15 drops of marijuana tincture or 1 to 3 drops of fluid extract. The prescription product dronabinol (Marinol) is used in doses of 5 to 15 mg/m2 every 2 for 4 hours for cancer chemotherapy-induced nausea and vomiting, and 2.5 to 10 mg twice daily for appetite stimulation in people with AIDS (14).
INHALATION: People typically use 1 to 3 grains (65 to 195 mg) of cannabis for smoking. Hashish, the plant resin, is smoked in a dose of up to 1 grain (16 to 65 mg). Potency may vary. The drug deteriorates rapidly, requiring ascending doses to produce its effect (5267).

Comments

Avoid confusion with hemp, a distinct variety of Cannabis sativa cultivated for its fiber and seeds, which contains less than 1% THC. Marijuana is classified as a Schedule I controlled substance, making possession illegal (6). In March 1999, the Institute of Medicine released a report, titled "Marijuana and Medicine: Assessing the Science Base," which concludes: "Until a non-smoked, rapid-onset cannabinoid drug delivery system becomes available, we acknowledge that there is no clear alternative for people suffering from chronic conditions that might be relieved by smoking marijuana, such as pain or AIDS wasting. One possible approach is to treat patients as n-of-1 clinical trials, in which patients are fully informed of their status as experimental subjects using a harmful drug delivery system, and in which their condition is closely monitored and documented under medical supervision, thereby increasing the knowledge base of the risks and benefits of marijuana use under such conditions."

British health authorities authorized clinical trials of marijuana-based drugs for patients with multiple sclerosis (MS) and severe pain. Participants in these studies will use sublingual formulations manufactured by GW Pharmaceuticals, designed to maximize pain relief. The manufacturer claims that the results of these studies might influence the future legal status of marijuana in Britain (5046).

MARJORAM

Also Known As

Garden Marjoram, Gartenmajoran, Knotted Marjoram, Majoran, Majorana aetheroleum oil, Majorana herb, Marjolaine, Mejorana, Sweet Marjoram.
CAUTION: See separate listing for Oregano.

Scientific Names

Origanum majorana, synonym Majorana hortensis.
Family: Lamiaceae or Labiatae.

People Use This For

Orally, marjoram is used for rhinitis and colds in infants, rhinitis in toddlers, and gastritis (2,18). Marjoram oil is used for coughs, gall bladder complaints, and gastrointestinal cramps (18).

In combination products, marjoram leaf, flower, or oil are used for stimulating appetite, as a digestive aid, antispasmodic, antiflatulent, astringent, for "strengthening of the stomach," acute and chronic gastritis, ulcus ventriculi, colic-like nervous gastrointestinal disorders, and diathermic effect for circulatory deficiencies in the abdominal regions. Marjoram is also used in combination products as a support of intestinal activity; purification of the system; supportive for acute inflammatory liver diseases; managing gallstones; dry, irritating coughs; swellings of the nasal and pharyngeal mucosa; inflammation of the ears; headaches; reducing blood glucose levels; promoting milk secretion; and as a nerve, heart, and circulation system tonic. Combination products with marjoram are used for promoting healthy sleep, treating mood swings, a tonic during convalescence, a blood builder, anorexia, sprains, bruises, lumbago, dysmenorrhea, climacteric complaints, strengthening of the female organs, an adjuvant for vaginal discharge, adnexitis, menstrual disturbances, urogenital bleeding, and as a diuretic (2).

In folk medicine, the marjoram leaf and flower are used for cramps, depression, dizziness, gastrointestinal disorders, migraines, nervous headaches, neurasthenia, paralysis, paroxysmal coughs, rhinitis, and as a diuretic (18).

For food uses, marjoram is a culinary spice and commonly used in foods (11). The oil and oleoresin are used as flavor ingredients in foods and beverages (11).

In manufacturing, the oil is used as a fragrance component in soaps and cosmetics (11).

Safety

LIKELY SAFE ...when the flower, leaf, and oil are consumed in amounts commonly found in food (11). Marjoram has Generally Recognized as Safe (GRAS) status in the US (11).

POSSIBLY SAFE ...when the leaf is used orally for medicinal purposes (12) on a short-term basis (2). ...when marjoram oil is used orally and appropriately (11).

POSSIBLY UNSAFE ...when the flower, leaf, and oil are used long-term because marjoram contains arbutin and hydroxyquinone. Some information suggests hydroxyquinone might cause cancer (2). ...when using fresh marjoram topically because it can cause eye and skin inflammation (11).

CHILDREN: LIKELY SAFE ...when the flower, leaf, and oil are used orally in food amounts. POSSIBLY UNSAFE ...when larger amounts are used in children; avoid using (2).

PREGNANCY: LIKELY SAFE ...when used orally in food amounts (11,12). POSSIBLY UNSAFE ...when used in greater amounts because it has the potential for stimulating menstruation (19).

LACTATION: Insufficient reliable information available; avoid using in amounts larger than those found in foods.

Effectiveness

There is insufficient reliable information available about the effectiveness of marjoram.

Mechanism of Action

The applicable parts of marjoram are the flower, leaf and oil. Marjoram has antiflatulent, antispasmodic, diaphoretic, and diuretic properties (11). The volatile oil demonstrates antimicrobial and insecticidal activity (18). There is some evidence that marjoram has antibacterial activity and antiviral activity against the herpes simplex virus (11). The constituents of marjoram include small amounts of arbutin and hydroxyquinone (2). Arbutin, an antibacterial principle, is poorly absorbed from the gastrointestinal tract (7). Marjoram is a rich source of calcium and iron (19).

Adverse Reactions

Topically, fresh marjoram can cause eye and skin inflammation (11). Hydroxyquinone can cause skin depigmentation (2); however, this adverse effect has not been reported with the use of the marjoram ointment (2).

Interactions with Herbs & Other Dietary Supplements

Insufficient reliable information available.

Interactions with Drugs

No interactions are known to occur, and there is no known reason to expect a clinically significant interaction with marjoram.

Interactions with Foods

No interactions are known to occur, and there is no known reason to expect a clinically significant interaction with marjoram.

Interactions with Lab Tests

No interactions are known to occur, and there is no known reason to expect a clinically significant interaction with marjoram.

Interactions with Diseases or Conditions

CROSS-ALLERGENICITY: Marjoram can cause allergic reactions in people allergic to the Lamiaceae family plants, which include basil, hyssop, lavender, mint, oregano, and sage (3705).

Dosage and Administration

ORAL: The typical dose of marjoram is one to two cups of the tea throughout the day (18). The tea is prepared by steeping 1-2 teaspoons of the flower or leaf in 250 mL boiling water for 5 minutes and then straining.
TOPICAL: Marjoram is commonly used as a poultice or mouthwash (18).

Comments

In early Greek mythology, the goddess of love, Aphrodite, was believed to have grown marjoram, and marjoram has since been used in various love potions (6002). Avoid confusion with oregano (Origanum vulgare), also referred to as wild marjoram and winter marjoram (2,18).

MARSH BLAZING STAR

Also Known As

Backache Root, Blazing-Star, Button Snakeroot, Colic Root, Devil's Bite Prairie-Pine, Gayfeather, Gay-Feather.

Scientific Names

Liatris spicata, synonym Laciniaria spicata; Liatris callilepis; Serratula spicata.
Family: Compositae or Asteraceae.

People Use This For

Orally, marsh blazing star root is used for kidney disorders, dysmenorrhea, gonorrhea, and as a diuretic (18).

Safety

There is insufficient reliable information available about the safety of marsh blazing star.
Pregnancy and Lactation: Insufficient reliable information available; avoid using.

Effectiveness

There is insufficient reliable information available about the effectiveness of marsh blazing star.

Mechanism of Action

The applicable part of marsh blazing star is the root. Marsh blazing star contains coumarin as its active principle (18). However, coumarin itself is not an anticoagulant. It has only 0.1%-0.02% of the anticoagulant effect of bishydroxy-coumarin (295). Some studies suggest coumarin might be effective in reducing edemas and inflammations by increasing venous and lymphatic return (295).

Adverse Reactions

Orally, use of marsh blazing star, which contains coumarin, can be associated with nausea and vomiting (286), diarrhea, dizziness, insomnia (287), asymptomatic SGOT elevations (286), and liver toxicity (6,18,4501).
Topically, handling the plant can cause contact dermatitis (3837).
Marsh blazing star can cause an allergic reaction in individuals sensitive to the Asteraceae/Compositae family. Members of this family include ragweed, chrysanthemums, marigolds, daisies, and many other herbs.

Interactions with Herbs & Other Dietary Supplements

Insufficient reliable information available.

Interactions with Drugs

No interactions are known to occur, and there is no known reason to expect a clinically significant interaction with marsh blazing star.

Interactions with Foods

No interactions are known to occur, and there is no known reason to expect a clinically significant interaction with marsh blazing star.

Interactions with Lab Tests

No interactions are known to occur, and there is no known reason to expect a clinically significant interaction with marsh blazing star.

Interactions with Diseases or Conditions

CROSS-ALLERGENICITY: Can cause an allergic reaction in individuals sensitive to the Asteraceae/Compositae family. Members of this family include ragweed, chrysanthemums, marigolds, daisies, and many other herbs.

Dosage and Administration

ORAL: The ground root is used as a tea.

Comments

None.

MARSH MARIGOLD

Also Known As

Bull's Eyes, Cowslip, Horse Blobs, Kingcups, Leopard's Foot, Meadow Routs, Palsy Root, Solsequia, Sponsa Solis, Verrucaria, Water Blobs, Water Dragon.

Scientific Names

Caltha palustris.
Family: Ranunculaceae.

People Use This For

Orally, marsh marigold is used to stop pain and cramps, for menstrual disorders and bronchial inflammation. Historically, it was used orally for jaundice, and liver and biliary disorders. Marsh marigold was also used as a laxative, diuretic, and to lower cholesterol levels and raise blood sugar.
Some Native Americans and Russians used marsh marigold topically for cleaning skin lesions and sores (18).

Safety

LIKELY UNSAFE …when the fresh above ground parts are used orally or topically because they cause severe local irritation (18).
There is insufficient reliable information about the safety of the medicinal use of the dried above ground parts.

PREGNANCY AND LACTATION: LIKELY UNSAFE …when the fresh above ground parts are used orally or topically (18). There is insufficient reliable information available about the safety of the dried above ground parts during pregnancy and lactation.

Effectiveness
There is insufficient reliable information available about the effectiveness of marsh marigold.

Mechanism of Action
The applicable parts of marsh marigold are the above ground parts of the flowering plant. When the fresh plant is crushed or cut into small pieces, the glycoside ranunculin is enzymatically changed into a severely irritating protoanemonin, which, in turn, rapidly degrades into the less toxic anemonin (18). Both protoanemonin and ranunculin are destroyed to an unknown extent during the drying process (2).

Adverse Reactions
Orally, ingestion of marsh marigold can cause severe irritation of the gastrointestinal tract, with colic and diarrhea. Irritation of the urinary tract can also occur.
Topically, skin contact with the fresh plant can cause blisters and burns that are difficult to heal (18).

Interactions with Herbs & Other Dietary Supplements
Insufficient reliable information available.

Interactions with Drugs
No interactions are known to occur, and there is no known reason to expect a clinically significant interaction with marsh marigold.

Interactions with Foods
No interactions are known to occur, and there is no known reason to expect a clinically significant interaction with marsh marigold.

Interactions with Lab Tests
No interactions are known to occur, and there is no known reason to expect a clinically significant interaction with marsh marigold.

Interactions with Diseases or Conditions
No interactions are known to occur, and there is no known reason to expect a clinically significant interaction with marsh marigold.

Dosage and Administration
No typical dosage.

Comments
None.

MARSH TEA

Also Known As
James' Tea, Labrador Tea, Ledi palustris herba, Marsh Citrus, Moth Herb, Romarin Sauvage, Sumpfporst, Swamp Tea, Wild Rosemary.
CAUTION: See separate listing for Labrador Tea.

Scientific Names
Ledum palustre.
Family: Lamiaceae.

People Use This For
Orally, marsh tea is used for rheumatic discomforts, whooping cough (2), for bronchitis, cold, cough, whitlow (herpes infection of the finger), relieving chest and lung ailments, stimulating milk flow, as a diaphoretic, diuretic, abortifacient (2), expectorant, and narcotic.

Safety

LIKELY UNSAFE …when large amounts are used orally to try to cause abortion (2). The essential oil of marsh tea causes severe gastrointestinal tract irritation, kidneys and urinary tract damage, and central nervous system excitation followed by paralysis (2).

There is insufficient reliable information available about the safety of marsh tea for its other uses.

PREGNANCY: LIKELY UNSAFE …when used orally; contraindicated (2,19). Marsh tea is considered to be a potential uterine stimulant (19).

LACTATION: Insufficient reliable information available; avoid using.

Effectiveness

There is insufficient reliable information available about the effectiveness of marsh tea.

Mechanism of Action

Some evidence suggests marsh tea might have antitussive and anti-inflammatory activity. It might also inhibit motility (2) and stimulate uterine activity (19).

Adverse Reactions

Orally, ingestion of large amounts of marsh tea can cause poisoning (2). The essential oil of marsh tea can cause severe irritation of the gastrointestinal tract, vomiting, diarrhea, irritation and damage to the kidneys and urinary tract, heavy perspiration, myalgias, arthralgias, and central nervous system excitation with narcotic intoxication, followed by paralysis (2).

Interactions with Herbs & Other Dietary Supplements

Insufficient reliable information available.

Interactions with Drugs

CNS DEPRESSANTS: Marsh tea can potentiate effects of barbiturates and alcohol (2).

Interactions with Foods

No interactions are known to occur, and there is no known reason to expect a clinically significant interaction with marsh tea.

Interactions with Lab Tests

No interactions are known to occur, and there is no known reason to expect a clinically significant interaction with marsh tea.

Interactions with Diseases or Conditions

KIDNEY DYSFUNCTION: Contraindicated in individuals with kidney dysfunction (2).
GI IRRITATION: Theoretically, might exacerbate gastrointestinal tract inflammation or irritation (2).
URINARY TRACT IRRITATION: Theoretically, might exacerbate urinary tract irritation and inflammation (2).

Dosage and Administration

No typical dosage.

Comments

Marsh tea essential oil is unsafe: avoid using.

MARSHMALLOW

Also Known As

Alteia, Althaeae folium, Althaeae radi, Althea, Herba Malvae , Mallards, Mortification Root, Racine De Guimauve, Sweet Weed, Wymote.
CAUTION: See separate listings for Mallow flower and Mallow leaf.

Scientific Names

Althaea officinalis.
Family: Malvaceae.

People Use This For

Orally, marshmallow leaf and root are used for irritation or inflammation of the mouth and oral pharynx and the associated dry cough (1,2,4,5,6,8,9,11,18), and for inflammation of the gastric mucosa (1,2,4,8,11,18).

Topically, marshmallow leaf and root are used for abscesses (4,18), for varicose and thrombotic ulcers (4), as a poultice for skin inflammation or burns (8,18), and for other wounds (4,18). Marshmallow leaf is used topically as a poultice for insect bites (8). Marshmallow root is used topically in ointments for chapped skin (6,11) and chilblains (11).

In folk medicine, the marshmallow leaf and root have been used for respiratory tract mucous membrane inflammation (4,18), diarrhea (18), peptic ulcers (4), constipation (18), urinary tract inflammation (4,18), and urinary calculus (4).

For food uses, marshmallow leaf is used as a flavoring agent (4).

In manufacturing, the marshmallow root is used in foods and beverages (4,6,11).

Safety

LIKELY SAFE ...when consumed in amounts commonly found in foods (4,11). The leaf and root are approved for use in foods in the US (11). ...when taken orally for medicinal purposes (2,4,12).

POSSIBLY SAFE ...when used topically (4).

PREGNANCY AND LACTATION: Insufficient reliable information available.

Effectiveness

POSSIBLY EFFECTIVE ...when marshmallow leaf or root is taken orally for soothing irritation of the mouth and pharynx (1,2,4,5,6,7,8,9,11), for dry cough (1,2,8), and for irritation of the gastric mucosa (2).

There is insufficient reliable information available about the effectiveness of marshmallow leaf or root for its other uses.

Mechanism of Action

The applicable parts of marshmallow are the leaves and the root. Marshmallow leaf and root contain mucilage polysaccharides (1,4,6,7,11,18) that can soothe and protect mucous membranes from local irritation by forming a protective layer (1,2,4,6,7,9,18). The mucilage can inhibit mucociliary transport (1,2,6,18), stimulate phagocytosis (1,2,18) and other immune system activities (1,18), suppress cough (1,6,8,11), increase the anti-inflammatory effects of topical dexamethasone (1,6,18), and have hypoglycemic activity (1,4). The mucilage can also have antimicrobial (4,6), spasmolytic, antisecretory (6), diuretic, antilithic, and wound-healing (4) effects.

Adverse Reactions

Orally, marshmallow can cause hypoglycemia (4,11,18).

Interactions with Herbs & Other Dietary Supplements

HERBS AND SUPPLEMENTS: Concomitant use of marshmallow can retard the absorption of other herbs or supplements (1,2,11,12).

Interactions with Drugs

DEXAMETHASONE: Theoretically, marshmallow can increase the topical anti-inflammatory effects of dexamethasone (6,18).

HYPOGLYCEMIC DRUGS: Theoretically, due to claims of hypoglycemic effects, marshmallow might interfere with hypoglycemic therapy (4).

ORAL DRUGS: The fiber in marshmallow might impair absorption of oral drugs (1,2,11,12,19).

Interactions with Foods

No interactions are known to occur, and there is no known reason to expect a clinically significant interaction with marshmallow.

Interactions with Lab Tests

BLOOD GLUCOSE: Theoretically, marshmallow could lower blood glucose and test results (4,11,18).

Interactions with Diseases or Conditions

DIABETES: Theoretically, marshmallow could interfere with blood sugar control (4). Marshmallow syrup also contains sugar (2).

Dosage and Administration

ORAL: For irritation of the mouth or pharynx and associated dry cough, the typical dose of marshmallow is 2-5 grams of the dried leaf, 5 grams of the dried root or one cup of either leaf or root tea three times daily (4). The leaf tea is prepared by steeping 2-5 grams of the dried leaf in 150 mL boiling water for 5-10 minutes and then straining. The root tea is prepared by steeping 2-5 grams of the dried root in 150 mL cold water for 1-1.5 hours, straining, and then warming before consumption. The maximum dose of marshmallow is 5 grams of the dried leaf or 6 grams to 15 grams of the dried root daily (1,2,4,11). The usual dose of the liquid leaf or root extract (1:1 in 25% alcohol) is 2-5 mL three times daily (4). For irritation of oral or pharyngeal mucosa and the associated cough, the common dose of the marshmallow root syrup is 2-10 mL up to three times daily. The root syrup should not be used for any other indication (1,2,4). The syrup does contain sugar (2).

TOPICAL: The 5% powdered leaf in an ointment base is commonly applied three times daily (4).

Comments
Avoid confusion with the mallow (Malva sylvestris) flower and leaf.

MARTAGON

Also Known As
Purple Turk's Cap Lily, Turk's Cap.

Scientific Names
Lilium martagon.

People Use This For
Orally, martagon is used as a diuretic and for dysmenorrhea (18).
Topically, martagon is used for ulcers (18).

Safety
There is insufficient reliable information available about the safety of martagon.
Pregnancy and Lactation: Insufficient reliable information available; avoid using.

Effectiveness
There is insufficient reliable information available about the effectiveness of martagon.

Mechanism of Action
The applicable parts of martagon are the leaf, stem, and flower. Lilium martagon contains varied constituents including starch, soluble polysaccharides, gamma-methylene glutamic acid, and tuliposide (18).

Adverse Reactions
None reported.

Interactions with Herbs & Other Dietary Supplements
Insufficient reliable information available.

Interactions with Drugs
No interactions are known to occur, and there is no known reason to expect a clinically significant interaction with martagon.

Interactions with Foods
No interactions are known to occur, and there is no known reason to expect a clinically significant interaction with martagon.

Interactions with Lab Tests
No interactions are known to occur, and there is no known reason to expect a clinically significant interaction with martagon.

Interactions with Diseases or Conditions
No interactions are known to occur, and there is no known reason to expect a clinically significant interaction with martagon.

Dosage and Administration
ORAL: It is used in powdered form for tea (18).
TOPICAL: It is used in powdered form for poultices (18).

Comments

There is very little scientific information about this product. Our staff is continually analyzing the available information on natural medicines and will add data here as it becomes available.

MASTERWORT

Also Known As

Cow Cabbage, Cow Parsnip, Hogweed, Madnep, Radix Pimpinelle Franconiae, Woolly Parsnip, Youthwort. CAUTION: See separate listing for Goutweed (Aegopodium podagraria).

Scientific Names

Heracleum sphondylium, synonym Heracleum lanatum.
Family: Apiaceae.

People Use This For

In folk medicine, masterwort is used orally for relief of muscle cramps, stomach disorders, digestive problems, diarrhea, and mucous membrane inflammation of the GI tract (18).

Safety

POSSIBLY UNSAFE ...when used orally. Masterwort can cause phototoxicity (19) and some of the furocoumarin constituents can be carcinogenic (4).
PREGNANCY: LIKELY UNSAFE ...when used orally; contraindicated for use in early pregnancy, due to the reported ability to stimulate menstruation (19).
LACTATION: POSSIBLY UNSAFE ...when used orally (4); avoid using.

Effectiveness

There is insufficient reliable information available about the effectiveness of masterwort.

Mechanism of Action

Masterwort is considered to be a mild expectorant, although this effect remains unproven (18). It contains furocoumarins (bergapten, isopimpinellin, pimpinellin, isoberapten, spondin) and a volatile oil containing n-octylacetate (18). Bergapten, also known as 5-methoxypysoralen, is phototoxic and may also be carcinogenic (4).

Adverse Reactions

Orally, use increases skin sensitivity to UV light and can lead to phototoxicity (19).
Topically, application of the fresh plant can cause photodermatitis (3835).
Masterwort may also be carcinogenic.

Interactions with Herbs & Other Dietary Supplements

Insufficient reliable information available.

Interactions with Drugs

PSORALEN THERAPY: Contraindicated due to additive photosensitizing effect (19).

Interactions with Foods

No interactions are known to occur, and there is no known reason to expect a clinically significant interaction with masterwort.

Interactions with Lab Tests

No interactions are known to occur, and there is no known reason to expect a clinically significant interaction with masterwort.

Interactions with Diseases or Conditions

ULTRAVIOLET LIGHT THERAPY: Contraindicated due to photosensitizing effect (19); avoid excessive periods in sun (19).

Dosage and Administration

No typical dosage.

Comments

Masterwort is reportedly used as a replacement/adulterant for greater burnet-saxifrage (Pimpinella major) (7).

MASTIC

Also Known As

Lentisk, Mastich, Mastix.

Scientific Names

Pistacia lentiscus.

People Use This For

Orally, mastic is used for gastric and duodenal ulcers, respiratory conditions, muscle aches, and to improve circulation. It is also used for bacterial and fungal infections (6).

Topically, mastic is used as skin care for cuts, as an insect repellent, to improve adhesive strength in surgical tapes, and as a drug releasing vehicle (6).

In dentistry, mastic resin is used as a material for fillings (18). The masticated resin releases substances that freshen the breath and tighten the gums (18).

In manufacturing, mastic resin is used in the food and drink industries (18) and in the production of chewing gum (18).

Safety

POSSIBLY SAFE ...when used orally (18).

PREGNANCY AND LACTATION: Insufficient reliable information available; avoid using.

Effectiveness

There is insufficient reliable information available about the effectiveness of mastic.

Mechanism of Action

The applicable part of mastic is the resin. Mastic tree contains resins including the triterpenes mastic acid, isomastic acid, oleanlic acid, and tirucallol. It also contains a volatile oil containing alpha-pinene as a constituent. The volatile oil and the resin are both thought to have astringent and aromatic effects (18). For prevention of gastric and duodenal ulcers, some researchers think mastic might have antisecretory and possibly cytoprotective effects. Animal models show that it seems to help protect the gastric mucosa during aspirin, phenylbutazone, or reserpine therapy (4142). This effect has not yet been found in humans. There is some in vitro evidence that mastic extract has antimicrobial and antifungal activity (4141). There is also preliminary evidence that mastic might have hypotensive and antioxidant effects (6).

Adverse Reactions

Children who ingest mastic tree resin might develop diarrhea (18). The pollen of mastic tree is allergenic (4140). Exposure to mastic tree can cause allergic reactions in individuals allergic to Schinus terebintifolious and other Pistacia species (4140).

Interactions with Herbs & Other Dietary Supplements

CROSS-ALLERGENICITY: Individuals allergic to mastic tree might also have an allergic reaction to Schinus terebintifolious and other Pistacia species (4140).

Interactions with Drugs

No interactions are known to occur, and there is no known reason to expect a clinically significant interaction with mastic.

Interactions with Foods

No interactions are known to occur, and there is no known reason to expect a clinically significant interaction with mastic.

Interactions with Lab Tests

No interactions are known to occur, and there is no known reason to expect a clinically significant interaction with mastic.

Interactions with Diseases or Conditions

No interactions are known to occur, and there is no known reason to expect a clinically significant interaction with mastic.

Dosage and Administration

No typical dosage.

Comments

Mastic resin is the resin from the trunk of Pistacia lentiscus.

MATE

Also Known As

Hervea, Ilex, Jesuit's Brazil Tea, Jesuit's Tea, Maté Folium, Paraguay Tea, St. Bartholemew's Tea, Yerba Maté, Yerba Mate.
CAUTION: See separate listing for Caffeine.

Scientific Names

Ilex paraguariensis.
Family: Aquifoliaceae.

People Use This For

Orally, mate is used as a stimulant to relieve mental and physical fatigue (2,6,8).
In folk medicine, it has been used as a diuretic (4,6,8), for modifying mood or affective disorders, as a mild analgesic for headache and rheumatic pains (4), and as a laxative in large amounts (13). It has also been used for depression (4), weight loss (8), urinary tract infection, cardiac insufficiency, arrhythmias, nervous heart complaints, kidney and bladder stones (18), and to promote cleansing and excretion of waste (6).
In foods, the use of mate includes a tea-like beverage (5,6,9,13).

Safety

POSSIBLY SAFE ...when used orally and appropriately on a short-term basis (2,12).
POSSIBLY UNSAFE ...when mate is used orally in large amounts or for prolonged periods of time. Chronic use of the caffeine contained in mate can sometimes produce tolerance, habituation, and psychological dependence (15). The abrupt discontinuation can sometimes result in physical withdrawal symptoms (15).
CHILDREN: POSSIBLY UNSAFE ...when used orally. The adverse effects of caffeine can be more severe in children than adults (15).
PREGNANCY: Insufficient reliable information available. Although the caffeine content of a typical dose should not cause concern, other constituents could be unsafe.
LACTATION: POSSIBLY UNSAFE ...when used orally; avoid using. The caffeine is secreted in breast milk and can cause sleep disturbances in breast-fed infants (18).

Effectiveness

POSSIBLY EFFECTIVE ...when used orally for relief of mental and physical fatigue (2), as a central nervous system stimulant (12,15,18), as a diuretic (15,18), for headache (15), for increasing blood pressure in hypotension (15), and for weight loss (caffeine/ephedrine) (695,696,1704).
There is insufficient reliable information available about the effectiveness of mate for its other uses.

Mechanism of Action

The applicable parts of mate are the leaf and leaf stem. Mate is thought to have appetite suppressant (4), lipolytic, and glycogenolytic activity (2,18). It contains 0.2-2% caffeine (compared to 1-2% in coffee) (4,5,6,7,9,12,13,18) which acts as a central nervous system stimulant (12,15,18), increases heart rate and contractility (7,18), increases blood pressure (6663), inhibits platelet aggregation (6,18), stimulates gastric acid secretion, causes diuresis (15,18), relaxes extracerebral vascular and bronchial smooth muscle, stimulates the release of catecholamines (18), and might indirectly inhibit histamine release (6130). It also contains theophylline and theobromine, which have actions similar to caffeine (4,6). Mate contains 4-16% tannins (4,12) with possible carcinogenic and hepatotoxic properties (12).

Adverse Reactions

Large amounts, or the prolonged use of mate is associated with an increased risk of cancers of the esophagus (4,6), mouth, larynx (1528), kidney (1529), bladder (1530), and lung (1531). There is one report of venous occlusive disease associated with excessive, long-term mate consumption (4,5614). The caffeine constituent of mate can cause insomnia, nervousness, restlessness, agitation (7,15), gastric irritation (7), nausea, vomiting, diuresis (15), fast heartbeat, arrhythmias, increased respiratory rate, muscle spasms, ringing in the ears, headache, delirium, and convulsions (15,505). High doses of mate providing 250 mg of caffeine can also increase blood pressure. This doesn't seem to occur in people who habitually consume caffeine products (6663). The adverse effects of caffeine are usually more severe in children than adults (15). Some evidence shows caffeine is associated with fibrocystic breast disease in women; other evidence disputes this (14,15). The chronic use of caffeine, especially in large amounts, can produce tolerance, habituation, and psychological dependence (15). The abrupt discontinuation of caffeine can result in physical withdrawal symptoms, including irritability, anxiety, headaches, and dizziness (15).

Combining ephedra with mate increases the risk of adverse effects, due to the caffeine contained in mate (2729). One unpublished report associated jitteriness, hypertension, seizures, temporary loss of consciousness, and hospitalization requiring life support with the use of a combination ephedra and guarana (caffeine) product (1380). There is one report of ischemic stroke in an athlete who consumed ephedra 40-60 mg, creatine monohydrate 6 grams, caffeine 400-600 mg, and a variety of other supplements daily for six weeks (1275).

Interactions with Herbs & Other Dietary Supplements

CAFFEINE CONTAINING HERBS/SUPPLEMENTS: Concomitant use of mate and caffeine-containing herbs/supplements constitutes therapeutic duplication (due to the caffeine contained in mate) which increases the risk of caffeine-related adverse effects. Other natural products which contain caffeine include black tea, cocoa, coffee, cola nut, green tea, and guarana.

EPHEDRA (Ma Huang): Concomitant use can increase the risk of stimulatory adverse effects, due to the caffeine contained in mate (7). One unpublished report associated jitteriness, hypertension, seizures, temporary loss of consciousness, and hospitalization requiring life support with the use of a combination ephedra and guarana (caffeine) product (1380).

Interactions with Drugs

ACETAMINOPHEN (Tylenol): Theoretically, concomitant use might increase the pain-relieving activity of acetaminophen, due to the caffeine contained in mate. Caffeine increases the pain-relieving activity of acetaminophen by up to 40% (512).

ASPIRIN: Theoretically, concomitant use might increase the pain-relieving activity of aspirin, due to the caffeine contained in mate. Caffeine increases the pain-relieving activity of aspirin by up to 40% (512).

BENZODIAZEPINES: Theoretically, concomitant use might reduce the sedative and anxiolytic effects of benzodiazepines, due to the caffeine contained in mate (14).

BETA-ADRENERGIC AGONISTS: Theoretically, concomitant use might increase the cardiac inotropic effects of beta agonists, due to the caffeine contained in mate (15). Beta-adrenergic agonists include albuterol (Proventil, Ventolin), metaproterenol (Alupent), terbutaline (Brethine), and isoproterenol (Isuprel).

CIMETIDINE (Tagamet): Theoretically, concomitant use might increase serum caffeine concentrations and the risk of adverse effects, due to the caffeine contained in mate. Cimetidine decreases the rate of caffeine clearance by 30-50% (14).

CLOZAPINE (Clozaril): Theoretically, co-administration might acutely exacerbate psychotic symptoms, due to the caffeine contained in mate. Caffeine can increase the effects and toxicity of clozapine (151). Caffeine doses of 400-1000 mg per day inhibit clozapine metabolism (5051).

CNS STIMULANTS: Concomitant use might increase the risk of stimulant adverse effects, due to the caffeine contained in mate (151,2719). CNS stimulants include nicotine, cocaine, sympathomimetic amines, and amphetamines.

DIABETES THERAPY: Theoretically, concomitant use of mate and diabetes drugs might interfere with blood glucose control, due to the caffeine contained in coffee. This is based in the claim that caffeine might have hyperglycemic effects (19).

DISULFIRAM (Antabuse): Theoretically, concomitant use might increase serum caffeine concentrations and the risk of adverse effects, due to the caffeine contained in mate. Disulfiram decreases the rate of caffeine clearance (15).

EPHEDRINE: Concomitant use might increase the risk of stimulatory adverse effects, due to the caffeine contained in mate (7,19). An unpublished report associated jitteriness, hypertension, seizures, temporary loss of consciousness, and hospitalization requiring life support with the use of a combination ephedra (ephedrine) and guarana (caffeine) product (1380).

ESTROGEN (Estrace): Theoretically, concomitant use might increase serum caffeine concentrations and the risk of adverse effects, due to the caffeine contained in mate. Estrogen inhibits caffeine metabolism (2714).

ERGOTAMINE: Theoretically, concomitant use might increase the GI absorption of ergotamine, due to the caffeine contained in mate. Caffeine increases the GI absorption of ergotamine (15).

LITHIUM (Eskalith, Lithobid): Theoretically, abrupt mate withdrawal might increase serum lithium levels, due to the caffeine contained in mate. There are two case reports of lithium tremor that worsened upon abrupt coffee withdrawal (609,610).

MEXILETINE (Mexitil): Theoretically, concomitant use might increase serum caffeine concentrations and the risk of adverse effects, due to the caffeine contained in mate. Mexiletine reduces caffeine metabolism (14).

MONOAMINE OXIDASE INHIBITORS (MAOIs): Theoretically, concomitant intake of large amounts of mate with MAOIs might precipitate a hypertensive crisis, due to the caffeine contained in mate. This is based on the claim that intake of large amounts of caffeine with MAOIs might precipitate a hypertensive crisis (19).

ORAL CONTRACEPTIVES (OCs): Theoretically, concomitant use might increase serum caffeine concentrations and the risk adverse effects, due to the caffeine contained in mate. OCs decrease the rate of caffeine clearance by 40-65% (14).

PHENYLPROPANOLAMINE (Dexatrim, Propagest): Theoretically, concomitant use might cause an additive increase in blood pressure and serum caffeine concentrations, due to the caffeine contained in mate (14). Concomitant use of caffeine and phenylpropanolamine can cause an additive increase in blood pressure, and increase serum caffeine concentrations (14).

QUINOLONES: Theoretically, concomitant use might increase serum caffeine concentrations and the risk of adverse effects, due to the caffeine contained in mate. Quinolones decrease caffeine clearance (606,607,608). Quinolones (also referred to as fluoroquinolones) include ciprofloxacin (Cipro), enoxacin (Penetrex), gatifloxacin (Tequin), levofloxacin (Levaquin), lomefloxacin (Maxaquin), moxifloxacin (Avelox), norfloxacin (Noroxin), ofloxacin (Floxin), sparfloxacin (Zagam), and trovafloxacin (Trovan).

RILUZOLE (Rilutek): Theoretically, concomitant use might increase serum caffeine and riluzole concentrations and the risk of adverse effects of both caffeine and riluzole, due to the caffeine contained in mate. Caffeine and riluzole are both metabolized by cytochrome P450 1A2 and concomitant use might reduce metabolism of one or both agents (14).

TERBINAFINE (Lamisil): Theoretically, concomitant use might increase serum caffeine concentrations and the risk of adverse effects, due to the caffeine contained in mate. Terbinafine decreases the rate of caffeine clearance (14).

THEOPHYLLINE (Theo-Dur): Theoretically, concomitant use might increase serum theophylline concentrations and the risk of adverse effects, due to the caffeine contained in mate. Large amounts of caffeine might inhibit theophylline metabolism (14).

VERAPAMIL (Calan, Isoptin, Verelan): Theoretically, concomitant use might increase plasma caffeine concentrations and the risk of adverse effects, due to the caffeine contained in mate. Verapamil increases plasma caffeine concentrations by 25% (14).

Interactions with Foods

GRAPEFRUIT JUICE: Concomitant use can increase caffeine levels and the risk of adverse effects (504).

Interactions with Lab Tests

BLEEDING TIME: Mate might prolong bleeding time and increase test results, due to its caffeine content (1701).

BLOOD PRESSURE: Mate might increase blood pressure and blood pressure readings, due to its caffeine content (4).

URATE: Mate might falsely increase serum urate test results determined by the Bittner method, due to its caffeine content. Caffeine causes false elevations in serum urate test results determined by the Bittner method (15).

CATECHOLAMINES: Mate might increase urine catecholamine concentrations and test results, due to its caffeine content. Caffeine can increase urine catecholamine concentrations (15).

CREATINE: Mate might increase urine creatine concentrations and test results, due to its caffeine content (1701).

DIPYRIDAMOLE THALLIUM IMAGING: Mate might interfere with dipyridamole thallium imaging studies, due to its caffeine content. Caffeine attenuates the characteristic cardiovascular responses to dipyridamole and has altered test results (14).

5-HYDROXYINDOLEACETIC ACID: Mate might increase urine 5-hydroxyindoleacetic acid concentrations and test results, due to its caffeine content. Caffeine can increase urine catecholamine concentrations (15).

VANILLYLMANDELIC ACID (VMA): Mate might increase urine VMA concentrations and test results, due to its caffeine content. Caffeine can increase urine VMA concentrations (15).

TESTS FOR NEUROBLASTOMA: Mate, due to its caffeine content, might cause false-positive diagnosis of neuroblastoma, when diagnosis is based on tests of urine vanillylmandelic acid (VMA) or catecholamine concentrations. Caffeine can increase urine catecholamine and VMA concentrations (15).

TESTS FOR PHEOCHROMOCYTOMA: Mate, due to its caffeine content, might cause false-positive diagnosis of pheochromocytoma, when diagnosis is based on tests of urine vanillylmandelic acid (VMA) or catecholamine concentrations. Caffeine can increase urine catecholamine and VMA concentrations (15).

Interactions with Diseases or Conditions

DEPRESSION, ANXIETY DISORDERS: The caffeine in mate might aggravate these conditions (14).

HEART CONDITIONS: The caffeine in mate might induce cardiac arrhythmias in sensitive individuals (14,16).

HYPERTENSION: The caffeine in mate might increase blood pressure in people with high blood pressure (2272). Consumption of 250 mg caffeine can increase blood pressure in healthy people. But this doesn't seem to occur in people who habitually consume caffeine products (6663).

KIDNEY DISEASE: The diuretic effect of the caffeine in mate can aggravate certain kidney disorders (19).

ULCERS: The caffeine in mate can aggravate gastric and peptic ulcers; avoid using (14,16).

Dosage and Administration

ORAL: The typical dose of mate is 2-4 grams of the dried leaf or one cup of the tea three times daily (4,18). The tea is prepared by steeping 2-4 grams of the dried leaf in 150 mL boiling water for 5-10 minutes and then straining. Some authorities suggest a maximum of 3 grams of the dried leaf per day (2,18). The usual dose of the liquid extract (1:1 in 25% alcohol) is 2-4 mL three times per day (4).

Comments

Mate, also known as Yerba Maté, is a popular beverage, much like coffee or tea, in Brazil, Paraguay, and Argentina (6002). The beverage is often prepared from leaves of Ilex paraguariensis, also referred to as Jesuit's tea, Jesuit's Brazil tea, Paraguay tea, and St. Bartholemew's tea. The herbal tea has caused multiple anticholinergic poisonings. However, belladonna alkaloids were identified and the poisonings were traced to a single contaminated lot of imported herbs (785).

MEADOWSWEET

Also Known As

Bridewort, Dolloff, Dropwort, Filipendula, Lady Of The Meadow, Meadow Queen, Meadow Sweet, Meadow-Wart, Queen Of The Meadow, Spiraeae flos, Spireae herba, Ulmaria.

Scientific Names

Filipendula ulmaria, synonym Spiraea ulmaria.
Family: Rosaceae.

People Use This For

Orally, meadowsweet is used as supportive therapy for colds (2,7,8,18).

In folk medicine, it is used for cough, bronchitis (18), dyspepsia, heartburn, peptic ulcer disease (4), and rheumatic disorders including gout (4,8,9,18). It is also used in folk medicine as a diuretic (8,9,18) and urinary antiseptic for acute cystitis (4).

Safety

POSSIBLY SAFE ...when used orally and appropriately (2,12).
POSSIBLY UNSAFE ...when an aqueous extract (tea) is used in large amounts or for prolonged periods of time because it contains high amounts of tannins (4).
PREGNANCY: LIKELY UNSAFE ...when used orally. Some evidence suggests meadowsweet might stimulate uterine activity (4).
LACTATION: Insufficient reliable information available; avoid using.

Effectiveness

There is insufficient reliable information available about the effectiveness of meadowsweet.

Mechanism of Action

The applicable parts of meadowsweet are the above ground parts and flower. Meadowsweet has stomachic, mild urinary antiseptic, antirheumatic, astringent, and antacid activities (4). It contains tannins, and the volatile oil contains low concentrations of salicylates (2,7,18). In animals, the above ground parts of meadowsweet decrease motor activity, lower temperature, induce muscle relaxation, and potentiate the effect of narcotics (4). In animals, the flower extract increases life expectancy, decreases vascular permeability, increases bronchial, intestinal, and uterine tone, and promotes uric acid excretion. In vitro, it has bacteriostatic activity (4). Meadowsweet aqueous extracts contain high concentrations of tannins (4) with strong astringent effects and potential adverse effects.

Adverse Reactions

Orally, meadowsweet can cause nausea and other stomach complaints (18). Bronchospastic activity has occurred with its use (4). Meadowsweet contains a salicylate constituent. There is insufficient reliable information available to know if the side effects and toxicity normally associated with salicylates could occur. The adverse reactions associated with salicylates include gastric and renal irritation, hypersensitivity, blood in stool, tinnitus, nausea, and vomiting. Salicin has been associated with skin rashes (4).

Interactions with Herbs & Other Dietary Supplements

SALICYLATE-CONTAINING HERBS: Theoretically, concomitant use of meadowsweet could potentiate the therapeutic and adverse effects of other herbs containing salicylate constituents. These herbs include black cohosh, poplar, sweet birch, white willow, and wintergreen (19).

Interactions with Drugs

NARCOTICS: Theoretically, meadowsweet can potentiate the narcotic effects (4).

SALICYLATE INTERACTIONS: Meadowsweet contains a salicylate constituent. There is insufficient reliable information available to determine if enough salicylate is present to cause drug interactions common to salicylates or aspirin. Aspirin can impair the effectiveness of beta-adrenergic blockers, probenecid, and sulfinpyrazone. It can increase the effects, side effects, or toxicity of alcohol, anticoagulants, carbonic anhydrase inhibitors, heparin, methotrexate, sulfonylureas, and valproic acid (151).

Interactions with Foods

No interactions are known to occur, and there is no known reason to expect a clinically significant interaction with meadowsweet.

Interactions with Lab Tests

There are no reports of lab interactions with this product. However, because it contains salicylates, use caution in interpreting test results known to be affected by salicylates.

Interactions with Diseases or Conditions

ASTHMA: Meadowsweet can exacerbate asthma and can have bronchospastic effects. Use cautiously in individuals with asthma (4).

ASPIRIN ALLERGY: Use cautiously in individuals with aspirin allergy; contains salicylate constituent.

Dosage and Administration

ORAL: For adults, the typical dose is one cup of the tea several times per day (2,8,18). The tea is prepared by steeping 2.5-3.5 grams of the dried flower or 4-5 grams of the above ground parts in 150 mL boiling water for 10 minutes and then straining. The usual dose of the liquid extract (1:1 in 25% alcohol) is 1.5-6 mL three times per day (4). The common dose of the tincture (1:5 in 45% alcohol) is 2-4 mL three times per day (4).

Comments

None.

MEDIUM CHAIN TRIGLYCERIDES (MCT)

Also Known As

MCT, MCT's, Medium-Chain Triglycerides.

Scientific Names

Medium chain triglycerides.

People Use This For

Orally, medium chain triglycerides (MCTs) are used as adjunctive therapy for malabsorption syndromes including diarrhea, steatorrhea (fat indigestion), gastrectomy, lymphatic abnormalities, and intestinal resection (14). MCTs are also used for chyluria and chylothorax, and for seizures in children, including akinetic, clonic, and petit mal (14). MCTs are also used for nutritional support of athletic training (1900), and decreasing body fat and increasing lean muscle mass (2272).

Intravenously, MCTs are used as a source of fat in total parenteral nutrition (14).

Safety

LIKELY SAFE ...when used orally and appropriately (14). ...when used intravenously and appropriately as part of total parenteral nutrition. Intravenous MCTs are a FDA approved-prescription product (14).

PREGNANCY AND LACTATION: LIKELY SAFE ...when used orally and appropriately (14).

Effectiveness

EFFECTIVE ...when used orally for malabsorption syndromes. These include diarrhea, steatorrhea, gastrectomy, lymphatic abnormalities, and intestinal resection (14). ...when used as an intravenous (IV) fat source in total parenteral nutrition preparations (2275,2276,2277,2278).

POSSIBLY EFFECTIVE ...when used orally for treating chyluria (14). ...when used orally for treating chylothorax (14). ...when used to treat seizures in children, including akinetic, clonic, and petit mal types (14,2273,2274).

POSSIBLY INEFFECTIVE ...when used orally to improve the absorption of calcium and magnesium. Although there is some conflicting evidence, most studies have shown that MCTs do not increase calcium and magnesium

absorption in healthy adults (6059), or in patients with small bowel resection (6050).
There is insufficient reliable information available about the effectiveness of MCTs for other uses.

Mechanism of Action
Medium chain triglycerides (MCTs) are semi-synthetic lipids composed of fatty acids with a chain length of six to twelve carbon atoms (14). They are primarily used for patients who cannot effectively absorb conventional long chain fats. They are normally substituted for only 50 to 70% of dietary fat since MCTs do not contain essential fatty acids (14). MCTs improve symptoms associated with malabsorption syndromes. They decrease diarrhea, protein loss, fecal fat, nitrogen excretion, steatorrhea (fat indigestion), and creatorrhea (14). They also increase fat absorption, body weight, and serum albumin; and promote a return to normal levels of phosphorus and uric acid (14). In healthy individuals, single doses of MCT oil can reduce blood triglyceride levels (834).

Adverse Reactions
Orally, MCTs can cause diarrhea, vomiting, irritability (2274), nausea, abdominal discomfort, intestinal gas noises, and essential fatty acid deficiency (14).

Interactions with Herbs & Other Dietary Supplements
Insufficient reliable information available.

Interactions with Drugs
No interactions are known to occur, and there is no known reason to expect a clinically significant interaction with MCTs.

Interactions with Foods
FOOD: Concomitant administration of MCTs with food can reduce the adverse effects associated with MCT (2273).

Interactions with Lab Tests
TRIGLYCERIDES: MCTs can lower blood triglyceride levels and test results (834).

Interactions with Diseases or Conditions
HEPATIC ENCEPHALOPATHY, CIRRHOSIS: MCTs in individuals with hepatic cirrhosis can cause narcosis and coma (14); use with caution.
DIABETES: MCTs can cause hyperketonemia (14); use with caution.
STEATORRHEA: MCTs can cause decreased fecal water, sodium, and potassium excretion (14). Some reports indicate that MCTs can also increase absorption of calcium and magnesium; however, this effect has not been supported in studies (6050,6059).
MECHANICAL VENTILATION: MCTs can cause increased oxygen consumption (14).

Dosage and Administration
ORAL: MCT oil contains 8.3 calories per gram, and one tablespoon provides 115 calories and weighs 14 grams (14). For malabsorption syndromes, initially 1 tablespoon is typically taken three to four times per day mixed with fruit juices, salads, and vegetables; incorporated into sauces for use on fish, chicken, or lean meats; or used in cooking or baking (14). For improving seizure control in children, 60% of the caloric intake is from MCT oil (2274).
INTRAVENOUS (IV): As a fat source in total parenteral nutrition formulations, a fat mixture containing 50% MCT and 50% long chain triglycerides is commonly used (2275,2276,2278).

Comments
MCTs ingested with food reduces the adverse effects (2273). Essential fatty acids must be also included in the diet to avoid essential fatty acid deficiency (14).

MELANOTAN-II

Also Known As
Melanotan II, MT-II.
CAUTION: See separate listing for Melatonin.

Scientific Names
Melanotan-II.

People Use This For

Subcutaneously, melanotan-II has been used to evaluate its effects on psychogenic erectile dysfunction (5687,5689), organic erectile dysfunction (5688,5689), and its effects after unilateral nerve-sparing radical prostatectomy (5689). It has also been used subcutaneously to evaluate its effects on tanning of the skin and for the prevention of sunlight-induced skin cancers (5683).

Safety

POSSIBLY SAFE ...when used subcutaneously to initiate penile erections in men with psychogenic or organic erectile dysfunction (5687,5688). Controlled clinical studies suggest mild to moderate adverse effects such as decreased appetite, facial flushing and nausea might occur with a dosage of 0.025 mg/kg (5685,5687,5688).

There is insufficient reliable information available about the safety of melanotan-II for its other uses or at other dosages.

PREGNANCY AND LACTATION: Insufficient reliable information available; avoid using.

Effectiveness

POSSIBLY EFFECTIVE ...when used subcutaneously to initiate penile erections in men with psychogenic or organic erectile dysfunction (5687,5688). Preliminary clinical trials have shown melanotan-II is superior to placebo for initiating spontaneous sustained penile erections (5685,5687,5688). ...when used subcutaneously for visible tanning of the skin (5685). A controlled clinical pilot study demonstrated melanotan-II caused increased pigmentation in the face, upper body, and buttocks. (5685).

There is insufficient reliable information available about the effectiveness of melanotan-II for its other uses.

Mechanism of Action

Melanotan-I and Melanotan-II are two alpha-melanocyte-stimulating-hormone analogues currently being extensively studied (5686). Both analogues have the ability to darken and tan the skin (5686) and were developed to not only promote skin pigmentation but also to possibly prevent sunlight-induced skin cancers (5683,5686). Compared to alpha-melanocyte-stimulating-hormone, melanotan-I and melanotan-II have increased melanotropic potency (26-100-fold) and increased resistance to degradation by plasma enzymes due to two amino acid substitutions (norleucine for methionine at position 4 and racemization of D-phenylalanine at position 7) in the alpha-melanocyte-stimulating-hormone peptide sequence (5685,5686). Melanotan-II is a cyclic heptapeptide containing a lactam bridge between the amino acids lysine and aspartic acid, enabling it to have even greater melanotropic potency than melanotan-I, a linear tridecapeptide (5685,5686). During a pilot phase-I clinical study, it was discovered by observers that melanotan-II not only caused increased visible tanning but also spontaneous penile erections with use (5685). Subsequent controlled clinical trials have shown melanotan-II initiates erections in men with psychogenic and organic dysfunction (5687,5688). The exact mechanism of action is unknown, but it is hypothesized that melanotan-II acts on pro-erectile pathways at the level of the central nervous system (5687). There are distinct melanocortin receptors found primarily in the brain (5686) and animal data suggests melanotropic peptides act in the hypothalamic regions surrounding the third ventricle (5687). Since dopamine agonists also induce penile erections (and yawning), evidence suggests the central mechanism involves a dopamine-oxytocin pathway (5687). Further clinical trials are in progress evaluating the pharmacokinetics, safety, and efficacy of melanotan-II (5689).

Adverse Reactions

Subcutaneously, melanotan-II can cause gastrointestinal cramping (5685), nausea (5685,5687,5688), decreased appetite (5687), facial flushing (5685,5688), fatigue, somnolence (5685), yawning, stretching and spontaneous penile erections (5685,5687,5688). It can also cause increased pigmentation of the face, upper body, and buttocks (5685).

Interactions with Herbs & Other Dietary Supplements

Insufficient reliable information available.

Interactions with Drugs

No interactions are known to occur, and there is no known reason to expect a clinically significant interaction with melanotan-II.

Interactions with Foods

No interactions are known to occur, and there is no known reason to expect a clinically significant interaction with melanotan-II.

Interactions with Lab Tests

No interactions are known to occur, and there is no known reason to expect a clinically significant interaction with melanotan-II.

Interactions with Diseases or Conditions

No interactions are known to occur, and there is no known reason to expect a clinically significant interaction with melanotan-II.

Dosage and Administration

SUBCUTANEOUS: The typical dosage is 0.025 mg/kg (5685,5687,5688). There is no frequency or other dosage information available.

Comments

Melanotan-II is not yet commercially available and is presently being studied in phase-II clinical trials (5689). Commercial dosage forms of melanotan-II such as a nasal spray or as an eyedrop are being investigated (5684,5687,5690).

MELATONIN

Also Known As

MEL, MLT, Pineal Hormone.

Scientific Names

N-acetyl-5-methoxytryptamine.

People Use This For

Orally, melatonin is used for jet lag, insomnia, shift-work disorder, circadian rhythm disorders in the blind, and benzodiazepine and nicotine withdrawal. Melatonin is also used orally for Alzheimer's disease; tinnitus; depression; migraine and cluster headache; hypertension; hyperpigmentation; osteoporosis; cancer of the breast, brain, lung, prostate, head, neck, and gastrointestinal tract; thrombocytopenia associated with cancer chemotherapy; and for cachexia in people with cancer. It is also used orally for epilepsy, as an anti-aging agent, for menopause, as preanesthetic medication, and for birth control. Transbuccal and sublingual forms of melatonin are also used for insomnia, shift-work disorder, and as preanesthetic medication.
Topically, melatonin is used as a skin protectant against ultraviolet (UV) light and sunburn.
Intramuscularly, melatonin is used for treating cancer.

Safety

LIKELY SAFE ...when used orally or parenterally and appropriately, short-term. Melatonin seems to be safe when used for up to 2 months (1049,1068,1077,1085,1738,1754,5854,5855,5857).
POSSIBLY SAFE ...when used orally and appropriately, long-term. There is some evidence melatonin can be used safely for up to 9 months in some patients (7040,7043).
CHILDREN: POSSIBLY UNSAFE ...when used orally or parenterally. Melatonin supplementation might adversely effect children. Young people, up to the age of 20 years produce melatonin endogenously in high levels (1740). Melatonin levels are inversely related to gonadal development (1739,1742,1743). Theoretically, exogenously administered melatonin might adversely effect gonadal development. Use with caution.
PREGNANCY: POSSIBLY UNSAFE ...when used orally or parenterally. High doses might have a contraceptive effect (214,1740). It is not known if lower doses cause this effect. Until more is known, advise pregnant patients to avoid using melatonin at any dose.
LACTATION: Insufficient reliable information available; avoid using.

Effectiveness

LIKELY EFFECTIVE ...when used orally for circadian rhythm sleep disorders in blind children and adults. Melatonin has a FDA orphan drug status for this indication (1082,1691,1744,1749,6585). ...when used orally for sleep-wake cycle disturbances in children and adolescents with mental retardation, autism, and other central nervous system disorders (1056,1745,1746,1747,1771).
POSSIBLY EFFECTIVE ...when used orally for jet lag. The effectiveness of melatonin for jet lag is controversial due to conflicting findings (6496). However, the majority of evidence shows that melatonin can modestly improve certain symptoms of jet lag such as alertness and psychomotor performance. Melatonin does not seem to be as helpful for other symptoms such as daytime sleepiness or fatigue (1049,1077,1079,1085,1722). ...when used orally for primary insomnia. Melatonin supplementation seems to be most beneficial for elderly patients with insomnia related to melatonin deficiency (1072,1729,1738,1754,7081). Melatonin might also improve subjective quality of sleep in non-elderly patients, but probably will not improve objective measures such as the time it takes to fall asleep (sleep latency) or total sleep time (1068,1070,1083). Sustained-release melatonin preparations seem to be better for improving sleep maintenance (1738,1754), and immediate-release preparations seem to be more beneficial for decreasing sleep latency (1738). ...when used orally for secondary insomnia. There is some evidence that melatonin can improve insomnia

related to depression (1053,1729) or Alzheimer's disease (1729). ...when used orally for tardive dyskinesia (TD). Melatonin 10 mg daily seems to decrease symptoms by 24-30% in some patients with TD after 6 weeks of treatment (7082). ...when used orally for thrombocytopenia. There is some evidence that melatonin can improve thrombocytopenia associated with cancer, cancer treatment, or certain other disorders. There is also some evidence melatonin can prevent thrombocytopenia induced by chemotherapy or interleukin-2 (IL-2) (1694,1695,1696,1697,2564). ...when used orally as adjunct treatment for advanced solid tumors. There is some evidence that combining high-dose melatonin with conventional chemotherapy or with interleukin-2 (IL-2) might improve tumor regression rate and one-year survival rate in patients with cancer of the breast, lung, kidney, liver, pancreas, stomach, or colon (1692,5854,5855,5857,7040,7043). Melatonin plus chemotherapy in patients with metastatic solid tumors seems to increase regression rate and one-year survival rate by approximately 50% compared to chemotherapy alone (7040). ...when used orally or intramuscularly for advanced solid tumors resistant to conventional treatment. There is some preliminary evidence that melatonin alone can improve stabilization rate and possibly one-year survival rate in patients with resistant or untreatable neoplasms of the lung, liver, pancreas, colon, breast, or brain (1080,1688,1693,2566). ...when used orally in combination with radiotherapy for glioblastoma. There is some evidence that melatonin can prolong survival time in patients with glioblastoma (14). ...when used orally in combination with the luteinizing hormone-releasing hormone (LHRH) analogue triptorelin for metastatic prostate cancer. There is evidence that 20 mg of oral melatonin used daily in combination with 37.5 mg of intramuscular triptorelin injected every 28 days can significantly decrease levels of prostate-specific antigen (PSA) and growth factors for prostate cancer, prolactin (PRL) and insulin-like growth factor-1 (IGF-1) (7255). ...when used orally for benzodiazepine withdrawal in elderly people with insomnia. So far, this benefit has only been demonstrated with a controlled-release formulation of melatonin (349,1751). ...when used sublingually for preoperative anxiety and sedation. Sublingual melatonin in doses of 0.05, 0.1, or 0.2 mg per kilogram appears to be as effective as comparable doses of midazolam and superior to placebo as a preanesthetic agent (1125). In some cases, melatonin might be preferable to midazolam because melatonin does not seem to cause anterograde amnesia or impair cognitive and psychomotor skills (1125). ...when used orally for prevention of episodic cluster headache (1127). ... when used orally to reduce some of the symptoms of acute nicotine withdrawal. A single oral dose of melatonin 0.3 mg 3.5 hours after nicotine withdrawal in smokers reduces subjective symptoms of anxiety, restlessness, irritability, depression, and cigarette craving over the next 10 hours (2424). ...when used topically to prevent erythema (sunburn) from ultraviolet (UV) light exposure. When applied prior to UV light exposure, melatonin seems to significantly decrease erythema (1051,1066,1768,1769).
POSSIBLY INEFFECTIVE ...when used orally to improve sleep and adjustment to rotating shift work (1052,1054,1721).
LIKELY INEFFECTIVE ...when used orally for depression. Although melatonin might help improve insomnia in some patients with depression, it does not seem to improve objective measures of depression (1053,1764,1766). There is also some concern that melatonin can worsen symptoms in some patients (1764). Tell patients with depression to avoid melatonin.
There is insufficient reliable information available about the effectiveness of melatonin for its other uses.

Mechanism of Action

Melatonin is a hormone synthesized endogenously in the pineal gland and secreted into the blood and cerebrospinal fluid (1123). It is produced from tryptophan, which is converted to 5-hydroxytryptophan, then to serotonin, then to N-acetylserotonin, and finally to melatonin (1773).

Melatonin's primary role seems to be regulation of the body's circadian rhythm, endocrine secretions, and sleep patterns (1773,7043). Melatonin production is influenced by day/night cycles. Light inhibits melatonin secretion and darkness stimulates secretion (1773). Endogenous melatonin is involved in several other functions including growth hormone secretion and sexual maturation, pain control, balance, and sexual activity (1776,1777,1778,6497). Melatonin release peaks between one to three years of age (507). Although it is commonly thought that melatonin levels naturally decline with age, this is controversial. More recent evidence seems to indicate that melatonin secretion does not decline with age after adolescence, and that melatonin suppression by light is not affected by age (1775,1781). However, there is good evidence that melatonin levels can be abnormally low in certain conditions or disease states. For example, insomniacs of all ages can have decreased melatonin levels. Patients with sleep disorders related to other conditions, such as fibromyalgia and depression, can also have low levels (6498). In other conditions, melatonin's response to light can be altered. For example, in patients with bipolar I disorder, melatonin response to light appears to be abnormal, but is not affected in less severe bipolar II disorder or unipolar depression(1123).

When exogenous melatonin is administered, it has a rapid, transient, and mild sleep-inducing effect. It can lower alertness, body temperature, and performance for 3-4 hours after oral administration. However, there is not usually a "hangover" effect the following day (1068,1132,1753,1756,1757,1758,1759,1760,1774). People try melatonin for cluster headache due to its effects on body temperature. People with cluster headache seem to have a rise in body heat and melatonin can lower core body temperature (1128,1129,1132). There is a lot of interest in using melatonin for patients with cancer. This all started due to the "Melatonin Hypothesis" that suggests that people with decreased pineal gland function are at an increased risk for developing cancer. Some researchers predicted that increased exposure to light would lower melatonin production and increase risk for some cancers (7042). Population studies have in fact found that blind patients and people living in arctic regions have relatively lower rates of breast cancer (7041,7042). There is also evidence that patients with advanced cancer have pineal gland hypofunction and low melatonin levels. Researchers now think supplemental melatonin might help treat certain cancers due to several pharmacological effects including antioxidant, immunomodulatory, and oncostatic effects. Melatonin seems to have very potent antioxidant effects. It might reduce chemotherapy toxicity by scavenging free radicals produced by treatment. Melatonin seems to also affect immune function by activating monocytes and increasing interleukin 2 (IL-2) activity. It appears to enhance IL-2-induced lymphocytosis (2568). Some researchers theorize it might improve survival in patients with cancer by preventing the immunosuppression caused by chemotherapy (7040). It may also help prevent thrombocytopenia associated with cancer chemotherapy by preventing chemotherapy-induced apoptosis of bone marrow cells, and acting synergistically with cytokines to stimulate platelet generation (2564).

Other pineal hormones, such as 5-methoxytryptamine, may also contribute to the thrombopoietic effects of melatonin (2565). Melatonin also seems to have oncostatic effects. Melatonin slows growth of breast cancer cells in vitro and inhibit melanoma cell growth in vitro and in animal models (1064,5856). Researchers think it has direct oncostatic effects possibly by controlling oncogene expression and inducing cancer cell apoptosis (7040).

Melatonin can also affect hormones that influence cancer cell growth. For example, it seems to reduce levels of insulin-like growth factor 1 (IGF-1) and prolactin (PRL), which have a role in breast cancer and prostate cell proliferation (1064,5854,5855,5857,7043,7255).

Melatonin has a variety of other effects. Melatonin is thought to be 6-10 times more effective than vitamin E as an antioxidant. Some researchers are interested in using melatonin for tardive dyskinesia (TD). Melatonin is theorized to work in TD due to a potential antioxidant effect on dopaminergic neurons. There is also some evidence that patients with TD have pineal gland calcification and low endogenous melatonin levels (7082).

Melatonin seems to promote osteoblast differentiation and matrix mineralization in bone (3265). There is preliminary evidence that very high melatonin doses plus norethisterone can have additive or synergistic effects on inhibiting ovarian function in women and possibly act as a contraceptive (769,1740). There is also interest in using melatonin for menopausal symptoms. Melatonin seems to reverse or reduce menopause related changes in thyroid hormone, luteinizing hormone (LH), and follicle stimulating hormone (FSH), and to improve mood in menopausal women (2425). There is some interest in melatonin for its antimicrobial effects. Preliminary evidence shows that melatonin alone or in combination with isoniazid (INH) is active against some Mycobacterium species (330). Some people use melatonin for improving sexual performance. In animal models, melatonin has dose dependent effects on sexual function. Repeated high doses seem to decrease sexual behavior. However, a single low dose of melatonin does seem to increase sexual behavior (6497). Exogenous melatonin undergoes extensive and rapid first pass metabolism. It is first hydroxylated and then undergoes sulphate conjugation (1773,6498). There is also some evidence that cytochrome P450 1A2 and 2C19 catalyze melatonin hydroxylation (6498).

Orally melatonin has an absolute bioavailability of 15% for doses of 2 and 4 mg (1126). Half-life is about 30-60 minutes in humans (1385,1772). Melatonin can be absorbed transdermally, but time to peak levels is delayed (1058). The timing of melatonin administration appears to be important for best therapeutic effect; however, the optimal timing for jet lag and insomnia has not been established (1772). For cancer, researchers theorize that evening doses are best because melatonin might have the greatest activity in the evening (1064).

Adverse Reactions

Orally, melatonin can cause headache, transient depressive symptoms, daytime fatigue and drowsiness, dizziness, abdominal cramps and irritability (14,169), and reduced alertness (14,1078). People should not drive or use machinery for 4 to 5 hours after taking melatonin (1772). Aircraft crew undergoing multiple time zone travel might experience further disruption in circadian rhythms (1722). Melatonin has exacerbated dysphoria in depressed patients (1764). Whether chronic administration of melatonin suppresses endogenous production of melatonin by the pineal gland is unknown (1772).

Interactions with Herbs & Other Dietary Supplements

HERBS/SUPPLEMENTS WITH SEDATIVE PROPERTIES: Theoretically, concomitant use with herbs that have sedative properties might enhance therapeutic and adverse effects. These include 5-HT, calamus, calendula, California poppy, catnip, capsicum, celery, couch grass, elecampane, Siberian ginseng, German chamomile, goldenseal, gotu kola, hops, Jamaican dogwood, kava, lemon balm, sage, sassafras, scullcap, shepherd's purse, stinging nettle, valerian, wild carrot, wild lettuce, ashwaganda root, yerba mansa (4,19), and others.

Interactions with Drugs

BENZODIAZEPINES: A controlled-release melatonin preparation demonstrates effectiveness for benzodiazepine withdrawal in elderly people with insomnia (349). However, benzodiazepine withdrawal should only be done under the supervision of a health care provider.

BETA BLOCKERS: Melatonin can reverse the negative effects of propranolol (Inderal) and atenolol (Tenormin), but not carvedilol (Coreg), on nocturnal sleep (1062,1780).

CNS DEPRESSANTS: Theoretically, concomitant use of melatonin with alcohol, benzodiazepines, or other sedative drugs might cause additive sedation.

FLUOXETINE (Prozac): Concomitant use with melatonin is reported to improve the sleep of some patients with major depressive disorder taking fluoxetine (1053).

FLUVOXAMINE (Luvox): Fluvoxamine can significantly increase melatonin levels. In some cases, fluvoxamine might increase bioavailability of exogenously administered melatonin by up to 20 times (5038,6499). Some researchers think this might be a beneficial interaction and be potentially useful for cases of refractory insomnia (6499). However, this interaction might also cause unwanted excessive drowsiness and possibly other adverse effects. Fluvoxamine is known to increase endogenous melatonin secretion (6498). However, it also seems to increase serum levels of exogenously administered melatonin, possibly by decreasing melatonin metabolism. This effect has been found in healthy people taking fluvoxamine 50-75 mg and melatonin 5 mg (5038,6499). It is not known exactly how fluvoxamine increases melatonin levels, but it might decrease melatonin metabolism by inhibiting cytochrome P450 (CYP450) 1A2 and 2C19 metabolism (5038,6498,6499).

IMMUNOSUPPRESSANTS: Melatonin can stimulate immune function and might interfere with immunosuppressive therapy (7040); avoid using. Immunosuppressant drugs include azathioprine (Imuran), basiliximab (Simulect), cyclosporine (Neoral, Sandimmune), daclizumab (Zenapax), muromonab-CD3 (OKT3, Orthoclone OKT3), mycophenolate (CellCept), tacrolimus (FK506, Prograf), sirolimus (Rapamune), prednisone (Deltasone, Orasone), and other corticosteroids (glucocorticoids).

ISONIAZID (INH): Theoretically, melatonin might enhance the effects of isoniazid against some Mycobacterium species (330).

NIFEDIPINE GITS (Procardia XL): Melatonin can decrease the effectiveness of nifedipine GITS. Immediate-release melatonin 5 mg at night in combination with nifedipine GITS 30-60 mg daily increases systolic blood pressure an average of 6.5 mmHg and diastolic by an average of 4.9 mmHg. Melatonin also increases heart rate by 3.9 bpm (6436). The mechanism of this interaction is not known.

VERAPAMIL (Calan, Isoptin, Verelan): Concomitant use can increase melatonin excretion (1063).

Interactions with Foods

No interactions are known to occur, and there is no known reason to expect a clinically significant interaction with melatonin.

Interactions with Lab Tests

BLOOD PRESSURE: Melatonin can increase blood pressure in patients treated with antihypertensive medications. Immediate-release melatonin 5 mg at night in combination with nifedipine GITS (Procardia XL) increases systolic blood pressure an average of 6.5 mmHg and diastolic by an average of 4.9 mmHg (6436).

HEART RATE: Melatonin in combination with antihypertensive medications can increase heart rate. Immediate-release melatonin 5 mg at night in combination with nifedipine GITS (Procardia XL) increases heart rate by an average of 3.9 bpm (6436).

HUMAN GROWTH HORMONE: Melatonin supplementation can increase human growth hormone serum levels and test results (1076,1779).

LUTEINIZING HORMONE: Melatonin supplementation can decrease serum luteinizing hormone levels and test results (1741).

OXYTOCIN: Melatonin can produce dose-dependent changes in plasma oxytocin concentrations and test results. A 500 mcg melatonin dose increases oxytocin levels; a 5 mg melatonin dose reduces oxytocin levels (1779).

VASOPRESSIN: Melatonin can produce dose-dependent changes in plasma vasopressin concentrations and test results. A 500 mcg melatonin dose increases vasopressin levels; a 5 mg melatonin dose reduces vasopressin levels (1779).

Interactions with Diseases or Conditions

CANCER: Melatonin can decrease the incidence of cytokine (interleukin II and tumor necrosis factor) induced hypotension in cancer patients (1069).

CEREBRAL PALSY: There is one case of dyskinesias and akathisia in a cerebral palsy patient who abruptly discontinued nightly use of melatonin (14).

DEPRESSION: Melatonin can worsen dysphoria in some people with depression (1764).

HYPERTENSION: Melatonin can worsen blood pressure in patients who are taking antihypertensive medications. Immediate-release melatonin 5 mg at night in combination with nifedipine GITS (Procardia XL) increases systolic blood pressure an average of 6.5 mmHg and diastolic by an average of 4.9 mmHg. Melatonin also increases heart rate by 3.9 bpm (6436). The mechanism of this interaction is not known.

LIVER DISEASE: Melatonin is metabolized by the liver. Use in liver disease might increase plasma melatonin concentrations and lead to adverse effects. There is one report of auto-immune hepatitis (14); use with caution.

SEIZURE DISORDERS: Melatonin increased the incidence of seizures in one study (14); use with caution.

Dosage and Administration

ORAL: For insomnia, a typical dose of 0.3-5 mg at bedtime has been used (1072,1729,1738,1754,7081). Both immediate

---

release and sustained release preparations have been used. For jet lag, 5 mg is commonly taken at bedtime for one week beginning three days before the flight (1049,1077,1079,1085,1722). For tardive dyskinesia, 10 mg daily of a controlled release formulation has been used (7082). As adjunctive treatment for solid tumors, 10-50 mg in combination with radiotherapy, chemotherapy, or interleukin 2 (IL-2) has been used in clinical studies. Melatonin is typically started 7 days prior to start of chemotherapy and continued throughout full treatment course (1773,7040,7043). For treatment of metastatic prostate cancer resistant to triptorelin used alone, 20 mg taken daily has been used in combination with 3.75 mg of triptorelin injected intramuscularly every 28 days (7255). For prevention and treatment of thrombocytopenia associated with cancer chemotherapy, a dose of 20 mg each evening has been used (2564) For benzodiazepine withdrawal in elderly people with insomnia, 2 mg of controlled-release melatonin taken at bedtime for 6 weeks (the benzodiazepine dosage is reduced 50% during the second week, 75% during weeks 3 and 4, and stopped during weeks 5 and 6) and continued up to 6 months, has been used (349). For prevention of cluster headache, an evening dose of 10 mg has been used (1127). As premedication for surgery in adults, 0.05 mg/kg sublingually has been used (1125,1768,1769). For reducing the symptoms of acute nicotine withdrawal, 0.3 mg orally 3.5 hours after stopping smoking has been used (2424).

TOPICAL: No typical dosage.

Comments

Most commercial melatonin is synthesized in the laboratory. However, in rare cases it can be derived from animal pineal gland. Melatonin from animal sources should be avoided due to the possibility of contamination (1772). The controlled-released product, Circadin (not available in the US), is undergoing a multi-center Phase III clinical study in France for the indication of sleep. The manufacturer, Neurim Pharmaceutical Labs (Israel), is preparing to apply for approval of Circadin as a prescription drug in Canada and Europe (364). Safety concerns about melatonin have lead to banning of melatonin in Japan and restricted sale in the UK (1126).

MENTZELIA

Also Known As
None.

Scientific Names
Mentzelia cordifolia.
Family: Loasaceae.

People Use This For
Traditionally, mentzelia branch tips, stems, and roots have been used orally for gastritis, gastrointestinal mucous membrane inflammation, nervous gastric disorders and digestive symptoms, hyperacidity, gastric spasms, feeling of fullness, pressure on the stomach, upset stomach, gastric irritation due to alcohol abuse, innate digestive weakness, and gastric pain (2).

Safety
There is insufficient reliable information available about the safety of mentzelia.
Pregnancy and Lactation: Insufficient reliable information available; avoid using.

Effectiveness
There is insufficient reliable information available about the effectiveness of mentzelia.

Mechanism of Action
The applicable parts of mentzelia are the branch tips, stems and roots. There is insufficient reliable information available about the possible mechanism of action and active ingredients.

Adverse Reactions
None reported.

Interactions with Herbs & Other Dietary Supplements
Insufficient reliable information available.

Interactions with Drugs
No interactions are known to occur, and there is no known reason to expect a clinically significant interaction with mentzelia.

Interactions with Foods

No interactions are known to occur, and there is no known reason to expect a clinically significant interaction with mentzelia.

Interactions with Lab Tests

No interactions are known to occur, and there is no known reason to expect a clinically significant interaction with mentzelia.

Interactions with Diseases or Conditions

No interactions are known to occur, and there is no known reason to expect a clinically significant interaction with mentzelia.

Dosage and Administration

No typical dosage.

Comments

There is very little scientific information about this product. Our staff is continually analyzing the available information on natural medicines and will add data here as it becomes available.

MERCURY HERB

Also Known As

None.

Scientific Names

Mercurialis annua.
Family: Euphorbiaceae.

People Use This For

Orally, the flowering plant of mercury herb is used for inflammation with pus, as a laxative, a diuretic, and as an adjuvant treatment for gastrointestinal and urinary tract disease (18).

Safety

LIKELY UNSAFE ...when the fresh plant, particularly the root and rhizome are used orally (18). Small amounts might cause symptoms no worse than diarrhea.
PREGNANCY AND LACTATION: LIKELY UNSAFE ...when used orally (18); avoid using.

Effectiveness

There is insufficient reliable information available about the effectiveness of mercury herb.

Mechanism of Action

Mercury herb contains saponins, a small amount of cyanogenic glycosides, pyridone derivatives including hermidin, amines including methylamine, and flavonoids including rutin, narcissin, and isorhamnetin (18). The root and stock of mercury herb act as strong laxatives (18). There is no information regarding the toxic compound in the plant (18). The insignificant amount of cyanogenic glycosides cannot account for the plant's toxicity (18).

Adverse Reactions

Orally, ingestion might cause diarrhea and overactive bladder (18). Symptoms of poisoning might include nerve paralysis, liver and kidney failure, as well as death (18). The pollen has shown to be allergenic (4143,4144), and may be responsible for rhinitis and asthmatic symptoms (4143). Mercury herb might also cause allergic reactions in individuals allergic to Olea europaea, Fraxinus elatior, Ricinus communis, Salsola kali, Parietaria judaica, and Artemisia vulgaris (4143).

Interactions with Herbs & Other Dietary Supplements

CROSS-ALLERGENICITY: Individuals allergic to mercury herb might also be allergic to Mercurialis annua and Olea europaea, Fraxinus elatior, Ricinus communis, Salsola kali, Parietaria judaica, and Artemisia vulgaris (4143).

Interactions with Drugs

No interactions are known to occur, and there is no known reason to expect a clinically significant interaction with mercury herb.

Interactions with Foods

No interactions are known to occur, and there is no known reason to expect a clinically significant interaction with mercury herb.

Interactions with Lab Tests

No interactions are known to occur, and there is no known reason to expect a clinically significant interaction with mercury herb.

Interactions with Diseases or Conditions

No interactions are known to occur, and there is no known reason to expect a clinically significant interaction with mercury herb.

Dosage and Administration

ORAL: The mercury herb is administered as an extract or in juice (18).

Comments

None.

MESOGLYCAN

Also Known As

Aortic Glycosaminoglycans, Aortic GAGs, Glycosaminoglycans, Heparinoid Fraction, Heparinoids, Mucopolysaccharide, Sulfomucopolysaccharide.
CAUTION: See separate listing for Chondroitin Sulfate.

Scientific Names

None.

People Use This For

Orally, mesoglycan is used for treating atherosclerosis, varicose veins, hemorrhoids, phlebitis, thrombophlebitis (6645), lower limb ischemia (6629), deep vein thrombosis, hyperlipidemia, peripheral obliterative arterial disease, venous insufficiency (14), cerebrovascular disease (6637,6639), and stroke (6641).
Topically, mesoglycan is used for treating leg ulcers (6627).
Intramuscularly, mesoglycan is used for treating venous insufficiency, cerebrovascular disease (14), stroke (6641), and cutaneous necrotizing venulitis (6627).
Intravenously, mesoglycan is used for treating lower limb ischemia (6629).

Safety

POSSIBLY SAFE …when used orally or parenterally and appropriately (14). Although some evidence suggests these products are safe, since they are derived from animals there is concern about contamination with diseased animal parts (see Adverse Reactions) (1825). However, there are no reports of disease transmission to humans due to use of contaminated mesoglycan.
There is insufficient information available about the safety of mesoglycan for its other uses.
PREGNANCY AND LACTATION: Insufficient reliable information available; avoid using.

Effectiveness

POSSIBLY EFFECTIVE …when used orally or parenterally for treating venous insufficiency. There is some evidence from uncontrolled trials that mesoglycan can improve the subjective and objective symptoms associated with various venous conditions including varicose syndromes, post-phlebitic syndromes, and thrombophlebitis when used over a 1-3 month period (6630,6638,6644,6645). …when used orally and intravenously for treating acute episodes of lower limb ischemia. Evidence from an uncontrolled trial shows that an alternating schedule of intravenous and oral mesoglycan (see Dosage and Administration) can improve walking distance in patients with acute episodes of lower limb ischemia (6629). …when used orally for reducing triglycerides in patients with hypertriglyceridemia. There is some evidence that mesoglycans can reduce total and VLDL triglycerides in patients with hypertriglyceridemia (6646). …when used orally for treating cerebrovascular disease (6635,6637,6639). Mesoglycan seems to reduced ischemic events, improved quality of life, and provide subjective improvement when used over a 6 month period in patients with cerebrovascular disease (6637,6639). There is some evidence that mesoglycan might be comparable to standard antiplatelet drug therapy (6639). …when used topically for treating leg ulcers in patients with chronic venous insufficiency (6627).

POSSIBLY INEFFECTIVE ...when used orally for preventing long-term sequelae of deep vein thrombosis (DVT) (6640). Oral mesoglycan plus compression stockings appears to be no better than placebo, following standard DVT therapy, for preventing recurrent DVT and/or pulmonary embolism during a follow-up period ranging from 5 to 48 months (6640). ...when used intramuscularly and orally for treating patients with acute cerebral infarction (6641). There seems to be no difference in outcome between patients treated with intravenous dexamethasone alone, or in combination with intramuscular mesoglycan for 5 days followed by 25 days of oral mesoglycan (6641). There is insufficient reliable information available about the effectiveness of mesoglycan for its other uses. However, there is some preliminary human evidence that intramuscular mesoglycan might be useful for treating cutaneous necrotizing venulitis in patients with reduced fibrinolytic activity (6634). There is also some early evidence that mesoglycan might slow the progression of atherosclerosis by decreasing the rate of carotid and femoral artery intima-media thickening (6628). More evidence is needed to rate mesoglycan for these uses.

Mechanism of Action

Mesoglycan belongs to a broad class of compounds called glycosaminoglycans (GAG). GAGs, also called mucopolysaccharides, are amino hexose polysaccharides contained in mucoproteins, glycoproteins, and blood group substances (6626). GAGs are a heparinoid (non-heparin) byproduct of heparin extraction from cow lung tissue or aorta, and pig intestinal mucosa (15,6622,6623). Mesoglycan specifically is composed of dermatan sulfate and heparan sulfate, with smaller concentrations of chondroitin sulfate, hyaluronic acid, and related hexosaminoglycans (6614,6622,6623). The concentrations of these substances can vary depending on the origin of the product. People try it for vascular conditions because it seems to have numerous pharmacological effects on the vascular system. Mesoglycan exhibits profibrinolytic activity without influencing hemaglutination in humans after oral administration (6631,6642). It seems to also decrease plasma fibrinogen concentrations without affecting prothrombin time, partial thromboplastin time, or antithrombin III (6633). However, mesoglycan has been shown to prolong activated partial thromboplastin time (aPTT) (6629). Preliminary human evidence suggests that mesoglycan might restore normal fibrinolysis in patients with reduced cutaneous fibrinolytic activity (6634). It also reduces pericapillary connective tissue edema, and capillary and venule dilation, in patients with primary venous insufficiency (6630). It also improves arterial wall elasticity, trancutaneous oxygen perfusion, and blood flow (6643,6644). Mesoglycan reduces total and VLDL triglyceride concentrations and increases lipoprotein lipase activity in patients with hypertriglyceridemia (6646). It reduces total cholesterol and triglyceride concentrations, and increases HDL cholesterol concentrations in patients recovering from cerebral ischemic episode (6633).

Adverse Reactions

Orally, nausea, vomiting, epigastric pain, heartburn (14), headache, diarrhea (6629), and local cutaneous reactions (14) have been reported.

Intramuscularly, reactions at the site of injection can occur (14).

There is some concern about potential contamination. Mesoglycan is derived from raw animal tissues gathered from slaughterhouses, possibly from sick or diseased animals (6616). Products made from contaminated or diseased organs might present a human health hazard. There is also concern that mesoglycan produced from cows in countries where bovine spongiform encephalitis (BSE) has been reported might be contaminated with diseased tissue. Countries where BSE has been reported include Great Britain, France, The Netherlands, Portugal, Luxembourg, Ireland, Switzerland, Oman, and Belgium (1825). However, there have been no reports of BSE transfer to humans from contaminated mesoglycan products. Until more is known, tell patients to avoid these products unless country of origin can be determined. Patients should avoid products that are produced in countries where BSE has been found.

Interactions with Herbs & Other Dietary Supplements

Insufficient reliable information available.

Interactions with Drugs

ANTICOAGULANTS: Theoretically, combined use might increase bleeding risk (14). However, human evidence suggests that mesoglycan has profibrinolytic activity without affecting coagulation (6631,6642). These agents include aspirin, clopidogrel (Plavix), dalteparin (Fragmin), enoxaparin (Lovenox), heparin, ticlopidine (Ticlid), warfarin (Coumadin) and others.

THROMBOLYTIC DRUGS: Theoretically, combined use might increase bleeding risk (14). These drugs include alteplase (Activase), anistreplase (Eminase), reteplase (Retevase), streptokinase (Streptase), and urokinase (Abbokinase).

Interactions with Foods

No interactions are known to occur, and there is no known reason to expect a clinically significant interaction with mesoglycan.

Interactions with Lab Tests
ACTIVATED PARTIAL THROMBOPLASTIN TIME (aPTT): Intravenous mesoglycan prolongs activated partial thromboplastin time (6629).
CHOLESTEROL: Intramuscular mesoglycan reduces total cholesterol and increases HDL cholesterol concentrations and test results (6633).
FIBRINOGEN: Intramuscular mesoglycan decreases plasma fibrinogen concentrations and test results (6633).
TRIGLYCERIDES: Intramuscular mesoglycan decreases plasma triglyceride concentrations and test results (6633).

Interactions with Diseases or Conditions
COAGULATION DISORDERS: Mesoglycan might cause bleeding in people with coagulation disorders (14).
HEPARINOID HYPERSENSITIVITY: Mesoglycan might cause allergic reactions in people hypersensitive to heparin or heparinoid derivatives (14); contraindicated.

Dosage and Administration
ORAL: A typical dose is 100 mg per day (6614). For cerebrovascular disease, 100-144 mg per day has been used (6635,6639,6641). For deep vein thrombosis (DVT), 72 mg per day has been used (6640). For hypertriglyceridemia, 96 mg per day has been used (6646). For venous insufficiency, 50 mg three times daily has been used (6638).
INTRAMUSCULAR: For cerebrovascular disease, 30 mg once or twice daily has been used (14). For venous insufficiency, 30 mg per day has been used (14).

Comments
None.

METHIONINE

Also Known As
DL-Methionine, DL Methionine, L-Methionine.

Scientific Names
L-2-amino-4-(methylthio)butyric acid.

People Use This For
Orally, methionine is used for liver function support (2408) and preventing liver damage in acetaminophen poisoning (2413).

Safety
POSSIBLY SAFE ...when used orally to treat acetaminophen poisoning (2413).
POSSIBLY UNSAFE ...when used orally for self-medication in amounts greater than those found in foods (2409,2410,2411).
PREGNANCY AND LACTATION: POSSIBLY UNSAFE ...when used orally for self-medication in amounts greater than found in food (2409,2410,2411).

Effectiveness
POSSIBLY EFFECTIVE ...when taken orally for preventing liver damage in cases of acetaminophen poisoning and when administered within ten hours of acetaminophen ingestion (2413).

Mechanism of Action
Methionine is a sulfur-containing essential amino acid (9) found in meat, fish, and dairy products (2408). In children of short stature, methionine can potentiate growth hormone and its releasing hormone secretion (2412). In humans, it can increase serum homocysteine levels (2410,2411). To detoxify, excessive methionine requires glycine; thus, methionine supplementation can compete with the glycine needed for other metabolic processes (2415). In humans, supplementing with methionine prior to nitrous oxide anesthesia can counter the anesthesia-induced reduction in methionine-synthase enzyme activity (2414); however, the clinical significance for this is unknown.

Adverse Reactions
Orally, methionine increases plasma homocysteine levels and can promote atherosclerosis (2410,2411).

Interactions with Herbs & Other Dietary Supplements
Insufficient reliable information available.

Interactions with Drugs
ACETAMINOPHEN: Methionine can decrease liver damage in cases of acetaminophen poisoning (2413).

Interactions with Foods
SALT AND NITRITE: A diet rich in methionine, salt, and nitrite can increase the risk of gastric cancer (2409).
GLYCINE: Excess methionine intake can place a competitive demand on the body's availability of glycine (2415).

Interactions with Lab Tests
HOMOCYSTEINE: Methionine can increase plasma homocysteine levels and test results (2410,2411).

Interactions with Diseases or Conditions
ACETAMINOPHEN POISONING: Methionine can decrease liver damage in cases of acetaminophen poisoning (2413).
ATHEROSCLEROSIS: Theoretically, methionine supplementation can promote or exacerbate atherosclerosis by increasing homocysteine levels (2410).

Dosage and Administration
ORAL: People also typically take a 500 mg capsule containing the free form of L-methionine with a meal or glass of water (5026).

Comments
Methionine is possibly unsafe, and should only be used by emergency room personnel for medical emergencies.

MEXICAN SCAMMONY ROOT

Also Known As
Ipomoea, Orizaba Jalap.
CAUTION: See separate listings for Pokeweed berry, Pokeweed root, and Jalap.

Scientific Names
Ipomoea orizabensis.
Family: Convolvulaceae.

People Use This For
Orally, Mexican scammony root is used as a purgative (18).

Safety
There is insufficient reliable information available about the safety of Mexican scammony root.
PREGNANCY: LIKELY UNSAFE ...when used orally; contraindicated (18).
LACTATION: Insufficient reliable information available; avoid using.

Effectiveness
POSSIBLY EFFECTIVE ...when taken orally as a purgative (18).

Mechanism of Action
Mexican scammony root exerts a potent stimulant laxative effect on the intestines. It contains 12-15% resinous polymeric ester glycosides (18).

Adverse Reactions
Orally, it can cause intestinal colic, and in large amounts, vomiting (18).

Interactions with Herbs & Other Dietary Supplements
STIMULANT LAXATIVE HERBS: Theoretically, concomitant use with other stimulant laxative herbs may increase the risk of potassium depletion. (19).
HORSETAIL/LICORICE: Theoretically, concomitant use with horsetail plant or licorice rhizome increases the risk of potassium depletion (19).
CARDIAC GLYCOSIDE-CONTAINING HERBS: Overuse/abuse may increase the risk of cardiac glycoside toxicity (2,18,19,500).

Interactions with Drugs
CARDIAC GLYCOSIDE DRUGS: Theoretically, overuse/abuse of this product increases the risk of adverse effects of cardiac glycoside drugs, e.g., digoxin.

Interactions with Foods
No interactions are known to occur, and there is no known reason to expect a clinically significant interaction with Mexican scammony root.

Interactions with Lab Tests
No interactions are known to occur, and there is no known reason to expect a clinically significant interaction with Mexican scammony root.

Interactions with Diseases or Conditions
GI CONDITIONS: Contraindicated; may have GI irritant effects (19). Stimulant laxatives are contraindicated in individuals with symptoms of appendicitis (abdominal pain, nausea and vomiting) (272).

Dosage and Administration
ORAL: People typically take 3 to 12 grains (195 to 780 mg) of the powdered root. The powdered resin from the root is dosed 3 to 8 grains (195 to 520 mg) (5267).

Comments
Ipomoea orizabensis is no longer used as a purgative because of the adverse effect of vomiting.

MEZEREON

Also Known As
Camolea, Daphne, Dwarf Bay, Spurge Flax, Spurge Laurel, Spurge Olive, Wild Pepper.

Scientific Names
Daphne mezereum.
Family: Thymelaeaceae.

People Use This For
Traditionally, the mezereon root has been used orally to relieve headaches and toothaches (18). It has also been used topically for joint pains, and to increase circulation in rheumatic conditions (18).

Safety
POSSIBLY UNSAFE ...when used topically (18). Prolonged skin contact can lead to necrosis (18).
LIKELY UNSAFE ...when used orally. The plant is poisonous and can cause death (18).
PREGNANCY AND LACTATION: LIKELY UNSAFE ...when used orally or topically (18); avoid using.

Effectiveness
There is insufficient reliable information available about the effectiveness of mezereon.

Mechanism of Action
The applicable part of mezereon is the bark. Mezereon contains diterpenes including mezerein and daphnetoxin. It possesses powerful skin stimulating effects and can be hallucinogenic (18).

Adverse Reactions
Ingesting mezereon can cause reddening and swelling of the oral mucous membranes, salivation, thirst, stomach pains, vomiting (18), severe diarrhea (18,4145), and blood in the urine (4145). Symptoms can also include headache, dizziness, stupor, tachycardia, spasms, and death through circulatory collapse (18). Skin contact with mezereon can cause red, painful swelling of the skin, blister formation, and shedding of the epidermis (18). Extended exposure can cause necrosis (18). Contact with the eyes can cause severe conjunctivitis (18).

Interactions with Herbs & Other Dietary Supplements
Insufficient reliable information available.

Interactions with Drugs

No interactions are known to occur, and there is no known reason to expect a clinically significant interaction with mezereon.

Interactions with Foods

No interactions are known to occur, and there is no known reason to expect a clinically significant interaction with mezereon.

Interactions with Lab Tests

No interactions are known to occur, and there is no known reason to expect a clinically significant interaction with mezereon.

Interactions with Diseases or Conditions

No interactions are known to occur, and there is no known reason to expect a clinically significant interaction with mezereon.

Dosage and Administration

TOPICAL: Used as a 20% ointment (18).

Comments

Mezereon is a protected species (18). It is seldom used medicinally today (18).

MGN-3

Also Known As

Biobran, Hemicellulose Complex with Arabinoxylane.

Scientific Names

None.

People Use This For

Orally, MGN-3 is used for boosting immune function, preventing and treating cancer, treating AIDS, hepatitis, diabetes, chronic fatigue syndrome and other immunodeficiency disorders (3114,3115).

Safety

There is insufficient reliable information available about the safety of MGN-3.
PREGNANCY AND LACTATION: Insufficient reliable information available; avoid using.

Effectiveness

There is insufficient reliable information available about the effectiveness of MGN-3.

Mechanism of Action

MGN-3 is a hemicellulose complex containing arabinoxylane as a major component. It is produced by hydrolyzing rice bran using enzymes from mycelia of Shiitake, Kawaratake, and Suehirotake mushrooms (3114). Some studies suggest it might improve immunity by enhancing natural killer cell activity, increasing interferon-gamma production by peripheral blood mononuclear cells, and acting synergistically with interleukin-2 (aldesleukin) to increase natural killer cell activity and production of tumor necrosis factor alpha (3116,3117). Other evidence suggests that MGN-3 has activity against HIV (3113). Results from three small studies of healthy individuals and individuals with cancer suggest that MGN-3 also enhances natural killer cell activity (3118,3119,3120).

Adverse Reactions

None reported.

Interactions with Herbs & Other Dietary Supplements

Insufficient reliable information available.

Interactions with Drugs

No interactions known to occur, and there is no known reason to expect a clinically significant interaction with MGN-3.

Interactions with Foods

No interactions known to occur, and there is no known reason to expect a clinically significant interaction with MGN-3.

Interactions with Lab Tests

No interactions known to occur, and there is no known reason to expect a clinically significant interaction with MGN-3.

Interactions with Diseases or Conditions

No interactions known to occur, and there is no known reason to expect a clinically significant interaction with MGN-3.

Dosage and Administration

ORAL: A dose of 3 grams per day has been used in cancer patients (3119,3120).

Comments

The FDA is seeking a permanent injunction against the marketing of MGN-3 by Lane Labs. The complaint charges that MGN-3 is an unapproved drug product promoted as treatment for cancer and HIV infection (387).

MICROALGAE

Also Known As

Astaxanthin.
CAUTION: See separate listing for Beta-Carotene.

Scientific Names

3,3'-dihydroxy-4,4'-diketo-beta-carotene, 3S, 3'S-astaxanthin; 3R, 3'R-astaxanthin; 3R,3'S-astaxanthin.

People Use This For

Orally, the microalgae constituent astaxanthin is used to treat or prevent macular degeneration in the eyes, for Alzheimer's and Parkinson's disease, to aid in stroke recovery, to protect against cancer, and to reduce LDL cholesterol (4322). It is also used to reduce skin damage from ultraviolet light (4334).
Orally as a nutritional supplement, the microalgae constituent astaxanthin is used to cause coloration in farm-raised fish (4326,4328) and as a nutritional supplement for poultry (4329).

Safety

LIKELY SAFE ...when the microalgae constituent astaxanthin is used orally in food amounts.
POSSIBLY SAFE ...when the microalgae constituent astaxanthin is used orally in medicinal amounts up to 14.4 mg/day for two weeks (4322).
There is insufficient reliable information available about the safety of the microalgae constituent astaxanthin orally in amounts greater than 14.4 mg/day or for longer than two weeks.
PREGNANCY AND LACTATION: LIKELY SAFE ...when the microalgae constituent astaxanthin is used orally in food amounts.
There is insufficient reliable information about the safety of using the microalgae constituent in larger amounts.

Effectiveness

There is insufficient reliable information about the effectiveness of the microalgae constituent astaxanthin.

Mechanism of Action

The microalgae constituent astaxanthin is a reddish carotenoid pigment that is a powerful antioxidant (4322,4326,4332). The richest natural source of the microalgae constituent astaxanthin is Haematococcus pluvialis; but salmon, trout, red seabream, shrimp, lobster, fish eggs, and many bird species also contain substantial amounts (4322). Although plants contain astaxanthin, it is usually in the form of the 3S,3'S isomer. In contrast, the astaxanthin found in Atlantic or Pacific salmon consists of three isomeric forms (4326). Some evidence suggests the microalgae constituent astaxanthin might stimulate immunity (4335,4336) or reduce age-related macular degeneration (4330). Other evidence suggests it might protect against mammary, liver, bladder, or oral cancers (4337,4338,4339,4340). It also might have gastroprotective effects against Helicobacter pylori (4341). In farm-raised fish, supplementation can produce pigmentation that cannot be distinguished from that of ocean fish on a natural diet (4331).

Adverse Reactions
None reported.

Interactions with Herbs & Other Dietary Supplements
Insufficient reliable information available.

Interactions with Drugs
No interactions are known to occur, and there is no known reason to expect a clinically significant interaction with the microalgae constituent astaxanthin.

Interactions with Foods
No interactions are known to occur, and there is no known reason to expect a clinically significant interaction with the microalgae constituent astaxanthin.

Interactions with Lab Tests
No interactions are known to occur, and there is no known reason to expect a clinically significant interaction with the microalgae constituent astaxanthin.

Interactions with Diseases or Conditions
No interactions are known to occur, and there is no known reason to expect a clinically significant interaction with the microalgae constituent astaxanthin.

Dosage and Administration
ORAL: A typical dose is 2 capsules Haematococcus microalgae per day. Each capsule contains 2.5 mg astaxanthin (4395).

Comments
The Aquasearch company patented a novel process for cultivating microalgae and has been successful in defending that patent. A recent court decision affirmed that the Cyanotech company's method for cultivating microalgae infringed on the patent and that Cyanotech violated the Uniform Trade Secrets Act (4396).

MILK THISTLE

Also Known As
Cardui mariae fructus, Cardui mariae herba, Holy Thistle, Lady's Thistle, Legalon, Marian Thistle, Mariendistel, Mary Thistle, Milk Thistle Above Ground Parts, Milk Thistle Fruit, Milk Thistle Seed, Our Lady's Thistle, St. Mary Thistle, Silybin, Silybum, Silymarin.
CAUTION: See separate listing for Blessed Thistle.

Scientific Names
Silybum marianum, synonyms Carduus marianum, Carduus marianus.
Family: Asteraceae or Compositae.

People Use This For
Orally, milk thistle is used as a liver protectant to lessen damage from potentially hepatotoxic drugs, and for treating liver disorders including toxic liver damage caused by chemicals, Amanita phalloides mushroom poisoning, jaundice, chronic inflammatory liver disease, hepatic cirrhosis, and chronic hepatitis. It is also used orally for loss of appetite, dyspeptic and gallbladder complaints, hangover, and diseases of the spleen. Milk thistle is used orally for prostate cancer, pleurisy, malaria, depression, uterine complaints, stimulating breast milk flow, and stimulating menstrual flow. Intravenously, it is used as a supportive treatment for Amanita phalloides mushroom poisoning.
For food use, the leaves and flower are eaten as a vegetable and seeds are roasted for use as a coffee substitute.

Safety
POSSIBLY SAFE ...when used orally and appropriately. Milk thistle extracts standardized to contain 70-80% of the silymarin constituent seems to be safe when used for up to 41 months (2614,2616).
There is insufficient reliable information available about the safety of intravenous formulations of milk thistle and its constituents.
PREGNANCY AND LACTACTION: Insufficient reliable information available; avoid using.

Effectiveness

POSSIBLY EFFECTIVE …when used orally for hepatic cirrhosis. A specific milk thistle extract (Legalon) standardized to contain 70-80% of the constituent silymarin seems to reduce hepatic cirrhosis-related mortality when used long-term over 41 months (2616). …when used orally to treat hepatotoxicity from organic solvents. A specific milk thistle extract (Legalon) standardized to contain 70-80% of the constituent silymarin seems to improve liver function tests (LFTs) in patients with hepatotoxicity resulting from long-term exposure to organic solvents (2614). …when used orally for chronic hepatitis. A specific preparation of silybin, an active constituent extracted from milk thistle, complexed with phosphatidylcholine (Silipide), seems to improve liver function tests (LFTs), including bilirubin, alkaline phosphatase, gammaglutamyl transpeptidase (GGTP), alanine aminotransferase (ALT, formerly SGPT) and aspartate aminotransferase (AST, formerly SGOT) after 7 days in patients with chronic active hepatitis. Silybin is complexed with phosphatidylcholine to improve the bioavailability of silybin (7356). …when used intravenously (IV) as supportive treatment for liver damage due to Amanita phalloides mushroom poisoning (2615).

Most clinical studies of milk thistle's effectiveness have used a specific extract standardized to 70-80% silymarin (Legalon). In the US, this formulation is found in the brand name product Thisilyn (Nature's Way). There is insufficient reliable information available to rate the effectiveness of milk thistle for its other uses. However, there is preliminary evidence that milk thistle might also be helpful for treating alcoholic liver disease (2613,2618,7321,7322,7355). There is also some clinical evidence that the milk thistle constituent silymarin can reduce insulin resistance in people with diabetes and alcoholic cirrhosis (2617). More evidence is needed to rate milk thistle for these uses.

Mechanism of Action

The applicable parts of milk thistle are the fruit (seed), and above ground parts. The seed is most commonly used medicinally. Silymarin, the active constituent of the milk thistle seed, consists of four flavonolignans called silibinin (silybin), isosilybinin, silichristin (silychristin), and silidianin. Silibinin makes up about 50% to 70% of silymarin (7318). When ingested silymarin undergoes enterohepatic recirculation and has higher concentrations in liver cells. Several activities seem to contribute to the therapeutic effect of silymarin in liver disease. Silymarin seems to cause an alteration of the outer hepatocyte cell membrane that prevents toxin penetration. It also stimulates nucleolar polymerase A resulting in increased ribosomal protein synthesis, which can stimulate liver regeneration and the formation of new hepatocytes. There is also some evidence that silymarin might have antifibrotic, anti-inflammatory, and immunomodulating effects that could also be beneficial in liver disease (6879). Silymarin and silybin inhibit beta-glucuronidase, which might help protect against hepatic injury and possibly colon cancer. Inhibition of beta-glucuronidase is thought to reduce the hydrolyis of glucuronides into toxic metabolites in the liver and intestine (7354). There is also preliminary research that milk thistle constituents might protect against kidney damage. In vitro, silibinin and silicristin can protect the kidney cells from nephrotoxic drugs such as acetaminophen, cisplatin, and vincristine. Silibinin and silicristin also appear to have a regenerative effect on kidney cells, similar to the effects on hepatic cells (7320).

There is some interest in using milk thistle for prostate cancer. In vitro research shows that silymarin and silibinin have antiproliferative effects on androgen-responsive prostate cancer cells (7319).

The milk thistle plant above ground parts seems to have some estrogenic activity. A milk thistle plant extract appears to enhance estradiol binding to estrogen receptors, induce transcription activity in estrogen-responsive cells, and enhance estradiol-induced transcription activity in estrogen-responsive cells (6180).

There is preliminary evidence that milk thistle might affect drug metabolism. In vitro, silymarin and its flavonolignan, silibinin, inhibit cytochrome P450 2C9 (CYP2C9) and cytochrome P450 3A4 (CYP3A4), the major phase 1 hepatic enzyme, and uridine diphosphoglucuronosyl transferase (UGT), the major phase 2 enzyme that is responsible for glucuronidation (6450,7089,7318).

Adverse Reactions

Orally, milk thistle is usually well-tolerated (6879). It can cause an occasional laxative effect (795). Other less common gastrointestinal effects include nausea, diarrhea, dyspepsia, flatulence, abdominal bloating, fullness or pain, and anorexia (6879).

There is one case of a woman who experienced intermittent episodes of sweating, nausea, abdominal pain, vomiting, diarrhea, weakness and collapse, requiring hospitalization (3525).

Some patients can have allergic reactions to milk thistle including pruritus, rash, urticaria, eczema and anaphylaxis (6879). Allergic reactions are may be more likely to occur in patients sensitive to the Asteraceae/Compositae family. Members of this family include ragweed, chrysanthemums, marigolds, daisies, and many other herbs.

Interactions with Herbs & Other Dietary Supplements

Insufficient reliable information available.

Interactions with Drugs

ESTROGEN: Theoretically, silymarin, an active constituent of milk thistle, might increase the clearance of estrogen by inhibiting beta-glucuronidase (6879).

GLUCURONIDATED DRUGS: Theoretically, silymarin, an active constituent of milk thistle, might decrease the clearance of drugs that undergo glucuronidation, such as lorazepam (Ativan), lamotrigine (Lamictal), entacapone (Comtan) and others (7318,7354).

OTHER DRUGS: There's preliminary evidence that milk thistle might inhibit the cytochrome P450 2C9 (CYP2C9) and cytochrome P450 3A4 (CYP3A4) enzyme (6450,7089,7318). Theoretically, it might increase levels of drugs metabolized by CYP2C9 and CYP3A4. However, so far, this interaction has not been reported in humans. Some drugs metabolized by CYP2C9 include amitriptyline (Elavil), clopidogrel (Plavix), clozapine (Clozaril), diazepam (Valium), estradiol (Estrace), grepafloxacin (Raxar), mirtazepine (Remeron), ondansetron (Zofran), tacrine (Cognex), verapamil (Calan), warfarin (Coumadin), zileuton (Zyflo), and others. Some drugs metabolized by CYP3A4 include lovastatin (Mevacor), ketoconazole (Nizoral), itraconazole (Sporanox), fexofenadine (Allegra), triazolam (Halcion), and numerous others. Use milk thistle cautiously or avoid in patients taking these drugs.

Interactions with Foods

No interactions are known to occur, and there is no known reason to expect a clinically significant interaction with milk thistle.

Interactions with Lab Tests

No interactions are known to occur, and there is no known reason to expect a clinically significant interaction with milk thistle.

Interactions with Diseases or Conditions

CROSS-ALLERGENICITY: Can cause an allergic reaction in individuals sensitive to the Asteraceae/Compositae family. Members of this family include ragweed, chrysanthemums, marigolds, daisies, and many other herbs.
HORMONE SENSITIVE CANCERS/CONDITIONS: Because milk thistle plant extract might have estrogenic effects (6180), women with hormone sensitive conditions should avoid milk thistle above ground parts. Some of these conditions include breast, uterine, and ovarian cancer, and endometriosis and uterine fibroids. The more commonly used milk thistle seed extracts are not known to have estrogenic effects.

Dosage and Administration

ORAL: For hepatic cirrhosis, a milk thistle extract containing 70-80% silymarin (Legalon), 420 mg per day has been used (2616). For chronic active hepatitis, a milk thistle constituent, silibinin (Silibide), 240 mg twice daily as been used (7356). Some people make a milk thistle tea, but the active ingredients are not very soluble in water (515).
INTRAVENOUS: For Amanita phalloides mushroom poisoning, the common dose is 20-50 mg/kg over 24 hours, divided into four infusions, each administered over a two hour period. This is usually started within 48 hours after mushroom ingestion (7,2615). Intravenous silibinin is unavailable in the US.

Comments

The broken leaves of the milk thistle plant exude of milky sap (6). The leaves have distinctive white markings which, according to legend, were the Virgin Mary's milk (7161). The plant was once grown in Europe as a vegetable for salads and as a substitute for spinach (6). Avoid confusion with blessed thistle (Cnicus benedictus).

MONEYWORT

Also Known As

Creeping Jenny, Creeping Joan, Herb Two-Pence, Meadow Runagates, Running Jenny, Serpentaria, String Of Sovereigns, Twopenny Grass, Wandering Jenny, Wandering Tailor.

Scientific Names

Lysimachia nummularia.
Family: Primulaceae.

People Use This For

Topically, moneywort is used for acute and chronic eczema and as a constituent of dermatologic gels, ointments, and drops. It is also used topically as an astringent and antibacterial agent (18).
Historically, moneywort was used orally for diarrhea, to increase salivation, and as a cough expectorant.

Safety

There is insufficient reliable information available about the safety of moneywort.
Pregnancy and Lactation: Insufficient reliable information available; avoid using.

Effectiveness

There is insufficient reliable information available about the effectiveness of moneywort.

Mechanism of Action

There is insufficient reliable information available about the possible mechanism of action and active ingredients.

Adverse Reactions

None reported.

Interactions with Herbs & Other Dietary Supplements

Insufficient reliable information available.

Interactions with Drugs

No interactions are known to occur, and there is no known reason to expect a clinically significant interaction with moneywort.

Interactions with Foods

No interactions are known to occur, and there is no known reason to expect a clinically significant interaction with moneywort.

Interactions with Lab Tests

No interactions are known to occur, and there is no known reason to expect a clinically significant interaction with moneywort.

Interactions with Diseases or Conditions

No interactions are known to occur, and there is no known reason to expect a clinically significant interaction with moneywort.

Dosage and Administration

ORAL: One cup of tea is taken 2-3 times daily with honey for cough. The tea is prepared by steeping 2 heaping teaspoons of dried herb in 250 mL of boiling water for 5 minutes and straining (18).
TOPICAL: No typical dosage.

Comments

There is very little scientific information about this product. Our staff is continually analyzing the available information on natural medicines and will add data here as it becomes available.

MORINDA

Also Known As

Indian Mulberry, Noni, Hog Apple, Menkoedoe, Mulberry, Ruibarbo Caribe, Wild Pine, Tahitian Noni Juice, Bois Douleur, Pau-Azeitona, Mora De La India, Mengkudu, Nhau, Nonu, Nono.
CAUTION: See separate listing for Ba Ji Tian.

Scientific Names

Morinda citrifolia.
Family: Rubiaceae.

People Use This For

Orally, morinda is used for berberi, colic, convulsions, cough, diabetes, dysuria, stimulating menstrual flow (emmenagogue), fever, hepatosis, constipation (laxative), leukorrhea (whitish vaginal discharge), malarial fever, nausea, sapraemia (general reaction to circulating toxins from saprophytic, non-pathogenic, organisms), smallpox, splenomegaly, swelling (513), asthma, bone and joint problems, cancer, cataracts, colds, depression, digestive problems, gastric ulcers, heart trouble, high blood pressure, infections, kidney disorders, migraine, premenstrual syndrome, stroke (439), analgesia, and sedation (4119).
Topically, morinda is used as an emollient and to reduce signs of aging (437).

Traditionally in Polynesia and the Pacific Islands, the fruit is used for aging, diabetes, bad breath, mouth ulcers, hemorrhoids, tumors, tuberculosis, ciguatera fish poisoning, and high blood pressure (6,438). The leaves have been used in medicines for rheumatic aches and swelling of the joints, stomachache, dysentery, and swelling caused by the parasitic disease filariasis (6,438). The bark has been used in a preparation to aid childbirth (6,435,438). The leaves are used topically for arthritis by wrapping around the affected joint, for headache by applying to the forehead, and for direct application to burns, sores and leprotic lesions (6,438). A mixture of leaves and fruit is applied to abcesses, and preparations of the root are used on stonefish and sting-ray wounds, and as a smallpox salve (438).
The fruit, leaf, root, seed, and bark are also used as food (6,435,438).

Safety
POSSIBLY SAFE ...when used orally or topically and appropriately for medicinal purposes (6). ...when the fruit is used as food (6).
PREGNANCY AND LACTATION: Insufficient reliable information available; avoid using.

Effectiveness
There is insufficient reliable information available about the effectiveness of morinda.

Mechanism of Action
The applicable parts of morinda are the fruits, leaves, and roots. The fruit of Morinda citrifolia contains essential oils, hexoic and octoic acids, paraffin, and esters of ethyl and methyl alcohols (6). Ripe fruit contains n-caproic acid (6). Anthraquinones, morindone, alizarin, xeronine, and damnacanthal have also been isolated from various parts of morinda (6). Xeronine is claimed to work at a molecular level to repair damaged cells and regulate their function (6). Xeronine is mainly present in the plant as an inactive precursor called proxeronine, together with an inactive form of the enzyme required to convert it to xeronine. This conversion takes place in the intestines provided the proenzyme is not destroyed by stomach acid (440). The fruit juice contains a polysaccharide-rich substance which increases survival in mice with Lewis lung carcinoma, possibly by activating the host immune system (441). Damnacanthal, an anthraquinone isolated from the roots of morinda inhibits tyrosine kinase, has a stimulatory effect on ultraviolet-induced apoptosis, and induces normal morphology in ras-transformed cells (442,443). The fruit juice also contains a significant amount of potassium, approximately 56 mEq/L (1298). In mice, lyophilized aqueous extracts of morinda roots have sedative and central analgesic effects, the latter blocked by naloxone (444). Alcoholic extracts of the leaves have anthelmintic activity in vitro (6). Capsules containing morinda extract are reported to contain proteins, fats, carbohydrates, vitamin A, vitamin C, niacin, calcium, iron, sodium, and potassium (440).

Adverse Reactions
None reported.

Interactions with Herbs & Other Dietary Supplements
Insufficient reliable information is available.

Interactions with Drugs
POTASSIUM-SPARING DIURETICS (Spironolactone, Triamterene): Theoretically, concomitant use of morinda fruit juice (noni juice) and potassium sparing diuretics might increase the risk of hyperkalemia. Morinda fruit juice contains approximately 56 mEq/L of potassium (1298).

Interactions with Foods
FOOD: It is claimed that the increase in stomach acid caused by food ingestion will cause destruction of the enzyme required for formation of the active ingredient xeronine in the intestine (440).

Interactions with Lab Tests
URINE COLOR: The anthraquinone constituents can discolor urine from pink to rust and interfere with diagnostic tests, due to anthraquinone content (275).

Interactions with Diseases or Conditions
CHRONIC RENAL INSUFFICIENCY: Use of morinda fruit juice (noni juice) can increase the risk of hyperkalemia; use with caution. One reported case associates the use on morinda fruit juice with hyperkalemia in a patient with chronic renal insufficiency (1298). Morinda fruit juice contains approximately 56 mEq/L of potassium (1298).
HYPERKALEMIA: Caution, use of morinda fruit juice (noni juice) can contribute to elevated potassium levels; contraindicated. Morinda fruit juice contains approximately 56 mEq/L of potassium (1298).

Dosage and Administration
ORAL: One to 10 ounces daily of juice prepared from the fruit has been used (436,439). Capsules containing 200

to 620 mg of Morinda citrifolia extract are also marketed. It is claimed that 1200 mg from capsules is equivalent to one ounce of juice (439).

Comments

The smell and taste of Morinda citrifolia fruit juice (noni juice) are unpleasant (440). Capsules containing dried plant extracts are marketed to overcome this, but it is not known what effect the drying process has on the constituents. Morinda juice is imported to the US from the islands of French Polynesia. It is very expensive, about $100 a bottle.

MORMON TEA

Also Known As

Brigham Tea, Desert Tea, Popotillo, Teamster's Tea, Squaw Tea.
CAUTION: See separate listing for Ephedra.

Scientific Names

Ephedra nevadensis.
Family: Ephedraceae.

People Use This For

Historically, Mormon tea has been used for syphilis, gonorrhea, colds, kidney disorders, and as a "spring" tonic (515). It has also been used as a beverage (6).

Safety

LIKELY SAFE ...when consumed in food amounts (12).
There is insufficient reliable information about the safety of Mormon tea for medicinal uses.
PREGNANCY AND LACTATION: Insufficient reliable information available; avoid using in amounts greater than those found in foods.

Effectiveness

There is insufficient reliable information available about the effectiveness of Mormon tea.

Mechanism of Action

Mormon tea contains large amounts of tannins (515). Tannin constituents exert an astringent effect on the mucosal tissue. This effect dehydrates the tissue, reducing internal secretions, and forming external cells into a protective layer (12). Plants with at least 10% tannins can cause gastrointestinal disturbances, kidney damage, and necrotic conditions of the liver (12). Some animal experiments show that tannins might cause cancer. Others show they might prevent it (12). Regular consumption of herbs with high tannin concentrations correlates to an increase in esophageal or nasal cancer (12). Despite the "ephedra" in the scientific name, Mormon tea contains no ephedrine or other alkaloids (515). An aqueous extract demonstrates mild diuresis and constipation (515).

Adverse Reactions

None reported.

Interactions with Herbs & Other Dietary Supplements

TANNIN-CONTAINING HERBS: Theoretically, herbs that contain high percentages of tannins might cause precipitation of constituents of other herbs (19).

Interactions with Drugs

ORAL DRUGS: Theoretically, concomitant oral administration may cause precipitation of some drugs due to the high tannin content of Mormon tea (19). Separate administration of oral drugs and tannin-containing herbs by the longest period of time practical (19).

Interactions with Foods

No interactions are known to occur, and there is no known reason to expect a clinically significant interaction with Mormon tea.

Interactions with Lab Tests

No interactions are known to occur, and there is no known reason to expect a clinically significant interaction with Mormon tea.

Interactions with Diseases or Conditions

No interactions are known to occur, and there is no known reason to expect a clinically significant interaction with Mormon tea.

Dosage and Administration

ORAL: People prepare and consume Mormon tea by steeping the dried branches in 150 mL boiling water for five to ten minutes and then straining (5008).

Comments

None.

MOTHERWORT

Also Known As

Leonuri cardiacae herba, Leonurus, Lion's Ear, Lion's Tail, Roman Motherwort, Throw-Wort.

Scientific Names

Leonurus cardiaca and other Leonurus species.
Family: Laminaceae or Labiatae.

People Use This For

Orally, motherwort is used for cardiac symptoms of neurosis (2,4,9,18), cardiac insufficiency (4,18), fast heart rate or other arrhythmias (4,18), and hyperthyroidism (2,9,18).
In Chinese medicine, motherwort is used topically for itching and shingles. The seeds of Leonurus artemisia or Leonurus heterophyllus are used to improve eyesight and as a general tonic (1532).
In folk medicine, uses of motherwort include treating amenorrhea (4) and flatulence (18).

Safety

POSSIBLY SAFE ...when used orally and appropriately (2,12).
PREGNANCY: LIKELY UNSAFE ...when used orally because it might have uterine-stimulating effects (4,12,19).
LACTATION: Insufficient reliable information available; avoid using.

Effectiveness

There is insufficient reliable information available about the effectiveness of motherwort.

Mechanism of Action

The applicable parts of motherwort are the above ground parts. Motherwort has sedative (4,18), negative chronotropic, hypotonic (18), cardiac-inhibitory, and antispasmodic effects (4). Constituents include leonurine and stachydrine, which can stimulate uterine tone and blood flow (4,12,19). Ursolic acid can have antiviral, tumor-inhibiting, and cytotoxic activity (4). The intravenous administration of a Leonurus heterophyllus extract can decrease blood viscosity by decreasing platelet aggregation, decreasing fibrinogen, and increasing erythrocyte deformability (1533).

Adverse Reactions

Using motherwort in amounts greater than 3 grams can cause diarrhea, stomach irritation, and uterine bleeding (12). The leaves can cause contact dermatitis, and the oil can cause photosensitivity (4). Motherwort can also cause allergic reactions in sensitive individuals (4).

Interactions with Herbs & Other Dietary Supplements

CARDIAC GLYCOSIDE-CONTAINING HERBS: Contraindicated; concomitant use can increase the risk of cardiac glycoside toxicity. Cardiac glycoside-containing herbs include black hellebore, Canadian hemp roots, digitalis leaf, hedge mustard, figwort, lily of the valley roots, oleander leaf, pheasant's eye plant, pleurisy root, squill bulb leaf scales, strophanthus seeds, and uzara (2,18,19,500).

Interactions with Drugs

CNS DEPRESSANTS: Concomitant use of motherwort can potentiate the sedative and tranquilizing effects of these drugs, including the sedative effects of antihistamines (19).

Interactions with Foods

No interactions are known to occur, and there is no known reason to expect a clinically significant interaction with motherwort.

Interactions with Lab Tests

THYROID FUNCTION: Motherwort might improve thyroid function and thyroid function test results in patients with thyroid hyperfunction (2).

Interactions with Diseases or Conditions

CARDIAC DISORDERS: Excessive use of motherwort can interfere with the treatment of cardiac disorders (4).
UTERINE BLEEDING CONDITIONS: Theoretically, it can exacerbate uterine bleeding due to its possible stimulation of uterine blood flow (4,12,19).

Dosage and Administration

ORAL: The typical dose of motherwort is 2 grams of the dried above ground parts or 1 cup of the tea 3 times per day (4). To prepare tea steep 2 grams of the dried above ground parts in 150 mL boiling water for 5-10 minutes, then strain. The average amount used is 4.5 grams per day (2).

Comments

None.

MOUNTAIN ASH

Also Known As

Eberesche, Ebereschenbeeren, European Mountain-Ash, Quickbeam, Rowan Tree, Sorb Apple, Sorbi acupariae fructus, Witchen.

Scientific Names

Sorbus aucuparia.
Family: Rosaceae.

People Use This For

Orally, mountain ash berries are used for kidney diseases, diabetes, arthritis, disorders of uric acid metabolism, dissolution of uric acid deposits, mucous membrane inflammation, internal inflammations, vitamin C deficiency, alkalizing the blood, increasing metabolism, purifying the blood (2,18) and for menstrual complaints (18). A berry puree is used for diarrhea (18). Fresh squeezed berry juice is used for lung conditions, especially those associated with fever (18).
In manufacturing, fresh berries are used as an ingredient in marmalade, stewed fruit, juice, liqueur and vinegar. Dried fruit is used in tea mixtures (18).

Safety

POSSIBLY UNSAFE …when large amounts of fresh berries are ingested. The constituent, parasorbic acid is an irritant and large amounts can cause gastric irritation and kidney damage (18).
There is insufficient reliable information available about the safety of the oral use of dried or cooked berries.
PREGNANCY AND LACTATION: POSSIBLY UNSAFE …when large amounts of fresh berries are ingested (18).
There is insufficient reliable information available about the safety of dried or cooked berries; avoid using.

Effectiveness

There is insufficient reliable information available about the effectiveness of mountain ash.

Mechanism of Action

The applicable part of mountain ash is the berry used fresh, dried, or cooked then dried. Mountain ash berry contains parasorbic acid, cyanogenic glycosides, fruit acids (malic acid, tartaric acid), tannins, and vitamin C (18). The parasorbic acid that is contained in the fresh berry can cause local irritation. However, the compound is partially degraded by drying and completely destroyed by cooking (2).

Adverse Reactions

Ingestion of large amounts of fresh berries may cause gastroenteritis, vomiting, queasiness, gastric pain, diarrhea, kidney damage (albuminuria, glycosuria), and polymorphic xanthomas due to parasorbic acid (18).

Interactions with Herbs & Other Dietary Supplements

Insufficient reliable information available.

Interactions with Drugs

No interactions are known to occur, and there is no known reason to expect a clinically significant interaction with mountain ash.

Interactions with Foods

No interactions are known to occur, and there is no known reason to expect a clinically significant interaction with mountain ash.

Interactions with Lab Tests

No interactions are known to occur, and there is no known reason to expect a clinically significant interaction with mountain ash.

Interactions with Diseases or Conditions

No interactions are known to occur, and there is no known reason to expect a clinically significant interaction with mountain ash.

Dosage and Administration

No typical dosage.

Comments

None.

MOUNTAIN FLAX

Also Known As

Dwarf Flax, Fairy Flax, Mill Mountain, Purging Flax.

Scientific Names

Linum catharticum.
Family: Linaceae.

People Use This For

Orally, mountain flax is used as an emetic and purgative to cause bowel elimination (18).

Safety

POSSIBLY UNSAFE …when used orally, particularly with long-term use (18).
PREGNANCY AND LACTATION: UNSAFE …when used orally; contraindicated due to possible emetic effects (18).

Effectiveness

There is insufficient reliable information available about the effectiveness of mountain flax.

Mechanism of Action

The applicable parts of mountain flax are the above ground flowering parts. Mountain flax is thought to have laxative effects at 0.5 grams. It contains the lignan achromatin, tannins and a volatile oil (18).

Adverse Reactions

Orally, mountain flax can cause vomiting, gastrointestinal tract inflammation and diarrhea (18).

Interactions with Herbs & Other Dietary Supplements

Insufficient reliable information available.

Interactions with Drugs

No interactions are known to occur, and there is no known reason to expect a clinically significant interaction with mountain flax.

Interactions with Foods

No interactions are known to occur, and there is no known reason to expect a clinically significant interaction with mountain flax.

Interactions with Lab Tests

No interactions are known to occur, and there is no known reason to expect a clinically significant interaction with mountain flax.

Interactions with Diseases or Conditions

No interactions are known to occur, and there is no known reason to expect a clinically significant interaction with mountain flax.

Dosage and Administration

No typical dosage.

Comments

None.

MOUNTAIN LAUREL

Also Known As

Broad-Leafed Laurel, Calico Bush, Lambkill, Laurel, Mountain Ivy, Rose Laurel, Sheep Laurel, Spoon Laurel.

Scientific Names

Kalmia latifolia.

People Use This For

Historically, mountain laurel has been used topically for tinea capitis, psoriasis, herpes, and secondary syphilis (18).

Safety

UNSAFE ...when used orally. Mountain laurel leaf is not only an irritant, but can also lead to cardiac arrest, respiratory failure and death (18).
There is insufficient reliable information available about safety of the topical use of mountain laurel.
PREGNANCY AND LACTATION: UNSAFE ...when used orally (18). There is insufficient reliable information available about safety of mountain laurel for topical use; avoid using.

Effectiveness

There is insufficient reliable information available about the effectiveness of mountain laurel.

Mechanism of Action

The applicable part of mountain laurel is the fresh or dried leaf. Mountain laurel contains andromedan derivatives, flavonoids, and acylphloroglucinols (18). Andromedan derivatives act on the sodium channels, inhibiting conduction by preventing closure of the excitable cells (18). The andromedan derivative Grayanotoxin I and the acylphloroglucinol constituents can be cytotoxic (4145).

Adverse Reactions

Orally, mountain laurel can result in painful oral and gastric mucous membranes, increased salivation, cold sweat, nausea, vomiting, diarrhea, and paresthesias (18). Dizziness, headache, fever attacks, and intoxicated states with temporary loss of vision, muscle weakness, coordination disorders, and spasms can also develop. Bradycardia, cardiac arrhythmias, drop in blood pressure, eventual cardiac arrest and respiratory failure can lead to death (18).

Interactions with Herbs & Other Dietary Supplements

Insufficient reliable information available.

Interactions with Drugs

No interactions are known to occur, and there is no known reason to expect a clinically significant interaction with mountain laurel.

Interactions with Foods

No interactions are known to occur, and there is no known reason to expect a clinically significant interaction with mountain laurel.

Interactions with Lab Tests

No interactions are known to occur, and there is no known reason to expect a clinically significant interaction with mountain laurel.

Interactions with Diseases or Conditions

No interactions are known to occur, and there is no known reason to expect a clinically significant interaction with mountain laurel.

Dosage and Administration

TOPICAL: Mountain laurel is only available in homeopathic preparations (18).

Comments

None.

MOUSE EAR

Also Known As

None.
CAUTION: See separate listing for Cudweed.

Scientific Names

Pilosella officinarum.
Family: Asteraceae.

People Use This For

Orally, mouse ear is used for asthma, bronchitis, coughs and whooping cough. It is also used orally as a diuretic, to promote sweating, and to relieve flatulence and colic.
Topically, mouse ear is used for wounds (18).

Safety

There is insufficient reliable information available about the safety of mouse ear.
Pregnancy and Lactation: Insufficient reliable information available; avoid using.

Effectiveness

There is insufficient reliable information available about the effectiveness of mouse ear.

Mechanism of Action

The applicable parts of mouse ear are the above ground flowering plant parts. There is insufficient reliable information available about the possible mechanism of action and active ingredients.

Adverse Reactions

Mouse ear can cause an allergic reaction in individuals sensitive to the Asteraceae/Compositae family. Members of this family include ragweed, chrysanthemums, marigolds, daisies, and many other herbs.

Interactions with Herbs & Other Dietary Supplements

Insufficient reliable information available.

Interactions with Drugs

No interactions are known to occur, and there is no known reason to expect a clinically significant interaction with mouse ear.

Interactions with Foods

No interactions are known to occur, and there is no known reason to expect a clinically significant interaction with mouse ear.

Interactions with Lab Tests

No interactions are known to occur, and there is no known reason to expect a clinically significant interaction with mouse ear.

Interactions with Diseases or Conditions
CROSS-ALLERGENICITY: Can cause an allergic reaction in individuals sensitive to the Asteraceae/Compositae family. Members of this family include ragweed, chrysanthemums, marigolds, daisies, and many other herbs.

Dosage and Administration
ORAL: Mouse ear is used as a liquid extract (18).
TOPICAL: It is used as a liquid extract (18).

Comments
None.

MSM (METHYLSULFONYLMETHANE)

Also Known As
Crystalline DMSO, Dimethyl Sulfone, DMSO2, Methylsulfonyl Methane, Methyl Sulfonyl Methane, MSM, OptiMSM, Sulfonyl Sulfur.

Scientific Names
Methylsulfonylmethane; Dimethylsulfone.

People Use This For
Orally and topically, MSM is used for chronic pain, arthritis, joint inflammation, rheumatoid arthritis, osteoporosis, bursitis, tendinitis, tenosynovitis, musculoskeletal pain, muscle cramps, scleroderma, scar tissue, stretch marks, wrinkles, protection against sun/wind burn, eye inflammation, oral hygiene, periodontal disease, wounds, cuts, and abrasions/accelerated wound healing (3500).

Orally, MSM is also used for relief of allergies (allergic rhinitis, allergic sinusitis, allergy-induced asthma, inhalant allergens, environmental allergens), drug hypersensitivity, gastrointestinal upset, chronic constipation, gastric hyperacidity, ulcers, diverticulosis, premenstrual syndrome (PMS), mood elevation, obesity, poor circulation, hypertension, and elevated serum cholesterol. It is also used orally for diabetes mellitus type 2 (NIDDM), interstitial cystitis, hepatic dysfunction, Alzheimer's disease, snoring, lung dysfunction/emphysema, pneumonia, chronic fatigue syndrome, auto-immune disorders (systemic lupus erythematous), HIV infection/AIDS, and cancer (breast cancer and colon cancer). Other oral uses of MSM include eye inflammation, mucous membrane inflammation, myositis ossificans generalis, temporomandibular joint dysfunction, leg cramps, connective tissue disorders, migraine, headaches, hangover, parasitic infections of the intestinal and urogenital tracts including Trichomonas vaginalis and Giardia, Candida albicans and other yeast infections, insect bites, radiation poisoning (3500), and as an immunostimulant (6).

Safety
There is insufficient reliable information available about the safety of MSM.
Pregnancy and Lactation: Insufficient reliable information available; avoid using.

Effectiveness
There is insufficient reliable information available about the effectiveness of MSM.

Mechanism of Action
MSM is a precursor source of sulfur for cysteine and methionine. Incorporation of MSM-derived sulfur into methionine is regulated by a limiting step involving micro-organisms in the intestinal lumen (3501). It is an odorless breakdown product of dimethyl sulfoxide (DMSO) (6). MSM delays chemically-induced colon cancer tumor onset in animals (3502). A four percent (4%) MSM solution delays the latency period between induction and onset of chemically induced mammary tumors or cancers in rats (3503). MSM does not affect expression of auto-immune diabetes in spontaneously diabetic mice (3504).

Adverse Reactions
Orally, MSM can cause nausea, diarrhea, and headache in some patients.

Interactions with Herbs & Other Dietary Supplements
Insufficient reliable information available.

Interactions with Drugs
No interactions are known to occur, and there is no known reason to expect a clinically significant interaction with MSM.

Interactions with Foods
No interactions are known to occur, and there is no known reason to expect a clinically significant interaction with MSM.

Interactions with Lab Tests
No interactions are known to occur, and there is no known reason to expect a clinically significant interaction with MSM.

Interactions with Diseases or Conditions
No interactions are known to occur, and there is no known reason to expect a clinically significant interaction with MSM.

Dosage and Administration
ORAL: People typically use 1000 to 3000 mg daily with meals. One product suggests 400 mg per 50 pounds of body weight daily (6006). Some people take 250-500 mg per day for adult dietary supplementation (3500).
TOPICAL: No typical dosage.

Comments
MSM occurs naturally in green plants such as field horsetail (Equisetum arvense), certain species of algae, fruits, vegetables, grains, and both bovine and human adrenal glands, milk and urine. It is destroyed with heat or dehydration (6).

MUGWORT

Also Known As
Armoise Commune, Artemisia, Artemisiae vulgaris herba, Artemisiae vulgaris radix, Carline Thistle, Felon Herb, Gemeiner Beifuss, Hierba de San Juan, Sailor's Tobacco, St. John's Plant, Wild Wormwood.
CAUTION: See separate listings for Tarragon, Wormseed, and Wormwood.

Scientific Names
Artemisia vulgaris.
Family: Asteraceae or Compositae.

People Use This For
Orally, mugwort above ground parts are used for gastrointestinal problems, such as colic, diarrhea, constipation, cramps, weak digestion, stimulation of gastric juice and bile secretion, as a laxative in cases of obesity and "for the liver", for worm infestations, for hysteria, epilepsy, persistent vomiting, convulsions in children, menstrual problems and irregular periods, promoting circulation, and as a sedative (2).
Orally, mugwort root is used as a tonic in individuals with diminished strength and energy (2).
In combination with other ingredients, mugwort root is used for psychoneuroses, neurasthenia, depression, hypochondria, autonomic neuroses, general irritability, restlessness, insomnia, and anxiety (2).

Safety
There is insufficient reliable information available about the safety of mugwort.
PREGNANCY: LIKELY UNSAFE ...when used orally. Mugwort is said to be an abortifacient and a menstrual and uterine stimulant (2,12).
LACTATION: Insufficient reliable information available; avoid using.

Effectiveness
There is insufficient reliable information available about the effectiveness of mugwort.

Mechanism of Action

The applicable parts of mugwort are the above ground parts and root. Mugwort contains sesquiterpene lactones, lipophilic flavonoids, polyenes, umbelliferone and aesculetin. It also contains a complex volatile oil with constituents of 1,8 cineole, camphor, linalool or thujone (18). Some evidence suggests mugwort can stimulate uterine activity (19), possibly due to the thujone content (19). Other evidence suggests the aqueous extract and the volatile oil have antimicrobial properties (18).

Adverse Reactions

Orally, mugwort can cause an allergic reaction in individuals sensitive to the Asteraceae/Compositae family. Members of this family include ragweed, chrysanthemums, marigolds, daisies, and many other herbs. Mugwort pollen can cause reactions in people who are allergic to tobacco (3716). Theoretically, mugwort might cause allergic reaction in people allergic to honey or royal jelly (3717).

Interactions with Herbs & Other Dietary Supplements

Insufficient reliable information available.

Interactions with Drugs

No interactions are known to occur, and there is no known reason to expect a clinically significant interaction with mugwort.

Interactions with Foods

No interactions are known to occur, and there is no known reason to expect a clinically significant interaction with mugwort.

Interactions with Lab Tests

No interactions are known to occur, and there is no known reason to expect a clinically significant interaction with mugwort.

Interactions with Diseases or Conditions

CROSS-ALLERGENICITY: Can cause an allergic reaction in individuals sensitive to the Asteraceae/Compositae family. Members of this family include ragweed, chrysanthemums, marigolds, daisies, and many other herbs. Theoretically, mugwort might cause allergic reactions in individuals with allergies to honey or royal jelly (3717). Mugwort pollen might cause reactions in people allergic to tobacco (3716).

Dosage and Administration

ORAL: People use 5 mL of mugwort tincture 30 minutes before bedtime or 1-4 mL of the tincture up to three times daily (5008). Some people use 10 to 25 drops per dose of mugwort tincture (1:5, 50% alcohol) (5013) or prepare and consume mugwort tea by steeping 15 grams of the dried herb in 500 mL of boiling water and straining (5008). Two to three cups of tea is consumed daily before meals (5008).

Comments

Mugwort has a pleasant, tangy taste. The plant is indigenous to Asia, North America, and Northern Europe (18).

MUIRA PUAMA

Also Known As

Muira-Puama, Muirapuama, Potency Wood, Ptychopetali lignum.

Scientific Names

Ptychopetalum olacoides; Ptychopetalum unicatum.
Family: Olacaeae.

People Use This For

Orally, muira puama is used for preventing sexual disorders, and as an aphrodisiac (2,5,18). It is also used orally as a nerve stimulant, for dyspepsia, menstrual irregularities, rheumatism, paralysis caused by poliomyelitis, a general tonic, and as an appetite stimulant (5).
Topically, it is used as an aphrodisiac, for rheumatism, and muscle paralysis (5).
In combination with other herbs, muira puama is used as a remedy for sexual impotence (5).

Safety

There is insufficient reliable information available about the safety of muira puama.

Pregnancy and Lactation: Insufficient reliable information available; avoid using.

Effectiveness

There is insufficient reliable information available about the effectiveness of muira puama.

Mechanism of Action

The applicable parts of muira puama are the wood and root. No constituents in muira puama are known to exhibit any pronounced physiological activity (5).

Adverse Reactions

None reported.

Interactions with Herbs & Other Dietary Supplements

Insufficient reliable information available.

Interactions with Drugs

No interactions are known to occur, and there is no known reason to expect a clinically significant interaction with muira puama.

Interactions with Foods

No interactions are known to occur, and there is no known reason to expect a clinically significant interaction with muira puama.

Interactions with Lab Tests

No interactions are known to occur, and there is no known reason to expect a clinically significant interaction with muira puama.

Interactions with Diseases or Conditions

No interactions are known to occur, and there is no known reason to expect a clinically significant interaction with muira puama.

Dosage and Administration

ORAL: People typically use 1 to 2 mL of the muira puama extract in water two to three times daily. The number of drops recommended varies among products. The labeling on one product says one dropperful equals 1 mL and contains 500 mg muira puama. Other products do not specify the concentration of the active ingredient. Shake well before using; contains alcohol (6006).

TOPICAL: No typical dosage.

Comments

Previously, Liriosma ovata and Acanthea virilis were each thought to be the source of muira puama. They continue to be sold as muira puama in the herb trade (5).

MULLEIN

Also Known As

Aaron's Rod, Adam's Flannel, American Mullein, Beggar's Blanket, Blanket Herb, Blanket Leaf, Bouuillon Blanc, Candleflower, Candlewick, Clot-Bur, Clown's Lungwort, Cuddy's Lungs, Duffle, European Mullein, Feltwort, Flannelflower, Fluffweed, Golden Rod, Hag's Taper, Hare's Beard, Hedge Taper, Higtaper, Jacob's Staff, Longwort, Orange Mullein, Our Lady's Flannel, Rag Paper, Shepherd's Club, Shepherd's Staff, Torches, Torch Weed, Velvet Plant, Verbasci flos, Wild Ice Leaf, Woolen.

CAUTION: See separate listing for Goldenrod.

Scientific Names

Verbascum densiflorum; Verbascum phlomides; Verbascum thapiforme; Verbascum thapsus.

Family: Scrophulariaceae.

People Use This For

Orally, mullein is used for respiratory tract mucous membrane inflammation (2,18) and cough (5,6,7,8,18).

Topically, it is used for wounds (8,18), burns, hemorrhoids, bruises (5,6), frostbite, erysipelas (5), and inflamed mucosa (8). The leaves are used topically to soften and protect the skin (6).

In folk medicine, it is used internally for earaches (5,6), colds, chills and flu (6,7,8), tracheitis (8), asthma (5,6), diarrhea, gastrointestinal bleeding, migraines (5), gout (6), and tuberculosis (5,6). The root is used for croup (6), and the leaf and stem are used for bronchitis (8,18). In folk medicine, mullein is also used as a sedative, narcotic (5), diuretic, and antirheumatic (8,18).

In manufacturing, mullein is used as a flavoring component in alcoholic beverages (12).

Safety

POSSIBLY SAFE ...when used orally and appropriately (2,5,12).

There is insufficient reliable information available about the safety of the topical use of mullein.

PREGNANCY AND LACTATION: Insufficient reliable information available; avoid using.

Effectiveness

POSSIBLY EFFECTIVE ...when used orally for treating respiratory tract mucous membrane inflammation, cough, and sore throat (2,5).

There is insufficient reliable information available about the effectiveness of mullein for its other uses.

Mechanism of Action

The applicable part of mullein is the flower. Mullein contains mucilage which alleviates local irritation (2,5,6,18). The saponins in mullein have an expectorant effect (2,5,8,18), and the extract can have activity against influenza and herpes simplex viruses (1534).

Adverse Reactions

None reported.

Interactions with Herbs & Other Dietary Supplements

Insufficient reliable information available.

Interactions with Drugs

No interactions are known to occur, and there is no known reason to expect a clinically significant interaction with mullein.

Interactions with Foods

No interactions are known to occur, and there is no known reason to expect a clinically significant interaction with mullein.

Interactions with Lab Tests

No interactions are known to occur, and there is no known reason to expect a clinically significant interaction with mullein.

Interactions with Diseases or Conditions

No interactions are known to occur, and there is no known reason to expect a clinically significant interaction with mullein.

Dosage and Administration

ORAL: The typical dose of mullein is 1.5-2 grams of the dry petals or one cup of tea. up to 3-4 grams dry petals per day (2,7,8,18). The tea is prepared by steeping 1.5-2 grams of the finely chopped, dry petals in 150 mL boiling water for 10-15 minutes and then strain.

TOPICAL: No typical dosage.

Comments

Avoid confusion with goldenrod (Solidago species), also known as Aaron's rod. There is confusion as to which Verbascum species are associated with the name American mullein and which are associated with the name European mullein.

MUSK

Also Known As
Deer Musk, Tonquin Musk.

Scientific Names
Moschus moschiferus.
Family: Moschidae.

People Use This For
In Chinese medicine, musk is used for stroke, coma, neurasthenia, convulsions, heart pains, and ulcerous sores (11).
For food use, musk is often used with nut, caramel, and fruit-type flavors (11).
In manufacturing, it is also used as a constituent of fragrances and a fixative in perfumes (6).

Safety
LIKELY SAFE ...when used orally at low concentrations, generally below 0.00001%. It has Generally Recognized as Safe (GRAS) status in the US.
There is insufficient reliable information available about the safety of the oral use of larger amounts of musk.
PREGNANCY AND LACTATION: Insufficient reliable information available; avoid using.

Effectiveness
There is insufficient reliable information available about the effectiveness of musk.

Mechanism of Action
Musk contains muscone (0.3%-2%) and normuscone, steroids, paraffins, triglycerides, waxes, mucopyridine, and fatty acids, which may have anti-inflammatory and antihistaminic activity (6).

Adverse Reactions
Musk components are known to cause a variety of dermal hypersensitivity reactions (6).

Interactions with Herbs & Other Dietary Supplements
Insufficient reliable information available.

Interactions with Drugs
No interactions are known to occur, and there is no known reason to expect a clinically significant interaction with musk.

Interactions with Foods
No interactions are known to occur, and there is no known reason to expect a clinically significant interaction with musk.

Interactions with Lab Tests
No interactions are known to occur, and there is no known reason to expect a clinically significant interaction with musk.

Interactions with Diseases or Conditions
No interactions are known to occur, and there is no known reason to expect a clinically significant interaction with musk.

Dosage and Administration
No typical dosage.

Comments
Musk is the secretion from the musk gland of the male musk deer. Avoid confusion with sumbul, which is also known as musk root (Ferula sumbul, Family: Apiaceae), which is sometimes substituted for musk (6).

MYRRH

Also Known As
Abyssinian Myrrh, African Myrrh, Arabian Myrrh, Bal, Balsamodendron Myrrha, Bdellium, Bol, Bola, Commiphora, Didin, Didthin, Guggal Gum and Resin, Gum Myrrh, Heerabol, Opopanax, Somalien Myrrh, Yemen Myrrh.

Scientific Names
Commiphora molmol, synonyms Commiphora abyssinica, Commiphora madagascariensis; Commiphora myrrha; other Commiphora species; Commiphora erythraea.
Family: Burseraceae.

People Use This For
Topically, myrrh is used for mild inflammation of the oral and pharyngeal mucosa (2,5,8,9,11,13,18), aphthous ulcers (4), gingivitis (4,8,11), and chapped lips (11).
In folk medicine it is used orally for indigestion (4,5,8,9,11,13,18), ulcers (5), colds (4), cough, asthma (11), bronchial congestion (4,5,8,11,18), arthritic pain (11), cancer, leprosy, and syphilis (5,6). It is also used as a stimulant (11,13), antispasmodic (11), and to increase menstrual flow (5,6,11). Topically, myrrh is used in folk medicine for hemorrhoids (5,11), bedsores (5,8,11), wounds (5,11,19), abrasions, furunculosis (4), bad breath, and loose teeth (11).
In foods and beverages, myrrh is used as a flavoring component (11).
In manufacturing, myrrh is used as a fragrance and fixative in cosmetics (11).
It is also used in embalming and as incense (5,13).

Safety
LIKELY SAFE ...when consumed in amounts commonly found in food (11). Myrrh is approved for use in foods in the US (11).
POSSIBLY SAFE ...when used orally and appropriately (12). ...when used topically and appropriately (2,4,5,11,18).
POSSIBLY UNSAFE ...when used orally in excessive doses (12).
PREGNANCY: LIKELY UNSAFE ...when used orally because myrrh stimulates uterine tone and blood flow, and possibly has an abortifacient effect (4,12,19). There is insufficient reliable information available about the safety of the topical use of myrrh during pregnancy.
LACTATION: Insufficient reliable information available; avoid using.

Effectiveness
POSSIBLY EFFECTIVE ...when used topically for mild inflammation of the mouth and throat (2).
There is insufficient reliable information available about the effectiveness of myrrh for its other uses.

Mechanism of Action
The applicable part of myrrh is resin. Myrrh resin contains a volatile oil and mucilage that have antimicrobial (4,5,6,8,11,18), deodorizing (8), anti-inflammatory (4,8), and antitumor properties (1536). In animals, it exhibits antipyretic (4) and hypoglycemic (4) effects, as well as protects against the development of gastric ulcers (1535). Myrrh can stimulate smooth muscle (6,12) and possibly peristalsis (6). It stimulates uterine tone (6,12) and promotes uterine blood flow (12,19). Most authorities report myrrh has astringent activity (2,4,5,6,9,11,18), although some experts disagree with this (8).

Adverse Reactions
Dermatitis has been reported with the use of myrrh (6). Amounts greater than 2-4 grams can cause kidney irritation and diarrhea (12). Large amounts can affect the heart rate (19).

Interactions with Herbs & Other Dietary Supplements
Insufficient reliable information available.

Interactions with Drugs
DIABETES THERAPY: The use of myrrh in diabetics can interfere with their therapy (4).

Interactions with Foods
No interactions are known to occur, and there is no known reason to expect a clinically significant interaction with myrrh.

Interactions with Lab Tests
BLOOD GLUCOSE: Theoretically, myrrh can lower blood glucose and test results.

Interactions with Diseases or Conditions

DIABETES: Theoretically, myrrh can interfere with diabetes therapy (4).

HEART CONDITIONS: Use myrrh with caution in individuals with heart conditions, because large amounts can affect the heart rate (19).

OTHER: Use myrrh with caution because it can exacerbate uterine bleeding (12,19), fever, and systemic inflammation (19).

Dosage and Administration

TOPICAL: For mild mouth and throat irritation, dab the undiluted tincture of myrrh on affected areas two to three times daily. Myrrh is also commonly used as a rinse or gargle with 5-10 drops in a glass of water (2,8). A typical mouthwash can contain 30-60 drops in a glass of water also (8). The tooth powder contains 10% powdered resin (2,18).

Comments

Myrrh is the oelogum resin exuded from fissures or cuts in the bark of Commiphora species trees. While there is confusion about the sources of myrrh, most authorities include Commiphora molmol and other Commiphora species as sources. However, authorities consider Commiphora mukul to be a related species, but not a source of myrrh (8).

MYRTLE

Also Known As

Myrti aetherolum, Myrti folium.

Scientific Names

Myrtus communis.
Family: Myrtaceae.

People Use This For

Orally, myrtle is used for treating acute and chronic respiratory infections including bronchitis, whooping cough, tuberculosis, bladder conditions, diarrhea, and worm infestation (18).

Safety

LIKELY UNSAFE ...when the undiluted oil is used orally because it contains cineole. Ingesting more than 10 grams of cineole can result in respiratory failure and collapse (18).

There is insufficient reliable information available about the safety of myrtle leaf and branch.

CHILDREN: LIKELY UNSAFE ...when used orally. Avoid facial contact with myrtle oil preparations which may cause glottal spasm, bronchospasm, asthma-like attacks, or respiratory failure in infants or small children (18).

PREGNANCY AND LACTATION: LIKELY UNSAFE ...when used orally (18); avoid using.

Effectiveness

There is insufficient reliable information available about the effectiveness of myrtle.

Mechanism of Action

The applicable parts of myrtle are the leaf and branch. Myrtle contains a volatile oil, tannins, and acylphloroglucinols. Myrtol, a volatile oil, stimulates mucous membranes of the stomach and deodorizes the breath. It might also have fungicidal, disinfectant, and antibacterial properties (18). The volatile oil contains between 15-45% of 1,8-cineole, a constituent responsible for toxicity (18).

Adverse Reactions

Orally, myrtle can cause nausea, vomiting, and diarrhea (18). Consumption of large amounts might lead to low blood pressure, circulatory disorders, respiratory failure and collapse (18).

Topically, facial contact with myrtle oil preparations may cause glottal or bronchial spasm, asthma-like attacks or respiratory failure in infants and children (18).

Interactions with Herbs & Other Dietary Supplements

Insufficient reliable information available.

Interactions with Drugs

No interactions are known to occur, and there is no known reason to expect a clinically significant interaction with myrtle.

Interactions with Foods
No interactions are known to occur, and there is no known reason to expect a clinically significant interaction with myrtle.

Interactions with Lab Tests
No interactions are known to occur, and there is no known reason to expect a clinically significant interaction with myrtle.

Interactions with Diseases or Conditions
No interactions are known to occur, and there is no known reason to expect a clinically significant interaction with myrtle.

Dosage and Administration
ORAL: A typical dose is 200 mg one time only (18).

Comments
Myrtle leaves resemble the leaves of Bux semper-virens and Vaccinium vitisidaea (18).

N-ACETYL CYSTEINE

Also Known As
Acetylcysteine, L-Cysteine, NAC, N-Acetylcysteine, N-Acetyl-B-Cysteine, N-Acetyl-L-Cysteine, N-Acetyl L-Cysteine, N-Acetyl-Cysteine.

Scientific Names
N-acetyl-L-cysteine.

People Use This For
Orally, N-acetyl cysteine (NAC) is used as an antidote for acetaminophen poisoning (14,15), unstable angina, carbon monoxide poisoning, common bile duct obstruction in infants, lyosomal storage disorders, amyotrophic lateral sclerosis (ALS, Lou Gehrig's disease), phenytoin-induced hypersensitivity, and keratoconjunctivitis. It is also used for reducing lipoprotein (a) levels (14,2244), reducing homocysteine levels (2256), and for chronic bronchitis (6176). NAC is also used orally for myoclonus epilepsy; otitis media (14); hemodialysis-related pseudoporphyria (5052); Sjogren's syndrome; preventing sports injury complications; radiation therapy; increasing immunity to flu; detoxifying heavy metals such as mercury, lead, and cadmium; preventing alcoholic liver damage; protecting against environmental pollutants, including carbon monoxide, chloroform, urethanes and certain herbicides (2244); reducing toxicity of ifosfamide and doxorubicin (14,2244); as a hangover remedy (6179); and for preventing nonionic, low-osmolality contrast agent-induced reduction of renal function in patients with renal insufficiency (6611).

By inhalation or intratracheal installation, NAC is used as a mucolytic agent in acute and chronic lung disorders such as pneumonia, bronchitis, emphysema, cystic fibrosis, and others (15).

Topically, NAC is used for reducing dental plaque (14).

Rectally, NAC is used for meconium ileus and meconium ileus equivalent (14).

Intravenously, NAC is used for acetaminophen overdose, acrylonitrile poisoning, amyotrophic lateral sclerosis (ALS, Lou Gehrig's disease), hepatorenal syndrome, and for unstable angina in combination with nitroglycerin (14,1752).

Safety
LIKELY SAFE ...when used orally, intratracheally, or by inhalation and appropriately. N-acetyl cysteine (NAC) is a FDA-approved prescription drug (15).

PREGNANCY: POSSIBLY SAFE ...when used orally, intratracheally, or by inhalation. N-acetyl cysteine (NAC) crosses the placenta, but has not been associated with adverse effects to the fetus or mothers (1711). However, NAC should only be used in pregnant women when clearly indicated such as in cases of acetaminophen toxicity.

LACTATION: Insufficient reliable information available; avoid using.

Effectiveness
EFFECTIVE ...when used orally or intravenously for treating acetaminophen poisoning (15,17). The oral and intravenous routes of administration are equally effective in preventing mortality and permanent sequelae of acetaminophen poisoning (17). ...when used by inhalation as a mucolytic for adjunctive treatment of acute and chronic bronchopulmonary disorders (15). ...when used for atelectasis caused by mucus obstruction (15). ...when used for post-traumatic chest conditions (15). ...when used for pulmonary complications of surgery and cystic fibrosis (15). ...when used for preparing people for bronchial diagnostic studies (15). ...when used as an adjunct for preventing endotracheal

crusting in tracheostomy care (15). ...when used for inhalation injury (15). ...when used intravenously for acrylonitrile poisoning (14).

POSSIBLY EFFECTIVE ...when used orally or intravenously for treating unstable angina pectoris in combination with nitroglycerin (14,2245,2246). Concurrent intravenous administration of N-acetyl cysteine also seems to reduce development of nitroglycerin tolerance (832,2245). However, severe headache can occur when N-acetyl cysteine and nitroglycerin are administered together and may limit feasibility of concomitant use (2245). ...when used orally for preventing acute exacerbations of chronic bronchitis. Chronic oral use of N-acetyl cysteine seems to reduce the risk of acute exacerbations of chronic bronchitis when used over a 3-6 month period (6176). ...when used orally for preventing ifosfamide (Ifex) toxicity (14,5808). ...when used orally for preventing nonionic, low-osmolality contrast agent-induced reduction of renal function in patients with renal insufficiency. Oral administration of N-acetyl cysteine on the day before and day of iopromide (Ultravist-300) administration, plus hydration with intravenous saline, prevents reduction of renal function in patients with chronic renal insufficiency undergoing elective computed tomography (CT) (6611). ...when used orally for reducing homocysteine levels (2256,2258). ...when used orally for treating myoclonus epilepsy (2259). ...when used orally for reducing symptoms of influenza (2260). ...when used topically for reducing dental plaque (14). ...when used rectally for treating meconium ileus and meconium ileus equivalent (a bowel obstruction associated with cystic fibrosis) (14).

POSSIBLY INEFFECTIVE ...when used orally for preventing or reversing doxorubicin-induced cardiac toxicity (2252,2253). ...when used for treating Sjogren's syndrome (14). ...when used orally to prevent second primary tumors in patients with head, neck, or lung cancer (1710). N-acetyl cysteine alone or in combination with retinyl palmitate also has no effect on survival or event-free survival in patients with head, neck, or lung cancer (1705,1710). ...when used intravenously for treating amyotrophic lateral sclerosis (ALS) (14,2254).

LIKELY INEFFECTIVE ...when used for reducing lipoprotein (a) levels (2256,2257). ...when used orally for reducing nitroglycerin tolerance (2281,2282).

There is insufficient reliable information about the effectiveness of N-acetyl cysteine for its other uses. However, there is some preliminary clinical evidence that intravenous N-acetyl cysteine might improve renal function in hepatorenal syndrome (1752). There is also some evidence that topical N-acetyl cysteine might be useful for lamellar ichthyosis, a congenital skin disease (3974,3975). There is also preliminary evidence that oral N-acetyl cysteine might be helpful for some patients with HIV who have low glutathione levels (1539,1750,5063). More evidence is needed to rate N-acetyl cysteine for these uses.

Mechanism of Action

N-acetyl cysteine is the N-acetyl derivative of the amino acid L-cysteine (15,1705). N-acetyl cysteine (NAC) is a good source of sulfhydryl (SH) groups, and is metabolized into compounds that can stimulate glutathione synthesis and act as antioxidants and free radical scavengers (1761). The antioxidant effect of NAC may explain its apparent ability to prevent adverse effects caused by toxic chemicals, drug reactions, and nonionic, low-osmolality contrast agents (1762,6611). The antioxidant and free radical properties might also make NAC useful in the treatment of HIV, pulmonary, and cardiac disease (1539,1705,1765,5063). NAC also appears to reduce cellular production of pro-inflammatory mediators such as tumor necrosis factor-alpha and interleukin 1 (1763). NAC has mucolytic properties that result from several mechanisms. NAC ruptures mucous disulfide bonds which reduces mucous viscosity. NAC also has an irritating effect on mucosa that stimulates mucociliary clearance (14). NAC works for acetaminophen hepatotoxicity by restoring glutathione levels in the liver and acting as an alternative substrate for conjugation of toxic acetaminophen metabolites (15). NAC might be helpful in the congenital skin disease lamellar ichthyosis due to antiproliferative effects on skin cells (3975). In HIV patients, NAC might restore glutathione levels. Glutathione deficiency in HIV has been associated with poor survival (1750). In vitro, NAC also seems to improve T-cell function and reduce HIV expression (5063). NAC may also have anticarcinogenic properties by inhibiting the invasive activity of tumor cells and angiogenesis (1767).

Adverse Reactions

Orally, N-acetyl cysteine (NAC) can cause nausea, vomiting, and diarrhea, particulary when used in high doses (17). NAC has an unpleasant odor that sometimes makes it difficult for patients to take orally. Using a straw to drink NAC solutions can improve tolerability (17). In some cases, placement of a nasogastric or duodenal tube and administration of metoclopramide or ondansetron can also be helpful for patients unable to tolerate oral NAC (17). Rarely, generalized urticaria with mild fever, sulfhemoglobinemia, headache, hypotension, rash, and hepatotoxicity have occurred (15,17). Intravenously, NAC can sometimes cause allergic reactions including anaphylactoid reactions (17,1716). For less severe allergic reactions, diphenhydramine can be administered and the NAC infusion can be continued. For more severe reactions (e.g., angioedema, respiratory symptoms), the infusion should be temporarily discontinued and resumed an hour after diphenhydramine administration (1716).

By inhalation, NAC has been associated with stomatitis, nausea, vomiting, drowsiness, clamminess, and severe rhinorrhea (15). Fever, chills, chest tightness, and bronchoconstriction have been reported rarely (15). Sensitization and dermal eruptions has been reported. However, sensitization has not been confirmed by patch testing (15).

In cases of NAC overdose, symptoms typically resemble a severe anaphylactoid reaction (17).

Interactions with Herbs & Other Dietary Supplements
Insufficient reliable information available.

Interactions with Drugs
ACTIVATED CHARCOAL: There is some concern that using oral N-acetyl cysteine in combination with activated charcoal in patients with acetaminophen overdose decreases the effectiveness of N-acetyl cysteine. However, researchers have found that concurrent use of activated charcoal does not reduce the effectiveness of N-acetyl cysteine (1755).
CARBAMAZEPINE: Concomitant use can reduce carbamazepine (Tegretol) serum levels and therapeutic effects (14).
NITROGLYCERIN: Concomitant administration of N-acetyl cysteine and intravenous nitroglycerin use can cause severe hypotension (14,2246); concomitant use of oral NAC and nitroglycerin can cause intolerable headaches (2245,2280).

Interactions with Foods
No interactions are known to occur, and there is no known reason to expect a clinically significant interaction with NAC.

Interactions with Lab Tests
BLOOD PRESSURE: Concomitant administration of intravenous NAC and nitroglycerin can lower blood pressure and reduce blood pressure readings (2246).
CHLORIDE: NAC can cause false-positive serum chloride test results measured with the Beckman Synchron CX3 analyzer (275).
CREATININE: Intravenous NAC can cause falsely low serum creatinine test results when measured by single-slide method on Kodak Ektachem systems (275).
CYSTEINE (FREE): Intravenous NAC can increase free cysteine plasma concentrations and test results (275).
GOLD: Intravenous NAC can increase urinary gold excretion (concentration) and test results in patients previously given gold (275).
KETONES: NAC can cause false-positive urine ketone test results when measured with Chemstrips (Boehringer Mannheim) or Multistix (Miles) (275). NAC can cause false-positive blood or urine ketone test results in procedures using nitroprusside (14).
LIPOPROTEIN A: Used orally, NAC might reduce serum lipoprotein A concentrations and test results in some patients (275).
LITHIUM: Very high serum NAC concentrations might cause falsely low serum lithium test results when measured with Kodak Ektachem systems (275).
LIVER FUNCTION TESTS: NAC might increase liver enzyme (AST, ALT) concentrations and test results. Liver function tests were markedly elevated on two occasions in a child with cystic fibrosis after receiving large NAC doses by rectal and naso-gastric tube administration (15).
PROTHROMBIN TIME (PT): Intravenous NAC can decrease PT and test results (1341).
SALICYLATE: Serum NAC concentrations of 50 mg/dL (occurring with intravenous NAC administration) can cause falsely low serum salicylate test results when measured with Kodak Ektachem systems. Serum NAC concentrations of 10 mg/dL (occurring with oral NAC administration) do not interfere with serum salicylate results measured with Kodak Ektachem systems (275). NAC can interfere with serum salicylate assays measured by colorimetric methods which rely on the reagent 4-aminophenol for the color change (14).

Interactions with Diseases or Conditions
ALLERGY: Contraindicated in individuals with acetylcysteine allergy (15).
ASTHMA: Oral NAC inhalation or intratracheal administration might cause bronchospasm, monitor closely (15).
HEMODIALYSIS-ASSOCIATED PSEUDOPORPHYRIA: NAC might improve pseudoporphyria skin lesions associated with hemodialysis. Two cases are reported in which pseudoporphyria skin lesions healed with oral NAC administration in patients on chronic hemodialysis (5052).
SEPTIC SHOCK: NAC might depress cardiac function (14).

Dosage and Administration
ORAL: For acetaminophen overdose, an oral loading dose of 140 mg/kg of a 5% solution should be administered. The commercially available 10 and 20% solutions may be diluted with water or carbonated or non-carbonated beverages, and administered through a straw to lessen the disagreeable odor of N-acetyl cysteine (NAC). Seventeen additional doses of 70 mg/kg as a 5% solution should be given every 4 hours, for a total dose of 1330 mg/kg over 72 hours (17). A typical dose for unstable angina is 600 mg three times daily with transdermal nitroglycerin (2245). For preventing acute exacerbations of chronic bronchitis, doses of 200 mg twice daily, 200 mg three times daily, 300 mg slow-release twice daily, and 600 mg controlled-release twice daily have been used (6176). For ifosfamide toxicity prophylaxis, 2 grams every 6 hours has been used (5808). For reducing plasma homocysteine levels, 1.2 grams daily has been used (2258). For myoclonus epilepsy, 4-6 grams daily has been used (2259). For reducing symptoms of influenza, 600 mg twice daily has

been used (2260). For hemodialysis-associated pseudoporphyria skin lesions, 200 mg four times daily or 600 mg twice daily has been used (5052). For preventing iopromide (Ultravist-300)-induced reduction of renal function in patients with chronic renal insufficiency, 600 mg NAC twice daily on the day before and day of iopromide administration plus IV saline (0.45%) 1 mL/kg body weight per hour for 12 hours before and 12 hours after iopromide administration has been used (6611).

TOPICAL: For reducing dental plaque, a 10% aqueous acetylcysteine solution has been used (14).

RECTAL: For meconium ileus equivalent, a typical adult dose is 4-6% acetylcysteine enema every 6 to 12 hours (14); for meconium ileus or meconium ileus equivalent in pediatric patients, a typical dose is 10% acetylcysteine enema every 3 to 12 hours (14).

INTRAVENOUS: There are 2 dosage regimens for intravenous NAC. For patients presenting 10 to 24 hours after acetaminophen ingestion, particularly if large doses were taken, the following 48-hour regimen should be used (17). Administer a loading dose of 140 mg IV NAC as a 3% solution over 1 hour. The 3% solution is prepared by diluting the 20% IV solution with 5% dextrose. Twelve additional doses of 70 mg/kg IV NAC should be administered over 1 hour every 4 hours thereafter. The alternative 20-hour regimen consists of IV administration of 150 mg/kg NAC in 200 ml of 5% dextrose solution, administered over 15 minutes. Follow this dose with 50 mg/kg NAC in 500 ml 5% dextose over 4 hours and 100 mg/kg in 1 liter 5% dextrose over 16 hours. The total dose is 300 mg/kg over 20 hours. This regimen is most effective if begun within 8 hours of acetaminophen ingestion (17).

Comments
None.

N-ACETYL GLUCOSAMINE

Also Known As
Acetylglucosamine, Glucosamine N-Acetyl, N-Acetyl D-Glucosamine, N-Acetyl-D-Glucosamine, NAG, N-A-G, Poly-NAG.
CAUTION: See separate listings for Glucosamine Sulfate and Glucosamine Hydrochloride.

Scientific Names
2-acetamido-2-deoxyglucose.

People Use This For
Orally, N-acetyl glucosamine is used for ulcerative colitis, Crohn's disease (2610,2609), and osteoarthritis (2611).

Safety
There is insufficient reliable information available about the safety of N-acetyl glucosamine.
Pregnancy and Lactation: Insufficient reliable information available; avoid using.

Effectiveness
There is insufficient reliable information available about the effectiveness of N-acetyl glucosamine.

Mechanism of Action
N-acetyl glucosamine is a glycoprotein derived from marine exoskeletons or produced synthetically (6). In inflammatory bowel disease (IBD), N-acetylation of glucosamine is relatively deficient, possibly reducing the synthesis of the gastric and intestinal mucosa's protective glycoprotein cover (2609). Theoretically, supplementation with N-acetyl glucosamine could remedy this deficiency and restore the glycoprotein cover (2609). However, no human studies to date have evaluated this claim. Similarly, no human studies have evaluated N-acetyl glucosamine for treating osteoarthritis. Preliminary evidence suggests glucosamine decreases glucose-induced insulin secretion by inhibiting pancreatic glucokinase in the beta cells of the islet of Langerhans (371,372,3406). Evidence also suggests glucosamine impairs insulin-mediated glucose uptake and metabolism in skeletal muscle. It is hypothesized that glucosamine desensitizes cell membranes to the effects of insulin (372,3406). Evidence suggests that type 2 diabetes and glucosamine induce insulin resistance by acting on a common pathway (3405) and glucosamine-induced insulin resistance might be dose-dependent (3406).

Adverse Reactions
Orally, there is concern that use of N-acetyl glucosamine products derived from marine exoskeletons might cause reactions in people allergic to shellfish, although no reactions have been reported. Until more is known, and because the source of N-acetyl glucosamine products is not listed on product labels, use N-acetyl glucosamine with caution in people with shellfish allergy.

Interactions with Herbs & Other Dietary Supplements
Insufficient reliable information available.

Interactions with Drugs
ANTIDIABETES DRUGS: Theoretically, N-acetyl glucosamine might decrease the hypoglycemic effects of insulin and oral antidiabetes agents by increasing insulin resistance and/or decreasing insulin production.

Interactions with Foods
No interactions are known to occur, and there is no known reason to expect a clinically significant interaction with N-acetyl glucosamine.

Interactions with Lab Tests
BLOOD GLUCOSE: Theoretically, N-acetyl glucosamine might increase blood glucose levels and test results, by increasing insulin resistance and/or decreasing insulin production. There are also anecdotal reports of poorer control in people with diabetes who take glucosamine (22,1203,1204,3405,3406).

Interactions with Diseases or Conditions
DIABETES: Theoretically, N-acetyl glucosamine might exacerbate diabetes by increasing insulin resistance and/or decreasing insulin production.
SHELLFISH ALLERGY: There is concern that N-acetyl glucosamine products derived from marine exoskeletons might cause reactions in people allergic to shellfish, although no reactions have been reported. Until more is known, and because the source of N-acetyl glucosamine products is not listed on product labels, use N-acetyl glucosamine with caution in people with shellfish allergy.

Dosage and Administration
ORAL: Most products recommend a daily dosage of 1500 mg, although the suggested dosage ranges from 500 mg to 3000 mg per day in divided doses (5261).

Comments
Avoid confusion with glucosamine sulfate and glucosamine hydrochloride. Read glucosamine product labels carefully for their content. Although glucosamine sulfate or glucosamine hydrochloride are marketed together in combination products with N-acetyl glucosamine, no human studies have evaluated these combinations for treating osteoarthritis. Only glucosamine sulfate has been studied in humans for osteoarthritis. Chitosan is the deacylated polymer of N-acetyl glucosamine (see separate listing for Chitosan).

NADH

Also Known As
B-DPNH, BNADH, Coenzyme 1, Enada, NAD, Reduced DPN, Reduced Nicotinamide Adenine Dinucleotide.

Scientific Names
NADH.

People Use This For
Orally, NADH is used for improving mental clarity, alertness and concentration; improving memory; cellular energy; for antioxidant effects; chronic fatigue syndrome; depression; jet lag; hypertension; Alzheimer's disease; Parkinson's disease; improving athletic endurance; enhancing energy; improving DNA repair; enhancing immune function; reducing aging; protecting the liver from alcohol damage; preventing alcohol-induced inhibition of testosterone; lowering cholesterol levels; and protecting against zidovudine (AZT) toxicity (3075,3076,3077).
Intravenously, NADH is used as an IM or IV injection for Parkinson's disease (3085,3086,3089,3090) and depression (3076).

Safety
There is insufficient reliable information available about the safety of NADH.
Pregnancy and Lactation: Insufficient reliable information available; avoid using.

Effectiveness
There is insufficient reliable information available about the effectiveness of NADH.

Mechanism of Action
NADH is the reduced form of NAD (nicotinamide adenine dinucleotide), a coenzyme necessary to dehydrogenate

primary and secondary alcohols (3082). In dehydrogenation, NAD acts as a hydrogen acceptor, forming NADH. NADH, in turn, serves as a hydrogen donor in the respiratory chain (3082). NADH is an essential intermediate in the cellular processes that generate energy from glucose in the form of ATP (3008). Some evidence suggests oral NADH reduces blood pressure, total cholesterol, and LDL (3083). Preliminary evidence suggests that NADH might help people with chronic fatigue syndrome by triggering energy production through ATP generation (229,3084). Other evidence suggests that NADH might benefit people with Alzheimer's disease (3087). NADH has been proposed as a therapeutic agent for people with Parkinson's disease because evidence suggests it might increase tyrosine hydroxylase activity and dopamine production (3085,3086,3088,3091). However, while two open trials found it was beneficial (3086,3089), one small double-blind study showed it was not (3090).

Adverse Reactions
None reported.

Interactions with Herbs & Other Dietary Supplements
Insufficient reliable information available.

Interactions with Drugs
No interactions are known to occur, and there is no known reason to expect a clinically significant interaction with NADH.

Interactions with Foods
No interactions are known to occur, and there is no known reason to expect a clinically significant interaction with NADH.

Interactions with Lab Tests
No interactions are known to occur, and there is no known reason to expect a clinically significant interaction with NADH.

Interactions with Diseases or Conditions
No interactions are known to occur, and there is no known reason to expect a clinically significant interaction with NADH.

Dosage and Administration
ORAL: For nutrition and energy enhancement, a typical dose is 2.5-5 mg daily or every other day (3462). For therapeutic support of Alzheimer's disease, Parkinson's disease and chronic fatigue syndrome, a typical dose is 10-15 mg daily or every other day (3462). Some people recommend the disodium salt form of NADH, taken with water either 30 minutes before or 2 hours after meals (3462).

Comments
None.

NASTURTIUM

Also Known As
Indian Cress.
CAUTION: See separate listing for Watercress.

Scientific Names
Tropaeolum majus.
Family: Tropaeolaceae.

People Use This For
Orally and in combination with other herbs, nasturtium is used for urinary tract infection, respiratory tract mucous membrane inflammation (2,18), and cough and bronchitis (18).
Topically, it is used in combination with other herbs for mild muscular pain (2).

Safety
POSSIBLY SAFE ...when used topically (2). ...when used orally in combination with other herbs (2).
There is insufficient reliable information available about the safety of nasturtium used orally as a single entity.
CHILDREN: LIKELY UNSAFE ...when used orally in combination with other herbs. Contraindicated (2,18).

There is insufficient reliable information about the safety of the topical use of nasturtium by children.
PREGNANCY AND LACTATION: Insufficient reliable information available; avoid using nasturtium by itself or in combination with other herbs.

Effectiveness

There is insufficient reliable information available about the effectiveness of nasturtium.

Mechanism of Action

The applicable parts of nasturtium are the above ground parts. Nasturtium contains 300 mg vitamin C per 100 grams of fresh plant (18). Benzyl mustard oil (benzyl isothiocyanate), the principal active constituent of nasturtium, may have bacteriostatic, virustatic, antimycotic (2,18), and antitumor (1537) activity. It is accumulated and excreted mainly in the respiratory and the urinary tracts (2,18). Applied topically, benzyl mustard oil has rubifacient activity (2,18).

Adverse Reactions

Orally, large amounts of nasturtium or benzyl mustard oil can cause GI tract irritation (2,18); one case of urticarial exanthema is reported (2). Large amounts of nasturtium can cause albuminuria due to glomerular and tubular damage (2).
Topically, long term intensive contact with the plant can cause skin irritation (18); benzyl mustard oil can cause skin and mucosal irritation (2). Benzyl mustard oil is a contact allergen if applied to the skin (2).

Interactions with Herbs & Other Dietary Supplements

Insufficient reliable information available.

Interactions with Drugs

No interactions are known to occur, and there is no known reason to expect a clinically significant interaction with nasturtium.

Interactions with Foods

No interactions are known to occur, and there is no known reason to expect a clinically significant interaction with nasturtium.

Interactions with Lab Tests

No interactions are known to occur, and there is no known reason to expect a clinically significant interaction with nasturtium.

Interactions with Diseases or Conditions

KIDNEY DISEASE: Contraindicated in individuals with kidney disease.
GI ULCERS: Contraindicated in individuals with gastric or intestinal ulcers (2,18).

Dosage and Administration

ORAL: No typical dosage.
TOPICAL: When used in combination with other herbs, the dose varies according to the combination (2).

Comments

None.

NEEM

Also Known As

Bead Tree, Holy Tree, Indian Lilac, Margosa, Nim, Nimba, Persian Lilac, Pride of China.

Scientific Names

Azadirachta indica.
Family: Meliaceae.

People Use This For

Orally, neem is used for fever, dyspepsia, respiratory conditions, and infectious diseases (6422). The bark is used for malaria and skin diseases. The leaves are used for worm infections, ulcers, cardiovascular disease, diabetes and gingivitis. The stem, root bark, and fruit are used as a tonic and astringent (6).
Topically, neem is used to treat head lice (6421), for skin diseases (6422), and as a mosquito repellent (1740).

Intravaginally, neem is used as a contraceptive (6).
Neem is also used as an insecticide (6).

Safety
POSSIBLY SAFE ...when the oil is used orally (6).
LIKELY UNSAFE ...when large amounts of seeds are used orally. It can cause poisoning (6).
There is insufficient reliable information available about the safety of the above ground parts of neem.
CHILDREN: LIKELY UNSAFE ...when the oil or seeds are taken orally. There are reports of infants who were
severely poisoned and died (3473,3474,3476).
PREGNANCY AND LACTATION: Insufficient reliable information available; avoid using.

Effectiveness
There is insufficient reliable information available about the effectiveness of neem.

Mechanism of Action
The applicable parts of neem are the above ground parts. Neem has varied constituents and pharmacological activity.
Neem bark and leaves contain tannin and oil (18). Neem seeds yield a fixed oil composed primarily of glycerides and
bitter compounds including nimbin, nimbinin and nimbidol (6). A small study in women demonstrated neem oil has
spermicidal and contraceptive properties when used intravaginally (6). In animals, oral administration of oil reduced
blood glucose levels by up to 48%, which lends some credence to the folk use for diabetes (6). In vitro studies
suggest neem oil possesses antibacterial activity against varied organisms (6). A toothpaste containing neem extract
exhibited antimicrobial activity and low levels of abrasiveness (6). Leaves of neem may be useful in preventing plaque
formation (3). Constituents gedunin and nimbolide show in vitro antimalarial activity (6). Though neem oil is toxic to
infants and children, the toxic constituent is unknown (3473,3475). Researchers speculate that a long-chain
monounsaturated free acid may be responsible (3475).

Adverse Reactions
Severe poisoning in infants and small children characterized by vomiting, loose stools, drowsiness, metabolic acidosis,
anemia, polymorphonuclear leukocytosis, seizure, loss of consciousness, coma, cerebral edema, Reye-like syndrome
symptoms and death have been reported to occur within hours after ingestion of neem oil (3473,3474,3476). Liver and renal
biopsy reports have revealed pathologic findings seen typically in Reye's syndrome (3473,3474,3475).

Interactions with Herbs & Other Dietary Supplements
Insufficient reliable information available.

Interactions with Drugs
No interactions are known to occur, and there is no known reason to expect a clinically significant interaction
with neem.

Interactions with Foods
No interactions are known to occur, and there is no known reason to expect a clinically significant interaction
with neem.

Interactions with Lab Tests
No interactions are known to occur, and there is no known reason to expect a clinically significant interaction
with neem.

Interactions with Diseases or Conditions
No interactions are known to occur, and there is no known reason to expect a clinically significant interaction
with neem.

Dosage and Administration
ORAL: Used as a tincture (18).

Comments
Azadirachtin, the insecticide constituent of seeds, is effective in concentrations as low as 0.1 ppm. It is biodegradable,
non-mutagenic and nontoxic to fish, birds and "warm-blooded animals" (6). The Environmental Protection Agency has
approved the use of a neem formulation (Margosan-O) as a pesticide for limited use on nonfood crops (6).

NERVE ROOT

Also Known As
American Valerian, Bleeding Heart, Cypripedium, Lady's Slipper, Moccasin Flower, Monkey Flower, Noah's Ark, Shoe, Slipper Root, Venus Shoe, Yellows.

Scientific Names
Cypripedium pubescens, synonym Cypripedium calceolus.
Family: Orchidaceae.

People Use This For
Orally, nerve root is used for menorrhagia and diarrhea (18).
Topically, it is used to treat pruritus vulvae (18).
In folk medicine, it is used for insomnia, emotional tension, hysteria, anxiety states (4), agitation, nervousness (18) and specifically anxiety states associated with insomnia.

Safety
POSSIBLY UNSAFE ...when the root or rhizome is used orally. Nerve root is reported to cause hallucinations (4).
PREGNANCY AND LACTATION: POSSIBLY UNSAFE ...when used orally; avoid using.

Effectiveness
There is insufficient reliable information available about the effectiveness of nerve root.

Mechanism of Action
The applicable parts of nerve root are the rhizome and root. Nerve root contains tannins, glycosides, resins, quinones and a volatile oil (4,18), and is said to have astringent and styptic properties (18). The quinone constituent of nerve root is thought to be responsible for its sensitizing properties (4).

Adverse Reactions
Orally, nerve root can cause hallucinations (4). Large doses are associated with giddiness, restlessness, headache, mental excitement and visual hallucinations (4).
Topically, it can cause contact dermatitis (4).

Interactions with Herbs & Other Dietary Supplements
Insufficient reliable information available.

Interactions with Drugs
No interactions are known to occur, and there is no known reason to expect a clinically significant interaction with nerve root.

Interactions with Foods
No interactions are known to occur, and there is no known reason to expect a clinically significant interaction with nerve root.

Interactions with Lab Tests
No interactions are known to occur, and there is no known reason to expect a clinically significant interaction with nerve root.

Interactions with Diseases or Conditions
No interactions are known to occur, and there is no known reason to expect a clinically significant interaction with nerve root.

Dosage and Administration
ORAL: 2-4 grams dried rhizome/root or as tea (steep 2-4 grams dried rhizome/root in 150 mL of boiling water for 5-10 minutes, strain), three times daily (4). Liquid extract (1:1 in 45% alcohol) 2-4 mL three times daily (4).

Comments
Avoid confusion with Calypso bulbosa (Cypripedium bulbosum) and Cypripedium parviflorum, related species also known as lady's slipper.

NEW JERSEY TEA

Also Known As
Jersey Tea, Mountain-Sweet, Redroot, Red Root, Walpole Tea, Wild Snowball.

Scientific Names
Ceanothus americanus.
Family: Rhamnaeceae.

People Use This For
Historically, New Jersey tea has been used as an expectorant, antispasmodic, clotting agent, and astringent and for gonorrhea, syphilis, colds, fever, and chills (18).

Safety
LIKELY SAFE ...when used orally (12,18).
PREGNANCY AND LACTATION: Insufficient reliable information available; avoid using.

Effectiveness
There is insufficient reliable information available about the effectiveness of New Jersey tea.

Mechanism of Action
The applicable parts of New Jersey tea are the root, root bark, and leaf. New Jersey tea contains cyclic peptide alkaloids and triterpenes (18). An aqueous-ethanol extract of New Jersey tea is said to reduce the blood-clotting time by 25% in blood taken from young rats (18).

Adverse Reactions
None reported.

Interactions with Herbs & Other Dietary Supplements
Insufficient reliable information available.

Interactions with Drugs
No interactions are known to occur, and there is no known reason to expect a clinically significant interaction with New Jersey tea.

Interactions with Foods
No interactions are known to occur, and there is no known reason to expect a clinically significant interaction with New Jersey tea.

Interactions with Lab Tests
No interactions are known to occur, and there is no known reason to expect a clinically significant interaction with New Jersey tea.

Interactions with Diseases or Conditions
No interactions are known to occur, and there is no known reason to expect a clinically significant interaction with New Jersey tea.

Dosage and Administration
ORAL: Used as an extract (18).

Comments
None.

NEW ZEALAND GREEN-LIPPED MUSSEL

Also Known As
New Zealand Green Lipped Mussel, NZGLM.

Scientific Names
Perna canaliculus.
Family: Mytilidae.

People Use This For
Orally, New Zealand green-lipped mussel is used for symptoms of rheumatoid arthritis and osteoarthritis (6).

Safety
POSSIBLY SAFE ...when used orally. There is only limited information available (6).
PREGNANCY: POSSIBLY UNSAFE ...when used orally; avoid using. May cause retarded fetal development and delay in parturition (936).
LACTATION: Insufficient reliable information available; avoid using.

Effectiveness
LIKELY INEFFECTIVE ...when taken orally for treating rheumatoid arthritis (6,935); an early report of effectiveness was not reproduced in subsequent studies (6,935).
There is insufficient reliable information available about the effectiveness of New Zealand green-lipped mussel for its other uses.

Mechanism of Action
The dried New Zealand green-lipped mussels may contain a prostaglandin inhibitor that exerts an anti-inflammatory effect (932,933). Researchers report that an extract of New Zealand green-lipped mussel reduced symptoms in dogs with advanced arthritis. The results of this unpublished study were presented at the Experimental Biology 2000 conference (5055).

Adverse Reactions
Orally, New Zealand green-lipped mussel can cause diarrhea, nausea, and flatulence (6). One case was reported of reversible, granulomatous hepatitis (6).

Interactions with Herbs & Other Dietary Supplements
Insufficient reliable information available.

Interactions with Drugs
No interactions are known to occur, and there is no known reason to expect a clinically significant interaction with New Zealand green-lipped mussel.

Interactions with Foods
No interactions are known to occur, and there is no known reason to expect a clinically significant interaction with New Zealand green-lipped mussel.

Interactions with Lab Tests
No interactions are known to occur, and there is no known reason to expect a clinically significant interaction with New Zealand green-lipped mussel.

Interactions with Diseases or Conditions
No interactions are known to occur, and there is no known reason to expect a clinically significant interaction with New Zealand green-lipped mussel.

Dosage and Administration
ORAL: New Zealand green-lipped mussel extract 300-350 mg three times per day was used in human studies for rheumatoid arthritis; except for one early trial, studies found New Zealand green-lipped mussels ineffective (6,935).

Comments
New Zealand green-lipped mussels are available commercially as a freeze dried, ground, and encapsulated product.

NIACIN AND NIACINAMIDE (VITAMIN B3)

Also Known As

3-Pyridine Carboxamide, Anti-Blacktongue Factor, Antipellagra Factor, B Complex Vitamin, Niacin, Niacin-Niacinamide, Niacin/Niacinamide, Niacinamide, Nicamid, Nicosedine, Nicotinamide, Nicotinic Acid, Nicotinic Acid Amide, Nicotylamidum, Pellagra Preventing Factor, Vitamin B-3, Vitamin PP.
CAUTION: See separate listings for Inositol Nicotinate (Inositol Hexaniacinate) and Tryptophan.

Scientific Names

Niacin; Niacinamide; Vitamin B3.

People Use This For

Orally, niacin is used with diet therapy for treating hyperlipoproteinemia. It is also used in conjunction with other therapies for peripheral vascular disease, vascular spasm, migraine headache, Meniere's syndrome, vertigo (15), and to reduce the diarrhea associated with cholera (14).
Orally, niacin or niacinamide is used for preventing vitamin B3 deficiency, treating pellagra, schizophrenia, drug-induced hallucinations, chronic brain syndrome, hyperkinesis, depression, motion sickness, alcohol dependence, vasculitis associated with skin lesions and edema, acne, leprosy (15), preventing premenstrual headache, improving digestion, for protection from toxins and pollutants, for reducing the effects of aging, memory loss, arthritis, lowering blood pressure, improving circulation, promoting relaxation, improving orgasm (3035,3036,3037), and preventing cataracts (6378).
Orally, niacinamide is used for treating diabetes, and the skin conditions bullous pemphigoid and granuloma annulare (14).
Topically, niacinamide is used for treating inflammatory acne vulgaris (5940).

Safety

LIKELY SAFE ...when used orally and appropriately (15). Niacin and niacinamide are FDA-approved products.
POSSIBLY SAFE ...when niacinamide is used topically and appropriately up to 12 weeks (5940).
PREGNANCY AND LACTATION: LIKELY SAFE ...when used orally in amounts that do not exceed the recommended dietary allowance (3094). There is insufficient reliable information available about the safety of larger oral amounts of niacin, niacinamide, or topical niacinamide used during pregnancy or lactation; avoid using.

Effectiveness

EFFECTIVE ...when niacin or niacinamide is used orally for preventing niacin deficiency and treating pellagra. Both niacin and niacinamide are FDA-approved for prevention and treatment of niacin deficiency and pellagra. Niacinamide is sometimes preferred for this indication because it lacks the vasodilating effects of niacin (see Adverse Reactions) (15). ...when niacin is used orally as an adjunct to diet therapy for hyperlipidemia. Niacin is FDA-approved for hyperlipidemia not responding to diet therapy alone. However, niacin is generally considered second-line therapy. It is also used in combination with other cholesterol-lowering drugs when diet and single-drug therapy are not adequately ineffective (1327,4867). Niacin reduces cholesterol at least as well as "statins" and bile acid sequestrants. Niacin is especially good for mixed hyperlipidemia. It is effective for reducing low-density lipoprotein (LDL) cholesterol, total cholesterol, triglycerides, and increasing high-density lipoprotein (HDL) cholesterol. Niacin also seems to be effective for isolated hypoalphalipoproteinemia (4817). However, niacin's use is limited due to a higher incidence of adverse effects and lower patient tolerance (4818,4867,4886,4887,4888,4889,4890).
POSSIBLY EFFECTIVE ...when niacin is used orally for secondary prevention of myocardial infarction. In a large scale, long-term study, high dose niacin significantly reduced the risk of a second heart attack in men; however, there was not a significant decrease in overall or cause-specific mortality (4847). ...when niacin is used orally in combination with a bile acid sequestrant for atherosclerosis in high-risk men with existing cardiovascular disease. In a large-scale trial, niacin plus colestipol significantly decreased coronary atherosclerosis progression; increased frequency of atherosclerosis regression; and decreased incidence of cardiovascular events; including death, myocardial infarction, and revascularization procedures (4848). ...when niacin is used to control fluid loss due to cholera (4868). In a randomized controlled study divided doses of 2 grams of nicotinic acid daily reduced diarrhea in adults with cholera (4868). Laboratory evidence supports the use of nicotinic acid, but not niacinamide, to reduce intestinal secretion induced by cholera toxin (4869). ...when niacinamide is used to prevent the development of diabetes in high-risk children (4874,4875). High-dose niacinamide was effective in preventing type 1 diabetes in a large trial of high-risk children (4874). Following the success of this trial, a very large, multinational, long-term study was begun to determine whether regular use of niacinamide can prevent diabetes (4876). Preliminary results released by a German group found no protective effect, but the authors cautioned that their findings did not exclude the possibility that niacinamide might be effective (4875). ...when niacinamide is used to preserve residual beta-cell function in newly diagnosed type 1 diabetes (4877,4878,4879,4880). Clinical trials, including one placebo-controlled trial and one vitamin E-comparison study showed niacinamide might prolong the "honeymoon period" in newly-diagnosed type 1 diabetes when the pancreas is

still capable of producing some insulin (4877,4878,4879,4800). The clinical studies to date have been performed by one group of Italian investigators. Concerns about potential concurrent induction of insulin resistance have been raised (4881). ...when niacinamide is used orally for protecting residual beta-cell function and improving glycemic control in adults with type 2 diabetes (4882). In a small, placebo-controlled, single-blind study, niacinamide increased C-peptide release and improved insulin secretion in lean diabetics who had failed sulfonylurea therapy (4882). ...when niacinamide is used orally for osteoarthritis (4883). Niacinamide 3 grams daily in divided doses improved joint flexibility and reduced inflammation better than placebo, and allowed for reduction in standard anti-inflammatory drug doses in a double-blind, 12-week study. Adverse effects were mild, but more frequent in the niacinamide group (4883). ...when used orally to reduce the occurrence of cataracts. A large-scale population-based study found high dietary intake of niacin is associated with a reduced risk of nuclear cataracts (6378).

LIKELY INEFFECTIVE ...when niacinamide is used orally for treating schizophrenia (14) and hyperlipidemia (15,4849).

There is insufficient reliable information available about the effectiveness of niacin and niacinamide for its other uses.

Mechanism of Action

Vitamin B3 includes niacin (nicotinic acid) and niacinamide (nicotinamide) (4849). The term niacin refers specifically to nicotinic acid, but is also used collectively to refer to both nicotinic acid and nicotinamide (niacinamide). Niacin is converted to niacinamide when ingested in amounts that do not exceed physiological requirements. The pharmacological effects of niacin and niacinamide are indistinguishable. Niacin is a water-soluble vitamin which is well absorbed when used orally (4849). Dietary sources include meats, beans, and various niacin-fortified foods. In addition, dietary tryptophan is biosynthetically converted to niacin (60 mg tryptophan equals 1 mg of niacin or one niacin equivalent) (4849). Niacinamide is required for lipid metabolism, tissue respiration, and glycogenolysis. Niacinamide is incorporated into the coenzymes, nicotinamide adenine dinucleotide (NAD) and nicotinamide adenine dinucleotide phosphate (NADP). These coenzymes act as hydrogen-carrier molecules. Niacin deficiency causes pellagra, a condition that affects the gastrointestinal tract, skin, and central nervous system (4849). Pellagra was common in the early twentieth century, but niacin-fortified foods have virtually eliminated this deficiency disease except in conditions such as chronic alcoholism (4850). Some researchers think that sleep deprivation-induced dermatitis might be caused by niacin depletion because of similarities between this condition and pellagra (1350). Causes of niacin deficiency include poor diet, isoniazid therapy, carcinoid tumors that decrease endogenous production, and Hartnup disease, an autosomal recessive disorder that interferes with tryptophan absorption (4849). Conditions that increase niacin requirements, such as hyperthyroidism, diabetes mellitus, liver cirrhosis, pregnancy, and lactation, rarely cause deficiency (4969). When doses of niacin or niacinamide greater than 300-800 mg daily are administered different pharmacological effects occur. Niacin 1000 mg or more per day decreases serum low-density lipoprotein (LDL) by 10 to 25%, increases serum high-density lipoprotein (HDL) concentrations by 15 to 35%, and decreases triglycerides by 20 to 50% (4867). The exact mechanism for the beneficial effects on serum lipids is unknown, but niacin inhibits free fatty acid release from adipose tissue; inhibits cyclic AMP accumulation which controls the activity of triglyceride lipase and hence lipolysis; decreases the rate of liver synthesis of LDL and VLDL; and, increases the rate of chylomicron triglyceride removal from plasma secondary to increased lipoprotein lipase activity (15,4849). Niacin also produces vasodilation of cutaneous blood vessels of the face, neck, and chest, probably mediated by prostaglandins, such as prostacyclin. In most individuals, tolerance to these effects occurs within two weeks (15). Preliminary clinical data suggest that some people with schizophrenia do not experience the characteristic vasodilatory response to niacin, suggesting an impaired response to phospholipid-dependent signaling (4870). Niacin also causes the release of histamine, which increases gastric motility and acid secretion (15). A review of cancer patients taking supplemental multivitamins suggests that niacin in combination with riboflavin might reduce the incidence of cataract development in older people (4885). Preliminary clinical research indicates that niacin reduces the fibrinogen concentration in plasma and stimulates fibrinolysis in hyperlipidemic men (4871). Large amounts of niacin can decrease uric acid excretion and impair glucose tolerance (15). Niacinamide has no beneficial effect on lipids and should not be used for treating hyperlipidemia (4849). Niacinamide does not cause the vasodilation associated with niacin (4849). High-dose niacinamide prevents or delays insulin deficiency in laboratory models of type 1 diabetes and protects islet cells from cytotoxic actions (4872,4873). Niacinamide is a free radical scavenger and might alter the auto-immune processes in type 1 diabetes that cause beta-cell destruction (4872,4873). Niacinamide is hypothesized to inhibit induction of nitric oxide synthase by interleukin 1 in chondrocytes, leading researchers to speculate about its potential use in destructive joint diseases (4884).

Adverse Reactions

Naturally occurring niacin in foods causes no known adverse effects (4849). Small amounts of niacin and niacinamide used for dietary supplementation can cause minor adverse reactions. Doses of niacin as low as 30 mg per day are associated with flushing, characterized by a burning, tingling, and itching sensation as well as erythema on the face, arms, and chest (4849). Flushing may be accompanied by itching, headache, increased intracranial blood flow, and occasionally, pain (4849). Onset is highly variable, from within 30 minutes to as long as 6 weeks after the initial dose (4849).

At higher doses, side effects distinguish niacin and niacinamide (4849). Niacinamide in large amounts is associated with headache, dizziness, nausea and vomiting, diarrhea, blurred vision, hepatotoxicity, hyperglycemia, abnormal prothrombin times, and hypoalbuminemia (14,15). Niacin in large amounts is associated with flushing, pruritus, burning sensations, stinging or tingling of the skin, nausea, bloating, flatulence, hunger pains, vomiting, heartburn, diarrhea, increased sebaceous gland activity, hypotension, dizziness, tachycardia, arrhythmias, syncope, vasovagal attacks, headache, and blurred vision (14,15). Dental and gingival pain have also been reported (4862). In most people taking niacin, flushing and other skin sensations, increased sebaceous gland activity, and increased gastrointestinal motility disappear within two weeks; however, adverse effects have been reported to appear up to 2 years after initiation of therapy (4851). Some evidence suggests that extended-release formulations may reduce the occurrence of these side effects (4857). Slow dose titration, pretreatment with 325 mg aspirin, and taking niacin with meals or the sustained release product at bedtime may reduce flushing (4852,4853,4854,4858). Flushing tends to decrease over time, despite dosage elevation (4864). Niacin, particularly at doses of 3 to 9 grams per day, might cause jaundice and elevated serum transaminases (4849). The drug should be discontinued if liver function tests rise to three times the upper limit of normal (4863). Severe hepatotoxicity with fulminant hepatitis and subsequent liver transplant has been reported (4849). Whether sustained release niacin is more hepatotoxic than immediate release formulations is controversial (4855,4856). High doses of niacin should not be used without medical supervision. Chronic use of large amounts of niacin have been associated with rash, hyperpigmentation resembling acanthosis nigricans, dry skin, xerostomia, hyperuricemia, gout, peptic ulcer, amblyopia, proptosis, loss of central vision secondary to an atypical form of cystoid macular edema, nervousness, panic, hyperglycemia, abnormal glucose tolerance and glycosuria, hepatotoxicity, abnormal prothrombin times and hypoalbuminemia (14,15). Niacin in higher doses can significantly raise homocysteine levels; 17% increase with 1000 mg niacin per day and 55% with 3000 mg per day (1733). Elevated homocysteine levels are an independent risk factor for arterial occlusive disease (490); however, the clinical significance of the effect of niacin on homocysteine is not yet known.

Interactions with Herbs & Other Dietary Supplements

BORAGE: Theoretically, concomitant use might have additive hepatotoxic effects; avoid concurrent use.
CHAPARRAL: Theoretically, concomitant use might have additive hepatotoxic effects; avoid concurrent use.
VALERIAN: Theoretically, concomitant use might have additive hepatotoxic effects; avoid concurrent use.
UVA URSI: Theoretically, concomitant use might have additive hepatotoxic effects; avoid concurrent use.

Interactions with Drugs

ANTIDIABETES DRUGS: Concomitant use with niacin or niacinamide can interfere with blood glucose control, requiring drug dosing adjustment (15). Monitor blood glucose levels carefully.
CARBAMAZEPINE (Tegretol): Concomitant use with niacinamide can decrease the clearance of carbamazepine and increase the risk of toxicity (14).
GANGLIONIC BLOCKING DRUGS: Concomitant use with niacin can potentiate the hypotensive effects of these drugs (15).
HMG-CoA REDUCTASE INHIBITORS: Concomitant use of niacin with HMG-CoA reductase inhibitors can increase the risk of myopathy. HMG-CoA reductase inhibitors include atorvastatin (Lipitor), cerivastatin (Baycol), fluvastatin (Lescol), lovastatin (Mevacor), pravastatin (Pravachol), and simvastatin (Zocor) (14,15). NCEP guidelines suggest combination therapy only when diet and single drug therapy is not sufficiently effective (4867).
BILE ACID SEQUESTRANTS: Concomitant use of cholestyramine (Questran) or colestipol (Colestid) reduces niacin absorption (14).
ISONIAZID (INH, Laniazid): Isoniazid inhibits the conversion of tryptophan to niacin and might induce pellagra, particularly in poorly nourished patients (4865,4866).
TRANSDERMAL NICOTINE (Nicoderm, Nicotrol): Concomitant use can increase the risk of flushing and dizziness with niacin (14).

Drug Influences on Nutrient Levels and Depletion

SOME DRUGS CAN AFFECT NIACIN AND NIACINAMIDE LEVELS:
ANTIBIOTICS: Destruction of normal gastrointestinal flora by antibiotics can cause decreased production of B vitamins. The clinical significance of this decreased production is not known. Consider supplementation only if clinical judgment warrants it (4434,4435,4436,4437,4438,4439,4440,4441,4442,4443).

Interactions with Foods

ETHANOL: Niacin should be used with caution in heavy alcohol drinkers. Both niacin and ethanol can increase the risk of hepatotoxicity. Niacin-induced flushing can be magnified by concomitant ingestion of ethanol (alcohol) (14,15,1289).
HOT DRINKS: Concomitant ingestion of niacin and hot drinks can magnify niacin-induced flushing (14,15,1289).

Interactions with Lab Tests

CATECHOLAMINES: Niacin can falsely increase some urinary catecholamine fluorometric assay results. Niacin produces fluorescent substances in the urine, which can falsely elevate test results (15).

GLUCOSE: Niacin can increase blood glucose levels and test results. Niacin can also cause false-positive reactions with urine glucose tests which rely on cupric sulfate solution (Benedict's reagent) (15).

CHOLESTEROL: Niacin reduces serum total cholesterol, LDL cholesterol, and VLDL cholesterol concentrations and test results. Niacin increases HDL cholesterol concentrations and test results (15).

HOMOCYSTEINE: At higher doses, niacin can increase homocysteine levels. Doses of 1000 mg and 3000 mg per day reportedly increase homocysteine levels by 17% and 55% respectively (1733).

LIVER FUNCTION TESTS: Both niacin and niacinamide can increase serum bilirubin, alanine aminotransferase (ALT), aspartate aminotransferase (AST), and lactate dehydrogenase (LDH) concentrations and test results. Liver function tests should be monitored regularly, particularly early in the course of therapy and in patients receiving long-term treatment with high doses of niacin or niacinamide (15). Niacin should be discontinued if liver function tests rise to three times the upper limit of normal (4863).

TRIGLYCERIDES: Niacin reduces serum triglyceride concentrations and test results (15).

Interactions with Diseases or Conditions

ALLERGIES: Niacin and niacinamide might exacerbate allergies by causing histamine release (14,15).

CROHN'S DISEASE: Nicotinic acid (niacin) serum levels decrease with increases in the Crohn's disease activity index in patients who do not receive nutritional treatments (6269).

CORONARY ARTERY DISEASE/UNSTABLE ANGINA: Large amounts of niacin can increase the risk of cardiac arrhythmias. One study showed an increased incidence of cardiac arrhythmias when niacin was used in patients with coronary artery disease (15); use with caution.

DIABETES: Niacin and niacinamide can interfere with blood glucose control requiring dosing adjustment of antidiabetic agents. Niacin and niacinamide can cause hyperglycemia, abnormal glucose tolerance, and glycosuria. Increased blood glucose monitoring may be necessary, particularly early in the course of treatment (15,4859,4860).

GALLBLADDER DISEASE: Niacin or niacinamide might exacerbate gallbladder disease (14,15); use with caution.

GOUT: Large amounts of niacin or niacinamide might precipitate gout. Niacin and niacinamide can cause hyperuricemia (14,15); use with caution.

ARTERIAL HEMORRHAGE: Contraindicated; niacin can cause hypotension, and might exacerbate hypotension associated with arterial hemorrhage (15).

SEVERE HYPOTENSION: Contraindicated; niacin can cause hypotension (15).

KIDNEY DISEASE: Niacin is excreted unchanged in the urine and might accumulate in patients with kidney disease (14,15); use with caution.

LIVER DISEASE: Contraindicated; niacin and niacinamide have been associated with liver damage. Avoid large amounts in patients with a history of liver disease (15).

PEPTIC ULCER DISEASE: Contraindicated in patients with active peptic ulcer disease. Large amounts of niacin or niacinamide might activate peptic ulcer disease (14,15); use with caution in patients with a history of peptic ulcer disease.

Dosage and Administration

ORAL: The typical dose of niacin as a dietary supplement is 10-20 mg daily (15). Higher doses may be required for liver cirrhosis, carcinoid syndrome, or prolonged isoniazid therapy (4849). Additionally, people with malabsorption syndrome, those undergoing hemodialysis or peritoneal dialysis, pregnant women with multiple fetuses, and women breast-feeding more than one infant may require more niacin (4849). For preventing and treating vitamin B3 deficiency, doses of nicotinic acid and niacinamide are considered equivalent (15). For mild vitamin B3 deficiency, niacin or niacinamide 50-100 mg per day is used (14). For pellagra in adults, niacin or niacinamide 300-500 mg daily is given in divided doses. For pellagra in children, niacin or niacinamide 100-300 mg daily is given in divided doses. For Hartnup disease, niacin or niacinamide 50-200 mg daily is used. For hyperlipoproteinemia niacin is begun at 125 mg twice daily and gradually titrated to 1.5 to 3 grams per day to minimize side effects (4867). Some people can require up to 9 grams of niacin daily for an adequate response (15). To prevent coronary events in people with hyperlipidemia, niacin 4 grams daily has been used (4848). For reducing fluid loss induced by cholera toxin, niacin 2 grams daily has been used (4868). To prevent type 1 diabetes in high-risk children, sustained-release niacinamide 1.2 grams/m2 (body surface area) per day has been used (4875). To slow disease progression of newly diagnosed type 1 diabetes, niacinamide 25 mg/kg daily has been used (4878). For treating osteoarthritis, niacinamide 3 grams per day in divided doses has been used (4883). A daily dietary intake of approximately 44 mg of niacin has been associated with reduced risk of nuclear cataracts (6378). The daily recommended dietary allowances (RDAs) of niacin are: Infants 0-6 months, 2 mg; Infants 7-12 months, 4 mg; Children 1-3 years, 6 mg; Children 4-8 years, 8 mg; Children 9-13 years, 12 mg; Men 14 years and older, 16 mg; Women 14 years and older, 14 mg; Pregnant women, 18 mg; and Lactating women, 17 mg (3094,4849). The maximum daily dose of niacin is: Children 1-3 years, 10 mg; Children 4-8 years, 15 mg; Children 9-13 years, 20 mg; Adults, including Pregnant and Lactating women, 14-18 years, 30 mg; and Adults, including pregnant and lactating women, older than 18 years, 35 mg (3094,4849).

Comments

Vitamin B3 is present in many foods including yeast, meat, fish, milk, eggs, green vegetables, and cereal grains (15). The term niacin is used to refer specifically to nicotinic acid, but is also used collectively to refer to both nicotinic acid and nicotinamide (niacinamide). Niacin and niacinamide are frequently used in combination with other B vitamins in vitamin B complex formulations. Vitamin B complex generally includes vitamin B1 (Thiamine), vitamin B2 (Riboflavin), vitamin B3 (Niacin/Niacinamide), vitamin B5 (pantothenic acid), vitamin B6 (pyridoxine), vitamin B12 (cyanocobalamin), and folic acid. However, some products do not contain all of these ingredients and some may include others, such as biotin, para-aminobenzoic acid (PABA), choline bitartrate, and inositol (3022,3060,3061).

NIAULI OIL

Also Known As

Caje Oil, Niauli Aetheroleum.
CAUTION: See separate listings for Tea Tree Oil and Cajeput Oil.

Scientific Names

Melaleuca viridiflora.
Family: Myrtaceae.

People Use This For

Orally and topically, niauli oil is used for upper respiratory tract mucous membrane inflammation (2,18), cough and bronchitis (18).

Safety

POSSIBLY SAFE ...when used orally and appropriately (2,18). ...when used topically and appropriately (12,18).
LIKELY UNSAFE ...when greater than 10 grams of oil is ingested orally. Can cause hypotension, circulatory disorders, and respiratory failure (18).
CHILDREN: LIKELY UNSAFE ...when used topically in the nasal and facial areas because it could cause bronchospasm, asthma-like symptoms and respiratory failure (2,18).
PREGNANCY AND LACTATION: Insufficient reliable information available; avoid using.

Effectiveness

POSSIBLY EFFECTIVE ...when used orally or topically for upper respiratory tract mucous membrane inflammation (2).
There is insufficient reliable information available about the effectiveness of niauli oil for its other uses.

Mechanism of Action

It contains cineole (7,9), which has in vitro antibacterial activity and stimulates circulation (2,18). Cineole has actions similar to that of eucalyptus oil (9). Cineole induces liver enzymes involved with drug metabolism (18).

Adverse Reactions

Orally, niauli oil can cause nausea, vomiting, and diarrhea (2). The consumption of amounts greater than 10 grams can cause hypotension, circulatory disorders, collapse, and respiratory failure (18). It can cause glottal spasm, bronchospasm, and respiratory failure when applied to facial and nasal areas of infants and small children (2,18).

Interactions with Herbs & Other Dietary Supplements

Insufficient reliable information available.

Interactions with Drugs

LIVER- METABOLIZED DRUGS: Theoretically, concomitant use of niauli oil can reduce or shorten the effect of some drugs due to induction of hepatic enzymes (2).

Interactions with Foods

No interactions are known to occur, and there is no known reason to expect a clinically significant interaction with niauli oil.

Interactions with Lab Tests

No interactions are known to occur, and there is no known reason to expect a clinically significant interaction with niauli oil.

Interactions with Diseases or Conditions
GI TRACT DISEASE: Niauli oil is contraindicated in individuals with inflammatory diseases of the GI tract.
LIVER DISEASE: Contraindicated in individuals with severe liver disease or bile duct inflammation (2,18).

Dosage and Administration
ORAL: The typical dose of niauli oil is 200 mg per administration, up to 2 grams per day (2,18).
TOPICAL: Niauli oil is commonly used as oily nose drops, consisting of 2-5% niauli oil in vegetable oil (2,18). Other topical preparations contain 10-30% niauli oil in an oil base (2,18).

Comments
Niauli oil consists of the essential oil distilled from leaves of Melaleuca viridiflora. Avoid confusion with tea tree oil (Maleleuca alternifolia) and cajeput oil (Melaleuca leucodendra and Melaleuca quinquenervia).

NORTHERN PRICKLY ASH

Also Known As
Angelica Tree, Pepper Wood, Prickly Ash, Toothache Bark, Xanthoxylum, Yellow Wood, Zanthoxylum.
CAUTION: See separate listings for Ash and Southern Prickly Ash.

Scientific Names
Zanthoxylum americanum.
Family: Rutaceae.

People Use This For
Orally, northern prickly ash is used for cramps, intermittent claudication, Raynaud's syndrome, chronic rheumatic conditions, peripheral circulatory insufficiency associated with rheumatic symptoms (4), for low blood pressure, fever, and inflammation (18).
Traditionally, it has been used as a tonic, stimulant, for toothache, sores, ulcers, as a diaphoretic in fever, and cancer (as an ingredient in Hoxsey cure) (11).
In manufacturing, northern prickly ash is used as a flavoring agent in foods and beverages (11).

Safety
POSSIBLY SAFE …when used orally in food flavoring (4). Northern prickly ash is listed by the Council of Europe as a natural source of food flavoring without toxicity assessment. …when the bark is used orally and appropriately in medicinal amounts (12).
There is insufficient reliable information available about the safety of the oral use of northern prickly ash berry.
PREGNANCY: POSSIBLY UNSAFE …when the bark is used orally (12); avoid using. There is insufficient reliable information available about the safety of the berry during pregnancy; avoid using.
LACTATION: Insufficient reliable information available; avoid using.

Effectiveness
There is insufficient reliable information available about the effectiveness of northern prickly ash (4).

Mechanism of Action
The applicable parts of northern prickly ash are the bark and berry. There is insufficient reliable information available about the possible mechanism of action and active ingredients. Contains coumarins and alkaloids which may be pharmacologically active (4).

Adverse Reactions
None reported.

Interactions with Herbs & Other Dietary Supplements
HERBS WITH ANTICOAGULANT/ANTIPLATELET POTENTIAL: Concomitant use of herbs that have coumarin constituents or affect platelet aggregation could theoretically increase the risk of bleeding in some people. These herbs include: angelica, anise, arnica, asafoetida, bogbean, boldo, capsicum, celery, chamomile, clove, danshen, fenugreek, feverfew, garlic, ginger, ginkgo, ginseng Panax, horse chestnut, horseradish, licorice, meadowsweet, onion, papain, passionflower, poplar, quassia, red clover, turmeric, wild carrot, wild lettuce, willow, and others (4,19).

Interactions with Drugs
ACID-INHIBITING DRUGS: Theoretically, due to claims that northern prickly ash increases stomach acid, it might interfere with antacids, sucralfate (Carafate), H-2 antagonists, and proton pump inhibitors (19).
ANTICOAGULANTS: Theoretically, excessive ingestion might interfere with anticoagulant therapy (4).

Interactions with Foods
No interactions are known to occur, and there is no known reason to expect a clinically significant interaction with northern prickly ash.

Interactions with Lab Tests
No interactions are known to occur, and there is no known reason to expect a clinically significant interaction with northern prickly ash.

Interactions with Diseases or Conditions
GASTROINTESTINAL ULCERS: Contraindicated. Northern prickly ash can stimulate gastrointestinal secretions (19).
GI CONDITIONS: Northern prickly ash can irritate the gastrointestinal tract. It is contraindicated in individuals with infectious or inflammatory gastrointestinal conditions (19).

Dosage and Administration
ORAL, Bark: 1-3 grams dried bark, or drink as decoction (boil 1-3 grams dry bark 10-15 minutes, strain), three times daily; liquid bark extract (1:1 in 45% alcohol) 1-3 mL three times daily; bark tincture (1:5 in 45% alcohol) 2-5 mL three times daily (4).
ORAL, Berry: Liquid berry extract (1:1 in 45% alcohol) 0.5-1.5 mL (4).

Comments
None.

NUTMEG AND MACE

Also Known As
Mace, Macis, Muscadier, Muskatbuam, Muskatnuss, Myristica, Myristicae Aril, Myristicae Semen, Noix Muscade, Nuez Moscada, Nutmeg, Nux Moschata.

Scientific Names
Myristica fragrans, synonym Myristica officinalis.
Family: Myristicaceae.

People Use This For
Orally, nutmeg and mace are used for diarrhea, nausea, gastric spasms, flatulence, and gastric mucosal inflammation. They are also used for cancer, kidney disease, insomnia, increasing menstrual flow, inducing abortion, as a hallucinogen, and a general tonic.
Topically, nutmeg and mace are used as an analgesic, especially for rheumatism, mouth sores, and toothache.
In foods, nutmeg and mace are used as culinary spices. In foods and beverages, nutmeg, nutmeg oil, mace, and mace oil are used as flavor components.
In manufacturing, nutmeg oil is used as a fragrance component in soaps and cosmetics.

Safety
LIKELY SAFE ...when used orally in amounts found in foods. The maximum use level is 0.3% (11). Nutmeg, mace, nutmeg oil and mace oil have Generally Recognized as Safe (GRAS) status in the US (11).
LIKELY UNSAFE ...when used orally for self-medication in amounts larger than found in foods (12).
There is insufficient reliable information available about the safety of the topical use of nutmeg and mace.
PREGNANCY: LIKELY SAFE ...when used orally in amounts found in foods. Larger amounts might have abortifacient activity (2) and safrole content might be mutagenic (2,12).
LACTATION: LIKELY SAFE ...when used orally in amounts found in foods. There is insufficient reliable information available for larger amounts; avoid using.

Effectiveness
There is insufficient reliable information available for the effectiveness of nutmeg and mace.

Mechanism of Action

Both nutmeg and mace contain volatile oils with constituents that include myristicin, elemicin, eugenol, isoeugenol, gerinol, pinese, cineole, borneol, and safrole (2563). Volatile oil constituents of nutmeg and mace have a variety of individual pharmacological effects, some of which oppose others. For example, the volatile oil borneol is thought to be responsible for CNS stimulant effects, whereas several others such as methyleugenol, isoeugenol, safrole, myristicin, 1,8-cineole, geranyl acetate, and 1,8-p-methadiene seem to have sedative effects (2563). Alpha- and beta-pinene, and 1,8-cineole seem to have convulsant activity, whereas safrole, eugenol, and methyleugenol have anticonvulsant activity (2563). Nutmeg also has psychoactive effects and can cause hallucinations, feelings of unreality, euphoria, and delusions (2563). The constituents myristicin and elemicin are thought to be metabolized to amphetamine-related compounds (6), but this has not yet been verified (2563). Myristicin and elemicin might also have effects on serotonergic systems and possibly have an antidepressant effect (2563). Some constituents have anesthetic activity such as myristicin, methyleugenol, methylisoeugenol, safrole, and 1,8-cineole (2563). Antihistaminic effects have been found with elemicin and methylisoeugenol (2563). High doses of nutmeg can cause anticholinergic side effects (14), but the constituents 1,8-cineole and alpha-terpinene are reported to have anticholinesterase activity (2563). Nutmeg and mace and their oils have a variety of other effects including antispasmodic (2,6), antioxidant (11), hypotensive (2563), emetic (6), antibacterial, antifungal (6) and larvicidal effects (11). Calcium antagonist activity has been reported with myristicin, eugenol, and safrole (2563). Myristicin, eugenol, and isoeugenol inhibit prostaglandin activity (6), might have anti-inflammatory properties, and possibly inhibit platelet aggregation (14). Safrole found in nutmeg oil promotes liver carcinomas in mice (6). Animal studies suggest myristicin acts as an inducer of cytochrome P-450 enzyme systems (3492,3493) and may inhibit tumor formation (3492).

Adverse Reactions

Orally, nutmeg and mace can cause significant side effects when used in amounts greater than those found in foods. Atropine-like (anticholinergic) effects can occur with doses of nine teaspoons of nutmeg powder such as flushing, tachycardia, and dry mouth (14). Higher doses can cause more significant side effects. For example, ingestion of 5 grams or more of powdered nutmeg or mace can cause thirst, dry mouth, nausea and vomiting, burning epigastric pain, urgency, weak pulse, tachycardia, hypotension, flushing, feeling of pressure in the chest or lower abdomen, hot and cold sensations, sweating, hypothermia, dizziness, blurred vision, double and triple vision, miosis, nystagmus, headache, numbness, weakness, unsteady gait, drowsiness, stupor, disorientation, euphoria, anxiety, panic, mild to intense visual hallucinations, often with sensation of limb loss and fear of impending death, auditory hallucinations, agitation, hyperactivity, aimless wandering, incoherent and irrelevant speech, combativeness (12,2563,3492,3494), seizures (9), shock, coma (2492), and occasionally death (12). Many of these symptoms are attributed to excessive anticholinergic activity (14). Symptoms generally occur 2-6 hours after ingestion and recovery usually occurs within 24 hours, but can take several days, depending on the dose used (14,3492). In pregnant women, large amounts can also cause abortion (2).

Topically, nutmeg can cause allergic dermatitis (6,18).

Interactions with Herbs & Other Dietary Supplements

SAFROLE-CONTAINING HERBS: Avoid concomitant use with other safrole-containing herbs due to potential for additive toxicity (12). Other herbs that contain safrole include basil, camphor, and cinnamon (12).

Interactions with Drugs

MAOIs: Theoretically, concomitant use might potentiate monoamine oxidase inhibitor activity (12,19).
PHENOBARBITAL: Theoretically, concomitant use may decrease the therapeutic effects of phenobarbital (3492). Studies suggest myristicin acts as an inducer of cytochrome P-450 enzyme systems (3492,3493).
OTHER DRUGS: Theoretically, concomitant use may affect drugs metabolized by cytochrome P450 enzyme systems (3493). Use caution when considering concomitant use of nutmeg or mace with other drugs affected by cytochrome P450 enzyme systems.

Interactions with Foods

No interactions are known to occur, and there is no known reason to expect a clinically significant interaction with nutmeg and mace.

Interactions with Lab Tests

No interactions are known to occur, and there is no known reason to expect a clinically significant interaction with nutmeg and mace.

Interactions with Diseases or Conditions

No interactions are known to occur, and there is no known reason to expect a clinically significant interaction with nutmeg and mace.

Dosage and Administration

ORAL: Typical dose for antiflatulent effect is 0.03 mL nutmeg oil (17). For nausea, gastric upset, or chronic diarrhea, the common dose is 3-5 drops of the essential oil on a sugar lump or in honey (6002). For diarrhea, 4-6 tablespoons of the powder has been used daily (14,6002) (Note: this may be in the range associated with toxicity - see adverse effects section).

TOPICAL: For toothache, 1 to 2 drops of essential oil are applied to the surrounding gum (6002).

Comments

Nutmeg is the shelled, dried seed of Myristica fragrans (11). Nutmeg oil is distilled from worm-eaten nutmeg seeds; the worms remove much of the starch and fat leaving portions of the seed rich in volatile oil (11). Mace is the dried aril (netlike covering) surrounding the shell of the seed of Myristica fragrans (11). Ingestion of 5-20 grams of nutmeg powder (1-3 whole seeds) might cause psychoactive effects (6). Because nutmeg and mace are so similar, high doses of mace might also have psychoactive effects but as yet this has not been proven (6).

NUX VOMICA

Also Known As

Brechnusssamen, Poison Nut, Quaker Buttons, Strychni Semen, Strychnos Seed.

Scientific Names

Strychnos nux-vomica.
Family: Loganiaceae.

People Use This For

Nux vomica is used for impotence and for glycine encephalopathy (14). It is also used in combination for diseases of the gastrointestinal tract, organic and functional disorders of the heart and circulatory system, diseases of the eye, nervous conditions, depression, migraine, climacteric complaints, facial neuralgias (Sympatalgien), and Raynaud's disease (2). Historically, it has been thought of as an oral tonic, and used as an appetite-stimulant. It has also been used for diseases of the respiratory tract, anemia, and geriatric complaints (18). Nux vomica contains strychnine and brucine (13) and has, therefore, been used in manufacturing. It is used as a rodenticide (505).

Safety

UNSAFE ...when used orally (2,13,14,18,505). Nux vomica in doses of 30-50 mg contains approximately 5 mg of strychnine, and can cause severe adverse effects. 1-2 grams of nux vomica contains 60-90 mg of strychnine, and can be fatal (13,18). Chronic ingestion of lesser amounts can cause death after a period of weeks (18).

PREGNANCY AND LACTATION: UNSAFE ...when used orally; avoid using (2,13,14,18,505).

Effectiveness

LIKELY INEFFECTIVE ...when used orally for any therapeutic effect (14).

Mechanism of Action

The applicable part of nux vomica is the seed. Nux vomica contains strychnine and brucine (13). These are centrally-acting neurotoxins. Strychnine competitively antagonizes post-synaptic binding of the inhibitory transmitter glycine, which leads to heightened reflex excitability of muscles. External irritations or centrally-acting stimulants can trigger convulsions (2,14,505). Nux vomica can selectively inhibit the spinal cord in subconvulsive amounts (2). However, strychnine accumulates with extended administration, particularly in individuals with liver damage (2). Chronic use of subconvulsive amounts can cause death after a period of weeks (18). Strychnine causes convulsions by leading to a full contraction of all voluntary muscles. Death is secondary to impaired respiration or exhaustion (13,14,18,505).

Adverse Reactions

When taken orally 30-50 mg nux vomica (5 mg strychnine) can cause restlessness, feelings of anxiety, heightening of sense perception, enhanced reflexes, equilibrium disorders, painful neck and back stiffness, followed later by twitching, tonic spasms of jaw and neck muscles, painful convulsions of the entire body triggered by visual or tactile stimulation with possible opisthotonos, muscle hypertonicity and agitation. Dyspnea may follow spasm of the respiratory muscles (14,18). Seizures occur within 15 minutes of ingestion (or 5 minutes of inhalation) and may result in hyperthermia, metabolic and respiratory acidosis, rhabdomyolysis, and myoglobinuric renal failure (14,17). 1-2 grams of nux vomica (60-90 mg strychnine) can be fatal (13,505); most deaths occur 3-6 hours post-ingestion from respiratory and subsequent cardiac arrest, anoxic brain damage, or multiple organ failure secondary to hyperthermia (14,18,505). Strychnine accumulates with extended administration, particularly in individuals with liver damage (2). Chronic use of subconvulsive amounts can cause death after a period of weeks (18).

Interactions with Herbs & Other Dietary Supplements

Insufficient reliable information available.

Interactions with Drugs

ANALEPTICS, PHENOTHIAZINES: Contraindicated in individuals with symptoms of poisoning (18).

Interactions with Foods

No interactions are known to occur, and there is no known reason to expect a clinically significant interaction with nux vomica.

Interactions with Lab Tests

No interactions are known to occur, and there is no known reason to expect a clinically significant interaction with nux vomica.

Interactions with Diseases or Conditions

LIVER DISEASE: Contraindicated. Strychnine accumulates in individuals with liver damage (2). Also, strychnine accumulation can cause liver damage (18).

Dosage and Administration

Toxic, avoid using.

Comments

Strychnine may be detected by thin-layer chromatography (qualitative analysis) and high performance liquid chromatography (quantitative analysis). Urine and gastric aspirate are most useful in confirming poisoning (17). Nux vomica powder may be confused with the powder of date nuts, olive stones, and by-products of stone-nut processing (18).

OAK bark

Also Known As

Common Oak, Durmast Oak, Eichenrinde, English Oak, Pedunculate Oak, Quercus cortex, Sessile Oak, Stave Oak, Stone Oak, Tanner's Bark, Tanner's Oak.

Scientific Names

Quercus robur; Quercus petraea; Quercus alba.
Family: Fagaceae.

People Use This For

Orally, oak bark is used for diarrhea (2), colds, fever, cough and bronchitis, and for stimulating appetite and improving digestion (18).
Topically, oak bark is used for inflammatory skin conditions; mild inflammation of the mouth, throat, genital, and anal region (2,7); and for chilblains (8).

Safety

POSSIBLY SAFE ...when used orally (2,12) for up to 3-4 days for treating diarrhea (7). ...when used topically up to 2-3 weeks on intact skin (2).
LIKELY UNSAFE ...when used topically on extensive areas of damaged skin or for longer than 2-3 weeks (2).
PREGNANCY AND LACTATION: Insufficient reliable information available; avoid using.

Effectiveness

POSSIBLY EFFECTIVE ...when used orally for nonspecific acute diarrhea (2). ...when used topically for inflammatory skin diseases, mild inflammation of the mouth, throat, genital and anal region (2,7).
There is insufficient reliable information available about the effectiveness of oak bark for its other uses.

Mechanism of Action

Oak bark contains 8-20% tannins, including gallotannins (7,8). Gallotannins are extensively hydrolyzed in the upper small intestine and are unlikely to produce astringent activity in the colon (7,3901). Some studies suggest tannins might have antiviral and antimicrobial effects, and CNS depressant and cariostatic effects (11). Other studies suggest they can depress growth. Tannins exert an astringent effect on mucosal tissue. This effect dehydrates the tissue, internally reducing secretions, and externally forming a protective layer of harder, constricted cells (12). Plants with at least 10% tannins can cause gastrointestinal disturbances, kidney damage, and necrotic conditions of the liver (12). Some evidence suggests that tannins might cause cancer. Others information suggests they might prevent it (12). Regular consumption of herbs with high tannin concentrations correlates to an increased incidence of esophageal or nasal cancer (12).

Adverse Reactions
Oak bark can cause gastrointestinal disturbances, kidney damage, and necrotic conditions of the liver (12).

Interactions with Herbs & Other Dietary Supplements
ALKALINE CONSTITUENTS: Theoretically, herbs that contain high percentages of tannins such as oak bark may precipitate alkaloids and alkaline constituents of herbs (19).
IRON: Theoretically, concomitant administration might precipitate iron salts due to tannin content (19).

Interactions with Drugs
ALKALOID DRUGS: Theoretically, avoid concomitant administration due to potential of oak bark's tannin content to precipitate alkaloids and other alkaline drugs (19). Separate administration of oral drugs and tannin-containing herbs by the longest period of time practical (19).
IRON: Theoretically, concomitant administration may precipitate iron salts due to tannin content (19).

Interactions with Foods
No interactions are known to occur, and there is no known reason to expect a clinically significant interaction with oak bark.

Interactions with Lab Tests
No interactions are known to occur, and there is no known reason to expect a clinically significant interaction with oak bark.

Interactions with Diseases or Conditions
KIDNEY DYSFUNCTION: Theoretically, oral use of oak bark might worsen kidney dysfunction (12).
LIVER DYSFUNCTION: Theoretically, oral use of oak bark might worsen liver dysfunction (12).
ECZEMA: Oak bark baths are contraindicated in individuals with weeping eczema or large areas of skin damage (2).
INFECTION: Oak bark baths are contraindicated in individuals with febrile or infectious diseases (2).
CARDIAC CONDITIONS: Oak bark baths are contraindicated in individuals with cardiac insufficiency (2).
HYPERTONIA: Oak bark baths are contraindicated in individuals with hypertonia (2).

Dosage and Administration
ORAL: A typical dose of oak bark for diarrhea is one cup tea up to three times a day for up to 3-4 days. To make tea, add 1 gram coarsely powdered bark to 150 mL cold water, boil for a short period of time, strain (8).
TOPICAL: For rinses, compresses, poultices, and gargles, prepare with 20 grams bark in 1 L of water (18). For baths, prepare with 5 grams of bark in 1 L of water, added to bath water (18). Oak bark should not be used topically longer than 2-3 weeks (2).

Comments
None.

OAK MOSS

Also Known As
Lichen Oak Moss, Tree Moss.
CAUTION: See separate listing for Usnea.

Scientific Names
Evernia prunastri.
Family: Usneaceae.

People Use This For
In folk medicine, oak moss is used as an intestinal tonic.
In manufacturing, it is used as a fragrance component in perfumes (4023).

Safety

POSSIBLY SAFE ...when used orally in prepared teas or aqueous forms for short periods of time (12). Although water extracts of oak moss contain the constituent thujone that is known to cause adverse effects, the amount of thujone is low (2).

LIKELY UNSAFE ...when used orally long-term, in large amounts of tea, or as a hot alcoholic extract (12) because enough thujone might be consumed to cause renal damage (4,12).

There is insufficient reliable information available about the safety of oak moss for its other uses.

PREGNANCY AND LACTATION: POSSIBLY UNSAFE ...when used orally. The constituent thujone shows evidence of uterine stimulant activity (19).

Effectiveness

There is insufficient reliable information available about the effectiveness of oak moss.

Mechanism of Action

Oak moss contains thujone, a ketone that shows evidence of neurotoxicity. Thujone intoxication causes psychoactivity resembling that of cannabinoid intoxication (12). Some data suggest thujone-containing volatile oils have uterine stimulant effects (19). Other information suggests thujone might exacerbate liver conditions, e.g., porphyria (12).

Adverse Reactions

Orally, large amounts or long-term use of thujone-containing products can cause restlessness, vomiting, vertigo, tremors, renal damage, and convulsions (12).

Topically, use can cause contact sensitivity (4034,4039) and allergic reaction in people with lichen and moss allergy (4023,4033).

Interactions with Herbs & Other Dietary Supplements

THUJONE CONTAINING HERBS: Avoid; concomitant use may increase the risk of thujone toxicity. Thujone-containing herbs include: oriental arborvitae (12), sage (2,4,12), tansy (2,4,12), thuja (cedar) (11,12), tree moss (12), and wormwood (2,12).

Interactions with Drugs

No interactions are known to occur, and there is no known reason to expect a clinically significant interaction with oak moss.

Interactions with Foods

No interactions are known to occur, and there is no known reason to expect a clinically significant interaction with oak moss.

Interactions with Lab Tests

No interactions are known to occur, and there is no known reason to expect a clinically significant interaction with oak moss.

Interactions with Diseases or Conditions

PORPHYRIA: Can exacerbate porphyria in patients with underlying defects in hepatic heme synthesis (12).
RENAL DYSFUNCTION: Can exacerbate this condition (12).
CROSS-ALLERGENICITY: Can cause reaction in people allergic to lichens and mosses (4023,4033).

Dosage and Administration

No typical dosage.

Comments

Avoid confusing oak moss (Evernia prunastri) with other usnea species. Many, including oak moss, are referred to as tree moss.

OAT above ground parts

Also Known As
Avenae herba, Oat Herb, Wild Oat Herb.
CAUTION: See separate listings for Oat Bran, Oat Straw, and Oats.

Scientific Names
Avena sativa.
Family: Gramineae or Poaceae.

People Use This For
Orally, the above ground parts of oats are used for acute or chronic anxiety, excitation and stress, neurasthenia and pseudoneurasthenia syndromes, weak bladder, connective tissue disorders (2), for gout, kidney ailments, old age syndromes, opium and nicotine withdrawal, rheumatism, skin diseases (18), and as a tonic (2).
In combination with other herbs, oat above ground parts are used orally for cardiovascular, respiratory, and metabolic diseases, diseases and discomforts of old age, anemia, hypothyroidism, neuralgias and neuritis, hematoma, pulled muscles, sexual disorders, tobacco abuse, spasms, increasing milk production, and for increasing performance capacity (2).

Safety
POSSIBLY SAFE ...when the spikelet, the top of the herb, is used orally or topically (12).
PREGNANCY AND LACTATION: Insufficient reliable information available; avoid using.

Effectiveness
There is insufficient reliable information available about effectiveness of oat above ground parts.

Mechanism of Action
The above ground parts of oat contain soluble oligosaccharides and polysaccharides including saccharose, kestose, neokestose, beta-glucans, galactoarabinoxylans, silicic acid, steroid saponins, avenic acid A and B and flavonoids (18).

Adverse Reactions
None reported.

Interactions with Herbs & Other Dietary Supplements
Insufficient reliable information available.

Interactions with Drugs
MORPHINE: Theoretically, concomitant use might antagonize morphine (19).
NICOTINE: Theoretically, concomitant use might reduce the hypertensive response from nicotine (19).

Interactions with Foods
No interactions are known to occur, and there is no known reason to expect a clinically significant interaction with oat above ground parts.

Interactions with Lab Tests
No interactions are known to occur, and there is no known reason to expect a clinically significant interaction with oat above ground parts.

Interactions with Diseases or Conditions
No interactions are known to occur, and there is no known reason to expect a clinically significant interaction with oat above ground parts.

Dosage and Administration
ORAL: A typical oral dose is 1 cup tea used repeatedly throughout the day and shortly before bedtime. To make tea, boil 3 grams above ground parts in 250 mL water, and strain (18).

Comments
None.

OAT BRAN

Also Known As
Dietary Fiber.
CAUTION: See separate listings for Oat above ground parts, Oat Straw, Oats, and Wheat Bran.

Scientific Names
Avena sativa.
Family: Poaceae.

People Use This For
Orally, oat bran is used for reducing the risk of heart disease, as part of a diet low in saturated fat and cholesterol(4960,4962,4963,4964,4965,4966,4967,4968), lowering blood cholesterol (4960,4961,4963,4965,4971,4972,4973,4975,4976,4977,4978), reducing postprandial blood glucose in people with diabetes (4961,4980,4981,4982,4983), blocking fat absorption (4970), preventing gallstones (4984), reducing risk of colon cancer, treating irritable bowel syndrome (IBS), diverticulosis, and inflammatory bowel disease (5103,5105,5106).

Safety
LIKELY SAFE ...when used orally and appropriately (4960,4969). Oat bran has Generally Recognized as Safe (GRAS) status in the US (4912).
PREGNANCY AND LACTATION: Insufficient reliable information available; avoid using in amounts greater than those found in foods.

Effectiveness
EFFECTIVE ...when used orally as part of a diet low in saturated fat and cholesterol for reducingthe risk of heart disease and lowering total and LDL blood cholesterol (4960,4961,4962,4963,4964,4965,4966,4967,4968,4971,4972) (4973,4974,4975,4976,4977,4978,6188). Oat bran products (oat bran muffins, oat bran flakes, oat bran Os, etc.) may vary in their ability to lower cholesterol, depending on the total soluble fiber content and other dietary variables (6188).
POSSIBLY EFFECTIVE ...when used orally for reducing postprandial blood glucose in people with diabetes (4960,4980,4982,6266). In a randomized crossover study of 13 people with type 2 diabetes, a high fiber diet that included oat bran was more effective in lowering preprandial blood glucose and the area under the curve for 24-hour plasma glucose and glucose (measured every 2 hours), and improving cholesterol and triglyceride levels than the standard ADA diet (6266). ...when used orally as part of a high fiber diet for reducing risk factors associated with cardiovascular disease. In a large-scale epidemiological study, consumption of large amounts of dietary fiber was associated with reduction of cardiovascular disease risk factors including reduction in body weight, fasting and postprandial insulin secretion, blood pressure, and improved lipid profile (2737).
LIKELY INEFFECTIVE ...when used orally for reducing risk of colon cancer (5104,6267). A large well-designed study showed that fiber, including oat-bran fiber, does not prevent the recurrence of colorectal adenomas.
There is insufficient reliable information available about the effectiveness of oat bran for its other uses.

Mechanism of Action
Oat bran decreases serum cholesterol and dependent cardiovascular risk by decreasing absorption of cholesterol or fatty acids and decreasing absorption of biliary cholesterol or bile acids (4974,4960,4963). Dietary fiber, including oat bran, is also thought to decrease the risk of cardiovascular disease by decreasing fasting insulin levels, resulting in decreased obesity, hypertension, and improved lipid profile (2737). Beta-glucan (oat gum), a constituent of oat bran, increases the viscosity of food in the small intestine and delays absorption, thereby reducing peak postprandial plasma glucose and insulin levels both in people with diabetes and normal people (4961,4980,4981,4982,4983). Oat bran combines with intestinal water which forms a gum (4961), increases stool weight, and stool fat excretion (4970). Beta-glucan may help control appetite by slowing stomach emptying, prolonging the feeling of fullness and stabilizing blood sugar (5078). Oat bran alters the metabolism of bile acids (4984). Although earlier studies did not differentiate between types of fiber (5105,5106,5108), later studies indicate that oat bran, unlike wheat bran, does not protect against colon cancer (5104,5107).

Adverse Reactions
Oat bran may cause bezoars (concretions) and intestinal obstruction, especially in people who have difficulty chewing or swallowing food, or have conditions that decrease small bowel motility (4979,4985). Oat bran can cause reactions in people with gluten allergy, due to its gluten content (2).

Interactions with Herbs & Other Dietary Supplements
CHOLESTEROL-REDUCING HERBS: Theoretically, concomitant use might cause additive cholesterol-lowering effects.

Interactions with Drugs

No interactions are known to occur, and there is no known reason to expect a clinically significant interaction with oat bran.

Interactions with Foods

FATTY FOODS: Concomitant use of foods high in saturated fats or cholesterol can interfere with the cholesterol-lowering effect of oat bran (4960).

Interactions with Lab Tests

CHOLESTEROL: Oat bran lowers blood levels total and low density lipoprotein (LDL) cholesterol and test results (4971).
BLOOD GLUCOSE: Oat bran lowers postprandial blood glucose and test results (4961).
INSULIN: Oat bran lowers postprandial insulin levels and test results (4961).

Interactions with Diseases or Conditions

CELIAC DISEASE: Contraindicated in individuals with celiac disease due to gluten content (6).
GI CONDITIONS: Contraindicated in people with intestinal ulcerations, stenosis, disabling adhesions, cathartic colon or other conditions that may result in intestinal or esophageal obstruction (4921). Use with caution or avoid in people with difficulty chewing or swallowing food, or conditions that decrease small bowel motility (4921).

Dosage and Administration

ORAL: A typical dose for lowering plasma cholesterol, cardiovascular risk and post-prandial glucose is 3 grams of soluble fiber per day (4960). Thirty-eight grams of oat bran or 75 grams of dry oatmeal contains about 3 grams of beta-glucan (4961,4971).

Comments

Oat bran is milled from the outer layer of hulled whole oats and is made up of both soluble and insoluble fiber (4960,4961,4970). Oat bran contains oat gum or beta-glucan, a soluble polysaccharide (4961,4981). The FDA allows medical claims for foods containing over 51% whole grains. Therefore, certain breads and cereals, etc., can claim to reduce the risk of certain medical conditions such as heart disease.

OAT STRAW

Also Known As

Avenae stramentum, Oatstraw, Straw.
CAUTION: See separate listings for Oat Bran, Oats, and Oat above ground parts.

Scientific Names

Avena sativa.
Family: Gramineae or Poaceae.

People Use This For

Topically, oat straw is used for skin inflammation, irritation, injury, pruritus, seborrhea (2), warts (18), arthritis, paralysis, and liver disorders (6).
In folk medicine, oat straw is used as a tea for flu and coughs, abdominal fatigue, bladder and rheumatic disorders, eye ailments, frostbite, gout, impetigo, and metabolic diseases. It has also been used in foot baths for chronically cold or tired feet (18).

Safety

POSSIBLY SAFE ...when used topically and appropriately (2).
There is insufficient reliable information available about the safety of the oral use of oat straw.
PREGNANCY AND LACTATION: Insufficient reliable information available.

Effectiveness

POSSIBLY EFFECTIVE ...when used topically for inflammatory skin conditions (2).
There is insufficient reliable information available about the effectiveness of oat straw for its other uses.

Mechanism of Action

There is insufficient reliable information available about the possible mechanism of action and active ingredients.

Adverse Reactions
None reported.

Interactions with Herbs & Other Dietary Supplements
Insufficient reliable information available.

Interactions with Drugs
No interactions are known to occur, and there is no known reason to expect a clinically significant interaction with oat straw.

Interactions with Foods
No interactions are known to occur, and there is no known reason to expect a clinically significant interaction with oat straw.

Interactions with Lab Tests
No interactions are known to occur, and there is no known reason to expect a clinically significant interaction with oat straw.

Interactions with Diseases or Conditions
No interactions are known to occur, and there is no known reason to expect a clinically significant interaction with oat straw.

Dosage and Administration
TOPICAL: To use as a bath additive, simmer 100 grams of chopped straw in 3 liters of water for 20 minutes, strain, and add to bath water (2,18).

Comments
Oat straw consists of the dried threshed, leaf and stem of the oat plant (Avena sativa).

OATS

Also Known As
Avena Fructus, Dietary Fiber, Groats, Oat Fruit, Oat Grain, Oatmeal.
CAUTION: See separate listings for Oat Bran, Oat above ground parts, and Oat Straw.

Scientific Names
Avena sativa.
Family: Gramineae or Poaceae.

People Use This For
Orally, oat fruit is used for disorders of the gastrointestinal tract (2,18), gallbladder, kidney, and cardiovascular systems (18). It is used for constipation, diarrhea, rheumatism, throat and chest complaints (18), physical fatigue, diabetes (2,18), hypercholesterolemia (6), neurasthenia and neurasthenia syndrome (2), colon cancer prevention (6267), nicotine withdrawal (2,6), and in tonics (2).
Topically, oats are used for managing dry, itchy skin (6), weeping eczema, contact dermatitis, chickenpox, and to enhance skin hydration (272).
In folk medicine, the oat fruit has been used as a sedative, for lowering uric acid levels, and as a diuretic (6).
In traditional Ayurvedic medicine, oats are used for opium withdrawal (6).
For food uses, they are used as a grain or cereal (6).
In manufacturing, oats are a component of bath products and soaps (6).

Safety
LIKELY SAFE …when used orally (6).
PREGNANCY AND LACTATION: LIKELY SAFE …when used orally (6).

Effectiveness
POSSIBLY EFFECTIVE …when used orally for reducing postprandial blood glucose in people with diabetes (6266). In a randomized crossover study of 13 people with type 2 diabetes, a high fiber diet that included oatmeal was more effective in lowering preprandial blood glucose and the area under the curve for 24-hour plasma glucose and glucose (measured every 2 hours), and improving cholesterol and triglyceride levels than the standard ADA diet (6266).

POSSIBLY INEFFECTIVE ...when used orally for reducing risk of colon cancer (6267). A large well-designed study showed that fiber does not prevent the recurrence of colorectal adenomas (6267).

There is insufficient reliable information available about the effectiveness of oats for other uses (2,272). However, oatmeal might enhance the cholesterol lowering effect of a low-fat diet. In an unpublished study, oatmeal increased the cholesterol lowering effect of an American Heart Association's Step 1 diet in a group of post-menopausal women with initial cholesterol levels above 200 mg/dl. After three weeks of the low-fat diet, cholesterol was lowered by 12 mg/dl. When 1 1/2 cups of cooked oatmeal daily was added to the low fat diet, cholesterol levels were reduced by an additional 8-9 mg/dl (6100).

Preliminary clinical evidence suggests that oatmeal containing 3.5 grams of beta-glucan consumed with a high fat meal might prevent acute fat-induced endothelial dysfunction and benefit cardiovascular health (318).

Researchers report that a group of people who ate a high soluble-fiber oatmeal breakfast experienced a greater feeling of fullness and consumed 30% fewer calories at lunch, compared with a group who ate nonfiber sugared corn flakes for breakfast. The results of this unpublished study were presented at the Experimental Biology 2000 meeting (5078).

Mechanism of Action

Oats contain oat gluten (6), gel-forming dietary fiber (7), and beta-glucans (18). The dietary fiber found in oat bran acts as a bulk-forming laxative. By stretching the intestinal wall it stimulates increased peristalsis (6).

Researchers think that the beta-glucan contained in oats helps control appetite by slowing stomach emptying, prolonging the feeling of fullness, and stabilizing blood sugar (5078). Beta-glucans increase bile acid secretion and some evidence suggests they reduce serum lipids (6). Preliminary information suggests oat tea might aid in opium withdrawal (6). Some information also suggests that an alcoholic oat extract might reduce cigarette use, but a second study failed to reproduce this result (6). Oat bran, milled from the outer layer of hulled whole oats, reduces serum cholesterol (6).

Adverse Reactions

Allergic reactions to oat gluten are rare (2). The fiber content in large amounts of oats can cause flatulence, and anal irritation (6).

Interactions with Herbs & Other Dietary Supplements

Insufficient reliable information available.

Interactions with Drugs

ORAL DRUGS: Theoretically, large amounts of oatmeal might interfere with drug absorption (19).
MORPHINE: Theoretically, a green seed extract of oat might antagonize the analgesic effect of morphine (19).
NICOTINE: Theoretically, a green seed extract of oat might antagonize the hypertensive effect of nicotine (19).

Interactions with Foods

No interactions are known to occur, and there is no known reason to expect a clinically significant interaction with oat fruit.

Interactions with Lab Tests

No interactions are known to occur, and there is no known reason to expect a clinically significant interaction with oat fruit.

Interactions with Diseases or Conditions

CELIAC DISEASE: Contraindicated due to gluten content (6).

Dosage and Administration

ORAL: No typical dosage.
TOPICAL: The oat fruit is commonly applied once or twice daily (6002).

Comments

None.

OCTACOSANOL

Also Known As

Hexacosanol (26-C), Tetracosanol (24-C), Triacontanol (30-C).
CAUTION: See separate listing for Policosanol.

Scientific Names
1-Octacosanol; N-octacosanol; Octacosyl alcohol.

People Use This For
Orally, octacosanol is used for improving strength, stamina, and reaction times (17,2922,2926), for herpes infections (6), for treating inflammatory skin diseases (6), for Parkinson's disease (2920), for amyotrophic lateral sclerosis (ALS) (2921), for hyperlipidemia (2923), and for atherosclerosis (2923).

Safety
There is insufficient reliable information available about the safety of octacosanol.
Pregnancy and Lactation: Insufficient reliable information available; avoid using.

Effectiveness
POSSIBLY INEFFECTIVE ...when used orally for treating amyotrophic lateral sclerosis (ALS) (2922).
There is insufficient reliable information available about the effectiveness of octacosanol for its other uses.

Mechanism of Action
Octacosanol is a 28-carbon waxy alcohol, related to vitamin E (2922). It is hypothesized that octacosanol could improve oxygen utilization during anaerobic glycolysis and aid in lactic acid removal by increasing the efficiency of the tricarboxylic acid cycle (17). In rats, octacosanol suppresses lipid accumulation in adipose tissue and increases the mobilization of free fatty acids from the fat cells in muscle (2924,2925).

Adverse Reactions
The use of octacosanol can cause position-related or nonrotational dizziness, increased nervous tension, and worsening of dyskinesias caused by levodopa or carbidopa (6).

Interactions with Herbs & Other Dietary Supplements
Insufficient reliable information available.

Interactions with Drugs
LEVODOPA/CARBIDOPA: Octacosanol can worsen dyskinesias associated with the use of levodopa or carbidopa (6).

Interactions with Foods
No interactions are known to occur, and there is no known reason to expect a clinically significant interaction with octacosanol.

Interactions with Lab Tests
No interactions are known to occur, and there is no known reason to expect a clinically significant interaction with octacosanol.

Interactions with Diseases or Conditions
PARKINSON'S DISEASE: Octacosanol can worsen dyskinesias associated with the levodopa or carbidopa treatment of Parkinson's disease (6).

Dosage and Administration
ORAL: For Parkinson's disease, the typical dose of octacosanol is 5 mg three times a day with meals (6,17). For amyotrophic lateral sclerosis (ALS), the usual dose is 40 mg per day (2921).

Comments
Octacosanol refers specifically to a 28-carbon alcohol, but it is commonly used to denote a mixture of 24- to 36-carbon alcohols, including tetracosanol (24-C), hexacosanol (26-C), and triacontanol (30-C) (6,268,269,270). It is found in a variety of plant sources, including sugar cane (Saccharum officinarum) (6,2923) and wheat germ oil (2922). Avoid confusion with policosanol.

OLEANDER

Also Known As
Common Oleander, Oleanderblatter, Oleandri folium, Rose Bay, Rose Laurel, Yellow Oleander.

Scientific Names

Nerium oleander; Thevetia peruviana
Family: Apocynaceae.

People Use This For

Orally, oleander is used for cardiac conditions (2,18), asthma, epilepsy, cancer, and dysmenorrhea (214). A fixed combination of oleander leaf powdered extract, pheasant's eye fluid extract, lily-of-the-valley fluid extract, and squill powdered extract has been used for treating mild limited heart failure with circulatory instability (2,7). Topically, oleander is used to treat skin eruptions (2,18,214) and warts (214).

Traditionally, oleander is used to treat leprosy, malaria, ringworm, indigestion, venereal disease, and as an abortifacient (5000). In Sri Lanka, yellow oleander seeds have been used orally for deliberate self-poisoning and suicide, particularly in women and children (2532).

Safety

LIKELY UNSAFE ...when used orally. Ingestion of oleander leaf, oleander leaf tea, and oleander seeds has led to fatal poisonings (2,9,3495).

There is insufficient reliable information available about the safety of the topical use of oleander.

PREGNANCY AND LACTATION: LIKELY UNSAFE ...when used orally. Oleander has been reported to have abortifacient properties (5000). There is insufficient reliable information available about the safety of topical use of oleander during pregnancy and lactation; avoid using.

Effectiveness

There is insufficient reliable information available about the effectiveness of oleander.

Mechanism of Action

All parts of the oleander plant contain the cardiac glycosides oleandrin, oleandroside, nerioside, digitoxigenin, which have positive inotropic and negative chronotropic actions (2,3495). They bind to sodium- and potassium-sensitive membrane-bound enzymes called ATPases and inhibit enzyme activities, resulting in increased intracellular sodium ions and calcium ions and increased extracellular potassium levels (3477,5000). At toxic levels, the sodium and calcium ions depolarize the cell after repolarization, causing late afterdepolarization and increased automaticity. Severe toxicity produces bradycardia and heart block (3477). Oleander leaf also contains other biologically active constituents that have antimitotic and insecticidal properties (5000). In folk medicine, oleander is also reported to have emetogenic, cathartic, insecticidic, parasiticidic, anthelmintic, menstrual stimulant, and abortifacient activities (214).

Adverse Reactions

Orally, oleander can cause bitter taste, burning sensation in mouth, nausea, vomiting, diarrhea, weakness, headache, stupor (17,18,3495), mucus membrane irritation, increased salivation, abdominal pain, buccal erythema, visual disturbances, mydriasis, peripheral neuritis (3495,5000), malignant dysrhythmias, ventricular ectopy, cardiovascular collapse, cardiac arrest (17), hyperkalemia (2532,3495) and death (3495). Oleander poisoning resembles digitoxin poisoning. Predominant symptoms are nausea and vomiting (onset in several hours), and cardiac toxicity, with conduction delays lasting for 3-6 days (17). Yellow oleander toxicity has been reported to be reversed with anti-digoxin Fab fragments. The majority of patients with yellow oleander toxicity who received anti-digoxin Fab fragments converted from an oleander-induced arrhythmia to normal sinus rhythm within 8 hours. A dose of 800 mg anti-digoxin Fab fragments was used intravenously. Associated hyperkalemia reversed within the first two hours (2532). A recurrence of arrhythmia can occur 48 hours post-exposure from any seed fragments remaining in the gastrointestinal tract (2532).

Interactions with Herbs & Other Dietary Supplements

CALCIUM: Contraindicated (18).

CARDIAC GLYCOSIDE-CONTAINING HERBS: Contraindicated, and concomitant use can increase the risk of cardiac glycoside toxicity. Cardiac glycoside-containing herbs include black hellebore, Canadian hemp roots, digitalis leaf, hedge mustard, figwort, lily of the valley roots, motherwort, pheasant's eye plant, pleurisy root, squill bulb leaf scales, strophanthus seeds, and uzara (2,18,19,500).

OTHER CARDIOACTIVE HERBS: Avoid concomitant use with other cardioactive herbs due to unpredictability of effects (4).

STIMULANT LAXATIVE HERBS: Theoretically, overuse or misuse of stimulant laxatives with cardiac glycoside-containing herbs increases the risk of cardiac toxicity due to potassium depletion (19).

LICORICE/HORSETAIL: Theoretically, overuse/misuse of licorice rhizome or horsetail plant with cardiac glycoside-containing herbs increases the risk of cardiac toxicity due to potassium depletion (19).

Interactions with Drugs

DIGOXIN: Contraindicated; therapeutic duplication increases risk of cardiac glycoside toxicity (2).

CARDIAC DRUGS: Theoretically, concomitant use may increase risk of cardiac toxicity (152).
STIMULANT LAXATIVES: Theoretically, overuse/misuse may increase risk of cardiac glycoside toxicity due to potassium depletion (2).
POTASSIUM-DEPLETING DIURETICS: Theoretically, concomitant use may increase risk of cardiac glycoside toxicity due to potassium depletion (2,506).
QUININE: Theoretically, concomitant use may increase risk of cardiac toxicity (2,506).
TETRACYCLINES AND MACROLIDE ANTIBIOTICS: Theoretically, concomitant use may increase risk of cardiac glycoside toxicity (152,17).
CALCIUM: Calcium salts may enhance effects (18).

Interactions with Foods
No interactions are known to occur, and there is no known reason to expect a clinically significant interaction with oleander.

Interactions with Lab Tests
No interactions are known to occur, and there is no known reason to expect a clinically significant interaction with oleander.

Interactions with Diseases or Conditions
HEART DISEASE: Self-use contraindicated; requires diagnosis, treatment, and monitoring (515).
ELECTROLYTE IMBALANCE: Theoretically, based on digitalis glycosides (15), contraindicated in individuals with potassium deficiency states and hypercalcemia.

Dosage and Administration
No typical dosage.

Comments
The annual incidence of oleander poisoning in Sri Lanka exceeds 150 per 100,000. Approximately 10% of these ingestions are fatal (2532). Abbott TDx Digoxin II assay can be used for rapid confirmation of the ingestion of oleander (17).

OLIVE leaf

Also Known As
Oleae folium, Olivier.
CAUTION: See separate listing for Olive Oil.

Scientific Names
Olea europaea.
Family: Oleaceae.

People Use This For
Orally, olive leaf extract is used for treatment of conditions caused by, or associated with, a virus, retrovirus, bacterium, or protozoan including influenza, the common cold, meningitis, Epstein-Barr Virus (EBV), encephalitis, herpes I and II, human herpes virus 6 and 7, shingles, HIV/ARC/AIDS, chronic fatigue, hepatitis B, pneumonia, tuberculosis, gonorrhea, malaria, dengue, bacteremia, severe diarrhea, blood poisoning, and dental, ear, urinary tract and surgical infections (290).
In folk medicine, olive leaf is used for lowering high blood pressure (2,7,18), treating diabetes (810), to enhance renal and digestive function (514), and as a diuretic (2,18) antipyretic (514).

Safety
There is insufficient reliable information available about the safety of olive leaf.
Pregnancy and Lactation: Insufficient reliable information available; avoid using.

Effectiveness
POSSIBLY EFFECTIVE ...when used orally for lowering blood pressure in people with hypertension (1540).
There is insufficient reliable information available about the effectiveness of olive leaf for its other uses.

Mechanism of Action
In animal experiments, olive leaf preparations demonstrate multiple properties including antispasmodic, hypotensive,

antiarrhythmic and arrhythmogenic (2,18), hypoglycemic (810), bronchodilator, coronary dilator, antipyretic, and diuretic (2). The constituent, oleuropein, has bacteriostatic (1541) and antioxidant (514) activity. Constituent flavonoids have serum complement-inactivating activity (1542). An aqueous olive leaf extract reduced blood pressure in one small, uncontrolled trial of people with hypertension (1540).

Adverse Reactions
Olive tree pollen causes seasonal respiratory allergy (1543).

Interactions with Herbs & Other Dietary Supplements
Insufficient reliable information available.

Interactions with Drugs
DRUGS AFFECTING BLOOD PRESSURE: Theoretically, concomitant use may enhance blood pressure-lowering effects (1540) and may interfere with blood pressure-increasing effects (1540).

Interactions with Foods
No interactions are known to occur, and there is no known reason to expect a clinically significant interaction with olive leaf.

Interactions with Lab Tests
BLOOD PRESSURE: Olive leaf might reduce blood pressure and blood pressure readings (1540).

Interactions with Diseases or Conditions
HYPOTENSION: Theoretically, may exacerbate this condition due to blood pressure-reducing effects (1540).

Dosage and Administration
ORAL: One cup tea (steep 2 teaspoons dried leaf in 150 mL boiling water 30 minutes, strain) three to four times per day (18).

Comments
None.

OLIVE OIL

Also Known As
Monounsaturated Fatty Acid, n-9 Fatty Acid, Olivae oleum, Omega-9 Fatty Acid, Salad Oil, Sweet Oil, Unsaturated Fatty Acid.
CAUTION: See separate listing for Olive leaf.

Scientific Names
Olea europaea.
Family: Oleaceae.

People Use This For
Orally, olive oil is commonly used for preventing cardiovascular disease (2219), hypertension, hypercholesterolemia, and diabetes (2219,2220). It is also used orally for breast cancer (2222) and rheumatoid arthritis (3454). Olive oil is used orally for migraine headache in adolescents (5097); firming the breasts; treating bile duct and gallbladder inflammation, gallstones, jaundice, flatulence, and meteorism (swelling of the abdomen due to intestinal or peritoneal gas); prevention of colorectal cancer (3362,3363); as a mild laxative for constipation; and Roemheld syndrome. Some people also use olive oil to boost bacteria in the gut and as a "cleanser" or "purifier" (2,14,16).
Topically, olive oil is used for softening ear wax (14), treating ringing and pain in the ears (2), as nose drops, for wound dressing, treating minor burns and psoriasis, preventing and treating stretch marks due to pregnancy (2), and for protecting the skin from ultraviolet (UV) damage after sun exposure (3364).
For food use, olive oil is used as a cooking and salad oil (13).
In manufacturing, olive oil is used to make soaps (13), commercial plasters and liniments, and as a setting-retardant in dental cements (13).

Safety
LIKELY SAFE ...when used orally in the amounts found in foods.

There is insufficient reliable information available about the safety of olive oil used in amounts greater than those used in food preparation.

PREGNANCY AND LACTATION: LIKELY SAFE ...when consumed in food amounts; avoid using in amounts greater than those found in foods (18).

Effectiveness
LIKELY EFFECTIVE ...when used orally as a mild laxative for constipation (14,16).

POSSIBLY EFFECTIVE ...when used orally for hypercholesterolemia. Increasing dietary olive oil consumption can significantly reduce total serum cholesterol levels (2219,2220,3285,3286,3287,3288,3289,3290). ...when used orally for hypertension. Consuming a modified diet including high amounts of extra virgin olive oil over 6 months, in conjunction with conventional treatments for hypertension, can significantly improve blood pressure. In some cases, patients with mild to moderate hypertension can decrease doses or discontinue use of antihypertensive medications (2219,2220,3289,5091). ...when used orally for reducing the risk of breast cancer. People who have higher dietary intake of olive oil seem to have a lower risk of developing breast cancer (2221,2222,2223). ...when used orally for reducing the risk of rheumatoid arthritis. There is some evidence that people consuming high amounts of dietary olive oil have a decreased risk of developing rheumatoid arthritis (3454). ...when used orally for migraine headache prophylaxis in adolescents. Taking olive oil preparations containing oleic acid 1,382 mg daily over a 2 month period seems to reduce frequency, duration, and severity of migraine headaches in adolescents (5097). ...when used orally for reducing the risk of colorectal cancer. There is some evidence that people with higher intakes of dietary olive oil have a decreased risk of developing colorectal cancer. Olive oil intake also seems to reduce colorectal mucosal changes and polyp formation, which are two factors involved in the sequence of developing colorectal cancer (3362).

POSSIBLY INEFFECTIVE ...when used topically for softening ear wax (3274). ...when used topically for treating ear pain in children with acute otitis media (3276).

There is insufficient reliable information available about the effectiveness of olive oil for its other uses.

Mechanism of Action
Olive oil contains the monounsaturated fatty acids oleic acid (56-83%), palmitic acid (8-20%), and linoleic acid (4-20%) (18). People use olive oil to prevent coronary heart disease and atherogenesis because it seems to lower certain cardiac risk factors. Olive oil seems to increase low-density lipoprotein (LDL) cholesterol resistance to oxidation and possibly decrease its contribution to atherogenesis (2219,2220,2224). Olive oil might also have anti-inflammatory effects by decreasing pro-inflammatory omega-6 fatty acid concentrations, and increasing anti-inflammatory omega-3 fatty acid concentrations (3289). Metabolites of oleic acid in olive oil, an omega-9 monounsaturated fatty acid, seems to competitively inhibit production of the omega-6 fatty acid metabolites which are inflammatory prostaglandins and leukotrienes. Oleic acid metabolites might also suppress production of inflammatory cytokines (3454). Some researchers think olive oil might have a role in preventing colon cancer. Consumption of olive oil seems to reduce production of deoxycholic acid, a bile acid thought to be involved in the development of mucosal changes and polyp formation preceding colorectal cancer (3362). Other compounds in olive oil called secoiridoides (oleuropein and derivatives) have broad spectrum antimicrobial activity in vitro (3284).

Adverse Reactions
Orally, olive oil may cause biliary colic in people with gallstones (2,18,19).

Topically, olive oil may cause allergic reactions (rare) (2). May irritate eyes; avoid eye contact (19). Delayed hypersensitivity and contact dermatitis are reported with topical use (289,3275).

Interactions with Herbs & Other Dietary Supplements
Insufficient reliable information available.

Interactions with Drugs
DIABETES THERAPY: Monitor blood glucose levels closely due to claims that olive oil has hypoglycemic effects (19).

Interactions with Foods
No interactions are known to occur, and there is no known reason to expect a clinically significant interaction with olive oil.

Interactions with Lab Tests
No interactions are known to occur, and there is no known reason to expect a clinically significant interaction with olive oil.

Interactions with Diseases or Conditions
GALLSTONES: Contraindicated; may trigger gallbladder colic (2,18,19).

Dosage and Administration
ORAL: As adjunctive therapy in hypertension, 30-40 grams per day of extra-virgin olive oil has been used as part of the diet (5091). As a laxative, 30 mL has been used (16).
TOPICAL: No typical dosage.

Comments
Olive oil consists of the fatty oil pressed from the drupes (fruit) of olive trees (Olea europaea). It is classified, in part, according to oleic acid content. Extra virgin olive oil contains a maximum of 1% free oleic acid, virgin olive oil contains 2% and ordinary olive oil contains 3.3%. Unrefined olive oils with more than 3.3% free oleic acid are considered "unfit for human consumption" (3273). The American Heart Association recommends a maximum 30% of dietary calories from fat (2224). Some studies show beneficial effects when olive oil is the main source of dietary fat intake (2224).

OMEGA-6 FATTY ACIDS

Also Known As
N-6, N-6 EFAs, N-6 Essential Fatty Acids, Omega 6, Omega-6, Omega 6 Fatty Acids, Omega-6 Oils, Omega 6 Oils, Polyunsaturated Fatty Acids, PUFAs.
CAUTION: See separate listings for Gamma Linolenic Acid, Evening Primrose Oil, Borage Seed Oil, and Black Currant Seed Oil.

Scientific Names
Omega-6 polyunsaturated fatty acids.

People Use This For
Orally, omega-6 fatty acids are used for reducing the risk of coronary heart disease, lowering total cholesterol and LDL cholesterol levels, increasing HDL cholesterol levels, and reducing cancer risk (3507).
Arachidonic acid, an omega-6 fatty acid, is used as a supplement in infant formulas (424).

Safety
There is insufficient reliable information available about the safety of omega-6 fatty acids for therapeutic purposes.
Pregnancy and Lactation: Insufficient reliable information available; avoid using for therapeutic purposes.

Effectiveness
POSSIBLY INEFFECTIVE ...when arachidonic acid (an omega-6 fatty acid) is used as a supplement in infant formula for improving cognitive and mental development or growth up to 18 months of age (424).
There is insufficient reliable information available about the effectiveness of omega-6 fatty acids for its other uses.

Mechanism of Action
Preliminary studies suggest that omega-6 fatty acids might play a role in breast cancer development (3508); however, it is unclear whether omega-6 fatty acids are associated with breast cancer in humans (3508,3511). A low-fat diet with reduced omega-6 fatty acid content can decrease sex steroid hormone levels, alter eicosanoid biosynthesis, and play a role in preventing and treating breast and prostate cancers (3510). Long-chain polyunsaturated fatty acids, such as arachidonic acid (an omega-6 fatty acid) make up a third of all lipids in the brain's grey matter (425). Arachidonic acid is a membrane component in the central nervous system, and may have a role as a neurotransmitter (424,425). Arachidonic acid is present in human breast milk but not in standard infant formulas. Formula-fed infants have lower plasma arachidonic acid levels than breast milk-fed infants; the clinical significance of this, if any, is unknown (424).

Adverse Reactions
Orally, use of the omega-6 fatty acids can elevate triglycerides (3509).

Interactions with Herbs & Other Dietary Supplements
Insufficient reliable information available.

Interactions with Drugs
No interactions are known to occur, and there is no known reason to expect a clinically significant interaction with omega-6 fatty acids.

Interactions with Foods

No interactions are known to occur, and there is no known reason to expect a clinically significant interaction with omega-6 fatty acids.

Interactions with Lab Tests

No interactions are known to occur, and there is no known reason to expect a clinically significant interaction with omega-6 fatty acids.

Interactions with Diseases or Conditions

HYPERTRIGLYCERIDEMIA: Avoid the use of the omega-6 fatty acids, because they can elevate triglyceride levels (3509).

Dosage and Administration

ORAL: As a supplement in infant formula, 0.3% of arachidonic acid (an omega-6 fatty acid) has been used (424).

Comments

Omega-6 fatty acids include linoleic acid (LA), gamma-linolenic acid (GLA), and arachidonic acid. Linoleic acid is found in vegetable oils, including corn, evening primrose seed, safflower, and soybean oils (512,3507). Gamma-linolenic acid is found in black currant seed, borage seed, and evening primrose oils (512). Information on omega-6 fatty acid dietary supplementation derives from studies using specific omega-6 fatty acids or plant oils containing omega-6 fatty acids. See separate listings for black currant seed oil, borage seed oil, and evening primrose oil.

ONION

Also Known As

Allii cepae bulbus, Green Onion, Onions.

Scientific Names

Allium cepa.
Family: Alliaceae, Amaryllidaceae or Liliaceae.

People Use This For

Orally, onion is used for loss of appetite, preventing atherosclerosis (2), for treating dyspepsia, fever, colds, cough, bronchitis, hypertension, tendency toward infection, and inflammation of the mouth and pharynx (18).
In folk medicine, it has been used for cough, whooping cough, bronchitis, asthma, angina, stimulation of gallbladder, dehydration, and as a menstruation aid. Onion has also been used for hypertension, diabetes, insect bites, wounds, light burns, furuncles, warts, bruises (18), as an antiflatulent (11), anthelmintic (11,18), and diuretic (6,11).
For food uses, onion is considered a culinary food and condiment (11).
In manufacturing, the oil is used as a flavoring agent in foods (11).

Safety

LIKELY SAFE ...when consumed in amounts commonly found in food and has Generally Recognized as Safe (GRAS) status for food use in the US (11).
POSSIBLY SAFE ...when used orally and appropriately (2). A maximum of 35 mg of the diphenylamine constituent is recommended per day if onion preparations are used over several months (2).
There is insufficient reliable information available about the safety of onion for its other uses.
PREGNANCY AND LACTATION: Insufficient reliable information available; avoid amounts greater than used in foods.

Effectiveness

There is insufficient reliable information available about the effectiveness of onion.

Mechanism of Action

The applicable part of the onion is the bulb. Onion contains essential oils (2), sulfur compounds, and cysteine sulfoxide compounds. One of the sulfur compounds, thiosulphinate, exhibits antimicrobial effects (18). The methyl and propyl compounds of cysteine sulfoxide are primarily responsible for onion flavor and lacrimation (7,11). Diphenylamine is also a constituent of onion (513). Diphenylamine is referred to as a dose standard (2). The mechanism of the diuretic effect of onion is unknown. In people with asthma, an ethanolic onion extract significantly reduced bronchial constriction (18). In sensitized guinea pigs, onion juice provided protection from asthma attacks (18). In humans, eating onions reversed the effect of a fatty meal, restoring fibrinolytic activity (7). In humans, onion also inhibits platelet aggregation (7). Onions show hypoglycemic actions, and in animals, both cholesterol lowering effects and antifungal activities have been noted (11).

Adverse Reactions
The consumption of large quantities of onions can cause stomach distress (18). Hand eczema can occur with frequent contact (18).

Interactions with Herbs & Other Dietary Supplements
HERBS WITH ANTICOAGULANT/ANTIPLATELET POTENTIAL: Concomitant use of herbs that have coumarin constituents or affect platelet aggregation could theoretically increase the risk of bleeding in some people. These herbs include: angelica, anise, arnica, asafoetida, bogbean, boldo, capsicum, celery, chamomile, clove, danshen, fenugreek, feverfew, garlic, ginger, ginkgo, ginseng (Panax), horse chestnut, horseradish, licorice, meadowsweet, prickly ash, papain, passionflower, poplar, quassia, red clover, turmeric, wild carrot, wild lettuce, willow, and others (4,19).

Interactions with Drugs
ANTIDIABETES DRUGS: Theoretically, concomitant use might enhance antidiabetes drug effects and alter blood sugar control (19).
ANTIPLATELET DRUGS: Theoretically, concomitant use might enhance antiplatelet drug activity and increase bleeding risk (19).
ASPIRIN: Concomitant intake might augment onion allergy. One case is reported of severe urticaria and swelling in a person with a known mild onion allergy after consuming onion and aspirin (5054).

Interactions with Foods
No interactions are known to occur, and there is no known reason to expect a clinically significant interaction with onion.

Interactions with Lab Tests
BLOOD GLUCOSE: Onions can decrease blood glucose levels and test results (19).

Interactions with Diseases or Conditions
DIABETES: Theoretically, therapeutic amounts of onions can interfere with blood sugar control. Monitor blood sugar carefully when using onion for medicinal purposes (19).

Dosage and Administration
ORAL: The typical dose is 50 grams of fresh onion per day. The juice of 50 grams fresh onion or 20 grams dried onion is also used per day (2). A maximum of 35 mg diphenylamine per day is recommended if onion preparations are used over several months (2).
TOPICAL: An onion slice is typically placed on the skin, or the juice is used as a poultice (18).

Comments
Onions are rich in vitamin C (19) and in folk medicine, were cooked in milk and used as a mucolytic to clear congested airways (7).

OPIUM ANTIDOTE

Also Known As
Combretum, Jungle Weed.

Scientific Names
Combretum micranthum.
Family: Combretaceae.

People Use This For
Historically, opium antidote has been used orally for gallbladder disease, dyspepsia, and liver disease. It is no longer used as a single entity, only in combination preparations (18).

Safety
There is insufficient reliable information available about the safety of opium antidote (18).
Pregnancy and Lactation: Insufficient reliable information available; avoid using.

Effectiveness

There is insufficient reliable information available about the effectiveness of opium antidote.

Mechanism of Action

The applicable parts of opium antidote are the leaf and stem. Opium antidote is said to possess mild bile-stimulating properties and astringent effects. It contains catechin tannins, flavonoids, and pyrrolidine alkaloid betaines. A methanolic extract shows some evidence of activity against HSV-1 and HSV-2 (18). Activity was present only in the extract dissolved 7 days before assay, but not in the freshly prepared extract (5001).

Adverse Reactions

None reported.

Interactions with Herbs & Other Dietary Supplements

Insufficient reliable information available.

Interactions with Drugs

No interactions are known to occur, and there is no known reason to expect a clinically significant interaction with opium antidote.

Interactions with Foods

No interactions are known to occur, and there is no known reason to expect a clinically significant interaction with opium antidote.

Interactions with Lab Tests

No interactions are known to occur, and there is no known reason to expect a clinically significant interaction with opium antidote.

Interactions with Diseases or Conditions

No interactions are known to occur, and there is no known reason to expect a clinically significant interaction with opium antidote.

Dosage and Administration

No typical dosage.

Comments

There is very little scientific information about this product. Our staff is continually analyzing the available information on natural medicines and will add data here as it becomes available.

ORCHIC EXTRACT

Also Known As

Bovine Orchic Extract, Bovine Testicle Extract, Bull Balls Extract, Orchic, Orchic Concentrate, Orchic Factors, Orchic Substance.

Scientific Names

None.

People Use This For

Orally, men use orchic extract to maintain healthy testicular function (1319).

Safety

There is insufficient reliable information available to rate the safety of orchic extract. However, since orchic extract preparations are derived from animals, there is concern about contamination with diseased animal parts (see Adverse Reactions) (1825). So far, there are no reports of disease transmission to humans due to use of contaminated orchic extract.

Pregnancy and Lactation: Insufficient reliable information available; avoid using.

Effectiveness

There is insufficient reliable information available about the effectiveness of orchic extract.

Mechanism of Action

Orchic extract is obtained from bovine testicles (1319). Marketers imply that orchic extracts are a good source of testosterone. However, there is no evidence to support this claim.

Adverse Reactions

Adverse effects for orchic extract have not been reported. However, there are concerns about possible product contamination. Orchic extract is derived from raw bovine testes gathered from slaughterhouses, possibly from sick or diseased animals (1319,6616). Products made from contaminated or diseased organs might present a human health hazard. There is also concern that orchic extracts produced from cows in countries where bovine spongiform encephalitis (BSE) has been reported might be contaminated with diseased tissue. Countries where BSE has been reported include Great Britain, France, The Netherlands, Portugal, Luxembourg, Ireland, Switzerland, Oman, and Belgium (1825). However, there have been no reports of BSE transfer to humans from contaminated orchic extract products. Until more is known, tell patients to avoid these products unless country of origin can be determined. Patients should avoid products that are produced in countries where BSE has been found.

Interactions with Herbs & Other Dietary Supplements

Insufficient reliable information available.

Interactions with Drugs

No interactions are known to occur, and there is no known reason to expect a clinically significant interaction with orchic extract.

Interactions with Foods

No interactions are known to occur, and there is no known reason to expect a clinically significant interaction with orchic extract.

Interactions with Lab Tests

ANABOLIC STEROIDS: Theoretically, orchic extract might cause a positive anabolic steroid screening test result (1320). However, this effect has not been demonstrated.

Interactions with Diseases or Conditions

No interactions are known to occur, and there is no known reason to expect a clinically significant interaction with orchic extract.

Dosage and Administration

No typical dosage.

Comments

None.

OREGANO

Also Known As

Carvacrol, Dostenkraut, European Oregano, Mediterranean Oregano, Mountain Mint, Oil of Oregano, Oregano Oil, Organy, Origani vulgaris herba, Origano, Origanum, Phytoprogestin, Wild Marjoram, Winter Marjoram, Wintersweet. CAUTION: See separate listing for Marjoram.

Scientific Names

Origanum vulgare.
Family: Lamiaceae or Labiatae.

People Use This For

Orally, oregano is used for respiratory tract disorders such as coughs, asthma, croup, and bronchitis.
Oregano is also used orally for gastrointestinal disorders, such as dyspepsia and bloating.
It is also used orally for dysmenorrhea, rheumatoid arthritis, urinary tract disorders including urinary tract infections (UTIs), headaches, and heart conditions.
The oil of oregano is also used orally for intestinal parasites, allergies, sinusitis, arthritis, cold and flu, earaches, and fatigue.
Topically, oregano oil is used for acne, athlete's foot, dandruff, insect and spider bites, canker sores, gum disease, toothaches, psoriasis, seborrhea, ringworm, rosacea, muscle pain, varicose veins, and warts.

It is also used topically as an insect repellent.

In foods and beverages, oregano is used as a culinary spice and a food preservative.

Safety
LIKELY SAFE ...when used orally in amounts found in foods (11). Oregano leaf and oil have Generally Recognized as Safe (GRAS) status in the US (11).

POSSIBLY SAFE ...when used orally or topically and appropriately in medicinal amounts (2,12,14,18). There is insufficient reliable information available to rate the safety of oregano oil when used in medicinal amounts.

PREGNANCY: LIKELY SAFE ...when used orally in amounts found in foods (11). POSSIBLY UNSAFE ...when used in medicinal amounts. Oregano is thought to have abortifacient and emmenagogue effects (19,7122).

LACTATION: LIKELY SAFE ...when used orally in amounts found in foods (11). There is insufficient reliable information available about the safety of oregano when used in medicinal amounts while nursing.

Effectiveness
POSSIBLY EFFECTIVE ...when used orally for intestinal parasitic infection. The emulsified oil of oregano 200 mg three times daily for 6 weeks can eradicate the parasites Blastocystis hominis, Entamoeba hartmanni, and Endolimax nana from the stools of infected patients (6878).

There is insufficient reliable information available about the effectiveness of oregano for its other reported uses.

Mechanism of Action
The applicable part of oregano is the leaf and oil. Oregano contains the constituents carvacrol and thymol which have anthelmintic, fungicidal, and irritant properties (11,2129). The essential oil is thought to have diuretic, expectorant, and antispasmodic properties. It might also stimulate bile production (11). Oregano oil also has in vitro activity against a variety of common gram positive and gram negative organisms, including Acinetobacter calcoacetica, Enterococcus faecalis, Escherichia coli, Klebsiella pneumoniae, Pseudomonas aeruginosa, Salmonella species, Serratia marcescens, Staphylococcus aureus, and the yeast Candida albicans (316,2129,2130,3702,3703,3704,6113). The carvacrol and thymol constituents also inhibit bacterial growth, with additive or possibly synergistic activity in oregano oil (2130). Carvacrol has a bacteriocidal effect on Bacillus cereus, a common food pathogen, by altering bacterial membrane permeability (165). Oregano oil seems to inhibit the growth intestinal parasites in vivo (6878). There is preliminary evidence that oregano may contain phytoprogestins that bind the progesterone receptor (3701).

Adverse Reactions
Orally, large amounts of oregano can cause gastrointestinal upset (14). Concentrated, non-emulsified oil of oregano can cause localized irritation of the gastrointestinal tract (6878). Oregano might also cause systemic allergic reactions (3705). Individuals allergic to Lamiaceae family plants including basil, hyssop, lavender, marjoram, mint, and sage, might also demonstrate an allergic reaction to oregano (3705).

Interactions with Herbs & Other Dietary Supplements
Insufficient reliable information available.

Interactions with Drugs
No interactions are known to occur, and there is no known reason to expect a clinically significant interaction with oregano.

Interactions with Foods
No interactions are known to occur, and there is no known reason to expect a clinically significant interaction with oregano.

Interactions with Lab Tests
No interactions are known to occur, and there is no known reason to expect a clinically significant interaction with oregano.

Interactions with Diseases or Conditions
CROSS-ALLERGENICITY: Oregano can cause reactions in people allergic to Lamiaceae family plants, including basil, hyssop, lavender, marjoram, mint, and sage (3705).

Dosage and Administration
ORAL: A typical dose is one cup of tea. To make tea, steep 1 heaping teaspoon of leaf in 250 mL boiling water 10 minutes, strain. Tea may be sweetened with honey (18). Emulsified oil of oregano has been used in a dose of 200 mg three times daily for 6 weeks for eradication of intestinal parasites (6878).

TOPICAL: Unsweetened tea is used as a gargle or mouthwash (18). To use oregano as a bath additive, steep 100 grams dried leaf in 1 L water for 10 minutes, strain, and add to a full bath (18).

Comments

Oregano oil has been tested as an insect repellent for Culicodoides imicola, a pathogen-bearing species of insects commonly known as no-see-ums or biting midges. Oregano oil is not as effective as DEET for protecting horses (and presumably, people) from C. imicola (2119).

OREGON FIR BALSAM

Also Known As

Balsam, Balsam Fir Oregon, Balsam Oregon, Coastal Douglas Fir, Douglas Fir, Douglas Spruce, Oregon Balsam, Red Fir.

Scientific Names

Pseudotsuga menziesii, synonym Pseudotsuga douglasii; Pseudotsuga mucronata; Pseudotsuga taxifolia.
Family: Pinaceae.

People Use This For

In traditional medicine, Oregon fir balsam has been used for burns, sores, cuts, relieving heart and chest pain, and for treating tumors (11).

Safety

There is insufficient reliable information available about the safety of Oregon fir balsam.
Pregnancy and Lactation: Insufficient reliable information available; avoid using.

Effectiveness

There is insufficient reliable information available about the effectiveness of Oregon fir balsam.

Mechanism of Action

There is insufficient reliable information available about the possible mechanism of action and active ingredients.

Adverse Reactions

None reported.

Interactions with Herbs & Other Dietary Supplements

Insufficient reliable information available.

Interactions with Drugs

No interactions are known to occur, and there is no known reason to expect a clinically significant interaction with Oregon fir balsam.

Interactions with Foods

No interactions are known to occur, and there is no known reason to expect a clinically significant interaction with Oregon fir balsam.

Interactions with Lab Tests

No interactions are known to occur, and there is no known reason to expect a clinically significant interaction with Oregon fir balsam.

Interactions with Diseases or Conditions

No interactions are known to occur, and there is no known reason to expect a clinically significant interaction with Oregon fir balsam.

Dosage and Administration

No typical dosage.

Comments

Oregon fir balsam is an oleoresin (rather than a true balsam) collected from the trunk of the Oregon fir tree. Oregon fir balsam has been detected as an adulterant in Canada balsam (Abies balsamea) (11).

There is very little scientific information about this product. Our staff is continually analyzing the available information on natural medicines and will add data here as it becomes available.

OREGON GRAPE

Also Known As

Barberry, Blue Barberry, Creeping Barberry, Holly Barberry, Holly-Leaved Berberis, Holly Mahonia, Mountain-Grape, Oregon Barberry, Oregon-Grape, Oregon Grape-Holly, Scraperoot, Trailing Mahonia, Water-Holly. CAUTION: See separate listing for European Barberry.

Scientific Names

Mahonia aquifolium, synonym Berberis aquifolium; Mahonia nervosa, synonym Berberis nervosa; Mahonia repens, synonyms Berberis repens, Berberis sonnei.
Family: Beberidaceae.

People Use This For

Topically, Oregon grape is used for psoriasis (515).

In folk medicine, it is used for ulcers, heartburn, stomach problems, as a bitter tonic, and as a cathartic (515). The American Indians used Oregon grape for general debility and as an appetite stimulant (515).

Safety

POSSIBLY SAFE ...when used topically and appropriately (854,857). Canada has approved a Mahonia aquifolium product for topical use based on safety data (855,856). ...when used orally. Amounts of less than 500 mg per day of berberine, a constituent of Oregon grape, are usually considered safe (2,12).

LIKELY UNSAFE ...when more than 500 mg per day berberine is consumed (2,12). Berberine is considered moderately toxic (12). The human LD50 for berberine is reported to be 27.5 mg/kg (12).

PREGNANCY: LIKELY UNSAFE ...when used orally (12) due to potential uterine stimulant activity of berberine (11,19).

LACTATION: Insufficient reliable information available; avoid using.

Effectiveness

There is insufficient reliable information available about the effectiveness of Oregon grape.

Mechanism of Action

The applicable parts of Oregon grape are the rhizome and root. Oregon grape root contains 2.4-4.5% of isoquinoline alkaloid constituents including berberine, berbamine, and oxyacanthine (18,515). Berberine and oxyacanthine show evidence of antibacterial activity (11). Berberine has anticonvulsant, sedative, hypotensive, antifibrillatory, and bile-stimulating effects. In low doses, it is a cardiac and respiratory stimulant. In high doses it is a depressant (11,12,515). Some evidence suggests berberine sulfate might be amebicidal and trypanocidal (11). Other information suggests the constituent berbamine might have anti-arrhythmic, hypotensive, spasmolytic, and immunostimulating activity (11,515). In an open clinical trial, an extract of dried stem, branch bark, and branch tips of Mahonia aquifolium in an ointment base improved psoriasis symptoms and quality of life (857). In another trial, some patients treated with Mahonia aquifolium bark extract in an ointment base found it more useful than placebo for treating mild to moderate psoriasis (854). However, more than half of the other participants and their physicians rated the treatment as ineffective (854).

Adverse Reactions

No reports of adverse effects associated with Oregon grape. Ingesting more than 500 mg berberine, a constituent of Oregon grape, can cause lethargy, nosebleed, skin and eye irritation, kidney irritation (12), hemorrhagic nephritis (2), dyspnea, hypotension, cardiac damage (12), nausea, vomiting, diarrhea, respiratory spasms and arrest, and death (2). When used topically, Oregon grape can cause itching, burning, skin irritation, and allergic reactions (854).

Interactions with Herbs & Other Dietary Supplements

BERBERINE-CONTAINING HERBS: Concomitant use can increase the risk of berberine toxicity. Berberine-containing herbs include bloodroot, goldenseal, celandine, Chinese goldthread, goldthread, Oregon grape (Mahonia species), amur cork tree, Chinese corktree (12).

Interactions with Drugs

No interactions are known to occur, and there is no known reason to expect a clinically significant interaction with Oregon grape.

Interactions with Foods

No interactions are known to occur, and there is no known reason to expect a clinically significant interaction with Oregon grape.

Interactions with Lab Tests

No interactions are known to occur, and there is no known reason to expect a clinically significant interaction with Oregon grape.

Interactions with Diseases or Conditions

KIDNEY IRRITATION: CAUTION, berberine may exacerbate kidney irritation. It can cause kidney irritation and nephritis (2).

Dosage and Administration

ORAL: The common dose of the tincture is 2-4 mL three times daily, and the usual dose of the powder is 0.5 to 1 gram three times daily (6002).
TOPICAL: Psoriasis, 10% Mahonia aquifolium bark extract ointment applied to affected areas two to three times daily (854). Mahonia aquifolium 10% root extract cream massaged into affected areas three times daily or as directed by physician (855).

Comments

A Mahonia aquifolium root extract product, Prime Relief, received a Drug Identification Number (DIN) from Health Canada (855). The DIN allows this product to be labeled and marketed for treating psoriasis in Canada (855,856).

ORIENTAL ARBORVITAE

Also Known As

Chinese Arborvitae.

Scientific Names

Platycladus orientalis, synonyms Biota orientalis, Thuja orientalis.
Family: Cupressaceae.

People Use This For

Orally, Oriental arborvitae is used orally for headache, apprehension, calming nervous disorders and excitement, for cancer, constipation, convulsions, dysmenorrhea, ejaculation problems, narrowing of intestine, fever, vomiting blood, bloody stools, blood in urine, hemorrhage, insomnia, painful menses, heavy menstrual flow, irregular and variable menstrual bleeding, nausea, neurasthenia, palpitation, perspiration, rheumatism, tumors, and as a tonic. It is also used for diuretic, laxative, menstrual-stimulant, pain-reliever, parasiticide, and sedative effects.
Topically, it is used for nosebleed, piles, for burns and scalds, and as a hair tonic. It is also used for its astringent and antiperspirant properties.

Safety

POSSIBLY SAFE ...when the seed is used orally (12) ...when the leafy twigs are used orally in tea. It is important to use it short-term and not to exceed the usual dose (12).
PREGNANCY AND LACTATION: POSSIBLY UNSAFE ...when used orally because it contains thujone (12) which shows some evidence of uterine stimulant activity (19); avoid using.

Effectiveness

There is insufficient reliable information is available about the effectiveness of oriental arborvitae.

Mechanism of Action

The applicable parts of oriental arborvitae are the seed and the cacumen (leafy twigs) (12). Oriental arborvitae contains thujone in the volatile oil. Alcoholic extracts and essential oils containing thujone can cause neurotoxicity including convulsions and hallucinations (12). Some evidence suggests Thuja orientalis might have antibacterial activity (4041).

Adverse Reactions

Thujone intoxication can cause psychoactivity similar to tetrahydrocannibinol, the active constituent in marijuana. Long-term or high dosages of plants containing thujone can cause restlessness, vomiting, dizziness, tremors, renal damage, and convulsions (12).

Interactions with Herbs & Other Dietary Supplements

THUJONE CONTAINING HERBS: Avoid; concomitant use may increase the risk of thujone toxicity. Thujone-containing herbs include: oak moss (12), sage (2,4,12), tansy (2,4,12), thuja (cedar) (11,12), tree moss (12), and wormwood (2,12).

Interactions with Drugs

No interactions are known to occur, and there is no known reason to expect a clinically significant interaction with oriental arborvitae.

Interactions with Foods

No interactions are known to occur, and there is no known reason to expect a clinically significant interaction with oriental arborvitae.

Interactions with Lab Tests

No interactions are known to occur, and there is no known reason to expect a clinically significant interaction with oriental arborvitae.

Interactions with Diseases or Conditions

PORPHYRIA: Can exacerbate porphyria in patients with underlying defects in hepatic heme synthesis (12).
RENAL DYSFUNCTION: Can exacerbate this condition (12).

Dosage and Administration

ORAL: A standard dose for the leafy twigs is 5-15 grams of raw or charred, daily as tea (12). No typical dosage for the seed.

Comments

None.

ORNITHINE

Also Known As

L-Ornithine.
CAUTION: See separate listing for Ornithine Ketoglutarate.

Scientific Names

L-5-aminorvaline; L-2,5-diaminovaleric acid.

People Use This For

Orally, ornithine is used for improving athletic performance and for wound healing (2416).

Safety

There is insufficient reliable information available about the safety of ornithine used for medicinal purposes.
Pregnancy and Lactation: Insufficient reliable information available; avoid using.

Effectiveness

POSSIBLY INEFFECTIVE ...when taken orally for enhancing athletic performance (2417,2418).
There is insufficient reliable information available for the effectiveness of ornithine for wound healing.

Mechanism of Action

Ornithine is a non-essential amino acid produced in the body by hydrolysis of arginine (9,511). By supplementing ornithine, people believe they can increase their anabolic hormone levels, reducing skeletal muscle hypertrophy (2147). However, supplemental ornithine has no effect on insulin secretion (2147,2148) or serum human growth hormone (hGH) levels in bodybuilders (2148).

Adverse Reactions

None reported.

Interactions with Herbs & Other Dietary Supplements
Insufficient reliable information available.

Interactions with Drugs
No interactions are known to occur, and there is no known reason to expect a clinically significant interaction with ornithine.

Interactions with Foods
No interactions are known to occur, and there is no known reason to expect a clinically significant interaction with ornithine.

Interactions with Lab Tests
No interactions are known to occur, and there is no known reason to expect a clinically significant interaction with ornithine.

Interactions with Diseases or Conditions
No interactions are known to occur, and there is no known reason to expect a clinically significant interaction with ornithine.

Dosage and Administration
ORAL: Take one 500 mg capsule containing L-ornithine daily on an empty stomach before bedtime (5020).

Comments
Avoid confusion with ornithine alpha-ketoglutarate (OKG).
There is very little scientific information about this product. Our staff is continually analyzing the available information on natural medicines and will add data here as it becomes available.

ORNITHINE KETOGLUTARATE

Also Known As
OKG, Ornicetil, Ornithine Alphaketoglutarate, L-Ornithine Alpha-Ketoglutarate, Ornithine Alpha Ketoglutarate.
CAUTION: See separate listing for Ornithine.

Scientific Names
L(+)-ornithine alpha-ketoglutarate.

People Use This For
Orally, ornithine ketoglutarate is used for enhancing athletic performance and wound healing (2442).
Intravenously, it is used as a component in total parenteral nutrition for preventing growth retardation in children receiving long-term total parenteral nutrition (2444). It is also used intravenously for improving skeletal muscle protein synthesis after surgery (2446), preventing decreases in muscle free glutamine concentrations, and preserving protein synthesis after total hip replacement (2448) or stroke (2447).

Safety
POSSIBLY SAFE ...when use intravenously and appropriately (2444,2445,2446,2448).
There is insufficient reliable information available about the safety of the oral use of ornithine ketoglutarate.
PREGNANCY AND LACTATION: Insufficient reliable information available; avoid using.

Effectiveness
POSSIBLY EFFECTIVE ...when used orally for wound healing in burn patients (2443). ...when used intravenously for preventing growth retardation in children receiving long-term total parenteral nutrition (2444), reducing loss of muscle glutamine after surgical trauma (2445), improving skeletal muscle protein synthesis after surgery (2446), preventing a decrease in the muscle free glutamine concentration, and preservation of protein synthesis after total hip replacement (2448).
POSSIBLY INEFFECTIVE ...when used orally for enhancing athletic performance (2452).
LIKELY INEFFECTIVE ...when used intravenously for treating encephalopathy in patients with acute and chronic liver disease (2449,2450).
There is insufficient reliable information available about the effectiveness of ornithine ketoglutarate for its other uses.

Mechanism of Action

Ornithine ketoglutarate modifies amino acid metabolism and increases blood insulin and glucagon levels in healthy people (2415).

Adverse Reactions

None reported.

Interactions with Herbs & Other Dietary Supplements

Insufficient reliable information available.

Interactions with Drugs

No interactions are known to occur, and there is no known reason to expect a clinically significant interaction with ornithine ketoglutarate.

Interactions with Foods

No interactions are known to occur, and there is no known reason to expect a clinically significant interaction with ornithine ketoglutarate.

Interactions with Lab Tests

No interactions are known to occur, and there is no known reason to expect a clinically significant interaction with ornithine ketoglutarate.

Interactions with Diseases or Conditions

No interactions are known to occur, and there is no known reason to expect a clinically significant interaction with ornithine ketoglutarate.

Dosage and Administration

ORAL: For athletic support, 2-4 grams of ornithine ketoglutarate is commonly taken three times per day with meals (2442). For the healing of burn wounds, 30 grams is taken daily as an enteral bolus (2443).
INTRAVENOUS: For preventing growth retardation in children receiving long-term total parenteral nutrition (TPN), 15 grams of ornithine ketoglutarate is typically added to the daily TPN (2444). For improving skeletal muscle protein synthesis after surgery, 350 mg/kg per day is added to the TPN (2446). For preventing decreases in muscle free glutamine concentrations and preserving protein synthesis after total hip replacement, 280 mg/kg per day is added to the TPN (2448).

Comments

Avoid confusion with ornithine.

ORRIS

Also Known As

Blue Flag, Daggers, Flag, Flaggon, Flag Lily, Fliggers, Florentine Iris, Gladyne, Iris, Jacob's Sword, Liver Lily, Myrtle Flower, Poison Flag, Rhizoma iridis, Segg, Sheggs, Snake Lily, Water Flag, White Dragon Flower, Wild Iris, Yellow Flag, Yellow Iris.
CAUTION: See separate listing for Blue Flag.

Scientific Names

Iris germanica; Iris florentina, synonym Iris x germanica var. florentina; Iris pallida, synonym Rhizoma iridis.
Family: Iridaceae.

People Use This For

Orally, orris root is used for "blood-purifying", "gland-stimulating", increasing kidney activity, skin diseases (2), bronchitis, cold, cancer, stimulating appetite and digestion, stimulating bile flow, sciatica, sclerosis, splenitis. It is also used for diuretic, emetic, laxative, purgative, and stimulant properties (513).
Topically, orris root is used for halitosis, nasal polyps, teething, and as a dentifrice (513).
In combination with other herbs, orris root is used orally for headache, toothache, muscle and joint pain, migraine, neuralgia, acute and chronic respiratory tract mucous membrane inflammation, bronchitis, bronchial asthma, cough, mucous congestion, nasal mucous membrane inflammation, hoarseness, for improving bronchial and mucous membrane blood supply, interval therapy of asthma, care of heart, nerves, and stomach, for nervous disturbances of cardiovascular function, loss of appetite, gastrointestinal disturbances, bowel sluggishness, feeling of fullness,bloating,

ailments of gallbladder, liver and pancreas, diabetes, relief of irritations caused by urinary tract inflammatory diseases, skin diseases, and as a sedative (2).

In combination with other herbs, orris root is used topically for tumors, swelling of the lymph glands, uric acid sedimentation, kyphosis, keloid formation, rheumatic disorders, burns, and cuts (2).

Safety

POSSIBLY SAFE ...when used orally (12). Orris root must be carefully peeled and dried before using (2). Fresh root and juice can cause severe mucosal and skin irritation (12).

There is insufficient reliable information available about the safety of the topical use of orris.

PREGNANCY AND LACTATION: Insufficient reliable information available; avoid using.

Effectiveness

There is insufficient reliable information available about the effectiveness of orris.

Mechanism of Action

The applicable parts of orris are the rhizome and root. Orris root contains triterpenes, including irigermanal, and isoflavonoids, including irilon, irisolone, irigenine, and tectoridine. It also contains C-glucosylxanthones and a volatile oil. The chief constituents of the volatile oil are irones, particularly alpha-, beta-, and gamma-irone. Some think orris root has mild expectorant effects (18).

Adverse Reactions

No adverse effects are reported when orris root has been carefully peeled and dried. However, taken orally the fresh plant juice or root can cause severe mucosal irritation, abdominal pain, vomiting, and bloody diarrhea (18). Used topically, the fresh plant juice or root can cause severe skin and mucosal irritation (12,18).

Interactions with Herbs & Other Dietary Supplements

Insufficient reliable information available.

Interactions with Drugs

No interactions are known to occur, and there is no known reason to expect a clinically significant interaction with orris.

Interactions with Foods

No interactions are known to occur, and there is no known reason to expect a clinically significant interaction with orris.

Interactions with Lab Tests

No interactions are known to occur, and there is no known reason to expect a clinically significant interaction with orris.

Interactions with Diseases or Conditions

No interactions are known to occur, and there is no known reason to expect a clinically significant interaction with orris.

Dosage and Administration

No typical dosage.

Comments

Orris root is generally used in combination with other herbs and can be found in homeopathic dilutions and tea preparations (18). Historically, orris root was highly prized in the perfume industry. Upon drying, the root develops a pleasant violet-like scent. This scent continues to improve in storage, reaching its peak in about three years. Orris root was widely used in face powders and other cosmetics until it was determined to cause allergic reactions. Orris root powder is still used extensively in potpourris, sachets, and pomanders. It is one of the most effective fixatives and it prolongs the scent of the more transient volatile oils. Of the two orris species, Iris x germanica var. florentina root is considered superior to Iris pallida (4081).

OSHA

Also Known As
Bear Root, Chuchupate, Colorado Cough Root, Indian Parsley, Mountain Lovage, Porter's Licorice Root, Wild Celery Root.
CAUTION: See separate listings for Lovage and Licorice.

Scientific Names
Ligusticum porteri.
Family: Apiaceae (Umbelliferae).

People Use This For
Orally, osha is used for sore throat, bronchitis, cough, common cold, influenza, pneumonia, and indigestion. (6728,6730,6731). Osha is also used orally to treat other viral infections including herpes and AIDS/HIV (6731). Topically, osha is used to prevent infections of skin wounds (6728).
Traditionally, osha has also been used by Native American and Hispanic cultures for pneumonia, colds, bronchitis, influenza, tuberculosis, hay fever, and coughs (6731,6732,6737).

Safety
POSSIBLY SAFE ...when used orally and appropriately (12).
PREGNANCY: LIKELY UNSAFE ...when used orally. Osha has been used to stimulate menstruation and is reported to have abortifacient activity (12,19); contraindicated.
LACTATION: Insufficient reliable information available; avoid using.

Effectiveness
There is insufficient reliable information available about the effectiveness of osha.

Mechanism of Action
The applicable part of osha is the root (12). Osha contains the compound ligustilide, which might have antimicrobial and antiviral activities (6733,6734,6736). Preliminary evidence indicates that osha might have viral protease inhibitory effects. It might also inhibit the influenza virus (6733). To date, there are no studies published of osha use in humans or animals.

Adverse Reactions
None reported.

Interactions with Herbs & Other Dietary Supplements
Insufficient reliable information available.

Interactions with Drugs
No interactions are known to occur, and there is no known reason to expect a clinically significant interaction with osha.

Interactions with Foods
No interactions are known to occur, and there is no known reason to expect a clinically significant interaction with osha.

Interactions with Lab Tests
No interactions are known to occur, and there is no known reason to expect a clinically significant interaction with osha.

Interactions with Diseases or Conditions
No interactions are known to occur, and there is no known reason to expect a clinically significant interaction with osha.

Dosage and Administration
ORAL: As a tincture, osha is commonly taken as 20-60 drops up to 5 times daily. These are usually prepared as a 1:2 tincture with the fresh root or 1:5 tincture with the dried root (6729). Osha is often combined with other herbs and supplements and sold as a multi-ingredient product.

Comments
The leaves of osha are similar in appearance to the very toxic poison hemlock (6728,6732). Osha must be identified by the

root, which is described as malodorous with a strong celery-like odor, or should be obtained from reputable commercial sources (6728,6732). Osha, which grows at higher elevations in the western US, is difficult to cultivate (6732). The popularity of Osha has led to over harvesting of the wild plant (6732,6735). Osha has been designated an endangered plant by conservationists (6735).

OSTRICH FERN

Also Known As
None.

Scientific Names
Matteucccia struthiopteris.
Family: Aspleniaceae.

People Use This For
Ostrich fern is used for food. It is regarded as a seasonal delicacy (6).

Safety
LIKELY SAFE ...when used as a food if prepared appropriately (6,5002).
LIKELY UNSAFE ...when not cooked properly (6). May cause severe food poisoning.
PREGNANCY AND LACTATION: Insufficient reliable information available; avoid using.

Effectiveness
There is insufficient reliable information available about the effectiveness of ostrich fern (6).

Mechanism of Action
The applicable part of ostrich fern is the young shoot top. One field guide states wild ostrich fern greens have laxative properties (6). Toxins responsible for poisonings have not been identified, but they are believed deactivated by boiling. The CDC recommends thorough cooking (e.g. boiling for 10 minutes) before eating (5002).

Adverse Reactions
Centers for Disease Control and Prevention (CDC) links outbreaks of severe food poisoning to consumption of raw or lightly cooked fiddlehead ferns (6,5002). Ostrich fern can cause nausea, vomiting, abdominal cramping (6), diarrhea, and headaches after ingestion (5002).

Interactions with Herbs & Other Dietary Supplements
Insufficient reliable information available.

Interactions with Drugs
No interactions are known to occur, and there is no known reason to expect a clinically significant interaction with ostrich fern.

Interactions with Foods
No interactions are known to occur, and there is no known reason to expect a clinically significant interaction with ostrich fern.

Interactions with Lab Tests
No interactions are known to occur, and there is no known reason to expect a clinically significant interaction with ostrich fern.

Interactions with Diseases or Conditions
No interactions are known to occur, and there is no known reason to expect a clinically significant interaction with ostrich fern.

Dosage and Administration
ORAL: Cook young shoots of ostrich fern (fiddleheads) thoroughly (e.g. boiling for 10 minutes) before eating (5002).

Comments
The tops of the young shoots of ostrich fern, known as fiddleheads, are regarded as a seasonal delicacy.
They are available canned, frozen or fresh (6). Boil at least 10 minutes before eating.

OSWEGO TEA

Also Known As

Bee Balm, Bergamot, Blue Balm, High Balm, Low Balm, Monarda, Mountain Balm, Mountain Mint, Scarlet Monarda. CAUTION: See separate listings for Bergamot Oil, Bitter Orange peel, Sweet Orange, and Bitter Orange flower.

Scientific Names

Monarda didyma.
Family: Labitae or Lamiaceae.

People Use This For

Orally, oswego tea is used for digestive disorders including flatulence and premenstrual syndrome. It is also used as an antispasmodic and diuretic.
In Europe, oswego tea is used for decreasing fever and as a fragrance (18).

Safety

There is insufficient reliable information available about the safety of oswego tea.
PREGNANCY: UNSAFE ...when used orally because it may possibly promote menstruation and stimulate menstrual flow (12).
LACTATION: Insufficient reliable information available; avoid using.

Effectiveness

There is insufficient reliable information available about the effectiveness of oswego tea.

Mechanism of Action

There is insufficient reliable information available about the possible mechanism of action and active ingredients.

Adverse Reactions

None reported.

Interactions with Herbs & Other Dietary Supplements

Insufficient reliable information available.

Interactions with Drugs

No interactions are known to occur, and there is no known reason to expect a clinically significant interaction with oswego tea.

Interactions with Foods

No interactions are known to occur, and there is no known reason to expect a clinically significant interaction with oswego tea.

Interactions with Lab Tests

No interactions are known to occur, and there is no known reason to expect a clinically significant interaction with oswego tea.

Interactions with Diseases or Conditions

No interactions are known to occur, and there is no known reason to expect a clinically significant interaction with oswego tea.

Dosage and Administration

ORAL: Oswego tea is taken as tea prepared from the powdered herb (18).

Comments

Oswego tea got the alternate name bergamot because of the similarity of its pleasant scent to that of the oil of bergamot oranges (see separate listing). During the period of the Boston tea party, it was drunk in place of black tea. Lemon balm is also known as bee balm, a common name for oswego tea, and may be confused with it.

OX-EYE DAISY

Also Known As
Butter Daisy, Dun Daisy, Golden Daisy, Goldenseal, Great Ox-Eye, Herb Margaret, Horse Daisy, Horse Gowan, Marguerite, Maudlin Daisy, Maudlinwort, Moon Daisy, Moon Flower, Moon Penny, Ox Eye Daisy, Poverty Weed, White Daisy, White Weed.
CAUTION: See separate listing for Goldenseal (Hydrastis canadensis).

Scientific Names
Chrysanthemum leucanthemum.
Family: Compositae.

People Use This For
Orally, ox-eye daisy is used for indications similar to German chamomile. These uses include the common cold, cough, bronchitis, fever, mouth and pharynx inflammation, liver and gallbladder complaints, loss of appetite, and susceptibility to infection. It is also used as an antispasmodic, diuretic, and tonic (18).
Topically, ox-eye daisy is used for skin inflammation, wounds and burns.

Safety
There is insufficient reliable information available about the safety of ox-eye daisy.
Pregnancy and Lactation: Insufficient reliable information available; avoid using.

Effectiveness
There is insufficient reliable information available about the effectiveness of ox-eye daisy.

Mechanism of Action
The applicable parts of ox-eye daisy are the above ground flowering parts. There is insufficient reliable information available about the possible mechanism of action and active ingredients.

Adverse Reactions
Ox-eye daisy can cause an allergic reaction in individuals sensitive to the Asteraceae/Compositae family. Members of this family include ragweed, chrysanthemums, marigolds, daisies, and many other herbs.

Interactions with Herbs & Other Dietary Supplements
Insufficient reliable information available.

Interactions with Drugs
No interactions are known to occur, and there is no known reason to expect a clinically significant interaction with ox-eye daisy.

Interactions with Foods
No interactions are known to occur, and there is no known reason to expect a clinically significant interaction with ox-eye daisy.

Interactions with Lab Tests
No interactions are known to occur, and there is no known reason to expect a clinically significant interaction with ox-eye daisy.

Interactions with Diseases or Conditions
CROSS-ALLERGENICITY: Can cause an allergic reaction in individuals sensitive to the Asteraceae/Compositae family. Members of this family include ragweed, chrysanthemums, marigolds, daisies, and many other herbs.

Dosage and Administration
ORAL: The daily dose is equivalent to 10-15 grams dried herb, taken as tea. The tea is prepared by steeping 3 grams dried leaf in 150 mL of boiling water for 10-15 minutes and straining (18).
TOPICAL: A tea is prepared by steeping 2 teaspoons of dried leaf in 1 cup of boiling water for 15 minutes, straining and applied topically. As a bath additive, 50 grams of dried herb is added to 1 L bath water (18).

Comments
Ox-eye daisy is alternately known as goldenseal, but it is unrelated to the more commonly known goldenseal (Hydrastis canadensis).

PAGODA TREE

Also Known As
None.

Scientific Names
Sophora japonica.
Family: Leguminosae or Fabaceae.

People Use This For
Orally, pagoda tree is used in dilutions for dysentery (18).

Safety
POSSIBLY UNSAFE …when the seeds are used orally (18). Regular use of seed meal can cause facial edema or even death. High doses could cause cystine poisoning (18).
PREGNANCY AND LACTATION: POSSIBLY UNSAFE …when used orally (18); avoid using.

Effectiveness
There is insufficient reliable information available about the effectiveness of pagoda tree.

Mechanism of Action
The applicable parts of the pagoda tree are the seeds. Cystine poisoning may occur with high dosages (18).

Adverse Reactions
None reported with short term use. Using pagoda tree seed long term may cause edema and death (18).

Interactions with Herbs & Other Dietary Supplements
Insufficient reliable information available.

Interactions with Drugs
No interactions are known to occur, and there is no known reason to expect a clinically significant interaction with pagoda tree.

Interactions with Foods
No interactions are known to occur, and there is no known reason to expect a clinically significant interaction with pagoda tree.

Interactions with Lab Tests
No interactions are known to occur, and there is no known reason to expect a clinically significant interaction with pagoda tree.

Interactions with Diseases or Conditions
No interactions are known to occur, and there is no known reason to expect a clinically significant interaction with pagoda tree.

Dosage and Administration
No typical dosage.

Comments
None.

PANAX PSEUDOGINSENG

Also Known As
Field Seven, Pseudoginseng Root, Samch'il, San Qi, San Qui, Sanshichi, Three Seven, Tian Qi.
CAUTION: See separate listing for Ginseng Panax.

Scientific Names
Panax pseudodinseng; Panax notoginseng; Panax zingiberensis.

People Use This For

In Chinese medicine, Panax pseudoginseng root is used orally to stop bleeding, i.e., vomiting blood, coughing up blood, blood in the urine or stool, or nosebleed. It is also used to treat blood stasis, to relieve pain and reduce swelling, and to reduce blood cholesterol level. It is also used for angina and hemorrhagic disease (5558,5559). The flower of Panax pseudoginseng is sometimes used to reduce blood pressure, for dizziness, and acute sore throat (5559).

Topically, Panax pseudoginseng is used to stop bleeding (5559).

In combination with seven other herbs (PC-SPES), Panax pseudoginseng is used to treat prostate cancer (5548).

Safety

POSSIBLY SAFE ...when used orally in a specific herbal combination (PC-SPES) (5548).

There is insufficient reliable information available about the safety of Panax pseudoginseng for its other uses.

PREGNANCY AND LACTATION: LIKELY UNSAFE ...when used orally; contraindicated (5559).

Effectiveness

POSSIBLY EFFECTIVE ...when used orally in a specific herbal combination for prostate cancer. Studies using Panax pseudoginseng in combination with seven other herbs (PC-SPES), found that it significantly decreases prostate-specific antigen (PSA) levels (3576,5122,5548,6284,6286), causes clinically significant reductions in serum testosterone (5548), improves quality of life, and reduces pain (6286) in patients with prostate cancer. In two reports, PSA levels fell significantly within one month of treatment (5122,5548).

There is insufficient reliable information available about the effectiveness of Panax pseudoginseng for its other uses.

Mechanism of Action

The Panax pseudoginseng root contains 12% saponins. Water hydrolysis of the saponins produces panaxadiol and panaxatriol that are the genins of arasaponin. Panax pseudoginseng is believed to dilate the coronary vessels, reduce vascular resistance, and improve the coronary collateral circulation. This could increase blood flow while reducing blood pressure. It would also reduce the heart metabolic rate and oxygen consumption. Some evidence suggests Panax pseudoginseng also has an antiarrhythmic effect (5558). Trilinolein, a triacylglycerol purified from Panax pseudoginseng, might have antioxidant activity (6289).

Adverse Reactions

Orally, Panax pseudoginseng can cause dry mouth, flushed skin, nervousness, insomnia, nausea, and vomiting (5558).

Interactions with Herbs & Other Dietary Supplements

CARDIOACTIVE HERBS: Avoid concomitant use with other cardioactive herbs due to unpredictability of effects and adverse effects. Cardioactive herbs include: calamus, cereus, cola, coltsfoot, devil's claw, European mistletoe, fenugreek, fumitory, ginger, Panax ginseng, hawthorn, white horehound, mate, parsley, quassia, Scotch broom flower, shepherd's purse, and wild carrot (4). Cardiac glycoside containing herbs, include black hellebore, Canadian hemp roots, digitalis leaf, hedge mustard, figwort, lily of the valley roots, motherwort, oleander leaf, pheasant's eye plant, pleurisy root, squill bulb leaf scales, and strophanthus seeds (2,18,19,500).

Interactions with Drugs

CARDIOACTIVE DRUGS: Theoretically, Panax pseudoginseng could interfere with cardiovascular therapy; avoid using.

Interactions with Foods

No interactions are known to occur, and there is no known reason to expect a clinically significant interaction with Panax pseudoginseng.

Interactions with Lab Tests

CARDIAC FUNCTION: Panax pseudoginseng might improve tests of cardiovascular function.

Interactions with Diseases or Conditions

No interactions are known to occur, and there is no known reason to expect a clinically significant interaction with Panax pseudoginseng.

Dosage and Administration

ORAL: A typical dose is 1-1.5 grams divided into three doses per day (5558).
TOPICAL: No typical dosage.

Comments

None.

PANCREATIN

Also Known As

Pancreatinum, Pancreatis pulvis.

Scientific Names

Pancreatin.

People Use This For

Orally, pancreatin is used to treat malabsorption syndromes associated with pancreatic insufficiency in cystic fibrosis, chronic pancreatitis, or pancreas removal (15). It is also used for flatulence (14) or as a digestive aid.

Safety

LIKELY SAFE ...when used orally and appropriately for replacement therapy by individuals with pancreatic insufficiency (15). Some pancreatin products contaminated by Salmonella have caused illness (14). Use only products from reputable manufacturers.
PREGNANCY: Insufficient reliable information available; avoid using unless essential for replacement therapy (15).
LACTATION: Insufficient reliable information available; avoid using unless essential for replacement therapy (15).

Effectiveness

EFFECTIVE ...when used orally as replacement therapy in pancreatic insufficiency due to cystic fibrosis, chronic pancreatitis, or pancreas removal (14,15).
LIKELY INEFFECTIVE ...when used to treat digestive disorders not related to pancreatic insufficiency, including flatulence (15,16).

Mechanism of Action

Pancreatin contains digestive enzymes, principally lipase, protease, and amylase obtained from pork or beef pancreas (14,15). These enzymes catalyze the hydrolysis of fat into glycerol and fatty acids; peptides into proteoses, peptides, and derived substances; and starches into dextrins and sugars (14). They act principally in the duodenum and small intestine (14). Pancreatin is inactivated when acid, including gastric acid, is present in more than trace amounts (15).

Adverse Reactions

Orally, excessive doses of pancreatin can cause nausea, vomiting, diarrhea or other transient intestinal upset, and perianal soreness (14,15). Extremely high doses have been associated with high uric acid level in blood and urine, and colon strictures (14,15).
Topically, pancreatin preparations that are held in the mouth prior to swallowing can cause irritation of the mucosa, including ulceration and stomatitis (15). Pancreatin powder is irritating to the skin, eyes, mucus membranes, and respiratory tract. Skin contact with or inhalation of the powder should be avoided (14). Hypersensitivity reactions, e.g., sneezing, lacrimation, skin rash, have been reported (14,15). Inhalation of dust containing pancreatin has been associated with pulmonary hypersensitivity reactions, allergic rhinitis, bronchospasm, and asthma (14).

Interactions with Herbs & Other Dietary Supplements

FOLIC ACID: Pancreatin can decrease absorption of folic acid (14).

Interactions with Drugs

ACARBOSE (Precose): Enzymes present in pancreatin can decrease the efficacy of acarbose (14).
GASTRIC ACID INHIBITORS: Pancreatin activity ceases in gastric acid. For this reason, concomitant use of antacids, H-2 receptor antagonists, or other drugs that reduce stomach acidity can increase pancreatin activity (14).

Interactions with Foods
ACIDIC FOODS: Concomitant intake of acidic foods or fruit juices can break down pancreatin enzymes, reducing the activity of pancreatin preparations that are not enteric-coated (14).
ALKALINE FOODS: Mixing enteric-coated granules into alkaline foods, e.g. chicken, veal, green beans, might destroy the coating (14).

Interactions with Lab Tests
URIC ACID: Pancreatin can cause an increase in serum and urine uric acid levels (14).

Interactions with Diseases or Conditions
No interactions are known to occur, and there is no known reason to expect a clinically significant interaction with pancreatin.

Dosage and Administration
ORAL: For pancreatic replacement therapy, the initial dose of pancreatin is usually 8,000 to 24,000 USP units of lipase activity taken before or with each meal or snack. To control steatorrhea, dose can be increased as needed or until nausea, vomiting or diarrhea occurs (15). Pancreatin is available as enteric-coated tablets; powder; or capsules containing powder or enteric-coated granules (14). The powder or contents of the capsules can be mixed with food prior to administration, but should not be allowed to stand for more than an hour (14).

Comments
Each mg of pancreatin contains not less than 25 USP units of amylase activity, not less than 2 USP units of lipase activity, and not less than 25 USP units of protease activity (15,16). Pancreatin that is more potent is labeled as a multiple of these three minimum activities, e.g. pancreatin 4X (10,16).

PANGAMIC ACID

Also Known As
Calcium Chloride, Calcium Gluconate, Calcium Pangamate, Di-calcium Phosphate, Di-isopropylamine Dichloroacetate, Dicalcium Phosphate, Dimethyl Glycine, Dimethylglycine, DMG, Gluconic Acid, Glycine, Pangamate, Russian Formula, Sodium Gluconate, Vitamin B15.
CAUTION: See separate listing for Dimethylglycine.

Scientific Names
None.

People Use This For
Orally, pangamic acid is used for detoxifying the body; treating asthma and allied diseases; conditions of the skin and respiratory tract; painful nerve and joint afflictions; cell proliferation like cancer; eczema; arthritis; neuritis; and improving the oxygenation of the heart, brain, and other vital organs (5). It is also used for alcoholism, hangovers, fatigue, protecting against urban air pollutants, extending cell life, stimulating increased immune system response, lowering blood cholesterol levels, and assisting in hormone regulation (2643).

Safety
POSSIBLY UNSAFE ...when used orally (5,2623). There is no standard chemical identity for pangamic acid. Dichloroacetate, present in some formulations, is mutagenic, possibly carcinogenic. Dimethylglycine, present in some formulations, can react with nitrites in the intestines to form the potent carcinogen, dimethylnitrosamine (5).
PREGNANCY AND LACTATION: POSSIBLY UNSAFE ...when used orally because it is difficult to know what constituents are present. Dichloroacetate, present in some formulations, is mutagenic according to the Ames test (5).

Effectiveness
POSSIBLY INEFFECTIVE ...when used orally for improving exercise endurance (2645).
There is insufficient reliable information available about the effectiveness of pangamic acid for its other uses.

Mechanism of Action
There is no standard chemical identity for pangamic acid. Formulations can include one or more of the following: sodium gluconate, calcium gluconate, glycine, diisopropylamine dichloroacetate, dimethylglycine, calcium chloride, dicalcium phosphate, stearic acid, cellulose, or other constituents (5). Diisopropylamine acts on the smooth muscle to reduce blood pressure (5). In the intestines, dimethylglycine reacts with nitrates to form the potent carcinogen,

dimethylnitrosamine (5). The high phosphate content of dicalcium phosphate has been blamed for upper gastrointestinal lesions and deaths in experimental animals (2644).

Adverse Reactions
Orally, pangamic acid can be potentially carcinogenic (2623).

Interactions with Herbs & Other Dietary Supplements
CARDIAC GLYCOSIDE-CONTAINING HERBS: Theoretically, concomitant use of these herbs with large amounts of calcium salts, including calcium chloride and dicalcium phosphate, can increase the inotropic effects of cardiac glycosides and the risk of arrhythmias. Cardiac glycoside-containing herbs include black hellebore (19), Canadian hemp roots (19), digitalis leaf (500), figwort (4), lily of the valley roots (19,500), motherwort (4) oleander leaf (19), pheasant's eye plant (2,19), pleurisy root (19), squill bulb leaf scales (19,500), and strophanthus seeds (19).

Interactions with Drugs
DIGOXIN: Theoretically, concomitant use of digoxin with large amounts of calcium salts, such as calcium chloride and dicalcium phosphate, can increase the inotropic effects of digoxin and the risk of arrhythmias (15).
THIAZIDE DIURETICS: Theoretically, concomitant use of these diuretics with calcium salts like calcium chloride and dicalcium phosphate can result in hypercalcemia (15).
VERAPAMIL: Theoretically, concomitant use of verapamil with calcium salts, including calcium chloride and dicalcium phosphate, can decrease the drug's effects (506).

Interactions with Foods
No interactions are known to occur, and there is no known reason to expect a clinically significant interaction with pangamic acid.

Interactions with Lab Tests
No interactions are known to occur, and there is no known reason to expect a clinically significant interaction with pangamic acid.

Interactions with Diseases or Conditions
KIDNEY DYSFUNCTION: Use pangamic acid with caution, because it can cause oxalate stones and other kidney problems (5).

Dosage and Administration
No typical dosage.

Comments
There is no standard chemical identity for pangamic acid. Pangamic acid is the name given to a product originally claimed to contain D-gluconodimethyl aminoacetic acid, which was obtained from apricot kernels and later from rice bran (5,14). The name pangamic acid comes from the Greek: pan = universal, and gamic = seed, due to its presence in almost all seeds (14). It is also referred to as vitamin B15, but pangamic acid is not generally recognized as a vitamin (2623). Research by Soviet sports scientists focused attention on pangamic acid (2643), but little, if any, research has been conducted in the US (2643). The claims of pangamic acid's effectiveness are controversial (5). Natural sources for D-gluconodimethyl aminoacetic acid include brewer's yeast, whole brown rice, sesame seeds, and pumpkin seeds (2643).

PANTOTHENIC ACID (VITAMIN B5)

Also Known As
B Complex Vitamin, Calcii Pantothenas, Calcium Pantothenate, D-Calcium Pantothenate, D-Panthenol, D-Pantothenyl Alcohol, Dexpanthenol, Dexpanthenolum, Pantothenic, Pantothenol, Pantothenylol, Vitamin B-5, Vitamin B5.

Scientific Names
D-pantothenic acid; Pantothenic acid.

People Use This For
Orally, pantothenic acid is used for treating dietary deficiencies, acne, alcoholism, allergies, alopecia, asthma, autism, burning feet syndrome, candidiasis, cardiac failure, carpal tunnel syndrome, respiratory disorders, celiac disease, colitis, conjunctivitis, convulsions, and cystitis. It is also used orally for dandruff, depression, diabetic neuropathy, enhancing immune function, glossitis, gray hair, headache, hyperactivity, hypoglycemia, insomnia,

irritability, low blood pressure, multiple sclerosis, muscular dystrophy, muscular cramps in the legs associated with pregnancy or alcoholism, neuralgia, and obesity. Pantothenic acid is also used orally for osteoarthritis, rheumatoid arthritis, Parkinson's disease, peripheral neuritis, premenstrual syndrome (PMS), prostatitis, protection against mental and physical stress and anxiety, reducing adverse effects of thyroid therapy in congenital hypothyroidism, reducing signs of aging, reducing susceptibility to colds and other infections, retarded growth, shingles, skin disorders, stimulating adrenal glands, stomatitis, chronic fatigue syndrome, salicylate toxicity, streptomycin neurotoxicity, vertigo, and wound healing.

Topically, dexpanthenol, an analog of pantothenic acid, is used for itching, promoting healing of mild eczemas and dermatoses, insect stings, bites, poison ivy, diaper rash, acne, and preventing and treating acute radiotherapy skin reactions.

Intramuscularly or by intravenous infusion, dexpanthenol is used for stimulating intestinal peristalsis, to minimize the possibility of paralytic ileus after major abdominal surgery, for intestinal atony causing abdominal distension, postoperative or postpartum flatus, for postoperative delay in resumption of intestinal motility, and for treating paralytic ileus.

Safety

LIKELY SAFE …when used orally and appropriately. Amounts up to 10 grams have been ingested without significant adverse effects (14,15). …when used topically and appropriately short-term (14).
PREGNANCY: LIKELY SAFE …when used orally in amounts not exceeding the recommended daily allowance (RDA). The RDA during pregnancy is 6 mg (3094). There is insufficient reliable information about the safety of using pantothenic acid in amounts exceeding the RDA during pregnancy; avoid using.
LACTATION: LIKELY SAFE …when used orally in amounts not exceeding the recommended daily allowance (RDA). The RDA during lactation is 7 mg (3094). There is insufficient reliable information available about the safety of using pantothenic acid in amounts exceeding the RDA during lactation; avoid using.

Effectiveness

EFFECTIVE …when used orally to treat and prevent pantothenic acid deficiency (14).
POSSIBLY INEFFECTIVE …when used topically to treat or prevent skin reactions from radiation therapy. Twice daily topical application of dexpanthenol, an analog of pantothenic acid, to areas of irradiated skin does not seem to reduce erythema, desquamation, itching, or pain following radiation treatment (7192).
There is insufficient reliable information available about the effectiveness of pantothenic acid for its other uses.

Mechanism of Action

Pantothenic acid is required for intermediary metabolism of carbohydrates, proteins, and lipids (15). It is a precursor of coenzyme A which is required for acetylation reactions in gluconeogenesis, in the release of energy from carbohydrates, the synthesis and degradation of fatty acids, and the synthesis of sterols, steroid hormones, porphyrins, acetylcholine, and other compounds (15). Pantothenic acid also appears to be essential to normal epithelial function (15). Dietary deficiency of pantothenic acid has not been identified, but experimentally-induced deficiency has been associated with somnolence, fatigue, headache, paresthesia of the hands and feet followed by hyperreflexia and muscle weakness in the legs, cardiovascular instability, GI complaints, changes in disposition, and increased susceptibility to infections (15). Dexpanthenol is converted in the body to pantothenic acid, then coenzyme A which is a cofactor in acetylcholine synthesis. In large parenteral doses, dexpanthenol has been reported to increase gastrointestinal peristalsis by stimulating acetylation of choline to acetylcholine, but efficacy has not been proven (14,15). Some evidence suggests that dexpanthenol stimulates fibroblast proliferation and epithelialization (14).

Adverse Reactions

Orally, large amounts of pantothenic acid can cause diarrhea (14). There is also one case of eosinophilic pleuropericardial effusion in a patient taking pantothenic acid 300 mg per day in combination with biotin 10 mg per day for 2 months (3914).
Topically, dexpanthenol, an alcohol analog of pantothenic acid, can cause chronic dermatitis (14).

Interactions with Herbs & Other Dietary Supplements

Insufficient reliable information available.

Interactions with Drugs

PARASYMPATHOMIMETICS: Theoretically, administration of dexpanthenol, the alcohol analog of pantothenic acid, within 12 hours after administration of parasympathomimetics, e.g., neostigmine, might cause additive effects (15). Theoretically, this interaction might also occur with pantothenic acid and calcium pantothenate.
ANTICHOLINESTERASE EYE DROPS: Dexpanthenol might potentiate the miotic effects of echothiophate iodide or isoflurophate eye drops, but the clinical significance is not known (15).

Drug Influences on Nutrient Levels and Depletion
SOME DRUGS CAN AFFECT PANTOTHENIC ACID LEVELS:
ANTIBIOTICS: Destruction of normal gastrointestinal flora by antibiotics can cause decreased production of B vitamins. The clinical significance of this decreased production is not known. Consider supplementation only if clinical judgment warrants it (4434,4435,4436,4437,4438,4439,4440,4441,4442,4443).

Interactions with Foods
No interactions are known to occur, and there is no known reason to expect a clinically significant interaction with pantothenic acid.

Interactions with Lab Tests
No interactions are known to occur, and there is no known reason to expect a clinically significant interaction with pantothenic acid.

Interactions with Diseases or Conditions
HEMOPHILIA: Dexpanthenol (alcohol analog of pantothenic acid) may prolong bleeding time (15).
GI OBSTRUCTION: Dexpanthenol (alcohol analog of pantothenic acid) injection is contraindicated in individuals with gastrointestinal obstruction (15).

Dosage and Administration
ORAL: As a dietary supplement, 5-10 mg pantothenic acid (15) has been used. Recommended daily intakes for vitamin B5 are as follows; Infants 0-6 months, 1.7 mg; Infants 7-12 months, 1.8 mg; Children 1-3 years, 2 mg; Children 4-8 years, 3 mg; Children 9-13 years, 4 mg; Men and women 14 years and older, 5 mg (3094); Pregnant women, 6 mg; and Lactating women, 7 mg (3094).
TOPICAL: Dexpanthenol 2% cream applied to the affected areas once or twice daily (15). Dexpanthenol is the alcohol analog of pantothenic acid.
INJECTION: Dexpanthenol for injection is a FDA-approved prescription drug.

Comments
Only the dextrorotatory isomer of pantothenic acid has biologic activity (15). Vitamin B5 is commercially available as D-pantothenic acid and the synthetic derivatives, dexpanthenol and calcium pantothenate (15). Pantothenic acid is widely distributed in plant and animal tissues; rich sources include meat, vegetables, cereal grains, legumes, eggs, and milk (15). Calcium pantothenate 10 mg is equivalent to pantothenic acid 9.2 mg (15). Pantothenic acid is frequently used in combination with other B vitamins in vitamin B complex formulations. Vitamin B complex generally includes vitamin B1 (thiamine), vitamin B2 (riboflavin), vitamin B3 (niacin/niacinamide), vitamin B5 (pantothenic acid), vitamin B6 (pyridoxine), vitamin B12 (cyanocobalamin), and folic acid. However, some products do not contain all of these ingredients and some may include others, such as biotin, para-aminobenzoic acid (PABA), choline bitartrate, and inositol (3022,3060,3061).

PAPAIN

Also Known As
Papainum Crudum, Plant Protease Concentrate, Vegetable Pepsin.
CAUTION: See separate listings for Bromelain, Papaya, and American Pawpaw.

Scientific Names
Carica papaya.
Family: Caricacea.

People Use This For
Orally, papain is used for inflammation and edema following trauma and surgery, as a digestive aid, for treating parasitic worms (2), inflammation of the throat and pharynx (964,968,969), herpes zoster symptoms (965), chronic diarrhea, hay fever, nasal drainage, and psoriasis. Papain is also used as an adjuvant treatment for tumors.
Topically, it is used to treat infected wounds, sores, and ulcers (11).
In manufacturing, papain is a component of cosmetics, dentifrices, enzymatic soft contact lens cleaners, meat tenderizers, and meat products. It is also used for stabilizing and chillproofing beer (11).

Safety
LIKELY SAFE ...when used orally in amounts commonly found in foods. Papain has Generally Recognized as Safe (GRAS) status in the US (11).

POSSIBLY SAFE ...when used orally and appropriately for medicinal purposes (964,968,969).
POSSIBLY UNSAFE ...when used orally in large amounts. In excessive doses, papain can cause significant side effects including esophageal perforation (6) ...when raw papain is used topically. Raw papain or papaya latex is a severe irritant and vesicant (6).
PREGNANCY: POSSIBLY UNSAFE ...when used orally. There is some concern that crude papain is teratogenic and embryotoxic (6).
LACTATION: Insufficient reliable information available; avoid using.

Effectiveness

POSSIBLY EFFECTIVE ...when used orally in combination with other agents for treating inflammation and swelling in patients with pharyngitis (964,968,969). ...when used orally for treating symptoms of herpes zoster (965).
LIKELY INEFFECTIVE ...when used as a vermifuge (2).
There is insufficient reliable information available about the effectiveness of papain for its other uses.

Mechanism of Action

Papain is actually a mixture of the proteolytic enzymes papain, chymopapain A, chymopapain B, and papaya peptidase A isolated from the fruit of Carica papaya. Chymopapain A and B have a similar proteolytic spectrum to papain but are less potent (6). There is some evidence that a multi-enzyme preparation containing papain can increase the release of reactive oxygen species (ROS) by polymorphonuclear cells (PMNs). ROS are thought to have tumoricidal effects (962). The multi-enzyme preparation also seems to induce the cytokines tumor necrosis factor (TNF)-alpha, interleukin-1 (IL-1)-beta, and interleukin-6 (IL-6) in a time and dose dependent manner (1364).

Adverse Reactions

Orally, large amounts of papain can cause esophageal perforation (6). Ingestion of papaya latex (raw papain) can cause severe gastritis.
Topically, papaya latex can cause severe irritation and blisters (6). Topical use of papain can cause itching (966). Severe allergic reactions have been reported in sensitive individuals (6,967). One case report suggests that there may be cross-sensitivity between papain, fig, and kiwi (963).

Interactions with Herbs & Other Dietary Supplements

HERBS WITH ANTICOAGULANT/ANTIPLATELET POTENTIAL: Concomitant use of herbs that have coumarin constituents or affect platelet aggregation could theoretically increase the risk of bleeding in some people. These herbs include: angelica, anise, arnica, asafoetida, bogbean, boldo, capsicum, celery, chamomile, clove, danshen, fenugreek, feverfew, garlic, ginger, ginkgo, ginseng (Panax), horse chestnut, horseradish, licorice, meadowsweet, prickly ash, onion, passionflower, poplar, quassia, red clover, turmeric, wild carrot, wild lettuce, willow, and others (4,19).

Interactions with Drugs

ANTICOAGULANT, ANTIPLATELET DRUGS: Theoretically, concomitant use may increase risk of bleeding. There is one case report of increased International Normalization Ratio (INR) associated with concomitant use of warfarin (Coumadin) and papaya extract (papain) (613).

Interactions with Foods

POTATO PROTEIN: May inhibit papain proteolytic activity (958).
FIG, KIWI: Cross sensitivity to papain may occur in individuals sensitive to fig and kiwi (963).

Interactions with Lab Tests

INTERNATIONAL NORMALIZATION RATIO (INR): Concomitant use of papaya extract (papain) and warfarin may increase INR (613).

Interactions with Diseases or Conditions

CLOTTING DISORDERS: Avoid; theoretically, may increase bleeding risk (2).

Dosage and Administration

ORAL: 1500 mg (2520 FIP units) per day have been used in clinical trials to treat inflammation and swelling following trauma and surgery (2).
TOPICAL: No typical dosage.

Comments

None.

PAPAYA

Also Known As
Caricae papayae folium, Mamaerie, Melon Tree, Melonenbaumblaetter, Papaw, Papayas.
CAUTION: See separate listings for Papain and American Pawpaw.

Scientific Names
Carica papaya.
Family: Caricaceae.

People Use This For
In folk medicine, papaya is used orally for preventing and treating gastrointestinal tract disorders, intestinal parasite infections, and as sedative and diuretic (2). Papaya is used topically in folk medicine for nervous pains and elephantoid growths (4009).

Safety
LIKELY SAFE ...when consumed in amounts commonly found in foods (11). Papaya has Generally Recognized as Safe (GRAS) status in the US (11).
POSSIBLY SAFE ...when used orally and appropriately (6).
POSSIBLY UNSAFE ...when used orally in large amounts because papaya may cause esophageal perforation (6). ...when used topically because papaya latex (raw papain) is a severe irritant and vesicant (6).
PREGNANCY: POSSIBLY UNSAFE ...when used orally; avoid using. Crude papain shows evidence that it is teratogenic and embryotoxic (6); however, this might be due to extraneous substances rather than papain (11).
LACTATION: Insufficient reliable information available; avoid using.

Effectiveness
There is insufficient reliable information available about the effectiveness of papaya.

Mechanism of Action
The applicable part of papaya is the leaf. Papaya leaf contains 2% papain and carpain (6). Papain is a mixture of enzymes that degrade protein, carbohydrates, and fats (515). Papain is unstable in digestive juices, which raises questions about whether it can be effective when used orally (515). Carpain is thought to be amebicidal. It might cause bradycardia (4009) or have central nervous system depressant or paralytic effects.

Adverse Reactions
Ingestion of large amounts of papain might cause esophageal perforation. Severe allergic reactions can occur in individuals sensitive to papain (6,515).

Interactions with Herbs & Other Dietary Supplements
PAPAIN: Concomitant use of papain and papaya can increase the effects and adverse effects of papain.

Interactions with Drugs
WARFARIN: Concomitant use might potentiate the effects of warfarin (Coumadin) increasing the international normalization ratio (INR) (613).

Interactions with Foods
No interactions are known to occur, and there is no known reason to expect a clinically significant interaction with papaya.

Interactions with Lab Tests
INTERNATIONAL NORMALIZATION RATIO (INR): Papain, which is in papaya leaf, can increase INR in people maintained on warfarin (Coumadin) (613).

Interactions with Diseases or Conditions
No interactions are known to occur, and there is no known reason to expect a clinically significant interaction with papaya.

Dosage and Administration
ORAL: People typically use papaya with enzyme chewable tablets which contain 250 mg of papaya powder, 150 mg of dried pineapple juice powder, and 10 mg of papain (5024). One tablet is chewed up to three times daily, preferably after a meal (5024).

Comments

Fermenting papaya leaves may make more potent, richer brewed teas (515).

PARA-AMINOBENZOIC ACID (PABA)

Also Known As

4-Aminobenzoic Acid, ABA, Aminobenzoate Potassium, Aminobenzoic Acid, Ethyl Dihydroxypropyl Aminobenzoate, Glyceryl Paraaminobenzoate, Octyl Diemthyl PABA, PABA, Padamate O, P-Aminobenzoic Acid, Para Amino Benzoic Acid, Para Aminobenzoic Acid, Paraaminobenzoic Acid, Vitamin B10, Vitamin H.

Scientific Names

Para-aminobenzoic acid.

People Use This For

Orally, PABA is used for vitiligo, pemphigus, dermatomyositis, morphea, scleroderma, and Peyronie's disease (10,266,1050). PABA is also used orally to treat female infertility, arthritis, anemia, rheumatic fever, constipation, and headaches (16,1050,1057). It is also used orally to darken gray hair, prevent hair loss, rejuvenate the skin, and prevent phototoxic reactions (1050,1061).
Topically, PABA is used as a sunscreen (266).
Historically, PABA was used for disseminated systemic lupus erythematosus and lymphoblastoma cutis (16).

Safety

LIKELY SAFE ...when used topically and appropriately. PABA is FDA approved for topical use and there have not been reports of significant toxicity (266,272).
POSSIBLY SAFE ...when used orally and appropriately (10). PABA is a FDA-approved drug, but some potentially serious side effects have been reported (10).
POSSIBLY UNSAFE ...when used orally in high doses. Doses greater than 12 grams per day have been associated with leukopenia (1061).
CHILDREN: LIKELY SAFE ...when used topically and appropriately (266,272). POSSIBLY SAFE ...when used orally and appropriately (10). PABA is a FDA-approved drug for use in children, but serious side effects have been reported (10). POSSIBLY UNSAFE ...when used orally in high doses. Doses greater than 220 mg/kg/day have been associated with fatal toxic effects (1061).
PREGNANCY AND LACTATION: LIKELY SAFE ...when used topically and appropriately (266,272). There is insufficient reliable information available about the safety of the oral use of PABA during pregnancy and breast-feeding; avoid using.

Effectiveness

EFFECTIVE ...when used topically and appropriately as a sunscreen. PABA is a FDA approved sunscreen (266). PABA seems to be effective during sweating, but will lose effectiveness if the skin is immersed in water (272).
POSSIBLY INEFFECTIVE ...when used orally to treat scleroderma (1074). Although PABA is FDA approved for scleroderma, evidence supporting PABA for scleroderma is limited. Some retrospective studies suggest it might help for some symptoms of scleroderma (1071,1073,1075), but the most convincing evidence shows that it does not help (1074). There is insufficient reliable information available about the effectiveness of PABA for its other uses. Although PABA is a FDA-approved drug for use in vitiligo, pemphigus, dermatomyositis, morphea, and Peyronie's disease (10), there is very limited evidence to support these uses (10,1067). More evidence is needed to rate PABA for these uses.

Mechanism of Action

Para-aminobenzoic Acid (PABA) is a part of the folic acid molecule (16) and is found naturally in several foods including grains, eggs, milk, and meat (266). PABA was once considered to be a B vitamin, but is now thought to be a nonessential nutrient (16). Interestingly, pathogenic bacteria require PABA to synthesize folic acid. Sulfonamide antibiotics exert their antibacterial effect by inhibiting folic acid synthesis from PABA (16). Although blood, urine, sweat, and spinal fluid contain detectable amounts of PABA, deficiency of PABA has not been described in humans. (266). Endogenous PABA seems to be involved in a number of biologic processes, but its precise role is not known (10,266). PABA is exogenously administered for fibrotic diseases such as dermatomyositis, morphea, pemphigus, Peyronie's disease, and scleroderma because these conditions might be caused by an imbalance of serotonin and monoamine oxidase (MAO) activity. PABA might enhance MAO activity by increasing tissue oxygenation. MAO requires significant tissue oxygenation to function properly (10,266). Topically, PABA is used as a sunscreen because it can block transmission of ultraviolet (UV) radiation to the epidermis (272). PABA primarily blocks UVB sunlight, but may give some protection against UVA radiation at higher concentrations (272).

Adverse Reactions

Orally, nausea, vomiting, dyspepsia, diarrhea, and anorexia are the most common side effects of PABA (10,1074). PABA should be discontinued if adverse effects prevent the patient from eating (10). In one report up to 25% of patients discontinued PABA due to intolerance of side effects (1074). Allergic reactions including fever and skin rash have also occurred (10,1074). Liver toxicity, including fatal hepatitis has been reported in patients taking high doses (12-48 grams per day) (1061,1094). In one case 12 grams per day for 2 months caused liver toxicity (1094). Although PABA is sometimes used to treat vitiligo, it has also been reported to cause vitiligo (1086). High dose PABA (up to 48 grams per day) can also cause decreased white blood count below 4,000 mm3 in approximately 30% of patients (1061). Death has also been reported in 3 children treated with 24 grams of PABA per day for rheumatic fever or arthritis. At autopsy, all had fatty changes in the liver, kidney, and myocardium (1061).

Topically, PABA can cause contact dermatitis and sometimes paradoxical photosensitivity (272). Some forms of PABA may stain clothing with a yellow discoloration (266).

Interactions with Herbs & Other Dietary Supplements

Insufficient reliable information available.

Interactions with Drugs

DAPSONE (Avlosulfon): PABA might inhibit the antibacterial effects of dapsone; avoid concurrent use (266).
SULFONAMIDE ANTIBIOTICS: PABA inhibits the antimicrobial activity of sulfonamide antibiotics. Sulfonamide antibiotics exert antibacterial effect by competitively inhibiting folic acid synthesis from PABA. Excess PABA may overcome the folate depleting effect of the sulfonamides (10). Avoid using PABA concurrently with sulfonamide antibiotics. Sulfonamide antibiotics include sulfadiazine, sulfisoxazole (Gantrisin), sulfamethoxazole (Gantanol), sulfamethizole (Thiosulfil Forte), sulfasalazine (Azulfidine), and co-trimoxazole (trimethoprim-sulfamethoxazole, Bactrim, Septra).

Interactions with Foods

No interactions are known to occur, and there is no known reason to expect a clinically significant interaction with PABA.

Interactions with Lab Tests

LEUKOPENIA: White blood cell count might be transiently reduced when PABA is initiated, especially with high doses, but normalizes with continued administration (10).
LIVER FUNCTION TESTS: PABA has been reported to elevate liver function tests (1084). Monitor liver function tests at baseline, one month after initiating PABA therapy, and every 3 to 6 months thereafter (1084).

Interactions with Diseases or Conditions

RENAL DISEASE: PABA is renally excreted and might accumulate in patients with renal dysfunction (10); use cautiously. Dose adjustments may be necessary.

Dosage and Administration

ORAL: For vitiligo, pemphigus, dermatomyositis, morphea, scleroderma, and Peyronie's disease, the FDA approved dose for adults is 12 grams daily in 4 to 6 divided doses of the potassium salt of PABA (10). In children, the FDA approved dose is 220 mg/kg per day in 4 to 6 divided doses. PABA should be taken with meals or a snack to avoid stomach upset (10). Since PABA is renally excreted, dosage adjustments might be necessary in renal dysfunction.
TOPICAL: PABA sunscreens come in concentrations of 1 to 15% (272).

Comments

PABA appears to have fallen into disuse due to lack of proven efficacy and fears of significant toxicity (1061,1065,1084). However, lower doses of PABA, typically 100 mg per tablet, are included in some multivitamins (1050).

PAREIRA

Also Known As

Ice Vine, Pereira Brava, Velvet Leaf.
CAUTION: See separate listing for Abuta.

Scientific Names

Chondrodendron tomentosum.
Family: Menispermaceae.

People Use This For
Orally, pareira is used as a diuretic and to promote menstruation (18).
Parenterally, the component tubocurarine is used as a neuromuscular blocking agent (18,505).

Safety
There is insufficient reliable information available about the safety of pareira.
PREGNANCY: UNSAFE ...when used orally or parenterally because it may promote menstruation (19).
LACTATION: Insufficient reliable information available; avoid using.

Effectiveness
There is insufficient reliable information available about the effectiveness of pareira.

Mechanism of Action
The applicable part of pareira is the root. Pareira contains tubocurarine, which is used in modern anesthetics. It competitively inhibits acetylcholine binding at the nicotinic receptors at the neuromuscular junction, resulting in skeletal muscle paralysis. Tubocurarine and the other curare-like alkaloids contained in pareira are quaternary alkaloids and carry a positive charge that is not altered by pH. For this reason, they are poorly absorbed when taken orally and therefore have little neuromuscular blocking activity (505).

Adverse Reactions
None reported when pareira is used orally (18). Tubocurarine can cause hypotension due to histamine release and ganglionic blockade if IV administration is too rapid. The histamine release can also cause increased salivation, and bronchospasm. The ganglionic blockade can cause decreased GI motility and tone. Tubocurarine can also cause allergic reactions in susceptible patients (15).

Interactions with Herbs & Other Dietary Supplements
Insufficient reliable information available.

Interactions with Drugs
No interactions are known to occur, and there is no known reason to expect a clinically significant interaction with pareira.

Interactions with Foods
No interactions are known to occur, and there is no known reason to expect a clinically significant interaction with pareira.

Interactions with Lab Tests
No interactions are known to occur, and there is no known reason to expect a clinically significant interaction with pareira.

Interactions with Diseases or Conditions
No interactions are known to occur, and there is no known reason to expect a clinically significant interaction with pareira.

Dosage and Administration
No typical dosage.

Comments
Tubocurarine, a constituent of pareira, is unsafe for parenteral self-medication (15,505).

PARSLEY leaf, root

Also Known As
Common Parsley, Garden Parsley, Hamburg Parsley, Persely, Persil, Petersylinge, Petroselini herba, Petrosilini radix, Rock Parsley.
CAUTION: See separate listings for Fool's Parsley, Parsley Piert, and Parsley seed.

Scientific Names

Carum petroselinum; Petroselinum crispum, synonym Apium petroselinum; Petroselinum hortense; Petroselinum sativum.
Family: Apiaceae or Umbelliferae.

People Use This For

Orally, parsley leaf/root is used as a breath freshener, for urinary tract infections, and kidney or bladder stones (2,11,18). Topically, parsley leaf/root is used for cracked or chapped skin (11), bruises, tumors, insect bites, lice, parasites, and to stimulate hair growth (6).
Traditionally, parsley is used for gastrointestinal disorders (6,18); constipation (6); jaundice (6,18); flatulence; indigestion; colic; bronchitic cough (4,6,11); asthma; general edema; rheumatism (11); anemia; hypotension; diseases of the prostate, liver, and spleen; and to promote menstrual flow (4,6,11,18). It has also been used as an aphrodisiac (6).
In foods and beverages, parsley leaf/root is widely used as a garnish, condiment, food, and as a flavoring (11).

Safety

LIKELY SAFE ...when used orally in amounts used in foods. Parsley has Generally Recognized as Safe (GRAS) status in the US (11).
POSSIBLY SAFE ...when used orally and appropriately in amounts larger than those found in foods (2,12).
LIKELY UNSAFE ...when used orally in very large amounts (i.e. 200 grams) the apiole constituent could cause toxicity. Apiole can cause blood dyscrasias and kidney and liver toxicity (4). ...when parsley oil is ingested orally due to the amount of the potentially toxic constituents, apiole and myristicin, in the oil (2,11). Myristicin can cause giddiness and hallucinations (4).
There is insufficient reliable information available about the safety of the topical use of parsley leaf/root.
PREGNANCY: LIKELY SAFE ...when parsley is used in food amounts. LIKELY UNSAFE ...when larger amounts are used orally due to potential abortifacient, uterine or menstrual flow stimulant effects (4,12,515).
LACTATION: Insufficient reliable information available; avoid using.

Effectiveness

There is insufficient reliable information available about the effectiveness of parsley leaf and root.

Mechanism of Action

Parsley leaf/root contains a volatile oil, carotene, vitamin B1, vitamin B2, and vitamin C (515). The volatile oil contains apiole, myristicin, and photosensitizing furanocoumarins (psoralens) (512); however, the amounts vary significantly among varieties of parsley (512). Parsley has antiflatulent, antispasmodic, antirheumatic, expectorant, antimicrobial (4), and aquaretic effects (6,18,512). Aquaretics increase urine volume (water loss) but not sodium excretion (512). The constituent apiole appears to be associated with antispasmodic, vasodilator, and menstrual flow-stimulant effects. Apiole can also increase smooth muscle contractibility in the bladder and intestines (11). Both the apiole and myristicin constituents are believed to have aquaretic and uterine stimulant effects (512). The mechanism of aquaresis is that parsley irritates the kidney epithelium which increases renal blood flow and glomerular filtration rate (512). Apiole and myristicin have a structure similar to safrole. Safrole is considered carcinogenic and hepatotoxic (4).

Adverse Reactions

Parsley leaf/root can occasionally cause allergic skin or mucous membrane reactions (2). Adverse effects specifically associated with more than 10 grams of the constituent, apiole, include hemolytic anemia, thrombocytopenia purpura, nephrosis, hepatic dysfunction, and kidney irritation (4). Adverse effects specifically associated with the constituent, myristicin, include giddiness, deafness, hallucinations, hypotension, bradycardia, paralysis, and fatty degeneration of the liver and kidneys (4). Parsley oil can cause contact photodermatitis with sun exposure (4).

Interactions with Herbs & Other Dietary Supplements

Insufficient reliable information available.

Interactions with Drugs

ANTICOAGULANTS: Theoretically, large amounts of parsley leaf/root might interfere with oral anticoagulant therapy, due to the vitamin K contained in parsley (19).
ASPIRIN: Concomitant intake might augment parsley allergy. One case is reported of severe urticaria and swelling in a person with a known mild parsley allergy after consuming parsley and aspirin (5054).
DIURETICS: Theoretically, parsley leaf/root might interfere with diuretic therapy by enhancing sodium retention (512).
MAOIs: Theoretically, concomitant use of large amounts of parsley leaf/root or parsley oil might potentiate monoamine oxidase inhibitor drug therapy, due to the myristicin contained in parsley (4).

Interactions with Foods

No interactions are known to occur, and there is no known reason to expect a clinically significant interaction with parsley leaf and root.

Interactions with Lab Tests

No interactions are known to occur, and there is no known reason to expect a clinically significant interaction with parsley leaf and root.

Interactions with Diseases or Conditions

EDEMA: Theoretically, parsley leaf/root might increase sodium retention and worsen edema (512).
HYPERTENSION: Theoretically, parsley leaf/root might increase sodium retention and worsen hypertension (512).
KIDNEY DISEASE: Contraindicated in individuals with kidney disease or inflammation. Parsley leaf/root can aggravate these conditions (4,19).

Dosage and Administration

ORAL: A typical dose for use as a mild diuretic is one cup tea two to three times daily. To make tea, steep 2 grams finely chopped dried root in 150 mL boiling water 10-15 minutes, strain (8). Maximum daily dose is 6 grams root/leaf (2). When used to flush the kidneys, large amounts of water should be consumed (2).
TOPICAL: No typical dosage.

Comments

None.

PARSLEY PIERT

Also Known As

Field Lady's Mantle, Parsley Breakstone, Parsley Piercestone.
CAUTION: See separate listings for Fool's Parsley, Parsley leaf, root and Parsley seed.

Scientific Names

Aphanes arvensis.
Family: Rosaceae.

People Use This For

Orally, parsley piert is used for reducing fever, urinary tract disorders such as kidney and bladder stones, and as a diuretic (18).

Safety

There is insufficient reliable information available about the safety of parsley piert.
Pregnancy and Lactation: Insufficient reliable information available; avoid using.

Effectiveness

There is insufficient reliable information available about the effectiveness of parsley piert.

Mechanism of Action

The applicable parts of parsley piert are the above ground parts. There is insufficient reliable information available about the possible mechanism of action and active ingredients of parsley piert.

Adverse Reactions

None reported.

Interactions with Herbs & Other Dietary Supplements

Insufficient reliable information available.

Interactions with Drugs

No interactions are known to occur, and there is no known reason to expect a clinically significant interaction with parsley piert.

Interactions with Foods

No interactions are known to occur, and there is no known reason to expect a clinically significant interaction with parsley piert.

Interactions with Lab Tests

No interactions are known to occur, and there is no known reason to expect a clinically significant interaction with parsley piert.

Interactions with Diseases or Conditions

No interactions are known to occur, and there is no known reason to expect a clinically significant interaction with parsley piert.

Dosage and Administration

ORAL: People typically prepare parsley piert as a tea with 1 to 2 teaspoons of the dried herb added to 1 cup boiling water. The usual dose is 3 cups per day. In tincture form, the usual dose is 2 to 4 mL three times daily (5253).

Comments

Avoid confusion with parsley (Petroselinum crispum) and fool's parsley (Aethusa cynapium).
There is very little scientific information about this product. Our staff is continually analyzing the available information on natural medicines and will add data here as it becomes available.

PARSLEY seed

Also Known As

Common Parsley, Garden Parsley, Parsley Fruit, Persil, Petroselini fructus.
CAUTION: See separate listings for Fool's Parsley, Parsley leaf, root and Parsley Piert.

Scientific Names

Petroselinum crispum, synonym Apium petroselinum; Carum petroselinum; Petroselinum hortense; Petroselinum sativum.
Family: Apiaceae or Umbelliferae.

People Use This For

Orally, parsley seed is used for ailments of the gastrointestinal tract and urinary tract (2,18), stimulating appetite and improving digestion, treating flatulence, and stimulating menstrual flow (515).
Traditionally, parsley seed has been used orally for inducing abortion (11,515), treating jaundice, menstrual difficulties, asthma, coughs, indigestion, and edema (11).
In foods, parsley seed oil is used as a flavoring (11).
In manufacturing, parsley seed oil is used as a fragrance in soaps, cosmetics, and perfumes (11).

Safety

LIKELY SAFE ...when used orally in amounts found in foods.
POSSIBLY UNSAFE ...when parsley seed is used orally in tea. The volatile oil of parsley has toxic constituents, and the tea might have a low volatile oil content (2).
LIKELY UNSAFE ...when parsley seed or seed oil is used orally in amounts greater than found in foods. The volatile oil constituent has been associated with renal epithelium irritation and cardiac arrhythmias (2). ...when parsley seed oil is used topically, it can cause photodermatitis upon sun exposure (4).
PREGNANCY: LIKELY UNSAFE ...when used orally (2,19). Might have abortifacient, uterine, and menstrual flow-stimulating effects (4,515).
LACTATION: Insufficient reliable information available; avoid using.

Effectiveness

There is insufficient reliable information available about the effectiveness of parsley seed.

Mechanism of Action

It is thought that parsley seed's effects can cause mild aquaresis, stimulate appetite, and improve digestion, as a result of the volatile oil content (515). Aquaretics increase urine volume (water loss) but not sodium excretion (512). The constituent apiole is thought to be responsible for antispasmodic, vasodilator, and menstrual flow-stimulant effects. Apiole can increase smooth muscle contractibility in the bladder and intestines (11). Both the apiole and myristicin constituents are believed to have aquaretic and uterine stimulant effects (512). Researchers think aquaretic effects of parsley result from irritation of the kidney epithelium that increases renal blood flow and glomerular filtration rate (512). Apiole and myristicin are documented to have a structure similar to safrole which is known to be carcinogenic and hepatotoxic (4). Parsley seed oil is reported to stimulate hepatic regeneration (4).

Adverse Reactions
Orally, parsley seed oil can cause renal damage and cardiac arrhythmias (2). Adverse effects specifically associated greater than 10 grams of the constituent apiole include hemolytic anemia, thrombocytopenia purpura, nephrosis, hepatic dysfunction, and kidney irritation (4). Adverse effects specifically associated with the constituent myristicin include giddiness, deafness, hallucinations, hypotension, bradycardia, paralysis, and fatty degeneration of the liver and kidneys (4). External use of parsley seed oil can cause contact photodermatitis upon exposure to the sun (4).

Interactions with Herbs & Other Dietary Supplements
Insufficient reliable information available.

Interactions with Drugs
DIURETICS: Theoretically, parsley seed might increase sodium retention and interfere with diuretic therapy (512).
MAOIs: Theoretically, concomitant use of large amounts of parsley seed or seed oil can potentiate monoamine oxidase inhibitor drug therapy due to the constituent myristicin (4).

Interactions with Foods
No interactions are known to occur, and there is no known reason to expect a clinically significant interaction with parsley seed.

Interactions with Lab Tests
No interactions are known to occur, and there is no known reason to expect a clinically significant interaction with parsley seed.

Interactions with Diseases or Conditions
EDEMA: Theoretically, parsley seed might increase sodium retention and worsen edema (512).
HYPERTENSION: Theoretically, parsley seed might increase sodium retention and worsen hypertension (512).
KIDNEY DISEASE: Contraindicated in individuals with kidney disease or inflammation. Parsley seed can aggravate these conditions (4,19).

Dosage and Administration
ORAL: A typical oral dose is one cup tea up to 2-3 times per day. To make tea, steep 1 gram of fresh crushed seed in 150 mL boiling water for 10 minutes, strain (18).

Comments
Parsley seed oil is distilled from the seeds of parsley (Petroselinum crispum).

PARSNIP above ground parts

Also Known As
Pastinacae herba.
CAUTION: See separate listing for Parsnip root.

Scientific Names
Pastinaca sativa.
Family: Apiaceae.

People Use This For
Orally, parsnip above ground parts are used for digestive and kidney disorders (18).

Safety
There is insufficient reliable information available about the safety of the above ground parts of parsnip.
Pregnancy and Lactation: Insufficient reliable information available; avoid using.

Effectiveness
There is insufficient reliable information available about the effectiveness of the above ground parts of parsnip.

Mechanism of Action

Parsnip contains furocoumarins angelicin, bergapten, xanthotoxin and psoralen. Furocoumarins are photoxoxic and mutagenic (2), photosensitizing and are responsible for adverse dermatological reactions (6,11,19,515).

Adverse Reactions

Contact dermatitis and phototoxic reactions (including skin blisters) are possible following topical exposure to fresh parsnip plant and exposure to sunlight (6). Light-skinned people may be particularly susceptible to these reactions (18).

Interactions with Herbs & Other Dietary Supplements

Insufficient reliable information available.

Interactions with Drugs

No interactions are known to occur, and there is no known reason to expect a clinically significant interaction with parsnip above ground parts.

Interactions with Foods

No interactions are known to occur, and there is no known reason to expect a clinically significant interaction with parsnip above ground parts.

Interactions with Lab Tests

No interactions are known to occur, and there is no known reason to expect a clinically significant interaction with parsnip above ground parts.

Interactions with Diseases or Conditions

No interactions are known to occur, and there is no known reason to expect a clinically significant interaction with parsnip above ground parts.

Dosage and Administration

ORAL: Eight ounces (240 mL) of tea taken orally three times daily for the first 8 days, and then 360 mL is taken orally daily. The daily dose may be increased to as much as 2 L daily, and is taken for a total of 4-6 weeks. The tea is prepared by simmering one handful of dried herb in 1 L of boiling water for 10 minutes and straining (18).

Comments

There is very little scientific information about this product. Our staff is continually analyzing the available information on natural medicines and will add data here as it becomes available.

PARSNIP root

Also Known As

Pastinacae Radix.
CAUTION: See separate listing for Parsnip above ground parts.

Scientific Names

Pastinaca sativa.
Family: Apiaceae.

People Use This For

Orally, parsnip root is used for kidney complaints, fever, and as an analgesic and a diuretic (18).

Safety

LIKELY SAFE ...when used orally in food amounts (18).
There is insufficient reliable information available about the safety of using parsnip root in medicinal amounts.
PREGNANCY AND LACTATION: LIKELY SAFE ...when used orally in food amounts. There is insufficient reliable information available about the safety of using medicinal amounts during pregnancy and breast-feeding; avoid using.

Effectiveness

There is insufficient reliable information available about the effectiveness of parsnip.

Mechanism of Action

Parsnip contains furocoumarins angelicin, bergapten, xanthotoxin, and psoralen. Furocoumarins are phototoxic and mutagenic (2), photosensitizing, and are responsible for adverse dermatological reactions (6,11,19,515).

Adverse Reactions

Topically, contact dermatitis and phototoxic reactions (including skin blisters) are possible following exposure to fresh parsnip plant and exposure to sunlight (6). Light-skinned people may be particularly susceptible to these reactions (18).

Interactions with Herbs & Other Dietary Supplements

Insufficient reliable information available.

Interactions with Drugs

No interactions are known to occur, and there is no known reason to expect a clinically significant interaction with parsnip root.

Interactions with Foods

No interactions are known to occur, and there is no known reason to expect a clinically significant interaction with parsnip root.

Interactions with Lab Tests

No interactions are known to occur, and there is no known reason to expect a clinically significant interaction with parsnip root.

Interactions with Diseases or Conditions

No interactions are known to occur, and there is no known reason to expect a clinically significant interaction with parsnip root.

Dosage and Administration

ORAL: One teaspoon of freshly grated parsnip root taken three times daily (18).

Comments

Parsnip root closely resembles and can be confused with the parsley root. Avoid confusing parsnip root with similar appearing hemlock and bear's breech (or hogweed) root, both of which are toxic (18).

PASSIONFLOWER

Also Known As

Apricot Vine, Corona De Cristo, Fleischfarbige, Fleur De La Passion, Flor De Passion, Madre Selva, Maypop, Maypop Passion Flower, Passiflora, Passiflora incarnata, Passiflorae herba, Passiflore, Passiflorina, Passion Flower, Passion Vine, Passionaria, Passionblume, Passionflower Herb, Passionsblumenkraut, Purple Passion Flower, Water Lemon, Wild Passion Flower.

Scientific Names

Passiflora incarnata.
Family: Passifloraceae.

People Use This For

Orally, passionflower is used for nervous restlessness (2), mild insomnia (1,18), and nervous GI complaints (18).
Topically, passionflower is used in bath preparations (11), for hemorrhoids, burns, and inflammation (6).
Traditionally, passionflower is used orally for neuralgia, generalized seizures, hysteria, spasmodic asthma (4), climacteric symptoms, pediatric attention disorders, pediatric nervousness and excitability, palpitations, cardiac rhythm abnormalities, high blood pressure, and pain relief.
In foods and beverages, the extract is used as a flavoring (11).

Safety

LIKELY SAFE ...when used orally in food amounts. Passionflower is approved for food use in the US. The maximum level of the extract used is 0.32% in nonalcoholic beverages (11).
POSSIBLY SAFE ...when used orally and appropriately for medicinal purposes (1,2,4,12).
POSSIBLY UNSAFE ...when used orally in excessive amounts (4).
There is insufficient reliable information available about the safety of the topical use of passionflower.

PREGNANCY: UNSAFE ...when used orally. Harman alkaloid constituents show evidence of uterine stimulation (4,6).
LACTATION: Insufficient reliable information available; avoid using.

Effectiveness

POSSIBLY EFFECTIVE...when used orally for nervous restlessness (2). In a double-blind, placebo-controlled trial of 182 outpatients, a 6-ingredient combination product that included passionflower was statistically superior for relieving symptoms of adjustment disorder with anxious mood, as scored on the Hamilton Anxiety Rating Scale (6250). Other herbs in the product were crataegus, ballota, valerian, which have mild sedative effects, and cola and paullinia with stimulant properties (6250). ...when used orally for mild insomnia (1).
There is insufficient reliable information available about the effectiveness of passionflower for its other uses.

Mechanism of Action

The applicable parts of passionflower are the above ground parts. Passionflower has sedative, hypnotic (4,5), and antispasmodic effects (4,11). It also relieves pain (4). Some evidence suggests the passionflower constituent apigenin binds to central benzodiazepine receptors (4001), possibly causing anxiolytic effects without impairing memory or motor skills (4001). Other evidence suggests passionflower extracts might reduce amphetamine-induced hypermotility, aggressiveness, and restlessness; and raise the pain threshold (1,4,11). Although animal data suggest the constituents maltol and ethylmaltol can reduce spontaneous motor activity, prolong barbiturate-induced sleep time, and show anticonvulsant activity (1,4), not enough maltol is found in passionflower preparations to cause these effects (1).
The harman (harmala) alkaloids identified in passionflower include harmine, harmaline, harmalol, harman, and harmin (6). Some evidence suggests the harman alkaloids have central stimulant activity via a monoamine oxidase mechanism (4,4002); however, the sedative effects of maltol and ethylmaltol can mask these effects (4). The constituent passicol shows some evidence of antibacterial and antifungal activity (4). The experts do not agree about whether passionflower contains the cyanogenic glycoside gynocardine (3,11,19).

Adverse Reactions

Orally, passionflower can cause vasculitis and altered consciousness. This has been reported with use of an herbal product (Relaxir) produced mainly from the fruits of passionflower (6). A case report was recently published of toxicity in a 34-year-old woman following passionflower use at therapeutic doses (6251). The patient developed severe nausea, vomiting, drowsiness, prolonged QT interval, and episodes of nonsustained ventricular tachycardia, requiring hospitalization for IV hydration and cardiac monitoring (6251). Although there is disagreement about whether passionflower contains cyanogenic glycosides, several related Passiflora species do contain them (3), including Passiflora edulis, which is associated with liver and pancreas toxicity (7).

Interactions with Herbs & Other Dietary Supplements

HERBS WITH SEDATIVE PROPERTIES: Theoretically, concomitant use with herbs that have sedative properties might enhance therapeutic and adverse effects. These include calamus, calendula, California poppy, catnip, capsicum, celery, couch grass, elecampane, Siberian ginseng , German chamomile, goldenseal, gotu kola, hops, Jamaican dogwood, kava, lemon balm, sage, St. John's wort, sassafras, scullcap, shepherd's purse, stinging nettle, valerian, wild carrot, wild lettuce, ashwaganda root, and yerba mansa (4,19).
HERBS WITH ANTICOAGULANT/ANTIPLATELET POTENTIAL: Concomitant use of herbs that have coumarin constituents or affect platelet aggregation could theoretically increase the risk of bleeding in some people. These herbs include: angelica, anise, arnica, asafoetida, bogbean, boldo, capsicum, celery, chamomile, clove, danshen, fenugreek, feverfew, garlic, ginger, ginkgo, Panax ginseng, horse chestnut, horseradish, licorice, meadowsweet, prickly ash, onion, papain, poplar, quassia, red clover, turmeric, wild carrot, wild lettuce, willow, and others (4,19).

Interactions with Drugs

MONOAMINE OXIDASE INHIBITORS (MAOIs): Theoretically, concomitant use of passionflower can potentiate MAOI activity (4).
BARBITURATES: Theoretically, concomitant use can increase drug-induced sleep time (1).
SEDATIVES, TRANQUILIZERS: Theoretically, concomitant use can potentiate the effects of these drugs, including the sedative effects of antihistamines (19).

Interactions with Foods

No interactions are known to occur, and there is no known reason to expect a clinically significant interaction with passionflower.

Interactions with Lab Tests

No interactions are known to occur, and there is no known reason to expect a clinically significant interaction with passionflower.

Interactions with Diseases or Conditions

No interactions are known to occur, and there is no known reason to expect a clinically significant interaction with passionflower.

Dosage and Administration

ORAL: The typical dose of passionflower is 0.25-2 grams of the dried above ground parts three times daily or one cup of the tea two to three times daily and 30 minutes before bedtime (1,4,18). The tea is prepared by steeping 0.25-2 grams of the dried above ground parts in 150 mL boiling water for 10-15 minutes and then straining. The average amount of passionflower is 4-8 grams per day. The usual dose of the liquid extract (1:1 in 25% alcohol) is 0.5-1.0 mL three times daily. The common dose of the tincture (1:8 in 45% alcohol) is 0.5-2 mL three times daily (4).
TOPICAL: Passionflower is typically used as a hemorrhoid rinse, which is prepared by simmering 20 grams of the dried above ground parts in 200 mL water, straining, and cooling before use (18).

Comments

In 1569, Spanish explorers discovered passionflower in Peru. They believed the flowers symbolized Christ's passion and indicated his approval for their exploration (6). Passionflower is found in combination herbal sedative products, some of which include German chamomile, hops, kava, scullcap, and valerian. Passionflower was formerly approved as an OTC sedative and sleep aid in the US, but it was taken off the market in 1978 because safety and effectiveness had not been proven (11,515).

PATCHOULY OIL

Also Known As

Huo xiang, Patchouli, Patchouly, Putcha-Pat.

Scientific Names

Pogostemon cablin, synonyms Pogostemon heyneanus, Pogostemon patchouly.
Family: Labiatae or Lamiaceae.

People Use This For

In Chinese medicine, patchouly oil is used orally for colds, headaches, nausea, vomiting, diarrhea, and abdominal pain. It is also used to treat bad breath, particularly when it is associated with alcohol ingestion. The leaf, fruit and flower are used to treat tumors (11).
In foods and beverages, patchouly oil is used as a flavor ingredient (11).
In manufacturing, patchouly oil is used in perfumes and cosmetics (18).

Safety

LIKELY SAFE ...when used orally in amounts found in foods. It is approved for use in foods, and the maximum use is 0.0002% (11).
There is insufficient reliable information available about the safety of patchouly oil for its other uses.
PREGNANCY AND LACTATION: Insufficient reliable information available; avoid using in amounts greater than those typically found in foods.

Effectiveness

There is insufficient reliable information available about the effectiveness of patchouly oil.

Mechanism of Action

Patchouly oil is the oil distilled from the dried leaf, young leaves, and shoots of the Pogostemon cablin plant. Animal data suggests that patchouly oil is nontoxic with short term oral use. Patchouly oil may have bactericidal activity, and the component pogostone appears to have antibacterial and antifungal activities. The components eugenol, cinnamaldehyde, and benzaldehyde may have insecticidal activity against insects in stored grain (11).

Adverse Reactions

None reported.

Interactions with Herbs & Other Dietary Supplements

Insufficient reliable information available.

Interactions with Drugs
No interactions are known to occur, and there is no known reason to expect a clinically significant interaction with patchouly oil.

Interactions with Foods
No interactions are known to occur, and there is no known reason to expect a clinically significant interaction with patchouly oil.

Interactions with Lab Tests
No interactions are known to occur, and there is no known reason to expect a clinically significant interaction with patchouly oil.

Interactions with Diseases or Conditions
No interactions are known to occur, and there is no known reason to expect a clinically significant interaction with patchouly oil.

Dosage and Administration
No typical dosage.

Comments
Patchouly oil can be adulterated with other oils, including gurjun balsam oil, copaiba balsam oil, and cedarwood oil (11).

PAU D'ARCO

Also Known As
Ipe, Ipe Roxo, Ipes, Lapacho, Lapacho Colorado, Lapacho Morado, Pau dArco, Pau de Arco, Purple Lapacho, Red Lapacho, Taheebo, Taheebo Tea, Trumpet Bush.

Scientific Names
Tabebuia impetiginosa, synonym Tabebuia avellanedae; Tabebuia heptaphylla.
Family: Bignoniaceae.

People Use This For
Orally, pau d'arco is used for Candida yeast infections; viral respiratory infections, including the common cold and flu; infectious diarrhea; bladder infections; and parasitic infections (3564,6006). It has also been used orally for cancer (6,515,6006).
Topically, pau d'arco is used for Candida infections (6).
In folk medicine, pau d'arco has been used orally for cancer, diabetes, ulcers, gastritis, liver ailments, asthma, bronchitis, cystitis, prostatitis, ringworm, rheumatism, hernias, gonorrhea (515), syphilis, chlorosis, boils, wounds, Candida infections, and as a "tonic and blood builder" (6).

Safety
POSSIBLY UNSAFE ...when used orally in typical doses. Significant evaluation of the safety of pau d'arco in typical doses has not been conducted; however, serious toxicities have been found with higher doses (6,515,3564). Pau d'arco should be used with caution.
LIKELY UNSAFE ...when used orally in large doses. In studies in cancer patients, when doses were elevated to provide therapeutic plasma levels of the active constituent lapachol, patients experienced significant toxicities, including increased risk of bleeding (6,515). Doses of pau d'arco providing greater than 1.5 grams per day of the lapachol constituent have been associated with the most risk (6).
There is insufficient reliable information available about the safety of pau d'arco for its other uses.
PREGNANCY: POSSIBLY UNSAFE ...when used orally in typical doses; avoid using. LIKELY UNSAFE ...when used orally in large doses; contraindicated. Significant evaluation of the safety of pau d'arco in typical doses has not been conducted; however, serious toxicities have been found with higher doses (6,515,3564).
There is insufficient reliable information available about the safety of pau d'arco used topically in pregnancy.
LACTATION: Insufficient reliable information; avoid using.

Effectiveness
There is insufficient reliable information available about the effectiveness of pau d'arco.

Mechanism of Action

The applicable parts of pau d'arco are the bark and the wood. The active constituents are thought to be a naphthoquinone derivative, lapachol, and its derivatives. The wood contains lapachol and the bark contains mostly lapachol derivatives. Lapachol and its derivatives are thought to have similar pharmacological activities (515). Lapachol is thought to be responsible for increasing the risk of bleeding by prolonging prothrombin time. Its effects on clotting are reversible by vitamin K (6). Preliminary data suggests that lapachol also has anti-inflammatory, antimalarial, antibacterial, antifungal, antiparasitic, and immunomodulatory activity (6,515). Some evidence suggests that lapachol is active against sarcomas, but at potentially effective levels, adverse effects are severe enough to prevent its use for that indication (515).

Adverse Reactions

In high doses, pau d'arco causes severe nausea, vomiting, diarrhea, dizziness, anemia, and increases the risk of bleeding (515). Doses of pau d'arco providing greater than 1.5 grams per day of the lapachol constituent have been associated with the most risk (6).

Interactions with Herbs & Other Dietary Supplements

HERBS WITH ANTICOAGULANT/ANTIPLATELET POTENTIAL: Certain herbs have the potential to contribute to bleeding because they have coumarin constituents, or they affect platelet aggregation, or they have high vitamin K content. Theoretically, concomitant use of more than one of these herbs could increase the chance of bleeding in susceptible individuals. These herbs include: alfalfa, angelica, anise, arnica, asafoetida, bogbean, boldo, capsicum, celery, Roman and German chamomile, clove, danshen, fenugreek, feverfew, garlic, ginger, ginkgo, ginseng Panax, horse chestnut, horseradish, licorice, meadowsweet, nettle, northern and southern prickly ash, onion, papain, parsley, passionflower, poplar, quassia, red clover, turmeric, wild carrot, wild lettuce, and willow (4,19).

Interactions with Drugs

ANTICOAGULANT, ANTIPLATELET DRUGS: Theoretically, concomitant use with pau d'arco might increase clotting time and increase the risk for bleeding (515).

Interactions with Foods

No interactions are known to occur, and there is no known reason to expect a clinically significant interaction with pau d'arco.

Interactions with Lab Tests

PROTHROMBIN TIME (PT)/INTERNATIONAL NORMALIZED RATION (INR): Pau d'arco can increase PT and INR test results and increase the risk of bleeding (6,515).

Interactions with Diseases or Conditions

COAGULATION DISORDERS: Pau d'arco can increase bleeding time and might interfere with therapy in patients with coagulation disorders (6,515); use with caution.

Dosage and Administration

ORAL: People typically use 1 to 4 grams daily in 2 to 3 divided doses. One manufacturer warns that the product should not be used for more than 7 days; however, the reason for this warning is not known. The contents of pau d'arco capsules may also be emptied and prepared as a tea. A tincture in the amount of 0.5 to 1 mL and a glycerin-based liquid in the amount of 1 to 3 mL, are used 3 times daily (6006).

Comments

Pau d'arco wood is extremely hard and almost indestructible (515). In South America, the Indians used the tree to make bows for hunting. Pau d'arco is the Spanish name for "bow stick" (6002). Teas, labeled as pau d'arco or lapacho, do not always contain the Tabebuia species; in some cases they have contained the related species, Tecoma curialis (515). Some report that the inner-bark preparations of pau d'arco are preferred because they are the most effective. Some products may use the outer-bark and mislabel the product as true inner-bark pau d'arco (3564). The anticancer activity of the pau d'arco constituent lapachol was extensively researched in the 1960s. The research was abandoned due to its toxicity (6).

PEANUT OIL

Also Known As

Arachis, Earth-Nut, Groundnuts, Monkey Nuts.

Scientific Names

Arachis hypogaea.
Family: Leguminosae or Fabaceae.

People Use This For

Orally, peanut oil is used to lower cholesterol and prevent heart disease (18). It is also used orally to aid in weight loss and decrease appetite, and to help prevent cancer (4262).
Topically, it is used for arthritis and joint pain, scalp crusting and scaling without hair loss, dry skin, eczema and ichthyosis (noninflammatory skin disorders that cause scaling) (18).
Rectally, peanut oil is used in ointments and medicinal oils for treating constipation.
It is also used as a vehicle for external, enteral and parenteral pharmaceutical formulations (16,18).
In manufacturing, peanut oil is used in skin care products and baby care products (18).

Safety

LIKELY SAFE ...when used orally in amounts found in foods. ...when used orally, topically, or rectally in medicinal amounts.
PREGNANCY AND LACTATION: LIKELY SAFE ...when used orally in amounts found in foods.

Effectiveness

There is insufficient reliable information available about the effectiveness of peanut oil.

Mechanism of Action

Peanuts contain beta-sitosterol and resveratrol, which may contribute to cardioprotective and cancer protective activity (4262,4267,4263). The high monounsaturated, low saturated fat content of peanut oil is thought to prevent heart disease and lower cholesterol (4262). Population studies suggest people who eat nuts have a lower risk of developing heart disease (4264). This benefit must be weighed against animal evidence that suggests peanut oil is atherogenic, perhaps due to the triglyceride content or the presence of a lectin (4265,4266).

Adverse Reactions

Peanut oil can cause a severe allergic reaction in individuals allergic to the Fabaceae family. Members of this family include peanuts and soybeans (4079,4080).

Interactions with Herbs & Other Dietary Supplements

Insufficient reliable information available.

Interactions with Drugs

No interactions are known to occur, and there is no known reason to expect a clinically significant interaction with peanut oil.

Interactions with Foods

No interactions are known to occur, and there is no known reason to expect a clinically significant interaction with peanut oil.

Interactions with Lab Tests

No interactions are known to occur, and there is no known reason to expect a clinically significant interaction with peanut oil.

Interactions with Diseases or Conditions

CROSS-ALLERGENICITY: Peanut oil can cause a severe allergic reaction in individuals sensitive to the Fabaceae family. Members of this family include peanuts and soybeans (4079,4080).

Dosage and Administration

ORAL: No typical dosage.
TOPICAL: For bath use, 4 mL peanut oil is added to 10 L water. Adults bathe for 15-20 minutes 2-3 times daily. Children bathe for a few minutes 2-3 times weekly (18).
RECTAL: As an enema, 130 mL of room temperature peanut oil has been used.

Comments

Sometimes the less expensive soya oil is added to peanut oil (18).

PEAR

Also Known As
None.

Scientific Names
Pyrus communis.
Family: Rosaceae.

People Use This For
Orally, pear fruit is used for mild digestive disorders (18), cholera, colic, diarrhea, nausea, liver sclerosis, spasms, tumors, and for reducing fevers (18). It is used also for its laxative, bactericidal, calmative, and diuretic properties (18). Topically, pear fruit is used as an astringent.
For food use, pears are eaten as fresh fruit, preserved fruit, and used in cooking.

Safety
LIKELY SAFE …when used orally (18).
There is insufficient reliable information available about the safety of pear fruit for its other uses.
PREGNANCY AND LACTATION: LIKELY SAFE ...when used orally in food amounts (18).

Effectiveness
There is insufficient reliable information available about the effectiveness of pear fruit.

Mechanism of Action
The applicable part of the pear is the fruit. Pear fruit contains pectin (18) that might contribute to antidiarrheal activity (7).

Adverse Reactions
None reported.

Interactions with Herbs & Other Dietary Supplements
Insufficient reliable information available.

Interactions with Drugs
No interactions are known to occur, and there is no known reason to expect a clinically significant interaction with pear fruit.

Interactions with Foods
No interactions are known to occur, and there is no known reason to expect a clinically significant interaction with pear fruit.

Interactions with Lab Tests
No interactions are known to occur, and there is no known reason to expect a clinically significant interaction with pear fruit.

Interactions with Diseases or Conditions
No interactions are known to occur, and there is no known reason to expect a clinically significant interaction with pear fruit.

Dosage and Administration
No typical dosage.

Comments
None.

PECTIN

Also Known As
Pectinic Acid.

Scientific Names
Pectin.

People Use This For
Orally, pectin is used as an adsorbent (6,14,15,16), for reducing high cholesterol and triglycerides, for reducing the risk of colon cancer, for reducing damage from radiation (6), for treating diabetes (1900), and as an antibacterial (2211).
Topically, pectin is used for protecting raw or ulcerated mouth and throat sores (2218).
In combination with kaolin (Kaopectate) (13) or paregoric (Parepectolin) (15), pectin is used to treat diarrhea.
In food manufacturing, it is used as a thickening agent in cooking and baking (11).
In manufacturing, pectin is used as a denture adhesive component (272).

Safety
LIKELY SAFE ...when consumed in amounts commonly found in foods (11). Pectin has Generally Recognized as Safe (GRAS) status for food use in the US (11). ...when used orally for medicinal purposes in 10% concentration mixtures with kaolin (16).
PREGNANCY AND LACTATION: LIKELY SAFE ...when consumed in amounts found in foods (11).

Effectiveness
EFFECTIVE ...when used orally as an adsorbent for treating diarrhea, usually in combination with kaolin or other ingredients (6,14,15).
POSSIBLY EFFECTIVE ...when used orally as a cholesterol-lowering agent (2214,2215,2216,2217).
There is insufficient reliable information available about the effectiveness of pectin for its other uses.

Mechanism of Action
Pectin is a soluble fiber (polysaccharide) obtained from the inner portion of the rind of citrus fruits and apple pomace (14). It is found in the cell walls of plant tissue and helps give plants rigidity (6). Pectin acts as an adsorbent and bulk-forming agent (14) and can interfere with drug and nutrient absorption (6,14,19).

Adverse Reactions
The occupational inhalation of pectin dust can cause asthma (580,581,582,583,584).

Interactions with Herbs & Other Dietary Supplements
NUTRITIONAL SUPPLEMENTS: Concomitant use of pectin can interfere with the absorption of nutritional supplements (6).
BETA-CAROTENE: Concomitant use of pectin can significantly reduce beta-carotene absorption (2225).

Interactions with Drugs
BETA-CAROTENE (Solatene): Concomitant use of pectin can significantly reduce beta-carotene absorption (2225).
DIGOXIN (Lanoxin), LOVASTATIN (Mevacor), TETRACYCLINE (Achromycin, Sumycin): Concomitant use of pectin can interfere with the intestinal absorption of these drugs (14,615,2212,2213).
ORAL DRUGS: Concomitant use of pectin can interfere with the absorption of other oral drugs (14).

Interactions with Foods
NUTRIENTS: Pectin can interfere with the absorption of dietary nutrients (6).

Interactions with Lab Tests
CHOLESTEROL: Pectin can decrease serum cholesterol and test results (275).

Interactions with Diseases or Conditions
PECTIN HYPERSENSITIVITY: Contraindicated.

Dosage and Administration
ORAL: As an adsorbent, 30 mL of 10% pectin in a mixture with kaolin is taken as needed (16).
As an antihyperlipidemic, 15 grams per day was used in one study (2214).
TOPICAL: No typical dosage.

Comments

Commercial pectin can contain sugars of organic acids and other additives, but pharmaceutical grade pectin contains no impurities or additives (13). The FDA is currently reevaluating the effectiveness of pectin combinations for diarrhea (272).

PELLITORY

Also Known As
None.
CAUTION: See separate listing for Pellitory-of-the-Wall.

Scientific Names
Anacyclus pyrethrum.
Family: Asteraceae.

People Use This For
Orally, pellitory is used for arthritis and as a digestive aid.
Topically, pellitory is used for toothaches and as an insecticide (18).

Safety
There is insufficient reliable information available about the safety of pellitory.
Pregnancy and Lactation: Insufficient reliable information available; avoid using.

Effectiveness
There is insufficient reliable information available about the effectiveness of pellitory.

Mechanism of Action
The applicable part of pellitory is the root. Application of pellitory to skin may stimulate nerve endings and result in redness and irritation, which is felt as a hot, burning sensation. Alkylamines may possibly contribute, since they may stimulate mucous membranes (18).

Adverse Reactions
Signs of skin irritation may occur with overuse (18). Pellitory can cause an allergic reaction in individuals sensitive to the Asteraceae/Compositae family. Members of this family include ragweed, chrysanthemums, marigolds, daisies, and many other herbs.

Interactions with Herbs & Other Dietary Supplements
Insufficient reliable information available.

Interactions with Drugs
No interactions are known to occur, and there is no known reason to expect a clinically significant interaction with pellitory.

Interactions with Foods
No interactions are known to occur, and there is no known reason to expect a clinically significant interaction with pellitory.

Interactions with Lab Tests
No interactions are known to occur, and there is no known reason to expect a clinically significant interaction with pellitory.

Interactions with Diseases or Conditions
CROSS-ALLERGENICITY: Can cause an allergic reaction in individuals sensitive to the Asteraceae/Compositae family. Members of this family include ragweed, chrysanthemums, marigolds, daisies, and many other herbs.

Dosage and Administration
No typical dosage.

Comments
Avoid confusing with the similar sounding pellitory-of-the-wall.

PELLITORY-OF-THE-WALL

Also Known As
Lichwort, Pellitory of the Wall.
CAUTION: See separate listing for Pellitory.

Scientific Names
Parietaria officinalis.
Family: Urticaceae.

People Use This For
Orally, pellitory-of-the-wall is used as a diuretic, laxative, and as a demulcent. It is also used for chronic cough and for a variety of kidney disorders including urinary tract infections (UTIs) and pyelonephritis, renal pain, and kidney stones. Topically, pellitory-of-the-wall is used for treating burns and wounds.

Safety
POSSIBLY SAFE ...when used orally (12).
PREGNANCY AND LACTATION: Insufficient reliable information available; avoid using.

Effectiveness
There is insufficient reliable information available about the effectiveness of pellitory-of-the-wall.

Mechanism of Action
The applicable parts of pellitory-of-the-wall are the aerial parts. It contains flavonoids and tannins (7161).

Adverse Reactions
Pellitory-of-the-wall pollen has been associated with seasonal allergy (7161).

Interactions with Herbs & Other Dietary Supplements
Insufficient reliable information available.

Interactions with Drugs
No interactions are known to occur, and there is no known reason to expect a clinically significant interaction with pellitory-of-the-wall.

Interactions with Foods
No interactions are known to occur, and there is no known reason to expect a clinically significant interaction with pellitory-of-the-wall.

Interactions with Lab Tests
No interactions are known to occur, and there is no known reason to expect a clinically significant interaction with pellitory-of-the-wall.

Interactions with Diseases or Conditions
No interactions are known to occur, and there is no known reason to expect a clinically significant interaction with pellitory-of-the-wall.

Dosage and Administration
No typical dosage.

Comments
The name pellitory-of-the-wall comes from its habit of growing in old walls and dry, stony areas (7161). Avoid confusion between pellitory-of-the-wall and the similar sounding pellitory.

PENNYROYAL leaf

Also Known As
American Pennyroyal, European Pennyroyal, Lurk-In-The-Ditch, Mosquito Plant, Penny Royal, Piliolerial, Pudding Grass, Pulegium, Run-By-The-Ground, Squaw Balm, Squawmint, Stinking Balm, Tickweed. CAUTION: See separate listing for Pennyroyal oil.

Scientific Names
Hedeoma pulegioides, synonym Melissa pulegioides; Mentha pulegium, synonym Pulegium vulgare. Family: Lamiaceae or Labiatae.

People Use This For
Orally, pennyroyal leaf is used as an antispasmodic, antiflatulent, diaphoretic (4), stimulant, for bowel disorders, pneumonia, stomach pains, weakness (6), and as a diuretic (14). It is also used orally as an abortifacient (4,5,6,9,12), menstrual stimulant or regulator (4,6,14), for intestinal disorders, colds (4,6,18), digestive disorders, liver and gall bladder disorders (18), and respiratory ailments (6).

Safety
LIKELY UNSAFE …when the alcoholic extract is used orally. Repeated use of the alcoholic extract over a period of two weeks was linked to a death (650).
There is insufficient reliable information available about the safety of the oral use of pennyroyal leaf as tea (4,650).
CHILDREN: UNSAFE …when used orally. Two infants developed severe hepatic and neurologic injuries and one infant died (4,291).
PREGNANCY: LIKELY UNSAFE …when used orally as pennyroyal leaf tea. Reported to cause onset of menses (650). UNSAFE …when used as oil, considered to be an abortifacient and can cause death (4).
LACTATION: LIKELY UNSAFE ...when used orally as an alcoholic extract or oil (650). There is insufficient reliable information available for oral use of pennyroyal leaf tea; avoid using (4,6).

Effectiveness
There is insufficient reliable information available about the effectiveness of pennyroyal leaf.

Mechanism of Action
Both American and European pennyroyal leaf contain 1-2% of essential oils (12,14), tannins and flavonoids (18). The volatile oil, pulegone and its metabolite, menthofuran, or methofuran's metabolites might be responsible for hepatotoxicity, neurotoxicity, and bronchiolar epithelial cell destruction (6,650). The oxidative metabolites of pulegone and menthofuran are thought to cause cell damage by binding to target proteins (650). Some metabolites of pulegegone also extensively deplete hepatic glutathione levels (650,291), which allows metabolite accumulation and direct cellular damage similar to acetaminophen toxicity (291). In addition, pulegegone is isomerized to isopulegone, which can be toxic to the lungs and liver (14). Pulegone is less concentrated in the American species (30%) than in European species (62-97%) (12,14).

Adverse Reactions
Orally, pennyroyal leaf can cause abdominal cramping and pain, fever, nausea (4,6,650), vomiting (possibly bloody), lethargy alternating with agitation, confusion, delirium, restlessness, seizures, dizziness (14), weakness, syncope (650), auditory and visual hallucinations (6), elevated blood pressure and pulse rate, bilateral lung congestion, hepatic failure, renal failure, acidosis, disseminated intravascular coagulation (DIC) (14), abortion (14,18), respiratory failure (18), shock (6), and death (14,650). Topically, it can cause an urticarial rash (4) and dermatitis (6).

Interactions with Herbs & Other Dietary Supplements
Insufficient reliable information available.

Interactions with Drugs
No interactions are known to occur, and there is no known reason to expect a clinically significant interaction with pennyroyal leaf.

Interactions with Foods
No interactions are known to occur, and there is no known reason to expect a clinically significant interaction with pennyroyal leaf.

Interactions with Lab Tests

No interactions are known to occur, and there is no known reason to expect a clinically significant interaction with pennyroyal leaf.

Interactions with Diseases or Conditions

KIDNEY DISEASE: The volatile oil can cause kidney irritation (19).

Dosage and Administration

No typical dosage.

Comments

American pennyroyal and European pennyroyal are historically interchangeable as a source of pennyroyal oil (12). About 50-100 grams of leaves are required to produce 1 ml of pennyroyal oil (4).

PENNYROYAL oil

Also Known As

American Pennyroyal, European Pennyroyal, Lurk-In-The-Ditch, Mosquito Plant, Penny Royal, Piliolerial, Pudding Grass, Pulegium, Run-By-The-Ground, Squaw Balm, Squawmint, Stinking Balm, Tickweed. CAUTION: See separate listing for Pennyroyal leaf.

Scientific Names

Hedeoma pulegioides, synonym Melissa pulegioides; Mentha pulegium, synonym Pulegium vulgare. Family: Lamiaceae or Labiatae.

People Use This For

Orally, pennyroyal oil is used as an antispasmodic, antiflatulent, diaphoretic (4), stimulant, pneumonia, for stomach pains, weakness (6), and as a diuretic (14).

Topically, it is used as an antiseptic, insect repellent (4,6), and for skin diseases (18).

Historically, it has been used orally as an abortifacient (4,5,6,9,12), menstrual stimulant or regulator (4,6,14), for intestinal disorders, colds, respiratory ailments (4,6,18), digestive disorders, and liver and gallbladder disorders (18).

Historically, it has been used topically for tactile hallucinations, gout (4), venomous bites, mouth sores, as a flea-killing bath, and counterirritant (6).

In foods it is used as a flavoring agent (4,6).

In manufacturing, it is used as a dog and cat flea repellent (6,515), and a fragrance for detergents, perfumes and soaps (6).

Safety

POSSIBLY SAFE ...when used orally as food flavoring. Pulegone-free American pennyroyal is allowed only in alcoholic beverages in Canada (4). The Council of Europe lists pennyroyal as a natural source of food flavoring, without assessment of toxicity (4).

LIKELY UNSAFE ...when used orally or topically; contraindicated (4). Neurologic injury reported in adults consuming 2.5-5.0 mL of pennyroyal oil (5,6,9). Nephrotoxicity, hepatotoxicity, and death have been reported after ingestion of 15-30 mL (4,5,6,12,5601). Some evidence suggests oil can be absorbed systemically (6,14,292).

PREGNANCY: LIKELY UNSAFE ...when used orally or topically. Pennyroyal oil is an abortifacient (4).

LACTATION: LIKELY UNSAFE ...when used orally or topically; contraindicated.

Effectiveness

LIKELY EFFECTIVE ...when used orally as abortifacient only when lethal or near-lethal amounts (15-30 mL) are ingested (4,5,6,18).

There is insufficient reliable information available about the effectiveness of pennyroyal oil for its other uses.

Mechanism of Action

Pennyroyal oil contains pulegone, which may cause hepatotoxicity, neurotoxicity, and bronchiolar epithelial cell destruction (6). The oxidative metabolites of pulegone and its metabolite menthofuran may cause cell damage by binding to target proteins (650), depleting hepatic glutathione levels (650,292), and direct cellular damage similar to acetaminophen toxicity (291). In addition, pulegone is isomerized to isopulegone, which can be toxic to the lungs and liver (14). Its abortifacient effect might be due to uterine contractions triggered by genito-urinary tract irritation (4,6,19). In the American species, pulegone is less concentrated (30%) than in European species (62-97%) (12,14).

Adverse Reactions

Orally, pennyroyal oil can cause abdominal pain and tenderness (5601), nausea (4,6), vomiting (possibly bloody) (14,5601), burning of the throat (17), fever (4,6), lethargy alternating with agitation, confusion, delirium, restlessness, seizures, dizziness (14,5601), auditory and visual hallucinations (6), elevated blood pressure and pulse rate, bilateral lung congestion, acidosis, disseminated intravascular coagulation (DIC) (14,5601), abortion (14,18), hepatic failure, renal failure (14,5601), respiratory failure (18,5601), shock (6), and death (14,5601).
Topically, it can cause a urticarial rash (4,5601) and dermatitis (6).

Interactions with Herbs & Other Dietary Supplements

Insufficient reliable information available.

Interactions with Drugs

No interactions are known to occur, and there is no known reason to expect a clinically significant interaction with pennyroyal oil.

Interactions with Foods

No interactions are known to occur, and there is no known reason to expect a clinically significant interaction with pennyroyal oil.

Interactions with Lab Tests

No interactions are known to occur, and there is no known reason to expect a clinically significant interaction with pennyroyal oil.

Interactions with Diseases or Conditions

KIDNEY DISEASE: The volatile oil can cause kidney irritation (19).

Dosage and Administration

No typical dosage.

Comments

Historically, American pennyroyal and European pennyroyal are interchangeable as sources of pennyroyal oil. (12).

PEONY flower

Also Known As

European Peony, Paeonia, Paeoniae flos, Piney.
CAUTION: See separate listing for Peony root.

Scientific Names

Paeonia mascula; Paeonia officinalis.
Family: Paeoniaceae.

People Use This For

Orally, peony flowers are used for gout, arthritis, respiratory tract ailments (2,18), and as a cough remedy (8).
Topically, peony flowers are used for skin and mucous membrane diseases, and for healing fissures, especially anal fissures associated with hemorrhoids (2,18)
In herb combinations, peony flowers are used orally for heart trouble and gastritis (2).
In folk medicine, peony flowers are used for epilepsy, bowel complaints, as an emetic, and for inducing menstruation or miscarriage (18).
In manufacturing, peony flowers are also used commercially to color cough syrups (18). They are used in herbal teas to improve their appearance (2,8).

Safety

There is insufficient reliable information available about the safety of peony flower.
PREGNANCY: LIKELY UNSAFE ...when used orally, due to historical use as an abortifacient and menstruation-inducing agent (18).
LACTATION: Insufficient reliable information available; avoid using.

Effectiveness

There is insufficient reliable information available about the effectiveness of peony flower.

Mechanism of Action

Hypertonia has been reported in animal tests, but the peony part(s)/product used were not specified (18).

Adverse Reactions

Overdose has reportedly led to gastroenteritis with vomiting, colic, and diarrhea (8,18).

Interactions with Herbs & Other Dietary Supplements

Insufficient reliable information available.

Interactions with Drugs

No interactions are known to occur, and there is no known reason to expect a clinically significant interaction with peony flower.

Interactions with Foods

No interactions are known to occur, and there is no known reason to expect a clinically significant interaction with peony flower.

Interactions with Lab Tests

No interactions are known to occur, and there is no known reason to expect a clinically significant interaction with peony flower.

Interactions with Diseases or Conditions

No interactions are known to occur, and there is no known reason to expect a clinically significant interaction with peony flower.

Dosage and Administration

ORAL: One cup tea (steep 1 gram flowers in 150 mL boiling water 5-10 minutes, strain) daily (8,18).
TOPICAL: No typical dosage.

Comments

Avoid confusion with peony root.

PEONY root

Also Known As

European Peony, Paeonia, Paeoniae Radix, Piney.
CAUTION: See separate listing for Peony flower.

Scientific Names

Paeonia mascula; Paeonia officinalis.
Family: Paeoniaceae.

People Use This For

Orally, peony is used for spasms (2).
In herbal combinations, peony root is used for arthritis, GI tract diseases, the heart and circulatory system, neuralgia, migraines, as a tonic, and for neurasthenia (characterized by vague fatigue accompanying or following depression, believed to be brought about by psychological factors) (2,18).
In folk medicine, peony is used for epilepsy, excitability, whooping cough, arthritis, bowel complaints, as an emetic, and for inducing menstruation (8).

Safety

There is insufficient reliable information available about the safety of peony root.
PREGNANCY: LIKELY UNSAFE ...when used orally. Historically, it has been used to induce menstruation (18,19).
LACTATION: Insufficient reliable information available; avoid using.

Effectiveness

There is insufficient reliable information available about the effectiveness of peony.

Mechanism of Action
Peony root extract exhibits neuroprotective activity and prevents experimentally induced brain neuron spike discharges in rats (3818). Researchers attribute neuroprotection to the constituent gallotannins and paeoniflorin (3818). Hypertonia reported in animal tests (peony part(s)/product used not specified) (18) (18).

Adverse Reactions
Orally, peony root overdose can result in gastroenteritis with vomiting, colic, and diarrhea (8,18).

Interactions with Herbs & Other Dietary Supplements
Insufficient reliable information.

Interactions with Drugs
No interactions are known to occur, and there is no known reason to expect a clinically significant interaction with peony root.

Interactions with Foods
No interactions are known to occur, and there is no known reason to expect a clinically significant interaction with peony root.

Interactions with Lab Tests
No interactions are known to occur, and there is no known reason to expect a clinically significant interaction with peony root.

Interactions with Diseases or Conditions
No interactions are known to occur, and there is no known reason to expect a clinically significant interaction with peony root.

Dosage and Administration
ORAL: People typically use 1 ounce of the powdered root added to two cups of boiling water. The dose is a cup three or four times daily (5267). One source advises against the use of peony root without medical supervision (5263).

Comments
Avoid confusion with peony flower.

PEPPERMINT leaf

Also Known As
Brandy Mint, Lamb Mint, Menthae piperitae folium, Menthe poivree.
CAUTION: See separate listing for Peppermint Oil.

Scientific Names
Mentha piperita.
Family: Labiatae.

People Use This For
Orally, peppermint leaf is used for loss of appetite (18), spasms of the gastrointestinal tract, gallbladder, and bile ducts (2), for flatulence, gastritis, and enteritis (1).
In folk medicine, it has been used to treat nausea, vomiting, morning sickness, respiratory infections, and dysmenorrhea (18).
In foods and in herbal teas, peppermint is used as a culinary spice (11).

Safety
LIKELY SAFE ...when consumed in amounts commonly found in foods. Peppermint has Generally Recognized as Safe (GRAS) status for food use in the US (11).
POSSIBLY SAFE ...when used orally and appropriately for medicinal purposes and used appropriately (1,12).
CHILDREN: POSSIBLY UNSAFE ...when used in infants and small children because its menthol content can cause unpleasant choking sensations (512).
PREGNANCY: LIKELY SAFE ...when used in food amounts. POSSIBLY UNSAFE ...when used orally in larger amounts due to its potential to induce menstrual bleeding (19).
LACTATION: Insufficient reliable information available; avoid using amounts greater than those found in foods.

Effectiveness

POSSIBLY EFFECTIVE ...when used orally for gastrointestinal, gallbladder, and bile duct spasms (2).
There is insufficient reliable information available about the effectiveness of peppermint leaf for its other uses.

Mechanism of Action

Peppermint has spasmolytic and antiflatulent activities. It also stimulates bile production (2,18). The constituents include the volatile oil menthol (7,11,18), flavonoids (11,18), and azulene (11). In vitro and in animals, menthol's antispasmodic effects result from a direct action on the digestive tract smooth muscle that is characteristic of calcium antagonist activity (1,7). Flavonoids have bile-stimulating effects. In animals, azulene has anti-inflammatory and anti-ulcer effects (11). Peppermint's soothing effect in coughs or colds results from the stimulation of salivation, which increases the swallowing reflex and suppresses cough (3).

Adverse Reactions

Orally, peppermint leaf can increase colic in people with gallstones (2,18,19). It can also cause an unpleasant choking sensation in infants and small children (512).

Interactions with Herbs & Other Dietary Supplements

Insufficient reliable information available.

Interactions with Drugs

No interactions are known to occur, and there is no known reason to expect a clinically significant interaction with peppermint leaf.

Interactions with Foods

No interactions are known to occur, and there is no known reason to expect a clinically significant interaction with peppermint leaf.

Interactions with Lab Tests

No interactions are known to occur, and there is no known reason to expect a clinically significant interaction with peppermint leaf.

Interactions with Diseases or Conditions

GALLSTONES: Physician consultation is advised before the use of the peppermint leaf in individuals with gallstones (2), because it can increase symptoms of colic (18).
HIATAL HERNIA: Theoretically, peppermint can exacerbate hernia symptoms due to its relaxation of the lower esophageal sphincter (500).

Dosage and Administration

ORAL: For upset stomach, the typical dose of peppermint leaf is one cup of the tea three to four times daily between meals (1,512). The tea is prepared by steeping 1 tablespoon of the dried leaf in 150 mL boiling water for 10 minutes and then straining. It can also be consumed at meal times or as needed (7). The average daily amount of the peppermint leaf is 3-6 grams (18). Peppermint tea is contraindicated in infants and small children because its menthol content can cause an unpleasant choking sensation (512). The usual dose of the tincture (1:5 in 45% ethanol) is 2-3 mL three times daily (1).

Comments

None.

PEPPERMINT OIL

Also Known As

Menthae piperitae Aetheroleum, Menthe Poivree.
CAUTION: See separate listing for Peppermint leaf.

Scientific Names

Mentha piperita.
Family: Lamiaceae.

People Use This For

Orally, peppermint oil is used for colds, coughs, inflammation of the mouth and pharynx, liver and gallbladder complaints, irritable bowel syndrome (IBS), cramps of the upper gastrointestinal (GI) tract and bile ducts, dyspepsia, as an antipyretic and antiflatulent, and for tension headache. It is also used orally for nausea, vomiting, morning sickness, respiratory infections, dysmenorrhea, indigestion, diarrhea, and as a stimulant.

Topically, the peppermint oil is used for headache, myalgias, neuralgias, toothache, oral mucosa inflammation, rheumatic conditions, pruritus, urticaria, as an antibacterial and antiviral agent, as an antispasmodic in barium enemas, and for repelling mosquitoes.

As an inhalant, peppermint oil is used as an aromatic, for symptomatic treatment of cough and colds, and as an analgesic for pain.

In foods and beverages, peppermint oil is a common flavoring agent.

In manufacturing, it is used as a fragrance component in soaps and cosmetics, and as a flavoring agent in pharmaceuticals.

Safety

LIKELY SAFE ...when used orally in amounts commonly found in foods. Peppermint oil has Generally Recognized as Safe (GRAS) status in the US. The maximum level is 0.104% in candy (11).

POSSIBLY SAFE ...when used orally or topically and appropriately for medicinal purposes (1,8006). Tell patients not to use peppermint oil on the face, particularly around the nose (8006). ...when used by inhalation as aromatherapy (7107).

LIKELY UNSAFE ...when used orally in large amounts. High doses of peppermint oil have been associated with interstitial nephritis and acute renal failure (7). Menthol, a major constituent, is considered lethal at a dose of 2-9 grams (7).

CHILDREN: LIKELY SAFE ...when used orally in amounts commonly found in foods (11). LIKELY UNSAFE ...when used orally in medicinal amounts. Oral peppermint oil has caused tongue spasms and respiratory arrest in infants and small children (8006). ...when applied topically to the facial, nasal, and chest areas of infants and small children. Peppermint oil can cause bronchospasm, spasms of the tongue, or respiratory arrest (2,6,11,8006). ...when inhaled for medicinal purposes by small children (502).

PREGNANCY: LIKELY SAFE ...when used orally in food amounts (11). LIKELY UNSAFE ...when used orally in large amounts. High doses of peppermint oil can induce menstruation (19).

LACTATION: Insufficient reliable information available; avoid using.

Effectiveness

POSSIBLY EFFECTIVE ...when used orally for treating irritable bowel syndrome (IBS). There is some evidence that enteric coated peppermint oil capsules can reduce abdominal pain, distention, flatulence, and bowel movements in 70-80% of patients with IBS (3802,3803). Since peppermint oil seems to decrease bowel movements, it may be most appropriate for IBS patients with diarrhea-predominant symptoms. ...when used orally for postoperative nausea (3804). ...when used orally in combination with caraway oil for non-ulcer dyspepsia (6740,6741). The combination of enteric-coated peppermint oil 90 mg and caraway oil 50 mg appears to be superior to placebo and similar to cisapride for relieving dyspepsia (6740,6741). ...when used topically for myalgias and neuralgias (11). ...when used topically for treating tension headaches (3801,6190). ...when used rectally to reduce colonic spasm during radiologic exam (6739,6749). Peppermint oil added as an ingredient in barium enema preparations seems to relax the colon during barium enema examination (6739,6749).

There is insufficient reliable information available about the effectiveness of peppermint oil for its other uses.

Mechanism of Action

Peppermint oil is obtained by steam distillation of the fresh above ground parts of the flowering peppermint plant (4800). Peppermint oil is a complex mixture of compounds, including menthol (28-29%), menthone (20-31%), and menthyl acetate (3-10%) (1,6,11,7,18,3582). However, pharmaceutical grade peppermint oil is typically standardized to contain at least 44% menthol. Peppermint oil is thought to work for respiratory tract symptoms found in the common cold by increasing salivation, which increases the swallowing reflex and suppresses the cough reflex (3,7), reduces bronchial secretions, and can have nasal decongestant activity (1). Peppermint oil is used for irritable bowel syndrome (IBS) due to antispasmodic effects. The antispasmodic activity appears to results from direct relaxing effects on gastrointestinal (GI) tract smooth muscle, characteristic of calcium antagonist action (1,7,6744). This is thought to prevent hypercontractility that is commonly found in patients with IBS. Peppermint oil is thought to be helpful for gaseousness and flatulence by relaxing the lower esophageal sphincter, equalizing the intraluminal pressures between the stomach and esophagus (7,3582), which increases belching (512). Preliminary evidence suggests that peppermint oil in combination with caraway oil can reduce gastroduodenal motility when administered orally in enteric-coated capsules (6742). For pain in myalgias and neuralgias, topical peppermint oil is thought to have counterirritant effects (3582). Preliminary unpublished research suggests that peppermint oil might be an effective mosquito repellent with potential for reducing transmission of malaria and other mosquito-borne diseases, and might be useful for killing mosquito larva (1263). Peppermint oil has antimicrobial and antiviral activities in vitro (11).

Adverse Reactions

Orally, peppermint oil can cause heartburn (1) and allergic reactions including flushing and headache (6). Enteric-coated capsules might reduce the incidence of heartburn (3582,3802). Oral peppermint oil has also been associated with burning mouth syndrome and chronic mouth ulceration in people with contact sensitivity to peppermint (6743). Theoretically, the oil can worsen the symptoms of a hiatal hernia due to its relaxation of gastrointestinal (GI) smooth muscle (6). When applied externally, the oil can cause skin irritation (1) and contact dermatitis (6). Application of the oil to facial, nasal or chest areas of babies and small children can cause laryngeal and bronchial spasms and instant respiratory collapse (1,6,11). When inhaled, peppermint oil can cause allergic reactions including flushing and headache (6). When used orally in combination with caraway oil, it has caused belching, heartburn, and diarrhea (6740).

Interactions with Herbs & Other Dietary Supplements

Insufficient reliable information available.

Interactions with Drugs

ANTACIDS: Drugs that decrease stomach acid and raise gastric pH can cause premature dissolution of enteric-coated peppermint oil (787). Separate dose administration times by at least 2 hours.
GASTRIC ACID BLOCKING DRUGS (H2 antagonists): cimetidine, ranitidine, famodidine, nizatidine; proton pump inhibitors: omeprazole, lansoprazole, rabeprazole, pantoprazole; and misoprostil. Drugs that decrease stomach acid and raise gastric pH can cause premature dissolution of enteric-coated peppermint oil (787).

Interactions with Foods

FOOD: Enteric-coated peppermint oil capsules used for treating irritable bowel syndrome (IBS) are contraindicated with food, and should be taken between meals (787).

Interactions with Lab Tests

No interactions are known to occur, and there is no known reason to expect a clinically significant interaction with peppermint oil.

Interactions with Diseases or Conditions

ACHLORHYDRIA: Enteric-coated peppermint oil should not be used when the stomach is not producing hydrochloric acid. Achlorhydria increases gastric pH and may cause premature dissolution of the enteric coating (787).

Dosage and Administration

ORAL: The typical dose of peppermint oil for digestive disorders is 0.2-0.4 mL diluted in liquid three times daily (1), and the average daily amount is 6-12 drops (2). For irritable bowel syndrome (IBS), the usual dose is 0.2-0.4 mL three times daily in enteric-coated capsules (1,2,3802). It's usually taken between meals (787).
TOPICAL: Peppermint oil is commonly applied as 5-20% semi-solid and oily preparations, 5-10% aqueous-ethanol preparations, and 1-5% nasal ointments. Rub a small amount into affected skin (2). For tension headaches, a 10% peppermint oil in ethanol solution applied across forehead and temples, repeated after 15 and 30 minutes, has been used (6190).
INHALATION: Typical dose is 3-4 drops of the oil in hot water. A lozenge containing 2-10 mg is also used (1,2).

Comments

Avoid confusion with peppermint leaf and rectified mint oil (18). In 1990, the FDA banned the sale of peppermint oil as an over-the-counter drug for use as a digestive aid due to lack of proof of efficacy (512). Peppermint is grown commercially in Indiana, Wisconsin, Oregon, Washington, and Idaho (6738).

PERILLA

Also Known As

Beefsteak Plant, Wild Coleus.
CAUTION: See separate listing for Alpha-Linolenic Acid.

Scientific Names

Perilla frutescens.
Family: Lamiaceae.

People Use This For

Orally, perilla is used for treating asthma. It is also used orally for nausea, sunstroke, inducing sweating, and as an antispasmodic.

In foods, perilla is used as a flavoring.

In manufacturing, perilla seed oil is used commercially in the production of varnishes, dyes, and inks.

Safety

POSSIBLY SAFE …when used orally and appropriately. There is some evidence perilla can be safely used for up to 4 weeks (1338).

PREGNANCY AND LACTATION: Insufficient reliable information available; avoid using.

Effectiveness

There is insufficient reliable information available to rate the effectiveness of perilla. However, there is preliminary evidence that perilla seed oil might improve pulmonary function in people with asthma (1338). More evidence is needed to rate perilla for this use.

Mechanism of Action

The applicable parts of perilla are the leaf and seed. Perilla contains multiple flavones. The major flavones apigenin and luteolin are found in the leaves and seeds, along with other flavones including shishonin (6). Perilla seed oil is also high in the fatty acid alpha-linolenic acid. Alpha-linolenic acid is thought decrease serum cholesterol and triglyceride levels, increase the concentration of the fatty acids eicosapentaenoic acid and arachidonic acid and inhibit production of inflammatory leukotrienes. Perilla seed oil is thought to help asthma because of the alpha-linolenic acid effects on leukotrienes (1338). Animal and in vitro studies suggest perilla oil may have antitumor effects (6). Perilla extract may have an immunosuppressant effect by preferentially attenuating IgE production (6). Patch testing suggests 1-perillaldehyde and perillalcohol contained in perilla oil are responsible for the occurrence of dermatitis (6). Cell studies have shown luteolin to have anti-proliferative activity (5003). Animals grazing on perilla have developed pulmonary edema and respiratory distress. Animal studies show the oil constituent, perilla ketone, induces pulmonary edema. Aldehyde antioxide contained in perilla oil may be toxic (6).

Adverse Reactions

Topically, perilla used topically may cause contact dermatitis (6).

Interactions with Herbs & Other Dietary Supplements

Insufficient reliable information available.

Interactions with Drugs

No interactions are known to occur, and there is no known reason to expect a clinically significant interaction with perilla.

Interactions with Foods

No interactions are known to occur, and there is no known reason to expect a clinically significant interaction with perilla.

Interactions with Lab Tests

No interactions are known to occur, and there is no known reason to expect a clinically significant interaction with perilla.

Interactions with Diseases or Conditions

No interactions are known to occur, and there is no known reason to expect a clinically significant interaction with perilla.

Dosage and Administration

ORAL: For asthma, perilla seed oil 10 to 20 grams per day has been used (1338).

Comments

None.

PERIWINKLE

Also Known As

Common Periwinkle, Earlyflowering, Evergreen, Lesser Periwinkle, Myrtle, Periwinkle, Small Periwinkle, Vincae minoris herba, Wintergreen.

CAUTION: See separate listing for Madagascar Periwinkle.

Scientific Names
Vinca minor.
Family: Apocynaceae.

People Use This For
Orally, periwinkle is used for "brain health" (increasing cerebral circulation, supporting brain metabolism, increasing mental productivity, preventing memory and concentration impairment and feebleness, improving memory and thinking capacity, preventing premature aging of brain cells and geriatric support). It also is used orally for mucous membrane inflammation, diarrhea, vaginal discharge, "blood-purification," throat ailments, tonsillitis, angina, sore throat, intestinal inflammation, toothache, edema, promoting wound healing, improving immune function, and as a diuretic, sedative, antihypertensive, and hemostatic remedy (2).

Safety
UNSAFE ...when used orally (2,17). Periwinkle contains pharmacologically active toxic alkaloids that can cause nerve, liver, and kidney damage (17).
PREGNANCY AND LACTATION: UNSAFE ...when used orally; avoid using.

Effectiveness
There is insufficient reliable information available about the effectiveness of periwinkle.

Mechanism of Action
The applicable parts of periwinkle are the above ground parts. Periwinkle contains pharmacologically active, toxic alkaloids including vincristine which have cytotoxic and neurological actions and can injure liver and kidneys (513). Periwinkle may have astringent activity (19). Constituent, vincamine, has hypotensive activity (19). In animals, periwinkle causes leukocytopenia, lymphocytopenia, and lowers alpha-1, alpha-2, and gamma-globulin levels presumably due to immune suppression (2).

Adverse Reactions
Orally, periwinkle may cause cytotoxic, neurologic, liver and kidney damage are possible due to vinca alkaloid constituents (17). Periwinkle may also potentially cause GI complaints and skin flushing (18). Consuming large amounts may cause severe drop in blood pressure (18).

Interactions with Herbs & Other Dietary Supplements
Insufficient reliable information available.

Interactions with Drugs
ANTIHYPERTENSIVE, ANTIHYPOTENSIVE DRUGS: Theoretically, concomitant use may interfere with blood pressure control (12,19).

Interactions with Foods
No interactions are known to occur, and there is no known reason to expect a clinically significant interaction with periwinkle.

Interactions with Lab Tests
No interactions are known to occur, and there is no known reason to expect a clinically significant interaction with periwinkle.

Interactions with Diseases or Conditions
HYPOTENSION: Contraindicated, due to potential hypotensive effects (12,19).
CONSTIPATION: Contraindicated, due to astringent activity (12,19).

Dosage and Administration
ORAL: People typically add 3 to 10 drops of the extract to water and use two to three times daily. Periwinkle extract contains glycerin and alcohol (6006).

Comments
The periwinkle constituent, vincamine, can be converted in the laboratory to the compound vinpocetine which is marketed as a dietary supplement (14,1799) (see separate listing for Vinpocetine). Avoid confusing periwinkle with Madagascar periwinkle (Catharanthus roseus).

PERU BALSAM

Also Known As
Balsam, Balsam of Peru, Balsam Peru, Balsamum Peruvianum, Black Balsam, Indian Balsam, Peruvian Balsam.
CAUTION: See separate listing for Tolu Balsam.

Scientific Names
Myroxylon pereirae, synonym Myroxylon balsamum pereirae.
Family: Leguminosae or Fabaceae.

People Use This For
Topically, Peru balsam is used for infected and poorly healing wounds, burns, decubitus ulcers (bed sores), frost bite, ulcus cruris, bruises caused by prosthetics, hemorrhoids, anal pruritus, diaper rash, and intertrigo (2,11).
In dentistry, peru balsam is a component of dental preparations for treating dry socket and as an ingredient in some dental impression materials. It is also used in toothpaste and toothpowder (11).
In traditional medicine, it has been used for cancer (11), to stop bleeding, promoting wound healing, as a diuretic, and to expel worms (6).
In manufacturing, Peru balsam is utilized as a fixative or fragrance in soaps and cosmetics (11) and as a food flavoring agent (11).

Safety
POSSIBLY SAFE ...when balsam preparations are applied topically and used for less than 1 week (2). In some individuals, peru balsam is a contact allergen (11).
LIKELY UNSAFE ...when used orally; avoid using. Peru balsam is for external use only (2,6). Kidney damage can occur with internal consumption of large doses (18).
PREGNANCY: Insufficient reliable information available; avoid using.
LACTATION: POSSIBLY UNSAFE ...when used topically because systemic toxicity to babies can occur following application of Peru balsam to the nipples of nursing mothers (6).

Effectiveness
POSSIBLY EFFECTIVE ...when used topically for healing wounds, burns, decubitus ulcers (bed sores), frost bite, ulcus cruris, bruises caused by prosthetics, hemorrhoids, and scabies (2).
There is insufficient reliable information available about the effectiveness of Peru balsam for its other uses.

Mechanism of Action
The applicable part of peru balsam is the oleo resin. Peru balsam's volatile oil consists mainly of benzoic and cinnamic acid esters, including benzyl benzoate (11). Benzyl benzoate is an effective scabicide (19). Peru balsam also has mild antiseptic and antibacterial properties and is believed to promote epithelial cell growth (11).

Adverse Reactions
Orally, Peru balsam can cause kidney damage with consumption of large amounts (18).
Topically, it can cause allergic skin reactions and contact dermatitis, including urticaria, recurring aphthoid oral ulcers, Quincke's disease, and diffuse purpurea (2,18). It has the potential to cause photodermatitis and phototoxicity (18).
Kidney damage can also occur with the external use of large amounts (18).

Interactions with Herbs & Other Dietary Supplements
Insufficient reliable information available.

Interactions with Drugs
No interactions are known to occur, and there is no known reason to expect a clinically significant interaction with Peru balsam.

Interactions with Foods
No interactions are known to occur, and there is no known reason to expect a clinically significant interaction with Peru balsam.

Interactions with Lab Tests
No interactions are known to occur, and there is no known reason to expect a clinically significant interaction with Peru balsam.

Interactions with Diseases or Conditions

KIDNEY DISEASE: Use with caution or avoid due to its potential to cause kidney damage.

Dosage and Administration

TOPICAL: Preparations of Peru balsam usually contain 5-20% Peruvian balsam (2). The maximum concentration for extensive surface application is 10% Peruvian balsam (2).

Comments

Peru balsam is the oleo resin exuded from scorched tree stems of Myroxylon balsamum.

PEYOTE

Also Known As

Devil's Root, Dumpling Cactus, Mescal Buttons, Mescaline, Pellote, Sacred Mushroom.

Scientific Names

Lophophora williamsii.
Family: Cactaceae.

People Use This For

Orally, peyote is used for treating fevers, rheumatism, and paralysis.
Topically, peyote is used for treating fractures, wounds, and snake bite.
Recreationally, peyote is used as a hallucinogen.

Safety

UNSAFE ...when used orally. Peyote is illegal in the US. It is a FDA schedule I controlled substance (14).
PREGNANCY AND LACTATION: UNSAFE ...when used orally due to potential for adverse effects (14).

Effectiveness

There is insufficient reliable information available about the effectiveness of peyote.

Mechanism of Action

The applicable parts of peyote are the above ground parts after the hair tufts are removed. The clinical effects of peyote are due to mescaline, which is structurally similar to amphetamines, and similar in activity to LSD, and the mushroom hallucinogens psilocybin and psilocin. In fact, people who take mescaline have a cross-tolerance to these other hallucinogens. Mescaline causes central nervous system and sympathetic stimulation and hallucinations. It's not clear exactly how mescaline causes hallucinations. However, its effects can be blocked by either serotonin antagonist methysergide or dopamine antagonist haloperidol. The hallucinogenic dose of peyote is about 5 mg/kg (14), or 4 to 12 slices of sprouts cut into 3-4.5 cm diameter pieces. Amphetamine-like or sympathomimetic effects are more common with higher doses (18).

Adverse Reactions

Nausea and vomiting are usually the first symptoms to occur after peyote ingestion. They usually resolve 2 hours after ingestion. Hallucinogenic effects peak at 3.5 to 4 hours, and resolve 15 hours post-ingestion. The hallucinations include visual, aural, taste, smell, touch, and abnormal perception of time and space. Anxiety, paranoia, fear and emotional instability may also occur. Common physiologic effects include mild elevations in heart rate, blood pressure and respiration rate. Sometimes slow heart beat occurs instead in response to elevated blood pressure. Mydriasis, blurred vision, palpitations, salivation, headache, dizziness, difficulty with walking, and drowsiness may also occur. Ingestion of peyote is rarely fatal. However, people can die as a result of homicidal, psychotic or suicidal behavior associated with their hallucinations. Flashbacks may also occur (14).

Interactions with Herbs & Other Dietary Supplements

Insufficient reliable information available.

Interactions with Drugs

INSULIN: Mescaline can increase the toxic effects of an insulin overdose.
PHYSOSTIGMINE: If given with mescaline, it can increase the risk of death.
METHYSERGIDE, HALOPERIDOL: Block mescaline's hallucinogenic effects.
VERAPAMIL: Can counteract mescaline-induced cerebral vasospasm.
METHADONE, ALCOHOL: Concomitant administration with mescaline can lead to seizures, kidney damage due to protein overload from the seizures (rhabdomyolysis), and prolonged coma (14).

Interactions with Foods

No interactions are known to occur, and there is no known reason to expect a clinically significant interaction with peyote.

Interactions with Lab Tests

No interactions are known to occur, and there is no known reason to expect a clinically significant interaction with peyote.

Interactions with Diseases or Conditions

No interactions are known to occur, and there is no known reason to expect a clinically significant interaction with peyote.

Dosage and Administration

No typical dosage.

Comments

Peyote is considered unsafe and illegal. It should not be used (see Safety) (14). Mescaline is also available as a crystalline powder, tablets, and powder. However, tablets which are perceived as mescaline often contain LSD, PCP, amphetamines, aspirin, STP, and/or strychnine instead. A previous 10 year survey found that 76% of "mescaline" tablets were altered in this manner (14).

PHEASANT'S EYE

Also Known As

Adonis herba, False Hellebore, Oxeye, Pheasants Eye, Red Morocco, Rose-A-Rubie, Sweet Vernal, Yellow Pheasant's Eye, Yellow Pheasants Eye.
CAUTION: See separate listings for American Hellebore, Black Hellebore, and White Hellebore.

Scientific Names

Adonis vernalis.
Family: Ranunculaceae.

People Use This For

Orally, pheasant's eye is used for mild heart failure (2,7,18), arrhythmia (18), and nervous heart complaints (18).
In folk medicine, pheasant's eye is used for dehydration, cramps, fever, and menstrual disorders (18).

Safety

POSSIBLY SAFE …when the standardized extract is used orally under the supervision of a medical professional trained in the appropriate use of pheasant's eye (2).
LIKELY UNSAFE …when the standardized extract is used orally without appropriate medical supervision (18,512). Pheasant's eye contains cardiac glycosides and monitoring is required to minimize serious adverse effects.
UNSAFE …when the plant is ingested. Pheasant's eye is highly poisonous (18).
PREGNANCY AND LACTATION: LIKELY UNSAFE …when used orally for self-medication (512).

Effectiveness

There is insufficient reliable information available about the effectiveness of pheasant's eye.

Mechanism of Action

The applicable parts of pheasant's eye are the above ground parts. Pheasant's eye contains cardioactive glycosides (2,7,18). It has cardiac effects similar to digoxin, including positive inotropic and negative chronotropic effects (7). In experimental animals, pheasant's eye demonstrates a tonic effect on veins (2).

Adverse Reactions

Symptoms of pheasant's eye overdose include nausea, vomiting, and arrhythmias (2).

Interactions with Herbs & Other Dietary Supplements

CALCIUM: Concomitant use with calcium can increase the risk of cardiac toxicity (2,3805).

CARDIAC GLYCOSIDE-CONTAINING HERBS: Contraindicated. Concomitant use can increase the risk of cardiac glycoside toxicity. Cardiac glycoside-containing herbs include black hellebore, Canadian hemp roots, digitalis leaf, hedge mustard, figwort, lily of the valley roots, motherwort, oleander leaf, pleurisy root, squill bulb leaf scales, strophanthus seeds, and uzara (2,18,19,500).

CARDIOACTIVE HERBS: Avoid concomitant use with cardioactive herbs due to unpredictability of effects and adverse effects. These include: calamus, cereus, cola, coltsfoot, devil's claw, European mistletoe, fenugreek, fumitory, ginger, ginseng Panax, hawthorn, white horehound, mate, parsley, quassia, scotch broom flower, shepherd's purse, and wild carrot (4).

LICORICE/HORSETAIL: The overuse or misuse of licorice rhizome or horsetail plant increases the risk of cardiac toxicity due to potassium depletion. (19).

STIMULANT LAXATIVE HERBS: The overuse or misuse of stimulant laxatives increases the risk of cardiac toxicity due to potassium depletion. Stimulant laxative herbs include: aloe dried leaf sap, blue flag rhizome, alder buckthorn, European buckthorn, butternut bark, cascara bark, castor oil, colocynth fruit pulp, gamboge bark exudate, jalap root, black root, manna bark exudate, podophyllum root, rhubarb root, senna leaves and pods, wild cucumber fruit (Ecballium elaterium), and yellow dock root (19).

Interactions with Drugs

CALCIUM: Concomitant use of pheasant's eye with calcium can increase the risk of cardiac glycoside arrhythmias (2,3805).

CORTICOSTEROIDS: Concomitant use of pheasant's eye can increase the therapeutic and adverse effects of long-term corticosteroid use (2).

DIGOXIN: Concomitant use is contraindicated due to an increased risk of cardiac glycoside toxicity (2,4).

POTASSIUM DEPLETING DIURETICS, STIMULANT LAXATIVES: Concomitant use of pheasant's eye can increase the risk of cardiac glycoside toxicity due to potassium loss (2).

QUINIDINE: Concomitant use can increase cardiac effects and adverse effects (2).

Interactions with Foods

No interactions are known to occur, and there is no known reason to expect a clinically significant interaction with pheasant's eye.

Interactions with Lab Tests

No interactions are known to occur, and there is no known reason to expect a clinically significant interaction with pheasant's eye.

Interactions with Diseases or Conditions

HYPOKALEMIA: Contraindicated (2,3805).

HYPERCALCEMIA: Contraindicated (2,3805).

Dosage and Administration

ORAL: The average amount of pheasant's eye is 600 mg of the standardized adonis powder (DAB9) per day (2). The maximum single dose is 1 gram (2), and the maximum daily amount is 3 grams (2).

Comments

Pheasant's eye is considered a poisonous plant (18).

PHENYLALANINE

Also Known As

DLPA, D-Phenylalanine, DL-Phenylalanine, L-Phenylalanine.

Scientific Names

Alpha-aminohydrocinnamic acid; Beta-phenyl-alanine.

People Use This For

Orally, phenylalanine is used for depression, Parkinson's disease, chronic pain, osteoarthritis, rheumatoid arthritis, alcohol withdrawal symptoms, and vitiligo.
Topically, it is used for vitiligo (2461).

Safety

LIKELY SAFE …when L-phenylalanine is consumed orally in amounts typically found in foods (2022).
POSSIBLY SAFE …when L-phenylalanine is used orally for therapeutic purposes (2455,2456,2461,2463,2465,2466,2467,2468,2469).
There is insufficient reliable information available about the oral safety of D-phenylalanine.
There is insufficient reliable information available about the topical safety of phenylalanine.
PREGNANCY: LIKELY SAFE …when L-phenylalanine is consumed in amounts typically found in foods by pregnant women with normal phenylalanine metabolism and serum levels (2020,2022). UNSAFE …when L-phenylalanine is consumed in amounts typically found in foods by pregnant women with serum phenylalanine concentrations greater than 360 micromol/L, which increases the risk of birth defects (1402). The risk for facial defects is highest at gestation weeks 10-14, neurological and growth abnormalities between 3-16 weeks, and cardiovascular defects at 3-8 weeks. Experts recommend that women with high phenylalanine serum concentrations follow a low phenylalanine diet for at least 20 weeks prior to conception to decrease the risk for birth defects (1402). In addition, some experts recommend screening in women not tested for phenylketonuria (PKU) at birth (1401).
There is insufficient reliable information available about the safety of oral, therapeutic amounts of L-phenylalanine in pregnant women with normal phenylalanine metabolism and serum concentrations; avoid using.
There is insufficient reliable information available about the safety of oral D-phenylalanine in pregnant women; avoid using.
LACTATION: LIKELY SAFE …when L-phenylalanine is consumed in amounts typically found in foods by breast-feeding women with normal phenylalanine metabolism (2020,2022).
There is insufficient reliable information available about the safety of oral, therapeutic amounts of L-phenylalanine in lactating women with normal phenylalanine metabolism; avoid using.
There is insufficient reliable information available about the safety of oral D-phenylalanine during lactation; avoid using.

Effectiveness

POSSIBLY EFFECTIVE …when D-phenylalanine is used orally for treating the symptoms of Parkinson's disease (2455) and for enhancing acupuncture anesthesia for tooth extraction (2456). …when DL-phenylalanine is used orally for treating depression (2468). …when L-phenylalanine is used orally and combined with UVA exposure for treating vitiligo in adults (2461,2463,2464,2466) and in children (2467). …when used orally for unipolar depression combined with selegiline (Eldepryl) (2469). …when L-phenylalanine is applied topically and combined with UVA exposure for treating vitiligo (2461).
POSSIBLY INEFFECTIVE …when D-phenylalanine is used orally for enhancing acupuncture analgesia for chronic low back pain (2456) and as analgesia for chronic pain of varied etiology (2459). …when DL-phenylalanine is used orally for treating Parkinson's disease (2454).
There is insufficient reliable information available about the effectiveness of phenylalanine for its other uses.

Mechanism of Action

Phenylalanine exists as two enantiomers, D-phenylalanine and L-phenylalanine. DL-phenylalanine is a mixture of these two forms. D-phenylalanine is non-nutritive (not an essential human amino acid) and its role in humans is not currently understood. L-phenylalanine is an essential human amino acid, and is the only form of phenylalanine found in proteins. L-phenylalanine is normally metabolized to tyrosine (9). Human data suggests that about one-third of a D-phenylalanine dose is converted to L-phenylalanine (2051,2052). L-phenylalanine exacerbates tardive dyskinesia in people with schizophrenia (2457) and can contribute to the development and severity of tardive dyskinesia in people with unipolar depression treated with neuroleptics (2458). L-phenylalanine does not alter pain tolerance to burns in healthy people (2460). D-phenylalanine increases the pain threshold in animals, inducing a naloxone-reversible analgesia by blocking enzymatic degradation of enkephalin (2459). Large neutral amino acids (LNAAs) including DL-phenylalanine, leucine, and isoleucine can exacerbate tremor, rigidity, and the "on-off" syndrome in people with Parkinson's disease who have used levodopa for more than 5-10 years (2454,3291). The amount of dietary LNAAs appears to affect the severity of "on-off" symptoms and may be independent of dietary protein-induced alterations in oral levodopa bioavailability (3291,3292,3293,3294). DL-phenylalanine and other LNAAs might worsen symptoms by decreasing the amount of levodopa that crosses the blood-brain barrier (3291,3294). Preliminary evidence suggests that L-phenylalanine, given with the non-selective monoamine oxidase (MAO-A/MOA-B) inhibitor pargyline, might prevent the elimination of tyramine, increasing the risk of hypertensive crisis (2021). However, hypertensive crisis was not reported in a small number of patients who used L-phenylalanine with the partially selective monoamine oxidase B (MAO-B) inhibitor, selegiline (Eldepryl) (2469).

Adverse Reactions

Orally, L-phenylalanine can exacerbate tardive dyskinesia in people with schizophrenia (2457). Large neutral amino acids (LNAAs) including DL-phenylalanine, leucine and isoleucine, exacerbate tremor, rigidity, and the "on-off" syndrome in patient's with Parkinson's disease using levodopa (2454,3291,3292,3293,3294). Birth defects associated with elevated maternal phenylalanine concentrations include severe mental retardation, microcephaly (a smaller than normal head), abnormal facial features and congenital heart disease (1401,1402). The risk of birth defects during pregnancy increases when maternal phenylalanine serum concentrations exceed 360 micromol/L (1402). Preliminary data suggest that L-phenylalanine supplements might cause hypertension or increase the risk of stroke in certain genetically predisposed people (2084).

Interactions with Herbs & Other Dietary Supplements

Insufficient reliable information available.

Interactions with Drugs

NON-SELECTIVE MONOAMINE OXIDASE INIHIBTORS (MAOIs): Theoretically, concomitant use of L-phenylalanine and non-selective MAOI drugs might increase the risk of hypertensive crisis. Some evidence suggests that L-phenylalanine, given with the non-selective MAOI drug pargyline, might prevent the elimination of tyramine, increasing the risk of hypertensive crisis (2021).
SELEGILINE (Eldepryl): Concomitant use of L-phenylalanine with selegiline (selective monoamine oxidase type-B inhibitor) might be effective for treating unipolar depression (2469).
LEVODOPA: Concomitant use of DL-phenylalanine and levodopa can exacerbate tremor, rigidity, and the "on-off" syndrome in patients with Parkinson's disease (2454,3291,3292,3293,3294).
NEUROLEPTIC DRUGS: Concomitant use of L-phenylalanine and neuroleptics can contribute to the development and severity of tardive dyskinesia in patients with neuroleptic-treated unipolar depression (2458).

Interactions with Foods

No interactions are known to occur, and there is no known reason to expect a clinically significant interaction with phenylalanine.

Interactions with Lab Tests

No interactions are known to occur, and there is no known reason to expect a clinically significant interaction with phenylalanine.

Interactions with Diseases or Conditions

ALKAPTONURIA: Contraindicated (2470); alkaptonuria is an inherited disorder involving the inability to metabolize phenylalanine and tyrosine, leading to ochre pigment deposits in the connective tissues. There are no clinical manifestations until mid-adulthood, when the pigment deposits lead to progressive degenerative joint diseases (2050,2053,2055).
HYPERTENSION: Use with caution in patients at risk for hypertension. Some evidence suggests that L-phenylalanine might cause hypertension in genetically predisposed patients (2084).
PHENYLKETONURIA (PKU): Contraindicated (2470); phenylketonuria is an inherited disorder involving the inability to metabolize phenylalanine, leading to toxic serum levels of phenylalanine and its metabolites (2050,2053).
SCHIZOPHRENIA: Use with caution. L-Phenylalanine can exacerbate tardive dyskinesia in people with schizophrenia (2457).
STROKE: Use with caution in patients at risk for stroke. Some evidence suggests that L-phenylalanine might increase the risk of stroke in genetically predisposed patients (2084).
TYROSINEMIA/TYROSINURIA: Contraindicated (2470); tyrosinemia is an inherited disorder involving the inability to metabolize tyrosine leading to toxic serum levels of tyrosine and its metabolites. Because phenylalanine is metabolized to tyrosine, it can also cause toxic tyrosine levels in people with tyrosinemia (2053,2054).

Dosage and Administration

ORAL: For Parkinson's disease, the dose of D-phenylalanine is typically 200 to 500 mg per day (2455). As an adjunct to acupuncture anesthesia or analgesia in tooth extraction: 4 grams of D-phenylalanine is usually taken 30 minutes before acupuncture (2456). For depression, the usual dose of L-phenylalanine is 250 mg with 5-10 mg L-deprenyl per day (2469), and the common dose of DL-phenylalanine is 150 to 200 mg per day (2468). For vitiligo in adults, 50-100 mg/kg of L-phenylalanine is typically used per day along with UVA exposure (2461,2463,2464,2465,2466).
TOPICAL: A 10% L-phenylalanine cream along with UVA exposure is commonly used for vitiligo (2461).

Comments

Phenylalanine exists as two enantiomers, D and L. These molecules are mirror images of each other. The racemic mix DL-phenylalanine (50% D-, 50% L-phenylalanine) is produced by laboratory synthesis. Phenylalanine products are available which contain pure L-phenylalanine (an essential amino acid), pure D-phenylalanine (biological activity unknown), or DL-phenylalanine (2050,2051). Major dietary sources of L-phenylalanine include meat, fish, eggs, cheese, and milk (2023).

PHOSPHATE SALTS

Also Known As
Aluminum Phosphate;
Calcium Phosphate: Bone Ash, Bone Phosphate, Calcium Orthophosphate, Calcium Phosphate Dibasic Anhydrous, Calcium Phosphate Dibasic Dihydrate, Calcium Phosphate Tribasic, Di-Calcium Phosphate, Dicalcium Phosphate, Dicalcium Phosphates, Neutral Calcium Phosphate, Precipitated Calcium Phosphate, Tertiary Calcium Phosphate, Tricalcium Phosphate, Whitlockite;
Potassium Phosphate: Dibasic Potassium Phosphate, Dipotassium Hydrogen Orthophosphate, Dipotassium Monophosphate, Dipotassium Phosphate, Monobasic Potassium Phosphate, Potassium Acid Phosphate, Potassium Biphosphate, Potassium Dihydrogen Orthophosphate;
Sodium Phosphate: Anhydrous Sodium Phosphate, Dibasic Sodium Phosphate, Disodium Hydrogen Orthophosphate, Disodium Hydrogen Orthophosphate Dodecahydrate, Disodium Hydrogen Phosphate, Disodium Phosphate, Phosphate of Soda, Sodium Orthophosphate.
CAUTION: Do not confuse Phosphate Salts with toxic substances such as Organophosphates, or with Tribasic Sodium Phosphates and Tribasic Potassium Phosphates which are strongly alkaline (14).

Scientific Names
Aluminum phosphate; Calcium phosphate; Potassium phosphate; Sodium phosphate.

People Use This For
Orally, phosphate salts are used for treating hypophosphatemia and hypercalcemia (14,3372), hypophosphatemic rickets or osteomalacia (14), and for prevention of recurrent nephrolithiasis (kidney stones) (14,3372). Phosphate salts are also used orally for enhancing exercise performance (2499,8300,8301), as an antacid for gastroesophageal reflux disease (GERD), and as a laxative for presurgical bowel preparation (15).
Topically, phosphate salts are used with calcium in dentistry for sensitive teeth (1237).
Rectally, phosphate salts are used as a laxative for presurgical bowel preparation (15).
Intravenously, potassium phosphate is used for hypophosphatemia and hypokalemia, preventing hypophosphatemia in people receiving parenteral nutrition, and treating hypercalcemia (9,14,15).

Safety
LIKELY SAFE ...when sodium, potassium, aluminum, and calcium phosphates are used orally and appropriately short-term (15). ...when sodium phosphate is used rectally and appropriately short-term (14,15). Long-term use or high doses used orally or rectally require monitoring of serum electrolytes (14,2494,2495,2496,2497,2498,3092). ...when used intravenously, potassium phosphate is a FDA-approved prescription drug.
PREGNANCY AND LACTATION: LIKELY SAFE ...when used at recommended dietary allowances (RDAs) of 1250 mg daily for mothers between 14-18 years of age and 700 mg daily for those over 18 years of age (3094).

Effectiveness
EFFECTIVE ...when sodium and potassium phosphates are used orally for preventing and treating hypophosphatemia (14). ...when sodium phosphates are used orally and appropriately as a laxative and bowel prep for surgery, x-ray, or endoscopy (15). ...when calcium phosphate is used orally as a calcium supplement (14,15). ...when sodium phosphates are used rectally as a laxative and bowel prep for surgery, x-ray, or endoscopy (14,15). ...when the FDA-approved IV product is used for the correction of hypophosphatemia (8302,8303).
LIKELY EFFECTIVE ...when sodium and potassium phosphates are used orally for treating hypercalcemia (14).
POSSIBLY EFFECTIVE ...when used orally to improve aerobic exercise performance by increasing capacity to use oxygen (VO2 max) (217). ...when used orally for prevention of calcium oxalate kidney stones. Potassium and sodium phosphate salts may be an acceptable alternative to conventional thiazide diuretics for kidney stones in patients with hypercalciuria (14,2209,6470).
LIKELY INEFFECTIVE ...when phosphates are used orally for enhancing anaerobic exercise performance (2499,8300,8301).
There is insufficient information available to rate the effectiveness of phosphate salts for their other uses.
However, there is preliminary unpublished research suggesting that calcium and phosphate together might be used to treat people with sensitive teeth (1237). More evidence is needed to rate phosphate salts for this use.

Mechanism of Action

Phosphate is the most abundant intracellular anion in the body. It is critical for membrane structure, transport, and energy storage (3092). Normal plasma concentrations range from 0.8-1.6 mmol/L, or 2.5-5 mg/dL (0.032 mmol phosphate = 1 mg) (14). Phosphate plays an important role in buffering body fluids, and plays a primary role in the renal excretion of hydrogen ions (14). It is present in carbohydrates, proteins, lipids and various enzymes involved in energy transfer (14). It is required for utilization of many B vitamins (14). Vitamin D3 and its metabolites influence phosphate absorption from the gut and also affect renal tubular reabsorption of phosphate (14,3092,3372). Dietary phosphate deprivation lowers the serum phosphate levels, which are inversely related to serum calcium levels (14,3372). Hypophosphatemia causes an increase in intestinal calcium absorption and increased calcium in the blood, which can inhibit formation of new bone (14,3372), and potentially lead to a greater risk of renal calcium stone formation (3372). Hyperphosphatemia can occur with excessive intake of vitamin D (3092). Sodium phosphates are used as saline laxatives. They cause influx of fluids in the intestine by an osmotic action and increase peristalsis (14). Aluminum phosphate used orally neutralizes gastric acid (15). Oral ingestion of large amounts of sodium dihydrogen phosphate can lower urine pH (1).

Adverse Reactions

All phosphate salts, used orally can cause gastrointestinal irritation, fluid and electrolyte disturbances including hyperphosphatemia and hypocalcemia, and extraskeletal calcification (14). Potassium phosphates can cause hyperkalemia (14). Sodium phosphates can cause hypernatremia and hypokalemia (14,2494,2495,2496,2497). Sodium and potassium phosphates can cause diarrhea (14). Aluminum phosphate can cause constipation (14). Phosphate salts used rectally can cause fluid and electrolyte disturbances including hyperphosphatemia and hypocalcemia, gastrointestinal irritation, and perforation of the rectum (14).

Interactions with Herbs & Other Dietary Supplements

Insufficient reliable information available.

Interactions with Drugs

ANTACIDS: Antacids containing aluminum, calcium, or magnesium can bind phosphate in the gut and prevent its absorption (14,3371). Some patients with phosphate depletion due to chronic antacid abuse might also present with recurrent nephrolithiasis and ureter obstruction (3371).

COLESTIPOL (Colestid): Concomitant administration of colestipol and phosphate can decrease oral absorption of phosphate (14).

Drug Influences on Nutrient Levels and Depletion

SOME DRUGS CAN AFFECT PHOSPHATE LEVELS:

ALUMINUM SALTS: Use of aluminum salts can bind phosphate in the gut and reduce serum phosphate levels. Avoid prolonged administration of large doses of aluminum-containing drugs, which might lead to hypophosphatemia (3371,4400).

Interactions with Foods

No interactions are known to occur, and there is no known reason to expect a clinically significant interaction with phosphate salts.

Interactions with Lab Tests

ACID PHOSPHATASE: Phosphates can cause a false-decrease in serum test results. High substrate concentrations can inhibit the analytic reaction (275).

ALKALINE PHOSPHATASE: Phosphates can cause a false-decrease in serum test results. High substrate concentrations can inhibit the analytic reaction (275).

AMMONIA: Phosphates can cause a false-decrease in plasma test results by inhibiting formation of indophenol color in Berthelot reaction (275).

CALCIUM: Phosphates can increase fecal levels and test results (275). Phosphates can cause a false-decrease in serum and urine test results by inhibiting emission in some flame methods and by competing with EDTA for calcium (275).

LIPID GLYCEROL: Phosphates can cause a false-decrease in serum test results by inhibiting phospholipase with method of Horney (275).

MAGNESIUM: Phosphates can decrease urine levels and test results by reducing increased excretion with bed rest (275).

PARATHYROID HORMONE: Phosphates can increase plasma levels and test results (275).

PHOSPHATE: Phosphates increase fecal, serum, and urine levels and test results (275).

POTASSIUM: Phosphates (except potassium phosphate) can decrease serum levels and test results (275).

PYRUVATE KINASE: Phosphates can cause a false-increase in red blood cell test results by activating analytic enzyme (275).

Interactions with Diseases or Conditions

HYPERCALCEMIA: Use cautiously in individuals with high serum calcium levels. The product of serum phosphate and calcium levels should not exceed 60 to prevent precipitation of calcium phosphate and soft tissue calcification (6479).

HYPOPHOSPHATEMIA: Low phosphate levels can be associated with many conditions, including poor oral intake or absorption, reduced renal tubular reabsorption, respiratory alkalosis, excessive insulin use, certain malignancies, diabetic ketoacidosis, and chronic alcoholism (14,3092).

HYPERPHOSPHATEMIA: People with Addison's disease, severe cardiopulmonary, renal, or hepatic disease are at risk for hyperphosphatemia and hypocalcemia when phosphates are used (14,2497). Hyperphosphatemia might also occur in people with renal insufficiency, hypoparathyroidism, severe hyperthyroidism, untreated adrenal insufficiency (due to volume contraction, metabolic acidosis and reduced glomerular permeability), metabolic, lactic or respiratory acidosis, rhabdomyolysis, infarction, hemolysis, or tumor lysis syndrome (3092).

EDEMA: Use phosphates with caution in people with cirrhosis, heart failure, or other edematous conditions (14).

KIDNEY DYSFUNCTION: Closely monitor serum electrolytes when phosphates are used by people with mild to moderate renal impairment (14).

Dosage and Administration

ORAL: For bowel preparation for diagnostic tests, a typical dose is dibasic sodium phosphate 3.42 to 7.56 grams and monobasic sodium phosphate 9.1-20.2 grams daily given as a single dose (15). Phosphate laxative preparations should be taken on an empty stomach and with plenty of water (14). For use as an antacid, a typical dose of aluminum phosphate gel is 10-30 mL every 2 hours (14). As a calcium supplement the usual dose of dibasic calcium phosphate is 4.4 grams daily in divided doses (14). The usual dose of tribasic calcium phosphate as a calcium supplement is 1.6 grams twice daily (14). Treating hypophosphatemia or hypercalcemia with oral phosphates requires monitoring of serum electrolyte levels and medical supervision (14). For kidney stones, potassium and sodium phosphate salts providing 1200-1500 mg of elemental phosphate have been used (14,2209,6470). As a supplement, the recommended daily dietary allowances (RDAs) of phosphate (expressed as phosphorus) are: Children 1-3 years, 460 mg; Children 4-8 years, 500 mg; Males and females 9-18 years, 1250 mg; Males and females over 18 years, 700 mg (3094). The adequate intakes (AI) for infants are: 100 mg for infants 0-6 months old and 275 mg for infants 7-12 months of age (3094).

RECTAL: For bowel preparation for diagnostic tests, a typical dose is dibasic sodium phosphate 6.84-7.56 grams and monobasic sodium phosphate 18.24-20.16 grams daily, administered as a single dose (15). Treating hypophosphatemia with rectal phosphates requires monitoring of serum electrolyte levels (14).

INTRAVENOUS: Injectable potassium phosphate is a FDA-approved prescription product.

Comments

Foods high in phosphate include milk, whole grain cereals, nuts, dried fruits and vegetables, and some meats (14). Phosphates present in dairy products and meats are soluble and readily absorbed, whereas those in cereal grains are bound and insoluble, and may be poorly absorbed (3092). Cola drinks contain significant amounts of phosphate and excessive intake can result in hyperphosphatemia and hypocalcemia (14).

PHOSPHATIDYLCHOLINE

Also Known As

Phosphatidyl Choline.
CAUTION: See separate listings for Choline, Lecithin, Phosphatidylserine, and Soy.

Scientific Names

None.

People Use This For

Orally, phosphatidylcholine is used for treating anxiety (5154), eczema (5154), gallbladder disease (5154,5227), hepatitis (5154,5224,5225,5226,5227), manic-depressive illness (5154), peripheral vascular disorders (9), hyperlipidemias (9,5227), improving ultrafiltration in peritoneal dialysis (5222), tardive dyskinesia (5223), premenstrual syndrome (5227), memory loss (5227,5228), Alzheimer's disease (5227), immunodepression (5227), and preventing aging (5227).

Safety

LIKELY SAFE ...when used orally and appropriately (4914). Even large amounts, 30 grams per day for 6 weeks, have been well tolerated (5223). Lecithin, which contains a substantial amount of phosphatidylcholine, has Generally Recognized as Safe (GRAS) status in the US (4912).

PREGNANCY AND LACTATION: Insufficient reliable information available; avoid using.

Effectiveness

POSSIBLY EFFECTIVE ...when the polyunsaturated form of phosphatidylcholine is used orally in combination with interferon for chronic hepatitis C (5226).

POSSIBLY INEFFECTIVE ...when used orally for hepatitis A (5225). Studies regarding hepatitis B show conflicting results (5224,5226). ...when used orally for improving ultrafiltration in peritoneal dialysis (5222). ...when used orally for treating tardive dyskinesia (5223).

There is insufficient reliable information available about the effectiveness of phosphatidylcholine for its other uses.

Mechanism of Action

Phosphatidylcholine is a phospholipid and a major constituent of lecithin (9). Egg lecithin contains 69% phosphatidylcholine, while soybean lecithin contains 24% phosphatidylcholine (4914). Phosphatidylcholine is a precursor to acetylcholine (5228). In a clinical trial, a single dose of 25 grams improved explicit memory 90 minutes later (5228).

Adverse Reactions

Orally, use of phosphatidylcholine can increase sweating (5229). Ingesting large amounts (30 grams per day) can cause gastrointestinal upset and diarrhea (5223).

Interactions with Herbs & Other Dietary Supplements

Insufficient reliable information available.

Interactions with Drugs

No interactions are known to occur, and there is no known reason to expect a clinically significant interaction with phosphatidylcholine.

Interactions with Foods

No interactions are known to occur, and there is no known reason to expect a clinically significant interaction with phosphatidylcholine.

Interactions with Lab Tests

No interactions are known to occur, and there is no known reason to expect a clinically significant interaction with phosphatidylcholine.

Interactions with Diseases or Conditions

No interactions are known to occur, and there is no known reason to expect a clinically significant interaction with phosphatidylcholine.

Dosage and Administration

ORAL: For hepatitis C, 1.8 grams of lecithin used daily with hepatitis C interferon (5226).

Comments

The term "phosphatidylcholine" is sometimes used interchangeably with "lecithin" although the two are different. Choline is a component of phosphatidylcholine, which is a component of lecithin (16). Although closely related, these terms are not synonymous. However, in the clinical literature, they are often confused. Brand names are PhosChol (9,5153), Ultracholine (9).

PHOSPHATIDYLSERINE

Also Known As

BC PS, BC-PS, Bovine Cortex Phosphatidylserine, Bovine Phosphatidylserine, Cephalin, Kephalin, LECI PS, LECI-PS, Lecithin Phosphatidylserine, Phosphatidyl Serine, PS, PtdSer, Soy PS, Soy-PS, Soy Phosphatidylserine. CAUTION: See separate listings for Choline, Lecithin, Phosphatidylcholine, and Soy.

Scientific Names

Phosphatidylserine.

People Use This For

Orally, phosphatidylserine is used for Alzheimer's disease and other dementias, age-related decline in mental function, improving cognitive function in young people, attention deficit hyperactivity disorder (ADHD), depression, preventing exercise-induced stress, and improving athletic performance (2436,7117,7121).

Safety

POSSIBLY SAFE ...when used orally and appropriately. Phosphatidylserine seems to be safe when used for up to 6 months (2255,2437,2438,2439,2440,2441,7118). Most studies have used bovine cortex derived phosphatidylserine. Since these preparations are derived from animals, there is some concern about contamination with diseased animal parts (see Adverse Reactions) (1825). So far, there are no reports of disease transmission to humans due to use of contaminated phosphatidylserine preparations. Most manufacturers now only produce soy or cabbage derived phosphatidylserine (1825,7115).
CHILDREN: POSSIBLY SAFE ...when used orally and appropriately (7117).
PREGNANCY AND LACTATION: Insufficient reliable information available; avoid using.

Effectiveness

POSSIBLY EFFECTIVE ...when used orally for Alzheimer's disease and senile dementia, short-term. Phosphatidylserine can increase cognitive function, global improvement rating scales, and improve behavioral rating scales over 6-12 weeks of treatment (2255,2437,2438,2439,7114,7118). Phosphatidylserine seems to be most effective in patients with less severe symptoms (2437,2439), but phosphatidylserine seems to lose its effectiveness with extended use. After 16 weeks of treatment, progression of Alzheimer's disease seems to overcome any benefit of phosphatidylserine (2255). ...when used orally for improving age-related cognitive and memory impairment (2440,2441,7119,7120). Phosphatidylserine seems to improve attention and arousal, verbal fluency, and memory in aging people with intellectual deterioration (7119,7120).

Most clinical studies have used phosphatidylserine derived from bovine cortex. However, most supplements now use soy or cabbage derived phosphatidylserine. Clinical studies have not yet evaluated phosphatidylserine from soy or other sources. It is not known if phosphatidylserine from soy and other sources is as effective as bovine derived products.

There is insufficient reliable information available to rate the effectiveness of phosphatidylserine for its other uses. However, there is some preliminary evidence that phosphatidylserine might improve depression in geriatric patients (7113). There is also some evidence that phosphatidylserine might reduce exercise-induced stress. Athletes taking phosphatidylserine during over-training seem to have the perception of well-being and reduced muscle soreness (2264). More research is needed to rate phosphatidylserine for these uses.

Mechanism of Action

Phosphatidylserine is a fat-soluble phospholipid that occurs endogenously in humans. It is the most abundant phospholipid in the human brain and is important in neuronal membrane functions such as maintenance of the cell's internal environment, signal transduction, secretory vesicle release, cell-to-cell communication, and cell growth regulation (2437,7115). Phosphatidylserine is also a component of the mitochondrial membrane, where it might function as a metabolic reservoir for other phospholipids (7121). Although the body is able to synthesize phosphatidylserine through an elaborate series of reactions and substantial energy expenditure, the body obtains most phosphatidylserine from dietary sources. Phosphatidylserine is present in small quantities in most foods (7116). It is not clear how phosphatidylserine works for dementia such as Alzheimer's disease and age-related memory impairment. However, one theory is that patients with dementia or age-related memory impairment have structural or functional abnormalities in neuronal membranes that cause changes in neurotransmitter functioning. For example, people with cognitive dysfunction often have changes in acetylcholine, norepinephrine, and serotonin levels. Some researchers think the abnormal neuronal function can be attributed to changes in lipid composition of the brain. It is thought that exogenous administration of phosphatidylserine might then normalize brain lipid content and return neuronal function to normal (2441). Phosphatidylserine has been shown to increase acetylcholine, norepinephrine, serotonin, and dopamine levels in animal models and patients with Alzheimer's disease. In an animal model, phosphatidylserine also seems to minimize age-related neuronal dendrite loss and atrophy of cholinergic neurons (2437). There is some interest in phosphatidylserine for decreasing exercise-induced stress. Some preliminary evidence shows that phosphatidylserine might blunt the rise in cortisol following strenuous over-training (2264).

Adverse Reactions

Orally, phosphatidylserine is typically well tolerated. Some patients can experience gastrointestinal upset or insomnia. These side effects are more likely to occur with higher doses, 300 mg for gastrointestinal upset and 600 mg for insomnia (7116,7121). Most phosphatidylserine supplements used to be derived from bovine cortex, so there has been some concern about possible contamination from sick or diseased animals, including those harboring bovine spongiform encephalopathy (BSE, mad cow disease). Using supplements produced from diseased animals might present a human health hazard. So far there are no reports of BSE or other disease transmission to humans from dietary supplements containing animal materials and the risk of potential disease transmission is thought to be low. However, because of this concern most manufacturers now only produce soy or cabbage derived phosphatidylserine.

Interactions with Herbs & Other Dietary Supplements

Insufficient reliable information available.

Interactions with Drugs

No interactions are known to occur, and there is no known reason to expect a clinically significant interaction with phosphatidylserine.

Interactions with Foods

No interactions are known to occur, and there is no known reason to expect a clinically significant interaction with phosphatidylserine.

Interactions with Lab Tests

URIC ACID: Phosphatidylserine 300 mg daily can reduce uric acid levels (7116).

ALANINE AMINOTRANSFERASE (ALT, SGPT): Phosphatidylserine 300 mg daily can reduce alanine aminotransferase levels (7116).

Interactions with Diseases or Conditions

No interactions are known to occur, and there is no known reason to expect a clinically significant interaction with phosphatidylserine.

Dosage and Administration

ORAL: For Alzheimer's disease, senile dementia, and age-related cognitive or memory impairment, 100 mg three times daily has been used in clinical studies (2437,2438,2440,2441). For treatment of attention deficit hyperactivity disorder (ADHD) in children, people typically use 200 to 300 mg daily (7117).

Comments

Cephalin (synonym kephalin) is the term formerly used to refer to what are now known as phosphatidylserine and phosphatidylethanolamine (511).

PIMPINELLA above ground parts

Also Known As

Bibernellkraut, Burnet Saxifrage, Pimpernell, Pimpinellae herba, Saxifrage.
CAUTION: See separate listing for Pimpinella root.

Scientific Names

Pimpinella saxifraga, synonym Pimpinella major.
Family: Apiaceae.

People Use This For

Orally, pimpinella above ground parts are used for lung ailments and stimulating gastrointestinal activity (2).
Topically, pimpinella above ground parts are used for varicose veins (2).

Safety

There is insufficient reliable information available about the safety of pimpinella above ground parts.
Pregnancy and Lactation: Insufficient reliable information available; avoid using.

Effectiveness

There is insufficient reliable information about the effectiveness of pimpinella above ground parts.

Mechanism of Action

There is insufficient reliable information available about the possible mechanism of action and active ingredients.

Adverse Reactions

None reported.

Interactions with Herbs & Other Dietary Supplements

Insufficient reliable information available.

Interactions with Drugs

No interactions are known to occur, and there is no known reason to expect a clinically significant interaction with pimpinella above ground parts.

Interactions with Foods

No interactions are known to occur, and there is no known reason to expect a clinically significant interaction with pimpinella above ground parts.

Interactions with Lab Tests

No interactions are known to occur, and there is no known reason to expect a clinically significant interaction with pimpinella above ground parts.

Interactions with Diseases or Conditions

No interactions are known to occur, and there is no known reason to expect a clinically significant interaction with pimpinella above ground parts.

Dosage and Administration

No typical dosage.

Comments

There is very little scientific information about this product. Our staff is continually analyzing the available information on natural medicines and will add data here as it becomes available.

PIMPINELLA root

Also Known As

Burnet Saxifrage, Greater Burnet-Saxifrage, Pimpernell, Pimpinellae radix, Saxifrage.
CAUTION: See separate listing for Pimpinella above ground parts.

Scientific Names

Pimpinella major; Pimpinella saxifraga.
Family: Apiaceae.

People Use This For

Orally, pimpinella root is used for upper respiratory tract mucous membrane inflammation (2).
Topically, pimpinella root is used for inflammation of the oral and pharyngeal mucous membranes, and as a bath additive for poorly healing wounds (18).
In folk medicine, pimpinella root is used for urinary tract disorders and inflammation, bladder and kidney stones, edema, and "flushing out" therapy for urinary tract bacterial inflammation (18).

Safety

POSSIBLY SAFE ...when used orally and appropriately (2).
There is insufficient reliable information available about the safety of the topical use of pimpinella root.
PREGNANCY AND LACTATION: Insufficient reliable information available; avoid using.

Effectiveness

POSSIBLY EFFECTIVE ...when used orally for treating upper respiratory tract mucous membrane inflammation (2).
There is insufficient reliable information available about the effectiveness of pimpinella root for its other uses.

Mechanism of Action

Pimpinella root is reported to loosen and aid in moving bronchial secretions (18).

Adverse Reactions

None reported. However, it may cause photosensitivity in fair-skinned individuals (18).

Interactions with Herbs & Other Dietary Supplements

Insufficient reliable information available.

Interactions with Drugs

No interactions are known to occur, and there is no known reason to expect a clinically significant interaction with pimpinella root.

Interactions with Foods

No interactions are known to occur, and there is no known reason to expect a clinically significant interaction with pimpinella root.

Interactions with Lab Tests

No interactions are known to occur, and there is no known reason to expect a clinically significant interaction with pimpinella root.

Interactions with Diseases or Conditions

No interactions are known to occur, and there is no known reason to expect a clinically significant interaction with pimpinella root.

Dosage and Administration

ORAL: One cup tea (briefly steep 3 grams finely cut root in 150 mL boiling water, strain) 3 to 4 times daily (8); up to 6-12 grams root per day (2). Tincture (1:5), 6-15 mL per day (8).
TOPICAL: No typical dosage.

Comments

Pimpinella root is often adulterated with other herbs including Hercaleum sphondylium, Heracleum mantegazianum, and Pastinaca sativa (8,18).

PINE

Also Known As

Dwarf-Pine, Pini Turiones, Pix Liquida, Pumilio Pine, Scotch Fir, Scotch Pine, Swiss Mountain Pine.
CAUTION: See separate listings for Dwarf Pine Needle, Fir, Fir Needle Oil, Poplar, and Scotch Pine Needle.

Scientific Names

Pinus sylvestris.
Family: Pinaceae.

People Use This For

Orally, pine is used for upper and lower respiratory tract mucous membrane inflammation (2), blood pressure problems, common cold, cough or bronchitis, fevers, and a tendency towards infection (18).
Topically, pine is used for mild muscular pain and neuralgia (2,18).
In folk medicine, pine has been used to treat uncomplicated coughs and acute bronchial disease, nasal congestion, and hoarseness (18).

Safety

POSSIBLY SAFE ...when used orally and ppropriately (2). ...when used topically and appropriately (2).
PREGNANCY AND LACTATION: Insufficient reliable information available; avoid using.

Effectiveness

There is insufficient reliable information available about the effectiveness of pine.

Mechanism of Action

The applicable part of pine is the sprout. Pine sprouts can dry secretions. They demonstrate mild antiseptic effects and stimulate peripheral circulation (2,18). Pine sprouts contain an essential oil that can stimulate serous bronchial gland function, suppress mucous gland function (7), and aid with expectoration (7).

Adverse Reactions

None reported.

Interactions with Herbs & Other Dietary Supplements

Insufficient reliable information available.

Interactions with Drugs

No interactions are known to occur, and there is no known reason to expect a clinically significant interaction with pine.

Interactions with Foods

No interactions are known to occur, and there is no known reason to expect a clinically significant interaction with pine.

Interactions with Lab Tests

No interactions are known to occur, and there is no known reason to expect a clinically significant interaction with pine.

Interactions with Diseases or Conditions

RESPIRATORY CONDITIONS: Pine sprout is contraindicated for oral use in individuals with bronchial asthma or whooping cough (18).
SKIN CONDITIONS: It is contraindicated as a bath additive in individuals with extensive skin injury or acute skin diseases.
FEVER, INFECTIOUS DISEASE, CARDIAC INSUFFICIENCY, OR HYPERTONIA: Contraindicated as a bath additive (18).

Dosage and Administration

ORAL: The average daily amount of pine sprout is 2-9 grams (2,18) as teas, syrups, or tinctures.
TOPICAL: It is applied topically as a 20-50% pine sprout extract in an alcoholic solution, oil, ointment, liquid, or semi-solid preparation (2,18). As a bath, 100 grams of the alcoholic extract is usually added to the bath water (18).

Comments

Avoid confusion with fir shoots (Picea bies or Abies alba) or pine oil.

PINK ROOT

Also Known As

American Wormgrass, Carolina Pink, Indian Pink, Maryland Pink, Pinkroot, Starbloom, Wormgrass.

Scientific Names

Spigelia marilandica.
Family: Loganiaceae.

People Use This For

Orally, pink root is used to treat worm infestation.

Safety

POSSIBLY SAFE …when used orally and appropriately, short-term (12).
POSSIBLY UNSAFE …when fresh root is used or when use is not accompanied by catharsis (12).
PREGNANCY: LIKELY UNSAFE ...when used orally. For pink root to be effective, it must be used along with a purgative laxative. However, purgative laxative use is contraindicated during pregnancy (272). For this reason, pink root should not be used in pregnancy.
LACTATION: Insufficient reliable information available; avoid using.

Effectiveness

There is insufficient reliable information available about the effectiveness of pink root.

Mechanism of Action

The applicable parts of pink root are the dried rhizome and root. Pink root has anthelmintic actions (18). Although there has been no recent research involving pink root, older sources identify the chief constituents as acidic resins, volatile oil, tannins, waxes, and a volatile base (presumably identical to isoquinoline) (18).

Adverse Reactions

Pink root allegedly contains a toxin that can paralyze the spinal marrow and lead to death by asphyxiation (18). Theoretically, prolonged use of pink root can cause depressive effects on the heart (19).

Interactions with Herbs & Other Dietary Supplements

Insufficient reliable information available.

Interactions with Drugs

No interactions are known to occur, and there is no known reason to expect a clinically significant interaction with pink root.

Interactions with Foods

No interactions are known to occur, and there is no known reason to expect a clinically significant interaction with pink root.

Interactions with Lab Tests

No interactions are known to occur, and there is no known reason to expect a clinically significant interaction with pink root.

Interactions with Diseases or Conditions

No interactions are known to occur, and there is no known reason to expect a clinically significant interaction with pink root.

Dosage and Administration

ORAL: A typical adult dose is 2-5 grams twice daily (12). A common dose for children over 4 years is 0.5-4 grams twice daily (12). A strong purgative laxative (e.g., senna) should always be used with pink root (12).

Comments

As late as 1955, pink root was commonly used throughout the country as an anthelmintic. Various unpleasant symptoms have been reported from use of the fresh root or when use is not accompanied by catharsis (12).

PINUS BARK

Also Known As

Canada Pitch, Canadian Hemlock, Eastern Hemlock, Hemlock Bark, Hemlock Gum, Hemlock Spruce, Hemlocktanne, Pruche de l'Est.

Scientific Names

Tsuga canadensis.
Family: Pinaceae or Abietaceae.

People Use This For

Orally, pinus bark is used for digestive disorders, diarrhea, and diseases of the mouth and throat. Historically, pinus bark was used to treat scurvy (18).

Safety

There is insufficient reliable information available about the safety of pinus bark.
Pregnancy and Lactation: Insufficient reliable information available; avoid using.

Effectiveness

There is insufficient reliable information available about the effectiveness of pinus bark.

Mechanism of Action

Pinus bark is reputed to have astringent, anti-inflammatory, and diuretic properties. It is also thought to induce sweating. The astringent effects of pinus bark are attributed to its tannin content (18). Tannins dehydrate the mucous membrane tissue, reducing internal secretions and causing external cells to form a protective layer. Plants with at least 10% tannins may cause gastrointestinal disturbances, kidney damage, and necrotic conditions of the liver. Some animal experiments show that tannins may cause cancer; others show they may prevent it. Regular consumption of herbs with high tannin concentrations correlates with increased incidence of esophageal or nasal cancer (12).

Adverse Reactions

None reported.

Interactions with Herbs & Other Dietary Supplements

TANNIN-CONTAINING HERBS: Theoretically, herbs that contain high percentages of tannins (such as pinus bark) may cause precipitation of constituents of other herbs (19).

Interactions with Drugs

ORAL DRUGS: Theoretically, concomitant oral administration may cause precipitation of some drugs due to the high tannin content of pinus bark [19]. Separate administration of oral drugs and tannin-containing herbs by the longest period of time practical [19].

Interactions with Foods

No interactions are known to occur, and there is no known reason to expect a clinically significant interaction with pinus bark.

Interactions with Lab Tests

No interactions are known to occur, and there is no known reason to expect a clinically significant interaction with pinus bark.

Interactions with Diseases or Conditions

No interactions are known to occur, and there is no known reason to expect a clinically significant interaction with pinus bark.

Dosage and Administration

No typical dosage.

Comments

Pinus bark is seldom used [18].

PIPSISSEWA

Also Known As

Bitter Winter, Bitter Wintergreen, Chimaphila, Ground Holly, Holly, King's Cure, King's Cureall, Love in Winter, Prince's Pine, Rheumatism Weed, Spotted Wintergreen, Umbellate Wintergreen.

Scientific Names

Chimaphila umbellata synonym Chimaphila corymbosa.
Family: Ericaceae.

People Use This For

Orally, pipsissewa is used as a urinary antiseptic [18]. It is also used orally as a diuretic, astringent, mild disinfectant, antispasmodic, for bladder stones, epilepsy, nervous disorders, and cancer.
Topically, pipsissewa is used for treating ulcerous sores and blisters.
In food and beverages, pipsissewa extracts are used as flavor components [11].

Safety

LIKELY SAFE ...when used in amounts typically found in foods. It has Generally Recognized as Safe (GRAS) status in the US; maximum use is 0.03% [11].
POSSIBLY SAFE ...when used orally short-term [12].
POSSIBLY UNSAFE ...for prolonged oral use because it can cause hydroquinone toxicity [18].
There is insufficient reliable information available about the topical use of pipsissewa.
PREGNANCY AND LACTATION: POSSIBLY SAFE ...when used in food amounts [11]; avoid using larger amounts.

Effectiveness

There is insufficient reliable information available about the effectiveness of pipsissewa.

Mechanism of Action

The applicable parts of pipsissewa are the above ground plant parts. The component chimaphilin has a weak sensitizing effect. It is not suitable for long term use due to its hydroquinone glycoside content [18]. Chimaphilin may have urinary antiseptic, bacteriostatic, and astringent activity [11]. Animal data suggests pipsissewa may elicit hypoglycemia. Arbutin may have urinary antiseptic properties due to hydrolysis to its hydroquinone by the intestinal flora [7,11].

Adverse Reactions

Chronic use may lead to hydroquinone toxicity. Symptoms of toxicity include tinnitus, vomiting, delirium, convulsions, and collapse [11].

Interactions with Herbs & Other Dietary Supplements
Insufficient reliable information available.

Interactions with Drugs
No interactions are known to occur, and there is no known reason to expect a clinically significant interaction with pipsissewa.

Interactions with Foods
No interactions are known to occur, and there is no known reason to expect a clinically significant interaction with pipsissewa.

Interactions with Lab Tests
No interactions are known to occur, and there is no known reason to expect a clinically significant interaction with pipsissewa.

Interactions with Diseases or Conditions
No interactions are known to occur, and there is no known reason to expect a clinically significant interaction with pipsissewa.

Dosage and Administration
No typical dosage.

Comments
Pipsissewa is used similarly to uva ursi (18).

PITCHER PLANT

Also Known As
Eve's Cups, Fly-Catcher, Fly-Trap, Huntsman's Cup, Pitcher Plant, Purple Pitcher Plant, Purple Side-Saddle Flower, Sarapin, Side-Saddle Plant, Smallpox Plant, Water-cup.

Scientific Names
Sarracenia purpurea.
Family: Sarraceniaceae.

People Use This For
Orally, pitcher plant is used for digestive disorders, particularly constipation, urinary tract diseases, as a diuretic, a cure for smallpox, and to prevent scar formation (5944).

By injection, pitcher plant extract (Sarapin) is used as a trigger point injection to treat pain including sciatic pain, intercostal pain, alcoholic or occipital neuritis, brachial plexus neuralgia, meralgia paresthetica, and lumbar or trigeminal neuralgia (5971). Pitcher plant extract (Sarapin) has been used by injection in combination with bupivacaine hydrochloride 0.5% (Marcaine) and gamma globulin to treat the omohyoideus myofascial pain syndrome (5972). It has been used in combinations by injection (extract triamcinolone and lidocaine with adrenalin) to treat migraine cephalagia (5973), for diagnosis and treatment of forms of sciatic pain including piriformis syndrome (extract and lidocaine), quadratus lumborum syndrome (extract and corticosteroid) (5974), and in combination with physiotherapy and an intraoral splint to treat the Ernest Syndrome that is often mistaken for temporomandibular joint problems (5978). It is also used in prolotherapy (phenol and extract) to cause inflammation at the site where the ligaments and tendons attach to the bone to stimulate the body to proliferate stronger, shorter, and less painful ligaments and/or tendons (5977).

Safety
LIKELY SAFE ...when the extract of pitcher plant, Sarapin (a prescription product), is used appropriately by injection by a qualified health professional (5971).

POSSIBLY UNSAFE ...when the extract of pitcher plant, Sarapin (a prescription product), is injected in areas of inflammation (5971).

There is insufficient reliable information available about the safety of the oral use of pitcher plant.

PREGNANCY AND LACTATION: Insufficient reliable information available; avoid using.

Effectiveness

There is insufficient reliable information available about the effectiveness of the extract of pitcher plant (Sarapin) injection (5971). Sarapin was "grandfathered" to prescription drug status in the United States from the time when it was not necessary to prove effectiveness.
There is insufficient reliable information available about the effectiveness of the pitcher plant for its other uses..

Mechanism of Action

The pitcher plant leaf and root contain sarracenia acid, tannin, resin, and the alkaloid sarracenin (5944). The extract has an effect on sensory nerves without changing skin sensation or affecting motor nerves. Some evidence suggests that pitcher plant extract affects only C nerve fibers, perhaps containing a biological antagonist that potentiates the action of the ammonium ion (5975). This could be beneficial in chronic neuropathic pain.

Adverse Reactions

Used by injection, pitcher plant extract can cause a local sensation of heaviness. Some individuals experience a local sensation of heat or aggravation of symptoms.

Interactions with Herbs & Other Dietary Supplements

Insufficient reliable information available.

Interactions with Drugs

No interactions are known to occur, and there is no known reason to expect a clinically significant interaction with pitcher plant.

Interactions with Foods

No interactions are known to occur, and there is no known reason to expect a clinically significant interaction with pitcher plant.

Interactions with Lab Tests

No interactions are known to occur, and there is no known reason to expect a clinically significant interaction with pitcher plant.

Interactions with Diseases or Conditions

No interactions are known to occur, and there is no known reason to expect a clinically significant interaction with pitcher plant.

Dosage and Administration

INJECTION: Pitcher plant extract (Sarapin) is given by nerve block or local infiltration. Doses are as follows: 2-3 mL cervical, 5-10 mL dorsal, 5-10 mL lumbar, 3-5 mL sacral, 10 mL caudal canal, 10 mL sciatic nerve, 5-10 mL local infiltration. Following injection, patients should be maintained in recumbent position for 15 minutes (5971). For use in migraine, 4 mg triamcinolone, 0.75 mL Sarapin and 0.15 mL lidocaine with adrenalin drawn into a syringe in that order have been administered at the trigger points in both temples using a 28 gauge, 5/8 inch needle (5973).
Sarapin is an FDA approved prescription product. For additional information, contact the manufacturer, High Chemical Company, 1-800-447-8792.

Comments

None.

PLEURISY ROOT

Also Known As

Butterfly Weed, Canada Root, Flux Root, Orange Milkweed, Orange Swallow-Wort, Pleurisy, Swallow-Wort, Tuber Root, White Root, Wind Root.

Scientific Names

Asclepias tuberosa.
Family: Asclepiadaceae.

People Use This For

Orally, pleurisy root is used for coughs, pleurisy, uterine disorders, to ease breathing, as an analgesic, expectorant, antispasmodic, and to promote sweating. It is also used orally for bronchitis, pneumonitis, and influenza.

Safety

POSSIBLY UNSAFE ...when the root is used orally because it contains digitalis-like cardenolide glycosides (4). It can cause vomiting (12). Canadian regulations do not allow pleurisy root as a non-medicinal ingredient for oral use products (12).
PREGNANCY: UNSAFE ...when used orally (12) because it might have uterine stimulant and estrogenic activity (19).
LACTATION: POSSIBLY UNSAFE ...when used orally (12); avoid using.

Effectiveness

There is insufficient reliable information available about the effectiveness of pleurisy root.

Mechanism of Action

Pleurisy root contains digitalis-like cardenolide glycosides (18). Animal data suggest that pleurisy root does not affect blood pressure, respiration, or heart muscle (4).

Adverse Reactions

Pleurisy root may cause dermatitis. It is also a gastrointestinal irritant and emetic, and can cause nausea and vomiting (19). At higher doses, it may cause digitalis-like poisoning symptoms (18).

Interactions with Herbs & Other Dietary Supplements

CARDIAC GLYCOSIDE-CONTAINING HERBS: Contraindicated. Concomitant use can increase the risk of cardiac glycoside toxicity. Cardiac glycoside-containing herbs include black hellebore, Canadian hemp roots, digitalis leaf, hedge mustard, figwort, lily of the valley roots, motherwort, oleander leaf, pheasant's eye plant, squill bulb leaf scales, strophanthus seeds, and uzara (2,18,19,500).

Interactions with Drugs

DIGOXIN: Because pleurisy root contains cardenolide glycosides, it could have additive effects with digoxin (19).
ANTIDEPRESSANTS: Theoretically, excessive amounts of pleurisy root might interfere with antidepressant therapy (4).
HORMONES: Theoretically, excessive amounts of pleurisy root might interfere with hormone drug therapy (4).

Interactions with Foods

No interactions are known to occur, and there is no known reason to expect a clinically significant interaction with pleurisy root.

Interactions with Lab Tests

No interactions are known to occur, and there is no known reason to expect a clinically significant interaction with pleurisy root.

Interactions with Diseases or Conditions

CARDIAC CONDITIONS: Pleurisy root may worsen or interfere with cardiac drug therapy (4).

Dosage and Administration

No typical dosage.

Comments

None.

PODOPHYLLUM

Also Known As

American Mandrake, Devil's Apple, Duck's Foot, Ground Lemon, Himalayan Mayapple, Hog Apple, Indian Apple, Indian Podophyllum, Mandrake, Mayapple, Podophylli pelati rhizoma/resina, Podophyllum peltatum, Raccoon Berry, Vegetable Mercury, Wild Lemon, Wild Mandrake.
CAUTION: See separate listings for Bryonia (English Mandrake) and European Mandrake.

Scientific Names

Podophyllum hexandrum, synonym Podophyllum emodi; Podophyllum peltatum.
Family: Berberidaceae.

People Use This For

Topically, podophyllum resin is used for removal of topical warts (6,5617), including plantar warts (9), condyloma acuminata (venereal warts) (2,6,7,9,11,5617), and other papillomas (11).

Historically, podophyllum resin has been used orally as a cathartic, for jaundice and liver ailments, fever, syphilis, and cancer (11,5617). The resin has also been used orally as an anthelmintic and an antidote for snake bites (6). It has also been used orally as an abortifacient (5618).

Safety

POSSIBLY SAFE ...when used topically and appropriately (9,12). Podophyllum must be applied in low concentration solutions (0.5% podophyllotoxin) (6,9) to small surface areas (25 square cm or less) (2,7,18) with protection of adjacent skin (2,7) and washed off within 1-4 hours (6,9). Contact with skin should not exceed 6 hours (6). Risk of systemic toxicity increases if applied to large areas, open lesions, normal skin or mucous membranes, with prolonged use (9) and use of ointment form (6).

LIKELY UNSAFE ...when used orally; potentially lethal (2,6,9,5617). ...when used topically near the eyes (19), on cervical or urethral warts (9). Contraindicated for use on moles, birthmarks, or inflamed warts because it can cause permanent skin damage (19). Fatalities have been reported from oral ingestion and topical application (6,9,5617).

PREGNANCY: LIKELY UNSAFE ...when used orally or topically for self-medication; avoid using. Considered potentially embryotoxic and teratogenic (2,7,9,11,12,5618). Fetal intrauterine death and multiple birth deformities associated with oral and topical podophyllum use have been reported (5618).

LACTATION: LIKELY UNSAFE ...when used orally or topically for self-medication (2,6,9,5617); avoid using.

Effectiveness

LIKELY EFFECTIVE ...when used topically for removal of benign epithelial growths, including warts, fibroids, papillomas (15), and anogenital condylomata acuminata (2). ...when used orally as a laxative (6,7,9,11,13,15), but it is unsafe for oral ingestion (2,6,9).

There is insufficient reliable information available about the effectiveness of podophyllum for its other uses.

Mechanism of Action

The applicable parts of podophyllum are the root, rhizome, and resin. The major active constituents in podophyllum are lignan derivatives (6,9,11), including podophyllotoxin (2,6,7,9,11), which is antimitotic (9,11,13,18) and antineoplastic (6,11). It induces catharsis through irritation of the intestinal mucosa (6,9), it induces lymphocyte activating factor/interleukin 1, it stimulates macrophage proliferation, and it modulates other cytokines (11). Significant absorption occurs through the skin (6) and the gastrointestinal tract (5617). Etoposide and teniposide, semisynthetic analogs of podophyllotoxin, are active against testicular cancer, small cell lung cancer, leukemia, lymphoma (6,11,13), Kaposi's sarcoma, neuroblastoma (13), rheumatoid arthritis (6,11), and psoriasis (11). Podophyllotoxin exposure during pregnancy is considered to be highly embryotoxic (6,7,11,5618); teratogenicity has been reported (6,5618) but not confirmed by studies in experimental animals (7,11).

Adverse Reactions

Oral ingestion and topical application can cause severe abdominal pain (18), nausea, vomiting (6,5617), bloody-watery diarrhea, vomiting of bile, dizziness, headache, coordination disorders, spasms, nephritis (18), fever, altered mental status, visual hallucinations, confusion, tachypnea, peripheral neuropathy, muscle paralysis, hypotension, bone marrow suppression, renal failure (6,5617), coma, respiratory failure, and death (6,18,5617). Chronic use as a cathartic can cause hypokalemia and metabolic alkalosis (6,5617). Oral or topical use of podophyllum in pregnant women can cause fetal congenital malformations and death (6,5618). Podophyllum can cause severe local irritation, especially to eyes and mucous membranes (9,11,18). It might also cause transformation of condyloma to squamous cell carcinoma (9). Symptoms of toxicity usually do not appear for a period of time, ranging from a few to 13 hours after ingestion or absorption (5617). Neurologic changes may progress rapidly after onset of symptoms (6).

Interactions with Herbs & Other Dietary Supplements

CARDIAC GLYCOSIDE-CONTAINING HERBS: Contraindicated; concomitant use may increase the risk of cardiac glycoside toxicity. Cardiac glycoside-containing herbs include: black hellebore, Canadian hemp roots, digitalis leaf, hedge mustard, figwort, lily of the valley roots, motherwort, oleander leaf, pheasant's eye plant, pleurisy root, squill bulb leaf scales, and strophanthus seeds (2,18,19,500).

STIMULANT LAXATIVE HERBS: Theoretically, concomitant use with other stimulant laxative herbs may increase the risk of potassium depletion. Stimulant laxative herbs include: aloe dried leaf sap, wild cucumber fruit (Ecballium elaterium), blue flag rhizome, alder buckthorn, European buckthorn, butternut bark, cascara bark, castor oil, colocynth fruit pulp, gamboge bark exudate, jalap root, black root, manna bark exudate, rhubarb root, senna leaves and pods, and yellow dock root (19).

POTASSIUM-DEPLETING HERBS: Theoretically, concomitant use with horsetail plant or licorice rhizome increases the risk of potassium depletion.

Interactions with Drugs
No interactions are known to occur, and there is no known reason to expect a clinically significant interaction with podophyllum.

Interactions with Foods
No interactions are known to occur, and there is no known reason to expect a clinically significant interaction with podophyllum.

Interactions with Lab Tests
No interactions are known to occur, and there is no known reason to expect a clinically significant interaction with podophyllum.

Interactions with Diseases or Conditions
GALLSTONES: Contraindicated. Theoretically, podophyllum can stimulate bile secretion (19).
GI CONDITIONS: Contraindicated. Podophyllum can irritate the gastrointestinal tract, exacerbating infectious or inflammatory conditions (19).

Dosage and Administration
TOPICAL: 1.5-3 grams root or fluid extract, or 2.5-7.5 grams tincture (5-25% in benzoin), applied once or twice per week to an area no more than 25 square cm, with protection of surrounding skin (2,6,7,13,18). Alternatively, 0.5% solution applied twice per day for three days, washed off after 1-6 hours (6-9), or 0.15% cream applied twice per day for three days (9). Lower concentrations applied twice per day are at least as effective as higher concentrations applied twice per week (6,7,9). Should not be used for self-treatment; requires supervision.

Comments
Podophyllum resin is prepared from the root and rhizome of the plant. Podophyllum toxicity has been successfully treated using charcoal hemoperfusion (6,5617).

POINSETTIA

Also Known As
Christmas Flower, Easter Flower, Lobster Flower Plant, Lobsterplant, Mexican Flame Leaf, Mexican Flameleaf, Paintedleaf, Papagallo.

Scientific Names
Euphorbia pulcherrima; Euphorbia poinsettia; Poinsettia pulcherrima.
Family: Euphorbiaceae.

People Use This For
Orally, poinsettia is used as an antipyretic, to stimulate milk production, and as an abortifacient (6). The latex is taken orally as an analgesic, antibacterial, and emetic (6).
Topically, the latex is used as a depilatory (6).
In folk medicine, it has been used as a skin remedy, for warts, and toothaches (6).

Safety
POSSIBLY UNSAFE ...when used orally or topically, but toxicity is limited to local irritation, contact dermatitis, mucosal burns, and keratoconjunctivitis (17).
CHILDREN: POSSIBLY UNSAFE ...when used orally or topically. Poinsettia was implicated in the poisoning death of a 2 year old child (6).
PREGNANCY AND LACTATION: POSSIBLY UNSAFE ...when used orally or topically; avoid using.

Effectiveness
There is insufficient reliable information available about the effectiveness of poinsettia.

Mechanism of Action
The applicable parts of poinsettia are the whole plant and latex. There is insufficient reliable information available about the possible mechanism of action and active ingredients of poinsettia.

Adverse Reactions
Toxicity is limited to local irritation, contact dermatitis, mucosal burns, and keratoconjunctivitis (17).

Interactions with Herbs & Other Dietary Supplements
Insufficient reliable information available.

Interactions with Drugs
No interactions are known to occur, and there is no known reason to expect a clinically significant interaction with poinsettia.

Interactions with Foods
No interactions are known to occur, and there is no known reason to expect a clinically significant interaction with poinsettia.

Interactions with Lab Tests
No interactions are known to occur, and there is no known reason to expect a clinically significant interaction with poinsettia.

Interactions with Diseases or Conditions
GI IRRITATION, INFLAMMATION: Euphorbia species are said to have GI irritant effects (19); avoid using.

Dosage and Administration
No typical dosage.

Comments
Recent studies indicate that the plant is less toxic than once believed (6). American Association of Poison Control Centers reported 22,793 cases of poisoning with no fatalities and 92.4% with no toxicity (3838).

POISON IVY

Also Known As
Markweed, Poison Vine, Three-Leafed Ivy.

Scientific Names
Toxicodendron radicans; Rhus Toxicodendron (Rhus radicans).
Family: Anacardiaceae.

People Use This For
In folk medicine, poison ivy has been used as a narcotic (18).

Safety
LIKELY UNSAFE ...when used orally or topically (6).
PREGNANCY AND LACTATION: LIKELY UNSAFE ...when used orally or topically (6); avoid using.

Effectiveness
There is insufficient reliable information available about the effectiveness of poison ivy.

Mechanism of Action
Poison ivy is a severe skin irritant that stimulates the immune system (18). Contact sensitivity is due to the urushiols, which bind to skin proteins, sensitizing the individual (6). Once sensitized, re-exposure leads to allergic reactions (6).

Adverse Reactions
Orally, the plant can cause severe mucous membrane irritation, nausea, vomiting, intestinal colic, diarrhea, dizziness, stupor, nephritis, hematuria, fever, and unconsciousness (18).
Topically, the plant can cause contact dermatitis, reddening, swelling, herpes-like blisters (18), and erythema multiforme (3839). Eye contact can cause severe conjunctivitis, corneal inflammations, or loss of sight (18).
Inhalation due to burning of the plant can result in fever, major lung infection, and death from throat swelling (6).

Interactions with Herbs & Other Dietary Supplements
GINKGO BILOBA: Fruit pulp can cause cross-reactivity in people allergic to poison ivy (6).

Interactions with Drugs

No interactions are known to occur, and there is no known reason to expect a clinically significant interaction with poison ivy.

Interactions with Foods

MANGO: Fruit skin can cause cross-reactivity in people allergic to poison ivy (6,735).
CASHEW: Nut shell oil can cause cross-reactivity in people allergic to poison ivy (6,735).

Interactions with Lab Tests

No interactions are known to occur, and there is no known reason to expect a clinically significant interaction with poison ivy.

Interactions with Diseases or Conditions

No interactions are known to occur, and there is no known reason to expect a clinically significant interaction with poison ivy.

Dosage and Administration

No typical dosage.

Comments

To prevent poison ivy from causing skin irritation, wash exposed area with water within 5 to 10 minutes (6). Use soap and water first, then ether or alcohol (18).

POISONOUS BUTTERCUP

Also Known As

Celery-Leafed Crowfoot, Cursed Crowfoot.
CAUTION: See separate listings for Buttercup and Bulbous Buttercup.

Scientific Names

Ranunculus sceleratus.
Family: Ranunculaceae.

People Use This For

Topically, poisonous buttercup is used as a stimulant for skin diseases (e.g., scabies) and leucoderma (18).

Safety

LIKELY UNSAFE ...when the above ground parts are used orally or topically. The fresh plant causes severe local irritation (18).
There is insufficient reliable information about the safety of the oral or topical use of the dried, cut leaf.
PREGNANCY AND LACTATION: LIKELY UNSAFE ...when used orally or topically (18,19). Oral use might possibly stimulate uterine activity (19).

Effectiveness

There is insufficient reliable information available about the effectiveness of poisonous buttercup.

Mechanism of Action

The applicable parts of poisonous buttercup are the above ground parts. Poisonous buttercup contains ranunculin, anemonin, and protoanemonin. Protoanemonin is a potent topical irritant (18). It causes pain and burning sensations, severe tongue inflammation, and increases salivation. When the freshly harvested plant is cut into small pieces or perhaps when it is dried, protoanemonin changes into a pungent, volatile intermediate that quickly dimerizes to a form that does not irritate the mucous membrane. In vitro, leaf extracts have shown a wide fungicidal spectrum of activity (3836).

Adverse Reactions

Topically, extended contact with fresh or bruised plant can lead to blisters and burns that are difficult to heal (18). Some species of Ranunculus can cause photodermatitis. Avoid excessive sunlight or ultraviolet light exposure while using this product (19).

Interactions with Herbs & Other Dietary Supplements
Insufficient reliable information available.

Interactions with Drugs
No interactions are known to occur, and there is no known reason to expect a clinically significant interaction with poisonous buttercup.

Interactions with Foods
No interactions are known to occur, and there is no known reason to expect a clinically significant interaction with poisonous buttercup.

Interactions with Lab Tests
No interactions are known to occur, and there is no known reason to expect a clinically significant interaction with poisonous buttercup.

Interactions with Diseases or Conditions
No interactions are known to occur, and there is no known reason to expect a clinically significant interaction with poisonous buttercup.

Dosage and Administration
TOPICAL: Poisonous buttercup is used as a tincture (18).

Comments
None.

POKEWEED berry

Also Known As
American Nightshade, American Spinach, Bear's Grape, Branching Phytolacca, Cancer Jalap, Chongras, Coakum, Coakum-Chorngras, Cokan, Crowberry, Fitolaca, Garget, Hierba Carmín, Inkberry, Jalap, Kermesbeere, Phytolacca Berry, Pigeonberry, Pocan, Poke, Pokeberry, Raisin d'Amérique, Red-Ink Plant, Red Plant, Red Weed, Scoke, Skoke, Teinturière, Virginian Poke.
CAUTION: See separate listings for Jalap, Mexican Scammony Root, and Pokeweed root.

Scientific Names
Phytolacca americana, synonym Phytolacca decandra.
Family: Phytolaccaceae.

People Use This For
Pokeweed is used as a food, red food coloring (18), and wine coloring agent (6).
In manufacturing, it is used to make ink and dye (6).

Safety
LIKELY UNSAFE ...when the fresh berry is ingested. One berry can be toxic to a child; 10 berries to an adult (6,18). Green berries are considered more toxic than mature, red berries (4). ...when pokeweed berry and juice comes in contact with broken skin or is ingested, it can cause hematological changes (4,3477,3481,3482). Protective gloves should be used to handle the plant (6,3477). All parts of the pokeweed plant, especially the root, are considered to be toxic (3477,3479,3483). Severe poisoning has been reported from ingesting tea brewed from pokeweed root (6,3478) and pokeweed leaves (3480). Poisoning also has resulted from ingestion of pokeberry wine and pokeberry pancakes (3479).
CHILDREN: UNSAFE ...when used orally. Consumption of even one berry can be toxic. Children have died after ingesting pokeweed berries (3479,3483).
PREGNANCY AND LACTATION: LIKELY UNSAFE ...when the fresh berry is ingested. Evidence suggests the berry has uterine stimulant and abortifacient effects (4,19).

Effectiveness
There is insufficient reliable information about the effectiveness of pokeweed berry.

Mechanism of Action
Pokeweed contains saponin glycosides, proteinaceous mitogens (3477,3478), tannin, and resin (6). The toxicity of pokeweed is attributed to proteinaceous mitogens and the saponin glycosides which include phytolaccatoxin and

phytolaccagenin. The saponin glycosides cause gastrointestinal irritation and the proteinaceous mitogens are thought to affect thymus-dependent (T) cells and thymus-independent (B) lymphocytes (3477,3478).

Adverse Reactions

Orally, all parts of the pokeweed plant can cause nausea, vomiting, cramping, abdominal pain, diarrhea, burning sensation in mouth and throat, weakness, bloody emesis, hypotension, bloody diarrhea, tachycardia, difficulty in breathing, salivation, urinary incontinence, spasm, convulsion (4,3477,3478,3479), severe thirst, somnolence, transient blindness, respiratory failure (18,3477,3479), and death (4,18,3477,3483). Plasmacytosis, mitotic changes in peripheral blood cells, eosinophilia, thrombocytopenia, abnormal platelet morphology and other hematologic abnormalities may result from topical exposure (especially in individuals with cuts or abrasions on hands or other extremities) and ingestion of pokeweed plant, berries, or root (3477,3478,3481,3482).

Interactions with Herbs & Other Dietary Supplements

Insufficient reliable information available.

Interactions with Drugs

No interactions are known to occur, and there is no known reason to expect a clinically significant interaction with pokeweed berry.

Interactions with Foods

No interactions are known to occur, and there is no known reason to expect a clinically significant interaction with pokeweed berry.

Interactions with Lab Tests

No interactions are known to occur, and there is no known reason to expect a clinically significant interaction with pokeweed berry.

Interactions with Diseases or Conditions

No interactions are known to occur, and there is no known reason to expect a clinically significant interaction with pokeweed berry.

Dosage and Administration

No typical dosage.

Comments

Avoid confusion with jalap (Ipomoea orizabensis). All parts of the pokeweed plant are considered toxic except the above ground leaves grown in early spring (6). The immature leaves are canned and marketed as the food product, "poke salad" (6). In folk medicine, the leaves have been used for rheumatism, arthritis, emesis, and purging (6). Ongoing research is investigating the use of pokeweed in flu, HSV-1, and polio (4,18). The United Kingdom allows pokeweed in medicinal products provided toxic constituents are absent and the product adheres to mandated limits (4).

POKEWEED root

Also Known As

American Nightshade, American Spinach, Bear's Grape, Branching Phytolacca, Cancer Jalap, Chongras, Coakum, Coakum-Chorngras, Cokan, Crowberry, Fitolaca, Garget, Hierba Carmín, Inkberry, Jalap, Kermesbeere, Phytolacca Berry, Pigeonberry, Pocan, Poke, Poke Root, Pokeberry, Raisin d'Amérique, Red-Ink Plant, Red Plant, Red Weed, Scoke, Skoke, Teinturière, Virginian Poke.
CAUTION: See separate listings for Jalap, Mexican Scammony Root, and Pokewood berry.

Scientific Names

Phytolacca americana, synonym Phytolacca decandra.
Family: Phytolaccaceae.

People Use This For

Orally, pokeweed root is used as an emetic (18).
Historically, it has been used for rheumatism, mucous membrane inflammation of upper and lower respiratory tract, tonsillitis, laryngitis, adenitis, mastitis, mumps, skin infections (scabies, tinea, sycosis, ringworm, acne), mammary abscesses (4), edema, skin cancers, dysmenorrhea, and syphilis (6).

Safety

LIKELY UNSAFE ...when used orally. All parts of the pokeweed plant, especially the root, are considered to be toxic (3477,3479,3483). The Herb Trade Association recommends against selling pokeweed root as an herbal beverage or food (4,3478). Severe poisoning has been reported from ingesting tea brewed from pokeweed root (6,3478) and pokeweed leaves (3480). ...when root comes in contact with broken skin or is ingested, it can cause hematological changes (3477,3481,3482). Protective gloves should be used to handle the plant (6,3477).
PREGNANCY AND LACTATION: LIKELY UNSAFE ...when used orally. Evidence suggests it might have uterine stimulant and abortifacient effects (4,19).

Effectiveness

There is insufficient reliable information available about the effectiveness of pokeweed root.

Mechanism of Action

Pokeweed contains saponin glycosides, proteinaceous mitogens (3477,3478), tannin, and resin (6). The toxicity of pokeweed is attributed to proteinaceous mitogens and the saponin glycosides which include phytolaccatoxin and phytolaccagenin. The saponin glycosides cause gastrointestinal irritation and the proteinaceous mitogens are thought to affect thymus-dependent (T) cells and thymus-independent (B) lymphocytes (3477,3478).

Adverse Reactions

Orally, all parts of the pokeweed plant can cause nausea, vomiting, cramping, abdominal pain, diarrhea, burning sensation in mouth and throat, weakness, bloody emesis, hypotension, bloody diarrhea, tachycardia, difficulty in breathing, salivation, urinary incontinence, spasm, convulsion (4,3477,3478,3479), severe thirst, somnolence, transient blindness, respiratory failure (18,3477,3479), and death (4,18,3477,3483). Plasmacytosis, mitotic changes in peripheral blood cells, eosinophilia, thrombocytopenia, abnormal platelet morphology and other hematologic abnormalities may result from topical exposure (especially in individuals with cuts or abrasions on hands or other extremities) and ingestion of pokeweed plant, berries or root (3477,3478,3481,3482).

Interactions with Herbs & Other Dietary Supplements

Insufficient reliable information available.

Interactions with Drugs

No interactions are known to occur, and there is no known reason to expect a clinically significant interaction with pokeweed root.

Interactions with Foods

No interactions are known to occur, and there is no known reason to expect a clinically significant interaction with pokeweed root.

Interactions with Lab Tests

No interactions are known to occur, and there is no known reason to expect a clinically significant interaction with pokeweed root.

Interactions with Diseases or Conditions

No interactions are known to occur, and there is no known reason to expect a clinically significant interaction with pokeweed root.

Dosage and Administration

No typical dosage.

Comments

Avoid confusion with jalap (Ipomoea orizabensis). All parts of the pokeweed plant are considered toxic except the above ground leaves grown in early spring (6). The immature leaves are canned and marketed as the food product, "poke salad" (6). In folk medicine, the leaves have been used for rheumatism, arthritis, emesis, and purging (6). Ongoing research is investigating the use of pokeweed in flu, HSV-1, and polio (4,18). The United Kingdom allows pokeweed in medicinal products provided toxic constituents are absent and the product adheres to mandated limits (4).

POLICOSANOL

Also Known As
Dotriacontanol, Heptacosanol, Hexacosanol, Nonacosanol, Octacosanol, Tetracosanol, Tetratriacontanol, and Triacontanol, 32-C.
CAUTION: See separate listing for Octacosanol.

Scientific Names
Policosanol.

People Use This For
Orally, policosanol is used for hyperlipidemia (2923,2942), for intermittent claudication (2931), for decreasing myocardial ischemia in patients with coronary heart disease (2941), and as an anti-plaque agent (2942).

Safety
POSSIBLY SAFE ...when used orally and appropriately. Policosanol seems to be safe when used in doses of 10-20 mg per day for up to 2 years (2927,2928,2929,2930,2931,2943,2944).
PREGNANCY AND LACTATION: Insufficient reliable information available; avoid using.

Effectiveness
POSSIBLY EFFECTIVE ...when used orally for treating hypercholesterolemia. Policosanol significantly decreases total cholesterol and low-density lipoprotein (LDL) cholesterol, and increases high-density lipoprotein (HDL) cholesterol (2927,2928,2929,2930,2943,2944). ...when used orally for intermittent claudication. Policosanol seems to significantly improve walking distance (2931).
There is insufficient reliable information available about the effectiveness of policosanol for its other uses.

Mechanism of Action
Policosanol is derived from sugar cane (2942) and refers to a mixture of 24-34 carbon alcohols comprised primarily of octacosanol (28-C) and also including tetracosanol (24-C), hexacosanol (26-C), heptacosanol (27-C), nonacosanol (29-C), triacontanol (30-C), dotriacontanol (32-C), and tetratriacontanol (268,269,270,2942). Policosanol lowers cholesterol levels by inhibiting hepatic cholesterol synthesis (2934,2939) and seems to increase the degradation of low-density lipoprotein (LDL) cholesterol (2939). Policosanol also decreases arachidonic acid and collagen-induced platelet aggregation (2933,2935,2936,2937,2938). Policosanol 20 mg per day reduces platelet aggregation about as much as aspirin 100 mg per day (2937), but it does not seem to significantly affect coagulation time (2935,2937).

Adverse Reactions
Orally, policosanol can cause erythema (2929), migraines, insomnia, somnolence, irritability, dizziness, upset stomach, polyphagia, dysuria, weight loss, skin rash, and nose and gum bleeding (786,2937).

Interactions with Herbs & Other Dietary Supplements
Insufficient reliable information available.

Interactions with Drugs
ANTICOAGULANT/ANTIPLATELET DRUGS: Policosanol can inhibit platelet aggregation (2949,2950,2951,2952,2961). Theoretically, taking policosanol with other antiplatelet or anticoagulant drugs might increase the risk of bruising and bleeding. Some of these drugs include aspirin; clopidogrel (Plavix); nonsteroidal anti-inflammatory drugs (NSAIDs) such as diclofenac (Voltaren, Cataflam, others), ibuprofen (Advil, Motrin, others), naproxen (Anaprox, Naprosyn, others); and anticoagulant drugs such as dalteparin (Fragmin), enoxaparin (Lovenox), heparin, warfarin (Coumadin) and others.

Interactions with Foods
No interactions are known to occur, and there is no known reason to expect a clinically significant interaction with policosanol.

Interactions with Lab Tests
CHOLESTEROL: Policosanol can decrease serum total cholesterol and low-density lipoprotein (LDL) cholesterol levels and increase high density lipoprotein (HDL) cholesterol levels (2927,2928,2943).

Interactions with Diseases or Conditions
No interactions are known to occur, and there is no known reason to expect a clinically significant interaction with policosanol.

Dosage and Administration

ORAL: For hypercholesterolemia, the typical dose of policosanol is 5-10 mg twice daily (2927,2928,2929,2930). For intermittent claudication, 10 mg twice daily has been used (2931).

Comments

None.

POMEGRANATE

Also Known As

Granada, Grenadier, Shi Liu Gen Pi, Shi Liu Pi.

Scientific Names

Punica granatum.
Family: Punicaceae.

People Use This For

Orally, pomegranate is used for tapeworm infestations and opportunistic intestinal worms. It is also used as an astringent, for diarrhea and dysentery, and as an abortive.
Topically, it is used as a gargle for sore throat and to treat hemorrhoids (18).

Safety

POSSIBLY SAFE ...when the fruit rind is used orally (12).
UNSAFE ...when the root is used orally. The root contains the toxic alkaloid pelletierine (12). ...when the fruit rind is used in individuals with diarrhea (12).
There is insufficient reliable information available about the topical safety of pomegranate bark and root.
PREGNANCY: UNSAFE ...when used orally. The bark, root, and fruit rind can stimulate menstruation or uterine contractions (12,19).
LACTATION: UNSAFE ...when the bark or root is used orally (12).
There is insufficient reliable information available about the safety of pomegranate during pregnancy and breast-feeding when used topically; avoid using.

Effectiveness

There is insufficient reliable information available about the effectiveness of pomegranate.

Mechanism of Action

The applicable parts of the pomegranate are the bark, rind, root, seed, and stem (18,1287). The seed oil contains polyphenols and fatty acids, including punicic acid, palmitic acid, stearic acid, oleic acid, and linoleic acid (1287). Fermented pomegranate juice and cold pressed seed oil demonstrate antioxidant activity, possibly due to their flavonoid content (1287). Pomegranate root and stem contain the piperidine alkaloids isopelletierine, N-methyliospelletierine, and pseudopelletierin. The root contains up to 25% tannins, and the fruit rind contains up to 28% tannins (18). Tannins can exert an astringent effect on mucosal tissues, dehydrating the tissue, reducing internal secretions and forming a hardened, external protective layer of cells. Plants with at least 10% tannins can cause gastrointestinal disturbances, kidney damage, and necrotic conditions of the liver. Some preliminary data suggest that tannins might cause cancer; other data suggest tannins may prevent it. Regular consumption of herbs with high tannin concentrations correlates with increased incidence of esophageal or nasal cancer (12).

Adverse Reactions

Orally, overdoses can cause strychnine-like effects in the form of heightened reflex arousal that can escalate to paralysis. At amounts greater than 80 grams, people experience vomiting, including bloody emesis, followed by dizziness, chills, vision disorders, collapse, and possibly death due to respiratory failure. Total blindness can occur within a few hours to a few days after ingestion, and resolves after several weeks (18).

Interactions with Herbs & Other Dietary Supplements

TANNIN-CONTAINING HERBS: Theoretically, herbs that contain high percentages of tannins (such as pomegranate) may cause precipitation of constituents of other herbs (19).

Interactions with Drugs
ORAL DRUGS: Theoretically, concomitant oral administration may cause precipitation of some drugs due to the high tannin content of pomegranate (19). Separate administration of oral drugs and tannin-containing herbs by the longest period of time practical (19).

Interactions with Foods
No interactions are known to occur, and there is no known reason to expect a clinically significant interaction with pomegranate.

Interactions with Lab Tests
No interactions are known to occur, and there is no known reason to expect a clinically significant interaction with pomegranate.

Interactions with Diseases or Conditions
No interactions are known to occur, and there is no known reason to expect a clinically significant interaction with pomegranate.

Dosage and Administration
No typical dosage.

Comments
The root and stem bark are unsafe for self-medication (12). When used to treat parasites, the fruit rind should not be taken with fats or oils (12).

POPLAR

Also Known As
Balm of Gilead, Balsam Poplar Buds, Pappelknospen, Populi Gemma.
CAUTION: See separate listings for Dwarf Pine Needle, Fir Needle Oil, Fir, Pine, and Scotch Pine Needle.

Scientific Names
Populus tacamahacca; Populus balsamifera; Populus candicans.
Family: Salicaceae.

People Use This For
Orally, poplar is used as an ingredient in herbal cough preparations. It is also used as a stimulant and expectorant (11). Topically, it is used for sores, bruises, cuts, pimples (11), external hemorrhoids, frostbite, and sunburn (2).

Safety
LIKELY SAFE ...when applied topically and used appropriately (2,12). ...when used in alcoholic beverages in amounts that have been approved in the US (11).
There is insufficient reliable information available about the safety of poplar for its other uses.
PREGNANCY AND LACTATION: Insufficient reliable information available; avoid using.

Effectiveness
POSSIBLY EFFECTIVE ...when used topically for the of treatment of superficial skin injuries, external hemorrhoids, frostbite, and sunburn (2).
There is insufficient reliable information available about the effectiveness of poplar for its other uses.

Mechanism of Action
The applicable parts of the poplar are the dried unopened leaf buds. Poplar contains salicin (11).

Adverse Reactions
Topically, occasional allergic skin reactions can occur with the use of poplar (2).
There are no reports of aspirin-type allergic reactions with the use of salicin-rich plants (12).

Interactions with Herbs & Other Dietary Supplements
Insufficient reliable information available.

Interactions with Drugs

No interactions are known to occur, and there is no known reason to expect a clinically significant interaction with poplar.

Interactions with Foods

No interactions are known to occur, and there is no known reason to expect a clinically significant interaction with poplar.

Interactions with Lab Tests

No interactions are known to occur, and there is no known reason to expect a clinically significant interaction with poplar.

Interactions with Diseases or Conditions

ALLERGIES: Contraindicated in people allergic to poplar buds, propolis, Peru balsam, or salicylates (2,18).

Dosage and Administration

ORAL: No typical dosage.
TOPICAL: The common application of poplar is 5 grams of the dried buds per day or semi-solid preparations equivalent to 20-30% dried buds per day (2,18).

Comments

Available information supports only the external use of poplar. Avoid confusion with spruce (Picea excelsa) and Canada balsam (Abies balsamea), also known as balm of Gilead.

PORIA MUSHROOM

Also Known As

Fu Ling, FuShen, Hoelen, Indian Bread, Matsuhodo, Polyporus, Poria, Tuckahoe.

Scientific Names

Wolfiporia cocos, synonym Poria cocos.
Family: Polyporaceae.

People Use This For

Traditionally, poria mushroom filaments have been used for amnesia, anxiety, restlessness, fatigue, tension, nervousness, dizziness, dysuria and urination problems, edema, insomnia, splenitis, stomach problems, diarrhea, tumors, and as an antitussive (847). In herbal combinations, poria filaments have been used as a component of various herbal combinations for treating diarrhea (3731,3732), chronic glomerulonephritis (3733), tinnitus (3734), and for decreasing upper gastrointestinal tract bleeding (3735).

Safety

POSSIBLY SAFE …when used orally (12).
PREGNANCY AND LACTATION: Insufficient reliable information available; avoid using.

Effectiveness

There is insufficient reliable information available about the effectiveness of poria mushroom.

Mechanism of Action

The applicable part of poria mushroom is the sclerotium (filament). Poria contains pachyman which prevents urinary protein excretion, serum cholesterol elevation, and reduces the degree of histopathological changes in nephritic rats (3727). Some evidence suggests a hydroalcoholic extract (3728) and isolated triterpene constituents (3729,3736,3737) might have anti-inflammatory activity. Other evidence suggests poria extracts might also have immunosuppressive effects (3726). In addition, isolated triterpene constituents show evidence that they might have antitumor (3729) and anti-emetic effects (3730).

Adverse Reactions

None reported.

Interactions with Herbs & Other Dietary Supplements

Insufficient reliable information available.

Interactions with Drugs

No interactions are known to occur, and there is no known reason to expect a clinically significant interaction with poria mushroom.

Interactions with Foods

No interactions are known to occur, and there is no known reason to expect a clinically significant interaction with poria mushroom.

Interactions with Lab Tests

No interactions are known to occur, and there is no known reason to expect a clinically significant interaction with poria mushroom.

Interactions with Diseases or Conditions

No interactions are known to occur, and there is no known reason to expect a clinically significant interaction with poria mushroom.

Dosage and Administration

ORAL: People typically use 10 to 15 grams per day (1663).

Comments

Various combination herbal mixtures containing poria are reported to be effective for treating diarrhea (3731,3732), chronic glomerulonephritis (3733), tinnitus (3734), and decreasing upper gastrointestinal tract bleeding (3735). Further studies are needed to verify these results.

POTASSIUM

Also Known As

Potassium Acetate, Potassium Bicarbonate, Potassium Chloride, Potassium Citrate, Potassium Gluconate, Potassium Phosphate.

Scientific Names

Potassium; K; atomic number 19.

People Use This For

Orally, potassium is used for treating and preventing hypokalemia, hypertension, Menière's disease, thallium poisoning, hypercalciuria, insulin resistance, myocardial infarction, stroke prevention, symptoms of menopause, and infant colic. It is also used orally for allergies, headaches, acne, alcoholism, Alzheimer's disease, arthritis, blurred vision, cancer, chronic fatigue syndrome, colitis, confusion, constipation, dermatitis, edema, fever, gout, insomnia, irritability, mononucleosis, muscle weakness, muscular dystrophy, stress, and as an adjunct for treating myasthenia gravis.

Intravenously, potassium is used for treating and preventing hypokalemia, cardiac arrhythmias including atrial tachycardia and ventricular arrhythmias, and myocardial infarction.

Safety

LIKELY SAFE ...when consumed orally in amounts up to 80-90 mEq total potassium (supplements and diet) per day by individuals with normal renal function (14,15,16). Larger amounts increase the risk of hyperkalemia (15). ...when used intravenously (IV). Parental potassium is a FDA-approved prescription product.

UNSAFE ...when use results in blood levels above 7 mEq/L. This is potentially life-threatening (14).

PREGNANCY AND LACTATION: LIKELY SAFE ...when used orally at the normal dietary intake of 40-80 mEq per day, which is adequate to maintain the mother's serum potassium between 3.5-5 mEq/L (14). When the mother's serum potassium levels are in the normal range, levels in breast milk are generally low (14).

Effectiveness

EFFECTIVE ...when used orally or intravenously for treating and preventing hypokalemia (14,15). ...when used orally to alkalinize the urine (14).

POSSIBLY EFFECTIVE ...when used orally for treating hypertension. Potassium supplementation seems to reduce systolic blood pressure by about 2-4 mm Hg and diastolic blood pressure by about 0.5-3.5 mm Hg (3385). Potassium seems to be most effective for people with low potassium levels, high daily sodium intake, and for African Americans (3384,3385,3386). ...when used orally from dietary sources for preventing hypertension and stroke. There is some evidence that foods that provide at least 350 mg of potassium per serving and that are low in sodium, saturated fat, and cholesterol might help reduce the risk of developing high blood pressure and stroke (1310). However, there is no proof that taking potassium supplements has this same effect. ...when used orally for hypercalciuria (2208,2209).

Mechanism of Action

The potassium mineral plays a role in many body functions including acid-base balance, electrodynamic characteristics of the cell, isotonicity, and various enzymatic reactions (15). It is essential in physiological processes including nerve impulse transmission, cardiac, smooth, and skeletal muscle contraction, gastric secretion, renal function, tissue synthesis, and carbohydrate synthesis (15). Evidence suggests that inadequate dietary intake of potassium can play a role in the development of hypertension. A potassium intake of 48-90 mEq/day can benefit people with hypertension (14,15).

Adverse Reactions

Orally or intravenously (IV), potassium can cause stomach upset, nausea, diarrhea, vomiting, belching, flatulence, and ulcerations (15,16,3385). Hyperkalemia, typically serum potassium above 5 mEq/L, can cause paresthesia, generalized weakness, flaccid paralysis, listlessness, vertigo, mental confusion, hypotension, blood in the stool, cardiac arrhythmias, heart block, and death (15,16,3385).

Interactions with Herbs & Other Dietary Supplements

Insufficient reliable information available.

Interactions with Drugs

ACE INHIBITORS, POTASSIUM-SPARING DIURETICS: Concomitant use with these drugs can increase potassium levels and the risk of hyperkalemia adverse effects (15).

Drug Influences on Nutrient Levels and Depletion

SOME DRUGS CAN AFFECT POTASSIUM LEVELS:
LOOP DIURETICS and THIAZIDE DIURETICS: Use of loop diuretics and thiazide diuretics increases urine potassium excretion and can cause hypokalemia. Monitor potassium serum levels and give potassium supplements when appropriate (15,4412,4425,4449).
BISACODYL (Dulcolax): Bisacodyl can cause potassium loss in patients undergoing bowel-cleansing regimens. Use caution in patients who are predisposed to hypokalemia (i.e., diuretic therapy), monitor potassium serum levels, and give potassium supplements when appropriate (4411,4412).
STIMULANT LAXATIVES: Excessive use of stimulant laxatives can result in potassium loss and hypokalemia. Limit stimulant laxatives to short-term use (4411,4412,4425,4453).

Interactions with Foods

POTASSIUM-CONTAINING FOODS: Theoretically, concomitant use can increase potassium levels and the risk of adverse effects, especially in individuals with renal dysfunction, ACE inhibitor or potassium-sparing diuretic therapy. Potassium-containing foods include fruits (especially dried), cereals, beans, milk, and vegetables (16).
POTASSIUM-CONTAINING SALT SUBSTITUTES: Theoretically, concomitant use can increase potassium levels and the risk of adverse effects, especially in individuals with renal dysfunction, ACE inhibitor, or potassium-sparing diuretic therapy.

Interactions with Lab Tests

POTASSIUM: Potassium supplementation increases serum and urine potassium concentrations and test results (15).
BLOOD PRESSURE: Potassium taken orally can reduce blood pressure and blood pressure readings (14).

Interactions with Diseases or Conditions

ELECTROLYTE IMBALANCES: Potassium is contraindicated in individuals with untreated Addison's disease, heat cramps, acute dehydration, hyperkalemia from any cause (14,15,16), adynamia episodica hereditaria (14,16), severe renal impairment with oliguria, anuria, or azotemia (14,15), or who have extensive tissue breakdown, e.g., severe burns (15). Use potassium with caution in people with heart and kidney disease (15,16), GI disease with risk of bleeding (14,15), and sickle cell anemia (14).
GI MOTILITY CONDITIONS: Oral potassium tablets and capsules are contraindicated in individuals with gastrointestinal motility conditions (15).
ASPIRIN OR TARTRAZINE SENSITIVITY: Avoid oral potassium products that contain tartrazine (15).

Dosage and Administration

ORAL: Potassium supplementation must be individualized and based on the person's serum potassium level, which should be maintained between 3.5-5 mEq/L (14). The normal adult daily requirement and usual dietary intake is 40-80 mEq daily (15). For preventing hypokalemia, 20 mEq is typically taken daily (15). The common dose of potassium for treating hypokalemia is 40-100 mEq or more daily, in two to four divided amounts (15).

For hypercalciuria, 1 mEq/kg is taken daily (14) or four tablets of Urophos-K are taken twice a day (2209). The typical dose for hypertension is 48-90 mEq daily (14,15). The common dose of potassium citrate for urinary alkalinization is 20-30 mEq four times daily (14).

INTRAVENOUS (IV): IV potassium products are prescription products.

Comments

Potassium tablets or capsules are available as food supplements and are not required to meet the rigorous standards for prescription medications.

POTATO

Also Known As

Irish Potato, White Potato.
CAUTION: See separate listing for African Wild Potato.

Scientific Names

Solanum tuberosum.
Family: Solanaceae.

People Use This For

Orally, raw potato juice is used for gastritis and stomach disorders (6). A purified protein extract from potato is used as an appetite suppressant for weight loss (473).

Topically, raw potato is used as a poultice for arthritis, infections, boils, burns, and sore eyes (6).

Traditionally, brewed potato peel tea is used orally for edema and to soothe bodily swelling (6).

Potato is eaten as a food, used as a source of starch, and fermented into alcohol (6).

Safety

LIKELY SAFE ...when unblemished, ripe potatoes are used as food (6).

POSSIBLY SAFE ...when the purified protein extract from potato is used orally and appropriately (473). ...when unblemished, ripe potatoes are used orally for medicinal purposes (6).

LIKELY UNSAFE ...when damaged, green potatoes and sprouts are consumed. These contain toxic solanum alkaloids that cannot be destroyed by cooking and can cause serious adverse effects (See Adverse Reactions). There is insufficient reliable information available about the safety of potato for its other uses.

PREGNANCY AND LACTATION: LIKELY SAFE ...when unblemished, ripe potatoes are used orally in food amounts. There is insufficient reliable information available about the safety of oral or topical use of potato in pregnancy and lactation for medicinal purposes.

Effectiveness

There is insufficient reliable information available about the effectiveness of potato.

Mechanism of Action

The applicable part of the potato is the tuber. Potatoes are a source of vitamin C, iron, riboflavin, and are rich in carbohydrates (6). A proteinase inhibitor isolated from potatoes is claimed to increase the effects of cholecystokinin (CCK), by blocking the effects of the enzymes chymotrypsin and trypsin, which break down CCK (473). CCK produces satiety and has been shown to play a role in the short-term inhibition of food intake (476,477,6255). It has been reported by the manufacturer of a purified protein extract from potato (Satietrol), which contains this proteinase inhibitor and other nutrients and minerals claimed to affect CCK, that the product reduced feelings of hunger by 30-32% 3.5 hours after a fixed calorie meal. These effects were also found in a group of people who lost weight on a calorie-controlled diet (473). Damaged, green potatoes, and sprouts contain toxic solanum alkaloids that cannot be destroyed by cooking (see Adverse Reactions). Researchers report that a potato peel extract inhibited bacterial adhesion to host cells without killing the bacteria. They believe this activity might be due to polyphenol oxidase, a compound known to have anti-adhesive properties. This unpublished research was presented at the 2000 Annual Meeting of the American Society for Microbiology (6107).

Adverse Reactions

Adverse reactions have not been reported with unblemished, ripe potatoes. Solanum glycosides found in damaged, green potatoes and sprouts can cause headache, flushing, nausea, vomiting, diarrhea, abdominal pain, thirst, and restlessness. Deaths have been reported in malnourished individuals who may not have received adequate medical care (17). Twenty mg solanine per 100 grams potato is the maximum concentration considered safe. Solanum glycosides cannot be destroyed by cooking (6). Exposure to potato dust is associated with a high-incidence of respiratory symptoms due to bacterial and fungal contaminants (6).

Interactions with Herbs & Other Dietary Supplements
Insufficient reliable information available.

Interactions with Drugs
DIABETES THERAPY: Concomitant use of potato may interfere with blood sugar control and insulin levels (6).
THROMBOLYTICS (tPA, Alterplase): Theoretically, concomitant use of potato may enhance thrombolytic effects. A carboxypeptidase inhibitor isolated from potato tubers may have inhibitory effects on thrombin-activatable thrombolysis inhibitor, and thereby enhance the activity of thrombolytic agents (474,475).

Interactions with Foods
No interactions are known to occur, and there is no known reason to expect a clinically significant interaction with potato.

Interactions with Lab Tests
No interactions are known to occur, and there is no known reason to expect a clinically significant interaction with potato.

Interactions with Diseases or Conditions
DIABETES: Potatoes can affect blood sugar control. They should be consumed as appropriate carbohydrate equivalents (6).

Dosage and Administration
ORAL: For appetite suppression and weight loss, a purified protein extract from potato (Satietrol) containing a proteinase inhibitor, is marketed as a powder to be mixed with 8 ounces of water and taken 15 minutes before meals (473). There is no typical dosage of potato juice.
TOPICAL: Raw potato is used as a poultice (6).

Comments
The potato is one of the main food crops of the world (6).

POTENTILLA

Also Known As
Crampweed, Goosegrass, Goose Tansy, Goosewort, Moor Grass, Prince's Feathers, Silverweed, Trailing Tansy, Wild Agrimony.
CAUTION: See separate listings for Agrimony, Tormentil, and Jewelweed.

Scientific Names
Potentilla anserina.
Family: Rosacea.

People Use This For
Orally, potentilla flower and leaf are used for premenstrual syndrome (PMS), mild dysmenorrhea, and diarrhea (2,18). Topically, potentilla flower and leaf are used for the local treatment of oropharyngeal inflammation (2,7,18).

Safety
POSSIBLY SAFE ...when used orally and appropriately (2).
PREGNANCY AND LACTATION: Insufficient reliable information available; avoid using.

Effectiveness
POSSIBLY EFFECTIVE ...when applied topically for treatment of oropharyngeal inflammation (7).
There is insufficient reliable information available about the effectiveness of potentilla for its other uses.

Mechanism of Action
The applicable parts of potentilla are the flower and leaf. The tannin constituents of potentilla have astringent effects (2) and are likely responsible for antidiarrheal and local anti-inflammatory activity. Potentilla also increases tonus and the contraction frequency of isolated animal uterus (2,7).

Adverse Reactions
Orally, potentilla can cause stomach irritation (7,12).

Interactions with Herbs & Other Dietary Supplements
Insufficient reliable information available.

Interactions with Drugs
No interactions are known to occur, and there is no known reason to expect a clinically significant interaction with potentilla.

Interactions with Foods
No interactions are known to occur, and there is no known reason to expect a clinically significant interaction with potentilla.

Interactions with Lab Tests
No interactions are known to occur, and there is no known reason to expect a clinically significant interaction with potentilla.

Interactions with Diseases or Conditions
No interactions are known to occur, and there is no known reason to expect a clinically significant interaction with potentilla.

Dosage and Administration
ORAL: For premenstrual syndrome (PMS), dysmenorrhea, and acute diarrhea, the typical dose is 4-6 grams per day (2,18). Potentilla is often prepared as a tea and given in a dose of one cup 2-3 times daily. The tea is prepared by steeping 2 grams of the finely cut flower or leaf in 150 mL boiling water for 10 minutes and then straining (18).
TOPICAL: No typical dosage.

Comments
Avoid confusion with agrimony (Agrimonia eupratoria) and tormentil (Potentilla erecta), also referred to as potentilla. Avoid confusion with jewelweed, also known as silverweed.

PRECATORY BEAN

Also Known As
Bead Vine, Black-Eyed Susan, Buddhist Rosary Bead, Crab's Eye, Indian Bead, Jequirity Bean, Jequirity Seed, Legume, Love Bean, Lucky Bean, Ojo De Pajaro, Prayer Beads, Prayer Head, Rosary Pea, Seminole Bead, Weather Plant.

Scientific Names
Abrus pecatorius.
Family: Leguminosae or Fabaceae.

People Use This For
In folk medicine, precatory bean has been used to quicken labor, as an abortifacient, oral contraceptive, and as an analgesic in terminally-ill patients (6). The whole plant has been used for ophthalmic inflammations (6).

Safety
LIKELY UNSAFE ...when used orally; 5 mg of abrin, a constituent of precatory bean, is considered toxic to humans (6). Significant precatory bean ingestion causes severe gastroenteritis, followed by diarrhea and vomiting that can become bloody. Symptoms may not appear for several days (3499). Fatalities can occur after 3-4 days of persistent gastroenteritis (17,3499).
CHILDREN: UNSAFE ...when used orally. Ingestion of one seed in young children can be fatal (6,3499,5607). Older children (ages 9-12) have been reported to experience severe abdominal pain, vomiting and bloody stools after ingestion of one or more seeds (5607).
PREGNANCY AND LACTATION: LIKELY UNSAFE ...when used orally (6); avoid using.

Effectiveness
There is insufficient reliable information available about the effectiveness of precatory bean.

Mechanism of Action

The precatory bean plant contains the indole alkaloids abrine, abrus agglutinin, hyaphorine, and precatorine (6). Abrin, isolated from the seeds, is a potent inhibitor of protein synthesis and moderate inhibitor of DNA synthesis. In vitro, ethanol extracts of the seeds causes irreversible impairment in human sperm motility (3842), and aqueous extracts of the seeds agglutinate human red blood corpuscles (6369). Some isoflavanquinone constituents isolated from the root inhibit platelet aggregation; others possess potent anti-inflammatory and antiallergic effects (3841).

Adverse Reactions

Orally, the seeds that are chewed or with cracked shells can cause stomach cramping, nausea (6), vomiting, severe diarrhea (possibly bloody) (3499), cold sweat (6), fever, weakness (3499), tachycardia, coma, circulatory collapse (6,3499), cerebral edema (3499), and death (17,3499,5608). Signs of toxicity, including gastroenteritis usually occurs several hours after ingestion of the seeds, followed by the development of bloody diarrhea. Fatalities have usually occurred 3-4 days after ingestion of the seeds. Symptoms may last for up to 10 days (17). Topically, the seeds when used as a necklace can cause dermatitis (6). Eye contact with the seed's contents can cause necrotizing conjunctivitis (3499).
TOXICITY MANAGEMENT: There is no known antidote. There is no method for enhancing elimination. Patients seen within 4 hours of seed ingestion should be treated with usual decontamination methods including lavage, charcoal, and cathartics. In cases of diarrhea, the need for cathartics may be unnecessary (17).

Interactions with Herbs & Other Dietary Supplements

Insufficient reliable information available.

Interactions with Drugs

No interactions are known to occur, and there is no known reason to expect a clinically significant interaction with precatory bean.

Interactions with Foods

No interactions are known to occur, and there is no known reason to expect a clinically significant interaction with precatory bean.

Interactions with Lab Tests

No interactions are known to occur, and there is no known reason to expect a clinically significant interaction with precatory bean.

Interactions with Diseases or Conditions

No interactions are known to occur, and there is no known reason to expect a clinically significant interaction with precatory bean.

Dosage and Administration

No typical dosage.

Comments

Children are attracted to the bright colors of the seed (17). The hard coat of a mature seed may resist digestion when swallowed but treatment for suspected poisoning should begin as soon as possible (3499). Abrin, a constituent of precatory bean, is being investigated for the treatment of experimental cancers and is used as a "molecular probe" to investigate cell function (6).

PREGNENOLONE

Also Known As

None.
CAUTION: See separate listings for Progesterone and Wild Yam.

Scientific Names

Pregnenolone; (3 beta)-3-hydroxypregn-5-en-20-one; delta 5-pregnen-3 beta-ol-20-one; 17 beta-(1-ketoethyl)- delta 5-androsten-3 beta-ol.

People Use This For

Orally, pregnenolone is used for slowing or reversing aging, for arthritis, depression, endometriosis, fatigue, fibrocystic breast disease, memory enhancement, menopause, premenstrual syndrome (PMS), stress, increasing energy, and improving immunity. It is also used for strengthening the heart, Alzheimer's disease, allergic reactions, detoxification, lupus, multiple sclerosis, prostate disorders, psoriasis, scleroderma, seizures, trauma, and injuries (3000-3004).

Safety

There is insufficient reliable information available about the safety of pregnenolone.
Pregnancy and Lactation: Insufficient reliable information available; avoid using.

Effectiveness

There is insufficient reliable information available about the effectiveness of pregnenolone.

Mechanism of Action

Pregnenolone is produced by the body from cholesterol and is the precursor for all the steroid hormones, including progesterone, aldosterone, cortisol, dehydroepiandrosterone (DHEA), testosterone, and estrogens (3008). Lower cerebrospinal fluid (CSF) levels of pregnenolone are reported in people with affective disorders, particularly during episodes of active depression (3005). Pregnenolone has antagonist activity at GABA-A receptors in the brain and induces changes in the sleep EEG by increasing the time spent in slow wave sleep (3007). Higher pregnenolone concentrations in the luteal phase serum are associated with more severe PMS symptoms (3006). Reliable information on the effects of exogenously administered pregnenolone is not available (3005).

Adverse Reactions

Orally, supplemental pregnenolone may cause steroid-related adverse effects. There have been warnings of overstimulation, insomnia, irritability, anger, anxiety, acne, headache, negative mood changes, facial hair growth, hair loss, and arrhythmias (3004).

Interactions with Herbs & Other Dietary Supplements

Insufficient reliable information available.

Interactions with Drugs

STEROID HORMONE DRUGS: Theoretically, pregnenolone can enhance the effects of steroid hormone drugs (see Mechanism of Action).

Interactions with Foods

No interactions are known to occur, and there is no known reason to expect a clinically significant interaction with pregnenolone.

Interactions with Lab Tests

No interactions are known to occur, and there is no known reason to expect a clinically significant interaction with pregnenolone.

Interactions with Diseases or Conditions

HORMONE SENSITIVE CANCERS/CONDITIONS: Because pregnenolone is converted to estrogens (3008), women with hormone sensitive conditions should avoid pregnenolone. Some of these conditions include breast, uterine, and ovarian cancer, and endometriosis and uterine fibroids.

Dosage and Administration

No typical dosage.

Comments

Pregnenolone was studied for stress, fatigue, and arthritis in the 1940s before synthetic hormones became available (3000).

PREMORSE

Also Known As

Devil's Bit, Ofbit, Premorse Scaboius.

Scientific Names
Scabiosa succisa.
Family: Dipsacaceae.

People Use This For
Orally, premorse is used for febrile colds and coughs, and to promote sweating (18).

Safety
There is insufficient reliable information available about the safety of premorse.
Pregnancy and Lactation: Insufficient reliable information available; avoid using.

Effectiveness
There is insufficient reliable information available about the effectiveness of premorse.

Mechanism of Action
The applicable parts of the premorse are the above ground parts. There is insufficient reliable information available about the possible mechanism of action and active ingredients of premorse.

Adverse Reactions
None reported.

Interactions with Herbs & Other Dietary Supplements
Insufficient reliable information available.

Interactions with Drugs
No interactions are known to occur, and there is no known reason to expect a clinically significant interaction with premorse.

Interactions with Foods
No interactions are known to occur, and there is no known reason to expect a clinically significant interaction with premorse.

Interactions with Lab Tests
No interactions are known to occur, and there is no known reason to expect a clinically significant interaction with premorse.

Interactions with Diseases or Conditions
No interactions are known to occur, and there is no known reason to expect a clinically significant interaction with premorse.

Dosage and Administration
ORAL: Premorse is used as a tea (18).

Comments
There is very little scientific information about this product. Our staff is continually analyzing the available information on natural medicines and will add data here as it becomes available.

PRICKLY PEAR CACTUS

Also Known As
Cactus Flowers, Gracemere-Pear, Tuna Cardona, Opuntia, Nopal, Nopol, Prickly Pear, Westwood-Pear.

Scientific Names
Opuntia ficus indica; Opuntia hyptiacantha; Opuntia lasciacantha; Opuntia macrocentra; Opuntia megacantha; Opuntia puberula; Opuntia streptacantha; Opuntia velutina.
Family: Cactaceae.

People Use This For

Orally, prickly pear cactus is used for diabetes (5951,7028), hypercholesterolemia (5952), obesity, and as an antiviral agent (5952). It is also used for colitis, diarrhea, and benign prostatic hypertrophy (BPH) (5953).
In foods, the prickly pear juice is used in jellies and candies.

Safety

LIKELY SAFE ...when used orally as a food (5951,5969).
POSSIBLY SAFE ...when the leaves, stems, or standardized product are used short-term (5951,5959,5960,5963).
Although the prickly pear cactus reduces blood sugar it does not appear to cause hypoglycemia.
There is insufficient reliable information available about the safety of prickly pear cactus used long-term.
PREGNANCY AND LACTATION: Insufficient reliable information available; avoid using.

Effectiveness

POSSIBLY EFFECTIVE ...when used orally, short-term to reduce blood glucose levels in patients with type 2 diabetes. There is some preliminary clinical evidence that prickly pear cactus can decrease blood glucose levels in patients with type 2 diabetes. Single doses can decrease blood glucose levels by 17-46% in some patients (5951,5959,5961,5962,5964). However, it is not known if extended daily use can consistently lower blood glucose levels and decrease HbA1c levels. Only the broiled stems of the specific species Opuntia streptacantha seem to be beneficial. Raw or crude stems don't seem to decrease glucose levels (5961). Other prickly pear cactus species also do not seem to significantly lower blood glucose levels (5970,7028).
There is insufficient reliable information about the effectiveness of prickly pear cactus for its other uses.

Mechanism of Action

The applicable parts of prickly pear cactus are the leaves and stems. Prickly pear cactus is often consumed as part of the diet. Ingesting 500 grams of prickly pear cactus provides 14.3 grams carbohydrate, 8.25 grams protein, 1.05 grams lipids, 18.85 grams cellulose (fibrous polysaccharide), 455.75 grams water, and 99.75 kilocalories (7028). Some species of prickly pear cactus can lower blood glucose and lipid levels (5952,5958,5959,5960,5963). This effect is often attributed to the high fibrous polysaccharide content, including pectin (5952,5958). Fiber can slow carbohydrate absorption and decrease lipid absorption from the gut. However, some researchers suspect prickly pear might also have an insulin sensitizing effect (7028). There is also some evidence that the pectin component can also alter the liver metabolism of cholesterol and affect cholesterol levels (5958). Broiled stems seem to be more effective for reducing blood glucose levels than raw stems (5961,5964). The reason for this difference is not known. The hypoglycemic effects of prickly pear cactus peak 3-4 hours after ingestion and can last for up to 6 hours. There is some preliminary evidence that prickly pear has antiviral activity against the herpes simplex virus (HSV), respiratory syncytial virus (RSV), and human immunodeficiency virus (HIV) (5956).

Adverse Reactions

Orally, prickly pear cactus is usually well-tolerated. However, prickly pear cactus can cause some side effects including mild diarrhea, nausea, increased stool volume, increased stool frequency, abdominal fullness, and headache (5951,7028).

Interactions with Herbs & Other Dietary Supplements

Insufficient reliable information available.

Interactions with Drugs

CHLORPROPAMIDE (Diabinese): Using chlorpropamide and prickly pear cactus together can have additive effects on blood glucose and insulin levels in patients with type 2 diabetes (5968). There is some concern that people taking both chlorpropamide or other hypoglycemic drugs and prickly pear cactus might be at an increased risk for hypoglycemia. Advise patients to monitor glucose levels closely. Dose adjustments may be necessary. Other hypoglycemic drugs include glimepiride (Amaryl), glipizide (Glucotrol), glyburide (Diabeta, Micronase), tolazamide (Tolinase), tolbutamide (Orinase), and others.

Interactions with Foods

No interactions are known to occur, and there is no known reason to expect a clinically significant interaction with prickly pear cactus.

Interactions with Lab Tests

BLOOD GLUCOSE: Prickly pear cactus can reduce blood glucose levels and lab tests (5957).
CHOLESTEROL: There is some evidence that prickly pear cactus might reduce total and low-density lipoprotein (LDL) cholesterol levels (5958).

Interactions with Diseases or Conditions

DIABETES: Prickly pear cactus can reduce blood glucose in patients with type 2 diabetes (5957). Prickly pear cactus might have additive effects with diabetes medications and potentially cause hypoglycemia (see Interactions with Drugs). Advise patients to closely monitor glucose levels after starting prickly pear cactus. Dose adjustments to diabetes medications may be necessary.

Dosage and Administration

ORAL: For diabetes, broiled stems 100-500 grams daily is typically used (5964). Doses are often divided and given three times daily. For colitis, diarrhea, and benign prostatic hypertrophy (BPH), prickly pear cactus flowers 0.3-1 grams or as a tea has been used. A typical dose of the liquid extract of dried flowers is 0.3-1 mL of 1:1 in 25% alcohol (5953).

Comments

Prickly pear cactus is primarily used in Mexican and Mexican-American cultures as a part of the diet and as a treatment for type 2 diabetes. Most research on this product has been performed in Mexico. The immature form of prickly pear cactus is used. Mature stems are fibrous and tough and not appropriate for consumption (7028).

PROCAINE

Also Known As

Gero-Vita, Gerovital, Gerovital-H3, GH-3, KH-3, Procaine Hydrochloride.

Scientific Names

2-Dietylaminoethyl p-aminobenzoate monohydrochloride.

People Use This For

Orally or parenterally, procaine is used for arthritis, cerebral atherosclerosis, dementia, depression, hair loss, hypertension, sexual dysfunction, and an overall rejuvenating effect (6).
Parenterally, prescription-only procaine is used for local anesthesia (6).

Safety

LIKELY SAFE ...when the prescription-only product is used parenterally as a local anesthetic (15).
There is insufficient reliable information available about the safety of the oral use of procaine.
PREGNANCY: LIKELY UNSAFE ...when used for self-medication; avoid using (6).
LACTATION: Insufficient reliable information available for self-medication; avoid using.

Effectiveness

EFFECTIVE ...when the parenteral, prescription-only product is used for local anesthesia (15).
LIKELY INEFFECTIVE ...when used orally (6).

Mechanism of Action

Procaine has poor oral absorption, and there is no evidence that pharmacologic levels are achieved with oral administration (6). Hematoporphyrin is added to some oral preparations to increase procaine absorption (6), although no evidence supports this effect.

Adverse Reactions

Orally, procaine can cause heartburn, migraines, and systemic lupus erythematosus (SLE) (6).

Interactions with Herbs & Other Dietary Supplements

DIGITALIS: Intravenous use of procaine hydrochloride is contraindicated with concurrent use of digitalis (15).

Interactions with Drugs

AMINOSALICYLIC ACID, SULFONAMIDES: The procaine metabolite aminobenzoic acid can antagonize activity of these drugs. Avoid concomitant use (15).
ANTICHOLINESTERASE DRUGS, DIGOXIN, SUCCINYLCHOLINE: Intravenous use of procaine hydrochloride is contraindicated (15).

Interactions with Foods

No interactions are known to occur, and there is no known reason to expect a clinically significant interaction with procaine.

Interactions with Lab Tests

No interactions are known to occur, and there is no known reason to expect a clinically significant interaction with procaine.

Interactions with Diseases or Conditions

MYASTHENIA GRAVIS: The intravenous use of procaine is contraindicated in individuals with myasthenia gravis, which is progressive muscular weakness (15).
SYSTEMIC LUPUS ERYTHEMATOSUS (SLE): Contraindicated. Theoretically, procaine might exacerbate this condition (6).
PSEUDOCHOLINESTERASE DEFICIENCY: Contraindicated (6).

Dosage and Administration

ORAL: People typically take procaine in a cyclical regimen: 200 mg procaine once or twice daily for 25 days, then no drug for 5 days, then repeat the cycle (5274).

Comments

None.

PROGESTERONE

Also Known As

Corpus Luteum Hormone, Luteal Hormone, Luteohormone, Lutine, NSC-9704, Pregnancy Hormone, Pregnanedione, Progestational Hormone, Progesteronum.
CAUTION: See separate listings for Pregnenolone and Wild Yam.

Scientific Names

Progesterone; 4-Pregnene-3; 20-Dione.

People Use This For

Orally, progesterone is used for treating secondary amenorrhea (15,226,1215,1217), abnormal uterine bleeding associated with hormonal imbalance (15), treating severe symptoms of premenstrual syndrome (PMS) (1220), and treating benzodiazepine dependence and withdrawal (1221). Oral progesterone preparations are also used in combination with estrogens as part of hormone replacement therapy to prevent irregular bleeding and the increased risk of endometrial carcinoma associated with estrogen monotherapy (15,226,228,1215,1216,1217).
Topically, progesterone is used as an alternative to oral treatment as a component of hormone replacement therapy and for treating menopausal vasomotor symptoms (224,2031). Topical progesterone is also used for treating or preventing hormone-mediated allergies, bloating, breast tenderness, decreased sex drive, depression, fatigue, fibrocystic breasts, headaches, hypoglycemia, increased blood clotting, infertility, irritability, memory loss, miscarriages, osteoporosis, premenopausal bone loss, symptoms of premenstrual syndrome, thyroid dysfunction, unclear thinking, uterine cancer, uterine fibroids, water retention, weight gain (1209), and treating vulval lichen sclerosis (1210).
Intravaginally, progesterone is used for cervical ripening (15), mastodynia in women with benign breast disease (1223), and to prevent and treat endometrial hyperplasia (2031,2033). Progesterone is also used intravaginally or intramuscularly for treating infertility in women (9,2032), anovulatory bleeding, and treating symptoms of premenstrual syndrome (PMS) (9).

Safety

LIKELY SAFE ...when used orally and appropriately. Micronized progesterone (Prometrium) is a FDA-approved prescription product. Micronized progesterone (Prometrium) has been safely used in multiple clinical trials lasting up to 3 years (15,226,228,1216,1220,1221,1224). ...when used intravaginally and appropriately, short-term (1225,2031,2032,2033,2034). Progesterone intravaginal gel (Crinone) is a FDA-approved prescription product. Progesterone intravaginal gel (Crinone) has been safely used in trials lasting up to 3 months (1225,2031,2033,2034,2041). ...when used intramuscularly and appropriately, short-term (227,1218,1225,2034). Progesterone oil for intramuscular injection is a FDA-approved prescription product (227,1218,1225,2034). ...when used transdermally and appropriately. Transdermal progesterone has been used safely in clinical trials lasting up to a year (224,1229).
There is insufficient reliable information available about the safety of other progesterone preparations.
PREGNANCY: LIKELY SAFE ...when used intravaginally and appropriately as part of infertility treatment. Intravaginal progesterone gel (Crinone 8%) is FDA-approved for use in conjunction with infertility treatment (1225).
LIKELY UNSAFE ...when used orally, intramuscularly, intravaginally, or transdermally for purposes other than medically supervised adjunctive treatment for infertility; contraindicated (15).
LACTATION: Insufficient reliable information available; avoid using.

Effectiveness

LIKELY EFFECTIVE ...when used orally in combination with estrogen as a component of hormone replacement therapy in women with a uterus. Micronized progesterone (Prometrium) is FDA-approved for use with estrogen as a component of hormone replacement therapy. Micronized progesterone (Prometrium) has been shown to provide the same protection against the effects of unopposed estrogen therapy as medroxyprogesterone (226,228,1216,1217,1226,1230). In one trial, micronized progesterone (Prometrium) did not reduce the beneficial lipid effects of estrogen therapy as much as medroxyprogesterone (226); however, this effect was not seen in another trial (1216). ...when used orally for secondary amenorrhea in premenopausal women. Micronized progesterone is FDA-approved for the treatment of secondary amenorrhea (15). ...when used intravaginally in infertile women as a component of infertility treatment. Intravaginal progesterone gel (Crinone 8%) is FDA-approved for use as a component of infertility treatment in women. Clinical trials have shown that intravaginal progesterone achieves pregnancy rates comparable to oral progesterone in women infertile due to various etiologies (1225,2032,2087,2088,2091). Clinical trials comparing intravaginal progesterone to intramuscular progesterone have shown varying relative efficacy results (1218,2086,2089). ...when used intravaginally for secondary amenorrhea in premenopausal women. Intravaginal progesterone gel (Crinone 4%) is FDA-approved for the treatment of secondary amenorrhea. Several open-label clinical trials have shown intravaginal progesterone gel (Crinone 4%) to be effective for restoring menses when used in conjunction with estrogen replacement therapy (2041,2088,2091).

POSSIBLY EFFECTIVE ...when used intravaginally to prevent endometrial hyperplasia associated with estrogen replacement therapy. One short-term clinical trial has shown that intravaginal progesterone (Crinone) prevents endometrial hyperplasia in women with an intact uterus taking estrogen replacement therapy (2031). ...when used intravaginally for treating mastodynia. One clinical trial has shown that intravaginal progesterone gel (Crinone) is superior to placebo for reducing breast pain and tenderness in women with benign breast disease (1223). ...when used topically for treating menopausal vasomotor symptoms. One clinical trial has shown that topical progesterone cream (Progest) is superior to placebo for reducing vasomotor symptoms such as hot flashes in menopausal women (224). ...when used intravaginally for treatment of benign endometrial hyperplasia. One short term, open label clinical trial has shown that a specific intravaginal progesterone cream may help reverse endometrial hyperplasia and decrease vaginal bleeding in premenopausal women with benign hyperplasia (2033). ...when used intramuscularly in infertile women as a component of infertility treatment. Clinical trials have shown that intramuscular progesterone achieves pregnancy rates comparable to oral progesterone (227), and with varying efficacy relative to intravaginal progesterone in infertile women (1218,2086).

POSSIBLY INEFFECTIVE ...when used orally for treating symptoms of premenstrual syndrome (PMS). One clinical trial has shown that oral micronized progesterone is comparable to placebo and inferior to alprazolam for relieving symptoms associated with PMS (9,1220). ...when used orally for benzodiazepine dependence and withdrawal. One clinical trial has shown that oral micronized progesterone is comparable to placebo for relieving symptoms of withdrawal and for helping patients remain drug-free from diazepam (1221). ...when used topically for treating vulval lichen sclerosis. One clinical trial has shown that topical progesterone is comparable to placebo and inferior to clobetasol (Temovate) for treating the signs and symptoms of vulval lichen sclerosis (225). ...when used topically for preventing postmenopausal bone loss. One clinical trial has shown that topical progesterone is comparable to placebo for increasing bone mineral density in postmenopausal women (224).

There is insufficient reliable information available about the effectiveness of progesterone for its other uses.

Mechanism of Action

Progesterone is an endogenous progestin secreted by the corpus luteum. It is primarily secreted during the luteal phase of the menstrual cycle, but small amounts are also secreted during the follicular phase (15). The normal physiological effects of progesterone are responsible for its therapeutic benefit when administered exogenously. Progesterone transforms proliferative endometrium into a secreting endometrium. This effect is beneficial in preventing and treating endometrial hyperplasia. It may also be beneficial in infertility because progesterone is necessary for implantation of the fertilized ovum and for maintaining pregnancy (15). In premenstrual syndrome (PMS), progesterone has been proposed as a therapy because the symptoms of PMS are thought to correlate with physiological fluctuations in endogenous progesterone (1220). It was thought to be beneficial for preventing benzodiazepine withdrawal because metabolites of progesterone have been found to have sedative-hypnotic properties (1221). Other effects of progesterone include growth of mammary tissue and uterine smooth muscle relaxation. Progesterone also has mild estrogenic and androgenic effects (15). Intravaginal, topical, and intramuscular administration of progesterone may be advantageous over oral dosing because it avoids first-pass effect and may achieve greater concentrations in the uterus (2033,2034).

Adverse Reactions

Orally, progesterone can cause gastrointestinal disturbances, changes in appetite, weight gain, fluid retention and edema, fatigue (14,1224), acne, drowsiness or insomnia, allergic skin rashes, hives, fever, headache, depression, breast discomfort or enlargement (14), PMS-like syndrome, altered menstrual cycles, or irregular bleeding (14).
Topically, progesterone can cause vaginal spotting (224).

Interactions with Herbs & Other Dietary Supplements
Insufficient reliable information available.

Interactions with Drugs
CONJUGATED EQUINE ESTROGENS (Premarin): Concomitant use can cause breast tenderness (228). Use of conjugated equine estrogens with oral micronized progesterone in postmenopausal women may blunt the beneficial effects of estrogen on the lipoprotein profile (1216), although it might not affect estrogen-induced reduction in plasma lipoprotein (a) (1217).

Interactions with Foods
No interactions are known to occur, and there is no known reason to expect a clinically significant interaction with progesterone.

Interactions with Lab Tests
ALANINE AMINOTRANSFERASE (ALT): Can increase serum levels and test results due to hepatotoxicity (275).
ALBUMIN: May increase serum levels and test results (275).
ALKALINE PHOSPHATASE (Alk Phos): Can increase serum levels and test results due to hepatotoxicity (275).
ASPARTATE AMINOTRANSFERASE (AST): Progesterone can decrease serum levels and test results in healthy people or increase serum levels and test results due to hepatotoxicity (275).
BILE: Can increase urine levels and test results due to hepatotoxicity (275).
BILIRUBIN: Can increase serum levels and test results due to hepatotoxicity (275).
CHOLESTEROL: Might decrease serum levels and test results (275).
GLOBULIN: Can decrease serum levels and test results (275).
GAMMA-GLOBULIN: Can increase serum levels and test results (275).
GLUCARIC ACID: Can increase urine level and test results (275).
17-HYDROXYCORTICOSTEROIDS: Can decrease urine level and test results (275).
16-ALPHA-HYDROXYPROGESTERONE: Can cause increase in plasma test results (275).
LUTEINIZING HORMONE (LH): Can decrease peak plasma level and test results (275).
MAGNESIUM: Can increase serum level and test results (275).
PREGNANEDIOL: Can decrease urine level and test results (275).
PROGESTERONE: Can decrease plasma levels and test results (275).
PROSTAGLANDIN: Can decrease urine levels and test results (275).
PROTEIN: Can increase serum levels and test results (275).
SODIUM: Can increase serum and test results due to sodium retention (275). Large doses of progesterone can increase urine levels and test results (275).
THYROXINE (T4) BINDING GLOBULIN: Can increase serum levels and test results due to increased synthesis (275).

Interactions with Diseases or Conditions
ARTERIAL DISEASE: Contraindicated in individuals with high risk arterial disease (9).
BREAST CANCER: Should be avoided except as part of the management of breast cancer (9).
DEPRESSION: Use cautiously in individuals with a history of major depression (9).
FLUID RETENTION PROBLEMS: Use cautiously in individuals with conditions that can be aggravated by fluid retention (14), including cardiovascular or renal impairment, diabetes mellitus, asthma, epilepsy, and migraine.
LIVER DISEASE: Contraindicated. Progesterone has been associated with attacks of acute porphyria (9).
VAGINAL BLEEDING: Contraindicated in women who have undiagnosed vaginal bleeding (9).

Dosage and Administration
ORAL: For hormone replacement therapy, 200 mg micronized progesterone (Prometrium) orally per day is given for 12 days of a 25 day cycle with 0.625 mg conjugated estrogens (1215,1217).
TOPICAL: For menopausal vasomotor symptoms, 20 mg progesterone cream (equivalent to 1/4 teaspoon Progest cream) is applied daily to rotating sites including upper arms, thighs or breasts (224).
INTRAMUSCULAR: As a component of in vitro fertilization, 50 mg is used intramuscularly (227,1218,1225,2034).
INTRAVAGINAL: For mastodynia associated with benign breast disease, a dose of 4 grams of vaginal cream containing 2.5% natural progesterone is placed intravaginally from the 19th to the 25th day of a 28 day cycle (1223). As a component of in vitro fertilization, one applicator (90 mg) of progesterone gel (Crinone 8%) is placed intravaginally 1-2 times daily (2032,2036). For secondary amenorrhea, one applicator (90 mg) of progesterone gel (Crinone 4% or 8%) is placed intravaginally every other day for 6 days per month (2041).
For hormone replacement therapy, one applicator (90 mg) of progesterone gel (Crinone 4% or 8%) is placed intravaginally on days 17, 19, 21, 23, 25, and 27 of a 28 day cycle with 0.625 mg conjugated equine estrogens (2031). For reducing intravaginal bleeding and reversal of hyperplasia in premenopausal

women with benign endometrial hyperplasia, a dose of 100 mg progesterone cream placed intravaginally daily from day 10 to day 25 of a 28 day cycle has been used (2033).

Comments

The term "natural progesterone" is really a misnomer. Products marketed as natural progesterone are those products that are structurally identical to endogenous progesterone. However, these products must be prepared in a laboratory. "Natural progesterones," including the prescription products Crinone and Prometrium, are synthesized from the constituent diosgenin, isolated from wild yam. In the laboratory, this constituent is converted to pregnenolone and then to progesterone. The human body is not capable of synthesizing progesterone from diosgenin in vivo (515). OTC progesterone products may not contain progesterone concentrations as labeled. According to a British report, two-ounce jars of Progest cream used in a clinical trial contained 100 mg progesterone per ounce rather than the 465 mg claimed by the manufacturer (848,1228,1231). Topical progesterone products marketed as cosmetics require no FDA approval prior to marketing (853). There is currently no limit on the amount of progesterone allowed in cosmetic products. In 1993 the FDA proposed, but never finalized, a rule limiting progesterone-containing cosmetic products to a maximum level of 5 mg/oz with the product label specifying consumer usage not to exceed 2 oz per month (365).

PROPIONYL-L-CARNITINE

Also Known As

L-carnitine Propionyl, Propionyl L Carnitine, LPC, PLC, Propionylcarnitine.
CAUTION: See separate listings for Acetyl-L-Carnitine and L-Carnitine.

Scientific Names

Propionyl-L-carnitine.

People Use This For

Orally, propionyl-L-carnitine is used for treating peripheral vascular disease (PVD), atherosclerotic and diabetic angiopathies, intermittent claudication, and congestive heart failure (14,1434,1435,1436).
Intravenously, propionyl-L-carnitine has been used for treating peripheral vascular disease and intermittent claudication (1437); to improve healing of ulcerative lesions in people with peripheral vascular disease (1574); and to treat ischemic heart disease, angina, and congestive heart failure (1571,1572,1573,1575).

Safety

LIKELY SAFE ...when used orally and appropriately (1434,1435,1436,1437). ...when single intravenous doses are used under appropriate medical supervision (1571,1572,1573,1575).
PREGNANCY AND LACTATION: Insufficient reliable information available; avoid using.

Effectiveness

POSSIBLY EFFECTIVE ...when used orally for improving physical functioning and quality of life in people with peripheral vascular disease and intermittent claudication characterized by a maximal walking distance less than 250 meters (14,1434,1435,1436,1576). ...when used orally to produce small improvements in myocardial ischemia and exercise capacity in people with chronic, stable angina (1579,1580,1581). ...when used orally to improve left ventricular function and exercise capacity in people with class II or III congestive heart failure (1575,1582,1583). ...when single doses are used intravenously for improving maximal walking capacity in people with peripheral vascular disease (14,1437). ...when single doses are given intravenously to produce short-term increases in left ventricular function and cardiac output, and a reduction in myocardial ischemia in people with chronic ischemic heart disease (1571,1572,1573).
LIKELY INEFFECTIVE ...when used orally for improving physical functioning in people with peripheral vascular disease (PVD) characterized by a maximal walking distance greater than 250 meters (1434,1435,1436).
There is insufficient reliable information about the effectiveness of propionyl-L-carnitine for its other uses.

Mechanism of Action

L-carnitine is an essential cofactor in skeletal muscle and myocardium for transfer of long-chain fatty acids to intramitochondrial beta-oxidation sites where they are transformed into energy. There may be altered homeostasis and reduced levels of L-carnitine in peripheral vascular disease, myocardial ischemia, and heart failure (14,1572). Propionyl-L-carnitine may be hydrolyzed in the blood to L-carnitine and acetyl-L-carnitine, and also converted to L-carnitine and propionyl coenzyme A in the mitochondria of cells (14). Within cells, propionyl-L-carnitine helps to maintain mitochondrial acyl-CoA/CoA ratios which are increased in L-carnitine deficiency states, leading to deficient metabolism of fatty acids and urea synthesis (1439). Propionyl-L-carnitine also increases pyruvate flux into the Krebs cycle, stimulates pyruvate dehydrogenase activity, has free radical scavenging activity, improves homeostasis in the coagulation cascade, and has positive effects on blood viscosity (1578). Compared with L-carnitine, propionyl-L-carnitine may produce greater increases in cellular L-carnitine concentrations, possibly by being transported more easily into muscle fibers, and may provide additional substrates for muscle-cell energy production (14). Heart tissues may be able to utilize exogenous propionyl-L-carnitine to stimulate the tricarboxylic acid cycle and protect against ischemia (1439).

Treatment with intravenous propionyl-L-carnitine has been reported to restore levels of muscle L-carnitine which are deficient in people with peripheral vascular disease (14). Intravenous and oral treatment may improve physical functioning in some people with peripheral vascular disease (1434,1435,1436,1437,1576), but a study suggesting that propionyl-L-carnitine was superior to L-carnitine in this regard used only single intravenous doses, and the clinical significance of the difference was questionable (14,1437).

Propionyl-L-carnitine improves energy, metabolism, and myocardial contractility in experimental models of heart failure (1577). Small studies suggest that propionyl-L-carnitine may have a positive inotropic effect and improve ventricular function and cardiac output in chronic heart failure (1571,1572,1573). It reduces myocardial ischemia, as measured by ST segment depression, in people with angina (1573,1579).

Adverse Reactions
Orally, nausea, vomiting, gastric pain, asthenia, and angina have been reported (14).

Interactions with Herbs & Other Dietary Supplements
Insufficient reliable information available.

Interactions with Drugs
No interactions are known to occur, and there is no known reason to expect a clinically significant interaction with propionyl-L-carnitine.

Interactions with Foods
No interactions are known to occur, and there is no known reason to expect a clinically significant interaction with propionyl-L-carnitine.

Interactions with Lab Tests
No interactions are known to occur, and there is no known reason to expect a clinically significant interaction with propionyl-L-carnitine.

Interactions with Diseases or Conditions
GASTROINTESTINAL DISORDERS: Might be exacerbated by propionyl-L-carnitine (14).
HYPERSENSITIVITY: Contraindicated in people with known hypersensitivity to propionyl-L-carnitine or L-carnitine (14).

Dosage and Administration
ORAL: For peripheral vascular disease (PVD), atherosclerotic or diabetic arteriopathies, and intermittent claudication, 500-1500 mg propionyl-L-carnitine twice daily has been used (14,1434,1435,1436). One study in peripheral vascular disease used 1000 mg three times daily (1576). A dose of 500 mg three times daily has been used in congestive heart failure and stable angina (1579,1580,1581,1583).
INTRAVENOUS: A 1500 mg bolus followed by 1 mg/kg/minute infused for 30 minutes has been used to restore muscle L-carnitine levels in people with peripheral vascular disease (14). Single 600 mg bolus doses have also been tested in people with peripheral vascular disease (14,1437), and infusions of 2000 mg twice daily have been used to improve healing of ulcerative lesions in people with peripheral vascular disease (1574). Single doses of 15 to 30 mg/kg have been used in people with chronic ischemic heart disease or congestive heart failure (1571,1572,1573,1575).

Comments
None.

PROPOLIS

Also Known As
Bee Glue, Bee Propolis, Hive Dross, Propolis Balsam, Propolis Resin, Propolis Wax, Russion Penicillin.

Scientific Names
Propolis.

People Use This For

Orally, propolis is used for tuberculosis, bacterial and fungal infections, protozoal infections, nasopharyngeal carcinoma, improving immune response, and gastrointestinal disturbances including duodenal ulcer (5). Propolis is also used orally for treating Helicobacter pylori infection in peptic ulcer disease (6109) and treating the common cold (6602). It is also used as an antioxidant and anti-inflammatory agent (5,6).

Topically, propolis is used for wound cleansing (5,6), genital herpes (1926), and as a mouth rinse for enhancing healing following oral surgery (799).

In manufacturing, it is used as an ingredient in cosmetics (6).

Safety

There is insufficient reliable information available about the safety of propolis.

Pregnancy and Lactation: Insufficient reliable information available; avoid using.

Effectiveness

POSSIBLY EFFECTIVE ...when used as a mouth rinse for sulcoplasty. Propolis mouth rinse following sulcoplasty seems to improve healing and reduce pain and inflammation (799). ...when used topically for recurrent herpetic genital lesions. A 3% propolis ointment seems to significantly improve healing of genital lesions caused by herpes simplex virus type 2 (HSV-2). There is some evidence that it might help heal lesions faster and more completely than 5% acyclovir ointment (1926).

There is insufficient reliable information available to rate the effectiveness of propolis for its other uses. However, there is some evidence that propolis might help for treating the common cold. There is some evidence that propolis might decrease the duration of cold symptoms by 2.5 times compared to placebo in patients with rhinovirus infection (6602). More evidence is needed to rate propolis for this use.

Mechanism of Action

Propolis is a resinous material from poplar and conifer buds. It is used by bees for maintaining their hives. Since propolis is incorporated into bee hives, harvesting the pure product is difficult. Many propolis preparations are frequently contaminated with bee hive by-products (3574). Therapeutic uses of propolis are primarily attributed to antiviral, antibacterial, and antimycotic effects. Propolis contains flavonoids including pinocembrin, galangin, pinobanksin, and pinobanksin-3-acetate which are thought to be responsible for the propolis' antimicrobial effects (5,1926). Propolis extracts that contain the constituents pinocembrim and galagin have been shown to inhibit the growth and enzyme activity of Streptococcus mutans, an organism which causes dental caries (2631). Propolis also seems to have in vitro activity against a variety of strains of Helicobacter pylori (H. pylori) (6109). Propolis might also have anti-inflammatory effects. There is preliminary evidence that it might suppress the lipoxygenase pathway of arachidonic acid metabolism and decrease the synthesis of prostaglandins and leukotrienes involved in inflammation (2630). Topically applied propolis also seems to help accelerate epithelial repair in animal models (800). Propolis also contains caffeic acid phenethyl esters (CAPE) which might have cancer chemopreventive properties (2629). These same constituents seem to also be contact allergens (2633). Propolis also has weak free radical-scavenging properties (6).

Adverse Reactions

Orally, propolis can cause allergic reactions (6,2632) and acute oral mucositis with ulceration from the use of the propolis-containing lozenges (2632). Patients allergic to bees or bee products may be more likely to experience allergic reactions.

Topically, propolis-containing products, including some cosmetics can cause eczematous contact dermatitis (6,2632).

Interactions with Herbs & Other Dietary Supplements

Insufficient reliable information available.

Interactions with Drugs

No interactions are known to occur, and there is no known reason to expect a clinically significant interaction with propolis.

Interactions with Foods

No interactions are known to occur, and there is no known reason to expect a clinically significant interaction with propolis.

Interactions with Lab Tests

No interactions are known to occur, and there is no known reason to expect a clinically significant interaction with propolis.

Interactions with Diseases or Conditions

ASTHMA: Some sources suggest allergens in propolis may worsen asthma (3574); avoid using.
HYPERSENSITIVITY: Avoid using propolis in people hypersensitive to bee by-products including honey, conifers, poplars, Peruvian balsam, and salicylates (19).

Dosage and Administration

ORAL: No typical dosage.
TOPICAL: As a mouth rinse after sulcoplasty, a 5% aqueous alcohol solution of propolis is commonly used (799). For herpetic lesions, 3% propolis ointment applied to the lesions 4 times daily has been used (1926).

Comments

Propolis has a long history of medicinal use, dating back to 350 B.C., the time of Aristotle. Greeks have used propolis for abscesses; Assyrians have used it for healing wounds and tumors; and Egyptians have used it for mummification (3574).

PUFF BALL

Also Known As

Bovista, Deer Balls, Hart's Truffle Puffball.

Scientific Names

Lycoperdon spp.
Family: Gasteromycetes.

People Use This For

Orally, puff ball is used for nosebleeds and skin disorders (18).
For food uses young puff ball mushrooms are edible (18).

Safety

LIKELY SAFE ...when young puff ball mushrooms are consumed orally (18).
There is insufficient reliable information available about the safety of the oral use of puff ball for medicinal purposes.
PREGNANCY AND LACTATION: Insufficient reliable information available; avoid using.

Effectiveness

There is insufficient reliable information available about the effectiveness of puff ball.

Mechanism of Action

The applicable parts of puff ball are the aerial parts and spores. Puff ball contains amino acids, glucosamine, sterol, enzymes, and approximately 3% urea (18).

Adverse Reactions

Inhaling the spores can cause respiratory illness, pneumonia-like symptoms, and widespread lung densities (3846,3847).

Interactions with Herbs & Other Dietary Supplements

Insufficient reliable information available.

Interactions with Drugs

No interactions are known to occur, and there is no known reason to expect a clinically significant interaction with puff ball.

Interactions with Foods

No interactions are known to occur, and there is no known reason to expect a clinically significant interaction with puff ball.

Interactions with Lab Tests

No interactions are known to occur, and there is no known reason to expect a clinically significant interaction with puff ball.

Interactions with Diseases or Conditions
No interactions are known to occur, and there is no known reason to expect a clinically significant interaction with puff ball.

Dosage and Administration
ORAL: Puff ball is used in pulverized form or in alcoholic extracts (18).

Comments
None.

PULSATILLA

Also Known As
Easter Flower, European Pasqueflower, Meadow Anenome, Meadow Windflower, Pasque Flower, Pasqueflower, Passe Flower, Wind Flower.

Scientific Names
Anemone pulsatilla, synonym Pulsatilla vulgaris; Anemone pratensis, synonym Anemone nigricans; Pulsatilla nigricans; Pulsatilla pratensis.
Family: Ranunculacaeae.

People Use This For
Orally, pulsatilla is used for painful conditions of the male or female reproductive system, such as dysmenorrhea, orchitis, ovaralgia, or epididymitis. Pulsatilla is used for tension headache, hyperactive states, insomnia, boils, asthma and pulmonary disease, earache (4), migraines, neuralgia, general restlessness, diseases and functional disorders of the GI and urinary tract.
Topically, pulsatilla is used for boils, skin eruptions associated with bacterial infection, and inflammatory and infectious diseases of the skin and mucosa (2).

Safety
LIKELY UNSAFE ...when fresh above ground parts are used orally or topically because pulsatilla is a severe local irritant (4).
There is insufficient reliable information available about the safety of the use of dried pulsatilla.
PREGNANCY: LIKELY UNSAFE ...when used orally. The fresh or dried above ground parts are contraindicated because they might cause abortifacient and teratogenic effects (2). ...when the fresh above ground parts are used topically. There is insufficient reliable information available about the safety of the topical use of dried pulsatilla during pregnancy.
LACTATION: LIKELY UNSAFE ...when the fresh above ground parts are used for oral or topical use (19). There is insufficient reliable information available about the safety of dried pulsatilla during breast-feeding.

Effectiveness
There is insufficient reliable information available about the effectiveness of pulsatilla.

Mechanism of Action
The applicable parts of pulsatilla are the above ground parts. Pulsatilla has analgesic, antispasmodic, sedative, and antibacterial properties. It exhibits both uterine stimulant and depressant activities. Pulsatilla contains ranunculin, which hydrolyzes to toxic, unstable protoanemonin, which readily dimerizes to nontoxic anemonin (4). Protoanemonin causes central nervous system stimulation, then paralysis in experimental animals. It also has antimicrobial activity (2). Both anemonin and protoanemonin show some evidence of sedative and antipyretic activity (4). Irritation of the kidney and urinary tract might be due to the alkylating action of protoanemonin (2). Some evidence suggests anemonin might be cytotoxic (4).

Adverse Reactions
Orally, fresh pulsatilla is a toxic gastrointestinal irritant (4,19). It can cause kidney and urinary tract irritation (2).
Topically, contact with the fresh plant can cause skin irritation, mucous membrane irritation, itching and pustule formation known as ranunculus dermatitis (2).
Inhalation of protoanemonin-containing volatile oil may cause nasal mucosal and conjunctival irritation (4). Allergic reactions have been documented with patch tests (4).

Interactions with Herbs & Other Dietary Supplements
Insufficient reliable information available.

Interactions with Drugs
No interactions are known to occur, and there is no known reason to expect a clinically significant interaction with pulsatilla.

Interactions with Foods
No interactions are known to occur, and there is no known reason to expect a clinically significant interaction with pulsatilla.

Interactions with Lab Tests
No interactions are known to occur, and there is no known reason to expect a clinically significant interaction with pulsatilla.

Interactions with Diseases or Conditions
No interactions are known to occur, and there is no known reason to expect a clinically significant interaction with pulsatilla.

Dosage and Administration
ORAL: A typical oral dose is 120-300 mg dried above ground parts three times daily. Alternatively one cup tea consumed three times daily. To make tea, steep or simmer 120-300 mg dried above ground parts in 150 mL water 5-10 minutes, strain (4). Liquid extract (1:1 in 25% alcohol) has been used 0.12-0.3 mL three times daily (4). Tincture (1:10 in 40% alcohol) has been used 0.3-1 mL three times daily (4).
TOPICAL: No typical dosage.

Comments
None.

PUMPKIN

Also Known As
Cucurbitea peponis semen, Field Pumpkin, Pepo, Pumpkin Seed.

Scientific Names
Cucurbita pepo.
Family: Cucurbitaceae.

People Use This For
Orally, pumpkin is used for dysuria secondary to benign prostatic hyperplasia (BPH), bladder irritation (2,5,7,18), and treating intestinal worms (515).
In combination, pumpkin is used in a herbal combination to treat symptoms of BPH (5093).
In folk medicine, pumpkin has been used to treat pyelonephritis (18).
The roasted pumpkins seeds are considered a snack food (6002).

Safety
POSSIBLY SAFE ...when used orally and appropriately (2,7,18).
PREGNANCY AND LACTATION: Insufficient reliable information available; avoid using amounts greater than those found in food.

Effectiveness
POSSIBLY EFFECTIVE ...when used orally for dysuria associated with BPH and bladder irritation (2).
POSSIBLY INEFFECTIVE ...when an herbal blend containing pumpkin seed oil extract is used orally for treating symptoms of BPH. In a double-blind placebo controlled trial, an herbal product containing pumpkin seed oil extract 160 mg, saw palmetto lipodal extract 106 mg, nettle root extract 80 mg, lemon bioflavonoid extract 33 mg, and vitamin A (100% as beta-carotene) 190 IU used three times daily for six months failed to significantly improve symptoms in a group of men with BPH (5093).
There is insufficient reliable information available about the effectiveness of pumpkin for its other uses.

Mechanism of Action

The applicable part of pumpkin is the seed. Pumpkin seeds contain as much as 50% fatty oil (515). Pumpkin seeds are also rich in carotenoids, including lutein, carotene, and beta carotene (6,515). The seed oil is rich in unsaturated fatty acids, including 55% linoleic acid and 25% oleic acid (6). The oil is also rich in vitamin E, primarily gamma-tocopherol (6). Pumpkin seed oil can exhibit a diuretic effect, which can relieve bladder discomfort, causing the perception of reduced prostate gland swelling without reducing the gland size. The phytosterol constituents are also believed to affect urine flow. Another constituent, cucurbitin, has anthelmintic effects. Concentration of cucurbitin varies significantly among Cucurbita species (515).

Adverse Reactions

One case is reported of decreased ejaculatory volume associated with an herbal blend product containing pumpkin seed oil extract, saw palmetto extract, nettle root extract, lemon bioflavonoid extract, and beta-carotene (5093).

Interactions with Herbs & Other Dietary Supplements

Insufficient reliable information available.

Interactions with Drugs

No interactions are known to occur, and there is no known reason to expect a clinically significant interaction with pumpkin.

Interactions with Foods

No interactions are known to occur, and there is no known reason to expect a clinically significant interaction with pumpkin.

Interactions with Lab Tests

No interactions are known to occur, and there is no known reason to expect a clinically significant interaction with pumpkin.

Interactions with Diseases or Conditions

No interactions are known to occur, and there is no known reason to expect a clinically significant interaction with pumpkin.

Dosage and Administration

ORAL: For dysuria secondary to benign prostatic hyperplasia and bladder irritation, the typical dose is 5 grams of the ground seeds two times daily (2,7,18). As an anthelmintic, 20-167 grams of the seeds are commonly taken three times daily (515).

Comments

Seeds of autumn squash (Cucurbita maxima) and Canadian pumpkin (crooked neck squash, Cucurbita moschata) have properties similar to Cucurbita pepo seed (515).

PUNCTURE VINE

Also Known As

Abrojos, Caltrop, Cat's-Head, Common Dubbletjie, Devil's-Thorn, Devil's-Weed, Espigón, Goathead, Gokhru, Nature's Viagra, Puncturevine, Tribule terrestre, Tribulis, Tribulis Terrestris, Tribulus, Tribulus Terrestris.

Scientific Names

Tribulus terrestris.
Family: Zygophyllaceae.

People Use This For

Orally, puncture vine is used for angina pectoris (3931), male impotence, enhancing athletic performance (817), treating anemia, Bright's disease, cancer, coughs, improving digestion, treating flatulence, gonorrhea, headache, hepatitis, inflammation, stomatitis, vertigo, leprosy, nasal tumors, neurasthenia, painful urination, childbirth, psoriasis, rheumatism, scabies, sore throat, and spermatorrhea. It is also used as a gentle laxative, for stimulating appetite and milk flow, as an abortifacient, aphrodisiac, astringent, diuretic, tonic, and vermifuge (3919).

Safety

LIKELY UNSAFE ...when the spine-covered fruit is used orally. There has been one report of a bilateral pneumothorax adverse effect (818).

There is insufficient reliable information available about the safety of the parts of puncture vine other than the fruit.

PREGNANCY: POSSIBLY UNSAFE ...when used orally; avoid using. It has been used as an abortifacient (3919).

LACTATION: Insufficient reliable information available; avoid using.

Effectiveness

There is insufficient reliable information available about the effectiveness of puncture vine.

Mechanism of Action

Puncture vine contains diosgenin and other saponins (3929). An unidentified saponin of Tribulus terrestris is reported effective for treating angina pectoris in people with coronary heart disease (3931).

Adverse Reactions

Orally there is one case report of bilateral pneumothorax following the removal of a puncture vine fruit with sharp spines (818).

Interactions with Herbs & Other Dietary Supplements

Insufficient reliable information available.

Interactions with Drugs

No interactions are known to occur, and there is no known reason to expect a clinically significant interaction with puncture vine.

Interactions with Foods

No interactions are known to occur, and there is no known reason to expect a clinically significant interaction with puncture vine.

Interactions with Lab Tests

No interactions are known to occur, and there is no known reason to expect a clinically significant interaction with puncture vine.

Interactions with Diseases or Conditions

No interactions are known to occur, and there is no known reason to expect a clinically significant interaction with puncture vine.

Dosage and Administration

ORAL: Puncture vine is used as an extract (817).

Comments

Puncture vine was so named because its sharp seeds can flatten bicycle tires (817).

PURPLE LOOSESTRIFE

Also Known As

Blooming Sally, Flowering Sally, Long Purples, Loosestrife, Lythrum, Milk Willow-Herb, Purple Willow-Herb, Rainbow Weed, Salicare, Soldiers, Spiked, Spiked Loosestrife, Willow Sage.

CAUTION: See separate listings for Loosestrife and Sage.

Scientific Names

Lythrum salicaria.

Family: Lythraceae.

People Use This For

Orally, purple loosestrife is used for diarrhea, chronic intestinal inflammation, and menstrual complaints. It is also used as an anti-inflammatory, astringent, and antibiotic.

Topically, it is used for varicose veins, bleeding gums, hemorrhoids, and eczema.

Safety

There is insufficient reliable information available about the safety of purple loosestrife.

Pregnancy and Lactation: Insufficient reliable information available; avoid using.

Effectiveness

There is insufficient reliable information available about the effectiveness of purple loosestrife.

Mechanism of Action

The applicable parts of purple loosestrife are the above ground flowering parts. The astringent effects are attributed to tannins and salicarin. Salicarin may also have antimicrobial effects against intestinal bacteria (18).

Adverse Reactions

None reported.

Interactions with Herbs & Other Dietary Supplements

Insufficient reliable information available.

Interactions with Drugs

No interactions are known to occur, and there is no known reason to expect a clinically significant interaction with purple loosestrife.

Interactions with Foods

No interactions are known to occur, and there is no known reason to expect a clinically significant interaction with purple loosestrife.

Interactions with Lab Tests

No interactions are known to occur, and there is no known reason to expect a clinically significant interaction with purple loosestrife.

Interactions with Diseases or Conditions

No interactions are known to occur, and there is no known reason to expect a clinically significant interaction with purple loosestrife.

Dosage and Administration

ORAL: The daily dose is 2-3 cups of tea. The tea is prepared by steeping 3 grams dried herb in 100 mL of boiling water for 10-15 minutes and straining. Alternately, 2-3 teaspoons of tincture are taken daily. The tincture is taken by adding 20 grams dried herb to 100 mL of a 20% alcohol solution and straining after 5 days (18).
TOPICAL: No typical dosage.

Comments

There is very little scientific information about this product. Our staff is continually analyzing the available information on natural medicines and will add data here as it becomes available.

PYCNOGENOL

Also Known As

Condensed Tannins, French Marine Pine Bark Extract, French Maritime Pine Bark Extract, Leucoanthocyanidins, Oligomeric Proanthocyanidins, OPC, OPCs, Pine Bark, Pine Bark Extract, Procyandiol Oligomers, Procyanodolic Oligomers, PCO, PCOs, Pygenol.

Scientific Names

Pinus pinaster, synonyms Pinus maritima, Pinus marittima.
Family: Pinaceae.

People Use This For

Orally, pycnogenol is used for treating chronic venous insufficiency; preventing vascular conditions such as heart disease and varicose veins; slowing the aging process; treating allergies, hypertension, muscle soreness, pain, diabetes, chronic pelvic pain associated with endometriosis and dysmenorrhea; and preventing and treating diabetic and other retinopathies. It is also used orally for preventing stroke, arthritis, maintaining skin health, treating attention deficit hyperactivity disorder (ADHD), improving athletic endurance, and improving sperm morphology in subfertile men . Topically, pycnogenol is used as a component of "antiaging" creams.

Safety

POSSIBLY SAFE ...when used orally and appropriately. Pycnogenol has been safely used in doses of 200 to 450 mg daily for up to 3 months (2451,2462,2553,2556).

PREGNANCY AND LACTATION: Insufficient reliable information available; avoid using.

Effectiveness

POSSIBLY EFFECTIVE ...when used orally to reduce the symptoms of chronic venous insufficiency (CVI, varicose veins). Pycnogenol seems to significantly reduce symptoms of leg pain and heaviness, and edema when used for 3 to 12 weeks. Most studies have used doses of 100-120 mg three times daily. (2451,2462,2493). But a lower dose of 45 mg to 90 mg once daily also seems to be effective (2435). ...when used orally for diabetic and other retinopathies (2536). Pycnogenol 50 mg three times daily for 2 months seems to slow or prevent further deterioration in retinal function in patients with retinopathy caused by diabetes, atherosclerosis, or central venous thrombosis. Patients can have some improvement in visual acuity and retinal vascularization (2536). ...when used orally to increase exercise capacity in athletes (2554). Pycnogenol 200 mg daily for 30 days seems to improve treadmill exercise capacity in recreational athletes aged 20 to 35 years (2554).

There is insufficient reliable information to rate the effectiveness of pycnogenol for its other uses. However, there is some preliminary evidence pycnogenol might be helpful for patients with coronary artery disease. There is some evidence that pycnogenol 150mg 3 times daily for 4 weeks might improve certain factors such as microcirculation, myocardial ischemia, and the potential for platelet aggregation (2553). There is also preliminary evidence that pycnogenol might help reduce pelvic pain in women with endometriosis or dysmenorrhea (2555). There is evidence that pycnogenol in combination with dextroamphetamine might help certain symptoms in patients with attention deficit hyperactivity disorder (ADHD) (6558). More evidence is needed to rate pycnogenol for these uses.

Mechanism of Action

Pycnogenol is an extract from the bark of the French maritime pine tree (2431). Pycnogenol contains several active constituents including flavonoid monomers such as catechin, epicatechin, and taxifolin. It also contains condensed procyanidins (also called flavonoids or proanthocyanidins) such as procyanidin B1, B3, B6, B7 which are dimers, oligomers, and polymers of catechin and epicatechin (2431,2433). Pycnogenol also contains phenolic acids including gallic, ferulic, caffeic, vanillic, p-coumaric, protocatechuic, and p-hydroxybenzoic acids, and their glucosides and glucose esters (2431,2433,2435,2543).

In chronic venous insufficiency (CVI, varicose veins) procyanidins in pycnogenol reduce capillary permeability, which contributes to edema and microbleeding, by cross-linking capillary wall proteins such as collagen and elastin (2435,2544). There is also some evidence that procyanidins make elastin more resistant to degradation by elastase (2451,2635), and that pycnogenol might inhibit elastase and collagenase released by activated macrophages (2462). Pycnogenol might also help prevent capillary permeability due to the antioxidant effects of several of its constituents (2433,2435,2636,2542,2451). Pycnogenol also seems to recycle ascorbyl and tocopheryl radicals, helping to maintain vitamin C and E levels (2542). Benefits for other uses including diabetic retinopathy and improving athletic performance are also thought to be due to the antioxidant effects of pycnogenol (2536,2554).

There is interest in using pycnogenol for prevention of cardiovascular disease. In vitro, pycnogenol prevents oxidation of low-density lipoprotein (LDL) cholesterol and protects DNA from damage by free radicals (2433). It also seems to prevent free-radical induced endothelial in vitro (2433). Pycnogenol inhibits epinephrine-induced platelet aggregation, such as that seen in smokers (2435,3285). But pycnogenol does not appear to increase bleeding risk or affect smoking-related increases in blood pressure or heart rate (3283). Pycnogenol might also increase production of nitric oxide from vascular endothelial cells by stimulating nitric oxide synthetase. This can lead to vasodilatation and possibly reduce the potential for atherogenesis and thrombus formation (2433,2451,2545,2637).

There is preliminary evidence that pycnogenol might stimulate the immune system. It seems to boost natural killer cell activity (2435) and improves T- and B-cell function, as in animal models (2636). There is also some interest in pycnogenol for Alzheimer's disease. In vitro, pycnogenol protects animal brain cells from the toxic effects of high levels of glutamate, and also from the toxic effects of amyloid-beta-protein, which is found in the plaques characteristic of Alzheimer's Disease (2435).

Pycnogenol inhibits angiotensin converting enzyme (ACE) in-vitro, but is unlikely to have clinically significant hypotensive effects when used orally in humans (2435).

Constituents of pycnogenol are metabolized through glucuronide and sulfate conjugation. Ferulic acid and taxifolin conjugates are excreted in the urine within 18 hours. Conjugated metabolites of the procyanidin fraction are excreted within 28 to 34 hours (2431,2543).

Adverse Reactions

None reported.

Interactions with Herbs & Other Dietary Supplements

Insufficient reliable information available.

Interactions with Drugs
IMMUNOSUPPRESSANTS: Theoretically, pycnogenol may interfere with immunosuppressant therapy because of its immunostimulating activity (2435,2636). Immunosuppressant drugs include azathioprine (Imuran), basiliximab (Simulect), cyclosporine (Neoral, Sandimmune), daclizumab (Zenapax), muromonab-CD3 (OKT3, Orthoclone OKT3), mycophenolate (CellCept), tacrolimus (FK506, Prograf), sirolimus (Rapamune), prednisone (Deltasone, Orasone), and other corticosteroids (glucocorticoids).

Interactions with Foods
No interactions are known to occur, and there is no known reason to expect a clinically significant interaction with pycnogenol.

Interactions with Lab Tests
No interactions are known to occur, and there is no known reason to expect a clinically significant interaction with pycnogenol.

Interactions with Diseases or Conditions
No interactions are known to occur, and there is no known reason to expect a clinically significant interaction with pycnogenol.

Dosage and Administration
ORAL: For chronic venous insufficiency, 45 to 360 mg daily, or 100 mg three times daily have been used (2435,2451,2462,2493). For diabetic and other retinopathies, 50 mg three times daily has been used (2536). For coronary artery disease, 150 mg three times daily has been used (2553). To improve exercise capacity in athletes, 200 mg daily has been used (2554). For chronic pelvic pain, dysmenorrhea, and endometriosis in women, 30 to 60 mg daily has been used (2555). To improve sperm morphology in subfertile men, 200 mg daily has been used (2556).
TOPICAL: No typical dosae.

Comments
Pycnogenol is the US registered trademark for an extract derived from French Maritime Pine Bark (Pinus pinaster) which contains procyanidins, a group of bioflavonoids. Originally, the term pycnogenol was used as a generic term for procyanidins. Procyanidins are also referred to as condensed tannins, leucoanthocyanidins, proanthocyanidins, oligomeric proanthocyanidins (OPCs), and procyandiol oligomers (PCOs). They are derived from various other sources besides French maritime pine bark, including peanut skins (Arachis hypogaea), grape seed (Vitis vinifera) (515), and witch hazel bark (Hamamelis virginiana) (2641).

PYGEUM

Also Known As
African Plum Tree.

Scientific Names
Prunus africana, previously referred to as Pygeum africanum.
Family: Rosaceae.

People Use This For
Orally, pygeum bark is used for treating functional symptoms of benign prostatic hyperplasia (BPH) (nocturia, dysuria, pollakiuria micturitional disorders, and bladder fullness) (6,7,3902,3903) and prostatic adenoma (3904).
Traditionally, pygeum bark has been used orally for inflammation, kidney disease, urinary problems, malaria, stomachache, fever, difficult urination, fever, madness, prostate gland inflammation, and as an aphrodisiac (515).

Safety
LIKELY SAFE ...when used orally and appropriately (6,7,3902,3903,6368).
PREGNANCY AND LACTATION: Insufficient reliable information available; avoid using.

Effectiveness
LIKELY EFFECTIVE ...when used orally for treating functional symptoms of benign prostatic hyperplasia (BPH) (6,7,3902,3903,4302). Effects and improvement of symptoms appear similar when pygeum extract is given orally as 100 mg once daily or 50 mg twice daily (6368).
POSSIBLY EFFECTIVE ...when used orally for functional symptoms of prostatic adenoma (3904).
There is insufficient reliable information available about the effectiveness of pygeum for its other uses.

Mechanism of Action

The applicable part of pygeum is the bark. Scientists theorize that fibroblast proliferation plays a key role in development of BPH. Some information suggests that pygeum extracts can have antiproliferative effects on fibroblasts (4301). Pygeum bark contains varied constituents that demonstrate benefit in individuals with benign prostatic hyperplasia (BPH) (6,7). Ferulic acid esters of fatty acids reduce prostatic cholesterol levels, limiting synthesis of testosterone (6,7). Theoretically the phytosterols, including beta-sitosterol, beta-sitosterone and campesterol (6,7), compete with androgen precursors and inhibit prostaglandin biosynthesis (7). Some evidence suggests that the triterpenes, including oleanolic, crataegolic and ursolic acid, might have anti-inflammatory activity in prostrate connective tissue (6,7). Pygeum bark extract also increases prostatic secretions and improves seminal fluid composition (6). Multiple clinical trials demonstrate that pygeum bark extract improves symptoms of BPH (6,7). However, not all symptoms are improved in every patient. More trials reported nocturia and maximum flow improved than report reduction in residual volume (4302). Pygeum bark extract also appears to offer similar benefits to individuals with prostatic adenoma (3904).

Adverse Reactions

Orally, pygeum bark can cause nausea and abdominal pain (6,7).

Interactions with Herbs & Other Dietary Supplements

Insufficient reliable information available.

Interactions with Drugs

No interactions are known to occur, and there is no known reason to expect a clinically significant interaction with pygeum.

Interactions with Foods

No interactions are known to occur, and there is no known reason to expect a clinically significant interaction with pygeum.

Interactions with Lab Tests

No interactions are known to occur, and there is no known reason to expect a clinically significant interaction with pygeum.

Interactions with Diseases or Conditions

No interactions are known to occur, and there is no known reason to expect a clinically significant interaction with pygeum.

Dosage and Administration

ORAL: A typical dose used for functional symptoms of BPH is 100-200 mg standardized lipophilic extract (14% triterpenes, 0.5 % n-docosanol) per day in 6-8 week cycles (6,7). Dosages of pygeum extract given as 50 mg twice daily or 100 mg once daily appear to be equally safe and effective for functional symptoms of BPH (6368).

Comments

Some think saw palmetto is a better choice for treating BPH than pygeum. In one study it was more effective in treating functional symptoms of BPH and had fewer adverse effects (6). Pygeum is more expensive than saw palmetto. Also, overharvesting of the bark of pygeum is threatening the survival of the species (515).

PYRETHRUM

Also Known As

Dalmation Insect Flowers, Dalmation Pellitory.

Scientific Names

Chrysanthemum cinerariifolium.
Family: Asteraceae.

People Use This For

Topically, pyrethrum is used as an insecticide, particularly for head lice, crablice and their nits, and as an antiscabies agent (18).

Safety

LIKELY SAFE ...when the commercially available combination of pyrethrins (0.17-0.33%) and piperonyl butoxide (2-4%) are used topically and appropriately in a nonaerosol preparation (272).
POSSIBLY SAFE ...when pyrethrins are used topically in amounts less than 2 grams (18).
CHILDREN: POSSIBLY UNSAFE ...when used in children under the age of 2 years (4084).
PREGNANCY AND LACTATION: Insufficient reliable information available; avoid using.

Effectiveness

EFFECTIVE ...when pyrethrins are used topically and appropriately in concentrations of 0.17-.0.33% for 12-24 hours. They are usually combined with piperonyl butoxide (2-4%) (272). Brand names include: A-200 Pyrinate, Barc, Lice-Enz, Licetrol, Pronto, R and C, RID, Tisit, Tisit Blue, Triple X.
There is insufficient reliable information available about the effectiveness of pyrethrum flowers for lice infections.
INEFFECTIVE ...when pyrethrum flowers are used to treat scabies (4084).

Mechanism of Action

The applicable part of pyrethrum is the flower head. Pyrethrum is also the name of the crude extract obtained from flowers of Chrysanthemum cinerariifolium. Pyrethrin refers to more refined extract containing several naturally occurring pyrethrins (505). The active constituents, the pyrethrins, are toxic to insect nervous systems (18).

Adverse Reactions

Pyrethrum has limited toxicity. The symptoms of overdose include headache, tinnitus, nausea, tingling of fingers and toes, respiratory disturbances, and other symptoms of neurotoxicity (18). The pyrethrum flower or derivatives of it might cause an allergic reaction in individuals sensitive to the Asteraceae/Compositae family. Members of this family include ragweed, chrysanthemums, marigolds, daisies, and many other herbs.

Interactions with Herbs & Other Dietary Supplements

Insufficient reliable information available.

Interactions with Drugs

No interactions are known to occur, and there is no known reason to expect a clinically significant interaction with pyrethrum.

Interactions with Foods

No interactions are known to occur, and there is no known reason to expect a clinically significant interaction with pyrethrum.

Interactions with Lab Tests

No interactions are known to occur, and there is no known reason to expect a clinically significant interaction with pyrethrum.

Interactions with Diseases or Conditions

ASTHMA: Exposure to pyrethrin might severely exacerbate asthma; avoid using. There is one case report of fatal asthma in a child with a history of asthma after bathing a pet dog with a 0.2% pyrethrin shampoo. There is speculation that this might have been due to allergenic impurities from the pyrethrin extraction process (6654).
CROSS-ALLERGENICITY: Can cause an allergic reaction in individuals sensitive to the Asteraceae/Compositae family. Members of this family include ragweed, chrysanthemums, marigolds, daisies, and many other herbs.

Dosage and Administration

TOPICAL: Externally as a liquid extract, rinse after use (18). In general, the OTC combination of pyrethrins (0.17-0.33%) and piperonyl butoxide (2-4%) are applied to the infested area and allowed to remain for not less than 10 minutes. It is then thoroughly washed off with warm water (272).

Comments

To treat lice, the OTC combination products with piperonyl butoxide are preferred for safety and effectiveness (272).

PYRIDOXINE (VITAMIN B6)

Also Known As

Adermine Hydrochloride, B Complex Vitamin, B-6, B6, Pyridoxal, Pyridoxamine, Pyridoxine Hydrochloride, Vitamin B-6.

Scientific Names

Pyridoxine; Vitamin B6.

People Use This For

Orally, pyridoxine is used most commonly for treating premenstrual syndrome (PMS), vitamin B6 deficiency, "morning sickness" in pregnancy, depression associated with pregnancy or oral contraceptive use, primary homocystinuria, hyperhomocysteinemia, and preventing neuritis associated with isoniazid or penicillamine. Pyridoxine is also used orally for boosting immunity, muscle cramps, protection against cancer, diuresis, conjunctivitis, cystitis primary hyperoxaluria preventing kidney stones, carpal tunnel syndrome (CTS), night leg cramps, arthritis, and allergies. It is used for attention deficit hyperactivity disorder (ADHD), asthma, pyridoxine-responsive sideroblastic anemia, xanthurenic aciduria, primary cystathioninuria, acne, various skin conditions, stimulating appetite, hyperlipidemia, heart disease, radiation sickness, menopausal symptoms, infertility, amenorrhea-galactorrhea syndrome, and suppressing postpartum lactation. Pyridoxine is also used orally for dizziness, motion sickness, psychosis, autism, hyperkinesis, acute chorea, chronic progressive hereditary chorea, tardive dyskinesia, absence (petit mal) seizures, febrile convulsions, gyrate atrophy of the choroid and retina, diabetes, diabetic neuropathy, alcohol intoxication, preventing leukopenia secondary to mitomycin, reversing procarbazine neurotoxicity, preventing anemia due to pyridoxine deficiency, preventing seizures associated with cycloserine, fluorouracil-induced erythrodysesthesia, and acute hydrazine toxicity.

Intravenously, pyridoxine is used for seizures in infants unresponsive to other therapies, acute toxicity due to isoniazid, cycloserine or hydrazine overdose, and acute poisoning from mushrooms of the genus Gyromitra.

Safety

LIKELY SAFE ...when used orally and appropriately (15). ...when used parenterally and appropriately. Injectable pyridoxine is a FDA-approved prescription product (15).

POSSIBLY UNSAFE ...when used orally in excessive doses, long-term. Use for two months or longer in doses of 50 mg per day or greater can increase the risk of neurotoxic side effects (15,4610).

PREGNANCY: LIKELY SAFE ...when used orally in doses not exceeding the recommended dietary allowance (RDA). The RDA for pregnant women is 1.9 mg per day (3094). POSSIBLY SAFE ...when used orally and appropriately in amounts exceeding the recommended dietary allowance. A special sustained-release product providing pyridoxine 75 mg per day is FDA-approved for use in pregnancy. However, it should not be used long-term or without medical supervision and close monitoring. POSSIBLY UNSAFE ...when used orally in excessive doses. There is some concern that high-dose maternal pyridoxine can cause neonatal seizures (4609,6397).

LACTATION: LIKELY SAFE ...when used orally in doses not exceeding the recommended dietary allowance (RDA) (3094). The RDA in lactating women is 2 mg per day. There is insufficient reliable information about the safety of pyridoxine when used in higher doses in lactating women.

Effectiveness

EFFECTIVE ...when used orally for preventing and treating vitamin B6 deficiency (15). ...when used orally for hereditary sideroblastic anemia (15). ...when used orally for treating some people with metabolic disorders, including xanthurenic aciduria, primary cystathioninuria, primary hyperoxaluria, and primary homocystinuria (15).

POSSIBLY EFFECTIVE ...when used orally for treating pregnancy-induced nausea and vomiting. Pyridoxine 25 mg every 8 hours for 72 hours improves vomiting and severe nausea in pregnancy. However, it doesn't seem to improve mild-moderate nausea (6168). Lower doses, pyridoxine 10 mg every 8 hours, improves nausea, but not vomiting in pregnancy (6167). ...when used orally for premenstrual syndrome (PMS). There is some evidence that pyridoxine can improve symptoms of PMS such as breast pain or tenderness (mastalgia) and PMS-related depression in some patients. Although some clinicians advocate higher doses of pyridoxine for PMS, such as 200-500 mg per day, lower doses of 50-100 mg per day seem to work just as well. There is no apparent dose-response curve for PMS, so the lowest effective dose should be used. Higher doses might increase the risk of side effects (3093). ...when used orally in combination with folic acid and vitamin B12 for hyperhomocysteinemia (3047,3886,6883,6884). Pyridoxine plus vitamin B12 and folic acid can lower homocysteine levels, but it's not clear if this results in lower cardiovascular morbidity and mortality. Using pyridoxine alone does not seem to reduce homocysteine levels (3047). ...when used orally for improving biochemical parameters and behavior in conjunction with other therapies in autism (14). ...when used orally for partially reversing fluorouracil-induced erythrodysesthesia in metastatic colon cancer patients so that further therapy with fluorouracil is possible (14). ...when used orally for attention deficit hyperactivity disorder (ADHD) in children with low serotonin levels (41). However, there is no evidence pyridoxine works in children without low serotonin levels. ...when used orally for hyperkinetic cerebral dysfunction syndrome. There is preliminary evidence that pyridoxine may have a beneficial effect on hyperkinetic children who have low levels of blood serotonin (3351). ...when used orally for decreasing the risk of recurring kidney stones. There is some evidence that pyridoxine alone, or in combination with magnesium, can decrease urinary oxalate levels in people with hyperoxaluria and who have previously had kidney stones (1201,6437,6438,6439,6440). However, it's unclear if this effect translates into a significantly reduced incidence of kidney stones. There is also some evidence that higher pyridoxine intake in women is associated with decreased risk of kidney stone formation (6441), but this effect is not found in men (6442).

POSSIBLY INEFFECTIVE ...when used orally in combination with magnesium for treating children with autism. Ten weeks of high-dose oral pyridoxine and magnesium failed to ameliorate autistic behaviors in a group of ten children with autism (5049).

LIKELY INEFFECTIVE ...when used orally for diabetic neuropathy (14). ...when used orally for familial hypercholesterolemia (14). ...when used orally for suppressing lactation (14).

There is insufficient reliable information available to rate the effectiveness of pyridoxine for its other uses. However, there is some interest in using pyridoxine for asthma in patients who take theophylline. Theophylline seems to lower pyridoxine levels (4522,7066). Some clinicians are trying pyridoxine 200-300 mg daily to see if it improves symptoms, but the effectiveness of supplementation is questionable. Many patients don't seem to benefit and studies show conflicting results (7064,7065). More evidence is needed to rate pyridoxine for this use.

Mechanism of Action

Pyridoxine is required for amino acid metabolism. It is also involved in carbohydrate and lipid metabolism (15). In the body, pyridoxine is converted to pyridoxal phosphate and pyridoxamine phosphate, which are coenzymes in a wide variety of metabolic reactions. These reactions include transamination of amino acids, conversion of tryptophan to niacin, synthesis of gamma-aminobutyric acid (GABA) in the CNS, metabolism of serotonin, norepinephrine and dopamine, metabolism of polyunsaturated fatty acids and phospholipids, and the synthesis of heme, a hemoglobin constituent (14,15). Pyridoxine is involved with several of the reactions important for the overall metabolism of nitrogen; therefore, pyridoxine requirements are related to the total amino acid nitrogen burden to be metabolized (14). Pyridoxine deficiency in adults principally affects the peripheral nerves, skin, mucous membranes, and hematopoietic system. In children, the CNS is also affected. Deficiency can occur in people with uremia, alcoholism, cirrhosis, hyperthyroidism, malabsorption syndromes, and congestive heart failure; and in those receiving certain drugs (15). Pyridoxine is a cofactor for enzymes involved in one of two pathways for the metabolism of homocysteine, and high levels of homocysteine are a risk factor for atherosclerosis (1483,3047). Pyridoxine deficiency has been associated with elevated plasma homocysteine levels, but pyridoxine supplements alone are unlikely to reduce fasting plasma homocysteine levels, and it is not known whether they affect the incidence of atherosclerosis (1483,3047,3048,3049,3050). For kidney stones, pyridoxine is thought to be beneficial by decreasing urinary excretion of oxalate. Most kidney stones are composed of calcium oxalate and high urinary oxalate has been associated with development and recurrence of kidney stones (6437,6438,6439,6440,6441,6442). In attention-deficit hyperactivity disorder (ADHD), some kids can have low serotonin levels (41); however, this is controversial (6444). It's thought that pyridoxine can increase serotonin levels and might improve symptoms in some kids with low serotonin levels (41). It has been suggested that large doses of vitamin B6 may be useful in carpal tunnel syndrome, based on an observation of low vitamin B6 tissue levels in autopsy specimens from people who had the syndrome (6885). However, tissue levels decline in dead or infarcted tissue and the existence of vitamin B6 deficiency during life cannot be deduced from these observations (6885).

Adverse Reactions

Orally or by injection, pyridoxine can cause nausea, vomiting, abdominal pain, loss of appetite, headache, paresthesia, somnolence, increased serum aspartate transaminase (AST, SGOT), decreased serum folic acid concentrations, skin reactions and other allergic reactions, breast soreness or enlargement, and photosensitivity (14,15). Long-term use of two months or longer with large amounts of pyridoxine (as little as 50 mg per day, but usually 2 grams or more per day) can cause sensory neuropathy or neuronopathy syndromes (14,15). The mechanism of the neurotoxicity is unknown, but it is characterized by impairment of the sense of position and vibration of the distal limbs and gradual, progressive sensory ataxia. Improvement is gradual when pyridoxine is stopped (15). There is some concern that long-term dietary pyridoxine intake in small amounts ranging from 3.56-6.59 mg daily can increase the risk of developing ulcerative colitis (3350). However, this is preliminary. It is too soon to suggest that patients cut back on pyridoxine intake. Injectable pyridoxine can also cause burning or stinging at the injection site, seizures after intravenous administration of large amounts (15), and hypotonia and respiratory distress in infants (14).

Interactions with Herbs & Other Dietary Supplements

Insufficient reliable information available.

Interactions with Drugs

AMIODARONE (Cordarone): Concomitant use can increase the risk of amiodarone-induced photosensitivity (14).

LEVODOPA (Larodopa): Concomitant use accelerates peripheral metabolism of levodopa, reversing the therapeutic effects. This interaction does not occur when carbidopa is used concurrently with levodopa (Sinemet) (15).

PHENYTOIN (Dilantin), PHENOBARBITAL: Concomitant use can decrease the serum concentrations of phenytoin and phenobarbital (15).

Drug Influences on Nutrient Levels and Depletion

SOME DRUGS CAN AFFECT PYRIDOXINE LEVELS:

ANTIBIOTICS: Destruction of normal gastrointestinal flora by antibiotics can cause decreased production of B vitamins. The clinical significance of this decreased production is not known. Consider supplementation only if clinical judgment warrants it (4434,4435,4436,4437,4438,4439,4440,4441,4442,4443).

ESTROGENS and ESTROGEN-CONTAINING ORAL CONTRACEPTIVES: Use of estrogens and estrogen-containing oral contraceptives can interfere with pyridoxine metabolism, reducing serum pyridoxine levels. The need for pyridoxine supplementation has not been adequately studied (4498).

HYDRALAZINE (Apresoline): Hydralazine can increase pyridoxine requirements. The need for pyridoxine supplementation has not been adequately studied (14,4453,4531,4533).

ISONIAZID (INH, Rifamate): Isoniazid can increase pyridoxine requirements. Patients receiving more than 10 mg/kg/day of INH should be supplemented with 50-100 mg of pyridoxine per day (14,4481,4482).

PENICILLAMINE (Cuprimine): Penicillamine can increase pyridoxine requirements. The need for pyridoxine supplementation has not been adequately studied (14,4453,4531).

THEOPHYLLINE (Theo-Dur): Theophylline interferes with pyridoxine metabolism and can reduce serum pyridoxine levels (4522,7066). However, the clinical significance of this is not known. Some clinicians try supplementing with pyridoxine 200-300 mg daily in asthmatic patients taking theophylline (7064,7065), but the effectiveness of supplementation is questionable. Many patients don't seem to benefit and studies show conflicting results (7064,7065).

Interactions with Foods

No interactions are known to occur, and there is no known reason to expect a clinically significant interaction with pyridoxine.

Interactions with Lab Tests

UROBILINOGEN: Pyridoxine can cause a false positive result in the spot test with Ehrlich's reagent (15).

Interactions with Diseases or Conditions

No interactions are known to occur, and there is no known reason to expect a clinically significant interaction with pyridoxine.

Dosage and Administration

ORAL: As a dietary supplement, 2 mg per day of pyridoxine is generally considered sufficient in individuals with normal gastrointestinal (GI) absorption (14,15). For vitamin B6 deficiency in adults, the typical dose is 2.5-25 mg daily for three weeks, then 1.5-2.5 mg per day as maintenance therapy (14,15). For vitamin B6 deficiency in women taking oral contraceptives, the dose is 25-30 mg per day (15). For symptoms associated with premenstrual syndrome (PMS), the daily dose is 50-100 mg. Doses as high as 500 mg per day have been used, but daily doses over 100 mg don't appear to have additional benefit, and may increase the risk for adverse effects (3093). For hereditary sideroblastic anemia, initially 200-600 mg per day is used, decreasing to 30-50 mg daily after an adequate response (15). For metabolic disorders, including xanthurenic aciduria, primary cystathioninuria, primary hyperoxaluria, or primary homocystinuria, 100-500 mg daily is generally effective (15). For kidney stones, 25-500 mg daily has been used (6437,6439). When used with magnesium for preventing kidney stones, pyridoxine 10 mg daily has been used in combination with magnesium 300 mg daily (1201). For preventing anemia due to pyridoxine deficiency or neuritis in people receiving isoniazid or penicillamine, the typical dose is 10-50 mg daily (15). For premenstrual syndrome, 50-100 mg is commonly used per day (3093). For preventing seizures in people receiving cycloserine, 100-300 mg is taken daily in divided doses (15). For nausea during pregnancy, 10-25 mg pyridoxine every eight hours has been used (6167,6168); alternatively, 75 mg of sustained-release pyridoxine combined with 12 mcg vitamin B12 (cyanocobalamin), 1 mg folic acid, and 200 mg calcium (PremesisRx) is used daily as a FDA-approved prescription supplement for nausea during pregnancy (23). For hyperkinetic cerebral dysfunction syndrome in children, 300 mg daily has been used in a clinical trial. However, some children can require larger dosages ranging from 500 mg to 2 grams daily (3351). The daily recommended dietary allowances (RDAs) of vitamin B6 are: Infants 0-6 months, 0.1 mg; Infants 7-12 months, 0.3 mg; Children 1-3 years, 0.5 mg; Children 4-8 years, 0.6 mg; Children 9-13 years, 1 mg; Males 14-50 years, 1.3 mg; Men over 50 years, 1.7 mg; Females 14-18 years, 1.2 mg; Women 19-50 years, 1.3 mg; Women over 50 years, 1.5 mg; Pregnant women, 1.9 mg; and Lactating women, 2 mg (3094). The recommended maximum daily intake is: Children 1-3 years, 30 mg; Children 4-8 years, 40 mg; Children 9-13 years, 60 mg; Adults, pregnant and lactating women, 14-18 years, 80 mg; and Adults, pregnant and lactating women, over 18 years, 100 mg (3094).

INJECTION: This is a FDA-approved prescription product that is available as a 100 mg/mL injection.

Comments

Pyridoxine is present in many foods including cereal grains, legumes, vegetables, liver, meat, and eggs (15). Pyridoxine is frequently used in combination with other B vitamins in vitamin B complex formulations. Vitamin B complex generally includes vitamin B1 (thiamine), vitamin B2 (riboflavin), vitamin B3 (niacin/niacinamide), vitamin B5 (pantothenic acid), vitamin B6 (pyridoxine), vitamin B12 (cyanocobalamin), and folic acid. However, some products do not contain all of these ingredients and some may include others, such as biotin, para-aminobenzoic acid (PABA), choline bitartrate, and inositol (3022,3060,3061).

PYRUVATE

Also Known As
2-Oxypropanoic Acid, Acetylformic Acid, Alpha-Ketopropionic Acid, Calcium Pyruvate, Magnesium Pyruvate, Potassium Pyruvate, Proacemic Acid, Sodium Pyruvate.

Scientific Names
2-Oxopropanoate (pyruvate); 2-oxopropanoic acid (pyruvic acid).

People Use This For
Orally, pyruvate is used for weight loss, improving exercise endurance, and inhibiting tumor growth (2471).

Safety
There is insufficient reliable information available about the safety of pyruvate.
Pregnancy and Lactation: Insufficient reliable information available; avoid using.

Effectiveness
POSSIBLY EFFECTIVE …when used orally for enhancing weight loss (2472,2474).
There is insufficient reliable information available about the effectiveness of pyruvate for its other uses.

Mechanism of Action
Some evidence suggests that pyruvate reduces free radical production (2487), increases lipid oxidation and decreases carbohydrate oxidation (2488). Very small clinical trials suggest dietary supplementation with dihydroxyacetone and pyruvate increases arm and leg exercise endurance (807,808). Very preliminary evidence also suggests a liquid diet supplemented with pyruvate might inhibit tumor growth (806).

Adverse Reactions
Orally, ingesting large amounts of pyruvate can cause GI upset, including gas, bloating, and diarrhea (2471). One death was associated with intravenous use in a child with restrictive cardiomyopathy (2473).

Interactions with Herbs & Other Dietary Supplements
Insufficient reliable information available.

Interactions with Drugs
No interactions are known to occur, and there is no known reason to expect a clinically significant interaction with pyruvate.

Interactions with Foods
No interactions are known to occur, and there is no known reason to expect a clinically significant interaction with pyruvate.

Interactions with Lab Tests
No interactions are known to occur, and there is no known reason to expect a clinically significant interaction with pyruvate.

Interactions with Diseases or Conditions
CARDIOMYOPATHY: One death was associated with intravenous use in a child with restrictive cardiomyopathy (2473).

Dosage and Administration
ORAL: A typical dose used for weight loss is 22 to 44 grams per day, as a supplement to a low-cholesterol, low-fat diet (2474).

Comments
None.

QUASSIA

Also Known As

Amargo, Bitter-Ash, Bitter Wood, Bitterwood, Jamaican Quassia, Picrasma, Quassia Bark, Ruda, Surinam Quassia, Surinam Wood.

Scientific Names

Quassia amara; Picrasma excelsa.
Family: Simaroubaceae.

People Use This For

Orally, quassia is used for anorexia; indigestion; constipation (7); fever (11); as an anthelmintic for thread worms, nematodes, and ascaris (4,18); as a tonic or purgative (18); and as a mouthwash (6).
Topically, quassia is used for pediculosis (4).
Rectally, quassia is used for nematode infestation (4).
In manufacturing, quassia is used as a flavoring agent in foods, beverages, pastilles, lozenges, and laxatives (4,11). The bark and wood have been used as an insecticide (6,11).

Safety

POSSIBLY SAFE ...when consumed in amounts found in foods and beverages. It has Generally Recognized as Safe (GRAS) status in the US (4). Maximum reported use level is 0.007% in nonalcoholic beverages (11).
POSSIBLY UNSAFE ...when used orally in therapeutic amounts. Quassia wood contains cardioactive glycosides (4), but toxicity is likely limited by emetic effects of large doses (4).
There is insufficient reliable information available about the safety of the topical or rectal use of quassia.
PREGNANCY AND LACTATION: LIKELY UNSAFE ...when used orally; contraindicated. Quassia has cytotoxic and emetic properties (4,18,19). There is insufficient reliable information available about the safety of rectal or topical use during pregnancy or lactation; avoid using.

Effectiveness

POSSIBLY EFFECTIVE ...when used in a tincture as a scalp lotion to treat head lice (4).
There is insufficient reliable information available about the effectiveness of quassia for its other uses.

Mechanism of Action

The applicable part of quassia is the wood (4,8,11). Quassia leaves are also reportedly used (6). Quassia contains quassinoids that have potent bitter properties (11). Quassia also contains beta-carboline alkaloids, quassin, quassimarin, canthin-6-one (4), and small amounts of the coumarin scopoletin (4). The quassinoid constituents increase gastric acid and bile secretions, perhaps accounting for appetite stimulant and digestive effects (18,19,4). There is evidence that the beta-carboline alkaloids might have positive inotropic activity (4). The constituent canthin-6-one is reported to have antibacterial, antifungal, and cytotoxic activity (4). Quassimarin demonstrates evidence of antileukemic (11) and antitumor effects (18,4). Quassin demonstrates antilarval activity against Culex quinquefasciatus (mosquito) (3302).

Adverse Reactions

Quassia can cause mucous membrane irritation, nausea, and vomiting (4,18). Long-term use can cause vision changes and blindness (18).

Interactions with Herbs & Other Dietary Supplements

CARDIOACTIVE GLYCOSIDE-CONTAINING HERBS: Theoretically, concomitant use with other cardiac glycoside-containing herbs might increase risk of cardiac toxicity. Cardiac glycoside containing herbs, including black hellebore, Canadian hemp roots, digitalis leaf, hedge mustard, figwort, lily of the valley roots, motherwort, oleander leaf, pheasant's eye plant, pleurisy root, squill bulb leaf scales, and strophanthus seeds (2,18,19).
CARDIOACTIVE HERBS: Avoid concomitant use with other cardioactive herbs due to unpredictability of effects and adverse effects. Other cardioactive herbs include: calamus, cereus, cola, coltsfoot, devil's claw, European mistletoe, fenugreek, fumitory, ginger, Panax ginseng, hawthorn, white horehound, mate, parsley, scotch broom flower, shepherd's purse, and wild carrot (4).
HORSETAIL/LICORICE: Theoretically, abuse of licorice or horsetail might increase risk of cardiac toxicity due to potassium loss (4).
STIMULANT LAXATIVE HERBS: Theoretically, abuse might increase risk of cardiac toxicity due to potassium depletion. Stimulant laxative herbs include: aloe dried leaf sap, blue flag rhizome, alder buckthorn, European buckthorn, butternut bark, cascara bark, castor oil, colocynth fruit pulp, gamboge bark exudate, jalap root, black root, manna bark exudate, podophyllum root, rhubarb root, senna leaves and pods, wild cucumber fruit (Ecballium elaterium), and yellow dock root (19).

HERBS WITH ANTICOAGULANT/ANTIPLATELET POTENTIAL: Concomitant use of herbs that have coumarin constituents or affect platelet aggregation could theoretically increase the risk of bleeding in some people. These herbs include: angelica, anise, arnica, asafoetida, bogbean, boldo, capsicum, celery, chamomile, clove, danshen, fenugreek, feverfew, garlic, ginger ginkgo, Panax ginseng, horse chestnut, horseradish, licorice, meadowsweet, prickly ash, onion, papain, passionflower, poplar, red clover, turmeric, wild carrot, wild lettuce, willow, and others (4,19).

Interactions with Drugs
ACID INHIBITORS: Theoretically, because quassia stimulates gastric acid, it might oppose effect of antacids and H-2 antagonists (11,19).
CARDIAC THERAPY: Theoretically, concomitant use with cardiac medications increases risk of cardiac effects and adverse effects (4).
POTASSIUM-DEPLETING DRUGS: Theoretically, concomitant use of potassium-depleting diuretics or stimulant laxative abuse might increase risk of cardiac glycoside toxicity due to potassium loss (13).
ANTICOAGULANTS: Theoretically, excessive doses might have additive effects with anticoagulant therapy with warfarin (Coumadin) (4).

Interactions with Foods
No interactions are known to occur, and there is no known reason to expect a clinically significant interaction with quassia.

Interactions with Lab Tests
No interactions are known to occur, and there is no known reason to expect a clinically significant interaction with quassia.

Interactions with Diseases or Conditions
GI IRRITATION/INFLAMMATION: In large amounts quassia can irritate the gastrointestinal tract; avoid using (8).

Dosage and Administration
ORAL: A typical dose is one cup tea 2-3 times daily (12). To make tea, simmer 1-2 grams of wood in 150 mL boiling water 10-15 minutes, strain (12).
RECTAL: As an enema (1:20): 150 mL rectally every morning for 3 days with 16 gram magnesium sulfate orally (4).
TOPICAL: No typical dosage.

Comments
Quassia bark has been used as an insecticide (11).

QUEBRACHO

Also Known As
Quebracho Blanco, White Quebracho.

Scientific Names
Aspidosperma quebracho-blanco.
Family: Apocynaceae.

People Use This For
Orally, quebracho is used for asthma and conditions of the lower respiratory tract. It is also used as an expectorant and respiratory tract stimulant (18). Sometimes it is used to lower blood pressure (particularly arterial hypertension), as a spasmolytic, diuretic, peripheral vasoconstrictor, uterine sedative and local anesthetic.
In folk medicine, quebracho is used orally to decrease fever and as an aphrodisiac.
In foods and beverages, it is used as a flavoring agent (11).

Safety
LIKELY SAFE ...whe used in amounts found in foods. It is approved for food use in the US (11).
There is insufficient reliable information available about the oral use of quebracho bark in amounts exceeding those found in foods.
PREGNANCY AND LACTATION: Avoid using in amounts greater than those typically found in foods.

Effectiveness
There is insufficient reliable information available about the effectiveness of quebracho.

Mechanism of Action

The applicable part of quebracho is the bark. There is insufficient reliable information available about the possible mechanism of action and active ingredients.

Adverse Reactions

People who take quebracho bark orally may experience side effects including salivation, headache, outbreaks of sweating, vertigo, stupor and sleepiness. In large doses, it can cause nausea and vomiting (18).

Interactions with Herbs & Other Dietary Supplements

Insufficient reliable information available.

Interactions with Drugs

No interactions are known to occur, and there is no known reason to expect a clinically significant interaction with quebracho.

Interactions with Foods

No interactions are known to occur, and there is no known reason to expect a clinically significant interaction with quebracho.

Interactions with Lab Tests

No interactions are known to occur, and there is no known reason to expect a clinically significant interaction with quebracho.

Interactions with Diseases or Conditions

No interactions are known to occur, and there is no known reason to expect a clinically significant interaction with quebracho.

Dosage and Administration

ORAL: It is used as an extract or powder and in combination bronchial preparations (18).

Comments

The bark is odorless and has a bitter taste. Quebracho Colorado or red quebracho is also known as quebracho, but is chemically distinct from white quebracho. Be careful not to confuse these two plants (11).

QUEEN'S DELIGHT

Also Known As

Cockup Hat, Marcory, Queens Delight, Queen's Root, Queens Root, Silver Leaf, Stillingia, Yaw Root.

Scientific Names

Stillingia sylvatica, synonym Stillingia treculeana.
Family: Euphorbiaceae.

People Use This For

Orally, queen's delight is used as a "blood purifier", for digestive disorders, treatment of hepatic, gallbladder and skin diseases, and as an emetic and laxative (18).
Historically, it has been used orally for bronchitis, laryngitis, laryngismus stridulus, and constipation (4). It has also been used topically for cutaneous eruptions, hemorrhoids, and exudative skin eruptions with lymphatic involvement (4).

Safety

POSSIBLY UNSAFE ...when used orally in medicinal amounts because the dried root preparations contain diterpene esters that are highly irritating (4,12). Queen's delight might activate latent viruses, and there is some evidence it might be carcinogenic (18). ...when the dried or fresh root preparations are used topically (4).
LIKELY UNSAFE ...when the fresh root is used orally because it contains caustic white latex that is highly irritating to mucous membranes (12).
PREGNANCY: POSSIBLY UNSAFE ...when the dried root preparations are used orally or when the dried or fresh root are used topically; avoid using (4). LIKELY UNSAFE ...when the fresh root preparations are used orally (12).
LACTATION: POSSIBLY UNSAFE ...when the dried or fresh root are used topically. LIKELY UNSAFE ...when used orally; contraindicated (4,12,19).

Effectiveness

There is insufficient reliable information available about the effectiveness of queen's delight.

Mechanism of Action

The applicable part of queen's delight is the root. Queen's delight contains a volatile oil and diterpenes including prostatin, gnidilatidin, and others (18). Diterpene esters, isolated in the latex (or milky juice) of the fresh or green root, are potent irritants that cause swelling of the skin and mucous membranes (4,18). Diterpenes may also be carcinogenic agents; they are believed able to activate latent viruses (18).

Adverse Reactions

Orally, queen's delight can cause vomiting, diarrhea (18), and nausea (19). In large amounts, it may cause a burning sensation of the mouth, throat, diarrhea, nausea, vomiting, dysuria, aches and pains, pruritus, skin eruptions, cough, depression, fatigue, and perspiration (4). Topically, it may cause inflammation, swelling (18), and contact dermatitis (19).

Interactions with Herbs & Other Dietary Supplements

Insufficient reliable information available.

Interactions with Drugs

No interactions are known to occur, and there is no known reason to expect a clinically significant interaction with queen's delight.

Interactions with Foods

No interactions are known to occur, and there is no known reason to expect a clinically significant interaction with queen's delight.

Interactions with Lab Tests

No interactions are known to occur, and there is no known reason to expect a clinically significant interaction with queen's delight.

Interactions with Diseases or Conditions

GI CONDITIONS: Contraindicated in individuals with gastrointestinal irritation, inflammation, nausea or vomiting (19).

Dosage and Administration

ORAL: People typically prepare queen's delight as a liquid, boiling 1 teaspoon of the dried root with one cup of water. The suggested dose is a cup a day, taken a mouthful at a time. As a tincture, queen's delight is taken in a dose of 5 to 20 drops (5263).

Comments

None.

QUERCETIN

Also Known As

Citrus Bioflavonoid, Citrus Bioflavonoids, Meletin, Sophretin.

Scientific Names

3,3',4'5,7-Penthydroxyflavone.

People Use This For

Orally, quercetin is used for treating atherosclerosis (1900,2006), hypercholesterolemia (1900), coronary heart disease (1995), diabetes (1995), cataracts (1900,2006), allergies (1900,2006), peptic ulcer (1900), schizophrenia (1996), inflammation, asthma, gout, viral infections, preventing cancer (483), and for treating chronic, bacterial prostatitis (481).
Intravenously and intraperitoneally, quercetin is used for treating cancer (2006).

Safety

POSSIBLY SAFE ...when used orally in amounts up to 500 mg twice daily for up to one month (481). There is insufficient reliable information available about the safety of larger oral doses or longer periods of oral use. ...when used intravenously in amounts less than 945 mg/m2 (2007).

LIKELY UNSAFE ...when used intravenously in amounts greater that 945 mg/m2 which are reported to cause nephrotoxicity (2007).

There is insufficient reliable information available about the safety of intraperitoneal quercetin.

PREGNANCY AND LACTATION: Insufficient reliable information available; avoid using.

Effectiveness

POSSIBLY EFFECTIVE ...when used orally for treating symptoms of chronic, nonbacterial prostatitis (481). In one clinical trial, quercetin reduced pain and improved quality of life, but had no effect on voiding dysfunction (481). There is insufficient reliable information available about the effectiveness of quercetin for its other uses.

Mechanism of Action

Quercetin is a dietary flavonoid found in many plants (481,483,1995). It has antioxidant, anti-inflammatory, nitric oxide inhibitor, and tyrosine kinase inhibitor (leading to inhibition of the division and growth of T-cells and some cancer cells) activity (481,1995). The anti-inflammatory effects of quercetin might be due to inhibition of the production and activity of leukotrienes and prostaglandins, and inhibition of histamine release by basophils and mast cells (483). Quercetin appears to reduce capillary fragility and it might offer some protection against diabetic cataracts, possibly by inhibiting aldose reductase in the lens (483,2006). The anti-inflammatory and antioxidant effects might be responsible for the observed benefits in men with chronic, nonbacterial prostatitis (481). Scientists theorize that quercetin might reduce cancer risk by inactivating malignant precursors or by inhibiting carcinogenesis (2006). Preliminary studies suggest it might have inhibitory effects on various cancer types, including breast, leukemia, colon, ovary, oral squamous cell, endometrial, gastric and non-small-cell lung (483,485). Quercetin has antiestrogenic effects in cultures of breast cancer cells (484). It also inhibits estrone sulfatase and estrogen synthesis in liver cells (489). Existing evidence suggests quercetin alters intestinal cell homeostasis of copper, iron, and manganese (1997). Although researchers believe quercetin might protect against heart disease (1995), short term supplementation does not show affect on any of the known risk factors for heart disease (1998,1999). Preliminary evidence suggests that quercetin might inhibit collagen- and ADP-induced platelet aggregation, but at concentrations much higher than those achieved with typical oral dosing (1999). Evidence suggests that quercetin might benefit some people with schizophrenia when used in combination with other antioxidants, polysorb, and conventional therapy (1996). Quercetin demonstrates activity against retroviruses, Herpes simplex, polio, parainfluenza and respiratory syncytial viruses (483). The oral absorption of quercetin is highly variable, depending on the source. The degree of glycosylation and plasma protein binding, as well as absorption, affect the activity of quercetin (481,486,487).

Adverse Reactions

Orally, quercetin can cause headache and tingling of the extremities (481). Intravenous administration of quercetin is associated with flushing, sweating, dyspnea, nausea, and vomiting (2007). Injection pain can be minimized by premedicating patient with 10 mg of morphine and administering amounts greater than 945 mg/m2 over 5 minutes (2007). Nephrotoxicity has been reported with use of amounts greater than 945 mg/m2 (2006,2007).

Interactions with Herbs & Other Dietary Supplements

PAPAIN, BROMELAIN: Concomitant administration of quercetin with papain or bromelain might increase GI absorption of quercetin (481).

VITAMIN C: Concurrent use enhances the antioxidant activity of quercetin (2006).

Interactions with Drugs

QUINOLONE ANTIBIOTICS: Quercetin might competitively inhibit quinolone antibiotics by binding to the DNA gyrase site on bacteria (481).

Interactions with Foods

No interactions are known to occur, and there is no known reason to expect a clinically significant interaction with quercetin.

Interactions with Lab Tests

No interactions are known to occur, and there is no known reason to expect a clinically significant interaction with quercetin.

Interactions with Diseases or Conditions

KIDNEY DYSFUNCTION: Theoretically, intravenous quercetin may exacerbate kidney dysfunction (2006).

Dosage and Administration
ORAL: 400-500 mg three times daily is a common dose (483). For prostatitis, 500 mg twice daily has been used (481).
INTRAVENOUS: For treating cancer, 420-1400 mg/m2 by IV bolus weekly or in 3-week intervals has been used (2007).
INTRAPERITONEAL: No typical dosage.

Comments
Quercetin is a dietary flavonoid that occurs abundantly in red wine, onions, green tea, apples, berries and brassica vegetables (481,483,1995). Quercetin is found in Ginkgo biloba, St. John's Wort (Hypericum perforatum) and American Elder (Sambucus canadensis) (483).

QUILLAIA

Also Known As
China Bark, Murillo Bark, Panama Bark, Quillaja, Soapbark, Soap Tree, Soap Tree Bark.

Scientific Names
Quillaja saponaria.
Family: Rosaceae.

People Use This For
Orally, quillaia inner bark is used for cough, bronchitis (6), and pulmonary ailments (11).
Topically, quillaia extract is used to treat skin sores, athletes foot (11), itchy scalp (6), in shampoos for dandruff (6,11), in hair tonic preparations, in douches (11), and for leukorrhea (12).
For food uses, quillaia is used in frozen dairy desserts, candy, baked goods, gelatins, and puddings (11).
In manufacturing, quillaia extracts are used in dermatological creams, as foaming agents in root beer (11), in beverages, and cocktails (6). Quillaia is also used as a foaming agent in fire extinguishers (11).

Safety
LIKELY SAFE ...when used orally and in food amounts. Approved for food use in the US (11). The maximum level used is 0.01% in beverages (11).
POSSIBLY UNSAFE ...when used orally in medicinal amounts. Quillaia is a gastrointestinal tract irritant that contains oxalates and tannins. Large amounts can cause liver damage, respiratory failure, convulsions, and coma (12). There is insufficient reliable information available about the safety of the topical or vaginal use of quillaia.
PREGNANCY AND LACTATION: LIKELY SAFE ...when used orally in food amounts. POSSIBLY UNSAFE ...when used orally in amounts larger than those found in foods; avoid using.

Effectiveness
There is insufficient reliable information available about the effectiveness of quillaia.

Mechanism of Action
The applicable part of quillaia is the inner bark. Quillaia contains tannins, oxalates, and saponins. Tannins possess strong astringent properties (7,12). Upon contact, they dehydrate the external layer of tissue, reducing internal secretions, and forming external cells into a protective layer (12). Plants with at least 10% tannins, like quillaia (19) can cause gastrointestinal disturbances, kidney damage, and necrotic conditions of the liver (12). Some evidence suggests that tannins might cause cancer; other evidence shows they might prevent it (12). Regular consumption of herbs with high tannin concentrations correlates with increased incidence of esophageal or nasal cancer (12). When ingested, oxalates combine with calcium in the blood forming insoluble oxalates and depleting available calcium, potentially to deficiency levels. Insoluble calcium oxalate, deposited in the kidneys can cause mechanical damage. Precipitation of calcium oxalate in renal tubules can result in acute renal failure (12). Some evidence suggests saponins might cause red blood cell hemolysis and GI irritation (11). Other evidence suggests they might have anti-inflammatory, antimicrobial, and cytotoxic effects (11). They also possess expectorant properties, can induce sneezing, and can depress cardiac and respiratory activity (6,11). Preliminary information suggests quillaia saponins can reduce the rate of absorption of bile salts (3850), suggesting they might be effective in reducing cholesterol levels (11). QS-21, an isolated saponin from the bark, appears to be a potent immuno-stimulatory complex adjuvant when administered with vaccines (6). It shows evidence that it might augment both antibody and cell-mediated immune responses (3851), significantly increasing antibody levels (6). For this reason it is being evaluated in HIV patients (11). Another purified saponin, DS-1, is being investigated as a pharmaceutical excipient in nasal and ocular delivery of insulin (3852), and also as a transmucosal delivery agent for the aminoglycoside antibiotics (3853).

Adverse Reactions

Orally, large amounts are associated with liver damage, diarrhea, respiratory failure, stomach pain, convulsions, coma (12), red blood cell hemolysis (11), and renal failure (12). If inhaled, the powder can cause sneezing (6). It also can be caustic to mucosa (12).

Interactions with Herbs & Other Dietary Supplements

CALCIUM, IRON, ZINC: Concurrent use might decrease mineral absorption. Quillaia contains oxalate (7,12), which can bind multivalent metal ions in the gastrointestinal tract and decrease mineral absorption.

Interactions with Drugs

ORAL MEDICATION: Theoretically, the tannin content might delay absorption of sedatives, hypnotics, antidepressants, and tranquilizers due to tannin content (19,7).
METFORMIN: Quillaia might reduce efficacy of metformin (Glucophage) (7).

Interactions with Foods

CALCIUM, IRON, ZINC: Concurrent use might decrease mineral absorption from foods. Quillaia contains oxalate (7,12), which can bind multivalent metal ions in the gastrointestinal tract and decrease mineral absorption.

Interactions with Lab Tests

No interactions are known to occur, and there is no known reason to expect a clinically significant interaction with quillaia.

Interactions with Diseases or Conditions

KIDNEY DISEASE: Contraindicated in individuals with kidney disease or a history of kidney stones due to oxalate content (12,19).
GI CONDITIONS: Contraindicated in individuals with gastrointestinal inflammation or irritation due to irritant properties (18).

Dosage and Administration

ORAL: A typical dose is 200 mg prepared as tea (12).
TOPICAL: No typical dosage.

Comments

In South America, quillaia bark is used to wash clothes (6).

QUINCE

Also Known As

None.

Scientific Names

Cydonia oblongata.
Family: Rosaceae.

People Use This For

Orally, quince seed is used for digestive disorders, diarrhea, coughs, and gastrointestinal inflammation. Topically, it is used as a compress or poultice for injuries, inflammation of the joints, injuries of the nipples, and gashed or deeply cut fingers. A topical lotion is used to soothe the eyes (18).

Safety

There is insufficient reliable information available about the safety of quince.
Pregnancy and Lactation: Insufficient reliable information available; avoid using.

Effectiveness

There is insufficient reliable information available about the effectiveness of quince.

Mechanism of Action

The applicable part of quince is the seed. The seeds contain cyanogenic glycosides as amygdalin at 0.4-1.5%, or 27-75 mg cyanide per 100 grams of seeds, suggesting potential toxicity (18).

Adverse Reactions
None reported.

Interactions with Herbs & Other Dietary Supplements
Insufficient reliable information available.

Interactions with Drugs
ORAL DRUGS: May impair absorption of concomitantly administered medications due to possible binding by the high water-soluble fiber content of quince seed (19).

Interactions with Foods
May reduce serum nutrient levels due to possible binding by the high water-soluble fiber content of quince seed (19).

Interactions with Lab Tests
No interactions are known to occur, and there is no known reason to expect a clinically significant interaction with quince.

Interactions with Diseases or Conditions
No interactions are known to occur, and there is no known reason to expect a clinically significant interaction with quince.

Dosage and Administration
ORAL: Quince seed is taken as a powder, extract, or tea. The tea is prepared by steeping 1 teaspoon of whole seeds in 150 mL of boiling water for 10-15 minutes and straining (18).
TOPICAL: A viscous poultice is prepared from the ground seeds (18).

Comments
None.

RADISH

Also Known As
Radis, Raphani sativi radix, Small Radish, Turnip Radish.

Scientific Names
Raphanus sativus.
Family: Brassicaceae.

People Use This For
Orally, radish is used for peptic disorders, dyskinesia of the bile ducts, loss of appetite, inflammation of the mouth and pharynx, tendency towards infections, inflammation or excessive mucus of the respiratory tract, bronchitis, fever, colds, and cough (2,18).

Safety
LIKELY SAFE ...when used orally in moderate amounts (2,18). Large amounts may lead to gastrointestinal irritation (18).
PREGNANCY AND LACTATION: Insufficient reliable information available; avoid very large doses.

Effectiveness
POSSIBLY EFFECTIVE ...when used orally for peptic disorders involving bile duct motility conditions and for respiratory tract mucous membrane inflammation (2).
There is insufficient reliable information available about the effectiveness of radish for its other uses.

Mechanism of Action
The applicable part of radish is the root. Radish root stimulates secretions in the upper GI tract, promotes motility, stimulates bile flow, and has antimicrobial effects (2,18).

Adverse Reactions
Orally, large amounts of radish may cause irritation of the gastrointestinal mucus membrane (18).

Interactions with Herbs & Other Dietary Supplements
Insufficient reliable information available.

Interactions with Drugs
No interactions are known to occur, and there is no known reason to expect a clinically significant interaction with radish.

Interactions with Foods
No interactions are known to occur, and there is no known reason to expect a clinically significant interaction with radish.

Interactions with Lab Tests
No interactions are known to occur, and there is no known reason to expect a clinically significant interaction with radish.

Interactions with Diseases or Conditions
CHOLELITHIASIS: Contraindicated, might cause biliary colic [2,18].

Dosage and Administration
ORAL: 0.5 tablespoons pressed root juice, several times daily; up to 50-100 mL per day [2,18].

Comments
None.

RASPBERRY leaf

Also Known As
Framboise, Red Raspberry, Rubi idaei folium, Rubus.
CAUTION: See separate listing for Blackberry leaf.

Scientific Names
Rubus idaeus, synonym Rubus strigosus.
Family: Rosaceae.

People Use This For
Orally, raspberry leaf is used for GI tract disorders, upper and lower respiratory tract disorders, cardiovascular system disorders, influenza, fever, diabetes, vitamin deficiency, as a diaphoretic or diuretic, for stimulating bile production, "purification of skin and blood" [2], diarrhea, dysmenorrhea, menorrhagia, morning sickness associated with pregnancy, preventing miscarriage, and facilitating labor and delivery [3,4,5].
Topically, it is used for inflammation of the mouth and throat [2,8], and skin rash and inflammation [2].
For food uses, raspberry leaf in small quantities is a source of natural flavoring in Europe [4].

Safety
LIKELY SAFE ...when used orally in amounts found in foods. Very small quantities of raspberry leaf are used as food flavoring [4].
POSSIBLY SAFE ...when used orally or topically and appropriately in medicinal amounts [2,12].
PREGNANCY: LIKELY SAFE ...when used orally in amounts found in foods [4]. POSSIBLY SAFE ...when used orally and appropriately in medicinal amounts during late pregnancy and under the supervision of a health care provider. Raspberry leaf is commonly used by nurse midwives to facilitate delivery. There is some evidence that raspberry leaf can be safely used for this purpose [6481]. However, it is not known if raspberry leaf works for this use; avoid using. Make sure patients do not use raspberry leaf without the guidance of a health care professional. LIKELY UNSAFE ...when used orally in medicinal amounts throughout pregnancy or for self-treatment. Raspberry leaf can cause uterine contractions [4,19] and might have estrogenic effects [6180]. These effects can adversely effect pregnancy. Tell pregnant patients not to use raspberry leaf at any time during pregnancy without the close supervision of a health care provider.
LACTATION: LIKELY SAFE ...when used orally in amounts found in foods [4]. There is insufficient reliable information available about the safety of larger amounts of raspberry leaf while breast-feeding; avoid using.

Effectiveness
There is insufficient reliable information available about the effectiveness of raspberry leaf.

Mechanism of Action

Raspberry leaf contains a high tannin content (13-15%), which is responsible for its astringent properties (4). When applied topically to skin or mucous membranes tannins cause capillary vasoconstriction, decreased vascular permeability, and a local anti-inflammatory effect (7). The effects of raspberry leaf on smooth muscle, such as that found in the uterus seems to be variable. Different constituents found in raspberry leaf seem to either stimulate or contract uterine smooth muscle. When used in humans, raspberry leaf might have either stimulatory or spasmolytic effects. There is some evidence that these effects might be dose and tissue dependent. For example, in low doses raspberry leaf might cause more contraction, while higher doses might have spasmolytic effects and decrease contraction. Also, raspberry might decrease contraction of tonic tissues and increase contraction of relaxed tissues (1096,1122). Raspberry leaf might also have some estrogenic effects. In an animal model, raspberry leaf seems to increase serum ceruloplasmin oxidase activity, which is a measure of estrogenic activity in the liver (6180).

Adverse Reactions

None reported.

Interactions with Herbs & Other Dietary Supplements

IRON, CALCIUM, MAGNESIUM: Theoretically, concomitant use may decrease mineral absorption due to tannin content (7).

Interactions with Drugs

ORAL MEDICATION: Theoretically, tannin content of raspberry leaf may modify absorption of sedatives, hypnotics, antidepressants, and tranquilizers (7,19).
METFORMIN (Glucophage): Theoretically, concomitant use may reduce effectiveness (7).

Interactions with Foods

No interactions are known to occur, and there is no known reason to expect a clinically significant interaction with raspberry leaf.

Interactions with Lab Tests

No interactions are known to occur, and there is no known reason to expect a clinically significant interaction with raspberry leaf.

Interactions with Diseases or Conditions

HORMONE SENSITIVE CANCERS/CONDITIONS: Because raspberry leaf might have estrogenic effects (6180), women with hormone sensitive conditions should avoid raspberry leaf. Some of these conditions include breast, uterine, and ovarian cancer, and endometriosis and uterine fibroids.

Dosage and Administration

ORAL: For facilitating labor, midwives typically prescribe raspberry leaf tea prepared by steeping 2 grams dried leaf in 240 mL of boiling water for 5 minutes and then straining (1122). Doses for other uses are typically one cup of tea up to 6 times daily. The tea is prepared by steeping 1.5 grams (approximately 2 teaspoons) of finely cut leaves in 150 mL boiling water 5 minutes and then straining (3,8,18). Alternatively, soak finely cut leaves in cold water for 2 hours and then strain (3). A liquid extract (1:1 in 25% alcohol) is also often used and dosed as 4-8 mL three times daily (4).

Comments

Raspberry leaf extract has been used in Europe for centuries. The therapeutic use of raspberry leaf was first described in 1597 in The Herbal, or a General History of Plants (1096).

RED BUSH TEA

Also Known As

Kaffree Tea, Red Bush, Rooibos Tea.

Scientific Names

Aspalathus linearis, synonyms Aspalathus contaminata, Borbonia pinfolia, Psoralea linearis.
Family: Leguminosae or Fabaceae.

People Use This For

Orally, red bush tea is used as a nonstimulating, nonsedating beverage.

Safety

LIKELY SAFE …when used orally as a beverage (6,4120).
PREGNANCY AND LACTATION: Insufficient reliable information available; avoid using.

Effectiveness

There is insufficient reliable information available for the effectiveness of red bush tea.

Mechanism of Action

Red bush tea contains almost no active constituents (5,6). It contains acid polysaccharides (4120,4121), flavonoids (6,4122), a low amount of tannins (less than 5%) (5,6), and a relatively high amount of vitamin C (9.4%) (6). Some evidence suggests daily intake of acid polysaccharides found in the extracts of red bush tea might suppress HIV infection (4120,4121). Other information suggests the tea could prevent age-related changes to the central nervous system (4123) or suppress mutagenic activity (6).

Adverse Reactions

One report of salmonella contamination has occurred, possibly from lizard origin (6).

Interactions with Herbs & Other Dietary Supplements

Insufficient reliable information available.

Interactions with Drugs

No interactions are known to occur, and there is no known reason to expect a clinically significant interaction with red bush tea.

Interactions with Foods

No interactions are known to occur, and there is no known reason to expect a clinically significant interaction with red bush tea.

Interactions with Lab Tests

No interactions are known to occur, and there is no known reason to expect a clinically significant interaction with red bush tea.

Interactions with Diseases or Conditions

No interactions are known to occur, and there is no known reason to expect a clinically significant interaction with red bush tea.

Dosage and Administration

ORAL: Brewed like normal tea (5).

Comments

Tea is made from the branches and twigs of Aspalathus linearis. The fragrant, caffeine-free tea is the national drink of South Africa (5,6,7).

RED CLOVER

Also Known As

Beebread, Cow Clover, Daidzein, Genistein, Isoflavone, Isoflavones, Meadow Clover, Phytoestrogen, Phytoestrogens, Purple Clover, Trefoil, Trifolium, Wild Clover.
CAUTION: See separate listings for Soy and Sweet Clover.

Scientific Names

Trifolium pratense.
Family: Leguminosae or Fabaceae.

People Use This For

Orally, red clover is used for symptoms of menopause (3376,4734), cancer prevention, indigestion (4734), whooping cough (4,18), cough, asthma, bronchitis (11), and sexually transmitted diseases (STDs) (5).
Topically, red clover is used for cancerous growths (5), skin sores, burns, sore eyes, and chronic skin diseases including eczema and psoriasis (4,18).
In foods and beverages, the solid extract of red clover is used as a flavoring ingredient (11).

Safety

LIKELY SAFE ...when used orally in amounts commonly used in foods (4).

POSSIBLY SAFE ...when used orally and appropriately in medicinal amounts. Red clover extracts seem to be safe when used for up to one year (12,3375,6127).

There is insufficient reliable information available about the safety of the topical use of red clover.

PREGNANCY AND LACTATION: LIKELY SAFE ...when used orally in amounts commonly used in foods (4). LIKELY UNSAFE ...when used orally in medicinal amounts; red clover has estrogenic activity (4,12); avoid using. There is insufficient reliable information available about the safety of the topical use of red clover during pregnancy and lactation.

Effectiveness

POSSIBLY EFFECTIVE ...when used orally for prevention of osteoporosis. There is some evidence that taking red clover isoflavones 40 mg daily for one year can significantly reduce the loss of spinal bone mineral density (BMD) and bone mineral content (BMC) in pre- and perimenopausal women. But red clover isoflavones don't seem to have this effect in postmenopausal women. Red clover also does not seem to effect hipbone density or mineral content (6127). ...when used orally for symptoms of benign prostatic hyperplasia (BPH). Red clover isoflavones 40-80 mg daily for 3 months seems to decrease nocturnal urinary frequency, international prostate symptom scores (IPSS), and improved quality of life in men with BPH. However, red clover isoflavones do not seem to effect urine flow rate, prostate-specific antigen (PSA) values, or prostate size (6128). More evidence is needed to rate red clover for these uses.

POSSIBLY INEFFECTIVE ...when used orally for hypercholesterolemia in postmenopausal women. Red clover extract given over a 12 week period does not seem to significantly lower cholesterol in postmenopausal women with moderately elevated cholesterol levels (3375).

There is insufficient reliable information available about the effectiveness of red clover for its other uses.

Mechanism of Action

The applicable part of red clover is the flower top. The flower top contains more than 100 different chemicals (4744). Red clover contains isoflavones, a class of phytoestrogens, which are structurally similar to those of estrogens. The principal isoflavones found in red clover are biochanin A and formononetin. When ingested biochanin A and formononetin are metabolized to the isoflavones genistein and daidzen, respectively (3375,3376). The isoflavones are hydrolyzed by beta-glucosidases in the jejunum, releasing genistein and daidzein (3982). These are widely distributed in the body with peak concentrations at 4 to 8 hours after dietary intake and excretion within 24 hours (3982). The absorption of isoflavones from food may be saturable, suggesting improved effect if ingested throughout the day (3982). Isoflavone bioavailability does not seem to be affected by food source of isoflavones or other foods in the diet (3982). Red clover isoflavone constituents might act as selective estrogen-receptor modulators (SERMs) (3376). In premenopausal women with normal endogenous estrogen levels, isoflavones may have an anti-estrogen effect. In postmenopausal women with low endogenous estrogens, isoflavones are likely to act as weak estrogens (3387,3988,3989,3990,3994,6029). Isoflavones have a higher affinity for the beta estrogen receptor than the classical alpha estrogen receptor (3376,3983,3992,6029). The beta estrogen receptor predominates in the heart, vasculature, bone, and bladder, which may account for some of red clover's beneficial effects. Osteoporosis in postmenopausal women is related to declining estrogen levels. Red clover is thought to be beneficial for preventing osteoporosis due to its weak estrogenic effects (3376,6029,6127). For lowering cholesterol, estrogenic effects of red clover isoflavones might be involved in modulating lipid metabolism. Red clover can also increase bile acid excretion and might up-regulate low-density lipoprotein (LDL) receptors (6029,6030,4738). Some researchers think red clover may have a role in preventing cardiovascular disease due to its potential effects on cholesterol levels and preliminary evidence that it might improve systemic arterial compliance (836,3375). Red clover isoflavones might have anticarcinogenic activity (4740,4742) possibly due to both estrogenic and nonestrogenic mechanisms (4741). Red clover also contains the constituent coumestrol, which seems to have activity similar to diethylstilbestrol (DES) (4743,4744). The coumarin constituents contained in red clover can cause anticoagulant effects (4). Red clover is also thought to have antispasmodic, expectorant, and astringent activity (4,11).

There is some evidence that red clover isoflavones can inhibit oxidative and conjugative metabolism (4736). Isoflavones might also affect drug absorption and biliary excretion by interacting with multi-drug transporters such as P-glycoprotein (4736). Given the wide range of drugs and metabolites whose pharmacokinetics depend on these mechanisms, drug interactions with isoflavones might be more common than literature reports suggest.

Adverse Reactions

Orally, red clover can cause rash-like reactions (4). Theoretically, it can cause estrogenic-type activity.

Interactions with Herbs & Other Dietary Supplements

HERBS WITH ANTICOAGULANT/ANTIPLATELET POTENTIAL:

Concomitant use of herbs that have coumarin constituents or affect platelet aggregation could theoretically increase the risk of bleeding in some people. Some of these herbs are angelica, anise, arnica, asafoetida, bogbean, boldo, capsicum, celery, chamomile, clove, danshen, fenugreek, feverfew, garlic, ginger, ginkgo, ginseng Panax, horse chestnut, horseradish, licorice, meadowsweet, prickly ash, onion, papain, passionflower, poplar, quassia, turmeric, wild carrot, wild lettuce, willow, and others (4,19).

HERBS WITH ESTROGENIC ACTIVITY: Theoretically, red clover could be additive or possibly antagonistic with other herbs with estrogenic activity. These herbs include black cohosh, ipriflavone, and soy.

Interactions with Drugs

ANTICOAGULANT DRUGS: Theoretically, concomitant use of large amounts of red clover can increase the anticoagulant effects and bleeding risk of these drugs due to its coumarin content (4).

ESTROGEN OR ORAL CONTRACEPTIVES: Theoretically, concomitant use of large amounts of red clover might interfere with hormone replacement therapy or oral contraceptives through competition for estrogen receptors (4737,4743).

OTHER DRUGS: There's preliminary evidence that red clover can inhibit the cytochrome P450 (CYP450) 3A4 enzyme (6450). Theoretically, red clover might increase levels of drugs metabolized by CYP450 3A4. However, so far, this interaction has not been reported in humans. Some drugs metabolized by CYP450 3A4 include lovastatin (Mevacor), ketoconazole (Nizoral), itraconazole (Sporanox), fexofenadine (Allegra), triazolam (Halcion), and numerous others. Use red clover cautiously or avoid in patients taking these drugs.

Interactions with Foods

No interactions are known to occur, and there is no known reason to expect a clinically significant interaction with red clover.

Interactions with Lab Tests

No interactions are known to occur, and there is no known reason to expect a clinically significant interaction with red clover.

Interactions with Diseases or Conditions

COAGULATION DISORDERS: Use red clover with caution and avoid large amounts due to its coumarin content, which might increase the risk of bleeding (4).

HORMONE SENSITIVE CANCERS/CONDITIONS: Because isoflavones in red clover have estrogenic effects (4,11,4741), women with hormone sensitive conditions should avoid red clover. Some of these conditions include breast, uterine, and ovarian cancer, and endometriosis and uterine fibroids.

Dosage and Administration

ORAL: The typical dose of red clover is 4 grams of the flower tops three times daily or one cup of the tea three times daily (4). The tea is prepared by steeping 4 grams of the flower tops in 150 mL boiling water for 10-15 minutes, and then straining (4). The liquid extract (1:1 in 25% alcohol) is commonly taken 1.5-3 mL three times per day (4,18). The tincture (1:10 in 45% alcohol) is usually dosed as 1-2 mL three times daily (4).

TOPICAL: No typical dosage.

Comments

Red clover in large quantities induces sterility in livestock (4743). The cheetah population in zoos was threatened by reproductive failure and liver disease, thought to be caused by diets high in isoflavones (4735).

RED MAPLE

Also Known As

Bird's Eye Maple, Sugar Maple, Swamp Maple.

Scientific Names

Acer rubrum.
Family: Aceraceae.

People Use This For

In Native American folk medicine, red maple was used topically for eye conditions and as an astringent (18).

Safety

There is insufficient reliable information available about the safety of red maple.
Pregnancy and Lactation: Insufficient reliable information available; avoid using.

Effectiveness

There is insufficient reliable information available about the effectiveness of red maple.

Mechanism of Action

The applicable part of red maple is the bark. There is insufficient reliable information available about the possible mechanism of action and active ingredients.

Adverse Reactions

None reported.

Interactions with Herbs & Other Dietary Supplements

Insufficient reliable information available.

Interactions with Drugs

No interactions are known to occur, and there is no known reason to expect a clinically significant interaction with red maple.

Interactions with Foods

No interactions are known to occur, and there is no known reason to expect a clinically significant interaction with red maple.

Interactions with Lab Tests

No interactions are known to occur, and there is no known reason to expect a clinically significant interaction with red maple.

Interactions with Diseases or Conditions

No interactions are known to occur, and there is no known reason to expect a clinically significant interaction with red maple.

Dosage and Administration

TOPICAL: Red maple is used as dried, powdered herb (18).

Comments

There is very little scientific information about this product. Our staff is continually analyzing the available information on natural medicines and will add data here as it becomes available.

RED SANDALWOOD

Also Known As

Red Sanderswood, Red Saunders, Rubywood, Sandalwood Padauk, Santali lignum rubrum, Sappan.
CAUTION: See separate listings for White Sandalwood oil and White Sandalwood wood.

Scientific Names

Pterocarpus santalinus.
Family: Leguminosae or Fabaceae.

People Use This For

Orally, red sandalwood is used for ailments of the gastrointestinal tract, as a diuretic or astringent, for "blood purification," and coughs (2).
In manufacturing, it is used as a flavoring in alcoholic beverages (12).

Safety

LIKELY SAFE ...when used as flavoring in alcoholic beverages (12).
POSSIBLY SAFE ...when used orally for medicinal purposes (12,18).
PREGNANCY AND LACTATION: Insufficient reliable information available; avoid using.

Effectiveness

There is insufficient reliable information available about the effectiveness of red sandalwood.

Mechanism of Action

The applicable part of red sandalwood is the heartwood (18). Red sandalwood contains the constituent santalins A and B, neoflavonoids, stilbene derivatives, and a volatile oil with traces of pterocarpol, isopterocarpol, and eudesmol (18). It is said to have diuretic and astringent effects (18).

Adverse Reactions

None reported.

Interactions with Herbs & Other Dietary Supplements

Insufficient reliable information available.

Interactions with Drugs

No interactions are known to occur, and there is no known reason to expect a clinically significant interaction with red sandalwood.

Interactions with Foods

No interactions are known to occur, and there is no known reason to expect a clinically significant interaction with red sandalwood.

Interactions with Lab Tests

No interactions are known to occur, and there is no known reason to expect a clinically significant interaction with red sandalwood.

Interactions with Diseases or Conditions

No interactions are known to occur, and there is no known reason to expect a clinically significant interaction with red sandalwood.

Dosage and Administration

No typical dosage.

Comments

Avoid confusion with white sandalwood (Santalum album).
There is very little scientific information about this product. Our staff is continually analyzing the available information on natural medicines and will add data here as it becomes available.

RED SOAPWORT

Also Known As

Bouncing-Bet, Saponariae rubrae radix, Soapwort.
CAUTION: See separate listing for White Soapwort.

Scientific Names

Saponaria officinalis.
Family: Caryophyllaceae.

People Use This For

Orally, red soapwort is used for inflammation of mucous membranes in the upper and lower respiratory tract (2).
Topically, it is used as a remedy for poison ivy, acne, psoriasis, eczema, and boils (6).
It is used as a foaming agent in beer (6).
In manufacturing, red soapwort is used as an ingredient in soaps, herbal shampoos (6002), and detergents (6).

Safety

LIKELY SAFE ...when used topically. Red soapwort is widely used in soaps and shampoos (6) without reports of adverse effects.
POSSIBLY SAFE ...when used orally (2).
PREGNANCY AND LACTATION: Insufficient reliable information available; avoid using.

Effectiveness

POSSIBLY EFFECTIVE ...when taken orally for inflammation of the mucous membranes in the upper and lower respiratory tract (2).
There is insufficient reliable information available about the effectiveness of red soapwort for its other uses.

Mechanism of Action

The applicable part of red soapwort is the root. The root contains saponin constituents that have expectorant effects. Saponins irritate the gastric mucosa, which then stimulate bronchial mucous secretion via the parasympathetic sensory pathways (7). In large amounts, red soapwort is cytotoxic (2).

Adverse Reactions

Orally, red soapwort can cause stomach irritation (2), nausea, and vomiting (7).

Interactions with Herbs & Other Dietary Supplements

Insufficient reliable information available.

Interactions with Drugs

No interactions are known to occur, and there is no known reason to expect a clinically significant interaction with red soapwort.

Interactions with Foods

No interactions are known to occur, and there is no known reason to expect a clinically significant interaction with red soapwort.

Interactions with Lab Tests

No interactions are known to occur, and there is no known reason to expect a clinically significant interaction with red soapwort.

Interactions with Diseases or Conditions

GI MUCOSAL IRRITATION (e.g. ulcers, etc.): Red soapwort is contraindicated, because it can exacerbate existing GI mucosal irritation due to its saponin content (6).

Dosage and Administration

ORAL: The typical dose of red soapwort is 1.5 grams of the dried root per day as a tea or equivalent preparation (2).

Comments

In the Middle Ages, Franciscan and Dominican monks viewed soapwort as a divine gift that was meant to keep them clean (6). Avoid confusion with white soapwort root.

RED-SPUR VALERIAN

Also Known As

Bouncing Bess, Bovis and Soldier, Delicate Bess, Drunken Sailor, Pretty Betsy, Red Spur Valerian.

Scientific Names

Centranthus ruber.

People Use This For

In traditional medicine, red-spur valerian is used as a sedative (18).

Safety

There is insufficient reliable information available about the safety of red-spur valerian.
Pregnancy and Lactation: Insufficient reliable information available; avoid using.

Effectiveness

There is insufficient reliable information available about the effectiveness of red-spur valerian.

Mechanism of Action

The applicable part of red-spur valerian is the root. Red-spur valerian contains valepotriate, that may have sedative and equilibrate properties (18).

Adverse Reactions

None reported.

Interactions with Herbs & Other Dietary Supplements

Insufficient reliable information available.

Interactions with Drugs

No interactions are known to occur, and there is no known reason to expect a clinically significant interaction with red-spur valerian.

Interactions with Foods

No interactions are known to occur, and there is no known reason to expect a clinically significant interaction with red-spur valerian.

Interactions with Lab Tests

No interactions are known to occur, and there is no known reason to expect a clinically significant interaction with red-spur valerian.

Interactions with Diseases or Conditions

No interactions are known to occur, and there is no known reason to expect a clinically significant interaction with red-spur valerian.

Dosage and Administration

ORAL: People typically use 0.3 to 1 mL valerian liquid extract or 4 to 8 mL valerian tincture (5264).

Comments

There is very little scientific information about this product. Our staff is continually analyzing the available information on natural medicines and will add data here as it becomes available.

RED YEAST

Also Known As

Hong Qu, Monascus, Red Rice Yeast, Red Yeast Rice, Xue Zhi Kang, Zhi Tai.
CAUTION: See separate listing for Beta-Sitosterol.

Scientific Names

Monascus purpureus Went; other Monascus species.
Family: Monascaceae.

People Use This For

Orally, red yeast is used for maintaining desirable cholesterol levels in healthy people (796) and reducing cholesterol in people with hyperlipidemia (6,512,2624).
In Chinese medicine, red yeast is used for indigestion, diarrhea, improving blood circulation, and for spleen and stomach health (6,512).
For food uses, red yeast is used as a food coloring for Peking duck and other foods (512).

Safety

POSSIBLY SAFE ...when used orally and appropriately, short-term. Red yeast has been safely used in studies lasting up to 12 weeks (512,2624,6988,6989,6990,6995,6996).
There is insufficient reliable information available about the safety of red yeast when used long-term.
CHILDREN: POSSIBLY UNSAFE ...when used orally. Safety has not been established in children under 18 years of age and questions remain about the benefit of lowering cholesterol in children (512).
PREGNANCY: LIKELY UNSAFE ...when used orally. The red yeast constituent, lovastatin, has induced fetal skeletal malformations in animals (2619); avoid using.
LACTATION: Insufficient reliable information available; avoid using.

Effectiveness

LIKELY EFFECTIVE ...when used orally for lowering cholesterol and triglyceride levels (2624,6988,6989,6990). Several studies have shown that red yeast can significantly lower total and low-density lipoprotein (LDL) cholesterol levels, and triglycerides when used for 8-12 weeks (2624,6989,6990). Most studies have used 2.4 grams per day, but benefits have also been found with 1.2 grams per day (6988). In one study, red yeast was similar to simvastatin (Zocor) for improving lipid profiles (6993). Most studies used a specific proprietary red yeast product (Cholestin, Pharmanex). There is insufficient reliable information available about the effectiveness of red yeast for its other uses.

Mechanism of Action

Red yeast is the product of rice fermented with Monascus purpureus yeast (512). Red yeast supplements are different than red yeast rice sold in Chinese grocery stores (6994). Supplements are manufactured by culturing M. purpureus on rice at carefully controlled temperature and growing conditions to increase the concentration of mevinic acids (6994). Red yeast contains eight mevinic acids (statins), primarily lovastatin (also referred to as monacolin K or mevinolin) (512,2624,6988). These compounds, which constitute about 0.4% of red rice, competitively inhibit 3-hydroxy-3-methyl-glutaryl-coenzyme A (HMG-CoA) reductase, blocking cholesterol biosynthesis (512,2624). Red yeast also contains sterols, including beta-sitosterol, campesterol, stigmasterol, and sapogenin; isolfavones and isoflavone glycosides, and monounsaturated fatty acids (2624,6988). Although the cholesterol lowering effect is likely partially caused by the lovastatin content, it is unclear to what extent. The overall cholesterol-lowering effect of red yeast is likely also the result of the combination of lovastatin, mevinic acids, and other constituents.

Adverse Reactions

Orally, red yeast can cause gastritis, abdominal discomfort, and elevated liver enzymes (512). In clinical studies, heartburn, flatulence, and dizziness were reported infrequently and did not result in study withdrawal (6988). Anaphylaxis following inhalation of red yeast has also been reported (6997). Theoretically, similar reactions caused by HMG-CoA reductase inhibitor (Statins) drugs can be caused by red yeast; however, all of those adverse reactions have not yet been reported for red yeast.

Interactions with Herbs & Other Dietary Supplements

CHOLESTEROL LOWERING HERBS/SUPPLEMENTS: Theoretically, red yeast might enhance the effects of herbs and supplements that also lower cholesterol.

COENZYME Q10 (CoQ10, Ubiquinone): Theoretically, red yeast can lower coenzyme Q10 levels. Red yeast contains the constituent, lovastatin, and related compounds, which can lower coenzyme Q10 levels (6983,6984,6985,6986).

GRAPEFRUIT: Concomitant use of red yeast (Cholestin) and grapefruit products can increase the serum levels of lovastatin, a constituent of red yeast (527). Grapefruit and grapefruit seed extract products can inhibit cytochrome P450 metabolism of lovastatin (6,527,5858).

HEPATOTOXIC HERB & SUPPLEMENTS: Theoretically, red yeast might enhance the adverse effects of potentially hepatotoxic herbs/supplements such as borage, chaparral, niacin, valerian, and uva ursi.; avoid concurrent use.

HERBS/SUPPLEMENTS WITH THYROID ACTIVITY: Theoretically, red yeast might interfere with effects of herbs/supplements that affect thyroid function, including bugleweed, balm leaf, tiratricol, and wild thyme. Concomitant use of levothyroxine with lovastatin can cause thyroid function abnormalities (15). Avoid concurrent use.

ST. JOHN'S WORT: Theoretically, St. John's wort might reduce serum levels of red yeast. St. John's wort induces cytochrome P450 3A4 enzyme that can lower serum levels of the lovastatin constituent (1290,1291).

Interactions with Drugs

ALCOHOL: Theoretically, alcohol may adversely affect liver function in patients taking red yeast, due to the lovastatin constituent (15).

CYCLOSPORINE: Theoretically, red yeast in combination with cyclosporine might increase the risk of myopathy due to the red yeast lovastatin constituent (15); use with caution.

GEMFIBROZIL (Lopid): Theoretically, red yeast in combination with gemfibrozil might increase the risk of myopathy due to the red yeast lovastatin constituent (15).

HMG-CoA REDUCTASE INHIBITORS ("Statins"): Using red yeast with these drugs might increase the risk of adverse effects without necessarily improving therapeutic benefit; avoid concomitant use. HMG-CoA reductase inhibitors include atorvastatin (Lipitor), cerivastatin (Baycol), fluvastatin (Lescol), lovastatin (Mevacor), pravastatin (Pravachol), and simvastatin (Zocor) (14,15).

LEVOTHYROXINE (Synthroid): Theoretically, concomitant use of levothyroxine with red yeast might cause thyroid function abnormalities due to the red yeast lovastatin constituent (15).

NIACIN: Theoretically, red yeast in combination with high-dose niacin might increase the risk of myopathy due to the red yeast lovastatin constituent (15).

OTHER DRUGS: Theoretically, drugs that inhibit the cytochrome P450 3A4 enzyme might increase serum levels of red yeast constituents such as lovastatin and increase the risk of adverse effects. Drugs with this interaction include clarithromycin, erythromycin, itraconazole, ketoconazole, cimetidine, nefazodone, protease inhibitors, and others (6987).

Interactions with Foods

ALCOHOL: Theoretically, alcohol may adversely affect liver function in patients taking red yeast due to the lovastatin constituent (15).

FOOD: Food enhances the bioavailability of lovastatin (15), a constituent of red yeast.

GRAPEFRUIT JUICE: Concomitant use of grapefruit juice and lovastatin, a constituent of red yeast, can increase serum lovastatin levels and the risk of adverse effects (794).

Interactions with Lab Tests

LIVER ENZYMES: Red yeast might increase serum liver transaminase concentrations and test results due its lovastatin content. Lovastatin can increase serum liver transaminase concentrations and test results (15).

CREATINE KINASE (CK): Red yeast might increase serum creatine kinase concentrations and test results due its lovastatin content. Lovastatin can increase serum creatine kinase concentrations and test results (15).

SERUM CHOLESTEROL: Red yeast can reduce serum cholesterol concentrations and test results. Red yeast contains a mixture of lovastatin and other HMG-CoA reductase inhibitors (6,15,512,2624).

Interactions with Diseases or Conditions

LIVER DYSFUNCTION: Red yeast is contraindicated in people with liver dysfunction, risk of liver dysfunction, or abnormal liver function test results (512,2619).

THYROID DYSFUNCTION: Concomitant use of lovastatin with levothyroxine can interfere with thyroid therapy (15).

Dosage and Administration

ORAL: Most clinical studies have used a specific brand product (Cholestin). However, most other red yeast brands contain a similar amount of red yeast, 600 mg. For hypercholesterolemia, a typical dose of red yeast is 1200 mg two times daily with food (2624). A total daily dose of 2400 mg red yeast contains approximately 9.6 mg total statins, of which 7.2 mg is lovastatin (2624).

Comments

Red yeast is the product of rice fermented with the Monascus purpureus yeast that contains monacolin K (lovastatin, mevinolin) and other HMG-CoA reductase inhibiting compounds (512). Red yeast is marketed as a dietary supplement, Cholestin (Pharmanex). The FDA is currently investigating whether red yeast should be classified as a drug or a dietary supplement. In May 1998, the FDA banned the sale of Cholestin in the US, claiming it was an unregulated drug (2625). In February 1999, a US Federal judge overrode the FDA decision, saying Cholestin could be sold as a food supplement (2626). In July 2000 the 10th Circuit Court of Appeals in Denver decided that the ruling was in error and restored the FDAs ability to regulate Cholestin as a drug (6610). Until more clinical information is available, red yeast should be treated as a HMG-CoA reductase inhibitor, with all the possible side effects, drug interactions, and precautions associated with this drug class. The American Heart Association has cautioned against using red yeast pending the results of long-term studies (6991).

REED HERB

Also Known As
Reed.

Scientific Names
Phragmites communis.

People Use This For
Orally, reed herb stem and rhizome are used for digestive disorders (18).
Topically, the juice of reed herb is used to relieve insect bites (18).
In Oriental medicine, reed herb is used for diabetes, leukemia, and breast cancer (18).

Safety
There is insufficient reliable information available about the safety of reed herb.
Pregnancy and Lactation: Insufficient reliable information available; avoid using.

Effectiveness
There is insufficient reliable information available about the effectiveness of reed herb.

Mechanism of Action

The applicable parts of reed herb are the stem and rhizome. Reed herb contains vitamin A, vitamin C, and several vitamins of the B-group (18). It also contains triterpenes (beta-amyrin and taraxerol) and several flavonoids including chrysoeriol, isoquercitrin, luteolin, rutin, and tricin (18). The plant is thought to have diuretic effects and stimulate sweating (18).

Adverse Reactions

None reported.

Interactions with Herbs & Other Dietary Supplements

Insufficient reliable information available.

Interactions with Drugs

No interactions are known to occur, and there is no known reason to expect a clinically significant interaction with reed herb.

Interactions with Foods

No interactions are known to occur, and there is no known reason to expect a clinically significant interaction with reed herb.

Interactions with Lab Tests

No interactions are known to occur, and there is no known reason to expect a clinically significant interaction with reed herb.

Interactions with Diseases or Conditions

No interactions are known to occur, and there is no known reason to expect a clinically significant interaction with reed herb.

Dosage and Administration

Reed herb is prepared as a tea for oral or topical use (18).

Comments

None.

REISHI MUSHROOM

Also Known As

Ling Chih, Ling Zhi, Mannentake, Mushroom Of Immortality, Mushroom of Spiritual Potency, Reishi, Rei-Shi, Spirit Plant.

Scientific Names

Ganoderma lucidum.
Family: Ganodermataceae.

People Use This For

Orally, reishi mushroom is used for enhancing the immune system, lowering blood pressure and cholesterol, treating and preventing viral infections and tumors, treating inflammatory disease, cardiovascular disease, asthma and bronchial diseases. It is used for reducing stress, providing a kidney tonic, treating hepatitis and liver disease, supporting HIV disease, treating or preventing altitude sickness, and supporting chemotherapy. Other oral uses include preventing fatigue, treating insomnia, gastric ulcers, neurasthenia, poisoning (5472,5473,5474,5475,5493), post-herpeticneuralgia, and herpes zoster pain (5485).
It is also used in combination with seven other herbs (PC-SPES) to treat prostate cancer (5548).

Safety

POSSIBLY SAFE ...when used orally and appropriately (12). ...when used orally in a specific herbal combination (PC-SPES) (5548).
PREGNANCY AND LACTATION: Insufficient reliable information available; avoid using.

Effectiveness

POSSIBLY EFFECTIVE ...when used orally in a specific herbal combination for prostate cancer. Studies using reishi mushroom in combination with seven other herbs (PC-SPES), found that it significantly decreases prostate-specific antigen (PSA) levels (3576,5122,5548,6284,6286), causes clinically significant reductions in serum testosterone (5548), improves quality of life, and reduces pain (6286) in patients with prostate cancer. In two reports, PSA levels fell significantly within one month of treatment (5122,5548).
There is insufficient reliable information available about the effectiveness of reishi mushroom for its other uses.

Mechanism of Action

The applicable parts of reishi mushrooms are the fruiting body and mycelium (12). Reishi mushrooms have a long history in folk medicine, but researchers are just beginning to isolate and identify medicinal substances in reishi that have antitumor, immune modulating, anti-aging, cardiovascular, anticoagulant, cholesterol lowering, hypoglycemic, hepatoprotective, antiviral, and antibacterial effects (5476,5477,5481,5482,5483,5484,5485,5486,5487,5488,5489) (5490,5491,5492). Protease inhibitors and other anti-HIV substances have been found in reishi mushrooms (5479,5480). Studies of these compounds have not been performed in humans. Reishi mushroom extracts contain high levels of adenosine (5478).

Adverse Reactions

Reishi mushroom, when taken orally can cause dryness of the mouth, throat, and nasal area, itchiness, stomach upset, nosebleed, and bloody stools which have occurred with extended oral use (3 to 6 months) (12). Also, a rash with the consumption of reishi wine and respiratory allergy to reishi spores can occur (12,5479).

Interactions with Herbs & Other Dietary Supplements

HERBS WITH ANTICOAGULANT/ANTIPLATELET POTENTIAL: Concomitant use of with herbs that have anticoagulant or antiplatelet activity could theoretically increase the risk of bleeding in some people (5476). These herbs include: angelica, anise, arnica, asafoetida, bogbean, boldo, capsicum, celery, chamomile, clove, danshen, fenugreek, feverfew, garlic, ginger, ginkgo, ginseng Panax, horse chestnut, horseradish, licorice, meadowsweet, prickly ash, onion, papain, passionflower, poplar, quassia, red clover, turmeric, wild carrot, wild lettuce, willow, and others (4,19).
HERBS/SUPPLEMENTS WITH HYPOTENSIVE ACTIVITY: Theoretically, concurrent use might increase risk of hypotension with herbs that lower blood pressure (5488), including black cohosh, celery seed, Panax ginseng, and others (4).

Interactions with Drugs

ANTICOAGULANT/ANTIPLATELET DRUGS: Reishi seems to have anticoagulant effects (5476). Theoretically, taking reishi with other anticoagulant or antiplatelet drugs might increase the risk of bruising and bleeding. Some of these drugs include aspirin, clopidogrel (Plavix), nonsteroidal anti-inflammatory drugs (NSAIDs) such as diclofenac (Voltaren, Cataflam, others), ibuprofen (Advil, Motrin, others), naproxen (Anaprox, Naprosyn, others), dalteparin (Fragmin), enoxaparin (Lovenox), heparin, warfarin (Coumadin) and others.
ANTIHYPERTENSIVE DRUGS: Theoretically, concurrent use might increase risk of hypotension with drugs that lower blood pressure (5488).

Interactions with Foods

No interactions are known to occur, and there is no known reason to expect a clinically significant interaction with reishi mushroom.

Interactions with Lab Tests

BLEEDING TIME: Theoretically, reishi mushroom use might prolong coagulation and bleeding time results (5476).

Interactions with Diseases or Conditions

THROMBOCYTOPENIA: Theoretically, reishi mushroom use might increase the risk of bleeding in people with thrombocytopenia (5476).
HYPOTENSION: Theoretically, reishi mushroom use might worsen hypotension or interfere with drug therapy to increase blood pressure (5488).

Dosage and Administration

ORAL: People typically use 1.5-9 grams orally per day of the crude dried mushroom, 1-1.5 grams per day of reishi powder, or 1 mL per day of reishi tincture (5473). Reishi tea is also used therapeutically (5473).

Comments

Reishi mushroom is used medicinally but not eaten. The flesh is described as "tough" and "woody" with a bitter taste (353).

RESVERATROL

Also Known As
Cis-Resveratrol, Kojo-Kon, Phytoestrogen, Protykin, Resveratrols, Trans-Resveratrol.
CAUTION: See separate listings for Grape seed, Grape Skin Extract, Quercetin, and Wine.

Scientific Names
3,4',5-stilbenetriol; 3,5,4'-trihydroxystilbene; 3,4',5-trihydroxystilbene.

People Use This For
Orally, resveratrol is used for atherosclerosis (2945), lowering cholesterol levels (2946,2957), increasing HDL cholesterol levels (2946), and preventing cancer (2945,2947,2956,2957).
In Japanese and Chinese folk medicine, it is used for several disorders, including atherosclerosis (2946).

Safety
LIKELY SAFE ...when consumed in amounts found in foods (2030).
There is insufficient reliable information available about the safety of resveratrol when used in supplemental doses in amounts greater than those found in foods.
PREGNANCY AND LACTATION: LIKELY SAFE ...when used in amounts found in some foods (2030). Resveratrol is found in grape skins, grape juice, wine, and other food sources. Wine should not be used as a source of resveratrol during pregnancy and lactation.

Effectiveness
There is insufficient reliable information available about the effectiveness of resveratrol.

Mechanism of Action
Resveratrol is a polyphenolic compound that exists in nature as cis- and trans- stereoisomers. The biological activity of cis-resveratrol is not entirely known, but preliminary data suggests that it has antiplatelet activity (2030,2950). Preliminary evidence suggests that trans-resveratrol has antioxidant, antimutagenic (2948), antitumor (2958,2959) and phytoestrogenic activity (2960). Preliminary evidence also suggest that trans-resveratrol inhibits cyclooxygenases 1 and 2, hydroperoxidases, 5-lipoxygenase (2030,2948), platelet aggregation (2949,2950,2951,2952,2961), and causes blood vessel dilation (2954). Early research suggests resveratrol might reduce the risk of cancer (2948,2959). Biological activity in humans has not yet been described (2030). Resveratrol is primarily found in red wine, red grape skins, purple grape juice, mulberries, and in smaller amounts in peanuts (513,2030,2956). Other sources include eucalyptus (Eucalyptus wandoo, Eucalyptus sideroxylon), spruce (Picea excelsa), and Bauhinia racemosa (2030). Polygonum cuspidatum, the roots of which are used in Chinese and Japanese traditional medicine, is considered to be one of the richest sources of trans-resveratrol (2030). The trans-resveratrol content of wine is highly dependent on grape type, climate, and practices used to make the wine (9). White wines have very low trans-resveratrol concentrations. Pinot Noir consistently has the highest concentrations of trans-resveratrol, regardless of climate. Other red wines, including Cabernet Sauvignon, produced in cold, humid climates, such as Bordeaux and Canada, have higher trans-resveratrol content than those produced in hot, dry climates (2030).

Adverse Reactions
None reported.

Interactions with Herbs & Other Dietary Supplements
HERBS WITH ANTICOAGULANT/ANTIPLATELET POTENTIAL: Theoretically, concomitant use of resveratrol with herbs that have anticoagulant or antiplatelet activity could increase the risk of bleeding in some people (2949,2950,2951,2952,2961). These herbs include: angelica, anise, arnica, asafoetida, bogbean, boldo, capsicum, celery, chamomile, clove, danshen, fenugreek, feverfew, garlic, ginger, ginkgo, ginseng Panax, horse chestnut, horseradish, licorice, meadowsweet, prickly ash, onion, papain, passionflower, poplar, quassia, red clover, turmeric, wild carrot, wild lettuce, willow, and others (4,19).

Interactions with Drugs
ANTICOAGULANT/ANTIPLATELET DRUGS: Resveratrol seems to have antiplatelet effects (2949,2950,2951,2952,2961). Theoretically, taking resveratrol with other antiplatelet or anticoagulant drugs might increase the risk of bruising and bleeding. Some of these drugs include aspirin, clopidogrel (Plavix), nonsteroidal anti-inflammatory drugs (NSAIDs) such as diclofenac (Voltaren, Cataflam, others), ibuprofen (Advil, Motrin, others), naproxen (Anaprox, Naprosyn, others), dalteparin (Fragmin), enoxaparin (Lovenox), heparin, warfarin (Coumadin), and others.

Interactions with Foods

No interactions are known to occur, and there is no known reason to expect a clinically significant interaction with resveratrol.

Interactions with Lab Tests

No interactions are known to occur, and there is no known reason to expect a clinically significant interaction with resveratrol.

Interactions with Diseases or Conditions

HORMONE SENSITIVE CANCERS/CONDITIONS: Because resveratrol might have estrogenic effects (2960), women with hormone sensitive conditions should avoid resveratrol. Some of these conditions include breast, uterine, and ovarian cancer, and endometriosis and uterine fibroids.

Dosage and Administration

ORAL: Resveratrol is frequently given in combination with other products, such as grape seed extract. Supplemental doses of resveratrol are typically 200-600 mcg per day and may be divided and given twice daily (2945,5021). One glass of red wine provides approximately 640 mcg and a handful of peanuts provides approximately 73 mcg of resveratrol (2945).

Comments

There is very little scientific information about this product. Our staff is continually analyzing the available information on natural medicines and will add data here as it becomes available.

RHATANY

Also Known As

Brazilian Rhatany, Krameria, Mapato, Peruvian Rhatany, Pumacuchu, Raiz Para Los Dientes, Ratanhiawurzel, Red Rhatany, Rhatanhia, Rhatania, Ratanhiae radix.

Scientific Names

Krameria triandra; Krameria argentea.
Family: Krameriaceae.

People Use This For

Orally, rhatany is used as an antidiarrheal agent for enteritis and angina.
Topically, rhatany is used for mild inflammation of the oral and pharyngeal mucosa, inflammation of the gums, fissures of the tongue, stomatitis, pharyngitis, non-infectious canker sores, chilblains, and leg ulcers.

Safety

POSSIBLY SAFE ...when used topically for short-term use (2,12). Use should be limited to two weeks unless medical evaluation determines that there is no problem and use can continue. (2).
There is insufficient reliable information available about the safety of rhatany for its other uses.
PREGNANCY AND LACTATION: Insufficient reliable information available; avoid using.

Effectiveness

POSSIBLY EFFECTIVE ...when used topically for mild inflammation of the oral and pharyngeal mucosa (2).
There is insufficient reliable information available about the effectiveness of rhatany for its other uses.

Mechanism of Action

The applicable part of rhatany is the root. Rhatany contains high concentrations of proanthocyanidin tannins (10-15%), which are responsible for the observed astringent properties (2,3,18,4100). The alcohol in the tincture preparation may enhance astringent effects (4102). Astringents precipitate the surface proteins of cells decreasing the cell size (4101) and secretions from the inflamed tissues (4102), diminishing inflammation. Astringents also have the ability to alleviate inflammation by constricting the blood vessels and reducing the supply of blood to the affected area (4102).

Adverse Reactions

Orally, rhatany taken can cause digestive complaints (18). Rarely, allergic mucous membrane reactions have occurred (2,18).

Interactions with Herbs & Other Dietary Supplements

Insufficient reliable information available.

Interactions with Drugs

ORAL DRUGS: Theoretically, concomitant oral administration may cause precipitation of some drugs due to the high tannin content of rhatany. Separate administration of oral drugs and tannin-containing herbs by the longest period of time practical (19).

Interactions with Foods

No interactions are known to occur, and there is no known reason to expect a clinically significant interaction with rhatany.

Interactions with Lab Tests

No interactions are known to occur, and there is no known reason to expect a clinically significant interaction with rhatany.

Interactions with Diseases or Conditions

ALLERGY: Contraindicated if rhatany allergy.

Dosage and Administration

ORAL: Rhatany is sometimes taken as a decoction of 1 gram of the herb in 1 cup of water or as 5-10 drops of the tincture in one glass of water (6002).
TOPICAL: As mouth wash or gargle (simmer 1-1.5 grams of powdered root in 150 mL boiling water 10-15 minutes, strain) two to three times daily (8). As mouth wash or gargle, 5-10 drops of rhatany tincture in one glass of water two to three times daily (8). Undiluted rhatany tincture (oral paint) used directly on the affected area two to three times daily (2). Limit rhatany use to maximum two weeks without medical evaluation (2).

Comments

Avoid confusion with roots of other Krameria species (18). Rhatany (Krameria triandra) root is difficult to find and adulteration is common with other Krameria species (8).

RHUBARB

Also Known As

Chinese Rhubarb, Da Huang, Garden Rhubarb, Himalayan Rhubarb, Indian Rhubarb, Medicinal Rhubarb, Rhei, Rhei radix, Turkey Rhubarb.

Scientific Names

Rheum officinale; Rheum palmatum; Rheum tanguticum; Rheum australe, synonym Rheum emodi; Rheum x cultorum, synonym Rheum rhabarbarum.
Family: Polygonaceae.

People Use This For

Orally, rhubarb root or rhizome is used for constipation (2,4,12,18), diarrhea (4,7), dyspepsia, gastritis (7), preparation for gastrointestinal diagnostic procedures after recto-anal surgery, for bowel movement relief when anal fissures are present, and for hemorrhoids (18).
For food uses, rhubarb stems are edible. Rhubarb is also used as a flavoring agent.

Safety

LIKELY SAFE ...when the root or rhizome are used in food amounts. The maximum use is 0.05% (11). Chinese and garden rhubarb are approved for food use in the US (11).
POSSIBLY SAFE ...when used orally and appropriately in medicinal amounts for less than eight days.
CHILDREN: POSSIBLY UNSAFE ...when used orally. Rhubarb root or rhizome should not be used in children under age 12 (2,12). There is one report of a 4-year-old who ingested rhubarb leaves (containing oxalic acid) and died (17).
PREGNANCY AND LACTATION: LIKELY SAFE ...when used in food amounts. POSSIBLY UNSAFE ...when used in larger amounts because it is a stimulant laxative; avoid using (2,4,12).

Effectiveness

POSSIBLY EFFECTIVE ...when used orally for constipation at high doses (2,4,7,12). ...when used orally for diarrhea at low doses (4,7,12).

There is insufficient reliable information available about the effectiveness of rhubarb for its other uses.

Mechanism of Action

The applicable parts of rhubarb are the rhizome and root. Rhubarb contains anthraquinones, tannins and calcium oxalate (4,7,12,18). At low doses, the tannin effects predominate and have an astringent effect on the gastrointestinal tract that relieves diarrhea (4,7). At higher doses, anthraquinone effects seem to predominate, producing a stimulant laxative effect that relieves constipation (4,7). Anthroid laxative use is not associated with an increased risk of developing colorectal ademoma or carcinoma (6138).

Adverse Reactions

With short-term use, rhubarb can cause cramp-like or spasmodic gastrointestinal discomforts, watery diarrhea, uterine contractions, and there has been one report of anaphylaxis (2,4,12,18). Chronic use or abuse of rhubarb can cause electrolyte loss (especially potassium), hyperaldosteronism, accelerated bone deterioration, albuminuria, hematuria, dehydration, inhibition of gastric motility, pseudomelanosis coli, arrhythmias, muscular weakness, nephropathies, and edema (2,12). Chronic use of anthroid laxatives can cause pseudomelanosis coli (pigment spots in intestinal mucosa) which is harmless, usually reverses with discontinuation (2), and is not associated with an increased risk of developing colorectal ademoma or carcinoma (6138).

Interactions with Herbs & Other Dietary Supplements

CALCIUM, IRON, ZINC: Concurrent use might decrease mineral absorption. Rhubarb contains oxalate (7,12), which can bind multivalent metal ions in the gastrointestinal tract and decrease mineral absorption.

CARDIAC GLYCOSIDE-CONTAINING HERBS: Overuse of rhubarb might cause potassium depletion, increasing the risk of cardiac toxicity. Cardiac glycoside-containing herbs include black hellebore, Canadian hemp root, digitalis leaf, hedge mustard, figwort, lily of the valley roots, motherwort, oleander leaf, pheasant's eye plant, pleurisy root, squill bulb leaf scales, and strophanthus seeds (2,18,19,500).

CARDIOACTIVE HERBS: Overuse of rhubarb might cause potassium depletion increasing risk of toxicity of cardioactive herbs. These include calamus, cereus, cola, coltsfoot, devil's claw, European mistletoe, fenugreek, fumitory, ginger, ginseng Panax, hawthorn, mate, parsley, quassia, scotch broom flower, shepherd's purse, white horehound, and wild carrot (4).

STIMULANT LAXATIVE HERBS: Theoretically, concomitant use with other stimulant laxative herbs may increase the risk of potassium depletion. Stimulant laxative herbs include aloe dried leaf sap, blue flag rhizome, alder buckthorn, European buckthorn, butternut bark, cascara bark, castor oil, colocynth fruit pulp, gamboge bark exudate, jalap root, black root, manna bark exudate, podophyllum root, senna leaves and pods, wild cucumber fruit (Ecballium elaterium), and yellow dock root (19).

LICORICE/HORSETAIL: Theoretically, concomitant use with horsetail plant or licorice rhizome increases the risk of potassium depletion (19).

Interactions with Drugs

ANTIARRHYTHMIC DRUGS: Overuse of rhubarb might cause potassium depletion, increasing the risk of antiarrhythmic drug toxicity (664).

CORTICOSTEROIDS: Overuse of rhubarb might compound corticosteroid-induced potassium loss (2).

DIGOXIN: Overuse of rhubarb might cause potassium depletion, increasing the risk of digoxin toxicity (2).

LAXATIVE DRUGS: Concomitant use might compound fluid and electrolyte loss.

POTASSIUM-DEPLETING DIURETICS: Overuse of rhubarb might compound diuretic-induced potassium loss (2).

ORAL DRUGS: Concomitant use might reduce absorption of drugs due to reduced GI transit time (500).

CARDIAC GLYCOSIDES: Theoretically, overuse of rhubarb increases the risk of adverse effects of cardiac glycoside drugs, e.g. digoxin (Lanoxin).

Interactions with Foods

CALCIUM, IRON, ZINC: Concurrent use might decrease mineral absorption from foods. Rhubarb contains oxalate (7,12), which can bind multivalent metal ions in the gastrointestinal tract and decrease mineral absorption.

Interactions with Lab Tests

URINE TESTS: Rhubarb might discolor urine and interfere with diagnostic tests (2).

Interactions with Diseases or Conditions

CONSTIPATION, DIARRHEA: Can exacerbate diarrhea or constipation (4,12).

KIDNEY STONES: Rhubarb contains calcium oxalate. Use it with caution in people with a history of kidney stones (4,12).

GI CONDITIONS: Contraindicated in cases of intestinal obstruction, appendicitis, abdominal pain of unknown origin, inflammatory conditions of the intestine including Crohn's disease, colitis, and irritable bowel syndrome (IBS) (2,12).

Dosage and Administration

ORAL: Use is individualized to the smallest amount that is effective to normalize bowel movements (2). Rhubarb is used for short term use only, ideally less than eight days (2,12). When rhubarb is used for constipation, 1-4 grams of the dried root are used per day (7). When rhubarb is used for diarrhea, 100-300 mg of the dried root are used per day (7).

Comments

None.

RIBOFLAVIN (VITAMIN B2)

Also Known As

B Complex Vitamin, Flavin, Flavine, Lactoflavin, Riboflavine, Vitamin B-2, Vitamin G.

Scientific Names

Riboflavin; Vitamin B2.

People Use This For

Orally, riboflavin is used for preventing riboflavin deficiency, treating ariboflavinosis, preventing migraine headaches, treating acne, congenital methemoglobinemia, muscle cramps, burning feet syndrome, carpal tunnel syndrome, red blood cell aplasia, multiple acylcoenzyme A dehydrogenase deficiency (14,15), eye fatigue, cataracts, and glaucoma. It is also used orally for increasing energy levels; boosting immune system function; maintaining healthy hair, skin, mucous membranes, and nails; for slowing aging; canker sores; memory loss including Alzheimer's disease; ulcers; boosting athletic performance; promoting healthy reproductive function; burns; alcoholism; liver disease; sickle cell anemia (3031,3032,3033,3034); and for treating lactic acidosis induced by nucleoside analog reverse transcriptase inhibitor (NRTI) drugs (2024,6132).

Safety

LIKELY SAFE ...when used orally. No toxic effects have been reported (15,1396,1397,1398).

PREGNANCY: LIKELY SAFE ...when used orally at the recommended dietary allowance (RDA) of 1.4 mg per day (3094). There is insufficient reliable information about the safety of using larger amounts during pregnancy.

LACTATION: LIKELY SAFE ...when used orally at the recommended dietary allowance (RDA) of 1.6 mg per day (3094). There is insufficient reliable information about the safety of using larger amounts during lactation.

Effectiveness

EFFECTIVE ...when used orally for preventing riboflavin deficiency (15) and for treating ariboflavinosis (15).

POSSIBLY EFFECTIVE ...when used orally for preventing migraine headaches (1397,1398). In one human trial, riboflavin reduced headache frequency similar to the beta-blockers, bisoprolol (Zebeta) and metoprolol (Lopressor) (1396). ...when used orally to reduce the occurrence of cataracts. A large-scale population-based study found that high dietary intake of riboflavin is associated with a reduced risk of nuclear cataracts (6378).

POSSIBLY INEFFECTIVE ...when used orally for reducing severity or duration of migraine headaches, acute anti-migraine drug consumption, or migraine-associated gastrointestinal symptoms (1398).

There is insufficient reliable information available about the effectiveness of riboflavin for its other uses.

Mechanism of Action

Riboflavin is required for tissue respiration (15). It is converted to the coenzyme riboflavin 5-phosphate (flavin mononucleotide, FMN) and then to the coenzyme flavin adenine dinucleotide (FAD) (15). These act as hydrogen carriers for several enzymes known as flavoproteins, which are involved in oxidation-reduction reactions of organic substrates and in intermediary metabolism (15). Riboflavin is a cofactor for various respiratory enzymes such as glutaryl coenzyme A dehydrogenase, erythrocyte glutathione reductase, sarcosine dehydrogenase, electron-transferring flavoprotein, ETF dehydrogenase, and NADH dehydrogenase (14). It is also indirectly involved in maintaining erythrocyte integrity (15). Riboflavin deficiency, or ariboflavinosis, is characterized by cheilosis, angular stomatitis, glossitis, sore throat, keratitis, scrotal skin changes, neuropathy, and seborrheic dermatitis (14,15). In severe cases there is a normocytic and normochromic anemia (15). Riboflavin deficiency can occur in people with long-standing infections such as HIV-1, liver disease, alcoholism, malignancy, and in those taking probenecid (15). Researchers think that riboflavin deficiency might contribute to lactic acidosis that can occur in HIV patients taking stavudine (d4T, Zerit), zidovudine (AZT, Retrovir) and similar nucleoside analog reverse transcriptase inhibitor (NRTI) drugs (2024). Although NRTI-induced lactic acidosis has been considered irreversible and fatal, riboflavin reportedly can reverse this condition in some patients (2024).

Adverse Reactions

Orally, large doses of riboflavin (400 mg per day) might cause diarrhea and polyuria (1398). Riboflavin can cause a yellow-orange discoloration of the urine (14).

Interactions with Herbs & Other Dietary Supplements

Insufficient reliable information available.

Interactions with Drugs

ASPIRIN: Concomitant use might cause gastric intolerance. One participant taking riboflavin 400 mg/day plus aspirin 75 mg/day withdrew from a study after two weeks due to gastric intolerance (1397).
BETA-BLOCKERS: Theoretically, concomitant use of riboflavin and beta-blockers might enhance migraine prevention without increasing adverse effects. Clinical data suggest that riboflavin and the beta-blockers, bisoprolol and metoprolol, might prevent migraines by two different pathophysiological mechanisms (1396). Beta-blockers include atenolol (Tenormin), bisoprolol (Zebeta), metoprolol (Lopressor), nadolol (Corgard), propranolol (Inderal), and timolol (Blocadren).
LAMIVUDINE (3TC, Epivir), STAVUDINE (d4T, Zerit), ZIDOVUDINE (AZT, Retrovir): Riboflavin is reported to reverse the lactic acidosis caused by nucleoside reverse transcriptase inhibitor (NRTI)-type antiretroviral drugs, including lamivudine, stavudine, and zidovudine (2024,6132).
PROBENECID (Benemid): Decreases riboflavin absorption (15).
PROPANTHELINE (Pro-Banthine): Delays and increases riboflavin absorption (15).

Drug Influences on Nutrient Levels and Depletion

SOME DRUGS CAN AFFECT RIBOFLAVIN LEVELS:
ANTIBIOTICS: Destruction of normal gastrointestinal flora by antibiotics can cause decreased production of B vitamins. The clinical significance of this decreased production is not know. Consider supplementation only if clinical judgment warrants it (4434,4435,4436,4437,4438,4439,4440,4441,4442,4443).
METOCLOPRAMIDE (Reglan, Maxeran): Concomitant use can decrease riboflavin absorption in the gastrointestinal tract. The need for supplementation has not been adequately studied. Consider supplementation only if clinical judgment warrants it (4561).
ORAL CONTRACEPTIVES: Use of oral contraceptives can reduce serum vitamin B2 levels. The mechanism of this interaction is unknown. The need for supplementation has not been adequately studied (4548).
PHENOTHIAZINES: Use of phenothiazines can increase urinary vitamin B2 excretion and reduce serum vitamin B2 levels. The need for supplementation has not been adequately studied, although doses of 2-5 mg/day of riboflavin have been used (4425).
PROBENECID (Benemid): Probenecid inhibits dietary vitamin B2 absorption. The clinical relevance and the need for supplementation has not been adequately studied (15).
PROPANTHELINE BROMIDE (Pro-Banthine): Propantheline bromide delays and increases supplemental riboflavin absorption (15). The clinical relevance of this interaction has not been adequately studied (15).

Interactions with Foods

FOOD: Increases riboflavin absorption (15).

Interactions with Lab Tests

ACETOACETATE DECARBOXYLASE: Riboflavin can falsely increase serum acetoacetate decarboxylase test results, due to enzyme activation (275).
CATECHOLAMINES: Riboflavin can falsely elevate plasma and urine fluorometric catecholamine test results, due to fluorescent substances it produces in the plasma and urine (15,275).
COLORIMETRIC TESTS: Large amounts of riboflavin can interfere with urinalysis based on spectrometry or color reactions. Large amounts of riboflavin cause bright yellow urine (15,275).
DIAGNEX BLUE EXCRETION: Riboflavin can falsely increase urine diagnex blue excretion test results, by color interference (275).
DRUGS-OF-ABUSE ASSAYS: Large doses of riboflavin (200 mg twice daily) cause errors in Abbott TDx drugs-of-abuse urine assays. Riboflavin produces a fluorophore that competes with the fluorescein-labeled antibody used in the assay (1266).
UROBILINOGEN: Riboflavin can falsely increase plasma and urine fluorometric urobilinogen test results, due to fluorescent substances it produces in the plasma and urine (15,275).

Interactions with Diseases or Conditions
HEPATITIS, CIRRHOSIS, BILIARY OBSTRUCTION: Riboflavin absorption is decreased in these conditions (15).

Dosage and Administration
ORAL: As a dietary supplement, 1-4 mg a day is generally sufficient (15). For riboflavin deficiency in adults, 5-30 mg is taken daily in divided doses (15). For multiple acylcoenzyme A dehydrogenase deficiency, the usual dose is 100 mg one to three times daily (14). For preventing migraine headaches, a dose of 400 mg per day has been used (1396,1397,1398), and maximum benefit might take up to three months to achieve (1398). A daily dietary intake of approximately 2.6 mg of riboflavin has been associated with reduced risk of nuclear cataracts (6378).

The daily recommended dietary allowances (RDAs) of riboflavin are: Infants 0-6 months, 0.3 mg; Infants 7-12 months, 0.4 mg; Children 1-3 years, 0.5 mg; Children 4-8 years, 0.6 mg; Children 9-13 years, 0.9 mg; Men 14 years or older, 1.3 mg; Women 14-18 years, 1 mg; Women over 18 years, 1.1 mg; Pregnant women, 1.4 mg; and Lactating women, 1.6 mg (3094). For treating stavudine or zidovudine-induced lactic acidosis, 50 mg per day has been used (2024,6132).

Comments
Riboflavin is found in many foods including milk, meat, eggs, nuts, enriched flour, and green vegetables (15). Riboflavin is frequently used in combination with other B vitamins in vitamin B complex formulations. Vitamin B complex generally includes vitamin B1 (thiamine), vitamin B2 (riboflavin), vitamin B3 (niacin/niacinamide), vitamin B5 (pantothenic acid), vitamin B6 (pyridoxine), vitamin B12 (cyanocobalamin), and folic acid. However, some products do not contain all of these ingredients and some may include others, such as biotin, para-aminobenzoic acid (PABA), choline bitartrate, and inositol (3022,3060,3061).

RIBOSE

Also Known As
D-ribose.

Scientific Names
Beta-D-ribofuranose.

People Use This For
Orally, ribose is used to increase muscle function (5673), recovery (5671,5672,5673), athletic performance (5672,5673,5675), boost muscle tissue energy (5670,5671), and enhance effectiveness of creatine, maximize ribose production, replenish ATP stores (5668,5671), and improve or maintain nucleotide salvage and/or synthesis in heart and skeletal muscles following high intensity exercise (5668,5674). It has also been used to improve exercise tolerance (5669), maintain or increase energy stores in the heart or muscle cells (5667), and improve quality of life (5668) in individuals with reduced myocardial blood flow such as improving the heart's tolerance to ischemia in patients with coronary artery disease (5664). Oral ribose has been used to prevent symptoms such as cramping, pain and stiffness after exercise in patients with myoadenylate deaminase deficiency (MAD) (5676,5677,5679,5680), also known as AMP deaminase deficiency (AMPD deficiency) (5681). Ribose has also been used to improve exercise tolerance in patients with McArdle's disease (5678).
Intravenously, ribose has been used to facilitate thallium-201 redistribution and improve imaging of ischemic myocardium in patients with coronary artery disease (5661,5662,5663). It has also been used intravenously in patients with MAD to prevent symptoms such as cramping, pain and stiffness (5676).

Safety
POSSIBLY SAFE ...when used orally or intravenously and appropriately, short-term (5661,5662,5663,5664,5676,5677,5679,5680). There is insufficient reliable information available about the safety of ribose for its other uses.
PREGNANCY AND LACTATION: Insufficient reliable information available; avoid using.

Effectiveness
LIKELY EFFECTIVE ...when used intravenously to facilitate thallium-201 redistribution and improve imaging of ischemic myocardium in patients with coronary artery disease. Studies show ribose accelerates clearance of thallium-201 from normal, nonischemic regions of coronary arteries (5661,5662,5663).
POSSIBLY EFFECTIVE ...when used orally to improve the heart's tolerance to ischemia in patients with coronary artery disease. A small randomized and placebo controlled study showed increased time to onset of moderate angina and time to ST depression during treadmill walking exercise testing in patients with coronary artery disease (5664).
...when used orally or intravenously to prevent symptoms such as cramping, pain and stiffness after exercise in patients with myoadenylate deaminase deficiency (MAD), also known as AMP deaminase deficiency (AMPD deficiency). One case report and a small clinical study suggest symptoms can be prevented with administration of ribose before and

during exercise (5677,5679).

LIKELY INEFFECTIVE ...when used orally to improve exercise tolerance in patients with McArdle's disease. A double blind placebo controlled crossover trial reported no benefit to patients with McArdle's disease (5678). There is insufficient reliable information available about the effectiveness of ribose for its other uses.

Mechanism of Action

Ribose, a pentose sugar which is usually supplied by the oxidative pentose phosphate pathway (PPP) (also known as the hexose monophosphate shunt), is rapidly taken up by cells and phosphorylated to ribose-5-phosphate (5653). Ribose is rate-limiting in the production of phosphoribosyl-pyrophosphate (PRPP) (5652,5653,5682), a precursor for the salvage and de-novo adenine nucleotide synthetic pathways which maintain adenine, ADP, and AMP levels for the resynthesis of ATP (5651,5652,5665,5682). High energy bonds of ATP are the direct source for myocardial contractions (5652). During ischemia, the levels of ATP in the myocardium fall as the rate of oxidative phosphorylation decreases (5651,5653) and do not recover if the period of no perfusion is too long (5651). ADP and AMP levels rise transiently during ischemia but decrease as they are dephosphorylated into metabolites (adenine, inosine and hypoxanthine) which easily diffuse through the cell membrane and are washed out of the myocardium during reperfusion (5652,5653). Since the metabolites which use the salvage synthetic pathway are no longer available as precursors for ATP resynthesis, the de-novo synthetic pathway is activated (5652). Restoration of ATP levels via this pathway is slow in comparison to the salvage pathway (5652,5664) due to the short supply of PRPP which is usually supplied by the oxidative pentose phosphate pathway (5664). Studies suggest that this also occurs during ischemic events after high intensity exercise in skeletal muscle (5656,5657,5658). Evidence suggests exogenous ribose bypasses the PPP when it is converted to ribose-5-phosphate, increasing the amount of PRPP available for the de-novo synthetic pathway and ultimately resulting in the repletion of ATP levels in the myocardium (5652). Animal studies suggest exogenous ribose with adenine improves myocardial ATP, ADP and adenine nucleotide recovery after moderate periods of ischemia and improves recovery of contractile myocardial function (5652,5653). Other animal studies suggest exogenous ribose given during both periods of ischemia and reperfusion significantly increases ATP levels (5659) and may shorten ATP recovery time (5654,5659,5660). There have been no human studies done to confirm these findings. Laboratory evidence also suggests ribose may have a role in preserving hearts for transplantation by maintaining ATP levels (5666). Controlled human studies have established that infusion of ribose facilitates the distribution and accelerates the clearance of thallium-201 from normal (nonischemic) regions of the coronary artery, leaving only thallium-201 in ischemic myocardium (5661,5662,5663). The mechanism of action on how this occurs is unknown (5662). A small, randomized, placebo study controlled reported oral ribose given to patients with coronary artery disease may improve their tolerance to ischemia during exercise (5664). Other studies suggest oral ribose may prevent exercise-induced muscle pain and stiffness in patients with myoadenylate deaminase deficiency (5677,5676,5679,5680). Randomized, prospective controlled human studies are needed to establish the mechanism of action and the effectiveness of exogenous ribose when used to improve tolerance to exercise-induced ischemia in healthy individuals and patients with unstable cardiac condition such as coronary artery disease.

Adverse Reactions

Orally, ribose can cause diarrhea (5676), decreased blood glucose levels (5667), gastrointestinal discomfort, nausea and headache (5664). Hypoglycemia (5650,5662,5676), slightly increased serum insulin levels (5663) and decreased serum phosphate (5650) have been reported after infusion of ribose.

Interactions with Herbs & Other Dietary Supplements

Insufficient reliable information available.

Interactions with Drugs

INSULIN: Theoretically, ribose may increase the hypoglycemic effect of insulin and should be avoided by people taking insulin.

ORAL ANTIHYPERGLYCEMIC AGENTS: Theoretically, ribose may increase the hypoglycemic effect of oral antihyperglycemic agents such at the sulfonylureas, biguanides, alfa-glucosidase inhibitors, thiazolidinediones and meglitinides.

SALICYLATES: Theoretically, ribose may enhance the hypoglycemic effects of salicylates.

MAOIs: Theoretically, ribose may enhance the hypoglycemic effects of MAOIs.

OTHER AGENTS WHICH MAY CAUSE HYPOGLYCEMIA: Theoretically, ribose may increase the hypoglycemic effect of other agents such as ethanol and propranolol. Individuals taking any agents which may cause hypoglycemia should avoid taking ribose.

Interactions with Foods

No interactions are known to occur, and there is no known reason to expect a clinically significant interaction with ribose.

Interactions with Lab Tests

GLUCOSE: Ribose may decrease serum glucose levels (5650,5662,5667,5676).
PHOSPHATE: Ribose may decrease serum phosphate levels (5650).
INSULIN: Ribose may increase serum insulin levels (5663).

Interactions with Diseases or Conditions

HYPOGLYCEMIA: Theoretically, ribose should be avoided in patients who have hypoglycemia, or diseases or conditions that may increase their risk for hypoglycemia.
DIABETES: Theoretically, ribose should be avoided in patients with diabetes since it may interfere and enhance the glucose lowering effects of insulin or any oral antihyperglycemic agents.

Dosage and Administration

ORAL: People typically take 2.2 grams per day 30 minutes following exercise or before bedtime on days with no scheduled exercise. Individuals who feel they are overly tired or are concerned about their energy stores typically take 2.2-3.0 grams twice per day or adjust to perceived benefit. A dose typically may be taken before exercise and additional doses of 1.0-2.2 grams may be taken every hour of exercise (5668).
To improve exercise tolerance in patients with coronary artery disease, 15 grams four times per day has been used (5664). Beginning 1 hour before exercise until the end of the exercise session, 3 grams every 10 minutes has been used to reduce exercise-induced symptoms such as muscle stiffness and cramps associated with myoadenylate deaminase deficiency (5679).
INTRAVENOUS: For imaging of coronary arteries using thallium-201, a 30 minute 3.3 mg/kg/minute infusion of ribose as a 10% solution has been used (5662,5663).
No typical dosage information is available for other indications.

Comments

There are some preparations available containing both ribose and creatine (5673).

RICE BRAN

Also Known As

Dietary Fiber, Stabilized Rice Bran, Ricebran Oil, Rice Bran Oil.
CAUTION: See separate listings for Oat Bran and Wheat Bran.

Scientific Names

Oryza sativa.

People Use This For

Orally, rice bran is used for diabetes, hypertension, hyperlipidemia, alcoholism, weight loss, AIDS, preventing cancer, strengthening the immune system, increasing energy, enhancing athletic performance, aiding and improving liver function, preventing cardiovascular disease, and as an antioxidant (863). Rice bran oil is also used orally for hyperlipidemia (1354).
Topically, rice bran is used for ectopic dermatitis (872).

Safety

LIKELY SAFE ...when used orally and appropriately. Rice bran and rice bran oil have been used safely in studies lasting up to 5 years (865,876,877,880,1354).
POSSIBLY SAFE ...when used as a bath additive. There is some evidence that a therapeutic bath containing rice bran broth can be safely used (872).
PREGNANCY AND LACTATION: LIKELY SAFE ...when used orally in amounts found in foods (272). There is insufficient reliable information available about the safety of rice brand when used for medicinal purposes during pregnancy and lactation; avoid using.

Effectiveness

POSSIBLY EFFECTIVE ...when used orally for moderate hypercholesterolemia (865,877). In one study, rice bran was compared to oat and wheat bran for decreasing serum cholesterol. Each fiber was given as part of the diet at 11.8 grams per day for 4 weeks. Only oat bran significantly lowered total cholesterol, but rice bran exerted a mild effect (877). In another study, a higher dose of 84 grams per day was used and full-fat rice bran was compared to oat bran and placebo administered over 6 weeks in combination with a low-fat diet. Rice bran significantly lowered low-density lipoprotein (LDL) and total cholesterol. Triglycerides and high-density lipoprotein (HDL) levels were not affected. Oat bran produced a slightly greater decrease in cholesterol (877). Rice bran oil has also been shown to be beneficial for hypercholesterolemia. In a one-year clinical trial, rice bran oil non-saponifiables reduced total cholesterol by 14%, LDL cholesterol by 20%, triglycerides by 20%, and increased HDL cholesterol by 41% (1354). Lipid lowering effects have not been demonstrated in men without high lipid levels (873). ...when used orally to reduce urine calcium excretion and stone formation in people with hypercalciuria (876,878,880,881,882). ...when used orally in combination with cholestyramine to increase fecal excretion of polychlorinated biphenyl (PCB) and polychlorinated dibenzofuran (PCDF) in people who have ingested these chemicals (867,870). ...when rice bran broth is used topically to treat symptoms of atopic dermatitis (872).

There is insufficient reliable information available about the effectiveness of rice bran for its other uses.

Mechanism of Action

Rice bran contains 21% fiber, 21% lipids, 13% amino acids, and a wide variety of vitamins and minerals (864,884,885). Rice bran oil contains gamma oryzanol (871,879), tocopherols, tocotrienols, unsaturated fatty acids (877), and other non-saponifiable constituents (1354). The hypercholesterolemic effect of fiber has been attributed primarily to soluble forms of fiber. It is thought that soluble fiber adsorbs bile, preventing bile acid reabsorption, and decreasing cholesterol absorption. This results in upregulation of low-density lipoprotein (LDL) receptors and increased catabolism of LDL cholesterol (877). However, most of the fiber in rice bran is insoluble. Rice bran contains significantly less soluble fiber than oat bran. The unusually high amount of oil contained in rice bran is thought to contribute significantly to its antihypercholesterolemic effects, due to non-saponifiable constituents or the fatty acid content (877). Rice bran can increase stool size by several mechanisms, including water retention (871,879). Scientists think increased fecal bulk reduces risk of cancer because it dilutes carcinogens, especially tumor promoters such as secondary bile acids (871). Diets high in fiber have resulted in lower insulin levels, less weight gain, and a reduction in cardiovascular disease risk factors such as hypertension and adverse cholesterol profile (2737). Rice bran reduces the risk of recurrent urinary stone disease, perhaps because the phytin in rice bran reduces calcium absorption (881). Healthy women on a calcium-rich diet, who added rice bran to their diets decreased renal excretion of calcium and increased renal excretion of oxalic acid (874). A rice bran isolate designated as Compound X shows evidence of antihistamine activity. It also inhibits bacterial growth (884). A modified rice bran isolate, MGN-3 (see separate listing), exhibits anti-HIV activity (866).

Adverse Reactions

Increasing the amount of bran in the diet can cause erratic bowel habits, flatulence, and abdominal discomfort during the first few weeks (272). Topical use of rice bran broth baths can cause itching and skin redness (872). Rash and itching from rice bran has been associated in rare cases from contact infestation with Pyemotes tritici, an arthropod commonly called straw itch mite (2284).

Interactions with Herbs & Other Dietary Supplements

HERBS AND SUPPLEMENTS: Theoretically, a diet high in rice bran might slow or reduce the absorption of some herbs and supplements.

Interactions with Drugs

ORAL DRUGS: Theoretically, a diet high in rice bran might slow or reduce the absorption of some oral drugs.
DIGOXIN: Theoretically, rice bran may interfere with digoxin absorption (156).

Interactions with Foods

NUTRIENTS: Theoretically, a diet high in rice bran might slow or reduce the absorption of nutrients in foods.
IRON: Fiber inhibits dietary iron absorption (156).

Interactions with Lab Tests

No interactions are known to occur, and there is no known reason to expect a clinically significant interaction with rice bran.

Interactions with Diseases or Conditions

HYPOCALCEMIA: Rice bran can decrease dietary absorption of calcium (272); avoid concurrent administration of rice bran and calcium replacement therapy.
LOW IRON LEVELS: Rice bran can decrease dietary absorption of iron (272); avoid concurrent administration of rice bran and iron replacement therapy.
GASTROINTESTINAL CONDITIONS: Contraindicated in people with intestinal ulcerations, stenosis, disabling adhesions, cathartic colon or other conditions that may result in intestinal or esophageal obstruction (272). Use with caution or avoid in people with difficulty chewing or swallowing food, or conditions that decrease small bowel motility (272).

Dosage and Administration

ORAL: For reducing cholesterol, 12-84 grams rice bran per day (865,877), or 4.8 grams rice bran oil (providing 312 mg tocotrienols, 360 mg tocopherols, and 2.4 grams other non-saponifiables) per day has been used (1354). For reducing the risk of kidney stones, 10 grams rice bran twice daily has been used (881,882). For decontamination of ingested polychlorinated biphenyl (PCB) and polychlorinated dibenzofuran (PCDF), 10 grams rice bran with a dietary fiber content 50% and 4 grams cholestyramine (Questran) three times a dayhas been used (870).

Comments
Rice bran is the outer grain hull of rice (Oryza sativa) (515) and is also referred to as stabilized rice bran.

RNA AND DNA

Also Known As
DNA, DeoxyNucleic Acid, Nuclei Acids, Nucleic, Nucleic Acid, Nucleic Acids, Nucleotides, Purines, Pyrimidines, RNA, RNA-DNA, RNA/DNA.

Scientific Names
Deoxyribonucleic Acid; Ribonucleic Acid.

People Use This For
Orally, RNA/DNA combinations are used to improve memory and mental sharpness (5529), to treat or prevent Alzheimer's disease (5528), to treat depression, increase energy, tighten skin, increase sex drive, and to counteract the effects of aging (5529,5530,5901).
Enterally, RNA is used in nutrition formulations that include omega-3 fatty acids and arginine for reducing the time needed for recovery after surgery (5531,5534), to boost immune response (5532,5533), and to improve outcomes of burn patients (5535) and intensive care patients (5536).
In Chinese medicine, RNA is used as a subcutaneous injection to treat eczema, psoriasis, hives, and shingles (5538).

Safety
LIKELY SAFE ...when RNA and DNA are consumed in food. ...when RNA is used in enteral nutrition along with omega-3 fatty acids and arginine (5531,5533,5534,5535,5536).
POSSIBLY SAFE ...when RNA is injected subcutaneously (5538).
There is insufficient reliable information available about the safety of oral RNA/DNA supplement combinations.
CHILDREN: LIKELY SAFE ...when infant formulas contain nucleotide supplements (5900).
PREGNANCY AND LACTATION: LIKELY SAFE ...when RNA and DNA are consumed in food. POSSIBLY UNSAFE ...when used orally as supplements. Some evidence suggests some orally ingested DNA might cross the placenta and be mutagenic (5539).

Effectiveness
POSSIBLY EFFECTIVE ...when RNA is used enterally to reduce the recovery time after surgery or serious illness and to boost the immune response (5531,5532,5533). ...when nucleotide supplements are used in infant formula to boost immune response (5900).
POSSIBLY INEFFECTIVE ...in producing better outcome in burn patients than standard nutritional formulas (5535).

Mechanism of Action
Although most organisms can synthesize nucleotides (5900), dietary nucleotides (derived from DNA and RNA) appear to be essential under conditions of rapid growth such as intestinal development, liver resection or injury and also during challenges to the immune system. When preformed nucleotides are consumed, they are degraded to free bases in the intestine before absorption. Experimental evidence shows they are incorporated into the hepatic pyrimidine nucleotide pool (5900) and that they affect the hepatic RNA content. The hepatic RNA content, in turn, affects the recovery time from liver injury. In protein-deprived animals, dietary nucleotides appear to benefit the intestinal tract. They can also restore immune function, while restoring the nitrogen balance (protein intake) does not (5543). In the absence of nucleotides, normal T-lymphocyte maturation is blocked (5543). A Crohn's disease model in rats shows RNA has a highly significant effect upon the healing intestinal ulcerations (5900). Supplementing an enteral diet with arginine, RNA, and omega-3 fatty acids can reduce concentrations of tumor necrosis factor alpha, and interleukin-6 and accelerate the recovery in the concentration of interleukin-1 beta and interleukin-2 alpha receptor (5532).

Adverse Reactions
A subcutaneous injection of RNA can cause itching, redness, and swelling at the injection site (5538).

Interactions with Herbs & Other Dietary Supplements
Insufficient reliable information available.

Interactions with Drugs

No interactions are known to occur, and there is no known reason to expect a clinically significant interaction with RNA and DNA.

Interactions with Foods

No interactions are known to occur, and there is no known reason to expect a clinically significant interaction with RNA and DNA.

Interactions with Lab Tests

No interactions are known to occur, and there is no known reason to expect a clinically significant interaction with RNA and DNA.

Interactions with Diseases or Conditions

No interactions are known to occur, and there is no known reason to expect a clinically significant interaction with RNA and DNA.

Dosage and Administration

ORAL: A typical oral dose of RNA/DNA is 1-1.5 grams/day (5530).
ENTERAL: A typical enteral dose of RNA is 30 mg/kg/day along with arginine and omega-3 fatty acids (5533,5534).
INJECTION: A typical dose is 10 mg injectable RNA every other day for 2-4 weeks (5538).

Comments

RNA/DNA can be derived from cultivated brewer's yeast (5529) or salmon (5530).

ROMAN CHAMOMILE

Also Known As

Chamomile, Chamomilla, Chamomillae ramane flos, English Chamomile, Fleur De Camomille Romaine, Flores Anthemidis, Garden Chamomile, Grosse Kamille, Ground Apple, Low Chamomile, Manzanilla, Römische Kamille, Sweet Chamomile, Whig Plant.
CAUTION: See separate listing for German Chamomile.

Scientific Names

Chamaemelum nobile, synonym Athemis nobilis.
Family: Asteraceae or Compositae.

People Use This For

Orally, Roman chamomile is used for indigestion, nausea and vomiting, anorexia, morning sickness, painful menstrual periods, flatulent indigestion associated with mental stress, inflammation of the oral and pharyngeal cavities, nasal mucous membrane inflammation, and sinusitis.

Topically, Roman chamomile is used for eczema, wounds, and inflammation. The extract of Roman chamomile is used topically in antiseptic ointments, creams, and gels to treat cracked nipples, sore gums, inflammations, and irritation of the skin and mucosa.

In oral herbal combinations, Roman chamomile is used for liver and gallbladder disease, gallstones, fatty liver, chronic heartburn, loss of appetite, bloating, upset stomach, digestive disturbances, Roemheld's syndrome, flatulent indigestion, indigestion in infants, and in spastic constipation. It is used as a "blood purification" remedy, a general tonic during puberty and menopause, a preventative for menstrual discomforts, for missed periods, and insufficient or irregular periods.

In herbal inhalation therapy, Roman chamomile is used as steam baths for frontal sinus mucous membrane inflammation, hay fever, nasal and pharyngeal mucosal swelling, and inflammation of the ears.

In topical herbal combinations, Roman chamomile is used for wounds, burns, frostbite, diaper rash on infants and toddlers, decubitus ulcers, and hemorrhoids.

In aromatherapy, chamomile is used topically and by inhalation as an analgesic.

Historically, Roman chamomile has been used to treat digestive and rheumatic disorders. Teas have also been used as a hair tint and conditioner, and to treat parasitic worm infections.

In foods and beverages, the essential oil and extract are used as flavor components.

In manufacturing, the volatile oil of Roman chamomile is used as a fragrance component in soaps, cosmetics, and perfumes; and to flavor cigarette tobacco. The extract is also used in cosmetics, soaps, and other personal care products.

Safety

LIKELY SAFE ...when used orally in amounts found in foods. It has Generally Recognized as Safe (GRAS) status in the US (11). The maximum use level is 0.002% for the oil (11).
POSSIBLY SAFE ...when used orally and appropriately in medicinal amounts (2,12). ...when the essential oil is inhaled or used topically as aromatherapy (7107).
PREGNANCY: LIKELY UNSAFE ...when used orally in medicinal amounts. Roman chamomile is believed to be an abortifacient (4). There is insufficient reliable information available about the safety of the topical use of Roman chamomile during pregnancy; avoid using.
LACTATION: Insufficient reliable information available; avoid using (4).

Effectiveness

There is insufficient reliable information available about the effectiveness of Roman chamomile.

Mechanism of Action

The applicable part of Roman chamomile is the flowerhead. Roman chamomile possesses antiflatulent, antispasmodic, and sedative properties (4). Large amounts of Roman chamomile can act as an emetic while small amounts act as an anti-emetic (4). In cosmetics, Roman chamomile is considered a deodorant and a stimulant to skin metabolism (11). Roman chamomile contains the coumarin scopoletin-7-glucoside and varied flavonoids, their glycosides (including rutin and volatile oils), as well as other constituents (4). Some evidence suggests azulene constituents contained in volatile oils exert anti-allergy and anti-inflammatory effects by inhibiting histamine release. However, the constituent nobilin, a sesquiterpene lactone, is thought to trigger allergy in sensitive individuals (4). Some evidence suggests Roman chamomile acts on the central nervous system, possibly reducing aggressive behavior (18). Experimental evidence suggests the volatile oil could have anti-inflammatory, antidiuretic, and sedative effects (4). The essential oil is active against gram-positive bacteria and dermatomyces (18). The sesquiterpinoids nobilin, 1,10-epoxynobilin, and 3-dehydronobilin show some evidence of antitumor activity (4). Although the constituents of Roman chamomile are not identical to those of German chamomile both plants are similarly used (512).

Adverse Reactions

Orally, large amounts of Roman chamomile might cause vomiting (11), although this is disputed (12).
Topically, Roman chamomile can cause contact dermatitis (4,567). Allergic skin reactions occur in up to 20% of individuals (19). It can cause an allergic reaction in individuals sensitive to the Asteraceae/Compositae family. Members of this family include ragweed, chrysanthemums, marigolds, daisies, and many other herbs. It can also cause rhinitis in individuals with atopic allergy to mugwort (2).

Interactions with Herbs & Other Dietary Supplements

HERBS WITH ANTICOAGULANT/ANTIPLATELET POTENTIAL: Concomitant use of herbs that have coumarin constituents or affect platelet aggregation could theoretically increase the risk of bleeding in some people. These herbs include: angelica, anise, arnica, asafoetida, bogbean, boldo, capsicum, celery, clove, danshen, fenugreek, feverfew, garlic, ginger, ginkgo, ginseng (Panax), horse chestnut, horseradish, licorice, meadowsweet, prickly ash, onion, papain, passionflower, poplar, quassia, red clover, turmeric, wild carrot, wild lettuce, willow, and others (4,19).

Interactions with Drugs

ANTICOAGULANTS: Theoretically, concomitant use might potentiate effects and adverse effects of anticoagulants (4).

Interactions with Foods

No interactions are known to occur, and there is no known reason to expect a clinically significant interaction with Roman chamomile.

Interactions with Lab Tests

No interactions are known to occur, and there is no known reason to expect a clinically significant interaction with Roman chamomile.

Interactions with Diseases or Conditions

ASTHMA: May exacerbate asthma (4).
CROSS-ALLERGENICITY: Can cause an allergic reaction in individuals sensitive to the Asteraceae/Compositae family. Members of this family include ragweed, chrysanthemums, marigolds, daisies, and many other herbs. Can cause rhinitis in individuals with atopic allergy to mugwort (2).

Dosage and Administration

ORAL: A typical dose is 1-4 grams dried flowerheads three times daily, or one cup tea. To make tea, steep 1-4 grams dried flowerheads in 150 mL of boiling water for 5-10 minutes, strain (4). Liquid extract (1:1 in 70% alcohol), 1-4 mL three times daily (4).

TOPICAL: A 3% steeped tea is prepared for topical use (8).

Comments

Though widely used, there is very little information about Roman chamomile. Most of the existing information concerns German chamomile (4,7) but it is extrapolated to Roman chamomile.

ROSE GERANIUM

Also Known As

Aetheroleum Pelargonii, Algerian Geranium Oil, Bourbon Geranium Oil, Moroccan Geranium Oil, Oleum Geranii, Pelargonium Oil.

Scientific Names

Pelargonium graveolens.
Family: Geraniaceae.

People Use This For

In African traditional medicine, the roots of various Pelargoinum species are used as astringents and for diarrhea.

In foods and beverages, rose geranium oil is used as a flavoring agent (11).

In manufacturing, rose geranium oil is used as an inexpensive substitute for rose oil (11). It is also used as a fragrance component in soaps, cosmetics, and perfumes (11).

Safety

LIKELY SAFE ...when used in amounts found in foods (11). It has Generally Recognized as Safe (GRAS) status in the US (11).

PREGNANCY AND LACTATION: Insufficient reliable information; avoid amounts greater than found in foods.

Effectiveness

There is insufficient reliable information about the effectiveness of rose geranium.

Mechanism of Action

The applicable part of rose geranium is the oil that is distilled from the stem and leaf. The geranium oil constituents citronellol, citronellyl acetate, citronellyl formate, and geraniol exhibit marginal antitumor activity (3751). The essential oils from Pelargonium species show some indication of antibacterial and antifungal activity (3752,3753).

Adverse Reactions

Geranium oil has been associated with dermatitis in hypersensitive individuals (11), however, geranium is generally considered to be nonsensitizing, nonirritating, and nonphototoxic to human skin (11).

Interactions with Herbs & Other Dietary Supplements

Insufficient reliable information available.

Interactions with Drugs

No interactions are known to occur, and there is no known reason to expect a clinically significant interaction with rose geranium.

Interactions with Foods

No interactions are known to occur, and there is no known reason to expect a clinically significant interaction with rose geranium.

Interactions with Lab Tests

No interactions are known to occur, and there is no known reason to expect a clinically significant interaction with rose geranium.

Interactions with Diseases or Conditions

No interactions are known to occur, and there is no known reason to expect a clinically significant interaction with rose geranium.

Dosage and Administration

No typical dosage.

Comments

Avoid confusing rose geranium oil with East Indian or Turkish geranium oil (known as palmorosa oil) that is derived from a different plant (11).

ROSE HIP

Also Known As

Cynosbatos, Dog Rose, Heps, Hip, Hip Fruit, Hip Sweet, Hipberry, Hop Fruit, Rosa de castillo, Rosae pseudofructus cum semen, Rose Hip with seed, Rose Hips, Rosehips, Wild Boar Fruit.
CAUTION: See separate listings for Acerola, Vitamin C, and Cherokee Rosehip.

Scientific Names

Rosa canina; other Rosa species including Rosa alba, Rosa centifolia, Rosa damascena; Rosa gallica; Rosa rugosa; Rosa villosa, synonym Rosa pomifera.
Family: Rosaceae.

People Use This For

Orally, rose hip is used as a supplemental source of dietary vitamin C (6,11) and for preventing and treating colds, influenza-like infections, infectious diseases, vitamin C deficiencies, fever, increasing immune function during exhaustion, gastric spasms, gastric acid deficiency, preventing gastric mucosal inflammation and gastric ulcers, and as a "stomach tonic" for intestinal diseases. It is also used orally for diarrhea, gallstones, gallbladder ailments, lower urinary tract and kidney disorders, dropsy (edema), gout, disorders of uric acid metabolism, arthritis, sciatica, diabetes, increasing peripheral circulation, for reducing thirst (6), and as a laxative and diuretic (2).
In folk medicine, rose hip is used to treat chest ailments (6).
In foods and in manufacturing, it is used for rose hip tea, jam and soup (5,8), and as a natural source of vitamin C (11).

Safety

LIKELY SAFE ...when consumed in amounts commonly found in foods (11). Rosa alba, Rosa centifiolia, Rosa damascena, and Rosa gallica have Generally Recognized as Safe (GRAS) status for food use in the US (11).
POSSIBLY SAFE ...when used orally and appropriately for medicinal purposes (12).
PREGNANCY AND LACTATION: Insufficient reliable information available; avoid using in amounts greater than those found in foods.

Effectiveness

POSSIBLY INEFFECTIVE ...when the dry rose hips and powder are used orally as sources of vitamin C for treating or preventing vitamin C deficiency and other uses (2). Much of the vitamin C is destroyed during drying, processing, and in storage (2,11).
There is insufficient reliable information available about the effectiveness of rose hip for its other uses.

Mechanism of Action

Rose hip contains pectin, citric acid, and malic acid, which can have laxative and diuretic activities (5,18). The diuretic activity is controversial (8). Fresh rose hip contains between 0.5-1.7% vitamin C (5,8) and is estimated to contain 1250 mg vitamin C per 100 grams of rose hip (6). However, much of the vitamin C is destroyed during drying and processing (11), and declines rapidly with storage (2). Vitamin C is required for collagen formation and tissue repair (15). It is an enzyme cofactor in the synthesis of collagen, carnitine, norepinephrine, and peptide hormones, and in tyrosine metabolism (3042). Vitamin C is also involved in oxidation-reduction reactions, conversion of folic acid to folinic acid, carbohydrate metabolism, synthesis of lipids and proteins, iron metabolism, resistance to infections, and cellular respiration (15). It acts as an antioxidant, decreasing oxidants in gastric juice, decreasing lipid peroxidation, and decreasing oxidative DNA and protein damage (3042). Vitamin C deficiency that lasts for three to five months results in symptomatic scurvy that affects collagenous structures, bones, and blood vessels (15). Vitamin C enhances the absorption of soluble non-heme iron, either by reducing it (converting ferric to ferrous) or by preventing chelation by phytates or other food ligands (14,3042). The interaction between iron salts and vitamin C can be variable (14).

Adverse Reactions

Orally, the adverse effects of vitamin C are related to the amount of vitamin C actually contained in the rose hip product (see Effectiveness). The adverse reactions include nausea, vomiting, esophagitis, heartburn, abdominal cramps, GI obstruction, fatigue, flushing, headache, insomnia, sleepiness, diarrhea, hyperoxaluria, precipitation of urate, oxalate, or cysteine stones or drugs in the urinary tract (14,15). Large amounts are associated with deep vein thrombosis (15). The inhalation of the rose hip dust is reportedly a respiratory allergen in production workers. It can cause mild to moderate anaphylaxis (6).

Topically, the rose hip dust ("itching powder") can cause itching by mechanical irritation (6).

Interactions with Herbs & Other Dietary Supplements

IRON: Concomitant use interacts with the vitamin C in rose hip; 200 mg of vitamin C per 30 mg of elemental iron increases oral iron absorption, especially ferric iron (14,15,3042).

Interactions with Drugs

Rose hip interactions depend on the amount of vitamin C present (see Effectiveness).

ASPIRIN AND OTHER SALICYLATES: Concomitant use interacts with the vitamin C in rose hip and can increase urinary excretion of ascorbic acid and decrease excretion of salicylates, but this may not have a clinically significant effect on salicylate plasma levels (15,3046).

ALUMINUM-CONTAINING ANTACIDS: Concomitant use interacts with the vitamin C in rose hip and can increase aluminum absorption, but the clinical significance of this is unknown (3046). Administer rose hip with vitamin C two hours before or four hours after antacids (3046).

IRON: Concomitant use interacts with the vitamin C in rose hip; 200 mg of vitamin C per 30 mg of elemental iron increases iron absorption, especially ferric iron (14,15,3042).

WARFARIN (Coumadin): Concomitant use interacts with the vitamin C in rose hip. Large amounts of vitamin C can impair the warfarin response (3046).

INCREASED VITAMIN C REQUIREMENTS: Estrogens, oral contraceptives, barbiturates, tetracyclines, and salicylates increase the vitamin C requirements (15).

Interactions with Foods

Rose hip interactions depend on the amount of vitamin C present (see Effectiveness).

IRON: Concomitant use interacts with the vitamin C in rose hip and can increase the absorption of dietary (ferric) iron (14,3042).

Interactions with Lab Tests

Rose hip interactions depend on the amount of vitamin C present (see Effectiveness).

ACETAMINOPHEN: The vitamin C in rose hip can cause false negative urine results with methods based on hydrolysis and formation of an indophenol blue chromagen (14).

ASPARTATE AMINOTRANSFERASE (AST, SGOT): Large amounts of the vitamin C in rose hip can cause a false increase in results of serum tests relying on color reactions (Redox reactions) and Technicon SMA 12/60 (14).

BILIRUBIN: Large amounts of the vitamin C in rose hip can cause a false increase in serum test results measured by Technicon SMA 12/60 or colorimetric methods (14).

CALCIUM/SODIUM: 3-6 grams of vitamin C daily can cause a true increase in urinary calcium and test results (15) and a true decrease in urinary sodium and test results.

CARBAMAZEPINE (Tegretol): Large amounts of the vitamin C in rose hip can cause falsely increased serum assay results measured by Ames ARIS method (14).

CREATININE: The vitamin C in rose hip can cause a false increase in serum creatinine or urine test results (14).

GLUCOSE: Large amounts of the vitamin C in rose hip can cause false increases in urine test results measured by copper reduction methods (e.g. Clinitest) and false decreases in results measured by glucose oxidase methods (e.g. Clinistix, Tes-Tape) (14,15).

LDH: The vitamin C in rose hip can cause a false decrease measured by Technicon SMA 12/60 and Abbott 100 methods (14).

OCCULT BLOOD: The vitamin C in rose hip may cause false negative guaiac results to occur with 250 mg or more of vitamin C per day (3042).

THEOPHYLLINE: Large amounts of the vitamin C in rose hip can cause falsely decreased serum assay results when measured by the ARIS system or Ames Seralyzer photometer (14).

URIC ACID: Large amounts of the vitamin C in rose hip can cause a true decrease in serum uric acid concentrations and test results with enzymatic method assays (15) and a false increase in test results with assays based on other methods (14).

Interactions with Diseases or Conditions

DIABETES: The vitamin C in rose hip might affect glycogenolysis and the control of diabetes, but not all experts agree on this (15).

GLUCOSE-6-PHOSPHATE DEHYDROGENASE DEFICIENCY: Large amounts of the vitamin C in rose hip might increase the risk of oxalate stone formation (15).

SICKLE CELL DISEASE: The vitamin C in rose hip rarely can decrease the blood pH, precipitating sickle cell crisis (15).

HEMOCHROMATOSIS, THALASSEMIA, SIDEROBLASTIC ANEMIA: Use rose hip with caution, because the vitamin C content can increase iron absorption, which could worsen this condition (14,15).

INCREASED NEEDS: Vitamin C requirements increase in pregnancy, lactation, hyperthyroidism, stress, fever, infection, trauma, burns, smoking, and cold exposure (15).

Dosage and Administration

ORAL: The typical dose of rose hips is as a tea, which is prepared by steeping 2-2.5 grams of the crushed rose hips in 150 mL boiling water for 10-15 minutes and then straining (8).

Comments

Rose hip with seed is the ripe, dried receptacle (hip) with fruit (seed) of various Rosa species, including dog rose (Rosa canina), white rose (Rosa alba), provence rose (Rosa centifolia), and damask rose (Rosa damascena). Avoid confusion with Cherokee rosehip, rose flower, and vitamin C. CAUTION: Sometimes rose hip seeds or plain rose hip receptacles without seeds are sold. These are different than rose hip with seed. Fresh rose hips contain a high concentration of vitamin C; however, much of the vitamin C is destroyed during drying and processing (11) and declines rapidly with storage (2). Many rose hip-derived "natural" vitamin C products are supplemented with synthetic vitamin C (6,11), but may not be clearly labeled accordingly (6).

ROSEMARY

Also Known As

Compass Plant, Compass-Weed, Old Man, Polar Plant.

Scientific Names

Rosmarinus officinalis.
Family: Labiatae or Lamiaceae.

People Use This For

Orally, rosemary is used for dyspepsia, flatulence (2,4,5,18,400), inducing abortion, increasing menstrual flow (5,6), gout, cough, headache (4), liver and gallbladder complaints, loss of appetite, and for cardiovascular conditions such as high blood pressure (18).

Topically, rosemary is used for preventing baldness (5,6); alopecia areata (5177); circulatory disturbances; toothache; eczema; joint or musculoskeletal pain (2,5,18,7107) such as myalgia, sciatica and intercostal neuralgia (4); balneotherapy (18); wound healing; and as an insect repellent (6).

In foods, rosemary is used as a spice (5,6). The leaf and oil are used in foods, and the oil in beverages (11).

In manufacturing, rosemary oil is used as a fragrant component in soaps and perfumes (11).

Safety

LIKELY SAFE ...when used orally in amounts typically found in foods. Rosemary has Generally Recognized as Safe (GRAS) status in the US (11). The maximum use level of the leaves is 0.41% in baked goods. The maximum level of oil used is 0.003% (4,11).

POSSIBLY SAFE ...when used orally and appropriately in medicinal amounts (18). ...when used topically and appropriately (18,5177). Rosemary oil has been used safely for up to 7 months (5177). ...when used by inhalation as aromatherapy (7107).

LIKELY UNSAFE ...when the essential oil is used orally. Ingestion of undiluted oil from rosemary can cause significant adverse effects (515).

PREGNANCY: LIKELY SAFE ...when used orally in amounts typically found in foods (11).

POSSIBLY UNSAFE ...when used orally in medicinal amounts. Rosemary might have uterine and menstrual flow stimulant effects (4,12,18); avoid using. There is insufficient reliable information available about the safety of the topical use of rosemary during pregnancy.

LACTATION: LIKELY SAFE ...when used orally in amounts typically found in foods (11). There is insufficient reliable information available about the safety of using rosemary in medicinal amounts during lactation; avoid using.

Effectiveness

POSSIBLY EFFECTIVE ...when used topically in combination with other essential oils for alopecia areata. Rosemary oil in combination with the essential oils from thyme, lavender, and cedarwood seem to improve hair growth by 44% after 7 months of treatment (5177).

POSSIBLY INEFFECTIVE ...when used orally as an abortifacient (5,6).
There is insufficient reliable information available about the effectiveness of rosemary for its other uses.

Mechanism of Action

The applicable part of rosemary is the leaf. The active constituent of rosemary leaves is the essential oil. Dried leaves contain from 1-2.5% of the essential oil (4,5,18). The oil consists primarily of cineole, borneol, camphor, and pinenes (4,6). The essential oil might have a spasmolytic effect on smooth muscle of the gastrointestinal tract and in the ducts of the gallbladder (2,4). Rosemary might also have a positive inotropic effect on the heart and increases coronary blood flow (2). It's not clear how rosemary oil works in alopecia areata (5177). However, there is some evidence that topical use of rosemary might irritate the skin and increase blood circulation (2). Rosemary also seems to have antibacterial, antifungal (4), and antioxidant properties (4,6).

Adverse Reactions

Orally, large amounts of leaves containing rosemary oil might cause deep coma, spasm, vomiting, gastroenteritis, uterine bleeding, kidney irritation, pulmonary edema, and death (18). Ingestion of undiluted oil might cause stomach and intestinal irritation, kidney damage, and seizures (5,6). The camphor constituent can sometimes lead to seizures (4). Rosemary used topically can lead to photosensitivity, erythema, and dermatitis in hypersensitive individuals (4,6). Asthma due to repeated occupational exposure (occupational asthma) can occur (783).

Interactions with Herbs & Other Dietary Supplements

Insufficient reliable information available.

Interactions with Drugs

No interactions are known to occur, and there is no known reason to expect a clinically significant interaction with rosemary.

Interactions with Foods

No interactions are known to occur, and there is no known reason to expect a clinically significant interaction with rosemary.

Interactions with Lab Tests

No interactions are known to occur, and there is no known reason to expect a clinically significant interaction with rosemary.

Interactions with Diseases or Conditions

SEIZURE DISORDERS: Theoretically, rosemary might potentiate seizure activity (4,7107); avoid using.

Dosage and Administration

ORAL: A typical dose is 1-2 grams of crude leaf. Rosemary is often prepared as a tea. A typical dose is one cup tea three times daily, prepared by steeping 1-2 grams leaf in 150 mL boiling water for 5-10 minutes then straining (2,4,18). A liquid extract (1:1 in 45% alcohol) has also been used in a dose of 2-4 mL three times daily (4).
TOPICAL: Typically, semi-solid or liquid preparations containing 6-10% of the essential oil are used (2,18). For a rosemary bath, 50 grams crude leaf in 1 L hot water is commonly added to bath water (18). For the treatment of alopecia areata, a combination of the essential oils including rosemary 3 drops or 114 mg, thyme 2 drops or 88 mg, lavender 3 drops or 108 mg, and cedarwood 2 drops or 94 mg, all mixed with 3 mL jojoba oil and 20 mL grapeseed oil has been used. Each night, the mixture is massaged into the scalp for 2 minutes with a warm towel placed around the head to increase absorption (5177).

Comments

None.

ROSEROOT

Also Known As

Arctic Root, Golden Root, King's Crown, Rose Root, Rose Root Extract, Rosenroot, Rodia riza, Lignum rhodium.

Scientific Names

Rhodiola rosea, synonyms Sedum rhodiola, Sedum rosea.
Family: Crassulaceae.

People Use This For

Orally, roseroot is used for increasing energy, stamina, strength and mental capacity; and as a so-called "adaptogen" to help the body adapt to and resist physical, chemical, and environmental stress. It is also used for improving athletic performance, improving sexual function, depression, cardiac disorders such as arrhythmias, and hyperlipidemia. Roseroot is also used for treating cancer, tuberculosis, and diabetes; preventing cold and flu, aging, and liver damage; improving hearing; strengthening the nervous system; enhancing immunity; and shortening recovery time after prolonged workouts.

Safety

There is insufficient reliable information about the safety of roseroot.
Pregnancy and Lactation: Insufficient reliable information available; avoid using.

Effectiveness

There is insufficient reliable information available to rate the effectiveness of roseroot. However, there is preliminary evidence that a standardized roseroot extract 170 mg daily might help for fatigue in night shift workers. Roseroot extract seems to improve cognitive performance after the first treatment, but its effects don't seem to continue after the second treatment (6877). More evidence is needed to rate roseroot for this use.

Mechanism of Action

The applicable part of roseroot is the root. Roseroot contains a phenylpropanoid glycoside called salidroside (synonyms: rhodioloside, rhodosine), which is reported to have stimulant, anti-stress, and adaptogenic actions (increasing resistance to the harmful effects of stressors) (6877). Animal studies are reported to show protection from stressors such as cold and radiation, increased work capacity, decreased fatigue and improved learning and memory (6877). Roseroot extracts demonstrate antiarrhythmic properties and protection against reperfusion injury after ischemia. These effects can be abolished by naloxone infusion, suggesting that the mechanism might involve an increase in endogenous opioids (3191,3192,3195). Roseroot extracts might also prevent stress-induced cardiac damage by preventing rises in cardiac catecholamines and cyclic-AMP (3193). Roseroot extract reduces experimentally induced mutations, possibly by increasing the efficiency of intracellular DNA repair mechanisms (3190). Roseroot extracts also demonstrate hepatoprotective (3196) and myeloprotective effects (3197). Roseroot extracts also demonstrate potential for improving learning and memory (3198,6877). Preliminary research in a small number of patients with superficial bladder cancer suggests that roseroot extract might improve cell characteristics and reduce relapses (3194).

Adverse Reactions

None reported.

Interactions with Herbs & Other Dietary Supplements

Insufficient reliable information available.

Interactions with Drugs

No interactions are known to occur, and there is no known reason to expect a clinically significant interaction with roseroot.

Interactions with Foods

No interactions are known to occur, and there is no known reason to expect a clinically significant interaction with roseroot.

Interactions with Lab Tests

No interactions are known to occur, and there is no known reason to expect a clinically significant interaction with roseroot.

Interactions with Diseases or Conditions

No interactions are known to occur, and there is no known reason to expect a clinically significant interaction with roseroot.

Dosage and Administration

Typical doses range from 50-250 mg of roseroot extract 1 to 3 times daily (3188,3189). For improving well-being and psychomotor function during stress, roseroot extract 50 mg twice daily has been used (1927).

Comments

Roseroot is native to the arctic regions of eastern Siberia, Scandinavia, Lapland, and Alaska (3187,3189). It has a long history of use as a medicinal plant in Iceland, Sweden, France, Russia, and Greece, where it is mentioned by

Dioscorides in the first century A.D. (6877). It is reported that Chinese emperors sent expeditions to Siberia to collect the plant in the hope that it would bring long life or immortality (3187). Roseroot has been used as an ingredient in folk medicine love potions (3189). The green aerial parts of the plant have been used as a food ingredient (6877).

ROSINWEED

Also Known As
Compass Weed, Pilot Weed, Polar Plant.
CAUTION: See separate listing for Cup Plant.

Scientific Names
Silphium laciniatum.

People Use This For
Orally, rosinweed is only used in homeopathy for digestive disorders (18).

Safety
There is insufficient reliable information available about the safety of rosinweed.
Pregnancy and Lactation: Insufficient reliable information available; avoid using.

Effectiveness
There is insufficient reliable information available about the effectiveness of rosinweed.

Mechanism of Action
The applicable part of rosinweed is the root. Rosinweed root is stated to have antispasmodic, diaphoretic, and diuretic effects (18).

Adverse Reactions
None reported.

Interactions with Herbs & Other Dietary Supplements
Insufficient reliable information available.

Interactions with Drugs
No interactions are known to occur, and there is no known reason to expect a clinically significant interaction with rosinweed.

Interactions with Foods
No interactions are known to occur, and there is no known reason to expect a clinically significant interaction with rosinweed.

Interactions with Lab Tests
No interactions are known to occur, and there is no known reason to expect a clinically significant interaction with rosinweed.

Interactions with Diseases or Conditions
No interactions are known to occur, and there is no known reason to expect a clinically significant interaction with rosinweed.

Dosage and Administration
ORAL: People typically use 2 to 4 mL of rosinweed liquid extract (5264).

Comments
Avoid confusion with cup plant (Silphium perfoliatum), also referred to as rosinweed.
There is very little scientific information about this product. Our staff is continually analyzing the available information on natural medicines and will add data here as it becomes available.

ROYAL JELLY

Also Known As
Bee saliva, Bee Spit, Honey Bee Milk, Honey Bee's Milk.
CAUTION: See separate listings for Bee Pollen, Bee Venom, and Honey.

Scientific Names
Apis mellifera.
Family: Apidae.

People Use This For
Orally, royal jelly is used as a general health tonic, for rejuvenation, potentiating the immune system, treating bronchial asthma, liver disease, pancreatitis, insomnia, stomach ulcers, kidney disease, bone fractures, skin disorders, and hyperlipidemia.
Topically, royal jelly is used as a skin tonic and hair growth stimulant.

Safety
There is insufficient reliable information available about the safety of royal jelly.
Pregnancy and Lactation: Insufficient reliable information available; avoid using.

Effectiveness
There is insufficient reliable information available to rate the effectiveness of royal jelly. However, there is preliminary evidence that royal jelly might lower cholesterol levels in people with hyperlipidemia (3515). More evidence is needed to rate royal jelly for this use.

Mechanism of Action
Royal jelly is a milky secretion produced by glands in the heads of nurse honey bees (Apis mellifera). The composition of royal jelly varies with geographical areas and climatic conditions. It typically contains about 60 to 70 % water, 12 to 15% crude proteins, 10 to16 % sugar, 3 to 6 % lipids, and 2 to 3% low molecular weight compounds such as vitamins, salts, and free amino acids (7313). Royal jelly is used for the development and nurturing of queen bees (6). There is very little scientific information available about its effects in humans. In animal models, royal jelly seems to have some antitumor activity (6) and antiatherogenic activity (3515).

Adverse Reactions
Orally, royal jelly appears to cause few side effects in nonallergic people (7314). However, in people with a history of atopy or asthma, royal jelly appears to cause a high rate of allergic symptoms including pruritus, urticaria, eczema, eyelid and facial edema, conjunctivitis, rhinorrhea, dyspnea, and asthma (7314,7315,7316). In severe cases, royal jelly can cause status asthmaticus, anaphylaxis, and death (792,7315,7316). Allergic symptoms have been associated with IgE-mediated hypersensitivity reactions (3513). Tell people with a history of allergy or asthma not to use royal jelly.
There is also one case report of hemorrhagic colitis with abdominal pain, bloody diarrhea with concomitant hemorrhagic and edematous mucosa of the sigmoid colon after ingestion of royal jelly. Symptoms resolved within 2 weeks following discontinuation of royal jelly and conservative treatment (3516).
Topically, skin irritation, exacerbation of dermatitis, or contact dermatitis may occur (791).

Interactions with Herbs & Other Dietary Supplements
Insufficient reliable information available.

Interactions with Drugs
No interactions are known to occur, and there is no known reason to expect a clinically significant interaction with royal jelly.

Interactions with Foods
No interactions are known to occur, and there is no known reason to expect a clinically significant interaction with royal jelly.

Interactions with Lab Tests
No interactions are known to occur, and there is no known reason to expect a clinically significant interaction with royal jelly.

Interactions with Diseases or Conditions

ASTHMA, ATOPY: In patients with asthma or atopy, royal jelly causes a high rate of allergic symptoms including pruritus, urticaria, eczema, eyelid and facial edema, conjunctivitis, rhinorrhea, dyspnea, and asthma (7314,7315,7316). In severe cases, royal jelly can cause status asthmaticus, anaphylaxis, and death (792,7315,7316). Allergic symptoms have been associated with IgE-mediated hypersensivity reactions (3513). Advise people with asthma or allergies not to use royal jelly.
DERMATITIS: Royal jelly might exacerbate dermatitis; avoid using (791).

Dosage and Administration

ORAL: For hyperlipidemia, 50-100 mg per day has been used (3515).

Comments

Avoid confusion with bee pollen and bee venom.

RUE

Also Known As

Common Rue, Garden Rue, German Rue, Herb-of-Grace, Herbygrass, Raute, Ruda, Rue Officinale, Ruta graveolens, Rutae folium, Rutae herba.
CAUTION: See separate listing for Goat's Rue.

Scientific Names

Ruta graveolens.
Family: Rutaceae.

People Use This For

Orally, the above ground parts of rue are used for menstrual disorders and discomforts, as a uterine stimulant and abortifacient, for loss of appetite, dyspepsia, circulatory disorders, arteriosclerosis, heart palpitations, nervousness, hysteria, fever (2), feverish infectious diseases, cramps, hepatitis, diarrhea (18), pleurisy, headaches, neuralgic afflictions, and weakness of the eyes. It is also used orally for respiratory complaints, arthritis (2), intestinal worm infestations, epilepsy, multiple sclerosis, Bell's palsy, and cancer of the mouth (2). Rue is used orally as an antispasmodic, diuretic (2), antibacterial, antifungal (6), hemostatic (11), or contraceptive agent (18).
Topically, rue is used for arthritis, dislocations, sprains, injuries of the bone, inflammation of the skin, oral and pharyngeal cavities, earaches, toothaches (18), headaches (515), tumors and warts, and as an insect repellent (6).
In foods and beverages, rue and its oil are used as flavor components (11).
In manufacturing, rue oil is used as a fragrance ingredient in soaps and cosmetics (11).

Safety

LIKELY SAFE ...when consumed in amounts commonly found in foods. Rue and its oil have Generally Recognized as Safe (GRAS) status for food use in the US. The maximum level is 0.001% for rue and 0.0002% for the oil (11).
LIKELY UNSAFE ...when the fresh rue is used orally for medicinal purposes (2). Fresh rue can cause severe kidney and liver damage (2). ...when more than 120 grams of leaves or 100 mL oil are ingested. Can cause severe gastrointestinal upset, systemic complications, and death (2,6). Dried rue leaf contains less volatile oil than fresh rue, and it has milder effects (515). Canadian regulations prohibit the use of rue as a non-medicinal ingredient in oral products (12). ...when fresh rue is applied topically (2), because it can cause contact dermatitis and severe photodermatitis (2,6,11,19).
PREGNANCY: LIKELY UNSAFE ...when used orally because it might cause uterine stimulant and abortifacient effects (12); avoid using. Deaths have been reported in women who used rue as an abortifacient (2).
LACTATION: POSSIBLY SAFE ...when used orally in food amounts. LIKELY UNSAFE ...when used orally in larger amounts than those found in food.

Effectiveness

There is insufficient reliable information available about the effectiveness of rue.

Mechanism of Action

The applicable parts of rue are the above ground parts. Rue contains the alkaloids arborine, arborinine, and gamma-fagarine, and the furocoumarins rutamarin, bergapten, and xanthotoxin. The alkaloids and the furocoumarins show evidence of reversible spasmolytic activity and anti-inflammatory and antihistaminic properties (6,11,515). The furocoumarins also have photosensitizing, phototoxic, and mutagenic effects (2) and they are responsible for adverse skin reactions (6,11,19,515). The constituent, chalepensin, shows some evidence of antifertility and anti-implantation effects. The rutin constituent shows evidence of antispasmodic activity, and it might decrease capillary permeability and fragility. Rue oil has anthelmintic activities, possibly due to the constituent 2-undecanone (11). It can also cause abortions (11). Although rue oil caused fatal adrenal gland, liver, and kidney hemorrhage in animals (11), 30 mg per day for three months did not affect liver function in humans (11). Rue extract's effect on neuromuscular conditions is thought to result from potassium channel-blocking in myelinated nerve cells (6).

Adverse Reactions
Orally, rue can cause GI irritation (12), melancholic mood, sleep disorders, tiredness, dizziness, spasms, and severe kidney and liver damage (2). The fresh leaf juice can cause painful stomach and intestinal irritation, fainting, lethargy, bradycardia, abortion, swelling of the tongue, and clammy skin (2). Rue oil causes severe stomach pain, vomiting, exhaustion, confusion, and convulsions (11). Large amounts, over 100 mL of the oil or 120 grams of the leaf, can cause vomiting, violent gastric pain, systemic complications, and death (2,6). Contact dermatitis (2) and phototoxic reactions including skin blisters have occurred with topical exposure to the fresh plant and rue-containing products followed by exposure to sunlight (2,6). There is one case report of increased phototoxic response to PUVA therapy associated with ingestion of a rue remedy (6177).

Interactions with Herbs & Other Dietary Supplements
GOLDENSEAL: Reports that the effects of large amounts of rue can be overcome by administering goldenseal are unsubstantiated (515).

Interactions with Drugs
PUVA: Rue might increase the phototoxic response to PUVA therapy due to its 5-methoxypsoralen content. There is one case report of increased phototoxic response to PUVA therapy associated with ingestion of a rue remedy (6177). Drugs used in PUVA therapy include, methoxsalen (8-methoxypsoralen, 8-MOP, Oxsoralen) and Trioxsalen (Trisoralen).

Interactions with Foods
No interactions are known to occur, and there is no known reason to expect a clinically significant interaction with rue.

Interactions with Lab Tests
No interactions are known to occur, and there is no known reason to expect a clinically significant interaction with rue.

Interactions with Diseases or Conditions
KIDNEY OR LIVER DYSFUNCTION: Contraindicated (2,12).
GASTROINTESTINAL TRACT PROBLEMS: Rue can exacerbate pre-existing inflammation or irritation of the gastrointestinal tract (19).
URINARY TRACT PROBLEMS: Rue can exacerbate kidney inflammation and urinary tract discomfort (19).

Dosage and Administration
ORAL: People typically use 500 mg crushed rue. A maximum dose of 1 gram per day is recommended. As a tea, 1 cup of boiling water is poured over 1 teaspoon of the herb. The tea is taken cold, 1 cup per day (5252,5254).
TOPICAL: No typical dosage.

Comments
Avoid confusion with goat's rue (Galega officinalis) and meadow rue (Thalictrum species).

RUPTUREWORT

Also Known As
Bruchkraut, Flax weed, Herniariae herba, Herniary.

Scientific Names
Herniaria glabra; Herniaria hirsuta.
Family: Rutaceae.

People Use This For
Orally, rupturewort is used for disorders of the urinary and respiratory tracts, nerve inflammation, gout, arthritis, rheumatism, for "purifying the blood" (2,18), and as a diuretic (8).

Safety

There is insufficient reliable information available about the safety of rupturewort.

Pregnancy and Lactation: Insufficient reliable information available; avoid using.

Effectiveness

There is insufficient reliable information available about the effectiveness of rupturewort.

Mechanism of Action

The applicable parts of rupturewort are the above ground parts. The constituents triterpene saponins, flavonoids, coumarins, and tannins seem to have mild spasmolytic and diuretic activity [18], but these effects have not been scientifically proven [18].

Adverse Reactions

None reported.

Interactions with Herbs & Other Dietary Supplements

Insufficient reliable information available.

Interactions with Drugs

No interactions are known to occur, and there is no known reason to expect a clinically significant interaction with rupturewort.

Interactions with Foods

No interactions are known to occur, and there is no known reason to expect a clinically significant interaction with rupturewort.

Interactions with Lab Tests

No interactions are known to occur, and there is no known reason to expect a clinically significant interaction with rupturewort.

Interactions with Diseases or Conditions

No interactions are known to occur, and there is no known reason to expect a clinically significant interaction with rupturewort.

Dosage and Administration

ORAL: As a diuretic, take one cup tea (simmer 1.5 grams finely cut above ground parts in 150 mL boiling water for 5 minutes, strain) 2-3 times daily [8].

Comments

None.

RUSTY-LEAVED RHODODENDRON

Also Known As

Rhododendri Ferruginei Folium, Rosebay, Rust-Red Rhododendron, Rusty Leaved Rhododendron, Snow Rose.

Scientific Names

Rhododendron ferrugineum.
Family: Ericaceae.

People Use This For

In combination with other herbs, rusty-leaved rhododendron is used for extreme tension of the muscles or arteries (hypertonia), muscle and joint rheumatism, joint disease, hardening of muscles, muscular pain, weak connective tissue, neuralgia, sensitivity to weather change, sciatica, trigeminal neuralgia, migraine, headaches, intercostal neuralgia, gout, biliary or urinary stones, and geriatric and aging disorders [2].

In folk medicine, rusty-leaved rhododendron has been used for stones, geriatric complaints, gout, hypertension, migraine, muscular pain, and rheumatic complaints [18].

Safety

LIKELY UNSAFE ...when used orally [2]. The entire plant is considered poisonous [2,7,18,3477,3496]. Hydroquinone toxicity is also a potential risk with long-term use (2). Most poisonings result from the consumption of honey made from rhododendron nectar (3477).

PREGNANCY AND LACTATION: LIKELY UNSAFE ...when used orally; avoid using.

Effectiveness

There is insufficient reliable information available about the effectiveness of rusty-leaved rhododendron (2).

Mechanism of Action

The applicable part of rusty-leaved rhododendron is the leaf. Rusty-leaved rhododendron contains grayanotoxins and arbutin (2). Grayanotoxins lower blood pressure (7). Grayanotoxins also prevent nerve conduction by inhibiting the closure of sodium channels on cell membranes, which increases sodium conductance and causes cellular depolarization (18,3477). Grayanotoxin toxicity includes muscular and respiratory paralysis (7). Arbutin is hydrolyzed to hydroquinone by the intestinal flora (7). As a result, long-term use may to lead to hydroquinone toxicity (2).

Adverse Reactions

Adverse effects of ingestion include weakness, dizziness, nausea, vomiting hypotension, bradycardia, transient A-V dissociation (17,3496) and blurred vision (17). Symptoms of poisoning due to the constituent grayanotoxin include sweating, impaired consciousness (2,3496) chills, fainting (2), shock (3496), seizure (3477), cardiac and respiratory arrest (2,3477), severe stupor (18), and possibly death (18,3477). Chronic use may lead to hydroquinone toxicity (2). Hydroquinone toxicity is characterized by a gastroenteritis-like syndrome (17).

Interactions with Herbs & Other Dietary Supplements

Insufficient reliable information available.

Interactions with Drugs

No interactions are known to occur, and there is no known reason to expect a clinically significant interaction with rusty-leaved rhododendron.

Interactions with Foods

No interactions are known to occur, and there is no known reason to expect a clinically significant interaction with rusty-leaved rhododendron.

Interactions with Lab Tests

No interactions are known to occur, and there is no known reason to expect a clinically significant interaction with rusty-leaved rhododendron.

Interactions with Diseases or Conditions

No interactions are known to occur, and there is no known reason to expect a clinically significant interaction with rusty-leaved rhododendron.

Dosage and Administration

No typical dosage.

Comments

Rusty-leaved rhododendron is considered likely unsafe; avoid using. Rusty-leaved rhododendron is considered a poisonous plant (2,7,18). Rhododendron honey is also known as "mad honey" (3477,3496).

RUTIN

Also Known As

Citrus Bioflavonoid, Citrus Bioflavonoids, Eldrin, Oxerutin, Quercetin-3-rhamnoglucoside, Quercetin-3-rutinoside, Rutine, Rutinum, Rutosid, Rutoside, Rutosidum, Sclerutin, Sophorin.

Scientific Names

Rutin, rutoside.

People Use This For

Orally, rutin is used as a vascular protectant (14); for reducing capillary permeability, fragility, and bleeding (3,9,11,14); for treating varicose vein symptoms (3,14); and prophylaxis of mucositis associated with cancer treatments (2199). In combination with trypsin and bromelain, rutin is used orally for osteoarthritis (6252).

In Chinese medicine, rutin has been used orally to treat internal bleeding and bleeding hemorrhoids, and to prevent strokes (11).

Safety
LIKELY SAFE ...when used orally in amounts present in fruits and vegetables.
POSSIBLY UNSAFE ...when used orally in amounts greater than those found in foods. Although rutin is generally considered nontoxic, there are reports of rutin forming an obstructive mass in the gastrointestinal tract (11). There is also concern that flavonoids, including rutin, could become mutagenic and play a role in the etiology of gastric cancer (3106).
PREGNANCY AND LACTATION: Insufficient reliable information available; avoid using amounts greater than those found in foods.

Effectiveness
POSSIBLY EFFECTIVE ...when used orally in combination with trypsin and bromelain for treating osteoarthritis (6252). In a double-blind trial, 73 patients with painful osteoarthritis of the knee were randomly assigned the combination enzyme product (Phlogenzym) or diclofenac (Voltaren) 50 mg three times daily during the first week and then twice daily in weeks 2 and 3. The enyzme product was similar to diclofenac in relieving pain and improving knee function (6252).
There is insufficient reliable information about the effectiveness of rutin for its other uses.

Mechanism of Action
Rutin is thought to be an antioxidant, a free radical scavenger, and an iron-chelator (209,3100). It has been reported to decrease capillary fragility and permeability, although the existing evidence is inconclusive (11). Some studies suggest rutin might offer protection from damage induced by asbestos (209,3103), cytotoxic effects of oxidized low density lipoproteins (11,3105), and gastric injury from ethanol (3107). Other evidence suggests it might be beneficial in inflammatory bowel disease (3101,3102). When added to the diet, rutin appears to offer some protection against DNA damage caused by hepatocarcinogens (3104). However, limited preliminary evidence suggests rutin might worsen the progression of melanoma (211).

Adverse Reactions
Orally, rutin may cause headache, flushing, rashes, or mild gastrointestinal disturbance (313).

Interactions with Herbs & Other Dietary Supplements
IRON: Some information suggests that rutin might have iron-chelating properties (209).

Interactions with Drugs
No interactions are known to occur, and there is no known reason to expect a clinically significant interaction with rutin.

Interactions with Foods
No interactions are known to occur, and there is no known reason to expect a clinically significant interaction with rutin.

Interactions with Lab Tests
No interactions are known to occur, and there is no known reason to expect a clinically significant interaction with rutin.

Interactions with Diseases or Conditions
No interactions are known to occur, and there is no known reason to expect a clinically significant interaction with rutin.

Dosage and Administration
ORAL: As a supplement, a common dose of rutin is 500 mg per day (312). For relieving symptoms of edema associated with chronic venous insufficiency, a typical dose is 500 mg twice daily (313). For osteoarthritis, a combination enzyme product (Phlogenzym), which contains rutin 100 mg, trypsin 48 mg, and bromelain 90mg, 2 tablets 3 times daily has been used (6252).

Comments
Rutin (rutoside) is a flavonoid present in numerous plants. The major sources of rutin for medical use include buckwheat, Japanese pagoda tree, and Eucalyptus macrorhyncha (11). Other sources of rutin include the leaves of several species of eucalyptus (9), lime tree flowers, elder flowers (8), hawthorn leaves and flowers (2,3,8), rue (2), St. John's Wort (3), Ginkgo biloba (3), apples (3100), and other fruits and vegetables (3108).

RYE GRASS

Also Known As
Grass Pollen, Grass Pollen Extract, Rye, Rye Grass Pollen, Rye Grass Pollen Extract, Rye Pollen Extract.

Scientific Names
Secale cereale.
Family: Poaceae or Gramineae.

People Use This For
Orally, rye grass is used for shrinking prostate size; relieving the symptoms of benign prostatic hyperplasia (BPH) including frequency, nocturia, urgency, decreased urine flow rate, dribbling, painful urination, and residual volume after voiding (5292,5293,5294,5295). It is also used orally for chronic prostatitis and prostate pain (5296), promoting men's health, and prostate health (5291).

Safety
POSSIBLY SAFE …when products of good quality are used orally. There are no reports of toxicity in clinical trials (5292,5293,5294,5296).
PREGNANCY AND LACTATION: Insufficient reliable information available; avoid using.

Effectiveness
POSSIBLY EFFECTIVE …when used orally for the management of BPH symptoms that include frequency, nocturia, urgency, decreased urine flow rate, dribbling, painful urination, residual urine volume after voiding. …when used for shrinking prostate size (5292,5293,5294,5295). …when used for prostatitis and prostatodynia (5296). Studies have used Cernilton brand rye grass pollen extract (5292,5293,5294).

Mechanism of Action
The applicable part of rye grass is the pollen extract. Rye grass pollen extract is prepared by microbial digestion of the pollen, followed by water and acetone extraction (5290,5295). The extract does not affect luteinizing hormone, follicle-stimulating hormone, testosterone, or dihydrotestosterone (5292). Some evidence suggests that rye grass pollen extract might inhibit prostate cancer cell growth (5297). Other evidence suggests that it might interfere with inflammation by inhibiting the biosynthesis of prostaglandins and leukotrienes (5298).

Adverse Reactions
Orally, rye grass can cause abdominal distention, heartburn, and nausea (5293).

Interactions with Herbs & Other Dietary Supplements
Insufficient reliable information available.

Interactions with Drugs
No interactions are known to occur, and there is no known reason to expect a clinically significant interaction with rye grass.

Interactions with Foods
No interactions are known to occur, and there is no known reason to expect a clinically significant interaction with rye grass.

Interactions with Lab Tests
No interactions are known to occur, and there is no known reason to expect a clinically significant interaction with rye grass.

Interactions with Diseases or Conditions
No interactions are known to occur, and there is no known reason to expect a clinically significant interaction with rye grass.

Dosage and Administration
ORAL: The typical dose of rye grass pollen is 126 mg three times daily (5294). Clinical studies have used Cerniltin, a brand manufactured by Cernitin.

Comments

Clinical evidence for the effectiveness of rye grass extract is limited. For BPH, there was one double-blind, placebo-controlled study (5292) that showed marginal benefit and two open trials (5293,5294). For treating prostatitis and prostatodynia, the evidence is limited to one open trial (5296).

SACCHAROMYCES BOULARDII

Also Known As

Probiotics, S boulardii, S. boulardii, Saccharomyces.
CAUTION: See separate listings for Bifidobacteria, Brewer's Yeast (Hansen CBS 5926), Lactobacillus.

Scientific Names

Saccharomyces boulardii.

People Use This For

Orally, Saccharomyces boulardii is used for treating and preventing diarrhea, including infectious types such as rotaviral diarrhea in children and traveler's diarrhea. It is also used orally to prevent and treat antibiotic-associated diarrhea. Saccharomyces boulardii is also used orally for general digestion problems, irritable bowel syndrome (IBS), inflammatory bowel syndrome (IBD, Crohn's disease, ulcerative colitis), relapsing Clostridium difficile colitis, and bacterial overgrowth in short bowel syndrome. It is also used orally for lactose intolerance, urinary tract infections (UTIs), vaginal and Candida-related (yeast) infections, high cholesterol levels, hives, fever blisters, canker sores, and adolescent acne.

Safety

LIKELY SAFE ...when used orally and appropriately (4353).
CHILDREN: POSSIBLY SAFE ...when used orally and appropriately (4347,4356).
PREGNANCY AND LACTATION: Insufficient reliable information available; avoid using.

Effectiveness

POSSIBLY EFFECTIVE ...when used orally to prevent diarrhea associated with use of antibiotics (4353,4355). Although there is one conflicting report (4351), the majority of evidence shows that Saccharomyces boulardii can be useful for preventing antibiotic-associated diarrhea (4353,4355). ...when used in tube feedings to prevent diarrhea (4349). ...when used orally to prevent traveler's diarrhea (155). ...when used orally to treat acute diarrhea in infants (4347). ...when used orally to treat HIV-associated diarrhea (4347).
POSSIBLY INEFFECTIVE ...when used orally in combination with vancomycin or metronidazole (Flagyl) to treat recurrent Clostridium difficile disease (4352,4354). For people with an initial episode of Clostridium difficile, Saccharomyces boulardii in combination with vancomycin or metronidazole seems to be no more effective than vancomycin or metronidazole alone (4352).
There is insufficient reliable information available about the effectiveness of Saccharomyces boulardii for its other uses.

Mechanism of Action

Saccharomyces boulardii is typically a non-pathogenic yeast (4363). Saccharomyces boulardii is used as a probiotic agent to help colonize the gastrointestinal tract. It is used therapeutically in cases where disease is thought to occur due to depleted intestinal normal flora or colonization with pathogenic organisms. Saccharomyces boulardii typically reaches a maximum steady state in 3 days when taken orally. It does not multiply in the gut. Less than 1% of the ingested dose is recovered from stools (4363). Saccharomyces boulardii is thought to help for Clostridium difficile infection by producing proteases that might decrease the toxicity of Clostridium difficile toxins A and B (4348,4361). There is also some evidence that Saccharomyces boulardii might cause an increase in the intestinal chloride resorption (4362). Individuals who have low stool concentrations of Saccharomyces boulardii after repeated use are most likely to have Clostridium difficile recurrence (4360). In addition to its effect on Clostridium difficile, Saccharomyces boulardii also shows evidence of interaction with cholera toxin (4363).

Adverse Reactions

Orally, side effects are usually infrequent. Rarely, oral use has been associated with fungemia in both immunocompromised and immunocompetent people (1247,4357,4358,4360). Fungemia with a closely related strain, Saccharomyces cerevisiae, has been reported in a neutropenic baby treated with Saccharomyces boulardii. However, it is also possible that the yeast isolated was Saccharomyces boulardii (7329). Most laboratories are unable to differentiate between Saccharomyces boulardii and Saccharomyces cerevisiae (7353).

Interactions with Herbs & Other Dietary Supplements
Insufficient reliable information available.

Interactions with Drugs
ANTIFUNGALS: Antifungals can cause Saccharomyces boulardii to be ineffective (14).

Interactions with Foods
No interactions are known to occur, and there is no known reason to expect a clinically significant interaction with Saccharomyces boulardii.

Interactions with Lab Tests
SACCHAROMYCES CEREVISIAE: In patients that experience fungemia following use of Saccharomyces boulardii, cultures can indicate fungemia from Saccharomyces cerevisiae (7329). Most laboratories are unable to distinguish between Saccharomyces cerevisiae and Saccharomyces boulardii (7353).

Interactions with Diseases or Conditions
IMMUNOSUPPRESSION: There is some concern that immunocompromised patients taking Saccaromyces boulardii might be at an increased risk for fungemia. Although Saccaromyces is generally a nonpathogenic organism, there have been cases of fungemia following its use (1247,4357,4358,4360).
YEAST ALLERGY: Patients with yeast allergy can be allergic to products containing Saccharomyces boulardii (14).

Dosage and Administration
ORAL: A typical dose to prevent diarrhea is 250-500 mg two to four times a day (4355). A typical dose to treat recurrent diarrhea in adults is 1 gram daily for four weeks along with antibiotic therapy (4352). To treat AIDS-related diarrhea, people typically begin with a dose of 3 grams per day, reducing dose to 1 gram/day as symptoms lessen (4364,4365). Infants: 250 mg two to four times a day according to age (4356). To prevent contamination of indwelling catheters, open packets or capsules with gloves, outside the individual's room (4359). Refrigerate after opening to preserve potency (4366).

Comments
Saccharomyces boulardii was previously identified as a unique species of yeast, but is now believed to be a strain of Saccharomyces cerevisiae (baker's yeast) (1227,1251,1282,7353).

SAFFLOWER

Also Known As
American Saffron, Bastard Saffron, Dyer's Saffron, Fake Saffron, False Saffron, Hing Hua, Honghua, Zaffer, Zafran.

Scientific Names
Carthamus tinctorius.
Family: Asteraceae or Compositae.

People Use This For
Orally, safflower seed oil is used for reducing the risk of cardiovascular disease (6) and preventing atherosclerosis (18). In Chinese medicine, safflower flower is used for hyperemia in women (18) and hair growth (11).
In folk medicine, safflower is used orally for fever (6), tumors, coughs, bronchial conditions (18), blood stasis, pain, blood invigoration, amenorrhea, painful menses, stimulating menstruation, coronary heart disease, chest pain, traumatic injuries (11,18), inducing sweating (6), as a laxative (6), purgative, stimulant, antiperspirant, abortifacient, and expectorant (18).
For food uses, safflower seed oil is used as a cooking oil (6).
In manufacturing, safflower flower is used to color cosmetics and dye fabrics. Safflower seed oil is used as a paint solvent (6).

Safety
LIKELY SAFE ...when safflower seed oil is used orally (6).
POSSIBLY SAFE ...when safflower flower is used orally and appropriately as safflower flower (6,12,18).
PREGNANCY: LIKELY SAFE ...when safflower seed oil is used orally in food amounts. LIKELY UNSAFE ...when safflower flower is used because it has abortifacient, menstrual stimulant, and uterine stimulant effects (11,12).
LACTATION: LIKELY SAFE ...when safflower seed oil is used orally. There is insufficient reliable information available about the safety of safflower flower during lactation; avoid using.

Effectiveness

POSSIBLY EFFECTIVE …when safflower oil is used as a dietary supplement to reduce the risk of cardiovascular disease (6).

There is insufficient reliable information available about the effectiveness of safflower for its other uses.

Mechanism of Action

The applicable parts of safflower are the flower and seed oil. Safflower flower contains a complex mixture of red and yellow pigments (11,18). The constituent, safflower yellow, has immunosuppressive and anticoagulant activity (11). Safflower polysaccharide has immunopotentiating effects (11). Safflower extracts exhibit cardiac stimulant, vasodilating, hypolipemic, hypotensive, and uterine stimulant properties (11). Safflower seed oil is a rich source of the essential unsaturated fatty acid, linoleic acid (6). It also contains linolenic acid (18). Some evidence suggests essential fatty acids are necessary to maintain the integrity of the central nervous system (6). Other evidence suggests that diets high in unsaturated and polyunsaturated fatty acids reduce atherosclerosis and the risk of heart disease (6). A diet rich in safflower oil can increase platelet linoleic acid levels, reduce serum cholesterol, particularly low-density lipoprotein (LDL) cholesterol, and apolipoprotein B levels (6) without affecting serum triglyceride, high-density (HDL) lipoprotein cholesterol or apolipoprotein A-1 levels (6). However, recent research suggests that improving the lipid profile might not be as important to reducing the risk of cardiovascular disease as previously suggested (6).

Adverse Reactions

Safflower can cause an allergic reaction in individuals sensitive to the Asteraceae/Compositae family. Members of this family include ragweed, chrysanthemums, marigolds, daisies, and many other herbs.

Interactions with Herbs & Other Dietary Supplements

HERBS WITH ANTICOAGULANT/ANTIPLATELET POTENTIAL: Concomitant use of herbs that have coumarin constituents or affect platelet aggregation could theoretically increase the risk of bleeding in some people. These herbs include: angelica, anise, arnica, asafoetida, bogbean, boldo, capsicum, celery, chamomile, clove, danshen, fenugreek, feverfew, garlic, ginger, ginkgo, ginseng (Panax), horse chestnut, horseradish, licorice, meadowsweet, prickly ash, onion, papain, passionflower, poplar, quassia, red clover, turmeric, wild carrot, wild lettuce, willow, and others (4,19).

Interactions with Drugs

ANTICOAGULANTS: Theoretically concomitant use with safflower might increase effects and adverse effects of anticoagulants.

Interactions with Foods

No interactions are known to occur, and there is no known reason to expect a clinically significant interaction with safflower.

Interactions with Lab Tests

No interactions are known to occur, and there is no known reason to expect a clinically significant interaction with safflower.

Interactions with Diseases or Conditions

BLEEDING DISORDERS: Contraindicated in people with hemorrhagic diseases, peptic ulcers, or clotting disorders. Safflower can prolong coagulation time (12).

CROSS-ALLERGENICITY: Safflower can cause an allergic reaction in individuals sensitive to the Asteraceae/Compositae family. Members of this family include ragweed, chrysanthemums, marigolds, daisies, and many other herbs.

Dosage and Administration

ORAL: A typical dose is one cup of tea up to three times daily. To make tea, simmer 1 gram dried flower in 150 mL boiling water, 5-10 minutes, strain (18).

Comments

Although safflower seed oil is a rich source of linoleic acid, some experts contend gamma-linolenic acid might be more useful as a physiologic source of essential fatty acids. To be useful in the body, linoleic acid must be converted to dihomo-gamma-linolenic acid (DHGA) and arachidonic acid (6). Gamma-linolenic acid does not require this conversion before it can be used in the body.

SAFFRON

Also Known As
Autumn Crocus, Azafran, Croci stigma, Indian Saffron, Saffron Crocus, Safran, Spanish Saffron, True Saffron.

Scientific Names
Crocus sativus.
Family: Iridaceae.

People Use This For
Orally, saffron is used for asthma, insomnia, cancer (11), atherosclerosis (6), cough, whooping cough, stomach gas (11), and as a sedative (2).
In combination with opium and quinine, it is used for premature ejaculation (6).
In combination with salicylic acid and vegetable oils, an extract of saffron is used topically for treating baldness (6,11).
In Chinese medicine, saffron is used for depression, fright, shock, spitting up blood, pain and difficulties in menstruation and after childbirth (11).
In folk medicine, saffron is used as a digestive stimulant (11,18), an aphrodisiac (6,11), a pain reliever, and a sedative (2), for stimulating menstruation (11), for dry skin (6), to induce sweating, and as an expectorant.
In food, saffron is used as a culinary spice, yellow food coloring (11), and as a flavoring agent (11).
In manufacturing, saffron extracts are used as fragrance in perfumes (11) and as a dye for cloth (6).

Safety
LIKELY SAFE ...when used orally in amounts typically found in foods. Saffron has Generally Recognized as Safe (GRAS) status in the US (11). The maximum use level is 0.1% (11).
POSSIBLY SAFE ...when used orally and appropriately for medicinal purposes. There is some evidence that amounts up to 1.5 grams per day can be used safely (11,12).
LIKELY UNSAFE ...when used orally in excessive amounts. Doses of 5 grams or more can cause severe side effects (2,12). Doses of 12-20 grams can be lethal (18).
PREGNANCY: LIKELY SAFE ...when used orally in amounts typically found in foods (11). LIKELY UNSAFE ...when used orally in amounts exceeding those found in foods. Larger amounts of saffron have uterine stimulant and abortifacient effects (2,18); avoid using.
LACTATION: Insufficient reliable information available; avoid using.

Effectiveness
There is insufficient reliable information available about the effectiveness of saffron.

Mechanism of Action
Saffron constituents include crocin, picrocrocin, and crocetin (6,11). Picrocrocin is responsible for the characteristic bitter taste of saffron and crocin for the yellow-red color used for coloring food and cloth (11). In rabbits, crocetin appears to improve atherosclerosis by increasing plasma oxygen diffusion (6,11,18) and decreasing cholesterol and triglyceride levels (4110). In addition, crocetin binds to albumin (4109), potentially increasing oxygen diffusion and improving atherosclerosis (4109). Small amounts of saffron stimulate gastric secretions (18); larger amounts appear to stimulate uterine smooth muscle, contributing to abortifacient affects (18). Saffron extracts limit the in vitro growth of experimental tumor colony cells by inhibiting cellular nucleic acid synthesis (4104,4105).

Adverse Reactions
Orally, no adverse effects have been reported with up to 1.5 grams of saffron per day (2,11,12). Poisoning can occur with 5 grams (2,11,18), symptoms include: yellow appearance of the skin, sclera, and mucous membranes (mimicking icterus), vomiting, vertigo, bloody diarrhea, hematuria, bleeding from the nose, lips, eyelids or uterus, numbness, uremic collapse, and thrombocytopenic purpura leading to severe necrosis of the nose (2,11). 10 grams can induce abortion (2), 12-20 grams is reportedly lethal (2,12,18).
ALLERGY: Rhinoconjunctivitis and allergy induced asthma reported (4106). Anaphylactic reactions can occur within minutes of eating food prepared with saffron (4107).

Interactions with Herbs & Other Dietary Supplements
CROSS-SENSITIVITY: Cross-reactivity exists between saffron and Lolium, Olea (includes olive), and Salsola species plants (4106).

Interactions with Drugs
No interactions are known to occur, and there is no known reason to expect a clinically significant interaction with saffron.

Interactions with Foods

No interactions are known to occur, and there is no known reason to expect a clinically significant interaction with saffron.

Interactions with Lab Tests

No interactions are known to occur, and there is no known reason to expect a clinically significant interaction with saffron.

Interactions with Diseases or Conditions

CROSS-ALLERGENICITY: Cross-reactivity reported between saffron and Lolium, Olea (includes olive), and Salsola species plants (4106).

Dosage and Administration

ORAL: People typically use 12 to 15 stigmas (the thread-like pistils) in a cup of boiling water and drink one cup daily (5250).

Comments

None.

SAGE

Also Known As

Common Sage, Dalmatian Sage, Garden Sage, Meadow Sage, Sauge, Scarlet Sage, Spanish Sage, True Sage.
CAUTION: See separate listings for Boneset, Clary Sage, Danshen, German Sarsaparilla, Purple Loosestrife, Spearmint, and Wood Sage.

Scientific Names

Salvia officinalis; Salvia lavandulaefolia.
Family: Labiatae or Lamiaceae.

People Use This For

Orally, sage is used for loss of appetite, excessive perspiration (2,6), dysmenorrhea, diarrhea, gastritis (6), galactorrhea, reduction of saliva secretion and digestive problems including flatulence, bloating, and dyspepsia (4,7,18).
Topically, sage is used as a gargle for laryngitis, pharyngitis, stomatitis, gingivitis, glossitis, minor oral injuries (4,7,18), and inflammation of the nasal mucosa (2).
As an inhalant, sage is used for asthma (6).
In foods, it is used as a culinary spice (4,5,6).
In manufacturing, sage is used as a fragrance component in soaps and cosmetics (11).

Safety

LIKELY SAFE ...when used orally in amounts typically found in foods (11). Sage is approved for use in foods in the US (11).
POSSIBLY UNSAFE ...when used orally in amounts greater than those found in foods, or when used long-term (4,5,12). Sage contains thujone constituent that can be toxic if enough is consumed (12).
LIKELY UNSAFE ...when used orally as sage oil (2,4).
There is insufficient reliable information about the safety of sage for its other uses.
PREGNANCY: LIKELY UNSAFE ...when used orally because the constituent, thujone, can have menstrual stimulant and abortifacient effects (2,4,5,6,12,19).
LACTATION: POSSIBLY UNSAFE ...when used orally because it is thought to reduce mother's milk supply (12,19).

Effectiveness

POSSIBLY EFFECTIVE ...when used orally for flatulence, bloating, dyspepsia, and excessive perspiration (2,6).
...when used topically for nose and throat mucous membrane inflammation (2,5).
There is insufficient reliable information available about the effectiveness of sage for its other uses.

Mechanism of Action

The applicable part of sage is the leaf. Sage contains 1-2.8% of volatile oil that may be responsible for pharmacological activity. The volatile oil contains camphor and thujone which are potentially toxic (4,5). Sage seems to have antiflatulent, antispasmodic, astringent (4), antibacterial, fungistatic, virustatic, antiperspirant, secretion promoting (2), and blood sugar lowering (5) activities.

Adverse Reactions

Orally, sage can cause cheilitis, stomatitis, dry mouth, local irritation (6), and mental and physical deterioration (5). Large amounts or prolonged use of sage leaf, or ingestion of sage oil, may cause restlessness, vomiting, vertigo, tachycardia, tremors, seizures, and kidney damage (2,4,5,12,18). Poisoning was reported following ingestion of sage oil (4).

Interactions with Herbs & Other Dietary Supplements

HERBS WITH SEDATIVE PROPERTIES: Theoretically, concomitant use with herbs that have sedative properties might enhance therapeutic and adverse effects. These include calamus, calendula, California poppy, catnip, capsicum, celery, couch grass, elecampane, Siberian ginseng, German chamomile, goldenseal, gotu kola, hops, Jamaican dogwood, kava, lemon balm, St. John's wort, sassafras, scullcap, shepherd's purse, stinging nettle, valerian, wild carrot, wild lettuce, ashwaganda root, and yerba mansa (4,19).

Interactions with Drugs

ANTICONVULSANTS: Some species of sage can cause convulsions. Theoretically, this might interfere with anticonvulsant drug therapy (4).
HYPOGLYCEMIC DRUGS: Theoretically, due to claims of hypoglycemic activity, sage might have additive effects and adverse effects with hypoglycemic drugs (4).
DRUGS WITH SEDATIVE PROPERTIES: Theoretically, concomitant use with drugs with sedative properties might cause additive effects and side effects (4).

Interactions with Foods

No interactions are known to occur, and there is no known reason to expect a clinically significant interaction with sage.

Interactions with Lab Tests

No interactions are known to occur, and there is no known reason to expect a clinically significant interaction with sage.

Interactions with Diseases or Conditions

DIABETES: Sage might interfere with blood sugar control (4).
SEIZURE DISORDERS: Avoid, due to the potential for causing seizures (2,4,5,12).

Dosage and Administration

ORAL: 1-2 grams leaf three times daily, or, one cup tea (steep 1-2 grams leaf in 150 mL boiling water 5-10 minutes, strain) three times daily (2,4); up to 4-6 grams leaf per day (2); not for long term use (12). Liquid extract (1:1 in 45% alcohol), 1-4 mL three times daily (4).
TOPICAL: For gargles and rinses, 2.5 grams leaf or 2-3 drops essential oil in 100 mL of water, or 5 grams alcohol extract in 1 glass of water (2).

Comments

Sage is a rich source of beta-carotene (19).

SALEP

Also Known As

Cuckoo Flower, Levant Salep, Orchid, Sahlep, Saloop, Satyrion.

Scientific Names

Orchis morio.
Family: Orchidaceae.

People Use This For

Orally, salep is used for diarrhea (particularly in children), heartburn, flatulence, and indigestion (18).

Safety

POSSIBLY SAFE ...when used orally (18).
PREGNANCY AND LACTATION: Insufficient reliable information available; avoid using.

Effectiveness

There is insufficient reliable information available about the effectiveness of salep.

Mechanism of Action

The applicable part of salep is the tuber. Salep contains up to 40% mucilage including glucans, glucomannans, starch, and protein (18).

Adverse Reactions

None reported.

Interactions with Herbs & Other Dietary Supplements

Insufficient reliable information available.

Interactions with Drugs

No interactions are known to occur, and there is no known reason to expect a clinically significant interaction with salep.

Interactions with Foods

No interactions are known to occur, and there is no known reason to expect a clinically significant interaction with salep.

Interactions with Lab Tests

No interactions are known to occur, and there is no known reason to expect a clinically significant interaction with salep.

Interactions with Diseases or Conditions

No interactions are known to occur, and there is no known reason to expect a clinically significant interaction with salep.

Dosage and Administration

ORAL: Used as a powdered formulation in medicinal preparations. Taken in water before or after meals (18).

Comments

None.

SAMe

Also Known As

Ademetionine, Adenosylmethionine, S-Adenosyl Methionine, S-Adenosyl-L-Methionine, S-Adenosylmethionine, S-Adenosyl-Methionine, SAM-e, Sammy.

Scientific Names

S-adenosyl-L-methionine.

People Use This For

Orally, SAMe is used for depression, heart disease (5182), fibromyalgia, osteoarthritis, bursitis, tendonitis, chronic low back pain, dementia, Alzheimer's disease, Parkinson's disease, improving intellectual performance, slowing the aging process (5187), multiple sclerosis (5232), spinal cord injury (6), seizures, migraine headache, chronic lead poisoning, disorders of porphyrin, and bilirubin metabolism (5231).
Intravenously, SAMe is used for treating depression (5231), osteoarthritis (5188), AIDS-related myelopathy (5232), fibromyalgia (5221), liver disease, cirrhosis, and intrahepatic cholestasis (5198,5219,5231).
Intramuscularly, SAMe is injected for fibromyalgia (5231), depression (5193), and Alzheimer's disease (5220).

Safety

LIKELY SAFE ...when used orally, intravenously, or intramuscularly and appropriately (5231,5232). Serious toxicity has not been reported in multiple clinical studies involving as many as 22,000 patients and lasting from a few days to 2 years (5189,5201,5202,5209,5219,5231).
PREGNANCY: POSSIBLY SAFE ...when used intravenously short-term during the third trimester of pregnancy. In two small-scale trials, SAMe 800 mg daily was used intravenously for 14-20 days during the third trimester of pregnancy for intrahepatic cholestasis. No adverse effects in the mother or fetus were observed (5219,5231,5240). Large-scale trials are needed to confirm the safety of SAMe use in pregnancy. Use of SAMe in pregnancy should only be considered when benefits clearly outweigh the potential risks. There is insufficient reliable information available about the use of SAMe at

higher doses, for extended periods of time, or during the earlier trimesters of pregnancy.
LACTATION: Insufficient reliable information available; avoid using.

Effectiveness

LIKELY EFFECTIVE ...when used orally for relieving symptoms of osteoarthritis. Multiple clinical trials have shown that SAMe is superior to placebo and comparable to NSAIDs for decreasing symptoms associated with osteoarthritis in studies lasting from several weeks to 2 years (5188,5199,5203,5204,5205,5206,5207,5208,5209,5215). Significant symptom relief with SAMe may require up to 30 days of treatment compared to only 15 days with NSAIDs. Some evidence suggests that intravenous loading doses of SAMe given over 5 days, followed by oral treatment, can speed symptom relief to 14 days (5188). ...when used intravenously or intramuscularly for short-term treatment of major depression. Several small-scale clinical trials have shown that parenterally administered SAMe is superior to placebo and possibly as effective as intravenous or oral tricyclic antidepressants in studies lasting up to 30 days (2082,3562,5184,5189,5200,5231). Significantly more studies have been done with parenteral SAMe than oral SAMe. In some trials, the antidepressant effect occurred rapidly, within 1-2 weeks of initiation of treatment (5200); however, this benefit is likely the result of the parenteral route of administration (3562). Parenteral SAMe has been used successfully in combination with an oral tricyclic antidepressant to speed the onset of antidepressant action (5193). Available studies are limited by small numbers of patients, inconsistent diagnostic criteria, and short treatment periods (5189,5231). Further study is needed to clarify benefit of extended treatment with parenteral SAMe compared to conventional antidepressant therapy.

POSSIBLY EFFECTIVE ...when used orally for short-term treatment of major depression. Several studies have shown that orally administered SAMe is superior to placebo and possibly as effective as tricyclic antidepressants in trials lasting up to 42 days (2082,2083,5189,5190,5192,5195,5196,5231). Available studies are limited by small numbers of patients, inconsistent diagnostic criteria, short treatment periods, and flawed study designs (3562,5189,5231). Well designed, large scale studies are needed to clarify the benefit of orally administered SAMe in major depression. ...when used orally for treating fibromyalgia. Two clinical trials demonstrated significant improvement in symptoms of fibromyalgia compared to placebo (5211,5241). ...when used orally or intravenously for treating intrahepatic cholestasis associated with acute or chronic liver disease. Multiple clinical trials have shown that short-term SAMe therapy is superior to placebo in decreasing pruritus, fatigue, alkaline phosphatase levels, and total and conjugated bilirubin (5219,5238,5239,5240). Trials have more frequently used injectable dosage forms than oral formulations (5219). ...when used intravenously for treating intrahepatic cholestasis due to pregnancy (ICP). One clinical trial using intravenous SAMe during the third trimester of pregnancy demonstrated significant benefit compared to placebo for normalizing liver function tests, decreasing associated symptoms, and preventing premature labor and low infant birthweight in pregnant women with ICP (5219,5240). ...when used intravenously for AIDS-related myelopathy. SAMe has investigational orphan drug status for this use (5217,5185,5218). ...when used orally to improve mortality and delay liver transplantation in patients with early stages of alcoholic liver cirrhosis. In one study, there was a significant decrease in overall mortality and transplantation rate when only patients with early stages of liver disease were included (1712). ...when used orally or intravenously for decreasing signs and symptoms of chronic liver disease due to medications, alcoholism, or lead poisoning. Multiple clinical trials have shown that SAMe can normalize liver enzymes, decrease bilirubin, and decrease symptoms associated with various forms of chronic liver disease. Most trials have enrolled small numbers of patients and have been short duration (5198,5231,5235,5236,5238). Large-scale studies are needed to confirm SAMe's potential benefit in liver disease.

POSSIBLY INEFFECTIVE ...when used intravenously for treating fibromyalgia (5221). ...when used orally to improve mortality and delay liver transplantation in patients with advanced alcoholic liver cirrhosis. In one trial, there was not a significant difference in mortality and transplantation rate in patients with alcoholic liver cirrhosis compared to placebo when the patient population included patients with advanced liver disease (1712).

There is insufficient reliable information available about the effectiveness of SAMe for its other uses.

Mechanism of Action

S-adenosylmethionine (SAMe) is a naturally occurring molecule that is distributed throughout virtually all body tissues and fluids (5231). It plays an essential role in many biochemical reactions involving enzymatic transmethylation. It contributes to the synthesis, activation and/or metabolism of hormones, neurotransmitters, nucleic acids, proteins, phospholipids, and some drugs (5231,5232). SAMe is produced endogenously from methionine and adenosine triphosphate (ATP). SAMe synthesis is closely linked to vitamin B12 and folate metabolism (5231). Deficiencies of these vitamins can result in decreased SAMe concentrations in the central nervous system (5231). SAMe supplementation may be beneficial in osteoarthritis due to analgesic and anti-inflammatory effects. Preliminary evidence suggests SAMe might also stimulate articular cartilage growth and repair (5209). The mechanism of antidepressant effect is unknown, but SAMe is associated with increased serotonin turnover and elevated dopamine and norepinephrine levels (5196,5232). SAMe may also work by altering cellular membrane fluidity. Changes in neuronal membrane fluidity might facilitate signal transduction across membranes and increase the efficiency of receptor-effector coupling (5196). In liver disease, exogenously administered SAMe might act as an essential nutrient by restoring biochemical factors that are depleted in people with liver dysfunction. People with acute or chronic liver disease lose the ability to synthesize SAMe from methionine, which can lead to deficiencies in cysteine and choline. It can also lead to depletion of glutathione, which plays a major role in liver detoxification and antioxidant reactions. This depletion may in turn exacerbate liver disease (5198,5219,5236). SAMe may also be beneficial in AIDS-related myelopathy, by replenishing depleted endogenous SAMe. Epidemiological data suggests that people with AIDS have a deficiency of SAMe in their cerebrospinal fluid, and this may lead to myelopathy by impairing SAMe dependent myelin and oligodendrocyte repair mechanisms (5185,5217,5218). Some evidence suggests that SAMe might also have a gastric cytoprotective effect (5213). Exogenously administered SAMe has low oral bioavailability, presumably the result of significant first-pass effect and rapid hepatic metabolism (5231). It achieves peak plasma concentrations 3 to 5 hours after ingestion of an enteric-coated tablet (5231), has a half-life of about 100 minutes and is excreted in urine and feces (5231). SAMe crosses the blood-brain barrier (5231). SAMe is metabolized to s-adenosylhomocysteine, which can be metabolized to homocysteine (5232). Homocysteine is remethylated to form methionine, which can form more SAMe, or converted via transsulfuration to the antioxidant, glutathione (5232). These reactions require folate, cyanocobalamin, and pyridoxine (5231). Elevated levels of homocysteine have been linked to cardiovascular and renal disease (1698). The long-term effect of SAMe administration on atherosclerotic and thrombotic vascular disorders is unknown, although there was no difference in cardiovascular mortality in a study of people with cirrhosis taking SAMe 1200 mg daily for 2 years (1712). Low levels of SAMe have been correlated with coronary artery disease (1714). Administration of SAMe to healthy people has shown a positive effect on 5-methyltetrahydrofolate, a key cofactor in homocysteine metabolism. SAMe supplementation has been suggested as a remedy for elevated homocysteine levels (1713).

Adverse Reactions

Orally, SAMe can cause flatulence, vomiting, diarrhea, headache (347), and nausea. These side effects are more common with higher doses (5231). Anxiety has occurred in people with depression (5231) and hypomania in people with bipolar disorder (5231). When used as an injection, SAMe has caused mania in people with bipolar disorder (5216,5231).

Interactions with Herbs & Other Dietary Supplements

Insufficient reliable information available.

Interactions with Drugs

ANTIDEPRESSANTS: Concurrent use may cause additive serotonergic effects and serotonin syndrome-like effects, including agitation, tremors, anxiety, tachycardia, tachypnea, diarrhea, hyperreflexia, shivering, and diaphoresis (3521,5193). In a case report, SAMe 100 mg intramuscularly was given daily along with clomipramine (Anafranil) 25 mg per day. The clomipramine dose was later increased to 75 mg per day, and 48-72 hours later the patient experienced side effects similar to serotonin syndrome, requiring hospitalization (3521). Theoretically, this may also occur when SAMe is used with other tricyclic antidepressants and with non-tricyclic antidepressants (5193). Concurrent use of SAMe with imipramine (Tofranil) has resulted in a more rapid onset of antidepressant action (5193,5231). Theoretically, this effect may also occur with other antidepressants.
HEPATOTOXIC DRUGS: SAMe protects against hepatic dysfunction caused by acetaminophen, alcohol, estrogens, monoamine oxidase inhibitors, phenobarbital, phenytoin, and steroids (5231).
MONOAMINE OXIDASE INHIBITORS (MAOIs): Theoretically, because SAMe affects serotonin and other neurotransmitters in a way similar to conventional antidepressants (5196,5232), concomitant use might have additive adverse effects, including hypertension, hyperthermia, agitation, confusion, coma, etc. SAMe should be avoided in patients taking MAOIs or within 2 weeks of discontinuation of an MAOI.

Interactions with Foods

No interactions are known to occur, and there is no known reason to expect a clinically significant interaction with SAMe.

Interactions with Lab Tests

No interactions are known to occur, and there is no known reason to expect a clinically significant interaction with SAMe.

Interactions with Diseases or Conditions

BIPOLAR DISORDER: Use of SAMe can cause patients to convert from a depressed state to a hypomanic or manic state (3523).

Dosage and Administration

ORAL: For depression, an oral dose of 400-1600 mg per day has been used (5231). Doses of 1600 mg per day are the most commonly used in clinical trials (5189). For osteoarthritis, an oral dose of 200 mg three times daily is typically used (5188). For alcoholic liver disease or cirrhosis, oral doses of 1200-1600 mg per day have been used (1712,5231,5238,5241). For intrahepatic cholestasis, an oral dose of 800 mg twice daily is typically used (5219,5231,5239).

For fibromyalgia, an oral dose of 800 mg per day is typically used (5241).
PARENTERAL: For depression, an intravenous or intramuscular injection of 200-400 mg per day is typically used (5231). For speeding the onset of antidepressant effect in combination with a tricyclic antidepressant, SAMe 200 mg intramuscularly for the first 2 weeks of tricyclic antidepressant therapy has been used (5193). For osteoarthritis, an intravenous dose of 400 mg per day has been used (5188). For intrahepatic cholestasis, an intravenous dose of 800 mg per day is typically used (9,5219,5231). For intrahepatic cholestasis of pregnancy (ICP), an intravenous dose of 800 mg per day has been used (5219,5231,5240). For AIDS-related myelopathy, an intravenous dose of 800 mg daily for 14 days has been used (5217).

Comments

Early studies utilized parenteral SAMe before an oral formulation was available (5231). Currently, several oral salt forms of SAMe are available: sulfate, sulfate-p-toluenesulfonate (also labeled as tosylate), and butanedisulfonate (5231,5444,5447). The tosylate salt has a 1% oral bioavailability and the butanedisulfonate salt has a 5% oral bioavailability, presumably due to a large first pass effect (1896,1897). Concerns about the stability of the tosylate formulation have been expressed (5446), while the butanedisulfonate salt is stable for 2 years at room temperature (1896,5444).

SAMPHIRE

Also Known As
Crest Marine, Peter's Cress, Pierce-Stone, Sampier, Sea Fennel.

Scientific Names
Crithum maritimum.
Family: Umbelliferae.

People Use This For
Orally, samphire is used for "states of general resistance" and scurvy (18).

Safety
POSSIBLY SAFE ...when used orally (18).
PREGNANCY AND LACTATION: Insufficient reliable information available; avoid using.

Effectiveness
There is insufficient reliable information available about the effectiveness of samphire.

Mechanism of Action
The applicable parts of samphire are the above ground parts. Samphire is thought to be a diuretic (18). It contains vitamin C (ascorbic acid) (18), which is used to treat and prevent scurvy (16).

Adverse Reactions
None reported.

Interactions with Herbs & Other Dietary Supplements
Insufficient reliable information available.

Interactions with Drugs
No interactions are known to occur, and there is no known reason to expect a clinically significant interaction with samphire.

Interactions with Foods
No interactions are known to occur, and there is no known reason to expect a clinically significant interaction with samphire.

Interactions with Lab Tests
No interactions are known to occur, and there is no known reason to expect a clinically significant interaction with samphire.

Interactions with Diseases or Conditions

No interactions are known to occur, and there is no known reason to expect a clinically significant interaction with samphire.

Dosage and Administration

ORAL: Samphire is used as an extract and a food additive (18).

Comments

There is very little scientific information about this product. Our staff is continually analyzing the available information on natural medicines and will add data here as it becomes available.

SANDY EVERLASTING

Also Known As

Common Shrubby Everlasting, Eternal Flower, Everlasting, Fleur de Pied de Chat, Goldilocks, Harnblumen, Helichrysum, Katzenpfotchenbluten, Yellow Chaste Weed.
CAUTION: See separate listing for Immortelle.

Scientific Names

Helichrysum augustifolium, synonym Helichrysum italicum; Helichrysum oriental; Helichrysum stoechas.
Family: Asteraceae or Compositae.

People Use This For

Orally, sandy everlasting is used for peptic discomforts (2), (e.g., dyspepsia) (18), liver complaints, chronic cholecystitis, and gallbladder complaints with accompanying cramps (18).
Historically, sandy everlasting has been used as a diuretic (18), for chronic bronchitis, asthma, whooping cough, psoriasis, burns, rheumatism, headache, migraine, allergies, and liver ailments (11).
In foods, beverages, and tobacco, the extract is used as a flavoring component (11).
In manufacturing, it is used in perfumes, and before- and after-sun products (11).

Safety

LIKELY SAFE ...when used in amounts typically found in foods (11). Sandy everlasting has Generally Recognized as Safe (GRAS) status in the US (11).
POSSIBLY SAFE ...when used orally and appropriately (2).
PREGNANCY AND LACTATION: Insufficient reliable information available; avoid using in amounts greater than those generally found in foods and beverages.

Effectiveness

POSSIBLY EFFECTIVE ...when used orally for treating peptic discomforts such as dyspepsia (2,18).
There is insufficient reliable information available about the effectiveness of sandy everlasting for its other uses.

Mechanism of Action

The applicable part of sandy everlasting is the dried flower. Sandy everlasting contains flavonoids, quercitrin, kaempferol, naringenin, and isohelichrysin. These components might increase bile secretion. They have been shown to increase bile secretion in animals (11). The flavonoids also absorb UV light (11). Quercitrin increases the detoxifying function of the liver and exhibits anti-inflammatory activity (11). The constituent arenarin has antibacterial activity and promotes gastric and pancreatic secretions (8). The volatile oil of Helichrysum italicum flowers seems to have some antibacterial and antifungal activity (11).

Adverse Reactions

Sandy everlasting can cause an allergic reaction in individuals sensitive to the Asteraceae/Compositae family. Members of this family include ragweed, chrysanthemums, marigolds, daisies, and many other herbs.

Interactions with Herbs & Other Dietary Supplements

Insufficient reliable information available.

Interactions with Drugs

No interactions are known to occur, and there is no known reason to expect a clinically significant interaction with sandy everlasting.

Interactions with Foods

No interactions are known to occur, and there is no known reason to expect a clinically significant interaction with sandy everlasting.

Interactions with Lab Tests

No interactions are known to occur, and there is no known reason to expect a clinically significant interaction with sandy everlasting.

Interactions with Diseases or Conditions

BILIARY OBSTRUCTION: Sandy everlasting is contraindicated, due to bile stimulating effects (2,18).
GALLSTONES: Sandy everlasting might complicate therapy (2,18).
CROSS-ALLERGENICITY: Sandy everlasting can cause an allergic reaction in individuals sensitive to the Asteraceae/Compositae family. Members of this family include ragweed, chrysanthemums, marigolds, daisies, and many other herbs.

Dosage and Administration

ORAL: One cup fresh tea (made by steeping 1 gram dried flower in 150 mL boiling water 5-10 minutes, strain) several times per day (8,18); average amount 3 grams of dried flower per day (2).
TOPICAL: No typical dosage.

Comments

None.

SANGRE DE GRADO

Also Known As

Blood of the Dragon, Drago, Dragon's Blood, Lan-Hiqui, Laniqui, Sangre de Drago, Sangre de Dragon, Sangue de Agua, Sangue de Drago, SP 303, SP-303, Taspine.
CAUTION: See also Dragon's Blood (Draconis resina) and Herb Robert (Geranium robertianum).

Scientific Names

Croton lechleri.
Family: Euphorbiaceae.

People Use This For

Orally, sangre de grado or its constituent, SP-303, is used for treating diarrhea associated with cholera, AIDS, traveling, cancer treatment, Clostridium difficile infection, and irritable bowel syndrome (IBS) (2784,2785,2801). It is also used orally for supporting the body's tissue repair mechanisms (2800) and treating viral respiratory infection (2789,2804). Topically, sangre de grado or its constituent, SP-303, is used for treating herpes simplex virus (types 1 and 2) (2787,2788). Traditionally, sangre de grado has been used for oropharyngeal and gastrointestinal ulcers, fever, hemorrhage, bleeding gums, fractures, wound healing, hemorrhoids, eczema, insect bites and stings, vaginitis, for vaginal baths before childbirth, and as a general tonic (2802,2803,2804).

Safety

POSSIBLY SAFE ...when SP-303, a derivitive of sangre de grado, is used orally or topically and appropriately (2784,2787,2788).
There is insufficient reliable information available about the safety of sangre de grado.
PREGNANCY AND LACTATION: Insufficient reliable information available; avoid using.

Effectiveness

POSSIBLY EFFECTIVE ...when a standardized resin extract containing SP-303 (SB-Normal Stool Formula, ShamanBotanicals.com) is used orally for reducing stool weight and frequency in people with AIDS-related diarrhea (2784) and symptomatic treatment of traveler's diarrhea (2806). ...when a standardized resin extract containing SP-303 (currently unavailable in the US), is used topically for treating genital and anal herpes simplex lesions in people with AIDS (2788).
POSSIBLY INEFFECTIVE ...when a standardized resin extract containing SP-303 is used topically for treating acyclovir-unresponsive mucocutaneous herpes simplex lesions in people with AIDS (2787).
There is insufficient reliable information available about the effectiveness of sangre de grado for its other uses. However, topically applied sangre de grado resin alleviated the symptoms of insect bites (fire ants, wasps, bees) and

plant reactions in a group of pest control workers. The results of this unpublished study were presented at the Pediatric Academic Societies and the American Academy of Pediatrics 2000 Joint Meeting (6114).

Mechanism of Action

Sangre de grado is a tree native to the Amazon regions of South America (2805,2784). The resin, a viscous red latex, and bark have a long history of oral and topical medicinal use (2784,2797). Sangre de grado is reported to have anti-inflammatory (2804,6114), antibacterial, anti-hemorrhagic, antiseptic, and anti-tumor properties (2804). Topically, it has been shown to reduce vasodilation, swelling, and secretory response to irritants, promote mucosal healing, and prevent hyperalgesic responses in the laboratory (6114). Several active constituents of sangre de grado have been isolated, including SP-303 and tapsine (2786,2796). All published human experience has been with SP-303 (see Effectiveness). Preliminary evidence suggests that the constituent SP-303 might control diarrhea by inhibiting cyclic adenosine monophosphate (cAMP), which causes chloride and fluid secretion (2786). SP-303 shows activity against types 1 and 2 herpes simplex viruses, respiratory syncytial virus (RSV), and influenza A virus, possibly by inhibiting viral penetration of cells (2790,2791,2792,2793,2794). Tapsine demonstrates anti-inflammatory and wound healing properties when applied topically (2795,2796). Sangre de grado does not stimulate cell proliferation and has not shown carcinogenic activity after 17 months of treatment in experimental models (2796,2797,2798). Preliminary evidence suggests that sangre de grado resin is not cytotoxic, and has antibacterial and pro-oxidant activity (2798,2799).

Adverse Reactions

Orally, no serious adverse reactions or lab abnormalities have been reported in clinical studies using the sangre de grado derivative, SP-303 (2784,2806).
Topically, SP-303 can cause local pain and burning (2787). Topical sangre de grado resin can cause scarring (2803).

Interactions with Herbs & Other Dietary Supplements

Insufficient reliable information available.

Interactions with Drugs

No interactions are known to occur, and there is no known reason to expect a clinically significant interaction with sangre de grado.

Interactions with Foods

No interactions are known to occur, and there is no known reason to expect a clinically significant interaction with sangre de grado.

Interactions with Lab Tests

No interactions are known to occur, and there is no known reason to expect a clinically significant interaction with sangre de grado.

Interactions with Diseases or Conditions

No interactions are known to occur, and there is no known reason to expect a clinically significant interaction with sangre de grado.

Dosage and Administration

ORAL: For treating AIDS-related diarrhea, a sangre de grado extract containing 500 mg of SP-303 (SB-Normal Stool Formula, ShamanBotanicals.com) every 6 hours has been used (2784). For treating traveler's diarrhea, a sangre de grado extract containing 125-500 mg SP-303 (SB-Normal Stool Formula, ShamanBotanicals.com) 4 times daily for 2 days has been used (2806).

Comments

SP-303 was in Phase III clinical trials with "fast track" designation for treatment of AIDS-related diarrhea and Phase II trials for traveler's diarrhea (2807). After the FDA rejected a new drug application and requested additional clinical testing, the manufacturer, Shaman Pharmaceuticals, became Shaman Botanicals.com and elected to market SP-303 as a dietary supplement, SB-Normal Stool Formula (2807).

SANICLE

Also Known As

European Sanicle, Poolroot, Saniculae herba, Self-Heal, Wood Sanicle.
CAUTION: See separate listing for Self-Heal.

Scientific Names
Sanicula europaea.
Family: Apiaceae.

People Use This For
Orally, sanicle is used for mild respiratory tract mucous membrane inflammation (2), cough, and bronchitis (18).

Safety
POSSIBLY SAFE ...when used orally and appropriately (2,12).
PREGNANCY AND LACTATION: Insufficient reliable information available; avoid using.

Effectiveness
POSSIBLY EFFECTIVE ...when used orally for mild respiratory tract mucous membrane inflammation (2).

Mechanism of Action
The applicable parts of sanicle are the above ground parts. Sanicle contains triterpene saponins, caffeine derivatives, and flavonoids such as rutin, isoquercitrin, astragalin. It seems to have astringent and expectorant effects (18). The expectorant effect seems to result from the irritation caused by the saponins on the gastric mucosa that reflexly stimulates the bronchial mucous glands via parasympathetic sensory pathways (7). Large amounts of saponins may cause stomach upset, nausea, and vomiting (7). In animals, sanicle demonstrates edema reduction (18).

Adverse Reactions
Orally, large amounts of sanicle may cause upset stomach, nausea, and vomiting due to saponin content (7).

Interactions with Herbs & Other Dietary Supplements
Insufficient reliable information available.

Interactions with Drugs
No interactions are known to occur, and there is no known reason to expect a clinically significant interaction with sanicle.

Interactions with Foods
No interactions are known to occur, and there is no known reason to expect a clinically significant interaction with sanicle.

Interactions with Lab Tests
No interactions are known to occur, and there is no known reason to expect a clinically significant interaction with sanicle.

Interactions with Diseases or Conditions
GI MUCOSAL IRRITATION (e.g., ulcers, etc.): Theoretically, may exacerbate existing GI mucosal irritation due to saponin content (6); contraindicated.

Dosage and Administration
ORAL: A typical dose is 4-6 grams dried above ground parts per day (2).

Comments
Avoid confusion with Prunella vulgaris, also referred to as self-heal. In commerce, sanicle may be mixed with leaves of Cardamine enneaphylos, and Astrantia major is sometimes labeled as sanicle (18).

SARSAPARILLA

Also Known As
Ecuadorian Sarsaparilla, Honduras Sarsaparilla, Jamaican Sarsaparilla, Mexican Sarsaparilla, Salsaparilha, Salsepareille, Sarsa, Sarsaparillae radix, Sarsaparillewurzel, Smilax.
CAUTION: See separate listings for Couch Grass, German Sarsaparilla, and Tormentil.

Scientific Names

Smilax febrifuga; Smilax medica, synonyms Smilax aristolochiifolia, Smilax aristolochiaefolii; Smilax regelii, synonym Smilax officinalis; other Smilax species.
Family: Smilacaceae.

People Use This For

Orally, sarsaparilla is used for psoriasis (2,4) and other skin diseases (2), rheumatoid arthritis (2,4), kidney disease, as an anabolic for performance enhancement or body-building in athletes (5,11), and as a diuretic and diaphoretic (2). Mexican and Honduran sarsaparilla is used for treating gonorrhea, fevers, and digestive disorders (11).
Traditionally, sarsaparilla is used as an adjunct for treating leprosy (4) and for syphilis (3,5,11).
In manufacturing, sarsaparilla is used as a flavoring agent in foods, beverages (2,11), and pharmaceuticals (3,4).

Safety

LIKELY SAFE ...when used in the amounts commonly found in foods (11). It is approved for food use in the US (11).
POSSIBLY SAFE ...when used orally and appropriately for medicinal purposes (12).
POSSIBLY UNSAFE ...when used in excessive amounts and should be avoided due to the possible gastrointestinal irritation of its saponin constituents (4).
PREGNANCY AND LACTATION: Insufficient reliable information available and excessive amounts can have irritant effects; avoid using (4).

Effectiveness

There is insufficient reliable information available about the effectiveness of sarsaparilla.

Mechanism of Action

The applicable part of sarsaparilla is the root. Sarsaparilla can have antirheumatic, antiseptic, and antipruritic activity (4). It contains about 2% saponins and other varied constituents, including quercetin and phytosterols (beta-sitosterol, stigmasterol, pollinastanol). The saponins, including sarsasapogenin and smilagenin (3,4,5,11), exhibit diuretic, diaphoretic, expectorant, and laxative effects (5). The sterols contained in sarsaparilla are not anabolic steroids nor are they converted in vivo to anabolic steroids (3,11). Testosterone has never been detected in any plant, including sarsaparilla (3,5). Sarsaparilla also improves appetite and digestion (4), and its extracts can improve psoriasis symptoms (4). Sarsaparilla shows liver-protective and anti-inflammatory activity in rats (4).

Adverse Reactions

Orally, sarsaparilla can cause gastric irritation with excessive amounts or temporary kidney impairment (11). Large doses can lead to European cholera, worsened diuresis, and shock (18). Occupational exposure to sarsaparilla root dust can cause rhinitis and asthma symptoms (4111).

Interactions with Herbs & Other Dietary Supplements

DIGITALIS: Sarsaparilla can increase digitalis glycoside absorption (2,11).
OTHER HERBS: Theoretically, sarsaparilla can alter the absorption or elimination of simultaneously administered herbs, which will effect the herbs' actions (2).

Interactions with Drugs

DIGOXIN: Sarsaparilla can increase digitalis glycoside absorption (2,11).
ORAL DRUGS: Theoretically, sarsaparilla increases the absorption or elimination of simultaneously administered drugs, resulting in unpredictable effects (2).
HYPNOTIC DRUGS: Sarsaparilla can accelerate the elimination of these drugs (2,11).

Interactions with Foods

No interactions are known to occur, and there is no known reason to expect a clinically significant interaction with sarsaparilla.

Interactions with Lab Tests

No interactions are known to occur, and there is no known reason to expect a clinically significant interaction with sarsaparilla.

Interactions with Diseases or Conditions

ASTHMA: Sarsaparilla root dust can cause the symptoms of asthma (4111).
KIDNEY DYSFUNCTION: Theoretically, sarsaparilla can exacerbate kidney impairment (2,11).

Dosage and Administration

ORAL: The typical oral dose of sarsaparilla is 1-4 grams of the dried root or one cup of the tea three times daily. The tea is prepared by simmering 1-4 grams of the dried root in boiling water for 5-10 minutes and then straining (4). The typical dose of the liquid extract (1:1 in 20% alcohol, 10% glycerol) is 8-15 mL (4).

Comments

In the Old West of the United States, sarsaparilla was the most popular drink of the cowboys (6002). Avoid confusion with Indian or false sarsaparilla (Hemidesmus indicus, Family: Asclepiadaceae), reportedly a widespread adulterant of sarsaparilla (3,5,11). False sarsaparilla contains none of the saponins or other principal constituents found in sarsaparilla (5).

SASSAFRAS

Also Known As

Ague Tree, Cinnamon Wood, Common Sassafras, Kuntze Saloop, Sassafrax, Saxifrax.

Scientific Names

Sassafras ablidum, synonyms Sassafras officinale, Sassafras varifolium.
Family: Lauraceae.

People Use This For

Orally, sassafras is used for urinary tract disorders, mucous membrane inflammation, syphilis (18), and as a tonic and "blood purifier"(3).
Topically, it is used to treat skin eruptions, rheumatism, eye inflammation, sprains, swelling, and for relief of insect bites or stings (6). Sassafras oil is also used topically as an antiseptic and pediculicide (4).
In folk medicine, it is used for bronchitis, geriatric high blood pressure, gout, arthritis, skin problems, kidney disorders, and cancers (11).
In beverages and candy, a safrole-free bark extract has limited use as a flavoring agent (11).

Safety

POSSIBLY SAFE ...when consumed in amounts found in foods and beverages if safrole-free (11). Safrole-free sassafras is approved for food use in the US (11). The maximum level used is 0.22% extract in nonalcoholic beverages.
POSSIBLY UNSAFE ...when safrole-free sassafras is used in amounts larger than food. Some studies link even safrole-free sassafras extracts to tumors (515).
LIKELY UNSAFE ...when used orally as an medicinal agent; avoid using (3,4). Sassafras root bark and oil contain safrole and related compounds that are carcinogenic and hepatotoxic in animals (4,12,17). Consumption of 5 mL sassafras oil can be fatal in adults (4). ...when used topically; avoid external use due to toxic safrole content (4).
CHILDREN: LIKELY UNSAFE ...when used orally. A few drops of sassafras oil can be fatal (4).
PREGNANCY AND LACTATION: LIKELY UNSAFE ...when used orally (12). Sassafras oil has abortifacient effects (4).

Effectiveness

POSSIBLY INEFFECTIVE ...as a tonic and "blood purifier"(3).
There is insufficient reliable information available about the effectiveness of sassafras for its other uses.

Mechanism of Action

The applicable part of sassafras is the root bark. The major constituent of the volatile oil, safrole, is carcinogenic (causes malignant liver tumors in experimental animals) (6,11). Safrole and its metabolite, L-hydroxysafrole, are neurotoxic (6).

Adverse Reactions

Orally, sassafras can cause diaphoresis and hot flashes (11). Consumption of large amounts of sassafras oil can cause hallucinations lasting for several days (4). In adults, 5 mL sassafras oil can cause shakes, vomiting, dilated pupils, hypertension, tachycardia, stupor, collapse (6), abortion, paralysis, liver cancer, and death (4,6). A few drops of sassafras oil may be fatal in children (4).
Topically, sassafras can result in contact dermatitis (6).

Interactions with Herbs & Other Dietary Supplements

SAFROLE-CONTAINING HERBS: Avoid concomitant use with other safrole-containing herbs due to potential for additive toxicity (12). Other herbs that contain safrole include basil, camphor, cinnamon, and nutmeg (12).

HERBS WITH SEDATIVE PROPERTIES: Theoretically, concomitant use with herbs that have sedative properties might enhance therapeutic and adverse effects. These include calamus, calendula, California poppy, catnip, capsicum, celery, couch grass, elecampane, Siberian ginseng, German chamomile, goldenseal, gotu kola, hops, Jamaican dogwood, kava, lemon balm, sage, St. John's wort, scullcap, shepherd's purse, stinging nettle, valerian, wild carrot, wild lettuce, ashwaganda root, and yerba mansa (4,19).

Interactions with Drugs
BARBITURATES: Theoretically, concomitant use with barbiturates may cause additive effects (19).
OTHER DRUGS WITH SEDATIVE PROPERTIES: Theoretically, concomitant use with drugs with sedative properties may cause additive effects (19).

Interactions with Foods
No interactions are known to occur, and there is no known reason to expect a clinically significant interaction with sassafras.

Interactions with Lab Tests
PHENYTOIN: Sassafras oil may cause false-positive blood phenytoin test results (6).

Interactions with Diseases or Conditions
URINARY CONDITIONS: Sassafras can aggravate urinary irritation (19).

Dosage and Administration
No typical dosage.

Comments
Use only safrole-free extract and leaves. Sassafras was used in the past to flavor root beer (11). In 1976, the FDA banned marketing of sassafras for sassafras tea (4). One study estimates that safrole 0.66 mg/kg could be toxic. One cup of tea made with 2.5 grams of sassafras is estimated to contain 200 mg of safrole (approximately 3 mg/kg) (4).

SAVIN TOPS

Also Known As
Sabina, Savin, Savine.

Scientific Names
Juniperus sabina.

People Use This For
Orally, the branches and leaves of savin tops are used to induce abortions (18).
Topically, they are used as a powder to treat fig warts (18).

Safety
POSSIBLY UNSAFE ...when used topically. Savin tops can cause severe irritation of skin and mucous membranes (18).
UNSAFE ...when used orally. Savin tops may be fatal if ingested as a powder or tea; 6 drops of the volatile oil can cause death (18).
PREGNANCY AND LACTATION: UNSAFE ...when used orally and topically due to overall toxicity as well as ability to induce abortions (19); avoid using.

Effectiveness
There is insufficient reliable information available about the effectiveness of savin tops.

Mechanism of Action
The applicable parts of savin tops are the branches and leaves. Savin tops contains ligans (thujone, podophyllotoxin, and others), hydroxycoumarins, and volatile oil (3-5%) including sabinyl acetate and sabinene (18). The ligans may have antineoplastic and antiviral properties (18). Savin tops has powerful irritant properties that can cause inflammation of the skin and mucous membranes (18,19).

Adverse Reactions

Orally, symptoms of poisoning include queasiness, cardiac rhythm disorders, spasm, kidney damage, hematuria, central paralysis, unconsciousness and death (18). Ingestion can also cause irritation of the mucous membranes resulting in gastroenteritis, hepatitis, pneumonitis, and nephritis (19).
Topically, the volatile oil can cause skin irritation, blisters, necroses, and resorbent poisoning (18).

Interactions with Herbs & Other Dietary Supplements

Insufficient reliable information available.

Interactions with Drugs

No interactions are known to occur, and there is no known reason to expect a clinically significant interaction with savin tops.

Interactions with Foods

No interactions are known to occur, and there is no known reason to expect a clinically significant interaction with savin tops.

Interactions with Lab Tests

No interactions are known to occur, and there is no known reason to expect a clinically significant interaction with savin tops.

Interactions with Diseases or Conditions

INFLAMMATION: Components of the essential oil (sabinene and sabinyl acetate) may increase irritation of the skin or mucous membranes (19).

Dosage and Administration

ORAL: No typical dosage.
TOPICAL: Powder applied twice daily (amount unspecified); "put bandages into skin folds" (18).

Comments

Use only safrole-free extract and leaves. The toxicity of the oil depends on how long it has been stored. Toxicity of oil develops over time through terpene peroxide formation (18). The toxicity of fresh branch tips is apparently low.

SAW PALMETTO

Also Known As

American Dwarf Palm Tree, Cabbage Palm, Ju-Zhong, Palmier Nain, Sabal, Sabal Fructus, Saw Palmetto Berry.

Scientific Names

Serenoa repens, synonyms Serenoa serrulata, Sabal serrulata.
Family: Arecaceae/Palmaceae.

People Use This For

Orally, saw palmetto is used for symptoms of benign prostatic hyperplasia (BPH) (2,4). It is also used as a mild diuretic (6), a sedative, an anti-inflammatory, and as an antiseptic.
In combination with seven other herbs (PC-SPES), saw palmetto is used to treat prostate cancer (5548).
Historically, saw palmetto has been used to increase breast size, to improve sexual vigor, and as an aphrodisiac (6,515). It has also been used orally to stimulate hair growth (515), treat colds, coughs, irritated mucous membranes, sore throat, asthma, chronic bronchitis, migraines, and cancer. The powdered fruit has been used as a uterine and vaginal tonic suppository (11).

Safety

LIKELY SAFE ...when used orally and appropriately. Saw palmetto has been safely used in clinical studies lasting up to 48 weeks (2,4,12,2732,2735).
POSSIBLY SAFE ...when used orally in a specific herbal combination (PC-SPES) (5548).
PREGNANCY AND LACTATION: LIKELY UNSAFE ...when used orally. Saw palmetto has anti-androgen and estrogenic activity (4,6,11); avoid using.

Effectiveness

LIKELY EFFECTIVE ...when used orally for reducing the symptoms of benign prostatic hyperplasia (BPH). Multiple clinical studies lasting up to 48 weeks have shown that saw palmetto significantly improves urinary symptoms such as frequent urination, painful urination, hesitancy, urgency, and perineal heaviness. It also decreases nocturia, improves peak and mean urinary flow, and lowers residual urine volume in patients with BPH (2732,5094,6750,6751,6752,6762,6764,6772,6773,6777,6778). Saw palmetto seems to be comparable in efficacy to finasteride (Proscar), but saw palmetto might be better-tolerated (6424). The combination of a specific brand formulation containing saw palmetto and stinging nettle root (PRO 160/120) also seems to be comparable to finasteride (Proscar) for relieving symptoms of BPH (6763). However, saw palmetto does not reduce prostate size or prostate-specific antigen (PSA) levels like finasteride (6424). Alpha-adrenergic blockers such as prazosin (Minipress) seem to be superior to saw palmetto for relieving symptoms of BPH (6775,6776). Treatment for 1-2 months with saw palmetto is usually necessary before significant symptomatic improvement occurs (2732,6750,6778). Most clinical studies have used a liposterolic extract of saw palmetto berry containing 80-90% fatty acids. This formulation is similar to Quanterra Prostate (Warner-Lambert), Super Saw Palmetto (Enzymatic Therapy), ProstaPro (Phytopharmica), Saw Palmetto (Centrum), Standardized Saw Palmetto Extract (Nature's Way), and others.
POSSIBLY EFFECTIVE ...when used orally in a specific herbal combination for prostate cancer. Studies using saw palmetto in combination with seven other herbs (PC-SPES) in prostate cancer patients, found that it significantly decreases prostate-specific antigen (PSA) levels (5122,5548), causes tumor cell death, and causes clinically significant reductions in testosterone (5548). In two reports, PSA levels fell significantly within one month of treatment (5122,5548).
POSSIBLY INEFFECTIVE ...when used orally as part of a unique herbal blend for treating symptoms of benign prostatic hyperplasia (BPH). A combination product containing saw palmetto lipid extract 106 mg, nettle root extract 80 mg, pumpkin seed oil extract 160 mg, lemon bioflavonoid extract 33 mg, and beta-carotene 190 IU taken 3 times daily for 6 months failed to significantly improve symptoms in a group of men with BPH (5093).
There is insufficient reliable information available about the effectiveness of saw palmetto for its other uses.

Mechanism of Action

The applicable part of saw palmetto is the ripe fruit. The lipid fraction of the volatile oil and fatty oils contains the constituents active in treating benign prostatic hyperplasia (BPH) (3,6). Many saw palmetto products are standardized based on this fatty acid content. The most effective saw palmetto products seem to be whole berries or berry extracts prepared with lipophilic nonpolar solvents. Water extraction, including brewed tea, probably does not adequately extract fat-soluble active constituents (512). Saw palmetto has antiandrogenic, antiproliferative, and anti-inflammatory properties that seem to be responsible for improving symptoms of benign prostatic hyperplasia (BPH). Saw palmetto appears to noncompetitively inhibit 5 alpha-reductase types 1 and 2 and to prevent the conversion of testosterone to dihydrotestosterone (DHT) in vitro, which would reduce prostate growth (6765,6769,6770,6773). However, 5 alpha-reductase levels in prostatic tissue and serum testosterone, DHT, and PSA are not significantly reduced by saw palmetto in vivo (4,2735,6771). Saw palmetto does not seem to affect overall prostate size, but shrinks the inner prostatic epithelium (12,2736,5093). Saw palmetto, which appears to exert prostate-specific activity, might slow prostate cell proliferation by inhibiting fibroblast growth factor and epidermal growth factor and stimulating apoptosis (6765,6769,6770). Inflammatory mediators appear to contribute to the etiology of BPH, and laboratory evidence suggests that saw palmetto inhibits lipoxygenase and cyclo-oxygenase, which are involved in inflammation (6769,6779). Saw palmetto might also have antiestrogen, antispasmodic, and alpha-adrenergic inhibitory properties (5095,6766,6780). Laboratory fertility studies indicate that saw palmetto has no effect on oocytes or sperm motility, but it might induce metabolic changes in sperm (4239,4240).

Adverse Reactions

Adverse effects of saw palmetto are generally mild and comparable to placebo. Dizziness, gastrointestinal complaints such as nausea, vomiting, constipation, and diarrhea have been reported most often (6751,6752,6762). There is one case report of cholestatic hepatitis associated with the use of the multi-ingredient product that contains saw palmetto (Prostata) (598). Some clinicians are concerned that saw palmetto might cause erectile dysfunction, ejaculatory disturbance, or altered libido because of saw palmetto's potential effects on 5-alpha-reductase. There is one case report of decreased ejaculatory volume associated with an herbal blend product containing saw palmetto extract, nettle root extract, pumpkin seed oil extract, lemon bioflavonoid extract, and beta-carotene (5093). However, clinical studies indicate that the occurrence of impotence in men taking saw palmetto is similar to placebo and significantly less than finasteride (Proscar) (2732,6424,6762).

Interactions with Herbs & Other Dietary Supplements

Insufficient reliable information available.

Interactions with Drugs

ORAL CONTRACEPTIVES, HORMONE THERAPY: Concomitant use with saw palmetto can interfere with oral contraceptives and hormone therapy (4).

Interactions with Foods

No interactions are known to occur, and there is no known reason to expect a clinically significant interaction with saw palmetto.

Interactions with Lab Tests

PROSTATE-SPECIFIC ANTIGEN: Contrary to earlier concerns, saw palmetto extract appears to have no significant effect on serum prostate-specific antigen (PSA) levels (764).

Interactions with Diseases or Conditions

No interactions are known to occur, and there is no known reason to expect a clinically significant interaction with saw palmetto.

Dosage and Administration

ORAL: For treating symptoms of benign prostatic hyperplasia (BPH), the recommended daily dose is 1-2 grams of whole berries. Clinical studies have used 160 mg twice daily or 320 mg once daily of a lipophilic extract containing 80-90% fatty acids (2,512). A liquid extract is commonly dosed as 0.6-1.5 mL (4). A tea prepared by simmering 0.5-1 grams of dried berry in 150 mL boiling water for 5-10 minutes and then straining is taken three times daily (4). However, brewed teas or other hydrophilic preparations might not contain adequate active constituents (512).

Comments

In the first half of the twentieth century, saw palmetto tea was included in the United States Pharmacopeia and the National Formulary (4229).

SCARLET PIMPERNEL

Also Known As

Adder's Eyes, Phytoestrogen, Poor Man's Weatherglass, Red Chickweed, Red Pimpernel, Shepherd's Barometer.

Scientific Names

Anagallis arvensis.
Family: Primulaceae.

People Use This For

Orally, scarlet pimpernel is used for depression, mucous membrane disorders, liver disorders, herpes, and as supportive therapy for carcinomas. It is also used orally for painful kidney disorders, particularly those with inflammation and an increase in urination.
Topically, scarlet pimpernel is used for poorly healing wounds and pruritus.
It is used both orally and topically to treat painful joints (18).

Safety

POSSIBLY UNSAFE ...when used orally or topically long-term (18).
There is insufficient reliable information available about the safety of scarlet pimpernel for short-term oral or topical use.
PREGNANCY: LIKELY UNSAFE ... when used orally or topically long-term. Scarlet pimpernel shows evidence of uterine stimulant activity (18).
LACTATION: POSSIBLY UNSAFE ...when used orally or topically long-term; avoid using.

Effectiveness

There is insufficient reliable information available about the effectiveness of scarlet pimpernel.

Mechanism of Action

The applicable parts of scarlet pimpernel are the above ground flowering plant parts. In vitro data suggests that the aqueous extract has fungitoxic activity, and the isolated components triterpenglycoside, anagalloside and aglycon anagalligenone have bacsteriostatic activity. Animal and human tissue data suggests uterine contracting activity. Triterepene saponins isolated from scarlet pimpernel may have activity against human sperm and may have estrogenic activity. A methanolic extract has hemolytic activity in human blood, and has activity against herpes simplex I, adenovirus type II, and polio type II. The gastrointeritis and nephritis that occurs with large doses or long-term administration is probably due to the cucurbitacins that are present in scarlet pimpernel (18).

Adverse Reactions

Orally, gastrointeritis and nephritis may occur with large doses or long-term administration (18).

Interactions with Herbs & Other Dietary Supplements

Insufficient reliable information available.

Interactions with Drugs

No interactions are known to occur, and there is no known reason to expect a clinically significant interaction with scarlet pimpernel.

Interactions with Foods

No interactions are known to occur, and there is no known reason to expect a clinically significant interaction with scarlet pimpernel.

Interactions with Lab Tests

No interactions are known to occur, and there is no known reason to expect a clinically significant interaction with scarlet pimpernel.

Interactions with Diseases or Conditions

HORMONE SENSITIVE CANCERS/CONDITIONS: Because scarlet pimpernel might have estrogenic effects (18), women with hormone sensitive conditions should not use scarlet pimpernel. Some of these conditions include breast, uterine, and ovarian cancer, and endometriosis and uterine fibroids.
INFERTILITY: Scarlet pimpernel might have activity against sperm (18). Use cautiously or avoid in women trying to conceive and in men with fertility problems.

Dosage and Administration

ORAL: One cup of tea is commonly taken throughout the day. The tea is prepared by steeping teaspoons of dried plant in 150 mL of boiling water for 10 minutes and straining. The usual daily dosage can be up to 1.8 grams 4 times daily (18).
TOPICAL: No typical dosage.

Comments

None.

SCHISANDRA

Also Known As

Bac Ngu Vi Tu, Bei Wu Wei Zi, Beiwuweizi, Chinesischer Limonenbaum, Chosen-Gomischi, Five-Flavor-Fruit, Five-Flavor-Seed, Gomishi, Hoku-Gomishi, Kita-Gomishi, Limonnik Kitajskij, M Mei Gee, Magnolia Vine, Matsbouza, Nanwuweizi, Ngu Mei Gee, Northern Schisandra, Omicha, Schisandrae, Schisandra Berry, Schizandra, Schizandrae, Southern Schisandra, Wu Wei Zi, Wu-Wei-Zi, Wuweizi, Western Shisandra, Xiwuweizi.

Scientific Names

Schisandra chinensis; Schisandra splenanthera; other Schisandra species.
Family: Schisandraceae.

People Use This For

Orally, schisandra is used as an adaptogen for increasing resistance to disease and stress, increasing energy (515), and increasing physical performance and endurance (3559). Schisandra is also used orally for improving vision, boosting muscular activity, improving cellular energy, for hepatitis, liver protection, preventing premature aging, increasing lifespan, for premenstrual syndrome, stimulating the immune system, speeding recovery after surgery, protecting against radiation, counteracting the effects of sugar, preventing motion sickness, normalizing blood sugar and blood pressure, reducing high cholesterol, preventing infection, improving adrenal health, and energizing RNA-DNA to rebuild cells (515).
In traditional Chinese medicine, schisandra is used for coughs, asthma, insomnia, neurasthenia, chronic diarrhea, dysentery, night sweats, spontaneous sweating, involuntary seminal discharge, thirst, impotence, physical exhaustion, excessive urination (11), depression, irritability, and memory loss (6).
Schisandra fruit is eaten as a food (11).

Safety

POSSIBLY SAFE ...when used orally and appropriately (12,3559).
PREGNANCY: POSSIBLY UNSAFE ...when used orally; avoid using. Some evidence suggests schisandra fruit is a uterine stimulant (11,3559).
LACTATION: Insufficient reliable information; avoid using.

Effectiveness

POSSIBLY EFFECTIVE ...when schisandra fruit extract is used orally for improving liver function in patients with hepatitis (3559). Schisandra fruit extracts reduce serum glutamic-pyruvic transaminase (SGPT) levels in patients with viral or drug-induced hepatitis (3559). ...when schisandra fruit extract is used orally for improving concentration, coordination, and endurance (3559).
There is insufficient reliable information available about the effectiveness of schisandra for its other uses.

Mechanism of Action

The applicable part of schisandra is the fruit. A variety of active constituents including schizandrins, schizandrols, gomisins, schizandrers, schisantherins, wuweizisus, and many others, collectively known as lignans, have been isolated from schisandra (11,3559). Some schisandra extracts are standardized based on specific lignan content (3559). Schisandra improves liver function by increasing hepatic glutathione, glucose-6-phosphate, and glutathione-reductase activity. It might also have a hepatoprotective effect by inhibiting lipid peroxidation, increasing liver glycogen production, inducing the hepatic microsomal cytochrome P-450 system, and promoting hepatocyte growth (11,3559). Schisandra is referred to as an adaptogen; it increases concentration, coordination, and endurance in workers and athletes (3559). The mechanism(s) for these effects is not known. Schisandra also has antioxidant and anti-inflammatory properties (3559). Other reported properties of various schisandra lignans include antitussive (6), anticonvulsant, antidepressant, antifatigue, tranquilizing, respiratory stimulant (11), and platelet activating factor (PAF) inhibition (3767).

Adverse Reactions

Orally, schisandra can cause heartburn, acid indigestion, decreased appetite, stomach pain, allergic skin rashes, and urticaria in some patients (11,3559).

Interactions with Herbs & Other Dietary Supplements

Insufficient reliable information available.

Interactions with Drugs

HEPATICALLY METABOLIZED DRUGS: Theoretically, concurrent administration may interfere with metabolism of some drugs, due to the hepatic enzyme-activating effects of schisandra (6).

Interactions with Foods

No interactions are known to occur, and there is no known reason to expect a clinically significant interaction with schisandra.

Interactions with Lab Tests

SERUM GLUTAMIC-PYRUVIC TRANSAMINASE (SGPT)/ALANINE AMINOTRANSFERASE (ALT): Schisandra might lower serum SGPT/ALT levels and test results (11,3559).

Interactions with Diseases or Conditions

GASTROESOPHAGEAL REFLUX DISEASE (GERD), PEPTIC ULCER DISEASE (PUD): Schisandra might exacerbate GERD or PUD by increasing gastric acidity (3559).
EPILEPSY: One source recommends avoiding use in these patients (3559). The reason for this warning is not clear, but it may be due to schisandra's potential CNS stimulating effects (6).
HIGH INTRACRANIAL PRESSURE: One source recommends avoiding use in these patients (3559). The reason for this warning is not clear, but it may be due to schisandra's potential CNS stimulating effects (6).

Dosage and Administration

ORAL: For hepatitis, schisandra extract standardized to 20 mg lignan content (equivalent to 1.5 grams crude schisandra) given daily has been used (3559). For improving mental and physical performance, schisandra extract 500 mg to 2 grams daily or crude schisandra 1.5-6 grams daily have been used (3559); Crude schisandra decoction (boiled tea) 5-15 grams daily has also been used (3559). People have also taken schisandra extract 100 mg twice daily (6002). Appropriate dosing may vary depending on extract type and standardization.

Comments

Some evidence suggests that nigranoic acid, isolated from the stem of Schisandra sphaerandra, might be useful in HIV therapy. In vitro it exhibits anti-HIV reverse transcriptase and polymerase activity (3768). An antihepatotoxic drug known as DBD has been developed in China derived from the schisandra constituent schisandrin C (3559).

SCOPOLIA

Also Known As

Belladonna, Belladonna Scopola, Glockenbilsenkraut, Japanese Belladonna, Russian Krainer Tollkraut, Scopola, Scopoliae Rhizoma.

Scientific Names

Scopolia carniolica.
Family: Solanaceae.

People Use This For

Orally, scopolia used for spasms of the gastrointestinal (GI) tract, bile ducts, and urinary tract (2), and for liver and gallbladder complaints (18).
In folk medicine, scopolia is used orally as a diuretic, sedative, hypnotic, narcotic, for dilating pupils, and pain relief.

Safety

LIKELY UNSAFE ...when used orally for self-medication (12). Use of scopolia requires monitoring (12). The lethal adult dose is considered to be 100 mg of atropine which is approximately 20-50 grams of scopolia root or rhizome depending on its alkaloid content (18).
PREGNANCY AND LACTATION: LIKELY UNSAFE ...when used orally for self-medication (12); avoid using.

Effectiveness

LIKELY EFFECTIVE ...when used for spasms of the gastrointestinal (GI) tract, bile ducts, and urinary tract for adults and children older than 6 years (2).
There is insufficient reliable information available about the effectiveness of scopolia for its other uses.

Mechanism of Action

The applicable parts of scopolia are the rhizome and root. Scopolia root or rhizome contains 0.3-0.8% alkaloids, primarily L-hyoscyamine and lesser amounts of atropine and scopolamine (2). L-Hyoscyamine, the levorotatory isomer of atropine, is considered the active principle (2). Scopolia root has parasympatholytic activity. It is a competitive antagonist of acetylcholine, acting preferentially at the muscarinic receptors (2). Scopolia has antispasmodic effects, relaxing the smooth muscle of the gastrointestinal tract and bile ducts (2). Scopolia root can eliminate muscular tremors and muscular rigidity caused by central nervous impulses. It also has positive chronotropic and dromotropic effects (2).

Adverse Reactions

Orally, scopolia root can cause dry mouth, dry and reddened skin, hyperthermia, disturbance of ocular accommodation, tachycardia, difficulty urinating, glaucoma attacks (2), and constipation (18). Early symptoms of poisoning include reddened skin, dry mouth, and tachycardiac arrhythmias (18). Ingestion of large amounts can cause central excitation including restlessness, compulsive speech, hallucinations, delirium, manic episodes, followed by exhaustion and sleep, and asphyxiation (18).

Interactions with Herbs & Other Dietary Supplements

ANTICHOLINERGIC HERBS: Scopolia can potentiate the effects and adverse effects of other herbs with anticholinergic activity including belladonna, henbane, mandrake, and jimson weed (12).

Interactions with Drugs

ANTICHOLINERGIC DRUGS: The alkaloid constituents, hyoscyamine, scopolamine, and atropine could potentiate the effects and adverse effects of anticholinergic drugs (15).
TRICYCLIC ANTIDEPRESSANTS: Concomitant use with scopolia can potentiate anticholinergic effects and adverse effects (2).
AMANTADINE: Concomitant use with scopolia might increase effects (2).
QUINIDINE: Concomitant use with scopolia might increase effects (2).

Interactions with Foods
No interactions are known to occur, and there is no known reason to expect a clinically significant interaction with scopolia.

Interactions with Lab Tests
No interactions are known to occur, and there is no known reason to expect a clinically significant interaction with scopolia.

Interactions with Diseases or Conditions
CONGESTIVE HEART FAILURE (CHF): Contraindicated; scopolia might cause tachycardia and exacerbate CHF due to its hyoscyamine (atropine) and scopolamine content (15).
CONSTIPATION: Contraindicated; scopolia might cause constipation due to its hyoscyamine (atropine) and scopolamine content (15).
DOWN SYNDROME: Caution, patients with Down syndrome might be hypersensitive to the antimuscarinic effects (mydriasis, positive chronotropic heart effects, etc.) of hyoscyamine (atropine) and scopolamine contained in scopolia (15).
ESOPHAGEAL REFLUX: Contraindicated; scopolia might delay gastric emptying and decrease lower esophageal pressure, promoting gastric retention and exacerbating reflux due to its hyoscyamine (atropine) and scopolamine content (15).
FEVER: Contraindicated; scopolia might increase the risk of hyperthermia in patients with fever due to its hyoscyamine (atropine) and scopolamine content (15).
GASTRIC ULCER: Contraindicated; scopolia might delay gastric emptying and exacerbate gastric ulcers due to its hyoscyamine (atropine) and scopolamine content (15).
GI INFECTIONS: Contraindicated; scopolia might suppress GI motility causing retention of infecting organisms or toxins due to its hyoscyamine (atropine) and scopolamine content (15).
HIATAL HERNIA: Contraindicated; scopolia might delay gastric emptying and decrease lower esophageal pressure, promoting gastric retention and exacerbating reflux due to its hyoscyamine (atropine) and scopolamine content (15).
TOXIC MEGACOLON: Contraindicated; scopolia might suppress intestinal motility, which might produce paralytic ileus and exacerbate toxic megacolon, due to its hyoscyamine (atropine) and scopolamine content (2,15).
NARROW-ANGLE GLAUCOMA: Contraindicated; scopolia might increase ocular tension in patients with narrow-angle (angle-closure) glaucoma due to its hyoscyamine (atropine) and scopolamine content (2,15).
OBSTRUCTIVE GI TRACT DISEASE: Contraindicated; scopolia might exacerbate obstructive GI tract diseases (including atony, paralytic ileus, and stenosis) due to its hyoscyamine (atropine) and scopolamine content (15).
TACHYARRHYTHMIAS: Contraindicated; scopolia might cause tachycardia due to its hyoscyamine (atropine) and scopolamine content (2,15).
URINARY RETENTION: Contraindicated; scopolia might increase urinary retention due to its hyoscyamine (atropine) and scopolamine content (2,15).
ULCERATIVE COLITIS: Contraindicated; scopolia might suppress intestinal motility, which might produce paralytic ileus and precipitate toxic megacolon, due to its hyoscyamine (atropine) and scopolamine content (15).

Dosage and Administration
ORAL: The average daily dose is 0.25 mg total alkaloids calculated as hyoscyamine (2). The maximum single dose is 1 mg total alkaloids calculated as hyoscyamine (2). The maximum daily dose is 3 mg total alkaloids calculated as hyoscyamine. Scopolia is administered as pulverized root, powder, or other preparations (2).

Comments
None.

SCOTCH BROOM flower

Also Known As
Bannal, Besenginaterkraut, Broom Tops, Butcher's-Broom, Cystisi scoparii flos, Genet a Balais, Ginsterkraut, Herbe de Hogweed, Hogweed, Irish Broom Tops, Scoparius.
CAUTION: See separate listings for Butcher's Broom, Scotch Broom herb, and Spanish Broom.

Scientific Names
Cytisus scoparius, synonyms Sarothamnus scoparius, Sarothamnus vulgaris, Spartium scoparium.
Family: Leguminosae or Fabaceae.

People Use This For

Orally, scotch broom flower is used as a mild diuretic (9) and for improving circulation (6).

Topically, scotch broom flower is used for sore muscles, abscesses, and swelling (11). It is used in hair rinses to lighten and brighten hair (11).

Historically, it has been used as a cathartic and emetic (6), for cardiac dropsy, tachycardia, and profuse menstruation (4).

Safety

POSSIBLY SAFE ...when consumed in food amounts. It is listed as a flavoring agent by Council of Europe without safety assessment (4).

LIKELY UNSAFE ...when used orally for self-medication in amounts greater than those found in foods (4,12). Contains sparteine, an alkaloid with cardiac depressant activities similar to quinidine (4).

There is insufficient reliable information available about the safety of scotch broom flower for topical use.

PREGNANCY: LIKELY UNSAFE ...when used orally because it appears to be an abortifacient (5,9,12).

LACTATION: POSSIBLY SAFE ...when used orally in food amounts. LIKELY UNSAFE ...when used orally in amounts greater than those found in foods; avoid using (4,12).

Effectiveness

There is insufficient reliable information available about the effectiveness of scotch broom flower.

Mechanism of Action

Scotch broom flower contains sparteine, an alkaloid, which has curare-like properties and mimics quinidine's anti-arrhythmic effect (4). Sparteine extends diastole without a positive inotropic effect (8). The diuretic effect of the herb may be due to the flavone glycoside, scoparoside (5). It also contains tyramine (4,6,11).

Adverse Reactions

Orally, it may cause nausea, diarrhea, vertigo, stupor, tachycardia with circulatory collapse, and respiratory arrest (4). Smoking scotch broom cigarettes may cause headaches and uterine stimulation (6), and may risk contracting pulmonary aspergillosis (5,6).

Interactions with Herbs & Other Dietary Supplements

Insufficient reliable information available.

Interactions with Drugs

MONOAMINE OXIDASE INHIBITORS (MAOIs): The tyramine content of scotch broom flower can cause hypertensive crisis (2).

Interactions with Foods

No interactions are known to occur, and there is no known reason to expect a clinically significant interaction with scotch broom flower.

Interactions with Lab Tests

No interactions are known to occur, and there is no known reason to expect a clinically significant interaction with scotch broom flower.

Interactions with Diseases or Conditions

HYPERTENSION: Contraindicated due to vasoconstrictive effect (2,4).

CARDIAC DISEASE: Contraindicated due to negative inotropic and negative chronotropic effects (2,4).

KIDNEY DISORDERS: The component, scoparin, might have diuretic activity which could aggravate kidney disorders (19).

SPLEEN AND LIVER DISORDERS: Contraindicated (19).

Dosage and Administration

ORAL: Drink as tea (steep 1-2 grams in boiling water 5-10 minutes, strain) three times daily (4). Liquid extract (1:1 in 25% alcohol), 1-2 mL (4) Tincture: (1:5 in 45% alcohol) 0.5-2 mL (4).

Comments

Avoid confusion with butcher's broom root, scotch broom herb, and Spanish broom flower. Scotch broom seeds used as a coffee substitute are dangerous (6).

SCOTCH BROOM herb

Also Known As

Bannal, Basam, Besom, Bizzom, Broom, Browme, Breeam, Brum, Cytisi scoparii herba, Hogweed, Irish Broom, Scoparium, Scoparius.
CAUTION: See separate listings for Butcher's Broom, Scotch Broom flower, and Spanish Broom.

Scientific Names

Cytisus scoparius, synonyms Sarothamnus scoparius, Sarothamnus vulgaris, Spartium scoparium.
Family: Leguminosae or Fabaceae.

People Use This For

Orally, scotch broom herb is used for heart and circulatory disorders (2).
Historically, people used scotch broom herb for edema, cardiac arrhythmia, racing heartbeat, low blood pressure, heavy menstruation, hemorrhaging after birth, as a contraction stimulant, for bleeding gums, hemophilia, gout, rheumatism, sciatica, gallbladder and kidney stones, enlarged spleen, jaundice, bronchial conditions, and snake bites (18).

Safety

POSSIBLY SAFE ...when the aqueous-ethanolic extract is used orally and appropriately (2).
LIKELY UNSAFE …when used orally in excessive amounts. Toxicity has been reported with ingestion of more than 300 mg sparteine (30 grams of above ground parts) (18).
PREGNANCY: POSSIBLY UNSAFE ...when used orally due to potential for uterine contractions (6,18).
LACTATION: Insufficient reliable information available; avoid using.

Effectiveness

POSSIBLY EFFECTIVE ...when used orally for cardiac and circulatory disorders (2). Functional heart and circulatory disorders require medical management rather than self-medication.
There is insufficient reliable information available about the effectiveness of scotch broom for its other uses.

Mechanism of Action

The constituent, sparteine, has negative inotropic and chronotropic effects, which are responsible for its cardiac activity. It also seems to stimulate uterine contractions (6). The constituent tyramine, acts as an indirect vasoconstrictor and hypertensive (18).

Adverse Reactions

Orally, sparteine toxicity can occur with doses greater than 300 mg of sparteine, which is roughly equivalent to 30 grams of scotch broom. Symptoms of this toxicity include dizziness, headache, palpitations, prickling in the extremities, feeling of weakness in the legs, sweating, sleepiness, pupil dilation, and ocular palsy (18).

Interactions with Herbs & Other Dietary Supplements

Insufficient reliable information available.

Interactions with Drugs

MONOAMINE OXIDASE INHIBITORS (MAOIs): Scotch broom contains tyramine. It should not be used with monoamine oxidase inhibitors because it might cause a hypertensive crisis (2,18)
METABOLISM INHIBITORS: Quinidine (Quinidex) and haloperidol (Haldol) inhibit sparteine metabolism, which is found in scotch broom herb, increasing the risk of adverse effects including circulatory collapse (17).

Interactions with Foods

No interactions are known to occur, and there is no known reason to expect a clinically significant interaction with scotch broom herb.

Interactions with Lab Tests

No interactions are known to occur, and there is no known reason to expect a clinically significant interaction with scotch broom herb.

Interactions with Diseases or Conditions

A-V BLOCK: Contraindicated (18).
HIGH BLOOD PRESSURE: Contraindicated (18).

Dosage and Administration

ORAL: One cup freshly brewed tea 3-4 times daily. To make tea, steep 1 level teaspoon (1-2 grams) above ground parts in 150 mL boiling water 5-10 minutes , strain (7). Liquid extract: 1-2 mL daily (18). Tincture: 0.5-2 mL daily (18). Aqueous-ethanolic extracts: 1-1.5 grams of above ground parts (7).

Comments

Avoid confusion with butcher's broom, scotch broom flower, and Spanish broom.

SCOTCH PINE NEEDLE

Also Known As

Pine Oils, Pini Atheroleum.
CAUTION: See separate listings for Dwarf Pine Needle, Fir Needle Oil, Poplar, Fir, and Pine.

Scientific Names

Pinus sylvestris.
Family: Pinaceae.

People Use This For

Orally or by inhalation, scotch pine needle is used for the common cold, cough, and bronchitis.
Orally, scotch pine needle is used for fever, inflammation of the mouth and pharynx, and the tendency for infection (18).
Topically, scotch pine needle is used for rheumatic and neuralgic ailments (18).

Safety

There is insufficient reliable information available about the safety of scotch pine needle.
Pregnancy and Lactation: Insufficient reliable information available; avoid using.

Effectiveness

There is insufficient reliable information available about the effectiveness of scotch pine needle.

Mechanism of Action

The applicable part of scotch pine needle is the oil. The essential oil includes alpha-pinene, delta3-carene, camphene, beta-pinene, limonene, myrcene, and terpinolene. People think scotch pine needle oil has hyperemic, weak antiseptic, and secretolytic properties (18).

Adverse Reactions

Orally, scotch pine needle can worsen bronchospasms (18).
Topically, scotch pine needle can be irritating to the skin and mucous membranes (18).

Interactions with Herbs & Other Dietary Supplements

Insufficient reliable information available.

Interactions with Drugs

No interactions are known to occur, and there is no known reason to expect a clinically significant interaction with scotch pine needle.

Interactions with Foods

No interactions are known to occur, and there is no known reason to expect a clinically significant interaction with scotch pine needle.

Interactions with Lab Tests

No interactions are known to occur, and there is no known reason to expect a clinically significant interaction with scotch pine needle.

Interactions with Diseases or Conditions

CARDIAC DISORDERS: Avoid using as a bath additive in individuals with a history of cardiac insufficiency (18).
INFECTION: Avoid using as a bath additive in individuals with fever or infectious diseases (18).
HYPERTONIA: Avoid using as a bath additive (18).

RESPIRATORY ILLNESS: Contraindicated in individuals with asthma and whooping cough because scotch pine needle oil might cause or worsen bronchospasms (18).
SKIN CONDITIONS: Avoid using as a bath additive when extensive skin injuries or acute skin diseases are present (18).

Dosage and Administration

ORAL: An average daily dose is 5 grams (18).
INHALATION: Place several drops in hot water and breathe in the vapors (18).
TOPICAL: Several drops or semi-solid preparation containing 10-50 % drug may be rubbed onto the affected area (18).
As a bath additive 25 mg drug per liter water is used in bubble bath or bath salts (18).
The essential oil is administered in alcoholic solutions, ointments, gels, emulsions, oils, or as an inhalant (18).

Comments

Avoid confusion with "pine oils" that are synthetically produced (18).

SCOTCH THISTLE

Also Known As
Woolly Thistle.

Scientific Names
Onopordum acanthium.
Family: Asteraceae.

People Use This For
Orally, scotch thistle is used as a cardiac stimulant (18).

Safety
There is insufficient reliable information available about the safety of scotch thistle.
Pregnancy and Lactation: Insufficient reliable information available; avoid using.

Effectiveness
There is insufficient reliable information available about the effectiveness of scotch thistle.

Mechanism of Action
There is insufficient reliable information available about the possible mechanism of action and active ingredients.

Adverse Reactions
Scotch thistle can cause an allergic reaction in individuals sensitive to the Asteraceae/Compositae family. Members of this family include ragweed, chrysanthemums, marigolds, daisies, and many other herbs.

Interactions with Herbs & Other Dietary Supplements
Insufficient reliable information available.

Interactions with Drugs
No interactions are known to occur, and there is no known reason to expect a clinically significant interaction with scotch thistle.

Interactions with Foods
No interactions are known to occur, and there is no known reason to expect a clinically significant interaction with scotch thistle.

Interactions with Lab Tests
No interactions are known to occur, and there is no known reason to expect a clinically significant interaction with scotch thistle.

Interactions with Diseases or Conditions
CROSS-ALLERGENICITY: Scoth thistle can cause an allergic reaction in individuals sensitive to the Asteraceae/Compositae family. Members of this family include ragweed, chrysanthemums, marigolds, daisies, and many other herbs.

Dosage and Administration

ORAL: Scotch thistle is available in Europe as Cardiodoron (18).

Comments

Scotch thistle sounds and looks similar to milk thistle. Be careful not to confuse the two. There is very little scientific information about this product. Our staff is continually analyzing the available information on natural medicines and will add data here as it becomes available.

SCULLCAP

Also Known As

Blue Pimpernel, Helmet Flower, Hoodwort, Mad Weed, Mad-Dog Herb, Mad-Dog Weed, Quaker Bonnet, Scutelluria, Skullcap.
CAUTION: See separate listing for Baikal Skullcap.

Scientific Names

Scutellaria lateriflora.
Family: Labiatae or Lamiaceae.

People Use This For

Orally or by injection, scullcap is used for cerebral thrombosis or embolism and paralysis caused by stroke (4). Traditionally, scullcap is used for fever (18), "female weakness" (5,6), rabies, and as a tonic (5,6,18). It has also been used for grand mal seizures (4), chorea, epilepsy, hysteria, insomnia, nervous tension, spasms (4), and as a tranquilizer (5,6). In traditional Chinese medicine, scullcap has been used for hyperlipidemia and atherosclerosis, allergic conditions, dermatitis, and for inflammation (4).

Safety

POSSIBLY SAFE …when used orally and appropriately (12).
PREGNANCY AND LACTATION: Insufficient reliable information available; avoid using.

Effectiveness

POSSIBLY EFFECTIVE …when the constituent scutellarin is used orally, intravenously, or intramuscularly for cerebral thrombosis or embolism and paralysis caused by stroke (4).
There is insufficient reliable information available about the effectiveness of scullcap for its other uses.

Mechanism of Action

The applicable parts of scullcap are the above ground parts. Scullcap contains flavonoids including scutellarin, catalpol, lignin, resin, tannin, and volatile oil (4,18). Pharmacological activity of scullcap flavonoids has primarily been demonstrated in vitro and in animals. Scullcap has been shown to inhibit mast cell histamine release in vitro. In animals, scullcap has been shown to inhibit lipid peroxidation and have a hypolipidemic effect (4). These effects have not been demonstrated in humans. Although scullcap is purported to have sedative and antispasmodic activity, one study did not find these effects (4). Scullcap might have anti-inflammatory effects by inhibition of cyclo-oxygenase pathways; however, this effect has only been found in vitro. Scullcap is also purported to have anticonvulsant activity (4,18), but this has not been verified.

Adverse Reactions

Orally, large amounts of scullcap can cause giddiness, stupor, confusion, limb twitching, seizures (4,6), "intermission" of the pulse, and other symptoms consistent with epilepsy (6). There are four reports of hepatotoxicity, one of which led to a fatality. However, it is uncertain whether hepatotoxicity resulted from scullcap, or an adulterant e.g. germander, or a combination of scullcap with valerian (515).

Interactions with Herbs & Other Dietary Supplements

HERBS WITH SEDATIVE PROPERTIES: Theoretically, concomitant use with herbs that have sedative properties might enhance therapeutic and adverse effects. These include calamus, calendula, California poppy, catnip, capsicum, celery, couch grass, elecampane, Siberian ginseng, German chamomile, goldenseal, gotu kola, hops, Jamaican dogwood, kava, lemon balm, sage, St. John's wort, sassafras, shepherd's purse, stinging nettle, valerian, wild carrot, wild lettuce, ashwaganda root, and yerba mansa (4,19).

Interactions with Drugs
No interactions are known to occur, and there is no known reason to expect a clinically significant interaction with scullcap.

Interactions with Foods
No interactions are known to occur, and there is no known reason to expect a clinically significant interaction with scullcap.

Interactions with Lab Tests
No interactions are known to occur, and there is no known reason to expect a clinically significant interaction with scullcap.

Interactions with Diseases or Conditions
LIVER DISORDERS: Avoid use in individuals with liver disorders. Scullcap has been associated with some reports of liver toxicity, though adulterants might be responsible (515).

Dosage and Administration
ORAL: A typical dose is 1-2 grams or as a tea three times daily (4). To make tea, steep 1-2 grams above ground parts in 150 mL of boiling water for 5-10 minutes, strain. Extract: 2-4 mL (1:1 in 25% alcohol) three times daily. Tincture: 1-2 mL (1:5 in 45 % alcohol) three times daily (4).

Comments
Scullcap has been commonly adulterated with germander and teucrium (4,5,12).

SCURVY GRASS

Also Known As
Scrubby Grass, Spoonwort.
CAUTION: See separate listing for Watercress.

Scientific Names
Cochlearia officinalis.
Family: Brassicaceae.

People Use This For
Orally, scurvy grass is used for vitamin C deficiency, gout, arthritis, stomach ache, as a diuretic, and as a blood purifier.
Topically, scurvy grass is used for skin irritations, canker sores, and gum disease.
Historically, scurvy grass was used to remove undesirable agents from the blood.

Safety
There is insufficient reliable information available about the safety of scurvy grass.
Pregnancy and Lactation: Insufficient reliable information available; avoid using.

Effectiveness
There is insufficient reliable information available about the effectiveness of scurvy grass.

Mechanism of Action
The applicable parts of scurvy grass are the leaves and aerial parts or pressed juice. Alcohol extracts of scurvy grass are used topically. Scurvy grass contains glucosilinates, an unidentified volatile oil and bitter principle, tannin, and vitamin C. It might have antiseptic, diuretic, and mild laxative actions (7122). The mustard oils in scurvy grass can irritate the mucous membranes (18).

Adverse Reactions
Orally, large amounts of scurvy grass can cause symptoms of gastrointestinal irritation.
Topically, skin irritation may occur with topical application.

Interactions with Herbs & Other Dietary Supplements
Insufficient reliable information available.

Interactions with Drugs

No interactions are known to occur, and there is no known reason to expect a clinically significant interaction with scurvy grass.

Interactions with Foods

No interactions are known to occur, and there is no known reason to expect a clinically significant interaction with scurvy grass.

Interactions with Lab Tests

No interactions are known to occur, and there is no known reason to expect a clinically significant interaction with scurvy grass.

Interactions with Diseases or Conditions

No interactions are known to occur, and there is no known reason to expect a clinically significant interaction with scurvy grass.

Dosage and Administration

No typical dosage.

Comments

Scurvy grass was once used by sailors to prevent scurvy (7122). Scurvy grass is also known as watercress (see separate listing). Be careful not to confuse these two plants. The scurvy grass flowers have a strong fragrance and taste when they are rubbed (18).

SEA BUCKTHORN

Also Known As

Argasse, Argousier, Buckthorn, Dhar-Bu, Espino Armarillo, Espino Falso, Finbar, Grisset, Meerdorn, Oblepikha, Purging Thorn, Rokitnik, Sallow Thorn, Sanddorn, Sceitbezien, Sea Buckhorn, Sea-Buckthorn, Seabuckthorn, Seedorn, Star-Bu, Tindved.
CAUTION: See separate listings for Alder Buckthorn, European Buckthorn, and Cascara (California Buckthorn).

Scientific Names

Hippophae rhamnoides.
Family: Elaeagnaceae.

People Use This For

Orally, sea buckthorn leaves and flowers are used for treating arthritis, gastrointestinal ulcers, gout, and exanthemata (4500,4501). A tea containing sea buckthorn leaves is used as a source of vitamins, flavones, amino acids, fatty acids and minerals; for improving blood pressure and blood lipids; preventing and controlling blood vessel diseases; removing free radicals; and boosting immunity (461).
Orally, sea buckthorn berries are used for preventing infections, improving sight, and inhibiting sclerosis and aging (18). Orally, sea buckthorn seed or berry oil is used as an expectorant, for treating asthma, cardiac disorders including angina, for lowering cholesterol, preventing atheroma, and as an antioxidant. It is also used orally for postponing senility; reducing cancer morbidity and the toxicity of chemotherapy; balancing the immune system; stomach and intestinal diseases including ulcers and reflux esophagitis (459,462,464,478,479,480); treating night blindness (463); and as a supplemental source of vitamins C, A, and E, beta carotene, flavonoids, superoxide dismutase, minerals, amino acids, and fatty acids (459,460,462).
Topically, sea buckthorn berries, berry concentrate, and berry or seed oil are used as a sunscreen, for treating radiation damage from x-rays and sunburns (18,458,462,4500); healing wounds including bedsores, burns, and cuts (18,458,462,4501); for acne, dermatitis, dry skin, eczema, skin ulcers, postpartum pigmentation (458,459), and for protecting mucus membranes (463).
In foods, sea buckthorn berries are used to make jellies, juices, purees, and sauces (4500,4501,4503).
In manufacturing, sea buckthorn is used in cosmetics and anti-aging preparations.

Safety

LIKELY SAFE ...when consumed in amounts found in foods.
POSSIBLY SAFE ...when used orally and appropriately. There are no published reports of toxicity (18,4501).
PREGNANCY AND LACTATION: Insufficient reliable information available; avoid using in amounts greater than those found in foods.

Effectiveness

There is insufficient reliable information about the effectiveness of sea buckthorn.

Mechanism of Action

The applicable parts of sea buckthorn are the flowers, fruit, seeds, and leaves. Sea buckthorn contains ascorbic acid (vitamin C) (18,4504), fruit acids (malic acid, acetic acid, and quinic acid), flavonoids (kaempferol, isorhamnetin, quercetin tri- and tetra-glycosides), carotenoids (beta-carotene, gamma-carotene, lycopene), fatty oils (oleic acid, isolinol acid, linolenic acid, and stearic acid), and sugar alcohols (mannitol and quebrachit) (18). A volatile oil in the fruit contains vitamins A, B1, B2, B6, in addition to vitamin C (4501). Preliminary evidence suggests that sea buckthorn extract (plant part not specified) and two constituents of the seed oil (beta-sitosterol-beta-D-glucoside and aglycone) might have activity against gastric ulcers (466,472). The fruit juice reduces the incidence and growth of experimentally-induced tumors (468). The seed oil might protect against carbon tetrachloride, ethyl alcohol and acetaminophen-induced liver damage (469,470). Some data suggest that sea buckthorn extract (plant part not specified) might protect cells from lipid peroxidation injury (471) and might increase the rate and extent of wound tissue epithelialization and granulation (467). Preliminary human evidence indicates that sea buckthorn seed oil might reduce the toxicity of chemotherapy on the blood, gastrointestinal tract and immune system (478), improve symptoms of reflux esophagitis (479), and improve the symptoms and cure rate of peptic ulcers (480).

Adverse Reactions

None reported.

Interactions with Herbs & Other Dietary Supplements

Insufficient reliable information available.

Interactions with Drugs

No interactions are known to occur, and there is no known reason to expect a clinically significant interaction with sea buckthorn.

Interactions with Foods

No interactions are known to occur, and there is no known reason to expect a clinically significant interaction with sea buckthorn.

Interactions with Lab Tests

No interactions are known to occur, and there is no known reason to expect a clinically significant interaction with sea buckthorn.

Interactions with Diseases or Conditions

No interactions are known to occur, and there is no known reason to expect a clinically significant interaction with sea buckthorn.

Dosage and Administration

ORAL: 1-2 cups of a tea prepared from the leaves is typically consumed daily (461). 1-3 seed oil capsules (500 mg per capsule) are commonly used three times daily (462,464). 3-5 mL of the seed oil is commonly used three times daily (478,479). Up to 2 dropperfuls of the berry oil is commonly used three times daily (463).
TOPICAL: The berry or seed oil is typically applied three or four times per day (462,463).

Comments

Avoid confusion with alder buckthorn (Rhamnus frangula). The fatty oil of sea buckthorn seeds and berries is harvested from August until the first snow of December (18). The fruit juices and purees are popular due to their flavor (4504).

SECRETIN

Also Known As

None.

Scientific Names

Secretin; Oxykrinin.

People Use This For
Sublingually, secretin is used for treating autism.

Intravenously, secretin is used for autism and pervasive developmental disorder, diagnosing Zollinger-Ellison syndrome, pancreatic dysfunction, hyperparathyroidism, preventing stress ulcers, treating duodenal ulcers, gastrointestinal bleeding, pancreatitis, and cardiac failure.

Safety
LIKELY SAFE ...when used parenterally and appropriately. Secretin is a FDA-approved, prescription product (2917,6136,6636).

There is insufficient reliable information available about the safety of secretin when used sublingually.

PREGNANCY AND LACTATION: Insufficient reliable information available; avoid using.

Effectiveness
LIKELY EFFECTIVE ...when used intravenously as a diagnostic agent. Secretin is a FDA-approved prescription product for use in diagnosing pancreatic exocrine disease and Zollinger-Ellison syndrome (gastrinoma) (15).

LIKELY INEFFECTIVE ...when used intravenously for autism or pervasive developmental disorder. The use of secretin for autism is controversial. There have been some anecdotal and preliminary reports showing subjective improvement in gastrointestinal function, social and behavioral function, and language skills after single infusions of secretin (2917,6632). However, the majority of evidence shows that secretin, both synthetic human and porcine-derived preparations, is no better than placebo for any outcome measure when given in single or repeated doses (5247,6136,6636,7052).

There is insufficient reliable information available to rate the effectiveness of secretin for its other uses. However, there is some preliminary evidence that secretin might help prevent post-surgical stress ulcers (2912,2913). There's also preliminary evidence secretin might help symptoms of chronic recurrent pancreatitis (2918). More evidence is needed to rate secretin for these uses.

Mechanism of Action
Secretin is an endogenously occurring gastrointestinal hormone in humans. Secretin is in a family of hormones that also includes glucagon, glucose-dependent insulin releasing peptide (GIP), vasoactive intestinal polypeptide (VIP), and others. Normal fasting serum levels are 3-15 pg/mL. Secretin is released from S cells in the duodenum and proximal jejunum when duodenal pH falls below 4.5. Serum levels can increase to 30 pg/mL after stimulation. The primary action of secretin is to stimulate release of bicarbonate and water from the pancreas. Intravenous administration of secretin in physiological doses has the same effect. The concurrent presence of cholecystokinin (CCK) potentiates the action of secretin on the pancreas. Administration in pharmacological doses also causes decreased release of meal-stimulated gastrin and decreases gastric acid secretion (7053). Exogenously administered secretin is given intravenously because orally administered secretin is inactivated by proteolytic enzymes (15). Many people use secretin for autism, but a potential mechanism of action in autism is not known. Secretin began being used for autism based on anecdotal cases showing improvement in symptoms (2917,6632). Some researchers have speculated that certain autistic patients might have abnormally low secretin levels, but this has not been verified. Reliable clinical evidence now shows that secretin probably does not have a viable role in treating autism (5247,6136,6636,7052).

Adverse Reactions
Intravenously, the most common adverse reaction is flushing of the face, neck, and chest immediately after infusion (6007,7052). Less common potential adverse effects are vomiting (6007,7052), diarrhea, fainting, venous thrombosis (15), fever, and tachycardia (7052). Some patients can have allergic reactions including urticaria, erythema, and anaphylaxis (15,7052). Because of the potential for these hypersensitivity reactions, a 0.1 mL test dose is often administered prior to giving a full dose (7052).

Interactions with Herbs & Other Dietary Supplements
Insufficient reliable information available.

Interactions with Drugs
ANTICHOLINERGIC MEDICATIONS: Concomitant use with secretin injection can cause hyporesponsiveness to a secretin stimulation test (15,2916).

Interactions with Foods
No interactions are known to occur, and there is no known reason to expect a clinically significant interaction with secretin.

Interactions with Lab Tests

No interactions are known to occur, and there is no known reason to expect a clinically significant interaction with secretin.

Interactions with Diseases or Conditions

No interactions are known to occur, and there is no known reason to expect a clinically significant interaction with secretin.

Dosage and Administration

INTRAVENOUS: For autism, a wide variety of doses have been used. Due to the potential for hypersensitivity reactions, a 0.1 CU test dose is often given prior to administration of the full dose. Clinical studies have used either single infusions or repeated infusions for 2 or more doses separated by 6 weeks or more. Doses are most often 2 CU/kg (5247,5256,7052), but clinicians use a wide range of doses (6007). So far, clinical research does not support the use of secretin for autism. No dosage regimen has yet been proven to improve the symptoms of autism.

Comments

In some countries, secretin doses are expressed in Crick-Harper-Raper (CHR) units (14). In the United States and other countries, secretin doses are expressed in clinical units (CU) (14), where 4 CHR units = 1 CU (14). Secretin products are available in the forms of purified porcine secretin and synthetic human secretin (6136).

SELENIUM

Also Known As

L-Selenomethionine, Selenite, Selenium Dioxide, Selenized Yeast, Selenomethionine.

Scientific Names

Selenium; Se; atomic number 34.

People Use This For

Orally, selenium is used for treating HIV/AIDS, preventing cancer, heart disease, osteoarthritis, rheumatoid arthritis, abnormal pap smears, atherosclerosis, macular degeneration, infertility, gray hair, Osgood-Schlatter disease, and Keshan disease (1900,2619,2661,2662,2671,3342,3343).

Safety

LIKELY SAFE ...when used orally in amounts up to 400 mcg daily (4896).
LIKELY UNSAFE ...when used orally in doses greater than 400 mcg. Blood selenium levels can be used to assess the degree of toxicity from dietary selenium. Levels below 1000 mcg/L are not usually associated with serious damage, whereas levels above 2000 mcg/L are predictive of serious damage (14,4896). Supplemental selenium toxicity is less predictable (4896). The chemical form of selenium, e.g., selenite, selenomethionine, affects blood and tissue levels in varying degrees (4896).
PREGNANCY: LIKELY SAFE ...when used orally at the recommended dietary allowance (RDA) of 60 mcg per day (4896). Some evidence suggests larger amounts might be teratogenic or associated with miscarriage (14).
LACTATION: LIKELY SAFE ...when used orally at the recommended dietary allowance (RDA) of 70 mcg per day; avoid using larger amounts (4896).

Effectiveness

POSSIBLY EFFECTIVE ...when used orally for reducing total cancer mortality, total cancer incidence, and the incidence of lung, colorectal, and prostate cancers (2664,2667,2673,3341).
There is insufficient reliable information available about the effectiveness of selenium for its other uses.

Mechanism of Action

Selenium is an antioxidant that regulates the activity of glutathione peroxidase enzymes. These enzymes catalyze the detoxification of hydrogen peroxide and organic hydroperoxides. Selenium's protection against cardiovascular diseases and cancers is hypothesized to result from this detoxification, through an increased resistance of low-density lipoproteins (LDLs) against oxidative modification, modulation of prostaglandin synthesis and platelet aggregation, and protection against toxic heavy metals. Selenium deficiency has been implicated in the etiology of Keshan disease, an endemic cardiomyopathy observed in China, and congestive cardiomyopathy in people on artificial nutrition (2676,3341). Selenium is used for arthritis due to its antioxidant effects. The antioxidants reduce inflammation by reducing the cellular production or concentration of toxic oxygen species (2662). Selenium also seems to inhibit tumorigenesis via antioxidant pathways. In large amounts, it seems to inhibit tumor growth and stimulate apoptosis (2664). There are different varieties of selenium. Some people think that organic selenium (selenomethionine) is better absorbed than inorganic selenium (selenite). So some practitioners recommend organic selenium from sources such as selenium enriched yeast. However, there is no basis for this recommendation. Inorganic selenium seems to be just as well absorbed as organic selenium (6485).

Adverse Reactions

Orally, selenium can cause symptoms of acute toxicity including nausea, vomiting, nail changes, fatigue, and irritability (17). Chronic toxicity resembles arsenic toxicity, with symptoms including hair loss, white horizontal streaking on fingernails, paronychia, fatigue, irritability, hyperreflexia, nausea, vomiting, garlic odor on breath, and a metallic taste. Muscle tenderness, tremor, lightheadedness, and facial flushing are also observed in selenium poisoning (17). Selenium can cause thrombocytopenia and moderate hepatorenal dysfunction (17). Blood selenium levels can be used to assess the degree of toxicity. Levels below 1000 mcg/L are not usually associated with serious damage, whereas levels above 2000 mcg/L are predictive of serious damage (14). In one rare situation in Italy, 2,065 individuals were exposed to an inorganic selenium (selenite) supply present in the local water over an eleven-year period. Selenium levels were between 3-13 mcg/L in the water supply, and the study showed the melanoma incidence was 3.9 times greater in this area when compared to the remainder of the Italian province with a normal water supply (3343).

Interactions with Herbs & Other Dietary Supplements

Insufficient reliable information available.

Interactions with Drugs

CISPLATIN (Platinol-AQ): Concomitant use of selenium can increase the cytotoxic effects of cisplatin in the presence of the chelate ethylenediaminetetraacetic acid (EDTA), in comparison to cisplatin treatment alone (2668).

Interactions with Foods

No interactions are known to occur, and there is no known reason to expect a clinically significant interaction with selenium.

Interactions with Lab Tests

BLOOD SELENIUM ASSAYS: Avoid powdered gloves when drawing blood for selenium and other trace element assays due to the potential for sample contamination (2663).
CREATININE KINASE: Selenium toxicity can elevate serum creatinine kinase levels (17).
EKG: Selenium toxicity can elevate the ST segment and cause T-wave changes characteristic of myocardial infarction (17).

Interactions with Diseases or Conditions

No interactions are known to occur, and there is no known reason to expect a clinically significant interaction with selenium.

Dosage and Administration

ORAL: For cancer prevention, the typical dose of selenium is 200 mcg per day (2664,3341). In humans, 30 mcg per day is considered necessary to prevent Keshan disease, which is associated with selenium deficiency (2671).
The daily recommended dietary allowances (RDAs) of selenium are: Infants 0-12 months, not determined; Children 1-3 years, 20 mcg; Children 4-8 years, 30 mcg; Children 9-13 years, 40 mcg; People over 13 years, 55 mcg; Pregnant women, 60 mcg; and Lactating women, 70 mcg (3341,4896). The tolerable upper limit for adults is 400 mcg per day (4896).

Comments

Dietary selenium deficiency has been linked to diseases as diverse as cancer, heart disease, arthritis, and AIDS; epidemiological evidence is now emerging for the beneficial effects of selenium supplementation (2662). Most selenium enters the human body via the diet; therefore, the amount of selenium in food depends on where it is grown or raised. Crab, liver, fish, poultry, and wheat are generally good selenium sources; however, natural selenium levels in the soil are highly variable throughout the world (2671,3341). In the US, the Eastern Coastal Plain, and the Pacific Northwest have the lowest selenium levels, and people in these regions naturally ingest about 60 to 90 mcg per day (2671). The average daily intake in the US is 125 mcg, ranging between 60 to 200 mcg (2671).

SELF-HEAL

Also Known As
All-Heal, Blue Curls, Brownwort, Carpenter's Herb, Carpenter's Weed, Heal-All, Heart of the Earth, Hercules Woundwort, Hock-Heal, Prunella, Self Heal, Sicklewort, Siclewort, Slough-Heal, Woundwort.
CAUTION: See other listing for Sanicle.

Scientific Names
Prunella vulgaris.
Family: Labiatae or Lamiaceae.

People Use This For
Orally, self-heal is used for inflammatory bowel disease (Crohn's disease and ulcerative colitis), HIV/AIDS, fever, headache, vertigo, liver disease, diarrhea, and gastroenteritis. It is also used for mouth and throat ulcers, sore throat, and internal hemorrhaging.
Topically, self-heal is used for leukorrhea and gynecological disorders.

Safety
POSSIBLY SAFE …when used orally (12).
PREGNANCY AND LACTATION: Insufficient reliable information available; avoid using.

Effectiveness
There is insufficient reliable information available about the effectiveness of self-heal.

Mechanism of Action
Self-heal contains entacyclic triterpenes, tannins, caffeic and rosmarinic acids, thiamine, and vitamins C and K. It has antioxidant and astringent properties (7122). Laboratory evidence suggests that an aqueous extract of self-heal has activity against HIV and might work synergistically with zidovudine (AZT, Retrovir) and didanosine (ddI, Videx) (7234,7286).

Adverse Reactions
None reported.

Interactions with Herbs & Other Dietary Supplements
Insufficient reliable information available.

Interactions with Drugs
No interactions are known to occur, and there is no known reason to expect a clinically significant interaction with self-heal.

Interactions with Foods
No interactions are known to occur, and there is no known reason to expect a clinically significant interaction with self-heal.

Interactions with Lab Tests
No interactions are known to occur, and there is no known reason to expect a clinically significant interaction with self-heal.

Interactions with Diseases or Conditions
No interactions are known to occur, and there is no known reason to expect a clinically significant interaction with self-heal.

Dosage and Administration
ORAL: One cup of tea is commonly used. The tea is prepared by simmering one teaspoon of the dried plant in 150 mL of boiling water for 10-15 minutes and straining. For a gargle, the tea is simmered for 9 minutes (18).

Comments
Sanicle is also known as self-heal. Be careful not to confuse these two plants.

SENEGA

Also Known As

Chinese Senega, Flax, Klapperschlangen, Milkwort, Mountain Polygala, Polygalae radix, Rattlesnake Root, Senaga Snakeroot, Seneca, Seneca Snakeroot, Senega, Senega Snakeroot, Seneka, Snake Root.
CAUTION: See separate listings for Asarabacca and Bitter Milkwort.

Scientific Names

Polygala glomerata; Polygala japonica; Polygala reinii; Polygala senega, synonym Polygala senega latifolia; Polygala tenuifolia.
Family: Polygalaceae.

People Use This For

Orally, senega is used for respiratory tract mucous membrane inflammation (2), bronchial asthma, chronic bronchitis (4,515), emphysema (8), for inducing sweating, increasing saliva, as an expectorant, and an emetic (515).
Topically, senega is used as a gargle for pharyngitis (4).
Historically, senega was a cure for rattlesnake bite (515).

Safety

POSSIBLY SAFE ...when used orally and appropriately short-term (12).
LIKELY UNSAFE ...when used orally, long-term. Prolonged use can cause gastrointestinal irritation (12).
There is insufficient reliable information available about the safety of the topical use of senega.
PREGNANCY: LIKELY UNSAFE ...when used orally because it appears to have uterine and menstrual flow stimulant effects (12,19). There is insufficient reliable information available about the safety of the topical use of senega during pregnancy.
LACTATION: Insufficient reliable information available; avoid using.

Effectiveness

POSSIBLY EFFECTIVE ...when used orally for inflammation of respiratory tract mucous membrane (2).
There is insufficient reliable information available about the effectiveness of senega for its other uses.

Mechanism of Action

The applicable part of senega is the root. Senega root contains salicylic acid, methyl salicylate, and a saponin mixture referred to as senegin (4). People claim senega has expectorant and emetic activity, and that it can stimulate sweating and saliva (2,4,515). The active expectorant principles are triterpenoid saponins (515). Researchers think the saponins irritate the gastrointestinal tract mucosa and cause reflex secretion of mucous in the bronchioles (515). A French patent based on human studies states that a triterpenic acid extract has anti-inflammatory activity, and is effective against graft rejection, eczema, psoriasis, and multiple sclerosis (4).

Adverse Reactions

Orally, prolonged use of senega can cause gastrointestinal irritation (2). Large amounts can cause diarrhea, dizziness (8), queasiness (18), vomiting, and purging (4).

Interactions with Herbs & Other Dietary Supplements

Insufficient reliable information available.

Interactions with Drugs

No interactions are known to occur, and there is no known reason to expect a clinically significant interaction with senega.

Interactions with Foods

No interactions are known to occur, and there is no known reason to expect a clinically significant interaction with senega.

Interactions with Lab Tests

No interactions are known to occur, and there is no known reason to expect a clinically significant interaction with senega.

Interactions with Diseases or Conditions

FEVER: Contraindicated due to CNS depressant effects (19).

GI CONDITIONS: Contraindicated in individuals with gastrointestinal conditions including inflammation and gastritis or gastric ulcers (4,12) due to local stimulant activity and intestinal irritant effects (19).

Dosage and Administration

ORAL: A typical oral dose is 0.5-1 grams dried root or 1 cup of tea three times daily. To make tea, steep 0.5-1 grams dried root in 150 mL boiling water 5-10 minutes, and strain (4).

TOPICAL: No typical dosage.

Comments

Avoid confusion with Polygala sibirica, also referred to as polygala.

SENNA

Also Known As

Alexandrian Senna, Alexandrinische Senna, Casse, Indian Senna, Khartoum Senna, Sena Alejandrina, Séné d'Egypte, Senna Alexandrina, Sennae folium, Sennae fructus, Sennae fructus acutifoliae, Sennae fructus angustifolia, Tinnevelly Senna, True Senna.

Scientific Names

Senna alexandrina, synonyms Cassia acutifolia, Cassia angustifolia, Cassia senna.

People Use This For

Orally, senna used as a laxative for constipation, after anorectal surgery, for hemorrhoids, evacuating the GI tract to facilitate diagnostic tests, evacuation relief in individuals with anal fissures, and in "slimming" and "cleansing" teas.

Safety

LIKELY SAFE ...when used orally and appropriately short-term (2,12,272).

POSSIBLY UNSAFE ...when used orally for longer than one to two weeks (2,12). Frequent use causes the colon to function poorly, creating laxative dependence (6,272).

CHILDREN: LIKELY SAFE ...when the standardized nonprescription products are used orally and appropriately (272). If senna is used to treat constipation, only standardized products should be used.

PREGNANCY: POSSIBLY UNSAFE ...when used orally. Constipation in pregnancy should not be self-medicated (2,6,12).

LACTATION: POSSIBLY UNSAFE ...when used orally. Anthraquinone constituents cross into breast milk and can cause loose stools in some breast-fed infants (272).

Effectiveness

LIKELY EFFECTIVE ...when used orally for constipation (2,6). ...when used for bowel evacuation regimens (6). There is insufficient reliable information available about the effectiveness of senna for its other uses.

Mechanism of Action

The applicable parts of senna are the leaf and fruit. Senna leaf and fruit are stimulant laxatives (272). The cathartic properties of the leaf are greater than the fruit (4). Senna contains anthraquinones including dianthrone that consists mostly of sennosides A and B and minor amounts of sennosides C and D (6,11). Senna also contains small amounts of free anthraquinones. The dianthrone glycosides are not present in the fresh leaf, but appear to form during the drying process (11). Although it is not known exactly how the anthraquinone laxatives work, the cathartic action is limited primarily to the colon (272). Sennosides irritate the lining of the large intestine, causing contraction. Sennosides A and B also seem to induce fluid secretion in the colon. Prostaglandins might be involved in the laxative effect (6). Anthroquinone laxatives produce an effect 8-12 hours after administration, though sometimes up to 24 hours can be required (272). Anthroid laxative use is not associated with an increased risk of developing colorectal ademoma or carcinoma (6138).

Adverse Reactions

Orally, senna can cause abdominal discomfort, colic, and cramps (4). Excessive use or abuse is associated with potassium depletion, finger clubbing, development of cachexia, decreased serum globulin concentrations (4), heart function disorders, muscular weakness (2), osteomalacia, arthropathy, hepatitis, coma, neuropathy, asthma, allergy symptoms, and rhinoconjunctivitis (6). Chronic use can cause pseudomelanosis coli (pigment spots in intestinal mucosa) which is harmless, usually reverses with discontinuation (2), and is not associated with an increased risk of developing colorectal ademoma or carcinoma (6138). Prolonged senna use can cause "laxative-dependency syndrome" characterized by poor gastric motility (6), non-functioning colon (4) and laxative-induced diarrhea (6). Occupational exposure has been linked to asthma and allergy symptoms, including rhinoconjunctivitis (6).

Interactions with Herbs & Other Dietary Supplements

STIMULANT LAXATIVE HERBS: Theoretically, concomitant use with other stimulant laxative herbs increases the risk of potassium depletion. Stimulant laxative herbs include aloe dried leaf sap, wild cucumber fruit (Ecballium elaterium), blue flag rhizome, alder buckthorn, European buckthorn, butternut bark, cascara bark, castor oil, colocynth fruit pulp, gamboge bark exudate, jalap root, black root, manna bark exudate, podophyllum root, rhubarb root, and yellow dock root (19).

HORSETAIL/LICORICE: Theoretically, concomitant use with horsetail plant or licorice rhizome increases the risk of potassium depletion (19).

Interactions with Drugs

CARDIAC GLYCOSIDE DRUGS: Theoretically, overuse/abuse of this product increases the risk of adverse effects of cardiac glycoside drugs, e.g. digoxin (Lanoxin).

Interactions with Foods

No interactions are known to occur, and there is no known reason to expect a clinically significant interaction with senna.

Interactions with Lab Tests

COLORIMETRIC TESTS: Senna can discolor urine (pink, red, purple, orange, rust), interfering with diagnostic tests that depend on a color change, due to its anthraquinone content (1,4,12,275).

POTASSIUM: Excessive use of senna can cause potassium depletion, reducing serum potassium concentrations and test results (1,2,4,12,19).

Interactions with Diseases or Conditions

GI CONDITIONS: Use of senna is contraindicated in people with abdominal pain, intestinal obstruction, and acute intestinal inflammation including Crohn's disease, ulcerative colitis, appendicitis (2), stomach inflammation, anal prolapse, hemorrhoids (19), or undiagnosed abdominal pain (2,4).

HEART DISEASE: Overuse of senna can cause electrolyte disturbances and exacerbate these conditions.

ELECTROLYTE DISTURBANCES, POTASSIUM DEFICIENCY: Overuse of senna can exacerbate these conditions (2).

FLUID DEPLETION: Use of senna is contraindicated in individuals with dehydration, diarrhea, or loose stools. It can exacerbate these conditions.

Dosage and Administration

ORAL: A typical dose is 15-30 mg hydroxyanthracene derivatives daily, calculated as sennoside B (1,2). Senna leaf is used as a tea, one cup in the morning and/or at bedtime. To make tea, steep 0.5-2 grams finely chopped leaf in warm but not boiling water for 10 minutes, and strain (8). Alternatively, a cold water tea might have less adverse GI effects. To make cold water tea, steep 0.5-2 grams finely chopped leaf in cold water for 10-12 hours, and strain (8). Liquid leaf extract (1:1 in 25% alcohol), 0.5-2.0 mL (frequency unspecified) (4). One cup of fruit tea is taken in the morning and/or at bedtime. To make tea, steep 1/2 flat teaspoon of senna fruit in 150 mL warm, but not boiling water, for ten minutes, and strain (8). Individualize senna dosing to the smallest amount necessary to maintain a soft stool (2). Senna leaf should not be used continuously for more than one to two weeks (2). Use of standardized OTC senna leaf preparations reduces variability and improves dosing control (4,515).

Comments

Because senna fruit is gentler than senna leaf, the American Herbal Products Association only warns against long-term use for senna leaf, not senna fruit (12). The AHPA recommends that senna leaf products be labeled "Do not use this product if you have abdominal pain or diarrhea. Consult a health care provider prior to use if you are pregnant or nursing. Discontinue use in the event of diarrhea or watery stools. Do not exceed recommended dose. Not for long-term use." (12).

SHARK CARTILAGE

Also Known As

AE-941, MSI-1256F, Shark Cartilage Extract, Shark Cartilage Powder.
CAUTION: See separate listings for Bovine Cartilage, Chondroitin, and Squalamine.

Scientific Names
Squalus acanthias.

People Use This For
Orally, shark cartilage is used for preventing and treating cancer (840,2013,2014,2015,2019,6714,6715), arthritis (2014,2019), psoriasis (2014,2019), enteritis (2014), diabetic retinopathy (2014), and wound-healing (2015,2019).
Topically, it is used for arthritis (2014,2019).
Rectally, it is used for cancer (2013,2014).

Safety
POSSIBLY SAFE …when used orally and appropriately, short-term. Shark cartilage has been safely used in studies lasting up to 20 weeks (2015,6709,6716,6717). There is insufficient reliable information available about the safety of shark cartilage for its other uses.
PREGNANCY AND LACTATION: Insufficient reliable information available; avoid using.

Effectiveness
POSSIBLY INEFFECTIVE …when used orally for treating cancer. Shark cartilage appears to offer no benefit in people with advanced, previously treated cancer, including breast, colorectal, lung, prostate, non-Hodgkin's lymphoma, and brain cancer (1206,2015,6716,6717). However, studies of shark cartilage in people with less advanced cancer or in combination with other cancer treatments have not been published.
There is insufficient reliable information available about the effectiveness of shark cartilage for its other uses.

Mechanism of Action
The use of shark cartilage attracted popular attention after some publications suggested that sharks don't get cancer and implied that shark cartilage could prevent cancer in humans (2014,6922). Since then researchers have found that renal cell carcinoma, lymphoma, and cartilage tumors have been identified in sharks (5045,6714). However, there is still some preliminary evidence that shark cartilage might have some potential as an anticancer agent. Shark cartilage is about 40% proteins, 5-20% glycosaminoglycans, and calcium salts (2019). Chondroitin, a glycosaminoglycan in cartilage, might be an active constituent (6714). Researchers theorize that shark cartilage might inhibit angiogenesis, preventing new vessel growth required for solid tumor proliferation (2013). Some preliminary clinical evidence also shows that shark cartilage given orally appears to inhibit wound angiogenesis (6709). Early laboratory research suggests that shark cartilage might also have antimutagenic, antioxidant, anti-inflammatory, and analgesic activity (6723,6724,6725). The anti-tumor effects of shark cartilage derivatives, squalamine lactate, AE-941, and U-995, are being investigated in preclinical and phase 1 to 3 clinical trials (6718,6719,6720,6721,6726,6727).

Adverse Reactions
Orally, people taking shark cartilage have had a bad taste in the mouth, nausea, vomiting, dyspepsia, constipation, hypotension, dizziness, hyperglycemia, hypercalcemia, altered consciousness, decreased motor strength, decreased sensation, generalized weakness, fatigue, and decreased performance (2014,2015,2019,6716). It might also cause signs of acute hepatitis, including low-grade fever, jaundice, yellowing of eyes, right upper quadrant tenderness, and elevated liver enzymes (2012). Some shark cartilage products have an offensive odor and taste (2014).

Interactions with Herbs & Other Dietary Supplements
CALCIUM: Shark cartilage might cause hypercalcemia (2015,6716). Theoretically, concomitant use with supplemental calcium might exacerbate this adverse effect.

Interactions with Drugs
No interactions are known to occur, and there is no known reason to expect a clinically significant interaction with shark cartilage.

Interactions with Foods
FRUIT JUICE: Acidic fruit juice such as orange, apple, grape, or tomato, can decrease potency of shark cartilage over time. If shark cartilage is added to a fruit juice, it should be mixed immediately prior to use (2014).

Interactions with Lab Tests
CALCIUM: Shark cartilage might increase serum calcium levels and test results (2015,6716).

Interactions with Diseases or Conditions
HYPERCALCEMIA: Shark cartilage is reported to cause hypercalcemia (2015,6716) and might exacerbate this condition; avoid using.

Dosage and Administration

ORAL: For treatment of cancer, some studies have used 1 gram of shark cartilage per kg of body weight given in three to four divided doses daily (2015,6716). Typical doses suggested by commercially available products range from 500 mg to 4.5 grams given in 2-6 divided doses daily (6002). Liquid concentrates of shark cartilage are usually taken as 1 to 2 tablespoons daily (6002). Administer with meals (2015).

Comments

Shark cartilage is obtained from sharks caught in the Pacific Ocean (6). The National Cancer Institute is conducting clinical trials on shark cartilage for non-small cell lung cancer and metastatic kidney cancer (6715). Phase II clinical trials of shark cartilage for use in prostate cancer and AIDS-related Kaposi's sarcoma (KS) reported in 1995 (2013) were not completed (840).

SHARK LIVER OIL

Also Known As

Basking Shark Liver Oil, Deep Sea Shark Liver Oil, Dog Fish Liver Oil, Shark Liver, Shark Oil.
CAUTION: See separate listings for Cod Liver Oil, Fish Oils, Liver Extract, Shark Cartilage, and Squalamin

Scientific Names

Cetorhinus maximus; Centroporus squamosus; Sqaulus acanthias.

People Use This For

Orally, shark liver oil is used as an adjunctive treatment for leukemia and other cancers (6,2552), to prevent radiation illness from cancer X-ray therapy, to prevent the common cold and flu, and for general immunostimulation. It is also used orally for increasing leukocyte and thrombocyte counts during chemotherapy (6,2552).
Topically, shark liver oil is used for skin conditions, skin cancer, and as a topical protectant (6,2551).

Safety

There is insufficient reliable information available about the safety of shark liver oil.
Pregnancy and Lactation: Insufficient reliable information available; avoid using.

Effectiveness

There is insufficient reliable information available about the effectiveness of shark liver oil.

Mechanism of Action

Shark liver oil is a major source of squalene and alkylglycerols (6). Shark liver oil is classified as topical protectant(6,2551). Alkoxyglycerol derived from shark liver oil may decrease irradiation damage patients undergoing treatment of uterine cancer (2552). It is thought that the radioprotective properties of alkoxyglyce may stem from its incorporation into a pool of platelet-activating factors, and resulting in biosynthesis (2550). Alkoglycerol may also increase leukocyte and thrombocyte counts within specific dose ranges (2552). Shark liver oil h been shown in animals to have antiangiogenesis properties in certain cancers, including cutaneous lesions, kidney car and urinary bladder cancer including L-1 syngeneic (2549). However, other findings are contradictory (2552).

Adverse Reactions

Both shark liver oil and the constituent squalene have been associated with cases of aspirar and subsequent lipoid pneumonia (2546,2547,2548).

Interactions with Herbs & Other Dietary Supplements

Insufficient reliable information available.

Interactions with Drugs

No interactions are known to occur, and there is no known reason to expect a clinically nificant interaction with shark liver oil.

Interactions with Foods

No interactions are known to occur, and there is no known reason to expect a clinic significant interaction with shark liver oil.

Interactions with Lab Tests

No interactions are known to occur, and there is no known reason to expect a clinically significant interaction with shark liver oil.

Interactions with Diseases or Conditions

No interactions are known to occur, and there is no known reason to expect a clinically significant interaction with shark liver oil.

Dosage and Administration

No typical dosage.

Comments

Shark liver oil is commercially derived from the livers of three species of shark: the deep sea shark (Centrophorus squamosus), the dogfish (Sqaulus acanthias) and the basking shark (Cetorhinus maximus) (6). The liver constitutes 25% of the total shark body weight (6).

SHELLAC

Also Known As

Gommelaque, Lac, Lacca.

Scientific Names

Laccifer.
Family: Coccidae.

People Use This For

In dentistry, shellac is used as a binding agent for dentures, restorations, moldings, and as a constituent in "artificial calculus" in dental schools (6).
In the pharmaceutical industry, shellac is used in tablet coating formulations, enteric coating, microencapsulation, matrix formulation, humidity tolerance, and for its binding ability (6).
In manufacturing, shellac is used as a finish for furniture, an ingredient in hair spray and in other cosmetics (6).

Safety

LIKELY SAFE ...when used orally. It has Generally Recognized as Safe (GRAS) status in the US (6).
PREGNANCY AND LACTATION: Insufficient reliable information available.

Effectiveness

There is insufficient reliable information available about the effectiveness of shellac.

Mechanism of Action

Aleuretic acid, r-butolic acid, shellolic acid, and jalaric acid are the major constituents of shellac (6).

Adverse Reactions

There is one report of contact cheilitis associated with shellac (6).

Interactions with Herbs & Other Dietary Supplements

Insufficient reliable information available.

Interactions with Drugs

No interactions are known to occur, and there is no known reason to expect a clinically significant interaction with shellac.

Interactions with Foods

No interactions are known to occur, and there is no known reason to expect a clinically significant interaction with shellac.

Interactions with Lab Tests

No interactions are known to occur, and there is no known reason to expect a clinically significant interaction with shellac.

Interactions with Diseases or Conditions

SHELLAC ALLERGY: Contraindicated.

Dosage and Administration

No typical dosage.

Comments

Shellac is derived from the secretions of the insect Laccifer. Although shellac has been used for years in pharmacy, dentistry, and as a finish for furniture, it has fallen into disfavor for some products because it ages over time (6).

SHEPHERD'S PURSE

Also Known As

Blind Weed, Bursae Pastoris Herba, Capsella, Caseweed, Cocowort, Lady's Purse, Mother's-Heart, Pepper-And-Salt, Pick-Pocket, Poor Man's Parmacettie, Rattle Pouches, Sanguinary, Shepherd's Heart, Shepherd's Purse Herb, Shepherd's Scrip, Shepherd's Sprout, Shepherds Purse, Shovelweed, St. James' Weed, Toywort, Witches' Pouches.

Scientific Names

Capsella bursa-pastoris.
Family: Brassicaceae.

People Use This For

Orally, shepherd's purse is used for headache, mild cardiac insufficiency, hypotension, nervous heart complaints, premenstrual complaints (18), prolonged or painful menstrual periods (2,4), vomiting blood, blood in urine, diarrhea, and acute catarrhal cystitis (4).
Topically, it is used for nosebleeds, superficial burns, and bleeding skin injuries (2,18).

Safety

POSSIBLY SAFE ...when preparations of the above ground parts are used orally and appropriately (2,4,12). ...when used topically (2,4).
POSSIBLY UNSAFE ...when large amounts of shepherd's purse are ingested. It can cause heart palpitations (12).
PREGNANCY: LIKELY UNSAFE ...when used orally or topically because it seems to cause uterine stimulation, menstrual flow stimulation, and might cause miscarriage (12).
LACTATION: Insufficient reliable information available; avoid excessive use (4).

Effectiveness

There is insufficient reliable information available about the effectiveness of shepherd's purse.

Mechanism of Action

The applicable parts of shepherd's purse are the above ground parts. Shepherd's purse has constituents that cause positive and negative inotropic effects, and positive and negative chronotropic effects. It also seems to cause hypertensive and sometimes antihypertensive effects. It stimulates smooth muscle and increases uterine contraction. It also has abortifacient effects, and antihemorrhagic and urinary antiseptic effects (2,4,18). One constituent in shepherd's purse is sinigrin, which can be broken down to allyl isothiocyanate. Allyl isothiocyanate is associated with abnormal thyroid function and goiter (4).

Adverse Reactions

Orally, shepherd's purse can cause sedation, hypertension, hypotension, abnormal thyroid function, abnormal menstruation (4), palpitations (12). Toxic doses in animals have caused sedation, paralysis, respiratory depression, and death (4).

Interactions with Herbs & Other Dietary Supplements

HERBS WITH SEDATIVE PROPERTIES: Theoretically, concomitant use with herbs that have sedative properties might enhance therapeutic and adverse effects. These include calamus, calendula, California poppy, catnip, capsicum, celery, couch grass, elecampane, Siberian ginseng, German chamomile, goldenseal, gotu kola, hops, Jamaican dogwood, kava, lemon balm, sage, St. John's wort, sassafras, scullcap, stinging nettle, valerian, wild carrot, wild lettuce, ashwaganda root, and yerba mansa (4,19).

Interactions with Drugs

ANTIHYPERTENSIVE, ANTIHYPOTENSIVE DRUGS: Theoretically, concomitant use may interfere with blood

pressure control (4).
CARDIOVASCULAR DRUGS: Theoretically, concomitant use may interfere with cardiovascular therapy (4).
THYROID THERAPY: Theoretically, concomitant use may interfere with thyroid dysfunction therapy (4).
DRUGS WITH SEDATIVE PROPERTIES: Theoretically, concomitant use with drugs with sedative properties may cause additive effects and side effects (4).

Interactions with Foods
No interactions are known to occur, and there is no known reason to expect a clinically significant interaction with shepherd's purse.

Interactions with Lab Tests
No interactions are known to occur, and there is no known reason to expect a clinically significant interaction with shepherd's purse.

Interactions with Diseases or Conditions
KIDNEY STONES: Contains oxalate, use with caution in people with a history of kidney stones (12).
CARDIOVASCULAR CONDITIONS: Use with caution, may interfere with therapy (4).
THYROID CONDITIONS: Use with caution, may interfere with therapy (4).

Dosage and Administration
ORAL: 1-4 grams dried above ground parts three times daily, or one cup tea (steep 1-4 grams dried above ground parts in 150 mL boiling water 10-15 minutes, strain) three times daily (4); up to 10-15 grams dried above ground parts per day (2). Liquid extract (1:1 in 25% alcohol), 1-4 mL three times daily (4). Avoid excessive amounts (12).
TOPICAL: Apply tea (steep 3-5 grams dried above ground parts in 180 mL boiling water 10-15 minutes, strain) topically (2).

Comments
None.

SHIITAKE MUSHROOM

Also Known As
Forest Mushroom, Hua Gu, Lentinula, Pasania Fungus, Shiitake, Shitake, Snake Butter.
CAUTION: See separate listing for Lentinan.

Scientific Names
Lentinus edodes, synonyms Lenticus edodes, Lentinan edodes, Lentinula edodes, Tricholomopsis edodes.
Family: Polyporaceae.

People Use This For
Orally, shiitake mushrooms are used for boosting the immune system, reducing serum cholesterol levels, and as an anti-aging agent (1156).
For food uses, the edible mushroom is used in Japanese cooking (6).

Safety
LIKELY SAFE ...when consumed in food amounts (6).
POSSIBLY UNSAFE ...when used orally for medicinal purposes; ingestion of 4 grams shiitake powder daily for 10 weeks can cause eosinophilia (1149).
PREGNANCY AND LACTATION: Insufficient reliable information available; avoid using in amounts greater than those found in foods.

Effectiveness
There is insufficient reliable information available about the effectiveness of shiitake mushroom.

Mechanism of Action
Shiitake contains very low concentrations of lentinan (0.02%), which has antitumor effects (6). Shiitake may reduce plasma levels of free cholesterol, triglycerides, and phospholipids. (1155).

Adverse Reactions
Orally, shiitake mushrooms can cause abdominal discomfort, eosinophilia (1149), "shiitake" dermatitis (1148,1152), and

possibly photosensitivity (1148). There is one report of abdominal obstruction and death due to ingestion of a whole shiitake mushroom (1147). Ingestion of 4 grams shiitake powder daily for 10 weeks caused eosinophilia in 5 of 10 healthy humans (1149). An allergic contact dermatitis can be induced by shiitake hyphae (filaments) (1153). In mushroom workers, hypersensitivity pneumonitis due to shiitake spore inhalation has occurred (1150,1151).

Interactions with Herbs & Other Dietary Supplements
Insufficient reliable information available.

Interactions with Drugs
No interactions are known to occur, and there is no known reason to expect a clinically significant interaction with shiitake mushrooms.

Interactions with Foods
No interactions are known to occur, and there is no known reason to expect a clinically significant interaction with shiitake mushrooms.

Interactions with Lab Tests
No interactions are known to occur, and there is no known reason to expect a clinically significant interaction with shiitake mushrooms.

Interactions with Diseases or Conditions
EOSINOPHILIA: Contraindicated, may exacerbate condition (1149).

Dosage and Administration
No typical dosage.

Comments
None.

SILVER LINDEN

Also Known As
Tiliae tormentosae flos.
CAUTION: See separate listings for Linden Charcoal, Linden dried flower, Linden dried leaf, and Linden dried sapwood.

Scientific Names
Tilia tormentosa, synonym Tilia argentea.
Family: Tiliaceae.

People Use This For
Orally, silver linden is used for respiratory tract mucous membrane inflammation, for its antispasmodic effects, as an expectorant, a diaphoretic, and for its diuretic effects (2).

Safety
There is insufficient reliable information available about the safety of silver linden.
Pregnancy and Lactation: Insufficient reliable information available; avoid using.

Effectiveness
There is insufficient reliable information available about the effectiveness of silver linden.

Mechanism of Action
The applicable part of silver linden is the dried flower. Pharmacologically active benzodiazepine receptor ligands have been isolated from silver linden (6).

Adverse Reactions
None reported.

Interactions with Herbs & Other Dietary Supplements
Insufficient reliable information available.

Interactions with Drugs

No interactions are known to occur, and there is no known reason to expect a clinically significant interaction with silver linden.

Interactions with Foods

No interactions are known to occur, and there is no known reason to expect a clinically significant interaction with silver linden.

Interactions with Lab Tests

No interactions are known to occur, and there is no known reason to expect a clinically significant interaction with silver linden.

Interactions with Diseases or Conditions

CARDIAC CONDITIONS: Avoid with existing cardiac conditions (4,6).

Dosage and Administration

ORAL: 2 grams of flowertops as tea (steeped in boiling water for 5 to 10 minutes) (18). 2-4 grams daily dose (2,4,18) Tincture (1:5 in 45% alcohol) 2-4 mL or liquid extract (1:1 in 25% alcohol) 1-2 mL (4).
TOPICAL: No typical dosage.

Comments

Avoid confusion with linden charcoal, linden flower, linden leaf and linden wood.
There is very little scientific information about this product. Our staff is continually analyzing the available information on natural medicines and will add data here as it becomes available.

SIMARUBA

Also Known As

Bitter Damson, Dysentery Bark, Mountain Damson, Slave Wood, Stave Wood, Sumaruba.

Scientific Names

Simaruba amara.

People Use This For

Orally, simaruba is used to treat diarrhea, dysentery, malaria, water-retention, fever, unspecified gastrointestinal upset, as a tonic, and to cause abortion (18,4500).

Safety

There is insufficient reliable information available about the safety of simaruba.
PREGNANCY AND LACTATION: LIKELY UNSAFE …when used orally due to apparent abortifacient effects (18,4500); avoid using.

Effectiveness

There is insufficient reliable information available about the effectiveness of simaruba.

Mechanism of Action

The applicable part of simaruba is the bark. Simaruba contains the following active ingredients: 20-27% tannins, simarubin, essential oil, and fat (18,4500). It also contains the following bitter substances: quassinoids including simarolide, simarubidin, 13,18-dehydro-glaucarubinone; 0.1-0.2% 5-hydroxy-canthin-6-one a volatile oil; and unspecified alkaloids (18).

Adverse Reactions

Orally, large amounts of simaruba can cause vomiting (18).

Interactions with Herbs & Other Dietary Supplements

Insufficient reliable information available.

Interactions with Drugs

No interactions are known to occur, and there is no known reason to expect a clinically significant interaction with simaruba.

Interactions with Foods

No interactions are known to occur, and there is no known reason to expect a clinically significant interaction with simaruba.

Interactions with Lab Tests

No interactions are known to occur, and there is no known reason to expect a clinically significant interaction with simaruba.

Interactions with Diseases or Conditions

No interactions are known to occur, and there is no known reason to expect a clinically significant interaction with simaruba.

Dosage and Administration

ORAL: A typical dose is 1 gram (18).

Comments

Simaruba amara grows in the Caribbean islands and in the northern parts of South America (18).

SITOSTANOL

Also Known As

24-alpha-ethylcholestanol, Beta-sitostanol, Dihydro-beta-sitosterol, Fucostanol, Phytostanol, Plant Stanol, Stigmastanol.
CAUTION: See separate listing for Beta-sitosterol.

Scientific Names

3-beta,5-alpha-stigmastan-3-ol.

People Use This For

Orally, sitostanol is used for prevention of heart disease and hypercholesterolemia (1886,3888,6668,7193,7194).

Safety

LIKELY SAFE ...when used orally and appropriately. Sitostanol has been safely used in studies lasting up to one year (5429,5430,5431,5432,5433,5434,5435,5436,5437,5438,5439) (5441,5442,5443,5814).
CHILDREN: LIKELY SAFE ...when used orally and appropriately, short-term. Sitostanol has been safely used in children in studies lasting for up to 3 months (3888,3889,5438,7193,7194). There is insufficient reliable information available about the safety of long-term use of sitostanol in children.
PREGNANCY AND LACTATION: Insufficient reliable information available; avoid using.

Effectiveness

LIKELY EFFECTIVE ...when used orally for hypercholesterolemia (1886,3888,5429,5430,5431,5432,5433,5434,5435,5437,5438) (5439,5441,5442,5443,7103). Sitostanol is usually taken as a component of a sitostanol-enriched food such as margarine. It is effective in about 88% of patients when used alone or in combination with a low-fat diet or HMG-CoA reductase inhibitor ("statin") for reducing total and low-density lipoprotein cholesterol (3888,5431,5433,5435,5437,5814,7195). Sitostanol alone can reduce total and LDL cholesterol levels by 10 to 15% (5443). Peak cholesterol lowering effects occur at about 2 grams per day. Higher doses do not seem to offer any additional benefit (5814,6185,7195). When added to a statin such as pravastatin (Pravachol) or simvastatin (Zocor), sitostanol reduces total cholesterol by an additional 3-11% and LDL cholesterol by another 7-16% (5431,5433). Treatment with sitostanol for 2-3 weeks is usually necessary before cholesterol levels decrease significantly. If sitostanol is discontinued, cholesterol levels tend to rise within 2-3 weeks (7105).
POSSIBLY EFFECTIVE ...when used orally for familial hypercholesterolemia in children (3888,3889,5438). ...when used orally for reducing cholesterol levels in healthy children. There is some evidence that ingesting sitostanol in margarine can reduce cholesterol levels in healthy children (7193,7194). However, there is no known benefit to lowering cholesterol in children with normal cholesterol levels. Treating children is not recommended unless low-density lipoprotein (LDL) levels are greater than 190 mg/dL or greater than 160 mg/dL in the presence of other coronary risk factors.

Mechanism of Action

Sitostanol is a saturated form of plant sterols that structurally resembles cholesterol. It is prepared commercially from vegetable oils or the oil from pine tree wood pulp and is then made fat-soluble with canola oil (5435,5430,5814). Sitostanol is unabsorbable and tasteless. It competitively inhibits both dietary and biliary cholesterol absorption by competing with cholesterol for the limited space in mixed micelles (5435,5439,5443,5814,7196). However, sitostanol doesn't have to be taken with meals to lower cholesterol blood levels. Some researchers think sitostanol remains in the intestinal lumen or in the enterocytes after ingestion. So administration of sitostanol at any time of day seems to be as effective as multiple daily doses with meals (7103). Cholesterol levels decrease within 2 to 3 weeks of initiation of sitostanol, and return to pretreament levels within 2 to 3 weeks of discontinuation (7105) which also suggests a prolonged effect. Sitostanol may not have the same effect in all people. Preliminary clinical evidence suggests that sitostanol might work better in people with apolipoprotein E4 alleles, a genetic predisposition to hypercholesterolemia (7105,7195). About 12% of patients do not respond to sitostanol. In certain patients, hepatic cholesterol synthesis might increase in response to decreased availability of cholesterol, resulting in no change in cholesterol levels (5430,5443). There is some concern that sitostanol might decrease absorption of some nutrients since it decreases fat absorption. Sitostanol does seem to reduce the absorption of dietary beta-carotene. However, when corrected for lower levels of LDL, the major carrier of beta-carotene, the reduction in beta-carotene levels may not be clinically significant (7103,7104,7105). Sitostanol does not seem to affect retinol, vitamin D, or lycopene (5434,7104,7105).

Adverse Reactions

Orally, sitostanol seems to be very well tolerated. Adverse effects have not been reported in clinical trials in adults or children (5429,5430,5431,5432,5433,5434,5435,5436,5437,5438,5439) (5441,5442,5443,7103,7104,7105,7193,7194). However, because sitostanol decreases cholesterol absorption in the gut, it might be expected to produce some gastrointestinal symptoms like diarrhea and excess amounts of fat in the stool (steatorrhea).

Interactions with Herbs & Other Dietary Supplements

BETA-CAROTENE: Sitostanol can reduce absorption and blood levels of beta-carotene (3888,5434,5814,7103,7104,7105). Sitostanol lowers blood levels of low-density lipoprotein (LDL) cholesterol, which is a major carrier of fat-soluble antioxidants (7103,7104,7105). When corrected for lower LDL levels the reduction in beta-carotene levels does not seem to be clinically significant (7103,7104,7105). Supplementation with beta-carotene is probably not necessary. Suggest that concerned patients increase dietary consumption of beta-carotene rich vegetables or take a multivitamin that contains beta-carotene (7104).

CHOLESTEROL LOWERING HERBS/SUPPLEMENTS: Sitostanol might enhance the effects of herbs and supplements that also lower cholesterol levels. Some of these herbs and supplements include chromium, flaxseed, garlic, guar gum, niacin, oat bran, psyllium, red yeast, and others.

Interactions with Drugs

HMG-COA REDUCTASE INHIBITORS ("Statins"): Combining sitostanol and the statin drugs pravastatin (Pravachol) or simvastatin (Zocor) has additive cholesterol lowering effects (3888,5431,5433). Combining sitostanol with other cholesterol lowering drugs likely also has additive effects. Some of these other drugs include cholestyramine (Questran), colestipol (Colestid), clofibrate (Atromid-S), fenofibrate (Tricor), gemfibrozil (Lopid), niacin, and others.

Interactions with Foods

BETA-CAROTENE: Sitostanol can reduce absorption and blood levels of beta-carotene (3888,5434,5814,7103,7104,7105). Sitostanol lowers blood levels of low-density lipoprotein (LDL) cholesterol, which is a major carrier of fat-soluble antioxidants (7103,7104,7105). When corrected for lower LDL levels the reduction in beta-carotene levels does not seem to be clinically significant (7103,7104,7105). Supplementation with beta-carotene is probably not necessary. Suggest that concerned patients increase dietary consumption of beta-carotene rich vegetables or take a multivitamin that contains beta-carotene (7104).

Interactions with Lab Tests

SERUM CHOLESTEROL: Sitostanol decreases total and low-density lipoprotein (LDL) cholesterol and test results (5429,5431,5432,5433,5435,5437,5438,5439,5441,5442).

Interactions with Diseases or Conditions

No interactions are known to occur, and there is no known reason to expect a clinically significant interaction with sitostanol.

Dosage and Administration

ORAL: For hypercholesterolemia, clinical studies have used from 800 mg to 4 grams per day (5814). However, doses above 2 grams per day do not seem to provide additional benefit (7195). Effectiveness is not dependent on administration schedule. Single daily doses seem to be as effective as divided doses administered twice or three times daily (7195). For familial hypercholesterolemia in children, clinical studies have used 2-6 grams daily initially and then tapered down to 1.5 grams daily (3888,3889,5438).

Comments

Sitostanol is an ingredient in the functional food product Benecol margarine and in some salad dressings. The FDA authorized the use of labeling health claims for foods containing plant stanol esters, including sitostanol, for reducing the risk of coronary heart disease (CHD). This rule is based on the FDA's conclusion that plant stanol esters in conjunction with a diet low in saturated fat and cholesterol might reduce the risk of CHD by lowering blood cholesterol levels (6668). Although there is plenty of evidence that sitostanol does lower cholesterol levels, so far there is no proof that long-term use actually lowers the risk of developing CHD. Do not confuse sitostanol with beta-sitosterol, an unsaturated plant sterol in the cholesterol-lowering margarine Take Control (5443). Both sitostanol and beta-sitosterol are used for lower cholesterol levels in people with hypercholesterolemia and appear to be equally effective (7196).

SKIRRET

Also Known As
None.

Scientific Names
Sium sisarum.
Family: Apiaceae.

People Use This For
Orally, skirret is used for digestive disorders and loss of appetite.
Historically, it was used orally for chest complaints (18).

Safety
There is insufficient reliable information available about the safety of skirret.
Pregnancy and Lactation: Insufficient reliable information available; avoid using.

Effectiveness
There is insufficient reliable information available about the effectiveness of skirret.

Mechanism of Action
The applicable part of skirret is the root. There is insufficient reliable information available about the possible mechanism of action and active ingredients.

Adverse Reactions
None reported.

Interactions with Herbs & Other Dietary Supplements
Insufficient reliable information available.

Interactions with Drugs
No interactions are known to occur, and there is no known reason to expect a clinically significant interaction with skirret.

Interactions with Foods
No interactions are known to occur, and there is no known reason to expect a clinically significant interaction with skirret.

Interactions with Lab Tests
No interactions are known to occur, and there is no known reason to expect a clinically significant interaction with skirret.

Interactions with Diseases or Conditions
No interactions are known to occur, and there is no known reason to expect a clinically significant interaction with skirret.

Dosage and Administration
ORAL: Skirret is used in powdered form (18).

Comments

There is very little scientific information about this product. Our staff is continually analyzing the available information on natural medicines and will add data here as it becomes available.

SKUNK CABBAGE

Also Known As

Dracontium, Meadow Cabbage, Polecatweed, Skunkweed, Spathyema Foetida, Swamp Cabbage.

Scientific Names

Symplocarpus foetidus, synonym Dracontium foetidum.
Family: Araceae.

People Use This For

Orally, skunk cabbage is used to treat bronchitis, asthma (18), and whooping cough (4).

In folk medicine, it is used as a gastrointestinal stimulant (12); and to treat catarrh, cancer, chorea, convulsions, cough, edema, epilepsy (4500,4502), headache, hemorrhage, hysteria, pregnancy, labor, worms (4500,4502), rheumatism, ringworm, scabies, snakebite, skin sores, spasms, splinters, swellings, toothache, and wounds (4500,4502).

As a food, American Indians boil and eat young leaves, roots, and stalks (4500,4501,4502).

Safety

POSSIBLY SAFE ...when used orally and appropriately; the boiled leaves, roots, and stalks are used as food (4500,4501,4502) without reports of serious adverse effects (4).

PREGNANCY AND LACTATION: POSSIBLY UNSAFE ...when used orally; avoid using. May affect the menstrual cycle (4), and irritant properties may stimulate uterine contractions (4,12).

Effectiveness

There is insufficient reliable information available about the effectiveness of skunk cabbage.

Mechanism of Action

Skunk cabbage contains a variety of constituents, including an acrid principle, unspecified alkaloids, an essential oil, a fatty oil, phenolic compounds, and tannin (4,4502). The seeds are reported to contain a narcotic (4502). The root contains calcium oxalate which could irritate the kidney or promote kidney stones in sensitive individuals (12,4502). The leaves contain n-hydroxytryptamine (4).

Adverse Reactions

Orally, large amounts of skunk cabbage are reported to cause nausea, vomiting, headache, vertigo, and dimness of vision (18,4502). Excessive use of gastrointestinal irritants can cause abdominal cramps, burning, blistering in the mouth and throat, nausea, colic, and watery or bloody diarrhea (12).

Topically, the fresh plant can cause severe itching, inflammation, and blistering (4,4502).

Interactions with Herbs & Other Dietary Supplements

CALCIUM, IRON, ZINC: Concurrent use might decrease mineral absorption. Skunk cabbage contains oxalate (7,12), which can bind multivalent metal ions in the gastrointestinal tract and decrease mineral absorption.

Interactions with Drugs

No interactions are known to occur, and there is no known reason to expect a clinically significant interaction with skunk cabbage.

Interactions with Foods

CALCIUM, IRON, ZINC: Concurrent use might decrease mineral absorption from foods. Skunk cabbage contains oxalate (7,12), which can bind multivalent metal ions in the gastrointestinal tract and decrease mineral absorption.

Interactions with Lab Tests

No interactions are known to occur, and there is no known reason to expect a clinically significant interaction with skunk cabbage.

Interactions with Diseases or Conditions

KIDNEY STONES: Individuals with a history of oxalate kidney stones should avoid or use cautiously (12,4502).

GI CONDITIONS: May aggravate GI ulcers, GI inflammation or irritation (12,19).

Dosage and Administration
ORAL: Powdered rhizome/root: 0.5-1 mg three times daily mixed with honey or by infusion or decoction. Liquid extract: (1:1 in 25% alcohol) 0.5-1 mL three times daily. Tincture: (1:10 in 45% alcohol) 2-4 mL three times daily (4).

Comments
Skunk cabbage is a common name for members of the toxic Veratrum family (4501). Skunk cabbage gets it name from a volatile oil emitted by the plant that has a disagreeable odor (18).

SLIPPERY ELM

Also Known As
Indian Elm, Moose Elm, Red Elm, Sweet Elm.

Scientific Names
Ulmus rubra; Ulmus fulva.
Family: Ulmaceae.

People Use This For
Orally, slippery elm is used for coughs, sore throat, colic, diarrhea, constipation, hemorrhoids, irritable bowel syndrome (IBS), cystitis, urinary inflammation, urinary tract infections, syphilis, herpes, and for expelling tapeworms. It is also used orally for protecting against stomach and duodenal ulcers, for colitis, diverticulitis, GI inflammation, and acidity. Slippery elm is used orally as an abortifacient (4,6121).

Topically, slippery elm is used for wounds, burns (18), gout, rheumatism, cold sores, boils, abscesses, ulcers, toothaches, sore throat, and as a lubricant to ease labor (6).

In manufacturing, slippery elm is used in some baby foods and adult nutritionals, and in some oral lozenges used for soothing throat pain (6).

Safety
LIKELY SAFE ...when used orally and appropriately (4,12,512).
PREGNANCY: POSSIBLY SAFE ...when the inner bark is used orally in amounts used in foods (4). **LIKELY UNSAFE** ...when the whole bark is used. Use of the whole bark is contraindicated because it is an abortifacient (4,6).
LACTATION: Insufficient reliable information available; avoid using.

Effectiveness
POSSIBLY EFFECTIVE ...when used orally as a lozenge for sore throat. Slippery elm has demulcent properties and can soothe sore throats (512,1740,4102).
There is insufficient reliable information available about the effectiveness of slippery elm for its other uses.

Mechanism of Action
The applicable part of slippery elm is the inner bark rind. The mucilages are considered the principal constituent. They are responsible for slippery elm's demulcent and emollient effects (4,18). Used internally, slippery elm preparations cause reflex stimulation of nerve endings in the GI tract, leading to mucous secretion (6). This induced mucous may protect the GI tract against ulcers, excess acidity, etc. Tannin constituents have astringent properties (4). Oleoresins of some species are responsible for contact dermatitis (6).

Adverse Reactions
Orally, the whole bark is an abortifacient (4).
Topically, slippery elm extracts can cause contract dermatitis (6). The pollen is an allergen (6).

Interactions with Herbs & Other Dietary Supplements
Insufficient reliable information available.

Interactions with Drugs
ORAL DRUGS: Theoretically, may slow the absorption and reduce serum levels of orally administered drugs due to mucilage content (19).

Interactions with Foods
No interactions are known to occur, and there is no known reason to expect a clinically significant interaction with slippery elm.

Interactions with Lab Tests

No interactions are known to occur, and there is no known reason to expect a clinically significant interaction with slippery elm.

Interactions with Diseases or Conditions

No interactions are known to occur, and there is no known reason to expect a clinically significant interaction with slippery elm.

Dosage and Administration

ORAL: Powdered inner bark (1:8 as a decoction) 4-16 mL three times daily (4). Nutritional supplement, 4 grams powdered inner bark in 500 mL boiling water, three times daily (4). Alcohol extract (1:1 in 60% alcohol), 5 mL three times daily (4).
TOPICAL: As a poultice, coarse powdered inner bark mixed with boiling water (4).

Comments

Avoid confusing whole bark with inner bark. Commercial lozenges containing slippery elm are preferred to the native herb when used for cough and sore throat, because they provide sustained release of mucilage to the throat (3).

SMARTWEED

Also Known As

Arsesmart, Water Pepper.

Scientific Names

Polygonum hydropiper.

People Use This For

Orally, smartweed is used to treat bleeding of the womb, menstrual bleeding, bleeding hemorrhoids, and diarrhea (18). Topically, smartweed is used to wash bloody wounds (18).

Safety

There is insufficient reliable information available about the safety of smartweed.
Pregnancy and Lactation: Insufficient reliable information available; avoid using.

Effectiveness

There is insufficient reliable information available about the effectiveness of smartweed.

Mechanism of Action

The applicable parts of smartweed are the leaf, and the entire plant during flowering season. Smartweed contains tannins, hydropiperoside, sesquiterpenealdehydes, and flavonoids (18). Smartweed is reported to stop bleeding. It is also thought to influence the elimination of urine and to have some effect on rheumatic pain (18).

Adverse Reactions

Orally, smartweed can cause gastrointestinal irritation (19).
Topically, the fresh plant can cause inflammatory reactions due to chemical irritation (18).

Interactions with Herbs & Other Dietary Supplements

Insufficient reliable information available.

Interactions with Drugs

WARFARIN: Concomitant use can decrease the anticoagulant effects of warfarin (Coumadin), possibly increasing the risk of clotting (19).

Interactions with Foods

No interactions are known to occur, and there is no known reason to expect a clinically significant interaction with smartweed.

Interactions with Lab Tests

No interactions are known to occur, and there is no known reason to expect a clinically significant interaction with smartweed.

Interactions with Diseases or Conditions
GASTROINTESTINAL DISORDERS: Smartweed can exacerbate inflammatory conditions by irritating the mucous membranes (19).

Dosage and Administration
ORAL: A small amount of the powdered drug three times a day or one cup tea (one teaspoon of the drug per cup, boil) three times per day (18).

Comments
Smartweed has an extraordinary hot pepper-like taste (18).

SMOKELESS TOBACCO

Also Known As
Chaw, Chew, Chewing Tobacco, Dip, Snuff, Tobacco.

Scientific Names
Nicotiana tabacum.

People Use This For
Recreationally, smokeless tobacco is used as "snuff" by buccal and nasal routes (6).

Safety
LIKELY UNSAFE ...when used recreationally (6). Nicotine, a constituent, is lethal at 40-100 mg, though the lethal level might be elevated through habituation (18). Nicotine is associated with increased risk of cancer and cardiovascular complications (6).
PREGNANCY: LIKELY UNSAFE ...when used recreationally (19,4125). Nicotine is a teratogen and it is likely to reduce infant birth weight and size as well as increase the risk of miscarriage, prematurity, and neurologic impairment of baby (19).
LACTATION: LIKELY UNSAFE ...when used recreationally (19,4125); avoid using.

Effectiveness
There is no medicinal use for smokeless tobacco.

Mechanism of Action
The main active constituent of smokeless tobacco is nicotine (18). Small doses increase blood pressure (6,18) and gastric mucosal activity (18). Larger doses can reduce blood pressure, lower gastrointestinal muscle tone (18), produce tachycardia, and may be vasoconstrictive (6). Tobacco stimulates respiratory and tremor centers (18). In human studies, tobacco is known to decrease the level of high-density lipoproteins (HDLs) (19). Evidence suggests that nitrosamines found in tobacco might cause tumors (6).

Adverse Reactions
Nausea and dizziness are common with initial recreational use (6). Use of "snuff" affects blood pressure and heart rate (6,18), causes loss of taste and smell, gingival recession, periodontal tissue destruction, tooth loss, soft tissue erythema, oral leukoplakia, epidermoid carcinoma, and oropharyngeal cancer (6). A single case of thromboangiitis obliterans has been linked to chronic use (6). The saccharin found in flavored tobacco might increase the risk of bladder cancer (6). Bad breath and discolored teeth are common problems associated with smokeless tobacco (6). The symptoms of nicotine poisoning are dizziness, salivation, vomiting, diarrhea, trembling, weak legs, spasms, unconsciousness, cardiac arrest, and respiratory failure (18,4125).

Interactions with Herbs & Other Dietary Supplements
OATS: Theoretically, oats might decrease the hypertensive response to nicotine (19).

Interactions with Drugs
ACETAMINOPHEN: Interacts with the nicotine in smokeless tobacco and decreases the blood levels of acetaminophen (Tylenol) (19).
ADENOSINE: Interacts with the nicotine in smokeless tobacco and increases the circulatory effects of adenosine (19).
AMOBARBITOL: Interacts with the nicotine in smokeless tobacco and increases the elimination of amobarbital (Amytal) (19).
BENZODIAZEPINES: Interact with the nicotine in smokeless tobacco and increases the elimination of

benzodiazepines (19).
BETA-BLOCKERS: Interact with the nicotine in smokeless tobacco and decreases the effectiveness of beta-blockers (19).
CAFFEINE: Interacts with the nicotine in smokeless tobacco and increases the elimination of caffeine (19).
CIMETIDINE: Interacts with the nicotine in smokeless tobacco and decreases the blood levels of cimetidine (Tagamet). Cimetidine reduces the metabolic breakdown of nicotine (19).
DIFLUNISAL: Interacts with the nicotine in smokeless tobacco and increases the elimination of diflunisal (Dolobid) (19).
ESTROGEN: Interacts with the nicotine in smokeless tobacco and increases the metabolism of estrogen (19).
FUROSEMIDE: Interacts with the nicotine in smokeless tobacco and decreases the effectiveness of furosemide (Lasix) (19).
GLUTETHIMIDE: Interacts with the nicotine in smokeless tobacco and enhances the effects of glutethimide (19).
HALOPERIDOL: Interacts with the nicotine in smokeless tobacco and increases the metabolism of haloperidol (Haldol) (19).
HEPARIN: Interacts with the nicotine in smokeless tobacco and increases the elimination of heparin (19).
INSULIN: Interacts with the nicotine in smokeless tobacco and decreases the effectiveness of insulin (19).
ORAL CONTRACEPTIVES: Interact with the nicotine in smokeless tobacco and increases the risk of blood clots in women over age 30 using oral contraceptives (19).
PHENOTHIAZINES: Interact with the nicotine in smokeless tobacco and increases the metabolism of phenothiazines (19).
PENTAZOCINE: Interacts with the nicotine in smokeless tobacco and increases the elimination of pentazocine (Talwin)(19).
PHENYLBUTAZONE: Interacts with the nicotine in smokeless tobacco; nicotine increases the metabolism of phenylbutazone (19).
PROPOXYPHENE: Interacts with the nicotine in smokeless tobacco and decreases the effectiveness of propoxyphene (Darvon) (19).
QUININE: Interacts with the nicotine in smokeless tobacco and increases the metabolism of quinine (19).
RANITIDINE: Ranitidine (Zantac) reduces the metabolic breakdown of nicotine, a constituent of smokeless tobacco (19).
TACRINE: Interacts with the nicotine in smokeless tobacco and increases the metabolism of tacrine (Cognex) (19).
THEOPHYLLINE: Interacts with the nicotine in smokeless tobacco and increases the metabolism of theophylline (19).
THIOTHIXENE: Interacts with the nicotine in smokeless tobacco and increases the metabolism of thiothixene (Navane) (19).
TRICYCLIC ANTIDEPRESSANTS: Interact with the nicotine in smokeless tobacco and increases the elimination of tricyclic antidepressants (19).
VITAMIN B12: Interacts with the nicotine in smokeless tobacco and decreases the blood levels of vitamin B12 (19).
VITAMIN C: Interacts with the nicotine in smokeless tobacco and increases the elimination of vitamin C (19).
ZOLPIDEM: Interacts with the nicotine in smokeless tobacco and increases the metabolism of zolpidem (Ambien) (19).

Interactions with Foods
No interactions are known to occur, and there is no known reason to expect a clinically significant interaction with smokeless tobacco.

Interactions with Lab Tests
No interactions are known to occur, and there is no known reason to expect a clinically significant interaction with smokeless tobacco.

Interactions with Diseases or Conditions
DIABETES: Persistent hyperglycemia has been observed in diabetic patients who use "candified" chewing tobacco and regularly swallow the salivary juices (6). Long term nicotine use leads to insulin resistance (4133).
GASTROINTESTINAL ULCERS: The nicotine in smokeless tobacco stimulates gastric acid secretion, causing ulcer exacerbation (19).
HEART DISEASE: The nicotine in smokeless tobacco decreases HDL level and increases blood pressure (19). High doses of nicotine can increase heart rate and potentiate cardiac arrhythmia or ischemia (4132).
OSTEOPOROSIS: The nicotine in smokeless tobacco causes further deterioration of bone disease (19,4126).

Dosage and Administration
No typical dosage.

Comments
None.

SMOOTH ALDER

Also Known As
Hazel Alder, Tag Alder.

Scientific Names
Alnus serrulata.
Family: Betulaceae.

People Use This For
Orally, smooth alder is used for pharyngitis and intestinal bleeding.

Safety
There is insufficient reliable information available about the safety of smooth alder.
Pregnancy and Lactation: Insufficient reliable information available; avoid using.

Effectiveness
There is insufficient reliable information about the effectiveness of smooth alder.

Mechanism of Action
The applicable part of smooth alder is the bark. There is insufficient reliable information available about the possible mechanism of action and active ingredients.

Adverse Reactions
None reported.

Interactions with Herbs & Other Dietary Supplements
Insufficient reliable information available.

Interactions with Drugs
No interactions are known to occur, and there is no known reason to expect a clinically significant interaction with smooth alder.

Interactions with Foods
No interactions are known to occur, and there is no known reason to expect a clinically significant interaction with smooth alder.

Interactions with Lab Tests
No interactions are known to occur, and there is no known reason to expect a clinically significant interaction with smooth alder.

Interactions with Diseases or Conditions
No interactions are known to occur, and there is no known reason to expect a clinically significant interaction with smooth alder.

Dosage and Administration
No typical dosage.

Comments
There is very little scientific information about this product. Our staff is continually analyzing the available information on natural medicines and will add data here as it becomes available.

SNEEZEWORT

Also Known As
None.

Scientific Names
Achillea ptarmica.

People Use This For
Orally, sneezewort is used for rheumatic and painful disorders, toothache, diarrhea, nausea, vomiting, and flatulence (18).
Topically, sneezewort is used for toothache (18).
In folk medicine, sneezewort is used for tiredness, urinary tract complaints, and as an appetite stimulant (18).

Safety
There is insufficient reliable information available about the safety of sneezewort.
Pregnancy and Lactation: Insufficient reliable information available; avoid using.

Effectiveness
There is insufficient reliable information available about the effectiveness of sneezewort.

Mechanism of Action
The applicable part of sneezewort is the dried root. Sneezewort contains alkamides, polyynes, and volatile oil (18).

Adverse Reactions
Orally, sneezewort may cause an allergic reaction (18).

Interactions with Herbs & Other Dietary Supplements
Insufficient reliable information is available.

Interactions with Drugs
No interactions are known to occur, and there is no known reason to expect a clinically significant interaction with sneezewort.

Interactions with Foods
No interactions are known to occur, and there is no known reason to expect a clinically significant interaction with sneezewort.

Interactions with Lab Tests
No interactions are known to occur, and there is no known reason to expect a clinically significant interaction with sneezewort.

Interactions with Diseases or Conditions
SNEEZEWORT ALLERGY: Contraindicated.

Dosage and Administration
ORAL: A typical dose is two cups of tea daily. To make tea, simmer 2 teaspoons of the cut root in 2 cups of water (18).
TOPICAL: The fresh root can be chewed (18).

Comments
None.

SOLOMON'S SEAL

Also Known As
Dropberry, Lady's Seals, Ladys Seals, Sealroot, Sealwort, Solomons Seal, St Marys Seal, St. Mary's Seal.

Scientific Names
Polygonatum multiflorum.
Family: Liliaceae.

People Use This For
Historically, Solomon's seal was used for respiratory and lung disorders, and as an astringent and anti-inflammatory. It has also been used topically for bruises, furuncles, ulcers or boils on the fingers, hemorrhoids, skin redness, edema, and hematoma (18).

Safety
POSSIBLY SAFE ...when used orally, short-term (12).
PREGNANCY AND LACTATION: Insufficient reliable information available; avoid using.

Effectiveness
There is insufficient reliable information available about the effectiveness of Solomon's seal.

Mechanism of Action
There is insufficient reliable information available about the active ingredients or possible mechanism of action for Solomon's seal. Solomon's seal may cause hypoglycemia (19).

Adverse Reactions
Long-term use may cause gastrointestinal irritation. Use of large doses or overdoses may cause nausea, diarrhea, gastric complaints, and nausea (18).

Interactions with Herbs & Other Dietary Supplements
HYPOGLYCEMIC HERBS: Theoretically, concomitant use with other hypoglycemic herbs may have additive effects (19).

Interactions with Drugs
DIABETES THERAPY: Theoretically, concomitant use may enhance hypoglycemic drug effects and alter blood glucose control (19). Monitor blood glucose.
INSULIN: Insulin dosage adjustments may be necessary, due to the possible hypoglycemic effects of Solomon's seal (19).
CHLORPROPAMIDE (Diabinese): Concomitant use may cause additive hypoglycemic effects (19).

Interactions with Foods
No interactions are known to occur, and there is no known reason to expect a clinically significant interaction with Solomon's seal.

Interactions with Lab Tests
No interactions are known to occur, and there is no known reason to expect a clinically significant interaction with Solomon's seal.

Interactions with Diseases or Conditions
DIABETES: Theoretically may interfere with blood glucose control (19).

Dosage and Administration
No typical dosage.

Comments
Solomon's seal is obsolete as a medicinal herb.

SORREL

Also Known As
Acedera Común, Azeda-Brava, Garden Sorrel, Sorrel Dock, Sour Dock, Wiesensauerampfer.

Scientific Names
Rumex acetosa.
Family: Polygonaceae.

People Use This For
Orally, sorrel is used for acute and chronic inflammation of the nasal passages and respiratory tract, and as an adjunct to antibacterial therapy. It is also used as a diuretic and to stimulate secretions (18).

In combination with gentian root, European elder flower, verbena, and cowslip flower, sorrel is used orally for maintaining healthy sinuses (373) and treating sinusitis (7,374,379).

Safety
POSSIBLY SAFE ...when used orally in food amounts (4247). ...when used orally in combination with gentian root, European elder flower, verbena, and cowslip flower (Quanterra Sinus Defense, Sinupret) (7,374,379).

LIKELY UNSAFE ...when used in large amounts. A 53 year old died after ingesting 500 grams of sorrel in soup (17). There is insufficient reliable information available about the safety of sorrel used in medicinal amounts.

CHILDREN: POSSIBLY UNSAFE ...when used orally because it contains oxalic acid. A four-year old child died after consuming rhubarb leaves, which are also a source of oxalic acid (17).

PREGNANCY AND LACTATION: LIKELY SAFE ...when used orally in food amounts. There is insufficient reliable information available about the safety of sorrel in amounts larger than those found in foods during pregnancy and lactation; avoid using.

Effectiveness
POSSIBLY EFFECTIVE ...when used orally in combination with gentian root, European elder flower, verbena, and cowslip flower (Quanterra Sinus Defense, Sinupret) for treating acute or chronic sinusitis (7,374,379).

There is insufficient reliable information available about the effectiveness of sorrel for its other uses.

Mechanism of Action
Sorrel contains 7-15% tannins (11), which exert an astringent effect on the mucosal tissue. This effect dehydrates the tissue, reducing internal secretions and forming the external cells into a protective layer. Plants with at least 10% tannins may cause gastrointestinal disturbances, kidney damage, and necrotic conditions of the liver. Some animal data show that tannins may cause cancer; other data show they may prevent it. Regular consumption of herbs with high tannin concentrations correlates with increased incidence of esophageal or nasal cancer (12). Sorrel leaf has a 0.3% oxalate content (12). Once absorbed, the oxalic acid reacts with calcium in plasma and resulting insoluble calcium oxalate may precipitate in the kidneys, blood vessels, heart, lungs, and liver. This may also cause hypocalcemia (12,17). Oxalate crystals damage mucosal tissue, resulting in severe irritation and possible damage. The systemic absorption of oxalates may result in kidney damage, both in people with pre-existing kidney disease and in healthy kidneys (19).

Adverse Reactions
Consuming excessive amounts of sorrel can cause diarrhea, nausea, polyuria (6), dermatitis (4) and gastrointestinal symptoms. Oxalic acid (constituent) poisoning affects skin, eyes, respiratory system, and kidneys. Oral symptoms of oxalate irritation include swelling of the mouth, tongue, and throat, with difficulty in speaking and suffocation. It has a corrosive effect on the digestive tract and can lead to oxalic acid crystals in the kidneys, blood vessels, heart, lungs, liver, and/or hypocalcemia (17).

Interactions with Herbs & Other Dietary Supplements
CALCIUM, IRON, ZINC: Concurrent use might decrease mineral absorption. Sorrel contains oxalate (7,12), which can bind multivalent metal ions in the gastrointestinal tract and decrease mineral absorption.

TANNIN-CONTAINING HERBS: Theoretically, herbs that contain high percentages of tannins (such as sorrel) may cause precipitation of constituents of other herbs (19).

Interactions with Drugs
ORAL DRUGS: Theoretically, concomitant oral administration may cause precipitation of some drugs due to the high tannin content of sorrel (19). Separate administration of oral drugs and tannin-containing herbs by the longest period of time practical (19).

DOXYCYCLINE (Vibramycin): Concurrent use of sorrel, gentian root, European elder flower, verbena, and cowslip flower (Quanterra Sinus Defense, Sinupret) with doxycycline and a topical decongestant might improve the outcome of conventional (antibiotic/decongestant) therapy for acute bacterial sinusitis (374).

Interactions with Foods
CALCIUM, IRON, ZINC: Concurrent use might decrease mineral absorption from foods. Sorrel contains oxalate (7,12), which can bind multivalent metal ions in the gastrointestinal tract and decrease mineral absorption.

Interactions with Lab Tests
No interactions are known to occur, and there is no known reason to expect a clinically significant interaction with sorrel.

Interactions with Diseases or Conditions
COAGULATION DISORDERS: Oxalate constituents can alter the calcium concentrations and decrease coagulation time (4,12).
GI CONDITIONS: Theoretically, sorrel can exacerbate stomach and intestinal ulcers due to mucosal irritant effect (19).
KIDNEY DISEASE: Can damage kidneys with formation of insoluble oxalate; use with caution or avoid in individuals with history of kidney stones (12,19).

Dosage and Administration
ORAL: For acute or chronic sinusitis, two Sinupret tablets three times daily for up to two weeks has been used in clinical trials (7,374,379), equivalent to gentian root 12 mg, European elder flower 36 mg, verbena 36 mg cowslip flower 36 mg and sorrel 36 mg three times daily. For maintaining healthy sinuses, a typical dose is one tablet of Quanterra Sinus Defense three times daily with water, equivalent to gentian root 9 mg, European elder flower 29 mg, verbena 29 mg, cowslip flower 29 mg, and sorrel 29 mg three times daily (373). Each tablet of Quanterra Sinus Defense contains 125 mg of the herbal combination found in Sinupret (373).

Comments
Roselle (Hibiscus sabdariffa) is also known as Jamaica sorrel or Guinea sorrel. It could be confused with sorrel (11,18).

SOUR CHERRY

Also Known As
Cerezo Acido, Cerisier Acide, English Morello, Ginjeira, Griottier, Guindo, Montmorency Cherry, Morello Cherry, Pie Cherry, Red Cherry, Richmond, Sauerkirsche, Sauerkirschenbaum, Tart Cherry.

Scientific Names
Prunus Cerasus, synonyms Cerasus vulgaris, Prunus vulgaris.
Family: Rosaceae.

People Use This For
In traditional medicine, the fruit of sour cherry has been used orally for arthritis and gout (6).
In folk medicine, the stem of the sour cherry is used to cause diuresis and facilitate digestion (4284).
In food use, sour cherries are eaten as a food or flavoring, and used in pies and other baked goods (6).
In manufacturing, sour cherry fruit is used to make cherry syrup USP, a vehicle for drugs with unpleasant taste (6).

Safety
LIKELY SAFE …when the fruit is used orally for food or medicinal use.
There is insufficient reliable information available about the safety of the oral use of sour cherry stem.
PREGNANCY AND LACTATION: LIKELY SAFE …when the fruit is consumed in typical food amounts. There is insufficient reliable information available about the safety of sour cherry stem use during pregnancy or lactation.

Effectiveness
There is insufficient reliable information about the effectiveness of sour cherry.

Mechanism of Action
Sour cherry fruit contains vitamin C, vitamin A, alpha-linolenic acid, and traces of vitamin E, beta-carotene, folacin thiamine, as well as other constituents (4282). It contains varied antioxidants including kaempferol and quercetin (4282,4283). A preliminary study at Michigan State University suggests compounds found in the sour cherry have anti-inflammatory effects that are ten times stronger than aspirin but without aspirin's

side effects (6). The stem of the sour cherry contains an isoflavone constituent, prunetin 5-O-beta-D-glycopyranoside (4284).

Adverse Reactions
None reported.

Interactions with Herbs & Other Dietary Supplements
Insufficient reliable information available.

Interactions with Drugs
No interactions are known to occur, and there is no known reason to expect a clinically significant interaction with sour cherry.

Interactions with Foods
No interactions are known to occur, and there is no known reason to expect a clinically significant interaction with sour cherry.

Interactions with Lab Tests
No interactions are known to occur, and there is no known reason to expect a clinically significant interaction with sour cherry.

Interactions with Diseases or Conditions
No interactions are known to occur, and there is no known reason to expect a clinically significant interaction with sour cherry.

Dosage and Administration
No typical dosage.

Comments
Of the more than 270 varieties of sour cherry, only a few are important commercially. These include the Montmorency, Richmond, and English morello (6).

SOUTHERN PRICKLY ASH

Also Known As
Prickly Ash, Prickly Yellow Wood, Sea Ash, Toothache Tree, Xanthoxylum, Zanthoxylum.
CAUTION: See separate listings for Ash and Northern Prickly Ash.

Scientific Names
Zanthoxylum clava-herculis.
Family: Rutaceae.

People Use This For
Orally, southern prickly ash is used for cramps, intermittent claudication, Raynaud's syndrome, chronic rheumatic conditions, and peripheral circulatory insufficiency associated with rheumatic symptoms (4).
In folk medicine, southern prickly ash is used as a tonic, stimulant, for toothache, sores, ulcers, as a diaphoretic in fever, and for cancer (as an ingredient in Hoxsey cure) (11).

Safety
POSSIBLY SAFE ...when used orally and appropriately in food flavoring (4). It is listed by the Council of Europe as a natural source of food flavoring. ...when the bark is used orally in medicinal amounts (12).
There is insufficient reliable information about the safety of the oral use of the berry.
PREGNANCY: LIKELY UNSAFE ...when used orally (12) because it might have menstrual stimulant effects (19).
There is insufficient reliable information about the safety of the berry during pregnancy; avoid using.
LACTATION: LIKELY UNSAFE ...when used orally because it might cause colic in nursing infants (19).

Effectiveness
There is insufficient reliable information available about the effectiveness of southern prickly ash.

Mechanism of Action

The applicable parts of southern prickly ash are the bark and berry. Southern prickly ash contains nitidine (hypotensive, antileukemic, hepatic enzyme inhibitor), chelerythrine (anti-inflammatory, antibiotic against gram positive bacteria, potentiates barbiturate induced sleep, hepatic enzyme inhibitor), asarinin (antitubercular), and neoherculin (insecticidal, salivation stimulant) (4). Reports of death after ingestion by cattle, chickens, and fish attributed to the neuromuscular blocking properties of the bark (4).

Adverse Reactions

None reported.

Interactions with Herbs & Other Dietary Supplements

DIGITALIS: May interfere with cardiac glycoside therapy (4).
HERBS WITH ANTICOAGULANT/ANTIPLATELET POTENTIAL: Certain herbs have the potential to contribute to bleeding because they have coumarin constituents, or they affect platelet aggregation, or they have high vitamin K content. Theoretically, concomitant use of more than one of these herbs could increase the chance of bleeding in susceptible individuals. These herbs include: alfalfa, angelica, anise, arnica, asafoetida, bogbean, boldo, capsicum, celery, Roman and German chamomile, clove, danshen, fenugreek, feverfew, garlic, ginger, ginkgo, ginseng (Panax), horse chestnut, horseradish, licorice, meadowsweet, nettle, onion, papain, parsley, passionflower, poplar, quassia, red clover, turmeric, wild carrot, wild lettuce, and willow (4,19).

Interactions with Drugs

ACID-INHIBITING DRUGS: Theoretically, due to claims that southern prickly ash increases stomach acid, it might interfere with antacids, sucralfate (Carafate), H-2 antagonists, and proton pump inhibitors (19).

Interactions with Foods

No interactions are known to occur, and there is no known reason to expect a clinically significant interaction with southern prickly ash.

Interactions with Lab Tests

No interactions are known to occur, and there is no known reason to expect a clinically significant interaction with southern prickly ash.

Interactions with Diseases or Conditions

LIVER DISEASE: Theoretically, may inhibit hepatic enzymes.

Dosage and Administration

ORAL (Bark): 1-3 grams dried bark, or drink as decoction (boil 1-3 grams dry bark 10-15 minutes, strain), three times daily; liquid bark extract (1:1 in 45% alcohol) 1-3 mL three times daily; bark tincture (1:5 in 45% alcohol) 2-5 mL three times daily (4).
ORAL (Berry): 0.5-1.5 grams dried berry; liquid berry extract (1:1 in 45% alcohol) 0.5-1.5 mL (4).

Comments

None.

SOY

Also Known As

Daidzein, Edamame, Frijol de Soya, Genistein, Haba Soya, Hydrolyzed Soy Protein, Isoflavone, Isoflavones, Legume, Miso, Natto, Phytoestrogen, Plant Estrogen, Shoyu, Soja, Sojabohne, Soy Fiber, Soy Milk, Soy Protein, Soy Protein Extract, Soy-Protein, Soya, Soybean, Soybean Curd, Tempeh, Texturized Vegetable Protein, Tofu.

Scientific Names

Glycine max, synonym Glycine soja.
Family: Leguminosae or Fabaceae.

People Use This For

Orally, soy is used for hyperlipidemia, menopausal symptoms, and for preventing osteoporosis and breast cancer. It is also used orally for cyclic breast pain, hypertension, constipation, diarrhea, slowing the progression of kidney disease, decreasing urine protein excretion, preventing hot flashes in breast cancer survivors, and for preventing endometrial and prostate cancer.

Intravenously, soy is used as a source of calories and fatty acids in fat emulsions.

In foods, soy is used as a milk substitute for infant feeding formulas and as an alternative to cow's milk in vegetarian diets. Soybeans are eaten boiled or roasted. Soy flour and soy oil are used as ingredients in foods, beverages, and condiments.

Safety

LIKELY SAFE ...when soy protein is used orally and appropriately. Soy protein products in doses up to 60 grams per day providing up to 90 mg isoflavones have been safely used in studies lasting up to 2 months (842,2293,2294,2296,3025,3402,3977,4755,6412). ...when soy protein is used intravenously as an emulsion (15).

POSSIBLY SAFE ...when soy extracts are used orally and appropriately. There is some evidence that soy extracts containing concentrated isoflavones 50 mg daily can be safely used for up to 12 weeks (4751,6455).

CHILDREN: LIKELY SAFE ...when used orally in amounts found in foods. Soy in amounts found in food or as a component of infant formula seems to be safe (3400,7331). Exposure to soy formula in infancy does not appear to cause health or reproductive problems later in life (7331). POSSIBLY UNSAFE ...when used orally as an alternative to cow's milk in children with severe milk allergy. Although soy-protein based infant formulas are often promoted for children with milk allergy, children with a severe allergy to cow's milk are also frequently sensitive to soy protein (14). There is insufficient reliable information available about the safety of soy products when used in amounts higher than typical food quantities for children.

PREGNANCY: LIKELY SAFE ...when used orally in amounts found in foods (14). POSSIBLY UNSAFE ...when used orally in medicinal amounts. Soy contains mildly estrogenic constituents (3373,3988,3989,3990,3994,6029). Theoretically, therapeutic use of soy might adversely effect fetal development; avoid using.

LACTATION: LIKELY SAFE ...when used orally in amounts found in foods. A single 20 gram dose of roasted soybeans, containing 37 mg isoflavones, produces 4-6 times less isoflavones in breast milk than provided in a soy-based infant formula (2290). There is insufficient reliable information available about the safety of long-term use of therapeutic amounts of soy during lactation.

Effectiveness

LIKELY EFFECTIVE ...when used orally for hyperlipidemia. Soy protein preparations reduce total cholesterol and low-density lipoprotein (LDL) levels in both hypercholesterolemic and normocholesterolemic men and women (842,2293,2294,2296,2585,3402,4755,6412,7346). Replacement of dietary animal protein with soy protein decreases serum total cholesterol by 9%, LDL cholesterol by 13%, and triglycerides by 11% after 1-2 months. Soy protein does not seem to effect serum high-density lipoprotein (HDL) cholesterol (2560,3401). Some of the beneficial effects might be attributed to the isoflavone content of soy protein, since preparations providing higher concentrations of isoflavones seem to produce more significant effects (3402,6413). The FDA has approved labeling soy products for cholesterol reduction when used in combination with a diet low in saturated fat and cholesterol. To be eligible for this labeling, soy products must provide at least 6.25 grams of soy protein per serving, which is 25% of the effective amount of 25 grams per day (3977). Tell patients not to rely on concentrated soy extracts or purified isoflavone supplements for lowering lipids. They lack the fiber and beneficial fatty acids of soy protein and don't seem to be as effective as isoflavone rich foods like soy protein for lowering serum cholesterol concentrations (851,4738,7345). ...when used intravenously as a source of calories and fatty acids in soy fat emulsions (15). ...when used orally as an alternative for providing nutrition in term infants in isolated soy protein-based formula (3400).

POSSIBLY EFFECTIVE ...when used orally for hot flashes related to menopause. Asian women who eat a high-soy diet have fewer hot flashes. Soy protein 20-60 grams providing 34-76 mg of isoflavones daily modestly decreases the frequency and severity of hot flashes in menopausal women (2296,2297,3978,3986,3987). Soy extracts in tablet form, providing 50 mg of isoflavones daily, seem to have similar beneficial effects (4751,6455). ...when used orally to reduce the risk of osteoporosis in perimenopausal and postmenopausal women (842,6449). There is some evidence that postmenopausal Asian women consuming 54.3 mg soy isoflavones per day in the diet have higher bone mineral density (BMD) (7342). Supplementing the diet with soy protein also seems to boost BMD in perimenopausal and postmenopausal women. Soy protein containing higher amounts of the constituent isoflavones seems to have a greater effect. In postmenopausal women, 40 grams daily of soy protein containing 90 mg isoflavones (2.25 mg per gram) produces significant increases in spinal bone mineral content and density after 6 months of treatment. This effect is not found when soy protein providing only 56 mg isoflavones (1.39 mg per gram) is used for 6 months in postmenopausal women (842). In perimenopausal women, 40 grams daily of soy protein providing 80 mg isoflavones (2 mg per gram) produces significant improvement in bone mineral content and density after 6 months of treatment. This effect is not found when soy protein providing only 4 mg isoflavones (0.1 mg per gram) is used in perimenopausal women for 6 months (6449). ...when used orally for reducing the risk of breast cancer. There is some evidence from population studies that Asian women who eat a diet high in soy have a reduced risk of developing breast cancer (5939,7334,7335,7336). Soy food intake during adolescence seems to correlate with decreased incidence of breast cancer among Chinese women. This benefit persists even when Asian women immigrate to the western cultures where soy is less likely to be a regular component of the diet (7335,7336). This suggests that early exposure to soy might be important for protection against breast cancer later in life. ...when soy fiber is used orally for reducing the duration of diarrhea in infants (2291,2292). ...when isolated soy protein-based formula is used orally in infants with galactosemia, hereditary lactase deficiency, or lactose intolerance (3400). ...when soy protein is used orally for reducing proteinuria in people with kidney disease (2286,2287,2288). ...when soymilk is used orally for reducing the risk of prostate cancer in men (2298). Consumption of soymilk at least once a day seems to reduce the risk of prostate cancer (2298). ...when soy protein is used to lower blood pressure in perimenopausal women (2296).

POSSIBLY INEFFECTIVE ...when used to prevent hot flashes in breast cancer survivors (3991).

There is insufficient reliable information available to rate the effectiveness of soy for its other uses. However, there is preliminary clinical evidence that soy might improve lipid profiles in patients with diabetes and potentially slow the development of diabetic nephropathy (7348). There is also some epidemiological evidence that increasing soy intake might lower the risk endometrial cancer. Endometrial cancer incidence is lower in Japan, China, and other Asian countries where the typical diet is low in calories and high in soy and whole grain foods, vegetables, and fruits (7338). There is also some preliminary evidence that soymilk (34 grams soy protein/day) might reduce cyclical breast pain in some women (2428). More evidence is needed to rate soy for these uses.

Mechanism of Action

Soybeans are legumes that contain up to 25% oil, 24% carbohydrates, and 50% protein, as well as stearic, linoleic, and palmitic acids. They are also rich in calcium, iron, potassium, amino acids, vitamins, and fiber. Soy protein is produced from raw soybeans by removing the lipid and indigestible components and concentrating the protein, which is then used in the manufacture of meat replacement products. Soy protein contains all of the essential amino acids in sufficient quantities to support human life (2426).

Non-fortified soy beverages such as soymilk contain only about 10 mg of calcium per serving. Calcium-fortified soymilk can contain from 80-500 mg of calcium per serving in the form of tricalcium phosphate (6414). However, calcium from cow's milk is significantly better absorbed than calcium from fortified soymilk (6414). Fermented soy foods, such as soy sauce, miso, tempeh, and natto, have higher amounts of calcium and vitamin K2 (7342).Soybeans and soy foods contain the most significant dietary source of phytoestrogens called isoflavones (3387,3978,4753,6029). Soy protein usually contains 1 to 3 mg of isoflavones per gram of protein (7333). When ingested, the isoflavone glucosides (IFGs) genistin and daidzin are hydrolyzed by beta-glucosidases in the jejunum, releasing the isoflavone aglycones (IFAs) genistein and daidzein (3982,5937). These are widely distributed in the body and undergo enterohepatic recycling (7330). Peak concentrations appear at 4 to 8 hours after dietary intake, and excretion is within 24 hours (3982). The absorption of isoflavones from food may be saturable, suggesting improved effect if ingested throughout the day, but there is considerable variation in absorption from person to person (3380,3982,7344). There is some variation in how isoflavones are absorbed from different soy products. Soy germ products result in higher plasma levels of daidzein and lower levels of genistein. Soy protein products result in higher levels of genistein. Soy foods such as tofu produce less dramatic rises of daidzein and genistein. From soy food sources genistein appears to be more bioavailable than daidzein (7330). Isoflavone bioavailability is similar for most soy foods (4750).

Soy isoflavones are heterocyclic phenols with structural similarity to estradiol and selective estrogen-receptor modulators (SERMs). The phenolic ring allows soy isoflavones to bind to both the estrogen receptors alpha and beta, but with a higher affinity for the beta estrogen receptor (3983,3992,6029,7344). The beta estrogen receptor predominates in the heart, vasculature, bone, and bladder, which may account for some of soy's beneficial effects. Actions at the cellular level depend on the target tissue, receptor status of the tissue, and the level of endogenous estrogen (7344). Soy phytoestrogens might act as selective SERMs (3387,3990). In premenopausal women with normal endogenous estrogen levels, soy phytoestrogens may have an anti-estrogen effect. In postmenopausal women with low endogenous estrogens, soy phytoestrogens are more likely to act as weak estrogens (3373,3988,3989,3990,3994,6029).

Soy has several pharmacological effects that might be beneficial for preventing cardiovascular disease (6029). The estrogenic effects of soy isoflavones are thought to play a role in modulating lipid metabolism (2426). Soy might also increase bile acid excretion, up-regulate low-density lipoprotein (LDL) receptors, inhibit cholesterol absorption in the small bowel, and prevent the oxidation of LDL cholesterol (2426,2594,6029,6030,7344,7347). Soy is also thought to have weak antioxidant effects (2586,6029) and may possibly inhibit platelet aggregation (3992). Soy also seems to improve arterial compliance in perimenopausal women (851) and there is some preliminary evidence that it might prevent progression of coronary artery atherosclerosis (7333). However, lipoprotein (a), which has been identified as an independent risk factor for coronary heart disease, does not seem to be affected by soy (7347).

For preventing postmenopausal osteoporosis, soy is thought to be beneficial due to its weak estrogenic effects on bone (5598,6029). However, soy proteins and isoflavones do not seem to influence calcium absorption or calcium retention (7343).

Estrogenic effects of soy have also been attributed to benefit menopausal symptoms such as hot flashes. However, the incidence of hot flashes does not seem to correlate with serum levels of the phytoestrogens genistein, daidzein, and equol. Components of soy other than phytoestrogens may be responsible for reduction in hot flashes (4752).

In cancer, soy is thought to be beneficial due to preliminary evidence that suggests isoflavones in soy have antioxidant, antiproliferative, and antiangiogenic activity (2296,3983). There is a lot of controversy about soy and its potential role in breast cancer. Some researchers think that soy is protective against breast cancer. Asian women who eat a traditional diet high in soy seem to have a lower risk of developing of breast cancer (4590,5939). This benefit persists even when Asian women immigrate to the western cultures where soy is less likely to be a regular component of the diet. This suggests that exposure to soy early in life (i.e., before menopause), provides the most benefit against breast cancer. It is theorized that isoflavones found in soy enhance early cellular differentiation and maturation of mammary glands. More mature mammary glands seem to be less susceptible to carcinogens (4590). Animal models show that soy protein can prevent chemically induced breast cancer (3976). There is also some evidence that the soy isoflavone, genistein, can suppress breast cancer cell growth by stimulating apoptosis (3378). Other research suggests that genistein influences enzymes involved in signal transduction that regulate cell growth and replication (7337). There is also evidence that drinking soymilk daily can reduced serum 17-beta-estradiol and progesterone levels in premenopausal women. Higher serum estradiol levels is associated with increase risk of breast cancer (2429). Soy consumption also seems to alter the ratios of various estrogen metabolites in the urine, reducing excretion of potentially carcinogenic estrogen metabolites, which suggests that soy might cause a shift in estrogen metabolism to produce more benign metabolites (2430). However, some researchers suggest that, due to the estrogenic effects of soy, it might actually increase the risk of breast cancer (6030). There is also preliminary in vitro data that soy can stimulate proliferation of normal human breast tissue (3980,3981).

In prostatic diseases, soy phytoestrogens are thought to potentially be beneficial due to estrogenic mechanisms as well as inhibition of 5-alpha-reductase and 17-beta-hydroxysteroid dehydrogenase (3984,3985). A diet high in soy foods seems to reduce serum estradiol levels and possibly testosterone levels (7339).

The soy isoflavones, genistein and daidzein, seem to be responsible for effects on thyroid hormones. The isoflavones seem to block production of thyroid hormone by interfering with thyroid peroxidase catalyzed iodination of thyroglobulin. This can result in increased thyroid stimulating hormone (TSH) and goiter. However, these clinical results appear most likely to occur in people with low iodine levels (6466).

There is some evidence that isoflavones can inhibit oxidative and conjugative metabolism of drugs (4736). Isoflavones might also affect drug absorption and biliary excretion by interacting with drug transporters such as P-glycoprotein and the canalicular multispecific organic anion transporter (4736). Given the wide range of drugs and metabolites whose pharmacokinetics depends on these mechanisms, drug interactions with isoflavones might be more common than literature reports suggest.

Adverse Reactions

Orally, soy most commonly causes gastrointestinal side effects, such as constipation, bloating, and nausea (2297). Soy can also cause allergic reactions in some people (2280), such as skin rash and itching (6412). Inhaled soy dust and soy hull aeroallergen can trigger symptoms of asthma. The risk and severity increase with exposure (5084). Inhaled soy dust was reported as the cause of an asthma epidemic in Spain (5084,5085,5086).

Soy products have also been associated with goiter and hypothyroidism in children taking soy formula. However, this seems to only occur in people with iodine deficiency (6466). There have also been concerns about the effects of phytoestrogens in infants fed soy-based formulas (7332). Isoflavone consumption can cause infertility in some animals (7344), but this has not been described in humans. Adults who received soy formulas as infants have not experienced any adverse health or reproductive outcomes compared with people who received cow milk formulas as infants (7331). There is controversy about the role of soy in breast cancer. Population studies suggest that soy is protective against breast cancer. Asian women who eat a traditional diet high in soy seem to have a lower risk of developing of breast cancer (4590,5939). However, some researchers suggest that, due to the estrogenic effects of soy, it might actually increase the risk of breast cancer (6030). Some preliminary research suggests that soy can stimulate proliferation of normal human breast tissue (3980,3981). More research is needed to define to role of soy in breast cancer. Since soy has a mild estrogenic effect some clinicians are concerned that soy might increase the risk of endometrial hyperplasia. However, soy does not seem to have a proliferative effect on endometrial cells (7358). Population studies suggest that soy might actually reduce the risk of endometrial cancer (7338).

There is some concern about consumption of large amounts of fermented soy products (e.g., misso, tempeh). There is preliminary evidence that fermented soy products might be associated with an increased risk of stomach cancer. However, stomach cancer risk seems to be reduced if intake of nonfermented soy foods is high. These epidemiological findings need to be verified. These associations might be confounded by the higher salt and N-nitroso content of fermented soy foods or other dietary factors such as fruit and vegetable intake. More research is required to determine if soy products have any role in stomach cancer (7340,7341).

There is preliminary evidence showing an association between tofu ingestion and cognitive functioning. Data collected from the Honolulu-Asia Aging Study and the Honolulu Heart Program shows that two or more servings per week of tofu during midlife might be associated with cognitive impairment in late life (6415). Of the 3,734 Japanese-American men participating, cognitive impairment was identified in 19% of the high tofu users versus 4% of the low tofu users approximately 30 years later when the men were between 71-93 years of age. However, numerous other factors, such as lifestyle and health of the participants, may be involved. A larger percentage of the high tofu users were immigrants from Japan, had fewer years of education, and had worked at low complexity jobs. The high tofu users had also experienced a greater incidence of strokes (6416). These findings are too preliminary to be used as a basis for clinical recommendations.

Interactions with Herbs & Other Dietary Supplements
Insufficient reliable information available.

Interactions with Drugs
ESTROGEN: Theoretically, soy might competitively inhibit the effects of estrogen replacement therapy (3860).
TAMOXIFEN (Nolvadex): There is some concern that soy might interfere with tamoxifen because of its potential estrogenic effects. There is preliminary evidence that soy isoflavones might antagonize the antitumor effects of tamoxifen (7072). Tell patients taking tamoxifen to avoid therapeutic use of soy products.

Interactions with Foods
PLANT-BASED FOODS: Soy protein isolate reduces the absorption of non-heme iron from foods (5053). Non-heme iron is found in plant-based foods.

Interactions with Lab Tests
THYROID STIMULATING HORMONE (TSH): Theoretically, soy might increase TSH levels. Soy can inhibit thyroid hormone synthesis resulting in increased secretion of TSH, and might potentially cause goiter. However, this seems to occur primarily in people with low iodine levels (6466).

Interactions with Diseases or Conditions
ASTHMA: People with asthma are at increased risk for soy hull allergy. The risk and severity of symptoms increase with increased exposure (5084).
ALLERGIC RHINITIS: People with allergic rhinitis are at increased risk for soy hull allergy. The risk and severity of symptoms increase with increased exposure (5084).
BREAST CANCER: Soy isoflavones have estrogenic properties. Some experts are concerned about the use of soy in women with breast cancer because estrogens can increase this risk. However, some preclinical studies show that soy may have protective effects for breast cancer (3976), while others suggest soy might increase breast cell proliferation (3980,3981). Because there is insufficient reliable information about the effects of soy preparations in patients with breast cancer, a history of breast cancer, or a family history of breast cancer, therapeutic use of soy should be done with caution in these patients (956).
CYSTIC FIBROSIS: Children with cystic fibrosis may develop hypoproteinemia when fed soymilk (368).
HYPOTHYROIDISM: Theoretically, soy might worsen hypothyroidism. Soy can inhibit thyroid hormone synthesis, increase thyroid stimulating hormone (TSH), and possibly cause goiter. However, this seems to occur primarily in people with low iodine levels (6466). Use with caution.
HYPERBILIRUBINEMIA: Large amounts of soybean oil (2-3 g/kg) might worsen hyperbilirubinemia in infants (14).
KIDNEY STONES (Nephrolithiasis): There is some concern that soy products might increase the risk of kidney stones because of its high oxalate content. Soy products can contain from 0.5 mg to 14 mg oxalate per gram or approximately 43 mg to 640 mg per soy serving, depending on soy food type (7073). Tell patients with a history of kidney stones to avoid excessive consumption of soy.
MILK ALLERGY: Children who are severely allergic to cow's milk are frequently sensitive to soy as well (14); use with caution or avoid.

Dosage and Administration
ORAL: For lowering cholesterol, a typical dose is 20-50 grams per day of soy protein (2293,2295,2296,3401,6412,7346). For preventing osteoporosis, 40 grams per day soy protein containing 2-2.25 mg isoflavones per gram has been used in clinical studies (842,6449). For reducing the severity and number of hot flashes, 20-60 grams per day of soy protein providing 34-76 mg isoflavones has been used in studies (2296,2297). Soy extract tablets providing 50 mg soy isoflavones per day have also been used (4751,6455). For reducing the risk of prostate cancer, two or more glasses of soymilk daily has been used (2298). For proteinuria, a diet limited to 700-800 mg/kg soy protein daily has been used (2287). For reducing cyclical breast pain in premenopausal women, 34 grams soy protein daily (as soymilk) has been used (2428). For diarrhea in infants, soy fiber fortified formula containing 18-20 grams of soy protein per liter has been used (2291,2292). Soy foods contain variable amounts of isoflavones: Soy flour contains 2.6 mg isoflavones per gram of soy flour, fermented soy beans contain 1.3 mg per gram, boiled soybeans contain 0.6 mg per gram, soymilk contains 0.4 mg per gram, soybean curd contains 0.5 mg per gram, fried soybean curd contains 0.7 mg per gram, soybean paste contains 0.4 mg per gram, and soy sauce contains 0.016 mg per gram (7342).

Comments
None.

SOYBEAN OIL

Also Known As
Intralipid, Legume, Soy, Soybean, Soyca, Travmulsion.

Scientific Names
Glycine soja.
Family: Leguminosae or Fabaceae.

People Use This For
Parenterally, soybean oil is used in nutrient formulas. It is also used as a source of lecithin (4077).
Plant sterols, derived from soybean oil, are used to lower total and LDL cholesterol without affecting HDL (4086).
Soybean oil has been used as a filler in some breast implants (see Comments) (6125).

Safety
LIKELY SAFE ...when soybean oil or the plant sterols from soybean oil are used orally and appropriately in margarine. ...when soybean oil is used in pharmaceutical grade parenteral formulas. Soybean oil is listed in the United States Pharmacopeia (10).
PREGNANCY: LIKELY SAFE ...when used orally in amounts found in foods. Avoid using in amounts greater than those typically found in foods. Theoretically, parenteral use of lipids like soybean oil during pregnancy might lead to hypertriglyceridemia, ketonemia, premature labor, and placental infection. However, women have used parenteral nutrition with lipids to treat severe morning sickness without any adverse effects (4084).
LACTATION: LIKELY SAFE ...when used orally in amounts found in foods. Avoid using in amounts greater than those typically found in foods.

Effectiveness
EFFECTIVE ...when soybean oil is used as a parenteral nutrient (16).
POSSIBLY EFFECTIVE ...when the plant sterols from soybean oil are used in margarine to lower total and LDL cholesterol without affecting HDL (4086). The FDA has approved such labeling for the products Take Control and Benecol as a structure/function claim under the Dietary Supplement Health Education Act, not as a drug (4087).

Mechanism of Action
Soybean oil is used in parenteral nutrition as a source of fatty acids (16). In a comparison between diets with 20% fat from butter or soybean oil, people using soybean oil demonstrated a 12% decrease in LDL and a 3% reduction in HDL (4085). People using a margarine containing plant sterols from soybean oil reduced total and LDL cholesterol by 8-13% compared to a control group (4086).

Adverse Reactions
Soybean oil can cause an allergic reaction in individuals allergic to the Fabaceae family. Members of this family include peanuts and soybeans (4079,4080).

Interactions with Herbs & Other Dietary Supplements
Insufficient reliable information available.

Interactions with Drugs
No interactions are known to occur, and there is no known reason to expect a clinically significant interaction with soybean oil.

Interactions with Foods
No interactions are known to occur, and there is no known reason to expect a clinically significant interaction with soybean oil.

Interactions with Lab Tests
CHOLESTEROL: Soybean oil sterols can reduce serum total cholesterol and LDL cholesterol concentrations, and test results (4086).

Interactions with Diseases or Conditions
CROSS-ALLERGENICITY: Soybean oil can cause an allergic reaction in individuals sensitive to the Fabaceae family. Members of this family include peanuts and soybeans (4079,4080).

Dosage and Administration

ORAL: In the form of a plant sterol-enriched margarine, such as Take Control, a serving size is one tablespoon, or 14 grams.
PARENTERAL: No typical dosage.

Comments

Soybean oil is obtained by cold pressing the seeds of the Glycine soja (18).
The British Health Ministry recommends that women with soybean oil filled (Trilucent) breast implants have them removed as a precautionary measure. While there is currently no evidence of any serious medical problems, tests reveal that the soybean oil filler can break down, producing aldehydes which might be toxic to the implant recipient or to a developing fetus (6125).

SPANISH BROOM

Also Known As

Genet, Weaver's Broom.
CAUTION: See separate listings for Butcher's Broom, Scotch Broom flower, and Scotch Broom herb.

Scientific Names

Spartium junceum, synonym Genista juncea.
Family: Leguminosae or Fabaceae.

People Use This For

Historically, Spanish broom has been used as a laxative and diuretic (11).
In foods and beverages, Spanish broom extracts are used as a flavor component. (11).
In manufacturing, an extract is used as a fragrance in soaps and cosmetics (11).

Safety

LIKELY SAFE ...when used orally in amounts found in foods. Spanish broom is approved for food use in the US (11).
PREGNANCY AND LACTATION: **POSSIBLY UNSAFE** ...when used orally. Large amounts of the alkaloid constituent sparteine can stimulate menstrual flow (19). The most common Spanish broom extract, Genet absolute, should not contain alkaloids because of the extraction method used, however, other extracts might (11).

Effectiveness

There is insufficient reliable information about the effectiveness of Spanish broom.

Mechanism of Action

The applicable part of Spanish broom is the flower. Sparteine seems to hasten childbirth (11).

Adverse Reactions

None reported.

Interactions with Herbs & Other Dietary Supplements

Insufficient reliable information available.

Interactions with Drugs

No interactions are known to occur, and there is no known reason to expect a clinically significant interaction with Spanish broom.

Interactions with Foods

No interactions are known to occur, and there is no known reason to expect a clinically significant interaction with Spanish broom.

Interactions with Lab Tests

No interactions are known to occur, and there is no known reason to expect a clinically significant interaction with Spanish broom.

Interactions with Diseases or Conditions
No interactions are known to occur, and there is no known reason to expect a clinically significant interaction with Spanish broom.

Dosage and Administration
No typical dosage.

Comments
Avoid confusion with butcher's broom, scotch broom flower, and scotch broom herb. Spanish broom stems have appeared as an adulterant to scotch broom (Cytisus scoparius).

SPANISH ORIGANUM OIL

Also Known As
Origanum Oil, Sicilian Thyme, Spanish Origanum, Spanish Thyme.
CAUTION: See separate listings for Thyme oil, Thyme, and Wild Thyme.

Scientific Names
Satureja capitata; Thymus capitatus, synonym Coridothymus capitatus; carvacrol-rich Origanum species.
Family: Labiatae or Lamiaceae.

People Use This For
Spanish origanum oil has no reported medicinal uses.
In food and beverages, Spanish origanum oil is used as a flavor component (11).
In manufacturing, it is used as a fragrance component in soaps, cosmetics, and perfumes.

Safety
LIKELY SAFE ...when used in amounts found in foods. Spanish origanum is approved for food use in the US. The maximum use level is 0.01% (11).
PREGNANCY AND LACTATION: Insufficient reliable information available; avoid using in amounts greater than those found in foods.

Effectiveness
There is insufficient reliable information available about the effectiveness of Spanish origanum oil.

Mechanism of Action
Spanish origanum oil is characterized by its carvacrol content (11). It contains carvacrol and thymol (11) which show some evidence of anthelmintic (11), antifungal (4059,4060,4062,4063), and antibacterial (4064,4065,4066) activity. These constituents also demonstrate some evidence of antioxidant activity, including decreased Fe (III) catalyzed phospholipid liposome peroxidation and peroxy radical scavenging activity (4067).

Adverse Reactions
None reported.

Interactions with Herbs & Other Dietary Supplements
Insufficient reliable information available.

Interactions with Drugs
No interactions are known to occur, and there is no known reason to expect a clinically significant interaction with Spanish origanum oil.

Interactions with Foods
No interactions are known to occur, and there is no known reason to expect a clinically significant interaction with Spanish origanum oil.

Interactions with Lab Tests
No interactions are known to occur, and there is no known reason to expect a clinically significant interaction with Spanish origanum oil.

Interactions with Diseases or Conditions

No interactions are known to occur, and there is no known reason to expect a clinically significant interaction with Spanish origanum oil.

Dosage and Administration

No typical dosage.

Comments

Spanish origanum oil is distilled from the flowering tops of Thymus capitatus and carvacrol-rich Origanum species.

SPEARMINT

Also Known As

Curled Mint, Fish Mint, Garden Mint, Green Mint, Lamb Mint, Mackerel Mint, Our Lady's Mint, Sage of Bethlehem, Spire Mint, Yerba buena.
CAUTION: See separate listing for Sage.

Scientific Names

Mentha spicata, synonym M. viridis.
Family: Labiatae or Lamiaceae.

People Use This For

Orally, spearmint is used for digestive disorders, including flatulence (18), indigestion, nausea, sore throat, diarrhea, colds, headaches, toothaches, cramps, and cancer.

Topically, it is used for oral mucosal inflammation, arthritis, local muscle and nerve pain, and skin conditions including pruritus and urticaria.

In Europe, it is used orally under the direction of a physician for bile duct and gallbladder inflammation, gallstones, upper gastrointestinal tract spasms, flatulence, irritable bowel syndrome (IBS), and inflammation of respiratory tract. It is also used as an aromatic, stimulant, antiseptic, local anesthetic, and antispasmodic.

In foods and beverages, spearmint is used as a flavoring agent.

In manufacturing, it is used in health food products, cosmetics, and oral hygiene products such as mouthwash and toothpaste (11).

Safety

LIKELY SAFE ...when used in amounts found in foods and consumed in appropriate amounts. It has Generally Recognized as Safe (GRAS) status in the US and its maximum use is 0.132% (11).
POSSIBLY SAFE ...when used orally and topically for medicinal reasons (11,12).
PREGNANCY AND LACTATION: Avoid using in amounts greater than those typically found in foods.

Effectiveness

There is insufficient reliable information available about the effectiveness of spearmint leaf and oil.

Mechanism of Action

The applicable parts of spearmint are the leaf and oil. There is insufficient reliable information available about the possible mechanism of action and active ingredients.

Adverse Reactions

None reported.

Interactions with Herbs & Other Dietary Supplements

Insufficient reliable information available.

Interactions with Drugs

No interactions are known to occur, and there is no known reason to expect a clinically significant interaction with spearmint.

Interactions with Foods

No interactions are known to occur, and there is no known reason to expect a clinically significant interaction with spearmint.

Interactions with Lab Tests

No interactions are known to occur, and there is no known reason to expect a clinically significant interaction with spearmint.

Interactions with Diseases or Conditions

No interactions are known to occur, and there is no known reason to expect a clinically significant interaction with spearmint.

Dosage and Administration

ORAL: Spearmint is used in tea, and is also available in tablets, capsules, tinctures and other oral formulations (11).

Comments

None.

SPINACH

Also Known As

Spinaciae folium, Spinatblatter.

Scientific Names

Spinacia oleracea.
Family: Chenopodiaceae.

People Use This For

Orally, spinach is used for gastrointestinal complaints and fatigue. It is also used as a blood-builder, an appetite stimulant, for stimulating growth in children, and during convalescence (2).
For food uses, spinach is a commonly consumed vegetable.

Safety

LIKELY SAFE ...when consumed in food amounts.
CHILDREN: LIKELY UNSAFE ...when used orally in infants under 4 months old because the nitrate content can cause methemoglobinemia (18).
PREGNANCY AND LACTATION: LIKELY SAFE ...when consumed in food amounts; avoid using in amounts greater than those consumed in food.

Effectiveness

There is insufficient reliable information available about the effectiveness of spinach.

Mechanism of Action

The applicable part of spinach is the leaf. Spinach contains vitamin C (18), vitamin E, vitamin K, magnesium (19), and nitrates (18). It also contains triterpene saponins including oxalic acid (18). Spinach is thought to have hypoglycemic effects (19). Consumption of fresh spinach is associated with a decreased risk of stomach cancer in humans (4112). Preliminary research suggests that compounds contained in spinach might slow aging effects on the nervous system (1418,1419).

Adverse Reactions

Orally, spinach may cause methemoglobinemia in infants younger than 4 months old (18).

Interactions with Herbs & Other Dietary Supplements

CALCIUM, IRON, ZINC: Concurrent use might decrease mineral absorption. Spinach contains oxalate (7,12), which can bind multivalent metal ions in the gastrointestinal tract and decrease mineral absorption.

Interactions with Drugs

ANTICOAGULANTS: Spinach contains vitamin K. Individuals using anticoagulants should consume a consistent daily amount to maintain the effect of anticoagulant therapy (19).
DIABETES THERAPY: Monitor blood glucose level closely due to claims that spinach leaves have hypoglycemic effects (19).

Interactions with Foods

CALCIUM, IRON, ZINC: Concurrent use might decrease mineral absorption from foods. Spinach contains oxalate (7,12), which can bind multivalent metal ions in the gastrointestinal tract and decrease mineral absorption.

Interactions with Lab Tests

No interactions are known to occur, and there is no known reason to expect a clinically significant interaction with spinach.

Interactions with Diseases or Conditions

KIDNEY DISEASE: May cause formation of insoluble oxalate crystals in the kidneys causing further damage (19).
DIABETES: Theoretically, may interfere with blood glucose control (19).

Dosage and Administration

No typical dosage.

Comments

Spinach is rich in beta-carotene, vitamin E, vitamin K, and magnesium (19).

SPINY RESTHARROW

Also Known As

Cammock, Ground Furze, Hauhechelwurzel, Land Whin, Ononidis radix, Petty Whin, Restharrow, Stay Plough, Stinking Tommy, Wild Liquorice.

Scientific Names

Ononis spinosa.
Family: Fabacea.

People Use This For

Orally, spiny restharrow is used for gout, kidney and bladder stones, rheumatic complaints, urinary tract infections (18), irrigation therapy for inflammatory disease of the lower urinary tract, and prevention and treatment of kidney gravel (2,18).

Safety

POSSIBLY SAFE ...when used orally and appropriately (2).
PREGNANCY AND LACTATION: Insufficient reliable information available; avoid using.

Effectiveness

There is insufficient reliable information available about the effectiveness of spiny restharrow.

Mechanism of Action

The applicable part of spiny restharrow is the root. The drug contains isoflavonoids including ononin (2,18), triterpenes including alphaonoceradiendiol (18), and volatile oil (18). The volatile oil contains anethole, carvone, and menthol (18). Spiny restharrow is reported to have a diuretic effect (2,18).

Adverse Reactions

None reported.

Interactions with Herbs & Other Dietary Supplements

Insufficient reliable information available.

Interactions with Drugs

No interactions are known to occur, and there is no known reason to expect a clinically significant interaction with spiny restharrow.

Interactions with Foods

No interactions are known to occur, and there is no known reason to expect a clinically significant interaction with spiny restharrow.

Interactions with Lab Tests

No interactions are known to occur, and there is no known reason to expect a clinically significant interaction with spiny restharrow.

Interactions with Diseases or Conditions

EDEMA: Contraindicated in individuals with edema resulting from cardiac or kidney impairment (2,18).

Dosage and Administration

ORAL: A typical oral dose is 6-12 grams daily or as a tea (2,18). To prepare tea, pour boiling water over 2-2.5 grams of ground drug, strain after 20-30 minutes (18). Drink with plenty of liquid (2,18).

Comments

None.

SPLEEN EXTRACT

Also Known As

Bovine Spleen, Hydrolyzed Spleen Extract, Predigested Spleen Extract, Raw Spleen, Spleen, Spleen Concentrate, Spleen Factors, Spleen Peptides, Spleen Polypeptides, Splenopentin, Tuftsin.

Scientific Names

None.

People Use This For

Orally, spleen extract is used as replacement therapy after splenectomy or in people with inadequate spleen function (6614). It is also used orally for treating people with low white blood cell counts, enhancing general immune function and immune function in people with cancer, and for treating bacterial infections (6614). Spleen extract is also used orally for treating celiac disease, dermatitis herpetiformis, glomerulonephritis, HIV-related bacterial infections, rheumatoid arthritis, systemic lupus erythematosus, thrombocytopenia, ulcerative colitis, and vasculitis (6614).

Safety

There is insufficient reliable information available to rate the safety of spleen extract. However, since spleen extract preparations are derived from animals, there is concern about contamination with diseased animal parts (see Adverse Reactions) (1825). So far, there are no reports of disease transmission to humans due to use of contaminated spleen extract.

Pregnancy and Lactation: Insufficient reliable information available; avoid using.

Effectiveness

There is insufficient reliable information available about the effectiveness of spleen extract.

Mechanism of Action

Spleen extract is derived from fresh animal spleens. Spleen extract contains the peptides tuftsin and splenopentin (6614). Tuftsin stimulates phagocytosis, motility, and immunogenic response of phagocytic cells, and has bactericidal and tumoricidal activities (6659,6660). Tuftsin activity correlates inversely with splenic function (6662). Spleen extracts are tried in people with HIV disease because some patients have significantly lower tuftsin activity than healthy people (6662). There is preliminary evidence that spleen extract might protect against radiation. Spleen extract seems to shorten the time to regain normal immune response in animals exposed to sublethal doses of radiation (6661).

Adverse Reactions

Adverse reactions have not been reported. However, there is some concern about contamination. Spleen extract is derived from raw animal spleens gathered from slaughterhouses, possibly from sick or diseased animals (6616). Products made from contaminated or diseased organs might present a human health hazard. There is also concern that spleen extracts produced from cows in countries where bovine spongiform encephalitis (BSE) has been reported might be contaminated with diseased tissue. Countries where BSE has been reported include Great Britain, France, The Netherlands, Portugal, Luxembourg, Ireland, Switzerland, Oman, and Belgium (1825). There have been no reports of BSE transfer to humans from contaminated spleen extract products. Until more is known, tell patients to avoid these products unless country of origin can be determined. Patients should avoid products that are produced in countries where BSE has been found.

Interactions with Herbs & Other Dietary Supplements
Insufficient reliable information available.

Interactions with Drugs
No interactions are known to occur, and there is no known reason to expect a clinically significant interaction with spleen extract.

Interactions with Foods
No interactions are known to occur, and there is no known reason to expect a clinically significant interaction with spleen extract.

Interactions with Lab Tests
No interactions are known to occur, and there is no known reason to expect a clinically significant interaction with spleen extract.

Interactions with Diseases or Conditions
No interactions are known to occur, and there is no known reason to expect a clinically significant interaction with spleen extract.

Dosage and Administration
ORAL: A typical dose is approximately 1.5 grams total spleen peptides (equivalent to 50 mg of tuftsin and splenopentin) per day (6614).

Comments
None.

SQUALAMINE

Also Known As
Spiny Dogfish Shark.

Scientific Names
Squalus acanthias.

People Use This For
Orally, squalamine has been used experimentally as an antibiotic (6).
Topically, synthetic squalamine compounds have been investigated as antibiotics (4138).
In combination with captopril, oral squalamine is being investigated as an anti-angiogenic therapy for diabetic retinopathy (1269).
Squalamine is also being investigated as a possible treatment for pediatric solid tumors (5043).

Safety
There is insufficient reliable information available about the safety of squalamine or its derivative SM-7.
Pregnancy and Lactation: Insufficient reliable information available.

Effectiveness
There is insufficient reliable information available about the effectiveness of squalamine or its derivative SM-7.

Mechanism of Action
Squalamine was first isolated from the spiny dogfish shark and later synthesized synthetically. It shows evidence that it might have fungicidal and antiprotozoal activity (4139). Squalamine has also demonstrated significant activity against gram (-) and gram (+) bacteria (4139). Some compounds that mimic the structure of squalamine show promise in their activity against gram (-) rods, gram (+) cocci including methicillin-resistant Staphylococcus aureus, vancomycin-resistant Enterococcus faecium, and fungi (4138). In addition to antibiotic activity, squalamine also shows promise in inhibiting angiogenesis, and preventing formation and growth of tumors (4137,5043). Researchers report that squalamine demonstrates activity in breast, lung, and neuroblastoma cancer models. This unpublished research was reported at the American Association for Cancer Research 91st Annual Meeting (5043).

Adverse Reactions
None reported.

Interactions with Herbs & Other Dietary Supplements

Insufficient reliable information available.

Interactions with Drugs

CISPLATIN: Theoretically, concomitant use might inhibit growth and promote shrinkage of neuroblastomas. Preclinical data suggest that squalamine used in combination with cisplatin might inhibit tumor growth and promote tumor shrinkage in the treatment of neuroblastomas. This unpublished research was reported at the American Association for Cancer Research 91st Annual Meeting (5043).

Interactions with Foods

No interactions are known to occur, and there is no known reason to expect a clinically significant interaction with squalamine.

Interactions with Lab Tests

No interactions are known to occur, and there is no known reason to expect a clinically significant interaction with squalamine.

Interactions with Diseases or Conditions

No interactions are known to occur, and there is no known reason to expect a clinically significant interaction with squalamine.

Dosage and Administration

No typical dosage.

Comments

Squalamine has been isolated from the stomach and liver tissues of the spiny dogfish shark. Synthetic products that mimic the structure of squalamine appear to be good candidates for further development as topical antimicrobial agents. They have broad spectrum antimicrobial activity, but their potential for systemic toxicity limits their use (4138). Avoid confusion with shark cartilage, which is prepared from the cartilage of spiny dogfish shark, hammerhead shark (Sphyrna lewini), and other shark species (6).

Researchers at Georgetown University Medical Center plan a study of squalamine as an antiangiogenic therapy in combination with captopril for diabetic retinopathy (1269).

Magainin, the manufacturer of an investigational squalamine drug product plans a clinical study of squalamine in the treatment of pediatric solid tumors (5043).

SQUAWVINE

Also Known As

Checkerberry, Deerberry, Hive Vine, Noon Kie Oo Nah Yeah, One-Berry, Partridgeberry, Running Box, Squaw Berry, Squaw Vine, Twinberry, Two-Eyed Berry, Winter Clover.

Scientific Names

Mitchella repens.
Family: Rubiaceae.

People Use This For

Orally, squawvine is used for amenorrhea (absence of menstruation), anxiety, diarrhea, edema, excessive menstruation, fibrocystic disease of the breast, oliguria (lack of urination), painful menstruation, postpartum depression, varicose veins (3199), pregnancy (to make labor less difficult) (407,3199), improving lactation, insomnia, congestive heart failure, kidney failure, liver failure (407), chronic dysentery, spermatorrhea (involuntary discharge of semen without orgasm), as an emmenagogue (to promote menstruation), as an astringent for treating colitis, and reducing mucous membrane and leukorrheal (whitish vaginal) discharges (411).

Topically, squawvine is used for treating sore nipples (410).

Traditionally, squawvine was used by American Indians for promoting easy childbirth (taken during the last few weeks of pregnancy only), and as an abortifacient (408).

Safety

POSSIBLY SAFE ...when used orally and appropriately (12).

There is insufficient reliable information about the safety of squawvine for its other uses.

PREGNANCY: POSSIBLY UNSAFE ...when used orally due to reported abortifacient properties (12).
LACTATION: Insufficient reliable information available; avoid using.

Effectiveness
There is insufficient reliable information available about the effectiveness of squawvine.

Mechanism of Action
The applicable parts of squawvine are the above ground parts. Squawvine is reported to contain resin, wax, mucilages, dextrin, saponins, and unspecified alkaloids, glycosides and tannins (407,410,411).

Adverse Reactions
None reported.

Interactions with Herbs & Other Dietary Supplements
Insufficient reliable information available.

Interactions with Drugs
No interactions are known to occur, and there is no known reason to expect a clinically significant interaction with squawvine.

Interactions with Foods
No interactions are known to occur, and there is no known reason to expect a clinically significant interaction with squawvine.

Interactions with Lab Tests
No interactions are known to occur, and there is no known reason to expect a clinically significant interaction with squawvine.

Interactions with Diseases or Conditions
No interactions are known to occur, and there is no known reason to expect a clinically significant interaction with squawvine.

Dosage and Administration
ORAL: A typical dose is 20-50 mg.

Comments
None.

SQUILL

Also Known As
European Squill, Indian Squill, Mediterranean Squill, Red Squill, Scilla, Sea Onion, Sea Squill Bulb, White Squill.

Scientific Names
Urginea indica, synonyms Drimia indica, Scilla indica; Urginea maritima, synonyms Drimia maritima, Scilla maritima, Urginea scilla.
Family: Liliaceae.

People Use This For
Orally, squill is used for mild heart failure (2,7,18), arrhythmias, nervous heart complaints, some venous conditions (18), edema, inducing emesis, as an expectorant (6), for chronic bronchitis, asthma with bronchitis, and whooping cough (4). Historically, squill has been used as a diuretic (6,11,13), expectorant, abortifacient, emetic, heart tonic, and a rat poison (3488,3489).
In manufacturing, squill has been used in pest control as a rodenticide (red squill) (11,13).

Safety
UNSAFE ...when used orally (4,6,18,512). Squill contains cardiac glycosides that can cause adverse effects (512).
PREGNANCY: UNSAFE ...when used orally because it can have an abortifacient effect (4).
LACTATION: UNSAFE ...when used orally (4).

Effectiveness

There is insufficient reliable information available about the effectiveness of squill.

Mechanism of Action

Squill contains cardioactive glycosides, including bufadienolides, scillaren A, and proscillaridin A (2,4,6,18). Squill seems to have cardiac effects similar to digoxin, including positive inotropic and negative chronotropic effects (4,7). The aglycones in squill are poorly absorbed from the gastrointestinal tract and are therefore less potent than digitalis cardiac glycosides. Squill has additional cardiovascular properties that include reducing left ventricular diastolic pressure, and reducing pathologically elevated venous pressure (2,18). Large amounts of squill can induce vomiting due to gastric irritation and central action (4). In lesser amounts squill causes an expectorant-like effect (6).

Adverse Reactions

Orally, squill can cause gastric irritation, loss of appetite, diarrhea, vomiting, stomach disorders, headache, irregular pulse (2,18), and convulsions (6). Skin contact with the fresh bulb can cause dermatitis (18). Signs of overdose include restlessness, nausea, vomiting, life-threatening arrhythmias (ventricular tachycardia, atrial tachycardia with atrioventricular block, ventricular fibrillation), stupor, vision disorders, depression, confusion, hallucinations, psychosis, seizure, cardiac arrest, asphyxiation, and death (18,3488). A fatality has been reported after ingestion of squill bulb (3488).

Interactions with Herbs & Other Dietary Supplements

CALCIUM: Concomitant use of calcium may increase risk of cardiac toxicity (2,3805).
CARDIAC GLYCOSIDE-CONTAINING HERBS: Contraindicated, and concomitant use can increase the risk of cardiac glycoside toxicity. Cardiac glycoside-containing herbs include black hellebore, Canadian hemp roots, digitalis leaf, hedge mustard, figwort, lily of the valley roots, motherwort, oleander leaf, pheasant's eye plant, pleurisy root, strophanthus seeds, and uzara (2,18,19,500).
OTHER CARDIOACTIVE HERBS: Avoid concomitant use with other cardioactive herbs due to unpredictability of effects and adverse effects. Other cardioactive herbs include: calamus, cereus, cola, coltsfoot, devil's claw, European mistletoe, fenugreek, fumitory, ginger, Panax ginseng, hawthorn, white horehound, mate, parsley, quassia, scotch broom flower, shepherd's purse, and wild carrot (4). See individual product listings.
STIMULANT LAXATIVE HERBS: Theoretically, overuse or misuse of stimulant laxatives with cardiac glycoside-containing herbs increases the risk of cardiac toxicity due to potassium depletion. Stimulant laxative herbs include: aloe dried leaf sap, blue flag rhizome, alder buckthorn, European buckthorn, butternut bark, cascara bark, castor oil, colocynth fruit pulp, gamboge bark exudate, jalap root, black root, manna bark exudate, podophyllum root, rhubarb root, senna leaves and pods, wild cucumber fruit (Ecballium elaterium), and yellow dock root (19).
LICORICE/HORSETAIL: Theoretically, overuse/misuse of licorice rhizome or horsetail plant with cardiac glycoside-containing herbs increases the risk of cardiac toxicity due to potassium depletion (19).

Interactions with Drugs

ARRHYTHMOGENIC AGENTS: Increased risk of arrhythmias when used with sympathomimetics, methylxanthines and phosphodiesterase inhibitors (18).
CALCIUM: Concomitant use may increase risk of cardiac toxicity (2,3805).
CORTICOSTEROIDS: Concomitant use may increase effects and adverse effects of long-term corticosteroid use (2).
DIGOXIN: Concomitant use contraindicated, due to increased risk of cardiac glycoside toxicity (2,4).
POTASIUM DEPLETING DIURETICS, STIMULANT LAXATIVES: Concomitant use may increase risk of cardiac glycoside toxicity due to potassium loss (2).
QUINIDINE: Concomitant use may increase cardiac effects and adverse effects (2).

Interactions with Foods

No interactions are known to occur, and there is no known reason to expect a clinically significant interaction with squill.

Interactions with Lab Tests

No interactions are known to occur, and there is no known reason to expect a clinically significant interaction with squill.

Interactions with Diseases or Conditions

ELECTROLYTE IMBALANCE: Contraindicated in individuals with hypokalemia or hypercalcemia.
CARDIAC CONDITIONS: Contraindicated in individuals with second or third degree atrioventricular block, hypertrophic cardiomyopathy, carotid sinus syndrome, ventricular tachycardia, or thoracic aortic aneurysm Wolff-Parkinson-White syndrome (18).

GI CONDITIONS: Can irritate gastrointestinal tract. Contraindicated in individuals with infectious or inflammatory gastrointestinal conditions (19).

Dosage and Administration

ORAL: Mild heart failure (NYHA stage I and II heart disease), 100-500 mg standardized squill bulb powder per day (2,7).

Comments

Unsafe for self-medication (512). New York Heart Association (NYHA) stage I and II heart disease refers to people with heart disease who do not have limitations of physical activity. They are comfortable at rest but ordinary physical activity results in fatigue, palpitation, trouble breathing, or anginal pain (2).

ST. JOHN'S WORT

Also Known As

Amber, Amber Touch-and-Heal, Demon Chaser, Fuga Daemonum, Goatweed, Hardhay, Hypereikon, Hyperici Herba, Hypericum, Johns Wort, Klamath Weed, Millepertuis, Rosin Rose, Saint Johns Wort, Saint John's Wort, Saynt Johannes Wort, SJW, St Johns Wort, St John's Wort, Tipton Weed.

Scientific Names

Hypericum perforatum.
Family: Hypericaceae.

People Use This For

Orally, St. John's wort is used for depression, dysthymia, anxiety, exhaustion, fibrositis, headache, heart palpitations, lack of drive, mood disturbances associated with menopause, migraine headache, muscle pain, neuralgia, obsessive-compulsive disorder (OCD), and sciatica. St. John's wort is also used orally for secondary symptoms associated with depression such as fatigue, loss of appetite, insomnia, and anxiety or nervous unrest. It is also used orally for cancer, vitiligo, HIV/AIDS, and as a diuretic. Oily St. John's wort preparations are used orally for gastric indigestion. Topically, oily St. John's wort preparations are used for treating bruises and abrasions, inflammation and muscle pain, first degree burns and wound healing, hemorrhoids, vitiligo, and neuralgia.

In manufacturing, the hypericin-free extracts of St. John's wort are used in the making of alcoholic beverages.

Safety

LIKELY SAFE ...when used orally and appropriately, short-term. St. John's wort extracts seem to be safe when used for up to 8 weeks (12,3547,3548,3549,3550,3551,3552,5087,5096,6400) (6434,7047).

POSSIBLY UNSAFE ...when used orally in large doses. Doses of 1800 mg or more per day of St. John's wort extract can be unsafe because of the risk of severe phototoxic skin reactions (7,758). People with severe depression, HIV, or AIDS are more likely to use these larger doses (758).

PREGNANCY: POSSIBLY UNSAFE ...when used orally. St. John's wort can increase muscle tone of the uterus (4); avoid using.

LACTATION: POSSIBLY UNSAFE ...when used orally. Nursing infants can experience colic, drowsiness, and lethargy (1377); avoid using.

Effectiveness

LIKELY EFFECTIVE ...when used orally for treating mild to moderate depression. St. John's wort extracts, standardized based on hypericin content, are superior to placebo (203,204,205,376,3548,3549,3551,3552,4899,6428), likely as effective as low-dose tricyclic antidepressants (3548,3549,3551,6434), and possibly as effective as the selective serotonin reuptake inhibitors (SSRIs) fluoxetine (Prozac) (3550,4897) and sertraline (Zoloft) (6400). There is not as much evidence to support extracts standardized based on constituents other than hypericin. However, extracts based on hyperforin content also seem to be effective (761). The value of St. John's wort for depression has been called into question based on equivocal findings of one well-conducted study (5096). However, the overwhelming majority of evidence shows that St. John's wort can work for many patients. Consider St. John's wort as another option along with conventional antidepressants for treatment of mild to moderate depression (5087). However, St. John's wort is not appropriate for more severely depressed patients.

Most clinical studies on the effectiveness of St. John's wort have used preparations containing the specific standardized extract Lichtwer LI 160, containing 0.3% hypericin (382). LI 160 is contained in the product Kira (Lichtwer Pharma US, Inc.). Lichtwer LI 160 WS is the hyperforin stabilized version of LI 160. LI 160 WS is contained in the product Quanterra Emotional Balance (Warner-Lambert). Some studies have also used the extract ZE 117, containing 0.2% hypericin (4897,6434). ZE 117 is contained in the product Remotiv (Zeller). One study also used the extract WS 5572, containing 3-7% hyperforin (761). WS 5572 is contained in the product Movana (Pharmaton).

POSSIBLY INEFFECTIVE ...when used orally as an antiretroviral agent in HIV-infected adults (206). ...when used orally for polyneuropathy. St. John's wort does not seem to relieve most measures of pain in diabetic and non-diabetic patients with polyneuropathy (7047).

There is insufficient reliable information available about the effectiveness of St. John's wort for its other uses. However, early evidence suggests St. John's wort might be useful for obsessive-compulsive disorder (OCD). A special extended-release formulation of St. John's wort standardized to 0.3% hypericin for 12 weeks seems to significantly improve symptoms in some patients with OCD (5075). There is also preliminary clinical evidence that St. John's wort might be beneficial for premenstrual syndrome (PMS). St. John's wort extract standardized to 0.3% hypericin seems to improve symptoms of PMS by approximately 50% in some women (6429). Although these findings look promising, further evidence is needed to rate the effectiveness of St. John's wort for these uses.

Mechanism of Action

The applicable parts of St. John's wort are the dried, above ground parts. Several active constituents have been isolated. Two constituents that play a significant role are hypericin and hyperforin (761). Hypericin inhibits catechol-O-methyl transferase (COMT) and monoamine oxidase (MAO) in vitro. However, hypericin does not seem to reach adequate concentrations in human tissue to achieve these effects (167,759). Hypericin also has affinity for sigma receptors and acts as a receptor antagonist at adenosine, benzodiazepine, GABA-A, GABA-B, and inositol triphosphate receptors (759). Recently hyperforin was also identified as a probable major player in St. John's wort's antidepressant activity (762,763). Hyperforin modulates the effects of serotonin, possibly through serotonin reuptake inhibition (763,3553,6474) and 5-HT3 and 5-HT4 receptor antagonism (762). Hyperforin also inhibits synaptosomal uptake of gamma-butyric acid (GABA) and L-glutamate (3553). Extracts of St. John's wort inhibit reuptake of serotonin, norepinephrine, and dopamine in vitro (763,6427) and down-regulate beta-adrenergic and 5-HT2 receptors when used chronically in animals (763). It is likely that constituents other than hypericin and hyperforin also contribute to the antidepressant action of St. John's wort preparations (762). St. John's wort extracts can also prolong narcotic-induced sleep time, decrease barbiturate-induced sleep time, and antagonize the effects of reserpine (758). There is preliminary evidence that St. John's wort can enhance the analgesic effect of morphine, but St. John's wort alone does not have analgesic effects (1279). St. John's wort and its constituents, hypericin and pseudohypericin, have activity against viruses and bacteria including influenza virus, herpes simplex virus types I and II, Sindbis virus, poliovirus, retrovirus, murine cytomegalovirus (CMV), hepatitis C, and Gram negative and Gram positive bacteria (6). Hyperforin can also inhibit growth of penicillin- and methicillin-resistant Staphylococcus aureus and other Gram positive organisms, but not Gram negative organisms (3554). Hypericin is photodynamically active and is thought to be the constituent responsible for phototoxic reactions (3547). Topical preparations are thought to be beneficial for inflammatory skin conditions and superficial wounds by inhibiting epidermal inflammatory response. Both hypericin and hyperforin constituents likely contribute to this effect (6426). In vitro, several St. John's wort extracts can inhibit cytochrome P450 (CYP450) enzymes, including 2C9, 2C19, 2D6, and 3A4 (1379,6476). This is contradictory to what has been found in vivo. When used in humans, St. John's wort seems to induce many of these enzymes rather than inhibit them (1291,1292,1293,1303,3570,3599,6425). St. John's wort extract seems to induce CYP3A4 activity by 98%, CYP2D6 activity by 23%, and CYP1A2 activity by 34%. St. John's wort's effects on CYP2D6 and CYP1A2 seem to be greater in females than males (1303). The reason for the discrepancy between in vitro and in vivo findings might be due to St. John's wort's in vivo effects on production of metabolizing enzymes. The hyperforin constituent in St. John's wort seems to bind to a nuclear receptor called the pregnane X receptor (PXR). PXR regulates expression of CYP3A4. Stimulation of PXR by St. John's wort causes increased expression of CYP3A4 and explains how St. John's wort can induce metabolism of drugs that are CYP3A4 substrates (6463,6475). St. John's wort also induces the intestinal P-glycoprotein/multi-drug resistance 1(MDR-1) drug transporter (1340). Induction of both intestinal P-glycoprotein/MDR-1 and intestinal and hepatic CYP3A4 decreases the intestinal absorption and increases hepatic first pass clearance of numerous drugs such as cyclosporine, indinavir, and amitriptyline (382,1340). St. John's wort does not appear to affect N-acetyltransferase (NAT2) (3571).

Adverse Reactions

Orally, St. John's wort is usually well tolerated. Side effects can include insomnia, vivid dreams, restlessness, anxiety, agitation, irritability (3569), gastrointestinal discomfort, fatigue, dry mouth, dizziness (394,758,3547), headache (3547), skin rash (7404), paresthesia (5073), and delayed hypersensitivity (4). St. John's wort can induce hypomania in depressed patients (325,3524,3568) and mania in depressed patients with occult bipolar disorder (3555). Insomnia seems to be one of the most common side effects. Insomnia can often be alleviated by decreasing the dose or taking St. John's wort in the morning (3569). There is also some concern that St. John's wort might cause sexual dysfunction like conventional antidepressants. There is one report of loss of sexual libido in a man who took St. John's wort for 9 months (7312). There is a report of a serotonin-like syndrome (extreme anxiety, nausea, hypertension, tachycardia) in a patient taking no other medicines and with no history of psychiatric or cardiac disease (6201). St. John's wort can cause intermenstrual bleeding or abnormal menstrual bleeding (1292). However, this effect has occurred in patients who were also taking an oral contraceptive. Changes in menstrual bleeding might be the result of a drug interaction (see Interactions with Drugs) (1292). Overall, St. John's wort extracts seem to be better tolerated than tricyclic antidepressants (3548,3549), but

similarly or better tolerated than fluoxetine (Prozac) (3550) and sertraline (Zoloft) (4897,6400). St. John's wort extracts do not seem to adversely affect cardiac conduction measures on ECG, as has been found with tricyclic antidepressants (3552). Topical use or chronic oral use of St. John's wort can cause significant photodermatitis (206,620,758,6477). Photosensitivity has occurred with oral doses of St. John's wort extract 1800 mg per day for 15 days (758). Lower doses might not cause this effect. For example, a single dose of St. John's wort extract 1800 mg (5.4 mg hypericin) followed by 900 mg (2.7 mg hypericin) daily does not seem to produce skin hypericin concentrations thought to be high enough to cause phototoxicity (3539). Light or fair-skinned people should employ protective measures against direct sunlight when using St. John's wort either topically or orally (2,11,628). Neuropathy can also occur with use of St. John's wort (621). There is some speculation that St. John's wort might be associated with a higher incidence of cataracts (223). The hypericin constituent is photoactive and, in the presence of light, may damage lens proteins, leading to cataracts (1296); however, this effect has not been verified in humans. Some preliminary evidence suggests that high doses of St. John's wort might reduce male and female fertility (4239,4240), but this effect has not been demonstrated in humans. St. John's wort might lead to withdrawal effects similar to those found with conventional antidepressants, including headache, nausea, dizziness, insomnia, paresthesias, confusion, and fatigue. Withdrawal effects are most likely to occur within 2 days after discontinuation, but can occur one week or more after stopping treatment in some people. Occurrence of withdrawal symptoms does not appear to relate to dose or duration of use (3569).
Topically, St. John's wort oil may irritate the skin (4).

Interactions with Herbs & Other Dietary Supplements

HERBS WITH SEDATIVE PROPERTIES: Theoretically, concomitant use with herbs that have sedative properties might enhance therapeutic and adverse effects. These include calamus, calendula, California poppy, catnip, capsicum, celery, couch grass, elecampane, Siberian ginseng, German chamomile, goldenseal, gotu kola, hops, Jamaican dogwood, kava, lemon balm, sage, sassafras, scullcap, shepherd's purse, stinging nettle, valerian, wild carrot, wild lettuce, ashwaganda root, and yerba mansa (4,19).
DIGITALIS: Concomitant use might reduce the therapeutic effects of digitalis. St. John's wort extract (LI 160) decreases digoxin serum levels in healthy people. St. John's wort seems to lower digoxin serum concentrations about 25% (382).

Interactions with Drugs

5-HT1 AGONISTS (Triptans): Theoretically, concomitant use of St. John's wort with selective serotonin agonists can increase the risk of serotonergic adverse effects and possibly serotonin syndrome. Concomitant use should be avoided (3572). The "triptans" include frovatriptan (Miguard), naratriptan (Amerge), rizatriptan (Maxalt), sumatriptan (Imitrex), and zolmitriptan (Zomig).
AMITRIPTYLINE (Elavil): Concomitant use can reduce serum concentrations of amitriptyline and its metabolite, nortriptyline (1378). St. John's wort induces intestinal and hepatic cytochrome P450 3A4 (CYP3A4) and intestinal P-glycoprotein/MDR-1, a drug transporter, which increases amitriptyline clearance (1340).
ANTIDEPRESSANTS: Concomitant use can lead to increased adverse effects (4,12,16,166) and increase the risk of serotonergic side effects, including serotonin syndrome (166,542,3569). Although this effect has only been reported with nefazodone (Serzone), paroxetine (Paxil), and sertraline (Zoloft) (see Nefazodone, Paroxetine, and Sertraline below), it might also occur with other antidepressants. Use of St. John's wort with other antidepressants should only be done with close supervision.
BARBITURATES: St. John's wort can decrease barbiturate-induced sleep time (6,758).
CARBAMAZEPINE (Tegretol): Researchers used to think St. John's wort could decrease carbamazepine levels since St. John's wort is an inducer of cytochrome P450 3A4 (CYP3A4) drug metabolism. But research now shows that St. John's wort does not seem to significantly effect carbamazepine levels (1339). St. John's wort may not be a potent enough enzyme inducer to affect auto-inducing drugs such as carbamazepine (1339).
CYCLOSPORINE (Neoral, Sandimmune): Concomitant use can decrease plasma cyclosporine levels by 61% (1234). Using St. John's wort with cyclosporine in patients with heart, kidney, or liver transplants can cause subtherapeutic cyclosporine levels and acute transplant rejection (1234,1293,1301,6112,6435). This interaction has occurred with a St. John's wort extract standardized to 0.3% hypericin and dosed at 300-600 mg per day (6435). Withdrawal of St. John's wort can result in increased cyclosporine levels by 64% (1234). St. John's wort induces cytochrome P450 3A4 (CYP3A4) and the multi-drug transporter, P-glycoprotein/MDR-1, which increases cyclosporine clearance (1291,1293,1340).
DIGOXIN (Lanoxin): Concomitant use can reduce serum levels and the therapeutic effects of digoxin, requiring dosing adjustments when St. John's wort is started or stopped. St. John's wort extract 900 mg daily can reduce serum digoxin levels by 25% after 10 days in healthy people (382,6473). St. John's wort is thought to affect the multidrug transporter, P-glycoprotein, which mediates digoxin and other drugs' absorption and elimination (382).
FENFLURAMINE (Pondimin): Concomitant use with St. John's wort can increase the risk of serotonergic side effects and serotonin syndrome-like symptoms. St. John's wort 600 mg per day with fenfluramine can cause nausea, headache, and anxiety (3569).
MONOAMINE OXIDASE INHIBITORS (MAOIs): Theoretically, because St. John's wort might affect serotonin

similar to conventional antidepressants (763,3553), concurrent use might cause additive adverse effects, including hypertension, hyperthermia, agitation, confusion, coma, etc. St. John's wort should be avoided in patients taking MAOIs or within 14 days of MAOI discontinuation.

NARCOTICS: St. John's wort can increase narcotic-induced sleep time (6,758) and might also increase analgesic effects (1279).

NEFAZODONE (Serzone): Concomitant use has been associated with serotonergic side effects, including nausea, vomiting, and restlessness (5074).

NONNUCLEOSIDE REVERSE TRANSCRIPTASE INHIBITORS (NNRTIs): Concomitant use might decrease serum levels of NNRTIs. St. John's wort can substantially decrease plasma concentrations of the protease inhibitor indinavir (Crixivan) (1290). Since NNRTIs and protease inhibitors are metabolized through similar routes, NNRTIs might also be affected. Subtherapeutic concentrations are associated with therapeutic failure, development of viral resistance, and development of drug class resistance. St. John's wort induces intestinal and hepatic cytochrome 3A4 (CYP3A4) and intestinal P-glycoprotein/MDR-1, a drug transporter (1290,1291,1340). NNRTI-type antiretroviral drugs include nevirapine (Viramune), delavirdine (Rescriptor), and efavirenz (Sustiva).

NORTRIPTYLINE (Pamelor, Aventyl): Concomitant use can reduce serum concentrations of amitriptyline and its metabolite, nortriptyline (1378).

ORAL CONTRACEPTIVES: Concomitant use may decrease steroid concentrations resulting in breakthrough bleeding and irregular menstrual bleeding. Bleeding irregularities usually occurred after one week of starting St. John's wort and regular cycles returned when St. John's wort was discontinued. St. John's wort is thought to induce the cytochrome P450 3A4 enzymes, which are responsible for steroid metabolism (1292). Women taking St. John's wort and oral contraceptives concurrently should use an additional or alternative form of birth control.

PAROXETINE (Paxil): Concomitant use with St. John's wort may increase the risk of adverse effects and serotonin syndrome-like symptoms. People taking St. John's wort and paroxetine together can experience nervousness, hyperactivity, diaphoresis, nausea, weakness, fatigue, lethargy, and incoherence (542,3569).

PHOTOSENSITIZING DRUGS: Theoretically, concomitant use might result in increased photosensitivity (166). Some drugs that cause photosensitivity include amitriptyline, quinolones, sulfa drugs, and tetracycline.

PROTEASE INHIBITORS (PIs): Concomitant use can reduce serum concentrations of protease inhibitors. In healthy volunteers, St. John's wort can reduce the serum indinavir (Crixivan) area under the curve (AUC) by 57% and the extrapolated trough by 81%. Subtherapeutic concentrations are associated with therapeutic failure, development of viral resistance, and development of drug class resistance. St. John's wort is thought to induce cytochrome P450 enzymes and might also affect other protease inhibitor-type antiretroviral drugs (1290,1291), including amprenavir (Agenerase), nelfinavir (Viracept), ritonavir (Norvir), and saquinavir (Fortovase, Invirase).

RESERPINE: St. John's wort can antagonize the effects of reserpine (758).

SERTRALINE (Zoloft): Concomitant use can cause serotonergic side effects, including dizziness, nausea, vomiting, epigastric pain, headache, anxiety, confusion, and feelings of restlessness and irritability (5074).

THEOPHYLLINE: Concomitant use might decrease serum levels and the therapeutic effects of theophylline, requiring dose adjustment. St. John's wort 300 mg daily can cause a clinically significant decrease in serum theophylline levels. Discontinuation of St. John's wort can then result in increased serum levels of theophylline (3556).

WARFARIN (Coumadin): Concomitant use might decrease the therapeutic effects of warfarin (1292). St. John's wort seems to significantly decrease International Normalized Ratio (INR) (1292). St. John's wort is thought to induce the cytochrome P450 2C9 enzyme, which is involved in warfarin's metabolism (1292).

OTHER DRUGS: Based on St. John's wort's effects on cytochrome P450 (CYP450) enzymes; its documented effects on drugs metabolized by CYP450 3A4, 2C9, and 2D6 enzymes; and St. John's wort's effects on P-glycoprotein (1290,1292,1293,6425,6473), use caution when considering concomitant use of St. John's wort and other drugs affected by these systems. Drugs which might be affected include some calcium channel blockers (diltiazem, nicardipine, verapamil), chemotherapeutic agents (etoposide, paclitaxel, vinblastine, vincristine, vindesine), antifungals (ketoconazole, itraconazole), glucocorticoids, cisapride (Propulsid), alfentanil (Alfenta), f entanil (Sublimaze), losartan (Cozaar), fluoxetine (Prozac), midazolam (Versed), omeprazole (Prilosec), ondansetron (Zofran), fexofenadine (Allegra), and others.

Interactions with Foods

TYRAMINE-CONTAINING FOODS: Theoretically, concomitant use of large amounts of St. John's wort and tyramine-containing foods might cause a hypertensive crisis (166). St. John's wort has weak monoamine oxidase inhibitory activity. This interaction has not been described in the literature.

Interactions with Lab Tests

PROTHROMBIN TIME (PT), INTERNATIONAL NORMALIZED RATIO (INR): St. John's wort can decrease PT/INR test results in patients treated with warfarin (Coumadin) (1292).

Interactions with Diseases or Conditions

ALZHEIMER'S DISEASE: St. John's wort might induce psychosis in patients with Alzheimer's dementia. In one case, psychotic delirium developed in an elderly woman within three weeks of starting a low dose (75 mg per day) of St. John's wort extract standardized to 0.3% hypercin (St. John's wort, Pharmanex). Symptoms resolved within several days after discontinuing St. John's wort and starting medications for treatment of Alzheimer's disease. Although it is not clear if St. John's wort caused the delirium or contributed to the underlying dementia, there is concern that St. John's wort might contribute to dementia in patients with Alzheimer's disease (5249).

BIPOLAR DISORDER: St. John's wort can induce hypomania or mania when used in patients with bipolar disorder or depressed patients with occult bipolar disorder (3555,3568). In some cases, mania occurred after 2-8 weeks of treatment with St. John's wort and was effectively managed by decreasing the dose of St. John's wort and increasing the dose of mood stabilizers such as lithium (3568). Theoretically, like other antidepressants, St. John's wort may also induce rapid cycling between depression and mania in patients with bipolar disorder (3555).

DEPRESSION: St. John's wort can induce hypomania with typical doses in patients with major depression (325,3524,3568). In one case hypomania occurred after 4-8 weeks of treatment with St. John's wort and was effectively managed by decreasing the dose and initiating valproic acid (3568).

INFERTILITY: Preliminary evidence suggests that St. John's wort might inhibit oocyte fertilization and alter sperm DNA (4239,4240). This effect has not yet been demonstrated in humans; however, until more is known, use with caution in couples attempting to conceive and avoid use in couples having difficulty conceiving.

SCHIZOPHRENIA: St. John's wort might induce psychosis in patients with schizophrenia. There are two cases of relapse in non-medicated schizophrenia patients in remission who started taking St. John's wort. Psychotic symptoms resolved with readministration of antipsychotics and discontinuation of St. John's wort (6478).

Dosage and Administration

ORAL: For mild to moderate depression, most clinical trials have used St. John's wort extract standardized to 0.3% hypericin content. Doses were most commonly 300 mg three times daily (7,3548,3549). Doses of 1200 mg daily have also been used (5096). Some studies have also used a 0.2% hypericin extract dosed at 250 mg twice daily (4897,6434). A St. John's wort extract standardized to 5% hyperforin and dosed at 300 mg three times daily has also been used (761,6400). In cases of long-term maintenance therapy, daily doses of 300-600 mg have been used (7). For obsessive-compulsive disorder, one study used an extended-release preparation of St. John's wort extract standardized to 0.3% hypericin content, dosed at 450 mg twice daily (5075). For premenstrual syndrome (PMS), one study used St. John's wort extract standardized to 0.3% hypericin dosed at 300 mg once daily (6429). For somatic symptoms associated with depression, 300 mg three times daily of the standardized hypericin extract has been used (376). The typical daily dose of the crude drug is 2-4 grams of the above ground parts per day or 0.2-1 mg of total hypericin in other forms (2). One cup of the tea is usually taken one to three times per day and is prepared by steeping 2-4 grams of the dried herb in 150 mL of boiling water for 5-10 minutes and then straining (4). The liquid extract (1:1 in 25% alcohol) is typically taken as 2-4 mL three times daily (4). The tincture (1:10 in 45% alcohol) is commonly dosed 2-4 mL three times daily (4). Advise patients to avoid abrupt discontinuation of St. John's wort due to the risk of adverse withdrawal effects (see Adverse Reactions) (3569).

Comments

St. John's wort is a natural source of food flavoring in Europe, limited to a final concentration of 0.1 mg/kg hypericin in the finished product, except in pastilles or lozenges (1 mg/kg hypericin) and alcoholic beverages (2 mg/kg hypericin) (4). St. John's wort is native to Europe but is commonly found in the US and Canada in the dry ground of roadsides, meadows, and woods (6). Although not indigenous to Australia and long considered a weed, St. John's wort is now grown as a cash crop and produces 20 percent of the world's supply (6200). The flowers of St. John's wort can have the brightest appearance on June 24th, the birthday of John the Baptist (6). Hypericin, a constituent of St. John's wort, has been identified by the FDA as an investigational new drug, now being studied and developed by VIMRx Pharmaceuticals for the treatment of HIV (6). The Federal Institute for Drugs and Medical Products in Germany no longer bases dose recommendations on the hypericin content of St. John's wort products (7).

STAR ANISE

Also Known As

Aniseed Stars, Anisi stellati fructus, Badiana, Chinese Anise, Chinese Star Anise, Eight-Horned Anise, Eight Horns, Illicium.
CAUTION: See separate listing for Anise.

Scientific Names

Illicium verum.
Family: Illiciacae.

People Use This For

Orally, star anise is used for respiratory tract mucous membrane inflammation, peptic discomfort (2,18), flatulence (11), loss of appetite, cough, and bronchitis (18).

As an inhalant, it is used for respiratory tract congestion (11).

In Chinese medicine, star anise is used for increasing milk secretion, promoting menstruation, facilitating childbirth, increasing libido, and treating symptoms of male climacteric (11).

In foods and beverages, star anise is considered a culinary spice; both the seed and oil are used as flavoring (11).

In manufacturing, the oil is used as a fragrance component in soaps, cosmetics, perfumes, and toothpaste, and to mask undesirable odors in drug products (11).

Safety

LIKELY SAFE ...when consumed in amounts commonly found in foods (11). It has Generally Recognized as Safe (GRAS) status in the US for food use (11).

POSSIBLY SAFE ...when used orally for medicinal purposes and used appropriately (12).

There is insufficient reliable information available about the safety of star anise as an inhalant.

PREGNANCY AND LACTATION: Insufficient reliable information available; avoid using.

Effectiveness

POSSIBLY EFFECTIVE ...when used orally for respiratory tract mucous membrane inflammation and peptic discomfort (2).

There is insufficient reliable information available about the effectiveness of star anise for its other uses.

Mechanism of Action

The applicable part of star anise is the seed. Star anise seed contains a volatile oil (11,18), of which the chief constituent is anethole (80-90%). Anethole has antiflatulent and expectorant effects. It also can have insecticidal and antifungal activity (11). At one time anethole was considered the active estrogenic agent in the essential oil. However, more recent information suggests the active estrogenic compounds are the anethole polymers, dianethole and photoanethole (11). Anethole might be mutagenic (11).

Adverse Reactions

Topically, use of the constituent anethole can cause dermatitis, including erythema, scaling, and vesiculation (11). Sensitization rarely occurs (18).

Interactions with Herbs & Other Dietary Supplements

Insufficient reliable information available.

Interactions with Drugs

No interactions are known to occur, and there is no known reason to expect a clinically significant interaction with star anise.

Interactions with Foods

No interactions are known to occur, and there is no known reason to expect a clinically significant interaction with star anise.

Interactions with Lab Tests

No interactions are known to occur, and there is no known reason to expect a clinically significant interaction with star anise.

Interactions with Diseases or Conditions

HORMONE SENSITIVE CANCERS/CONDITIONS: Because star anise might have estrogenic effects (11), women with hormone sensitive conditions should avoid star anise. Some of these conditions include breast, uterine, and ovarian cancer; endometriosis; and uterine fibroids.

Dosage and Administration

ORAL: The typical dose of star anise is one cup of tea (8) prepared by steeping 0.5-1 grams of the powdered seed in 150 mL boiling water for 10 minutes; then strain. The average amount of star anise is 3 grams of the seed or 300 mg of the essential oil per day (2,8).

Comments

Star anise oil is the distilled oil of the seed (fruit) of star anise (Illicium verum). Avoid confusing star anise with Japanese star anise (Illicium lanceolatum), a highly poisonous species (11). In the US, star anise oil (derived from

Illicium verum) and anise oil (derived from Pimpinella anisum) are used interchangeably and both are recognized as "anise oil" in the USP (11).

STAVESACRE

Also Known As
Lousewort.

Scientific Names
Delphinium staphisagria.

People Use This For
Topically, stavesacre seeds are used to treat lice infestation (18).
Historically, the stavesacre plant was used for neuralgia (18).

Safety
LIKELY UNSAFE ...when used orally. The seeds are poisonous (18).
There is insufficient reliable information available about the safety of the topical use of stavesacre and the use of stavesacre extracts.
PREGNANCY AND LACTATION: LIKELY UNSAFE ...when used orally; avoid using.

Effectiveness
There is insufficient reliable information available about the effectiveness of stavesacre (18).

Mechanism of Action
Stavesacre contains diterpene alkaloids including delphinine, staphisine, and staphisagroine, which are reported to have effects similar to aconitine (18). Aconitine is a nor-diterpene alkaloid found in Monkshood, a highly toxic plant.

Adverse Reactions
Ingesting a stavesacre extract can cause inflammation of the alimentary tract (18,19), nausea, pruritus, urinary and stool urgency (18). Ingesting 2 teaspoons of seeds can cause weakened pulse, stomach pain, labored breathing, and collapse (18). Topical use of stavesacre can cause inflammation, eczema, and reddening of the skin (18).

Interactions with Herbs & Other Dietary Supplements
Insufficient reliable information available.

Interactions with Drugs
No interactions are known to occur, and there is no known reason to expect a clinically significant interaction with stavesacre.

Interactions with Foods
No interactions are known to occur, and there is no known reason to expect a clinically significant interaction with stavesacre.

Interactions with Lab Tests
No interactions are known to occur, and there is no known reason to expect a clinically significant interaction with stavesacre.

Interactions with Diseases or Conditions
GASTROINTESTINAL IRRITATION: Can aggravate inflammation of the alimentary tract by irritating mucosal membranes (19).

Dosage and Administration
ORAL: No typical dosage.
TOPICAL: Washes and ointments are used to treat lice.

Comments
None.

STEVIA

Also Known As
Azucacaa, Ca-A-Jhei, Ca-A-Yupi, Caa-He-É, Capim Doce, Eira-Caa, Erva Doce, Kaa Jhee, Paraguayan Sweet Herb, Sweetleaf, Sweet Leaf of Paraguay, Yerba Dulce.

Scientific Names
Stevia rebaudiana, synonym Stevia eupatorium.
Family: Asteraceae/Compositae.

People Use This For
Orally, stevia is used as a weight loss aid (6).
Traditionally, stevia is used for treating diabetes, as a contraceptive (11), for hypertension, heartburn, lowering uric acid levels, as a cardiotonic and diuertic (3918).
For food uses, stevia is used as a non-caloric sweetener in South America and Asia (6,11).

Safety
POSSIBLY SAFE ...when used orally in small amounts as an occasional food or beverage sweetener (12).
There is insufficient reliable information about the safety of stevia used in larger amounts or long-term. The FDA, regulatory agencies in Europe, and the World Health Organization have not approved stevia due to unanswered questions regarding chronic use and toxicity (5037).
PREGNANCY AND LACTATION: Insufficient reliable information available; avoid using.

Effectiveness
There is insufficient reliable information available about the effectiveness of stevia leaf.

Mechanism of Action
The applicable part of stevia is the leaf. Stevia leaf contains the glycoside stevioside which is non-caloric, heat and acid stable, and 100 times sweeter than sucrose at 10% sucrose concentration (11). Stevioside increases hepatic glycogen synthesis in animal experiments (3750). It might also have androgenic activity, perhaps without effect on male fertility (14). Stevia extract and stevioside decrease blood pressure (3745,3747), and stevia extract has vasodilating and diuretic activity in rats (3746,3747). Preliminary evidence suggests that the stevia constituents, stevioside and steviol, might stimulate insulin secretion via a direct action on beta cells (5032). Additional evidence suggests that steviol might inhibit GI glucose absorption (5035). An aqueous stevia leaf extract increased glucose tolerance and reduced plasma glucose levels in a small group of healthy people (3301), but has not been studied in people with diabetes. A fermented aqueous extract of stevia is bactericidal against many food-borne pathogenic bacteria in vitro, including E. coli 0157:H7, the enterohemorrhagic E. coli responsible for outbreaks of severe food poisoning in recent years (3300). Stevioside shows no evidence of mutagenic, genotoxic, antifertility, or teratogenic effects (11). However, the stevia constituent steviol, and metabolized steviol, are mutagenic in vitro (3748,3749). Some evidence suggests that stevia might adversely affect reproduction. An aqueous stevia extract reduced sperm production and testis weight in male rats (5033). Steviol fed to female hamsters reduced the number and birth weight of offspring (5036).

Adverse Reactions
Theoretically, stevia might cause allergic reactions in individuals sensitive to Asteraceae/Compositae family plants. Members of this family include ragweed, chrysanthemums, marigolds, daisies, and many other herbs.

Interactions with Herbs & Other Dietary Supplements
Insufficient reliable information available.

Interactions with Drugs
DIABETES DRUGS: Theoretically, stevia might enhance blood glucose control requiring dosing adjustment of diabetes drug therapy in patients with type 2 diabetes (3301,5032,5035).
VERAPAMIL (Calan, Isoptin, Verelan): Theoretically, stevia and verapamil might have additive antihypertensive activity. Preliminary evidence suggests that concomitant use might have additive blood pressure lowering effects, due to the stevioside contained in stevia (5031).

Interactions with Foods
No interactions are known to occur, and there is no known reason to expect a clinically significant interaction with stevia.

Interactions with Lab Tests

BLOOD PRESSURE: Theoretically, stevia might reduce blood pressure and blood pressure readings. Preliminary evidence suggests that stevia extract and stevioside, contained in stevia, might lower blood pressure (3745,3747,5031).
GLUCOSE: Theoretically, stevia might decrease blood glucose concentrations and test results (3301,5032,5035).

Interactions with Diseases or Conditions

CROSS-ALLERGENICITY: Theoretically, stevia might cause allergic reactions in individuals sensitive to Asteraceae/Compositae family plants. Members of this family include ragweed, chrysanthemums, marigolds, daisies, and many other herbs.
DIABETES: Theoretically, stevia might reduce blood glucose and alter blood glucose control in patients with type 2 diabetes (3301,5032,5035).
KIDNEY DISEASE: Theoretically, stevia might cause kidney damage. Preliminary evidence suggests that large amounts of steviol, contained in stevia, might cause acute renal damage (5034).

Dosage and Administration

ORAL: A typical dose of powdered stevia leaf is 1000 mg per day (342,343).

Comments

Avoid confusion with Stevia salifolia, commonly referred to as ronion or roninowa, which contains the bitter glycoside stevisalioside (14).
In a 1991 import alert, the FDA identified stevia as an "unsafe food additive" (12) and banned importation (11). The alert was revised in 1995 to allow stevia to be imported "explicitly labeled as a dietary supplement or for use as a dietary ingredient of a dietary supplement" (12). Canada and the European Community prohibit stevia as a food additive (5030). The FDA, regulatory agencies in Europe, and the World Health Organization have not approved stevia due to unanswered safety questions (5037).

STINGING NETTLE above ground parts

Also Known As

Common Nettle, Great Stinging Nettle, Nettle, Nettles, Ortie, Small Nettle, Urtica, Urticae herba et folium.
CAUTION: See separate listings for Stinging Nettle root and White Dead Nettle Flower.

Scientific Names

Urtica dioica; Urtica urens; and hybrid species.
Family: Urticaceae.

People Use This For

Orally, stinging nettle above ground parts is used for allergies, allergic rhinitis (6,11,7035), and musculoskeletal aches and pains such as osteoarthritis (1,2,5,6,8,9,11,18). It is also used orally in conjunction with copious fluid intake in so-called "irrigation therapy" for urinary tract infections (UTI), and urinary tract inflammation (1,2,5,6,9,11,18), and kidney stones (nephrolithiasis) (2,6,11,18). People also use stinging nettle for internal bleeding, including uterine bleeding, epistaxis, and melena (4,11); anemia (8,11,18); poor circulation; splenomegaly (11); diabetes (4,6,8,18) and other endocrine disorders (11); gastric hyperacidity (6,8); biliary complaints (8); diarrhea and dysentery (11); asthma (5,6); pulmonary congestion (5,6,11); rash and eczema (4,6); cancer; prevention of signs of aging (6); blood purification (11); wound-healing (6,8); and as a general tonic (5).
Topically, stinging nettle above ground parts is used for musculoskeletal aches and pains (2,5,6,18), scalp seborrhea and oily hair (6,8,18), and hair loss (alopecia) (5,6).
In foods, young stinging nettle above ground parts is eaten as a cooked vegetable (11).
In manufacturing, stinging nettle extract is used as an ingredient in hair and skin products (11).

Safety

POSSIBLY SAFE ...when used orally and appropriately (1,2,12). There is insufficient reliable information available about the safety of the topical use of stinging nettle above ground parts.
PREGNANCY: LIKELY UNSAFE ...when used orally due to possible abortifacient and uterine-stimulant effects (4,6,19).
LACTATION: There is insufficient reliable information available about the safety of stinging nettle above ground parts during lactation; avoid using.

Effectiveness

POSSIBLY EFFECTIVE ...when used orally for osteoarthritis. There is some evidence that stinging nettle leaf

extract might improve symptoms of pain in patients with osteoarthritis (1,2,6500). Some clinicians use stinging nettle leaf extract in combination with conventional non-steroidal anti-inflammatory drugs (NSAIDs) or other analgesics. There is some evidence that adding stinging nettle might allow for using lower analgesic doses in some patients (6500).
There is insufficient reliable information available about the effectiveness of stinging nettle for its other uses. However, there is some evidence that stinging nettle might improve symptoms of allergic rhinitis. Starting stinging nettle at the first sign of symptoms seems to provide subjective improvement (7035). More evidence is needed to rate stinging nettle for this use.

Mechanism of Action

Stinging nettle leaf contains several nutrients and active constituents. The plant has traditionally been used as a food because of significant amounts of nutrients including carotene, vitamin C, vitamin K, potassium (2,8,11,18,19), and calcium (2,11). There is about as much vitamin C and carotene in stinging nettle as spinach and other greens (5). Stinging nettle is also a good source of chlorophyll. Stinging nettle contains the sterol beta-sitosterol and the flavonoids quercetin, rutin, kaempferol, and others. Stinging nettle seems to have a variety of pharmacological effects including analgesic (1,4), anti-inflammatory (19), local anesthetic (1), hemostatic (4), antibacterial (11), antiviral (6), and hyperglycemic effects (4). For osteoarthritis and other musculoskeletal conditions, stinging nettle might work due to potential analgesic and anti-inflammatory effects. Some researchers think that stinging nettle might be beneficial for allergic rhinitis due to quercetin content. Quercetin is thought to have anti-inflammatory and mast-cell stabilizing effects. It decreases histamine release from basophils and mast cells (483). There is evidence that it might inhibit adrenergic stimulation, tumor necrosis factor (TNF), and platelet activation factor (PAF) (1). Stinging nettle seems to also act as a diuretic. The leaf juice can increase urine output and slightly decrease systolic blood pressure and body weight in people with venous insufficiency (1,11). Because of these effects, some people use stinging nettle for urinary tract disorders, including urinary tract infections (UTIs) and kidney stones. Stinging nettle also seems to lower body temperature and have CNS depressant (4,6,11) and anti-seizure activity (4). When given intravenously stinging nettle also seems to decrease blood pressure and heart rate (1,4). Stinging nettle leaf is well known to cause skin irritation when touched. The stinging nettle hairs of the leaf contain histamine, acetylcholine (1,4,5,8,11,18), and serotonin (1,4,8,11,18), that can cause local irritation.

Adverse Reactions

Orally, stinging nettle is typically well tolerated. The stinging nettle juice can sometimes cause diarrhea (1).
Topically, fresh stinging nettle leaves applied or touched accidentally can cause local irritation (4,19).

Interactions with Herbs & Other Dietary Supplements

HERBS WITH SEDATIVE PROPERTIES: Theoretically, concomitant use with herbs that have sedative properties might enhance therapeutic and adverse effects. These include calamus, calendula, California poppy, catnip, capsicum, celery, couch grass, elecampane, Siberian ginseng, German chamomile, goldenseal, gotu kola, hops, Jamaican dogwood, kava, lemon balm, sage, St. John's wort, sassafras, scullcap, shepherd's purse, valerian, wild carrot, wild lettuce, ashwaganda, and yerba mansa (4,19).
HERBS WITH CLOTTING POTENTIAL: Excessive use of herbs that contain vitamin K, an essential coagulation factor, can increase the risk of clotting in people using anticoagulants. These herbs include: alfalfa, parsley, nettle, plantain, and others.

Interactions with Drugs

ANTICOAGULANTS: There is some concern that stinging nettle might decrease the effects of anticoagulant drugs such as warfarin (Coumadin). Stinging nettle contains a significant amount of vitamin K (19); use cautiously. Dose adjustment of anticoagulants may be needed.
ANTIDIABETES DRUGS: There is some evidence that stinging nettle can increase blood glucose levels. Theoretically, concomitant use of excessive amounts of stinging nettle might interfere with blood glucose control (4).
ANTIHYPERTENSIVE AGENTS: There is some evidence that stinging nettle might have blood pressure lowering effects. Theoretically, concomitant use of excessive amounts of stinging nettle might have additive effects with antihypertensive drugs on blood pressure (4).
CENTRAL NERVOUS SYSTEM (CNS) DEPRESSANTS: There is some evidence that stinging nettle preparations might have CNS depressant activity. Theoretically, concomitant use of excessive amounts of stinging nettle might have additive effects with CNS depressant drugs (4).

Interactions with Foods

No interactions are known to occur, and there is no known reason to expect a clinically significant interaction with stinging nettle above ground parts.

Interactions with Lab Tests

No interactions are known to occur, and there is no known reason to expect a clinically significant interaction with stinging nettle above ground parts.

Interactions with Diseases or Conditions

CONGESTIVE HEART FAILURE (CHF): Stinging nettle tea is often given as "irrigation therapy" and given in conjunction with large amounts of fluids. This should be avoided in patients with CHF. Large amounts of fluids might worsen symptoms of CHF (2,18).

DIABETES: There is some evidence stinging nettle above ground parts can increase blood glucose levels (4). Theoretically, stinging nettle might worsen blood glucose control in patients with diabetes; use with caution.

HYPERTENSION: There is some evidence that stinging nettle above ground parts might have blood pressure lowering effects (4). Theoretically, stinging nettle might have additive effects with medications used to treat high blood pressure; use with caution.

RENAL INSUFFICIENCY: Stinging nettle tea is often used as "irrigation therapy" and given in conjunction with large amounts of fluids. This should be avoided in patients with kidney dysfunction. Large amounts of fluids might worsen this condition (2,18).

Dosage and Administration

ORAL: For osteoarthritis, people typically use crude stinging nettle leaf 9 grams daily (6500). For allergic rhinitis, people typically use stinging nettle extract 300 mg three times daily. However, in some cases, 300 mg up to seven times daily has been used (7035). Stinging nettle is often taken as a tea. One cup of tea is made by steeping 1.5-5 grams above ground parts in 150 mL boiling water for 10 minutes and then straining. Tea is typically taken in doses of one cup up to three times per day (1,2,4,8). Fresh juice from stinging nettle, 10-15 mL three times daily has been used (1). A dried extract of stinging nettle (7:1), 770 mg twice daily has also been used (1). Liquid extract of stinging nettle (1:1 in 25% alcohol), 3-4 mL three times daily has also been used (1,4).
TOPICAL: Tincture/spirit (1:10) has been used (18).

Comments

Stinging nettle leaf has a long history of use. It was used primarily as a diuretic and laxative as early as the times of the Greek physicians Dioscorides and Galen.

STINGING NETTLE root

Also Known As

Common Nettle, Great Stinging Nettle, Nettle, Nettles, Small Nettle, Urtica, Urticae Radix.
CAUTION: See separate listing for Stinging Nettle above ground parts and White Dead Nettle Flower.

Scientific Names

Urtica dioica; Urtica urens; hybrid species.
Family: Urticaceae.

People Use This For

Orally, stinging nettle root is used for urination disorders associated with benign prostatic hyperplasia (BPH), including nocturia, frequency, dysuria, urinary retention, and irritable bladder (1,2,5,6,7,8,18).
In folk medicine, stinging nettle root is used for joint ailments (6,7), as a diuretic (6,7,8), and an astringent (8).

Safety

POSSIBLY SAFE ...when used orally and appropriately (1,2).
PREGNANCY AND LACTATION: Insufficient reliable information available; avoid using.

Effectiveness

POSSIBLY EFFECTIVE ...when used orally for symptoms associated with benign prostatic hyperplasia (BPH) Stages I and II (1,2).
POSSIBLY INEFFECTIVE ...when an herbal blend containing nettle root extract is used orally for treating symptoms of BPH. In a double-blind, placebo controlled trial, an herbal product containing nettle root extract 80 mg, saw palmetto lipoidal extract 106 mg, pumpkin seed oil extract 160 mg, lemon bioflavonoid extract 33 mg, and vitamin A (100% as beta-carotene) 190 IU taken three times daily for six months failed to significantly improve symptoms in a group of men with BPH (5093).
There is insufficient reliable information available about the effectiveness of stinging nettle root for its other uses.

Mechanism of Action

Stinging nettle root contains polysaccharides with immunomodulating (1,18) and weak anti-inflammatory (1,7) effects. Hydroalcoholic extracts decrease binding capacity of sex hormone binding globulin (1,7,8) and might suppress prostatic cell metabolism (1,7). In several clinical trials of varying design quality, hydroalcoholic root extracts increased urine output (1,2,7), decreased nocturia (1,6,11), and decreased urinary frequency (1). In some clinical trials urine flow increased (1,7), and in other trials residual volume decreased (1,2,7), although in one well-designed study there was no improvement in subjective symptoms, urine flow, or residual volume (7). Studies investigating the effect of nettle root on prostate size have produced contradictory results (1,2,18).

Adverse Reactions

Oral use of stinging nettle root can cause gastrointestinal complaints (1,2,7,18), sweating (7), and allergic skin reactions (1,7). One case is reported of decreased ejaculatory volume associated with an herbal blend product containing nettle root extract, saw palmetto extract, pumpkin seed oil extract, lemon bioflavonoid extract, and beta-carotene (5093).

Interactions with Herbs & Other Dietary Supplements

Insufficient reliable information available.

Interactions with Drugs

No interactions are known to occur, and there is no known reason to expect a clinically significant interaction with stinging nettle root.

Interactions with Foods

No interactions are known to occur, and there is no known reason to expect a clinically significant interaction with stinging nettle root.

Interactions with Lab Tests

No interactions are known to occur, and there is no known reason to expect a clinically significant interaction with stinging nettle root.

Interactions with Diseases or Conditions

No interactions are known to occur, and there is no known reason to expect a clinically significant interaction with stinging nettle root.

Dosage and Administration

ORAL: Symptomatic treatment of benign prostatic hyperplasia (BPH): Dried hydroalcoholic extract (5:1, extracted with 20% methanol), 600-1200 mg per day (1). Liquid extract (1:1 in 45% alcohol), 1.5-7.5 mL three times per day (1). Ethanolic extract (1:5 in 40% alcohol), 5 mL per day (1). Tea, (steep 1.5 grams dried, powdered root in 150 mL boiling water 5-10 minutes, strain) up to 4-6 grams per day (1,2,8,18).

Comments

Avoid confusing stinging nettle with white dead nettle. Stinging nettle root is used predominantly for urinary disorders, including BPH. White dead nettle herb is used for gastrointestinal complaints. White dead nettle flower is used for inflammation of the mucous membranes of the upper respiratory tract and vaginal discharge.

STONE ROOT

Also Known As

Citronella, Colinsonia, Hardback, Hardhack, Heal-all, Horse Balm, Horseweed, Knob Grass, Knob Root, Knobweed, Richleaf, Rich Weed.
CAUTION: See separate listings for Citronella Oil and Lemongrass.

Scientific Names

Collinsonia canadensis.
Family: Labiatae.

People Use This For

Orally stone root is used to treat bladder inflammation (18), edema (18), gastrointestinal disorders (18), headaches (4501), hyperuricuria (4), indigestion (4501), kidney stones (4,18), urea "bladder semolina" (18), urinary calculus (4,18), water retention (4501), and as a tonic (18,4501).

Safety

POSSIBLY SAFE ...when used orally and appropriately. There are no reports of serious adverse effects (4,12,18).
PREGNANCY AND LACTATION: Insufficient reliable information available; avoid using (4).

Effectiveness

There is insufficient reliable information available about the effectiveness of stone root.

Mechanism of Action

The applicable parts of stone root are the rhizome and root. Stone root rhizome or root contains a volatile oil, caffeic acid derivatives including rosmaric acid (18), saponins, tannin, mucilage, and resin (4,4501). Constituents of the volatile oil include caryophyllene, germacrene D, limonene, alpha- and beta-pinenes (18). Although no pharmacologic data is documented (4), stone root is said to have antifungal effects (4501), diuretic effects (4,6,18,4501), stimulate stomach function (18), cause sweating (4), and reduce occurrence of urinary stones and help rid the body of stones (4).

Adverse Reactions

Orally, ingesting large amounts of stone root can cause intestinal tract irritation and colic-like pain, dizziness, nausea, and painful urination (18).

Interactions with Herbs & Other Dietary Supplements

HERBS WITH DIURETIC PROPERTIES: Theoretically, due to the diuretic effects of stone root (4,6,18,4501), there may be additive effects and side effects with herbs having diuretic activity.

Interactions with Drugs

DIURETICS: Theoretically, due to the diuretic effects of stone root (4,6,18,4501), there may be additive effects and side effects with drugs having diuretic activity.

Interactions with Foods

No interactions are known to occur, and there is no known reason to expect a clinically significant interaction with stone root.

Interactions with Lab Tests

No interactions are known to occur, and there is no known reason to expect a clinically significant interaction with stone root.

Interactions with Diseases or Conditions

No interactions are known to occur, and there is no known reason to expect a clinically significant interaction with stone root.

Dosage and Administration

ORAL: A typical dose of dried root is 1-4 grams or as tea three times daily (4). To make tea, simmer 1-4 grams root or rhizome in 150 mL of boiling water for 5-10 minutes, strain. As liquid extract: (1:1 in 25% alcohol) 1-4 mL three times daily (4). Tincture, (1:5 in 40% alcohol) 2-8 mL three times daily (4); tincture of Collinsonia, 2-8 mL (4).

Comments

This aromatic perennial herb has a strong, unpleasant smell that is reported to be numbing in large amounts (18).

STORAX

Also Known As

American Storax, Balsam Styracis, Balsamum Styrax Liquidus, Copalm, Estoraque Liquido, Gum Tree, Levant Storax, Liquid Amber, Liquid Storax, Opossum Tree, Red Gum, Styrax, Sweet Gum, White Gum.

Scientific Names

Liquidamber orientalis; Liquidambar styraciflua.
Family: Hamamelidaceae or Atlingiaceae.

People Use This For

Orally, storax is used for cancer (11), coughs (11), colds (11), diarrhea (6), epilepsy (11), sore throats (6), and parasitic infections (6).
Topically, storax is used to protect wounds (6,11), for ulcers (18), and scabies.

Storax is an ingredient in Compound Benzoin Tincture (6,11).
As an inhalant, it is placed in a vaporizer and used to treat coughs (6) and bronchitis (18).
Historically, storax was used for parasitic skin diseases (9).
For food uses, it is used as a flavoring component or fixative (6,11).
In manufacturing, storax is used as a fragrance component or fixative in soaps and perfumes (6,11). Storax is also used as a fumigant and imbedding material in microscopy (4501).

Safety

LIKELY SAFE ...when the balsam is used in food amounts. Storax is approved for food use and the maximum level used is 0.002% (11).
POSSIBLY SAFE ...when used orally. There are no published reports of toxicity from oral use (6,18,4501). ...when used topically. Storax should not be used topically on large, open wounds (18).
POSSIBLY UNSAFE ...when large amounts are ingested. ...when applied to large open wounds. Systemic absorption can cause poisoning including kidney damage, e.g., albuminuria and hemorrhagic nephritis (18).
PREGNANCY AND LACTATION: Insufficient reliable information available; avoid using.

Effectiveness

There is insufficient reliable information available about the effectiveness of storax.

Mechanism of Action

The applicable part of storax is the balsam. American storax balsam and Levant storax balsam are very similar chemically. Both contain aromatic alcohols (18), cinnamic acid (18,4503), cinnamic acid esters (6,18), storesins (13,4501), styrene (6,18,4503), a volatile oil (11,13), vanillin (6,11,18) and triterpenes (18). However, the amount of constituents varies between the species. In Levant storax, the volatile oil is usually less than 1%. In American storax, it ranges from 7 to over 20% (11). Storax has stimulant, antiseptic, and expectorant properties (11,13). It is also reported to have antimicrobial and anti-inflammatory properties (11).

Adverse Reactions

Orally, storax balsam can cause diarrhea (18).
Topically, storax balsam can cause skin sensitization and contact allergies (9,18). When applied to large, open wounds, systemic absorption can cause kidney damage (e.g., albuminuria and hemorrhagic nephritis) (18).

Interactions with Herbs & Other Dietary Supplements

Insufficient reliable information available.

Interactions with Drugs

No interactions are known to occur, and there is no known reason to expect a clinically significant interaction with storax.

Interactions with Foods

No interactions are known to occur, and there is no known reason to expect a clinically significant interaction with storax.

Interactions with Lab Tests

No interactions are known to occur, and there is no known reason to expect a clinically significant interaction with storax.

Interactions with Diseases or Conditions

No interactions are known to occur, and there is no known reason to expect a clinically significant interaction with storax.

Dosage and Administration

ORAL: No typical dosage.
TOPICAL/INHALATION: Storax is applied topically and administered by inhalation via a vaporizer (6,18).
It is available commercially in combination products.

Comments

Storax is a medicinal balsam obtained from the tree trunks of Liquidambar orientalis (Levant storax) or Liquidambar styraciflua (American storax) (13,4503). It is obtained by traumatizing the bark of the tree in early summer and stripping the bark later, perhaps as late as autumn. The bark is pressed in cold water, alternating with boiling water, and the crude liquid storax is collected (6). Storax is considered to be similar to Peru balsam in its effects (9,4501).

STRAWBERRY

Also Known As

Alpine Strawberry, Fragariae folium, Mountain Strawberry, Strawberries, Virginian Strawberry, Wild Strawberry, Wood Strawberry.

Scientific Names

Fragaria vesca; Fragaria virginiana; Fragaria viridis.
Family: Rosaceae.

People Use This For

Orally, strawberry is used for GI tract mucous membrane inflammation, diarrhea, intestinal sluggishness, liver disease, jaundice, upper and lower respiratory tract mucous membrane inflammation, gout, arthritis, nervous tension, kidney ailments involving gravel and stones, diuretic, supportive for heart and circulatory ailments, fever, night sweats, blood purification, for stimulating metabolism, anemia, as a tonic, for inhibiting menstruation, and supporting "natural weight loss" (2).
Topically, strawberry is used as a compress for rashes (2).

Safety

POSSIBLY SAFE ...when used orally and appropriately (12).
PREGNANCY AND LACTATION: Insufficient reliable information available; avoid using.

Effectiveness

There is insufficient reliable information available about the effectiveness of strawberry.

Mechanism of Action

The applicable part of strawberry is the leaf and fruit. Strawberry leaf contains ellagic acid tannins, oligomeric proanthocyanidins, and flavonoids including rutin and quercetin. People claim that strawberry leaf has astringent and diuretic activity (18); however, there are no data to support these claims (18). Strawberry leaves are rich in vitamin C (19). Preliminary research suggests that compounds contained in strawberry fruit might slow aging effects on the nervous system (1418,1419).

Adverse Reactions

Orally, allergic reactions may occur in people sensitive to strawberries (2).

Interactions with Herbs & Other Dietary Supplements

Insufficient reliable information available.

Interactions with Drugs

No interactions are known to occur, and there is no known reason to expect a clinically significant interaction with strawberry.

Interactions with Foods

No interactions are known to occur, and there is no known reason to expect a clinically significant interaction with strawberry.

Interactions with Lab Tests

No interactions are known to occur, and there is no known reason to expect a clinically significant interaction with strawberry.

Interactions with Diseases or Conditions

STRAWBERRY HYPERSENSITIVITY: Contraindicated (18).

Dosage and Administration

ORAL: Diarrhea, one cup tea (steep 1 gram dried leaf in 250 mL boiling water 5-10 minutes, strain); several cups daily (18).

Comments

None.

STROPHANTHUS

Also Known As
Kombe, Kombe-Strophanthus Seeds, Strophanthi Grati Semen, Strophanthi Kombe Semen, Strophanthus Seeds.

Scientific Names
Strophanthus gratus; Strophanthus kombe.
Family: Apocynaceae.

People Use This For
Orally, strophanthus is used for arteriosclerosis, cardiac insufficiency, gastrocardial symptoms, hypertension, and neurodystonia [18].

Safety
UNSAFE ...when used orally for self-medication [12,4077].
PREGNANCY: UNSAFE ...when used orally due to possible uterine stimulating effects [19]; avoid using.
LACTATION: UNSAFE ...when used orally; avoid using [4077].

Effectiveness
There is insufficient reliable information available about the effectiveness of strophanthus.

Mechanism of Action
The applicable part of strophanthus is the seed. Strophanthus gratus contains a cardiac glycoside strophanthin-G (ouabain) which has digitalis-like effects, but milder. The cardiac glycoside in Strophanthus kombe, strophanthin-K (strophoside), has milder effects than strophanthin-G [18,4077].

Adverse Reactions
Side effects include nausea, vomiting, headache, stupor, disturbance of color vision, and cardiac arrhythmias, particularly when strophanthin-G is administered parenterally and during overdose [18].

Interactions with Herbs & Other Dietary Supplements
ANTHROQUINONE-CONTAINING HERBS AND LAXATIVE HERBS: Anthroquinone-containing herbs such as aloe, alder buckthorn, European buckthorn, cascara sagrada, frangula, rhubarb, and senna; laxative herbs such as castor bean can worsen strophanthus seed toxicity, particularly with long-term use, due to electrolyte loss [19].
LICORICE: Can worsen effects of strophanthus seed due to hypokalemia [19].
CARDIAC GLYCOSIDE-CONTAINING HERBS: Contraindicated, and concomitant use can increase the risk of cardiac glycoside toxicity. Cardiac glycoside-containing herbs include black hellebore, Canadian hemp roots, digitalis leaf, hedge mustard, figwort, lily of the valley roots, motherwort, oleander leaf, pheasant's eye plant, pleurisy root, squill bulb leaf scales, and uzara [2,18,19,500].
CINCHONA, EPHEDRA: Use with strophanthus seed may increase risk of toxicity [18,19].

Interactions with Drugs
CARDIAC MEDICATIONS: Cardiac medications, including quinidine (and related noncardiac medication quinine) may increase risk of toxicity; contraindicated [18].
DIGOXIN: Therapeutic duplication, avoid using [2].
LAXATIVES: Overuse/misuse may cause electrolyte depletion and increase risk of strophanthus seed toxicity [18,19].
POTASSIUM DEPLETING DIURETICS, GLUCOCORTICOIDS: May cause electrolyte depletion and increase risk of strophanthus seed toxicity [18,19].
CALCIUM SALTS: Contraindicated [18].

Interactions with Foods
No interactions are known to occur, and there is no known reason to expect a clinically significant interaction with strophanthus.

Interactions with Lab Tests
No interactions are known to occur, and there is no known reason to expect a clinically significant interaction with strophanthus.

Interactions with Diseases or Conditions
CARDIAC CONDITIONS: CAUTION, strophanthus seed may cause arrhythmias [18].

Dosage and Administration

No typical dosage.

Comments

Strophanthus seeds can be confused with other African Strophanthus species (18). Strophanthus is used as an arrow poison in Africa (4077).

SUMA

Also Known As

Brazilian Ginseng, Pfaffia.

Scientific Names

Pfaffia paniculata.
Family: Amaranthaceae.

People Use This For

Orally, suma is used as an immune enhancer or adaptogen, which is a substance that is thought to help the body adapt to all types of stress by enhancing or restoring the immune system.

In the Amazon, people use it orally for cancer, diabetes, tumors, and as a tonic, which is an agent used to invigorate, refresh, or restore body function. They also use it topically for wounds and skin problems (515).

Safety

POSSIBLY SAFE …when used orally short-term (12).

There is insufficient reliable information available about the safety of the topical use of suma.

PREGNANCY AND LACTATION: Insufficient reliable information available; avoid using.

Effectiveness

There is insufficient reliable information available about the effectiveness of suma.

Mechanism of Action

The applicable part of suma is the root. Cell culture data suggests that isolated constituents pfaffic acid, a nortriterpene, and saponin derivatives pfaffosiges A through F inhibit melanoma growth. An ethanolic extract had mild anti-inflammatory and analgesic effect, but did not relieve noninflammatory pain (515). At present, we don't know how these components relate to the uses of suma.

Adverse Reactions

Powdered suma root can cause occupational asthma during industrial exposure to the root powder (515).

Interactions with Herbs & Other Dietary Supplements

Insufficient reliable information available.

Interactions with Drugs

No interactions are known to occur, and there is no known reason to expect a clinically significant interaction with suma.

Interactions with Foods

No interactions are known to occur, and there is no known reason to expect a clinically significant interaction with suma.

Interactions with Lab Tests

No interactions are known to occur, and there is no known reason to expect a clinically significant interaction with suma.

Interactions with Diseases or Conditions

No interactions are known to occur, and there is no known reason to expect a clinically significant interaction with suma.

Dosage and Administration

No typical dosage.

Comments

Suma is called Brazilian ginseng, presumably to present the herb in terms that consumers understand. It is unrelated to the ginsengs (American ginseng and Panax Ginseng) or other plants which use ginseng as an alternate common name (Blue Cohosh, Canaigre, Codonopsis, Siberian Ginseng, Ashwaganda), but may be confused with them (515).

SUMBUL

Also Known As
Ferrula, Musk Root.

Scientific Names
Ferula sumbul.
Family: Apiaceae.

People Use This For
Orally, sumbul is used for asthma and bronchitis. It is also used as an antispasmodic and sedative (18).

Safety
There is insufficient reliable information available about the safety of sumbul.
Pregnancy and Lactation: Insufficient reliable information available; avoid using.

Effectiveness
There is insufficient reliable information available about the effectiveness of sumbul.

Mechanism of Action
The applicable part of sumbul is the root/rhizome. There is insufficient reliable information available about the possible mechanism of action and active ingredients.

Adverse Reactions
None reported.

Interactions with Herbs & Other Dietary Supplements
Insufficient reliable information available.

Interactions with Drugs
No interactions are known to occur, and there is no known reason to expect a clinically significant interaction with sumbul.

Interactions with Foods
No interactions are known to occur, and there is no known reason to expect a clinically significant interaction with sumbul.

Interactions with Lab Tests
No interactions are known to occur, and there is no known reason to expect a clinically significant interaction with sumbul.

Interactions with Diseases or Conditions
No interactions are known to occur, and there is no known reason to expect a clinically significant interaction with sumbul.

Dosage and Administration
ORAL: Sumbul is used as a liquid extract or tincture (18).

Comments
There is very little scientific information about this product. Our staff is continually analyzing the available information on natural medicines and will add data here as it becomes available.

SUMMER SAVORY

Also Known As
Bean Herb, Bohnenkraut, Savory.
CAUTION: See separate listing for Winter Savory.

Scientific Names
Satureja hortensis, synonym Calamintha hortensis.
Family: Labiatae or Lamiaceae.

People Use This For
Orally, summer savory is used as an appetite stimulant or expectorant, for coughs, flatulence (5), intestinal disorders including cramps, indigestion, diarrhea, nausea (5,6,11,18), and to relieve frequent thirst in people with diabetes (5). Topically, summer savory is used for insect bites (11). Traditionally, summer savory is used as a tea for sore throats (11), as a tonic, astringent (6,11), antiflatulent (5,6,11), and as an aphrodisiac (6,11).
For food uses, summer savory is used in cooking as a culinary spice (5,6). The oil is used as a flavoring agent (5,6,11).

Safety
LIKELY SAFE ...when used orally in amounts found in food (6,11). The maximum use level is 0.519 % for summer savory spice and 0.036 % for the oil (11). Summer savory has Generally Recognized as Safe (GRAS) status in the US (11).
POSSIBLY SAFE ...when used orally and appropriately in medicinal amounts (5,6,18). ...when used topically as dilute oil (6,11), summer savory is nonirritating and nonsensitizing (11). Undiluted oil is a severe topical irritant (6).
PREGNANCY AND LACTATION: Insufficient reliable information available; avoid using amounts in excess of foods.

Effectiveness
There is insufficient reliable information available about the effectiveness of summer savory.

Mechanism of Action
The applicable parts of summer savory are the leaves and stem. Summer savory contains tannins (18), and a volatile oil (0.2-3.0 %) including thymol, carvacrol, p-cymene, limonene, and camphene (5,6,11,18). Other constituents also present include vitamin A, calcium, potassium, and proteins (11). Summer savory oil has antifungal, antibacterial, and spasmolytic properties (6,11). The mild antiseptic activity is due to cymene and carvacrol (5,18). A mild antidiarrheal effect is reportedly due to the astringent activity of the tannins (5,6,18).

Adverse Reactions
Topically, summer savory can cause skin eruptions (12). The concentrated oil of summer savory is strongly irritating (6).

Interactions with Herbs & Other Dietary Supplements
Insufficient reliable information available.

Interactions with Drugs
No interactions are known to occur, and there is no known reason to expect a clinically significant interaction with summer savory.

Interactions with Foods
No interactions are known to occur, and there is no known reason to expect a clinically significant interaction with summer savory.

Interactions with Lab Tests
No interactions are known to occur, and there is no known reason to expect a clinically significant interaction with summer savory.

Interactions with Diseases or Conditions
No interactions are known to occur, and there is no known reason to expect a clinically significant interaction with summer savory.

Dosage and Administration
ORAL: A typical dose is 3 teaspoons. In making the drink, do not boil, allow plant to soak (18).
TOPICAL: No typical dosage.

Comments

Summer savory is prized both for its value as a spice and in folk medicine as an aphrodisiac. Many sources agree that it adds flavor to beans and other legumes (5), but there is no information to support other uses.

SUNDEW

Also Known As

Dew Plant, Drosera, Lustwort, Red Rot, Round-Leafed Sundew, Youthwort.

Scientific Names

Drosera intermedia; Drosera longifolia; Drosera ramentacea; Drosera rotundifolia.
Family: Droseraeae.

People Use This For

Orally, sundew is used for bronchitis, asthma, pertussis, tracheitis, gastric ulceration (4), cancer (20), coughing fits, and dry cough (2).

Safety

POSSIBLY SAFE ...when used orally and appropriately (2,4).
PREGNANCY AND LACTATION: Insufficient reliable information available; avoid using.

Effectiveness

There is insufficient reliable information available about the effectiveness of sundew.

Mechanism of Action

Sundew seems to cause antispasmodic, demulcent, and expectorant effects (4). Researchers wonder if the antitussive effect demonstrated in animals is due to naphthoquinone constituents (4). Antimicrobial activity reported in vitro for naphthaquinone constituents (4).

Adverse Reactions

None reported.

Interactions with Herbs & Other Dietary Supplements

Insufficient reliable information available.

Interactions with Drugs

No interactions are known to occur, and there is no known reason to expect a clinically significant interaction with sundew.

Interactions with Foods

No interactions are known to occur, and there is no known reason to expect a clinically significant interaction with sundew.

Interactions with Lab Tests

No interactions are known to occur, and there is no known reason to expect a clinically significant interaction with sundew.

Interactions with Diseases or Conditions

No interactions are known to occur, and there is no known reason to expect a clinically significant interaction with sundew.

Dosage and Administration

ORAL: 1-2 grams dried plant three times daily, or one cup tea (made by steeping 1-2 grams dried plant in 150 mL boiling water 5-10 minutes, strain) three times daily (4); 3 grams dried plant is the average daily dose (2).
Liquid extract (1:1 in 25% alcohol), 0.5-2 mL three times daily (4). Tincture (1:5 in 60% alcohol), 0.5-1 mL three times daily (4).

Comments

None.

SUNFLOWER OIL

Also Known As
Corona Solis, Helianthi Annui Oleum, Marigold of Peru, Sunflower, Sunflower Oils, Sunflower Seed Oil.

Scientific Names
Helianthus annuus.
Family: Asteraceae.

People Use This For
Orally, sunflower oil is used for constipation.
Topically, it is used for poorly healing wounds, skin lesions, psoriasis, arthritis, and as a massage oil (18).
For food use, sunflower oil is used as a cooking oil.

Safety
LIKELY SAFE ...when used in amounts found in foods.
There is insufficient reliable information available about the safety of oral or topical medicinal uses for sunflower oil.
PREGNANCY AND LACTATION: Insufficient reliable information available; avoid using.

Effectiveness
There is insufficient reliable information available about the effectiveness of sunflower oil.

Mechanism of Action
Sunflower oil is cold pressed from the seeds of Helianthus annuus (18). There is insufficient reliable information available about the possible mechanism of action and active ingredients.

Adverse Reactions
Sunflower oil can cause an allergic reaction in individuals sensitive to the Asteraceae/Compositae family. Members of this family include ragweed, chrysanthemums, marigolds, daisies, and many other herbs.

Interactions with Herbs & Other Dietary Supplements
Insufficient reliable information available.

Interactions with Drugs
No interactions are known to occur, and there is no known reason to expect a clinically significant interaction with sunflower oil.

Interactions with Foods
No interactions are known to occur, and there is no known reason to expect a clinically significant interaction with sunflower oil.

Interactions with Lab Tests
No interactions are known to occur, and there is no known reason to expect a clinically significant interaction with sunflower oil.

Interactions with Diseases or Conditions
CROSS-ALLERGENICITY: Can cause an allergic reaction in individuals sensitive to the Asteraceae/Compositae family. Members of this family include ragweed, chrysanthemums, marigolds, daisies, and many other herbs.

Dosage and Administration
No typical dosage.

Comments
None.

SUPEROXIDE DISMUTASE

Also Known As
Orgotein, S.O.D., SOD, Super-Oxide Dismutase, Super Dioxide Dismutase.

Scientific Names
Superoxide dismutase.

People Use This For
Orally, superoxide dismutase is used for removing wrinkles (6), regenerating tissue (2227), and extending the length of life (6).

As an injection, superoxide dismutase is used for inflammatory diseases including osteoarthritis, sports injuries, rheumatoid arthritis (6), radiation-induced or interstitial cystitis (6), hyperuricemic syndromes (6), acute paraquat poisoning (6), for improving tolerance to radiation therapy (6), treating cancer (2226), improving rejection rates in kidney transplantation (6), managing reperfusion injury in acute myocardial infarction (6), and treating respiratory distress syndrome (6).

Safety
There is insufficient reliable information available to rate the safety of superoxide dismutase. However, there have been no reports of toxicity. Some evidence suggests SOD is not teratogenic (6).

Pregnancy and Lactation: Insufficient reliable information available; avoid using.

Effectiveness
POSSIBLY EFFECTIVE ...when used as an injection for treating osteoarthritis (2228,2229) or rheumatoid arthritis (2230,2231,2232). ...when used as an injection for reducing bronchopulmonary dysplasia in neonates with respiratory distress syndrome (2242). ...when used as an injection for interstitial cystitis (2233).

LIKELY INEFFECTIVE ...when used orally (6). ...when used as an injection for managing reperfusion injury in acute myocardial infarction (2241,2243).

There is insufficient reliable information available about the effectiveness of superoxide dismutase for its other uses.

Mechanism of Action
Superoxide dismutase is an essential enzyme found in all living cells. It catalyzes the conversion of toxic superoxide to oxygen and hydrogen peroxide (6,511). The action of SOD is believed to prevent oxygen-related damage to body tissues (6). SOD isoenzymes contain copper and zinc, or manganese (511). They are acid-labile and appear to have no oral bioavailability even when administered as enteric coated capsules (6). SOD deficiency is associated with amyotrophic lateral sclerosis (511). Results of two clinical trials suggest SOD can prevent or reduce radiation-induced cystitis (2234,2236), but a third trial suggests SOD is ineffective and allergenic (2235). Results of two clinical trials suggest SOD can improve rejection rates as adjunct therapy in kidney transplantation (2239,2240), but a third trial suggests it has no significant effect (2238).

Adverse Reactions
SOD used orally has no reported adverse reactions. Given as an injection, SOD can cause pain or allergic reactions at injection site (6).

Interactions with Herbs & Other Dietary Supplements
Insufficient reliable information available.

Interactions with Drugs
No interactions are known to occur, and there is no known reason to expect a clinically significant interaction with superoxide dismutase.

Interactions with Foods
No interactions are known to occur, and there is no known reason to expect a clinically significant interaction with superoxide dismutase.

Interactions with Lab Tests
No interactions are known to occur, and there is no known reason to expect a clinically significant interaction with superoxide dismutase.

Interactions with Diseases or Conditions
No interactions are known to occur, and there is no known reason to expect a clinically significant interaction with superoxide dismutase.

Dosage and Administration
ORAL: No typical dosage.

INJECTION: For osteoarthritis, 16 mg as an intra-articular injection is used twice (2228,2229). For rheumatoid arthritis a typical dose is 4 mg as an intra-articular injection per week (2230,2232). A typical dose for interstitial or radiation-induced cystitis is 12 mg injected into the bladder wall, up to 6 times (2233). For radiation-induced cystitis, a typical dose is 8 mg injected intramuscularly per day (2234). For reducing rejection risk in kidney transplantation, a typical dose is 200 mg intravenously during surgery (2239). For reducing bronchopulmonary dysplasia in neonatal respiratory distress syndrome, 0.25 mg/kg subcutaneously twice daily until ventilator support is no longer required (2242).

Comments
Oral SOD products purchased in health food stores might not have any of the activity stated on the label because they are acid labile and break down before absorption (6). However, bovine or recombinant (rh-SOD) source parenteral SOD products are available (2238).

SWAMP MILKWEED

Also Known As
Rose-Colored Silkweed, Swamp Silkweed.

Scientific Names
Asclepias incarnata.
Family: Asclepiadaceae.

People Use This For
Orally, swamp milkweed is used for digestive disorders (18).

Safety
LIKELY UNSAFE ...when used orally. Contains cardenolides, a type of cardioactive steroid. Digitalis-like poisonings are possible (18).
PREGNANCY AND LACTATION: LIKELY UNSAFE ...when used orally due to presence of cardioactive steroids (18); avoid using.

Effectiveness
There is insufficient reliable information available about the effectiveness of swamp milkweed.

Mechanism of Action
The applicable parts of swamp milkweed are the root and rhizome. Swamp milkweed contains cardioactive steroids known as cardenolides. In swamp milkweed, they have little therapeutic significance (18), but the concentration of the specific cardenolide present is not reported. In large amounts, swamp milkweed has an emetic effect (18).

Adverse Reactions
Orally, large amounts of swamp milkweed can cause vomiting (18). Handling the plant can cause local inflammation (19).

Interactions with Herbs & Other Dietary Supplements
CARDIAC GLYCOSIDE-CONTAINING HERBS: Contraindicated; concomitant use increases the risk of cardiac glycoside toxicity. Cardiac glycoside-containing herbs, include black hellebore, Canadian hemp roots, digitalis leaf, hedge mustard, figwort, lily of the valley roots, motherwort, oleander leaf, pheasant's eye plant, pleurisy root, squill bulb leaf scales, and strophanthus seeds (2,18,19,500).
OTHER CARDIOACTIVE HERBS: Avoid concomitant use with other cardioactive herbs due to unpredictability of effects and adverse effects. Other cardioactive herbs include calamus, cereus, cola, coltsfoot, devil's claw, European mistletoe, fenugreek, fumitory, ginger, Panax ginseng, hawthorn, white horehound, mate, parsley, quassia, scotch broom flower, shepherd's purse, and wild carrot (4).
STIMULANT LAXATIVE HERBS: Theoretically, overuse or misuse of stimulant laxatives with cardiac glycoside-containing herbs increases the risk of cardiac toxicity due to potassium depletion. Stimulant laxative herbs include: aloe dried leaf sap, blue flag rhizome, alder buckthorn, European buckthorn, butternut bark, cascara bark, castor oil, colocynth fruit pulp, gamboge bark exudate, jalap root, black root, manna bark exudate, podophyllum root, rhubarb root, senna leaves and pods, wild cucumber fruit (Ecballium elaterium), and yellow dock root (19).
LICORICE/HORSETAIL: Theoretically, overuse/misuse of licorice rhizome or horsetail plant with cardiac glycoside-containing herbs increases the risk of cardiac toxicity due to potassium depletion (19).

Interactions with Drugs
DIGOXIN: Contraindicated; therapeutic duplication increases risk of cardiac glycoside toxicity (2).

CARDIAC DRUGS: Theoretically, concomitant use may increase risk of cardiac toxicity (152).
STIMULANT LAXATIVES: Theoretically, overuse/misuse may increase risk of cardiac glycoside toxicity due to potassium depletion (2).
POTASSIUM-DEPLETING DIURETICS: Theoretically, concomitant use might increase risk of cardiac glycoside toxicity due to potassium depletion (2,506).
QUININE: Theoretically, concomitant use might increase risk of cardiac toxicity (2,506).
TETRACYCLINES AND MACROLIDE ANTIBIOTICS (erythromycin-like drugs): Theoretically, concomitant use might increase risk of cardiac glycoside toxicity (152,17).

Interactions with Foods
No interactions are known to occur, and there is no known reason to expect a clinically significant interaction with swamp milkweed.

Interactions with Lab Tests
No interactions are known to occur, and there is no known reason to expect a clinically significant interaction with swamp milkweed.

Interactions with Diseases or Conditions
HEART DISEASE: Contraindicated; theoretically the cardiac glycosides contained in swamp milkweed (18) might exacerbate the condition or interfere with existing drug therapy.

Dosage and Administration
No typical dosage.

Comments
None.

SWEET ALMOND

Also Known As
Almond, Almond Oil, Amygdala Dulcis, Expressed Almond Oil, Fixed Almond Oil, Sweet Almond Oil.
CAUTION: See separate listing for Bitter Almond.

Scientific Names
Prunus amygdalus dulcis.
Family: Rosaceae.

People Use This For
Orally, sweet almond is used as a mild laxative (11).
Topically, it is used as an emollient for chapped skin, to soothe mucous membranes (as a demulcent), and as a weak antibacterial (11).
Parenterally, sweet almond is also used as a solvent for injectable drugs (11).
In folk medicine, sweet almond has been used as a remedy for cancer of the bladder, breast, mouth, spleen, and uterus (11).
Sweet almonds, themselves, are a familiar food.
In manufacturing, sweet almond is used widely in cosmetics.

Safety
LIKELY SAFE ...when used orally (11). Unlike bitter almond oil, sweet almond oil contains no benzaldehyde and no (or only trace) poisonous hydrocyanic acid HCN (11,12). ...when used topically. Almond oil is nonirritating and nonsensitizing to skin (11).
PREGNANCY AND LACTATION: Insufficient reliable information available; avoid using.

Effectiveness
POSSIBLY EFFECTIVE ...when used orally as a laxative (11). ...when used topically as an emollient and demulcent (11).

Mechanism of Action
The applicable part of sweet almond is the fixed oil. Researchers believe the effects of sweet almond oil are due to the presence of many triglycerides (largely triolein and dioleolinolein) and fatty acids (oleic, linoleic, palmitic, stearic,

lauric, myristic and palmitoleic acids) (11). A Japanese patent claims isolation of low molecular weight peptides with analgesic and anti-inflammatory properties (11).

Adverse Reactions
None reported.

Interactions with Herbs & Other Dietary Supplements
Insufficient reliable information available.

Interactions with Drugs
No interactions are known to occur, and there is no known reason to expect a clinically significant interaction with sweet almond.

Interactions with Foods
No interactions are known to occur, and there is no known reason to expect a clinically significant interaction with sweet almond.

Interactions with Lab Tests
No interactions are known to occur, and there is no known reason to expect a clinically significant interaction with sweet almond.

Interactions with Diseases or Conditions
No interactions are known to occur, and there is no known reason to expect a clinically significant interaction with sweet almond.

Dosage and Administration
ORAL: As a laxative in doses up to 30 mL (11).

Comments
Avoid confusion between volatile almond oil and fixed almond oil. Fixed almond oil (sweet almond oil) is prepared by pressing the kernels of both sweet almond and bitter almond. It does not contain benzaldehyde or hydrocyanic acid (HCN). Sweet almond does not yield a volatile oil. Volatile almond oil (bitter almond oil) contains 95% benzaldehyde and 2-4% poisonous HCN. It is made by water maceration and steam distillation of partially defatted bitter almond (Prunus dulcis amara), apricot (Prunus armeniaca), peach (Prunus persica), and plum (Prunus domestica) kernels (11).

SWEET ANNIE

Also Known As
Annual Mugwort, Annual Wormwood, Artemisinin, Chinese Wormwood, Ching-hao, Qing Hao, Qinghao, Qinghaosu, Sweet Wormwood.

Scientific Names
Artemisia annua.
Family: Asteraceae or Compositae.

People Use This For
Orally, sweet Annie is used for dysentery, dyspepsia, fever (antipyretic), jaundice, night-sweats, scabies, tuberculosis (1277), cryptosporidiosis in people with AIDS (3173), preventing pneumocystis carinii infections in people with AIDS (3177), psoriasis, systemic lupus erythematosus and other auto-immune disorders (3175), bacterial and fungal infections, malaria, inflammatory conditions (3176), anorexia, circulatory disorders, common cold, constipation, gallbladder disorders, gastritis, nematode infestation, painful menstruation, and rheumatism (3179). Topically, sweet Annie is used for bacterial and fungal infections (3176), arthritis, rheumatism, bruises, neuralgia, and sprains (3179).
In Chinese medicine, sweet Annie is used orally for infections, fever, and malaria (3177,3178).

Safety
POSSIBLY SAFE ...when used orally and appropriately (12).
There is insufficient reliable information available about the safety of sweet Annie for its other uses.
PREGNANCY: LIKELY UNSAFE ...when used orally; avoid using (12,19).
LACTATION: Insufficient reliable information available; avoid using.

Effectiveness

EFFECTIVE ...when the sweet Annie extract, artemisinin, is used orally and by injection for treating malaria (14,3180). There is insufficient reliable information available about the effectiveness of sweet Annie for its other uses.

Mechanism of Action

The applicable parts of sweet Annie are the above ground parts (12). The constituent, artemisinin (qinghaosu), is a sesquiterpene lactone with antimalarial activity (14,3178). Preliminary evidence suggests that artemisinin and quercetagetin 6,7,3',4'-tetramethyl ether might have cytotoxic effects against some types of tumor cells (3183). Extracts of sweet Annie are reported to have antipyretic, anti-inflammatory, and bacteriostatic properties (3184). Evidence suggests that sweet Annie promotes cell-mediated immunity and inhibits antibody responses (3177). Preliminary research suggests that capsules containing sweet Annie herb might have antimalarial activity (3185).

Adverse Reactions

The use of artemether, the semisynthetic derivative of artemisinin, which is a constituent of sweet Annie, has been associated with hypoglycemia, prolongation of the QT interval on the electrocardiogram, abdominal pain, and local injection site pain (3180). Artesunate has been associated with prolonged ataxic gait and slurred speech (450). Sweet Annie might cause an allergic reaction in people sensitive to the Asteraceae/Compositae family. Members of this family include ragweed, chrysanthemums, marigolds, daisies, and many other herbs.

Interactions with Herbs & Other Dietary Supplements

Insufficient reliable information available.

Interactions with Drugs

No interactions are known to occur, and there is no known reason to expect a clinically significant interaction with sweet Annie.

Interactions with Foods

No interactions are known to occur, and there is no known reason to expect a clinically significant interaction with sweet Annie.

Interactions with Lab Tests

No interactions are known to occur, and there is no known reason to expect a clinically significant interaction with sweet Annie.

Interactions with Diseases or Conditions

CROSS-ALLERGENICITY: Sweet Annie might cause an allergic reaction in people sensitive to the Asteraceae/Compositae family. Members of this family include ragweed, chrysanthemums, marigolds, daisies, and many other herbs.

Dosage and Administration

ORAL: Daily doses of 3-9 grams of sweet Annie above ground parts have been used (3176,3177).

Comments

The semisynthetic derivatives of artemisinin (a constituent of sweet Annie); artemether, arteether, and artesunate, are used as prescription antimalarial drugs in Asia, Africa, and Europe (14,3178,3181,3182).

SWEET BAY

Also Known As

Bay, Bay Laurel, Bay Leaf, Bay Tree, Daphne, Grecian Laurel, Laurel, Mediterranean Bay, Noble Laurel, Roman Laurel, True Bay.

Scientific Names

Laurus nobilis.
Family: Lauraceae.

People Use This For

Orally, sweet bay is used to treat cancer, and as a bile and general stimulant, antiflatulent, diaphoretic (11), and herb for foods (11).
Topically, sweet bay is used as an anti-dandruff agent (11), as a counterirritant, and to treat rheumatic conditions (18).

In veterinary medicine, sweet bay is used as an udder ointment (18).

Historically, the fruit essential and fatty oils of sweet bay have been used for treating furuncles, a localized infection of hair follicles (18).

For food uses, sweet bay is used as a seasoning.

In food manufacturing, it is used as an herb and oil in processed foods (11).

In manufacturing, the oil is used in cosmetics, soaps, and detergents (11).

Safety

LIKELY SAFE ...when used orally in amounts found in foods (12). The highest levels of sweet bay used in food are 0.1% as a herb and 0.02% as an oil (11).

LIKELY UNSAFE ...when the whole, intact leaf is swallowed. The whole leaf is indigestible and can become lodged in the esophagus, hypopharynx (132,133,134,137), or perforate the intestinal lining (135,136).

PREGNANCY AND LACTATION: Insufficient reliable information available; avoid using in amounts exceeding those commonly found in foods.

Effectiveness

There is insufficient reliable information available about the effectiveness of sweet bay.

Mechanism of Action

The applicable part of sweet bay is the dried leaf. The sweet bay constituent, methyl eugenol, has sedative and narcotic properties in mice. The essential oil has bactericidal and fungicidal properties (11). The other constituents of sweet bay include proanthocyanidins, alkaloids, and plant acids (11).

Adverse Reactions

Sweet bay can cause allergic reactions, including contact dermatitis (11). The whole, intact leaf is indigestible and can become lodged in the esophagus and hypopharynx (132,133,134,137) and perforate the intestinal lining (135,136).

Interactions with Herbs & Other Dietary Supplements

Insufficient reliable information available.

Interactions with Drugs

SEDATIVE DRUGS AND NARCOTIC ANALGESICS: Because sweet bay theoretically can enhance the therapeutic and adverse effects of sedatives and narcotics, concomitant use should be avoided.

Interactions with Foods

No interactions are known to occur, and there is no known reason to expect a clinically significant interaction with sweet bay.

Interactions with Lab Tests

No interactions are known to occur, and there is no known reason to expect a clinically significant interaction with sweet bay.

Interactions with Diseases or Conditions

SWEET BAY ALLERGY: Because of contact dermatitis, sweet bay should be avoided in those having sensitivity to it.

Dosage and Administration

TOPICAL: An extract of sweet bay is typically used in baths and soaks (5008).

ORAL: No typical dosage.

Comments

The ancient Greeks and Romans crowned their victors with the leafy branches of sweet bay (11).

SWEET CICELY

Also Known As

British Myrrh, Shepherd's Needle, Sweet Bracken, Sweet Chervil, Sweet-Cus, Sweet-Fern, Sweet-Humlock, Sweets, The Roman Plant.

Scientific Names

Myrrhis odorata.
Family: Apiaceae.

People Use This For

Orally, sweet cicely is used for breathing difficulties, asthma, as an expectorant, digestive aid, and blood purifier. It is also used orally for chest and throat complaints, and for urinary tract complaints [18].
Topically, sweet cicely is used for gout swelling and indurations.

Safety

There is insufficient reliable information available about the safety of sweet cicely.
Pregnancy and Lactation: Insufficient reliable information available; avoid using.

Effectiveness

There is insufficient reliable information available about the effectiveness of sweet cicely.

Mechanism of Action

There is insufficient reliable information available about the possible mechanism of action and active ingredients.

Adverse Reactions

None reported.

Interactions with Herbs & Other Dietary Supplements

Insufficient reliable information available.

Interactions with Drugs

No interactions are known to occur, and there is no known reason to expect a clinically significant interaction with sweet cicely.

Interactions with Foods

No interactions are known to occur, and there is no known reason to expect a clinically significant interaction with sweet cicely.

Interactions with Lab Tests

No interactions are known to occur, and there is no known reason to expect a clinically significant interaction with sweet cicely.

Interactions with Diseases or Conditions

No interactions are known to occur, and there is no known reason to expect a clinically significant interaction with sweet cicely.

Dosage and Administration

Sweet cicely is used as a tea or tonic [18].

Comments

There is very little scientific information about this product. Our staff is continually analyzing the available information on natural medicines and will add data here as it becomes available.

SWEET CLOVER

Also Known As

Common Melilot, Field Melilot, Hart's Tree, Hay Flower, King's Clover, Melilot, Meliloti herba, Melilotus, Sweet Lucerne, Sweet Melilot, Tall Melilot, Wild Laburnum, Yellow Melilot, Yellow Sweet Clover.
CAUTION: See separate listings for Red Clover and Hay Flower.

Scientific Names

Melilotus altissimus; Melilotus officinalis.
Family: Leguminosae or Fabaceae.

People Use This For

Orally, sweet clover is used for symptoms of chronic venous insufficiency and varicose veins, including leg pain and heaviness, night cramps, pruritus and edema (1,2,18), supportive treatment of thrombophlebitis (2,8,18), hemorrhoids (2,18), post-thrombotic syndromes, and lymphatic congestion (2).

Topically, sweet clover is used for contusions and ecchymoses (2,18).

Historically, sweet clover has been used as a diuretic (8,18).

Safety

LIKELY SAFE ...when preparations of the flowering branch and leaf are used orally in moderate amounts (1,2,18).

LIKELY UNSAFE …when large amounts are used orally because it can cause transient liver injury (18).

PREGNANCY: Insufficient reliable information available. A study of 30 second and third trimester pregnant women did not report any adverse effects (1).

LACTATION: Insufficient reliable information available; avoid using.

Effectiveness

POSSIBLY EFFECTIVE ...when used orally for problems associated with chronic venous insufficiency (1,2), including leg pain and heaviness, nighttime leg cramps, itching and swelling, for supportive treatment of thrombophlebitis, lymphatic congestion, post-thrombotic syndromes, and hemorrhoids (2). ...when used for contusions and ecchymoses (2). ...when used intravenously for treating symptoms of varicose veins (1).

There is insufficient reliable information available about the effectiveness of sweet clover for its other uses.

Mechanism of Action

The applicable parts of sweet clover are the flowering branch and leaf. Fresh herb contains coumarinic acids (18), which are converted to free coumarins during drying (1,8,18). Dicoumarol, which has anticoagulant activity, can be formed if the fresh herb is allowed to spoil (1). There is some evidence to suggest that sweet clover aids wound healing (2,8), and a locally perfused sweet clover extract might eliminate adrenaline-induced vasoconstriction. This would indicate peripheral vasodilation (1). Coumarin isolated from sweet clover reduces experimentally-induced paw inflammation in rats (1). Intravenous administration decreases pain, edema, and improves wound healing in people with phlebitis, and relieves symptoms of varicose veins (1). Sweet clover seems to increase venous reflux and improve lymphatic kinetics, and therefore reduces edema (2).

Adverse Reactions

Orally, headaches are rare (1,2,18), and large amounts can cause stupor and transient liver injury in susceptible individuals (18). There was one case report of bleeding diathesis following two months ingestion of large amounts of a multi-herb, "seasonal tonic" tea containing melilot, sweet woodruff, and tonka bean (all coumarin-containing herbs) (809).

Interactions with Herbs & Other Dietary Supplements

HERBS WITH ANTICOAGULANT/ANTIPLATELET POTENTIAL: Concomitant use of herbs that have coumarin constituents or affect platelet aggregation could theoretically increase the risk of bleeding in some people. These herbs include: angelica, anise, arnica, asafoetida, bogbean, boldo, capsicum, celery, chamomile, clove, danshen, fenugreek, feverfew, garlic, ginger, ginkgo, ginseng Panax, horse chestnut, horseradish, licorice, meadowsweet, prickly ash, onion, papain, passionflower, poplar, quassia, red clover, turmeric, wild carrot, wild lettuce, willow, and others (4,19).

Interactions with Drugs

ANTICOAGULANT, ANTIPLATELET DRUGS: Theoretically, concomitant use might increase bleeding risk (19).

HEPATOTOXIC DRUGS: Theoretically, concomitant use might increase risk of hepatotoxicity (see Adverse Reactions).

Interactions with Foods

No interactions are known to occur, and there is no known reason to expect a clinically significant interaction with sweet clover.

Interactions with Lab Tests

LIVER ENZYMES: Sweet clover might cause an increase in liver enzymes and test results, indicating liver damage; monitor (18).

Interactions with Diseases or Conditions

LIVER DISEASE: Theoretically, sweet clover might exacerbate liver disease (see Adverse Reactions) (18); avoid using.

Dosage and Administration

ORAL: Average amount, sweet clover preparations equivalent to 3-30 mg coumarin per day [1,2]. Phlebitis or varicose veins, one cup (made by steeping 1-2 teaspoons finely chopped sweet clover in 150 mL boiling water 5-10 minutes, strain) two to three cups per day [8,18]; 6 mL Melilotus/rutin preparation (600 mg Melilotus extract containing 3 mg coumarin and 150 mg rutin) per day reported in one clinical trial [1]. CAUTION: Monitor liver enzymes with oral use [18], especially in people at risk for liver damage.
TOPICAL: Sweet clover extract in semi-solid preparations containing 3-5 mg/g coumarin [2,8,18]. As a poultice for sores and hemorrhoids, wrap sweet clover in linen, thoroughly soak with hot water, place on the affected area [8].
INJECTION: Liquid forms for parenteral use corresponding to 1-7.5 mg coumarin per day [2,8].

Comments

Avoid confusion with red clover (Trifolium pratense) and hay flower, the sieved flower and fruit from cut hay grass (Poaceae family) plants.

SWEET GALE

Also Known As

Bayberry, Bog Myrtle, Dutch Myrtle.
CAUTION: See separate listing for Bayberry.

Scientific Names

Myrica gale.
Family: Myricaceae.

People Use This For

Orally, sweet gale is used for digestive disorders.
In Sweden, a strong brew of sweet gale dried bark is used as an anthelmintic and to cure itching [18].

Safety

There is insufficient reliable information available about the safety of sweet gale. The volatile oil of sweet gale is considered toxic [18].
Pregnancy and Lactation: Insufficient reliable information available; avoid using.

Effectiveness

There is insufficient reliable information available about the effectiveness of sweet gale.

Mechanism of Action

The applicable parts of sweet gale are the leaf, branch, and wax from catkin. Sweet gale contains 0.4-0.7% of a volatile oil that contains alpha-pinene, delta-cadinene, gamma-cadinene, limonene, beta-myrcene, beta-phellandrene, and 1,8 cineole. It also contains flavonoids including myricitrin [18]. Sweet gale is thought to have astringent and aromatic properties [18].

Adverse Reactions

None reported. The volatile oil is considered toxic.

Interactions with Herbs & Other Dietary Supplements

Insufficient reliable information available.

Interactions with Drugs

No interactions are known to occur, and there is no known reason to expect a clinically significant interaction with sweet gale.

Interactions with Foods

No interactions are known to occur, and there is no known reason to expect a clinically significant interaction with sweet gale.

Interactions with Lab Tests

No interactions are known to occur, and there is no known reason to expect a clinically significant interaction with sweet gale.

Interactions with Diseases or Conditions

No interactions are known to occur, and there is no known reason to expect a clinically significant interaction with sweet gale.

Dosage and Administration

No typical dosage.

Comments

In the Middle ages, sweet gale was mixed with beer, and is said to have led to periods of extreme excitation (18).

SWEET ORANGE

Also Known As

Citri Sinensis, Jaffa Orange, Navel Orange, Pericarpium, Valencia Orange.
CAUTION: See separate listings for Bergamot Oil, Oswego Tea, Bitter Orange flower, and Bitter Orange peel.

Scientific Names

Citrus sinensis, synonyms Citrus aurantium sinensis, Citrus aurantium dulcis.
Family: Rutaceae.

People Use This For

Orally, sweet orange peel is used as an appetite stimulant (2).
In Chinese medicine, sweet orange peel is used to reduce phlegm, treat coughs, colds, anorexia, and malignant breast sores (11).
Historically, it has been used as a tonic, antiflatulent, and for dyspepsia (11).

Safety

LIKELY SAFE ...when used orally or topically. The volatile oil of sweet orange peel has a low potential for sensitizing skin (18).
CHILDREN: LIKELY UNSAFE ...when used orally in large amounts; avoid using. There are reports of intestinal colic, convulsions, and death (11).
PREGNANCY AND LACTATION: Insufficient reliable information available; avoid using.

Effectiveness

POSSIBLY EFFECTIVE ...when the juice is consumed for preventing hypertension and stroke. Some sweet orange juice products that provide at least 350 mg of potassium per serving and that are low in sodium, saturated fat, and cholesterol are permitted by the FDA to make labeling claims that they might reduce the risk of developing high blood pressure and stroke (1308). ...when used orally as an appetite stimulant and for dyspeptic ailments (2).
There is insufficient reliable information available about the effectiveness of sweet orange for its other uses. However, there is some evidence that consumption of vitamin C-rich citrus fruits, including sweet orange and others, might improve lung function in people with asthma. Intake of citrus fruits 1-2 times per week has produced this benefit in some studies (6049,6055,6056). However, other studies have not found this benefit (6057,6058). More evidence is needed to rate the effectiveness of sweet orange for this use.

Mechanism of Action

The applicable parts of sweet orange are the peel and juice. Orange peel contains essential oil and bitter principles (11). The constituents naringin and nobiletin might have anti-inflammatory activity (11,1281). The flavonoid and pectin constituents have antibacterial and antifungal activities. Pectin also seems to lower blood cholesterol levels (11). There is also some preliminary evidence that flavonoids contained in sweet orange juice might inhibit growth of human prostate, lung, melanoma, and colon cancer cells (5042). Potential benefits of sweet orange in asthma have been attributed to antioxidant properties of vitamin C or other fruit constituents (6049,6054,6055). For preventing high blood pressure and stroke, sweet orange juice is thought to be beneficial due to high concentrations of potassium. Potassium consumption seems to reduce the risk of developing hypertension and stroke (1310).

Adverse Reactions

There have been reports of intestinal colic, convulsions, and death in children following ingestion of large amounts of sweet orange peel (11).

Interactions with Herbs & Other Dietary Supplements

Insufficient reliable information available.

Interactions with Drugs

FEXOFENADINE (Allegra): Sweet orange juice can significantly decrease oral absorption and blood levels of fexofenadine when used together. Sweet orange decreases bioavailability of fexofenadine by about 72%. Sweet orange juice seems to inhibit organic anion transporting polypeptide (OATP), which is a drug transporter in the gut, liver, and kidney (7046). It's not yet known how long sweet orange juice inhibits OATP. Separating administration times might not prevent this interaction. Tell patients it's best to take their medications with a plain glass of water.

Interactions with Foods

No interactions are known to occur, and there is no known reason to expect a clinically significant interaction with sweet orange.

Interactions with Lab Tests

No interactions are known to occur, and there is no known reason to expect a clinically significant interaction with sweet orange.

Interactions with Diseases or Conditions

No interactions are known to occur, and there is no known reason to expect a clinically significant interaction with sweet orange.

Dosage and Administration

ORAL: 10-15 grams fresh or dry peel (free of white pulp layer) per day as a digestive aid (2). Peel may be used to prepare a tea (steep peel in boiling water 10-15 minutes, strain) or in other herbal preparations (2). Store peel away from children, due to reported death after ingestion of large amounts (11).

Comments

Researchers report that drinking three glasses of orange juice daily might increase HDL cholesterol in people with high cholesterol (346). Further research is needed to verify this finding. Avoid confusion with bergamot oil, oswego tea, bitter orange flower, and bitter orange peel.

SWEET SUMACH

Also Known As

None.

Scientific Names

Rhus aromatica.
Family: Anacardiaceae.

People Use This For

Orally, sweet sumach is used for irritable bladder, urinary incontinence, bed-wetting, kidney and bladder disorders, and uterine hemorrhages (18).

Safety

There is insufficient reliable information available about the safety of sweet sumach.
Pregnancy and Lactation: Insufficient reliable information available; avoid using.

Effectiveness

There is insufficient reliable information available about the effectiveness of sweet sumach.

Mechanism of Action

The applicable part of sweet sumach is the root bark. There is insufficient reliable information available about the possible mechanism of action and active ingredients.

Adverse Reactions

Topically, sweet sumach can cause contact allergic dermatitis in susceptible individuals (4078).

Interactions with Herbs & Other Dietary Supplements

Insufficient reliable information available.

Interactions with Drugs
No interactions are known to occur, and there is no known reason to expect a clinically significant interaction with sweet sumach.

Interactions with Foods
No interactions are known to occur, and there is no known reason to expect a clinically significant interaction with sweet sumach.

Interactions with Lab Tests
No interactions are known to occur, and there is no known reason to expect a clinically significant interaction with sweet sumach.

Interactions with Diseases or Conditions
No interactions are known to occur, and there is no known reason to expect a clinically significant interaction with sweet sumach.

Dosage and Administration
No typical dosage.

Comments
Sweet sumach belongs to the same family as poison ivy, and can cause similar dermal reactions (4078).
There is very little scientific information about this product. Our staff is continually analyzing the available information on natural medicines and will add data here as it becomes available.

SWEET VERNAL GRASS

Also Known As
Grass, Spring Grass.

Scientific Names
Anthoxanthum odoratum.

People Use This For
Orally, sweet vernal grass is used for headache (18), nausea (18), sleeplessness (18), and conditions of the urinary tract (route unspecified).
In Russia, sweet vernal grass is used as an ingredient in certain brandies (6).
For food uses, sweet vernal grass is used as a flavoring agent.

Safety
LIKELY UNSAFE ...when used orally for medicinal use. ...when the whole plant is used orally as a flavoring or in larger amounts. Sweet vernal grass contains the constituent, dicumarol that has anticoagulant properties (6,18). It also contains the constituent coumarin, which the FDA has banned for flavoring purposes. Coumarin has been associated with hepatotoxicity ranging from elevated liver enzymes to severe hepatic damage (6,18,297,4501).
There is insufficient reliable information available about the safety of the topical use of sweet vernal grass.
PREGNANCY AND LACTATION: LIKELY UNSAFE ...when used orally (6,18); avoid using.

Effectiveness
There is insufficient reliable information available about the effectiveness of sweet vernal grass (18).

Mechanism of Action
Sweet vernal grass contains hydroxycinnamic acid glycosides that form coumarin (up to 1.5%) when the harvested plant is dehydrated (18). After an outbreak of hemorrhagic diathesis in cattle fed sweet vernal grass hay, veterinary experiments identified dicumarol, a known anticoagulant, in the hay (6). There is some evidence that coumarin can reduce edema and inflammation by increasing venous and lymphatic return (295).

Adverse Reactions
Use of high levels of sweet vernal grass can cause headaches and dizziness (18). The oral use of sweet vernal grass when the harvested plant is dehydrated can be associated with nausea and vomiting (286), diarrhea, dizziness, insomnia (287), asymptomatic SGOT elevations (286), and rarely, liver toxicity (6,18,297,4501).

Cattle poisoned by sweet vernal hay showed characteristically rapid onset of symptoms including progressive weakness, mucosal pallor, stiff gait, tachypnea, tachycardia, and hematomata, quickly resulting in death (6).

Interactions with Herbs & Other Dietary Supplements
HERBS WITH ANTICOAGULANT/ANTIPLATELET POTENTIAL: Concomitant use of herbs that have coumarin constituents or affect platelet aggregation could theoretically increase the risk of bleeding in some people. These herbs include: angelica, anise, arnica, asafoetida, bogbean, boldo, capsicum, celery, chamomile, clove, danshen, fenugreek, feverfew, garlic, ginger, ginkgo, ginseng Panax, horse chestnut, horseradish, licorice, meadowsweet, prickly ash, onion, papain, passionflower, poplar, quassia, red clover, turmeric, wild carrot, wild lettuce, willow, and others (4,19).

Interactions with Drugs
ANTICOAGULANTS/ANTIPLATELETS: Theoretically, sweet vernal grass might cause additive effects and side effects with drugs having anticoagulant or antiplatelet properties (19).

Interactions with Foods
No interactions are known to occur, and there is no known reason to expect a clinically significant interaction with sweet vernal grass.

Interactions with Lab Tests
No interactions are known to occur, and there is no known reason to expect a clinically significant interaction with sweet vernal grass.

Interactions with Diseases or Conditions
LIVER DISEASE: Although it is rare, coumarin can cause liver toxicity (298).

Dosage and Administration
ORAL: No typical dosage.
TOPICAL: Used as an extract (18).

Comments
This aromatic plant has been used as a flavoring agent due to its vanilla-like aroma (6).

SWEET VIOLET

Also Known As
Garden Violet, Sweet Violet Herb, Sweet Violet Root, Violae Odoratae Rhizoma, Herba, Violet.
CAUTION: See separate listing for Garden Violet.

Scientific Names
Viola odorata.
Family: Violaceae.

People Use This For
Orally, sweet violet is used for calming and relaxing nerves (2), physical and mental exhaustion (2), physical and psychological symptoms associated with menopause (hot flashes), metabolic imbalances, and to "detoxify blood". It is also used orally for depression, irritability, anxiety (2), GI complaints, abdominal pain, gallbladder complaints, mucous membrane inflammation of the stomach and intestines, enteritis, duodenitis, digestion problems caused by improper diet, flatulence, heartburn, and loss of appetite (2).
Topically, it is used for skin impurities and disorders (2), and as a skin cleanser (18).
In herbal combinations, sweet violet is used for acute and chronic bronchitis, bronchial asthma, acute and chronic mucous inflammations of the upper and lower respiratory tract, cold symptoms of the upper respiratory tract, hoarseness, cough, mucous congestion, bronchial inflammation, and late "flu" symptoms. It is also used for chesty, spastic and whooping coughs, emphysema, "dust-damaged" lung (2), urinary incontinence due to senility, irritable bladder, enuresis nocturna or prostate condition (2), insomnia, and improving deep sleep.
In folk medicine, the root has been used for respiratory tract conditions, particularly dry mucous membrane inflammation, rheumatism of the minor joints, fever, skin diseases, inflammation of the oral mucosa, nervous strain, headache, and insomnia (18). In folk medicine, the herb has been used for coughs, hoarseness, tuberculosis, throat inflammation, bronchitis accompanied by fixed mucous, nervous strain, insomnia, and hysteria (18).

Safety

POSSIBLY SAFE ...when used orally in appropriate amounts (2,18).

There is insufficient reliable information available about the safety of the topical use of sweet violet.

PREGNANCY AND LACTATION: Insufficient reliable information available; avoid using.

Effectiveness

There is insufficient reliable information available about the effectiveness of sweet violet.

Mechanism of Action

The applicable parts of sweet violet are the root and above ground parts. Sweet violet contains saponins (2), which have expectorant properties, and in high doses irritate mucous membranes (2).

Adverse Reactions

None reported.

Interactions with Herbs & Other Dietary Supplements

Insufficient reliable information available.

Interactions with Drugs

No interactions are known to occur, and there is no known reason to expect a clinically significant interaction with sweet violet.

Interactions with Foods

No interactions are known to occur, and there is no known reason to expect a clinically significant interaction with sweet violet.

Interactions with Lab Tests

No interactions are known to occur, and there is no known reason to expect a clinically significant interaction with sweet violet.

Interactions with Diseases or Conditions

No interactions are known to occur, and there is no known reason to expect a clinically significant interaction with sweet violet.

Dosage and Administration

ORAL: The typical dose of sweet violet as an herb is one cup tea (steep 2 teaspoons herb in 250 mL boiling water 10-15 minutes, strain) 2-3 times daily (18). As a root (5% w/v), take 1 tablespoon 5-6 times daily (simmer 20 grams in boiling water for 10-15 minutes, and strain) (18).

Comments

None.

SWEET WOODRUFF

Also Known As

Galii odorati herba, Master of the Wood, Waldmeister, Woodruff, Wordward.

Scientific Names

Galium odorata, synonym Asperula odorata.
Family: Rubiaceae.

People Use This For

Orally, sweet woodruff is used for preventing and treating respiratory tract, gastrointestinal tract, liver, gallbladder, and urinary tract disorders; for blood purification, venous complaints, weak veins, hemorrhoids, vasodilation; spasms, abdominal discomforts; strengthening the nervous system (2), agitation, hysteria, nervous menstrual disorders (18), restlessness, insomnia, neuralgia (11); strengthening heart function (2), cardiac irregularity (18); stomachache, migraine, and bladder stones (11). Sweet woodruff is also used orally for inducing sweating, as an antispasmodic, diuretic (11), or expectorant (6).

Topically, sweet woodruff is used for skin diseases, treating wounds (2), venous conditions, hemorrhoids, and for reducing inflammation (11).

In foods and beverages, sweet woodruff is used as a flavoring component (11).

In manufacturing, the extracts of sweet woodruff above ground parts are used as fragrance components in perfumes (11).

Safety

LIKELY SAFE …when used orally in amounts found in alcoholic beverages (11). Approved only for use in alcoholic beverages in the US (11).

POSSIBLY SAFE …when used orally and appropriately for medicinal uses on a short-term basis (12,18).

There is insufficient reliable information available about the safety of the topical use of sweet woodruff.

PREGNANCY AND LACTATION: Insufficient reliable information available; avoid using.

Effectiveness

There is insufficient reliable information available about the effectiveness of sweet woodruff.

Mechanism of Action

The applicable parts of sweet woodruff are the above ground parts. Sweet woodruff leaves and the constituent asperuloside show evidence of anti-inflammatory activity (11). Sweet woodruff also demonstrates antibacterial activity (4009). The fresh plant contains up to 1% coumarin as a bound glycoside. Coumarin is supposedly enzymatically released during dehydration (11). Interestingly, one investigation failed to detect any coumarins in sweet woodruff (11). The coumarin constituent is thought to have anti-inflammatory, anti-edema, spasmolytic, and lymphokinetic effects, but the levels found in sweet woodruff are so low that therapeutic effects are doubtful (18). Other constituents present in sweet woodruff include monotopein, tannins, anthracene and naphthalene derivatives, plus traces of nicotinic acid, a fixed oil, and a bitter principle (11).

Adverse Reactions

Orally, sweet woodruff above ground parts can be associated with headache (12), and in larger amounts, stupor (18). Long-term usage can cause liver damage (18).

Interactions with Herbs & Other Dietary Supplements

Insufficient reliable information available.

Interactions with Drugs

No interactions are known to occur, and there is no known reason to expect a clinically significant interaction with sweet woodruff.

Interactions with Foods

No interactions are known to occur, and there is no known reason to expect a clinically significant interaction with sweet woodruff.

Interactions with Lab Tests

No interactions are known to occur, and there is no known reason to expect a clinically significant interaction with sweet woodruff.

Interactions with Diseases or Conditions

No interactions are known to occur, and there is no known reason to expect a clinically significant interaction with sweet woodruff.

Dosage and Administration

ORAL: A typical dose is one cup tea. To make tea, use 2 teaspoons (1.8 grams) in a glass of water (18). The average single dose is 1 gram during the day or shortly before bedtime (18).

Comments

Sweet woodruff root contains a red dye (6). Sweet woodruff is considered obsolete for medicinal use in many countries (18). Avoid confusing sweet woodruff, Galium odoratum, with Asperula odorata which is also referred to as woodruff.

TAGETES

Also Known As

African Marigold, Aztec Marigold, Big Marigold, Chinchilla Enana, Dwarf Marigold, French Marigold, Huacatay, Mexican Marigold, Muster John Henry, Saffron Marigold, Stinking-Roger, Tagetes.

Scientific Names

Tagetes erecta; Tagetes minuta , synonym Tagetes glandulifera; Tagetes patula.
Family: Asteraceae or Compositae.

People Use This For

Orally, the flowerheads and foliage of African marigold have been used as an anthelmintic, a menstrual flow stimulant, and for treating colic (11). African marigold is also used orally in treating whooping cough, cough, colds, mumps, mastitis, and sore eyes (11).

The Mexican marigold is used orally for improving digestion, stimulating appetite, inducing sweating, as an anthelmintic, a bile flow stimulant, a sedative in gastric pain, an antiflatulent, a diuretic, and antiabortifacient (11). The French marigold is used orally for coughs and dysentery (11).

Topically, the African marigold leaf is used for treating sores and ulcers (11). The juice of the leaf is used topically for eczema (11). Topically, the oil of the Mexican marigold is used for treating wound maggots (11).

In foods and beverages, Mexican marigold is used as a flavor component (11).

In manufacturing, oil from the Mexican marigold is used as fragrance in perfumes (11). The flowers of the African marigold are useful as mosquito repellent (11). The dried, ground flowers of marigolds are used as chicken feed to enhance the characteristic yellow color of chicken skin and egg yolk (11).

Safety

LIKELY SAFE ...when used orally in amounts found in foods. Tagetes oil has Generally Recognized as Safe (GRAS) status in the US (11). The maximum use level of the oil in foods is 0.003% (11).

There is insufficient reliable information available about the safety of tagetes used in amounts greater than those found in foods.

PREGNANCY AND LACTATION: Insufficient reliable information available; avoid amounts greater than found in foods.

Effectiveness

There is insufficient reliable information available about the effectiveness of tagetes.

Mechanism of Action

The applicable parts of tagetes are the above ground parts. Some evidence suggests tagetes oil might have tranquilizing, hypotensive, bronchodilatory, spasmolytic, and anti-inflammatory properties (11). The constituent ocimenone demonstrates cidal activity against mosquito larvae (11). Alpha-terthienyl, isolated from the African marigold, exhibits nematocidal and larvicidal activity (11). Patulin, isolated from the French marigold is antispasmodic, reduces capillary permeability, and increases blood pressure (11).

Adverse Reactions

Topically, tagetes can cause contact dermatitis (11). Tagetes can also cause an allergic reaction in individuals sensitive to the Asteraceae/Compositae family. Members of this family include ragweed, chrysanthemums, marigolds, daisies, and many other herbs.

Interactions with Herbs & Other Dietary Supplements

Insufficient reliable information available.

Interactions with Drugs

No interactions are known to occur, and there is no known reason to expect a clinically significant interaction with tagetes.

Interactions with Foods

No interactions are known to occur, and there is no known reason to expect a clinically significant interaction with tagetes.

Interactions with Lab Tests

No interactions are known to occur, and there is no known reason to expect a clinically significant interaction with tagetes.

Interactions with Diseases or Conditions
CROSS-ALLERGENICITY: Can cause an allergic reaction in individuals sensitive to the Asteraceae/Compositae family. Members of this family include ragweed, chrysanthemums, marigolds, daisies, and many other herbs.

Dosage and Administration
No typical dosage.

Comments
Tagetes oil is distilled from the above ground parts of Tagetes erecta, minuta, and patula (11).

TAMARIND

Also Known As
Imlee, Tamarindo.
CAUTION: See separate listing for Garcinia.

Scientific Names
Tamarindus indica.
Family: Leguminosae or Fabaceae.

People Use This For
Orally, tamarind is used for chronic or acute constipation, liver and gallbladder disorders, and to decrease fever (18).
Topically, a thick paste of the seeds is used as a cast for broken bones.
In China, tamarind is used to treat pregnancy-related nausea and as an anthelmintic in children.
In Arabia, it is used for stomach disorders, colds, and fevers.
In foods and beverages, tamarind is used as a flavoring agent . It is also widely used in Asian cuisine for chutneys and curries (11).

Safety
LIKELY SAFE ...when used orally and appropriately in amounts found in foods. It has Generally Recognized as Safe (GRAS) status in the US, and its maximum use is 0.81% (11).
There is insufficient reliable information available about the safety of tamarind used in amounts greater than those found in food.
PREGNANCY AND LACTATION: Insufficient reliable information available; avoid using in amounts greater than found in foods.

Effectiveness
There is insufficient reliable information available about the effectiveness of tamarind.

Mechanism of Action
The partially dried, fruit/pod of tamarind is used medicinally. It contains plant acids, largely d-tartaric acid, sugars, pectin, protein, vitamins, and minerals. The volatile oil contains over 60 compounds including methyl salicylate and safrole. The fruit pulp has mild laxative properties, but heat causes loss of this effect. Some evidence suggests an aqueous extract is highly toxic to the trematode Schistosoma mansoni, and the parasite-carrying snail Bulinus trucatus. Other evidence suggests that the tamarind constituent, tamarindienal might have antifungal activity against Aspergillus niger and Candida albicans, and antibacterial activity against Bacillus subtilis, Staphylococcus aureus, Escherichia coli, and Pseudomonas aeruginosa (11).

Adverse Reactions
None reported.

Interactions with Herbs & Other Dietary Supplements
Insufficient reliable information available.

Interactions with Drugs
No interactions are known to occur, and there is no known reason to expect a clinically significant interaction with tamarind.

Interactions with Foods

No interactions are known to occur, and there is no known reason to expect a clinically significant interaction with tamarind.

Interactions with Lab Tests

No interactions are known to occur, and there is no known reason to expect a clinically significant interaction with tamarind.

Interactions with Diseases or Conditions

No interactions are known to occur, and there is no known reason to expect a clinically significant interaction with tamarind.

Dosage and Administration

ORAL: As a laxative, 10-50 grams of tamarind paste is used orally as fruit cubes (18). This is a paste prepared from the fermented fruit of Tamarindus indica (18).

Comments

None.

TANNIC ACID

Also Known As

None.

Scientific Names

Tannic acid.

People Use This For

Topically, tannic acid is used for cold sores and fever blisters (272), diaper rash and prickly heat (272), poison ivy (272), ingrown toenails (272), sore throat, inflamed tonsils, spongy or receding gums, acute dermatitis, and as a styptic.
Vaginally, tannic acid is used as a douche for leukorrhea (12).
In Chinese medicine, nutgalls that contain a high concentration of tannic acid have been used to treat cancer.
In folk medicine, tannic acid has been used orally and topically for bleeding, chronic diarrhea, dysentery, bloody urine, painful joints, persistent coughs, and cancer (11).
In foods and beverages, tannic acid is used as a flavoring agent (11).
In manufacturing, it has been used in hemorrhoidal ointments and suppositories (11), for tanning hides and manufacturing ink (11), and to kill dust mites on furniture (272).

Safety

LIKELY SAFE ...when used orally in amounts found in foods. Tannic acid has Generally Recognized as Safe (GRAS) status in the US. The maximum use level is 0.018% (11).
POSSIBLY UNSAFE ...when used topically to treat diaper rash and prickly heat (272), and minor burn or sunburn (272). There is insufficient reliable information available about the safety of the topical use of tannic acid to treat cold sores and fever blisters. The FDA's concern about potential oral absorption and toxicity has prompted requests for further data (272).
PREGNANCY AND LACTATION: LIKELY UNSAFE ...when used topically on damaged skin or large areas of skin (2). There is insufficient reliable information available about the safety of the oral use of tannic acid during pregnancy and lactation; avoid using amounts greater than those found in foods.

Effectiveness

POSSIBLY INEFFECTIVE ...when used topically to treat cold sores and fever blisters (272). ...when used topically to treat diaper rash or prickly heat (272). ...when used topically to treat minor burn or sunburn (272).
There is insufficient reliable information available about the effectiveness of tannic acid for its other uses.

Mechanism of Action

Tannic acid is a mixture of glycosides of phenolics, mainly gallic acid (11). Pharmaceutical grade tannic acid is generally considered to be pentadigalloylglucose (11). Tannic acid has astringent effects (11,12). It dehydrates tissue, internally reducing secretions, and externally forming a protective layer of harder, constricted cells (12). Tannins show some evidence of antiviral, antimicrobial, CNS depressant, and cariostatic effects (11). Some evidence suggests that tannins might cause cancer, but other evidence shows tannins might prevent it (12). Regular consumption of herbs with high tannin concentrations correlates with increased incidence of esophageal or nasal cancer (12).

Adverse Reactions

Orally, large amounts of tannic acid can cause gastric irritation, nausea, and vomiting (11). Tannins have been associated with fatal liver damage from extensive use on burns or in enemas (11). However, the toxicity may be due to an impurity, digallic acid, rather than the tannins themselves (11).

Interactions with Herbs & Other Dietary Supplements

ORAL HERBS: Theoretically, herbs that contain high percentages of tannins (such as oak bark) might precipitate alkaloids and other alkaline constituents of herbs (19).

Interactions with Drugs

ORAL DRUGS: Theoretically, avoid concomitant administration due to potential of tannic acid to precipitate alkaloids and other basic drugs (19). Separate administration of oral drugs and tannic acid by the longest period of time practical (19).

Interactions with Foods

No interactions are known to occur, and there is no known reason to expect a clinically significant interaction with tannic acid.

Interactions with Lab Tests

No interactions are known to occur, and there is no known reason to expect a clinically significant interaction with tannic acid.

Interactions with Diseases or Conditions

KIDNEY DYSFUNCTION: Theoretically, oral use of tannic acid is contraindicated in individuals with kidney dysfunction. Tannic acid can cause kidney damage, potentially exacerbating a pre-existing condition (12).
LIVER DYSFUNCTION: Theoretically, oral of tannic acid is contraindicated in individuals with liver dysfunction. Tannic acid can cause liver damage, potentially exacerbating a pre-existing condition (12).
SKIN CONDITIONS: Full baths with tannic acid tea are contraindicated in individuals with weeping eczema and extensive skin damage (12).
PRE-EXISTING CONDITIONS: Theoretically, full baths are contraindicated in individuals with fever or infectious diseases, NYHA III and IV heart failure, or hypertonia stage IV (WHO) (2).

Dosage and Administration

No typical dosage.

Comments

New York Heart Association (NYHA) stage I and II heart disease refers to people with heart disease without resulting limitations of physical activity and who are comfortable at rest and in whom ordinary physical activity results in fatigue, palpitation, trouble breathing, or anginal pain (2). Tannic acid is extracted from the nutgalls formed on twigs of certain oak trees by insects (Quercus infectoria and other Quercus species). The "universal antidote," formerly used for poisoning, contained tannic acid, activated charcoal, and magnesium oxide. These three ingredients in combination were believed to synergistically reduce the absorption of poisons. Unfortunately, tannic acid was instead adsorbed by activated charcoal, which diminished the benefit of the combination (272).

TANSY

Also Known As

Bitter Buttons, Buttons, Chrysanthemi vulgaris flos, Chrysanthemi vulgaris herba, Daisy, Hindheal, Parsley Fern, Tansy Flower, Tansy Herb, Scented Fern, Stinking Willie.

Scientific Names

Tanacetum vulgare, synonym Chrysanthemum vulgare.
Family: Asteraceae or Compositae.

People Use This For

Topically, tansy is used for scabies, pruritus ani (4), bruises, sores, sprains, swelling, freckles, inflammation, leukorrhea, sunburn, swelling, toothache, tumors, and as an insect repellent (515,4009).

Traditionally, tansy is used orally for stimulating menstrual flow (5,6), as an abortifacient (2), an anthelmintic (2,18,515), for roundworm or threadworm infestation in children (4), migraines, neuralgia (4,6), epilepsy (4009), rheumatism, improving digestion and stimulating appetite (4009), as an antispasmodic (4,6), for flatulence (4), bloating due to intestinal or peritoneal gas (2,18), stomach and duodenal ulcers, noninflammatory gallbladder conditions, palpitation, sciatica, stomachache (4009), edema associated with weak heart, colds, fever, inducing sweating, hysteria, calming nerves, gout, kidney problems, or tuberculosis. Tansy above ground parts have also been used as an antioxidant, antiseptic, bactericide, cordial, narcotic, pediculicide, tonic, and stimulant (4009).

In foods and manufacturing, the extracts are used in perfume (6), as a flavoring agent in foods and beverages (4,515), and a source of green dye (6).

Safety

POSSIBLY UNSAFE ...when used topically. Tansy can cause severe contact dermatitis (6,18,19).

LIKELY UNSAFE ...when varieties containing the toxic constituent thujone are used orally (2,6,515). Fatalities have been associated with ingestion of as little as 10 drops of tansy oil, although one individual recovered after ingesting 15 mL (6). Fatalities have also been reported from prepared teas or powdered forms (4,6). However, thujone concentration varies widely amongst tansy species (4,6,515).

PREGNANCY: LIKELY UNSAFE ...when used topically due to potential abortifacient, menstrual flow, and uterine stimulant effects (12,19).

LACTATION: POSSIBLY UNSAFE ...when used topically due to thujone content (2,6).

Effectiveness

There is insufficient reliable information available about the effectiveness of tansy.

Mechanism of Action

The applicable parts of tansy are the above ground parts. The activity and toxicity of the above ground parts of tansy vary greatly according to the subspecies (515). Thujone, a constituent with both activity and toxicity ranging from a concentration of 0-95% in the volatile oil (4,515). The thujone constituent causes an increase in salivation and an increase in blood flow to the mucous membranes and pelvic viscera (7). Researchers think thujone has a mind-altering effect similar to tetrahydrocannabinol (THC), the active principle in marijuana (515). Thujone also shows evidence of neurotoxicity (2), hepatotoxicity, and it might be harmful to individuals with defects in hepatic heme synthesis (4,12). Chronic thujone poisoning leads to seizures, delirium, and hallucinations (7). Tansy extracts have demonstrated effects in alleviating pain, stimulating bile, and increasing appetite in individuals with liver and gallbladder disorders (4). Some evidence suggests tansy extracts might also have antispasmodic activity (4). Other evidence suggests the constituent, caffeic acid, might have a role in the bile-stimulating effects (4). Tansy shows evidence that it might reduce serum lipid levels and has some hypoglycemic effects (4). Tansy demonstrates antifungal activity (4). Some evidence suggests tansy oil has antibacterial activity (6). In addition, tansy oil, ether extract, and the constituent beta-thujone show evidence of anthelmintic activity (4). Aqueous extracts of tansy can partially inactivate tick-borne encephalitis in vitro. They also induce resistance in experimental animals (6). Preliminary studies suggest tansy has some antitumor effects (4). The constituents believed to be responsible for allergic contact dermatitis are the sesquiterpene lactones (4,6,19).

Adverse Reactions

Orally, large amounts of thujone or using thujone-containing products long-term can cause restlessness, vomiting, vertigo, tremors, renal damage, and convulsions (12). Symptoms of toxicity include rapid, feeble pulse (4,6), severe gastroenteritis (2), severe spasms (4), convulsions (2,4), rapid breathing (2), vomiting, abdominal pain, facial flushing, loss of consciousness, irregular heartbeat, dilated pupils, pupillary rigidity, uterine bleeding, abortion, kidney damage, and liver damage (2,18). Death can occur 1-3.5 hours after ingestion (18).

Topically, tansy is associated with severe contact dermatitis (6,19) and local mucosal membrane irritation (19). It can cause an allergic reaction in individuals sensitive to the Asteraceae/Compositae family. Members of this family include ragweed, chrysanthemums, marigolds, daisies, and many other herbs.

Interactions with Herbs & Other Dietary Supplements

THUJONE-CONTAINING HERBS: Concomitant use of herbs containing thujone can increase the risk of thujone toxicity. Thujone-containing herbs include oak moss, oriental arborvitae, sage, wormwood, thuja (cedar), and tree moss (12); avoid using.

Interactions with Drugs

ALCOHOL: The constituent, thujone, heightens and alters the effect of alcohol (7).

HYPOGLYCEMIC DRUGS: Theoretically, might interfere with hypoglycemic therapy and blood sugar control (4).

Interactions with Foods

No interactions are known to occur, and there is no known reason to expect a clinically significant interaction with tansy.

Interactions with Lab Tests

No interactions are known to occur, and there is no known reason to expect a clinically significant interaction with tansy.

Interactions with Diseases or Conditions

PORPHYRIA: Theoretically, can exacerbate porphyria in people with underlying defects in hepatic heme synthesis (12).

CROSS-ALLERGENICITY: Can cause an allergic reaction in individuals sensitive to the Asteraceae/Compositae family. Members of this family include ragweed, chrysanthemums, marigolds, daisies, and many other herbs.

Dosage and Administration

No typical dosage.

Comments

The name tansy is derived from the Greek word, athanasia, for immortality. Tansy was thought to impart mortality and it was used for embalming (6). Avoid confusion with tansy ragwort (Senecio species) and other plants generically referred to as "tansy".

TANSY RAGWORT

Also Known As

Cankerwort, Common Ragwort, Dog Standard, European Ragwort, Ragweed, Ragwort, St. James Wort, Staggerwort, Stammerwort, Stinking Nanny.
CAUTION: See separate listing for Golden Ragwort.

Scientific Names

Senecio jacoboea.
Family: Asteraceae/Compositae.

People Use This For

Orally, tansy ragwort is used for cancer, colic, wound-healing, spasms, as a laxative, to induce sweating and menstruation, and for "cleansing and purification".

Safety

UNSAFE …when used orally. Tansy ragwort contains hepatotoxic unsaturated pyrrolizidine alkaloids (UPAs) (12,19). Repeated exposure to low concentrations of UPAs linked to veno-occlusive disease, a serious condition (4,12). UPAs may also be carcinogenic and mutagenic (12). Topical use on abraded or broken skin might be unsafe due to potential for systemic absorption (12,19).

PREGNANCY: UNSAFE …when used orally because of possible menstruation promoting and oxytocic activity, and teratogenic effects (19).

LACTATION: UNSAFE …when used orally due to pyrrolizidine alkaloid (19).

Effectiveness

There is insufficient reliable information available about the effectiveness of tansy ragwort.

Mechanism of Action

The applicable parts of tansy ragwort are the above ground flowering parts. Some pyrrolizidine alkaloids have shown carcinogenic and mutagenic properties, and there are reports of renal toxicity. However, the primary concern is veno-occlusive disease (12). Unsaturated pyrrolizidine alkaloids are known to be hepatotoxic in animals and humans (4).

Adverse Reactions

Chronic exposure to plants containing UPA constituents has been associated with veno-occlusive disease (4021). Symptoms of acute veno-occlusive disease are characterized by a dull, dragging ache in the right upper abdomen and marked distention of the abdomen. These symptoms are sometimes accompanied by reduced urine output. Subacute veno-occlusive disease is associated with vague symptoms and persistent liver enlargement (4021). Tansy ragwort can cause an allergic reaction in individuals sensitive to the Asteraceae/Compositae family. Members of this family include ragweed, chrysanthemums, marigolds, daisies, and many other herbs.

Interactions with Herbs & Other Dietary Supplements

EUCALYPTUS: Theoretically, concomitant use might increase the risk of unsaturated pyrrolizidine alkaloid toxicity due to enzyme induction by eucalyptus (19).

PYRROLIZIDINE ALKALOID-CONTAINING HERBS: Concomitant use is contraindicated due to the risk of additive toxicity. Herbs containing unsaturated pyrrolizidine alkaloids include: alkanna (12), borage (271), gravel root (4), hemp agrimony (271), hound's tongue (19), petasites (19), comfrey (271), coltsfoot, and the Senecio species plants; dusty miller (19), alpine ragwort (19), groundsel (271), golden ragwort (19), and tansy ragwort (271).

Interactions with Drugs

No interactions are known to occur, and there is no known reason to expect a clinically significant interaction with tansy ragwort.

Interactions with Foods

No interactions are known to occur, and there is no known reason to expect a clinically significant interaction with tansy ragwort.

Interactions with Lab Tests

No interactions are known to occur, and there is no known reason to expect a clinically significant interaction with tansy ragwort.

Interactions with Diseases or Conditions

LIVER DISEASE: Contraindicated.

CROSS-ALLERGENICITY: Can cause an allergic reaction in individuals sensitive to the Asteraceae/Compositae family. Members of this family include ragweed, chrysanthemums, marigolds, daisies, and many other herbs.

Dosage and Administration

No typical dosage.

Comments

Both tansy ragwort and golden ragwort are known as ragweed and can therefore be confused (see separate listing). American Herbal Products Association recommends labeling all botanical products that contain toxic pyrrolizidine alkaloids "For external use only. Do not apply to broken or abraded skin; do not use when nursing" (12).

TARRAGON

Also Known As

Estragon, Little Dragon, Mugwort.
CAUTION: See separate listing for Mugwort (Artemisia vulgaris).

Scientific Names

Artemisia dracunculus.
Family: Asteraceae or Compositae.

People Use This For

Orally, tarragon is used for digestive disorders, toothache, to promote menstruation, as a diuretic, appetite stimulant, and hypnotic.
In foods and beverages, it is used as a culinary herb and a flavor component.
In manufacturing, tarragon is used as a fragrance component in soaps and cosmetics (11).

Safety

LIKELY SAFE ...when used in amounts found in foods. It has Generally Recognized as Safe (GRAS) status in the US. The maximum use level is 0.27% (11).
POSSIBLY SAFE ...when used orally short-term in medicinal amounts (12).
POSSIBLY UNSAFE ...for extended oral use due to estragole, which can be carcinogenic (12).
PREGNANCY AND LACTATION: LIKELY SAFE ...when used in food amounts. LIKELY UNSAFE ...when used in larger amounts due to possible menstrual promoting effects (11); avoid using.

Effectiveness

There is insufficient reliable information available about the effectiveness of tarragon.

Mechanism of Action

The applicable parts of tarragon are the above ground parts. Estragole is the main constituent of tarragon's essential oil (81%). The constituent estragole is a procarcinogen but the carcinogenic risk is minimal. It is not directly hepatotoxic or hepatocarcinogenic but requires activation by liver enzymes to reach full toxicity. In the liver other enzymes inactivate the carcinogenic metabolites, limiting possible damage to the liver (12). Tarragon shows evidence of antibacterial activity, but estragole does not appear to be responsible. Some information suggests undiluted tarragon oil can irritate the skin, but a concentration of 4% in petrolatum appears to be nonirritating and nonsensitizing (11).

Adverse Reactions

Tarragon can cause an allergic reaction in individuals sensitive to the Asteraceae/Compositae family. Members of this family include ragweed, chrysanthemums, marigolds, daisies, and many other herbs.

Interactions with Herbs & Other Dietary Supplements

Insufficient reliable information available.

Interactions with Drugs

No interactions are known to occur, and there is no known reason to expect a clinically significant interaction with tarragon.

Interactions with Foods

No interactions are known to occur, and there is no known reason to expect a clinically significant interaction with tarragon.

Interactions with Lab Tests

No interactions are known to occur, and there is no known reason to expect a clinically significant interaction with tarragon.

Interactions with Diseases or Conditions

CROSS-ALLERGENICITY: Can cause an allergic reaction in individuals sensitive to the Asteraceae/Compositae family. Members of this family include ragweed, chrysanthemums, marigolds, daisies, and many other herbs.

Dosage and Administration

No typical dosage.

Comments

Tarragon is also known as mugwort. Be careful not confuse it with mugwort (Artemisia vulgaris). Tarragon is a rich plant source of potassium (19). Adulteration of tarragon oil is common (11).

TAUMELLOOLCH

Also Known As

Bearded Darnel, Cheat, Darnel, Drake, Ray-Grass, Tare.

Scientific Names

Lolium temulentum.
Family: Poaceae.

People Use This For

Orally, taumelloolch is used for blood poisoning (4502), cancer (4502), cysts (4502), dizziness (18), eczema (4502), hemorrhage (4502), idiocy (4502), indurations (4502), "knots" (4502), leprosy (4502), migraine (4502), nerve pain (18), nose bleeds (18), putrid flesh (4502), sleeplessness (18), stomach cramps (18), involuntary dyskinetic movements (4502), toothache (4502), tumors (4502), and urinary incontinence (4502).
In children, taumelloolch is used orally for colic (4502).
Topically, taumelloolch is used as a poultice for skin diseases, to draw out splinters, and for broken bones (4502).
In folk medicine taumelloolch is used orally for gangrene (4502), headache (4502), meningitis (4502), neuralgia (4502), rheumatism (4502), and sciatica (4502).

Safety

LIKELY UNSAFE …when used orally. Symptoms of toxicity range from confusion and giddiness to weakness and death from respiratory failure (18,4502).

There is insufficient reliable information available about the safety of the topical use of taumelloolch.

PREGNANCY AND LACTATION: LIKELY UNSAFE (18,4502); avoid using.

Effectiveness

There is insufficient reliable information available about the effectiveness of taumelloolch.

Mechanism of Action

The applicable part of taumelloolch is the seed. The active agents of taumelloolch are temulentin, temultin acid, tannin, and glycoside (18). It has analgesic and narcotic properties, as well as toxicity (4502). Much of what is known about the toxicity of taumelloolch is anecdotal. Poisoning has been reported from ingestion of the grain, the berries mixed with grains, and the seed infected with a bacterial toxin (18,4502). To date, the toxic principle has not been identified (18,4502). No cases of poisonings have been reported in recent times, although the plant has become extremely rare through intensive seed-corn purification (18).

Adverse Reactions

Symptoms of taumelloolch toxicity include colic, confusion, giddiness, weakness, dizziness, dilated pupils, headache, confusion, staggering, somnolence, trembling, vision and speech disorders, vomiting, delirium, and death from respiratory failure (18,4502).

Interactions with Herbs & Other Dietary Supplements

Insufficient reliable information available.

Interactions with Drugs

No interactions are known to occur, and there is no known reason to expect a clinically significant interaction with taumelloolch.

Interactions with Foods

No interactions are known to occur, and there is no known reason to expect a clinically significant interaction with taumelloolch.

Interactions with Lab Tests

No interactions are known to occur, and there is no known reason to expect a clinically significant interaction with taumelloolch.

Interactions with Diseases or Conditions

No interactions are known to occur, and there is no known reason to expect a clinically significant interaction with taumelloolch.

Dosage and Administration

No typical dosage.

Comments

Taumelloolch is believed to be the tares of the biblical parable of the wheat and the tares (4502). Some information suggests that an ergot component extracted from the grass and seeds of taumelloolch is used by a mystic cult to induce religious ecstasy (4502).

TAURINE

Also Known As

Aminoethanesulfonate, L-Taurine.

Scientific Names

2-Aminoethane sulfonic acid.

People Use This For

Orally, taurine is used for the treatment of congestive heart failure (CHF) (5248), high blood pressure, high cholesterol (hypercholesterolemia), seizure disorders (epilepsy), and as an antioxidant (3467).

Safety

POSSIBLY SAFE ...when used orally and appropriately (5271). Taurine has been used safely in studies lasting 4 to 6 weeks (5248,5271).

PREGNANCY AND LACTATION: Insufficient reliable information available; avoid using.

Effectiveness

POSSIBLY EFFECTIVE ...when used orally for the treatment of congestive heart failure (CHF). Supplementation with taurine seems to improve left ventricular function (5248,5271) and symptoms of heart failure (5271,5306) in patients with New York Heart Association (NYHA) functional class II to IV. In some patients with severe heart failure NYHA functional class improved from IV to II after treatment for 4-8 weeks (5306).

There is insufficient reliable information about the effectiveness of taurine for its other uses.

Mechanism of Action

Taurine is a conditionally essential amino acid present in high amounts in meat and fish. The most common dietary source of taurine is human breast milk (272,3467). Taurine is normally synthesized in the human body in adequate amounts from cysteine and hypotaurine (272,3467) During prolonged times of insufficient intake, such as during parenteral nutrition, the body cannot maintain adequate levels of taurine and supplementation becomes necessary (3467). Supplementation is also necessary in non-breast-fed infants because their ability to synthesize taurine is undeveloped and cow's milk does not provide a sufficient amount (272,3467). Taurine is often added to human infant formulas, enteral products, and some parenteral nutritional solutions (272). Excess taurine is excreted by the kidneys (272,3467). Endogenous taurine is involved in retinal photoreceptor activity, bile acid conjugation, white blood cell antioxidant activity, central nervous system neuromodulation, platelet aggregation, cardiac contractility, sperm motility, growth, insulin activity (272), and osmoregulation (272,5280). Taurine is thought to be beneficial in the treatment of congestive heart failure (CHF) because some patients have lower levels of taurine in the heart muscle (3467). However, this is controversial (5315). Taurine seems to be involved in the regulation of intracellular calcium homeostasis (3467,5315). Taurine might also help because it seems to lower blood pressure and might normalize excessive sympathetic nervous system activity that often occurs in people with hypertension and CHF. Preliminary studies also suggest taurine might have natriuretic and diuretic activity (3467). Taurine might also have a cholesterol-lowering effect. Taurine seems to stimulate bile acid synthesis (3467). There is some evidence that taurine might also have antioxidant and free radical scavenging activity (3467). Platelets normally have high levels of taurine, and can become more prone to aggregation during taurine depletion. However, it is unknown if taurine supplementation has any effect on platelet coagulation (3467).

Adverse Reactions

None reported.

Interactions with Herbs & Other Dietary Supplements

Insufficient reliable information available.

Interactions with Drugs

No interactions are known to occur, and there is no known reason to expect a clinically significant interaction with taurine.

Interactions with Foods

No interactions are known to occur, and there is no known reason to expect a clinically significant interaction with taurine.

Interactions with Lab Tests

No interactions are known to occur, and there is no known reason to expect a clinically significant interaction with taurine.

Interactions with Diseases or Conditions

No interactions are known to occur, and there is no known reason to expect a clinically significant interaction with taurine.

Dosage and Administration

ORAL: For the treatment of congestive heart failure, 2-4 grams per day has been used in clinical studies (3467,5248,5306).

Comments

None.

TEA TREE OIL

Also Known As

Australian Tea Tree Oil, Melaleuca Oil, Oil of Melaleuca, Oleum Melaleucae.
CAUTION: See separate listings for Cajeput Oil and Niauli Oil.

Scientific Names

Melaleuca alternifolia.
Family: Myrtaceae.

People Use This For

Topically, tea tree oil is commonly used for skin and skin surface infections such as acne, onychomycosis, lice, scabies, athletes foot (4031), and ringworm (9,11,515,4028). It is also used topically as a local antiseptic for cuts and abrasions, for burns, insect bites and stings, boils, vaginal infections, infections of the mouth and nose, sore throat (9,11,515), and for ear infections such as otitis media and otitis externa (7025).
It is also used as a bath additive to treat cough, bronchial congestion, and pulmonary inflammation (11).

Safety

POSSIBLY SAFE ...when used topically and appropriately (11,512,4028).
LIKELY UNSAFE ...when used orally. Like other essential oils, tea tree oil can cause significant toxicity if used orally (17,515,4028).
CHILDREN: POSSIBLY SAFE ...when used topically and appropriately (11,512). LIKELY UNSAFE ...when used orally. Ingestion of tea tree oil can be toxic (17,515,4030).
PREGNANCY AND LACTATION: POSSIBLY SAFE ...when used topically and appropriately (11,512). LIKELY UNSAFE ...when used orally. Ingestion of tea tree oil can be toxic (17,515).

Effectiveness

POSSIBLY EFFECTIVE ...when used topically for treating acne vulgaris (11,515,6006). Daily application of a 5% tea tree oil gel for 3 months seems to significantly reduce the average number of acne lesions. Improvement seems to be similar to treatment with 5% benzoyl peroxide (6006). ...when used topically for tinea pedis (athlete's foot). Application of a 10% tea tree oil cream seems comparable to tolnaftate 1% cream (Genaspor, Tinactin, Ting, and others) for relieving symptoms of athlete's foot, including scaling, inflammation, itching, and burning. However, application of 10% tea tree oil cream appears no more effective than placebo in producing a mycological cure for tinea pedis (4031,6006). ...when used topically for onychomycosis. There is some evidence that highly concentrated tea tree oil can be helpful for onychomycosis. Application of 100% tea tree oil solution twice daily for 6 months can produce a mycological cure in about 18% of patients with toenail infections. It can also improve nail appearance and symptoms in about 56% of patients after 3 months and 60% of patients after 6 months of treatment. It seems to be comparable to twice daily application of clotrimazole 1% solution (Fungoid, Lotrimin, Lotrimin AF) (7031). Lower concentrations of tea tree oil do not seem to be as effective. For example, there is some evidence that a 5% tea tree oil cream applied three times daily for 2 months has no beneficial effect (7032). There is insufficient reliable information available about the effectiveness of tea tree oil for its other uses.

Mechanism of Action

Tea tree oil is obtained by the distillation of the leaves of the tea tree. The oil contains more than 100 monoterpenoid, sesquiterpenoid and alcohol compounds. Up to 90% is made up of terpinen-4-ol, 1,8-cineole, alpha-terpineol, terpinolene, and alpha- and gamma-terpinene (4027,7111). The primary constituent terpinen-4-ol is active against numerous pathogenic bacteria (5,6,9,11,515) and fungi (6,9) but seems to spare normal skin flora (6). The constituents, alpha-terpineol and linalool, may also contribute to its antimicrobial activity (515). Tea tree oil has in vitro activity against Enterococcus faecium and Enterococcus faecalis, including vancomycin-resistant strains, Klebsiella pneumoniae, including gentamicin-resistant strains, Stenotrophomonas maltophilia, and methicillin-sensitive Staphylococcus aureus. Tea tree oil seems to have less activity against Methicillin-resistant Staphylococcus aureus and Pseudomonas aeruginosa. Oils produced with increased concentrations of terpinen-4-ol seem to have greater activity against these organisms (7111). The constituent alpha-limonene may be responsible for the adverse effect of contact eczema (6).

Adverse Reactions

Orally, tea tree oil and other essential oils can cause significant toxicity. Tea tree oil can cause confusion, inability to walk, disorientation, ataxia, systemic contact dermatitis, and a eucalyptus-like odor on the breath (17,4028). There is at least one case of coma following ingestion of 120 mL of tea tree oil (4028). Ingestion of as little as 2.5 mL of tea tree oil can cause petechial body rash and neutrophil leukocytosis. It can take up to a week for symptoms to resolve (6). In young children, ingestion of 10 mL or less of tea tree oil might cause significant ataxia and drowsiness (4030). Topically, tea tree oil is usually well tolerated; however, it can cause local irritation and inflammation (5), allergic contact eczema, and allergic contact dermatitis in some patients (658,4027,4029). There is some concern that topical use of tea tree oil in the middle ear for treatment of ear infections might cause ototoxicity. There is preliminary evidence that preparations of 100% tea tree oil can cause ototoxicity and impaired hearing. However, so far there are no reports of ototoxicity in humans. Until more is known, tell patients to avoid such highly concentrated tea tree oil preparations. Lower concentrations of 2% tea tree oil seem less likely to have this effect (7025).

Interactions with Herbs & Other Dietary Supplements
Insufficient reliable information available.

Interactions with Drugs
No interactions are known to occur, and there is no known reason to expect a clinically significant interaction with tea tree oil.

Interactions with Foods
No interactions are known to occur, and there is no known reason to expect a clinically significant interaction with tea tree oil.

Interactions with Lab Tests
No interactions are known to occur, and there is no known reason to expect a clinically significant interaction with tea tree oil.

Interactions with Diseases or Conditions
No interactions are known to occur, and there is no known reason to expect a clinically significant interaction with tea tree oil.

Dosage and Administration
TOPICAL: For acne, 5% tea tree oil gel applied daily has been used (6006). For tinea pedis (athlete's foot), 10% tea tree oil cream applied twice daily for 1 month has been used (4031,6006). For onychomycosis, 100% tea tree oil solution applied twice daily for 6 months has been used (7031).

Comments
Tea tree oil has the aroma of nutmeg (515). The tea tree was named by eighteenth century sailors who made an aromatic tea from the leaves of the tree growing on the swampy southeast Australian coast (515). Do not confuse the tea tree with the unrelated common tea plant that is used to make black and green teas. Tea tree oil was used during World War II to treat skin injuries of workers in munitions factories and was commonly used in surgery and dentistry in the mid 1920s (6). Avoid confusion with cajeput oil and niauli oil.

TEAZLE

Also Known As
Barber's Brush, Brushes and Combs, Card Thistle, Church Broom, Teasel, Venus' Basin.

Scientific Names
Dipsacus silvestris.
Family: Dipsacaceae.

People Use This For
Topically, teazle is used for small wounds, fistulae, psoriasis, and as a rub for arthritis (18).

Safety
There is insufficient reliable information available about the safety of teazle.
Pregnancy and Lactation: Insufficient reliable information available; avoid using.

Effectiveness
There is insufficient reliable information available about the effectiveness of teazle.

Mechanism of Action
The applicable part of teazle is the root. There is insufficient reliable information available about the possible mechanism of action and active ingredients.

Adverse Reactions
None reported.

Interactions with Herbs & Other Dietary Supplements
Insufficient reliable information available.

Interactions with Drugs
No interactions are known to occur, and there is no known reason to expect a clinically significant interaction with teazle.

Interactions with Foods
No interactions are known to occur, and there is no known reason to expect a clinically significant interaction with teazle.

Interactions with Lab Tests
No interactions are known to occur, and there is no known reason to expect a clinically significant interaction with teazle.

Interactions with Diseases or Conditions
No interactions are known to occur, and there is no known reason to expect a clinically significant interaction with teazle

Dosage and Administration
TOPICAL: Teazle is used as an alcoholic extract (18).

Comments
Avoid confusing teazle with boneset, which is also called teasel. (18).
There is very little scientific information about this product. Our staff is continually analyzing the available information on natural medicines and will add data here as it becomes available.

TERMINALIA

Also Known As
Arjuna, Axjun Argun, Bahera, Bahira, Bala Harade, Balera, Behada, Beleric Myrobalan, Bihara, Chebulic Myrobalan, Hara, Harada, Haritaki, He Zi, Hirala, Indian Almond, Myrobalan.

Scientific Names
Terminalia arjuna; Terminalia bellirica, synonym Terminalia belerica; Terminalia chebula.
Family: Combretaceae.

People Use This For
Orally, Terminalia arjuna is used for cardiovascular conditions, including ischemic heart disease and angina, hypertension, and hyperlipidemia (6,33). It is also used orally as a diuretic, for earaches, dysentery, venereal and urogenital diseases, and as an aphrodisiac (6,33,3565).
Orally, Terminalia belerica and Terminalia chebula are used for hyperlipidemia (2527,2519) and digestive disorders, including both diarrhea and constipation, and indigestion (6,33). They have also been used for HIV infection (2518). Terminalia belerica is also used orally as a hepatoprotectant and for respiratory conditions, including respiratory tract infections, cough, and sore throat (6,33). Terminalia chebula is also used orally for dysentery (33).
Topically, Terminalia belerica and Terminalia chebula are used as a lotion for sore eyes. Terminalia chebula is also used topically as a mouthwash and gargle (6,33).
Intravaginally, Terminalia chebula is used as a douche for treating vaginitis (6,33).
In traditional Ayurvedic medicine, Terminalia belerica has been used as a "health-harmonizer" in combination with Terminalia chebula and Emblica officinalis (6). This combination is also used to lower cholesterol and to prevent necrosis of cardiac tissue (6). In traditional Ayurvedic medicine, Terminalia arjuna has been used to balance the three humors, kapha, pitta, and vata (6,33). It has also been used for asthma, bile duct disorders, scorpion stings, and for poisonings (33).

Safety
POSSIBLY SAFE ...when used orally and appropriately, short term. Several small studies have used the powdered bark of Terminalia arjuna safely in cardiac patients in trials lasting from 2 weeks to 3 months (2502,2503,2504); however,

patients should avoid self-treatment with this product, due to the potentially significant cardiovascular effects. Further study is needed to determine the safety of Terminalia arjuna for long-term use.

There is insufficient reliable information available about the safety of Terminalia belerica and Terminalia chebula (6).

PREGNANCY: POSSIBLY UNSAFE ...when used orally. One source warns against using Terminalia belerica and Terminalia chebula during pregnancy; however, the reason for this warning is not described (33); avoid using.

There is insufficient reliable information available about the safety of Terminalia arjuna in pregnancy; avoid using.

LACTATION: Insufficient reliable information available; avoid using.

Effectiveness

POSSIBLY EFFECTIVE ...when used orally as a short-term adjunct to conventional therapy for treating postmyocardial infarction angina. In one small clinical trial, postmyocardial infarction patients with angina received the standard therapy of nitrates, aspirin, and/or a calcium channel blocker plus the powdered bark of Terminalia arjuna or the standard therapy alone for 3 months. Patients receiving Terminalia arjuna experienced significantly less angina, improved left ventricular ejection fractions, and decreased left ventricular mass compared to patients receiving the standard therapy alone (2502,2503). ...when Terminalia arjuna is used as a short-term adjunct to conventional therapy for treating severe congestive heart failure. In a small cross-over trial, patients with severe, refractory congestive heart failure had significant reductions in symptoms and improved left ventricular function after 2 weeks of treatment (2504). Large-scale, long-term trials are necessary to clarify Terminalia arjunas' potential role in the treatment of cardiovascular conditions.

There is insufficient reliable information available for the effectiveness of Terminalia belerica and Terminalia cebula for any medicinal use.

Mechanism of Action

There are three species of terminalia of medicinal interest: Terminalia arjuna, Terminalia belerica and Terminalia chebula (6,33). The applicable part of Terminalia arjuna is the bark. The bark contains several active constituents, including Terminalia arjuna gallic acid, ethyl gallate, and the flavone luteolin. Luteolin may have anticancer properties (2506). The bark of Terminalia arjuna is reported to be beneficial in cardiovascular conditions; however, the exact mechanism is not known. Terminalia arjuna is reported to lower serum cholesterol and low-density lipoprotein (LDL) levels (2505,2517,2519). It is also thought to have an antihypertensive effect and act as a cardiac stimulant. However, studies have been conflicting; some indicating that it may actually increase blood pressure (33). The applicable part of Terminalia belerica and Terminalia chebula is the fruit (6). These species also have been reported to improve lipid profiles, but to a lesser degree than Terminalia arjuna. Terminalia chebula is reported to have a greater effect on lipids than Terminalia belerica (2517,2519). The astringent properties of Terminalia belerica and Terminalia chebula are attributed to their beneficial effects in bowel irregularity and indigestion (33). Terminalia belerica also contains gallic acid, and is thought to have hepatoprotective properties (2507). An ethanolic extract of Terminalia chebula containing gallic acid and its ethyl ester may have activity against methicillin-resistant Staphylococcus aureus (2508). Terminalia chebula may also have activity against cytomegalovirus (CMV), herpes simplex I, Streptococcus mutans, Salmonella sp., Shigella, and retroviral reverse transcriptase (2509,2510,2511,2512,2513,2514). Both Terminalia belerica and Terminalia chebula may have activity against HIV (2518). The gallic acid and chebulagic acid in Terminalia chebula may have immunosuppressive effects against cytotoxic T lymphocytes (2515).

Adverse Reactions

None reported in humans. In animal studies, Terminalia chebula has caused hepatic and renal lesions (2516).

Interactions with Herbs & Other Dietary Supplements

Insufficient reliable information available.

Interactions with Drugs

No interactions are known to occur, and there is no known reason to expect a clinically significant interaction with terminalia.

Interactions with Foods

No interactions are known to occur, and there is no known reason to expect a clinically significant interaction with terminalia.

Interactions with Lab Tests

No interactions are known to occur, and there is no known reason to expect a clinically significant interaction with terminalia.

Interactions with Diseases or Conditions

No interactions are known to occur, and there is no known reason to expect a clinically significant interaction with terminalia.

Dosage and Administration

ORAL: For improving left ventricular function, treating postmyocardial infarction anginal pain as an adjunct to conventional therapy, and congestive failure, a dose of the powdered bark of Terminalia arjuna 500 mg every 8 hours has been used (2502,2503,2504).

Comments

The bark of Terminalia arjuna has been used in India for more than 3000 years, primarily as a heart remedy. An Indian physician named Vagbhata has been credited as the first to use this product for heart conditions in the seventh century A.D. Research on Terminalia has been going on since the 1930s, but pharmacological studies have provided mixed results. Its role in heart disease remains unclear.

THIAMINE (VITAMIN B1)

Also Known As

Antiberiberi Factor, Antiberiberi Vitamin, Antineuritic Factor, Antineuritic Vitamin, Anurine, Aneurine Hydrochloride, B complex Vitamin, Thiamin Chloride, Thiamin Hydrochloride, Thiamine Chloride, Thiamine Hydrochloride, Thiaminium Chloride Hydrochloride.

Scientific Names

Thiamine; Thiamin; Vitamin B1; Vitamin B-1.

People Use This For

Orally, thiamine is used for thiamine deficiency syndromes, including beriberi, peripheral neuritis associated with pellagra, and neuritis of pregnancy. It is used for poor appetite, ulcerative colitis, chronic diarrhea, GI disorders, cerebellar syndrome, an insect repellent (15), diabetic neuropathy, AIDS (14), maintaining a positive mental attitude, enhancing learning abilities, heart disease, alcoholism, stress, and aging. Thiamine is also used orally for canker sores, immunodepression, memory loss including Alzheimer's disease, vision problems such as cataracts and glaucoma, motion sickness, and increasing energy (3027,3028,3029,3030).

By injection, thiamine is used for Wernicke's encephalopathy syndrome, other thiamine deficiency syndromes in critically ill people, acute alcohol withdrawal, and coma or hypothermia of unknown origin (14,15).

Safety

LIKELY SAFE ...when used orally and is generally considered nontoxic; although, rare hypersensitivity reactions have occurred (15). ...when used appropriately as the injectable FDA-approved prescription product.

PREGNANCY AND LACTATION: LIKELY SAFE ...when used orally at the recommended dietary allowance (RDA) of 1.4 mg per day (3094). There is insufficient reliable information available about the safety of using larger amounts during pregnancy or lactation.

Effectiveness

EFFECTIVE ...when used orally for the treatment of thiamine deficiency syndromes including beriberi and peripheral neuritis associated with pellagra or neuritis of pregnancy. ...when used orally as a dietary supplement to prevent deficiency in people with malabsorption conditions such as alcoholism, cirrhosis, and GI diseases, in those with inadequate intake due to severe anorexia, nausea, or vomiting, and in those with increased requirements due to pregnancy, increased carbohydrate intake, increased physical activity, hyperthyroidism, infection, and hepatic disease, although deficiency is rare with these conditions. ...when used orally for temporary correction of metabolic disorders associated with genetic diseases such as subacute necrotizing encephalopathy (SNE, Leigh's disease), maple syrup urine disease (branched-chain aminoacidopathy), and lactic acidosis associated with pyruvate carboxylase deficiency and hyperalaninemia (15). ...when used as the FDA-approved, prescription-only, injectable (IM, IV) product.

POSSIBLY EFFECTIVE ...when used orally for diabetic neuropathy (14). ...when used orally to reduce the occurrence of cataracts. A large-scale population-based study found high dietary intake of thiamine was associated with a reduced risk of nuclear cataracts (6378).

There is insufficient reliable information available about the effectiveness of thiamine for its other uses.

Mechanism of Action

Thiamine is required for carbohydrate metabolism (15). It combines with adenosine triphosphate (ATP) to form thiamine diphosphate, a coenzyme in carbohydrate metabolism, wherein the decarboxylation of pyruvic acid and alpha-ketoglutaric acid occurs. This coenzyme is also a part of transketolation reactions (15). Thiamine is also a coenzyme in the utilization of pentose in the hexose monophosphate shunt (15). Thiamine deficiency leads to decreased transketolase activity in erythrocytes and to increased pyruvic acid concentration in the blood, both of which can be used to diagnose deficiency (15). Pyruvic acid is converted to lactic acid, and lactic acidosis can therefore occur in vitamin B1 deficiency (15). Syndromes associated with vitamin B1 deficiency are beriberi and Wernicke-Korsakoff syndrome (3041). Beriberi is characterized by anorexia; abdominal discomfort; constipation; peripheral neurologic changes; sleep disturbance; poor memory; and sometimes cardiovascular symptoms, including dyspnea, edema, palpitations, vasodilation, warm extremities, and high output cardiac failure. Wernicke-Korsakoff syndrome is characterized by confusion, aphonia, confabulation, nystagmus, ophthalmoplegia, and coma. In Crohn's disease, decreased serum thiamine levels have been reported (6269).

Adverse Reactions

Orally, thiamine rarely can cause dermatitis and other hypersensitivity reactions (14).
Injection of thiamine can cause feelings of warmth, tingling, pruritus, pain, urticaria, weakness, sweating, nausea, restlessness, tightness of the throat, angioedema, respiratory distress, cyanosis, pulmonary edema, GI bleeding, transient vasodilation and hypotension, vascular collapse, and death. Tenderness and induration can occur at IM injection sites (15).

Interactions with Herbs & Other Dietary Supplements

HORSETAIL: Theoretically, it might cause the breakdown of thiamine (19).

Interactions with Drugs

NEUROMUSCULAR BLOCKING AGENTS: Concomitant use of thiamine can enhance the effects of neuromuscular blocking agents (15).

Drug Influences on Nutrient Levels and Depletion

SOME DRUGS CAN AFFECT THIAMINE LEVELS:
ANTIBIOTICS: Destruction of normal gastrointestinal flora by antibiotics can cause decreased production of B vitamins. The clinical significance of this decreased production is not known. Consider supplementation only if clinical judgment warrants it (4434,4435,4436,4437,4438,4439,4440,4441,4442,4443).
LOOP DIURETICS: Use of loop diuretics can increase urinary thiamine excretion resulting in thiamine depletion. Thiamine depletion might contribute to impaired heart function in some patients with congestive heart failure (CHF) treated long-term with furosemide. Supplementation with 200 mg thiamine (orally or intravenously) per day can replete thiamine, and in some cases, improve left ventricular function in patients with congestive heart failure (CHF) treated with furosemide. Consider thiamine supplementation in patients using loop diuretics, especially long-term (1282,1283,1284,1285,1286).

Interactions with Foods

No interactions are known to occur, and there is no known reason to expect a clinically significant interaction with thiamine.

Interactions with Lab Tests

URIC ACID: Thiamine can cause false positive results in the phosphotungstate method for uric acid determination (15).
UROBILINOGEN: Thiamine can cause false positive results in the urine spot test with Ehrlich's reagent for urobilinogen (15).
SERUM THEOPHYLLINE: Large amounts of thiamine can interfere with Schack and Waxler spectrophotometric determination of serum theophylline concentrations (15).

Interactions with Diseases or Conditions

ALCOHOLISM, CIRRHOSIS, MALABSORPTION SYNDROMES: Thiamine absorption is decreased in these conditions (15).

Dosage and Administration

ORAL: As a dietary supplement in adults, 1-2 mg per day is commonly used. For mild thiamine deficiency syndromes in adults, the usual dose of thiamine is 5-30 mg daily in either a single dose or divided doses for one month (14,15). The typical dose for severe deficiency can be up to 300 mg per day (14). Parenteral thiamine is recommended for critically ill people (15). For genetic enzyme deficiency disorders, 10-20 mg daily is recommended, although 600-4000 mg daily in divided doses may be needed for Leigh's disease (14,15). For maple syrup urine disease, 100-200 mg daily is recommended, although up to 1000 mg has been used (14). A daily dietary intake of approximately 10 mg of thiamine has been associated with reducing the risk of nuclear cataracts (6378).

The daily recommended dietary allowances (RDAs) of thiamine are: Infants 0-6 months, 0.2 mg; Infants 7-12 months, 0.3 mg; Children 1-3 years, 0.5 mg; Children 4-8 years, 0.6 mg; Males 9-13 years, 0.9 mg; Males 14 years and older, 1.2 mg; Females 9-13 years, 0.9 mg; Women 14-18 years, 1 mg; Women over 18 years, 1.1 mg; Pregnant women, 1.4 mg; and Lactating women, 1.5 mg (3094).
INJECTION: IM or slow IV.

Comments

Thiamine is present in many foods including yeast, cereal grains, legumes, nuts, and meat (15). Thiamine is frequently used in combination with other B vitamins in vitamin B complex formulations. Vitamin B complex generally includes vitamin B1 (thiamine), vitamin B2 (riboflavin), vitamin B3 (niacin/niacinamide), vitamin B5 (pantothenic acid), vitamin B6 (pyridoxine), vitamin B12 (cyanocobalamin), and folic acid. However, some products do not contain all of these ingredients and some may include others, such as biotin, para-aminobenzoic acid (PABA), choline bitartrate, and inositol (3022,3060,3061).

THUNDER GOD VINE

Also Known As

Huang-T'eng Ken, Lei Gong Teng, Lei-Kung T'eng, Taso-Ho-Hua, Threewingnut, Yellow Vine.

Scientific Names

Tripterygium wilfordii.
Family: Celastraceae.

People Use This For

Orally, thunder god vine is used for rheumatoid arthritis, excessive menstrual periods, multiple sclerosis, and as a male contraceptive (6). In Chinese medicine, it is used for abscesses, boils, fever, inflammation (6), systemic lupus erythematosus (SLE), psoriasis, and Behcet's disease (1442).
Thunder god vine has also been used non-medicinally as an insecticide against maggots or larvae, and as a rat and bird poison (6).

Safety

LIKELY UNSAFE ...when used orally. Use of thunder god vine has been associated with significant side effects (see Adverse Reactions) (6).
PREGNANCY: LIKELY UNSAFE ...when used orally. Thunder god vine is thought to be teratogenic (6,4047); avoid using.
LACTATION: Insufficient reliable information available; avoid using.

Effectiveness

POSSIBLY EFFECTIVE ...when used orally as a male contraceptive. Thunder god vine seems to reversibly inhibit sperm motility and production. Normalization of sperm function typically returns six weeks after discontinuation of treatment (6,4046). ...when used orally as adjunctive treatment for rheumatoid arthritis. There is some evidence that thunder god vine produces additive symptom relief in patients concurrently taking nonsteroidal anti-inflammatory drugs (NSAIDs) (4046).
There is insufficient reliable information available about the effectiveness of thunder god vine for its other uses.

Mechanism of Action

The applicable parts of thunder god vine are the leaf and root. Thunder god vine leaf and root are reported to have antifertility effects in males, and immunosuppressive, antiviral, and antitumor activities (6). Thunder god vine appears to inhibit spermatogenesis and reduce sperm motility without affecting testosterone levels. These activities are attributed to triptolide and tripdiolide, and possibly four other compounds (6). Male fertility appears to return to normal six weeks after discontinuation (6). The immunosuppressive effects of thunder god vine are attributed to the constituents tripchlorolide, tribromolide, and demethylzeylasteral (6). Thunder god vine shows evidence of multiple mechanisms of immunosuppression. It inhibits production of cytokine IL2 and gamma interferon; it inhibits response of human mononuclear cells; and it inhibits generation of cytotoxic T-cells (6). T-2, an alcoholic extract that contains triptolide and tripdiolide, inhibits T-cell and B-cell proliferation, as well as immunoglobulin production by B-cells (6,1442). Several diterpenes, including triptolide and tripdiolide show evidence of anti-inflammatory and immunosuppressive effects (6). Low doses of triptolide show evidence of antitumor and antileukemic effects (6). The isolated constituent, triterene, inhibits antibody response and granuloma growth in rats (6). Demethylzeylasteral has anti-angiogenic effects (6). Neotripteriforidin, tripteriforidin, and salaspermic acid exhibit potent anti-HIV replication activity in vitro (6,4048,4049).

Adverse Reactions

Oral use of thunder god vine is associated with gastrointestinal upset, infertility, lymphocytes suppression (6), and skin reactions (4046). Women using the extract "T2" developed amenorrhea (6). Adverse effects appear to be more prevalent with immediate-release products than with sustained release products (6). There is one report of a young male with some evidence of pre-existing heart damage who developed vomiting, diarrhea, leukopenia, renal failure, hypotension, shock, and died three days after ingestion (6). There is also one report of an infant born with meningoencephalocele after the mother used thunder god vine for rheumatoid arthritis during pregnancy (4047).

Interactions with Herbs & Other Dietary Supplements

Insufficient reliable information available.

Interactions with Drugs

IMMUNOSUPPRESSANTS: Theoretically, concomitant use might enhance drug effects. Immunosuppressant drugs include azathioprine (Imuran), basiliximab (Simulect), cyclosporine (Neoral, Sandimmune), daclizumab (Zenapax), muromonab-CD3 (OKT3, Orthoclone OKT3), mycophenolate (CellCept), tacrolimus (FK506, Prograf), sirolimus (Rapamune), prednisone (Deltasone, Orasone), and other corticosteroids (glucocorticoids).

Interactions with Foods

No interactions are known to occur, and there is no known reason to expect a clinically significant interaction with thunder god vine.

Interactions with Lab Tests

No interactions are known to occur, and there is no known reason to expect a clinically significant interaction with thunder god vine.

Interactions with Diseases or Conditions

IMMUNE SYSTEM COMPROMISE: Theoretically, thunder god vine might exacerbate these conditions (6).

Dosage and Administration

ORAL: Rheumatoid arthritis, 30 mg thunder god vine polyglycoside extract per day was used in one study (6).

Comments

None.

THYME flower, leaf

Also Known As

Common Thyme, French Thyme, Garden Thyme, Rubbed Thyme, Spanish Thyme, Thymi herba.
CAUTION: See separate listings for Thyme Oil and Wild Thyme.

Scientific Names

Thymus vulgaris; Thymus zygis.
Family: Lamiaceae.

People Use This For

Orally, thyme is used for bronchitis, pertussis (2,18), sore throat, colic, and dyspnea (6121).
Topically, thyme is used for upper respiratory tract mucous membrane inflammation, laryngitis, tonsillitis (2,18), stomatitis, and halitosis (1).
In folk medicine, thyme was used as an appetite stimulant (11), for dyspepsia, chronic gastritis, diarrhea in children, enuresis in children (4), as an antiflatulent, diuretic, urinary disinfectant, anthelmintic (18), and for rheumatic and skin disorders (11).
In foods, thyme is used as a culinary herb (4,11).

Safety

LIKELY SAFE ...when used in the amounts found in foods (11). Thyme has Generally Recognized as Safe (GRAS) status in the US (11). Maximum use of thyme in foods is 0.172%. Maximum use of thyme oil is 0.003% (11).
POSSIBLY SAFE ...when used orally and appropriately (1,2,12). ...when used topically and appropriately (18). There is insufficient reliable information available about the safety of thyme in larger amounts; avoid using (4).

PREGNANCY: LIKELY SAFE ...when used in food amounts. UNSAFE ...when used in larger amounts because it might induce menstruation (4,19).
LACTATION: LIKELY SAFE ...when used in food amounts.

Effectiveness
POSSIBLY EFFECTIVE ...when used for symptoms of bronchitis and pertussis (1,2). ...when used topically for upper respiratory tract mucous inflammation (2), stomatitis, and halitosis (1).
There is insufficient reliable information available about the effectiveness of thyme for its other uses.

Mechanism of Action
Thyme contains thymol, carvacrol, and flavonoid constituents, which are responsible for the antispasmodic, antitussive, and expectorant effects (4). This explains why thyme is used as an antiflatulent, antispasmodic, antitussive, astringent, expectorant, antibacterial, anthelmintic, and to stimulate saliva (2,4,18). There may also be phenolic compounds of the volatile oil and flavonoids associated with antispasmodic activity. This mechanism may involve calcium channel blockade. However, some scientists question whether the phenolic components are involved (4). The antibacterial and antifungal activity is associated with the thymol and carvacrol (1). Thymol also demonstrates anthelmintic activity (4). The constituent, rosmarinic acid, reduces experimentally-induced edema, inhibits passive cutaneous anaphylaxis, and impairs experimental activation of macrophages in vivo (1). In animals, the thyme extract seems to have analgesic and antipyretic effects (4). The thymus vulgaris also has antithyrotropic activity (11). The fluid extracts show antispasmodic activity in smooth muscle, but the active constituents causing this activity have not been identified (11).

Adverse Reactions
Topically thyme oil can lead to irritation (4). There is a low potential for sensitization (18).

Interactions with Herbs & Other Dietary Supplements
Insufficient reliable information available.

Interactions with Drugs
No interactions are known to occur, and there is no known reason to expect a clinically significant interaction with thyme.

Interactions with Foods
No interactions are known to occur, and there is no known reason to expect a clinically significant interaction with thyme.

Interactions with Lab Tests
No interactions are known to occur, and there is no known reason to expect a clinically significant interaction with thyme.

Interactions with Diseases or Conditions
URINARY TRACT INFLAMMATION: CAUTION, use might exacerbate inflammation (19).
GI IRRITATION (e.g., ulcers, etc.): CAUTION, use might exacerbate inflammation (19).
CROSS-ALLERGENICITY: CAUTION, cross-reactivity to oregano and other Labiatae species reported in an individual allergic to thyme (3808).
OTHER: When used as a bath, be cautious in cases of extensive skin injuries or disease, or in cases involving high fever or infectious disease, cardiac insufficiency or hypertonia (18).

Dosage and Administration
ORAL: 1-2 grams dried leaf/flower several times daily, or one cup tea (steep 1-2 grams dried leaf/flower in 150 mL boiling water for 10 minutes, strain) several times daily as needed (1,2,18); not to exceed 10 grams dried leaf with 0.03% phenol (calculated as thymol) per day (18). Fluid extract, 1-2 grams up to three times daily (2).
TOPICAL: Gargle (1) or compress (2,18), steep 5 grams dried leaf per 100 mL boiling water 10 minutes, strain (1,2,18).

Comments
Thyme is a plant rich in iron (19).

THYME OIL

Also Known As

Common Thyme, Red Thyme Oil, Spanish Thyme, Thyme Aetheroleum, Thyme Oil, White Thyme Oil.
CAUTION: See separate listings for Thyme, Spanish Origanum oil, and Wild Thyme.

Scientific Names

Thyme vulgaris, Thymus vulgaris, Thymus zygis.
Family: Lamiaceae.

People Use This For

Orally, thyme oil is used for bedwetting in children, and as an antispasmodic and antiflatulent.
Topically, thyme oil is used as a counterirritant, an antiseptic in mouthwashes and liniments, and as a counterirritant in douche products. Thyme oil is also used for alopecia areata.
Otically, it is used as an antibacterial and antifungal ingredient.
In foods, thyme oil is used as a flavoring agent.
In manufacturing, red thyme oil is used in perfumes. Thyme oil is also used in soaps, cosmetics, toothpastes.

Safety

LIKELY SAFE ...when used in amounts found in foods (11). It has Generally Recognized as Safe (GRAS) status in the US. The maximum use levels are less than 0.003% (11).
POSSIBLY SAFE ...when used topically and appropriately (5177). Thyme oil has been used safely for up to 7 months (5177).
LIKELY UNSAFE ...when used orally in medicinal amounts (4). ...when used topically unless it is diluted (4).
PREGNANCY: LIKELY SAFE ...when used orally in food amounts. LIKELY UNSAFE ...when used orally in larger amounts because it might induce menstruation (4,12); avoid using.
LACTATION: LIKELY SAFE ...when used orally in food amounts. There is insufficient reliable information available about the safety of thyme oil for larger amounts; avoid using.

Effectiveness

POSSIBLY EFFECTIVE ...when used topically in combination with other essential oils for alopecia areata. Thyme oil in combination with the essential oils from rosemary, lavender, and cedarwood seem to improve hair growth by 44% after 7 months of treatment (5177).
There is insufficient reliable information available about the effectiveness of thyme oil for its other uses.

Mechanism of Action

Thyme oil contains the volatile oils thymol and carvacrol. These constituents may have antispasmodic, antitussive, and expectorant effects (4). Thymol has fungicidal, antibacterial, anthelmintic (especially hookworms), and counterirritant properties (4,11). It's not clear how thyme oil works in alopecia areata (5177); however, it may be related to its effects as a counterirritant.

Adverse Reactions

Orally, thyme oil can cause nausea, vomiting, gastric pain, headache, dizziness, convulsions, coma, and cardiac and respiratory arrest (4). Topically, it can cause skin or mucous membrane irritation, cheilitis, and glossitis (4).

Interactions with Herbs & Other Dietary Supplements

Insufficient reliable information available.

Interactions with Drugs

No interactions are known to occur, and there is no known reason to expect a clinically significant interaction with thyme oil.

Interactions with Foods

No interactions are known to occur, and there is no known reason to expect a clinically significant interaction with thyme oil.

Interactions with Lab Tests

No interactions are known to occur, and there is no known reason to expect a clinically significant interaction with thyme oil.

Interactions with Diseases or Conditions

SKIN INJURIES: Medical consultation needed before use in individuals with extensive skin injuries/disease (18).

INFECTION: Medical consultation needed before use in individuals with high fever or infectious disease.

CARDIAC INSUFFICIENCY AND HYPERTONIA: Medical consultation needed before use in individuals with cardiac insufficiency or hypertonia (18).

Dosage and Administration

ORAL: A typical dose is 2 to 3 drops on a sugar cube, 2 or 3 times a day (5263).

TOPICAL: Must be diluted (4). Thyme oil is commonly applied as needed in 1% to 2% ointments (6002). For the treatment of alopecia areata, a combination of the essential oils including thyme 2 drops or 88 mg, rosemary 3 drops or 114 mg, lavender 3 drops or 108 mg, and cedarwood 2 drops or 94 mg, all mixed with 3 mL jojoba oil and 20 mL grapeseed oil has been used. Each night, the mixture is massaged into the scalp for 2 minutes with a warm towel placed around the head to increase absorption (5177).

Comments

Thyme oil is obtained by distillation of the leaves and flowering tops of thyme (Thymus vulgaris and/or Thymus zygis). White thyme oil (redistilled red thyme oil) is often adulterated (11).

THYMUS EXTRACT

Also Known As

Predigested Thymus Extract, Pure Thymic Extract, Thymomodulin, Thymosin, Thymostimulin, Thymus, Thymus Acid Lysate Derivative, Thymus Complex, Thymus Concentrate, Thymus-Derived Polypeptides, Thymus Factors, Thymus Polypeptides, Thymus Substance.

Scientific Names

None.

People Use This For

Orally, thymus extract is used for infectious diseases including recurrent respiratory infections, colds, flu, hepatitis B, hepatitis C, Epstein-Barr virus (EBV), mononucleosis, herpes and shingles, sinusitis (6614,6665,6666), and AIDS/HIV (6614). It is also used orally for asthma, hay fever, food allergies (6614), cancer (6665), rheumatoid arthritis, chronic fatigue syndrome (CFS), and systemic lupus erythematosus (SLE) (6666). It is also used orally for maintaining white cell production in cancer patients treated with radiation or chemotherapy (6614,6665), and preventing the effects of aging (6665).

Safety

POSSIBLY SAFE …when used orally and appropriately. No adverse effects have been reported in human studies with purified thymus extract (938,1010,1175,1176,1177,1178) (6691,6694,6696,6697,6698,6699). Although some evidence suggests these products are safe, since they are derived from animals, there is concern about contamination with diseased animal parts (see Adverse Reactions) (1825). However, so far there are no reports of disease transmission to humans due to use of contaminated thymus extract.

PREGNANCY AND LACTATION: Insufficient reliable information available; avoid using.

Effectiveness

POSSIBLY EFFECTIVE …when used orally for reducing acute asthma attacks in children with asthma. Thymomodulin (calf thymus extract) seems to improve immune function and reduce the number of asthma attacks up to one year after discontinuing intermittent treatment in a group of children with asthma (6694). …when used orally for treating adults and children with recurrent respiratory infections (938,6696,6697,6698,6699). Thymomodulin (calf thymus extract) treatment seems to reduce the number of infections or coughing attacks in patients with recurrent respiratory infections (6697,6698,6699). Thymomodulin (calf thymus extract) alone, or in combination with vaccine, seems to be more effective than vaccine alone or antibiotics in reducing the number and duration of infections in adults with recurrent respiratory infections (938). …when used orally for preventing allergic episodes in patients with perennial allergic rhinitis (1010). There is some evidence that treatment for 4 months with thymomodulin (calf thymus extract) might reduce the frequency of allergic episodes in patients with perennial allergic rhinitis (1010). …when used orally in combination with an elimination diet for preventing allergic reactions in children with food allergies. Thymomodulin (calf thymus extract) plus an elimination diet might prevent allergic reactions to allergenic foods after completion of the elimination diet, compared to an elimination diet alone (1175,1176).

There is insufficient reliable information available about the effectiveness of thymus extract for its other uses.

Mechanism of Action

Thymus extract is derived from bovine thymus glands (6614). Purified thymus extract induces immune response in spleen cells from athymic animals in vitro (6688). Preliminary human data suggests that a semipurified calf thymus extract might be useful for treating immunodeficiency conditions, bone marrow failure, auto-immune disorders, chronic skin diseases, recurrent viral and bacterial infections, and some cancers (6677).

Thymomodulin is a purified acid lysate derivative of calf thymus extract containing several polypeptides (6614,6689). It induces T-lymphocyte maturation, enhances the function of mature T-cells, and has indirect effects on B-cell and macrophage functions in vitro (6689). Thymomodulin improves immune function in patients with asthma, chronic bronchitis, recurrent respiratory infections, perennial allergic rhinnitis, food allergies, chronic active hepatitis B, and HIV infection (938,1010,1175,1176,1178,6694,6696,6697,6698,6699). It reduces airway hyperresponsiveness to methacholine in atopic patients with asthma (6695). Limited human data suggest that thymomodulin might be useful for treating chronic active hepatitis B (1015,1177) and improving symptoms in patients with HIV infection (1178). Thymomodulin demonstrates activity when administered orally in elderly patients (6691).

Thymosin is a polypeptide extracted from fetal calf thymus glands that stimulates in vitro T-cell proliferation when incubated with T-lymphocytes from people with low T-cell counts (511,6687).

Thymostimulin is a polypeptide extracted from bovine thymus glands (14,6680). Preliminary human evidence suggests that parenteral thymostimulin might be useful for improving immune function in infants with inadequate B-lymphocyte or T-lymphocyte function (6682,6683), children with recurrent respiratory infections (6679,6684), and patients with primary immunodeficiencies (6685). Limited human evidence also suggests that parenteral thymostimulin might be useful for preventing recurrent herpes simplex labialis (HSL) episodes (6678), preventing exacerbations in patients with chronic obstructive pulmonary disease (COPD) (6681), and preventing cystitis, conjunctivitis, stomatomucositis, and myelotoxicity in women with breast cancer treated with chemotherapy (6680). Thymostimulin is not beneficial for treating patients with auto-immune chronic active hepatitis (6686).

Adverse Reactions

Adverse effects have not been reported. However, there is some concern about potential contamination. Thymus extract is derived from raw bovine thymus glands gathered from slaughterhouses, possibly from sick or diseased animals (6616,6620). Products made from contaminated or diseased organs might present a human health hazard (6692). There is also concern that thymus extract produced from cows in countries where bovine spongiform encephalitis (BSE) has been reported might be contaminated with diseased tissue. Countries where BSE has been reported include Great Britain, France, The Netherlands, Portugal, Luxembourg, Ireland, Switzerland, Oman, and Belgium (1825). However, there have been no reports of BSE transfer to humans from contaminated thymus extract products. Until more is known, tell patients to avoid these products unless country of origin can be determined. Patients should avoid products that are produced in countries where BSE has been found.

Interactions with Herbs & Other Dietary Supplements

Insufficient reliable information available.

Interactions with Drugs

IMMUNOSUPPRESSANTS: Patients using immunosuppressive drugs are cautioned to avoid thymus extract products, unless they are certified pathogen-free (see Disease Interactions). Immunosuppressant drugs include azathioprine (Imuran), basiliximab (Simulect), cyclosporine (Neoral, Sandimmune), daclizumab (Zenapax), muromonab-CD3 (OKT3, Orthoclone OKT3), mycophenolate (CellCept), tacrolimus (FK506, Prograf), sirolimus (Rapamune), prednisone (Deltasone, Orasone), and other corticosteroids (glucocorticoids).

Interactions with Foods

No interactions are known to occur, and there is no known reason to expect a clinically significant interaction with thymus extract.

Interactions with Lab Tests

No interactions are known to occur, and there is no known reason to expect a clinically significant interaction with thymus extract.

Interactions with Diseases or Conditions

IMMUNE COMPROMISE, IMMUNOSUPPRESSION: Patients with compromised immune systems or using immunosuppressive drugs should be cautioned to avoid thymus extract products, unless they are certified pathogen-free, to reduce their risk of infection. This includes patients with HIV/AIDS and organ transplant recipients using immunosuppressive drugs.

Dosage and Administration

ORAL: A typical daily dose is 750 mg of crude thymus polypeptide fraction or 120 mg of pure thymus polypetides (thymomodulin) (6614).

Comments

The quality and potency of thymus extract products can vary greatly (6614).

TIRATRICOL

Also Known As

Triac, triiodothyroacetic acid.

Scientific Names

3,3',5-triiodothyroacetic acid.

People Use This For

Orally, tiratricol is used for treating pituitary resistance to thyroid hormone (PRTH) (1607,1608,1609,1610,1615), treating thyroid cancer (orphan drug designation) (1604,1616,1617,1618), treating fetal hypothyroidism (1613,1614), increasing metabolic rate for weight loss, and reducing cellulite (1601,1602,1606,1611,1612).

Safety

LIKELY SAFE ...when used orally under medical supervision for treating thyroid cancer (1604,1616,1617,1618). ...when used orally under medical supervision for treating pituitary resistance to thyroid hormone (PRTH) (1607,1608,1609,1610,1615).
POSSIBLY SAFE ...when used orally under medical supervision for treating fetal hypothyroidism (1613,1614).
POSSIBLY UNSAFE ...when used orally in the elderly, tiratricol might aggravate occult cardiac disease (15); avoid using.
LIKELY UNSAFE ...when used orally for increasing metabolic rate for weight loss or reducing cellulite (1620,1621,1622,1623,1624,1625). The FDA has issued a warning against tiratricol use for weight loss (1605).
PREGNANCY: POSSIBLY SAFE ...when used orally under medical supervision for treating fetal hypothyroidism (1613,1614). LIKELY UNSAFE ...when used orally for other purposes during pregnancy due to possible risk of fetal heart damage (1627,1628); avoid using.
LACTATION: Insufficient reliable information available; avoid using.

Effectiveness

LIKELY EFFECTIVE ...when used orally for treating pituitary resistance to thyroid hormone (PRTH) (1607,1608,1609,1610,1615).
POSSIBLY EFFECTIVE ...when used orally for treating fetal hypothyroidism (1613,1614). ...when used orally for thyroid cancer in combination with levo-thyroxine (1616,1617,1618). Tiratricol is an FDA designated orphan drug under study for use in combination with levo-thyroxine to suppress thyroid stimulating hormone (TSH) in patients with well-differentiated thyroid cancer who are intolerant to adequate doses of levo-thyroxine alone (1604).
LIKELY INEFFECTIVE ...when used orally for increasing metabolic rate for weight loss in people with normal thyroid function (1611,1612).
There is insufficient reliable information available about the effectiveness of tiratricol for its other uses.

Mechanism of Action

Tiratricol is a naturally occurring metabolite of T4 (thyroxine) and a structural analog of T3 (triiodothyronine) (1633,1634). Low concentrations of tiratricol are found in plasma, but tiratricol has no known role in thyroid physiology (1633). Tiratricol has a high affinity for T3 receptors and suppresses thyroid stimulating hormone (TSH) secretion at therapeutic doses without causing significant peripheral effects, such as increased basal metabolism rate and heart rate (1634). Tiratricol might lower total and LDL cholesterol, and stimulate bone formation (1632). About 67% of an oral dose of tiratricol is absorbed; the half-life is 6 hours (1631).

Adverse Reactions

Orally, tiratricol can cause severe diarrhea, fatigue, lethargy, and profound weight loss (1605). Heart attacks and strokes are possible, as well as symptoms of hyperthyroidism, including increased appetite, abdominal cramps, tremors, menstrual irregularities, nervousness, insomnia, sweating, intolerance to heat, fever, palpitations, tachycardia, increased pulse and blood pressure, chest pain, and cardiac arrhythmias (15,1605). Case reports have implicated tiratricol in centrally-mediated hypothyroidism, pseudohypothyroidism, internuclear ophthalmoplegia, and hepatotoxicity (1621,1623,1624,1625).

Interactions with Herbs & Other Dietary Supplements

HERBS WITH THYROID ACTIVITY: Theoretically, tiratricol might enhance the effects and adverse effects of herbs that affect thyroid function, including bugleweed, balm leaf, and wild thyme.

HERBS & SUPPLEMENTS WITH SYMPATHOMIMETIC ACTIVITY: Theoretically, large doses of tiratricol might enhance the effects and adverse effects of herbs and supplements that have sympathomimetic activity, including caffeine, guarana, and ephedra (15).

VITAMIN K: Theoretically, tiratricol might antagonize the prothrombinemic effects of vitamin K by increasing catabolism of vitamin K-dependent clotting factors (15).

Interactions with Drugs

ANTICOAGULANTS: Theoretically, tiratricol might potentiate the hypoprothrombinemic effects of oral anticoagulants, including warfarin (Coumadin), by increasing catabolism of vitamin K-dependent clotting factors (15).

ANTI-DIABETES DRUGS: Theoretically, tiratricol might interfere with blood glucose control requiring adjustment of diabetes drug therapy (15); monitor closely.

CHOLESTYRAMINE (Questran): Theoretically, cholestyramine might decrease tiratricol absorption (15).

SYMPATHOMIMETIC DRUGS: Theoretically, large doses of tiratricol might enhance the effects and adverse effects of sympathomimetic drugs (15).

THYROID HORMONES: Concurrent use of tiratricol with thyroid hormones can have additive effects (1617); use only under medical supervision.

VITAMIN K: Theoretically, tiratricol might antagonize the prothrombinemic effects of vitamin K by increasing catabolism of vitamin K-dependent clotting factors (15).

Interactions with Foods

No interactions are known to occur, and there is no known reason to expect a clinically significant interaction with tiratricol.

Interactions with Lab Tests

THYROID FUNCTION TESTS: Abnormalities have been reported in people taking tiratricol (1604).

THYROID-STIMULATING HORMONE (TSH): Tiratricol reduces serum TSH levels, and test results (1631).

THYROTRPIN-RELEASING HORMONE (TRH) STIMULATION: Triatricol reduces TSH secretion, serum levels and test results, to exogenous TRH stimulation (1609,1611,1617,1623,1633).

PROTHROMBIN TIME (PT), INTERNATIONAL NORMALIZATION RATIO (INR): Theoretically, tiratricol might increase prothrombin time, increasing PT and INR test results, by increasing catabolism of vitamin K-dependent clotting factors (15).

Interactions with Diseases or Conditions

ADRENAL INSUFFICIENCY, DIABETES, HYPOPITUITARISM: Theoretically, tiratricol might unmask symptoms of these conditions in patients with untreated hypothyroidism (15).

ANGINA, CARDIOVASCULAR DISEASE, HYPERTENSION: Theoretically, tiratricol might aggravate symptoms of these conditions (15); avoid using.

PROLONGED CLOTTING TIME: Theoretically, tiratricol might increase the risk of bleeding in people with prolonged clotting time by increasing catabolism of vitamin K-dependent clotting factors (15).

DIABETES: Theoretically, tiratricol might interfere with blood glucose control requiring adjustment of diabetes drug therapy (15), monitor closely.

MYXEDEMA: Patients with myxedema might be particularly sensitive to thyroid agents, including tiratricol (15).

LIVER DISEASE: Tiratricol is potentially hepatotoxic and might worsen liver disease (1624); avoid using.

Dosage and Administration

ORAL: The oral dose for TSH suppression tests used in clinical trials is 10-24 mcg twice daily initially, titrated to a TSH concentration of less than 0.1 mU/L (1632,1633). The oral dose typically used for weight loss is 1 mg twice daily (1601).

Comments

Tiratricol is a thyroid supplement and should not be used by anyone with normal thyroid function (1605). The drug, which is available by prescription in France, has been studied since the fifties, mostly for thyroid disease (9,1629,1630). The FDA has determined that the product Triax (TRIAC, tiratricol) is not a dietary supplement but an unapproved new drug containing a potent thyroid hormone, which may cause serious health consequences. The State of Missouri embargoed the product at its distributor (Syntrax) and the Utah-based manufacturer (Pharmatech) has agreed to stop distributing any product containing the ingredient TRIAC. The FDA has issued recalls for other tiratricol-containing products, including Tricana Metabolic Hormone Analogue, Tria-Cutz Thyroid Stimulator Dietary Supplement Capsules, and Sci-Fi-Tri-Cuts Dietary Supplement Capsules (6675).

TOLU BALSAM

Also Known As

Balsam, Balsam of Tolu, Balsam Tolu, Balsamum Tolutanum, Opobalsam, Resin Tolu, Resina Tolutana, Thomas Balsam, Tolu, Toluiferum Balsamum.
CAUTION: See separate listing for Peru Balsam.

Scientific Names

Myroxylon balsamum, synonym Myroxylon balsamum genuinum; Toliufera balsamum, synonyms Myroxylan balsamum, Myroxylan toluiferum.
Family: Leguminosae or Fabaceae.

People Use This For

Orally, tolu balsam is used for cough, bronchitis (18), inflammation of respiratory tract mucous membranes (2), and as a flavoring and expectorant ingredient in cough medicines (11).
Topically, it is used as an ingredient in Compound Benzoin Tincture, for treatment of bedsores, cracked nipples, lips, and minor skin cuts.
As an inhalant, tolu balsam is used to treat laryngitis and croup (11).
Historically, tolu balsam has been used for cancer (11).
For food uses, tolu balsam is also used to flavor chewing gum, foods, and beverages (11).
In manufacturing, balsam and balsam oil are used as fixatives or as fragrances in soaps and cosmetics (11).

Safety

LIKELY SAFE ...when the oleo resin is used orally in the very low amounts found in foods. Tolu balsam has been approved for food use in the US (11).
POSSIBLY SAFE ...when used orally and appropriately for medicinal purposes (2).
There is insufficient reliable information available about the safety of the topical use of tolu balsam.
PREGNANCY AND LACTATION: Insufficient reliable information available; avoid using.

Effectiveness

POSSIBLY EFFECTIVE ...when used orally to treat inflammation of respiratory tract mucous membranes (2).
There is insufficient reliable information available about the effectiveness of tolu balsam for its other uses.

Mechanism of Action

The applicable part of tolu balsam is the oleo resin. Tolu balsam has mild antiseptic action and expectorant properties (11).

Adverse Reactions

Orally, tolu balsam may cause kidney irritation (12).
Topically, it may cause allergic reactions (11).

Interactions with Herbs & Other Dietary Supplements

Insufficient reliable information available.

Interactions with Drugs

No interactions are known to occur, and there is no known reason to expect a clinically significant interaction with tolu balsam.

Interactions with Foods

No interactions are known to occur, and there is no known reason to expect a clinically significant interaction with tolu balsam.

Interactions with Lab Tests

No interactions are known to occur, and there is no known reason to expect a clinically significant interaction with tolu balsam.

Interactions with Diseases or Conditions

FEVER: Theoretically, tolu balsam is contraindicated in individuals with fever or inflammation (12,19).
KIDNEY DISEASE: Theoretically, tolu balsam might exacerbate kidney disease.
TOLU BALSAM ALLERGY: Avoid use of tolu balsam (11).

Dosage and Administration
ORAL: A typical dosage is 500-600 mg per day (2,18).
TOPICAL: No typical dosage.

Comments
Avoid confusion with Peru balsam. Tolu balsam is the oleo resin exuded from slits cut in the trunk of Myroxylon balsamum.

TOMATO

Also Known As
Love Apple.
CAUTION: See seperate listing for Lycopene.

Scientific Names
Lycopersicon esculentum.
Family: Solanaceae.

People Use This For
Orally, tomato fruit is used orally for reducing the risk of cancer (2404,2405,2406,2407).
Orally, tomato leaf and vine are used for treating arthritis, colds, chills and digestive disorders (18).

Safety
LIKELY SAFE …when the tomato fruit or its products are consumed in amounts found in foods (2406).
POSSIBLY UNSAFE …when the leaf is used orally (18).
There is insufficient reliable information about the safety of the tomato vine.
PREGNANCY AND LACTATION: LIKELY SAFE …when the tomato fruit or its products are consumed in typical food amounts. Avoid using amounts greater than those typically consumed in foods.

Effectiveness
POSSIBLY EFFECTIVE…when tomato fruit products are used orally for reducing the risk of prostate cancer. Epidemiological studies suggest that the risk of prostate cancer is decreased in men who consume four or more weekly servings of tomato products, including tomatoes, tomato sauce, pizza, and tomato juice (2406).
POSSIBLY INEFFECTIVE …when tomato fruit products are used orally for reducing the risk of bladder cancer. Epidemiological studies find no association between consumption of tomatoes and tomato-based products, and the risk of bladder cancer (2407).
There is insufficient reliable information available about the effectiveness of tomato fruit for its other uses. Epidemiological studies of consumption of tomatoes and tomato-based products, and the risk of cancers of the breast, cervix, colon, esophagus, larynx, lungs, oral cavity, ovaries, pancreas, pleura, rectum, and stomach, are inconclusive (1444,2404,2407).
There is insufficient reliable information available about the effectiveness of tomato leaf and vine.

Mechanism of Action
The applicable parts of tomato are the fruit, leaf, and vine. Tomatoes are the major dietary source of the carotenoid, lycopene. Lycopene is better absorbed from tomato products, such as tomato paste, than from fresh tomatoes (1497). Consumption of tomato juice can also significantly increase serum lycopene levels (1498,6607). One cup (240 mL) of tomato juice contains approximately 23 mg lycopene, depending on the brand (1499). Decreased serum or tissue lycopene concentrations are associated with an increased risk of prostate cancer (1447,1496,2405,2406,2407). Researchers have speculated that tomato products might stimulate immune function. However, there is evidence that long-term consumption of tomato juice has no effect on cell-mediated immune function (6607).

Adverse Reactions
Orally, symptoms of toxicity may include severe mucous membrane irritation, including vomiting, diarrhea, and colic. This is followed by dizziness, stupor, headache, bradycardia, respiratory disturbances, and mild spasms. In very severe cases, death by respiratory failure might occur (18). Signs of oral poisoning are not expected with ingestion of less than 100 grams of tomato leaves.

Interactions with Herbs & Other Dietary Supplements
Insufficient reliable information available.

Interactions with Drugs

No interactions are known to occur, and there is no known reason to expect a clinically significant interaction with tomato.

Interactions with Foods

No interactions are known to occur, and there is no known reason to expect a clinically significant interaction with tomato.

Interactions with Lab Tests

No interactions are known to occur, and there is no known reason to expect a clinically significant interaction with tomato.

Interactions with Diseases or Conditions

No interactions are known to occur, and there is no known reason to expect a clinically significant interaction with tomato.

Dosage and Administration

ORAL: For preventing prostate cancer, four or more servings of tomato products per week (equivalent to a dietary lycopene intake of greater than 6 mg daily) has been used (2406).

Comments

US Department of Agriculture (USDA) and Purdue University researchers are developing a tomato that contains more than twice as much lycopene and has a longer shelf life than currently available tomatoes (6671). The tomato, which is still in development, is modified with a yeast gene that slows the ripening process, allowing more time for lycopene to accumulate. Researchers think it will be several years before the tomato is commercially available.

TONKA BEAN

Also Known As

Coumarouna Odorata, Cumaru, Dutch Tonka, English Tonka, Legume, Tonka, Tonka Seed, Tonquin Bean, Torquin Bean.

Scientific Names

Dipteryx odorata.
Family: Leguminosae or Fabaceae.

People Use This For

Orally, tonka bean is used as a tonic (6,4500), an aphrodisiac, to treat cachexia (4502), cramps (4502,4507), lymphedema (4507), nausea (4502,4507), cough (4500), schistosomiasis (6,4502), spasms (4502), and tuberculosis (4500).
Topically, tonka bean is used for mouth ulcers (4500,4502), earache (4502), and sore throat (4502).
In manufacturing, coumarin, one of the active constituents is used as a flavoring and fragrance in various products in the food, liquor, tobacco, soap, and cosmetic industries (6,13,4502,4507).
In foods, the seeds are used to make a nutty-flavored beverage (6,4502).

Safety

LIKELY UNSAFE …when used orally. The FDA deems any food containing tonka bean or tonka bean extract to be impure (6). Rarely, coumarin, a constituent, has been associated with hepatotoxicity ranging from elevated liver enzymes to severe hepatic damage (6,18,297,4501). In a number of countries, coumarin-containing products have been removed from the market (4501).
There is insufficient reliable information available about the safety of the topical use of tonka bean.
PREGNANCY AND LACTATION: LIKELY UNSAFE …when used orally (6,18,297,4501); avoid using.

Effectiveness

There is insufficient reliable information available about the effectiveness of tonka bean.

Mechanism of Action

The applicable parts of tonka bean are the fruit and seed. Tonka bean seeds usually contain 1-3% coumarin but may contain up to 10% (6,4501,4502). Tonka bean seeds also contain coumaric-acid-beta-glucoside, o-coumaric acid, linoleic acid, oleic-acid, sitosterol, stearic acid, stigmasterol, and umbelliferone (296). The fruit contains melilotoside-1-p-coumaryl-beta-d-glucose (296). There is some evidence that coumarin can reduce edema and inflammation by increasing venous and lymphatic return (295). Other information suggests tonka bean might have narcotic and spasmolytic properties (4502,18).

Adverse Reactions

Orally, coumarin can be associated with nausea, vomiting (286), diarrhea, dizziness, insomnia (287), asymptomatic SGOT elevations (286), and rarely, liver toxicity (6,18,297,4501). Large doses of the extract can paralyze the heart (4502).

Interactions with Herbs & Other Dietary Supplements

HERBS WITH ANTICOAGULANT/ANTIPLATELET POTENTIAL: Concomitant use of herbs that have coumarin constituents or affect platelet aggregation could theoretically increase the risk of bleeding in some people. These herbs include angelica, anise, arnica, asafoetida, bogbean, boldo, capsicum, celery, chamomile, clove, danshen, fenugreek, feverfew, garlic, ginger, ginkgo, ginseng Panax, horse chestnut, horseradish, licorice, meadowsweet, prickly ash, onion, papain, passionflower, poplar, quassia, red clover, turmeric, wild carrot, wild lettuce, willow, and others (4,19).

Interactions with Drugs

ANTICOAGULANTS/ANTIPLATELETS: Theoretically, tonka bean might cause additive effects and side effects with drugs having anticoagulant or antiplatelet properties (19).

Interactions with Foods

No interactions are known to occur, and there is no known reason to expect a clinically significant interaction with tonka bean.

Interactions with Lab Tests

No interactions are known to occur, and there is no known reason to expect a clinically significant interaction with tonka bean.

Interactions with Diseases or Conditions

LIVER DISEASE: Although it is rare, the tonka bean constituent, coumarin, can cause liver toxicity (298).

Dosage and Administration

ORAL: Some people use an amount of tonka bean based on its coumarin content, and the typical dose of coumarin used is 60 mg daily (5008).
TOPICAL: No typical dosage.

Comments

A number of countries have removed coumarin-containing products from the market (4501). The term coumarin is derived from Coumarou, the Caribbean name for the tonka tree (13). In plants, more than 700 different coumarins have been identified. Coumarin, itself, is widely distributed and has the characteristic odor of new-mown hay (13). Do not confuse coumarin with the potent anticoagulants bishydroxycoumarin, dicumarol, (13,295) or warfarin (a derivative of 4-hydroxycoumarin) (16).

TORMENTIL

Also Known As

Biscuits, Bloodroot, Cinquefoil, Earthbank, English Sarsaparilla, Ewe Daisy, Flesh And Blood, Potentilla, Septfoil, Shepherd's Knapperty, Shepherd's Knot, Thormantle, Tormentilla, Tormentillae rhizoma.
CAUTION: See separate listings for Couch Grass, Potentilla, German Sarsaparilla, and Sarsaparilla.

Scientific Names

Potentilla erecta.
Family: Rosaceae.

People Use This For

Orally, tormentil is used to treat diarrhea (2,18), acute and subacute gastroenteritis (18), and fever (400).
Topically, tormentil is used for reducing superficial bleeding (400) and treating mild inflammation of the oral and pharyngeal mucous membranes (2,18).

Safety

POSSIBLY SAFE ...when used orally or topically and appropriately (2,12).
PREGNANCY AND LACTATION: Insufficient reliable information available; avoid using.

Effectiveness

POSSIBLY EFFECTIVE ...when used orally for diarrhea (2,7,12,18). ...when applied topically for mild oral and pharyngeal mucus membrane inflammation (2,7,12,18).
There is insufficient reliable information available about the effectiveness of tormentil root for its other uses.

Mechanism of Action

The applicable part of tormentil is the root. It contains 17-22% tannins, proanthocyanidins, flavonoids, and triterpenes (18). The astringent effect of tannins relieves diarrhea and soothes mucus membrane inflammation. Tannins reduce superficial bleeding by causing skin and superficial capillary contraction (400). Tannins also show some evidence of antiviral, antimicrobial, CNS depressant, and cariostatic effects (11). Some evidence suggests that tannins might cause cancer but other evidence shows tannins might prevent it (12). Regular consumption of herbs with high tannin concentrations correlates with increased incidence of esophageal or nasal cancer (12).

Adverse Reactions

Orally, tormentil can cause nausea, vomiting (7,12,18), and stomach complaints (2). Tormentil contains more than 10% tannins and theoretically has the potential to cause kidney damage and necrotic conditions of the liver (12).

Interactions with Herbs & Other Dietary Supplements

Insufficient reliable information available.

Interactions with Drugs

No interactions are known to occur, and there is no known reason to expect a clinically significant interaction with tormentil.

Interactions with Foods

MILK: When added to tormentil tea, milk can bind to the tannins and decrease their astringent and adverse effects (12).

Interactions with Lab Tests

No interactions are known to occur, and there is no known reason to expect a clinically significant interaction with tormentil.

Interactions with Diseases or Conditions

No interactions are known to occur, and there is no known reason to expect a clinically significant interaction with tormentil.

Dosage and Administration

ORAL: For diarrhea, a typical dose is one cup of the tea 2 to 4 times daily between meals, up to 4-6 grams of root per day. The tea is prepared by steeping 2-3 grams of the finely cut or powdered root in 150 mL boiling water for 10-15 minutes and then straining (2,7,18). Diarrhea lasting longer than 3 to 4 days should be medically evaluated (2).
TOPICAL: The usual daily dose of the tincture (1:10) is 10-20 drops in one glass of water used as a mouth or throat rinse (2,18).

Comments

Avoid confusion with potentilla (Potentilla anserina).

TRAGACANTH

Also Known As

Goat's Thorn, Green Dragon, Gum Dragon, Gum Tragacanth, Gummi Tragacanthae, Hog Gum, Syrian Tragacanth, Tragacanth Gum.
CAUTION: See separate listing for Astragalus.

Scientific Names

Astragalus gummifera; other Astragalus species.
Family: Leguminosae or Fabaceae.

People Use This For

Orally, tragacanth is used both for diarrhea (6) and as a laxative (18).

Topically, it is an ingredient in toothpastes, hand lotions, and vaginal creams and jellies (11).

For food uses, it is important for stabilizing, thickening, and suspending ingredients in salad dressings, foods, and beverages (11).

In pharmaceutical preparations, it is used as an emulsifier, binding agent, and demulcent (11). Tragacanth is also a component of denture adhesives (6).

Safety

LIKELY SAFE ...when used orally in amounts found in foods. It has Generally Recognized as Safe (GRAS) status in the US. The maximum level used is 1.3% (11). ...when used topically, in the amounts found in cosmetics. Tragacanth is not considered to be irritating, sensitizing, or phototoxic (4072).

POSSIBLY SAFE ...when used orally in greater amounts for medicinal purposes (4068). However, insufficient fluid intake with tragacanth might lead to esophageal closure or obstruction ileus (18).

PREGNANCY AND LACTATION: Insufficient reliable information available; avoid using amounts greater than those found in foods.

Effectiveness

There is insufficient reliable information available about the effectiveness of tragacanth.

Mechanism of Action

Tragacanth contains water-soluble tragacanthin and water-insoluble bassorin (11). When added to water, tragacanthin dissolves to form a viscous colloidal solution; bassorin swells to form a thick gel (11). Among plant gums, tragacanth produces the most viscous solution (11). When ingested, the bulk of tragacanth stretches the intestinal wall, increasing peristalsis (18). Although tragacanth increases stool weight and decreases GI transit time, it does not appear to affect cholesterol, triglyceride, or phospholipid levels as do other soluble fibers (6). Some preliminary data indicate that people with diabetes who ingest tragacanth along with a high sugar load have lower peak serum glucose and insulin levels (4069). However this effect has not been consistent (6). The mucilaginous, adhesive properties of tragacanth justify its use as a component in denture adhesives (6). Tragacanth appears to inhibit growth of cancer cells (11). Preliminary evidence suggests tragacanthin polysaccharides might offer some protection from hantavirus infections (4070). Tragacanth is highly susceptible to bacterial digestion, even in the presence of preservatives (11).

Adverse Reactions

Orally, use of tragacanth requires ample fluid intake. Insufficient fluid intake can lead to obstruction ileus and esophageal closure (18). Tragacanth can cause asthma symptoms in people who are sensitive to quillaia bark (6).

Interactions with Herbs & Other Dietary Supplements

HERBS AND SUPPLEMENTS: Theoretically, concomitant administration might reduce absorption of supplements and/or herbs due to hydrocolloidal fiber content of tragacanth (19).

Interactions with Drugs

ORAL DRUGS: Theoretically, concomitant administration of oral drugs might reduce drug absorption due to hydrocolloidal fiber content of tragacanth (19).

Interactions with Foods

NUTRIENTS: Theoretically, concomitant administration might impair nutrient absorption from foods due to hydrocolloidal fiber content of tragacanth (19).

Interactions with Lab Tests

No interactions are known to occur, and there is no known reason to expect a clinically significant interaction with tragacanth.

Interactions with Diseases or Conditions

QUILLAIA ALLERGY: Tragacanth can cause asthma symptoms in individuals sensitive to quillaia bark (19).

Dosage and Administration

No typical dosage.

Comments

Karaya gum is a common adulterant in tragacanth (16). It is important to use any amount with adequate fluid intake to prevent esophageal closure or obstruction of the ileus (18).

TRAILING ARBUTUS

Also Known As
Gravel Plant, Ground Laurel, Mountain Pink, Water Pink, Winter Pink.

Scientific Names
Epigaea repens.
Family: Ericaceae.

People Use This For
Orally, trailing arbutus is used for urinary tract conditions, as an astringent, and a diuretic (18).

Safety
POSSIBLY SAFE …when the leaves are used orally short-term (12).
UNSAFE …when the fresh or dried leaves are used orally long-term because they could cause hydroquinone toxicity (18).
PREGNANCY AND LACTATION: Insufficient reliable information available; avoid using.

Effectiveness
There is insufficient reliable information available about the effectiveness of trailing arbutus.

Mechanism of Action
The applicable parts of trailing arbutus are the above ground parts. Trailing arbutus is not suitable for long term use due to its hydroquinone glycoside content (18). Arbutin may have urinary antiseptic properties due to hydrolysis to its hydroquinone by the intestinal flora (7,11). As a result, long term use is stated to lead to hydroquinone toxicity (18).

Adverse Reactions
Orally, chronic use of trailing arbutus may lead to hydroquinone toxicity. Symptoms of toxicity include tinnitus, vomiting, delirium, convulsions, and collapse (11). Liver damage, cachexia, hemolytic anemia, and hair depigmentation may also occur with long term use (18). Overdosage could lead to inflammation of the mucous membranes of the bladder and urinary tract, and may be accompanied by bloody urine, difficulty with urination, and painful urination (18).

Interactions with Herbs & Other Dietary Supplements
Insufficient reliable information available.

Interactions with Drugs
No interactions are known to occur, and there is no known reason to expect a clinically significant interaction with trailing arbutus.

Interactions with Foods
No interactions are known to occur, and there is no known reason to expect a clinically significant interaction with trailing arbutus.

Interactions with Lab Tests
No interactions are known to occur, and there is no known reason to expect a clinically significant interaction with trailing arbutus.

Interactions with Diseases or Conditions
No interactions are known to occur, and there is no known reason to expect a clinically significant interaction with trailing arbutus.

Dosage and Administration
ORAL: Trailing arbutus is taken as a tea or extract (18).

Comments
Trailing arbutus's alternate name of gravel plant is similar to that of gravel root. Be careful not to confuse the two.

TRANSFER FACTOR

Also Known As

Bovine Dialyzable Leukocyte Extract, Bovine Dialyzable Transfer Factor, Bovine Transfer Factor, Dialyzable Leukocyte Extract, Dialyzable Transfer Factor, DLE, TFd.
CAUTION: See separate listing for Bovine Colostrum.

Scientific Names

Transfer Factor

People Use This For

Orally and parenterally, transfer factor is used for infectious diseases in both immunocompetent and immunosuppressed patients, including cryptosporidiosis (1410,1445,1480), septicemia, sinusitis and bronchitis, influenza, the common cold, herpes (1400), varicella, hepatitis B infections, cytomegalovirus (CMV), Pneumocystis carinii, Mycobacterium tuberculosis, Mycobacterium fortuitum, Mycobacterium avium, and coccidiomycosis, candidiasis, leishmaniasis, and lepromatous leprosy (1420,1476,1507). Transfer factor is also used for diabetes, autism, infertility, systemic lupus erythematosus (SLE), fibromyalgia, chronic fatigue syndrome (CFS) (1400), Behcet's syndrome, pemphigus vegetans, Wiskott-Aldrich syndrome, alopecia totalis, Alzheimer's disease, retinitis pigmentosa, amyotrophic lateral sclerosis (ALS, Lou Gehrig's disease), osteosarcoma, bone metastasis, epidermal dysplasia, food and chemical hypersensitivity, myasthenia gravis, subacute sclerosis panencephalitis, atopic dermatitis, and bronchial asthma (1507).

Safety

POSSIBLY SAFE ...when used orally or parenterally and appropriately, short-term. Both human-derived transfer factor and bovine-derived transfer factor have been safely used in small studies lasting up to 3 months (1445,1507). Some evidence suggests these products are safe, however, some preparations are derived from animals and there is concern about contamination with diseased animal parts (see Adverse Reactions) (1825). There are no reports of disease transmission to humans due to use of contaminated bovine transfer factor.
PREGNANCY AND LACTATION: Insufficient reliable information available; avoid using.

Effectiveness

There is insufficient reliable information available to rate the effectiveness of transfer factor for its uses. However, there is some preliminary evidence that oral transfer factor might be beneficial for people with cryptosporidiosis related to AIDS. Transfer factor from bovine sources seems to improve stool frequency and help eradicate oocysts in some patients (1445,1480).

Mechanism of Action

Transfer factor refers to a variety of dialyzable polypeptide molecules extracted from leukocytes of humans and animals, such as cows and mice (1493,1494). Transfer factors are derived from sources that have developed immunity to a certain infectious diseases. For example, bovine transfer factor for cryptosporidiosis is prepared by first inoculating calves with cryptosporidium and then harvesting of lymph nodes (1410,1420,1445,1480). Human transfer factor is prepared from blood of donors with antigen-specific immune responses (1476,1507). The theory is that use of transfer factor from sensitized donors, human or animal, can cause deficient recipients to express cell-mediated immunity (1493). This effect is antigen-specific and results in expression of delayed type hypersensitivity and production of lymphokines (1493,1495,1507). Animal studies indicate that transfer factor prepared from bovine lymphocytes or bovine colostrum confer cell-mediated immunity to specific antigens on recipients of different species (1475,1477,1478). The exact mechanism of action of transfer factors is unknown; however, antigen specificity is well-established (1475,1477,1478). There is no evidence that non-specific transfer factor products, such as those marketed on the Internet, are effective for any indication.

Adverse Reactions

Orally or parenterally, transfer factor might cause fever in some patients (1507). There is also some concern that bovine-derived transfer factor that is produced from cows in countries where bovine spongiform encephalitis (BSE) has been reported might be contaminated with diseased tissue. Countries where BSE has been reported include Great Britain, France, The Netherlands, Portugal, Luxembourg, Ireland, Switzerland, Oman, and Belgium (1825). However, there have been no reports of BSE transfer to humans from contaminated transfer factor products. Until more is known, tell patients to avoid these products unless country of origin can be determined. Patients should avoid products that are produced in countries where BSE has been found.

Interactions with Herbs & Other Dietary Supplements

Insufficient reliable information available.

Interactions with Drugs
No interactions are known to occur, and there is no known reason to expect a clinically significant interaction with transfer factor.

Interactions with Foods
No interactions are known to occur, and there is no known reason to expect a clinically significant interaction with transfer factor.

Interactions with Lab Tests
No interactions are known to occur, and there is no known reason to expect a clinically significant interaction with transfer factor.

Interactions with Diseases or Conditions
No interactions are known to occur, and there is no known reason to expect a clinically significant interaction with transfer factor.

Dosage and Administration
ORAL: For cryptosporidiosis, clinical studies used bovine transfer factor 1 unit (5 x 108 lymph node cell equivalents) weekly for 1-1/2 to 3 months (1420,1445).

Comments
None.

TRAVELER'S JOY

Also Known As
Travelers Joy.
CAUTION: See separate listings for Clematis and Woodbine.

Scientific Names
Clematis vitalba.
Family: Ranunculaceae.

People Use This For
Orally, traveler's joy is used for diseases of the male genitals and migraine headaches.
Topically, traveler's joy is used for poorly healing wounds and migraine headaches.

Safety
LIKELY UNSAFE …when used orally or topically for any reason due to protoanemonin, a severe local irritant (18).
PREGNANCY AND LACTATION: LIKELY UNSAFE …when used orally or topically (18).

Effectiveness
There is insufficient reliable information available about the effectiveness of traveler's joy.

Mechanism of Action
The applicable part of traveler's joy is the fresh leaf. When the fresh plant is crushed or cut into small pieces, the glycoside ranunculin is enzymatically changed into a severely irritating protoanemonin, which, in turn, rapidly degrades into the less toxic anemonin (18). Both protoanemonin and ranunculin are destroyed to an unknown extent during the drying process (2).

Adverse Reactions
Orally, traveler's joy can cause severe irritation of the gastrointestinal tract, including colic and diarrhea. Irritation of the urinary tract can also occur.
Topically, skin contact can cause blisters and burns that are difficult to heal (18).

Interactions with Herbs & Other Dietary Supplements
Insufficient reliable information available.

Interactions with Drugs

No interactions are known to occur, and there is no known reason to expect a clinically significant interaction with traveler's joy.

Interactions with Foods

No interactions are known to occur, and there is no known reason to expect a clinically significant interaction with traveler's joy.

Interactions with Lab Tests

No interactions are known to occur, and there is no known reason to expect a clinically significant interaction with traveler's joy.

Interactions with Diseases or Conditions

No interactions are known to occur, and there is no known reason to expect a clinically significant interaction with traveler's joy.

Dosage and Administration

No typical dosage.

Comments

None.

TREE OF HEAVEN

Also Known As

A-Lan-Thus, Ailanthus Glandulosa, Ailanto, Chinese Sumach, Copal Tree, Heaven Tree, Paradise Tree, Varnish Tree, Vernis de Japon.

Scientific Names

Ailanthus altissima.
Family: Simaroubaceae.

People Use This For

In Chinese medicine, tree of heaven is used for pathological leukorrhea, diarrhea, chronic diarrhea, chronic dysentery, and dysmenorrhea (18).
In Africa, tree of heaven is used to treat asthma, cramps, epilepsy, fast heart rate, gonorrhea, malaria, and tapeworms (18). It has also been used as a bitter and a tonic (4500).
For food uses, the young leaves of the tree are eaten (4500).
In manufacturing, tree of heaven is used as insecticide (4500,4501).

Safety

There is insufficient reliable information available about the safety of tree of heaven. However, fatal poisonings have been reported in animal experiments (18).
Pregnancy and Lactation: Insufficient reliable information available; avoid using.

Effectiveness

There is insufficient reliable information about the effectiveness of tree of heaven.

Mechanism of Action

The applicable parts of tree of heaven are the dried trunk and root bark. The bark of the tree of heaven is said to have astringent, antipyretic, and antispasmodic properties (18). Some evidence suggests the quassionoid constituents, including ailanthone and quassin, have antiprotozoan, anthelmintic, antileukemic, and cytotoxic properties (18,4501). The bark also contains tannins and indole alkaloids of the beta-carboline type (18).

Adverse Reactions

Orally, large amounts of the tree of heaven bark can cause queasiness, dizziness, headache, limb tingling, and diarrhea (18). Skin contact with the leaves can cause dermatitis (4501).

Interactions with Herbs & Other Dietary Supplements

Insufficient reliable information available.

Interactions with Drugs

No interactions are known to occur, and there is no known reason to expect a clinically significant interaction with tree of heaven.

Interactions with Foods

No interactions are known to occur, and there is no known reason to expect a clinically significant interaction with tree of heaven.

Interactions with Lab Tests

No interactions are known to occur, and there is no known reason to expect a clinically significant interaction with tree of heaven.

Interactions with Diseases or Conditions

No interactions are known to occur, and there is no known reason to expect a clinically significant interaction with tree of heaven.

Dosage and Administration

Daily dose is 6-9 grams (18). No further information available.

Comments

Although native to China, the tree of heaven has been naturalized to the United States (4501). Until recently, it was used only in folk medicine. Currently, it is being investigated as a potential drug (18).

TRYPSIN

Also Known As

Proteinase, Proteolytic Enzyme, Tripsin.

Scientific Names

Trypsin.

People Use This For

Orally, trypsin is used for digestive enzyme supplementation in conjunction with lipase, amylase, and other proteases (801,2647).

In combination with bromelain and rutin, trypsin is used for osteoarthritis (6252).

Topically, it is used for wound and ulcer cleansing to remove necrotic tissue and debris (13). Also, the prescription aerosol products containing trypsin, Peru balsam, and castor oil are applied topically for enzymatic debridement, promotion of normal wound healing (506), and promoting the healing of necrotic oral mucosa ulcers (2644).

Safety

POSSIBLY SAFE ...when used topically by health care professionals trained in wound debridement (506). The topical combination containing trypsin, Peru balsam, and castor oil is a FDA-approved prescription aerosol product.
There is insufficient reliable information available about the safety of trypsin for its other uses.
PREGNANCY AND LACTATION: Insufficient reliable information available; avoid using.

Effectiveness

POSSIBLY EFFECTIVE ...when used orally in combination with bromelain and rutin for treating osteoarthritis (6252). In a double-blind trial, 73 patients with painful osteoarthritis of the knee were randomly assigned the combination enzyme product (Phlogenzym) or diclofenac (Voltaren) 50 mg three times daily during the first week and then twice daily in weeks 2 and 3. The enzyme product was similar to diclofenac in relieving pain and improving knee function (6252). ...when used topically for cleansing wounds of necrotic material and enhancing wound healing (2643,2645).
There is insufficient reliable information available about the effectiveness of trypsin for its other uses.

Mechanism of Action

Trypsin is a proteolytic enzyme formed in the small intestines by the action of enteropeptidase on trypsinogen (511). It is used to remove dead tissue that remains after trauma, infections such as decubitus ulcers, and surgical procedures. The removal of dead cells allows the growth of healthy tissues (13). Some topical preparations that are available contain balsam of Peru and castor oil to protect the skin and prevent premature epithelial destruction (13). Evidence from in vitro studies of necroses and purulent exudates (2648) and a human study (2649) shows streptokinase-streptodornase can have better proteolytic activity than trypsin alone.

Adverse Reactions
Topically, trypsin can cause localized pain (2643) and transient burning (506).

Interactions with Herbs & Other Dietary Supplements
Insufficient reliable information available.

Interactions with Drugs
No interactions are known to occur, and there is no known reason to expect a clinically significant interaction with trypsin.

Interactions with Foods
No interactions are known to occur, and there is no known reason to expect a clinically significant interaction with trypsin.

Interactions with Lab Tests
No interactions are known to occur, and there is no known reason to expect a clinically significant interaction with trypsin.

Interactions with Diseases or Conditions
No interactions are known to occur, and there is no known reason to expect a clinically significant interaction with trypsin.

Dosage and Administration
ORAL: For osteoarthritis, a combination enzyme product (Phlogenzym), which contains rutin 100 mg, trypsin 48 mg, and bromelain 90 mg, was given 2 tablets 3 times daily (6252).
TOPICAL: Wound debridement products (Dermuspray, Granulderm, Granulex, and GranuMed) containing trypsin, Peru balsam, and castor oil (506) are FDA-approved prescription products.

Comments
Commercial trypsin is prepared from animal sources, such as ox pancreas (13).

TUNG SEED

Also Known As
Balucanat, Candle-berry, Candleberry Tree, Candlenut, China-Wood Oil, Country Walnut, Indian Walnut, Kukui, Otaheite Walnut, Tung, Varnish Tree.

Scientific Names
Aleurites moluccana or Aleurites cordata.
Family: Euphorbiaceae.

People Use This For
Orally, tung seed is used for asthma (6), bloody diarrhea (4502), dysentery (4502), sprue (4502), and as a bowel stimulant (6,4502).
Topically, tung seed is used to stimulate hair growth and for constipation (4502).
In manufacturing, the oil of tung seed is used in soaps, rubber substitutes, linoleum, and insulation (6,4502). The seed cake of tung seed is used as a fertilizer (6). The seed is also the source of the oil that is widely used as a wood preservative and varnish (4502).

Safety
LIKELY UNSAFE ...when used orally (6,4501). Tung seed is believed to contain toxalbumin and hydrogen cyanide (6). Toxicity ranges from severe gastrointestinal irritation to death (6,4501,4502). Even a single seed might cause severe poisoning (4502).
There is insufficient reliable information available about the safety of the topical use of tung seed.
PREGNANCY AND LACTATION: LIKELY UNSAFE ...when used orally (6,4501); avoid using.

Effectiveness
There is insufficient reliable information available about the effectiveness of tung seed.

Mechanism of Action
Tung seed contains an oil that consists of eleostearic acid, linolenic, linoleic and oleic acid. It is also thought to contain a toxalbumin and hydrogen cyanide (6). Internally, tung seed has cathartic effects (6,4502). The kernels have laxative and stimulant effects. They also promote sweating (4502).

Adverse Reactions
Orally, tung seed can cause severe stomach pain, violent vomiting, debility, diarrhea, slowed reflexes, slowed breathing, and possibly death (6,4501,4502). Skin contact with tung seed can cause acute dermatitis (4501,4502).

Interactions with Herbs & Other Dietary Supplements
Insufficient reliable information available.

Interactions with Drugs
No interactions are known to occur, and there is no known reason to expect a clinically significant interaction with tung seed.

Interactions with Foods
No interactions are known to occur, and there is no known reason to expect a clinically significant interaction with tung seed

Interactions with Lab Tests
No interactions are known to occur, and there is no known reason to expect a clinically significant interaction with tung seed.

Interactions with Diseases or Conditions
No interactions are known to occur, and there is no known reason to expect a clinically significant interaction with tung seed.

Dosage and Administration
No typical dosage.

Comments
The seeds of the fruit from this plant resemble a walnut, and the term walnut is applied to this species (4501). Tung seed should never be confused with the common walnut. Unlike the walnut, if tung seeds are eaten raw they are toxic. When roasted, the kernels are reported to be edible (6,4501). It is said that fishermen throw tung seeds into the water to stupefy the fish (6,4502).

TURKEY CORN

Also Known As
Bleeding Heart, Corydalis, Dutchman's Breeches, Squirrel Corn, Staggerweed.
CAUTION: See separate listing for Corydalis.

Scientific Names
Dicentra cucullaria.
Family: Furnariaceae.

People Use This For
Orally, turkey corn is used for digestive and menstrual disorders, urinary tract diseases, and skin rashes (18).

Safety
POSSIBLY UNSAFE …when used orally. Theoretically, the constituent bicuculline, an antagonist of gamma-aminobutyric acid (GABA), could cause poisoning (18).
PREGNANCY AND LACTATION: POSSIBLY UNSAFE …when used orally; avoid using.

Effectiveness
There is insufficient reliable information available about the effectiveness of turkey corn.

Mechanism of Action

The applicable part of turkey corn is the dried tuber. Turkey corn is thought to have diuretic and tonic properties (18). It contains various isoquinoline alkaloids, including bicuculline, corlumine, protopine, cryptopine, and cularine. Bicuculline is a centrally-acting, spasmogenic antagonist of GABA (18).

Adverse Reactions

None reported.

Interactions with Herbs & Other Dietary Supplements

Insufficient reliable information available.

Interactions with Drugs

No interactions are known to occur, and there is no known reason to expect a clinically significant interaction with turkey corn.

Interactions with Foods

No interactions are known to occur, and there is no known reason to expect a clinically significant interaction with turkey corn

Interactions with Lab Tests

No interactions are known to occur, and there is no known reason to expect a clinically significant interaction with turkey corn.

Interactions with Diseases or Conditions

No interactions are known to occur, and there is no known reason to expect a clinically significant interaction with turkey corn.

Dosage and Administration

ORAL: Turkey corn is used as a liquid extract (18).

Comments

None.

TURMERIC

Also Known As

Curcuma, Curcumae longae rhizoma, Curcumin, Indian Saffron, Tumeric, Turmeric Root.
CAUTION: See separate listings for Javanese Turmeric, Zedoary, and Goldenseal.

Scientific Names

Curcuma longa, synonyms Curcuma domestica, Curcuma aromatica.
Family: Zingiberaceae.

People Use This For

Orally, turmeric is used for dyspepsia (2,18), hemorrhage, jaundice, hepatitis (6), flatulence (6,18), abdominal bloating, feelings of fullness after meals, loss of appetite, liver and gallbladder complaints, headaches, abdominal pains, chest infections, fever, diarrhea, amenorrhea, "blood rushes" (18), and colorectal cancer.
Topically, turmeric is used for analgesia, ringworm (6), bruising, leech bites, festering eye infections, inflammatory skin conditions, inflammation of the oral mucosa, and infected wounds (18).
In folk medicine, turmeric root is used for diarrhea, intermittent fever, edema, bronchitis, colds, worms, leprosy, kidney inflammation, cystitis (18), and as an anticancer treatment (6).
In food and manufacturing, the essential oil is used in perfumes (11), and turmeric and its resin are used as a flavor and color component in foods (11). Turmeric is also a culinary spice and a major ingredient in curry powder (6).

Safety

LIKELY SAFE ...in amounts commonly found in foods (11). It has Generally Recognized as Safe (GRAS) status in the US as a food product (11). Maximum amount used in food is 22%, maximum amount used as a spice is 0.883%.
POSSIBLY SAFE ...when used orally or topically in medicinal amounts (2,12).
PREGNANCY: LIKELY SAFE ...when used as a spice. LIKELY UNSAFE ...when used orally in larger amounts because it might stimulate menstrual flow and the uterus (12).

LACTATION: LIKELY SAFE ...when used in amounts in food as a spice. There is insufficient reliable information available about the safety of larger amounts of turmeric during lactation.

Effectiveness
There is insufficient reliable information available about the effectiveness of turmeric.

Mechanism of Action
The applicable part of turmeric is the root. Turmeric is rich in potassium and iron (19). Turmeric root contains volatile oil and diarylheptanoids, including curcumin. The constituents of the oil show evidence of anti-inflammatory and antiarthritic activity (11). In preliminary research, turmeric-containing products demonstrate anti-inflammatory effects, but fail to show antipyretic activity (6131). Curcumin can have bile-stimulating, liver-protectant, antioxidant, and anticancer effects (6,18). Aqueous extracts also show some evidence of hypotensive effects and antispasmodic activity (11). Some evidence suggests they might also lower serum cholesterol and triglycerides. Curcuminoid constituents are responsible for the yellow color of turmeric (512).

Adverse Reactions
Orally, overuse or long-term use of turmeric can cause GI disturbances and complaints (18,512).

Interactions with Herbs & Other Dietary Supplements
HERBS WITH ANTICOAGULANT/ANTIPLATELET POTENTIAL: Concomitant use of herbs that have coumarin constituents or affect platelet aggregation could theoretically increase the risk of bleeding in some people. These herbs include: angelica, anise, arnica, asafoetida, bogbean, boldo, capsicum, celery, chamomile, clove, danshen, fenugreek, feverfew, garlic, ginger, ginkgo, ginseng (Panax), horse chestnut, horseradish, licorice, meadowsweet, prickly ash, onion, papain, passionflower, poplar, quassia, red clover, wild carrot, wild lettuce, willow, and others (4,19).

Interactions with Drugs
ANTIPLATELET DRUGS: Theoretically, turmeric might increase the effects and adverse effects of antiplatelet drugs (19).
RESERPINE AND INDOMETHACIN: Theoretically, turmeric root might reduce the frequency of reserpine and indomethacin induced gastric/duodenal ulcers (19).

Interactions with Foods
No interactions are known to occur, and there is no known reason to expect a clinically significant interaction with turmeric.

Interactions with Lab Tests
No interactions are known to occur, and there is no known reason to expect a clinically significant interaction with turmeric.

Interactions with Diseases or Conditions
OBSTRUCTION/GALLSTONES: Turmeric is contraindicated in individuals with bile duct obstruction (2,12) or gallstones.
GI DISORDERS: Turmeric is contraindicated in individuals with stomach ulcers or hyperacidity disorders (12).

Dosage and Administration
ORAL: The typical dose of turmeric is 0.5-1 grams of the powdered root several times daily between meals (8) up to 1.5-3 grams per day (2). Standardized preparations are preferred to tea preparations due to the low aqueous solubility of the volatile oil and the other active constituents (8). The tincture (1:10) is commonly dosed as 10-15 drops two to three times daily (18).
TOPICAL: No typical dosage.

Comments
Turmeric has a warm, bitter taste and a yellow color, and it is frequently used to flavor or color curry powders, mustards, butters, and cheeses (6,6002). Avoid confusion with Javanese tumeric root.

TURPENTINE OIL

Also Known As
Purified Turpentine Oil, Spirits Of Turpentine, Terebinthinae aetheroleum, Turpentine.

Scientific Names

Pinus palustris, synonym Pinus australis; Pinus pinaster; other Pinus species.
Family: Pinaceae.

People Use This For

Topically, turpentine oil is used for rheumatic and neuralgic ailments (2), muscle pain, toothaches, and disseminated sclerosis (6).
By inhalation, the vapors of turpentine oil are used to reduce the thickened secretions associated with chronic diseases of the bronchi (2).
In foods and beverages, distilled turpentine oil is used as a flavoring ingredient (11).
In manufacturing, turpentine oil is used as an ingredient in soap and cosmetics (11). Turpentine oil is also used as a paint solvent (6).

Safety

LIKELY SAFE ...when used orally in the very small amounts found in foods. In the US, turpentine oil is approved for food use, and the maximum level is 0.002% (11).
POSSIBLY SAFE ...when used topically and appropriately (2). ...when the vapors are inhaled appropriately (2).
POSSIBLY UNSAFE ...when applied topically to large areas (2).
LIKELY UNSAFE ...when used orally for medicinal purposes. 2 mL/kg of turpentine oil is considered toxic (17). 120-180 mL is potentially lethal in adults (17). Pulmonary aspiration can cause hemorrhagic pulmonary edema (17).
CHILDREN: LIKELY UNSAFE ...when used orally, 15 mL is potentially lethal (17). There is insufficient reliable information available about the safety of turpentine oil applied topically or inhaled as vapors in children.
PREGNANCY AND LACTATION: LIKELY UNSAFE ...when used orally. It might be an abortifacient (19). There is insufficient reliable information available about the safety of turpentine oil applied topically or inhaled as vapors during pregnancy and lactation.

Effectiveness

POSSIBLY EFFECTIVE ...when used as inhalation therapy for chronic diseases of the bronchi with heavy secretion (2). ...when used topically for rheumatic and neuralgic ailments (2).
There is insufficient reliable information available about the effectiveness of turpentine oil for its other uses.

Mechanism of Action

Turpentine oil is a central nervous system depressant and a pulmonary aspiration hazard. When applied topically, turpentine oil is irritating and exhibits rubefacient and counterirritant effects (6,11). When inhaled, turpentine oil can have a decongestant effect, possibly by stimulating the cold receptors, which results in reflex vasoconstriction (7).

Adverse Reactions

Orally, turpentine oil can cause headache, insomnia, coughing, vomiting, hematuria, albuminuria (6), urinary tract inflammation (17), coma (6), and death (17). Pulmonary aspiration produces hemorrhagic pulmonary edema (17). As inhalation therapy, it can cause mild respiratory tract inflammation (17). Turpentine oil can exacerbate bronchial spasms in people with asthma and whooping cough (7).
Topically, it can cause skin irritation, contact allergies, and hypersensitivity (6). Symptoms of poisoning can occur when turpentine oil is applied extensively, including kidney and central nervous system damage (2).

Interactions with Herbs & Other Dietary Supplements

Insufficient reliable information available.

Interactions with Drugs

No interactions are known to occur, and there is no known reason to expect a clinically significant interaction with turpentine oil.

Interactions with Foods

No interactions are known to occur, and there is no known reason to expect a clinically significant interaction with turpentine oil.

Interactions with Lab Tests

No interactions are known to occur, and there is no known reason to expect a clinically significant interaction with turpentine oil.

Interactions with Diseases or Conditions

ACUTE RESPIRATORY TRACT INFLAMMATION: Inhalation of turpentine is contraindicated (2).

ASTHMA, WHOOPING COUGH: Turpentine can exacerbate bronchial spasms (7).
HYPERSENSITIVITY: Contraindicated (2).

Dosage and Administration
TOPICAL: Several drops of the oil are typically rubbed onto the affected area. The liquid and semi-solid preparations are commonly made in concentrations of 10-50% (2). Application of turpentine should not exceed three to four times per day (3).
INHALATION: The vapors of turpentine are often inhaled as several drops of the oil in hot water (2).

Comments
Turpentine oil is obtained by the distillation of the oleoresin (gum turpentine) of longleaf pine (Pinus palustris) and other Pinus species. Terpin hydrate is a semi-synthetic derivative of turpentine (6). Turpentine oil has been used to adulterate juniper berry oil (512). Avoid confusion with gum turpentine, which is the oleoresin (6).

TURTLE HEAD

Also Known As
Balmony, Bitter Herb, Chelone, Hummingbird Tree, Salt-rheum Weed, Shellflower, Snakehead, Turtlebloom.

Scientific Names
Chelone glabra.
Family: Scrophulariaceae.

People Use This For
Orally, turtle head above ground parts and roots are used as a cathartic tonic (4500).

Safety
POSSIBLY SAFE …when used orally (12,18).
PREGNANCY AND LACTATION: Insufficient reliable information available; avoid using.

Effectiveness
There is insufficient reliable information available about the effectiveness of turtle head.

Mechanism of Action
The applicable parts of turtle head are the above ground parts and root. Turtle head contains iridoide monoterpenes including catalpol and a bitter-tasting resin (18).

Adverse Reactions
None reported.

Interactions with Herbs & Other Dietary Supplements
Insufficient reliable information available.

Interactions with Drugs
No interactions are known to occur, and there is no known reason to expect a clinically significant interaction with turtle head.

Interactions with Foods
No interactions are known to occur, and there is no known reason to expect a clinically significant interaction with turtle head.

Interactions with Lab Tests
No interactions are known to occur, and there is no known reason to expect a clinically significant interaction with turtle head.

Interactions with Diseases or Conditions
No interactions are known to occur, and there is no known reason to expect a clinically significant interaction with turtle head.

Dosage and Administration
No typical dosage.

Comments
Avoid confusion with Chelone obliqua commonly known as red turtle head (4500).

TYROSINE

Also Known As
L-tyrosine, Tyr, Tyrosinum.

Scientific Names
2-amino-3-(4-hydroxyphenyl)propionic acid.

People Use This For
Orally, tyrosine is used for depression, attention deficit disorder (ADD/ADHD), hyperactivity disorder, phenylketonuria, and improving alertness following sleep depravation. It is also used for stress, premenstrual syndrome (PMS), Parkinson's disease, chronic fatigue syndrome (CFS), narcolepsy, alcohol and cocaine withdrawal, Alzheimer's disease, cardiovascular disease, impotence, loss of libido, schizophrenia, and as a suntan agent and appetite suppressant.

Safety
LIKELY SAFE …when used orally in amounts found in foods. Tyrosine has Generally Recognized as Safe (GRAS) status in the US (7218).
POSSIBLY SAFE …when used orally and appropriately, short-term. Tyrosine seems to be safe when used in doses up to 150 mg/kg per day for up to 3 months (7210,7211,7215).
CHILDREN: LIKELY SAFE …when used orally in amounts found in foods (7218). There is insufficient reliable information available about the safety of tyrosine in children when used in higher amounts.
PREGNANCY AND LACTATION: LIKELY SAFE …when used orally in amounts found in foods (7218). There is insufficient reliable information available about the safety of tyrosine during pregnancy and lactation when used in larger amounts.

Effectiveness
EFFECTIVE …when used orally for phenylketonuria (PKU). Tyrosine is used as a component of protein supplements for people with phenylketonuria (PKU), a genetic disorder in which there is an inability to metabolize phenylalanine, a precursor of tyrosine (7212,7213,7232). The current recommendation for people with PKU is the incorporation of 6 grams of tyrosine per 100 grams of protein. However, additional separate supplementation with free tyrosine is not recommended because it can produce wide variations in tyrosine plasma concentrations and potential side effects (7212).
POSSIBLY EFFECTIVE …when used orally for improving alertness following sleep depravation (7215). Tyrosine 150 mg/kg seems to delay performance decline in psychomotor tests by about 3 hours after loss of a night's sleep (7215).
POSSIBLY INEFFECTIVE …when used orally for moderate depression (7208). …when used orally for adult attention deficit disorder (ADD). Some patients might have transient improvement in symptoms after starting tyrosine, but adult patients quickly grow tolerant to its effects (7210,7211). …when used orally for childhood attention deficit disorder (ADD) (7209).
There is insufficient reliable information available about the effectiveness of tyrosine for its other uses.

Mechanism of Action
Tyrosine is a nonessential amino acid that the body synthesizes from phenylalanine. For people with phenylketonuria (PKU) who cannot synthesize tyrosine from phenylalanine, tyrosine is an essential amino acid (7212). Tyrosine can also be obtained from dietary proteins in dairy products, meats, fish, eggs, nuts, beans, oats, and wheat. When dietary intake of tyrosine is inadequate, more phenylalanine is converted to tyrosine (7217). Dietary needs of tyrosine are dependent on phenylalanine. When phenylalanine intake is adequate (about 9 mg/kg/day), dietary tyrosine intake should be about 7 mg/kg/day (7214). Inadequate tyrosine intake is rare in developed nations.
Tyrosine is incorporated into all proteins. It is a precursor of thyroxine and melanin (7212) and a precursor for the synthesis of the catecholamines, norepinephrine, epinephrine, and dopamine (7215,7217). Tyrosine is classified as a large neutral amino acid (LNAA) and is transported across the blood brain barrier by the LNAA transporter. Tyrosine competes with other LNAAs, such as tryptophan, to get into the brain (7217). There is interest in tyrosine for preventing the negative effects related to stress. Some scientists think that the brain may not be able to synthesize enough tyrosine from phenylalanine to meet its needs under stressful conditions (7217). Tyrosine is needed for synthesizing

catecholamines like epinephrine, norepinephrine, and dopamine that can become depleted during stress. There is speculation that increasing the availability of tyrosine to the brain allows increased catecholamine synthesis, and avoidance of the negative effects of stress. There is some evidence in animals and humans that supplemental tyrosine might improve performance, memory, and learning under extreme environmental conditions, intense exercise, or psychological stress (7215,7217).

Adverse Reactions
Orally, tyrosine can cause some side effects including nausea, headache, fatigue, heartburn, and arthralgia (7211).

Interactions with Herbs & Other Dietary Supplements
Insufficient reliable information available.

Interactions with Drugs
LEVODOPA (L-DOPA) (Sinemet): There is some concern that tyrosine might decrease the effectiveness of L-dopa. Tyrosine and levodopa compete for absorption in the proximal duodenum by the large neutral amino acid (LNAA) transport system (1289). Advise patients to separate doses of tyrosine and L-dopa by at least 2 hours.
THYROID HORMONE MEDICATIONS: There is some concern that tyrosine might have additive effects with thyroid hormone medications. Tyrosine is a precursor to thyroid hormone and might boost levels (7212). These drugs include Levothyroxine (Synthroid, Levoxyl) and liothyroxine (Cytomel).

Interactions with Foods
No interactions are known to occur, and there is no known reason to expect a clinically significant interaction with tyrosine.

Interactions with Lab Tests
THYROID STIMULATING HORMONE (TSH): Theoretically, tyrosine might decrease TSH levels. Tyrosine is a precursor of thyroxine and might boost thyroid hormone levels, which can decrease TSH results (7212).

Interactions with Diseases or Conditions
HYPERTHYROIDISM, GRAVES' DISEASE: Theoretically, tyrosine might exacerbate hyperthyroidism and Grave's disease. Tyrosine is a precursor of thyroxine and might boost levels (7212). Tell patients with hyperthyroidism or Grave's disease not to take tyrosine supplements.

Dosage and Administration
ORAL: For improving alertness after sleep depravation, 150 mg/kg/day of tyrosine has been used (7215).

Comments
None.

USNEA

Also Known As
Beard Moss, Old Man's Beard, Tree Moss, Tree's Dandruff, Usnea Lichen, Woman's Long Hair.
CAUTION: See separate listing for Oak Moss.

Scientific Names
Usnea species, including Usnea barbata, Usnea florida, Usnea hirta, Usnea plicata.
Family: Usneaceae.

People Use This For
Topically, usnea is used for mild inflammation of the mouth and pharynx (2,18).

Safety
POSSIBLY SAFE ...when used topically and appropriately (2,12).
PREGNANCY AND LACTATION: Insufficient reliable information available; avoid using.

Effectiveness
POSSIBLY EFFECTIVE ...when used topically for mild inflammation of the oral and pharyngeal mucosa (2).

Mechanism of Action

The applicable part of usnea is the plant body. Usnea contains a variety of lichen acids including usnic acid, thamnolic acid, lobaric acid, stictinic acid, evernic acid, barbatic acid, diffractaic acid, protocetraric acid. However, the exact composition varies significantly amongst species. Usnea is considered to have antimicrobial activity (2). The hydroalcoholic extracts of Usnea barbata and Usnea hirta have anti-inflammatory, analgesic, and antipyretic activity (852).

Adverse Reactions

Topically, poisoning can be possible, although signs of poisoning have not yet been described (18). Adverse reactions are uncommon in appropriate amounts.

Interactions with Herbs & Other Dietary Supplements

Insufficient reliable information available.

Interactions with Drugs

No interactions are known to occur, and there is no known reason to expect a clinically significant interaction with usnea.

Interactions with Foods

No interactions are known to occur, and there is no known reason to expect a clinically significant interaction with usnea.

Interactions with Lab Tests

No interactions are known to occur, and there is no known reason to expect a clinically significant interaction with usnea.

Interactions with Diseases or Conditions

No interactions are known to occur, and there is no known reason to expect a clinically significant interaction with usnea.

Dosage and Administration

TOPICAL: The typical dose of usnea is one lozenge three to six times per day. Each lozenge usually contains the equivalent of 100 mg dried usnea (2).

Comments

Usnea species are whitish, reddish, or black lichens that grow on a variety of trees. Avoid confusion with oak moss (Evernia prunastri), also referred to as tree moss.

UVA URSI

Also Known As

Arberry, Arcostaphylos, Bear's Grape, Bearberry, Beargrape, Bearsgrape, Common Bearberry, Hogberry, Kinnikinnik, Manzanita, Mountain Box, Mountain Cranberry, Ptarmigan Berry, Raisin D'Ours, Red Bearberry, Redberry, Rockberry, Sagackhomi, Sandberry, Uva-Ursi, Uvae ursi folium.
CAUTION: See separate listings for Alpine Cranberry, Cramp Bark, and Cranberry.

Scientific Names

Arctostaphylos uva-ursi, synonym Arbutus uva-ursi.
Family: Ericacea.

People Use This For

Orally, uva ursi is used for urinary tract infections (UTIs) (4,5,6,18), inflammatory conditions of the efferent urinary tract (2,5,6,18), cystitis, urethritis, diuresis, constipation (4,5,6), lithuria, dysuria, acidic urine, pyelonephritis (4), and bronchitis (11).
In combination, an herbal preparation containing uva ursi, hops, and peppermint is used to treat people with compulsive, strangury enuresis and painful urination (4).

Safety

POSSIBLY SAFE ...when used orally and appropriately, short-term (2,4,12).
POSSIBLY UNSAFE ...when used orally for extended periods. There is some concern about the safety of long-term

use because of the hydroquinone constituent of uva ursi. Hydroquinone can have mutagenic and carcinogenic effects, and long-term use might result in significant adverse effects. Tell patients to avoid using uva ursi for more than one week or more than five times per year (2,7,18).

CHILDREN: LIKELY UNSAFE ...when used orally due to the risk of hepatotoxicity in children less than 12 years old (2,7,18).

PREGNANCY: LIKELY UNSAFE ...when used orally (2,4,6,7,12,18). Uva ursi can have oxytocic effects (19); avoid using.

LACTATION: Insufficient reliable information available; avoid using (2).

Effectiveness

POSSIBLY EFFECTIVE ...when used orally for treating inflammatory disorders of the efferent urinary tract, including urinary tract infections (UTIs) (2,4,4800). ...when used orally in combination with dandelion to prevent recurrent urinary tract infections (UTIs) (1932). A combination product containing both uva ursi and dandelion seems to significantly reduce the recurrence rate of UTIs in women (1932). However, since it is not clear if this kind of extended use is safe, tell patients not to use uva ursi product for long-term prevention of UTIs.

There is insufficient reliable information available about the effectiveness of uva ursi for its other uses.

Mechanism of Action

The applicable part of uva ursi is the leaf. Uva ursi can have urinary antiseptic and astringent effects (4). Some references report diuretic activity, but others disagree (6,8). Its constituents include arbutin (a phenol), tannins, and hydroquinone (4,6,7). The tannins can be responsible for adverse gastrointestinal tract effects (5) and limit the duration of use (4). Uva ursi and the constituent, arbutin, exhibit antimicrobial activity in vitro (2,4). Arbutin is absorbed from the gastrointestinal tract unchanged and is hydrolyzed to hydroquinone in alkaline urine. There it can exert antiseptic and astringent effects (4,5,7). Hydroquinone is cytotoxic in vitro (4). Crude uva ursi extract can be more effective than the constituent arbutin as an astringent and antiseptic (4). In rats, uva ursi shows anti-inflammatory activity against experimentally-induced inflammation (4). Large amounts of uva ursi are reported to be oxytocic, although in vitro studies show no uteroactivity (4).

Adverse Reactions

Orally, uva ursi can cause nausea, vomiting (2), gastrointestinal discomfort, and a greenish-brown discoloration of the urine (4). Large amounts can be oxytocic, increasing the rapidity of labor (4). One gram of hydroquinone, equivalent to 6-20 grams of uva ursi, can cause tinnitus, nausea, vomiting, shortness of breath, cyanosis, convulsions, delirium, and collapse (4). Five grams of hydroquinone, equivalent to 30-100 grams of uva ursi, can cause death (4). Other adverse effects due to uva ursi include hepatotoxicity and irritation and inflammation of the urinary tract mucous membranes (18). Chronic use, especially in children (18), can cause liver impairment due to its tannin content (4).

Interactions with Herbs & Other Dietary Supplements

URINE-ACIDIFIERS: Theoretically, concomitant use of uva ursi with products that acidify the urine, including vitamin C, can reduce the antibacterial activity of uva ursi (2,12,19).

URINE-ALKALINIZERS: Theoretically, concomitant use of uva ursi with products that alkalinize the urine, including sodium bicarbonate, can enhance the antibacterial activity of uva ursi (8).

Interactions with Drugs

URINE-ACIDIFYING DRUGS: Concomitant use with drugs that acidify the urine can reduce the antibacterial efficacy of uva ursi (2,19).

URINE-ALKALINIZING DRUGS: Theoretically, concomitant use with drugs that alkalinize the urine can enhance the antibacterial activity of uva ursi (2,19).

Interactions with Foods

URINE-ACIDIFYING FOODS: Foods that acidify urine, including acidic fruits and juices, can reduce the antibacterial activity of uva ursi (2,5,19).

URINE-ALKALINIZING FOODS: Foods that alkalinize urine can enhance the antibacterial activity of uva ursi (7,8).

Interactions with Lab Tests

COLORIMETRIC URINE TESTS: Theoretically, uva ursi can interfere with colorimetric urine tests and can turn urine greenish-brown (4).

Interactions with Diseases or Conditions

KIDNEY DISORDERS: Contraindicated (12,19).

GI IRRITATION: Because excessive use of uva ursi can lead to stomach distress due to its tannin content, its use is contraindicated in patients with GI irritation (12,19).

Dosage and Administration

ORAL: The typical dose of dried herb is 1.5-4 grams daily (4). It's also commonly used as a tea. The tea is prepared by steeping 3 grams of the dried leaf in 150 mL cold water for 12-24 hours and then straining. One cup of tea is usually taken up to 4 times daily (2,7,515). Uva ursi leaf teas should be prepared with cold water to minimize the tannin content (515). The hydroquinone derivative, calculated as water-free arbutin, is commonly dosed as 100-210 mg up to 4 times daily (2,7,515). The fluid extract (1:1 in 25% alcohol) is given 1.5-4 mL three times daily (4). Medical consultation is needed for urinary tract symptoms persisting longer than 48 hours (4). Uva ursi should not be used longer than one week without monitoring due to its potential risks (7). Limit its use to less than five times per year (7).

Comments

Bears are particularly fond of the fruit, which is implied in the Latin name "uva ursi", which means "bear's grape." Most authorities refer to Arctostaphylos uva-ursi as uva ursi. However, the related plants, Arctostaphylos adentricha and Arctostaphylos coactylis, have also been termed uva ursi by some authors (6).

UZARA

Also Known As

Uzara, Uzarae radix.

Scientific Names

Xysmalobium undulatum.
Family: Asclepiadaceae.

People Use This For

Orally, uzara is used for diarrhea (2,18).

Safety

POSSIBLY SAFE ...when used orally for short-term use (2). Medical consultation is needed for diarrhea persisting more than three to four days (2).
LIKELY UNSAFE ...when used parenterally. Deaths have occurred after administration of uzara products (18).
PREGNANCY AND LACTATION: Insufficient reliable information available; avoid using.

Effectiveness

There is insufficient reliable information available about the effectiveness of uzara.

Mechanism of Action

The applicable part of uzara is the root. It inhibits intestinal motility (2), and in larger amounts, it can have digitalis-like effects on the heart (2). Uzara contains a cardiac glycoside mixture of cardenolides, which include uzarone, xysmalobin, and uzarin. The glycosides can be poorly absorbed (2,18).

Adverse Reactions

Orally, there have been no reports of adverse reactions associated with white uzara, but it is theoretically possible due to the cardiac glycoside content (2,18).
Parenterally, deaths have occurred after administration of uzara products (18).

Interactions with Herbs & Other Dietary Supplements

CARDIAC GLYCOSIDE-CONTAINING HERBS: Uzara is contraindicated with these herbs, and concomitant use can increase the risk of cardiac glycoside toxicity. Cardiac glycoside containing herbs include black hellebore, Canadian hemp roots, digitalis leaf, hedge mustard, figwort, lily of the valley roots, motherwort, oleander leaf, pheasant's eye plant, pleurisy root, squill bulb leaf scales, and strophanthus seeds (2,18,19,500).
OTHER CARDIOACTIVE HERBS: Avoid concomitant use of uzara with other cardioactive herbs due to the unpredictability of therapeutic and adverse effects. Other cardioactive herbs include calamus, cereus, cola, coltsfoot, devil's claw, European mistletoe, fenugreek, fumitory, ginger, ginseng panax, hawthorn, white horehound, mate, parsley, quassia, scotch broom flower, shepherd's purse, and wild carrot (4).
STIMULANT LAXATIVE HERBS: Theoretically, overuse or misuse of stimulant laxatives with cardiac glycoside-containing herbs, like uzara, increases the risk of cardiac toxicity due to potassium depletion. Stimulant laxative herbs include the dried leaf sap of aloe, blue flag rhizome, alder buckthorn, European buckthorn, butternut bark, cascara bark, castor oil, colocynth fruit pulp, gamboge bark exudate, jalap root, black root, manna bark exudate, podophyllum root, rhubarb root, senna leaves and pods, wild cucumber fruit (Ecballium elaterium), and yellow dock root (19).

LICORICE/HORSETAIL: Theoretically, overuse or misuse of the licorice rhizome or horsetail plant with cardiac glycoside-containing herbs, like uzara, increases the risk of cardiac toxicity due to potassium depletion (19).

Interactions with Drugs

DIGOXIN: Uzara is contraindicated with digoxin because therapeutic duplication increases the risk of cardiac glycoside toxicity (2).
CARDIAC DRUGS: Theoretically, concomitant use with uzara can increase the risk of cardiac toxicity (152).
STIMULANT LAXATIVES: Theoretically, overuse or misuse can increase the risk of cardiac glycoside toxicity due to potassium depletion (2).
POTASSIUM-DEPLETING DIURETICS: Theoretically, concomitant use with uzara can increase the risk of cardiac glycoside toxicity due to potassium depletion (2,506).
QUININE: Theoretically, concomitant use can increase the risk of cardiac toxicity (2,506).
TETRACYCLINES and MACROLIDE ANTIBIOTICS (erythromycin-like drugs): Theoretically, concomitant use with uzara can increase the risk of cardiac glycoside toxicity (152,17).

Interactions with Foods

No interactions are known to occur, and there is no known reason to expect a clinically significant interaction with uzara.

Interactions with Lab Tests

No interactions are known to occur, and there is no known reason to expect a clinically significant interaction with uzara.

Interactions with Diseases or Conditions

HEART DISEASE: Uzara is contraindicated in individuals with heart disease (2,18). Theoretically, the cardiac glycosides contained in uzara can exacerbate this condition or interfere with existing drug therapy.
HYPOKALEMIA: Theoretically, the use of uzara can increase the risk of cardiac toxicity in hypokalemic patients.

Dosage and Administration

ORAL: Uzara is commonly taken as liquid ethanol-water extracts or dry extracts obtained from methanol-water extractions (2). The initial dose is 75 mg of the total glycosides calculated as uzarin or the equivalent to 1 gram of the dried root (2). Then the dose is 45-90 mg per day of the total glycosides calculated as uzarin (2). Seek medical consultation for diarrhea persisting more than three to four days (2).

Comments

None.

VALERIAN

Also Known As

Amantilla, All-Heal, Baldrian, Baldrianwurzel, Belgium Valerian, Common Valerian, Fragrant Valerian, Garden Heliotrope, Garden Valerian, Indian Valerian, Mexican Valerian, Pacific Valerian, Valeriana, Valeriana officinalis, Valeriana rhizome, Valerianae radix, Valeriane.

Scientific Names

Valeriana edulis; Valeriana jatamansii, synonym Valeriana wallichii; Valeriana officinalis; Valeriana sitchensis. Family: Valerianaceae.

People Use This For

Orally, valerian is used as a sedative-hypnotic for insomnia and as an anxiolytic for restlessness and sleeping disorders associated with anxiety (2). It has also been used for mood disorders such as depression (7), infantile convulsions, mild tremors, epilepsy, and attention deficit hyperactivity disorder (ADHD). It is also used orally for muscle and joint pain (6121), conditions associated with anxiety and psychological stress including nervous asthma, headaches, and stomach upset. Valerian is also used for menstrual cramps and symptoms associated with menopause, including hot flashes and anxiety (304,3484).
Topically, valerian is used as a bath additive for restlessness and sleep disorders (2,18).
Traditionally, valerian is used for hysterical states, excitability, hypochondria, and migraine (4).
In manufacturing, the extracts and essential oil are used as flavoring in foods and beverages (11).

Safety

LIKELY SAFE ...when used in amounts found in foods. The maximum use level in foods is 0.01% for the extract and 0.002% for the essential oil. Valeriana officinalis is approved for food use in the US and has Generally Recognized as Safe (GRAS) status in the US (11,3484).

POSSIBLY SAFE ...when used orally and appropriately, short-term for medicinal purposes (12). Clinical studies have reported safe use of valerian in over 12,000 patients in trials lasting up to 28 days (304,2074,3484,3485,6480).

POSSIBLY UNSAFE ...when used orally long term or in high doses. Extended use has been associated with a benzodiazepine-like withdrawal syndrome when discontinued. Long-term use of valerian has been associated with hepatotoxicity in four cases (304); however, some suggest that hepatotoxicity may be an idiosyncratic reaction to valerian rather than dose-related (304). There is insufficient reliable information available about the safety the topical use of valerian.

PREGNANCY AND LACTATION: Insufficient reliable information available; avoid using (4).

Effectiveness

POSSIBLY EFFECTIVE ...when used orally for insomnia. Several small-scale studies have shown consistent benefit in reducing the time to sleep onset (sleep latency) and subjective improvement in sleep quality in patients using valerian compared to placebo (7,304,3485,6248,6249). Valerian seems to be comparable to low-dose benzodiazepines (6480); however, valerian does not always relieve insomnia as fast as benzodiazepines. Sometimes several days to 4 weeks of continuous nightly use is required for significant relief (7,6249). ...when used orally for subjective improvement in restlessness and sleep disorders associated with behavioral disorders and anxiety (2,7,304). ...when used orally for improving mood (7). Significant improvement can require 2-4 weeks of treatment (7). ...when used orally for subjective improvement in ability to concentrate (304,2074).

Clinical studies have used a variety of valerian root extracts including some that were standardized to contain 0.4-0.6% valerenic acid (7,304,3485).

There is insufficient reliable information available about the effectiveness of valerian for its other uses.

Mechanism of Action

The applicable part of valerian is the root. Valerian is reported to have sedative-hypnotic, anxiolytic, antidepressant, anticonvulsant, and antispasmodic effects (7,3484,3485). Valerian might also have hypotensive and mild analgesic properties (4). The pharmacological effects of valerian have primarily been attributed to constituents known as valepotriates and volatile oils, including monoterpenes and sesquiterpenes. The primary monoterpene is berneol and the primary sesquiterpenes are valerenic acid, valerenone, and kessyl glycol (4,7,3484,3486). However, because valerian extracts without some of these constituents have similar effects, it is likely that multiple constituents are responsible for its pharmacological effects (304). Valepotriate constituents are known to have sedative-hypnotic and spasmolytic effects. Valepotriates have also been shown to decrease benzodiazepine withdrawal in an animal model and to bind dopamine receptors (3484,3486). The valepotriates might possibly act as prodrugs. They are thought to rapidly decompose to homobaldrinal in the intestine after ingestion (3486). Valepotriates are highly unstable and rapidly decompose in acid or alkaline environments and at high temperatures. Although there are published reports of toxicity due to the valepotriate constituents, because these constituents are poorly absorbed and quickly degraded to less toxic metabolites, they are not likely to cause acute adverse reactions (12). Commercial preparations are thought to rarely contain valepotriates (2,7,304). The presence of an epoxide group on the valepotriates has raised concern about possible cytotoxicity and carcinogenicity (7,3485,3486); however, in vivo studies to date have failed to show any carcinogenic effects (3486). The sesquiterpenes, valerenic acid and kessyl glycol, have been shown to cause sedation in animals (3486). Valerenic acid also appears to inhibit the enzyme system responsible for the central catabolism of GABA, increasing GABA concentrations and decreasing CNS activity (4,3486). There is some evidence that valerian might also contain other constituents such as lignans and GABA which may also be responsible for the sedative effects of valerian (304,3486).

Adverse Reactions

Orally, valerian can cause headache, excitability, uneasiness, cardiac disturbances, and insomnia (6,12,3484). Occasionally, valerian causes morning drowsiness (2074). Although most reports describe a lack of residual morning effects on alertness and concentration, a few reports suggest that impaired alertness and information processing does occur (12,2074). Impairment is dose-dependent and peaks within the first few hours after an oral valerian dose (304,2074). Patients should be warned against driving or operating dangerous machinery after taking valerian (304). Signs of valerian toxicity include trouble walking, hypothermia, and increased muscle relaxation (6). Side effects are rare in products without valepotriate constituents (7). In one individual, 20 times the normal dose caused fatigue, tight chest, abdominal cramping, and tremor of the hand and foot (659). Extended use can cause benzodiazepine-like withdrawal symptoms when treatment is discontinued (304,3487). Patients should taper doses slowly after extended use. There have been several case reports of hepatotoxicity associated with use of multi-ingredient preparations containing valerian. In these cases, it is thought that the preparations may have been adulterated with hepatotoxic agents (304). Four other cases of hepatotoxicity involving long-term use of single-ingredient valerian preparations have also been reported (304,3484).

Because a variety of doses were used in the cases reported and many people have used higher doses safely, some suggest these hepatotoxic reactions might have been idiosyncratic (304).

Interactions with Herbs & Other Dietary Supplements
HERBS AND SUPPLEMENTS WITH SEDATIVE PROPERTIES: Use of valerian with other herbs and supplements that have sedative properties might enhance therapeutic and possibly adverse effects. Some of these products include calamus, calendula, California poppy, catnip, capsicum, celery, couch grass, elecampane, ginseng Siberian, German chamomile, goldenseal, gotu kola, hops, Jamaican dogwood, kava, L-tryptophan, lemon balm, melatonin, sage, SAMe, St. John's wort, sassafras, scullcap, shepherd's purse, stinging nettle, wild carrot, wild lettuce, ashwaganda root, and yerba mansa (4,19).

Interactions with Drugs
ALCOHOL: Theoretically, valerian can potentiate the sedative effects of alcohol (4).
BARBITURATES: Theoretically, concomitant use of valerian with barbiturates can cause additive therapeutic and adverse effects (19).
BENZODIAZEPINES: Theoretically, concomitant use with benzodiazepines can cause additive therapeutic and adverse effects (19).
OTHER DRUGS WITH SEDATIVE PROPERTIES: Theoretically, concomitant use of valerian and drugs with sedative properties can cause additive therapeutic and adverse effects (4,19).
OTHER DRUGS: There is preliminary evidence that valerian can inhibit the cytochrome P450 (CYP450) 3A4 enzyme (6450). Theoretically, valerian might increase levels of drugs metabolized by CYP450 3A4. However, so far, this interaction has not been reported in humans. Some drugs metabolized by CYP450 3A4 include lovastatin (Mevacor), ketoconazole (Nizoral), itraconazole (Sporanox), fexofenadine (Allegra), triazolam (Halcion), chemotherapeutic agents (etoposide, paclitaxel, vinblastine, vincristine, vindesine), and numerous others. Use valerian cautiously or avoid in patients taking these drugs.

Interactions with Foods
ALCOHOL: Theoretically, valerian can potentiate the sedative effects of alcohol (4).

Interactions with Lab Tests
No interactions are known to occur, and there is no known reason to expect a clinically significant interaction with valerian.

Interactions with Diseases or Conditions
No interactions are known to occur, and there is no known reason to expect a clinically significant interaction with valerian.

Dosage and Administration
ORAL: The typical dose of valerian is one cup of the tea taken one to several times per day. The tea is prepared by steeping 2-3 grams of the root in 150 mL of boiling water for 5-10 minutes and then straining (2). The maximum dose of valerian is 15 grams of the root per day (18). The simple tincture is commonly taken as 1-3 mL once to several times per day (2,18). The tincture (1:5) is typically dosed as 15-20 drops in water several times per day (18). Extracts in amounts equivalent to 2-3 grams of the root have been taken several times per day (2). For decreasing sleep latency and improving sleep quality, most studies have used 400-900 mg valerian extract up to 2 hours before bedtime for as long as 28 days (7,304,2074,3484,6480). Other studies have used valerian extract 45 mg given 3 to 9 times daily or 450 mg three times daily (304,3484).
TOPICAL: Prepared by mixing 100 grams of the root with 2 L of hot water, and adding to one full bath (2,18).

Comments
In Germany, one specific tincture is required to carry a label warning of reduced ability to drive or operate machinery (12). Even though there is some evidence that valepotriate constituents might be mutagenic, they are rarely found in commercial products because they are unstable and heat labile (304).

VANADIUM

Also Known As
Metavanadate, Orthovanadate, Vanadate, Vanadium Pentoxide, Vanadyl, Vanadyl Sulfate.

Scientific Names
Vanadium; V; atomic number 23.

People Use This For

Orally, vanadium is used for diabetes, hypoglycemia, hyperlipidemia, heart disease, edema, improving athletic performance in weight training, and preventing cancer. Vanadium is also used for treating tuberculosis, diabetes, syphilis, and a form of microcytic anemia (chlorosis).

Safety

LIKELY SAFE ...when used orally and appropriately. Vanadium is safe when taken in amounts below the tolerable upper intake level (UL) of 1.8 mg per day (7135).

POSSIBLY UNSAFE ...when used orally in high doses. Taking more than the tolerable upper intake level (UL) of 1.8 mg per day can increase the risk of gastrointestinal side effects and theoretically, renal toxicity (7135). In some cases, patients with diabetes have used very high doses (100 mg per day) safely for up to 4 weeks (3055,3056,3057). However, there is concern that prolonged use of high doses might cause serious side effects including kidney damage (7135). Tell patients to avoid exceeding the UL.

CHILDREN: LIKELY SAFE ...when used orally in amounts found in foods (7135). There is insufficient reliable information available about the safety of vanadium when used in children in amounts greater than those typically found in foods.

PREGNANCY AND LACTATION: LIKELY SAFE ...when used orally in amounts found in foods (7135). There is insufficient reliable information available about the safety of vanadium when used in pregnant or breast-feeding women in amounts greater than those typically found in foods.

Effectiveness

POSSIBLY EFFECTIVE ...when used orally for type 2 diabetes. There is some evidence that high doses of vanadyl sulfate (100 mg daily, 31 mg elemental vanadium), can improve hepatic and peripheral insulin sensitivity in patients with type 2 diabetes and possibly reduce blood glucose levels (3055,3056,3057); however, prolonged used of these high doses might not be safe (7135). It's not known if lower doses have the same benefit. Until more is known, tell patients not to use vanadium for treating type 2 diabetes.

There is insufficient reliable information available about the effectiveness of vanadium for its other uses.

Mechanism of Action

Vanadium is a trace mineral. Good sources of dietary vanadium include mushrooms; shellfish; black pepper; parsley; dillseed; grains and grain products; and beverages such as beer, wine, and artificially sweetened drinks (7135). Drinking water can also contain trace amounts of vanadium (3011). Several forms of vanadium are available, including vanadyl sulfate and salts of metavanadate and orthovanadate. The vanadium pentoxide form, which is considered toxic, is not found in foods or supplements. An average diet provides 6 to 18 mcg vanadium per day. Only about 5% of ingested vanadium is absorbed. In vivo, vanadium is converted to the vanadyl cation, which can form complexes with ferritin and transferrin. Highest concentrations are found in the liver, kidney, and bone (7135).

Vanadium appears to be important in normal bone growth and as a cofactor for various enzyme reactions. Vanadium inhibits ATPases, phosphatases, and phosphoryl-transfer enzymes (7135).

Vanadium also seems to have cardiovascular effects. There is some evidence that prolonged administration might be associated with dose-dependent increases in blood pressure (3012). Vanadium also seems to have digitalis-like effects on heart muscle, producing positive inotropic effects, diuresis, and natriuresis (14). Vanadium also inhibits cholesterol synthesis from mevalonic acid (3012).

Some evidence suggests that vanadium can mimic the actions of insulin, possibly by causing phosphorylation of insulin receptor proteins. Vanadium activates the receptor; stimulates glucose oxidation and transport; inhibits lipolysis in adipose tissue; stimulates glycogen synthesis in the liver; inhibits hepatic gluconeogenesis; inhibits intestinal glucose transport; and increases glucose uptake, utilization, and glycogen synthesis in skeletal muscle (3012,3013). It appears to augment the effects of insulin in insulin-resistant type 2 diabetes, but might not have an effect in type 1 diabetes (482). Preliminary evidence suggests that L-glutamic acid gamma-monohydroxamate might activate endogenous vanadium, facilitating glucose metabolism through conversion of intracellular vanadium into an active insulinomimetic compound (388).

There is also some evidence that vanadium might protect against dental caries (3012). A few preliminary studies suggest vanadium might offer protection against hematological toxicity and the development of hepatic carcinoma (3014,3016), but others suggest that vanadium is potentially mutagenic, carcinogenic (3019), and might interfere with mitosis and chromosome distribution (3051).

Adverse Reactions

Orally, vanadium most commonly causes mild gastrointestinal upset (7135). There is concern that taking doses exceeding the tolerable upper intake level (UL) of 1.8 mg per day can increase the risk of gastrointestinal side effects and possibly lead to more severe toxicity. In some cases, patients with diabetes have used very high doses (100 mg per day) safely for up to 4 weeks (3055,3056,3057). However, there is concern that prolonged use of high doses might cause serious side effects including kidney damage (7135). Doses of 22.5 mg daily for five months can cause cramps and diarrhea (3012). Vanadium has also been associated with green discoloration of tongue, fatigue, lethargy, and focal neurological lesions, which were unrelated to dose (7135).

Significant toxic effects have been observed in animal studies of vanadium including decreased weight gain, deterioration in health, pro-oxidant effects, alteration in renal function, increased serum urea and creatinine levels, tissue vanadium accumulation, and some deaths (3017,3018,3021). High body levels of vanadium have been associated with an increased incidence of renal stone disease, distal renal tubular acidosis, hypokalemic periodic paralysis, sudden unexplained nocturnal death, and malnutrition-related diabetes mellitus (3020).

Ingestion of vanadium pentoxide form of vanadium can cause significant toxicity. It has been associated with gastrointestinal disturbances, abnormalities of renal function tests, and nervous system effects (3011). Severe and chronic respiratory tract disorders have been reported from occupational exposure to vanadium dusts (17). This form of vanadium is not found in foods or vanadium supplements.

Toxic effects from systemic exposure to industrial vanadium-containing compounds include peripheral vasoconstriction, arrhythmias, CNS depression, tremors, headaches, neuropathy, abdominal cramping, diarrhea, anemia, and neutropenia (14).

Interactions with Herbs & Other Dietary Supplements

Insufficient reliable information available.

Interactions with Drugs

ANTICOAGULANTS: Theoretically, the sodium orthovanadate form of vanadium might potentiate anticoagulant therapeutic and adverse effects (3054).

ANTIDIABETES DRUGS: The vanadyl sulfate form of vanadium might have additive effects with diabetes drug therapy. The vanadyl sulfate form of vanadium increases insulin sensitivity (3055,3056,3057) and might lower blood glucose (3057) in individuals with type 2 diabetes. Monitor carefully.

DIGOXIN: Theoretically, concomitant use with vanadium might increase the therapeutic and adverse effects of digoxin, due to digitalis-like effects of vanadium (14).

Interactions with Foods

No interactions are known to occur, and there is no known reason to expect a clinically significant interaction with vanadium.

Interactions with Lab Tests

BLOOD GLUCOSE: The vanadyl sulfate form of vanadium might lower blood glucose levels and test results in people with type 2 diabetes (3057).

SERUM CREATININE: There is preliminary evidence that vanadium might adversely affect renal function (7135). Theoretically, renal function tests might be altered in people taking high doses of vanadium for extended periods.

Interactions with Diseases or Conditions

DIABETES: The vanadyl sulfate form of vanadium might alter blood glucose control in patients with type 2 diabetes. The vanadyl sulfate form of vanadium increases insulin sensitivity (3055,3056,3057) and might lower blood glucose (3057) in individuals with type 2 diabetes. Monitor carefully.

RENAL DYSFUNCTION: There is preliminary evidence that vanadium might cause nephrotoxicity (7135). People with renal dysfunction should avoid vanadium supplements.

Dosage and Administration

ORAL: For type 2 diabetes, the vanadyl sulfate form of vanadium 50 mg twice daily has been used (3055,3056,3057). The National Institute of Medicine has set the tolerable upper intake level (UL) of vanadium at 1.8 mg per day of elemental vanadium for adults (7135). No UL has been set for infants, children, and pregnant or lactating women (7135). Vanadium intake should be limited to food or infant formula in these groups (7135). An average diet provides 6 to 18 mcg vanadium per day (7135). Vanadyl sulfate contains 31% elemental vanadium. Sodium metavanadate contains 42% elemental vanadium. Sodium orthovanadate contains 28% elemental vanadium (16).

Comments

Vanadium was named for the Norse goddess of beauty, Vanadis, because of its beautiful multicolored compounds. Some dental and orthopedic implants can contain vanadium (14).

VANILLA

Also Known As
Bourbon Vanilla, Common Vanilla, Madagascar Vanilla, Mexican Vanilla, Réunion Vanilla, Tahiti Vanilla, Tahitian Vanilla, Vanillin.

Scientific Names
Vanilla planifolia, synonym V. fragrans; Vanilla tahitensis.
Family: Orchidaceae.

People Use This For
Traditionally, vanilla is used orally as an aphrodisiac, antiflatulent, antipyretic, and stimulant (6).
In foods and beverages, vanilla is used as a flavoring agent (11). It is added to foods to reduce the amount of sugar needed for sweetening and inhibit the development of dental caries (6).
In manufacturing, vanilla is used as a flavoring agent in syrups for pharmaceutical use (11). It is also used as a fragrance in perfumes (11).

Safety
LIKELY SAFE …when used orally (12). It has Generally Recognized as Safe (GRAS) status in the US (11). Maximum use level in baked goods is about 0.964% (11).
PREGNANCY AND LACTATION: Insufficient reliable information available; avoid amounts in excess of those found in foods.

Effectiveness
There is insufficient reliable information available about the effectiveness of vanilla.

Mechanism of Action
The applicable part of vanilla is the fruit. Although the constituent vanillin is primarily responsible for the flavor of vanilla (11), over 150 aromatic compounds contribute to its fragrance (11,6). The catechin content of vanilla shows evidence of an anti-caries effect (6). In controlled studies, meals flavored with vanilla provided a higher degree of satisfaction than identical meals without vanilla flavoring (6). Contact dermatitis associated with the vanilla plant is thought to be due to the calcium oxalate crystals in the plant (6).

Adverse Reactions
Oral and topical use of vanilla has been associated with allergic responses including contact dermatitis (6,11). Workers preparing vanilla have reported headache, dermatitis, and insomnia, characterized as "vanillism."

Interactions with Herbs & Other Dietary Supplements
Insufficient reliable information available.

Interactions with Drugs
No interactions are known to occur, and there is no known reason to expect a clinically significant interaction with vanilla.

Interactions with Foods
No interactions are known to occur, and there is no known reason to expect a clinically significant interaction with vanilla.

Interactions with Lab Tests
No interactions are known to occur, and there is no known reason to expect a clinically significant interaction with vanilla.

Interactions with Diseases or Conditions
No interactions are known to occur, and there is no known reason to expect a clinically significant interaction with vanilla.

Dosage and Administration
No typical dosage.

Comments
Synthetically-produced vanillin is often used as a substitute for vanilla (6), even though the fragrance, rather than the

vanillin content, determines the value of vanilla (11). Vanilla extracts have been extensively adulterated (11). Extracts of Mexican origin have been adulterated with coumarin, often due to tonka beans (6). Since 1954, the FDA has prohibited the use of coumarin in food (6).

VERBENA

Also Known As

Blue Vervain, Common Verbena, Common Vervain, Eisenkraut, Enchanter's Plant, European Vervain, Herb of Grace, Herb of the Cross, Holywort, Juno's Tears, Pigeon's Grass, Pigeonweed, Simpler's Joy, Turkey Grass, Verbenae herba, Vervain.
CAUTION: See separate listing for Lemon Verbena.

Scientific Names

Verbena officinalis.
Family: Verbenaceae.

People Use This For

Orally, verbena is used for sore throats and other oral and pharyngeal inflammation, respiratory tract diseases such as asthma and whooping cough, and angina (2).
Topically, verbena is used for poorly healing wounds, abscesses and burns (2), as a gargle for cold symptoms and oral/pharyngeal cavity diseases, arthritis, rheumatism, dislocations, contusions, itching, and minor burns (18).
In combination with gentian root, European elder flower, verbena, cowslip flower, and sorrel, it is used orally for maintaining healthy sinuses (373) and treating sinusitis (7,374,379).
In folk medicine, verbena is used orally for depression, melancholia, hysteria, generalized seizure, gallbladder pain, fever, debility of convalescence after fevers (4), pains, spasms, exhaustion, angina, nervous conditions, digestive disorders, liver and gallbladder diseases, jaundice, kidney and lower urinary tract ailments and diseases, menopausal complaints, irregular menstruation, for lactation during nursing, arthritic conditions, gout, metabolic disorders, anemia, and edema associated with weak heart (2,18).
In manufacturing, the flowers are used as a flavoring agent in alcoholic beverages (4,12).

Safety

LIKELY SAFE …when used orally in amounts used as flavoring. In the US, the flowers are allowable as a flavoring agent only in alcoholic beverages (12).
POSSIBLY SAFE …when used orally and appropriately in therapeutic amounts (12). …when verbena is used orally in a combination with gentian root, European elder flower, cowslip flower, and sorrel (Quanterra Sinus Defense, Sinupret) (7,374,379).
LIKELY UNSAFE …when used orally in excessive amounts because the constituent, verbenalin, can cause stupor and convulsions (4).
There is insufficient reliable information available about the safety of the topical use of verbena.
PREGNANCY: LIKELY UNSAFE …when used orally because verbena is believed to be an abortifacient and oxytoxic agent (4). There is insufficient reliable information available about the safety of the topical use of verbena during pregnancy.
LACTATION: Insufficient reliable information available; avoid using.

Effectiveness

POSSIBLY EFFECTIVE …when used orally in combination with gentian root, European elder flower, cowslip flower, and sorrel (Quanterra Sinus Defense, Sinupret) for treating acute or chronic sinusitis (7,374,379).
There is insufficient reliable information available about the effectiveness of verbena for its other uses.

Mechanism of Action

The applicable parts of verbena are the above ground parts. They contain the iridoid glycosides verbascoside (acetoside), verbenalin, and verbenin (aucubin) (4). Verbena possesses weak parasympathetic properties and can cause a slight contraction of the uterus. The herb shows evidence of luteinizing activity, perhaps by inhibiting the gonadotrophic activity of the posterior pituitary (4). Some evidence indicates the iridoid glycosides have a mild laxative effect. Small amounts of the constituent, verbenin, appear to stimulate sympathetic activity. Larger amounts of verbenin inhibit sympathetic activity (4). Preliminary evidence suggests verbenin might also stimulate milk secretion (4). The constituent, verbenalin, shows evidence of uterine stimulant activity (4). The constituent verbascoside shows evidence of analgesic and antihypertensive activity. Verbascoside also appears to enhance the antitremor action of levodopa (4).

VERONICA

Adverse Reactions
Excessive amounts of the constituent, verbenalin, can cause CNS paralysis, stupor, and convulsions (4).

Interactions with Herbs & Other Dietary Supplements
Insufficient reliable information available.

Interactions with Drugs
DOXYCYCLINE (Vibramycin): Concurrent use of verbena, gentian root, European elder flower, cowslip flower, and sorrel (Quanterra Sinus Defense, Sinupret) with doxycycline and a topical decongestant might improve the outcome of conventional (antibiotic/decongestant) therapy for acute bacterial sinusitis (374).
LEVODOPA: Theoretically, concomitant use might enhance the antitremor effects of levodopa (4).
HYPERTENSIVE, HYPOTENSIVE DRUGS: Theoretically, excessive amounts of verbena can interfere with drug therapy for hypertension or hypotension (4).
HORMONE THERAPY: Theoretically, excessive amounts of verbena can interfere with hormone therapies (4).

Interactions with Foods
No interactions are known to occur, and there is no known reason to expect a clinically significant interaction with verbena.

Interactions with Lab Tests
No interactions are known to occur, and there is no known reason to expect a clinically significant interaction with verbena.

Interactions with Diseases or Conditions
HYPERTENSION: Theoretically, excessive amounts of verbena might reduce blood pressure (4).
HYPOTENSION: Theoretically, excessive amounts of verbena might exacerbate this condition (4).

Dosage and Administration
ORAL: A typical dose is one cup tea three times daily (4). To make tea, steep 2-4 grams dried above ground parts in 150 mL boiling water for 5 10 minutes and strain (4). Liquid extract (1:1 in 25% ethanol), 2-4 mL three times daily has been used (4). Tincture (1:1 in 40% ethanol), 5-10 mL three times daily has also been used (4).
For acute or chronic sinusitis, two Sinupret tablets three times daily for up to two weeks has been used in clinical trials (7,374,379), equivalent to gentian root 12 mg, European elder flower 36 mg, verbena 36 mg, cowslip flower 36 mg, and sorrel 36 mg three times daily. For maintaining healthy sinuses, a typical dose is one tablet of Quanterra Sinus Defense three times daily with water, equivalent to gentian root 9 mg, European elder flower 29 mg, verbena 29 mg, cowslip flower 29 mg, and sorrel 29 mg three times daily (373). Each tablet of Quanterra Sinus Defense contains 125 mg of the herbal combination found in Sinupret (373).
TOPICAL: No typical dosage.

Comments
None.

VERONICA

Also Known As
Ehrenpreiskraut, Gypsyweed, Speedwell, Veronica Herb, Veronicae herba.
CAUTION: See separate listings for Black Root (Leptandra virginica) and Brooklime (Veronica beccabungo) which are both known also as Speedwell.

Scientific Names
Veronica officinalis.
Family: Scrophulariaceae.

People Use This For
Orally, veronica is used for diseases and discomforts of the respiratory tract, gastrointestinal tract, liver, kidney, and lower urinary tract; gout; arthritis; rheumatic complaints; diseases of the spleen; scrofulosis; as an appetite stimulant and tonic; and to induce sweating (2).
Topically, veronica is used as a gargle for inflammation of the oral and pharyngeal mucosa, for perspiration of the feet, stimulation of wound healing, chronic skin conditions, and itching (2).
In folk medicine, veronica is used orally for nervous irritation, "blood purification," and promotion of metabolism (2,18).

Safety

LIKELY SAFE ...when consumed in amounts found in alcoholic beverages; allowable flavoring agent in alcoholic beverages in the US (12).
POSSIBLY SAFE ...when used orally and appropriately as a medicinal agent (12).
There is insufficient reliable information available about the safety of the topical use of veronica.
PREGNANCY AND LACTATION: Insufficient reliable information available; avoid using.

Effectiveness

There is insufficient reliable information available about the effectiveness of veronica.

Mechanism of Action

The applicable parts of veronica are the above ground parts. Extracts protected against ulcers induced by indomethacin. May enhance gastric mucosa regeneration (4010).

Adverse Reactions

None reported.

Interactions with Herbs & Other Dietary Supplements

Insufficient reliable information available.

Interactions with Drugs

NONSTEROIDAL ANTI-INFLAMMATORY DRUGS (NSAIDs): Theoretically, concomitant use with veronica may protect against NSAID-induced ulcerogenic activity (4010).

Interactions with Foods

No interactions are known to occur, and there is no known reason to expect a clinically significant interaction with veronica.

Interactions with Lab Tests

No interactions are known to occur, and there is no known reason to expect a clinically significant interaction with veronica.

Interactions with Diseases or Conditions

GASTRIC ULCERS: Theoretically, veronica may enhance ulcer healing (4010).

Dosage and Administration

ORAL: As an expectorant, 1 cup tea (steep 1.5 grams finely cut above ground parts in 150 mL boiling water 10 minutes, strain) 2-3 times daily is commonly used (18).
TOPICAL: For lavages and compresses for eczema, ulcers, wounds, boil 1 handful above ground parts in 1 L water for 10 minutes) (18).

Comments

Avoid confusion with other Veronica species, including Veronica allionii and Veronica chamaedrys (18).

VETIVER

Also Known As

Chiendent Odorant, Cuscus, Cuscus Grass, Khas-khas, Khus Khus, Khus-khus Grass, Vétiver, Vetivergras, Zacate Violeta.

Scientific Names

Vetiveria zizanoides.
Family: Poaceae.

People Use This For

Orally, vetiver is used as a uterine stimulant to promote menses and to cause abortion (12). It is also used orally for nervous and circulatory problems (5279).
Topically, it is used for stress relief, recovery from emotional traumas and shocks (5283), treatment of lice (5279), and as an insect repellent (513).

As an inhalant, vetiver is used for "aroma therapy" for nervousness, insomnia, rheumatism, and muscle relaxation (5281,5282).

In manufacturing, vetiver is used as a flavoring in alcoholic beverages (12).

Safety

LIKELY SAFE ...when used in amounts found in alcoholic beverages. It is approved as a flavoring additive in alcoholic beverages in the US (308).

POSSIBLY SAFE ...when used orally (12).

PREGNANCY: LIKELY UNSAFE ...when used orally because it is a potential abortifacient and it has menstrual and uterine stimulant effects (12).

LACTATION: Insufficient reliable information available: avoid using.

Effectiveness

There is insufficient reliable information about the effectiveness of vetiver.

Mechanism of Action

The applicable part of vetiver is the root. Vetiver root contains numerous constituents including limonene, p-cymene, palmitic acid, benzoic acid, delta-3-carene (513). Vetiver may contain a volatile oil which accounts for its use as a repellent to flies, cockroaches, bedbugs, and clothes moths (5279).

Adverse Reactions

None reported.

Interactions with Herbs & Other Dietary Supplements

Insufficient reliable information available.

Interactions with Drugs

No interactions are known to occur, and there is no known reason to expect a clinically significant interaction with vetiver.

Interactions with Foods

No interactions are known to occur, and there is no known reason to expect a clinically significant interaction with vetiver.

Interactions with Lab Tests

No interactions are known to occur, and there is no known reason to expect a clinically significant interaction with vetiver.

Interactions with Diseases or Conditions

No interactions are known to occur, and there is no known reason to expect a clinically significant interaction with vetiver.

Dosage and Administration

No typical dosage.

Comments

None.

VINPOCETINE

Also Known As

AY-27255, Cavinton, Ethyl Apovincaminate, Ethylapovincaminoate, RGH-4405, TCV-3b.

Scientific Names

Eburnamenine-14-carboxylic acid, ethyl ester.

People Use This For

Orally, vinpocetine is used for enhancing memory (1782,1783,1796,1797), improving cerebral blood flow, improving cerebral oxygen and glucose utilization (1782,1783), protecting against age-related cognitive decline and Alzheimer's disease (14,1783,1784), treating cerebrovascular disease (14,1789,1793), preventing post-stroke morbidity and mortality (14,1785),

treating organic psychosyndromes (1787), treating intractable tumoral calcinosis in people undergoing hemodialysis (14,1788), decreasing stroke risk (14,1790,1791), treating menopausal symptoms (1792), seizure disorders (1795), and preventing motion sickness (1798).
Intravenously, vinpocetine is injected for treating seizure disorders (1794) and stroke (1786).

Safety

POSSIBLY SAFE ...when used orally and appropriately (14,1784). No significant adverse effects were reported in a study of people with Alzheimer's disease treated with large doses of vinpocetine (60 mg per day) for one year (1784).
PREGNANCY AND LACTATION: Insufficient reliable information available; avoid using.

Effectiveness

POSSIBLY EFFECTIVE ...when vinpocetine is used orally for cerebrovascular diseases (14,1787,1789,1793). ...when used orally for enhancing memory (1796,1797).
POSSIBLY INEFFECTIVE ...when used orally for preventing post-stroke morbidity and mortality (14,1785).
There is insufficient reliable information available about the effectiveness of vinpocetine for its other uses.

Mechanism of Action

Vinpocetine is a synthetic derivative of vincamine, a compound derived from the periwinkle plant, Vinca minor (see separate listing for Periwinkle) (14). Vinpocetine appears to have many varied pharmacologic effects, but mechanisms of action are unclear, and well-designed clinical studies to substantiate activity have not been published (14). A few studies using vinpocetine for poorly-defined cerebrovascular diseases have indicated some efficacy, but faulty study design limits interpretation (14,1787,1789,1793). Vinpocetine had no effect on dementia progression in 15 people with Alzheimer's disease treated for one year with gradually increasing doses up to 60 mg/day (1784). Vinpocetine does not appear to be effective for preventing post-stroke debility or death (14,1785). Some studies indicate that vinpocetine might enhance cerebral blood flow without affecting peripheral blood flow (14,1786,1793). Preliminary evidence indicates that vinpocetine stimulates cerebral metabolism (14). Vinpocetine improves memory in healthy subjects and healthy volunteers with benzodiazepine-induced memory impairment (1796,1797). Potential mechanisms for the nootropic-like effects of vinpocetine include indirect or direct cholinergic activity, augmented norepinephrine effects on cortical cyclic adenosine monophosphate (AMP), increased turnover of brain catecholamines, and inhibition of adenosine reuptake (14,1800). Other pharmacological effects of vinpocetine include increased cerebral glucose utilization, anticonvulsant activity, neuronal protectant activity, adenosine-like effects, and phosphodiesterase inhibition (14). Vinpocetine inhibits drug-induced platelet aggregation (14,1801). The bioavailability of vinpocetine varies from 7% to 57%, and food significantly enhances absorption (14,1802). Vinpocetine undergoes hepatic metabolism to inactive compounds (14). The elimination half-life of vinpocetine is 1-2.5 hours (14). Vinpocetine has been shown not to interact with desipramine, imipramine, glyburide, and oxazepam (14).

Adverse Reactions

Orally, adverse effects include stomach pressure, upper abdominal pain, nausea, facial flushing, slight reductions in systolic and diastolic blood pressure, sleep disturbances, and headache (14).

Interactions with Herbs & Other Dietary Supplements

HERBS WITH ANTICOAGULANT/ANTIPLATELET POTENTIAL: Theoretically, concomitant use of herbs that have coumarin constituents or affect platelet aggregation might increase the risk of bleeding in some people. These herbs include angelica, anise, arnica, asafoetida, bogbean, boldo, capsicum, celery, chamomile, clove, danshen, fenugreek, feverfew, garlic, ginger, ginkgo, ginseng Panax, horse chestnut, horseradish, licorice, meadowsweet, prickly ash, onion, papain, passionflower, poplar, quassia, red clover, turmeric, wild carrot, wild lettuce, willow, and others (4,19).

Interactions with Drugs

ANTI-PLATELET DRUGS: Theoretically, concomitant use with vinpocetine might enhance anti-platelet effects and increase bleeding risk (14,1801).
WARFARIN (Coumadin): Concomitant use with vinpocetine might increase anticoagulant effects and increase bleeding risk; monitor INR (14).
BLOOD PRESSURE LOWERING DRUGS: Theoretically, concomitant use with vinpocetine might enhance blood pressure lowering effects; monitor blood pressure (14).

Interactions with Foods

FOODS: Administration of oral vinpocetine with food enhances its absorption (1802).

Interactions with Lab Tests

PROTHROMBIN TIME (PT), INTERNATIONAL NORMALIZATION RATIO (INR): Vinpocetine might increase PT and INR (14). It has been reported to modestly increase warfarin AUC, PT, and factor VII clotting time (14).

BLOOD PRESSURE: Theoretically, vinpocetine might lower blood pressure and blood pressure measurements (14).

BLOOD GLUCOSE: Theoretically, vinpocetine might reduce blood sugar levels and test results (14).

Interactions with Diseases or Conditions

COAGULOPATHIES: Vinpocetine should not be used by people with blood-clotting disorders because it might increase bleeding risk (14,1801).

Dosage and Administration

ORAL: The dose commonly used for cerebrovascular disorders is 5-10 mg three times daily (14). People typically take 10 mg three times daily with food (1799).

Comments

Vinpocetine is a synthetic derivative of apovincamine which is found in periwinkle. Vinpocetine synthesis requires considerable laboratory manipulation, stretching the Dietary Supplement Health and Education Act (DSHEA) definition of a "dietary supplement" (14,1799). Vinpocetine is sold by prescription in Germany under the brand name, Cavinton (9). It has also been referred to generically as cavinton (9). Although website advertising claims that "more than a hundred" safety and effectiveness studies have been funded by the Hungarian manufacturer Gedeon Richter, few double-blind controlled clinical studies have been published (14,1782,1785).

VITAMIN A

Also Known As

3-Dehydroretinol, Antixerophthalmic Vitamin, Axerophtholum, Dehydroretinol, Oleovitamin A, Retinoids, Retinol, Retinol Acetate, Retinol Palmitate, Retinyl Acetate, Retinyl Palmitate, Vitamin A1, Vitamin A2, Vitaminum A. CAUTION: See separate listings for Beta-Carotene and Lutein.

Scientific Names

Vitamin A.

People Use This For

Orally, vitamin A is most commonly used to prevent and treat the symptoms of vitamin A deficiency; promote good vision; prevent glaucoma and cataracts; prevent and speed recovery from infections; improve immune function; and for skin conditions including acne, eczema, psoriasis, cold sores, wounds and burns, sunburn, keratosis follicularis (Darier's disease), ichthyosis (noninflammatory skin scaling), lichen planus pigmentosus, and pityriasis rubra pilaris (14,15,3062,3064,3065). Vitamin A is also used orally to prevent and treat vitamin A deficiency due to abnormal storage and transport of vitamin A in people with abetalipoproteinemia, protein deficiency, diabetes mellitus, hyperthyroidism, fever, liver disease, or cystic fibrosis with liver involvement. It is also used orally for heavy menses, premenstrual syndrome, atrophic vaginitis, candidiasis, fibrocystic breast disease, reduced sperm count, gastrointestinal ulcers, Crohn's disease, periodontal disease, diabetes, Hurler syndrome (mucopolysaccharidosis), sinusitis, urinary tract infections, reducing complications of measles, with antibiotics for hastening clinical shigellosis cure, atrophic rhinitis, loss of sense of smell, asthma, persistent headaches, kidney stones, hyperthyroidism, anemia, deafness, tinnitus, cataracts, glaucoma, leukoplakia, preventing and treating cancer, degenerative diseases of the nervous system, protecting the heart and cardiovascular system (antioxidant effects), and slowing the aging process (14,15,3062,3064,3065). Vitamin A is used orally to decrease morbidity associated with malaria in children (1464), and to reduce morbidity and mortality from pneumonia and HIV in children with vitamin A deficiency (1465,1466). Vitamin A is also used orally to decrease the risk of HIV transmission to the fetus during pregnancy and to the newborn during childbirth and early breast-feeding periods (6376).

Topically, Vitamin A is used to improve wound healing, reduce wrinkles, and to protect the skin against UV radiation (14,1468,3063).

As an intramuscular injection, Vitamin A is used for preventing and treating the symptoms of vitamin A deficiency, including xerophthalmia and night blindness; preventing vitamin A deficiency in people with malabsorption; preventing bronchopulmonary dysplasia in premature infants; and preventing stress ulcers in severely ill hospitalized patients (14,15).

Safety

LIKELY SAFE ...when used orally or intramuscularly and appropriately. Vitamin A is safe in adults when used in doses less than 10,000 units per day (7135).

POSSIBLY UNSAFE ...when used orally in excessive doses. Prolonged use of excessive doses can cause significant side effects such as hypervitaminosis A. The risk for developing hypervitaminosis A is related to total cumulative dose of vitamin A rather than a specific daily dose (5,1467,1469). Tell patients to avoid doses greater than 10,000 units per day (7135).

There is insufficient reliable information about the safety of the topical use of vitamin A.

CHILDREN: LIKELY SAFE ...when used orally or intramuscularly and appropriately. The amount of vitamin A that is safe depends on age. For children up to 3 years of age, doses less than 2,000 units per day seem to be safe. For children ages 4 to 8, doses less than 3,000 units per day seem to be safe. For children ages 9 to 13, doses less than 5,700 units per day seem to be safe. For children 14 to 18, doses of 9,300 units per day seems to be safe (7135). POSSIBLY UNSAFE ...when used orally in excessive doses. For children up to 3 years of age, avoid doses greater than 2,000 units per day. For children ages 4 to 8, avoid doses greater than 3,000 units per day. For children ages 9 to 13, avoid doses greater than 5,700 units per day. For children 14 to 18, avoid doses greater than 9,300 units per day (7135).

There is insufficient reliable information about the safety of the topical use of vitamin A in children.

PREGNANCY AND LACTATION: LIKELY SAFE ...when used orally or intramuscularly and appropriately. Vitamin A is safe during pregnancy and lactation when used in doses less than 10,000 units per day (7135). POSSIBLY UNSAFE ...when used orally or intramuscularly in excessive doses. Daily intake of greater than 10,000 units can cause fetal malformations (3066,7135). The first semester of pregnancy seems to be the critical period for susceptibility to vitamin A-associated birth defects such as craniofacial abnormalities and abnormalities of the central nervous system (7135). Pregnant women should monitor vitamin A intake from all sources. Forms of vitamin A are found in several foods including animal products, primarily liver, some fortified breakfast cereals, and dietary supplements (3066).

There is insufficient reliable information about the safety of the topical use of vitamin A during pregnancy and lactation.

Effectiveness

EFFECTIVE ...when used orally for preventing and treating the symptoms of vitamin A deficiency, including xerophthalmia and night blindness (15). ...when used orally for preventing and treating vitamin A deficiency due to abnormal storage and transport of vitamin A in people with abetalipoproteinemia, protein deficiency, diabetes mellitus, hyperthyroidism, fever, liver disease, or cystic fibrosis with liver involvement (15).

POSSIBLY EFFECTIVE ...when used orally for reducing the complications of measles in children with vitamin A deficiency (7135). ...when used orally in large amounts for treating acne vulgaris, though other retinoids have largely replaced retinol for this use (14). ...when used orally for decreasing malaria symptoms in children under 3 years of age living in endemic areas (1464). ...when used orally as an adjunct for decreasing mortality from HIV and diarrhea in children with vitamin A deficiency (1465). ...when used orally for reducing risk of breast cancer. Epidemiological evidence shows an association between increasing amounts of dietary vitamin A and reduced risk of breast cancer risk among premenopausal women with a positive family history of breast cancer (1444). However, it's not known if supplemental vitamin A has a similar benefit. ...when used orally by malnourished women to reduce pregnancy-related mortality. In one trial, 23,300 IU retinyl acetate taken weekly before, during and after pregnancy by malnourished women reduced pregnancy-related mortality by 40% (6153). ...when used orally by malnourished women to reduce the occurrence of pregnancy-related night blindness, and post-partum diarrhea and fever. Retinyl acetate taken weekly before, during, and after pregnancy by malnourished women in Nepal reduced, but did not eliminate, the occurrence of pregnancy-related night blindness, diarrhea, and fever (2581,6154). ...when used orally to reduce the occurrence of cataracts. A large-scale population-based study found dietary intake of vitamin A was associated with a reduced risk of nuclear cataracts (6378).

POSSIBLY INEFFECTIVE ...when vitamin A is used orally by malnourished women to reduce fetal and early infant mortality. In one trial, 23,300 IU retinyl acetate weekly taken before, during, and after pregnancy by malnourished women in Nepal failed to reduce fetal and early infant mortality (6152). ...when used orally to decrease the risk of HIV transmission to the fetus during pregnancy and to the newborn during delivery and early breast-feeding periods (6376).

LIKELY INEFFECTIVE ...when used orally for decreasing the severity of pneumonia in children living in developing countries (1466). ...when used orally to reduce the risk of second primary tumors and tumor reoccurrence in patients with head and neck or lung cancer. A large scale randomized intervention study also found no significant differences in survival and event-free survival in patients taking or not taking supplemental vitamin A (6379).

There is insufficient reliable information available about the effectiveness of vitamin A for its other uses.

Mechanism of Action

Vitamin A is a fat-soluble vitamin. Vitamin A includes a family of molecules containing a 20-carbon structure with various chemical groups at the 15 carbon position. Variations at the 15 carbon position yield different vitamin A forms, including retinol, retinal, retinoic acid, and retinyl ester. These different forms of vitamin A are often collectively referred to as "retinoids". The vitamin A family also includes provitamin A carotenoids, which are dietary precursors to retinol. Vitamin A is found in foods in several forms. Retinol, also called preformed vitamin A, is present in esterified form in animal-derived products including eggs, whole milk, butter, fortified margarine, meat, and oily salt-water fish (7135). Fresh water fish contain a form of vitamin A called 3-dehydroretinol, but has only 30-40% of the biologic activity of retinol (15). The primary dietary source is plants, which synthesize carotenoids that are converted to vitamin A in the body (7135). Carotenoid pigments (including alpha-, beta-, and gamma-carotene and cryptoxanthin) are present in green and yellow vegetables, especially carrots, and fruits (15). Ingested vitamin A is stored in the body as retinol, predominantly in the liver, but also in the retina, kidneys, lungs, adrenal glands, and intraperitoneal fat (1467). Retinol-binding protein (RBP) is required to transport retinol from the liver and accumulates in the liver during periods of vitamin A deficiency (6377). When vitamin A as retinol is available, it binds to accumulated RBP and is promptly released into the blood when needed (6377). Transport protein levels can be reduced in people with protein malnutrition, causing signs of vitamin A deficiency. In alcoholism, vitamin A deficiency is common since alcohol accelerates the breakdown of retinol through induction of cytochrome isoenzymes and interferes with the conversion of beta-carotene to retinol (1488,7139). Vitamin A toxicity can occur when RBP capacity is exceeded and unbound retinol enters the circulation resulting in vitamin A excess, called hypervitaminosis A (15). The majority of vitamin A is primarily excreted in the urine. Lesser amounts are lost through the breath and feces, as inactive metabolites (7135). In vitamin A excess, biliary excretion increases (7135). Vitamin A is required for growth and bone development, vision, reproduction, and the integrity of mucosal and epithelial surfaces. Retinoic acid is thought to be the active form of vitamin A in processes involving growth and cellular differentiation (14). Retinoic acid regulates the expression of various genes that encode for structural proteins, such as keratins in the skin; enzymes, such as alcohol dehydrogenase; extracellular matrix proteins, such as the basement membrane protein laminin; and retinol binding proteins and receptors (7135). Vitamin A acts as a cofactor in mucopolysaccharide synthesis, cholesterol synthesis, hydroxysteroid metabolism, and glycoprotein glycosylation (14,15). Vitamin A is also important for immune function. Retinoic acid is required in maintaining sufficient levels of natural killer cells, and preliminary evidence suggests that retinoic acid might increase the production of cytokines, such as interleukin 1 (IL-1) (7135). Additionally, B lymphocyte growth, differentiation, and activation are dependent on retinol. In embryonic development, vitamin A plays an important role in neural development, and is also involved in the development of the limbs, heart, eyes, and ears. In the retina, retinol is converted to cis-retinal, which combines with opsin to form rhodopsin, the visual pigment. Retinal is required by the eye for the transduction of light into the neural signals that produce vision. The most specific indicator of vitamin A deficiency is xerophthalmia, which is initially manifested by night blindness that progresses to complete visual loss if untreated. Vitamin A deficiency is also associated with follicular hyperkeratosis and increased risk of infectious morbidity and mortality (7135). In vitro studies suggest retinoids might help prevent cancer by inducing tumor suppressor genes known as retinoic acid receptors (RAR). Tumor suppressor gene RAR-beta2 is absent in many malignant tumor cells, possibly due to methylation of the gene. When demethylated, the RAR-beta2 gene can be induced by retinoic acid to function and suppress growth of cancer cells (6380,6381). Ethanol may compete with retinol for alcohol dehydrogenase and inhibit retinoic acid synthesis, interfering with normal retinoid signaling of RAR genes and cause malignant transformation of hepatic cells (6377). Preliminary evidence suggests that all-trans-retinoic acid applied topically might help protect the skin against UV radiation damage (1468).

Adverse Reactions

With chronic use of large amounts, early symptoms of vitamin A overdose include fatigue, malaise, lethargy, irritability, psychiatric changes mimicking severe depression or schizophrenic disorder, anorexia, abdominal discomfort, nausea and vomiting, mild fever, and excessive sweating (14,15). Slow growth, premature epiphyseal closure, painful hyperostosis of the long bones, osteosclerosis, joint pain, muscle pain, hypercalcemia, and hypercalciuria have been reported (14,15). CNS symptoms of hypervitaminosis include increased intracranial pressure, pseudotumor cerebri, bulging fontanelles in infants, headache, swelling of the optic disk, bulging eyeballs, dizziness, and visual disturbances. Other symptoms include dry skin and lips; cracking, scaling, and itchy skin; skin redness, hyperpigmentation, and massive skin peeling. Hypervitaminosis A can cause brittle nails, cheilitis, gingivitis, hair loss, reduced menstrual flow, hepatosplenomegaly, cirrhosis, jaundice, ascites, spider angiomas, elevated serum AST (SGOT) and ALT (SGPT) concentrations, anemia, leukopenia, leukocytosis, and thrombocytopenia (14,15). Long term chronic use of vitamin A can cause hepatic congestion and fibrosis, especially around the central vein (6377). Sometimes children fail to gain weight normally while adults lose weight (14,15). Toxicity from a single ingestion of a large dose of vitamin A is more common in young children than adults (15). Approximately 25,000 units/kg can cause irritability, drowsiness, dizziness, delirium, coma, vomiting, diarrhea (15), increased intracranial pressure with bulging fontanelles in infants, headache, swelling of the optic disk, bulging eyeballs, and visual disturbances (15). Skin redness and generalized peeling of the skin occur a few days later and may last for several weeks (15).

Interactions with Herbs & Other Dietary Supplements

VITAMIN E: Concomitant use can increase the absorption, utilization, and storage of vitamin A, and may protect against hypervitaminosis A, although these effects are controversial (15).

MINERAL OIL: Concomitant use can decrease oral vitamin A absorption (15).

Interactions with Drugs

CHEMOTHERAPEUTIC AGENTS: Theoretically, concomitant use might decrease the effectiveness of chemotherapy. Preliminary evidence from an unpublished study suggests that antioxidants such as vitamin E and vitamin A may decrease the effectiveness of chemotherapy (14,391).

MINOCYCLINE (Minocin): Concomitant, long-term administration increases the risk of pseudotumor cerebri (benign intracranial hypertension) (14).

NEOMYCIN (Neo-Fradin): Concomitant use of neomycin can reduce supplemental vitamin A absorption (14,15).

Drug Influences on Nutrient Levels and Depletion

SOME DRUGS CAN AFFECT VITAMIN A LEVELS:

ALCOHOL (Ethanol): Chronic and excessive alcohol consumption can deplete hepatic vitamin A stores and potentially cause vitamin A deficiency (1488,7135,7139). There is preliminary evidence that chronic ethanol intake induces cytochrome P450 2E1 (CYP2E1), which increases vitamin A metabolism and depletes vitamin A stores (1488).

CHOLESTYRAMINE (Questran): Cholestyramine can reduce dietary vitamin A absorption and serum levels. Supplementation with water-miscible vitamin A is recommended for patients during long-term cholestyramine therapy (15,4455,4456).

COLESTIPOL (Colestid): Colestipol can reduce dietary vitamin A absorption and serum levels (4460).

MINERAL OIL: Use of mineral oil can reduce dietary vitamin A absorption and serum levels. Avoid long-term use of mineral oil (4495). Vitamin A refers to beta-ionone derivatives, with the biological activity of retinol (511). Vitamin A does not include provitamin A carotenoids.

ORLISTAT (Xenical): Orlistat can reduce vitamin A levels (1725,1726,1727,1730). Consider a multivitamin with fat-soluble vitamins, taken at least 2 hours before or after orlistat, or at bedtime.

Interactions with Foods

FAT: Dietary fat increases vitamin A absorption (7135).

Interactions with Lab Tests

CHOLESTEROL: There are unsubstantiated reports that vitamin A can produce false increases in serum cholesterol test results measured by the Zlatkis-Zak reaction (15).

BILIRUBIN: Vitamin A can cause false increase in bilirubin test results using Ehrlich's reagent (15).

Interactions with Diseases or Conditions

ALCOHOLISM: Chronic alcohol ingestion might potentiate the adverse effects of vitamin A, particularly hepatotoxicity (7135,7139). There is some evidence that chronic and excessive ethanol intake induces cytochrome P450 2E1 (CYP2E1) metabolism of vitamin A, which can increase production of hepatotoxic and carcinogenic vitamin A metabolites (1488,7135,7139).

ANEMIA: Anemia may not be adequately treated by iron supplements alone in patients with vitamin A deficiency. Vitamin A deficiency impairs iron mobilization from body stores. Combining vitamin A with iron supplementation in anemic patients with concurrent vitamin A deficient seems to improve hemoglobin concentrations better than iron alone (7135).

FAT MALABSORPTION DISORDERS: Oral vitamin A absorption is decreased in conditions where fat absorption is reduced, such as celiac disease, short gut syndrome, obstructive jaundice, cystic fibrosis, pancreatic disease, and cirrhosis of the liver (7135). Water-miscible oral vitamin A preparations should be used in patients with fat malabsorption disorders.

HYPERLIPIDEMIA: Type V hyperlipoproteinemia increases risk of vitamin A hypervitaminosis (7135).

INTESTINAL INFECTIONS AND INFESTATIONS: Ascariasis, giardiasis, hookworm, salmonellosis, schistosomiasis, and other intestinal infections and infestations can reduce oral vitamin A absorption (7135).

LIVER DISEASE: Pre-existing liver disease increases risk of hypervitaminosis and hepatotoxicity (7135).

MALNUTRITION: In severe protein energy malnutrition (marasmus and kwashiorkor), there is reduced release of retinol from the liver. Until nutrition status is normalized, there is increased risk of vitamin A hypervitaminosis (7135).

Dosage and Administration

ORAL: The typical dose for treatment of deficiency in adults without corneal changes is 10,000 to 25,000 units daily until clinical improvement occurs, usually 1-2 weeks. Individuals with fat malabsorption, low protein intake, or hepatic or pancreatic disease might benefit from water-miscible oral preparations. If oral absorption is still insufficient, parenteral administration may be necessary. For prevention of nuclear cataracts, 10,000 units per day has been used (6378). Adequate Intake (AI) levels of vitamin A for infants have been established: birth to 6 months, 400 mcg/day (1300 units); 7 to 12 months, 500 mcg/day (1700 units). Recommended Dietary Allowance (RDA) levels for children and adults have been established: children 1 to 3 years, 300 mcg/day (1000 units); 4 to 8 years, 400 mcg/day (1300 units); 9 to 13 years, 600 mcg/day (2000 units); men 14 years and older, 900 mcg/day (3000 units); women 14 years and older, 700 mcg/day (2300 units); pregnancy 14 to 18 years, 750 mcg/day (2500 units); 19 years and older, 770 mcg/day (2600 units); lactation 14 to 18 years, 1200 mcg/day (4000 units); 19 years and older 1300 mcg/day (4300 units) (7135). Tolerable Upper Intake Levels (UL) for vitamin A have also been established. The UL is the highest level of intake that is likely to pose no risk of adverse effects. The ULs for vitamin A are for preformed vitamin A (retinol) and do not include provitamin A carotenoids: infants and children from birth to 3 years, 600 mcg/day (2000 units); children 4 to 8 years, 900 mcg/day (3000 units); 9 to 13 years 1700 mcg/day (6000 units); 14 to 18 years (including pregnancy and lactation) 2800 mcg/day (9000 units); adults age 19 and older (including pregnancy and lactation) 3000 mcg/day (10,000 units). Vitamin A dosage is most commonly expressed in units, but dosage in micrograms is sometimes used. One mcg of vitamin A equals 3.33 units of vitamin A. Vitamin A recommendations are for retinol, or preformed vitamin A. Formerly, vitamin A RDA recommendations were expressed as retinol equivalents (RE) to account for the differences in bioconversion of the various vitamin A forms to retinol. Retinol activity equivalents (RAE) are now used: 1 mcg of retinol equals 1 RAE which equals 2 mcg supplemental beta-carotene, 12 mcg of dietary beta-carotene, and 24 mcg dietary alpha-carotene or beta-cryptoxanthin. Either preformed vitamin A from animal products (retinol) or provitamin A carotenoids from plant products is an acceptable vitamin A source, although provitamin A carotenoids must be consumed in larger quantities (7135). Consumption of 5 servings of fruits and vegetables per day supplies 5 to 6 mg per day of provitamin A carotenoids, which provides about 50-65% of the adult RDA for vitamin A (7135).

PARENTERAL: Injectable vitamin A is available as a FDA-approved prescription product.

Comments
None.

VITAMIN B12

Also Known As
B-12, B Complex, B Complex Vitamin, Bedumil, Cobamin, Cobalamin, Cobalamins, Cyanocobalamin, Cyanocobalaminum, Cycobemin, Hydroxocobalamin, Hydroxocobalaminum, Hydroxocobemine, Idrossocobalamina, Methylcobalamin, Vitadurin, Vitamin B-12.
CAUTION: See separate listing for Dibencozide.

Scientific Names
Vitamin B12; Cyanocobalamin; Hydroxocobalamin; Methylcobalamin.

People Use This For
Orally, vitamin B12 is used for treating pernicious anemia and preventing and treating vitamin B12 deficiency. It is also used orally for treating primary hyperhomocystinemia, heart disease, male infertility, diabetes, memory loss, circadian rhythm sleep disorders, Alzheimer's disease, depression, psychiatric disorders, osteoporosis, tendonitis, immunosuppression, AIDS, inflammatory bowel disease, asthma, allergies, vitiligo, and seborrheic dermatitis. It is also used orally for thyrotoxicosis, amyotrophic lateral sclerosis (Lou Gehrig's disease), multiple sclerosis, periodontal disease, tinnitus, hemorrhage, malignancy, and liver and kidney disease. Vitamin B12 is also used orally for aging, improving concentration, mood elevation, boosting energy, maintaining fertility, and protection against the toxins and allergens from tobacco smoke.

Topically, a vitamin B12 nasal gel is applied for pernicious anemia and preventing and treating vitamin B12 deficiency.

Parenterally, vitamin B12 is used for pernicious anemia and preventing and treating vitamin B12 deficiency. It is also used parenterally for tremor associated with shaky-leg syndrome or orthostatic tremor. Vitamin B12 is also used parenterally to treat chronic fatigue syndrome, thyrotoxicosis, hemorrhage, malignancy, and liver and kidney disease.

Safety
LIKELY SAFE ...when used orally, intravenously, or intranasally and appropriately. Vitamin B12 is generally considered safe, even in large doses (15).

PREGNANCY: LIKELY SAFE ...when used orally in amounts that do not exceed the recommended dietary allowance (RDA). The RDA for vitamin B12 in pregnant women is 2.6 mcg per day (3094). There is insufficient reliable information available about the safety of larger amounts of vitamin B12 during pregnancy.

LACTATION: LIKELY SAFE ...when used orally in amounts that do not exceed the recommended dietary allowance (RDA). The RDA of vitamin B12 during lactation is 2.8 mcg per day (3094). There is insufficient reliable information available about the safety of larger amounts of vitamin B12 while nursing.

Effectiveness
EFFECTIVE ...when used intramuscularly or intranasally for pernicious anemia. Both the cyanocobalamin and hydroxocobalamin forms of vitamin B12 are used intramuscularly. Cyanocobalamin is used for intranasal administration (15) ...when used orally, intramuscularly, or intranasally for prevention and treatment of dietary vitamin B12 deficiency. People at risk for vitamin B12 deficiency include strict vegetarians and people with increased vitamin B12 requirements associated with pregnancy, thyrotoxicosis, hemolytic anemia, hemorrhage, malignancy, and

hepatic and renal disease. Vitamin B12 deficiency is especially common in older adults (2915,2919). Oral therapy is as effective as intramuscular administration, even in patients with malabsorption disorders (2900,2901,2911,2915). However, oral preparations should not be used in patients with diarrhea or vomiting, severe neurologic involvement, and in patients likely to be nonadherent (2900). ...when used intramuscularly for familial selective vitamin B12 malabsorption (Imerslund-Grasbeck disease) (15).

LIKELY EFFECTIVE ...when used orally for pernicious anemia. Oral vitamin B12 seems to be as effective as intramuscular administration (2900,2902,2909,2910,3024). However, oral preparations should not be used in patients with diarrhea or vomiting, severe neurologic involvement, and in patients likely to be nonadherent (2900). ...when used orally in combination with folic acid and other vitamins for hyperhomocysteinemia in patients with end-stage renal disease (1489,7289,6884). Vitamin B12 in combination with folic acid and other vitamins seems to significantly reduce homocysteine levels (1489,6883,6884). Vitamin B12 supplementation is most likely to have an effect on homocysteine levels in people who have low vitamin B12 levels (3047).

POSSIBLY INEFFECTIVE ...when used orally in methylcobalamin form for delayed sleep phase syndrome. Methylcobalamin, with or without bright light therapy, doesn't seem to help people with primary circadian rhythm sleep disorders (1344,1345,1346,1347,1348).

LIKELY INEFFECTIVE ...when used orally for treating psychiatric disorders. In non-vitamin B12 deficiency patients, vitamin B12 supplements are ineffective for psychiatric disorders (15).

There is insufficient reliable information available to rate the effectiveness of vitamin B12 for its other uses. However, there are some preliminary clinical reports that the cyanocobalamin form of vitamin B12 can help relieve tremor associated with shaky-leg syndrome (6358). More evidence is needed to rate the effectiveness of vitamin B12 for this use.

Mechanism of Action

Vitamin B12 is a naturally occurring B complex vitamin that is formed by microorganisms. It is also found in some foods from animal origin (e.g., meat, fish, shellfish, liver) in coenzyme form, mainly adenosylcobalamin and methylcobalamin. Cyanocobalamin and hydroxocobalamin are synthetic forms of vitamin B12. Vitamin B12 is required for nucleoprotein and myelin synthesis, cell reproduction, normal growth, and normal erythropoiesis. Synthetic vitamin B12 can be converted to coenzyme B12, which is essential for the conversion of methylmalonate to succinate, and the synthesis of methionine from homocysteine. Vitamin B12 is involved in maintaining sulfhydryl groups in the reduced form required by enzymes involved in fat and carbohydrate metabolism and protein synthesis. Vitamin B12 is essential for folate utilization, and its absence results in a functional folate deficiency (15). Vitamin B12 deficiency can take months to years to become symptomatic due to large body stores. Normal serum vitamin B12 levels range between 200-900 pg/mL. Serum concentrations less than 200 pg/mL indicate deficiency, and concentrations less than 100 pg/mL usually result in megaloblastic anemia or neurologic damage (15). Vitamin B12 deficiency results in megaloblastic anemia, gastrointestinal lesions, and neurologic damage, beginning with an inability to produce myelin and progressing to degeneration of the axon and nerve head (15). Vitamin B12 deficiency can also cause neurologic symptoms including neuropsychiatric disorders such as depression (6357), paresthesias, ataxia, memory loss, weakness, and personality and mood changes without anemia (1484,1485,3235,5646). Some neurologic symptoms and elevated homocysteine levels can occur without any signs of B12 deficiency anemia (1484,1485,3235). Elevated methylmalonate or methylmalonic acid (MMA) levels occur early in vitamin B12 deficiency, and may precede other symptoms (1484,1485,5646). In combination with homocysteine levels, MMA levels can be used to diagnose vitamin B12 deficiency (5646). The risk for vitamin B12 deficiency increases with age, male gender, and in people of Caucasian and Latin American descent. Deficiency in vitamin B12 results from insufficient intake, malabsorption from food, and other medical conditions (1484,1485). The classic mechanism of absorption involves a transport system in the terminal ileum and intrinsic factor, a glycoprotein produced by the stomach. At normal gastric pH, vitamin B12 is cleaved from proteins in food, binds to intrinsic factor, and is absorbed by ileal transport. Absorption can be reduced by conditions that cause increased gastric pH such as in atrophic gastritis, use of acid-suppressing drugs, or partial gastrectomy. Reduced absorption also occurs with loss of intrinsic factor in conditions such as pernicious anemia (an autoimmune disorder in which the ability to produce intrinsic factor is lost) and total gastrectomy. Intramuscular administration is often used to avoid these absorption problems. However, there is also a lesser-known transport system for vitamin B12 that does not rely on either intrinsic factor or the terminal ileum. Absorption is more efficient by the intrinsic factor route (about 60%), but 1% of an oral dose of vitamin B12 can be absorbed without intrinsic factor or stomach acid. Large oral doses (300 to 1000 mcg) can provide sufficient absorption to treat pernicious anemia and malabsorption from food (2900,2901,2909). Folic acid, particularly in large doses, can mask vitamin B12 deficiency. Folate will improve vitamin B12 associated anemia, but it will allow the neurologic abnormalities to progress. There is some concern that food fortified with folic acid can cause under-recognition of vitamin B12 deficiency, particularly in the elderly (5646). Vitamin B12 deficiency is independently associated with elevated homocysteine levels, although not as strongly as folic acid deficiency. Elevated homocysteine concentrations are in turn associated with an increased risk of cardiovascular disease (1483,3234), and possibly other conditions such as Alzheimer's disease and vascular dementia (5646). Homocysteine is metabolized by two pathways, one of which (the remethylation pathway) requires folate and also uses the methylcobalamin form of vitamin B12 as a cofactor (3047). A deficiency of vitamin B12 can therefore inhibit metabolism of homocysteine by this pathway (3047). Low vitamin B12 levels are also associated with other conditions such as hearing loss in elderly women (1482) and possibly chronic fatigue syndrome. Some researchers think that vitamin B12 supplements could help symptoms of chronic fatigue syndrome by correcting red blood cell abnormalities and improving oxygen delivery to tissues (6082). The methylcobalamin form of vitamin B12 might also influence melatonin levels. Methylcobalamin seems to improve alertness and reduce sleep time in humans with normal sleep patterns, possibly due to affects on melatonin (1349).

Adverse Reactions

Orally and intramuscularly, vitamin B12 does not usually cause adverse effects, even in large doses (15,7290). In some people, vitamin B12 can cause diarrhea, peripheral vascular thrombosis, itching, transitory exanthema, urticaria, feelings of swelling of the entire body, and anaphylaxis, possibly due to impurities in vitamin B12 preparations. Treatment of vitamin B12 deficiency can unmask polycythemia vera, which is an increase in blood volume and the number of red blood cells (15).

Interactions with Herbs & Other Dietary Supplements

FOLIC ACID: Folic acid, particularly in large doses, can mask vitamin B12 deficiency (5646).
VITAMIN C: Large amounts of vitamin C can destroy vitamin B12 and should not be taken within an hour of oral vitamin B12 (15).

Interactions with Drugs

CHLORAMPHENICOL (Chloromycetin): Chloramphenicol can impair hematopoietic response to supplemental vitamin B12 (15).

Drug Influences on Nutrient Levels and Depletion

SOME DRUGS CAN AFFECT VITAMIN B12 LEVELS:

ALCOHOL, ETHANOL: Excessive consumption of alcohol for greater than 2 weeks can decrease absorption of vitamin B12 (14,15).

ANTIBIOTICS: Destruction of normal gastrointestinal flora by antibiotics can cause decreased production of B vitamins. The clinical significance of this decreased production is not known. Consider supplementation only if clinical judgment warrants it (4434,4435,4436,4437,4438,4439,4440,4441,4442,4443).

COBALT IRRADIATION: Cobalt irradiation of the small bowel can decrease gastrointestinal (GI) absorption of vitamin B12 (14,15).

COLCHICINE: Use of colchicine can reduce dietary vitamin B12 absorption. The significance of this and need for supplementation has not been adequately studied (4543,4544,4545).

COLESTIPOL (Colestid), CHOLESTYRAMINE (Questran): These drugs can decrease gastrointestinal (GI) absorption of vitamin B12 (14,15); separate administration.

METFORMIN (Glucophage): Metformin may reduce serum folic acid and vitamin B12 levels (32,4490). A multivitamin preparation may be valuable in some patients.

H2-BLOCKERS; Cimetidine (Tagamet), Ranitidine (Zantac), Famotidine (Pepcid), and others: Long-term use of high-dose H2-blockers may lead to iron and B12 malabsorption (4539,4540,4541). The mechanism of this is thought to be through the inhibition of gastric acid secretion necessary for absorption of iron and B12. Monitor for signs/symptoms of anemia. This interaction is theoretically possible with proton pump inhibitors.

PROTON PUMP INHIBITORS; Lansoprazole (Prevacid), Omeprazole (Prilosec, Losec), Rabeprazole (Aciphex), Pantoprazole (Protonix, Pantoloc): Proton pump inhibitors might decrease dietary, but not supplemental, vitamin B12 absorption and resulting serum levels. The need for vitamin B12 supplementation has not been adequately studied. Vitamin B12 depletion may be particularly important in patients with inadequate diet, poor stores of the vitamin, and in patients receiving continuous, long-term therapy (see H2-Blockers above).

ORAL CONTRACEPTIVES: Use of oral contraceptives can increase vitamin B12 metabolism, decrease binding capacity, and reduce vitamin B12 serum levels. The significance of this and the need for vitamin B12 supplementation has not been adequately studied (4547).

POTASSIUM CHLORIDE, EXTENDED RELEASE (K-Dur): Use of extended release potassium chloride can reduce dietary vitamin B12 absorption and serum levels. The need for supplementation has not been adequately studied (4511,4512).

NICOTINE: Nicotine can reduce vitamin B12 blood levels. The need for vitamin B12 supplementation has not been adequately studied (19).

ZIDOVUDINE (AZT, Combivir, Retrovir): Patients with HIV disease taking zidovudine may have subnormal B12 concentrations, possibly predisposing them to hematologic toxicity, especially anemia (30). Give supplements of B12 only if clinical judgment warrants it.

Interactions with Foods

No interactions are known to occur, and there is no known reason to expect a clinically significant interaction with vitamin B12.

Interactions with Lab Tests

INTRINSIC FACTOR: Vitamin B12 can cause a false-positive test result for intrinsic factor antibodies (15).

Interactions with Diseases or Conditions

POLYCYTHEMIA VERA: The treatment of vitamin B12 deficiency can unmask the symptoms of polycythemia vera (15).

MEGALOBLASTIC ANEMIA: Use vitamin B12 with caution. The correction of megaloblastic anemia with vitamin B12 can result in fatal hypokalemia and gout in susceptible individuals, and it can obscure folate deficiency in megaloblastic anemia (15); use with caution.

COBALAMIN OR COBALT HYPERSENSITIVITY: Contraindicated (15).

LEBER'S DISEASE: Vitamin B12 is contraindicated in early Leber's disease, which is hereditary optic nerve atrophy. Vitamin B12 can cause severe and swift optic atrophy (15).

OTHER: The therapeutic response to vitamin B12 can be impaired by concurrent infections, uremia, and folic acid or iron deficiency (15).

Dosage and Administration

ORAL: For malabsorption of vitamin B12 from food or pernicious anemia, cyanocobalamin doses of 300 to 2000 mcg daily have been used (2900,2901,2909). For primary circadian rhythm sleep disorders, 0.5-1 mg of the methylcobalamin form of vitamin B12 three times daily has been used, with or without bright light therapy (1345,1347). The typical general supplemental dose of vitamin B12 is 1-25 mcg per day (15). For strict vegetarians, 6 mcg per day is often used (14). The recommended dietary allowances (RDAs) of vitamin B12 are: Infants 0-6 months, 0.4 mcg;

Infants 7-12 months, 0.5 mcg; Children 1-3 years, 0.9 mcg; Children 4-8 years, 1.2 mcg; Children 9-13 years, 1.8 mcg; Older children and adults, 2.4 mcg; Pregnant women 2.6 mcg; and Lactating women, 2.8 mcg (3094). Because 10-30% of older people do not absorb food-bound vitamin B12 efficiently, those over 50 years should meet the RDA by eating foods fortified with B12 or take a vitamin B12 supplement (3094,7290). Oral supplementation of 100 mcg per day has been used to maintain vitamin B12 levels in older people (2911).

INTRAMUSCULAR (IM): For treatment of vitamin B12 deficiency, the usual dose is 30 mcg daily for 5-10 days. For maintenance therapy, 100-200 mcg once monthly is commonly used. Both cyanocobalamin and hydroxocobalamin forms are used (15). For familial selective vitamin B12 malabsorption, cyanocobalamin 1000 mcg weekly for 3 weeks, followed by 250 mcg monthly is commonly used (15). For relief of tremor associated with shaky-leg syndrome, injections of 1000 mcg of the cyanocobalamin form of vitamin B12 daily for two weeks, then weekly for two months, and once a month thereafter has been used (6358).

Comments

Vitamin B12 is frequently used in combination with other B vitamins in vitamin B complex formulations. Vitamin B complex generally includes vitamin B1 (Thiamine), vitamin B2 (Riboflavin), vitamin B3 (Niacin/Niacinamide), vitamin B5 (Pantothenic Acid), vitamin B6 (Pyridoxine), vitamin B12 (Cyanocobalamin), and folic acid. However, some products do not contain all of these ingredients and some may include others, such as biotin, para-aminobenzoic acid (PABA), choline bitartrate, and inositol (3022,3060,3061).

VITAMIN C (ASCORBIC ACID)

Also Known As

Antiscorbutic Vitamin, Ascorbate, Ascorbic Acid, Calcium Ascorbate, Cevitamic Acid, Iso-Ascorbic Acid, Sodium Ascorbate, Vitamin C.
CAUTION: See separate listings for Acerola, Cherokee Rosehip, and Rose Hip.

Scientific Names

Ascorbic acid.

People Use This For

Orally, vitamin C is used for preventing and treating scurvy; preventing deficiency in people with gastrointestinal diseases and those on chronic total parenteral nutrition or chronic hemodialysis; increasing iron absorption from the gastrointestinal tract; and increasing the healing rate of wounds, burns, fractures, ulcers, and pressure sores. It is used for urine acidification, treating idiopathic methemoglobinemia, correcting tyrosinemia in premature infants on high-protein diets, increasing iron excretion (in combination with deferoxamine), preventing and treating the common cold and other viral infections, tuberculosis, dysentery, furunculosis, hematuria, retinal hemorrhages, hemorrhagic states, and anemia. Vitamin C is also used orally for atherosclerosis, preventing vascular thrombosis, myocardial infarction, stroke, hypertension, lowering cholesterol, glaucoma, preventing cataracts, preventing gallbladder disease, dental caries, pyorrhea, gum infections, constipation, peptic ulcer, acne, dermatitis, improving immune function, hay fever, asthma, bronchitis, cystic fibrosis, cystitis, prostatitis, infertility, and diabetes. It is also used orally for mental depression; cognitive impairment; stress; fatigue; attention deficit-hyperactivity disorder (ADHD); autism; collagen disorders; arthritis and bursitis; back pain and disc inflammation; cancer; osteogenesis imperfecta; improving physical endurance; reducing aging; heat prostration; for counteracting the side effects of cortisone and related drugs; aiding drug withdrawal in addiction; and treatment of levodopa, succinylcholine, and arsenic toxicity.

Topically, vitamin C is used for improving skin conditions, protecting against free radicals and pollutants, and photo-aged skin. It is also applied topically for ulcerative mucositis associated with radiation therapy.

In combination with vitamin K3, vitamin C is also used for treating prostate and breast cancers.

Parenterally, vitamin C is used for preventing and treating vitamin C deficiency and correcting tyrosinemia in premature infants on high-protein diets.

Safety

LIKELY SAFE ...when used orally and appropriately. Vitamin C is safe when used in doses below the tolerable upper intake level (UL). Tell patients not to exceed the UL of 2000 mg per day (6268). ...when used intravenously or intramuscularly and appropriately. Injectable vitamin C is a FDA-approved prescription product (15).

POSSIBLY UNSAFE ...when used orally in excessive doses. Doses greater than the tolerable upper intake level (UL) of 2000 mg per day can increase the risk of significant adverse effects such as osmotic diarrhea and gastrointestinal upset (6268).

CHILDREN: LIKELY SAFE ...when used orally and appropriately (6268). POSSIBLY UNSAFE ...when used orally in excessive amounts. Tell patients not to use doses above the tolerable upper intake level (UL) of 400 mg per day for children ages 1 to 3 years, 650 mg per day for children 4 to 8 years, 1200 mg per day for children 9 to 13 years, and 1800 mg per day for adolescents 14 to 18 years. Higher doses can cause osmotic diarrhea and gastrointestinal upset (6268).

PREGNANCY AND LACTATION: LIKELY SAFE ...when used orally and appropriately (6268). POSSIBLY UNSAFE ...when used orally in excessive doses. Tell patients not to use doses exceeding the of 2000 mg per day for pregnant or breast-feeding women over age 19 and 1800 mg per day for pregnant and breast-feeding women 14 to 18 years. Higher doses can cause osmotic diarrhea and gastrointestinal upset. Large doses of vitamin C during pregnancy can also cause newborn scurvy (6268); avoid using.

Effectiveness

EFFECTIVE ...when taken orally or given intramuscularly for preventing and treating vitamin C deficiency, including scurvy. Vitamin C administration can reverse complications of scurvy within two days to three weeks (15).

LIKELY EFFECTIVE ...when taken orally for improving iron absorption. Concurrent administration of at least 200 mg vitamin C per 30 mg iron can increase iron absorption (15,3042). ... when used orally or intramuscularly for tyrosinemia in premature infants on high protein diets (15).

POSSIBLY EFFECTIVE ...when used orally from dietary sources for reducing cancer risk. People consuming fruits and vegetables that provide vitamin C 200 mg per day may have a decreased risk of developing cancers of the mouth, esophagus, stomach, colon, and lung (1444,3042); however, this benefit is not found with vitamin C supplements (3042). ...when used orally from dietary sources for reducing cancer risk. Mortality from cancer seems to be reduced in men (but not women) who eat a diet high in fruits and vegetables containing vitamin C. Researchers project that plasma ascorbic acid increases to protective levels when the average man increases his fruit and vegetable consumption by one serving per day (3910). ...when used orally to promote regression of premalignant gastric lesions in people at high risk for gastric cancer. Vitamin C 1 gram twice daily seems to cause regression of intestinal metaplasia and multifocal nonmetaplastic atrophy (2579). ...when used orally for treating the common cold. There is a lot of controversy about the effectiveness of vitamin C for treating the common cold (1969,1989,7100). However, the majority of evidence shows that high doses of vitamin C can decrease the duration of symptoms by 1-1.5 days in some patients (1966,1967,1968,1987,6458,7102). Tell patients that the high doses used for treating the common cold, 1-3 grams daily, can increase the risk of side effects. Some patients might not think the modest benefit is worth the risk. ...when used orally with vitamin E for preventing pre-eclampsia in high-risk pregnancies (3236). ...when used orally from dietary sources to reduce mortality from cardiovascular disease. Men and women whose plasma ascorbic acid levels are higher as a result of a diet high in fruits and vegetables appear to have a 30% lower risk of death from cardiovascular disease and ischemic heart disease compared with people with lower plasma ascorbic acid levels. Increasing fruit and vegetable intake by one serving per day in the average person could boost plasma ascorbic acid to protective levels (3910). It's not known if vitamin C from supplements has this benefit. ...when used orally as an adjunct for hypertension. Vitamin C added to a conventional antihypertensive medication regimen appears to decrease both systolic and mean blood pressure, but does not seem to decrease diastolic readings (2044). ...when used orally from dietary sources for reducing the risk of stroke. Population studies show that increasing vitamin C intake in the diet seems to decrease the relative risk of both ischemic and hemorrhagic stroke (1957,1958). It's not known if supplemental vitamin C has this effect. ...when used orally in combination with vitamin E to slow progression of atherosclerosis in men. Slow release vitamin C 250 mg in combination with 91 mg (136 IU) of vitamin E twice daily for 3 years seems to slow the progression of atherosclerosis of the carotid artery in men. The combination appears to benefit both smoking and nonsmoking men, but has no effect in women (1918). ...when used orally to reduce the risk of gallbladder disease. There is some evidence that vitamin C supplement use and increased vitamin C serum levels decreases the risk of developing gallbladder disease in women. However, it doesn't seem to have this effect in men (5877). ...when used orally in combination with vitamin E to protect against vascular dementia. There some evidence from a population study that use of both vitamin C and E can lower the risk of developing vascular dementia. However, the combination does not seem to have a protective effect against Alzheimer's dementia (4636). ...when used orally in combination with zinc and other antioxidant vitamins to slow progression of intermediate and advanced age-related macular degeneration (ARMD). Taking vitamin C 500 mg plus elemental zinc 80 mg, vitamin E 400 IU, and beta-carotene 15 mg daily seems to provide a risk reduction of 27 % for visual acuity loss and a risk reduction of 28% for progression to more advanced ARMD in patients with intermediate and advanced ARMD (7303). There isn't enough evidence to know if this combination is beneficial for people with less advanced disease or for preventing AMD. Vitamin C with antioxidants, but without zinc doesn't seem to have any effect on AMD (7303,7304). ...when taken orally from dietary sources to reduce risk of cartilage loss and disease progression in osteoarthritis. There is some evidence that increasing dietary vitamin C intake reduces osteoarthritis progression and cartilage loss (5881). ...when used orally to decrease the risk of developing reflex sympathetic dystrophy (RSD) after wrist fracture. Patients given vitamin C supplements for 50 days after a wrist fracture seem to be significantly less likely to develop RSD (2045). ...when taken orally from dietary sources to lower blood lead levels (3097,3098,3099). ...when taken orally to prevent the development of nitrate tolerance in patients taking sublingual nitroglycerin. There is some evidence that short-term vitamin C supplementation can prevent attenuation of tolerance to the vasodilatory effects of nitrates (1441,1961). ....when used topically for improving photo-aged or wrinkled skin. Topical preparations containing from 5-10% vitamin C seem to improve the appearance of wrinkled skin. In one trial, a topical preparation containing 10% vitamin C as L-ascorbic acid, acetyl tyrosine, zinc sulfate, sodium hyaluronate, and bioflavonoids (Cellex-C High Potency Serum) used for 3 months and applied to photo-aged facial skin improved fine and coarse wrinkling, yellowing and sallowness, roughness, and skin tone compared to placebo (6155). In an unpublished study, a 5% vitamin C cream significantly reduced large, deep wrinkles after 6 months of treatment (1325). ...when used orally in combination with vitamin E to prevent ultraviolet (UV) radiation-induced erythema (sunburn) (4715,4716). Vitamin C in combination with high dose oral RRR-alpha-tocopherol (natural vitamin E) seems to protect against skin inflammation after exposure to ultraviolet (UV) radiation (1416,4715). This effect is not found when vitamin C is used without vitamin E (1417). ...when used topically in combination with vitamin E and melatonin to prevent ultraviolet (UV) radiation-induced erythema (sunburn). Topically applied vitamin C in combination with topical vitamin E and melatonin seems to provide modest photoprotective effects when used prior to UV exposure. However, it has no effect when used during or after UV exposure (4713,4714). ...when used topically to prevent erythema following laser resurfacing. There is some evidence that an aqueous formulation of topical vitamin C can decrease the degree and duration of erythema following cutaneous carbon dioxide laser resurfacing for scar and wrinkle removal (1959).

POSSIBLY INEFFECTIVE ...when taken orally for preventing the common cold. There is a lot of controversy about the effectiveness of using vitamin C for prevention of the common cold. However, the majority of evidence shows that vitamin C supplementation does not decrease the risk of developing a cold (1966,1967,1968,1987,3042,6458,7101). ...when used orally as an urinary acidifier (14,15). ...when used topically to prevent radiation dermatitis. A 10% vitamin C solution does not appear to have a protective effect when applied to the scalp of patients treated with radiation for intracranial tumors (789).

LIKELY INEFFECTIVE ...when used orally to treat cancer (4842,4843). High dose vitamin C 10 grams daily in patients with advanced cancer, regardless of prior chemotherapy, does not improve survival or decrease disease progression (4842,4843).

There is insufficient reliable information available to rate the effectiveness of vitamin C for its other uses. However, there is some evidence that low levels of vitamin C are associated with certain conditions. Vitamin C levels might be decreased in some asthmatics (5873). Some clinical evidence suggests that oral vitamin C might decrease exercise-induced asthma (1443). Vitamin C in combination with aged garlic extract and vitamin E might also be useful for sickle cell disease (5056). There's also some evidence that the combination of vitamins C and E might help prevent cardiac transplant-associated arteriosclerosis (5197). There is conflicting information about the use of vitamin C to prevent cataracts. Vitamin C plus vitamin E and beta-carotene doesn't seem to have any significant effect on age-related loss of vision due to cataracts in well-nourished people who took the supplement for an average of 6.3 years (7304). But population research suggests that vitamin C use in multivitamins or any supplement containing vitamin C for 10 years appears to reduce the incidence of nuclear and cortical cataracts by 60%. Use of supplements for shorter periods doesn't appear to reduce the risk for cataract development (4208). More evidence is needed to rate the effectiveness of vitamin C for these uses.

Mechanism of Action

Vitamin C is a commonly used water-soluble vitamin. Although many mammals can produce vitamin C, humans must obtain vitamin C from foods (1964). It's contained in the high concentration in fresh fruits and vegetables, especially the citrus fruits. Vitamin C is labile, and the amount in foods can decrease significantly with cooking and storage (3042). Vitamin C has a role in several physiological functions. It is involved in tyrosine metabolism and is a cofactor in the synthesis of carnitine, thyroxin, norepinephrine, dopamine, and tryptophan (3042). Vitamin C is also involved in a variety of metabolic processes including oxidation-reduction reactions and cellular respiration, carbohydrate metabolism, synthesis of lipids and proteins, catabolism of cholesterol to bile acids, conversion of folic acid to folinic acid, and iron metabolism (5877). Vitamin C is probably best known for its effects as an antioxidant and its role in maintaining proper immune function (15). Normal plasma vitamin C levels typically exceed 0.3 mg/dL. When plasma levels exceed 1.4 mg/dL, excretion of vitamin C greatly increases (1965,1969). Concentrations below 0.2 mg/dL indicate significant deficiency (1964). Vitamin C deficiency can cause personality changes, fatigue, and decline in psychomotor performance and motivation within 84 to 97 days. Sustained vitamin C deficiency over 3 to 5 months results in symptomatic scurvy characterized by gingival swelling and bleeding; loosening of the teeth; hyperkeratosis; perifollicular hemorrhages; petechial hemorrhages in the viscera; and hemorrhages into the muscles of the arms, legs, and joints (1964). Severe scurvy may progress to neuritis, jaundice, fever, dyspnea, and death. In infants, vitamin C deficiency is initially manifested by listlessness, anorexia, irritability, and failure to thrive. Later symptoms result from hemorrhage and collagen deficiency, with seizures, shock, and death if left untreated (1965). Wound healing is also delayed in people with vitamin C deficiency; however, there is no evidence to indicate that vitamin C supplementation improves healing in people with normal nutritional status (14). Because of vitamin C's role in maintaining normal immune function, a lot of people use it for treating and preventing infectious conditions such as the common cold. T-lymphocyte activity, phagocyte function, leukocyte mobility, and possibly antibody and interferon production seem to be increased by vitamin C (1963,1965). Vitamin C levels in phagocytes and lymphocytes are up to 100 times greater than in plasma (7101). Some researchers think that vitamin C levels in white blood cells decrease at the onset of a cold and that boosting vitamin C intake might be beneficial. There is some evidence vitamin C might have other effects in patients with the common cold. Vitamin C might protect normal tissues against reactive oxygen species that are produced by phagocytes during a viral infection. It might also enhance the proliferative responses of T-lymphocytes (1988). There is some evidence that vitamin C might also have weak antihistamine properties (1969). There is preliminary evidence vitamin C excretion might actually decrease during a cold, indicating that patients may retain vitamin C. However, absorption of vitamin C is unchanged during a cold (1986). Other potentially beneficial effects of vitamin C are attributed primarily to its role as an antioxidant and free radical scavenging effects. Vitamin C readily undergoes reversible oxidation and reduction in the body (1963). Vitamin C decreases oxidants in gastric juice, lipid peroxidation, and oxidative DNA and protein damage (3042). Damage by reactive oxygen species are thought to be a contributing factor to a number of diseases, including dementia, asthma, hypertension, osteoarthritis, and cancer. Researchers theorized that antioxidants such as vitamin C might protect against some diseases associated with oxidative damage. For example, in hypertension, endothelium-derived nitric oxide (NO), which causes vasodilation, might be inhibited by superoxide anions. Vitamin C can scavenge the superoxide anions and theoretically might help patients with hypertension. However, in this case there is some evidence that oral doses might not reach concentrations high enough for this effect (5879). In people with chronic heart failure, intra-arterial vitamin C seems to improve endothelial dysfunction and flow-dependent dilation of the arteries. Vitamin C appears to prevent inactivation of NO-mediated vasodilation. Four weeks of oral vitamin C one gram twice daily appears to produce a similar effect (2434). Intracoronary infusion of vitamin C has been shown to enhance the inotropic response to dobutamine (Dobutrex), possibly by reducing oxidative stress caused by beta-adrenergic stimulation of the ventricle (2432). In smokers, supplemental vitamin C appears to restore coronary microcirculatory responsiveness and impaired coronary flow reserve induced by the oxidant effects of smoking. Vitamin C might reduce oxidative stress caused by the large number of oxidants in cigarette smoke (1956). Pulmonary function is positively related to dietary vitamin C intake in smokers and nonsmokers (2400). For radiation-induced oral mucositis, the reduced form of vitamin C might be beneficial due to its antioxidant effect and role in maintaining connective tissue integrity (6103). Vitamin C may also reduce toxicity to normal tissues from reactive oxygen during radio-immunotherapy due to its antioxidant effects (5878). Free radicals are also generated in the skin by exposure to ultraviolet light and cause photo-aging. Vitamin C in the skin is believed to play a key role in neutralizing these free radicals and reducing UV skin damage. Topical application of vitamin C is thought prevent skin damage when applied prior to UV exposure due to antioxidant effects (6062,6155). Topical preparations are thought to help treat photo-aged and wrinkled skin due to antioxidant properties and possibly by increasing collagen production and improving collagen organization (1325,6155). Topical preparations containing 10% vitamin C might be most effective for increasing vitamin C concentrations in the skin. Because vitamin C is water soluble, oral supplementation of vitamin C might not produce high enough concentrations in the skin to treat photo-aged skin (6064,6155).

Adverse Reactions

Orally, the adverse effects of vitamin C are dose-related (3042) and include nausea; vomiting; esophagitis; heartburn; abdominal cramps; gastrointestinal obstruction; fatigue; flushing; headache; insomnia; sleepiness; diarrhea;

hyperoxaluria; and the precipitation of urate, oxalate, or cysteine stones or drugs in the urinary tract (14,15). Hyperoxaluria, hyperuricosuria, hematuria, and crystalluria have occurred in people taking 1 gram or more per day (14,3042).

Large amounts of vitamin C are associated with deep vein thrombosis. Prolonged use of large amounts of vitamin C can also result in increased metabolism of vitamin C and scurvy can occur when vitamin C intake is reduced (15). Oral supplementation with vitamin C has also been associated with an increased rate of carotid inner wall thickening in men. There is preliminary evidence that supplemental intake of vitamin C 500 mg daily for 18 months can cause a 2.5-fold increased rate of carotid inner wall thickening in non-smoking men and a 5-fold increased rate in men who smoked. The men in this study were 40-60 years old. This effect was not associated with vitamin C from dietary sources (1355).

There is also some concern that supplements of vitamin C 200 mg might increase production reactive oxygen molecules capable of damaging DNA. This is based on very preliminary in vitro evidence that vitamin C can induce decomposition of lipid hydroperoxides to reactive molecules. More evidence is needed to know if this is clinically relevant in humans taking vitamin C supplements (7088)

Topically, vitamin C might cause tingling or irritation at the site of application (6166).

Interactions with Herbs & Other Dietary Supplements

IRON: Concomitant use of 200 mg of vitamin C per 30 mg of elemental iron increases oral iron absorption, especially ferric iron (14,15,3042). Ascorbic acid reduces iron to its reduced (ferrous) and best absorbed form (1960).

Interactions with Drugs

ACETAMINOPHEN (Tylenol): High doses of vitamin C (3 grams or more) can decrease elimination rate of acetaminophen by approximately 75% and might increase the risk of acetaminophen side effects. Vitamin C seems to competitively inhibit sulfate conjugation of acetaminophen (6451).

ALUMINUM-CONTAINING ANTACIDS: Concomitant use might increase aluminum absorption. Clinical significance is unknown (3046). Administer vitamin C two hours before, or four hours after taking an antacid (3046).

ASPIRIN AND OTHER SALICYLATES: Concomitant use can increase urinary excretion of ascorbic acid and decrease excretion of salicylates. However, it might not have a clinically significant effect on salicylate plasma levels (3046).

DOBUTAMINE (Dobutrex): There is some evidence that vitamin C might increase the inotropic effect of dobutamine. In preclinical research, an intracoronary infusion of vitamin C appears to increase the effect of dobutamine on left ventricular contractility in people with normal heart function (2432).

ETHINYL ESTRADIOL (Estinyl, Ortho-Novum, Loestrin, Ovral, and many other oral contraceptives): Vitamin C was previously thought to interfere with the metabolism of ethinyl estradiol, resulting in higher blood levels. However, pharmacokinetic research has shown that vitamin C doesn't have any clinically important effect on ethinyl estradiol metabolism (3712).

HEPARIN: There is some evidence that high dose vitamin C might decrease the effectiveness of heparin (1962,6452). However, vitamin C in combination with B vitamin infusion appears to have no effect on the anticoagulant effects of heparin when mixed together in the same IV bag (1962).

IRON: 200 mg vitamin C per 30 mg of elemental iron increases iron (especially ferric iron) absorption (3042). Ascorbic acid reduces iron to its reduced (ferrous) and best absorbed form (1960).

WARFARIN (Coumadin): Concomitant use with large amounts of vitamin C might impair response to warfarin (3046); use with caution.

Drug Influences on Nutrient Levels and Depletion

SOME DRUGS CAN AFFECT VITAMIN C LEVELS.

ASPIRIN AND OTHER SALICYLATES: Concomitant use can increase urinary excretion of vitamin C. However, there is no evidence of vitamin C deficiency associated with use of aspirin and other salicylates. Consider supplementation only in patients on long-term salicylate therapy with signs of vitamin C deficiency (15,3046).

ESTROGEN AND ORAL CONTRACEPTIVES: Estrogens can increase elimination of vitamin C (15,19). Consider supplementation only if clinical judgment warrants it.

NICOTINE AND SMOKING: Nicotine can increase elimination of vitamin C (19). Smokers have been reported to have lower plasma levels of vitamin C than nonsmokers with similar diets. These low levels can be corrected with moderate supplementation or by an increasing fruit and vegetable intake to recommended dietary levels (5875). Consider supplementation only if clinical judgment warrants it.

Interactions with Foods

COPPER: Vitamin C can decrease the absorption of dietary copper (1964).

IRON: Vitamin C can increase the absorption of dietary ferric iron (14,3042).

Interactions with Lab Tests

ACETAMINOPHEN: Vitamin C can cause false-negative urine results with methods based on hydrolysis and formation of an indophenol blue chromagen (14).

ASPARTATE AMINOTRANSFERASE (AST, SGOT): Large amounts of ascorbic acid can cause a false increase in results of serum tests relying on color reactions (Redox reactions) and Technicon SMA 12/60 (14).

BILIRUBIN: Large amounts of vitamin C can cause a false increase in serum test results measured by Technicon SMA 12/60 or colorimetric methods (14).

CALCIUM/SODIUM: 3-6 grams of vitamin C daily can cause an increase in urinary calcium and test results (15), and a decrease in urinary sodium and test results.

CARBAMAZEPINE (Tegretol): Large doses of vitamin C can cause falsely increased serum assay results measured by Ames ARIS method (14).

CREATININE: Vitamin C can cause a false increase in serum creatinine or urine test results (14).

GLUCOSE: Large amounts of vitamin C can cause false increases in urine test results measured by copper reduction methods (e.g., Clinitest), and false decreases in results measured by glucose oxidase methods (e.g., Clinistix, Tes-Tape) (14,15).

LACTIC DEHYDROGENASE (LDH): Vitamin C can cause a false decrease measured by Technicon SMA 12/60 and Abbott 100 methods (14).

OCCULT BLOOD: False-negative guaiac results occur with 250 mg or more of vitamin C per day (3042).

THEOPHYLLINE: Large amounts of vitamin C can cause falsely decreased serum assay results when measured by the ARIS system or Ames Seralyzer photometer (14).

URIC ACID: Large amounts of vitamin C can cause a decrease in serum uric acid concentrations and test results with enzymatic method assays (15), and a false increase in test results with assays based on other methods (14).

VITAMIN B12: Large amounts of vitamin C can interfere with vitamin B12 assay, resulting in falsely low vitamin B12 levels (1965).

Interactions with Diseases or Conditions

ANGIOPLASTY: There is some concern that when antioxidant vitamins, including vitamin C, are used together they might have harmful effects in patients after angioplasty. A combination of beta-carotene 30,000 IU, vitamin C 500 mg, and vitamin E 700 IU daily started 30 days before angioplasty, and continued for 6 months thereafter, seems to prevent beneficial vascular remodeling in patients after angioplasty by promoting fibrosis at the site of angioplastic intervention (1317). Tell patients to avoid taking supplements of these vitamins immediately before and following angioplasty without the supervision of a health care professional.

CANCER: Cancerous cells accumulate high concentrations of vitamin C. Cancer cells uptake the oxidized form of vitamin C, dehydroascorbic acid, then convert it back to vitamin C (4838,4839,4840,4841). However, it is not yet known if this benefits growth of cancer cells or has any detrimental effect of cancer treatments. Until more is known, patients with cancer should only use high doses of vitamin C under the direction of their oncologist.

DIABETES: Vitamin C can affect glycogenolysis and increase blood sugar, but this effect remains controversial (15).

GLUCOSE-6-PHOSPHATE DEHYDROGENASE DEFICIENCY: Large amounts of vitamin C can cause hemolysis in individuals with glucose-6-phosphate dehydrogenase deficiency (15).

IRON OVERLOAD, HEMOCHROMATOSIS, THALASSEMIA, SIDEROBLASTIC ANEMIA: Use vitamin C with caution, because it can increase iron absorption, which could worsen these conditions (14,15,1960).

KIDNEY STONES: Large amounts of vitamin C can increase the risk of oxalate stone formation (15). Tell patients prone to kidney stone formation to avoid high doses of vitamin C.

MYOCARDIAL INFARCTION (MI): Vitamin C levels are significantly reduced during the acute phase after a MI. However, low plasma levels of vitamin C have not been associated with an increased risk of MI (5876).

SICKLE CELL DISEASE: Vitamin C can decrease blood pH, which can rarely precipitate sickle cell crisis (15).

INCREASED NEEDS: Vitamin C requirements are increased in pregnancy, lactation, hyperthyroidism, stress, fever, infection, trauma, burns, smoking, and cold exposure (15).

Dosage and Administration

ORAL: For scurvy, 100-250 mg once or twice daily for several days is commonly used (15). Alternatively, vitamin C deficiency is sometimes treated with 100 mg three times daily for one week and then once daily until tissue saturation is normal (14). For treating the common cold, 1-3 grams daily has been used (6458). For chronic hemodialysis in adults, 100-200 mg per day is recommended (15). For preventing nitrate tolerance, 3-6 grams of vitamin C daily has been used (1961). For preventing sunburn, 2 grams of vitamin C in combination with RRR-alpha-tocopherol (natural vitamin E) 1000 IU has been used (4716). For treatment of premalignant gastric lesions, vitamin C 1 gram twice daily has been used (2579). For slowing progression of atherosclerosis, slow release vitamin C 250 mg in combination with 91 mg (136 IU) of vitamin E has been given twice daily (1918). For tyrosinemia in premature infants on high protein diets, 100 mg of vitamin C has been used (15). The daily recommended dietary allowances (RDAs) are: Infants 0 to 12 months, human milk content (older recommendations specified 30 to 35 mg); Children 1 to 3 years, 15 mg; Children 4 to 8 years, 25 mg; Children 9 to 13 years, 45 mg; Adolescents 14 to 18 years, 75 mg for boys and 65 mg for girls; Adults age 19 and greater, 90 mg for men and 75 mg for women; Pregnancy and Lactation: age 18 or younger, 115 mg; ages 19 to 50 years 120 mg (7135). People who use tobacco should take an additional 35 mg per day (4844). The tolerable upper intake levels (UL) for vitamin C are 400 mg per day for children ages 1 to 3 years, 650 mg per day for children 4 to 8 years, 1200 mg per day for children 9 to 13 years, and 1800 mg per day for adolescents and pregnant and lactating women 14 to 18 years, and 2000 mg per day for adults and pregnant and lactating women (7135).

TOPICAL: Most topical preparations used for aged or wrinkled skin are applied daily. Studies have used creams containing 5-10% vitamin C and applied daily (1325,6155). In one study of a specific vitamin C formulation (Cellex-C High Potency Serum) used 3 drops applied daily to areas of facial skin (6155). Avoid application to eye area or eye-lids. Also avoid contact with hair or clothes. It can cause discoloration (6166).

PARENTERAL: For scurvy, 100 to 250 mg twice daily has been used intravenously, intramuscularly, or subcutaneously (15). For tyrosinemia in premature infants on high protein diets, 100 mg of vitamin C has been used intramuscularly (15).

Comments

Most experts recommend getting antioxidants, including vitamin C, from a diet high in fruits, vegetables, and whole grains rather than taking supplements (1440,3042). A recent review by an independent laboratory found that 15% of the vitamin C in products tested did not meet labeled potency, including one product that claimed to meet USP standards (4845).

VITAMIN D

Also Known As
Calcifediol: 25-hydroxyvitamin D3, 25-hydroxycholecalciferol, 25-HCC, 25-OHCC, 25-OHD3.
Calcitriol: 1,25-dihydroxyvitamin D3, 1,25-dihydroxycholecalciferol, 1,25-DHCC, 1,25-diOHC, 1,25(0H)2D3.
Cholecalciferol: vitamin D3, activated 7-dehydrocholesterol, colecalciferol. Dihydrotachysterol: DHT, dichysterol, dihydrotachysterol 2.
Ergocalciferol: vitamin D2, calciferol, activated ergosterol, viosterol, ergocalciferolum, irradiated ergosterol.
Calcipotriene: calcipotriol. Paricalcitol: paracalcin, 19-nor-1,25-dihydroxyvitamin D2.
Alfacalcidol: 1-alpha-hydroxycholecalciferol, 1 alpha (OH)D3.

Scientific Names
Vitamin D; calcifediol; 25-hydroxycholecalciferol; calcitriol; 1,25-dihydroxycholecalciferol; cholecalciferol; dihydrotachysterol; ergocalciferol; calcipotriene; paricalcitol; alfacalcidol.

People Use This For
Orally, vitamin D is used for building bone mass and preventing bone loss; protecting against muscle weakness; promoting strong teeth (3058,3059); reducing risk of colon, breast, and prostate cancer (15); treating cancer; enhancing immune function; preventing auto-immune diseases (3058,3059); and rheumatoid arthritis (14,15). It is also used orally for preventing and treating rickets, postmenopausal osteoporosis (14,15), to prevent falls and fractures in people at risk for osteoporosis (6363), corticosteroid-induced osteoporosis, osteomalacia, anticonvulsant-induced osteomalacia, renal osteodystrophy, osteitis fibrosa in people on dialysis, hepatic osteodystrophy, osteogenesis imperfecta, preventing and treating hypocalcemia and tetany in premature infants, hypocalcemic tetany, bone disorders in people with familial hypophosphatemia, hypophosphatemia associated with Fanconi syndrome, hypocalcemia associated with postoperative or idiopathic hypoparathyroidism or pseudohypoparathyroidism, plaque-type psoriasis, actinic keratoses, lupus vulgaris, squamous cell carcinomas, vitiligo, scleroderma, myelodysplastic syndrome (14,15), and treating multiple sclerosis (5083). Vitamin D is also used orally to treat severe proximal myopathy associated with vitamin D deficiency (6359) and to maintain bone density in prostatic cancer patients at risk for osteoporosis when treated with luteinizing hormone-releasing hormone analogue (LHRH-a) (6360,6361).
Topically, vitamin D is used as calcitriol or calcipotriene for plaque-type psoriasis (14).
Intravenously, vitamin D, administered as calcitriol, is used for hypocalcemic tetany in premature infants, hypocalcemia and hyperparathyroidism in renal dialysis patients, and osteitis fibrosa (14,15).
Intramuscularly, vitamin D is administered as ergocalciferol for hepatic osteodystrophy, as an injectable source of vitamin D (14,15) and to treat severe proximal myopathy associated with vitamin D deficiency (6359).

Safety
LIKELY SAFE ...when used orally and appropriately (15). Therapeutic amounts do not differ much from amounts that can cause hypercalcemia.
PREGNANCY: LIKELY SAFE ...when used orally at the recommended adequate intake of 200 units daily, and in amounts up to 400 units daily found in many prenatal vitamin supplements (15); avoid larger amounts (15).

Hypercalcemia during pregnancy due to vitamin D intake can lead to suppression of parathyroid hormone, hypocalcemia, tetany, seizures, aortic valve stenosis, retinopathy, and mental and/or physical retardation in the infant (15).

LACTATION: LIKELY SAFE ...when used orally at amounts up to 400 units daily (15); avoid larger amounts.

Effectiveness

EFFECTIVE ...when oral calcifediol is used for treating osteomalacia secondary to liver disease (hepatic osteodystrophy). ...when oral calcifediol is used for managing hypocalcemia and preventing renal osteodystrophy in people with chronic renal failure undergoing dialysis. ...when oral calcifediol is used for preventing corticosteroid-induced osteopenia and osteoporosis (14,15). ...when oral calcitriol is used for preventing tetany in vitamin D-deficient premature infants with hypocalcemia. ...when oral calcitriol is used in conjunction with phosphate supplements for treating bone disorders in people with familial hypophosphatemia. ...when oral calcitriol is used for vitamin D-dependent rickets. ...when oral calcitriol is used for managing hypocalcemia and preventing renal osteodystrophy in people with chronic renal failure undergoing dialysis. ...when oral calcitriol is used for treating osteitis fibrosa. ...when oral calcitriol is used for anticonvulsant-induced rickets. ...when oral calcitriol is used for plaque-type psoriasis. ...when oral calcitriol is used for increasing serum calcium concentrations in people with hypoparathyroidism or pseudohypoparathyroidism (14,15). ...when topical calcitriol is used for treating plaque-type psoriasis (14). ...when oral cholecalciferol is used for treating nutritional rickets and osteomalacia. ...when oral cholecalciferol is used for preventing corticosteroid-induced osteopenia and osteoporosis (15). ...when oral dihydrotachysterol is used in conjunction with phosphate supplements for treating bone disorders in people with familial hypophosphatemia. ...when oral dihydrotachysterol is used for renal osteodystrophy and osteitis fibrosa. ...when oral dihydrotachysterol is used for managing hypocalcemia and preventing renal osteodystrophy in people with chronic renal failure undergoing dialysis. ...when oral dihydrotachysterol is used for increasing serum calcium concentrations in people with hypoparathyroidism or pseudohypoparathyroidism. ...when oral dihydrotachysterol is used for preventing and treating hypocalcemic tetany (14,15). ...when oral ergocalciferol is used for treating nutritional rickets and osteomalacia due to malabsorption syndromes. ...when oral ergocalciferol is used for neonatal rickets. ...when oral ergocalciferol is used in very large doses and in conjunction with phosphate supplements for bone disorders in people with familial hypophosphatemia. ...when oral ergocalciferol is used for hypophosphatemia associated with Fanconi syndrome. ...when oral ergocalciferol is used in large amounts for vitamin D-dependent rickets. ...when oral ergocalciferol is used in high doses for increasing serum calcium concentrations in people with hypoparathyroidism or pseudohypoparathyroidism (14,15). ...when calcipotriene is used topically for treating moderate plaque psoriasis (14).

POSSIBLY EFFECTIVE ...when oral alfacalcidol is used to maintain bone density in prostatic carcinoma patients at risk for osteoporosis when treated with luteinizing hormone-releasing hormone analogue (LHRH-a). Alfacalcidol maintains but does not increase bone mineral density (6360). ...when oral calcifediol is used for anticonvulsant-induced osteomalacia. ...when oral calcifediol is used for postmenopausal osteoporosis (14). ...when oral calcitriol is used with isotretinoin for treating actinic keratoses and early squamous cell carcinomas. ...when oral calcitriol is used for myelodysplastic syndrome. ...when oral calcitriol is used for postmenopausal osteoporosis (14). ...when oral dihydrotachysterol is used in conjunction with calcium supplements and sodium fluoride supplements for treating osteoporosis. ...when oral dihydrotachysterol is used for osteogenesis imperfecta (14,15). ...when oral ergocalciferol is used in conjunction with calcium supplements and sodium fluoride supplements for treating postmenopausal osteoporosis. ...when oral ergocalciferol is used for preventing and treating anticonvulsant-induced rickets and osteomalacia. ...when oral ergocalciferol is used for preventing corticosteroid-induced osteomalacia. ...when oral ergocalciferol is used for hepatic osteodystrophy (14,15). ...when topical calcipotriene is used for treating vitiligo and scleroderma (14). ...when cholecalciferol is used orally for decreasing secondary hyperparathyroidism and bone turnover in black women. In one study, supplementation with cholecalciferol resulted in increased serum levels of 25-hydroxyvitamin D, reduced levels of parathyroid hormone, and decreased production of markers of bone turnover (3463). ...when cholecalciferol is given orally in breast-fed infants for increasing bone mineral density. In a retrospective study, prepubertal girls who received cholecalciferol in infancy had significantly greater bone mineral density at some skeletal sites compared to girls that did not receive vitamin D during infancy (3464). ...when ergocalciferol is used orally or intramuscularly to treat severe proximal myopathy associated with severe vitamin D deficiency. Several case reports suggest vitamin D therapy can provide prompt relief of muscle weakness and restore mobility (6359). ...when vitamin D with calcium is administered orally to prevent falls and decrease risk of nonvertebral fractures in elderly women. Vitamin D in combination with calcium, but not calcium alone may prevent falls and decrease risk of fractures in individuals at risk for osteoporosis by decreasing body sway and systolic blood pressure instead of increasing bone mass strength (6362,6363).

POSSIBLY INEFFECTIVE ...when used orally for preventing bone loss associated with long-term renal transplantation (4823). Calcitriol 0.25 mcg per day in combination with calcium carbonate 500 mg per day did not significantly improve bone loss in renal transplant patients; however, the treatment group had less osteoclast suppression and there was a trend to maintenance of trabecular bone volume and wall thickness, and some improvement in axial bone mineral density (4823). ...when used orally for multiple sclerosis (5083).

LIKELY INEFFECTIVE ...when oral calcitriol is used for corticosteroid-induced osteoporosis (14).

Mechanism of Action

The term vitamin D is used to refer to several vitamin D analogs which are closely related to sterol compounds that occur in nature or are prepared synthetically (9). Dietary sources include eggs; fatty fish such as herrings, mackerel, sardines, and tuna; and vitamin D fortified foods. But these are relatively minor sources. Skin exposure to the sun provides as much as 80 to 90% of the body's vitamin D stores (7133). Full-body sun exposure can lead to the synthesis of as much as 10,000 units of vitamin D per day (6855). Vitamin D is stored in body fat for use during periods without sun exposure (15). Conversely, excessive sun exposure causes photodegradation of vitamin D produced in the skin, limiting the risk of vitamin D toxicity from such exposure (15). Use of sunscreens can reduce vitamin D synthesis in the body, although this is unlikely to lead to deficiencies since exposure of the face and arms to the sun for 5 to 10 minutes, 2 to 3 times per week ensures adequate synthesis (6855). However, vitamin D supplements may be needed by elderly people with limited sun exposure, people living in northern latitudes, dark-skinned African Americans, Asian Indians living in the western hemisphere, as well as people with gastrointestinal diseases leading to malabsorption of vitamin D from the diet (6855,7133). The elderly, who generally have less sun exposure and less dietary vitamin D intake, may be at the greatest risk for insufficient vitamin D. Elderly people more often have impaired renal function, impaired skin synthesis of vitamin D, and possibly also a decreased number of vitamin D receptors (7133). Dark-skinned people need increased exposure to sunlight to produce the same amount of vitamin D as fair-skinned people, because the skin pigment melanin competes with vitamin D precursors in the skin for photons from UV-B light (6857). This also affects vitamin D in breast milk. For example, breast milk from African Americans is generally lower in vitamin D content than that from Caucasian women (35 units/L compared with 68 units/L, respectively) (6857). African American infants who are exclusively breast-fed are therefore at risk for vitamin D deficiency and rickets, even if they live in sunny climates such as the southern US (6857). People who are obese (body mass index >30kg/m2) may have reduced serum vitamin D levels and reduced bioavailability of vitamin D from both cutaneous synthesis and gastrointestinal absorption. In response to similar UV-B exposures, the increase in serum vitamin D levels can be 57% less in obese people than in those who were slim. The content of vitamin D precursors in the skin are similar in both groups, suggesting that vitamin D synthesis is not affected in obese people, but that vitamin D is sequestered into body fat, reducing its availability (6856). Regardless of the source, sun or diet, vitamin D undergoes two reactions to become biologically active (7133). Cholecalciferol is hydroxylated to calcifediol, also known as 25-hydroxyvitamin D, 25-hydroxycholecalciferol, in the liver, and then to calcitriol, also known as 1,25-dihydroxyvitamin D, 1,25-dihydroxycholecalciferol, in the kidneys (14,15). The active forms of vitamin D work with parathyroid hormone and calcitonin to regulate serum calcium and phosphorus concentrations, principally by enhancing intestinal absorption of these minerals. Vitamin D is sometimes referred to as a hormone since it is activated in the body and regulates calcium and phosphate homeostasis and bone mineralization. Vitamin D deficiency causes increased parathyroid hormone activity, which acts to maintain serum calcium and phosphate concentrations, at the expense of skeletal calcium (15). Provided permanent skeletal deformities have not occurred, supplementing vitamin D in the form of ergocalciferol or cholecalciferol will correct deficiency in people who can activate and utilize them. Since part of the activation process, namely the 1-hydroxylation, occurs in the kidneys, people with chronic renal failure might not be able to activate these forms of vitamin D. Instead, they require calcitriol, dihydrotachysterol, or calcifediol (15). Alfacalcidol, a synthetic derivative of cholecalciferol, is hydroxylated in the liver to calcitriol and does not require renal hydroxylation. It is considered equal in biological activity to calcitriol and has been used to treat renal osteodystrophy (505). Liver disease can prevent 25-hydroxylation of vitamin D. Therefore, people with liver disease might need supplemental 25-hydroxylated vitamin D derivatives, e.g., calcifediol (14). Since vitamin D is important for calcium homeostasis and for bone health, it is used to help prevent osteoporosis. Some researchers suggest that postmenopausal women need serum levels of 25-hydroxy-vitamin D (calcifediol) of at least 40 mmol/L for optimal bone health (6854). Osteopenia in elderly men also seems to correlate with circulating levels of vitamins D and K (7132). There is some preliminary evidence that people with vitamin D deficiency might be at an increased risk of colon, breast, and prostate cancer (15). Some researchers think vitamin D might have antiproliferative effects in these cancers (6855).

Adverse Reactions

Early symptoms of vitamin D toxicity are those of hypercalcemia. They include weakness, fatigue, sleepiness, headache, loss of appetite, dry mouth, metallic taste, nausea, vomiting, abdominal cramps, constipation, diarrhea, dizziness, ringing in the ears, trouble walking, skin eruptions, hypotonia in infants, muscle pain, bone pain, and irritability. Advanced symptoms may include runny nose, itching, decreased libido, and kidney insufficiency due to precipitation of calcium phosphate in the tubules. Symptoms of renal impairment include frequency, nighttime awakening to urinate, thirst, inability to concentrate urine, and proteinuria. Other symptoms include osteoporosis in adults, decreased growth in children, weight loss, anemia, calcific conjunctivitis, photophobia, metastatic calcification, pancreatitis, generalized vascular calcification, and seizures. Rarely, people develop hypertension and psychosis. Lab values of urinary calcium, phosphate, albumin, blood urea nitrogen, serum cholesterol, aspartate aminotransferase, and alanine aminotransferase concentrations might increase (15). Serum alkaline phosphatase concentrations can decrease (15). Serum electrolyte imbalances, along with mild acidosis, might result in cardiac arrhythmias (15). Topical use of calcipotriene can cause hypercalcemia, hypercalciuria, burning, itching, skin irritation, erythema, dry skin, peeling, rash, dermatitis, and hyperpigmentation (14).

Interactions with Herbs & Other Dietary Supplements
CARDIAC GLYCOSIDE-CONTAINING HERBS: Vitamin D should be administered with caution to people taking cardiac glycosides, because hypercalcemia can cause cardiac arrhythmias (15). Cardiac glycoside-containing herbs include black hellebore, Canadian hemp, digitalis, hedge mustard, figwort, lily-of-the-valley, motherwort, oleander, pheasant's eye, pleurisy, squill, and strophanthus (2,18,19,500).
MINERAL OIL: Excessive use can interfere with intestinal absorption of vitamin D (15).

Interactions with Drugs
CORTICOSTEROIDS: Corticosteroids increase the need for supplemental vitamin D (15).
DIGOXIN: Vitamin D should be administered with caution to people taking cardiac glycosides, because hypercalcemia can cause cardiac arrhythmias (15).
THIAZIDE DIURETICS: Concomitant use of thiazides and pharmacologic amounts of vitamin D in people with hypoparathyroidism might result in hypercalcemia (15).
PHENYTOIN (Dilantin), PHENOBARBITAL: Concomitant use might reduce plasma concentrations of the active 25-hydroxylated vitamin D analogs and increase metabolism to inactive metabolites. Vitamin D analogs that require 25-hydroxylation in the body for activity might be ineffective when used with phenobarbital or phenytoin (14,15).
HEPATIC ENZYME INDUCERS: Concomitant use of drugs that induce hepatic enzymes might reduce plasma concentrations of the active 25-hydroxylated vitamin D analogs and increase metabolism to inactive metabolites (15).
MINERAL OIL: It can reduce supplemental vitamin D absorption. Avoid long-term use of mineral oil (4495).

Drug Influences on Nutrient Levels and Depletion
SOME DRUGS CAN AFFECT VITAMIN D LEVELS:
CHOLESTYRAMINE (Questran, LoCholest, Prevalite): Concomitant use can decrease vitamin D absorption in the gastrointestinal tract. However, there is no clinical evidence that supplementation is necessary (4454,4455,4456,4457,4458,4459).
COLESTIPOL (Colestid): Concomitant use can decrease vitamin D absorption in the gastrointestinal tract. In some cases, supplementation may be appropriate (4460,4461).
RIFAMPIN (Rimactane): Rifampin increases vitamin D metabolism and reduces vitamin D serum levels. The need for vitamin D supplementation has not been adequately studied (4514).
CARBAMAZEPINE (Tegretol): Carbamazepine increases vitamin D metabolism and reduces vitamin D serum levels. The necessity for supplementation with vitamin D has not been adequately studied (4430,4431).
PHENYTOIN (Dilantin) and FOSPHENYTOIN (Cerebyx): Use of phenytoin and fosphenytoin can cause vitamin D deficiency when used long-term. Some authors suggest that patients receiving long-term phenytoin therapy should receive 400-800 IU/day of vitamin D and maintain a diet rich in calcium (4475).
PHENOBARBITAL (Luminal): Phenobarbital can cause vitamin D deficiency when used long-term. Some authors recommended that patients receiving long-term phenobarbital therapy take 400-800 IU/day of vitamin D and maintain a diet rich in calcium. Other authors suggest that vitamin D should be supplemented only if deficiencies are noted (4453,4531).
MINERAL OIL: Mineral oil can reduce dietary vitamin D absorption. Avoid long-term use of mineral oil (4495).
ORLISTAT (Xenical): Orlistat can reduce vitamin D levels (1725,1726,1727,1730). Consider a multivitamin with fat-soluble vitamins, taken at least 2 hours before or after orlistat, or at bedtime.
STIMULANT LAXATIVES: Stimulant laxatives can reduce dietary vitamin D absorption. Limit stimulant laxatives to short-term use (4425). Some stimulant laxatives include cascara (CitraMax Plus), senna (Senokot), bisacody (Dulcolax), and others.
CORTICOSTEROIDS: Use of corticosteroids can cause osteoporosis and calcium depletion with long-term administration. This calcium depletion creates a greater need for both supplemental calcium and vitamin D, which is necessary for calcium absorption. It might be prudent to supplement calcium and vitamin D (calcitriol) before, during, and after long-term and/or high-dose corticosteroid therapy (4462,4463,4464,4465,4466,4467).

Interactions with Foods
No interactions are known to occur, and there is no known reason to expect a clinically significant interaction with vitamin D.

Interactions with Lab Tests
SERUM CHOLESTEROL: Vitamin D might cause false increases in serum cholesterol test results measured by the Zlatkis-Zak reaction (15).

Interactions with Diseases or Conditions
HYPERCALCEMIA: Contraindicated (14,15).
SARCOIDOSIS, HYPOPARATHYROIDISM: These conditions might predispose individuals to increased sensitivity to vitamin D (15).

RENAL DISEASE: Use ergocalciferol with extreme caution in individuals with renal failure or renal stones, if at all (15).

ARTERIOSCLEROSIS, HEART DISEASE: Use ergocalciferol with extreme caution in individuals with arteriosclerosis (15).

Dosage and Administration

ORAL: A typical dose of calcifediol, calcitriol, cholecalciferol, and ergocalciferol is present in many multivitamin supplements. Amounts used as dietary supplements must not exceed the recommended dietary allowance (RDA) of 400 units daily (14). Larger amounts require supervision, and must be individualized to maintain serum calcium concentrations of 9-10 mg/dL and avoid hypercalcemia (15). Daily recommended dietary allowances (RDAs) of vitamin D are no longer published because both sunlight exposure and dietary intake of vitamin D in the general population vary (15). The National Academy of Sciences now publishes an Adequate Intake (AI) which is an estimate of the amount of vitamin D that appears to sustain normal functioning (15). The current daily AI of vitamin D used as cholecalciferol or ergocalciferol to prevent rickets in healthy children and osteomalacia in adults is based on age. Birth through 50 years of age, 5 mcg (200 units); Adults (ages 51 to 70), 10 mcg (400 units); Adults (greater than 70 years of age), 15 mcg (600 units) daily (15). The upper intake levels (UL) for vitamin D are 25 mcg for infants 0-12 months and 50 mcg for everyone over one year of age (3094).

Other vitamin D analogs and vitamin D products for other routes of administration are available as FDA-approved prescription drugs.

Comments

The main dietary sources of vitamin D are fish liver oils, butter, eggs, and fortified milk and cereals (15). One unit of vitamin D equals the biologic activity of 25 mg of ergocalciferol or cholecalciferol (15).

Alfacalcidol is used for experimental purposes in the United States (505), and is available commercially in Canada (6365). Cholecalciferol is available only in combination products commercially (15).

VITAMIN E

Also Known As

All Rac-Alpha-Tocopherol, Alpha-Tocopherol, d-Alpha-Tocopherol, d-Alpha-Tocopheryl, d-Alpha-Tocopheryl Acetate, d-Alpha-Tocopheryl Succinate, dl-Alpha-Tocopherol, dl-Alpha-Tocopheryl, dl-Alpha-Tocopheryl Acetate, d-Tocopherol, dl-Tocopherol, d-Beta-Tocopherol, d-Delta-Tocopherol, d-Gamma-Tocopherol, Mixed Tocopherols, RRR-Alpha-Tocopherol, Tocopherol, Tocopheryl Acetate, Tocopheryl Acid Succinate, Tocopheryl Succinate, Tocotrienol, Tocotrienol Concentrate from Vitamin E.

Scientific Names

Alpha-tocopherol; alpha tocotrienol; beta-tocopherol; beta tocotrienol; delta-tocopherol; delta tocotrienol; gamma-tocopherol; gamma tocotrienol.

People Use This For

Orally, vitamin E is used for replacement therapy in vitamin E deficiency, treating and preventing cardiovascular disease, including slowing atherogenesis and preventing heart attacks. It is used orally for angina, thrombophlebitis, intermittent claudication, hypertension, and preventing ischemia-reperfusion injury after coronary artery bypass surgery. Vitamin E is also used orally for treating diabetes and its complications. Vitamin E is used orally for preventing cancer, particularly lung and oral cancer in smokers; colorectal cancer and polyps; and gastric, prostate, and pancreatic cancer. Vitamin E is used orally for Alzheimer's disease and other dementias, Parkinson's disease, night cramps, restless leg syndrome, and as an adjunct in the treatment of epilepsy. Vitamin E is also used orally for preventing pre-eclampsia in high-risk women, for improving physical endurance, increasing energy, preventing allergies, for asthma and infections, for protecting against negative effects of air pollution, preventing aging, preventing cataracts, and improving healing after photoreactive keratectomy. It is also used orally for inflammatory skin disorders, aging skinburns, cystic fibrosis, oral leukoplakia, premenstrual syndrome, habitual abortion, menopausal syndrome, hot flashes associated with breast cancer, infertility, impotence, chronic cystic mastitis, mammary dysplasia, peptic ulcers, porphyria, tardive dyskinesia, neuromuscular disorders, Huntington's chorea, chronic progressive hereditary chorea, and myotonic dystrophy. Additionally, vitamin E is used orally for preventing vitamin E deficiency in people with malabsorption syndromes or abetalipoproteinemia, treating hemolytic anemia caused by vitamin E deficiency in premature neonates, preventing retinopathy of prematurity, preventing bronchopulmonary dysplasia secondary to oxygen therapy in neonates, and preventing intraventricular hemorrhage in premature neonates. Vitamin E is used orally for correcting erythrocyte membrane abnormalities in people with beta-thalassemia, for hereditary spherocytosis, glucose-6-phosphate dehydrogenase deficiency or sickle-cell anemia, treating anemia in conjunction with erythropoietin in people on dialysis, reducing doxorubicin-induced hair loss, reducing amiodarone-induced pulmonary toxicity, and for radiation-induced fibrosis. Vitamin E is also used orally to treat retinitis pigmentosa, osteoarthritis, nonalcoholic steatohepatitis in children, reduce muscle damage after exercise, and improve muscle strength.

Topically, vitamin E is used for dermatitis, aging skin, granuloma annulare, and protecting against skin ulceration caused by extravasation of chemotherapy drugs.

Safety

LIKELY SAFE ...when used orally and appropriately (14). Vitamin E is generally considered non-toxic, even at doses exceeding the recommended dietary allowance (RDA); however, adverse effects are more likely to occur with higher doses (see Adverse Reactions) (15). The recommended tolerable upper limit of vitamin E is 1000 mg per day, equivalent to 1100 IU of synthetic vitamin E and 1500 IU of natural vitamin E (4729).

POSSIBLY UNSAFE ...when used orally in excessive amounts (4729). Repeated administration of doses exceeding the recommended tolerable upper limit has been associated with significant side effects (see Adverse Reactions) (3582,4729). The recommended tolerable upper limit of vitamin E is 1000 mg per day, equivalent to 1100 IU of synthetic vitamin E and 1500 IU of natural vitamin E (4729). Mega-dosing should be avoided. ...when used intravenously in large doses. Large repeated intravenous doses of all-rac-alpha-tocopherol (synthetic vitamin E) were associated with decreased activity of clotting factors and bleeding in one report (See Adverse Reactions) (3074).

PREGNANCY: LIKELY SAFE ...when used orally in amounts that do not exceed the recommended dietary allowance (RDA) (15); however, maternal supplementation is not generally recommended unless dietary vitamin E falls below the RDA (4260). POSSIBLY SAFE ...when used orally and appropriately in amounts exceeding the recommended diatary allowance (RDA). No adverse effects were reported with oral intake of 400 IU per day starting at weeks 18-22 of pregnancy in women at high risk for pre-eclampsia (3236) or with 600-900 IU daily during the last two months of pregnancy (4260). There is insufficient reliable information available about the safety of the topical use of vitamin e during pregnancy.

LACTATION: LIKELY SAFE ...when used orally in amounts that do not exceed the recommended dietary allowance (RDA) (15). There is insufficient reliable information about the safety of vitamin E supplementation in amounts greater than the RDA while nursing.

Effectiveness

EFFECTIVE ...when used orally for preventing and treating vitamin E deficiency (10,15). However, vitamin E deficiency is rare in humans. It most commonly occurs in people with malabsorption disorders such as abetalipoproteinemia; cystic fibrosis; gastrectomy; hepatitic-biliary tract disease including chronic cholestasis, hepatic cirrhosis, biliary atresia, and obstructive jaundice; in infants receiving formula with insufficient vitamin E; intestinal diseases including celiac and tropical sprue; and regional enteritis (10). Vitamin E supplementation may be of most benefit in this population.

POSSIBLY EFFECTIVE ...when used orally from dietary sources for primary prevention of heart disease. There is some evidence from population studies that increasing dietary consumption of vitamin E might significantly reduce the relative risk of developing heart disease and cardiovascular events such as myocardial infarction (3898,3933,3934), but vitamin E supplements do not seem to have this benefit. The majority of controlled clinical trials show that vitamin E supplements offer no benefit for preventing heart disease (3896,3897,3899,3907,3935,3937). Tell patients not to rely on supplements. Recommend increasing dietary intake of vitamin E instead. ...when used orally for treating tardive dyskinesia. Vitamin E can significantly improve Abnormal Involuntary Movement Scale (AIMS) scores in people with tardive dyskinesia. It seems to be more effective in higher doses and in people who have had tardive dyskinesia for less than 5 years (3942,3943,3944,3945,3946,3948). In the largest study to date conflicting findings have been reported; however, this study has not yet been published, preventing further evaluation of its findings (3947). Both RRR-alpha-tocopherol (natural vitamin E) and unspecified forms were used in clinical trials. ...when used orally for reducing the incidence of prostate cancer (3959,4643,4644,4645,4646). In one study, 29,133 smokers taking 50 mg per day of all-rac-alpha-tocopherol (synthetic vitamin E), either alone or in combination with beta-carotene, had a significantly lower incidence of prostate cancer and mortality associated with prostate cancer (3959). Epidemiological studies also support an inverse relationship between vitamin E consumption and the risk of prostate cancer. These epidemiological studies did not distinguish between different forms of vitamin E (4644,4645,4646). ...when used orally for slowing cognitive decline in Alzheimer's disease (4635,4636). There's some evidence that all-rac-alpha-tocopherol (synthetic vitamin E) 2000 IU per day is similar to selegiline (Eldepryl) and superior to placebo for slowing cognitive function decline in patients with moderately severe Alzheimer's disease. However, there is no additive effect when vitamin E was used in combination with selegiline (Eldepryl) (4635). ...when used orally with vitamin C for protecting against development of vascular and mixed dementias. A longitudinal cohort study of 3,385 elderly men aged 71 to 93 years found that men who consumed supplemental vitamin E and vitamin C had a decreased risk of developing vascular and mixed or other dementias; however, there was no protective effect for Alzheimer's dementia. This study did not distinguish between different forms of vitamin E (4636). ...when used to delay neurologic symptoms in early Huntington's chorea (4686). RRR-alpha-tocopherol (natural vitamin E) can significantly improve symptoms in patients with early Huntington's disease, but this benefit is not seen in patients with more advanced disease (4686). ...when used orally as an adjunct to conventional therapy for pain associated with rheumatoid arthritis. Vitamin E in conjunction with standard therapy is superior to standard therapy alone for reducing pain, but not inflammation in patients with rheumatoid arthritis (4723). ...when used orally for improving sperm function and fertilization rates (3583,4693,4695). In one study, males with asthenospermia or oligoasthenospermia receiving vitamin E supplementation achieved impregnation at a rate of 21% compared to none for similar patients receiving placebo (4695). In another study, males enrolled in an in vitro fertilization program who had previously had low fertilization rates were treated with vitamin E for 3 months. Fertilization rates increased significantly from 19% to 29% after 1 month of treatment (3583). In a crossover trial, males found to have elevated reactive oxygen species in their semen, which might be associated with infertility, were treated with vitamin E. After treatment, in vitro sperm binding to the zona pellucida was significantly increased (4693). Interestingly, high-dose vitamin E in combination with vitamin C does not seem to offer any benefit to sperm functionality (4696). Vitamin E plus selenium seems to improve sperm functionality, but doesn't improve fertilization rates (3585). Although vitamin E preparations used alone appear to offer some benefit in men with asthenospermia or oxidative damage to sperm, combining vitamin E with vitamin C or selenium does not appear to be beneficial. Studies did not differentiate between different forms of vitamin E. ...when used orally to normalize retinal blood flow and improve renal function in type 1 diabetes patients. In a crossover trial, patients with type 1 diabetes of less than ten years were given vitamin E 1800 IU daily for 4 months. At the end of the treatment period, retinal blood flow was similar to controls without diabetes and creatinine clearance was significantly decreased (4725). ...when used orally in combination with vitamin C to treat uveitis (4730). Vitamin E plus vitamin C seems to improve visual acuity in patients with acute anterior uveitis, but does not seem to decrease inflammation measured by laser flare (4730). ...when used orally in combination with vitamin A to improve healing after photoreactive keratectomy. High dose (50,000 to 75,000 units) vitamin A in the form of retinol palmitate taken daily with 230 mg vitamin E (alpha-tocopheryl nicotinate) seems to accelerate re-epithelialization, reduce haze formation, and improve visual acuity in patients undergoing laser surgery for myopia (348). ...when used orally in combination with zinc and other antioxidant vitamins to slow progression age-related macular degeneration (ARMD). Taking vitamin E 400 IU, plus elemental zinc 80 mg, vitamin C 500 mg, and beta-carotene 15 mg daily seems to provide a risk reduction of 27% for visual acuity loss and a risk reduction of 28% for progression to more advanced ARMD in patients with intermediate and advanced ARMD (7303). ...when used orally to prevent nitrate tolerance in patients with ischemic heart disease (4705). In a small placebo-controlled study, patients with ischemic heart disease and healthy volunteers receiving vitamin E had a decreased attenuation of response to nitroglycerin compared to placebo (4705). ...when used orally in conjunction with erythropoietin for anemia in patients on dialysis. Two small studies in adults and children on chronic hemodialysis showed improved response to erythropoietin with vitamin E supplementation (4640,4647). In one study, children given vitamin E 15 mg/kg in combination with erythropoietin had significantly increased hemoglobin (Hgb) and hematocrit (Hct) levels after 2 weeks of combination treatment compared to 8 and 5 weeks in patients without combination treatment (4640). In a study of adults, concurrent supplementation with vitamin E 500 mg daily allowed dose reductions of erythropoietin from an average of 93 U/kg/week to 74 U/kg/week with the same results on Hgb levels (4647). ...when used orally to treat focal segmental glomerulosclerosis in children (4675). A small, open-label study showed vitamin E reduced proteinuria in children refractory to standard medical management (4675). ...when used orally for correcting erythrocyte membrane abnormalities in people with beta-thalassemia and low vitamin E plasma concentrations (4642). ...when used to control hemolysis in adults and children with glucose-6-phosphate dehydrogenase (G6PD) deficiency (4682,4683). There is renewed interest in vitamin E for G6PD deficiency (4685). In two open studies, vitamin E 800 IU alone or in combination with selenium reduced hemolysis and reticulocytosis and increased red blood cell (RBC) half-life and vitamin E levels in patients with G6PD deficiency (4682,4683). In one study, vitamin E plus selenium 25 mcg daily offered significantly more improvement compared to vitamin E alone (4683). These findings are contrary to an earlier study that found no effect with vitamin E at 2000 to 2400 IU per day (4684). ...when used orally with vitamin C for preventing pre-eclampsia in high-risk women (3236). Combination vitamin E 400 IU and vitamin C 1000 mg daily significantly reduced the risk of proteinuric hypertension when started in weeks 16 to 22 of pregnancy (3236). Other researchers using vitamin E in combination with vitamin C and allopurinol beginning at 24 to 32 weeks gestation found the combination similar to placebo (4718). ...when used to reduce the symptoms of premenstrual syndrome (PMS) (4719,4720). Vitamin E seems to reduce symptoms of anxiety, craving, and depression in patients with PMS (4719,4720). ...when used orally for retrolental fibroplasia, intracranial hemorrhage, and intraventricular hemorrhage in premature neonates (10,4655,4656). ...when used orally in combination with pentoxifylline (Trental) to treat radiation-induced fibrosis (4672,4673). Vitamin E 1000 IU plus pentoxifylline 800 mg daily seems to reverse radiation-induced fibrosis (4672,4673). Regression of radiation-induced fibrosis becomes significant after 3 months of treatment and continues to improve thereafter. After 12 months of treatment, mean surface area of fibrosis can decrease by 66% (4672). ...when used orally in combination with vitamin C to prevent ultraviolet-induced erythema (sunburn) (4715,4716). High dose oral RRR-alpha-tocopherol (natural vitamin E) in combination with vitamin C protected against skin inflammation after exposure to ultraviolet (UV) radiation in two small, double-blind, placebo-controlled studies (4715,1416). Alpha-tocopherol acetate 400 IU alone does not seem to offer this benefit (1417). ...when used topically in combination with vitamin C and melatonin to prevent ultraviolet-induced erythema (sunburn). In one study, topically applied vitamin E in combination with topical vitamin C and melatonin provided modest photoprotective effect when used prior to UV exposure, but had no effect when used during or after UV exposure (4713,4714).

...when used topically in combination with dimethyl sulfoxide (DMSO) for treating chemotherapy extravasation (4668). ...when used topically to treat granuloma annulare (4681). Topical vitamin E seems to clear granuloma annulare lesions within 1-3 weeks (4681). ...when used in combination with vitamin C and allopurinol to reduce ischemia reperfusion injury during coronary artery bypass surgery. When vitamin E, vitamin C, and allopurinol were given 2 days prior to surgery and 1 day postoperatively, patients had fewer perioperative infarctions and less creatine kinase-MB release (4699); however, this benefit was not found when using vitamin E alone or in combination with vitamin C without allopurinol (4697,4698). ...when used orally in combination with beta-carotene and selenium for prevention of gastroesophageal cancer. In a large-scale study of 29,584 people in China, the combination of vitamin E, beta-carotene, and selenium over 5.25 years significantly reduced total mortality, total cancer mortality, and stomach cancer mortality. However, this population has a high risk of gastric cancer, which is thought to be related to poor vitamin and mineral intake (4679). It is unknown if supplementation with these vitamins and minerals would be beneficial in people with adequate nutrition. Although there has been some conflicting evidence (4677), vitamin E alone does not seem to offer this benefit (3960,4676). ...when used orally from dietary sources to slow progression of gastric cancer. There is preliminary evidence that increasing dietary consumption of vitamin E can slow progression of gastric carcinoma (3360). ...when used orally in combination with vitamin A and vitamin C or multivitamin to prevent colorectal adenoma. Vitamin E, in combination with vitamins A and C, has shown a protective effect in patients with previous colorectal adenomas (3954,3956). A retrospective study has also associated vitamin E and multivitamin use with a lower incidence of colorectal cancer (3958); however, vitamin E alone has not been shown to be beneficial (3953,3955,3957). ...when used orally to enhance immune function in elderly people (4687,4689,4690,4691). Vitamin E supplementation 100-200 mg daily improved immune system function in elderly people (4687,4689,4690,4691), but lower doses do not seem to provide this benefit (4692). ...when used orally to prevent progression of osteoarthritis. Vitamin E does not seem to prevent developing osteoarthritis, but might slow progression (5881).

POSSIBLY INEFFECTIVE ...when used orally for preventing heart disease and cardiovascular events such as myocardial infarction (MI). Using antioxidants like vitamin E for preventing heart disease is controversial. Several large population studies show that increasing dietary intake of vitamin E might help reduce the risk of developing heart disease (3898,3933,3934), but with few exceptions (3357,3936), large-scale controlled clinical trials show that vitamin E supplements offer no benefit for primary prevention in high risk patients (3907,3935,3937) or secondary prevention of heart disease and cardiovascular events such as MI, stroke, and death (3896,3897,3899). Based on these findings, the FDA has refused to allow labeling claims for vitamin E supplements for prevention of cardiovascular disease (3939). Tell patients not to rely on vitamin E supplements for preventing heart disease. Recommend increasing dietary vitamin E consumption instead. ...when used to treat atherosclerosis. RRR-alpha-tocopherol (natural vitamin E) doesn't appear to have any effect on atherosclerosis progression or mortality in patients with atherosclerosis (3899,3936). However, there is preliminary evidence that a combination of vitamin E and vitamin C, might help prevent the progression of atherosclerosis in men, particularly smokers (1918). ...when used to reduce angina. Although vitamin E may have some effect on endothelial dysfunction, it has not benefited nonsmokers or smokers with angina (3896,4634,4649,4650,4651,4652). ...when used to treat intermittent claudication in male smokers (4732). All rac-alpha-tocopherol (synthetic vitamin E) doesn't appear to have any effect when used alone or in combination with beta-carotene on symptoms or disease progression (4732). ...when used to treat congestive heart failure (CHF). Vitamin E taken for 12 weeks doesn't seem to improve prognostic or functional indices of CHF or improve quality-of-life measurements (3906). ...when used to treat hypertension. Vitamin E taken for 3 to 4 years doesn't seem to provide any additive benefit on clinic or ambulatory blood pressure in patients already on hypertension treatment (5210). ...when used to treat osteoarthritis. Vitamin E 500 IU per day doesn't appear to improve pain, stiffness, or function in symptomatic knee osteoarthritis (5264). ...when used orally in combination with vitamin C to prevent development of Alzheimer's disease in elderly men. A longitudinal cohort study of 3,385 elderly men aged 71 to 93 years found that men who consumed supplemental vitamin E and vitamin C developed Alzheimer's dementia at the same rate as those men who did not (4636). ...when used orally for reducing the risk of lung cancer in male smokers (3949). In a large Finnish study, 29,133 male smokers taking all rac-alpha-tocopherol (synthetic vitamin E) 50 mg per day for five to eight years were as likely to be diagnosed with lung cancer as those receiving placebo (3949). ...when used to prevent oral mucosal lesions in smokers. Although there is some conflicting evidence (3951,4708), the largest and most significant controlled trial indicates that supplementation with all rac-alpha-tocopherol (synthetic vitamin E) 50 mg daily for five to seven years has no effect on the incidence of oral lesions in male cigarette smokers (3951). ...when used to prevent carcinoma of the pancreas or reduce mortality associated with pancreatic cancer in male smokers (3961). All rac-alpha-tocopherol (synthetic vitamin E) 50 mg daily supplements taken for five to eight years by male smokers did not affect the incidence or mortality of carcinoma of the pancreas (3961). ...when used to prevent age-related maculopathy in men who smoke (4667). ...when used to reduce oxidative stress in smokers. In one small study, a 400 IU daily vitamin E supplementation was effective in reducing copper-catalyzed LDL oxidizability; however, the more relevant PMN function was unaffected (3355). ...when used to treat retinitis pigmentosa (83). All rac-alpha-tocopherol (synthetic vitamin E) does not appear to slow visual decline is people with retinitis pigmentosa and has been associated with more rapid loss of visual acuity, although the validity of the study with these findings has been questioned (83,84,85,86,87,88). ...when used in combination with penicillamine for slowing progression of Duchenne muscular dystrophy (4703). A double-blind study in 106 boys for 18 months found no difference between placebo and combination vitamin E and

penicillamine for slowing disease progression (4703). ...when used orally in combination with selenium for myotonic dystrophy. A small study comparing placebo to combination vitamin E and selenium showed no difference in functional deterioration over two years (4704). ...when used orally for Parkinson's disease (4709,4710,4711). A large double-blind, placebo-controlled study using all rac-alpha-tocopherol (synthetic vitamin E) 2000 IU daily showed no delay in disease progression, benefit to cognitive performance, or amelioration of levodopa side effects (4709,4710,4711). However, preliminary evidence suggests that dietary vitamin E might be useful for preventing Parkinson's disease. In one epidemiological study, high dietary vitamin E intake was associated with a decreased occurrence of Parkinson's disease (4712). ...when used for hemolytic anemia associated with vitamin E deficiency in premature infants. Vitamin E 25 IU per day given to premature infants for six weeks had no beneficial effects on hemolytic anemia (4648). ...when used for bronchopulmonary dysplasia in premature infants. In one study, vitamin E had no benefit in premature infants weighing less than 1500 grams at birth (4657). ...when used to reduce hot flashes in breast cancer survivors (454). Supplemental vitamin E appears to have little effect on reducing hot flashes in women who have had breast cancer (454). There have been no clinical trials using vitamin E supplementation for postmenopausal symptoms. ...when used topically to reduce surgical wound scarring (4721,4722). ...when used orally to increase muscle strength (6693).
LIKELY INEFFECTIVE ...when used to prevent breast cancer (4658,4659). Neither dietary nor supplemental vitamin E intake has shown any protective effect for breast cancer (4658,4659). ...when used for benign breast disease (4660,4661). Three well-designed studies of supplemental vitamin E 600 mg per day found no effect on mammary dysplasia (4660,4661,4662).

There is insufficient reliable information available to rate the effectiveness of vitamin E for other its other uses. However, limited evidence suggests vitamin E might offer some benefit for nocturnal leg cramps (4700,4701), but there is conflicting evidence (4702). There is also preliminary evidence that vitamin E might reduce seizure frequency in refractory epilepsy; however, trials have been few and contradictory (4670,4671,6066). Preliminary small-scale clinical studies have also indicated that vitamin E might be beneficial in diabetes and diabetic neuropathy. Some evidence suggests it improves glucose disposal in type 2 diabetics (4726,4727), improves monocyte function, which lessens atherogenesis (95), and improves nerve conduction in diabetic neuropathy (4724). In type 1 diabetes, clinical research indicates that vitamin E might have a role in the management of early vascular disease by improving endothelial vasodilator function (94). One study has shown that 750 IU (503 mg) RRR-alpha-tocopherol daily for 1 year decreased lipoprotein susceptibility to copper oxidization in type 1 diabetics (3358). There's some evidence that rac-alpha-tocopherol (synthetic vitamin E) might reduce the risk of ischemic stroke in male smokers with hypertension and diabetes (3359). There is conflicting information about the use of vitamin E to prevent cataracts. Vitamin E alone or in combination with other vitamins does not seem to prevent the development and progression of age-related cataracts and vision loss (4666,7304). Vitamin E plus vitamin C and beta-carotene doesn't seem to have any significant effect on age-related loss of vision due to cataracts in well-nourished people when taken for an average of 6.3 years (7304), but most population research suggests a beneficial effect of vitamin E (2395,4208,4663,4664,4665,4759). Vitamin E use in multivitamins or any supplement containing vitamin E for 10 years appears to reduce the incidence of nuclear and cortical cataracts by 60%, according to epidemiological research. Use of supplements for shorter periods doesn't appear to reduce the risk for cataract development (4208). Preliminary clinical evidence also indicates that vitamin E may be helpful in nonalcoholic steatohepatitis in children; however, long-term studies have not been performed (89). There's also some early evidence that vitamin E might decrease muscle damage associated with weight lifting (6693). Vitamin E in combination with aged garlic extract and vitamin C might be useful for sickle cell disease (5056). There's also some evidence that the combination of vitamins E and C might help prevent cardiac transplant-associated arteriosclerosis (5197). More evidence is needed to rate the effectiveness of vitamin E for these uses.

Mechanism of Action

Vitamin E is a fat-soluble vitamin present in many foods including vegetable oils, cereal grains, animal fats, meat, poultry, eggs, fruits, and vegetables (96). Wheat germ oil is a particularly rich source. Maximum vitamin E intake from diet alone typically reaches about 60 IU per day (97). Vitamin E deficiency is rare and most typically seen in genetic abnormalities that prevent maintenance of normal blood concentrations of vitamin E or conditions that prevent absorption. Vitamin E deficiency does not cause specific disease in adults, although creatinuria, ceroid deposition, muscle weakness, and decreased erythrocyte survival are associated with low serum vitamin E concentrations. In adults, total body stores of vitamin E, found in adipose tissue, have been estimated to be 3-8 grams and are sufficient to meet the body's requirements for 4 or more years of a deficient diet. In premature infants, vitamin E deficiency can cause irritability, edema, thrombosis, and hemolytic anemia (15). Unlike most nutrients, vitamin E does not appear to have a specific role in a required metabolic process. The major function of vitamin E is probably that of a chain-breaking antioxidant that prevents the formation of free radicals. Vitamin E's therapeutic benefits have primarily been attributed to its antioxidant effects. Vitamin E exists in eight forms, including alpha-, beta-, gamma-, and delta-tocopherols and four tocotrienols. Although vitamin E exists in numerous forms, supplemental vitamin E usually refers to alpha-tocopherol. For biological activity, vitamin E is dependent on hepatic alpha-tocopherol transfer protein (alpha-TTP) for distribution. Although the typical diet contains other forms of vitamin E (beta-, gamma-, and delta- tocopherols), these have very limited systemic bioavailability because they do not bind with alpha-TTP. Supplemental beta-, gamma-, and delta-tocopherols, and tocotrienols appear to have little in vivo activity in humans and do not contribute toward meeting established vitamin E requirements (4844). Only the alpha-tocopherol form of vitamin E is maintained in plasma and thought to be therapeutically useful. Alpha-tocopherol exists as eight stereoisomers. The RRR-alpha-tocopherol isomer, formerly called d-alpha-tocopherol, has the greatest affinity for alpha-TTP and the most biologic activity (4844). RRR-alpha-tocopherol is sometimes called natural vitamin E and occurs naturally in foods (3940,4844). The racemic mixture of all eight alpha-tocopherol isomers, or all rac-alpha-tocopherol, was formerly known as dl-alpha-tocopherol (4844). All rac-alpha-tocopherol, sometimes called synthetic vitamin E, is found in vitamin E-fortified foods. Both forms of vitamin E, natural and synthetic, can be found in vitamin E supplements. All rac-alpha-tocopherol has lower affinity for alpha-TTP and thus has less biologic activity than RRR-alpha-tocopherol (4627,4844). Based on weight, 15 mg of RRR-alpha tocopherol is approximately equivalent in potency to 30 mg of all rac-alpha-tocopherol (99,200,218,4844). Although higher bioavailability for the natural form is well-known, the relative potency of natural and synthetic vitamin E is controversial. Some researchers cite the potency of the natural to synthetic form as 1.36, rather than 2.0 (100,202,247,248). Therapeutic benefits of vitamin E have largely been attributed to its role as an antioxidant. Oxidative damage has been attributed to many conditions for which vitamin E is used, including lipid peroxidation in heart disease (6204). Some preliminary research suggests that vitamin E might inhibit the local inflammatory process and oxidation of low-density lipoprotein (LDL) cholesterol that is associated with atherosclerosis (97,249). But when this theory was tested in healthy adults without heart disease, RRR-alpha-tocopherol, even at 2000 IU per day, did not produce markers that indicate a reduction in lipid oxidation (3370). This appears to be another case where promising laboratory data turns out to be clinically irrelevant. In tardive dyskinesia, it is thought that some patients may have increased dopamine turnover resulting in increased production of free radicals and structural damage. Additionally, people with tardive dyskinesia may have decreased levels of vitamin E and vitamin C (3598). Oxidative damage has also been associated with diabetes and related complications. Oxidative damage has also long been associated with the development of cancers. Vitamin E and other antioxidants are theorized to minimize this damage. Preliminary evidence also suggests vitamin E and other antioxidants can decrease oxidative damage associated with tumor-directed radio-immunotherapy (5882). Vitamin E is used for photo-aged skin and to prevent oxidative skin damage related to ultraviolet (UV) radiation (e.g., sunburn) due to it's antioxidant effects. However, some researchers think that this benefit requires concomitant use with other antioxidants such as vitamin C to prevent degradation of vitamin E (6062,6064). Chemotherapy and radiation therapy also adversely affect vitamin E status (98). Vitamin E status may also decline with standard parenteral nutrition formulas. Lipid emulsions and amino acid solutions appear to be susceptible to oxidative degradation with storage (98). In dementia, preliminary data suggest vitamin E might improve cognitive function by decreasing beta-amyloid damage (4637,4638,4639). Some evidence links asthma to increased oxidative stress and vitamin E deficiency (315,401,409,422,6058). Epidemiological and case-control studies have associated asthma with lower vitamin E intake, lower vitamin E serum levels, and lower vitamin levels in lung lining fluid, but clinical studies using vitamin E supplementation for asthma have not been performed (315,401,409,422,6058). Lower vitamin E serum levels have also been associated with higher IgE levels and positive allergen skin tests (5275). In addition to its antioxidant function, vitamin E inhibits protein kinase C activity, which is involved in cell proliferation and differentiation in several cell types, including smooth muscle, platelets, and monocytes (4844). Large amounts of vitamin E interfere with vitamin K-dependent clotting factor production, producing hypoprothrombinemic effects, especially in people with vitamin K deficiency or those who are taking oral anticoagulants (3046,3072,3073,3074). For immune function in the elderly, vitamin E supplementation might replenish an unapparent deficiency. Deficiency of vitamin E and other micronutrients are common in apparently well-nourished people over age 90 and might affect the number and function of natural killer cells in old age (4688). In the treatment of epilepsy, vitamin E is primarily used because some patients taking anti-epileptic drugs have decreased blood levels of vitamin E. Vitamin E might also act as a membrane stabilizer and enzyme repressor in these patients (3356,6066). Although biological activity of other forms is significantly less and current guidelines do not include forms of vitamin E other than alpha-tocopherol for meeting dietary requirements (4844), the other forms, such as gamma-tocopherol and the tocotrienols, have been associated with some pharmacological activity. For example, gamma-tocopherol appears to decrease the programmed death of human coronary artery endothelial cells, possibly by decreasing LDL oxidation (4092). Gamma-tocopherol inhibits prostate cancer cell growth in vitro (4089). Gamma-tocopherol also appears to prolong prothrombin and partial thromboplastin times and has caused hemorrhage in experimental animals (4098). Beta- and delta-tocopherol have also been shown to prolong prothrombin and partial thromboplastin times in laboratory animals (4098). RRR-alpha-tocopheryl succinate, known as vitamin E succinate (VES), is currently being researched for its chemotherapeutic and chemopreventive potential. VES has been shown to inhibit tumor cell growth, primarily by triggering apoptosis in human prostate carcinoma (3361). The tocotrienols from rice and barley bran might lower total cholesterol and LDL, possibly by decreasing activity of HMG CoA reductase, but in a different way than "statin" drugs (3237,3238,3239,3240,3241). Tocotrienols might also be capable of decreasing carotid artery plaque size in some people, possibly by decreasing platelet aggregation (3239). Some people think that taking vitamin E with a high fat meal is necessary to increase absorption. However, vitamin E (d-alpha-tocopherol) is similarly absorbed when taken with high-fat (36 grams) or low-fat (3 grams fat) meals (6133).

Adverse Reactions

Orally, vitamin E seldom causes adverse effects. In uncommon cases, vitamin E can cause nausea, diarrhea, intestinal cramps, fatigue, weakness, headache, blurred vision, rash, gonadal dysfunction, and creatinuria. Vitamin E has been associated with the development of thrombophlebitis and pulmonary embolism, but this is controversial (14). It is unclear if vitamin E contributes to increased risk of hemorrhagic stroke. One study suggested a higher incidence of hemorrhagic stroke in male smokers taking all rac-alpha-tocopherol (synthetic vitamin E), but several other studies lasting from 1.4 years to 4.5 years with study participants taking either all rac-alpha-tocopherol (synthetic vitamin E) or RRR-alpha-tocopherol (natural vitamin E) showed no increased risk for stroke (3896,3897,3936,3949,4635). High doses of vitamin E might increase the risk of bleeding due to antagonism of vitamin K-dependent clotting factors and platelet aggregation. Patients with vitamin K deficiencies or taking anticoagulant or antiplatelet drugs are at a greater risk for bleeding (4844). Although only certain isomers of vitamin E are included for determination of dietary requirements, all isomers are considered for determining safe intake levels. All the isomers are thought to potentially contribute to toxicity. Topically, vitamin E has been associated with contact dermatitis, inflammatory reactions, and eczematous lesions (14,15).

Interactions with Herbs & Other Dietary Supplements

IRON: Concomitant use of vitamin E in amounts greater than 10 units/kg per day can delay the response to iron therapy in children with iron-deficiency anemia (15).

MINERAL OIL: Concomitant use can decrease the absorption of vitamin E and other fat-soluble vitamins (14,15).

OMEGA-6 FATTY ACIDS: Increased intake of omega-6 fatty acids may increase vitamin E requirements, particularly at higher doses (4844).

VITAMIN A: Concomitant use can increase the absorption, utilization and storage of vitamin A. Vitamin E might also protect against hypervitaminosis A (15).

VITAMIN C: Concomitant use helps reduce the risk of pre-eclampsia in high-risk women (3236). Laboratory evidence suggests that vitamin C might help recycle oxidized alpha-tocopherol (4844).

HERBS WITH ANTICOAGULANT/ANTIPLATELET POTENTIAL: Concomitant use of herbs that have coumarin constituents or affect platelet aggregation could theoretically increase the risk of bleeding in some people. These herbs include: angelica, anise, arnica, asafoetida, bogbean, boldo, capsicum, celery, chamomile, clove, danshen, fenugreek, feverfew, garlic, ginger, ginkgo, Panax ginseng, horse chestnut, horseradish, licorice, meadowsweet, prickly ash, onion, papain, passionflower, poplar, quassia, red clover, turmeric, wild carrot, wild lettuce, willow, and others (4,19).

Interactions with Drugs

ANTICOAGULANT/ANTIPLATELET AGENTS: Concomitant use of vitamin E and anticoagulant or antiplatelet agents might increase the risk of bleeding, possibly through inhibition of platelet aggregation and antagonism of vitamin K-dependent clotting factors (4733,4844). These agents include aspirin, clopidogrel (Plavix), dalteparin (Fragmin), enoxaparin (Lovenox), heparin, ticlopidine (Ticlid), warfarin (Coumadin) and others.

CHEMOTHERAPY: Preliminary evidence suggests antioxidants such as vitamin E and vitamin A might reduce the effectiveness of cancer chemotherapy (391). Patients undergoing chemotherapy should not use vitamin E and other antioxidants without the supervision of a health care provider.

NITRATES: Vitamin E might prevent tolerance to nitrates (4705).

WARFARIN (Coumadin): Use of more than 400 IU of vitamin E per day with warfarin might prolong prothrombin time (PT), INR, and increase the risk of bleeding, due to interference with production of vitamin K-dependent clotting factors (91,92,93,3046,3072). However, there's some evidence that doses up to 1200 IU can be used safely in patients taking warfarin (90). The risk for vitamin E interaction with warfarin is greater in people who are already deficient in vitamin K (91,92,93). Limited clinical evidence suggests that doses up to 1200 IU daily may be used safely by patients taking warfarin, but this may not be applicable in all patient populations (90). Monitor INR closely in patients taking warfarin who start vitamin E in doses of 400 IU or more.

Drug Influences on Nutrient Levels and Depletion

SOME DRUGS CAN AFFECT VITAMIN E LEVELS.

CHOLESTYRAMINE (Questran): Cholestyramine can reduce dietary vitamin E absorption and serum levels (4455,4456).

COLESTIPOL (Colestid): Colestipol can reduce dietary vitamin E absorption and serum levels (4460,4461).

GEMFIBROZIL (Lopid): Gemfibrozil can decrease serum levels of both alpha- and gamma- tocopherol, but the clinical significance of this is not known (4096).

MINERAL OIL: Mineral oil can reduce dietary vitamin E absorption and serum levels. Avoid long-term use of mineral oil (4495,4496).

ETHANOL: Theoretically, ethanol might decrease serum levels of alpha- and gamma-tocopherol, contributing to liver injury (4097).

ORLISTAT (Xenical): Orlistat can reduce the absorption of beta-carotene and some fat-soluble vitamins (1725,1726,1727,1730). Consider a multivitamin with fat-soluble vitamins, taken at least 2 hours before or after orlistat, or at bedtime.

Interactions with Foods
FOODS HIGH IN FAT: High-fat meals might increase vitamin E absorption; however, the amount of fat required to facilitate vitamin E absorption has not been established (4844).

Interactions with Lab Tests
CHOLESTEROL: In rare cases, vitamin E can increase serum cholesterol and triglycerides levels (15).
CREATINE PHOSPHOKINASE (CPK): In rare cases, vitamin E can increase serum creatine phosphokinase (15).
PROTHROMBIN TIME (PT)/INTERNATIONAL NORMALIZED RATIO (INR): High dose vitamin E might increase PT and INR in patients concurrently taking warfarin or other anticoagulant agents (4844). People with vitamin K deficiency are at greater risk for vitamin E interference with clotting and increased PT and INR (91,92,93).
URINE HORMONES: In rare cases, vitamin E can increase urinary estrogens and androgens (15).
THYROXINE AND TRIIODOTHYRONINE: In rare cases, vitamin E can decrease serum thyroxine and triiodothyronine (15).

Interactions with Diseases or Conditions
ANGIOPLASTY: There is some concern that when antioxidant vitamins, including vitamin E, are used together they might have harmful effects in patients after angioplasty. A combination of beta-carotene 30,000 IU, vitamin C 500 mg, and vitamin E 700 IU daily started 30 days before angioplasty, and continued for 6 months thereafter, seems to prevent beneficial vascular remodeling in patients after angioplasty by promoting fibrosis at the site of angioplastic intervention (1317). Tell patients to avoid taking supplements of these vitamins immediately before and following angioplasty without the supervision of a health care professional.
PRE-ECLAMPSIA: Vitamin E with vitamin C helps prevent pre-eclampsia in high-risk women (3236).
RETINITIS PIGMENTOSA: All rac-alpha-tocopherol (synthetic vitamin E) 400 IU has been associated with accelerated visual decline in people with retinitis pigmentosa. However, much lower doses (3 IU) does not seem to produce this effect (83).
VITAMIN K DEFICIENCY: Vitamin E might worsen coagulation defects in people with vitamin K deficiency (15); use cautiously.

Dosage and Administration
ORAL: A typical dose for vitamin E deficiency in adults is RRR-alpha tocopherol (natural vitamin E) 60-75 IU per day (15). For tardive dyskinesia, most studies used RRR-alpha-tocopherol (natural vitamin E) 1600 IU daily (3942,3943,3944). For preventing prostate cancer, vitamin E (type unspecified) 59 to 100 IU daily has been used (3959,4646). For improving male fertility, vitamin E (type unspecified) 200 to 600 IU daily has been used (3584,4693). A typical dose for Alzheimer's disease is up to 2000 IU daily (15). For early Huntington's chorea one study used RRR-alpha-tocopherol (natural vitamin E) 3000 IU (4686). Rheumatoid arthritis pain has been treated with vitamin E (type unspecified) 600 IU twice daily (4723). For diabetic neuropathy, vitamin E (type unspecified) 900 mg daily has been used (4724). For improving retinal blood flow and creatinine clearance in type 1 diabetes, vitamin E (type unspecified) 1800 IU has been used (4725). For enhancing immune function in elderly people, vitamin E (type unspecified) 100 to 200 mg daily has been used (4687,4689,4690). For preventing nitrate tolerance, vitamin E (type unspecified) 200 mg three times daily has been used (4705). For improving response to erythropoietin in people on dialysis, adults have received vitamin E (type unspecified) 300 to 500 mg daily, and children have received 15 mg per kg per day (4640,4641,4647). For children with focal segmental glomerulosclerosis, vitamin E (type unspecified) 200 IU has been used to reduce proteinuria (4675). For G6PD deficiency, vitamin E (type unspecified) 800 IU daily has been used (4682,4683). Premenstrual syndrome (PMS) has been treated with RRR-alpha-tocopherol (natural vitamin E) 400 IU daily (4719). For accelerating re-epithelialization following photoreactive keratectomy, 230 mg vitamin E (alpha-tocopheryl nicotinate) and vitamin A (retinol palmitate) 25,000 units have been used 3 times daily for 30 days, followed by twice daily for 2 months (348). In premature neonates, oral vitamin E (type unspecified) 15 to 30 IU per kg per day has been used to prevent retinopathy and bronchopulmonary dysplasia (15). For nocturnal leg cramps, vitamin E (type unspecified) 400 IU at bedtime has been used (4701). Radiation-induced fibrosis has been treated with vitamin E (type unspecified) 1000 IU daily in combination with pentoxifylline 800 mg (4672,4673). For beta-thalassemia, vitamin E 750 IU daily has been used (15). For preventing sunburn, RRR-alpha-tocopherol 1000 IU in combination with 2 grams of ascorbic acid has been used (4716). For reducing the risk of cancer, heart disease, and cataracts, people have used multiple forms of vitamin E 200-800 IU per day (839). For sickle cell anemia, 450 IU daily has been used (15). For preventing pre-eclampsia in high risk women, vitamin E 400 IU with vitamin C 1000 mg daily has been used (3236). The oral dose of palm oil tocotrienols (Palmvitee) used to reduce lipids is 200-260 mg per day (3238,3239,3240). For restless leg syndrome, 400 IU twice daily has been used (6670).
TOPICAL: For treating chemotherapy extravasation, 10% vitamin E (type unspecified) has been used topically in

combination with 90% dimethyl sulfoxide (DMSO) (4713).

The recommended daily intake of vitamin E for adults was recently increased. Both women and men should consume 15 mg of vitamin E from food (4844). This is equivalent to 22 IU of the RRR-alpha-tocopherol (natural vitamin E) or 33 IU of the all rac-alpha-tocopherol (synthetic vitamin E) (4729). For Infants 7-12 months, 6 mg; Children 1-3 years, 7 mg; Children 4 -8 years, 11 mg; Older children and adults, 15 mg; Pregnant women, 15 mg; Lactating women, 19 mg (4844). The recommended upper dosage limit for all forms of supplemental alpha-tocopherol is 1000 mg (4729). Dosing for vitamin E can be confusing. Some sources and clinical studies choose to express vitamin E dosing based on mg or International Units (IU). Current guidelines have expressed recommended dietary allowance (RDA) and upper tolerable limits for vitamin E in milligrams. However most products are still labeled in IUs. It becomes important to understand how to convert between IUs and milligrams of vitamin E. The appropriate method for doing this depends of the formulation of vitamin E being considered and whether or not you are determining RDA or tolerable upper limit. For conversions related to RDA and to convert IUs of RRR-alpha-tocopherol (natural vitamin E) to milligrams of alpha-tocopherol, multiply by a factor of 0.67. For example, 30 IU of RRR-alpha-tocopherol is 20 mg RRR-alpha-tocopherol (natural vitamin E). To convert IUs of all-rac-tocopherol (synthetic vitamin E) to milligrams of alpha-tocopherol, multiply by a factor of 0.45. For example, 30 IU all rac-tocopherol equals 13.5 mg of all rac-alpha-tocopherol (synthetic vitamin E). The tolerable upper limit conversion factor for racemic and RRR-alpha tocopherol assumes that all isomers of vitamin E might contribute to toxicity so the conversion factor for all rac-alpha tocopherol (synthetic vitamin E) is different. For conversions related to upper limit and to convert IUs all rac-alpha tocopherol (synthetic vitamin E), multiply by a factor of 0.91. For example, 2000 IUs all rac-alpha tocopherol (synthetic vitamin E) is equivalent to 1820 mg. The conversion factor of 0.67 is the same for calculating upper limit for RRR-alpha tocopherol (natural vitamin E). The same factors are used for either acetate or succinate salts because the content has been adjusted for the molecular weights of the salts (4844). Natural vitamin E (d-alpha-tocopherol) is similarly absorbed when taken with high-fat (36 grams) or low-fat (3 grams fat) meals (6133). Synthetic vitamin E (all rac-alpha-tocopherol) should be taken with food for best absorption (6405).

Comments

The American Heart Association recommends obtaining antioxidants, including vitamin E, by eating a well-balanced diet high in fruits, vegetables, and whole grains rather than from supplements until more is known about the risks and benefits of supplementation (1440).

VITAMIN K

Also Known As

Vitamin K1: Methylphytyl Naphthoquinone, Phylloquinone, Phytomenadione, Phytonadione, 2-Methyl-3-Phytyl-1, 4-Naphthoquinone.
Vitamin K2: Menaquinone, Menatetrenone, MK-1, MK-2, MK-4, MK-5, MK-6, MK-7, MK-8, MK-9, MK-10, MK-11, MK-12, MK-13.
Vitamin K3: Menadione, Menadione Sodium Bisulfite, 2-Methyl-1,4-Naphthoquinone.
Vitamin K4: Menadiol Diacetate, Menadiol Sodium Diphosphate, Menadiol Sodium Phosphate, Menadiolum Solubile Methylnaphthohydroquinone.
Vitamin K5: 4-Amino-2-Methyl-1-Naphthol.

Scientific Names

Phytonadione (K1); menaquinone (K2); menadione (K3); menadiol acetate (K4); 4-amino-2-methyl-1-naphthol (K5).

People Use This For

Orally, vitamin K1 (phytonadione) is used for preventing and treating hypoprothrombinemia caused by vitamin K deficiency; to counteract excessive doses of oral anticoagulants; to prevent hemorrhagic disease of the newborn; to treat hypoprothrombinemia induced by salicylates, sulfonamides, quinine, quinidine, or broad-spectrum antibiotic therapy; to prevent and treat osteoporosis; and relieve itching associated with primary biliary cirrhosis. Vitamin K2 (menaquinone) is used orally to treat osteoporosis and steroid-induced bone loss, and to lower total cholesterol in dialysis patients. Vitamin K3 (menadiol acetate) is used orally in combination with vitamin C for treating prostate and breast cancers. Vitamin K4 (menadiol sodium diphosphate) is used orally for treating hypoprothrombinemia resulting from impaired absorption or synthesis of vitamin K.
Topically, vitamin K1 (phytonadione) is used for eliminating spider veins, bruises, scars, stretch marks and burns, treating rosacea, speeding healing, and reducing postoperative bruising and swelling.
Parenterally, vitamin K1 (phytonadione) is used to prevent and treat hypoprothrombinemia caused by vitamin K deficiency, especially that associated with malabsorption syndromes or prolonged parenteral nutrition; to counteract excessive doses of oral anticoagulants; to prevent and treat hemorrhagic disease of the newborn; and to treat

hypoprothrombinemia induced by salicylates, sulfonamides, quinine, quinidine, or broad-spectrum antibiotic therapy. Vitamin K4 (menadiol sodium diphosphate) is injected for treating hypoprothrombinemia resulting from impaired absorption or synthesis of vitamin K.

Safety

LIKELY SAFE …when vitamin K1 is used orally or parenterally, and appropriately. Vitamin K1 (phytonadione) in oral and injectable form is a FDA-approved drug (14,15).
CHILDREN: LIKELY SAFE …when vitamin K1 is used orally or parenterally and appropriately.
Vitamin K1 (phytonadione) in oral and injectable form is FDA approved for use in children (15). LIKELY UNSAFE …when vitamin K4 is used orally or parenterally in neonates. Vitamin K4 (menadiol sodium diphosphate) has been associated with a higher incidence of hyperbilirubinemia and kernicterus than with vitamin K1 (phytonadione) (14). Menadiol sodium diphosphate is no longer available in the US.
PREGNANCY: LIKELY SAFE ...when used orally in amounts that do not exceed the recommended dietary allowance (RDA) (15). POSSIBLY UNSAFE ...when used orally in amounts exceeding the recommended dietary allowance (RDA). Large doses of vitamin K, particularly as vitamin K4 (menadiol sodium diphophate), when administered to mothers near term are associated with hyperbilirubinemia and kernicterus in newborn infants (14).
LACTATION: LIKELY SAFE ...when used orally in amounts not exceeding the recommended dietary allowance (RDA) (15). There's insufficient reliable information available about the safety of using higher amounts in breast-feeding women.

Effectiveness

EFFECTIVE …when vitamin K1 (phytonadione) is used orally or parenterally for preventing and treating hypoprothrombinemia caused by vitamin K deficiency (15). …when vitamin K1 (phytonadione) is used orally or parenterally to counteract excessive oral anticoagulation (15). …when vitamin K1 (phytonadione) is used orally for preventing hemorrhagic disease of newborns. …when vitamin K1 (phytonadione) is used orally or parenterally for treating hypoprothrombinemia induced by salicylates, sulfonamides, quinine, quinidine, or broad-spectrum antibiotic therapy (15). …when vitamin K4 (menadiol sodium diphosphate) is used orally for treating hypoprothrombinemia resulting from impaired absorption or synthesis of vitamin K (14).
There is insufficient reliable information available to rate the effectiveness of vitamin K for its other uses. However, there is some preliminary clinical evidence that vitamin K2 (menaquinone) might help to treat osteoporosis, by slowing bone loss and possibly decreasing fractures (54,55). But vitamin K2 (menaquinone) seems to be ineffective for preventing osteoporosis in postmenopausal women (58). Vitamin K2 (menaquinone) might also decrease steroid induced osteoporosis (6799). There is also preliminary clinical evidence that vitamin K2 (menaquinone) might reduce serum cholesterol in patients on continuous ambulatory peritoneal dialysis with elevated cholesterol levels (59). More evidence is needed to rate vitamin K for these uses.

Mechanism of Action

Vitamin K is a generic term for a group of related compounds. Vitamin K compounds have a common central ring structure, which results in similar activity. Varying side chains differentiate the compounds in terms of intestinal absorption, transport, tissue distribution, and bioavailability (57). Only small amounts of vitamin K are stored in body tissues (64). Vitamin K1 (phytonadione) is obtained from dietary sources, such as leafy green vegetables, broccoli, Brussels sprouts, plant oils, and margarine (14,57,7135). Vitamin K2 (menaquinone) is obtained from meat and cheeses and synthesis by bacteria in the colon (64). Vitamin K4 (menadiol sodium diphosphate) is a synthetic, water-soluble salt of vitamin K3 (menadione) and is converted to vitamin K3 in the liver (14). Bile salts are required for oral absorption of vitamin K1 (phytonadione) and vitamin K2 (menaquinone), but not vitamin K4 (menadiol sodium diphosphate) (14,15). Vitamin K is a coenzyme for the hepatic synthesis of blood coagulation factors II (prothrombin), VII (proconvertin), IX (Christmas factor or plasma thromboplastin component), and X (Stuart-Prower factor), and proteins C and S in the liver (57,7131,7135). Vitamin K is also involved in carboxylation of gamma-carboxyglutamate (Gla) proteins that facilitate binding of coagulation factors to platelets (57). In adequate doses, vitamin K reverses the inhibitory effects of coumarin and warfarin derivatives on the synthesis of clotting factors (15). Besides its classic role in blood coagulation, vitamin K is involved in other physiologic processes. People try supplementing vitamin K for osteoporosis because there is evidence that low vitamin K intake or serum levels are associated with reduced bone mineral density and fractures in people with osteoporosis (55,60,61,62,837,6193,7131). Osteopenia in elderly men seems to correlate with circulating levels of vitamins K and D (7132). Whether people taking vitamin K antagonists or oral anticoagulants are at increased risk of fracture is controversial (51,52,63,7134). Oral anticoagulants might have some effect on the bone mineral density of the radius of the arm, but no effect on the bones of the hip and back (7135).The most pronounced effects of vitamin K antagonists appear to be on rapidly growing bone (7133). Endogenous vitamin K is responsible for activation of osteocalcin (bone Gla protein) that provides calcium-attracting properties to bone (6797,7130). Supplementing vitamin K increases osteocalcin levels in postmenopausal women (56,6797,6798). Vitamin K is known to act as a cofactor for carboxylation of osteocalcin, leading to the suggestion that undercarboxylated osteocalcin (ucOC) levels could be used as an indicator of vitamin K nutritional status (7130,7131,7135). However, variations in testing methodology and inconsistent clinical findings indicate that the usefulness of ucOC levels is undecided (7135). Higher ucOC levels are seen in elderly women with hip fracture, and supplemental vitamin K1 normalizes ucOC levels and increases bone mass (7130). Preliminary evidence suggests that vitamin K may affect calcium balance, urinary calcium excretion, and the production of prostaglandin E2 and interleukin 6 (7131). Vitamin K might also play a role in prevention of atherosclerosis (53,57). Atherosclerosis has been linked to low serum vitamin K levels (53). Laboratory evidence suggests vitamin K supplementation might protect against atherosclerosis (65). There is new research that the combination of vitamin K3 and vitamin C might play a role in treating prostate and breast cancer. The combination appears to cause a unique type of tumor cell death (1257).

Adverse Reactions

Few adverse effects are reported from oral vitamin K (14,15). Vitamin K4 (menadiol sodium diphosphate) has been associated with gastrointestinal irritation (14). There have been very rare cases of hemolytic anemia and thrombocytopenia, usually in neonates. The rare cases of thrombosis usually occur in people with other predisposing factors (14). Contact dermatitis has been reported with occupational exposure to vitamin K3 (menadione) and vitamin K4 (menadiol) (14).

Interactions with Herbs & Other Dietary Supplements

COENZYME Q10: Coenzyme Q10 is chemically similar to vitamin K2 (menaquinone) and might have vitamin K-like effects (2128,6048). Concomitant use might cause additive effects and increase the risk of clotting in people taking anticoagulants.

HERBS WITH CLOTTING POTENTIAL: Concomitant use of vitamin K with herbs that contain vitamin K can have additive effects and increase the risk of clotting in people using anticoagulants. Some of these products include alfalfa, cabbage, parsley, nettle, plantain, and others.

VITAMIN E: Higher doses of vitamin E can antagonize the effects of vitamin K (7135). Vitamin E appears to reduce the absorption of vitamin K and to inhibit vitamin K dependent enzymes (7135).

Interactions with Drugs

WARFARIN: Vitamin K antagonizes the effects of oral anticoagulants such as warfarin (Coumadin) (15). Excessive vitamin K intake, either from supplements or from changes in the diet, can reduce anticoagulation effect (15).

Drug Influences on Nutrient Levels and Depletion

SOME DRUGS CAN AFFECT VITAMIN K LEVELS:

CHOLESTYRAMINE (Questran): Cholestyramine might reduce dietary vitamin K absorption and serum levels (15,4455).

CHOLESTIPOL (Colestid): Colestipol might reduce dietary vitamin K absorption and serum levels (15,4460,4461).

ORAL ANTIBIOTICS: Various beneficial intestinal bacteria are eliminated when oral antibiotics are taken. Some of these intestinal bacteria are responsible for producing vitamin K. The nutritional importance of the quantity of vitamin K produced by these organisms can vary between individuals (4439).

MINERAL OIL: Mineral oil reduces gastrointestinal absorption of vitamin K (14). Avoid prolonged use.

ORLISTAT (Xenical): Orlistat can reduce the absorption of some fat-soluble vitamins, although the effect of orlistat on nutritionally derived vitamin K is unknown (1725,1726,1727,1730). Consider a multivitamin with fat-soluble vitamins, taken at least 2 hours before or after orlistat, or at bedtime.

Interactions with Foods

No interactions are known to occur, and there is no known reason to expect a clinically significant interaction with vitamin K.

Interactions with Lab Tests

BILIRUBIN: Large amounts of vitamin K can increase serum bilirubin and test results in neonates or people with G-6-PD deficiency (275).

CALCIUM: Can reduce urinary calcium excretion and test results (275).

ERYTHROCYTES: Can decrease blood erythrocyte levels and test results (275).

HEMATOCRIT: Vitamin K3 and vitamin K4 might decrease hematocrit and test results, especially in people with G-6-PD deficiency (275).

HEMOGLOBIN: Vitamin K3 and vitamin K4 might decrease blood hemoglobin level and test results, especially in people with G-6-PD deficiency (275).

HEMOGLOBIN: Can increase urine hemoglobin levels and test results (275).

17-HYDROXYCORTICOSTEROIDS: Might cause false increase in urine test results due to in vitro interference with Reddy method (275).

HYDROXYPROLINE: Can decrease urine levels and test results (275).

LEUKOCYTES, PLATELETS: Vitamin K3 and vitamin K4 can decrease blood levels and test results due to pancytopenia (275).
OSTEOCALCIN: Can increase serum levels and test results in postmenopausal women (275).
PORPHYRINS: Can increase urine levels and test results (275).
PROTEIN: Can increase urine levels and test results (275).
PROTHROMBIN TIME (PT): Can decrease PT due to procoagulation effects of vitamin K (275).
UROBILINOGEN: May increase urine levels and test results due to hemolytic anemia in G-6-PD deficiency (275).

Interactions with Diseases or Conditions
BILIARY FISTULA, OBSTRUCTIVE JAUNDICE: Menadiol sodium diphosphate should be used with caution (14).
REDUCED BILE SECRETION: People with decreased bile secretion may require co-administration of supplemental bile salts to ensure adequate vitamin K absorption (15).
G6-PD DEFICIENCY: Menadiol sodium diphosphate should be used with caution in individuals with glucose-6-phosphate dehydrogenase deficiency due to an increased risk of hemolysis (14).
HEMODIALYSIS: Excessive vitamin K intake has been associated with soft tissue calcification (14).
LIVER DISEASE: Vitamin K should be discontinued promptly in people with liver disease and hypoprothrombinemia who do not respond to initial treatment with vitamin K; continued treatment may further decrease prothrombin concentrations (14).
VITAMIN K HYPERSENSITIVITY: Contraindicated (14).

Dosage and Administration
ORAL: There is no typical dose for vitamin K. Doses should be individualized and medically supervised (15). People with decreased bile secretion might require co-administration of supplemental bile salts to ensure adequate vitamin K absorption (15). Efficient absorption of vitamin K from the intestine requires dietary fat, although the amount needed for optimal absorption has not been determined (7135). For osteoporosis, clinical studies used vitamin K2 (menaquinone) 45 mg per day (54,55,59). Vitamin K2 (menaquinone) is not currently available in the US. There is insufficient information to determine recommended dietary allowances (RDAs) for vitamin K, so daily adequate intake (AI) recommendations have been formed: Infants 0-6 months, 2 mcg; Infants 6-12 months, 2.5 mcg; Children 1-3 years, 30 mcg; Children 4-8 years, 55 mcg; Children 9-13 years, 60 mcg; Adolescents 14-18 years (including those pregnant or lactating), 75 mcg; Men over 19 years, 120 mcg; Women over 19 years (including those pregnant and lactating), 90 mcg (7135).
PARENTERAL: Injectable vitamin K is a FDA-approved prescription product.

Comments
The name vitamin K comes from the German word Koagulationsvitamin (57). Vitamin K1 (phytonadione) is the only form of vitamin K available in the US. Vitamin K1 (phytonadione) is generally the preferred form of vitamin K, due to lower toxicity, rapid effects, greater potency, and superior efficacy in some indications, such as oral anticoagulant-induced hypoprothrombinemia (14). Vitamin K3 (menadione) is no longer used therapeutically because it has been linked to hepatic toxicity (7135). Vitamin K4 (menadiol), which was marketed as Synkavite tablets and injection, is no longer available in the US (14). A specific form of vitamin K2 (menaquinone), MK-4, is an accepted treatment for osteoporotic osteopenia in Japan (57,58). An increased understanding of the physiologic role of vitamin K beyond blood coagulation has led some researchers to suggest that the guidelines for nutritional intake of vitamin K should be increased (57). The 2001 National Institute of Medicine Food and Nutrition Board slightly increased recommendations for adequate intake, but cited insufficient conclusive evidence for substantial increases (7135).

VITAMIN O

Also Known As
Liquid Oxygen, Stabilized Liquid Oxygen, Stabilized Oxygen.

Scientific Names
None.

People Use This For
Orally, vitamin O is used for increasing energy; improving immune function; eliminating bacteria, viruses, fungi and parasites; treating yeast infections; eliminating toxins and poisons from the body; and healing mouth sores. Vitamin O is also used for improving concentration, memory and alertness; calming the nervous system; easing depression, irritability, unexplained hostility and dizziness; relieving arthritis, muscle aches and pains, asthma, bronchial problems, emphysema and lung disease, sinus infection, diabetes, body weakness, chronic fatigue, and heart and circulation problems. Vitamin O has been used for obesity; constipation; gas and bloating; loss of appetite; poor digestion;

stomach acid; premenstrual syndrome (PMS); menopause; sexual dysfunction; headaches; migraines; premature aging; rashes; skin problems; itchy ears, nose and anus; and tumors and deposit buildup (5316,5317,5318,5319).
Topically, it is used as an antiseptic (5316).

Safety

There is insufficient reliable information available about the safety of vitamin O.
Pregnancy and Lactation: Insufficient reliable information available; avoid using.

Effectiveness

There is insufficient reliable information available about the effectiveness of vitamin O.

Mechanism of Action

The chemical formula of the oxygen compound in vitamin O is not disclosed in promotional information. One supplier describes its product as a mildly buffered solution of deionized water and sodium chloride with a pH of 7.2 (5318). Another supplier lists magnesium peroxide as the active ingredient (5320). Still another claims the ingredients are secret (5321).

Adverse Reactions

None reported.

Interactions with Herbs & Other Dietary Supplements

Insufficent reliable information available.

Interactions with Drugs

No interactions are known to occur, and there is no known reason to expect a clinically significant interaction with vitamin O.

Interactions with Foods

No interactions are known to occur, and there is no known reason to expect a clinically significant interaction with vitamin O.

Interactions with Lab Tests

No interactions are known to occur, and there is no known reason to expect a clinically significant interaction with vitamin O.

Interactions with Diseases or Conditions

No interactions are known to occur, and there is no known reason to expect a clinically significant interaction with vitamin O.

Dosage and Administration

ORAL: In capsule form of unspecified strength, the dose is typically two capsules three times per day with water (5320). Various quantities, usually measured in drops, of solutions are recommended (e.g., 6 drops in 8 ounces of water, juice, milk, etc; 20 drops 3 times a day in a glass of water; 20 drops per gallon of water) (5321).

Comments

Although vitamin O is called liquid oxygen, remember that oxygen only exists in a liquid form at temperatures below -183 degrees C and that water, by weight, is about 88% oxygen (16). The FTC states that Vitamin O appears to be nothing more than saltwater (311).
In May 2000, Rose Creek Health Products agreed to pay $375,000 to settle Federal Trade Commission charges that they made false and unsubstantiated health claims in their advertising for "Vitamin O". The settlement prohibits the company from making unsupported representations that "Vitamin O" is an effective treatment for any life-threatening diseases, or that the effectiveness of "Vitamin O" is established by medical or scientific research or studies (5076).

WAFER ASH

Also Known As
Pickaway Anise, Prairie Grub, Scubby Trefoil, Stinking Prairie Bush, Swamp Dogwood, Three-Leaved Hop Tree, Wingseed.

Scientific Names
Ptelea trifoliata.
Family: Rutaceae.

People Use This For
Orally, wafer ash is used for stomach complaints, gallstones, rheumatism, as an appetite stimulant and a tonic (18). Topically, wafer ash is used as a wound dressing (18).

Safety
There is insufficient reliable information available about the safety of wafer ash.
Pregnancy and Lactation: Insufficient reliable information is available; avoid using.

Effectiveness
There is insufficient reliable information available about the effectiveness or wafer ash.

Mechanism of Action
The applicable part of wafer ash is the root bark. Wafer ash contains furoquinoline alkaloids including kokusaginin, skimmianine, ptelein, and dictamnine. It also contains furocoumarins (18). Scientists think the alkaloid, pteleatinium chloride, is the active constituent of wafer ash. Pteleatinium chloride shows evidence of antimicrobial activity (3854), particularly against mycobacterium tuberculosis and yeast fungus (18).

Adverse Reactions
Topically, skin contact with the wafer ash plant can trigger phototoxic reactions (18).

Interactions with Herbs & Other Dietary Supplements
Insufficient reliable information available.

Interactions with Drugs
No interactions are known to occur, and there is no known reason to expect a clinically significant interaction with wafer ash.

Interactions with Foods
No interactions are known to occur, and there is no known reason to expect a clinically significant interaction with wafer ash.

Interactions with Lab Tests
No interactions are known to occur, and there is no known reason to expect a clinically significant interaction with wafer ash.

Interactions with Diseases or Conditions
No interactions are known to occur, and there is no known reason to expect a clinically significant interaction with wafer ash.

Dosage and Administration
ORAL: Wafer ash is used as an extract.
TOPICAL: No typical dosage.

Comments
There is very little scientific information about this product. Our staff is continually analyzing the available information on natural medicines and will add data here as it becomes available.

WAHOO

Also Known As

Arrowwood, Bitter Ash, Bleeding Heart, Burning Bush, Bursting Heart, Eastern Burning Bush, Fish Wood, Fusanum, Fusoria, Gadrose, Gatten, Gatter, Indian Arrowroot, Indian Arrowwood, Pegwood, Pigwood, Prickwood, Skewerwood, Spindle Tree, Strawberry Bush, Strawberry Tree.

Scientific Names

Euonymus atropurpureus.
Family: Celastraceae.

People Use This For

Orally, wahoo root bark is used orally for indigestion, to stimulate bile production, and as a laxative, diuretic, or tonic (18).

Safety

LIKELY UNSAFE …when the bark, seeds or berries are used orally. Ingesting 36 berries can be fatal (18). The poisonous principle has not been identified (17).
PREGNANCY AND LACTATION: LIKELY UNSAFE …when used orally (18).

Effectiveness

There is insufficient reliable information available about the effectiveness of wahoo.

Mechanism of Action

The applicable parts of wahoo are the trunk, root bark, and fruit. The seeds contain cardioactive steroids known as cardenolides. The trunk, root bark, and fruit also contain varied alkaloids, caffeine, and theobromine (18). Wahoo is thought to stimulate bile flow and have laxative effects. In larger amounts, it can affect the heart (18).

Adverse Reactions

Wahoo is considered poisonous (17). Several hours after ingesting wahoo seeds, people experience severe upset stomach, sometimes with bloody diarrhea, fever, shortness of breath, circulatory problems, signs of collapse, stupor increasing to unconsciousness, alternating with motor restlessness, severe tonic-clonic spasms with locked jaw muscles and coma.

Interactions with Herbs & Other Dietary Supplements

CARDIAC GLYCOSIDE-CONTAINING HERBS: Contraindicated; concomitant use increases the risk of cardiac glycoside toxicity. Cardiac glycoside containing herbs include black hellebore, Canadian hemp roots, digitalis leaf, hedge mustard, figwort, lily of the valley roots, motherwort, oleander leaf, pheasant's eye plant, pleurisy root, squill bulb leaf scales, and strophanthus seeds (2,18,19,500).
OTHER CARDIOACTIVE HERBS: Avoid concomitant use with other cardioactive herbs due to unpredictability of effects and adverse effects. Other cardioactive herbs include: calamus, cereus, cola, coltsfoot, devil's claw, European mistletoe, fenugreek, fumitory, ginger, panax ginseng, hawthorn, white horehound, mate, parsley, quassia, scotch broom flower, shepherd's purse, and wild carrot (4).
STIMULANT LAXATIVE HERBS: Theoretically, use of stimulant laxatives can have additive effects and adverse effects. Use also increases the risk of cardiac toxicity due to potassium depletion. Stimulant laxative herbs include: aloe dried leaf sap, blue flag rhizome, alder buckthorn, European buckthorn, butternut bark, cascara bark, castor oil, colocynth fruit pulp, gamboge bark exudate, jalap root, black root, manna bark exudate, podophyllum root, rhubarb root, senna leaves and pods, wild cucumber fruit (Ecballium elaterium), and yellow dock root (19).
LICORICE/HORSETAIL: Theoretically, overuse/misuse of licorice rhizome or horsetail plant with wahoo increases the risk of cardiac toxicity due to potassium depletion (19).

Interactions with Drugs

DIGOXIN: Contraindicated. Using cardenolide constituents with digoxin increases risk of cardiac glycoside toxicity (2).
CARDIAC DRUGS: Theoretically, concomitant might increase risk of cardiac toxicity (152).
STIMULANT LAXATIVES: Theoretically, use of stimulant laxatives can have additive effects and adverse effects. It can also increase risk of cardiac glycoside toxicity due to potassium depletion (2).
POTASSIUM-DEPLETING DIURETICS: Theoretically, concomitant use increases risk of cardiac glycoside toxicity due to potassium depletion (2,506).
QUININE: Theoretically, concomitant use might increase risk of cardiac toxicity (2,506).

TETRACYCLINES and MACROLIDE ANTIBIOTICS (erythromycin-like drugs): Theoretically, concomitant use can increase risk of cardiac glycoside toxicity (152,17).

Interactions with Foods

No interactions are known to occur, and there is no known reason to expect a clinically significant interaction with wahoo.

Interactions with Lab Tests

No interactions are known to occur, and there is no known reason to expect a clinically significant interaction with wahoo.

Interactions with Diseases or Conditions

GI CONDITIONS: Theoretically, wahoo can increase gastric secretions and stimulate peristalsis. These effects might exacerbate gastrointestinal irritation or inflammation (18).
HEART DISEASE: Contraindicated; theoretically cardiac glycosides contained in wahoo seed can exacerbate the condition or interfere with existing drug therapy.

Dosage and Administration

No typical dosage.

Comments

Avoid confusion with Euonymus europaeus (18).

WALLFLOWER

Also Known As

Beeflower, Gillyflower, Giroflier, Handflower, Keiri, Wallstock-Gillofer.

Scientific Names

Cheiranthus cheiri.
Family: Brassicaceae.

People Use This For

Orally, wallflower is used for cardiac insufficiency, to encourage menstruation, and as a laxative. It was also used for liver and gallbladder diseases because of its bitter taste.

Safety

POSSIBLY UNSAFE …when used orally (18).
PREGNANCY AND LACTATION: POSSIBLY UNSAFE …when used orally due to its possible toxic effects; avoid using (18).

Effectiveness

There is insufficient reliable information available about the effectiveness of wallflower.

Mechanism of Action

The applicable parts of wallflower are the above ground parts. It does contain cardiac glycosides, but they may be poorly absorbed when wallflower is taken orally (18).

Adverse Reactions

Poisoning may occur with parenteral administration, but is expected to be low with oral administration due to poor absorption of the cardiac glycosides (18).

Interactions with Herbs & Other Dietary Supplements

STIMULANT LAXATIVE HERBS: Theoretically, overuse or misuse of stimulant laxatives with cardiac glycoside-containing herbs increases the risk of cardiac toxicity due to potassium depletion. Stimulant laxative herbs include: aloe dried leaf sap, blue flag rhizome, alder buckthorn, European buckthorn, butternut bark, cascara bark, castor oil, colocynth fruit pulp, gamboge bark exudate, jalap root, black root, manna bark exudate, podophyllum root, rhubarb root, senna leaves and pods, wild cucumber fruit (Ecballium elaterium), and yellow dock root (19).
LICORICE/HORSETAIL: Theoretically, overuse/misuse of licorice rhizome or horsetail plant with cardiac glycoside-containing herbs increases the risk of cardiac toxicity due to potassium depletion (19).

CARDIAC GLYCOSIDE-CONTAINING HERBS: Contraindicated, concomitant use may increase the risk of cardiac glycoside toxicity. Cardiac glycoside-containing herbs include: black hellebore, Canadian hemp roots, digitalis leaf, hedge mustard, figwort, lily-of-the-valley roots, motherwort, oleander leaf, pheasant's eye plant, pleurisy root, squill bulb leaf scales, and strophanthus seeds (2,18,19,500).

OTHER CARDIOACTIVE HERBS: Avoid concomitant use with other cardioactive herbs due to unpredictability of effects and adverse effects. Other cardioactive herbs include: calamus, cereus, cola, coltsfoot, devil's claw, European mistletoe, fenugreek, fumitory, ginger, ginseng Panax, hawthorn, white horehound, mate, parsley, quassia, scotch broom flower, shepherd's purse, and wild carrot (4). See individual product listings.

CHINCHONA, EPHEDRA: Use with wallflower seed may increase risk of toxicity (18,19).

Interactions with Drugs

CARDIAC MEDICATIONS: Cardiac medications, including quinidine (and related noncardiac medication quinine) may increase risk of toxicity; contraindicated (18).

DIGOXIN: Therapeutic duplication, avoid (2).

LAXATIVES: Overuse/misuse may cause electrolyte depletion and increase risk of wallflower seed toxicity (18,19).

POTASSIUM DEPLETING DIURETICS, GLUCOCORTICOIDS: May cause electrolyte depletion and increase risk of wallflower seed toxicity (18,19).

CALCIUM SALTS: Contraindicated (18).

Interactions with Foods

No interactions are known to occur, and there is no known reason to expect a clinically significant interaction with wallflower.

Interactions with Lab Tests

No interactions are known to occur, and there is no known reason to expect a clinically significant interaction with wallflower.

Interactions with Diseases or Conditions

CARDIAC CONDITIONS: CAUTION, wallflower seed may cause arrhythmias (18).

Dosage and Administration

No typical dosage.

Comments

Canadian hemp is also known as wallflower (Cheiranthus cheiri). Wallflower is considered obsolete as a medicinal herb (18).

WATER AVENS

Also Known As

Chocolate Root, Cure All, Indian Chocolate, Throat Root, Water Chisch, Water Flower.

Scientific Names

Geum rivale.
Family: Rosaceae.

People Use This For

Orally, water avens underground parts, and the fresh, flowering plant are used orally for diarrhea (4), catarrhal colitis (4), passive uterine hemorrhage (4), intermittent fevers (4), and ulcerative colitis (4).

Safety

There is insufficient reliable information is available about the safety of water avens.
Pregnancy and Lactation: Insufficient reliable information is available; avoid using.

Effectiveness

There is insufficient reliable information available about the effectiveness of water avens.

Mechanism of Action

The applicable parts of water avens are the underground parts, fresh flowering plant, and root. High tannin content of water avens is probably responsible for astringent action. The freshly harvested rhizome and root contain trace amounts of the volatile oil eugenol (18).

Adverse Reactions

None reported.

Interactions with Herbs & Other Dietary Supplements

MINERALS: Theoretically, can decrease absorption of iron, calcium, and magnesium, due to tannin content (7).

Interactions with Drugs

ORAL MEDICATION: Theoretically, the tannin content might delay absorption of sedatives, hypnotics, antidepressants, and tranquilizers (7,19).
METFORMIN: Theoretically, water avens might reduce the efficacy of metformin (7).

Interactions with Foods

No interactions are known to occur, and there is no known reason to expect a clinically significant interaction with water avens.

Interactions with Lab Tests

No interactions are known to occur, and there is no known reason to expect a clinically significant interaction with water avens.

Interactions with Diseases or Conditions

No interactions are known to occur, and there is no known reason to expect a clinically significant interaction with water avens.

Dosage and Administration

No typical dosage.

Comments

There is very little scientific information about this product. Our staff is continually analyzing the available information on natural medicines and will add data here as it becomes available.

WATER DOCK

Also Known As

None.

Scientific Names

Rumex aquaticus.
Family: Polygaceae.

People Use This For

Orally, water dock is used for "blood purification" and constipation (18).
Topically, it is used for mouth ulcers, skin sores, scorbutic conditions, and for cleaning the teeth (18).
For food uses, the leaves are used in salads (18).

Safety

There is insufficient reliable information available about the safety of water dock.
Pregnancy and Lactation: Insufficient reliable information is available; avoid using.

Effectiveness

There is insufficient reliable information available about the effectiveness of water dock.

Mechanism of Action

The applicable part of water dock is the dried root. Water dock contains anthracene derivatives, oxalic acid and calcium oxalate, and tannins (18), an essential oil, fat, protein, quercitrin, starch, and tannin. Water dock is considered to have digestive properties (18).

Adverse Reactions
None reported.

Interactions with Herbs & Other Dietary Supplements
CALCIUM, IRON, ZINC: Concurrent use might decrease mineral absorption. Water dock contains oxalate (7,12), which can bind multivalent metal ions in the gastrointestinal tract and decrease mineral absorption.

Interactions with Drugs
No interactions are known to occur, and there is no known reason to expect a clinically significant interaction with water dock.

Interactions with Foods
CALCIUM, IRON, ZINC: Concurrent use might decrease mineral absorption from foods. Water dock contains oxalate (7,12), which can bind multivalent metal ions in the gastrointestinal tract and decrease mineral absorption.

Interactions with Lab Tests
No interactions are known to occur, and there is no known reason to expect a clinically significant interaction with water dock.

Interactions with Diseases or Conditions
COAGULATION DISORDERS: Oxalate constituents can alter serum calcium concentrations, possibly decreasing coagulation time (12).
KIDNEY DISEASE: Use with caution in individuals with a history of kidney stones. Insoluble oxalate crystals may form in the kidneys, causing further damage (12).

Dosage and Administration
ORAL: Water dock is used orally or topically as a liquid extract or as a powder.

Comments
None.

WATER FENNEL

Also Known As
Horsebane, Water Dropwort.

Scientific Names
Oenanthe aquatica.

People Use This For
Orally, the ripe seeds of water fennel are used orally as an expectorant, for the relief of coughs, as a diuretic, and as an antiflatulent (18).

Safety
There is insufficient reliable information available about the safety of water fennel.
Pregnancy and Lactation: Insufficient reliable information is available; avoid using.

Effectiveness
There is insufficient reliable information available about the effectiveness of water fennel.

Mechanism of Action
The applicable part of water fennel is the ripe seed. The active agents include fatty oil, volatile oil (including (+)-beta-phellandrene, dillapiol, myristicin, androle), resin, wax, galacton, mannan, and rubber substances (18), resin, wax, galacton, mannan, and rubber substances (18).

Adverse Reactions
None reported.

Interactions with Herbs & Other Dietary Supplements
Insufficient reliable information available.

Interactions with Drugs
No interactions are known to occur, and there is no known reason to expect a clinically significant interaction with water fennel.

Interactions with Foods
No interactions are known to occur, and there is no known reason to expect a clinically significant interaction with water fennel.

Interactions with Lab Tests
No interactions are known to occur, and there is no known reason to expect a clinically significant interaction with water fennel.

Interactions with Diseases or Conditions
No interactions are known to occur, and there is no known reason to expect a clinically significant interaction with water fennel.

Dosage and Administration
ORAL: A typical dose of water fennel is 1 gram as a tea or extract (18).

Comments
There is very little scientific information about this product. Our staff is continually analyzing the available information on natural medicines and will add data here as it becomes available.

WATER GERMANDER

Also Known As
None.

Scientific Names
Teucrium scordium.
Family: Lamiaceae.

People Use This For
Water germander is used for bronchial asthma, diarrhea, fever, intestinal parasites, hemorrhoids, and festering and inflamed wounds (18).

Safety
There is insufficient reliable information available about the safety of water germander.
Pregnancy and Lactation: Insufficient reliable information is available; avoid using.

Effectiveness
There is insufficient reliable information available about the effectiveness of water germander.

Mechanism of Action
The applicable parts of water germander are the above ground parts. There is insufficient reliable information available about the possible mechanism of action and active ingredients.

Adverse Reactions
None reported.

Interactions with Herbs & Other Dietary Supplements
Insufficient reliable information available.

Interactions with Drugs
No interactions are known to occur, and there is no known reason to expect a clinically significant interaction with water germander.

Interactions with Foods
No interactions are known to occur, and there is no known reason to expect a clinically significant interaction with water germander.

Interactions with Lab Tests

No interactions are known to occur, and there is no known reason to expect a clinically significant interaction with water germander.

Interactions with Diseases or Conditions

No interactions are known to occur, and there is no known reason to expect a clinically significant interaction with water germander.

Dosage and Administration

ORAL/TOPICAL: A typical dose is four teaspoons (7.2 grams) above ground parts per day, as a prepared tea (18). The same preparation can be used internally or externally (18).

Comments

There is very little scientific information about this product. Our staff is continually analyzing the available information on natural medicines and will add data here as it becomes available.

WATER HEMLOCK

Also Known As

Beaver Poison, Brook-Tongue, Carotte a Moreau, Children's Bane, Cique Vireuse, Cowbane, Death-of-Man, European Water Hemlock, False Parsley, Fever Root, Mockeel Root, Muskrat Weed, Musquash Root, Poison Parsnip, Snake Weed, Snakeroot, Spotted Cowbane, Spotted Hemlock, Spotted Parsley, Wasser-Schierling, Wild Carrot, Wild Dill, Wild Parsnip.
CAUTION: See separate listings for Hemlock and Hemlock Water Dropwort.

Scientific Names

Cicuta virosa; Cicuta maculata; Cicuta douglasii, Cicuta occidentalis; Cicuta bulbifera; Cicuta vagans.
Family: Umbelliferae.

People Use This For

Orally, water hemlock is used for migraine headaches, painful menstruation, and worm infestations (18).
Topically, water hemlock is used for inflammation of the skin (18,6348,6351).

Safety

UNSAFE ...when used orally (18). Water hemlock is considered to be the most poisonous plant growing in North America (6349). Intoxication can result from chewing or ingestion of all plant parts (6348). Usual lethal adult dose is one rhizome (6347) or a 2-3 cm portion of root (6349). ...when used topically (6348). Death can result when hemlock is applied topically (6348,6349).
CHILDREN: UNSAFE ...when used orally or topically (6347,6351,6355,). Fatalities have resulted when hollow stems of water hemlock are used as whistles (6347), when hemlock is ingested (6355), or when hemlock has been applied topically (6351).
PREGNANCY AND LACTATION: UNSAFE ...when used orally or topically (18). Water hemlock is toxic; avoid using (18).

Effectiveness

There is insufficient reliable information available about the effectiveness of water hemlock.

Mechanism of Action

All parts of water hemlock at all stages of growth, including leaves and stems, are considered poisonous and can be lethal if ingested (6346,6349). The freshly harvested root is considered most toxic in early spring (6346). All plant parts contain the toxin cicutoxin, but it is especially concentrated in the root (6350). Cicutoxin is a highly unsaturated aliphatic alcohol (6346,6347,6348) that is found in a yellow oily liquid of roots and stems (6354). Water hemlock poisoning consists of cholinergic effects such as salivation, perspiration, diaphoresis, abdominal discomfort, and nausea (6350); and occurs almost immediately after ingestion (6346). Convulsions, seizures, and spastic-tonic movements follow (6346,6350,6353) which are believed to be due to cholinergic stimulation of the brain stem (reticular formation) or the basal ganglia (6346,6350). Narrow pupils, most likely due to the cholinergic effects of the toxin, and dilated pupils, due to brain hypoxia or ischemia, have been reported (6346). Increases in creatine phosphokinase occur indicating the severity of muscle rigors, rigidity and convulsions, and increases in serum lactic dehydrogenase also may occur that indicate possible liver or skeletal muscle damage (6347). Cicutoxin can also be absorbed through the skin (6349). Death usually results from cyanosis, exhaustion, and respiratory paralysis (6347,6348,6350).

Adverse Reactions

Toxic effects occur immediately after ingestion (6350). Prompt medical attention is advised after ingestion of water hemlock (6346). Death can result 15 minutes to 8 hours after ingestion (6351,6353). The usual lethal adult dose is one rhizome (6347) or a 2-3 cm portion of root (6349). The first symptoms of water hemlock poisoning are nausea (6346), vomiting, wheezing (6347), salivation, sweating, dizziness, abdominal pain (6346), flushing (6349), lethargy (6350), delirium (6349), and defecation (6351). These symptoms are followed by respiratory distress; muscle spasms; restless movements; bronchial secretions (6346); convulsions (6345,6346,6348); mydriasis; miosis; eyeball protrusion (6346); glycosuria; proteinuria; abnormal EEG; elevated serum CPK, LDH, AST and alkaline phosphatase levels (6346); metabolic acidosis (6347,6348,6349); hypertension (6346); supraventricular tachycardia (6347); hypotension; bradycardia (6346); muscle rigidity; tremors (6437); grinding of teeth (6346); tonic-clonic movements; grand-mal seizures (6353); rhabdomyolysis; acute renal failure (6348,6349,6351); cerebral edema (6350); unconsciousness (6346,6347); and coma (6346). Death can occur during convulsions (18) and from respiratory paralysis, exhaustion (6347,6348,6350), or heart failure (18).

Interactions with Herbs & Other Dietary Supplements

Insufficient reliable information available.

Interactions with Drugs

No interactions are known to occur, and there is no known reason to expect a clinically significant interaction with water hemlock.

Interactions with Foods

No interactions are known to occur, and there is no known reason to expect a clinically significant interaction with water hemlock.

Interactions with Lab Tests

SERUM MUSCLE ENZYMES: Ingestion of water hemlock can cause elevations in serum muscle enzymes such as creatine phosphokinase (CPK) and lactic dehydrogenase (LDH isoenzyme fraction 5) levels (6346,6347).
SERUM LIVER ENZYMES: Ingestion of water hemlock can cause elevations in serum liver enzymes such as lactic dehydrogenase (LDH), aspartate aminotransferase (AST), and alkaline phosphatase (6346,6347).

Interactions with Diseases or Conditions

No interactions are known to occur, and there is no known reason to expect a clinically significant interaction with water hemlock.

Dosage and Administration

No typical dosage.

Comments

Water hemlock is found in marshy, swampy areas of meadows (6346) and along banks of streams (6339,6346), pools, or rivers (6345). Accidental ingestion usually occurs when water hemlock is mistaken for edible plants such as artichokes, celery, sweet potatoes, sweet anise, and wild parsnip (6346). There are approximately 20 species of water hemlock (Cicuta) and most are found in North America (6339). The most commonly encountered are Cicuta maculata in southern Missouri and the eastern United States, Cicuta vagans in the Pacific Northwest, Cicuta bulbifera in the Middle Northwest, Cicuta occidentalis in the Rocky Mountain region (6351,) and Cicuta virosa which is found throughout the United States and is known as the common European water hemlock (6346,6347,6348). All species of water hemlock are considered poisonous (6351). The rhizome has an extremely unpleasant smell and is extremely toxic (18).

WATER PLANTAIN

Also Known As

Mad-Dog Weed.
CAUTION: See separate listings for Great Plantain, Buckhorn Plantain, Blond Psyllium, Black Psyllium.

Scientific Names

Alisma plantago-aquatica.
Family: Alismataceae.

People Use This For

Orally, water plantain is used for bladder and urinary tract diseases (18).

Safety
POSSIBLY UNSAFE …when used orally (18).
PREGNANCY AND LACTATION: POSSIBLY UNSAFE …when used orally due to its toxic potential; avoid using (18).

Effectiveness
There is insufficient reliable information available about the effectiveness of water plantain.

Mechanism of Action
The applicable part of water plantain is the root/rhizome. The fresh rootstock is thought to be poisonous. It contains the cyanogenic chlorogenic acid sulfate (18).

Adverse Reactions
None reported.

Interactions with Herbs & Other Dietary Supplements
Insufficient reliable information available.

Interactions with Drugs
No interactions are known to occur, and there is no known reason to expect a clinically significant interaction with water plantain.

Interactions with Foods
No interactions are known to occur, and there is no known reason to expect a clinically significant interaction with water plantain.

Interactions with Lab Tests
No interactions are known to occur, and there is no known reason to expect a clinically significant interaction with water plantain.

Interactions with Diseases or Conditions
No interactions are known to occur, and there is no known reason to expect a clinically significant interaction with water plantain.

Dosage and Administration
No typical dosage.

Comments
Water plantain is considered possibly unsafe; avoid using (18). Water plantain rootstock is said to be bitter in taste (18). It sounds similar to either the common or species names of great plantain, and buckhorn plantain. Be careful not to confuse them.

WATERCRESS

Also Known As
Agrião, Berro, Berro Di Agua, Brunnenkresse, Crescione Di Fonte, Cresson au Poulet, Cresson D'eau, Cresson De Fontaine, Indian Cress, Mizu-Garashi, Nasilord, Nasturtii herba, Oranda-Garashi, Scurvy Grass, Selada-Air, Tall Nasturtium, Wasserkresse, Waterkres.
CAUTION: See separate listings for Nasturtium and Scurvy Grass.

Scientific Names
Nasturtium officinale.
Family: Brassicaceae.

People Use This For
Orally, watercress is used for respiratory tract mucous membrane inflammation (2).
Topically, watercress is used for arthritis, rheumatoid arthritis (18), earache, eczema, scabies, and warts.
In folk medicine, watercress is used orally for coughs, bronchitis, as a spring tonic, an appetite stimulant (18), improving digestion and stimulating appetite (8), alopecia, cancer, flu, goiter, polyps, scurvy, tuberculosis, gland tumors, as an

abortifacient, aphrodisiac, bactericide, laxative, restorative, stimulant, and anthelmintic.
For food uses, watercress is widely used in leaf salads and as a culinary spice (12).

Safety
LIKELY SAFE …when used orally in food amounts (18).
POSSIBLY SAFE …when used orally short-term oral medicinal use (2,8,12).
POSSIBLY UNSAFE ...when used orally in large amounts or for extended use. Can cause gastric mucosal irritation (8,12) or damage (19).
There is insufficient reliable information available about the safety of watercress for its other uses.
CHILDREN: LIKELY SAFE ...when used orally in amounts commonly found in food. LIKELY UNSAFE ...when used orally in larger amounts. Contraindicated in children younger than 4 years old (2,12,19).
PREGNANCY: LIKELY SAFE ...when used orally in amounts commonly found in foods. LIKELY UNSAFE ...when used orally in larger amounts. Might stimulate menstruation or have abortifacient effects (19).
LACTATION: Insufficient reliable information available; avoid using.

Effectiveness
POSSIBLY EFFECTIVE …when used orally for respiratory tract mucous membrane inflammation (2).
There is insufficient reliable information available about the effectiveness of watercress for its other uses.

Mechanism of Action
The applicable parts of watercress are the above ground parts. Watercress is thought to have antibiotic and diuretic activity (18). The above ground parts contain mustard oil (18), vitamin C, and beta-carotene, and vitamin K (19). Mustard oil is believed responsible for diuretic effects and gastrointestinal irritation after consumption of large amounts of watercress (18). The constituent, phenethyl isothiocyanate, released by chewing watercress, inhibits metabolic activation of a lung carcinogen (4019).

Adverse Reactions
Orally, large amounts of watercress can cause gastrointestinal irritation (18). Theoretically, excessive or prolonged use might cause kidney damage (19). No adverse effects are reported from topical use.

Interactions with Herbs & Other Dietary Supplements
Insufficient reliable information available.

Interactions with Drugs
CHLORZOXAZONE: Concomitant use may potentiate effects of chlorzoxazone (Paraflex) due to reduced metabolism and elimination (4018).
WARFARIN: Theoretically, consuming large amount amounts of watercress with its high vitamin K content might antagonize the anticoagulant effects of warfarin (Coumadin) (19).

Interactions with Foods
No interactions are known to occur, and there is no known reason to expect a clinically significant interaction with watercress.

Interactions with Lab Tests
COAGULATION TESTS: Might decrease prothrombin time, INR, and test results due to high vitamin K content (19).

Interactions with Diseases or Conditions
GASTRIC OR DUODENAL ULCERS: Contraindicated (2,12,19).
INFLAMMATORY KIDNEY DISEASES: Contraindicated (2,12,19).

Dosage and Administration
ORAL: A typical dose is one cup of tea before meals, 2-3 times daily. To make tea, pour 150 mL boiling water over 2 grams above ground parts, cover for 10 minutes, strain (18). A daily dose ranges to 4-6 grams dried herb, 20-30 grams fresh herb, or 60-150 grams freshly pressed juice (2).
TOPICAL: Watercress is used topically as a poultice or compress (18).

Comments
Avoid confusing watercress with nasturtium (Tropaeolum majus).

WHEAT BRAN

Also Known As
Bran, Dietary Fiber.
CAUTION: See separate listings for Oat Bran and Rice Bran.

Scientific Names
Triticum aestrivum.
Family: Poaceae.

People Use This For
Orally, wheat bran is used as a supplemental source of dietary fiber for preventing colon diseases (including cancer), reducing the risk of hemorrhoids and hiatus hernia, reducing cholesterol and blood sugar levels (5), reducing the risk of breast cancer (160) and gallbladder disease (162), and to improve glycemic control in type 2 diabetes (6266).

Safety
LIKELY SAFE ...when used orally (5).
PREGNANCY AND LACTATION: LIKELY SAFE ...when used orally (5).

Effectiveness
LIKELY EFFECTIVE ...when used orally as a source of fiber (163).
POSSIBLY EFFECTIVE ...when used for treating constipation and restoring normal bowel function, reducing risk of hemorrhoids or hiatus hernia, preventing GI diseases (5,162,163), lowering blood pressure (4963), and reducing plasma estradiol level when used in conjunction with a low fat diet (160). ...when used to improve glycemic control in type 2 diabetes (6266). In a randomized crossover study of 13 people with type 2 diabetes, a high fiber diet that included wheat bran was more effective in lowering preprandial blood glucose and the area under the curve for 24-hour plasma glucose and glucose (measured every 2 hours), and improving cholesterol and triglyceride levels than the standard ADA diet (6266).
POSSIBLY INEFFECTIVE ... when used to reduce the risk of colorectal cancer (4819,4820,4821). Several large well-designed studies showed that fiber, including wheat-bran fiber, does not prevent the recurrence of colorectal adenomas, despite earlier evidence that suggested a beneficial effect (160,4819,4820,4821).
There is insufficient reliable information available about the effectiveness of wheat bran for its other uses.

Mechanism of Action
The applicable part of wheat bran is the outer hull of the grain, which is largely composed of insoluble fiber (4963). The laxative effect of wheat bran is dependent on particle size; larger particles have a greater laxative effect than smaller particles (6265). Wheat bran has negligible water-holding capacity and no stool softening effect in people with normal stools (6265). Wheat bran increases colonic transit time, stool output, and bowel movement frequency (6265). It might reduce breast cancer risk by lowering plasma estrogen levels by interfering with enterohepatic circulation and increasing the rate of fecal estrogen excretion (162). Wheat bran might be beneficial in controlling insulin-resistance syndrome (162). Preliminary evidence suggests consumption of wheat bran might move the digestion site of foods from the proximal to distal portion of the colon (375). In the distal colon, butyrate produced from digestion of grains and starches reduces ammonia produced by fermentation of foods high in fat and sugar, possibly preventing cell damage and reducing the risk of colon cancer (375).

Adverse Reactions
Orally, wheat bran may cause flatulence and GI discomfort, especially with initial use. One carefully controlled study designed to look at side effects noted no increase in GI symptoms in subjects taking 20 to 40 grams of wheat bran per day (6265).

Interactions with Herbs & Other Dietary Supplements
Insufficient reliable information available.

Interactions with Drugs
DIGOXIN: Theoretically, may interfere with absorption (156).

Interactions with Foods
IRON: Wheat fiber inhibits dietary iron absorption (156).

Interactions with Lab Tests

BLOOD PRESSURE: Wheat bran might lower blood pressure and blood pressure readings in individuals with hypertension (4963).

Interactions with Diseases or Conditions

No interactions are known to occur, and there is no known reason to expect a clinically significant interaction with wheat bran.

Dosage and Administration

ORAL: Adults: 20-35 grams per day or 10-13 grams dietary fiber per 1000 kcal. In one study, 40 grams per day was no more effective than 20 grams for laxative effect (6265). Children 2 years of age and older: fiber intake equal to their age plus 5 grams (163). For best results, slowly increase fiber intake while reducing intake of foods high in fat, salt and sugar (5).

Comments

Wheat bran is the outer grain hull of wheat (Triticum aestrivum).

WHEATGRASS

Also Known As

Couchgrass, Doggrass, Quackgrass, Twitchgrass, Wheat Grass.
CAUTION: See separate listing for Chlorophyll.

Scientific Names

Agropyron repens, synonym Elytrigia repens.

People Use This For

Orally, wheatgrass is primarily used as a concentrated source of nutrients. It is used therapeutically for increasing hemoglobin production, improving blood sugar disorders such as diabetes, preventing tooth decay, improving wound healing, and preventing bacterial infections (5285). It is also used orally for removing deposits of drugs, heavy metals, and carcinogens from the body and neutralizing toxins, removing toxins from the liver and removing toxins from the blood stream (5285). Wheatgrass is used for cancer in alternative cancer treatment programs (6981).
Traditionally, wheatgrass has been used for preventing gray hair, reducing high blood pressure, aiding in the prevention and cure of cancer, improving digestion (5285), and blocking intestinal cholesterol absorption (5281).

Safety

LIKELY SAFE …when consumed in food amounts (5286).
There is insufficient reliable information available about the safety of wheatgrass used in larger amounts.
PREGNANCY AND LACTATION: Insufficient reliable information available; avoid using.

Effectiveness

There is insufficient reliable information available about the effectiveness of wheatgrass.

Mechanism of Action

The applicable part of wheatgrass are the above ground parts. Wheatgrass contains large amounts of chlorophyll. High-chlorophyll beverages are sometimes included in diets purported to treat diseases such as cancer and rheumatoid arthritis (6981,6982). Wheatgrass juice is a popular health drink, but clinical studies supporting its use as a health tonic, vegetable substitute, or disease modifier have not been performed.

Adverse Reactions

None reported.

Interactions with Herbs & Other Dietary Supplements

Insufficient reliable information available.

Interactions with Drugs

WARFARIN: Theoretically, due to the vitamin K content, wheatgrass might decrease the anticoagulant effect of warfarin (Coumadin) (15). One manufacturer reports that a 3.5 gram dose of wheatgrass contains 35 mcg vitamin K (5287).

Interactions with Foods

No interactions are known to occur, and there is no known reason to expect a clinically significant interaction with wheatgrass.

Interactions with Lab Tests

No interactions are known to occur, and there is no known reason to expect a clinically significant interaction with wheatgrass.

Interactions with Diseases or Conditions

No interactions are known to occur, and there is no known reason to expect a clinically significant interaction with wheatgrass.

Dosage and Administration

ORAL: A typical oral wheatgrass dose is 3.5 grams, 1 teaspoon or 7 tablets (5281,5287). Wheatgrass juice 2-4 ounces has also been used (5289).

Comments

There are at least 25 varieties of wheatgrass in the following plant families: Agropyron, Elytrigia, Eremopyrum, Pascopyrum, Pseudoroegneria (5284). Wheatgrass juice or tablets are used as a part of an uncooked vegan diet, also known as a "living food" diet (5286). Wheatgrass products claim nutritional benefits similar to dark green salad (5281), e.g., seven 500 mg tablets or 1 teaspoon powder wheatgrass to a serving of a 1/3 to 1 cup leafy dark green salad (5287,5288); however, this claim has not been verified.

WHEY PROTEIN

Also Known As

Bovine Whey Protein Concentrate.

Scientific Names

None.

People Use This For

Orally, whey protein is used as a food supplement, for promoting positive nitrogen balance (4924,4941), as an alternative to milk for people with lactose intolerance, for protein allergy, asthma, high cholesterol, obesity (4925), replacing or supplementing milk-based infant formulas (4921), decreasing the risk of developing atopic disease in infants genetically predisposed to allergy (4927,4929), treating metastatic carcinoma (4930,4933), preventing colon cancer (4928), and reversing weight loss and increasing glutathione (GSH) in people with HIV disease (4926,4932,4935,4936).

Safety

LIKELY SAFE ...when quality products are used orally and appropriately. There are no reports of toxicity in clinical trials (4926,4927,4929,4930,4932,4935,4936,4941).
PREGNANCY AND LACTATION: LIKELY SAFE ...when quality products are used orally and appropriately (4921,4929).

Effectiveness

EFFECTIVE ...when used orally as a replacement for, or in addition to, milk-based infant formulas (4921).
POSSIBLY EFFECTIVE ...when used orally for reversing weight loss and increasing glutathione (GSH) in people with HIV disease (4926,4932,4935,4936). ...when used orally to decrease the risk of developing atopic disease in infants genetically predisposed to allergy (4927,4929). ...when used for treating metastatic carcinoma (4930).
There is insufficient reliable information available about the effectiveness of whey protein for its other uses.

Mechanism of Action

Whey is a by-product of cheese making which contains carbohydrates including lactose; minerals including calcium, sodium, phosphorus, and potassium (2640,4923); proteins including alpha-lactalbumin, beta-lactoglobulin, lactoferrin, serum albumin, lysozyme, and immunoglobulins A, G, and M (2640,4921); and cysteine (4937). The concentrations of whey protein, lactose, and minerals can be increased or reduced as required for the intended use of the product (4923). Whey products may vary in the amount and activity of immunoglobulins and other proteins present, depending on the production methods used (2640). Whey protein typically contains 24% branched chain amino acids which are readily oxidized as an energy source during stress. Whey protein is also a source of gamma-glutamylcysteine, a precursor of glutathione (GSH), which acts as an intracellular antioxidant (2640). GSH is depleted by oxidative stress, which occurs in infections, trauma, or major surgery (2640). Low levels of GSH in patients with HIV have been associated with impaired T-cell function (2640). A specific whey protein formulation (Immunocal) might enhance the reduced-to-oxidized glutathione ratio (GSH/GSSG) in lymphocytes, a marker of oxidative stress in reactive oxygen species (ROS)-mediated diseases, including AIDS-related wasting (1382). It also has anti-HIV and anti-apoptotic effects in vitro (4937). In patients with HIV infection, whey protein increases body weight (4926,4935,4936), elevates GSH in mononuclear cells (4926), increases albumin, increases CD4 and CD8 counts (4935), and reduces diarrhea (4932,4936). Whey protein has immunomodulating activity (4939,4940). It's thought that immunoglobulins in whey protein may bind antigens in the gut and prevent their absorption (2640). Whey protein formulations can be produced that are high in specific immunoglubulins. For example, whey proteins derived from the milk of cows infected with Cryptosporidium may be a rich source of antibodies against Cryptosporidium (2640). These whey protein formulation can reduce gastrointestinal Cryptosporidium parvum infection in animal models (4934). Some researchers are interested in using whey protein to prevent cancer. It's thought that whey protein might prevent cancer by providing GSH substrates and increasing tissue GSH levels (4943). Whey protein might exert antitumor effects by depleting tumor cells of GSH, making them more vulnerable to chemotherapy (2640,4930). Animal models of cancer indicated that whey protein diets might protect against certain cancers (3976,4928,4933). Researchers are also interested in whey protein for cardiovascular conditions. There is preliminary evidence that a unique combination of hydrolyzed whey protein isolates inhibits angiotensin converting enzyme (ACE) (6171).

Adverse Reactions

Orally, whey protein is usually well tolerated. High doses from 2.3 to 6.5 g/kg/day can cause increased stool frequency, nausea, thirst, bloating, cramps, reduced appetite, fatigue, and headache. Whey protein can also increase blood urea nitrogen (BUN) levels twofold (2640).

Interactions with Herbs & Other Dietary Supplements

Insufficient reliable information available.

Interactions with Drugs

LEVODOPA: Theoretically, concomitant use might decrease levodopa (Laradopa) absorption (10,4944).
MINERAL/DRUG INTERACTIONS: Theoretically, concomitant use of fluoride (Fluoritab), fluoroquinolones, tetracyclines, and alendronate (Fosamax) can decrease absorption of these drugs, due to whey protein mineral content (9). To avoid interaction, separate administration by at least two hours.

Interactions with Foods

No interactions are known to occur, and there is no known reason to expect a clinically significant interaction with whey protein.

Interactions with Lab Tests

BLOOD UREA NITROGEN (BUN): Whey protein in amounts of 2.3 g/kg/day or more, in addition to a normal diet, can produce twofold increases in BUN concentrations (2640). However, whey protein does not change serum creatinine, indicating that the effect is due to protein loading, rather than reduced renal function (2640).

Interactions with Diseases or Conditions

MILK ALLERGY: Individuals allergic to bovine milk products should avoid using whey protein (4942).

Dosage and Administration

ORAL: A typical dose as a dietary supplement in people with HIV disease is 8.4-84 grams per day (4926,4935), or 2.4 g/kg per day in a calorie-enriched formula (4941), or 42-84 grams per day in a glutamine enriched formula (4935). A dose for treating metastatic carcinoma is 30 grams per day (4930).

Comments

Whey protein is the soluble protein contained in whey, the watery portion of milk that separates from the curds in the process of cheese making (516,5121). A bovine whey protein concentrate product (Immuno-C) was investigated for treating Cryptosporidium infection in immunocompromised or immunocompetent people (FDA orphan drug status) (14); the product has not been approved for this use and no published clinical data are available.

WHITE COHOSH

Also Known As

Baneberry, Coralberry, Doll's Eye, Snakeberry, White Baneberry.
CAUTION: See separate listings for Black Cohosh, Blue Cohosh, and European Baneberry.

Scientific Names

Actaea alba, synonym Actaea pachypoda; Actaea rubra.
Family: Ranunculaceae.

People Use This For

Historically, white cohosh has been used to stimulate menstruation and to treat other female disorders. The root has been used for colds and cough, urogenital disorders, stomach disorders, reviving those near death, as a purgative, in childbirth, and for curing itching (6).

Safety

LIKELY UNSAFE ...when used orally. The entire plant is toxic (6,14).
PREGNANCY AND LACTATION: LIKELY UNSAFE ...when used orally due to toxicity (6); avoid using.

Effectiveness

There is insufficient reliable information available about the effectiveness of white cohosh.

Mechanism of Action

The constituent protoanemonin is believed to cause irritant effects (6). The fruit and berries are especially toxic. They contain toxic glycosides and an essential oil (6).

Adverse Reactions

Orally, white cohosh can cause gastrointestinal irritation (19), acute stomach cramping, headache, tachycardia, vomiting, delirium, circulatory failure (6), bloody diarrhea, dysuria, hematuria, visual hallucinations, and incoherence (14).
Topically, the application of white cohosh can lead to inflammation and skin blistering (6).

Interactions with Herbs & Other Dietary Supplements

Insufficient reliable information available.

Interactions with Drugs

No interactions are known to occur, and there is no known reason to expect a clinically significant interaction with white cohosh.

Interactions with Foods

No interactions are known to occur, and there is no known reason to expect a clinically significant interaction with white cohosh.

Interactions with Lab Tests

No interactions are known to occur, and there is no known reason to expect a clinically significant interaction with white cohosh.

Interactions with Diseases or Conditions

GI CONDITIONS: Can irritate the gastrointestinal tract. Contraindicated in individuals with infectious or inflammatory gastrointestinal conditions (19).

Dosage and Administration

No typical dosage.

Comments

White cohosh appears to be a substance with no reliable evidence to support its use, yet with documented toxicity. It should not be confused with black cohosh, used for symptoms of menopause, nor with blue cohosh, a substance used as a uterine stimulant and antispasmodic (6). White cohosh is also known as baneberry but it should not be confused with European baneberry.

WHITE DEAD NETTLE FLOWER

Also Known As
Archangel, Bee Nettle, Blind Nettle, Deaf Nettle, Dumb Nettle, Lamii Albi Flos, Stingless Nettle, White Archangel.
CAUTION: See separate listings for Stinging Nettle above ground parts and Stinging Nettle root.

Scientific Names
Lamium album.
Family: Lamiaceae.

People Use This For
Orally, white dead nettle is used for simple inflammation of mucous membranes in the upper respiratory tract (2,8).
Topically, it is used for mild inflammation of the mouth, throat, and skin (2,18), and for non-specific vaginal discharge (2,18).
In folk medicine, white dead nettle has been used as an ingredient in sedative herbal teas (8).

Safety
LIKELY SAFE ...when used orally and appropriately (2,18).
There is insufficient reliable information available about the safety of white dead nettle flower for its other uses.
PREGNANCY AND LACTATION: Insufficient reliable information available; avoid using.

Effectiveness
POSSIBLY EFFECTIVE ...when used orally for simple inflammation of mucous membranes in the upper respiratory tract (2). ...when used topically for mild inflammation of the oropharynx and skin (2).
There is insufficient reliable information available about the effectiveness of white dead nettle flower for its other uses.

Mechanism of Action
Nettle flowers contain tannin, mucilage, and saponins (2). These give nettle expectorant and astringent effects.

Adverse Reactions
None reported.

Interactions with Herbs & Other Dietary Supplements
Insufficient reliable information available.

Interactions with Drugs
No interactions are known to occur, and there is no known reason to expect a clinically significant interaction with white dead nettle flower.

Interactions with Foods
No interactions are known to occur, and there is no known reason to expect a clinically significant interaction with white dead nettle flower.

Interactions with Lab Tests
No interactions are known to occur, and there is no known reason to expect a clinically significant interaction with white dead nettle flower.

Interactions with Diseases or Conditions
No interactions are known to occur, and there is no known reason to expect a clinically significant interaction with white dead nettle flower.

Dosage and Administration
ORAL: The average daily dose is 3 grams (2).
TOPICAL: 5 grams of the white dead nettle flower is commonly added to a sitz bath (2).

Comments
Avoid confusion with stinging nettle herb and stinging nettle root.

WHITE HELLEBORE

Also Known As
European Hellebore, European White Hellebore, Langwort.
CAUTION: See separate listings for Black Hellebore, American Hellebore, Pheasant's Eye (false hellebore).

Scientific Names
Veratrum album.
Family: Liliaceae.

People Use This For
Orally, white hellebore is used to treat cholera, gout, and hypertension (6).
Topically, it is used for herpetic lesions (6).
In Roman times, it was used as a poison. An extract has been used as an arrow tip poison (6).
It has also been used as an insecticide against flies and mosquitoes (6).

Safety
LIKELY UNSAFE ...when used orally. All plant parts are considered toxic (6). Between 10-20 mg of alkaloids (1-2 grams of rhizome/root) are lethal (6,18). ...when used topically. Toxic alkaloids can be absorbed through intact skin (6,18).
PREGNANCY: LIKELY UNSAFE ...when used orally or topically because it could be teratogenic (6); avoid using.
LACTATION: LIKELY UNSAFE ...when used orally or topically; avoid using.

Effectiveness
There is insufficient reliable information available about the effectiveness of white hellebore.

Mechanism of Action
The applicable parts of white hellebore are the rhizome and root. White hellebore contains the toxic ester-alkaloids protoveratirine A and B (13), which are sensory nerve irritants (18). These alkaloids inhibit the inactivation of the sodium ion channels and thus have a paralyzing effect on many excitable cells, including those of the heart (18).

Adverse Reactions
Orally, white hellebore can cause mucous membrane irritation (18), a burning sensation in upper abdomen, salivation, vomiting, gastric erosion, severe hypotension, bradycardia, and shock (6,553). Large doses may cause central respiratory depression, blindness, paralysis, convulsions, cardiac arrhythmias, and death (6).
Topically, it can cause skin irritation (18) and the toxic alkaloids could be absorbed.
By inhalation, the powdered root induces violent sneezing and runny nose (6).

Interactions with Herbs & Other Dietary Supplements
Insufficient reliable information available.

Interactions with Drugs
No interactions are known to occur, and there is no known reason to expect a clinically significant interaction with white hellebore.

Interactions with Foods
No interactions are known to occur, and there is no known reason to expect a clinically significant interaction with white hellebore.

Interactions with Lab Tests
No interactions are known to occur, and there is no known reason to expect a clinically significant interaction with white hellebore.

Interactions with Diseases or Conditions
No interactions are known to occur, and there is no known reason to expect a clinically significant interaction with white hellebore.

Dosage and Administration
No typical dosage.

Comments
Crude white hellebore is not used therapeutically (13), though it is sometimes used in homeopathic dilutions (18).

WHITE HOREHOUND

Also Known As
Common Hoarhound, Hoarhound, Horehound, Houndsbane, Marrubii herba, Marrubium, Mastranzo.
CAUTION: See separate listing for Black Horehound.

Scientific Names
Marrubium vulgare.
Family: Lamiaceae.

People Use This For
Orally, white horehound is used for loss of appetite (2), cough and bronchitis, respiratory tract mucous membrane inflammation, indigestion, bloating and flatulence, and liver and gallbladder complaints (4,18,512).
Topically, white horehound is used for skin damage, ulcers, and wounds (18).
In traditional medicine, white horehound is used orally for whooping cough, asthma, tuberculosis, diarrhea, jaundice, debility, painful menstruation, as a laxative (18), an anthelmintic (515), as a diuretic, and to induce sweating (6).
In manufacturing, the extracts of white horehound are used as flavoring in foods and beverages (11), and as an expectorant in cough syrups and lozenges (515).

Safety
LIKELY SAFE ...when used orally in amounts found in foods. It has Generally Recognized as Safe (GRAS) status in the US (11). The maximum use level is 0.073% for the extract.
POSSIBLY SAFE ...when used orally and appropriately (2,12).
POSSIBLY UNSAFE ...when used orally in excessive amounts because it can have a purgative effect (4,12).
There is insufficient reliable information available about the safety of the topical use of white horehound.
PREGNANCY: LIKELY UNSAFE ...when used orally. It might have abortifacient effect (19), or stimulate menstrual flow and the uterus (12). There is insufficient reliable information available about the safety of topical use during pregnancy; avoid using.
LACTATION: There is insufficient reliable information available about the safety of oral use during lactation; avoid amounts greater than found in foods. There is insufficient reliable information available about the safety of topical useduring lactation; avoid using.

Effectiveness
POSSIBLY EFFECTIVE ...when used orally to stimulate appetite. ...when used orally for bloating (2). ...when used orally for coughs and colds (8,11,515).
There is insufficient reliable information available about the effectiveness of white horehound for its other uses.

Mechanism of Action
The applicable parts of white horehound are the above ground parts. White horehound contains marrubiin, bitter ingredients, volatile oil, and tannins (515). The constituent, marrubiin does not exist in the fresh plant; it is formed from premarrubiin during processing (515). The volatile oil of white horehound exhibits vasodilation, expectorant (11), and antischistosomal activity (4). Some evidence suggests the hydroxycinnamic derivatives might have weak antioxidant activity (11). Other evidence suggests marrubinic acid stimulates bile secretion (515). Marrubiin's expectorant effect results from direct stimulation of bronchial mucosal secretions (512). Marrubiin shows some evidence it can normalize extrasystolic arrhythmias (4,11), but large amounts might cause arrhythmias (4). An alcoholic extract reduces spasms of gastrointestinal tract (515). An aqueous extract demonstrates evidence that it can antagonize serotonin (11) and exerts anti-inflammatory activity (4,11).

Adverse Reactions
Orally, large amounts of white horehound can cause purgative effects (4,12). Skin contact with the irritant in plant juice can cause contact dermatitis (4).

Interactions with Herbs & Other Dietary Supplements
Insufficient reliable information available.

Interactions with Drugs
No interactions are known to occur, and there is no known reason to expect a clinically significant interaction with white horehound.

Interactions with Foods

No interactions are known to occur, and there is no known reason to expect a clinically significant interaction with white horehound

Interactions with Lab Tests

No interactions are known to occur, and there is no known reason to expect a clinically significant interaction with white horehound.

Interactions with Diseases or Conditions

HEART CONDITIONS: Theoretically, large amounts of white horehound might cause arrhythmias (4).

Dosage and Administration

ORAL: A typical dose is 1-2 grams dried above ground parts or one cup tea three times daily before meals to stimulate bile secretion or during the day as an expectorant (8). To make tea, steep 1-2 grams dried above ground parts in 150 mL boiling water 5-10 minutes, and strain (4,8). Up to 4.5 grams dried above ground parts or 2-6 tablespoons of pressed juice (or equivalent preparations) are used per day (2). A typical dose of pressed juice is 30-60 mL daily (18). Liquid extract (1:1 in 25% ethanol), 1-3 mL three times daily (4). Tincture (1:10 in 45% alcohol), 1-2 mL three times daily (4).
TOPICAL: No typical dosage.

Comments

White horehound derives its name from ancient Greece where it was used for treating mad-dog bites (515).

WHITE LILY

Also Known As

Baurenlilien, Farmer's Lily, Madonna Lily, Meadow Lily, White Pond Lily.

Scientific Names

Lilium candidium.
Family: Liliaceae.

People Use This For

Orally, white lily is used for gynecological disorders.
Topically, it is used for ulcers, inflammation, furuncles, finger ulcers, reddened skin, burns, and injuries.
Historically, it has been used as an astringent, anti-inflammatory, softener, pain reliever, diuretic, antihemorrhagic, and expectorant (18).

Safety

There is insufficient reliable information available about the safety of white lily.
Pregnancy and Lactation: Insufficient reliable information available; avoid using.

Effectiveness

There is insufficient reliable information available about the effectiveness of white lily.

Mechanism of Action

The applicable part of white lily is the root and bulb. There is insufficient reliable information available about the possible mechanism of action and active ingredients.

Adverse Reactions

None reported.

Interactions with Herbs & Other Dietary Supplements

Insufficient reliable information available.

Interactions with Drugs

No interactions are known to occur, and there is no known reason to expect a clinically significant interaction with white lily.

Interactions with Foods
No interactions are known to occur, and there is no known reason to expect a clinically significant interaction with white lily.

Interactions with Lab Tests
No interactions are known to occur, and there is no known reason to expect a clinically significant interaction with white lily.

Interactions with Diseases or Conditions
No interactions are known to occur, and there is no known reason to expect a clinically significant interaction with white lily.

Dosage and Administration
ORAL: No typical dosage.
TOPICAL: A thick paste made from the fresh or cooked root is placed in the middle of a compress or poultice and applied to the affected area several times throughout the day (18).

Comments
There is very little scientific information about this product. Our staff is continually analyzing the available information on natural medicines and will add data here as it becomes available.

WHITE MUSTARD

Also Known As
Sinapis albae semen, Weibe Senfsamen.
CAUTION: See separate listings for Black Mustard, Black Mustard Oil, and Hedge Mustard.

Scientific Names
Brassica alba; Sinapis alba.
Family: Cruciferae or Brassicaceae.

People Use This For
Orally, white mustard is used "to brighten and clear" the voice and for those with a tendency for infection (18). Topically, white mustard is used for cough and colds (11,18), pulmonary congestion (2,11), bronchitis (18), joint and soft tissue inflammation, rheumatism (2,18), arthritis (2,11,18), lumbago (11), inflammation of the mouth and pharynx, and hyperemization of the skin (18).
Traditionally, it has been used orally as an emetic, diuretic, and appetite stimulant (6,11) and topically as a counterirritant (6) and a bath to treat paralytic symptoms (18).
In foods and condiments, white mustard is a common flavoring agent (11), and is considered a culinary spice (11).

Safety
LIKELY SAFE ...when used orally in the amounts commonly found in foods (11,12). It has Generally Recognized as Safe (GRAS) status in the US. The maximum level used is 12.4% (11).
POSSIBLY SAFE ...when used orally and appropriately for medicinal purposes (12). ...when used topically and appropriately (12,19).
LIKELY UNSAFE ...when used orally as an emetic because mustard is an irritant. Used as an emetic, the esophageal tissue is twice exposed to the corrosive effects of white mustard (19). Ingestion of a large quantity can cause irritant poisoning (12,19). ...when used topically for more than 15-30 minutes because severe burns can occur (12,19). ...when used topically on a regular basis for more than 2 weeks (2,12,19).
CHILDREN: LIKELY SAFE ...when used orally in food amounts. LIKELY UNSAFE ...when used orally in larger amounts. ...when used topically in children under 6 years of age (2,12,19).
PREGNANCY: LIKELY SAFE ...when used orally in food amounts. LIKELY UNSAFE ...when used orally in larger amounts because white mustard can have abortifacient and menstrual-stimulant properties (19).
LACTATION: Insufficient reliable information available; avoid using.

Effectiveness
POSSIBLY EFFECTIVE ...when used topically for pulmonary congestion and for inflammation of the joints and soft tissue (2).
There is insufficient reliable information available about the effectiveness of white mustard for its other uses.

Mechanism of Action

The applicable part of white mustard is the seed. White mustard seeds contain mustard oil glycosides and mustard oils (2). White mustard contains the glucosinolate sinalbin, which on hydrolysis yields p-hydroxybenzyl isothiocyanate, p-hydroxybenzylamine, and other constituents, such as proteins, fatty oil, and sinapine (11,18). These products of hydrolysis possess irritant and bacteriostatic properties (18). White mustard's pungent taste comes from p-hydroxybenzyl isothiocyanate (11). Some evidence suggests the glucosinolate products can have protective effects against carcinogens (11).

Adverse Reactions

Orally, long-term use of white mustard can increase the risk of nerve damage (2,18). Isothiocyanates, such as those in mustard, can cause endemic goiters (6,11).
Topically, white mustard can cause blistering and skin ulceration, as well as nerve damage (2,12,18,19).

Interactions with Herbs & Other Dietary Supplements

Insufficient reliable information available.

Interactions with Drugs

No interactions are known to occur, and there is no known reason to expect a clinically significant interaction with white mustard.

Interactions with Foods

No interactions are known to occur, and there is no known reason to expect a clinically significant interaction with white mustard.

Interactions with Lab Tests

No interactions are known to occur, and there is no known reason to expect a clinically significant interaction with white mustard.

Interactions with Diseases or Conditions

KIDNEY DISEASE: Irritant poisoning from white mustard can occur in people with kidney disorders (12,19).

Dosage and Administration

ORAL: The average amount of white mustard is 60-150 grams daily (18). To "brighten and clear" the voice, mustard flour, or powdered mustard, is stirred with honey to form balls (18). One or two of these honey balls are taken on an empty stomach (18).
TOPICAL: As a foot bath, 20 to 30 grams of mustard flour is typically mixed in 1 liter of water (18). For a mustard bath, 150 grams of mustard flour in a pouch is commonly placed in the bath (18). For local application, 4 tablespoons (50-70 grams) of the powdered seeds are usually mixed with warm water to form a soft material, which is applied for 10-15 minutes for adults and 5-10 minutes for children older than 6 years of age (2,18). Decrease the application time in individuals with sensitive skin (2). Treatment should not exceed two weeks (2,12,18,19).

Comments

Avoid confusion with other Sinapis or Brassica species (black mustard, Brassica nigra; brown mustard, Brassica juncea).

WHITE SANDALWOOD oil

Also Known As

East Indian Sandalwood Oil, Sanderswood, Santal Oil, White Saunders Oil, Yellow Sandalwood Oil, Yellow Saunders Oil.
CAUTION: See separate listings for Red Sandalwood and White Sandalwood wood.

Scientific Names

Santalum album.
Family: Santalaceae.

People Use This For

Orally, white sandalwood oil is used as an adjuvant therapy for lower urinary tract infection (2), common cold, cough/bronchitis, fevers, urinary tract inflammatory conditions, mouth and pharynx inflammation, liver and gallbladder complaints, and infection (18).

In folk medicine, white sandalwood oil is used orally, for stomachache, vomiting, gonorrhea, pains, "strengthening the heart" (11), headache, urogenital disorders (6), to reduce libido, for heatstroke, sunstroke, and resulting fever (18).
In food and beverages, it is used as a flavor component (11).
In manufacturing, white sandalwood oil is used as a fragrance ingredient in soaps, cosmetics, and perfumes (11).

Safety

LIKELY SAFE ...when used orally in amounts found in food. Approved for food use in the US. The average level used is less than 0.001% (11). ...when used topically in amounts found in cosmetics unless allergic to white sandalwood oil. The maximum use level is 1% in perfumes (11).
POSSIBLY SAFE ...when used orally for short-term medicinal use as enteric-coated products (2).
POSSIBLY UNSAFE ...when used orally for longer than 6 weeks, condition should be medically evaluated (2,19). There is insufficient reliable information available about the safety of the topical use of white sandalwood oil in amounts greater than those found in cosmetics.
PREGNANCY: POSSIBLY SAFE ...when used as a flavoring. LIKELY UNSAFE ...when used orally in medicinal amounts because it might have an abortifacient effect (19); avoid using. There is insufficient reliable information available about the safety of topical use during pregnancy.
LACTATION: Insufficient reliable information available; avoid using amounts greater than those found in foods.

Effectiveness

There is insufficient reliable information available about the effectiveness of white sandalwood oil.

Mechanism of Action

White sandalwood oil is reported to have antifungal, antiseptic, diuretic (11), antibacterial, and spasmolytic activity (2). It is considered to be a kidney irritant (19). Although some evidence suggests it is not irritating, sensitizing, or phototoxic when applied to the skin, the constituent, santolol, can cause contact dermatitis (11).

Adverse Reactions

Orally, use of white sandalwood oil can cause itching, nausea, gastrointestinal complaints, and blood in the urine (18). Topically, use can cause contact dermatitis in sensitive individuals (11).

Interactions with Herbs & Other Dietary Supplements

Insufficient reliable information available.

Interactions with Drugs

No interactions are known to occur, and there is no known reason to expect a clinically significant interaction with white sandalwood oil.

Interactions with Foods

No interactions are known to occur, and there is no known reason to expect a clinically significant interaction with white sandalwood oil

Interactions with Lab Tests

No interactions are known to occur, and there is no known reason to expect a clinically significant interaction with white sandalwood oil.

Interactions with Diseases or Conditions

KIDNEY DISEASE: Contraindicated in kidney disease, particularly in individuals with diseases of the kidney parenchyma (2,19).

Dosage and Administration

ORAL: A typical oral dose is 1-1.5 grams of oil per day in an enteric-coated form; maximum use 6 weeks without medical evaluation (2).

Comments

None.

WHITE SANDALWOOD wood

Also Known As
East Indian Sandalwood, Sandalwood, Santali Lignum Albi, Tan Xiang, White Saunders, Yellow Sandalwood, Yellow Saunders.
CAUTION: See separate listings for Red Sandalwood and White Sandalwood oil.

Scientific Names
Santalum album.
Family: Santalaceae.

People Use This For
Orally, white sandalwood wood is used as an adjunct therapy for lower urinary tract infections (2,18), treating colds, cough, bronchitis, fevers, inflammatory conditions of the mouth, pharynx, or efferent urinary tract, and for liver and gallbladder complaints (18).
In folk medicine, white sandalwood wood is used for heat stroke, sun stroke and associated fever, gonorrhea, and as an anti-aphrodisiac (18).

Safety
POSSIBLY SAFE ...when the wood is used orally and appropriately short-term, for less than 6 weeks (2,12).
POSSIBLY UNSAFE ...when used orally longer than 6 weeks (2,12,18).
PREGNANCY: LIKELY UNSAFE ...when used orally because it is believed to have abortifacient effects (19); avoid using.
LACTATION: Insufficient reliable information available; avoid using.

Effectiveness
There is insufficient reliable information available about the effectiveness of white sandalwood wood.

Mechanism of Action
White sandalwood wood has antibacterial, spasmolytic, and urinary disinfectant activities (2,18).

Adverse Reactions
Orally, white sandalwood wood can cause nausea, gastrointestinal complaints, itching, and hematuria (blood in the urine) (2,18). High doses or use longer than six weeks can cause kidney toxicity (2,12,18). White sandalwood has minimal potential for sensitization (18).

Interactions with Herbs & Other Dietary Supplements
Insufficient reliable information available.

Interactions with Drugs
No interactions are known to occur, and there is no known reason to expect a clinically significant interaction with white sandalwood wood.

Interactions with Foods
No interactions are known to occur, and there is no known reason to expect a clinically significant interaction with white sandalwood wood.

Interactions with Lab Tests
No interactions are known to occur, and there is no known reason to expect a clinically significant interaction with white sandalwood wood.

Interactions with Diseases or Conditions
KIDNEY DISEASE: White sandalwood wood is contraindicated in diseases of kidney parenchyma (2,12,18).

Dosage and Administration
ORAL: The typical dose is 10-20 grams of the wood per day, brewed as a tea or other preparations (2).
White sandalwood wood should not be used for more than a six-week duration (2,12).

Comments
Sandalwood has a very dense composition and is valued as a wood for carving (6). Avoid confusion with red sandalwood (Pterocarpus santalinus) and white sandalwood oil.

WHITE SOAPWORT

Also Known As
Gypsophilae radix, Soapwort.
CAUTION: See separate listing for Red Soapwort.

Scientific Names
Gypsophila paniculata and other Gypsophila species.
Family: Caryophyllaceae.

People Use This For
Orally, white soapwort is used for cough, bronchitis (18), and inflammation of the mucous membrane in the upper and lower respiratory tract (2).
In folk medicine, white soapwort is used topically for chronic skin disorders and eczema (18).

Safety
POSSIBLY SAFE ...when used orally and appropriately (2).
PREGNANCY AND LACTATION: Insufficient reliable information; avoid using.

Effectiveness
POSSIBLY EFFECTIVE ...when used orally for upper and lower respiratory tract mucous membrane inflammation (2).
There is insufficient reliable information available about the effectiveness of white soapwort for its other uses.

Mechanism of Action
The applicable part of white soapwort is the root. White soapwort has expectorant, emetic, antibiotic, and insecticidal effects (18). In large amounts, it is cytotoxic (2). The saponin constituents exhibit expectorant effects (2), and they irritate the gastric mucosa to stimulate the bronchial mucous glands via parasympathetic sensory pathways (7). Saponins can cause stomach upset, nausea, and vomiting (7).

Adverse Reactions
Orally, white soapwort can cause stomach irritation (2), nausea, and vomiting (7).

Interactions with Herbs & Other Dietary Supplements
Insufficient reliable information available.

Interactions with Drugs
No interactions are known to occur, and there is no known reason to expect a clinically significant interaction with white soapwort.

Interactions with Foods
No interactions are known to occur, and there is no known reason to expect a clinically significant interaction with white soapwort.

Interactions with Lab Tests
No interactions are known to occur, and there is no known reason to expect a clinically significant interaction with white soapwort.

Interactions with Diseases or Conditions
GI IRRITATION: Theoretically, the saponin content of white soapwort can exacerbate existing gastrointestinal mucosal irritation (6).

Dosage and Administration
ORAL: The typical dose of white soapwort is 30-150 mg per day of the dried root or 3-15 mg per day of the gysophila saponin or equivalent preparations (2).

Comments
In the Middle Ages, Franciscan and Dominican monks viewed soapwort as a divine gift that was meant to keep them clean (6). Avoid confusion with the red soapwort root.

WILD CARROT

Also Known As
Beesnest Plant, Bird's Nest Root, Daucus, Queen Anne's Lace.
CAUTION: See separate listings for Hemlock and Water Hemlock.

Scientific Names
Daucus carota L. subspecies carota.
Family: Apiaceae or Umbelliferae.

People Use This For
Orally, wild carrot is used for urinary calculus or stones, high uric acid in urine, cystitis, and gout (4).
Traditionally, wild carrot seed oil has been used for dysentery, indigestion, uterine pain, gout, heart disease, cancer, kidney problems, as a nerve tonic, a diuretic, an antiflatulent, an aphrodisiac, to induce menstruation, and as an anthelmintic (6,11).
For food uses, wild carrot is used as a flavoring agent in alcoholic and non-alcoholic beverages, frozen dairy desserts, candy, baked goods, gelatins, puddings, meat and meat products, condiments relishes, and soups (4,11).
In manufacturing, wild carrot seed oil is used as a fragrance in soaps, detergents, creams, lotions, and perfumes (11).

Safety
LIKELY SAFE ...when wild carrot seed oil is used in food. It has Generally Recognized as Safe (GRAS) status in the US (11). Maximum amount found in foods is less than 0.003% (11).
POSSIBLY SAFE ...when wild carrot seed oil is used orally and appropriately in medicinal amounts (4,11).
LIKELY UNSAFE ...when an excessive amount of wild carrot seed oil is used orally, it can cause renal irritation (4). Theoretically, high doses of oil could cause neurological effects (6) because the seed contains the psychoactive agent myristicin.
There is insufficient reliable information available about the safety of the oral use of the above ground parts of wild carrot.
PREGNANCY: LIKELY UNSAFE ...when used orally. The seeds, oil, and above ground parts can cause uterine stimulant, abortifacient, and menstrual stimulant effects (19).
LACTATION: POSSIBLY UNSAFE ...when the seed oil is used orally. Wild carrot seed oil has mild estrogenic activity and irritant effects (4). There is insufficient reliable information available about the safety of the oral use of the seeds or above ground parts during lactation.

Effectiveness
There is insufficient reliable information available about the effectiveness of wild carrot.

Mechanism of Action
The applicable parts of wild carrot are the fruit and seed. Wild carrot fruit/seed contains flavones including apigenin, chrysin, luteolin; flavonols including kaempferol and quercetin and various glycosides. The amount and composition of the volatile oil contained in the fruit/seed varies between different cultivars. The furanocoumarins, 8-methoxypsoralen and 5 methoxypsoralen are found in the plant (4). Some evidence suggests that wild carrot might have significant antifertility activity (4,3858). Other evidence suggests that wild carrot has cholinergic-type actions, perhaps due to the choline constituents (4). Wild carrot seed oil shows some evidence of vasodilation, cardiac depressant, and smooth muscle relaxation effects (11). Terpinen-4-ol, a component of the seed oil, is a renal irritant and believed to cause a diuretic effect (4). A tertiary base isolated from wild carrot seed appears to have papaverine-like antispasmodic activity.

Adverse Reactions
Orally, ingesting excessive doses can cause renal irritation or neurological effects. Hypersensitivity reactions and increased sensitivity to UV light and sunburn might occur (19,4).
Topically, contact with the plant can cause dermatitis (4).

Interactions with Herbs & Other Dietary Supplements
HERBS WITH SEDATIVE PROPERTIES: Theoretically, concomitant use with herbs that have sedative properties might enhance therapeutic and adverse effects. These include calamus, calendula, California poppy, catnip, capsicum, celery, couch grass, elecampane, Siberian ginseng, German chamomile, goldenseal, gotu kola, hops, Jamaican dogwood, kava, lemon balm, sage, St. John's wort, sassafras, scullcap, shepherd's purse, stinging nettle, valerian, wild lettuce, ashwaganda root, and yerba mansa (4,19).
HERBS WITH ANTICOAGULANT/ANTIPLATELET POTENTIAL: Concomitant use of herbs that have coumarin constituents or affect platelet aggregation could theoretically increase the risk of bleeding in some people. These herbs include: angelica, anise, arnica, asafoetida, bogbean, boldo, capsicum, celery, chamomile, clove, danshen,

fenugreek, feverfew, garlic, ginger, ginkgo, Panax ginseng, horse chestnut, horseradish, licorice, meadowsweet, prickly ash, onion, papain, passionflower, poplar, quassia, red clover, turmeric, wild lettuce, willow, and others (4,19).

Interactions with Drugs
HORMONES: Theoretically, excessive use of the above ground parts of wild carrot might interfere with hormonal therapy (4).
CARDIAC OR BLOOD PRESSURE MEDICATIONS: Theoretically, excessive doses of wild carrot seed oil might affect therapy (4).
PSORALENS: Concomitant use of psoralens is contraindicated due to the potential of an additive, photosensitizing effect (19).

Interactions with Foods
No interactions are known to occur, and there is no known reason to expect a clinically significant interaction with wild carrot.

Interactions with Lab Tests
No interactions are known to occur, and there is no known reason to expect a clinically significant interaction with wild carrot.

Interactions with Diseases or Conditions
UV LIGHT THERAPY: Contraindicated due to photosensitizing effect; avoid excessive periods in the sun (19).
RENAL INFLAMMATION/IRRITATION: Contraindicated due to renal irritant properties (4,19).

Dosage and Administration
ORAL: Dried above ground parts: 2-4 grams or as tea three times daily. To make tea, steep 2-4 grams of above ground parts in boiling water for 5-10 minutes, strain (4). Liquid extract (1:1 in 25% alcohol) 2-4 mL three times daily (4).

Comments
Carrot seed oil is steam-distilled from the dried root of both the familiar vegetable known as carrot, and the wild carrot. Avoid confusing wild carrot (which has an inedible white tap root) with the common carrot (Daucus carota subspecies sativus) (4).

WILD CHERRY

Also Known As
Black Cherry, Black Choke, Choke Cherry, Rum Cherry Bark, Virginian Prune, Wild Black Cherry.
CAUTION: See separate listing for Cherry Laurel Water.

Scientific Names
Prunus serotina; Prunus virginiana.
Family: Rosaceae.

People Use This For
Orally, wild cherry is used for colds, whooping cough, bronchitis and other lung problems, diarrhea, gout, digestive disorders, pain, and cancer. It is also used in cough syrups because of its sedative, expectorant, astringent, and antitussive effects.
In foods and beverages, wild cherry is used as a flavoring agent.

Safety
LIKELY SAFE ...when used orally in amounts found in foods and beverages. It has Generally Recognized as Safe (GRAS) status in the US (11).
POSSIBLY SAFE ...when used orally and appropriately short-term, in limited amounts (12).
POSSIBLY UNSAFE ...when used orally and long-term or in excessive amounts (12,19). The constituent, prunasin, hydrolyzes to hydrocyanic acid (HCN) (11,12,13,18).
PREGNANCY: LIKELY UNSAFE ...when used orally because prunasin is potentially teratogenic (19).
LACTATION: Insufficient reliable information available; avoid using.

Effectiveness
There is insufficient reliable information available about the effectiveness of wild cherry.

Mechanism of Action

The applicable part of wild cherry is the stem bark. Wild cherry bark has astringent, antitussive, and sedative effects (18). It contains prunasin, a cyanogenic glycoside that is hydrolyzed to toxic hydrocyanic acid (HCN) and benzaldehyde (11). Bark collected in the fall has a higher HCN yield (approximately 0.15%) than bark collected in the spring (approximately 0.05%). Leaves collected in the spring have the highest HCN yield (approximately 0.25%) (11).

Adverse Reactions

Orally, large amounts of wild cherry can lead to fatal poisonings (18).

Interactions with Herbs & Other Dietary Supplements

Insufficient reliable information available.

Interactions with Drugs

DRUGS METABOLIZED BY CYTOCHROME P450 3A4: There's preliminary evidence that wild cherry can inhibit the cytochrome P450 (CYP450) 3A4 enzyme (6450). Theoretically, wild cherry might increase levels of drugs metabolized by CYP450 3A4. However, so far, this interaction has not been reported in humans. Some drugs metabolized by CYP450 3A4 include lovastatin (Mevacor), ketoconazole (Nizoral), itraconazole (Sporanox), fexofenadine (Allegra), triazolam (Halcion), and numerous others. Use wild cherry cautiously or avoid in patients taking these drugs.

Interactions with Foods

No interactions are known to occur, and there is no known reason to expect a clinically significant interaction with wild cherry.

Interactions with Lab Tests

No interactions are known to occur, and there is no known reason to expect a clinically significant interaction with wild cherry.

Interactions with Diseases or Conditions

No interactions are known to occur, and there is no known reason to expect a clinically significant interaction with wild cherry.

Dosage and Administration

ORAL: People use 5 to 12 drops of the liquid extract containing wild cherry bark (12-14% by volume) in water two to three times daily (5023).

Comments

Avoid confusion with cherry laurel water. In Chinese medicine, the stem and bark of related species (Prunus armeniaca) may be effective as an antidote for apricot kernel poisoning (18).

WILD DAISY

Also Known As

Bruisewort.

Scientific Names

Bellis perennis.
Family: Asteraceae.

People Use This For

In folk medicine, wild daisy is used orally for coughs, bronchitis, disorders of the liver and kidneys, inflammation, and as an expectorant and astringent. It is used topically in folk medicine for wounds and skin diseases. Historically, it was used as a "blood purifier" (18).

Safety

There is insufficient reliable information available about the safety of wild daisy.
Pregnancy and Lactation: Insufficient reliable information available; avoid using.

Effectiveness

There is insufficient reliable information available about the effectiveness of wild daisy.

Mechanism of Action
There is insufficient reliable information available about the possible mechanism of action and active ingredients.

Adverse Reactions
Wild daisy can cause an allergic reaction in individuals sensitive to the Asteraceae/Compositae family. Members of this family include ragweed, chrysanthemums, marigolds, daisies, and many other herbs.

Interactions with Herbs & Other Dietary Supplements
Insufficient reliable information available.

Interactions with Drugs
No interactions are known to occur, and there is no known reason to expect a clinically significant interaction with wild daisy.

Interactions with Foods
No interactions are known to occur, and there is no known reason to expect a clinically significant interaction with wild daisy.

Interactions with Lab Tests
No interactions are known to occur, and there is no known reason to expect a clinically significant interaction with wild daisy.

Interactions with Diseases or Conditions
CROSS-ALLERGENICITY: Can cause an allergic reaction in individuals sensitive to the Asteraceae/Compositae family. Members of this family include ragweed, chrysanthemums, marigolds, daisies, and many other herbs.

Dosage and Administration
ORAL: One cup of tea taken orally 2-4 times daily. The tea is prepared by steeping 2 teaspoons of dried herb in 300 mL of boiling water for 20 minutes and straining (18).
TOPICAL: No typical dosage.

Comments
There is very little scientific information about this product. Our staff is continually analyzing the available information on natural medicines and will add data here as it becomes available.

WILD INDIGO

Also Known As
American Indigo, Baptista Tinctoria, False Indigo, Horsefly Weed, Indigo Broom, Rattlebush, Yellow Broom, Yellow Indigo.

Scientific Names
Baptista tinctoria.
Family: Leguminosae or Fabaceae.

People Use This For
Orally, wild indigo is used for diphtheria, influenza, malaria, septic angina, and typhoid fever with prostration. It is also used for upper respiratory tract infections, common head cold, tonsillitis, stomatitis, inflammation of the mouth and throat mucous membranes, fever, lymphadenitis, furunculosis (18), and Crohn's disease (392).
Topically, wild indigo is used for painless ulcers, inflamed nipples, and as a douche for leukorrhea.
Historically, it has been used as an oral tea for fever, scarlet fever, typhoid, and pharyngitis in North America. It has been used topically for cleaning open and inflamed wounds (18).

Safety
UNSAFE …when used orally or topically, long-term; contraindicated due to potential toxicity (12,19).
PREGNANCY AND LACTATION: UNSAFE …when used orally or topically due to its toxic potential (12,19).

Effectiveness
There is insufficient reliable information available about the effectiveness of wild indigo.

Mechanism of Action
The applicable part of wild indigo is the root. Preliminary evidence suggests that glycoprotein constituents might have lymphocyte stimulating activity (393). Quinolizidine alkaloids cause gastrointestinal symptoms with high doses (18).

Adverse Reactions
Orally, large doses can cause vomiting, diarrhea, gastrointestinal complaints, and spasms (12).

Interactions with Herbs & Other Dietary Supplements
Insufficient reliable information available.

Interactions with Drugs
No interactions are known to occur, and there is no known reason to expect a clinically significant interaction with wild indigo.

Interactions with Foods
No interactions are known to occur, and there is no known reason to expect a clinically significant interaction with wild indigo.

Interactions with Lab Tests
No interactions are known to occur, and there is no known reason to expect a clinically significant interaction with wild indigo.

Interactions with Diseases or Conditions
GASTRIC DISORDERS: Use of wild indigo is contraindicated in patients with inflammatory gastrointestinal conditions, particularly with accompanying capillary congestion (19).

Dosage and Administration
ORAL: One cup of tea taken orally 3 times daily. The tea is prepared by simmering 0.5-1 grams dried root in 150 mL of boiling water for 10-15 minutes and straining (18).
TOPICAL: An ointment is prepared using one part of liquid extract to 8 parts of ointment base and applied to the affected area (18).

Comments
None.

WILD LETTUCE

Also Known As
Acrid Lettuce, Bitter Lettuce, German Lactucarium, Green Endive, Lactucarium, Lettuce Opium, Poison Lettuce, Strong-Scented Lettuce.

Scientific Names
Lactuca virosa.
Family: Asteraceae or Compositae.

People Use This For
Orally, wild lettuce is used for whooping cough, mucous inflammations of the bronchial tract, asthma, urinary tract diseases (18), and irritable cough (4). The seed oil is used orally for arteriosclerosis and as a substitute for wheat germ oil (18).
Topically, wild lettuce latex is used as an antiseptic.
Traditionally, wild lettuce is used for insomnia, restlessness, and excitability in children, priapism, painful menses, nymphomania, muscular or joint pains (4), for aiding circulation, swollen genitals, and opium substitute in cough preparations (6).
By inhalation, wild lettuce is used for a recreational "high" or hallucinogenic effect (6).

Safety
POSSIBLY SAFE …when used orally and appropriately (12,4).
LIKELY UNSAFE …when used orally in large doses because they can cause stupor, depressed respiration, and even death (4).
PREGNANCY AND LACTATION: Insufficient reliable information available; avoid using.

Effectiveness

There is insufficient reliable information available about the effectiveness of wild lettuce.

Mechanism of Action

The applicable parts of wild lettuce are the latex and leaf. Wild lettuce is thought to have mild sedative, analgesic, and hypnotic or tranquilizing effects (4,18). Wild lettuce contains lactucin and lactupicrin (4). The milky latex, known as lactucarium, can cause mydriasis (4). This effect is theorized to be due to the presence of hyoscyamine (4); however, the dried sap contains no hyoscyamine (4). Wild lettuce has sedative activity (4). Lactucin, lactupicrin, and hyoscyamine have all been proposed responsible for this activity, but the active constituent(s) has not been identified (4). Low concentrations (nanogram amounts) of morphine have been found in Lactuca species and are considered too low to have a pharmacological effect (4).

Adverse Reactions

Orally, large amounts can cause sweating, increased respiration, tachycardia, pupil dilation, dizziness, ringing in the ears, vision disorders, pressure in the head, somnolence, excitatory states (18), respiratory depression, coma, and death (4).

Topically, wild lettuce can cause contact dermatitis (4). It can cause an allergic reaction in individuals sensitive to the Asteraceae/Compositae family. Members of this family include ragweed, chrysanthemums, marigolds, daisies, and many other herbs.

Interactions with Herbs & Other Dietary Supplements

HERBS WITH SEDATIVE PROPERTIES: Theoretically, concomitant use with herbs that have sedative properties might enhance therapeutic and adverse effects. These include: calamus, calendula flowers, California poppy plant, catnip leaves, capsicum fruit, celery, couch grass, elecampane, Siberian ginseng, German chamomile, goldenseal, gotu kola, hops, Jamaican dogwood bark, kava root, lemon balm, passionflower, sage, St. John's wort, sassafras bark, scullcap plant, shepherd's purse, stinging nettle, valerian root/rhizome, wild carrot, ashwaganda root, and yerba mansa (4,19).

HERBS WITH ANTICOAGULANT/ANTIPLATELET POTENTIAL: Concomitant use of herbs that have coumarin constituents or affect platelet aggregation could theoretically increase the risk of bleeding in some people. These herbs include: angelica, anise, arnica, asafoetida, bogbean, boldo, capsicum, celery, chamomile, clove, danshen, fenugreek, feverfew, garlic, ginger, ginkgo, ginseng (Panax), horse chestnut, horseradish, licorice, meadowsweet, prickly ash, onion, papain, passionflower, poplar, quassia, red clover, turmeric, wild carrot, willow, and others (4,19).

Interactions with Drugs

DRUGS WITH SEDATIVE PROPERTIES: Theoretically, concomitant use with drugs with sedative effects might cause additive effects and adverse effects (19).

Interactions with Foods

No interactions are known to occur, and there is no known reason to expect a clinically significant interaction with wild lettuce.

Interactions with Lab Tests

No interactions are known to occur, and there is no known reason to expect a clinically significant interaction with wild lettuce.

Interactions with Diseases or Conditions

BENIGN PROSTATIC HYPERPLASIA (BPH): Contraindicated in prostate enlargement (12). Wild lettuce might contain hyoscyamine (4) which is contraindicated in conditions involving urinary retention, including BPH (15).

CROSS-ALLERGENICITY: Wild lettuce can cause an allergic reaction in individuals sensitive to members of the Asteraceae/Compositae plant family. Members of this family include ragweed, chrysanthemums, marigolds, daisies, and many other herbs.

NARROW-ANGLE GLAUCOMA: Contraindicated (12). Wild lettuce might contain hyoscyamine (4) which can exacerbate narrow-angle (closed-angle) glaucoma (15).

Dosage and Administration

ORAL: A typical dose is 0.5-3 grams dried leaves or as tea three times daily. To make tea, steep 0.5 - 3 grams dried leaves in 150 mL of boiling water, strain (4). As the liquid extract (1:1 in 25% alcohol), 0.5 - 3 mL three times daily (4). For the dried latex extract, lactucarium, 0.3 -1 grams three times daily (4). Also available as a soft extract, with the usual dose of 0.3 - 1 grams three times daily (4).

Comments

None.

WILD MINT

Also Known As

Hairy Mint, Marsh Mint, Water Mint.

Scientific Names

Mentha aquatica.
Family: Labiatae or Lamiaceae.

People Use This For

Orally, wild mint is used for diarrhea and painful menstruation. It is also used as an astringent and stimulant (18).

Safety

There is insufficient reliable information available about the safety of wild mint.
Pregnancy and Lactation: Insufficient reliable information available; avoid using.

Effectiveness

There is insufficient reliable information available about the effectiveness of wild mint.

Mechanism of Action

The applicable part of wild mint is the leaf. There is insufficient reliable information available about the possible mechanism of action and active ingredients.

Adverse Reactions

None reported.

Interactions with Herbs & Other Dietary Supplements

Insufficient reliable information available.

Interactions with Drugs

No interactions are known to occur, and there is no known reason to expect a clinically significant interaction with wild mint.

Interactions with Foods

No interactions are known to occur, and there is no known reason to expect a clinically significant interaction with wild mint.

Interactions with Lab Tests

No interactions are known to occur, and there is no known reason to expect a clinically significant interaction with wild mint.

Interactions with Diseases or Conditions

No interactions are known to occur, and there is no known reason to expect a clinically significant interaction with wild mint.

Dosage and Administration

ORAL: One small cup of tea is taken orally throughout the day.

Comments

There is very little scientific information about this product. Our staff is continually analyzing the available information on natural medicines and will add data here as it becomes available.

WILD RADISH

Also Known As
Joint-Podded Charlock.

Scientific Names
Raphanus raphanistrum.
Family: Brassicaceae.

People Use This For
Orally, wild radish is used for skin conditions and stomach disorders (18).

Safety
There is insufficient reliable information available about the safety of wild radish.
Pregnancy and Lactation: Insufficient reliable information available; avoid using.

Effectiveness
There is insufficient reliable information available about the effectiveness of wild radish.

Mechanism of Action
The applicable part of wild radish is the fresh plant before flowering. Wild radish contains glucosinolates (glucopurtranjivine) in freshly harvested, unbruised plants that produce isopropyl mustard oil upon aging (18).

Adverse Reactions
Orally, use of the wild radish plant at high doses can cause mucous membrane irritation of the GI tract (18).

Interactions with Herbs & Other Dietary Supplements
Insufficient reliable information available.

Interactions with Drugs
No interactions are known to occur, and there is no known reason to expect a clinically significant interaction with wild radish.

Interactions with Foods
No interactions are known to occur, and there is no known reason to expect a clinically significant interaction with wild radish.

Interactions with Lab Tests
No interactions are known to occur, and there is no known reason to expect a clinically significant interaction with wild radish.

Interactions with Diseases or Conditions
No interactions are known to occur, and there is no known reason to expect a clinically significant interaction with wild radish.

Dosage and Administration
ORAL: Wild radish plant is used ground or as an alcoholic extract (18).

Comments
There is very little scientific information about this product. Our staff is continually analyzing the available information on natural medicines and will add data here as it becomes available.

WILD THYME

Also Known As
Mother of Thyme, Serpyllum, Shepherd's Thyme.
CAUTION: See separate listings for Thyme, Spanish Origanum oil, and Thyme Oil.

Scientific Names

Thymus serpyllum.
Family: Labiatae or Lamiaceae.

People Use This For

Orally, wild thyme is used for cough, bronchitis, and inflammation of the respiratory tract.
In folk medicine, it is used orally for kidney and bladder disorders, to relieve flatulence and colic, as a digestive aid, expectorant, aromatic, and antimicrobial. It is used topically in folk medicine for arthritis and sprains (18).

Safety

LIKELY SAFE ...when used in amounts found in foods. Wild thyme has Generally Recognized as Safe (GRAS) status in the US (4083).
POSSIBLY SAFE ...when preparations of the above ground flowering parts are used orally and appropriately (12).
PREGNANCY AND LACTATION: LIKELY SAFE ...when used orally in food amounts; avoid using in amounts greater than those typically found in foods.

Effectiveness

There is insufficient reliable information available about the effectiveness of wild thyme.

Mechanism of Action

The applicable parts of wild thyme are the above ground, flowering parts. There is insufficient reliable information available about the possible mechanism of action and active ingredients.

Adverse Reactions

None reported.

Interactions with Herbs & Other Dietary Supplements

Insufficient reliable information available.

Interactions with Drugs

No interactions are known to occur, and there is no known reason to expect a clinically significant interaction with wild thyme.

Interactions with Foods

No interactions are known to occur, and there is no known reason to expect a clinically significant interaction with wild thyme.

Interactions with Lab Tests

No interactions are known to occur, and there is no known reason to expect a clinically significant interaction with wild thyme.

Interactions with Diseases or Conditions

THYROID DISORDERS: Can suppress thyroid function by decreasing hormone production and/or release (19).

Dosage and Administration

ORAL: One cup of tea taken orally before meals. The tea is prepared by steeping 1.5-2 grams dried plant in 150 mL of boiling water for 10 minutes and straining. The daily dose is equivalent to 4-6 grams dried herb (18).

Comments

None.

WILD YAM

Also Known As

Atlantic Yam, Barbasco, China Root, Colic Root, Devil's Bones, Dioscorea, Dioscoreae, Mexican Yam, Natural DHEA, Phytoestrogen, Rheumatism Root, Wild Mexican Yam, Yam, Yuma.
CAUTION: See separate listings for Pregnenolone and Progesterone.

Scientific Names

Discorea composita; Discorea floribunda; Discorea mexicana, synonym Dioscorea macrostachya; Discorea villosa. Family: Dioscoreaceae.

People Use This For

Orally, wild yam is used as a "natural alternative" for estrogen replacement therapy (515), postmenopausal vaginal dryness (5121), premenstrual syndrome, osteoporosis (5125), increasing energy and libido in men and women (5127), and for breast enlargement (5121). Wild yam is also used orally for treating diverticulosis (5121), gallbladder colic, painful menstruation, cramps (18), rheumatoid arthritis (5124), and for increasing energy (5126).
The constituent of wild yam root, diosgenin, is used as a precursor for commercial chemical synthesis of human steroidal hormones (515,816).

Safety

POSSIBLY SAFE ...when used orally (12).
There is insufficient reliable information available about the safety of the topical use of wild yam.
PREGNANCY AND LACTATION: Insufficient reliable information available; avoid using.

Effectiveness

There is insufficient reliable information available about the effectiveness of wild yam.

Mechanism of Action

The applicable part of wild yam is the root/rhizome. The tubers of Dioscorea species contain the glycoside diosgenin, a steroid precursor that was used in the first commercial production of oral contraceptives, topical hormones, systemic corticosteroids, androgens, estrogens, progestogens, and other sex hormones (515). Dioscorea continues to be used as the precursor for manufacturing progesterone contained in some "natural progesterone" cosmetic products. The chemical transformation of diosgenin to estrogen, progesterone, or any other steroidal compound does not occur in the human body (515). Diosgenin prevents estrogen-induced bile flow suppression (5129). It shows some evidence that it might stimulate growth of mammary tissue (5130), and attenuate indomethacin-induced intestinal inflammation (5131). A wild yam extract enhances estradiol binding to estrogen receptors and induces transcription activity in estrogen-responsive cells (6180).

Adverse Reactions

Orally, ingestion of large amounts of wild yam tincture has caused emesis (12).

Interactions with Herbs & Other Dietary Supplements

Insufficient reliable information is available.

Interactions with Drugs

No interactions are known to occur, and there is no known reason to expect a clinically significant interaction with wild yam.

Interactions with Foods

No interactions are known to occur, and there is no known reason to expect a clinically significant interaction with wild yam.

Interactions with Lab Tests

No interactions are known to occur, and there is no known reason to expect a clinically significant interaction with wild yam.

Interactions with Diseases or Conditions

HORMONE SENSITIVE CANCERS/CONDITIONS: Because wild yam might have estrogenic effects (6180), women with hormone sensitive conditions should avoid wild yam. Some of these conditions include breast, uterine, and ovarian cancer; and endometriosis and uterine fibroids.

Dosage and Administration

No typical dosage.

Comments

Diosgenin, a component of wild yam, is promoted as a natural precursor to dehydroepiandosterone (DHEA) (see separate listing for DHEA). Some wild yam products are promoted as "natural DHEA." Although diosgenin can be converted to steroidal compounds, including DHEA, in the laboratory, this chemical synthesis does not occur in the human body. So taking wild yam extract will not increase DHEA levels in humans (515,2112). People interested in taking DHEA should avoid wild yam products labeled as "natural DHEA."

WILLARD WATER

Also Known As

Biowater, Carbonaceous Activated Water, Catalyst Altered Water, Williard's Water.

Scientific Names

None.

People Use This For

Orally, Willard water is used for arthritis, acne, anxiety, nervous stomach, hypertension, ulcers, and hair growth. In manufacturing, it has been used as a food preserver, laundry aid, and a treatment for bovine and feline leukemia (6).

Safety

There is insufficient reliable information available about the safety of Willard water.
Pregnancy and Lactation: Insufficient reliable information available; avoid using.

Effectiveness

There is insufficient reliable information available about the effectiveness of Willard water.

Mechanism of Action

The formula for Willard water has changed over time. Some of the ingredients found in products analyzed by the FDA included rock salt in various combinations, lignite, sodium metasilicate, sulfated castor oil, calcium chloride, and magnesium sulfate (18).

Adverse Reactions

None reported.

Interactions with Herbs & Other Dietary Supplements

Insufficient reliable information available.

Interactions with Drugs

No interactions are known to occur, and there is no known reason to expect a clinically significant interaction with Willard water.

Interactions with Foods

No interactions are known to occur, and there is no known reason to expect a clinically significant interaction with Willard water

Interactions with Lab Tests

No interactions are known to occur, and there is no known reason to expect a clinically significant interaction with Willard water.

Interactions with Diseases or Conditions

No interactions are known to occur, and there is no known reason to expect a clinically significant interaction with Willard water.

Dosage and Administration

No typical dosage.

Comments
Willard water was developed in the early twentieth century at the South Dakota School of Mines by a chemistry professor named John Wesley Willard, Ph.D. It was developed and patented as an industrial cleanser to clean and degrease train parts. However, it became legendary among townsfolk who used Williard water to treat almost every disease known to humans and animals, and as a plant fertilizer. It is not recognized as safe or effective by the FDA (6).

WILLOW BARK

Also Known As
Basket Willow, Bay Willow, Brittle Willow, Crack Willow, Daphne Willow, Knackweide, Laurel Willow, Lorbeerweide, Osier Rouge, Pupurweide, Purple Osier, Purple Osier Willow, Reifweide, Salicis cortex, Silberweide, Violet Willow, Weidenrinde, White Willow, White Willow Bark, Willowbark.

Scientific Names
Salix alba; Salix daphnoides; Salix fragilis; Salix pentandra; Salix purpurea; other Salix species.
Family: Salicaeae.

People Use This For
Orally, willow bark is used for mild feverish colds and infections, headaches (8), pain (512), pain caused by inflammation (8), muscle and joint aches, influenza, respiratory tract mucous membrane inflammation, gouty arthritis, ankylosing spondylitis, rheumatoid arthritis, and other systemic connective tissue disorders characterized by inflammatory changes (4), and diseases accompanied by fever, and rheumatic ailments (2).
Historically, willow bark has been used for gout and inflammatory joint disease (7).

Safety
POSSIBLY SAFE ...when used orally and appropriately, short-term (2,12,6456). Willow bark has been used safely up to 4 weeks in one study (6456).
CHILDREN: POSSIBLY UNSAFE ...when used orally for viral infections. Although Reye's syndrome has not been reported (12), the salicin constituent in willow bark is similar to aspirin and might pose the same risk (15).
PREGNANCY: Insufficient reliable information available; avoid using.
LACTATION: POSSIBLY UNSAFE ...when used orally. Willow bark contains salicylates which are excreted in breast milk and have been linked to macular rashes in breast-fed infants (4).

Effectiveness
POSSIBLY EFFECTIVE ...when used orally for treating low back pain. There's some evidence that a willow bark extract providing 120-240 mg of the salicin constituent daily can reduce back pain in some patients. The higher concentration of 240 mg salicin is more effective. However, it can take up to 1 week for significant relief (6456). ...when used orally for conditions accompanied by fever, rheumatic ailments, and headaches (2), although the effectiveness of specific products depends on the actual salicin content (8,18).
There is insufficient reliable information available about the effectiveness of willow bark for its other uses.

Mechanism of Action
Willow bark constituents include flavonoids, tannins, and salicylates. Most of the information about willow bark is based on documented pharmacology for salicylates. These actions include anti-inflammatory, antipyretic, dose-dependent hyperglycemic/hypoglycemic, uricosuric/antiuricosuric activities, and increase in blood clotting time and plasma-albumin binding (4). Though researchers long believed salicin was the active principle, studies have shown that a series of phenolic glycosides designated salicortin, fragilin, tremulacin, and others are present, some in larger amounts than true salicin (512). These phenolic glycosides are heat labile and they convert to salicin if willow bark is dried (512). Salicin is a prodrug that is metabolized to saligenin in the gastrointestinal tract and to salicylic acid after absorption (4). Because time is required for the prodrugs to convert to salicylic acid, the properties of willow bark have a slower onset and a longer effectiveness than salicylate itself (3). In vitro tests show that salicin and salicortin inhibit cyclooxygenase. This means irreversible inhibition of thrombocytes is unlikely and there should be no increased interaction with blood coagulants (8). The tannins constituents have astringent properties (4). Tannins also show some evidence of antiviral, antimicrobial, non-specific CNS depressant and cariostatic effects (11). Tannins exert an astringent effect on mucosal tissue. This effect dehydrates the tissue, internally reducing secretions, and externally forming a protective layer of harder, constricted cells (12). Plants with at least 10% tannins can cause gastrointestinal disturbances, kidney damage, and necrotic conditions of the liver (12). Some evidence suggests that tannins might cause cancer, while other evidence shows they may prevent it (12). Regular consumption of herbs with high tannin concentrations correlates with increased incidence of esophageal or nasal cancer (12).

Adverse Reactions

Orally, no adverse reactions have been reported from the use of willow bark. Theoretically, gastrointestinal disturbances, kidney damage, and necrotic conditions of the liver are possible due to the tannin content (12). Theoretically, adverse reactions associated with salicylates are possible including gastric and renal irritation, hypersensitivity, blood in stool, tinnitus, nausea, and vomiting.
Topically, salicin has been associated with skin rashes (4).

Interactions with Herbs & Other Dietary Supplements

SALICYLATE-CONTAINING HERBS: Theoretically, concomitant use may potentiate salicylate effects and adverse effects. Salicylate-containing herbs include aspen bark, black cohosh, poplar, sweet birch, and wintergreen (19).
HERBS WITH ANTICOAGULANT/ANTIPLATELET POTENTIAL: Concomitant use of herbs that have coumarin constituents or affect platelet aggregation could theoretically increase the risk of bleeding in some people. These herbs include: angelica, anise, arnica, asafoetida, bogbean, boldo, capsicum, celery, chamomile, clove, danshen, fenugreek, feverfew, garlic, ginger, ginkgo, ginseng (Panax), horse chestnut, horseradish, licorice, meadowsweet, prickly ash, onion, papain, passionflower, poplar, quassia, red clover, turmeric, wild carrot, wild lettuce, and others (4,19).
TANNIN-CONTAINING HERBS: Theoretically, herbs such as willow bark contain high percentages of tannins, which might cause precipitation of constituents of other herbs (19).

Interactions with Drugs

ANTICOAGULANTS/ANTIPLATELETS: Theoretically, data suggests irreversible inhibition of thrombocytes is unlikely and there should be no increased interaction with blood coagulants (8).
SALICYLATE INTERACTIONS: There is insufficient reliable information available to determine if enough salicylate is present in willow bark to cause drug interactions common to salicylates or aspirin. Aspirin can impair the effectiveness of beta-adrenergic blockers, probenecid, and sulfinpyrazone. It can increase the effects, side effects, or toxicity of alcohol, anticoagulants, carbonic anhydrase inhibitors, heparin, methotrexate, NSAIDS, sulfonylureas, and valproic acid (151).
ORAL DRUGS: Theoretically, concomitant oral administration might cause precipitation of some drugs due to the high tannin content of willow bark (19). Separate administration of oral drugs and tannin-containing herbs by the longest period of time practical (19).

Interactions with Foods

No interactions are known to occur, and there is no known reason to expect a clinically significant interaction with willow bark.

Interactions with Lab Tests

There are no lab interactions reported with willow bark; however, due to the variable salicylate content, use caution in interpreting test results known to be affected by salicylates.

Interactions with Diseases or Conditions

SALICYLATE PRECAUTIONS: Avoid or use cautiously in individuals with aspirin hypersensitivity, asthma, active peptic ulcer disease, diabetes, gout, hemophilia, hypoprothrombinemia, kidney or liver disease (4).
KIDNEY OR LIVER DYSFUNCTION: Theoretically, oral use of willow bark is contraindicated in people with kidney or liver dysfunction because it might exacerbate these conditions. Plants with at least 10% tannins are reported to have the potential to cause kidney damage and liver necrosis (12).

Dosage and Administration

ORAL: For back pain, willow bark extract providing 120-240 mg salicin has been used in a clinical study. The higher 240 mg dose might be more effective (6456). A typical dose for other uses is 1-3 grams dried bark 3-4 times daily, or one cup tea. Or, an average daily dose equivalent to 60-120 mg salicin is commonly used (2).
To make tea, steep 1-3 grams bark in 150 mL of boiling water for 5 minutes, and strain (4,8). Liquid extract (1:1 in 25% alcohol), 1-3 mL three times daily has been used (4).

Comments

Salicylate concentrations vary greatly among Salix species (4,12,512). Salix alba bark is reported to contain 0.49-0.98% salicin (4); Salix purpurea bark contains 3-9%; Salix daphnoides 4.9-5.6%; Salix fragilis 3.9-10.2% (8).
Based on a willow bark content of 7% salicin (superior quality willow bark), 1.5 gallons of willow bark tea per day would have to be consumed to obtain the pain relief of 4.5 grams of aspirin, the average daily dose used to treat arthritic-rheumatic disorders (512).

WINE

Also Known As
None.
CAUTION: See separate listing for Resveratrol.

Scientific Names
Vitis vinifera.
Family: Vitaceae.

People Use This For
Orally, wine is used for reducing the risk of cardiovascular disease, including coronary heart disease, atherosclerosis, and myocardial infarction, and for reducing the risk of ischemic stroke and type 2 diabetes. It is also used orally to prevent cognitive decline in later life and to prevent Alzheimer's disease. Wine is also used orally for anxiety, achlorhydria, malabsorption syndromes, and as an appetite stimulant.
Topically, wine is used to stimulate wound healing and improve rheumatoid skin ulcerations.

Safety
LIKELY SAFE ...when used orally; up to 240mL/day (6,14).
POSSIBLY UNSAFE ...when used orally in excess of 240mL/day. Larger amounts can cause minimal to significant adverse effects (6,14).
PREGNANCY: LIKELY UNSAFE ...when used orally because alcohol is a teratogen. Use during pregnancy, especially during the first two months after conception, is associated with significant risk of spontaneous abortion, as well as fetal alcohol syndrome, and developmental and behavioral dysfunction in infants and children exposed to alcohol in utero (4260).
LACTATION: LIKELY UNSAFE ...when used orally because alcohol is secreted in breast milk. It can cause abnormal psychomotor development, pseudo-Cushing syndrome, alcohol poisoning, and potentiate severe hypoprothrombic bleeding in infants (4260).

Effectiveness
LIKELY EFFECTIVE ...when used orally for preventing cardiovascular disease, including coronary heart disease, atherosclerosis, and myocardial infarction. Consuming alcoholic drinks, including wine, in moderation, one to two drinks per day, seem to reduce the risk of coronary heart disease by approximately 30-50% (2058,2060,2261,2267,2268,2270,2271,6835,6837,6840) (6841,6888,6892). Tell patients not to exceed two drinks per day. More than two drinks daily can increase the risk of cardiovascular and overall mortality (841,2060,2261,6173,6889,6890). Alcoholic beverage consumption does not seem to reduce morbidity and mortality in people with established cardiovascular disease (6173).
POSSIBLY EFFECTIVE ...when used orally for reducing the risk of all-cause mortality. There is some evidence that moderate consumption of alcoholic drinks, including wine, one to two drinks per day, can reduce the risk of all-cause mortality in people who are middle-aged or older (2261,6823,6835,6837,6843). Tell patients not to exceed more than two drinks per day. More than two drinks per day can increase the risk of all-cause mortality (841,2261). ...when used orally in moderation to reduce mortality in people with ischemic left ventricular (LV) dysfunction. Consumption of 1 to 14 drinks per week is associated with reduced all-cause mortality compared with non-drinkers in people with ischemic LV dysfunction. This benefit did not seem to occur for those patients with non-ischemic LV dysfunction (6827). ...when used orally in moderation for reducing the risk of type 2 diabetes in healthy men. Light to moderate alcohol consumption (from 2 drinks per week, up to 3 or 4 drinks per day), from wine and other sources, is associated with a reduced risk of type 2 diabetes in healthy male health professionals (6172,6891). ...when used orally for preventing ischemic stroke. Moderate alcohol consumption (up to 2 drinks per day) appears to reduce the risk of having an ischemic stroke (841,2271,2279,6834,6842,6893). Tell patients to avoid heavy consumption of alcohol. Seven or more drinks per day seems to increase the risk of ischemic stroke (6842). There is also some evidence that any alcohol consumption can increase the risk of hemorrhagic stroke (841,2271). ...when used orally in moderation to maintain cognitive function in later life. Elderly men who have a history of consuming up to one alcoholic drink per day seem to maintain better general cognitive function during their late 70's and 80's compared to non-drinkers (6824,6829). However, consumption of more than 4 drinks per day during middle age seems to be associated with significantly poorer cognitive function in later life (6824).
POSSIBLY INEFFECTIVE ...when used orally for reducing morbidity and mortality in men with established coronary heart disease (CHD) (6173). Consumption of 1-14 alcoholic drinks per week, including wine, has no effect on CHD, cardiovascular disease, or all-cause mortality compared to drinking less than 1 drink per week. More than 3 drinks per day is associated with increased mortality in men with a history of heart attacks (6173).
There is insufficient reliable information available to rate the effectiveness of wine for its other uses. However, there is some evidence that 1-2 drinks per day can reduce the risk of developing Alzheimer's disease in both men and women

compared to non-drinkers (6603). There is also some preliminary evidence that moderate alcohol consumption, equivalent to 1 to 3 glasses of wine per day, in postmenopausal women, is associated with increased bone mineral density in the trochanter and spine (predominantly trabecular bone which is metabolically more active) (6825,6836). There does not appear to be an effect on sites such as the femoral neck which are predominantly cortical bone (6825,6836), and women who drink may still be at increased risk for hip fractures due to falls (6836). There is also some preliminary evidence that intake of up to 21 alcoholic drinks per week, including wine, might slightly reduce the risk of cancer-related mortality (6823). The effect of alcohol on anxiety is complex and may be affected by the psychological state of the user. It sometimes reduces anxiety, sometimes increases it, and sometimes has no effect (2266). More evidence is needed to rate the effectiveness of wine for these uses.

Mechanism of Action

Wine is the natural yeast fermentation product of the juice of sun-ripened grapes, the fruit of Vitis vinifera. Wine normally contains 10-14% alcohol, predominantly as ethanol, which is a central nervous system depressant (2263). Several mechanisms have been proposed for the protective effects of alcohol against coronary heart disease, including increased high-density lipoprotein (HDL) cholesterol levels, lowered low-density lipoprotein (LDL) cholesterol, lowered fibrinogen, increased prostacyclin/thromboxane ratio, and inhibitory effects on platelets and blood clotting (2060,2261,2268,2270,6838,6840,6841). One to two alcoholic drinks per day increases HDL cholesterol by about 12% (6892). This increase in HDL cholesterol levels might account for about 50% of the cardioprotective effect of moderate alcohol consumption (2261,6838,6841). A further 18% of the effect has been attributed to a decrease in LDL cholesterol, but this is counterbalanced by a 17% increase in risk due to increases in blood pressure (6841). The explanation for the remainder of the protective effect is unknown but may include effects on clotting and thrombosis (6841). Effects of alcohol on blood clotting include a reduction in clotting potential and enhancement of clot breakdown (2261). Alcohol consumption decreases platelet aggregation, possibly via inhibition of prostaglandin synthesis (6892). Moderate alcohol consumption is also associated with an increase in plasma levels of tissue-type plasminogen activator, an indicator of fibrinolytic capacity (6894). Moderate alcohol consumption produces a reduction in coronary narrowing due to atherosclerosis (2261,6840). The loss of any protective effect of alcohol against cardiovascular disease at higher intakes may be due to an increase in hypertension, fatal arrhythmias, and direct damage to heart muscle (alcoholic cardiomyopathy) (2060,2261,2267,2270). It has been speculated that some alcoholic beverages, in particular red wine, may be more protective than others against coronary heart disease, but there is no conclusive evidence of this from clinical studies (2267,2268,6892). The speculation is based on the higher concentrations of polyphenolic compounds found in red wine than in other alcoholic drinks, and the antioxidant properties of these polyphenols, which may contribute to protection against CHD by reducing oxidation of LDL cholesterol (2268). The polyphenolic compounds in red wine include trans-resveratrol, proanthocyanidins, and flavonoids such as quercetin, kaempferol, and catechins (1262,2057), but the polyphenol content of wine is highly dependent on grape type, climate, and practices used to make the wine (2057). Unlike red wines, white wines have very low polyphenol concentrations (2030). The antioxidant potential of plasma and erythrocytes is increased for up to 4.5 hours after red wine consumption (6828). However, there is some evidence that the increase of polyphenols in plasma after red wine consumption is not sufficient to acutely influence lipoprotein oxidation (1262,6826). Several red wine components also have in vitro antiplatelet effects, including trans-resveratrol, quercetin, and catechin (2057). However, red wine and white wine seem to have similar activity on platelets (2057,2949). Human data also suggest rebound hypercoagulability can normally occur when acute or chronic alcohol consumption stops, but that red wine attenuates this effect (2060,2061). Red wine might also reduce mutagenic DNA damage and improve endothelial function when added to a high fat diet. Red wine also might have additive vasorelaxing benefits with a low-fat, high plant material diet (2059). Possible mechanisms by which alcohol could have a protective effect against ischemic stroke include increasing HDL and prostacyclin, decreasing fibrinogen, and inhibiting platelet aggregation (6842). Moderate alcohol intake may be protective against the development of type 2 diabetes due to an increase in insulin sensitivity (6891). Moderate alcohol consumption may be protective against postmenopausal bone loss due to an increase in estrogen levels, increased calcitonin secretion and reduced parathyroid hormone secretion (6825,6836). However, heavy and chronic alcohol consumption reduces bone mineral density, possibly due to increased calcium and magnesium excretion, increased cortisol secretion, and reduced osteoblast activity (6836). Chronic alcoholics also often have other risk factors for osteoporosis, including poor nutrition, smoking, sedentary lifestyle, and lower body weight (6825,6836).

Adverse Reactions

Wine can cause a variety of side effects, depending on the amount ingested. They include flushing, confusion, emotional lability, perceptual and sensational disturbances, possible blackout spells, incoordination, trouble walking, central nervous system depression, seizures, drowsiness, respiratory depression, hypothermia, hypoglycemia, lacticacidosis or ketoacidosis, hypokalemia, anemia, thrombocytopenia, nausea, vomiting, diarrhea, abdominal pain and bleeding, and arrhythmias (14). The effects of chronic heavy ethanol ingestion (3 or more alcoholic drinks per day) vary with individuals, but include physical dependence, malnutrition, amnesia, dementia, somnolence, cardiac myopathy, hepatotoxicity, cirrhosis, pancreatitis, hypomagnesemia, acute and chronic skeletal myopathies, Wernicke's encephalopathy, Korsakoff's psychosis, chronic cerebellar syndrome (14), and cancers of the mouth, esophagus, pharynx, larynx, and liver (14,6843). Chronic intake of three or more drinks per day is associated with an increased risk of all-cause mortality, ischemic stroke, and hypertension (2261,6892). Consumption of any amount of alcohol can increase the risk of hemorrhagic stroke (841,2271). Consuming more than one alcoholic drink daily might increase mortality from breast cancer by as much as 30% in women (6843). Repeated topical use of wine can dry the skin (14). Wine is associated with triggering asthmatic reactions in people with a history of asthma, possibly due to salicylates and/or added sulfites contained in wines (6174). People who are allergic to sulfites and/or yeast might react to wine.

Interactions with Herbs & Other Dietary Supplements

HERBS/SUPPLEMENTS WITH SEDATIVE PROPERTIES: Theoretically, concomitant use with herbs that have sedative properties might enhance adverse effects. These include 5-HTP, calamus, calendula, California poppy, catnip, capsicum, celery, couch grass, elecampane, Siberian ginseng, German chamomile, goldenseal, gotu kola, hops, Jamaican dogwood, kava, lemon balm, melatonin, sage, St. John's wort, sassafras, scullcap, shepherd's purse, stinging nettle, valerian, wild carrot, wild lettuce, ashwaganda root, yerba mansa, and others (4,19).

Interactions with Drugs

ASPIRIN/NSAIDs: Concomitant use of aspirin or nonsteroidal anti-inflammatory drugs with alcohol can increase the risk of gastrointestinal bleeding (2262).
BENZODIAZEPINES, BARBITURATES, NARCOTICS: Concomitant consumption of large amounts of alcohol may decrease metabolism of narcotics, barbiturates, and benzodiazepines (15,2262).
CISAPRIDE: Concomitant use of cisapride (Propulsid) might increase blood alcohol levels and effects, due to the alcohol in wine (2262). Red wine increases plasma cisapride concentrations, possibly by reducing metabolism (1383).
CNS DEPRESSANTS: Concomitant use of antihistamines, barbiturates, benzodiazepines, and tricyclic antidepressants with alcohol may increase sedative and other adverse effects (2262).
CYCLOSPORINE: Red wine reduces plasma cyclosporine concentrations, possibly by reducing cyclosprine absorption. In one study, red wine reduced cyclosporine AUC by 36% in caucasian males and 8% in Asian males (1384,1387).
DRUGS THAT CAUSE DISULFIRAM-LIKE REACTIONS: Disulfiram-like reactions can occur when alcohol is used concomitantly with chlorpropamide (Diabinese) (506), disulfiram (Antabuse), tolbutamide (Orinase), metronidazole (Flagyl), sulfonamides, griseofulvin (Fulvicin), cefoperazone (Cefobid), and cefamandole (Mandol) (2262).
ERYTHROMYCIN: Concomitant use of erythromycin with alcohol can increase blood alcohol levels and effect (2262).
H2-RECEPTOR ANTAGONISTS: Concomitant use of cimetidine (Tagamet) and ranitidine (Zantac) with alcohol may increase blood alcohol levels and adverse effects (2262).
HEPATOTOXIC DRUGS: Concomitant use with acetaminophen, isoniazid, and phenylbutazone can increase the risk of hepatotoxicity (2262).
HYPOGLYCEMIC DRUGS: Alcohol may cause hypoglycemia secondary to decreased gluconeogenesis (2263), and concomitant use may increase the risk of hypoglycemia with long-acting sulfonylureas such as chlorpropamide (Diabinese) (2262).
MONOAMINE OXIDASE INHIBITORS (MAOIs): Concomitant use of monoamine oxidase inhibitors with red wine can cause hypertensive crisis due to tyramine content (506).
METFORMIN: Concomitant consumption of large amounts of alcohol may increase the risk of lactic acidosis with metformin (Glucophage) (2262).
PHENYTOIN: Concomitant consumption of large amounts of alcohol may induce metabolism, reducing therapeutic effectiveness of phenytoin (Dilantin) (15,2262).
WARFARIN: Acute alcohol intoxication can decrease metabolism and increase effects of warfarin (Coumadin) (15,2262). In contrast, chronic intoxication can induce metabolism of warfarin, reducing therapeutic effectiveness (15,2262).

Interactions with Foods

FOOD: Concomitant chronic use of alcohol might interfere with absorption of B vitamins and other nutrients (2263).

Interactions with Lab Tests

FOLATE: Chronic alcohol ingestion may decrease folate levels and test results (2263).
LIVER FUNCTION TESTS: Chronic alcohol ingestion can increase alkaline phosphatase (Alk phos), alanine aminotransferase (ALT), aspartate aminotransferase (AST), gamma-glutamyltransferase (GGT), and bilirubin test results (2263).
MEAN CORPUSCULAR VOLUME (MCV): Chronic alcohol ingestion can increase MCV (2263).
TRIGLYCERIDES: Chronic alcohol ingestion can increase triglycerides (2263).

Interactions with Diseases or Conditions

ASTHMA: Wine is associated with triggering asthma reactions, possibly due to salicylates and/or added sulfites contained in wines (6174).

GOUT: Alcohol use can exacerbate gout (2263).

HEART CONDITIONS: Alcohol use can exacerbate variant angina (14), congestive heart failure (2261,2263,6889), and idiopathic cardiomyopathy (6889).

HIGH BLOOD PRESSURE: Consuming three or more alcoholic drinks a day can increase blood pressure and exacerbate hypertension (2261).

HYPERTRIGLYCERIDEMIA: Alcohol use can exacerbate hypertriglyceridemia (2261,2263,6892).

INSOMNIA: Alcohol use can exacerbate insomnia (2263).

LIVER DISEASE: Alcohol use can exacerbate liver disease (2261).

NEUROLOGICAL CONDITIONS: Alcohol use can exacerbate degenerative neurological conditions (6889).

PANCREATITIS: Alcohol use can exacerbate pancreatitis (2261).

PEPTIC ULCER DISEASE (PUD)/GASTROESOPHAGEAL REFLUX DISEASE (GERD): Alcohol use can exacerbate PUD and GERD (2261,2263).

PORPHYRIA: Alcohol use can exacerbate porphyria (2261).

PSYCHIATRIC DISORDERS: Consuming three or more drinks of alcohol a day can exacerbate psychiatric disorders and increase cognitive impairment (2261).

Dosage and Administration

ORAL: For reducing the risk of cardiovascular disease, ischemic stroke, and all-cause mortality, 1-2 glasses (120-240 mL) per day has been used (2261,2271,6835,6837,6840,6841,6842,6888,6892,6893). Up to one drink per day has been associated with less cognitive decline in older men (6824,6829). Between 2 drinks per week and 3 or 4 drinks per day has been associated with reduced risk of type 2 diabetes in healthy men (6172,6891). Alcohol intake is often measured in number of "drinks". One drink is equivalent to a 4 oz (120 mL) glass of wine, 12 oz of beer, or 1 oz of spirits (14).

Comments

A recent report disputes the "French paradox" and suggests that reduced risk of heart disease in the French population is not due to red wine consumption, but due to the traditional French diet, which is low in animal fat (835).

WINTER CHERRY

Also Known As

Cape Gooseberry, Coqueret, Strawberry Tomato.
CAUTION: See separate listing for Ashwaganda.

Scientific Names

Physalis alkekengi.
Family: Solanaceae.

People Use This For

Orally, winter cherry is used for arthritis, gout, and as a diuretic in kidney and bladder conditions (18).

Safety

There is insufficient reliable information available about the safety of winter cherry.
Pregnancy and Lactation: Insufficient reliable information available; avoid using.

Effectiveness

There is insufficient reliable information available about the effectiveness of winter cherry.

Mechanism of Action

The applicable part of winter cherry is the ripe fruit. There is insufficient reliable information available about the possible mechanism of action and active ingredients.

Adverse Reactions

None reported in humans. The unripe fruit has caused poisoning in animals (18).

Interactions with Herbs & Other Dietary Supplements

Insufficient reliable information available.

Interactions with Drugs
No interactions are known to occur, and there is no known reason to expect a clinically significant interaction with winter cherry.

Interactions with Foods
No interactions are known to occur, and there is no known reason to expect a clinically significant interaction with winter cherry.

Interactions with Lab Tests
No interactions are known to occur, and there is no known reason to expect a clinically significant interaction with winter cherry.

Interactions with Diseases or Conditions
No interactions are known to occur, and there is no known reason to expect a clinically significant interaction with winter cherry.

Dosage and Administration
ORAL: Winter cherry is used either in ground form or as an extract (18).

Comments
Avoid confusing this product with ashwaganda, which is also known as winter cherry. There is very little scientific information about this product. Our staff is continually analyzing the available information on natural medicines and will add data here as it becomes available.

WINTER SAVORY

Also Known As
Savory.
CAUTION: See separate listing for Summer Savory.

Scientific Names
Satureja montana, synonyms Satureja obovata, Calamintha montana.
Family: Labiatae or Lamiaceae.

People Use This For
Orally, winter savory is used for intestinal disorders including cramps, indigestion, diarrhea, nausea, flatulence (11), sore throat, as a tonic, and as an expectorant.
In folk medicine, winter savory is used to decrease libido (5).
In manufacturing, the oleoresin of winter savory oil is used as a flavoring agent (11).

Safety
LIKELY SAFE …when used appropriately as food. Maximum level used in food is 0.013 % for winter savory oleoresin (11).
There is insufficient reliable information available about the safety of the medicinal use of winter savory.
PREGNANCY AND LACTATION: Insufficient reliable information available; avoid using.

Effectiveness
There is insufficient reliable information available about the effectiveness of winter savory.

Mechanism of Action
The applicable parts of winter savory are the leaf and stem. Winter savory contains flavonoids (11), ursolic and oleanolic acids, and 1.6% volatile oil. Constituents of the volatile oil include carvacrol, p-cymene, and thymol (6,11). Some evidence suggests the flavonoid, eriodictyol, might have a vasodilator effect (4124). Other information indicates carvacrol, found in both savories, might have diuretic effects (6,11).

Adverse Reactions
None reported.

Interactions with Herbs & Other Dietary Supplements
Insufficient reliable information available.

Interactions with Drugs

No interactions are known to occur, and there is no known reason to expect a clinically significant interaction with winter savory.

Interactions with Foods

No interactions are known to occur, and there is no known reason to expect a clinically significant interaction with winter savory.

Interactions with Lab Tests

No interactions are known to occur, and there is no known reason to expect a clinically significant interaction with winter savory.

Interactions with Diseases or Conditions

No interactions are known to occur, and there is no known reason to expect a clinically significant interaction with winter savory.

Dosage and Administration

No typical dosage.

Comments

Although summer savory and winter savory are both used as spices, in the United States summer savory is the most common (6).

WINTER'S BARK

Also Known As

Pepper Bark, Wintera, Wintera Aromatica, Winters Bark, Winter's Cinnamon, Winters Cinnamon.

Scientific Names

Drimys winteri.

People Use This For

Orally, winter's bark is used for digestive disorders, flatulence, colic, and stomachache (18).
Topically, it is used for toothaches and dermatitis (18).

Safety

There is insufficient reliable information available about the safety of winter's bark.
Pregnancy and Lactation: Insufficient reliable information available; avoid using.

Effectiveness

There is insufficient reliable information available about the effectiveness of winter's bark.

Mechanism of Action

Winter's bark contains sesquiterpenes and volatile oils (eugenol, caryophyllene, 1,8-cineole, and pines), which have carminative, stomachic, and tonic properties (18).

Adverse Reactions

None reported.

Interactions with Herbs & Other Dietary Supplements

Insufficient reliable information available.

Interactions with Drugs

No interactions are known to occur, and there is no known reason to expect a clinically significant interaction with winter's bark.

Interactions with Foods

No interactions are known to occur, and there is no known reason to expect a clinically significant interaction with winter's bark.

Interactions with Lab Tests

No interactions are known to occur, and there is no known reason to expect a clinically significant interaction with winter's bark.

Interactions with Diseases or Conditions

No interactions are known to occur, and there is no known reason to expect a clinically significant interaction with winter's bark.

Dosage and Administration

ORAL: People typically use 30 grains (1950 mg) of the powdered bark (5267).

Comments

There is very little scientific information about this product. Our staff is continually analyzing the available information on natural medicines and will add data here as it becomes available.

WINTERGREEN leaf

Also Known As

Boxberry, Canada Tea, Checkerberry, Deerberry, Ground Berry, Hilberry, Mountain Tea, Partridge Berry, Spiceberry, Teaberry, Wax Cluster.
CAUTION: See separate listing for Wintergreen oil.

Scientific Names

Gaultheria procumbens.
Family: Ericaceae.

People Use This For

In folk medicine, wintergreen leaf has been used orally for headache; stomachache; flatulence; fever; kidney disorders (11); asthma (18); neuralgia (particularly sciatica); pleurisy (and pain associated with); ovarian pain; inflammation of the testis, epididymis, or diaphragm; gouty arthritis; and dysmenorrhea (18).
Topically, wintergreen leaf has been used as a wash for rheumatism, sore muscles, and lumbago (11).
In manufacturing, wintergreen leaf is used as a flavoring agent in food, candies (6), teas (11) and pharmaceutical products (3800).

Safety

LIKELY SAFE ...when used orally and appropriately in medicinal amounts (12). ...when consumed as a flavoring agent in amounts found in foods (12).
CHILDREN: POSSIBLY UNSAFE ...when used orally; potentially toxic to small children (19).
PREGNANCY: Insufficient reliable information; avoid using in amounts greater than those found in foods.
LACTATION: POSSIBLY UNSAFE ...when used orally or topically; potentially toxic to infants (19).

Effectiveness

There is insufficient reliable information available about the effectiveness of wintergreen leaf.

Mechanism of Action

When freshly harvested, the plant contains galutherin that changes into methyl salicylate as the plant is dried (18). The leaves contain 0.5-0.8% wintergreen oil (6).

Adverse Reactions

Topically, use of wintergreen leaf can cause contact dermatitis due to the essential oils (18). Symptoms of toxicity (salicylism) include tinnitus, nausea, vomiting (6), diarrhea, headache, stomach pain, and confusion (3805).

Interactions with Herbs & Other Dietary Supplements

Insufficient reliable information available.

Interactions with Drugs

No interactions are known to occur, and there is no known reason to expect a clinically significant interaction with wintergreen leaf.

Interactions with Foods

No interactions are known to occur, and there is no known reason to expect a clinically significant interaction with wintergreen leaf.

Interactions with Lab Tests

No interactions are known to occur, and there is no known reason to expect a clinically significant interaction with wintergreen leaf.

Interactions with Diseases or Conditions

GI CONDITIONS: Contraindicated; may aggravate gastrointestinal irritation or inflammation (19).

Dosage and Administration

ORAL: People typically prepare wintergreen leaf as a tea with 1 teaspoon of the dried leaves added to 1 cup boiling water. The tea is taken cold, 1 cup per day (5253,5254).
TOPICAL: No typical dosage.

Comments

None.

WINTERGREEN oil

Also Known As

Boxberry, Canada Tea, Checkerberry, Deerberry, Gaultheria Oil, Ground Berry, Hilberry, Mountain Tea, Partridge Berry, Spiceberry, Teaberry, Wax Cluster.
CAUTION: See separate listing for Wintergreen leaf.

Scientific Names

Gaultheria procumbens.
Family: Ericaceae.

People Use This For

Orally, small doses of wintergreen oil have been used to stimulate gastric secretion and aid digestion (6).
Topically, wintergreen oil is used as a counterirritant (272), for musculoskeletal pain, and as an antiseptic (3800).
In manufacturing, the oil is used as a flavoring agent in food, candies (6), teas (11), and in pharmaceutical products (3800).

Safety

LIKELY SAFE ...when consumed as a flavoring agent in amounts commonly found in foods (12). The maximum level of methyl salicylate is 0.04% in candy flavoring (6). ...when used topically and appropriately (272).
LIKELY UNSAFE ...when used orally for medicinal purposes, unless the methyl salicylate content is highly diluted (6,272).
CHILDREN: LIKELY UNSAFE ...when used orally. 4-10 mL can be lethal (159). ...when used topically in children less than 2 years old (272). Children can be poisoned by ingesting topical liniment. One teaspoon of topical liniment contains 7 grams salicylates or approximately 22 adult aspirin tablets (159). Child-resistant containers are required for topical liquid preparations containing more than 5% methyl salicylate (6,272).
PREGNANCY: LIKELY SAFE ...when used in amounts commonly found in foods. There is insufficient reliable information available about the safety of the oral use of wintergreen oil in large amounts; avoid using in amounts greater than those found in foods.
LACTATION: LIKELY UNSAFE ...when used orally. It might be toxic to nursing infants (19).

Effectiveness

LIKELY EFFECTIVE ...when used as a counterirritant in adults and children older than 2 years of age, according to a FDA Advisory Panel (272).
There is insufficient reliable information available about the effectiveness of wintergreen oil for its other uses.

Mechanism of Action

Wintergreen oil contains 98% methyl salicylate (6). It has antipyretic, anti-inflammatory, and analgesic properties (11), possibly due to its counterirritant effect (6).

Adverse Reactions

Topically, contact dermatitis can occur due to the essential oils (18). Other symptoms of toxicity (salicylism) include tinnitus, nausea, vomiting (6), diarrhea, headache, stomach pain, and confusion (3805). When applied topically and covered with an occlusive dressing, 12-20% of methyl salicylate was absorbed systemically over ten hours (272).

Interactions with Herbs & Other Dietary Supplements
Insufficient reliable information available.

Interactions with Drugs
WARFARIN (Coumadin): Concomitant use of topical wintergreen oil-containing products and warfarin can increase INR and bleeding risk due to systemic absorption of the methyl salicylate contained in wintergreen oil (3811,6181). Topical analgesic gels, lotions, creams, ointments, liniments, and sprays can contain up to 55% methyl salicylate (6181).
ASPIRIN: Topical use of wintergreen oil in large amounts, with occlusive dressings, or for prolonged periods of time, can cause additive salicylate toxicity (159,272).

Interactions with Foods
No interactions are known to occur, and there is no known reason to expect a clinically significant interaction with wintergreen oil.

Interactions with Lab Tests
No interactions are known to occur, and there is no known reason to expect a clinically significant interaction with wintergreen oil.

Interactions with Diseases or Conditions
GASTROINTESTINAL INFLAMMATION: Oral use is contraindicated because it can aggravate inflammation (19).
SALICYLATE ALLERGY/ASTHMA: Individuals with salicylate allergy, asthma, or nasal polyps should use cautiously due to its potential for allergic reaction (272).

Dosage and Administration
TOPICAL: Apply as gels, lotion, ointments, or liniments (containing 10-60% methyl salicylate) 3-4 times daily (3). Heat can increase skin absorption; do not apply after strenuous exercise or use a heating pad after application (3).

Comments
Wintergreen oil is obtained by steam distillation of warmed, water-macerated leaves.

WITCH HAZEL

Also Known As
Hamamelis, Hazel, Snapping Tobacco Wood, Spotted Elder, Winter Bloom, Witchazel.

Scientific Names
Hamamelis virginiana.
Family: Hamamelidaceae.

People Use This For
Orally, witch hazel is used for diarrhea, mucus colitis, vomiting blood, coughing up blood (4,6), tuberculosis, colds, and fevers (6).
Topically, witch hazel is used for itching, skin inflammation, eye inflammation (6), skin injury, mucous membrane inflammation, varicose veins (2), hemorrhoids, and bruises (4).
Rectally, witch hazel is used as an enema for bleeding "piles" (6).
Traditionally, witch hazel is used orally for tumors (6) and cancer (11). Traditionally, witch hazel is used topically for insect bites, minor burns, and other skin irritations (11).
In manufacturing, witch hazel leaf extract, bark extract, and witch hazel water are used as astringents and hemostatics in preparations for insect bites, stings, teething (13), hemorrhoids, itching, irritations, and minor pain (11).

Safety
LIKELY SAFE ...when witch hazel water is used topically and appropriately (6,272).
POSSIBLY SAFE ...when used orally and appropriately (2,12). In high doses, tannins in bark can cause liver damage (8). The volatile oil contains safrole, a known carcinogen, but in amounts too small for concern (4).
PREGNANCY AND LACTATION: Insufficient reliable information; avoid using.

Effectiveness

LIKELY EFFECTIVE ...when witch hazel water is used topically for temporary relief of itching, discomfort, irritation, and burning associated with anorectal disorders (272).

POSSIBLY EFFECTIVE ...when bark, leaf or witch hazel water is used for treating mild skin injury, local skin and mucous membrane inflammation, varicose veins (2), or as a styptic (7,8).

There is insufficient reliable information available about the effectiveness of witch hazel for its other uses.

Mechanism of Action

The applicable parts of witch hazel are the leaf and bark. Witch hazel leaf and bark possess astringent, styptic, and anti-inflammatory properties (4). Researchers attribute astringent and hemostatic properties to the tannin constituents (4). The leaf contains 8-10% tannins (512). The bark contains up to 12% tannins (7). Tannins, applied topically to broken skin or mucous membranes induce protein precipitation. They tighten up superficial cell layers and shrink colloidal structures thereby causing capillaries to constrict. The decrease in vascular permeability approximates an anti-inflammatory effect. The astringent activity of tannins also causes an indirect antibacterial effect (7). Tannins are not without adverse effects. Plants with at least 10% tannins can cause gastrointestinal disturbances, kidney damage, and necrotic conditions of the liver (12). Some evidences suggests that tannins might cause cancer. Other evidence shows tannins may prevent it (12). Regular consumption of herbs with high tannin concentrations correlates with increased incidence of esophageal or nasal cancer (12). Steam distillation used for producing Hamamelis water removes the tannins (13). Thus, the astringent properties of Hamamelis water result from its 14-15% alcohol content (13).

Adverse Reactions

Orally, witch hazel might infrequently cause stomach irritation. Rarely, it might cause liver damage (8). Because of the tannins, ingestion of 1 gram witch hazel can cause nausea, vomiting, and possibly impactions (6). Topically, witch hazel can cause contact dermatitis (6).

Interactions with Herbs & Other Dietary Supplements

Insufficient reliable information is available.

Interactions with Drugs

No interactions are known to occur, and there is no known reason to expect a clinically significant interaction with witch hazel.

Interactions with Foods

No interactions are known to occur, and there is no known reason to expect a clinically significant interaction with witch hazel.

Interactions with Lab Tests

No interactions are known to occur, and there is no known reason to expect a clinically significant interaction with witch hazel.

Interactions with Diseases or Conditions

No interactions are known to occur, and there is no known reason to expect a clinically significant interaction with witch hazel.

Dosage and Administration

ORAL: A typical dose is 2 grams of dried leaves three times daily or as tea. To make tea, steep 2 grams in 150 mL of boiling water for 5-10 minutes, and strain (4). Hamamelis Liquid Extract (1:1 in 45% alcohol), 2-4 mL three times daily has also been used (4).

TOPICAL: For compresses and irrigations, simmer 5-10 grams leaf and bark per 250 mL of water (2). For poultice, use witch hazel water (Hamamelis water) undiluted or diluted 1:3 with water. Semi-solid preparations 20-30% (2). Extracts, semi solid and liquid preparations corresponding to 5-10% leaf and bark (2).

RECTAL: Suppositories, corresponding to 0.1-1 grams leaf and bark applied 1-3 times daily (2). Anorectal disorders, Hamamelis water applied externally up to six times a day or after each bowel movement (272).

Comments

Witch hazel water (Hamamelis water, distilled witch hazel extract) is distilled from dried leaves, bark, and partially dormant twigs of Hamamelis virginiana (11).

WOOD ANEMONE

Also Known As
Crowfoot, Smell Fox, Wind Flower.

Scientific Names
Anemone nemorosa.
Family: Ranunculaceae.

People Use This For
In Russian folk medicine, the aerial parts of wood anemone are used orally for stomach pains, delayed menstruation, gout, whooping cough, and asthma (18).

Safety
LIKELY UNSAFE …when the fresh plant is used orally. Freshly harvested wood anemone can cause severe irritation to the gastrointestinal tract. Ingesting 30 freshly harvested plants is believed to be fatal (18).
There is insufficient reliable information available about the safety of the dried, cut above ground parts.
PREGNANCY AND LACTATION: LIKELY UNSAFE …when the fresh plant is used orally or topically (18). There is insufficient reliable information available about the safety of the oral or topical use of the dried, cut plant during pregnancy and lactation; avoid using.

Effectiveness
There is insufficient reliable information available about the effectiveness of wood anemone.

Mechanism of Action
The applicable parts of wood anemone are the above ground parts. When the fresh plant is crushed or cut into small pieces, the glycoside ranunculin is enzymatically changed into a severely irritating protoanemonin, which, in turn, rapidly degrades into the less toxic anemonin (18). Both protoanemonin and ranunculin are destroyed to an unknown extent during the drying process (2).

Adverse Reactions
Orally, the ingestion of freshly harvested wood anemone can cause colic, diarrhea, and severe irritation to the gastrointestinal tract and the urinary drainage passages (18).
Topically, wood anemone can cause slow-healing blisters and burns after prolonged skin contact (18).

Interactions with Herbs & Other Dietary Supplements
Insufficient reliable information is available.

Interactions with Drugs
No interactions are known to occur, and there is no known reason to expect a clinically significant interaction with wood anemone.

Interactions with Foods
No interactions are known to occur, and there is no known reason to expect a clinically significant interaction with wood anemone.

Interactions with Lab Tests
No interactions are known to occur, and there is no known reason to expect a clinically significant interaction with wood anemone.

Interactions with Diseases or Conditions
No interactions are known to occur, and there is no known reason to expect a clinically significant interaction with wood anemone.

Dosage and Administration
No typical dosage.

Comments
Avoid confusion with the poisonous plant, pasque flower (Pulsatilla pratensis). Although the two plants are from the same botanical family and have similar pharmacological compounds, they are not synonymous (2,18).

WOOD SAGE

Also Known As
Ambroise, Garlic Sage, Hind Heal, Large-Leaved Germander.
CAUTION: See separate listing for Sage.

Scientific Names
Teucrium scorodonia.
Family: Lamiaceae.

People Use This For
Orally, wood sage is used for gastrointestinal tract disorders, tuberculosis, mucous membrane inflammation of the bronchi and nose, throat spasms, hypertension, healing wounds, and liver disorders (18).

Safety
There is insufficient reliable information available about the safety of wood sage.
Pregnancy and Lactation: Insufficient reliable information is available; avoid using.

Effectiveness
There is insufficient reliable information available about the effectiveness of wood sage.

Mechanism of Action
The applicable parts of wood sage are the above ground parts. Wood sage is thought to have spasmolytic and expectorant properties (18). It contains flavonoids, a volatile oil, diterpenes, and iridoide monoterpenes (18).

Adverse Reactions
None reported.

Interactions with Herbs & Other Dietary Supplements
Insufficient reliable information available.

Interactions with Drugs
No interactions are known to occur, and there is no known reason to expect a clinically significant interaction with wood sage.

Interactions with Foods
No interactions are known to occur, and there is no known reason to expect a clinically significant interaction with wood sage.

Interactions with Lab Tests
No interactions are known to occur, and there is no known reason to expect a clinically significant interaction with wood sage.

Interactions with Diseases or Conditions
No interactions are known to occur, and there is no known reason to expect a clinically significant interaction with wood sage.

Dosage and Administration
ORAL: A typical dose for bronchitis is one cup of tea. To make tea, steep 2 teaspoons of dried herb in 150 mL water for 10-15 minutes, and strain.

Comments
Wood sage smells faintly of leeks when being dried. In most countries, wood sage is obsolete as a drug (18).

WOOD SORREL

Also Known As
Common Sorrel, Cuckoo Bread, Cuckowes Meat, Fairy Bells, Green Sauce, Hallelujah, Mountain Sorrel, Shamrock, Sour Trefoil, Stickwort, Stubwort, Surelle, Three-Leaved Grass, White Sorrel, Wood Sour.

Scientific Names
Oxalis acetosella.
Family: Oxalidaceae.

People Use This For
Orally, wood sorrel is used for liver and digestive disorders.
Historically, it was used to treat scurvy, wounds, and inflammation of the gums (18).

Safety
POSSIBLY UNSAFE …when used orally, particularly in large amounts (6,17).
CHILDREN: POSSIBLY UNSAFE …when used orally. One four-year old child died after consuming rhubarb leaves, which is also a source of oxalic acid (17).
PREGNANCY: LIKELY UNSAFE …when used orally because it might stimulate menses (19): avoid using.
LACTATION: POSSIBLY UNSAFE …when used orally (6,17); avoid using.

Effectiveness
There is insufficient reliable information available about the effectiveness of wood sorrel.

Mechanism of Action
The applicable part of wood sorrel is the whole flowering plant. It contains 0.3-1.25% oxalic acid (18). Oxalate content is high in fresh leaves and roots (17,19). Once absorbed, the oxalic acid reacts with calcium in plasma and resulting insoluble calcium oxalate may precipitate in the kidneys, blood vessels, heart, lungs, and liver. This may also cause hypocalcemia (12,17). Oxalate crystals damage mucosal tissue, resulting in severe irritation and possible damage. The systemic absorption of oxalates may result in kidney damage, both in people with pre-existing kidney disease and in healthy kidneys (19).

Adverse Reactions
Orally, consuming excessive amounts of wood sorrel can cause diarrhea, nausea, polyuria (6), dermatitis (4) and gastrointestinal symptoms due to its oxalic acid content. Oxalic acid poisoning affects skin, eyes, respiratory system and kidneys. Oral symptoms of oxalate irritation include swelling of the mouth, tongue and throat, with difficulty in speaking and suffocation. It has a corrosive effect on the digestive tract. It can lead to oxalic acid crystals in the kidneys, blood vessels, heart, lungs, liver, and/or hypocalcemia (17).

Interactions with Herbs & Other Dietary Supplements
CALCIUM, IRON, ZINC: Concurrent use might decrease mineral absorption. Wood sorrel contains oxalate (7,12), which can bind multivalent metal ions in the gastrointestinal tract and decrease mineral absorption.

Interactions with Drugs
No interactions are known to occur, and there is no known reason to expect a clinically significant interaction with wood sorrel.

Interactions with Foods
CALCIUM, IRON, ZINC: Concurrent use might decrease mineral absorption from foods. Wood sorrel contains oxalate (7,12), which can bind multivalent metal ions in the gastrointestinal tract and decrease mineral absorption.

Interactions with Lab Tests
No interactions are known to occur, and there is no known reason to expect a clinically significant interaction with wood sorrel.

Interactions with Diseases or Conditions
COAGULATION DISORDERS: Oxalate constituents can alter the calcium concentrations and decrease coagulation time (4,12).
GI CONDITIONS: Theoretically can exacerbate stomach and intestinal ulcers due to mucosal irritant effect (19).
KIDNEY DISEASE: Can damage kidneys with formation of insoluble oxalate; use with caution or avoid in individuals with history of kidney stones (12,19).

Dosage and Administration
No typical dosage.

Comments
Wood sorrel is also called common sorrel, and could be confused with sorrel.

WOODBINE

Also Known As

Clematis, Devil's-Darning-Needle, Old-Man's Beard, Traveler's-Joy, Vine Bower, Virgin's Bower.
CAUTION: See separate listings for Clematis and Traveler's Joy.

Scientific Names

Clematis virginiana.
Family: Rananculaceae.

People Use This For

Historically, woodbine has been used orally for skin sores, cuts, itching, venereal disorders, cancer, tumors, itching, fever, nephrosis, ulcers, diuretic, purgative, tuberculosis, and cervical lymphadenitis (6).

Safety

LIKELY UNSAFE ...when used orally or topically because it is a powerful irritant (6).
PREGNANCY AND LACTATION: LIKELY UNSAFE ...when used orally or topically; avoid using.

Effectiveness

There is insufficient reliable information available about the effectiveness of woodbine.

Mechanism of Action

The applicable part of woodbine is the leaf. There is insufficient reliable information available about the possible mechanism of action and active ingredients.

Adverse Reactions

Orally, the juice derived from the woodbine leaf is said to be a powerful local irritant (6).

Interactions with Herbs & Other Dietary Supplements

Insufficient reliable information available.

Interactions with Drugs

No interactions are known to occur, and there is no known reason to expect a clinically significant interaction with woodbine.

Interactions with Foods

No interactions are known to occur, and there is no known reason to expect a clinically significant interaction with woodbine.

Interactions with Lab Tests

No interactions are known to occur, and there is no known reason to expect a clinically significant interaction with woodbine.

Interactions with Diseases or Conditions

No interactions are known to occur, and there is no known reason to expect a clinically significant interaction with woodbine.

Dosage and Administration

ORAL: People typically make a liquid preparation of woodbine, combining one heaping teaspoon of leaves and flowers with one cup of water and allowing the mixture to stand for 30 minutes. The dose is one tablespoon 4 to 6 times daily (5263).

Comments

Avoid confusion with American ivy, gelsemium or honeysuckle, which are also known as woodbine.

WORMSEED

Also Known As
Levant, Santonica, Sea Wormwood, Worm Seed.
CAUTION: See separate listings for Chenopodium Oil, Levant Berry, Mugwort. Wormwood, and Wormwood Oil.

Scientific Names
Artemisia cina.
Family: Asteraceae.

People Use This For
Orally, wormseed is used for ascaris and oxyuris infestations [18].

Safety
UNSAFE ...when used orally due to its highly toxic adverse effects [18].
PREGNANCY AND LACTATION: UNSAFE ...when used orally due to potential for toxicity [18]; avoid using.

Effectiveness
There is insufficient reliable information available about the effectiveness of wormseed.

Mechanism of Action
The anthelmintic activity is attributed to the sesquiterpene lactone beta-santonin. When wormseed is used with a laxative, it appears to paralyze the muscles of ascarids and facilitate their elimination from the body . Some data suggest wormseed lowers body temperature when a fever is present [18].

Adverse Reactions
Orally, death has been reported with less than 10 grams of herb. Symptoms of poisoning are possible in amounts used to treat parasitic infestations. Symptoms may include kidney irritation, gastroenteritis, stupor, visual disorders, muscle twitching, and epileptiform spasms [18]. It can cause an allergic reaction in individuals sensitive to the Asteraceae/Compositae family. Members of this family include ragweed, chrysanthemums, marigolds, daisies, and many other herbs.

Interactions with Herbs & Other Dietary Supplements
Insufficient reliable information available.

Interactions with Drugs
No interactions are known to occur, and there is no known reason to expect a clinically significant interaction with wormseed.

Interactions with Foods
No interactions are known to occur, and there is no known reason to expect a clinically significant interaction with wormseed.

Interactions with Lab Tests
No interactions are known to occur, and there is no known reason to expect a clinically significant interaction with wormseed.

Interactions with Diseases or Conditions
CROSS-ALLERGENICITY: Can cause an allergic reaction in individuals sensitive to the Asteraceae/Compositae family. Members of this family include ragweed, chrysanthemums, marigolds, daisies, and many other herbs.

Dosage and Administration
No typical dosage.

Comments
Avoid confusing wormseed with chenopodium oil (or wormseed oil), wormwood oil, or wormwood. Avoid confusing wormseed, also referred to as levant, with levant berry.

WORMWOOD above ground parts

Also Known As

Absinth, Absinthe, Absinthii Herba, Absinthites, Absinthium, Ajenjo, Armoise, Artesian Absinthium, Artemisia, Common Wormwood, Green Ginger, Herbe d'Absinthe, Wermut, Wermutkraut, Wurmkraut.
CAUTION: See separate listings for Wormwood oil and Mugwort.

Scientific Names

Artemisia absinthium.
Family: Asteraceae or Compositae.

People Use This For

Orally, wormwood above ground parts is used for loss of appetite, indigestion, biliary dyskinesia (2), and gastrointestinal complaints such as low acidity gastritis (8).
Topically, wormwood above ground parts is used for healing wounds and insect bites (18).
In combination with other herbs, wormwood above ground parts is used for indigestion, particularly functional disorders of the gallbladder drainage system, loss of appetite, and discomfort due to fullness and flatulence (2).
Historically, wormwood above ground parts was used as an anthelmintic, aphrodisiac, tonic (515), antispasmodic (8), and to stimulate sweating.
In manufacturing, wormwood above ground parts is used for flavoring alcoholic bitters and vermouth (11).

Safety

LIKELY SAFE ...when used orally in the amount found in bitters and vermouth. Approved for food use in the US provided finished products are thujone-free (11). The maximum use level is 0.024% (11).
POSSIBLY SAFE ...when used orally and appropriately short-term (12). Although aqueous extracts or brewed teas are reported to contain the toxic constituent thujone, the amount is low (12).
LIKELY UNSAFE ...when used orally long-term or in excessive amounts.
There is insufficient reliable information available about the safety of the topical use of wormwood above ground parts.
PREGNANCY: UNSAFE ...when used orally. Thujone has potential uterine and menstrual stimulant effects (12). There is insufficient reliable information available about the safety of the topical use of wormwood above ground parts during pregnancy.
LACTATION: Insufficient reliable information available; avoid using.

Effectiveness

There is insufficient reliable information available about the effectiveness of wormwood above ground parts.

Mechanism of Action

Wormwood contains bitter principles (absinthin and anabsinthin) and a volatile oil composed of up to 70% thujone (7). In small doses, wormwood acts as an aromatic bitter (7). As the amount ingested increases, the toxic effects of thujone become more pronounced leading to increased salivation and increased blood flow to mucous membranes and pelvic viscera (7). Thujone heightens and alters the effect of alcohol (7). Chronic thujone poisoning leads to seizures, delirium, and hallucinations (7). Researchers think thujone has a mind-altering effect similar to tetrahydrocannabinol, the active principle in marijuana (515). Some evidence suggests that thujone exposure might be harmful to individuals with underlying defects in hepatic heme synthesis (12). Thujone also induces synthesis of a rate-controlling enzyme for the 5-aminolevulinic acid synthase pathway. This effect is similar to that of phenobarbital and glutethimide, drugs with known porphyrinogenic activity (12). Thujone shows evidence of antioxidant, antimicrobial and antifungal activity (12).

Adverse Reactions

Orally, habitual use of large amounts of wormwood can cause restlessness, insomnia, nightmares, vomiting, stomach and intestinal cramps (8), dizziness, tremors (11,12), urine retention (8), renal damage, and convulsions (11,12).
Absinthism, a group of neurological symptoms, is characterized by digestive disorders, thirst, restlessness, vertigo, tremor, numbness of extremities, diminished intellect, delirium, paralysis, and death (17).
Topically, skin contact with fresh wormwood can cause contact dermatitis (19). Wormwood can also cause an allergic reaction in people sensitive to the Asteraceae/Compositae family. Members of this family include ragweed, chrysanthemums, marigolds, daisies, and many other herbs.

Interactions with Herbs & Other Dietary Supplements

THUJONE-CONTAINING HERBS: Concomitant use with other herbs that contain thujone might increase risk of thujone toxicity. Thujone-containing herbs include: oak moss, oriental arborvitae, sage, tansy, thuja (cedar), and tree moss (12).

Interactions with Drugs

ACID-INHIBITING DRUGS: Theoretically, due to claims that wormwood increases stomach acid, it might interfere with antacids, sucralfate (Carafate), H-2 antagonists, or proton pump inhibitors (19).

ANTICONVULSANTS: Theoretically, concomitant use might interfere with the effectiveness of anticonvulsant drugs due to wormwood's potential to cause seizures (8,11,12).

Interactions with Foods

No interactions are known to occur, and there is no known reason to expect a clinically significant interaction with wormwood above ground parts.

Interactions with Lab Tests

No interactions are known to occur, and there is no known reason to expect a clinically significant interaction with wormwood above ground parts.

Interactions with Diseases or Conditions

ULCERS: Contraindicated in individuals with gastric or duodenal ulcers due to potential for stomach irritation and intestinal tract stimulation (8,19).

CROSS-ALLERGENICITY: Wormwood can cause an allergic reaction in people sensitive to the Asteraceae/Compositae family. Members of this family include ragweed, chrysanthemums, marigolds, daisies, and many other herbs (4).

Dosage and Administration

ORAL: A typical dose is one cup tea before eating as an appetite stimulant or after meals as a bile flow stimulant (8). To make tea, steep 1-1.5 grams (1 teaspoon) finely chopped above ground parts in 150 mL boiling water 10 minutes, and strain. Total daily dose is up to 3 grams per day (2). Do not exceed 1.5 grams above ground parts per dose (8).

Comments

Wormwood is the principal flavor ingredient in absinthe, a 136-proof alcoholic beverage popular at the turn of the century (515). Absinthe is historically associated with addiction, acts of violence (515), damage to the nervous system and mental deterioration (17). Vincent van Gogh's self-amputation of his left ear is attributed to his absinthe addiction (11,515). Absinthe was banned in many countries by 1915, including the US (11).

WORMWOOD oil

Also Known As

Artemisia.
CAUTION: See separate listing for Wormwood above ground parts.

Scientific Names

Artemisia absinthium.
Family: Asteraceae/Compositae.

People Use This For

Topically, wormwood oil is used as a counterirritant (11).
In foods, it is used as a flavoring agent (11).
In manufacturing, wormwood oil is used as a fragrance component in soaps, cosmetics, and perfumes.

Safety

LIKELY SAFE ...when used topically. Amounts found in cosmetics are considered nontoxic. The maximum level used is 0.25% in perfumes (11).

POSSIBLY SAFE ...when used orally in very small, thujone-free amounts. Thujone-free wormwood oil is approved for use in foods in the US (11). The maximum use level for the thujone-free oil is 0.0006% (11).

LIKELY UNSAFE ...when thujone-containing wormwood oil is used orally. One-half ounce of thujone-containing volatile oil can cause convulsions and unconsciousness (17,515).

There is insufficient reliable information available about the safety of wormwood oil when used topically in amounts greater than those found in cosmetics.

PREGNANCY: LIKELY UNSAFE ...when used topically; avoid using. Wormwood oil might have uterine and menstrual stimulant effects (12,19) and thujone could be toxic.

LACTATION: LIKELY UNSAFE ...when used topically; avoid using. There is concern about the toxic potential of thujone.

Effectiveness

There is insufficient reliable information available about the effectiveness of wormwood oil.

Mechanism of Action

The volatile oil of wormwood is considered an active narcotic poison (17). The major constituents of the oil are azulenes (11,515) but it also contains 3-12% thujone (11,515). The azulene constituents have anti-inflammatory and antipyretic activity (11). They also have antibacterial effects against Staphylococcus aureus, the penicillin-resistant strain S. aureus, Klebsiella pneumoniae and Pseudomonas aeruginosa (11). The constituent, thujone is chemically related to camphor (12). As the amount of thujone ingested is increased, the toxic effect becomes pronounced, leading to increased salivation and erythema of the mucous membranes and pelvic viscera. Thujone heightens and alters the effect of alcohol. Researchers think thujone has a mind-altering effect similar to tetrahydrocannabinol, the active constituent marijuana (4). Chronic thujone poisoning leads to epileptic seizures, delirium, and hallucinations (7). Some evidence suggests thujone might be harmful to individuals with underlying defects in hepatic heme synthesis. Other evidence suggests thujone induces synthesis of a rate-controlling enzyme for the 5-aminolevulinic acid synthase pathway. Phenobarbital and glutethimide have similar effects, suggesting thujone might have porphyrinogenic activity (12).

Adverse Reactions

Orally, wormwood oil can cause nausea, vomiting, diffuse muscle aches, acute renal toxicity, seizures, rhabdomyolysis, and acute renal failure (661,662). Wormwood oil can cause an allergic reaction in people sensitive to the Asteraceae/Compositae family. Members of this family include ragweed, chrysanthemums, marigolds, daisies, and many other herbs.

Interactions with Herbs & Other Dietary Supplements

THUJONE-CONTAINING HERBS: Concomitant use might increase the risk of thujone toxicity. Thujone-containing herbs include: oak moss, oriental arborvitae, sage, tansy, thuja (cedar), and tree moss (12); avoid using.

Interactions with Drugs

No interactions are known to occur, and there is no known reason to expect a clinically significant interaction with wormwood oil.

Interactions with Foods

No interactions are known to occur, and there is no known reason to expect a clinically significant interaction with wormwood oil.

Interactions with Lab Tests

No interactions are known to occur, and there is no known reason to expect a clinically significant interaction with wormwood oil.

Interactions with Diseases or Conditions

CROSS-ALLERGENICITY: Wormwood oil can cause an allergic reaction in individuals sensitive to the Asteraceae/Compositae family. Members of this family include ragweed, chrysanthemums, marigolds, daisies, and many other herbs.

Dosage and Administration

No typical dosage.

Comments

Wormwood oil is distilled from leaves and flowers of Artemisia absinthium just before or during flowering. Thujone-containing wormwood oil is highly toxic.

XANTHAN GUM

Also Known As

Corn Sugar Gum, Xanthan.

Scientific Names

Xanthomonas campestris.

People Use This For

Orally, xanthan gum is used for lowering blood glucose and total plasma cholesterol in people with diabetes (4916). It is also used as a laxative (4917,4918).

Topically, xanthan gum is used as a saliva substitute in people with Sjogren's syndrome (4915).

In manufacturing, xanthan gum is used as a thickening, suspending, emulsifying, and stabilizing agent in foods, toothpastes, and pharmaceutical products (13,16).

Safety

LIKELY SAFE ...when used in amounts found in foods, up to 10 mg/kg per day (4914). It has Generally Recognized as Safe (GRAS) status in the US (4912). ...when used orally for medicinal use in amounts up to 15 grams per day (4914,4916,4917,4918). ...when used topically and appropriately (4914).

PREGNANCY AND LACTATION: Insufficient reliable information is available; avoid using in amounts greater than found in foods.

Effectiveness

POSSIBLY EFFECTIVE ...when used orally as a bulk-forming laxative (4917,4918). ...when used for lowering blood glucose and cholesterol in people with diabetes (4916). ...when used topically as a saliva substitute in people with Sjogren's syndrome (4915).

Mechanism of Action

Xanthan gum is a bulk-forming laxative. In the body it forms an emollient gel that stimulates peristalsis and passage of intestinal contents (4917,4921). Xanthan gum slows gastric emptying and intestinal absorption of glucose (4916). It mimics saliva as a lubricating and wetting agent in humans (4915), and shows evidence that it might reduce demineralization of tooth enamel (4920). Xanthan gum demonstrates antitumor activity, and shows evidence of synergism with 5-fluorouracil and bleomycin (11).

Adverse Reactions

Orally, xanthan gum can cause flatulence and abdominal distention (4916,4918). Occupational exposure in workers handling xanthan gum powder can cause flu-like symptoms, nose and throat irritation without acute or chronic loss of pulmonary function (4913).

Interactions with Herbs & Other Dietary Supplements

BULK-FORMING LAXATIVE HERBS AND SUPPLEMENTS: Theoretically, concomitant use may increase likelihood of flatulence and abdominal distention.

HERBS THAT CAN CAUSE HYPOGLYCEMIA: Theoretically, concomitant use with pharmacologically active amounts of xanthan gum could result in excessive lowering of blood glucose.

Interactions with Drugs

BULK-FORMING LAXATIVES: Theoretically, concomitant use may increase likelihood of flatulence and abdominal distension.

DRUGS THAT CAN CAUSE HYPOGLYCEMIA: Theoretically, concomitant use with pharmacologically active amounts of xanthan gum could result in excessive lowering of blood glucose.

Interactions with Foods

No interactions are known to occur, and there is no known reason to expect a clinically significant interaction with xanthan gum.

Interactions with Lab Tests

BLOOD GLUCOSE: Might lower blood glucose and test results (4916).

CHOLESTEROL: Might lower serum cholesterol and test results (4916).

Interactions with Diseases or Conditions

CONTRAINDICATIONS: Bulk forming laxative are contraindicated in individuals with nausea, vomiting, or other symptoms of appendicitis, acute surgical abdomen, fecal impaction, intestinal obstruction, or undiagnosed abdominal pain (506,4921).

INTESTINAL STENOSIS: Avoid xanthan gum in amounts greater than found in foods (4921).

Dosage and Administration

ORAL: The World Health Organization (WHO) has set the maximum acceptable intake for xanthan gum as a food additive at 10 mg/kg per day (4914), and as a laxative at 15 grams per day (4918). For safety and effectiveness, bulk laxatives require adequate fluid intake (4921). For diabetes a typical dose is 12 grams per day as an ingredient in muffins (4916).

TOPICAL: Saliva substitutes, 0.018% or 0.092% aqueous solutions with added electrolytes and peppermint flavoring (4915).

Comments

Xanthan gum is a polysaccharide produced by fermenting carbohydrate with the bacterium Xanthomonas campestris (13,16). Xanthan gum is an ingredient in some sustained release matrix tablets (4914).

XYLITOL

Also Known As

Birch Sugar, E967, Meso-Xylitol, Xylit, Xylite.

Scientific Names

Xylitol; xylo-pentane-1,2,3,4,5-pentol.

People Use This For

Orally, xylitol is used to prevent acute otitis media in young children (14,6816), to prevent dental caries and dry mouth (6814), and as a sugar substitute for people with diabetes (6814,6819).
Intravenously, xylitol is used as an energy source in parenteral nutrition (6819).
In foods, xylitol is used as a sweetener, including sugar-free preparations (9).

Safety

LIKELY SAFE ...when used orally in amounts found in foods (14).
POSSIBLY SAFE ...when used orally and appropriately in medicinal amounts. Xylitol has been used safely in doses from 20-53 grams per day for up to 3 years (14,6815,6819,6821).
POSSIBLY UNSAFE ...when used orally in very high doses, long-term. There is some concern that very high doses for extended periods of use can induce tumor growth (14,6815,6820). However, this effect has not yet been demonstrated in humans.
CHILDREN: POSSIBLY SAFE ...when used orally and appropriately in medicinal amounts. Xylitol has been used safely in children in doses up to 20 grams per day for up to 3 years (14,6815,6819).
PREGNANCY AND LACTATION: Insufficient reliable information available; avoid using.

Effectiveness

LIKELY EFFECTIVE ...when used orally for preventing dental caries. Use of xylitol containing products such as foods, chewing gum, candies, soluble dragees, and toothpaste that provide 1-20 grams of xylitol per day can significantly reduce the rate of cavity formation in both adults and children (6815,6819,6822). Xylitol products appear to be more effective than products containing sorbitol for preventing cavity formation (6822).
POSSIBLY EFFECTIVE ...when used orally for reducing the incidence of acute otitis media in preschool children. Xylitol 8.4 to 10 grams per day given as a chewing gum, lozenge, or syrup 5 times a day after meals to preschool children, significantly reduced the number of episodes of acute otitis media and the usage of antibiotics (14,6816,6817).

Mechanism of Action

Xylitol is a polyhydric alcohol (polyol) related to the pentose sugar, xylose (9). Its sweetness and caloric content are comparable to sucrose, but it has little effect on blood glucose or insulin levels (14). In the body, it is produced during metabolism of glucose in the liver (268). Ingested xylitol is absorbed slowly from the gut and metabolized in the liver. The unabsorbed fraction is broken down by colonic bacteria (6814). Xylitol has several properties that might be useful against dental caries. Xylitol is not fermented by plaque flora to the low pH associated with caries. Xylitol lowers plaque and salivary levels of Streptococcus mutans and lactobacilli which cause caries. Xylitol also reduces bacterial adhesiveness. Xylitol increases salivary flow rates and calcium and phosphate concentrations in saliva, which promote buffering and remineralization of tooth surfaces. Xylitol also stimulates activity of the antimicrobial enzyme lactoperoxidase in saliva (6815,6819). Since habitual xylitol consumption selects for mutans streptococci with impaired adhesion properties, which shed more easily from plaque to saliva, this can lead to early colonization of infant's teeth with these organisms from their mother's saliva (6818). This has been associated with a higher incidence of dental caries in the infants, but was reduced in one study when mothers used xylitol chewing gum 2 to 3 times a day while their children were between 3 months and 2 years of age (6818).

Due to its five carbon structure, xylitol is not a substrate for growth of most bacteria and it may inhibit some bacterial enzymes and interfere with their metabolism of six carbon sugars (14,6819). In the prevention of acute otitis media, xylitol may work by inhibiting growth of bacteria including Streptococcus pneumoniae, and preventing adhesion of pneumococci and Haemophilus influenzae to nasopharyngeal cells (14,6819). However, it does not seem to inhibit growth of Haemophilus influenzae (14). There is also some preliminary evidence from animal models that suggests xylitol might increase the calcium and phosphorus content of bone and protect against osteoporosis (6819).

Adverse Reactions

Orally, acute administration of large amounts of xylitol (30 to 40 grams) can cause osmotic diarrhea and flatulence. However, if the dose is increased gradually, tolerance to this effect can occur and prevent development of diarrhea and flatulence (9,14). Both topical and oral administration has been associated with allergic reactions (14). Intravenous infusion of high doses has been associated with hyperuricemia, changes in liver-function tests, and acidosis, including lactic acidosis (9,6815).

Interactions with Herbs & Other Dietary Supplements

Insufficient reliable information available.

Interactions with Drugs

No interactions are known to occur, and there is no known reason to expect a clinically significant interaction with xylitol.

Interactions with Foods

No interactions are known to occur, and there is no known reason to expect a clinically significant interaction with xylitol.

Interactions with Lab Tests

No interactions are known to occur, and there is no known reason to expect a clinically significant interaction with xylitol.

Interactions with Diseases or Conditions

No interactions are known to occur, and there is no known reason to expect a clinically significant interaction with xylitol.

Dosage and Administration

ORAL: For acute otitis media, total daily doses of 8.4 to 10 grams have been used in chewing gum, lozenges, or syrup given in 5 divided doses, after meals for prevention (14). A wide range of doses have been used in the prevention of dental caries in adults and children. Typically, doses are from 7 to 20 grams per day divided into 3-5 doses, usually given as candies or chewing gum (6815,6819).
INTRAVENOUS: No typical dosage.

Comments

Xylitol is a naturally occurring pentose alcohol found in almost all plant material, including fruits such as raspberries, strawberries and plums, vegetables and mushrooms. Commercial preparations are extracted from birch wood (14,6814).

YARROW

Also Known As

Achilee, Achillea, Acuilee, Band Man's Plaything, Bauchweh, Birangasifa, Bloodwort, Carpenter's Weed, Civan Percemi, Common Yarrow, Devil's Nettle, Devil's Plaything, Erba Da Cartentieri, Erba Da Falegname, Gemeine Schafgarbe, Green Arrow, Herbe Aux Charpentiers, Katzenkrat, Milefolio, Milfoil, Millefeuille, Millefolii flos, Millefolii herba, Millefolium, Millegoglie, Noble Yarrow, Nosebleed, Old Man's Pepper, Roga Mari, Sanguinary, Soldier's Wound Wort, Staunchweed, Tausendaugbram, Thousand-Leaf, Wound Wort.

Scientific Names

Achillea millefolium.
Family: Asteraceae/Compositae.

People Use This For

Orally, yarrow is used for fever, common cold, amenorrhea, dysentery, diarrhea (4,8), loss of appetite, mild or spastic gastrointestinal tract discomfort (2), inducing sweating (6), and specifically for thrombotic conditions with hypertension, including cerebral and coronary thromboses (4).
Fresh leaves of yarrow are chewed to relieve toothache (6).
Topically, yarrow is used as a styptic (4), for wounds (7), and as a sitz bath for painful, lower pelvic, cramp-like conditions of psychosomatic origin in women (2).

In combination with other herbs, yarrow is used for bloating, flatulence, mild gastrointestinal cramping, and nervous gastrointestinal complaints (7).

In folk medicine, yarrow is used as a styptic for bleeding hemorrhoids (18).

For food uses, the young leaves and flowers of yarrow are used in salads.

In manufacturing, yarrow is also used as a cosmetic cleanser (6) and in snuff (6). Yarrow oil is used in shampoos (6).

Safety

LIKELY SAFE ...when used orally in typical food amounts (11). Approved for use only in alcoholic beverages in the US (11). Finished products must be thujone-free (11), although the volatile oil of yarrow is believe to contain only a trace of thujone (11).

POSSIBLY SAFE ...when used orally and appropriately for medicinal purposes (2,12).

PREGNANCY: LIKELY UNSAFE ...when used orally because it is believed to be an abortifacient and affect the menstrual cycle (12).

LACTATION: Insufficient reliable information available; avoid excessive amounts during lactation (4).

Effectiveness

There is insufficient reliable information available about the effectiveness of yarrow.

Mechanism of Action

The applicable parts of yarrow are the above ground parts. Yarrow has diaphoretic, antipyretic, hypotensive, astringent, diuretic, urinary antiseptic, spasmolytic, and antiflatulent effects (4). Yarrow contains amino acids, fatty acids, ascorbic acid, caffeic acid, folic acid, salicylic acid and succinic acid; alkaloids; flavonoids including rutin; tannins; a volatile oil, an unknown cyanogenetic compound, and sugars (4). The volatile oil contains chamazulene, other azulenes (11), and trace amounts of thujone (4,11) The volatile oil content, and especially the azulene content, varies considerably depending on the source (11). Some evidence suggests that achilleine, an alkaloid constituent, might decrease clotting time (4). The alkaloid fraction has shown evidence of antipyretic and hypotensive effects (4). An aqueous extract shows some evidence of anti-inflammatory and diuretic activity (4). Researchers think that anti-inflammatory and anti-allergy activities are associated with the constituent chamazulene (6). Not all species contain azulene constituents (6).

An ethanolic extract shows moderate antibacterial activity against Staphylococcus aureus, Bacillus subtilis, Mycobacterium smegmatis, Escherichia coli, Shigella sonnei, and Shigella flexneri (4). Some evidence suggests that the volatile oil of yarrow might have CNS depressant activity (4).

Adverse Reactions

Orally, large amounts of yarrow might cause sedative and diuretic effects (4,5).

Topically, yarrow can cause dermatitis (4). It can cause an allergic reaction in individuals sensitive to the Asteraceae/Compositae family. Members of this family include ragweed, chrysanthemums, marigolds, daisies, and many other herbs.

Interactions with Herbs & Other Dietary Supplements

SEDATIVE HERBS: Theoretically, concomitant use might enhance sedative effects of other herbs with sedative properties, including German chamomile, hops, kava, scullcap, and valerian (19).

THUJONE CONTAINING HERBS: Avoid; concomitant use can increase the risk of thujone toxicity. Thujone-containing herbs include: oak moss, oriental arborvitae, sage, tansy, thuja (cedar), tree moss, and wormwood (2,4,11,12).

Interactions with Drugs

ACID-INHIBITING DRUGS: Theoretically, due to claims that yarrow increases stomach acid, it might interfere with antacids, sucralfate (Carafate), H-2 antagonists, or proton pump inhibitors (19).

ANTICOAGULANTS: Theoretically, concomitant use might cause increased effects and adverse effects (4).

BARBITURATES: Theoretically, concomitant use might prolong barbiturate-induced sleep time (4).

HYPERTENSIVE or HYPOTENSIVE DRUG THERAPY: Theoretically, concomitant use might interfere with drug therapy (4).

Interactions with Foods

No interactions are known to occur, and there is no known reason to expect a clinically significant interaction with yarrow.

Interactions with Lab Tests

No interactions are known to occur, and there is no known reason to expect a clinically significant interaction with yarrow.

Interactions with Diseases or Conditions

CROSS-ALLERGENICITY: Can cause an allergic reaction in individuals sensitive to the Asteraceae/Compositae family. Members of this family include ragweed, chrysanthemums, marigolds, daisies, and many other herbs.

Dosage and Administration

ORAL: A typical oral dose is 2-4 grams dried flowerheads or one cup tea three times daily. To make tea, steep 2-4 grams dried flowerhead or 2 grams finely cut above ground parts in 150 mL of boiling water for 10-15 minutes, and strain (4). A daily dose is up to 4.5 grams above ground parts, 3 grams flowerheads, 3 teaspoons pressed juice from fresh plants, or equivalent preparations per day. Liquid extract (1:1 in 25% alcohol), 2-4 mL three times daily has been used (4). Tincture (1:5 in 45% alcohol), 2-4 mL three times daily has also been used (4).
TOPICAL: As a sitz bath, add 100 grams above ground parts per 20 L of water (2).

Comments

None.

YELLOW DOCK

Also Known As

Broad-Leaved Dock, Curled Dock, Curly Dock, Field Sorrel, Narrow Dock, Rumex, Sheep Sorrel, Sorrel, Sour Dock, Yellowdock.

Scientific Names

Rumex crispus; Rumex obtusifolius.
Family: Polygonaceae.

People Use This For

Orally, yellow dock is used for acute and chronic inflammation of nasal passages and the respiratory tract, as an adjunct to antibacterial therapy (18), a laxative (4,5,6), tonic (6), and for treating venereal diseases (5,6).
Topically, yellow dock is used as a dentifrice (6).
Historically, it has been used for chronic skin diseases (4,6,18), dermatitis, rashes (6), scurvy (18), obstructive jaundice, and psoriasis with constipation (4).
For food uses, the leaf stalks are used in salads (6).

Safety

POSSIBLY SAFE ...when consumed in amounts commonly found in foods. Young leaves must be boiled to remove the oxalate content; death has occurred after consuming uncooked leaves (6,18). ...when used orally and appropriately for medicinal purposes.
PREGNANCY: POSSIBLY UNSAFE ...when used orally; avoid using. Contains anthraquinone glycosides, and unstandardized laxatives are not desirable during pregnancy (4).
LACTATION: POSSIBLY UNSAFE ...when used orally; avoid using. Anthraquinones are secreted into breast milk (4,5).

Effectiveness

There is insufficient reliable information available about the effectiveness of yellow dock.

Mechanism of Action

The applicable parts of yellow dock are the root and rhizome. Yellow dock contains anthraquinone glycosides (chrysophanic acid, emodin, physcion), oxalates (oxalic acid and calcium oxalate), and tannins (4,5,6,12). Oxalate content is high in the leaves and low in the stalks (17). The anthroquinones (2-4%) have a mild stimulant laxative effect (4,6,12). Anthroid laxative use is not associated with an increased risk of developing colorectal ademoma or carcinoma (6138). The tannins (12-20%) (12,19) are responsible for the astringent effect (5). Yellow dock is reported to stimulate bile production (4). The leaves of yellow dock contain provitamin A (beta-carotene) and iron (19).

Adverse Reactions

Orally, vomiting may occur after ingestion of fresh rhizome (18). Consuming excessive amounts can cause diarrhea, nausea, polyuria (6), or dermatitis (4). Excessive oral use can also cause abdominal cramps, hypokalemia, and intestinal atrophy (4). There is one report of a death, preceded by vomiting, diarrhea, coma, respiratory depression, liver and kidney failure, severe metabolic acidosis, and ventricular fibrillation, after ingestion of 500 g of yellow dock (17). Oxalic acid reacts with calcium in plasma, forming insoluble calcium oxalate, which can cause hypocalcemia; the crystals may precipitate in the kidneys, blood vessels, heart, lungs, and liver. Individuals with a history of kidney stones should use yellow dock cautiously (12).

Topically, contact with the plant may cause dermatitis in people sensitive to yellow dock (6). Older or uncooked leaves should be avoided (6). Yellow dock can cause allergic reaction in individuals allergic to ragweed (4117).

Interactions with Herbs & Other Dietary Supplements

CALCIUM, IRON, ZINC: Concurrent use might decrease mineral absorption. Yellow dock contains oxalate (7,12), which can bind multivalent metal ions in the gastrointestinal tract and decrease mineral absorption.

CARDIAC-GLYCOSIDE-CONTAINING HERBS: Theoretically, concomitant use may increase the risk of cardiac glycoside toxicity because of the presence of stimulant laxatives in yellow dock, which can decrease serum potassium (19).

STIMULANT LAXATIVE HERBS: Theoretically, concomitant use of yellow dock with other stimulant laxative herbs can increase the risk of potassium depletion. Stimulant laxative herbs include aloe dried leaf sap, blue flag rhizome, alder buckthorn, European buckthorn, butternut bark, cascara bark, castor oil, colocynth fruit pulp, gamboge bark exudate, jalap root, black root, manna bark exudate, podophyllum root, rhubarb root, senna leaves and pods, and wild cucumber fruit (19).

Interactions with Drugs

DIGOXIN: Toxic effects due to hypokalemia (4) are possible when yellow dock is used chronically or in large amounts (19).

Interactions with Foods

CALCIUM, IRON, ZINC: Concurrent use might decrease mineral absorption from foods. Yellow dock contains oxalate (7,12), which can bind multivalent metal ions in the gastrointestinal tract and decrease mineral absorption.

Interactions with Lab Tests

COLORIMETRIC TESTS: Yellow dock might discolor urine (pink, red, purple, orange, rust), interfering with diagnostic tests that depend on a color change, due to its anthraquinone content (12,275).

SERUM POTASSIUM: Excessive use of yellow dock might cause potassium depletion, reducing serum potassium concentrations and test results (4,19).

Interactions with Diseases or Conditions

COAGULATION DISORDERS: Oxalate constituents of yellow dock can alter calcium concentrations and decrease coagulation time (4,12).

GI CONDITIONS: Avoid use in individuals with intestinal obstruction (4). Theoretically, yellow dock can exacerbate stomach and intestinal ulcers due to its mucosal irritant effect (19).

KIDNEY DISEASE: Yellow dock can damage kidneys with formation of insoluble oxalate; use with caution or avoid in individuals with a history of kidney stones (12,19). Yellow dock contains oxalates, and thus should be avoided in individuals with kidney disease (12).

Dosage and Administration

ORAL: Typical dose of the dried root is 2-4 grams or as a tea (Simmer 2-4 grams root in 150 mL of boiling water for 5-10 minutes, strain) 3 times daily (4). The liquid extract 2-4 mL (1:1 in 25% alcohol) 3 times daily (4) and a tincture 1-2 mL (1:5 in 45% alcohol) have also been used (4).

Comments

None.

YELLOW LUPIN

Also Known As

None.

Scientific Names

Lupinus luteus.
Family: Leguminosae or Fabaceae.

People Use This For

Orally, yellow lupin is used for urinary tract disorders, as an anthelmintic for worm infestations, and as a diuretic. Topically, it is used for ulcers.

Safety
POSSIBLY UNSAFE ...when the seeds or above ground parts are used orally (18).
There is insufficient reliable information available about the topical safety of yellow lupin.
PREGNANCY AND LACTATION: POSSIBLY UNSAFE ...when used orally; avoid using.

Effectiveness
There is insufficient reliable information available about the effectiveness of yellow lupin.

Mechanism of Action
Yellow lupin contains 0.6-1.6% quinolizidine alkaloids in the above ground plant parts, including sparteine, 13-hydroxylupanine, lupinines and p-cumaroyllupinine. The seed contain 0.4-3.3% quinolizidine alkaloids, including lupinines, sparteine, and in some cultivated strains, gramine. At present, we don't know how these components relate to the uses of lupin. Poisoning has been seen in animals, and is known as "lupinosis." It is due to the presence of mycotoxins that are produced by the fugus Phomopsis leptostromiformis, which sometimes lives in lupins (18).

Adverse Reactions
Orally, the symptoms of poisoning following ingestion include salivation, vomiting, dysphagia, cardiac arrhythmias, ascending paralysis and possibly death due to respiratory failure (18).

Interactions with Herbs & Other Dietary Supplements
Insufficient reliable information available.

Interactions with Drugs
No interactions are known to occur, and there is no known reason to expect a clinically significant interaction with yellow lupin.

Interactions with Foods
No interactions are known to occur, and there is no known reason to expect a clinically significant interaction with yellow lupin.

Interactions with Lab Tests
No interactions are known to occur, and there is no known reason to expect a clinically significant interaction with yellow lupin.

Interactions with Diseases or Conditions
No interactions are known to occur, and there is no known reason to expect a clinically significant interaction with yellow lupin.

Dosage and Administration
No typical dosage.

Comments
None.

YELLOW TOADFLAX

Also Known As
Brideweed, Butter and Eggs, Buttered Hayhocks, Calves' Snout, Churnstaff, Devil's Head, Devil's Ribbon, Doggies, Dragon-Bushes, Eggs and Bacon, Eggs and Collops, Flaxweed, Fluelli, Gallwort, Larkspur Lion's Mouth, Monkey Flower, Pattens and Clogs, Pedlar's Basket, Pennywort, Rabbits, Ramsted, Snapdragon, Toadpipe, Yellow Rod.

Scientific Names
Linaria vulgaris.
Family: Scrophulariaceae.

People Use This For
Orally, yellow toadflax is used for digestive and urinary tract disorders. It is also used as an anti-inflammatory, diuretic, and to stimulate sweating (18).
Topically, yellow toadflax is used for hemorrhoids, festering wounds, skin rashes, and ulcus cruris (18).

Safety

There is insufficient reliable information available about the safety of yellow toadflax.

Pregnancy and Lactation: Insufficient reliable information available; avoid using.

Effectiveness

There is insufficient reliable information available about the effectiveness of yellow toadflax.

Mechanism of Action

The applicable part of yellow toadflax is the whole flowering plant. There is insufficient reliable information available about the possible mechanism of action and active ingredients.

Adverse Reactions

None reported.

Interactions with Herbs & Other Dietary Supplements

Insufficient reliable information available.

Interactions with Drugs

No interactions are known to occur, and there is no known reason to expect a clinically significant interaction with yellow toadflax.

Interactions with Foods

No interactions are known to occur, and there is no known reason to expect a clinically significant interaction with yellow toadflax.

Interactions with Lab Tests

No interactions are known to occur, and there is no known reason to expect a clinically significant interaction with yellow toadflax.

Interactions with Diseases or Conditions

No interactions are known to occur, and there is no known reason to expect a clinically significant interaction with yellow toadflax.

Dosage and Administration

ORAL: One batch of tea taken over the course of one day. The tea is prepared by steeping 2 teaspoons dried herb in 300-600 mL of boiling water for 18 minutes and straining (18).

TOPICAL: Yellow toadflax is used in a poultice (18).

Comments

There is very little scientific information about this product. Our staff is continually analyzing the available information on natural medicines and will add data here as it becomes available.

YERBA MANSA

Also Known As

Lizard's Tail, Swamp Root, Yerba Manza.

Scientific Names

Anemopsis californica.
Family: Saururaceae.

People Use This For

Orally, yerba mansa is used for cancer; catarrh; common cold; cough; gastrointestinal disturbances; orthopedic, skin, and throat ailments; tuberculosis; venereal diseases; and women's ailments. It is also used orally as an analgesic, disinfectant, emetic, laxative, tonic, and to induce sweating (4206).

Safety

There is insufficient reliable information available about the safety of yerba mansa.

Pregnancy and Lactation: Insufficient reliable information is available; avoid using.

Effectiveness

There is insufficient reliable information available about the effectiveness of yerba mansa.

Mechanism of Action

The applicable parts of yerba mansa are the root and rhizome. Yerba mansa is believed to have sedative effects. It is also a urinary irritant (19). In animals, methyleugenol, a constituent of the volatile oil, prolongs the hypnotic effect of barbiturates and CNS depressant effects of chlorpromazine (19).

Adverse Reactions

None reported.

Interactions with Herbs & Other Dietary Supplements

HERBS WITH SEDATIVE PROPERTIES: Theoretically, concomitant use with herbs that have sedative properties might enhance therapeutic and adverse effects. These include calamus, calendula, California poppy, catnip, capsicum, celery, couch grass, elecampane, Siberian ginseng, German chamomile, goldenseal, gotu kola, hops, Jamaican dogwood, kava, lemon balm, sage, St. John's wort, sassafras, scullcap, shepherd's purse, stinging nettle, valerian, wild carrot, wild lettuce, and ashwaganda root (4,19).

Interactions with Drugs

DRUGS WITH SEDATIVE PROPERTIES: Theoretically, concomitant use might cause additive or prolonged sedative effects (19).
BARBITURATES: Theoretically, methyleugenol, a constituent of the volatile oil might prolong the hypnotic effect of barbiturates (19).
CHLORPROMAZINE: Theoretically, methyleugenol, a constituent of the volatile oil might prolong the CNS depressant effects of chlorpromazine (Thorazine) (19).

Interactions with Foods

No interactions are known to occur, and there is no known reason to expect a clinically significant interaction with yerba mansa.

Interactions with Lab Tests

No interactions are known to occur, and there is no known reason to expect a clinically significant interaction with yerba mansa.

Interactions with Diseases or Conditions

URINARY TRACT INFLAMMATION: Contraindicated due to urinary irritant effects (19).

Dosage and Administration

No typical dosage.

Comments

There is very little scientific information about this product. Our staff is continually analyzing the available information on natural medicines and will add data here as it becomes available.

YERBA SANTA

Also Known As

Bear's Weed, Consumptive's Weed, Eriodictyon, Gum Bush, Gum Plant, Hierba Santa, Holy Herb, Holy Weed, Mountain Balm, Sacred Herb, Tarweed.

Scientific Names

Eriodictyon californicum; Eriodictyon glutinosum; Wigandia californicum.
Family: Hydrophyllaceae.

People Use This For

Orally, yerba santa is used for coughs, colds, tuberculosis (6), asthma (6,11,18), and chronic bronchitis (11).
Topically, the herb is used as a poultice to treat bruises (6,11), sprains, wounds, insect bites (11), and to relieve rheumatism (6).
In folk medicine, it has been used as an antispasmodic, a tonic (11), an antipyretic, and an expectorant (6,11).
In foods and beverages, a fluid extract of yerba santa is used as a flavoring component (6,11).

In manufacturing, the herb is also used as a pharmaceutical flavoring agent to mask the bitter taste of other drugs (6,11,18).

Safety

LIKELY SAFE ...when consumed in food amounts (11). ...when used as an oral medicinal (6,12,18). There is insufficient reliable information about the safety of the topical use of yerba santa.

PREGNANCY AND LACTATION: Insufficient reliable information available.

Effectiveness

There is insufficient reliable information available about the effectiveness of yerba santa.

Mechanism of Action

The applicable part of yerba santa is the leaf. Yerba santa contains several flavonoids including eriodictyonine (6%), eriodictyol (0.5%) (6,11,18), chrysoeriol, and cirsimaritin (4118); tannins (11,18); and a trace amount of volatile oil (6,11,18). Yerba santa may have a mild diuretic effect (18). Eriodictyol is reported to exert an expectorant effect (6,11).

Adverse Reactions

None reported.

Interactions with Herbs & Other Dietary Supplements

Insufficient reliable information available.

Interactions with Drugs

No interactions are known to occur, and there is no known reason to expect a clinically significant interaction with yerba santa.

Interactions with Foods

No interactions are known to occur, and there is no known reason to expect a clinically significant interaction with yerba santa.

Interactions with Lab Tests

No interactions are known to occur, and there is no known reason to expect a clinically significant interaction with yerba santa.

Interactions with Diseases or Conditions

No interactions are known to occur, and there is no known reason to expect a clinically significant interaction with yerba santa.

Dosage and Administration

ORAL: People typically prepare yerba santa using 1 teaspoon of the leaves added to 1 cup boiling water. The liquid is taken warm, 30 minutes before bedtime or a mouthful taken 3 times a day (5254).

Comments

None.

YEW

Also Known As

Chinwood, Common Yew, English Yew, Pacific Yew, Western Yew.

Scientific Names

Taxus bacatta; Taxus brevifolia; and other Taxus species.
Family: Taxaceae.

People Use This For

In folk medicine, yew is used for promoting menstruation, inducing abortion, treating diphtheria, tapeworm infestation, tonsillitis, epilepsy (18), rheumatism, urinary tract conditions, and liver conditions (6).
Yew is FDA-approved for the treatment of breast and ovarian cancer.

Safety

LIKELY UNSAFE ...when used orally (6,18). All parts of the yew plant are considered poisonous (5604). Ingestion of 50-100 grams of yew needles can cause death (18,5604). Yew can cause severe gastrointestinal irritation and can cause heart rate to slow dangerously (17,159). Many of the reported fatalities have occurred after ingestion of large amounts of plant material, especially yew needles (5603,5604,5605).

CHILDREN: UNSAFE ...when the berries are used orally. One chewed berry is potentially lethal (159).

PREGNANCY AND LACTATION: UNSAFE ...when the needles are used orally. Yew needles have been used as an abortifacient (16,18).

Effectiveness

There is insufficient reliable information available about the effectiveness of yew.

Mechanism of Action

The applicable parts of yew are the bark, branch tip, and needle. The yew bark is reported to have antispasmodic, nerve toxicant, and cardiac metabolism effects (6,18). It contains many alkaloids of which taxine A and B are considered to be cardiotoxic (5603,5604). Taxine B affects myocardial cells of the heart by inhibiting both calcium and sodium transport across cell membranes (5604). Yew also contains flavonoids (18). Old growth Pacific yew bark contains 0.01% paclitaxel (13,512). Initially, the small yield from the bark limited the amount of drug that could be produced. Efforts to increase the drug without decimating the supply of the Pacific yew resulted in a semi-synthetic process that produces larger yields (512). English yew needles can be used to isolate 10 desacetylbaccatin III which is converted to paclitaxel (13,512). Paclitaxel is available as the prescription drug, Taxol, for treating advanced ovarian cancer, non-small cell lung cancer, metastatic breast cancer, esophageal cancer, bladder cancer, head and neck cancer, and AIDS-related Kaposi's sarcoma (15).

Adverse Reactions

Death has occurred with ingestion of 50-100 grams of yew needles (18,5604). Symptoms of poisoning include queasiness, dry mouth, (18) vomiting, vertigo, severe abdominal pain, weakness (5604), nervousness, trembling, dyspnea, incoordination (5603), tachycardia, bradycardia, arrhythmias, hypotension, unconsciousness, coma (5604), mydriasis, reddening of the lips, pale and cyanotic skin (6,18), and death secondary to cardiac arrest (5604).

Interactions with Herbs & Other Dietary Supplements

Insufficient reliable information available.

Interactions with Drugs

No interactions are known to occur, and there is no known reason to expect a clinically significant interaction with yew.

Interactions with Foods

No interactions are known to occur, and there is no known reason to expect a clinically significant interaction with yew.

Interactions with Lab Tests

No interactions are known to occur, and there is no known reason to expect a clinically significant interaction with yew.

Interactions with Diseases or Conditions

No interactions are known to occur, and there is no known reason to expect a clinically significant interaction with yew.

Dosage and Administration

No typical dosage.

Comments

None.

YIN CHEN

Also Known As

Armoise Capillaire, Capillary Wormwood, Chiu, In Chen, Inchin-Ko-To, Inchinko, Kawara-Yomogi, Kyunchinho, Rumput Roman, Shih Yin Ch'en, Yin Ch'en, Yin Ch'en Hao, Yin Chen Hao.

Scientific Names
Artemisia capillaris; Artemisia scoparia.
Family: Asteraceae or Compositae.

People Use This For
In Chinese and Japanese medicine, yin chen is used orally to treat hepatitis, infectious cholecystitis, and hyperlipidemia (4343). Yin chen is used to stimulate the bile flow, liver, and gallbladder (4342,4343). Yin chen is also used orally for newborn kernicterus (4343), for symptoms of intermittent fever and chills, bitter taste in the mouth, chest constriction, flank pain, dizziness, nausea, and loss of appetite (4342,4343). In addition, it is used for headache, constipation, painful urination, fever (4327), itching, tumors, catarrh, rheumatism, painful menses, malaria, and spasms (4327).

In Chinese and Japanese herbal combinations, yin chen is used orally for jaundice with fever, urinary dysfunction, constipation, and abdominal distention.

Yin chen is contained in inchin-ko-to, a Kampo (Chinese/Japanese) medicine (4343) used to treat hepatitis C (4333).

Safety
POSSIBLY SAFE ...when the above ground parts are used orally and appropriately (12,4342). However, serious conditions such as hepatitis require medical management by a physician and should not be self-treated.

CHILDREN: POSSIBLY UNSAFE ...when used orally. Children under the age of 12 years should not use except under care of physician (4344).

PREGNANCY AND LACTATION: LIKELY UNSAFE ...when used orally; avoid using (12).

Effectiveness
POSSIBLY EFFECTIVE ...when used orally to treat acute hepatitis, jaundice, and gallstone-related illness (4342,4343). There is insufficient reliable information available about the effectiveness of yin chen for its other uses.

Mechanism of Action
The applicable parts of yin chen are the above ground parts which contain varied constituents. Scoparone, chlorogenic acid, and caffeic acid have demonstrated effects in stimulating bile secretion and protecting the liver against carbon tetrachloride injury (4343). The essential oils cause yin chen to have antipyretic (4343) and antifungal properties (4344). Yin chen is also believed to have bactericide, anti-inflammatory, and diuretic properties (4342,4343,4344). Some evidence suggests yin chen can reduce blood pressure, cholesterol levels, and act as an antiasthmatic agent (4342,4343). Inchin-ko-to, a medicine that contains yin chen, shows evidence that it can prevent apoptosis that is believed to be the mechanism of cell death in viral and fulminant hepatitis (4345). Genepin, a metabolite of inchin-ko-to, appears to be responsible for therapeutic effects (4346).

Adverse Reactions
Orally, use of yin chen is associated with nausea, abdominal distention, and dizziness (4343). One study using yin chen and da zao (Fructus Zizyphi Jujubae) orally to treat infectious hepatitis reported 2 women developed Adams-Stokes syndrome. This syndrome is usually associated with heart block (4342). Yin chen can cause an allergic reaction in individuals sensitive to the Asteraceae/Compositae family. Members of this family include ragweed, chrysanthemums, marigolds, daisies, and many other herbs.

Interactions with Herbs & Other Dietary Supplements
Insufficient reliable information available.

Interactions with Drugs
No interactions are known to occur, and there is no known reason to expect a clinically significant interaction with yin chen.

Interactions with Foods
No interactions are known to occur, and there is no known reason to expect a clinically significant interaction with yin chen.

Interactions with Lab Tests
No interactions are known to occur, and there is no known reason to expect a clinically significant interaction with yin chen.

Interactions with Diseases or Conditions
No interactions are known to occur, and there is no known reason to expect a clinically significant interaction with yin chen.

Dosage and Administration

ORAL: A typical dose of yin chen is 9-15 grams. In very serious conditions up to 30 grams might be used three times daily (4342). Yin chen is most often used in herbal combinations.

Comments

Traditional Chinese medicine nearly always uses herbal combinations. A well accepted motto in herbal medicine translates as "One ruler, two ministers, three aides, and four guides." In this expression, the active principle is the ruler and the other nine are helpers with different degrees of strength (4343).

YLANG YLANG OIL

Also Known As

Ylang Ylang.
CAUTION: See separate listing for Cananga Oil (Cananga odorata macrophylla).

Scientific Names

Cangana odorata genuina, synonym Canangium odoratum genuina.
Family: Annonaceae.

People Use This For

There are no medicinal uses described for ylang ylang oil (11).
In foods and beverages, ylang ylang oil is used as a flavoring agent.
In manufacturing, it is used as a fragrance for cosmetics (maximum levels 1% in perfumes) and soaps (11).

Safety

LIKELY SAFE ...when consumed in amounts found in foods (11). It has Generally Recognized as Safe (GRAS) status in the US. ...when applied topically in amounts found in cosmetics and soaps (11) it is nonirritating and nonsensitizing to skin, and no phototoxicity is reported (11).
PREGNANCY AND LACTATION: Insufficient reliable information available; avoid using.

Effectiveness

There is insufficient reliable information available about the effectiveness of ylang ylang oil.

Mechanism of Action

There is insufficient reliable information available about the possible mechanism of action and active ingredients.

Adverse Reactions

None reported.

Interactions with Herbs & Other Dietary Supplements

Insufficient reliable information available.

Interactions with Drugs

No interactions are known to occur, and there is no known reason to expect a clinically significant interaction with ylang ylang oil.

Interactions with Foods

No interactions are known to occur, and there is no known reason to expect a clinically significant interaction with ylang ylang oil.

Interactions with Lab Tests

No interactions are known to occur, and there is no known reason to expect a clinically significant interaction with ylang ylang oil.

Interactions with Diseases or Conditions

No interactions are known to occur, and there is no known reason to expect a clinically significant interaction with ylang ylang oil.

Dosage and Administration

No typical dosage.

Comments

Ylang ylang oil is the distilled oil from freshly harvested Cangana odorata genuina flower.

YOGURT

Also Known As

Acidophilus Milk, Bulgarian Yogurt, Live Culture Yogurt, Probiotics, Yoghurt.
CAUTION: See separate listings for Bifidobacteria, Brewer's Yeast (Hansen CBS 5926), Lactobacillus, and Saccharomyces Boulardii.

Scientific Names

None.

People Use This For

Orally, yogurt is used for restoring gastrointestinal normal flora after antibiotic therapy (6,3589), reducing antibiotic-associated diarrhea (1255,3589), acute diarrhea in children (1253), treating and preventing vaginal candidiasis, bacterial vaginosis (6,1245), and preventing urinary tract infections (6761). Yogurt is also used orally for reducing the risk of colorectal cancer, treating hyperlipidemia (6,3590), eradicating Helicobacter pylori infection in peptic ulcer disease (6110), and preventing sunburns.
Intravaginally, yogurt is used by women for treating vaginal candidiasis (6) and bacterial vaginosis in pregnancy (1248). Yogurt is also eaten as a food and used as an alternative to milk in lactose-intolerant individuals (6).

Safety

LIKELY SAFE ...when used in food amounts. ...when used orally for medicinal purposes (6).
POSSIBLY SAFE ...when used intravaginally. There are no adverse reactions reported in a small clinical study (1248).
PREGNANCY: LIKELY SAFE ...when used orally in food amounts (6). There is insufficient reliable information available about the safety of the intravaginal use of yogurt (6), although no adverse reactions were reported in a small clinical study of pregnant women with bacterial vaginosis (1248).
LACTATION: LIKELY SAFE ...when used orally in food amounts (6). There is insufficient reliable information available about the safety of the intravaginal use of yogurt.

Effectiveness

POSSIBLY EFFECTIVE ...when used orally as a component of nutritional support for children with acute diarrheal illnesses (1242,1246,1253). ...when used orally for promoting recovery from persistent diarrhea in children (1250,1254). ...when used orally for borderline to moderate hyperlipidemia (1240,1241,3590). Fermented milk or yogurt products fermented with specific organisms including Lactobacillus acidophilus and a combination of Enterococcus faecium and Streptococcus thermophilus have been shown to produce mild to moderate reductions in serum cholesterol (1240,1241,3590). In one crossover study, four weeks of treatment with a human strain of Lactobacillus acidophilus resulted in a significant 3.2% reduction in total serum cholesterol (1240). In another small crossover study, a milk preparation fermented with Lactobacillus acidophilus plus added fructo-oligosaccharides was tested in men. After three weeks of treatment, there was a significant decrease in total cholesterol (4.4%), low-density lipoprotein (LDL) levels (5.4%), and the LDL/high-density lipoprotein (HDL) ratio (5.3%). There were not significant changes in triglyceride or HDL levels (1241). In a larger study, borderline hyperlipidemic men and women taking a specific yogurt fermented with a strain of Enterococcus faecium and two strains of Streptococcus thermophilus (CAUSIDO culture) for eight weeks had a significant average LDL reduction of 8.4% after adjusting for changes in body mass. Yogurts in this study fermented with a Streptococcus thermophilus/Lactobacillus acidophilus combination and a Streptococcus thermophilus/lactobacillus rhamnosus combination did not significantly reduce LDL cholesterol (3590). ...when used orally for reducing symptoms of antibiotic-associated diarrhea. There is some preliminary clinical evidence that a specific yogurt product fermented with Lactobacillus rhamnosus GG can significantly decrease symptoms of diarrhea, abdominal distress, stomach pain, and flatulence in people taking erythromycin (1255,3589). It's not known if other yogurt products offer the same benefits. ...when used orally as an alternative to milk for lactose-intolerant individuals (6). ...when used orally for preventing vaginal candidiasis (1245,1249). ...when used orally for bacterial vaginosis (1245). ...when used intravaginally for treating bacterial vaginosis in pregnancy (1248).
POSSIBLY INEFFECTIVE ...when used orally as an adjunctive treatment for asthma (1244,3589).
There is insufficient reliable information about the effectiveness of yogurt for its other uses. However, preliminary unpublished research indicates that consuming yogurt (a milk drink containing Lactobacillus) does not seem to prevent recurrent urinary tract infections (UTIs) when used up to 6 months in women with a history of UTIs (6761).

Mechanism of Action

Yogurt is a dairy preparation produced by fermenting milk using one or more of a variety of specific organisms such as

Lactobacillus acidophilus, Lactobacillus rhamnosus, Lactobacillus bulgaricus, Enterococcus faecium, Streptococcus thermophilus, and others (1240,1241,3586,3589,3590). Yogurt is a good dietary source of calcium (6,3586), protein, phosphorus, and riboflavin (3586). However, yogurt's medicinal benefit has primarily been attributed to the live cultures it contains as a source of probiotics. Probiotics are symbiotic bacteria similar to the human gastrointestinal normal flora that, when ingested, can pass through the stomach and potentially colonize the lower gastrointestinal tract. It is thought that this colonization might restore the normal flora after antibiotic therapy and maintain the balance of flora to prevent or minimize antibiotic-associated diarrhea (3587,3589). Probiotics contained in yogurt are also thought to help restore normal flora and normal bowel function in other cases of diarrhea (3587). For candidal vaginal infections, probiotics, particularly Lactobacillus acidophilus strains, are thought to be beneficial by helping to restore the normal flora of the vagina. Lactobacillus strains are normal flora in the vagina. Lactobacillus acidophilus has also been found to inhibit growth of Candida albicans. Presence of Lactobacillus species in the rectum has been associated with Lactobacillus colonization in the vagina (3588). For lowering cholesterol in hyperlipidemia, it is thought that certain culture strains found in yogurt might deconjugate bile salts (3590). People with lactase deficiency sometimes tolerate pasteurized yogurt or live culture yogurt better than milk (6). However, lactose absorption is probably greater with live culture yogurt than pasteurized yogurt (1256). Enzymes contained in live culture yogurt are thought to help in the breakdown and absorption of lactose (3586). The lactic acid bacteria found in yogurt can also suppress growth of pathogenic bacteria (3589) such as Salmonella typhimurium (6). Bulgaricum, a compound produced by some Lactobacillus bulgaricus strains, has also been shown to inhibit Gram positive and Gram negative bacteria (6). Preliminary evidence indicates that a yogurt-like fermented milk has activity against Helicobacter pylori (H. pylori). In one report, a liquid fraction of milk fermented overnight with Lactobacillus casei killed H. pylori bacteria. Although this mixture is essentially yogurt, commercial yogurt preparations did not demonstrate the same anti-H. pylori activity. The results of this unpublished study were reported at the 2000 annual meeting of the American Society for Microbiology (6110). Yogurt also shows some evidence that it might stimulate the immune system (6,3589). In vitro studies have produced an increase of immune related substances after yogurt consumption or exposure to lactic acid bacteria (3589). Other components of yogurt, such as whey protein, short peptides, and conjugated linoleic acid, may contribute to its proposed immune effects (3589). Yogurt may have an effect on IgE-mediated diseases such as asthma by decreasing IgE production, but human studies have produced conflicting results (3589). Yogurt may reduce nitrite concentrations in the gastrointestinal tract (3589). In animals, nitrites lead to the formation of carcinogenic compounds. In healthy infants, milk fermented with Lactobacillus casei increases fecal lactobacilli and decreases potentially harmful beta-glucosidase enzyme activity. Beta-glucosidase is a bacterial enzyme that has been associated with enterohepatic circulation of toxins and carcinogens. Beta-glucosidase has been shown to be elevated in diets high in meat (1243).

Adverse Reactions
Contamination of yogurt can cause adverse effects. A batch of yogurt contaminated with a toxic strain of E. coli caused hemolytic uremic syndrome (6).

Interactions with Herbs & Other Dietary Supplements
Insufficient reliable information is available.

Interactions with Drugs
CIPROFLOXACIN: Concomitant administration can significantly reduce absorption of ciprofloxacin (Cipro) (1252).
ERYTHROMYCIN: Concomitant use might reduce erythromycin-associated diarrhea (1255,3589).
TETRACYCLINES: Concomitant administration can reduce the absorption of tetracyclines (15).

Interactions with Foods
No interactions are known to occur, and there is no known reason to expect a clinically significant interaction with yogurt.

Interactions with Lab Tests
No interactions are known to occur, and there is no known reason to expect a clinically significant interaction with yogurt.

Interactions with Diseases or Conditions
SHORT BOWEL SYNDROME: People with short bowel syndrome absorb lactose from yogurt better than from milk (6).

Dosage and Administration
ORAL: Yogurt should be labeled with a "Live and Active Cultures" seal from the National Yogurt Association, indicating the product reliably contains at least 100 million active cultures per gram of yogurt (e.g., Dannon, Yoplait). For preventing antibiotic-induced diarrhea, 125 mL (approximately 4 ounces) of yogurt containing Lactobacillus GG taken twice daily throughout the antibiotic treatment course has been used (1255). Some researchers recommend

taking 240 mL (8 ounces) of other yogurt preparations twice daily (1736). Separate antibiotic administration and yogurt by at least two hours (1740). For acute diarrhea, 125 grams of yogurt containing Lactobacillus casei twice daily has been used (1253). For reducing cholesterol, several different doses have been tried depending on the preparation. A typical dose of 200 mL of yogurt containing Lactobacillus acidophilus per day has been used (1240). A combination product of 125 mL Lactobacillus acidophilus yogurt with 2.5% fructo-oligosaccharides three times daily has also been used (1241). A dose of 450 mL daily of yogurt containing the CAUSIDO culture has also been used (3590). For preventing vaginal candidiasis and bacterial vaginosis, a typical dose is 150 mL Lactobacillus acidophilus yogurt per day (1245).
INTRAVAGINAL: No typical dosage.

Comments

Yogurt is milk that has been fermented with Lactobacillus acidophilus, Lactobacillus bulgaricus, Streptococcus lactis, Streptococcus thermophilus, or other bacteria (6,511). Bulgarian yogurt is concentrated by a factor of 1.5 and contains the highest amount of lactose (6).

YOHIMBE

Also Known As

Johimbi, Yohimbehe, Yohimbehe cortex.

Scientific Names

Pausinystalia yohimbe, synonyms Pausinystalia johimbe, Corynanthe johimbi, Corynanthe yohimbi.
Family: Rubiaceae.

People Use This For

Orally, yohimbe is used as an aphrodisiac (2), for impotence (3305), exhaustion (2), angina, hypertension (19), diabetic neuropathy, and postural hypotension (505). Yohimbe is also used for general sexual dysfunction in men and women, sexual dysfunction caused by selective-serotonin reuptake inhibitors (SSRI) (3306,3970,3971), and as an adjunct to conventional antidepressants for refractory depression (3304).
Yohimbe bark is also smoked or snuffed for its hallucinogenic effects (6,515).

Safety

POSSIBLY SAFE ...when used orally and appropriately with medical supervision. The primary active constituent, yohimbine has been shown to be safe in several clinical trials lasting up to 10 weeks (3305,3307,3311,3313). However, yohimbe is not appropriate for self-treatment.
LIKELY UNSAFE ...when used orally in excessive doses or without medical supervision. The primary active ingredient, yohimbine, is considered unsafe for unmonitored nonprescription use (515). Large doses can cause significant toxicity including severe hypotension, heart conduction disorders, and death (18).
There is insufficient reliable information available about the safety of inhaling yohimbe bark.
CHILDREN: LIKELY UNSAFE ...when used orally. Children can be extra sensitive to the adverse effects of yohimbe (19).
PREGNANCY AND LACTATION: LIKELY UNSAFE ...when used orally. Yohimbe might have uterine relaxant effects and also cause fetal toxicity (19).

Effectiveness

POSSIBLY EFFECTIVE ...when used orally for impotence. There is some evidence that the primary constituent, yohimbine, can be helpful for impotence. Yohimbine seems to help men with organic, psychogenic, mixed, and unknown vascular erectile dysfunction (6,11,3305,3307,3311,3313). Some herbalists suggest that the yohimbe bark actually works better than the isolated yohimbine constituent; however, yohimbe bark has not been evaluated in studies.
...when used orally for selective-serotonin reuptake inhibitor (SSRI) induced sexual dysfunction. There is evidence from multiple clinical trials that the primary constituent, yohimbine, can improve sexual dysfunction associated with SSRIs (3305,3306,3307,3311,3313,3970,3971,3972,3973). However, this benefit has not been described specifically for the yohimbe bark.
There is insufficient reliable information available about the effectiveness of yohimbe for its other uses.

Mechanism of Action

The applicable part of yohimbe is the bark. The constituent thought to be responsible for yohimbe's effects is the alkaloid yohimbine (6,11). Yohimbe bark contains approximately 6% yohimbine (6). Aphrodisiac activity of yohimbe has been attributed to genital blood vessel dilation, nerve impulse transmission to genital tissue, and increased reflex excitability in the sacral region of the spinal cord (11). The yohimbine constituent readily penetrates the central nervous system and works primarily through alpha 2-adrenergic receptor blockade (6,11,3305). It also has monoamine oxidase inhibiting, calcium channel blocking, and peripheral serotonin receptor blocking effects (6,11). Yohimbine likely works several ways to affect impotence since it has been effective in men with organic, psychogenic, mixed, and unknown vascular erectile dysfunction (6,11,3305,3310,3311). Yohimbine's effect on impotence might be mediated through both increased penile blood flow and increased central sympathetic excitatory impulses to the genital tissue (11,3305,3309). In women, a nitric oxide-enhanced form of yohimbine (NMI-870) is theorized to improve sexual arousal by increasing vaginal blood flow by dilating vaginal blood vessels (6198).

Adverse Reactions

Orally, yohimbe and the constituent yohimbine in typical doses can cause excitation, tremor, insomnia, anxiety, hypertension, tachycardia, dizziness, gastric intolerance, salivation, sinusitis, irritability, headache, urinary frequency, fluid retention, nausea, and vomiting (2,11,3303,3304,3305,3309,3311,3313). Although low doses can stimulate respiration, high doses can cause respiratory depression (11). High doses can also cause other severe toxicities including paralysis, severe hypotension, cardiac conduction disorders, cardiac failure, and death (6,18). There is also one report of a hypersensitivity reaction including fever; chills; malaise; itchy, scaly skin; progressive renal failure; and lupus-like syndrome associated with ingestion of a one-day dose of yohimbine (6169).

Interactions with Herbs & Other Dietary Supplements

CAFFEINE-CONTAINING HERBS: Theoretically, concomitant use of yohimbe with large amounts of caffeine-containing herbs or products can increase the risk of hypertensive crisis (12). Caffeine-containing herbs include coffee, cola, guarana, mate, and tea.

EPHEDRA: Theoretically, concomitant use of large amounts of ephedra can increase the risk of hypertensive crisis due to ephedrine content (12).

HERBS WITH MONOAMINE OXIDASE INHIBITING (MAOI) ACTIVITY: Theoretically, concomitant use of these herbs with yohimbe can have additive therapeutic and adverse effects (12). Herbs with MAOI activity include California poppy, ginkgo, mace, and St. John's wort (12).

Interactions with Drugs

ALPHA 2-ADRENERGIC-BLOCKING DRUGS: Yohimbe is contraindicated due to the risk of increased alpha-adrenergic blockade (19).

ANTIDIABETES DRUGS: Theoretically, concomitant use of yohimbe can interfere with antidiabetes drugs due to MAOI activity (15,515).

ANTIHYPERTENSIVE DRUGS: Concomitant use of yohimbe can interfere with blood pressure control and should be used with caution (6,11).

BETA-BLOCKING DRUGS: Theoretically, these drugs can protect against yohimbine toxicity (19).

CLONIDINE (Catapres), GUANABENZ (Wytensin): Avoid concomitant use of these drugs because yohimbine antagonizes their effects (11,19).

MONOAMINE OXIDASE INHIBITORS (MAOIs): Concomitant use with yohimbe can result in additive effects (6,11,12).

NALOXONE (Narcan): Concomitant use can have additive therapeutic and adverse effects (19).

PHENOTHIAZINES: Yohimbe is contraindicated with phenothiazines due to the risk of increased alpha 2-adrenergic antagonism (19).

SYMPATHOMIMETIC DRUGS: Yohimbe is contraindicated because concomitant use increases the risk of hypertensive crisis due to yohimbe MAOI activity (5,6).

TRICYCLIC ANTIDEPRESSANTS: Yohimbe is contraindicated due to its potential to increase or decrease blood pressure (19).

Interactions with Foods

TYRAMINE-CONTAINING FOODS: Avoid concomitant consumption of large amounts of tyramine-containing foods, due to the risk of hypertensive crisis (5,6,11). Tyramine-containing foods include aged cheeses, fermented meats, red wines, and others (506).

VASOPRESSOR-CONTAINING FOODS: Avoid concomitant consumption of large amounts of vasopressor-containing foods due to the risk of hypertensive crisis (5,6,11). Vasopressor-containing foods include overripe fava beans, coffee, tea, colas, and chocolate (506).

Interactions with Lab Tests

No interactions are known to occur, and there is no known reason to expect a clinically significant interaction with yohimbe.

Interactions with Diseases or Conditions

ANGINA, HEART DISEASE: Contraindicated, due to the cardiovascular effects of the yohimbe constituent, yohimbine (6,11,19,515).

ANXIETY: Avoid; the yohimbe constituent, yohimbine, might cause anxiety (19,515).
BENIGN PROSTATIC HYPERPLASIA (BPH): Contraindicated. Theoretically, yohimbe might exacerbate symptoms of BPH due to the presynaptic alpha-2 blocking activity of the constituent yohimbine (14).
DIABETES: Avoid, due to the monoamine oxidase inhibiting (MAOI) activity of yohimbe (15,515). Use of MAO inhibitors in patients receiving insulin or oral antidiabetes drugs has been associated with hypoglycemic episodes (15).
DEPRESSION: Contraindicated. The constituent yohimbine might elicit manic-like symptoms in individuals with bipolar depression or suicidal tendencies in individuals with endogenous depression (19).
HYPERTENSION: Avoid; small amounts of yohimbine can increase blood pressure (6,19).
HYPOTENSION: Contraindicated; large amounts of yohimbine can cause hypotension (6,515).
KIDNEY DISEASE: Contraindicated (2,6,11,12,18,19,515). Theoretically, yohimbine might have antidiuretic effects (19).
LIVER DISEASE: Contraindicated (2,6,11,12,19,515). Theoretically, liver disease might alter metabolism of the constituent yohimbine (19).
POST-TRAUMATIC STRESS DISORDER (PTSD): Avoid; the constituent yohimbine has been associated with triggering acute symptoms in four individuals with PTSD (1294).
PROSTATE INFLAMMATION: Contraindicated (11,12). Theoretically, yohimbe might exacerbate symptoms of prostate inflammation due to the presynaptic alpha-2 blocking activity of the constituent yohimbine (14).
SCHIZOPHRENIA: Caution, the constituent yohimbine might activate psychoses in patients with schizophrenia (19,515).
YOHIMBE HYPERSENSITIVITY: Contraindicated (19).

Dosage and Administration

ORAL: For sexual dysfunction, including impotence, a typical dose of the constituent yohimbine is 15-30 mg daily (3303,3305,3307,3313). Doses of yohimbine up to 100 mg daily have been tried (3312). However, significantly more severe adverse effects would be expected with such a high dose. Yohimbe typically contains 6% yohimbine (6). Yohimbe bark 250-500 mg would typically contain 15-30 mg of the yohimbine constituent. A tincture of the bark is sometimes used in the amount of 5-10 drops three times per day (3895).

Comments

Yohimbe is the name of an evergreen tree that is native to Zaire, Cameroon, and Gabon. The bark of the yohimbe tree contains the alkaloid, yohimbine (6,4201).

YUCCA

Also Known As

Adam's Needle, Aloe Yucca, Bear Grass, Dagger Plant, Joshua Tree, Mohave Yucca, Our-Lord's-Candle, Soapweed, Spanish Bayonet.

Scientific Names

Yucca aloifolia; Yucca brevifolia, synonym Yucca arborescens; Yucca filamentosa; Yucca glauca; Yucca schidigera, synonym Yucca mohavensis; Yucca whipplei; and other Yucca species.
Family: Liliaceae or Agavaceae.

People Use This For

Orally, yucca is used to treat arthritis (4,5,6,11), hypertension, migraine headaches, colitis, hypercholesterolemia (6), stomach disorders, diabetes, poor circulation (4), and liver and gallbladder disorders (18).
Topically, yucca is used for sores, skin diseases, inflammation, preventing bleeding, sprains, broken limbs, dandruff, baldness (11), joint pain, and as a hair wash (4).
Traditionally, yucca is used by American Indians as a foodstuff (4).
In manufacturing, yucca extract is used as a foaming and flavoring agent in carbonated beverages (6,11), and compounds within the plant have been used in the synthesis of new drugs (6).

Safety

LIKELY SAFE ...when consumed in amounts commonly found in foods (11). Mojave yucca and Joshua tree are both approved for food use in the US (11).
POSSIBLY SAFE ...when used orally and appropriately, short-term (12).
There is insufficient reliable information available about the safety of the topical or long-term oral use use of yucca.
PREGNANCY AND LACTATION: POSSIBLY SAFE ...when used orally in amounts found in foods (yucca saponins are thought not to be absorbed from the GI tract) (4); avoid using in amounts greater than those found in foods (4).

Effectiveness

POSSIBLY EFFECTIVE ...when used orally in combination with diet and exercise for lowering high blood pressure and correcting abnormal triglycerides and high cholesterol (4,6).

There is insufficient reliable information available about the effectiveness of yucca for its other uses.

Mechanism of Action

Yucca contains saponins that are believed responsible for the pharmacologic activity of the plant (4,6,11).

In experimental animals, yucca extracts exhibit anti-inflammatory, antitumor, and antiviral activity (4,6,11).

A twelve-week study of Mohave yucca extract in rats showed no evidence of toxicity (11). In vitro, the extract had hemolytic activity (6,11). A human study of "saponin extract" of the "desert yucca plant" provides inconclusive evidence that it may reduce arthritic symptoms of pain, swelling, and stiffness (4,6). It may also reduce high blood pressure, high triglyceride and cholesterol levels, and incidence of migraine headaches (4,6). The mechanism for these effects is unknown because researchers do not believe yucca saponins are absorbed from the gastrointestinal tract (4).

Adverse Reactions

Orally, yucca can cause stomach upset (7,18), mucous membrane irritation, bitter taste, nausea, and vomiting (7). Intravenous yucca administration may result in hemolysis (6).

Interactions with Herbs & Other Dietary Supplements

Insufficient reliable information available.

Interactions with Drugs

No interactions are known to occur, and there is no known reason to expect a clinically significant interaction with yucca.

Interactions with Foods

No interactions are known to occur, and there is no known reason to expect a clinically significant interaction with yucca.

Interactions with Lab Tests

No interactions are known to occur, and there is no known reason to expect a clinically significant interaction with yucca.

Interactions with Diseases or Conditions

No interactions are known to occur, and there is no known reason to expect a clinically significant interaction with yucca.

Dosage and Administration

ORAL: People typically use 380 to 490 mg of the powdered yucca stalk or root two to three times daily.

One yucca supplier suggests three daily doses based on body weight: under 100 pounds, 380 mg per dose; 100 to 175 pounds, 760 mg; and over 175 pounds, 1140 mg. Yucca can be prepared as a liquid by boiling one-fourth ounce of the root in 16 ounces of water for 15 minutes. People typically drink 3 to 5 cups of the liquid per day (6006).

TOPICAL: No typical dosage.

Comments

None.

ZEDOARY

Also Known As

Cedoaria, Cetoal, E Zhu, E-Zhu, Indian Arrowroot, Kua, Shoti, Temu Kuning, Temu Putih, Turmeric, Zedoaire, Zedoária, Zedoarie rhizoma, Zitwer, Zitwerwirtzelstock.

CAUTION: See separate listings for Turmeric, Goldenseal, and Javanese Turmeric.

Scientific Names

Curcuma zedoaria.

Family; Zingiberaceae.

People Use This For

Orally, zedoary is used for colic, spasms, stimulating appetite, improving digestion (2), stimulating bile flow, and as an anti-inflammatory (512).

In combination herbal products, zedoary extracts are used for gastrointestinal complaints and stimulating bile flow (18). In folk medicine, zedoary is used for nervous diseases (18).

Safety

POSSIBLY SAFE …when used orally and appropriately (12).

PREGNANCY: LIKELY UNSAFE …when used orally; avoid using (12) due to potential abortifacient effects (19).

LACTATION: Insufficient reliable information available; avoid using.

Effectiveness

There is insufficient reliable information available about the effectiveness of zedoary.

Mechanism of Action

The applicable part of zedoary is the rhizome. Zedoary contains a volatile oil and curcuminoids (18). Zedoary is thought to stimulate bile production and gallbladder emptying (512). The volatile oil contains sesquiterpene ketones known as turmerones that are believed responsible for increasing bile production (512). The curcuminoid constituents are believed to be responsible for gallbladder emptying effects (512). The isolated sesquiterpene constituent dehydrocurdione shows some evidence of anti-inflammatory activity (4011). Experimental evidence suggests other sesquiterpenes isolated from zedoary might be hepatoprotective (4012). Compounds isolated from zedoary demonstrate some evidence of antifungal (4013) and cytotoxic (4014) activity.

Adverse Reactions

None reported.

Interactions with Herbs & Other Dietary Supplements

Insufficient reliable information is available.

Interactions with Drugs

No interactions are known to occur, and there is no known reason to expect a clinically significant interaction with zedoary.

Interactions with Foods

No interactions are known to occur, and there is no known reason to expect a clinically significant interaction with zedoary.

Interactions with Lab Tests

No interactions are known to occur, and there is no known reason to expect a clinically significant interaction with zedoary.

Interactions with Diseases or Conditions

HEAVY MENSES: Some experts suggest that zedoary should not be used by women who have heavy menstrual periods (12).

Dosage and Administration

ORAL: One cup of tea three times daily at meals. To make tea, steep 1-1.5 grams powdered dried rhizome in 150 mL boiling water, 5-10 minutes, and strain (18).

Comments

Traditional methods for preparing zedoary involve prolonged washing with water to remove most of the protein, water-soluble nutrients, and presumably, an unidentified toxic constituent (4015).

ZINC

Also Known As

Zinc Acetate, Zinc Acexamate, Zinc Aspartate, Zinc Citrate, Zinc Gluconate, Zinc Methionine, Zinc Monomethionine, Zinc Oxide, Zinc Picolinate, Zinc Sulfate.

Scientific Names

Zinc; Zn; atomic number 30.

People Use This For

Orally, zinc is used for treatment and prevention of zinc deficiency. It is also used orally for treating the common cold, recurrent ear infections, macular degeneration, night blindness, cataracts, diabetes, hypertension, AIDS, psoriasis, eczema, and acne. It is also used orally for anorexia nervosa, acute diarrhea in children with zinc deficiency, blunted sense of taste (hypogeusia), aphthous ulcers, Crohn's disease, ulcerative colitis, and peptic ulcers. Other oral uses include benign prostatic hyperplasia (BPH), male infertility, male impotence, osteoporosis, rheumatoid arthritis, and muscle cramps in patients with cirrhosis. It is also used orally for sickle cell anemia, thalassemia, Alzheimer's disease, Down syndrome, Wilson's disease, Hansen's disease, acrodermatitis enteropathica, and delayed wound healing associated with zinc deficiency. Zinc is also used orally for improving athletic performance and strength, improving immune function, improving growth and health in zinc-deficient stunted children, tinnitus, and severe head injuries. It is also used orally and locally for parasitic infections.

Topically, zinc is used for treating acne, herpes simplex infections, resistant trichomonas infection, and speeding wound healing. Zinc citrate is used in toothpaste and mouthwash to prevent dental plaque formation and gingivitis. Intranasally, zinc is used for treating the common cold.

Ophthalmically, zinc sulfate is used in products for eye irritation.

Intravenously, zinc is used as a component of total parenteral nutrition and for improving outcomes in burn patients.

Safety

LIKELY SAFE ...when used orally and appropriately. Zinc is safe in amounts that do not exceed the tolerable upper intake level (UL) of 40 mg per day (7135). ...when used topically and appropriately on intact skin. Although topical absorption can occur, as much as 2 grams/kg of topical zinc oxide has been well tolerated (14).

POSSIBLY SAFE ...when used orally and appropriately in doses higher than the tolerable upper intake level (UL). There is some concern that doses higher than the UL of 40 mg per day might decrease copper absorption and result in anemia. However, there is some evidence doses of elemental zinc as high as 80 mg daily in combination with copper 2 mg can be used safely for approximately 6 years without significant adverse effects (7303).

LIKELY UNSAFE ...when taken orally in excessive amounts. Chronic intake of 450-1600 mg daily of a zinc supplement can cause sideroblastic anemia. Ingestion of 10-30 grams of zinc sulfate can be lethal in adults (7135).

CHILDREN: LIKELY SAFE ...when used orally and appropriately (7135). Zinc is safe in amounts that do not exceed the tolerable upper intake level (UL). The UL for children is based on age. It is 4 mg per day for infants birth to 6 months, 5 mg per day for infants 7 to 12 months, 7 mg per day for children 1 to 3 years, 12 mg per day for children 4 to 8 years, 23 mg per day for children 9 to 13 years, and 34 mcg per day for adolescents 14 to 18 years (7135). POSSIBLY UNSAFE ...when used orally in high doses. Taking amounts greater than the tolerable upper intake level (UL) can cause sideroblastic anemia and copper deficiency (7135).

PREGNANCY: LIKELY SAFE ... when used orally and appropriately. Zinc is safe in amounts that do not exceed the tolerable upper intake level (UL) of 40 mg per day or 34 mg per day for pregnant women 14 to 18 years (7135). LIKELY UNSAFE ...when used orally in high doses. Tell pregnant patients not to exceed the tolerable upper intake level (UL) (7135). Taking higher doses during the third trimester can cause premature births and stillbirths (332).

LACTATION: LIKELY SAFE ...when used orally and appropriately. Zinc is safe in amounts that do not exceed the tolerable upper intake level (UL) of 40 mg per day or 34 mg per day for lactating women 14 to 18 years (7135). POSSIBLY UNSAFE ...when used orally in high doses. Tell breast-feeding patients not to exceed the tolerable upper intake level (UL). Higher doses can cause zinc-induced copper deficiency in nursing infants (7135).

Effectiveness

EFFECTIVE ...when used orally or intravenously for preventing and treating zinc deficiency (2619). However, routine zinc supplementation is not recommended (403). Zinc deficiency requiring supplementation may occur in severe diarrhea, malabsorption syndromes, liver cirrhosis and alcoholism, after major surgery, and during long-term administration of total parenteral nutrition (3539). ...when used orally for Wilson's disease (822,823,2693).

LIKELY EFFECTIVE ...when used orally for reducing the duration and severity of acute diarrhea in malnourished or zinc-deficient children (825,826,827,3455,3456).

POSSIBLY EFFECTIVE ...when used as a lozenge for decreasing the duration of the common cold in adults. The majority of studies show a significant decrease in the duration of symptoms of the common cold when adults take zinc gluconate or acetate lozenges providing 9-24 mg elemental zinc per dose. Lozenges should be taken every 2 hours while awake starting within 48 hours of symptom onset (333,334,335,337,6703,6705). However, not all studies have been positive (333,338,339,6521,6522,6700). The reason for these different findings is not clear, but might be due to differences in zinc formulations and study methodologies. In some cases, flavoring agents such as citric acid, mannitol, and sorbitol might chelate zinc and decrease zinc ionization. Since zinc ionization is thought to be important for benefit, this could decrease effectiveness (300,340,6522). Some of the positive studies have also been criticized for inadequately blinding the unpleasant, distinctive taste of zinc (6522,6706). Overall, zinc products seem to be beneficial for reducing duration of symptoms of the common cold in adults. Products containing flavoring agents such as citric acid, mannitol, or sorbitol might decrease effectiveness and should be avoided. So far, zinc lozenges do not seem to be effective for children (341). ...when used intranasally for reducing the duration of symptoms of the common cold. If started within 24 hours of cold onset, a specific zinc nasal spray (Zicam Cold Remedy, Gel Tech) seems to reduce the duration of symptoms. Preliminary clinical evidence suggests it might reduce the duration of cold symptoms by around 75% (1278,6471). ...when used orally for hypogeusia (6542,6543,6544,6545,6546). Zinc may be effective for taste dysfunction in some patients with zinc depletion (6542,6546). Zinc has also been effective for hypogeusia conditions unrelated to zinc deficiency, such as gustin/carbonic anhydrase VI deficiency, captopril-induced taste disturbances, hypogeusia secondary to head and neck radiation, and post-traumatic olfactory disorder (6543,6544,6545,6547). In uremic adults, zinc supplementation, orally or via dialysate, might improve taste acuity, but appears to be ineffective for pediatric dialysis patients (6548,6549,6550). ...when used orally in combination with antioxidant vitamins to slow progression age-related macular degeneration (ARMD). Taking elemental zinc 80 mg plus vitamin C 500 mg, vitamin E 400 IU, and beta-carotene 15 mg daily seems to provide a risk reduction of 27 % for visual acuity loss and a risk reduction of 28% for progression to more advanced ARMD in patients with intermediate and advanced ARMD (7303). There isn't enough evidence to know if zinc plus antioxidants is beneficial for people with less advanced disease or for preventing ARMD. Zinc from the diet or zinc supplements alone does not seem to have any effect on ARMD progression (6583,6584,7303). ...when used orally for anorexia nervosa (6905,6906). Zinc supplementation can increase weight gain and improve depressive symptoms in patients with anorexia nervosa (6905,6906). ...when used to treat or prevent peptic ulcers (6588,6589,6590,6591). Zinc acexamate (not available in the US) has shown efficacy for peptic ulcers when compared to placebo or H2 receptor antagonist drugs (6589). It is not known if other zinc salts are effective. ...when used orally for acrodermatitis enteropathica (821,2689,2690,2691). ...when used orally for increasing birth weight and head circumference by pregnant women with mildly low plasma zinc levels (301). ...when given orally for improving growth and overall health in zinc-deficient stunted infants (6191). ...when used orally to treat sickle cell disease in people with zinc deficiency (6594,6595,6596). Zinc might decrease the incidence of sickle-cell crisis and infections (6594,6596). Although zinc has reduced the number of hospitalizations for sickle cell crisis, the severity of a crisis does not appear to be reduced, based on length of hospital stay (6594,6596). ...when used orally for treating muscle cramps in zinc-deficient patients with cirrhosis (1352). ...when used orally for treating acne. Some research suggests that zinc levels might be lower in the serum and skin of people with acne (2686,6507,6508,6509). Clinical trials have been small, but most suggest that zinc can improve acne (6297,6298,6299,6501,6502,6503,6504). So far, it is not clear how zinc compares to traditional treatments. Comparative trials with tetracycline yielded conflicting results (6505,6506). ...when used topically with erythromycin for treating acne (819,820,2687,2688). ...when used orally in combination with anti-leprosy drugs for Hansen's disease (14,6534,6535,6536,6537). Zinc levels appear to be reduced in people with leprosy. Early clinical evidence suggests that the addition of zinc to the anti-leprosy drug regimen might allow lowering or eliminating steroid doses in a severe form of leprosy, erythema nodosum leprosum (6534,6535,6536). ...when used as a toothpaste or mouthwash alone or in combination with triclosan to prevent plaque accumulation, development of gingivitis, and formation of calculus (6523,6524,6525,6526,6527,6528,6529). However, most studies used zinc citrate in combination with triclosan, which is not available in the US (6523). ...when used topically for herpes simplex infection (14,6538,6539,6540). Zinc sulfate seems to reduce severity and duration of symptoms in both orolabial and genital herpes (6538,6539,6540). ...when used parenterally immediately post-head trauma for improving rate of neurological recovery (2696). ...when used intravenously in combination with other minerals for improving outcomes in burn patients (6520). Supplementation with zinc, copper, and selenium significantly reduced pulmonary infections and shortened intensive care unit stay in patients with serious burns (6520). ...when used topically to treat leg ulcers (2694,6901). ...when used orally to treat arterial and venous leg ulcers in people with low zinc levels (6903). However, zinc is not beneficial for people without depleted zinc levels (6902). ...when used orally for recurring aphthous ulcers in people with low zinc levels (6593). However, it's not helpful for people with adequate zinc levels (6592,6593).

POSSIBLY INEFFECTIVE ...when used orally for improving iron status in pregnant women taking supplemental iron and folic acid (6104). ...when used orally to treat eczema (6911). Zinc levels appear to be normal in children with eczema. Oral zinc does not appear to improve the surface area affected and degree of erythema, symptom scores of itch and sleep disturbance, or topical steroid use in children with eczema (6911). ...when used orally to treat psoriasis (6513,6514,6912). Zinc epidermal levels are reportedly lower in people with psoriasis (6509). However, zinc has no effect on the psoriasis area and severity index (6513,6514). ...when used orally to treat psoriatic arthritis (6514). Oral zinc, alone or in combination with non-steroidal anti-inflammatory drugs (NSAIDs), has no effect on the course of psoriatic arthritis (14,6514,6515). ...when used orally to treat rheumatoid arthritis (14,2823,6516,6517,6518,6519). ...when used orally to prevent or treat aphthous ulcers (6592,6593). ...when used to treat inflammatory bowel disease (6913,6915,6916). ...when used to treat tinnitus (6914,6917,6921). ...when used to treat alopecia. Although there is some preliminary evidence that zinc in combination with biotin might be helpful for alopecia areata (6932), most studies indicate that zinc is not effective for alopecia areata, alopecia totalis, or alopecia universalis (6931,6932). ...when used orally to prevent age-related macular degeneration (ARMD). Dietary zinc or zinc supplementation alone does not seem to reduce the risk of developing of ARMD (6579,6580,6581). ...when used orally in combination with antioxidant vitamins for cataracts. Taking elemental zinc 80 mg plus vitamin C 500 mg, vitamin E 400 IU, and beta-carotene 15 mg daily does not seem to have any effect on the development or progression of age-related lens opacities (cataracts) or the need for cataract surgery in well-nourished people (7304). ...when used orally in combination with vitamins for AIDS diarrhea-wasting syndrome (6564). ...when used orally in combination with selenium for decreasing the occurrence of infectious disease in the elderly. Although zinc and selenium supplementation in elderly people seems to increase antibody titres in those receiving influenza vaccination, supplementation does not seem to reduce the occurrence rate of infections (6553). There is insufficient reliable information available about the effectiveness of zinc for its other uses. However, there is some preliminary clinical evidence that zinc supplementation in combination with zidovudine (AZT, Retrovir, component of Combivir) can reduce opportunistic infections with Pneumocystis carinii and Candida (6566). However, zinc supplementation might adversely effect overall survival in people with AIDS (6565). Zinc has also been used to treat male impotence secondary to disease or medical treatment, with varying results (6568,6569,6570,6571,6572,6708). Preliminary clinical evidence shows modest slowing of cognitive decline in patients with Alzheimer's disease who take zinc supplements (2824). More evidence is needed to rate zinc for these uses.

Mechanism of Action

Zinc is a biologically essential trace element (511). It is a cofactor in many biological processes, including DNA, RNA, and protein synthesis. Zinc also plays a role in immune function and wound healing, reproduction, growth and development, behavior and learning, taste and smell, blood clotting, thyroid hormone function, and is associated with insulin action (331,403). Nearly 100 specific enzymes depend on zinc as a catalyst (7135). Meat, seafood, dairy products, nuts, legumes, and whole grains contain relatively high concentrations of zinc (331). Many breakfast cereals contain added zinc (7135). Zinc is absorbed from foods at a rate of 15-40%. Bioavailability is influenced by zinc status. Most zinc is absorbed in the small intestine, particularly the jejunum (7135). More zinc is absorbed in states of zinc deficiency. More than 85% of the total body zinc is in skeletal muscle and bone, with plasma zinc tightly regulated at about 10 to 15 micromol/L (7135). Most zinc is excreted in the feces, with a small amount eliminated in the urine (7135). Zinc deficiency is characterized by growth retardation, low insulin levels, anorexia, mental lethargy, irritability, low sperm count, generalized hair loss, rough and dry skin, skin lesions, slow wound healing, decreased thyroid function, delayed onset of puberty, poor sense of smell and taste, diarrhea, and nausea. Deficiency is rare in the United States; most diets provide more than the recommended dietary allowance (RDA) (3539). Zinc is responsible for neutrophil, natural killer cell, and T-lymphocyte function (6551). Even mild zinc deficiency might adversely affect T cell functions (6552). Supplemental zinc seems to improved cell-mediated immune response in older people (824). For the common cold, zinc supplementation is theorized to be beneficial by inhibiting viral replication and boosting immune function (3581). The amount of available ionized zinc seems to determine the effectiveness of zinc (336). The extent of zinc ionization varies with different lozenge formulations (340). The addition of flavoring agents such as citric acid, mannitol or sorbitol to zinc gluconate lozenge preparations decreases the extent of zinc ionization, while the addition of glycine to zinc gluconate lozenges does not (300). Zinc ions might have effects against other viruses. There's some evidence that zinc ions also have antiviral activity against the herpes virus (6538,6539,6541). For wound healing, topical zinc might enhance re-epithelialization, decrease inflammation, and inhibit bacterial growth, thus enhancing wound healing (2699). Topical zinc might be effective for treating acne (819,820,2687,2688) due to anti-inflammatory activity resulting from inhibition of polymorphonuclear leukocyte chemotaxis induced by decreased granulocyte zinc levels (2686). Some researchers try zinc supplementation in the elderly for boosting immune function. Since many elderly are zinc deficient, the theory is that zinc supplementation might increase immune response. So far, there's contradictory information about supplementation's effects on immune function in the elderly. In some cases, it has increased antibody response to vaccination, and in some cases it seems to have no effect (6553,6563). Zinc may also inhibit conversion of testosterone to dihydrotestosterone (DHT), which has been associated with acne (3581). Zinc blocks copper absorption and increases copper elimination in the stool of people with Wilson's disease (2692). In acrodermatitis enteropathica, zinc seems to regulate linoleic acid and serum lipoprotein metabolism (2689). The role of zinc in Alzheimer's disease, might be both protective and causative. Laboratory studies suggest that zinc might contribute to aggregation of amyloid beta peptide, but protect against subsequent neurotoxicity as an antioxidant (6510,6511,6512). In children with thalassemia major, zinc deficiency is common (6597,6598,6599). Zinc supplementation in addition to transfusion increases the growth rate in children with thalassemia (14). Preliminary research suggests some people with type 2 diabetes might be zinc deficient, possibly as a result of altered zinc metabolism (6531,6532). In type 1 diabetes with zinc deficiency, zinc supplementation might reduce lipid peroxidation (6533). Zinc levels appear to be reduced in some people with major depression (6562). Male fertility appears to be influenced by zinc (6573,6574,6575,6576). Infertile males have lower seminal plasma zinc, with normal or reduced blood zinc (6575,6577). Clinical research suggests that short term dietary zinc depletion results in reduced serum testosterone concentrations, seminal volume, and total seminal zinc loss per ejaculate (6576). Supplementation with zinc improves sperm parameters in men with reduced sperm mobility (6578). Excess zinc might reduce sperm motility (6573). Zinc levels appear to decrease in the prostate tissue and prostatic fluid in men with prostatic carcinoma (6909,6910). In people with osteoporosis, urinary zinc excretion is increased, possibly as a result of bone resorption (6918). Serum zinc levels have been variably reported as normal or decreased in osteoporosis (6918,6920). Early clinical evidence suggests that zinc in combination with copper, manganese, and calcium might slow bone loss (1994). Zinc sulfate ophthalmic solution acts as a mild astringent, precipitating protein and clearing mucus from the outer surface of the eye (15). Zinc oxide absorption is best in an acidic environment (2809). Zinc acetate is absorbed over a wide pH range and might be a better choice in people with reduced stomach acid (2809). An enteric-coated zinc aspartate preparation (Taurizine) showed no absorption (2740). Zinc uptake in human intestinal epithelial cells was similar with zinc chloride, zinc methionine, or zinc propionate (2739).

Adverse Reactions

Orally, zinc can cause nausea and vomiting (2619). There is concern that high daily doses above the tolerable upper intake level (UL) of 40 mg per day might increase the risk of copper deficiency (7135). To prevent copper deficiency some clinicians give a small dose of copper when zinc is used in high doses, long-term. (7303).

In overdose, zinc can cause watery diarrhea, irritation and corrosion of the gastrointestinal tract, acute renal tubular necrosis, and interstitial nephritis (331,1352). Other symptoms of toxicity include flu-like and central nervous system symptoms including fever; coughing; nausea; vomiting; diarrhea; epigastric pain; lethargy; fatigue and neuropathy (2663,2681); dehydration; severe vomiting; and zinc-induced copper deficiency with symptoms including sideroblastic anemia, neutropenia, impaired immune function, and an increase in the ratio of low-density-lipoprotein to high-density-lipoprotein (LDL/HDL) cholesterol (2619,2681).

Daily doses of 300 mg of supplemental zinc for six weeks appear to impair immune response (7135). Chronic intake of 450-1600 mg daily of a zinc supplement has been associated with sideroblastic anemia (14).

There is preliminary evidence that higher dietary zinc intake might increase the risk for benign prostatic hyperplasia (BPH) (6908).

Occupational inhalation of zinc oxide fumes can cause metal fume fever with symptoms including fatigue, chills, fever, myalgias, cough, dyspnea, leukocytosis, thirst, metallic taste, and salivation (331).

Interactions with Herbs & Other Dietary Supplements

COPPER: Concomitant use may impair copper absorption (2693).

COFFEE: Concomitant use may decrease zinc absorption up to 50% (14).

IP-6 (Phytic Acid): IP-6 in foods can decrease zinc absorption (7135). Theoretically IP-6 supplements could also interfere with zinc absorption. IP-6 chelates multivalent metal ions in the gastrointestinal tract, preventing absorption (1858).

IRON: Non-heme iron might decrease zinc absorption. Non-heme Iron and zinc compete for a common absorption pathway in the gut. However, when iron and zinc are taken concomitantly with food, this interaction is not likely to occur. When taken with food, zinc absorption is facilitated by proteins in food through an alternate pathway that does not compete with iron (7357). Protein bound heme iron (found in red meats) does not affect zinc absorption (7135).

Interactions with Drugs

CAPTOPRIL (Capoten): Concomitant use can interfere with zinc supplementation by increasing urinary zinc elimination (25,26). There is no data on other ACE-Inhibitors. The clinical consequence of urinary zinc loss in hypertensive patients is unknown (25,26). Give supplements of zinc only if clinical judgment warrants it.

CHLORTHALIDONE (Hygroton): Concomitant use might increase serum and hair zinc levels, and also increase urinary zinc elimination (275).

CISPLATIN (Platinol-AQ): Concomitant use with zinc might increase the cytotoxicity of cisplatin when in the presence of the chelate ethylenediaminetetraacetic acid (EDTA), as compared to cisplatin treatment alone (2668).

TETRACYCLINES: Concomitant use decreases absorption and serum levels of demeclocycline (Declomycin), minocycline (Minocin), and tetracycline (Achromycin) due to zinc binding (15,506). Concomitant use can also reduce the effects of zinc supplementation due to reduced zinc absorption. Doxycycline (Vibramycin) does not interact with zinc (15,506).

FLUOROQUINOLONES: Concomitant use reduces drug absorption and serum levels of fluoroquinolones due to zinc binding (506,828,2682). Concomitant use can also reduce the effects of zinc supplementation due to reduced zinc absorption.

INTERFERON ALFA-2B (Intron A): Concomitant use might be effective for treating necrolytic acral erythema associated with hepatitis C (6192). There is one case report of oral zinc sulfate 225 mg twice daily plus interferon alfa-2b for six months resolving all lesions in a woman with necrolytic acral erythema and hepatitis C (6192). Necrolytic acral erythema is categorized in the family of necrolytic erythemas which includes acrodermatitis enteropathica (see Effectiveness) (6192).

PENICILLAMINE (Cuprimine): Concomitant use can reduce the effects of supplemental zinc (2678).

POTASSIUM-SPARING DIURETICS: Concomitant use can lead to zinc accumulation and increase risk of adverse effects (830).

THIAZIDE DIURETICS: Concomitant use can interfere with zinc supplementation by increasing urinary zinc elimination (830,831).

Drug Influences on Nutrient Levels and Depletion

SOME DRUGS CAN AFFECT ZINC LEVELS:

AMILORIDE (Midamor): Amiloride reduces urinary zinc excretion and can increase zinc levels (830).

CAPTOPRIL (Capoten): Captopril might increase urinary zinc excretion in patients with hypertension. There is no data on other ACE-inhibitors (ACEIs). The clinical consequence of urinary zinc loss in hypertensive patients is unknown (25,26). Patients receiving high-doses (greater than 200 mg daily), long-term have developed taste disturbances which resolved in some patients with zinc supplementation (6543).

DEFEROXAMINE (Desferal): Deferoxamine increases urinary zinc elimination (6597,6598).

FLUOROQUINOLONES: Treatment with fluoroquinolones can reduce dietary zinc absorption. The clinical significance is yet to be determined, and the need for supplementation has not been adequately studied. Consider zinc supplementation in patients on long-term fluoroquinolone therapy (506,828,2682).

PENICILLAMINE (Cuprimine): Penicillamine can reduce serum zinc levels and might cause zinc depletion in some patients (4453,4531,4534).

LOOP DIURETICS and THIAZIDE DIURETICS: Use of loop diuretics and thiazide diuretics can increase urinary zinc loss and reduce serum levels. This is more likely with higher doses or when used in combination with diuretics of another class (4412,4425).

TETRACYCLINES: Tetracyclines, except doxycycline (Vibramycin), can reduce dietary zinc absorption and serum levels due to zinc binding. The clinical significance is yet to be determined, and the need for supplementation has not been adequately studied. Consider zinc supplementation in patients on long-term tetracycline therapy (15,506).

Interactions with Foods

FOODS: Concomitant administration with foods containing bran, phytates, calcium, or phosphorus may decrease supplemental zinc absorption (506).

COFFEE: Concomitant use might decrease zinc absorption up to 50% (14).

VEGETARIANISM: Absorption of zinc from vegetarian diets is lower than from nonvegetarian diets most likely due to the higher amount of phytate, calcium, and other inhibitors of zinc absorption (7135). Dietary zinc requirements, particularly in strict vegetarians, may be 50% greater when the major food sources are grains and legumes (7135).

Interactions with Lab Tests

BLOOD ZINC ASSAYS: Avoid using powdered gloves when drawing blood for zinc assays, due to potential for sample contamination (2663).

HEMOGLOBIN A1C (HgbA1c): Supplementation with elemental zinc 50 mg per day has increased HgbA1c in type 1 diabetics (6530).

LIPID PROFILES: Zinc supplementation might reduce high-density lipoprotein (HDL) cholesterol levels and test results (2681). Zinc supplementation might increase the ratio of low-density-lipoprotein to high-density-lipoprotein (LDL/HDL) cholesterol and test results (2681).

Interactions with Diseases or Conditions

ALCOHOLISM: Long-term excessive alcohol consumption is associated with impaired zinc absorption and increased excretion of zinc in the urine (7135).

ALLERGY: Contraindicated in people with known hypersensitivity to zinc compounds (14).

HEMOCHROMATOSIS: Use caution in people who are homozygous for hemochromatosis (14).

HIV: Contraindicated in people with human immunodeficiency virus infection. Some evidence suggests association between higher intakes of zinc and reduced survival time (14).

GLAUCOMA: Avoid, or use zinc-containing ophthalmic solutions with caution (14).

MALABSORPTION SYNDROMES (SPRUE, CROHN'S DISEASE, SHORT BOWEL SYNDROME, ETC.): People with malabsorption syndromes may be zinc deficient due to decreased zinc absorption and increased urinary zinc losses (7135).

RHEUMATOID ARTHRITIS: Zinc absorption is reduced in people with rheumatoid arthritis (2823).

Dosage and Administration

ORAL: The typical dose for treating the common cold is one zinc gluconate or acetate lozenge, providing 9-24 mg elemental zinc, dissolved in the mouth every 2 hours while awake when cold symptoms are present (333,335,336). The zinc nasal spray (Zicam Cold Remedy, Gel Tech) is sprayed into each nostril 4 times daily until symptoms resolve (6471). For acute diarrhea in malnourished or zinc-deficient children, 10-40 mg elemental zinc is given daily (825,826,827,3455,3456). For hypogeusia, 25-100 mg oral zinc has been used in clinical trials (6542). Anorexia nervosa has been treated with 100 mg of zinc gluconate daily (6905). For treating gastric ulcers, zinc sulfate 200 mg three times daily has been used (6591). For muscle cramps in zinc deficient patients with cirrhosis, zinc sulfate 220 mg twice daily has been used (1352). For Hansen's disease, 220 mg oral zinc sulfate has been used (14). Sickle cell anemia has been treated with zinc sulfate 220 mg three times daily (6594). For treating acne, clinical trials have used 30 to 135 mg elemental zinc daily (6297,6298,6299,6500,6501,6502). For treating age-related macular degeneration, elemental zinc 80 mg plus vitamin C 500 mg, vitamin E 400 IU, and beta-carotene 15 mg has been given daily (7303). The National Institute of Medicine has established Adequate Intake (AI) levels of zinc for infants birth to 6 months at 2 mg/day (7135). For older infants, children, and adults, Recommended Dietary Allowance (RDA) quantities of zinc have been established: infants and children 7 months to 3 years, 3 mg/day; 4 to 8 years, 5 mg/day; 9 to 13 years, 8 mg/day; girls 14 to 18 years, 9 mg/day; boys and men age 14 and older, 11 mg/day; women 19 and older, 8 mg/day; pregnant women 14 to 18, 13 mg/day; pregnant women 19 and older, 11 mg/day; lactating women 14 to 18, 14 mg/day; lactating women 19 and older, 12 mg/day (7135). The typical North American male consumes about 13 mg/day of dietary zinc; women

consume approximately 9 mg/day (7135). The Tolerable Upper Intake Levels (UL) for zinc for people who are not receiving zinc under medical supervision are: Infants birth to 6 months, 4 mg/day; 7 to 12 months, 5 mg/day; children 1 to 3 years, 7 mg/day; 4 to 8 years, 12 mg/day; 9 to 13 years, 23 mg/day; 14 to 18 years (including pregnancy and lactation), 34 mg/day; adults 19 years and older (including pregnancy and lactation), 40 mg/day (7135). Different salt forms provide different amounts of elemental zinc: Zinc sulfate contains 23% elemental zinc (220 mg zinc sulfate contains 50 mg zinc). Zinc gluconate contains 14.3% elemental zinc (10 mg zinc gluconate contains 1.43 mg zinc) (506).
TOPICAL: For acne vulgaris, zinc acetate 1.2% with erythromycin 4% as a lotion has been applied twice daily (819). For herpes simplex infections, zinc sulfate 0.25% applied 8 to 10 times daily has been used (14). Lower concentrations have shown variable efficacy (14,6538).

Comments
Zinc acetate (Galzin) is a FDA-approved orphan drug for treating Wilson's disease.

REFERENCE CITATIONS

1 Monographs on the medicinal uses of plant drugs. Exeter, UK: European Scientific Co-op Phytother, 1997.

2 Blumenthal M, et al. ed. The Complete German Commission E Monographs: Therapeutic Guide to Herbal Medicines. Trans. S. Klein. Boston, MA: American Botanical Council, 1998.

3 Tyler VE. Herbs of Choice. Binghamton, NY: Pharmaceutical Products Press, 1994.

4 Newall CA, Anderson LA, Philpson JD. Herbal Medicine: A Guide for Healthcare Professionals. London, UK: The Pharmaceutical Press, 1996.

5 Foster S, Tyler VE. Tyler's Honest Herbal: A Sensible Guide to the Use of Herbs and Related Remedies. 3rd ed., Binghamton, NY: Haworth Herbal Press, 1993.

6 The Review of Natural Products by Facts and Comparisons. St. Louis, MO: Wolters Kluwer Co., 1999.

7 Schulz V, Hansel R, Tyler VE. Rational Phytotherapy: A Physician's Guide to Herbal Medicine. Terry C. Telger, transl. 3rd ed. Berlin, GER:Springer, 1998.

8 Wichtl MW. Herbal Drugs and Phytopharmaceuticals. N.M. Bisset, Ed. Stuttgart: Medpharm GmbH Scientific Publishers, 1994.

9 Martindale W. Martindale the Extra Pharmacopoeia. Pharmaceutical Press, 1999.

10 United States Pharmacopeial Convention, Inc., ed. Drug Information for the Health Care Professional. 19th ed. Englewood, CO: Micromedex Inc., 1999.

11 Leung AY, Foster S. Encyclopedia of Common Natural Ingredients Used in Food, Drugs and Cosmetics. 2nd ed. New York, NY: John Wiley & Sons, 1996.

12 McGuffin M, et al., ed. American Herbal Products Association's Botanical Safety Handbook. Boca Raton, FL: CRC Press, 1997.

13 Robbers JE, Speedie MK, Tyler VE. Pharmacognosy and Pharmacobiotechnology. Baltimore, MD: Williams & Wilkins, 1996.

14 Micromedex Healthcare Series. Englewood, CO: MICROMEDEX Inc.

15 McKevoy GK, ed. AHFS Drug Information. Bethesda, MD: American Society of Health-System Pharmacists, 1998.

16 Gennaro A. Remington: The Science and Practice of Pharmacy. 19th ed. Lippincott: Williams & Wilkins, 1996.

17 Ellenhorn MJ, et al. Ellenhorn's Medical Toxicology: Diagnoses and Treatment of Human Poisoning. 2nd ed. Baltimore, MD: Williams & Wilkins, 1997.

18 Gruenwald J, et al. PDR for Herbal Medicines. 1st ed. Montvale, NJ: Medical Economics Company, Inc., 1998.

19 Brinker F. Herb Contraindications and Drug Interactions. 2nd ed. Sandy, OR: Eclectic Medical Publications, 1998.

20 Anon. The Body Physical: Herbal Suggestions for Cancer. http://www.temenos-nj.com/docs/cncrherb.html (Accessed 14 August 2000).

21 Miller LG. Herbal medicinals: selected clinical considerations focusing on known or potential drug-herb interactions. *Arch Int Med* 1998;158(20):2200-11.

22 Adams ME. Hype about glucosamine. *Lancet* 1999;354(9176):353.

23 O'Mara NB. PremesisRx. Therapeutic Research Faculty. *Pharmacist's Letter/Prescriber's Letter* 1999;15(12):151206.

24 Cheung D. Is Diclectin safe for morning sickness? Therapeutic Research Faculty. *Pharmacist's Letter/Prescriber's Letter* 2000;16(3):160316.

25 Golik A, Zaidensttein R, Dishi V, et al. Effects of captopril and enalapril on zinc metabolism in hypertensive patients. *J Am Coll Nutr* 1998;17:75-8.

26 Golik A, Modai D, Averbukh Z, et al. Zinc metabolism in patients treated with captopril versus enalapril. *Metabolism* 1990;39:665-7.

27 Kung AWC, Pun KK. Bone mineral density in premenopausal women receiving long-term physiological doses of levothyroxine. *JAMA* 1991;265:2688-91.

28 Schneider DL, Barrett-Connor EL, Morton DJ. Thyroid hormone use and bone mineral density in elderly men. *Arch Intern Med* 1995;155:2005-7.

29 Franklyn AJ, Bettenridge J, Daykin J, et al. Long-term thyroxine treatment and bone mineral density. *Lancet* 1992;340:9-13.

30 Paltiel O, Falutz J, Veilleux M, et al. Clinical correlates of subnormal vitamin B12 levels in patients infected with the human immunodeficiency virus. *Am J Hematol* 1995;49:318-22.

31 Tang G, Serfaty-Lacrosniere C, Camilo ME, et al. Gastric acidity influences the blood response to a beta-carotene dose in humans. *Am J Clin Nutr* 1996;64:622-6.

32 Carlsen SM, Folling I, Grill V, et al. Metformin increases total homocysteine levels in non-diabetic male patients with coronary heart disease. *Scand J Clin Lab Invest* 1997;57:521-7.

33 Chevallier A. Encyclopedia of Medicinal Plants. New York, NY: DK Publishing, 1996.

34 Leatherdale B, et al. Improvement in glucose tolerance due to Momordica charantia. *Br Med J (Clin Res Ed)* 1981;282:1823-4.

35 Welihinda J, et al. Effect of Momordica charantia on the glucose tolerance in maturity onset diabetes. *J Ethnopharmacol* 1986;17:277-82.

36 Srivastava Y, et al. Antidiabetic and adaptogenic properties of Momordica charantia extract: An experimental and clinical evaluation. *Phytother Res* 1993;7:285-9.

37 Raman A, et al. Anti-diabetic properties and phytochemistry of Momordica charantia L. (Cucurbitaceae). *Phytomedicine* 1996;294.

38 Baldwa VS, Bhandari CM, Pangaria A, Goyal RK. Clinical trial in patients with diabetes mellitus of an insulin-like compound obtained from plant sources. *Upsala J Med Sci* 1977;82:39-41.

39 Perossini M, et al. Diabetic and hypertensive retinopathy therapy with Vaccinium myrtillus anthocyanosides (Tegens). Double blind, placebo-controlled clinical trial. *Ann Ottalmol Clin Ocul* 1987;113:1173.

40 Scharrer A, Ober M. Anthocyanosides in the treatment of retinopathies. *Kiln Monastbl Augenheilkd* 1981;178:386-9.

41 Coleman M, Steinberg G, Tippett J, et al. A preliminary study of the effect of pyridoxine administration in a subgroup of hyperkinetic children: A double-blind crossover comparison with methylphenidate. *Biol Psych* 1979;14:741-51.

42 Cucinotta D, Passeri M, Ventura S, et al. Multicenter clinical placebo-controlled study with acetyl-L-carnitine (ALC) in the treatment of mildly demented elderly patients. *Drug Development Res* 1988;14:213-6.

43 Kidd PM. A review of nutrients and botanicals in the integrative management of cognitive dysfunction. *Altern Med Rev* 1999;4(3):144-61.

44 Mayeux R, Sano M. Treatment of Alzheimer's Disease. *N Engl J Med* 1999;341(22):1670-9.

45 Shanmugasundaram ER, Rajeswari G, Baskaran K, et al. Use of Gymnema sylvestre leaf extract in the control of blood glucose in insulin-dependent diabetes mellitus. *J Ethnopharmacol* 1990;30:281-94.

46 Baskaran K, Kizar-Ahamath B, Shanmugasundaram MR, Shanmugasundaram ERB. Antidiabetic effect of leaf extract from Gymnema sylvestre in non-insulin-dependent diabetes mellitus patients. *J Ethnopharmacol* 1990;30:295-300.

47 Head KA. Type 1 diabetes: prevention of the disease and its complications. *Townsend Letter for Doctors & Patients* 1998;180:72-84.

48 Sinsheimer JE, Subba-Rao G, McIlhenny HM. Constitents from G sylvestre leaves: isolation and preliminary characterization of the gymnemic acids. *J Pharmacol Sci* 1970;59:622-8.

49 Awang DV. Parthenocide: demise of a facile theory of feverfew activity. *J Herbs Spices Med Plants* 1998;5:95-8.

50 Murch SJ, Simmons CB, Saxena PK. Melatonin in feverfew and other medicinal plants. *Lancet* 1997;350:1598-9.

51 Matsunaga S, Ito H, Sakou T. The effect of vitamin K and D supplementation on ovariectomy-induced bone loss. *Calcif Tissue Int* 1999;65:285-9.

52 Caraballo PJ, Heit JA, Atkinson EJ, et al. Long-term use of oral anticoagulants and the risk of fracture. *Arch Intern Med* 1999;159:1750-6.

53 Jie KG, Bots ML, Vermeer C, et al. Vitamin K status and bone mass in women with and without aortic atherosclerosis: a population-based study. *Calcif Tissue Int* 1996;59:352-6.

54 Shiraki M, Shiraki Y, Aoki C, Miura M. Vitamin K2 (menatetrenone) effectively prevents fractures and sustains lumbar bone mineral density in osteoporosis. *J Bone Miner Res* 2000;15:515-21.

55 Olson RE. Osteoporosis and vitamin K intake. *Am J Clin Nutr* 2000;71:1031-2.

56 Vermeer C, Gijsbers BL, Craciun AM, et al. Effects of vitamin K on bone mass and bone metabolism. *J Nutr* 1996;126:1187S-91S.

57 Vermeer C, Schurgers LJ. A comprehensive review of vitamin K and vitamin K antagonists. *Hematol Oncol Clin North Am* 2000;14:339-53.

58 Iwamoto I, Kosha S, Noguchi S, et al. A longitudinal study of the effect of vitamin K2 on bone mineral density in postmenopausal women a comparative study with vitamin D3 and estrogen-progestin therapy. *Maturitas* 1999;31:161-4.

59 Nagasawa Y, Fujii M, Kajimoto Y, et al. Vitamin K2 and serum cholesterol in patients on continuous ambulatory peritoneal dialysis. *Lancet* 1998;351:724.

60 Bitensky L, Hart JP, Catterall A, et al. Circulating vitamin K levels in patients with fractures. *J Bone Joint Surg Br* 1988;70:663-4.

61 Hart JP, Shearer MJ, Klenerman L, et al.

Electrochemical detection of depressed circulating levels of vitamin K1 in osteoporosis. *J Clin Endocrinol Metab* 1985;60:1268-9.

62 Hodges SJ, Akesson K, Vergnaud P, et al. Circulating levels of vitamins K1 and K2 decreased in elderly women with hip fracture. *J Bone Miner Res* 1993;8:1241-5.

63 Kanai T, Takagi T, Masuhiro K, et al. Serum vitamin K level and bone mineral density in post-menopausal women. *Int J Gynaecol Obstet* 1997;56:25-30.

64 Shearer MJ, Bach A, Kohlmeier M. Chemistry, nutritional sources, tissue distribution and metabolism of vitamin K with special reference to bone health. *J Nutr* 1996;126:1181S-6S.

65 Kawashima H, Nakajima Y, Matubara Y, et al. Effects of vitamin K2 (menatetrenone) on atherosclerosis and blood coagulation in hypercholesterolemic rabbits. *Jpn J Pharmacol* 1997;75:135-43.

66 Rosen HM, Yoshimura N, Hodgman JM, Fischer JE. Plasma amino acid patterns in hepatic encephalopathy of differing etiology. *Gastroenterology* 1977;72:483-7.

67 MacLean D, Vissing J, Vissing SF, Haller RG. Oral branched-chain amino acids do not improve exercise capacity in McArdle disease. *Neurology* 1998;51:1456-9.

68 O'Keefe SJ, Ogden J, Dicker J. Enteral and parenteral branched chain amino acid-supplemented nutritional support in patients with encephalopathy due to alcoholic liver disease. *JPEN J Parenter Enteral Nutr* 1987;11:447-53.

69 Marchesini G, Bianchi G, Rossi B, et al. Nutritional treatment with branched-chain amino acids in advanced liver cirrhosis. *J Gastroenterol* 2000;35:7-12.

70 Vorgerd M, Grehl T, Jager M, et al. Creatine therapy in myophosphorylase deficiency (McArdle disease): a placebo-controlled crossover trial. *Arch Neurol* 2000;57:956-63.

71 Cangiano C, Laviano A, Meguid MM, et al. Effects of administration of oral branched-chain amino acids on anorexia and caloric intake in cancer patients. *J Natl Cancer Inst* 1996;88:550-2.

72 Richardson MA, Bevans ML, Weber JB, et al. Branched chain amino acids decrease tardive dyskinesia symptoms. *Psychopharmacology (Berl)* 1999;143:358-64.

73 Mori N, Adachi Y, Takeshima T, et al. Branched-chain amino acid therapy for spinocerebellar degeneration: a pilot clinical crossover trial. *Intern Med* 1999;38:401-6.

74 Stein TP, Schluter MD, Leskiw MJ, Boden G. Attenuation of the protein wasting associated with bed rest by branched-chain amino acids. *Nutrition* 1999;15:656-60.

75 National Institute of Medicine. The role of protein and amino acids in sustaining and enhancing performance. URL: http://books.nap.edu/books/0309063469/html/309.html#pagetop (Accessed 27 September 2000).

76 Supplement Watch. Branched-chain amino acids. www.supplementwatch.com/sup-atoz/b/bcaa.html. (Accessed 27 September 2000).

77 Blomstrand E, Ek S, Newsholme EA. Influence of ingesting a solution of branched-chain amino acids on plasma and muscle concentrations of amino acids during prolonged submaximal exercise. *Nutrition* 1996;12:485-90.

78 Suryawan A, Hawes JW, Harris RA, et al. A molecular

model of human branched-chain amino acid metabolism. *Am J Clin Nutr* 1998;68:72-81.

79   Branchey L, Branchey M, Shaw S, Lieber CS. Relationship between changes in plasma amino acids and depression in alcoholic patients. *Am J Psychiatry* 1984;141:1212-5.

80   Majumdar SK, Shaw GK, Thomson AD, et al. Changes in plasma amino acid patterns in chronic alcoholic patients during ethanol withdrawal syndrome: their clinical implications. *Med Hypotheses* 1983;12:239-51.

81   Naylor CD, O'Rourke K, Detsky AS, Baker JP. Parenteral nutrition with branched-chain amino acids in hepatic encephalopathy. A meta-analysis. *Gastroenterology* 1989;97:1033-42.

82   Fabbri A, Magrini N, Bianchi G, et al. Overview of randomized clinical trials of oral branched-chain amino acid treatment in chronic hepatic encephalopathy. *JPEN J Parenter Enteral Nutr* 1996;20:159-64.

83   Berson EL, Rosner B, Sandberg MA, et al. A randomized trial of vitamin A and vitamin E supplementation for retinitis pigmentosa. *Arch Ophthalmol* 1993;111:761-72.

84   Gamel JW, Barr CC. A randomized trial of vitamin A and vitamin E supplementation for retinitis pigmentosa. *Arch Ophthalmol* 1993;111:1462-3.

85   Fielder AR. A randomized trial of vitamin A and vitamin E supplementation for retinitis pigmentosa. *Arch Ophthalmol* 1993;111:1463; discussion 1463-6.

86   Clowes DD. A randomized trial of vitamin A and vitamin E supplementation for retinitis pigmentosa. *Arch Ophthalmol* 1993;111:1461-2.

87   Norton EW. A randomized trial of vitamin A and vitamin E supplementation for retinitis pigmentosa. *Arch Ophthalmol* 1993;111:1460.

88   Marmor MF. A randomized trial of vitamin A and vitamin E supplementation for retinitis pigmentosa. *Arch Ophthalmol* 1993;111:1460-1.

89   Lavine JE. Vitamin E treatment of nonalcoholic steatohepatitis in children: a pilot study. *J Pediatr* 2000;136:734-8.

90   Kim JM, White RH. Effect of vitamin E on the anticoagulant response to warfarin. *Am J Cardiol* 1996;77:545-6.

91   Corrigan JJ Jr. The effect of vitamin E on warfarin-induced vitamin K deficiency. *Ann N Y Acad Sci* 1982;393:361-8.

92   Corrigan JJ Jr. Coagulation problems relating to vitamin E. *Am J Pediatr Hematol Oncol* 1979;1:169-73.

93   Corrigan JJ Jr, Marcus FI. Coagulopathy associated with vitamin E ingestion. *JAMA* 1974;230:1300-1.

94   Skyrme-Jones RA, O'Brien RC, Berry KL, Meredith IT. Vitamin E supplementation improves endothelial function in type I diabetes mellitus: a randomized, placebo-controlled study. *J Am Coll Cardiol* 2000;36:94-102.

95   Devaraj S, Jialal I. Low-density lipoprotein postsecretory modification, monocyte function, and circulating adhesion molecules in type 2 diabetic patients with and without macrovascular complications: the effect of alpha-tocopherol supplementation. *Circulation* 2000;102:191-6.

96   Surai PF, MacPherson A, Speake BK, Sparks NH. Designer egg evaluation in a controlled trial. *Eur J Clin Nutr* 2000;54:298-305.

97   Meydani M. Effect of functional food ingredients: vitamin E modulation of cardiovascular diseases and immune status in the elderly. *Am J Clin Nutr* 2000;71:1665S-8S.

98   Jonas CR, Puckett AB, Jones DP, et al. Plasma antioxidant status after high-dose chemotherapy: a randomized trial of parenteral nutrition in bone marrow transplantation patients. *Am J Clin Nutr* 2000;72:181-9.

99   Burton GW, Traber MG, Acuff RV, et al. Human plasma and tissue alpha-tocopherol concentrations in response to supplementation with deuterated natural and synthetic vitamin E. *Am J Clin Nutr* 1998;67:669-84.

100   Vatassery GT, Bauer T, Dysken M. On the biological activity of vitamin E. Am J Clin Nutr 2000;72:202-3.

101   Klein AD, Penneys NS. Aloe vera. *J Am Acad Dermatol* 1988 Apr;18(4 Pt 1):714-20.

102   Lyss G, et al. Helenalin, an antiinflammatory sesquiterpene lactone from Arnica, selectively inhibits transcription factor NF-kappa B. *Biol Chem* 1997;378(9):951-61.

103   Baillargeon L, et al. The effects of Arnica montana on blood coagulation. Radomized controlled trial. *Can Fam Physician* 1993;39:2362-7.

104   Schroder H, et al. Helenalin and 11 alpha, 13-dihydrohelenalin, two constituents from Arnica montana L., inhibit human platelet function via thiol-dependent pathways. *Thromb Res* 1990;57(6):839-45.

105   Sabeel AI, Kurkus J, Lindholm T. Intensive Hemodialysis and Hemoperfusion Treatment of Amanita Mushroom Poisoning. *Mycopathologia* 1995;131(2):107-114.

106   Bustamante J, et al. Alpha-lipoic acid in Liver Metabolism and Disease. *Free Radic Biol Med* 1998;24(6):1023-39.

107   Ehren I, et al. Effects of L-arginine treatment on symptoms and bladder nitric oxide levels in patients with interstitial cystitis. *Urology* 1998; 52(6):1026-9.

108   Bode-Boger SM, et al. L-arginine-induced vasodilation in healthy humans: pharmacokinetic-pharmacodynamic relationship. *Br J Clin Pharmacol* 1998; 46(5):489-97.

109   Sandrini G, et al. Effectiveness of ibuprofen-arginine in the treatment of acute migraine attacks. *Int J Clin Pharmacol Res* 1998; 18(3):145-50.

110   Lerman A, et al. Long-term L-arginine supplementation improves small-vessel coronary endothelial function in humans. *Circulation* 1998;97(21):2123-8.

111   Chuntrasakul C, et al. Metabolic and immune effects of dietary arginine, glutamine, and omega-3 fatty acids supplementation in immunocompromised patients. *J Med Assoc Thai* 1998;81(5):334-43.

112   Andres A, et al. L-arginine reverses the antinatriuretic effect of cyclosporin in renal transplant patients. *Nephrol Dial Transplant* 1997 Jul;12(7):1437-40.

113   Pichard C, et al. A randomized double-blind controlled study of 6 months of oral nutritional supplementation with arginine and omega-3 fatty acids in HIV-infected patients. Swiss HIV Cohort Study. *AIDS* 1998;12(1):53-63.

114   Wheeler MA, et al. Effect of long-term oral L-arginine on the nitric oxide synthase pathway in the urine from patients with interstitial cystitis. *J Urol* 1997;158(6):2045-50.

115   Saffle JR, et al. Randomized trial of immune-enhancing enteral nutrition in burn patients. *J Trauma* 1997;42(5):793-800, discussion 800-2.

116   Adams MR, et al. Oral L-arginine improves

endothelium-dependent dilatation and reduces monocyte adhesion to endothelial cells in young men with coronary artery disease. *Atherosclerosis* 1997;129(2):261-9.

117 Takano H, et al. Oral administration of L-arginine potentiates allergen-induced airway inflammation and expression of interleukin-5 in mice. *J Pharmacol Exp Ther* 1998;286(2):767-71.

118 Hibbard MK, Sandri-Goldin, RM. Arginine-rich regions succeeding the nuclear localization region of the herpes simplex virus type 1 regulatory protein ICP27 are required for efficient nuclear localization and late gene expression. *J Virol* 1995;69(8):4656-7.

119 Griffith RS, DeLong DC, Nelson JD. Relation of arginine-lysine antagonism to herpes simplex growth in tissue culture. *Chemotherapy* 1981; 27(3):209-13.

120 McCaffrey MJ, et al. Effect of L-arginine infusion on infants with persistent pulmonary hypertension of the newborn. *Biol Neonate* 1995;67(4):240-3.

121 Sapienza MA, et al. Effect of inhaled L-arginine on exhaled nitric oxide in normal and asthmatic subjects. *Thorax* 1998 Mar;53(3):172-5.

122 Saijyo T, et al. Autonomic nervous system activity during infusion of L-arginine in patients with liver cirrhosis. *Liver* 1998 Feb;18(1):27-31.

123 Newcomer AD, et al. Response of patients with irritable bowel syndrome and lactase deficiency using unfermented acidophilus milk. *Am J Clin Nutr* 1983 Aug;38(2):257-63.

124 Gotz V, et al. Prophylaxis against ampicillin-associated diarrhea with a lactobacillus preparation. *Am J Hosp Pharm* 1979 Jun;36(6):754-7.

125 Contardi I. [Oral bacterial therapy in prevention of antibiotic-induced diarrhea in childhood]. [Article in Italian]. *Clin Ter* 1991 Mar 31;136(6):409-13.

126 Kaaja RJ, et al. Treatment of cholestasis of pregnancy with peroral activated charcoal. A preliminary study. *Scand J Gastroenterol* 1994 Feb;29(2):178-81.

127 Bowry VW, Ingold KU, Stocker R. Vitamin E in human density lipoprotein. When and how this antioxidant becomes a pro-oxidant. *Biochem J* 1992; 288(Pt 2):341-4.

128 Kagan VE, et al. Recycling of vitamin E in human low density lipoproteins. *J Lipid Res* 1992;33(3):385-97.

129 Back DJ, et al. Interaction of ethinyloestradiol with ascorbic acid in man. *Br Med J (Clin Res Ed)* 1981;282:1516.

130 Morris JC, et al. [Letter] *Br Med J (Clin Res Ed)* 1981;283:503.

131 Levine M, et al. Vitamin C pharmacokinetics in healthy volunteers: evidence for recommended dietary allowance. *Proc Natl Acad Sci USA* 1996;93(8):3704-9.

132 Buto SK, et al. Bay Leaf Impaction in the Esophagus and Hypopharynx. Ann Intern Med 1990;113(1):82-3.

133 Johns AN. Beware of the Bay Leaf. *Br Med J* 1980;281:1682.

134 Belitsos NJ. Bay Leaf Impaction. *Ann Intern Med* 1990;113(6):483-4.

135 Bell CD, Mustar, RA. Bay Leaf Perforation of Meckel's Diverticulum. *JCC* 1997;40(2):146.

136 Palin WE, Richardson JD. Complications From Bay Leaf Ingestions. *JAMA* 1983;289(6):729-30.

137 Brokaw SA. Complications of bay leaf ingestion [letter]. *JAMA* 1983;250(6):729.

138 Price JF. Antioxidant vitamins in the prevention of

cardiovascular disease. The epidemiological evidence. *Eur Heart J* 1997;18:719-27.

139 Omenn GS. Chemoprevention of lung cancer: the rise and demise of beta-carotene. *Annu Rev Public Health* 1998;19:73-99.

140 Giuliano AR, Gapstur S. Can cervical dysplasia and cancer be prevented with nutrients? *Nutr Rev* 1998;56(1):9-16.

141 Lieberman S. A Review of the effectiveness of cimicifuga racemosa (Black Cohosh) for the symptoms of menopause. *J Womens Health* 1998;7(5):525-9.

142 Jarboe CH, et al. Uterine relaxant properties of Viburnium. *Nature* 1966;212:837.

143 Soderling E, et al. Betaine-containing toothpaste relieves subjective symptoms of dry mouth. *Acta Odontol Scand* 1998;56(2):65-9.

144 Barak AJ, Beckenhauer HC, Tuma DJ. Betaine, ethanol, and the liver, a review. *Alcohol* 1996;13(4):395-8.

145 Wilcken DE, et al. Homocystinuria - the effects of betaine in the treatment of patients not responsive to pyridoxine. *N Engl J Med* 1983;309(8):448-53.

146 Duell PG, Malinow MR. Homocysteine: An important risk factor for atherosclerotic vascular disease. *Curr Opin Lipidol* 1997;8(1):28-34.

147 Bakker RC, Brandjes DP. Hyperhomocysteinaemia and associated disease. *Pharm World Sci,* 1997; 19(3):126-32.

148 Daviglus ML, et al. Dietary beta-carotene, vitamin C, and risk of prostate cancer: results from the Western Electric Study. *Epidemiology* 1996;7(5):472-7.

149 Simopoulos AP, Leaf A, Salem N. Workshop statement on the essentiality of and recommended dietary intakes for Omega-6 and Omega-3 fatty acids. *Prostaglandins Leukot Essent Fatty Acids* 2000;63:119-21.

150 Johnson JA, Lalonde RL. Congestive Heart Failure. Eds. DiPiro JT, et al. Pharmacotherapy, third ed. Stamford: Appleton and Lange, 1997.

151 Sklar S. et al. Drug therapy screening system. Indianapolis, IN:First Data Bank 99.1-99.2 eds.

152 Bourgoin BP, et al. Lead content in 70 brands of dietary calcium supplements. *Am J Public Health* 1993;83(8):1155-60.

153 Elmer GW, Surawicz CM, McFarland LV. Biotherapeutic Agents, A neglected modality for the treatment and prevention of selected intestinal and vaginal infections. *JAMA* 1996;275(11): 870-5.

154 Renk BZ. Probiotic bifidobacterium strains. In: Wisconsin Alumni Res Foundation. www.wisc.edu/warf.boi/p98062us.html (Accessed 29 January 1999).

155 Scarpignato C, Rampal P. Prevention and treatment of traveler's diarrhea: A clinical pharmacological approach. *Chemotherapy* 1995;41(suppl 1):48-81.

156 Chiesara E, Borghini R, Marabini. Dietary fibre and drug interactions. *Eur J Clin Nutr* 1995;49(suppl 3):S123-8.

157 Drug Facts and Comparisons. Olin BR, Ed. St. Louis, MO: Facts and Comparisons. (updated monthly).

158 Pandya DP Nutrition and Coronary Heart Disease. *Comp Ther* 1998;24(4):198-204.

159 Gossel TA, Bricker JD. Principles of Clinical Toxicology. New York, NY:Raven Press, 1994.

160 ECP consensus panel on cereals and cancer. *Eur J Cancer Prev* 1998;7(suppl 2):S1-S2.

161 Saavedra JM, et al. Feeding of bifidobacterium bifidum and streptococcus thermophilus to infants in hospital for prevention of diarrhea and shedding of rotavirus. *Lancet*

1994;344:1046-9.

162 Bouhnik Y, et al. Fecal recovery in humans of viable bifidobacterium ingested in fermented milk. *Gastroenterology* 1992;102:875-8.

163 Sauvaire Y, et al. 4-hydroxyisoleucine. A novel amino acid potentiator of insulin secretion. *Diabetes* 1998;47:206-10.

164 Madar Z, Thorne R. Dietary fiber. *Prog Food Nutr Sci* 1987;11:153-74.

165 Ultee A, Kets EP, Smid EJ. Mechanisms of action of carvacrol on the food-borne pathogen Bacillus cereus. *Appl Environ Microbiol* 1999;65:4606-4610.

166 Miller LG. Herbal Medicinals. Selected clinical considerations focusing on known or potential drug-herb interactions. *Arch Intern Med* 1998;158:2200-11.

167 Bennett DA Jr, Phun L, Polk JF, et al. Neuropharmacology of St. John's Wort (Hypericum). *Ann Pharmacother* 1998 Nov;32(11):1201-8.

168 Hippius H. St. John's Wort (Hypericum perforatum) an herbal antidepressant. *Curr Med Res Opin* 1998;14(3):171-84.

169 Wagner J, Wagner ML, Hening WA. Beyond benzodiazepines: alternative pharmacologic agents for the treatment of insomnia. *Ann Pharmacother* 1998;32(6):680-91.

170 Henry JG, Sobki S, Afafat N. Interference by biotin therapy on measurement of TSH and FT4 by enzyme immunoassay on Boehringer Mannheim ES 700 analyzer. *Ann Clin Biochem* 1996;33:162-3.

171 Hochman LG, Scher RK, Meyerson MS. Brittle nails: response to daily biotin supplementation. *Cutis* 1993;51:303-5.

172 Said HM, Redha R, Nylander W. Biotin transport in the human intestine: inhibition by anticonvulsant drugs. *Am J Clin Nutr* 1989;49:127-31.

173 Bonjour JP. Biotin in human nutrition. *Ann N Y Acad Sci* 1985;447:97-104.

174 Nyhan WL. Clinical problems relating to biotin. *Ann N Y Acad Sci* 1985;447:222-4.

175 Krause KH, et al. Biotin Status of Epileptics. *Ann N Y Acad Sci* 1985;447:297-313.

176 Mock DM, et al. Disturbances in biotin metabolism in children undergoing long-term anticonvulsant therapy. *J Pediatr Gastroenterol Nutr* 1998;26(3):245-50.

177 Coggeshall JC, et al. Biotin status and plasma glucose in diabetics. *Annals New York Academy of Sciences* 1985;447:389-92.

178 Arvill A, Bodin L. Effect of short-term ingestion of konjac glucomannan on serum cholesterol in healthy men. *Am J Clin Nutr* 1995;61(3):585-9.

179 Vido L, et al. Childhood obesity treatment: double blinded trial on dietary fibres (glucomannan) versus placebo. *Padiatr Padol* 1993;28(5):133-6.

180 Livieri C, Novazi F, Lorini R. [The use of highly purified glucomannan-based fibers in childhood obesity]. [Article in Italian] *Pediatr Med Chir* 1992;14(2):195-8.

181 Vita PM, et al. [Chronic use of glucomannan in the dietary treatment of severe obesity]. [Article in Italian] *Minerva Med* 1992;83(3):135-9.

182 Walsh DE, Yaghoubian V, Behforooz A. Effect of glucomannan on obese patients: a clinical study. *Int J Obes* 1984;8(4):289-93.

183 Cairella M, Marchini GAD. [Evaluation of the action of glucomannan on metabolic parameters and on the sensation of satiation in overweight and obese patients]. [Article in Italian] *Clin Ter,* 1995; 146:269-74.

184 Koshy KM, Griswold E, Schneeberger EE. Interstitial nephritis in a patient taking creatine. *N Engl J Med* 1999;340(10):814-5.

185 Kubota K, et al. [Effect of green tea on iron absorption in elderly patients with iron deficiency anemia]. [Article in Japanese] *Nippon Ronen Igakkai Zasshi* 1990;27(5):555-8.

186 Barker G, et al. The effects of sucralfate suspension and diphenhydramine syrup plus kaolin-pectin on radiotherapy-induced mucositis. *Oral Surg Oral Med Oral Pathol* 1991;71(3):288-93.

187 Carnel SB, et al. Treatment of radiation- and chemotherapy-induced stomatitis. *Otolaryngol Head Neck Surg* 1990;102(4):326-30.

188 Epstein WL. Topical prevention of poison ivy/oak dermatitis. *Arch Dermatol* 1989;125(4):499-501.

189 Juch RD, et al. Pharmazeutische Praparate, Egerkingen, Schweiz. Pastes: what do they contain? How do they work? *Dermatology* 1994;189(4):373-7.

190 Tart RP, et al. Enteric MRI contrast agents: comparative study of five potential agents in humans. *Magn Reson Imaging* 1991;9(4):559-68.

191 Mitchell DG, et al. Comparison of Kaopectate with barium for negative and positive enteric contrast at MR imaging. *Radiology* 1991;181(2):475-80.

192 Despotis GJ, et al. DG Response of kaolin ACT to heparin: evaluation with an automated assay and higher heparin doses. *Ann Thorac Surg* 1996;61(3):795-9.

193 Paquet C. Assessment of kaolin agglutination test. *Tuber Lung Dis* 1994; 75(5):397.

194 Sarnaik RM, et al. Serodiagnosis of tuberculosis: assessment of kaolin agglutination test. *Tuber Lung Dis* 1993;74(6):405-6.

195 Levin JL, et al. Kaolinosis in a cotton mill worker. *Am J Ind Med* 1996;29(2):215-21.

196 Chaudhary BA, Kanes GJ, Pool WH. Pleural thickening in mild kaolinosis. *South Med J* 1997; 90(11):1106-9.

197 Altekruse EB, et al. Kaolin dust concentrations and pneumoconiosis at a kaolin mine. *Thorax* 1984;39(6):436-41.

198 Rodin SM, Johnson BF. Pharmacokinetic interactions with digoxin. *Clin Pharmacokinet* 1988;15(4):227-44.

199 Babhair SA, Tariq M. Effect of magnesium trisilicate and kaolin-pectin on the bioavailability of trimethoprim. *Res Commun Chem Pathol Pharmacol* 1983;40(1):165-8.

200 Kayden HJ, Wisniewski T. On the biological activity of vitamin E. *Am J Clin Nutr* 2000;72:201-3.

201 Dobelis IN, Dwyer J, Rattray D, et al., Eds. Magic and Medicine of Plants. Pleasantville, NY: The Reader's Digest Assn. Inc., 1986.

202 Cohn W. Evaluation of vitamin E potency. *Am J Clin Nutr* 1999;69:156-8.

203 Vorbach EU, Arnoldt KH, Hubner WD. Efficacy and tolerability of St. John's wort extract LI 160 versus imipramine in patients with severe depressive episodes according to ICD- 10. *Pharmacopsychiatry* 1997;30(Suppl 2):81-5.

204 Wheatley D. LI 160, an extract of St. John's wort, versus amitriptyline in mildly to moderately depressed outpatients - a controlled 6-week clinical trial. *Pharmacopsychiatry* 1997;30 Suppl 2:77-80.

205 Volz HP. Controlled clinical trials of hypericum extracts

REFERENCES

in depressed patients - an overview. *Pharmacopsychiatry* 1997;30 Suppl 2:72-6.

206 Gulick RM, McAuliffe V, Holden-Wiltse J, et al. Phase I studies of hypericin, the active compound in St. John's Wort, as an antiretroviral agent in HIV-infected adults. AIDS Clinical Trials Group Protocols 150 and 258. *Ann Intern Med* 1999;130(6):510-4.

207 Ashton AK, Ahrens K, Gupta S, Masand PS. Antidepressant-induced sexual dysfunction and Ginkgo Biloba. *Am J Psychiatry* 2000;157:836-837.

208 Davydov L, Stirling AL. Stevens-Johnson syndrome with Ginkgo biloba. *J Herb Pharmacother* 2001;1:65-69.

209 Kostyuk VA, Potapovich AI. Antiradical and chelating effects in flavonoid protection against silica-induced cell injury. *Arch Biochem Biophys* 1998;355(1):43-8.

210 SR Vitamins. The Wild Oregano Oil Miracle website: http://www.srvitamins.com/articles/ thewildoreganooilmiracle.htm (Accessed April 2001).

211 Drewa G, Schachtschabel DO, Palgan K, et al. The influence of rutin on the weight, metastasis and melanin content of B16 melanotic melanoma in C57BL/6 mice. *Neoplasma* 1998;45(4):266-71.

212 Kehoe, WA. Ginkgo biloba for SSRI-induced sexual dysfunction. Therapeutic Research Center. *Pharmacist's Letter* 1997;13(9):130916.

213 Paick J, Lee J. An experimental study of the effect of ginkgo biloba extract on the human and rabbit corpus cavernosum tissue. *J Urol* 1996;156:1876-80.

214 Fetrow CW, Avala JR. Professional's Handbook of Complementary and Alternative Medicines. Springhouse Corporation, 1999.

215 Osol and Farar. The Dispensatory of the United States of America. 25th ed. JB Lippincott Co., 1955.

216 Dorland's Illustrated Medical Dictionary, 25th ed. WB Saunders Company, 1974.

217 Pheatt N, ed. *Sport's Supplements Pharmacist's Letter Continuing Education Booklet* 1999;99(2):1-56.

218 Horwitt MK, Elliott WH, Kanjananggulpan P, Fitch CD. Serum concentrations of alpha-tocopherol after ingestion of various vitamin E preparations. *Am J Clin Nutr* 1984;40:240-5.

219 Pratt S. Dietary prevention of age-related macular degeneration. *J Am Optom Assoc* 1999;70:39-47.

220 Hertog MGL, Sweetnam PM, Fehily AM, et al. Antioxidant flavonols and ischemic heart disease in a Welsh population of men: the Caerphilly Study. *Am J Clin Nutr* 1997;65:1489-94.

221 Drew S, Davies E. Effectiveness of Ginkgo biloba in treating tinnitus: double blind, placebo controlled trial. *BMJ* 2001;322:73.

222 Chen J, Wollman Y, Chernichovsky T, et al. Effect of oral administration of high-dose nitric oxide donor L-arginine in men with organic erectile dysfunction: results of a double-blind, randomized, placebo-controlled study. *BJU Int* 1999;83:269-73.

223 Johnson N. Sun trap. 24 July 1999. URL: http:// www.newscientist.com/ns/1990724/newsstory9.html (Accessed 20 August 1999).

224 Leonetti HB, Longo S, Anasti JN. Transdermal progesterone cream for vasomotor symptoms and postmenopausal bone loss. *Obstet Gynecol* 1999;94:225-8.

225 Bracco GL, Carli P, Sonni L, et al. Clinical and histologic effects of topical treatments of vulval lichen sclerosus. A critical evaluation. *J Reprod Med* 1993;38(1):37-40.

226 Langer RD. Micronized progesterone: a new therapeutic option. *Int J Fertil Womens Med* 1999;44(2):67-73.

227 Licciardi FL, Kwiatkoski A, Noyes NL, et al. Oral versus intramuscular progesterone for in vitro fertilization: a prospective randomized study. *Fertil Steril* 1999;71(4):614-8.

228 Greendale GA, Reboussin BA, Hogan P, et al. Symptom relief and side effects of postmenopausal hormones: results from the Postmenopausal Interventions Trial. *Obstet Gynecol* 1998;92(6):982-8.

229 Jellin J, ed. Dietary Supplements. *Pharmacist's Letter* 1999;14(4):22.

230 Sloane P. Advances in the treatment of Alzheimer's disease. *Am Fam Physician* 1998;58:1577-86, 1589-90.

231 Morris M, Beckett L, Scherr P, et al. Vitamin E and vitamin C supplement use and risk of incident Alzheimer's disease. *Alzheimer Dis Assoc Disord* 1998;12:121-6.

232 Sano M, Ernesto C, Thomas R, et al. A controlled trial of selegiline, alpha-tocopherol, or both as treatment for Alzheimer's disease. The Alzheimer's Disease Cooperative Study. *N Engl J Med* 1997;336:1216-22.

233 Chakravarty N. Inhibition of histamine release from mast cells by nigellone. *Ann Allergy* 1993;70(3):237-42.

234 Haq A, Abdullatif M, Lobo PI, et al. Black seed: effect on human lymphocytes and polymorphonuclear leukocyte phagocytic activity. *Immunopharmacology* 1995;30(2):147-55.

235 Houghton PJ, Zarka R, de las Heras B, Hoult JR. Fixed oil of Black seed and derived thymoquinone inhibit eicosanoid generation in leukocytes and membrane lipid peroxidation. *Planta Med* 1995;61(1):33-6.

236 Salomi NJ, Nair SC, Jayawardhanan KK, et al. Antitumour principles from Black seed seeds. *Cancer Lett* 1992;63(1):41-6.

237 Daba MH, Abdel-Rahman MS. Hepatoprotective activity of thymoquinone in isolated rat hepatocytes. *Toxicol Lett* 1998;95(1):23-9.

238 Worthen DR, Ghosheh OA, Crooks PA. The in vitro anti-tumor activity of some crude and purified components of blackseed, Black seed L. *Anticancer Res* 1998;18(3A):1527-32.

239 Badary OA, Al-Shabanah OA, Nagi MN, et al. Inhibition of benzo(a)pyrene-induced forestomach carcinogenesis in mice by thymoquinone. *Eur J Cancer Prev* 1999;8(5):435-40.

240 Nagi MN, Alam K, Badary OA, et al. Thymoquinone protects against carbon tetrachloride hepatotoxicity in mice via an antioxidant mechanism. *Biochem Mol Biol Int* 1999;47(1):153-9.

241 Aqel M, Shaheen R. Effects of the volatile oil of Black seed seeds on the uterine smooth muscle of rat and guinea pig. *J Ethnopharmacol* 1996;52(1):23-6.

242 Keshri G, Singh MM, Lakshmi V, Kamboj VP. Post-coital contraceptive efficacy of the seeds of Black seed in rats. *Indian J Physiol Pharmacol* 1995;39(1):59-62.

243 Hanafy MS, Hatem ME. Studies on the antimicrobial activity of Black seed seed (black cumin). *J Ethnopharmacol* 1991;34(2-3):275-8.

244 Benjamin J, Muir T, Briggs K, Pentland B. A case of cerebral haemorrhage-can Ginkgo biloba be implicated? *Postgrad Med J* 2001;77:112-3.

245 Tennekoon KH, Jeevathayaparan S, Kurukulasooriya AP, Karunanayake EH. Possible hepatotoxicity of Black seed

seeds and Dregea volubilis leaves. *J Ethnopharmacol* 1991;31(3):283-9.

246 Medenica RD. Use of Black seed to increase immune function. U.S. Patent 5,482,711, issued January 9, 1996. Obtained from US Patent and Trademark Ofc on April 12, 2000. www.uspto.gov/patft/index.htm.

247 Kiyose C, Muramatsu R, Kameyama Y, et al. Biodiscrimination of alpha-tocopherol stereoisomers in humans after oral administration. *Am J Clin Nutr* 1997;65:785-9.

248 Baker H, Handelman GJ, Short S, et al. Comparison of plasma alpha and gamma tocopherol levels following chronic oral administration of either all-rac-alpha-tocopheryl acetate or RRR-alpha-tocopheryl acetate in normal adult male subjects. *Am J Clin Nutr* 1986;43:382-7.

249 van Tits LJ, Demacker PN, de Graaf J, et al. Alpha-tocopherol supplementation decreases production of superoxide and cytokines by leukocytes ex vivo in both normolipidemic and hypertriglyceridemic individuals. *Am J Clin Nutr* 2000;71:458-64.

250 Bucci AJ, et al. In vitro interaction of quinidine with kaolin and pectin. *J Pharm Sci* 1981;70(9):999-1002.

251 Allen MD, et al. Effect of magnesium-aluminum hydroxide and kaolin-pectin on absorption of digoxin from tablets and capsules. *J Clin Pharmacol* 1981;21(1):26-30.

252 Albert KS, et al. Influence of kaolin-pectin suspension on digoxin bioavailability. *J Pharm Sc* 1978;67(11):1582-6.

253 Albert KS, et al. Pharmacokinetic evaluation of a drug interaction between kaolin-pectin and clindamycin. *J Pharm Sci* 1978 67(11):1579-82.

254 Huyzen RJ, et al. Alternative perioperative anticoagulation monitoring during cardiopulmonary bypass in aprotinin-treated patients. *J Cardiothorac Vasc Anesth* 1994;8(2):153-6.

255 Grim W, Muller H. A randomized controlled trial of the effect of fluid extract of Echinacea purpurea on the incidence and severity of colds and respiratory infections. *Am J Med* 106:138-43.

256 He K, et al. Additional bioactive annonaceous acetogenins from Asminia triloba (Annonaceae). *Bioorg Med Chem* 1997;5(3):501-6.

257 Ratnayake S, et al. Evaluation of various parts of the paw paw tree, Asmina triloba (Annonaceae), as commercial sources for the pesticidal annonaceous acetogenins. *J Econ Entomol* 1992;85(6):2353-6.

258 Zhao GX, et al. Asimin, asimininacin, and asiminecin: novel highly cytotoxic asimicin isomers from Asiminia triloba. *J Med Chem* 1994;37(13):1971-6.

259 Salonen JT, Seppanen K, Nyyssonen K, et al. Intake of mercury from fish, lipid peroxidation, and the risk of myocardial infarction and coronary, cardiovascular, and any death in eastern Finnish men. *Circulation* 1995;91:645-55.

260 Cone EH, Lange R, Darwin WD. In vivo adulteration: excess fluid ingestion causes false-negative marijuana and cocaine urine test results. *J Anal Toxicol* 1998;22(6):460-73.

261 Wu AH, et al. CEDIA for screening drugs of abuse in urine and the effect of adulterants. *J Forensic Sci* 1995;40(4):614-8.

262 Rabbani GH, et al. Randomized controlled trial of berberine sulfate therapy for diarrhea due to

enterotoxigenic Escherichia coli and Vibrio cholerae. *J Infect Dis* 1987;155(5):979-84.

263 Sheng WD, et al. Treatment of chloroquine-resistant malaria using pyrimethamine in combination with berberine, tetracycline, or cotrimoxazole. *East Afr Med J* 1997;74(5):283-4.

264 Khosla PG, et al. Berberine, a potential drug for trachoma. *Rev Int Trach Pathol Ocul Trop Subtrop Sante Publique* 1992;69:147-65.

265 Tamminga C, et al. Depression associated with oral choline. [letter] *Lancet* 1976;2(7991):905.

266 Facts and Comparisons staff. Drug Facts and Comparisons. St Louis: Wolters Kluwar Company (updated monthly).

267 Pharmacist's Letter Chaparral. February, 1999.

268 Merck Index, 12th ed. Whitehouse Station: Merck Research Laboratories, 1996.

269 Neal H. Dictionary of Chemical Names and Synonyms. Chelsea: Lewis Publishers, 1992.

270 Parker SP, ed. McGaw Hill Dictionary of Chemistry. New York: McGraw-Hill Book Company 1984.

271 Bruneton J. Pharmacognosy, Phytochemistry, Medicinal Plants. Paris: Lavoisier Publishing, 1995.

272 Covington TR, et al. Handbook of Nonprescription Drugs. Washington, DC: Am Pharmaceutical Assn, 1996.

273 FDA. FDA warns about GBL-related products. FDA Talk Paper. vm.cfsan.fda.gov/~1rd/ (Accessed 11 May 1999).

274 Chenoy R, et al. Effect of oral gamolenic acid from evening primrose oil on menopausal flushing. *BMJ* 19 Feb 1994; 308(6927):501-3.

275 Young DS. Effects of Drugs on Clinical Laboratory Tests 4th ed. Washington: AACC Press, 1995.

276 Balch JF, Balch PA. Prescription for Nutritional Healing. Garden City Park: Avery Publishing Group, 1997.

277 Silagy CA, Neil HA. A meta-analysis of the effect of garlic on blood pressure. *J Hypertension* 1994;12(4):463-8.

278 McMahon FG, Vargas R. Can garlic lower blood pressure? A pilot study. *Pharmacotherapy* 1993;13(4):406-7.

279 Auer W, Eiber A, Hertkorn E, et al. Hypertension and hyperlipidaemia: garlic helps in mild cases. *Br J Clin Pract Symp Suppl* 1990;69:3-6.

280 Hentschel C, Dressler S, Hahn EG. Fumaria officinalis (fumitory)-clinical applications. *Fortschr Med* 1995;113(19):291-2.

281 Pittler MH, Ernst E. Horse-chestnut seed extract for chronic venous insufficiency. A criteria-based systematic review. *Arch Dermatol* 1998;134(11):1356-60.

282 Greeske K, Pohlmann BK. Horse chestnut seed extract-an effective therapy principle in general practice. Drug therapy of chronic venous insufficiency. *Fortschr Med* 1996;114(15):196-200.

283 Diehm C, et al. Comparison of leg compression stocking and oral horse-chestnut seed extract in patients with chronic venous insufficiency. *Lancet* 1996;347(8997):292-4.

284 Diehm C, et al. Medical edema protection-clinical benefit in patients with chronic deep vein incompetence. *Vasa* 1992;21(2):188-92.

285 Bisler H, et al. Effects of horse-chestnut seed on transcapillary filtration in chronic venous insufficiency. *Dtsch Med Wochenschr* 1986;111(35):1321-9.

286 Mohler JL, et al. Phase II evaluation of coumarin (1,2-benzopyrone) in metastatic prostatic carcinoma. *Prostate* 1992;20(2):123-31.

287 Marshall ME, Butler K, Fried A. Phase I evaluation of coumarin (1,2 benzopyrone) and cimetidine in patients with advanced malignancies. *Mol Biother* 1991;3(3):170-8.

288 Howanitz JH, Howanitz PJ, eds. Renal Function by D.O. Rogerson Laboratory Medicine Test Selection and Interpretation. New York: Churchill Livingstone, 1991.

289 van Joost T, Smitt JH, van Ketel WG. Sensitization to olive oil (olea europeae). *Contact Dermatitis* 1981;7(6):309-10.

290 Privitera JR. Olive Leaf Extract: A new/old healing bonanza for mankind. www.oliveleafextract.com/contents.html (Accessed 23 Jun 1999).

291 Bakerink JA, Gospe SM Jr, Dimand RJ, Eldridge MW. Multiple organ failure after ingestion of pennyroyal oil from herbal tea in two infants. *Pediatrics* 1996;98(5):944-7.

292 Sudekum M, Poppenga RH, Raju N, Braselton WE Jr. Pennyroyal oil toxicosis in a dog. *J Am Vet Med Assoc* 1992;200(6):817-8.

293 Gittleman AL. Eat Fat, Lose Weight. Los Angeles: Keat's Publishing 1999.

294 Werbach M. Healing Through Nutrition. A Natural Approach to Treating 50 Common Illnesses with Diet and Nutrients. New York: Harper Collins 1993.

295 Ritschel WA, Brady ME, Tan HIS, et al. Pharmacokinetics of Coumarin and its 7-hyroxy-metabolites upon intravenous and peroral administration of coumarin in man. *Eur J Clin Pharmacol* 1997;12:457-61.

296 Agriculture Res Svc. Dr. Duke's phytochemical and ethnobotanical databases. www.ars-grin.gov/duke/ (Accessed 7 July 1999).

297 Cox D, O'Kennedy R, Thornes RD. The rarity of toxicity in patients treated with coumarin (1,2-benzopyrone). *Hum Toxicol* 1989;8(6):501-6.

298 Mann J, Truswell AS, eds. Essentials of Human Nutrition. Oxford: Oxford Univ Press 1998.

299 Rozanova IA, et al. Effect of antiatherosclerotic diet, containing polyunsaturated fatty acids of the omega-3 family from flax oil, on fatty acid composition of cell membranes of patients with ischemic heart disease. Hypertensive disease and hyperlipoproteinemia. *Vopr Pitan* 1997;(5):15-7.

300 Zarembo JE, Godfrey JC, Godfrey NJ. Zinc(II) in saliva: determination of concentrations produced by different formulations of zinc gluconate lozenges containing common excipients. *J Pharm Sci* 1992;81(2):128-30.

301 Goldenberg RL, Tamura T, Neggers Y, et al. The effect of zinc supplementation on pregnancy outcome. *JAMA* 1995;274(6):463-8.

303 Upton R, Ed. Astragalus Root: analytical, quality control, and therapeutic monograph. Santa Cruz, CA: Am Herbal Pharmacopoeia; 1999:1-25.

304 Upton R, Ed. Valerian Root: analytical, quality control, and therapeutic monograph. Santa Cruz, CA: Am Herbal Pharmacopoeia; 1999:1-25.

305 Life Extension Foundation. URL: http://lef.org/prod_desc/item132.html (Accessed 7 September 1999).

306 Nature's Life. www.natlife.com/pancreat.htm (Accessed 7 September 1999).

307 Huggins C. Calcium-rich food at each meal ensures intake. New York, NY: Reuters Health, 1999. www.reutershealth.com/eline/open/1999100109.html (Accessed 4 October 1999).

308 FDA. Ofc Regulatory Affairs Food Additive Status List. www.fda.gov/ora/inspect-ref/iom/exhibits/ApA2.html (Accessed 5 October 1999).

309 Fatty acid may be key to new treatment for cystic fibrosis. Reuters Health. www.reutershealth.com/eline/open/1999100810.html (Accessed 10 October 1999).

310 Penzak SR, Gubbins PO, Gurley BJ, et al. Grapefruit juice decreases the systemic availability of itraconazole capsules in healthy volunteers. *Ther Drug Monit* 1999;21(3):304-9.

311 FTC charges marketer of vitamin O of making false claims. Fed Trade Comm. www.ftc.gov/opa/1999/9903/rosecreek.htm (Accessed 12 October 1999).

312 MedicineShoppe. www.medicineshoppe.com (Accessed 14 October 1999).

313 Mehta DK (Ex Ed). British National Formulary, Number 37. British Medical Association and Royal Pharmaceutical Society of Great Britain: London, England, March 1999.

314 Herbs for milk production. Breastfeeding/Nursing/Parenting. www.gentlebirth.org/archives/breastfeed.html#Herbs (Accessed 18 October 1999).

315 Baker JC, Tunnicliffe WS, Duncanson RC, Ayres JG. Dietary antioxidants and magnesium in type 1 brittle asthma: a case control study. *Thorax* 1999;54:115-8.

316 Hammer KA, Carson CF, Riley TV. Antimicrobial activity of essential oils and other plant extracts. *J Appl Microbiol* 1999;86:985-990.

317 Fernandez-Anaya S, Crespo JF, Rodriguez JR, et al. Beer anaphylaxis. *J Allergy Clin Immunol* 1999;103(5 Pt 1):959-60.

318 Katz DL. Acute nutrient effects in endothelial function: a randomized, single-blind, crossover trial in healthy adults. Am Coll of Nutr 40th Ann Meeting. Oct 1999, Wash, DC.

321 Traditional uses for medicinal mushrooms. Garuda Int. URL: garudaint.com/amush.htm#cordyceps (Accessed 9 September 1999).

322 Morreale P, Manopulo R, Galati M, et al. Comparison of the anti-inflammatory efficacy of chondroitin sulfate and diclofenac sodium in patients with knee osteoarthritis. *J Rheumatol* 1996;23(8):1385-91.

323 Conrozier T. [Anti-arthrosis treatments: efficacy and tolerance of chondroitin sulfates]. [Article in French]. *Presse Med* 1998;27(36):1862-5.

324 Mazieres B, Loyau G, Menkes CJ, et al. [Chondroitin sulfate in the treatment of gonarthrosis and coxarthrosis. 5-months result of a multicenter double-blind controlled prospective study using placebo]. [Article in French]. *Rev Rhum Mal Osteoartic* 1992;59(7-8):466-72.

325 O'Breasail AM, Argouarch S. Hypomania and St John's wort. *Can J Psychiatry* 1998;43(7):746-7.

326 Trivedy C, Warnakulasuriya S, Peters TJ. Areca nuts can have deleterious effects. *BMJ* 1999;318(7193):1287.

327 Cox SC, Walker DM. Oral submucous fibrosis. A review. *Aust Dent J* 1996;41(5):294-9.

328 Gupta PC, Sinor PN, Bhonsle RB, et al. Oral submucous fibrosis in India: a new epidemic? *Natl Med J India* 1998;11(3):113-6.

329 VanWyk CW. Oral submucous fibrosis. The South African experience. *Indian J Dent Res* 1997 8(2):39-45.

330 Wiid I, Hoal-van Helden E, Hon D, et al. Potentiation of

isoniazid activity against Mycobacterium tuberculosis by melatonin. *Antimicrob Agents Chemother* 1999;43(4):975-7.

331   Barceloux DG. Zinc. *J Toxicol Clin Toxicol* 1999;37(2):279-92.

332   Anon. Zinc for the common cold. *Med Lett Drugs Ther* 1997;39(993):9-10.

333   Mossad SB, Macknin ML, Medendorp SV, Mason P. Zinc gluconate lozenges for treating the common cold. A randomized, double-blind, placebo-controlled study. *Ann Intern Med* 1996;125(2):81-8.

334   Godfrey JC, Conant Sloane B, Smith DS, et al. Zinc gluconate and the common cold: a controlled clinical study. *J Int Med Res* 1992;20(3):234-6.

335   Al-Nakib W, Higgins PG, Barrow I, et al. Prophylaxis and treatment of rhinovirus colds with zinc gluconate lozenges. *J Antimicrob Chemother* 1987;20(6):893-901.

336   Eby GA, Davis DR, Halcomb WW. Reduction in duration of common colds by zinc gluconate lozenges in a double-blind study. *Antimicrob Agents Chemother* 1984;25(1):20-4.

337   Farr BM, Conner EM, Betts RF, et al. Two randomized controlled trials of zinc gluconate lozenge therapy of experimentally induced rhinovirus colds. *Antimicrob Agents Chemother* 1987;31(8):1183-7.

338   Smith DS, Helzner EC, Nuttall CE Jr, et al. Failure of zinc gluconate in treatment of acute upper respiratory tract infections. *Antimicrob Agents Chemother* 1989;33(5):646-8.

339   Weismann K, Jakobsen JP, Weismann JE, et al. Zinc gluconate lozenges for common cold. A double-blind clinical trial. *Dan Med Bull* 1990;37(3):279-81.

340   Eby GA. Zinc ion availability—the determinant of efficacy in zinc lozenge treatment of common colds. *J Antimicrob Chemother* 1997;40(4):483-93.

341   Macknin ML, Piedmonte M, Calendine C, et al. Zinc gluconate lozenges for treating the common cold in children: a randomized, controlled trial. *JAMA* 1998;279(24):1962-7.

342   VitaminShoppe.com. www.vitaminshoppe.com/ product.asp?dispmode=quick&tab=1&sku=ON-1028 (Accessed 3 November 1999).

343   Stevia. MotherNature. www.mothernature.com/ency/ Herb/Stevia.asp (Accessed 3 November 1999).

344   Mother's intake of soy may affect development of fetus. Reuters health. www.reutershealth.com/ frame_eline.html (Accessed 5 November 1999).

345   Carta A, Calvani M, Bravi D, Bhuachalla SN. Acetyl-L-carnitine and Alzheimer's disease: pharmacological considerations beyond the cholinergic sphere. *Ann NY Acad Sci* 1993;695:324-6.

346   Orange juice raises good cholesterol. Reuters Health. www.reutershealth.com/frame_elinehtml (Accessed 9 November 1999).

347   SAMe for depression. *Medical Letter* 1999;41:107-8.

348   Vetrugno M, Maino A, Cardia G, et al. A randomised, double masked, clinical trial of high dose vitamin A and vitamin E supplementation after photorefractive keratectomy. *Br J Ophthalmol* 2001;85:537-9.

349   Garfinkel D, Zisapel N, Wainstein J, Laudon M. Facilitation of benzodiazepine discontinuation by melatonin, a new clinical approach. *Arch Intern Med* 1999;159(20):2456-60.

351   Black walnut hull capsules. VitaminShoppe.com. www.vitaminshoppe.com/

product.asp?dispmode=quick&tab=1&sku=NW-1035 (Accessed 16 November 1999).

352   Black walnut hull liquid extract. VitaminShoppe.com. www.vitaminshoppe.com/ product.asp?dispmode=quick&tab=1&sku=NW-2263 (Accessed 16 November 1999).

353   Reishi: Ancient medicine is modern hope. URL: home.pacific.net.hk/~gng/reishi.html (Accessed 20 November 1999).

354   Kobashi Y, Nakajima M, Niki Y, Matsushima T. [A case of acute eosinophilic pneumonia due to Sho-saiko-to]. [Article in Japanese]. *Nippon Kyobu Shikkan Gakkai Zasshi* 1997;35(12):1372-7.

355   Wada Y, Kubo M. [Acute lymphoblastic leukemia complicated by type C hepatitis during treatment and further by acute interstitial pneumonia due to sho-saiko-to in 7-year-old]. [Article in Japanese]. *Arerugi* 1997;46(11):1148-55.

356   Sato A, Toyoshima M, Kondo A, et al. [Pneumonitis induced by the herbal medicine Sho-saiko-to in Japan]. [Article in Japanese]. *Nippon Kyobu Shikkan Gakkai Zasshi* 1997;35(4):391-5.

357   Daibo A, Yoshida Y, Kitazawa S, et al. [A case of pneumonitis and hepatic injury caused by a herbal drug (sho-saiko-to)]. [Article in Japanese]. *Nippon Kyobu Shikkan Gakkai Zasshi* 1992;30(8):1583-8.

358   Sugiyama H, Nagai M, Kotajima F, et al. [A case of interstitial pneumonia with chronic hepatitis C following interferon-alfa and sho-saiko-to therapy]. [Article in Japanese]. *Arerugi* 1995;44(7):711-4.

359   Ishizaki T, Sasaki F, Ameshima S, et al. Pneumonitis during interferon and/or herbal drug therapy in patients with chronic active hepatitis. *Eur Respir J* 1996;9(12):2691-6.

360   Nakagawa A, Yamaguchi T, Takao T, Amano H. [Five cases of drug induced pneumonitis due to Sho-saiko-to or interferon-alpha or both]. [Article in Japanese]. *Nippon Kyobu Shikkan Gakkai Zasshi* 1995;33(12):1361-6.

361   Miyazaki E, Ando M, Ih K, et al. [Pulmonary edema associated with the Chinese medicine shosaikoto]. [Article in Japanese]. *Nihon Kokyuki Gakkai Zasshi* 1998;36(9):776-80.

362   Piras G, Makino M, Baba M. Sho-saiko-to, a traditional Kampo medicine, enhances the anti-HIV-1 activity of lamivudine (3TC) in vitro. *Microbiol Immunol* 1997;41(10):835-9.

363   Benninger J, Schneider HT, Schuppan D, et al. Acute hepatitis induced by greater celandine (Chelidonium majus). *Gastroenterol* 1999;117(5):1234-7.

364   Pipeline. Paladin Labs, Inc. www.pharmanex.com/e/ index.html (Accessed 21 November 1999).

365   FDA. Guide to inspections cosmetic prod mfgrs: products containing estrogenic hormones, placental extract or vitamins. www.fda.gov/ora/inspect_ref/igs/ cosmet.html (Accessed 22 November 1999).

366   Nityanand S, Srivastava JS, Asthana OP. Clinical trials with gugulipid. A new hypolipidaemic agent. *J Assoc Phys India* 1989;37(5):323-8.

367   Arandjelovic C. Canadian health officials pull Chinese herbal drugs. (Reprinted from Reuters). Richters HerbLetter 23 November 1999.

368   Skopnik H, Heimann G. [Manifestation of intolerance to cow's milk protein in mucoviscidosis with the symptom triad of hypoproteinemia, edema and anemia]. [Article in

German]. *Klin Padiatr* 1987;199(6):453-6.

369 New health claim proposed for relationship of soy protein and coronary heart disease. FDA. www.fda.gov/ bbs/topics/ANSWERS/ANS00923.html (Accessed 16 November 1999).

370 Benowitz LI, Goldberg DE, Madsen JR, et al. Inosine stimulates extensive axon collateral growth in the rat corticospinal tract after injury. *Proc Natl Acad Sci USA* 1999;96(23:13486-90.

371 Balkan B, Dunning BE. Glucosamine inhibits glucokinase in vitro and produces a glucose-specific impairment of in vivo insulin secretion in rats. *Diabetes* 1994;43(10):1173-9.

372 Giaccari A, Morviducci L, Zorretta D, et al. In vivo effects of glucosamine on insulin secretion and insulin sensitivity in the rat: possible relevance to the maladaptive responses to chronic hyperglycaemia. *Diabetologia* 1995;38(5):518-24.

373 Sinupret. www.takeyourq.com/secondary/ sinus_copy.html (Accessed 29 November 1999).

374 Neubauer N, Marz RW. Placebo-controlled, randomized, double-blind, clincal trial with Sinupret sugar coated tablets on the basis of a therapy with antibiotics and decongestant nasal drops in acute sinusitis. *Phytomedicine* 1994;1:177-81.

375 Govers MJ, Gannon NJ, Dunshea FR, et al. Wheat bran affects the site of fermentation of resistant starch and luminal indexes related to colon cancer risk: a study in pigs. *Gut* 1999;45:840-7.

376 Hubner WD, Lande S, Podzuweit H. Hypericum treatment of mild depressions with somatic symptoms. *J Geriatr Psychiatry Neurol* 1994;7 Suppl 1:S12-4.

377 Stevinson C, Dixon M, Ernst E. Hypericum for fatigue. *Phytomedicine* 1998;5(6):443-7.

378 Heavy cocaine use puts rate of coronary aneurysms at 30%. Reuters Health 1999 Nov 29. www.reutershealth.com/frame_mednews.html(Accessed 29 November 1999).

379 Marz RW, Ismail C, Popp MA. Action profile and efficacy of a herbal combination preparation for the treatment of sinusitis. *Wien Med Wochenschr* 1999;149(8-10):202-8.

380 Dupuis C. Poison ivy. *Pharmacy Practic* 1995;11(5):51-2,54-5.

381 Malinow MR, Bardana EJ Jr, Goodnight SH Jr. Pancytopenia during ingestion of alfalfa seeds. *Lancet* 1981 March;14(8220 Pt1):615.

382 Johne A, Brockmoller J, Bauer S, et al. Pharmacokinetic interaction of digoxin with an herbal extract from St John's wort (Hypericum perforatum). *Clin Pharmacol Ther* 1999;66(4):338-45.

383 Dalvi SS, Nayak VK, Pohujani SM, et al. Effect of gugulipid on bioavailability of diltiazem and propranolol. *J Assoc Phys India* 1994;42(6):454-5.

384 JointFlex. www.jointflex.com/products.html (Accessed 4 December 1999).

385 Zicam. www.zicam.com/home.html (Accessed 9 December 1999).

387 FDA Talk Paper: FDA takes action against firm marketing unapproved drugs. www.fda.gov/bbs/topics/ ANSWERS/ANS00988.html (Accessed 14 December 1999).

388 Goldwaser I, Li J, Gershonov E, et al. L-Glutamic acid gamma-monohydroxamate. A potentiator of vanadium-evoked glucose metabolism in vitro and in vivo. *J Biol*

Chem 1999;274(37):26617-24.

389 Duda RB, Zhong Y, Navas V, et al. American ginseng and breast cancer therapeutic agents synergistically inhibit MCF-7 breast cancer cell growth. *J Surg Oncol* 1999;72(4):230-9.

390 Strahl S, Ehret V, Dahm HH, Maier KP. [Necrotizing hepatitis after taking herbal medication]. [Article in German]. *Dtsch Med Wochenschr* 1998;123(47):1410-4.

391 Vitamins may interfere with cancer chemotherapy. Reuters Health. www.reutershealth.com/ frame_eline.html (Accessed 15 December 1999).

392 Wild Indigo. MotherNature. www.mothernature.com/ ency/Herb/Wild_Indigo.asp (Accessed 18 December 1999).

393 Beuscher N, Scheit KH, Bodinet C, Kopanski L. [Immunologically active glycoproteins of Baptisia tinctoria]. [Article in German]. *Planta Med* 1989;55(4):358-63.

394 Anon. A better treatment for depression? *UC Berkeley Wellness Letter* 1997;13(12):1-2.

395 Subrahmanyam M. A prospective randomized, clinical and histological study of superficial burn wound healing with honey and silver sulfadiazine. *Burns* 1998;24(2):157-61.

396 Subrahmanyam M. Honey dressing vs boiled potato peel in the treatment of burns: a prospective randomized study. *Burns* 1996;22(6):491-3.

397 Subrahmanyam M. Honey impregnated gauze vs amniotic membrane in the treatment of burns. *Burns* 1994;20(4):331-3.

398 Subrahmanyam M. Honey impregnated gauze versus polyurethane film (OpSite) in the treatment of burns- a prospective randomized study. *Br J Plast Surg* 1993;46(4):322-3.

399 Subrahmanyam M. Topical application of honey in treatment of burns. *Br J Surg* 1991;78(4):497-8.

400 Magic and Medicine of Plants. 7th ed. New York, NY: Readers Digest Assn, 1993.

401 Kelly FJ, Mudway I, Blomberg A, et al. Altered lung antioxidant status in patients with mild asthma. *Lancet* 1999;354:482-3.

402 Covington TR, ed. The Handbook of Non-Prescription Drugs. Washington, DC: APhA, 1996.

403 Whitney E, Cataldo CB, Rolfes SR, eds. Understanding Normal and Clinical Nutrition. Belmont, CA: Wadsworth, 1998.

404 Kehoe WA. Grapefruit juice and lovastatin: Is this an important interaction? Pharmacists Letter, Dec. 1998:Detail Document #141204.

405 Cook IJ, et al. Effect of dietary fiber on rectosigmoid motility in patients with irritable bowel syndrome: A controlled, crossover study. *Gastroenterol* 1990;98:66-72.

406 Upton R, Ed. Hawthorn leaf with flower: quality control, analytical and therapeutic monograph. Santa Cruz, CA: Am Herbal Pharmacopoeia, 1999:1-29.

407 Thrive online website. thriveonline.com/health/Library/ vitamins/vitamin215.html (Accessed 22 November 1999).

408 Native Am Indian Res. URL: http://indy4.fdl.cc.mn.us/ ~isk/food/parttrib.html (Accessed 22 November 1999).

409 Powell CV, Nash AA, Powers HJ, Primhak RA. Antioxidant status in asthma. *Pediatr Pulmonol* 1994;18:34-8.

410 A Modern Herbal (Mrs.M.Grieve) website. URL: http://

botanical.com/botanical/mgmh/s/squawv85.html (Accessed 25 November 1999).

411 HolisticOnLine. URL: http://holisticonline.com/Herbal-Med/_scripts/getHerb_Dir.idc?Herb_Names=275 (Accessed 25 November 1999).

412 Woo KS, Chook P, Lolin YI, et al. Folic acid improves arterial endothelial function in adults with hyperhomocysteinemia. *J Am Coll Cardiol* 1999;34:2002-6.

413 Horticopia plant info. www.horticopia.com/p&a.htm (Accessed 5 December 1999).

414 Common poisonous or irritating plants. Star Nursery. www.starnursery.com/005.htm (Accessed 18 December 1999).

415 MotherNature Health Encyclopedia. www.mothernature.com/ency/Herb/Ligustrum.asp (Accessed 5 December 1999).

416 Pajaron MJ, Vila L, Prieto I, et al. Cross-reactivity of Olea europaea with other Oleaceae species in allergic rhinitis and bronchial asthma. *Allergy* 1997;52(8):829-35.

417 Batanero E, Gonzalez De La Pena MA, Villalba M, et al. Isolation, cDNA cloning and expression of Lig v 1, the major allergen from privet pollen. *Clin Exp Allergy* 1996;26(12):1401-10.

418 Khoo KS, Ang PT. Extract of astragalus membranaceus and ligustrum lucidum does not prevent cyclophosphamide-induced myelosuppression. *Singapore Med J* 1995;36(4):387-90.

419 Lau BH, Ruckle HC, Botolazzo T, Lui PD. Chinese medicinal herbs inhibit growth of murine renal cell carcinoma. *Cancer Biother* 1994;9(2):153-61.

420 Niikawa M, Hayashi H, Sato T, et al. Isolation of substances from glossy privet (Ligustrum lucidum Ait.) inhibiting the mutagenicity of benzo[a]pyrene in bacteria. *Mutat Res* 1993;319(1):1-9.

421 Rittenhouse JR, Lui PD, Lau BH. Chinese medicinal herbs reverse macrophage suppression induced by urological tumors. *J Urol* 1991;146(2):486-90.

422 Kalayci O, Besler T, Kilinc K, et al. Serum levels of antioxidant vitamins (alpha tocopherol, beta carotene, and ascorbic acid) in children with bronchial asthma. *Turk J Pediatr* 2000;42:17-21.

423 Sun Y, Hersh EM, Talpaz M, et al. Immune restoration and/or augmentation of local graft versus host reaction by traditional Chinese medicinal herbs. *Cancer* 1983;52(1):70-3.

424 Lucas A, Stafford M, Morley R, et al. Efficacy and safety of long-chain polyunsaturated fatty acid supplementation of infant-formula milk: a randomized trial. *Lancet* 1999;354(9194):1948-54.

425 Gibson RA. Long-chain polyunsaturated fatty acids and infant development (editorial). *Lancet* 1999;354(9194):1919.

426 Arjmandi BH, Birnbaum RS, Juma S, et al. The synthetic phytoestrogen, ipriflavone, and estrogen prevent bone loss by different mechanisms. *Calcif Tissue Int* 2000;66(1):61-5.

427 Melis GB, Paoletti AM, Bartolini R, et al. Ipriflavone and low doses of estrogens in the prevention of bone mineral loss in climacterium. *Bone Miner* 1992;19,Suppl 1:S49-56.

428 Agnusdei D, Adami S, Cervetti R, et al. Effects of ipriflavone on bone mass and calcium metabolism in postmenopausal osteoporosis. *Bone Miner* 1992;19,Suppl 1:S43-8.

429 Sato Y, Kuno H, Kaji M, et al. Effect of ipriflavone on bone in elderly hemiplegic stroke patients with hypovitaminosis D. *Am J Phys Med Rehabil* 1999;78(5):457-63.

430 Ohta H, Komukai S, Makita K, et al. Effects of 1-year ipriflavone treatment on lumbar bone mineral density and bone metabolic markers in postmenopausal women with low bone mass. *Horm Res* 1999;51(4):178-83.

431 Head KA. Ipriflavone: an important bone-building isoflavone. *Altern Med Rev* 1999;4(1):10-22.

432 Agnusdei D, Bufalino L. Efficacy of ipriflavone in established osteoporosis and long-term safety. *Calcif Tissue Int* 1997;61,Suppl 1:S23-7.

433 Gennari C, Adami S, Agnusdei D, et al. Effect of chronic treatment with ipriflavone in postmenopausal women with low bone mass. *Calcif Tissue Int* 1997;61,Suppl 1:S19-22.

434 Petilli M, Fiorelli G, Benvenuti S, et al. Interactions between ipriflavone and the estrogen receptor. *Calcif Tissue Int* 1995;56(2):160-5.

435 History and tradition of Morinda Citrifolia. www.freeyellow.com/members2/rsscomp/morindacitrifoliastory.htm (Accessed 6 December 1999).

436 Brunner Prof Svcs. Tahitian Noni prod overview. www.brunnerbiz.com/noni/fact3.html (Accessed 6 December 1999).

437 Brunner Prof Svcs. Tahitian Noni skin supplement info. www.brunnerbiz.com/noni/skinsupp.html (Accessed 6 December 1999).

438 Herbex Ltd. Use of Noni in the Pac Islands. URL http://4-u-veges.com/noni_use.html (Accessed 6 December 1999).

439 Maui Noni. www.timewealth.com/story.htm (Accessed 6 December 1999).

440 Herb's herbs, Noni info. www.hookele.com/noni/ (Accessed 1 January 2000).

441 Hirazumi A, Furusawa E. An immunomodulatory polysaccharide-rich substance from the fruit juice of Morinda citrifolia (noni) with antitumour activity. *Phytother Res* 1999;13(5):380-7.

442 Hiwasa T, Arase Y, Chen Z, et al. Stimulation of ultraviolet-induced apoptosis of human fibroblast UVr-1 cells by tyrosine kinase inhibitors. *FEBS Lett* 1999;444(2-3):173-6.

443 Hiramatsu T, Imoto M, Koyano T, Umezawa K. Induction of normal phenotypes in ras-transformed cells by damnacanthal from Morinda citrifolia. *Cancer Lett* 1993;73(2-3):161-6.

444 Younos C, Rolland A, Fleurentin J, et al. Analgesic and behavioural effects of Morinda citrifolia. *Planta Med* 1990;56(5):430-4.

445 Nature's Sunshine. www.parentzone.com/sunshine/morinda.htm (Accessed 6 December 1999).

446 Samra Health and Beauty. www.samra.com/herb.htm (Accessed 6 December 1999).

447 Herbal Marketplace. URL: http://members.aol.com/genery/morinda.htm (Accessed 6 December 1999).

448 Yoshikawa M, Yamaguchi S, Nishisaka H, et al. Chemical constituents of Chinese natural medicine, morindae radix, the dried roots of morinda officinalis how: structures of morindolide and morofficinaloside. *Chem Pharm Bull* (Tokyo) 1995;43(9):1462-5.

449 Cui C, Yang M, Yao Z, et al. [Antidepressant active constituents in the roots of Morinda officinalis how].

[Article in Chinese]. *Chung Kuo Chung Yao Tsa Chih* 1995;20(1):36-9, 62-3.

450 Miller LG, Panosian CB. Ataxia and slurred speech after artesunate treatment for falciparum malaria [Letter]. *N Engl J Med* 1997;336(18):1328.

451 Yang YJ, Shu HY, Min ZD. [Anthraquinones isolated from Morinda officinalis and Damnacanthus indicus]. [Article in Chinese]. *Yao Hsueh Hsueh Pao* 1992;27(5):358-64.

452 Li S, Ouyang Q, Tan X, et al. [Chemical constituents of Morinda officinalis how]. [Article in Chinese]. *Chung Kuo Chung Yao Tsa Chih* 1991;16(11):675-6, 703.

453 Qiao ZS, Wu H, Su ZW. [Comparison with the pharmacological actions of Morinda officinalis, Damnacanthus officinarum and Schisandra propinqua]. [Article in Chinese]. *Chung Hsi I Chieh Ho Tsa Chih* 1991;11(7):390,415-7.

454 Barton DL, Loprinzi CL, Quella SK, et al. Prospective evaluation of vitamin E for hot flashes in breast cancer survivors. *J Clin Oncol* 1998;16:495-500.

455 Nagao T, Ibayashi S, Fujii K, et al. Treatment of warfarin-induced hair loss with ubidecarenone. *Lancet* 1995;346:1104-5.

456 Henriksen JE, Andersen CB, Hother-Nielsen O, et al. Impact of ubiquinone (coenzyme Q10) treatment on glycaemic control, insulin requirement and well-being in patients with Type 1 diabetes mellitus. *Diabet Med* 1999;16:312-8.

457 Weis M, Mortensen SA, Rassing MR, et al. Bioavailability of four oral coenzyme Q10 formulations in healthy volunteers. *Mol Aspects Med* 1994;15:s273-80.

458 Canada Seabuckthorn Ent Ltd. www.seabuckthorn.com (Accessed 10 January 2000).

459 Seabuckthorn seminar news release from Okanagan Univ Coll, 3333 College Way, Kelowna, BC, Canada. V1V 1V7. Dec 29, 1998. www.ouc.bc.ca/update/news82.htm (Accessed 10 January 2000).

460 Sneddon Ent. www.sneddonenterprises.com/Seabuckthornhome.html (Accessed 10 January 2000).

461 KeDi High-Tech Ind Co (Xiamen Office). www.eckorea.net/co/kedi/3.asp (Accessed 10 January 2000).

462 Seabuckthorn seed oil. RichNature Inc. www.richnature.com/products/herbal/seaseed.htm (Accessed 10 January 2000).

463 Seabuckthorn berry oil. RichNature Inc. www.richnature.com/products/herbal/seaberry.htm (Accessed 10 January 2000).

464 Shineway. www.shineway.com/seabuckt.htm (Accessed 10 January 2000).

465 Floraleads GR. URL: http://floraleads.com/OILSEA.HTM (Accessed 10 January 2000).

466 Amosova EN, Zueva EP, Razina TG, et al. [The search for new anti-ulcer agents from plants in Siberia and the Far East]. [Article in Russian]. *Eksp Klin Farmakol* 1998;61(6):31-5.

467 Ianev E, Radev S, Balutsov M, et al. [The effect of an extract of sea buckthorn (Hippophae rhamnoides L.) on the healing of experimental skin wounds in rats]. [Article in Bulgarian]. *Khirurgiia (Sofiia)* 1995;48(3):30-3.

468 Li Y, Liu H. Prevention of tumour production in rats fed aminopyrine plus nitrite by sea buckthorn juice. *IARC Sci Publ* 1991;(105):568-70.

469 Cheng TJ, Pu JK, Wu LW, et al. [A preliminary study on hepato-protective action of seed oil of Hippophae rhamnoides L. (HR) and mechanism of the action]. [Article in Chinese]. *Chung Kuo Chung Yao Tsa Chih* 1994;19(6):367-70, 384.

470 Cheng TJ. [Protective action of seed oil of Hippophae rhamnoides L. (HR) against experimental liver injury in mice]. [Article in Chinese]. *Chung Hua Yu Fang I Hsueh Tsa Chih* 1992;26(4):227-9.

471 Wang Y, Lu Y, Liu X, et al. [The protective effect of Hippophae rhamnoides L. on hyperlipidemic serum cultured smooth muscle cells in vitro]. [Article in Chinese]. *Chung Kuo Chung Yao Tsa Chih* 1992;17(10):601, 624-6 (inside back cover).

472 Xiao M, Yang Z, Jiu M, et al. [The antigastroulcerative activity of beta-sitosterol-beta-D-glucoside and its aglycone in rats]. [Article in Chinese]. *Hua Hsi I Ko Ta Hsueh Hsueh Pao* 1992;23(1):98-101.

473 Satietrol press releases. PacificHealth Labs, Inc., Woodbridge, NJ. www.satietrol.com/press.htm and www.satietrol.com/press1.htm (Accessed 10 January 2000).

474 Klement P, Liao P, Bajzar L. A novel approach to arterial thrombolysis. *Blood* 1999;94(8):2735-43.

475 Redlitz A, Nicolini FA, Malycky JL, et al. Inducible carboxypeptidase activity. A role in clot lysis in vivo. *Circulation* 1996;93(7):1328-30.

476 Kopin AS, Mathes WF, McBride EW, et al. The cholecystokinin-A receptor mediates inhibition of food intake yet is not essential for the maintenance of body weight. *J Clin Invest* 1999;103(3):383-91.

477 Lam WF, Gielkens HA, de Boer SY, et al. Influence of hyperglycemia on the satiating effect of CCK in humans. *Physiol Behav* 1998;65(3):505-11.

478 Zhongrui L, Shuzhen T. [Clinical observation on curative effect of oral seabuckthorn seed oil on cancers under chemotherapy]. [Article in Chinese] . *Hippophae* 1993;6(4):39-41.

479 Changshun L, Xinming C, Fenrong W, et al. [Clinical observation on reflux esophagitis treated with seabuckthorn seed oil]. [Article in Chinese]. *Hippophae* 1996;9(4):40-1.

480 Gengquan Q, Xiang Q. [A clinical report on the therapeutics of seabuckthorn oil softgels on peptic ulcer in 30 cases]. [Article in Chinese]. *Hippophae* 1997;10(4):39-41.

481 Shoskes DA, Zeitlin SI, Shahed A, Rajfer J. Quercetin in men with category III chronic prostatitis: A preliminary prospective, double-blind, placebo-controlled trial. *Urol* 1999;54:960-3.

482 Aharon Y, Mevorach M, Shamoon H. Vanadyl sulfate does not enhance insulin action in patients with type 1 diabetes. *Diabetes Care* 1998;21(12):2194-5.

483 Anon. Quercetin. *Alt Med Rev* 1998;3(2):140-3.

484 Miodini P, Fioravanti L, Di Fronzo G, Cappelletti V. The two phyto-oestrogens genistein and quercetin exert different effects on oestrogen receptor function. *Br J Cancer* 1999;80(8):1150-5.

485 El Attar TM, Virji AS. Modulating effect of resveratrol and quercetin on oral cancer cell growth and proliferation. *Anticancer Drugs* 1999;10(2):187-93.

486 Wiseman H. The bioavailability of non-nutrient plant factors: dietary flavonoids and phyto-oestrogens. *Proc Nutr Soc* 1999;58(1):139-46.

487 McAnlis GT, McEneny J, Pearce J, Young IS.

REFERENCES

Absorption and antioxidant effects of quercetin from onions, in man. *Eur J Clin Nutr* 1999;53(2):92-6.

488 Hansten PD, Horn JR. Hansten and Horn's Drug Interactions Analysis and Management. Vancouver, CAN:Appl Therapeut, 1999.

489 Huang Z, Fasco MJ, Kaminsky LS. Inhibition of estrone sulfatase in human liver microsomes by quercetin and other flavonoids. *J Steroid Biochem Mol Biol* 1997;63(1-3):9-15.

490 Garg R, Malinow MR, Pettinger M, et al. Niacin treatment increases plasma homocysteine levels. *Am Heart J* 1999;138:1082-7.

491 The Way Up website. www.thewayup.com/products/0187.htm (Accessed 3 February 2000).

492 Eriksson JG, Forsen TJ, Mortensen SA, Rohde M. The effect of coenzyme Q10 administration on metabolic control in patients with type 2 diabetes mellitus. *Biofactors* 1999;9:315-8.

493 Intermittent claudication info from MotherNature. www.mothernature.com/ency/Concern/Intermittent_Claudication.asp (Accessed 3 February 2000).

494 Alternatives Natl Prod. www.alternativesnatural.com/vs/ (Accessed 3 February 2000).

495 Prevention home page. www.prevention.com/healing/vitamin/ail/raynauds/more2.html (Accessed 3 February 2000).

496 Anon. Inositol hexaniacinate. *Altern Med Rev* 1998;3(3):222-3.

497 Mehta DK (Executive Editor). British National Formulary 38. British Medical Association and Royal Pharmaceutical Society of Great Britain, London, UK, 1999. pg 104.

498 Sunderland GT, Belch JJ, Sturrock RD, et al. A double-blind, randomized, placebo-controlled trial of hexopal in primary Raynaud's disease. *Clin Rheumatol* 1988;7(1):46-9.

499 Hutt V, Wechsler JG, Klor HU, Ditschuneit H. [Effect of a clofibrate-inositol nicotinate combination on lipids and lipoproteins in primary hyperlipoproteinemia of types IIa, IV and V]. [Article in German]. *Arzneimittelforschung* 1983;33(5):776-9.

500 Brinker F. Herb Contraindications and Drug Interactions. Sandy, OR: Eclectic Medical Publ, 1997.

501 De Smet PAGM, Keller K, Hansel R, Chandler RF, Eds. Adverse Effects of Herbal Drugs 1. Verlag, Berlin: Springer, 1992.

502 De Smet PAGM, Keller K, Hansel R, Chandler RF, Eds. Adverse Effects of Herbal Drugs 2. Verlag, Berlin: Springer, 1993.

503 Duke, JA. The Green Pharmacy. Emmaus, PA: Rodale Press, 1997.

504 Holt GA. Food & Possible Interactions with Drugs: Revised and Expanded Ed. Chicago, IL: Precept Press, 1998.

505 Hardman JG, Limbird LL, eds. Goodman and Gillman's The Pharmacological Basis of Therapeutics, 9th ed. New York, NY: McGraw-Hill, 1996.

506 Burnham TH, ed. Drug Facts and Comparisons, Updated Monthly. Facts and Comparisons, St. Louis, MO.

507 Pheatt N, ed. Nonherbal Dietary Supplements. *Pharmacist's Letter Continuing Education Booklet* 1998;98(4):1-51.

508 Lieberman S. The Real Vitamin and Mineral Book.

Honesdale, PA: Paragon Press, 1997.

509 Dukes, MNG. Meyler's Side Effects of Drugs. 13th ed. Elsevier: Amsterdam, 1997.

510 Meuss AR, transl. Phytotherapy in Paediatrics - Handbook for Physicians and Pharmacists by H Schilcher. 2nd edition. Stuttgart, Germany: Medpharm GmbH Scientific Publishers, 1997.

511 Spraycar M, Ed. Stedman's Medical Dictionary. 26th ed. Baltimore, MD: Williams & Wilkins, 1995.

512 Robbers JE, Tyler VE. Tyler's Herbs of Choice: The Therapeutic Use of Phytomedicinals. New York, NY: The Haworth Herbal Press, 1999.

513 Agri Res Svc: Dr. Duke's phytochemical and ethnobotanical databases. www.ars-grin.gov/duke (Accessed 3 November 1999).

514 Bruneton J. Pharmacognosy, Phytochemistry, Medicinal Plants. Paris, FR: Lavoisier Publishing, 1995.

515 Foster S, Tyler VE. Tyler's Honest Herbal, 4th ed., Binghamton, NY: Haworth Herbal Press, 1999.

516 Morrix W, ed. The American Heritage Dictionary of the English Language. New York, NY: Am Heritage Publ, 1969.

517 Duke JA, Vasquez R. Amazonian Ethnobotanical Dictionary. Boca Raton, FL: CRC Press, 1994.

518 Schultes RE, Raffauf RF. The Healing Forest, Medicinal and Toxic Plants of the Northwest Amazonia. Portland, OR: Dioscorides Press, 1990.

519 Foster S, Duke JA. Eastern/Central Medicinal Plants. New York, NY: Houghton Mifflin Co., 1990.

520 Richter W, et al. Interaction between fibre and lovastatin. *Lancet* 1991;338:706.

521 Kantola T, et al. Grapefruit juice greatly increases serum concentrations of lovastatin and lovastatin acid. *Clin Pharmacol Ther* 1998;63:397-402.

522 Ioannides-Demos LL, et al. Dosing implications of a clinical interaction between grapefruit juice and cyclosporine and metabolite concentrations in patients with autoimmune diseases. *J Rheumatol* 1997;24:49-54.

523 Josefsson M, et al. Effect of grapefruit juice on the pharmacokinetics of amlodipine in healthy volunteers. *Eur J Clin Pharmacol* 1996;51:189-93.

524 Garg SK, et al. Effect of grapefruit juice on carbamazepine bioavailability in patients with epilepsy. *Clin Pharmacol Ther* 1998;64:286-8.

525 Weber A, et al. Can grapefruit juice influence ethinylestradiol bioavailability? *Contraception* 1996;53:41-7.

526 Schubert W, et al. Inhibition of 17 beta-estradiol metabolism by grapefruit juice in ovariectomized women. *Maturitas* 1994;20:155-63.

527 Kantola T, et al. Grapefruit juice greatly increases serum concentrations of lovastatin and lovastatin acid. *Clin Pharmacol Ther* 1998 63:397-402.

528 Bailey DG, et al. Interaction of citrus juices with felodipine and nifedipine. *Lancet* 1991;337:268-9.

529 Bailey DG, et al. Effect of grapefruit juice and naringin on nisoldipine pharmacokinetics. *Clin Pharmacol Ther* 1993;54:589-94.

530 Rau SE, et al. Grapefruit juice-terfenadine single-dose interaction: magnitude, mechanism, and relevance. *Clin Pharmacol Ther* 1997 61:401-9.

531 Robbins RC, et al. Ingestion of grapefruit lowers elevated hematocrits in human subjects. *Int J Vitam Nutr Res* 1988;58:414-7.

532 Gin H, et al. The influence of Guar gum on absorption

REFERENCES

of metformin from the gut in healthy volunteers. *Horm Metab Res* 1989;21:81-3.

533 Huupponen R, et al. Effect of guar gum, a fibre preparation, on digoxin and penicillin absorption in man. *Eur J Clin Pharmacol* 1984;26:279-81.

534 Spillane PK, et al. Neurological manifestations of kava intoxication. *Med J Aust* 1997;167:172-3.

535 Swensen JN. Man convicted of driving under the influence of kava. Salt Lake City, UT: Deseret News, 1996.

536 Almeida JC, et al. Coma from the health food store: interaction between kava and alprazolam. *Ann Intern Med* 1996;125:940-1.

537 Bano G, et al. The effect of piperine on pharmacokinetics of phenytoin in healthy volunteers. *Planta Med* 1987;53:568-9.

538 Bano G, et al. Effect of piperine on bioavailability and pharmacokinetics of propranolol and theophylline in healthy volunteers. *Eur J Clin Pharmacol* 1991;41;615-7.

539 Etman M. Effect of a bulk forming laxative on the bioavailablility of caramazepine in man. *Drug Dev Ind Pharm* 1995;21:1901-6.

540 Perlman BB. Interaction between lithium salts and ispaghula husk. *Lancet* 1990; 35:416.

541 Amabeoku, GJ, et al. Pharmacokinetic interaction of single doses of quinine and carbamazepine, phenobarbitone and phenytoin in healthy volunteers. *East Afr Med J* 1993;70:90-3.

542 Gordon JB. SSRIs and St. John's Wort: possible toxicity? *Am Fam Physician* 1998;57(5):950,953.

543 McRae S. Elevated serum digoxin levels in a patient taking digoxin and Siberian ginseng. *CMAJ* 1996;155:293-5.

544 Tatro D, Ed. Anticoagulants-Vitamin E: in Drug Interaction Facts, Facts and Comparisons. St. Louis, MO, January 1997.

545 Dunbain DW, et al. Lead poisoning from Indian herbal medicine (Ayurveda). *Med J Aust* 1992;157:835-6.

546 Sheerin NS, et al. Simultaneous exposure to lead, arsenic and mercury from Indian ethnic remedies. *Br J Clin Pract* 1994;48:332-3.

547 Markowitz SB, et al. Lead poisoning due to Hai Ge Fan, the porphyrin content of individual erythrocytes. *JAMA* 1994;271:932-4.

548 Tay CH, et al. Arsenic Poisoning from anti-asthmatic herbal preparations. *Med J Aust* 1975;2:424-8.

549 Colgrove ML, et al. Lead poisoning-associated death from Asian Indian folk remedies, Florida. *MMWR Morb Mortal Wkly Rep* 1984;33:642-5.

550 Schaumburg HH, et al. Alopecia and sensory polyneuropathy from thallium in a Chinese herbal medication. *JAMA* 1992;268:3430-1.

551 Espinoza EO, et al. Toxic metals in selected traditional Chinese medicinals. *J Forensic Sci* 1996;41:453-6.

552 Takegoshi K, et al. A case of Venoplant-induced hepatic injury. *Gastroenterol Jpn* 1986;21:62-5.

553 Jaspersen-Schib R, et al. [Serious plant poisonings in Switzerland 1966-1994. Case analysis from the Swiss Toxicology Information Center]. [Article in German]. *Schweiz Med Wochenschr* 1996;126:1085-98.

554 Cerulli J, et al. Chromium picolinate toxicity. *Ann Pharmacother* 1998;32:428-31.

555 Lin JL, et al. Flavonoid-induced acute nephropathy. *Am J Kidney Dis* 1994;23:433-40.

556 Becker BN. Ginseng-induced diuretic resistance. *JAMA* 1996 276:606-7.

557 Tao SH, Bolger, PM. Hazard assessment of germanium supplements. *Regul Toxicol Pharmacol* 1997;25:211-9.

558 Tai YT. Adverse effects from traditional Chinese medicine. *Lancet* 1993;341:892.

559 Tai YT, et al. Cardiotoxicity after accidental herb-induced aconite poisoning. *Lancet* 1992;340:1254-6.

560 Osher HL, Katz KH, Wagner DJ. Khellin in the treatment of angina pectoris. *N Engl J Med* 1951;244:315-21.

561 Fatovich DM. Aconite: a lethal Chinese herb. *Ann Emerg Med* 1992;21:309-11.

562 Tomlinson B, et al. Herb-induced aconite poisoning. *Lancet* 1993;341:370-1.

563 Chan TYK, et al. Aconitine poisoning following the ingestion of Chinese herbal medicines: a report of eight cases. *Aust N Z J Med* 1993;23:268-71.

564 van Ypersele de Strihou C, et al. The tragic paradigm of Chinese herbs nephropathy. *Nephrol Dial Transplant* 1995;10:157-60.

565 Blumenthal HJ, et al. Chewing gum headaches. *Headache* 1997;37:665-6.

566 Jones TK, et al. Profound neonatal congestive heart failure caused by maternal consumption of blue cohosh herbal medication. *J Pediatr* 1998;132:550-2.

567 Subiza J, et al. Anaphylactic reaction after the ingestion of chamomile tea; a study of cross-reactivity with other composite pollens. *J Allergy Clin Immunol* 1989;84:353-8.

568 Smith BC, et al. Acute hepatitis induced by ingestion of the herbal medication chaparral. *Aust NZ Med J* 1993;23:526.

569 Gordon DW, et al. Chaparral ingestion: the broadening spectrum of liver injury caused by herbal medications. *JAMA* 1995;273:489-90.

570 Batchelor WB, et al. Chaparral-induced hepatic injury. *Am J Gastroenterol* 1995;90:831-3.

571 Katz M, et al. Herbal hepatitis: subacute hepatic necrosis secondary to chaparral leaf. *J Clin Gastroenterol* 1990;12:203-6.

572 Ko RJ, et al. Lethal ingestion of Chinese herbal tea containing ch'an su. *West J Med* 1996;164:71-5.

573 Chan JCN, et al. Anticholinergic poisoning from Chinese herbal medciines. *Aust N Z J Med* 1994;24:317-8.

574 Sperl W, et al. Reversible hepatic veno-occlusive disease in an infant after consumption of pyrrolizidine-containing herbal tea. *Eur J Pediatr* 1995;154:112-6.

575 Roulet M, et al. Hepatic veno-occlusive disease in newborn infant of a woman drinking herbal tea. *J Pediatr* 1988;112:433-4.

576 Matthews, MK. Association of Ginkgo biloba with intracerebral hemorrhage. *Neurology* 1998;50:1934.

577 Gilbert GJ. Ginkgo biloba. *Neurology* 1997;48:1137.

578 Rowin J, Lewis SL. Spontaneous bilateral subdural hemotomas with chronic Gingko biloba ingestion. *Neurology* 1996;46:1775-6.

579 Rosenblatt M, Mindel T. Spontaneous hyphema associated with ingestion of Gingko biloba extract. *N Engl J Med* 1997;336:1108.

580 Jaakkola MS, et al. Asthma caused by occupational exposure to pectin. *J Allergy Clin Immunol* 1997;100:575-6.

581 Westphal W, et al. [Exogenous allergic asthma following pectin exposure-a new occupational allergen].[Article in

German]. *Pneumologie* 1990;44(Suppl 1):337-8.

582 Baldwin JL, et al. Pectin-induced occupational asthma. *Chest* 1993;104:1936-7.

583 Cohen AJ, et al. Occupational asthma caused by pectin inhalation during the manufacture of jam. *Chest* 1993;103:309-11.

584 Kraut A, et al. Christmas candy maker's asthma. IgG4-mediated pectin allergy. *Chest* 1992;102:1605-7.

585 Garty BZ. Garlic burns. *Pediatrics* 1993;91:658-9.

586 Rose KD, et al. Spontaneous spinal epidural hematoma with associated platelet dysfunction from excessive garlic ingestion: a case report. *Neurosurg* 1990;26:880-2.

587 Burnham BE. Garlic as a possible risk for postoperative bleeding. *Plast Reconstr Surg* 1995;95:213.

588 Shuster J. Black cohosh root? Chasteberry Tree? Seizures! *Hosp Pharm* 1996;31:1553-4.

589 Scaglione F, et al. Efficacy and safety of the standardized Ginseng extract G115 for potentiating vaccination against the influenza syndrome and protection against the common cold. *Drugs Exp Clin Res* 1996;22:65-72.

590 Palmer BV, et al. Gin Seng and mastalgia. *BMJ* 1978;1:1284.

591 Hopkins MP, et al. Ginseng face cream and unexplained vaginal bleeding. *Am J Obstet Gynecol* 1988;159:1121-2.

592 Greenspan EM. Ginseng and vaginal bleeding. *JAMA* 1983;249:2018.

593 Koren G, et al. Maternal ginseng use associated with neonatal androgenization. *JAMA* 1990;264:2866.

594 Gonzalez-Seijo JC, et al. Manic episode and ginseng: Report of a possible case. *J Clin Psychopharmacol* 1995;15:447-8.

595 Ryu S, Chien Y. Ginseng-associated cerebral arteritis. *Neurology* 1995;45:829-30.

596 Dega H, et al. Ginseng as a cause of Stevens-Johnson syndrome. *Lancet* 1996;313:756.

597 Brown R. Potential interactions of herbal medicines with antipsychotics, antidepressants and hypnotics. *Eur J Herbal Med* 1997;3:25-8.

598 Hamid S, et al. Protracted cholestatic hepatitis after the use of Prostata. *Ann Intern Med* 1997;127:169-70.

599 Cohen AJ. Long term safety and efficacy of ginkgo biloba extract in the treatment of anti-depressant-induced sexual dysfunction. Psychiatry Online. www.priory.com/pharmol/gingko.htm. (Accessed 24 July 1999).

600 Malo JL, et al. Prevalence of occupational asthma and immunologic sensitization to guar gum among employees at a carpet-manufacturing plant. *J Allergy Clin Immunol* 1990;86(4 Pt 1):562-9.

601 Lagier F, et al. Occupational asthma caused by guar gum. *J Allergy Clin Immunol* 1990;85:785-90.

602 Lewis JH. Esophageal and small bowel obstruction from guar gum-containing diet pills: analysis of 26 cases reported to the FDA. *Am J Gastroenterol* 1992;87:1424-8.

603 Norton SA, et al. Kava dermopathy. *J Am Acad Dermatol* 1994;31(1):89-97.

604 Agha FP, et al. Giant colonic bezoar: a medication bezoar due to psyllium seed husks. *Am J Gastroenterol* 1984;79:319-21.

605 Brown R. Potential interactions of herbal medicines with antipsychotics, antidepressants and hypnotics. *Eur J Herbal Med* 1997;3:25-8.

606 Harder S, et al. Ciprofloxacin-caffeine: a drug interaction established using in vivo and in vitro investigations. *Am J Med* 1989;87(Suppl 5A):89S-91S.

607 Carbo M, et al. Effect of quinolones on caffeine disposition. *Clin Pharmacol Ther* 1989;45:234-40.

608 Healy DP, et al. Interaction between oral ciprofloxacin and caffeine in normal volunteers. *Antimicrob Agents Chemother* 1989;33:474-8.

609 Mester R, et al. Caffeine withdrawal increases lithium blood levels. *Biol Psychiatry* 1995;37:348-50.

610 Jefferson JW. Lithium tremor and caffeine intake: two cases of drinking less and shaking more. *J Clin Psychiatry* 1988;49 72-3.

611 Yu CM, et al. Chinese herbs and warfarin potentiation by Danshen. *J Intern Med* 1997;241:337-9.

612 Tam LS, et al. Warfarin interacions with Chinese traditional medicines: danshen and methyl salicylate medicated oil. *Aust N Z J Med* 1995;25:258.

613 Shaw D, et al. Traditional remedies and food supplements: a 5-year toxicological study (1991-1995). *Drug Safety* 1997;17:342-56.

614 Personal correspondence. Efamol Nutraceuticals, Boston, MA, 22 January 1998.

615 Richter WO, Jacob BG, Schwandt P. Interaction between fibre and lovastatin. *Lancet* 1991;338:706.

616 Sunter WH. Warfarin and garlic. *Pharm J* 1991;246:722.

617 Shader RI, Greenblatt DJ. Phenylzine and the dream machine-ramblings and reflections. *J Clin Psychopharmacol* 1985;5:65.

618 Jones BD, Runikis AM. Interaction of ginseng with phenelzine. *J Clin Psychopharmacol* 1987;7:201-2.

619 Janetzky K, et al. Probable interaction between warfarin and ginseng. *Am J Health Syst Pharm* 1997;54:692-3.

620 Golsch S, et al. [Reversible increase in photosensitivity to UV-B caused by St. John's wort extract]. [Article in German]. *Hautarzt* 1997;48:249-52.

621 Bove GM. Acute neuropathy after exposure to sun in a patient treated with St. John's Wort. *Lancet* 1998;352:1121-2.

622 Sharma RD, et al. Effect of fenugreek seeds on blood glucose and serum lipids in type I diabetes. *Eur J Clin Nutr* 1990;44:301-6.

623 Thys-Jacobs S, et al. Calcium carbonate and the premenstrual syndrome: Effects on premenstrual and menstrual symptoms. *Am J Obstet Gynecol* 1998;179:444-52.

624 Chang T, et al. The effect of water-soluble vitamin E on cyclosporine pharmacokinetics in healthy volunteers. *Clin Pharmacol Ther* 1996;59:297-303.

625 Pan SH, et al. Enhanced oral cyclosporine absorption with water-soluble vitamin E early after liver transplantation. *Pharmacother* 1996;16:59-65.

626 Lasswell WL Jr., et al. In vitro interaction of neuroleptics and tricylic antidepressants with coffee, tea, and gallotannic acid. *J Pharm Sci* 1984; 73:1056-8.

627 Kulhanek F, et al. Precipitation of Antipsychotic drugs in interaction with coffee or tea. *Lancet* 1979;2:1130.

628 Brockmoller J, et al. Hypericin and pseudohypericin: pharmacokinetics and effects on photosensitivity in humans. *Pharmacopsych* 1997;30(Suppl 2):94-101.

629 Kang-yum E, et al. Chinese patent medicine as a potential source of mercury poisoning. *Vet Hum Toxicol* 1992;34:235-8.

630 Prussick R, et al. The protective effect of vitamin E on

REFERENCES

the hemolysis associated with Dapsone treatment in patients with dermatitis herpetiformis. *Arch Dermatol* 1992;128:210-3.

631 Merhav H, et al. Tea drinking and microcytic anemia in infants. *Am J Clin Nutr* 1985;41:1210-3.

632 Ridker PM, et al. Comfrey herb tea and hepatic veno-occlusive disease. *Lancet* 1989;2:657-8.

633 Weston CFM, et al. Veno-occlusive disease of the liver secondary to ingestion of comfrey. *BMJ* 1987;295:183.

634 Bach N, et al. Comfrey herb tea-induced heapatic veno-occlusive disease. *Am J Med* 1989;87:97-9.

635 Yeong ML, et al. Hepatic veno-occlusive disease associated with comfrey ingestion. *J Gastroenterol Hepatol* 1990;5:211-4.

636 Hassell LH, et al. Acute anticholinergic syndrome following ingestion of Angel's trumpet tea. *Hawaii Med J* 1995;54:669-70.

637 Kamiyama T, et al. Autoimmune hepatitis triggered by administration of an herbal medicine. *Am J Gastroenterol* 1997;92:703-4.

638 Mullins RJ. Echinacea-associated anaphylaxis. *Med J Aust* 1998;168:170-1.

639 Doyle H, et al. Herbal stimulant containing ephedrine has also caused psychosis. *BMJ* 1996;313:756.

640 Castot A, et al. [Pharmacovigilance off the beaten track: herbal surveillance or pharmacovigilance of medicinal plants]. [Article in French]. *Therapie* 1997;52:97-103.

641 Mostefa-Kara N, et al. Fatal hepatitis after herbal tea. *Lancet* 1992;340:674.

642 Larrey D, et al. Hepatitis after germander (Teucrium chamaedrys) administration: another instance of herbal medicine hepatotoxicity. *Ann Intern Med* 1992;117:129-32.

643 Woolf, GM. Jin Bu Huan toxicity in adults- Los Angeles, 1993. *MMWR Morb Mortal Wkly Rep* 1993;42:920-2.

644 Horowitz RS, et al. Jin Bu Huan toxicity in children- Colorado, 1993. *MMWR Morb Mortal Wkly Rep* 1993;42:633-5.

645 Pye KG, et al. Severe dyserythropoeisis and autoimmune thrombocytopenia associated with ingestion of kelp supplement. *Lancet* 1992;339:1540.

646 Spiller HA, et al. Retrospective study of mistletoe ingestion. *J Toxicol Clin Toxicol* 1996;34:405-8.

647 Harvey J, et al. Mistletoe hepatitis. *Br Med J (Clin Res Ed)* 1981;282:186-7.

648 Krenzelok EP, et al. American mistletoe exposures. *Am J Emerg Med* 1997;15:516-20.

649 Solbakken AM, et al. [Nature medicine as intoxicant]. [Article in Norwegian] *Tidsskr Nor Laegeforen* 1997;117:1140-1.

650 Anderson IB, et al. Pennyroyal toxicity: measurement of toxic metabolite levels in two cases and review of the literature. *Ann Intern Med* 1996;124:726-34.

651 Takahashi M, et al. Contact dermatitis due to honeybee royal jelly. *Contact Dermatitis* 1983;9:452-5.

652 Bullock RJ, et al. Fatal royal jelly-induced asthma. *Med J Aust* 1994;160:44.

653 Thien FCK, et al. Royal jelly-induced asthma. *Med J Aust* 1993;159:639.

654 Beuers U. Hepatitis after chronic abuse of senna. *Lancet* 1991;337:372-3.

655 Ortiz Cansado A, et al. [Veno-occlusive liver disease due to intake of Senecio vulgaris tea]. [Article in Spanish]. *Gastroenterol Hepatol* 1995;18:413-6.

656 Tomioka M, et al. [Hepatic veno-occlusive disease associated with ingestion of Senecio tephrosioides]. [Article in Spanish]. *Rev Gastroenterol Peru* 1995;15:299-302.

657 But PP, Tomlinson B, Lee KL. Hepatitis related to the Chinese medicine Shou-wu-pian manufactured from Polygonum multiflorum. *Vet Hum Toxicol* 1996;38:280-2.

658 De Groot AC. Airborn allergic contact dermatitis from tea tree oil. *Contact Dermatitis* 1996;35:304-5.

659 Willey LB, et al. Valerian overdose: a case report. *Vet Hum Toxicol* 1995;37:364-5.

660 Cahill DJ, et al. Multiple follicular development associated with herbal medicine. *Hum Reprod* 1994;9:1469-70.

661 Berlin R, et al. Wormwood: Oregon Poison Ctr. Portland, OR: Oregon Health Sci Univ 1996.

662 Weisbord SD, Soule JB, Kimmel PL. Poison on line-acute renal failure caused by oil of wormwood purchased through the internet. *N Engl J Med* 1997;337:825-7.

663 Graedon J, Graedon T. The People's Guide to Deadly Possible Interactions with Drugs. New York, NY: St. Martin's Press, 1995.

664 Blumenthal M. Herb and Conventional Possible Interactions with Drugs. Austin, TX: Am Botanical Council, 1997.

665 LoVecchio F, Curry SC, Bagnasco T. Butyrolactone-induced central nervous system depression after ingestion of RenewTrient, a dietary supplement. *N Engl J Med* 1998;339(12):847-8.

666 Personal correspondence. Dave Kanyer, Asst. Director of Pharmacy, Community Hospital of the Monterey Peninsula, Dec 1998.

667 Blickstein D, et al. Warfarin antagonism by avocado. *Lancet* 1991;337(8746):914-5.

668 Colquhoun DM, et al. Comparison of the effects on lipoproteins and apolipoproteins of a diet high in monounsaturated fatty acids, enriched with avocado, and a high-carbohydrate diet. *Am J Clin Nutr* 1992;56(4):671-77.

669 Lopez Ledesma R, et al. Monounsaturated fatty acid (avocado) rich diet for mild hypercholesterolemia. *Arch Med Res* 1996;27(4):519-23.

670 Carranza J, et al. [Effects of avocado on the level of blood lipids in patients with phenotype II and IV dyslipidemias].[Article in Spanish]. *Arch Inst Cardiol Mex* 1995;65(4):342-8.

671 Lerman-Garber I, et al. Effect of a high-monounsaturated fat diet enriched with avocado in NIDDM patients. *Diabetes Care* 1994;17(4):311-5.

672 van Weerden WM, et al. Effects of adrenal androgens on the transplantable human prostate tumor PC-82. *Endocrinol* 1992;131(6):2909-13.

673 Mecenas CA, et al. Production of premature delivery in pregnant rhesus monkeys by androstenedione infusion. *Nat Med* 1996;2(4):443-8.

674 Anon. Creatine and androstenedione, two dietary supplements. *Med Lett Drugs Ther* 1998;40(1039):105-6.

675 Alvizouri-Munoz M, et al. Effects of avocado as a source of monounsaturated fatty acids on plasma lipid levels. *Arch Med Res* 1992;23(4):163-7.

676 Chen Z, et al. Identification of hevein (Hev b 6.02) in Hevea latex as a major cross- reacting allergen with avocado fruit in patients with latex allergy. *J Allergy Clin Immunol* 1998;102(3):476-81.

677 Diehl HW, May EL. Cetyl myristoleate isolated from Swiss albino mice: an apparent protective agent against adjuvant arthritis in rats. *J Pharm Sci* 1994;83(3):296-9.

678 Plaitakis A, et al. Pilot trial of branched-chain aminoacids in amyotrophic lateral sclerosis. *Lancet* 1988;1(8593):1015-8.

679 Branched-chain amino acids and amyotrophic lateral sclerosis: a treatment failure? The Italian ALS Study Group. *Neurology* 1993;43(12):2466-70.

680 Testa D, Caraceni T, Fetoni V. Branched-chain amino acids in the treatment of amyotrophic lateral sclerosis. *J Neurol* 1989;236(8):445-7.

681 Tandan R, et al. A controlled trial of amino acid therapy in amyotrophic lateral sclerosis: I. Clinical, functional, and maximum isometric torque data. *Neurology* 1996;47(5):1220-6.

682 FDA. FDA warns about products containing gamma butyrolactone or GBL and asks companies to issue a recall. Talk Paper, 21 January 1999.

683 Leclercq I, Desager JP, Horsmans Y. Inhibition of chlorzoxazone metabolism, a clinical probe for CYP2E1, by a single ingestion of watercress. *Clin Pharmacol Ther* 1998 64(2):144-9.

684 Plauth M, et al. Long-term treatment of latent portosystemic encephalopathy with branched-chain amino acids. A double-blind placebo-controlled crossover study. *J Hepatol* 1993;17(3):308-14.

685 Egberts EH, et al. Branched chain amino acids in the treatment of latent portosystemic encephalopathy. A double-blind, placebo-controlled, crossover study. *Gastroenterol* 1985;88(4):887-95.

686 Rossi Fanelli F, et al. Use of branched chain amino acids for treating hepatic encephalopathy: clinical experiences. *Gut* 1986; 27(Suppl 1):111-5.

687 Wahren J, et al. Is intravenous administration of branched chain amino acids effective in the treatment of hepatic encephalopathy? A multicenter study. *Hepatol* 1983;3(4):475-80.

688 Michel H, et al. Treatment of acute hepatic encephalopathy in cirrhotics with a branched-chain amino acids enriched versus a conventional amino acids mixture. A controlled study of 70 patients. *Liver* 1985 5(5):282-9.

689 Vilstrup H, et al. Branched chain enriched amino acid versus glucose treatment of hepatic encephalopathy. A double-blind study of 65 patients with cirrhosis. *J Hepatol* 1990;10(3):291-6.

690 Marchesini G, et al. Long-term oral branched-chain amino acid treatment in chronic hepatic encephalopathy. A randomized double-blind casein-controlled trial. The Italian Multicenter Study Group. *J Hepatol* 1990;11(1):92-101.

691 Chuah SY, Ellis BJ, Mayberry JF. Exacerbation of hepatic encephalopathy by branched-chain amino acids-a case report. *J Hum Nutr Diet* 1992;5(1):53-6.

692 Blomstrand E, et al. Influence of ingesting a solution of branched-chain amino acids on perceived exertion during exercise. *Acta Physiol Scand* 1997;159(1):41-9.

693 MacLean DA, Graham TE. Branched-chain amino acid supplementation augments plasma ammonia responses during exercise in humans. *J Appl Physiol* 1993;74(6):2711-7.

694 MacLean DA, Graham TE, Saltin B. Branched-chain amino acids augment ammonia metabolism while attenuating protein breakdown during exercise. *Am J Physiol* 1994;267(6 Pt 1):E1010-22.

695 Breum L, et al. Comparison of an ephedrine/caffeine combination and dexfenfluramine in the treatment of obesity. A double-blind multi-centre trial in general practice. *Int J Obes Relat Metab Disord* 1994;18(2):99-103.

696 Toubro S, et al. The acute and chronic effects of ephedrine/caffeine mixtures on energy expenditure and glucose metabolism in humans. *Int J Obes Relat Metab Disord* 1993;17(Suppl 3):S73-7.

697 Toubro S, et al. Safety and efficacy of long-term treatment with ephedrine, caffeine and an ephedrine/ caffeine mixture. *Int J Obes Relat Metab Disord* 1993;17(Suppl 1):S69-72.

698 Cystadane (betaine anhydrous for oral solution) Package insert, Orphan Med, rev. 10/96.

699 Feldman J, et al. [Double-blind study of the treatment of disc lumbosciatica by chemonucleolysis]. [Article in French]. *Rev Rhum Mal Osteoartic* 1986; 53(3):147-52.

700 Nordby EJ. A comparison of discectomy and chemonucleolysis. *Clin Orthop* 1985;(200):279-83.

701 Javid MJ. Chemonucleolysis versus laminectomy. A cohort comparison of effectiveness and charges. *Spine* 1995;20(18):2016-22.

702 Kuthan F. [Bee Venom Treatment of Rheumatic disorders. (Summary of paper presented concerning apitherapy at the Int Apicult Congress Apimondia in Bucharest, Romania)]. [Article in German]. www.beesting.com/kuthan.html. May 1999. (Accessed 23 July 1999)

703 Clarkson PM, Haymes EM. Trace mineral requirements for athletes. *Int J Sport Nutr* 1994;4(2):104-19.

704 Clarkson PM. Minerals: exercise performance and supplementation in athletes. *J Sports Sci* 1991;9:91-116.

705 Campbell WW, Anderson RA. Effects of aerobic exercise and training on the trace minerals chromium, zinc and copper. *Sports Med* 1987 4(1):9-18.

706 Broun ER, et al. Excessive zinc ingestion. A reversible cause of sideroblastic anemia and bone marrow depression. *JAMA* 1990;264(11):1441-3.

707 Sandstead HH. Requirements and toxicity of essential trace elements, illustrated by zinc and copper. *Am J Clin Nutr* 1995 61(3 Suppl):621S-4S.

708 Brewer GJ, et al. Treatment of Wilson's disease with zinc: XV long-term follow-up studies. *J Lab Clin Med* 1998;132(4):264-78.

709 Weight LM, et al. Vitamin and mineral status of trained athletes including the effects of supplementation. *Am J Clin Nutr* 1988;47(2):186-91.

710 Finley EB, Cerklewski FL. Influence of ascorbic acid supplementation on copper status in young adult men. *Am J Clin Nutr* 1983;37(4):553-6.

711 Scharf MB, et al. Effect of gamma-hydroxybutyrate on pain, fatigue, and the alpha sleep anomaly in patients with fibromyalgia. Preliminary report. *J Rheumatol* 1998;25(10):1986-90.

712 Chin RL, et al. Clinical course of gamma-hydroxybutyrate overdose. *Ann Emerg Med* 1998;31(6):716-22.

713 Tunnicliff, G. Sites of action of gamma-hydroxybutyrate (GHB)-a neuroactive drug with abuse potential. *J Toxicol Clin Toxicol* 1997;35(6):581-90.

714 FDA Talk Paper. FDA re-issues warning on GHB. 18 February 1997.

715 Latha B, et al. The efficacy of trypsin: chymotrypsin

REFERENCES

preparation in the reduction of oxidative damage during burn injury. *Burns* 1998;24(6):532-8.

716 Latha B, et al. Serum enzymatic changes modulated using trypsin: chymotrypsin preparation during burn wounds in humans. *Burns* 1997;23(7-8):560-4.

717 Shaw PC. The use of a trypsin-chymotrypsin formulation in fractures of the hand. *Br J Clin Pract* 1969;23(1):25-6.

718 McCue FC, Webster TM, Gieck J. Clinical effects of proteolytic enzymes after reconstructive hand surgery. *Int Surg* 1972;57(6):479-82.

719 Patil SP, Niphadkar PV, Bapat MM. Allergy to fenugreek (Trigonella foenum graecum). *Ann Allergy Asthma Immunol* 1997;78(3):297-300.

720 Ahsan SK, et al. Effect of Trigonella foenum-graecum and Ammi majus on calcium oxalate urolithiasis in rats. *J Ethnopharmacol* 1989;26(3):249-54.

721 Fischer-Rasmussen W, Kjaer SK, Dahl C, Asping U. Ginger treatment of hyperemesis gravidarum. *Eur J Obstet Gynecol Reprod Biol* 1991;38(1):19-24.

722 Phillips S, Ruggier R, Hutchinson SE. Zingiber officinale (ginger)-an antiemetic for day case surgery. *Anaesthesia* 1993;48(8):715-7.

723 Bone ME, et al. Ginger root-a new antiemetic. The effect of ginger root on postoperative nausea and vomiting after major gynaecological surgery. *Anaesthesia* 1990;45(8):669-71.

724 Foster S. Feverfew, Tanacetum parthenium, botanical series #310. Austin, TX: Am Botanical Council, 1996.

725 Awang, DVC. Feverfew effective in Migraine prevention. *HerbalGram* 1998;42:18.

726 Awang, DVC. Feverfew trials: the promise of- and the problem with standardized extracts. *HerbalGram* 1997;41:16-7.

727 Kuritsky A, et al. Feverfew in the treatment of migraine: its effect on serotonin uptake and platelet activity. *Neurology* 1994:44(Suppl 2):A201. (Abstract 293P)

728 Heymsfield SB, et al. Garcinia cambogia (hydroxycitric acid) as a potential antiobesity agent: a randomized controlled trial. *JAMA* 1998;280(18):1596-600.

729 Natural Remedies. Garcinia cambogia. Natural Remedies Pvt. Ltd. www.indianherbs.com/gar_cal.htm. (Accessed 16 July 1999)

730 Latest research reveals new native asian fruit has the ability to reduce body-fat production by 40-70%. Quick Results. www.quickresults.com.au/weightloss/asianf.htm (Accessed 16 July 1999).

731 Isaacsohn JL, et al. Garlic powder and plasma lipids and lipoproteins, a multicenter, randomized, placebo-controlled trial. *Arch Intern Med* 1998;158:1189-94.

732 Berthold HK, Sudhop T, von Bergmann K. Effect of a garlic oil preparation on serum lipoproteins and cholesterol metabolism. *JAMA* 1998;279(23):1900-2.

733 Mitscher LA, et al. Chemoprotection: a review of the potential therapeutic antioxidant properties of green tea (Camellia sinensis) and certain of its constituents. *Med Res Rev* 1997;17(4):327-65.

734 Kono S, et al. Green tea consumption and serum lipid profiles: a cross-sectional study in northern Kyushu, Japan. *Prev Med* 1992;21(4):526-31.

735 Kingsbury JM. Poison ivy, poison sumac, and other rash-producing plants. York State Coll of Agri, Life Sci, Info Bull. #105;1976.

736 Liu JH, et al. Angelol-type coumarins from Angelica pubescence F. biserrata and their inhibitory effect on platelet aggregation. *Phytochem* 1995;39(5):1099-101.

737 Lo ACT, et al. Danggui (Angelica sinensis) affects the pharmacodynamics but not the pharmacokinetics of warfarin in rabbits. *Eur J Drug Metab Pharmacokinet* 1995;20:55-60.

738 Hirata JD, et al. Does dong quai have estrogenic effects in postmenopausal women? A double-blind, placebo-controlled trial. *Fertil Steril* 1997;68(6):981-6.

739 Cooper RL, Cooper MM. Red pepper-induced dermatitis in breast-fed infants. *Dermatol* 1996;93(1):61-2.

740 Stone-Dorshow T, Levitt MD. Gaseous response to ingestion of a poorly absorbed fructo-oligosaccharide sweetener. *Am J Clin Nutr* 1987;46:61-5.

741 Bornet FR. Undigestible sugars in food products. *Am J Clin Nutr* 1994;59(Suppl):763S-9S.

742 Roberfroid MB. Prebiotics and synbiotics: concepts and nutritional properties. *Br J Nutr* 1998;80:S197-202.

743 Schaafsma G, et al. Effects of a milk product, fermented by Lactobacillus acidophilus and with fructo-oligosaccharides added, on blood lipids in male volunteers. *Eur J Clin Nutr* 1998;52:436-40.

744 Roberfroid M. Dietary fiber, inulin, and oligofructose: a review comparing their physiological effects. *Crit Rev Food Sci Nutr* 1993;33:103-48.

745 Briet F, et al. Symptomatic response to varying levels of fructo-oligosaccharides consumed occasionally or regularly. *Eur J Clin Nutr* 1995;49:501-7.

746 Mitsouka T, Hidaka H, Eida T. Effect of fructo-oligosaccharides on intestinal microflora. *Nahrung* 1987;31:427-36.

747 Alles MS, et al. Fate of fructo-oligosaccharides in the human intestine. *Br J Nutr* 1996;76:211-21.

748 Pierre F, et al. Short-chain fructo-oligosaccharides reduced the occurrence of colon tumors and develop gut-associated lymphoid tissue in Min mice. *Cancer Res* 1997;57:225-8.

749 Gibson GR. Dietary modulation of the human gut microflora using prebiotics. *Br J Nutr* 1998;80:S209-12.

750 Bouhnik Y, et al. Short-chain fructo-oligosaccharide administration dose-dependently increases fecal bifidobacteria in healthy humans. *J Nutr* 1999;129:113-6.

751 Fry AC, et al. The effects of gamma-oryzanol supplementation during resistance exercise training. *Int J Sport Nutr* 1997;7:318-29.

752 Sasaki J, et al. Effects of gamma-oryzanol on serum lipids and apolipoproteins in dyslipidemic schizophrenics receiving major tranquilizers. *Clin Ther* 1990;12:263-8.

753 Shimomura Y, et al. Effect of gamma-oryzanol on serum TSH concentrations in primary hypothyroidism. *Endocrinol Jpn* 1980;27:83-6.

754 Sugano M, Tsuji E. Rice bran oil and human health. *Biomed Environ Sci* 1996;9:242-6.

755 Wheeler KB, Garleb KA. Gamma oryzanol-plant sterol supplementation: metabolic, endocrine, and physiologic effects. *Int J Sport Nutr* 1991;1:170-7.

756 Seetharamaiah GS, Chandrasekhara N. Effect of oryzanol on cholesterol absorption and biliary and fecal bile acids in rats. *Indian J Med Res* 1990;92:471-5.

757 Ishihara M, et al. [Clinical effect of gamma-oryzanol on climacteric disturbance- on serum lipid peroxides]. [Article in Japanese]. *Nippon Sanka Fujinka Gakkai Zasshi* 1982;34:243-51.

758 Upton R, ed. St. John's wort, Hypericum perforatum: quality control, analytical and therapeutic monograph.

759 Chavez ML, Chavez PI. Saint John's wort. *Hosp Pharm* 1997;32(12):1621-32.

760 Chavez ML. Glucosamine sulfate and chondroitin sulfates. *Hosp Pharm* 1997;32(9):1275-85.

761 Laakmann G, et al. St. John's wort in mild to moderate depression: the relevance of hyperforin for the clinical efficacy. *Pharmacopsych* 1998;31(Suppl 1):54-9.

762 Chatterjee SS, et al. Antidepressant activity of hypericum perforatum and hyperforin: the neglected possibility. *Pharmacopsych* 1998;31(Suppl 1):7-15.

763 Muller WE, et al. Hyperforin represents the neurotransmitter reuptake inhibiting constituent of hypericum extract. *Pharmacopsych* 1998;31(Suppl 1):16-21.

764 Gerber GS, et al. Saw palmetto (Serenoa repens) in men with lower urinary tract symptoms: effects on urodynamic parameters and voiding symptoms. *Urol* 1998;51(6):1003-7.

765 FDA. Unapproved over-the-counter (OTC) drugs still marketed? FDA Med Bull, 1996;26(1). www.fda.gov/medbull/january96/otc.html (Accessed 23 July 1999).

766 Young at Heart. AL-CO-EZE. www.yatheartmktg.com/yath8.html (Accessed 16 July 1999).

767 Shiroky JB, et al. Low-dose methotrexate with leucovorin (folinic acid) in the management of rheumatoid arthritis. Results of a multicenter randomized, double-blind, placebo-controlled trial. *Arthritis Rheum* 1993;36(6):795-803.

768 Duhra P. Treatment of gastrointestinal symptoms associated with methotrexate therapy for psoriasis. *J Am Acad Dermatol* 1993;28(3):466-9.

769 Voordouw BC, et al. Melatonin and melatonin-progestin combinations alter pituitary-ovarian function in women and can inhibit ovulation. *J Clin Endocrinol Metab* 1992;74(1):108-17.

770 Becker BN. Ginseng-induced diuretic resistance. *JAMA* 1996;276(8):606-7.

771 Walaszek Z. Potential use of D-glucarate derivatives in cancer prevention. *Cancer Lett* 1990;54:1-8.

772 Dwivedi C, et al. Effect of calcium glucarate on B-glucuronidase activity and glucarate content on certain vegetables and fruits. *Biochem Med Metab Bio* 1990;43:83-92.

773 Heerdt AS, Young CW, Borgen PI. Calcium glucarate as a chemopreventive agent in breast cancer. *Isr J Med Sci* 1995;31:101-5.

774 Walaszek Z, et al. Metabolism, uptake and excretion of D-glucaric acid salt and its potential use in cancer prevention. *Cancer Detect Prev* 1997;21(2):178-90.

775 Walaszek Z, et al. Dietary glucarate as anti-promter of 7,12-dimethylbenz(a)anthracene-induced mammary tumorigenesis. *Carcinogenesis* 1986;7(9):1463-6.

776 Curley RW Jr., et al. Activity of D-glucarate analogues: synergistic antiproliferative effects with retinoid in cultured human mammary tumor cells appear to specifically require the D-glucarate structure. *Life Sci* 1994;54(18):1299-303.

777 Furuno K, et al. Preventive effect of D-glucarate against renal damage induced by kanamycin. *J Antibiot (Tokyo)* 1976;29(9):950-3.

778 Kampf D, Roots I, Hildenbrandt AG. Urinary excretion of D-glucarate, an indicator of drug metabolizing enzyme activity, in patients with impaired renal function. *Eur J Clin Pharmacol* 1980;18(3):255-61.

779 Mezey E. Increased urinary excretion of D-glucarate acid in alcoholism. *Res Commun Chem Pathol Pharmacol* 1976;15(4):735-42.

780 Pointel JP, et al. Titrated extract of Centella asiatica (TECA) in the treatment of venous insufficiency of the lower limbs. *Angiol* 1987;38(1 Pt 1):46-50.

781 Farese RV Jr., et al. Licorice-induced hypermineralocorticoidism. *N Engl J Med* 1991;325(17):1223-7.

782 Singh YN, Blumenthal M. Kava an overview. *HerbalGram* 1997;39:33-44, 46-55.

783 Cartier LC, Lehrer A, Malo JL. Occupational asthma caused by aromatic herbs. *Allergy* 1996;51:647-9.

784 Joy JE, Watson SJ Jr, Benson JA Jr, et al. Marijuana and medicine: assessing the science base. A summary of the 1999 Inst of Med report. *Arch Gen Psychiatr* 2000 Jun;57:547-52.

785 Hsu CK, et al. Anticholinergic poisoning associated with herbal tea. *Arch Intern Med* 1995;155(20):2245-8.

786 GVI Sourcing. www.gvisourcing.com/pharmaceuticals/ppg/default.html (Accessed 16 July 1999).

787 Foster S. Peppermint, Menta x piperita, botanical series #306. Austin, TX: Am Botanical Council, 1990.

788 Kapil A, Moza N. Anticomplementary activity of boswellic acids-an inhibitor of C3-convertase of the classical complement pathway. *Int J Immunopharmacol* 1992;14(7):1139-43.

789 Halperin EC, Gaspar L, George S, et al. A double-blind, randomized, prospective trial to evaluate topical vitamin C solution for the prevention of radiation dermatitis. *Int J Radiat Oncol Biol Phys* 1993;26:413-6.

790 Wslbling RH, Leonhardt K. Local therapy of herpes simplex with dried extract from Melissa officinalis. *Phytomedicine* 1994;1:25-31.

791 Takahashi M, Matsuo I, Ohkido M. Contact dermatitis due to honeybee royal jelly. *Contact Dermatitis* 1983;9:452-5.

792 Bullock RJ, et al. Fatal royal jelly-induced asthma. *Med J Aust* 1994;160:44.

793 Reiter WJ, et al. Dehydroepiandosterone in the treatment of erectile dysfunction: A prospective, double-blind, randomized, placebo-controlled study. *Urol* 1999;53(3):590-5.

794 Kantola T, Kivisto KT, Neuvonen PJ. Grapefruit juice greatly increases serum concentrations of lovastatin and lovastatin acid. *Clin Pharmacol Ther* 1998;63(4):397-402.

795 Foster S. Milk Thistle, Silybum marianum, botanical series #305. Austin, TX: Am Botanical Council, 1996.

796 Cholestin. Pharmanex.com. www.pharmanex.com/products/heart_health/cholestin.html (Accessed 21 November 1999).

797 Awang DVC. Siberian ginseng toxicity may be case of mistaken identity. [Letter]. *CMAJ* 1996;155(9):1237.

798 Moretti S. Effect of L-carnitine on human immunodeficiency virus-1 infection-associated apoptosis: a pilot study. *Blood* 1998;91(10):3817-24.

799 Magro-Filho O, de Carvalho AC. Topical effect of propolis in the repair of sulcoplasties by the modified Kazanjian technique. Cytological and clinical evaluation. *J Nihon Univ Sch Dent* 1994;36(2):102-11.

800 Magro-Filho O, de Carvalho AC. Application of propolis to dental sockets and skin wounds. *J Nihon Univ Sch Dent* 1990;32(1):4-13.

801 Emerson Ecologics new products

Santa Cruz, CA: Am Herbal Pharmacopoeia; 1997;1-32.

www.emersonecologics.com/homepage/Promotions/ Hot1.html (Accessed 19 July 1999).

802 Pycnogenol. Robar Health Res. URL: cybermontana.com/robar/pycnogenol.html. (Accessed 19 July 1999).

803 The wonders of Pycnogenol. HealthTrak. www.healthtrak.com/whatispyc.html. (Accessed 19 July 1999).

804 Brookland Botanic Garden. Highbush Blueberry. www.bbg.org/research/nymf/encyclopedia/eri/ vac0050a.htm#medicinaluses (Accessed 12 October 2000).

805 Bartram T. Encyclopedia of Herbal Medicine. Dorset: Grace Publishers; 1995.

806 Stanko RT, Mullick P, Clarke MR, et al. Pyruvate inhibits growth of mammary adenocarcinoma 13762 in rats. *Cancer Res* 1994;54(4):1004-7.

807 Stanko RT, Robertson RJ, Galbreath RW, et al. Enhanced leg exercise endurance with a high-carbohydrate diet and dihydroxyacetone and pyruvate. *J Appl Physiol* 1990;69(5):1651-6.

808 Stanko RT, Robertson RJ, Spina RJ, et al. Enhancement of arm exercise endurance capacity with dihydroxyacetone and pyruvate. J *Appl Physiol* 1990;68(1):119-24.

809 Hogan RP III. Hemorrhagic diathesis caused by drinking an herbal tea. *JAMA* 1983;249:2679-80.

810 Gonzalez M, Zarzuelo A, Gamez MJ, et al. Hypoglycemic activity of olive leaf. *Planta Med* 1992;58(6):513-5.

811 Heimann SW. Pycnogenol for ADHD? *J Am Acad Child Adolesc Psychiatr* 1999;38(4):357-8.

812 Mash DC, Kovera CA, Buck BE, et al. Medication development of ibogaine as a pharmacotherapy for drug dependence. *Ann NY Acad Sci* 1998;844:274-92.

813 Glick SD, Maisonneuve IS. Mechanisms of antiaddictive actions of ibogaine. *Ann NY Acad Sci* 1998;844:214-26.

814 Natural Medicines- blueberry. Rx.com. www.rx.com/ reference/natural/Blueberry.jhtml (Accessed 12 October 2000).

815 Royal Botanical Gardens Kew online databases. www.rbgkew.org.uk/web.dbs/webdbsintro.html.

816 Germplasm Resources Info. www.ars-grin.gov/npgs (Accessed 3 November 1999).

817 Harrington C. Plant dubbed nature's Viagra. Calgary, CAN: Canadian Press; 15 Nov. 1998.

818 Dudley JP. Bilateral pneumothorax resulting from the bronchoscopic removal of a puncture vine fruit. *Ann Otol Rhinol Laryngol* 1983;92(4 Pt 1):396-7.

819 Pierard-Franchimont C, Goffin V, Visser JN, et al. A double-blind controlled evaluation of the sebosuppressive activity of topical erythromycin-zinc complex. *Eur J Clin Pharmacol* 1995;49(1-2):57-60.

820 Feucht CL, Allen BS, Chalker DK, et al. Topical erythromycin with zinc in acne. A double-blind controlled study. *J Am Acad Dermatol* 1980;3(5):483-91.

821 Mostafa WZ, al-Zayer AA. Acrodermatitis enteropathica in Saudi Arabia. *Int J Dermatol* 1990;29(2):134-8.

822 Hoogenraad TU, Van Hattum J, Van den Hamer CJ. Management of Wilson's disease with zinc sulphate. Experience in a series of 27 patients. *J Neurol Sci* 1987;77(2-3):137-46.

823 Anderson LA, Hakojarvi SL, Boudreaux SK. Zinc acetate treatment in Wilson's disease. *Ann*

Pharmacother 1998;32(1):78-87.

824 Fortes C, Forastiere F, Agabiti N, et al. The effect of zinc and vitamin A supplementation on immune response in an older population. *J Am Geriatr Soc* 1998;46(1):19-26.

825 Faruque AS, Mahalanabis D, Haque SS, et al. Double-blind, randomized, controlled trial of zinc or vitamin A supplementation in young children with acute diarrhea. *Acta Paediatr* 1999;88(2):154-60.

826 Roy SK, Tomkins AM, Akramuzzaman SM, et al. Randomized, controlled trial of zinc supplementation in malnourished Bangladeshi children with acute diarrhea. *Arch Dis Child* 1997;77(3):196-200.

827 Sazawal S, Black RE, Bhan MK, et al. Zinc supplementation in young children with acute diarrhea in India. *N Engl J Med* 1995;333(13):839-44.

828 Blondeau JM. Expanded activity and utility of the new fluoroquinolones: a review. *Clin Ther* 1999;21(1):3-40.

829 Mountokalakis T, Dourakis S, Karatzas N, et al. Zinc deficiency in mild hypertensive patients treated with diuretics. *J Hypertens Suppl* 1984;2(3):S571-2.

830 Reyes AJ, Olhaberry JV, Leary WP, et al. Urinary zinc excretion, diuretics, zinc deficiency and some side-effects of diuretics. *S Afr Med J* 1983;64(24):936-41.

831 Cohanim M, Yendt ER. The effects of thiazides on serum and urinary zinc in patients with renal calculi. *Johns Hopkins Med J* 1975;136(3):137-44.

832 Ghio S, de Servi S, Perotti R, et al. Different susceptibility to the development of nitroglycerin tolerance in the arterial and venous circulation in humans- effects of N-acetylcysteine administration. *Circulation* 1992;86:798-802.

833 Blueberry. Eat 5 a day for better health. www.5aday.com/ (Accessed 12 October 2000).

834 Calabrese C, Myer S, Munson S, et al. A cross-over study of the effect of a single oral feeding of medium chain triglyceride oil vs canola oil on post-ingestion plasma triglyceride levels in healthy men. *Altern Med Rev* 1999;4(1):23-8.

835 Law M, Wald N. Why heart disease mortality is low in France: the time lag explanation. *BMJ* 1999;318(7196):1471-80.

836 Nestel PJ, Pomeroy S, Kay S, et al. Isoflavones from red clover improve systemic arterial compliance but not plasma lipids in menopausal women. *J Clin Endocrinol Metab* 1999;84(3):895-8.

837 Feskanich D, Weber P, Willett WC, et al. Vitamin K intake and hip fractures in women: a prospective study. *Am J Clin Nutr* 1999;69(1):74-9.

838 Zheng GQ, Kenney PM, Lam LK. Sesquiterpenes from clove (Eugenia caryophyllata) as potential anticarcinogenic agents. *J Nat Prod* 1992;55(7):999-1003.

839 Anon. The wellness guide to dietary supplements. *UC Berkeley Wellness Letter* 1998;14(11):WNL SUPP.

840 Personal correspondence. Lane Labs, Inc. Allendale, NJ, June 28, 1999.

841 Hart CL, Smith GD, Hole DJ, Hawthorne VM. Alcohol consumption and mortality from all causes, coronary heart disease, and stroke: results from a prospective cohort study of Scottish men with 21 years of follow up. *BMJ* 1999;318(7200):1725-9.

842 Potter SM, Baum JA, Teng H, et al. Soy protein and isoflavones: their effects on blood lipids and bone density in postmenopausal women. *Am J Clin Nutr*

1998;68(6 Suppl):1375S-9S.

843 Flaxseed oil: filling a vital need. Barleans Organic Oils. URL: barleans.com/vital.html (Accessed 23 July 1999).

844 Flaxseed oil. MotherNature.com www.mothernature.com/ency/Supp/Flaxseed.asp (Accessed 23 July 1999).

845 Allman MA, Pena MM, Pang D. Supplementation with flaxseed oil versus sunflower seed oil in healthy young men consuming a low fat diet: effects on platelet composition and function. *Eur J Clin Nutr* 1995;49(3):169-78.

846 Personal correspondence: Paddock Laboratories, Inc., Minneapolis, MN, July 6, 1999.

847 Poria Cocos - Fu Ling. www.go-symmetry.com/poria-cocos.html (Accessed 16 July 1999).

848 Personal correspondence: Transitions for Health, Inc., Portland, OR, June 5, 1999.

849 Tritrungtasna O, Jerasutus S, Suvanprakorn P. Treatment of alopecia areata with khellin and UVA. *Int J Dermatol* 1993;32:690.

850 Waller DP, et al. Lack of androgenicity of Siberian ginseng. *JAMA* 1992;267(17):2329.

851 Nestel PJ, Yamashita T, Sasahara T, et al. Soy isoflavones improve systemic arterial compliance but not plasma lipids in menopausal and perimenopausal women. *Arterioscler Thromb Vasc Biol* 1997;17(12):3392-8.

852 Dobrescu D, Tanasescu M, Mezdrea A, et al. Contributions to the complex study of some lichens-Usnea genus. Pharmacological studies on Usnea barbata and Usnea hirta species. *Rom J Physiol* 1993;30(1-2):101-7.

853 FDA Ctr Food Safety, Applied Nutr, Ofc Cosmetics Fact Sheet, 1995 Feb 23. URL: vm.cfsan.fda.gov/~dms/cos-210.html (Accessed 14 July 1999).

854 Wiesenauer M, Lydtke R. Mahonia aquifolium in patients with Psoriasis vulgaris; an intraindividual study. *Phytomedicine* 1996;3(3):231-5.

855 Personal correspondence. Prime Pharmaceutical Corporation, Toronto, Ontario, Canada, June 28, 1999.

856 Natural Health Remedies. Health Canada. URL: hc-sc.gc.ca/english/archives/96-97/herbnae.html (Accessed 16 July 1999).

857 Gieler U, von der Weth A, Heger M. Mahonia aquifolium- a new type of topical treatment for psoriasis. *J Dermatol Treatment* 1995;6:31-4.

858 Hiermann A, Bucar F. Studies of Epilobium angustifolium extracts on growth of accessory sexual organs in rats. *J Ethnopharmacol* 1997;55(3):179-83.

859 Hiermann A, Reidlinger M, Juan H, Sametz W. [Isolation of the antiphlogistic principle from Epilobium angustifolium]. [Article in German]. *Planta Med* 1991;57(4):357-60.

860 Hiermann A, Juan H, Sametz W. Influence of Epilobium extracts on prostaglandin biosynthesis and carrageenin induced edema of the rat paw. *J Ethnopharmacol* 1986;17(2):161-9.

861 AA. Cramp bark. Myst herb & tea. www.mystherb.com (Accessed 19 July 1999).

862 FDA List of orphan designations and approvals. www.fda.gov/orphan/designat/list.html (Accessed 20 July 1999).

863 Via-Bran. www.viabran.com (Accessed 20 July 1999).

864 USDA nutrient database for standard reference, release 12 (March 1998), crude rice bran. www.nal.usda.gov/fnic/cgi-bin/list_nut.pl (Accessed 20 July 1999).

865 Gerhardt AL, Gallo NB. Full-fat rice bran and oat bran similarly reduce hypercholesterolemia in humans. *J Nutr* 1998;128(5):865-9.

866 Ghoneum M. Anti-HIV activity in vitro of MGN-3, an activated arabinoxylane from rice bran. Biochem Biophys *Res Commun* 1998;243(1):25-9.

867 Iida T, Nakagawa R, Hirakawa H, et al. Clinical trial of a combination of rice bran fiber and cholestyramine for promotion of fecal excretion of retained polychlorinated dibenzofuran and polychlorinated biphenyl in Yu-Cheng patients. *Fukuoka Igaku Zasshi* 1995;86(5):226-33.

868 Abdel-Fattah A, Aboul-Enein MN, Wassel GM, El-Menshawi BS. An approach to the treatment of vitiligo by khellin. *Dermatologica* 1982;165:136-40.

869 Duarte J, Torres AI, Zarzuelo A. Cardiovascular effects of visnagin on rats. *Planta Med* 2000;66:35-9.

870 Iida T, Hirakawa H, Matsueda T, et al. [Therapeutic trials for promotion of faecal excretion of PCDFs by the administration of rice bran fiber and cholestyramine in Yusho patients]. [Article in Japanese]. *Fukuoka Igaku Zasshi* 1993;84(5):257-62.

871 Weisburger JH, Reddy BS, Rose DP, et al. Protective mechanisms of dietary fibers in nutritional carcinogenesis. *Basic Life Sci* 1993;61:45-63.

872 Fujiwaki T, Furusho K. The effects of rice bran broth bathing in patients with atopic dermatitis. *Acta Paediatr Jpn* 1992;34(5):505-10.

873 Sanders TA, Reddy S. The influence of rice bran on plasma lipids and lipoproteins in human volunteers. *Eur J Clin Nutr* 1992;46(3):167-72.

874 Jahnen A, Heynck H, Gertz B, et al. Dietary fibre: the effectiveness of a high bran intake in reducing renal calcium excretion. *Urol Res* 1992;20(1):3-6.

875 Cara L, Dubois C, Borel P, et al. Effects of oat bran, rice bran, wheat fiber, and wheat germ on postprandial lipemia in healthy adults. *Am J Clin Nutr* 1992;55(1):81-8.

876 Ebisuno S, Morimoto S, Yasukawa S, Ohkawa T. Results of long-term rice bran treatment on stone recurrence in hypercalciuric patients. *Br J Urol* 1991;67(3):237-40.

877 Kestin M, Moss R, Clifton PM, Nestel PJ. Comparative effects of three cereal brans on plasma lipids, blood pressure, and glucose metabolism in mildly hypercholesterolemic men. *Am J Clin Nutr* 1990;52(4):661-6.

878 Noronha IL, Andriolo A, Lucon AM, et al. [Rice bran in the treatment of idiopathic hypercalciuria in patients with urinary calculosis]. [Article in Portugese]. *Rev Paul Med* 1989;107(1):19-24.

879 Tomlin J, Read NW. Comparison of the effects on colonic function caused by feeding rice bran and wheat bran. *Eur J Clin Nutr* 1988;42(10):857-61.

880 Ebisuno S, Morimoto S, Yoshida T, et al. Rice-bran treatment for calcium stone formers with idiopathic hypercalciuria. *Br J Urol* 1986;58(6):592-5.

881 Ohkawa T, Ebisuno S, Kitagawa M, et al. Rice bran treatment for patients with hypercalciuric stones: experimental and clinical studies. *J Urol* 1984;132(6):1140-5.

882 Ohkawa T, Ebisuno S, Kitagawa M, et al. Rice bran treatment for hypercalciuric patients with urinary calculous disease. *J Urol* 1983;129(5):1009-11.

883 Tsuda M. Purification and characterization of a lectin from rice bran. *J Biochem (Tokyo)* 1979;86(5):1451-61.

884 Kumar B, Chaudhuri DK. Isolation, partial characterization of antithiamine factor present in rice-bran and its effect on TPP-transketolase system and Staphylococcus aureus. *Int J Vitam Nutr Res* 1976;46(2):154-9.

885 Guerra MJ, Jaffe WG [Nutritional studies with rice bran]. [Article in Spanish]. *Arch Latinoam Nutr* 1975;25(4):401-17.

886 Herb.com. www.herb.com/materia.htm (Accessed 30 July 1999).

887 Fessenden JM, Wittenborn W, Clarke L. Gingko biloba: a case report of herbal medicine and bleeding postoperatively from a laparoscopic cholecystectomy. *Am Surg* 2001;67:33-5.

888 Bomser J, Madhavi DL, Singletary K, Smith MA. In vitro anticancer activity of fruit extracts from Vaccinium species. *Planta Med* 1996;62:212-6.

889 Joseph JA, Shukitt-Hale B, Denisova NA, et al. Reversals of age-related declines in neuronal signal transduction, cognitive, and motor behavioral deficits with blueberry, spinach, or strawberry dietary supplementation. *J Neurosci* 1999;19:8114-21.

900 Youdim KA, Shukitt-Hale B, MacKinnon S, et al. Polyphenolics enhance red blood cell resistance to oxidative stress: in vitro and in vivo (1). *Biochim Biophys Acta* 2000 Sep 1;1519(1):117-22.

901 Birdsall TC. 5-Hydroxytryptophan: A Clinically-Effective Serotonin Precursor. *Altern Med Rev* 1998;3(4):271-80.

902 Michelson D, Page SW, Casey R, et al. An eosinophilia-myalgia syndrome related disorder associated with exposure to L-5-hydroxytryptophan. *J Rheumatol* 1994;21(12):2261-5.

903 Nakajima T, Kudo Y, Kaneko Z. Clinical evaluation of 5-hydroxy-L-tryptophan as an antidepressant drug. *Folia Psychiatr Neurol Jpn* 1978;32(2):223-30.

904 Coppen A, Whybrow PC, Noguera R, et al. The comparative antidepressant value of L-tryptophan and imipramine with and without attempted potentiation by liothyronine. *Arch Gen Psychiatr* 1972;26(3):234-41.

905 AMA Health Insight. Personal nutritionist, the food guide pyramid. www.ama-assn.org/insight/gen_hlth/pernutri/fdpyrami.htm (Accessed 16 October 2000).

906 Rao B, Broadhurst AD. Tryptophan and depression. [letter] *Br Med J* 1976; 1(6007):460.

907 Cao G, Shukitt-Hale B, Bickford PC, et al. Hyperoxia-induced changes in antioxidant capacity and the effect of dietary antioxidants. *J Appl Physiol* 1999;86:1817-22.

908 Bickford PC, Gould T, Briederick L, et al. Antioxidant-rich diets improve cerebellar physiology and motor learning in aged rats. *Brain Res* 2000;866:211-7.

909 Cignarella A, Nastasi M, Cavalli E, Puglisi L. Novel lipid-lowering properties of Vaccinium myrtillus L. leaves, a traditional antidiabetic treatment, in several models of rat dyslipidaemia: a comparison with ciprofibrate. *Thromb Res* 1996;84:311-22.

910 Vorberg G. Ginkgo biloba extract (GBE): A long-term study of chronic cerebral insufficiency in geriatric patients. *Clin Trials J* 1985;22:149-157.

911 Zheng GQ, Kenney PM, Lam LK. Anethofuran, carvone, and limonene: potential cancer chemopreventive agents from dill weed oil and caraway oil. *Planta Med* 1992;58:338-41.

912 Van Hiele LJ. L-5-hydroxytryptophan in depression: the first substitution therapy in psychiatry: the treatment of 99 out-patients with therapy-resistant depressions. *Neuropsychobiol* 1980;6:230-40.

913 Puttini PS, Caruso I. Primary fibromyalgia syndrome and 5-hydroxy-L-tryptophan: a 90-day open study. *J Int Med Res* 1992;20(2):182-9.

914 Cangiano C, Ceci F, Cancino A, et al. Eating behavior and adherence to dietary prescriptions in obese adult subjects treated with 5-hydroxytryptophan. *Am J Clin Nutr* 1992;56(5):863-7.

915 Kahn RS, Westenberg HGM. L-5-hydroxytryptophan in the treatment of anxiety disorders. *J Affect Disord* 1985;8:197-200.

916 Trouillas P, Brudon F, Adeleine P. Improvement of cerebellar ataxia with levorotatory form of 5-hydroxytryptophan: a double-blind study with quantified data processing. *Arch Neurol* 1988;45:1217-22.

917 Williams A, Goodenberger D, Caline DB, et al. Palatal myclonus following herpes zoster amellorated by 5-hydroxytryptophan and carbidopa. *Neurology* 1978;28:358-9.

918 Meyer JS, Welch KM, Deshmukh VD, et al. Neurotransmitter precursor amino acids in the treatment of multi-infarct dementia and Alzheimer's disease. *J Amer Geriat Soc* 1977;25:289-98.

919 FDA talk paper. Impurities confirmed in dietary supplement 5-hydroxy-L-tryptophan. August 31, 1998. URL: http://vm.cfsan.fda.gov/~lrd/tp5htp.html (Accessed 17 September 1999).

920 Kaplan PW, Tusa RJ, Shankroff J, et al. Visual evoked potentials in adrenoleukodystrophy: a trial with glycerol trioleate and Lorenzo oil. *Ann Neurol* 1993;34(2):169-74.

921 Poulos A, Gibson R, Sharp P, et al. Very long chain fatty acids in X-linked adrenoleukodystrophy brain after treatment with Lorenzo's oil. *Ann Neurol* 1994;36(5):741-6.

922 Duchesne N, Dufour M, Bouchard G, et al. Adrenoleukodystrophy: magnetic resonance follow-up after Lorenzo's oil therapy. *Can Assoc Radiol J* 1995;46(5):386-91.

923 Moser HW. Clinical and therapeutic aspects of adrenoleukodystrophy and adrenomyeloneuropathy. *J Neuropathol Exp Neurol* 1995;54(5):740-5.

924 Aubourg P, Adamsbaum C, Lavallard-Rousseau MC, et al. A two-year trial of oleic and erucic acids (Lorenzo's oil) as treatment for adrenomyeloneuropathy. *N Engl J Med* 1993;329(11):745-52.

925 Kickler TS, Zinkham WH, Moser A, et al. Effect of erucic acid on platelets in patients with adrenoleukodystrophy. *Biochem Mol Med* 1996;57(2):125-33.

926 Chai BC, Etches WS, Stewart MW, Siminoski K. Bleeding in a patient taking Lorenzo's oil: evidence for a vascular defect. *Postgrad Med J* 1996;72(844):113-4.

927 Revell P, Green A, Green S. Platelets in treated adrenoleukodystrophy: a brief report. *J Inherit Metab Dis* 1995;18(5):635-7.

928 Moser HW. Komrower Lecture. Adrenoleukodystrophy: natural history, treatment and outcome. *J Inherit Metab Dis* 1995;18(4):435-47.

929 Maeda K, Suzuki Y, Yajima S, et al. Improvement of clinical and MRI findings in a boy with adrenoleukodystrophy by dietary erucic acid therapy. *Brain Dev* 1992;14(6):409-12.

930 Wong V. Adrenoleukodystrophy in a Chinese boy. *Brain*

Dev 1992;14(4):276-7.

931 Rasmussen M, Moser AB, Borel J, et al. Brain, liver, and adipose tissue erucic and very long chain fatty acid levels in adrenoleukodystrophy patients treated with glyceryl trierucate and trioleate oils (Lorenzo's oil). *Neurochem Res* 1994;19(8):1073-82.

932 Miller TE, Dodd J, Ormrod DJ, Geddes R. Anti-inflammatory activity of glycogen extracted from Perna canaliculus (NZ green-lipped mussel). *Agents Actions* 1993;38 Spec No:C139-42.

933 Couch RA, Ormrod DJ, Miller TE, Watkins WB. Anti-inflammatory activity in fractionated extracts of the green-lipped mussel. *N Z Med J* 1982;95(720):803-6.

934 Miller TE, Ormrod D. The anti-inflammatory activity of Perna canaliculus (NZ green lipped mussel). *N Z Med J* 1980;92(667):187-93.

935 Larkin JG, Capell HA, Sturrock RD. Seatone in rheumatoid arthritis: a six-month placebo-controlled study. *Ann Rheum Dis* 1985;44(3):199-201.

936 Miller T, Wu H. In vivo evidence for prostaglandin inhibitory activity in New Zealand green-lipped mussel extract. *N Z Med J* 1984;97(757):355-7.

937 Naghii MR, Samman S. The effect of boron supplementation on its urinary excretion and selected cardiovascular risk factors in healthy male subjects. *Biol Trace Elem Res* 1997;56(3):273-86.

938 Vettori G, Lazzaro A, Mazzanti P, Cazzola P. [Prevention of recurrent respiratory infections in adults]. [Article in Italian]. *Minerva Med* 1987;78(17):1281-9.

939 Usuda K, Kono K, Iguchi K, et al. Hemodialysis effect on serum boron level in the patients with long term hemodialysis. *Sci Total Environ* 1996;191(3):283-90.

940 Meacham SL, Taper LJ, Volpe SL. Effect of boron supplementation on blood and urinary calcium, magnesium, and phosphorus, and urinary boron in athletic and sedentary women. *Am J Clin Nutr* 1995;61(2):341-5.

941 Newnham RE. Essentiality of boron for healthy bones and joints. *Environ Health Perspect* 1994;102(Suppl 7):83-5.

942 Meacham SL, Taper LJ, Volpe SL. Effects of boron supplementation on bone mineral density and dietary, blood, and urinary calcium, phosphorus, magnesium, and boron in female athletes. *Environ Health Perspect* 1994;102(Suppl 7):79-82.

943 Penland JG. Dietary boron, brain function, and cognitive performance. *Environ Health Perspect* 1994;102(Suppl 7):65-72.

944 Green NR, Ferrando AA. Plasma boron and the effects of boron supplementation in males. *Environ Health Perspect* 1994;102(Suppl 7):73-7.

945 Shils M, Olson A, Shike M. Modern Nutrition in Health and Disease. 8th ed. Philadelphia, PA: Lea and Febiger, 1994.

946 Wyatt RJ, Engelman K, Kupfer DJ, et al. Effects of L-tryptophan (a natural sedative) on human sleep. *Lancet* 1970;2(7678):842-6.

947 Hunt MJ, Barnetson R. A comparative study of gluconolactone versus benzoyl peroxide in the treatment of acne. *Australas J Dermatol* 1992;33(3):131-4.

948 Thueson DO, Chan EK, Oechsli LM, Hahn GS. The roles of pH and concentration in lactic acid-induced stimulation of epidermal turnover. *Dermatol Surg Jun* 1998;24(6):641-5.

949 Kempers S, Katz HI, Wildnauer R, Green B. An evaluation of the effect of an alpha hydroxy acid-blend skin cream in the cosmetic improvement of symptoms of moderate to severe xerosis, epidermolytic hyperkeratosis, and ichthyosis. *Cutis* 1998;61(5):347-50.

950 Berardesca E, Distante F, Vignoli GP, et al. Alpha hydroxyacids modulate stratum corneum barrier function. *Br J Dermatol* 1997;137(6):934-8.

951 Rawlings AV, Davies A, Carlomusto M, et al. Effect of lactic acid isomers on keratinocyte ceramide synthesis, stratum corneum lipid levels and stratum corneum barrier function. *Arch Dermatol Res* 1996;288(7):383-90.

952 Stiller MJ, Bartolone J, Stern R, et al. Topical 8% glycolic acid and 8% L-lactic acid creams for the treatment of photodamaged skin. A double-blind, vehicle-controlled clinical trial. *Arch Dermatol* 1996;132(6):631-6.

953 Piacquadio D, Dobry M, Hunt S, et al. Short contact 70% glycolic acid peels as a treatment for photodamaged skin. A pilot study. *Dermatol Surg* 1996;22(5):449-52.

954 Ditre CM, Griffin TD, Murphy GF, et al. Effects of alpha-hydroxy acids on photoaged skin: a pilot clinical, histologic, and ultrastructural study [see comments]. *J Am Acad Dermatol* 1996;34(2 Pt 1):187-95.

955 Wehr R, Krochmal L, Bagatell F, Ragsdale W. A controlled two-center study of lactate 12 percent lotion and a petrolatum-based creme in patients with xerosis. *Cutis* 1986;37(3):205-7, 209.

956 Barnes S. Phytoestrogens and breast cancer. *Baillieres Clin Endocrinol Metab* 1998;12(4):559-79.

957 Hotz G, Frank T, Zoller J, Wiebelt H. [Antiphlogistic effect of bromelaine following third molar removal]. [Article in German]. *Dtsch Zahnarztl Z* 1989;44(11):830-2.

958 Valueva TA, Revina TA, Mosolov VV. Potato tuber protein proteinase inhibitors belonging to the Kunitz soybean inhibitor family. *Biochemistry (Mosc)* 1997;62(12):1367-74.

959 Tanabe S, Tesaki S, Watanabe M, Yanagihara Y. [Cross-reactivity between bromelain and soluble fraction from wheat flour]. [Article in Japanese]. *Arerugi* 1997;46(11):1170-3.

960 Masson M. [Bromelain in blunt injuries of the locomotor system. A study of observed applications in general practice]. [Article in German]. *Fortschr Med* 1995;113(19):303-6.

961 Zimacheva AV, Mosolov VV. [Cysteine proteinase inhibitors from soy seeds]. [Article in Russian]. *Biokhimiia* 1995;60(1):118-23.

962 Zavadova E, Desser L, Mohr T. Stimulation of reactive oxygen species production and cytotoxicity in human neutrophils in vitro and after oral administration of a polyenzyme preparation. *Cancer Biother* 1995;10(2):147-52.

963 Diez-Gomez ML, Quirce S, Aragoneses E, Cuevas M. Asthma caused by Ficus benjamina latex: evidence of cross-reactivity with fig fruit and papain. *Ann Allergy Asthma Immunol* 1998;80(1):24-30.

964 Raus I. [Clinical studies on Frubienzyme in a controlled double-blind trial]. [Article in German]. *Fortschr Med* 1976;94(28):1579-82.

965 Billigmann P. [Enzyme therapy-an alternative in treatment of herpes zoster. A controlled study of 192 patients]. [Article in German]. *Fortschr Med* 1995;113(4):43-8.

966 Shuttleworth D, Hill S, Marks R, Connelly DM. Relief of experimentally induced pruritus with a novel eutectic mixture of local anaesthetic agents. *Br J Dermatol* 1988;119(4):535-40.

967 Mansfield LE, Ting S, Haverly RW, Yoo TJ. The incidence and clinical implications of hypersensitivity to papain in an allergic population, confirmed by blinded oral challenge. *Ann Allergy* 1985;55(4):541-3.

968 Bienen H, Raus I. [Therapeutic comparison of throat lozenges; (author's transl)]. [Article in German]. *MMW Munch Med Wochenschr* 1981;123(18):745-7.

969 Reinecke M. [Treatment of inflammatory diseases of the mouth and throat with Larypront in ENT practice; (author's transl)]. [Article in German]. *MMW Munch Med Wochenschr* 1976;118(39):1253-4.

970 Baron JA, Beach M, Mandel JS, et al. Calcium supplements for the prevention of colorectal adenomas. Calcium Polyp Prev Study Group. *N Engl J Med* 1999;340(2):101-7.

971 Levine RJ, Hauth JC, Curet LB, et al. Trial of calcium to prevent preeclampsia. *N Engl J Med* 1997;337(2):69-76.

972 Whelton PK, Kumanyika SK, Cook NR, et al. Efficacy of nonpharmacologic interventions in adults with high-normal blood pressure: results from phase 1 of the trials of hypertension prevention (TOHP). Trials of Hypertension Prev (TOHP) Collab Res Group. *Am J Clin Nutr* 1997;65(2 Suppl):652S-60S.

973 Purwar M, Kulkarni H, Motghare V, Dhole S. Calcium supplementation and prevention of pregnancy induced hypertension. *J Obstet Gynaecol Res* 1996;22(5):425-30.

974 Yamamoto ME, Applegate WB. Klag MJ, et al. Lack of blood pressure effect with calcium and magnesium supplementation in adults with high-normal blood pressure. Results from phase I of the trials of hypertension prevention (TOHP). Trials of Hypertension Prev (TOHP) Collab Res Group. *Ann Epidemiol* 1995;5(2):96-107.

975 Petersen LJ, Rudnicki M, Hojsted J. Long-term oral calcium supplementation reduces diastolic blood pressure in end stage renal disease. A randomized, double-blind, placebo-controlled study. *Int J Artif Organs* 1994;17(1):37-40.

976 Weinberger MH, Wagner UL, Fineberg NS. The blood pressure effects of calcium supplementation in humans of known sodium responsiveness. *Am J Hypertens* 1993;6(9):799-805.

977 Storm D, Eslin R, Porter ES, et al. Calcium supplementation prevents seasonal bone loss and changes in biochemical markers of bone turnover in elderly New England women: a randomized, placebo-controlled trial. *J Clin Endocrinol Metab* 1998;83(11):3817-25.

978 Baeksgaard L, Andersen KP, Hyldstrup L. Calcium and vitamin D supplementation increases spinal BMD in healthy, postmenopausal women. *Osteoporos Int* 1998;8(3):255-60.

979 Riggs BL, et al. Long-term effects of calcium supplementation on serum parathyroid hormone level, bone turnover, and bone loss in elderly women. *J Bone Miner Res* 1998;13(2):168-74.

980 Dawson-Hughes B, et al. Effect of calcium and vitamin D supplementation on bone density in men and women 65 years of age or older. *N Engl J Med* 1997;337(10):670-6.

981 Devine A, et al. A 4-year follow-up study of the effects of calcium supplementation on bone density in elderly postmenopausal women. *Osteoporos Int* 1997;7(1):23-8.

982 Bernstein CN, et al. A randomized, placebo-controlled trial of calcium supplementation for decreased bone density in corticosteroid-using patients with inflammatory bowel disease: a pilot study. *Aliment Pharmacol Ther* Oct. 1996;10(5):777-86.

983 Ilich-Ernst JZ, et al. Iron status, menarche, and calcium supplementation in adolescent girls. *Am J Clin Nutr* Oct. 1998;68(4):880-7.

984 Dwyer JH, et al. Dietary calcium, calcium supplementation, and blood pressure in African American adolescents. *Am J Clin Nutr* 1998 Sep;68(3):648-55.

985 Thys-Jacobs S, et al. Calcium carbonate and the premenstrual syndrome: effects on premenstrual and menstrual symptoms. Premenstrual Syndrome Study Group. Am J Obstet Gynecol Aug.1998;179(2):444-52.

986 Reid IR. The roles of calcium and vitamin D in the prevention of osteoporosis. *Endocrinol Metab Clin North Am* 1998;27(2):389-98.

987 Ricci TA, et al. Calcium supplementation suppresses bone turnover during weight reduction in postmenopausal women. *J Bone Miner Res* 1998;13(6):1045-50.

988 Kalkwarf HJ, et al. The effect of calcium supplementation on bone density during lactation and after weaning. *N Engl J Med* 1997;337(8):523-8.

989 McKenna AA, et al. Zinc balance in adolescent females. *Am J Clin Nutr* 1997;65(5):1460-4.

990 Gupta SK, et al. Reversal of fluorosis in children. *Acta Paediatr Jpn* 1996;38(5):513-9.

991 Steinbach G, et al. Calcium carbonate treatment of diarrhea in intestinal bypass patients. *Eur J Gastroenterol Hepatol* 1996;8(6):559-62.

992 Lupton JR, et al. Calcium supplementation modifies the relative amounts of bile acids in bile and affects key aspects of human colon physiology. *J Nutr* 1996;126(5):1421-8.

993 Alberts DS, et al. Randomized, double-blind, placebo-controlled study of effect of wheat bran fiber and calcium on fecal bile acids in patients with resected adenomatous colon polyps. *J Natl Cancer Inst* 1996;88(2):81-92.

994 Baron JA, et al. Calcium supplementation and rectal mucosal proliferation: a randomized controlled trial. *J Natl Cancer Inst* 1995;87(17):1303-7.

995 Gallagher JC, Riggs BL, DeLuca. Effect of estrogen on calcium absorption and serum vitamin D metabolites in postmenopausal osteoporosis. *J Clin Endocrinol Metab* 1980;51(6):1359-64.

996 Whiting SJ. Safety of some calcium supplements questioned. *Nutr Rev* 1994;52(3):95-7.

997 Roberts HJ. Potential toxicity due to dolomite and bonemeal. *South Med J* 1983;76(5):556-9.

998 Dietary Reference Intakes (DRI's), Institute Med of Natl Acad Sci, 1997.

999 Akedo I, et al. Three cases with familial adenomatous polyposis diagnosed as having malignant lesions in the course of a long-term trial using docosahexanoic acid (DHA)-concentrated fish oil capsules. *Jpn J Clin Oncol* 1998;28(12):762-5.

1000 Danno K, Sugie N. Combination therapy with low-dose etretinate and eicosapentaenoic acid for psoriasis vulgaris. *J Dermatol* 1998;25(11):703-5.

1001 Prisco D, et al. Effect of medium-term supplementation with a moderate dose of n-3 polyunsaturated fatty acids on blood pressure in mild hypertensive patients. *Thromb Res* 1998;1(3):105-12.

1002 Gans RO, et al. Fish oil supplementation in patients with stable claudication. *Am J Surg* 1990;160(5):490-5.

1003 Vognild E, et al. Effects of dietary marine oils and olive oil on fatty acid composition, platelet membrane fluidity, platelet responses, and serum lipids in healthy humans. *Lipids* 1998;33(4):427-36.

1004 Mayser P, Mrowietz U, Arenberger P, et al. Omega-3 fatty acid-based lipid infusion in patients with chronic plaque psoriasis: results of a double-blind, randomized, placebo-controlled, multicenter trial [published erratum appears in *J Am Acad Dermatol* 1998;38(3):421]. J Am Acad Dermatol 1998;38(4):539-47.

1005 Campan P, Planchand PO, Duran D. Pilot study on n-3 polyunsaturated fatty acids in the treatment of human experimental gingivitis. *J Clin Periodontol* 1997;24(12):907-13.

1006 Thies N. The effect of 12 months' treatment with eicosapentaenoic acid in five children with cystic fibrosis. *J Paediatr Child Health* 1997;33(4):349-51.

1007 Singh RB, et al. Randomized, double-blind, placebo-controlled trial of fish oil and mustard oil in patients with suspected acute myocardial infarction: the Indian experiment of infarct survival-4. *Cardiovasc Drugs Ther* 1997;11(3):485-91.

1008 Sagar PS, et al. Cytotoxic action of cis-unsaturated fatty acids on human cervical carcinoma (HeLa) cells: relationship to free radicals and lipid peroxidation and its modulation by calmodulin antagonists. *Cancer Lett* 1992;63(3):189-98.

1009 Grimsgaard S, et al. Highly purified eicosapentaenoic acid and docosahexaenoic acid in humans have similar triacylglycerol-lowering effects but divergent effects on serum fatty acids. *Am J Clin Nutr* 1997;66(3):649-59.

1010 Marzari R, Mazzanti P, Cazzola P, Pirodda E. [Perennial allergic rhinitis. Prophylaxis of acute episodes using thymomodulin]. [Article in Italian]. *Minerva Med* 1987;78(22):1675-81.

1011 Allard JP, et al. Lipid peroxidation during n-3 fatty acid and vitamin E supplementation in humans. *Lipids* 1997;32(5):535-41.

1012 Andreassen AK, et al. Hypertension prophylaxis with omega-3 fatty acids in heart transplant recipients. *J Am Coll Cardiol* 1997;29:1324-31.

1013 Badalamenti S, et al. Lack of renal effects of fish oil administration in patients with advanced cirrhosis and impaired glomerular filtration. *Hepatol* 1997;25(2):313-6.

1014 Agren JJ, et al. Fish diet, fish oil and docosahexaenoic acid rich oil lower fasting and postprandial plasma lipid levels. *Eur J Clin Nutr* 1996;50(11):765-71.

1015 Zeman K, Dworniak D, Tchorzewski H, et al. Effect of thymic extract on allogeneic MLR and mitogen-induced responses in patients with chronic active hepatitis B. *Immunol Invest* 1991;20(7):545-55.

1016 Saynor R, Gillott T. Changes in blood lipids and fibrinogen with a note on safety in a long term study on the effects of n-3 fatty acids in subjects receiving fish oil supplements and followed for seven years. *Lipids* 1992;27(7):533-8.

1017 van der Tempel H, et al. Effects of fish oil supplementation in rheumatoid arthritis. *Ann Rheum Dis* 1990;49(2):76-80.

1018 Vuksan V, et al. American ginseng (Panax quinquefolius L) reduces postprandial glycemia in nondiabetic subjects and subjects with type 2 diabetes mellitus. *Arch Intern Med* 2000;160:1009-13.

1019 Behan PO, Behan WM, Horrobin D. Effect of high doses of essential fatty acids on the postviral fatigue syndrome. *Acta Neurol Scand* 1990;82(3):209-16.

1020 Toft I, et al. Effects of n-3 polyunsaturated fatty acids on glucose homeostasis and blood pressure in essential hypertension. A randomized, controlled trial. *Ann Intern Med* 1995;123(12):911-8.

1021 Badalamenti S, Salerno F, Lorenzano E. Renal effects of dietary supplementation with fish oil in cyclosporine-treated liver transplant recipients. *Hepatol* 1995;22(6):1695-71.

1022 Sacks FM, et al. Controlled trial of fish oil for regression of human coronary atherosclerosis. HARP Res Group. *J Am Coll Cardiol* 1995;25(7):1492-8.

1023 Sakakibara H, et al. Effect of supplementation with eicosapentaenoic acid ethylster MND- 21, on generation of leukotrienes by calcium ionophore-activated leukocytes in bronchial asthma. *Nihon Kyobu Shikkan Gakkai Zasshi* 1995;33(4):395-402.

1024 Eritsland J, et al. Long-term metabolic effects of n-3 polyunsaturated fatty acids in patients with coronary artery disease. *Am J Clin Nutr* 1995;61(4):831-6.

1025 Shimizu H, et al. Long-term effect of eicosapentaenoic acid ethyl (EPA-E) on albuminuria of non-insulin dependent diabetic patients. *Diabetes Res Clin Pract* 1995;28(1):35-40.

1026 Onwude JL, et al. A randomised double blind placebo controlled trial of fish oil in high risk pregnancy. *Br J Obstet Gynaecol* 1995;102(2):95-100.

1027 Bulstra-Ramakers MT, et al. The effects of 3g eicosapentaenoic acid daily on recurrence of intrauterine growth retardation and pregnancy induced hypertension. *Br J Obstet Gynaecol* 1995;102(2):123-6.

1028 Leaf A, et al. Do fish oils prevent restenosis after coronary angioplasty? *Circulation* 1994;90(5):2248-57.

1029 McVeigh GE, et al. Fish oil improves arterial compliance in non-insulin-dependent diabetes mellitus. *Arterioscler Thromb* 1994;14(9):1425-9.

1030 Sacks FM, et al. Short report: the effect of fish oil on blood pressure and high-density lipoprotein-cholesterol levels in phase I of the trials of hypertension prevention. *J Hypertens* 1994;12(2):209-13.

1031 Lau CS, Morley KD, Belch JJ. Effects of fish oil supplementation on non-steroidal anti-inflammatory drug requirement in patients with mild rheumatoid arthritis- a double-blind, placebo-controlled study. *Br J Rheumatol* 1993;32:982-9.

1032 Rossi E, Costa M. Fish oil derivatives as a prophylaxis of recurrent miscarriage associated with antiphospholipid antibodies (APL): a pilot study. *Lupus* 1993;2(5):319-23.

1033 Vandongen R, Mori TA, Burke V, et al. Effects on blood pressure of omega 3 fats in subjects at increased risk of cardiovascular disease. *Hypertension* 1993;22(3):371-9.

1034 Grimminger F, et al. A double-blind, randomized, placebo-controlled trial of n-3 fatty acid based lipid infusion in acute, extended guttate psoriasis. Rapid improvement of clinical manifestations and changes in neutrophil leukotriene profile. *Clin Invest*

REFERENCES

REFERENCES

1993;71(8):634-43.

1035 Soyland E, et al. Effect of dietary supplementation with very-long-chain n-3 fatty acids in patients with psoriasis. *N Engl J Med* 1993;328(25):1812-6.

1036 Thien FC, Mencia-Huerta J, Lee TH. Dietary fish oil effects on seasonal hay fever and asthma in pollen-sensitive subjects. *Am Rev Respir Dis* 1993;147(5):1138-43.

1037 Greenfield SM, et al. A randomized controlled study of evening primrose oil and fish oil in ulcerative colitis. *Aliment Pharmacol Ther* 1993;7(2):159-66.

1038 Bellamy CM, et al. Can supplementation of diet with omega-3 polyunsaturated fatty acids reduce coronary angioplasty restenosis. *Eur Heart J* 1992;13(12):1626-31.

1039 Kjeldsen-Kragh J, et al. Dietary omega-3 fatty acid supplementation and naproxen treatment in patients with rheumatoid arthritis. *J Rheumatol* 1992;19(10):1531-6.

1040 Hawthorne AB, et al. Treatment of ulcerative colitis with fish oil supplementation: a prospective 12 month randomised controlled trial. *Gut* 1992;33(7):922-8.

1041 Astorga G, et al. Active rheumatoid arthritis: effect of dietary supplementation with omega-3 oils. A controlled double-blind trial. *Rev Med Chil* 1991;119(3):267-72.

1042 D'Almeida A, et al. Effects of a combination of evening primrose oil (gamma linolenic acid) and fish oil (eicosapentaenoic + docahexaenoic acid) versus magnesium, and versus placebo in preventing pre-eclampsia. *Women Health* 1992;19(2-3):117-31.

1043 Hamazaki T, et al. The effect of docosahexaenoic acid on aggression in young adults. A placebo-controlled double-blind study. *J Clin Invest* 1996;97(4):1129-33.

1044 Conquer JA, Holub BJ. Supplementation with an algae source of docosahexaenoic acid increases (n-3) fatty acid status and alters selected risk factors for heart disease in vegetarian subjects. *J Nutr* 1996;126(12):3032-9.

1045 Carlson SE, Werkman SH. A randomized trial of visual attention of preterm infants fed docosahexaenoic acid until two months. *Lipids* 1996;31(1):85-90.

1046 Buckley LM, et al. Calcium and vitamin D3 supplementation prevents bone loss in the spine secondary to low-dose corticosteroids in patients with rheumatoid arthritis. A randomized double-blind, placebo-controlled trial. *Ann Intern Med* 1996;125(12):961-8.

1047 White E, Shannon JS, Patterson RE. Relationship between vitamin and calcium supplement use and colon cancer. *Cancer Epidemiol Biomarkers Prev* 1997;6(10):769-74.

1048 Mindell E. Earl Mindell's Supplement Bible. New York, NY: Simon and Schuster, 1998.

1049 Suhner A, et al. Comparative study to determine the optimal melatonin dosage form for the alleviation of jet lag. *Chronobiol Int* 1998;15(6):655-6.

1050 MotherNature. PABA website. www.mothernature.com/ency/supp/paba.asp (Accessed 19 October 2000).

1051 Dreher F, et al. Topical melatonin in combination with vitamins E and C protects skin from ultraviolet-induced erythema: a human study in vivo. *Br J Dermatol* 1998;139(2):332-9.

1052 Wright SW, et al. Randomized clinical trial of melatonin after night-shift work: efficacy and neuropsychologic effects. *Ann Emerg Med* 1998 32(3 Pt 1):334-40.

1053 Dolberg OT, Hirschmann S, Grunhaus L. Melatonin for the treatment of sleep disturbances in major depressive disorder. *Am J Psychiatr* 1998;155(8):1119-21.

1054 James M, et al. Can melatonin improve adaptation to night shift? *Am J Emerg Med* 1998;16(4):367-70.

1055 Arunachalam K, Gill HS, Chandra RK. Enhancement of natural immune function by dietary consumption of Bifidobacterium lactis (HN019). *Eur J Clin Nutr* 2000;54:263-267.

1056 McArthur AJ, Budden S. Sleep dysfunction in Rett syndrome: a trial of exogenous melatonin treatment. *Dev Med Child Neurol* 1998;40(3):186-92.

1057 Healthgate.com. Complete guide to vitamins, minerals & supplements. www.healthgate.com/vit/vit85.shtml (Accessed 19 October 2000).

1058 Benes L, et al. Transmucosal, oral controlled-release, and transdermal drug administration in human subjects: a crossover study with melatonin. *J Pharm Sci* 1997;86(10):1115-9.

1059 Leibenluft E, et al. Effects of exogenous melatonin administration and withdrawal in five patients with rapid-cycling bipolar disorder. *J Clin Psychiatr* 1997;58(9):383-8.

1060 Lievin V, Peiffer I, Hudault S, et al. Bifidobacterium strains from resident infant human gastrointestinal microflora exert antimicrobial activity. *Gut* 2000;47:646-52.

1061 Worobec S, LaChine A. Dangers of orally administered para-aminobenzoic acid. *JAMA* 1984;251:2348.

1062 Van Den Heuvel CJ, Reid KJ, Dawson D. Effect of atenolol on nocturnal sleep and temperature in young men: reversal by pharmacological doses of melatonin. *Physiol Behav* 1997;61(6):795-802.

1063 Wikner J, Wetterberg L, Rojdmark S. Does hypercalcaemia or calcium antagonism affect human melatonin secretion or renal excretion? *Eur J Clin Invest* 1997;27(5):374-9.

1064 Lissoni P, et al. Adjuvant therapy with the pineal hormone melatonin in patients with lymph node relapse due to malignant melanoma. *J Pineal Res* 1996;21(4):239-42.

1065 Zarafonetis CJ, Dabich L, DeVol EB, et al. Potassium para-aminobenzoate and liver function test findings. *J Am Acad Dermatol* 1986;15:144-9.

1066 Bangha E, Elsner P, Kistler GS. Suppression of UV-induced erythema by topical treatment with melatonin (N-acetyl-5-methoxytryptamine). A dose response study. *Arch Dermatol Res* 1996;288(9):522-6.

1067 Carson CC. Potassium para-aminobenzoate for the treatment of Peyronie's disease: is it effective? *Tech Urol* 1997;3:135-9.

1068 Attenburrow ME, Cowen PJ, Sharpley AL. Low dose melatonin improves sleep in healthy middle-aged subjects. *Psychopharmacol (Berl)* 1996;126(2):179-81.

1069 Lissoni P, et al. Prevention of cytokine-induced hypotension in cancer patients by the pineal hormone melatonin. *Support Care Cancer* 1996;4(4):313-6.

1070 Ellis CM, Lemmens G, Parkes JD. Melatonin and insomnia. *J Sleep Res* 1996;5(1):61-5.

1071 Zarafonetis CJ, Dabich L, Skovronski JJ, et al. Retrospective studies in scleroderma: skin response to potassium para-aminobenzoate therapy. *Clin Exp Rheumatol* 1988;6:261-8.

1072 Garfinkel D, et al. Improvement of sleep quality in elderly people by controlled-release melatonin. *Lancet* 1995 Aug 26;346(8974):541-44.

1073 Zarafonetis CJ, Dabich L, Negri D, et al. Retrospective studies in scleroderma: effect of potassium para-aminobenzoate on survival. *J Clin Epidemiol* 1988;41:193-205.

1074 Clegg DO, Reading JC, Mayes MD, et al. Comparison of aminobenzoate potassium and placebo in the treatment of scleroderma. *J Rheumatol* 1994 Jan;21:105-10.

1075 Zarafonetis CJ, Dabich L, Devol EB, et al. Retrospective studies in scleroderma: pulmonary findings and effect of potassium p-aminobenzoate on vital capacity. *Respiration* 1989;56:22-33.

1076 Valcavi R, et al. Melatonin stimulates growth hormone secretion through pathways other than the growth hormone-releasing hormone. *Clin Endocrinol (Oxf)* 1993;39(2):193-9.

1077 Petrie K, et al. A double-blind trial of melatonin as a treatment for jet lag in international cabin crew. *Biol Psychiatr* 1993;33(7):526-30.

1078 Dollins AB, et al. Effect of pharmacological daytime doses of melatonin on human mood and performance. *Psychopharmacol* (Berl) 1993;112(4):490-6.

1079 Claustrat B, et al. Melatonin and jet lag: confirmatory result using a simplified protocol. *Biol Psychiatr* 1992;32(8):705-11.

1080 Lissoni P, et al. Randomized study with the pineal hormone melatonin versus supportive care alone in advanced nonsmall cell lung cancer resistant to a first-line chemotherapy containing cisplatin. *Oncol* 1992;49(5):336-9.

1081 Dahlitz M, et al. Delayed sleep phase syndrome response to melatonin. *Lancet* 1991;337(8750):1121-4.

1082 Sack RL, et al. Melatonin administration to blind people: phase advances and entrainment. *J Biol Rhythms* 1991;6(3):249-61.

1083 James SP, et al. Melatonin administration in insomnia. *Neuropsychopharmacol* 1990;3(1):19-23.

1084 Ludwig G. Evaluation of conservative therapeutic approaches to Peyronie's disease (fibrotic induration of the penis). *Urol Int* 1991;47:236-9.

1085 Petrie K, et al. Effect of melatonin on jet lag after long haul flights. *BMJ* 1989;298(6675):705-7.

1086 Hughes CG. Oral PABA and vitiligo. *J Am Acad Dermatol* 1983;9:770.

1087 Carnielli VP, Da Riol R, Montini G. Iron supplementation enhances response to high doses of recombinant human erythropoietin in preterm infants. *Arch Dis Child Fetal Neonatal Ed* 1998;79(1):F44-8.

1088 Silva J, et al. Iron supplementation in haemodialysis-practical clinical guidelines. *Nephrol Dial Transplant* 1998;13(10):2572-7.

1089 Brolin RE, et al. Prophylactic iron supplementation after Roux-en-Y gastric bypass: a prospective, double-blind, randomized study. *Arch Surg* 1998;133(7):740-4.

1090 Fudin R, et al. Correction of uremic iron deficiency anemia in hemodialyzed patients: a prospective study. *Nephron* 1998;79(3):299-305.

1091 Sowade O, et al. The estimation of efficacy of oral iron supplementation during treatment with epoetin beta (recombinant human erythropoietin) in patients undergoing cardiac surgery. *Eur J Haematol* 1998;60(4):252-9.

1092 Andrews CM, Lane DW, Bradley JG. Iron pre-load for major joint replacement. *Transfus Med* 1997;7(4):281-6.

1093 Sever Y, et al. Iron treatment in children with attention deficit hyperactivity disorder. A preliminary report. *Neuropsychobiol* 1997;35(4):178-80.

1094 Kantor GR, Ratz JL. Liver toxicity from potassium para-aminobenzoate. *J Am Acad Dermatol* 1985;13:671-2.

1095 Bruner AB, et al. Randomized study of cognitive effects of iron supplementation in non- anaemic iron-deficient adolescent girls. *Lancet* 1996;348(9033):992-6.

1096 Bamford DS, Percival RC, Tothill AU. Raspberry leaf tea: a new aspect to an old problem. *Br J Pharmacol* 1970;40:161P+.

1097 Corti MC, et al. Serum iron level, coronary artery disease, and all-cause mortality in older men and women. *Am J Cardiol* 1997;79(2):120-7.

1098 Ullen H, et al. Supplementary iron intake and risk of cancer: reversed causality? *Cancer Lett* 1997;114(1-2):215-6.

1099 Reunanen A, et al. Body iron stores, dietary iron intake and coronary heart disease mortality. *J Intern Med* 1995;238(3):223-30.

1100 Lund EK, et al. Oral ferrous sulfate supplements increase the free radical-generating capacity of feces from healthy volunteers. *Am J Clin Nutr* 1999;69(2):250-5.

1101 Schumann K, Elsenhans B, Maurer A. Iron supplementation. *J Trace Elem Med Biol* 1998;12(3):129-40.

1102 Rehman A, et al. The effects of iron and vitamin C co-supplementation on oxidative damage to DNA in healthy volunteers. *Biochem Biophys Res Comm* 1998;246(1):293-8.

1103 Recommended Dietary Allowances. Inst Med of Natl Acad Sci, 1989.

1104 Soewondo S. The effect of iron deficiency and mental stimulation on Indonesian children's cognitive performance and development. *Kobe J Med Sci* 1995;41(1-2):1-17.

1105 Budeiri D, Li Wan Po A, Dornan JC. Is evening primrose oil of value in the treatment of premenstrual syndrome? *Control Clin Trials* 1996;17(1):60-8.

1106 Khoo SK, Munro C, Battistutta D. Evening primrose oil and treatment of premenstrual syndrome. *Med J Aust* 1990;153(4):189-92.

1107 Gordon M, et al. A phase II controlled study of a combination of the immune modulator, lentinan, with didanosine (ddI) in HIV patients with CD4 cells of 200-500/mm3. *J Med* 1995;26(5-6):193-207.

1108 Yoshiyuki T, et al. Treatment for peritoneal dissemination of gastric cancer by intraperitoneal administration of CDDP through Infuse-a-Port. *Gan To Kagaku Ryoho* 1994;21(13):2323-5.

1109 Tari K, et al. Effect of lentinan for advanced prostate carcinoma. *Hinyokika Kiyo* 1994;40(2):119-23.

1110 Nishihira T, Akimoto M, Mori S. Anti-cancer effects of BRMs associated with nutrition in cancer patients. *Gan To Kagaku Ryoho* 1988;15(4 Pt 2-3):1615-20.

1111 Wada T, et al. A comparative clinical trial with tegafur plus lentinan treatment at two different doses in advanced cancer. *Gan To Kagaku Ryoho* 1987;14(8):2509-11.

1112 Kosaka A, et al. Synergistic action of lentinan (LNT) with endocrine therapy of breast cancer in rats and humans. *Gan To Kagaku Ryoho* 1987;14(2):516-22.

1113 Taguchi T. Clinical efficacy of lentinan on patients with stomach cancer: end point results of a four-year follow-up survey. *Cancer Detect Prev Suppl* 1987;1:333-49.

REFERENCES

1114 Thein DJ, Hurt WC. Lysine as a prophylactic agent in the treatment of recurrent herpes simplex labialis. *Oral Surg Oral Med Oral Pathol* 1984;58(6):659-66.

1115 McCune MA, et al. Treatment of recurrent herpes simplex infections with L-lysine monohydrochloride. *Cutis* 1984;34(4):366-73.

1116 DiGiovanna JJ, Blank H. Failure of lysine in frequently recurrent herpes simplex infection. Treatment and prophylaxis. *Arch Dermatol* 1984;120(1):48-51.

1117 Chiang BL, Sheih YH, Wang LH, et al. Enhancing immunity by dietary consumption of a probiotic lactic acid bacterium (Bifidobacterium lactis HN019): optimization and definition of cellular immune responses. *Eur J Clin Nutr* 2000;54:849-855.

1118 Milman N, Scheibel J, Jessen O. Lysine prophylaxis in recurrent herpes simplex labialis: a double-blind, controlled crossover study. *Acta Derm Venereol* 1980;60(1):85-7.

1119 Griffith RS, Norins A, Kagan C. A multicentered study of lysine therapy in Herpes simplex infection. *Dermatologica* 1978;156(5):257-67.

1120 Griffith RS, et al. Success of L-lysine therapy in frequently recurrent herpes simplex infection. Treatment and prophylaxis. *Dermatologica* 1987;175(4):183-90.

1121 Lo JC, et al. Fanconi's syndrome and tubulointerstitial nephritis in association with L-lysine ingestion. *Am J Kidney Dis* 1996;28(4):614-7.

1122 McFarlin BL, Gibson MH, O'Rear J, Harman P. A national survey of herbal preparation use by nurse-midwives for labor stimulation. Review of the literature and recommendations for practice. *J Nurse Midwifery* 1999;44:205-16.

1123 Nurnberger JI Jr, Adkins S, Lahiri DK, et al. Melatonin suppression by light in euthymic bipolar and unipolar patients. *Arch Gen Psychiatr* 2000;57:572-9.

1124 Flodin NW. The metabolic roles, pharmacology, and toxicology of lysine. *J Am Coll Nutr* 1997;16(1):7-12.

1125 Naguib M, Samarkandi AH. The comparative dose-response effects of melatonin and midazolam for premedication of adult patients: a double-blinded, placebo-controlled study. *Anesth Analg* 2000;91:473-9.

1126 DeMuro RL, Nafziger AN, Blask DE, et al. The absolute bioavailability of oral melatonin. *J Clin Pharmacol* 2000;40:781-4.

1127 Leone M, D'Amico D, Moschiano F, et al. Melatonin versus placebo in the prophylaxis of cluster headache: a double-blind pilot study with parallel groups. *Cephalalgia* 1996;16:494-6.

1128 Peres MF, Seabra ML, Zukerman E, Tufik S. Cluster headache and melatonin. *Lancet* 2000;355:147.

1129 Blau JN, Engel HO. A new cluster headache precipitant: increased body heat. *Lancet* 1999;354:1001-2.

1130 Hall SL, Greendale GA. The relation of dietary vitamin C intake to bone mineral density: results from the PEPI study. *Calcif Tissue Int* 1998;63(3):183-9.

1131 Civitelli R, et al. Dietary L-lysine and calcium metabolism in humans. *Nutr* 1992;8(6):400-5.

1132 Cagnacci A, Krauchi K, Wirz-Justice A, Volpe A. Homeostatic versus circadian effects of melatonin on core body temperature in humans. *J Biol Rhythms* 1997;12:509-17.

1133 Smith KA, Fairburn CG, Cowen PJ. Symptomatic relapse in bulimia nervosa following acute tryptophan depletion. *Arch Gen Psychiatr* 1999;56(2):171-6.

1134 Sharma RP, Shapiro LE, Kamath SK. Acute dietary tryptophan depletion: effects on schizophrenic positive and negative symptoms. *Neuropsychobiol* 1997;35(1):5-10.

1135 van Hall G, Raaymakers JS, Saris WH. Ingestion of branched-chain amino acids and tryptophan during sustained exercise in man: failure to affect performance. *J Physiol (Lond)* 1995;486(pt 3):789-94.

1136 Delgado PL, Price LH, Miller HL. Serotonin and the neurobiology of depression. Effects of tryptophan depletion in drug-free depressed patients. *Arch Gen Psychiatr* 1994;51(11):865-74.

1137 Macfarlane GT, Cummings JH. Probiotics and prebiotics: can regulating the activities of intestinal bacteria benefit health? *BMJ* 1999;318:999-1003.

1138 Bowen DJ, Spring B, Fox E. Tryptophan and high-carbohydrate diets as adjuncts to smoking cessation therapy. *J Behav Med* 1991;14(2):97-110.

1139 Etzel KR, Stockstill JW, Rugh JD. Tryptophan supplementation for nocturnal bruxism: report of negative results. *Rugh JDJ Craniomandib Disord* 1991;5(2):115-20.

1140 Stockstill JW, McCall D Jr., Gross AJ. The effect of L-tryptophan supplementation and dietary instruction on chronic myofascial pain. *J Am Dent Assoc* 1989;118(4):457-60.

1141 Messiha FS. Fluoxetine: adverse effects and drug-drug interactions. *J Toxicol Clin Toxicol* 1993;31(4):603-30.

1142 Devoe LD, Castillo RA, Searle NS. Maternal dietary substrates and human fetal biophysical activity. The effects of tryptophan and glucose on fetal breathing movements. *Am J Obstet Gynecol* 1986;155(1):135-9.

1143 Lieberman HR, Corkin S, Spring BJ. The effects of dietary neurotransmitter precursors on human behavior. *Am J Clin Nutr* 1985;42(2):366-70.

1144 Schmidt HS. L-tryptophan in the treatment of impaired respiration in sleep. *Bull Eur Physiopathol Respir* 1983;19(6):625-9.

1145 Seltzer S, Dewart D, Pollack R. The effects of dietary tryptophan on chronic maxillofacial pain and experimental pain tolerance. *J Psychiatr Res* 1982-83;17(2):181-6.

1146 Hartmann E, Spinweber CL. Sleep induced by L-tryptophan. Effect of dosages within the normal dietary intake. *J Nerv Ment Dis* 1979;167(8):497-9.

1147 Hitosugi M, et al. Autopsy case of duodenal obstruction from impacted mushroom. *J Gastroenterol* 1998;33(4):562-5.

1148 Hanada K, Hashimoto I. Flagellate mushroom (Shiitake) dermatitis and photosensitivity. *Dermatol* 1998;197(3):255-7.

1149 Levy AM, et al. Eosinophilia and gastrointestinal symptoms after ingestion of shiitake mushrooms. *J Allergy Clin Immunol* 1998;101(5):613-20.

1150 Murakami M, et al. Decreased pulmonary perfusion in hypersensitivity pneumonitis caused by Shiitake mushroom spores. *J Intern Med* 1997;241(1):85-8.

1151 Matsui S, et al. Hypersensitivity pneumonitis induced by Shiitake mushroom spores. *Intern Med* 1992;31(10):1204-6.

1152 Nakamura T. Shiitake (Lentinus edodes) dermatitis. *Contact Dermatitis* 1992;27(2):65-70.

1153 Ueda A, et al. Allergic contact dermatitis in shiitake (Lentinus edodes (Berk) Sing) growers. *Contact Dermatitis* 1992;26(4):228-33.

1154 Hirayama K, Rafter J. The role of probiotic bacteria in cancer prevention. *Microbes Infect* 2000;2:681-6.

1155 Otsuka M, et al. Influences of a shiitake (Lentinus edodes)-fructo-oligosaccharide mixture (SK-204) on experimental pulmonary thrombosis in rats. *Yakugaku Zasshi* 1996;116(2):169-73.

1156 Shitake Components. www.rainforest-mushrooms.com/ ShitakeComponents.html (Accessed 23 July 1999).

1157 Colloidal minerals in brief. www.colloidal.com.au/ (Accessed 23 July 1999).

1158 Wallach J. Dr. Joel Wallach's colloidal minerals. www.elementsofhealth.com/b1.html (Accessed 23 July 1999).

1159 Schauss A. Colloidal minerals: Clinical implications of clay suspension products sold as dietary supplements. *Amer J of Nat Med* 1997;4(1):5-10.

1160 Sposito G, Skipper NT, Sutton R, et al. Surface geochemistry of the clay minerals. *Proc Natl Acad Sci USA* 1999;96(7):3358-64.

1161 Schrauzer G. An overview of liquid mineral supplements. *Int J of Integrative Med* 1999;1(2):18-22.

1162 Branton SL, Lott BD, Maslin WR, et al. Fatty liver-hemorrhagic syndrome observed in commercial layers fed diets containing chelated minerals. *Avian Dis* 1995;39(3):631-5.

1163 Infinity2 product question and answers. www.infinity2.net/ChelatedMineralsQuestionF.html (Accessed 23 July 1999).

1164 Chelated minerals. www.netmins.com/chelndx.html (Accessed 23 July 1999).

1165 Youngevity. www.ciya.com/13.html (Accessed 23 July 1999).

1166 Reach for Life quality products.. www.reach4life.com/ 1111.html (Accessed 23 July 1999).

1167 Durlach J, Bac P, Durlach V, et al. Magnesium status and ageing: an update. *Magnes Res* 1998;11(1):25-42.

1168 Scheen AJ. Perspective in the treatment of insulin resistance. *Hum Reprod* 1997;12(Suppl 1):63-71.

1169 Ziment I. Alternative therapies for asthma. *Curr Opin Pulm Med* 1997;3(1):61-7.

1170 Preuss HG, Gondal JA, Lieberman S. Association of macronutrients and energy intake with hypertension. *J Am Coll Nutr* 1996;15(1):21-35.

1171 de Valk HW, Verkaaik R, van Rijn HJ, et al. Oral magnesium supplementation in insulin-requiring Type 2 diabetic patients. *Diabet Med* 1998;15(6):503-7.

1172 Lima M, Cruz T, Pousada JC, et al. The effect of magnesium supplementation in increasing doses on the control of type 2 diabetes. *Diabetes Care* 1998;21(5):682-6.

1173 Hill J, Micklewright A, Lewis S, et al. Investigation of the effect of short-term change in dietary magnesium intake in asthma. *Eur Respir J* 1997;10(10):2225-9.

1174 Zehender M, Meinertz T, Faber T, et al. Antiarrhythmic effects of increasing the daily intake of magnesium and potassium in patients with frequent ventricular arrhythmias. Magnesium in Cardiac Arrhythmias (MAGICA)Investigators. *J Am Coll Cardiol* 1997;29(5):1028-34.

1175 Cavagni G, Piscopo E, Rigoli E, et al. Food allergy in children: an attempt to improve the effects of the elimination diet with an immunomodulating agent (thymomodulin). A double-blind clinical trial. *Immunopharmacol Immunotoxicol* 1989;11(1):131-42.

1176 Genova R, Guerra A. Thymomodulin in management of food allergy in children. *Int J Tissue React*

1986;8(3):239-42.

1177 Galli M, Crocchiolo P, Negri C, et al. Attempt to treat acute type B hepatitis with an orally administered thymic extract (thymomodulin): preliminary results. *Drugs Exp Clin Res* 1985;11(9):665-9.

1178 Valesini G, Barnaba V, Benvenuto R, et al. A calf thymus acid lysate improves clinical symptoms and T-cell defects in the early stages of HIV infection: second report. *Eur J Cancer Clin Oncol* 1987;23(12):1915-9.

1179 Withanachchi J, Al-Faleh H, Griffiths J, Senaratne MP. Dichotomous and modest response to folic acid and lack of additional effect of vitamin B-12 in hyperhomocystinemia. *Clin Invest Med* 2000;23(4):S5.

1180 Witteman JC, Grobbee DE, Derkx FH, et al. Reduction of blood pressure with oral magnesium supplementation in women with mild to moderate hypertension. *Am J Clin Nutr* 1994 60(1):129-35.

1181 Lasserre B, Spoerri M, Moullet V, et al. Should magnesium therapy be considered for the treatment of coronary heart disease? II. Epidemiological evidence in outpatients with and without coronary heart disease. *Magnes Res* 1994;7(2):145-53.

1182 Yamori Y, Nara Y, Mizushima S, et al. Nutritional factors for stroke and major cardiovascular diseases: international epidemiological comparison of dietary prevention. *Health Rep* 1994;6(1):22-7.

1183 Mauskop A, Altura BT, Cracco RQ, et al. Deficiency in serum ionized magnesium but not total magnesium in patients with migraines. Possible role of ICa2+/IMg2+ ratio. *Headache* 1993;33(3):135-8.

1184 Mauskop A, Altura BT, Cracco RQ, et al. Intravenous magnesium sulfate relieves cluster headaches in patients with low serum ionized magnesium levels. *Headache* 1995;35(10):597-600.

1185 Mauskop A, Altura BT, Cracco RQ, Altura BM. Intravenous magnesium sulphate relieves migraine attacks in patients with low serum ionized magnesium levels: a pilot study. *Clin Sci (Colch)* 1995;89(6):633-6.

1186 Facchinetti F, Sances G, Borella P, et al. Magnesium prophylaxis of menstrual migraine: effects on intracellular magnesium. *Headache* 1991; 31(5):298-301.

1187 Facchinetti F, Borella P, Sances G, et al. Oral magnesium successfully relieves premenstrual mood changes. *Obstet Gynecol* 1991;78(2):177-81.

1188 Walker AF, De Souza MC, Vickers MF, et al. Magnesium supplementation alleviates premenstrual symptoms of fluid retention. *J Womens Health* 1998;7(9):1157-65.

1189 Starobrat-Hermelin B, Kozielec T. The effects of magnesium physiological supplementation on hyperactivity in children with attention deficit hyperactivity disorder (ADHD). Positive response to magnesium oral loading test. *Magnes Res* 1997;10(2):149-56.

1190 Thel MC, Armstrong AL, McNulty SE, et al. Randomised trial of magnesium in in-hospital cardiac arrest. Duke Internal Medicine Housestaff. *Lancet* 1997;350(9087):1272-6.

1191 Lichodziejewska B, Klos J, Rezler J, et al. Clinical symptoms of mitral valve prolapse are related to hypomagnesemia and attenuated by magnesium supplementation. *Am J Cardiol* 1997;79(6):768-72.

1192 Sanjuliani AF, de Abreu Fagundes VG, Francischetti EA. Effects of magnesium on blood pressure and intracellular ion levels of Brazilian hypertensive patients. *Int J Cardiol* 1996;56(2):177-83.

1193 Hoogerbrugge N, Cobbaert C, de Heide L, et al. Oral physiological magnesium supplementation for 6 weeks with 1 g/d magnesium oxide does not affect increased Lp(a) levels in hypercholesterolaemic subjects. *Magnes Res* 1996;9(2):129-32.

1194 Dahle LO, Berg G, Hammar M, et al. The effect of oral magnesium substitution on pregnancy-induced leg cramps. *Am J Obstet Gynecol* 1995;173(1):175-80.

1195 Plum-Wirell M, Stegmayr BG, Wester PO. Nutritional magnesium supplementation does not change blood pressure nor serum or muscle potassium and magnesium in untreated hypertension. A double-blind crossover study. *Magnes Res* 1994;7(3-4):277-83.

1196 Alexandersen P, Toussaint A, Christiansen C, et al. Ipriflavone in the treatment of postmenopausal osteoporosis: A randomized comtrolled trial. *JAMA* 2001;285:1482-8.

1197 Purvis JR, Cummings DM, Landsman P, et al. Effect of oral magnesium supplementation on selected cardiovascular risk factors in non-insulin-dependent diabetics. *Arch Fam Med* 1994;3(6):503-8.

1198 Galloe AM, Rasmussen HS, Jorgensen LN, et al. Influence of oral magnesium supplementation on cardiac events among survivors of an acute myocardial infarction. *BMJ* 1993;307(6904):585-7.

1199 Widman L, Wester PO, Stegmayr BK, et al. The dose-dependent reduction in blood pressure through administration of magnesium. A double blind placebo controlled cross-over study. *Am J Hypertens* 1993;6(1):41-5.

1200 Anon. Moderate alcohol consumption prevents bone loss in postmenopausal women. Reuters Health. www.medscape.com/reuters/prof/2000/09/09.28/20000927epid005.html (Accessed 28 September 2000).

1201 Rattan V, Sidhu H, Vaidyanathan S. Effect of combined supplementation of magnesium oxide and pyridoxine in calcium-oxalate stone formers. *Urol Res* 1994;22(3):161-5.

1202 Brodsky MA, Orlov MV, Capparelli EV, et al. Magnesium therapy in new-onset atrial fibrillation. *Am J Cardiol* 1994;73(16):1227-9.

1203 Holmang A, Nilsson C, Niklasson M, et al. Induction of insulin resistance by glucosamine reduces blood flow but not interstitial levels of either glucose or insulin. *Diabetes* 1999;48:106-11.

1204 Kim YB, Zhu JS, Zierath JR, et al. Glucosamine infusion in rats rapidly impairs insulin stimulation of phosphoinositide 3-kinase but does not alter activation of Akt/protein kinase B in skeletal muscle. *Diabetes* 1999;48:310-20.

1205 Attias J, Weisz G, Almog S, et al. Oral magnesium intake reduces permanent hearing loss induced by noise exposure. *Am J Otolaryngol* 1994;15(1):26-32.

1206 Anon. Shark cartilage no use in cancer treatment. Reuters Health. www.reutershealth.com/frame2/eline.html (Accessed 2 October 2000).

1207 Wright IM. Neonatal effects of maternal consumption of blue cohosh. *J Pediatr* 1999;134:384-5.

1208 Skorodin MS, Tenholder MF, Yetter B, et al. Magnesium sulfate in exacerbations of chronic obstructive pulmonary disease. *Arch Intern Med* 1995;155(5):496-500.

1209 Menopause Help Online. Natural progesterone for hormonal balance in women. www.menopause-help-online.com (Accessed 23 July 1999).

1210 Chang R. Functional properties of edible mushrooms. *Nutr Rev* 1996;54(11 Pt 2):S91-3.

1211 Kubo K, Nanba H. The effect of maitake mushrooms on liver and serum lipids. *Alt Ther Health Med* 1996;2(5):62-6.

1212 Kubo K, Aoki H, Nanba H. Anti-diabetic activity present in the fruit body of Grifola frondosa (Maitake). I. *Biol Pharm Bull* 1994;17(8):1106-10.

1213 Kabir Y, Kimura S. Dietary mushrooms reduce blood pressure in spontaneously hypertensive rats (SHR). *J Nutr Sci Vitaminol (Tokyo)* 1989;35(1):91-4.

1214 Kabir Y, Yamaguchi M, Kimura S. Effect of shiitake (Lentinus edodes) and maitake (Grifola frondosa) mushrooms on blood pressure and plasma lipids of spontaneously hypertensive rats. *J Nutr Sci Vitaminol* (Tokyo) 1987;33(5):341-6.

1215 Espeland MA, Hogan PE, Fineberg SE, et al. Effect of postmenopausal hormone therapy on glucose and insulin concentrations. PEPI Investigators. Postmenopausal Estrogen/Progestin Interventions. *Diabetes Care* 1998;21(10):1589-95.

1216 Chen FP, Lee N, Soong YK. Changes in the lipoprotein profile in postmenopausal women receiving hormone replacement therapy. Effects of natural and synthetic progesterone. *J Reprod Med* 1998;43(7):568-74.

1217 Espeland MA, Marcovina SM, Miller V, et al. Effect of postmenopausal hormone therapy on lipoprotein(a) concentration. Postmenopausal Estrogen/Progestin Interventions (PEPI) Investigators. *Circulation* 1998;97(10):979-86.

1218 Perino M, Brigandi FG, Abate FG, et al. Intramuscular versus vaginal progesterone in assisted reproduction: a comparative study. *Clin Exp Obstet Gynecol* 1997;24(4):228-31.

1219 Steingrub JS, Lopez T, Teres D, et al. Amniotic fluid embolism associated with castor oil ingestion. *Crit Care Med* 1988;16:642-3.

1220 Freeman EW, Rickels K, Sondheimer SJ, et al. A double-blind trial of oral progesterone, alprazolam, and placebo in treatment of severe premenstrual syndrome. *JAMA* 1995;274(1):51-7.

1221 Schweizer E, Case WG, Garcia-Espana F, et al. Progesterone co-administration in patients discontinuing long-term benzodiazepine therapy: effects on withdrawal severity and taper outcome. *Psychopharmacol (Berl)* 1995;117(4):424-9.

1222 Simon JA, Robinson DE, Andrews MC, et al. The absorption of oral micronized progesterone: the effect of food, dose proportionality, and comparison with intramuscular progesterone. *Fertil Steril* 1993;60(1):26-33.

1223 Nappi C, Affinito P, Di Carlo C, et al. Double-blind controlled trial of progesterone vaginal cream treatment for cyclical mastodynia in women with benign breast disease. *J Endocrinol Invest* 1992;15(11):801-6.

1224 Freeman EW, Weinstock L, Rickels K, et al. A placebo-controlled study of effects of oral progesterone on performance and mood. *Br J Clin Pharmacol* 1992;33(3):293-8.

1225 Smitz J, Devroey P, Faguer B, et al. A prospective randomized comparison of intramuscular or intravaginal natural progesterone as a luteal phase and early pregnancy supplement. *Hum Reprod* 1992;7(2):168-75.

1226 Darj E, Nilsson S, Axelsson O, et al. Clinical and endometrial effects of oestradiol and progesterone in post-menopausal women. *Maturitas* 1991;13(2):109-15.

1227 Bassetti S, Frei R, Zimmerli W. Fungemia with Saccharomyces cerevisiae after treatment with Saccharomyces boulardii. *Am J Med* 1998;105:71-2.

1228 Cooper A, Spencer C, Whitehead MI et al. Systemic absorption of progesterone cream from Progest cream in postmenopausal women. *Lancet* 1998;351:1255-6.

1229 Burry KA, Paton PE, Hermsmeyer K. Percutaneous absorption of progesterone in postmenopausal women treated with transdermal estrogen. *Am J Obstet Gynecol* 1999;180(6Part 1):1504-11.

1230 FDA. www.verity.fda.gov/default.html.

1231 Cooper AJ, Whitehead MI. Correspondence. *Lancet* 1998;352:906.

1232 Grifon Maitake caplet. www.maitake.com/qm caplet.html (Accessed 23 July 1999).

1233 Colombel JF, Cortot A, Neut C, Romond C. Yoghurt with Bifidobacterium longum reduces erythromycin-induced gastrointestinal effects. *Lancet* 1987;2:43.

1234 Abul-Ezz SR, Barone GW, Gurley BJ, et al. Effect of herbal supplements on cyclosporine blood levels and associated acute rejection. *Am Soc of Nephrol Ann Mtg, Toronto, CAN* 2000;Oct. 11-16:abstract A3754. www.abstracts-on-line.com/abstracts/ASN/search/results.asp?Num=0%2E3418788 (Accessed 17 October 2000).

1235 Belchak AM. Wine drinking may reduce colon cancer risk. Reuters Health. www.reutershealth.com/frame2/eline.html (Accessed 17 October 2000).

1236 Ha GY, Yang CH, Kim H, Chong Y. Case of sepsis caused by Bifidobacterium longum. *J Clin Microbiol* 1999;37:1227-1228.

1237 Hendry J. Dentists use natural materials to treat sensitive teeth. Reuters Health. www.reutershealth.com/frame2/eline.html (Accessed 19 October 2000).

1238 Ascherio A, Zhang SM, Hernan MA, et al. Prospective study of caffeine intake and risk of Parkinson's disease in men and women. Proceedings 125th Ann Mtg Am Neurological Assn, Boston, MA 2000;Oct 15-18:42 (abstract 53).

1239 Bryant M. Too much iron may rust blood vessels. Reuters Health. www.reutershealth.com/frame2/eline.html (Accessed 27 October 2000).

1240 Anderson JW, Gilliland SE. Effect of fermented milk (yogurt) containing Lactobacillus acidophilus L1 on serum cholesterol in hypercholesterolemic humans. *J Am Coll Nutr* 1999;18(1):43-50.

1241 Schaafsma G, Meuling WJ, van Dokkum W L, et al. Effects of a milk product, fermented by Lactobacillus acidophilus and with fructo-oligosaccharides added, on blood lipids in male volunteers. *Eur J Clin Nutr* 1998;52(6):436-40.

1242 Bhatnagar S, Singh KD, Sazawal S, et al. Efficacy of milk versus yogurt offered as part of a mixed diet in acute noncholera diarrhea among malnourished children. *J Pediatr* 1998;132(6):999-1003.

1243 Guerin-Danan C, Chabanet C, Pedone C, et al. Milk fermented with yogurt cultures and Lactobacillus casei compared with yogurt and gelled milk: influence on intestinal microflora in healthy infants. *Am J Clin Nutr* 1998;67(1):111-7.

1244 Wheeler JG, Shema SJ, Bogle ML, et al. Immune and clinical impact of Lactobacillus acidophilus on asthma.

Ann Allergy Asthma Immunol 1997;79(3):229-33.

1245 Shalev E, Battino S, Weiner E, et al. Ingestion of yogurt containing Lactobacillus acidophilus compared with pasteurized yogurt as prophylaxis for recurrent candidal vaginitis and bacterial vaginosis. *Arch Fam Med* 1996;5(10):593-6.

1246 Nizami SQ, Bhutta ZA, Molla AM. Efficacy of traditional rice-lentil-yogurt diet, lactose free milk protein-based formula and soy protein formula in management of secondary lactose intolerance with acute childhood diarrhea. *J Trop Pediatr* 1996;42(3):133-7.

1247 Niault M, Thomas F, Prost J, et al. Fungemia due to Saccharomyces species in a patient treated with enteral Saccharomyces boulardii. *Clin Infect Dis* 1999;28:930.

1248 Neri A, Sabah G, Samra Z. Bacterial vaginosis in pregnancy treated with yogurt. *Acta Obstet Gynecol Scand* 1993;72(1):17-9.

1249 Hilton E, Isenberg HD, Alperstein P, et al. Ingestion of yogurt containing Lactobacillus acidophilus as prophylaxis for candidal vaginitis. *Ann Intern Med* 1992;116(5):353-7.

1250 Touhami M, Boudraa G, Mary JY, et al. Clinical consequences of replacing milk with yogurt in persistent infantile diarrhea. *Ann Pediatr (Paris)* 1992;39(2):79-86.

1251 McCullough MJ, Clemons KV, McCusker JH, Stevens DA. Species identification and virulence attributes of Saccharomyces boulardii (nom. inval.). *J Clin Microbiol* 1998;36:2613-7.

1252 Neuvonen PJ, Kivisto KT, Lehto P. Interference of dairy products with the absorption of ciprofloxacin. *Clin Pharmacol Ther* 1991;50(5 Pt 1):498-502.

1253 Isolauri E, Juntunen M, Rautanen T, et al. A human Lactobacillus strain (Lactobacillus casei sp strain GG) promotes recovery from acute diarrhea in children. *Pediatrics* 1991;8(1):90-7.

1254 Boudraa G, Touhami M, Pochart P, et al. Effect of feeding yogurt versus milk in children with persistent diarrhea. *J Pediatr Gastroenterol Nutr* 1990;11(4):509-12.

1255 Siitonen S, Vapaatalo H, Salminen S, et al. Effect of Lactobacillus GG yogurt in prevention of antibiotic associated diarrhea. *Ann Med* 1990;22(1):57-9.

1256 Lerebours E, N'Djitoyap NC, Lavoine A, et al. Yogurt and fermented-then-pasteurized milk: effects of short-term and long-term ingestion on lactose absorption and mucosal lactase activity in lactase-deficient subjects. *Am J Clin Nutr* 1989;49(5):823-7.

1257 Vitamins C plus K3 cause unique type of tumor apoptosis. Reuters Health. www.reutershealth.com/cgi-bin/ssi/framethis?catalog=mednews&file=1991227scc.html (Accessed 27 December 1999).

1258 Alexandrakis G, Tse DT, Rosa RH Jr, Johnson TE. Nasolacrimal duct obstruction and orbital cellulitis associated with chronic intranasal cocaine abuse. *Arch Ophthalmol* 1999;117(12):1617-22.

1259 Ros JJ, Pelders MG, De Smet PA. A case of positive doping associated with a botanical food supplement. *Pharm World Sci* 1999;21(1):44-6.

1260 Joeres R, Klinker H, Heusler H, et al. Influence of mexiletine on caffeine elimination. *Pharmacol Ther* 1987;33(1):163-9.

1261 Cooper RA, Molan PC, Harding KG. Antibacterial activity of honey against strains of Staphylococcus aureus from infected wounds. *J R Soc Med* 1999;92(6):283-5.

1262 Caccetta RA, Croft KD, Beilin LJ, Puddey IB. Ingestion of red wine significantly increases plasma phenolic acid concentrations but does not acutely affect ex vivo lipoprotein oxidizability. *Am J Clin Nutr* 2000;71:67-74.

1263 Richter's Herb Letter. www.richters.com/ newdisplay.cgi?page=./HL/ HerbLett.html&cart_id=3085578.5928. (Accessed 31 December 1999).

1264 Cignarella A, Nastasi M, Cavalli E, Puglisi L. Novel lipid-lowering properties of Vaccinium myrtillus L. leaves, a traditional antidiabetic treatment, in several models of rat dyslipidaemia: a comparison with ciprofibrate. *Thromb Res* 1996;84(5):311-22.

1265 Fraisse D, Carnat A, Lamaison JL. [Polyphenolic composition of the leaf of bilberry]. [Article in French]. *Ann Pharm Fr* 1996;54(6):280-3.

1266 Kunsman GW, Levine B, Smith ML. Vitamin B2 interference with TDx drugs-of-abuse assays. *J Forensic Sci* 1998;43(6):1225-7.

1267 Personal correspondence. David Winston, Herbalist AHG. Herbal Therapeutics Inc. Research Library Washington, NJ. January 2000.

1268 Merritt JC, Crawford WJ, Alexander PC, et al. Effect of marihuana on intraocular and blood pressure in glaucoma. *Ophthalmol* 1980;87(3):222-8.

1269 Magainin Pharmaceuticals announces new research program for anti-angiogenesis agent - Squalamine - at Georgetown Univ Med Ctr. PRNewswire. www.prnewswire.com (Accessed 22 January 2000).

1270 Okada S, Rohan PJ, Miller FW, et al. Myopathies following ingestion of special nutritional products. *Arthritis Rheum* 1996;39(9):349.

1271 Zaacks SM, Klein L, Tan CD, et al. Hypersensitivity myocarditis associated with ephedra use. *J Toxicol Clin Toxicol* 1999;37(4):485-9.

1272 Powell T, Hsu FF, Turk J, Hruska K. Ma-huang strikes again: ephedrine nephrolithiasis. *Am J Kidney Dis* 1998;32(1):153-9.

1273 Nadir A, Agrawal S, King PD, Marshall JB. Acute hepatitis associated with the use of a Chinese herbal product, ma-huang. *Am J Gastroenterol* 1996;91(7):1436-8.

1274 Theoharides TC. Sudden death of a healthy college student related to ephedrine toxicity from a ma-huang containing drink. *J Clin Psychopharmacol* 1997;17(5):437-9.

1275 Vahedi K, Domingo V, Amarenco P, Bousser MG. Ischemic stroke in a sportsman who consumed MaHuang extract and creatine monohydrate for bodybuilding. *J Neurol Neurosurg Psychiatr* 2000;68:112-3.

1276 Doyle H, Kargin M. Herbal stimulant containing ephedrine has also caused psychosis. *BMJ* 1996;313(7059):756.

1277 Agri Res Svc: Dr.Duke's phytochemical and ethnobotanical databases. www.ars-grin.gov/duke (Accessed 25 January 2000).

1278 Zicam reduces length of common cold. Medscape. www.medscape.com/reuters/eline/wed/t0201-1f.html (Accessed 2 February 2000).

1279 Hussain MD, Teixeira MG. Saint John's wort and analgesia: effect of Saint John's wort on morphine induced analgesia. AAPS Ann Mtg & Expo Indianapolis,

IN:2000;Oct 29- Nov 2:presentation #3453. URL: view.abstractonline.com/aaps/abstractViewer.asp (Accessed 30 October 2000)

1280 Baur A, Harrer T, Peukert M, et al. Alpha-lipoic acid is an effective inhibitor of human immuno-deficiency virus (HIV-1) replication. *Klin Wochenschr* 1991;69(15):722-4.

1281 Ishiwa J, Sato T, Mimaki Y, et al. A citrus flavonoid, nobiletin, suppresses production and gene expression of matrix metalloproteinase 9/gelatinase B in rabbit synovial fibroblasts. *J Rheumatol* 2000;27(1):20-5.

1282 McFarland LV. Saccharomyces boulardii is not Saccharomyces cerevisiae. *Clin Infect Dis* 1996;22:200-1.

1283 Brady JA, Rock CL, Horneffer MR. Thiamin status, diuretic medications, and the management of congestive heart failure. *J Am Diet Assoc* 1995;95(5):541-4.

1284 Shimon I, Almog S, Vered Z, et al. Improved left ventricular function after thiamine supplementation in patients with congestive heart failure receiving long-term furosemide therapy. *Am J Med* 1995;98(5):485-90.

1285 Pfitzenmeyer P, Guilland JC, d'Athis P, et al. Thiamine status of elderly patients with cardiac failure including the effects of supplementattion. *Int J Vitam Nutr Res* 1994;64(2):113-8.

1286 Seligmann H, Halkin H, Rauchfleisch S, et al. Thiamine deficiency in patients with congestive heart failure receiving long-term furosemide therapy: a pilot study. *Am J Med* 1991;91(2):151-5.

1287 Schubert SY, Lansky EP, Neeman I. Antioxidant and eicosanoid enzyme inhibition properties of pomegranate seed oil and fermented juice flavonoids. *J Ethnopharmacol* 1999;66(1):11-7.

1288 Cheng TO. Ginseng-warfarin interaction. *ACC Current Journal Review* 2000;9(1):84.

1289 DiPiro JT, Talbert RL, Yee GC, et al, eds. Pharmacotherapy: A pathophysiologic approach. 4th ed. Stamford, CT: Appleton & Lange, 1999.

1290 Piscitelli SC, Burstein AH, Chaitt D, et al. Indinavir concentrations and St. John's wort. *Lancet* 2000;355(9203):547-8.

1291 Risk of drug interactions with St. John's wort and indinavir and other drugs. www.fda.gov/cder/drug/ advisory/stjwort.html (Accessed 11 February 2000).

1292 Yue QY, Bergquist C, Gerden B. Safety of St John's wort (Hypericum perforatum). *Lancet* 2000;355(9203):576-7.

1293 Ruschitzka F, Meier PJ, Turina M, et al. Acute heart transplant rejection due to Saint John's wort. *Lancet* 2000;355(9203):548-9.

1294 Southwick SM, Morgan CA III, Charney DS, High JR. Yohimbine use in a natural setting: effects on post-traumatic stress disorder. *Biol Psychiatr* 1999;46(3):442-4.

1295 Androgenic hormone improves symptoms, improves bone density in lupus. www.medscape.com/reuters/prof/ 2000/02/02.15/cl02150p.html (Accessed 15 February 2000).

1296 Roberts JE, Wang RH, Tan IP, et al. Hypericin (active ingredient in St. John's wort) photo-oxidation of lens proteins. *Photochem Photobiol* 1999;69(S):42S.

1297 Frieling UM, Schaumberg DA, Kupper TS, et al. A randomized, 12-year primary-prevention trial of beta carotene supplementation for nonmelanoma skin cancer in the physicians' health study. *Arch Dermatol* 2000;136(2):179-84.

1298 Mueller BA, Scott MK, Sowinski KM, Prag KA. Noni juice (Morinda citrifolia): hidden potential for hyperkalemia? *Am J Kidney Dis* 2000;35(2):310-2.

1299 Speetjens JK, Collins RA, Vincent JB, Woski SA. The nutritional supplement chromium(III) tris(picolinate) cleaves DNA. *Chem Res Toxicol* 1999;12(6):483-7.

1300 Weiss W, Huber G, Engel KH, et al. Identification and characterization of wheat grain albumin/globulin allergens. *Electrophoresis* 1997;18(5):826-33.

1301 Gurley BJ, Barone GW. Herb-drug interaction involving St. John's wort and cyclosporine. AAPS Ann Mtg & Expo Indianapolis, IN:2000;Oct29- Nov2: presentation #3443. URL: view.abstractonline.com/aaps/ abstractViewer.asp (Accessed 30 October 2000).

1302 Singh AK, Granley K, Misrha U, et al. Screening and confirmation of drugs in urine: interference of hordenine with the immunoassays and thin layer chromatography methods. *Forensic Sci Int* 1992; 54(1):9-22.

1303 Gurley BJ, Gardner SF, Hubbard MA. Clinical assessment of potential cytochrome P450-mediated herb-drug interactions. AAPS Ann Mtg & Expo Indianapolis, IN: 2000; Oct29- Nov2:presentation #3460.

1304 Millet Y, Jouglard J, Steinmetz MD, et al. Toxicity of some essential plant oils. Clinical and experimental study. *Clin Toxicol* 1981;18(12):1485-98.

1305 Gohla SH, Haubeck HD, Neth RD. Mitogenic activity of high molecular polysaccharide fractions isolated from the Cupressaceae Thuja occidentale L. I. Macrophage-dependent injection of CD-4-positive T-helper (Th+) lymphocytes. *Leukemia* 1988;2(8):528-33.

1306 Offergeld R, Reinecker C, Gumz E, et al. Mitogenic activity of high molecular polysaccharide fractions isolated from the cuppressaceae Thuja occidentalis L. enhanced cytokine-production by thyapolysaccharide, g-fraction (TPSg). *Leukemia* 1992;6(Suppl 3):189S-91S.

1307 Wu ZL, Chen JK, Ong T, et al. Antitransforming activity of chlorophyllin against selected carcinogens and complex mixtures. *Teratog Carcinog Mutagen* 1994;14(2):75-81.

1308 Anon. Tropicana orange juice to carry FDA-approved health claim. Reuters Health. www.medscape.com/ reuters/prof/2000/10/10.31/20001030rglt001.html (Accessed 31 October 2000).

1309 Dashwood RH, Breinholt V, Bailey GS. Chemopreventive properties of chlorophyllin: Inhibition of aflatoxin B1 (AFB1)-DNA binding in vivo and anti-mutagenic activity against AFB1 and two heterocyclic amines in the Salmonella mutagenicity assay. *Carcinogenesis* 1991;12(5):939-42.

1310 Anon. FDA approved potassium health claim notification for potassium containing foods. FDA www.cfsan.fda.gov/~dms/hclm-k.html (Accessed 1 November 2000).

1311 Sarkar D, Sharma A, Talukder G. Clastogenic activity of pure chlorophyll and anticlastogenic effects of equivalent amounts of crude extract of Indian spinach leaf and chlorophyllin following dietary supplementation to mice. *Environ Mol Mutagen*, 1996; 28(2):121-6.

1312 Amara-Mokrane YA, Lehucher-Michel MP, Balansard G, et al. Protective effects of alpha-hederin, chlorophyllin and ascorbic acid towards the induction of micronuclei by doxorubicin in cultured human lymphocytes. *Mutagenesis*, 1996; 11(2):161-7.

1313 Lewis CJ. Letter regarding dietary supplement health claim for omega-3 fatty acids and coronary heart disease.

FDA URL: vm.cfsan.fda.gov/~dms/ds-ltr11.html#let (Accessed 13 November 2000)

1314 Dai R, Shoemaker R, Farrens D, et al. Characterization of silkworm chlorophyll metabolites as an active photosensitizer for photodynamic therapy. *J Nat Prod*, 1992; 55(9):1241-51.

1315 Lee WY, Park JH, Kim BS, et al. Chlorophyll derivatives (CpD) extracted from silk worm excreta are specifically cytotoxic to tumor cells in vitro. *Yonsei Med J*, 1990; 31(3):225-33.

1316 Foerster KK, Schmid K, Rovati LC. Efficacy of glucosamine sulfate in osteoarthritis of the lumbar spine: a placebo-controlled, randomized, double-blind study. Am Coll Rheumatol 64th Ann Scientific Mtg, Philadelphia, PA: 2000;Oct 29- Nov 2:abstract 1613. www.abstracts-on-line.com/abstracts/ACR/search/ results.asp?Num=0%2E732551 (Accessed 2 November 2000).

1317 Anon. High-dose multivitamins adversely affect coronary plaque composition. Reuters Health. www.medscape.com/reuters/prof/2000/11/11.02/ 20001101clin013.html (Accessed 2 November 2000).

1318 Smith SW, Zvosec DL. Death and central nervous system depression after ingestion of 1.4-butanediol, a gamma-hydroxybutyrate-related dietary supplement. *Ann Emerg Med* 2000;36(4):S85.

1319 ORCHIC PMG (Protomorphogen). Natural Health Cod. www.nbizz.com/naturalhealthdoc/listings/184.html (Accessed 9 November 2000).

1320 Gambos J. Fooling the bladder cops: the complete drug testing guide. www.csun.edu/~hbcsc096/dt/ftbc.txt (Accessed 9 November 2000).

1321 Young RW, Beregi JS Jr. Use of chlorophyllin in the care of geriatric patients. *J Am Geriatr Soc*, 1980; 28(1):46-7.

1322 Christiansen SB, Byel SR, Stromsted H, et al. [Can chlorophyll reduce fecal odor in colostomy patients]? [Article in Danish]. *Ugeskr Laeger*, 1989; 151(27):1753-4.

1323 Nahata MC, Slencsak CA, Kamp J. Effect of chlorophyllin on urinary odor in incontinent geriatric patients. *Drug Intell Clin Pharm*, 1983;17(10):732-4.

1324 Yoshida A, Yokono O, Oda T. Therapeutic effect of chlorophyll-a in the treatment of patients with chronic pancreatitis. *Gastroenterol Jpn*, 1980; 15(1):49-61.

1325 Anon. Vitamin C Cream Improves Collagen Quality of Skin. Reuters Health. www.medscape.com/reuters/prof/ 2000/11/11.13/20001110clin020.html (Accessed 13 November 2000).

1326 Mathews-Roth MM. Carotenoids in erythropoietic protoporphyria and other photosensitivity diseases. *Ann N Y Acad Sci*, 1993; 691:127-38.

1327 Anon. Statin Plus Niacin Brings CAD Progression to A 'Standstill'. Reuters health. www.medscape.com/reuters/ prof/2000/11/11.14/20001113clin018.html (Accessed 14 November 2000).

1328 Anon. Tea may benefit blood vessels. Reuters Health. www.reutershealth.com/frame2/eline.html (Accessed 14 November 2000).

1329 Cardiovascular Benefits Claimed For Cocoa Flavonoids. www.medscape.com/reuters/prof/2000/02/02.21/ dd02210b.html (Accessed 21 February 2000).

1330 Rindone JP, Hiller D, Collacott E, et al. Randomized, controlled trial of glucosamine for treating osteoarthritis of the knee. *West J Med*, 2000;172(2):91-4.

1331 Duker EM, Kopanski L, Jarry H, Wuttke W. Effects of

extracts from Cimicifuga racemosa on gonadotropin release in menopausal women and ovariectomized rats. *Planta Med* 1991;57(5):420-4.

1332 Hamerski D, Schmitt D, Matern U. Induction of two prenyltransferases for the accumulation of coumarin phytoalexins in elicitor-treated Ammi majus cell suspension cultures. *Phytochemistry* 1990;29:1131-5.

1333 Bourinbaiar AS, Tan X, Nagorny R. Inhibitory effect of coumarins on HIV-1 replication and cell-mediated or cell-free viral transmission. *Acta Virol* 1993;37:241-50.

1334 Harvei S, Bjerve KS, Tretli S, et al. Prediagnostic level of fatty acids in serum phospholipids: omega-3 and omega-6 fatty acids and the risk of prostate cancer. *Int J Cancer* 1997;71:545-51.

1335 Giovannucci E, Leitzmann M, Spiegelman D, et al. A prospective study of physical activity and prostate cancer in male health professionals. *Cancer Res* 1998;58:5117-22.

1336 Gann PH, Hennekens CH, Sacks FM, et al. Prospective study of plasma fatty acids and risk of prostate cancer. *J Natl Cancer Inst* 1994;86:281-6.

1337 Kolonel LN, Nomura AM, Cooney RV. Dietary fat and prostate cancer: current status. *J Natl Cancer Inst* 1999;91:414-28.

1338 Okamoto M, Mitsunobu F, Ashida K, et al. Effects of perilla seed oil supplementation on leukotriene generation by leucocytes in patients with asthma associated with lipometabolism. *Int Arch Allergy Immunol* 2000;122:137-142.

1339 Burstein AH, Horton RL, Dunn T, et al. Lack of effect of St John's Wort on carbamazepine pharmacokinetics in healthy volunteers. *Clin Pharmacol Ther* 2000;68:605-2.

1340 Durr D, Stieger B, Kullak-Ublick GA, et al. St John's Wort induces intestinal P-glycoprotein/MDR1 and intestinal and hepatic CYP3A4. *Clin Pharmacol Ther* 2000;68:598-604.

1341 Jepsen S, Hansen AB. The influence of N-acetylcysteine on the measurement of prothrombin time and activated partial thromboplastin time in healthy subjects. *Scand J Clin Lab Invest* 1994;54(7):543-7.

1342 Leeb BF, Schweitzer H, Montag K, Smolen JS. A meta-analysis of chondroitin sulfate in the treatment of osteoarthritis. *J Rheumatol* 2000;27(1):205-11.

1343 Mosbech H, Muller U. Side-effects of insect venom immunotherapy: results from an EAACI multicenter study. *Allergy* 2000;55:1005-10.

1344 Yamadera W, Sasaki M, Itoh H, et al. Clinical features of circadian rhythm sleep disorders in outpatients. *Psychiatry Clin Neurosci* 1998;52(3):311-6.

1345 Okawa M, Uchiyama M, Ozaki S, et al. Circadian rhythm sleep disorders in adolescents: clinical trials of combined treatments based on chronobiology. *Psychiatry Clin Neurosci* 1998;52(5):483-90.

1346 Okawa M, Takahashi K, Egashira K, et al. Vitamin B12 treatment for delayed sleep phase syndrome: a multi-center double-blind study. *Psychiatry Clin Neurosci* 1997;51(5):275-9.

1347 Yamadera H, Takahashi K, Okawa M. A multicenter study of sleep-wake rhythm disorders: therapeutic effects of vitamin B12, bright light therapy, chronotherapy and hypnotics. *Psychiatry Clin Neurosci* 1996;50(4):203-9.

1348 Ohta T, Ando K, Iwata T, et al. Treatment of persistent sleep-wake schedule disorders in adolescents with methylcobalamin (vitamin B12). *Sleep* 1991;14(5):414-8.

1349 Mayer G, Kroger M, Meier-Ewert K. Effects of vitamin B12 on performance and circadian rhythm in normal subjects. *Neuropsychopharmacology* 1996;15(5):456-64.

1350 Reimund E. Sleep deprivation-induced dermatitis: further support of nicotinic acid depletion in sleep deprivation. *Med Hypotheses* 1991;36(4):371-3.

1351 Shad JA, Chinn CG, Brann OS. Acute hepatitis after ingestion of herbs. *South Med J* 1999;92(11):1095-7.

1352 Kugelmas M. Preliminary observation: oral zinc sulfate replacement is effective in treating muscle cramps in cirrhotic patients. *J Am Coll Nutr* 2000;19(1):13-5.

1353 Grubben MJ, Boers GH, Blom HJ, et al. Unfiltered coffee increases plasma homocysteine concentrations in healthy volunteers: a randomized trial. *Am J Clin Nutr* 2000;71(2):480-4.

1354 Watkins TR, Geller M, Kooyenga DK, Bierenbaum ML. Hypocholesterolemic and antioxidant effect of rice bran oil non-saponifiables in hypercholesterolemic subjects. *Environmental & Nutritional Interactions* 1999;3:115-22.

1355 Dwyer JH, Merz NB, Shirocre AM, et al. Progression of early atherosclerosis and intake of vitamin C and vitamin E from supplements and food. The Los Angeles Atherosclerosis Study. 41st Annual Conference on Cardiovascular Disease Epidemiology and Prevention - Abstract P77. *Circulation* 2001;103:1365d.

1356 Marijuana Use by Middle-Aged Adults Linked to Increased Risk of MI. www.medscape.com/reuters/prof/2000/03.03.03/ep03030b.html (Accessed 3 March 2000).

1357 Feigin A, Kieburtz K, Como P, et al. Assessment of coenzyme Q10 tolerability in Huntington's disease. *Mov Disord* 1996;11(3):321-3.

1358 Mullins RJ. Allergic reactions to Echinacea. *J Allergy Clin Immunol* 2000;104(1 part 2):S340-341 (Abstract 1003).

1360 McGuire JK, Kulkarni MS, Baden HP. Fatal hypermagnesemia in a child treated with megavitamin/megamineral therapy. *Pediatrics* 2000;105(2):e18 (electronic article). www.pediatrics.org/cgi/content/abstract/105/2/e18 (Accessed 8 March 2000).

1361 Blum A, Hathaway L, Mincemoyer R, et al. Effects of oral L-arginine on endothelium-dependent vasodilation and markers of inflammation in healthy postmenopausal women. *J Am Coll Cardiol* 2000;35(2):271-6.

1362 Creager MA, Gallagher SJ, Girerd XJ, et al. L-arginine improves endothelium-dependent vasodilation in hypercholesterolemic humans. *J Clin Invest* 1992;90(4):1248-53.

1363 Clarkson P, Adams MR, Powe AJ, et al. Oral L-arginine improves endothelium-dependent dilation in hypercholesterolemic young adults. *J Clin Invest* 1996;97(8):1989-94.

1364 Desser L, Rehberger A, Paukovits W. Proteolytic enzymes and amylase induce cytokine production in human peripheral blood mononuclear cells in vitro. *Cancer Biother* 1994;9:253-63.

1365 Wallace MB, Lim J, Cutler A, Bucci L. Effects of dehydroepiandrosterone vs androstenedione supplementation in men. *Med Sci Sports Exerc* 1999;31:1788-92.

1366 Phan TG, Estell J, Duggin G, et al. Lead poisoning from drinking Kombucha tea brewed in a ceramic pot. *Med J*

Aust 1998;169(11-12):644-6.

1367 Schilling BK, Stone MH, Utter A, et al. Creatine supplementation and health variables: a retrospective study. *Med Sci Sports Exerc* 2001;33:183-8.

1368 Greenhaff P. Renal dysfunction accompanying oral creatine supplements. *Lancet* 1998;352:233-4.

1369 Ferraro S, Codella C, Palumbo F, et al. Hemodynamic effects of creatine phosphate in patients with congestive heart failure: a double-blind comparison trial versus placebo. *Clin Cardiol* 1996;19:699-703.

1370 Lyon MJ, Shaw JC. Allergic Contact Dermatitis Reaction to Henna. *Arch Dermatol* 2000;136(1):124-5.

1371 Leppala JM, Virtamo J, Fogelholm R, et al. Controlled trial of alpha-tocopherol and beta-carotene supplements on stroke incidence and mortality in male smokers. *Arterioscler Thromb Vasc Biol.* 2000;20(1):230-5.

1372 Sigurjonsdottir HA, Ragnarsson J, Franzson L, Sigurdsson G. Is blood pressure commonly raised by moderate consumption of liquorice? *J Hum Hypertens,* May 1995;9(5):345-8.

1373 Baron AM, Donnerstein RL, Samson RA, et al. Hemodynamic and electrophysiologic effects of acute chocolate ingestion in young adults. *Am J Cardiol* 1999;84(3):370-3.

1374 Friedman G. Diet and the irritable bowel syndrome. *Gastroenterol Clin North Am* 1991;20(2):313-24.

1375 Blue-Green Algae Protein Is a Promising Anti-HIV Microbicide Candidate. www.medscape.com/reuters/prof/2000/03/03.16/dd03160g.html (Accessed 16 March 2000).

1376 Anderson JW, Allgood LD, Lawrence A, et al. Cholesterol-lowering effects of psyllium intake adjunctive to diet therapy in men and women with hypercholesterolemia: meta-analysis of 8 controlled trials. *Am J Clin Nutr* 2000;71(2):472-9.

1377 Lee A, Minhas R, Ito S, et al. Safety of St. John's wort during breastfeeding. *Clin Pharmacol Ther* 2000;67(2):130 (abstract PII-64).

1378 Roots I, Johne A, Schmider, Brockmoller J, et al. Interaction of a herbal extract from St. John's wort with amitriptyline and its metabolites. *Clin Pharmacol Ther* 2000;67(2):159 (abstract PIII-69).

1379 Carson SW, Hill-Zabala CE, Roberts SH, Hawke RL. Inhibitory effect of methanolic solution of St. John's wort (hypericum perforatum) on cytochrome p450 3A4 activity in human liver microsomes. *Clin Pharmacol Ther* 2000;67(2):99 (abstract PI-39).

1380 For Dieter, Nearly the Ultimate Loss. www.washingtonpost.com/wp-dyn/articles/A33421-2000Mar17.html (Accessed 19 March 2000).

1381 FDA Takes Aim at Ephedra. www.washingtonpost.com/wp-dyn/articles/A33439-2000Mar17.html (Accessed 19 March 2000).

1382 Dallas S, Stempak D, Koren G, et al. Whey protein concentrate (WPC) modulation of lymphocyte glutathione levels in vitro. *Clin Pharmacol Ther* 2000;67(2):156 (abstract PIII-56).

1383 Offman EM, Freeman DJ, Dresser GK, et al. Cisapride interaction with grapefruit juice and red wine. *Clin Pharmacol Ther* 2000;67(2):110 (abstract PI-83).

1384 Tsunoda SM, Christians U, Velez RL, et al. Red wine (RW) effects on cyclosporine (CyA) metabolites. *Clin Pharmacol Ther,* 2000;67(2):150 (abstract PIII-35).

1385 Bertino JS, Demuro RL, Blask DE, et al. Absolute bioavailability (F) of oral melatonin (M). *Clin*

1386 Veronese M, Burke J, Dorval E, et al. Grapefruit juice (GFJ) inhibits hepatic and intestinal CYP3A4 dose-dependently. *Clin Pharmacol Ther* 2000;67(2):151 (abstract PIII-37).

1387 Tsunoda SM, Harris RZ, Velez RL, et al. Red wine (RW) effects on cyclosporine (CyA) Pharmacokinetics. *Clin Pharmacol Ther,* 1998;65(2):159 (abstract PII-51).

1388 Bailey DG, Dresser GK, Kreeft JH, et al. Grapefruit juice-felodipine interaction: Effect of segments and an extract from unprocessed fruit. *Clin Pharmacol Ther* 2000;67(2):107 (abstract PI-71).

1389 Frye RF, Kroboth PD, Folan MM, et al. Effect of DHEA on CYP3A-mediated metabolism of triazolam. *Clin Pharmacol Ther* 2000;67(2):109 (abstract PI-82).

1390 Soldner A, Christians U, Susanto M, et al. Grapefruit juice exerts stimulatory effects on p-glycoprotein. *Clin Pharmacol Ther* 1998;65(2): (abstract OIII-B-4).

1391 Zaidenstein R, Avni B, Dishi V, et al. Effect of grapefruit juice on the pharmacokinetics of losartan in healthy volunteers. *Clin Pharmacol Ther,* 1998;65(2): (abstract PI-60).

1392 Dresser GK, Bailey DG, Carruthers SG. Grapefruit juice-felodipine interaction in healthy seniors. *Clin Pharmacol Ther* 1998;65(2): (abstract PIII-63).

1393 Martin KJ, Chen SF, Clark GM, et al. Evaluation of creatine analogues as a new class of anticancer agents using freshly explanted human tumor cells. *J Natl Cancer Inst* 1994;86:608-13.

1394 John Mendelson J, Tolliver B, Delucchi K, Berger P. Capsaicin increases the lethality of cocaine. *Clin Pharmacol Ther,* 1998;65(2): (abstract PII-27).

1395 Johnson MA, Robin P, Smith RP, Morrisona D, et al. Large lung bullae in marijuana smokers. *Thorax,* 2000;55(4):340-2.

1396 Sandor PS, Afra J, Ambrosini A, Schoenen J. Prophylactic treatment of migraine with beta-blockers and riboflavin: differential effects on the intensity dependence of auditory evoked cortical potentials. *Headache,* 2000;40:30-5.

1397 Schoenen J, Lenaerts M, Bastings E. High-dose riboflavin as a prophylactic treatment of migraine: results of an open pilot study. *Cephalalgia,* 1994;14(5):328-9.

1398 Schoenen J, Jacquy J, Lenaerts M. Effectiveness of high-dose riboflavin in migraine prophylaxis. A randomized controlled trial. *Neurology* 1998;50(2):466-70.

1399 Synthetic DHEA enhances post-burn skin graft re-epithelialization rate. www.medscape.com/reuters/prof/2000/03/03.27/cl03270m.html (Accessed 27 March 2000).

1400 Natural Health Consultants. Transfer Factor. http://www.naturalhealthconsult.com/Monographs/TF.html (Accessed 15 November 2000).

1401 Jardim LB, Palma-Dias R, Silva LC, et al. Maternal hyperphenylalaninaemia as a cause of microcephaly and mental retardation. *Acta Paediatr* 1996;85(8):943-6.

1402 Rouse B, Azen C, Koch R, et al. Maternal phenylketonuria collaborative Study (MPKUCS) offspring: facial anomalies, malformations, and early neurological sequelae. *Am J Med Genet,* 1997;69:89-95.

1403 Sternberg EM, Van Woert MH, Young SN, et al. Development of a scleroderma-like illness during therapy with L-5-hydroxytryptophan and carbidopa. *N*

REFERENCES

Engl J Med 1980;303:782-7.

1404 Joly P, Lampert A, Thomine E, et al. Development of pseudobullous morphea and scleroderma-like illness during therapy with L-5-hydroxytryptophan and carbidopa. *J Am Acad Dermatol* 1991;25(2 Pt 1):332-3.

1405 Anderson JW, Allgood LD, Turner J, et al. Effects of psyllium on glucose and serum lipid responses in men with type 2 diabetes and hypercholesterolemia. *Am J Clin Nutr* 1999;70:466-73.

1406 Miller EE, Evans AE, Cohn M. Inhibition of rate of tumor growth by creatine and cyclocreatine. *Proc Natl Acad Sci U S A* 1993;90:3304-8.

1407 O'Brien PM, Pipkin FB. The effect of essential fatty acid and specific vitamin supplements on vascular sensitivity in the mid trimester of human pregnancy. *Clin Exp Hypertens B* 1983;2:247-54.

1408 O'Brien PM, Morrison R, Pipken FB. Effect of dietary supplementation with linoleic and gammalinolenic acids on the pressor response to angiotensin II—possible role in pregnancy induced hypertension? *Br J Clin Pharmacol* 1985;19:335-42.

1409 Laivuori H, Hovatta O, Viinikka L, et al. Dietary supplementation with primrose oil or fish oil does not change urinary excretion of prostacyclin and thromboxane metabolites in pre-eclamptic women. *Prostaglandins Leukot Essent Fatty Acids* 1993;49:691-4.

1410 Ritchie DJ, Becker ES. Update on the management of intestinal cryptosporidiosis in AIDS. *Ann Pharmacother* 1994;28:767-78.

1411 Dove D, Johnson P. Oral evening primrose oil: its effect on length of pregnancy and selected intrapartum outcomes in low-risk nulliparous women. *J Nurse Midwifery* 1999;44:320-4.

1412 Brinkeborn RM, Shah DV, Degenring FH. Echinaforce and other Echinacea fresh plant preparations in the treatment of the common cold. A randomized, placebo controlled, double-blind clinical trial. *Phytomedicine* 1999;6:1-6.

1413 Mengs U, Clare CB, Poiley JA. Toxicity of Echinacea purpurea. Acute, subacute and genotoxicity studies. *Arzneimittelforschung* 1991;41:1076-81.

1414 Awang DVC, Kindack DG. Echinacea. *Can Pharm J* November 1999:512-6.

1415 D'Avanzo B, La Vecchia C, Franceschi S, et al. Coffee consumption and bladder cancer risk. *Eur J Cancer* 1992;28A(8-9):1480-4.

1416 Pannelli F, La Rosa F, Saltalamacchia G, et al. Tobacco smoking, coffee, cocoa and tea consumption in relation to mortality from urinary bladder cancer in Italy. *Eur J Epidemiol* 1989;5(6):392-7.

1417 Slattery ML, West DW, Robison LM. Fluid intake and bladder cancer in Utah. *Int J Cancer* 1988;42(1):17-22.

1418 Joseph JA, Shukitt-Hale B, Denisova NA, et al. Long-term dietary strawberry, spinach, or vitamin E supplementation retards the onset of age-related neuronal signal-transduction and cognitive behavioral deficits. *J Neurosci* 1998;18(19):8047-55.

1419 Joseph JA, Shukitt-Hale B, Denisova NA, et al. Reversals of age-related declines in neuronal signal transduction, cognitive, and motor behavioral deficits with blueberry, spinach, or strawberry dietary supplementation. *J Neurosci* 1999;19(18):8114-21.

1420 Chng HH, Shaw D, Klesius P, Saxon A. Inability of oral bovine transfer factor to eradicate cryptosporidial infection in a patient with congenital dysgammaglobulinemia. *Clin Immunol Immunopathol* 1989;50:402-6.

1421 Gebhardt R. Hepatoprotection with artichoke extract. *Pharm Ztg* 1995;140:34-7.

1422 Gebhardt R. Antioxidative and protective properties of extracts from leaves of the artichoke (Cynara scolymus L.) against hydroperoxide-induced oxidative stress in cultured rat hepatocytes. *Toxicol Appl Pharmacol* 1997;144:279-86.

1423 Hammerl WH, Kindler K, Kranzl C, et al. Effect of cynarin (cynarine) on hyperlipidemia, especially on hypercholesterolemia. *Wien Med Wochenschr* 1973;123:601-5.

1424 Heckers H, Dittmar K, Schmahl FW, et al. Inefficiency of cynarin as therapeutic regimen in familial type II hyperlipoproteinaemia. *Atherosclerosis* 1977;26:249-53.

1425 Gebhardt R. Inhibition of cholesterol biosynthesis in primary cultured rat hepatocytes by artichoke (Cynara scolymus L.) extracts. *J Pharmacol Exp Therap* 1998;386:1122-8.

1426 Brown JE, Rice-Evans CA. Luteolin-rich artichoke extract protects low density lipoprotein from oxidation in vitro. *Free Radic Res* 1998;29:247-55.

1427 Vogler BK, Pittler MH, Ernst E. The efficacy of ginseng. A systemic review of randomized clinical trials. *Eur J Clin Pharmacol* 1999;55:567-75.

1428 Osato MS, Reddy SG, Graham DY. Osmotic effect of honey on growth and viability of Helicobacter pylori. *Dig Dis Sci* 1999;44(3):462-4.

1429 Leonetti HB, Longo S, Anasti JN. Transdermal progesterone cream for vasomotor symptoms and postmenopausal bone loss. *Obstet Gynecol,* 1999;94:225-8.

1430 Anon. Adverse events associated with ingestion of gamma-butyrolactone—Minnesota, New Mexico, and Texas, 1998-1999. *MMWR Morb Mortal Wkly Rep* 1999;48(7):137-40.

1431 Harrington RD, Woodward JA, Hooton TM, et al. Life-threatening interactions between HIV-1 protease inhibitors and the illicit drugs MDMA and gamma-hydroxybutyrate. *Arch Intern Med* 1999;159:2221-4.

1432 Bergnes G, Yuan W, Khandekar VS, et al. Creatine and phosphocreatine analogs: anticancer activity and enzymatic analysis. *Oncol Res* 1996;8:121-30.

1433 Ellaway CM, Williams K, Leonard H, et al. Rett syndrome: randomized controlled trial of L-carnitine. *J Child Neurol,* 1999;14:162-7.

1434 Brevetti G, Diehm C, Lambert D, et al. European multicenter study on propionyl-L-carnitine in intermittent claudication. *J Am Coll Cardiol,* 1999;34:1618-24.

1435 Brevetti G, Perna S, Sabba C, et al. Propionyl-L-carnitine in intermittent claudication: double-blind, placebo-controlled, dose titration, multicenter study. *J Am Coll Cardiol,* 1995;26:1411-6.

1436 Brevetti G, Perna S, Sabba C, et al. Effect of propionyl-L-carnitine on quality of life in intermittent claudication. *Am J Cardiol,* 1997;79:777-80.

1437 Brevetti G, Perna S, Sabba C, et al. Superiority of L-propionylcarnitine vs L-carnitine in improving walking capacity in patients with peripheral vascular disease: an acute, intravenous, double-blind, cross-over study. *Eur Heart J,* 1992;13(2):251-5.

1438 Ishikura H, Matsuo N, Matsubara M, et al. Valproic acid overdose and L-carnitine therapy. *J Anal Toxicol* 1996;20(1):55-58.

1439 Siliprandi N, Di Lisa F, Menabo R. Propionyl-L-carnitine: biochemical significance and possible role in cardiac metabolism. *Cardiovasc Drugs Ther,* 1991;5 Suppl 1:11-5.

1440 Tribble DL. AHA Science Advisory. Antioxidant consumption and risk of coronary heart disease: emphasis on vitamin C, vitamin E, and beta-carotene: A statement for healthcare professionals from the American Heart Association. *Circulation* 1999;99:591-5.

1441 Watanabe H, Masaaki K, Ohtsuka S, et al. Randomized, double-blind, placebo-controlled study of the preventative effect of supplemental oral vitamin C on attenuation of development of nitrate tolerance. *J Am Coll Cardiol* 1998;31:1323-9.

1442 Tao X, Davis LS, Lipsky PE. Effect of an extract of the Chinese herbal remedy Tripterygium wilfordii Hook F on human immune responsiveness. *Arthritis Rheum* 1991;34:1274-81.

1443 Cohen HA, Neuman I, Nahum H. Blocking effect of vitamin C in exercise-induced asthma. *Arch Pediatr Adolesc Med* 1997;151(32):103-9.

1444 Zhang S, Hunter DJ, Forman MR, et al. Dietary carotenoids and vitamins A, C, and E and risk of breast cancer. *J Natl Cancer Inst* 1999;91(6):547-56.

1445 Louie E, Borkowsky W, Klesius PH, et al. Treatment of cryptosporidiosis with oral bovine transfer factor. *Clin Immunol Immunopathol* 1987;44:329-34.

1446 Klipstein-Grobusch K, Launer LJ, Geleijnse JM, et al. Serum carotenoids and atherosclerosis. The Rotterdam Study. *Atherosclerosis* 2000;148:49-56.

1447 Gann PH, Ma J, Giovannucci E, et al. Lower prostate cancer risk in men with elevated plasma lycopene levels: results of a prospective analysis. *Cancer Res* 1999;59:1225-30.

1448 Lee IM, Cook NR, Manson JE, et al. Beta-carotene supplementation and incidence of cancer and cardiovascular disease: the Women's Health Study. *J Natl Cancer Inst* 1999;91(24):2102-6.

1449 Ascherio A, Rimm EB, Hernan MA, et al. Relation of consumption of vitamin E, vitamin C, and carotenoids to risk for stroke among men in the United States. *Ann Intern Med,* 1999;130:963-70.

1450 Caffeine Content of Foods and Drugs. Center for Science in the Public Interest www.cspinet.org/new/cafchart.htm (Accessed 9 December 1999).

1451 Wakabayashi K, Kono S, Shinchi K, et al. Habitual coffee consumption and blood pressure: A study of self-defense officials in Japan. *Eur J Epidemiol* 1998;14(7):669-73.

1452 Hodgson JM, Puddey IB, Burke V, et al. Effects on blood pressure of drinking green and black tea. *J Hypertens* 1999;17(4):457-63.

1453 Dulloo AG, Duret C, Rohrer D, et al. Efficacy of a green tea extract rich in catechin polyphenols and caffeine in increasing 24-h energy expenditure and fat oxidation in humans. *Am J Clin Nutr* 1999;70:1040-5.

1454 Garbisa S, Biggin S, Cavallarin N, et al. Tumor invasion: molecular shears blunted by green tea. *Nat Med* 1999;5:1216.

1455 Cao Y, Cao R. Angiogenesis inhibited by drinking tea. *Nature* 1999;398:381.

1456 L'Allemain G. [Multiple actions of EGCG, the main component of green tea]. [Article in French] *Bull Cancer* 1999;86:721-4.

1457 Bushman JL. Green tea and cancer in humans: a review of the literature. *Nutr Cancer* 1998;31(3):151-9.

1458 Wakai K, Ohno Y, Obata K. Prognostic significance of selected lifestyle factors in urinary bladder cancer. *Jpn J Cancer Res* 1993;84(12):1223-9.

1459 Ohno Y, Aoki K, Obata K, et al. Case-control study of urinary bladder cancer in metropolitan Nagoya. *Natl Cancer Inst Monogr* 1985;69:229-34.

1460 Booth SL, Madabushi HT, Davidson KW, et al. Tea and coffee brews are not dietary sources of vitamin K-1 (phylloquinone). *J Am Diet Assoc* 1995;95:82-3.

1461 Lou FQ, Zhang MF, Zhang XG, et al. A study on tea-pigment in prevention of atherosclerosis. *Chin Med J (Engl)* 1989;102:579-83.

1462 Ali M, Afzal M. A potent inhibitor of thrombin stimulated platelet thromboxane formation from unprocessed tea. *Prostaglandins Leukot Med* 1987;27:9-13.

1463 Graham HN. Green tea composition, consumption, and polyphenol chemistry. *Prev Med* 1992;21:334-50.

1464 Shankar AH, Genton B, Semba RD, et al. Effect of vitamin A supplementation on morbidity due to Plasmodium falciparum in young children in Papua New Guinea: a randomised trial. *Lancet* 1999;354(9174):203-9.

1465 Fawzi WW, Mbise RL, Hertzmark E, et al. A randomized trial of vitamin A supplements in relation to mortality among human immunodeficiency virus-infected and uninfected children in Tanzania. *Pediatr Infect Dis J* 1999;18(2):127-33.

1466 Fawzi WW, Mbise RL, Fataki MR, et al. Vitamin A supplementation and severity of pneumonia in children admitted to the hospital in Dar es Salaam, Tanzania. *Am J Clin Nutr* 1998;68(1):187-92.

1467 Kowalski TE, Falestiny M, Furth E, Malet PF. Vitamin A hepatotoxicity: a cautionary note regarding 25,000 IU supplements. *Am J Med* 1994;97(6):523-8.

1468 Wang Z, Boudjelal M, Kang S, et al. Ultraviolet irradiation of human skin causes functional vitamin A deficiency, preventable by all-trans retinoic acid pre-treatment. *Nat Med* 1999;5(4):418-22.

1469 Meyers DG, Maloley PA, Weeks D. Safety of antioxidant vitamins. *Arch Intern Med* 1996;156(9):925-35.

1470 Cooper DA, Eldridge AL, Peters JC. Dietary carotenoids and certain cancers, heart disease, and age-related macular degeneration: a review of recent research. *Nutr Rev* 1999;57(7):201-14.

1471 Cooper DA, Eldridge AL, Peters JC. Dietary carotenoids and lung cancer: a review of recent research. *Nutr Rev* 1999;57(5 Pt 1):133-45.

1472 Garewal HS, Katz RV, Meyskens F, et al. Beta-carotene produces sustained remissions in patients with oral leukoplakia: results of a multicenter prospective trial. *Arch Otolaryngol Head Neck Surg* 1999;125(12):1305-10.

1473 Cook NR, Stampfer MJ, Ma J, et al. Beta-carotene supplementation for patients with low baseline levels and decreased risks of total and prostate carcinoma. *Cancer* 1999;86(9):1783-92.

1474 Neuman I, Nahum H, Ben-Amotz A. Prevention of exercise-induced asthma by a natural isomer mixture of beta-carotene. *Ann Allergy Asthma Immunol* 1999;82(6):549-53.

1475 Radosevich JK, Scott GH, Olson GB. Delayed-type hypersensitivity responses induced by bovine colostral components. *Am J Vet Res* 1985;46:875-8.

1476 Sharma MK, Foroozanfar N, Ala FA. Progressive BCG infection in an immunodeficient child treated with transfer factor. *Clin Immunol Immunopathol* 1978;10:369-80.

1477 Klesius PH, Fudenberg HH. Bovine transfer factor: in vivo transfer of cell-mediated immunity to cattle with alcohol precipitates. *Clin Immunol Immunopathol* 1977;8:238-46.

1478 Klesius PH, Qualls DF, Elston AL, Fudenberg HH. Effects of bovine transfer factor (TFd) in mouse coccidiosis (Eimeria ferrisi). *Clin Immunol Immunopathol* 1978;10:214-21.

1479 Devaraj S, Jialal I. Alpha-tocopherol decreases interleukin-1 beta release from activated human monocytes by inhibition of 5-lipoxygenase. *Arterioscler Thromb Vasc Biol* 1999;19(4):1125-33.

1480 McMeeking A, Borkowsky W, Klesius PH, et al. A controlled trial of bovine dialyzable leukocyte extract for cryptosporidiosis in patients with AIDS. *J Infect Dis* 1990;161:108-12.

1481 Lillie JW, O'Keefe M, Valinski H, et al. Cyclocreatine (1-carboxymethyl-2-iminoimidazolidine) inhibits growth of a broad spectrum of cancer cells derived from solid tumors. *Cancer Res* 1993;53:3172-3178.

1482 Houston DK, Johnson MA, Nozza RJ, et al. Age-related hearing loss, vitamin B-12, and folate in elderly women. *Am J Clin Nutr* 1999;69(3):564-71.

1483 Selhub J, Jacques PF, Wilson PW, et al. Vitamin status and intake as primary determinants of homocysteinemia in an elderly population. *JAMA* 1993;270(22):2693-8.

1484 Carmel R, Green R, Jacobsen DW, et al. Serum cobalamin, homocysteine, and methylmalonic acid concentrations in a multiethnic elderly population: ethnic and sex differences in cobalamin and metabolite abnormalities. *Am J Clin Nutr* 1999;70(5):904-10.

1485 Stabler SP, Allen RH, Fried LP, et al. Racial differences in prevalence of cobalamin and folate deficiencies in disabled elderly women. *Am J Clin Nutr* 1999;70(5):911-9.

1486 Laser Reutersward A, Skog K, Jagerstad M. Mutagenicity of pan-fried bovine tissues in relation to their content of creatine, creatinine, monosaccharides and free amino acids. *Food Chem Toxicol* 1987;25:755-762.

1487 Manabe S, Kurihara N, Wada O, et al. Formation of PhIP in a mixture of creatinine, phenylalanine and sugar or aldehyde by aqueous heating. *Carcinogenesis* 1992;13:827-830.

1488 Liu C, Russell RM, Seitz HK, et al. Ethanol enhances retinoic acid metabolism into polar metabolites in rat liver via induction of cytochrome P4502E1. *Gastroenterol* 2001;120:179-89.

1489 Bostom AG, Gohh RY, Beaulieu AJ, et al. Treatment of hyperhomocysteinemia in renal transplant recipients. A randomized, placebo-controlled trial. *Ann Intern Med* 1997;127(12):1089-92.

1492 Klipstein-Grobusch K, Grobbee DE, den Breeijen JH, et al. Dietary iron and risk of myocardial infarction in the Rottersam Study. *Am J Epidemiol* 1999;149:421-8.

1493 Kirkpatrick CH. Structural nature and functions of transfer factors. *Ann N Y Acad Sci* 1993;685:362-8.

1494 Kirkpatrick CH. Biological response modifiers. Interferons, interleukins, and transfer factor. *Ann Allergy* 1989;62:170-6.

1495 Hassner A, Adelman DC. Biologic response modifiers in primary immunodeficiency disorders. *Ann Intern Med* 1991;115:294-307.

1496 Clinton SK, Emenhiser C, Schwartz SJ, et al. Cis-trans lycopene isomers, carotenoids, and retinol in the human prostate. *Cancer Epidemiol Biomarkers Prev* 1996;5(10):823-33.

1497 Gartner C, Stahl W, Sies H. Lycopene is more bioavaiable from tomato paste than from fresh tomatoes. *Am J Clin Nutr,* 1997;66(1):116-22.

1498 Paetau I, Khachik F, Brown ED, et al. Chronic ingestion of lycopene-rich tomato juice or lycopene supplements significantly increases plasma concentrations of lycopene and related tomato carotenoids in humans. *Am J Clin Nutr* 1998;68(6):1187-95.

1499 USDA Cartenoids chart. www.nal.usda.gov/fnic/ foodcomp/Data/car98/car_tble.pdf1499 (Accessed 20 January 2000).

1500 Rueff F, Schoepf P, Pfuetzner W, Przybilla B. Sensitization to condurango bark is frequent in patients with allergy to natural rubber latex. *J Allergy Clin Immunol,* 1998; 101(1 Pt 2):S207.

1501 Pfutzner W, Thomas P, Rueff F, Przybilla B. Anaphylactic reaction elicited by condurango bark in a patient allergic to natural rubber latex. *J Allergy Clin Immunol,* 1998; 101(2 Pt 1):281-2.

1502 Medicinal Plants. Springer Verlag: Lavoisier, NY, 1995.

1503 Reichert R. Sedative Effects of California Poppy and Corydalis. *Quarterly Review of Natural Medicine,* Winter 1996:256.

1504 Brown D, Gaby A, Reichert R. *Quarterly Review of Natural Medicine,* Winter 1997:337.

1505 Trivedi CP, et al. Bronchodilator and anti-inflammatory effect of glycosidal fraction of Acacia farnesiana. *Indian J Physiol Pharmacol,* 1986; 30(3):267-8.

1506 Leung A. Better Health with (Mostly) Chinese Herbs and Foods. AYSL, Glen Rock, NJ, 1995.

1507 Fudenberg HH. Transfer factor: past, present and future. *Annu Rev Pharmacol Toxicol* 1989;29:475-516.

1508 Zhang H, et al. [Preliminary study of traditional Chinese medicine treatment of minimal brain dysfunction: analysis of 100 cases]. [Article in Chinese].*Chung Hsi I Chieh Ho Tsa Chih* 1990 May;10(5):278-9, 260.

1509 Zneg XL, et al. [Immunological and hematopoietic effect of Codonopsis pilosula on cancer patients during radiotherapy]. [Article in Chinese] *Chung Kuo Chung Hsi I Chieh Ho Tsa Chih* 1992 Oct;12(10):607-8, 581.

1510 O'Brien LW. Interactions and Toxicities of Drugs for HIV Disease. *Arch Intern Med,* 1991;151:2281-8.

1512 Anon. In vitro screening of traditional medicines for anti-HIV activity: memorandum from a WHO meeting. *Bull World Health Organ* 1989;67(6):613-8.

1513 Zhu SC. [Clinical observations on 36 cases of viral myocarditis treated with Epimedium grandiflorum Moor and vitamin C]. [Article in Chinese]. *Chung Hsi I Chieh Ho Tsa Chih* 1984 Sep;4(9):523-4, 514.

1514 Le Bars PL, et al. A placebo-controlled, double-blind, randomized trial of an extract of Ginkgo biloba for dementia. North American EGb Study Group. *JAMA* 1997 Oct 22; 278:1327-32.

1515 Oken BS, et al. The efficacy of Ginkgo biloba on cognitive function in Alzheimer disease. *Arch Neurol.* 1998 Nov;55(11):1409-15.

1516 Akhtar MS, et al. Field trial of Saussurea lappa roots against nematodes and Nigella sativa seeds against cestodes in children. *JPMA J Pak Med Assoc* 1991 Aug;41(8)185-7.

1517 Froohlich HH, et al. [Physical investigations into the thermotherapeutic action of the Kneipp hay flower sack].[Article in German] *MMW Munch Med Wochenschr* 1975 Mar 14; 117(11):443-8.

1518 Frohlich HH, et al. [The sedative effect of the Kneipp hay sack and balneological preparations of hay (author's translation)]. [Article in German] *MMW Munch Med Wochenschr* 1976 Mar 12;118(11):317-20.

1519 Tona L, et al. Antiamoebic and phytochemical screening of some Congolese medicinal plants. *J Ethnopharmacol* 1998 May, 61(1):57-65.

1520 Houpt JB, McMillan R, Wein C, Paget-Dellio SD. Effect of glucosamine hydrochloride in the treatment of pain of osteoarthritis of the knee. *J Rheumatol* 1999;26:2423-30.

1522 Park HJ, et al. Effects of dietary supplementation of lipophilic fraction from Panax ginseng on cGMP and cAMP in rat platelets and on blood coagulation. *Biol Pharm Bull.* 1996 Nov;19(11):1434-9.

1523 Lin RC, et al. Effects of isoflavones on alcohol pharmacokinetics and alcohol-drinking behavior in rats. *Am J Clin Nutr* 1998 Dec;68(6 Suppl):1512S-5S.

1524 Xie CI, et al. Daidzin, an antioxidant isoflavonoid, decreases blood alcohol levels and shortens sleep time induced by ethanol intoxication. *Alcohol Clin Exp Res* 1994 Dec;18(6):1443-7.

1525 Avalos J, et al. Guinea pig maximization test of the bark extract from pawpaw, Asimina triloba (Annonaceae). *Contact Dermatitis* 1993 Jul;29(1):33-5.

1526 Tomoda M, et al. Plant mucilages. XLII. An anti-complementary mucilage from the leaves of Malva sylvestris var. mauritiana. *Chem Pharm Bull (Tokyo)* 1989 Nov;37(11):3029-32.

1527 Stefanova Z, et al. Effect of a total extract from Fraxinus ornus stem bark and esculin on zymosan- and carrageenan-induced paw oedema in mice. *J Ethnopharmacol* 1995 May;46(2):101-6.

1528 Pintos J, et al. Mate, coffee, and tea consumption and risk of cancers of the upper aerodigestive tract in southern Brazil. *Epidemiology* 1994 Nov;5(6):583-90.

1529 De Stefani E, et al. Meat intake, 'mate' drinking and renal cell cancer in Uruguay: a case-control study. *Br J Cancer* 1998 Nov;78(9):1239-43.

1530 De Stefani E, et al. Black tobacco, mate, and bladder cancer. A case-control study from Uruguay. *Cancer* 1991 Jan 15;67(2):536-40.

1531 De Stefani E, et al. Mate drinking and risk of lung cancer in males: a case-control study from Uruguay. *Cancer Epidemiol Biomarkers Prev* 1996 Jul;5(7):515-9.

1532 Kong YC, et al. Isolation of the uterotonic principle from Leonurus artemisia, the Chinese motherwort. *Am J Chin Med* 1976 WINTER;4(4):373-82.

1533 Zou QZ, et al. Effect of motherwort on blood hyperviscosity. *Am J Chin Med* 1989;17(1-2):65-70.

1534 Zgorniak-Nowosielska I, et al. Antiviral activity of Flos verbasci infusion against influenza and Herpes simplex viruses. *Arch Immunol Ther Exp (Warsz)* 1991;39(1-2):103-8.

1535 al-Harbi MM, et al. Gastric antiulcer and cytoprotective effect of Commiphora molmol in rats. *J Ethnopharmacol* 1997 Jan;55(2):141-50.

1536 al-Harbi MM, et al. Anticarcinogenic effect of Commiphora molmol on solid tumors induced by Ehrlich carcinoma cells in mice. *Chemotherapy* 1994 Sep-Oct;40(5):337-47.

1537 Pintao AM, et al. In vitro and in vivo antitumor activity of benzyl isothiocyanate: a natural product from Tropaeolum majus. *Planta Med* 1995 Jun;61(3):233-6.

1538 Buck DS, et al. Comparison of two topical preparations for the treatment of onychomycosis: Melaleuca alternifolia (tea tree) oil and clotrimazole. *J Fam Pract* 1994 Jun;38(6):601-5.

1539 De Rosa SC, Zaretsky MD, Dubs JG, et al. N-acetylcysteine replenishes glutathione in HIV infection. *Eur J Clin Invest* 2000;30:915-29.

1540 Cherif S, et al. [A clinical trial of a titrated Olea extract in the treatment of essential arterial hypertension]. *J Pharm Belg* 1996 Mar-Apr;51(2):69-71.

1541 Aziz NH, et al. Comparative antibacterial and antifungal effects of some phenolic compounds. *Microbios* 1998;93(374):43-54.

1542 Pieroni A, et al. In vitro anti-complementary activity of flavonoids from olive (Olea europaea L.) leaves. *Pharmazie* 1996 Oct;51(10):765-8.

1543 Liccardi G, et al. Oleaceae pollinosis: a review. *Int Arch Allergy Immunol* 1996 Nov;111(3):210-7.

1544 Holti G. An experimentally controlled evaluation of the effect of inositol nicotinate upon the digital blood flow in patients with Raynaud's phenomenon. *J Int Med Res* 1979;7(6):473-83.

1545 Ring EF, Bacon PA. Quantitative thermographic assessment of inositol nicotinate therapy in Raynaud's phenomena. *J Int Med Res* 1977;5(4):217-22.

1546 Wilke H, Frahm H. [Treatment of hyperlipoproteinaemia types IIa, IIb, IV and V with a combination of clofibrate and inositol nicotinate]. [Article in German]. *Dtsch Med Wochenschr* 1976;101(11):401-5.

1547 Anon. Alpha-lipoic acid. *Altern Med Rev* 1998;3(4):308-10.

1548 Berkson BM. Thioctic acid in treatment of hepatotoxic mushroom (Phalloides) poisoning [Letter]. *N Engl J Med* 1979;300(7):371.

1549 Roldan EJ, Perez Lloret A. Thioctic acid in Amanita poisoning (letter). *Crit Care Med* 1986;14(8):753-4.

1550 Biewenga GP, Haenen GR, Bast A. The pharmacology of the antioxidant lipoic acid. *Gen Pharmacol* 1997;29(3):315-31.

1551 Filina AA, Davydova NG, Endrikhovskii SN, Shamshinova AM. [Lipoic acid as a means of metabolic therapy of open-angle glaucoma]. [Article in Russian]. *Vestn Oftalmol* 1995;111(4):6-8.

1552 Filina AA, Davydova NG, Kolomoitseva EM. [The effect of lipoic acid on the components of the glutathione system in the lacrimal fluid of patients with open angle glaucoma]. [Article in Russian]. *Vestn Oftalmol* 1993;109(5):5-7.

1554 Matalon R, Stumpf DA, Michals K, et al. Lipoamide dehydrogenase deficiency with primary lactic acidosis: favorable response to treatment with oral lipoic acid. *J Pediatr* 1984;104:65-9.

1555 Yoshida I, Sweetman L, Kulovich S, et al. Effect of lipoic acid in patient with defective activity of pyruvate dehydrogenase, 2-oxoglutarate dehydrogenase, and branched-chain keto acid dehydrogenase. *Pediatr Res* 1990;27:75-9.

REFERENCES

1556   Dana Consortium on the therapy of HIV dementia and related cognitive disorders. A randomized, double-blind, placebo-controlled trial of deprenyl and thioctic acid in human immunodeficiency virus-associated cognitive impairment. *Neurology* 1998;50:645-51.

1557   Maesaka H, Komiya K, Misugi K, Tada K. Hyperalaninemia hyperpyruvicemia and lactic acidosis due to pyruvate carboxylase deficiency of the liver; treatment with thiamine and lipoic acid. *Eur J Pediatr* 1976;122(2):159-68.

1561   Packer L, Tritschler HJ, Wessel K. Neuroprotection by the metabolic antioxidant alpha-lipoic acid. *Free Radic Biol Med* 1997;22(1-2):359-78.

1562   Merin JP, Matsuyama M, Kira T, et al. Alpha-lipoic acid blocks HIV-1 LTR-dependent expression of hygromycin resistance in THP-1 stable transformants. *FEBS Lett* 1996;394(1):9-13.

1563   Suzuki YJ, Aggarwal BB, Packer L. Alpha-lipoic acid is a potent inhibitor of NF-kappa B activation in human T cells. *Biochem Biophys Res Commun* 1992;189(3):1709-15.

1570   The Natural Pharmacist. Lipoic acid. www.tnp.com/substance.asp?ID=149. (Accessed 17 February 2000).

1571   Chiddo A, Gaglione A, Musci S, et al. Hemodynamic study of intravenous propionyl-L-carnitine in patients with ischemic heart disease and normal left ventricular function. *Cardiovasc Drugs Ther,* 1991;5 Suppl 1:107-11.

1572   Bartels GL, Remme WJ, Pillay M, et al. Acute improvement of cardiac function with intravenous L-propionylcarnitine in humans. *J Cardiovasc Pharmacol,* 1992;20(1):157-64.

1573   Bartels GL, Remme WJ, Pillay M, et al. Effects of L-propionylcarnitine on ischemia-induced myocardial dysfunction in men with angina pectoris. *Am J Cardiol,* 1994;74(2):125-30.

1574   Persico G, Amato B, Aprea G, et al. The early effects of intravenous L-propionyl carnitine on ulcerative trophic lesions of the lower limbs in arteriopathic patients: a controlled randomized study. *Drugs Exp Clin Res,* 1995;21(5):187-98.

1575   Anand I, Chandrashekhan Y, De Giuli F, et al. Acute and chronic effects of propionyl-L-carnitine on the hemodynamics, exercise capacity, and hormones in patients with congestive heart failure. *Cardiovasc Drugs Ther,* 1998;12(3):291-9.

1576   Dal Lago A, De Martini D, Flore R, et al. Effects of propionyl-L-carnitine on peripheral arterial obliterative disease of the lower limbs: a double-blind clinical trial. *Drugs Exp Clin Res,* 1999;25(1):29-36.

1577   Ferrari R, De Giuli F. The propionyl-L-carnitine hypothesis: an alternative approach to treating heart failure. *J Card Fail,* 1997;3(3):217-24.

1578   Wiseman LR, Brogden RN. Propionyl-L-carnitine. *Drugs Aging,* 1998;12(3):243-8; discussion 249-50.

1579   Cherchi A, Lai C, Onnis E, et al. Propionyl carnitine in stable effort angina. *Cardiovasc Drugs Ther,* 1990;4(2):481-6.

1580   Bartels GL, Remme WJ, den Hartog FR, et al. Additional anti-ischemic effects of long-term L-propionylcarnitine in anginal patients treated with conventional antianginal therapy. *Cardiovasc Drugs Ther,* 1995;9(6):749-53.

1581   Bartels GL, Remme WJ, Holwerda KJ, Kruijssen DA. Anti-ischaemic efficacy of L-propionylcarnitine - a promising novel metabolic approach to ischaemia? *Eur Heart J,* 1996;17(3):414-20.

1582   Caponnetto S, Canale C, Masperone MA, et al. Efficacy of L-propionylcarnitine treatment in patients with left ventricular dysfunction. *Eur Heart J,* 1994;15(9):1267-73.

1583   Mancini M, Rengo F, Lingetti M, et al. Controlled study on the therapeutic efficacy of propionyl-L-carnitine in patients with congestive heart failure. *Arzneimittelforschung,* 1992;42(9):1101-4.

1584   Anon. Acetyl-L-Carnitine. MotherNature.com website. URL: www.mothernature.com/ency/Supp/Acetyl-L-Carnitine.asp (Accessed 27 February 2000).

1585   James JS. AIDS treatment news archives. URL: http://aids.org/immunet/atn.nsf/page/a-267-(Accessed 27 February 2000).

1586   Anon. Acetylcarnitine. iHerb Ltd website. URL / www.iherb.com/acetyl1.html (Accessed 27 February 2000).

1587   Anon. ProXeed Fact Sheet. URL www.proxeed.com/physicians/studies/abstract.asp (Accessed 27 February 2000).

1588   De Falco FA, D'Angelo E, Grimaldi G, et al. [Effect of the chronic treatment with L-acetylcarnitine in Down's syndrome]. [Article in Italian] *Clin Ter* 1994;144(2):123-7.

1589   Tempesta E, Troncon R, Janiri L, et al. Role of acetyl-L-carnitine in the treatment of cognitive deficit in chronic alcoholism. *Int J Clin Pharmacol Res,* 1990;10(1-2):101-7.

1590   Mezzina C, De Grandis D, Calvani M, et al. Idiopathic facial paralysis: new therapeutic prospects with acetyl-L-carnitine. *Int J Clin Pharmacol Res,* 1992;12(5-6):299-304.

1591   Postiglione A, Soricelli A, Cicerano U, et al. Effect of acute administration of L-acetyl carnitine on cerebral blood flow in patients with chronic cerebral infarct. *Pharmacol Res,* 1991;23(3):241-6.

1592   Rosadini G, Marenco S, Nobili F, et al. Acute effects of acetyl-L-carnitine on regional cerebral blood flow in patients with brain ischaemia. *Int J Clin Pharmacol Res,* 1990;10(1-2):123-8.

1593   Onofrj M, Fulgente T, Melchionda D, et al. L-acetylcarnitine as a new therapeutic approach for peripheral neuropathies with pain. *Int J Clin Pharmacol Res,* 1995;15(1):9-15.

1594   Thal LJ, Carta A, Clarke WR, et al. A 1-year multicenter placebo-controlled study of acetyl-L-carnitine in patients with Alzheimer's Disease. *Neurology* 1996;47:705-11.

1595   Sano M, Bell K, Cote L, et al. Double-blind parallel design pilot study of acetyl levocarnitine in patients with Alzheimer's Disease. *Arch Neurol,* 1992;49:1137-41.

1596   Spagnoli A, Lucca U, Menasce G, et al. Long-term acetyl-L-carnitine treatment in Alzheimer's Disease. *Neurology,* 1991;41:1726-32.

1597   Brooks JO, Yesavage JA, Carta A, Bravi D. Acetyl L-carnitine slows decline in younger patients with Alzheimer's disease: a reanalysis of a double-blind, placebo-controlled study using the trilinear approach. *Int Psychoger,* 1998;10(2):193-203.

1598   Pettegrew JW, Klunk WE, Panchalingam K, et al. Clinical and neurochemical effects of acetyl-L-carnitine in Alzheimer's disease. *Neurobiol Aging,* 1995;16(1):1-4.

1599   Rai G, Wright G, Scott L, et al. Double-blind, placebo controlled study of acetyl-l-carnitine in patients with Alzheimer's dementia. *Curr Med Res Opin,* 1990;11(10):638-47.

1600 Dong Y, Yang MM, Kwan CY. In vitro inhibition of proliferation of HL-60 cells by tetrandrine and coriolus versicolor peptide derived from Chinese medicinal herbs. *Life Sci,* 1997;60(8):PL135-40.

1601 Netrition. "Triax" website: www.netrition.com/ triax_page.html (Accessed 14 November 1999).

1602 Get Huge. "The Triac Story" website: www.gethuge.net/ triac (Accessed 14 November 1999).

1604 FDA Orphan Drug List. http://www.fda.gov/orphan/ designat/list.htm (Accessed 14 November 1999).

1605 FDA warns against consuming triax metabolic accelerator. FDA website, URL: www.fda.gov/bbs/ topics/ANSWERS/ANS00984.html (Accessed 15 November 1999).

1606 Precision Athletics. "Triarcanna" website: www.precisionathletics.com/triac.html (Accessed 15 November 1999).

1607 McDermott MT, Ridgway EC. Central hyperthyroidism. *Endocrinol Metab Clin North Am* 1998;27(1):187-203.

1608 Takeda T, Suzuki S, Liu RT, et al. Triiodothyroacetic acid has unique potential for therapy of resistance to thyroid hormone. *J Clin Endocrinol Metab* 1995;80(7):2033-40.

1609 Kunitake JM, Hartman N, Henson LC, et al. 3,5,3'-triiodothyroacetic acid therapy for thyroid hormone resistance. *J Clin Endocrinol Metab* 1989;69(2):461-6.

1610 Dulgeroff AJ, Geffner ME, Koyal SN, et al. Bromocriptine and Triac therapy for hyperthyroidism due to pituitary resistance to thyroid hormone. *J Clin Endocrinol Metab* 1992;75(4):1071-5.

1611 Beck-Peccoz P, Sartorio A, De Medici C, et al. Dissociated thyromimetic effects of 3, 5, 3'-triiodothyroacetic acid (TRIAC) at the pituitary and peripheral tissue levels. *J Endocrinol Invest* 1988;11(2):113-8.

1612 Lind P, Langsteger W, Koltringer P, et al. 3,5,3'-Triiodothyroacetic acid (TRIAC) effects on pituitary thyroid regulation and on peripheral tissue parameters. *Nuklearmedizin* 1989;28(6):217-20.

1613 Nicolini U, Venegoni E, Acaia B, et al. Prenatal treatment of fetal hypothyroidism: is there more than one option? *Prenat Diagn* 1996;16(5):443-8.

1614 Asteria C, Rajanayagam O, Collingwood TN, et al. Prenatal diagnosis of thyroid hormone resistance. *J Clin Endocrinol Metab* 1999;84(2):405-10.

1615 Radetti G, Persani L, Molinaro G, et al. Clinical and hormonal outcome after two years of triiodothyroacetic acid treatment in a child with thyroid hormone resistance. *Thyroid* 1997;7(5):775-8.

1616 Jaffiol C, Daures JP, Nsakala N, et al. [Long term follow up of medical treatment of differentiated thyroid cancer]. [Article in French] *Ann Endocrinol (Paris)* 1995;56(2):119-26.

1617 Mueller-Gaertner HW, Schneider C. 3,5,3'-Triiodothyroacetic acid minimizes the pituitary thyrotrophin secretion in patients on levo-thyroxine therapy after ablative therapy for differentiated thyroid carcinoma. *Clin Endocrinol (Oxf)* 1988;28(4):345-51.

1618 Mechelany C, Schlumberger M, Challeton C, et al. TRIAC (3,5,3'-triiodothyroacetic acid) has parallel effects at the pituitary and peripheral tissue levels in thyroid cancer patients treated with L-thyroxine. *Clin Endocrinol (Oxf)* 1991;35(2):123-8.

1620 Chow WS, Lam KS. An overweight woman with galactorrhoea. *Postgrad Med J* 1998;74:121-2.

1621 Lledo Carreres M, Lajo Garrido JL, Gonzalez Rico M, et al. Toxic internuclear ophthalmoplegia related to antiobesity treatment. *Ann Pharmacother* 1992;26(11):1457-8.

1622 Ferner RE, Burnett A, Rawlins MD. Triiodothyroacetic acid abuse in a female body builder. *Lancet* 1986;1:383.

1623 Heim J. [Hypothyroidism of central origin corrected by the cessation of Triac therapy]. [Article in French]. *Ann Med Interne (Paris)* 1982;133(8):588-9.

1624 Jean-Pastor MJ, Jean P, Biour M, et al. [Hepatopathies from treatment with a specialty drug combination of tiratricol-cyclovalone-retinol]. [Article in French]. *J Toxicol Clin Exp* 1986;6(2):115-21.

1625 Bentin J, Desir D, Mockel J. Triac (3,5,3'-triiodo-thyroacetic acid) induced "pseudohypothyroidism". *Acta Clin Belg* 1984;39(5):285-9.

1627 Hawkey CM, Olsen EG, Symons C. Production of cardiac muscle abnormalities in offspring of rats receiving triiodothyroacetic acid (triac) and the effect of beta adrenergic blockade. *Cardiovasc Res* 1981;15(4):196-205.

1628 Olsen EG, Symons C, Hawkey C. Effect of triac on the developing heart. *Lancet* 1977;2(8031):221-3.

1629 Pitt-Rivers R. Physiological activity of the acetic acid analogues of some iodinated thyronines. *Lancet* 1953;2:234.

1630 Lerman JL, Pitt-rivers R. Physiological activity of triiodo and tetraiodothyroacetic acid on blood-cholesterol levels. *Lancet* 1956;1:885-9.

1631 Menegay C, Juge C, Burger AG. Pharmacokinetics of 3,5,3'-triiodothyroacetic acid and its effects on serum TSH levels. *Acta Endocrinol (Copenh)* 1989;121(5):651-8.

1632 Sherman SI, Ringel MD, Smith MJ, et al. Augmented hepatic and skeletal thyromimetic effects of tiratricol in comparison with levothyroxine. *J Clin Endocrinol Metab* 1997;82(7):2153-8.

1633 Sherman SI, Ladenson PW. Organ-specific effects of tiratricol: a thyroid hormone analog with hepatic, not pituitary, superagonist effects. *J Clin Endocrinol Metab* 1992;75(3):901-5.

1634 Bracco D, Morin O, Schutz Y, et al. Comparison of the metabolic and endocrine effects of 3,5,3'-triiodothyroacetic acid and thyroxine. *J Clin Endocrinol Metab* 1993;77(1):221-8.

1635 Ng TB. A review of research on the protein-bound polysaccharide (polysaccharopeptide, PSP) from the mushroom Coriolus versicolor (Basidiomycetes: Polyporaceae). *Gen Pharmacol* 1998;30(1):1-4.

1636 Mizutani Y, Yoshida O. Activation by the protein-bound polysaccharide PSK (krestin) of cytotoxic lymphocytes that act on fresh autologous tumor cells and T24 human urinary bladder transitional carcinoma cell line in patients with urinary bladder cancer. *J Urol,* 1991;145(5):1082-7.

1637 Kobayashi H, Matsunaga K, Oguchi Y. Antimetastatic effects of PSK (Krestin), a protein-bound polysaccharide obtained from basidiomycetes: an overview. *Cancer Epidemiol Biomarkers Prev,* 1995;4(3):275-281.

1638 Dong Y, Kwan CY, Chen ZN, et al. Antitumor effects of a refined polysaccharide peptide fraction isolated from Coriolus versicolor: in vitro and in vivo studies. *Res*

Commun Mol Pathol Pharmacol, 1996;92(2):140-8.

1639 Kanoh T, Saito K, Matsunaga K, et al. Enhancement of the antitumor effect by the concurrent use of a monoclonal antibody and the protein bound polysaccharide PSK in mice bearing a human cancer cell line. *In Vivo*, 1994;8(2):241-5.

1640 Maehara Y, Inutsuka S, Takeuchi H, et al. Postoperative PSK and OK-432 immunochemotherapy for patients with gastric cancer. *Cancer Chemother Pharmacol*, 1993;33(2):171-5.

1641 Harada M, Matsunaga K, Oguchi Y, et al. Oral administration of PSK can improve the impaired anti-tumor CD4+ T-cell response in gut associated lymphoid tissue (GALT) of specific-pathogen-free mice. *Int J Cancer*, 1997;70(3):362-72.

1642 Tsukagoshi S, Hashimoto Y, Fujii G, et al. Krestin (PSK). *Cancer Treat Rev*, 1984;11(2):131-55.

1643 Collins RA, Ng TB. Polysaccharopeptide from Coriolus versicolor has potential for use against human immunodeficiency virus type 1 infection. *Life Sci* 1997;60(25):PL383-7.

1644 Tochikura TS, Nakashima H, Hirose K, et al. A biological response modifier, PSK, inhibits human immunodeficiency virus infection in vitro. *Biochem Biophys Res Commun*, 1987;148(2):726-33.

1645 Gong S, Zhang HQ, Yin WP, et al. Involvement of interleukin-2 in analgesia produced by Coriolus versicolor polysaccharide peptides. *Chung Kuo Yao Li Hsueh Pao*, 1998;19(1):67-70.

1646 Ng TB, Chan WY. Polysaccharopeptide from the mushroom Coriolus versicolor possesses analgesic activity but does not produce adverse effects on female reproductive or embryonic development in mice. *Gen Pharmacol*, 1997;29(2):269-73.

1647 Yeung JH, Chiu LC, Ooi VE. Effect of polysaccharide peptide (PSP) on glutathione and protection against paracetamol-induced hepatotoxicity in the rat. *Methods Find Exp Clin Pharmacol*, 1994;16(10):723-9.

1648 Iino Y, Yokoe T, Maemura M, et al. Immunochemotherapies versus chemotherapy as adjuvant treatment after curative resection of operable breast cancer. *Anticancer Res*, 1995;15(6B):2907-11.

1649 Ogoshi K, Satou H, Isono K, et al. Immunotherapy for esophageal cancer. A randomized trial in combination with radiotherapy and radiochemotherapy. Cooperative Study Group for Esophageal Cancer in Japan. *Am J Clin Oncol*, 1995;18(3):216-22.

1650 Yokoe T, Iino Y, Takei H, et al. HLA antigen as predictive index for the outcome of breast cancer patients with adjuvant immunochemotherapy with PSK. *Anticancer Res*, 1997;17(4A):2815-8.

1651 Nakazato H, Koike A, Saji S, et al. Efficacy of immunochemotherapy as adjuvant treatment after curative resection of gastric cancer. Study Group of Immunochemotherapy with PSK for Gastric Cancer. *Lancet*, 1994;343(8906):1122-6.

1652 Sugimachi K, Maehara Y, Ogawa M, et al. Dose intensity of uracil and tegafur in postoperative chemotherapy for patients with poorly differentiated gastric cancer. *Cancer Chemother Pharmacol*, 1997;40(3):233-8.

1653 Hayakawa K, Mitsuhashi N, Saito Y, et al. Effect of Krestin as adjuvant treatment following radical radiotherapy in non-small cell lung cancer patients. *Cancer Detect Prev*, 1997;21(1):71-7.

1654 Morimoto T, Ogawa M, Orita K, et al. Postoperative adjuvant randomised trial comparing chemoendocrine therapy, chemotherapy and immunotherapy for patients with stage II breast cancer: 5-year results from the Nishinihon Cooperative Study Group of Adjuvant Chemoendocrine Therapy for Breast Cancer (ACETBC) of Japan. *Eur J Cancer*, 1996;32A(2):235-42.

1655 Suto T, Fukuda S, Moriya N, et al. Clinical study of biological response modifiers as maintenance therapy for hepatocellular carcinoma. *Cancer Chemother Pharmacol*, 1994;33 Suppl:S145-8.

1656 Toi M, Hattori T, Akagi M, et al. Randomized adjuvant trial to evaluate the addition of tamoxifen and PSK to chemotherapy in patients with primary breast cancer. 5-Year results from the Nishi-Nippon Group of the Adjuvant Chemoendocrine Therapy for Breast Cancer Organization. *Cancer*, 1992;70(10):2475-83.

1657 Mitomi T, Tsuchiya S, Iijima N, et al. Randomized, controlled study on adjuvant immunochemotherapy with PSK in curatively resected colorectal cancer. The Cooperative Study Group of Surgical Adjuvant Immunochemotherapy for Cancer of Colon and Rectum (Kanagawa). *Dis Colon Rectum*, 1992;35(2):123-30.

1658 Nio Y, Tsubono M, Tseng CC, et al. Immunomodulation by orally administered protein-bound polysaccharide PSK in patients with gastrointestinal cancer. *Biotherapy*, 1992;4(2):117-28.

1659 Kondo T, Sakamoto J, Nakazato H. Alternating immunochemotherapy of advanced gastric carcinoma: a randomized comparison of carbazilquinone and PSK to carbazilquinone in patients with curative gastric resection. *Biotherapy*, 1991;3(4):287-95.

1660 Torisu M, Hayashi Y, Ishimitsu T, et al. Significant prolongation of disease-free period gained by oral polysaccharide K (PSK) administration after curative surgical operation of colorectal cancer. *Cancer Immunol Immunother*, 1990;31(5):261-8.

1661 Go P, Chung CH. Adjuvant PSK immunotherapy in patients with carcinoma of the nasopharynx. *J Int Med Res*, 1989;17(2):141-149.

1662 Fukushima M. Adjuvant therapy of gastric cancer: the Japanese experience. *Semin Oncol*, 1996;23(3):369-78.

1663 Healthlink. "Monograph: Poria", URL: www.healthlink.us-inc.com/publiclibrary/htm-data/htm-herb/bhp985.htm (Accessed 22 November 1999).

1664 Life Extension Vitamin Supplies, Inc. "DMAE" website: www.lifeextensionvitamins.com/lifeextensionvitamins/dmae.html (Accessed 23 November 1999).

1665 Mothernature.com Health Encyclopedia. "DMAE" website: www.mothernature.com/ency/supp/dmae.asp (Accessed 23 November 1999).

1666 Smart Basic. "Glossary: DMAE" website: www.smartbasic.com/glos.nutrients/dmae.glos.html. (Accessed 23 November 1999).

1667 Life Link. "DMAE" website: www.west.net/~lifelink/dmae2.htm (Accessed 23 November 1999).

1668 Davies C, Maidment S, Hanley P, et al. Dimethylaminoethanol (DMAE). HSE. Risk assessment document; EH72/2;1997. (TOXLINE).

1669 Re O. 2-Dimethylaminoethanol (deanol): a brief review of its clinical efficacy and postulated mechanism of action. *Curr Ther Res Clin Exp* 1974;16(11):1238-42.

1670 Rimland B. Controversies in the treatment of autistic children: vitamin and drug therapy. *J Child Neurol* 1988;3 Suppl:S68-72.

1671 Pieralisi G, Ripari P, Vecchiet L. Effects of a standardized ginseng extract combined with dimethylaminoethanol bitartrate, vitamins, minerals, and trace elements on physical performance during exercise. *Clin Ther* 1991;13(3):373-82.

1672 George J, Pridmore S, Aldous D. Double blind controlled trial of deanol in tardive dyskinesia. *Aust N Z J Psychiatry* 1981;15(1):68-71.

1673 Penovich P, Morgan JP, Kerzner B, et al. Double-blind evaluation of deanol in tardive dyskinesia. *JAMA* 1978;239(19):1997-8.

1674 de Montigny C, Chouinard G, Annable L. Ineffectiveness of deanol in tardive dyskinesia: a placebo controlled study. *Psychopharmacology (Berl)* 1979;65(3):219-23.

1675 Lindeboom SF, Lakke JP. Deanol and physostigmine in the treatment of L-dopa-induced dyskinesias. *Acta Neurol Scand* 1978;58(2):134-8.

1676 Jus A, Villeneuve A, Gautier J, et al. Deanol, lithium and placebo in the treatment of tardive dyskinesia. A double-blind crossover study. *Neuropsychobiology* 1978;4(3):140-9.

1677 Oettinger L Jr. Pediatric psychopharmacology. A review with special reference to deanol. *Dis Nerv Syst* 1977;38(12 Pt 2):25-31.

1678 Lewis JA, Lewis BS. Deanol in minimal brain dysfunction. *Dis Nerv Syst* 1977;38(12 Pt 2):21-4.

1679 Lewis JA, Young R. Deanol and methylphenidate in minimal brain dysfunction. *Clin Pharmacol Ther* 1975;17(5):534-40.

1680 Fisman M, Mersky H, Helmes E. Double-blind trial of 2-dimethylaminoethanol in Alzheimer's disease. *Am J Psychiatry* 1981;138(7):970-2.

1681 Ferris SH, Sathananthan G, Gershon S, et al. Senile dementia: treatment with deanol. *J Am Geriatr Soc* 1977;25(6):241-4.

1682 Cherkin A, Exkardt MJ. Effects of dimethylaminoethanol upon life-span and behavior of aged Japanese quail. *J Gerontol* 1977;32(1):38-45.

1683 Stenback F, Weisburger JH, Williams GM. Effect of lifetime administration of dimethylaminoethanol on longevity, aging changes, and cryptogenic neoplasms in C3H mice. *Mech Ageing Dev* 1988;42(2):129-38.

1684 Haug BA, Holzgraefe M. Orofacial and respiratory tardive dyskinesia: potential side effects of 2-dimethylaminoethanol (deanol)? *Eur Neurol* 1991;31(6):423-5.

1685 Casey DE. Mood alterations during deanol therapy. *Psychopharmacology (Berl)* 1979;62(2):187-91.

1686 Sergio W. Use of DMAE (2-dimethylaminoethanol) in the induction of lucid dreams. *Med Hypotheses* 1988;26(4):255-7.

1687 Consumer Guide to Melatonin. MotherNature.com website, URL: www.mothernature.com/cg/melatonin.asp (Accessed 29 November 1999).

1688 Lissoni P, Barni S, Cattaneo G, et al. Clinical results with the pineal hormone melatonin in advanced cancer resistant to standard antitumor therapies. *Oncology* 1991;48(6):448-50.

1689 Claustrat B, Brun J, Geoffriau M, et al. Nocturnal plasma melatonin profile and melatonin kinetics during infusion in status migrainosus. *Cephalalgia* 1997;17(4):511-7; discussion 487.

1690 Mallo C, Zaidan R, Galy G, et al. Pharmacokinetics of melatonin in man after intravenous infusion and bolus injection. *Eur J Clin Pharmacol* 1990;38(3):297-301.

1691 FDA Ofc Orphan Prod Develop. List of orphan designations and approvals. www.fda.gov/orphan/designat/list.htm (Accessed 29 November 1999).

1692 Lissoni P, Tisi E, Barni S, et al. Biological and clinical results of a neuroimmunotherapy with interleukin-2 and the pineal hormone melatonin as a first line treatment in advanced non-small cell lung cancer. *Br J Cancer* 1992;66(1):155-8.

1693 Lissoni P, Barni S, Ardizzoia A, et al. A randomized study with the pineal hormone melatonin versus supportive care alone in patients with brain metastases due to solid neoplasms. *Cancer* 1994;73(3):699-701.

1694 Lissoni P, Tancini G, Paolorossi F, et al. Chemoneuroendocrine therapy of metastatic breast cancer with persistent thrombocytopenia with weekly low-dose epirubicin plus melatonin: a phase II study. *J Pineal Res* 1999;26(3):169-73.

1695 Lissoni P, Tancini G, Barni S, et al. The pineal hormone melatonin in hematology and its potential efficacy in the treatment of thrombocytopenia. *Recenti Prog Med* 1996;87(12):582-5.

1696 Lissoni P, Barni S, Brivio F, et al. A biological study on the efficacy of low-dose subcutaneous interleukin-2 plus melatonin in the treatment of cancer-related thrombocytopenia. *Oncology* 1995;52(5):360-2.

1697 Bregani ER, Lissoni P, Rossini F, et al. Prevention of interleukin-2-induced thrombocytopenia during the immunotherapy of cancer by a concomitant administration of the pineal hormone melatonin. *Recenti Prog Med* 1995;86(6):231-3.

1698 Perna AF, Castaldo P, Ingrosso D, et al. Homocysteine, a new cardiovascular risk factor, is also a powerful uremic toxin. *J Nephrol* 1999;12(4):230-40.

1699 Fauteck J, Schmidt H, Lerchl A, et al. Melatonin in epilepsy: first results of replacement therapy and first clinical results. *Biol Signals Recept* 1999;8(1-2):105-10.

1700 Brendler T. Herbal Remedies Disk. 1st ed. Berlin:1996.

1701 Wallach J. Interpretation of Diagnostic Tests. A synopsis of Laboratory Medicine:, Fifth ed; Boston, MA: Little Brown, 1992.

1704 Toubro S, Astrup A. Randomised comparison of diets for maintaining obese subjects' weight after major weight loss: ad lib, low fat, high carbohydrate diet v fixed energy intake. *BMJ* 1997;314(7073):29-34.

1705 van Zandwijk N. N-acetylcysteine for lung cancer prevention. *Chest* 1995;107:1437-41.

1706 Ammon HP, Safayhi H, Mack T, Sabieraj J. Mechanism of antiinflammatory actions of curcumine and boswellic acids. *J Ethnopharmacol* 1993;38(23):1139.

1707 De Smet PAGM, Keller K, Hansel R, Chandler RF. Adverse Effects of Herbal Drugs Vol. 3, Springer-Verlag, Berlin, 1997.

1708 Gupta I, Gupta V, Parihar A, et al. Effects of Boswellia serrata gum resin in patients with bronchial asthma: results of a double-blind, placebo-controlled, 6-week clinical study. *Eur J Med Res* 1998;3(11):511-4.

1709 Gupta I, Parihar A, Malhotra P, et al. Effects of Boswellia serrata gum resin in patients with ulcerative colitis. *Eur J Med Res* 1997;2(1):37-43.

1710 van Zandwijk N, Dalesio O, Pastorino U, et al. EUROSCAN, a randomized trial of vitamin A and N-acetylcysteine in patients with head and neck cancer or lung cancer. For the European Organization for Research and Treatment of Cancer Head and Neck and Lung

Cancer Cooperative Groups. *J Natl Cancer Inst* 2000;92:977-86.

1711 Horowitz RS, Dart RC, Jarvie DR, et al. Placental transfer of N-acetylcysteine following human maternal acetaminophen toxicity. *J Toxicol Clin Toxicol* 1997;35:447-51.

1712 Mato JM, Camara J, Fernandez de Paz J, et al. S-adenosylmethionine in alcoholic liver cirrhosis: a randomized, placebo-controlled, double-blind, multicenter clinical trial. *J Hepatol* 1999;30(6):1081-9.

1713 Loehrer FM, Schwab R, Angst CP, et al. Influence of oral S-adenosylmethionine on plasma 5-methyltetrahydrofolate, S-adenosylhomocysteine, homocysteine and methionine in healthy humans. J *Pharmacol Exp Ther* 1997;22(2):845-50.

1714 Loehrer FM, Angst CP, Haefeli WE, et al. Low whole-blood S-adenosylmethionine and correlation between 5-methyltetrahydrofolate and homocysteine in coronary artery disease. *Arterioscler Thromb Vasc Biol* 1996;16(6):727-33.

1715 Louis E. Tremor disorders: identification and treatment. *Medical Update for Psychiatrists* 1997;2:172-6.

1716 Bailey B, McGuigan MA. Management of anaphylactoid reactions to intravenous N-acetylcysteine. *Ann Emerg Med* 1998;31:710-5.

1719 American College of Rheumatology ad hoc committee on clinical guidelines. Guidelines for monitoring drug therapy in rheumatoid arthritis. *Arthritis Rheum* 1996;39:723-31.

1721 Jorgensen KM, Witting MD. Does exogenous melatonin improve day sleep or night alertness in emergency physicians working night shifts? *Ann Emerg Med* 1998;31(6):699-704.

1722 Sanders DC, Chaturvedi AK, Hordinsky JR. Melatonin: aeromedical, toxicopharmacological, and analytical aspects. *J Anal Toxicol* 1999;23(3):159-67.

1724 Arangino S, Cagnacci A, Angiolucci M, et al. Effects of melatonin on vascular reactivity, catecholamine levels, and blood pressure in healthy men. *Am J Cardiol* 1999;83(9):1417-9.

1725 Zhi J, Jelia AT, Koss-Twardy SG, et al. The effect of orlistat, an inhibitor of dietary fat absorption, on the pharmacokinetics of beta-carotene in healthy volunteers. *J Clin Pharmacol* 1996;36:152-9.

1726 James WP, Avenell A, Broom J, et al. A one-year trial to assess the value of orlistat in the management of obesity. *Int J Obes Relat Metab Disord* 1997;21:S24-S30.

1727 Melia AT, Loss-Twardy SG, Zhi J. The effect of orlistat, an inhibitor of dietary fat absorption, on the absorption of vitamins A and E in healthy volunteers. *J Clin Pharmacol* 1996;36:647-653.

1728 Brusco LI, Marquez M, Cardinali DP. Monozygotic twins with Alzheimer's disease treated with melatonin: Case report. *J Pineal Res* 1998;25(4):260-3.

1729 Brusco LI, Fainstein I, Marquez M, et al. Effect of melatonin in selected populations of sleep-disturbed patients. *Biol Signals Recept* 1999;8(1-2):126-31.

1730 Roche, Inc. Xenical package insert. Nutley, NJ:1999 May.

1731 Chen RM, Wu JJ, Lee SC, et al. Increase of intestinal Bifidobacterium and suppression of coliform bacteria with short-term yogurt ingestion. *J Dairy Sci* 1999:82:2308-14.

1733 Garg R, Malinow M, Pettinger M. Niacin treatment increases plasma homocyst(e)ine levels. *Am Heart J* 1999;138:1082-7.

1735 Dawson D, Rogers NL, van den Heuvel CJ, et al. Effect of sustained nocturnal transbuccal melatonin administration on sleep and temperature in elderly insomniacs. *J Biol Rhythms* 1998;13(6):532-8.

1736 Anon. Yogurt cuts down diarrhea. HealthNews, November 1999.

1738 Haimov I, Lavie P, Laudon M, et al. Melatonin replacement therapy of elderly insomniacs. *Sleep* 1995;18(7):598-603.

1739 Luboshitzky R, Wagner O, Lavi S, et al. Abnormal melatonin secretion in hypogonadal men: the effect of testosterone treatment. *Clin Endocrinol (Oxf)* 1997;47(4):463-469.

1740 Pierce A. The American Pharmaceutical Association Practical Guide to Natural Medicines. New York: The Stonesong Press, 1999:19.

1741 Nordlund JJ, Lerner AB. The effects of oral melatonin on skin color and on the release of pituitary hormones. *J Clin Endocrinol Metab* 1977;45(4):768-74.

1742 Cavallo A, Ritschel WA. Pharmacokinetics of melatonin in human sexual maturation. *J Clin Endocrinol Metab* 1996;81(5):1882-6.

1743 Commentz JC, Uhlig H, Henke A, et al. Melatonin and 6-hydroxymelatonin sulfate excretion is inversely correlated with gonadal development in children. *Horm Res* 1997;47(3):97-101.

1744 Palm L, Blennow G, Wetterberg L. Long-term melatonin treatment in blind children and young adults with circadian sleep-wake disturbances. *Dev Med Child Neurol* 1997;39(5):319-25.

1745 Lancioni GE, O'Reilly MF, Basili G. Review of strategies for treating sleep problems in persons with severe or profound mental retardation or multiple handicaps. *Am J Ment Retard* 1999;104(2):170-86.

1746 Jan JE, O'Donnell ME. Use of melatonin in the treatment of paediatric sleep disorders. *J Pineal Res* 1996;21(4):193-9.

1747 O'Callaghan FJ, Clarke AA, Hancock E, et al. Use of melatonin to treat sleep disorders in tuberous sclerosis. *Dev Med Child Neurol* 1999;41(2):123-6.

1749 Skene DJ, Lockley SW, Arendt J. Melatonin in circadian sleep disorders in the blind. *Biol Signals Recept* 1999;8(1-2):90-5.

1750 Herzenberg LA, De Rosa SC, Dubs JG, et al. Glutathione deficiency is associated with impaired survival in HIV disease. *Proc Natl Acad Sci U S A* 1997;94:1967-72.

1751 Dagan Y, Zisapel N, Nof D, et al. Rapid reversal of tolerance to benzodiazepine hypnotics by treatment with oral melatonin: a case report. *Eur Neuropsychopharmacol* 1997;7(2):157-60.

1752 Holt S, Goodier D, Marley R, et al. Improvement in renal function in hepatorenal syndrome with N-acetylcysteine. *Lancet* 1999;353:294-5.

1753 Waldhauser F, Saletu B, Trinchard-Lugan I. Sleep laboratory investigations on hypnotic properties of melatonin. *Psychopharmacology (Berl)* 1990;100(2):222-6.

1754 Garfinkel D, Laudon M, Nof D, et al. Improvement of sleep quality in elderly people by controlled-release melatonin. *Lancet* 1995;346(8974):541-4.

1755 Spiller HA, Krenzelok EP, Grande GA, et al. A prospective evaluation of the effect of activated charcoal before oral N-acetylcysteine in acetaminophen overdose. *Ann Emerg Med* 1994;23:519-23.

1756 Dollins AB, Zhdanova IV, Wurtman RJ, et al. Effect of inducing nocturnal serum melatonin concentrations in daytime on sleep, mood, body temperature, and performance. *Proc Natl Acad Sci USA* 1994;91(5):1824-8.

1757 Zhdanova IV, Wurtman RJ, Lynch HJ, et al. Sleep-inducing effects of low doses of melatonin ingested in the evening. *Clin Pharmacol Ther* 1995;57(5):552-8.

1758 Nave R, Peled R, Lavie P. Melatonin improves evening napping. *Eur J Pharmacol* 1995;275(2):213-6.

1759 Zhdanova IV, Wurtman RJ, Morabito C, et al. Effects of low oral doses of melatonin, given 2-4 hours before habitual bedtime, on sleep in normal young humans. *Sleep* 1996;19(5):423-31.

1760 Attenburrow ME, Cowen PJ, Sharpley AL. Low dose melatonin improves sleep in healthy middle-aged subjects. *Psychopharmacology (Berl)* 1996;126(2):179-81.

1761 Kelly GS. Clinical applications of N-acetylcysteine. *Altern Med Rev* 1998;3:114-27.

1762 Chyka PA, Butler AY, Holliman BJ, Herman MI. Utility of acetylcysteine in treating poisonings and adverse drug reactions. *Drug Saf* 2000;22:123-48.

1763 Gillissen A, Nowak D. Characterization of N-acetylcysteine and ambroxol in anti-oxidant therapy. *Respir Med* 1998;92:609-23.

1764 Carman JS, Post RM, Buswell R, et al. Negative effects of melatonin on depression. *Am J Psychiatry* 1976;133(10):1181-1186.

1765 Marchetti G, Lodola E, Licciardello L, Colombo A. Use of N-acetylcysteine in the management of coronary artery diseases. *Cardiologia* 1999;44:633-7.

1766 Leibenluft E, Feldman-Naim S, Turner EH, et al. Effects of exogenous melatonin administration and withdrawal in five patients with rapid-cycling bipolar disorder. *J Clin Psychiatry* 1997;58(9):383-8.

1767 Morini M, Cai T, Aluigi MG, et al. The role of the thiol N-acetylcysteine in the prevention of tumor invasion and angiogenesis. *Int J Biol Markers* 1999;14:268-71.

1768 Bangha E, Elsner P, Kistler GS. Suppression of UV-induced erythema by topical treatment with melatonin (N-acetyl-5-methoxytryptamine). Influence of the application time point. *Dermatology* 1997;195(3):248-52.

1769 Fischer T, Bangha E, Elsner P, et al. Suppression of UV-induced erythema by topical treatment with melatonin. Influence of the application time point. *Biol Signals Recept* 1999;8(1-2):132-5.

1770 Naguib M, Samarkandi AH. Premedication with melatonin: a double-blind, placebo-controlled comparison with midazolam. *Br J Anaesth* 1999;82(6):875-80.

1771 Jan JE, Freeman RD, Fast DK. Melatonin treatment of sleep-wake cycle disorders in children and adolescents. *Dev Med Child Neurol* 1999;41(7):491-500.

1772 Avery D, Lenz M, Landis C. Guidelines for prescribing melatonin. *Ann Med* 1998;30(1):122-30.

1773 Brzezinski A. Melatonin in humans. *N Engl J Med* 1997; 336(3):186-95.

1774 Arendt J. Melatonin. *BMJ* 1996;312(7041):1242-3.

1775 Nathan PJ, Burrows GD, Norman TR. The effect of age and pre-light melatonin concentration on the melatonin sensitivity to dim light. *Int Clin Psychopharmacol* 1999;14(3):189-92.

1776 Fraschini F, Cesarani A, Alpini D, et al. Melatonin influences human balance. *Biol Signals Recept* 1999;8(1-2):111-9.

1777 Meeking DR, Wallace JD, Cuneo RC, et al. Exercise-induced GH secretion is enhanced by the oral ingestion of melatonin in healthy adult male subjects. *Eur J Endocrinol* 1999;141(1):22-6.

1778 Ebadi M, Govitrapong P, Phansuwan-Pujito P, et al. Pineal opioid receptors and analgesic action of melatonin. *J Pineal Res* 1998;24(4):193-200.

1779 Forsling ML, Wheeler MJ, Williams AJ. The effect of melatonin administration on pituitary hormone secretion in man. *Clin Endocrinol (Oxf)* 1999;51(5):637-42.

1780 Stoschitzky K, Sakotnik A, Lercher P, et al. Influence of beta-blockers on melatonin release. *Eur J Clin Pharmacol* 1999;55(2):111-5.

1781 Zeitzer JM, Daniels JE, Duffy JF, et al. Do plasma melatonin concentrations decline with age? *Am J Med* 1999;107(5):432-6.

1782 Smartbasic.com. Glossary. www.smartbasic.com/glos.drugs/vinpocetine.glos.html (Accessed 16 December 1999).

1783 Life-enhancement.com. VincaClear. www.life-enhancement.com/vinca.html (Accessed 16 December 1999).

1784 Thal LJ, Salmon DP, Lasker B, et al. The safety and lack of efficacy of vinpocetine in Alzheimer's disease. *J Am Geriatr Soc* 1989;37(6):515-20.

1785 Bereczki D, Fekete I. A systematic review of vinpocetine therapy in acute ischaemic stroke. *Eur J Clin Pharmacol* 1999;55(5):349-52.

1786 Szakall S, Boros I, Balkay L, et al. Cerebral effects of a single dose of intravenous vinpocetine in chronic stroke patients: a PET study. *J Neuroimaging* 1998;8(4):197-204.

1787 Hindmarch I, Fuchs HH, Erzigkeit H. Efficacy and tolerance of vinpocetine in ambulant patients suffering from mild to moderate organic psychosyndromes. *Int Clin Psychopharmacol* 1991;6(1):31-43.

1788 Ueyoshi A, Ota K. Clinical appraisal of vinpocetine for the removal of intractable tumoral calcinosis in haemodialysis patients with renal failure. *J Int Med Res* 1992;20(5):435-43.

1789 Balestreri R, Fontana L, Astengo F. A double-blind placebo controlled evaluation of the safety and efficacy of vinpocetine in the treatment of patients with chronic vascular senile cerebral dysfunction. *J Am Geriatr Soc* 1987;35(5):425-30.

1790 Hayakawa M. Effect of vinpocetine on red blood cell deformability in stroke patients. *Arzneimittelforschung 1992;42(4):425-7.*

1791 Hayakawa M. Comparative efficacy of vinpocetine, pentoxifylline and nicergoline on red blood cell deformability. *Arzneimittelforschung* 1992;42(2):108-10.

1792 Kiss E. Adjuvant effect of cavinton in the treatment of climacteric symptoms. *Ther Hung* 1990;38(4):170-3.

1793 Miyazaki M. The effect of a cerebral vasodilator, vinpocetine, on cerebral vascular resistance evaluated by the Doppler ultrasonic technique in patients with cerebrovascular diseases. *Angiology* 1995;46(1):53-8.

1794 Dutov AA, Gal'tvanitsa GA, Volkova VA, et al. [Cavinton in the prevention of the convulsive syndrome in children after birth injury]. [Article in Russian] *Zh Nevropatol Psikhiatr Im S S Korsakova* 1991;91(8):21-2.

1795 Dutov AA, Tolpyshev BA, Petrov AP, et al. [Use of cavinton in epilepsy]. [Article in Russian] *Zh Nevropatol Psikhiatr Im S S Korsakova* 1986;86(6):850-5.

1796 Bhatti JZ, Hindmarch I. Vinpocetine effects on cognitive impairments produced by flunitrazepam. *Int Clin Psychopharmacol* 1987;2(4):325-31.

1797 Subhan Z, Hindmarch I. Psychopharmacological effects of vinpocetine in normal healthy volunteers. *Eur J Clin Pharmacol* 1985;28(5):567-71.

1798 Bodo D, Kotovskaia AR, Galle RR, et al. [Effectiveness of the preparation Gavinton in preventing motion sickness]. [Article in Russian]. *Kosm Biol Aviakosm Med* 1982;16(3):49-51.

1799 The Natural Pharmacist. Vinpocetine. www.tnp.com/substance.asp?ID=573. (Accessed 16 December 1999).

1800 Nicholson CD. Pharmacology of nootropics and metabolically active compounds in relation to their use in dementia. *Psychopharmacology (Berl)* 1990;101(2):147-59.

1801 Akopov SE, Gabrielian ES. Effects of aspirin, dipyridamole, nifedipine and cavinton which act on platelet aggregation induced by different aggregating agents alone and in combination. *Eur J Clin Pharmacol* 1992;42(3):257-9.

1802 Lohmann A, Dingler E, Sommer W, et al. Bioavailability of vinpocetine and interference of the time of application with food intake. *Arzneimittelforschung* 1992;42(7):914-7.

1803 McGrath JJ, Soares KVS. Cholinergic medication for neuroleptic-induced tardive dyskinesia (Cochrane Review). In: The Cochrane Library Update Software, Oxford,1999(4). www.imbi.uni-freiburg.de/mirrors/som.flinders.edu.au/FUSA/COCHRANE/cochrane/revabstr/ab000207.htm. (Accessed 4 January 2000).

1804 Soares KV, McGrath JJ. The treatment of tardive dyskinesia- a systematic review and meta-analysis. *Schizophr Res* 1999;39:1-16; discussion 17-18.

1805 Life Enhancement. DMAE: the mood-elevating smart nutrient. www.life-enhancement.com/n37/n37dmae.html (Accessed 4 January 2000).

1816 Allen LV. Nutritional Products. In: Covington TR, Ed. Handbook of Nonprescription Drugs. Washington, DC: American Pharmaceutical Association 1996:361-92.

1817 Valimaki MJ, Kinnunen K, Volin L, et al. A prospective study of bone loss and turnover after allogeneic bone marrow transplantation: effect of calcium supplementation with or without calcitonin. *Bone Marrow Transplant* 1999;23:355-61.

1818 Allender PS, Cutler JA, Follmann D, et al. Dietary calcium and blood pressure: a meta-analysis of randomized clinical trials. *Ann Intern Med* 1996;124:825-31.

1819 Bucher HC, Cook RJ, Guyatt GH, et al. Effects of dietary calcium supplementation on blood pressure. A meta-analysis of randomized controlled trials. *JAMA* 1996; 275:1016-22.

1820 Kawano Y, Yoshimi H, Matsuoka H, et al. Calcium supplementation in patients with essential hypertension: assessment by office, home and ambulatory blood pressure. *J Hypertens* 1998;16:1693-9.

1821 Griffith LE, Guyatt GH, Cook RJ, et al. The influence of dietary and nondietary calcium supplementation on blood pressure: an updated meta-analysis of randomized controlled trials. *Am J Hypertens* 1999;12:84-92.

1822 Thys-Jacobs S, Starkey P, Bernstein D, Tian J. Calcium carbonate and the premenstrual syndrome: effects on premenstrual and menstrual symptoms. Premenstrual Syndrome Study Group. *Am J Obstet Gynecol,* 1998;179:444-52.

1823 Alvir JM, Thys-Jacobs S. Premenstrual and menstrual symptom clusters and response to calcium treatment. *Psychopharmacol Bull,* 1991;27:145-8.

1824 Thys-Jacobs S, Ceccarelli S, Bierman A, et al. Calcium supplementation in premenstrual syndrome: a randomized crossover trial. *J Gen Intern Med* 1989;4:183-9.

1825 Lewis CJ. Letter to reiterate certain public health and safety concerns to firms manufacturing or importing dietary supplements that contain specific bovine tissues. FDA. www.cfsan.fda.gov/~dms/dspltr05.html (Accessed 29 November 2000).

1826 Steinbach G, Lupton J, Reddy BS, et al. Effect of calcium supplementation on rectal epithelial hyperproliferation in intestinal bypass subjects. *Gastroenterology* 1994;106:1162-7.

1827 Barsotti G, Cupisti A, Morelli E, et al. Secondary hyperparathyroidism in severe chronic renal failure is corrected by very-low dietary phosphate intake and calcium carbonate supplementation. *Nephron* 1998;79:137-41.

1828 Tsukamoto Y, Moriya R, Nagaba Y, et al. Effect of administering calcium carbonate to treat secondary hyperparathyroidism in nondialyzed patients with chronic renal failure. *Am J Kidney Dis* 1995;25:879-86.

1829 Rudnicki M, Hojsted J, Petersen LJ, et al. Oral calcium effectively reduces parathyroid hormone levels in hemodialysis patients: a randomized double-blind placebo-controlled study. *Nephron* 1993;65:369-74.

1830 Adachi JD, Ioannidis G. Calcium and vitamin D therapy in corticosteroid-induced bone loss: what is the evidence? *Calcif Tissue Int* 1999;65:332-6.

1831 Adachi JD, Bensen WG, Bianchi F, et al. Vitamin D and calcium in the prevention of corticosteroid induced osteoporosis: a 3 year followup. *J Rheumatol* 1996;23:995-1000.

1832 Recommendations for the prevention and treatment of glucocorticoid-induced osteoporosis. American College of Rheumatology Task Force on Osteoporosis Guidelines. *Arthritis Rheum* 1996;39:1791-801.

1833 Crowther CA, Hiller JE, Pridmore B, et al. Calcium supplementation in nulliparous women for the prevention of pregnancy-induced hypertension, preeclampsia and preterm birth: an Australian randomized trial. FRACOG and the ACT Study Group. *Aust N Z J Obstet Gynaecol,* 1999;39:12-8.

1834 Power ML, Heaney RP, Kalkwarf HJ, et al. The role of calcium in health and disease. *Am J Obstet Gynecol* 1999;181:1560-9.

1835 Dawson-Hughes B, Harris SS, Krall EA, Dallal GE. Effect of calcium and vitamin D supplementation on bone density in men and women 65 years of age or older. *N Engl J Med* 1997;337:670-6.

1836 Chapuy MC, Arlot ME, Duboeuf F, et al. Vitamin D3 and calcium to prevent hip fractures in the elderly women. *N Engl J Med* 1992;327(23):1637-42.

1837 Celotti F, Bignamini A. Dietary calcium and mineral/vitamin supplementation: a controversial problem. *J Int Med Res* 1999;27:1-14.

1838 Heller HJ, Stewart A, Haynes S, Pak CY.

Pharmacokinetics of calcium absorption from two commercial calcium supplements. *J Clin Pharmacol* 1999;39:1151-4.

1839 Fujita T, Ohue T, Fujii Y, et al. Heated oyster shell-seaweed calcium (AAA Ca) on osteoporosis. *Calcif Tissue Int* 1996;58:226-30.

1840 Fujita T, Ohue T, Fujii Y, et al. Effect of calcium supplementation on bone density and parathyroid function in elderly subjects. *Miner Electrolyte Metab* 1995;21:229-31.

1841 Talbot JR, Guardo P, Seccia S, etal. Calcium bioavailability and parathyroid hormone acute changes after oral intake of dairy and nondairy products in healthy volunteers. *Osteoporos Int* 1999;10:137-42.

1842 Heaney RP, Dowell MS, Barger-Lux MJ. Absorption of calcium as the carbonate and citrate salts, with some observations on method. *Osteoporos Int* 1999;9:19-23.

1843 Maton PN, Burton ME. Antacids revisited: a review of their clinical pharmacology and recommended therapeutic use. *Drugs* 1999;57:855-70.

1844 Clemens JD, Feinstein AR. Calcium carbonate and constipation: a historical review of medical mythopoeia. *Gastroenterology* 1977;72:957-61.

1845 Saunders D, Sillery J, Chapman R. Effect of calcium carbonate and aluminum hydroxide on human intestinal function. *Dig Dis Sci* 1988;33:409-13.

1846 Krall EA, Dawson-Hughes B. Smoking increases bone loss and decreases intestinal calcium absorption. *J Bone Miner Res* 1999;14:215-20.

1847 Praet JP, Peretz A, Mets T, Rozenberg S. Comparative study of the intestinal absorption of three salts of calcium in young and elderly women. *J Endocrinol Invest* 1998;21:263-7.

1848 Minihane AM, Fairweather-Tait SJ. Effect of calcium supplementation on daily nonheme-iron absorption and long-term iron status. *Am J Clin Nutr* 1998;68:96-102.

1849 Sokoll LJ, Dawson-Hughes B. Calcium supplementation and plasma ferritin concentrations in premenopausal women. *Am J Clin Nutr* 1992;56:1045-8.

1850 Kalkwarf HJ, Harrast SD. Effects of calcium supplementation and lactation on iron status. *Am J Clin Nutr* 1998;67:1244-9.

1851 Sam's General Store. IP-6, Inositol Hexaphosphate. www.samsstore.com/samsgeneralstore/ip6.html. (Accessed 11 January 2000).

1852 MotherNature.com. IP-6: new nutraceutical from fiber fights cancer. www.mothernature.com/news/ 1998_09_10/research_update.stm. (Accessed 11 January 2000).

1853 University of Maryland. Natural sugar-phosphate compound shows promise as cancer treatment. www.oea.umaryland.edu/Media/NewsSum/NewsDetail/ archive/1998_03/IP.htm. (Accessed 11 January 2000).

1854 Steinmetz KA, Potter JD. Vegetables, fruit, and cancer prevention: a review. *J Am Diet Assoc* 1996;96:1027-39.

1855 Graf E, Eaton JW. Antioxidant functions of phytic acid. *Free Radic Biol Med* 1990;8:61-69.

1857 Shamsuddin AM, Vucenik I, Cole KE. IP6: a novel anti-cancer agent. *Life Sci* 1997;61:343-54.

1858 Zhou JR, Erdman JW Jr. Phytic acid in health and disease. *Crit Rev Food Sci Nutr,* 1995;35:495-508.

1859 Shamsuddin AM. Metabolism and cellular functions of IP6: a review. *Anticancer Res* 1999;19:3733-6.

1860 Shamsuddin AM, Vucenik I. Mammary tumor inhibition by IP6: a review. *Anticancer Res* 1999;19:3671-4.

1861 Challa A, Rao DR, Reddy BS. Interactive suppression of aberrant crypt foci induced by azoxymethane in rat colon by phytic acid and green tea. *Carcinogenesis* 1997;18:2023-6.

1862 Saied IT, Shamsuddin AM. Up-regulation of the tumor suppressor gene p53 and WAF1 gene expression by IP6 in HT-29 human colon carcinoma cell line. *Anticancer Res* 1998;18:1479-84.

1863 Thompson LU, Zhang L. Phytic acid and minerals: effect on early markers of risk for mammary and colon carcinogenesis. *Carcinogenesis* 1991;12:2041-5.

1864 Vucenik I, Zhang ZS, Shamsuddin AM. IP6 in treatment of liver cancer. II. Intra-tumoral injection of IP6 regresses pre-existing human liver cancer xenotransplanted in nude mice. *Anticancer Res* 1998;18:4091-6.

1865 Shamsuddin AM, Yang GY. Inositol hexaphosphate inhibits growth and induces differentiation of PC-3 human prostate cancer cells. *Carcinogenesis* 1995;16:1975-9.

1866 Shamsuddin AM, Elsayed AM, Ullah A. Suppression of large intestinal cancer in F344 rats by inositol hexaphosphate. *Carcinogenesis* 1988;9:577-80.

1867 Vucenik I, Podczasy JJ, Shamsuddin AM. Antiplatelet activity of inositol hexaphosphate. *Anticancer Res* 1999;19:3689-93.

1868 Jariwalla RJ. Inositol hexaphosphate (IP6) as an anti-neoplastic and lipid-lowering agent. *Anticancer Res* 1999;19:3699-3702.

1869 Sandberg AS, Brune M, Carlsson NG, et al. Inositol phosphates with different numbers of phosphate groups influence iron absorption in humans. *Am J Clin Nutr* 1999;70:240-6.

1870 Sandstrom B, Sandberg AS. Inhibitory effects of isolated inositol phosphates on zinc absorption in humans. *J Trace Elem Electrolytes Health Dis* 1992;6:99-103.

1871 Ide N, Lau BH. Garlic compounds protect vascular endothelial cells from oxidized low density lipoprotein-induced injury. *J Pharm Pharmacol* 1997;49:908-11.

1872 Wakunaga Products. www.kyolic.com/green.htm. (Accessed 17 January 2000).

1873 Steiner M, Khan AH, Holbert D, Lin RI. A double-blind crossover study in moderately hypercholesterolemic men that compared the effect of aged garlic extract and placebo administration on blood lipids. *Am J Clin Nutr* 1996;64:866-70.

1874 Steiner M, Lin RS. Changes in platelet function and susceptibility of lipoproteins to oxidation associated with administration of aged garlic extract. *J Cardiovasc Pharmacol* 1998;31:904-8

1875 Lau BS, Lam F, Wang-Cheng R. Effect of an odor-modified garlic preparation on blood lipids. *Nutrition Research* 1987;7:139-49.

1876 Munday JS, James KA, Fray LM, et al. Daily supplementation with aged garlic extract, but not raw garlic, protects low density lipoprotein against in vitro oxidation. *Atherosclerosis* 1999;143:399-404.

1877 Imai J, Ide N, Nagae S, et al. Antioxidant and radical scavenging effects of aged garlic extract and its constituents. *Planta Med* 1994;60:417-20.

1878 Moriguchi T, Saito H, Nishiyama N. Aged garlic extract prolongs longevity and improves spatial memory deficit in senescence-accelerated mouse. *Biol Pharm Bull*

REFERENCES

1996;19:305-7.

1879 Efendy JL, Simmons DL, Campbell GR, Campbell JH. The effect of the aged garlic extract, 'Kyolic', on the development of experimental atherosclerosis. *Atherosclerosis* 1997;132:37-42.

1880 Ide N, Lau BH. Aged garlic extract attenuates intracellular oxidative stress. *Phytomedicine* 1999;6:125-31.

1881 Sigounas G, Hooker J, Anagnostou A, Steiner M. S-allylmercaptocysteine inhibits cell proliferation and reduces the viability of erythroleukemia, breast, and prostate cancer cell lines. *Nutr Cancer* 1997;27:186-91.

1882 Zhang Y, Moriguchi T, Saito H, Nishiyama N. Functional relationship between age-related immunodeficiency and learning deterioration. *N Eur J Neurosci* 1998;10:3869-75.

1883 Wang BH, Zuzel KA, Rahman K, Billington D. Treatment with aged garlic extract protects against bromobenzene toxicity to precision cut rat liver slices. *Toxicology* 1999;132:215-25.

1884 Gwilt PR, Lear CL, Tempero MA, et al. The effect of garlic extract on human metabolism of acetaminophen. *Cancer Epidemiol Biomarkers Prev* 1994;3:155-60.

1885 Horie T, Matsumoto H, Kasagi M, et al. Protective effect of aged garlic extract on the small intestinal damage of rats induced by methotrexate administration. *Planta Med* 1999;65:545-8.

1886 Nguyen TT, Dale LC, von Bergmann K, Croghan IT. Cholesterol-lowering effect of stanol ester in a US population of mildly hypercholesterolemic men and women: a randomized controlled trial. *Mayo Clin Proc* 1999;74:1198-206.

1888 Ostlund RE Jr, Spilburg CA, Stenson WF. Sitostanol administered in lecithin micelles potently reduces cholesterol absorption in humans. *Am J Clin Nutr* 1999;70:826-31.

1889 Mook-Jung I, Shin JE, Yun SH, et al. Protective effects of asiaticoside derivatives against beta-amyloid neurotoxicity. *J Neurosci Res* 1999;58:417-25.

1890 Maquart FX, Chastang F, Simeon A, et al. Triterpenes from Centella asiatica stimulate extracellular matrix accumulation in rat experimental wounds. *Eur J Dermatol* 1999;9:289-96.

1891 Refsum H, Ueland PM, Nygard O, Vollset SE. Homocysteine and cardiovascular disease. *Annu Rev Med* 1998;49:31-62.

1892 Malinow MR, Bostom AG, Krauss RM. Homocyst(e)ine, diet, and cardiovascular diseases: a statement for healthcare professionals from the Nutrition Committee, American Heart Association. *Circulation* 1999;99:178-82.

1893 Boushey CJ, Beresford SA, Omenn GS, Motulsky AG. A quantitative assessment of plasma homocysteine as a risk factor for vascular disease. Probable benefits of increasing folic acid intakes. *JAMA* 1995;274(13):1049-57.

1894 Personal Communication: Edwin W. Grimsley, MD. Savannah, GA. January, 2000.

1895 Personal correspondence, 3M Pharmaceuticals, Drug Surveillance and Information; January, 2000.

1896 Investigator's Brochure: Ademetionine 1,4-butanedisulfonate. Knoll Pharmaceuticals.

1897 Stramentinoli G, Gualano M, Galli-Kienle M. Intestinal absorption of S-adenosyl-L-methionine. *J Pharmacol Exp Ther* 1979;209(3):323-6.

1898 Morrow LE, Grimsley EW. Long-term diuretic therapy in hypertensive patients: effects on serum homocysteine, vitamin B6, vitamin B12, and red blood cell folate concentrations. *South Med J* 1999;92(9):866-70.

1899 Christensen B, Landaas S, Stensvold I, et al. Whole blood folate, homocysteine in serum, and risk of first acute myocardial infarction. *Atherosclerosis* 1999;147(2):317-26.

1900 Lininger SW. The Natural Pharmacy. 1st ed. Rocklin, CA: Prima Publishing; 1998.

1901 Brewster MA, Schedewie H. Trimethylaminuria. *Ann Clin Lab Sci,* Jan.-Feb. 1983; 13(1):20-4.

1902 Consumer Lab. www.consumerlab.com/results/ginseng.asp (Accessed 5 June 2001).

1903 Wesnes KA, Ward T, McGinty A, Petrini O. The memory enhancing effects of a Ginkgo biloba/Panax ginseng combination in healthy middle-aged volunteers. *Psychopharmacology* 2000;152:353-361.

1905 Broeder CE, Quindry J, Brittingham K, et al. The Andro Project: physiological and hormonal influences of androstenedione supplementation in men 35 to 65 years old participating in a high-intensity resistance training program. *Arch Intern Med* 2000;160:3093-104.

1906 Catlin DH, Leder BZ, Ahrens B, et al. Trace contamination of over-the-counter androstenedione and positive urine test results for a nandrolone metabolite. *JAMA* 2000;284:2618-21.

1907 Hudsin J, Towers GHN. Phytomedicines as antivirals. *Drugs Fut* 1999;24:295-320.

1908 Abdel-Fattah A, Aboul-Enein MN, Wassel G, El-Menshawi B. Preliminary report on the therapeutic effect of khellin in psoriasis. *Dermatologica* 1983;167:109-10.

1909 Clark RH, Feleke G, Din M, et al. Nutritional treatment for acquired immunodeficiency virus-associated wasting using beta-hydroxy beta-methylbutyrate, glutamine, and arginine: a randomized, double-blind, placebo-controlled study. *JPEN J Parenter Enteral Nutr* 2000;24:133-9.

1910 Thom H, Carter PE, Cole GF, et al. Ammonia and carnitine concentrations in children treated with sodium valproate compared with other anticonvulsant drugs. *Dev Med Child Neurol* 1991;33(9):795-802.

1911 Hug G, McGraw CA, Bates SR, et al. Reduction of serum carnitine concentrations during anticonvulsant therapy with phenobarbital, valproic acid, phenytoin, and carbamazepine in children. *J Pediatr* 1991;119(5):799-802.

1912 Riva R, Albani F, Gobbi G, et al. Carnitine disposition before and during valproate therapy in patients with epilepsy. *Epilepsia* 34(1):184-187.

1913 Zelnik N, Fridkis I, Gruener N. Reduced carnitine and antiepileptic drugs: cause relationship or co-existence? *Acta Paediatr* 1995;84(1):93-95.

1914 Bohles H, Sewell AC, Wenzel D. The effect of carnitine supplementation in valproate-induced hyperammonaemia. *Acta Paediatri* 1996;85(4):446-449.

1915 Altunbasak S, Baytok V, Tasouji M, et al. Asymptomatic hyperammonemia in children treated with valproic acid. *J Child Neurol* 1997;12(7):461-463.

1916 Coulter DL. Prevention of hepatotoxicity recurrence with valproate monotherapy and carnitine. *Ann Neurol* 1988;24:301.

1917 Vance CK, Vance H, Winter SC, et al. Control of valproate-induced hepatotoxicity with carnitine. *Ann Neurol* 1989;26(3):456.

1918 Salonen JT, Nyyssonen K, Salonen R, et al. Antioxidant Supplementation in Atherosclerosis Prevention (ASAP) study: a randomized trial of the effect of vitamins E and C on 3-year progression of carotid atherosclerosis. *J Intern Med* 2000;248:377-86.

1919 Ernst E, Pittler MH. Efficacy of ginger for nausea and vomiting: a systematic review of randomized clinical trials. *Br J Anaesth* 2000;84(3):367-71.

1920 Anon. Case problem: presenting conventional and complementary approaches for relieving nausea in a breast cancer patient undergoing chemotherapy. *J Am Diet Assoc* 2000;100(2):257-9.

1921 Wilkinson JM. What do we know about herbal morning sickness treatments? A literature survey. *Midwifery* 2000;16(3):224-8.

1922 Jewell D, Young G. Interventions for nausea and vomiting in early pregnancy. *Cochrane Database Syst Rev* 2000;(2):CD000145.

1923 Micklefield GH, Redeker Y, Meister V, et al. Effects of ginger on gastroduodenal motility. *Int J Clin Pharmacol Ther* 1999;37(7):341-6.

1924 Lumb AB. Mechanism of antiemetic effect of ginger. *Anaesthesia* 1993;48(12):1118.

1926 Vynograd N, Vynograd I, Sosnowski Z. A comparative multi-centre study of the efficacy of propolis, acyclovir and placebo in the treatment of genital herpes (HSV). *Phytomedicine* 2000;7(1):1-6.

1927 Spasov AA, Wikman GK, Mandrikov VB, et al. A double-blind, placebo-controlled pilot study of the stimulating and adaptogenic effect of Rhodiola rosea SHR-5 extract on the fatigue of students caused by stress during an examination period with a repeated low-dose regimen. *Phytomedicine* 2000;7(2):85-89.

1928 Rao AV, Agarwal S. Role of antioxidant lycopene in cancer and heart disease. *J Am Coll Nutr* 2000;19(5):563-9.

1929 Panton LB, Rathmacher JA, Baier S, et al. Nutritional supplementation of the leucine metabolite beta-hydroxy-beta-methylbutyrate (hmb) during resistance training. *Nutrition* 2000;16(9):734-9.

1930 Kelly GS. L-carnitine: therapeutic applications of a conditionally-essential amino acid. *Altern Med Rev,* 1998;3(5):345-60.

1931 Krahenbuhl S. Carnitine metabolism in chronic liver disease. *Life Sci,* 1996;59(19):1579-99.

1932 Larsson B, Jonasson A, Fianu S. Prophylactic effect of UVA-E in women with recurrent cystitis: a preliminary report. *Curr Ther Res* 1993;53:441-3.

1933 Brass E. Pharmacokinetic considerations for the therapeutic use of carnitine in hemodialysis patients. *Clin Ther,* Mar.-Apr. 1995; 17(2):176-85; discussion 175.

1934 Lee NA, Reasner CA. Beneficial effect of chromium supplementation on serum triglyceride levels in NIDDM. *Diabetes Care,* 1994;17(12):1449-52.

1935 Fox GN, Sabovic Z. Chromium picolinate supplementation for diabetes mellitus. *J Fam Pract* 1998 Jan;46(1):83-6.

1936 Reading SA. Chromium picolinate. *J Fla Med Assoc* 1996 Jan;83(1):29-31.

1937 Urberg M, Zemel MB. Evidence for synergism between chromium and nicotinic acid in the control of glucose tolerance in elderly humans. *Metabolism,* Sep. 1987; 36(9):896-9.

1938 Mohamedshah FY, Moser-Veillon PB, Yamini S, et al. Distribution of a stable isotope of chromium (53Cr) in serum, urine, and breast milk in lactating women. *Am J Clin Nutr* 1998 Jun;67(6):1250-5.

1939 Grant KE, Chandler RM, Castle AL, Ivy JL. Chromium and exercise training: effect on obese women. *Med Sci Sports Exerc,* Aug. 1997; 29(8):992-8.

1940 Felt O, Buri P, Gurny R. Chitosan: a unique polysaccharide for drug delivery. *Drug Dev Ind Pharm,* 1998;24(11)979-93.

1941 Illum L. Chitosan and its use as a pharmaceutical excipient. *Pharm Res,* 1998;15(9):1326-1331.

1942 Jing SB, Li L, Ji D, et al. Effect of chitosan on renal function in patients with chronic renal failure. *J Pharm Pharmacol,* 1997; 49(7):721-3.

1943 Rao SB, Sharma CP. Use of chitosan as a biomaterial: studies on its safety and hemostatic potential. *J Biomed Mater Res,* 1997;34(1):21-28.

1944 Biagini G, Bertani A, Muzzarelli R, et al. Wound management with N-carboxybutyl chitosan. *Biomaterials,* 1991; 12(3):281-6.

1945 Muzzarelli R, Biagini G, Pugnaloni A, et al. Reconstruction of parodontal tissue with chitosan. *Biomaterials,* 1989; 10(9):598-603.

1946 Tsoko M, Beauseigneur F, Gresti J, et al. Enhancement of activities relative to fatty acid oxidation in the liver of rats depleted of L-carnitine by D-carnitine and a gamma-butyrobetaine hydroxylase inhibitor. *Biochem Pharmacol,* 17 May 1995;49(10):1403-10.

1947 Colombani P, Wenk C, Kunz I, et al. Effects of L-carnitine supplementation on physical performance and energy metabolism of endurance-trained athletes: a double-blind crossover field study. *Eur J Appl Physiol,* 1996;73(5):434-9.

1948 Krahenbuhl S, Reichen J. Carnitine metabolism in patients with chronic liver disease. *Hepatology,* January 1997;25(1):148-53.

1949 Zeisel SH. Choline: needed for normal development of memory. *J Am Coll Nutr* 2000;19(5 Suppl):528S-531S.

1950 Hahn CJ, Evans GW. Absorption of trace metals in the zinc-deficient rat. *Am J Physiol,* 1975; 228(4):1020-3.

1951 Wasser WG, Feldman NS, D'Agati VD. Chronic renal failure after ingestion of over-the-counter chromium picolinate. [letter] *Ann Intern Med,* 1 Mar 1997; 126(5):410.

1952 Mertz W. Interaction of chromium with insulin: a progress report. *Nutr Rev, Jun.* 1998; 56(6):174-7.

1953 Anderson RA. Chromium, glucose intolerance and diabetes. *J Am Coll Nutr,* Dec. 1998; 17(6):548-55.

1954 Davydov M, Krikorian AD. Eleutherococcus senticosus (Rupr. & Maxim.) Maxim. (Araliaceae) as an adaptogen: a closer look. *J Ethnopharmacol* 2000;72(3):345-393.

1955 Morrison LM, Enrick N. Coronary heart disease: reduction of death rate by chondroitin sulfate A. *Angiology* 1973;24:269-87.

1956 Kaufmann PA, Gnecchi-Ruscone T, di Terlizzi M, et al. Coronary heart disease in smokers: vitamin C restores coronary microcirculatory function. *Circulation* 2000;102:1233-8.

1957 Yokoyama T, Date C, Kokubo Y, et al. Serum vitamin C concentration was inversely associated with subsequent 20-year incidence of stroke in a Japanese rural community : the shibata study. *Stroke* 2000;31:2287-94.

1958 Gale CR, Martyn CN, Winter PD, Cooper C. Vitamin C

REFERENCES

and risk of death from stroke and coronary heart disease in cohort of elderly people. *BMJ* 1995;310:1563-6.

1959 Alster TS, West TB. Effect of topical vitamin C on postoperative carbon dioxide laser resurfacing erythema. *Dermatol Surg* 1998;24:331-4.

1960 Slivka A, Kang JO, Cohen G. Ascorbic acid. *N Engl J Med* 1986;315:708-9.

1961 Daniel TA, Nawarskas JJ. Vitamin C in the prevention of nitrate tolerance. *Ann Pharmacother* 2000;34:1193-7.

1962 Hodby ED, Hirsh J, Adeniyi-Jones C. The influence of drugs upon the anticoagulant activity of heparin. *Can Med Assoc J* 1972;106:562-4.

1963 Leibovitz B, Siegel BV. Ascorbic acid and the immune response. *Adv Exp Med Biol* 1981;135:1-25.

1964 Kasa RM. Vitamin C: from scurvy to the common cold. *Am J Med Technol* 1983;49:23-6.

1965 Vilter RW. Nutritional aspects of ascorbic acid: uses and abuses. *West J Med* 1980;133:485-92.

1966 Martin NG, Carr AB, Oakeshott JG, Clark P. Co-twin control studies: vitamin C and the common cold. *Prog Clin Biol Res* 1982;103:365-73.

1967 Pitt HA, Costrini AM. Vitamin C prophylaxis in marine recruits. *JAMA* 1979;241:908-11.

1968 Anderson TW. Vitamin C and the common cold. *J Med Soc N J* 1979;76:765-6.

1969 Coulehan JL. Ascorbic acid and the common cold: reviewing the evidence. *Postgrad Med* 1979;66:153-60.

1970 Uebelhart D, Thonar EJ, Delmas PD, et al. Effects of oral chondroitin sulfate on the progression of knee osteoarthritis: a pilot study. *Osteoarthritis Cartilage*, May. 1998; 6 Suppl A:39-46.

1971 Bourgeois P, Chales G, Dehais J, et al. Efficacy and tolerability of chondroitin sulfate 1200 mg/day vs chondroitin sulfate 3 x 400 mg/day vs placebo. *Osteoarthritis Cartilage*, May 1998; 6 Suppl A:25-30.

1972 Bucsi L, Poor G. Efficacy and tolerability of oral chondroitin sulfate as a symptomatic slow-acting drug for osteoarthritis (SYSADOA) in the treatment of knee osteoarthritis. *Osteoarthritis Cartilage*, May 1998; 6 Suppl A:31-6.

1973 Kelly GS. The role of glucosamine sulfate and chondroitin sulfates in the treatment of degenerative joint disease. *Altern Med Rev*, Feb. 1998; 3(1):27-39.

1974 Limberg MB, McCaa C, Kissling GE, Kaufman HE. Topical application of hyaluronic acid and chondroitin sulfate in the treatment of dry eyes. *Am J Ophthalmol*, 15 Feb. 1987; 103(2):194-7.

1975 Fan YY, Chapkin RS. Importance of dietary gamma-linolenic acid in human health and nutrition. *J Nutr*, Sep. 1998; 128(9):1411-4.

1976 Johnson MM, Swan DD, Surette ME. Dietary supplementation with gamma-linolenic acid alters fatty acid content and eicosanoid production in healthy humans. *J Nutr*, Aug. 1997; 127(8):1435-44.

1977 Stainforth JM, Layton AM, Goodfield MJ. Clinical aspects of the use of gamma linolenic acid in systemic sclerosis. *Acta Derm Venereol*, Mar. 1996; 76(2):144-6.

1978 McCaul JA, Lamey PJ. Multiple oral mucoceles treated with gamma-linolenic acid: report of a case. *Br J Oral Maxillofac Surg*, Dec. 1994; 32(6):392-3.

1979 Guivernau M, Meza N, Barja P, Roman O. Clinical and experimental study on the long-term effect of dietary gamma-linolenic acid on plasma lipids, platelet aggregation, thromboxane formation, and prostacyclin production. *Prostaglandins Leukot Essent Fatty Acids*,

Nov. 1994; 51(5):311-6.

1980 Jamal GA. The use of gamma linolenic acid in the prevention and treatment of diabetic neuropathy. *Diabet Med* 1994 Mar;11(2):145-9.

1981 Horrobin DF. The use of gamma-linolenic acid in diabetic neuropathy. *Agents Actions Suppl* 1992;37:120-44.

1982 Cant A, Shay J, Horrobin DF. The effect of maternal supplementation with linoleic and gamma- linolenic acids on the fat composition and content of human milk: a placebo-controlled trial. *J Nutr Sci Vitaminol (Tokyo)* 1991 Dec;37(6):573-9.

1983 van der Merwe CF, Booyens J, Joubert HF, van der Merwe CA. The effect of gamma-linolenic acid, an in vitro cytostatic substance contained in evening primrose oil, on primary liver cancer. A double- blind placebo controlled trial. *Prostaglandins Leukot Essent Fatty Acids*, Jul. 1990; 40(3):199-202.

1984 Jamal GA, Carmichael H. The effect of gamma-linolenic acid on human diabetic peripheral neuropathy: a double-blind placebo-controlled trial. *Diabet Med*, May 1990; 7(4):319-23.

1985 Pullman-Mooar S, Laposata M, Lem D. Alteration of the cellular fatty acid profile and the production of eicosanoids in human monocytes by gamma-linolenic acid. *Arthritis Rheum*, Oct. 1990; 33(10):1526-33.

1986 Davies JE, Hughes RE, Jones E, et al. Metabolism of ascorbic acid (vitamin C) in subjects infected with common cold viruses. *Biochem Med* 1979;21:78-85.

1987 Hemila H. Does vitamin C alleviate the symptoms of the common cold?- a review of current evidence. *Scand J Infect Dis* 1994;26:1-6.

1988 Hemila H, Herman ZS. Vitamin C and the common cold: a retrospective analysis of Chalmers' review. *J Am Coll Nutr* 1995;14:116-23.

1989 Hemila H. Vitamin C, the placebo effect, and the common cold: a case study of how preconceptions influence the analysis of results. *J Clin Epidemiol* 1996;49:1079-84.

1990 Barrington WW, Angle CR, Willcockson NK, et al. Autonomic function in manganese alloy workers. *Environ Res*, Jul. 1998; 78(1):50-8.

1991 Greger JL. Dietary standards for manganese: overlap between nutritional and toxicological studies. *J Nutr*, Feb. 1998; 128(2 Suppl):368S-71S.

1992 Hauser RA, Zesiewicz TA, Martinez C, et al. Blood manganese correlates with brain magnetic resonance imaging changes in patients with liver disease. *Can J Neurol Sci*, May 1996; 23(2):95-8.

1993 Okano T. Effects of essential trace elements on bone turnover-in relation to the osteoporosis. *Nippon Rinsho* 1996 Jan;54(1):148-54.

1994 Strause L, Saltman P, Smith KT, et al. Spinal bone loss in postmenopausal women supplemented with calcium and trace minerals. *J Nutr*, Jul. 1994; 124(7):1060-4.

1995 Lean ME, Noroozi M, Kelly I. Dietary flavonols protect diabetic human lymphocytes against oxidative damage to DNA. *Diabetes* 1999 Jan;48(1):176-81.

1996 Rachkauskas GS. The efficacy of enterosorption and a combination of antioxidants in schizophrenics. *Lik Sprava* 1998 Jun;(4):122-4.

1997 Kuo SM, Leavitt PS, Lin CP. Dietary flavonoids interact with trace metals and affect metallothionein level in human intestinal cells. *Biol Trace Elem Res* 1998 Jun;62(3):135-53.

1998 Conquer JA, Maiani G, Azzini E, et al. Supplementation with quercetin markedly increases plasma quercetin concentration without effect on selected risk factors for heart disease in healthy subjects. *J Nutr* 1998 Mar;128(3):593-7.

1999 Janssen K, Mensink RP, Cox FJ, et al. Effects of the flavonoids quercetin and apigenin on hemostasis in healthy volunteers: results from an in vitro and a dietary supplement study. *Am J Clin Nutr* 1998 Feb;67(2):255-62.

2000 Freeland-Graves JH, Lin PH. Plasma uptake of manganese as affected by oral loads of manganese, calcium, milk, phosphorus, copper, and zinc. *J Am Coll Nutr*, Feb. 1991; 10(1):38-43.

2001 Krieger D, Krieger S, Jansen O, et al. Manganese and chronic hepatic encephalopathy. *Lancet*, 29 Jul. 1995; 346(8970):270-4.

2002 O'Dell BL. Mineral interactions relevant to nutrient requirements. *J Nutr*, Dec. 1989; 119(12 Suppl):1832-8.

2003 Moghissi KS. Risks and benefits of nutritional supplements during pregnancy. *Obstet Gynecol*, Nov. 1981; 58(5 Suppl):68S-78S.

2004 Penland JG, Johnson PE. Dietary calcium and manganese effects on menstrual cycle symptoms. *Am J Obstet Gynecol*, May 1993; 168(5):1417-23.

2005 Freeland-Graves JH, Turnlund JR. Deliberations and evaluations of the approaches, endpoints and paradigms for manganese and molybdenum dietary recommendations. *J Nutr*, Sep. 1996; 126(9 Suppl):2435S-40S.

2006 Li MK, et al. Effects of magnesium on calcium oxalate crystallization. *J Urol* 1985;133:123.

2007 Johansson G, Backman U, Danielson BG, et al. Biochemical and clinical effects of the prophylactic treatment of renal calcium stones with magnesium hydroxide. *J Urol* 1980;124:770-4.

2008 Freeland-Graves JH. Manganese: an essential nutrient for humans. *Nutr Today* 1988;23:13-9.

2009 Prudden JF, Balassa LL. The biological activity of bovine cartilage preparations. Clinical demonstration of their potent anti-inflammatory capacity with supplementary notes on certain relevant fundamental supportive studies. *Semin Arthritis Rheum* 1974 Summer;3(4):287-321.

2010 Prudden JF. The treatment of human cancer with agents prepared from bovine cartilage. *J Biol Response Mod* 1985 Dec;4(6):551-84.

2011 Durk H, Haase K, Saal J, et al. Nephrotic syndrome after injections of bovine cartilage and marrow extract. [letter] *Lancet* 1989 March 18;1(8638):614.

2012 Ashar B, Vargo E. Shark cartilage-induced hepatitis. [letter] *Ann Intern Med*, 1 Nov. 1996;125(9):780-1.

2013 Hunt TJ, Connelly JF. Shark cartilage for cancer treatment. *Am J Health Syst Pharm*, 15 Aug. 1995;52(16):1756-60.

2014 Lane IW, Comac L. Sharks don't get cancer. Garden City, NY: Avery Publishing Group; 1992.

2015 Miller DR, Anderson GT, Stark JJ, et al. Phase I/II trial of the safety and efficacy of shark cartilage in the treatment of advanced cancer. *J Clin Oncol* Nov. 1998;16(11):3649-55.

2016 Bovine cartilage, Vitamin Connection Website, URL: www.vitaminconnect.com (Accessed 24 June 1999).

2017 Bovine cartilage, ecoNugenics Website, URL: www.econugenics.com (Accessed 24 June 1999).

2018 Trial information, CenterWatch Website, URL: www.centerwatch.com (Accessed 24 June 1999).

2019 CancerNet, National Cancer Institute Website; URL: cancernet.nci.nih.gov (Accessed 28 June 1999).

2020 Sturtevant FM. Use of aspartame in pregnancy. *Int J Fertil* 1985;30(1):85-7.

2021 Silkaitis RP, Mosnaim AD. Pathways linking L-phenylalanine and 2-phenylethylamine with p-tyramine in rabbit brain. *Brain Res* 1976;114(1):105-15.

2022 Recommended Daily Allowances. USDA website, URL: www.nal.usda.gov/fnic/dga/rda.pdf (Accessed 8 March 2000).

2023 PKU - Dietary Treatment of the Untreated Adult PKU. National Society for Phenylketonuria (NSPKU) website, URL: web.ukonline.co.uk/nspku/untreatd.htm (Accessed 8 March 2000).

2024 Fouty B, Frerman F, Reves R. Riboflavin to treat nucleoside analogue-induced lactic acidosis. *Lancet* 1998;352(9124):291-2.

2025 Levine J, Mishori A, Susnosky M, et al. Combination of inositol and serotonin reuptake inhibitors in the treatment of depression. *Biol Psychiatry*, 1999;45(3):270-3.

2026 Levine J, Barak Y, Kofman O, Belmaker RH. Follow-up and relapse analysis of an inositol study of depression. *Isr J Psychiatry Relat Sci*, 1995;32(1):14-21.

2027 Souza FG, Mander AJ, Foggo M, et al. The effects of lithium discontinuation and the non-effect of oral inositol upon thyroid hormones and cortisol in patients with bipolar affective disorder. *J Affect Disord* 1991;22(3):165-70.

2028 Nestler JE, Jakubowicz DJ, Reamer P, et al. Ovulatory and metabolic effects of D-chiro-inositol in the polycystic ovary syndrome. *N Engl J Med*, 1999;340(17):1314-20.

2030 Soleas GJ, Diamandis EP, Goldberg DM. Resveratrol: a molecule whose time has come? And gone? *Clin Biochem* 1997;30(2):91-113.

2031 Ross D, Cooper AJ, Pryse-Davies J, et al. Randomized, double-blind, dose-ranging study of the endometrial effects of a vaginal progesterone gel in estrogen-treated postmenopausal women. *Am J Obstet Gynecol* 1997;177(4):937-41.

2032 Pouly JL, Bassil S, Frydman R, et al. Luteal support after in-vitro fertilization: Crinone 8%, a sustained release vaginal progesterone gel, versus Utrogestan, an oral micronized progesterone. *Hum Reprod* 1996;11(10):2085-9.

2033 Affinito P, Di Carlo C, Di Mauro P, et al. Endometrial hyperplasia: efficacy of a new treatment with a vaginal cream containing natural micronized progesterone. *Maturitas* 1994;20(2-3):191-8.

2034 Miles RA, Paulson RJ, Lobo RA, et al. Pharmacokinetics and endometrial tissue levels of progesterone after administration by intramuscular and vaginal routes: a comparative study. *Fertil Steril* 1994;62(3):485-90.

2041 Warren MP, Biller BMK, Shangold MM. A new clinical option for hormone replacement therapy in women with secondary amenorrhea: effects of cyclic administration of progesterone from the sustained-release vaginal gel Crinone (4% and 8%) on endometrial morphologic features and withdrawal bleeding. *Am J Obstet Gynecol* 1999;180(1 Pt 1):42-8.

2042 van den Berg H. Carotenoid interactions. *Nutr Rev*

REFERENCES

1999;57(1):1-10.

2043 Mazzotta G, Sarchielli P, Alberti A, Gallai V. Intracellular Mg++ concentration and electromyographical ischemic test in juvenile headache. *Cephalalgia* 1999;19(9):802-9.

2044 Duffy SJ, Gokce N, Holbrook M, et al. Treatment of hypertension with ascorbic acid. *Lancet* 1999;354(9195):2048-9.

2045 Zollinger PE, Tuinebreijer WE, Kreis RW, Breederveld RS. Effect of vitamin C on frequency of reflex sympathetic dystrophy in wrist fractures: a randomized trial. *Lancet* 1999;354(9195):2025-8.

2047 Colodny L, Hoffman RL. Inositol—clinical applications for exogenous use. *Altern Med Rev*, 1998;3(6):432-47.

2048 Nomenclature of Cyclitols. IUPAC Commission on the Nomenclature of Organic Chemistry (CNOC) and IUPAC-IUB Commission on Biochemical Nomenclature (CBN). URL: http://www.chem.qmw.ac.uk/iupac/cyclitol/ (Accessed 28 January 2000).

2049 Mori TA, Bao DQ, Burke V, et al. Dietary fish as a major component of a weight-loss diet: effect on serum lipids, glucose, and insulin metabolism in overweight hypertensive subjects. *Am J Clin Nutr* 1999;70(5):817-25.

2050 Stryer L. Biochemistry, third edition. W.H. Freeman and Co., New York, 1988.

2051 www.quest-iv-health.com/articles/amino.html (Accessed 2 February 2000).

2052 Lehmann WD, Theobald N, Fischer R, Heinrich HC. Stereospecificity of phenylalanine plasma kinetics and hydroxylation in man following oral application of a stable isotope-labelled pseudo-racemic mixture of L- and D-phenylalanine. *Clin Chim Acta* 1983;128(2-3):181-98.

2053 Disorders of amino-acid metabolism. Encyclopaedia Britannica website: www.britannica.com/bcom/eb/article/5/0,5716,118195+10,00.html (Accessed 3 February 2000).

2054 Tyrosinemia. Encyclopaedia Britannica website: www.britannica.com/bcom/eb/article/idxref/5/0,5716,507499,00.html (Accessed 3 February 2000).

2055 Alkaptonuria. Encyclopaedia Britannica website: www.britannica.com/bcom/eb/article/idxref/5/0,5716,507502,00.html (Accessed 3 February 2000).

2056 Kraft K. Artichoke leaf extract- recent findings reflecting effects on lipid metabolism, liver and gastrointestinal tracts. *Phytomedicine* 1997;4(4):369-78.

2057 Soleas GJ, Diamandis EP, Goldberg DM. Wine as a biological fluid: history, production, and role in disease prevention. *J Clin Lab Anal* 1997;11(5):287-313.

2058 Renaud SC, Gueguen R, Siest G, Salamon R. Wine, beer, and mortality in middle-aged men from eastern France. *Arch Intern Med* 1999;159(16):1865-70.

2059 Leighton F, Cuevas A, Guasch V, et al. Plasma polyphenols and antioxidants, oxidative DNA damage and endothelial function in a diet and wine intervention study in humans. *Drugs Exp Clin Res* 1999;25(2-3):133-41.

2060 Criqui MH. Alcohol and coronary heart disease: consistent relationship and public health implications. *Clin Chim Acta* 1996;246(1-2):51-7.

2061 Renaud SC, Ruf JC. Effects of alcohol on platelet functions. *Clin Chim Acta* 1996;246(1-2):77-89.

2063 Yun TK, Choi SY. Non-organ specific cancer prevention of ginseng: a prospective study in Korea. *Int J Epidemiol* 1998;27(3):359-64.

2064 Sorensen H, Sonne J. A double-masked study of the effects of ginseng on cognitive functions. *Curr Ther Res* 1996;57(12):959-68.

2065 Bitzan MM, Gold BD, Philpott DJ, et al. Inhibition of Helicobacter pylori and Helicobacter mustelae binding to lipid receptors by bovine colostrum. *J Infect Dis* 1998;177(4):955-61.

2067 Huppertz HI, Rutkowski S, Busch DH, et al. Bovine colostrum ameliorates diarrhea in infection with diarrheogenic Escherichia coli, shiga toxin-producing E. Coli, and E. coli expressing intimin and hemolysin. *J Pediatr Gastroenterol Nutr* 1999;29(4):452-6.

2068 Freedman DJ, Tacket CO, Delehanty A, et al. Milk immunoglobulin with specific activity against purified colonization factor antigens can protect against oral challenge with enterotoxigenic Escherichia coli. *J Infect Dis* 1998;177(3):662-7.

2069 Tacket CO, Losonsky G, Link H, et al. Protection by milk immunoglobulin concentrate against oral challenge with enterotoxigenic Escherichia coli. *N Engl J Med* 1988;318(19):1240-3.

2070 Tacket CO, Binion SB, Bostwick E, et al. Efficacy of bovine milk immunoglobulin concentrate in preventing illness after Shigella flexneri challenge. *Am J Trop Med Hyg* 1992;47(3):276-83.

2071 Tacket CO, Losonsky G, Livio S, et al. Lack of prophylactic efficacy of an enteric-coated bovine hyperimmune milk product against enterotoxigenic Escherichia coli challenge administered during a standard meal. *J Infect Dis* 1999 Dec;180(6):2056-9.

2072 Petschow BW, Talbott RD. Reduction in virus-neutralizing activity of a bovine colostrum immunoglobulin concentrate by gastric acid and digestive enzymes. *J Pediatr Gastroenterol Nutr* 1994;19(2):228-35.

2074 Kuhlmann J, Berger W, Podzuweit H, Schmidt U. The influence of valerian treatment on "reaction time, alertness and concentration" in volunteers. *Pharmacopsychiatry* 1999;32(6):235-41.

2075 Dev S. Ancient-modern concordance in Ayurvedic plants: some examples. *Environ Health Perspect* 1999;107(10):783-9.

2076 GRIN Taxonomy search page http://www.ars-grin.gov/cgi-bin/npgs/html/tax_search.pl? (Accessed 27 February 2000).

2077 Jacob A, Pandey M, Kapoor S, Saroja R. Effect of the Indian gooseberry (amla) on serum cholesterol levels in men aged 35-55 years. *Eur J Clin Nutr* 1988;42(11):939-44.

2078 Asmawi MZ, Kankaanranta H, Moilanen E, Vapaatalo H. Anti-inflammatory activities of Emblica officinalis Gaertn leaf extracts. *J Pharm Pharmacol* 1993;45(6):581-4.

2079 Ihantola-Vormisto A, Summanen J, Kankaanranta H, et al. Anti-inflammatory activity of extracts from leaves of Phyllanthus emblica. *Planta Med* 1997;63(6):518-24.

2080 Hu JF. [Inhibitory effects of Phyllanthus emblica juice on formation of N-nitrosomorpholine in vitro and N-nitrosoproline in rat and human]. [Article in Chinese] *Chung Hua Yu Fang I Hsueh Tsa Chih* 1990;24(3):132-5.

2081 Bhattacharya A, Chatterjee A, Ghosal S, Bhattacharya SK. Antioxidant activity of active tannoid principles of Emblica officinalis (amla). *Indian J Exp Biol*

1999;37(7):676-80.

2082 Janicak PG, Lipinski J, Davis JM, et al. S-adenosylmethionine in depression. A literature review and preliminary report. *Ala J Med Sci* 1988;25(3):306-13.

2083 De Vanna M, Rigamonti R. Oral S-adenosyl-L-methionine in depression. *Curr Ther Res* 1992;52(3):478-85.

2084 Zhao G. [Inherited metabolic aberration of phenylalanine in the family members of patients with essential hypertension and stroke]. [Article in Chinese]. *Chung Hua I Hsueh Tsa Chih (Taipei)* 1991;71(7):28, 388-90.

2085 Dr. Duke's Phytochemical and Ethnobotanical Databases; URL: www.ars-grin.gov/duke/ (Accessed 24 March 2000).

2086 Damario MA, Goudas VT, Session DR, et al. Crinone 8% vaginal progesterone gel results in lower embryonic implantation efficiency after in vitro fertilization-embryo transfer. *Fertil Steril,* 1999;72(5):830-6.

2087 Columbia Labs. HYPERLINK URL: http://www.columbialabs.com/html/crinhealth/progesterone/dosage.htm (Accessed 9 March 2000).

2088 Clinical Pharmacology. HYPERLINK URL: http://www.imc.gsm.com/scripts/frameset.asp (Accessed 9 March 2000).

2089 Gibbons WE, Toner JP, Hamacher P, Kolm P. Experience with a novel vaginal progesterone preparation in a donor oocyte program. *Fertil Steril* 1998;69(1):96-101.

2091 HYPERLINK URL: http://www.fda.gov/medwatch/safety/1998/may98.htm#crinon (Accessed 9 March 2000).

2092 Woelk H, Kapoula O, Lehrl S, et al. [Comparison of kava special extract WS 1490 and benzodiazepines in patients with anxiety]. [Article in German]. *Z Allg Med* 1993;69:271–7.

2093 Pittler MH, Ernst E. Efficacy of kava extract for treating anxiety: systematic review and meta-analysis. *J Clin Psychopharmacol* 2000;20(1):84-9.

2094 Volz HP, Kieser M. Kava-kava extract WS 1490 versus placebo in anxiety disorders—a randomized placebo-controlled 25-week outpatient trial. *Pharmacopsychiatry* 1997;30(1):1-5.

2095 Lehmann E, Kinzler E, Friedemann J. Efficacy of a special Kava extract (Piper methysticum) in patients with states of anxiety, tension and excitedness of non-mental origin- a double-blind placebo-controlled study of four weeks treatment. *Phytomedicine* 1996;3(2):113-9.

2096 Warnecke G. [Psychosomatic dysfunctions in the female climacteric. Clinical effectiveness and tolerance of Kava extract WS 1490]. [Article in German]. *Fortschr Med* 1991;109(4):119-22.

2097 Heinze HJ, Munthe TF, Steitz J, Matzke M. Pharmacopsychological effects of oxazepam and kava-extract in a visual search paradigm assessed with event-related potentials. *Pharmacopsychiatry* 1994;27(6):224-30.

2098 Munte TF, Heinze HJ, Matzke M, Steitz J. Effects of oxazepam and an extract of kava roots (Piper methysticum) on event-related potentials in a word recognition task. *Neuropsychobiology* 1993;27(1):46-53.

2099 Folic acid. SupraHealth, Inc. www.suprahealth.com/folic.htm. (Accessed 7 July 1999).

2100 Kreider RB, Ferreira M, Wilson M, et al. Effects of creatine supplementation on body composition, strength, and sprint performance. *Med Sci Sports Exerc* 1998;30(1):73-82.

2101 Vandenberghe K, Goris M, Van Hecke P, et al. Long-term creatine intake is beneficial to muscle performance during resistance training. *J Appl Physiol* 1997;83(6):2055-63.

2102 Earnest CP, Snell PG, Rodriguez R, et al. The effect of creatine monohydrate ingestion on aneробic power indices, muscular strength and body composition. *Acta Physiol Scand* 1995;153:207-9.

2103 Balsom PD, Soderland K, Ekblom B. Creatine in humans with special reference to creatine supplementation. *Sports Med* 1994;18(4):268-80.

2104 Hultman E, Soderlund K, Timmons JA, et al. Muscle creatine loading in men. *J Appl Physiol* 1996;81:232-7.

2105 Burke LM, Pyne DB, Telford RD. Oral creatine supplementation does not improve sprint performance in elite swimmers. *Med Sci Sports Exerc* 1995;27:S146.

2106 Mujika I, Chatard J, Lacoste L, et al. Creatine supplementation does not improve sprint performance in competitive swimmers. *Med Sci Sports Exerc* 1996;28(11):1435-41.

2107 Hanioka T, Tanaka M, Ojima M, et al. Effect of topical application of coenzyme Q10 on adult periodontitis. *Molec Aspects Med* 1994;15 (Suppl): S241-8.

2108 Watts TLP. Coenzyme Q10 and periodontal treatment: is there any beneficial effect? *Br Dent J* 1995;178:209-13.

2109 Malm C, Svensson M, Ekblom B, et al. Effects of ubiquinone-10 supplementation and high intensity training on physical performance in humans. *Acta Physiol Scand* 1997;161:379-84.

2110 Weston SB, Zhou S, Weatherby RP, et al. Does exogenous coenzyme Q10 affect aerobic capacity in endurance athletes? *Int J Sport Nutr* 1997;7:197-206.

2111 Kuritzky L. DHEA: Science or Wishful Thinking? *Hosp Pract* 1998; 33(5):85-6.

2112 Skolnick AA. Scientific verdict still out on DHEA. *JAMA* 1996;276(17):1365-7.

2113 Van Vollenhoven RF, Morabito LM, Engleman EG, et al. Treatment of Systemic Lupus Erythematosus with Dehydroepiandrosterone: 50 Patients Treated up to 12 Months. *J Rheumatol* 1998; 25:285-9.

2114 Van Vollenhoven RF, Engleman EG, McGurie JL. Dehydroepiandrosterone in Systemic Lupus Erythematosus. *Arth Rheum* 1995; 38(12):1826-31.

2115 Ebeling P, Koivisto VA. Physiological Importance of dehydroepiandrosterone. *Lancet* 1994; 343:1479-81.

2116 Dehydroepiandrosterone (DHEA). *Med Lett Drugs Ther* 1996; 38:91-2.

2117 Vandeberghe K, Gillis N, Van Leemputte M, et al. Caffeine counteracts the ergogenic action of muscle creatine loading. *J Appl Physiol* 1996;80(2):452-7.

2118 Pritchard NR, Kalra PA. Renal dysfunction accompanying oral creatine supplements. *Lancet* 1998;351(9111):1252-3.

2119 Braverman Y, Chizov-Ginzburg A. Repellency of synthetic and plant-derived preparations for Culicoides imicola. *Med Vet Entomol* 1997;11:355-60.

2120 Poortmans JR, Auquier H, Renaut V, et al. Effect of short-term creatine supplementation on renal responses in men. *Eur J Appl Physiol* 1997;76:566-7.

2121 Kamikawa T, Kobayashi A, Yamashita T, et al. Effects of coenzyme Q10 on exercise tolerance in chronic stable angina pectoris. *Am J Cardiol* 1985;56(4):247-51.

2122 Langsjoen P, Willis R, Folkers K. Treatment of essential hypertension with coenzyme Q10. *Mol Aspects Med* 1994;15 Suppl:S265-72.

2123 Folkers K, Hanioka T, Xia LJ, et al. Coenzyme Q10 increases T4/T8 ratios of lymphocytes in ordinary subjects and relevance to patients having the AIDS related complex. *Biochem Biophys Res Commun* 1991;176(2):786-91.

2124 Folkers K, Langsjoen P, Nara Y, et al. Biochemical deficiencies of coenzyme Q10 in HIV-infection and exploratory treatment. *Biochem Biophys Res Commun.* 1988;153(2):888-96.

2125 Suzuki S, Hinokio Y, Ohtomo M, et al. The effects of coenzyme Q10 treatment on maternally inherited diabetes mellitus and deafness, and mitochondrial DNA 3243 (A to G) mutation. *Diabetologia.* 1998;41(5):584-8.

2126 Andersen CB, Henriksen JE, Hother-Nielsen O, et al. The effect of coenzyme Q10 on blood glucose and insulin requirement in patients with insulin dependent diabetes mellitus. *Mol Aspects Med.* 1997;18 Suppl:S307-9.

2127 Folkers K, Simonsen R. Two successful double-blind trials with coenzyme Q10 (vitamin Q10) on muscular dystrophies and neurogenic atrophies. *Biochem Biophys Acta.* 1995;1271(1):281-6.

2128 Spigset O. Reduced effect of warfarin caused by ubidecarenone. *Lancet* 1994;334:1372-3.

2129 Daferera DJ, Ziogas BN, Polissiou MG. GC-MS analysis of essential oils from some Greek aromatic plants and their fungitoxicity on Penicillium digitatum. *J Agric Food Chem* 2000;48:2576-81.

2130 Dorman HJ, Deans SG. Antimicrobial agents from plants: antibacterial activity of plant volatile oils. *J Appl Microbiol* 2000;88:308-16.

2131 Buckle J. Use of aromatherapy as a complementary treatment for chronic pain. *Altern Ther Health Med* 1999;5:42-51.

2132 Degelau J, Guay D, Hallgren H. The effect of DHEAS on influenza vaccination in aging adults. *J Am Geriatr Soc* 1997;45(6):747-51.

2133 Yen SS, Morales AJ, Khorram O. Replacement of DHEA in aging men and women. Potential remedial effects. *Ann N Y Acad Sci* 1995;774:128-42.

2134 Greenberg S, Fishman WH. Coenzyme Q10: A New Drug for Cardiovascular Disease. *J Clin Pharmacol* 1990;30:596-608.

2135 Lewin A, Lavon H. The effect of coenzyme Q10 on sperm motility and function. *Mol Aspects Med* 1997;18 Suppl:S213-9.

2136 van Vollenhoven RF, Engleman EG, McGuire JL. Dehydroepiandrosterone in Systemic Lupus Erythematosus. *Arthritis Rheum* 1994;37(9):1305-10.

2138 Goodman GA, Rall TW, Nies AS, Taylor P. The Pharmacological Basis of Therapeutics 9th edition.

2139 Ma J, Stampfer MJ, Giovannucci E, et al. Methylenetetrahydrofolate reductase polymorphism, dietary interactions, and risk of colorectal cancer. *Cancer Res* 1997;57(6):1098-102.

2140 Lashner BA, Provencher KS, Seidner DL, et al. The effect of folic acid supplementation on the risk for cancer or dysplasia in ulcerative colitis. *Gastroenterol* 1997;112(1):29-32.

2141 La Vecchia C, Braga C, Negri E et al. Intake of selected micronutrients and risk of colorectal cancer. *Int J Cancer* 1997;73:525-30.

2142 Tseng M, Murray SC, Kupper LL, Sandler RS. Micronutrients and the risk of colorectal adenomas. *Am J Epidemiol* 1996;144(11):1005-14.

2143 Baron JA, Sandler RS, Haile RW, et al. Folate intake, alcohol consumption, cigarette smoking, and risk of colorectal adenomas. *J Natl Cancer Inst* 1998;90(1):57-62.

2144 Slattery ML, Schaffer D, Edwards SL, et al. Are dietary factors involved in DNA methylation associated with colon cancer? *Nutr Cancer* 1997;28(1):52-62.

2145 Freudenheim JL, Graham S, Marshall JR, et al. Folate intake and carcinogenesis of the colon and rectum. *Int J Epidemiol* 1991;20(2):368-74.

2146 Brouwer IA, van Dusseldorp M, Thomas CM, et al. Low-dose folic acid supplementation decreases plasma homocysteine concentrations: a randomized trial. *Am J Clin Nutr* 1999;69(1):99-104.

2147 Landgren F, Israelsson B, Lindgren A, et al. Plasma homocysteine in acute myocardial infarction: homocysteine-lowering effect of folic acid. *J Intern Med* 1995;237(4):381-8.

2148 Woodside JV, Yarnell JW, McMaster D, et al. Effect of B-group vitamins and antioxidant vitamins on hyperhomocysteinemia: a double-blind, randomized, factorial-design, controlled trial. *Am J Clin Nutr* 1998;67(5):858-66.

2149 Brattstrom LE, Israelsson B, Jeppsson JO, et al. Folic acid-an innocuous means to reduce plasma homocysteine. *Scand J Clin Lab Invest* 1988;48(3):215-21.

2150 Brown RS, Di Stanislao PT, Beaver WT, et al. The administration of folic acid to institutionalized epileptic adults with phenytoin-induced gingival hyperplasia. A double-blind, randomized, placebo-controlled, parallel study. *Oral Surg Oral Med Oral Pathol* 1991;70(5):565-8.

2151 Drew HJ, Vogel RI, Molofsky W, et al. Effect of folate on phenytoin hyperplasia. *J Clin Periodontol* 1987;14(6):350-6.

2152 Pack AR, Thomson ME. Effects of topical and systemic folic acid supplementation on gingivitis in pregnancy. *J Clin Periodontol* 1980;7(5):402-14.

2153 Juhlin L, Olsson MJ. Improvement of vitiligo after oral treatment with vitamin B12 and folic acid and the importance of sun exposure. *Acta Derm Venereol* 1997;77(6):460-2.

2154 Montes LF, Diaz ML, Lajous J, et al. Folic acid and vitamin B12 in vitiligo: a nutritional approach. *Cutis* 1992;50(1):39-42.

2155 Strom CM, Brusca RM, Pizzi WJ. Double-blind, placebo-controlled crossover study of folinic acid Leucovorin for the treatment of fragile X syndrome. *Am J Med Genet* 1992;44(5):676-82.

2156 Fisch GS, Cohen IL, Gross AC, et al. Folic acid treatment of fragile X males: a further study. *Am J Med Genet* 1988;30(1-2):393-9.

2157 Gillberg C, Wahlstrom J, Johansson R, et al. Folic acid as an adjunct in the treatment of children with the autism fragile-X syndrome (AFRAX). *Dev Med Child Neurol* 1986;28(5):624-7.

2158 Rosenblatt DS, Duschenes EA, Hellstrom FV, et al. Folic acid blinded trial in identical twins with fragile X syndrome. *Am J Hum Genet* 1985;37(3):543-52.

2159 Hagerman RJ, Jackson AW, Levitas A, et al. Oral folic acid versus placebo in the treatment of males with the fragile X syndrome. *Am J Med Genet* 1986;23(1-2):241-62.

2160 Brown WT, Cohen IL, Fisch GS, et al. High dose folic acid treatment of fragile (X) males. *Am J Med Genet* 1986;23(1-2):263-71.

2161 Muggia FM, Synold TW, Newman EM, et al. Failure of pretreatment with intravenous folic acid to alter the cumulative hematologic toxicity of lometrexol. *J Natl Cancer Inst* 1996;88(20):1495-6.

2162 Morgan SL, Baggott JE, Vaughn WH, et al. Supplementation with folic acid during methotrexate therapy for rheumatoid arthritis. A double-blind, placebo-controlled trial. *Ann Intern Med* 1994;121(11):833-41.

2163 Morgan SL, Baggott JE, Vaughn WH, et al. The effect of folic acid supplementation on the toxicity of low-dose methotrexate in patients with rheumatoid arthritis. *Arthritis Rheum* 1990;33(1):9-18.

2164 Ortiz Z, Shea B, Suarez-Almazor ME, et al. The efficacy of folic acid and folinic acid in reducing methotrexate gastrointestinal toxicity in rheumatoid arthritis. A metaanalysis of randomized controlled trials. *J Rheumatol* 1998;25(1):36-43.

2165 Kelly GS. Folates: supplemental forms and therapeutic applications. *Altern Med Rev* 1998;3(3):208-20.

2166 Pack AR. Effects of folate mouthwash on experimental gingivitis in man. *J Clin Periodontol* 1986;13(7):671-6.

2167 HMB Musclesoft. URL: musclesoft.com/hmb.htm (Accessed 24 July 1999).

2168 Nissen S, Sharp R, Ray M, et al. Effect of leucine metabolite beta-hydroxy-beta-methylbutyrate on muscle metabolism during resistance-exercise training. *J Appl Physiol* 1996;81(5):2095-104.

2169 Gennari C, Agnusdei D, Crepaldi G, et al. Effect of ipriflavone-a synthetic derivative of natural isoflavones-on bone mass loss in the early years after menopause. *Menopause* 1998;5(1):9-15.

2170 Agnusdei D, Crepaldi G, Isaia G, et al. A double blind, placebo-controlled trial of ipriflavone for prevention of postmenopausal spinal bone loss. *Calcif Tissue Int* 1997;61(2):142-7.

2171 Gambacciani M, Ciaponi M, Cappagli B, et al. Effects of combined low dose of the isoflavone derivative ipriflavone and estrogen replacement on bone mineral density and metabolism in postmenopausal women. *Maturitas* 1997;28(1):75-81.

2172 Agnusdei D, Gennari C, Bufalino L. Prevention of early postmenopausal bone loss using low doses of conjugated estrogens and the non-hormonal, bone-active drug ipriflavone. *Osteoporos Int* 1995;5(6):462-6.

2173 Valente M, Bufalino L, Castiglione GN, et al. Effects of 1-year treatment with ipriflavone on bone in postmenopausal women with low bone mass. *Calcif Tissue Int* 1994;54(5):377-80.

2174 Ushiroyama T, Okamura S, Ikeda A, et al. Efficacy of ipriflavone and 1 alpha vitamin D therapy for the cessation of vertebral bone loss. *Int J Gynaecol Obstet* 1995;48(3):283-8.

2175 Agnusdei D, Zacchei F, Bigazzi S, et al. Metabolic and clinical effects of ipriflavone in established post-menopausal osteoporosis. *Drugs Exp Clin Res* 1989;15(2):97-104.

2176 Agnusdei D, Camporeale A, Gonnelli S, et al. Short-term treatment of Paget's disease of bone with ipriflavone. *Bone Miner* 1992;19 Suppl 1:S35-42.

2177 Hyodo T, Ono K, Koumi T, et al. A study of the effects of ipriflavone administration on hemodialysis patients with renal osteodystrophy: preliminary report. *Nephron* 1991;58(1):114-5.

2178 Monostory K, Vereczkey L, Levai F, et al. Ipriflavone as an inhibitor of human cytochrome P450 enzymes. *Br J Pharmacol* 1998;123(4):605-10.

2179 Melis GB, Paoletti AM, Cagnacci A, et al. Lack of any estrogenic effect of ipriflavone in postmenopausal women. *J Endocrinol Invest* 1992;15(10):755-61.

2180 Inositol. Mmead Website. URL: www.mmeade.com/cheat/inositol.html (Accessed 24 July 1999).

2181 Inositol. CW Institute Website. URL: www.cwinstitute.com/cp/_disc16/00000009.htm (Accessed 24 July 1999).

2182 Inositol. Tell A Friend Website. URL: tellafriend.net/inositol.htm (Accessed 24 July 1999).

2183 Inositol. Mother Nature's Encyclopedia. URL: www.mothernature.com/ency/Supp/Inositol.asp (Accessed 24 July 1999).

2184 Benjamin J, Levine J, Fux M, et al. Double-blind, placebo-controlled, crossover trial of inositol treatment for panic disorder. *Am J Psychiatry* 1995;152(7):1084-6.

2185 Levine J, et al. Double-blind, controlled trial of inositol treatment of depression. *Am J Psychiatry,* 1995; 152(5):792-4.

2186 Fux M, et al. Inositol treatment of obsessive-compulsive disorder. *Am J Psychiatry,* 1996; 153(9):1219-21.

2187 Levine J. Controlled trials of inositol in psychiatry. *Eur Neuropsychopharmacol,* 1997; 7(2):147-55.

2188 Levine J, et al. CSF inositol in schizophrenia and high-dose inositol treatment of schizophrenia. *Eur Neuropsychopharmacol,* 1994; 4(4):487-90.

2189 Barak Y, et al. Inositol treatment of Alzheimer's disease: a double blind, cross-over placebo controlled trial. *Prog Neuropsychopharmacol Biol Psychiatry,* 1996; 20(4):729-35.

2190 Levine J, et al. Inositol treatment of autism. *J Neural Transm,* 1997; 104(2-3):307-10.

2191 Hallman M, et al. Inositol supplementation in premature infants with respiratory distress syndrome. *N Engl J Med,* 1992; 326(19):1233-9.

2192 Hallman M, Pohjavuori M, Bry K. Inositol supplementation in respiratory distress syndrome. *Lung,* 1990; 168 Suppl:877-82.

2193 Gregersen G, et al. Oral supplementation of myoinositol: effects on peripheral nerve function in human diabetics and on the concentration in plasma, erythrocytes, urine and muscle tissue in human diabetics and normals. *Acta Neurol Scand,* 1983; 67(3):164-72.

2194 Salway JG, Whitehead L, Finnegan JA. Effect of myo-inositol on peripheral-nerve function in diabetes. *Lancet,* 1978; 2(8103):1282-4.

2195 Gregersen G, et al. Myoinositol and function of peripheral nerves in human diabetics. A controlled clinical trial. *Acta Neurol Scand,* 1978; 58(4):241-8.

2196 Iodine. URL: www.suprahealth.com/iodine.htm (Accessed 19 July 1999).

2197 Ghent WR, et al. Iodine replacement in fibrocystic disease of the breast. *Can J Surg,* 1993; 36(5):453-60.

2198 Adamietz IA, et al. Prophylaxis with povidone-iodine against induction of oral mucositis by

REFERENCES

radiochemotherapy. *Support Care Cancer,* 1998; 6(4):373-7.

2199 Rahn R, Adamietz IA, Boettcher HD, et al. Povidone-iodine to prevent mucositis in patients during antineoplastic radiochemotherapy. *Dermatology* 1997;195(Suppl 2):57-61.

2200 Apelqvist J, Ragnarson Tennvall G. Cavity foot ulcers in diabetic patients: a comparative study of cadexomer iodine ointment and standard treatment. An economic analysis alongside a clinical trial. *Acta Derm Venereol,* 1996; 76(3):231-5.

2201 Vitamins etc. Potassium. URL: bookman.com.au/vitamins/potassium.html (Accessed 19 July 1999).

2202 Sequential Healing Health Services. Potassium. www.sequentialhealing.com/vit-min-nutrients/potassium.html (Accessed 19 July 1999).

2203 Poldinger W, Calanchini B, Schwarz W. A functional-dimensional approach to depression: serotonin deficiency as a target syndrome in a comparison of 5-hydroxytryptophan and fluvoxamine. *Psychopathology* 1991;24:53-81.

2204 Ribeiro CA. L-5-Hydroxytryptophan in the prophylaxis of chronic tension-type headache: a double-blind, randomized, placebo-controlled study. *Headache* 2000;40:451-6.

2205 Facts and Comparisons. Drug Facts and Comparisons. St. Louis: Wolters Kluwer Co., 1998.

2207 Ovrum E, et al. Conversion of postischemic ventricular fibrillation with intraaortic infusion of potassium chloride. *Ann Thorac Surg,* 1995; 60(1):156-9.

2208 Breslau NA, et al. Physiological effects of slow release potassium phosphate for absorptive hypercalciuria: a randomized double-blind trial. *J Urol,* 1998;160(3 Pt 1):664-8.

2209 Heller HJ, et al. Sustained reduction in urinary calcium during long-term treatment with slow release neutral potassium phosphate in absorptive hypercalciuria. *Urol* 1998;159(5):1451-5; discussion 1455-6.

2210 Singh RB, et al. Effect of treatment with magnesium and potassium on mortality and reinfarction rate of patients with suspected acute myocardial infarction. *Int J Clin Pharmacol Ther,* 1996; 34(5):219-25.

2211 Vitawise Inc. Pectin. URL: vitawise.com/apcc.htm

2212 Albert KS, Ayres JW, DiSanto AR, et al. Influence of kaolin-pectin suspension on digoxin bioavailability. *J Pharm Sci,* 1978;67(11):1582-6.

2213 Albert KS, Welch RD, DeSante KA, et al. Decreased tetracycline bioavailability caused by a bismuth subsalicylate antidiarrheal mixture. *J Pharm Sci,* 1979;68(5):586-8.

2214 Veldman FJ, Nair CH, Vorster HH, et al. Dietary pectin influences fibrin network structure in hypercholesterolaemic subjects. *Thromb Res,* 1997;86(3):183-96.

2215 Davidson MH, Dugan LD, Stocki J, et al. A low-viscosity soluble-fiber fruit juice supplement fails to lower cholesterol in hypercholesterolemic men and women. *J Nutr,* 1998;128(11):1927-32.

2216 Cerda JJ, Robbins FL, Burgin CW, et al. The effects of grapefruit pectin on patients at risk for coronary heart disease without altering diet or lifestyle. *Clin Cardiol,* 1988;11(9):589-94.

2217 Hillman LC, Peters SG, Fisher CA, et al. The effects of the fiber components pectin, cellulose and lignin on serum cholesterol levels. *Am J Clin Nutr,*

1985;42(2):207-13.

2218 Marti J. The Alternative Health & Medicine Encyclopedia. 2nd ed. Detroit, MI: Gale Research International Limited; 1998.

2219 Trevisan M, Krogh V, Freudenheim J, et al. Consumption of olive oil, butter, and vegetable oils and coronary heart disease risk factors. The Research Group ATS-RF2 of the Italian National Research Council. *JAMA,* 1990;263(5):688-92.

2220 Keys A, Menotti A, Karvonen MJ, et al. The diet and 15-year death rate in the seven countries study. *Am J Epidemiol,* 1986;124(6):903-15.

2221 Martin-Moreno JM, Willett WC, Gorgojo L, et al. Dietary fat, olive oil intake and breast cancer risk. *Int J Cancer,* 1994;58(6):774-80.

2222 la Vecchia C, Negri E, Franceschi S, et al. Olive oil, other dietary fats, and the risk of breast cancer (Italy). *Cancer Causes Control,* 1995;6(6):545-50.

2223 Trichopoulou A, Katsouyanni K, Stuver S, et al. Consumption of olive oil and specific food groups in relation to breast cancer risk in Greece. *Natl Cancer Inst,* 1995;87(2):110-6.

2224 Katan MB, Zock PL, Mensink RP. Dietary oils, serum lipoproteins, and coronary heart disease. *Am J Clin Nutr,* 1995;61(6 Suppl):1368S-73S.

2225 Rock CL, Swendseid ME. Plasma beta-carotene response in humans after meals supplemented with dietary pectin. *Am J Clin Nutr,* 1992;55(1):96-9.

2226 BC Cancer Agency. Superoxide dismutase (SOD). www.bccancer.bc.ca/uctm/36.html. (Accessed 19 July 1999).

2227 Medquest Pharmacy. Superoxide dismutase www.medquestpharmacy.com/store/prodtemplate.asp?product_id=76. (Accessed 19 July 1999).

2228 McIlwain H, Silverfield JC, Cheatum DE, et al. Intra-articular orgotein in osteoarthritis of the knee: a placebo-controlled efficacy, safety, and dosage comparison. *Am J Med,* 1989;87(3):295-300.

2229 Gammer W, Broback LG. Clinical comparison of orgotein and methylprednisolone acetate in the treatment of osteoarthrosis of the knee joint. *Scand J Rheumatol,* 1984;13(2):108-12.

2230 Goebel KM, Storck U, Neurath F. Intrasynovial orgotein therapy in rheumatoid arthritis. *Lancet,* 1981;1(8228):1015-7.

2231 Walravens M, Dequeker J. Comparison of gold and orgotein treatment in rheumatoid arthritis. *Curr Ther Res Clin Exp,* 1976; 20(1):62-9.

2232 Goebel KM, Storck U. Effect of intra-articular orgotein versus a corticosteroid on rheumatoid arthritis of the knees. *Am J Med,* 1983;74(1):124-8.

2233 Kadrnka F. [Results of a multicenter orgotein study in radiation induced and interstitial cystitis]. [Article in German]. *Eur J Rheumatol Inflamm,* 1981;4(2):237-43.

2234 Sanchiz F, Milla A, Artola N, et al. Prevention of radioinduced cystitis by orgotein: a randomized study. *Anticancer Res,* 1996;16(4A):2025-8.

2235 Nielsen OS, Overgaard J, Overgaard M, et al. Orgotein in radiation treatment of bladder cancer. A report on allergic reactions and lack of radioprotective effect. *Acta Oncol,* 1987;26(2):101-4.

2236 Marberger H, Bartsch G, Huber W, et al. Orgotein: a new drug for the treatment of radiation cystitis. *Curr Ther Res Clin Exp,* 1975;18(3):466-75.

2237   Chan TY. Interaction between warfarin and danshen (Salvia miltiorrhiza). *Ann Pharmacother* 2001;35:501-4.

2238   Pollak R, Andrisevic JH, Maddux MS, et al. A randomized double-blind trial of the use of human recombinant superoxide dismutase in renal transplantation. *Transplantation*, 1993 Jan;55(1):57-60.

2239   Land W, Schneeberger H, Schleibner S, et al. The beneficial effect of human recombinant superoxide dismutase on acute and chronic rejection events in recipients of cadaveric renal transplants. *Transplantation*, 1994;57(2):211-7.

2240   Schneeberger H, Schleibner S, Illner WD, et al. The impact of free radical-mediated reperfusion injury on acute and chronic rejection events following cadaveric renal transplantation. *Clin Transpl* 1993;:219-32.

2241   Flaherty JT, Pitt B, Gruber JW, et al. Recombinant human superoxide dismutase (h-SOD) fails to improve recovery of ventricular function in patients undergoing coronary angioplasty for acute myocardial infarction. *Circulation*, 1994;89(5):1982-91.

2242   Rosenfeld W, Evans H, Concepcion L, et al. Prevention of bronchopulmonary dysplasia by administration of bovine superoxide dismutase in preterm infants with respiratory distress syndrome. *J Pediatr*, 1984;105(5):781-5.

2243   Murohara Y, Yui Y, Hattori R, et al. Effects of superoxide dismutase on reperfusion arrhythmias and left ventricular function in patients undergoing thrombolysis for anterior wall acute myocardial infarction. *Am J Cardiol*, 1991;67(8):765-7.

2244   N-acetylcysteine. Smart Basics Inc. URL: webu5156.ntx.net/glos.news/feb_march1999/ immunityagainstflu.htm (Accessed 19 July 1999).

2245   Ardissino D, Merlini PA, Savonitto S, et al. Effect of transdermal nitroglycerin or N-acetylcysteine, or both, in the long-term treatment of unstable angina pectoris. *J Am Coll Cardiol*, 1997;29(5):941-7.

2246   Horowitz JD, Henry CA, Syrjanen ML, et al. Nitroglycerine/N-acetylcysteine in the management of unstable angina pectoris. *Eur Heart J*, 1988;9 Suppl A:95-100.

2247   Brown DM. Bile plug syndrome: successful management with a mucolytic agent. *Pediatr Surg* 1990;25(3):351-2.

2248   Evans JS, George DE, Mollit D. Biliary infusion therapy in the inspissated bile syndrome of cystic fibrosis. *J Pediatr Gastroenterol Nutr* 1991;12(1):131-5.

2249   Mulvaney WP, Quilter T, Mortera A. Experiences with acetylcysteine in cystinuric patients. *J Urol* 1975;114(1):107-8.

2250   Giovannucci E, et al. Multivitamin use, folate, and colon cancer in women in the Nurses' Health Study. *Ann Intern Med*, 1998; 129 (7):517-24.

2251   Drew HJ, Vogel RI, Molofsky W, et al. Effect of folate on phenytoin hyperplasia. *J Clin Periodontol* 1987;14(6):350-6.

2252   Unverferth DV, Jagadeesh JM, Unverferth Bj, et al. Attempt to prevent doxorubicin-induced acute human myocardial morphologic damage with acetylcysteine. *J Natl Cancer Inst*, 1983;71(5):917-20.

2253   Dresdale AR, Barr LH, Bonow RO, et al. Prospective randomized study of the role of N-acetyl cysteine in reversing doxorubicin-induced cardiomyopathy. *Am J Clin Oncol*, 1982;5(6):657-63.

2254   Louwerse ES, Weverling GJ, Bossuyt PM, et al. Randomized, double-blind, controlled trial of acetylcysteine in amyotrophic lateral sclerosis. *Arch Neurol*, 1995;52(6):559-64.

2255   Heiss WD, Kessler J, Mielke R, et al. Long-term effects of phosphatidylserine, pyritinol, and cognitive training in Alzheimer's disease. A neuropsychological, EEG, and PET investigation. *Dementia* 1994;5:88-98.

2256   Wiklund O, Fager G, Andersson A, et al. N-acetylcysteine treatment lowers plasma homocysteine but not serum lipoprotein(a) levels. *Atherosclerosis*, 1996;119(1):99-106.

2257   Kroon AA, Demacker PN, Stalenhoef AF. N-acetylcysteine and serum concentrations of lipoprotein(a). *J Intern Med*, 1991;230(6):519-26.

2258   Bostom AG, Shemin D, Yoburn D, et al. Lack of effect of oral N-acetylcysteine on the acute dialysis-related lowering of total plasma homocysteine in hemodialysis patients. *Atherosclerosis*, 1996;120(1-2):241-4.

2259   Hurd RW, Wilder BJ, Helveston WR, et al. Treatment of four siblings with progressive myoclonus epilepsy of the Unverricht-Lundborg type with N-acetylcysteine. *Neurology* 1996;47(5):1264-8.

2260   De Flora S, Grassi C, Carati L. Attenuation of influenza-like symptomatology and improvement of cell-mediated immunity with long-term N-acetylcysteine treatment. *Eur Respir J*, 1997;10(7):1535-41.

2261   Pearson TA. Alcohol and Heart Disease. *Circulation* 1996;94:3023-5.

2262   Fraser AG. Pharmacokinetic interactions between alcohol and other drugs. *Clin Pharmacokinet* 1997;33(2):79-90.

2263   Isselbacher KJ, Braunwald E, Wilson JD, et al. Harrison's Principles of Internal Medicine. 13th Ed. New York, NY: McGraw-Hill, 1994.

2264   Fahey TD, Pearl MS. The hormonal and perceptive effects of phosphatidylserine administration during two weeks of resistive exercise-induced overtraining. *Biol Sport* 1998;15:135-44.

2265   Kushner MG, Mackenzie TB, Fiszdon J, et al. The effects of alcohol consumption on laboratory-induced panic and state anxiety. *Arch Gen Psychiatry*, 1996;53(3):264-70.

2266   de Boer MC, Schippers GM, van der Staak. Alcohol and social anxiety in women and men: pharmacological and expectancy effects. *Addict Behav*, 1993;18(2):117-26.

2267   Kiechl S, Willeit J, Rungger G, et al. Alcohol consumption and atherosclerosis: what is the relation? Prospective results from the Bruneck Study. *Stroke*, 1998;29(5):900-7.

2268   Klatsky AL, Armstrong MA, Friedman GD. Red wine, white wine, liquor, beer, and risk for coronary artery disease hospitalization. *Am J Cardiol* 1997;80(4):416-20.

2269   Siscovick DS, Weiss NS, Fox N. Moderate alcohol consumption and primary cardiac arrest. *Am J Epidemiol*, 1986;123(3):499-503.

2270   Hennekens CH, Willett W, Rosner B, et al. Effects of beer, wine, and liquor in coronary deaths. *JAMA* 1979;242(18):1973-4.

2271   Stampfer MJ, Colditz GA, Willett WC, et al. A prospective study of moderate alcohol consumption and the risk of coronary disease and stroke in women. *N Engl J Med* 1988;319(5):267-73.

2272   Advanced medium chain triglycerides. Prolithic Sports. www.prolithic.com/hpages/efoods/mct.html. (Accessed 18 July 1999).

REFERENCES

2273 Sills MA, Forsythe WI, Haidukewych D, et al. The medium chain triglyceride diet and intractable epilepsy. *Arch Dis Child*, 1986;61(12):1168-72.

2274 Trauner DA. Medium-chain triglyceride (MCT) diet in intractable seizure disorders. *Neurology*, 1985;35(2):237-8.

2275 Nijveldt RJ, Tan AM, Prins HA, et al. Use of a mixture of medium-chain triglycerides and longchain triglycerides versus long-chain triglycerides in critically ill surgical patients: a randomized prospective double-blind study. *Clin Nutr*, 1998;17(1):23-9.

2276 Ball MJ. Parenteral nutrition in the critically ill: use of a medium chain triglyceride emulsion. *Intensive Care Med*, 1993;19(2):89-95.

2277 Jiang ZM, Zhang SY, Wang XR, et al. A comparison of medium-chain and long-chain triglycerides in surgical patients. *Ann Surg*, 1993;217(2):175-84.

2278 Clarke PJ, Ball MJ, Hands LJ, et al. Use of a lipid containing medium chain triglycerides in patients receiving TPN: a randomized prospective trial. *Br J Surg*, 1987;74(8):701-4.

2279 Truelsen T, Gronbaek M, Schnohr P, et al. Intake of beer, wine, and spirits and risk of stroke: the copenhagen city heart study. *Stroke* 1998;29(12):2467-72.

2280 Iversen HK. N-acetylcysteine enhances nitroglycerin-induced headache and cranial arterial responses. *Clin Pharmacol, Ther* 1992;52(2):125-33.

2281 Hogan JC, Lewis MJ, Henderson AH. N-acetylcysteine fails to attenuate haemodynamic tolerance to glyceryl trinitrate in healthy volunteers. *Br J Clin Pharmacol*, 1989;28(4):421-6.

2282 Hogan JC, Lewis MJ, Henderson AH. Chronic administration of N-acetylcysteine fails to prevent nitrate tolerance in patients with stable angina pectoris. *Br J Clin Pharmacol*, 1990;30(4):573-7.

2283 American Pharmaceutical Association. Handbook of Nonprescription Drugs. 11th Ed. Washington, DC: American Pharmaceutical Association; 1996.

2284 Uenotsuchi T, Satoh E, Kiryu H, Yano Y. Pyemotes dermatitis caused by indirect contact with husk rice. *Br J Dermatol* 2000;143:680-2.

2285 Phyto-soy. 1001Herbs. URL: www.1001herbs.com/phyto-soy/index.html (Accessed 19 July 1999).

2286 Soroka N, Silverberg DS, Greemland M, et al. Comparison of a vegetable-based (soya) and an animal-based low-protein diet in predialysis chronic renal failure patients. *Nephron*, 1998;79(2):173-80.

2287 Gentile MG, Fellin G, Cofano F, et al. Treatment of proteinuric patients with a vegetarian soy diet and fish oil. *Clin Nephrol*, 1993 Dec;40(6):315-20.

2288 D'Amico G, Gentile MG. Effect of dietary manipulation on the lipid abnormalities and urinary protein loss in nephrotic patients. *Miner Electrolyte Metab*, 1992;18(2-5):203-6.

2290 Franke AA, Custer LJ, Tanaka Y. Isoflavones in human breast milk and other biological fluids. *Am J Clin Nutr*, 1998;68(6 Suppl):1466-73.

2291 Brown KH, Perez F, Peerson JM, et al. Effect of dietary fiber (soy polysaccharide) on the severity, duration, and nutritional outcome of acute, watery diarrhea in children. *Pediatrics*, 1993;92(2):241-7.

2292 Vanderhoof JA, Murray ND, Paule CL, et al. Use of soy fiber in acute diarrhea in infants and toddlers. *Clin Pediatr (Phila)*, 1997;36(3):135-9.

2293 Wong WW, Smith EO, Stuff JE, et al. Cholesterol-lowering effect of soy protein in normocholesterolemic and hypercholesterolemic men. *Am J Clin Nutr*, 1998;68(6 Suppl):1385S-9.

2294 Nilausen K, Meinertz H. Variable lipemic response to dietary soy protein in healthy, normolipemic men. *Am J Clin Nutr*, 1998;68(6 Suppl):1380S-4.

2295 Bakhit RM, Klein BP, Essex-Sorlie D, et al. Intake of 25 g of soybean protein with or without soybean fiber alters plasma lipids in men with elevated cholesterol concentrations. *J Nutr*, 1994;124(2):213-22.

2296 Washburn S, Burke GL, Morgan T, et al. Effect of soy protein supplementation on serum lipoproteins, blood pressure, and menopausal symptoms in perimenopausal women. *Menopause* 1999;6(1):7-13.

2297 Albertazzi P, Pansini F, Bonaccorsi G, et al. The effect of dietary soy supplementation on hot flushes. *Obstet Gynecol*, 1998;91(1):6-11.

2298 Jacobsen BK, Knutsen SF, Fraser GE. Does high soy milk intake reduce prostate cancer incidence? The Adventist Health Study. *Cancer Causes Control*, 1998;9(6):553-7.

2299 Montori VM, Farmer A, Wollan PC, Dinneen SF. Fish oil supplementation in type 2 diabetes: a quantitative systemic review. *Diabetes Care* 2000;23(9):1407-15.

2300 Patti L, Maffettone A, Iovine C, et al. Long-term effects of fish oil on lipoprotein subfractions and low density lipoprotein size in non-insulin- dependent diabetic patients with hypertriglyceridemia. *Atherosclerosis* 1999;146(2):361-7.

2301 Yosefy C, Viskoper JR, Laszt A, et al. The effect of fish oil on hypertension, plasma lipids and hemostasis in hypertensive, obese, dyslipidemic patients with and without diabetes mellitus. *Prostaglandins Leukot Essent Fatty Acids* 1999;61(2):83-7.

2302 Eritsland J, Seljeflot I, Abdelnoor M, et al. Long-term effects of n-3 fatty acids on serum lipids and glycaemic control. *Scand J Clin Lab Invest* 1994;54(4):273-80.

2304 Daviglus ML, Stamler J, Orencia AJ, et al. Fish consumption and the 30-year risk of fatal myocardial infarction. *N Engl J Med* 1997;336(15):1046-53.

2305 Guallar E, Hennekens CH, Sacks FM, et al. A prospective study of plasma fish oil levels and incidence of myocardial infarction in U.S. male physicians. *J Am Coll Cardiol* 1995;25(2):387-94.

2306 Guallar E, Aro A, Jimenez FJ, et al. Omega-3 fatty acids in adipose tissue and risk of myocardial infarction: the EURAMIC study. *Arterioscler Thromb Vasc Biol* 1999;19(4):1111-8.

2307 Anon. Dietary supplementation with n-3 polyunsaturated fatty acids and vitamin E after myocardial infarction: results of the GISSI-Prevenzione trial. Gruppo Italiano per lo Studio della Sopravvivenza nell'Infarto miocardico. *Lancet* 1999;354(9177):447-55.

2308 Burr ML, Sweetham PM, Fehily AM. Diet and reinfarction. *Eur Heart J* 1994;15(8):1152-3.

2309 Ascherio A, Rimm EB, Stampfer MJ, et al. Dietary intake of marine n-3 fatty acids, fish intake, and the risk of coronary disease among men. *N Engl J Med* 1995;332(15):977-82.

2310 Pietinen P, Ascherio A, Korhonen P, et al. Intake of fatty acids and risk of coronary heart disease in a cohort of Finnish men. The Alpha-Tocopherol, Beta-Carotene Cancer Prevention Study. *Am J Epidemiol* 145(10):876-87.

2311 von Schacky C, Angerer P, Kothny W, et al. The effect of dietary omega-3 fatty acids on coronary atherosclerosis. A randomized, double-blind, placebo-controlled trial. *Ann Intern Med* 1999;130(7):554-62.

2312 Siscovick DS, Raghunathan TE, King I, et al. Dietary intake and cell membrane levels of long-chain n-3 polyunsaturated fatty acids and the risk of primary cardiac arrest. *JAMA* 1995;274(17):1363-7.

2313 Albert CM, Hennekens CH, O'Donnell CJ, et al. Fish consumption and risk of sudden cardiac death. *JAMA* 1998;279(1):23-8.

2314 Eritsland J, Amesen H, Gronseth K, et al. Effect of dietary supplementation with n-3 fatty acids on coronary artery bypass graft patency. *Am J Cardiol* 1996;77(1):31-6.

2315 Marckmann P, Bladbjerg EM, Jespersen J. Dietary fish oil (4 g daily) and cardiovascular risk markers in healthy men. *Arterioscler Thromb Vasc Biol* 1997;17(12):3384-91.

2317 Layne KS, Goh YK, Jumpsen JA, et al. Normal subjects consuming physiological levels of 18:3(n-3) and 20:5(n-3 from flaxseed or fish oils have characteristic differences in plasma lipid and lipoprotein fatty acid levels. *J Nutr* 1996;126(9):2130-40.

2318 Adler A, Holub BJ. Effect of garlic and fish-oil supplementation on serum lipid and lipoprotein concentrations in hypercholesterolemic men. *Am J Clin Nutr* 1997;65(2):445-50.

2319 Morcos NC. Modulation of lipid profile by fish oil and garlic combination. *J Natl Med Assoc* 1997;89(10):673-8.

2320 Cairns JA, Gill J, Morton B, et al. Fish oils and low-molecular-weight heparin for the reduction of restenosis after percutaneous transluminal coronary angioplasty. The EMPAR Study. *Circulation* 1996;94(7):1553-60.

2322 de Deckere EAM, Korver O, Verschuren PM, Katan MB. Health aspects of fish n-3 polyunsaturated fatty acids from plant and marine origin. *Eur J Clin Nutr* 1998;52(10):749-53.

2323 Higdon JV, Liu J, Du S, et al. Supplementation of postmenopausal women with fish oil rich in eicosapentaenoic acid and docosahexaenoic acid is not associated with greater in vivo lipid peroxidation compared with oils rich in oleate and linoleate as assessed by plasma malondialdehyde and F(2)-isoprostanes. *Am J Clin Nutr* 2000;72(3):714-22.

2331 Burton Goldberg Group. Alternative Medicine: The Definitive Guide. Puyallup, WA: Burton Goldberg Group, 1994.

2332 Cambridge Nutraceuticals, Glutamine. URL: www.cambridgenutra.com. (Accessed 19 July 1999).

2333 Balch JF, Balch PA. Prescription for Nutritional Healing. 2nd ed., Garden City Park, NY: Avery Publishing Group, 1997.

2334 Scolapio JS, et al. Effect of growth hormone, glutamine, and diet on adaptation in short-bowel syndrome: a randomized, controlled study. *Gastroenterology*, 1997; 113(4):1074-81.

2335 Shabert J, et al. Glutamine/antioxidant supplementation promotes gain in body cell mass in HIV patients with weight loss. *Int Conf AIDS* 1998;12:841(abstract no 42336).

2336 Anderson PM, Schroeder G, Skubitz KM. Oral glutamine reduces the duration and severity of stomatitis after cytotoxic cancer chemotherapy. *Cancer*, 1998; 83(7):1433-9.

2337 Noyer CM, et al. A double-blind placebo-controlled pilot study of glutamine therapy for abnormal intestinal permeability in patients with AIDS. *Am J Gastroenterol,* 1998; 93(6):972-5.

2338 Den Hond E, et al. Effect of long-term oral glutamine supplements on small intestinal permeability in patients with Crohn's disease. *J Parenter Enteral Nutr*, 1999; 23(1):7-11.

2339 Van Den Berg CJ, et al. Glutamine therapy of cystinuria. *Invest Urol*, 1980; 18(2):155-7.

2341 Haub MD, et al. Acute L-glutamine ingestion does not improve maximal effort exercise. *J Sports Med Phys Fitness*, 1998; 38(3):240-4.

2342 Castell LM, Newsholme EA. The effects of oral glutamine supplementation on athletes after prolonged, exhaustive exercise. *Nutrition,* 1997; 13(7-8):738-42.

2343 Shils ME, Young VR, eds. Modern Nutrition in Health and Disease. 7th ed., Philadelphia: Lea and Febiger, 1988.

2344 Alternative Medicines, "Histidine" URL: www.alternative medicines.com/herbdesc2/1histidi.htm (Accessed 19 July 1999).

2345 Staying Healthy With Nutrition, URL: www.healthy.net (Accessed 19 July 1999).

2346 Reference Guide for Amino Acids. URL: www.realtime.net/anr/aminoacd.html#hisidine (Accessed 19 July 1999).

2347 Gerber DA, Tanenbaum L, Ahrens M. Free serum histidine levels in patients with rheumatoid arthritis and control subjects following an oral load of free L-histidine. *Metabolism*, 1976; 25(6):655-7.

2348 Discontinued citation (see Ref 2352).

2349 Dixon JS, et al. The effect of drugs on serum histidine levels in rheumatoid arthritis. *Rheumatol Int,* 1983; 3(4):145-9.

2350 Pinals RS, et al. Treatment of rheumatoid arthritis with L-histidine: a randomized, placebo-controlled, double-blind trial. *J Rheumatol,* 1977; 4(4):414-9.

2351 Gerber DA, Tanenbaum L, Ahrens M. Free serum histidine levels in patients with rheumatoid arthritis and control subjects following an oral load of free L-histidine. *Metabolism*, 1976; 25(6):655-7.

2352 Blumenkrantz MJ, et al. Histidine supplementation for treatment of anaemia of uraemia. *Br Med J* 1975;2(5970):530-3.

2353 Reeves RD, et al. Failure of histidine supplementation to improve anemia in chronic dialysis patients. *Am J Clin Nutr,* 1977; 30(4):579-81.

2354 Bigwood EJ, ed. Protein and amino acid functions. Oxford, NY: Pergamon Press, 1972.

2355 Sacher RA, McPherson RA, eds. Widdmann's Clinical Interpretation of Laboratory Tests. 10th ed., Philadelphia: FA Davis Company, 1991.

2356 Asai K. Miracle Cure: Organic Germanium. New York: Japan Publications, 1980.

2357 Germanium. URL: www.tasqbase.com:80/german.htm (Accessed 19 July 1999).

2358 Germanium. URL: www.tellafriend.net/germanium.htm (Accessed 19 July 1999).

2359 Nutri-Mart Cyber Store, Organic Germanium Info. URL: www.nutrimart.com/ge-132.htm (Accessed 19 July 1999).

2360 Tao SH, Bolger PM. Hazard assessment of germanium supplements. *Regul Toxicol Pharmacol,* 1997;

25(3):211-9.

2361 Byrne TA, et al. A new treatment for patients with short-bowel syndrome. Growth hormone, glutamine, and a modified diet. *Ann Surg*, 1995; 222(3):243-54.

2362 Byrne TA, et al. Growth hormone, glutamine, and a modified diet enhance nutrient absorption in patients with severe short bowel syndrome. *JPEN J Parenter Enteral Nutr*, 1995; 19(4):296-302.

2363 Morlion BJ, et al. Total parenteral nutrition with glutamine dipeptide after major abdominal surgery: a randomized, double-blind, controlled study. *Ann Surg*, 1998; 227(2):302-8.

2364 Skubitz KM, Anderson PM. Oral glutamine to prevent chemotherapy induced stomatitis: a pilot study. *J Lab Clin Med*, 1996; 127(2):223-8.

2365 Jebb SA, et al. 5-fluorouracil and folinic acid-induced mucositis: no effect of oral glutamine supplementation. *Br J Cancer*, 1994; 70(4):732-5.

2366 Ziegler TR, et al. Clinical and metabolic efficacy of glutamine-supplemented parenteral nutrition after bone marrow transplantation. A randomized, double-blind, controlled study. *Ann Intern Med*, 1992; 116(10):821-8.

2368 Anderson PM, et al. Effect of low-dose oral glutamine on painful stomatitis during bone marrow transplantation. *Bone Marrow Transplant*, 1998; 22(4):339-44.

2369 Starling RD, et al. Effect of inosine supplementation on aerobic and anaerobic cycling performance. *Med Sci Sports Exerc*, 1996; 28(9):1193-8.

2370 Williams MH, et al. Effect of inosine supplementation on 3-mile treadmill run performance and VO2 peak. *Med Sci Sports Exerc*, 1990; 22(4):517-22.

2371 Ramirez FC, Lee K, Graham DY. All lactase preparations are not the same: results of a prospective, randomized, placebo-controlled trial. *Am J Gastroenterol*, 1994; 89(4):566-70.

2372 Sanders SW, Tolman KG, Reitberg DP. Effect of a single dose of lactase on symptoms and expired hydrogen after lactose challenge in lactose-intolerant subjects. *Clin Pharm*, 1992; 11(6):533-8.

2373 Lin MY, et al. Comparative effects of exogenous lactase (beta-galactosidase) preparations on in vivo lactose digestion. *Dig Dis Sci*, 1993; 38(11):2022-7.

2374 DairyEase product information. McNeil-PPC Inc. Fort Washington, PA 19034.

2375 Lami F, et al. Efficacy of addition of exogenous lactase to milk in adult lactase deficiency. *Am J Gastroenterol*, 1988; 83(10):1145-9.

2376 Horowitz M, et al. Lactose and calcium absorption in postmenopausal osteoporosis. *Arch Intern Med* 1987; 147(3):534-6.

2377 Newcomer AD, et al. Lactase deficiency: prevalence in osteoporosis. *Ann Intern Med*, 1978; 89(2):218-20.

2378 Mother Nature's Encyclopedia, Lipase. www.mothernature.com/ency/Supp/Lipase.asp (Accessed 19 July 1999).

2379 Lloyd-Still JD. Cystic fibrosis and colonic strictures. A new "iatrogenic" disease. *J Clin Gastroenterol*, 1995; 21(1):2-5.

2380 Croft NM, Marshall TG, Ferguson A. Gut inflammation in children with cystic fibrosis on high-dose enzyme supplements. *Lancet*, 1995; 346(8985):1265-267.

2381 Smyth RL, et al. Fibrosing colonopathy in cystic fibrosis: results of a case-control study. *Lancet*, 1995; 346(8985):1247-251.

2382 Smyth RL, et al. Strictures of ascending colon in cystic fibrosis and high-strength pancreatic enzymes. *Lancet*, 1994; 343(8889):85-86.

2383 Tursi JM, Phair PG, Barnes GL. Plant sources of acid stable lipases: potential therapy for cystic fibrosis. *J Paediatr Child Health*, 1994; 30(6):539-43.

2384 Malesci A. New enteric-coated high-lipase pancreatic extract in the treatment of pancreatic steatorrhea. *J Clin Gastroenterol*, 1994; 18(1):32-5.

2386 Mother Nature's Encyclopedia, Macular Degeneration. URL: www.mothernature.com/ency/CONCERN/ Macular_Degeneration.asp (Accessed 19 July 1999).

2388 Snodderly DM. Evidence for protection against age-related macular degeneration by carotenoids and antioxidant vitamins. *Am J Clin Nutr*, 1995; 62(6 Suppl):1448S-61S..

2389 Landrum JT, Bone RA, Joa H, et al. A one year study of the macular pigment: the effect of 140 days of a lutein supplement. *Exp Eye Res*, 1997; 65(1):57-62.

2390 van den Berg H, van Vliet T. Effect of simultaneous, single oral doses of beta-carotene with lutein or lycopene on the beta-carotene and retinyl ester responses in the triacylglycerol-rich lipoprotein fraction of men. *Am J Clin Nutr*, 1998; 68(1):82-9.

2391 Kostic D, White WS, Olson JA. Intestinal absorption, serum clearance, and interactions between lutein and beta-carotene when administered to human adults in separate or combined oral doses. *Am J Clin Nutr*, 1995; 62(3):604-10.

2392 Koonsvitsky BP, et al. "Olestra affects serum concentrations of alpha-tocopherol and carotenoids but not vitamin D or vitamin K status in free-living subjects. *J Nutr*, 1997; 127(8 Suppl):1636S-45S.

2394 Seddon JM, et al. Dietary carotenoids, vitamins A, C, and E, and advanced age-related macular degeneration. Eye Disease Case-Control Study Group. *JAMA*, 1994; 272(18):1413-20.

2395 Hankinson SE, et al. Nutrient intake and cataract extraction in women: a prospective study. *BMJ*, 1992; 305(6849):335-9.

2398 Lyle BJ, Mares-Perlman JA, Klein BE, et al. Antioxidant intake and risk of incident age-related nuclear cataracts in the Beaver Dam Eye Study. *Am J Epidemiol* 1999;149:801-9.

2400 Chen R, Tunstall-Pedoe H, Bolton-Smith C, et al. Association of dietary antioxidants and waist circumference with pulmonary function and airway obstruction. *Am J Epidemiol* 2001:153:157-63.

2401 Rao AV, Agarwal S. Bioavailability and in vivo antioxidant properties of lycopene from tomato products and their possible role in the prevention of cancer. *Nutr Cancer* 1998; 31(3): 199-203.

2403 Johnson EJ, et al. Ingestion by men of a combined dose of beta-carotene and lycopene does not affect the absorption of beta-carotene but improves that of lycopene. *J Nutr* 1997;127(9):1833-7.

2404 La Vecchia C. Mediterranean epidemiological evidence on tomatoes and the prevention of digestive-tract cancers. *Proc Soc Exp Biol Med* 1998;218(2):125-8.

2405 Tzonou A, Signorello LB, Lagiou P, et al. Diet and cancer of the prostate: a case-control study in Greece. *Int J Cancer* 1999;80(5):704-8.

2406 Giovannucci E, Ascherio A, Rimm EB, et al. Intake of carotenoids and retinol in relation to risk of prostate cancer. *J Natl Cancer Inst* 1995;87(23):1767-76.

2407 Giovannucci E. Tomatoes, tomato-based products, lycopene, and cancer: review of the epidemiologic literature. *J Natl Cancer Inst,* 1999;91(4):317-31.

2408 Mother Nature's Encyclopedia. Methionine. www.mothernature.com/ency/Supp/Methionine.asp (Accessed 16 July 1999).

2409 La Vecchia C, et al. Case-control study on influence of methionine, nitrite, and salt on gastric carcinogenesis in northern Italy. *Nutr Cancer,* 1997; 27(1): 65-8.

2410 Bellamy MF, et al. Hyperhomocysteinemia after an oral methionine load acutely impairs endothelial function in healthy adults. *Circulation* 1998;98(18):1848-52.

2411 Hladovec J, Sommerova Z, Pisarikova A. Homocysteinemia and endothelial damage after methionine load. *Thromb Res,* 1997; 88(4): 361-4.

2412 Bellone J, et al. Methionine potentiates both basal and GHRH-induced GH secretion in children. *Clin Endocrinol (Oxf)* 1997;47(1):61-4.

2413 Vale JA, Meredith TJ, Goulding R. Treatment of acetaminophen poisoning. The use of oral methionine. *Arch Intern Med,* 1981;141(3 Spec No): 394-6.

2414 Christensen B, et al. Preoperative methionine loading enhances restoration of the cobalamin-dependent enzyme methionine synthase after nitrous oxide anesthesia. *Anesthesiology,* 1994; 80(5): 1046-56.

2415 Meakins TS, Persaud C, Jackson AA. Dietary supplementation with L-methionine impairs the utilization of urea-nitrogen and increases 5-L-oxoprolinuria in normal women consuming a low protein diet. *J Nutr,* 1998; 128(4): 720-7.

2416 Mother Nature's Encyclopedia. Ornithine. www.mothernature.com/ency/Supp/Ornithine.asp.(Accessed 16 July 1999).

2417 Bucci LR, et al. Ornithine supplementation and insulin release in bodybuilders. *Int J Sport Nutr,* 1992; 2(3): 287-91.

2418 Fogelholm GM, et al. Low-dose amino acid supplementation: no effects on serum human growth hormone and insulin in male weightlifters. *Int J Sport Nutr,* 1993; 3(3): 290-7.

2419 Mother Nature's Encyclopedia. Lecithin. www.mothernature.com/ency/Supp/Lecithin.asp (Accessed 16 July 1999).

2424 Zhdanova IV, Piotrovskaya VR. Melatonin treatment attenuates symptoms of acute nicotine withdrawal in humans. *Pharmacol Biochem Behavior* 2000;67:131-5.

2425 Bellipanni G, Bianchi P, Pierpaoli W, et al. Effects of melatonin in perimenopausal and menopausal women: a randomized and placebo controlled study. *Exp Gerontol* 2001;36:297-310.

2426 Erdman JW. AHA Science Advisory: Soy protein and cardiovascular disease. A statement for healthcare professionals from the Nutrition Committee of the AHA. *Circulation* 2000;102:2555-9.

2427 Domino EF, et al. Lack of clinically significant improvement of patients with tardive dyskinesia following phosphatidylcholine therapy. *Biol Psychiatry,* 1985; 20(11): 1189-96.

2428 McFadyen IJ, Chetty U, Setchell KDR, et al. A randomized double blind, cross over trial of soya protein for the treatment of cyclical breast pain. *The Breast* 2000;9:271-6.

2429 Lu LJ, Anderson KE, Grady JJ, et al. Decreased ovarian hormones during a soya diet: implications for breast cancer prevention. *Cancer Res* 2000;60:4112-21.

2430 Xu X, Duncan AM, Wangen KE, Kurzer MS. Soy consumption alters endogenous estrogen metabolism in postmenopausal women. *Cancer Epidemiol Biomarkers Prev* 2000;9:781-6.

2431 Grosse Duweler K, Rohdewald P. Urinary metabolites of French maritime pine bark extract in humans. *Pharmazie* 2000;55:364-8.

2432 Mak S, Newton GE. Vitamin C augments the inotropic response to dobutamine in humans with normal left ventricular function. *Circulation* 2001;103:826-30.

2433 Packer L, Midori H, Toshikazu Y, eds. Antioxidant Food Supplements in Human Health. San Diego: Academic Press, 1999.

2434 Hornig B, Arakawa N, Kohler C, Drexler H. Vitamin C improves endothelial function of conduit arteries in patients with chronic heart failure. *Circulation* 1998;97:363-8.

2435 Rice-Evans CA, Packer L, eds. Flavonoids in Health and Disease. Manhattan, NY: Marcel Dekker, Inc., 1998.

2436 Mother Nature's Encyclopedia. Phosphatidylserine. URL: www.mothernature.com/ency/Supp/Phosphatidylserine.asp. (Accessed 16 July 1999).

2437 Crook T, et al. Effects of phosphatidylserine in Alzheimer's disease. *Psychopharmacol Bull* 1992;28(1):61-6.

2438 Delwaide PJ, et al. Double-blind, randomized, controlled study of phosphatidylserine in senile demented patients. *Acta Neurol Scand* 1986;73(2):136-40.

2439 Engel RR, et al. Double-blind cross-over study of phosphatidylserine vs. placebo in patients with early dementia of the Alzheimer type. *Eur Neuropsychopharmacol* 1992;2(2):149-55.

2440 Cenacchi T, et al. Cognitive decline in the elderly: a double-blind, placebo-controlled multicenter study on efficacy of phosphatidylserine administration. *Aging (Milano)* 1993;5(2):123-33.

2441 Crook TH, et al. Effects of phosphatidylserine in age-associated memory impairment. *Neurology* 1991;41(5):644-9.

2442 Mother Nature's Encyclopedia. OKG. www.mothernature.com/ency/Supp/OKG.asp. (Accessed 16 July 1999).

2443 De Bandt JP, et al. A randomized controlled trial of the influence of the mode of enteral ornithine alpha-ketoglutarate administration in burn patients. *J Nutr* 1998;128(3):563-9.

2444 Moukarzel AA, et al. Growth retardation in children receiving long-term total parenteral nutrition: effects of ornithine alpha-ketoglutarate. *Am J Clin Nutr* 1994;60(3):408-13.

2445 Wernerman J, et al. Glutamine and ornithine-alpha-ketoglutarate but not branched-chain amino acids reduce the loss of muscle glutamine after surgical trauma. *Metabolism* 1989;38(8 Suppl 1):63-6.

2446 Wernerman J, et al. Ornithine-alpha-ketoglutarate improves skeletal muscle protein synthesis as assessed by ribosome analysis and nitrogen use after surgery. *Ann Surg* 1987;206(5):674-8.

2447 Woollard ML, et al. Controlled trial of ornithine alpha ketoglutarate (OAKG) in patients with stroke. *Stroke* 1978;9(3):218-22.

2448 Blomqvist BI, et al. Glutamine and alpha-ketoglutarate prevent the decrease in muscle free glutamine concentration and influence protein synthesis after total hip replacement. *Metabolism* 1995;44(9):1215-22.

2449 Chainuvati T, Plengvanit U, Viranuvatti V. Ornicetil on encephalopathy. Effect of ornicetil (ornithine alpha-ketoglutarate) on encephalopathy in patients with acute and chronic liver disease. *Acta Hepatogastroenterol (Stuttg)* 1977;24(6):434-9.

2450 Gay G, et al. Effects of ornithine alphaketoglutarate on blood insulin, glucagon and aminoacids in alcoholic cirrhosis. *Biomedicine* 1979;30(3):173-7.

2451 Arcangeli P. Pycnogenol in chronic venous insufficiency. *Fitoterapia* 2000;71:236-44.

2452 Marconi C, Sassi G, Cerretelli P. The effect of an alpha-ketoglutarate-pyridoxine complex on human maximal aerobic and anaerobic performance. *Eur J Appl Physiol* 1982;49(3):307-17.

2454 Cotzias GC, Van Woert MH, Schiffer LM. Aromatic amino acids and modification of parkinsonism. *N Engl J Med,* 1967;276(7): 374-9.

2455 Heller B, Fischer BE, Martin R. Therapeutic action of D-phenylalanine in Parkinson's disease. *Arzneimittelforschung,* 1976;26(4):577-9.

2456 Kitade T, et al. Studies on the enhanced effect of acupuncture analgesia and acupuncture anesthesia by D-phenylalanine (2nd report)- schedule of administration and clinical effects in low back pain and tooth extraction. *Acupunct Electrother Res* 1990;15(2):121-35.

2457 Mosnik DM, et al. Tardive dyskinesia exacerbated after ingestion of phenylalanine by schizophrenic patients. *Neuropsychopharmacology,* 1997;16(2):136-46.

2458 Gardos G, et al. The acute effects of a loading dose of phenylalanine in unipolar depressed patients with and without tardive dyskinesia. *Neuropsychopharmacology,* 1992;6(4):241-7.

2459 Walsh NE, Ramamurthy S, Schoenfeld L, Hoffman J. Analgesic effectiveness of D-phenylalanine in chronic pain patients. *Arch Phys Med Rehabil* 1986;67(7):436-9.

2460 Mitchell MJ, Daines GE, Thomas BL. Effect of L-tryptophan and phenylalanine on burning pain threshold. *Phys Ther* 1987;67(2):203-5.

2461 Antoniou C, et al. Vitiligo therapy with oral and topical phenylalanine with UVA exposure. *Int J Dermatol,* 1989;28(8):545-7.

2462 Petrassi C, Mastromarino A, Spartera C. Pycnogenol in chronic venous insufficiency. *Phytomedicine* 2000;7:383-8.

2463 Siddiqui AH, et al. L-phenylalanine and UVA irradiation in the treatment of vitiligo. *Dermatology,* 1994; 188(3): 215-8.

2464 Thiele B, Steigleder GK. [Repigmentation treatment of vitiligo with L-phenylalanine and UVA irradiation]. [Article in German]. *Z Hautkr,* 1987; 62(7): 519-23.

2465 Cormane RH, et al. Phenylalanine and UVA light for the treatment of vitiligo. *Arch Dermatol Res,* 1985; 277(2): 126-30.

2466 Kuiters GR, et al. Oral phenylalanine loading and sunlight as source of UVA irradiation in vitiligo on the Caribbean island of Curacao NA. *J Trop Med Hyg,* 1986; 89(3): 149-55.

2467 Schulpis CH, et al. Phenylalanine plus ultraviolet light: preliminary report of a promising treatment for childhood vitiligo. *Pediatr Dermatol,* 1989; 6(4): 332-5.

2468 Beckmann H, et al. DL-phenylalanine versus imipramine: a double-blind controlled study. *Arch Psychiatr Nervenkr* 1979;227(1):49-58.

2469 Birkmayer W, et al. L-deprenyl plus L-phenylalanine in the treatment of depression. *J Neural Transm,* 1984; 59(1): 81-7.

2470 Henry JB, ed. Clinical Diagnosis and Management by Laboratory Methods. 19th ed. Philadelphia,PA: W.B. Saunders, 1996.

2471 Pyruvate. Mother Nature Website. URL: www.mothernature.com/ency/Supp/Pyruvate.asp (Accessed 16 July 1999).

2472 Stanko RT, Tietze DL, Arch JE. Body composition, energy utilization, and nitrogen metabolism with a 4.25-MJ/d low-energy diet supplemented with pyruvate. *Am J Clin Nutr* 1992;56(4):630-5.

2473 Matthys D, Van Coster R, Verhaaren H. Fatal outcome of pyruvate loading test in child with restrictive cardiomyopathy. *Lancet* 1991;338(8773):1020-1.

2474 Stanko RT, et al. Pyruvate supplementation of a low-cholesterol, low-fat diet: effects on plasma lipid concentrations and body composition in hyperlipidemic patients. *Am J Clin Nutr* 1994;59(2):423-7.

2475 Wagner DR. Hyperhydrating with glycerol: implications for athletic performance. *J Am Diet Assoc* 1999;99(2):207-12.

2476 Murray R, et al. Physiological responses to glycerol ingestion during exercise. *J Appl Physiol* 1991;71(1):144-9.

2477 Robergs RA, Griffin SE. Glycerol. Biochemistry, pharmacokinetics and clinical and practical applications. *Sports Med* 1998;26(3):145-67.

2478 Arnall DA, Goforth HW. Failure to reduce body water loss in cold-water immersion by glycerol ingestion. *Undersea Hyperb Med* 1993;20(4):309-20.

2479 Montner P, et al. Pre-exercise glycerol hydration improves cycling endurance time. *Int J Sports Med* 1996;17(1):27-33.

2480 Yu YL, et al. Treatment of acute cortical infarct with intravenous glycerol. A double-blind, placebo-controlled randomized trial. *Stroke* 1993;24(8):1119-24.

2481 Yu YL, et al. Treatment of acute cerebral hemorrhage with intravenous glycerol. A double-blind, placebo-controlled, randomized trial. *Stroke* 1992;23(7):967-71.

2482 Frei A, et al. Glycerol and dextran combined in the therapy of acute stroke. A placebo-controlled, double-blind trial with a planned interim analysis. *Stroke* 1987;18(2):373-9.

2483 Bayer AJ, Pathy MS, Newcombe R. Double-blind randomised trial of intravenous glycerol in acute stroke. *Lancet* 1987;1(8530):405-8.

2484 Friedli W, et al. [Treatment with 10% glycerin in acute ischemic cerebral infarct. Doubleblind study]. [Article in German]. *Schweiz Med Wochenschr,* 1979; 109(20): 737-42.

2485 Bjorvell H, Hylander B, Rossner S. Effects of glycerol addition to diet in weight-reducing clubs. *Int J Obes* 1984;8(2):129-33.

2486 Fawer R, et al. Intravenous glycerol in cerebral infarction: a controlled 4-month trial. *Stroke* 1978;9(5):484-6.

2487 Ivy JL, et al. Effects of pyruvate on the metabolism and insulin resistance of obese Zucker rats. *Am J Clin Nutr* 1994;59(2):331-7.

2488 DeBoer LW, et al. Pyruvate enhances recovery of rat hearts after ischemia and reperfusion by preventing free radical generation. *Am J Physiol* 1993;265(5 Pt 2):H1571-6.

2489 DMV International Nutritionals. Health benifits of lactoferrin. www.lfplus.com/s2/2.html. (Accessed 16 July 1999).

2490 Yamauchi K, et al. Effects of orally administered bovine lactoferrin on the immune system of healthy volunteers. *Adv Exp Med Biol* 1998;443:261-5.

2491 Bellamy W, et al. Antibacterial spectrum of lactoferricin B, a potent bactericidal peptide derived from the N-terminal region of bovine lactoferrin. *J Appl Bacteriol* 1992;73(6):472-9.

2492 Inder WJ, et al. The effect of glycerol and desmopressin on exercise performance and hydration in triathletes. *Med Sci Sports Exerc* 1998;30(8):1263-9.

2493 Schmidtke I, Schoop W. Pycnogenol: stasis oedema and its medical treatment. *Schweizerische Zeitschrift fur GanzheitsMedizin* 1995;3:114-5.

2494 Hill AG, et al. Cellular potassium depletion predisposes to hypokalaemia after oral sodium phosphate. *Aust N Z J Surg* 1998;68(12):856-8.

2495 Clarkston WK, et al. Oral sodium phosphate versus sulfate-free polyethylene glycol electrolyte lavage solution in outpatient preparation for colonoscopy: a prospective comparison. *Gastrointest Endosc* 1996;43(1):42-8.

2496 Fine A, Patterson J. Severe hyperphosphatemia following phosphate administration for bowel preparation in patients with renal failure: two cases and a review of the literature. *Am J Kidney Dis* 1997;29(1):103-5.

2497 DiPalma JA, et al. Biochemical effects of oral sodium phosphate. *Dig Dis Sci* 1996;41(4):749-53.

2498 Helikson MA, Parham WA, Tobias JD. Hypocalcemia and hyperphosphatemia after phosphate enema use in a child. *J Pediatr Surg* 1997;32(8):1244-6.

2499 Galloway SD, et al. The effects of acute phosphate supplementation in subjects of different aerobic fitness levels. *Eur J Appl Physiol* 1996;72(3):224-30.

2500 Uebelhack R, Franke L, Schewe HJ. Inhibition of platelet MAO-B by kava pyrone-enriched extract from Piper methysticum Forster (kava-kava). *Pharmacopsychiatry* 1998;31(5):187-92.

2501 Gleitz J, Beile A, Wilkens P, et al. Antithrombotic action of the kava pyrone (+)-kavain prepared from Piper methysticum on human platelets. *Planta Med* 1997;63(1):27-30.

2502 Dwivedi S, Jauhari R . Beneficial effects of Terminalia arjuna in coronary artery disease. *Indian Heart J* 1997;49(5):507-10.

2503 Dwivedi S, Agarwal MP. Antianginal and cardioprotective effects of Terminalia arjuna, an indigenous drug, in coronary artery disease. *J Assoc Physicians India* 1994;42(4):287-9.

2504 Bharani A, Ganguly A, Bhargava KD. Salutary effect of Terminalia Arjuna in patients with severe refractory heart failure. *Int J Cardiol* 1995;49(3):191-9.

2505 Ram A, Lauria P, Gupta R, et al. Hypocholesterolaemic effects of Terminalia arjuna tree bark. *J Ethnopharmacol* 1997;55(3):165-9.

2506 Pettit GR, Hoard MS, Doubek DL, et al. Antineoplastic agents 338. The cancer cell growth inhibitory. Constituents of Terminalia arjuna (Combretaceae). *J Ethnopharmacol* 1996;53(2):57-63.

2507 Anand KK, Singh B, Saxena AK, et al. 3,4,5-Trihydroxy benzoic acid (gallic acid), the hepatoprotective principle in the fruits of Terminalia belerica-bioassay guided activity. *Pharmacol Res* 1997;36(4):315-21.

2508 Sato Y, Oketani H, Singyouchi K, et al. Extraction and purification of effective antimicrobial constituents of Terminalia chebula RETS. against methicillin-resistant Staphylococcus aureus. *Biol Pharm Bull* 1997 Apr;20(4):401-4.

2509 Yukawa TA, Kurokawa M, Sato H, et al. Prophylactic treatment of cytomegalovirus infection with traditional herbs. *Antiviral Res* 1996;32(2):63-70.

2510 Shiraki K, Yukawa T, Kurokawa M, Kageyama S. [Cytomegalovirus infection and its possible treatment with herbal medicines]. [Article in Japanese]. *Nippon Rinsho* 1998;56(1):156-60.

2511 Suthienkul O, Miyazaki O, Chulasiri M, et al. Retroviral reverse transcriptase inhibitory activity in Thai herbs and spices: screening with Moloney murine leukemia viral enzyme. *Southeast Asian J Trop Med Public Health* 1993;24(4):751-5.

2512 Kurokawa M, Nagasaka K, Hirabayashi T, et al. Efficacy of traditional herbal medicines in combination with acyclovir against herpes simplex virus type 1 infection in vitro and in vivo. *Antiviral Res* 1995;27(1-2):19-37.

2513 Jagtap AG, Karkera SG. Potential of the aqueous extract of Terminalia chebula as an anticaries agent. *J Ethnopharmacol* 1999 Dec 15;68(1-3):299-306.

2514 Phadke SA, Kulkarni SD. Screening of in vitro antibacterial activity of Terminalia chebula, Eclapta alba and Ocimum sanctum. *Indian J Med Sci* 1989;43(5):113-7.

2515 Hamada S, Kataoka T, Woo JT, et al. Immunosuppressive effects of gallic acid and chebulagic acid on CTL-mediated cytotoxicity. *Biol Pharm Bull* 1997;20(9):1017-9.

2516 Arseculeratne SN, Gunatilaka AA, Panabokke RG. Studies of medicinal plants of Sri Lanka. Part 14: Toxicity of some traditional medicinal herbs. *J Ethnopharmacol* 1985;13(3):323-35.

2517 Shaila HP, Udupa SL, Udupa AL. Hypolipidemic activity of three indigenous drugs in experimentally induced atherosclerosis. *Int J Cardiol* 1998;67(2):119-214.

2518 el-Mekkawy S, Meselhy MR, Kusumoto IT, et al. Inhibitory effects of Egyptian folk medicines on human immunodeficiency virus (HIV) reverse transcriptase. *Chem Pharm Bull (Tokyo)* 1995;43(4):641-8.

2519 Thakur CP, Thakur B, Singh S, et al. The Ayurvedic medicines Haritaki, Amala and Bahira reduce cholesterol-induced atherosclerosis in rabbits. *Int J Cardiol* 1988;21(2):167-75.

2520 Kiistala R, Makinen-Kiljunen S, Heikkinen K, et al. Occupational allergic rhinitis and contact urticaria caused by bishop's weed (Ammi majus). *Allergy* 1999;54(6):635-9.

2521 Ossenkoppele PM, van der Sluis WG, van Vloten WA. [Phototoxic dermatitis following the use of Ammi majus fruit for vitiligo]. [Article in Dutch]. *Ned Tijdschr Geneeskd* 1991;135(11):478-80.

2522 Harvengt C, Desager JP. HDL-cholesterol increase in normolipaemic subjects on khellin: a pilot study. *Int J Clin Pharmacol Res* 1983;3(5):363-6.

2523 Durate J, Vallejo I, Perez-Vizcaino F, et al. Effects of visnadine on rat isolated vascular smooth muscles. *Planta Med* 1997;63(3):233-6.

2524 Duarte J, Perez-Vizcaino F, Torres AI, et al. Vasodilator effects of visnagin in isolated rat vascular smooth muscle. *Eur J Pharmacol* 1995;286(2):115-22.

2525 Rauwald HW, Brehm O, Odenthal KP. The involvement of a Ca2+ channel blocking mode of action in the pharmacology of Ammi visnaga fruits. *Planta Med* 1994;60(2):101-5.

2526 Ahsan SK, Tariq M, Ageel AM, et al. Effect of Trigonella foenum-graecum and Ammi majus on calcium oxalate urolithiasis in rats. *J Ethnopharmacol* 1989;26(3):249-54.

2527 Shlosberg A, Egyed MN. Examples of poisonous plants in Israel of importance to animals and man. *Arch Toxicol Suppl* 1983;6:194-6. .

2528 Bethea D, Fullmer B, Syed S, et al. Psoralen photobiology and photochemotherapy: 50 years of science and medicine. *J Dermatol Sci* 1999;19(2):78-88.

2529 McKevoy GK, ed. AHFS Drug Information. Bethesda, MD: American Society of Health-System Pharmacists, 2000.

2530 Rehman J, Dillow JM, Carter SM, et al. Increased production of antigen-specific immunoglobulins G and M following in vivo treatment with the medicinal plants Echinacea angustifolia and Hydrastis canadensis. *Immunol Lett* 1999;68(2-3):391-5.

2531 Zhu M, Chan KW, Ng LS, et al. Possible influences of ginseng on the pharmacodynamics of warfarin in rats. *J Pharm Pharmacol* 1999;51:175-80.

2532 Eddleston M, Rajapakse S, Rajakanthan K, et al. Anti-digoxin Fab fragments in cardiotoxicity induced by ingestion of yellow oleander: a randomized controlled trial. *Lancet* 2000;355(9208):967-72.

2533 McAlindon TE, LaValley MP, Gulin JP, Felson DT. Glucosamine and Chondroitin for Treatment of Osteoarthritis A Systematic Quality Assessment and Meta-analysis. *JAMA* 2000;283:1469-75.

2534 Jensen GS, Ginsberg DJ, Huerta P, et al. Consumption of Aphanizomenon flos-aquae has rapid effects on the circulation and function of immune cells in humans. A novel approach to nutritional mobilization of the immune system. *JANA* 2000;2(3):50;50-6.

2535 Kushak RI, Drapeau C, Van Cott EM, Winter HH. Favorable effects of blue-green algae Aphanizomenon flos-aquae on rat plasma lipids. *JANA* 2000;2(3):50;59-65.

2536 Spadea L, Balestrazzi E. Treatment of vascular retinopathies with pycnogenol. *Phytother Res* 2001;15(3):219-23.

2537 Choi HK, Jung GW, Moon KH, et al. Clinical study of SS-Cream in patients with lifelong premature ejaculation. *Urology* 2000;55(2):257-61.

2538 Kiesewetter H, Koscielny J, Kalus U, et al. Efficacy of orally administered extract of red vine leaf AS 195 (folia vitis viniferae) in chronic venous insufficiency (stages I-II). A randomized, double-blind, placebo-controlled trial. *Arzneimittelforschung* 2000;50(2):109-17.

2539 Xiao Dong S, Zhi Ping Z, Zhong Xiao W, et al. Possible enhancement of the first-pass metabolism of phenacetin by ingestion of grape juice in Chinese subjects. *Br J Clin Pharmacol* 1999;48(4):638-40.

2540 Ozturk HS, Kacmaz M, Cimen MY, Durak I. Red wine and black grape strengthen blood antioxidant potential. *Nutrition* 1999;15(11-12):954-5.

2541 Bombardelli E, Morazzoni P. Vitis vinifera L. *Fitoterapia* 1995; LXVI(4):291-317.

2542 Watson RR. Reduction of cardiovascular disease risk factors by French maritime pine bark extract. *CVR&R* 1999;June:326-9.

2543 Rohdewald P. Bioavailability and metabolism of pycnogenol. *Eur Bull Drug Res* 1999;7(2):5-7.

2544 Gulati OP. Pycnogenol in venous disorders: a review. *Eur Bull Drug Res* 1999;7(2):8-13.

2545 Rohdewald P. Reducing the risk for stroke and heart infarction with pycnogenol. *Eur Bull Drug Res* 1999;7(2):14-18.

2546 Lee JY, Lee KS, Kim TS, et al. Squalene-induced extrinsic lipoid pneumonia: serial radiologic findings in nine patients. *J Comput Assist Tomogr* 1999;23(5):730-5.

2547 Lee JS, Im JG, Song KS, et al. Exogenous lipoid pneumonia: high-resolution CT findings. *Eur Radiol* 1999;9(2):287-91.

2548 Asnis DS, Saltzman HP, Melchert A. Shark oil pneumonia. An overlooked entity. *Chest* 1993,103(3):976-7.

2549 Skopinska-Rozewska E, Krotkiewski M, Sommer E, et al. Inhibitory effect of shark liver oil on cutaneous angiogenesis induced in Balb/c mice by syngeneic sarcoma L-1, human urinary bladder and human kidney tumour cells. *Oncol Rep* 1999;6(6):1341-4.

2550 Hichami A, Duroudier V, Leblais V, et al. Modulation of platelet-activating-factor production by incorporation of naturally occurring 1-O-alkylglycerols in phospholipids of human leukemic monocyte-like THP-1 cells. *Eur J Biochem* 1997;250(2):242-8.

2551 Loftsson T, Petersen DS, Le Goffic F, Olafsson JH. Unsaturated glycerol monoethers as novel skin penetration enhancers. *Pharmazie* 1997;52(6):463-5.

2552 Hasle H, Rose C. [Shark liver oil (alkoxyglycerol) and cancer treatment]. [Article in Danish]. *Ugeskr Laeger* 1991;153(5):343-6.

2553 Wang S, Tan D, Zhao Y, et al. The effect of pycnogenol on the microcirculation, platelet function and ischemic myocardium in patients with coronary artery diseases. *Eur Bull Drug Res* 1999;7(2):19-25.

2554 Pavlovic P. Improved endurance by use of antioxidants. *Eur Bull Drug Res* 1999;7(2):26-29.

2555 Kohama T, Suzuki N. The treatment of gynecological disorders with pycnogenol. *Eur Bull Drug Res* 1999;7(2):30-2.

2556 Roseff SJ, Gulati R. Improvement of sperm quality by pycnogenol. *Eur Bull Drug Res* 1999;7(2):33-6.

2557 Bell L, Halstenson CE, Halstenson CJ, et al. Cholesterol-lowering effects of calcium carbonate in patients with mild to moderate hypercholesterolemia. *Arch Intern Med* 1992;152:2441-4.

2558 Ramon JM, Bou R, Romea S, et al. Dietary fat intake and prostate cancer risk: a case-control study in Spain. *Cancer Causes Control* 2000;11:679-85.

2559 Colditz GA. Changing dietary patterns and cancer prevention: alpha-linolenic acid health risks and benefits. *Cancer Causes Control* 2000;11:677-8.

2560 Costa RL, Summa MA. Soy protein in the management of hyperlipidemia. *Ann Pharmacother* 2000;34:931-5.

2561 Ezaki O, Takahashi M, Shigematsu T, et al. Long-term effects of dietary alpha-linolenic acid from perilla oil on serum fatty acids composition and on the risk factors of coronary heart disease in Japanese elderly subjects. *J Nutr Sci Vitaminol* 1999;45:759-72.

2562 Walker AF, Middleton RW, Petrowicz O. Artichoke leaf

extract reduces symptoms of irritable bowel syndrome in a post-marketing surveillance study. *Phytother Res* 2001;15:58-61.

2563 2563. Sangalli BC, Chiang W. Toxicology of nutmeg abuse. *Clin Toxicol* 2000;38:671-8.

2564 Lissoni P, Tancini G, Barni S, et al. Treatment of cancer chemotherapy-induced toxicity with the pineal hormone melatonin. *Support Care Cancer* 1997;5:126-9.

2565 Lissoni P, Bucovec R, Bonfanti A, et al. Thrombopoietic properties of 5-methoxytryptamine plus melatonin versus melatonin alone in the treatment of cancer-related thrombocytopenia. *J Pineal Res* 2001;30:123-6.

2566 Lissoni P, Giani L, Zerbini S, et al. Biotherapy with the pineal immunomodulating hormone melatonin versus melatonin plus Aloe vera in untreatable advanced solid neoplasms. *Nat Immun* 1998;16:27-33.

2567 Hammar M, Larsson L, Tegler L. Calcium treatment of leg cramps in pregnancy. Effect on clinical symptoms and total serum and ionized serum calcium concentrations. *Acta Obstet Gynecol Scand* 1981;60:345-7.

2568 Lissoni P. Modulation of anticancer cytokines IL-2 and IL-12 by melatonin and the other pineal indoles 5-methoxytryptamine and 5-methoxytryptophol in the treatment of human neoplasms. *Ann NY Acad Sci* 2000;917:560-7.

2569 Heaney RP. Calcium, dairy products and osteoporosis. *J Am Coll Nutr* 2000;19(2):83S-99S.

2570 Chiu KM. Efficacy of calcium supplements on bone mass in postmenopausal women. *J Gerontol Med Sci* 1999;54A(6):M275-80.

2571 McGarry KA, Kiel DP. Postmenopausal osteoporosis. Strategies for preventing bone loss, avoiding fracture. *Postgrad Med* 2000;108(3):79-82,85-88,91.

2572 Nieves JW, Komar L, Cosman F, Lindsay R. Calcium potentiates the effect of estrogen and calcitonin on bone mass: review and analysis. *Am J Clin Nutr* 1998;67:18-24.

2575 Deal C. Can calcium and vitamin D supplementation adequately treat most patients with osteoporosis? *Cleve Clin J Med* 2000;67(10):696-8.

2576 Kanis JA. The use of calcium in the management of osteoporosis. *Bone* 1999;24(4):279-90.

2577 Mackerras D, Lumley T. First- and second-year effects in trials of calcium supplementation on the loss of bone density in postmenopausal women. *Bone* 1997;21:527-33.

2578 Bryant RJ, Cadogan J, Weaver CM. The new dietary reference intakes for calcium: implications for osteoporosis. *J Am Coll Nutr* 1999;18(5):406S-412S.

2579 Correa P, Fontham ETH, Bravo JC, et al. Chemoprevention of gastric dysplasia: randomized trial of antioxidant supplements and anti-Helicobacter pylori therapy. *J Natl Cancer Inst* 2000;92:1881-8.

2580 Rautalahti M, Virtamo J, Haukka J, et al. The effect of alpha-tocopherol and beta-carotene supplementation on COPD symptoms. *Am J Respir Crit Care Med* 1997;156:1447-52.

2581 Christian P, West KP, Khatry SK, et al. Vitamin A or beta-carotene supplementation reduces symptoms of illness in pregnant and lactating Nepali women. *J Nutr* 2000;130:2675-82.

2582 Albanes D, Heinonen OP, Taylor PR, et al. Alpha-tocopherol and beta-carotene supplements and lung cancer incidence in the alpha-tocopherol, beta-carotene cancer prevention study: effects of baseline characteristics and study compliance. *J Natl Cancer Inst* 1996;88:1560-70.

2583 Sun D, Abraham SN, Beachey EH. Influence of berberine sulfate on synthesis and expression of Pap fimbrial adhesin in uropathogenic Escherichia coli. *Antimicrob Agents Chemother* 1988;32(8):1274-7.

2584 Sun D, Courtney HS, Beachey EH. Berberine sulfate blocks adherence of Streptococcus pyogenes to epithelial cells, fibronectin, and hexadecane. *Antimicrob Agents Chemother* 1988;32(9):1370-4.

2585 Takatsuka N, Nagata C, Kurisu Y, et al. Hypocholesterolemic effect of soymilk supplementation with usual diet in premenopausal normolipidemic Japanese women. *Prev Med* 2000;31:308-14.

2586 Wiseman H, O'Reilly JD, Adlercreutz H, et al. Isoflavone phytoestrogens consumed in soy decrease F2-isoprostane concentrations and increase resistance of low-density lipoprotein to oxidation in humans. *Am J Clin Nutr* 2000;72:395-400.

2587 Kaneda Y, Torii M, Tanaka T, Aikawa M. In vitro effects of berberine sulphate on the growth and structure of Entamoeba histolytica, Giardia lamblia and Trichomonas vaginalis. *Ann Trop Med Parasitol* 1991;85(4):417-25.

2588 Gupte S. Use of berberine in treatment of giardiasis. *Am J Dis Child* 1975; 129:866.

2589 Chan E. Displacement of bilirubin from albumin by berberine. *Biol Neonate* 1993;63(4):201-8.

2590 Winek CL, Elzein EO, Wahba WW, Feldman JA. Interference of herbal drinks with urinalysis for drugs of abuse. *J Anal Toxicol* 1993;17(4):246-7.

2591 Bhide MB, Shaven SR, Dutta NK. Absorption, distribution, and excretion of berberine. *Indian J Med Res* 1969;57(11):2128-31.

2592 van der Vliet A. Cigarettes, cancer and the carotenoids: a continuing, unresolved antioxidant paradox. *Am J Clin Nutr* 2000;72:1421-3.

2593 Alberg AJ, Chen JC, Zhao H, et al. Household exposure to passive cigarette smoking and serum micronutrient concentrations. *Am J Clin Nutr* 2000;72:1576-82.

2594 Normen L, Dutta P, Lia A, et al. Soy sterol esters and B-sitostanol ester as inhibitors of cholesterol absorption in human small bowel. *Am J Clin Nutr* 2000;71:908-13.

2595 Michaud DS, Feskanich D, Rimm EB, et al. Intake of specific carotenoids and risk of lung cancer in 2 prospective US cohorts. *Am J Clin Nutr* 2000;72:990-7.

2596 Osterhoudt KC, Lee SK, Callahan JM, Henretig FM. Catnip and the alteration of human consciousness. *Vet Hum Toxicol* 1997 Dec;39(6):373-5.

2597 Just MJ, Recio MC, Giner RM, et al. Anti-inflammatory activity of unusual lupane saponins from Bupleurum fruticescens. *Planta Med* 1998;64(5):404-7.

2598 Matsumoto T, Yamada H. Regulation of immune complexes binding of macrophages by pectic polysaccharide from Bupleurum falcatum L.: pharmacological evidence for the requirement of intracellular calcium/calmodulin on Fc receptor up-regulation by bupleuran 2IIb. *J Pharm Pharmacol* 1995;47(2):152-6.

2599 Green A, Williams G, Neale R, et al. Daily sunscreen applications and beta-carotene supplementation in prevention of basal-cell and squamous-cell carcinomas of the skin: a randomized controlled trial. *Lancet* 1999;354:723-9.

2600 Drovanti A, Bignamini AA, Rovati AA. Therapeutic

activity of oral glucosamine sulfate in osteoarthrosis: a placebo-controlled, double-blind investigation. *Clin Ther* 1980;3:260-72.

2601 da Camara CC, Dowless GV. Glucosamine sulfate for osteoarthritis. *Ann Pharmacother* 1998;32:580-7.

2602 Lopes Vaz AL. Double-blind, clinical evaluation of the relative efficacy of ibuprofen and glucosamine sulphate in the management of osteoarthrosis of the knee in out-patients. *Curr Med Res Opin* 1982;8:145-9.

2603 Pujalte JM, Llavore EP, Ylescupidez FR. Double-blind clinical evaluation of oral glucosamine sulphate in the basic treatment of osteoarthrosis. *Curr Med Res Opin* 1980;7:110-4.

2604 Qiu GX, et al. Efficacy and safety of glucosamine sulfate versus ibuprofen in patients with knee osteoarthritis. *Arzneimittelforschung* 1998;48:469-74.

2605 Reichelt A. Efficacy and safety of intramuscular glucosamine sulfate in osteoarthritis of the knee. A randomised, placebo-controlled, double-blind study. *Arzneimittelforschung* 1994;44:75-80.

2606 Forster KK, et al. Longer-term treatment of mild-to-moderate osteoarthritis of the knee with glucosamine sulfate- a randomized controlled, double-blind clinical study. *Euro J Clin Pharmacol* 1996;50:542.

2607 Setnikar I, et al. Pharmacokinetics of glucosamine in man. Arzneimittelforschung 1993;43:1109-13.

2608 Barclay TS, Tsourounis C, McCart GM. Glucosamine. *Ann Pharmacother* 1998;32:574-9.

2609 Burton AF, Anderson FH. Decreased incorporation of 14C-glucosamine relative to 3H-N-acetyl glucosamine in the intestinal mucosa of patients with inflammatory bowel disease. *Am J Gastroenterol* 1983;78:19-22.

2610 Goodman MJ, Kent PW, Truelove SC. Glucosamine synthetase activity of the colonic mucosa in ulcerative colitis and Crohn's disease. *Gut* 1977;18:219-28.

2611 Talent JM, Gracy RW. Pilot study of oral polymeric N-acetyl-D-glucosamine as a potential treatment for patients with osteoarthritis. *Clin Ther* 1996;18:1184M-90M.

2612 Leite JR, et al. Pharmacology of lemongrass (Cymbopogon citratus Stapf). III. Assessment of eventual toxic, hypnotic and anxiolytic effects on humans. *J Ethnopharmacol* 1986;17:75-83.

2613 Feher J, et al. [Liver-protective action of silymarin therapy in chronic alcoholic liver diseases]. [Article in Hungarian]. *Orv Hetil* 1989;130:2723-7.

2614 Szilard S, Szentgyorgyi D, Demeter I. Protective effect of Legalon in workers exposed to organic solvents. *Acta Med Hung* 1988;45:249-56.

2615 Hruby K, et al. Chemotherapy of Amanita phalloides poisoning with intravenous silibinin. *Hum Toxicol* 1983;2:183-95.

2616 Ferenci P, et al. Randomized controlled trial of silymarin treatment in patients with cirrhosis of the liver. *J Hepatol* 1989;9:105-13.

2617 Velussi M, et al. Long-term (12 months) treatment with an anti-oxidant drug (silymarin) is effective on hyperinsulinemia, exogenous insulin need and malondialdehyde levels in cirrhotic diabetic patients. *J Hepatol* 1997;26:871-9.

2618 Salmi HA, Sarna S. Effect of silymarin on chemical, functional, and morphological alterations of the liver. A double-blind, controlled study. *Scand J Gastroenterol* 1982;17:517-21.

2619 Hebel SK, ed. Drug Facts and Comparisons. 52nd ed. St. Louis: Facts and Comparisons, 1998.

2620 Tyrey L. Delta 9-Tetrahydrocannabinol: a potent inhibitor of episodic luteinizing hormone secretion. *J Pharmacol Exp Ther* 1980;213:306-8.

2621 Sallan SE, Zinberg NE, Frei E III. Antiemetic effect of delta-9-tetrahydrocannabinol in patients receiving cancer chemotherapy. *N Engl J Med* 1975;293:795-7.

2622 Schwartz RH, Beveridge RA. Marijuana as an antiemetic drug: how useful is it today? Opinions from clinical oncologists. *J Addict Dis* 1994;13:53-65.

2623 FDA/ORA CPG 7121.01. Sec. 457.100 Pangamic Acid and Pangamic Acid Products Unsafe for Food and Drug Use. (CPG 7121.01) www.fda.gov/ora/compliance_ref/cpg/cpgdrg/cpg457-100.html (Accessed 16 July 1999).

2624 Heber D, et al. Cholesterol-lowering effects of a proprietary Chinese red-yeast-rice dietary supplement. *Am J Clin Nutr* 1999;69:231-6.

2625 FDA talk paper. FDA determines Cholestin to be unapproved drug. www.fda.gov/bbs/topics/ANSWERS/ANS00871.html (Accessed 3 May 1999).

2626 Nando Media Web site. Judge rules against FDA in Cholestin challenge. www.nandotimes.com/healthscience/story/body/0,1079,19548-32099-232485-0,00.html (Accessed 3 May 1999).

2627 Puente S, et al. Eosinophilic gastroenteritis caused by bee pollen sensitization. *Med Clin (Barc)* 10 May 1997;108(18):698-700.

2628 Patrick L. Beta-carotene: the controversy continues. *Alt Med Rev* 2000;5:530-45.

2629 Lee SK, et al. Modulation of in vitro biomarkers of the carcinogenic process by chemopreventive agents. Anticancer Res 1999;19(1A):35-44.

2630 Mirzoeva OK, Calder PC. The effect of propolis and its components on eicosanoid production during the inflammatory response. *Prostaglandins Leukot Essent Fatty Acids* 1996;55:441-9.

2631 Park YK, et al. Antimicrobial activity of propolis on oral microorganisms. *Curr Microbiol* 1998;36:24-8.

2632 Hay KD, Greig DE. Propolis allergy: a cause of oral mucositis with ulceration. *Oral Surg Oral Med Oral Pathol* 1990;70:584-6.

2633 Hashimoto T, et al. Synthesis of two allergenic constituents of propolis and poplar bud excretion. *Z Naturforsch [C]* 1988;43:470-2.

2634 Yeih DF, Chiang FT, Huang SKS. Successful treatment of aconitine induced life threatening ventricular tachyarrhythmia with amiodarone. *Heart* 2000;84(4):E8.

2635 Tixier JM, et al. Evidence by in vivo and in vitro studies that binding of pycnogenols to elastin affects its rate of degradation by elastases. *Biochem Pharmacol* 1984;33:3933-9.

2636 Liu FJ, Zhang YX, Lau BH. Pycnogenol enhances immune and haemopoietic functions in senescence-accelerated mice. *Cell Mol Life Sci* 1998;54:1168-72.

2637 Fitzpatrick DF, Bing, Rohdewald P. Endothelium-dependent vascular effects of Pycnogenol. *J Cardiovasc Pharmacol* 1998;32:509-15.

2638 Practical Health. Pycnogenol. www.practicalhealth.com/pagebetweeneducationalandorder.htm (Accessed 16 July 1999).

2639 Thys-Jacobs S. Micronutrients and the premenstrual syndrome: The case for calcium. *J Am Coll Nutr* 2000;19(2):220-7.

2640 Bell SJ. Whey protein concentrates with and without immunoglobulins: a review. *J Med Food* 2000;3(1):1-13.

2641 Dauer A, Metzner P, Schimmer O. Proanthocyanidins from the bark of Hamamelis virginiana exhibit antimutagenic properties against nitroaromatic compounds. *Planta Med* 1998;64:324-7.

2642 Omenn GS, Goodman GE, Thornquist MD, et al. Effects of a combination of beta-carotene and vitamin A on lung cancer and cardiovascular disease. *N Engl J Med* 1996;334:1150-5.

2643 SmartBasics. Vitamin B15 or pangamic acid. URL: webu5156.ntx.net/glos.vitamins/vit.b15.glos.html (Accessed 18 May 1999).

2644 Wallner-Pendleton EA, et al. Toxicity of excess dicalcium phosphate in the diet of turkey poults. *Avian Dis* 1989;33:375-8.

2645 Gray ME, Titlow LW. The effect of pangamic acid on maximal treadmill performance. *Med Sci Sports Exerc* 1982;14(6):424-7.

2646 Hennekens CH, Buring JE, Manson JE, et al. Lack of effect of long-term supplementation with beta-carotene on the incidence of malignant neoplasms and cardiovascular disease. *N Engl J Med* 1996;334:1145-9.

2647 Prolyt formula. The Apothecary. www.intr.net/ apothecary/lyt.html. (Accessed 24 May 1999).

2648 Hellgren L, Vincent J. Degradation and liquefication effect of streptokinase-streptodornase and stabilised trypsin on tissue necroses, crusts of fibrinoid, purulent exudate and clotted blood from leg ulcers. *J Int Med Res* 1977;5:334-7.

2649 Suomalainen O. Evaluation of two enzyme preparations-Trypure and Varidase in traumatic ulcers. *Ann Chir Gynaecol* 1983;72:62-5.

2650 FDA talk paper. Food and Drug Administration Website. www.vm.cfsan.fda.gov/~lrd/TPMUSHRM.html (Accessed 24 May 1999).

2651 Sadjadi J. Anthrax associated with the Kombucha mushroom in Iran. *JAMA* 1998;280:1567-8.

2652 Kombucha-toxicity alert. *Crit Path AIDS Proj*, 1994;30:31-32 1994-5.

2653 Gamundi R, Valdivia M. The Kombucha mushroom: two different opinions. *Sidahora* 1995;90:34-5.

2654 Majchrowicz M. Kombucha: a dubious "cure". *GMHC Treat Issues* 1995;9:10.

2655 CDC. Unexplained severe illness possibly associated with consumption of Kombucha tea-Iowa, 1995. *MMWR Morb Mortal Wkly Rep* 1995;44:892-3,899-900.

2656 Srinivasan R, Smolinske S, Greenbaum DJ. Probable gastrointestinal toxicity of Kombucha tea: is this beverage healthy or harmful? *Gen Intern Med* 1997;12:643-4.

2657 Greenberg ER, Baron JA, Karagas MR, et al. Mortality associated with low plasma concentration of beta carotene and the effect of oral supplementation. *JAMA* 1996;275:699-703.

2658 Blot WJ, Li JY, Taylor PR. Nutritional intervention trials in Linxian, China: supplementation with specific vitamin/mineral combinations, cancer incidence, and disease-specific mortality in the general population. *J Natl Cancer Inst* 1993;85:1483-92.

2659 McLeod MN, Gaynes BN, Golden RN. Chromium potentiation of antidepressant pharmacotherapy for dysthymic disorder in 5 patients. *J Clin Psych* 1999;60(4):237-40.

2660 Logani S, Chen MC, Tran T, et al. Actions of Ginkgo Biloba related to potential utility for the treatment of conditions involving cerebral hypoxia. *Life Sciences* 2000;67:1389-96.

2661 May SW, Pollock SH. Selenium-based antihypertensives. Rationale and potential. *Drugs* 1998;56(6):959-64.

2662 Aaseth J, Haugen M, Forre O. Rheumatoid arthritis and metal compounds-perspectives on the role of oxygen radical detoxification. *Analyst* 1998;123:3-6.

2663 Chan S, Gerson B, Subramaniam S. The role of copper, molybdenum, selenium, and zinc in nutrition and health. *Clin Lab Med* 1998;18:673-85.

2664 Clark LC, Combs GF Jr, Turnbull BW, et al. Effects of selenium supplementation for cancer prevention in patients with carcinoma of the skin. A randomized controlled trial. *JAMA* 1996;276:1957-63.

2665 Wesnes K, Simmons D, Rook M, Simpson P. A double-blind placebo-controlled trial of Tanakan in the treatment of idiopathic cognitive impairment in the elderly. *Human Psychopharmacol* 1987;2:159-69.

2666 Hofferberth B. The efficacy of Egb 761 in patients with senile dementia of the Alzheimer type, A double-blind, palcebo-controlled study on different levels of investigation. *Human Psychopharmacol* 1994;9:215-22.

2667 Clark LC, Dalkin B, Krongrad A, et al. Decreased incidence of prostate cancer with selenium supplementation: results of a double-blind cancer prevention trial. *Br J Urol* 1998;81:730-4.

2668 Maier RH, Purser SM, Nicholson DL, Pories WJ. The cytotoxic interaction of inorganic trace elements with EDTA and cisplatin in sensitive and resistant human ovarian cancer cells. *In Vitro Cell Dev Biol Anim* 1997;33:218-21.

2671 Koller LD, Exon JH. The two faces of selenium-deficiency and toxicity-are similar in animals and man. *Can J Vet Res* 1986;50(3):297-306.

2673 Mark SD, Wang W, Fraumeni JF Jr, et al. Do nutritional supplements lower the risk of stroke or hypertension? *Epidemiology* 1998;9:9-15.

2674 Knoben JE, Anderson PO. Handbook of Clinical Drug Data. 7th ed. Hamilton, IL: Drug Intelligence Publications, Inc., 1993.

2676 Neve J. Selenium as a risk factor for cardiovascular diseases. *J Cardiovasc Risk* 1996;3(1):42-7.

2678 Brewer GJ, Yuzbasiyan-Gurkan V, Johnson V, et al. Treatment of Wilson's disease with zinc: XI. Interaction with other anticopper agents. *J Am Coll Nutr* 1993;12(1):26-30.

2679 Brewer GJ, Johnson V, Kaplan J. Treatment of Wilson's disease with zinc: XIV. Studies of the effect of zinc on lymphocyte function. *J Lab Clin Med* 1997;129(6):649-52.

2680 Fuchs GJ. Possibilities for zinc in the treatment of acute diarrhea. *Am J Clin Nutr* 1998;68(2 Suppl):480S-3.

2681 Fosmire GJ. Zinc toxicity. *Am J Clin Nutr*, 1990;51:225-7.

2682 Lomaestro BM, Bailie GR. Absorption interactions with fluoroquinolones. 1995 update. *Drug Saf*, 1995;12(5):314-33.

2686 Dreno B, Trossaert M, Boiteau HL, Litoux P. Zinc salts effects on granulocyte zinc concentration and chemotaxis in acne patients. *Acta Derm Venereol*, 1992;72(4):250-2.

2687 Schachner L, Eaglstein W, Kittles C, Mertz P. Topical erythromycin and zinc therapy for acne. *J Am Acad Dermatol*, 1990;22(2 Pt 1):253-60.

2688 Habbema L, Koopmans B, Menke HE, et al. A 4%

erythromycin and zinc combination (Zineryt) versus 2% erythromycin (Eryderm) in acne vulgaris: a randomized, double-blind comparative study. *Br J Dermatol* 1989;121(4):497-502.

2689 Walldius G, Michaelsson G, Hardell LI, Aberg H. The effects of diet and zinc treatment on the fatty acid composition of serum lipids and adipose tissue and on serum lipoproteins in two adolescent patients with acrodermatitis enteropathica. *Am J Clin Nutr,* 1983;38(4):512-22.

2690 Koletzko B, Bretschneider A, Bremer HJ. Fatty acid composition of plasma lipids in acrodermatitis enteropathica before and after zinc supplementation. *Eur J Pediatr,* 1985;143(4):310-4.

2691 Borroni G, Brazzelli V, Vignati G, et al. Bullous lesions in acrodermatitis enteropathica. Histopathologic findings regarding two patients. *Am J Dermatopathol,* 1992;14(4):304-9.

2692 Sturniolo GC, Mestriner C, Irato P, et al. Zinc therapy increases duodenal concentrations of metallothionein and iron in Wilson's disease patients. *Am J Gastroenterol,* 1999;94(2):334-8.

2693 Brewer GJ, Dick RD, Johnson VD, et al. Treatment of Wilson's disease with zinc: XV long-term follow-up studies. *J Lab Clin Med,* 1998;132(4):264-78.

2694 Rittenhouse T. The management of lower-extremity ulcers with zinc-saline wet dressings versus normal saline wet dressings. *Adv Ther,* 1996;13(2):88-94.

2696 Young B, Ott L, Kasarskis E, et al. Zinc supplementation is associated with improved neurologic recovery rate and visceral protein levels of patients with severe closed head injury. *J Neurotrauma,* 1996; 13(1):25-34.

2699 Agren MS. Studies on zinc in wound healing. *Acta Derm Venereol Suppl (Stockh),* 1990;154:1-36.

2700 Shukla A, Rasik AM, Jain GK, et al. In vitro and in vivo wound healing activity of asiaticoside isolated from Centella asiatica. *J Ethnopharmacol* 1999;65:1-11.

2701 FDA Orphan Drugs. List of orphan designations and approvals. www.fda.gov/orphan/DESIGNAT/list.htm (Accessed 19 January 2000).

2702 Shabert JK, Winslow C, Lacey JM, Wilmore DW. Glutamine-antioxidant supplementation increases body cell mass in AIDS patients with weight loss: a randomized, double-blind controlled trial. *Nutrition* 1999;15:860-4.

2703 Scolapio JS. Effect of growth hormone, glutamine, and diet on body composition in short bowel syndrome: a randomized, controlled study. *JPEN J Parenter Enteral Nutr* 1999;23:309-12.

2704 Rubio IT, Cao Y, Hutchins LF, et al. Effect of glutamine on methotrexate efficacy and toxicity. *Ann Surg* 1998;227:772-8.

2705 Yoshida S, Matsui M, Shirouzu Y, et al. Effects of glutamine supplements and radiochemotherapy on systemic immune and gut barrier function in patients with advanced esophageal cancer. *Ann Surg* 1998;227:485-91.

2706 Osol A, Hoover JE, eds. Remington's Pharmaceutical Science, 15th ed. Easton, PA: Mack Publishing Company, 1975.

2707 Zahn KA, Li RL, Purssell RA. Cardiovascular toxicity after ingestion of "herbal ecstacy". *J Emerg Med* 1999;17:289-91.

2708 Center for the evaluation of risks to human reproduction (CERHR). Caffeine. URL: http://cerhr.niehs.nih.gov/ genpub/topics/caffeine.html (Accessed 19 January 2000).

2709 Klebanoff MA, Levine RJ, DerSimonian R, et al. Maternal serum paraxanthine, a caffeine metabolite, and the risk of spontaneous abortion. *N Engl J Med* 1999;341:1639-44.

2710 Eskenazi B. Caffeine—filtering the facts. *N Engl J Med* 1999;341:1688-9.

2711 Fernandes O, Sabharwal M, Smiley T, et al. Moderate to heavy caffeine consumption during pregnancy and relationship to spontaneous abortion and abnormal fetal growth: a meta-analysis. *Reprod Toxicol* 1998;12:435-44.

2712 Stookey JD. The diuretic effects of alcohol and caffeine and total water intake misclassification. *Eur J Epidemiol* 1999;15:181-8.

2713 Wemple RD, Lamb DR, McKeever KH. Caffeine vs caffeine-free sports drinks: effects on urine production at rest and during prolonged exercise. *Int J Sports Med* 1997;18:40-6.

2714 Pollock BG, Wylie M, Stack JA, et al. Inhibition of caffeine metabolism by estrogen replacement therapy in postmenopausal women. *J Clin Pharmacol* 1999;39:936-40.

2715 Goldstein J, Hoffman HD, Armellino JJ, et al. Treatment of severe, disabling migraine attacks in an over-the-counter population of migraine sufferers: results from three randomized, placebo-controlled studies of the combination of acetaminophen, aspirin, and caffeine. *Cephalalgia* 1999;19:684-91.

2716 Lipton RB, Stewart WF, Ryan RE Jr, et al. Efficacy and safety of acetaminophen, aspirin, and caffeine in alleviating migraine headache pain: three double-blind, randomized, placebo-controlled trials. *Arch Neurol* 1998;55:210-7.

2717 Silberstein SD, Armellino JJ, Hoffman HD, et al. Treatment of menstruation-associated migraine with the nonprescription combination of acetaminophen, aspirin, and caffeine: results from three randomized, placebo-controlled studies. *Clin Ther* 1999;21:475-91.

2718 Migliardi JR, Armellino JJ, Friedman M, et al. Caffeine as an analgesic adjuvant in tension headache. *Clin Pharmacol Ther* 1994;56:576-86.

2719 DiPiro JT, Talbert RL, Yee GC, et al., Eds. Pharmacotherapy: A pathophysiologic approach. 4th ed. Stamford, CT: Appleton & Lange, 1999.

2720 Rees K, Allen D, Lader M. The influences of age and caffeine on psychomotor and cognitive function. *Psychopharmacology (Berl)* 1999;145:181-8.

2722 Nurminen ML, Niittynen L, Korpela R, Vapaatalo H. Coffee, caffeine and blood pressure: a critical review. *Eur J Clin Nutr* 1999;53:831-9.

2723 Dews PB, Curtis GL, Hanford KJ, O'Brien CP. The frequency of caffeine withdrawal in a population-based survey and in a controlled, blinded pilot experiment. *J Clin Pharmacol* 1999;39:1221-32.

2724 Akhtar S, Wood G, Rubin JS, et al. Effect of caffeine on the vocal folds: a pilot study. *J Laryngol Otol* 1999;113:341-5.

2725 Weber JG, Klindworth JT, Arnold JJ, et al. Prophylactic intravenous administration of caffeine and recovery after ambulatory surgical procedures. *Mayo Clin Proc* 1997;72:621-6.

2726 Hampl KF, Schneider MC, Ruttimann U, et al. Perioperative administration of caffeine tablets for prevention of postoperative headaches. *Can J Anaesth* 1995;42:789-92.

2727 Yucel A, Ozyalcin S, Talu GK, et al. Intravenous administration of caffeine sodium benzoate for postdural puncture headache. *Reg Anesth Pain Med* 1999;24:51-4.

2728 Camann WR, Murray RS, Mushlin PS, Lambert DH. Effects of oral caffeine on postdural puncture headache. A double-blind, placebo-controlled trial. *Anesth Analg* 1990;70:181-4.

2729 FDA. Proposed rule: dietary supplements containing ephedrine alkaloids. www.verity.fda.gov/ (Accessed 25 January 2000).

2732 Wilt TJ, Ishani A, Stark G, et al. Saw palmetto extracts for treatment of benign prostatic hyperplasia: a systematic review. *JAMA* 1998;280:1604-9.

2733 Gerber GS, Zagaja GP, Bales GT, et al. Saw palmetto (Serenoa repens) in men with lower urinary tract symptoms: effects on urodynamic parameters and voiding symptoms. *Urology* 1998;51:1003-7.

2734 Lowe FC, Fagelman E. Phytotherapy in the treatment of benign prostatic hyperplasia: an update. *Urology* 1999;53:671-8.

2735 Marks LS, Tyler VE. Saw palmetto extract: newest (and oldest) treatment alternative for men with symptomatic benign prostatic hyperplasia. *Urology* 1999;53:457-61.

2736 USRF Research. Clinical effects of saw palmetto extract in men with symptomatic BPH webpage: www.usrf.org/spepapers.html (Accessed 26 January 2000).

2737 Ludwig DS, Pereira MA, Kroenke CH, et al. Dietary fiber, weight gain, and cardiovascular disease risk factors in young adults. *JAMA*, 1999;282:1539-46.

2739 Beutler KT, Pankewycz O, Brautigan DL. Equivalent uptake of organic and inorganic zinc by monkey kidney fibroblasts, human intestinal epithelial cells, or perfused mouse intestine. *Biol Trace Elem Res* 1998;61:19-31.

2740 Duisterwinkel FJ, Wolthers BG, Koopman BJ, et al. Bioavailability of orally administered zinc, using Taurizine. *Pharm Weekbl Sci* 1986;8:85-8.

2742 Muscle Photos. ZMA for athletes. www.musclephotos.com/zma.html (Accessed 26 January 2000).

2743 Dr. Duke's Phytochemical and Ethnobotanical Databases. Ethnobotanical uses: Andrographis paniculata. www.ars-grin.gov/cgi-bin/duke/ethnobot.pl?andrographis%20pnaiculata (Accessed 27 January 2000).

2744 Caceres DD, Hancke JL, Burgos RA, et al. Use of visual analogue scale measurements (VAS) to assess the effectiveness of standardized Andrographis paniculata extract SHA-10 in reducing the symptoms of common cold. A randomized, double-blind, placebo study. *Phytomedicine* 1999;6:217-23.

2745 Ambrosia Herbals. Herbal extracts of therapuetic use. www.ambrosiaherbals.com/acorus_calamus.html (Accessed 27 January 2000).

2746 Indian Herbs. Andrographis paniculata. www.indianherbs.com/andro.htm (Accessed 27 January 2000).

2747 Kan Jang. Kang Jang herbal remedy for colds, flu, sinusitis, allergies from [sic] Swedish Herbal Institute. www.kanjang.com (Accessed 27 January 2000).

2748 Thamlikitkul V, Dechatiwongse T, Theerapong S, et al. Efficacy of Andrographis paniculata, Nees for pharyngotonsillitis in adults. *J Med Assoc Thai* 1991;74:437-42.

2749 Martz W. Plants with a reputation against snakebite. *Toxicon* 1992;30:1131-42.

2750 Madav S, Tripathi HC, Tandan SK, et al. Antiallergic activity of andrographolide. *Indian J Pharm Sci* 1998;60:176-8.

2751 Gupta PP, Tandon JS, Patnaik GK. Antiallergic activity of andrographolides isolated from Andrographis paniculata (Burm. F) Wall. *Pharm Biol* 1998;36:72-4.

2752 Kumar S, Gopal K. Screening of plant species for inhibition of bacterial population of raw water. *Journal of Environmental Science And Health Part A Toxic-Hazardous Engineering* 1999;34:975-87.

2753 Madav S, Tripathi HC, Tandan Mishra SK. Analgesic, antipyretic and antiulcerogenic effects of andrographolide. *Indian J Pharm Sci* 1995;57:121-5.

2754 Vedavathy S, Rao KN. Antipyretic activity of six indigenous medicinal plants of Tirumala Hills, Andhra Pradesh, India. *J Ethnopharmacol* 1991;33:193-6.

2755 Zhang CY, Tan BK. Mechanisms of cardiovascular activity of Andrographis paniculata in the anaesthetized rat. *J Ethnopharmacol* 1997;56:97-101.

2756 Guo ZL, Zhao HY, Zheng XH. The effect of andrographis paniculata nees (APN) in alleviating the myocardial ischemic reperfusion injury. *J Tongji Med Univ* 1994;14:49-51.

2757 Guo Z, Zhao H, Fu L. Protective effects of API0134 on myocardial ischemia and reperfusion injury. *J Tongji Med Univ* 1996;16:193-7.

2758 Zhao HY, Fang WY. Antithrombotic effects of Andrographis paniculata nees in preventing myocardial infarction. *Chin Med J (Engl)* 1991;104:770-5.

2759 Amroyan E, Gabrielian E, Panossian A, et al. Inhibitory effect of andrographolide from Andrographis paniculata on PAF-induced platelet aggregation. *Phytomedicine* 1999;6:27-31.

2760 Zhang C, Kuroyangi M, Tan BK. Cardiovascular activity of 14-deoxy-11,12-didehydroandrographolide in the anaesthetised rat and isolated right atria. *Pharmacol Res* 1998;38:413-7.

2761 Shukla B, Visen PK, Patnaik GK, Dhawan BN. Choleretic effect of andrographolide in rats and guinea pigs. *Planta Med* 1992;58:146-9.

2762 Visen PK, Shukla B, Patnaik GK, Dhawan BN. Andrographolide protects rat hepatocytes against paracetamol-induced damage. *J Ethnopharmacol* 1993;40:131-6.

2763 Rana AC, Avadhoot Y. Hepatoprotective effects of Andrographis paniculata against carbon tetrachloride-induced liver damage. *Arch Pharm Res* 1991;14:93-5.

2764 Leelarasamee A, Trakulsomboon S, Sittisomwong N. Undetectable anti-bacterial activity of Andrographis paniculata (Burma) wall. ex ness. *J Med Assoc Thai* 1990;73:299-304.

2765 Chang RS, Ding L, Chen GQ, et al. Dehydroandrographolide succinic acid monoester as an inhibitor against the human immunodeficiency virus. *Proc Soc Exp Biol Med* 1991;197:59-66.

2766 Puri A, Saxena R, Saxena RP, et al. Immunostimulant agents from Andrographis paniculata. *J Nat Prod* 1993;56:995-9.

2767 Raj RK. Screening of indigenous plants for anthelmintic action against human Ascaris lumbricoides:Part II. *Ind J Physiol Pharmacol* 1975;19(1):47-9.

2768 Matsuda T, Kuroyanagi M, Sugiyama S, et al. Cell differentiation-inducing diterpenes from Andrographis paniculata Nees. *Chem Pharm Bull (Tokyo)* 1994;42:1216-25.

2769 Akbarsha MA, Manivannan B, Hamid KS, Vijayan B. Antifertility effect of Andrographis paniculata (Nees) in male albino rat. *Indian J Exp Biol* 1990;28:421-6.

2770 Burgos RA, Caballero EE, Sanchez NS, et al. Testicular toxicity assessment of Andrographis paniculata dried extract in rats. *J Ethnopharmacol* 1997;58:219-24.

2771 Panossian A, Kochikian A, Gabrielian E, et al. Effect of Andrographis paniculata extract on progesterone in blood plasma of pregnant rats. *Phytomedicine* 1999;6:157-61.

2772 Caceres DD, Hancke JL, Burgos RA, Wikman GK. Prevention of common colds with Andrographis Paniculata dried extract: a pilot, double-blind trial. *Phytomedicine* 1997;4:101-4.

2773 Melchior J, Palm S, Wikman G. Controlled clinical study of standardized Andrographis paniculata in common cold- a pilot trial. *Phytomedicine* 1996;97;3:315-8.

2774 Hancke J, Burgos R, Caceres D, Wikman G. A double-blind study with a new monodrug kan jang: decrease of symptoms and improvement in the recovery from common colds. *Phytotherapy Res* 1995;9:559-62.

2775 GRIN/NPGS Taxonomy Info. Taxon: Andrographis paniculata (Burm. f.) www.ars-grin.gov/cgi-bin/npgs/html/taxon.pl?414228 (Accessed 27 January 2000).

2776 Zoha MS, Hussain AH, Choudhury SA. Antifertility effect of andrographis paniculata in mice. *Bangladesh Med Res Counc Bull* 1989;15:34-7.

2777 Gozalbes R, Galvez J, Garcia-Domenech R, Derouin F. Molecular search of new active drugs against Toxoplasma gondii. *SAR QSAR Environ Res* 1999;10:47-60.

2778 Kapil A, Koul IB, Banerjee SK, Gupta BD. Antihepatotoxic effects of major diterpenoid constituents of Andrographis paniculata. *Biochem Pharmacol* 1993;46:182-5.

2779 Gupta S, Yadava JN, Tandon JS. Antisecretory (antidiarrheal) activity of Indian medicinal plants against Escherichia coli enterotoxin-induced secretion in rabbit and guinea pig ileal loop models. *Int J Pharmacogn* 1993;31:198-204.

2780 Najib NA, Rahman N, Furuta T, et al. Antimalarial activity of extracts of Malaysian medicinal plants. *J Ethnopharmacol* 1999;64:249-54.

2781 Misra P, Pal NL, Guru PY, et al. Antimalarial activity of Andrographis paniculata (Kalmegh) against Plasmodium berghei NK 65 in Mastomys natalensis. *Int J Pharmacogn* 1992;30:263-74.

2782 Wang DW, Zhao HY. Prevention of atherosclerotic arterial stenosis and restenosis after angioplasty with Andrographis paniculata nees and fish oil. Experimental studies of effects and mechanisms. *Chin Med J (Engl)* 1994;107:464-70.

2783 Wang DW, Zhao HY. Experimental studies on prevention of atherosclerotic arterial stenosis and restenosis after angioplasty with Andrographis Paniculata Nees and fish oil. *J Tongji Med Univ* 1993;13:193-8.

2784 Holodniy M, Koch J, Mistal M, et al. A double blind, randomized, placebo-controlled phase II study to assess the safety and efficacy of orally administered SP-303 for the symptomatic treatment of diarrhea in patients with AIDS. *Am J Gastroenterol* 1999;94:3267-73.

2785 Shaman Botanicals. The ethnobotanical story behind shamanbotanicals.com Sb normal stool formula. www.shamanbotanicals.com/traditionaluse.htm (Accessed 31 January 2000).

2786 Gabriel SE, Davenport SE, Steagall RJ, et al. A novel plant-derived inhibitor of cAMP-mediated fluid and chloride secretion. *Am J Physiol* 1999;276:G58-G63.

2787 Safrin S, McKinley G, McKeough M, et al. Treatment of acyclovir-unresponsive cutaneous herpes simplex virus infection with topically applied SP-303. *Antiviral Res* 1994;25:185-92.

2788 Orozco-Topete R, Sierra-Madero J, Cano-Dominguez C, et al. Safety and efficacy of Virend for topical treatment of genital and anal herpes simplex lesions in patients with AIDS. *Antiviral Res* 1997;35:91-103.

2789 King SR, Tempesta MS. From shaman to human clinical trials: the role of industry in ethnobotany, conservation and community reciprocity. *Ciba Found Symp* 1994;185:197-206.

2790 Barnard DL, Smee DF, Huffman JH, et al. Antiherpesvirus activity and mode of action of SP-303, a novel plant flavonoid. *Chemotherapy* 1993;39:203-11.

2791 Wyde PR, Ambrose MW, Meyerson LR, Gilbert BE. The antiviral activity of SP-303, a natural polyphenolic polymer, against respiratory syncytial and parainfluenza type 3 viruses in cotton rats. *Antiviral Res* 1993;20:145-54.

2792 Barnard DL, Huffman JH, Meyerson LR, Sidwell RW. Mode of inhibition of respiratory syncytial virus by a plant flavonoid, SP-303. *Chemotherapy* 1993;39:212-7.

2793 Sidwell RW, Huffman JH, Moscon BJ, Warren RP. Influenza virus-inhibitory effects of intraperitoneally and aerosol-administered SP-303, a plant flavonoid. *Chemother* 1994;40:42-50.

2794 Gilbert BE, Wyde PR, Wilson SZ, Meyerson LR. SP-303 small-particle aerosol treatment of influenza A virus infection in mice and respiratory syncytial virus infection in cotton rats. *Antiviral Res* 1993;21:37-45.

2795 Perdue GP, Blomster RN, Blake DA, Farnsworth NR. South American plants II: taspine isolation and anti-inflammatory activity. *J Pharm Sci* 1979;68:124-6.

2796 Vaisberg AJ, Milla M, Planas MC, et al. Taspine is the cicatrizant principle in Sangre de Grado extracted from Croton lechleri. *Planta Med* 1989;55:140-3.

2797 Pieters L, de Bruyne T, Claeys M, et al. Isolation of a dihydrobenzofuran lignan from South American dragon's blood (Croton spp.) as an inhibitor of cell proliferation. *J Nat Prod* 1993;56:899-906.

2798 Chen ZP, Cai Y, Phillipson JD. Studies on the anti-tumour, anti-bacterial, and wound-healing properties of dragon's blood. *Planta Med* 1994;60:541-5.

2799 Desmarchelier C, Witting Schaus F, Coussio J, Cicca G. Effects of Sangre de Drago from Croton lechleri Muell.-Arg. on the production of active oxygen radicals. *J Ethnopharmacol* 1997;58:103-8.

2800 Ashaninka Imports, Inc. Sangre de Drago. www.ashaninka.com/sangre.htm (Accessed 31 January 2000).

2801 Shaman Botanicals. Types of diarrhea and Shamanbotanicals.com Sb normal stool formula. www.shamanbotanicals.com/dcmaster.htm (Accessed 31 January 2000).

2802 Dr. Duke's Syllabus. Module 8: Amazonian (Iberoamerican) website: www.ars-grin.gov/duke/syllabus/module8.htm (Accessed 31 January 2000).

2803 Iowa State University. Medicinal Plants of Ecuador medicinal plants of the Quijos - Quichua shamen, Ecuador website: www.public.iastate.edu/~cbutter/ethnobot.htm (Accessed 31 January 2000).

2804 Raintree Nutrition. Sangre de Grado website: www.raintree.com/sangre.htm (Accessed 31 January 2000).

2805 USDA, ARS, National Genetic Resources Program. Germplasm Resources Information Network - (GRIN). Taxon: Croton lechleri mull. Arg website: www.ars-grin.gov/cgi-bin/npgs/html/tax_search.pl?croton+lechleri (Accessed 31 January 2000).

2806 Dicesare D, Dupont HL, Mathewson JJ, et al. A double-blind randomized, placebo-controlled study of SP-303 (Provir) in the symptomatic treatment of acute diarrhea among travelers to Mexico and Jamaica. Infectious Diseases Society of America Annual Meeting, 1998 (abstract).

2807 BioWorld Today. Shaman will sidestep FDA by selling product over internet website: http://www.bioworld.com/index.html (Accessed 6 January 2000).

2808 FDA. List of orphan designations and approvals website: http://www.fda.gov/orphan/DESIGNAT/list.htm (Accessed 6 February 2000).

2809 Henderson LM, Brewer GJ, Dressman JB, et al. Effect of intragastric pH on the absorption of oral zinc acetate and zinc oxide in young healthy volunteers. JPEN J Parenter Enteral Nutr 1995;19:393-7.

2810 Dr. Duke's Phytochemical and Ethnobotanical Databases. website: www.ars-grin.gov/cgi-bin/duke/ethnobot.pl (Accessed 7 February 2000).

2811 Schlager TA, Anderson S, Trudell J, Hendley JO. Effect of cranberry juice on bacteriuria in children with neurogenic bladder receiving intermittent catheterization. J Pediatr 1999;135:698-702.

2812 Sobota AE. Inhibition of bacterial adherence by cranberry juice: potential use for the treatment of urinary tract infections. J Urol 1984;131:1013-6.

2813 Howell AB, Vorsa N, Foo LY, et al. Inhibition of the Adherence of P-Fimbriated Escherichia coli to Uroepithelial-Cell Surfaces by Proanthocyanidin Extracts from Cranberries (letter). N Engl J Med 1998;339:1085-6.

2814 Ahuja S, Kaack B, Roberts J. Loss of fimbrial adhesion with the addition of Vaccinum macrocarpon to the growth medium of P-fimbriated Escherichia coli. J Urol 1998;159:559-62.

2815 Habash MB, Van der Mei HC, Busscher HJ, Reid G. The effect of water, ascorbic acid, and cranberry derived supplementation on human urine and uropathogen adhesion to silicone rubber. Can J Microbiol 1999;45:691-4.

2816 Weiss EI, Lev-Dor R, Kashamn Y, et al. Inhibiting interspecies coaggregation of plaque bacteria with a cranberry juice constituent. J Am Dent Assoc 1998;129:1719-23.

2817 Saltzman JR, Kemp JA, Golner BB, et al. Effect of hypochlorhydria due to omeprazole treatment or atrophic gastritis on protein-bound vitamin B12 absorption. J Am Coll Nutr 1994;13:584-91.

2818 USDA, ARS, National Genetic Resources Program. Germplasm Resources Information Network - (GRIN) online database website: www.ars-grin.gov/cgi-bin/npgs/html/taxon.pl?41030 (Accessed 7 February 2000).

2819 USDA, ARS, National Genetic Resources Program. Germplasm Resources Information Network - (GRIN).

Online Database website: www.ars-grin.gov/cgi-bin/npgs/html/taxon.pl?41047 (Accessed 7 February 2000).

2820 The Natural History of the Northwoods. Small cranberry vaccinium oxycoccus website: www.rook.org/earl/bwca/nature/shrubs/vacciniumoxy.html (Accessed 4 February 2000).

2821 Wisconsin State Cranberry Growers Association. A history of cranberry growing website: www.wiscran.org/history.html (Accessed 7 February 2000).

2822 www.healthlink.com.au/nat_lib/htm-data/htm-herb/bhp770.htm (Accessed 8 February 2000).

2823 Naveh Y, Schapira D, Ravel Y, et al. Zinc metabolism in rheumatoid arthritis: plasma and urinary zinc and relationship to disease activity. J Rheumatol 1997;24:643-6.

2824 Potocnik FC, van Rensburg SJ, Park C, et al. Zinc and platelet membrane microviscosity in Alzheimer's disease. The in vivo effect of zinc on platelet membranes and cognition. S Afr Med J 1997;87:1116-9.

2825 de Haan A, van Doorn JE, Westra HG. Effects of potassium plus magnesium aspartate on muscle metabolism and force development during short intensive static exercise. Int J Sports Med 1985;6:44-9.

2826 Golf SW, Bender S, Gruttner J. On the significance of magnesium in extreme physical stress. Cardiovasc Drugs Ther 1998;12:197-202.

2827 Golf SW, Happel O, Graef V, Seim KE. Plasma aldosterone, cortisol and electrolyte concentrations in physical exercise after magnesium supplementation. J Clin Chem Clin Biochem 1984;22:717-21.

2828 Hagan RD, Upton SJ, Duncan JJ, et al. Absence of effect of potassium-magnesium aspartate on physiologic responses to prolonged work in aerobically trained men. Int J Sports Med 1982;3:177-81.

2829 Maughan RJ, Sadler DJ. The effects of oral administration of salts of aspartic acid on the metabolic response to prolonged exhausting exercise in man. Int J Sports Med 1983;4:119-23.

2830 Weller E, Bachert P, Meinck HM, et al. Lack of effect of oral Mg-supplementation on Mg in serum, blood cells, and calf muscle. Med Sci Sports Exerc 1998;30:1584-91.

2900 Kuzminski AM, Del Giacco EJ, et al. Effective treatment of cobalamin deficiency with oral cobalamin. Blood 1998;92:1191-1198.

2901 Andres E, Kurtz JE, Perrin AE, et al. Oral cobalamin therapy for the treatment of patients with food-cobalamin malabsorption. Am J Med 2001;111:126-129.

2902 Lederle FA. Oral cobalamin for pernicious anemia. Medicine's best kept secret? JAMA 1991;265:94-95.

2903 Gunnes P, Rasmussen K. Haemodynamic effects of pharmacological doses of secretin in patients with impaired left ventricular function. Eur Heart J, 1986; 7(2): 146-9.

2904 Gunnes P, et al. Cardiovascular effects of secretin infusion in man. Scand J Clin Lab Invest 1983;43(7):637-42.

2905 Tulassay Z, et al. [Secretin versus cimetidine in the therapy of active bleeding from peptic gastroduodenal lesions. A prospective, randomized, double-blind, multicentric study]. [Article in German]. Wien Med Wochenschr, 1990; 140(13): 361-4.

2906 Wagner PK, Rothmund M. [Effect of cimetidine and synthetic secretin as treatment of acute upper gastrointestinal bleeding-a prospective alternate trial].

[Article in German]. *Z Gastroenterol*, 1980; 18(6): 337-41.

2908 Rothmund M, Wagner PK. [Effect of cimetidine and secretin on acute bleedings from gastroduodenal ulcers and erosions: a prospective study]. [Article in German]. *Dtsch Med Wochenschr*, 1982; 107(7): 245-8.

2909 Elia M. Oral or parenteral therapy for B12 deficiency. *Lancet* 1998;352:1721-1722.

2910 Andres E, Goichot B, Schlienger JL. Food cobalamin malabsorption: a usual cause of vitamin B12 deficiency. *Arch Intern Med* 2000;160:2061-2062.

2911 Verhaeverbeke I, Mets T, Mulkens K, Vandewoude M. Normalization of low vitamin B12 serum levels in older people by oral treatment. *J Am Geriatr Soc* 1997;45:124-125.

2912 Spilker G, et al. [Long-acting secretin for the prevention of stress ulcers in surgery]. [Article in French]. *Nouv Presse Med*, 1982; 11(4): 267-9.

2913 Theisinger W, Spilker G, Bader M . [Prevention of stress ulcers with synthetic depot secretin]. [Article in German]. *Med Klin,* 1981; 76(10): 291-3.

2915 Allen LH, Casterline J. Vitamin B-12 deficiency in elderly individuals: diagnosis and requirements. *Am J Clin Nutr* 1994;60:12-14

2916 Product information. Secretin. Ferring Pharmaceticals, Tarrytown, NY; 6/88.

2917 Horvath K, Stefatos G, Sokolski KN. Improved social and language skills after secretin administration. *J Assoc Acad Minor Phys* 1998;9(1):9-15.

2918 Tympner F, Rosch W. The treatment of chronic recurrent pancreatitis with depot secretin-a preliminary report. *Hepatogastroenterology*, 1986; 33(4): 159-62.

2919 Lindenbaum J, Rosenberg IH, Wilson PW, et al. Prevalence of cobalamin deficiency in the Framingham elderly population. *Am J Clin Nutr* 1994;60:2-11.

2920 Snider SR. Octacosanol in parkinsonism. *Ann Neurol*, 1984; 16(6): 723.

2921 Norris FH, Denys EH, Fallat RJ. Trial of octacosanol in amyotrophic lateral sclerosis. *Neurology* 1986; 36(9): 1263-4.

2922 Nutrimart, Octacosonol website. URL: www.nutrimart.com/Bulk/Description/octacosonol.htm (Accessed 18 July 1999).

2923 Mother Nature's Encyclopedia, Octacosonol website: URL: www.mothernature.com/ency/supp/octacosanol.asp (Accessed 18 July 1999).

2924 Kato S, et al. Octacosanol affects lipid metabolism in rats fed on a high-fat diet. *Br J Nutr*, 1995; 73(3): 433-41.

2925 Kabir Y, Kimura S. Distribution of radioactive octacosanol in response to exercise in rats. *Nahrung*, 1994; 38(4): 373-7.

2926 Beltz SD, Doering PL. Efficacy of nutritional supplements used by athletes. *Clin Pharm*, 1993;12(12):900-8.

2927 Canetti M, et al. A two-year study on the efficacy and tolerability of policosanol in patients with type II hyperlipoproteinaemia. *Int J Clin Pharmacol Res*, 1995; 15(4): 159-65.

2928 Pons P, et al. Effects of successive dose increases of policosanol on the lipid profile of patients with type II hypercholesterolaemia and tolerability to treatment. *Int J Clin Pharmacol Res*, 1994; 14(1): 27-33.

2929 Torres O, et al. Treatment of hypercholesterolemia in NIDDM with policosanol. *Diabetes Care*, 1995; 18(3): 393-7.

2930 Batista J, et al. Effect of policosanol on hyperlipidemia and coronary heart disease in middle-aged patients. A 14-month pilot study. *Int J Clin Pharmacol Ther*, 1996; 34(3): 134-7.

2931 Castano G, et al. A double-blind, placebo-controlled study of the effects of policosanol in patients with intermittent claudication. *Angiology*, 1999; 50(2): 123-30.

2933 Arruzazabala ML, et al. Effect of policosanol on platelet aggregation in type II hypercholesterolemic patients. *Int J Tissue React*, 1998; 20(4): 119-24.

2934 Menendez R, et al. Cholesterol-lowering effect of policosanol on rabbits with hypercholesterolaemia induced by a wheat starch-casein diet. *Br J Nutr*, 1997; 77(6): 923-32.

2935 Arruzazabala ML, et al. Effect of policosanol successive dose increases on platelet aggregation in healthy volunteers. *Pharmacol Res*, 1996; 34(5-6): 181-5.

2936 Carbajal D, et al. Effect of policosanol on platelet aggregation and serum levels of arachidonic acid metabolites in healthy volunteers. *Prostaglandins Leukot Essent Fatty Acids*, 1998; 58(1): 61-4.

2937 Arruzazabala ML, et al. Comparative study of policosanol, aspirin and the combination therapy policosanol-aspirin on platelet aggregation in healthy volunteers. *Pharmacol Res*, 1997; 36(4): 293-7.

2938 Valdes S, Arruzazabala ML, Fernandez L. Effect of policosanol on platelet aggregation in healthy volunteers. *Int J Clin Pharmacol Res*, 1996; 16(2-3): 67-72.

2939 Menendez R, et al. Policosanol inhibits cholesterol biosynthesis and enhances low density lipoprotein processing in cultured human fibroblasts. *Biol Res*, 1994; 27(3-4): 199-203.

2941 Stusser R, et al. Long-term therapy with policosanol improves treadmill exercise-ECG testing performance of coronary heart disease patients. *Int J Clin Pharmacol Ther*, 1998; 36(9): 469-73.

2942 GVI Sourcing Website: URL: www.gvisourcing.com/pharmaceuticals/ppg/specs.html (Accessed 16 July 1999).

2943 Castano G, et al. Efficacy and tolerability of policosanol in elderly patients with type II hypercholesterolemia: A 12-month study. *Curr Ther Res*, 1995; 56(8): 819-23.

2944 Castano G, et al. Effects of policosanol in hypertensive patients with type II hypercholesterolemia. *Curr Ther Res*, 1996; 57(9): 691-5.

2945 Mother Nature's Encyclopedia Website, Resveratrol. URL: www.mothernature.com/ency/supp/resveratrol.asp (Accessed 16 July 1999).

2946 Resveratrol in wine. Resveratrol Website. URL: www.resveratrol.com/lib7.html (Accessed 16 July 1999).

2947 PanoLife Products, Inc. Website: URL: www.pano.com/science.html (Accessed 16 July 1999).

2948 Jang M, et al. Cancer chemopreventive activity of resveratrol, a natural product derived from grapes. *Science*, 1997; 275(5297): 218-20.

2949 Pace-Asciak CR, Rounova O, Hahn SE, et al. Wines and grape juices as modulators of platelet aggregation in healthy human subjects. *Clin Chim Acta*, 1996;246(1-2):163-82.

2950 Bertelli AA, et al. Antiplatelet activity of cis-resveratrol. *Drugs Exp Clin Res*, 1996; 22(2): 61-3.

2951 Pace-Asciak CR, et al. The red wine phenolics trans-resveratrol and quercetin block human platelet aggregation and eicosanoid synthesis: implications for protection against coronary heart disease. *Clin Chim Acta,* 1995; 235(2): 207-19.

2952   Bertelli A, et al. Plasma and tissue resveratrol concentrations and pharmacological activity. *Drugs Exp Clin Res,* 1998; 24(3): 133-8.

2954   Chen CK, Pace-Asciak CR. Vasorelaxing activity of resveratrol and quercetin in isolated rat aorta. *Gen Pharmacol,* 1996; 27(2): 363-6.

2956   Tyler VE. Grape expectations: Compound in grapes may fight cancer. Purdue Website. URL: www.purdue.edu/UNS/Clips/clips.7.97/9706.Prevention.html. (Accessed 16 July 1999).

2957   Hewitt D. Resveratrol. Immortality Website. URL: www.immortality.org/resveratrol.html (Accessed 16 July 1999).

2958   Huang C, et al. Resveratrol suppresses cell transformation and induces apoptosis through a p53-dependent pathway. *Carcinogenesis,* 1999; 20(2): 237-42.

2959   Carbo N, et al. Resveratrol, a natural product present in wine, decreases tumour growth in a rat tumour model. *Biochem Biophys Res Commun,* 1999;254(3):739-43.

2960   Gehm BD, et al. Resveratrol, a polyphenolic compound found in grapes and wine, is an agonist for the estrogen receptor. *Proc Natl Acad Sci U S A,* 1997; 94(25): 14138-43.

2961   Bertelli AA, et al. Antiplatelet activity of synthetic and natural resveratrol in red wine. *Int J Tissue React,* 1995; 17(1): 1-3.

2962   Blackshear J, Ebener MK. Leeching, hirudin, and coagulation tests. *Ann Intern Med* 1994;121(2):151-2.

2963   Haycox CL, et al. Indications and complications of medicinal leech therapy. *J Am Acad Dermatol* 1995;33(6):1053-5.

2964   Fenollar F, Fournier PE, Legre R. Unusual case of Aeromonas sobria cellulitis associated with the use of leeches. *Eur J Clin Microbiol Infect Dis* 1999;18(1):72-3.

2965   Mackay DR, et al. Aeromonas species isolated from medicinal leeches. Ann Plast Surg 1999;42(3):275-9.

2966   Varghese MR, et al. Vibrio fluvialis wound infection associated with medicinal leech therapy. *Clin Infect Dis* 1996;22(4):709-10.

2967   de Chalain TM. Exploring the use of the medicinal leech: a clinical risk-benefit analysis. *J Reconstr Microsurg* 1996;12(3):165-72.

2968   Lineaweaver WC, et al. Aeromonas hydrophila infections following use of medicinal leeches in replantation and flap surgery. *Ann Plast Surg* 1992;29(3):238-44.

2969   Dejobert Y, et al. Contact dermatitis from topical leech extract. *Contact Dermatitis,* 1991; 24(5): 366-7.

2970   Lineaweaver WC. Aeromonas hydrophila infections following clinical use of medicinal leeches: a review of published cases. *Blood Coagul Fibrinolysis,* 1991; 2(1): 201-3.

2971   Concannon MJ, Puckett CL. Microsurgical replantation of an ear in a child without venous repair. *Plast Reconstr Surg,* 1998; 102(6): 2088-93; discussion 2094-6.

2972   Utley DS, Koch RJ, Goode RL. The failing flap in facial plastic and reconstructive surgery: role of the medicinal leech. *Laryngoscope,* 1998; 108(8 Pt 1): 1129-35.

2973   Bapat RD, et al. Leech therapy for complicated varicose veins. *Indian J Med Res,* 1998; 107: 281-4.

2974   Daane S, Zamora S, Rockwell WB. Clinical use of leeches in reconstructive surgery. *Am J Orthop,* 1997; 26(8): 528-32.

2975   de Chalain T, Cohen SR, Burstein FD. Successful use of leeches in the treatment of purpura fulminans. *Ann Plast Surg,* 1995; 35(3): 300-04; discussion 304-6.

2976   Smeets IM, Engelberts I. The use of leeches in a case of post-operative life-threatening macroglossia. *J Laryngol Otol,* 1995; 109(5): 442-4.

2977   Iafolla AK. Medicinal leeches in the postoperative care of bladder exstrophy. *J Perinatol,* 1995;15(2):135-8.

2978   Soucacos PN, et al. The use of medicinal leeches, Hirudo medicinalis, to restore venous circulation in trauma and reconstructive microsurgery. *Int Angiol,* 1994; 13(3): 251-8.

2979   Soucacos PN, et al. Successful treatment of venous congestion in free skin flaps using medical leeches. *Microsurgery* 1994;15(7):496-501.

2980   Bergua A, et al. [Unavoidable epistaxis in the nasal infestation of leeches]. [Article in Spanish]. *Acta Otorrinolaringol Esp,* 1993; 44(5): 391-3.

2981   Seleznev KG, et al. Use of the medicinal leech in the treatment of ear diseases. *ORL J Otorhinolaryngol Relat Spe*c, 1992; 54(1): 1-4.

2982   Solomon E. Leech - an unusual cause of (laryngo-tracheal) obstruction. *Ethiop Med J,* 1991; 29(3): 141-2.

2983   Wade JW, Brabham RF, Allen RJ. Medicinal leeches: once again at the forefront of medicine. *South Med J,* 1990; 83(10): 1168-73.

2984   el-Awad ME, Patil K. Haematemesis due to leech infestation. *Ann Trop Paediatr,* 1990;10(1):61-2.

2985   Isgar B, Turner AG. Large scrotal haematoma treated with medicinal leeches. *Br J Urol* 1989;64(5):549-50.

2986   Golz A, et al. [Epistaxis caused by leeches]. [Article in Hebrew] *Harefuah,* 1989; 117(5-6): 141-3.

2987   Prasad SB, Sinha MR. Vaginal bleeding due to leech. *Postgrad Med J,* 1983; 59(690):272.

2988   Hernandez M, Ramirez Gutierrez RE. [Internal hirudiniasis: vaginal bleeding resulting from leech bite]. [Article in Spanish] *Ginecol Obstet Mex* 1998;66:284-6.

2989   Leeches USA Website, Leeches. URL: www.accurate-assi-leeches.com/leeches/leeches2.html (Accessed 16 July 1999).

2990   Biopharm Website, Leeches. URL: www.biopharm-leeches.com/uses.htm (Accessed 16 July 1999).

2991   Mortenson BW, Dawson KH, Murakami C. Medicinal leeches used to salvage a traumatic nasal flap. *Br J Oral Maxillofac Surg* 1998;36(6):462-4.

2992   Nazar PS, Doroshenko BH. [The leech therapy of infectious myocarditis]. [Article in Ukrainian]. *Lik Sprava,* 1998;6(6):146-8.

2993   Rigbi M, Orevi M, Eldor A. Platelet aggregation and coagulation inhibitors in leech saliva and their roles in leech therapy. *Semin Thromb Hemost* 1996;22(3):273-8.

2994   Orevi M, et al. A potent inhibitor of platelet activating factor from the saliva of the leech Hirudo medicinalis. *Prostaglandins,* 1992; 43(5): 483-95.

2995   Wallis RB. Hirudins: from leeches to man. *Semin Thromb Hemost,* 1996; 22(2): 185-96.

2996   Munro R, Jones CP, Sawyer RT. Calin-a platelet adhesion inhibitor from the saliva of the medicinal leech. *Blood Coagul Fibrinolysis,* 1991; 2(1): 179-84.

2997   Baskova IP. Inhibition of plasma kallikrein. Kininase and kinin-like activities of preparations from the medicinal leeches. *Thromb Res,* 1992; 67(6): 721-30.

REFERENCES

2998 Rigbi M, et al. The saliva of the medicinal leech Hirudo medicinalis-II. Inhibition of platelet aggregation and of leukocyte activity and examination of reputed anaesthetic effects. *Comp Biochem Physiol C,* 1987; 88(1): 95-8.

3000 Higher Ideals Website URL: www.healthy-u.com/ 17895/promise.html (10 April 1999).

3001 Johnson, LW. Conjugated linoleic acids for body fat mass reduction. *Integrative Medicine Consult* 2001;3(3):17,21.

3002 Medquest Pharmacy Website URL: www.medquest-pharmacy.com/store /prodtemplate. asp?product_id=59 (10 April 1999).

3003 Resource Development Specialists Website URL: www.intellex.com/~gilbert/pregmeta.html (Accessed 10 April 1999).

3004 Sahelian R. Pregnenolone: Natureõs Feel Good Hormone Website URL: www.raysahelian.com/ pregnenolone.html (10 April 1999).

3005 George MS, et al. CSF neuroactive steroids in affective disorders: pregnenolone, progesterone, and DBI. *Biol Psych,* 1994; 35(10): 775-80.

3006 Wang M, et al. Relationship between symptom severity and steroid variation in women with premenstrual syndrome: study on serum pregnenolone, pregnenolone sulfate, 5 alpha-pregnane-3,20-dione and 3 alpha-hydroxy-5 alpha-pregnan-20-one. *J Clin Endocrinol Metab,* 1996; 81(3): 1076-82.

3007 Steiger A, et al. Neurosteroid pregnenolone induces sleep-EEG changes in man compatible with inverse agonistic GABAA-receptor modulation. *Brain Res* 1993; 615(2): 267-74.

3008 Devlin TM, ed. Textbook of Biochemistry With Clinical Correlations. third ed. New York: Wiley-Liss Inc., 1992.

3009 Wallach J. Nutritional help for diabetes website URL: www.costarr.com/eze.htm (Accessed 10 April 1999).

3010 Kombucha Power Products Website URL: www.kombuchapower.com/diabetes.htm (Accessed 10 April 1999).

3011 Klaassen CD, ed. Casarett and Doull's Toxicology: The Basic Science of Poisons. fifth ed. New York: McGraw-Hill, 1996.

3012 Harland BF, Harden-Williams BA. Is vanadium of human nutritional importance yet? *J Am Diet Assoc,* 1994; 94(8): 891-4.

3013 Malabu UH, et al. Effects of chronic vanadate administration in the STZ-induced diabetic rat. *Diabetes,* 1994; 43: 9-15.

3014 Bishayee A, et al. Vanadium mediated chemoprotection against chemical hepatocarcinogenesis in rats: haematological and histological characteristics. *Eur J Cancer Prev,* 1997; 6(1): 58-70.

3016 Chakraborty A, Chatterjee M. Enhanced erythropoietin and suppression of gamma-glutamyl-transpeptidase (GGT) activity in murine lymphoma following administration of vanadium. *Neoplasma,* 1994; 41(5): 291-6.

3017 Domingo JL, et al. Oral vanadate and Tiron in treatment of diabetes mellitus in rats: improvement of glucose homeostasis and negative side effects. *Vet Human Toxicol,* 1993; 35(6): 495-500.

3018 Oster MH, et al. Vanadium treatment of diabetic Sprague-Dawley rats results in tissue vanadium accumulation and pro-oxidant effects. *Toxicology,* 1993; 83(1-3): 115-30.

3019 Stern A, et al. Vanadium as a modulator of cellular regulatory cascades and oncogene expression. *Biochem Cell Biol* 1993;71(3-4):103-12.

3020 Sitprija V, et al. Metabolic problems in northeastern Thailand: possible role of vanadium. *Mineral Electrolyte Metab,* 1998; 19(1): 51-6.

3021 Domingo JL, et al. Oral vanadium administration to streptozocin-diabetic rats has marked negative side-effects which are independent of the form of vanadium used. *Toxicology,* 1991; 66(3): 279-87.

3022 Kastrup EK. Drug Facts and Comparisons. 1998 ed. St. Louis, MO: Facts and Comparisons, 1998.

3023 Lacy C, et al. Drug Information Handbook. fifth ed. Hudson, OH: Lexi-Comp Inc., 1997.

3024 Hathcock JN, Troendle GJ. Oral cobalamin for treatment of pernicious anemia? *JAMA* 1991;265:96-97.

3025 Arai Y, Watanabe S, Kimira M, et al. Dietary intake of flavonols, flavones and isoflavones by Japanese women and the inverse correlation between quercetin intake and plasma LDL cholesterol concentration. *J Nutr* 2000;130:2243-50.

3026 Margolin KA, Green MR. Polymicrobial enteric septicemia from coffee enemas. *West J Med* 1984;140:460.

3027 BioSynergy Health Alternatives Website URL: www.biosynergy.com/b1.htm (Accessed 26 April 1999).

3028 WellBeings Website URL: www.americahealth.com/ B1.html (Accessed 26 April 1999).

3029 SupraHealth Inc. Website URL: www.suprahealth.com/ vit-b1.htm (Accessed 26 April 1999).

3030 Fresh Samantha Inc. Website URL: www.freshsamantha.com/vitamin_b1.htm (Accessed 26 April 1999).

3031 BioSynergy Health Alternatives Website URL: www.biosynergy.com/b2.htm (Accessed 26 April 1999).

3032 SupraHealth Inc. Website URL: www.suprahealth.com/ vit-b2.htm (Accessed 26 April 1999).

3033 WellBeings Website URL: www.americahealth.com/ B2.html (Accessed 26 April 1999).

3034 Vitamins Plus Website URL: www.vitaminsplus.com/ library/vitamins/vitaminb2.htm#BENEFITS (Accessed 26 April 1999).

3035 Cybervitamins USA Website URL: www.cybervitamins.com/niacin.htm (Accessed 3 May 1999).

3036 SupraHealth Inc. Website URL: www.suprahealth.com/ vit-b3.htm (Accessed 3 May 1999).

3037 Life Extension Foundation Website URL lef.org/ prod_desc/item412.html (Accessed 3 May 1999).

3038 WellBeings Website URL: www.americahealth.com/ B6.html (Accessed 9 May 1999).

3039 BioSynergy Health Alternatves Website URL: www.biosynergy.com/b6.htm (Accessed 9 May 1999).

3040 Life Extension Foundation Website URL: lef.org/ prod_desc/item417.html (Accessed 9 May 1999).

3041 Beers MH, Berkow R. The Merck Manual of Diagnosis and Therapy. 17th ed. West Point, PA: Merck and Co., Inc., 1999.

3042 Levine M, et al. Criteria and recommendations for vitamin C intake. *JAMA* 1999;281:1415-23.

3043 Monarch-One Website URL: www.monarch-one.com/ reviva.html (Accessed 13 May 1999).

3044 Enlightened Associates Website URL: enlightassoc.com/ antioxidants.html (Accessed 13 May 1999).

3045 Haas EM. Staying healthy with nutrition: vitamin C.

HealthWorld Online Website. URL: www.healthy.net/library/books/haas/vitamins/cvit.htm (Accessed 13 May 1999).

3046 Hansten PD, Horn JR. Drug Interactions Analysis and Management. Vancouver, WA: Applied Therapeutics Inc., 1997 and updates.

3047 Mayer EL, Jacobsen DW, Robinson K. Homocysteine and coronary atherosclerosis. *J Am Coll Cardiol* 1996;27:517-27.

3048 Robinson K, et al. Low circulating folate and vitamin B6 concentrations: Risk factors for stroke, peripheral vascular disease, and coronary artery disease. *Circulation* 1998;97:437-43.

3049 Omenn GS, Beresford SAA, Motulsky AG. Preventing coronary heart disease: B vitamins and homocysteine. *Circulation* 1998;97:421-4.

3050 Rimm EB, et al. Folate and vitamin B6 from diet and supplements in relation to risk of coronary heart disease among women. *JAMA* 1998;279:359-64.

3051 Leonard A, Gerber GB. Mutagenicity, carcinogenicity and teratogenicity of vanadium Compounds. *Mutat Res* 1994;317(1):81-8.

3052 Fawcett JP, et al. Oral vanadyl sulphate does not affect blood cells, viscosity or biochemistry in humans. *Pharmacol Toxicol,* 1997; 80(4): 202-6.

3053 Fawcett JP, et al. The effect of oral vanadyl sulfate on body composition and performance in weight-training athletes. *Int J Sport Nutr,* 1996; 6(4): 382-90.

3054 Funakoshi T, et al. Anticoagulant action of vanadate. *Chem Pharmaceut Bull,* 1992; 40(1): 174-6.

3055 Halberstam M, et al. Oral vanadyl sulfate improves insulin sensitivity in NIDDM but not in obese nondiabetic subjects. *Diabetes,* 1996; 45(5): 659-66.

3056 Cohen N, et al. Oral vanadyl sulfate improves hepatic and peripheral insulin sensitivity in patients with non-insulin-dependent diabetes mellitus. *J Clin Invest,* 1995; 95: 2501-9.

3057 Boden G, et al. Effects of vanadyl sulfate on carbohydrate and lipid metabolism in patients with non-insulin-dependent diabetes mellitus. *Metabolism,* 1996; 45(9): 1130-5.

3058 KCWeb Website URL: www.kcweb.com/herb/vit_d.htm (Accessed 30 May 1999).

3059 Smart Basics Inc Website URL: www.smartbasic.com/glos.vitamins/vit.d.glos.html (Accessed 30 May 1999).

3060 Quest Vitamins Website URL: www.questvitmains.co.uk/vitb.htm (Accessed 30 May 1999).

3061 Herbs 4 Us Website URL: www.herbs4us.com/vitaminb.htm (Accessed 30 May 1999).

3062 Smart Basics Inc. Website URL: www.smartbasic.com/glos.vitamins/vit.a.glos.html (Accessed 10 June 1999).

3063 Wells International Derma-E Natural Skin Care Website URL: www.derma-e/com/vitamina.html (Accessed 10 June 1999).

3064 SupraHealth Inc. Website URL: www.suprahealth.com/vit-a.htm (Accessed 10 June 1999).

3065 WellBeings Website URL: www.americahealth.com/A.html (Accessed 10 June 1999).

3066 FDA Talk Paper: Vitamin A and birth defects (T95-56). Food and Drug Administration, U.S.Department of Health and Human Services, Rockville, MD. 6 October 1995.

3067 Life Plus Website URL: enlightassoc.com/antioxidants.html (Accessed 20 June 1999).

3068 HerbsNow Website URL: www.herbsnow.com/vitamins.htm (Accessed 20 June 1999).

3069 Nature's Wonders Website URL: www.natureswonders.com/dermalk.html (Accessed 21 June 1999).

3070 Miner JL, Cederberg CA, Nielsen MK, et al. Conjugated linoleic acid (CLA), body fat, and apoptosis. *Obes Res* 2001;9:129-134.

3072 Tatro DS, ed. Drug Interactions Facts. Facts and Comparisons Inc., St.Louis, MO. 1999.

3073 Frank J, Weiser H, Biesalski HK. Interaction of vitamins E and K: effect of high dietary vitamin E on phylloquinone activity in chicks. *Int J Vit Nutr Res* 1997;67(4):242-7.

3074 Helson L. The effect of intravenous vitamin E and menadiol sodium diphosphate on vitamin K dependent clotting factors. *Thromb Res* 1984;35(1):11-8.

3075 Netrition Website URL: www.netrition.com/enada_page.html (Accessed 21 June 1999).

3076 Renascent Systems Inc. Website URL: www.nadh.com/index.html (Accessed 21 June 1999).

3077 The Healing Network Website URL: www.thehealingnetwork.com/nadh.htm (Accessed 21 June 1999).

3078 Hardman JG, Limbird LE, Eds. Goodman and Gilman's The Pharmacological Basis of Therapeutics. 9th ed. New York, NY:McGraw-Hill, 1996.

3079 Totally Natural Website URL: www.quickresults.com.au/foodsupps.b5.htm (Accessed 29 June 1999).

3080 Herbal Hope Website URL: www.herbalhope.com/ing/vitamin_b5.html (Accessed 29 June 1999).

3081 Sequential Healing Health Services Website URL: www.sequentialhealing.com/vit-min-nutrients/vit-b5.html (Accessed 29 June 1999).

3082 Budavari S, ed. The Merck Index. 12th ed. Whitehouse Station, NJ: Merck & Co., Inc. , 1996.

3083 Bushehri N, Jarrell ST, Lieberman S, et al. Oral reduced B-nicotinamide adenine dinucleotide (NADH) affects blood pressure, lipid peroxidation, and lipid profile in hypertensive rats (SHR). *Geriatr Nephrol Urol,* 1998; 8(2):95-100.

3084 Forsyth LM, Preuss HG, MacDowell AL, et al. Therapeutic effects of oral NADH on the symptoms of patients with chronic fatigue syndrome. *Ann All Asthma Immunol,* 1999; 82(2):185-91.

3085 Swerdlow RH. Is NADH effective in the treatment of Parkinson's disease?. *Drugs Aging,* 1998; 13(4):263-8.

3086 Kuhn W, Muller T, Winkel R, et al. Parenteral application of NADH in Parkinson's disease: clinical improvement partially due to stimulation of endogenous levodopa biosynthesis. *J Neural Transmiss (Budapest),* 1996; 103(10):1187-93.

3087 Birkmayer JG. Coenzyme nicotinamide adenine dinucleotide: new therapeutic approach for improving dementia of the Alzheimer type. *Ann Clin Lab Sci,* 1996; 26(1):1-9.

3088 Vrecko K, Birkmayer JG, Krainz J. Stimulation of dopamine biosynthesis in cultured PC 12 phaeochromocytoma cells by the coenzyme nicotinamide adeninedinucleotide (NADH). *J Neural Transmiss (Parkinsons Disease & Dementia Section),* 1993; 5(2):147-56.

3089 Birkmayer JG, Vrecko C, Volc D, Birkmayer W. Nicotinamide adenine dinucleotide (NADH) - a new therapeutic approach to Parkinson's disease. Comparison of oral and parenteral application. *Acta Neurol Scand Suppl,* 1993; 146:32-5.

3090 Dizdar N, Kagedal B, Lindvall B. Treatment of Parkinson's disease with NADH. *Acta Neurol Scand,* 1994; 90(5):345-7.

3091 Vrecko K, Storga D, Birkmayer JG, et al. NADH stimulates endogenous dopamine biosynthesis by enhancing the recycling of tetrahydrobiopterin in rat phaeochromocytoma cells. *Biochim Biophys Acta,* 1997; 1361(1):59-65.

3092 Fauci AS, Braunwald E, Isselbacher KJ, et al. Harrison's Principles of Internal Medicine, 14th ed. New York, NY: McGraw-Hill, 1998.

3093 Wyatt KM, Dimmock PW, Jones PW, O'Brien PM. Efficacy of vitamin B6 in the treatment of premenstrual syndrome. *BMJ* 1999;318:1375-81.

3094 Yates AA, Schlicker SA, Suitor CW. Dietary reference intakes: The new basis for recommendations for calcium and related nutrients, B vitamins, and choline. *J Am Diet Assoc* 1998;98:699-706.

3095 Song Z, Johansen HK, Faber V, et al. Ginseng treatment reduces bacterial load and lung pathology in chronic Pseudomonas aeruginosa pneumonia in rats. *Antimicrob Agents Chemother* 1997;41(5):961-4.

3096 Song Z, Kharazmi A, Wu H, et al. Effects of Ginseng treatment on neutrophil chemiluminescence and immunoglobulin G subclasses in a rat model of chronic Pseudomonas aeruginosa pneumonia. *Clin Diagn Lab Immunol* 1998;5(6):882-7.

3097 Simon JA, Hudes ES. Relationship of ascorbic acid to blood lead levels. *JAMA* 1999;281(24):2289-93.

3098 Dawson EB, Evans DR, Harris WA, et al. The effect of ascorbic acid supplementation on the blood lead levels of smokers. *J Am Coll Nutr* 1999;18(2):166-70.

3099 Cheng Y, Willett WC, Schwartz J, et al. Relation of nutrition to bone lead and blood lead levels in middle-aged to elderly men. *The Normative Aging Study. Am J Epidemiol* 1998;147(12):1162-74.

3100 Escarpa A, Gonzalez MC. High-performance liquid chromatography with diode-array detection for the determination of phenolic compounds in peel and pulp from different apple varieties. *J Chromatogr A* 1998;823(1-2):331-7.

3101 Cruz T, Galvez J, Ocete MA, et al. Oral administration of rutoside can ameliorate inflammatory bowel disease in rats. *Life Sci* 1998;62(7):687-95.

3102 Galvez J, Cruz T, Crespo E, et al. Rutoside as mucosal protective in acetic acid-induced rat colitis. *Planta Med* 1997;63(5):409-14.

3103 Kostyuk VA, Potapovich AI, Speransky SD, Maslova GT. Protective effect of natural flavonoids on rat peritoneal macrophages injury caused by asbestos fibers. *Free Radical Biol Med* 1996;21(4):487-93.

3104 Webster RP, Gawde MD, Bhattacharya RK. Protective effect of rutin, a flavonol glycoside, on the carcinogen-induced DNA damage and repair enzymes in rats. *Cancer Lett,* 1996;109(1-2):185-91.

3105 Schmitt A, Salvayre R, Delchambre J, Negre-Salvayre A. Prevention by alpha-tocopherol and rutin of glutathione and ATP depletion induced by oxidized LDL in cultured endothelial cells. *Br J Pharmacol* 1995;116(3):1985-90.

3106 Rueff J, Gaspar J, Laires A. Structural requirements for mutagenicity of flavonoids upon nitrosation. A structure-activity study. *Mutagenesis* 1995;10(4):325-8.

3107 Perez Guerrero C, Martin MJ, Marhuenda E. Prevention by rutin of gastric lesions induced by ethanol in rats: role of endogenous prostaglandins. *Gen Pharmacol* 1994;25(3):575-80.

3108 Deschner EE, Ruperto J, Wong G, Newmark HL. Quercetin and rutin as inhibitors of azoxymethanol-induced colonic neoplasia. *Carcinogenesis* 1991;12(7):1193-6.

3109 Lewis R, Wake G, Court G, et al. Non-ginsenoside nicotinic activity in ginseng species. *Phytother Res* 1999;13;59-64.

3110 Health Quest website URL www.healthquest4u.com/jcp/blindstudy.htm (Accessed 2 September 1999).

3111 Barnett ML, Kremer JM, St.Clair W, et al. Treatment of rheumatoid arthritis with oral type II collagen. *Arth Rheum* 1998;41(2):290-7.

3112 Barnett ML, Combitchi D, Trentham DE. A pilot trial of oral type II collagen in the treatment of juvenile rheumatoid arthritis. *Arth Rheum,* 1996; 39(4):623-8.

3113 Ghoneum M. Anti-HIV activity in vitro of MGN-3, an activated arabinoxylane from rice bran. *Biochem Biophys Res Commun* 1998;243(1):25-9.

3114 The Healing Network website URL: www.anaturalchoice.com/is.htm (Accessed 22 September 1999).

3115 CompassioNet Online website URL www.compassionet.com/mgn3.htm (Accessed 22 September 1999).

3116 Ghoneum M, Namatalla G, Kim C. Effect of MGN-3 on human natural killer cell activity and interferon-gamma synthesis in vitro. Abstract. Federation of American Societies for *Experimental Biology Journal,* 1996;10(6):26-32.

3117 Ghoneum M, Jewett A. Synergistic effect of modified arabinoxylane (MGN-3) and low dose of recombinant IL-2 on human NK cell activity and TNF production. Abstract. American Acadamy of Anti-Aging Medicine Educational Conference, August 15-6, 1998.

3118 Ghoneum M. Enhancement of human natural killer cell activity by modified arabinoxylane from rice bran (MGN-3). *Int J Immunotherapy,* 1998;14(2):89-99.

3119 Ghoneum M, Namatalla G. NK immunomodulatory function in 27 cancer patients by MGN-3, a modified arabinoxylane from rice bran. Abstract. 87th Annual Meeting of the American Association for Cancer Research. April 20-4, 1996.

3120 Ghoneum M. Immunomodulatory and anti-cancer properties of MGN-3, a modified xylose from rice bran, in 5 patients with breast cancer. Abstract. American Association for Cancer Research Special Conference. November 5-8, 1995.

3121 Belogortseva NI, Yoon JY, Kim KH. Inhibition of Helicobacter pylori hemagglutination by polysaccharide fractions from roots of Panax ginseng. *Planta Med* 2000;66:217-20.

3122 Shin HR, Kim JY, Yun TK, et al. The cancer-preventive potential of Panax ginseng: a review of human and experimental evidence. *Cancer Causes Control* 2000;11:565-76.

3123 Varis T, Kivisto KT, Neuvonen PJ. Grapefruit juice can increase the plasma concentration of methylprednisolone. *Eur J Clin Pharmacol* 2000;56:489-93.

3125 Kalden JR, Sieper J. Oral collagen in the treatment of rheumatoid arthritis [editorial]. *Arth Rheum,*

3125 1998;41(2):191-4.

3126 Trentham DE. Oral tolerization as a treatment of rheumatoid arthritis. *Rheum Dis Clin North Am,* 1998; 24(3):525-36.

3127 Mullins RJ, Richards C, Walker T. Allergic reactions to oral, surgical and topical bovine collagen. Anaphylactic risk for surgeons. *Aust N Z J Ophthalmol,* 1996; 24(3):257-60.

3128 AutoImmune Inc. announces phase III trial results for Colloral. URL http://www.autoimmune.com/clinic/coll.html (Accessed 24 October 1999).

3129 Wang XD, Zhang JM, Yang HH, Hu GY. Modulation of NMDA receptor by huperzine A in rat cerebral cortex. *Chung Kuo Yao Li Hsueh Pao,* 1999;20(1):31-5.

3130 DHM Inc. website. URL http://www.huperzine.net (Accessed 26 October 1999).

3131 Skolnick AA. Old Chinese herbal medicine used for fever yields possible new Alzheimer Disease therapy. *JAMA* 1997;277:776.

3132 Wang H, Tang XC. Anticholinesterase effects of huperzine A, E2020, and tacrine in rats. *Chung Kuo Yao Li Hsueh Pao,* 1998;19(1):27-30.

3133 Xiong ZQ, Cheng DH, Tang XC. Effects of huperzine A on nucleus basalis magnocellularis lesion-induced spatial working memory deficit. *Chung Kuo Yao Li Hsueh Pao,* 1998;19(2):128-32.

3134 Ye JW, Cai JX, Wang LM, Tang XC. Improving effects of huperzine A on spatial working memory in aged monkeys and young adult monkeys with experimental cognitive impairment. *J Pharmacol Exp Ther,* 1999;288(2):814-9.

3135 Wang T, Tang XC. Reversal of scopolamine-induced deficits in radial maze performance by (-)-huperzine A: comparison with E2020 and tacrine. *Eur J Pharmacol,* 1998;349(2-3):137-42.

3136 Cheng DH, Tang XC. Comparative studies of huperzine A, E2020, and tacrine on behavior and cholinesterase activities. *Pharmacol Biochem Behav,* 1998;60(2):377-86.

3137 Lallement G, Veyret J, Masqueliez C, et al. Efficacy of huperzine in preventing soman-induced seizures, neuropathological changes and lethality. *Fundam Clin Pharmacol,* 1997;11(5):387-94.

3138 Xu SS, Gao ZX, Weng Z, et al. Efficacy of tablet huperzine-A on memory, cognition, and behavior in Alzheimer's disease. *Zhongguo Yao Li Xue Bao* 1995;16(5):391-5.

3139 Grunwald J, Raveh L, Doctor BP, Ashani Y. Huperzine A as a pretreatment candidate drug against nerve agent toxicity. *Life Sci,* 1994;54(14):991-7.

3140 Zhang RW, Tang XC, Han YY, et al. [Drug evaluation of huperzine A in the treatment of senile memory disorders]. [Article in Chinese] *Chung Kuo Yao Li Hsueh Pao,* 1991;12(3):250-2.

3141 Tang XC, De Sarno P, Sugaya K, Giacobini E. Effect of huperzine A, a new cholinesterase inhibitor, on the central cholinergic system of the rat. *J Neurosci Res,* 1989;24(2):276-85.

3142 Safety Briefs, ISMP Medication Safety Alert, vol.4, #4. Institute for Safe Medication Practices, Warminster, PA. February 24, 1999.

3143 Potential new East-West combination drug for Alzheimer's shows promise. Reuters Health, URL: www.reutershealth.com/frame_eline.html (Accessed 2 November 1999).

3144 A Modern Herbal website. URL www.botanical.com/botanical/mgmh/m/mandra10.html (Accessed 9 November 1999).

3145 Health 4 Free web site. URL http://health4free.com/Product%20List/Bupleurum.htm (Accessed 26 October 1999).

3146 Yu D, et al. Treatment of primary thrombocytopenic purpura by modified minor decoction of bupleurum. *Journal of Traditional Chinese Medicine,* 1995;15(2):96-8. URL http://www.itppeople.com/articles/Bupleurum.htm (Acceessed 26 October 1999).

3147 Miller L, Murray WJ, eds. Herbal Medicinals: A Clinician's Guide. Pharmaceutical Products Press, Binghamton, NY, 1998.

3148 Bupleurum falcatum Bitter & cool. The Australian Naturopath Network web site. URL: www.comcen.com.au/~sburgess/herbs/Monographs/bupleuru.htm (Accessed 13 November 1999).

3149 Sequential Healing Health Services web site. URL http://www.sequentialhealing.com/herbs/bupleurum.html (Accessed 13 November 1999).

3150 PanoLife Products Inc. website. URL http://www.pano.com/huperzia.html (Accessed 26 October 1999).

3151 Jing H, Jiang Y, Luo S. [Chemical constituents of the roots of Bupleurum longicaule Wall. ex DC. var. franchetii de Boiss and B. chaishoui Shan et Sheh]. [Article in Chinese]. *Chung Kuo Chung Yao Tsa Chih,* 1996;21(12):739-41,762.

3152 Yen MH, Lin CC, Chuang CH, Liu SY. Evaluation of root quality of Bupleurum species by TLC scanner and the liver protective effects of xiao-chai-hu-tang prepared using three different Bupleurum species. *J Ethnopharmacol,* 1991;34(2-3):155-65.

3153 Blankson H, Stakkestad JA, Fagertun H, et al. Conjugated linoleic acid reduces body fat mass in overweight and obese humans. *J Nutr* 2000;130:2943-2948.

3154 Yamada H. [Structure and pharmacological activity of pectic polysaccharides from the roots of Bupleurum falcatum L]. [Article in Japanese] *Nippon Yakurigaku Zasshi,* 1995;106(3):229-37.

3155 Matsumoto T, Moriguchi R, Yamada H. Role of polymorphonuclear leucocytes and oxygen-derived free radicals in the formation of gastric lesions induced by HCl/ethanol, and a possible mechanism of protection by anti-ulcer polysaccharide. *J Pharm Pharmacol,* 1993;45(6):535-9.

3156 Hattori T, Ito M, Suzuki Y. [Studies on antinephritic effects of plant components in rats (1). Effects of saikosaponins original-type anti-GBM nephritis in rats and its mechanisms]. [Article in Japanese] *Nippon Yakurigaku Zasshi,* 1991;97(1):13-21.

3157 Ahn BZ, Yoon YD, Lee YH, et al. Inhibitory effect of bupleuri radix saponins on adhesion of some solid tumor cells and relation to hemolytic action: screening of 232 herbal drugs for anti-cell adhesion. *Planta Med,* 1998;64(3):220-4.

3158 Elias SL, Innis SM. Infant plasma trans, n-6, and n-3 fatty acids and conjugated linoleic acids are related to maternal plasma fatty acids, length of gestation, and birth weight and length. *Am J Clin Nutr* 2001;73:807-814.

3159 Chang WC, Hsu FL. Inhibition of platelet activation and endothelial cell injury by flavan-3-ol and saikosaponin compounds. *Prostaglandins Leukot Essent Fatty Acids*, 1991;44(1):51-6.

3160 Kato M, Pu MY, Isobe K, et al. Characterization of the immunoregulatory action of saikosaponin-d. *Cell Immunol*, 1994;159(1):15-25.

3161 Ushio Y, Oda Y, Abe H. Effect of saikosaponin on the immune responses in mice. *Int J Immunopharmacol*, 1991;13(5):501-8.

3162 Hoyos AB. Reduced incidence of necrotizing enterocolitis associated with enteral administration of Lactobacillus acidophilus and Bifidobacterium infantis to neonates in an intensive care unit. *Int J Infect Dis* 1999;3:197-202.

3163 Chiu HF, Lin CC, Yen MH, et al. Pharmacological and pathological studies on hepatic protective crude drugs from Taiwan (V): The effects of Bombax malabarica and Scutellaria rivularis. *Am J Chin Med*, 1992;20(3-4):257-64.

3164 Izumi S, Ohno N, Kawakita T, et al. Wide range of molecular weight distribution of mitogenic substance(s) in the hot water extract of a Chinese herbal medicine, Bupleurum chinense. *Biol Pharm Bull*, 1997;20(7):759-64.

3165 Guinea MC, Parellada J, Lacaille-Dubois MA, Wagner H. Biologically active triterpene saponins from Bupleurum fruticosum. *Planta Med*, 1994;60(2):163-7.

3166 Martin S, Padilla E, Ocete MA, et al. Anti-inflammatory activity of the essential oil of Bupleurum fruticescens. *Planta Med*, 1993;59(6):533-6.

3167 Lorente I, Ocete MA, Zarzuelo A, et al. Bioactivity of the essential oil of Bupleurum fruticosum. *J Nat Prod*, 1989;52(2):267-72.

3168 Bermejo Benito P, Abad Martinez MJ, Silvan Sen AM, et al. In vivo and in vitro antiinflammatory activity of saikosaponins. *Life Sci*, 1998;63(13):1147-56.

3169 Phuapradit P, Varavithya W, Vathanophas K, et al. Reduction of rotavirus infection in children receiving bifidobacteria-supplemented formula. *J Med Assoc Thai* 1999;82:S43-S48.

3170 Estevez-Braun A, Estevez-Reyes R, Moujir LM, et al. Antibiotic activity and absolute configuation of 8S-heptadeca-2(Z),9(Z)-diene-4,6-diyne-1,8-diol from Bupleurum salicifolium. *J Nat Prod*, 1994;57(8):1178-82.

3171 Zhang SL. [Therapeutic effects of huperzine A on the aged with memory impairment]. [Article in Chinese] *New Drugs and Clinical Remedies* 1986;5(5):260-2.

3172 Cheng YS, Lu CZ, Ying ZL, et al. [128 cases of myasthenia gravis treated with huperzine A]. [Article in Chinese] *New Drugs and Clinical Remedies* 1986;5(4):197-9.

3173 AIDS Treatment News Archive. URL: 4.17.177.49/immunet/atn.nsf/page/a-049-01 (Accessed 25 November 1999).

3174 Strictly Medicinal Herb Seeds website. URL: www.budget.net/~herbseed/sweetann.htm (Accessed 25 November 1999).

3175 Herb facts of the month. Herbal Connections website. URL: www.herbworld.com/snst/arc8-8.htm (Accessed 25 November 1999).

3176 HolisticOnLine website. URL: holisticonline.com/Herbal-Med/_scripts/getHerb_Dir.idc?Herb_Names=365 (Accessed 25 November 1999).

3177 Dharmananda S. PCP prophylaxis with drugs and herbs. Institute for Traditional Medicine Online. URL:

www.rdi.gpo.or.th/NetZine/V3N42/pcp.htm (Accessed 25 November 1999).

3178 Artemether/Artenam website. URL: www.arenco.be/ (Accessed 25 November 1999).

3179 Herbal Review, Sequential Healing Health Services website. URL: www.sequentialhealing.com/herbs/sweet-Annie.html (Accessed 25 November 1999).

3180 Pittler MH, Ernst E. Artemether for severe malaria: a meta-analysis of randomized clinical trials. *Clin Infect Dis* 1999;28(3):597-601.

3181 van Agtmael MA, Eggelte TA, van Boxtel CJ. Artemisinin drugs in the treatment of malaria: from medicinal herb to registered medication. *Trends Pharmacol Sci* 1999;20(5):199-205.

3182 Moneton P, Ducret JP. Positioning, labeling and control of medical information: artesunate strategy and Arsumax development story. *Med Trop (Mars)* 1998;58(3 Suppl):70-2.

3183 Zheng GQ. Cytotoxic terpenoids and flavonoids from Artemisia annua. *Planta Med* 1994;60(1):54-7.

3184 Huang L, Liu JF, Liu LX, et al. [Antipyretic and anti-inflammatory effects of Artemisia annua L]. [Article in Chinese]. *Chung Kuo Chung Yao Tsa Chih* 1993;18(1):44-48,63-4.

3185 Wan YD, Zang QZ, Wang JS. [Studies on the antimalarial action of gelatin capsule of Artemisia annua]. [Article in Chinese]. *Chung Kuo Chi Sheng Chung Hsueh Yu Chi Sheng Chung Ping Tsa Chih* 1992;10(4):290-4.

3186 Swedish Herbal Institute website. URL http://www.adaptogen.com/shi_np2.html (Accessed 22 November 1999).

3187 PlanetHerbs Online website. URL http://www.planetherbs.com/articles/rhodiola%20rosea.htm (Accessed 22 November 1999).

3188 Mother Nature's General Store, Inc. website. URL http://www.herbalphen.com/rhod.htm (Accessed 22 November 1999).

3189 Nutri-Mart Cyberstore. URL http://www.nutrimart.com/Bulk/Description/rhodiola_rosea.htm (Accessed 22 November 1999).

3190 Salikhova RA, Aleksandrova IV, Mazurik VK, et al. [Effect of Rhodiola rosea on the yield of mutation alterations and DNA repair in bone marrow cells]. [Article in Russian]. *Patol Fiziol Eksp Ter* 1997;(4):22-4.

3191 Lishmanov IB, Naumova AV, Afanas'ev SA, Maslov LN. [Contribution of the opioid system to realization of inotropic effects of Rhodiola rosea extracts in ischemic and reperfusion heart damage in vitro]. [Article in Russian]. *Eksp Klin Farmakol* 1997;60(3):34-6.

3192 Maimeskulova LA, Maslov LN, Lishmanov IB, Krasnov EA. [The participation of the mu-, delta- and kappa-opioid receptors in the realization of the anti-arrhythmia effect of Rhodiola rosea]. [Article in Russian]. *Eksp Klin Farmakol* 1997;60(1):38-9.

3193 Maslova LV, Kondrat'ev BI, Maslov LN, Lishmanov IB. [The cardioprotective and antiadrenergic activity of an extract of Rhodiola rosea in stress]. [Article in Russian]. *Eksp Klin Farmakol* 1994;57(6):61-3.

3194 Bocharova OA, Matveev BP, Baryshnikov AI, et al. [The effect of a Rhodiola rosea extract on the incidence of recurrences of a superficial bladder cancer]. [Article in Russian]. *Urol Nefrol (Mosk)* 1995;(2):46-7.

3195 Lishmanov IB, Maslova LV, Maslov LN, Dan'shina EN.

[The anti-arrhythmia effect of Rhodiola rosea and its possible mechanism]. [Article in Russian]. *Bull Eksp Biol Med* 1993;116(8):175-6.

3196 Udintsev SN, Krylova SG, Fomina TI. [The enhancement of the efficacy of adriamycin by using hepatoprotectors of plant origin in metastases of Ehrlich's adenocarcinoma to the liver in mice]. [Article in Russian]. *Vopr Onkol* 1992;38(10):1217-22.

3197 Udintsev SN, Shakhov VP. [Changes in clonogenic properties of bone marrow and transplantable mice tumor cells during combined use of cyclophosphane and biological response modifiers of adaptogenic origin]. [Article in Russian]. *Eksp Onko* 1990;12(6):55-6.

3198 Petkov VD, Yonkov D, Mosharoff A, et al. Effects of alcohol aqueous extract from Rhodiola rosea L. roots on learning and memory. *Acta Physiol Pharmacol Bulg* 1986;12(1):3-16.

3199 Sequential Healing Health Services website. URL www.sequentialhealing.com/herbs/squawvine.html (Accessed 22 November 1999).

3219 Brown L, Rimm EB, Seddon JM, et al. A prospective study of carotenoid intake and risk of cataract extraction in US men. *Am J Clin Nutr* 1999;70:517-24.

3220 Chasan-Taber L, Willett WC, Seddon JM, et al. A prospective study of carotenoid and vitamin A intakes and risk of cataract extraction in US women. *Am J Clin Nutr* 1999;70:509-16.

3221 Lyle BJ, Mares-Perlman JA, Klein BE, et al. Antioxidant intake and risk of incident age-related nuclear cataracts in the Beaver Dam Eye Study. *Am J Epidemiol* 1999;149:801-9.

3222 Teikari JM, Rautalahti M, Haukka J, et al. Incidence of cataract operations in Finnish male smokers unaffected by alpha tocopherol or beta carotene supplements. *J Epidemiol Community Health* 1998;52:468-72.

3223 Teikari JM, Virtamo J, Rautalahti M, et al. Long-term supplementation with alpha-tocopherol and beta-carotene and age-related cataract. *Acta Ophthalmol Scand* 1997;75:634-40.

3224 Sommerburg O, Keunen JE, Bird AC, et al. Fruits and vegetables that are sources for lutein and zeaxanthin: the macular pigment in human eyes. *Br J Ophthalmol* 1998;82:907-10.

3225 Hammond BR Jr, Wooten BR, Snodderly DM, et al. Density of the human crystalline lens is related to the macular pigment carotenoids, lutein and zeaxanthin. *Optom Vis Sci* 1997;74:499-504.

3226 Gross AS, Goh YD, Addison RS, et al. Influence of grapefruit juice on cisapride pharmacokinetics. *Clin Pharmacol Ther* 1999; 65:395-401.

3227 Lilja JJ, Kivisto KT, Neuvonen PJ. Grapefruit juice increases serum concentrations of atorvastatin and has no effect on pravastatin. *Clin Pharmacol Ther* 1999; 66:118-27.

3228 Ozdemir M, Aktan Y, Boydag BS. Interaction between grapefruit juice and diazepam in humans. *Eur J Drug Metab Pharmacokinet* 1998; 23:55-9.

3229 Grapefruit-drug interactions. URL: powernetdesign.com/ grapefruit (Accessed 26 September 1999).

3230 Zaidenstein R, Dishi V, Gips M, et al. The effect of grapefruit juice on the pharmacokinetics of orally administered verapamil. *Eur J Clin Pharmacol* 1998; 54:337-40.

3231 Arlt W, Callies F, van Vlijmen JC, et al. Dehydroepiandrosterone replacement in women with adrenal insufficiency. *N Engl J Med* 1999;341:1013-20.

3232 Oelkers W. Dehydroepiandrosterone for adrenal insufficiency (editorial). *N Engl J Med* 1999;341:1073-4.

3233 Selhub J, Jacques PF, Rosenberg IH, et al. Serum total homocysteine concentrations in the Third National Health and Nutrition Examination Survey (1991-4): population reference ranges and contribution of vitamin status to high serum concentrations. *Ann Intern Med* 1999;131(5):331-9.

3234 Murray M, Pizzorno J. Encyclopedia of Natural Medicine. 2nd ed. Rocklin, CA: Prima Health, 1998.

3235 Lindenbaum J, Healton EB, Savage DG, et al. Neuropsychiatric disorders caused by cobalamin deficiency in the absence of anemia or macrocytosis. *N Engl J Med,* 1988;318:1720-8.

3236 Chappell LC, Seed PT, Briley AL, et al. Effect of antioxidants on the occurrence of pre-eclampsia in women at increased risk: a randomized trial. *Lancet* 1999;354:810-6.

3237 Mensink RP, van Houwelingen AC, Kromhout D, Hornstra G. A vitamin E concentrate rich in tocotrienols had no effect on serum lipids, lipoproteins, or platelet function in men with mildly elevated serum lipid concentrations. *Am J Clin Nutr* 1999;69:213-9.

3238 Qureshi AA, Qureshi N, Wright JJ, et al. Lowering of serum cholesterol in hypercholesterolemic humans by tocotrienols (palmvitee). *Am J Clin Nutr* 1991;53(4 Suppl):1021S-6S.

3239 Tomeo AC, Geller M, Watkins TR, et al. Antioxidant effects of tocotrienols in patients with hyperlipidemia and carotid stenosis. *Lipids* 1995;30:1179-83.

3240 Qureshi AA, Bradlow BA, Brace L, et al. Response of hypercholesterolemic subjects to administration of tocotrienols. *Lipids* 1995;30:1171-7.

3241 Qureshi AA, Bradlow BA, Slaser WA, et al. Novel tocotrienols of rice bran modulate cardiovascular disease risk parameters of hypercholesterolemic humans. *Nutr Biochem* 1997;8:290-8.

3242 Conte A, de Bernardi M, Palmieri L, et al. Metabolic fate of exogenous chondroitin sulfate in man. *Arzneimittelforschung* 1991; 41:768-72.

3243 Pittler MH, Abbot NC, Harkness EF, et al. Randomized, double-blind trial of chitosan for body weight reduction. *Eur J Clin Nutr* 1999;53:379-81.

3244 Wuolijoki E, Hirvela T, Ylitalo P. Decrease in serum LDL cholesterol with microcrystalline chitosan. *Methods Find Exp Clin Pharmacol* 1999;21:357-61.

3245 Takahashi K, Yoshino K, Shirai T, et al. Effect of a traditional herbal medicine (shakuyaku-kanzo-to) on testosterone secretion in patients with polycystic ovary syndrome detected by ultrasound. *Nippon Sanka Fujinka Gakkai Zasshi* 1988;40:789-92.

3246 Armanini D, Bonanni G, Palermo M, et al. Reduction of serum testosterone in men by licorice. *N Engl J Med* 1999;341:1158.

3247 Abe Y, Ueda T, Kato T, Kohli Y. [Effectiveness of interferon, glycyrrhizin combination therapy in patients with chronic hepatitis C]. [Article in Japanese]. *Nippon Rinsho* 1994 Jul;52(7):1817-22.

3248 Sato H, Goto W, Yamamura J, et al. Therapeutic basis of glycyrrhizin on chronic hepatitis B. *Antiviral Res* 1996;30:171-7.

3249 Takahara T, Watanabe A, Shiraki K. Effects of glycyrrhizin on hepatitis B surface antigen: a

REFERENCES

biochemical and morphological study. *J Hepatol* 1994;21:601-9.

3250 Acharya SK, Dasarathy S, Tandon A, et al. A preliminary open trial on interferon stimulator (SNMC) derived from Glycyrrhiza glabra in the treatment of subacute hepatic failure. *Indian J Med Res* 1993;98:69-74.

3251 Eisenburg J. [Treatment of chronic hepatitis B. Part 2: Effect of glycyrrhizic acid on the course of illness]. [Article in German]. *Fortschr Med* 1992;110(21):395-8.

3252 Armanini D, Lewicka S, Pratesi C, et al. Further studies on the mechanism of the mineralocorticoid action of licorice in humans. *J Endocrinol Invest* 1996;19:624-9.

3253 Krahenbuhl S, Hasler F, Frey BM, et al. Kinetics and dynamics of orally administered 18 beta-glycyrrhetinic acid in humans. *J Clin Endocrinol Metab* 1994;78:581-5.

3254 Lee YS, Lorenzo BJ, Koufis T, et al. Grapefruit juice and its flavonoids inhibit 11 beta-hydroxysteroid dehydrogenase. *Clin Pharmacol Ther* 1996;59:62-71.

3255 Zhang YD, Lorenzo B, Reidenberg MM. Inhibition of 11 beta hydroxysteroid dehydrogenase obtained from guinea pig kidney by furosemide, naringenin and some other compounds. *J Steroid Biochem Mol Biol* 1994;49:81-5.

3256 Hiai S, Yokoyama H, Oura H, et al. Stimulation of pituitary-adrenocortical system by ginseng saponin. *Endocrinol Jpn* 1979;26:661-5.

3257 Kase Y, Saitoh K, Ishige A, et al. Mechanisms by which Hange-shashin-to reduces prostaglandin E2 levels. *Biol Pharm Bull* 1998;21:1277-81.

3259 Peters H, Noble NA. Dietary L-arginine in renal disease. *Semin Nephrol* 1996;16(6):567-75.

3260 Wang R, Ghahary A, Shen YJ, et al. Human dermal fibroblasts produce nitric oxide and express both constitutive and inducible nitric oxide synthase isoforms. *J Invest Dermatol* 1996;106:419-27.

3261 Venturi A, Gionchetti P, Rizzello F, et al. Impact on the composition of the faecal flora by a new probiotic preparation: preliminary data on maintenance treatment of patients with ulcerative colitis. *Aliment Pharmacol Ther* 1999;13:1103-8.

3262 Russell IJ, Michalek JE, Flechas JD, et al. Treatment of fibromyalgia syndrome with Super Malic: a randomized, double blind, placebo controlled, crossover pilot study. *J Rheumatol* 1995;22:953-8.

3263 Koo WK, Walters JC, Esterlitz J, et al. Maternal calcium supplementation and fetal bone mineralization. *Obstet Gynecol* 1999; 94:577-82.

3264 Raman L, Rajalakshmi K, Krishnamachari KAVR, et al. Effect of calcium supplementation to undernourished mothers during pregnancy on the bone density of the neonates. *Am J Clin Nutr* 1978; 31:466-9.

3265 Roth JA, Kim B-G, Lin W-L, et al. Melatonin promotes osteoblast differentiation and bone formation. *J Biol Chem* 1999;274(31):22041-7.

3267 Singh RB, Niaz MA, Ghosh S. Hypolipidemic and antioxidant effects of Commiphora mukul as an adjunct to dietary therapy in patients with hypercholesterolemia. *Cardiovasc Drugs Ther* 1994;8:659-64.

3268 Thappa DM, Dogra J. Nodulocystic acne: oral gugulipid versus tetracycline. *J Dermatol* 1994;21(10):729-31.

3269 Adzet T, Camarasa J, Laguna JC. Hepatoprotective activity of polyphenolic compounds from Cynara scolymus against CCl4 toxicity in isolated rat hepatocytes. *J Nat Prod* 1987;50:612-7.

3270 Wolkowitz OM, Reus VI, Keebler A, et al. Double-blind treatment of major depression with dehydroepiandosterone. *Am J Psychiat* 1999;156:646-9.

3272 Raintree Nutrition, Inc. URL http://www.rain-tree.com/index.html (Accessed 27 November 1999).

3273 The IOOC's Trade Standard Applying to Olive Oil and Olive Pomace Oil. URL: sovrana.com/ioocdef.htm (Accessed 20 November 1999).

3274 Kamien M. Practice tip. Which cerumenolytic? *Aust Fam Physician* 1999;28:817,828.

3275 Isaksson M, Bruze M. Occupational allergic contact dermatitis from olive oil in a masseur. *J Am Acad Dermatol* 1999;41(2 Pt 2):312-5.

3276 Hoberman A, Paradise JL, Reynolds EA, et al. Efficacy of Auralgan for treating ear pain in children with acute otitis media. *Arch Pediatr Adolesc Med* July 1997;151(7):675-8.

3278 Nutrimax Labs website, URL: www.nutramaxlabs.com/human/cosamin.htm (Accessed 19 November 1999).

3279 Chavez ML, Chavez PI. Echinacea. *Hosp Pharm* 1998;33(2):180-8.

3280 Gunning K. Echinacea in the treatment and prevention of upper respiratory tract infections. *West J Med* 1999;171:198-200.

3281 Barrett B, Vohmann M, Calabrese C. Echinacea for upper respiratory infection. *J Fam Pract* 1999;48:628-35.

3282 Grimm W, Muller HH. A randomized controlled trial of the effect of fluid extract of Echinacea purpurea on the incidence and severity of colds and respiratory infections. *Am J Med* 1999;106:138-43.

3283 Putter M, Grotemeyer KH, Wurthwein G, et al. Inhibition of smoking-induced platelet aggregation by aspirin and pycnogenol. *Thromb Res* 1999;95(4):155-61.

3284 Bisignano G, Tomaino A, Lo Cascio R, et al. On the in-vitro antimicrobial activity of oleuropein and hydroxytyrosol. *J Pharm Pharmacol* 1999;51:971-4.

3285 Mensink RP, Katan MB. An epidemiological and an experimental study on the effect of olive oil on total serum and HDL cholesterol in healthy volunteers. *Eur J Clin Nutr* 1989;43 Suppl 2:43-8.

3286 Mata P, Alvarez-Sala LA, Rubio MJ, et al. Effects of long-term monounsaturated- vs polyunsaturated-enriched diets on lipoproteins in healthy men and women. *Am J Clin Nutr* 1992;55:846-50.

3287 Lichtenstein AH, Ausman LM, Carrasco W, et al. Effects of canola, corn, and olive oils on fasting and postprandial plasma lipoproteins in humans as part of a National Cholesterol Education Program Step 2 diet. *Arterioscler Thromb* 1993;13:1533-42.

3288 Zambon A, Sartore G, Passera D, et al. Effects of hypocaloric dietary treatment enriched in oleic acid on LDL and HDL subclass distribution in mildly obese women. *J Intern Med* 1999;246:191-201.

3289 Ruiz-Gutierrez V, Muriana FJ, Guerrero A, et al. Plasma lipids, erythrocyte membrane lipids and blood pressure of hypertensive women after ingestion of dietary oleic acid from two different sources. *J Hypertens* 1996;14:1483-90.

3290 Tsimikas S, Philis-Tsimikas A, Alexopoulos S, et al. LDL isolated from Greek subjects on a typical diet or from American subjects on an oleate-supplemented diet induces less monocyte chemotaxis and adhesion when exposed to oxidative stress. *Arterioscler Thromb Vasc Biol* 1999;19:122-30.

3291 Nutt JG, Woodward WR, Hammerstad JP, et al. The "on-off" phenomenon in Parkinson's disease. Relation to levodopa absorption and transport. *N Engl J Med* 1984;310:483-8.

3292 Baruzzi A, Contin M, Riva R, et al. Influence of meal ingestion time on pharmacokinetics of orally administered levodopa in parkinsonian patients. *Clin Neuropharmacol* 1987;10(6):527-37.

3293 Juncos JL, Fabbrini G, Mouradian MM, et al. Dietary influences on the antiparkinsonian response to levodopa. *Arch Neurol* 1987;44:1003-5.

3294 Eriksson T, Granerus AK, Linde A, et al. "On-off" phenomenon in Parkinson's disease: relationship between dopa and other large neutral amino acids in plasma. *Neurology* 1988;38:1245-8.

3300 Tomita T, Sato N, Arai T, et al. Bactericidal activity of a fermented hot-water extract from Stevia rebaudiana Bertoni towards enterohemorrhagic Escherichia coli O157:H7 and other food-borne pathogenic bacteria. *Microbiol Immunol* 1997;41(12):1005-9.

3301 Curi R, Alvarez M, Bazotte RB, et al. Effect of Stevia rebaudiana on glucose tolerance in normal adult humans. *Braz J Med Biol Res*, 1986;19(6):771-4.

3302 Evans DA, Raj RK. Larvicidal efficacy of Quassin against Culex quinquefasciatus. *Indian J Med Res* 1991;93:324-7.

3303 Owen JA, Nakatsu SL, Fenemore J, et al. The pharmacokinetics of yohimbine in man. *Eur J Clin Pharmacol* 1987;3:877-82.

3304 Cappiello A, McDougle CJ, Malison RT, et al. Yohimbine augmentation of Fluvoxamine in refactory depression: a single blind study. *Biol Psychiatry* 1995;38:765-7.

3305 Montorsi F, Strambi LF, Guazzoni G, et al. Effect of yohimbine-trazodone on psychogenic impotence: a randomized, double-blind, placebo-controlled study. *Urology* 1994;44:732-6.

3306 Balon R. Fluoxetine-induced sexual dysfunction and yohimbine. *J Clin Psychiatry* 1993;54:161-2.

3307 Carey MP, Johnson BT. Effectiveness of yohimbine in the treatment of erectile disorder: four meta-analytic integrations. *Arch Sexual Behavior* 1996;25:341-60.

3309 Kunellius P, Hakkinen J, Lukkarinen O. Is high-dose yohimbine hydrochloride effective in the treatment of mixed-type impotence? A prospective, randomized, controlled, double-blind crossover study. *Urol* 1997;49:441-4.

3310 Wagner G, Saenz de Tejada IS. Update on male erectile dysfunction. *BMJ* 1998;316:678-82.

3311 Witt DK. Yohimbine for erectile dysfuntion. *J Fam Pract* 1998;46:282-3.

3312 Teloken C, Rhoden EL, Sogari P, et al. Therapeutic effects of high dose yohimbine hydrochloride on organic erectile dysfunction. *J Urol* 1998;159:122-4.

3313 Ashton AK. Yohimbine in the treatment of male erectile dysfunction. *Am J Psychiatr* 1994;151:1397.

3314 Anderson PO, Knoben JE, Troutman WG. Handbook of Clinical Drug Data. 9th ed. Stamford, CT: Appleton & Lange, 1999.

3315 Siegel G, Klubendorf D. The anti-atherosclerotic effect of Allium sativum: Statistics re-evaluated. *Atherosclerosis* 2000;150:437-8.

3316 Aydin A, Ersoz G, Tekesin O, et al. Garlic Oil and Helicobacter pylori Infection. *AJG* 2000;95:563-4.

3317 Fernandez-Vozmediano JM, Armario-Hita JC, Manrique-Plaza A. Allergic contact dermatitis from diallyl disulfide. *Contact Dermatitis* 2000;42:108-9.

3318 Stjernberg L, Berglund J. Garlic as an Insect Repellant. *JAMA* 2000;284:831.

3319 Bloch AS. Pushing the Envelope of Nutrition Support: Complementary Therapies. *Nutrition* 2000;16:236-9.

3320 Fleischauer AT, Poole C, Arab L. Garlic consumption and cancer prevention: meta-analyses of colorectal and stomach cancers. *Am J Clin Nutr* 2000;72:1047-52.

3321 Sato T, Miyata G. The Nutraceutical Benefit, Part IV: Garlic. *Nutrition* 2000;16:787-8.

3322 O'Gara EA, Hill DJ, Maslin DJ. Activities of Garlic Oil, Garlic Powder, and Their Diallyl Constituents against Helicobacter pylori. *Appl Environ Microbiol* 2000;66:2269-73.

3323 Voutilainen S, Lakka TA, Porkkala-Sarataho E, et al. Low serum folate concentrations are associated with an excess incidence of acute coronary events: the Kuopio Ischaemic Heart Disease Risk Factor Study. *Eur J Clin Nutr* 2000;54:424-8.

3324 Bostom AG, Shemin D, Bagley P, et al. Controlled Comparison of L-5-Methyltetrahydrofolate Versus Folic Acid for the Treatment of Hyperhomocysteinemia in the Hemodialysis Patients. *Circulation* 2000;101:2829-32.

3325 US Food and Drug Administration, Center for Food Safety, and Applied Nutrition, Office of Nutritional Products, Labeling, and Dietary Supplements. Letter regarding dietary supplement health claim for folic acid with respect to neural tube defects. 2000. http://vm.cfsan.fda.gov/~dms/ds-ltr7.html. (Accessed 16 October 2000).

3330 Tenebaum A, Fisman EZ, Motro M. L-Arginine: Rediscovery in Progress. *Cardiology* 1998;90:153-5.

3331 Brittenden J, Park KGM, Heys SD, et al. L-Arginine stimulates host defenses in patients with breast cancer. *Surgery* 1994;115:205-12.

3332 Oomen CM, van Erk MJ, Feskens E, et al. Arginine Intake and Risk of Coronary Heart Disease Mortality in Elderly Men. *Arterioscler Thromb Vasc Biol* 2000;20:2134-9.

3333 Harkins K. What's the use of cranberry juice? *Age Ageing* 2000;29:9-12.

3334 Jackson B, Hicks LE. Effect of cranberry juice on urinary pH in older aldults. *Home Healthc Nurse* 1997;15:199-202.

3335 Avorn J. The effect Of Cranberry Juice on the presence of bacteria and white blood cells in the urine of elderly women. What is the role of bacterial adhesion? *Adv Exp Med Biol* 1996;408:185-6.

3336 Kuzminski LN. Cranberry juice and urinary tract infections: Is there a beneficial relationship? *Nutr Rev* 1996;54:S87-S90.

3337 Fleet JC. New support for a folk remedy: Cranberry juice reduces bacteriuria and pyuria in elderly women. *Nutr Rev* 1994;52:168-70.

3338 Schmidt DR, Sobota AE. An examination of the anti-adherence activity of cranberry juice on urinary and nonurinary bacterial isolates. *Microbios* 1988;55:173-81.

3339 Kinney AB, Blount M. Effect of cranberry juice on urinary pH. *Nurs Res* 1979;28:287-90.

3341 Rayman MP. The importance of selenium to human health. *Lancet* 2000;356:233-41.

3342 Mark SD, Qiao YL, Dawsey SM, et al. Prospective study of serum selenium levels and incident esophageal and gastric cancers. *J Natl Cancer Inst* 2000;92:1753-63.

3343 Vinceti M, Rothman KJ, Bergomi KJ, et al. Excess melanoma incidence in a cohort exposed to high levels of environmental selenium. *Cancer Epidemiol Biomarkers Prev* 1998;7:853-6.

3344 Urgert R, Vliet TV, Zock PL, et al. Heavy coffee consumption and plasma homocysteine: a randomized controlled trial in healthy volunteers. *Am J Clin Nutr* 2000;72:1107-10.

3345 Leitzmann MF, Willett WC, Rimm EB, et al. A Prospective study of coffee consumption and the risk of symptomatic gallstone disease in men. *JAMA* 1999;281:2106-12.

3346 Ernst E. Colonic irrigation and the theory of autointoxication: A triumph of ignorance over science. *J Clin Gastroenterol* 1997;24:196-8.

3347 Green S. A critique of the rationale for cancer treatment with coffee enemas and diet. *JAMA* 1992;268:3224-7.

3348 Reed A, James N, Sikora K. Juices, coffee enemas, and cancer. *Lancet* 1990;336:677-8.

3349 Shils ME, Herman MG. Unproved dietary claims in the treatment of patients with cancer. *Bull N Y Acad Med* 1982;58:323-39.

3350 Geerling BJ, Dagnelie PC, Badart-Smook A, et al. Diet as a Risk Factor for the Development of Ulcerative Colitis. *Am J Gastroenterol* 2000;95:1008-13.

3351 Brenner A. The Effects of Megadoses of Selected B Complex Vitamins on Children with Hyperkinesis: Controlled Studies with Long-Term Follow-up. *J Learn Disabil* 1982;15:258-64.

3353 Siegel RK. Ginseng Abuse Syndrome. *JAMA* 1979;241:1614-5.

3354 Palop-Larrea V, Gonzalvez-Perales JL, Catalan-Oliver C, et al. Metrorrhagia and ginseng. *Ann Pharmacother* 2000;34:1347-8.

3355 Fuller CJ, May MA, Martin KJ. The effect of Vitamin E and Vitamin C supplementation on LDL oxidizability and neutrophil respiratory burst in young smokers. *J Am Coll Nutr* 2000;19:361-9.

3356 Sullivan C, Capaldi N, Mack G, et al. Seizures and natural Vitamin E. *Med J Aust* 1990;152:613-4.

3357 Boaz M, Smetana S, Weinstein T, et al. Secondary prevention with antioxidants of cardiovascular disease in endstage renal disease: randomised placebo-controlled trial. *Lancet* 2000;356:1213-8.

3358 Engelen W, Keenoy BM, Vertommen J, Leeuw ID. Effects of long-term supplementation with moderate pharmacologic doses of vitamin E are saturable and reversible in patients with type 1 diabetes. *Am J Clin Nutr* 2000;72:1142-9.

3359 Leppala JM, Virtamo J, Fogelholm R, et al. Vitamin E and Beta Carotene supplementation in high risk for stroke: a subgroup analysis of the alpha-tocopherol, beta-carotene cancer prevention study. *Arch Neurol* 2000;57:1503-9.

3360 Palli D, Russo A, Saieva C, et al. Dietary and familial determinants of 10-year survival among patients with gastric carcinoma. *Cancer* 2000;89:1205-13.

3361 Israel K, Yu W, Sanders BG, Kline K. Vitamin E succinate induces apoptosis in human prostate cancer succinate-triggered apoptosis. *Nutr Cancer* 2000;36:90-100.

3362 Stoneham M, Goldacre M, Seagroatt V, Gill L. Olive oil, diet and colorectal cancer: an ecological study and a

hypothesis. *J Epidemiol Community Health* 2000;54:756-60.

3363 Bartoli R, Fernandez-Bariares F, Navarro E, et al. Effect of olive oil on early and late events of colon carcinogenesis in rats: modulation of arachidonic acid metabolism and local prostaglandin E2 synthesis. *Gut* 2000;46:191-9.

3364 Hipkiss AR, Chana H. Carnosine protects proteins against methylglyoxal-mediated modifications. *Biochem Biophys Res Commun* 1998;248(1):28-32.

3365 Singh RB, Niaz MA, Rastogi SS, et al. Effect of hydrosoluble coenzyme Q10 on blood pressures and insulin resistance in hypertensive patients with coronary artery disease. *J Hum Hypertens* 1999;13:203-8.

3366 Rotig A, Appelkvist EL, Geromel V, et al. Quinone-responsive multiple respiratory-chain dysfunction due to widespread coenzyme Q10 deficiency. *Lancet* 2000;356:391-5.

3367 Laaksonen R, Jokelainen K, Sahi T, et al. Decreases in serum ubiquinone concentrations do not result in reduced levels in muscle tissue during short-term simvastatin treatment in humans. *Clin Pharmacol Ther* 1995;57:62-6.

3368 Kishi T, Watanabe T, Folkers K. Bioenergetics in clinical medicine. XV. Inhibition of coenzyme Q10 enzymes by clinically used adrenergic blockers of B-receptors. *Res Commun Chem Pathol Pharmacol* 1977;17:157-64.

3369 Kishi H, Kishi T, Folkers K. Bioenergetics in clinical medicine. III. Inhibition of coenzyme Q10 enzymes by clinically used anti-hypertensive drugs. *Res Commun Chem Pathol Pharmacol* 1975;12:533-40.

3370 Fuke C, Krikorian SA, Couris RR. Coenzyme Q10: A Review of essential functions and clinical trials. *US Pharmacist* 2000;28-41.

3371 Harmelin DL, Martin FR, Wark JD. Antacid-induced phosphate depletion syndrome presenting as nephrolithiasis. *Aust NZ J Med* 1990;20:803-5.

3372 Roberts DH, Knox FG. Renal phosphate handling and calcium nephrolithiasis: role of dietary phosphate and phosphate leak. *Semin Nephrol* 1990;10:24-30.

3373 Pino AM, Valladares LE, Palma MA, et al. Dietary isoflavones affect sex hormone-binding globulin levels in postmenopausal women. *J Clin Endocrinol Metab* 2000;85:2797-800.

3374 Nissen S, Sharp RL, Panton L, et al. B-Hydroxy-B-Methylbutyrate (HMB) supplementation in humans is safe and may decrease cardiovascular risk factors. *J Nutr* 2000;130:1937-45.

3375 Howes JB, Sullivan D, Lai N, et al. The effects of dietary supplementation with isoflavones from red clover on the lipoprotein profiles of postmenopausal women with mild to moderate hypercholesterolemia. *Atherosclerosis* 2000;152:143-7.

3376 Umland EM, Cauffield JS, Kirk JK, et al. Phytoestrogens as therapeutic alternatives to traditional hormone replacement in postmenopausal women. *Pharmacother* 2000;20:981-90.

3377 Pavelka K, Gatterova J, Olejarova M, et al. Glucosamine sulfate decreases progression of knee osteoarthritis in a long-term, randomized, placebo-controlled, independent, confirmatory trial. ACR Abstract Concurrent Session. OA- Advances in Management. November 1, 2000. Page S384, Abstract 1908.

3378 Nakagawa H, Yamamoto D, Kiyozuka Y, et al. Effects of genistein and synergistic action in combination with eicosapentaenoic acid on the growth of breast cancer cell lines. *J Cancer Res Clin Oncol* 2000;126:448-54.

3380 Lu LJ, Lin SN, Grady JJ, et al. Altered kinetics and extent of urinary daidzein and genistein excretion in women during chronic soya exposure. *Nutr Cancer* 1996;26:289-302.

3381 Kantha SS, Wada S, Tanaka H, et al. Carnosine sustains the retention of cell morphology in continuous fibroblast culture subjected to nutritional insult. *Biochem Biophys Res Commun* 1996;223(2):278-82.

3382 Anon. Black cohosh: was Lydia E. Pinkham on to something? *The Wellness Letter* 2001;17:5.

3383 Edmunds J. Blue cohosh and newborn myocardial infarction? *Midwifery Today Int Midwife* 1999;52:34-5.

3384 Davis BR, Oberman A, Blaufox MD, et al. Lack of effectiveness of a low-sodium/high-potassium diet in reducing antihypertensive medication requirements in overweight persons with mild hypertension. *Am J Hypertens* 1994;7:926-32.

3385 Whelton PK, He J, Cutler JA, et al. Effects of oral potassium on blood pressure. Meta-analysis of randomized controlled clinical trials. *JAMA* 1997;277:1624-32.

3386 Whelton PK, Buring J, Borhani NO, et al. The effect of potassium supplementation in persons with a high-normal blood pressure. Results from phase 1 of the trials of hypertension prevention (TOHP). *Ann Epidemiol* 1995;5:85-95.

3387 Zand RS, Jenkins DJ, Diamandis EP. Steroid hormone activity of flavonoids and related compounds. *Breast Cancer Res Treat* 2000;62:35-49.

3390 Zaloga GP, Roberts PR, Black KW, et al. Carnosine is a novel peptide modulator of intracellular calcium and contractility in cardiac cells. *Am J Physiol* 1997;272(1 Pt 2):H462-8.

3391 Maynard LM, Boissonneault GA, Chow CK, Bruckner GG. High levels of dietary carnosine are associated with increased concentrations of carnosine and histidine in rat soleus muscle. *J Nutr* 2001;131:287-90.

3392 Terkelsen LH, Eskild-Jensen A, Kjeldsen H, et al. Topical application of cod liver oil ointment accelerates wound healing: an experimental study in wounds in the ears of hairless mice. *Scand J Plast Reconstr Surg Hand Surg* 2000;34(1):15-20.

3393 Borchers AT, Stern JS, Hackman RM, et al. Mushrooms, tumors, and immunity. *Proc Soc Exp Biol Med* 1999;221(4):281-293.

3394 Ooi VE, Liu F. Immunomodulation and anti-cancer activity of polysaccharide-protein complexes. *Curr Med Chem* 2000;7(7):715-729.

3395 Veierod MB, Thelle DS, Laake P. Diet and risk of cutaneous malignant melanoma: a prospective study of 50,757 Norwegian men and women. *Int J Cancer* 1997;71(4):600-4.

3396 Dawson JK, Abernethy VE, Graham DR, Lynch MP. A woman who took cod-liver oil and smoked. *Lancet* 1996;347(9018):1804.

3397 Lombardo YB, Chicco A, D'Alessandro ME, et al. Dietary fish oil normalize dyslipidemia and glucose intolerance with unchanged insulin levels in rats fed a high sucrose diet. *Biochim Biophys Acta* 1996;1299(2):175-82.

3398 Stammers T, Sibbald B, Freeling P. Efficacy of cod liver oil as an adjunct to non-steroidal anti-inflammatory drug treatment in the management of osteoarthritis in general practice. *Ann Rheum Dis* 1992;51(1):128-9.

3399 Jensen T, Stender S, Goldstein K, et al. Partial normalization by dietary cod-liver oil of increased microvascular albumin leakage in patients with insulin-dependent diabetes and albuminuria. *N Engl J Med* 1989;321(23):1572-7.

3400 Committee on Nutr, Amer Acad of Pediatrics. Soy protein-based formulas: recommendations for use in infant feeding. *Pediatrics* 1998;101(1):148-53.

3401 Anderson JW, Johnstone BM, Cook-Newell ME. Meta-analysis of the effects of soy protein intake on serum lipids. *N Engl J Med* 1995;333(5):276-82.

3402 Crouse JR III, Morgan T, Terry JG, et al. A randomized trial comparing the effect of casein with that of soy protein containing varying amounts of isoflavones on plasma concentrations of lipids and lipoproteins. *Arch Intern Med* 1999;159(17):2070-6.

3403 Zhu JS, Halpern GM, Jones K. The scientific rediscovery of an ancient Chinese herbal medicine: Cordyceps sinensis: part I. *J Altern Complement Med* 1998;4(3):289-303.

3404 Zhu JS, Halpern GM, Jones K. The scientific rediscovery of a precious ancient Chinese herbal regimen: Cordyceps sinensis: part II. *J Altern Complement Med* 1998;4(4):429-57.

3405 Rossetti L, Hawkins M, Chen W, et al. In vivo glucosamine infusion induces insulin resistance in normoglycemic but not in hyperglycemic conscious rats. *J Clin Invest* 1995;96(1):132-40.

3406 Shankar RR, Zhu JS, Baron AD. Glucosamine infusion in rats mimics the beta-cell dysfunction of non-insulin-dependent diabetes mellitus. *Metabolism* 1998;47(5):573-7.

3407 Nakamura K, Yamaguchi Y, Kagota S, et al. Inhibitory effect of Cordyceps sinensis on spontaneous liver metastasis of Lewis lung carcinoma and B16 melanoma cells in syngeneic mice. *Jpn J Pharmacol* 1999;79(3):335-41.

3408 Zhang ZJ, Luo HL, Li JS. [Clinical and experimental studies on elimination of oxygen free radical of jinshuibao capsule in treating senile deficiency syndrome and its deoxyribonucleic acid damage repairing effects]. [Article in Chinese] *Chung Kuo Chung Hsi I Chieh Ho Tsa Chih* 1997;17(1):35-8.

3409 Chiu JH, Ju CH, Wu LH, et al. Cordyceps sinensis increases the expression of major histocompatibility complex class II antigens on human hepatoma cell line HA22T/VGH cells. *Am J Chin Med* 1998;26(2):159-70.

3410 Bok JW, Lermer L, Chilton J, et al. Antitumor sterols from the mycelia of Cordyceps sinensis. *Phytochemistry* 1999;51(7):891-8.

3411 Li LS, Zheng F, Liu ZH. [Experimental study on effect of Cordyceps sinensis in ameliorating aminoglycoside induced nephrotoxicity]. [Article in Chinese] *Chung Kuo Chung Hsi I Chieh Ho Tsa Chih* 1996;16(12):733-7.

3412 Wang SM, Lee LJ, Lin WW, Chang CM. Effects of a water-soluble extract of Cordyceps sinensis on steroidogenesis and capsular morphology of lipid droplets in cultured rat adrenocortical cells. *J Cell Biochem* 1998;69(4):483-9.

3414 Chen YJ, Shiao MS, Lee SS, Wang SY. Effect of Cordyceps sinensis on the proliferation and

REFERENCES

differentiation of human leukemic U937 cells. *Life Sci* 1997;60(25):2349-59.

3415 Kiho T, Yamane A, Hui J, et al. Polysaccharides in fungi. XXXVI. Hypoglycemic activity of a polysaccharide (CS-F30) from the cultural mycelium of Cordyceps sinensis and its effect on glucose metabolism in mouse liver. *Biol Pharm Bull* 1996;19(2):294-6.

3416 Kuo YC, Tsai WJ, Shiao MS, et al. Cordyceps sinensis as an immunomodulatory agent. *Am J Chin Med* 1996;24(2):111-25.

3417 Zhou DH, Lin LZ. [Effect of Jinshuibao capsule on the immunological function of 36 patients with advanced cancer]. [Article in Chinese] *Chung Kuo Chung Hsi I Chieh Ho Tsa Chih* 1995;15(8):476-8.

3418 Xu F, Huang JB, Jiang L, et al. Amelioration of cyclosporin nephrotoxicity by Cordyceps sinensis in kidney-transplanted recipients. *Nephrol Dial Transplant* 1995;10(1):142-3.

3419 Bao ZD, Wu ZG, Zheng F. [Amelioration of aminoglycoside nephrotoxicity by Cordyceps sinensis in old patients]. [Article in Chinese] *Chung Kuo Chung Hsi I Chieh Ho Tsa Chih* 1994;14(5):271-3, 259.

3420 Kuo YC, Lin CY, Tsai WJ, et al. Growth inhibitors against tumor cells in Cordyceps sinensis other than cordycepin and polysaccharides. *Cancer Invest* 1994;12(6):611-5.

3421 Kiho T, Hui J, Yamane A, Ukai S. Polysaccharides in fungi. XXXII. Hypoglycemic activity and chemical properties of a polysaccharide from the cultural mycelium of Cordyceps sinensis. *Biol Pharm Bull* 1993;16(12):1291-3.

3424 Chen JR, Yen JH, Lin CC, et al. The effects of Chinese herbs on improving survival and inhibiting anti-ds DNA antibody production in lupus mice. *Am J Chin Med* 1993;21(3-4):257-62.

3425 Liu C, Lu S, Ji MR. [Effects of Cordyceps sinensis (CS) on in vitro natural killer cells]. [Article in Chinese] *Chung Kuo Chung Hsi I Chieh Ho Tsa Chih* 1992;12(5):267-9, 259.

3427 Xu RH, Peng XE, Chen GZ, Chen GL. Effects of cordyceps sinensis on natural killer activity and colony formation of B16 melanoma. *Chin Med J (English)* 1992;105(2):97-101.

3428 Cheng Q. [Effect of cordyceps sinensis on cellular immunity in rats with chronic renal insufficiency]. [Article in Chinese] *Chung Hua I Hsueh Tsa Chih (Taipei)* 1992;72(1):27-9, 63.

3429 Zhao Y. [Inhibitory effects of alcoholic extract of Cordyceps sinensis on abdominal aortic thrombus formation in rabbits]. [Article in Chinese] *Chung Hua I Hsueh Tsa Chih (Taipei)* 1991; 71(11):612-5, 42.

3431 Chen GZ, Chen GL, Sun T, et al. Effects of Cordyceps sinensis on murine T lymphocyte subsets. *Chin Med J (English)* 1991; 104(1):4-8.

3432 Zhu XY, Yu HY. [Immunosuppressive effect of cultured Cordyceps sinensis on cellular immune response]. [Article in Chinese] *Chung Hsi I Chieh Ho Tsa Chih* 1990;10(8):485-7, 454.

3434 Yamaguchi N, Yoshida J, Ren LJ, et al. Augmentation of various immune reactivities of tumor-bearing hosts with an extract of Cordyceps sinensis. *Biotherapy* 1990;2(3):199-205.

3435 Zhou L, Yang W, Xu Y, et la. [Short-term curative effect of cultured Cordyceps sinensis (Berk.) Sacc. Mycelia in chronic hepatitis B]. [Article in Chinese] *Chung Kuo Chung Yao Tsa Chih* 1990;15(1):53-5, 65.

3436 Mei QB, Tao JY, Gao SB, et al. [Antiarrhythmic effects of Cordyceps sinensis (Berk.) Sacc]. [Article in Chinese] *Chung Kuo Chung Yao Tsa Chih* 1989;14(10):616-8, 640.

3437 Yoshida J, Takamura S, Yamaguchi N, et al. Antitumor activity of an extract of Cordyceps sinensis (Berk.) Sacc. against murine tumor cell lines. *Jpn J Exp Med* 1989;59(4):157-61.

3450 Geleijnse JM, Launer LJ, Hofman A, et al. Tea flavonoids may protect against atherosclerosis: the Rotterdam Study. Arch Intern Med 1999;159(18):2170-4.

3451 Schechter JO. Treatment of disequilibrium and nausea in the SRI discontinuation syndrome. *J Clin Psychiatry* 1998;59(8):431-2.

3452 Arfeen Z, Owen H, Plummer JL, et al. A double-blind randomized controlled trial of ginger for the prevention of postoperative nausea and vomiting. *Anaesth Intensive Care* 1995;23(4):449-52.

3453 Visalyaputra S, Petchpaisit N, Somcharoen K, Choavaratana R. The efficacy of ginger root in the prevention of postoperative nausea and vomiting after outpatient gynaecological laparoscopy. *Anaesthesia* 1998;53(5):506-10.

3454 Linos A, Kaklamani VG, Kaklamani E, et al. Dietary factors in relation to rheumatoid arthritis: a role for olive oil and cooked vegetables? *Am J Clin Nutr* 1999;70(6):1077-82.

3455 Penny ME, Peerson JM, Marin RM, et al. Randomized, community-based trial of the effect of zinc supplementation, with and without other micronutrients, on the duration of persistent childhood diarrhea in Lima, Peru. *J Pediatr* 1999;135(2 Pt 1):208-17.

3456 Bhutta ZA, Black RE, Brown KH, et al. Prevention of diarrhea and pneumonia by zinc supplementation in children in developing countries: pooled analysis of randomized controlled trials. *J Pediatr* 1999;135:689-97.

3457 Korschunov VM, Smeyanov VV, Efimov BA, et al. Therapeutic use of an antibiotic-resistant Bifidobacterium preparation in men exposed to high-dose gamma-irradiation. *J Med Microbiol* 1996;44:70-4.

3458 Isolauri E, Arvola T, Sutas Y, et al. Probiotics in the management of atopic eczema. *Clin Exp Allergy* 2000;30:1604-10.

3460 Korting GE, Smith SD, Wheeler MA, et al. A randomized double-blind trial of oral L-arginine for treatment of interstitial cystitis. *J Urol* 1999;161(2):558-65.

3461 Schweizer J, Hautmann C. Comparison of two dosages of Ginkgo biloba extract Egb 761 in patients with peripheral arterial occlusive disease Fontain's stage llb / a randomised, double-blind, multicentric clinical trial. *Arzneimittelforschung* 1999;49(11):900-4.

3462 Hawkins EB. NADH: Advanced supplementation for more energy and slower aging. *Natural Pharmacy* 1998 Jul;2(7):10.

3463 Kyriakidou-Himonas M, Aloia JF, Yeh JK. Vitamin D supplementation in postmenopausal black women. *J Clin Endocrinol Metab* 1999;84(11):3988-90.

3464 Zamora SA, Rizzoli R, Belli DC, et al. Vitamin D supplementation during infancy is associated with higher bone mineral mass in prepubertal girls. *J Clin Endocrinol Metab* 1999;84(12):4541-4.

3465 Boger RH, Bode-Boger SM, Thiele W, et al. Restoring vascular nitric oxide formation by L-arginine improves the symptoms of intermittent claudication in patients with peripheral arterial occlusive disease. *J Am Coll Cardiol* 1998;32(5):1336-44.

3466 Boger RH, Bode-Boger SM, Thiele W, et al. Biochemical evidence for impaired nitric oxide synthesis in patients with peripheral arterial occlusive disease. *Circ* 1997;95(8):2068-74.

3467 Niittynen L, Nurminen ML, Korpela R, et al. Role of arginine, taurine, and homocysteine in cardiovascular diseases. *Ann Med* 1999;31:318-26.

3469 Butland BK, Fehily AM, Elwood PC. Diet and lung function decline in a cohort of 2512 middle aged men. *Thorax* 2000;55(2):102-8.

3470 Le Marchand L, Murphy SP, Hankin JH, et al. Intake of flavonoids and lung cancer. *J Natl Cancer Inst* 2000;92(2):154-60.

3471 Gulyas A, Repges R, Dethlefsen U. Therapy of chronic obstructive pulmonary diseases in children. *Atemvegs und Lungenkrankheiten* 1997;23:291-4.

3472 Dekkers R. Apple juice and the chemical-contact softening of gallstones. *Lancet* 1999;354(9196):2171.

3473 Sinniah D, Baskaran G. Margosa oil poisoning as a cause of Reye's syndrome. *Lancet* 1981;1(8218):487-9.

3474 Sinniah D, Baskaran G, Looi LM, Leong KL. Reye-like syndrome due to margosa oil poisoning: report of a case with postmortem findings. *Am J Gastroenterol* 1982;77(3):158-61.

3475 Sinniah R, Sinniah D, Chia LS, Baskaran G. Animal model of margosa oil ingestion with Reye-like syndrome. Pathogenesis of microvesicular fatty liver. *J Pathol* 1989;159(3):255-64.

3476 Lai SM, Lim KW, Cheng HK. Margosa oil poisoning as a cause of toxic encephalopathy. *Singapore Med J* 1990;31(5):463-5.

3477 Furbee B, Wermuth M. Life-threatening plant poisoning. *Crit Care Clin* 1997;13(4):849-88.

3478 Lewis WH, Smith PR. Poke root herbal tea poisoning. *JAMA* 1979;242(25):2759-60.

3479 Roberge R, Brader E, Martin ML, et al. The root of evil-pokeweed intoxication. *Ann Emerg Med* 1986;15(4):470-3.

3480 Jaeckle KA, Freemon FR. Pokeweed poisoning. *South Med J* 1981;74(5):639-40.

3481 Barker BE, Farnes P, LaMarche PH. Haematological effects of pokeweed. *Lancet* 1967;1:437.

3482 Kell SO, Rosenberg SA, Conlon TJ, Spyker DA. A peek at poke: mitogenicity and epidemiology. *Vet Hum Toxicol* 1982;24(4):36.

3483 Anon. Toxic reactions to plant products sold in health food stores. *Med Lett Drugs Ther* 1979;21:29-32.

3484 Klepser TB, Klepser ME. Unsafe and potentially safe herbal therapies. *Am J Health Syst Pharm* 1999;56:125-38.

3485 Plushner SL. Valerian: Valerian officinalis. *Am J Health Syst Pharm* 2000;57:328,333,335.

3486 Houghton PJ. The scientific basis for the reputed activity of Valerian. *J Pharm Pharmacol* 1999;51(5):505-12.

3487 Garges HP, Varia I, Doraiswamy PM. Cardiac complications and delirium associated with Valerian root withdrawal. [Letter to the Editor] *JAMA* 1998;280(18):1566-7.

3488 Tuncok Y, Kozan O, Cavdar C, et al. Urginea maritima (squill) toxicity. *J Toxicol Clin Toxicol* 1995;33(1):83-6.

3489 Wax PM. Squill through the ages. *J Toxicol Clin Toxicol*, 1995;33(1):86.

3490 But PP, Tai YT, Young K. Three fatal cases of herbal aconite poisoning. *Vet Hum Toxicol* 1994;36(3):212-5.

3491 Feldkamp A, Koster B, Weber HP. [Fatal poisoning caused by aconite monk's hood]. [Article in German] *Monatsschr Kinderheilkd* 1991;139(6):366-7.

3492 Hallstrom H, Thuvander A. Toxicological evaluation of myristicin. *Nat Toxins* 1997;5(5):186-92.

3493 Jeong HG, Yun CH. Induction of rat hepatic cytochrome P450 enzymes by myristicin. *Biochem Biophys Res Commun* 1995;217(3):966-71.

3494 Dinakar HS. Acute psychosis associated with nutmeg toxicity. *Med Times* 1977;105(12):63-4.

3495 Haynes BE, Bessen HA, Wightman WD. Oleander tea: herbal draught of death. *Ann Emerg Med* 1985;14(4):350-3.

3496 Biberoglu S, Biberoglu K, Komsuoglu B. Mad honey. [Letter to the Editor] *JAMA* 1988;259(13):1943.

3497 Sheikh NM, Philen RM, Love LA. Chaparral-associated hepatotoxicity. *Arch Intern Med* 1997;157(8):913-9.

3499 Davies JH. Abrus precatorius (rosary pea). The most common lethal plant poison. *J Fla Med Assoc* 1978;65(3):188-91.

3500 Herschler R. Methylsulfonylmethane in dietary products. US patent no. 4,616,039; 1986.

3501 Richmond VL. Incorporation of methylsulfonylmethane sulfur into guinea pig serum proteins. *Life Sci* 1986;39(3):263-8.

3502 O'Dwyer PJ, et al. Use of polar solvents in chemoprevention of 1,2-dimethylhydrazine-induced colon cancer. *Cancer* 1988;62(5):944-8.

3503 McCabe D, et al. Polar solvents in the chemoprevention of dimethylbenzanthracene-induced rat mammary cancer. *Arch Surg* 1986;62(12):1455-9.

3504 Klandorf H, et al. Dimethyl sulfoxide modulation of diabetes onset in NOD mice. *Diabetes* 1998;62(2):194-7.

3507 IFIC Review: Sorting out the facts about fat website: ificinfo.health.org/review/ir-fat.htm (Accessed 16 July 1999).

3508 Godley PA. Essential fatty acid consumption and risk of breast cancer. *Breast Cancer Res Treat* 1995 Jul;35(1):91-5.

3509 Malloy MJ, Kane JP. Agents used in hyperlipidemia. In: B. Katzung, ed. Basic and Clinical Pharmacology. 4th ed. Norwald, CT: Appleton and Lange, 1989.

3510 Rose DP. The mechanistic rationale in support of dietary cancer prevention. *Prev Med* 1996; 25(1): 34-7.

3511 Noguchi M, et al. The role of fatty acids and eicosanoid synthesis inhibitors in breast carcinoma. *Oncology* 1995; 52(4): 265-71.

3512 Balch JF, Balch PA. Prescription for Nutritional Healing. Garden City Park, NY: Avery Publ Group.

3513 Thien FC, Leung R, Baldo BA, et al. Asthma and anaphylaxis induced by royal jelly. *Clin Exp Allergy* 1996;26(2):216-22.

3514 Roger A, Rubira N, Nogueiras C, et al. [Anaphylaxis caused by royal jelly]. [Article in Spanish]. *Allergol Immunopathol (Madr)* 1995;23(3):133-5.

3515 Vittek J. Effect of royal jelly on serum lipids in experimental animals and humans with atherosclerosis. *Experientia* 1995;51(9-10):927-35.

3516 Yonei Y, Shibagaki K, Tsukada N, et al. Case report:

REFERENCES

haemorrhagic colitis associated with royal jelly intake. *J Gastroenterol Hepatol* 1997;12(7):495-9.

3521 Iruela LM, et al. Toxic interaction of S-adenosylmethionine and clomipramine. *Am J Psych* 1993; 150:522.

3523 Carney MW, et al. The switch mechanism and the bipolar/unipolar dichotomy. *Br J Psychiatry* 1989;154:48-51.

3524 Schneck C. St. John's wort and hypomania. *J Clin Psychiatry* 1998; 59:689.

3525 Adverse Drug Reactions Advisory Committee. An adverse reaction to the herbal medication milk thistle (Silybum marianum). *Med J Aust* 1999;170:218-9.

3526 Page RL II, Lawrence JD. Potentiation of warfarin by dong quai. *Pharmacotherapy* 1999;19(7):870-6.

3527 Amaranthine Aromatics. Essential Oil Safety. http://www.amaranthine.com/product/esssafe.html (Accessed 6 November 1999).

3529 D'Adamo P. Larch arabinogalactan. *J Naturopath Med* 1996;6:33-7.

3530 Kelly GS. Larch arabinogalactan: Clinical relevance of a novel immune-enhancing polysaccharide. *Alt Med Rev* 1999;4:96-103.

3531 Anon. Best herb for fighting off colds. *Bottom Line* 1999;20:1.

3532 Priesnitz M. Blue green algae – superfood or pond scum? Natural Life, June 28, 1999; URL: www.life.ca/nl/68/algae.html (Accessed 5 December 1999).

3533 Anon. Spirulina. URL: www.go-symmetry.com/spirulina.htm (Accessed 5 December 1999).

3534 Anon. Earthrise Farms spirulina safety assurance. Earthrise Farms 1998; URL: www.spirulina.com/SPLSAssurance.html (Accessed 5 December 1999).

3535 Anon. Toxic algae in lake Sammamish. King County, WA. October 28, 1998; URL: splash.metrokc.gov/wlr/waterres/lakes/bloom.htm (Accessed 5 December 1999).

3536 Anon. Health Canada announces results of blue-green algal products testing – only Spirulina found Microcystin-free. Health Canada, September 27, 1999; URL: www.hc-sc.gc.ca/english/archives/releases/99_114e.htm (Accessed 27 October 1999).

3537 Anon. Butternut. Sequential Healing Health Services. http://www.sequentialhealing.com/herbs/butternut.html (Accessed 15 December 1999).

3538 Anon. Butternut. http://www.comcen.com.au~sburgess/herbs/Monographs/Juglans.htm. (Accessed 15 December 1999).

3539 Peirce A. The Amer Pharmaceutical Assn Practical Guide to Natural Medicines. New York,NY: The Stonesong Press, 1999.

3540 Ziegler D, Hanefeld M, Ruhnau K, et al. Treatment of symptomatic diabetic polyneuropathy with the antioxidant alpha-lipoic acid: A 7-month, multicenter, randomized, controlled trial (ALADIN III Study). *Diabetes Care* 1999;22:1296-301.

3541 Reljanovic M, Reichel G, Rett K, et al. Treatment of diabetic polyneuropathy with the antioxidant thioctic acid (alpha-lipoic acid): A 2-year, multicenter, randomized, double-blind, placebo-controlled trial (ALADIN II). Alpha Lipoic Acid in Diabetic Neuropathy [abstract]. *Free Radic Res* 1999;31:171-7.

3542 Ziegler D, Schatz H, Conrad F, et al. Effects of treatment with the antioxidant alpha-lipoic acid on cardiac autonomic neuropathy in NIDDM patients. *Diabetes Care* 1997;20:369-73.

3543 Obrosova I, Cao X, Greene DA, et al. Diabetes-induced changes in lens antioxidant status, glucose utilization and energy metabolism: Effect of DL-alpha-lipoic acid. *Diabetologia* 1998;41:1442-50.

3544 Streeper RS, Henriksen EJ, Jacob S, et al. Differential effects of lipoic acid stereoisomers on glucose metabolism in insulin-resistant skeletal muscle. *Am J Physiol* 1997;273:E185-91.

3545 Konrad T, Vicini P, Kusterer K, et al. Alpha-lipoic acid treatment decreases serum lactate and pyruvate concentrations and improves glucose effectiveness in lean and obese patients with Type 2 diabetes. *Diabetes Care* 1999;22:280-7.

3546 Packer L. Antioxidant properties of lipoic acid and its therapeutic effects in prevention of diabetes complications and cataracts. *Ann N Y Acad Sci* 1994;738:257-64.

3547 Schempp CM, Winghofer B, Langheinrich M, et al. Hypericin levels in human serum and interstitial skin blister fluid after oral single-dose and steady state administration of Hypericum perforatum extract (St. John's Wort). *Skin Pharmacol Appl Skin Physiol* 1999;12:299-304.

3548 Kim HL, Streltzer J, Goebert D. St. John's wort for depression: A meta analysis of well-defined clinical trials. *J Nerv Ment Dis* 1999;187:532-9.

3549 Linde K, Ramirez G, Mulrow CD, et al. St. John's wort for depression: an overview and meta-analysis of randomized clinical trials. *BMJ* 1996;313:253-8.

3550 Harrer G, et al. Comparison of equivalence between the St. John's wort extract LoHyp-57 and fluoxetine. *Arzneimittelforschung* 1999;49:289-96.

3551 Philipp M, Kohnen R, Hiller KO. Hypericum extract versus imipramine or placebo in patients with moderate depression: randomized mulicentre study of treatment for eight weeks. *BMJ* 1999;319:1534-9.

3552 Gaster B, Holroyd J. St John's wort for depression. *Arch Intern Med* 2000;160:152-6.

3553 Singer A, Wonnemann M, Muller WE. Hyperforin, a major antidepressant constituent of St. John's wort, inhibits serotonin uptake by elevating free intracellular Na+11. *J Pharmacol Exp Ther* 1999;290:1363-8.

3554 Schempp C, Pelz K, Wittmer A, et al. Antibacterial activity of hyperforin from St. John's wort, against multiresistant Stapylococcus aureus and gram-positive bacteria. *Lancet* 1999;353:2129.

3555 Nierenberg AA, Burt T, Matthews J, et al. Mania associated with St. John's wort. *Biol Psychiatry* 1999;46:1707-8.

3556 Nebel A, Schneider BJ, Baker RA, et al. Potential metabolic interaction between St. John's wort and theophylline. *Ann Pharmacother* 1999;33:502.

3557 Ziegler D, Hanefeld M, Ruhnau KJ, et al. Treatment of symptomatic diabetic peripheral neuropathy with the antioxidant alpha-lipoic acid: A 3-week, multicenter, randomized, controlled trial (ALADIN Study). *Diabetologia* 1995;38:1425-33.

3558 Huang KC. The Pharmacology of Chinese Herbs. 2nd ed. Boca Raton: CRC Press, 1999:267.

3559 Upton R, ed. Schisandra Berry: Analytical, Quality Control, and Therapeutic Monograph. Santa Cruz, CA: American Herbal Pharmacopoeia 1999;1-25

3561 Pepping J. Huperzine A. *Am J Health Syst Pharm* 2000;57:530-4.

3562 Gaster B. S-adenosylmethionine (SAMe) for treatment

of depression. *Alternative Medicine Alert,* 1999;12:133-5.

3563 Chevallier A. Encyclopedia of Medicinal Plants. New York, NY: DK Publishing 1996;202.

3564 Anon. Lapacho. The Natural Pharmacist 2000. http://www.tnp.com/substance.asp?ID=67 (Accessed 7 April 2000).

3565 Kumar DS, Prabhakar YS. On the ethnomedical significance of the Arjun tree, Terminalia arjuna (Roxb.) Wight & Arnot. *J Ethnopharmacol* 1987;20:173-90.

3566 Anon. Magnesium. The Natural Pharmacist. Prima Communications; 2000. http://www.tnp.com/substance.asp?ID=161#P5 (Accessed 4 May 2000).

3567 Anon. Colostrum. The Natural Pharmacist. Prima Communications, Inc., 2000. http://www.tnp.com/substance.asp?ID=121 (Accessed 5 May 2000).

3568 Moses EL, Mallinger AG. St. John's wort: Three cases of possible mania induction. *J Clin Psychopharmacol* 2000;20:115-7.

3569 Beckman SE, Sommi RW, Switzer J. Consumer use of St. John's wort: A survey of effectiveness, safety, and tolerability. *Pharmacotherapy* 2000;20:568-74.

3570 Ereshefsky B, Gewertz N, Lam YMF, et al. Determination of SJW differential metabolism at CYP2D6 and CYP3A4, using dextromethorphan probe methodology. Abstract Poster Presentations, 39th NCDEU Annual Meeting, 1999:Poster 130 128.

3571 Gewertz N, Ereshefsky B, Lam YWF, et al. Determination of the differential effects of St. John's wort on the CYP1A2 and NAT2 metabolic pathways using caffeine probe methodology. Abstract Poster Presentations, 39th NCDEU Annual Meeting, 1999:Poster 131.

3572 Brandes JL, Edvinsson L, Marcus D, et al. New treatment options for migraine. Medscape Neurology Treatment Updates 2000. http://www.medscape.com/medscape/Neurology/TreatmentUpdate/2000/tu05/TU05-05.html (Accessed 18 May 2000).

3573 Towheed TE, Anastassiades TP. Glucosamine and Chondriotin for treating symptoms of osteoarthritis. Evidence is widely touted but incomplete. *JAMA* 2000;238(11):1483-4.

3574 Anon. Bee Propolis. MotherNature.com 1999. http://www.mothernature.com/library/books/natmed/bee_propolis.asp (Accessed 28 May 2000).

3575 FDA. Special Nutritional Adverse Event Monitoring System. US FDA, 1998. http://vm.cfsan.fda.gov/~dms/aems.html (Accessed 12 June 2000).

3576 Ault A. Chinese herbal remedy holds promise for prostate cancer. Reuters Health May 23, 2000. http://www.medscape.com/reuters/prof/2000/05/05.23/20000523clin013.html (Accessed 2 June 2000).

3577 Anon. PC-SPES. UCSF Cancer Center Communications 2000. URL: http://cc.ucsf.edu/clinical/uro_pc-spes.html (Accessed 2 June 2000).

3578 Dillard J. Grape leaf for ADHD? OnHealth, Mar 19, 1999. http://onhealth.com/alternative/columnist/item,49799.asp (Accessed 3 June 2000).

3579 Meyer AS, Yi OS, Pearson DA, et al. Inhibition of human low-density lipoprotein oxidation in relation to composition of phenolic antioxidants in grapes (Vitis vinifera). *J Agric Food Chem* 1997;45:1638-43.

3580 Anon. OPCs (Oligomeric Proanthocyanidins). The Natural Pharmacist 2000. http://www.tnp.com/substance.asp?ID=181 (Accessed 3 June 2000).

3581 Murray MT. Natural Alternatives to Over-the-Counter and Prescription Drugs. New York, NY: Quill, 1994.

3582 Pizzorno JE, Murray MT, eds. Textbook of Natural Medicine. 2nd ed. New York, NY: Chuchill Livingstone, 1999.

3583 Geva E, Bartoov B, Zabludovsky N, et al. The effect of antioxidant treatment on human spermatozoa and fertilization rate in an in vitro fertilization program. *Fertil Steril* 1996;66:430-4.

3585 Vezina D, Mauffette F, Roberts KD, et al. Selenium-vitamin E supplementation in infertile men. Effects on semen parameters and micronutrient levels and distribution. *Biol Trace Elem Res* 1996;53:65-83.

3586 Anon. Health benefits of yogurt. Natl Yogurt Assn 1999. http://www.yaourt.org/healthbenefits.html (Accessed 6 June 2000).

3587 Gregory PJ. Probiotics for antibiotic-associated diarrhea. *Pharmacist's Letter* 2000;16(1):160103.

3588 Pizzorno JE, Murray MT, eds. Textbook of Natural Medicine. 2nd ed. Edinburgh: Churchill Livingstone, 1999.

3589 Meydani SN, Ha WK. Immunologic effects of yogurt. *Am J Clin Nutr* 2000;71:861-72.

3590 Agerholm-Larsen L, Raben A, Haulrik N, et al. Effect of 8 week intake of probiotic milk products on risk factors for cardiovascular diseases. *Eur J Clin Nutr* 2000;54:288-97.

3591 Anon. Female Viagra equivalent now available – Topical Natural Sensation from Strategic Science and Technologies, Inc. PRNewswire May 25, 2000.

3592 Anon. Arginine. The Natural Pharmacist 2000. http://www.tnp.com/substance.asp?ID=106. (accessed 14 June 2000).

3593 Blum A, Porat R, Rosenschein U, et al. Clinical and inflammatory effects of dietary L-arginine in patients with intractable angina pectoris. *Am J Cardiol* 1999;15:1488-90.

3594 Tentolouris C, Tousoulis D, Toutouzas P, et al. Effects of acute L-arginine administration in coronary atherosclerosis [letter]. *Circulation* 1999;99:1648.

3595 Rector TS, Bank AJ, Mullen KA, et al. Randomized, double-blind, placebo-controlled study of supplemental oral L-arginine in patients with heart failue. *Circulation* 1996;93:2135-41.

3596 Watanabe G, Tomiyama H, Doba N. Effects of oral administration of L-arginine on renal function in patients with heart failure. *J Hypertens* 2000;18:229-34.

3598 Kehoe WA. Vitamin E for neuroleptic-induced tardive dyskinesia. *Pharmacist's Letter* 1999;15(1):150105.

3599 Markowitz JS, DeVane CL, Boulton DW, et al. Effect of St. John's wort (Hypericum Perforatum) on cytochrome P-450 2D6 and 3A4 activity in healthy volunteers. *Life Sci* 2000;66:PL 133-9.

3600 Salvioli G, Neri M. L-acetylcarnitine treatment of mental decline in the elderly. *Drugs Exp Clin Res* 1994;20(4):169-76.

3601 Passeri M, Cucinotta D, Bonati PA, et al. Acetyl-L-carnitine in the treatment of mildly demented elderly patients. *Int J Clin Pharmacol Res,* 1990;10(1-2):75-9.

3602 Bella R, Biondi R, Raffaele R, Pennisi G. Effect of acetyl-L-carnitine on geriatric patients suffering from dysthymic disorders. *Int J Clin Pharmacol Res* 1990;10(6):355-60.

3603 Garzya G, Corallo D, Fiore A, et al. Evaluation of the effects of L-acetylcarnitine on senile patients suffering from depression. *Drugs Exp Clin Res* 1990;16(2):101-6.

3604 Tempesta E, Casella L, Pirrongelli C, et al. L-acetylcarnitine in depressed elderly subjects. A cross-over study vs placebo. *Drugs Exp Clin Res* 1987;13(7):417-23.

3605 Di Marzio L, Moretti S, D'Alo S, et al. Acetyl-L-carnitine administration increases insulin-like growth factor 1 levels in asymptomatic HIV-1-infected subjects: correlation with its suppressive effect on lymphocyte apoptosis and ceramide generation. *Clin Immunol* 1999;92(1):103-10.

3606 Famularo G, Moretti S, Marcellini S, et al. Acetyl-carnitine deficiency in AIDS patients with neurotoxicity on treatment with antiretroviral nucleoside analogues. *AIDS* 1997;11(2):185-90.

3607 Moncada ML, Vicari E, Cimino C, et al. Effect of acetylcarnitine treatment in oligoasthenospermic patients. *Acta Europ Fertil* 1992;23(5):221-4.

3608 Jeulin C, Lewin LM. Role of free L-carnitine and acetyl-L-carnitine in post-gonadal maturation of mammalian spermatozoa. *Hum Reprod Update* 1996;2(2):87-102.

3609 Jeulin C, Soufir JC, Marson J, et al. [Acetylcarnitine and spermatozoa: relationship with epididymal maturation and motility in the boar and man]. [Article in French]. *Reprod Nutr Develop* 1988;28(5):1317-27.

3610 Golan R, Weissenberg R, Lewin LM. Carnitine and acetylcarnitine in motile and immotile human spermatozoa. *Int J Androl* 1984;7(6):484-94.

3611 Kohengkul S, Tanphaichitr V, Muangmun V, Tanphaichitr N. Levels of L-carnitine and L-O-acetylcarnitine in normal and infertile human semen: a lower level of L-O-acetycarnitine in infertile semen. *Fertil Steril* 1977;28(12):1333-6.

3612 Tanphaichitr N. In vitro stimulation of human sperm motility by acetylcarnitine. *Int J Fertil* 1977;22(2):85-91.

3613 Anon. Carnitine. Supplementwatch.com. www.supplementwatch.com/sup-atoz/c/carnitine.html (Accessed 22 February 2000).

3614 Anon. L-carnitine. Vitaminbuzz, sponsored by the Vitamin Shoppe. www.vitaminbuzz.com/Supp/Carnitine-F.htm (Accessed 27 February 2000).

3615 Anon. L-carnitine. Whole Health Discount Center. www.wholehealthdiscountcenter.com/lc/ (Accessed 27 February 2000).

3616 Anon. Carnitor (levocarnitine) package insert. Sigma-Tau Pharmaceuticals Inc, Gaithersburg, MD. December 1999.

3617 Mintz M. Carnitine in human immunodeficiency virus type 1 infection/acquired immune deficiency syndrome. *J Child Neurol* 1995;10(Suppl 2):S40-4.

3618 Dalakas MC, Leon-Monzon ME, Bernardini I, et al. Zidovudine-induced mitochondrial myopathy is associated with muscle carnitine deficiency and lipid storage. *Ann Neurol* 1994;35(4):482-7.

3619 Georgala S, Schulpis KH, Georgala C, Michas T. L-carnitine supplementation in patients with cystic acne on isotretinoin therapy. *J Eur Acad Dermatol Venereol* 1999;13(3):205-9.

3620 Ramos AC, Barrucand L, Elias PR, et al. Carnitine supplementation in diphtheria. *Indian Pediatr* 1992;29(12):1501-5.

3621 Ramos AC, Elias PR, Barrucand L, Da Silva JA. The protective effect of carnitine in human diphtheric

myocarditis. *Pediatr Res* 1984;18(9):815-9.

3622 Plioplys AV, Kasnicka I. L-carnitine as a treatment for Rett syndrome. *South Med J* 1993;86(12):1411-2.

3623 Cacciatore L, Cerio R, Ciarimboli M, et al. The therapeutic effect of L-carnitine in patients with exercise-induced stable angina: a controlled study. *Drugs Exp Clin Res* 1991;17(4):225-35.

3624 Cherchi A, Lai C, Angelino F, et al. Effects of L-carnitine on exercise tolerance in chronic stable angina: a multicenter, double-blind, randomized, placebo-controlled, crossover study. *Int J Clin Pharmacol Ther Toxicol* 1985;23(10):569-72.

3625 Rizos I. Three-year survival of patients with heart failure caused by dilated cardiomyopathy and L-carnitine administration. *Am Heart J* 2000;139(2 Pt 3):S120-3.

3626 Ghidini O, Azzurro M, Vita G, Sartori G. Evaluation of the therapeutic efficacy of L-carnitine in congestive heart failure. *Int J Clin Pharmacol Ther Toxicol* 1988;26(4):217-20.

3627 Singh RB, Niaz MA, Agarwal P, et al. A randomized, double-blind, placebo-controlled trial of L-carnitine in suspected acute myocardial infarction. *Postgrad Med J* 1996;72(843):45-50.

3628 Iliceto S, Scrutinio D, Bruzzi P, et al. Effects of L-carnitine administration on left ventricular remodeling after acute anterior myocardial infarction: the L-Carnitine Ecocardiografia Digitalizzata Infarto Miocardico (CEDIM) Trial. *J Am Coll Cardiol* 1995;26(2):380-7.

3629 Davini P, Bigalli A, Lamanna F, Boem A. Controlled study on L-carnitine therapeutic efficacy in post-infarction. *Drugs Exp Clin Res* 1992;18(8):355-65.

3630 Plioplys AV, Plioplys S. Amantadine and L-carnitine treatment of Chronic Fatigue Syndrome. *Neuropsychobiology* 1997;35(1):16-23.

3631 Brevetti G, Chiariello M, Ferulano G, et al. Increases in walking distance in patients with peripheral vascular disease treated with L-carnitine: a double-blind, cross-over study. *Circ* 1988;77(4):767-73.

3632 Cifone MG, Alesse E, Di Marzio L, et al. Effect of L-carnitine treatment in vivo on apoptosis and ceramide generation in peripheral blood lymphocytes from AIDS patients. *Proc Assoc Am Physicians* 1997;109(2):146-53.

3633 Scaglia F, Longo N. Primary and secondary alterations of neonatal carnitine metabolism. *Semin Perinatol* 1999;23(2):152-61.

3634 Bonner CM, DeBrie KL, Hug G, et al. Effects of parenteral L-carnitine supplementation on fat metabolism and nutrition in premature neonates. *J Pediatr* 1995;126(2):287-92.

3635 Schmidt-Sommerfeld E, Penn D. Carnitine and total parenteral nutrition of the neonate. *Biol Neonate* 1990;58(Suppl 1):81-8.

3636 Melegh B, Kerner J, Sandor A, et al. Oral L-carnitine supplementation in low-birth-weight newborns: a study on neonates requiring combined parenteral and enteral nutrition. *Acta Paediatr Hung* 1986;27(3):253-8.

3637 Schmidt-Sommerfeld E, Penn D, Wolf H. Carnitine deficiency in premature infants receiving total parenteral nutrition: effect of L-carnitine supplementation. *J Pediatr* 1983;102(6):931-5.

3639 Heinonen OJ. Carnitine and physical exercise. *Sports Med* 1996;22(2):109-32.

3640 Berthillier G, Eichenberger D, Carrier HN, et al.

Carnitine metabolism in early stages of Duchenne muscular dystrophy. *Clin Chim Acta* 1982;122(3):369-75.

3641 Marthaler NP, Visarius T, Kupfer A, Lauterburg BH. Increased urinary losses of carnitine during ifosfamide chemotherapy. *Cancer Chemother Pharmacol* 1999;44(2):170-2.

3642 Heuberger W, Berardi S, Jacky E, et al. Increased urinary excretion of carnitine in patients treated with cisplatin. *Eur J Clin Pharmacol* 1998;54(7):503-8.

3643 Schoderbeck M, Auer B, Legenstein E, et al. Pregnancy-related changes of carnitine and acylcarnitine concentrations of plasma and erythrocytes. *J Perinat Med* 1995;23(6):477-85.

3644 Novak M. Carnitine supplementation in soy-based formula-fed infants. *Biol Neonate* 1990;58 Suppl 1:89-92.

3645 Goral S. Levocarnitine and muscle metabolism in patients with end-stage renal disease. *J Ren Nutr* 1998;8(3):118-21.

3646 Kletzmayr J, Mayer G, Legenstein E, et al. Anemia and carnitine supplementation in hemodialyzed patients. *Kidney Int* 1999;69Suppl:93-106.

3647 Ahmad S, Robertson HT, Golper TA, et al. Multicenter trial of L-carnitine in maintenance hemodialysis patients. II. Clinical and biochemical effects. *Kidney Int* 1990;38(5):912-8.

3648 Nuesch R, Rossetto M, Martina B. Plasma and urine carnitine concentrations in well-trained athletes at rest and after exercise. Influence of L-carnitine intake. *Drugs Exp Clin Res* 1999;25(4):167-71.

3649 Vecchiet L, Di Lisa F, Pieralisi G, et al. Influence of L-carnitine administration on maximal physical exercise. *Eur J Appl Physiol* 1990;61(5-6):486-90.

3650 Marconi C, Sassi G, Carpinelli A, Cerretelli P. Effects of L-carnitine loading on the aerobic and anaerobic performance of endurance athletes. *Eur J Appl Physiol* 1985;54(2):131-5.

3651 Mingrone G, Greco AV, Capristo E, et al. L-carnitine improves glucose disposal in type 2 diabetic patients. *J Am Coll Nutr* 1999;18(1):77-82.

3652 Capaldo B, Napoli R, Di Bonito P, et al. Carnitine improves peripheral glucose disposal in non-insulin-dependent diabetic patients. *Diabetes Res Clin Pract* 1991;14(3):191-5.

3653 Bertelli A, Ronca G. Carnitine and coenzyme Q10: biochemical properties and functions, synergism and complementary action. *Int J Tissue React* 1990;12(3):183-6.

3654 Anon. Moducare website. URL http://www.moducare.com/ (Accessed 30 March 2000).

3655 Anon. Seacoast Vitamins website. URL http://www.seacoastvitamins.com/NaturalBalance/Sterinol.html (Accessed 30 March 2000).

3656 Anon. Carmichael Wellness Products website. URL http://www.cwproducts.com/newpg/44490.asp (Accessed 30 March 2000).

3657 Coppen A, Bailey J. Enhancement of the antidepressant action of fluoxetine by folic acid: a randomised, placebo controlled trial. *J Affect Dis* 2000;60:121-31.

3658 Anon. W&B Associates Inc. website. URL http://www.wandb.com/cholesterol.6.htm (Accessed 30 March 2000).

3661 Patel SB, Honda A, Salen G. Sitosterolemia: exclusion of genes involved in reduced cholesterol biosynthesis. *J Lipid Res* 1998;39(5):1055-61.

3662 Salen G, Shore V, Tint GS, et al. Increased sitosterol absorption, decreased removal, and expanded body pools compensate for reduced cholesterol synthesis in sitosterolemia with xanthomatosis. *J Lipid Res* 1989;30(9):1319-30.

3663 Nguyen LB, Shefer S, Salen G, et al. Competitive inhibition of hepatic sterol 27-hydroxylase by sitosterol: decreased activity in sitosterolemia. *Proc Assoc Am Physicians* 1998;110(1):32-9.

3665 Jones PJ, MacDougall DE, Ntanios F, Vanstone CA. Dietary phytosterols as cholesterol-lowering agents in humans. *Can J Physiol Pharmacol* 1997;75(3):217-27.

3666 Heinemann T, Kullak-Ublick GA, Pietruck B, von Bergmann K. Mechanisms of action of plant sterols on inhibition of cholesterol absorption. Comparison of sitosterol and sitostanol. *Eur J Clin Pharmacol* 1991;40 Suppl 1:S59-63.

3667 Awad AB, von Holtz RL, Cone JP, et al. Beta-sitosterol inhibits growth of HT-29 human colon cancer cells by activating the sphingomyelin cycle. *Anticancer Res* 1998;18(1A):471-3.

3668 Awad AB, Chen YC, Fink CS, Hennessey T. Beta-sitosterol inhibits HT-29 human colon cancer cell growth and alters membrane lipids. *Anticancer Res* 1996;16(5A):2797-804.

3669 Bouic PJ, Etsebeth S, Liebenberg RW, et al. Beta-sitosterol and beta-sitosterol glucoside stimulate human peripheral blood lymphocyte proliferation: implications for their use as an immunomodulatory vitamin combination. *Int J Immunopharmacol* 1996;18(12):693-700.

3672 Hidaka H, Kojima H, Kawabata T, et al. Effects of an HMG-CoA reductase inhibitor, pravastatin, and bile sequestering resin, cholestyramine, on plasma plant sterol levels in hypercholesterolemic subjects. *J Atheroscler Thromb* 1995;2(1):60-5.

3673 Ntanios FY, Jones PJ, Frohlich JJ. Effect of 3-hydroxy-3-methylglutaryl coenzyme A reductase inhibitor on sterol absorption in hypercholesterolemic subjects. *Metabolism* 1999;48(1):68-73.

3677 Anon. LifeLink Products - Ultradiol website. URL www.lifelinknet.com/Ultra.htm (Accessed 9 April 2000).

3678 Anon. FDA alert on misuse of consumer products containing GHB, GBL and BD. Food and Drug Administration, Rockville, MD. Issued June 15, 1999. URL www.fda.gov/cder/graphics/ghb.gif (Accessed 9 April 2000).

3679 Anon. Important message for health professionals: Report serious adverse events associated with dietary supplements containing GBL, GHB or BD. Food and Drug Administration, Rockville, MD. August 25, 1999. URL http://vm.cfsan.fda.gov/~dms/mwgblghb.html (Accessed 9 April 2000).

3680 Otto A. Acquaintance rape drug may one day help instead of hurt (news). Pharmacy Today. American Pharmaceutical Association, Washington, DC. April 2000:17.

3681 Hillory J. Farias and Samantha Reid date-rape drug prohibition act of 2000. 106th Congress of the United States of America. HR 2130.

3682 Anon. Multistate outbreak of poisonings associated with illicit use of gamma hydroxy butyrate. *J Am Med Assoc* 1991;265(4):447-8.

3683 Kalra MA, Hart LL. Gammahydroxybutyrate in

narcolepsy. *Ann Pharmacother* 1992;26:647-8.

3684 Addolorato G, Cibin M, Caprista E, et al. Maintaining abstinence from alcohol with gamma hydroxybutyric acid. [Letter] *Lancet* 1998;351:38.

3685 Strong AJ. Gamma hydroxybutyric acid and intracranial pressure. [Letter] *Lancet* 1984;1(8389):1304.

3686 Gallimberti L, Canton G, Gentile N, et al. Gamma-hydroxybutyric acid for treatment of alcohol withdrawal syndrome. *Lancet* 1989;2(8666):787-9.

3687 Smith KM. Drugs used in acquaintance rape. *J Am Pharm Assoc* 1999;39:519-25.

3688 Dyer JE. Gamma-Hydroxybutyrate: a health-food product producing coma and seizure-like activity. *Am J Emerg Med* 1991;9(4):321-4.

3689 Scrima L, Hartman PG, Johnson FH Jr, et al. The effects of gamma-hydroxybutyrate on the sleep of narcolepsy patients: a double-blind study. *Sleep* 1990;13(6):479-90.

3690 Scrima L, Hartman PG, Johnson FH Jr, Hiller FC. Efficacy of gamma-hydroxybutyrate versus placebo in treating narcolepsy-cataplexy: double-blind subjective measures. *Biol Psychiatry* 1989;26(4):331-43.

3691 Scharf MB, Brown D, Woods M, et al. The effects and effectiveness of gamma-hydroxybutyrate in patients with narcolepsy. *J Clin Psychiatry* 1985;46(6):222-5.

3692 Broughton R, Mamelak M. The treatment of narcolepsy-cataplexy with nocturnal gamma-hydroxybutyrate. *Can J Neurol Sci* 1979;6(1):1-6.

3693 Hoes MJ, Vree TB, Guelen PJ. Gamma-hydroxybutyric acid as hypnotic. Clinical and pharmacokinetic evaluation of gamma-hydroxybutyric acid as hypnotic in man. *Encephale* 1980;6(1):93-9.

3694 Gallimberti L, Schifano F, Forza G, et al. Clinical efficacy of gamma-hydroxybutyric acid in treatment of opiate withdrawal. *Eur Arch Psychiatry Clin Neurosci* 1994;244(3):113-4.

3695 Gallimberti L, Cibin M, Pagnin P, et al. Gamma-hydroxybutyric acid for treatment of opiate withdrawal syndrome. *Neuropsychopharmacology* 1993;9(1):77-81.

3696 Gallimberti L, Ferri M, Ferrara SD, et al. Gamma-Hydroxybutyric acid in the treatment of alcohol dependence: a double-blind study. *Alcohol Clin Exp Res* 1992;16(4):673-6.

3697 Kleinschmidt S, Schellhase C, Mertzlufft F. Continuous sedation during spinal anaesthesia: gamma-hydroxybutyrate vs. propofol. *Eur J Anaesthesiol* 1999;16(1):23-30.

3698 Kleinschmidt S, Grundmann U, Knocke T, et al. Total intravenous anaesthesia with gamma-hydroxybutyrate (GHB) and sufentanil in patients undergoing coronary artery bypass graft surgery: a comparison in patients with unimpaired and impaired left ventricular function. *Eur J Anaesthesiol* 1998;15(5):559-64.

3699 Tunnicliff G. Significance of gamma-hydroxybutyric acid in the brain. *Gen Pharmacol* 1992;23(6):1027-34.

3700 Goodman LS, Gilman A. The Pharmacological Basis of Therapeutics. 5th ed. New York, NY: Macmillan Publ. Co., Inc., 1975.

3701 Zava DT, Dollbaum CM, Blen M. Estrogen and progestin bioactivity of foods, herbs, and spices. *Proc Soc Exp Biol Med* 1998;217(3):369-78.

3702 Rodriguez M, Alvarez M, Zayas M. [Microbiological quality of spices consumed in Cuba]. [Article in Spanish]. *Rev Latinoam Microbiol* 1991;33(2-3):149-51.

3703 Kivanc M, Akgul A, Dogan A. Inhibitory and stimulatory effects of cumin, oregano and their essential oils on growth and acid production of Lactobacillus plantarum and Leuconostoc mesenteroides. *Int J Food Microbiol* 1991;13(1):81-5.

3704 Akgul A, Kivanc M. Inhibitory effects of selected Turkish spices and oregano components on some foodborne fungi. *Int J Food Microbiol* 1988;6(3):263-8.

3705 Benito M, et al. Labiatae allergy: systemic reactions due to ingestion of oregano and thyme. *Ann Allergy Asthma Immunol* 1996; 76(5): 416-8.

3706 Krenzelok EP, Jacobsen TD, Aronis J. American mistletoe exposures. *Am J Emerg Med* 1997;15(5):516-20.

3707 Friess H, et al. Treatment of advanced pancreatic cancer with mistletoe: results of a pilot trial. *Anticancer Res* 1996 Mar-Apr;16(2):915-20.

3709 Kuttan G, et al. Anticarcinogenic and antimetastatic activity of Iscador. *Anticancer Drugs* 1997;8(Suppl 1):15-6.

3710 Upton R, ed. Ashwagandha root (Withania somnifera): Analytical, quality control, and therapuetic monograph. *American Herbal Pharmacopoeia* 2000;April:1-25.

3711 Davis L, Kuttan G. Effect of Withania somnifera on cyclophosphamide-induced urotoxicity. *Cancer Lett* 2000;148:9-17.

3712 Zamah NM, Humpel M, Kuhnz W, et al. Absence of an effect of high vitamin C dosage on the systemic availability of ethinyl estradiol in women using a combination oral contraceptive. *Contraception* 1993;48:377-91.

3713 Chu DT, Wong WL, Mavligit GM. Immunotherapy with Chinese medicinal herbs. II. Reversal of cyclophosphamide-induced immune suppression by administration of fractionated Astragalus membranaceus in vivo. *J Clin Lab Immunol* 1988;25:125-9.

3714 Thie NM, Prasad NG, Major PW. Evaluation of glucosamine sulfate compared to ibuprofen for the treatment of temporomandibular joint osteoarthritis: a randomized double blind controlled 3 month clinical trial. *J Rheumatol* 2001;28:1347-1355.

3715 Vehmeyer K, et al. Lectin-induced increase in clonogenic growth of haematopoietic progenitor cells. *Eur J Haematol* 1998 Jan;60(1):16-20.

3716 Ortega N, et al. Tobacco allergy: demonstration of cross-reactivity with other members of Solanaceae family and mugwort pollen. *Ann Allergy Asthma Immunol* 1999 Feb;82(2): 194-7.

3717 Lombardi C, et al. Allergic reactions to honey and royal jelly and their relationship with sensitization to compositae. *Allergol Immunopathol (Madr)* 1998;26(6):288-90.

3718 Westendorf J, Pfau W, Schulte A. Carcinogenicity and DNA adduct formation observed in ACI rats after long-term treatment with madder root, Rubia tinctorum L. *Carcinogenesis* 1998;19(12): 2163-8.

3719 Boozer CN, Nasser JA, Heymsfield SB, et al. An herbal supplement containing Ma Huang-Guarana for weight loss: a randomized, double-blind trial. *Int J Obes Relat Metab Disord* 2001;25:316-324.

3720 Bourinbaiar AS, Lee-Huang S. Potentiation of anti-HIV activity of anti-inflammatory drugs, dexamethasone and indomethacin, by MAP30, the antiviral agent from bitter melon. *Biochem Biophys Res Commun* 1995;208(2):779-85.

3721 Lee-Huang S, Huang PL, Chen HC, et al. Anti-HIV and

anti-tumor activities of recombinant MAP30 from bitter melon. *Gene* 1995;161(2):151-6.

3722 Cunnick JE, Sakamoto K, Chapes SK, et al. Induction of tumor cytotoxic immune cells using a protein from the bitter melon (Momordica charantia). *Cell Immunol* 1990;126(2):278-89.

3723 Jilka C, Strifler B, Fortner GW, et al. In vivo antitumor activity of the bitter melon (Momordica charantia). *Cancer Res* 1983;43(11):5151-5.

3724 Leung SO, Yeung HW, Leung KN. The immunosuppressive activities of two abortifacient proteins isolated from the seeds of bitter melon (Momordica charantia). *Immunopharmacol* 1987;13(3):159-71.

3726 Tseng J, Chang JG. Suppression of tumor necrosis factor-alpha, interleukin-1 beta, interleukin-6 and granulocyte-monocyte colony stimulating factor secretion from human monocytes by an extract of Poria cocos. *Chung Hua Min Kuo Wei Sheng Wu Chi Mien I Hsueh Tsa Chih* 1992;25(1):1-11.

3727 Hattori T, Hayashi K, Nagao T, et al. Studies on antinephritic effects of plant components (3): Effect of pachyman, a main component of Poria cocos Wolf on original-type anti-GBM nephritis in rats and its mechanisms. *Jpn J Pharmacol* 1992;59(1):89-96.

3728 Cuellar MJ, Giner RM, Recio MC, et al. Effect of the basidiomycete Poria cocos on experimental dermatitis and other inflammatory conditions. *Chem Pharm Bull (Tokyo)* 1997;45(3):492-4.

3729 Kaminaga T, Yasukawa K, Kanno H, et al. Inhibitory effects of lanostane-type triterpene acids, the components of Poria cocos, on tumor promotion by 12-O tetradecanoylphorbol-13-acetate in two-stage carcinogenesis in mouse skin. *Oncology* 1996;53(5):382-5.

3730 Tai T, Akita Y, Kinoshita K, et al. Anti-emetic principles of Poria cocos. *Planta Med* 1995;61(6):527-30.

3731 Wang SS, Yang S, Ma Y. [Efficacy of poria-polyporus anti-diarrhea oral liquor in treating infantile rotavirus diarrhea: a controlled study with smicta]. [Article in Chinese]. *Chung Kuo Chung Hsi I Chieh Ho Tsa Chih* 1995;15(5):284-6.

3732 Li YL. [Clinical and experimental study on the treatment of children diarrhea by granule of children-diarrhea fast-stopping]. [Article in Chinese]. *Chung Hsi I Chieh Ho Tsa Chih* 1991;11(2):79-82,67.

3733 Wang SQ, Du XR, Lu HW, et al. Experimental and clinical studies of Shen Yan Ling in treatment of chronic glomerulonephritis. *J Tradit Chin Med* 1989;9(2):132-4.

3734 Yang DJ. [Tinnitus treated with combined traditional Chinese medicine and Western medicine]. [Article in Chinese]. *Chung Hsi I Chieh Ho Tsa Chih* 1989;9(5):270-1,259-60.

3735 Gong QM, Wang SL, Gan C. [A clinical study on the treatment of acute upper digestive tract hemorrhage with wen-she decoction]. [Article in Chinese]. *Chung Hsi I Chieh Ho Tsa Chih* 1989;9(5):272-3,260.

3736 Yasukawa K, Kaminaga T, Kitanaka S, et al. 3 beta-p-hydroxybenzoyldehydrotumulosic acid from Poria cocos, and its anti-inflammatory effect. *Phytochemistry* 1998;48(8):1357-60.

3737 Nukaya H, Yamashiro H, Fukazawa H, et al. Isolation of inhibitors of TPA-induced mouse ear edema from Hoelen, Poria cocos. *Chem Pharm Bull (Tokyo)* 1996;44(4):847-9.

3740 Kouzi SA, McMurtry RJ, Nelson SD. Hepatotoxicity of germander (Teucrium chamaedrys L.) and one of its constituent neoclerodane diterpenes teucrin A in the mouse. *Chem Res Toxicol* 1994;7(6):850-6.

3741 Larrey D, Vial T, Pauwels A, et al. Hepatitis after germander (Teucrium chamaedrys) administration: another instance of herbal medicine hepatotoxicity. *Ann Intern Med* 1992;117(2):129-32.

3742 Pauwels A, Thierman-Duffaud D, Azanowsky JM, et al. [Acute hepatitis caused by wild germander. Hepatotoxicity of herbal remedies. Two cases]. [Article in French]. *Gastroenterol Clin Biol* 1992;16(1):92-5.

3743 Castot A, Djezzar S, Deleau N, et al. [Pharmacovigilance off the beaten track: herbal surveillance or pharmacovigilance of medicinal plants]. [Article in French]. *Therapie* 1997;52(2):97-103.

3744 Mostefa-Kara N, Pauwels A, Pines E, et al. Fatal hepatitis after herbal tea. *Lancet* 1992;340(8820):674.

3745 Chan P, Xu DY, Liu JC, et al. The effect of stevioside on blood pressure and plasma catecholamines in spontaneously hypertensive rats. *Life Sci* 1998;63(19):1679-84.

3746 Melis MS. A crude extract of Stevia rebaudiana increases the renal plasma flow of normal and hypertensive rats. *Braz J Med Biol Res* 1996;29(5):669-75.

3747 Melis MS. Chronic administration of aqueous extract of Stevia rebaudiana in rats: renal effects. *J Ethnopharmacol* 1995;47(3):129-34.

3748 Matsui M, Matsui K, Kawasaki Y, et al. Evaluation of the genotoxicity of stevioside and steviol using six in vitro and one in vivo mutagenicity assays. *Mutagenesis* 1996;11(6):573-9.

3749 Pezzuto JM, Compadre CM, Swanson SM, et al. Metabolically activated steviol, the aglycone of stevioside, is mutagenic. *Proc Natl Acad Sci, USA* 1985;82(8):2478-82.

3750 Hubler MO, Bracht A, Kelmer-Bracht AM. Influence of stevioside on hepatic glycogen levels in fasted rats. *Res Commun Chem Pathol Pharmacol* 1994;84(1):111-8.

3751 Fang HJ, Su XL, Liu HY, et al. [Studies on the chemical components and anti-tumor action of the volatile oils from Pelargonium graveoleus]. [Article in Chinese]. *Yao Hsueh Hsueh Pao* 1989;24(5):366-71.

3752 Lis-Balchin M, Buchbauer G, Hirtenlehner T, Resch M. Antimicrobial activity of Pelargonium essential oils added to a quiche filling as a model food system. *Lett Appl Microbiol* 1998;27(4):207-10.

3753 Pattnaik S, Subramanyam VR, Kole C. Antibacterial and antifungal activity of ten essential oils in vitro. *Microbios* 1996;86(349):237-46.

3754 Agarwal AK, Singh M, Gupta N, et al. Management of giardiasis by an immuno-modulatory herbal drug Pippali rasayana. *J Ethnopharmacol* 1994;44(3):143-6.

3755 Agarwal AK, Tripathi DM, Sahai R, et al. Management of giardiasis by a herbal drug Pippali Rasayana: a clinical study. *J Ethnopharmacol* 1997;56(3):233-6.

3756 Shah AH, Al-Shareef AH, Ageel AM, Qureshi S. Toxicity studies in mice of common spices, Cinnamomum zeylanicum bark and Piper longum fruits. *Plant Foods Hum Nutr* 1998;52(3):231-9.

3757 Khajuria A, Zutshi U, Bedi KL. Permeability characteristics of piperine on oral absorption-an active alkaloid from peppers and a bioavailability enhancer. *Indian J Exp Biol* 1998;36(1):46-50.

3758 Ghoshal S, Prasad BN, Lakshmi V. Antiamoebic activity

REFERENCES

of Piper longum fruits against Entamoeba histolytica in vitro and in vivo. *J Ethnopharmacol* 1996;50(3):167-70.

3759 el-Mofty MM, Khudoley VV, Shwaireb MH. Carcinogenic effect of force-feeding an extract of black pepper (Piper nigrum) in Egyptian toads (Bufo regularis). *Oncology* 1991;48(4):347-50.

3760 Singh A, Rao AR. Evaluation of the modulatory influence of black pepper (Piper nigrum, L.) on the hepatic detoxication system. *Cancer Lett* 1993; 72(1-2):5-9.

3761 Nalini N, Sabitha K, Viswanathan P, Menon VP. Influence of spices on the bacterial (enzyme) activity in experimental colon cancer. *J Ethnopharmacol* 1998;62(1):15-24.

3762 Day C, Cartwright T, Provost J, Bailey CJ. Hypoglycaemic effect of Momordica charantia extracts. *Planta Med* 1990;56(5):426-9.

3763 Ali L, Khan AK, Mamun MI, et al. Studies on hypoglycemic effects of fruit pulp, seed, and whole plant of Momordica charantia on normal and diabetic model rats. *Planta Med* 1993;59(5):408-12.

3764 Cakici I, Hurmoglu C, Tunctan B, et al. Hypoglycaemic effect of Momordica charantia extracts in normoglycaemic or cyproheptadine-induced hyperglycaemic mice. *J Ethnopharmacol* 1994;44(2):117-21.

3765 Sarkar S, Pranava M, Marita R. Demonstration of the hypoglycemic action of Momordica charantia in a validated animal model of diabetes. *Pharmacol Res* 1996;33(1):1-4.

3766 Hansson A, Veliz G, Naquira C, et al. Preclinical and clinical studies with latex from Ficus glabrata HBK, a traditional intestinal anthelminthic in the Amazonian area. *J Ethnopharmacol* 1986;17(2):105-38.

3767 Lee IS, Jung KY, Oh SR, et al. Structure-activity relationships of lignans from Schisandra chinensis as platelet activating antagonists. *Biol Pharm Bull* 1999;22(3): 265-7.

3768 Sun HD, Qiu SX, Lin LZ, et al. Nigranoic acid, a triterpenoid from Schisandra sphaerandra that inhibits HIV-1 reverse transcriptase. *J Nat Prod* 1996; 59(5):525-7.

3769 Fukuda K, Ohta T, Oshima Y, et al. Specific CYP3A4 inhibitors in grapefruit juice: furocoumarin dimers as components of drug interaction. *Pharmacogenetics* 1997; 7(5):391-6.

3770 Meagher EA, Barry OP, Lawson JA, et al. Effects of vitamin E on lipid peroxidation in healthy persons. *JAMA* 2001;285:1178-82.

3771 Lilja JJ, Kivisto KT, Backman JT, et al. Grapefruit juice substantially increases plasma concentrations of buspirone. *Clin Pharmacol Ther* 1998; 64(6):655-60.

3773 Kupferschmidt HH, Fattinger KE, Ha HR, et al. Grapefruit juice decreases the systemic availability of itraconazole capsules in healthy volunteers. *Br J Clin Pharmacol* 1998; 45(4):355-9.

3774 Lilja JJ, Kivisto KT, Neuvonen PJ. Grapefruit juice-simvastatin interaction: effect on serum concentrations of simvastatin, simvastatin acid, and HMG-CoA reductase inhibitors. *Clin Pharmacol Ther* 1998 ; 64(5):477-83.

3775 Ameer B, Weintraub RA. Drug interactions with grapefruit juice. *Clin Pharmacokinet* 1997; 33(2):103-21.

3800 Tyler VE, Brady LR, Robbers JE. Pharmacognosy. 7th ed. Philadelphia, PA: Lea & Febiger, 1976.

3801 Gobel H, Schmidt G, Soyka D. Effect of peppermint and eucalyptus oil preparations on neurophysiological and experimental algesimetric headache parameters. *Cephalalgia* 1994;14(3):228-34; discussion 182.

3802 Liu JH, Chen GH, Yeh HZ, et al. Enteric-coated peppermint-oil capsules in the treatment of irritable bowel syndrome: a prospective, randomized trial. *J Gastroenterol* 1997;32(6):765-8.

3803 Pittler MH, Ernst E. Peppermint oil for irritable bowel syndrome: a critical review and metaanalysis. *Am J Gastroenterol* 1998;93(7):1131-5.

3804 Tate S. Peppermint oil: a treatment for postoperative nausea. *J Adv Nurs* 1997;26(3):543-9.

3805 United States Pharmacopeial Convention I, editor. Drug Information for the Health Care Professional. 19th ed. Micromedex, 1999.

3807 Correa CM, Tibana A, Gontijo-Filho PP. Vegetables as a source of infection with Pseudomonas aeruginosa in a University and Oncology Hospital of Rio de Janeiro. *J Hosp Infect* 1991;18(4):301-6.

3808 Benito M, Jorro G, Morales C, et al. Labiatae allergy: systemic reactions due to ingestion of oregano and thyme. *Ann Allergy Asthma Immunol* 1996; 76(5):416-8.

3811 Chan TY. Potential dangers from topical preparations containing methyl salicylate. *Hum Exp Toxicol* 1996;15(9):747-50.

3818 Tsuda T, Sugaya A, Ohguchi H, et al. Protective effects of peony root extract and its components on neuron damage in the hippocampus induced by the cobalt focus epilepsy model. *Exp Neurol* 1997; 146(2):518-25.

3819 Croton, Botanical.com A Modern Herbal website. URL: www.botanical.com/botanical/mgmh/c/croto118.html. (Accessed 12 May 1999).

3820 Description and Natural History of the Periwinkle. URL: biotech.icmb.utexas.edu/botany/perihist.html

3821 Coolwort, Botanical.com A Modern Herbal website. URL: www.botanical.com/botanical/mgmh/c/coolwo97.html. (Accessed 12 May 1999).

3822 Mossa JS, Tariq M, Mohsin A, et al. Pharmacological studies on aerial parts of Calotropis procera. *Am J Chin Med* 1991;19(3-4):223-31.

3823 Kumar VL, Basu N. Anti-inflammatory activity of the latex of Calotropis procera. *J Ethnopharmacol* 1994;44(2):123-5.

3824 Mascolo N, Sharma R, Jain SC, et al. Ethnopharmacology of Calotropis procera flowers. *J Ethnopharmacol* 1988;22(2):211-21.

3825 Sen T, Basu A, Chaudhuri AK. Studies on the possible mechanism of the gastric mucosal protection by Calotropis procera - involvement of 5-lipoxygenase pathway. *Fund Clin Pharmacol* 1998;12(1):82-7.

3826 Levy L. The activity of chaulmoogra acids against Mycobacterium leprae. *Am Rev Respir Dis* 1975;111(5):703-5.

3827 Cowhage, Botanical.com A Modern Herbal website. URL: www.botanical.com/botanical/mgmh/c/cowha111.html. (Accessed 12 May 1999).

3828 Mascolo N, Autore G, Capasso F. Local anti-inflammatory activity of Tamus communis. *J Ethnopharmacol* 1987;19(1):81-4.

3829 Schmidt RJ, Moult SP. The dermatitic properties of black bryony (Tamus communis L.). *Contact Dermatitis* 1983;9(5):390-6.

3830 Carotenuto A, De Feo V, Fattorusso E, et al. The

flavonoids of Allium ursinum. *Phytochem* 1996;41(2):531-6.

3831 Rietz B, Isensee H, Strobach H, et al. Cardioprotective actions of wild garlic (allium ursinum) in ischemia and reperfusion. *Mol Cell Biochem* 1993;119(1-2):143-50.

3832 Rana BK, Singh UP, Taneja V. Antifungal activity and kinetics of inhibition by essential oil isolated from leaves of Aegle marmelos. *J Ethnopharmacol* 1997;57(1):29-34.

3833 Prakash D, Joshi BD, Pal M. Vitamin C in leaves and seed oil composition of the Amaranthus species. *Int J Food Sci Nutr* 1995;46(1):47-51.

3834 Sharma SR, Dwivedi SK, Swarup D. Hypoglycaemic, antihyperglycaemic and hypolipidemic activities of Caesalpinia bonducella seeds in rats. *J Ethnopharmacol* 1997;58(1):39-44.

3835 Ippen H. [Phytophotodermatitis caused by plant trimming (edger's rash)]. [Article in German]. *Derm Beruf Umwelt* 1990;38(6):190-2.

3836 Misra SB, Dixit SN. Antifungal properties of leaf extract of Ranunculus sceleratus L. *Experientia* 1978;34(11):1442-3.

3837 Goerz G, Wirth G, Maas B, et al. [Allergic contact dermatitis due to Asteraceae (Compositae). Cross reaction with Liatris spicata]. [Article in German]. *Derm Beruf Umwelt* 1985;33(3):95-8.

3838 Krenzelok EP, Jacobsen TD, Aronis JM. Poinsettia exposures have good outcomes...just as we thought. *Am J Emerg Med* 1996;14(7):671-4.

3839 Cohen LM, Cohen JL. Erythema multiforme associated with contact dermatitis to poison ivy: three cases and a review of the literature. *Cutis*, 1998; 62(3):139-42.

3841 Kuo SC, Chen SC, Chen LH, et al. Potent antiplatelet, anti-inflammatory and antiallergic isoflavanquinones from the roots of Abrus precatorius. *Planta Med* 1995;61(4):307-12.

3842 Wang JP, Hsu MF, Chang LC, et al. Inhibition of plasma extravasation by abruquinone A, a natural isoflavanquinone isolated from Abrus precatorius. *Eur J Pharmacol* 1995;273(1-2):73-81.

3846 Henriksen NT. Lycoperdonosis. *Acta Paediatr Scand* 1976;65(5):643-5.

3847 Respiratory illness associated with inhalation of mushroom spores - Wisconsin 1994. *Morb Mortal Wkly Rep* 1994;43(29):525-6.

3850 Sidhu GS, Oakenfull DG. A mechanism for the hypocholesterolaemic activity of saponins. *Br J Nutr* 1986;55(3):643-9.

3851 Wu JY, Gardner BH, Murphy CI, et al. Saponin adjuvant enhancement of antigen-specific immune responses to an experimental HIV-1 vaccine. *J Immunol* 1992;148(5):1519-25.

3852 Pillion DJ, Amsden JA, Kensil CR, et al. Structure-function relationship among Quillaja saponins serving as excipients for nasal and ocular delivery of insulin. *J Pharm Sci* 1996;85(5):518-24.

3853 Recchia J, Lurantos MH, Amsden JA, et al. A semisynthetic Quillajasaponin as a drug delivery agent for aminoglycoside antibiotics. *Pharm Res* 1995;12(12):1917-23.

3854 Mitscher LA, Bathala MS, Clark GW, et al. Antimicrobial agents from higher plants. The quaternary alkaloids of Ptelea trifoliata. *Lloydia* 1975;38(2):109-16.

3858 Majumder PK, Dasgupta S, Mukhopadhaya RK, et al. Anti-steroidogenic activity of the petroleum ether extract and fraction 5 (fatty acids) of carrot (Daucus carota L.) seeds in mouse ovary. *J Ethnopharmacol* 1997;57(3):209-12.

3859 Maher TJ. Chromium and other minerals in diabetes mellitus. *US Pharm* 1999 Nov:66-76.

3860 Nisley N, Klepser T. Phytoestrogens for the prevention and treatment of osteoporosis. *Alt Med Alert* 1999 Dec;138-42.

3861 Leder BZ, Longcope C, Catlin DH, et al. Oral androstenedione administration and serum testosterone concentrations in young men. *JAMA* 2000;283:779-82.

3862 Rasmussen BB, Volpi E, Gore DC, Wolfe RR. Androstenedione does not stimulate muscle anabolism in young healthy men. *J Clin Endocinol Metab* 2000;55-9.

3863 Tode T, Kikuchi Y, Hirata J, et al. Effect of Korean red ginseng on psychological functions in patients with severe climacteric syndromes. *Int J Gynaecol Obstet* 1999;67:169-74.

3864 Rabkin JG, Ferrando SJ, Wagner GJ, Rabkin R. DHEA treatment for HIV positive patients: effects on mood, androgenic and anabolic parameters. *Psychoneuroendocrinol* 2000;25:53-68.

3865 Dyner TS, Lang W, Geaga J, et al. An open-label, dose-escalation trial of oral dehydroepiandrosterone tolerance and pharmacokinetics in patients with HIV disease. *J Acq Immun Def Synd* 1993;6:459-65.

3866 Henderson E, Yang JY, Schwartz A. Dehydroepiandrosterone (DHEA) and synthetic DHEA analogs are modest inhibitors of HIV-1 IIIB replication. *AIDS Res Hum Retroviruses* 1992;8:625-31.

3867 Christeff N, Gherbi N, Mammes O, et al. Serum cortisol and DHEA concentrations during HIV infection. *Psychoneuroendocrinol* 1997;22:S11-8.

3868 Ruhnau KJ, Meissner HP, Finn JR, et al. Effects of 3-week oral treatment with the antioxidant thioctic acid (alpha-lipoic acid) in symptomatic diabetic polyneuropathy. *Diabet Med* 1999;16:1040-3.

3869 Sachse G, Willms B. Efficacy of thioctic acid in the therapy of peripheral diabetic neuropathy. *Hormone Metab Res Suppl* 1980;9:105-7.

3870 Gleiter CH, Schreeb KH, Freudenthaler S, et al. Lack of interaction between thioctic acid, glibenclamide and acarbose. *Br J Clin Pharmacol* 1999;48:819-25.

3871 Packer L, Witt EH, Tritschler HJ. Alpha-Lipoic acid as a biological antioxidant. *Free Rad Biol Med* 1995;19:227-50.

3872 Teichert J, Kern J, Tritschler HJ. Investigations on the pharmacokinetics of alpha-lipoic acid in healthy volunteers. *Int J Clin Pharmacol Ther* 1998;36:625-8.

3873 Nagamatsu M, Nickander KK, Schmelzer JD, et al. Lipoic acid improves nerve blood flow, reduces oxidative stress, and improves distal nerve conduction in experimental diabetic neuropathy. *Diabet Care* 1995;18:1160-7.

3874 Jacob S, Henriksen EJ, Tritschler HJ, et al. Improvement of insulin-stimulated glucose-disposal in type 2 diabetes after repeated parenteral administration of thioctic acid. *Exp Clin Endocrinol Diabet* 1996;104:284-8.

3875 Jacob S, Henriksen EJ, Schiemann AL, et al. Enhancement of glucose disposal in patients with type 2 diabetes by alpha-lipoic acid. *Arzneimittelforschung* 1995;45:872-4.

3876 Jacob S, Ruus P, Hermann R, et al. Oral administration of RAC-alpha-lipoic acid modulates insulin sensitivity in patients with type-2 diabetes mellitus: a placebo-controlled, pilot trial. *Free Rad Biol Med* 1999;27:309-14.

3877 Haramaki N, Assadnazari H, Zimmer G, et al. The influence of vitamin E and dihydrolipoic acid on cardiac energy and glutathione status under hypoxia-reoxygenation. *Biochem Mol Biol Int* 1995;37:591-7.

3878 Kishi Y, Schmelzer JD, Yao JK, et al. Alpha-lipoic acid: effect on glucose uptake, sorbitol pathway, and energy metabolism in experimental diabetic neuropathy. *Diabet* 1999;48:2045-51.

3879 Bustamante J, Lodge JK, Marcocci L, et al. Alpha-lipoic acid in liver metabolism and disease. *Free Rad Biol Med* 1998;24:1023-39.

3880 Marshall AW, Graul RS, Morgan MY, Sherlock S. Treatment of alcohol-related liver disease with thioctic acid: a six-month, randomized, double-blind trial. *Gut* 1982;23:1088-93.

3881 Conlon BJ, Aran JM, Erre JP, Smith DW. Attenuation of aminoglycoside-induced cochlear damage with the metabolic antioxidant alpha-lipoic acid. *Hear Res* 1999;128:40-4.

3882 Vilas GL, Aldonatti C, San Martin de Viale LC, Rios de Molina MC. Effect of Alpha-lipoic acid amide on hexachlorobenzene porphyria. *Biochem Mol Biol Int* 1999;47:815-23.

3883 Gurer H, Ozgunes H, Oztezcan S, Ercal N. Antioxidant role of alpha-lipoic acid in lead toxicity. *Free Rad Biol Med* 1999;27:75-81.

3884 Altenkirch H, Stoltenburg-Didinger G, Wagner HM, et al. Effects of lipoic acid in hexacarbon-induced neuropathy. *Neurotoxicol Teratol* 1990;12:619-22.

3885 Fuchs J, Schofer H, Milbradt R, et al. Studies on lipoate effects on blood redox state in human immunodeficiency virus infected patients. *Arzneimittelforschung* 1993;43:1359-62.

3886 Vermeulen EG, Stehouwer CD, Twisk JW, et al. Effect of homocysteine-lowering treatment with folic acid plus vitamin B6 on progression of subclinical atherosclerosis: a randomised, placebo-controlled trial. *Lancet* 2000;355:517-22.

3887 Bostom AG, Garber C. Endpoints for homocysteine-lowering trials. *Lancet* 2000;355:511-2.

3888 Vuorio AF, Gylling H, Turtola H, et al. Stanol ester margarine alone and with simvastatin lowers serum cholesterol in families with familial hypercholesterolemia caused by the FH-north karelia mutation. *Arterioscler Thromb Vasc Biol* 2000;20:500-6.

3889 Becker M, Staab D, Von Bergmann K. Treatment of severe familial hypercholesterolemia in childhood with sitosterol and sitostanol. *J Pediatr* 1993;122:292-6.

3890 American Diabetes Association. Nutrition and principles for people with diabetes mellitus. *Diabetes Care* 2000;23 (suppl 1). http://journal.diabetes.org/fulltext/supplements/diabetescare/supplement/243.html (Accessed 20 January 2000).

3891 Paice JA, Ferrans CE, Lashley FR, et al. Topical capsaicin in the management of HIV-associated peripheral neuropathy. *J Pain Symptom Manage* 2000;19:45-52.

3892 Bloch M, Schmidt PJ, Danaceau MA, et al. Dehydroepiandrosterone treatment of midlife dysthymia. *Biol Psychiatry* 1999;45:1533-41.

3893 Wolf OT, Neumann O, Hellhammer DH, et al. Effects of a two-week physiological dehydroepiandrosterone substitution on cognitive performance and well-being in healthy elderly women and men. *J Clin Endocrinol Metab* 1997;82:2363-7.

3894 MotherNature Encyclopedia. Alpha-lipoic acid website: www.mothernature.com (Accessed 29 February 2000).

3895 MotherNature. Yohimbe products website: www.mothernature.com (Accessed 29 February 2000).

3896 Yusuf S, Dagenais G, Pogue J, et al. Vitamin E supplementation and cardiovascular events in high-risk patients. The heart outcomes prevention evaluation study investigators. *N Engl J Med* 2000;342:154-60.

3897 GISSI-Prevenzione Investigators. Dietary supplementation with n-3 polyunsaturated fatty acids and vitamin E after myocardial infarction: results of the GISSI-Prevenzione trial. *Lancet* 1999;354:447-55.

3898 Stampfer MJ, Hennekens CH, Manson JE, et al. Vitamin E consumption and the risk of coronary disease in women. *N Engl J Med* 1993;328:1444-9.

3899 Lonn E, Yusuf S, Dzavik V, et al. Effects of ramipril and vitamin E on atherosclerosis: the study to evaluate carotid ultrasound changes in patients treated with ramipril and vitamin E (SECURE). *Circulation* 2001;103:919-25.

3900 Peirce A. The American Pharmaceutical Association Practical Guide to Natural Medicines. New York, NY: William Morrow and Co., 1999.

3901 Tyler VE, Brady LR, Robbers JB. Pharmacognosy. Philadelphia: Lea and Fibiger, 1981.

3902 Barlet A, et al. Efficacy of Pygeum africanum extract in the medical therapy of urination disorders due to benign prostatic hyperplasia: evaluation of objective and subjective parameters. A placebo-controlled, double-blind, multicenter study. *Wien Klin Wochenschr* 1990; 102(22):667-73.

3903 Breza J, et al. Efficacy and acceptability of tadenan (Pygeum africanum extract) in the treatment of benign prostatic hyperplasia (BPH): a multicentre trial in central Europe. *Curr Med Res Opin* 1998; 14(3):127-39.

3904 Dufour B, et al. Controlled study of the effects of Pygeum africanum extract on the functional symptoms of prostatic adenoma. *Ann Urol (Paris)* 1984; 18(3):193-5.

3905 Whitmore A. FDA warns consumers against dietary supplement products that may contain Digitalis mislabeled as Plantain. Food and Drug Administration, U.S. Department of the Interior, Washington DC, 1997.

3906 Keith ME, Jeejeebhoy KN, Langer A, et al. A controlled clinical trial of vitamin E supplementation in patients with congestive heart failure. +2001 Feb;73(2):219-24.

3907 Collaborative Group of the Primary Prevention Project. Low-dose aspirin and vitamin E in people at cardiovascular risk: a randomised trial in general practice. *Lancet* 2001 Jan 13;357(9250):89-95.

3908 Kleijnen J. Evening primrose oil. *BMJ* 1994;309:824-825.

3909 Head RJ, McLennan PL, Raederstorff D, et al. Prevention of nerve conduction deficit in diabetic rats by polyunsaturated fatty acids. *Am J Clin Nutr* 2000;71:386S-392S.

3910 Khaw KT, Bingham S, Welch A, et al. Relation between plasma ascorbic acid and mortality in men and women in EPIC-Norfolk prospective study: a prospective population study. European Prospective Investigation into Cancer and Nutrition. *Lancet* 2001;357:657-63.

3911 Singer P, Wirth M, Berger I. A possible contribution of decrease in free fatty acids to low serum triglyceride levels after diets supplemented with n-6 and n-3 polyunsaturated fatty acids. *Atherosclerosis* 1990; 83(2-3):167-75.

3912 Fischer S, et al. Results of linseed oil and olive oil therapy in hyperlipoproteinemia patients. *Dtsch Z Verdau Stoffwechselkr* 1984; 44(5):245-51.

3913 Castner JL, Timme SL, Duke JA. A Field Guide to Medicinal and Useful Plants of the Upper Amazon. Gainesville, FL: Feline Press, 1998.

3914 Debourdeau PM, Djezzar S, Estival JL, et al. Life-threatening eosinophilic pleuropericardial effusion related to vitamins B5 and H. *Ann Pharmacother* 2001;35:424-426.

3915 National Academy of Science, Institute of Medicine. Dietary Reference Intakes for Thiamin, Riboflavin, Niacin, Vitamin B6, Folate, Vitamin B12, Pantothenic Acid, Biotin, and Choline. http://books.nap.edu/books/ 0309065542/html/384.html#page_middle (Accessed 27 July 2001).

3916 Manabe H, et al. Effects of Catuaba extracts on microbial and HIV infection. *In Vivo* 1992; 6(2):161-5.

3917 Rain Tree Website, URL: www.rain-tree.com/ catuaba.htm. (Accessed 23 July 1999).

3918 Taylor L. Herbal Secrets of the Rainforest. Rocklin, CA: Prima Publishing, 1998.

3919 Agricultural Research Service. Dr. Duke's Phytochemical and Ethnobotanical Databases. URL: www.ars-grin.gov/duke/.

3920 Burkill JD. A Dictionary of the Economic Products of the Malay Peninsula. Kuala Lumpur: Art Printing Works, 1966.

3921 Calixto JB. Antispasmodic effects of an alkaloid extracted from Phyllanthus sellowianus: A comparative study with papaverine. *Braz J Med Biol Res* 1984; 17:313-21. [primary reference in Taylor].

3923 Calixto JB, et al. A review of the plants of the genus Phyllanthus: their chemistry, pharmacology, and therapeutic potential. *Med Res Rev* 1998; 18(4):225-58.

3924 Milne A, et al. Failure of New Zealand hepatitis B carriers to respond to Phyllanthus amarus. *N Z Med J* 1994; 107(980):243.

3925 Wang M, et al. Herbs of the genus Phyllanthus in the treatment of chronic hepatitis B: observations with three preparations from different geographic sites. *J Lab Clin Med* 1995; 126(4):350-2.

3927 Qian-Cutrone J, et al. Niruriside, a new HIV REV/RRE binding inhibitor from Phyllanthus niruri. *J Nat Prod* 1996; 59(2):196-9.

3928 Srividya N, Periwal S. Diuretic, hypotensive and hypoglycaemic effect of Phyllanthus amarus. *Indian J Exp Biol* 1995; 33:861-4.

3929 Wilkins AL, et al. Photosensitivity in South Africa. IX. Structure elucidation of a beta-glucosidase-treated saponin from Tribulus terrestis, and the identification of saponin chemotypes of South African T. terrestis. *Onderstepoort Journal Veterinary Res* 1996; 63:327-34.

3931 Wang B, Ma L, Liu T. 406 cases of angina pectoris in coronary heart disease treated with saponin of Tribulus terrestis. *Chung Hsi I Chieh Ho Tsa Chih* 1990; 10(2):85-7, 68.

3932 Harvey J, Colin-Jones DG. Mistletoe hepatitis. *Br Med J (Clin Res Ed)* 1981; 282:186-7.

3933 Rimm EB, Stampfer MJ, Ascherio A, et al. Vitamin E consumption and the risk of coronary heart disease in men. *N Engl J Med* 1993;328:1450-6.

3934 Kushi LH, Folsom AR, Prineas RJ, et al. Dietary antioxidant vitamins and death from coronary heart disease in postmenopausal women. *N Engl J Med* 1996;334:1156-62.

3935 Virtamo J, Rapola JM, Ripatti S, et al. Effect of vitamin E and beta carotene on the incidence of primary nonfatal myocardial infarction and fatal coronary heart disease. *Arch Intern Med* 1998;158:668-75.

3936 Stephens NG, Parsons A, Schofield PM, et al. Randomised controlled trial of vitamin E in patients with coronary disease: Cambridge Heart Antioxidant Study. *Lancet* 1996;347:781-6.

3937 Rapola JM, Virtamo J, Ripatti S, et al. Randomised trial of alpha-tocopherol and beta-carotene supplements on incidence of major coronary events in men with previous myocardial infarction. *Lancet* 1997;349:1715-20.

3938 Losonczy KG, Harris TB, Havlik RJ. Vitamin E and vitamin C supplement use and risk of all-cause and coronary heart disease mortality in older persons:epidemiologic studies of the elderly. *Am J Clin Nutr* 1996;64:190-6.

3939 Anon. Vitamin E health claim falls short of significant scientific agreement - FDA. FDC Reports: The Tan Sheet. January 24, 2000;10.

3940 Emmert DH, Kirchner JT. The role of vitamin E in the prevention of heart disease. *Arch Fam Med* 1999;8:537-42.

3942 Adler LA, Edson R, Lavori P, et al. Long-term treatment effects of vitamin E for tardive dyskinesia. *Biol Psychiatry* 1998;43:868-72.

3943 Sajjad SH. Vitamin E in the treatment of tardive dyskinesia: a preliminary study over 7 months at different doses. *Int Clin Psychopharmacol* 1998;13:147-55.

3944 Lohr JB, Caligiuri MP. A double-blind, placebo-controlled study of vitamin E treatment of tardive dyskinesia. *J Clin Psychiatry* 1996;57:167-73.

3945 Shriqui CL, Bradwejn J, Annable L, Jones BD. Vitamin E in the treatment of tardive dyskinesia: a double-blind, placebo-controlled study. *Am J Psychiatry* 1992;149:391-3.

3946 Dorfman-Etrog P, Hermesh H, Prilipko L, et al. The effect of vitamin E addition to acute neuroleptic treatment on the emergence of extrapyramidal side effects in schizophrenic patients: an open label study. *Eur Neuropsychopharmacol* 1999;9:475-7.

3947 Boomershine KH, Shelton PS, Boomershine JE. Vitamin E in the treatment of tardive dyskinesia. *Ann Pharmacother* 1999;33:1195-202.

3948 Dabiri LM, Pasta D, Darby JK, Mosbacher D. Effectiveness of vitamin E for treatment of long-term tardive dyskinesia. *Am J Psychiatry* 1994;151:925-6.

3949 The Alpha-Tocopherol, Beta Carotene Cancer Prevention Study Group. The effect of vitamin E and beta carotene on the incidence of lung cancer and other cancers in male smokers. *N Engl J Med* 1994;330:1029-35.

3951 Liede K, Hietanen J, Saxen L, et al. Long-term supplementation with alpha-tocopherol and beta-carotene and prevalence of oral mucosal lesions in smokers. *Oral Dis* 1998;4:78-83.

3952 Pantuck EJ, Pantuck CB, Anderson KE, et al. Effect of brussels sprouts and cabbage on drug conjugation. *Clin Pharmacol Ther* 1984;35:161-169.

REFERENCES

3953 Malila N, Virtamo J, Virtanen M, et al. The effect of alpha-tocopherol and beta-carotene supplementation on colorectal adenomas in middle-aged male smokers. *Cancer Epidemiol Biomarkers Prev* 1999;8:489-93.

3954 Roncucci L, Di Donato P, Carati L, et al. Antioxidant vitamins or lactulose for the prevention of the recurrence of colorectal adenomas. Colorectal Cancer Study Group of the Univ of Modena and the Health Care Dist 16. *Dis Colon Rectum* 1993;36:227-34.

3955 Greenberg ER, Baron JA, Tosteson TD, et al. A clinical trial of antioxidant vitamins to prevent colorectal adenoma. Polyp Prevention Study Group. *N Engl J Med* 1994;331:141-7.

3956 Paganelli GM, Biasco G, Brandi G, et al. Effect of vitamin A, C, and E supplementation on rectal cell proliferation in patients with colorectal adenomas. *J Natl Cancer Inst* 1992;84:47-51.

3957 McKeown-Eyssen G, Holloway C, Jazmaji V, et al. A randomized trial of vitamins C and E in the prevention of recurrence of colorectal polyps. *Cancer Res* 1988;48:4701-5.

3958 White E, Shannon JS, Patterson RE. Relationship between vitamin and calcium supplement use and colon cancer. *Cancer Epidemiol Biomarkers Prev* 1997;6:769-74.

3959 Heinonen OP, Albanes D, Virtamo J, et al. Prostate cancer and supplementation with alpha-tocopherol and beta-carotene: incidence and mortality in a controlled trial. *J Natl Cancer Inst* 1998;90:440-6.

3960 Varis K, Taylor PR, Sipponen P, et al. Gastric cancer and premalignant lesions in atrophic gastritis: a controlled trial on the effect of supplementation with alpha-tocopherol and beta-carotene. The Helsinki Gastritis Study Group. *Scand J Gastroenterol* 1998;33:294-300.

3961 Rautalahti MT, Virtamo JR, Taylor PR, et al. The effects of supplementation with alpha-tocopherol and beta-carotene on the incidence and mortality of carcinoma of the pancreas in a randomized, controlled trial. *Cancer* 1999;86:37-42.

3962 Slattery ML, Benson J, Curtin K, et al. Carotenoids and colon cancer. *Am J Clin Nutr* 2000;71:575-82.

3963 Steinmetz KA, Potter JD. Vegetables, fruit, and cancer. I. Epidemiology. *Cancer Causes Control* 1991;2:325-57.

3964 Slattery ML, Potter JD, Coates A, et al. Plant foods and colon cancer: an assessment of specific foods and their related nutrients (United States). *Cancer Causes Control* 1997;8:575-90.

3965 Cohen AJ, Bartlik B. Ginkgo biloba for antidepressant-induced sexual dysfunction. *J Sex Marital Ther* 1998;24:139-43.

3966 Balon R. Ginkgo biloba for antidepressant-induced sexual dysfunction? *J Sex Marital Ther* 1999;25:1-2.

3967 Ellison JM, DeLuca P. Fluoxetine-induced genital anesthesia relieved by Ginkgo biloba extract. *J Clin Psychiatry* 1998;59:199-200.

3968 Balon R. The effects of antidepressants on human sexuality: diagnosis and management update 1999. *Primary Psychiatry* 1999;6:40-54.

3969 Levine SB. Caution Recommended. *J Sex Marital Ther* 1999;25:2-5.

3970 Jacobsen FM. Fluoxetine-induced sexual dysfunction and an open trial of yohimbine. *J Clin Psychiatry* 1992;53:119-22.

3971 Hollander E, McCarley A. Yohimbine treatment of sexual side effects induced by serotonin reuptake blockers. *J Clin Psychiatry* 1992;53:207-9.

3972 Harvey KV, Balon R. Clinical implications of antidepressant drug effects on sexual function. *Ann Clin Psychiatry* 1995;7:189-201.

3973 Balon R. The effects of anitdepressants on human sexuality: diagnosis and management update 1999. *Primary Psychiatry* 1999;6:40-54.

3974 Redondo P, Bauza A. Topical N-acetylcysteine for lamellar ichthyosis. *Lancet* 1999;354:1880.

3975 Sekharam M, Trotti A, Cunnick JM, Wu J. Suppression of fibroblast cell cycle progression in G1 phase by N-acetylcysteine. *Toxicol Appl Pharmacol* 1998;149:210-6.

3976 Hakkak R, Korourian S, Shelnutt SR, et al. Diets containing whey proteins or soy protein isolate protect against 7,12-dimethylbenz(a)anthracene-induced mammary tumors in female rats. *Cancer Epidemiol Biomarkers Prev* 2000;9:113-7.

3977 FDA. Federal Register website: http://www.accessdata.fda.gov/scripts/oc/ohrms/index.cfm (Accessed 9 March 2000).

3978 Tham DM, Gardner CD, Haskell WL. Clinical review 97: Potential health benefits of dietary phytoestrogens: a review of the clinical, epidemiological, and mechanistic evidence. *J Clin Endocrinol Metab* 1998;83:2223-35.

3979 Setchell KD. Phytoestrogens: the biochemistry, physiology, and implications for human health of soy isoflavones. *Am J Clin Nutr* 1998;68:1333S-46S.

3980 McMichael-Phillips DF, Harding C, Morton M, et al. Effects of soy-protein supplementation on epithelial proliferation in the histologically normal human breast. *Am J Clin Nutr* 1998;68:1431S-5S.

3981 Petrakis NL, Barnes S, King EB, et al. Stimulatory influence of soy protein isolate on breast secretion in pre- and postmenopausal women. *Cancer Epidemiol Biomarkers Prev* 1996;5:785-94.

3982 Setchell KD. Absorption and metabolism of soy isoflavones-from food to dietary supplements and adults to infants. *J Nutr* 2000;130:654S-5S.

3983 Barnes S, Kim H, Darley-Usmar V, et al. Beyond ERalpha and ERbeta: Estrogen receptor binding is only part of the isoflavone story. *J Nutr* 2000;130:656S-7S.

3984 Evans BA, Griffiths K, Morton MS. Inhibition of 5 alpha-reductase in genital skin fibroblasts and prostate tissue by dietary lignans and isoflavonoids. *J Endocrinol* 1995;147:295-302.

3985 Adlercreutz H, Mazur W, Bartels P, et al. Phytoestrogens and prostate disease. *J Nutr* 2000;130:658S-9S.

3986 Brzezinski A, Adlercreutz H, Sheoul R, et al. Short-term effects of phytoestrogen-rich diet on postmenopausal women. *Menopause* 1997;4:89-94.

3987 Kurzer M. Hormonal effects of soy isoflavones: Studies in premenopausal and postmenopausal women. *J Nutr* 2000;130:660-1.

3988 Baird DD, Umbach DM, Lansdell L, et al. Dietary intervention study to assess estrogenicity of dietary soy among postmenopausal women. *J Clin Endocrinol Metab* 1995;80:1685-90.

3989 Duncan AM, Underhill KE, Xu X, et al. Modest hormonal effects of soy isoflavones in postmenopausal women. *J Clin Endocrinol Metab* 1999;84:3479-84.

3990 Ginsburg J, Prelevic GM. Lack of significant hormonal

effects and controlled trials of phyto-oestrogens. *Lancet* 2000;355:163-4.

3991 Quella SK, Loprinzi CL, Barton DL, et al. Evaluation of soy phytoestrogens for the treatment of hot flashes in breast cancer survivors: a North Central Cancer Treatment Group trial. *J Clin Oncol* 2000;18:1068.

3992 Anthony MS. Soy and cardiovascular disease: Cholesterol lowering and beyond. *J Nutr* 2000;130:662S-3S.

3993 Lockwood K, Moesgaard S, Yamamoto T, Folkers K. Progress on therapy of breast cancer with vitamin Q10 and the regression of metastases. *Biochem Biophys Res Commun* 1995;212:172-177.

3994 Hargreaves DF, Potten CS, Harding C, et al. Two-week dietary soy supplementation has an estrogenic effect on normal premenopausal breast. *J Clin Endocrinol Metab* 1999;84:4017-24.

3995 Lockwood K, Moesgaard S, Folkers K. Partial and complete regression of breast cancer in patients in relation to dosage of coenzyme Q10. *Biochem Biophys Res Commun* 1994;199:1504-1508.

3996 Poortmans JR, Francaux M. Long-term oral creatine supplementation does not impair renal function in healthy athletes. *Med Sci Sports Exerc* 1999;31:1108-10.

3997 Juhn MS, Tarnopolsky M. Potential side effects of oral creatine supplementation: a critical review. *Clin J Sport Med* 1998;8:298-304.

3998 Graham AS, Hatton RC. Creatine: a review of efficacy and safety. J Am Pharm Assoc (Wash) 1999;39:803-10.

3999 Pepping J. Creatine. *Am J Health Syst Pharm* 1999;56:1608-10.

4000 Medina JH, et al. Overview-flavonoids: a new family of benzodiazepine receptor ligands. *Neurochem Res* 1997; 22(4): 419-25.

4001 Salgueiro JB, et al. Anxiolytic natural and synthetic flavonoid ligands of the central benzodiazepine receptor have no effect on memory tasks in rats. *Pharmacol Biochem Behav,* 1997; 58(4): 887-91.

4002 Rommelspacher H, et al. (1-methyl-beta-carboline) is a natural inhibitor of monoamine oxidase type A in rats. *Eur J Pharmacol* 24 Jan. 1994; 252(1): 51-9.

4003 Anon. Licensed fish-oil concentrate versus cod-liver oil. *Lancet* 1987;2(8556):453.

4004 Henderson MJ, Jones RG. Cod liver oil or bust. *Lancet* 1987;2(8553):274-5.

4005 Landymore RW, MacAulay M, Sheridan B, Cameron C. Comparison of cod-liver oil and aspirin-dipyridamole for the prevention of intimal hyperplasia in autologous vein grafts. *Ann Thorac Surg* 1986;41(1):54-7.

4006 Neef H, et al. Inhibitory effects of Galega officinalis on glucose transport across monolayers of human intestinal epithelial cells (Caco-2). *Pharm Pharmacol Lett* 1996;6(2):86-9.

4007 Atanasov AT. Effect of Galega officinalis L. extract on platelet aggregation in rats. *J Herbs Spices Med Plants* 1995; 3(3): 71-6.

4008 Huxtable CR, Dorling RR, Colegate SM. Identification of galegine, an isoprenyl guanidine, as the toxic principle of Schoenus asperocarpus (poison sedge). *Aust Vet J* 1993;70(5):169-71.

4009 Dukes JA. CRC Handbook of Medicinal Herbs. first ed. Boca Raton, FL: CRC Press, Inc., 1985.

4010 Scarlat M, et al. Experimental anti-ulcer activity of Veronica officinalis L. extracts. *J Ethnopharmacol* 1985;

13(2): 157-63.

4011 Yoshioka T, Fujii E, Endo M, et al. Antiinflammatory potency of dehydrocurdione, a zedoary-derived sesquiterpene. *Inflamm Res* 1998; 47(12):476-81.

4012 Matsuda H, Ninomiya K, Morikawa T, et al. Inhibitory effect and action mechanism of sesquiterpenes from Zedoariae Rhizoma on D-galactosamine/ lipopolysaccharide-induced liver injury. *Bioorg Med Chem Lett* 1998; 8(4):339-44.

4013 Gupta SK, Banerjee AB, Achari B. Isolation of Ethyl p-methoxycinnamate, the major antifungal principle of Curcumba zedoaria. *Lloydia* 1976; 39(4):218-22.

4014 Syu WJ, Shen CC, Don MJ, et al. Cytotoxicity of curcuminoids and some novel compounds from Curcuma zedoaria. *J Nat Prod* 1998; 61(12):1531-4.

4015 Latif MA, Morris TR, Miah AH, et al. Toxicity of shoti (Indian arrowroot: Curcuma zedoaria) for rats and chicks. *Br J Nutr* 1979; 41(1):57-63.

4016 Wu D, Meydani M, Leka LS, et al. Effect of dietary supplementation with black currant seed oil on the immune response of healthy elderly subjects. *Am J Clin Nutr* 1999;70:536-43.

4017 Consumer Lab. www.consumerlab.com/results/ phytoestrogens2.asp (Accessed 16 August 2001).

4018 Leclercq I, Desager JP, Horsmans Y. Inhibition of chlorzoxazone metabolism, a clinical probe for CYP2E1, by a single ingestion of watercress. *Clin Pharmacol Ther* 1998; 64:144-9.

4019 Hecht SS, Chung FL, Richie JP Jr., et al. Effects of watercress consumption on metabolism of a tobacco-specific lung carcinogen in smokers. *Cancer Epidemiol Biomarkers Prev* 1995; 4:877-84.

4020 Habtemariam S. Cistifolin, an integrin-dependent cell adhesion blocker from the anti- rheumatic herbal drug, gravel root (rhizome of Eupatorium purpureum). *Planta Med* 1998 Dec;64(8):683-5.

4021 WHO working group. Pyrrolizidine alkaloids. Environmental Health Criteria, 80. WHO: Geneva, 1988.

4022 Landymore RW, Kinley CE, Cooper JH, et al. Cod-liver oil in the prevention of intimal hyperplasia in autogenous vein grafts used for arterial bypass. *J Thorac Cardiovasc Surg* 1985;89(3):351-7.

4023 Dahlquist I, Fregert S. Contact allergy to atranorin in lichens and perfumes. *Contact Dermatitis* 1980; 6:111-9.

4024 Lauterwein M, Oethinger M, Belsner K, et al. In vitro activities of the lichen secondary metabolites vulpinic acid, (+)-usnic acid, and (-)-usnic acid against aerobic and anaerobic microorganisms. *Antimicrob Agents Chemother* 1995; 39:2541-3.

4025 Brox JH, Killie JE, Gunnes S, Nordoy A. The effect of cod liver oil and corn oil on platelets and vessel wall in man. *Thromb Haemost.* 1981;46(3):604-11.

4026 Sanders TA, Vickers M, Haines AP. Effect on blood lipids and haemostasis of a supplement of cod-liver oil, rich in eicosapentainoic and docosahaenoic acids, in healthy young men. *Clin Sci (Colch)* 1981;61(3):317-24.

4027 Rubel DM, Freeman S, Southwell IA. Tea tree oil allergy: what is the offending agent? Report of three cases of tea tree oil allergy and review of the literature. *Australas J Dermatol* 1998;39:244-7.

4028 Carson CF, Riley TV, Cookson BD. Efficacy and safety of tea tree oil as a topical antimicrobial agent. *J Hosp Infect* 1998;40:175-8.

4029 Bhushan M, Beck MH. Allergic contact dermatitis from

tea tree oil in a wart paint. *Contact Dermatitis* 1997;36:117-8.

4030 Del Beccaro MA. Melaleuca oil poisoning in a 17-month old. *Vet Hum Toxicol* 1995;37:557-8.

4031 Tong MM, Altman PM, Barnetson RS. Tea tree oil in the treatment of tinea pedis. *Australas J Dermatol* 1992;33:145-9.

4033 Goncalo S. Contact sensitivity to lichens and compositae in Frullania dermatitis. *Contact Dermatitis* 1987 Feb;16(2):84-6.

4034 Goncalo S, Cabral F, Goncalo M. Contact sensitivity to oak moss. *Contact Dermatitis* 1988;19:355-7.

4039 Thune P, Solberg Y, McFadden N, et al. Perfume allergy due to oak moss and other lichens. *Contact Dermatitis* 1982;8:396-400.

4040 al-Bekairi AM, Qureshi S, Chaudhry MA, et al. Mitodepressive, clastogenic and biochemical effects of (+)-usnic acid in mice. *J Ethnopharmacol* 1991 Jul;33(3):217-20.

4041 Chen CP, Lin CC, Namba T. Screening of Taiwanese crude drugs for antibacterial activity against Streptococcus mutans. *J Ethnopharmacol* 1989;27:285-95.

4042 Akihisa T, Yasukawa K, Kimura Y, et al. Five D:C-friedo-oleanane triterpenes from the seeds of Trichosanthes kirilowii Maxim. and their anti-inflammatory effects. *Chem Pharm Bull (Tokyo)* 1994; 42:1101-5.

4043 Ozaki Y, Xing L, Satake M. Anti-inflammatory effect of Trichosanthes kirilowii Maxim, and its effective parts. *Biol Pharm Bull* 1996; 19:1046-8.

4044 Takano F, Yoshizaki F, Suzuki K, et al. Anti-ulcer effects of Trichosanthes fruits. *Chem Pharm Bull (Tokyo)* 1990; 38:1313-6.

4045 Hikino H, Yoshizawa M, Suzuki Y, et al. Isolation and hypoglycemic activity of trichosans A, B, C, D, and E: glycans of Trichosanthes kirilowii roots. *Planta Med* 1989; 55: 349-350.

4046 Tao XL, Sun Y, Dong Y, et al. A prospective, controlled, double-blind, cross-over study of tripterygium wilfodii hook F in treatment of rheumatoid arthritis. *Chin Med J (Engl)* 1989; 102:327-32.

4047 Nagashima G, Suzuki R, et al. Meningoencephalocele associated with Tripterygium wilfordii treatment. *Pediatr Neurosurg* 1997; 27:45-8.

4048 Chen K, Shi QA, Fujioka T, et al. Anti-AIDS agents, 4. Tripterifordin, a novel anti-HIV principle from Tripterygium wilfordii: isolation and structural elucidation. *J Nat Prod* 1992;55:88-92.

4049 Chen K, Shi Q, Kashiwada Y, et al. Anti-aids agents, 6. Salaspermic acid, an anti-HIV principle from Tripterygium wilfordii, and the structure-activity correlation with its related compounds. *J Nat Prod* 1992; 55:340-6.

4050 Attaguile G, Caruso A, Pennisi G, et al. Gastroprotective effect of aqueous extract of Cistus incanus L. in rats. *Pharmacol Res* 1995; 3: 29-32.

4051 Liu FJ, Sun DM. Studies on the active constituents lowering blood lipid in beeswax. *J Chin Mater Med (Zhongguo Zhongyao Zazhi)* 1996;21:553-4.

4052 Carbajal D, Molina V, Valdes S, et al. Anti-inflammatory activity of D-002: an active product isolated from beeswax. *Prostaglandins Leukot Essent Fatty Acids* 1998;59: 235-8.

4053 Carbajal D, Molina V, Valdes S, et al. Possible cytoprotective mechanism in rats of D-002, an anti-ulcerogenic product isolated from beeswax. *J Pharm Pharmacol* 1996; 48: 858-60.

4054 Carbajal D, Molina V, Valdes S, et al. Anti-ulcer activity of higher primary alcohols of beeswax. *J Pharm Pharmacol* 1995;47: 731-3.

4058 Roesyanto-Mahadi ID, Geursen-Reitsma AM, van Joost T, et al. Sensitization to fragrance materials in Indonesian cosmetics. *Contact Dermatitis* 1990; 22: 212-7.

4059 Arras G, Grella GE. Wild thyme, Thymus capitatus, essential oil seasonal changes and antimycotic activity. *J Hortic Sci* 1992;67:197-202.

4060 Thompson DP. Effect of phenolic compounds on mycelial growth of Fusarium and Penicillium species. *J Food Protection* 1997;60(10):1262-4.

4062 Stiles JC, Sparks W, Ronzio RA. The inhibition of Candida albicans by Oregano. *J Appl Nutrition* 1995;47:96-102.

4063 Viollon C, Chaumont JP. Antifungal properties of essential oils and their main components upon Cryptococcus neoformans. *Mycopathologia* 1994; 128: 151-3.

4064 Osawa K, Matsumoto T, Maruyama T, et al. Studies of the antibacterial activity of plant extracts and their constituents against periodontopathic bacteria. *Bull Tokyo Dent Coll* 1990; 31:17-21.

4065 Ultee A, Gorris LG, Smid EJ. Bactericidal activity of carvacrol towards the food-borne pathogen Bacillus cereus. *J Appl Microbiol* 1998; 85:211-8.

4066 Helander IM, Alakomi H-L, Latva-Kala K, et al. Characterization of the action of selected essential oil components on gram-negative bacteria. *J Agricultural and Food Chemistry* 1998; 46: 3590-5.

4067 Aeschbach R, Loliger J, Scott BC. Antioxidant actions of thymol, carvacrol, 6-gingerol, zingerone and hydroxytyrosol. *Food Chem Toxicol* 1994; 32: 31-6.

4068 Eastwood MA, Brydon WG, Anderson DM, et al. The effects of dietary gum tragacanth in man. *Toxicol Lett* 1984; 21: 73-81.

4069 Jenkins DJ, Wolever TM, Leeds AR, et al. Dietary fibres, fibre analogues, and glucose tolerance: importance of viscosity. *Br Med J* 1978; 1: 1392-4.

4070 Smee DF, Sidwell RW, Huffman JH, et al. Antiviral activities of tragacanthin polysaccharides on Punta Toro virus infections in mice. *Chemotherapy* 1996;42:286-93.

4071 FAO and WHO working groups. Tragacanth gum. *WHO Food Additives Series*, 1985;20:253-62.

4072 Anonymous. Final report on the safety assessment of Tragacanth Gum. *J Am Coll Toxicol* 1987;6:1-22.

4073 Vaswani SK, Hamilton RG, Carey RN, et al. Anaphylaxis recurrent urticaria and angioedema from grape hypersensitivity. *J All Clin Immunol* 1998;101(1 Part 2):S31.

4074 BIBRA working group. Anthocyanins. Toxicity profile. *BIBRA Toxicol Int* 1991;6.

4075 Garcia Ortiz JC, Cosmes Martin P, Lopez-Asunsolo A. Melon sensitivity shares allergens with Plantago and grass pollens. *Allergy (Copenhagen)* 1995;50:269-73.

4076 Hollis S. The Country Diary Herbal. New York, NY: Henry Holt and Company, 1990.

4077 Tyler VE, Brady LR, Robbers JE. Pharmacognosy, 9th ed. Philadelphia, PA: Lea & Febiger, 1988.

4078 Foster S, Duke JA. The Peterson Field Guide to Medicinal Plants: Eastern and Central North America.

Boston, MA: Houghton Mifflin Co., 1990.

4079 Eigenmann PA, Burks AW, Bannon GA, et al. Identification of unique peanut and soy allergens in sera adsorbed with cross-reacting antibodies. *J Allergy Clin Immunol* 1996; 98(5 Pt 1): 969-78.

4080 Bardare M, Magnolfi C, Zani G. Soy sensitivity: personal observation on 71 children with food intolerance. *Allerg Immunol (Paris)* 1988; 20:63-6.

4081 Van Hevelingen A. The orris iris. *The Herb Companion* 1992;4:32-5.

4082 Schmidt GD, Roberts LS. Foundations of Parasitology. St Louis: Times Mirror / Mosby College Publ, 1985.

4083 National Archives and Records Administration. Code of Federal Regulations: 21 CFR 182.10. www.access.gpo.gov/nara/cfr/ (Accessed 1 August 1999).

4084 Drugs in Pregnancy and Lactation. 4th ed. Baltimore, MD: Williams & Wilkens, 1994.

4085 Lichtenstein AH, Ausman LM, Jalbert SM, et al. Effects of different forms of dietary hydrogenated fats on serum lipoprotein cholesterol levels. *N Engl J Med* 1999;340: 1933-40.

4086 Weststrate JA, Meijer GW. Plant sterol-enriched margarines and reduction of plasma total- and LDL-cholesterol concentrations in normocholesterolaemic and mildly hypercholesterolaemic subjects. *Eur J Clin Nutr* 1998;52:334-43.

4087 FDA. Center for Science in the Public Interest. News Release: Statement on FDA Review of Take Control Margarine. May 5, 1999. Retrieved from URL: www.fda.gov. (Accessed 5 May 1999).

4089 Moyad MA, Brumfield SK, Pienta KJ. Vitamin E, alpha- and gamma-tocopherol, and prostate cancer. *Semin Urol Oncol* 1999;17:85-90.

4092 Li D, Saldeen T, Mehta JL. Gamma-tocopherol decreases ox-LDL-mediated activation of nuclear factor- kappaB and apoptosis in human coronary artery endothelial cells. *Biochem Biophys Res Commun* 1999;259:157-61.

4096 Aberg F, Appelkvist EL, Broijersen A, et al. Gemfibrozil-induced decrease in serum ubiquinone and alpha- and gamma- tocopherol levels in men with combined hyperlipidaemia. *Eur J Clin Invest* 1998;28:235-42.

4097 Sadrzadeh SM, Nanji AA, Meydani M. Effect of chronic ethanol feeding on plasma and liver alpha- and gamma-tocopherol levels in normal and vitamin E-deficient rats. Relationship to lipid peroxidation. *Biochem Pharmacol* 1994;47(11):2005-10.

4098 Takahashi O. Haemorrhagic toxicity of a large dose of alpha-, beta-, gamma- and delta-tocopherols, ubiquinone, beta-carotene, retinol acetate and L-ascorbic acid in the rat. *Food Chem Toxicol* 1995;33:121-8.

4100 Scholz E, Rimpler R. Proanthocyanidins from Krameria triandra root. *Planta Med* 1989;55(4):379-84.

4101 The Bantam Medical Dictionary. rev ed. New York, NY: Bantam Books, 1990.

4102 Covington TR, Berardi RR, Young LL. Handbook of Nonprescription Drugs. 11th ed. Washington, DC: American Pharmaceutical Assn, 1996.

4104 Abdullaev FI, Gonzalez de Mejia E. Antitumor activity of natural substances: lectins and saffron. *Arch Latinoam Nutr* 1997; 47(3): 195-202.

4105 Nair SC, Pannikar B, Panikkar KR. Antitumor activity of Saffron (Crocus sativus). *Cancer Lett* 1991;57(2):109-14.

4106 Feo F, et al. Occupational Allergy to Saffron Workers. *Allergy* 1997; 52(6): 633-41.

4107 Wuthrich B, Schmid-Grendelmeyer P, Lundberg M. Anaphylaxis to saffron. *Allergy* 1997;52(4):476-7.

4109 Miller TL, et al. Binding of crocetin to plasma albumin. *J Pharm Sci* 1982; 71(2): 173-7.

4110 Grainer JL, Jones JR. The Use of Crocetin in Experimental Atherosclerosis. *Experientia* 1975;31:548-9.

4111 Vandenplas O, Depelchin S, Toussaint G, et al. Occupational asthma caused by sarsaparilla root dust. *J Allergy Clin Immunol* 1996;97(6):1416-8.

4112 Ahn YO. Diet and stomach cancer in Korea. *Int J Cancer,* 1997;Suppl 10:7-9.

4113 Archana R, Namasivayam A. Antistressor effect of Withania somnifera. *J Ethnopharmacol* 1999;64(1):91-3.

4114 Davis L, Kuttan G. Suppressive effect of cyclophosphamide-induced toxicity by Withania somnifera extract in mice. *J Ethnopharmacol* 1998;62(3):209-14.

4116 Bhattacharya SK, Satyan KS, Ghosal S. Antioxidant activity of glycowithanolides from Withania somnifera. *Indian J Exp Biol* 1997; 35(3):236-9.

4117 Shen HD, Chang LY, Gong YJ, et al. A monoclonal antibody against ragweed pollen cross-reacting with yellow dock pollen. *Chung Hua Min Kuo Wei Sheng Wu Chi Mien I Hsueh Tsa Chih* 1985;18(4):232-9.

4118 Liu YL, Ho DK, Cassady JM, et al. Isolation of potential cancer chemopreventive agents from Eriodictyon californicum. *J Nat Prod* 1992;55(3):357-63.

4119 Younos C, Rolland A, Fleurentin J, et al. Analgesic and behavioural effects of Morinda citrifolia. *Planta Med* 1990;56(5):430-4.

4120 Nakano M, Nakashima H, Itoh Y. Anti-human immunodeficiency virus activity of oligosaccharides from rooibos tea (Aspalathus linearis) extracts in vitro. *Leukemia* 1997;11(3):128-30.

4121 Nakano M, Itoh Y, Mizuno T, Nakashima H. Polysaccharide from Aspalathus linearis with strong anti-HIV activity. *Biosci Biotechnol Biochem* 1997;61(2):267-71.

4122 Shimoi K, Masuda S, Shen B, et al. Radioprotective effects of antioxidative plant flavonoids in mice. *Mutat Res* 1996;350(1):153-61.

4123 Inanami O, Asanuma T, Inukai N, et al. The suppression of age-related accumulation of lipid peroxides in rat brain by administration of Rooibos tea (Aspalathus linearis). *Neurosci Lett* 1995;196(1-2):85-8.

4124 Sanchez de Rojas VR, Somoza B, Ortega T, et al. Vasodilatory effect in rat aorta of eriodictyol obtained from Satureja obovata. *Planta Med* 1999;65(3):234-8.

4125 Lacy CF, Armstrong LL, Ingrim NB, Lance LL. Drug Information Handbook. Hudson, OH: Lexi Comp Inc; 1998-9.

4126 Wolinsky-Friedland M. Drug-induced metabolic bone disease. *Endocrinol Metab Clin North Am* 1995; 24(2):395-420.

4132 Tzivoni D, Keren A, Meyler S, et al. Cardiovascular safety of transdermal nicotine patches in patients with coronary artery disease who try to quit smoking. *Cardiovasc Drugs Ther* 1998; 12(3):239-44.

4133 Eliasson B, Taskinen MR, Smith U. Long-term use of nicotine gum is associated with hyperinsulinemia and insulin resistance. *Circ* 1996;94(5):878-81.

4137 Sills AK Jr, Williams JI, Tyler BM, et al. Squalamine

REFERENCES

inhibits angiogenesis and solid tumor growth in vivo and perturbs embryonic vasculature. *Cancer Res* 1998;58(13):2784-92.

4138 Kikuchi K, Bernard EM, Sadownik A, et al. Antimicrobial activities of squalamine mimics. *Antimicrob Agents Chemother* 1997;41(7):1433-8.

4139 Moore KS, Wehrli S, Roder H, et al. Squalamine: an aminosterol antibiotic from the shark. *Proc Natl Acad Sci USA* 1993;90(4):1354-8.

4140 Keynan N, Tamir R, Waisel Y, et al. Allergenicity of the pollen of Pistacia. *Allergy* 1997;52(3):323-30.

4141 Iauk L, Ragusa S, Rapisarda A, et al. In vitro antimicrobial activity of Pistacia lentiscus L. extracts: preliminary report. *J Chemother* 1996; 8(3):207-9.

4142 Al-Said MS, Ageel AM, Parmar NS, Tariq M. Evaluation of mastic, a crude drug obtained from Pistacia lentiscus for gastric and duodenal anti-ulcer activity. *J Ethnopharmacol* 1986;15(3):271-8.

4143 Vallverdu A, Garcia-Ortega P, Martinez J, et al. Mercurialis annua: characterization of main allergens and cross- reactivity with other species. *Int Arch Allergy Immunol* 1997;112(4):356-64.

4144 Garcia-Ortega P, Martinez J, Martinez A, et al. Mercurialis annua pollen: a new source of allergic sensitization and respiratory disease. *J Allergy Clin Immunol* 1992;89(5):987-93.

4145 Mancini SD, Edwards JM. Cytotoxic principles from the sap of Kalmia latifolia. *J Nat Prod* 1979;42(5):483-8.

4146 Garcia Ortiz JC, Terron M, Bellido J. "Contact allergy to henna. "*Int Arch Allergy Immunol* 1997;114(3):298-9.

4147 Kandil HH, al-Ghanem MM, Sarwat MA, al-Thallab FS. Henna (Lawsonia inermis Linn.) inducing haemolysis among G6PD-deficient newborns. A new clinical observation. *Ann Trop Paediatr* 1996;16(4):287-91.

4148 Majoie IM, Bruynzeel DP. Occupational immediate-type hypersensitivity to henna in a hairdresser. *Am J Contact Dermat* 1996;7(1):38-40.

4149 Clarke DT, Jones GR, Martin MM. The anti-sickling drug lawsone (2-OH-1,4-naphthoquinone) protects sickled cells against membrane damage. *Biochem Biophys Res Commun* 1986;139(2):780-6.

4150 Sharma VK. Tuberculostatic activity of henna (Lawsonia inermis Linn.). *Tubercle* 1990;71(4):293-5.

4151 Van Damme EJ, Roy S, Barre A, et al. The major elderberry (Sambucus nigra) fruit protein is a lectin derived from a truncated type 2 ribosome-inactivating protein. *Plant J* 1997;12(6):1251-60.

4152 Todorov S, Philianos S, Petkov V, et al. Experimental pharmacological study of three species from genus Salvia. *Acta Physiol Pharmacol (Bulg)* 1984;10(2):13-20.

4200 Bak AA, Grobbee DE. The effect of serum cholesterol levels of coffee brewed by filtering or boiling. *N Engl J Med* 1989;321(21):1432-7.

4201 Chevallier A. The Encyclopedia of Medicinal Plants. London: Dorling Kindersley, Ltd., 1996.

4202 Andermann G, Dietz M. The influence of the route of administration on the bioavailability of an endogenous macromolecule: chondroitin sulphate (CSA). *Eur J Drug Metab Pharmacokinet* 1982;7:11-6.

4203 Ronca F, Palmieri L, Panicucci P, et al. Anti-inflammatory activity of chondroitin sulfate. *Osteoarthritis Cartilage* 1998;6 Suppl A:14-21.

4204 Conte A, Volpi N, Palmieri L, et al. Biochemical and pharmacokinetic aspects of oral treatment with

chondroitin sulfate. *Arzneimittelforschung* 1995;45:918-25.

4205 Silvestro L, Lanzarotti E, Marchi E, et al. Human pharmacokinetics of glycosaminoglycans using deuterium-labeled and unlabeled substances: evidence for oral absorption. *Semin Thromb Hemost* 1994;20(3):281-92.

4206 (http://www.herbweb.com/herbage/80.htm in CRC Ethnobotany Desk Reference, CRC Press, 1999).

4207 Vale S. Subarachnoid haemorrhage associated with Ginkgo biloba. *The Lancet* 1998;(352):36.

4208 Mares-Perlman JA, Lyle BJ, et al. Vitamin supplement use and incident cataracts in a population-based study. *Arch Ophthalmol* 2000;118:1556-63.

4209 Alic M. Green Tea for remission maintenance in Crohn's disease. *Am J Gastroenterol* 1999; 94(6):1710-1.

4210 Gupta S, Ahmad N, Mukhtar H. Prostate chemoprevention by green tea. *Semin Urol Oncol* 1999; 17(2):70-6.

4211 Taylor JR, Wilt VM. Probable antagonism of warfarin by green tea. *Ann Pharmacother* 1999; 33(4):426-8.

4212 Klaunig JE, Xu Y, Han C, et al. The effect of tea consumption on oxidative stress in smokers and nonsmokers. *Proc Soc Exp Biol Med* 1999;220(4):249-54.

4213 Li N, Sun Z, Han C, Chen J. The chemopreventive effects of tea on human oral precancerous mucosa lesions. *Proc Soc Exp Biol Med* 1999;220(4):218-24.

4214 Rasheed A, Haider M. Antibacterial activity of Camellia sinensis extracts against dental caries. *Arch Pharm Res* 1998; 21(3):348-52.

4215 Viereck EG. Alaska's Wilderness Medicines Healthful Plants of the Far North. Anchorage, AK: Alaska Northwest Books, 1998.

4216 Curhan GC, Willett WC, Speizer FE, Stamfer MJ. Beverage use and risk of kidney stones in women. *Ann Intern Med* 1998; 128(7):534-40.

4217 Lee IP, Kim YH, Kang MH, et al. Chemopreventive effect of green tea (Camellia sinensis) against cigarette smoke induced mutations in humans. *J Cell Biochem Suppl* 1997;27:68-75.

4218 Kaegi E. Unconventional therapies for cancer:2. Green tea. The Task Force on Alternative Therapies of the Canadian Breast Cancer Research Initiative. *CMAJ* 1998;158(8):1033-5.

4219 Hollman PC, Feskens EJ, Katan MB. Tea flavonols in cardiovascular disease and cancer epidemiology. *Proc Soc Exp Biol Med* 1999;220(4):198-202.

4221 Durlach PJ. The effects of a low dose of caffeine on cognitive performance. *Psychopharmacol* 1998;140(1):116-9.

4222 Sesso HD, Gaziano JM, Buring JE, et al. Coffee and tea intake and the risk of myocardial infarction. *Am J Epidemiol* 1999;149:162-7.

4223 Weisburger JH. Tea and health: the underlying mechanisms. *Proc Soc Exp Biol Med* 1999;220(4):271-5.

4224 Hindmarch I, Quinlan PT, Moore KL, Parkin C. The effects of black tea and other beverages on aspects of cognition and psychomotor performance. *Psychopharmacol* 1998; 139(3):230-8.

4225 Sotaniemi EA, Haapakoski E, Rautio A. Ginseng therapy in non-insulin dependent diabetic patients. *Diabetes Care* 1995;18(10):1373-5.

4226 http://www.uwcm.ac.uk/uwcm/dm/BoDD/

BotDermFolder/BotDermR/RANU.html (Accessed 6 October 1999).

4227 Lee BM, Lee SK, Kim HS. Inhibition of oxidative DNA damage, 8-OHdG, and carbonyl contents in smokers treated with antioxidants (vitamin E, vitamin C, beta-carotene and red ginseng.) *Cancer Lett* 1998;132(1-2):219-27.

4228 Oh M, Choi YH, Choi S, et al. Anti-proliferating effects of ginsenosider Rh2 on MCF-7 human breast cancer cells. *Int J Oncol* 1999;14(5):869-75.

4229 Fetrow CW, Avila JR. Professional's Handbook of Complementary and Alternative Medicines. Springhouse, PA: Springhouse Corporation, 1999.

4230 Allen JD, McLung J, Nelson AG, Welsch M. Ginseng supplementation does not enhance healthy young adult's peak aerobic exercise performance. *J Am Coll Nutr* 1998;17(5):462-6.

4231 Engels HJ, Wirth JC. No ergogenic effects of ginseng (Panax ginseng C.A. Meyer) during grades maximal aerobic exercise. *J Am Diet Assoc* 1997;97(10):1110-5.

4233 Wolkowitz OM, Reus VI, Manfredi F, et al. Dehydroepiandrosterone (DHEA) Treatment of Depression. *Biol Psychiatry* 1997;41:311-8.

4234 Salvati G, Genovesi G, Marcellini L, et al. Effects of Panax ginseng C.A. Meyer saponins on male fertility. *Panminerva Med* 1996; 38(4):249-54.

4235 Yun TK. Experimental and epidemiological evidence of the cancer-preventive effects of Panax ginseng C.A. Meyer. *Nutr Rev* 1996;54(11 Pt2): 71-81.

4236 Morris AC, Jacobs I, McLellan TM, et al. No ergogenic effect of ginseng ingestion. *Int J Sport Nutr* 1996;6(3):263-71.

4237 Leffler CT, Philippi AF, Leffler SG, et al. Glucosamine, chondroitin, and manganese ascorbate for degenerative joint disease of the knee or low back: a randomized, double-blind, placebo-controlled pilot study. *Mil Med* 1999;164:85-91.

4239 Ondrizek RR, Chan PJ, Patton WC, King A. Inhibition of human sperm motility by specific herbs used in alternative medicine. *J Assist Reprod Genet* 1999;16:87-91.

4240 Ondrizek RR, Chan PJ, Patton WC, King A. An alternative medicine study of herbal effects on the penetration of zona-free hamster oocytes and the integrity of sperm deoxyribonucleic acid. *Fertil Steril* 1999;71:517-22.

4242 Labrie F, Diamond P, Cusan L, et al. Effect of 12 month dehydroepiandrosterone replacement therapy on bone, vagina, and endometrium in postmenopausal women. *J Clin Endocrinol Metab* 1997;82(10):3498-505.

4243 Ding DZ, Shen TK, Cui YZ. Effects of red ginseng on the congestive heart failure and its mechanism. *Chung Kuo Chung His I Chieh Ho Tsa Chih* 1995; 15(6Z):325-7.

4244 Bahrke MS, Morgan WP. Evaluation of the ergogenic properties of ginseng. *Sports Med* 1994; 18(4):229-48.

4245 Tyler, V. Herb News. *Prevention* 1999; (9): 105.

4248 Kroboth PD, Salek FS, Pittenger AL, et al. DHEA and DHEA-S: A review. *J Clin Pharmacol* 1999;39:327-48.

4249 Casson PR, Faquin LC, Stentz FB. Replacement of dehydroepiandrosterone enhances T-lymphocyte insulin binding in postmenopausal women. *Fertil Steril* 1995;63(5):1027-31.

4250 Bates GW, Egerman RS, Umstot ES, et al. Dehydroepiandrosterone attenuates study-induced declines in insulin sensitivity in postmenopausal women. *Ann NY Acad Sci* 1995;774:291-3.

4251 Morales AJ, Haubrich RH, Hwang JY, et al. The effect of six months treatment with 100 mg daily dose of dehydroepiandrosterone (DHEA) on circulating sex steroids, body composition and muscle strength in age-advanced men and women. *Clin Endocrinol* 1998;49:421-32.

4252 Casson PR, Andersen RN, Herrod HG, et al. Oral dehyroepiandosterone in physiologic doses modulates immune function in postmenopausal women. *Am J Obstet Gynecol* 1995;1536-9.

4253 Arlt W, Justl H, Callies F, et al. Oral dehydroepiandrosterone for adrenal androgen replacement: pharmacokinetics and peripheral conversion to androgens and estrogens in young healthy females after dexamethasone suppression. *J Clin Endocrinol Metab* 1998; 83:1928-34.

4254 Kudielka BM, Hellhammer J, Hellhammer D, et al. Sex differences in endocrine and psychological responses to psychosocial stress in healthy elderly subjects and the impact of a 2 week dehydroepiandrosterone treatment. *J Clin Endocrinol Metab*, 1998;83:1756-61.

4255 Flynn MA, Weaver-Osterholtz D, Sharpe-Timms KL, et al. Dehydroepiandrosterone replacement in aging humans. *J Clin Endocrinol Metab*, 1999;84:1527-33.

4256 Wolkowitz O. Personal memo to Karen Davidson 10/18/99.

4257 Heinonen OP, Albanes D, Virtamo J, et al. Prostate cancer and supplementation with alpha-tocoherol and beta-carotene: incidence and mortality in a controlled trial. *J Natl Cancer Inst* 1998; 90(6):440-6.

4258 Young LY, Koda-Kimble MA. Applied Therapeutics: The Clinical Use of Drugs. 6th ed. Vancouver, CAN: Applied Thera, Inc. 1995.

4259 FDA Press Release. FDA Warns About GBL-Related Products. FDA website, URL: vm.cfsan.fda.gov/~lrd/tpgbl2.html (Accessed 11 May 1999).

4260 Briggs GB, Freeman RK, Yaffe SJ. Drugs in Pregnancy and Lactation. 5th ed. Philadelphia: Lippincott Williams & Wilkins;1998.

4261 FDA. http://www.fda.gov/orphan/designat/list.htm (Accessed 11 November 1999).

4262 http://www.peanut-institute.org/Equal_Olive_Oil_PR.html (Accessed 19 September 1999).

4263 Sobolev VS, Cole RJ, Dorner JW, et al. Isolation, Purification, and Liquid Chromatographic Determination of Stilbene Phytoalexins in Peanuts. *J AOAC Intl* 1995;78:1177-82.

4264 Stampfer J, Manson JE, Rimm EB, et al. Frequent nut consumption and risk of coronary heart disease study. *BMJ* 1998; 17:1341-5.

4265 Kritchevsky D, Tepper SA, Klurfeld DM. Lectin may contribute to the atherogenicity of peanut oil. *Lipids* 1998;33:821-3.

4266 Kritchevsky D. Cholesterol vehicle in experimental atherosclerosis. A brief review with special reference to peanut oil. *Arch Pathol Lab Med* 1988; 112:1041-4.

4267 la Vecchia C, Negri E, Franceschi S, et al. Olive oil, other dietary fats, and the risk of breast cancer. (Italy) *Cancer Causes Control* 1995 Nov 6(6):545-50.

4269 Muzzarelli RA, Biagini G, Bellardini, et al. Osteoconduction exerted by methylpyrrolidinone chitosan used in dental surgery. *Biomaterials*

1993;14(1):39-43.

4270 Muzzarelli R, Tarsi R, Fillippini O, et al. Antimicrobial properties of N-carboxybutyl chitosan. Antimicrob Agents Chemother 1990;34(10):2019-23.

4273 Prevention. http://www.prevention.com/healing/living/980929.lvg4.html. (Accessed 23 November 1999).

4274 Riordan SM, Williams R. Treatment of Hepatic Encephalopathy. N Engl J Med 1997;337(7):473-9.

4275 Shipochliev T. Uterotonic action of extracts from a group of medicinal plants. Vet Med Nauki 1981;18(4):94-8.

4276 http://www.pharmacotherapy.medscape.com/IMNG/SkinAllergyN<sum>/san2810.28.01.htm (Accessed 23 February 2000).

4277 http://www.senetekplc.com/sci-kinetin.html (Accessed 23 February 2000).

4278 Olsen A, Siboska GE, Clark BF, Rattan SI. N(6)-Furfuryladenine, kinetin, protects against Fenton reaction-mediated oxidative damage to DNA. Biochem Biophys Res Commun 1999;265(2):499-502.

4279 http://www.senetekplc.com/amhealth.html (Accessed 23 February 2000).

4280 http://www.keechstudio.com/osm/PRODUCTS/KINETIN/kinetin.html (Accessed 24 February 2000).

4282 National Genetics Resources Program. The Germplasm Resources Information Network http://www.ars-grin.gov/ (Accessed 24 February 2000).

4283 Wang H, Nair MG, Strasburg GM, et al. Novel antioxidant compounds from tart cherries (Prunus cerasus). J Nat Prod 1999;62(1):86-8.

4284 Bruneton J. Pharmacognosy Phytochemistry Medicinal Plants. 2nd ed. Paris, FR: Lavoisier, 1999:142.

4285 Phone conversation with Michelle, ICN Pharmaceuticals. 4:20 pm, 24 February 2000.

4286 http://www.youngagain2000.com/marcella75/kinetin.html (Accessed 25 February 2000).

4289 Protocol Title: A Phase 1B Dose-Range Study to Evaluate the Safety, Pharmacokinetics, and Effects of (+)-calaonlide A on surrogate markers in HIV-positive patients with no previous antiretroviral therapy. Protocol ID numbers: FDA 297A.

4290 Reuters Health. Anti-HIV herbal product shows therapeutic potential in phase I trial. November 1, 1999.

4291 Newman RA, Chen W, Madden TL. Pharmaceutical properties of related calanolide compounds with activity against human immunodeficiency virus. J Pharm Sci 1998;87:1077-80.

4292 Buckheit RW, White EL, Fliakas-Boltz V, et al. Unique anti-human immunodeficiency virus activities of the nonnucleoside reverse transcriptase inhibitors calanolide A, costatolide, and dihydrocostatolide. Antimicrob Agents Chemother 1999;43(8):1827-34.

4293 Boyer PL, Currens MH, McMahon JB. Analysis of nonnucleoside drug-resistant variants of human immunodeficiency virus type 1 reverse transcriptase. J Virol 1993;67(4):2412-20.

4294 Currens MJ, Nariner JM, McMahon JB, Boyd MR. Kinetic analysis of inhibition of human immunodeficiency virus type-a reverse transcriptase by calanolide A. J Pharmacol Exp Ther 1996;279(2):652-61.

4295 Currens MJ, Gulakowski RJ, Mariner JM, et al. Antiviral activity and mechanism of action of calanolide A against the human immunodeficiency virus type-1. J Pharmacol Exp Ther 1996;279(2):645-51.

4299 Kanth VR, Diwan PV. Analgesic, anti-inflammatory and hypoglycaemic activities of Sida cordifolia. Phytother Res 1999 Feb;13(1):75-7.

4300 Fuhr U. Drug Interactions with Grapefruit Juice. Drug Safety 1998;(4):251-72.

4301 Yablonsky F, et al. Antiproliferative effect of Pygeum africanum extract on rat prostatic fibroblasts. J Urol 1997;157:2881-7.

4302 Andro MC, Riffaud JP. Pygeum africanum extract for the treatment of patients with benign prostatic hyperplasia. A review of 25 years of published experience. Curr Ther Res 1995;56:796-817.

4303 Homer KA, Manji F, Beighton D. Inhibition of peptidase and glycosidase activities of Porphyromonas gingivalis, Bacteroides intermedius and Treponema denticola by plant extracts. J Clin Periodontol May 1992;19(5):305-10.

4304 Anon. Sida Cordifolia. http://metromkt.net/viable/1sidacor.shtml. (Accessed 9 March 2000).

4305 Anon. SinuS? For Soothing Sinus Support. http://www.djtrading.com/sinus.htm. (Accessed 9 March 2000).

4306 W&B Associates, Inc. Dr. Harris' Original Allergy Formula. http://www.wandb.com/sinus.htm. (Accessed 9 March 2000).

4307 Anon. Extreme Sports Nutrition. http://www.extremesn.com/sports/prolab/provate1.htm. (Accessed 9 March 2000).

4308 Anon. Spectrum Nutrition the Leader in Pro-hormonal supplementation. http://www.spectrumnutrition.com/spectrumnutrition/prolther60ca.html. (Accessed 9 March 2000).

4309 Anon. Concentrated Natural Supplement with Sida Cordifolia. http://www.customdirecttoyou.com/katieseyes/ther50.html. (Accessed 9 March 2000).

4310 Anon. Sida Cordifolia Linn. http://www.modern-natural.com/sida_cordifolia.htm. (Accessed 9 March 2000).

4311 International Cyberbusiness Services, Inc. Herb Information; 1999. http://www.holisticonline.com/Herbal-Med/w_herb_dir.htm. (Accessed 9 March 2000).

4312 Silesia Group, Inc. The oldest and most effective herbal mixtures from India. http://www.biznet1.com/herbs/india/index.htm. (Accessed 9 March 2000).

4313 Anon. Go with herbs. http://www.gowithherbs.com/1297-2.htm. (Accessed 9 March 2000).

4314 Anon. Strictly Medicinal Herb Seeds. http://www.chatlink.com/~herbseed/sida.html. (Accessed 9 March 2000).

4315 Anon. Ayurvedic Rasayanas. http://www.ayurveda-herbs.com/Aphrodisiac-Sex-Impotency.htm. (Accessed 9 March 2000).

4316 Dharma Group. Herbal Accelerator. http://www.dharmagroup.com/web/herbal.htm. (Accessed 9 March 2000).

4317 Anon. JNT-AV (100). http://www.herbwise.com:8001/encyclo/products/1296-1.htf. (Accessed 9 March 2000).

4318 Anon. Fastrak. http://members.tripod.com/~Roe/fastrak. (Accessed 9 March 2000).

4319 Prime Nutrition. Pyroclen Thermo Burn 100's. http://www.primenutrition.com/primen/sanpyrtherbu.html. (Accessed 9 March 2000).

4320 Anon. Pyruvate Formulas. http://www.undergroundsports.com/pyruvate.htm. (Accessed 9 March 2000).

4321 Maharishi Ayur-Ved Products Inc. 1998; Ayurvedic Herbs: Bala. http://www.mapi.com/cgi-local/shop.pl/page=herbbala.html/SID=1877132249. (Accessed 9 March 2000).

4322 Aquasearch Incorporated. Aquasearch Technology and Markets. 1999. URL. http://www.aqse.com/astax.htm. (Accessed 14 March 2000).

4323 Anon. Eat and lose weight. http://www.pricespower.com/eat&lose.htm. (Accessed 9 March 2000).

4324 Diet Gems. Fantastic products for weight loss. http://store.yahoo.net/dietgems/. (Accessed 9 March 2000).

4325 Anon. Ayurvedic Rasanas. http://www.ayurveda-herbs.com/Narayana-Massage-Oil-Pain.htm. (Accessed 9 March 2000).

4326 Goodwin TW. Metabolism, nutrition, and function of carotenoids. *Annu Rev Nutr* 1986;6:273-97.

4327 Duke J. ETHNOBOT. http://www.ars-grin.gov/duke (Accessed 14 March 2000).

4328 Igene Biotechnology Incorporated. Product Information. 2000. URL. http://www.igene.com/products.htm. (Accessed 14 March 2000).

4329 Cyanotech corporation. Natur Rose. 1999. URL. http://www.cyanotech.com. (Accessed 14 March 2000).

4330 Cyanotech. Cyanotech Launches Natural Astaxanthin as Human Dietary Supplement; Powerful Antioxidant Promises Key Benefits 2000. URL. http://www.npicenter.com/dailynewswire/archive/19990311/9/comt x-13365M3b921 161962.asp. (Accessed 14 March 2000).

4331 Storebakken, T. Utilization of astaxanthin from red yeast (Phaffia rhodozyma) in comparison with synthetic astaxanthin by Atlantic salmon. 1998. URL. http://www.igene.com/norway.html. (Accessed 14 March 2000).

4332 Kobayashi M, Kakizono T, Nishio N, et al. Antioxidant role of astaxanthin in the green alga Haematococcus pluvialis. *Appl Microbiol, Biotechnol* 1997;48(3):351-6.

4333 Dolan M. Hepatitis C-clinical background and treatment options. http://www.positivehealth.com/permit/Articles/Nutrition/hepc.htm. (Accessed 12 March 2000).

4334 Anon. Astaxanthin promoted as dietary supplement. 1999. URL. http://www.nzhealth.co.nz/nutrition/nutnews199903172.html. (Accessed 14 March 2000).

4335 Jyonouchi H, Sun S, Tomita Y, et al. Astaxathin, a carotenoid without vitamin A activity augments antibody responses in cultures including T-helpe cell clones and suboptimal doses of antigen. *J Nutr* 1995;125(10):2483-92.

4336 Chew BP, Wong MW, Park JS, et al. Dietary beta-carotene and astaxanthin but not canthaxanthin stimulate splenocyte function in mice. *Anticancer Res* 1999;19;5223-8.

4337 Chew BP, Park JS, Wong MW, et al. A comparison of the Anticancer activities of dietary beta-carotene, canthaxanthin and astaxanthin in mice in vivo. *Anticancer Res* 1999;19:1849-54.

4338 Tanaka T, Morishita Y, Suzui M, et al. Chemoprevention of mouse urinary bladder carcinogenesis by the naturally occurring carotenoid astaxanthin. *Carcinogenesis* 1994;15(1):15-9.

4339 Tanaka T, Makita H, Oshnishi M, et al. Chemoprevention of rat oral carcinogenesis by naturally occurring xanthophylls, astaxanthin, and canthaxanthin. *Cancer Res* 1995;55:4059-64.

4340 Gradelet S, Le Bon AM, Berges R, et al. Dietary carotenoids inhibit aflatoxin B1-induced liver preneoplastic foci and DNA damage in the rat: role of the modulation of aflatoxin B1 metabolism. *Carcinogenesis* 1998; 19(3):403-11.

4341 Bennedsen M, Wang X, Willen R, et al. Treatment of H. pylori infected mice with antioxidant astaxanthin reduces gastric inflammation, bacterial load and modulates cytokine release by splenocytes. *Immunol Lett*, 1999;70(3):185-9.

4342 Bensky D, Gamble A, Kaptchuk T. Chinese Herbal Medicine Materia Medica. Seattle, WA: Eastland Press, 1996:214-6.

4343 Huang KC. The Pharmacology of Chinese Herbs. 2nd ed. Boca Raton: CRC Press LLC., 1999:258.

4344 Chevallier A. The Encyclopedia of Medicinal Plants. New York: DK Publishing. 1996:170.

4345 Yamamoto M, Ogawa K, Morita M, et al. The herbal medicine Inchin-ko-to inhibits liver cell apoptosis induced by transforming growth factor beta 1. *Hepatology* 1996;23(3):552-9.

4346 Yamamoto M, Miura N, Ohtake N, et al. Genipin, a metabolite derived from the herbal medicine Inchin-ko-to, and suppression of fas-induced lethal liver apoptosis in mice. *Gastroenterol* 2000;118:380-9.

4347 Saavedra J. Probiotics and infectious diarrhea. *Am J Gastroenterol* 2000;95(1 Suppl):S16-8.

4348 Castagliuolo I, Riegler MF, Valenick L, et al. Saccharomyces boulardii protease inhibits the effects of clostridium difficile toxins A and B in human colonic mucosa. *Infection and Immun* 1999;67(1):302-7.

4349 Bleichner G, Blehaut H, Mentec H, et al. Saccharomyces boulardii prevents diarrhea in critically ill tube-fed patients. *Intensive Care Med* 1997;23:517-23.

4350 Lewis SJ, Potts LF, Barry RE. The lack of therapeutic effect of Saccharomyces boulardii in the prevention of antibiotic-related diarrhea in elderly patients. *J Infect* 1998;36:171-4.

4351 Elmer GW, McFarland LV. Comment on the lack of therapeutic effect of Saccharomyces boulardii in the prevention of antibiotic-related diarrhea in elderly patients. *J Infect* 1998;36(2):171-4.

4352 McFarland LV, Surawicz CM, Greenberg RN, et al. A randomized placebo-controlled trial of Saccharomyces boulardii in combination with standard antibiotics for Clostridium difficile disease. *JAMA* 1994;271(24):1913-8.

4353 McFarland LV, Surawicz CM, Greenberg RN, et al. Prevention of beta-lactam associated diarrhea by Saccharomyces boulardii compared with placebo. *Am J Gastroenterol* 1995;90(3):439-48.

4354 Surawicz CM, McFarland LV, Elmer G, et al. Treatment of recurrent clostridium difficile colitis with vancomycin and Saccharomyces boulardii. *Am J Gastroenterol* 1989;84(10):1285-7.

4355 Surawicz CM, Elmer GW, Speelman P, et al. Prevention of antibiotic-associated diarrhea by Saccharomyces boulardii: a prospective study. *Gastroenterol* 1989;96:981-8.

4356 Buts JP, Corthier G, Delmee M. Saccharomyces boulardii for Clostridium difficile-associated enteropathies in infants. *J of Pediatr Gastroenterol and Nutr* 1993;16(4):419-25.

4357 Pletinex M, Legein J, Vandenplas Y. Fungemia with

Saccharomyces boulardii in a 1-year-old girl with protracted diarrhea. *J Pediatric Gastroenterol and Nutr* 1995;21:113-5.

4358 Fredenucci I, Chomarat M, Boucaud C, et al. Saccharomyces boulardii fungemia in a patient receiving ultra-levure therapy. *CID* 1998;27:222-3.

4359 Hennequin C, Kauffmann-Lacroix C, Jobert A, et al. Possible role of catheters in Saccharomyces boulardii fungemia. *Eur J Clin Microbiol Infect Dis* 2000;19(1):16-20.

4360 Elmer GW, McFarland LV, Surawicz CM, et al. Behaviour of Saccharomyces boulardii in recurrent Clostridium difficile disease patients. *Alimen Pharmacol Ther* 1999;13(12):1663-8.

4361 Czerucka D, Roux I, Rampal P. Saccharomyces boulardii inhibits secretagogue-mediated adenosine 3',5'-cyclic monophosphate induction in intestinal cells. *Gastroenterol* 1994;106(1):65-72.

4362 Krammer M, Karbach U. Antidiarrheal action of the yeast Saccharomyces boulardii in the rat small and large intestine by stimulating chloride absorption. *Z Gastroenterol* 1993;31:73-7.

4363 Lewis SJ, Freedman AR. Review article: the use of biotherapeutic agents in the prevention and treatment of gastrointestinal disease. *Aliment Pharmacol Ther* 1998;12:807-22.

4364 PWA Health Group. Saccharomyces Boulardii Info Sheet. http://208.178.40.64/pwahg/info/sacc.html. (Accessed 16 March 2000).

4365 James JS. AIDS Treatment Archives. http://aids.org/immunet/atn.nsf/page/x-Saccharomyces-boulardii. (Accessed 16 March 2000).

4366 GN Gaines Nutrition Online Health Food Store. Saccromyces boulardii product information. URL: www.gaines.com/html/ARG/ARG71050info.html (Accessed 16 March 2000).

4367 Gorbach SL. Probiotics and gastrointestinal health. *Am J Gastroenterol* 2000;95(1 Suppl):S2-S4.

4368 Schultz M, Sartor RB. Probiotics and inflammatory bowel diseases. *Am J Gastroenterol* 2000;95(1):S19-S21.

4369 deRoos NM, Katan MB. Effects of probiotic bacteria on diarrhea, lipid metabolism, and carcinogenesis: a review of papers published between 1988 and 1998. *Am J Clin Nutr* 2000;71:405-11.

4370 Guandalini S, Pensabene L, Zikri MA, et al. Lactobacillus GG administered in oral rehydration solution to children with acute diarrhea: a multicenter European trial. *J Pediatr Gastroenterol Nutr* 2000;30:54.

4371 Vanderhoof JA, Whitney DB, Antonson DL, et al. Lactobacillus GG in the prevention of antibiotic-associated diarrhea in children. *J Pediatr* 1999;135(5):564-8.

4372 Arvola T, Laiho K, Torkkeli S, et al. Prophylactic Lactobacillus GG reduces antibiotic-associated diarrhea in children with respiratory infections: a randomized study. *Pediatrics* 1999;104(5):e64.

4373 Oberhelman RA, Gilman RH, Sheen P, et al. A placebo-controlled trial of Lactobacillus GG to prevent diarrhea in undernourished Peruvian children. *J Pediatr* 1999;134(1):15-20.

4374 Hilton E, Kolakowski P, Singer C, et al. Efficacy of Lactobacillus GG as a Diarrheal Preventative in Travelers. *J Travel Med* 1997;4(1):41-3.

4375 Vanderhoof JA, Young RJ, Murray N, et al. Treatment strategies for small bowel bacterial overgrowth in short bowel syndrome. *J Pediatr Gastroenterol Nutr* 1998;27(2):155-60.

4376 El-Nezami H, Kankaanpaa P, Salminen S, et al. Ability of dairy strains of lactic acid bacteria to bind a common food carcinogen, aflatoxin B1. *Food Chem Toxicol* 1998;36(4):321-6.

4377 Guarino A, Canani RB, Spagnuolo MI, et al. Oral bacterial therapy reduces the duration of symptoms and of viral excretion in children with mild diarrhea. *J Pediatr Gastroenterol Nutr* 1997;25(5):516-9.

4378 Hudault S, Lievin V, Bernet-Camard MF, et al. Antagonistic activity exerted in vitro and in vivo by Lactobacillus casei (strain GG) against Salmonella typhimurium C5 infection. *Appl Environ Microbiol* 1997;63(2):513-8.

4379 Sutas Y, Hurme M, Isolauri E. Down-regulations of anti-CD3 antibody-induced IL-4 production by bovine caseins hydrolyzed with Lactobacillus GG-derived enzymes. *Scand J Immunol* 1996;43(6):687-9.

4380 Saxelin M, Chuang NH, Chassy B, et al. Lactobacilli and bacteremia in southern Finland 1989-1992. *Clin Infect Dis* 1996;22(3):564-6.

4381 Malin M, Suomalainen H, Saxelin M, et al. Promotion of IgA immune response in patients with Crohn's disease by oral bacteriotherapy with Lactobacillus GG. *Ann Nutr Metab* 1996;40(3):137-45.

4382 Goldin BR, Gualtieri LJ, Moore RP. The effect of Lactobacillus GG on the initiation and promotion of DMH-induced intestinal tumors in the rat. *Nutr Cancer* 1996;25(2):197-204.

4383 Anon. Lactobacillus Rhamnosus strain GG for Diarrhea in infants? Inpharma Weekly 1999;1179. http://aids.medscape.com/adis/IP/1999/1179/ip1179.01.html (Accessed 18 March 2000).

4384 Anon. New dietary supplement with research-proven intestinal health benefits now available. 2000. URL. http://www.conagra.com/092398_2.html. (Accessed 18 March 2000).

4385 Anon. Lactobacillus GG and CRC. 2000. URL. http://www.geocities.com/HotSprings/Falls/4425/lgg.html (Accessed 18 March 2000).

4386 Valio. Valio Products. 2000. URL. http://www.valio.fi/english/products.html. (Accessed 18 March 2000).

4387 McIntosh GH, Royle PJ, Playne MJ. A probiotic strain of L. acidophilus reduces DMH-induced large intestinal tumors in male Sprague-Dawley rats. *Nutr Cancer* 1999;35(2):153-9.

4388 Mack DR, Michail S, Shu W, et al. Probiotics inhibit enteropathogenic E. coli adherence in vitro by inducing intestinal mucin gene expression. *Clin Exp Immunol* 1999;116(2):276-82.

4389 Tynkkynen S, Singh KV, Varmanen P. Vancomycin resistance factor of Lactobacillus rhamnosus GG in relation to enterococcal vancomycin resistance (van) genes. *Int J Food Microbiol* 1998; 41(3):195-204.

4390 Klein G, Zill E, Schindler R, et al. Peritonitis associated with vancomycin-resistant Lactobacillus rhamnosus in a continuous ambulatory peritoneal dialysis patient; organism identification, antibiotic therapy, and case report. *J Clin Microbiol* 1998;36(6):1781-3.

4391 Kalima P, Masterton RG, Roddie PH, et al. Lactobacillus rhamnosus infection in a child following bone marrow transplant. *J Infect* 1996;32(2):165-7.

4392 Pochapin M. The effect of probiotics on Clostridium difficile diarrhea. *Am J Gastroenterol* 2000;95(Suppl 1):S11-3.

4393 Goldin BR. Health Benefits of probiotics. *Br J Nutr* 1998;80(4):S203-7.

4394 Biller JA, Katz AJ, Flores AF, et al. Treatment of recurrent Clostridium difficile colitis with Lactobacillus GG. *J Pediatr Gastroenterol Nutr* 1995;21(2):224-6.

4395 Anon. Aquasearch Announces Launch of The AstaFactor(TM).2000.URL. http://www.aquasearch.com/whatsnew.htm (Accessed 20 March 2000).

4396 Anon. U.S. district court grants Aquasearch's motion for summary judgement. Court rules that Cyanotech infringed key Aquasearch patent, misappropriated Aquasearch trade secrets, and breached its contract with Aquasearch. 2000. URL. http://www.aquasearch.com/whatsnew.htm. (Accessed 20 March 2000).

4397 Hilton E, Rindos P, Isenberg HD. Lactobacillus GG Vaginal Suppositories and Vaginitis. *J Clin Microbiol* 1995;33(5):1433.

4398 Rautio M, Jousimies-Somer H, Kauma H, et al. Liver abscess due to Lactobacillus rhamnosus strain indistinguishable from L. rhamnosus strain GG. *Clin Infect Dis* 1999;28:1159-60.

4399 Pelto L, Ioslauri E, Lilius EM, et al. Probiotic bacteria down-regulate the milk-induced inflammatory response in milk-hypersensitive subjects but have an immunostimulatory effect in healthy subjects. *Clin Exp Allergy* 1998;28:1474-9.

4400 Spencer H, Menaham L. Adverse effects of aluminum-containing antacids on mineral metabolism. *Gastroenterology* 1979;76:603-6.

4404 Folkers K, Langsjoen P, Willis R, et al. Lovastatin decreases coenzyme Q levels in humans. *Proc Natl Acad Sci USA* 1990;87(22):8931.

4405 Mortensen SA, Leth A, Agner E, et al. Dose-related decrease of serum coenzyme Q10 during treatment with HMG-CoA reductase inhibitors. *Mol Aspects Med* 1997;18(Suppl):S137-44.

4406 Ghirlanda G, Oradei A, Manto A, et al. Evidence of plasma CoQ10-lowering effect by HMG-CoA reductase inhibitors: A double blind, placebo-controlled study. *J Clin Pharmacol* 1993;33(3):226-9.

4407 De Pinieux G, Chariot P, Ammi-Said M, et al. Lipid-lowering drugs and mitochondrial function: Effects of HMG-CoA Reductase inhibitors on serum ubiquinone and blood lactate/pyruvate ratio. *Br J Clin Pharmacol* 1996;42(3):333-7.

4408 Bargossi AM, Grossi G, Fiorella PL, et al. Exogenous CoQ10 supplementation prevents plasma ubiquinone reduction induced by HMG-CoA reductase inhibitors. *Mol Aspects Med* 1994;15(Suppl):187-93.

4409 Watts GF, Castelluccio C, Rice-Evans C, et al. Plasma coenzyme Q (ubiquinone) concentrations in patients treated with simvastatin. *J Clin Pathol* 1993;46(11):1055-7.

4410 Hanaki Y, Sugiyama S, Ozawa T, et al. Coenzyme Q10 and coronary artery disease. *Clin Investig* 1993;71(8 Suppl):112-5.

4411 Ritsema GH, Ellers G. Potassium supplements prevent serious hypokalemia in colon cleansing. *Clin Radiol* 1994;49(12);874-6.

4412 Murry JJ, Healy MD. Drug-mineral interactions: a new responsibility for the hospital dietician. *J Am Diet Assoc* 1991;91(1):66-73.

4425 Garabedian-Ruffalo SM, Ruffalo RL. Drug and nutrient interactions. *AFP* 1986;33(2):165-74.

4426 Kishi T, Fujita N, Eguchi T, et al. Mechanism for reduction of serum folate by antiepileptic drugs during prolonged therapy. *J Neurol Sci* 1997;145(1):109-12.

4427 Froscher W, Maier V, Laage M, et al. Folate deficiency, anticonvulsant drugs, and psychiatric morbidity. *Clin Neuropharmacol* 1995;18(2):165-82.

4428 Hendel J, Dam M, Gram L, et al. The effects of carbamazepine and valproate on folate metabolism in man. *Acta Neurol Scan* 1984;69(4):226-31.

4429 Traccis S, Monaco F, Sechi GP, et al. Long-term therapy with carbamazepine: Effects on nerve conduction velocity. *Eur Neurol* 1983;22(6):410-6.

4430 Hoikka V, Alhava EM, Karjalainen P, et al. Carbamazepine and bone mineral metabolism. *Acta Neurol Scand* 1984;70(2):77-80.

4431 Rajantie J, Lamberg-Allardt C, Wilska M. Does carbamazepine treatment lead to a need of extra vitamin D in some mentally retarded children? *Acta Paediatr Scand* 1984;73(3):325-8.

4434 Cummings JH, Macfarlane G. Role of intestinal bacteria in nutrient metabolism. *J Parenter Enteral Nutr* 1997;21(6):357-65.

4435 Honma N. The effect of lactic acid bacteria, Part 1: biological significance. *New Medicines and Clinics* 1986;35(12):1-3.

4436 Gorbach SL, Bengt E. Gustafsson memorial lecture. Function of the normal human microflora. *Scand J Infect Dis Suppl* 1986;49:17-30.

4437 Hill MJ. Intestinal flora and endogenous vitamin synthesis. *Eur J Cancer Prev* 1997;6(Suppl 1):S43-5.

4438 Conly J, Stein K. Reduction of vitamin K2 concentrations in human liver associated with the use of broad spectrum antimicrobials. *Clin Invest Med* 1994;17(6):531-9.

4439 Conly JM, Stein K, Worobetz L, Rutledge-Harding S. The contribution of vitamin K2 (menaquinones) produced by the intestinal microflora to human nutritional requirements for vitamin K. *Am J Gastroenterol* 1994;89(6):915-23.

4440 Cordes I, Buchmann S, Scheffner D. Vitamin K deficiency with erythromycin. Observation of a boy treated with valproate. *Monatsschr Kinderhdilkd* 1990;138(2):85-7.

4441 Lipsky JJ. Antibiotic-associated hypoprothrombinemia. *J Antimicrob Chemother* 1988;21(3):281-300.

4442 Alitalo R, Ruutu M, Valtonen V, et al. Hypoprothrombinemia and bleeding during administration of cefamandole and cefoperazone. Report of three cases. *Ann Clin Res* 1985;17(3):116-9.

4443 Shimada K, Matsuda T, Inamatsu T, et al. Bleeding secondary to vitamin K deficiency in patients receiving parenteral cephem antibiotics. *J Antimicrob Chemother* 1984;14(Suppl B):325-30.

4449 Robertson JI. Diuretics, potassium depletion and risk of arrhythmias. *Eur Heart J* 1984;5(Suppl A):25-8.

4452 Mountokalakis T, Dourakis S, Karatzas N, et al. Zinc deficiency in mild hypertensive patients treated with diuretics. *J Hypertens Suppl* 1984;2(3):S571-2.

4453 Thomas JA. Drug-nutrient interactions. *Nutr Rev* 1995;53(10):271-82.

4454 Hathcock JN. Metabolic mechanisms of drug-nutrient interactions. *Fed Proc* 1985;44(1 Pt 1):124-9.

REFERENCES

4455 West RJ, Lloyd JK. The effect of cholestyramine on intestinal absorption. *Gut* 1975;16(2):93-8.

4456 Cywes C, Millar AJ. Assessment of the nutritional status of infants and children with biliary atresia. *S Afr Med J* 1990;77(3):131-5.

4457 Elinder LS, Hadell K, Johansson J, et al. Probucol treatment decreases serum concentrations of diet-derived antioxidants. *Arterioscler Throm Vasc Biol* 1995;15(8):1057-63.

4458 Knodel LC, Talbert RL. Adverse effects of hypolipidaemic drugs. *Med Toxicol* 1987;2(1):10-32.

4459 Matsui MS, Rozovski SJ. Drug-nutrient interaction. *Clin Ther* 1982;4(6):423-40.

4460 Schwarz KB, Goldstein PD, Witztum JL, et al. Fat-soluble vitamin concentrations in hypercholestrolemic children treated with colestipol. *Pediatrics* 1980;65(2):243-50.

4461 Tonstad S, Silverstein M, Aksnes L, et al. Low dose colestipol in adolescents with familial hypercholesterolemia. *Arch Dis Child* 1996;74(2):157-60.

4462 Lems WF, Van Veen GJ, Gerrits MI, et al. Effect of low-dose prednisolone (with calcium and calcitriol supplementation) on calcium and bone metabolism in healthy volunteers. *Br J Rheumatol* 1998;37(1):27-33.

4463 Reid DM, Kennedy NS, Smith MA, et al. Total body calcium in rheumatoid arthritis: Effects of disease activity and corticosteroid treatment. *Br Med J (Clin Res Ed)* 1982;285(6338):330-2.

4464 Lems WF, Jacobs JW, Netelenbos JC, et al. Pharmacological prevention of osteoporosis in patients on corticosteroid medication, *Ned Tijdschr Geneeskd* 1998;142(34):1904-8.

4465 Gennari C. Differential effect of glucocorticoids on calcium absorption and bone mass. *Br J Rheumatol* 1993;32(Suppl 2):11-4.

4466 Need AG, Philcox JC, Hartley TF, et al. Calcium metabolism and osteoporosis in corticosteroid-treated postmenopausal women. *Aust N Z J Med* 1986;16(3):341-6.

4467 Reid IR, Ibbertson HK. Calcium supplements in the prevention of steroid-induced osteoporosis. *Am J Clin Nutr* 1986;44(2):287-90.

4470 Blum M, Kitai E, Ariel Y, et al. Oral contraceptive lowers serum magnesium. *Harefuah* 1991;121(10):363-4.

4471 Lewis DP, Van Dyke DC, Willhite LA, et al. Phenytoin-folic acid interaction. *Ann Pharmacother* 1995;29(7-8):726-35.

4472 Berg MJ, Stumbo PJ, Chenard CA, et al. Folic acid improves phenytoin pharmacokinetics. *J Am Diet Assoc* 1995;95(3):352-6.

4473 Berg MJ, Fincham RW, Ebert BE, et al. Phenytoin pharmacokinetics: Before and after folic acid administration. *Epilepsia* 1992;33(4):712-20.

4474 Zerwekh JE, Homan R, Tindall R, et al. Decreased serum 24,25-dihydroxy vitamin D concentration during long-term anticonvulsant therapy in adult epileptics. *Ann Neurol* 1982;12(2):184-6.

4475 Bell RD, Pak CY, Zerwekh J, et al. Effect of phenytoin on bone and mineral density in ambulatory epileptic children. *Brain Dev* 1994;16(5):382-5.

4477 Shafer RB, Nuttall FQ. Calcium and folic acid absorption in patients taking anticonvulsant drugs. *J Clin Endocrinol Metab* 1975;41(06):1125-9.

4479 Kishi T, Kishi H, Watanabe T, et al. Bioenergetics in clinical medicine. XI. Studies on coenzyme Q and diabetes mellitus. *J Med* 1976;7(3-4):307-21.

4481 Pellock JM, Howell J, Kendig EI Jr, et al. Pyridoxine deficiency in children treated with isoniazid. *Chest* 1985;87(5):658-61.

4482 Snider DE Jr. Pyridoxine supplementation during isoniazid therapy. *Tubercle* 1980;61(4):191-6.

4483 Termanini B, Gibril F, Sutliff VE, et al. Effect of long-term gastric acid suppressive therapy on serum vitamin B12 levels in patients with Zollinger-Ellison syndrome. *Am J Med* 1998;104(5):422-30.

4484 Bellou A, Aimone-Gastin I, De Korwin JD, et al. Cobalamin deficiency with megaloblastic anaemia in one patient under long-term omeprazole therapy. *J Intern Med* 1996;240(3):161-4.

4485 Saltzman JR, Kemp JA, Golner BB, et al. Effect of hypochlorhydria due to omeprazole treatment or atrophic gastritis on protein-bound vitamin B12 absorption. *J Am Coll Nutr* 1994;13(6):584-91.

4486 Marcuard SP, Albernaz L, Khazaine PG. Omeprazole therapy causes malabsorption of cyanocobalamin. *Ann Intern Med* 1994;120(3):211-5.

4490 Carpentier JL, Bury J, Luyckx A, et al. Vitamin B12 and folic acid serum levels in diabetics under various therapeutic regimens. *Diabete Metab,* 1976;2(4):187-90.

4491 Bristol-Myers Squibb Company. Glucophage package insert. Princeton, NJ; January 1999.

4492 Leeb BF, Witzmann G, Ogris E, et al. Folic acid cyanocobalamin levels in serum and erythrocytes during low-dose methotrexate therapy in rheumatoid arthritis and psoriatic arthritis patients. *Clin Exp Rheumatol,* 1995;13(4):459-63.

4493 Morgan SL, Baggott JE, Lee JY, et al. Folic acid supplementation prevents deficient blood folate levels and hyperhomocysteinemia during long-term, low dose methotrexate therapy for rheumatoid arthritis: Implications for cardiovascular disease prevention. *J Rheumatol* 1998;25(3):441-6.

4494 Dijkmans BA. Folate supplementation and methotrexate. *Br J Rheumatol* 1995;34(12):1172-4.

4495 Becker GL. The case against mineral oil. *Am J Digestive Dis* 1953;19:344-7.

4496 Clark JH, Russell GJ, Fitzgerald JF, et al. Serum beta-carotene, retinal, and alpha-tocopherol levels during mineral oil therapy for constipation. *Am J Dis Child* 1987;141(11):1210-2.

4498 Prasad AS, Lei KY, Moghissi KS, et al. Effect of oral contraceptives on nutrients. III. Vitamins B6, B12 and folic acid. *Am J Obstet Gynecol* 1976;125(8):1063-9.

4500 Hocking GM. A dictionary of natural products. 2nd ed. Medford, OR: Plexus Publishing, 1997.

4501 Micromedex Healthcare Series. Poisindex. Englewood, CO: Micromedex, Inc.

4502 Duke JA. CRC handbook of medicinal herbs. 1st ed. Boca Raton, LA: CRC Press, 1985.

4503 Bruneton J. Pharmacognosy, phytochemistry, medicinal plants. 2nd ed. Andover, MI: Intercept Ltd, 1995.

4504 Weiss RF. Herbal medicine. 5th ed. Beaconsfield: Beaconsfield Publishers Ltd, 1998.

4505 DeSmet P, ed. Adverse effects of herbal drugs. 1st ed. Berlin, Heidelberg: Springer-Verlag, 1993.

4506 Miller LG, Wallace JM, eds. Herbal medicinals a clinician's guide. 1st ed. New York, NY: Pharmaceutical Prod Press, 1998.

4507 Fetrow CW, Avila JR. Professional's handbook of complementary and alternative medicines. 1st ed. Springhouse: Springhouse Corp., 1999.

4511 Palva IP, Salokannel SJ, Timonen T, et al. Drug-induced malabsorption of vitamin B12. IV. Malabsorption and deficiency of B12 during treatment with slow-release potassium chloride. *Acta Med Scand* 1972;191(4):355-7.

4512 Salokannel SJ, Palva IP, Takkunen JT, et al. Malabsorption of vitamin B12 during treatment with slow-release potassium chloride. Preliminary report. *Acta Med Scand* 1970;187(5):431-2.

4514 D'Erasmo E, Ragno A, Raejntroph N, et al. Drug-induced osteomalacia. *Recenti Prog Med* 1998;89(10):529-33.

4515 Krogh-Jensen M, Ekelund S, Svendsen L. Folate and homocysteine status and haemolysis in patients treated with sulphasalazine for arthritis. *Scand J Clin Lab Invest* 1996;56(5):421-9.

4516 Logan EC, Williamson LM, Ryrie DR. Sulphasalazine associated pancytopenia may be caused by acute folate deficiency. *Gut* 1986;27(7):868-72.

4517 Grieco A, Caputo S, Bertoli A, et al. Megaloblastic anemia due to sulphasalazine responding to drug withdrawal alone. *Postgrad Med J* 1986;62(726):307-8.

4522 Delport R, Ubbink JB, Serfontein WJ, et al. Vitamin B6 nutritional status in asthma. The effect of theophylline therapy on plasma pyridoxal-5-phosphate and pyridoxal levels. *Int J Vitam Nutr Res* 1988;58(1):67-72.

4523 Van Wouwe JP. Carnitine deficiency during valproic acid treatment. *Int J Vitam Nutr Res* 1995;65(3):211-4.

4524 Matsuda I, Ohtani Y, Ninomiya N. Renal handling of carnitine in chlidren with carnitine deficiency and hyperammonemia associated with valproate therapy. *J Pediatr* 1986;109(1):131-4.

4525 Ohtani Y, Endo F, Matsuda I. Carnitine deficiency and hyperammonemia associated with valproic acid therapy. *J Pediatr* 1982;101(5):782-5.

4526 Opala G, Winter S, Vance C, et al. The effect of valproic acid on plasma carnitine levels. *Am J Dis Child* 1991;145(9):999-1001.

4527 Melegh B, Kerner J, Kispal G, et al. Effect of chronic valproic acid treatment on plasma and urine carnitine levels in children: Decreased urinary excretion. *Acta Paediatr Hung* 1987;28(2):137-42.

4528 De Vivo DC, Bohan TP, Coulter DL, et al. L-carnitine supplementation in childhood epilepsy: Current perspectives. *Epilepsia* 1998;39(11):1216-25.

4529 Coulter DL. Carnitine, valproate, and toxicity. *J Child Neurol* 1991;6(1):7-14.

4530 Taliani U, Camellini A, Bernardi P, et al. A clinical case of severe megaloblastic anemia during treatment with primidone. *Acta Biomed Ateneo Parmense* 1989;60(5-6):245-8.

4531 Segal S, Kaminski S. Drug-nutrient interactions. *American Druggist* 1996 Jul;42-8.

4532 Glaxo-Wellcome, Inc. Daraprim package insert. Research Triangle Park, NC; August, 1996.

4533 Raskin HN, Fishman RA. Pyridoxine-deficiency neuropathy due to hydralazine. *N Engl J Med* 1965;273(22):1182-5.

4534 Seelig MS. Auto-immune complications of D-penicillamine – A possible result of zinc and magnesium depletion and of pyridoxine inactivation. *J Am Coll Nutr* 1982;1(2):207-14.

4535 Jaffe IA. The antivitamin B6 effect of penicillamine. Clinical and immunological implications. *Adv Biochem Psypharmacol* 1972;4:217-26.

4536 Lambie DG, Johnson RH. Drugs and folate metabolism. *Drugs* 1985;30(2):145-55.

4537 Joosten E, Pelemans W. Megaloblastic anaemia in an elderly patient treated with triamterene. *Neth J Med* 1991;38(5-6):209-11.

4539 Aymard JP, Aymard B, Netter P, et al. Haematological adverse effects of histamine H2-receptor antagonists. *Med Toxicol Adverse Drug Exp*, 1988;3(6):430-48.

4540 Belaiche J, Zittoun J, Marquet J, et al. Effect of ranitidine on secretion of gastric intrinsic factor and absorption of vitamin B12. *Gastroenterol Clin Biol* 1983;7(4):381-4.

4541 Salom IL, Silvis SE, Doscherholmen A. Effect of cimetidine on the absorption of vitamin B12. *Scand J Gastroenterol* 1982;17(1):129-31.

4543 Race TF, Paes IC, Faloon WW. Intestinal malabsorption induced by oral colchicine. Comparison with neomycin and cathartic agents. *Am J Med Sci* 1970;259(1):32-41.

4544 Faloon WW, Chodos RB. Vitamin B12 absorption studies using cochicines, neomycin and continuous 57Co B12 administration. *Gastroenterolgy* 1969;56:1251.

4545 Webb DI, Chodos RB, Mahar CQ, et al. Mechanism of vitamin B12 malabsorption in patients receiving colchicine. *N Engl J Med* 1968;279(16):845-50.

4546 Amer College of Rheumatology ad hoc committee on clinical guidelines. Guidelines for monitoring drug therapy in rheumatoid arthritis. *Arthritis Rheum* 1996;39(5):723-31.

4547 Hielt K, Brynskov J, Hippe E, et al. Oral contraceptives and the cobalamin (vitamin B12) metabolism. *Acta Obstet Gynecol Scand* 1985;64(1):59-63.

4548 Sanpitak N, Chayutimonkul L. Oral contraceptives and riboflavin nutrition. *Lancet* 1974;1(7862):836-7.

4549 Leyden JJ. Absorption of minocycline hydrochloride and tetracycline hydrochloride. Effect of food, milk, and iron. *J Am Acad Dermatol* 1985;12(2 Pt 1):308-12.

4550 Neuvonen PJ, Pentikainen PJ, Gothoni G. Inhibition of iron absorption by tetracycline [letter]. *Br J Clin Pharmacol* 1975;2(1):94-6.

4556 Schwinger RH, Eromann E. Heart failure and electrolyte disturbances. *Methods Find Exp Clin Pharmacol* 1992;14(4):315-25.

4557 Paaby P, Norvin E. The absorption of vitamin B12 during treatment with paraminosalicylic acid. *Acta Med Scand* 1966;180(5):561-4.

4558 Toskes PP, Deren JJ. Selective inhibition of vitamin B12 absorption by para-aminosalicylic acid. *Gastroenterology* 1972;62(6):1232-7.

4559 Longsreth GF, Newcomer AD, Westbrook PR. Para-aminosalicylic acid-induced malabsorption. *Am J Dig Dis* 1972;17(8):731-4.

4560 Zimmerman J. Drug interactions in intestinal transport of folic acid and methotrexate. Further evidence for the heterogeneity of folate transport in the human small intestine. *Biochem Pharmacol* 1992;44(9):1839-42.

4561 Nimmo WS. Drugs, diseases, and altered gastric emptying. *Clin Pharmacokinet* 1967;1(3):189-203.

4562 Andrews R, Greenhaff P, Curtis S, et al. The effect of dietary creatine supplementation on skeletal muscle metabolism in congestive heart failure. *Eur Heart J* 1998;19:617-22.

4563 Gordon A, Hultman E, Kaijser L, et al. Creatine supplementation in chronic heart failure increases skeletal muscle creatine phosphate and muscle performance. *Cardiovasc Res* 1995;30:413-8.

4564 Tarnopolsky M, Martin J. Creatine monohydrate increases strength in patients with neuromuscular disease. *Neurology* 1999;52:854-7.

4565 Tarnopolsky MA, Roy BD, MacDonald JR. A randomized, controlled trial of creatine monohydrate in patients with mitochondrial cytopathies. *Muscle Nerve* 1997;20:1502-9.

4566 Klivenyi P, Ferrante RJ, Matthews RT, et al. Neuroprotective effects of creatine in a transgenic animal model of amyotrophic lateral sclerosis. *Nat Med* 1999;5:347-50.

4567 Matthews RT, Yang L, Jenkins BG, et al. Neuroprotective effects of creatine and cyclocreatine in animal models of Huntington's disease. *J Neurosci* 1998;18:156-63.

4568 Matthews RT, Ferrante RJ, Klivenyi P, et al. Creatine and cyclocreatine attenuate MPTP neurotoxicity. *Exp Neurol* 1999;157:142-9.

4569 Mihic S, MacDonald JR, McKenzie S, Tarnopolsky MA. Acute creatine loading increases fat-free mass, but does not affect blood pressure, plasma creatinine, or CK activity in men and women. *Med Sci Sports Exerc* 2000;32:291-6.

4570 Rawson ES, Clarkson PM. Acute creatine supplementation in older men. *Int J Sports Med* 2000;21:71-5.

4571 Bermon S, Venembre P, Sachet C, et al. Effects of creatine monohydrate ingestion in sedentary and weight-trained older adults. *Acta Physiol Scand* 1998;164:147-55.

4572 Rawson ES, Wehnert ML, Clarkson PM. Effects of 30 days of creatine ingestion in older men. *Eur J Appl Physiol* 1999;80:139-44.

4573 Earnest CP, Almada AL, Mitchell TL. High-performance capillary electrophoresis-pure creatine monohydrate reduces blood lipids in men and women. *Clin Sci (Colch)* 1996;91:113-8.

4574 Demant TW, Rhodes EC. Effects of creatine supplementation on exercise performance. *Sports Med* 1999;28:49-60.

4575 Williams MH, Branch JD. Creatine supplementation and exercise performance: an update. *J Am Coll Nutr* 1998;17:216-34.

4576 The Physician and Sportsmedicine. "Oral Creatine Supplementation" website: www.physsportsmed.com/issues/1999/05_99/juhn.htm (Accessed 17 March 2000).

4577 Heinanen K, Nanto-Salonen K, Komu M, et al. Creatine corrects muscle 31P spectrum in gyrate atrophy with hyperornithinaemia. *Eur J Clin Invest* 1999;29:1060-5.

4578 Sipila I, Rapola J, Simell O, Vannas A. Supplementary creatine as a treatment for gyrate atrophy of the choroid and retina. *N Engl J Med* 1981;304:867-70.

4579 Ingwall JS, Morales MF, Stockdale FE, Wildenthal K. Creatine: a possible stimulus skeletal cardiac muscle hypertrophy. *Recent Adv Stud Cardiac Struct Metab* 1975;8:467-81.

4580 Vandenberghe K, Van Hecke P, Van Leemputte M, et al. Phosphocreatine resynthesis is not affected by creatine loading. *Med Sci Sports Exerc* 1999;31:236-42.

4581 Baerheim A, Larsen E, Digranes A. Vaginal application of lactobacilli in the prophylaxis of recurrent lower urinary tract infection in women. *Scand J Prim Health Care* 1994;12:239-43.

4582 Febbraio MA, Flanagan TR, Snow RJ, et al. Effect of creatine supplementation on intramuscular TCr, metabolism and performance during intermittent, supramaximal exercise in humans. *Acta Physiol Scand* 1995;155:387-95.

4583 Harris RC, Soderlund K, Hultman E. Elevation of creatine in resting and exercised muscle of normal subjects by creatine supplementation. *Clin Sci (Colch)* 1992;83:367-74.

4584 Juhn MS, O'Kane JW, Vinci DM. Oral creatine supplementation in male collegiate athletes: a survey of dosing habits and side effects. *J Am Diet Assoc* 1999;99:593-5.

4585 FDA. "Special Nutritionals Adverse Event Monitoring System" website: http://vm.cfsan.fda.gov/cgi-bin/aems.cgi?QUERY=creatine&STYPE=EXACT (Accessed 17 March 2000).

4586 Cisowski M, Bochenek A, Kucewicz E, et al. The use of exogenous creatine phosphate for myocardial protection in patients undergoing coronary artery bypass surgery. *J Cardiovasc Surg (Torino)* 1996;37:75-80.

4587 Chambers DJ, Haire K, Morley N, et al. St. Thomas' Hospital cardioplegia: enhanced protection with exogenous creatine phosphate. *Ann Thorac Surg* 1996;61:67-75.

4588 Francaux M, Poortmans JR. Effects of training and creatine supplement on muscle strength and body mass. *Eur J Appl Physiol* 1999;80:165-8.

4589 Green AL, Hultman E, Macdonald IA, et al. Carbohydrate ingestion augments skeletal muscle creatine accumulation during creatine supplementation in humans. *Am J Physiol* 1996;271:E821-6.

4590 Lamartiniere CA. Protection against breast cancer with genistein: a component of soy. *Am J Clin Nutr* 2000;71:1705S-7S.

4591 Balsom PD, Soderlund K, Sjodin B, Ekblom B. Skeletal muscle metabolism during short duration high-intensity exercise: influence of creatine supplementation. *Acta Physiol Scand* 1995;154:303-10.

4592 Birch R, Noble D, Greenhaff PL. The influence of dietary creatine supplementation on performance during repeated bouts of maximal isokinetic cycling in man. *Eur J Appl Physiol* 1994;69:268-76.

4593 Dawson B, Cutler M, Moody A, et al. Effects of oral creatine loading on single and repeated maximal short sprints. *Aust J Sci Med Sport* 1995;27:56-61.

4594 Prevost MC, Nelson AG, Morris GS. Creatine supplementation enhances intermittent work performance. *Res Q Exerc Sport* 1997;68:233-40.

4595 Barnett C, Hinds M, Jenkins DG. Effects of oral creatine supplementation on multiple sprint cycle performance. *Aust J Sci Med Sport* 1996;28:35-9.

4596 Cooke WH, Barnes WS. The influence of recovery duration on high-intensity exercise performance after oral creatine supplementation. *Can J Appl Physiol* 1997;22:454-67.

4597 Vanakoski J, Kosunen V, Meririnne E, Seppala T. Creatine and caffeine in anaerobic and aerobic exercise: effects on physical performance and pharmacokinetic considerations. *Int J Clin Pharmacol Ther* 1998;36:258-62.

4598 Cooke WH, Grandjean PW, Barnes WS. Effect of oral creatine supplementation on power output and fatigue during bicycle ergometry. *J Appl Physiol* 1995;78:670-3.

4599 Odland LM, MacDougall JD, Tarnopolsky MA, et al. Effect of oral creatine supplementation on muscle [PCr] and short-term maximum power output *Med Sci Sports Exerc* 1997;29:216-9.

4600 Snow RJ, McKenna MJ, Selig SE, et al. Effect of creatine supplementation on sprint exercise performance and muscle metabolism. *J Appl Physiol* 1998;84:1667-73.

4601 Leenders NM, Lamb DR, Nelson TE. Creatine supplementation and swimming performance. *Int J Sport Nutr* 1999;9:251-62.

4602 Jones AM, Atter T, Georg KP. Oral creatine supplementation improves multiple sprint performance in elite ice-hockey players. *J Sports Med Phys Fitness* 1999;39:189-96.

4603 Theodorou AS, Cooke CB, King RF, et al. The effect of longer-term creatine supplementation on elite swimming performance after an acute creatine loading. *J Sports Sci* 1999;17:853-9.

4604 Kamber M, Koster M, Kreis R, et al. Creatine supplementation - part I: performance, clinical chemistry, and muscle volume. *Med Sci Sports Exerc* 1999;31:1763-9.

4605 McNaughton LR, Dalton B, Tarr J. The effects of creatine supplementation on high-intensity exercise performance in elite performers. *Eur J Appl Physiol* 1998;78:236-40.

4606 McKenna MJ, Morton J, Selig SE, Snow RJ. Creatine supplementation increases muscle total creatine but not maximal intermittent exercise performance. *J Appl Physiol* 1999;87:2244-52.

4607 Rossiter HB, Cannell ER, Jakeman PM. The effect of oral creatine supplementation on the 1000-m performance of competitive rowers. *J Sports Sci* 1996;14:175-9.

4608 Uc A, Bishop WP, Sanders KD. *Camphor Hepatotoxicity. South Med J* 2000;93(6):596-8.

4609 South M. Neonatal seizures after pyridoxine use — reply. *Lancet* 1999;354:2083.

4610 Parry GJ, Bredesen DE. Sensory neuropathy with low-dose pyridoxine. *Neurology* 1985;35:1466-8.

4611 Foster S. Black cohosh (Cimicifuga racemosa): a literature review. *Herbalgram* 1999;45:35-49.

4612 Enzymatic Therapy. "Remifemin" website: http://www.enzy.com/products/individual/eprod141.html (Accesssed 21 March 2000).

4613 Phytopharmica. "Remifemin" website: http://www.phytopharmica.com/consumer/products/1855-BP-remifemin.html (Accesssed 21 March 2000).

4614 Liske E, Wustenberg P. Therapy of climacteric complaints with Cimicifuga racemosa: herbal medicine with clinically proven evidence. *Menopause* 1998;5:250.

4615 Pepping J. Black cohosh: Cimicifuga racemosa. *Am J Health Syst Pharm* 1999;56:1400-2.

4616 Liske E. Therapeutic efficacy and safety of Cimicifuga racemosa for gynecologic disorders. *Adv Ther* 1998;15:45-53.

4618 Kruse SO, Lohning A, Pauli GF, et al. Fukiic and piscidic acid esters from the rhizome of Cimicifuga racemosa and the in vitro estrogenic activity of fukinolic acid. *Planta Med* 1999;65:763-4.

4619 Einer-Jensen N, Zhao J, Andersen KP, Kristoffersen K. Cimicifuga and Melbrosia lack oestrogenic effects in mice and rats. *Maturitas* 1996;25:149-53.

4620 Lehmann-Willenbrock E, Riedel HH. [Clinical and endocrinologic studies of the treatment of ovarian insufficiency manifestations following hysterectomy with intact adnexa]. [Article in German]. *Zentralbl Gynakol* 1988;110:611-8.

4621 Gruenwald J. Standardized black cohosh (Cimicifuga) extract clinical monograph. *Q Rev Nat Med* 1998;3:117-25.

4622 Huperzine Website. "Huperzine A (Cerebra): Memory and Alertness Enhancing Nutriceutical" website: www.hyperzine.net/about.htm (Accessed 24 March 2000).

4623 Consumer Lab. "Product Review: Glucosamine and Chondroitin" website: http://www.consumerlab.com/results/gluco.html (Accessed 24 March 2000).

4624 Xu SS, Cai ZY, Qu ZW, et al. Huperzine-A in capsules and tablets for treating patients with Alzheimer disease. *Zhongguo Yao Li Xue Bao* 1999;20:486-90.

4625 Camps P, Cusack B, Mallender WD, et al. Huprine X is a novel high-affinity inhibitor of acetylcholinesterase that is of interest for treatment of Alzheimer's disease. *Mol Pharmacol* 2000;57:409-17.

4626 Sun QQ, Xu SS, Pan JL, et al. Huperzine-A capsules enhance memory and learning performance in 34 pairs of matched adolescent students. *Chung Kuo Yao Li Hsueh Pao* 1999;20:601-3.

4627 Horwitt MK. My valedictory on the differences in biological potency between RRR-alpha-tocopheryl and all-rac-alpha-tocopheryl acetate. *Am J Clin Nutr* 1999;69:341-2.

4634 Neunteufl T, Priglinger U, Heher S, et al. Effects of vitamin E on chronic and acute endothelial dysfunction in smokers. *J Am Coll Cardiol* 2000;35:277-83.

4635 Sano M, Ernesto C, Thomas RG, et al. A controlled trial of selegiline, alpha-tocopherol, or both as treatment for Alzheimer's disease. The Alzheimer's Disease Cooperative Study. *N Engl J Med* 1997;336:1216-22.

4636 Masaki KH, Losonczy KG, Izmirlian G, et al. Association of vitamin E and C supplement use with cognitive function and dementia in elderly men. *Neurology* 2000;54:1265-72.

4637 Socci DJ, Crandall BM, Arendash GW. Chronic antioxidant treatment improves the cognitive performance of aged rats. *Brain Res* 1995;693:88-94.

4638 Yamada K, Tanaka T, Han D, et al. Protective effects of idebenone and alpha-tocopherol on beta-amyloid-(1-42)-induced learning and memory deficits in rats: implication of oxidative stress in beta-amyloid-induced neurotoxicity in vivo. *Eur J Neurosci* 1999;11:83-90.

4639 Joseph JA, Shukitt-Hale B, Denisova NA, et al. Long-term dietary strawberry, spinach, or vitamin E supplementation retards the onset of age-related neuronal signal-transduction and cognitive behavioral deficits. *J Neurosci* 1998;18:8047-55.

4640 Nemeth I, Turi S, Haszon I, Bereczki C. Vitamin E alleviates the oxidative stress of erythropoietin in uremic children on hemodialysis. *Pediatr Nephrol* 2000;14:13-7.

4641 Inal M, Kanbak G, Sen S, et al. Antioxidant status and lipid peroxidation in hemodialysis patients undergoing erythropoietin and erythropoietin-vitamin E combined therapy. *Free Rad Res* 1999;31:211-6.

4642 Suthutvoravut U, Hathirat P, Sirichakwal P, et al. Vitamin E status, glutathione peroxidase activity and the effect of vitamin E supplementation in children with thalassemia. *J Med Assoc Thai* 1993;76:146-52.

4643 Hartman TJ, Albanes D, Pietinen P, et al. The association between baseline vitamin E, selenium, and prostate cancer in the alpha-tocopherol, beta-carotene cancer prevention study. *Cancer Epidemiol Biomarkers Prev* 1998;7:335-40.

4644 Deneo-Pellegrini H, De Stefani E, Ronco A, Mendilaharsu M. Foods, nutrients and prostate cancer: a case-control study in Uruguay. *Br J Cancer* 1999;80:591-7.

4645 Kristal AR, Stanford JL, Cohen JH, et al. Vitamin and mineral supplement use is associated with reduced risk of prostate cancer. *Cancer Epidemiol Biomarkers Prev* 1999;8:887-92.

4646 Chan JM, Stampfer MJ, Ma J, et al. Supplemental vitamin E intake and prostate cancer risk in a large cohort of men in the United States. *Cancer Epidemiol Biomarkers Prev* 1999;8:893-9.

4647 Cristol JP, Bosc JY, Badiou S, et al. Erythropoietin and oxidative stress in haemodialysis: beneficial effects of vitamin E supplementation. *Nephrol Dial Transplant* 1997;12:2312-7.

4648 Zipursky A, Brown EJ, Watts J, et al. Oral vitamin E supplementation for the prevention of anemia in premature infants: a controlled trial. *Pediatrics* 1987;79:61-8.

4649 Ferns G, Williams J, Forster L, et al. Cholesterol standardized plasma vitamin E levels are reduced in patients with severe angina pectoris. *Int J Exp Pathol* 2000;81:57-62.

4650 Motoyama T, Kawano H, Kugiyama K, et al. Vitamin E administration improves impairment of endothelium-dependent vasodilation in patients with coronary spastic angina. *J Am Coll Cardiol* 1998;32:1672-9.

4651 Rapola JM, Virtamo J, Ripatti S, et al. Effects of alpha tocopherol and beta carotene supplements on symptoms, progression, and prognosis of angina pectoris. *Heart* 1998;79:454-8.

4652 Spencer AP, Carson DS, Crouch MA. Vitamin E and coronary artery disease. *Arch Intern Med* 1999;159:1313-20.

4655 Fish WH, Cohen M, Franzek D, et al. Effect of intramuscular vitamin E on mortality and intracranial hemorrhage in neonates of 1000 grams or less. *Pediatrics* 1990;85:578-84.

4656 Chiswick M, Gladman G, Sinha S, et al. Vitamin E supplementation and periventricular hemorrhage in the newborn. *Am J Clin Nutr* 1991;53:370S-2S.

4657 Watts JL, Milner R, Zipursky A, et al. Failure of supplementation with vitamin E to prevent bronchopulmonary dysplasia in infants less than 1,500 g birth weight. *Eur Resp J* 1991;4:188-90.

4658 Hunter DJ, Manson JE, Colditz GA, et al. A prospective study of the intake of vitamins C, E, and A and the risk of breast cancer. *N Engl J Med* 1993;329:234-40.

4659 Rohan TE, Howe GR, Friedenreich CM, et al. Dietary fiber, vitamins A, C, and E, and risk of breast cancer: a cohort study. *Cancer Causes Control* 1993;4:29-37.

4660 Ernster VL, Goodson WH III, Hunt TK, et al. Vitamin E and benign breast disease: a double-blind, randomized clinical trial. *Surgery* 1985;97:490-4.

4661 Meyer EC, Sommers DK, Reitz CJ, Mentis H. Vitamin E and benign breast disease. *Surgery* 1990 May;107(5):549-51.

4662 London RS, Sundaram GS, Murphy L, et al. The effect of vitamin E on mammary dysplasia: a double-blind study. *Obstet Gynecol* 1985;65:104-6.

4663 Leske MC, Chylack LT Jr, He Q, et al. Antioxidant vitamins and nuclear opacities: the longitudinal study of cataract. *Ophthalmol* 1998;105:831-6.

4664 Seddon JM, Christen WG, Manson JE, et al. The use of vitamin supplements and the risk of cataract among US male physicians. *Am J Publ Health* 1994;84:788-92.

4665 Tavani A, Negri E, La Vecchia C. Food and nutrient intake and risk of cataract. *Ann Epidemiol* 1996;6:41-6.

4666 Teikari JM, Rautalahti M, Haukka J, et al. Incidence of cataract operations in Finnish male smokers unaffected by alpha tocopherol or beta carotene supplements. *J Epidemiol Community Health* 1998;52:468-72.

4667 Teikari JM, Laatikainen L, Virtamo J, et al. Six-year supplementation with alpha-tocopherol and beta-carotene and age-related maculopathy. *Acta Ophthalmol Scand* 1998;76:224-9.

4668 Ludwig CU, Stoll HR, Obrist R, Obrecht JP. Prevention of cytotoxic drug induced skin ulcers with dimethyl sulfoxide (DMSO) and alpha-tocopherol. *Eur J Cancer Clin Oncol* 1987;23:327-9.

4670 Raju GB, Behari M, Prasad K, Ahuja GK. Randomized, double-blind, placebo-controlled, clinical trial of D-alpha-tocopherol (vitamin E) as add-on therapy in uncontrolled epilepsy. *Epilepsia* 1994;35:368-72.

4671 Ogunmekan AO, Hwang PA. A randomized, double-blind, placebo-controlled, clinical trial of D-alpha-tocopheryl acetate (vitamin E), as add-on therapy, for epilepsy in children. *Epilepsia* 1989;30:84-9.

4672 Delanian S, Balla-Mekias S, Lefaix JL. Striking regression of chronic radiotherapy damage in a clinical trial of combined pentoxifylline and tocopherol. *J Clin Oncol* 1999;17:3283-90.

4673 Delanian S. Striking regression of radiation-induced fibrosis by a combination of pentoxifylline and tocopherol. *Br J Radiol* 1998;71:892-4.

4675 Tahzib M, Frank R, Gauthier B, et al. Vitamin E treatment of focal segmental glomerulosclerosis: results of an open-label study. *Pediatr Nephrol* 1999;13:649-52.

4676 Varis K, Taylor PR, Sipponen P, et al. Gastric cancer and premalignant lesions in atrophic gastritis: a controlled trial on the effect of supplementation with alpha-tocopherol and beta-carotene. The Helsinki Gastritis Study Group. *Scand J Gastroenterol* 1998;33:294-300.

4677 Bukin YV, Draudin-Krylenko VA, Kuvshinov YP, et al. Decrease of ornithine decarboxylase activity in premalignant gastric mucosa and regression of small intestinal metaplasia in patients supplemented with high doses of vitamin E. *Cancer Epidemiol Biomarkers Prev* 1997;6:543-6.

4678 Dawsey SM, Wang GQ, Taylor PR, et al. Effects of vitamin/mineral supplementation on the prevalence of histological dysplasia and early cancer of the esophagus and stomach: results from the Dysplasia Trial in Linxian, China. *Cancer Epidemiol Biomarkers Prev* 1994;3:167-72.

4679 Wang GQ, Dawsey SM, Li JY, et al. Effects of vitamin/mineral supplementation on the prevalence of histological dysplasia and early cancer of the esophagus and stomach: results from the General Population Trial in Linxian, China. *Cancer Epidemiol Biomarkers Prev* 1994;3:161-6.

4681 Goldstein RK, Zillikens D, Miller K, Elsner P, Burg G. Local treatment of disseminated granuloma anulare with a vitamin E emulsion. *Hautarzt* 1991;42:176-8.

4682 Eldamhougy S, Elhelw Z, Yamamah G, et al. The vitamin E status among glucose-6 phosphate dehydrogenase deficient patients and effectiveness of oral vitamin E. *Int J Vita Nutr Res* 1988;58:184-8.

4683 Hafez M, Amar ES, Zedan M, et al. Improved erythrocyte survival with combined vitamin E and selenium therapy in children with glucose-6-phosphate dehydrogenase deficiency and mild chronic hemolysis. *J Pediatr* 1986;108:558-561.

4684 Johnson GJ, Vatassery GT, Finkel B, Allen DW. High-dose vitamin E does not decrease the rate of chronic hemolysis in glucose-6-phosphate dehydrogenase deficiency. *N Engl J Med* 1983;308:1014-7.

4685 Chan AC, Chow CK, Chiu D. Interaction of antioxidants and their implication in genetic anemia. *Proc Soc Exp Biol Med* 1999;222:274-82.

4686 Peyser CE, Folstein M, Chase GA, et al. Trial of d-alpha-tocopherol in Huntington's disease. *Am J Psychiatry* 1995;152:1771-5.

4687 Meydani SN, Meydani M, Blumberg JB, et al. Vitamin E supplementation and in vivo immune response in healthy elderly subjects. A randomized controlled trial. *JAMA* 1997;277:1380-6.

4688 Ravaglia G, Forti P, Maioli F, et al. Effect of micronutrient status on natural killer cell immune function in healthy free-living subjects aged >/=90 y. *Am J Clin Nutr* 2000;71:590-8.

4689 Pallast EG, Schouten EG, de Waart FG, et al. Effect of 50- and 100-mg vitamin E supplements on cellular immune function in noninstitutionalized elderly persons. *Am J Clin Nutr* 1999;69:1273-81.

4690 de la Fuente M, Ferrandez MD, Burgos MS, et al. Immune function in aged women is improved by ingestion of vitamins C and E. *Can J Physiol Pharmacol* 1998;76:373-80.

4691 Buzina-Suboticanec K, Buzina R, Stavljenic A, et al. Aging, nutritional status and immune response. *Int J Vita Nutr Res* 1998;68:133-41.

4692 De Waart FG, Portengen L, Doekes G, et al. Effect of 3 months vitamin E supplementation on indices of the cellular and humoral immune response in elderly subjects. *Br J Nutr* 1997;78:761-74.

4693 Kessopoulou E, Powers HJ, Sharma KK, et al. A double-blind, randomized, placebo, cross-over, controlled trial using the antioxidant vitamin E to treat reactive oxygen species associated male infertility. *Fertil Steril* 1995;64:825-31.

4695 Suleiman SA, Ali ME, Zaki ZM, et al. Lipid peroxidation and human sperm motility: protective role of vitamin E. *J Androl* 1996;17:530-7.

4696 Rolf C, Cooper TG, Yeung CH, Nieschlag E. Antioxidant treatment of patients with asthenozoospermia or moderate oligoasthenozoospermia with high-dose vitamin C and vitamin E: a randomized, placebo-controlled, double-blind study. *Hum Reprod* 1999;14:1028-33.

4697 Yau TM, Weisel RD, Mickle DA, et al. Vitamin E for coronary bypass operations. A prospective, double-blind, randomized trial. *J Thorac Cardiovasc Surg* 1994;108:302-10.

4698 Westhuyzen J, Cochrane AD, Tesar PJ, et al. Effect of preoperative supplementation with alpha-tocopherol and ascorbic acid on myocardial injury in patients undergoing cardiac operations. *J Thorac Cardiovasc Surg* 1997;113:942-8.

4699 Sisto T, Paajanen H, Metsa-Ketela T, et al. Pretreatment with antioxidants and allopurinol diminishes cardiac onset events in coronary artery bypass grafting. *Ann Thorac Surg* 1995;59:1519-23.

4700 Riley JD, Antony SJ. Leg cramps: differential diagnosis and management. *Am Fam Physician* 1995;52:1794-8.

4701 Roca AO, Jarjoura D, Blend D, et al. Dialysis leg cramps. Efficacy of quinine versus vitamin E. *ASAIO J* 1992;38:M481-5.

4702 Connolly PS, Shirley EA, Wasson JH, Nierenberg DW. Treatment of nocturnal leg cramps. A crossover trial of quinine vs vitamin E. *Arch Intern Med* 1992;152:1877-80.

4703 Fenichel GM, Brooke MH, Griggs RC, et al. Clinical investigation in Duchenne muscular dystrophy: penicillamine and vitamin E. *Muscle Nerve* 1988;11:1164-8.

4704 Orndahl G, Grimby G, Grimby A, et al. Functional deterioration and selenium-vitamin E treatment in myotonic dystrophy. A placebo-controlled study. *J Intern Med* 1994;235:205-10.

4705 Watanabe H, Kakihana M, Ohtsuka S, Sugishita Y. Randomized, double-blind, placebo-controlled study of supplemental vitamin E on attenuation of the development of nitrate tolerance. *Circulation* 1997;96:2545-50.

4706 Honegger UE, Scuntaro I, Wiesmann UN. Vitamin E reduces accumulation of amiodarone and desethylamiodarone and inhibits phospholipidosis in cultured human cells. *Biochem Pharmacol* 1995;49:1741-5.

4707 Kachel DL, Moyer TP, Martin WJ II. Amiodarone-induced injury of human pulmonary artery endothelial cells: protection by alpha-tocopherol. *J Pharmacol Exp Ther* 1990;254:1107-12.

4708 Benner SE, Winn RJ, Lippman SM, et al. Regression of oral leukoplakia with alpha-tocopherol: a community clinical oncology program chemoprevention study. *J Natl Cancer Inst* 1993;85:44-7.

4709 The Parkinson Study Group. Effects of tocopherol and deprenyl on the progression of disability in early Parkinson's disease. *N Engl J Med* 1993;328:176-83.

4710 Kieburtz K, McDermott M, Como P, et al. The effect of deprenyl and tocopherol on cognitive performance in early untreated Parkinson's disease. Parkinson Study Group. *Neurology* 1994;44:1756-9.

4711 Parkinson Study Group. Impact of deprenyl and tocopherol treatment on Parkinson's disease in DATATOP patients requiring levodopa. *Ann Neurol* 1996;39:37-45.

4712 de Rijk MC, Breteler MM, den Breeijen JH, et al. Dietary antioxidants and Parkinson disease. The Rotterdam Study. *Arch Neurol* 1997;54:762-5.

4713 Dreher F, Gabard B, Schwindt DA, Maibach HI. Topical melatonin in combination with vitamins E and C protects skin from ultraviolet-induced erythema: a human study in vivo. *Br J Dermatol* 1998;139:332-9.

4714 Dreher F, Denig N, Gabard B, et al. Effect of topical antioxidants on UV-induced erythema formation when administered after exposure. *Dermatol* 1999;198:52-5.

4715 Fuchs J, Kern H. Modulation of UV-light-induced skin inflammation by D-alpha-tocopherol and L-ascorbic

4716 Eberlein-Konig B, Placzek M, Przybilla B. Protective effect against sunburn of combined systemic ascorbic acid (vitamin C) and d-alpha-tocopherol (vitamin E). *J Am Acad Dermatol* 1998;38:45-8.

acid: a clinical study using solar simulated radiation. *Free Radic Biol Med* 1998;25:1006-12.

4718 Gulmezoglu AM, Hofmeyr GJ, Oosthuisen MM. Antioxidants in the treatment of severe pre-eclampsia: an explanatory randomised controlled trial. *Br J Obstet Gynacol* 1997;104:689-96.

4719 London RS, Murphy L, Kitlowski KE, Reynolds MA. Efficacy of alpha-tocopherol in the treatment of the premenstrual syndrome. *J Reprod Med* 1987;32:400-4.

4720 London RS, Sundaram GS, Murphy L, Goldstein PJ. The effect of alpha-tocopherol on premenstrual symptomatology: a double-blind study. *J Am Coll Nutr* 1983;2:115-22.

4721 Baumann LS, Spencer JS. The Effects of Topical Vitamin E on the Cosmetic Appearance of Scars. *Dermatol Surg* 1999;25:311-5.

4722 Jenkins M, Alexander JW, MacMillan BG, et al. Failure of topical steroids and vitamin E to reduce postoperative scar formation following reconstructive surgery. *J Burn Care Rehabil* 1986;7:309-12.

4723 Edmonds SE, Winyard PG, Guo R, et al. Putative analgesic activity of repeated oral doses of vitamin E in the treatment of rheumatoid arthritis. Results of a prospective placebo controlled double blind trial. *Ann Rheum Dis* 1997;56:649-55.

4724 Tutuncu NB, Bayraktar M, Varli K. Reversal of defective nerve conduction with vitamin E supplementation in type 2 diabetes: a preliminary study. *Diabetes Care* 1998;21:1915-8.

4725 Bursell SE, Clermont AC, Aiello LP, et al. High-dose vitamin E supplementation normalizes retinal blood flow and creatinine clearance in patients with type 1 diabetes. *Diabetes Care* 1999;22:1245-51.

4726 Paolisso G, D'Amore A, Giugliano D, et al. Pharmacologic doses of vitamin E improve insulin action in healthy subjects and non-insulin-dependent diabetic patients. *Am J Clin Nutr* 1993;57:650-6.

4727 Paolisso G, Di Maro G, Galzerano D, et al. Pharmacological doses of vitamin E and insulin action in elderly subjects. *Am J Clin Nutr* 1994;59:1291-6.

4729 National Academy of Science, Institute of Medicine. Dietary Reference Intakes for Vitamin C, Vitamin E, Selenium, and Carotenoids. http://www4.nas.edu/iom/iomhome.nsf/Pages/Recently+Released+Reports (Accessed 20 April 2000).

4730 van Rooij J, Schwartzenberg SG, Mulder PG, Baarsma SG. Oral vitamins C and E as additional treatment in patients with acute anterior uveitis: a randomised double masked study in 145 patients. *Br J Ophthalmol* 1999;83:1277-82.

4732 Tornwall ME, Virtamo J, Haukka JK, et al. The effect of alpha-tocopherol and beta-carotene supplementation on symptoms and progression of intermittent claudication in a controlled trial. *Atherosclerosis* 1999;147:193-7.

4733 Liede KE, Haukka JK, Saxen LM, Heinonen OP. Increased tendency towards gingival bleeding caused by joint effect of alpha-tocopherol supplementation and acetylsalicylic acid. *Ann Med* 1998;30:542-6.

4734 ARS-GRIN. "Herbalist's Desk Reference (HDR)" URL: www.ars-grin.gov (Accessed 25 April 2000).

4735 Setchell KD, Gosselin SJ, Welsh MB, et al. Dietary

estrogens—a probable cause of infertility and liver disease in captive cheetahs. *Gastroenterol* 1987;93:225-33.

4736 Evans AM. Influence of dietary components on the gastrointestinal metabolism and transport of drugs. *Ther Drug Monit* 2000;22:131-6.

4737 Anon. Phytoestrogens. *Med Letter* 2000;42:17-18.

4738 Hodgson JM, Puddey IB, Beilin LJ, et al. Supplementation with isoflavonoid phytoestrogens does not alter serum lipid concentrations: a randomized controlled trial in humans. *J Nutr* 1998;128:728-32.

4739 Hodgson JM, Puddey IB, Beilin LJ, et al. Effects of isoflavonoids on blood pressure in subjects with high-normal ambulatory blood pressure levels: a randomized controlled trial. *Am J Hypertens* 1999;12:47-53.

4740 Yanagihara K, Ito A, Toge T, Numoto M. Antiproliferative effects of isoflavones on human cancer cell lines established from the gastrointestinal tract. *Cancer Res* 1993;53:5815-21.

4741 Le Bail JC, Champavier Y, Chulia AJ, Habrioux G. Effects of phytoestrogens on aromatase, 3beta and 17beta-hydroxysteroid dehydrogenase activities and human breast cancer cells. *Life Sci* 2000;66:1281-91.

4742 Cassady JM, Zennie TM, Chae YH, et al. Use of a mammalian cell culture benzo(a)pyrene metabolism assay for the detection of potential anticarcinogens from natural products: inhibition of metabolism by biochanin A, an isoflavone from Trifolium pratense L. *Cancer Res* 1988;48:6257-61.

4743 Kurzer MS, Xu X. Dietary phytoestrogens. *Annu Rev Nutr* 1997;17:353-81.

4744 ARS-GRIN. Dr. Duke's Phytochemical and Ethnobotanical Databases URL: www.ars-grin.gov (Accessed 24 April 2000).

4745 Absolute Truth Hardcore Bodybuilding. "Ipriflavone" website: http://members.tripod.com/~absolutetruth/index2.htm (Accessed 26 April 2000).

4746 Gambacciani M, Cappagli B, Piaggesi L, et al. Ipriflavone prevents the loss of bone mass in pharmacological menopause induced by GnRH-agonists. *Calcif Tissue Int* 1997;61:S15-8.

4747 Yamazaki I, Shino A, Shimizu Y, et al. Effect of ipriflavone on glucocorticoid-induced osteoporosis in rats. *Life Sci* 1986;38:951-8.

4748 Cecchettin M, Bellometti S, Cremonesi G, et al. Metabolic and bone effects after administration of ipriflavone and salmon calcitonin in postmenopausal osteoporosis. *Biomed Pharmacother* 1995;49:465-8.

4749 Nozaki M, Hashimoto K, Inoue Y, et al. Treatment of bone loss in oophorectomized women with a combination of ipriflavone and conjugated equine estrogen. *Int J Gynaecol Obstet* 1998;62:69-75.

4750 Xu X, Wang HJ, Murphy PA, Hendrich S. Neither background diet nor type of soy food affects short-term isoflavone bioavailability in women. *J Nutr* 2000;130:798-801.

4751 Scambia G, Mango D, Signorile PG, et al. Clinical effects of a standardized soy extract in postmenopausal women: a pilot study. *Menopause* 2000;7:105-11.

4752 Albertazzi P, Pansini F, Bottazzi M, et al. Dietary soy supplementation and phytoestrogen levels. *Obstet Gynecol* 1999;94:229-31.

4753 Kurzer MS, Xu X. Dietary phytoestrogens. *Annu Rev Nutr* 1997;17:353-81.

4755 Sirtori CR, Pazzucconi F, Colombo L, et al. Double-blind study of the addition of high-protein soya milk v. cows' milk to the diet of patients with severe hypercholesterolemia and resistance to or intolerance of statins. *Br J Nutr* 1999;82:91-6.

4756 Maugeri D, Panebianco P, Russo MS, et al. Ipriflavone-treatment of senile osteoporosis: results of a multicenter, double-blind clinical trial of 2 years. *Arch Gerontol Geriatr* 1994;19:253-63.

4757 Scali G, Mansanti P, Zurlo A, et al. Analgesic effect of ipriflavone versus sCalcitonin in the treatment of osteoporotic vertebral pain. *Curr Ther Res* 1991;49:1004-10.

4759 Mares-Perlman JA, Brady WE, Klein BE, et al. Serum carotenoids and tocopherols and severity of nuclear and cortical opacities. *Invest Ophthalmol Vis Sci* 1995;36:276-88.

4760 MotherNature.Com. "The Consumer Guide to Garlic" and "Garlic" website: www.mothernature.com (Accessed 4 May 2000).

4761 Graham DY, Anderson SY, Lang T. Garlic or jalapeno peppers for treatment of Helicobacter pylori infection. *Am J Gastroenterol* 1999;94:1200-2.

4762 Ernst E. Is garlic an effective treatment for Helicobacter pylori infection? *Arch Intern Med* 1999;159:2484-5.

4763 Aydin A, Ersoz G, Tekesin O, et al. Garlic oil and Helicobacter pylori infection. *Am J Gastroenterol* 2000;95:563-4.

4764 O'Gara EA, Hill DJ, Maslin DJ. Activities of Garlic Oil, Garlic Powder, and Their Diallyl Constituents against Helicobacter pylori. *Appl Environ Microbiol* 2000;66:2269-73.

4765 Calvet X, Carod C, Gene E. Re: Peppers at treatment for Helicobacter pylori infection. *Am J Gastroenterol* 2000;95:820-1.

4766 Ledezma E, DeSousa L, Jorquera A, et al. Efficacy of ajoene, an organosulphur derived from garlic, in the short-term therapy of tinea pedis. *Mycoses* 1996;39:393-5.

4767 Ledezma E, Lopez JC, Marin P, et al. Ajoene in the topical short-term treatment of tinea cruris and tinea corporis in humans. Randomized comparative study with terbinafine. *Arzneimittelforschung* 1999;49:544-7.

4768 Ankri S, Mirelman D. Antimicrobial properties of allicin from garlic. *Microbes Infect* 1999;1:125-9.

4769 Weber ND, Andersen DO, North JA, et al. In vitro virucidal effects of Allium sativum (garlic) extract and compounds. *Planta Med* 1992;58:417-23.

4770 Steinmetz KA, Kushi LH, Bostick RM, et al. Vegetables, fruit, and colon cancer in the Iowa Women's Health Study. *Am J Epidemiol* 1994;139:1-15.

4771 Witte JS, Longnecker MP, Bird CL, et al Relation of vegetable, fruit, and grain consumption to colorectal adenomatous polyps. *Am J Epidemiol* 1996;144:1015-25.

4772 Le Marchand L, Hankin JH, Wilkens LR, et al. Dietary fiber and colorectal cancer risk. *Epidemiology* 1997;8:658-65.

4773 Dorant E, van den Brandt PA, Goldbohm RA. A prospective cohort study on the relationship between onion and leek consumption, garlic supplement use and the risk of colorectal carcinoma in The Netherlands. *Carcinogenesis* 1996;17:477-84.

4774 You WC, Zhang L, Gail MH, et al. Helicobacter pylori infection, garlic intake and precancerous lesions in a Chinese population at low risk of gastric cancer. *Int J Epidemiol* 1998;27:941-4.

4775 You WC, Blot WJ, Chang YS, et al. Allium vegetables and reduced risk of stomach cancer. *J Natl Cancer Inst* 1989;81:162-4.

4776 Takezaki T, Gao CM, Ding JH, et al. Comparative study of lifestyles of residents in high and low risk areas for gastric cancer in Jiangsu Province, China; with special reference to allium vegetables. *J Epidemiol* 1999;9:297-305.

4777 Key TJ, Silcocks PB, Davey GK, et al. A case-control study of diet and prostate cancer. *Br J Cancer* 1997;76:678-87.

4778 Dorant E, van den Brandt PA, Goldbohm RA. A prospective cohort study on Allium vegetable consumption, garlic supplement use, and the risk of lung carcinoma in The Netherlands. *Cancer Res* 1994;54:6148-53.

4779 Dorant E, van den Brandt PA, Goldbohm RA. Allium vegetable consumption, garlic supplement intake, and female breast carcinoma incidence. *Breast Cancer Res Treat* 1995;33:163-70.

4780 Mostafa MG, Mima T, Ohnishi ST, Mori K. S-allylcysteine ameliorates doxorubicin toxicity in the heart and liver in mice. *Planta Med* 2000;66:148-51.

4782 Holzgartner H, Schmidt U, Kuhn U. Comparison of the efficacy and tolerance of a garlic preparation vs. bezafibrate. *Arzneimittelforschung* 1992;42:1473-7.

4783 Jain AK, Vargas R, Gotzkowsky S, McMahon FG. Can garlic reduce levels of serum lipids? A controlled clinical study. *Am J Med* 1993;94:632-5.

4784 Mader FH. Treatment of hyperlipidaemia with garlic-powder tablets. Evidence from the German Association of General Practitioners' multicentric placebo-controlled double-blind study. *Arzneimittelforschung* 1990;40:1111-6.

4785 Rotzsch W, Richter V, Rassoul F, Walper A. [Postprandial lipemia under treatment with Allium sativum. Controlled double-blind study of subjects with reduced HDL2-cholesterol]. [Article in German] *Arzneimittelforschung* 1992;42:1223-7.

4786 Silagy C, Neil A. Garlic as a lipid lowering agent—a meta-analysis. J R Coll Physicians Lond 1994;28:39-45.

4787 Vorberg G, Schneider B. Therapy with garlic: results of a placebo-controlled, double-blind study. *Br J Clin Pract Symp Suppl* 1990;69:7-11.

4788 Warshafsky S, Kamer RS, Sivak SL. Effect of garlic on total serum cholesterol. A meta-analysis. *Ann Intern Med* 1993;119:599-605.

4789 Adler AJ, Holub BJ. Effect of garlic and fish-oil supplementation on serum lipid and lipoprotein concentrations in hypercholesterolemic men. *Am J Clin Nutr* 1997;65:445-50.

4790 Morcos NC. Modulation of lipid profile by fish oil and garlic combination. *J Natl Med Assoc* 1997;89:673-8.

4791 Kenzelmann R, Kade F. Limitation of the deterioration of lipid parameters by a standardized garlic-ginkgo combination product. A multicenter placebo-controlled double-blind study. *Arzneimittelforschung* 1993;43:978-81.

4792 Superko HR, Krauss RM. Garlic powder, effect on plasma lipids, postprandial lipemia, low-density lipoprotein particle size, high-density lipoprotein subclass distribution and lipoprotein(a). *J Am Coll Cardiol* 2000;35:321-6.

4793 Simons LA, Balasubramaniam S, von Konigsmark M, et

al. On the effect of garlic on plasma lipids and lipoproteins in mild hypercholesterolaemia. *Atherosclerosis* 1995;113:219-25.

4794 Luley C, Lehmann-Leo W, Moller B, et al. Lack of efficacy of dried garlic in patients with hyperlipoproteinemia. *Arzneimittelforschung* 1986;36:766-8.

4795 Neil HA, Silagy CA, Lancaster T, et al. Garlic powder in the treatment of moderate hyperlipidaemia: a controlled trial and meta-analysis. *J R Coll Physicians Lond* 1996;30:329-34.

4796 McCrindle BW, Helden E, Conner WT. Garlic extract therapy in children with hypercholesterolemia. *Arch Pediatr Adolesc Med* 1998;152:1089-94.

4797 Breithaupt-Grogler K, Ling M, Boudoulas H, Belz GG. Protective effect of chronic garlic intake on elastic properties of aorta in the elderly. *Circulation* 1997;96:2649-55.

4798 Koscielny J, Klussendorf D, Latza R, et al. The antiatherosclerotic effect of Allium sativum. *Atherosclerosis* 1999;144:237-49.

4799 Chutani SK, Bordia A. The effect of fried versus raw garlic on fibrinolytic activity in man. *Atherosclerosis* 1981;38:417-21.

4800 Blumenthal M, Goldberg A, Brinckmann J (eds). *Herbal Medicine* Expanded Commission E Monographs. Newton, MA: Integrative Medicine Communications, 2000.

4801 Kiesewetter H, Jung F, Jung EM, et al. Effects of garlic coated tablets in peripheral arterial occlusive disease. *Clin Investig* 1993;71:383-6.

4802 Kiesewetter H, Jung F, Jung EM, et al. Effect of garlic on platelet aggregation in patients with increased risk of juvenile ischaemic attack. *Eur J Clin Pharmacol* 1993;45:333-6.

4803 Legnani C, Frascaro M, Guazzaloca G, et al. Effects of a dried garlic preparation on fibrinolysis and platelet aggregation in healthy subjects. *Arzneimittelforschung* 1993;43:119-22.

4804 Ali M, Bordia T, Mustafa T. Effect of raw versus boiled aqueous extract of garlic and onion on platelet aggregation. *Prostaglandins Leukot Essent Fatty Acids* 1999;60:43-7.

4805 Morris J, Burke V, Mori TA, et al. Effects of garlic extract on platelet aggregation: a randomized placebo-controlled double-blind study. *Clin Exp Pharmacol Physiol* 1995;22:414-7.

4807 Arora RC, Arora S. Comparative effect of clofibrate, garlic and onion on alimentary hyperlipemia. *Atherosclerosis* 1981;39:447-52.

4808 Sasaki J, Kita T, Ishita K, et al. Antibacterial activity of garlic powder against Escherichia coli O-157. *J Nutr Sci Vitaminol (Tokyo)* 1999;45:785-90.

4809 Jepson RG, Kleijnen J, Leng GC. Garlic for peripheral arterial occlusive disease (Cochrane Review). In: The Cochrane Library, Issue 2, 2000. Oxford: Update Software.

4810 Gebhardt R, Beck H. Differential inhibitory effects of garlic-derived organosulfur compounds on cholesterol biosynthesis in primary rat hepatocyte cultures. *Lipids* 1996;31:1269-76.

4811 Qureshi AA, Din ZZ, Abuirmeileh N, et al. Suppression of avian hepatic lipid metabolism by solvent extracts of garlic: impact on serum lipids. *J Nutr* 1983;113:1746-55.

4812 Pedraza-Chaverri J, Tapia E, Medina-Campos ON, et al. Garlic prevents hypertension induced by chronic inhibition of nitric oxide synthesis. *Life Sci* 1998;62:71-7.

4813 Dirsch VM, Kiemer AK, Wagner H, Vollmar AM. Effect of allicin and ajoene, two compounds of garlic, on inducible nitric oxide synthase. *Atherosclerosis* 1998;139:333-9.

4814 American Academy of Pediatrics. Camphor revisited: focus on toxicity (RE9422). *Pediatrics* 1994;94(1):127-8.

4815 Ip C, Lisk DJ. Efficacy of cancer prevention by high-selenium garlic is primarily dependent on the action of selenium. *Carcinogenesis* 1995;16:2649-52.

4816 Anibarro B, Fontela JL, De La Hoz F. Occupational asthma induced by garlic dust. *J Allergy Clin Immunol* 1997;100:734-8.

4817 Zema MJ. Gemfibrozil, nicotinic acid and combination therapy in patients with isolated hypoalphalipoproteinemia: a randomized, open-label, crossover study. *J Am Coll Cardiol* 2000;35:640-6.

4818 Guyton JR, Blazing MA, Hagar J, et al. Extended-release niacin vs gemfibrozil for the treatment of low levels of high-density lipoprotein cholesterol. Niaspan-Gemfibrozil Study Group. *Arch Intern Med* 2000;160:1177-84.

4819 Alberts DS, Martinez ME, Roe DJ, et al. Lack of effect of a high-fiber cereal supplement on the recurrence of colorectal adenomas. Phoenix Colon Cancer Prevention Physicians' Network. *N Engl J Med* 2000;342:1156-62.

4820 Schatzkin A, Lanza E, Corle D, et al. Lack of effect of a low-fat, high-fiber diet on the recurrence of colorectal adenomas. Polyp Prevention Trial Study Group. *N Engl J Med* 2000;342:1149-55.

4821 Fuchs CS, Giovannucci EL, Colditz GA, et al. Dietary fiber and the risk of colorectal cancer and adenoma in women. *N Engl J Med* 1999;340:169-76.

4822 Iso H, Stampfer MJ, Manson JE, et al. Prospective study of calcium, potassium, and magnesium intake and risk of stroke in women. *Stroke* 1999;30:1772-9.

4823 Cueto-Manzano AM, Konel S, Freemont AJ, et al. Effect of 1,25-dihydroxyvitamin D3 and calcium carbonate on bone loss associated with long-term renal transplantation. *Am J Kidney Dis* 2000;35:227-36.

4824 Zittermann A, Bock P, Drummer C, et al. Lactose does not enhance calcium bioavailability in lactose-tolerant, healthy adults. *Am J Clin Nutr* 2000;71:931-6.

4825 Chan JM, Giovannucci E, Andersson SO, et al. Dairy products, calcium, phosphorous, vitamin D, and risk of prostate cancer. *Cancer Causes Control* 1998;9:559-66.

4827 Harvard School of Public Health Press Releases. "Higher Intake of Dairy Products May Be Linked to Prostate Cancer Risk" website: www.hsph.harvard.edu/press/releases/press04042000.html. (Accessed 5 May 2000).

4828 Mennella JA, Johnson A, Beauchamp GK. Garlic ingestion by pregnant women alters the odor of amniotic fluid. *Chem Senses* 1995;20:207-9.

4829 Mennella JA, Beauchamp GK. Maternal diet alters the sensory qualities of human milk and the nursling's behavior. *Pediatrics* 1991;88:737-44.

4830 Mennella JA, Beauchamp GK. The effects of repeated exposure to garlic-flavored milk on the nursling's behavior. *Pediatr Res* 1993;34:805-8.

4832 Cronin E. Dermatitis of the hands in caterers. *Contact*

4833 Lee TY, Lam TH. Contact dermatitis due to topical treatment with garlic in Hong Kong. *Contact Dermatitis* 1991;24:193-6.

Dermatitis 1987;17:265-9.

4838 Vera JC, Rivas CI, Zhang RH, et al. Human HL-60 myeloid leukemia cells transport dehydroascorbic acid via the glucose transporters and accumulate reduced ascorbic acid. *Blood* 1994;84:1628-34.

4839 Spielholz C, Golde DW, Houghton AN, et al. Increased facilitated transport of dehydroascorbic acid without changes in sodium-dependent ascorbate transport in human melanoma cells. *Cancer Res* 1997;57:2529-37.

4840 Vera JC, Rivas CI, Zhang RH, Golde DW. Colony-stimulating factors signal for increased transport of vitamin C in human host defense cells. *Blood* 1998;91:2536-46.

4841 Agus DB, Vera JC, Golde DW. Stromal cell oxidation: a mechanism by which tumors obtain vitamin C. *Cancer Res* 1999;59:4555-8.

4842 Moertel CG, Fleming TR, Creagan ET, et al. High-dose vitamin C versus placebo in the treatment of patients with advanced cancer who have had no prior chemotherapy. A randomized double-blind comparison. *N Engl J Med* 1985;312:137-41.

4843 Creagan ET, Moertel CG, O'Fallon JR, et al. Failure of high-dose vitamin C (ascorbic acid) therapy to benefit patients with advanced cancer. A controlled trial. *N Engl J Med* 1979;301:687-90.

4844 Food and Nutrition Board, Institute of Medicine. "Dietary Reference Intakes for Vitamin C, Vitamin E, Selenium, and Carotenoids" website: www.iom.edu/IOM/IOMHome.nsf/Pages/Recently+Released+Reports (Accessed 17 May 2000).

4845 Consumer Lab. "Product Review: Vitamin C" website: http://www.consumerlab.com/results/vitaminc.html (Accessed 17 May 2000).

4846 Jolliet P, Simon N, Barre J, et al. Plasma coenzyme Q10 concentrations in breast cancer: prognosis and therapeutic consequences. *Int J Clin Pharmacol Ther* 1998;36:506-509.

4847 Canner PL, Berge KG, Wenger NK, et al. Fifteen year mortality in Coronary Drug Project patients: long-term benefit with niacin. *J Am Coll Cardiol* 1986;8:1245-55.

4848 Zhao XQ, Brown BG, Hillger L, et al. Effects of intensive lipid-lowering therapy on the coronary arteries of asymptomatic subjects with elevated apolipoprotein B. *Circulation* 1993;88:2744-53.

4849 Institute of Medicine. Dietary Reference Intakes for Thiamin, Riboflavin, Niacin, Vitamin B6, folate, Vitamin B12, Pantothenic Acid, Biotin, and Choline. website: http://books.nap.edu/books/0309065542/html/123.html#pagetop (Accessed 24 May 2000).

4850 Park YK, Sempos CT, Barton CN, et al. Effectiveness of food fortification in the United States: the case of pellagra. *Am J Public Health* 2000;90:727-38.

4851 Gibbons LW, Gonzalez V, Gordon N, Grundy S. The prevalence of side effects with regular and sustained-release nicotinic acid. *Am J Med* 1995;99:378-85.

4852 Whelan AM, Price SO, Fowler SF, Hainer BL. The effect of aspirin on niacin-induced cutaneous reactions. *J Fam Pract* 1992;34:165-8.

4853 Jungnickel PW, Maloley PA, Vander Tuin EL, et al. Effect of two aspirin pretreatment regimens on niacin-induced cutaneous reactions. *J Gen Intern Med* 1997;12:591-6.

4854 Capuzzi DM, Guyton JR, Morgan JM, et al. Efficacy and safety of an extended-release niacin (Niaspan): a long-term study. *Am J Cardiol* 1998;82:74-81;disc. 85U-6U.

4855 Gray DR, Morgan T, Chretien SD, Kashyap ML. Efficacy and safety of controlled-release niacin in dyslipoproteinemic veterans. *Ann Intern Med* 1994;121:252-8.

4856 McKenney JM, Proctor JD, Harris S, Chinchili VM. A comparison of the efficacy and toxic effects of sustained- vs immediate-release niacin in hypercholesterolemic patients. *JAMA* 1994;271:672-7.

4857 Knopp RH, Alagona P, Davidson M, et al. Equivalent efficacy of a time-release form of niacin (Niaspan) given once-a-night versus plain niacin in the management of hyperlipidemia. *Metabolism* 1998;47:1097-104.

4858 Knopp RH. Clinical profiles of plain versus sustained-release niacin (Niaspan) and the physiologic rationale for nighttime dosing. *Am J Cardiol* 1998;82:24U-28U;discussion 39U-41U.

4859 Crouse JR III. New developments in the use of niacin for treatment of hyperlipidemia: new considerations in the use of an old drug. *Coron Artery Dis* 1996;7:321-6.

4860 Garg A, Grundy SM. Nicotinic acid as therapy for dyslipidemia in non-insulin-dependent diabetes mellitus. *JAMA* 1990;264:723-6.

4861 Misra MC, Parshad R. Randomized clinical trial of micronized flavonoids in the early control of bleeding from acute internal haemorrhoids. *Br J Surgery* 2000;87:868-72.

4862 Leighton RF, Gordon NF, Small GS, et al. Dental and gingival pain as side effects of niacin therapy. *Chest* 1998;114:1472-4.

4863 American Society of Health-System Pharmacists. ASHP Therapeutic Position Statement on the safe use of niacin in the management of dyslipidemias. *Am J Health Syst Pharm* 1997;54:2815-9.

4864 Goldberg AC. Clinical trial experience with extended-release niacin (Niaspan): dose-escalation study. *Am J Cardiol* 1998;82:35U-38U;discussion 39U-41U.

4865 Ishii N, Nishihara Y. Pellagra encephalopathy among tuberculous patients: its relation to isoniazid therapy. *J Neurol Neurosurg Psychiatry* 1985;48:628-34.

4866 Darvay A, Basarab T, McGregor JM, Russell-Jones R. Isoniazid induced pellagra despite pyridoxine supplementation. *Clin Exp Dermatol* 1999;24:167-9.

4867 National Cholesterol Education Program. Cholesterol Lowering in the Patient with Coronary Heart Disease. website: http://www.nhlbi.nih.gov/health/prof/heart/chol/chol_low.pdf (Accessed 25 May 2000).

4868 Rabbani GH, Butler T, Bardhan PK, Islam A. Reduction of fluid-loss in cholera by nicotinic acid: a randomized controlled trial. *Lancet* 1983;2:1439-42.

4869 Briend A, Nath SK, Heyman M, Desjeux JF. Comparative effects of nicotinic acid and nicotinamide on cholera toxin-induced secretion in rabbit ileum. *J Diarrhoeal Dis Res* 1993;11:97-100.

4870 Hudson CJ, Lin A, Cogan S, et al. The niacin challenge test: clinical manifestation of altered transmembrane signal transduction in schizophrenia? *Biol Psychiatry* 1997;41:507-13.

4871 Johansson JO, Egberg N, Asplund-Carlson A, Carlson LA. Nicotinic acid treatment shifts the fibrinolytic balance favourably and decreases plasma fibrinogen in hypertriglyceridaemic men. *J Cardiovasc Risk*

1997;4:165-71.

4872 Kolb H, Burkart V. Nicotinamide in type 1 diabetes. Mechanism of action revisited. *Diabetes Care* 1999;22:B16-20.

4873 Gale EA. Theory and practice of nicotinamide trials in pre-type 1 diabetes. *J Pediatr Endocrinol Metab* 1996;9:375-9.

4874 Elliott RB, Pilcher CC, Fergusson DM, Stewart AW. A population based strategy to prevent insulin-dependent diabetes using nicotinamide. *J Pediatr Endocrinol Metab* 1996;9:501-9.

4875 Lampeter EF, Klinghammer A, Scherbaum WA, et al. The Deutsche Nicotinamide Intervention Study: an attempt to prevent type 1 diabetes. DENIS Group. *Diabetes* 1998;47:980-4.

4876 Reimers JI, Andersen HU, Pociot F. [Nicotinamide and prevention of insulin-dependent diabetes mellitus. Rationale, effects, toxicology and clinical experiences. ENDIT Group]. [Article in Danish]. *Ugeskr Laeger* 1994;156:461-5.

4877 Pozzilli P, Visalli N, Cavallo MG, et al. Vitamin E and nicotinamide have similar effects in maintaining residual beta cell function in recent onset insulin-dependent diabetes. *Eur J Endocrinol* 1997;137:234-9.

4878 Visalli N, Cavallo MG, Signore A, et al. A multi-centre randomized trial of two different doses of nicotinamide in patients with recent-onset type 1 diabetes (the IMDIAB VI). *Diabetes Metab Res Rev* 1999;15:181-5.

4879 Pozzilli P, Visalli N, Signore A, et al. Double blind trial of nicotinamide in recent-onset IDDM (the IMDIAB III study). *Diabetologia* 1995;38:848-52.

4880 Pozzilli P, Browne PD, Kolb H. Meta-analysis of nicotinamide treatment in patients with recent-onset IDDM. The Nicotinamide Trialists. *Diabetes Care* 1996;19:1357-63.

4881 Greenbaum CJ, Kahn SE, Palmer JP. Nicotinamide's effects on glucose metabolism in subjects at risk for IDDM. *Diabetes* 1996;45:1631-4.

4882 Polo V, Saibene A, Pontiroli AE. Nicotinamide improves insulin secretion and metabolic control in lean type 2 diabetic patients with secondary failure to sulphonylureas. *Acta Diabetol* 1998;35:61-4.

4883 Jonas WB, Rapoza CP, Blair WF. The effect of niacinamide on osteoarthritis: a pilot study. *Inflamm Res* 1996;45:330-4.

4884 McCarty MF, Russell AL. Niacinamide therapy for osteoarthritis—does it inhibit nitric oxide synthase induction by interleukin 1 in chondrocytes? *Med Hypotheses* 1999;53:350-60.

4885 Sperduto RD, Hu TS, Milton RC, et al. The Linxian cataract studies. Two nutrition intervention trials. *Arch Ophthalmol* 1993;111:1246-53.

4886 Illingworth DR, Stein EA, Mitchel YB, et al. Comparative effects of lovastatin and niacin in primary hypercholesterolemia. A prospective trial. *Arch Intern Med* 1994;154:1586-95.

4887 Vacek JL, Dittmeier G, Chiarelli T, et al. Comparison of lovastatin (20 mg) and nicotinic acid (1.2 g) with either drug alone for type II hyperlipoproteinemia. *Am J Cardiol* 1995;76:182-4.

4888 Vega GL, Grundy SM. Lipoprotein responses to treatment with lovastatin, gemfibrozil, and nicotinic acid in normolipidemic patients with hypoalphalipoproteinemia. *Arch Intern Med* 1994 Jan 10;154(1):73-82.

4889 Guyton JR, Goldberg AC, Kreisberg RA, et al. Effectiveness of once-nightly dosing of extended-release niacin alone and in combination for hypercholesterolemia. *Am J Cardiol* 1998;82:737-43.

4890 Lal SM, Hewett JE, Petroski GF, et al. Effects of nicotinic acid and lovastatin in renal transplant patients: a prospective, randomized, open-labeled crossover trial. *Am J Kidney Dis* 1995;25:616-22.

4891 Peikert A, Wilimzig C, Kohne-Volland R. Prophylaxis of migraine with oral magnesium: results from a prospective, multi-center, placebo-controlled and double-blind randomized study. *Cephalalgia* 1996;16:257-63.

4895 Taubert K. [Magnesium in migraine. Results of a multicenter pilot study]. [Article in German]. *Fortschr Med* 1994;112:328-30.

4896 National Academy of Science, Institute of Medicine. "Dietary Reference Intakes for Vitamin C, Vitamin E, Selenium, and Carotenoids." http://www.nap.edu/pdf/0309069351/pdf_image/284.pdf. (Accessed 6 June 2000).

4897 Schrader E. Equivalence of St. John's wort extract (Ze 117) and fluoxetine: a randomized, controlled study in mild-moderate depression. *Int Clin Psychopharmacol* 2000;15:61-8.

4898 Thanapongsathorn W, Vajrabukka T. Clinical trial of oral diosmin (Daflon) in the treatment of hemorrhoids. *Dis Colon Rectum* 1992;35:1085-8.

4899 Linde K, Mulrow CD. St. John's wort for depression. *Cochrane Database Syst Rev* 2000;2:CD000448.

4900 Cospite M. Double-blind, placebo-controlled evaluation of clinical activity and safety of Daflon 500 mg in the treatment of acute hemorrhoids. *Angiology* 1994;45:566-73.

4901 Mero A, et al. Effects of bovine colostrum supplementation on serum IGF-I, IgG, hormone, and saliva IgA during training. *Appl Physiol* 1997;83(4):1144-51.

4902 Alternative Health Care, "Colostrum" Website. URL: www.healthalternative.org/colostrum/ (Accessed 16 July 1999).

4903 Sarker SA, et al. Successful treatment of rotavirus diarrhea in children with immunoglobulin from immunized bovine colostrum. *Pediatr Infect Dis J* 1998; 17(12): 1149-54.

4904 Mitra AK, et al. Hyperimmune cow colostrum reduces diarrhoea due to rotavirus: a double-blind, controlled clinical trial. *Acta Paediatr* 1995;84(9):996-1001.

4905 Greenberg PD, Cello JP. Treatment of severe diarrhea caused by Cryptosporidium parvum with oral bovine immunoglobulin concentrate in patients with AIDS. *J Acquir Immune Defic Syndr Hum Retrovirol* 1996;13(4):348-54.

4906 Plettenberg A, et al. A preparation of bovine colostrum in the treatment of HIV-positive patients with chronic diarrhea. *Clin Invest* 1993; 71(1): 42-5.

4907 Rump JA, et al. Treatment of diarrhea in human immunodeficiency virus-infected patients with immunoglobulins from bovine colostrum. *Clin Invest* 1992;70(7):588-94.

4908 Nord J, et al. Treatment with bovine hyperimmune colostrum of cryptosporidial diarrhea in AIDS patients. *AIDS* 1990;4(6):581-4.

4909 Ylitalo S, et al. Rotaviral antibodies in the treatment of acute rotaviral gastroenteritis. *Acta Paediatr* 1998;

87(3):264-7.

4910 Mother can transmit Lyme to fetus. *Reuters News* 8 May 1997.

4911 Playford RJ, et al. Bovine colostrum is a health food supplement which prevents NSAID induced gut damage. *Gut* 1999;44(5):653-8.

4912 FDA, Ctr for Food Safety and Applied Nutr, Ofc of Premarket Approval, EAFUS: A food additive database website: vm.cfsan.fda.gov/~dms/eafus.html (Accessed 20 July 1999).

4913 Sargent EV, Adolph J, Clemmons MK, et al. Evaluation of flu-like symptoms in workers handling xanthan gum powder. *Occup Med* 1990;32(7):625-30.

4914 Wade A, Weller PJ, eds. Handbook of Pharmaceutical Excipients. 2nd ed. Washington, DC: Am Pharmaceutical Assn, 1994.

4915 van der Reijden WA, et al. Treatment of xerostomia with polymer-based saliva substitutes in patients with Sjogren's syndrome. *Arthritis Rheum* 1996; 39(1): 57-63.

4916 Osilesi O, et al. Use of xanthan gum in dietary management of diabetes mellitus. *Am J Clin Nutr* 1985; 42(4): 597-603.

4917 Eastwood MA, Brydon WG, Anderson DM. The dietary effects of xanthan gum in man. *Food Addit Contam* 1987;4(1):17-26.

4918 Daly J, Tomlin J, Read NW. The effect of feeding xanthan gum on colonic function in man: correlation with in vitro determinants of bacterial breakdown. *Br J Nutr* 1993; 69(3): 897-902.

4919 Di Carlo G, Mascolo N, Izzo AA, Capasso F. Flavonoids: Old and new aspects of a class of natural therapeutic drugs. *Life Sci* 1999;65:337-53.

4920 van der Reijden WA, et al. Influence of polymers for use in saliva substitutes on de- and remineralization of enamel in vitro. *Caries Res* 1997;31(3):216-23.

4921 Covington TR, ed. Handbook of Nonprescription Drugs. 11th ed. Washington, DC: Am Pharmaceutical Assn, 1996.

4922 Dairy Managaemnt, Inc. "Whey" Website: URL: www.drymilk.com/infolib/factsht/factwhey.htm (Accessed 16 July 1999).

4923 Dairy Management, Inc. Website: URL: www.drymilk.com/infolib/order/orderwhey.htm (Accessed 16 July 1999).

4924 URL: www.creatine-glutamine.com/creatinecentral/whey.html

4925 URL: www.countryfreshfarms.com

4926 Bounous G, Baruchel S, Falutz J, et al. Whey proteins as a food supplement in HIV-seropositive individuals. *Clin Invest Med* 1993;16(3):204-9.

4927 Vandenplas Y, et al. Effect of a whey hydrolysate prophylaxis of atopic disease. *Ann Allergy* 1992; 68(5): 419-24.

4928 McIntosh GH. Colon cancer: dietary modifications required for a balanced protective diet. *Prev Med* 1993; 22(5): 767-74.

4929 Fukushima J, et al. Long-term consumption of whey hydrolysate formula by lactating women reduces the transfer of beta-lactoglobulin into human milk. *Nutr Sci Vitaminol (Tokyo)* 1997;43(6):673-8.

4930 Kennedy RS, et al. The use of a whey protein concentrate in the treatment of patients with metastatic carcinoma: a phase I-II clinical study. *Anticancer Res* 1995; 15(6B): 2643-9.

4932 Salomon SB, et al. An elemental diet containing medium-chain triglycerides and enzymatically hydrolyzed protein can improve gastrointestinal tolerance in people infected with HIV. *J Am Diet Assoc* 1998; 98(4): 460-2.

4933 Papenburg R, et al. Dietary milk proteins inhibit the development of dimethylhydrazine-induced malignancy. *Tumor Biol* 1990; 11(3): 129-36.

4934 Fayer R, Guidry A, Blagburn BL. Immunotherapeutic efficacy of bovine colostral immunoglobulins from a hyperimmunized cow against cryptosporidiosis in neonatal mice. *Infect Immun* 1990;58(9):2962-5.

4935 Vergel NR, Salvato P, Mooney M. Anabolic steroids, resistance exercise and protein supplementation effect on lean body mass in HIV+ patients. *Int Conf AIDS* 1998; 12: 557 (abstract # 32185).

4936 Voss T, et al. Management of HIV-related weight loss and diarrhea with an enteral formula containing whey peptides and medium-chain triglycerides. *Int Conf AIDS* 1991; 7(2): 223 (abstract # WB2165).

4937 Baruchel S, Olivier R, Wainberg M. Anti-HIV and anti-apoptotic activity of the whey protein concentrate: IMMUNOCAL. *Int Conf AIDS* 1994; 10(2): 32 (abstract # 421A).

4939 Wong CW, et al. Influence of whey and purified whey proteins on neutrophil functions in sheep. *J Dairy Res* 1997;64(2):281-8.

4940 Wong CW, Watson DL. Immunomodulatory effects of dietary whey proteins in mice. *J Dairy Res* 1995; 62(2): 359-68.

4941 Engelson ES, et al. Effect of a high protein diet upon protein metabolism in HIV-infected men and women. *Int Conf AIDS* 1998; 12: 553 (abstract # 32166).

4942 Laoprasert N, et al. Anaphylaxis in a milk-allergic child following ingestion of lemon sorbet containing trace quantities of milk. *J Food Prot* 1998;61(11):1522-4.

4943 Bounous G, Batist G, Gold P. Whey proteins in cancer prevention. *Cancer Lett* 1991; 57(2): 91-4.

4944 Semla TP, Beizer JL, Higbee MD. Geriatric Dosage Handbook. 4th ed. Hudson, OH: Lexicomp, 1998.

4945 Sherman RA, Tran JM, Sullivan R. Maggot therapy for venous stasis ulcers. *Arch Dermatol* 1996;132(3):254-6.

4946 Teich S, Myers RA. Maggot therapy for severe skin infections. *South Med J* 1986; 79(9): 1153-5.

4947 Reames MK, Christensen C, Luce EA. The use of maggots in wound debridement. *Ann Plast Surg* 1988; 21(4): 388-91.

4948 Mumcuoglu KY, et al. Maggot therapy for the treatment of diabetic foot ulcers. *Diabetes Care* 1998; 21(11): 2030-1.

4949 Sherman RA, Wyle F, Vulpe M. Maggot therapy for treating pressure ulcers in spinal cord injury patients. *J Spinal Cord Med* 1995;18(2):71-4.

4950 Thomas S, Andrews A, Jones M, et al. Maggots are useful in treating infected or necrotic wounds. *BMJ* 1999;318(7186):807-8.

4951 Sherman RA, Wyle FA. Low-cost, low-maintenance rearing of maggots in hospitals, clinics, and schools. *Am J Trop Med Hyg* 1996;54(1):38-41.

4952 Husain A, Sreevatsa Malaviya GN, Husain S, et al. Characterization of microbial flora of leprous ulcers infested with maggots. *Acta Leprol* 1993;8(3):143-7.

4953 Sherman RA. A new dressing design for use with maggot therapy. *Plast Reconstr Surg* 1997;100(2):451-6.

REFERENCES

4954 Villa P, Cova D, De Francesco L, et al. Protective effect of diosmetin on in vitro cell membrane damage and oxidative stress in cultured rat hepatocytes. *Toxicology* 1992;73:179-89.

4956 Koyuncu H, Berkarda B, Baykut F, et al. Preventive effect of hesperidin against inflammation in CD-1 mouse skin caused by tumor promoter. *Anticancer Res* 1999;19:3237-41.

4959 Craig WJ. Health-promoting properties of common herbs. *Am J Clin Nutr* 1999;70:491-9.

4960 FDA Talk Paper. FDA Allows Whole Oat Foods to make Claim on Reducing the Risk of Heart Disease. FDA Website: vm.cfsan.fda.gov/~lrd/tpoats.html (Accessed 16 July 1999).

4961 Wursch P, Pi-Sunyer FX. The role of viscous soluble fiber in the metabolic control of diabetes. A review with special emphasis on cereals rich in beta-glucan. *Diabetes Care* 1997; 20(11): 1774-80.

4962 Pietinen P, Rimm EB, Korhonen P, et al. Intake of dietary fiber and risk of coronary heart disease in a cohort of Finnish men. The alpha-tocopherol, beta-carotene cancer prevention study. *Circ* 1996;94(11):2720-7.

4963 Van Horn L. Fiber, lipids, and coronary heart disease. A statement for healthcare professionals from the Nutr Committee, Am Heart Assn. *Circulation* 1997;95(12):2701-4.

4964 Rimm EB, et al. Vegetable, fruit, and cereal fiber intake and risk of coronary heart disease among men. *JAMA* 1996;275(6):447-51.

4965 He J, et al. Oats and buckwheat intakes and cardiovascular disease risk factors in an ethnic minority of China. *Am J Clin Nutr* 1995;61(2):366-72.

4966 Khaw KT, Barrett-Connor E. Dietary fiber and reduced ischemic heart disease mortality rates in men and women: a 12-year prospective study. *Am J Epidemiol* 1987;126(6):1093-102.

4967 Morris JN, Marr JW, Clayton DG. Diet and heart: a postscript. *Br Med J* 1977;2(6098):1307-14.

4968 Kromhout D, de Lezenne C, Coulander C. Diet, prevalence and 10-year mortality from coronary heart disease in 871 middle-aged men. The Zutphen Study. *Am J Epidemiol* 1984;119(5):733-41.

4969 American Dietetic Association Website URL: www.eatright.org/adap1097.html (Accessed 16 July 1999).

4970 Chen HL, et al. Mechanisms by which wheat bran and oat bran increase stool weight in humans. *Am J Clin Nutr* 1998;68(3):711-9.

4971 Brown L, et al. Cholesterol-lowering effects of dietary fiber: a meta-analysis. *Am J Clin Nutr* 1999;69(1):30-42.

4972 Kwiterovich PO Jr. The role of fiber in the treatment of hypercholesterolemia in children and adolescents. *Pediatrics* 1995; 96(5 Pt 2):1005-9.

4973 Romero AL, et al. Cookies enriched with psyllium or oat bran lower plasma LDL cholesterol in normal and hypercholesterolemic men from Northern Mexico. *J Am Coll Nutr* 1998;17(6):601-8.

4974 Marlett JA, et al. Mechanism of serum cholesterol reduction by oat bran. *Hepatol* 1994;20(6):1450-7.

4975 Poulter N, et al. Lipid profiles after the daily consumption of an oat-based cereal: a controlled crossover trial. *Am J Clin Nutr* 1994;59(1):66-9.

4976 Braaten JT, et al. Oat beta-glucan reduces blood cholesterol concentration in hypercholesterolemic subjects. *Eur J Clin Nutr*, 1994;48(7):465-74.

4977 Ripsin CM, et al. Oat products and lipid lowering. A meta-analysis. *JAMA* 1992;267(2):3317-25.

4978 Davidson MH, et al. The hypocholesterolemic effects of beta-glucan in oatmeal and oat bran. A dose-controlled study. *JAMA* 1991;265(14):1833-9.

4979 Cooper SG, Tracey EJ. Small-bowel obstruction caused by oat-bran bezoar. *N Engl J Med* 1989;320(17):1148-9.

4980 Pick ME, et al. Oat bran concentrate bread products improve long-term control of diabetes: a pilot study. *J Am Diet Assoc* 1996;96(12):1254-61.

4981 Wood PJ, et al. Effect of dose and modification of viscous properties of oat gum on plasma glucose and insulin following an oral glucose load. *Br J Nutr* 1994;72(5):731-43.

4982 Braaten JT, et al. High beta-glucan oat bran and oat gum reduce postprandial blood glucose and insulin in subjects with and without type 2 diabetes. *Diabet Med* 1994;11(3):312-8.

4983 Braaten JT, et al. Oat gum lowers glucose and insulin after an oral glucose load. *Am J Clin Nutr* 1991;53(6):1425-30.

4984 Arffmann S, et al. Effect of oat bran on lithogenic index of bile and bile acid metabolism. *Digestion* 1983;28(3):197-200.

4985 Rosario PG, et al. Dentureless distention: oat bran bezoars cause obstruction. *J Am Geriatr Soc* 1990;38(5):608.

4986 Surgical Materials Testing Laboratory Website. URL: www.smtl.co.uk/WMPRC/Maggots/maggots.html (Accessed 22 March 1999).

4988 Council on Pharmacy and Chemistry. Surgical Maggots - Lederle. *JAMA* 1932;98(5):401.

4989 Livingston SK. Maggots in the treatment of chronic osteomyelitis, infected wounds, and compound fractures. *Surg Gyn Obstet* 1932;54:702-6.

4990 Buchman J, Blair JE. Maggots and their use in the treatment of chronic osteomyelitis. *Surg Gyn Obstet* 1932;55:177-90.

4991 Buchman J. The rationale of the treatment of chronic osteomyelitis with special reference to maggot therapy. *Ann Surg* 1934;99:251-9.

4992 Wilson EH, Doan CA, Miller DF. The Baer maggot treatment of osteomyelitis. *JAMA*,1932;98(14):1149-52.

4993 Baer WS. The treatment of chronic osteomyelitis with the maggot (larva of the blow fly). *J Bone Joint Surg* 1931;13:438-75.

4994 Livingston SK. The therapeutic active principle of maggots. *J Bone Joint Surg* 1936;18(3):751-6.

4995 Fine A, Alexander H. Maggot therapy - technique and clincial application. *J Bone Joint Surg* 1934;16:572-8.

4996 Robinson W. Progress of maggot therapy in the United States and Canada in the treatment of suppurative diseases. *Am J Surg* 1935;29(1):67-71.

4997 Ferguson LK, McLaughlin CW. Maggot therapy - a rapid method of removing necrotic tissues. *Am J Surg* 1935;29(1):72-84.

4998 Weil GS, Simon RJ, Sweadner WR. A biological, bacteriological and clinical study of larval or maggot therapy in the treatment of acute and chronic pyogenic infections. *Am J Surg* 1933;19(1):36-48.

4999 Horn KL. Maggot therapy for subacute mastoiditis. *Arch Otolaryngol* 1976;102:377-9.

5000 Langford SD, Boor PJ. Oleander toxicity: an examination of human and animal toxic exposures.

Toxicology 1996;109(1):1-13.

5001 Ferrea G, et al. In vitro activity of a Combretum micranthum extract against herpes simplex virus types 1 and 2. *Antiviral Res* 1993 Aug;21(4):317-25.

5002 Centers for Disease Control and Prev. Ostrich fern poisoning New York and western Canada, 1994. *JAMA* 1995 Mar 22-9;273(12):912-3.

5003 Makino T, et al. Inhibitory effect of Perilla frutescens and its phenolic constituents on cultured murine mesangial cell proliferation. *Planta Med,* 1998; 64(6): 541-45.

5004 Bruynzeel DP. Bulb dermatitis. Dermatological problems in the flower bulb industries. *Contact Dermatitis* 1997 Aug;37(2):70-7.

5005 Bruynzeel DP, de Boer EM, Brouwer EJ, et al. Dermatitis in bulb growers. *Contact Dermatitis* 1993 Jul;29(1):11-5.

5006 Middleton E. Some biological properties of plant flavonoids. *Ann Allergy* 1988;61:53-7.

5007 Moraes-Cerdeira RM, Burandt CL Jr, Bastos JK, Nanayakkara D, Mikell J, Thurn J, McChesney JD. Evaluation of four Narcissus.

5008 Fetrow CW, Avila JR. Professional's Handbook of Complementary and Alternative Medicines, Springhouse Corporation: Springhouse, PA 1999.

5009 Murray M, Pizzorno J. Encyclopedia of Natural Medicine, second ed. Prima Health, Rocklin, CA, 1998.

5010 Murray M. The Healing Power of Herbs, second ed. Prima Health, Rocklin, CA, 1995.

5011 Lininger S. The Natural Pharmacy, Prima Health, Rocklin, CA, 1998.

5012 Mother Nature Website, URL: www.mothernature.com.

5013 Moore M. Herbal Materia Medica fifth edition, Southwest School of Botanical Medicine: Bisbee, AZ 1995.

5014 Manufacturer: Aubrey Organics. Tampa, FL.

5015 Manufacturer: Lily of the Desert. Denton, TX.

5016 Manufacturer: Schiff Pharmaceuticals. Salt Lake City, UT.

5017 Manufacturer: Country Life.

5018 Manufacturer: Kal.

5019 Manufacturer: Nature's Way. Springville, UT.

5020 Manufacturer: Twinlab. Ronkonkoma, NY.

5021 Manufacturer: Vitaline Formulas. Ashland, OR.

5022 Manufacturer: Earthrise. Petaluma, CA.

5023 Manufacturer: Nature's Answer. Hanppange, NY.

5024 Manufacturer: Walgreens. Deerfield, IL.

5025 Manufacturer: Natrol. Chatsworth, CA

5026 Manufacturer: Solaray.

5027 Manufacturer: Atkins Nutritionals.

5028 Personal correspondence. Jaana Leppala, jleppala@ucla.edu (Accessed 4 March 2000).

5029 Cockerham MB, Weinberger BB, Lerchie SB. Oral glutamine for the prevention of oral mucositis associated with high-dose paclitaxel and melphalan for autologous bone marrow transplantation. *Ann Pharmacother,* 2000;34(3):300-3.

5030 Schardt D. Stevia, A Bittersweet Tale. Nutrition Action Healthletter April 2000- U.S. Edition. URL: www.cspinet.org/nah/4_00/stevia.html (Accessed 28 March 2000).

5031 Melis MS, Sainati AR. Effect of calcium and verapamil on renal function of rats during treatment with stevioside. *J Ethnopharmacol,* 1991;33(3):257-622.

5032 Jeppesen PB, Gregersen S, Poulsen CR, Hermansen K.

Stevioside acts directly on pancreatic beta cells to secrete insulin: actions independent of cyclic adenosine monophosphate and adenosine triphosphate-sensitive K+-channel activity. *Metabolism,* 2000;49(2):208-214.

5033 Melis MS. Effects of chronic administration of Stevia rebaudiana on fertility in rats. *J Ethnopharmacol,* 1999;67(2):157-161.

5034 Toskulkao C, Chaturat L, Temcharoen P, Glinsukon T. Acute toxicity of stevioside, a natural sweetener, and its metabolite, steviol, in several animal species. *Drug Chem Toxicol* 1997;20(1-2):31-44.

5035 Toskulkao C, Sutheerawatananon M, Wanichanon C, et al. Effects of stevioside and steviol on intestinal glucose absorption in hamsters. *J Nutr Sci Vitaminol (Tokyo)* 1995;41(1):105-13.

5036 Wasuntarawat C, Temcharoen P, Toskulkao C, et al. Developmental toxicity of steviol, a metabolite of stevioside, in the hamster. *Drug Chem Toxicol* 1998;21(2):207-22.

5037 Stevia: Not Ready For Prime Time. Ctr for Sci in the Public Interest. www.cspinet.org/additives/stevia (Accessed 28 March 2000).

5038 Hartter S, Grozinger M, Weigmann H, et al. Increased bioavailability of oral melatonin after fluvoxamine coadministration. *Clin Pharmacol Ther* 2000;67(1):1-6.

5039 Ravina A, Slezak L, Mirsky N, et al. Reversal of corticosteroid-induced diabetes mellitus with supplemental chromium. *Diabet Med,* 1999;16(2):164-7.

5040 Roeback JR Jr, Hla KM, Chambless LE, Fletcher RH. Effects of chromium supplementation on serum high-density lipoprotein cholesterol levels in men taking beta-blockers. A randomized, controlled trial. *Ann Intern Med* 1991;115(12):917-24.

5041 NBA Bans Androstenedione. URL: nba.com/news/ nba_androban_000330.html (Accessed 31 March 2000).

5042 Tangerine, Orange Juice May Inhibit Cancer Cell Growth. www.medscape.com/reuters/eline/mon/ t033120f.html (Accessed 3 April 2000).

5043 Magainin Presents Neuroblastoma Data for Squalamine at AACR Meeting. www.prnewswire.com (Accessed 3 April 2000).

5044 Iron chefs get nutritional boost cooking vegetables. American Chemical Society website. URL: center.acs.org/applications/news//story.cfm?story=347 (Accessed 6 April 2000).

5045 Sharks do get cancer, so shark cartilage unlikely to contain anticancer agent. www.medscape.com/reuters/ prof/2000/04.07/20000407clin011.html (Accessed 7 April 2000).

5046 UK patients to test cannabis medicines. www.medscape.com/reuters/eline/fri/t040630f.html (Accessed 7 April 2000).

5047 FDA announces the availability of new Ephedrine and street drug alternative docs. www.fda.gov (Accessed 6 April 2000).

5048 Cocaine use increases risk of hemorrhagic stroke. www.medscape.com (Accessed 13 April 2000).

5049 Findling RL, Maxwell K, Scotese-Wojtila L, et al. High-dose pyridoxine and magnesium administration in children with autistic disorder: an absence of salutary effects in a double-blind, placebo-controlled study. *J Autism Dev Disord* 1997;27(4):467-78.

5050 Coleman M. Infantile spasms associated with 5-hydroxytryptophan administration in patients with

Down's syndrome. *Neurology* 1971;21(9):911-9.

5051 Hagg S, Spigset O, Mjorndal T, Dahlqvist R. Effect of caffeine on clozapine pharmacokinetics in healthy volunteers. *Br J Clin Pharmacol* 2000;49(1):59-63.

5052 Vadoud-Seyedi J, de Dobbeleer G, Simonart T. Treatment of haemodialysis-associated pseudoporphyria with N-acetylcysteine: report of two cases. *Br J Dermatol* 2000;142(3):580-1.

5053 Lynch SR, Dassenko SA, Cook JD, et al. Inhibitory effect of a soybean-protein—related moiety on iron absorption in humans. *Am J Clin Nutr* 1994;60(4):567-72.

5054 Eberhard P, Gall HM, Muller I, Moller R. Dramatic augmentation of a food allergy by acetylsalicylic acid. *J Allergy Clin Immunol* 2000;105(4):844.

5055 Mundell EJ. Mussel extract helps arthritic dogs. www.reutershealth.com (Accessed 18 April 2000).

5056 Ohnishi ST, Ohnishi T, Ogunmola GB. Sickle cell anemia: a potential nutritional approach for a molecular disease. *Nutrition* 2000;16:330-8.

5057 Mundell EJ. Cocoa may help fight cholesterol. www.medscape.com (Accessed 18 April 2000).

5058 Researchers find potential additional health benefit of cranberries. www.prnewswire.com (Accessed 19 April 2000).

5059 Almada A, Harvey P, Platt K. Effects of chronic oral glucosamine sulfate on fasting insulin resistance index (FIRI) in non-diabetic individuals. *FASEB J* 2000;14 (4):A750.

5061 Antioxidant lozenge could help ward off flu. www.reutershealth.com (Accessed 19 April 2000).

5062 Mundell EJ. Sterol-enriched diets reduce cholesterol levels. www.medscape.com/reuters/prof/2000/04/04.21/20000421clin012.html (Accessed 21 April 2000).

5063 Bussey E. N-Acetylcysteine boosts T-cell function in HIV-infected patients. Medscape. www.medscape.com/reuters/prof/2000/04/04.28/20000428clin005.html (Accessed 28 April 2000).

5064 Oesterheld J, Kallepalli BR. Grapefruit juice and clomipramine: shifting metabolitic ratios. *J Clin Psychopharmacol* 1997;17(1):62-63.

5065 van Agtmael MA, Gupta V, van der Wosten TH, et al. Grapefruit juice increases the bioavailability of artemether. *Eur J Clin Pharmacol* 1999;55(5):405-10.

5066 van Agtmael MA, Gupta V, van der Graaf CA, van Boxtel CJ. The effect of grapefruit juice on the time-dependent decline of artemether plasma levels in healthy subjects. *Clin Pharmacol Ther* 1999;66(4):408-14.

5067 Damkier P, Hansen LL, Brosen K. Effect of diclofenac, disulfiram, itraconazole, grapefruit juice and erythromycin on the pharmacokinetics of quinidine. *Br J Clin Pharmacol* 1999;48(6):829-38.

5068 Takanaga H, Ohnishi A, Murakami H, et al. Relationship between time after intake of grapefruit juice and the effect on pharmacokinetics and pharmacodynamics of nisoldipine in healthy subjects. *Clin Pharmacol Ther* 2000:67(3):201-14.

5069 Takanaga H, Ohnishi A, Matsuo H, et al. Pharmacokinetic analysis of felodipine–grapefruit juice interaction based on an irreversible enzyme inhibition model. *Br J Clin Pharmacol* 2000;49(1):49-58.

5070 Dresser GK, Spence JD, Bailey DG. Pharmacokinetic-pharmacodynamic consequences and clinical relevance of cytochrome P450 3A4 inhibition. *Clin Pharmacokinet* 2000;38(1):41-57.

5071 Coreg monograph. In: Gillis MC, Ed. Compendium of Pharmaceuticals and Specialities (CPS). 34th ed. Ottawa, Ontario, CAN:Canadian Pharmacists Assn, 1999:395.

5072 He K, Iyer KR, Hayes RN, et al. Inactivation of cytochrome P450 3A4 by bergamottin, a component of grapefruit juice. *Chem Res Toxicol* 1998;11(4):252-9.

5073 Ernst E, Rand JI, Barnes J, Stevinson C. Adverse effects profile of the herbal antidepressant St. John's wort (Hypericum perforatum L.). *Eur J Clin Pharmacol* 1998;54(8):589-94.

5074 Lantz MS, Buchalter E, Giambanco V. St. John's wort and antidepressant drug interactions in the elderly. *J Geriatr Psychiatry Neurol* 1999;12(1):7-10.

5075 Taylor LH, Kobak KA. An open-label trial of St. John's wort (Hypericum perforatum) in obsessive-compulsive disorder. *J Clin Psychiatry* 2000 Aug;61(8):575-8.

5076 Fed Trade Comm. Marketers of Vitamin O settles FTC charges of making false health claims. www.ftc.gov/opa/2000/05/rosecreek2.htm (Accessed 1 May 2000).

5077 Ginkgo may protect against stroke damage. www.medscape.com/reuters/prof/2000/05/05.03/20000503scie003.html (Accessed 3 May 2000).

5078 Beta-glucan key to cardiovascular health benefits. www.medscape.com/MedscapeWire/2000/0500/medwire.0502.Beta.html (Accessed 3 May 2000).

5079 Lickteig MA. DUI charge for drinking tea. URL: 209.207.168.170/local/Wnews/03kavadui_a3empirea.html (Accessed 4 May 2000).

5080 McCrory DC, Matchar DB, Gray RN, et al. Evidence-based guidelines for migraine headache: overview of program description and methodology. US Headache Consortium, Apr 2000. www.aan.com/cgi-bin/whatsnewlink.pl?loc=/public/practiceguidelines (Accessed 3 May 2000).

5081 Butner LE, Fulco PP, Feldman G, et al. Calcium carbonate-induced hypothyroidism. *Ann Intern Med* 2000;132(4):595.

5082 Schneyer CR. Calcium carbonate and reduction of levothyroxine efficacy. *JAMA* 1998;279(10):750.

5083 Vitamin D does not benefit patients with relapsing-remitting MS. www.medscape.com/reuters/prof/2000/05/05.08/20000508clin009.html (Accessed 8 May 2000).

5084 Codina R, Ardusso L, Lockey RF, et al. Sensitization to soybean hull allergens in subjects exposed to different levels of soybean dust inhalation in Argentina. *J Allergy Clin Immunol* 2000;105(3):570-6.

5085 Anto JM, Sunyer J, Rodriguez-Roisin R, et al. Community outbreaks of asthma associated with inhalation of soybean dust. Toxicoepidemiological Committee. *N Engl J Med* 1989;320(17):1097-1102.

5086 White MC, Etzel RA, Olson DR, Goldstein IF. Re-examination of epidemic asthma in New Orleans, Louisianna, in relation to the presence of soy at the harbor. *Am J Epidemiol* 1997;145(5):432-8.

5087 Snow V, Lascher S, Mottur-Pilson C. Pharmacologic treatment of acute major depression and dysthymia. *Ann Intern Med* 2000;132(9):738-42.

5088 Schedules of controlled substances: addition of gamma-hydroxybutyric acid to Schedule I. *Federal Register* 2000;65(49):13235-8.

5089 Kachhi PN, Henderson SO. Priapism after androstenedione intake for athletic performance enhancement. *Ann Emerg Med* 2000;35(4):391-3.

5090 Khatta M, Alexander BS, Krichten CM, et al. The effect of coenzyme Q10 in patients with congestive heart failure. *Ann Intern Med* 2000;132(8):636-40.

5091 Ferrara LA, Raimondi AS, d'Episcopo L, et al. Olive oil and reduced need for antihypertensive medications. *Arch Intern Med* 2000;160(6):837-42.

5092 McEvoy AW, Kitchen ND, Thomas DG. Intracerebral haemorrhage in young adults: the emerging importance of drug misuse. *BMJ* 2000;320(7245):1322-4.

5093 Marks L, Partin AW, Epstein JI, et al. Effects of a saw palmetto herbal blend in men with symptomatic benign prostatic hyperplasia. *J Urol* 2000;163(5):1451-6.

5094 Gerber GS. Saw palmetto for the treatment of men with lower urinary tract symptoms. *J Urol* 2000;163(5):1408-12.

5095 Goepel M, Hecker U, Krege S, et al. Saw palmetto extracts potently and noncompetitively inhibit human alpha1-adrenoceptors in vitro. *Prostate* 1999;38(3):208-15.

5096 Shelton RC, Keller MB, Gelenberg A, et al. Effectiveness of St. John's wort in major depression: A randomized, placebo-controlled trial. *JAMA* 2001;285:1978-86.

5097 Harel Z, Gascon G, Riggs S, et al. Fish oil vs olive oil in the management of recurrent headaches in adolescents. Advancing Children's Health 2000. Joint Meeting of Pediatric Academic Soc and Am Acad of Pediatrics; Abstract 30. www.abstracts-on-line.com/abstracts/pas/aol.asp (Accessed 17 May 2000).

5098 Murray MT, Pizzorno JE Jr. Melaleuca alternifolia. In: Textbook of Natural Medicine. New York, NY:Churchill Livingstone 1999:817-20.

5099 Natl Org of Rare Diseases. Choline. www.stepstn.com/nord/db/dbsearch/search.htm (Accessed 20 July 1999).

5100 Pavillard ER, Wright EA. An antibiotic from maggots. *Nature* 1957;180:916-7.

5101 Robinson W. Stimulation of healing in non-healing wounds by allantoin occurring in maggot secretions and of wide biological distribution. *J Bone Joint Surg* 1935;17(2):267-71.

5102 Ziefren SW, et al. The secretion of collagenase by maggots and its implication. *Ann Surg* 1953;138(6):9332-4.

5103 Bennett WG, Cerda JJ. Benefits of dietary fiber. Myth or medicine? *Postgrad Med* 1996;99(2):153-6, 166-8, 171-2 passim.

5104 Reddy BS. Role of dietary fiber in colon cancer: an overview. *Am J Med* 1999;106(1A):16S-9S.

5105 Almy TP. Fiber and the gut. *Am J Med* 1981;71(2):193-5.

5106 Almy TP, Howell DA. Medical progress; Diverticular disease of the colon. *N Engl J Med* 1980;302(6):324-31.

5107 Kritchevsky D. Dietary fibre and cancer. *Eur J Cancer Prev* 1997;6(5):435-41.

5108 Dwyer JT, et al. Drug therapy reviews: dietary fiber and fiber supplements in the therapy of gastrointestinal disorders. *Am J Hosp Pharm* 1978;35(3):278-87.

5109 Kalant H, Roschlau WHE, Eds. Principles of Med. Pharmacology. New York, NY: Oxford Univ Press, 1998.

5110 Bloom FE, Kupfer DJ. Psychopharmacology: The Fourth Generation of Progress. New York, NY:Raven Press, Ltd., 1995.

5111 www.betterbodz.com.

5112 www.thewayup.com.

5113 Cocito L, et al. GABA and phosphatidylserine in human photosensitivity: a pilot study. *Epilepsy Res* 1994;17(1):49-53.

5114 Cavagnini F, et al. Effects of gamma aminobutyric acid (GABA) and muscimol on endocrine pancreatic function in man. *Metabolism* 1982;31(1):73-7.

5115 Cavagnini F, et al. Effect of acute and repeated administration of gamma aminobutyric acid (GABA) on growth hormone and prolactin secretion in man. *Acta Endocrinol (Copenh)* 1980;93(2):149-54.

5116 Nurnberger JI Jr, et al. Intravenous GABA administration is anxiogenic in man. *Psychiatry Res* 1986;19(2):113-7.

5117 Gamma-aminobutyric acid (GABA) www.axiom.net/conrucopia/gaba.html. (Accessed 15 June 1999).

5118 GABA Smart Basics Website. www.smartbasic.com/glos.aminos/gaba.glos.html. (Accessed 15 June 1999).

5119 Brown D. Encyclopedia of herbs and their uses. 1st ed. New York, NY: Dorland Kindersley Publ. Inc., 1995.

5120 Mcguffin M, et al, Ed. American Herbal Products Association's Botanical Safety Handbook. Boca Raton, FL:CRC Press LLC., 1997.

5121 Duke JA. The Green Pharmacy. Emmaus, PA: Rodale Press, 1997.

5122 Moyad MA, Pienta KJ, Montie JE. Use of PC-SPES, a commercially available supplement for prostate cancer, in a patient with hormone-naive disease. *Urology* 1999;54(2):319-28.

5123 Estronol; wild mexican yam. www.essentialcomputing.com/ams/estronol.htm (Accessed 16 July 1999).

5124 Wild Mexican Yam Website. www.nutrition-warehouse.com/Wild.Mexican.Yam.html (Accessed 16 July 1999).

5125 1st Choice Products Website: www.owasso.com/1sstchoice/index.htm (Accessed 16 July 1999).

5126 Dioscorea: wild mexican yam. www.usvitamin.com/fatigue/diosin.shtml (Accessed 16 July 1999).

5127 Men's wild yam efx . www.shop4value.com/hormone/manyam.htm (Accessed 16 July 1999).

5129 Accatino L, Pizarro M, Solis N, Koenig CS. Effects of diosgenin, a plant-derived steroid, on bile secretion and hepatocellular cholestasis induced by estrogens in the rat. *Hepatology* 1998;28(1):129-40.

5130 Aradhana AR, Rao AS, Kale RK. Diosgenin-a growth stimulator of mammary gland of ovariectomized mouse. *Indian J Exp Biol* 1992;30(5):367-70.

5131 Yamada T, et al. Dietary diosgenin attenuates subacute intestinal inflammation associated with indomethacin in rats. *Am J Physiol* 1997;273(2 Pt 1):G355-64.

5132 5Y6 Vitamin Stores Inc, Dibencozide. www.healthdepo.com/healthdepo/1457.htm (Accessed 20 July 1999).

5133 Beltz SD, Doering PL. Efficacy of nutritional supplements used by athletes. *Clin Pharm* 1993;12(12):900-8.

5134 Health & Science Research Institute. Anemia, anxiety, & depression. www.heath-science.com/anemia2.html (Accessed 20 July 1999).

5135 Clear Edge. Life Plus Website. www.staywellvitamins.com/clear.htm (Accessed 20 July 1999).

5136 Wagner JC. Use of chromium and cobamamide by athletes. *Clin Pharm* 1989;8:832-4.

REFERENCES

5137 Williams MH. Vitamin and mineral supplements to athletes: do they help? *Clin Sports Med* 1984;3(3):623-37.

5138 Vitamin B-12. Natl Acad Press website. URL: books.nap.edu/books/0309065542/html/199.html (Accessed 20 July 1999).

5139 Gilman AG, et al, Eds. Goodman and Gilman's The Pharmacological Basis of Therapeutics. 8th ed. New York, NY:Pergamon Press, 1990.

5140 Buchman AL, et al. Lecithin increases plasma free choline and decreases hepatic steatosis in long-term total parenteral nutrition patients. *Gastroenterology* 1992;102(4 Pt 1):1363-70.

5141 Wagenmakers A. Muscle amino acid metabolism at rest and during exercise: role in human physiology and metabolism. *Exerc Sport Sci Rev* 1998;26:287-314.

5142 Tuzhilin SA, et al. The treatment of patients with gallstones by lecithin. *Am J Gastroenterol* 1976; 65(3):231-5.

5143 Chan H, Abraham G, Oreopoulos DG. Oral lecithin improves ultrafiltration in patients on peritoneal dialysis. *Perit Dial Int* 1989;9(3):203-5.

5144 Lieber C.S. Alcohol and the liver: 1994 update. *Gastroenterol* 1994;106(4):1085-105.

5145 Cohen BM, Lipinski JF, Altesman RI. Lecithin in the treatment of mania: double-blind, placebo-controlled trials. *Am J Psychiatry* 1982;139(9):1162-4.

5146 Harris CM, et al. Effect of lecithin on memory in normal adults. *Am J Psychiatry* 1983;140(8):1010-2.

5147 Simons LA, Hickie JB, Ruys J. Treatment of hypercholesterolaemia with oral lecithin. *Aust N Z J Med* 1977;7(3):262-6.

5148 Oosthuizen W, et al. Lecithin has no effect on serum lipoprotein, plasma fibrinogen and macro molecular protein complex levels in hyperlipidaemic men in a double-blind controlled study. *Eur J Clin Nutr* 1998;52(6):419-24.

5149 Brinkman SD, et al. Lecithin and memory training in suspected Alzheimer's disease. *J Gerontol* 1982;37(1):4-9.

5150 Brinkman SD, et al. A dose-ranging study of lecithin in the treatment of primary degenerative dementia (Alzheimer disease). *J Clin Psychopharmacol* 1982;2(4):281-5.

5151 Pomara N, et al. Failure of single-dose lecithin to alter aspects of central cholinergic activity in Alzheimer's disease. *J Clin Psychiatry* 1983;44(8):293-5.

5152 Etienne P, et al. Alzheimer disease: lack of effect of lecithin treatment for 3 months. *Neurol* 1981;31(12):1552-4.

5153 Facts and Comparisons. Loose-leaf Ed. 1999.

5154 Lecithin/phosphatidylcholine? Mother Nature's Encyclopedia. www:mothernature.com/ency/supp/lecithin.asp (Accessed 20 July 1999).

5155 Holan KR, et al. Effect of oral administration of essential phospholipid, beta-glycerophosphate, and linoleic acid on biliary lipids in patients with cholelithiasis. *Digestion* 1979;19(4):251-8.

5156 Maltby N, et al. Efficacy of tacrine and lecithin in mild to moderate Alzheimer's disease: double-blind trial. *BMJ* 1994;308(6933):879-83.

5158 Portakal O, Ozkaya O, Erden Inal M, et al. Coenzyme Q10 concentrations and antioxidant status in tissues of breast cancer patients. *Clin Biochem* 2000;33:279-284.

5159 Lund EL, Quistorff B, Spang-Thomsen M, Kristjansen PE. Effect of radiation therapy on small-cell lung cancer is reduced by ubiquinone intake. *Folia Microbiol (Praha)* 1998;43:505-506.

5160 Grunewald KK, Bailey RS. Commercially marketed supplements for bodybuilding athletes. *Sports Med* 1993;15(2):90-103.

5161 Sehested P, Lund HI, Kristensen O. Oral choline in cerebellar ataxia. *Acta Neurol Scand* 1980;62(2):124-6.

5162 McNamara JO, et al. Effects of oral choline on human complex partial seizures. *Neurology* 1980;30 (12):1334-6.

5163 Shronts EP. Essential nature of choline with implications for total parenteral nutrition. *J Am Diet Assoc* 1997;97(6):639-46, 649.

5164 Spector SA, et al. Effect of choline supplementation on fatigue in trained cyclists. *Med Sci Sports Exerc* 1995;27(5):668-73.

5165 Gupta SK, Gaur SN. A placebo controlled trial of two dosages of LPC antagonist-choline in the management of bronchial asthma. *Indian J Chet Dis Allied Sci* 1997;39(3):149-56.

5166 Gaur SN, Agarwal G, Gupta SK. Use of LPC antagonist, choline, in the management of bronchial asthma. *Indian J Chest Dis Allied Sci* 1997;39(2):107-13.

5167 Growdon JH, Cohen EL, Wurtman RJ. Huntington's disease: clinical and chemical effects of choline administration. *Ann Neurol* 1977;1(5):418-22.

5168 Davis KL, et al. Cholinomimetics and memory. The effect of choline chloride. *Arch Neurol* 1980;37(1):49-52.

5169 Mohs RC, et al. Choline chloride treatment of memory deficits in the elderly. *Am J Psychiatry* 1979;136(10):1275-7.

5170 Mohs RC, et al. Choline chloride effects on memory in the elderly. *Neurobiol Aging* 1980;1(1):21-5.

5171 Davis KL, Berger PA. Pharmacological investigations of the cholinergic imbalance hypotheses of movement disorders and psychosis. *Biol Psychiatry* 1978;13(1):23-49.

5172 Davis KL, Hollister LE, Berger PA. Choline chloride in schizophrenia. *Am J Psychiatry* 1979;136(12):1581-4.

5173 Lawrence CM, et al. The use of choline chloride in ataxic disorders. *J Neurol Neurosurg Psychiatry* 1980;43(5):452-4.

5174 Buchman AL, et al. Choline deficiency: a cause of hepatic steatosis during parenteral nutrition that can be reversed with intravenous choline supplementation. *Hepatology* 1995;22(5):1399-403.

5175 Tan J, et al. Lack of effect of oral choline supplement on the concentrations of choline metabolites in human brain. *Magn Reson Med* 1998;39(6):1005-10.

5177 Hay IC, Jamieson M, Ormerod AD. Randomized trial of aromatherapy. Successful treatment for alopecia areata. *Arch Dermatol* 1998;134:1349-52.

5178 Albright CD, et al. Diet, apoptosis, and carcinogenesis. *Adv Exp Med Biol* 1997;422:97-107.

5179 Yen CL, Mar MH, Zeisel SH. Choline deficiency-induced apoptosis in PC12 cells is associated with diminished membrane phosphatdylcholine and sphingomyelin, accumulation of ceramide and diacylglycerol, and activiation of a caspase. *FASEB J* 1999;13(1):135-42.

5180 Zeisel SH. Choline: an important nutrient in brain development, liver function and carcinogenesis. *J Am Coll Nutr* 1992;11(5):473-81.

5182   Depression and Anxiety. Carmichael Wellness Products. www.cwinstitute.com/diseases3.asp (Accessed 20 July 1999).

5183   SAMe. Newsweek. www.newsweekinteractive.net/nw-sv/printed/us/st/he0112_1.htm (Accessed 20 July 1999).

5184   Fava M, et al. Rapidity of onset of the antidepressant effect of parenteral S-adenosyl-L-methionine. *Psychiatry Res* 1995;56(3):295-7.

5185   FDA Orphan Drug List Website: www.fda.gov/orphan/designat/list.htm. Orphan Drug Information S-adenosylmethionine Designated:Treatment of AIDS myelopathy. (Accessed 20 July 1999).

5186   Internet Grateful Med. "ChemID" Website: igm.nlm.nih.gov (Accessed 20 July 1999).

5187   The Way Up. S-adenosyl-methionine www.theway up.com/products/0235. (Accessed 20 July 1999).

5188   Bradley JD, et al. A randomized, double blind, placebo controlled trial of intravenous loading with S-adenosylmethionine (SAM) followed by oral SAM therapy in patients with knee osteoarthritis. *J Rheumatol* 1994;21(5):905-11.

5189   Bressa GM. S-adenosyl-l-methionine (SAMe) as antidepressant: meta-analysis of clinical studies. *Acta Neurol Scans Suppl* 1994;154:7-14.

5190   Bell KM, et al. S-adenosylmethionine blood levels in major depression: changes with drug treatment. *Acta Neurol Scand Suppl* 1994;154:15-8.

5191   Lambert J, Cormier J. Potential interaction between warfarin and boldo-fenugreek. *Pharmacotherapy* 2001; 21:509-512.

5192   Salmaggi P, et al. Double-blind, placebo-controlled study of S-adenosyl-L-methionine in depressed postmenopausal women. *Psychother Psychosom* 1993;59(1):34-40.

5193   Berlanga C, et al. Efficacy of S-adenosyl-L-methionine in speeding the onset of action of imipramine. *Psychiatry Res* 1992;44(3):257-62.

5195   Kagan BL, et al. Oral S-adenosylmethionine in depression: a randomized, double-blind, placebo-controlled trial. *Am J Psychiatry* 1990;147(5):591-5.

5196   Rosenbaum JF, et al. The antidepressant potential of oral S-adenosyl-l-methionine. *Acta Psychiatr Scand* 1990;81(5):432-6.

5197   Heartwire. Antioxidants get a vote of confidence in cardiac transplant patients. website: http://www.theheart.org/documents/lite/page.cfm?BJNOPIL (Accessed 13 December 2001).

5198   Chawla RK, Bonkovsky HL, Galambos JT. Biochemistry and pharmacology of S-adenosyl-L-methionine and rationale for its use in liver disease. *Drugs* 1990;40(Suppl 3):98-110.

5199   Domljan Z, et al. A double-blind trial of ademetionine vs naproxen in activated gonarthrosis. *Int J Clin Pharmacol Ther Toxicol* 1989;27(7):329-33.

5200   Bell KM, et al. S-adenosylmethionine treatment of depression: a controlled clinical trial. *Am J Psychiatry* 1988;145(9):1110-4.

5201   Vahora SA, Malek-Ahmasi P. S-adenosylmethionine in the treatment of depression. *Neurosci Biobehav Rev* 1988;12(2):139-41.

5202   Baldessarini RJ. Neuropharmacology of S-adenosyl-L-methionine. *Am J Med* 1987;83(5A):95-103.

5203   Konig B. A long-term (two years) clinical trial with S-adenosylmethionine for the treatment of osteoarthritis. *Am J Med* 1987;83(5a):78-80.

5204   Berger R, Nowak H. A new medical approach to the treatment of osteoarthritis. Report of an open phase IV study with ademetionine (Gumbaral). *Am J Med* 1987;83(5A):84-8.

5205   Muller-Fassbender H. Double-blind clinical trial of S-adenosylmethionine versus ibuprofen in the treatment of osteoarthritis. *Am J Med* 1987;83(5A):81-3.

5206   Vetter G. Double-blind comparative clinical trial with S-adenosylmethionine and indomethacin in the treatment of osteoarthritis. *Am J Med,* 1987; 83(5A):78-80.

5207   Maccagno A, et al. Double-blind controlled clinical trial of oral S-adenosylmethionine versus piroxicam in knee osteoarthritis. *Am J Med* 1987;83(5A):72-7.

5208   Caruso I, Pietrogrande V. Italian double-blind, multicenter study comparing S-adenosylmethionine, naproxen, and placebo in the treatment of degenerative joint disease. *Am J Med* 1987;83(5A):66-71.

5209   di Padova C. S-adenosylmethionine in the treatment of osteoarthritis. Review of the clinical studies. *Am J Med* 1987;83(5A):60-5.

5210   Palumbo G, Avanzini F, Alli C, et al. Effects of vitamin E on clinic and ambulatory blood pressure in treated hypertensive patients. Collaborative Group of the Primary Prevention Project (PPP)—Hypertension study. *Am J Hypertens* 2000;13:564-7.

5211   Tavoni A, et al. Evaluation of S-adenosylmethionine in primary fibromyalgia. A double-blind crossover study. *Am J Med* 1987;83(5A):107-10.

5213   Laudanno OM. Cytoprotective effect of S-adenosylmethionine compared with that of misoprostol against ethanol-, aspirin-, and strees-induced gastric damage. *Am J Med* 1987;83(5A):43-7.

5215   Glorioso S, et al. Double-blind, multicentre study of the activity of S-adenosylmethionine in hip and knee osteoarthritis. *Int J Clin Pharmacol Res* 1985;5(1):39-49.

5216   Lipinski JF, et al. Open trial of S-adenosylmethionine for treatment of depression. *Am J Psychiatry* 1984;141(3):448-50.

5217   Castagna A, et al. Cerebrospinal fluid S-adenosylmethionine (SAMe) and glutathione concentrations in HIV infection: effect of parenteral treatment with SAMe. *Neurol* 1995;45(9):1678-83.

5218   Tan SV, Guiloff RJ. Hypothesis on the pathogenesis of vacuolar myelopathy, dementia, and peripheral neuropathy in AIDS. *J Neurol Neurosurg Psychiatry* 1998;65(1):23-8.

5219   Almasio P, et al. Role of S-adenosyl-L-methionine in the treatment of intrahepatic cholestasis. *Drugs* 1990;40(Suppl 3):111-23.

5220   Cohen BM, Satlin A, Zubenko GS. S-adenosyl-L-methionine in the treatment of Alzheimer's disease. *J Clin Psychopharmacol* 1988;8(1):43-7.

5221   Volkmann H, et al. Double-blind, placebo-controlled cross-over study of intravenous S-adenosyl-L-methionine in patients with fibromyalgia. *Scand J Rheumatol* 1997;26(3):206-11.

5222   Chan PC, et al. Effect of phosphatidylcholine on ultrafiltration in patients on continuous ambulatory peritoneal dialysis. *Nephron* 1991;59(1):100-3.

5223   Domino EF, et al. Lack of clinically significant improvement of patients with tardive dyskinesia following phosphatidylcholine therapy. *Biol Psychiatry* 1985;20(11):1189-96.

5224   Jenkins PJ, et al. Use of polyunsaturated phosphatidyl

REFERENCES

REFERENCES

choline in HBsAg negative chronic active hepatitis: results of prospective double-blind controlled trial. *Liver* 1982;2(2):77-81.

5225 Guan R, et al. The effect of polyunsaturated phosphatidyl choline in the treatment of acute viral hepatitis. *Aliment Pharmacol Ther* 1995;9(6):699-703.

5226 Niederau C, et al. Polyunsaturated phosphatidyl-choline and interferon alpha for treatment of chronic hepatitis B and C: a multi-center, randomized, double-blind, placebo-controlled trial. Leich Study Group. *Hepatogastroenterol* 1998;45(21):797-804.

5227 Choline Website. SupraHealth. www.suprahealth.com/choline.htm.

5228 Ladd SL, et al. Effect of phosphatidylcholine on explicit memory. *Clin Neuropharmacol* 1993;16(6):540-9.

5229 Aronson PJ, Lorincz AL. Promotion of palmar sweating with oral phosphatidylcholine. *Acta Derm Venereol* 1985;65(1):19-24.

5231 Friedel HA, Goa KL, Benfield P. S-adenosyl-L-methionine. A review of its pharmacological properties and therapeutic potential in liver dysfunction and affective disorders in relation to its physiological role in cell metabolism. *Drugs* 1989;38(3):389-416.

5232 Bottiglieri T, Hyland K, Reynolds EH. The clinical potential of ademetionine (S-adenosylmethionine) in neurological disorders. *Drugs* 1994;48(2):137-52.

5234 U.S. Department of Agriculture, Agricultural Research Service. 2001. USDA Nutrient Database for Standard Reference, Release 14. Nutrient Data Laboratory Home Page, http://www.nal.usda.gov/fnic/foodcomp (Accessed 27 August 2001).

5235 Diaz BA, Dominguez HR, Uribe AF. Parenteral S-adenosylmethionine compared to placebos in the treatment of alcoholic liver diseases. *An Med Interna* 1996;13(1):9-15.

5236 Loguercio C, et al. Effect of S-adenosyl-L-methionine administration on red blood cell cysteine and glutathione levels in alcoholic patients with and without liver disease. *Alcohol* 1994;29(5):597-604.

5238 Podymova SD, Nadinskaia M. [Clinical trial of heptral in patients with chronic diffuse liver disease with intrahepatic cholestasis syndrome]. [Article in Russian]. *Klin Med* (Mosk) 1998;76(10):45-8.

5239 Frezza M, et al. Oral S-adenosylmethionine in the symptomatic treatment of intrahepatic cholestasis. A double-blind, placebo-controlled study. *Gastroenterol* 1990;99(1):211-5.

5240 Frezza M, et al. S-adenosylmethionine for the treatment of intrahepatic cholestasis of pregnancy. Results of a controlled clinical trial. *Hepatogastroenterol* 1990;37(Suppl 2):122-5.

5241 Jacobsen S, Danneskiold-Samsoe B, Andersen RB. Oral S-adenosylmethionine in primary fibromyalgia. Double-blind clinical evaluation. *Scand J Rheumatol* 1991;20(4):294-302.

5243 Heyman JA, et al. Failure of long term high-dose lecithin to retard progression of early-onset Alzheimer's disease. *Neural Transm Suppl* 1987;24:279-86.

5244 Botanical Dermatological Database. Annonaceae (Custard apple family). http://archive.uwcm.ac.uk/uwcm/dm/BoDD/BotDermFolder/BotDermA/ANNO.html. (Accessed 17 August 2001).

5245 Cavaliere H, Floriano I, Medeiros-Neto G. Gastrointestinal side effects of orlistat may be prevented by concomitant prescription of natural fibers (psyllium mucilloid). *Int J Obes Relat Metab Disord* 2001;25:1095-1099.

5246 Washington N, Harris M, Mussellwhite A, Spiller RC. Moderation of lactulose-induced diarrhea by psyllium: effects on motility and fermentation. *Am J Clin Nutr* 1998;67:317-321.

5247 Coniglio SJ, Lewis JD, Lang C, et al. A randomized, double-blind, placebo-controlled trial of single-dose intravenous secretin as treatment for children with autism. *J Pediatr* 2001;138:649-55.

5248 Azuma J, Sawamura A, Awata N. Usefulness of taurine in chronic congestive heart failure andits prospective application. *Jpn Circ J* 1992;56:95-9.

5249 Laird RD, Webb M. Psychotic episode during use of St. John's wort. *J Herb Pharmacother* 2001;1:81-7.

5250 Castleman M. The healing herbs, the ultimate guide to the curative power of nature's medicines. 2nd ed. New York, NY:Bantam Books, 1995.

5251 Reid D. A handbook of Chinese healing herbs. Boston, MA:Shambhala, 1995.

5252 Sifton D, ed. The PDR family guide to natural medicines & healing therapies. New York, NY:Three Rivers Press, 1999.

5253 Hoffman D. The herbal handbook: a user's guide to medical herbalism. rev ed. Rochester, VT:Healing Arts Press, 1998.

5254 Weiner MA, Weiner JA. Herbs that heal: prescription for herbal healing. Mill Valley, CA:Quantum Books, 1999.

5255 Raintree tropical plant database, Amazon plants. www.rain-tree.com/plants.htm (Accessed 30 July 1999).

5256 Autism Res Institute, Center for the Study of Autism websitewww.autism.com/ari/editorials/march99.html (Accessed 31 July 1999).

5259 HealthNotes Online. Herbal demo website: www.heatlhnotes.com/demopro/herb/elderberry.htm (Accessed 26 July 1999).

5260 Zakay-Rones Z, Varsano N, Zlotnik M, et al. Inhibition of several strains of influenza virus in vitro and reduction of symptoms by an elderberry extract (Sambucus nigra L.) during an outbreak of influenza B Panama. *J Altern Complement Med* 1995;1(4):361-9.

5261 Herbal products. VitaminShoppe.com. www.vitaminshoppe.com/a2z.asp?tab=1 (Accessed 23 July 1999).

5262 Herbs USA. Aphrodisiacs website: www.aphrodisiacs.net (Accessed 23 July 1999).

5263 Lust J. The herb book. New York, NY: Bantam Books, 1999.

5264 Brand C, Snaddon J, Bailey M, Cicuttini F. Vitamin E is ineffective for symptomatic relief of knee osteoarthritis: a six month double blind, randomised, placebo controlled study. *Ann Rheum Dis* 2001;60:946-9.

5265 Vitamin Power Products website: www.vitaminpower.com (Accessed 23 July 1999).

5266 Bear Paw Garlic, Health Source. www.health.source.tm/garlic2.htm (Accessed 31 July 1999).

5267 Botanical.Com A Modern Herbal. www.botanical.com (Accessed 31 July 1999).

5268 Herb Directory. HolisticOnLine. www.holisticonline.com (Accessed 1 August 1999).

5269 Herbal Monographs. Healthlink. www.healthline.com (Accessed 1 August 1999).

5271 Azuma J, Sawamura A, Awata N, et al. Therapeutic

effect of taurine in congestive heart failure: a double-blind crossover trial. *Clin Cardiol* 1985;8:276-82.

5272 Colostrum lactoferrin direct. www.colostrumdirect.com/lycopene/lactoferrin.html (Accessed 3 August 1999).

5273 Grifon Maitake Caplets. Maitake Products Inc.: www.maitake.com (Accessed 3 August 1999).

5274 GHS Gold. Gerovital Direct Prod. www:gerivital.co.uk (Accessed 3 August 1999).

5275 Fogarty A, Lewis S, Weiss S, Britton J. Dietary vitamin E, IgE concentrations, and atopy. Lancet 2000;356:1573-4.

5276 Herbal Materia Medica 4.0. website: www.herb.com/materia.htm (Acessed 6 August 1999).

5277 Aubourg P, Adamsbaum C, Lavallard-Rousseau MC, et al. A two-year trial of oleic and erucic acids (Lorenzo's oil) as treatment for adrenomyeloneuropathy. *N Engl J Med* 1993;329(11):745-52.

5278 DiGregorio VY, Schroeder DJ. Lorenzo's oil therapy of adrenoleukodystrophy. *Ann Pharmacother* 1995;29(3):312-3.

5279 Brown D. Encyclopedia of herbs and their uses. New York, NY:Dorland Kindersley Publ., Inc., 1995.

5280 Chesney RW. Taurine: its biological role and clinical implications. *Adv Pediatr* 1985;32:1-42.

5281 MotherNature.com. website: www.mothernature.com (Accessed 26 September 1999).

5282 Aromatherapy website. BOF's website. www.glink.net.hk/~aromatherapy (Accessed 26 September 1999).

5283 Moonmom Website. Essential oils website: www.provalue.net/users/moonmom/essentia.html (Accessed 26 September 1999).

5284 Gardenweb.com. plant database website: www.gardenweb.com/plants/nph/nph-ind.cgi. (Accessed 26 September 1999).

5285 Wheatgrass Express Inc., Wheatgrass website: www.wheat-grass.com (Accessed 26 September 1999).

5286 Rauma AL, Nenonen M, Helve T, et al. Effect of a strict vegan diet on energy and nutrient intakes by Finnish rheumatoid patients. *Eur J Clin Nutr* 1993;47(10):747-9.

5287 Pines Wheat Grass. Nutrional analysis website: www.wheatgrass.com/introtowg/factsheets/nutritionanalysis.html (Accessed 26 September 1999).

5288 Dole 5-A-Day. Spinach website: www.dole5aday.com/nut_center/veg/NUTVEG.html (Accessed 29 September 1999).

5289 Hawkhaven Greenhouse Int. Verdegrass nutritional information. www.hawkhaven.com/nutritionalinfo.html (Accessed 26 September 1999).

5290 Lowe FC, Dreikorn K, Borkowski A, et al. Review of recent placebo-controlled trials utilizing phytotherapeutic agents for treatment of BPH. *Prostate* 1998;37(3):187-93.

5291 Purple Mountain Products. AIM ReAssure for men1s prostate health. www.purplemountainproducts.com/reassurre.htm (Accessed 26 September 1999).

5292 Buck AC, Cox R, Rees RW, et al. Treatment of outflow tract obstruction due to benign prostatic hyperplasia with the pollen extract, cernilton. A double-blind, placebo-controlled study. *Br J Urol* 1990;66(4):398-404.

5293 Rugendorff EW, Weidner W, Ebeling L, Buck AC. Results of treatment with pollen extract (Cernilton N) in chronic prostatitis and prostatodynia. *Br J Urol* 1993;71(4):433-8.

5294 Yasumoto R, Kawanishi H, Tsujino T, et al. Clinical evaluation of long-term treatment using cernitin pollen extract in patients with benign prostatic hyperplasia. *Clin Ther* 1995;17(1):82-7.

5295 Lowe FC, Ku JC. Phytotherapy in treatment of benign prostatic hyperplasia: a critical review. *Urol* 1996;48(1):12-20.

5296 Buck AC, Rees RW, Ebeling L. Treatment of chronic prostatitis and prostatodynia with pollen extract. *Br J Urol* 1989;64(5):496-9.

5297 Habib FK, Ross M, Lewenstein A, et al. Identification of a prostate inhibitory substance in a pollen extract. *Prostate* 1995;26(3):133-9.

5298 Loschen G, Ebeling L. [Inhibition of arachidonic acid cascade by extract of rye pollen]. [Article in German]. *Arzneimittelforschung* 1991;41(2):162-7.

5299 Agri Res Svc: Dr. Duke's Phytochemical and Ethnobotanical databases: www.ars-grin.gov/duke (Accessed 27 September 1999).

5300 Peruvian Journey website: www.peruvian-journey.com/BHWS.htm (Accessed 30 September 1999).

5301 Al-Assmar SE. The seeds of the Hawaiian baby woodrose are a powerful hallucinogen. *Arch Intern Med* 1999;159(17):2090.

5302 Baby Hawaiian Woodrose. Tabu-smart. www.tabu-smart.com/woodrose.html (Accessed 4 October 1999).

5303 The list of psychoactive plants. Nature's Treasures. www.geocities.com.RainForest/3322naturetreasures.html (Accessed 4 October 1999).

5304 Shawcross WE. Recreational use of ergoline alkaloid from Argyreia nervosa. *J Psychoactive Drugs* 1983;15:251-9.

5305 Alpha-ketoglutaric acid, the way up website: www.thewayup.com/products.0048.htm (Accessed 6 October 1999).

5306 Azuma J, Hasegawa H, Sawamura A, et al. Therapy of congestive heart failure with orally administered taurine. *Clin Ther* 1983;5:398-408.

5307 Alpha-ketoglutaric acid. Smart basics website: www.smartbasic.com/cat.supplements/alpha.ketoglucaric.acid.html (Accessed 5 October 1999).

5308 Jeppsson A, Ekroth R, Friberg P, et al. Renal effects of alpha-ketoglutarate early after coronary operations. *Ann Thorac Surg* 1998;65(3):684-90.

5309 Wernerman J, Hammarqvist F, Vinnars E. Alpha-ketoglutarate and postoperative muscle catabolism. *Lancet* 1990;335(8691):701-3.

5310 Blomqvist BI, Hammarqvist F, von der Decken A, et al. Glutamine and alpha-ketoglutarate prevent the decrease in muscle free glutamine concentration and influence protein synthesis after total hip replacement. *Metabolism* 1995;44(9):1215-22.

5311 Riedel E, Nundel M, Hampl H. Alpha-Ketoglutarate application in hemodialysis patients improves amino acid metabolism. *Nephron* 1996;74(2):261-5.

5312 Kjellman U, Bjork K, Ekroth R, et al. Alpha-ketoglutarate for myocardial protection in heart surgery. *Lancet* 1995;345(8949):552-3.

5313 Kjellman UW, Bjork K, Ekroth R, et al. Addition of alpha-ketoglutarate to blood cardioplegia improves cardioprotection. *Ann Thorac Surg* 1997;63(6):1625-33.

5314 Aussel C, Coudray-Lucas C, Lasnier E, et al. Alpha-Ketoglutarate uptake in human fibroblasts. *Cell Biol Int* 1996;20(5):359-63.

5315 Huxtable RJ, Chubb J, Azari J. Physiological and experimental regulation of taurine content in the heart.

REFERENCES

Fed Proc 1980;39:2685-90.

5316 Stabilized liquid oxygen. HerbsNStuff. www.angelfire.com/biz2/herbsnstuff/oxy.html (Accessed 5 October 1999).

5317 Earth's Bounty Oxy-caps. Matrix Health. www.matrixhealth.com/product1.htm (Accessed 5 October 1999).

5318 Stabilized Oxygen. Portal Market. www.portalmarket.com/earthportals/Portal_Market/eathportals/portal_Ma_/oxygen.htm (Accessed 7 October 1999).

5319 Vitamin O fact sheet website. Technical White Paper: www.rgarden.com/vitamino.htm (Accessed 16 March 1999).

5320 Oxygen caps. Lifeplus vitamins. www.lifeplusvitamins.simpletnet.com/1p27p.html (Accessed 7 October 1999).

5321 How to use Oxy boost. O2oxyboost. www.o2xyboost.com/howto.htm (Accessed 7 October 1999).

5322 Beta sitosterol. Nutrimart. www.nutrimart.com/Bulk/Description/betasist.htm (Accessed 11 October 1999).

5323 Damiana. Nutrition House. www.nutritionhouse.com/page387.html (Accessed 11 October 1999).

5324 Beta sitosterol power. Mother Nature. www.mothernature.com/asp/product.asp?product+3005401103 (Accessed 11 October 1999).

5325 Saw palmetto & beta sitosterol power. Mother Nature. www.mothernature.com/asp/product.asp?product+3005401285 (Accessed 11 October 1999).

5326 Salen G, Shefer S, Nguyen L, et al. Sisterolemia. *J Lipid Res* 1992;33(7):945-55.

5327 Berges RR, Windeler J, Trampisch HJ, et al. Randomised, placebo-controlled, double-blind clinical trial of beta-sitosterol in patients with benign prostatic hyperplasia. Beta-sitosterol Study Group. *Lancet* 1995;345(8964):1529-32.

5328 Klippel KF, Hiltl DM, Schipp B. A multicentric, placebo-controlled, double-blind clinical trial of beta-sitosterol (phytosterol) for the treatment of benign prostatic hyperplasia. *Br J Urol* 1997;80(3):427-32.

5329 Wilt TJ, MacDonald R, Ishani A. beta-sitosterol for the treatment of benign prostatic hyperplasia: a systematic review. *BJU Int* 1999;83(9):976-83.

5330 Becker M, Staab D, Von Bergmann K. Treatment of severe familial hypercholesterolemia in childhood with sitosterol and sitostanol. *J Pediatr* 1993;122(2):292-6.

5331 Oster P, Schlierf G, Heuck CC, et al. [Sitosterol in familial hyperlipoproteinemia type II. A randomized, double-blind, cross-over study]. [Article in German] *Dtsch Med Wochenschr* 1976;101(36):1308-11.

5332 Schlierf G, Oster P, Heuck CC, et al. Sitosterol in juvenile type II hyperlipoproteinemia. *Atherosclerosis* 1978;30(4):245-8.

5333 Schwartzkopff W, Jantke HJ. [Dose-effect of beta-sitosterin in type IIa and IIb hypercholesterolemias]. [Article in German]. *MMW Munch Med Wochenschr* 1978;120(47):1575-8.

5334 Becker M, Staab D, Von Bergman K. Long-term treatment of severe familial hypercholesterolemia in children: effect of sitosterol and bezafibrate. *Pediatrics* 1992;89(1):138-42.

5335 Bouic PJ, Clark A, Lamprecht J, et al. The effects of B-sitosterol (BSS) and B-sitosterol glucoside (BSSG) mixture on selected immune parameters of marathon runners: inhibition of post marathon immune suppression and inflammation. *Int J Sports Med* 1999;20(4):258-62.

5336 Weststrate JA, Meijer GW. Plant sterol-enriched margarines and reduction of plasma total- and LDL-cholesterol concentrations in normocholesterolaemic and mildly hypercholesterolaemic subjects. *Eur J Clin Nutr* 1998;52(5):334-43.

5337 Donald PR, Lamprecht JH, Freestone M, et al. A randomised placebo-controlled trial of the efficacy of beta-sitosterol and its glucoside as adjuvants in the treatment of pulmonary tuberculosis. *Int J Tubercul Lung Dis* 1997;1(6):518-22.

5338 Gerolami A, Sarles H. Letter: Beta-sitosterol and chenodeoxycholic acid in the treatment of cholesterol gallstones. *Lancet* 1975;2(7937):721.

5339 Tangedahl TN, Thistle JL, Hofmann AF, et al. Effect of beta-sitosterol alone or in combination with chenic acid on cholesterol saturation of bile and cholesterol absorption in gallstone patients. *Gastroenterol* 1979;76(6):1341-6.

5340 Anon. Cholesterol-lowering Margarines. *Med Lett Drugs Ther* 1999;41(1055):56-8.

5341 Drug Info Line. Benecol, a cholesterol lowering margarine. www.pharminfo.com/pubs/druginfoline/druginfo1_22.html (Accessed 12 October 1999).

5342 Bouic PJ, Lamprecht JH, Plant sterols and sterolins: a review of their immune-modulating properties. *Altern Med Rev* 1999;4(3):170-7.

5343 Vutyavanich T, Kraisarin T, Ruangsri R. Ginger for nausea and vomiting in pregnancy: randomized, double-masked, placebo-controlled trial. *Obstet Gynecol* 2001;97:577-82.

5344 Lomaestro BM, Malone M. Glutathione in health and disease: pharmacotherapeutic issues. *Ann Pharmacother* 1995;29(12):1263-73.

5345 Flagg EW, Coates RJ, Jones DP, et al. Dietary glutathione intake and the risk of oral and pharyngeal cancer. *Am J Epidemiol* 1994;139(5):453-65.

5346 Walsh SW, Wang Y. Deficient glutathione peroxidase activity in preeclampsia is associated with increased placental production of thromboxane and lipid peroxides. *Am J Obstet Gynecol* 1993;169(6):1456-61.

5347 Knapen MF, Mulder TP, Van Rooij IA, et al. Low whole blood glutathione levels in pregnancies complicated by preeclampsia or the hemolysis, elevated liver enzymes, low platelets syndrome. *Obstet Gynecol* 1998;92(6):1012-5.

5348 Knapen MF, Peters WH, Mulder TP, et al. Glutathione and glutathione-related enzymes in decidua and placenta of controls and women with pre-eclampsia. *Placenta* 1999;20(7):541-6.

5349 Marshall KA, Reist M, Jenner P, el al. The neuronal toxicity of sulfite plus peroxynitrite is enhanced by glutathione depletion: implications for Parkinson's disease. *Free Radic Biol Med* 1999;27(5-6):515-20.

5350 Jenner P, Olanow CW. Understanding cell death in Parkinson's disease. *Ann Neurol* 1998;44(3 Suppl 1):S72-84.

5351 Jenner P. Oxidative mechanisms in nigral cell death in Parkinson's disease. *Mov Disord* 1998;(13 Suppl)1:24-34.

5352 Pearce RK, Owen A, Daniel S, et al. Alterations in the

distribution of glutathione in the substantia nigra in Parkinson's disease. *J Neural Transm* 1997;104(6-7):661-77.

5353 Merad-Boudia M, Nicole A, Santiard-Baron D, et al. Mitochondrial impairment as an early event in the process of apoptosis induced by glutathione depletion in neuronal cells: relevance to Parkinson's disease. *Biochem Pharmacol* 1998;56(5):645-55.

5354 Sechi G, Deledda MG, Bua G, et al. Reduced intravenous glutathione in the treatment of early Parkinson's disease. *Prog Neuropsychopharmacol Biol Psychiatry* 1996;20(7):1159-70.

5355 Mega L-glutathion. Life Ext Foundation. www.lef.org/prod_des/item56.html (Accessed 18 October 1999).

5356 L-Glutathione. Suprahealth. www.suprahealth.com/gluathi.htm (Accessed 18 October 1999).

5357 De Mattia G, Bravi MC, Laurenti O, et al. Influence of reduced glutathione infusion on glucose metabolism in patients with non-insulin-dependent diabetes mellitus. *Metabolism* 1998;47(8):993-7.

5358 Ciuchi E, Odetti P, Prando R. The effect of acute glutathione treatment on sorbitol level in erythrocytes from diabetic patients. *Diabetes Metab* 1997;23(1):58-60.

5359 Usberti M, Lima G, Arisi M, et al. Effect of exogenous reduced glutathione on the survival of red blood cells in hemodialyzed patients. *J Nephrol* 1997;10(5):261-5.

5360 Amano J, Suzuki A, Sunamori M. Salutary effect of reduced glutathione on renal function in coronary artery bypass operation. *J Am Coll Surg* 1994;179(6):714-20.

5361 Cook GC, Sherlock S. Results of a controlled clinical trial of glutathione in cases of hepatic cirrhosis. *Gut* 1965; 6(5):472-6.

5362 Witschi A, Reddy S, Stofer B, et al. The systemic availability of oral glutathione. *Eur J Clin Pharmacol* 1992;43(6):667-9.

5363 Hagen TM, Wierzbicka GT, Bowman BB, et al. Fate of dietary glutathione: disposition in the gastrointestinal tract. *Am J Physiol* 1990;259(4 Pt 1):G530-5.

5364 Aw TY, Wierzbicka G, Jones DP. Oral glutathione increases tissue glutathione in vivo. *Chem Biol Interact* 1991;80(1):89-97.

5365 Glossary - glutathione. Smart Basics. www.smartbasic.com/glos.aminos/glutathione.glos.html (Accessed 19 October 1999).

5366 Glutathione - Nutricology. MotherNature. http://www.mothernature.com/asp/product.asp?product=1394750140 (Accessed 19 October 1999).

5367 Roum JH, Borok Z, McElvaney NG, et al. Glutathione aerosol suppresses lung epithelial surface inflammatory cell-derived oxidants in cystic fibrosis. *J Appl Physiol* 1999;87(1):438-43.

5368 Holroyd KJ, Buhl R, Borok Z, et al. Correction of glutathione deficiency in the lower respiratory tract of HIV seropositive individuals by glutathione aerosol treatment. *Thorax* 1993;48(10):985-9.

5369 Borok Z, Buhl R, Grimes GJ, et al. Effect of glutathione aerosol on oxidant-antioxidant imbalance in idiopathic pulmonary fibrosis. *Lancet* 1991;338(8761):215-6.

5372 Marrades RM, Roca J, Barbera JA, et al. Nebulized glutathione induces bronchoconstriction in patients with mild asthma. *Am J Respir Crit Care Med* 1997;156(2 Pt 1):425-30.

5373 Smyth JF, Bowman A, Perren T, et al. Glutathione reduces the toxicity and improves quality of life of women diagnosed with ovarian cancer treated with cisplatin: results of a double-blind, randomised trial. *Ann Oncol* 1997;8(6):569-73.

5374 Cascinu S, Cordella L, Del Ferro E, et al. Neuroprotective effect of reduced glutathione on cisplatin-based chemotherapy in advanced gastric cancer: a randomized, double-blind, placebo-controlled trial. *J Clin Oncol* 1995;13(1):26-32.

5375 Links M, Lewis C. Chemoprotectants: a review of their clinical pharmacology and therapeutic efficacy. *Drugs* 1999;57(3):293-308.

5376 Leone R, Fracasso ME, Soresi E, et al. Influence of glutathione administration on the disposition of free and total platinum in patients after administration of cisplatin. *Cancer Chemother Pharmacol* 1992;29(5):385-90.

5377 Graziano F, Cardarelli N, Marcellini M, et al. A pilot clinical trial of postoperative intensive weekly chemotherapy using cisplatin, epi-doxorubicin, 5-fluorouracil, 6S-leucovorin, glutathione and filgrastim in patients with resected gastric cancer. *Tumori* 1998;84(3):368-71.

5378 Plaxe S, Freddo J, Kim S, et al. Phase I trial of cisplatin in combination with glutathione. *Gynecol Oncol* 1994;55(1):82-6.

5379 Locatelli MC, D'Antona A, Labianca R, et al. A phase II study of combination chemotherapy in advanced ovarian carcinoma with cisplatin and cyclophosphamide plus reduced glutathione as potential protective agent against cisplatin toxicity. *Tumori* 1993;79(1):37-9.

5380 Di Re F, Bohm S, Oriana S, et al. High-dose cisplatin and cyclophosphamide with glutathione in the treatment of advanced ovarian cancer. *Ann Oncol* 1993;4(1):55-61.

5381 Parnis FX, Coleman RE, Harper PG, et al. A randomised double-blind placebo controlled clinical trial assessing the tolerability and efficacy of glutathione as an adjuvant to escalating doses of cisplatin in the treatment of advanced ovarian cancer. *Eur J Cancer* 1995;31A(10):1721.

5382 Cascinu S, Frontini L, Comella G, et al. Intensive weekly chemotherapy is not effective in advanced pancreatic cancer patients: a report from the Italian Group for the Study of Dig. Tract Cancer (GISCAD). *Br J Cancer* 1999;79(3-4):491-4.

5383 Cascinu S, Labianca R, Alessandroni P, et al. Intensive weekly chemotherapy for advanced gastric cancer using fluorouracil, cisplatin, epi-doxorubicin, 6S-leucovorin, glutathione, and filgrastim: a report from the Italian Group for the Study of Digestive Tract Cancer. *J Clin Oncol* 1997;15(11):3313-9.

5384 Lenzi A, Culasso F, Gandini L, Placebo-controlled, double-blind, cross-over trial of glutathione therapy in male infertility. *Hum Reprod* 1993;8(10):1657-62.

5385 Coppola L, Grassia A, Giunta R, et al. Glutathione (GSH) improved haemostatic and haemorheological parameters in atherosclerotic subjects. *Drugs Exp Clin Res* 1992;18(11-12):493-8.

5386 Powers SK, Hamilton K. Antioxidants and exercise. *Clin Sports Med* 1999;18(3):525-36.

5387 Anderson ME. Glutathione: an overview of biosynthesis and modulation. *Chem Biol Interact* 1998;24;111-112:1-14.

5388 Lu SC. Regulation of hepatic glutathione synthesis: current concepts and controversies. *FASEB J*

REFERENCES

1999;13(10):1169-83.

5389 Amores-Sanchez MI, Medina MA. Glutamine, as a precursor of glutathione, and oxidative stress. *Mol Genet Metab* 1999;67(2):100-5.

5392 Ruffmann R, Wendel A. GSH rescue by N-acetylcysteine. *Klin Wochenschr* 1991;69(18):857-62.

5393 Droge W, Holm E. Role of cysteine and glutathione in HIV infection and other diseases associated with muscle wasting and immunological dysfunction. *FASEB J* 1997;11(13):1077-89.

5394 Herzenberg LA, De Rosa SC, Dubs JG, et al. Glutathione deficiency is associated with impaired survival in HIV disease. *Proc Natl Acad Sci USA* 1997;94(5):1967-72.

5395 Samiec PS, Drews-Botsch C, Flagg EW, et al. Glutathione in human plasma: decline in association with aging, age-related macular degeneration, and diabetes. *Free Radic Biol Med* 1998;24(5):699-704.

5396 Bains JS, Shaw CA. Neurodegenerative disorders in humans: the role of glutathione in oxidative stress-mediated neuronal death. *Brain Res Brain Res Rev* 1997;25(3):335-58.

5397 Loguercio C, Di Pierro M. The role of glutathione in the gastrointestinal tract: a review. *Ital J Gastroenterol Hepatol* 1999;31(5):401-7.

5398 Powers SK, Ji LL, Leeuwenburgh C. Exercise training-induced alterations in skeletal muscle antioxidant capacity: a brief review. *Med Sci Sports Exerc* 1999;31(7):987-97.

5429 Gylling H, Miettinen TA. Cholesterol reduction by different plant stanol mixtures and with variable fat intake. *Metabolism* 1999;48(5):575-80.

5430 Gylling H, Puska P, Vartiainen E, et al. Serum sterols during stanol ester feeding in a mildly hypercholesterolemic population. *J Lipid Res* 1999;40(4):593-600.

5431 Gylling H, Radhakrishnan R, Miettinen TA. Reduction of serum cholesterol in postmenopausal women with previous myocardial infarction and cholesterol malabsorption induced by dietary sitostanol ester margarine: women and dietary sitostanol. *Circ* 1997;96(12):4226-31.

5432 Gylling H, Miettinen TA. Serum cholesterol and cholesterol and lipoprotein metabolism in hypercholesterolaemic NIDDM patients before and during sitostanol ester-margarine treatment. *Diabetologia* 1994;37(8):773-80.

5433 Gylling H, Miettinen TA. Effects of inhibiting cholesterol absorption and synthesis on cholesterol and lipoprotein metabolism in hypercholesterolemic non-insulin-dependent diabetic men. *J Lipid Res* 1996;37(8):1776-85.

5434 Gylling H, Puska P, Vartiainen E, et al. Retinol, vitamin D, carotenes and alpha-tocopherol in serum of a moderately hypercholesterolemic population consuming sitostanol ester margarine. *Am J Cardiol* 1999;145(2):279-85.

5435 Hallikainen MA, Uusitupa MI. Effects of 2 low-fat stanol ester-containing margarines on serum cholesterol concentrations as part of a low-fat diet in hypercholesterolemic subjects. *Am J Clin Nutr* 1999;69(3):403-10.

5436 Heinemann T, Kullak-Ublick GA, Pietruck B, et al. Mechanisms of action of plant sterols on inhibition of cholesterol absorption. Comparison of sitosterol and sitostanol. *Eur J Clin Pharmacol* 1991;40 Suppl 1:S59-63.

5437 Jones PJ, Ntanios FY, Raeini-Sarjaz M, et al. Cholesterol-lowering efficacy of a sitostanol-containing phytosterol mixture with a prudent diet in hyperlipidemic men. *Am J Clin Nutr* 1999;69(6):1144-50.

5438 Gylling H, Siimes MA, Miettinen TA. Sitostanol ester margarine in dietary treatment of children with familial hypercholesterolemia. *J Lipid Res* 1995;36(8):1807-12.

5439 Miettinen TA, Puska P, Gylling H, et al. Reduction of serum cholesterol with sitostanol-ester margarine in a mildly hypercholesterolemic population. *N Engl J Med* 1995;333(20):1308-12.

5440 Lutjohann D, von Bergmann K. Phytosterolaemia: diagnosis, characterization and therapeutical approaches. *Ann Med* 1997;29(3):181-4.

5441 Vanhanen HT, Kajander J, Lehtovirta H. Serum levels, absorption efficiency, faecal elimination and synthesis of cholesterol during increasing doses of dietary sitostanol esters in hypercholesterolaemic subjects. *Clin Sci (Colch)* 1994;87(1):61-7.

5442 Weststrate JA, Meijer GW. Plant sterol-enriched margarines and reduction of plasma total- and LDL-cholesterol concentrations in normocholesterolaemic and mildly hypercholesterolaemic subjects. *Eur J Clin Nutr* 1998;52(5):334-43.

5443 Cholesterol-lowering margarines. *Medical Letter* 1999;41:56-8.

5444 Cowley G, Underwood A. Newsweek. July 5, 1999, 46-50.

5446 Czap A. Beware the son of SAMe. *Altern Med Rev,* 1999;4(2):73.

5447 Natrol. "SAM Sulfate" website: www.natrol.com (Accessed 3 November 1999).

5448 Powell-Tuck J, Jamieson CP, Bettany GE, et al. A double blind, randomised, controlled trial of glutamine supplementation in parenteral nutrition. *Gut* 1999;45(1):82-8.

5449 Houdijk AP, Rijnsburger ER, Jansen J, et al. Randomised trial of glutamine-enriched enteral nutrition on infectious morbidity in patients with multiple trauma. *Lancet* 1998; 352(9130):772-6.

5450 Jones C, Palmer TE, Griffiths RD. Randomized clinical outcome study of critically ill patients given glutamine-supplemented enteral nutrition. *Nutrition* 1999;15(2):108-15.

5451 Schloerb PR, Skikne BS. Oral and parenteral glutamine in bone marrow transplantation: a randomized, double-blind study. *JPEN J Parenter Enteral Nutr* 1999;23(3):117-22.

5452 Brown SA, Goringe A, Fegan C, et al. Parenteral glutamine protects hepatic function during bone marrow transplantation. *Bone Marrow Transplant* 1998;22(3):281-4.

5453 Ziegler TR, Bye RL, Persinger RL, et al. Effects of glutamine supplementation on circulating lymphocytes after bone marrow transplantation: a pilot study. *Am J Med Sci* 1998;315(1):4-10.

5454 Wilmore DW, Schloerb PR, Ziegler TR. Glutamine in the support of patients following bone marrow transplantation. *Curr Opin Clin Nutr Metab Care* 1999;2(4):323-7.

5455 Rohde T, Asp S, MacLean DA, et al. Competitive sustained exercise in humans, lymphokine activated killer cell activity, and glutamine - an intervention study.

Eur J Appl Physiol 1998;78(5):448-53.

5456 Rohde T, MacLean DA, Pedersen BK. Effect of glutamine supplementation on changes in the immune system induced by repeated exercise. *Med Sci Sports Exerc* 1998;30(6):856-62.

5457 Bowtell JL, Gelly K, Jackman ML, et al. Effect of oral glutamine on whole body carbohydrate storage during recovery from exhaustive exercise. *J Appl Physiol* 1999;86(6):1770-7.

5458 Decker-Baumann C, Buhl K, Frohmuller S, et al. Reduction of chemotherapy-induced side-effects by parenteral glutamine supplementation in patients with metastatic colorectal cancer. *Eur J Cancer* 1999;35(2):202-7.

5460 Niihara Y, Zerez CR, Akiyama DS, et al. Oral L-glutamine therapy for sickle cell anemia: I. Subjective clinical improvement and favorable change in red cell NAD redox potential. *Am J Hematol* 1998;58(2):117-21.

5461 Noyer CM, Simon D, Borczuk A, et al. A double-blind placebo-controlled pilot study of glutamine therapy for abnormal intestinal permeability in patients with AIDS. *Am J Gastroenterol* 1998;93(6):972-5.

5462 Okuno SH, Woodhouse CO, Loprinzi CL, et al. Phase III controlled evaluation of glutamine for decreasing stomatitis in patients receiving fluorouracil (5-FU)-based chemotherapy. *Am J Clin Oncol* 1999;22(3):258-61.

5464 Castell LM, Newsholme EA. Glutamine and the effects of exhaustive exercise upon the immune response. *Can J Physiol Pharmacol* 1998;76(5):524-32.

5465 Antonio J, Street C. Glutamine: a potentially useful supplement for athletes. *Can J Appl Physiol* 1999;24(1):1-14.

5466 Walsh NP, Blannin AK, Robson PJ, et al. Glutamine, exercise and immune function. Links and possible mechanisms. *Sports Med* 1998;26(3):177-91.

5467 Griffiths RD. Glutamine: establishing clinical indications. *Curr Opin Clin Nutr Metab Care* 1999;2(2):177-82.

5468 Sacks GS. Glutamine supplementation in catabolic patients. *Ann Pharmacother* 1999;33(3):348-54.

5469 Miller AL. Therapeutic considerations of L-glutamine: a review of the literature. *Altern Med Rev* 1999;4(4):239-48.

5470 Amores-Sanchez MI, Medina MA. Glutamine, as a precursor of glutathione, and oxidative stress. *Mol Genet Metab* 1999;67(2):100-5.

5471 FAQs about GABA. Betterbodz. www.betterbodz.com/library2/gabaquest.html (Accessed 4 November 1999).

5472 Mushrooms Nutraceuticals. Mushrooms, Nutrition and Health. www.gmushrooms.com/health/nmh.html. (Accessed 7 November 1999).

5473 Reishi. Mothernature encyclopedia. ww.mothernature.com/ency/herb/reishi.asp. (Accessed 7 November 1999).

5474 Reishi mushroom. Vitamin planet. www.vitaminplante.com/nutrition/reishi.htm. (Accessed 7 November 1999).

5475 Reishi: ancient medicine is modern hope. Health foods bus. www.home.pacific.net.hk/~gng/reishi.html. (Accessed 7 November 1999).

5476 Tao J, Feng KY. Experimental and clinical studies on inhibitory effect of ganoderma lucidum on platelet aggregation. *J Tongji Med Univ* 1990;10(4):240-3.

5477 Wasser SP, Weis AL. Therapeutic effects of substances occurring in higher Basidiomycetes mushrooms: a modern perspective. *Crit Rev Immunol* 1999;19(1):65-96.

5478 Gau JP, Lin CK, Lee SS, et al. The lack of antiplatelet effect of crude extracts from ganoderma lucidum on HIV-positive hemophiliacs. *Am J Chin Med* 1990;18(3-4):175-9.

5479 Singh AB, Gupta SK, Pereira BM, et al. Sensitization to Ganoderma lucidum in patients with respiratory allergy in India. *Clin Exp Allergy* 1995;25(5):440-7.

5480 Min BS, Nakamura N, Miyashiro H, et al. Triterpenes from the spores of Ganoderma lucidum and their inhibitory activity against HIV-1 protease. *Chem Pharm Bull (Tokyo)* 1998;46(10):1607-12.

5481 el-Mekkawy S, Meselhy MR, Nakamura N, et al. Anti-HIV-1 and anti-HIV-1-protease substances from Ganoderma lucidum. *Phytochem* 1998;49(6):1651-7.

5482 Kim RS, Kim HW, Kim BK. Suppressive effects of Ganoderma lucidum on proliferation of peripheral blood mononuclear cells. *Mol Cells* 1997;7(1):52-7.

5483 Wang SY, Hsu ML, Hsu HC, et al. The anti-tumor effect of Ganoderma lucidum is mediated by cytokines released from activated macrophages and T lymphocytes. *Int J Cancer* 1997;70(6):699-705.

5484 Kim HS, Kacew S, Lee BM. In vitro chemopreventive effects of plant polysaccharides (Aloe barbadensis miller, Lentinus edodes, Ganoderma lucidum and Coriolus versicolor). *Carcinogenesis* 1999;20(8):1637-40.

5485 Hijikata Y, Yamada S. Effect of Ganoderma lucidum on postherpetic neuralgia. *Am J Chin Med* 1998;26(3-4):375-81.

5486 Komoda Y, Shimizu M, Sonoda Y, et al. Ganoderic acid and its derivatives as cholesterol synthesis inhibitors. *Chem Pharm Bull (Tokyo)* 1989;37(2):531-3.

5487 Hikino H, Ishiyama M, Suzuki Y, et al. Mechanisms of hypoglycemic activity of ganoderan B: a glycan of Ganoderma lucidum fruit bodies. *Planta Med* 1989;55(5):423-8.

5488 Lee SY, Rhee HM. Cardiovascular effects of mycelium extract of Ganoderma lucidum: inhibition of sympathetic outflow as a mechanism of its hypotensive action. *Chem Pharm Bull (Tokyo)* 1990;38(5):1359-64.

5489 Kim DH, Shim SB, Kim NJ, et al. Beta-glucuronidase-inhibitory activity and hepatoprotective effect of Ganoderma lucidum. *Biol Pharm Bull* 1999;22(2):162-4.

5490 Yoon SY, Eo SK, Kim YS, et al. Antimicrobial activity of Ganoderma lucidum extract alone and in combination with some antibiotics. *Arch Pharm Res* 1994;17(6):438-42.

5491 Chen K, Li C. Recent advances in studies on traditional Chinese anti-aging materia medica. *J Tradit Chin Med* 1993;13(3):223-6.

5492 van der Hem LG, van der Vliet JA, Bocken CF, et al. Ling Zhi-8: studies of a new immunomodulating agent. *Transplantation* 1995;60(5):438-43.

5493 Wang WK, Chen HL, Hsu TL. Alteration of pulse in human subjects by three Chinese herbs. *Am J Chin Med* 1994;22(2):197-203.

5494 Wang HX, Ng TB, Liu WK, et al. Polysaccharide-peptide complexes from the cultured mycelia of the mushroom Coriolus versicolor and their culture medium activate mouse lymphocytes and macrophages. *Int J Biochem Cell Biol* 1996;28(5):601-7.

5495 Wellness MD webstore. Coriolus MRL. www.store.wellnessmd.com/store-welnessmd-com/MP1000chk. (Accessed 10 November 1999).

5496 Coriolus Versicolor introduction . JHS Natural Prod. website:www.jhsnaturals.com/history.html. (Accessed 10 November 1999).

5497 A polyspore named versicolor Mycoinfo. "www.mycoinfo.com/trametes.html. (Accessed 10 November 1999).

5498 Polysaccharide peptides, Inc. Coriolus-PSP. www.psp.bc.ca/e-coriolus-psp.htm. (Accessed 10 November 1999).

5499 Chem ID URL: http://igm.nlm.nih.gov/cgibin/doler?account=++&password=++&datafile=cheid (Accessed 10 November 1999).

5500 Alander M, Satokari R, Korpela R, et al. Persistence of colonization of human colonic mucosa by a probiotic strain, Lactobacillus rhamnosus GG, after oral consumption. *Appl Environ Microbiol* 1999;65(1):351-4.

5501 Bensky D, Gamble A, Kaptchuk T. Chinese Herbal Medicine Materia Medica. Seattle, WA: Eastland Press. 1996;483-5.

5502 Huang KC. The pharmacology of Chinese herbs. 2nd ed. Boca Raton, LA: CRC Press LLC. 1999;266-7.

5503 Kim HS, Lim HK, Park WK. Antinarcotic effects of the velvet antler water extract on morphine in mice. *J Ethnopharmacol* 1999;66(1):41-9.

5504 Goldsmith LA. The velvet case. *Arch Dermatol* 1988;124(5):768.

5505 Anon. Human clinical trials show significant results for New Zealand deer antler velvet's effect on sports performance. www.prnewswire.com (Accessed 7 March 2000).

5506 Elk Meadows Distributing. Start your family health tradition today with Vital-EX and feel great naturally. July 19, 1998. www.idsnowman.com/indexxx.htm. (Accessed 22 March 2000).

5507 Anon. Attributes of velvet deer antler. URL: http://angelfire.com/oh2/fountainofyouth/velvet.html. (Accessed 22 March 2000).

5508 DeerVelvet. org/GMTC Ltd. 2/21/99. URL: http://deervelvet.org/index.html. (Accessed 22 March 2000).

5509 Hart. January 30, 2000. URL: http://mysite.xtralco.nz/~BRAVEHART/ (Accessed 22 March 2000).

5510 Anon. Improve your health, revitalize your body with CERAVEL Deer Velvet TONIC. 2000. URL: http://www.ceravel.co.nz/. (Accessed 22 March 2000).

5511 Anon. Deer Velvet of New Zealand. 2000. http://www.comcen.com.u/~lawriedunn/deervelvet.html. (Accessed 22 March 2000).

5512 Anon. Immunostimulatory effects. 2000. http://www.countrylodge.co.nz/nutrition.html. (Accessed 22 March 2000).

5513 Anon. Deer Velvet Antler Nature's Superior Health Tonic. 2000. URL: http://www.gold-mountain.co.nz. (Accessed 22 March 2000).

5514 Suttie JM, Fennessy PR, Haines SR, et al. The Velvet Antler Industry: Background Research and Findings. 2000. http://www.healthy.net/library/articles/abdo/antler.htm (Accessed 22 March 2000).

5515 Mascot Enterprise. Super Nutrition Power-Herbal Supplement. 2000. URL: http://www.mascotsnp.com/ (Accessed 22 March 2000).

5516 Anon. 2000. URL. http://www.nutrisana.com/html/deer.velvet antler.html. (Accessed 22 March 2000).

5517 Sim JS, Sunwoo HH. Canadian Scientists Study Velvet Antler for Arthritis Treatment. 1999. URL. http://qeva.com/research/UofA.htm (Accessed 22 March 2000).

5518 Ko KM, Yip TT, Tsao SW, Kong YC, et al. Epidermal growth factor from deer (Cervus elaphus) submaxillary gland and velvet antler. *Gen Comp Endocrinol* 1986;3(3):431-40.

5519 Colloidal Silver Discovery Center. 2000. URL. http://colloidalsilver.net/info.html. (Accessed 24 March 2000).

5520 Anon. What is colloidal silver? 2000. URL. http://apothecary.hypermart.net/what_is_cs.htm. (Accessed 24 March 2000).

5521 Coburn DL. Colloidal Silver-A healthy silver lining. 1999. URL. http://www.colloidal-silver.com/ (Accessed 24 March 2000).

5522 Robey M, Medical and Non-medical uses. 1999. URL. http://www.colloidal-silver.com/ (Accessed 24 March 2000).

5523 Barrett S. Colloidal Silver: risk without benefit. November 5,1999. URL. http://www.quackwatch.com/01QuackeryRelated Topics/PhonyAds/silverad.html (Accessed 24 March 2000).

5524 Department of Health and Human Services. 21 CFR Part 310. Federal Register: August 17, 1999. URL. http://www.verity.fda.gov/search97cgi/s97_cgi.exe?action=View&VdkVgwKey=http (Accessed 21 March 2000).

5525 Fung MC, Bowen DL. Silver products for medical indications: risk-benefit assessment. *J Toxicol Clin Toxicol* 1996; 34(1):119-126. FDA, Ctr Drug Evaluation, Res. Rockville, MD.

5526 Fung MC, Weintraub M, Bowen DL. Colloidal silver proteins marketed as health supplements. *JAMA* 1995;274(15):1196-7.

5527 Anon. Life Plus, the very finest in health and nutrition supplements. www.lifeplusvitamins.com/colloidl.html. (Accessed 24 March 2000).

5528 Anon. 2000. Supplement explanations. URL: http://alzheimersmemory.com/supplement1.html. (Accessed 21 March 2000).

5529 Anon. 2000 www.angelfire.com/co2/slendermummie/madna.html. (Accessed 21 March 2000).

5530 Anon. 2000. www.moon-light.com/ (Accessed 21 March 2000).

5531 Daly JM, Lieberman MD, Goldfine J, et al. Enteral nutrition with supplemental arginine, RNA, and omega-3 fatty acids in patients after operation: immunologic, metabolic and clinical outcome. *Surgery* 1992;112(1):56-67.

5532 Senkal M, Kemen M, Homann HH, et al. Modulation of postoperative immune response by enteral nutrition with a diet enriched with arginine, RNA, and omega-3 fatty acids in patients with upper gastrointestinal cancer. *Eur J Surg* 1995;161:115-22.

5533 Kemen M, Senkal M, Homann HH, et al. Early postoperative enteral nutrition with arginine-omega-3 fatty acids and ribonucleic acid-supplemented diet vs placebo in cancer patients: an immunologic evaluation of impact. *Crit Care Med* 1995;23(4):652-9.

5534 Gianotti L, Braga M, Fortis C, et al. A prospective, randomized clinical trial on perioperative feeding with an arginine, omega-3-fatty acid, and RNA-enriched enteral diet: effect on host response and nutritional status. *Journal of Parenteral and Enteral Nutrition* 1999;23(6):314-20.

5535 Saffle JR, Wiebke G, Jennings K, et al. Randomized trial of immune-enhancing enteral nutrition in burn patients. *The Journal of Trauma, Injury, Infection and Critical Care* 1997;42(5):793-802.

5536 Bower RH, Cerra FB, Bershadsky B, et al. Early enteral administration of a formula (Impact) supplemented with arginine, nucleotides, and fish oil in intensive care unit patients: results of a multicenter, prospective, randomized clinical trial. *Crit Care Med* 1995;23(3):436-49.

5537 Wang T, Tang XC. Reversal of scopolamine-induced deficits in radial maze performance by (-)-huperzine A: comparison with E2020 and tacrine. *Eur J Pharmacol* 1998;349(2-3):137-42.

5538 Li L. Erythematous skin reaction to subcutaneous injection of ribonucleic acid. *Contact Dermatitis* 1999;41:239.

5539 Schubert R, Hohlweg U, Renz D, Doefler W. On the fate of orally ingested foreign DNA in mice: chromosomal association and placental transmission o the fetus. *Mol Gen Genet* 1998;259:569-76.

5541 Huang KC. The pharmacology of Chinese herbs. 2nd ed. New York, NY: CRC Press LLC. 1999;385-6, 400-1.

5542 Bruneton J. Pharmacognosy, Phytochemistry, Medicinal Plants. 2nd ed. Paris, FR: Lavoisier Publ. 1999;652.

5543 Van Buren CT, Rudolph F. Dietary nucleotides: a conditional requirement. *Nutr* 1997;13(5):470-2.

5544 Bensky D, Gamble A, Kaptchuk T. Chinese Herbal Medicine Materia Medica. Seattle, WA: Eastland Press 1996:107-8.

5545 Huang KC. The Pharmacology of Chinese Herbs. 2nd ed. New York: CRC Press LLC. 1999:113-114, 417.

5546 Chen SH, Yen YP, Chen XS. Effect of jiantangkang on blood glucose, sensitivity of insulin, and blood viscosity in non-insulin dependent diabetes mellitus. *Chung Kuo Chung His I Chieh Ho Tsa Chih* 1997;17(11):666-8.

5547 Wang HK, Xia Y, Yang ZY, et al. Recent advances in the discovery and development of flavonoids and their analogues as antitumor and anti-HIV agents. *Adv Exp Med Biol,* 1998;439:191-225.

5548 DiPaola RS, Zhang H, Lambert GH, et al. Clinical and biologic activity of an estrogenic herbal combination (PC-SPES) in prostate cancer. *N Engl J Med* 1998;339(12):785-91.

5549 Smol'ianinov ES, Gol'dberg VE, Matiash MG, et al. Effect of Scutellaria baicalensis extract on the immunologic status of patients with lung cancer receiving antineoplastic chemotherapy. *Eksp Klin Farmakol,* 1997;60(6):49-51.

5550 Gol'dberg VE, Ryzhakov VM, Matiash MG, et al. Dry extract of Scutellaria baicalensis as a hemostimulant in antineoplastic chemotherapy in patients with lung cancer. *Eksp Klin Farmakol,* 1997;60(6):28-30.

5551 Zhang H, Huang J. Preliminary study of traditional Chinese medicine treatment of minimal brain dysfunction: analysis of 100 cases. *Chung Hsi I Chieh Ho Tsa Chih,* 1990;10(5):278-9, 260.

5552 Kuno Y, Kawabe Y, Sakakibara S. Allergic contact dermatitis associated with photosensitivity, from alantolactone in a chrysanthemum farmer. *Contact Dermatitis* 1999;40(4):224-5.

5553 Paulsen E, Sogaard J, Andersen KE. Occupational dermatitis in Danish gardeners and greenhouse workers (III). Compositae-related symptoms. *Contact Dermatitis* 1998;38(3):140-6.

5554 deJong NW, Vermeulen AM, van Wijik RG, deGroot H.

Occupational allergy caused by flowers. *Allergy* 1998;53(2):204-9.

5555 Yu XY. A prospective clinical study on reversion of 200 precancerous patients with hua-sheng-ping. *Chung Kuo Chung His I Chieh Ho Tsa Chih* 1993;13(3):147-9.

5556 Camplimi P, Sertoli A, Fabbri P, Panconesi E. Alantolactone sensitivity in chrysanthemum contract dermatitis. *Contact Dermatitis,* 1978;4(2):93-102.

5557 Bleumink E, Mitchell JC, Geismann TA, Towers GH. Contact hypersensitivity to sesquiterpene lactones in Chrysanthemum dermatitis. *Contact Dermatitis* 1976;2(2):81-8.

5558 Huang KC. The Pharmacology of Chinese Herbs. 2nd ed. New York: CRC Press LLC. 1999:101-102.

5559 Bensky D, Gamble A, Kaptchuk T. Chinese Herbal Medicine Materia Medica. Seattle, WA: Eastland Press, 1996:359-60.

5598 Wangen TE, Duncan AM, Merz-Demlow BE, et al. Effects of soy isoflavones on markers of bone turnover in premenopausal and postmenopausal women. *J Clin Endocrinol Metab* 2000;85:3043-8.

5599 Lutz M, Bonilla S, Concha J, et al. Effect of dietary oils, cholesterol and antioxidant vitamin supplementation on liver microsomal fluidity and xenobiotic-metabolizing enzymes in rats. *Annals of Nutr and Metabolism* 1998;42(6):350-9.

5600 Farber JM, Carter AO, Varughese PV, et al. Listeriosis traced to the consumption of alfalfa tablets and soft cheese. [Letter to the Editor] *N Engl J Med* 1990;322:338.

5601 Sullivan JB Jr, Rumack BH, Thomas H Jr, et al. Pennyroyal oil poisoning and hepatotoxicity. *JAMA* 1979;242(26):2873-4.

5602 Anon. Toxic hypoglycemic syndrome - Jamaica, 1989-91. *MMWR Morb Mortal Wkly Rep* 1992;41(4):53-5.

5603 Sinn LE, Porterfield JF. Fatal taxine poisoning from yew leaf ingestion. *J Forensic Sci* 1991;36(2):599-601.

5604 Van IG, Visser R, Peltenburg H, et al. Sudden unexpected death due to Taxus poisoning. A report of five cases, with review of the literature. *Forensic Sci Int* 1992;56(1):81-7.

5605 Krenzelok EP, Jacobsen TD, Aronis J. Is the yew really poisonous to you? *J Toxicol Clin Toxicol* 1998;36(3):219-23.

5606 Fox DW, Hart MC, Bergeson PS, et al. Pyrrolizidine (Senecio) intoxication mimicking Reye syndrome. *J Pediatr* 1978;93(6):980-2.

5607 Sullivan G, Chavez PI. Mexican good-luck charm potentially dangerous. *Vet Hum Toxicol* 1981;23(4):259-60.

5608 Niyogi SK. Deadly crab's eye: Abrus precatorius poisoning. *N Engl J Med* 1969;281(1):51-2.

5609 Sherratt HS, Turnbull DM. Methylene blue and fatal encephalopathy from ackee fruit poisoning. *Lancet* 1999;353(9164):1623-4.

5610 Lebo DB, Ditto AM, Boxer MB, et al. Anaphylaxis to ackee fruit. *J Allergy Clin Immunol* 1996;98(5Pt1):997-8.

5611 Challoner KR, McCarron MM. Castor bean intoxication. *Ann Emerg Med* 1990;19(10):1177-83.

5612 Palatnick W, Tenenbein M. Hepatotoxicity from castor bean ingestion in a child. *J Toxicol Clin Toxicol* 2000;38(1):67-9.

5613 Aplin PJ, Eliseo T. Ingestion of castor oil plant seeds. *Med J Aust* 1997;167(5):260-1.

REFERENCES

5614 McGee J, Patrick RS, Wood CB, Blumgart LH. A case of veno-occlusive disease of the liver in Britain associated with herbal tea consumption. *J Clin Pathol* 1976;29(9):788-94.

5617 Cassidy DE, Drewry J, Fanning JP. Podophyllum toxicity: a report of a fatal case and a review of the literature. *J Toxicol Clin Toxicol* 1982;19(1):35-44.

5618 Rosenstein G, Rosenstein H, Freeman M, Weston N. Podophyllum- a dangerous laxative. *Pediatrics* 1976;57(3):419-21.

5619 Cohle SD, Trestrail JD III, Graham MA, et al. Fatal pepper aspiration. *Am J Dis Child* 1988;142(6):633-6.

5620 Sheahan K, Page DV, Kemper T, Suarez R. Childhood sudden death secondary to accidental aspiration of black pepper. *Am J Forensic Med Pathol* 1988;9(1):51-3.

5621 Anon. Plant Poisonings - New Jersey. *MMWR Morb Mortal Wkly Rep* 1981;30(6):65-7.

5622 Urich RW, Bowerman DL, Levisky JA, Pflug JL. Datura stramonium: a fatal poisoning. *J Forensic Sci* 1982;27(4):948-54.

5623 Anon. Jimson weed poisoning- Texas, New York, and California, 1994. *MMWR Morb Mortal Wkly Rep* 1995;44(3):41-4.

5624 McHenry LE, Hall RC. Angel's trumpet. Lethal and psychogenic aspects. *J Fla Med Assoc* 1978;65(3):192-6.

5625 Hall RC, Popkin MK, Mchenry LE. Angel's Trumpet psychosis: a central nervous system anticholinergic syndrome. *Am J Psychiatry* 1977;134(3):312-4.

5626 Greene GS, Patterson SG, Warner E. Ingestion of angel's trumpet: an increasingly common source of toxicity. *South Med J* 1996;89(4):365-9.

5627 Francis PD, Clarke CF. Angel trumpet lily poisoning in five adolescents: clinical findings and management. *J Paediatr Child Health* 1999;35(1):93-5.

5628 Anon. FDA Import Alert #53-03, 1991. www.verity.fda.gov/search97cgi/s97_cgi.exe?. (Accessed 9 May 2000).

5629 Pine, D. Cool tips for a hot season. FDA/CFSAN Cosmetics 1992. http://vm.cfsan.fda.gov/~dms/cos-815.html. (Accessed 9 May 2000).

5630 Anon. Color additives approved for use in human food. FDA/CFSAN/OPA 1988. http://vm.cfsan.fda.gov/~dms/opa-col2.html. (Accessed 9 May 2000).

5631 Jackson R. Quick suntan pills in Canada. *J Am Acad Dermatol* 1981;4(2):233.

5632 Lober CW. Canthaxanthin- the "tanning" pill. *J Am Acad Dermatol* 1985;13(4):660.

5633 Anon. A suntan in capsules - orobronze. *Drug Ther Bull* 1983;21(15):57.

5634 Rock GA, Decary F, Cole RS. Orange plasma from tanning capsules. *Lancet* 1981;1(8235):1419-20.

5635 Bluhm R, Branch R, Johnston P, Stein R. Aplastic anemia associated with canthaxanthin ingested for 'tanning' purposes. *JAMA* 1990;264(9):1141-2.

5636 Harnois C, Samson J, Malenfant M, Rousseau A. Canthaxanthin retinopathy. Anatomic and funtional reversibility. *Arch Ophthalmol* 1989;107(4):538-40.

5637 Herbert V. Canthaxanthin toxicity. *Am J Clin Nutr* 1991;53(2):573-4.

5638 White GL Jr, Beesley R, Thiese SM, Murdock RT. Retinal crystals and oral tanning agents. *Am Fam Physician* 1988;37(3):125-6.

5639 Chang TS, Aylward W, Clarkson JG, Gass JD. Asymmetric canthaxanthin retinopathy. *Am J Ophthalmol* 1995;119(6):801-2.

5640 Leyon H, Ros AM, Nyberg S, Algvere P. Reversibility of canthaxanthin deposits within the retina. *Acta Ophthalmol (Copenh)* 1990;68(5):607-11.

5641 Espaillat A, Aiello LP, Arrigg PG, et al. Canthaxanthine retinopathy. *Arch Ophtahalmol* 1999;117:412-3.

5642 Anon. Permitted colouring agents for use in medicinal products - E 161 Canthaxanthine. Health and Consumer Protection - The European Commission 1998. http://europa.eu.int/comm/dg24/health/sc/scmp/out10_en.html. (Accessed 9 May 2000).

5643 Durant J, Chantre P, Gonzalez G, et al. Efficacy and safety of Buxus sempervirens L. preparations (SPV30) in HIV-infected asymptomatic patients: a multicentre, randomized, double-blind, placebo-controlled trial. *Phytomedicine* 1998;5:1-10.

5644 Anon. Porphyria information for patients and their families. University of Cape Town / Medical Research Council - Liver Research Center 2000. www.uct.ac.za/depts/liver/porphpts.htm. (Accessed 9 May 2000).

5645 Mathews-Roth MM. Carotenoids in erythropoietic protoporphyria and other photosensitivity diseases. *Ann N Y Acad Sci* 1993;691:127-38.

5646 Clarke R. Prevention of vitamin B-12 deficiency in old age. *Am J Clin Nutr.* 2001;73:151-152.

5647 Vainio H, Rautalahti M. An international evaluation of the cancer preventive potential of carotenoids. *Cancer Epidemiol Biomarkers Prev* 1998;7(8):725-8.

5648 Huang DS, Odeleye OE, Watson RR. Inhibitory effects of canthaxanthin on in vitro growth of murine tumor cells. *Cancer Lett* 1992;65(3):209-13.

5649 Stahl W, Sies H. The role of carotenoids and retinoids in gap junctional communication. *Int J Vitam Nutr Res* 1998;68(6):354-9.

5650 Segal S, Foley J. The metabolism of D-ribose in man. *J Clin Invest* 1958;37:719-35.

5651 Foker JE, Einzig S, Wang T. Adenosine metabolism and myocardial preservation. Consequences of adenosine catabolism on myocardial high-energy compounds and tissue blood flow. *J Thorac Cardiovasc Surg* 1980;80(4):506-16.

5652 Pasque MK, Spray TL, Pellom GL, et al. Ribose-enhanced myocardial recovery following ischemia in the isolated working rat heart. *J Thorac Cardiovasc Surg* 1982;83(3):390-8.

5653 Pasque MK, Wechsler AS. Metabolic intervention to affect myocardial recovery following ischemia. *Ann Surg* 1984;200(1):1-12.

5654 Ward HB, St Cyr JA, Cogordan JA. Recovery of adenine nucleotide levels after global myocardial ischemia in dogs. *Surgery* 1984;96(2):248-55.

5655 Consumer Lab. www.consumerlab.com/results/sawpalmetto.asp (Accessed 5 June 2001).

5656 Stathis CG, Febbraio MA, Carey MF, et al. Influence of sprint training on human skeletal muscle purine nucleotide metabolism. *J Appl Physiol* 1994;76(4):1802-9.

5657 Tullson PC, Bangsbo J, Hellsten Y, et al. IMP metabolism in human skeletal after exhaustive exercise. *J Appl Physiol* 1995;78(1):146-52.

5658 Hellsten-Westing Y, Norman B, Balsom PD, et al. Decreased resting levels of adenine nucleotides in human skeletal muscle after high-intensity training. *J Appl Physiol* 1993;74(5):2523-8.

5659 Chatham JC, John Challiss RA, Radda GK, et al.

Studies of the protective effect of ribose in myocardial ischaemia by using P31-nuclear-magnetic-resonance spectroscopy. *Biochem Soc Trans* 1985;13:885-6.

5660 St Cyr JA, Bianco RW, Schneider JR, et al. Enhanced high energy phosphate recovery with ribose infusion after global myocardial ischemia in a canine model. *J Surg Res* 1989;46(2):157-62.

5661 Angello DA, Wilson RA, Gee D. Effect of ribose on thallium-201 myocardial redistribution. *J Nucl Med* 1988;29(12):1943-50.

5662 Perlmutter NS, Wilson RA, Angello DA, et al. Ribose facilitates thallium-201 redistribution in patients with coronary artery disease. *J Nucl Med* 1991;32(2):193-200.

5663 Hegewald MG, Palac RT, Angello DA, et al. Ribose infusion accelerates thallium redistribution with early imaging compared with late 24-hour imaging without ribose. *J Am Coll Cardiol* 1991;18(7):1671-81.

5664 Pliml W, von Arnim T, Stalein A, et al. Effects of ribose on excercise-induced ischaemia in stable coronary artery disease. *Lancet* 1992;340(8818):507-10.

5665 Geisbuhler TP, Schwager TL. Ribose-enhanced synthesis of UTP, CTP, and GTP from parent nucleosides in cardiac myocytes. *J Mol Cell Cardiol* 1998;30(4):879-87.

5666 Muller C, Zimmer HG, Gross M, et al. Effect of ribose on cardiac adenine nucleotides in a donor model for heart transplantation. *Eur J Med Res* 1998;3:554-8.

5667 Burke ER. D-Ribose What You Need To Know. Garden City Park, NY:Avery Publishing Group 1999: 1-43.

5668 Anon. Bioenergy Ribose-The Absolute Energy Source 2000. www.ribose.com (Accessed 16 May 2000).

5669 Almada AL. D-Ribose: Leave the sugar blues behind! *Alive* 1999;199:74,76.

5670 Anon. It's raining men...supplements, that is. Nutrition News September 30, 1999;1.

5671 Anon. Ribose size-the great genetic equalizer 2000. http://www.muscle-link.com/products/ribosesize.html (Accessed 24 May 2000).

5672 Anon. Liquid Ribose 2000. http:// www.performancebiolabs.com/liquid_ribose.htm (Accessed 24 May 2000).

5673 Anon. Ribose-C. George Stavrou's Bodysculpting 2000. http://www.bdsclpt.com/itm00003.htm (Accessed 24 May 2000).

5674 Anon. Ribose. Cutting Edge Nutrition 2000. http:// www.cuttingedgenutrition.com/cuttingedge/ribose.html (Accessed 16 May 2000).

5675 Blackwood JS. Supplement spotlight: ribose. Nutripeak.com 2000. http://www.nutripeak.com/ features/9910_spotlight3.asp (Accessed 16 May 2000).

5676 Gross M, Reiter S, Zollner N. Metabolism of D-ribose administered continuously to healthy persons and to patients with myoadenylate deaminase deficiency. *Klin Wochenschr* 1989;67(23):1205-13.

5677 Zollner N, Reiter S, Gross M, et al. Myoadenylate deaminase deficiency: successful symptomatic therapy by high dose oral administration of ribose. *Klin Wochenscher* 1986;64(24):1281-90.

5678 Steele IC, Patterson VH, Nicholls DP. A double blind, placebo controlled, crossover trial of D-ribose in McArdle's disease. *J Neurol Sci* 1996 136(1-2): 174-7.

5679 Wagner DR, Gresser U, Zollner N. Effects of oral ribose on muscle metabolism during bicycle ergometer in AMPD-deficient patients. *Ann Nutr Metab* 1991;35(5):297-302.

5680 Wagner DR, Felbel J, Gresser U, et al. Muscle metabolism and red cell ATP/ADP concentration during bicycle ergometer in patients with AMPdeficiency. *Klin Wochnescher* 1991;69(6):251-5.

5681 Gross M. Clinical heterogeneity and molecular mechanisms in inborn muscle AMP deaminase deficiency. *J Inherit Metab Dis* 1997;20(2):186-92.

5682 Fox IH, Kelley WN. Phosphoribosylpyrophosphate in man: biochemical and clinical significance. *Ann Intern Med* 1971;74:424-33.

5683 Lan EL, Ugwu SO, Blanchard J, et al. Preformulation studies with melanotan II: a potential skin cancer chemopreventive peptide. *J Pharm Sci* 1994;83(8):1081-4.

5684 Pinsuwan S, Myrdal PB, Yalkowsky SH. Systemic delivery of melanotan II through the ocular route in rabbits. *J Pharm Sci* 1997;86(3):396-7.

5685 Dorr RT, Lines R, Levine N, et al. Evaluation of melanotan-II, a superpotent cyclic melanotropic peptide in a pilot phase-I clinical study. *Life Sci* 1996;58(20):1777-84.

5686 Hadley ME, Hruby VJ, Blanchard J, et al. Discoverdevelopment of novel melanogenic drugs. Melanotan-I and -II. *Pharm Biotechnol* 1998;11:575-95.

5687 Wessells H, Fuciarelli K, Hansen J, et al. Synthetic melanotropic peptide initiates erections in men with psychogenic erectile dysfunction; double-blind, placebo controlled crossover study. *J Urol* 1998;160(2):389-93.

5688 Wessells H, Gralnek DR, Dorr RT, et al. Erectogenic properties of melanotan II in men with organic erectile dysfunction. 1999 Abstract Info-American Urological Association, Inc. http://www.auanet.org/meeting/ annual_meeting/abstractinfo/AUA99_1603.cfm. (Accessed 5 June 2000).

5689 Wessells H. Hunter Wessells, MD.,FACS. Impotence Specialists 2000. http://www.impotencespecialists.com/ drwessels/wessells.html (Accessed 4 June 2000).

5690 Rutz D. Tanning drug may find new life as Viagra alternatives. CNN 1999. http://cnn.com/HEALTH/men/ 9906/17/viagra.alternative/ (Accessed 2 June 2000).

5691 Wisniowski LA. FDA Import Alert #62-06 1992. website URL http://www.fda.gov/ora/fiars/ ora_import_ia6206.html. (Accessed 15 June 2000).

5692 Sant GR, LaRock DR. Standard intravesical therapies for interstitial cystitis. *Urol Clin North Am* 1994;21(1):73-83.

5693 Birder LA, Kanai AJ, de Groat WC. DMSO: effect on bladder afferent neurons and nitric oxide release. *J Urol* 1997;158(5):1989-95.

5694 Sant GR. Intravesical 50% dimethyl sulfoxide (Rimso-50) in treatment of interstitial cystitis. *Urology* 1987;29(4 Suppl):17-21.

5695 Barker SB, Matthews PN, Philip PF, Williams G. Prospective study of intravesical dimethyl sulphoxide in the treatment of chronic inflammatory bladder disease. *Br J Urol* 1987;59(2):142-4.

5696 Fowler JE Jr. Prospective study of intravesical dimthyl sulfoxide in treatment of suspected early interstitial cystitis. *Urology* 1981;18(1):21-6.

5697 Shirley SW, Stewart BH, Mirelman S. Dimethyl sulfoxide in treatment of inflammatory genitourinary disorders. *Urology* 1978;11(3):215-20.

5698 Bertelli G. Prevention and management of extravasation of cytotoxic drugs. *Drug Saf* 1995;12(4):245-55.

5699   Dorr RT. Antidotes to vesicant chemotherapy extravasations. *Blood Rev* 1990;4(1):41-60.

5701   Barber MD, Ross JA, Voss AC, et al. The effect of an oral nutritional supplement enriched with fish oil on weight-loss in patients with pancreatic cancer. *Br J Cancer* 1999;81(1):80-6.

5702   Goodfellow J, Bellamy MF, Ramsey MW, et al. Dietary supplementation with marine omega-3 fatty acids improve systemic large artery endothelial function in subjects with hypercholesterolemia. *J Am Coll Cardiol* 2000;35(2):265-70.

5703   Fenton WS, Hibbeln J, Knable M. Essential fatty acids, lipid membrane abnormalities, and the diagnosis and treatment of schizophrenia. *Biol Psychiatry* 2000;47(1):8-21.

5704   Nordoy A, Bonaa KH, Sandset PM, et al. Effect of omega-3 fatty acids and simvastatin on hemostatic risk factors and postprandial hyperlipemia in patients with combined hyperlipemia. *Arterioscler Thromb Vasc Biol* 2000;20(1):259-65.

5705   Hsu HC, Lee YT, Chen MF. Effect of n-3 fatty acids on the composition and binding properties of lipoproteins in hypertriglyceridemic patients. *Am J Clin Nutr* 2000 Jan;71(1):28-35.

5706   Roche HM, Gibney MJ. Effect of long-chain n-3 polyunsaturated fatty acids on fasting and postprandial triacylglycerol metabolism. *Am J Clin Nutr* 2000;71(1 Suppl):232S-7S.

5707   Nestel PJ. Fish oil and cardiovascular disease: lipids and arterial function. *Am J Clin Nutr* 2000;71(1 Suppl):228S-31S.

5708   Stordy BJ. Dark adaptation, motor skills, docosahexaenoic acid, and dyslexia. *Am J Clin Nutr* 2000;71(1 Suppl):323S-6S.

5709   Belluzzi A, Boschi S, Brignola C, et al. Polyunsaturated fatty acids and inflammatory bowel disease. *Am J Clin Nutr* 2000 Jan;71(1 Suppl):339S-42S.

5710   Navarro E, Esteve M, Olive A, et al. Abnormal fatty acid pattern in rheumatoid arthritis. A rationale for treatment with marine and botanical lipids. *J Rheumatol* 2000;27(2):298-303.

5711   Burgess JR, Stevens L, Zhang W, Peck L. Long-chain polyunsaturated fatty acids in children with attention-deficit hyperactivity disorder. *Am J Clin Nutr* 2000;71(1 Suppl):327S-30S.

5713   Su KP, Shen WW, Huang SY. Are omega3 fatty acids beneficial in depression but not mania? *Arch Gen Psychiatry* 2000;57(7):716-7.

5714   Siegers CP. Cytotoxicity of alkylphenols from Ginkgo biloba. *Phytomedicine* 1999;6(4):281-3.

5715   Ranchon I, Gorrand JM, Cluzel J, et al. Functional protection of photoreceptors from light-induced damage by dimethylurea and Ginkgo biloba extract. *Invest Ophthalmol Vis Sci* 1999;40(6):1191-9.

5716   Gardiner P, Wornham W. Recent review of complementary and alternative medicine used by adolescents. *Curr Opin Pediatr* 2000;12(4):298-302.

5717   Brautigam MR, Blommaert FA, Verleye G, et al. Treatment of age-related memory complaints with Gingko biloba extract: a randomized double blind placebo-controlled study. *Phytomedicine* 1998;5(6):425-34.

5718   Mix JA, Crews WD Jr. An examination of the efficacy of Ginkgo biloba extract EGb761 on the neuropsychologic functioning of cognitively intact older adults. *J Altern Complement Med* 2000;6(3):219-29.

5719   Kudolo GB. The effect of 3-month ingestion of Ginkgo biloba extract on pancreatic beta-cell function in response to glucose loading in normal glucose tolerant individuals. *J Clin Pharmacol* 2000;40(6):647-54.

5720   van Dongen MC, van Rossum E, Kessels AG, et al. The efficacy of ginkgo for elderly people with dementia and age-associated memory impairment: new results of a randomized clinical trial. *J Am Geriatr Soc* 2000;48(10):1183-94.

5721   Diamond BJ, Shiflett SC, Reiwel N, et al. Ginkgo biloba extract: mechanisms and clinical indications. *Arch Phys Med Rehabil* 2000;81(5):668-78.

5722   Kennedy DO, Scholey AB, Wesnes KA. The dose-dependent cognitive effects of acute administration of Ginkgo biloba to healthy young volunteers. *Psychopharmacology (Berl)* 2000;151(4):416-23.

5723   Marcilhac A, Dakine N, Bourhim N, et al. Effect of chronic administration of Gingko biloba extract or Ginkgolide on the hypothalamic-pituitary-adrenal axis in the rat. *Life Sci* 1998;62(25):2329-40.

5724   Amri H, Ogwuegbu SO, Boujrad N, et al. In vivo regulation of peripheral-type benzodiazepine and glucocorticoid synthesis by Gingko biloba extract EGb 761 and isolated ginkgolides. *Endocrinology* 1996;137(12):5707-18.

5725   Hoffman DL. Ginkgo biloba. Herbal Materia Medica 2000. www.healthy.net. (Accessed 9 November 2000).

5726   Chaitow L. The History of EDTA-Chelation Therapy. Health World Online 2000. www.healthy.net/asp/ templates/book.asp?PageType=Book&ID=586. (Accessed 17 November 2000).

5727   Blumer W, Cranton EM. Ninety Percent Reduction in Cancer Mortality After Chelation Therapy with EDTA. 1989. http://drcranton.com/chelation/study1.htm. (Accessed 17 November 2000).

5728   Heimbach J, Rieth S, Mohamedshah F, et al. Safety assessment of iron EDTA [sodium iron (Fe(3+) ethylenediaminetetraacetic acid]: summary of toxological fortification and exposure data. *Food Chem Toxicol* 2000;38(1):99-111.

5729   Schubert J. Chelation in medicine. *Sci Am* 1966;214(5):40-50.

5730   Zatlin GS, Senaldi EM, Bruckheim AH. Adult lead poisoning. *Am Fam Physician* 1985;32(4):137-43.

5731   Chisolm JJ Jr. BAL, EDTA, DMSA and DMPS in the treatment of lead poisoning in children. *J Toxicol Clin Toxicol* 1992;30(4):493-504.

5732   Lin JL, Ho HH, Yu CC. Chelation therapy for patients with elevated body lead burden and progressive renal insufficiency. A randomized, controlled trial. *Ann Intern Med* 1999;130(1):7-13.

5733   Mortensen ME, Walson PD. Chelation therapy for childhood lead poisoning. The changing scene in the 1990s. *Clin Pediatr (Phila)* 1993;32(5):284-91.

5734   Mehbod H. Treatment of lead intoxication. Combined use of peritoneal dialysis and edetate calcium disodium. *JAMA* 1967;201(12):972-4.

5735   Shrand H. Treatment of lead poisoning with intramuscular edathamil calcium-disodium. *Lancet* 1961;1:310-2.

5736   Gordon RA, Roberts G, Amin Z, et al. Aggressive approach in the treatment of acute lead encephalopathy with an extraordinarily high concentration of lead. *Arch Pediatr Adolesc Med* 1998;152(11):1100-4.

5737 Grier MT, Meyers DG. So much writing, so little science: a review of 37 years literature on edetate sodium chelation therapy. *Ann Pharmacother* 1993;27(12):1504-9.

5738 Chappell LT, Janson M. EDTA chelation therapy in the treatment of vascular disease. *J Cardiovasc Nurs* 1996;10(3):78-86.

5739 Kidd PM. Integrative cardiac revitalization: bypass surgery, angioplasty, and chelation. Benefits, risks, and limitations. *Altern Med Rev* 1998;3(1):4-17.

5740 Ernst E. Chelation therapy for coronary heart disease: An overview of all clinical investigations. *Am Heart J* 2000;140(1):139-41.

5741 Elihu N, Anandasbapathy S, Frishman WH. Chealtion therapy in cardiovascular disease: ethylenediaminetetraacetic acid, deferoxamine, and dexrazoxane. *J Clin Pharmacol* 1998;38(2):101-5.

5742 Ernst E. Chelation therapy for peripheral arterial occlusive disease: a systematic review. *Circulation* 1997;96(3):1031-3.

5743 Chappell LT. EDTA chelation therapy should be more commonly used in the treatment of vascular disease. *Altern Ther Health Med* 1995;1(2):53-7.

5744 Christensen K, Theilade D. Edta chelation therapy: an ethical problem. *Med Hypothesis* 1999;53(1):69-70.

5746 Gundling K, Ernst E. Complementary and alternative medicine in cardiovascular disease: what is the evidence it works? *WJM* 1999;171:191-4.

5747 Soffer A. Chelation therapy for arteriosclerosis. *JAMA* 1975;233(11):1206-7.

5749 Green S. Chelation therapy: unproven claims and unsound theories. Quackwatch 2000. www.quackwatch.com/cgi-bin/mfs/24/home/sbinfo/public_html/01.../chelation.html?23. (Accessed 17 November 2000).

5750 Kitchell JR, Palmon F, Aytan N, Meltzer LE. The treatment of coronary artery disease with disodium EDTA. A reappraisal. Am J Cardiology 1963;11:501-6.

5751 Olszewer E, Carter JP. EDTA chelation therapy in chronic degenerative disease. *Med Hypotheses* 1998;27(1):41-9.

5752 Sloth-Nielsen J, Guldager B, Mouritzen C, et al. Arteriographic findings in EDTA chelation therapy on peripheral arteriosclerosis. *Am J Surg* 1991;162(2):122-5.

5753 Guldager B, Jelnes R, Jorgensen SJ, et al. EDTA treatment of intermittent claudication—a double-blind, placebo-controlled study. *J Intern Med* 1992;231(3):261-7.

5754 van Rij AM, Solomon C, Packer SG, Hopkins WG. Chelation therapy for intermittent claudication. A double-blind, randomized, controlled trial. *Circulation* 1994;90(3):1194-9.

5756 Anon. Questions and Answers about chelation therapy. American Heart Association 2000. www.americanheart.org. (Accessed 17 November 2000).

5757 Neldner KH, Winkelmann RK, Perry HO. Scleroderma An evaluation of treatment with disodium edetate. *Arch Dermatol* 1962;86:95-9.

5758 Fuleihan FJ, Kurban AK, Abboud RT, et al. An objective evaluation of the treatment of systemic scleroderma with disodium EDTA, pyridoxine and reserpine. *Br J Dermatol* 1968;80(3):184-9.

5759 Barnett AJ, Coventry DA. Scleroderma. 1. Clinical features, course of illness and response to treatment in 61 cases. *Med J Aust* 1969;1(19):992-1001.

5760 Keech MK, McCann DS, Boyle AJ, Pinkus H. Effect of ethylenediaminetetra-acetic acid (EDTA) and tetrahyroxyquinone on sclerodermatous skin. Histologic and chemical studies. *J Invest Dermatol* 1966;47(3):235-46.

5761 Lyon Af, DeGraff AC. Reappraisal of digitalis. X. Treatment of digitalis toxicity. *Am Heart J* 1967;73(6):835-7.

5762 Surawica B. Use of the chelating agent, EDTA, in digitalis intoxication and cardiac arrhthymias. *Prog Cardiovasc Dis* 1960;2:432-43.

5763 Popovici A, Geschickter CF, Reinovsky A, Rubin M. Experimental control of serum calcium levels in vivo. *Proc Soc Exp Biol Med* 1950;74:415-7.

5764 Taweechaisupapong S, Doyle RJ. Sensitivity of bacterial coaggregation to chelating agents. *FEMS Immunol Med Microbiol* 2000;28(4):343-6.

5765 Beasley R, Fishwick D, Miles JF, Hendeles L. Preservatives in nebulizer solutions: risks without benefit. *Pharmacother* 1998;18(1):130-9.

5767 Anon. Ethylenediaminetetraacetic Acid, Trisodium Salt. NTP Chemical Repository Reports 2000. (Accessed 15 November 2000).

5768 Lamas GA, Ackermann A. Clinical evaluation of chelation therapy: is there any wheat amidst the chaff? *Am Heart J* 2000;140(1):4-5.

5769 Chappell LT, Wilson J, Ernst E. Chelation therapy for vascular disease. *Circulation* 1999; 99(1):164-5.

5770 Margolis S. Chelation therapy is ineffective for the treatment of peripheral vascular disease. Altern Ther Health Med 1995;1(2):53-6.

5771 Lacy CF, Armstrong LL, Ingrim NB, et al. Drug Information Handbook. 6th ed. Hudson, OH:Lexi-Comp Inc 1998:439-41.

5772 Ellsworth AJ, Witt DM, Dugdale DC, et al. Medical Drug Reference. Saint Louis, MO: Mosby-Year Book Inc 1998:302-3.

5773 Golan A, Savir H, Bar-Meir S, et al. Band keratopathy due to hyperparathyroidism. *Ophthalmologica* 1975;171(2):119-22.

5774 Yanoff M, Duker JS. Ophthalmology. Saint Louis, MO: Mosby-Year Book Inc., 1999.

5775 Carey CF, Lee HH, Woeltje KF. The Washington Manual of Medical Therapeutics. Philadelphia, PA: Lippincott-Raven Publishers, 1998.

5784 Melchoir J, Spasov AA, Ostrovskij OV, et al. Double-blind, placebo-controlled pilot and phase III study of activity of standardized Andrographis paniculata Herba Nees extract fixed combination (Kan jang) in the treatment of uncomplicated upper-respiratory tract infection. *Phytomedicine* 2000;7(5):341-50.

5798 Raskind JY, El-Chaar GM. The role of carnitine supplementation during valproic acid therapy. *Ann Pharmacother* 2000;34(5):630-638.

5799 Murakami K, Sugimoto T, Woo M, et al. Effect of L-carnitine supplementation on acute valproate intoxication. *Epilepsia* 1996;37(7):687-689.

5800 Cash CD. Gamma-hydroxybutyrate: an overview of the pros and cons for it being a neurotransmitter and/or a useful therapeutic agent. *Neurosci Biobehav Rev* 1994;18(2):291-304.

5801 Maitre M. The gamma-hydroxybutyrate signaling system in brain: organization and functional implications. *Prog Neurobiol* 1997;51(3):337-61.

REFERENCES

5802 Feigenbaum JJ, Howard SG. Gamma hydroxybutyrate is not a GABA agonist. *Prog Neurobiol* 1996;50(1):1-7.

5803 Mamelak M. Gammahydroxybutyrate: an endogenous regulator of energy metabolism. *Neurosci Biobehav Rev* 1989;13(4):187-98.

5804 Van Cauter E, Plat L, Scharf MB, et al. Simultaneous stimulation of slow-wave sleep and growth hormone secretion by gamma-hydroxybutyrate in normal young Men. *J Clin Invest* 1997;100(3):745-53.

5805 Cash CD. What is the role of the gamma-hydroxybutyrate receptor? *Med Hypotheses* 1996;47(6):455-9.

5806 Gerra G, Caccavari R, Fontanesi B, et al. Naloxone and metergoline effects on growth hormone response to gamma-hydroxybutyric acid. *Int Clin Psychopharmacol* 1995;10(4):245-50.

5807 Ferrara SD, Tedeschi L, Frison G, Rossi A. Fatality due to gamma-hydroxybutyric acid (GHB) and heroin intoxication. *J Forensic Sci* 1995;40(3):501-4.

5808 Holoye PY, Duelge J, Hansen RM, et al. Prophylaxis of Ifosamide toxicity with oral acetylcysteine. *Semin Oncol* 1983 Mar;10(1 Suppl 1):66-71.

5809 Consumer Lab. www.consumerlab.com/results/valerian.asp (Accessed 5 June 2001).

5810 Ellinwood EH Jr, Gonzalez AE, Dougherty GG Jr. Gamma-Butyrolactone effects on behavior induced by dopamine agonists. *Biol Psychiatry* 1983;18(9):1023-32.

5811 Dougherty GG, Ellinwood EH Jr. Influence of gamma-butyrolactone on behavior due to dopaminergic drugs. *Physiol Behav* 1983;30(4):607-12.

5812 Snead OC III, Bearden LJ. Naloxone overcomes the dopaminergic, EEG, and behavioral effects of gamma-hydroxybutyrate. *Neurol* 1980;30(8):832-8.

5813 Kohrs FP, Porter WH, et al. Gamma-hydroxybutyrate intoxication and overdose. [Letter and responses]. *Ann Emerg Med* 1999;33(4):475-6.

5814 Law M. Plant sterol and stanol margarines and health. *BMJ* 2000;320:861-4.

5815 Anon. Healing With Nutrition website. URL: www.healingwithnutrition.com/aminoacid.html#Dimethylglycine(DMG) (Accessed 20 May 2000).

5816 Kendall RV. N,N-Dimethylglycine (DMG): The Metabolic Enhancer that boosts the immune system, enhances performance and improves cardiovascular function. FoodScience of Vermont website. www.fslabs.com/dmg_tb.htm (Accessed 20 May 2000).

5817 Rimland B. Dimethylglycine (DMG), a nontoxic metabolite, and autism. Autism Res Institute website. www.autism.org/dmg.html (Accessed 20 May 2000).

5818 Anon. Natural Health Consultants website. www.naturalhealthconsult.com/Monographs/dmg.html (Accessed 20 May 2000).

5819 Bolman WM, Richmond JA. A double-blind, placebo-controlled, crossover pilot trial of low dose dimethylglycine in patients with autistic disorder. *J Autism Dev Disord* 1999;29(3):191-4.

5820 Reap EA, Lawson JW. Stimulation of the immune response by dimethylglycine, a nontoxic metabolite. *J Lab Clin Med* 1990;115(4):481-6.

5821 Tonda ME, Hart LL. N,N-dimthylglycine and L-carnitine as performance enhancers in athletes. *Ann Pharmacother* 1992;26:935-7.

5822 Weiss RC. Immunologic responses in healthy random-source cats fed N,N-dimethylglycine-supplemented diets. *Am J Vet Res* 1992;53(5):829-33.

5823 Gascon G, Patterson B, Yearwood K, Slotnick H. N,N-dimethylglycine and epilepsy. *Epilepsia* 1989;30(1):90-3.

5824 Freed WJ. Prevention of strychnine-induced seizures and death by the N-methylated glycine derivatives betaine, dimethylglycine and sarcosine. *Pharmacol Biochem Behav* 1985;22(4):641-3.

5825 Graber CD, Goust JM, Glassman AD, et al. Immunomodulating properties of dimethylglycine in humans. *J Infect Dis* 1981;143(1):101-5.

5826 Roach ES, Carlin L. N,N dimethylglycine for epilepsy [letter]. *N Engl J Med* 1982;307:1081-2.

5827 Herbert V. N,N-dimethylglycine for epilepsy [letter]. *N Engl J Med* 1983;308:527-8.

5828 Freed WJ. N,N-dimethylglycine, betaine and seizures [letter]. *Arch Neurol* 1984;41:1129-30.

5829 Ward TN, Smith EB, Reeves AG. Dimethylglycine and reduction of mortality in penicillin-induced seizures [letter]. *Ann Neurol* 1985;17(2):213.

5830 Kendall RV. Comment: N,N-dimethylglycine and L-carnitine as performance enhancers in athletes [letter]. *Ann Pharmacother* 1994;28:973.

5834 Anon. Natural Health Consultants website. www.naturalhealthconsult.com/Monographs/7Keto.html (Accessed 8 June 2000).

5835 Anon. Humanetics Corporation website. URL http://humaneticscorp.com/7keto.html (Accessed 8 June 2000).

5836 Anon. Chatham Health and Wellness Store website. URL http://www.chathamhealth.com/accord/twin7ketfuel.html (Accessed 8 April 2000).

5837 Lardy H, Partridge B, Kneer N, Wei Y. Ergosteroids: induction of thermogenic enzymes in liver of rats treated with steroids derived from dehydroepiandrosterone. *Proc Natl Acad Sci U S A* 1995;92(14):6617-9.

5838 Consumer Lab. www.consumerlab.com/results/ginkgobiloba.asp (Accessed 5 June 2001).

5839 Shi J, Schulze S, Lardy HA. The effect of 7-oxo-DHEA acetate on memory in young and old C57BL/6 mice. *Steroids* 2000;65(3):124-9.

5840 Davidson MH, Weeks C, Lardy H, et al. Clinical Safety and Endocrine Effects of 7-KETO-DHEA. Abstract presented at: Experimental Biology 98, April 19-22, 1998, San Francisco, CA. Abstract obtained from Humanetics Corporation website. URL http://humaneticscorp.com/7ketoabstracts.html (Accessed 8 June 2000).

5841 Nelson R, Herron M, Weeks C, Lardy H. Dehydroepiandrosterone and 7-KETO-DHEA augment Interleukin 2 (IL2) Production by Human Lymphocytes In Vitro. Abstract presented at: The 5th Conference on Retroviruses and Opportunistic Infections, February 1-5, 1998, Chicago, IL. Abstract obtained from Humanetics Corporation website. URL http://humaneticscorp.com/7ketoabstracts.html (Accessed 8 June 2000).

5842 Colker CM, Torina GC, Swain MA, Kalman DS. Double-Blind Study Evaluating the Effects of Exercise Plus 3-Acetyl-7-oxo-dehydroepiandrosterone on Body Composition and the Endocrine System in Overweight Adults. Abstract presented at 2nd ASEP Annual Meeting, October 14-16, 1999, and published in Journal of Exercise Physiology online, Volume 2 Number 4 October 1999.

5843 Anon. Natures Herbs website. URL: www.natures-herbs.com/chlorella.htm (Accessed 6 April 2000).

5844 Anon. Mother Nature.com website. URL www.mothernature.com/cg/chlorella.asp (Accessed 6 June 2000).

5845 Anon. Tisco website. URL www.sunchlorella.net/chlorellaindetail.htm (Accessed 6 June 2000).

5846 Peirce A. The American Pharmaceutical Association Practical Guide to Natural Medicines. William Morrow & Co.Inc., New York. 1999.

5847 Ng TP, Tan WC, Lee YK. Occupational asthma in a pharmacist induced by chlorella, a unicellular algae preparation. *Resp Med* 1994;88:555-7.

5848 Ruama AL, Torronen R, Hanninen O, Mykkanen H. Vitamin B12 status of long-term adherents of a strict uncooked vegan diet ("living food diet") is compromised. *J Nutr* 1995;125(10):2511-5.

5849 Davis DR. Some algae are potentially adequate sources of vitamin B-12 for vegans (letter, comment). *J Nutr* 1997;127(2):378,380.

5850 Morimoto T, Nagatsu A, Murakami N, et al. Anti-tumor-promoting glyceroglycolipids from the green alga, Chlorella vulgaris. *Phytochemistry* 1995;40(5):1433-7.

5851 Tyml R. Present state and possibilities of the medical use of chlorococcal algae. Acta Univ Palacki Olomuc Fac Med 1982;103:273-9.

5852 Jitsukawa K, Suizu R, Hidano A. Chlorella photosensitization. New phytophotodermatosis. *Int J Dermatol* 1984;23(4):263-8.

5853 Nelson AM, Neafie RC. Protothecosis. In: Strickland GT. Hunter's Tropical Medicine and Emerging Infectious Disease. 8th edition. WB Saunders Co., Philadelphia, PA. 2000:547.

5854 Lissoni P, Barni S, Cazzaniga M, et al. Efficacy of the concomitant administration of the pineal hormone melatonin in cancer immunotherapy with low-dose IL-2 in patients with advanced solid tumors who had progressed on Il-2 alone. *Oncology* 1994;51:344-7.

5855 Lissoni P, Barni S, Tancini G, et al. A randomised study with subcutaneous low-dose interleukin 2 alone vs. interleukin 2 plus the pineal neurohormone melatonin in advanced solid neoplasms other than renal cancer and melanoma. *Br J Cancer* 1994;69(1):196-9.

5856 Bubis M, Zisapel N. Modulation by melatonin of protein secretion from melanoma cells: is cAMP involved? *Molecular and Cellular Endocrinology* 1995;112:169-73.

5857 Lissoni P, Paolorossi F, Tancini G, et al. A phase II study of tamoxifen plus melatonin in metastatic solid tumour patients. *Br J Cancer* 1996;74(9):1466-8.

5858 Anon. NutriTeam website. URL www.nutriteam.com (Accessed 8 July 2000).

5859 Anon. Imhotep Inc. website. URL www.imhotepinc.com/GSE.htm (Accessed 8 July 2000).

5860 Code of Federal Regs, Title 21, Vol 3, Part 182: Substances Generally Recognized as Safe. FDA, Dept of Health and Human Svcs website. URL http://frwebgate3.access.gpo.gov/cgi-bin/waisgate.cgi?WAISdocID=362886791+3+0+0&WAISaction=retrieve (Accessed 11 July 2000).

5861 Citricidal Material Safety Data Sheet. NutriTeam website. URL http://nutriteam.com/msds.html (Accessed 11 July 2000).

5862 Xiong H, Li Y, Slavik MF, Walker JT. Spraying chicken skin with selected chemicals to reduce attached Salmonella typhimurium. *J Food Prot* 1998;61(3):272-5.

5863 Sakamoto S, Sato K, Maitani T, Yamada T. [Analysis of components in natural food additive "grapefruit seed extract" by HPLC and LC/MS]. [Article in Japanese]. *Eisei Shikenjo Hokoku* 1996;(114):38-42.

5864 Calori-Domingues MA, Fonseca H. Laboratory evaluation of chemical control of aflatoxin production in unshelled peanuts (Arachis hypogaea L.). *Food Addit Contam* 1995;12(3):347-50.

5865 Ranzani MR, Fonseca H. Mycological evaluation of chemically-treated unshelled peanuts. *Food Addit Contam* 1995;12(3):343-6.

5866 Ionescu G, Kiehl F, Wichmann-Kunz F, et al. Oral citrus seed extract in atopic eczema: in vitro and in vivo studies on intestinal microflora. *J Orthomolec Med* 1990;5(3):155-7.

5867 Von Woedtke T, Schluter B, Pflegel P, et al. Aspects of the antimicrobial efficacy of grapefruit seed extract and its relation to preservative substances contained. *Pharmazie* 1999;54(6):452-6.

5868 Reiter WJ, Pycha A, Schatzl G, et al. Serum dehydroepiandrosterone sulfate concentrations in men with erectile dysfunction. *Urology* 2000;55:755-8.

5869 Hayashi T, Teiji Esaki T, Emiko Muto E, et al. Dehydroepiandrosterone retards atherosclerosis formation through its conversion to estrogen: the possible role of nitric oxide. *Arterioscler Thromb Vasc Biol* 2000;20(3):782-92.

5870 Kline MD, Jaggers ED. Mania onset while using dehydroepiandrosterone (letter). *Am J Psychiatry* 1999;156(6):971.

5871 Moriyama Y, Yasue H, Yoshimura M, et al. The plasma levels of dehydroepiandrosterone sulfate are decreased in patients with chronic heart failure in proportion to the severity. *J Clin Endocrinol Metab* 2000;85:1834-40.

5872 Barry NN, McGuire JL, van Vollenhoven RF. Dehydroepiandrosterone in systemic lupus erythematosus: relationship between dosage, serum levels, and clinical response. *J Rheumatol* 1998;25:2352-6.

5873 Mainous AG, Hueston WJ, Connor MK. Serum vitamin C levels and use of health care resources for wheezing episodes. *Arch Fam Med* 2000;9:241-5.

5874 Moffat SD, Zonderman AB, Harman M, et al. The relationship between longitudinal declines in dehydroepiandrosterone sulfate concentrations and cognitive performance in older men. *Arch Int Med* 2000;160:2193-8.

5875 Lykkesfeldt J, Christen S, Wallock LM, et al. Ascorbate is depleted by smoking and replaced by moderate supplementation: a study in male smokers and nonsmokers with matched dietary antioxidant intakes. *Am J Clin Nutr* 2000;71:530-6.

5876 Riemersma RA, Carruthers KF, Elton RA, Fox KA. Vitamin C and the risk of acute myocardial infarction. *Am J Clin Nutr* 2000;71:1181-6.

5877 Simon JA, Hudes ES. Serum ascorbic acid and gallbladder disease prevalence among US adults. *Arch Intern Med* 2000;160:931-6.

5878 Loria CM, Klag MJ, Caulfield LE, Whelton PK. Vitamin C status and mortality in US adults. *Am J Clin Nutr* 2000;72:139-45.

5879 Sherman DL, Keaney JF, Biegelsen ES, et al. Pharmacological concentrations of ascorbic acid are required for the beneficial effect on endothelial vasomotor function in hypertension. *Hypertension* 2000;35:936-41.

5880 Daels-Rakotoarison DA, Seidel V, Gressier B, et al. Neurosedative and antioxidant activities of phenylpropanoids from Ballota nigra. *Arzneimittelforschung* 2000;50(1):16-23.

5881 McAlindon TE, Jacques P, Zhang Y, et al. Do antioxidant micronutrients protect against the development and progression of knee osteoarthritis? *Arthritis Rheum* 1996;39(4):648-56.

5882 Blumenthal RD, Lew W, Reising A, et al. Antioxidant vitamins reduce normal tissue toxicity induced by radio-immunotherapy. *Int J Cancer* 2000;86:276-80.

5883 Chan TY. Drug interactions as a cause of overanticoagulation and bleedings in Chinese patients receiving warfarin. *Int J Clin Pharmacol Ther* 1998;36(7):403-5.

5884 Izzat MB, Yim APC, El-Zufari MH. A taste of Chinese medicine! *Ann Thorac Surg* 1998;66:941-2.

5885 Millqvist E. Cough provocation with capsaicin is an objective way to test sensory hyperreactivity in patients with asthma-like symptoms. *Allergy* 2000;55:546-50.

5886 Sharma A, Gautam, Jadhav SS. Spice extracts as dose-modifying factors in radiation inactivation of bacteria. *J Agric Food Chem* 2000;48:1340-4.

5887 Galve-Roperh I, Sanchez C, Cortes ML, et al. Anti-tumoral action of cannabinoids: involvement of sustained ceramide accumulation and extracellular signal-regulated kinase activation. *Nat Medicine* 2000;6(3):313-9.

5888 Piomelli D. Pot of gold for glioma therapy. *Nat Medicine* 2000;6(3):255-6.

5889 Baker D, Pryce G, Croxford JL, et al. Cannabinoids control spasticity and tremor in a multiple sclerosis model. *Nature* 2000;404:84-7.

5890 Merchant RE, Carmack CA, Wise CM. Nutritional supplementation with Chlorella pyrenoidosa for patients with fibromyalgia syndrome: a pilot study. *Phytother Res* 2000;14:167-73.

5891 Konishi F, Tanaka K, Himeno K, et al. Antitumor effect induced by a hot water extract of Chlorella vulgaris (CE): resistance to Meth-A tumor growth mediated by CE-induced polymorphonuclear leukocytes. *Cancer Immunol Immunother* 1985;19(2):73-8.

5892 Miyazawa Y, Murayama T, Ooya N, et al. Immunomodulation by a unicellular green algae (Chlorella pyrenoidosa) in tumor-bearing mice. *J Ethnopharmacol* 1988 Dec;24(2-3):135-46.

5893 Haggans CJ, Hutchins AM, Olson BA, et al. Effect of flaxseed consumption on urinary estrogen metabolites in postmenopausal women. *Nutr Cancer* 1999;33(2):188-95.

5894 Nesbitt PD, Lam Y, Thompson LU. Human metabolism of mammalian lignan precursors in raw and processed flaxseed. *Am J Clin Nutr* 1999;69(3):549-55.

5895 Sung MK, Lautens M, Thompson LU. Mammalian lignans inhibit the growth of estrogen-independent human colon tumor cells. *Anticancer Res* 1998;18(3A):1405-8.

5896 Nestel PJ, Pomeroy SE, Sasahara T, et al. Arterial compliance in obese subjects is improved with dietary plant n-3 fatty acid from flaxseed oil despite increased LDL oxidizability. *Arterioscler Thromb Vasc Biol* 1997;17(6):1163-70.

5897 Thompson LU, Rickard SE, Cheung F, et al. Variability in anticancer lignan levels in flaxseed. *Nutr Cancer* 1997;27(1):26-30.

5898 Nordstrom DC, Honkanen VE, Nasu Y, et al. Alpha-linolenic acid in the treatment of rheumatoid arthritis. A double-blind, placebo-controlled and randomized study: flaxseed vs. safflower seed. *Rheumatol Int* 1995;14(6):231-4.

5899 Cunnane SC, Ganguli S, Menard C, et al. High alpha-linolenic acid flaxseed (Linum usitatissimum): some nutritional properties in humans. *Br J Nutr* 1993;69:443-53.

5900 Rudolph FB, Van Buren CT. The metabolic effects of enterally administered ribonucleic acids. *Current Opinion in Clinical Nutrition and Metabolic Care* 1998;1(6):527-30.

5901 Anon. 2000. Austin Nutritional Research. URL: http://www.realtime.net/anr/nutrient.html#Rnadna. (Accessed 9 May 2000).

5902 Kenny FS, Pinder SE, Ellis IO, et al. Gamma linolenic acid with tamoxifen as primary therapy in breast cancer. *Int J Cancer* 2000;85:643-8.

5903 Anon. 2000. Herbal Information Center General Store. URL:www.kcweb.com.herb/p_applecider.htm. (Accessed 10 May 2000).

5904 Anon. 2000. The book lovers' community for our community. URL: http://www.thathomesite.com/forums/load/health.msg0322241820838.html. (Accessed 10 May 2000).

5905 Anon. 2000. Apple Cider Vinegar with Centella for weight loss and so much more. URL: http://www.ageless.co.za/applecider.htm. (Accessed 10 May 2000).

5906 Good Health Organization International Ltd 2000. Organic Apple Cider Vinegar. URL: http://www.gho.co.nz/vinegar.html. (Accessed 10 May 2000).

5907 Anon. 2000. Apple Cider Vinegar. URL: http://www.go-symmetry.com/apple-vinegar.htm (Accessed 10 May 2000).

5908 Anon. 2000. Bragg Apple Cider Vinegar. URL:http://www.bragg.com/acvproduct.html. (Accessed 10 May 2000).

5909 Anon. Apple Cider Vinegar. URL:http://www.healthness.com/applecidervinegar.htm. (Accessed 10 May 2000).

5910 Duke J. The Green Pharmacy. Emmaus: Rodale Press, 1997

5911 Lhotta K, Hofle G, Gasser R, Finkenstedt G. Hypokalemia, hyperreninemia, and osteoporosis in a patient ingesting large amounts of cider vinegar. *Nephron* 1998;80:242-3.

5912 Nutrition Search. Nutrition Almanac, Revised Edition. New York: McGraw-Hill Book Company. 1979.

5913 Burton TM. In trials, potion of herbs slows prostate cancer. The Wall Street Journal, May 17, 2000, p.B-1.

5914 Anonymous. Pure Emu Oil and Emu Oil Products for Natural Healing and Better Health. 1999. URL: http://www.uniquelyemu.com (Accessed 18 May 2000).

5915 Anonymous. 2000. Welcome to Coopers Emu Oil Products. URL: http://www.coppersemuoilproducts.com/ (Accessed 18 May 2000).

5916 Anonymous. 2000. Aussiepol Trading Benefits of Emu Oil. URL. http://homepages.tig.com.au/~asuuipol/emuoil.html (Accessed 18 May 2000).

5917 Anonymous. 2000. Amazing Emu Oil. URL: http://

mars.ark.com/~emuzing/emuoil.html (Accessed 19 May 2000).

5918 Anonymous. 2000. Reported Uses of Em Oil. URL: http://www.gentleridge.com/emuoiluses.html (Accessed 19 May 2000).

5919 Anonymous. 1999. Chemical Analysis of Emu Oil. URL: http://www.emu-oil.com/analysis.htm (Accessed 19 May 2000).

5920 Hopkins L. 2000. Would you believe? URL. http://www.pureemuoil.com/pr6.htm (Accessed 19 May 2000).

5921 Anonymous. 2000. URL. http://turnagefarmsinc.com/emu2.htm (Accessed 19 May 2000).

5922 Anonymous. 2000. Moanui Natural Relief and Skin Care Products. URL http://www.moanui.co.nz/benefits.html. (Accessed 19 May 2000).

5923 Lopez A, Sims DE, Ablett RF, et al. Effect of emu oil on auricular inflammation with croton oil in mice. *Am J Vet Res* 1999;60(12):1558-61.

5924 Pariza M, Park Y, Cook ME. Conjugated linoleic acid and the control of cancer and obesity. *Toxicological Sciences* 1999;52 (Supplement) 107-10.

5925 Jiang J, Wolk A, Vessby B. Relation between the intake of milk fat and the occurrence of conjugated linoleic acid in human adipose tissue. *Am J Clin Nutr* 1999;70:21-7.

5926 O'Shea M, Stanton C, Devery R. Antioxidant enzyme defense responses of human MCF-7 and SW480 cancer cells to conjugated linoleic acid. *Anticancer Research* 1999;19:1953-60.

5927 Cesano Al, Visonneau S, Scimeca JA, et al. Opposite effects of linoleic acid and conjugated linoleic acid on human prostatic cancer in SCID mice. *Anticancer Res* 1998 May-Jun;18(3A):1429-34.

5928 West DB, Delany JP, Camet PM, et al. Effects of conjugated linoleic acid on body fat and energy metabolism in the mouse. *Am J Physiol (Regulatory Integrative Comp Physiol)* 1998;275:R667-72.

5929 DeLany JP, Blohm F, Truett AA, et al. Conjugated linoleic acid rapidly reduced body fat content in mice without affecting energy intake. *Am J Physiol (Regulatory Integrative Comp Physiol)* 1999;276:45:R1172-9.

5930 Clement I, Banni S, Andioni E, et al. Conjugated linoleic acid-enriched butter fat alters mammary gland morphogenesis and reduces cancer risk in rats. *J Nutr* 1999;129:2135-42.

5931 Banni S, Angioni E, Casu V, et al. An increase in vitamin A status by the feeding of conjugated linoleic acid. *Nutr Cancer* 1999;33(1):53-7.

5932 Kelly ML, Berry JR, Dwyer DA, et al. Dietary fatty acid sources affect conjugated linoleic acid concentrations in milk from lactating dairy cows. *J Nutr* 128:881-5.

5933 Herbel BK, McGuire MK, McGuire MA, Shultz TD. Safflower oil consumption does not increase plasma conjugated linoleic acid concentrations in humans. *Am J Clin Nutr* 1998;67:332-7.

5934 Sebedio JL, Gnaedig S, Chardigny JM. Recent advances in conjugated linoleic acid research. *Current Opinion in Clinical Nutrition and Metabolic Care* 1999;2(6):499-506.

5935 Scimeca JA. Toxicological evaluation of dietary conjugated linoleic acid in male Fischer 344 rats. *Food Chem Toxicol* 1998;36(5);391-5.

5936 McCarty MF. Toward a wholly nutritional therapy for type 2 diabetes. *Med Hypothesis* 2000;54(3):483-7.

5937 Izumi T, Piskula MK, Osawa S, et al. Soy isoflavone aglycones are absorbed faster and in higher amounts than their glucosides in humans. *J Nutr* 2000;130:1695-9.

5938 Faloon B. Conjugated linoleic acid-new studies 2000. URL: http:www.dietsexercise.com/CLAText.htm. (Accessed 27 May 2000).

5939 Murkies A, Dalais FS, Briganti EM, et al. Phytoestrogens and breast cancer in postmenopausal women: a case control study. *Menopause* 2000;7:289-96.

5940 Shalita AR, Smith JG, Parish LC, et al. Topical nicotinamide compared with clindamycin gel in the treatment of inflammatory acne vulgaris. *Int J Dermatol* 1995;34:434-7.

5941 Birch EE, Garfield S, Hoffman DR, et al. A randomized controlled trial of early dietary supply of long-chain polyunsaturated fatty acids and mental development in term infants. *Dev Med Child Neurol* 2000;42:174-81.

5942 Berges RR, Windeler J, Trampisch HJ, et al. Randomized, placebo-controlled, double-blind clinical trial of beta-sitosterol in patients with benign prostatic hyperplasia. *Lancet* 1995;345:1529-32.

5943 Bruneton J. Pharmacognosy Phytochemistry Medicinal Plants. 2nd ed. Paris:Lavoisier Publ, 1999:291-2.

5944 Fleming T, ed. PDR for Herbal Medicines, 2nd ed. Montvale: Medical Economics 2000.

5945 Anonymous. 2000. The power of healing plants. 2000 URL. http://www.african.savana.co.za/power.htm. (Accessed 30 May 2000).

5946 Anonymous. 2000. Research. 2000 URL. http://www.african-savana.co.za/research.htm (Accessed 30 May 2000).

5951 Frati A. 2000 Medical implications of prickly pear cactus. URL: http:www.tamuk.edu/webuser/cactus/cac_med.html. (Accessed 30 May 2000).

5952 Anonymous. 2000. Opticantha. URL. http://opticantha.com/ataglance.html. (Accessed 30 May 2000).

5953 Anonymous. 2000. Opuntia. URL. http:///www.healthlink.com.au/nat_lib/htm-herb/BPH691.HTM. (Accessed 30 May 2000).

5954 Bwititi P, Musabayane CT, Nhachi CF. Effects of Opuntia megacantha on blood glucose and kidney function in streptozotocin diabetic rats. *J Ethnopharmacol* 2000;69(3):247-52.

5955 Trejo-Gonzalez A, Gabriel-Ortiz G, Puebla-Perez A, et al. A purified extract from prickly pear cactus (Opuntia fuliginosa) controls experimentally induced diabetes in rats. *J Ethnopharmacol* 1996;55(1):27-33.

5956 Ahmad A, Davies J, Randall S, Skinner GR. Antiviral properties of extract of Opuntia streptacantha. *Antiviral Res* 1996;30(2-3):75-85.

5957 Roman-Ramos R, Flores-Saenz JL, Alarcon-Aguilar FJ. Anti-hyperglycemic effect of some edible plants. *J Ethnopharmacol* 1995;48(1):25-32.

5958 Fernandez ML, Lin EC, Trejo A, McNamara DJ. Prickly pear (Opuntia sp.) pectin alters hepatic cholesterol metabolism without affecting cholesterol absorption in guinea pigs fed a hypercholesterolemic diet. *J Nutr* 1994;124(6):817-24.

5959 Frati AC, Xilotl Diaz N, Altamirano P, et al. The effect of two sequential doses of Opuntia streptacantha upon glycemia. *Arch Invest Med (Mex)* 1991;22(3-4):333-6.

5960 Frati-Munari AC, Licona-Quesada R, Araiza-Andraca CR, et al. Activity of Opuntia streptocantha in healthy

REFERENCES

individuals with induced hyperglycemia. *Arch Invest Med (Mex)* 1990;21(2):99-102.

5961 Frati-Munari AC, Altamirano-Bustamante E, Rodrigues-Barcenas N, et al. Hypoglycemic action of Opuntia streptacantha Lemaire: study using raw extracts. *Arch Invest Med (Mex)* 1989;20(4):321-5.

5962 Frati-Munari AC, Del Valle-Martinez LM, Ariza-Andraca CR, et al. Hypoglycemic action of different doses of nopol (Opuntia streptacantha) in patients with type II diabetes mellitus. *Arch Invest Med (Mex)* 1989;20(2):197-201.

5963 Frati Munari AC, Quiroz Lazaro JL, Alramirano Bustamante P, et al. The effect of various doses of nopal (Opuntia streptacantha Lemaire) on the glucose tolerance test in healthy individuals. *Arch Invest Med (Mex)* 1988;19(2):143-8.

5964 Frati-Munari AC, Gordillo BE, Altamirano P, Ariza CR. Hypoglycemic effect of Opuntia streptacantha Lemaire in NIDDM. *Diabetes Care* 1988;11(1):63-6.

5968 Meckes-Lozyoa M, Roman-Ramos R. Opuntia streptacantha; a coadjutor in the treatment of diabetes mellitus. *Am J Chin Med* 1986;14(3-4):116-8.

5969 Frati-Munari AC, Roca-Vides RA, Lopez-Perez RJ, et al. The glycemic index of some foods common in Mexico. *Gac Med Mex* 1991;127(2):163-70.

5970 Frati Munari AC, Vera Lastra O, Ariza Andraca CR. Evaluation of nopol capsules in diabetes mellitus. *Gaeceta Medica de Mexico* 1992;128(4):431-6.

5971 Medical Economic. Physician's Desk Reference. Montvale:Medical Economics, 1999:1289.

5972 Rask MR. The Omohyoideus myofascial pain syndrome: report of four patients. *The Journal of Cranomandibular Practice* 1984;2(3):256-62.

5973 McCalla CX. Instantaneous cure of acute frontal cephalalgia. Manufacturer information from High Chemical Company; 1995.

5974 Vuturo AE, Executive Editor. Differential diagnosis and treatment of sciatica: the non-diskogenic causes. Advanced Clinical Updates; 1985.

5975 Manufacturer Information. Sarapin. Injection technique in pain control. High Chemical Company. Information not dated.

5976 Anon. Quarter Horse Woes. The Investigators. 2000. URL:http://www.kwtv.com/investigators/horse2.htm. (Accessed 19 June 2000).

5977 Gracer RI. A better method of pain management 2000. URL.http://www.tldp.com/issue/175-6/Prolong.html. (Accessed 19 June 2000).

5978 Wilk SJ. Pain disorders that are confused with TMJ. 2000. URL:http://tmjheadaches.com/conf.htm. (Accessed 19 June 2000).

5979 Consumer Lab. www.consumerlab.com/results/stjohnswort.asp (Accessed 5 June 2001).

5980 National Germplasm Resources Laboratory. National Genetic Resources Program 2000. Pitcher plant. URL:http:www.ars-grin.gov/cgi-bin/npgs/html. (Accessed 19 June 2000).

5991 Asero R. Detection and clinical characterization of patients with oral allergy syndrome caused by stable allergens in Rosaceae and nuts. *Ann Allergy Asthma Immunol* 1999;83(5):377-83.

5992 Durak I, Kacmaz M, Buyukkocak S, Cimen BM, Ozturk HS. Hazelnut supplementation enhances plasma antioxidant potential and lowers plasma cholesterol levels [letter]. *Clinica Chimica Acta* 1999; 284(1):113-5.

5993 Caballero T, Pascual C, Garcia-Ara MC, Ojeda JA, Martin-Esteban M. IgE crossreactivity between mugwort pollen (Artemisia vulgaris) and hazelnut (Abellana nux) in sera from patients with sensitivity to both extracts. *Clin Exp Allergy* 1997; 27(10):1203-11.

5994 Pumphrey RS, Wilson PB, Faragher EB, Edwards SR. Specific immunoglobulin E to peanut, hazelnut and brazil nut 731 patients: similar patterns found at all ages. *Clin Exp Allergy* 1999;29(9):1256-9.

5995 Savage GP, McNeil DL. Chemical composition of hazelnuts (Corylus avellana) grown in New Zealand. *Int J Food Sci Nutr* 1998;49(3):199-203.

5996 Caballero T, Martin-Esteban M. Association between pollen hypersensitivity and edible vegetable allergy: a review. *J Investig Allergol Clin Immunol* 1998;8(1):6-16.

5997 Sutherland MF, O'Hehir RE, Czarny D, Suphioglu C. Macadamia nut anaphylaxis: demonstration of specific IgE reactivity and partial cross-reactivity with hazelnut. *J Allergy Clin Immunol* 1999; 104 (4 Pt 1):889-90.

5998 Munoz MF, Lopez-Cazana JM, Villas F, et al. Exercise-induced anaphylactic reaction to hazelnut. *Allergy* 1994;49(5):314-6.

5999 O'Mahony M, Mitchell E, Gilbert RJ, Hutchinson DN, et al. An outbreak of foodborne botulism associated with contaminated hazelnut yoghurt. *Epidemiol Infect* 1990;104(3):389-95.

6000 King DS, et al. Effect of oral androstenedione on serum testosterone and adaptations to resistance training in young men. A randomized controlled trial. *JAMA*, 2 Jun. 1999; 281(21): 2020-8.

6001 Roche Laboratories, Inc. Package insert for Xenical. April 1999.

6002 Fetrow CW, Avila JR. Professional's Handbook of Complementary & Alternative Medicines. Springhouse, Pennsylvania: Springhouse Corporation, 1999.

6003 Offenbacher EG, Pi-Sunyer FX. Beneficial effect of chromium-rich yeast on glucose tolerance and blood lipids in elderly subjects. *Diabetes*, Nov. 1980; 29(11): 919-25.

6004 Rabinowitz MB, Gonick HC, Levin SR, Davidson MB. Effects of chromium and yeast supplements on carbohydrate and lipid metabolism in diabetic men. *Diabetes Care*, Jul-Aug 1983; 6(4): 319-27.

6006 Mother Nature Products website: www.mothernature.com (Accessed 23 July 1999).

6007 Kehoe WA. Secretin for the treatment of autism. *Pharmacist's Letter* Detail Document #141212. December, 1998.

6008 Gurley BJ, Gardner SF, Hubbard MA. Content versus label claims in ephedra-containing dietary supplements. *Am J Health Syst Pharm* 2000;57:963-9.

6009 White LM, Gardner SF, Gurley BJ, et al. Pharmacokinetics and Cardiovascular Effects of Ma-Huang (Ephedra sinica) in Normotensive Adults. *J Clin Pharmacol* 1997;37:116-22.

6010 Arlt W, Haas J, Callies F, et al. Biotransformation of Oral Dehydroepiandrosterone in Elderly Men: Significant Increase in Circulating Estrogens. *J Clin Endocrinol Metab* 1999;84(6):2170-6.

6011 Barnhart KT, Freeman E, Grisso JA, et al. The Effect of Dehydroepiandrosterone Supplementation to Symptomatic Perimenopausal Women on Serum Endocrine Profiles, Lipid Parameters, and Health-Related Quality of Life. *J Clin Endocrinol Metab* 1999;84(11):3896-902.

6012 Callies F, Arlt W, Siekmann L, et al. Influence of oral dehydroepiandrosterone (DHEA) on urinary steroid metabolites in males and females. *Steroids* 2000;65:98-102.

6013 Tilvis RS, Kahonen M, Harkonen M. Dehydroepiandrosterone Sulfate, Diseases and Mortality in a General Aged Population. *Aging (Milano)* 1999;11(1):30-4.

6014 Mazza E, Maccario M, Ramunni J, et al. Dehydroepiandrosterone Sulfate Levels in Women. Relationships With Age, Body Mass Index and Insulin Levels. *J Endocrinol Invest* 1999;22(9):681-7.

6015 Rossouw F, Kruger PE, Rossouw J. The Effect of Creatine Monohydrate Loading on Maximal Intermittent Exercise and Sport-Specific Strength in Well Trained Power-Lifters. *Nutrition Research* 2000;20(4):505-14.

6016 Timby N, Eriksson A. Gamma-Hydroxybutyrate-Associated Deaths. *Am J Med* 2000;108:518.

6017 Connor WE. Harbingers of coronary heart disease: dietary saturated fatty acids and cholesterol. Is chocolate benign because of its stearic acid content? *Am J Clin Nutr* 1999;70(6):951-2.

6018 Arts IC, Hollman PC, Kromhout D. Chocolate as a source of tea flavonoids (Letter). *Lancet* 1999;354:488.

6019 Bruinsma K, Taren DL. Chocolate: Food or Drug? *J Am Diet Assoc* 1999;99(10):1249-58.

6020 Mustad VA, Kris-Etherton PM, Derr J, et al. Comparison of the effects of diets rich in stearic acid versus myristic acid and lauric acid on platelet fatty acids and excretion of thromboxane A2 and PGI2 metabolites in healthy young men. *Metabolism* 1993;42(4):463-9.

6022 Ross GW, Abbott RD, Petrovitch H, et al. Association of coffee and caffeine intake with the risk of parkinson disease. *JAMA* 2000;283:2674-9.

6023 Tobias JD. Caffeine in the treatment of apnea associated with respiratory syncytial virus infection in neonates and infants. *South Med J* 2000;93(3):297-304.

6024 Watson JM, Jenkins EJ, Hamilton P, et al. Influence of caffeine on the frequency and perception of hypoglycemia in free-living patients with type 1 diabetes. *Diabetes Care* 2000;23(4):455-9.

6025 Lloyd T, Johnson-Rollings N, Eggli DF, et al. Bone status among postmenopausal women with different habitual caffeine intakes: a longitudinal investigation. *J Am Coll Nutr* 2000;19(2):256-61.

6026 The transfer of drugs and other chemicals into human milk (RE9403). Am Acad of Pediatrics. www.aap.org/policy/00026.html (Accessed 13 June 2000).

6027 Hu FB, Stampfer MJ, Manson JE, et al. Dietary saturated fats and their food sources in relation to the risk of coronary heart disease in women. *Am J Clin Nutr* 1999;70(6):1001-8.

6028 Hambrecht R, Hilbrich L, Erbs S, et al. Correction of endothelial dysfunction in chronic heart failure: additional effects of exercise training and oral L-arginine supplementation. *J Am Coll Cardiol* 2000;35(3):706-13.

6029 Setchell KD, Cassidy A. Dietary isoflavones: biological effects and relevance to human health. *J Nutr* 1999;129:758S-67S.

6030 Lissin LW, Cooke JP. Phytoestrogens and cardiovascular health. *J Am Coll Cardiol* 2000;35:1403-10.

6031 Nemecz G. Green tea. *U.S. Pharmacist* 2000;May:67-70.

6032 Leenen R, Roodenburg AJ, Tijburg LB, et al. A single dose of tea with or without milk increases plasma antioxidant activity in humans. *Eur J Clin Nutr* 2000;54:87-92.

6033 Hodgson JM, Puddey IB, Croft KD, et al. Acute effects of ingestion of black and green tea on lipoprotein oxidation. *Am J Clin Nutr* 2000;71:1103-7.

6034 Hardy ML. Herbs of special interest to women. *J Am Pharm Assoc* 200;40:234-42.

6035 Bendich A. The potential for dietary supplements to reduce premenstrual syndrome (PMS) symptoms. *J Am Coll Nutr* 2000;19(1):3-12.

6036 Belch J, Hill A. Evening primrose oil and borage oil in rheumatologic conditions. *Am J Clin Nutr* 2000;71(1):352S-6S.

6037 Watson PS, Scalia GM, Galbraith A, et al. Lack of effect of coenzyme Q on left ventricular function in patients with congestive heart failure. *J Am Coll Cardiol* 1999;33:1549-52.

6038 Permanetter B, Rossy W, Klein G, et al. Ubiquinone (coenzyme Q10) in the long-term treatment of idiopathic dilated cardiomyopathy. *Eur Heart J* 1992;13:1528-33.

6039 Vick JA, Shipman WH. Effects of whole bee venom and its fractions (apamin and melittin) of plasma cortisol levels in the dog. *Toxicon* 1972;10:377-80.

6040 Vick JA, Mehlman B, Brooks R, et al. Effect of bee venom and melittin on plasma cortisol in the unanesthetized monkey. *Toxicon* 1972;10:581-6.

6041 Hider RC. Honeybee venom: A rich source of pharmacologically active peptides. *Endeavour, New Series* 1988;12(2):60-5.

6042 Subbalakshmi C, Nagaraj R, Sitaram N. Biological activities of C-terminal 15-residue synthetic fragment of melittin: design of an analog with improved antibacterial activity. *FEBS Lett* 1999;448:62-6.

6043 de Jong NW, Vermeulen AM, de Groot H. Allergy to bumblebee venom. III. Immunotherapy follow-up study (safety and efficacy) in patients with occupational bumblebee-venom anaphylaxis. *Allergy* 1999;54:980-4.

6044 Cuende E, Fraguas J, Pena JE, et al. Beekeepers' arthropathy. *J Rheumatol* 1999;26:2684-90.

6045 Caldwell JR. Venoms, copper, and zinc in the treatment of arthritis. *Rheum Dis Clin North Am* 1999;25(4):919-28.

6046 Petroianu G, Liu J, Helfrich U, et al. Phosholipase A2-induced coagulation abnormalities after bee sting. *Am J Emerg Med* 2000;18:22-7.

6047 Langsjoen PH, Langsjoen PH, Folkers K. Long-term efficacy and safety of coenzyme Q10 therapy for idiopathic dilated cardiomyopathy. *Am J Cardiol* 1990;65:521-3.

6048 Heck AM, DeWitt BA, Lukes AL. Potential interactions between alternative therapies and warfarin. *Am J Health Syst Pharm* 2000;57:1221-7.

6049 Forastiere F, Pistelli R, Sestini P, et al. Consumption of fresh fruit rich in vitamin C and wheezing symptoms in children. *Thorax* 2000;55:283-8.

6050 Haderslev KV, Jeppesen PB, Mortensen PB, Staun M. Absorption of calcium and magnesium in patients with intestinal resections treated with medium chain fatty acids. *Gut* 2000;46:819-23.

6051 Rani PU, Naidu MU. Subjective and polysomnographic evaluation of a herbal preparation in insomnia. *Phytomedicine* 1998;5(4):253-7.

6052 Terjung RL, Clarkson P, Eichner ER, et al. The American College of Sports Medicine Roundtable on the physiological and health effects of oral creatine supplementation. *Med Sci Sports Exerc* 2000;32(3):706-17.

6053 Rico-Sanz J, Marco MT. Creatine enhances oxygen uptake and performance during alternating intensity exercise. *Med Sci Sports Exerc* 2000;32(2):379-85.

6054 Hatch GE. Asthma, inhaled oxidants, and dietary antioxidants. *Am J Clin Nutr* 1995;61:625S-30S.

6055 Carey IM, Strachan DP, Cook DG. Effects of changes in fresh fruit consumption on ventilatory function in healthy British adults. *Am J Respir Crit Care Med* 1998;158(3):728-33.

6056 Schwartz J, Weiss ST. Relationship between dietary vitamin C intake and pulmonary function in the First National Health and Nutrition Examination Survey (NHANES I). *Am J Clin Nutr* 1994;59:110-4.

6057 Butland BK, Fehily AM, Elwood PC. Diet, lung function, and lung function decline in a cohort of 2512 middle aged men. *Thorax* 2000;55:102-8.

6058 Troisi RJ, Willett WC, Weiss ST, et al. A prospective study of diet and adult-onset asthma. *Am J Respir Crit Care Med* 1995;151(5):1401-8.

6059 Griessen M, Ammann P, Selz L, et al. Comparison of the effect of medium-chain and long-chain triacylglycerols on calcium absorption in healthy subjects. *Am J Clin Nutr* 1999;69(6):1237-42.

6060 Wobenzym N media kit. Naturally Vitamins (Marlyn Nutraceuticals, Inc.): Scottsdale, AZ.

6061 Stricker PR. Other ergogenic agents. *Clin Sports Med* 1998;17(2):283-97.

6062 Keller KL, Fenske NA. Uses of vitamins A, C, and E and related compounds in dermatology: A review. *J Am Acad Dermatol* 1998;39:611-25.

6064 Kligman AM. Topical treatments for photoaged skin. Separating the reality from the hype. *Postgrad Med* 1997;102(2):115-26.

6065 Katiyar SK, Ahmad N, Mukhtar H. Green Tea and Skin. *Arch Dermatol* 2000;136:989-94.

6066 Caspi O, Greenfield RH, Gurgevich S. Case report in integrative medicine: a 24-year-old male with medically intractable seizures. *Int Med* 1998;1:173-6.

6067 Itil TM, Eralp E, Ahmed I, Kunitz A, et al. The pharmacological effects of ginkgo biloba, a plant extract, on the brain of dementia patients in comparison with tacrine. *Psychopharmacol Bull* 1998;34(3):391-7.

6068 Mease PJ, Merrill JT, Lahita RG, et al. GL701 (prasterone, dehydroepiandrosterone) improves systemic lupus erythematosus [abstract]. 2000 American College of Rheumatology Meeting. Philadelphia;29 October-2 November:1230.

6069 Mazzanti G, Mascellino MT, Battinelli L, Coluccia D, et al. Antimicrobial investigation of semipurified fractions of Ginkgo biloba leaves. *J Ethnopharmacol* 2000;71:83-8.

6070 Birnbaum J, Charpin D, Vervloet D. Rapid hymenoptera venom immunotherapy: comparative safety of three protocols. *Clin Exp Allergy* 1993;23:226-30.

6071 Bomalaski JS, Ford T, Hudson AP, Clark MA. Phospholipase A2-activating protein induces the synthesis of IL-1 and TNF in human monocytes. *J Immunol* 1995;154:4027-31.

6072 Somerfield SD. Bee venom and arthritis: magic, myth, or medicine? *NZ Med J* 1986;99:281-3.

6073 Nortier JL, Martinez MC, Schmeiser HH, et al. Urothelial carcinoma associated with the use of a Chinese herb (Aristolochia fangchi). *N Engl J Med* 2000;342:1686-92.

6074 Hollister-Stier Laboratories LLC. Instructions and dosing schedule for allergenic extracts hymenoptera venom prodcts. No. 355120-HD1.

6075 Li JT, Yunginger JW. Management of insect sting hypersensitivity. *Mayo Clin Proc* 1992;67(2):188-94.

6076 Golden DB, Kagey-Sobotka A, Lichtenstein LM. Survey of patients after discontinuing venom immunotherapy. *J Allergy Clin Immunol* 2000;105(2 Pt 1):385-90.

6077 Bousquet J, Muller UR, Dreboro S, et al. Immunotherapy with hymenoptera venoms. *Allergy* 1987;42:401-13.

6078 Ewan PW. ABC of allergies. Venom allergy. *BMJ* 1998;316:1365-8.

6079 Anon. Alpha Hydroxy Acids in Cosmetics. July 31, 1997. FDA. www.fda.gov/opacom/backgrounders/alphabg.html.

6080 Kurtzweil P. Alpha-hydroxy acids for skin care: Smooth sailing or rough seas? FDA 1999. www.fda.gov. (Accessed 18 August 2000).

6081 Sullivan RJ, Allen JS, Otto C, et al. Effects of chewing betel nut (Areca catechu) on the symptoms of people with schizophrenia in Palau, Micronesia. *Br J Psychiatry* 2000;177:174-8.

6082 Werbach MR. Nutritional strategies for treating chronic fatigue syndrome. *Altern Med Rev* 2000;5:93-108.

6083 Jacobson W, Saich T, Borysiewicz, LK, et al. Serum folate and chronic fatigue syndrome. *Neurol* 1993;43:2645-7.

6084 Borchers AT, Keen CL, Stern JS, Gershwin ME. Inflammation and Native American medicine: the role of botanicals. *Am J Clin Nutr* 2000;72:339-47.

6085 Dietrich R, Paglieroni TG, Wun T, et al. Cocoa inhibits platelet activation and function. *Am J Clin Nutr* 2000;72(1):30-5.

6086 Darouiche RO, Hull RA. Bacterial interference for prevention of urinary tract infection: an overview. *J Spinal Cord Med* 2000;23:136-40.

6087 Gionchetti P, Rizzello F, Venturi A, et al. Oral bacteriotherapy as maintenance treatment in patients with chronic pouchitis: a double-blind, placebo-controlled trial. *Gastroenterology* 2000;119:305-9.

6088 Reid G, Bruce AW, Cook RL, et al. Effect on urogenital flora of antibiotic therapy for urinary tract infection. *Scand J Infec Dis* 1990;22:43-7.

6089 McGroarty JA. Probiotic use of lactobacilli in the human female urogenital tract. *FEMS Immunol Med Microbiol* 1993;6:251-64.

6090 Velraeds MM, Van der Mei HC, Reid G, et al. Inhibition of initial adhesion of uropathogenic Enterococcus faecalis by biosurfactants from Lactobacillus isolates. *Appl Environ Microbiol* 1996;62:1958-63.

6091 Reid G, Cook RL, Bruce AW. Examination of strains of Lactobacilli for properties that may influence bacterial interference in the urinary tract. *J Urol* 1987;138:330-5.

6092 Chan RCY, Reid G, Irvin RT, et al. Competitive exclusion of uropathogens from human uroepithelial cells by Lactobacillus whole cells and cell wall fragments. *Infect Immun* 1985;47:84-9.

6093 Herthelius M, Gorbach SL, Mollby R, et al. Elimination of vaginal colonization with Escherichia coli by administration of indigenous flora. *Infect Immun* 1989;57:2447-51.

6094 Bruce AW, Reid G. Intravaginal instillation of Lactobacilli for prevention of recurrent urinary tract infections. *Can J Microbiol* 1988;34:339-43.

6095 Reid G, Bruce AW, Taylor M. Influence of three-day antimicrobial therapy and Lactobacillus vaginal suppositories on recurrence of urinary tract infections. *Clin Ther* 1992;14:11-6.

6096 Gupta K, Stapleton AE, Hooton TM, et al. Inverse association of H2O2-producing Lactobacilli and vaginal Escherichia coli colonization in women with recurrent urinary tract infections. *J Infect Dis* 1998;178:446-50.

6097 Mease PJ, Ginzler EM, Gluck OS, et al. Improvement in bone mineral density in steroid-treated SLE patients during treatment with GL701 (prasterone, dehydroepiandrosterone) [abstract]. 2000 American College of Rheumatology Meeting. Philadelphia;29 October - 2 November:835.

6098 van Vollenhoven RF. Dehydroepiandrosterone in systemic lupus erythematosus. *Rheum Dis Clin North Am* 2000;26(2):349-62.

6099 Roberfroid MB. Prebiotics and probiotics: are they functional foods? *Am J Clin Nutr* 2000;71:1682S-7S.

6100 Thumbs up for oats, but not for soy. www.healthscout.com/cgi-bin/WebObjects/Af.woa?id=95821&ap=24 (Accessed 19 May 2000).

6101 Jarrar D, Wang P, Cioffi WG, et al. Mechanisms of the salutary effects of dehydroepiandrosterone after trauma-hemorrhage. Direct or indirect effects on cardiac and hepatocellular functions? Arch Surg 2000;135(4):416-23.

6102 Markowitz JS, Carson WH, Jackson CW. Possible dihydroepiandrosterone-induced mania. *Biol Psychiatry* 1999;45(2):241-2.

6103 Israel RJ, Sonis ST. Topical dehydroascorbic acid (DHA) reduces moderate to severe mucositis in the hamster acute radiation model. 36th Am Soc Clin Oncol Ann Mtg Prog Proceedings/Abstracts: Abstract 2367. www.asco.org/prof/me/html/00abstracts/sm/m_2367.htm (Accessed 22 May 2000).

6104 Zavaleta N, Caulfield LE, Garcia T. Changes in iron status during pregnancy in peruvian women receiving prenatal iron and folic acid supplements with or without zinc. *Am J Clin Nutr* 2000;71(4):956-61.

6105 Gossage C, Deyhim M, Moser-Veillon PB, et al. Effect of beta-carotene supplementation and lactation on carotenoid metabolism and mitogenic T-lymphocyte proliferation. *Am J Clin Nutr* 2000;71(4):950-5.

6106 Thijs C, van Houwelingen A, Poorterman I, et al. Essential fatty acids in breast milk of atopic mothers: comparison with non-atopic mothers, and effect of borage oil supplementation. *Eur J Clin Nutr* 2000;54(3):234-8.

6107 Agrawal A. Potato peel extract holds potential as antiboitic. Reuters Health May 23, 2000. www.medscape.com/reuters/prof/2000/05/05.23/20000523drgd003.html (Accessed 23 May 2000).

6108 Ginseng effective in treating lung infection in mice. Reuters Health May 24 2000. www.reutershealth.com/frame/eline.html (Accessed 25 May 2000).

6109 Beehive material fights ulcer bacteria. Reuters Health May 25 2000. www.reutershealth.com/frame/eline.html (Accessed 26 May 2000).

6110 Fermented milk kills ulcer bug. Reuters Health May 25 2000. www.reutershealth.com/frame/eline.html (Accessed 26 May 2000).

6112 Breidenbach T, Hoffmann MW, Becker T, et al. Drug interaction of St John's wort with ciclosporin. *Lancet* May 2000;355(9218):1912.

6113 Oregano slows bacterial growth. Reuters Health May 26 2000. www.reutershealth.com/frame/eline.html (Accessed 30 May 2000).

6114 Miller MJ, Vergnolle N, Wallace JL, et al. Sangre de grado is a potent and unique inhibitor of neurogenic inflammation and promotes healing in experimental necrotizing enterocolitis. Pediatric Academic Soc and Am Acad Pediatrics Joint Mtg, May 12-6, 2000:Abstract 979. www.abstracts-on-line.com/abstracts/PAS (Accessed 30 May 2000).

6116 Blumenthal M, Goldberg A, Brinckmann J (eds). Herbal Medicine Expanded Commission E Monographs. Newton,MA;Integrative Medicine Communications, 2000.

6117 Creatine generally considered safe, but supplement's value still questioned. Reuters Health www.medscape.com/reuters/prof/2000/06/06.02/20000602clin014.html (Accessed 2 June 2000).

6118 Lewis CJ, Alpert S. Letter to health care professionals on FDA concerns about botanical prod, including dietary supplements, containing aristolochic acid. Ofc Nutr Prod, Labeling, Dietary Supplements, Ctr Food Safety Applied Nutr; FDA. May 31, 2000. URL: vm.cfsan.fda.gov/~dms/ds-botl2.html (Accessed 1 April 2000).

6119 Lewis CJ. Letter to industry on FDA concerns about botanical prod, including dietary supplements, containing aristolochic acid. Ofc of Nutr Prod, Labeling, Dietary Supplements; Ctr Food Safety and Applied Nutr. FDA. May 30, 2000. URL: vm.cdsan.fda.gov/~dms/ds-botl1.html (Accessed 1 June 2000).

6121 Gardiner P, Kemper KJ. Herbs in pediatric and adolescent medicine. *Pediatr Rev* 2000;21(2):44-57.

6122 Abramowicz M, ed. Calcium supplements. *Med Lett* 2000;42(1075):29-31.

6123 Beall DP, Scofield RH. Milk-alkali syndrome associated with calcium carbonate consumption. Report of 7 patients with parathyroid hormone levels and an estimate of prevalence among patients hospitalized with hypercalcemia. *Medicine (Baltimore)* 1995;74(2):89-96.

6124 Moser LR, Smythe MA, Tisdale JE. The use of calcium salts in the prevention and management of verapamil-induced hypotension. *Ann Pharmacother* 2000;34(5):622-9.

6125 Reaney P. UK women told to have soy breast implants removed. Reuters Health 2000;Jun 6. www.reutershealth.com/frame/eline.html (Accessed 7 June 2000).

6126 Consumer Lab. www.consumerlab.com/results/echinacea.asp (Accessed 5 June 2001).

6127 Atkinson C, Compston JE, Robins SP, Bingham SA. The effects of isoflavone phytoestrogens on bone; preliminary results from a large randomized, controlled trial. Endocrine Soc 82nd Ann Mtg, Toronto, CAN 2000;Jun 21-4:abstract 196.

6128 Gerber G, Lowe FC, Spigelman S. The use of a standardized extract of red clover isoflavones for the alleviation of BPH symptoms. Endocrine Soc 82nd Ann Mtg, Toronto, CAN 2000;Jun 21-4:abstract 2359.

6129 Mitchell S. Plant modification may enhance public consumption of omega-3 fatty acids. Reuters Health

REFERENCES

2000;Jun 8. www.medscape.com/reuters/prof/2000/06/06.08/20000608publ001.html (Accessed 8 June 2000).

6130 Pearson H. A real lifesaver, who says there's no cure for the summertime blues? *New Scientist* 2000;Jun 10. www.newscientist.com/nl/0610/coffee.html (Accessed 8 June 2000).

6131 Whitehouse MW. Turmeric has anti-inflammatory effects. 9th Asia Pacific League of Associations for Rheumatology Congress, 2001.

6132 Kulkarni PM, Schuman PC, Merlino NS, Kinzie JL. Lactic acidosis and hepatic steatosis in HIV seropositive patients treated with nucleoside analogues. Natl AIDS Treatment Advocacy Project. Dig Disease Week Liver Conf, San Diego,CA. 2000;May 21-4:Rep11. www.natap.org (Accessed 9 June 2000).

6133 Roodenburg AJ, Leenen R, van het Hof KH, et al. Amount of fat in the diet affects bioavailability of lutein esters but not of alpha-carotene, beta-carotene, and vitamin E in humans. *Am J Clin Nutr* 2000;71(5):1187-93.

6134 Stahl W, Heinrich U, Jungmann H, et al. Carotenoids and carotenoids plus vitamin E protect against ultraviolet light-induced erythema in humans. *Am J Clin Nutr* 2000;71(3):795-8.

6135 Zhu M, Wong PY, Li RC. Effect of oral administration of fennel (Foeniculum vulgare) on ciprofloxacin absorption and disposition in the rat. *J Pharm Pharmacol* 1999;51(12):1391-6.

6136 Sandler AD, Sutton KA, DeWeese J, et al. Lack of benefit of a single dose of synthetic human secretin in the treatment of autism and pervasive developmental disorder. *N Engl J Med* 1999;341(24):1801-6.

6137 Singh N, Singh PN, Hershman JM. Effect of calcium carbonate on the absorption of levothyroxine. *JAMA* 2000;283(21):2822-5.

6138 Nusko G, Schneider B, Schneider I, et al. Anthranoid laxative use is not a risk factor for colorectal neoplasia: results of a prospective case control study. *Gut* 2000;46(5):651-5.

6139 The international formula council clears up confusion on soy health claim . PRNewswire 2000;Jun 9. www.prnewswire.com (Accessed 12 June 2000).

6140 NCAA prohibits schools from supplying creatine to students. Reuters Health 2000;Jun 13. www.medscape.com/reuters/prof/2000/06/06.13/20000613publ004.html (Accessed 13 June 2000).

6143 Mori TA, Burke V, Puddey IB, et al. Purified eicosapentaenoic and docosahexaenoic acids have differential effects on serum lipids and lipoproteins, LDL particle size, glucose, and insulin in mildly hyperlipidemic men. *Am J Clin Nutr* 2000;71(5):1085-94.

6144 Lewin PK. Temporary henna tattoo with permanent scarification. *CMAJ* 1999;160(3):310.

6145 Lestringant GG, Bener A, Frossard PM. Cutaneous reactions to henna and associated additives. *Br J Dermatol* 1999;141(3):598-600.

6146 Etienne A, Piletta P, Hauser C, Pasche-Koo F. Ectopic contact dermatitis from henna. *Contact Dermatitis* 1997;(4):183.

6147 Wantke F, Gotz M, Jarisch R. Contact dermatitis due to henna, solvent red 1 and solvent red 3, a case report. *Contact Dermatitis* 1992;27(5):346-7.

6148 Nigam PK, Saxena AK. Allergic contact dermatitis from henna. *Contact Dermatitis* 1988;18(1):55-6.

6149 Gupta BN, Mathur AK, Agarwal C, Singh A. Contact sensitivity to henna. *Contact Dermatitis* 1986;15(5):303-4.

6150 Pasricha JS, Gupta R, Panjwani S. Contact dermatitis to henna (Lawsonia). *Contact Dermatitis* 1980;6(4):288-9.

6151 Cronin E. Immediate type hypersensitivity to henna. *Contact Dermatitis* 1979;5(3):198-9.

6152 Katz J, West KP Jr, Khatry SK, et al. Maternal low-dose vitamin A or {beta}-carotene supplementation has no effect on fetal loss and early infant mortality: a randomized, cluster trial in Nepal. *Am J Clin Nutr* 2000;71(6):1570-6.

6153 West KP Jr, Katz J, Khatry SK, et al. Double-blind cluster, randomised trial of low dose supplementation with vitamin A or beta carotene on mortality related to pregnancy in Nepal. The NNIPS-2 Study Group. *BMJ* 1999;318(7183):570-5.

6154 Christian P, West KP Jr, Khatry SK, et al. Vitamin A or beta-carotene supplementation reduces but does not eliminate maternal night blindness in Nepal. *J Nutr* 1998;128(9):1458-63.

6155 Traikovich SS. Use of topical ascorbic acid and its effects on photodamaged skin topography. *Arch Otolaryngol Head Neck Surg* 1999;125(10):1091-8.

6166 Cellex-C product information for professionals. Cellex-C. www.cellex-c.com/pro_side/navigator.html (Accessed 14 June 2000).

6167 Vutyavanich T, Wongtra-ngan S, Ruangsri R. Pyridoxine for nausea and vomiting of pregnancy: a randomized, double-blind, placebo-controlled trial. *Am J Obstet Gyneco*l 1995;173(3 Pt 1):881-4.

6168 Sahakian V, Rouse D, Sipes S, et al. Vitamin B6 is effective therapy for nausea and vomiting of pregnancy: a randomized, double-blind, placebo-controlled study. *Obstet Gynecol* 1991;78(1):33-6.

6169 Sandler B, Aronson P. Yohimbine-induced cutaneous drug eruption, progressive renal failure, and lupus-like syndrome. *Urol* 1993;41(4):343-5.

6170 Wang ZQ, Zhang XH, Baldor LC, et al. Chromium picolinate enhances insulin sensitivity in an animal model for the metabolic syndrome: the obese, insulin resistant JCR:LA-corpulent rat. Am Diabetes Assn's 60th Sci Sessions & Expo, San Antonio, TX 2000;Jun 9-13: abstract 291. www.diabetes.org/am2000/NumberResults.asp?idAbs=29 (Accessed 15 June 2000).

6171 Nelson L, Rao A, Olson P. Unique hydrolyzed whey protein isolates with antihypertensive activity. Institute of Food Tech 2000 Ann Mtg & Food Expo:abstract 38-6. URL: ift.confex.com/ift/2000/techprogram/paper_5129.htm (Accessed 15 June 2000)

6172 Ajani UA, Hennekens CH, Spelsberg, A, et al. Alcohol consumption and risk of type 2 diabetes mellitus among US male physicians. *Arch Intern Med* 2000;160(7):1025-30.

6173 Shaper AG, Wannamethee SG. Alcohol intake and mortality in middle aged men with diagnosed coronary heart disease. *Heart* 2000;83(4):394-9.

6174 Vally H, de Klerk N, Thompson PJ. Alcoholic drinks: important triggers for asthma. *J Allergy Clin Immunol* 2000;105(3):462-7.

6175 Lanthony P, Cosson JP. [The course of color vision in early diabetic retinopathy treated with ginkgo biloba extract. A preliminary, double-blind versus placebo study]. [Article in French]. *J Fr Ophthalmol* 1988;11(10):671-4.

6176 Grandjean EM, Berthet P, Ruffmann R, Leuenberger P. Efficacy of oral long-term N-acetylcysteine in chronic bronchopulmonary disease: a meta-analysis of published double-blind, placebo-controlled clinical trials. *Clin Ther* 2000;22(2):209-21.

6177 Puig L. Pharmacodynamic interaction with phototoxic plants during PUVA therapy. *Br J Dermatol* 1997;136(6):973-4.

6178 Gral N, Beani JC, Bonnot D, et al. [Plasma levels of psoralens after celery ingestion]. [Article in French]. *Ann Dermatol Venereol* 1993;120(9):599-603.

6179 Desperate remedies. New Scientist 1999;Nov 27:34-6.

6180 Eagon PK, Elm MS, Hunter DS, et al. Medicinal herbs: modulation of estrogen action. Era of Hope Mtg, Dept Defense; Breast Cancer Res Prog, Atlanta, GA 2000;Jun 8-11.

6181 Joss JD, LeBlond RF. Potentiation of warfarin anticoagulation associated with topical methyl salicylate. *Ann Pharmacother* 2000;34(6):729-33.

6182 Walter MC, Lochmuller H, Reilich P, et al. Creatine monohydrate in muscular dystrophies: A double-blind, placebo-controlled clinical study. *Neurology* 2000;54(9):1848-50.

6183 Gilliam JD, Hohzorn C, Martin D, Trimble MH. Effect of oral creatine supplementation on isokinetic torque production. *Med Sci Sports Exerc* 2000;32(5):993-6.

6185 Hallikainen MA, Sarkkinen ES, Uusitupa MI. Plant stanol esters affect serum cholesterol concentrations of hypercholesterolemic men and women in a dose-dependent manner. *J Nutr* 2000;130(4):767-76.

6186 Rome LA, Lippmann ML, Dalsey WC, et al. Prevalence of cocaine use and its impact on asthma exacerbation in an urban population. *Chest* 2000;117(5):1324-9.

6187 Potter SM, Zelazo PR, Stack DM, Papageorgiou AN. Adverse effects of fetal cocaine exposure on neonatal auditory information processing. *Pediatrics* 2000;105(3):E40

6188 Maier SM, Turner ND, Lupton JR. Serum lipids in hypercholesterolemic men and women consuming oat bran and amaranth products. *Cereal Chem* 2000:77(3);297-302.

6189 Pitchford P. Healing with whole foods. Berkeley, CA: North Atlantic Books, 1993.

6190 Gobel H, Fresenius J, Heinze A, et al. [Effectiveness of Oleum menthae piperitae and paracetamol in therapy of headache of the tension type]. [Article in German]. *Nervenarzt* 1996;67(8):672-81.

6191 Umeta M, West CE, Haidar J, et al. Zinc supplementation and stunted infants in Ethiopia: a randomised controlled trial. *Lancet* 2000;355(9220):2021-6.

6192 Khanna VJ, Shieh S, Benjamin J, et al. Necrolytic acral erythema associated with hepatitis C effective treatment with interferon alfa and zinc. *Arch Dermatol* 2000;136(6):755-7.

6193 Booth SL, Tucker KL, Chen H, et al. Dietary vitamin K intakes are associated with hip fracture but not with bone mineral density in elderly men and women. *Am J Clin Nutr* 2000;71(5):1201-8.

6196 Spinella P, De Palo CB, Scaroni C, et al. Effect of licorice on reduction of body fat mass. Endocrine Soc 82nd Annual Meeting, Toronto, CAN 2000;Jun21-4:abstract 2065. www.abstracts-on-line.com/abstracts/ENDO/search/results.asp?Num-0%2E2697367.

6197 Woznicki K. Eat honey after your workout. OnHealth 2000;Jun23: OnHealth. URL: onhealth.com/fitness/briefs/item,93168.asp (Accessed 26 June 2000).

6198 Varnell MA. Enhanced herb may help female sexual dysfunction. Reuters Health 2000;Jun 27. www.reutershealth.com/frame/eline.html Accessed 28 June 2000).

6199 Landbo C, Almdal TP. [Interaction between warfarin and coenzyme Q10]. [Article in Danish]. *Ugeskr Laeger* 1998;160(22):3226-7.

6200 Rey JM, Walter G. Hypericum perforatum (St. John's wort) in depression: pest or blessing? *Med J Aust* 1998;169:583-6.

6201 Brown TM. Acute St. John's wort toxicity. *Am J Emerg Med* 2000;18:231-2.

6203 Consumer Lab. www.consumerlab.com/results/vitamine.asp (Accessed 5 June 2001).

6204 Kehoe WA. Vitamin E and heart disease. *Pharmacist's Letter* 2000;16(3):160307.

6205 Consumer Lab. www.consumerlab.com/results/vitaminc.asp (Accessed 5 June 2001).

6206 Szolomicki S, Samochowiec L, Wojcicki J, Drozdzik M. The influence of active components of Eleutherococcus senticosus on cellular defense and physical fitness in man. *Phytother Res* 2000;14:30-5.

6207 Consumer Lab. www.consumerlab.com/results/multivit.asp (Accessed 5 June 2001).

6208 Diamond BJ, Shiflett SC, Feiwel N, et al. Ginkgo biloba extract: mechanisms and clinical indications. *Arch Phys Med Rehabil* 2000;81:668-78.

6209 Consumer Lab. www.consumerlab.com/results/calcium.asp (Accessed 5 June 2001).

6210 Consumer Lab. www.consumerlab.com/results/same.asp (Accessed 5 June 2001).

6211 Pittler MH, Ernst E. Ginkgo biloba extract for the treatment of intermittent claudication: a meta-analysis of randomized trials. *Am J Med* 2000,108:276-81.

6212 Li AL, Shi YD, Landsmann B, et al. Hemorheology and walking of peripheral arterial occlusive diseases patients during treatment with Ginkgo biloba extract. *Chung Kuo Yao Li Hsueh Pao* 1998;19:417-21.

6213 Peters H, Kieser M, Holscher U. Demonstration of the efficacy of ginkgo biloba special extract EGb 761 on intermittent claudication - a placebo-controlled, double-blind multicenter trial. *Vasa* 1998;27:106-10.

6214 Rigney U, Kimber S, Hindmarch I. The effects of acute doses of standardized Ginkgo biloba extract on memory and psychomotor performance in volunteers. *Phytother Res* 1999;13:408-15.

6215 Subhan Z, Hindmarch I. The psychopharmacological effects of Ginkgo biloba extract in normal healthy volunteers. *Int J Clin Pharmacol Res* 1984;4:89-93.

6216 Rai GS, Shovlin C, Wesnes KA. A double-blind, placebo-controlled study of Ginkgo biloba extract ('tanakan') in elderly outpatients with mild to moderate memory impairment. *Curr Med Res Opin* 1991;12:350-5.

6217 Consumer Lab. www.consumerlab.com/results/msm.asp (Accessed 5 June 2001).

6218 Holgers KM, Axelsson A, Pringle I. Ginkgo biloba extract for the treatment of tinnitus. *Audiol* 1994;33:85-92.

6219 Meyer B. [Multicenter, randomized, double-blind drug vs. placebo study of the treatment of tinnitus with Ginkgo biloba extract]. [Article in French]. *Presse Med* 1986;15:1562-4.

REFERENCES

6220 Cesarani A, Meloni F, Alpini D, et al. Ginkgo biloba (EGb 761) in the treatment of equilibrium disorders. *Adv Ther* 1998;15:291-304.

6221 Haguenauer JP, Cantenot F, Koskas H, Pierart H. [Treatment of equilibrium disorders with Ginkgo biloba extract. A multicenter, double-blind drug vs. placebo study]. [Article in French]. *Presse Med* 1986;15:1569-72.

6222 Hopfenmuller W. [Evidence for a therapeutic effect of Ginkgo biloba special extract. Meta-analysis of 11 clinical studies in patients with cerebrovascular insufficiency in old age]. [Article in German]. *Arzneimittelforschung* 1994;44:1005-13.

6223 Kleijnen J, Knipschild P. Ginkgo biloba for cerebral insufficiency. *Br J Clin Pharmacol* 1992;34:352-8.

6224 Wettstein A. Cholinesterase inhibitors and Gingko extracts- are they comparable in the treatment of dementia? Comparison of published, placebo-controlled efficacy studies of at least six months duration. *Phytomedicine* 2000;6:393-401.

6225 Kanowski S, Herrmann WM, Stephan K, et al. Proof of efficacy of the ginkgo biloba special extract (EGb 761) in outpatients suffering from mild to moderate primary degenerative dementia of the Alzheimer type or multi-infarct dementia. *Pharmacopsych* 1996;29:47-56.

6226 Natl Institute Health. Clinical trials. www.clinicaltrials.gov/ct/gui/c/r (Accessed 15 June 2000).

6227 Lebuisson DA, Leroy L, Rigal G. [Treatment of senile macular degeneration with Ginkgo biloba extract. A preliminary double-blind drug vs. placebo study]. [Article in French]. *Presse Med* 1986;15:1556-8.

6228 Evans JR. Ginkgo biloba extract for age-related macular degeneration. *Cochrane Database Syst Rev* 2000;(2):CD001775.

6229 Tamborini A, Taurelle R. [Value of standardized Ginkgo biloba extract (EGb 761) in the management of congestive symptoms of premenstrual syndrome]. [Article in French]. *Rev Fr Gynecol Obstet* 1993;88:447-57.

6230 Roncin JP, Schwartz F, D'Arbigny P. Ginkgo biloba (EGb 761) in control of acute mountain sickness and vascular reactivity to cold exposure. *Aviat Space Environ Med* 1996;67:445-52.

6231 Fowler JS, Wang GJ, Volkow ND et al. Evidence that gingko biloba extract does not inhibit MAO A and B in living human brain. *Life Sci* 2000;66:141-6.

6232 Porsolt RD, Roux S, Drieu K. Evaluation of a ginkgo biloba extract (EGb 761) in functional tests for monoamine oxidase inhibition. *Arzneimittelforschung* 2000;50:232-5.

6233 White HL, Scates PW, Cooper BR. Extracts of Ginkgo biloba leaves inhibit monoamine oxidase. *Life Sci* 1996;58:1315-21.

6234 Snowdon DA, Tully CL, Smith CD, et al. Serum folate and the severity of atrophy of the neocortex in Alzheimer disease: findings from the Nun study. *Am J Clin Nutr* 2000;71:993-8.

6235 Chao CL, Chien KL, Lee YT. Effect of short-term vitamin (folic acid, vitamins B6 and B12) administration on endothelial dysfunction induced by post-methionine load hyperhomocysteinemia. *Am J Cardiol* 1999;84:1359-61.

6236 Usui M, Matsuoka H, Miyazaki H, et al. Endothelial dysfunction by acute hyperhomocyst(e)inaemia: restoration by folic acid. *Clin Sci (Colch)* 1999;96:235-9

6237 Nelen WL, Blom HJ, Steegers EA, et al. Homocysteine and folate levels as risk factors for recurrent early pregnancy loss. *Obstet Gynecol* 2000;95:519-24.

6238 Ortega RM, Manas LR, Andres P, et al. Functional and psychic deterioration in elderly people may be aggravated by folate deficiency. *J Nutr* 1996;126:1992-9.

6239 Fava M, Borus JS, Alpert JE, et al. Folate, vitamin B12, and homocysteine in major depressive disorder. *Am J Psychiatry* 1997;154:426-8.

6240 Norton SA, Ruze P. Kava dermopathy. *J Am Acad Dermatol* 1994;31:89-97.

6241 Suitor CW, Bailey LB. Dietary folate equivalents: interpretation and application. *J Am Diet Assoc* 2000;100:88-94.

6242 Suitor CW, Bailey LB. Food folate vs synthetic folic acid: a comparison. *J Am Diet Assoc* 1999;99:285.

6243 Dietary reference intakes for thiamin, riboflavin, niacin, vitamin B6, folate, vitamin B12, pantothenic acid, biotin, and cholin. Institute of Medicine. http://books.nap.edu/books/0309065542/html/196.html#pagetop (Accessed 17 June 2000).

6244 Winther K, Randlov C, Rein E, Mehlsen J. Effects of ginkgo biloba extract on cognitive function and blood pressure in elderly subjects. *Curr Ther Res* 1998;59:881-8.

6245 Nardini M, De Stefano R, Iannuccelli M, et al. Treatment of depression with L-5-hydroxytryptophan combined with chlorimipramine, a double-blind study. *Int J Clin Pharmacol Res* 1983;3:239-50.

6246 Steinberg S, Annable L, Young SN, Liyanage N. A placebo-controlled study of the effects of L-tryptophan in patients with premenstrual dysphoria. *Adv Exp Med Biol* 1999;467:85-8.

6247 Ghadirian AM, Murphy BE, Gendron MJ. Efficacy of light versus tryptophan therapy in seasonal affective disorder. *J Affect Disord* 1998;50:23-7.

6248 Leathwood PD, Chauffard F, Heck E, Munoz-Box R. Aqueous extract of valerian root (Valeriana officinalis L.) improves sleep quality in man. *Pharmacol Biochem Behav* 1982;17:65-71.

6249 Donath F, Quispe S, Diefenbach K, et al. Critical evaluation of the effect of valerian extract on sleep structure and sleep quality. *Pharmacopsych* 2000;33:47-53.

6250 Bourin M, Bougerol T, Guitton B, Broutin E. A combination of plant extracts in the treatment of outpatients with adjustment disorder with anxious mood: controlled study vs placebo. *Fundam Clin Pharmacol* 1997;11:127-32.

6251 Fisher AA, Purcell P, Le Couteur DG. Toxicity of Passiflora incarnata L. *J Toxicol Clin Toxicol* 2000;38:63-6.

6252 Klein G, Kullich W. Short-term treatment of painful osteoarthritis of the knee with oral enzymes. *Clin Drug Invest* 2000;19:15-23.

6253 Kane S, Goldberg MJ. Use of bromelain for mild ulcerative colitis. *Ann Intern Med* 2000;132:680.

6254 Caso MA, Vargas RR, Salas VA, Begona IC. Double-blind study of a multivitamin complex supplemented with ginseng extract. *Drugs Exp Clin Res* 1996;22:323-9.

6255 Hill AJ, Peikin SR, Ryan CA, Blundell JE. Oral administration of proteinase inhibitor II from potatoes reduces energy intake in man. *Physiol Behav* 1990;48:241-6.

6256 Akobeng AK, Miller V, Stanton J, et al. Double-blind, randomized, controlled trial of glutamine-enriched polymeric diet in the treatment of active Crohn's disease. *J Pediatr Gastroenterol Nutr* 2000;30:78-84.

6257 Belluzzi A, Brignola C, Campieri M, et al. Effect of an enteric-coated fish-oil preparation on relapses in Crohn's disease. *N Engl J Med* 1996;334:1557-60.

6258 Belluzzi A, Brignola C, Campieri M, et al. Effects of new fish oil derivative on fatty acid phospholipid-membrane pattern in a group of Crohn's disease patients. *Dig Dis Sci* 1994;39:2589-94.

6259 Lorenz-Meyer H, Bauer P, Nicolay C, et al. Omega-3 fatty acids and low carbohydrate diet for maintenance of remission in Crohn's disease. A randomized controlled multicenter trial. Study Group Members (German Crohn's Disease Study Group). *Scand J Gastroenterol* 1996;31:778-85.

6260 Smith W, Mitchell P, Leeder SR. Dietary fat and fish intake and age-related maculopathy. *Arch Ophthalmol* 2000;118:401-4.

6261 Anderson JW, Davidson MH, Blonde L, et al. Long-term cholesterol-lowering effects of psyllium as an adjunct to diet therapy in the treatment of hypercholesterolemia. *Am J Clin Nutr* 2000;71:1433-8.

6262 Davidson MH, Maki KC, Kong JC, et al. Long-term effects of consuming foods containing psyllium seed husk on serum lipids in subjects with hypercholesterolemia. *Am J Clin Nutr* 1998;67:367-76.

6263 Olson BH, Anderson SM, Becker MP, et al. Psyllium-enriched cereals lower blood total cholesterol and LDL cholesterol, but not HDL cholesterol, in hypercholesterolemic adults: results of a meta-analysis. *J Nutr* 1997;127:1973-80.

6264 FDA, Ctr Food Safety, Applied Nutr. FDA allows foods containing psyllium to make health claim on reducing risk of heart disease. URL: http://vm.cfsan.fda.gov/~lrd/tpsylliu.html (Accessed 19 June 2000).

6265 McRorie J, Kesler J, Bishop L, et al. Effects of wheat bran and Olestra on objective measures of stool and subjective reports of GI symptoms. *Am J Gastroenterol* 2000;95:1244-52.

6266 Chandalia M, Garg A, Lutjohann D, et al. Beneficial effects of high dietary fiber intake in patients with type 2 diabetes mellitus. *N Engl J Med* 2000;342:1392-8.

6267 Schatzkin A, Lanza E, Corle D, et al. Lack of effect of a low-fat, high-fiber diet on the recurrence of colorectal adenomas. Polyp Prevention Trial Study Group. *N Engl J Med* 2000;342:1149-55.

6268 Natl Acad Sci, Institute of Medicine. Dietary reference intakes for vitamin C, vitamin E, selenium, and carotenoids. www.nap.edu/pdf/0309069351/pdf_image/325.pdf (Accessed 21 June 2000).

6269 Kuroki F, Iida M, Tominaga M, et al. Multiple vitamin status in Crohn's disease. Correlation with disease activity. *Dig Dis Sci* 1993;38:1614-8.

6270 Lashner BA, Provencher KS, Seidner DL, et al. The effect of folic acid supplementation on the risk for cancer or dysplasia in ulcerative colitis. *Gastroenterology* 1997;112:29-32.

6271 Lashner BA. Red blood cell folate is associated with the development of dysplasia and cancer in ulcerative colitis. *J Cancer Res Clin Oncol* 1993;119:549-54.

6278 Maherzi A, Galan P, Cezard JP, et al. Assessment of iron status in children and adolescents with Crohn's disease: value of basic red cell ferritin. *Ann Nutr Metab* 1996;40:331-5.

6279 Gasche C, Reinisch W, Lochs H, et al. Anemia in Crohn's disease. Importance of inadequate erythropoietin production and iron deficiency. *Dig Dis Sci* 1994;39:1930-4.

6280 Galland L. Magnesium and inflammatory bowel disease. *Magnesium* 1988;7:78-83.

6281 Geerling BJ, Badart-Smook A, Stockbrugger RW, Brummer RJ. Comprehensive nutritional status in patients with long-standing Crohn disease currently in remission. *Am J Clin Nutr* 1998;67:919-26.

6282 Englisch W, Beckers C, Unkauf M, et al. Efficacy of Artichoke dry extract in patients with hyperlipoproteinemia. *Arzneimittelforschung* 2000;50:260-5.

6284 de la Taille A, Hayek OR, Buttyan R, et al. Effects of a phytotherapeutic agent, PC-SPES, on prostate cancer: a preliminary investigation on human cell lines and patients. *BJU Int* 1999;84:845-50.

6285 Kubota T, Hisatake J, Hisatake Y, et al. PC-SPES: a unique inhibitor of proliferation of prostate cancer cells in vitro and in vivo. *Prostate* 2000;42:163-71.

6286 Pfeifer BL, Pirani JF, Hamann SR, Klippel KF. PC-SPES, a dietary supplement for the treatment of hormone-refractory prostate cancer. *BJU Int* 2000;85:481-5.

6287 Porterfield H. Survey of Us Too members and other prostate cancer patients to evaluate the efficacy and safety of PC-SPES. *Mol Urol* 1999;3(3):333-6.

6289 Chan P, Tomlinson B. Antioxidant effects of Chinese traditional medicine: focus on trilinolein isolated from the Chinese herb sanchi. *J Clin Pharmacol* 2000;40:457-61.

6290 Hui KM, Wang XH, Xue H. Interaction of flavones from the roots of Scutellaria baicalensis with the benzodiazepine site. *Planta Med* 2000;66:91-3.

6291 Liao JF, Wang HH, Chen MC, et al. Benzodiazepine binding site-interactive flavones from Scutellaria baicalensis root. *Planta Med* 1998;64:571-2.

6292 Nishioka T, Kawabata J, Aoyama Y. Baicalein, an alpha-glucosidase inhibitor from Scutellaria baicalensis. *J Nat Prod* 1998;61:1413-5.

6293 Gao Z, Huang K, Yang X, Xu H. Free radical scavenging and antioxidant activities of flavonoids extracted from the radix of Scutellaria baicalensis Georgi. *Biochim Biophys Acta* 1999;1472:643-50.

6294 Lee BH, Lee SJ, Kang TH, et al. Baicalein: an in vitro antigenotoxic compound from Scutellaria baicalensis. *Planta Med* 2000;66:70-1.

6295 Blaszczyk T, Krzyzanowska J, Lamer-Zarawska E. Screening for antimycotic properties of 56 traditional Chinese drugs. *Phytother Res* 2000;14:210-2.

6297 Goransson K, Liden S, Odsell L. Oral zinc in acne vulgaris: a clinical and methodological study. *Acta Derm Venereol* 1978;58:443-8.

6298 Hillstrom L, Pettersson L, Hellbe L, et al. Comparison of oral treatment with zinc sulphate and placebo in acne vulgaris. *Br J Dermatol* 1977;97:681-4.

6299 Meynadier J. Efficacy and safety study of two zinc gluconate regimens in the treatment of inflammatory acne. *Eur J Dermatol* 2000 May;10(4):269-73.

6300 Marshall LF, Camp PE, Bowers SA. Dimethyl sulfoxide for the treatment of intracranial hypertension: a

REFERENCES

preliminary trial. *Neurosurg* 1984;14(6):659-63.

6301 Karaca M, Bilgin UY, Akar M, de la Torre JC. Dimethyl sulphoxide lowers ICP after head trauma. *Eur J Clin Pharmacol* 1991;40(1):113-4.

6302 de la Torre JC. Role of dimethyl sulfoxide in prostaglandin-thromboxane and platelet systems after cerebral ischemia. *Ann N Y Acad Sci* 1983;411:293-308.

6303 Rosenstein ED. Topical agents in the treatment of rheumatic disorders. *Rheum Dis Clin North Am* 1999;25(4):899-918.

6304 Trice JM, Pinals RS. Dimethyl sulfoxide: a review of its use in the rheumatic disorders. *Semin Arthritis Rheum* 1985;15(1):45-60.

6305 Blumenthal LS, Fuchs M. The clinical use of dimethyl sulfoxide on various headaches, musculoskeletal, and other general medical disorders. *Ann N Y Acad Sci* 1967;141(1):572-85.

6306 Merlini G. Treatment of primary amyloidosis. *Semin Hematol* 1995;32(1):60-79.

6307 Rand-Luby L, Pommier RF, Williams ST, et al. Improved outcome of surgical flaps treated with topical dimethylsulfoxide. *Ann Surg* 1996;224(4):583-9.

6308 Thiers BH. Unusual treatments for herpesvirus infections II, herpes zoster. *J Am Acad Dermatol* 1983;8(3):433-6.

6309 Burton WJ, Gould PW, Hursthouse MW, et al. A multicentre trial of Zostrum (5 percent idoxuridine in dimethyl sulphoxide) in herpes zoster. *N Z Med J* 1981;94(696):384-6.

6310 MacCallum FO, Juel-Jensen BE. Herpes simplex virus skin infection in man treated with idoxuridine in dimethyl sulphoxide. Results of double-blind controlled trial. *Br Med J* 1966 (2(517):805-7.

6311 Juel Jensen BE, MacCallum FO, Mackenzie AM, Pike MC. Treatment of zoster with idoxuridine in dimethyl sulphoxide. Results of two double-blind controlled trials. *Br Med J* 1970;4(738):776-80.

6312 Wildenhoff KE, Esmann V, Ipsen J, Harving H, et al. Treatment of trigeminal and thoracic zoster with idoxuridine. *Scand J Infect Dis* 1981;13(4):257-62.

6313 Williams HJ, Furst DE, Dahl SL, et al. Double-blind, multicenter controlled trial comparing topical dimethyl sulfoxide and normal saline for treatment of hand ulcers in patients with systemic sclerosis. *Arthritis Rheum* 1985;28(3):308-14.

6314 Torres MA, Furst DE. Treatment of generalized systemic sclerosis. Rheum Dis Clin North Am 1990;16(1):217-41.

6315 Takacs T, Montet JC. In vitro dissolution of cholesterol biliary stones. *Gut* 1995;37(1):157-8.

6316 Takacs T. Lonovics J, Caroli-Bose FX, et al. Contact litholysis of common bile duct calculi. Study of 44 patients. *Gastroenterol Clin Biol* 1997;21(10):655-9.

6317 Kingery WS. A critical review of controlled clinical trials for peripheral neuropathic pain and complex regional pain syndromes. *Pain* 1997;73(2):123-39.

6318 Rowley SD. Hematopoietic stem cell processing and cryopreservation. *J Clin Apheresis* 1992;7(3):132-4.

6319 Lakota J, Fuchsberger P. Autologous stem cell transplatation with stem cells preserved in the presence of 4.5 and 2.2% DMSO. *Bone Marrow Transplant* 1996;18(1):262-3.

6320 Zambelli A, Poggi G, Da Prada G, et al. Clinical toxicity of cryopreserved circulation progenitor cells infusion. *Anticancer Res* 1998;18(6B):4705-8.

6321 Salim AS. The relationship between Helicobacter pylori and oxygen-derived free radicals in the mechanism of duodenal ulceration. *Intern Med* 1993;32(5):359-64.

6322 Kennedy R. DMSO (aka dimethylsulfoxide). The Doctors Medical Library 2000. www.medical-library.net/ sites/_dmso_(dimethylsulfoxide).html (Accessed 15 June 2000).

6323 Prior D, Mitchell A, Nebauer M, Smith M. Oncology nurses' experience of dimethyl sulfoxide odor. *Cancer Nurs* 2000;23(2):134-40.

6324 Rubin LF. Toxicologic update of dimethyl sulfoxide. *Ann N Y Acad Sci* 1983;411:6-10.

6325 Wolf P, Simon M. Dimethyl sulphoxide (DMSO) induced serum hyperosmolality. *Clin Biochem* 1983;16(4):261-2.

6326 Brayton CF. Dimethyl sulfoxide (DMSO): a review. *Cornell Vet* 1986;76(1):61-90.

6327 Spremulli EN, Dexter DL. Polar solvents: a novel class of antineoplastic agents. *J Clin Oncol* 1984;2(3):227-41.

6328 Toren A, Rechavi G. What really cures in autologous bone marrow transplantation? A possible role for dimethylsulfoxide. *Med Hypothesis* 1993;41(6):495-8.

6329 Evans MS, Reid KH, Sharp JB Jr. Dimethylsuloxide (DMSO) blocks conduction in peripheral nerve C fibers: a possible mechanism of analgesia. *Neurosci Lett* 1993;150(2):145-8.

6330 Jacob SW, Herschler R. Pharmacology of DMSO. *Cryobiology* 1986;23(1):14-27.

6331 Neulieb RL, Neulieb MK. The diverse actions of dimtheyl sulphoxide: an indicator of membrane transport activity. *Cytobios* 1990;63(254-255):139-65.

6332 Fitzgerald P, Moss N, O'Mahony S, Whelton MJ. Accidental hemlock poisoning. *Br Med J (Clin Res Ed)* 1987;295(6613):1657.

6333 Grieve M. Dropwort, hemlock water. A Modern Herbal 1931. www.botanical.com/botanical/mgmh/d/ drophe21.html. (Accessed 11 March 2000).

6334 Mitchell MI, Routledge PA. Hemlock water dropwort poisoning-a review. *Clin Toxicol* 1978;12(4):417-26.

6335 Ball MJ, Flather ML, Forfar JC. Hemlock water dropwort poisoning. *Postgrad Med J* 1987;63(739):363-5.

6336 Mitchell MI, Routledge PA. Poisoning by hemlock water dropwort [letter]. *Lancet* 1977;1(8008):423-4.

6337 Anger JP, Anger F, Chauvel Y, et al. [Fatal poisoning by water dropwort]. [Article in French]. *Eur J Toxicol Environ Hyg* 1976;9(2):119-25.

6338 Lopez TA, Cid MS, Bianchini ML. Biochemistry of hemlock (Conium maculatum L.) alkaloids and their acute and chronic toxicity in livestock. A review. *Toxicon* 1999;37(6):841-65.

6339 Panter KE, Keeler RF, Baker DC. Toxicosis in livestock from the hemlocks (Conium and Cicuta spp.). *J Anim Sci* 1988;66(9):2407-13.

6340 Drummer OH, Roberts AN, Bedford PJ, et al. Three deaths from hemlock poisoning. *Med J Aust* 1995;162(11):592-3.

6341 Frank BS, Panter KE. Ingestion of poison hemlock (Conium maculatum). *West J Med* 1995;163(6):573-4.

6342 Grieve M. Hemlock. A Modern Herbal 1931. www.botanicial.com/botanical/mgmh/h/hemloc18.html. (Accessed 11 March 2000).

6344 Krenzelok EP, Jacobsen TD, Aronis JM. Hemlock ingestions: the most deadly plant exposures. NACCT

Abstracts 1996: Abstract #131.

6345 Grieve M. Hemlock, Water. A Modern Herbal 1931. http://www.botanical.com/botanical/mgmh/h/hemat19.html. (Accessed 11 March 2000).

6346 Starreveld E, Hope E. Cicutoxin poisoning (water hemlock). *Neurol* 1975;25(8):730-4.

6347 Costanza DJ, Hoversten VW. Accidental ingestion of water hemlock. Report of two patients with acute and chronic effects. *Calif Med* 1973;119(2):78-82.

6348 Knutsen OH, Paszkowski P. New aspects in the treatment of water hemlock poisoning. *J Toxicol Clin Toxicol* 1984;22(2):157-66.

6349 Anon. Water hemlock poisoning-Maine, 1992. *MMWR Morb Mortal Wkly Rep* 1994;43(13):229-31.

6350 Applefeld JJ, Caplan ES. A case of water hemlock poisoning. *JACEP* 1979;8(10):401-3.

6351 Carlton BE, Tufts E, Girard DE. Water hemlock poisoning complicated by rhabdomyolysis and renal failure. *Clin Toxicol* 1979;14(1):87-92.

6352 Robson P. Water hemlock poisoning. *Lancet* 1965;2(7425):1274-5.

6353 Landers D, Seppi K, Blauer W. Seizures and death on a white river float trip. Report of water hemlock poisoning. *West J Med* 1985;142(5):637-40.

6354 Mutter L. Poisoning by western water hemlock. *Can J Public Health* 1976;67(5):386.

6355 Withers LM, Coler FR, Nelson RB. Water-hemlock poisoning. *N Engl J Med* 1969;281(10):566-7.

6356 Guillemant J, Le HT, Accarie C, et al. Mineral water as a source of dietary calcium: acute effects on parathyroid function and bone resorption in young men. *Am J Clin Nutr* 2000;71(4):999-1002.

6357 Penninx BW, Guralnik JM, Ferrucci L, et al. Vitamin B(12) deficiency and depression in physically disabled older women: epidemiologic evidence from the Women's Health and Aging Study. *Am J Psychiatry* 2000;157:715-21.

6358 Benito-Leon J, Porta-Etessam J. Shaky-leg syndrome and vitamin B12 deficiency. *N Engl J Med* 2000;342;(13):981.

6359 Prabhala A, Garg R, Dandona P. Severe myopathy associated with vitamin D deficiency in western New York. *Arch Intern Med* 2000;160(8):1199-203.

6360 Suzuki Y, Oishi Y, Yamazaki H, et al. How to avoid bone loss in patients with prostatic carcinoma receiving long-term LHRH-analogue. 2000 AbstractInfo-Am Urol Assn, Inc. www.abstracts-on-line.com/.../windowview.asp?abs=AUA0L1_707&Search. (Accessed 31 July 2000).

6361 Patten E. Vitamin D prevents bone loss in men undergoing treatment for prostate cancer. Doctor's Guide Dispatch 2000. www.docguide.com/dg.nsf/DGNews/. (Accessed 3 May 2000).

6362 Minne HW, Pfeifer M, Begerow B, et al. Vitamin D and calcium supplementation reduces falls in elderly women via improvement of body sway and normalization of blood pressure: a prospective, randomized, and double-blind study. Abstracts World Congress on Osteoporosis 2000. www.nof.org/for_professionals/world_congress/abstracts.pdf. (Accessed 31 July 2000).

6363 Thomasson WA. Vitamin D plus calcium prevents falls in elderly women. Doctor's Guide Dispatch 2000. www.docguide.com/dg.nsf/DGNews/ (Accessed 11 July 2000).

6365 Anon. Drug product database. Canadian Pharmacists' Assn 2000. www.hc-sc.gc.ca/hpb-dgps/therapeut/htmleng/dpd.html (Accessed 3 August 2000).

6366 Kauwell GP, Lippert BL, Wilsky CE, et al. Folate status of elderly women following moderate folate depletion responds only to a higher folate intake. *J Nutr* 2000;130(6):1584-90.

6367 Riddell LJ, Chisholm A, Williams S, Mann JI. Dietary strategies for lowering homocysteine concentrations. *Am J Clin Nutr* 2000;71(6):1448-54.

6368 Chatelain C, Autet W, Brackman F. Comparison of once and twice daily dosage forms of Pygeum africanum extract in patients with benign prostatic hyperplasia: a randomized, double-blind study, with long-term open label extension. *Urology* 1999;54(3):473-8.

6369 Niyogi SK. The toxicology of Abrus precatorius linnaeus. *J Forensic Sci* 1970;15(4):529-36.

6370 Sinclair CJ, Geiger JD. Caffeine use in sports. A pharmacological review. *J Sports Med Phys Fitness* 2000;40:71-9.

6371 Erenberg A, Leff RD, Haack DG, et al. Caffeine citrate for the treatment of apnea of prematurity: a double-blind, placebo-controlled study. *Pharmacother* 2000;20(6):644-52.

6372 Suleman A, Siddiqui NH. Haemodynamic and cardiovascular effects of caffeine. Medicine On Line Int J Medicine 2000. www.priory.com/pharmol/caffeine.htm (Accessed 14 April 2000).

6373 Bolla KI, Funderburk FR, Cadet JL. Differential effects of cocaine and cocaine alcohol on neurocognitive performance. *Neurology* 2000;54(12):2285-92.

6374 Heesch CM, Wilhelm CR, Ristich J, et al. Cocaine activates platelets and increases the formation of circulating platelet containing microaggregates in humans. *Heart* 2000;83(6):688-95.

6375 Vannemreddy PS, Nanda A. Relationship of active cocaine use with stroke mechanism and outcome. Am Assn Neurological Surgeons 68th Ann Mtg 2000. www.neurosurgery.org/abstractcenter/index.html. (Accessed 30 August 2000).

6376 Fawzi WW, Msamanga G, Hunter D, et al. Randomized trial of vitamin supplements in relation to vertical transmission of HIV-1 in Tanzania. *J Acquir Immune Defic Syndr* 2000;23(3):246-54.

6377 Russell RM. The vitamin A spectrum: from deficiency to toxicity. *Am J Clin Nutr* 2000;71(4):878-84.

6378 Cumming RG, Mitchell P, Smith W. Diet and cataract: the Blue Mountains Eye Study. *Ophthalmology* 2000;107(3):450-6.

6379 van Zandwijk N, Dalesio O, Pastorino U, et al. EUROSCAN, a randomized trial of vitamin A and N-acetylcysteine in patients with head and neck cancer or lung cancer. For the European Organization for Research and Treatment of Cancer Head and Neck and Lung Cancer Cooperative Groups. *J Natl Cancer Inst* 2000;92(12):977-86.

6380 Sporn MB. Retinoids and demethylating agents-looking for partners. *J Natl Cancer Inst* 2000;92(10):780-1.

6381 Widschwendter M, Berger J, Hermann M, et al. Methylation and silencing of the retinoic acid receptor-beta2 gene in breast cancer. *J Natl Cancer Inst* 2000;92(10):826-32.

6382 Omenn GS, Goodman GE, Thornquist MD, et al. Risk factors for lung cancer and for intervention effects in CARET, the Beta-Carotene and Retinol Efficacy Trial. *J Natl Cancer Inst* 1996;88(21):1550-9.

R
E
F
E
R
E
N
C
E
S

R E F E R E N C E S

6384 Lindenmuth GF, Lindenmuth EB. The efficacy of echinacea compound herbal tea preparation on the severity and duration of upper respiratory and flu symptoms: a randomized, double-blind, placebo-controlled study. *J Altern Complement Med* 2000;6(4):327-34.

6385 Dorn M, Knick E, Lewith G. Placebo-controlled, double-blind study of Echinaceae pallidae radix in upper respiratory tract infections. *Complement Ther Med* 1997;5:40-2.

6386 Melchart D, et al. Echinacea root extracts for the prevention of upper respiratory tract infections: a double-blind, placebo-controlled randomized trial. *Arch Fam Med* 1998;7(6):541-5.

6387 Parnham MJ. Benefit-risk assessment of the squeezed sap of the purple coneflower (Echinacea purpurea) for long-term oral immunostimulation. *Phytomedicine* 3(1):95-102.

6388 Luettig B, Steinmuller C, Gifford GE, et al. Macrophage activation by the polysaccharide arabinogalactan isolated from plant cell cultures of Echinacea purpurea. *J Natl Cancer Inst* 1989;81(9):669-75.

6389 Stimpel M, Proksch A, Wagner H, et al. Macrophage activation and inductio of macrophage cytotoxicity by purified polysaccharide fractions from the plant Echinacea purpurea. *Infect Immun* 1984;46(3):845-9.

6390 Binns SE, Purgina B, Bergeron C. Light-mediated antifungal activity of Echinacea extracts. *Plant Med* 2000;66(3):241-4.

6391 Perry NB, van Klink JW, Burgess EJ, et al. Alkamide levels in Echinacea purpurea: effects of processing, drying and storage. *Planta Med* 2000;66(1):54-6.

6392 Henneicke-von Zepelin H, Hentschel C, Schnitker J, et al. Efficacy and safety of a fixed combination phytomedicine in the treatment of the common cold (acute viral respiratory tract infection): results of a randomised, double blind, placebo-controlled, multicentre study. *Curr Med Res Opin* 1999;15(3):214-27.

6393 Pryor WA, Stahl W, Rock CL. Beta carotene: from biochemistry to clinical trials. *Nutr Rev* 2000;58(2Pt1):39-53.

6394 Westphal S, Orth M, Ambrosch A, et al. Postprandial chylomicrons VLDLs in severe hypertriacylglycerolemia are lowered more effectively than are chylomicron remnants after treatment with n-3 fatty acids. *Am J Clin Nutr* 2000;71(4):914-20.

6395 Norrish AE, Skeaff CM, Arribas GL, et al. Prostate cancer risk and consumption of fish oils: a dietary biomarker-based, case-control study. *Br J Cancer* 1999;81(7):1238-42.

6396 Kinrys G. Hypomania associated with omega3 fatty acids. *Arch Gen Psych* 2000;57(7):715-6.

6397 Baxter P, Aicardi J. Neonatal seizures after pyridoxine use. *Lancet* 1999;354:2082-3.

6398 Ogilvie GK, Fettman MJ, Mallinckrodt CH, et al. Effect of fish oil, arginine, and doxorubicin chemotherapy on remission and survival time for dogs with lymphoma: a double-blind, randomized, placebo-controlled study. *Cancer* 2000;88(8):1916-28.

6399 Stark KD, Park EJ, Maines VA, Holub BJ. Effect of a fish-oil concentrate on serum lipids in postmenopausal women receiving and not receiving hormone replacement therapy in a placebo-controlled, double-blind trial. *Am J Clin Nutr* 2000;72(2):389-94.

6400 Brenner R, Azbel V, Madhusoodanan S, et al. Comparison of an extract of Hypericum (LI 160) and sertraline in the treatment of depression: A double-blind, randomized pilot study. *Clin Ther* 2000;22:411-9.

6401 Pizzorno JE, Murray MT, eds. Textbook of Natural Medicine. 2nd ed. Edinburgh:Churchill Livingstone, 1999.

6402 Mathews JD, Riley MD, Fejo L, et al. Effects of heavy usage of kava on physical health: Summary of a pilot survey in an aboriginal community. *Med J Aust* 1988;148:548-55.

6403 Imai K. Nakachi K. Cross-sectional study of effects of drinking green tea on cardiovascular and liver diseases. *BMJ* 1995;310:693-6.

6404 Hegarty VM, May HM, Khaw K. Tea drinking and bone mineral density in older women. *Am J Clin Nutr* 2000;71:1003-7.

6405 Iuliano L, Micheletta F, Maranghi M, et al. Bioavailability of vitamin E as function of food intake in healthy subjects: effects on plasma peroxide-scavenging activity and cholesterol-oxidation products. *Arterioscler Thromb Vasc Biol* 2001;21:E34-7.

6406 Pye JK, Mansel RE, Hughes LE. Clinical experience of drug treatments for mastalgia. *Lancet* 1985;2(8451):373-7.

6407 Morisco C, Trimarco B, Condorelli M. Effect of coenzyme Q10 therapy in patients with congestive heart failure: A long-term, multicenter, randomized study. *Clin Investig* 1993;71(Suppl 8): S134–6.

6408 Hofman-Bang C, et al. Coenzyme Q10 as an adjunctive treatment of congestive heart failure. *J Card Fail* 1995;1:101-7.

6409 Baggio E, Gandini R, Plauncher AC, et al. Italian multicenter study on the safety and efficacy of coenzyme Q10 as adjunctive therapy in heart failure. CoQ10 Drug Surveillance Investigators. *Mol Aspects Med* 1994;(15 Suppl):S287-94.

6410 Pizzorno JE, Murray MT, eds. Textbook of Natural Medicine. 2nd Ed. New York: Churchill Livingston, 1999.

6411 Anon. Goldenseal. The Natural Pharmacist. 1999. www.tnp.com/propages.asp?ID=26. (Accessed 22 June 2000).

6412 Teixeira SR, Potter SM, Weigel R, et al. Effects of feeding 4 levels of soy protein for 3 and 6 wk on blood lipids and apolipoproteins in moderately hypercholesterolemic men. *Am J Clin Nutr* 2000;71:1077-84.

6413 Merz-Demlow BE, Duncan AM, Wangen KE, et al. Soy isoflavones improve plasma lipids in normocholesterolemic, premenopausal women. *Am J Clin Nutr* 2000;71:1462-9.

6414 Heaney RP, Dowell MS, Rafferty K, et al. Bioavailability of the calcium in fortified soy imitation milk, with some observations on method. *Am J Clin Nutr* 2000;71:1166-9.

6415 White LR, Petrovitch H, Ross GW, et al. Brain aging and midlife tofu consumption. *J Am Coll Nutr* 2000;19:242-55.

6416 Grodstein F, Mayeux R, Stampfer MJ. Tofu and cognitive function: food for thought. *J Am Coll Nutr* 2000;19:207-9.

6417 Giles JT, Palat CT III , Chien SH, et al. Evaluation of Echinacea for treatment of the common cold. *Pharmacother* 2000;20(6):690-7.

6418 Pepping J. Echinacea. *Am J Health Syst Pharm* 1999;56:121-3.

6419 Anon. Echinacea. The Natural Pharmacist 2000 www.tnp.com/propages.asp?ID=18#P8. (Accessed 23 June 2000).

6420 Anon. Horse Chestnut. The Natural Pharmacist 2000. www.tnp.com/substance.asp?ID=62. (Accessed 24 June 2000).

6421 Weil A. Losing sleep over lice? www.pathfinder.com/drweil/archiveqa/0,2283,1844,00.html. (Accessed 20 July 2000).

6422 Anon. Neem. The Natural Pharmacist 2000. www.tnp.com/substance.asp?ID=75 (Accessed 20 July 2000).

6423 Galluzzi S, Zanetti O, Binetti G, et al. Coma in a patient with Alzheimer's disease taking low dose trazodone and Ginkgo biloba. *J Neurol Neurosurg Psychiatry* 2000;68:679-80.

6424 Carraro JC, Raynaud JP, Koch G, et al. Comparison of phytotherapy (Permixon) with finasteride in the treatment of benign prostate hyperplasia: a randomized international study of 1,098 patients. *Prostate* 1996;29:231-40.

6425 Roby CA, Anderson GD, Kantor E, et al. St. John's wort: Effect on CYP3A4 activity. *Clin Pharmacol Ther* 2000;67:451-7.

6426 Schempp CM, Winghofer B, Ludtke R, et al. Topical application of St. John's wort (Hypericum perforatum L.) and its metabolite hyperforin inhibits the allostimulatory capacity of epidermal cells. *Br J Dermatol* 2000;142:979-84.

6427 Kleber E, Obry T, Hippeli S, et al. Biochemical activities of extracts from Hypericum perforatum L. *Arzneimittelforschung* 1999;49:106-9.

6428 Williams JW, Mulrow CD, Chiquette E, et al. A systematic review of newer pharmacotherapies for depression in adults: Evidence report summary. *Ann Intern Med* 2000;132:743-56.

6429 Stevinson C, Ernst E. A pilot study of Hypericum perforatum for the treatment of premenstrual syndrome. BJOG 2000;107:870-6.

6430 Anderson PO, Knoben JE. Handbook of Clinical Drug Data. 8th ed. Stamford, CT: Appleton & Lange, 1997.

6431 Zambon D, Sabate J, Munoz S, et al. Substituting walnuts for monounsaturated fat improves the serum lipid profile of hypercholesterolemic men and women. *Ann Intern Med* 2000;132:538-46.

6432 Kovacs DJ, Berk T. Recurrent Clostridium difficile-associated diarrhea and colitis treated with saccharomyces cerevisiae (baker's yeast) in combination with antibiotic therapy. A case report. *J Am Board Fam Pract* 2000;13(2):138-40.

6433 Savarese D, Boucher J, Corey B, et al. Glutamine treatment of paclitaxel-induced myalgias and arthralgias [letter]. *J Clin Oncol* 1998;16:3918-9.

6434 Woelk H. Comparison of St. John's wort and imipramine for treating depression: randomized controlled trial. *BMJ* 2000;321:536-9.

6435 Barone GW, Gurley BJ, Ketel BL, et al. Drug interaction between St. John's wort and cyclosporin. *Ann Pharmacother* 2000;34:1013-6.

6436 Lusardi P, et al. Cardiovascular effects of melatonin in hypertensive patients well controlled by nifedipine: a 24-hour study. *Br J Clin Pharmacol* 2000;49:423-7.

6437 Mitwalli A, Ayiomamitis A, Grass L, et al. Control of hyperoxaluria with large doses of pyridoxine in patients with kidney stones. *Int Urol Nephrol* 1988;20:353-9.

6438 Gill HS, Rose GA. Mild metabolic hyperoxaluria and its response to pyridoxine. *Urol Int* 1986;41:393-6.

6439 Yendt ER, Cohanim M. Response to physiologic dose of pyridoxine in type I primary hyperoxaluria. *N Engl J Med* 1985;312:953-7.

6440 Revusova V, Gratzlova J, Zvara V, et al. The evaluation of some biochemical parameters in pyridoxine-treated calcium oxalate renal stone formers. *Urol Int* 1977;32:348-52.

6441 Curhan GC, Willet WC, Speizer FE, et al. Intake of vitamin B6 and C and the risk of kidney stones in women. *J Am Soc Nephrol* 1999;10:840-5.

6442 Curhan GC, Willet WC, Rimm EB, et al. A prospective study of the intake of vitamins C and B6, and the risk of kidney stones in men. *J Urol* 1996;155:1847-51.

6443 Arnold LE, Kleykamp D, Votolato NA, et al. Gamma-linolenic acid for attention-deficit hyperactivity disorder: Placebo-controlled comparison to D-amphetamine. *Biol Psychiatry* 1989;25:222-8.

6444 Haslam RHA, et al. Is there a role for megavitamin therapy in attention deficit hyperactivity disorder? *Advances Neurol* 1992;58:303-10.

6445 Stoll BA. Dietary supplements of dehydroepiandrosterone in relation to breast cancer risk. *Eur J Clin Nutr* 1999;53:771-5.

6446 Baulieu EE, Thomas G, Legrain S, et al. Dehydroepiandrosterone (DHEA), DHEA sulfate, and aging. Contribution of the DHEAge study to a sociobiomedical issue. *Proc Natl Acad Sci USA* 2000;97:4279-84.

6447 van Vollenhoven RF, Park JL, Genovese MC, et al. A double-blind, placebo-controlled, clinical trial of dehydroepiandrosterone in severe lupus erythematosus. *Lupus* 1999;8:181-7.

6448 Jameson S. Statistical data support prediction of death within 6 months on low levels of coenzyme Q10 and other entities. *Clin Investig* 1993;71(8 Suppl):S137-9.

6449 Alekel DL, St. Germain A, Peterson CT et al. Isoflavone-rich soy protein isolate attenuates bone loss in the lumbar spine of perimenopausal women. *Am J Clin Nutr* 2000;72:844-52.

6450 Budzinski JW, Foster BC, Vandenhoek S, et al. An in vitro evaluation of human cytochrome P450 3A4 inhibition by selected commercial herbal extracts and tinctures. *Phytomedicine* 2000;7:273-82.

6451 Houston JB, Levy G. Drug biotransformation interactions in man VI: Acetaminophen and ascorbic acid. *J Pharm Sci* 1976;65:1218-21.

6452 Owen CA, Tyce GM, Flock EV, et al. Heparin-ascorbic acid antagonism. *Mayo Clin Proc* 1970;45:140-5.

6453 Dresser GK, Bailey DG, Carruthers SG. Grapefruit juice-felodipine interaction in the elderly. *Clin Pharmacol Ther* 2000;68:28-34.

6455 Upmalis DH, Lobo R, Bradley L, et al. Vasomotor symptom relief by soy isoflavone extract tablets in postmenopausal women: A multicenter, double-blind, randomized, placebo-controlled study. *Menopause* 2000;7:236-42.

6456 Chrubasik S, Eisenberg E, Balan E, et al. Treatment of low back pain exacerbations with willow bark extract: a randomized double-blind study. *Am J Med* 2000;109:9-14.

6457 Stevinson C, Pittler MH, Ernst E. Garlic for treating

REFERENCES

hypercholesterolemia: a meta-analysis of randomized clinical trials. *Ann Intern Med* 2000;133:420-9.

6458 Douglas RM, Chalker EB, Treacy B. Vitamin C for preventing and treating the common cold. *Cochrane Database Syst Rev* 2000;(2):CD000980.

6459 Ross EA, Szabo NJ, Tebbett IR. Lead content of calcium supplements. *JAMA* 2000;284:1425-29.

6460 Heaney RP. Lead in calcium supplements. Cause for alarm or celebration? *JAMA* 2000;284:1432-3.

6461 Vuksan V, et al. Similar postprandial glycemic reductions with escalation of dose and administration time of American ginseng in type 2 diabetes. *Diabetes Care* 2000 Sep;23(9):1221-6.

6462 Aman MG, Mitchell EA, Turbott SH. The effects of essential fatty acid supplementation by Efamol in hyperactive children. *J Abnorm Child Psychol* 1987;15:75-90.

6463 Moore LB, Goodwin B, Jones SA, et al. St. John's wort induces hepatic drug metabolism through activation of the pregnane X receptor. *Proc Natl Acad Sci U S A* 2000;97:7500-2.

6464 Cats A, Scholten P, Meuwissen SGM, et al. Acute Fasciola hepatica infection attributed to chewing khat. *Gut* 2000;47:584-5.

6465 Garlic: Effects on cardiovascular risks and disease, protective effects against cancer, and clinical adverse effects. Summary, evidence report/technol assessment: no 20. AHRQ Publ No. 01-E022, 2000;Oct. Agency for Healthcare Res and Quality. Rockville, MD. www.ahrq.gov/clinic/garlicsum.htm (Accessed 3 October 2000).

6466 Divi RL, Chang HC, Doerge DR. Anti-thyroid isoflavones from soybean: isolation, characterization, and mechanisms of action. *Biochem Pharmacol* 1997;54:1087-96.

6467 Anon. Product Review: Saw Palmetto. ConsumerLab.com 2000. www.consumerlab.com/results/sa palmetto.html (Accessed 2001 August 31).

6468 Anon. Herbal Rx for prostate problems. *Consumer Reports* 2000;Sep:60-2.

6470 Alvarez-Arroyo MV, Traba ML, Rapado TA, et al. Correlation between 1.25 dihydroxyvitamin D serum levels and fractional rate of intestinal calcium absorption in hypercalciuric nephrolithiasis. Role of phosphate. *Urol Res* 1992;20:96-7.

6471 Hirt M, Nobel S, Barron E, et al. Zinc nasal gel for the treatment of common cold symptoms: A double-blind, placebo-controlled trial. *ENT J* 2000;79:778-82.

6472 Chantre P, Cappelaere A, Leblan D, et al. Efficacy and tolerance or Harpagophytum procumbens versus diacerhein in treatment of osteoarthritis. *Phytomedicine* 2000;7:177-84.

6473 Cheng TO. St. John's wort interaction with digoxin [letter]. *Arch Intern Med* 2000;160:2548.

6474 Vormfelde SV, Poser W. Hyperforin in extracts of St. John's wort (Hypericum perforatum) for depression [letter]. *Arch Intern Med* 2000;160:2548.

6475 Wentworth JM, Agostini M, Love J, et al. St. John's wort, a herbal antidepressant, activates the steroid X receptor. *J Endocrinol* 2000;166:R11-6.

6476 Obach RS. Inhibition of human cytochrome P450 enzymes by constituents of St. John's wort, an herbal preparation used in the treatment of depression. *J Pharmacol Exp Ther* 2000;294:88-95.

6477 Lane-Brown MM. Photosensitivity associated with herbal preparations of St. John's wort (Hypericum perforatum). *Med J Aust* 2000;172:302.

6478 Lal S, Iskandar H. St. John's wort and schizophrenia. *CMAJ* 2000;163:262-3.

6479 Carey CF, Lee HH, Woeltje KF (eds). Washington Manual of Medical Therapeutics. 29th ed. New York, NY: Lippincott-Raven, 1998.

6480 Dorn M. [Efficacy and tolerability of Baldrian versus oxazepam in non-organic and non-psychiatric insomniacs: a randomized, double-blind, clinical, comparative study]. [Article in German]. *Forsch Komplementarmed Klass Naturheilkd* 2000;7:79-84.

6481 Parsons M, Simpson M, Ponton T. Raspberry leaf and its effects on labour: safety and efficacy. *J Aust Coll Midwives* 1999; Sep12:20-5.

6482 Heliovaara M, Aho K, Knekt P, et al. Coffee consumption, rheumatoid factor, and the risk of rheumatoid arthritis. *Ann Rheum Dis* 2000;59:631-5.

6483 De La Taille A, Buttyan R, Hayek O, et al. Herbal therapy PC-SPES: In vitro effects and evaluation of its efficacy in 69 patients with prostate cancer. *J Urol* 2000;164:1229-34.

6484 Small EJ, Frohlich MW, Bok R, et al. Prospective trial of the herbal supplement, PC-SPES, in patients with pregressive prostate cancer. *J Clin Oncol* 2000;18: 3595-603.

6485 Wen HY, Davis RL, Shi B, et al. Bioavailability of selenium from veal, chicken, beef, lamb, flounder, tuna, selenomethionine, and sodium selenite assessed in selenium-deficient rats. *Biol Trace Elem Res* 1997;58:43–53.

6486 Haller CA, Benowitz NL. Adverse cardiovascular and central nervous system events associated with dietary supplements containing ephedra alkaloids. *N Eng J Med* 2000;343(25):1833-8.

6487 Leikin JB, Klein L. Ephedra causes myocarditis. *Clin Toxicol* 2000;38:353-4.

6488 Gurley B. Extract versus herb: Effect of formulation on the absorption rate of botanical ephedrine from dietary supplements containing ephedra (ma huang). *Ther Drug Mon* 2000;22:497.

6489 Anon. Fibromyalgia. The Natural Pharmacist 2000. www.tnp.com/topic.asp?ID=305. (Accessed 14 November 2000).

6490 Le Bars PL, Kieser M, Itil KZ. A 26-week analysis of a double-blind, placebo-controlled trial of the Ginkgo biloba extract EGb 761 in dementia. *Dement Geriatr Cogn Disord* 2000;11:230-7.

6491 Forstl H. Clinical issues in current drug therapy for dementia. *Alzheimer's Dis Assoc Disord* 2000;14 (Suppl 1):S103-S108.

6492 Campos-Toimil M, Lugnier C, Droy-Lefaix M, et al. Inhibition of type 4 phosphodiesterase by rolipram and Ginkgo biloba extract (EGb 761) decreases agonist-induced rises in internal calcium in human endothelial cells. *Arterioscler Thromb Vasc Biol* 2000;20:e34-e40.

6493 Ritch R. Potential role for Ginkgo biloba extract in the treatment of glaucoma. *Med Hypoth* 2000;54:221-35.

6494 Bastianetto S, Ramassamy C, Dore S, et al. The ginkgo biloba extract (EGb 761) protects hippocampal neurons against cell death induced by beta-amyloid. *Eur J Neurosci* 2000;12:1882-90.

6495 Thal LJ, Calvani M, Amato A, et al. A 1-year controlled trial of acetyl-l-carnitine in early onset AD. *Neurol* 2000;55:805-10.

6496 Spitzer RL, Terman M, Williams JBW, et al. Jet lag: Clinical features, validation of a new syndrome-specific scale, lack of response to melatonin in a randomized, double-blind trial. *Am J Psychiatry* 1999;156:1392-6.

6497 Drago F, Busa L. Acute low doses of melatonin restore full sexual activity in impotent male rats. *Brain Res* 2000;878:98-104.

6498 von Bahr C, Ursing C, Yasui N, et al. Fluvoxamine but not citalopram increases serum melatonin in healthy subjects – an indication that cytochrome P450 CYP1A2 and CYP2C19 hydroxylate melatonin. *Eur J Clin Pharmacol* 2000;56:123-7.

6499 Grozinger M, Hartter S, Wang X, et al. Fluvoxamine strongly inhibits melatonin metabolism in a patient with low-amplitude melatonin profile. *Arch Gen Psychiatry* 2000 Aug;57:812-3.

6500 Mills S, Bone K. Principles and Practice of Phytotherapy. London: Churchill Livingstone 2000.

6501 Michaelsson G, Juhlin L, Vahlquist A. Effects of oral zinc and vitamin A in acne. *Arch Dermatol* 1977;113:31-6.

6502 Dreno B, Amblard P, Agache P, et al. Low doses of zinc gluconate for inflammatory acne. *Acta Derm Venereol* 1989;69:541-3.

6503 Orris L, Shalita AR, Sibulkin D, et al. Oral zinc therapy of acne. Absorption and clinical effect. *Arch Dermatol* 1978;114:1018-20.

6504 Weismann K, Wadskov S, Sondergaard J. Oral zinc sulphate therapy for acne vulgaris. *Acta Derm Venereol* 1977;57:357-60.

6505 Cunliffe WJ, Burke B, Dodman B, Gould DJ. A double-blind trial of a zinc sulphate/citrate complex and tetracycline in the treatment of acne vulgaris. *Br J Dermatol* 1979;101:321-5.

6506 Michaelsson G, Juhlin L, Ljunghall K. A double-blind study of the effect of zinc and oxytetracycline in acne vulgaris. *Br J Dermatol* 1977;97:561-6.

6507 Amer M, Bahgat MR, Tosson Z, et al. Serum zinc in acne vulgaris. *Int J Dermatol* 1982;21:481-4.

6508 Michaelsson G, Vahlquist A, Juhlin L. Serum zinc and retinol-binding protein in acne. *Br J Dermatol* 1977;96:283-6.

6509 Michaelsson G, Ljunghall K. Patients with dermatitis herpetiformis, acne, psoriasis and Darier's disease have low epidermal zinc concentrations. *Acta Derm Venereol* 1990;70:304-8.

6510 Huang X, Cuajungco MP, Atwood CS, et al. Alzheimer's disease, beta-amyloid protein and zinc. *J Nutr* 2000;130:1488S-92S.

6511 Lovell MA, Robertson JD, Teesdale WJ, et al. Copper, iron and zinc in Alzheimer's disease senile plaques. *J Neurol Sci* 1998;158:47-52.

6512 Lovell MA, Xie C, Markesbery WR. Protection against amyloid beta peptide toxicity by zinc. *Brain Res* 1999;823:88-95.

6513 Burrows NP, Turnbull AJ, Punchard NA, et al. A trial of oral zinc supplementation in psoriasis. *Cutis* 1994;54:117-8.

6514 Leibovici V, Statter M, Weinrauch L, et al. Effect of zinc therapy on neutrophil chemotaxis in psoriasis. *Isr J Med Sci* 1990;26:306-9.

6515 Clemmensen OJ, Siggaard-Andersen J, Worm AM, et al. Psoriatic arthritis treated with oral zinc sulphate. *Br J Dermatol* 1980;103:411-5.

6516 Dixon JS, Bird HA, Martin MF, et al. Biochemical and clinical changes occurring during the treatment of rheumatoid arthritis with novel antirheumatoid drugs. *Int J Clin Pharmacol Res* 1985;5:25-33.

6517 Rasker JJ, Kardaun SH. Lack of beneficial effect of zinc sulphate in rheumatoid arthritis. *Scand J Rheumatol* 1982;11:168-70.

6518 Zoli A, Altomonte L, Caricchio R, et al. Serum zinc and copper in active rheumatoid arthritis: correlation with interleukin 1 beta and tumour necrosis factor alpha. *Clin Rheumatol* 1998;17:378-82.

6519 Simkin PA. Oral zinc sulphate in rheumatoid arthritis. *Lancet* 1976;2:539-42.

6520 Berger MM, Spertini F, Shenkin A, et al. Trace element supplementation modulates pulmonary infection rates after major burns: a double-blind, placebo-controlled trial. *Am J Clin Nutr* 1998;68:365-71.

6521 Marshall I. Zinc for the common cold. *Cochrane Database Syst Rev* 2000;2:CD001364.

6522 Jackson JL, Lesho E, Peterson C. Zinc and the common cold: a meta-analysis revisited. *J Nutr* 2000;130(5S Suppl):1512S-5S.

6523 Guide to Clinical Preventive Services. 2nd ed. Natl Institute of Health, 1996. URL: http://text.nlm.nih.gov/cps/www/cps.67.html (Accessed 6 July 2000).

6524 Schaeken MJ, Van der Hoeven JS, Saxton CA, Cummins D. The effect of mouthrinses containing zinc and triclosan on plaque accumulation, development of gingivitis and formation of calculus in a 28-week clinical test. *J Clin Periodontol* 1996;23:465-70.

6525 Stephen KW, Saxton CA, Jones CL, et al. Control of gingivitis and calculus by a dentifrice containing a zinc salt and triclosan. *J Periodontol* 1990;61:674-9.

6526 Svatun B, Saxton CA, Rolla G. Six-month study of the effect of a dentifrice containing zinc citrate and triclosan on plaque, gingival health, and calculus. *Scand J Dent Res* 1990;98:301-4.

6527 Svatun B, Saxton CA, Huntington E, Cummins D. The effects of a silica dentifrice containing Triclosan and zinc citrate on supragingival plaque and calculus formation and the control of gingivitis. *Int Dent J* 1993;43:431-9.

6528 Williams C, McBride S, Mostler K, et al. Efficacy of a dentifrice containing zinc citrate for the control of plaque and gingivitis: a 6-month clinical study in adults. *Compend Contin Educ Dent* 1998;19:4-15.

6529 Polenik P. Zinc in etiology of periodontal disease. *Med Hypotheses* 1993;40:182-5.

6530 Cunningham JJ, Fu A, Mearkle PL, Brown RG. Hyperzincuria in individuals with insulin-dependent diabetes mellitus: concurrent zinc status and the effect of high-dose zinc supplementation. *Metabolism* 1994;43:1558-62.

6531 Rauscher AM, Fairweather-Tait SJ, Wilson PD, et al. Zinc metabolism in non-insulin dependent diabetes mellitus. *J Trace Elem Med Biol* 1997;11:65-70.

6532 Blostein-Fujii A, DiSilvestro RA, Frid D, et al. Short-term zinc supplementation in women with non-insulin-dependent diabetes mellitus: effects on plasma 5'-nucleotidase activities, insulin-like growth factor I concentrations, and lipoprotein oxidation rates in vitro. *Am J Clin Nutr* 1997;66:639-42.

6533 Faure P, Benhamou PY, Perard A, et al. Lipid peroxidation in insulin-dependent diabetic patients with early retina degeneration lesions: effects of an oral zinc supplementation. *Eur J Clin Nutr* 1995;49:282-8.

6534 Mahajan PM, Jadhav VH, Patki AH, et al. Oral zinc

therapy in recurrent erythema nodosum leprosum: a clinical study. *Indian J Lepr* 1994;66:51-7.

6535 Mathur NK, Bumb RA, Mangal HN. Oral zinc in recurrent Erythema Nodosum Leprosum reaction. *Lepr India* 1983;55:547-52.

6536 Mathur NK, Bumb RA, Mangal HN, Sharma ML. Oral zinc as an adjunct to dapsone in lepromatous leprosy. *Int J Lepr Other Mycobact Dis* 1984;52:331-8.

6537 George J, Bhatia VN, Balakrishnan S, Ramu G. Serum zinc/copper ratio in subtypes of leprosy and effect of oral zinc therapy on reactional states. *Int J Lepr Other Mycobact Dis* 1991;59:20-4.

6538 Brody I. Topical treatment of recurrent herpes simplex and post-herpetic erythema multiforme with low concentrations of zinc sulphate solution. *Br J Dermatol* 1981;104:191-4.

6539 Eby GA, Halcomb WW. Use of topical zinc to prevent recurrent herpes simplex infection: review of literature and suggested protocols. *Med Hypotheses* 1985;17:157-65.

6540 Kneist W, Hempel B, Borelli S. [Clinical, double-blind trial of topical zinc sulfate for herpes labialis recidivans]. [Article in German]. *Arzneimittelforschung* 1995;45:624-6.

6541 Arens M, Travis S. Zinc salts inactivate clinical isolates of herpes simplex virus in vitro. *J Clin Microbiol* 2000;38:1758-62.

6542 Heyneman CA. Zinc deficiency and taste disorders. *Ann Pharmacother* 1996;30:186-7.

6543 Abu-Hamdan DK, Desai H, Sondheimer J, et al. Taste acuity and zinc metabolism in captopril-treated hypertensive male patients. *Am J Hypertens* 1988;1:303S-8S.

6544 Henkin RI, Martin BM, Agarwal RP. Efficacy of exogenous oral zinc in treatment of patients with carbonic anhydrase VI deficiency. *Am J Med Sci* 1999;318:392-405.

6545 Henkin RI, Martin BM, Agarwal RP. Decreased parotid saliva gustin/carbonic anhydrase VI secretion: an enzyme disorder manifested by gustatory and olfactory dysfunction. *Am J Med Sci* 1999;318:380-91.

6546 Henkin RI, Schecter PJ, Friedewald WT, et al. A double-blind study of the effects of zinc sulfate on taste and smell dysfunction. *Am J Med Sci* 1976;272:285-99.

6547 Ripamonti C, Zecca E, Brunelli C, et al. A randomized, controlled clinical trial to evaluate the effects of zinc sulfate on cancer patients with taste alterations caused by head and neck irradiation. *Cancer* 1998;82:1938-45.

6548 Mahajan SK, Prasad AS, Lambujon J, et al. Improvement of uremic hypogeusia by zinc: a double-blind study. *Am J Clin Nutr* 1980;33:1517-21.

6549 Watson AR, Stuart A, Wells FE, et al. Zinc supplementation and its effect on taste acuity in children with chronic renal failure. *Hum Nutr Clin Nutr* 1983;37:219-25.

6550 Sprenger KB, Bundschu D, Lewis K, et al. Improvement of uremic neuropathy and hypogeusia by dialysate zinc supplementation: a double-blind study. Kidney Int Suppl 1983;16:S315-8.

6551 Shankar AH, Prasad AS. Zinc and immune function: the biological basis of altered resistance to infection. *Am J Clin Nutr* 1998;68:447S-63S.

6552 Prasad AS. Zinc and immunity. *Mol Cell Biochem* 1998;188:63-9.

6553 Girodon F, Galan P, Monget AL, et al. Impact of trace elements and vitamin supplementation on immunity and infections in institutionalized elderly patients: a randomized, controlled trial. MIN. VIT. AOX. geriatric network. *Arch Intern Med* 1999;159:748-54.

6554 Bjorksten B, Back O, Gustavson KH, et al. Zinc and immune function in Down's syndrome. *Acta Paediatr Scand* 1980;69:183-7.

6555 Licastro F, Chiricolo M, Mocchegiani E, et al. Oral zinc supplementation in Down's syndrome subjects decreased infections and normalized some humoral and cellular immune parameters. *J Intellect Disabil Res* 1994;38:149-62.

6556 Cahill DJ, Fox R, Wardle PG, et al. Multiple follicular development associated with herbal medicine. *Hum Reprod* 1994;9:1469-70.

6557 McCaleb RS, Leigh E, Morien K. The Encyclopedia of Popular Herbs. Roseville, CA: Prima Health, 2000.

6558 Heiman SW. Pycnogenol for ADHD? *J Am Acad Child Adolesc Psychiatry* 1999;38:357-8.

6559 Greenblatt J. Nutritional supplements in ADHD. *J Am Acad Child Adolesc Psychiatry* 1999;38:1209-10.

6562 Maes M, De Vos N, Demedts P, et al. Lower serum zinc in major depression in relation to changes in serum acute phase proteins. *J Affect Disord* 1999;56:189-94.

6563 Provinciali M, Montenovo A, Di Stefano G, et al. Effect of zinc or zinc plus arginine supplementation on antibody titre and lymphocyte subsets after influenza vaccination in elderly subjects: a randomized controlled trial. *Age Ageing* 1998;27:715-22.

6564 Kelly P, Musonda R, Kafwembe E, et al. Micronutrient supplementation in the AIDS diarrhea-wasting syndrome in Zambia: a randomized controlled trial. *AIDS* 1999;13:495-500.

6565 Tang AM, Graham NM, Saah AJ. Effects of micronutrient intake on survival in human immunodeficiency virus type 1 infection. *Am J Epidemiol* 1996;143:1244-56.

6566 Mocchegiani E, Veccia S, Ancarani F, et al. Benefit of oral zinc supplementation as an adjunct to zidovudine (AZT) therapy against opportunistic infections in AIDS. *Int J Immunopharmacol* 1995;17:719-27.

6568 Brook AC, Johnston DG, Ward MK, et al. Absence of a therapeutic effect of zinc in the sexual dysfunction of haemodialysed patients *Lancet* 1980;2:618-20.

6569 Goldiner WH, Hamilton BP, Hyman PD, Russell RM. Effect of the administration of zinc sulfate on hypogonadism and impotence in patients with chronic stable hepatic cirrhosis. *J Am Coll Nutr* 1983;2:157-62.

6570 Khedun SM, Naicker T, Maharaj B. Zinc, hydrochlorothiazide and sexual dysfunction. *Cent Afr J Med* 1995;41:312-5.

6571 Mahajan SK, Abbasi AA, Prasad AS, et al. Effect of oral zinc therapy on gonadal function in hemodialysis patients. A double-blind study. *Ann Intern Med* 1982;97:357-61.

6572 Rodger RS, Sheldon WL, Watson MJ, et al. Zinc deficiency and hyperprolactinaemia are not reversible causes of sexual dysfunction in uraemia. *Nephrol Dial Transplant* 1989;4:888-92.

6573 Fuse H, Kazama T, Ohta S, Fujiuchi Y. Relationship between zinc concentrations in seminal plasma and various sperm parameters. *Int Urol Nephrol* 1999;31:401-8.

6574 Henkel R, Bittner J, Weber R, et al. Relevance of zinc in human sperm flagella and its relation to motility. *Fertil*

Steril 1999;71:1138-43.

6575 Chia SE, Ong CN, Chua LH, et al. Comparison of zinc concentrations in blood and seminal plasma and the various sperm parameters between fertile and infertile men. *J Androl* 2000;21:53-7.

6576 Hunt CD, Johnson PE, Herbel J, Mullen LK. Effects of dietary zinc depletion on seminal volume and zinc loss, serum testosterone concentrations, and sperm morphology in young men. *Am J Clin Nutr* 1992;56:148-57.

6577 Mohan H, Verma J, Singh I, et al. Inter-relationship of zinc levels in serum and semen in oligospermic infertile patients and fertile males. *Indian J Pathol Microbiol* 1997;40:451-5.

6578 Omu AE, Dashti H, Al-Othman S. Treatment of asthenozoospermia with zinc sulphate: andrological, immunological and obstetric outcome. *Eur J Obstet Gynecol Reprod Biol* 1998;79:179-84.

6579 Mares-Perlman JA, Klein R, Klein BE, et al. Association of zinc and antioxidant nutrients with age-related maculopathy. *Arch Ophthalmol* 1996;114:991-7.

6580 Smith W, Mitchell P, Webb K, Leeder SR. Dietary antioxidants and age-related maculopathy: the Blue Mountains Eye Study. *Ophthalmology* 1999;106:761-77.

6581 VandenLangenberg GM, Mares-Perlman JA, Klein R, et al. Associations between antioxidant and zinc intake and the 5-year incidence of early age-related maculopathy in the Beaver Dam Eye Study. *Am J Epidemiol* 1998;148:204-14.

6582 Evans JR, Henshaw K. Antioxidant vitamin and mineral supplementation for preventing age-related macular degeneration. *Cochrane Database Syst Rev* 2000;(2):CD000253.

6583 Newsome DA, Swartz M, Leone NC, et al. Oral zinc in macular degeneration. *Arch Ophthalmol* 1988;106:192-8.

6584 Stur M, Tittl M, Reitner A, Meisinger V. Oral zinc and the second eye in age-related macular degeneration. *Invest Ophthalmol Vis Sci* 1996;37:1225-35.

6585 Sack RL, Brandes RW, Kendall AR, et al. Entrainment of free-running circadian rhythms by melatonin in blind people. *N Engl J Med* 2000;343:1070-7.

6586 Grazioso CF, Isalgue M, de Ramirez I, et al. The effect of zinc supplementation on parasitic reinfestation of Guatemalan schoolchildren. *Am J Clin Nutr* 1993;57:673-8.

6587 Sharquie KE, Najim RA, Farjou IB. A comparative controlled trial of intralesionally-administered zinc sulphate, hypertonic sodium chloride and pentavalent antimony compound against acute cutaneous leishmaniasis. *Clin Exp Dermatol* 1997;22:169-73.

6588 Rodriguez de la Serna A, Diaz-Rubio M. Multicenter clinical trial of zinc acexamate in the prevention of nonsteroidal antiinflammatory drug induced gastroenteropathy. Spanish Study Group on NSAID Induced Gastroenteropathy Prevention. *J Rheumatol* 1994;21:927-33.

6589 Jimenez E, Bosch F, Galmes JL, Banos JE. Meta-analysis of efficacy of zinc acexamate in peptic ulcer. *Digestion* 1992;51:18-26.

6590 Garcia-Plaza A, Arenas JI, Belda O, Diago A, et al. [A multicenter, clinical trial. Zinc acexamate vs famotidine in the treatment of acute duodenal ulcer. Study group of zinc acexamate]. [Article in Spanish]. *Rev Esp Enferm*

Dig 1996;88:757-62.

6591 Frommer DJ. The healing of gastric ulcers by zinc sulphate. *Med J Aust* 1975;2:793-6.

6592 Wray D. A double-blind trial of systemic zinc sulfate in recurrent aphthous stomatitis. *Oral Surg Oral Med Oral Pathol* 1982;53:469-72.

6593 Merchant HW, Gangarosa LP, Glassman AB, Sobel RE. Zinc sulfate supplementation for treatment of recurring oral ulcers. *South Med J* 1977;70:559-61.

6594 Gupta VL, Chaubey BS. Efficacy of zinc therapy in prevention of crisis in sickle cell anemia: a double blind, randomized controlled clinical trial. *J Assoc Physicians India* 1995;43:467-9.

6595 Leonard MB, Zemel BS, Kawchak DA, et al. Plasma zinc status, growth, and maturation in children with sickle cell disease. *J Pediatr* 1998;132:467-71.

6596 Prasad AS, Beck FW, Kaplan J, et al. Effect of zinc supplementation on incidence of infections and hospital admissions in sickle cell disease (SCD). *Am J Hematol* 1999;61:194-202.

6597 Aydinok Y, Coker C, Kavakli K, et al. Urinary zinc excretion and zinc status of patients with beta-thalassemia major. *Biol Trace Elem Res* 1999;70:165-72.

6598 Uysal Z, Akar N, Kemahli S, et al. Desferrioxamine and urinary zinc excretion in beta-thalassemia major. *Pediatr Hematol Oncol* 1993;10:257-60.

6599 Benso L, Gambotto S, Pastorin L, et al. Growth velocity monitoring of the efficacy of different therapeutic protocols in a group of thalassaemic children. *Eur J Pediatr* 1995;154:205-8.

6600 Sigurjonsdottir HA, Manhem K, Wallerstedt S. Liquorice-induced hypertension- a linear, dose-response relationship. Endocrine Soc 82nd Ann Mtg, Toronto, CAN, 2000; Jun 21-4:abstract 2279. www.abstracts-on-line.com/abstracts/ENDO/advanced_search/results.asp (Accessed 5 July 2000).

6601 Anon. Roasting process to pump up cancer fighting properties of coffee unveiled by oncology sciences corp. PRNewswire 2000; Jun 30. www.prnewswire.com (Accessed 3 July 2000).

6602 Szmeja Z, Kulczynski B, Sosnowski Z, Konopacki K. [Therapeutic value of flavonoids in Rhinovirus infections]. [Article in Polish]. *Otolaryngol Pol* 1989;43(3):180-4.

6603 Pennell MM. One to two drinks a day may reduce risk of Alzheimer dementia. Reuters Health. www.medscape.com/reuters/prof/2000/07/07.11/20000711epid005.html (Accessed 11 July 2000).

6604 Takahashi J, Kawakatsu K, Wakayama T, Sawaoka H. Elevation of serum theophylline levels by ipriflavone in a patient with chronic obstructive pulmonary disease. *Eur J Clin Pharmacol* 1992;43(2):207-8.

6606 Anon. Therapeutic marijuana use does not increase viral load in AIDS patients. Reuters Health. www.medscape.com/reuters/prof/2000/07/07.14/20000714clin001.html (Accessed 14 July 2000).

6607 Watzl B, Bub A, Blockhaus M, et al. Prolonged tomato juice consumption has no effect on cell-mediated immunity of well-nourished elderly men and women. *J Nutr* 2000;130:1719-23.

6608 Anon. FDA Grants orphan drug designation to Tishcon Corp UbiQGel (Coenzyme Q10). PRNewswire 2000; Jul 25. www.prnewswire.com (Accessed 25 July 2000).

6609 List of Orphan Designations and Approvals. FDA www.fda.gov/orphan/designat/list.htm (Accessed 25 July

2000).

6610 Anon. Court backs Food & Drug Administration's check of cholestin. NewsExcite.com. news.excite.com/news/ap/000723/19/cholesterol-dispute (Accessed 25 July 2000).

6611 Tepel M, van der Giet M, Schwarzfeld C, et al. Prevention of radiographic-contrast-agent-induced reductions in renal function by acetylcysteine. *N Engl J Med* 2000;343(3):180-4.

6612 Galloway GP, Frederick SL, Staggers FE Jr, et al. Gamma-hydroxybutyrate: an emerging drug of abuse that causes physical dependence. *Addiction* 1997;92(1):89-96.

6613 Price G. In-patient detoxification after GHB dependence. *Br J Psychiatry* 2000;177:181.

6614 Murray MT. Encyclopedia of Nutritional Supplements. Rocklin, CA: Prima Health, 1996.

6616 Murray M. Glandular extracts, what you must know. URL: darkwing.uoregon.edu/~sshapiro/Pemphigus/Glandulars.html (Accessed 2 August 2000).

6618 Adrenal cortex extract. www.thewayup.com/products/0076.htm (Accessed 7 August 2000).

6619 Tintera JW. The hypoadrenocortical state and its management. www.fred.net/slowup/tint01.html (Accessed 7 August 2000).

6620 Nationwide alert on hallmark labs injectable adrenal cortex extract. FDA. www.fda.gov/bbs/topics/NEWS/NEW00539.html (Accessed 7 August 2000).

6621 Anon. Aortic Glycosaminoglycans (GAG). Nutr dynamics. www.nutritiondynamics.com/cgi-bin/process.asp?product=Aortic+Glycosaminoglycans+%28GAG%29 (Accessed 02 August 2000).

6622 Heparinoids. Celsus Labs. www.heparin.com/heparinoids.html (Accessed 09 August 2000).

6623 Personal Correspondence. Alan Cardin, Ph.D., Celsus Laboratories, Cincinnnati, OH; 10.Aug.00.

6624 Fowler JF Jr. Systemic contact dermatitis caused by oral chromium picolinate. *Cutis* 2000;65(2):116.

6625 Pérez C, Domínguez E, Canal JR, et al. Hypoglycaemic activity of an aqueous extract from Ficus carica (fig tree) leaves in streptozotocin diabetic rats. Pharmaceutical Biology 2000;38(3):181-6. www.swets.nl/sps/journals/pb3803.html (Accessed 11 August 2000).

6626 Merriam-Webster Medical Dictionary. InteliHealth. www.intelihealth.com/IH/ihtIH/WSIHW000/331/9276.html?k=tnavx408x9276 (Accessed 9 August 2000).

6627 La Marca G, Pumilia G, Martino A. [Effectiveness of mesoglycan topical treatment of leg ulcers in subjects with chronic venous insufficiency]. [Article in Italian]. *Minerva Cardioangiol* 1999;47(9):315-9.

6628 Laurora G, Cesarone MR, Belcaro G, et al. [Control of the progress of arteriosclerosis in high risk subjects treated with mesoglycan. Measuring the intima media]. [Article in Italian]. *Minerva Cardioangiol* 1998;46(3):41-7.

6629 Raso AM, Maggio D, Trogolo M, et al. [Effectiveness of mesoglycan therapy in patients with ischemia of the lower limbs. Preliminary results of a new therapeutic protocol]. [Article in Italian]. *Minerva Cardioangiol* 1997;45(7-8):383-92.

6630 Scondotto G, Catena G, Aloisi D. [Use of mesoglycan in venous pathology]. [Article in Italian]. *Minerva Med* 1997;88(12):537-41.

6631 Blardi P, Messa G, Puccetti L, et al. [Effects on the coagulation-fibrinolysis system of a single oral dose of mesoglycan at the beginning and at the end of a prolonged treatment in man]. [Article in Italian]. *Recenti Prog Med* 1995;86(7-8):282-9.

6632 Lightdale JR, Hayer C, Duer A, et al. Effects of intravenous secretin on language and behavior of children with autism and gastrointestinal symptoms: a single-blinded, open-label pilot study. *Pediatrics* 2001 Nov;108(5):90.

6633 Vecchio F, Zanchin G, Maggioni F, et al. Mesoglycan in treatment of patients with cerebral ischemia: effects on hemorheologic and hematochemical parameters. *Acta Neurol (Napoli)* 1993;15(6):449-56.

6634 Lotti T, Celasco G, Tsampau D, et al. Mesoglycan treatment restores defective fibrinolytic potential in cutaneous necrotizing venulitis. *Int J Dermatol* 1993;32(5):368-71.

6635 Ambrosio LA, Marchese G, Filippo A, et al. The effect of mesoglycan in patients with cerebrovascular disease: a psychometric evaluation. *J Int Med Res* 1993;21(3):138-46.

6636 Schneider CK, Melmed RD, Martin CL, et al. Synthetic human secretin in the treatment of pervasive developmental disorders. World Congress of Pediatric Gastroenterol, Hepatol & Nutr. Boston, MA:2000; Aug 5-9:abstract 683. www.abstracts-on-line.com/abstracts/WCP/advanced_search/results.asp (Accessed 10 August 2000).

6637 Orlandi G, Viapiano F, Massetani R, et al. Clinical-instrumental evaluation of the effects of mesoglycan sulphate in chronic vascular encephalopathy. *Acta Neurol (Napoli)* 1991;13(3):255-60.

6638 Agrati AM, De Bartolo G, Palmieri G. [Heparan sulfate: efficacy and safety in patients with chronic venous insufficiency]. [Article in Italian]. *Minerva Cardioangiol* 1991;39(10):395-400.

6639 Abate G, Berenga A, Caione F, et al. [Controlled multicenter study on the therapeutic effectiveness of mesoglycan in patients with cerebrovascular disease]. [Article in Italian]. *Minerva Med* 1991;82(3):101-5.

6640 Prandoni P, Cattelan AM, Carta M. [Long-term sequelae of deep venous thrombosis of the legs. Experience with mesoglycan]. [Article in Italian]. *Ann Ital Med Int* 1989;4(4):378-85.

6641 Cazzato G, Zorzon M, Mase G, et al. [Mesoglycan in acute focal cerebral ischemia]. [Article in Italian]. *Riv Neurol* 1989;59(3):121-6.

6642 Vittoria A, Messa GL, Frigerio C, et al. Effect of a single dose of mesoglycan on the human fibrinolytic system, and the profibrinolytic action of nine daily doses. *Int J Tissue React* 1988;10(4):261-6.

6643 Andreozzi GM, Signorelli S, Lo Duca S, et al. Effects of mesoglycan sulfate on the arterial elastic module. *Angiology* 1987;38(8):593-600.

6644 Petruzzellis V, Velon A. [Therapeutic action of oral mesoglycan in the pharmacologic treatment of the varicose syndrome and its complications]. [Article in Italian]. *Minerva Med* 1985;76(12):543-8.

6645 Scondotto G, De Fabritiis A, Guastarobba A, et al. [Use of a minor fibrinolytic drug (mesoglycan) in phlebitis]. [Article in Italian] *Minerva Med* 1984;75(28-29):1733-8.

6646 Postiglione A, De Simone B, Rubba P, et al. Effect of oral mesoglycan on plasma lipoprotein concentration and on lipoprotein lipase activity in primary hyperlipoproteinemia. *Pharmacol Res Commun*

1984;16(1):1-8.

6647 Anon. Liver concentrate. Nutr Dynamics www.nutritiondynamics.com/cgi-bin/ (Accessed 2 August 2000).

6648 Aqeuous liver extract. www.thewayup.com/products/ 0158.htm (Accessed 11 August 2000).

6649 Liver extract. www.healthtalk.net/nutritionprofiles/ liver.asp (Accessed 11 August 2000).

6650 Fukuda Y, Sawata M, Washizuka M, et al. [Effect of liver hydrolysate on hepatic proliferation in regenerating rat liver]. [Article in Japanese]. *Nippon Yakurigaku Zasshi* 1999;114(4):233-8.

6651 Betz JM. Guidance for industry: labeling for dietary supplement products containing St. John's wort and saw palmetto. American Herbal Products Association, August 2000.

6652 Brown BT. Treating cancer with coffee enemas and diet. *JAMA* 1993;269:1635-6.

6653 Gerson M. The cure of advanced cancer by diet therapy: a summary of 30 years of clinical experimentation. *Physiol Chem & Physics* 1978;10:449-64.

6654 Wagner SL. Fatal asthma in a child after use of an animal shampoo containing pyrethrin. *West J Med* 2000;173(2):86-7.

6655 Carl W, Emrich LS. Management of oral mucositis during local radiation and systemic chemotherapy: a study of 98 patients. *J Prosthet Dent* 1991;66(3):361-9.

6656 Fidler P, Loprinzi CL, O'Fallon JR, et al. Prospective evaluation of a chamomile mouthwash for prevention of 5-FU-induced oral mucositis. *Cancer* 1996;77(3):522-5.

6657 Rostler S. Spoonful of cinnamon may help insulin go into cells. Reuters Health. www.reutershealth.com/ frame2/eline.html (Accessed 25 August 2000).

6659 Tuftsin. The On-line Medical Dictionary: www.graylab.ac.uk/cgi-bin/omd?query-Tuftsin&action=Search+OMD (Accessed 29 August 2000).

6660 Fridkin M, Najjar VA. Tuftsin: its chemistry, biology, and clinical potential. *Crit Rev Biochem Mol Biol* 1989;24(1):1-40.

6661 Volk HD, Eckert R, Diamantstein T, Schmitz H. [Immunorestitutive action of hydrolysates and ultrafiltrates of bovine spleen]. [Article in German]. *Arzneimittelforschung* 1991;41(12):1281-5.

6662 Corazza GR, Zoli G, Ginaldi L, et al. Tuftsin deficiency in AIDS. *Lancet* 1991;337(8732):12-3.

6663 Anon. Coffee drinking may damage blood vessels. Reuters Health. www.medscape.com/reuters/prof/2000/ 08/08.31/20000831clin018.html (Accessed 31 August 2000).

6665 Babal K. Thymic protein may enhance immunity. URL: people.we.mediaone.net/nutraceuticals/TPA.HTM (Accessed 2 August 2000).

6666 Weil A. Glandular extracts for hepatitis C? Ask Dr. Weil. www.pathfinder.com/drweil/archiveqa/ 0,2283,1538,00.html (Accessed 2 August 2000).

6667 Anon. Folic acid may help prevent second heart attack. Reuters Health. www.reutershealth.com/frame2/ eline.html (Accessed 5 September 2000).

6668 Anon. FDA authorizes new coronary heart disease health claim for plant sterol and plant stanol esters. FDA. www.fda.gov/bbs/topics/ANSWERS/ ANS01033.html (Accessed 7 September 2000).

6669 Anon. FDA takes action against firms marketing unapproved drugs. FDA. www.fda.gov/bbs/topics/

ANSWERS/ANS01032.html (Accessed 7 September 2000).

6670 Anon. Vitamin E can relieve sleep disorder that affects millions, medical specialists report. PR Newswire. www.prnewswire.com (Accessed 7 September 2000).

6671 Anon. New tomato has more antioxidant, longer shelf life. Reuters Health. www.reutershealth.com/frame2/ eline.html (Accessed 8 September 2000).

6672 Anon. Postscript on laetrile. FDA. www.fda.gov/bbs/ topics/ANSWERS/ANS00309.html (Accessed 8 September 2000).

6673 Anon. Laetrile (Amygdalin, other Names). FDA . www.fda.gov/ora/fiars/ora_import_ia6201.html (Accessed 8 September 2000).

6675 Anon. FDA warns against consuming dietary supplements containing tiratricol. FDA. www.fda.gov/ bbs/topics/ANSWERS/ANS01057.html (Accessed 22 November 2000).

6677 Skotnicki AB. Therapeutic application of calf thymus extract (TFX). *Med Oncol Tumor Pharmacother* 1989;6(1):31-43.

6678 Aiuti F, Sirianni MC, Fiorilli M, Paganelli R, et al. A placebo-controlled trial of thymic hormone treatment of recurrent herpes simplex labialis infection in immunodeficient host: results after a 1-year follow-up. *Clin Immunol Immunopathol* 1984;30(1):11-8.

6679 De Martino M, Rossi ME, Muccioli AT, Vierucci A. T lymphocytes in children with recurrent respiratory infections: effect of the use of thymostimulin on the alterations of T-cell subsets. *Int J Tissue React* 1984;6(3):223-8.

6680 Iaffaioli RV, Frasci G, Tortora G, et al. Effect of thymic extract thymostimulin on the incidence of infections and myelotoxicity during adjuvant chemotherapy for breast cancer. *Thymus* 1988-89;12(2):69-75.

6681 Banos V, Gomez J, Garcia A, et al. Effectiveness of immunomodulating treatment (thymostimulin) in chronic obstructive pulmonary disease. *Respiration* 1997;64(3):220-3.

6682 Lin CY, Hsu HC, Chen CL, Shen EY. Treatment of combined immunodeficiency with thymic extract (Thymostimulin). *Ann Allergy* 1987;58(5):379-84.

6683 Lin CY, Hsu CH, Liu KC, et al. Serial immunologic and histopathologic studies in the treatment of necrotizing fasciitis with combined immunodeficiency by a bovine thymic extract (thymostimulin). *J Pediatr Surg* 1986;21(11):1000-4.

6684 De Mattia D, Decandia P, Ferrante P, et al. Effectiveness of thymostimulin and study of lymphocyte-dependent antibacterial activity in children with recurrent respiratory infections. *Immunopharmacol Immunotoxicol* 1993;15(4):447-59.

6685 Aiuti F, Ammirati P, Fiorilli M, et al. Immunologic and clinical investigation on a bovine thymic extract. Therapeutic applications in primary immunoedificiencies. *Pediatr Res* 1979;13(7):797-802.

6686 Hegarty JE, Nouri Aria KT, Eddleston AL, Williams R. Controlled trial of a thymic hormone extract (Thymostimulin) in autoimmune chronic active hepatitis. *Gut* 1984;25(3):279-83.

6687 Kenady DE, Chretien PB, Potvin C, Simon RM. Thymosin reconstitution of T-cell deficits in vitro in cancer patients. *Cancer* 1977;39(2):575-80.

6688 Armerding D, Katz DH. Activation of T and B lymphocytes in vitro. IV. Regulatory influence on

REFERENCES

specific T cell functions by a thymus extract factor. *J Immunol* 1975;114(4):1248-54.

6689 Kouttab NM, Prada M, Cazzola P. Thymomodulin: biological properties and clinical applications. *Med Oncol Tumor Pharmacother* 1989;6(1):5-9.

6690 Burger O, Ofek I, Tabak M, et al. A high molecular mass constituent of cranberry juice inhibits helicobacter pylori adhesion to human gastric mucus. *FEMS Immunol Med Microbiol* 2000 Dec;29(4):295-301.

6691 Calsini P, Mocchegiani E, Fabris N. The pharmacodynamics of thymomodulin in elderly humans. *Drugs Exp Clin Res* 1985;11(9):671-4.

6692 James JS. Thymomodulin warning. AIDS Treatment News. Issue 203. www.immunet.org/immunet/atn.nsf/page/a-203-02. (Accessed 2 August 2000).

6693 Anon. Can vitamin E supplementation forestall muscle-damaging effects of a single bout of resistance training? Amer Physiological Soc press release. www.faseb.org/aps/meetings/mtg_pressrel6.htm (Accessed 26 September 2000).

6694 Genova R, Guerra A. [A thymus extract (thymomodulin) in the prevention of childhood asthma]. [Article in Italian]. *Pediatr Med Chir* 1983;5(5):395-402.

6695 Bagnato A, Brovedani P, Comina P, et al. Long-term treatment with thymomodulin reduces airway hyperresponsiveness to methacholine. *Ann Allergy* 1989;62(5):425-8.

6696 Maiorano V, Chianese R, Fumarulo R, et al. Thymomodulin increases the depressed production of superoxide anion by alveolar macrophages in patients with chronic bronchitis. *Int J Tissue React* 1989;11(1):21-5.

6697 Fiocchi A, Borella E, Riva E, et al. A double-blind clinical trial for the evaluation of the therapeutical effectiveness of a calf thymus derivative (Thymomodulin) in children with recurrent respiratory infections. *Thymus* 1986;8(6):331-9.

6698 Longo F, Lepore L, Agosti E, Panizon F. [Evaluation of the effectiveness of thymomodulin in children with recurrent respiratory infections]. [Article in Italian]. *Pediatr Med Chir* 1988;10(6):603-7.

6699 Galli L, de Martino M, Azzari C, et al. [Preventive effect of thymomodulin in recurrent respiratory infections in children]. [Article in Italian]. *Pediatr Med Chir* 1990;12(3):229-32.

6700 Douglas RM, Miles HB, Moore BW, et al. Failure of effervescent zinc acetate lozenges to alter the course of upper respiratory tract infections in Australian adults. *Antimicrob Agents Chemother* 1987;31:1263-5.

6703 Prasad AS, Fitzgerald JT, Bao B, et al. Duration of symptoms and plasma cytokine levels in patients with the common cold treated with zinc acetate. A randomized, double-blind, placebo-controlled trial. *Ann Intern Med* 2000;133:245-52.

6705 Petrus EJ, Lawson KA, Bucci LR, Blum K. Randomized, double-masked, placebo-controlled clinical study of the effectiveness of zinc acetate lozenges on common cold symptoms in allergy-tested subjects. *Curr Ther Res* 1998;59:595-607.

6706 Desbiens NA. Lessons learned from attempts to establish the blind in placebo-controlled trials of zinc for the common cold. *Ann Intern Med* 2000;133:302-3.

6708 Antoniou LD, Shalhoub RJ, Sudhakar T, Smith JC Jr. Reversal of uraemic impotence by zinc. *Lancet* 1977;2:895-8.

6709 Berbari P, Thibodeau A, Germain L, et al Antiangiogenic effects of the oral administration of liquid cartilage extract in humans. *J Surg Res* 1999;87:108-13.

6711 Pittler MH, Vogler BK, Ernst E. Feverfew for preventing migraine. *Cochrane Database Syst Rev* 2000;(3):CD002286.

6712 Brun J, Claustrat B, Saddier P, Chazot G. Nocturnal melatonin excretion is decreased in patients with migraine without aura attacks associated with menses. *Cephalalgia* 1995;15:136-9.

6713 Pugh WJ, Sambo K. Prostaglandin synthetase inhibitors in feverfew. *J Pharm Pmarmacol* 1988;40:743-5.

6714 Natl Cancer Institute CancerNet. Cartilage website: www.cancernet.nci.nih.gov/cam/cartilage.htm (Accessed 18 August 2000).

6715 Natl Institute of Health. Clinical Trials.URL: http://clinicaltrials.gov/ct/gui/c/r (Accessed 19 August 2000).

6716 Leitner SP, Rothkopf MM, Haverstick L, et al. Two phase II studies of oral dry shark cartilage powder (SCP) in patients (pts) with either metastatic breast or prostate cancer refractory to standard treatment. Proceedings of Amer Soc Clinical Oncol 1998;17:A240. www.asco.org/prof/me/html/98abstracts/asc/m_240.htm (Accessed 19 August 2000).

6717 Rosenbluth RJ, Jennis AA, Cantwell S, DeVries J. Oral shark cartilage in the treatment of patients with advanced primary brain tumors. A phase II pilot study. Proceedings of Amer Soc Clinical Oncol 1999;18:A554. www.asco.org/prof/me/html/99abstracts/cns/m_554.htm (Accessed 19 August 2000).

6718 Evans WK, Latreille J, Batist G, et al. AE-941, an inhibitor of angiogenesis: rationale for development in combination with induction chemotherapy/radiotherapy in patients with non small cell lung cancer (NSCLC). Proceedings of Amer Soc of Clinical Oncol 1999;18:A1938. www.asco.org/prof/me/html/99abstracts/luc/m_1938.htm (Accessed 19 August 2000).

6719 Patnaik A, Rowinsky E, Hammond L, et al. A phase I and pharmacokinetic (PK) study of the unique angiogenesis inhibitor, squalamine lactate (MSI-1256F). Proceedings of Amer Soc of Clinical Oncol 1999;18:A622. www.asco.org/prof/me/html/99abstracts/cp/m_622.htm (Accessed 19 August 2000).

6720 Kalidas M, Hammond LA, Patnaik P, et al. A phase I and pharmacokinetic (PK) study of the angiogenesis inhibitor, squalamine lactate (MSI-1256F). Proceedings of Amer Soc of Clinical Oncol 2000;19:A698. www.asco.org/prof/me/html/00abstracts/cp/m_698.htm (Accessed 19 August 2000).

6721 Bhargava P, Trocky N, Marshall J, et al. A phase I safety, tolerance and pharmacokinetic study of rising dose, rising duration continuous infusion of MSI-1256F (Squalamine Lactate) in patients with advanced cancer. Proceedings of Amer Soc Clinical Oncol 1999;18:A698. www.asco.org/prof/me/html/99abstracts/cp/m_623.htm (Accessed 19 August 2000).

6722 Mathews J. Media feeds frenzy over shark cartilage as cancer treatment. *J Natl Cancer Inst* 1993;85:1190-1.

6723 Gomes EM, Souto PR, Felzenszwalb I. Shark-cartilage containing preparation protects cells against hydrogen peroxide induced damage and mutagenesis. *Mutat Res* 1996;367:204-8.

6724 Fontenele JB, Araujo GB, de Alencar JW, Viana GS. The analgesic and anti-inflammatory effects of shark cartilage are due to a peptide molecule and are nitric oxide (NO) system dependent. *Biol Pharm Bull* 1997;20:1151-4.

6725 Fontenele JB, Viana GS, Xavier-Filho J, de-Alencar JW. Anti-inflammatory and analgesic activity of a water-soluble fraction from shark cartilage. *Braz J Med Biol Res* 1996;29:643-6.

6726 Sheu JR, Fu CC, Tsai ML, Chung WJ. Effect of U-995, a potent shark cartilage-derived angiogenesis inhibitor, on anti-angiogenesis and anti-tumor activities. *Anticancer Res* 1998;18:4435-41.

6727 Anon. AEterna announces the commencement of patient enrollment for the NIH - sponsored phase III clinical trial of AE-941/Neovastat in the treatment of lung cancer. Aeterna 2000 News Release 2000 May 17. http://micro.newswire.ca/releases/May2000/17/c5760.html/11884-0 (Accessed 19 August 2000).

6728 HerbSense. Essential herbs. www.herbsense.com/goodherbs.html (Accessed 22 August 2000).

6729 Herb.com. Herbal Materia Medica 4.0 website. URL: http://herb.com/materia.htm (Accessed 22 August 2000).

6730 Moore M. Specific indications for herbs in general use. Southwest School of Botanical Med. http://chili.rt66.com/hrbmoore/ManualsMM/SpecIndic3.txt htm (Accessed 22 August 2000).

6731 MotherNature.com. Consumer guide to OSHA. www.mothernature.com/cg/osha.asp (Accessed 22 August 2000).

6732 Herbnet. Herbnet Magazine. www.herbnet.com/magazine/mag0004_p02.htm (Accessed 22 August 2000).

6733 Colorado State Univ. Colorado AES project COL00271. 1999-2000 website. www.colostate.edu/depts/aes/projs/271.htm (Accessed 22 August 2000).

6734 Coulombe RA. Improve food safety through discovery and control of natural and induced toxicants and antitoxicants. Fedrip database, Natl Technical Info Svc (Ntis). Fedrip/1999/07801368.

6735 United Plant Savers. United Plant Savers at risk forum website. www.plantsavers.org/endanger2.html (Accessed 5 August 2000).

6736 Beck JJ, Stermitz FR. Addition of methyl thioglycolate and benzylamine to (Z)-ligustilide, a bioactive unsaturated lactone constituent of several herbal medicines. An improved synthesis of (Z)-ligustilide. *J Nat Prod* 1995;58:1047-55.

6737 Appelt GD. Pharmacological aspects of selected herbs employed in Hispanic folk medicine in the San Luis Valley of Colorado, USA: I. Ligusticum porteri (osha) and Matricaria chamomilla (manzanilla). *J Ethnopharmacol* 1985;13:51-5.

6738 American Botanical Council. Peppermint website. www.herbalgram.org/catalog/thirdparty/peppermint.html (Accessed 7 September 2000).

6739 Sparks MJ, O'Sullivan P, Herrington AA, Morcos SK. Does peppermint oil relieve spasm during barium enema? *Br J Radiol* 1995;68:841-3.

6740 Madisch A, Heydenreich CJ, Wieland V, et al. Treatment of functional dyspepsia with a fixed peppermint oil and caraway oil combination preparation as compared to cisapride. A multicenter, reference-controlled, double-blind equivalence study. *Arzneimittelforschung* 1999;49:925-32.

6741 May B, Kuntz HD, Kieser M, Kohler S. Efficacy of a fixed peppermint oil/caraway oil combination in non-ulcer dyspepsia. *Arzneimittelforschung* 1996;46:1149-53.

6742 Micklefield GH, Greving I, May B. Effects of peppermint oil and caraway oil on gastroduodenal motility. *Phytother Res* 2000;14:20-3.

6743 Morton CA, Garioch J, Todd P, et al. Contact sensitivity to menthol and peppermint in patients with intra-oral symptoms. *Contact Dermatitis* 1995;32:281-4.

6744 Beesley A, Hardcastle J, Hardcastle PT, Taylor CJ. Influence of peppermint oil on absorptive and secretory processes in rat small intestine. *Gut* 1996;39:214-9.

6745 Shwaireb MH. Caraway oil inhibits skin tumors in female BALB/c mice. *Nutr Cancer* 1993;19:321-5.

6746 Herb Info Canada. Caraway website. www.herb.plant.org/caraway.htm (Accessed 11 September 2000).

6747 FDA. EAFUS: A food additive database website. URL: http://vm.cfsan.fda.gov/~dms/eafus.html (Accessed 11 September 2000).

6748 Purdue Guide to Medicinal and Aromatic Plants, caraway website. www.hort.purdue.edu/newcrop/med-aro/factsheets/caraway.html (Accessed 11 September 2000).

6749 Leicester RJ, Hunt RH. Peppermint oil to reduce colonic spasm during endoscopy. *Lancet* 1982;2:989.

6750 Champault G, Patel JC, Bonnard AM. A double-blind trial of an extract of the plant Serenoa repens in benign prostatic hyperplasia. *Br J Clin Pharmacol* 1984;18:461-2.

6751 Braeckman J. The extract of serenoa repens in the treatment of benign prostatic hyperplasia: a multicenter open study. *Curr Ther Res* 1994;55:776-85.

6752 Reece-Smith H, Memon A, Smart CJ, Dewbury K. The value of permixon in benign prostatic hypertrophy. *Br J Urol* 1986;58:36-40.

6753 Lee YL, Owens J, Thrupp L, Cesario TC. Does cranberry juice have antibacterial activity? *JAMA* 2000;283:1691.

6754 Pedersen CB, Kyle J, Jenkinson AM, et al. Effects of blueberry and cranberry juice consumption on the plasma antioxidant capacity of healthy female volunteers. *Eur J Clin Nutr* 2000;54:405-8.

6755 Foo LY, Lu Y, Howell AB, Vorsa N. The structure of cranberry proanthocyanidins which inhibit adherence of uropathogenic P-fimbriated Escherichia coli in vitro. *Phytochemistry* 2000;54:173-81.

6756 Jepson RG, Mihaljevic L, Craig J. Cranberries for preventing urinary tract infections (Cochrane Review). In: The Cochrane Library 2000(3). Oxford: Update software.

6757 Ofek I, Goldhar J, Zafriri D, et al. Anti-Escherichia coli adhesin activity of cranberry and blueberry juices. *N Engl J Med.* 1991;324:1599.

6758 Haverkorn MJ; Mandigers J. Reduction of bacteriuria and pyuria using cranberry juice. *JAMA* 1994;272:590.

6759 Foda MMR, Middlebrook PF, Gatfield CT, et al. Efficacy of cranberry in prevention of urinary tract infection in a susceptible pediatric population. *Can J Urol* 1995;2:98-102.

6760 Walker EB, Barney DP, Mickelsen JN, et al. Cranberry concentrate: UTI prophylaxis. *J Fam Pract* 1997;45:167-8.

6761 Kontiokari T, Nuutinen M, Sundqvist K, et al. Cranberry-lingonberry juice and Lactobacillus GG drink for the prevention of urinary tract infections in women.

Abstract Poster Presentations, 38th Infectious Dis Soc of Am Mtg, 2000:Poster 179.

6762 Wilt T, Ishani A, Stark G, et al. Serenoa repens for benign prostatic hyperplasia (Cochrane Review). In: The Cochrane Library, Issue 3, 2000. Oxford: Update Software.

6763 Sokeland J. Combined sabal and urtica extract compared with finasteride in men with benign prostatic hyperplasia: analysis of prostate volume and therapeutic outcome. BJU Int 2000;86:439-42.

6764 Boyle P, Robertson C, Lowe F, Roehrborn C. Meta-analysis of clinical trials of permixon in the treatment of symptomatic benign prostatic hyperplasia. Urology 2000;55:533-9.

6765 Di Silverio F, Monti S, Sciarra A, et al. Effects of long-term treatment with Serenoa repens (Permixon) on the concentrations and regional distribution of androgens and epidermal growth factor in benign prostatic hyperplasia. Prostate 1998;37:77-83.

6766 Di Silverio F, D'Eramo G, Lubrano C, et al. Evidence that Serenoa repens extract displays an antiestrogenic activity in prostatic tissue of benign prostatic hypertrophy patients. Eur Urol 1992;21:309-14.

6767 Calabrese C, Berman SH, Babish JG, et al. A phase I trial of andrographolide in HIV positive patients and normal volunteers. Phytother Res 2000;14:333-8.

6769 Levin RM, Das AK. A scientific basis for the therapeutic effects of Pygeum africanum and Serenoa repens. Urol Res 2000;28:201-9.

6770 Bayne CW, Ross M, Donnelly F, Habib FK. The selectivity and specificity of the actions of the lipido-sterolic extract of serenoa repens (permixon) on the prostate. J Urol 2000;164:876-81.

6771 Strauch G, Perles P, Vergult G, et al. Comparison of finasteride (Proscar) and Serenoa repens (Permixon) in the inhibition of 5-alpha reductase in healthy male volunteers. Eur Urol 1994;26:247-52.

6772 Stepanov VN, Siniakova LA, Sarrazin B, Raynaud JP. Efficacy and tolerability of the lipidosterolic extract of Serenoa repens (Permixon) in benign prostatic hyperplasia: a double-blind comparison of two dosage regimens. Adv Ther 1999;16:231-41.

6773 Bayne CW, Donnelly F, Ross M, Habib FK. Serenoa repens (Permixon): a 5 alpha-reductase types I and II inhibitor-new evidence in a coculture model of BPH. Prostate 1999;40:232-41.

6774 Sokeland J, Albrecht J. [Combination of Sabal and Urtica extract vs. finasteride in benign prostatic hyperplasia (Aiken stages I to II). Comparison of therapeutic effectiveness in a one year double-blind study]. [Article in German]. Urologe A 1997;36:327-33.

6775 Grasso M, Montesano A, Buonaguidi A, et al. Comparative effects of alfuzosin versus Serenoa repens in the treatment of symptomatic benign prostatic hyperplasia. Arch Esp Urol 1995;48:97-103.

6776 Adriazola-Semino M, Lozano-Ortega JL, Garcia-Cobo E, et al. [Symptomatic treatment of benign hypertrophy of the prostate. Comparative study of prazosin and serenoa repens]. [Article in Spanish]. Arch Esp Urol 1992; 45:211-3.

6777 Carbin BE, Larsson B, Lindahl O. Treatment of benign prostatic hyperplasia with phytosterols. Br J Urol 1990;66:639-41.

6778 Descotes JL, Rambeaud JJ, Deschaseaux P, Faure G. Placebo-controlled evaluation of the efficacy and tolerability of Permixon in benign prostatic hyperplasia after exclusion of placebo responders Clin Drug Invest. 1995; 9:291-7.

6779 Paubert-Braquet M, Mencia Huerta JM, Cousse H, Braquet P. Effect of the lipidic lipidosterolic extract of Serenoa repens (Permixon) on the ionophore A23187-stimulated production of leukotriene B4 (LTB4) from human polymorphonuclear neutrophils. Prostaglandins Leukot Essent Fatty Acids 1997;57:299-304.

6780 Gutierrez M, Garcia de Boto MJ, Cantabrana B, Hidalgo A. Mechanisms involved in the spasmolytic effect of extracts from Sabal serrulata fruit on smooth muscle. Gen Pharmacol 1996;27:171-6.

6781 Roberts KL. A comparison of chilled cabbage leaves and chilled gelpaks in reducing breast engorgement. J Hum Lact 1995;11:17-20.

6782 Roberts KL, Reiter M, Schuster D. A comparison of chilled and room temperature cabbage leaves in treating breast engorgement. J Hum Lact 1995;11:191-4.

6783 Roberts KL, Reiter M, Schuster D. Effects of cabbage leaf extract on breast engorgement. J Hum Lact 1998;14:231-6.

6784 Nikodem VC, Danziger D, Gebka N, et al. Do cabbage leaves prevent breast engorgement? A randomized, controlled study. Birth 1993;20:61-4.

6785 Shifer P. Cabbage leaf enzymes. J Hum Lact 1995;11:264.

6786 Corrieri D. Cabbage leaves: an effective treatment for swollen tissues. J Hum Lact 1992;8:126-7.

6788 Lampe JW, King IB, Li S, et al. Brassica vegetables increase and apiaceous vegetables decrease cytochrome P450 1A2 activity in humans: changes in caffeine metabolite ratios in response to controlled vegetable diets. Carcinogenesis 2000;21:1157-62.

6789 Lust KD, Brown JE, Thomas W. Maternal intake of cruciferous vegetables and other foods and colic symptoms in exclusively breast-fed infants. J Am Diet Assoc 1996;96:46-8.

6790 Stoewsand GS. Bioactive organosulfur phytochemicals in Brassica oleracea vegetables-a review. Food Chem Toxicol 1995;33:537-43.

6791 Isbir T, Yaylim I, Aydin M, et al. The effects of Brassica oleraceae var capitata on epidermal glutathione and lipid peroxides in DMBA-initiated-TPA-promoted mice. Anticancer Res 2000;20:219-24.

6792 van Poppel G, Verhoeven DT, Verhagen H, Goldbohm RA. Brassica vegetables and cancer prevention. Epidemiology and mechanisms. Adv Exp Med Biol 1999;472:159-68.

6793 Yurtsever E, Yardimci KT. The in vivo effect of a Brassica oleracea var. capitata extract on Ehrlich ascites tumors of MUS musculus BALB/C mice. Drug Metabol Drug Interact 1999;15:215-22.

6794 Ballantyne CS, Phillips SM, MacDonald JR, et al. The acute effects of androstenedione supplementation in healthy young males. Can J Appl Physiol 2000;25:68-78.

6795 Brown GA, Vukovich MD, Reifenrath TA, et al. Effects of anabolic precursors on serum testosterone concentrations and adaptations to resistance training in young men. Int J Sport Nutr Exerc Metab 2000;10:340-59.

6796 Weber B, Lewicka S, Deuschle M, et al. Testosterone, androstenedione and dihydrotestosterone concentrations are elevated in female patients with major depression.

Psychoneuroendocrinology 2000;25:765-71.

6797 Douglas AS, Robins SP, Hutchison JD, et al. Carboxylation of osteocalcin in post-menopausal osteoporotic women following vitamin K and D supplementation. *Bone* 1995;17:15-20.

6798 Knapen MH, Hamulyak K, Vermeer C. The effect of vitamin K supplementation on circulating osteocalcin (bone Gla protein) and urinary calcium excretion. *Ann Intern Med* 1989;111:1001-5.

6799 Yonemura K, Kimura M, Miyaji T, Hishida A. Short-term effect of vitamin K administration on prednisolone-induced loss of bone mineral density in patients with chronic glomerulonephritis. *Calcif Tissue Int* 2000;66:123-8.

6800 Bierenbaum ML, Reichstein R, Watkins TR. Reducing atherogenic risk in hyperlipemic humans with flaxseed supplementation: a preliminary report. *J Am Coll Nutr* 1993;12(5):501-4.

6801 Lampe JW, Martini MC, Kurzer MS, et al. Urinary lignan and isoflavonoid excretion in premenopausal women consuming flaxseed powder. *Am J Clin Nutr* 1994;60:122-8.

6802 Clark WF, Parbtani A, Huff MW, et al. Flaxseed: a potential treatment for lupus nephritis. *Kidney Int* 1995;48:475-80.

6803 Cunnane SC, Hamadeh MJ, Liede AC, et al. Nutritional attributes of traditional flaxseed in healthy young adults. *Am J Clin Nutr* 1995;61:62-8.

6804 Merchant RE, Rice CD, Young HF. Dietary Chlorella pyrenoidosa for patients with malignant glioma: effects on immunocompetence, quality of life, and survival. *Phytother Res* 1990;4:220-31.

6805 Thompson LU, Rickard SE, Orcheson LJ, Seidl MM. Flaxseed and its lignan and oil components reduce mammary tumor growth at a late stage of carcinogenesis. *Carcinogenesis* 1996;17(6):1373-6.

6806 Prasad K. Dietary flax seed in prevention of hypercholesterolemic atherosclerosis. *Atherosclerosis* 1997;132:69-76.

6807 Prasad K, Mantha SV, Muir AD, Westcott ND. Reduction of hypercholesterolemic atherosclerosis by CDC-flaxseed with very low alpha-linolenic acid. *Atherosclerosis* 1998;136:367-75.

6808 Jenkins DJ, Kendall CWC, Vidgen E, et al. Health aspects of partially defatted flaxseed, including effects on serum lipids, oxidative measures, and ex vivo androgen and progestin activity: a controlled, crossover trial. *Am J Clin Nutr* 1999;69:395-402.

6809 Alonso L, Marcos ML, Blanco JG, et al. Anaphylaxis caused by linseed (flaxseed) intake. *J Allergy Clin Immunol* 1996;98(2):469-70.

6810 Brouwer IA, Verhoef P, Urgert R. Betaine supplementation and plasma homocysteine in healthy volunteers (letter). *Arch Intern Med* 2000;160(16):2546-7.

6811 Mar MH, Zeisel SH. Betaine in wine: answer to the French paradox? *Med Hypotheses* 1999 Nov;53(5):383-5.

6812 Soderling E, Le Bell A, Kirstila V, Tenovuo J. Betaine-containing toothpaste relieves subjective symptoms of dry mouth. *Acta Odontol Scand* 1998;56(2):65-9.

6813 Barak AJ, Beckenhauer HC, Tuma DJ. Betaine, ethanol, and the liver: a review. *Alcohol* 1996 ;13(4):395-8.

6814 Anon. General information on xylitol; and Makinen KK, History, Safety, and Dental Properties of Xylitol. Leaf Finland website: xylitol. www.xylifresh.com/english/ (Accessed 17 October 2000).

6815 Lee B, Sue D. Xylitol for prevention of dental caries. *DICP* 1989;23:691-2.

6816 Uhari M, Kontiokari T, Koskela M, Niemela M. Xylitol chewing gum in prevention of acute otitis media: double-blind, randomized trial. *BMJ* 1996;313:1180-4.

6817 Uhari M, Kontiokari T, Niemela M. A novel use of xylitol sugar in preventing acute otitis media. *Pediatrics* 1998;102:879-84.

6818 Soderling E, Isokangas P, Pienihakkinen K, Tenovuo J. Influence of maternal xylitol consumption on acquisition of mutans streptococci by infants. *J Dent Res* 2000;79(3):882-7.

6819 Makinen KK. Can the pentitol-hexitol theory explain the clinical observations made with xylitol? *Med Hypotheses* 2000;54:603-13.

6820 Crapo PA. Use of alternative sweeteners in diabetic diet. *Diabetes Care* 1988;11:174-82.

6821 Makinen KK. The rocky road of xylitol to its clinical application. *J Dent Res* 2000;79:1352-5.

6822 Gales MA, Nguyen TM. Sorbitol compared with xylitol in prevention of dental caries. *Ann Pharmacother* 2000;34:98-100.

6823 Gronbaek M, Becker U, Johnasen D, et al. Type of alcohol consumed and mortality from all causes, coronary heart disease, and cancer. *Ann Int Med* 2000;133:411-9.

6824 Galanis DJ, Joseph C, Masaki KH, et al. A longitudinal study of drinking and cognitive performance in elderly Japanese American men: the Honolulu-Asia aging study. *Am J Publ Health* 2000;90:1254-9.

6825 Ganry O, Baudoin C, Fardellone P. Effect of alcohol intake on bone mineral density in elderly women. *Am J Epidemiol* 2000;151:773-80.

6826 Caccetta RA, Croft KD, Beilin LJ, Puddey IB. Ingestion of red wine significantly increases plasma phenolic acid concentrations but does not acutely affect ex vivo lipoprotein oxidizability. *Am J Clin Nutr* 2000;71:67-74.

6827 Cooper HA, Exner DV, Domanski MJ. Light-to-moderate alcohol consumption and prognosis in patients with left ventricular systolic dysfunction. *J Am Coll Cardiol* 2000;35:1753-9.

6828 Durak I, Burak Cimen MY, Buyukkocak S, et al. The effect of red wine on blood antioxidant potential. *Curr Med Res Opin* 1999;15:208-13.

6829 Cervilla JA, Prince M, Joels S, et al. Long-term predictors of cognitive outcome in a cohort of older people with hypertension. *Br J Psychiatry* 2000;177:66-71.

6830 Loob W. Beer, an anticancer potion? www.panix.com/clay/nycbeer/special/hopshealth1.html (Accessed 31 October 2000)

6831 Anon. Bavarian Brewery Technologies website. http://bavarianbrewerytech.com/news/healthy.htm (Accessed 31 October 2000)

6832 Van der Gaag MS, Ubbink JB, Sillanaukee P, et al. Effect of consumption of red wine, spirits, and beer on serum homocysteine. *Lancet* 2000;355:1522.

6833 Arimoto-Kobayashi S, Sugiyama C, Harada N, et al. Inhibitory effects of beer and other alcoholic beverages on mutagenesis and DNA adduct formation induced by several carcinogens. *J Agri Food Chem* 1999;47(1):221-30.

REFERENCES

6834 Berger K, Ajani UA, Kase CS, et al. Light-to-moderate alcohol consumption and risk of stroke among US male physicians. *N Engl J Med* 1999;341(21):1557-64.

6835 Boffetta P, Garfinkel L. Alcohol drinking and mortality among men enrolled in an American Cancer Society prospective study. *Epidemiol* 1990;1(5):342-8.

6836 Feskanich D, Korrick SA, Greenspan SL, et al. Moderate alcohol consumption and bone density among postmenopausal women. *J Womens Health* 1999;8(1):65-73.

6837 Friedman LA, Kimball AW. Coronary heart disease mortality and alcohol consumption in Framingham. *Am J Epidemiol* 1986;124(3):481-9.

6838 Gaziano JM, Buring JE, Breslow JL, et al. Moderate alcohol intake, increased levels of high-density lipoprotein and its subfractions, and decreased risk of myocardial infarction. *N Engl J Med* 1993;329(25):1829-34.

6839 Gorinstein S, Zemser M, Berliner M, et al. Moderate beer consumption and positive biochemical changes in patients with coronary atherosclerosis. *J Intern Med* 1997;242(3):219-24.

6840 Kannel WB, Ellison RC. Alcohol and coronary heart disease: the evidence for a protective effect. *Clin Chim Acta* 1996;246(1-2):59-76.

6841 Langer RD, Criqui MH, Reed DM. Lipoproteins and blood pressure as biological pathways for effect of moderate alcohol consumption on coronary heart disease. *Circ* 1992;85(3):910-5.

6842 Sacco RL, Elkind M, Boden-Albala B, et al. The protective effect of moderate alcohol consumption on ischemic stroke. *JAMA* 1999;281(1):53-60.

6843 Thun MJ, Peto R, Lopez AD, et al. Alcohol consumption and mortality among middle-aged and elderly US adults. *N Engl J Med* 1997;337(24):1705-14.

6844 Swain R, Kaplan-Machlis B. Magnesium for the next millennium. *South Med J* 1999;92:1040-7.

6845 Meyer KA, Kushi LH, Jacobs DR, et al. Carbohydrates, dietary fiber, and incident type 2 diabetes in older women. *Am J Clin Nutr* 2000;71:921-30.

6846 Crosby V, Wilcock A, Corcoran R. The safety and efficacy of a single dose (500 mg or 1 g) of intravenous magnesium sulfate in neuropathic pain poorly responsive to strong opioid analgesics in patients with cancer. *J Pain Symptom Manage* 2000;19:35-9.

6847 Bendich A. The potential for dietary supplements to reduce premenstrual syndrome (PMS) symptoms. *J Am Coll Nutrition* 2000;19:3-12.

6848 Tramer MR, Schneider J, Marti RA, Rifat K. Role of magnesium sulfate in postoperative analgesia. *Anesthesiology* 1996;84:340-7.

6849 Vanpee D, Delgrange E, Gillet JB, Donckier J. Ingestion of antacid tablets (Rennie) and acute confusion. *J Emerg Med* 2000;19:169-71.

6850 Castelo-Branco C, Pons F, Vicente JJ, et al. Preventing postmenopausal bone loss with ossein-hydroxyapatite compounds. Results of a two-year, prospective trial. *J Reprod Med* 1999;44:601-5.

6851 Wolf RL, Cauley JA, Baker CE, et al. Factors associated with calcium absorption efficiency in pre- and perimenopausal women. *Am J Clin Nutr* 2000;72:466-71.

6852 Jorde R, Bonaa KH. Calcium from dairy products, vitamin D intake, and blood pressure: the Tromso study. *Am J Clin Nutr* 2000;71:1530-5.

6853 Dawson-Hughes B, Harris SS, Krall EA, Dallal GE. Effect of withdrawal of calcium and vitamin D supplements on bone mass in elderly men and women. *Am J Clin Nutr* 2000;72:745-50.

6854 Need AG, Horowitz M, Morris HA, Nordin BEC. Vitamin D status: effects on parathyroid hormone and 1,25-dihydroxyvitamin D in postmenopausal women. *Am J Clin Nutr* 2000;71:1577-81.

6855 Gesensway D. Vitamin D. *Ann Int Med* 2000;133:318.

6856 Wortsman J, Matsuoka LY, Chen TC, et al. Decreased bioavailability of vitamin D in obesity. *Am J Clin Nutr* 2000;72:690-3.

6857 Shah M, Salhab N, Patterson D, Seikaly MG. Nutritional rickets still afflict children in north Texas. *Tex Med* 2000;96:64-8.

6858 Liu VJ, Abernathy RP. Chromium and insulin in young subjects with normal glucose tolerance. *Am J Clin Nutr* 1982;35:661-7.

6859 Anderson RA, Polansky MM, Bryden NA, et al. Effects of supplemental chromium on patients with symptoms of reactive hypoglycemia. *Metabolism* 1987;36:351-5.

6860 Trent LK, Thieding-Cancel D. Effects of chromium picolinate on body composition. *J Sports Med Phys Fitness* 1995;35:273-80.

6861 Lukaski HC, Bolonchuk WW, Siders WA, Milne DB. Chromium supplementation and resistance training: effects on body composition, strength, and trace element status of men. *Am J Clin Nutr* 1996;63:954-65.

6862 Hallmark MA, Reynolds TH, DeSouza CA, et al. Effects of chromium and resistive training on muscle strength and body composition. *Med Sci Sports Exerc* 1996;28:139-44.

6863 Stearns DM, Belbruno JJ, Wetterhahn KE. A prediction of chromium (III) accumulation in humans from chromium dietary supplements. *FASEB J* 1995;9:1650-7.

6864 Kaats GR, Blum K, Fisher JA, Adelman JA. Effects of chromium picolinate supplementation on body composition: a randomized, double-masked, placebo-controlled study. *Curr Ther Res* 1996;57:747-56.

6865 Campbell WW, Beard JL, Joseph LJ, et al. Chromium picolinate supplementation and resistive training by older men: effects on iron status and hematologic indexes. *Am J Clin Nutr* 1997;66:944-9.

6866 McCarty MF. Chromium supplementation and iron metabolism (letter). *Am J Clin Nutr* 1997;65(3):890-2.

6867 Anderson RA, Cheng N, Bryden NA, et al. Elevated intakes of supplemental chromium improve glucose and insulin variables in individuals with type 2 diabetes. *Diabetes* 1997;46:1786-91.

6868 Kaats GR, Blum K, Pullin D, et al. A randomized, double-masked, placebo-controlled study of the effects of chromium picolinate supplementation on body composition: a replication and extension of a previous study. *Curr Ther Res* 1998;59:379-88.

6869 Vincent JB. The biochemistry of chromium. *J Nutr* 2000;130:715-8.

6870 Anon. Grapeseed Oil Corp. www.grapeseedoilcorp.com/everything.html (Accessed 14 January 2001).

6871 Mahan LK, Escott-Stump S. Krause's Food, Nutrition, and Diet Therapy. 9th edition. W.B.Saunders Co., Philadelphia, PA, 1996.

6872 Anon. Fish Oil: AHA Scientific Position Statement and Recommendation. American Heart Association website, URL www.americanheart.org/Heart_and_Stroke_A_Z_Guide/fish.html (Accessed 30

January 2001).

6873 Stone NJ. Fish consumption, fish oils, lipids and coronary heart disease. American Heart Association Medical/Scientific Statement. URL www.americanheart.org/Scientific/statements/1996/1102.html (Accessed 30 January 2001).

6874 Yetiv JZ. Clinical applications of fish oils. *JAMA* 1988;260:665-70.

6875 Israel DH, Gorlin R. Fish oils in the prevention of atherosclerosis. *J Am Coll Cardiol* 1992;19:174-85.

6876 Mueller BA, Talbert RL. Biological mechanisms and cardiovascular effects of omega omega-3 fatty acids. *Clin Pharm* 1988;7:795-807.

6877 Darbinyan V, Kteyan A, Panossian A, et al. Rhodiola rosea in stress induced fatigue - a double blind cross-over study of a standardized extract SHR-5 with a repeated low-dose regimen on the mental performance of healthy physicians during night duty. *Phytomedicine* 2000;7(5):365-71.

6878 Force M, Sparks WS, Ronzio RA. Inhibition of enteric parasites by emulsified oil of oregano in vivo. *Phytother Res* 2000;14:213-4.

6879 Anon. Milk thistle: effects on liver disease and cirrhosis and clinical adverse effects. Summary, Evidence Report/Technology Assessment: Number 21, September 2000. Agency for Healthcare Research and Quality, Rockville, MD. URL: www.ahrq.gov/clinic/milktsum.htm. (Accessed 8 January 2001).

6880 Liberto M, Cobrinik D. Growth-factor dependent induction of p21(CIP1) by the green tea polyphenol, epigallocatechin gallate. *Cancer Lett* 2000;154(2):151-61.

6881 Srivastava RC, Husain MM, Hasan SK, Athar M. Green tea polyphenols and tannic acid act as potent inhibitors of phorbol ester-induced nitric oxide generation in rat hepatocytes independent of their antioxidant properties. *Cancer Lett* 2000;153(1-2):1-5.

6882 Kao Y, Hiipakka RA, Liao S. Modulation of obesity by green tea catechin. *Am J Clin Nutr* 2000;72:1232-41.

6883 Booth GL, Wang EE. Preventive health care, 2000 update: screening and management of hyperhomocysteinemia for the prevention of coronary artery disease events. The Canadian Task Force on Preventive Health Care. *CMAJ* 2000;163:21-9

6884 Tremblay R, Bonnardeaux A, Geadah D, et al. Hyperhomocystinemia in hemodialysis patients: effects of 12-month supplementation with hydrosoluble vitamins. *Kidney Int* 2000;58:851-8.

6885 Boyde TRC. Pyridoxine supplements in the carpal tunnel syndrome [Letter]. *BMJ* 1995;311:631.

6886 Mukhtar H, Ahmad N. Tea polyphenols: prevention of cancer and optimizing health. *Am J Clin Nutr* 2000;71:1698S-1702S.

6887 Brinkhaus B, Lindner M, Schuppan D, Hahn EG. Chemical, pharmacological and clinical profile of the east Asian medical plant Centella asiatica. *Phytomedicine* 2000;7(5):427-48.

6888 Camargo CA, Stampfer MJ, Glynn RJ, et al. Moderate alcohol consumption and risk for angina pectoris or myocardial infarction in U.S. male physicians. *Ann Intern Med* 1997;126:372-5.

6889 Pearson TA. What to advise patients about drinking alcohol. The clinician's conundrum. *JAMA* 1994;272:967-8.

6890 Rehm JT, Bondy SJ, Sempos CT, Vuong CV. Alcohol consumption and coronary heart disease morbidity and mortality. *Am J Epidemiol* 1997;146:495-501.

6891 Rimm EB, Chan J, Stampfer MJ, et al. Prospective study of cigarette smoking, alcohol use and the risk of diabetes in men. *Br Med J* 1995;310:555-9.

6892 Goldberg I, Mosca L, Piano MR, Fisher EA. AHA Science Advisory: Wine and your heart: a science advisory for healthcare professionals from the Nutrition Committee, Council on Epidemiology and Prevention, and Council on Cardiovascular Nursing of the American Heart Association. *Circulation* 2001;103:472-5.

6893 Malarcher AM, Giles WH, Croft JB, et al. Alcohol intake, type of beverage, and the risk of cerebral infarction in young women. *Stroke* 2001;32:77-83.

6894 Ridker PM, Vaughan DE, Stampfer MJ, et al. Association of moderate alcohol consumption and plasma concentration of endogenous tissue-type plasminogen activator. *JAMA* 1994;272:929-33.

6895 Nadir A, Reddy D, Van Thiel DH. Cascara-sagrada induced intrahepatic cholestasis causing portal hypertension: case report and review of herbal hepatotoxicity. *Am J Gastroenterol* 2000;95:3634-7.

6896 Feskens EJM, Oomen CM, Hogendoorn E, et al. Arginine intake and 25-year CHD mortality: the seven countries study (letter). *Eur Heart J* 2001;22:611-2.

6897 Ackermann RT, Mulrow CD, Ramirez G, et al. Garlic shows promise for improving some cardiovascular risk factors. *Arch Intern Med* 2001;161:813-24.

6898 Anon. Epidemiological notes and reports: Macuna pruriens-associated pruritus, New Jersey. *MMWR* 1985;34(48):732-3.

6899 Nagashayana N, Sankarankutty P, Nampoothiri MRV, et al. Association of l-DOPA with recovery following Ayurveda medication in Parkinson's Disease. *J Neurol Sci* 2000;176:124-7.

6900 Houang ET, Ahmet Z, Lawrence AG. Successful treatment of four patients with recalcitrant vaginal trichomoniasis with a combination of zinc sulfate douche and metronidazole therapy. *Sex Transm Dis* 1997;24:116-9.

6901 Stromberg HE, Agren MS. Topical zinc oxide treatment improves arterial and venous leg ulcers. *Br J Dermatol* 1984;111:461-8.

6902 Wilkinson EA, Hawke CI. Oral zinc for arterial and venous leg ulcers. *Cochrane Database Syst Rev* 2000;(2):CD001273.

6903 Sandstrom B, Kivisto B, Cederblad A. Absorption of zinc from soy protein meals in humans. *J Nutr* 1987;117:321-7.

6905 Birmingham CL, Goldner EM, Bakan R. Controlled trial of zinc supplementation in anorexia nervosa. *Int J Eat Disord* 1994;15:251-5.

6906 Katz RL, Keen CL, Litt IF, et al. Zinc deficiency in anorexia nervosa. *J Adolesc Health Care* 1987;8:400-6.

6908 Lagiou P, Wuu J, Trichopoulou A, et al. Diet and benign prostatic hyperplasia: a study in Greece. *Urology* 1999;54:284-90.

6909 Zaichick VYe, Sviridova TV, Zaichick SV. Zinc in the human prostate gland: normal, hyperplastic and cancerous. *Int Urol Nephrol* 1997;29:565-74.

6910 Zaichick VY, Sviridova TV, Zaichick SV. Zinc concentration in human prostatic fluid: normal, chronic prostatitis, adenoma and cancer. *Int Urol Nephrol* 1996;28:687-94.

6911 Ewing CI, Gibbs AC, Ashcroft C, David TJ. Failure of

REFERENCES

oral zinc supplementation in atopic eczema. *Eur J Clin Nutr* 1991;45:507-10.

6912 David TJ, Wells FE, Sharpe TC, et al. Serum levels of trace metals in children with atopic eczema. *Br J Dermatol* 1990;122:485-9.

6913 Mulder TP, van der Sluys Veer A, Verspaget HW, et al. Effect of oral zinc supplementation on metallothionein and superoxide dismutase concentrations in patients with inflammatory bowel disease. *J Gastroenterol Hepatol* 1994;9:472-7.

6914 Sjogren A, Floren CH, Nilsson A. Evaluation of zinc status in subjects with Crohn's disease. *J Am Coll Nutr* 1988;7:57-60.

6915 Van de Wal Y, Van der Sluys Veer A, Verspaget HW, et al. Effect of zinc therapy on natural killer cell activity in inflammatory bowel disease. *Aliment Pharmacol Ther* 1993;7:281-6.

6916 Dronfield MW, Malone JD, Langman MJ. Zinc in ulcerative colitis: a therapeutic trial and report on plasma levels. *Gut* 1977;18:33-6.

6917 Naber TH, van den Hamer CJ, Baadenhuysen H, Jansen JB. The value of methods to determine zinc deficiency in patients with Crohn's disease. *Scand J Gastroenterol* 1998;33:514-23.

6918 Relea P, Revilla M, Ripoll E, et al. Zinc, biochemical markers of nutrition, and type I osteoporosis. *Age Ageing* 1995;24:303-7.

6920 Atik OS. Zinc and senile osteoporosis. *J Am Geriatr Soc* 1983;31:790-1.

6921 Paaske PB, Pedersen CB, Kjems G, Sam IL. Zinc in the management of tinnitus. Placebo-controlled trial. *Ann Otol Rhinol Laryngol* 1991;100:647-9.

6923 Allen LH, Rosado JL, Casterline JE, et al. Lack of hemoglobin response to iron supplementation in anemic Mexican preschoolers with multiple micronutrient deficiencies. *Am J Clin Nutr* 2000;71:1485-94.

6924 Mujika I, Padilla S, Ibanez J, et al. Creatine supplementation and sprint performance in soccer players. *Med Sci Sports Exerc* 2000;32:518-25.

6925 Francaux M, Demeure R, Goudemant JF, Poortmans JR. Effect of exogenous creatine supplementation on muscle PCr metabolism. *Int J Sports Med* 2000;21:139-45.

6926 Rico-Sanz J, Mendez Marco MT. Creatine enhances oxygen uptake and performance during alternating intensity exercise. *Med Sci Sports Exerc* 2000;32:379-85.

6927 Rico-Sanz J. Creatine reduces human muscle PCr and pH decrements and P(i) accumulation during low-intensity exercise. *J Appl Physiol* 2000;88:1181-91.

6928 Becque MD, Lochmann JD, Melrose DR. Effects of oral creatine supplementation on muscular strength and body composition. *Med Sci Sports Exerc* 2000;32:654-8.

6929 Willer B, Stucki G, Hoppeler H, et al. Effects of creatine supplementation on muscle weakness in patients with rheumatoid arthritis. *Rheumatology (Oxford)* 2000;39:293-8.

6930 Checking in on creatine: three studies shed light on physiological response to popular supplement. NCAA. 2000 Apr24. www.ncaa.org/news/20000424/active/ 3709n45.html (Accessed 19 July 2000).

6931 Ead RD. Oral zinc sulphate in alopacia areata- a double-blind trial. *Br J Dermatol* 1981;104:483-4.

6932 Camacho FM, Garcia-Hernandez MJ. Zinc aspartate, biotin, and clobetasol propionate in the treatment of alopecia areata in childhood. *Pediatr Dermatol*

1999;16:336-8.

6933 Pattrick M, Heptinstall S, Doherty M. Feverfew in rheumatoid arthritis: a double-blind, placebo-controlled study. *Ann Rheum Dis* 1989;48:547-9.

6934 Anon. Feverfew-a new drug or an old wives' remedy? *Lancet* 1985;1:1084.

6935 Awang DVC. Prescribing therapeutic feverfew [Tancetum pathrnium (L.) Schultz Bip., syn. Chrysanthemumparthenium (L.) Bernh.]. *Int Med* 1998;1:11-3.

6936 Heptinstall S, Groenewegen WA, Spangenberg P, Loesche W. Extracts of feverfew may inhibit platelet behaviour via neutralization of sulphydryl groups. *J Pharm Pharmacol* 1987;39:459-65.

6937 Wong HC. Is feverfew a pharmacologic agent? *CMAJ* 1999;160:21-2.

6938 de Weerdt GJ, Bootsman HPR, Hendriks H. Herbal medicines in migraine prevention. Randomized double-blind, placebo-controlled, crossover trial of a feverfew preparation. *Phytomedicine* 1996;3:225-30.

6939 Sumner H, Salan U, Knight DW, Hoult JR. Inhibition of 5-lipoxygenase and cyclo-oxygenase in leukocytes by feverfew. Involvement of sesquiterpene lactones and other components. *Biochem Pharmacol* 1992;43:2313-20.

6940 Health Canada. Labelling [sic] Standard: feverfew leaf. www.hc-sc.gc.ca/hpd-dgps/therapeut/zfiles/english/ guides/lebel/drug/feverfew_e.html (Accessed 24 July 2000).

6941 Williams CA, Hoult JR, Harborne JB, et al. A biologically active lipophilic flavonol from Tanacetum parthenium. *Phytochemistry* 1995;38:267-70.

6942 Heptinstall S, White A, Williamson L, Mitchell JR. Extracts of feverfew inhibit granule secretion in blood platelets and polymorphonuclear leucocytes. *Lancet* 1985;1:1071-4.

6943 Makheja AN, Bailey JM. A platelet phospholipase inhibitor from the medicinal herb feverfew (Tanacetum parthenium). *Prostaglandins Leukot Med* 1982;8:653-60.

6944 Groenewegen WA, Heptinstall S. A comparison of the effects of an extract of feverfew and parthenolide, a component of feverfew, on human platelet activity in-vitro. *J Pharm Pharmacol* 1990;42:553-7.

6945 Heptinstall S, Groenewegen WA, Spangenberg P, Losche W. Inhibition of platelet behaviour by feverfew: a mechanism of action involving sulphydryl groups. *Folia Haematol Int Mag Klin Morphol Blutforsch* 1988;115:447-9.

6946 Williams CA, Harborne JB, Geiger H, Hoult JR. The flavonoids of Tanacetum parthenium and T. vulgare and their anti-inflammatory properties. *Phytochemistry* 1999;51:417-23.

6947 Jain NK, Kulkarni SK. Antinociceptive and anti-inflammatory effects of Tanacetum parthenium L. extract in mice and rats. J Ethnopharmacol 1999;68:251-9.

6948 Barsby R, Salan U, Knight DW, Hoult JR. Irreversible inhibition of vascular reactivity by feverfew. *Lancet* 1991;338:1015.

6949 Barsby RW, Salan U, Knight DW, Hoult JR. Feverfew and vascular smooth muscle: extracts from fresh and dried plants show opposing pharmacological profiles, dependent upon sesquiterpene lactone content. *Planta Med* 1993;59:20-5.

6950 Barsby RW, Salan U, Knight DW, Hoult JR. Feverfew

extracts and parthenolide irreversibly inhibit vascular responses of the rabbit aorta. *J Pharm Pharmacol* 1992;44:737-40.

6951 Biggs MJ, Johnson ES, Persaud NP, Ratcliffe DM. Platelet aggregation in patients using feverfew for migraine. *Lancet* 1982;2:776.

6953 Makheja AN, Bailey JM. The active principle in feverfew. *Lancet* 1981;2:1054.

6954 Collier HO, Butt NM, McDonald-Gibson WJ, Saeed SA. Extract of feverfew inhibits prostaglandin biosynthesis. *Lancet* 1980;2:922-3.

6955 Heptinstall S, Awang DV, Dawson BA, et al. Parthenolide content and bioactivity of feverfew (Tanacetum parthenium (L.) Schultz-Bip.). Estimation of commercial and authenticated feverfew products. *J Pharm Pharmacol* 1992;44:391-5.

6956 Groenewegen WA, Heptinstall S. Amounts of feverfew in commercial preparations of the herb. *Lancet* 1986;1:44-5.

6957 Ross JJ, Arnason JT, Birnboim HC. Low concentrations of the feverfew component parthenolide inhibit in vitro growth of tumor lines in a cytostatic fashion. *Planta Med* 1999;65:126-9.

6958 Lamminpaa A, Estlander T, Jolanki R, Kanerva L. Occupational allergic contact dermatitis caused by decorative plants. *Contact Dermatitis* 1996;34:330-5.

6959 Johnson ES, Kadam NP, Hylands DM, Hylands PJ. Efficacy of feverfew as prophylactic treatment of migraine. *Br Med J (Clin Res Ed)* 1985;291:569-73.

6960 Murphy JJ, Heptinstall S, Mitchell JR. Randomized, double-blind, placebo-controlled trial of feverfew in migraine prevention. *Lancet* 1988;2:189-92.

6961 Palevitch D, Earon G, Carasso R. Feverfew (tanacetum parthenium) as a prophylactic treatment for migraine- a double-blind, placebo-controlled study. *Phytotherapy Res* 1997;11:508-11.

6962 Anderson D, Jenkinson PC, Dewdney RS, et al. Chromosomal aberrations and sister chromatid exchanges in lymphocytes and urine mutagenicity of migraine patients: a comparison of chronic feverfew users and matched non-users. *Hum Toxicol* 1988;7:145-52.

6964 Waller PC, Ramsay LE. Efficacy of feverfew as prophylactic treatment of migraine. *Br Med J (Clin Res Ed)* 1985;291:1128.

6965 Vogler BK, Pittler MH, Ernst E. Feverfew as a preventive treatment for migraine: a systematic review. *Cephalalgia* 1998;18:704-8.

6966 FDA. EAFUS: A food additive database. URL: http://vm.cfsan.fda.gov/~dms/eafus.html (Accessed 27 July 2000).

6967 Bodybuidling.com. Pinnacle Synephrinol. www.bodybuilding.com/store/pin/syn.html (Accessed 27 July 2000).

6968 Natl Lib of Med. Chem ID. URL: http://130.14.32.45/cgi-bin/VERSION_A/IGM-client?28890+detail+1 (Accessed 3 October 2000).

6969 Calapai G, Firenzuoli F, Saitta A, et al. Antiobesity and cardiovascular toxic effects of Citrus aurantium extracts in the rat: A preliminary report. Fitoterapia 1999;70:586-92.

6970 Sabinsa Corporation. Citrus Aurantium URL: http://sabinsa.com/products/citrus_aurant.htm (Accessed 31 July 2000).

6971 Carnat A, Carnat AP, Fraisse D, Lamaison JL. [Standardization of the sour orange flower and leaf]. [Article in French]. *Ann Pharm Fr* 1999;57:410-4.

6972 Ramadan W, Mourad B, Ibrahim S, Sonbol F. Oil of bitter orange: new topical antifungal agent. *Int J Dermatol* 1996;35:448-9.

6973 Mwaiko GL. Citrus peel oil extracts as mosquito larvae insecticides. *East Afr Med J* 1992;69:223-6.

6974 Satoh Y, Tashiro S, Satoh M, et al. [Studies on the bioactive constituents of Aurantii Fructus Immaturus]. [Article in Japanese]. *Yakugaku Zasshi* 1996;116:244-50.

6975 Huang YT, Wang GF, Chen CF, et al. Fructus aurantii reduced portal pressure in portal hypertensive rats. *Life Sci* 1995;57:2011-20.

6976 Kim DH, Song MJ, Bae EA, Han MJ. Inhibitory effect of herbal medicines on rotavirus infectivity. *Biol Pharm Bull* 2000;23:356-8.

6977 Hernandez L, Munoz RA, Miro G, et al. Use of medicinal plants by ambulatory patients in Puerto Rico. *Am J Hosp* Pharm 1984;41:2060-4.

6978 Zhao XW, Li JX, Zhu ZR, et al. Anti-shock effects of synthetic effective compositions of fructus aurantii immaturus. Experimental study and clinical observation. *Chin Med J (Engl)* 1989;102:91-3.

6979 Keogh AM, Baron DW. Sympathomimetic abuse and coronary artery spasm. *Br Med J* 1985;291:940.

6980 FDA. Special nutritionals adverse event monitoring system. URL: http://vm.cfsan.fda.gov/~dms/aems.html#search (Accessed 31 July 2000).

6981 Quackwatch. Unconventional cancer treatments: dietary treatments. www.quackwatch.com/01QuackeryRelatedTopics/OTA/ota03.html

6982 Nenonen MT, Helve TA, Rauma AL, Hanninen OO. Uncooked, lactobacilli-rich, vegan food and rheumatoid arthritis. *Br J Rheumatol* 1998;37:274-81.

6983 Bargossi AM, Battino M, Gaddi A, et al. Exogenous CoQ10 preserves plasma ubiquinone levels in patients treated with 3-hydroxy-3-methyglutaryl coenzyme A reductase inhibitors. *Int J Clin Lab Res* 1994;24:171-6.

6984 Folkers K, Langsjoen P, Willis R, et al. Lovastatin decreases coenzyme Q levels in humans. *Proc Natl Acad Sci USA* 1990;87:8931-4.

6985 Ghirlanda G, Oradei A, Manto A, et al. Evidence of plasma CoQ10-lowering effect by HMG-CoA reductase inhibitors: a double-blind, placebo-controlled study. *J Clin Pharmacol* 1993;33:226-9.

6986 Mortensen SA, Leth A, Agner E, Rohde M. Dose-related decrease of serum coenzyme Q10 during treatment with HMG-CoA reductase inhibitors. *Mol Aspects Med* 1997;18:S137-S144.

6987 Georgetown Univ Med Ctr. Cytochrome P450 drug interaction table. www.dml.georgetown.edu/depts/pharmacology/davetab.html (Accessed 8 August 2000).

6988 Wang J, Lu A, Chi J. Multicenter clinical trial of the serum lipid-lowering effects of a monascus purpureus (red yeast) rice preparation from traditional Chinese medicine. *Cur Ther Res* 1997;58:964-78.

6989 MedServ Medical News. Dietary supplement lowers cholesterol. www.medserv.dk/health/1999/03/26/story01.htm (Accessed 2 August 2000).

6990 Am Heart Assn. Am Heart Assn meeting report: Chinese condiment cuts blood cholesterol. www.americanheart.org/Whats_News/AHA_News_Releases/03-25-99-chinese.html (Accessed 2 August 2000).

6991 Am Heart Assn. Comment: the Am Heart Assn urges caution on cholestin. www.americanheart.org/ Whats_News/AHA_News_Releases/03-25-99-comment.htm (Accessed 2 August 2000).

6992 OnHealth with WebMD. www.onhealth.com/conditions/in-depth/item/item%2C2414_1_.asp (Accessed 2 August 2000).

6993 Kou W, Lu Z, Guo J. [Effect of xuezhikang on the treatment of primary hyperlipidemia]. [Article in Chinese]. *Chung Hua Nei Ko Tsa Chih* 1997;36:529-31.

6994 US Dept Health, Human Svcs, FDA. Pharmanex, Inc, administrative proceeding, public docket #97P-0441: final decision. www.fda.gov/ohrms/dockets/dockets/97p0441/ans0002.pdf (Accessed 10 August 2000).

6995 Havel R. Dietary supplement or drug? The case of Cholestin. *Am J Clin Nutr* 1000;69:175-6.

6996 Bliznakov EG. More on the Chinese red-yeast-rice supplement and its cholesterol-lowering effect. *Am J Clin Nutr* 2000;71:152-7.

6997 Wigger-Alberti W, Bauer A, Hipler UC, Elsner P. Anaphylaxis due to Monascus purpureus-fermented rice (red yeast rice). *Allergy* 1999;54 (1330-1).

6998 Jacobs KM, Hirsch KA. Psychiatric complications of Ma-huang. *Psychosomatics* 2000;41:58-62.

6999 Federal Trade Comm. FTC action against Lane Laboratories. www.ftc.gov/opa/2000/06/lanelabs.htm (Accessed 10 August 2000).

7000 Greenberg S, Frishman WH. Co-enzyme Q10: a new drug for cardiovascular disease. *J Clin Pharmacol* 1990;30:596-608.

7001 Consumer Lab. www.consumerlab.com/results/coenzymeq10.asp (Accessed 5 June 2001).

7002 Stockley I. Drug Interactions, 4th ed. London, UK: Pharmaceut Press, 1996.

7003 Fetrow CW, Avila JR. Complementary & alternative medicines. Springhouse, PA: Springhouse Corp, 1999.

7005 Locock RA. Capsicum. *Can Pharm J*, 1985; 118: 517-9.

7006 Visudhiphan S, Poolsuppasit S, Piboonnukarintr O, Timliang S. The relationship between high fibrinolytic activity and daily capsicum ingestion in Thais. *Am J Clin Nutr* 1982; 35: 1452-8.

7007 Cordell GA, Araujo OE. Capsaicin: identification, nomenclature, and pharmacotherapy. *Ann Pharmacother* 1993;27:330-6.

7008 Avorn J, Manone M, Gurwitz JH, et al. Reduction of bacteriuria and pyuria after ingestion of cranberry juice. *JAMA* 1994;271:751-4.

7009 Bomser J, Madhavi DL, Singletary K, Smith MAL. In vitro anticancer activity of fruit extracts from Vaccinium species. *Planta Medica* 1996;62:212-6.

7010 Brown D. Herbal Prescriptions for Better Health. Rocklin, CA: Prima Publishing, 1996.

7011 Amann W. [Akne vulgaris und agnus castus (Agnolyt)]. [Article in German]. *Z Allgemeinmed* 1975;14:1645-7.

7012 Du Mee C. Vitex agnus castus. *Aust J Med Herb* 1993;5(3):63-5.

7013 Brown D. Vitex agnus castus clinical monograph. *Qtrly Rev Natural Med* 1994;2(2):111-21.

7014 Wuttke W. Dopaminergic action of extracts of Agnus Castus. *Forschende Komplementarmedizen* 1996;3(6):329-30.

7015 Jarry H, Leonhardt S., Gorkow C, Wuttke W. In vitro prolactin but not LH and FSH release is inhibited by compounds in extracts of Agnus Castus: direct evidence for a dopaminergic principle by the dopamine receptor assay. *Exp Clin Endocrinol* 1994;102:448-54.

7016 Merz P, Gorkow C, Schroder A, et al. The effects of a special Agnus castus extract (BP1095el) on prolactin secretion in healthy male subjects. *Exp Clin Endocrinol Diabetes* 1996;104:447-53.

7020 HP-200 in Parkinson's Disease study group. An alternative medicine treatment for Parkinson's disease: Results of a multicenter clinical trial. *J Alt Comp Med* 1995;1:249-55.

7021 Infante ME, Perez AM, Simao MR, et al. Outbreak of acute toxic psychosis attributed to Mucuna pruriens. *Lancet* 1990;336:1129.

7022 Helbling A, Brander KA, Pichler WJ. Anaphylactic shock after subcutaneous injection of mandragora D3, a homeopathic drug. *J Allergy Clin Immunol* 2000;106 (5 pt 1):989-90.

7023 Dean CE. Prasterone (DHEA) and mania. *Ann Pharmacother* 2000;34:1419-22.

7024 Escher M, et al. Drug Points: hepatitis associated with kava, a herbal remedy for anxiety. *BMJ* 2001;322:139.

7025 Zhang SY, Robertson D. A study of tea tree oil ototoxicity. *Audiol Neurootol* 2000;5:64-8.

7026 Reginster JY, Deroisy R, Rovati LC, et al. Long-term effects of glucosamine sulfate on osteoarthritis progression: a randomized, placebo-controlled trial. *Lancet* 2001;357:251-6.

7027 Piscitelli SC, Burstein AH, Welden N, et al. Garlic supplements decrease saquinavir plasma concentrations [abstract]. 8th Conf on Retroviruses, Opportunistic Infections 2001.

7028 Rayburn K, Martinez R, Escobedo M, et al. Glycemic effects of various species of nopal (Opuntia sp.) in type 2 diabetes mellitus. *Texas J Rural Health* 1998;26(1):68-76.

7029 Malhotra S, Bailey DG, Paine MF, et al. Seville orange juice-felodipine interaction: comparison with dilute grapefruit juice and involvement of furocoumarins. *Clin Pharmacol Ther* 2001;69:14-23.

7030 Gregory PJ. Seizure associated with Ginkgo biloba? *Ann Intern Med* 2001;134:344.

7031 Buck DS, Nidorf DM, Addino JG. Comparison of two topical preparations for the treatment of onychomycosis: Melaleuca alternifolia (Tea Tree) oil and clotrimazole. *J Fam Pract* 1994;38:601-5.

7032 Syed TA, Qureshi ZA, Ali SM, et al. Treatment of toenail onychomycosis with 2% butenafine and 5% Melaleuca alternifolia (tea tree) oil in cream. *Trop Med Int Health* 1999;4:284-7.

7033 Tsubono Y, Nishino Y, Komatsu S, et al. Green tea and the risk of gastric cancer in Japan. *N Eng J Med* 2001;344:632-6.

7034 Sano T, Sasako M. Green tea and gastric cancer. *N Eng J Med* 2001;344:675-6.

7035 Mittman P. Randomized, double-blind study of freeze-dried Urtica dioica in the treatment of allergic rhinitis. *Planta Med* 1990;56:44-7.

7038 McCarty DJ, Csuka M, McCarthy G, et al. Treatment of pain due to fibromyalgia with topical capsaicin: A pilot study. *Semin Arthr Rheum* 1994;23:41-7.

7039 Natl Cancer Inst. Mistletoe (PDQ). CancerNet. www.cancernet.nci.nih.gov/cam/mistletoe.htm#7 (Accessed 30 March 2001).

7040 Lissoni P, Barni S, Mandala M, et al. Decreased toxicity and increased efficacy of cancer chemotherapy using the pineal hormone melatonin in metastatic solic tumor patients with poor clinical status. *Eur J Cancer* 1999;35:1688-92.

7041 Kliukiene J, Tynes T, Andersen A. Risk of breast cancer among Norwegian women with visual impairment. *Br J Cancer* 2001;84:397-9.

7042 Erren TC, Piekarski C. Does winter darkness in the arctic protect against cancer? The melatonin hypothesis revisited. *Med Hypotheses* 1999;53:1-5.

7043 Lissoni P, Barni S, Meregalli S, et al. Modulation of cancer endocrine therapy by melatonin: a phase II study of tamoxifen plus melatonin in metastatic breast cancer patients progressing under tamoxifen alone. *Br J Cancer* 1995;71:854-6.

7044 Kaegi E, et al. Unconventional therapies for cancer: 3. Iscador. *CMAJ* 1998;158:1157-9.

7045 Grossarth-Matichek R, Kiene H, Baumgartner SM, et al. Use of Iscador, an extract of European mistletoe (Viscum album), in cancer treatment: prospective nonrandomized and randomized matched-pair studies nested within a cohort study. *Alt Thera* 2001;7:57-78.

7046 Bailey DG, Dresser GK, Munoz C, et al. Reduction of fexofenadine bioavailability by fruit juices. *Clin Pharmacol Ther* 2001;69:P21.

7047 Sindrup SH, Madsen C, Bach FW, et al. St. John's wort has no effect on pain in polyneuropathy. *Pain* 2000;91:361-5.

7048 Bliddal H, Rosetzky A, Schlichting P, et al. A randomized, placebo-controlled, cross-over study of ginger extracts and ibuprofen in osteoarthritis. *Osteoarth Cartilage* 2000;8:9-12.

7049 Holtmann G, Madisch A, Juergen H, et al. A double-blind, randomized, placebo-controlled trial on the effects of an herbal preparation in patients with functional dyspepsia [Abstract]. Ann Mtg Digestive Disease Week 1999 May.

7050 Fabre N, Urizzi P, Souchard JP, et al. An antioxidant sinapic acid ester isolated from Iberis amara. *Fitoterapia* 2000;71:425-8.

7051 Steimer P. Iberogast therapy in gastroenterology. *Der Krankenhaus Arzt* 1983;56:1005-8.

7052 Roberts W, Weaver L, Brian J, et al. Repeated doses of porcine secretin in the treatment of autism: A randomized, placebo-controlled trial. *Pediatrics* 2001;107:e71.

7053 Mulvihill SJ, Debas HT. Regulatory peptides in the gut. In: Greenspan FS, Strewler GJ, Eds. Basic & Clinical Endocrinology. 5th ed. Stamford, CT: Appleton & Lange, 1997:581.

7054 Jacobson JS, Troxel AB, Evans J, et al. Randomized trial of black cohosh for the treatment of hot flashes among women with a history of breast cancer. *J Clin Oncol* 2001;19:2739-45.

7055 Schellenberg R. Treatment for the premenstrual syndrome with agnus castus fruit extract: prospective, randomized, placebo-controlled study. *Br Med J* 2001;322:134-7.

7056 Gallo M, Sarkar M, Au W, et al. Pregnancy outcome following gestational exposure to echinacea: A prospective controlled study. *Arch Intern Med* 2000;160:3141-3.

7057 Soon SL, Crawford RI. Recurrent erythema nodosum associated with echinacea herbal therapy. *J Am Acad Dermatol* 2001;44:298-9.

7058 Davies S, Howard JM, Hunnisett A, et al. Age-related decreases in chromium levels in 51,665 hair, sweat, and serum samples from 40,872 patients – implications for the prevention of cardiovascular disease and type II diabetes. *Metabolism* 1997;46:469-73.

7059 Melchart D, Linde K, Fischer P, Kaesmayr J. Echinacea for preventing and treating the common cold. *Cochrane Database Syst Rev* 2000;2:CD000530.

7060 Abraham AS, Brooks BA, Eylath U. The effects of chromium supplementation on serum glucose and lipids in patients with and without non-insulin dependent diabetes. *Metabolism* 1992;41:768-771.

7061 Gregory PJ. Minerals for diabetes. *Pharmacist's Letter* 2000;16:160212.

7062 Steben RE, Boudroux P. The effects of pollen and pollen extracts on selected blood factors and performance of athletes. *J Sports Med Phys Fitness* 1978;18:271-8.

7063 Maughan RJ, Evans SP. Effects of pollen extract upon adolescent swimmers. *Br J Sports Med* 1982;16:142-5.

7064 Sur S, Camara M, Buchmeier A, et al. Double-blind trial of pyridoxine (vitamin B6) in the treatment of steroid-dependent asthma. *Ann Allergy* 1993;70:147-52.

7065 Collipp PJ, Goldzier S III, Weiss N, et al. Pyridoxine treatment of childhood bronchial asthma. *Ann Allergy* 1975;35:93-7.

7066 Shimizu T, Maeda S, Mochizuki H, et al. Theophylline attenuates circulating vitamin B6 levels in children with asthma. *Pharmacol* 1994;49:392-7.

7067 FDA. Information paper on L-tryptophan and 5-hydroxy-L-tryptophan. Feb 2001. URL: http://vm.cfsan.fda.gov/~dms/ds-tryp1.html (Accessed 26 June 2001).

7068 Russmann S, Lauterberg BH, Hebling A. Kava hepatotoxicity [letter]. Ann Intern Med 2001;135:68.

7069 Hu X, et al. Antilipemic effect of Gynostemma pentaphyllum in patients. *Fujian Med J* 1988;10:4-6.

7070 Zhou H, et al. Treatment of hyperlipidemia with Gynostemma pentaphyllum jiaogulan. *Hunan Med J* 1991;8:259-60.

7071 Tan H, Liu ZL, Liu MJ. Antithrombotic effect of Gynostemma pentaphyllum. *Zhingguo Zhong Xi Yi Jie He Za Zhi* 1993;13:278-80.

7072 de Lemos ML. Effects of soy phytoestrogens genistein and daidzein on breast cancer growth. *Ann Pharmacother* 2001;35:1118-21.

7073 Massey LK, Palmer RG, Horner HT. Oxalate content of soybean seeds (Glycine max. Leguminosae), soyfoods, and other edible legumes. *J Agric Food Chem* 2001;49:4262-6.

7074 Terris MK, Issa MM, Tacker JR. Dietary supplementation with cranberry concentrate tablets may increase the risk of nephrolithiasis. *Urology* 2001;57:26-9.

7075 Gregory PJ. Does glucosamine increase serum lipid levels and blood pressure? *Pharmacist's Letter* 2001;17:17115.

7076 Lauritzen CH, Reuter HD, Repges R, et al. Treatment of premenstrual tension syndrome with Vitex agnus castus.: Controlled-double blind versus pyridoxine. *Phytomedicine* 1997;4:183-9.

7077 Gerhard II, Patek A, Monga B, et al. Mastodynon for female infertility. *Forsch Komplementarmed* 1998;5:272-8.

7078 Berger D. Schaffner W, Schrader E, et al. Efficacy of Vitex agnus castus L. extract Ze 440 in patients with premenstrual syndrome (PMS). *Arch Gynecol Obstet*

2000;264:150-3.

7079　Loch EG, Selle H, Boblitz N. Treatment of premenstrual syndrome with a phytopharmaceutical formulation containing Vitex agnus castus. *J Womens Health Gend Based Med* 2000;9:315-20.

7080　Shaver K. Potassium iodide for nuclear exposure. *Pharmacist's Letter/Prescriber's Letter* 2001;17:171214.

7081　Zhdanova IV, Wurtman RJ, Regan MM, et al. Melatonin treatment for age-related insomnia. *J Clin Endocrinol Metab* 2001;86:4727-30.

7082　Shamir E, Barak Y, Shalman I, et al. Melatonin treatment for tardive dyskinesia: A double-blind, placebo-controlled, crossover study. *Arch Gen Psychiatry* 2001;58:1049-52.

7083　Backon J. Ginger in preventing nausea and vomiting of pregnancy: a caveat due to its thromboxane synthetase activity and effect on testosterone binding. *Eur J Obstet Gynecol Reprod Biol* 1991;42:163-4.

7084　Altman RD, Marcussen KC. Effects of ginger extract on knee pain in patients with osteoarthritis. *Arthritis Rheum* 2001;44:2531-38.

7085　Marcus DM, Suarez-Almazor ME. Is there a role for ginger in the treatment of osteoarthritis? *Arthritis Rheum* 2001;44:2461-2.

7086　Shaver K. Liver toxicity with kava. *Pharmacist's Letter/Prescriber's Letter* 2001;18:180115.

7087　Vonau B, Chard S, Mandalia S, et al. Does the extract of the plant Echinacea purpurea influence the clinical course of recurrent genital herpes? *Int J STD AIDS* 2001;12:154-8..

7088　Lee SH, Oe T, Blair IA. Vitamin C-induced decomposition of lipid hydroperoxides to endogenous genotoxins. *Science* 2001;292:2083-4.

7089　Beckmann-Knopp S, Rietbrock S, Weyhenmeyer R, et al. Inhibitory effects of silibinin on cytochrome P-450 enzymes in human liver microsomes. *Pharmacol Toxicol* 2000;86:250-6.

7100　Gorman JF. The vitamin C controversy. *Postgrad Med* 1980;67:64,69.

7101　Hemila H. Vitamin C intake and susceptibility to the common cold. *Br J Nutr* 1997;77:59-72.

7102　Gorton HC, Jarvis K. The effectiveness of vitamin C in preventing and relieving the symptoms of virus-induced respiratory infections. *J Manipulative Physiol Ther* 1999;22:530-3.

7103　Plat J, van Onselen EN, van Heugten MM, Mensink RP. Effects on serum lipids, lipoproteins and fat soluble antioxidant concentrations of consumption frequency of margarines and shortenings enriched with plant stanol esters. *Eur J Clin Nutr* 2000;54:671-7.

7104　Hallikainen MA, Sarkkinen ES, Uusitupa MI. Effects of low-fat stanol ester enriched margarines on concentrations of serum carotenoids in subjects with elevated serum cholesterol concentrations. *Eur J Clin Nutr* 1999;53:966-9.

7105　Hallikainen MA, Sarkkinen ES, Gylling H, et al. Comparison of the effects of plant sterol ester and plant stanol ester-enriched margarines in lowering serum cholesterol concentrations in hypercholesterolaemic subjects on a low-fat diet. *Eur J Clin Nutr* 2000;54:715-25.

7106　Huber R, Barth H, Schmitt-Graff A, Klein R. Hypereosinophilia induced by high-dose intratumoral and peritumoral mistletoe application to a patient with pancreatic carcinoma. *J Altern Complement Med*

7107　Buckle J. Use of aromatherapy as a complementary treatment for chronic pain. *Altern Ther Health Med* 1999;5:42-51.

7109　FDA/CFSAN. Office of Special Nutritionals. http://vm.cfsan.fda.gov/cgi-bin/aems.html (Accessed 31 January 2001).

7110　American Health Consultants. Blue Cohosh: a word of caution. www.ahcpub.com/ahc_root_html/hot/archive/atwh1099.html (Accessed 31 January 2001).

7111　May J, Chan CH, King A, et al. Time-kill studies of tea tree oils on clinical isolates. *J Antimicrob Chemother* 2000;45:639-43.

7112　FDA Center for Food Safety and Applied Nutrition. Everything Added to Food in the US (EAFUS) Database. website: http://vm.cfsan.fda.gov/~dms/eafus.html (Accessed 31 January 2001).

7113　Maggioni M, Picotti GB, Bondiolotti GP, et al. Effects of phosphatidylserine therapy in geriatric patients with depressive disorders. *Acta Psychiatr Scand* 1990;81:265-70.

7114　Funfgeld EW, Baggen M, Nedwidek P, et al. Double-blind study with phosphatidylserine (PS) in parkinsonian patients with senile dementia of Alzheimer's type (SDAT). *Prog Clin Biol Res* 1989;317:1235-46.

7115　Blokland A, Honig W, Brouns F, Jolles J. Cognition-enhancing properties of subchronic phosphatidylserine (PS) treatment in middle-aged rats: comparison of bovine cortex PS with egg PS and soybean PS. *Nutrition* 1999;15:778-83.

7116　Pepping J. Phosphatidylserine. *Am J Health-Syst Pharm* 1999;56:2038,2043-4.

7117　Kidd PM. Attention Deficit/Hyperactivity disorder (ADHD) in children: rationale for its integrative management. *Altern Med Rev* 2000;5:402-28.

7118　Amaducci L. Phosphatidylserine in the treatment of Alzheimer's disease: results of a multicenter study. *Psychopharmacol Bull* 1988;24:130-4.

7119　Villardita C, Grioli S, Salmeri G, et al. Multicentre clinical trial of brain phosphatidylserine in elderly patients with intellectual deterioration. *Clin Trials J* 1987;24:84-93.

7120　Palmieri G, Palmieri R, Inzoli MR, et al. Double-blind controlled trial of phosphatidylserine in patients with senile mental deterioration. *Clin Trials J* 1987;24:73-83.

7121　Kidd PM. Phosphatidylserine; Membrane nutrient for memory. A clinical and mechanistic assessment. *Altern Med Rev* 1996;1:70-84.

7122　Chevallier A. Encyclopedia of Herbal Medicine. 2nd ed. New York, NY: DK Publ, Inc., 2000.

7123　Agricultural Research Service. Dr. Duke's phytochemical and ethnobotanical databases. www.ars-grin.gov/cgi-bin/duke/farmacy2.pl?575 (Accessed 31 January 2001).

7124　Cao GW, Yang WG, Du P. [Observation of the effects of LAK/IL-2 therapy combining with Lycium barbarum polysaccharides in the treatment of 75 cancer patients]. [Article in Chinese]. *Chung Hua Chung Liu Tsa Chih* 1994;16:428-31.

7125　Kim SY, Lee EJ, Kim HP, et al. LCC, a cerebroside from lycium chinense, protects primary cultured rat hepatocytes exposed to galactosamine. *Phytother Res* 2000;14:448-51.

7126　Huang KC. The Pharmacology of Chinese Herbs, KC Huang, 2nd ed. Boca Raton, FL: CRC Press,1999.

7127 Das SC, Isichei CO, Okwuasaba FK, et al. Chemical, pathological and toxicological studies of the effects of RICOM-1013-J of Ricinus communis var minor on women volunteers and rodents. *Phytother Res* 2000;14:15-9.

7128 Isichei CO, Das SC, Ogunkeye OO, et al. Preliminary clinical investigation of the contraceptive efficacy and chemical pathological effects of RICOM-1013-J of Ricinus communis var minor on women volunteers. *Phytother Res* 2000;14:40-2.

7129 Rodriguez J, Crespo JF, Lopez-Rubio A, et al. Clinical cross-reactivity among foods of the Rosaceae family. *J Allergy Clin Immunol* 2000;106:183-189.

7130 Price PA. Vitamin K nutrition and postmenopausal osteoporosis. *J Clin Invest* 1993;91:1268.

7131 Weber P. Management of osteoporosis: is there a role for vitamin K? *Int J Vitam Nutr Res* 1997;67:350-356.

7132 Tamatani M, Morimoto S, Nakajima M, et al. Decreased circulating levels of vitamin K and 25-hydroxyvitamin D in osteopenic elderly men. *Metabolism* 1998;47:195-9.

7133 Shearer MJ. The roles of vitamins D and K in bone health and osteoporosis prevention. *Proc Nutr Sci* 1997;56:915-37.

7134 Jamal SA, Browner WS, Bauer DC, Cummings SR. Warfarin use and risk for osteoporosis in elderly women. Study of Osteoporotic Fractures Research Group. *Ann Intern Med* 1998;128:829-832.

7135 Institute of Medicine. Dietary reference intakes for vitamin A, vitamin K, Arsenic, Boron, Chromium, Copper, Iodine, Iron, Manganese, Molybdenum, Nickel, Silicon, Vanadium, and Zinc. www.nap.edu/books/0309072794/html/ (Accessed 28 February 2001).

7136 Rubin MA, Miller JP, Ryan AS, et al. Acute and chronic resistive exercise increase urinary chromium excretion in men as measured with an enriched chromium stable isotope. *J Nutr* 1998;128:73-78.

7137 Rabinovitz H, Leibovitz A, Madar Z, et al. Blood glucose and lipid levels following chromium supplementation in diabetic elderly patients on a rehabilitation program. Program Abstracts, 53rd Annual Scientific Meeting, Gerontological Society of America. *Gerontologist* 2000;40:38.

7139 Leo MA, Lieber CS. Alcohol, vitamin A, and beta-carotene: adverse interactions, including hepatotoxicity and carcinogenicity. *Am J Clin Nutr* 1999;69:1071-85.

7140 Altmed.com. Alpha-Linolenic acid (ALA). www.altmed.com/resources/supps.cfm?ID=676 (Accessed 29 January 2001).

7141 Crawford M, Galli C, Visioli F, et al. Role of Plant-Derived Omega-3 Fatty Acids in Human Nutrition. *Ann Nutr Metab* 2000;44:263-5.

7142 Connor WE. Alpha-linolenic acid in health and disease. *Am J Clin Nutr* 1999;69:827-8.

7143 Connor WE. Importance of n-3 fatty acids in health and disease. *Am J Clin Nutr* 2000;71:171S-5S.

7144 Eritsland J. Safety considerations of polyunsaturated fatty acids. *Am J Clin Nutr* 2000;71:197S-201S.

7145 Gibson RA, Makrides M. n-3 polyunsaturated fatty acid requirements of term infants. *Am J Clin Nutr* 2000;71:251S-5S.

7146 Pang D, Allman-Farinelli MA, Wong T, et al. Replacement of linoleic acid with alpha-linolenic acid does not alter blood lipids in normolipidaemic men. *Br J Nutr* 1998;80:163-7.

7147 De Stefani E, Deneo-Pellegrini H, Boffetta P, et al. Alpha-linolenic acid and risk of prostate cancer: a case-control study in Uruguay. *Cancer Epidemiol Biomarkers Prev* 2000;9:335-8.

7148 Simopoulos AP. Essential fatty acids in health and chronic disease. *Am J Clin Nutr* 1999;70:560S-9S.

7149 Li D, Sinclair A, Wilson A, et al. Effect of dietary alpha-linolenic acid on thrombotic risk factors in vegetarian men. *Am J Clin Nutr* 1999;69:872-82.

7150 de Lorgeril M, Renaud S, Mamelle N, et al. Mediterranean alpha-linolenic acid-rich diet in secondary prevention of coronary heart disease. *Lancet* 1994;343:1454-9.

7151 Bemelmans WJ, Muskiet FA, Feskens EJ, et al. Associations of alpha-linolenic acid and linoleic acid with risk factors for coronary heart. *Eur J Clin Nutr* 2000;54:865-71.

7152 Ascherio A, Rimm EB, Giovannucci EL, et al. Dietary fat and risk of coronary heart disease in men: cohort follow up study in the United States. *BMJ* 1996;313:84-90.

7153 Hu FB, Stampfer MJ, Manson JE, et al. Dietary intake of alpha-linolenic acid and risk of fatal ischemic heart disease among women. *Am J Clin Nutr* 1999;69:890-7.

7154 Hu FB, Stampfer MJ, Manson JE, et al. Frequent nut consumption and risk of coronary heart disease in women: prospective cohort study. *BMJ* 1998;317:1341-5.

7155 Pedersen JI, Ringstad J, Almendingen K, et al. Adipose tissue fatty acids and risk of myocardial infarction-a case-control study. *Eur J Clin Nutr* 2000;54:618-25.

7156 Christensen JH, Christensen MS, Toft E, et al. Alpha-linolenic acid and heart rate variability. *Nutr Metab Cardiovasc Dis* 2000;10:57-61.

7157 Cunnane SC. The Canadian Society for Nutritional Sciences 1995 Young Scientist Award Lecture. Recent studies on the synthesis, beta-oxidation, and deficiency of linoleate and alpha-linolenate: are essential fatty acids more aptly named indispensable or conditionally dispensable fatty acids? *Can J Physiol Pharmacol* 1996;74:629-39.

7158 Lam AY, Elmer GW, Mohutsky MA. Possible interaction between warfarin and Lycium Barbarum. *Ann Pharmacother* 2001;35:1199-201.

7159 Lycos Health with WebMD. Khella. URL: http://webmd.lycos.com/content/article/3187.13434 (Accessed 26 February 2001).

7160 Thriveonline. Khella. www.thriveonline.com/medical/library/herbs/ame0305.html# (Accessed 26 February 2001).

7161 Chevallier A. Encyclopedia of Herbal Medicine. 2nd ed. New York, NY: DK Publ, Inc., 2000.

7162 Dr. Duke's phytochemical and ethnobotanical databases. www.ars-grin.gov/cgi-bin/duke/farmacy2.pl (Accessed 27 February 2001).

7163 Malhotra S, Bailey DG, Paine MF, Watkins PB. Seville orange juice-felodipine interaction: comparison with dilute grapefruit juice and involvement of furocoumarins. *Clin Pharmacol Ther* 2001 Jan;69(1):14-23.

7164 Royal Australian Coll of Gen Practitioners. Herbs and cardiovascular disease from past to present. http://afp.racgp.org.au/2000/december/pinn.htm (Accessed 27 February 2001).

7165 de Deckere EA, Korver O, Verschuren PM, Katan MB. Health aspects of fish and n-3 polyunsaturated fatty acids from plant and marine origin. *Eur J Clin Nutr* 1998;52:749-53.

7166 Allman-Farinelli MA, Hall D, Kingham K, et al. Comparison of the effects of two low fat diets with different alpha-linolenic:linoleic acid ratios on coagulation and fibrinolysis. *Atheroscler* 1999;142:159-68.

7167 Freeman VL, Meydani M, Yong S, et al. Prostatic levels of fatty acids and the histopathology of localized prostate cancer. *J Urol* 2000;164:2168-72.

7168 Klein V, Chajes V, Germain E, et al. Low alpha-linolenic acid content of adipose breast tissue is associated with an increased risk of breast cancer. *Eur J Cancer* 2000;36:335-40.

7169 Das A Jr, Hammad TA. Efficacy of a combination of FCHG49 glucosamine hydrochloride, TRH122 low molecular weight sodium chondroitin sulfate and manganese ascorbate in the management of knee osteoarthritis. *Osteoarth and Cartilage* 2000;8:343-50.

7170 Natl Inst Health, Natl Inst Environmental Health Sci. Indole-3-carbinol. URL: http://ntp-server.niehs.nih.gov/htdocs/Chem_Background/ExecSumm/IndoleCarbinol.html#CONTENTS (Accessed 5 March 2001).

7171 Dashwood RH. Indole-3-carbinol: anticarcinogen or tumor promoter in brassica vegetables? *Chem Biol Interact* 1998;110:1-5.

7172 Rosen CA, Woodson GE, Thompson JW, et al. Preliminary results of the use of indole-3-carbinol for recurrent respiratory papillomatosis. *Otolaryngol Head Neck Surg* 1998;118:810-5.

7173 Bell MC, Crowley-Nowick P, Bradlow HL, et al. Placebo-controlled trial of indole-3-carbinol in the treatment of CIN. *Gynecol Oncol* 2000;78:123-9.

7174 Wong GY, Bradlow L, Sepkovic D, et al. Dose-ranging study of indole-3-carbinol for breast cancer prevention. *J Cell Biochem Suppl* 1997;28-29:111-6.

7175 Michnovicz JJ. Increased estrogen 2-hydroxylation in obese women using oral indole-3-carbinol. *Int J Obes Relat Metab Disord* 1998;22:227-9.

7176 Balk JL. Indole-3-carbinol for cancer prevention. *Altern Med Alert* 2000; 3:105-7.

7177 Michnovicz JJ, Bradlow HL. Induction of estradiol metabolism by dietary indole-3-carbinol in humans. *J Natl Cancer Inst* 1990 June 6;82(11):947-9.

7178 Telang NT, Katdare M, Bradlow HL, et al. Inhibition of proliferation and modulation of estradiol metabolism: novel mechanisms for breast cancer prevention by the phytochemical indole-3-carbinol. *Proc Soc Exp Biol Med* 1997;216:246-52.

7179 Bradlow HL, Michnovicz J, Telang NT, Osborne MP. Effects of dietary indole-3-carbinol on estradiol metabolism and spontaneous mammary tumors in mice. *Carcinogenesis* 1991;12:1571-4.

7180 Grubbs CJ, Steele VE, Casebolt T, et al. Chemoprevention of chemically-induced mammary carcinogenesis by indole-3-carbinol. *Anticancer Res* 1995;15:709-16.

7181 Kojima T, Tanaka T, Mori H. Chemoprevention of spontaneous endometrial cancer in female Donryu rats by dietary indole-3-carbinol. *Cancer Res* 1994;54:1446-9.

7182 Yuan F, Chen DZ, Liu K, et al. Anti-estrogenic activities of indole-3-carbinol in cervical cells: implication for prevention of cervical cancer. *Anticancer Res* 1999;19:1673-80.

7183 Jin L, Qi M, Chen DZ, et al. Indole-3-carbinol prevents cervical cancer in human papilloma virus type 16 (HPV16) transgenic mice. *Cancer Res* 1999;59:3991-7.

7184 Kim DJ, Han BS, Ahn B, et al. Enhancement by indole-3-carbinol of liver and thyroid gland neoplastic development in a rat medium-term multiorgan carcinogenesis model. *Carcinogenesis* 1997;18:377-81.

7185 Pence BC, Buddingh F, Yang SP. Multiple dietary factors in the enhancement of dimethylhydrazine carcinogenesis: main effect of indole-3-carbinol. *J Natl Cancer Inst* 1986;77:269-76.

7186 Bailey GS, Dashwood RH, Fong AT, et al. Modulation of mycotoxin and nitrosamine carcinogenesis by indole-3-carbinol: quantitative analysis of inhibition versus promotion. *IARC Sci Publ* 1991;105:275-80.

7187 He YH, Friesen MD, Ruch RJ, Schut HA. Indole-3-carbinol as a chemopreventive agent in 2-amino-1-methyl-6-phenylimidazo[4,5-b]pyridine (PhIP) carcinogenesis: inhibition of PhIP-DNA adduct formation, acceleration of PhIP metabolism, and induction of cytochrome P450 in female F344 rats. *Food Chem Toxicol* 2000;38:15-23.

7188 Bradlow HL, Sepkovic DW, Telang NT, Osborne MP. Multifunctional aspects of the action of indole-3-carbinol as an antitumor agent. *Ann N Y Acad Sci* 1999;889:204-13.

7189 Srivastava B, Shukla Y. Antitumour promoting activity of indole-3-carbinol in mouse skin carcinogenesis. *Cancer Lett* 1998;134:91-5.

7190 Exon JH, South EH. Dietary indole-3-carbinol alters immune functions in rats. *J Toxicol Environ Health A* 2000;59:271-9.

7191 Garry D, Figueroa R, Guillaume J, Cucco V. Use of castor oil in pregnancies at term. *Altern Ther Health Med* 2000;6:77-9.

7192 Lokkevik E, Skovlund E, Reitan JB, et al. Skin treatment with bepanthen cream versus no cream during radiotherapy-a randomized, controlled trial. *Acta Onco* 1996;35:1021-6.

7193 Williams CL, Bollella MC, Strobino BA, et al. Plant stanol ester and bran fiber in childhood: effects on lipids, stool weight and stool frequency in preschool children. *J Am Coll Nutr* 1999;18:572-81.

7194 Tammi A, Ronnemaa T, Gylling H, et al. Plant stanol ester margarine lowers serum total and low-density lipoprotein cholesterol concentrations of healthy children: the STRIP project. Spec Turku Coronary Risk Factors Intervention Project. *J Pediatr* 2000;136:503-10.

7195 Lichtenstein AH, Deckelbaum RJ. Stanol/sterol ester-containing foods and blood cholesterol levels: a statement for healthcare professionals from Nutr Committee, Council on Nutr, Phys Activity, Metabolism of Am Heart Assn. *Circ* 2001;103:1177-9.

7196 Jones PJ, Raeini-Sarjaz M, Ntanios FY, et al. Modulation of plasma lipid levels and cholesterol kinetics by phytosterol versus phytostanol esters. *J Lipid Res* 2000;41:697-705.

7198 Berges RR, Kassen A, Senge T. Treatment of symptomatic benign prostatic hyperplasia with beta-sitosterol: an 18-month follow-up. *BJU Int* 2000;85:842-6.

7200 Fetrow CW, Avila JR. Professional's handbook of complementary and alternative medicines. 1st ed.

Springhouse: Springhouse Corp., 1999.

7201 Consumer Lab. www.consumerlab.com/results/ creatine.asp (Accessed 5 June 2001).

7202 Stoll AL, Severus WE, Freeman MP, et al. Omega 3 fatty acids in bipolar disorder: A preliminary double-blind, placebo-controlled trial. *Arch Gen Psychiatry* 1999;56:407-12.

7203 Vaidya AB, Rajagopalan TG, Mankodi NA, et al. Treatment of Parkinson's disease with the cowhage plant-Mucuna pruriens Bak. *Neurol India* 1978;26:171-6.

7204 Pras N, Woerdenbag HJ, Batterman S, et al. Mucuna pruriens: improvement of the biotechnological production of the anti-Parkinson drug L-dopa by plant cell selection. *Pharm World Sci* 1993;15:263-8.

7205 Vadivel V, Janardhanan K. Nutritional and anti-nutritional composition of velvet bean: an under-utilized food legume in south India. *Int J Food Sci Nutr* 2000;51:279-87.

7206 Vaidya RA, Aloorkar SD, Sheth AR, Pandya SK. Activity of bromoergocriptine, Mucuna pruriens and L-dopa in the control of hyperprolactinaemia. *Neurol India* 1978;26:179-182.

7207 Vaidya RA, Sheth AR, Aloorkar SD, et al. The inhibitory effect of the cowhage plant-Mucuna pruriens-and L-dopa on chlorpromazine-induced hyperprolactinaemia in man. *Neurol India* 1978;26:177-8.

7208 Gelenberg AJ, Wojcik JD, Falk WE, et al. Tyrosine for depression: a double-blind trial. *J Affect Disord* 1990;19:125-32.

7209 Eisenberg J, Asnis GM, van Praag HM, Vela RM. Effect of tyrosine on attention deficit disorder with hyperactivity. *J Clin Psychiatr* 1988;49:193-5.

7210 Reimherr FW, Wender PH, Wood DR, Ward M. An open trial of L-tyrosine in the treatment of attention deficit disorder, residual type. *Am J Psychiatr* 1987;144:1071-3.

7211 Wood DR, Reimherr FW, Wender PH. Amino acid precursors for the treatment of attention deficit disorder, residual type. *Psychopharmacol Bull* 1985;21:146-9.

7212 van Spronsen FJ, van Rijn M, Bekhof J. Phenylketonuria: tyrosine supplementation in phenylalanine-restricted diets. *Am J Clin Nutr.* 2001;73:153-7.

7213 Poustie VJ, Rutherford P. Tyrosine supplementation for phenylketonuria. *Cochrane Database Syst Rev* 2000;2:CD001507.

7214 Roberts SA, Thorpe JM, Ball RO, Pencharz PB. Tyrosine requirement of healthy men receiving a fixed phenylalanine intake determined by using indicator amino acid oxidation. *Am J Clin Nutr* 2001 Feb;73(2):276-82.

7215 Neri DF, Wiegmann D, Stanny RR, et al. The effects of tyrosine on cognitive performance during extended wakefulness. *Aviat Space Environ Med* 1995;66:313-9.

7216 Intelihealth. Tyrosine. http://www.intelihealth.com/IH/ihtIH/WSIHW000/8513/28412.html (Accessed 30 August 2001).

7217 Institute of Medicine. The Role of Protein and Amino Acids in Sustaining and Enhancing Performance. http://www.nap.edu/books/0309063469/html/ (Accessed 30 August 2001).

7218 U.S. Food and Drug Administration (FDA) Center for Food Safety and Applied Nutrition (CFSAN). EAFUS: A Food Additive Database. http://vm.cfsan.fda.gov/

~dms/eafus.html (Accessed 30 August 2001).

7219 Horning MS, Blakemore LJ, Trombley PQ. Endogenous mechanisms of neuroprotection: role of zinc, copper, and carnosine. *Brain Res* 2000;852(1):56-61.

7220 Grover JK, Vats V, Rathi SS, Dawar R. Traditional Indian anti-diabetic plants attenuate progression of renal damage in streptozotocin induced diabetic mice. *J Ethnopharmacol* 2001;76:233-8.

7221 Akhtar MS, Qureshi AQ, Iqbal J. Antidiabetic evaluation of Mucuna pruriens, Linn seeds. *J Pak Med Assoc* 1990;40:147-50.

7222 Guerranti R, Aguiyi JC, Errico E, et al. Effects of Mucuna pruriens extract on activation of prothrombin by Echis carinatus venom. *J Ethnopharmacol* 2001;75:175-80.

7223 Manyam BV. Paralysis agitans and levodopa in "Ayurveda": ancient Indian medical treatise. *Mov Disord* 1990;5:47-8.

7224 Sheng Y, Pero RW, Amiri A, Bryngelsson C. Induction of apoptosis and inhibition of proliferation in human tumor cells treated with extracts of Uncaria tomentosa. *Anticancer Res* 1998 Sep;18(5A):3363-8.

7225 Sandoval M, Charbonnet RM, Okuhama NN, et al. Cat's claw inhibits TNFalpha production and scavenges free radicals: role in cytoprotection. *Free Radic Biol Med* 2000;29:71-78.

7226 Mohamed AF, Matsumoto K, Tabata K, et al. Effects of Uncaria tomentosa total alkaloid and its components on experimental amnesia in mice: elucidation using the passive avoidance test. *J Pharm Pharmacol* 2000;52:1553-1561.

7227 Santa Maria A, Lopez A, Diaz MM, et al. Evaluation of the toxicity of Uncaria tomentosa by bioassays in vitro. *J Ethnopharmacol* 1997;57:183-7.

7229 Anon. Petasites hybridus. *Altern Med Rev* 2001;6:207-209.

7230 Grossmann WM, Schmidramsl H. An extract of Petasites hybridus is effective in the prophylaxis of migraine. *Int J Clin Pharmacol Ther* 2000;38:430-435.

7231 Mauz C, Candrian U, Luthy J, et al. Method for the reduction of pyrrolizidine alkaloids from medicinal plant extracts [Article in German; English abstract]. *Pharm Acta Helv.* 1985;60:256–259.

7232 NIH Consensus Statements. Phenylketonuria: Screening and Management. http://odp.od.nih.gov/consensus/cons/113/113_statement.htm#3 (Accessed 6 September 2001).

7233 Bozzetti F, Biganzoli L, Gavazzi C, et al. Glutamine supplementation in cancer patients receiving chemotherapy: a double-blind randomized study. *Nutrition* 1997;13:748-751.

7234 Yamasaki K, Nakano M, Otake T, et al. Anti-HIV-1 activity of Labiatae plants, especially aromatic plants. *Int Conf AIDS* 1996;11(1):65.

7235 Savarese D, Al-Zoubi A, Boucher J. Glutamine for irinotecan diarrhea. *J Clin Oncol* 2000;18:450-451.

7236 Brown GA, Vukovich MD, Martini ER, et al. Endocrine responses to chronic androstenedione intake in 30- to 56-year-old men. *J Clin Endocrinol Metab* 2000;85:4074-80.

7237 Ross GD, Vetvicka V, Yan J, et al. Therapeutic intervention with complement and beta-glucan in cancer. *Immunopharmacology* 1999;42(1-3):61-74.

7238 Muller A, Rice PJ, Ensley HE, et al. Receptor binding and internalization of a water-soluble (1—>3)-beta-D-glucan biologic response modifier in two monocyte/

REFERENCES

macrophage cell lines. *J Immunol* 1996;156(9):3418-3425.

7239 Yan J, Vetvicka V, Xia Y, et al. Beta-glucan, a "specific" biologic response modifier that uses antibodies to target tumors for cytotoxic recognition by leukocyte complement receptor type 3 (CD11b/CD18). *J Immunol* 1999;163(6):3045-3052.

7240 Penna C, Dean PA, Nelson H. Pulmonary metastases neutralization and tumor rejection by in vivo administration of beta glucan and bispecific antibody. *Int J Cancer* 1996;65(3):377-382.

7241 Williams DL, Pretus HA, McNamee RB, et al. Development, physicochemical characterization and preclinical efficacy evaluation of a water soluble glucan sulfate derived from Saccharomyces cerevisiae. *Immunopharmacology* 1991;22(3):139-155.

7242 Mueller A, Raptis J, Rice PJ, et al. The influence of glucan polymer structure and solution conformation on binding to (1—>3)-beta-D-glucan receptors in a human monocyte-like cell line. *Glycobiology* 2000;10(4):339-346.

7243 Sherwood ER, Williams DL, McNamee RB, et al. Enhancement of interleukin-1 and interleukin-2 production by soluble glucan. *Int J Immunopharmacol* 1987;9(3):261-267.

7244 Patchen ML, Liang J, Vaudrain T, et al. Mobilization of peripheral blood progenitor cells by Betafectin PGG-Glucan alone and in combination with granulocyte colony-stimulating factor. *Stem Cells* 1998;16(3):208-217.

7245 Turnbull JL, Patchen ML, Scadden DT. The polysaccharide, PGG-Glucan, enhances human myelopoiesis by direct action independent of an additive to early-acting cytokines. *Acta Hematol* 1999;102(2):66-71.

7246 Portera CA, Love EJ, Memore L, et al. Effect of macrophage stimulation on collagen biosynthesis in the healing wound. *Am Surg* 1997;63(2):125-131.

7247 Bowers GJ, Patchen ML, MacVittie TJ, et al. Glucan enhances survival in an inraabdominal infection model. *J Surg Res* 1989;47(2):183-188.

7248 Liang J, Melican D, Cafro L, et al. Enhanced clearance of a multiple antibiotic resistant Staphylococcus aureus in rats treated with PGG-glucan is associated with increased leukocyte counts and increased neutrophil oxidative burst activity. *Int J Immunopharmacol* 1998;20(11):595-614.

7249 Wakshull E, Brunke-Reese D, Lindermuth J, et al. PGG-Glucan, a soluble beta-(1,3)-glucan, enhances the oxidative burst response, microbicidal activity, and activates an NF-kappa B-like factor in human PMN: evidence for a glycosphingolipid beta-(1,3)-glucan receptor. *Immunopharmacology* 1999;4(2):89-107.

7250 Tsiapali E, Whaley S, Kalbfleisch J, et al. Glucans exhibit weak antioxidant activity, but stimulate macrophage free radical activity. *Free Radic Biol Med* 2001;30(4):393-402.

7251 Williams DL, Sherwood ER, Browder IW, et al. Pre-clinical safety evaluation of soluble glucan. *Int J Immunopharmac* 1988;10(4);405-414.

7252 Duvic M, Reisman M, Finley V, et al. Glucan-induced keratoderma in acquired immunodeficiency syndrome. *Arch Dermatol* 1987;123(6):751-756.

7253 Wan G, Li C, Guo S, et al. An airborne mold-derived product, beta-1,3-D-glucan, potentiates airway allergic responses. *Eur J Immunol* 1999;29(8):2491-2497.

7254 Yoshioka S, Ohno N, Miura T, et al. Immunotoxicity of soluble beta-glucans induced by indomethacin treatment. *FEMS Immunol Med Microbiol* 1998;21(3):171-179.

7255 Lissoni P, Cazzaniga M, Tancini G, et al. Reversal of clinical resistance to LHRH analogue in metastatic prostate cancer by the pineal hormone melatonin: efficacy of LHRH analogue plus melatonin in patients progressing on LHRH analogue alone. *Eur Urol* 1997;31(2):178-81.

7258 Amin AH, Subbaiah TV, Abbasi KM. Berberine sulfate: antimicrobial activity, bioassay, and mode of action. *Can J Microbiol* 1969;15(9):1067-76.

7259 Sun D, Courtney HS, Beachey EH. Berberine sulfate blocks adherence of Streptococcus pyogenes to epithelial cells, fibronectin, and hexadecane. *Antimicrob Agents Chemother* 1988;32(9):1370-4.

7260 Nishino H, Kitagawa K, Fujiki H, Iwashima A. Berberine sulfate inhibits tumor-promoting activity of teleocidin in two-stage carcinogenesis on mouse skin. *Oncology* 1986;(2):131-4.

7261 Okamura K, Suzuki M, Chihara T, et al. Clinical evaluation of schizophyllan combined with irradiation in patients with cervical cancer. A randomized controlled study. *Cancer* 1986;58(4):865-872.

7262 Mansell PW, Ichinose H, Reed RJ, et al. Macrophage-mediated destruction of human malignant cells in vivo. *J Natl Cancer Inst* 1975;54(3):571-580.

7263 Kimura Y, Tojima H, Fukase S, Takeda K. Clinical evaluation of sizofilan as assistant immunotherapy in treatment of head and neck cancer. *Acta Otolaryngol Suppl* 1994;511:192-195.

7264 Miyazaki K, Mizutani H, Katabuchi H, et al. Activated (HLA-DR+) T-lymphocyte subsets in cervical carcinoma and effects of radiotherapy and immunotherapy with sizofiran on cell-mediated immunity and survival. *Gynecol Oncol* 1995;56(3):412-420.

7265 Arinaga S, Karimine N, Takamuku K, et al. Enhanced induction of lymphokine-activated killer activity after lentinan administration in patients with gastric carcinoma. *Int J Immunopharmac* 1992;14(4):535-539.

7267 Gordon M, Bihari B, Goosby E, et al. A placebo-controlled trial of the immune modulator, lentinan, in HIV-positive patients: a phase I/II trial. *J Med* 1998;29(5-6):305-330.

7268 Browder W, Williams D, Pretus H, et al. Beneficial effect of enhanced macrophage function in the trauma patient. *Ann Surg* 1990;211(5):605-612; discussion 612-613.

7269 Babineau TJ, Marcello P, Swails W, et al. Randomized phase I/II trial of a macrophage-specific immunomodulator (PGG-glucan) in high-risk surgical patients. *Ann Surg* 1994;220(5):601-609.

7270 Babineau TJ, Hackford A, Kenler A, et al. A phase II multicenter, double-blind, randomized, placebo-controlled study of three dosages of an immunomodulator (PGG-glucan) in high-risk surgical patients. *Arch Surg* 1994;129(11):1204-1210.

7271 Dellinger EP, Babineau TJ, Bleicher P, et al. Effect of PGG-glucan on the rate of serious postoperative infection or death observed after high-risk gastrointestinal operations. Betafectin Gastrointestinal Study Group. *Arch Surg* 1999;134(9):977-983.

7272 Nicolosi R, Bell SJ, Bistrian BR, et al. Plasma lipid changes after supplementation with beta-glucan fiber from yeast. *Am J Clin Nutr* 1999;70(2):208-212.

7273 Bell S, Goldman VM, Bistrian BR, et al. Effect of beta-glucan from oats and yeast on serum lipids. *Crit Rev Food Sci Nutr* 1999;39(2):189-202.

7275 Genest K, Hughes DW. Natural products in Canadian pharmaceuticals IV. Hydrastis canadensis. *Can J Pharm Sci* 1969;4(2):41-5.

7277 Ammon HP, Muller AB. Forskolin: From a ayurvedic remedy to a modern agent. *Planta Med* 1985;6:473-7.

7278 Baumann G, Felix S, Sattelberger U, Klein G. Cardiovascular effects of forskolin (HL-362) in patients with idiopathic congestiv cardiomyopathy. A comparative study with dobutamine and sodium nitroprusside. *J Cardiovasc Pharmacol* 1990;16(1):93-100.

7279 Kramer W, Thormann J, Kindler M, Schlepper M. Effects of forskolin on left ventricular function in dilated cardiomyopathy. *Arzneimittleforschung* 1987;37(3):364-7.

7280 Lichey J, Friedrich T, Priesnitz M, et al. Effect of forskolin on methacholine-induced bronchoconstriction in extrinsic asthmatics. *Lancet* 1984;2:167.

7281 Bauer K, Dietersdorfer F, Kaspar S, et al. Pharmacodynamic effects of inhaled dry powder formulations of fenoterol and colforsin in asthma. *Clin Pharmacol Ther* 1993;53(1):76-83.

7282 Meyer BH, Stulting AA, Muller FO, et al. The effects of forskolin eye drops on intra-ocular pressure. *S Afr Med* 1987;71(9):570-1.

7283 Brubaker RF, Carlson KH, Kullerstrand LJ, et al. Topical forskolin (colforsin) and aqueous flow in humans. *Arch Ophthalmol* 1987;105(5):637-41.

7284 Seto C, Eguchi S, Araie M, et al. Acute effects of topical forskolin on aqueous humor dynamics in man. *Jpn J Ophthalmol* 30(3):238-44.

7285 Daniele B, Perrone F, Gallo C, et al. Oral glutamine in the prevention of fluorouracil induced intestinal toxicity: a double blind, placebo controlled, randomised trial. *Gut* 2001;48:28-33.

7286 John JF, Kuk R, Rosenthal A et al. Synergistic antiretroviral activities of the herb, Prunella vulgaris, with AZT, ddI, and ddC. *Abstr Gen Meet Am Soc Microbiol* 1994;94:481.

7288 Petit RG, French C. Phase III Clinical Trial Design Considerations for Oral Treatments of Chemotherapy-Induced Mucositis: AES-14 (Uptake-Facilitated L-Glutamine) Pivotal Studies. http://www.asco.org/prof/me/html/01abstracts/0037/2954.htm. (Accessed 2001 September 24).

7289 Manns B, Hyndman E, Burgess E, et al. Oral vitamin B(12) and high-dose folic acid in hemodialysis patients with hyper-homocyst(e)inemia. *Kidney Int* 2001;59:1103-1109.

7290 Dietary reference intakes for thiamine, riboflavin, niacin, vitamin B6, folate, vitamin B12, pantothenic acid, biotin, and choline (2000). Institute of Medicine. Accessed at National Academy Press Website:http://books.nap.edu/books/0309065542/html/306.html (accessed 10-5-01).

7291 Mebane AH. L-Glutamine and mania. *Am J Psychiatry* 984;141:1302-3.

7292 Meldrum BS. Glutamate as a neurotransmitter in the brain: review of physiology and pathology. *J Nutr* 2000;130:1007S-15S.

7293 Garlick PJ. Assessment of the safety of glutamine and other amino acids. *J Nutr* 2001;131:2556S-61S.

7294 Chapman AG. Glutamate and epilepsy. *J Nutr* 2000;130:1043S-5S.

7295 van Zaanen HC, van der Lelie H, Timmer JG, et al. Parenteral glutamine dipeptide supplementation does not ameliorate chemotherapy-induced toxicity. *Cancer* 1994;74:2879-84.

7296 Coghlin Dickson TM, Wong RM, Negrin RS, et al. Effect of oral glutamine supplementation during bone marrow transplantation. *JPEN J Parenter Enteral Nutr* 2000;24:61-6.

7297 Zoli G, Care M, Falco F, et al. Effect of oral glutamine on intestinal permeability and nutritional status in Crohn's disease [abstract]. *Gastroenterology* 1995;108:A766.

7298 Ribeiro Junior H, Ribeiro T, Mattos A, et al. Treatment of acute diarrhea with oral rehydration solutions containing glutamine. *J Am Coll Nutr* 1994;13:251-5.

7299 van der Hulst RR, van Kreel BK, von Meyenfeldt MF, et al. Glutamine and the preservation of gut integrity. *Lancet* 1993;341:1363-5.

7300 Jian ZM, Cao JD, Zhu XG, et al. The impact of alanyl-glutamine on clinical safety, nitrogen balance, intestinal permeability, and clinical outcome in postoperative patients: a randomized, double-blind, controlled study of 120 patients. *JPEN J Parenter Enteral Nutr* 1999;23:S62-6.

7303 Age-Related Eye Disease Study Research Group. A Randomized, Placebo-Controlled, Clinical Trial of High-Dose Supplementation With Vitamins C and E, Beta Carotene, and Zinc for Age-Related Macular Degeneration and Vision Loss. AREDS report no. 8. *Arch Ophthalmol* 2001;119:1417-36.

7304 Age-Related Eye Disease Study Research Group. A randomized, placebo-controlled, clinical trial of high-dose supplementation with vitamins C and E and beta carotene for age-related cataract and vision loss: AREDS report no. 9. *Arch Ophthalmol* 2001;119:1439-52.

7305 Jampol LM. Antioxidants, zinc, age-related macular degeneration: results and recommendations. *Arch Ophthalmol.* 2001;119:1533-4.

7306 Thomas MR, Litin SC, Osmon DR, et al. Lack of effect of Lactobacillus GG on antibiotic-associated diarrhea: a randomized, placebo-controlled trial. *Mayo Clin Proc* 2001;76:883-889.

7307 Lee SC, Park SW, Kim DK, et al. Iron supplementation inhibits cough associated with ACE inhibitors. *Hypertension* 2001;38:166-170.

7308 Hallberg L. Does calcium interfere with iron absorption? *Am J Clin Nutr* 1998 Jul;68(1):3-4.

7309 Chuntrasakul C, Siltharm S, Sarasombath S, et al. Metabolic and immune effects of dietary arginine, glutamine and omega-3 fatty acids supplementation in immunocompromised patients. *J Med Assoc Thai* 1998;81:334-43.

7310 Clark RH, Feleke G, Din M, et al. Nutritional treatment for acquired immunodeficiency virus-associated wasting using beta-hydroxy beta-methylbutyrate, glutamine, and arginine: a randomized, double-blind, placebo-controlled study. *JPEN J Parenter Enteral Nutr* 2000;24:133-9.

7311 Wahed A, Dasgupta A. Positive and negative in vitro interference of Chinese medicine dan shen in serum digoxin measurement. Elimination of interference by monitoring free digoxin concentration. *Am J Clin Pathol* 2001;116:403-408.

7312 Bhopal JS. St John's wort-induced sexual dysfunction. *Can J Psychiatry* 2001;46:456-457.

REFERENCES

REFERENCES

7313 Albert S, Bhattacharya D, Klaudiny J, et al. The family of major royal jelly proteins and its evolution. *J Mol Evol* 1999;49:290-297.

7314 Leung R, Ho A, Chan J, et al. Royal jelly consumption and hypersensitivity in the community. *Clin Exp Allergy* 1997;27:333-336.

7315 Harwood M, Harding S, Beasley R, Frankish PD. Asthma following royal jelly. *N Z Med J* 1996;109:325.

7316 Laporte JR, Ibaanez L, Vendrell L, Ballarin E. Bronchospasm induced by royal jelly. *Allergy* 1996;51:440.

7317 Piscoya J, Rodriguez Z, Bustamante SA, et al. Efficacy and safety of freeze-dried cat's claw in osteoarthritis of the knee: mechanisms of action of the species Uncaria guianensis. *Inflamm Res* 2001;50:442-448.

7318 Venkataramanan R, Ramachandran V, Komoroski BJ, et al. Milk thistle, a herbal supplement, decreases the activity of CYP3A4 and uridine diphosphoglucuronosyl transferase in human hepatocyte cultures. *Drug Metab Dispos* 2000;28:1270-3.

7319 Zhu W, Zhang JS, Young CY. Silymarin inhibits function of the androgen receptor by reducing nuclear localization of the receptor in the human prostate cancer cell line LNCaP. *Carcinogenesis* 2001;22:1399-403.

7320 Sonnenbichler J, Scalera F, Sonnenbichler I, Weyhenmeyer R. Stimulatory effects of silibinin and silicristin from the milk thistle Silybum marianum on kidney cells. *J Pharmacol Exp Ther* 1999;290:1375-83.

7321 Bunout D, Hirsch S, Petermann M. [Controlled study of the effect of silymarin on alcoholic liver disease.] [Article in Spanish] *Rev Med Chil* 1992;120:1370-5.

7322 Trinchet JC, Coste T, Levy VG. [Treatment of alcoholic hepatitis with silymarin. A double-blind comparative study in 116 patients]. [Article in French] *Gastroenterol Clin Biol* 1989;13:120-4.

7323 Paulova J, Dvorak M, Kolouch F, et al. [Verification of the hepatoprotective and therapeutic effect of silymarin in experimental liver injury with tetrachloromethane in dogs]. [Article in Czech] *Vet Med (Praha)* 1990;35:629-35.

7325 Malsch U, Kieser M. Efficacy of kava-kava in the treatment of non-psychotic anxiety, following pretreatment with benzodiazepines. *Psychopharmacology (Berl)* 2001;157:277-83.

7326 Blasiak J, Kowalik J. A comparison of the in vitro genotoxicity of tri- and hexavalent chromium. *Mutat Res* 2000;469:135-45.

7327 Genazzani AD, Stomati M, Strucchi C, et al. Oral dehydroepiandrosterone supplementation modulates spontaneous and growth hormone-releasing hormone-induced growth hormone and insulin-like growth factor-1 secretion in early and late postmenopausal women. *Fertil Steril* 2001;76:241-8.

7328 Robinzon B, Cutolo M. Should dehydroepiandrosterone replacement therapy be provided with glucocorticoids? *Rheumatology (Oxford)* 1999;38:488-95.

7329 Cesaro S, Chinello P, Rossi L, Zanesco L. Saccharomyces cerevisiae fungemia in a neutropenic patient treated with Saccharomyces boulardii. *Support Care Cancer* 2000;8:504-5.

7330 Setchell KD, Brown NM, Desai P, et al. Bioavailability of pure isoflavones in healthy humans and analysis of commercial soy isoflavone supplements. *J Nutr* 2001;131:1362S-75S.

7331 Strom BL, Schinnar R, Ziegler EE, et al. Exposure to soy-based formula in infancy and endocrinological and reproductive outcomes in young adulthood. *JAMA* 2001;286:807-14.

7332 Setchell KD, Zimmer-Nechemias L, Cai J, Heubi JE. Exposure of infants to phyto-oestrogens from soy-based infant formula. *Lancet* 1997;350:23-7.

7333 Clarkson TB, Anthony MS, Morgan TM. Inhibition of postmenopausal atherosclerosis progression: a comparison of the effects of conjugated equine estrogens and soy phytoestrogens. *J Clin Endocrinol Metab* 2001;86:41-7.

7334 Nomura A, Henderson BE, Lee J. Breast cancer and diet among the Japanese in Hawaii. *Am J Clin Nutr* 1978;31:2020-5.

7335 Lee HP, Gourley L, Duffy SW, et al. Dietary effects on breast-cancer risk in Singapore. *Lancet* 1991;337:1197-200.

7336 Shu XO, Jin F, Dai Q, et al. Soyfood intake during adolescence and subsequent risk of breast cancer among Chinese women. *Cancer Epidemiol Biomarkers Prev* 2001;10:483-88.

7337 Messina M, Barnes S, Setchell KD. Phyto-oestrogens and breast cancer. *Lancet* 1997;350:971-2.

7338 Goodman MT, Wilkens LR, Hankin JH, et al. Association of soy and fiber consumption with the risk of endometrial cancer. *Am J Epidemiol* 1997;146:294-306.

7339 Nagata C, Inaba S, Kawakami N, et al. Inverse association of soy product intake with serum androgen and estrogen concentrations in Japanese men. *Nutr Cancer* 2000;36:14-8.

7340 Wu AH, Yang D, Pike MC. A meta-analysis of soyfoods and risk of stomach cancer: the problem of potential confounders. *Cancer Epidemiol Biomarkers Prev* 2000;9:1051-8.

7341 Ji BT, Chow WH, Yang G, et al. Correspondence re: AH Wu et al, A meta-analysis of soyfoods and risk of stomach cancer: the problem of potential confounders. *Cancer Epidemiol Biomarkers Prev* 2001;10:570.

7342 Somekawa Y, Chiguchi M, Ishibashi T, Aso T. Soy intake related to menopausal symptoms, serum lipids, and bone mineral density in postmenopausal Japanese women. *Obstet Gynecol* 2001;97:109-15.

7343 Weaver CM, Elmore D, Spence LA, et al. Effects of soy isoflavones on calcium metabolism and bone resorption in postmenopausal women. *Altern Ther Health Med* 2001;7:S35.

7344 Vincent A, Fitzpatrick LA. Soy isoflavones: are they useful in menopause? *Mayo Clin Proc* 2000;75:1174-84.

7345 Lichtenstein AH. Got soy? *Am J Clin Nutr* 2001;73:667-8.

7346 Gardner CD, Newell KA, Cherin R, Haskell WL. The effect of soy protein with or without isoflavones relative to milk protein on plasma lipids in hypercholesterolemic postmenopausal women. *Am J Clin Nutr* 2001;73:728-35.

7347 Ashton EL, Dalais FS, Ball MJ. Effect of meat replacement by tofu on CHD risk factors including copper induced LDL oxidation. *J Am Coll Nutr* 2000;19:761-7.

7348 Stephenson TJ, Anderson JW, Fanti P. Soy protein use in early diabetic nephropathy. *Altern Ther Health Med* 2001;7:S31-2.

7349 US Department of Justice, Drug Enforcement Agency,

Diversion Control Program. Drugs and Chemicals of Concern: Salvia Divinorum, ska Maria Pastora, Salvia (Salvinorin A, Divinorin A). http://www.deadiversion.usdoj.gov/drugs_concern/salvia_d/summary.htm (Accessed 16 November 2001).

7350 Valdes LJ 3rd, Diaz JL, Paul AG. Ethnopharmacology of ska Maria Pastora (Salvia divinorum, Epling and Jativa-M.). *J Ethnopharmacol* 1983;7:287-312.

7351 Valdes LJ 3rd. Salvia divinorum and the unique diterpene hallucinogen, Salvinorin (divinorin) A. *J Psychoactive Drugs* 1994;26:277-83.

7352 Siebert DJ. Salvia divinorum and salvinorin A: new pharmacologic findings. *J Ethnopharmacol* 1994;43:53-6.

7353 Hennequin C, Thierry A, Richard GF, et al. Microsatellite typing as a new tool for identification of Saccharomyces cerevisiae strains. *J Clin Microbiol* 2001;39:551-9.

7354 Kim DH, Jin YH, Park JB, Kobashi K. Silymarin and its components are inhibitors of beta-glucuronidase. *Biol Pharm Bull* 1994;17:443-5.

7355 Pares A, Planas R, Torres M, et al. Effects of silymarin in alcoholic patients with cirrhosis of the liver: results of a controlled, double-blind, randomized and multicenter trial. *J Hepatol* 1998;28:615-21.

7356 Buzzelli G, Moscarella S, Giusti A, et al. A pilot study on the liver protective effect of silybin-phosphatidylcholine complex (IdB1016) in chronic active hepatitis. *Int J Clin Pharmacol Ther Toxicol* 1993;31:456-60.

7357 Whittaker P. Iron and zinc interactions in humans. *Am J Clin Nutr* 1998;68:442S-6S.

7358 Foth D, Cline JM. Effects of mammalian and plant estrogens on mammary glands and uteri of macaques. *Am J Clin Nutr* 1998;68:1413S-7S.

7359 Burr ML, Fehily AM, Gilbert JF, et al. Effects of changes in fat, fish, and fibre intakes on death and myocardial reinfarction: diet and reinfarction trial (DART). *Lancet* 1989;2:757-61.

7360 Sellmayer A, Witzgall H, Lorenz RL, Weber PC. Effects of dietary fish oil on ventricular premature complexes. *Am J Cardiol* 1995;76:974-7.

7361 Nilsen DW, Albrektsen G, Landmark K, et al. Effects of a high-dose concentrate of n-3 fatty acids or corn oil introduced early after an acute myocardial infarction on serum triacylglycerol and HDL cholesterol. *Am J Clin Nutr* 2001;74:50-6.

7362 Billman GE, Hallaq H, Leaf A. Prevention of ischemia-induced ventricular fibrillation by omega 3 fatty acids. *Proc Natl Acad Sci U S A* 1994;91:4427-30.

7363 Billman GE, Kang JX, Leaf A. Prevention of sudden cardiac death by dietary pure omega-3 polyunsaturated fatty acids in dogs. *Circulation* 1999;99:2452-7.

7364 Kromhout D, Bosschieter EB, de Lezenne Coulander C. The inverse relation between fish consumption and 20-year mortality from coronary heart disease. *N Engl J Med* 1985;312:1205-9.

7365 Kromhout D, Feskens EJ, Bowles CH. The protective effect of a small amount of fish on coronary heart disease mortality in an elderly population. *Int J Epidemiol* 1995;24:340-5.

7366 Sorensen NS, Marckmann P, Hoy CE, et al. Effect of fish-oil-enriched margarine on plasma lipids, low-density-lipoprotein particle composition, size, and susceptibility to oxidation. *Am J Clin Nutr* 1998;68:235-41.

7367 Rissanen T, Voutilainen S, Nyyssonen K, et al. Fish oil-derived fatty acids, docosahexaenoic acid and docosapentaenoic acid, and the risk of acute coronary events: the Kuopio ischaemic heart disease risk factor study. *Circulation* 2000;102:2677-9.

7368 Sirtori CR, Crepaldi G, Manzato E, et al. One-year treatment with ethyl esters of n-3 fatty acids in patients with hypertriglyceridemia and glucose intolerance: reduced triglyceridemia, total cholesterol and increased HDL-C without glycemic alterations. *Atherosclerosis* 1998;137:419-27.

7369 Luo J, Rizkalla SW, Vidal H, et al. Moderate intake of n-3 fatty acids for 2 months has no detrimental effect on glucose metabolism and could ameliorate the lipid profile in type 2 diabetic men. Results of a controlled study. *Diabetes Care* 1998;21:717-24.

7370 Gillum RF, Mussolino ME, Madans JH. The relationship between fish consumption and stroke incidence. The NHANES I Epidemiologic Follow-up Study (National Health and Nutrition Examination Survey). *Arch Intern Med* 1996;156:537-42.

7371 Keli SO, Feskens EJ, Kromhout D. Fish consumption and risk of stroke. The Zutphen Study. *Stroke* 1994;25:328-32.

7372 Yamori Y, Nara Y, Mizushima S, et al. Nutritional factors for stroke and major cardiovascular diseases: international epidemiological comparison of dietary prevention. *Health Rep* 1994;6:22-7.

7373 Iso H, Rexrode KM, Stampfer MJ, et al. Intake of fish and omega-3 fatty acids and risk of stroke in women. *JAMA* 2001;285:304-12.

7374 Orencia AJ, Daviglus ML, Dyer AR, et al. Fish consumption and stroke in men. 30-year findings of the Chicago Western Electric Study. *Stroke* 1996;27:204-9.

7375 Morris MC, Manson JE, Rosner B, et al. Fish consumption and cardiovascular disease in the physicians' health study: a prospective study. *Am J Epidemiol* 1995;142:166-75.

7376 US Food and Drug Administration. Center for Food Safety and Applied Nutrition. Letter Regarding Dietary Supplement Health Claim for Omega-3 Fatty Acids and Coronary Heart Disease. website: http://vm.cfsan.fda.gov/~dms/ds-ltr11.html (Accessed 30 November 2001).

7377 van Dam M, Stalenhoef AFH, Wittekoek J. Efficacy of Concentrated n-3 Fatty Acids in Hypertriglyceridaemia: A Comparison with Gemfibrozil. *Clin Drug Invest* 2001;21:175-81.

7378 Terry P, Lichtenstein P, Feychting M, et al. Fatty fish consumption and risk of prostate cancer. *Lancet* 2001;357:1764-6.

7379 Consumer Lab. Product Review: Omega-3 Fatty Acids (EPA and DHA) from Fish/Marine Oils. website: http://www.consumerlab.com/results/omega3.asp (Accessed 30 November 2001).

7380 Deslypere JP. Influence of supplementation with N-3 fatty acids on different coronary risk factors in men—a placebo controlled study. *Verh K Acad Geneeskd Belg* 1992;54:189-16.

7381 Hwang DH, Chanmugam PS, Ryan DH, et al. Does vegetable oil attenuate the beneficial effects of fish oil in reducing risk factors for cardiovascular disease? *Am J Clin Nutr* 1997;66:89-96.

7382 Vogel RA, Corretti MC, Plotnick GD. The postprandial

effect of components of the Mediterranean diet on endothelial function. *J Am Coll Cardiol* 2000;36:1455-60.

7383 Kelley DS, Rudolph IL. Effect of individual fatty acids of omega-6 and omega-3 type on human immune status and role of eicosanoids. *Nutrition* 2000;16:143-5.

7384 Meydani SN, Dinarello CA. Influence of dietary fatty acids on cytokine production and its clinical implications. *Nutr Clin Pract* 1993;8:65-72.

7400 Grontved A, Brask T, Kambskard J, Hentzer E. Ginger root against seasickness: a controlled trial on the open sea. *Acta Otolaryngol* 1998;105:45-9.

7401 Srivastava KC, Mustafa T. Ginger (Zingiber officinale) and rheumatic disorders. *Medical Hypotheses* 1989;29:25-8.

7402 Caprioli J, Sears M. Forskolin lowers intraocular pressure in rabbits, monkeys, and man. *Lancet* 1983;1(8331):958-60.

7403 Caprioli J, Sears M, Bausher L, et al. Forskolin lowers intraocular pressure by reducing aqueous inflow. *Invest Ophthamol Vis Sci* 1984;25(3):268-77.

7404 Sultana D, Peindl KS, Wisner KL. Rash associated with St. John's wort treatment in premenstrual dysphoric disorder. *Arch Women Ment Health* 2000;3:99-101.

7405 Burstein NL, Sears ML, Mead A. Aqueous flow in human eyes is reduced by forskolin, a potent adenylate cyclase activator. *Exp Eye Res* 1984;39(6):745-9.

7406 Metzger H, Lindner E. The positive inotropic-acting forskolin, a potent adenylatecyclase activator. *Arzneimittelforschung* 1981;31(8):1248-50.

7407 Lindner E, Metzger H. The action of forskolin on muscle cells is modified by hormones, calcium ions and calcium antagonists. *Arzneimittelforschung* 1983;33(10):1436-41.

7408 Seamon KB, Daly JW. Forskolin: a unique diterpene activator of cyclic AMP-generating systems. *J Cyclic Nucleotide Res* 1981;7(4):201-24.

7409 Kreutner W, Chapman RW, Gulbenkian A, Tozzi S. Bronchodilator and antiallergy activity of forskolin. *Eur J Pharmacol* 1985;111(1):1-8.

7410 Christenson JT, Thulesius O, Nazzal MM. The effect of forskolin on blood flow, platelet metabolism, aggregation and ATP release. *Vasa* 1995;24(1):56-61.

7411 Agarwal KC, Zielinski BA, Maitra RS. Significance of plasma adenosine in the antiplatelet activity of forskolin: potentiation by dipyridamole and dilazep. *Thromb Haemost* 1989;61(1):106-10.

7412 Agarwal KC, Parks RE. Forskolin: a potential antimetastatic agent. *Int J Cancer* 1983;32(6):801-4.

7413 Tzanakakis GN, Agarwal KC, Vezeridis MP. Inhibition of hepatic metastasis from a human pancreatic adenocarcinoma (RWP-2) in the nude mouse by prostacyclin, forskolin, and ketoconazole. *Cancer* 1990;65(3):446-51.

8000 Loprinzi CL, Goldberg RM, Burnham NL. Cancer-associated anorexia and cachexia. Implications for drug therapy. *Drugs* 1992;43(4):499-506.

8001 Loprinzi CL, Goldberg RM, Su JQ, et al. Placebo-controlled trial of hydrazine sulfate in patients with newly diagnosed non-small-cell lung cancer. *J Clin Oncol* 1994;12(6):1126-9.

8002 Loprinzi CL, Kuross SA, O'Fallon JR, et al. Randomized, placebo-controlled evaluation of hydrazine sulfate in patients with advanced colorectal cancer. *J Clin Oncol* 1994;12(6):1121-5.

8003 Kosty MP, Fleishman SB, Herndon JE II, et al. Cisplatin, vinblastine, and hydrazine sulfate in advanced, non-small-cell lung cancer: a randomized, placebo-controlled, double-blind phase III study of the cancer and leukemia Group B. *J Clin Oncol* 1994;12(6):1113-20.

8004 Chlebowski RT, Bulcavage L, Grosvenor M, et al. Hydrazine sulfate in cancer patients with weight loss. A placebo-controlled clinical experience. *Cancer* 1987;59(3):406-10.

8005 Kaegi E. Unconventional therapies for cancer: 4. Hydrazine sulfate. Task Force on Alternative Therapies of the Canadian Breast Cancer Research Initiative. *CMAJ* 1998;158(10):1327-30.

8300 Bredle DL, et al. Phosphate supplementation, cardiovascular function, and exercise performance in humans. *J Appl Physiol* 1988;65(4):1821-6.

8301 Duffy DJ, Conlee RK. Effects of phosphate loading on leg power and high intensity treadmill exercise. *Med Sci Sports Exerc* 1986;18(6):674-7.

8302 Perreault MM, Ostrop NJ, Tierney MG. Efficacy and safety of intravenous phosphate replacement in critically ill patients. *Ann Pharmacother* 1997;31(6):683-8.

8303 Rosen GH, et al. Intravenous phosphate repletion regimen for critically ill patients with moderate hypophosphatemia. *Crit Care Med* 1995;23(7):1204-10.

8304 Androstenediol 4AD. Vitanet. URL: store.yahoo.com/vitanet/vitan.html (Accessed 8 December 1999).

8305 Pittler MH, Ernst E. Guar gum for body weight reduction: Meta-analysis of randomized trials. *Am J Med* 2001;110:724-30.

Some Brand Name Natural Products - What they Contain
www.NaturalDatabase.com contains MANY more listings than appear here.

#100 Abc Acidophilus/Bifidum Complex - Systemic Formulas
Each capsule contains: A minimum of one billion Lactobacillus acidophilus (NAS strain) and one billion Bifidobacterium bifidum (Malyoth strain) uniquely suspended in an anaerobic, sunflower oil matrix containing vitamin E as a natural antioxidant.

#101 ACP VITAMIN ACP - Systemic Formulas
Rose Hips • Orange Peel • Bone Meal • Vitamin C • RNA/DNA Liver Factors • Lemon Bioflavonoid • Vitamin E • RNA/DNA Thymus Factors • Pedra Hume Ca • Acacia Gum flower • Vitamin A. See Editor's Note No. 14, page 1817.

#102 ACX VITAMIN DETOX - Systemic Formulas
Rose Hips • Vitamin C • RNA/DNA Liver Factors • Lemon Bioflavonoid • Pimiento • Vitamin E • Damiana • Pedra Hume Ca • RNA/DNA Thymus Factors • Vitamin A • Acacia Gum Flower • Hesperidin • RNA/DNA Spleen Factors • Peach Bark • Sun Dew. See Editor's Note No. 14, page 1817.

#111 AZV Multi-Vitamin and Mineral Supplement - Systemic Formulas
RNA/DNA Liver Factors • Rose Hips • Kelp • Linseed Oil • Vitamin A • Vitamin D • Vitamin E • Vitamin C • Calcium • Niacin • Phosphorus • Iron • Vitamin B1 (Thiamine) • Vitamin B2 (Riboflavin) • Magnesium • Vitamin B6 (Pyridoxine HCl) • Pantothenic Acid • Potassium • Zinc • Manganese • Vitamin B12 (Cyanocobalamin) • plus Lemon Bioflavonoid, Autolyzed RNA/DNA Yeast. See Editor's Note No. 14, page 1817.

#115 BSV VITAMIN B STRESS COMPLEX - Systemic Formulas
Abutua • Centaury • Red Bone Marrow • Nettle • Poke Root • Spearmint • RNA/DNA Liver Factors and Parotid Factors • Guarana • Vitamin B2 • Fringe Tree • Choline Bitartrate • Inositol • Niacinamide • PABA • Vitamin B1 • Calcium Pantothenate • Vitamin B6 • Niacin • Vitamin B12 • Folic Acid • Biotin. See Editor's Note No. 14, page 1817.

#12 B BRAIN - Systemic Formulas
RNA/DNA Brain Factors • Italian Pimiento • L-Alanine • Stevia • Tayuya • Vitamin B2 • Rutin • Niacin • Vitamin B6 • L-Glutamic Acid • Hydroxyproline • L-Proline • RNA/DNA Pituitary Factors • RNA/DNA Thalamus Factors. See Editor's Note No. 14, page 1817.

#120 CAL CALCIUM PLUS - Systemic Formulas
Calcium (from Citrate, Lactate, Hydroxide, Bone Meal, Bone Ash, Carbonate, Oyster Shell, Lysinate, Methionate, and Aspartate) • Lecithin • Magnesium Oxide • Vitamin C • Vitamin E • Trace Minerals • Iron Chelate • Copper Carbonate • Vitamin D • Betaine HCl • Boron Chelate.

#126 CTV VITAMIN C THERAPEUTIC - Systemic Formulas
Ascorbic Acid • Sodium Ascorbate • Beta-carotene (source of Vit. A) • Sago Palm • Calcium Ascorbate • Calcium Carbonate • Bioflavonoids • Potassium Bitartrate • Hesperidin • Rose Hips • Thymol Iodide.

#130 EZV 200 IU VITAMIN E - Systemic Formulas
Lactose • Fructose • Vitamin E • Honey Bake.

#132 FLX VEGETABLE OMEGA-3 FLAX SEED OIL - Systemic Formulas
Superunsaturate (Alphalinolenic Acid, Omega-3) • Polyunsaturate (Linoleic Acid, Omega-6) • Monounsaturate (Oleic Acid) • Saturated Fatty Acid • Beta Carotene • Vitamin E • Phytosterols • Lecithin and Traces of Fiber.

#134 LEV LECITHIN - Systemic Formulas
Lecithin • Inositol • Choline • Phospholipids.

#14 COLON - Systemic Formulas
Psyllium Husks • Cascara Sagrada • Licorice Root • Peach Bark • Stillingia • Dolomite • Calcium Carbonate • Citric Acid • Potassium Bicarbonate.

#140 Min Multi-Mineral Plus - Systemic Formulas
Great Salt Lake Water • Calcium Carbonate • Horse Tail • Magnesium Oxide • Calcium Lactate • Calcium Citrate • Irish Moss • Magnesium Chloride • Red Root • Zinc Chelate • Kelp • Manganese Chelate • Iron Chelate • Vitamin C • Iron Aspartate • Potassium Bitartrate • Copper Chelate • Manganese Picolinate • Zinc Picolinate • Molybdenum Chelate • Vanadium Chelate • Chromium Chelate • Selenium Chelate.

#150 PRO NUTRO PROTEIN - Systemic Formulas
Whey Protein • Pasteurized Saccharomyces Cerevisiae • Rice Protein • Green Lipped Mussel • RNA/DNA Trachea Factors • Dolomite • Dulse • Pimiento • Choline • Papain • Horse Tail (source of Silica) • Niacin • Pancreatin Enzyme • Vitamin C • Tyrosine • Valine • Aspartic Acid • Cystine • Methionine • Vitamin B6 • Vitamin E • RNA/DNA Thalamus Factors. See Editor's Note No. 14, page 1817.

#155 PTM Potassium Stabilizer - Systemic Formulas
Potassium Bitartrate • Potassium Chloride • Magnesium Oxide • Boldo • Pfaffia • Kelp • Maracuja • Chamomile.

#17 D DIGESTIVE - Systemic Formulas
Pancrelipase Enzyme • Golden Seal • RNA/DNA Oxbile Factors • Aspartic Acid • Betaine HCl • L-Glutamic Acid • Echinacea • Lipase • Amylase • Protease • Pepsin • Ammonium Chloride. See Editor's Note No. 14, page 1817.

#18 Ds DIGESTIVE STABILIZER - Systemic Formulas
Kola Nut • Pancrelipase Enzyme • RNA/DNA Oxbile Factors • Betaine HCl • Echinacea • Glutamic Acid • Spearmint • RNA/DNA Liver Factors • Calcium • Papaya Leaves • Golden Seal • Aspartic Acid • Ammonium Chloride • Pancreatin Enzyme • Gentian Root • Guava Powder • Bromelain • Pepsin 1/3000. See Editor's Note No. 14, page 1817.

#22 F+ Female Plus - Systemic Formulas
Sarsaparilla • Blue Cohosh • Dong Quai • Tayuya • False Unicorn • Cana do Brejo • Carrapichinho • Pfaffia • Motherwort • Balm Mint • Agoniada.

#31 GA ADRENAL - Systemic Formulas
RNA/DNA Adrenal Factors • Echinacea • Vitamin C • D-Calcium Pantothenate • Inositol • Ma Huang • Sete Sangrias • RNA/DNA Spleen Factors • Zinc Chelate • Selenium Aspartate. See Editor's Note No. 14, page 1817.

#32 GB PITUITARY - Systemic Formulas
RNA/DNA Brain Factors • Whey Protein • RNA/DNA Pituitary Factors • Peach Bark • Jaborandi • RNA/DNA Orchic Factors • L-Methionine • Vitamin B6 • Superoxidedismutase. See Editor's Note No. 14. page 1817.

#39 Gf THYROID - Systemic Formulas
Irish Moss • Thyroid-6x dilution • Pata de Vaca • Abutua Kelp • Cucurbita Pepo • RNA/DNA Lung Factors • RNA/DNA Thymus Factors. See Editor's Note No. 14, page 1817.

BRAND NAMES

Some Brand Name Natural Products - What they Contain
www.NaturalDatabase.com contains MANY more listings than appear here.

#400 APHA pH CONTROL - Systemic Formulas
Rhubarb Root • Spearmint • Calcium Carbonate • Nettle • Seaweed • Hyssop • Shave Grass • RNA/DNA Adrenal Factors • Potassium Bitartrate.
See Editor's Note No. 14, page 1817.

#402 ARTA ARTHRO SUPPORT - Systemic Formulas
Chapu de Couro • Spearmint Leaves • Pomegranate • Vitamin B2 • RNA/DNA Adrenal Factors • Potassium Bitartrate • Magnesium Sulfate • Vitamin B6 • Niacin • Chaparral • Mistletoe • Yucca • Tayuya • Burdock Seed • Lysine • Isoleucine • Methionine • Magnesium Chelate • RNA/DNA Pituitary Factors • Zinc Chelate • Chromium Chelate.
See Editor's Note No. 14, page 1817.

#403 ATAK SHIELD REJUVENATOR - Systemic Formulas
Pau d'Arco • Yarrow • Stevia • Calcium Carbonate • Betaine HCl • Tayuya • Gravel Root • Pimpinella Root • Yellow Dock • Echinacea • Rose Hips.

#405 BLDB BLOOD BUILDER - Systemic Formulas
RNA/DNA Blood Factors • Burdock • RNA/DNA Liver Factors • Wahoo • RNA/DNA Spleen Factors • L-Cystine • L-Leucine • Chlorophyll.
See Editor's Note No. 14, page 1817.

#408 CLNZ TOXIN CHELATOR - Systemic Formulas
Dandelion Root • Pfaffia • Cinquefoil • Milk Thistle • Mountain Mahogany • Yucca • Vitamin E • Wahoo • RNA/DNA Liver Factors • L-Methionine.
See Editor's Note No. 14, page 1817.

#41 GT THYMUS - Systemic Formulas
Vitamin C • Sweet Basil • Golden Seal • RNA/DNA Thymus Factors • Poke Root • Pau d'Arco • RNA/DNA Liver Factors and Lung Factors • Calcium Carbonate • Zinc Aspartate • RNA/DNA Spleen Factors • Magnesium Chloride • Bitter Root • Beta Carotene • Thymol Iodide • RNA/DNA Stomach Factors • Selenium Yeast • Chromium Chelate • Vitamin B2 • Inositol • Niacinamide • PABA • Vitamin B1 • Calcium Pantothenate • Vitamin B6 • Niacin • Vitamin B12 • Folic Acid • Biotin.
See Editor's Note No. 14, page 1817.

#425 DIJS STOMACH ANTACID - Systemic Formulas
Oregon Grape • Golden Seal • Spearmint • Sodium Bicarbonate • Potassium Bitartrate • Sodium Chloride • Spearmint Oil • Anise Oil • Potassium Bicarbonate • Sodium Citrate • Malt Diastase • Chlorophyll.

#428 DSIR DIGESTANT INTERNAL REGENERATOR - Systemic Formulas
RNA/DNA Stomach and Duodenal Factors • Echinacea • Rose Hips • Ma Huang • Stevia • Allantoin • RNA/DNA Thymus Factors • Hesperidin • Vitamin C • L-Methionine • Senna Pod • L-Glutamic Acid • Vitamin A • Pau d'Arco • Vitamin B6 • Spearmint Oil • Aloe Vera • Sodium Copper Chlorophyll.
See Editor's Note No. 14, page 1817.

#435 GOLD SHIELD PLUS - Systemic Formulas
Golden Seal • Niacin • Vitamin B6 • Rose Hips • Vitamin C • Fenugreek • Garlic • Vitamin B1 • Elder Berry • Spearmint Oil • Lomatium Dissecutim.

#44 H HEART - Systemic Formulas
RNA/DNA Heart Factors • Lecithin • Chromium Chelate • Phenylalanine • Sete Sangrias • Tayuya • RNA/DNA Thymus Factors • Woodruff • RNA/DNA Spleen Factors • Tyrosine • Vitamin B2 • Carnitine • Vitamin B1 • Niacin • Vitamin B6 •

Calcium (from Pantothenate) • Folic Acid • Biotin.
See Editor's Note No. 14, page 1817.

#45 Hcv HEART CARDIO VASCULAR - Systemic Formulas
Sete Sangrias • RNA/DNA Heart Factors • Pimiento • Cassia Bark • Stevia • Hawthorne Berries • Potassium Bitartrate.

#450 KDIR DIURETIC - Systemic Formulas
Manganese Chelate • Ch de Bugre • Juniper Berry • Peach Bark • Saw Palmetto • Zinc Aminoate • Magnesium Sulfate • Peach Leaves • Uva Ursi.

#46 Hn HEART NERVE - Systemic Formulas
RNA/DNA Brain and Spleen Factors • Hesperidin • RNA/DNA Lung Factors • Calcium Pantothenate • Niacin • Tayuya • Vitamin B2 • L-Threonine • RNA/DNA Aorta Factors • L-Methionine • Selenium Chelate • RNA/DNA Heart Factors • Beta Carotene • Chromium Chelate.
See Editor's Note No. 14, page 1817.

#460 KYRO MUSCLE/LIGAMENT/TISSUE STRENGTHENER - Systemic Formulas
Orange Peel • Beta Carotene • Collagen • Bone Meal • Pfaffia • Vitamin C • Manganese Chelate • Slippery Elm • RNA/DNA Liver Factors • Vitamin B12 • Sete Sangrias • Vitamin E • Lemon Bioflavonoid • Pimiento • RNA/DNA Heart Factors • Hesperidin • Stevia • Cassia Bark • Potassium Bitartrate • Vitamin A • Hawthorne Berry.

#481 OXAA CELL ORGANIZER - Systemic Formulas
Centaury Herb • Red Clover Blossom • Peach Bark • Stillingia • Buckthorn Bark • Oregon Grape • Cascara Sagrada • Prickly Ash Bark • Cinquefoil • Saw Palmetto • Burdock Root.

#482 OXCC CELL CLEANSER - Systemic Formulas
Choke Cherry • Irish Moss • Pimiento • Blessed Thistle • Peach Bark • Oregon Grape • Fringe Tree • Red Clover • Burdock Root.

#483 OXOX CELL ACTIVATOR - Systemic Formulas
Fenugreek • Cyani Petals • Pulsatilla • Mandrake • Myrrh Gum • Gentian Root • Primrose • Pfaffia • Bugleweed • Barberry • Prickly Ash • Golden Seal • Blue Vervain • Catnip • Allantoin • Comfrey Root.

#486 SENG RED GINSENG PLUS - Systemic Formulas
Red Ginseng • Pasteurized Saccharomyces Cerevisiae • Potassium Phosphate (Source of Phosphorous and Potassium) • Yucca • Chaparral.

#488 VIVI ANTI VIRO - Systemic Formulas
Pau D'Arco • Lomatium Dissecutim Oil • Vitamin E.

#491 VRM1 LARGE PATHOGENS - Systemic Formulas
Pau d'Arco • Rose Hips • Garlic • Valerian Root • Hops • Bromelain • Zapilopatle Beans • Hojas de Jalapa • Dolomite • Worm Seed Oil.

#492 VRM2 SMALL PATHOGENS - Systemic Formulas
Black Walnut Husks • Wormseed Herb • Kamala • Quassia Chips • Bromelain Enzyme • Bethyl Nut.

#493 VRM3 MICRO PATHOGENS - Systemic Formulas
Black Walnut Husks • Carrapichinho • Erva Tostao • Aniz Estrelado • Bromelain Enzyme • Worm Seed Oil • Yerba Santa.

#494 VRM4 CELLULAR PATHOGENS - Systemic Formulas
Kamala • Guarana • Carrapichinho • Maracuj • Wormseed Herb • Papain • Alfazema.

Some Brand Name Natural Products - What they Contain
www.NaturalDatabase.com contains MANY more listings than appear here.

#50 I EYES - Systemic Formulas
Rue Herb • Eye Bright • Vitamin A • Vitamin E • Chap,u de Couro •
Proline • Cystine • RNA/DNA Eye Factors • Vitamin B6 • Valine •
Niacin • RNA/DNA Brain Factors.
See Editor's Note No. 14, page 1817.

#58 Ks KIDNEY STABILIZER - Systemic Formulas
Rose Hips • Gelatin • RNA/DNA Kidney Factors • Magnesium
Sulfate • Juniper Berries • Vitamin C • Sete Sangrias • Spearmint Herb
• Calcium Carbonate, Hesperidin Complex • Serine • Phenylalanine •
RNA/DNA Adrenal and Thalamus Factors • Tyrosine • Vitamin A •
Sodium Copper Chlorophyll.
See Editor's Note No. 14, page 1817.

#60 L LIVER - Systemic Formulas
RNA/DNA Liver Factors • Mountain Mahogany • Spearmint Leaves •
Vitamin A • Vitamin D • Ragweed • Golden Seal • Quince Seed •
Boldo • Vitamin C • Vitamin E.
See Editor's Note No. 14, page 1817.

#61 LB LIVER NORMALIZER - Systemic Formulas
Red Beet • Betaine HCl • Choline Bitartrate • Lipase 24.

#62 LS LIVER STIMULANT - Systemic Formulas
Rose Hips • Vitamin C • Chromium Chelate • Magnesium Chelate •
Red Beet • Sete Sangrias • Ch de Bugre • Potassium Chelate • RNA/
DNA Adrenal Factors • Choline Bitartrate • Iron Chelate • RNA/DNA
Thymus Factors • Vitamin A • RNA/DNA Pituitary and Liver Factors.
See Editor's Note No. 14, page 1817.

#70 M+ MALE ENDOCRINE - Systemic Formulas
RNA/DNA Orchic Factors • Hops • Boldo (from Chile) • Cipó
Caboclo • Abacateiro • Agoniada • Chinese Bamboo • Cipó Cravo •
RNA/DNA Prostate Factors • African Yohimbe • Eucalyptus • Catuaba
• Muirapuama.
See Editor's Note No. 14, page 1817.

#72 Mpc Prostata Corrector - Systemic Formulas
Cucurbita Pepo Oil • Pau D'Arco • RNA/DNA Prostate Factors •
Gingko Leaves • Pau D'Alho • RNA/DNA Orchic, Thymus, Pituitary
& Hypothalamus Factors • Golden Seal • Echinacea Purpurea •
Thyme.
See Editor's Note No. 14, page 1817.

#73 Mpr Prostata Ovatum - Systemic Formulas
Cucurbita Pepo Oil.

#75 N3 ANTI-TENSIVE - Systemic Formulas
Tayuya • Blue Vervain • Valerian Root Extract • Senna Leaves •
L-Methionine • Passion Flower Extract • Calcium Chelate • Saw
Palmetto • Sete Sangrias • Mandrake Root • Ephedra • Tyrosine.

#77 NC CALM - Systemic Formulas
Calcium Carbonate • Dulse • Passion Flowers • Muirapuama • RNA/
DNA Brain Factors • Tayuya • Boldo • Selenium Chelate • RNA/DNA
Spleen and Lung Factors • Valerian • Niacin • Vitamin B12 • Vitamin
B2 • Vitamin B1.
See Editor's Note No. 14, page 1817.

#78 P PANCREAS - Systemic Formulas
RNA/DNA Pancreas Factors • Catuaba • Cynita Cactus • Japecanga •
Pata de Vaca • Pedra Hume Ca • Zinc Oxide.
See Editor's Note No. 14, page 1817.

#79 Ps PANCREAS STABILIZER - Systemic Formulas
RNA/DNA Pancreas Factors • Catuaba • Cynita Cactus • Japecanga •
Pata de Vaca • Pedra Hume Ca • Zinc Oxide.
See Editor's Note No. 14, page 1817.

#80 R Lung - Systemic Formulas
Golden Seal • RNA/DNA Lung Factors • Pancreatin 4x • RNA/DNA
Thymus Factors • L-Lysine • Aspartic Acid • Allantoin • Tayuya •
Aloe Vera.
See Editor's Notes No. 1 and No. 14, pages 1816 and 1817.

#82 S SPLEEN - Systemic Formulas
RNA/DNA Spleen Factors • Pedra Hume Ca • Nettle • Sweet Gum
Tree • RNA/DNA Liver Factors and Pancreas Factors • Lysine •
L-Methionine • Leucine • Isoleucine.
See Editor's Note No. 14, page 1817.

#FPMS Female Premenses Syndrome - Systemic Formulas
Vitamin B6 • Cystine • Vitamin A • Magnesium Sulfate • Vitamin E •
L-Thionine • Muirapuama • Blue Malva • Pata de Vaca • RNA/DNA
Pituitary Factors • L-Methionine • RNA/DNA Duodenal Factors •
Choline • Motherwort • Angelica • Cyani Blossoms • Niacin • Inositol
• Histidine • Superoxidedismutase • Dong Quai • Zinc Chelate •
Vitamin B12 • Octacosanol.
See Editor's Note No. 14, page 1817.

@zit.gone - Pacific BioLogic
Kochia fruit • Licorice root • Phellodendron bark • Coptis rhizome •
Chrysanthemum flower • Forsythia fruit • Ophiopogonis tuber •
Rehmannia root (fresh) • Trichosanthis root • Scrophularia root.

10 Mushroom Combination - Olympia Nutrition
Contains: Cordyceps, Reishi, Maitake, Shitake, Poria, Polyporus,
Coriolus, Tremella, Hericium, and Wood Ear mushrooms.

10% Plus Nighttime Cream - Jason
Alpha Hydroxy Acids.

100% Egg Protein - Healthy 'N Fit
100% pure extracted egg albumen (with a protein efficiency ratio of
3.9 or greater), enzymatic digest of egg albumia containing naturally
occurring amino acids, vanilla flavoring, bromelain and papain.

12-1/2% Plus with SPF 12-1/2 Protective Moisturizer - Jason
Antioxidant Ester-C • Vitamin E.

19-Nor 250 - AST Sports Science
Each capsule contains: 19-Norandrostenedione 250 mg.

19-Nor Andro 100 - Metabolic Response Modifiers
Each capsule contains: 19-norandrostenedione
(19-nor-4-androstene-3, 17-dione) 100 mg.

19-Nor Xtreme - Metabolic Response Modifiers
Two capsules contain: 19-norandrostenedione 100 mg •
19-nor-4-androstene-3, 17-diol 100 mg • 5-androstenediol 50 mg.

19-Nor-3-Andro - AST Sports Science
Each capsule contains: 19-Norandrostenedione 100 mg •
Androstenediol 100 mg • Androstenedione 100 mg.

2nd Wind - Resource Wellness
Two capsules contain: Proprietary Blend (698 mg/capsule):
Flammulina velutipes • Eleutherococcus senticosus (Siberian Ginseng
root extract) • Citrus reticulata (peel extract) • Ganoderma lucidum
• Panax Ginseng (root extract) • Cordyceps sinensis. Other
ingredients: Gelatin, Maltodextrin, Magnesium Stearate, Silicon
Dioxide, Sodium Lauryl Sulfate, Polysorbate 80.

2nd Wind - Sports Nutrition Source.com
Each scoop contains: Vitamin C 180 mg • Caffeine 20 mg • Ginseng
powdered root 10 mg • Chromium Picolinate 200 mcg.

BRAND NAMES

Some Brand Name Natural Products - What they Contain
www.NaturalDatabase.com contains MANY more listings than appear here.

BRAND NAMES

30 Day Beauty Secret - Futurebiotics
Formula I - Two tablets contain: • Royal Jelly (freeze dried) 50 mg • Horsetail (extract equivalent to) 300 mg • Dong Quai (extract equivalent to) 100 mg • Polygonum Multiflorum (extract equivalent to) 140 mg • Peony Root (extract equivalent to) 120 mg • Betaine HCl 75 mg • Selenium (Amino Acid Chelate) 50 mcg • Iodine (Kelp) 175 mcg • Iron (Amino Acid Chelate) 8 mg • Magnesium (Oxide, Amino Acid Chelate) 150 mg • Manganese (Amino Acid Chelate) 10 mg • Boron 3 mg • Zinc (Gluconate) 15 mg • Calcium (Carbonate, Phosphate, Casein) 300 mg • Phosphorus (Calcium Phosphate) 150 mg • Collagen 100 mg • Ribonucleic Acid (RNA) 50 mg • Sodium Phosphate 1 mg • Gelatin 200 mg • Papain 25 mg • Keratin 30 mg • Formula II - One caplet contains: Beta Carotene 10,000 IU • Vitamin C 150 mg • Vitamin B1 (Thiamin) 10 mg • Vitamin B2 (Riboflavin) 10 mg • Niacinamide 60 mg • Vitamin D (Fish Liver Oil) 200 IU • Vitamin E (Natural Mixed Tocopherols) 30 IU • Vitamin B6 (Pyridoxine) 10 mg • Vitamin B12 (Cyanocobalamin) 16 mcg • Folic Acid 400 mcg • Biotin 300 mcg • Pantothenic Acid 30 30 mg • Inositol 50 mg • Para Amino Benzoic Acid (PABA) 50 mg • Choline (Bitartrate) 150 mg.

30-Day Value Pack - Nature's Life
Mega-Vita-Min Vitamin C, 500 mg. Each tablet contains: Beta Carotene (Vitamin A equivalent to 5000 IU) 3 mg • Vitamin B1 (Thiamine HCl) 10 mg • Vitamin B2 (Riboflavin) 10 mg • Vitamin B6 (Pyridoxine HCl) 10 mg • Vitamin B12 (Cobalamin concentrate) 100 mcg • Niacin 10 mg • Pantothenic Acid (d-Calcium Pantothenate) 20 mg • Folic Acid 400 mcg • Choline (Bitartrate) 90 mg • Biotin (d-Biotin) 50 mcg • PABA (Para Aminobenzoic Acid) 20 mg • Lemon Bioflavonoids Complex (TESTLAB) 15 mg • Vitamin C 100 mg • Vitamin E (d-Alpha Tocopheryl with mixed Tocopherols) 10 IU • Boron (Full-Range Amino Acid Chelated) 25 mcg • Calcium (Full-Range Amino Acid Chelated) 50 mg • Chromium (Nutrition 21 Picolinate) 50 mcg • Copper (Full-Range Amino Acid Chelated) 200 mcg • Iodine (Icelandic Kelp) 225 mcg • Magnesium (Full-Range Amino Acid Chelated) 50 mg • Manganese (Full-Range Amino Acid Chelated) 2 mg • Molybdenum (Proteinate) 25 mcg • Phosphorus (Full-Range Amino Acid Chelated & Complexed) 19 mcg • Potassium (Proteinate) 15 mg • Selenium (Nutrition 21 Selenomethionine) 25 mcg • Silicon (Dioxide) 25 mcg • Vanadium (Full-Range Amino Acid Chelated) 25 mcg • Zinc (Nutrition 21 Picolinate) 2 mg • Betaine HCl 30 mg • Nuclei Acids (RNA & DNA from Yeast) 30 mg • Co Q10 (Co-enzyme Ubiquinone) 500 mcg • Essential Fatty Acids (Soy, Spirulina) 25 mg • Super Green Pro 96 (Soy Protein Super Food) 330 mg. In a natural base containing: Rose Hips concentrate, Acerola, Rutin, Hesperidin, Lecithin, Milk-Free Lactobacillus Acidophilus, Alfalfa Leaf, Watercress, Parsley, "72 Trace Minerals", Rice Bran, Spirulina, Barley Green, Psyllium, Apple Pectin, Oat Bran, Bromelain, Papain, Chlorella & Chlorophyll.

3-Daily - The Vitamin Shoppe
Three capsules contain: Vitamin A Activity 25000 IU • Vitamin E 400 IU • Green Tea extract 50 mg • L-Glutathione 10 mg • Vitamin D 400 IU • Vitamin C 500 mg • CoQ10 100 mcg • Selenium 50 mcg • Pycnogenol 100 mcg • N-Acetyl Cysteine 15 mg • Molybdenum 50 mcg • Vitamin B1 50 mg • Vitamin B2 50 mg • Niacinamide 50 mg • Vitamin B6 50 mg • Vitamin B12 500 mcg • Folic Acid 800 mcg • Inositol 50 mg • Choline 50 mg • PABA 50 mg • Vitamin K 30 mcg • Biotin 50 mcg • Pantothenic Acid 50 mg • Calcium 100 mg • Magnesium 50 mg • Zinc 15 mg • Iron 10 mg • Iodine 150 mcg • Potassium 50 mg • Manganese 5 mg • Chromium 100 mcg • Boron 3 mg • Apple Pectin 50 mg • Betaine HCl 25 mg • Glutamic Acid 25 mg • Papain 25 mg • Pepsin 25 mg • Amylase 10 mcg • Lipase 10 mcg • Chlorophyll 10 mg • Spirulina 45 mg • Chlorella 45 mg • Barley Grass 45 mg • Alfalfa concentrate 45 mg • Bee Pollen 45 mg • Rutin 50 mg • Bioflavonoids 50 mg • Shark Cartilage 50 mg • Siberian Ginseng 45 mg • Royal Jelly 15 mg • Echinacea/Golden Seal 50 mg • Shiitake/Reishi Mushrooms 45 mg • RNA/DNA 45 mg. A concentrated blend of: broccoli, tomato, garlic, onions, cauliflower, brussel sprouts, carrots, parsley, watercress, and pure dry cold-pressed borage.

4-Diol 250 - AST Sports Science
Each capsule contains: 4-Androstenediol 250 mg.

5 HTP Plus - Olympian Labs
Each capsule contains: 5-HTP (L-5 hydroxytryptophan) 100 mg • Vitamin B-6 10 mg • Magnesium Citrate 40 mg • Valerian powder 100 mg • Hops 50 mg • Calcium Citrate 80 mg.

50+ - Futurebiotics
Three capsules contain: Beta-carotene 10,000 IU • Vitamin C (buffered ascorbate) 300 mg • Vitamin E (natural) 100 IU • Vitamin D (as Vitamin D3) 400 IU • Vitamin B1 25 mg • Vitamin B2 25 mg • Vitamin B3 (niacinamide) 25 mg • Vitamin B6 25 mg • Vitamin B12 100 mcg • Pantothenic Acid 25 mg • Biotin 300 mcg • Folic Acid 400 mcg • PABA 25 mg • Choline Bitartrate 50 mg • Inositol 25 mg • Calcium (ascorbate, carbonate, chelate) 200 mg • Magnesium (oxide, chelate) 3 mg • Potassium (chloride, iodide) 20 mg • Zinc (gluconate) 15 mg • Copper (gluconate) 2 mg • Manganese (amino acid chelate) 3 mg • Iodine (potassium iodide) 150 mcg • Selenium (amino acid chelate) 150 mcg • Chromium (amino acid chelate) 200 mcg • Molybdenum (amino acid chelate) 50 mcg • Siberian Ginseng 50 mg • Ginkgo Biloba 25 mg • Turmeric 25 mg • Garlic (Pure-Gar 1500 deodorized concentrate) 200 mg • Cayenne 25 mg • Gotu Kola 100 mg • Alfalfa 50 mg.

5-Diol 250 - AST Sports Science
Each capsule contains: 5-Androstenediol 250 mg.

5-HTP - Swanson
Each capsule contains: L-5 HTP (L-5 hydroxytryptophan) 50 mg.

5-HTP - Metabolic Response Modifiers
Each capsule contains: 5-HTP (5-hydroxytryptophan) 100 mg.

7 Vitamin Treatment Cream - Orjene
Vitamin A • Vitamin B5 • Vitamin C • Vitamin D • Vitamin E • Vitamin F • Vitamin H • Antioxidants. Fortified with Beta Carotene.

7-Keto - Enzymatic Therapy/PhytoPharmica
Each capsule contains: DHEA (dehydroepiandrosterone; as 7-Keto) 25 mg.

7-Keto DHEA - PhysioLogics
Each softgel contains: 3-Acetyl-7-Oxo-Dehydroepiandrosterone 12.5 mg.

7-Keto Fuel - TwinLab
Each capsule contains: 7-Keto DHEA (3-Acetyl-7-Oxo-Dehydroepiandrosterone) 50 mg.

7-Keto Lean - PhytoPharmica
Each capsule contains: Iodine (potassium iodide) 100 mcg • Copper (gluconate) 500 mcg • Manganese (Krebs cycle chelate) 500 mcg • 7 KETO DHEA 100 mg • L-Tyrosine 100 mg • Asparagus (Asparagus officinalis) root (rhizome) extract (standardized to contain 4.0%-8.0% asparagosides) 100 mg • Choline Bitartrate 50 mg • Inositol (rice) 50 mg.

7-Keto Naturalean - Enzymatic Therapy
Each capsule contains: 7-Keto DHEA 100 mg • L-Tyrosine 100 mg • Asparagus root extract (Asparagus officinalis) standardized to contain 4.0-8.0% asparagosides 100 mg • Choline Bitartrate FCC 50 mg • Inositol 50 mg • Copper (Gluconate) 500 mcg • Manganese (Krebs Cycle Chelate) 500 mcg • Iodine (Potassium Iodine) 100 mcg. Other Ingredients: Magnesium stearate, Colloidal Silicon dioxide, and Gelatin capsule.

Some Brand Name Natural Products - What they Contain

www.NaturalDatabase.com contains MANY more listings than appear here.

8 Billion Acidophilus & Bifidus - Now
Each capsule contains: A guaranteed potency of: Lactobacillus Acidophilus 4 billion • Bifidobacterium Bifidum 3.2 billion •Bifidobacterium Longum 0.8 billion.

8% Plus Antioxidant Cuticle Cream - Jason
Vitamin A • Vitamin C • Vitamin E.

90% Protein Powder - Puritan's Pride
Two tablespoons (20 g) contain: Calories 70 • Protein 17 g • Total Fat 1 g • L-Isoleucine 850 mg • L-Leucine 1122 mg • L-Lysine 1092 mg • L-Methionine 225 mg • L-Threonine 659 mg • L-Phenylalanine 902 mg • L-Valine 867 mg • L-Histidine 451 mg • L-Arginine 1318 mg • L-Aspartic Acid 2012 mg • L-Cysteine 225 mg • L-Serine 902 mg • L-Glutamic Acid 3312 mg • L-Tryptophan 225 mg • L-Proline 884 mg • L-Glycine 728 mg • L-Alanine 746 mg • L-Tyrosine 659 mg.

A & D Natural Capsules - Progressive Labs
Each softgel contains: Vitamin A (from fish liver oil, Skip Jack liver oil) 10,000 IU • Vitamin D (from fish liver oil, Skip Jack liver oil) 400 IU.

A & D Vitamins - Puritan's Pride
Each softgel contains: Vitamin A 5,000 IU • Vitamin D 400 IU.

A Bonanza of B Vitamins - Swanson
Each capsule contains: Thiamin (as thiamin HCl)(vitamin B-1) 100 mg • Riboflavin (vitamin B-2) 100 mg • Niacinamide USP 100 mg • Vitamin B-6 USP (as pyridoxine HCl) 100 mg • Folic Acid 400 mcg • Vitamin B-12 (as cyanocobalamin) 100 mcg • Biotin USP 100 mcg • Pantothenic Acid (as d-calcium pantothenate) 100 mg • Choline (as choline bitartrate) 100 mg • Inositol 100 mg • PABA (para-aminobenzoic acid) 100 mg.

A Kid's Companion High Potency Chewable Multi-Vitamin Mineral Formula - Natrol
Two wafers contain: Vitamins/Minerals: Vitamin A Activity (Palmitate) 2500 IU • Vitamin A (Beta Carotene) 2500 IU • Vitamin D (Calciferol) 400 IU • Vitamin E (d-Alpha Tocopheryl Succinate) 30 IU • Vitamin C (Ascorbic Acid) 60 mg • Vitamin B1 (Thiamine HCl) 2.5 mg • Vitamin B2 (Riboflavin) 2.5 mg • Vitamin B6 (Pyridoxine HCl) 2.5 mg • Vitamin B12 (Cyanocobalamin) 10 mcg • Niacinamide 20 mg • Calcium (Carbonate) 200 mg • Iron (Gluconate) 5 mg • Folic Acid 400 mcg • Biotin 150 mcg • Pantothenic Acid (Calcium d-Pantothenate) 12.5 mg • Choline (Bitartrate) 10 mg • Inositol 10 mg • PABA (Para Amino Benzoic Acid) 5 mg • Iodine (Kelp) 150 mcg • Magnesium (Oxide) 50 mg • Zinc (Gluconate) 2.5 mg • Copper (Gluconate) 200 mcg • Vitamin K 25 mcg • Selenium, organically bound concentrate 5 mcg • Chromium (ChromeMate) 10 mcg • Manganese (Gluconate) 1 mg • Potassium (Chloride) 1 mg • Silica from standardized Horsetail extract 1.5 mg • Glycine 200 mg • Lemon Bioflavonoids 25 mg • Bee Pollen 25 mg • Acerola 25 mg • Black Currant 25 mg. Flavored with natural fruit extracts (Lemon, Orange) natural flavors (Butterscotch, Vanilla) & sweetened with Fructose.

A.S.A.P. - The Herbalist
Black Cohosh root • Passionflower herb • Scullcap herb • Valerian root • Lobelia leaf • Prickly Ash bark.

A+Zinc - Nutrilite
Each tablet contains: Vitamin A 10000 IU • Zinc Oxide 15 mg • Zinc Gluconate 15 mg.

A-25 Plex - Progressive Labs
Each softgel contains: Vitamin A (Beta Carotene) 15000 IU • Vitamin A (from fish liver oil) 10000 IU • Alfalfa 5 mg • Cranberry juice concentrate 5 mg • Carrot oil 6 mg • Lecithin 5 mg.

AARP Pharmacy Service Formula 502 (Seniors Vitamins) - Retired Persons Services, Inc.
Each caplet contains: Vitamin A (as vitamin A acetate and 3% as beta carotene) 5200 IU • Vitamin C (as ascorbic acid) 60 mg • Vitamin D (as cholecalciferol) 200 IU • Vitamin E (as dl-alpha tocopheryl acetate) 15 IU • Thiamin (vitamin b1as thiamine mononitrate) 1.2 mg • Riboflavin 1.4 mg • Niacin (as niacinamide) 16 mg • Vitamin B-6 (as pyridoxine hydrochloride) 2.2 mg • Folic Acid (folate) 400 mcg • Vitamin B-12 (as cyanocobalamin) 3 mcg • Pantothenic Acid (as d-calcium pantothenate) 10 mg • Calcium (as dicalcium phosphate and calcium carbonate) 100 mg • Iron (as ferrous fumarate) 10 mg • Phosphorous (as dicalcium phosphate) 77 mg • Iodine (as potassium iodide) 150 mcg • Magnesium (as magnesium oxide) 30 mg • Zinc (as zinc oxide) 15 mg • Copper (as cupric sulfate) 2 mg • Manganese (as manganese sulfate) 1 mg • Potassium (as potassium sulfate) 5 mg.
See Editor's Note No. 3, page 1816.

Absorbable Calcium with Vitamin D - Nature's Bounty
Two softgels contain: Vitamin D (as Cholecalciferol) 100 IU • Calcium (as Calcium Carbonate) 1000 mg. Other Ingredients: Soybean Oil, Gelatin, Glycerin, Lecithin, Titanium Dioxide Color.

Absorbable Iron with Hematinic Factors - The Vitamin Shoppe
Each tablet contains: Iron 50 mg • Heme Iron 25 mg • Vitamin C 75 mg • Copper 1 mg • Folic Acid 200 mcg • Vitamin B12 12.5 mcg.

AbsorbAid - Nature's Sources
Two capsules contain: Lipase 1145 LU • Amylase 8316 SKBU • Protease (from Bromelain) 36 GDU • Cellulase 299 CU • Lactase 900 LacU.

Absorbitol Fat Binder - Natrol
Two capsules contain: Chitosan Complex 900 mg. Other ingredients: Magnesium Stearate, Gelatin.

Acceleration - PhytoPharmica
Each capsule contains: Cola Nut extract (cola nitida) 250 mg (contains 35 mg of caffeine) • Green Tea extract (Camellia sinensis) 250 mg (contains 15 mg of caffeine) • Ma Huang extract (Ephedra sinensis) 250 mg (contains 15 mg of ephedrine). Contains no sugar, salt, yeast, wheat, corn, soy, dairy products, coloring, flavoring, or preservatives.

Accu-Mind & Memory - Leiner Health Products
Each caplet contains: Ginkgo Biloba extract (Ginkgo biloba) leaf 60 mg • Vinpocetine 5 mg. Other Ingredients: Dicalcium Phosphate, Cellulose, Silicon Dioxide, Croscarmellose Sodium, Stearic Acid, Dextrin, Crospovidone, Magnesium Stearate, Dextrose, Lecithin, Sodium Carboxymethylcellulose, Sodium Citrate.

ACE Antioxidant Complex - Nature's Life
Each tablet contains: Beta Carotene (Vitamin A equivalent to 5000 IU) 3 mg • Vitamin C 500 mg • Vitamin E (d-Alpha Tocopheryl Succinate) 200 IU • Selenium (Selenomax Selenomethionine) 25 mcg. In a natural base of Rose Hips powder & Nature's Life Greens (A proprietary blend of 24 vegetables & herbs, microalgae, sea vegetables & sprouts).

ACE Ultimate Antioxidant Plus - Nature's Life
Two capsules contain: Antioxidant Nutrients: Beta Carotene (Vitamin A equivalent to 25000 IU) 15 mg • Vitamin C 1000 mg • Vitamin E (d-Alpha Tocopheryl Succinate) 300 IU • Vitamin B2 (Riboflavin, Riboflavin-5-phosphate) 10 mg • Selenium (Selenite, Methionine) 200 mcg • Glutathione (Glutamine/Cysteine/Glycine Tripeptide) 100 mg • Superoxide Dismutase inducing Minerals: Zinc (Citrate, Picolinate) 10 mg • Manganese (Citrate) 10 mg • Copper (Citrate, Gluconate) 1 mg • Antioxidant Flavonoids: Lemon Bioflavonoids Complex (TESTLAB 50% total bioflavonoids as Flavanones,

Hesperidin, Naringenin & Eriocitrin = 50%) [Carbohydrate, Protein, Moisture & Fiber = 50%] 25 mg • Quercetin (Dimorphandra pod) 25 mg • Rutin (Saphora japonica) 25 mg • Hesperidin (citrus) 25 mg • Proanthocyanidins [(Pinus maritima) Pine bark extract] 5 mg • Epigallocatechin Gallate [(Camellia sinensis) Green Tea extract] 5 mg.

Acetabolan - Muscletech
Six capsules contain: Acetyl-L-Carnitine 1000 mg • Glutamine 2000 mg • L-Leucine 1000 mg • L-Valine 250 mg • L-Isoleucine 250 mg • OKG 100 mg • Zinc 60 mg • Taurine 1000 mg.

Acetabolan II - Muscletech
Six capsules contain: NAC (as N-Acetyl-Cysteine Hydrochloride) 400 mg. Ingredients: Acetyl-L-Carnitine • Tribulus terrestris • ZincTech: a unique blend of Chelated Zinc, Magnesium, & Vitamin B6.

Acetyl L-Carnitine - Source Naturals
Each tablet contains: Acetyl-l-Carnitine 500 mg.

Acid-A-Cal - Enzymatic Therapy
Each capsule contains: Calcium Chloride 96 mg • Calcium Phosphate 90 mg • Magnesium Glycerophosphate 51 mg • Vitamin C (Ascorbic Acid/Rose Hips) 50 mg • Vitamin B6 (Pyridoxine HCL) 25 mg • Other ingredients: Betaine HCL 96 mg • Ammonium Chloride 96 mg • Raw Kidney Tissue 30 mg • Citrus Bioflavonoids 30 mg. All organs & glands derived from bovine sources.
See Editor's Note No. 14, page 1817.

Acida-Zyme - Progressive Labs
Each capsule contains: Betaine HCl 200 mg • Glutamic Acid HCl 100 mg • Ammonium Chloride 35 mg • Pepsin USP/NF 25 mg • Protease (from plant enzymes) 150 Units.

Acidophilase - Wakunaga of America
Each caspule contains: Lactobacillus acidophilus 1 billion live cells • Food Enzyme complex 155 mg: Protease, Amylase, & Lactase in a vegetable starch complex.

Acidophilus - PhytoPharmica
Each capsule contains: Proprietary blend of active cultures 4 billion. Contains a specific mixture of Lactobacillus acidophilus, Lactobacillus rhamnosus, Bifidobacteria longum, Bifidobacteria breve.

Acidophilus E.C. - Progressive Labs
Each high potency capsule contains 2.8 billion live organisms from specially selected strains of lactobacillus acidophilus and lactobacillus casei subsp. Rhamnosus in a base of maltodextrin. Hypoallergenic, contains no milk, whey, soy, corn, wheat, yeast or preservatives. Product should be refrigerated to maintain maximum potency.

Acidophilus Xtra - Sundown Vitamins
Each caplet contains: Acidophilus • Bulgaricus • Thermophilus • Bifidum.

Ack-Nee with MAT - Olympian Labs
Two capsules contain: Vitamin A 10000 IU • Beta Carotene (pro-vitamin A) 500 IU • Vitamin E (d-a-tocopheryl acetate) 120 IU • L-Carnitine Fumarate 200 mg • Vitamin C 60 mg • Pantothenic Acid 20 mg • Vitamin B-6 (pyridoxine HCl) 5 mg • Chromium (picolinate, Cromax) 100 mcg • Selenium (l-selenomethionine) 70 mcg • Proprietary Blend: Goldenseal, Curcumin extract, Enyme blend (protease, lipase, amylase), MAT 500 mg.

Acne Support - Amazon Support
Each capsule contains: Abuta • Bitter Melon • Chuchuhuasi • Espinheira Santa • Fedegosa • Sarsaparilla • Tayuya.

Actilife Super Antioxidant - Crystal Springs
Two tablets contain: Red Grape extract seeds 100 mg • Polygonum cuspidatum extract root 100 mg • Trans-Resveratrol 20 mg • Total Resveratrols 24 mg • Emodin 10 mg • Zinc 30 mg.

Actisyn - SportPharma
Each packet contains: Calories 150 • Total Fat 1 g • Total Carbohydrate 8 g • Protein 27 g. Vanilla ingredients: Actipro Protein Substrate: Ion Exchanged Whey Protein Isolate, Whey Protein Concentrate, Enzymatically Hydrolyzed Whey Protein, Pepti-Lean Select Micro-Peptides • Actiplex: Specific Ratios of L-Glutamine, Taurine, L-Leucine, & N-Acetyl-L-Cysteine • Anticell Vitamins & Minerals: Ascorbic Acid, DL- Alpha Tocopheryl Acetate, Vitamin A Palmitate, Potassium Chloride, Magnesium Aspartate, Magnesium Fumerate, Magnesium Oxide, Pyridoxine HCL, Niacinamide, Calcium Phosphate, Magnesium Orotate, Sodium Chloride, Alpha Lipoic Acid, Calcium Alpha-Ketoglutarate, Zinc Gluconate, L-Selenomethionine • Maltodextrin • Actigen: Tri-Methyl Glycine, Specific Nucleotides including: Purine and Pyrimidine Isolates, RNA Hydrolysates • natural & artificial Vanilla & Cream Flavors • CMC Gum • Aspartame • Sunett Brand Sweetener (Acesulfame K).

Activated Quercetin - Source Naturals
Three tablets contain: Quercetin 1000 mg • Vitamin C (magnesium ascorbate) 600 mg • Magnesium (magnesium ascorbate) 47 mg • Bromelain (2000 GDU per g) 300 mg.

Active B-50 - The Vitamin Shoppe
Each capsule contains: Vitamin B1 (Thiamin) 50 mg • Vitamin B2 (Riboflavin) 50 mg • Vitamin B6 (Pyridoxine HCl) 50 mg • Vitamin B12 (Cobalamin Concentrate) 50 mcg • Niacinamide 50 mg • Folic Acid 400 mcg • Pantothenic Acid (d-Calcium Pantothenate) 50 mg • Biotin 50 mcg • Choline 50 mg • Inositol 50 mg • PABA (Para Amino Benzoic Acid) 50 mg. In a base of Alfalfa, Watercress, Parsley, Lecithin, and Rice Concentrate. No Yeast, Corn, Wheat, Soy, Salt, Sugar, Starch, Preservatives, Artificial Colors or Flavors added.

Active Booster Compound - Starlight International
Each caplet contains: Potassium (as Potassium Gluconate) 8.3 mg • Uva Ursi extract, 4:1 (Arctostaphylos uva ursi, leaf) 300 mg • Corn Silk Pistils extract, 4:1 (Zea mays, flower) 300 mg • Citric Acid 200 mg • Parsley leaf extract (Petroselinum crispum, leaf) 50 mg. Other Ingredients: Dicalcium Phosphate, Microcystalline Cellulose, Stearic Acid, Sodium Starch Glycolate, Croscarmellose Sodium, Magnesium Stearate, Silicon Dioxide, Pharmaceutical Shellac, Hydroxypropylmethylcellulose, Carbowax Powder, Calcium Carbonate, Mono & Diglycerides, Gum Acacia.

Active Joints - Health Smart Vitamins
Each caplet contains: Vitamin C (ascorbic acid) 60 mg • Manganese (as manganese glycinate) 2 mg • Glucosamine Sulfate 500 mg • Sea Cucumber 100 mg • Chondroitin Sulfate 400 mg.
See Editor's Note No. 15, page 1817.

Activin 50 Mg Grape Seed Extract - Natrol
One tablet contains: ActiVin (Grape Seed extract) 50 mg. Other ingredients: Dicalcium Phosphate, Microcrystalline Cellulose, Mono & Di-Glycerides, Stearic Acid, Silicon Dioxide, Magnesium Stearate.

Acti-Zyme - Nature's Plus
Two capsules contain: Live Food Enzymes: Aminogen (Aspergillus niger & Aspergillus oryzae proteolytic enzyme complex) 100 mg • Lugamase (Saccharamyces cerevisae & Aspergillus oryzae oligosaccharide enzyme complex) 100 mg • Amylase (30000 units/ gram) 50 mg • Lactase (1000 units/gram) 50 mg • Lipase (5000 units/ gram) 50 mg • Cellulase (5000 units/gram) 50 mg • Protease (100000 units/gram) 50 mg • Oxidase (5000 units/gram) 50 mg • Bromelain (2000 GDU/gram) 50 mg • Diastase (1000 units/gram) 5 mg • Maltase (1000 units/gram) 5 mg. Lactic Flora and Growth

Accelerants: FOS (Fructooligosaccharides), lactic flora growth accelerant 100 mg • Lactospor, micro-encapsulated pure culture of B.Coagulans, provides 300 million viable cells 50 mg. Bioavailability Enhancing Phytonutrient: Bioperine (Piper nigrum fruit) standardized 95% 1-piperoylpiperidine 5 mg. Contains no yeast, wheat, corn, soy, milk, salt, or starch.

Acutrim 16-Hour Steady Control - Ciba Self-Medication, Inc.
Each tablet contains: Active Ingredient: Phenylpropanolamine HCl 75 mg. Other Ingredients: Cellulose Acetate, Hydroxypropyl Methylcellulose, Stearic Acid.

Acutrim Maximum Strength - Ciba Self-Medication, Inc.
Each tablet contains: Active Ingredient: Phenylpropanolamine HCl 75 mg. Inactive Ingredients: Acacia • Calcium Carbonate • D&C Yellow #10 Aluminum Lake • FD&C Yellow #6 Aluminum Lake • Guar Gum • Hydroxypropyl Methylcellulose • Microcrystalline Cellulose • Silicon Dioxide • Stearic Acid.

Acutrim Natural A.M. - Heritage Consumers Products
Two tablets contain: Orange extract (4% synephrine) 100 mg • Niacin 100 mg • Guarana seed extract 300 mg • Polygonum cuspidatum root extract 25 mg • L-Arginine 450 mg • Guar Gum 200 mg • Citrus Pectin 50 mg.

Acutrim Natural P.M. - Heritage Consumer Products
Two tablets contain: Niacin 180 mg • L-Arginine 450 mg • Polygonum cuspidatum 30 mg • Inositol Hexanicotinate 100 mg • L-Glutamine 40 mg • Guar Gum 250 mg • Citrus Pectin 50 mg.

Adagin - Dazzle, Inc.
Each tablet contains: Calcium (as calcium carbonate) 36 mg • Proprietary Blend 520 mg: L-Arginine, Mucuna Pruriens 15% L-dopa, Ashwaganda, Alpha GPC, Tribulis Terrestris Extract 40%, Cordyceps Sinensis Extract, Optizine. Other Ingredients: Silicon Dioxide, Magnesium, Gelatin.

Adaptrin - Pacific BioLogic
Iceland Moss • Red Sandalwood • Hardy Orange • Vetiver • Margosa • Spiral Flag • White Sandalwood • Cloves • Columbine • Wild Lettuce • Marigold • Knotgrass • Licorice • Valerian • Camphor bark • Gypsum • Cardamom • Jamaican Pepper • Ribwort (plantain) • Heartleaved Sida • Myrobalan • Blackthorn • Golden Cinquefoil • Gingerlily • Homeopathic Monkshood.

AD-FX - HerbTech
Each capsule contains: American Ginseng (standardized extract HT-1001containing >15% ginsenosides) 125 mg • Ginkgo biloba standardized extract 29 mg (containing >4% terpenelactones).

Adipokinetix - Syntrax Innovations
Each capsule or tablet contains: Caffeine 100 mg • 1R, 2S Norephedrine HCL 25 mg • Yohimbine HCL 3 mg.

Adipo-Rx Fat Burning Kit - Athletic Technologies Inc.
Two capsules contain: Vitamin B6 (pyridoxine hcl) 50 mg • Chromium (picolinate) 200 mcg • Potassium (gluconate) 20 mg • Ma Huang (as extract providing 20 mg naturally occuring ephedrines) 340 mg • Kola Nut (as extract providing 120 mg naturally occuring caffeine) 1000 mg • Carnitine (as tartrate) 100 mg • White Willow Bark (as powder) 100 mg • Cayenne Pepper 50 mg • Buchu leaves (as powder) 50 mg • Uva Ursi leaves (as powder) 50 mg • Juniper berries (as powder) 50 mg • Proprietary Blend: Legume Protein Concentrate (Phaseo Vulgaris), Chitosan, Garcinia Cambogia (as 50% extract), Gymnema Sylvestre (as herb powder), Cider Vinegar (as powder), Cascara Sagrada (as herb powder), Aloe Vera (200:1 extract) 1300 mg.

Adrenal Chelate - Atrium Inc.
Each tablet contains: Raw Adrenal concentrate (not an extract) 80 mg • L-Leucine 10 mg • L-Isoleucine 20 mg • D-Calcium Pantothenate 60 mg • Sodium Ascorbate 120 mg • Potassium Aspartate 30 mg • Hesperidin Complex 150 mg • Bioflavonoid Complex 75 mg • Chlorophyll 10 mg. In a base of Alfalfa, Celery & Parsley.
See Editor's Note No. 14, page 1817.

Adrenal Plus - Futurebiotics
Raw Adrenal concentrate 80 mg* • Vitamin C (Ascorbic Acid) 150 mg • Pantothenic Acid 60 mg • Zinc (Gluconate) 5 mg • Manganese (Amino Acid Chelate) 1 mg • Schizandra (6:1) 20 mg** • Chinese Licorice (10:1) 12 mg** • Niacinamide 80 mg. *The freeze-dried adrenal concentrate in this product comes from imported range fed cattle growing naturally, unexposed to drugs or chemically influenced foods. **Extracts equivalent to Licorice & Schizandra powders 120 mg.
See Editor's Note No. 14, page 1817.

Adrenal Soluble Fractions - PhytoPharmica
Two capsules contain: Vitamin C (ascorbic acid/rose hip fruit) 250 mg • Vitamin B6 (pyridoxine HCl) 50 mg • Pantothenic Acid (calcium D-pantothenate) 100 mg • Adrenal extract (predigested soluble concentrate) 400 mg • Betaine 250 mg • L-Tyrosine 250 mg • Pituitary extract (freeze-dried) 120 mg • Adrenal cortex extract 33 mg.
See Editor's Note No. 14, page 1817.

Adrenal Support - PhytoPharmica
Two capsules contain: Vitamin C (ascorbic acid/rose hip fruit) 125 mg • Vitamin B6 (pyridoxine HCl) 25 mg • Pantothenic Acid (calcium D-pantothenate) 125 mg • L-Tyrosine 250 mg • Betaine 125 mg • Pituitary extract 60 mg • Adrenal extract (predigested soluble concentrate) 50 mg • Ginger (Zingiber officinale) root (rhizome) extract 6.5:1 50 mg • Adrenal cortex extract 17 mg.
See Editor's Note No. 14, page 1817.

Adrenal-Cortex Complex - Enzymatic Therapy
Each capsule contains: Adrenal-Cortex Complex 250 mg • Multi-Glandular Complex: Raw Liver, Raw Lung, Raw Pancreas, Raw Heart, Raw Kidney, Raw Spleen, & Raw Brain 100 mg. Contains no sugar, salt, yeast, wheat, corn, soy, dairy products, coloring, flavoring or preservatives.
See Editor's Note No. 14, page 1817.

Adrenal-Cortex Fractions - PhytoPharmica
Each capsule contains: Adrenal-Cortex Complex 250 mg • Multi-Glandular Complex containing: Raw Liver, Raw Lung, Raw Pancreas, Raw Heart, Raw Kidney, Raw Spleen, and Raw Brain 100 mg. Contains no sugar, salt, yeast, wheat, corn, soy, dairy products, coloring, flavoring, or preservatives. All organs & glands derived from bovine sources except raw pancreas (porcine).
See Editor's Note No. 14, page 1817.

Adren-Comp - Enzymatic Therapy
Each capsule contains: Chinese Thoroughwax extract (Bupleurum falcatum) 150 mg • Korean Ginseng root extract 3:1 (Panax ginseng) 100 mg • Siberian Ginseng extract (Eleutherococcus senticosus) standardized to contain greater than 1% eleutheroside E, 100 mg • Mexican Yam extract 10:1 (Dioscorea spinosa) standardized to contain 10% Diosgenin 100 mg • Licorice root extract (Glycyrrhiza glabra) standardized to contain 5% Glycyrrhizic acid 50 mg • Curcuma root extract 10:1 (Curcuma longa) 50 mg.

Adrenerlin - Bodyonics
Two capsules contain: Maca Pure (Lepidum meyenii)(Standardized to contain 0.6% macamides and macanes) 450 mg • Jeevani Botanical Complex (Tricopus zylanicus, Ashwanga (Withania somnifera), Piper Longum, Vishnukranthi (Evolvus alsinoies) 150 mg • Peptide GPX

250 mg • D-Ribose 10 mg • Acetyl-L-Carnitine 10 mg • Bitter Orange (Standardized 4% synephrine) 83.3 mg • Yerba Mate and Guarana Extract (Standardized) 200 mg Methylxanthines/ Caffeine 910 mg • Mucuna Pruriens (Standardized 15% L-Dopa) 33.3 mg • Calcium Pyruvate 10 mg. Other Ingredients: Magnesium Stearate, Gelatin.

Adreno Chelate - Progressive Labs
Each capsule contains: Calcium (Proteinate) 27 mg • Chloride (Proteinate) 50 mg • Sodium (Proteinate) 20 mg • Potassium (Proteinate) 20 mg • Raw Bovine Adrenal concentrate 40 mg • L-Isoleucine 10 mg • L-Leucine 10 mg.
See Editor's Note No. 14, page 1817.

Adreno Trophic - Progressive Labs
Each capsule contains: Pantothenic Acid (Calcium Pantothenate) 50 mg • Raw Bovine Adrenal concentrate 80 mg.
See Editor's Note No. 14, page 1817.

Adreno-Cortex - Atrium Inc.
Each tablet contains: Adrenal Cortex • Pituitary Anterior 20 mg • Pineal, bovine source 10 mg • Vitamin C (Calcium Ascorbate) 25 mg.
See Editor's Note No. 14, page 1817.

Adreno-Medulla Plus - Atrium Inc.
Each tablet contains: Adrenal Medulla 100 mg • Hypothalamus 15 mg • Pituitary Posterior Bovine Source 10 mg • Vitamin C (Calcium Ascorbate) 25 mg.
See Editor's Note No. 14, page 1817.

Adren-Plus - PhytoPharmica
Each capsule contains: Chinese Thoroughwax (Bupleurum chinense) root 150 mg • Korean Ginseng (Panax ginseng) root extract (standardized to contain 7% ginsenosides) 100 mg • Siberian Ginseng (Eleutherococcus senticosus) root extract (standardized to contain greater than 0.5% eleutheroside E) 100 mg • Wild (Mexican) Yam (Dioscorea villosa) root extract (standardized to contain 10% diosgenin) 100 mg • Licorice (Glycyrrhiza glabra) root extract (standardized to contain 5% glycyrrhizic acid) 50 mg • Curcuma (Curcuma longa) root (rhizome) extract (standardized to contain 85%-97% curcumin) 50 mg.

Adult Echinacea+C+Zinc Cherry Flavor - LiFizz Effervescent Vitamins
Each tablet contains: Vitamin C (Ascorbic Acid) 1500 mg • Zinc 15 mg • Echinacea extract (Echinacea purpurea) 100 mg. Other ingredients: Citric Acid, Sodium Bicarbonate, Sorbitol, Mannitol, Polyethylene Glycol 6000, Cherry Flavor, Povidone, Aspartame, Acesulfame Potassium, Magnesium Stearate, Silicon Dioxide, Simethicone.

Adult Echinacea+C+Zinc Lemon/Lime Flavor - LiFizz Effervescent Vitamins
Each tablet contains: Vitamin C (Ascorbic Acid) 1500 mg • Zinc 15 mg • Echinacea extract (Echinacea purpurea) 100 mg. Other Ingredients: Citric Acid, Sodium Bicarbonate, Sorbitol, Mannitol, Polyethylene Glycol 6000, Lemon Flavor, Povidone, Aspartame, Acesulfame Potassium, Lemon/Lime Flavor, Magnesium Stearate, Silicon Dioxide, Simethicone.

Adult Multi-Vitamin Orange Flavor - LiFizz Effervescent Vitamins
Each tablet contains: Vitamin A (Palmitate and Beta Carotene) 5000 IU • Vitamin C 60 mg • Vitamin D 400 IU • Vitamin E 15 IU • Thiamin 1.5 mg • Riboflavin 1.7 mg • Niacinamide 20 mg • Vitamin B6 2 mg • Folic Acid 400 mcg • Vitamin B12 6 mcg • Biotin 300 mcg • Pantothenic Acid 10 mg • Calcium 200 mg • Iron 6 mg • Magnesium 80 mg • Zinc 5 mg.

Adult-C-Vitamin Pink Grapefruit Flavor - LiFizz Effervescent Vitamins
Each tablet contains: Vitamin C (Ascorbic Acid) 500 mg. Other ingredients: Citric Acid, Sorbitol, Potassium Bicarbonate, Sodium Bicarbonate, Mannitol, Grapefruit Flavor, Polyethylene Glycol 6000, Orange Flavor, Aspartame, Acesulfame Potassium, Wild Berry Powder, Silicon Dioxide, Lemon/Lime flavor, Magnesium Stearate.

Adult-C-Vitamin Raspberry Flavor - LiFizz Effervescent Vitamins
Each tablets contains: Vitamin C (Ascorbic Acid) 500 mg. Other Ingredients: Citric Acid, Sodium Bicarbonate, Potassium Bicarbonate, Sorbitol, Mannitol, Polyethylen Glycol 6000, Red Beet Powder, Raspberry Flavor, Aspartame, Acesulfame Potassium, Magnesium Stearate.

AdvaCal - LaneLabs
Three capsules contain: Elemental Calcium (as calcium hydroxide, calcium oxide, combined with algae amino acid extract) 450 mg. Other Ingredients: Citric Acid, Gelatin, Water, Glycerine.

Advanced Chromium HCA - Health Smart Vitamins
Each capsule contains: Calcium (as calcium salt of hydroxy citric acid) 79 mg • Chromium (as chromium picolinate) 100 mcg • Garcinia cambogia fruit (50% (-) hydroxycitric acid [HCA], 250 mg) 500 mg.

Advanced C-Jointin - Puritan's Pride
Three softgels contain: Vitamin C (as Ascorbic Acid) 60 mg • Vitamin E (as d-Alpha-Tocopherol) 10 IU • Manganese (as Manganese Aspartate) 1 mg • Boron (as Boron Citrate) 1.5 mg • Evening Primrose Oil 250 mg • MSM (Methylsulfonylmethane) 750 mg • Chondroitin Sulfate 200 mg • Glucosamine Sulfate 1,000 mg.
See Editor's Note No. 15, page 1817.

Advanced Colloidal Chromium/Vanadium - Futurebiotics
One teaspoon contains: Chromium 0.18 ppm • Vanadium 0.18 ppm. Other ingredients: Deionized Water.

Advanced CoQ10 - Changes - TwinLab
One capsule contains: Coenzyme Q10 50 mg.

Advanced E + Grape Seed Extract - Leiner Health Products
Each softgel contains: Vitamin E (dl-Alpha Tocopherol) 400 IU • Grape Seed extract 20 mg. Other Ingredients: Gelatin, Vegetable Oil, Glycerin, Yellow Beeswax, Unbleached Lecithin, Titanium Dioxide, Carmine.

Advanced E with Alpha Lipoic Acid - Leiner Health Products
Each softgel contains: Vitamin C (Ascorbic Acid) 20 mg • Vitamin E (dl-Alpha Tocopherol, d-Alpha Tocopherol) 400 IU • Alpha Lipoic Acid 30 mg • Rice Bran oil 5 mg. Other Ingredients: Gelatin, Glycerin, Yellow Beeswax, Soybean Oil, Lecithin, Titanium Dioxide, Turmeric.

Advanced Formula - Biotech
Each tablet contains: Folate 400 mg • Pantothenic Acid 100 mg • Biotin 700 mcg • Iodine 75 mcg • Zinc 75 mg • Shen Min 225 mg • Shen Min (He Shou Wu root powder) 435 mg • Isoflavones 10 mg • Saw Palmetto berries standardized extract 160 mg • Silica 20 mg • Black Pepper extract 2.5 mg.

Advanced Geri-Max - Puritan's Pride
Each tablet contains: Vitamin A 10,000 IU • Vitamin C 250 mg • Vitamin D 400 IU • Vitamin E 150 IU • Thiamin 50 mg • Riboflavin 50 mg • Niacin 100 mg • Vitamin B6 50 mg • Folic Acid 400 mcg • Vitamin B12 50 mcg • Biotin 300 mcg • Pantothenic Acid 100 mg •

Calcium 10 mg • Iron 1 mg • Iodine 150 mcg • Magnesium 1.54 mg • Zinc 1.15 mg • Copper 0.25 mg • Manganese 0.61 mg • Potassium 1 mg • PABA 50 mg • Inositol 250 mg • Choline Bitartrate 250 mg • Rutin 25 mg • Citrus Bioflavonoid complex 25 mg • Hesperidin complex 25 mg • Betaine Hydrochloride 25 mg • L-Glutamic Acid 25 mg • Omega-3 EPA / DHA 50 mg. In a natural base of Alfalfa, Watercress, Parsley, Lecithin, and Rice Polishings.

Advanced Ginkgo 24% - Doctor's A-Z
Each softgel contains: Ginkgo Biloba leaf extract (24% flavone glycosides, 6% terpene lactones) 60 mg.

Advanced Joint Support - Futurebiotics
Four capsules supply: Glucosamine Sulfate 1000 mg • Vitamin C (Buffered Ascorbate) 750 mg • Vitamin E (natural) 400 IU • Calcium (Ascorbate) 185 mg • Selenium (Amino Acid Chelate) 100 mcg • Zinc (Amino Acid Chelate) 15 mg • Bovine Cartilage 200 mg • Pancreatin 4X (Quadruple Strength) 100 mg containing: (Lipase 1600 USP units, Amylase 10000 USP units, Protease 10000 USP units) • Papain 60 mg • Bromelain 50 mg • Turmeric (standardized Curcumin) 250 mg • Cayenne powder 15 mg • Ginger powder 100 mg • Boswellin (standardized for 65% Boswellic Acid) 100 mg • Devil's Claw 50 mg • Rutin 50 mg.
See Editor's Note No. 14, page 1817.

Advanced Lutein & Bilberry - Doctor's A-Z
Each softgel contains: Bilberry extract (25% anthocyanidins) 20 mg • FloraGLO® Lutein extract (from marigold) 6 mg.

Advanced Prostate Formula - Rx Vitamins
Three capsules contain: Saw Palmetto fruit 320 mg • Stinging Nettle root 100 mg • African Pygeum bark 50 mg • Zinc 50 mg • Glycine 50 mg • Alanine 50 mg • Glutamic Acid 50 mg • Vitamin B6 50 mg • Vitamin E 100 IU in Borage seed oil.

Advanced Strength Ginkgo Biloba - Leiner Health Products
Each caplet contains: Ginkgo Biloba extract (Ginkgo biloba) leaf 75 mg • Lecithin 15 mg. Other Ingredients: Dicalcium phosphate, Cellulose, Silicon Dioxide, Stearic Acid, Croscarmellose Sodium, Dextrin, Magnesium Stearate, Dextrose, Sodium Carboxymethylcellulose, Sodium Citrate.

Advanced Strength Kava Kava - Leiner Health Products
Each caplet contains: Kava Kava extract (Piper methysticum) root 400 mg. Other Ingredients: Dicalcium Phosphate, Cellulose, Talc, Stearic Acid, Croscarmellose Sodium, Silicon Dioxide, Magnesium Stearate, Crospovidone, Hydroxypropyl Methylcellulose, Hydroxypropyl Cellulose, Polysorbate 80, Polyethylene Glycol 3350.

Aflexa - McNeil Consumer Healthcare
One tablet contains: Glucosamine 340 mg (Glucosamine Sulfate, Glucosamine Hydrochloride). Other ingredients: Cellulose, Hydroxypropyl, Methylcellulose, Polyethylene Glycol, Silicon Dioxide, Propylene Glycol, Crospovidone, Hydroxypropyl Cellulose, Titanium Dioxide, Magnesium Stearate, Polysorbate 80, Povidone.

AfterFX Bar-Bavarian Mint - Nutripeak
Each bar contains: Protein 34 g • Vitamin A (Retinyl Palmitate) 5000 IU • Vitamin C (Ascorbic Acid) 120 mg • Vitamin D (Cholecalciferol) 400 IU • Vitamin E (dl-Alpha Tocopheryl Acetate) 60 IU • Thiamin Mononitrate (Vitamin B1) 1.5 mg • Riboflavin (Vitamin B2) 1.7 mg • Niacin (Niacinamide) 20 mg • Vitamin B6 (Pyridoxine Hydrochloride) 2 mg • Folic Acid 400 mcg • Vitamin B12 (Cyanocobalamin) 6 mcg • Biotin 300 mcg • Pantothenic Acid (Calcium D-Pantothenate) 10 mg • Calcium (Tricalcium Phosphate and Monocalcium Phosphate) 500 mg • Iron (Ferrous Fumarate) 18 mg • Phosphorus 300 mg • Iodine (Potassium Iodide) 150 mcg • Magnesium Oxide 100 mg • Zinc Amino Acid Chelate 15 mg • Copper Gluconate 2 mg • Sodium 75 mg • Potassium 250 mg • HMB (as calcium-b-hydroxy-b-methylbutyrate) 585 mg •

L-Glutamine 3 mg. Other Ingredients: Metamyosyn Protein Blend: Milk Protein Concentrate, Calcium Caseinate, Whey Protein Concentrate, Bovine Hydrolyzed Collagen, Cocoa (processed with alkali), Xanthan Gum, Soy Lecithin, Glycerin, Brown Rice Syrup, Cottonseed Oil, Soybean Oil, Maltodextrin, Sucralose, Acesulfame K, Natural and Artificial Flavors, Potassium Sorbate (preservative); Salt; Hydrogenated Cottonseed Oil.

Age Right Formula - Nature's Way
Four capsules contain: Acetylcarnitine 50 mcg • Acetylcysteine 50 mcg • Betaine Anhydrous 50 mg • Biotin (Biotin Triurate) 500 mcg • Boron (Amino Acid Chelate) 500 mcg • Calcium 43 mg • Calcium Pantethonate 175 mg • Caromix (Mixed Carotenoids) 2000 IU • Chromium Picolinate 100 mcg • Citrus Bioflavonoids 250 mg • Coenzyme Q10 (Ubiquinone) 15 mg • Copper (Amino Acid Chelate) 500 mcg • Fizyme Enzyme Formula 65 mg • Folic Acid (Folate) 250 mcg • Grape seed dried extract 15 mg • Green Tea (Polyphenol Catechin extract) 75 mg • Inositol 15 mg • Kelp (whole Thallus) 25 mg • Manganese (Amino Acid Chelate) 2.5 mg • Molybdenum Triuturate 25 mcg • Niacinamide 47.5 mg • Potassium (Aspartate, Chloride) 25 mg • Riboflavin (Vitamin B2) 25 mg • Selenium (l-Selenomethione) 25 mcg • Thiamine (Vitamin B1) 25 mg • Vitamin A (Retinol Palmitate) 2530 IU • Vitamin B12 (Cyanocobalamin) 250 mcg • Vitamin B6 (Pyridoxine HCL) 25 mg • Vitamin C (Ascorbic Acid) 250 mg • Vitamin D (as Vitamin D3) (Cholecalciferol) 200 IU • Vitamin E (d-Alpha Tocopheryl) 200 IU • Vitamin K (Phytonadione) 30 mcg • Zinc (Amino Acid Chelate) 5 mg. Other ingredients: Gelatin, Magnesium Stearate, Millet.

AgeErasers SAMe - Bodyonics
Each tablet contains: Vitamin B12 50 mcg • Folic Acid 100 mcg • SAMe 200 mg. Other Ingredients: Calcium Phosphate, Stearic Acid, Croscarmellose, Magnesium Strearate.

Air Power - Enzymatic Therapy
Each tablet contains: Active ingredient: Glycerol Guaiacolate 200 mg. Other ingredients: Fenugreek Powder 4:1 (Trigonella foenum-graecum) 350 mg • Marshmallow extract 4:1 mucilage content 30-40% (Althaea officinalis) 125 mg • PABA (Para-Aminobenzoic Acid) 50 mg • Mullein leaf (Verbascum nigrum) 50 mg. Contains no sugar, salt, yeast, wheat, corn, soy, dairy products, coloring, flavoring or preservatives.

Airborne - Knight-McDowell LAbs
Each tablet contains: Vitamin A 5000 IU • Vitamin C 1000 mg • Vitamin E 30 IU • Magnesium 40 mg • Zinc 8 mg • Selenium 15 mcg • Manganese 3 mg • Potassium 75 mg • Organic Herbal Extracts 350 mg: Lonicera, Forsythia, Schizonepeta, Ginger, Chinese Vitex, Isatis root, Echinacea • Amino Acids 50 mg (Glutamine, Lysine). Other Ingredients: Citric Acid, Sorbitol, Sodium Bicarbonate, Natural Orange Flavor, Polyethylene Glycol, Aspartame, Mineral and Canola Oil, Riboflavin.

AKG Fuel - TwinLab
Three capsules contain: Alpha-Ketoglutaric Acid (from Magnesium Alpha-Ketoglutarate) 1250 mg • Magnesium (from Magnesium Alpha-Ketoglutarate) 210 mg • L-Glutamine 1000 mg.

AKN Skin Care - Nature's Way
Two capsules contain: Burdock root • Capsicum root • Dandelion root • Echinacea purpurea root • Kelp (whole Thallus) • Licorice root • Plantain leaf • Sarsaparilla root • Yellow Dock root. Other ingredients: Gelatin.

ALC Fuel - TwinLab
Each capsule contains: Acetyl-L-Carnitine (ALC) 1000 mg.

Alert - PhytoPharmica
Each capsule contains: Cola Nut extract (Cola nitida; contains 35 mg caffeine) 250 mg • Green Tea extract (Camellia sinensis; contains

BRAND NAMES

15 mg caffeine) 250 mg • Oat Straw extract 10:1 (Avena sativa) 50 mg • Schisandra extract (standardized to contain 9% schizandrin) 50 mg • Siberian Ginseng extract (Eleutherococcus senticosus; (standardized to contain greater than 1% eleutheroside E) 50 mg • Ginger root extract 6.5:1 (Zingiber officinale) 25 mg • Korean Ginseng root extract (Panax ginseng; standardized to contain 7% saponis calculated as ginsenoside Rg1) 10 mg • Chromium (Polynicotinate) 100 mcg.

Alert Vitalizing Formula - Starlight International
Two capsules contain: Potassium (as potassium glycerophosphate) 35 mg • Schisandra extract 4:1 (schisandra chinensis, berry) 250 mg • Oriental Ginseng (panax ginseng, root) 300 mg • Guarana extract 6:1 (paulina cupana, seed) 600 mg • Caffeine 132 mg • Adrenal Substance 150 mg • Coenzyme Q10 5.0 mg • Siberian Ginseng (eicutherococcus senticosus, root) 1.0 mg • Spirulina 1.0 mg. Other Ingredients: Dicalcium Phosphate, Magnesium Stearate, Silicon Dioxide, Gelatin. See Editor's Note No. 14, page 1817.

Alertis Compound - The Herbalist
False Unicorn root • Squaw Vine herb • Cramp bark • Blue Cohosh root • Ginger root.

Alfalfa - Quest
Each tablet contains: Organic Alfalfa 650 mg. Other Ingredients: Terra Alba, Silica, Magnesium Stearate (vegetable source).

Alfalfa-Devil's Claw Formula - Quest
Each caplet contains: Alfalfa leaf powder (Medicago sativa) 70 mg • Alfalfa seed powder 70 mg • Burdock root powder (Arctium lappa) 70 mg • Celery seed powder (Apium graveolens) 70 mg • Devil's Claw root powder (Herpagophytum procumbens) 70 mg • Cayenne powder (Capsicum) 35 mg • Kelp powder (Fucus versiculosis) 35 mg • Queen of the Meadow root powder (Filipendula ulmaria) 5 mg • Sarsaparilla root powder (Smilax officinalis) 5 mg. Other Ingredients: Calcium Phosphate, Microcrystalline Cellulose, Vegetable Stearin, Croscarmellose Sodium, Magnesium Stearate (vegetable source).

Alka-Mine Coral Calcium - Ericssons
Coral Calcium • Magnesium • Ascorbic Acid • Silver.

All Purpose Multivitamin/Mineral - Leiner Health Products
Each tablet contains: Vitamin E (dl-Alpha Tocopheryl Acetate) 15 IU • Magnesium Oxide 100 mg • Calcium 160 mg • Phosphorus 125 mg • Folate (Folic Acid) 400 mcg • Iodine 150 mcg • Iron (Ferrous Fumarate) 18 mg • Niacin (Niacinamide) 20 mg • Riboflavin (Vitamin B2) 1.7 mg • Thiamin Mononitrate (Vitamin B1) 1.5 mg • Vitamin A Palmitate 5000 • Vitamin B12 (Cyanocobalamin - USP Method 2) 6 mcg • Vitamin B6 (Pyridoxine Hydrochloride) 2 mg • Vitamin C (Ascorbic Acid) 60 mg • Vitamin D (Ergocalciferol) 400 IU. Other ingredients: Dicalcium Phosphate, Gelatin, Hydroxypropyl Methylcellulose, Croscarmellose Sodium, Sodium Starch Glycolate, Niacinamide, dl-Alpha Tocopheryl Acetate, Cellulose, Tricalcium Phosphate, Silicon Dioxide, Titanium Dioxide, Starch, Polyethylene Glycol 3350, Hydroxypropyl Cellulose, Magnesium Stearate, Yeast, Pyridoxine Hydrochloride, Polysorbate 80, Pharmaceutical Glaze, Resin, Povidone, Potassium Iodide.

All-Day Complete - Swanson
Each rounded scoop (15 g) contains: Calories 44 • Calories from Fat 0 • Total Carbohydrate 2 g • Dietary Fiber 1 g • Protein 7 g • Vitamin A (as palmitate) 8000 IU • Vitamin A (as beta-carotene) 1000 IU • Vitamin C (as ascorbic acid) 1 g • Vitamin D (as cholecalciferol) 500 IU • Vitamin E (as d-alpha tocopheryl acetate) 400 IU • Vitamin K 5 mcg • Thiamin (as thiamin HCl; vitamin B-1) 25 mg • Riboflavin (vitamin B-2) 25 mg • Niacin (as niacinamide) 100 mg • Vitamin B-6 (as pyridoxine HCl) 25 mg • Folic Acid 400 mcg • Vitamin B-12 (as cyanocobalamin) 25mcg • Biotin 300 mcg • Pantothenic Acid (as d-calcium pantothenate) 100 mg • Calcium (from calcium carbonate and dicalcium phosphate) 500 mg • Iron (as ferrous gluconate) 18 mg

• Phosphorus (from d-calcium phosphate) 200 mg • Iodine (from potassium iodide) 150 mcg • Magnesium (from magnesium oxide) 200 mg • Zinc (from zinc oxide) 15 mg • Selenium (as proteinate) 50 mcg • Copper (from copper gluconate) 1 mg • Manganese (from manganese sulfate) 4 mg • Chromium (as chromium proteinate complex) 50 mcg • Molybdenum (as amino acid chelate) 50 mcg • Potassium (as potassium citrate) 99 mg • Lecithin 750 mg • Lemon Bioflavonoid complex 400 mg • Hesperidin complex 25 mg • PABA (para-aminobenzoic acid) 25 mg • Rutin (from buckwheat) 25 mg • Choline (from lecithin) 20 mg • Inositol (from lecithin) 15 mg • Betaine HCl 2 mg • Papain (from papaya) 2 mg • Kelp 1.5 mg.

All-Day Complete (for Seniors) - Swanson
Each rounded scoop (15 g) contains: Calories 40 • Calories from Fat 9 • Total Fat 1 g • Total Carbohydrate 4 g • Dietary Fiber 3 g • Protein 3 g • Vitamin A (as palmitate) 8000 IU • Vitamin A (as beta-carotene) 1000 IU • Vitamin C (as ascorbic acid) 1 g • Vitamin D (as cholecalciferol) 500 IU • Vitamin E (as d-alpha tocopheryl acetate) 400 IU • Vitamin K 5 mcg • Thiamin (as thiamin HCl; vitamin B-1) 25 mg • Riboflavin (vitamin B-2) 25 mg • Niacin (as niacinamide) 100 mg • Vitamin B-6 (as pyridoxine HCl) 25 mg • Folic Acid 400 mcg • Vitamin B-12 (as cyanocobalamin) 25 mcg • Biotin 300 mcg • Pantothenic Acid (as d-calcium pantothenate) 100 mg • Calcium (from calcium carbonate and dicalcium phosphate) 500 mg • Iron (as ferrous gluconate) 18 mg • Phosphorus (from d-calcium phosphate) 200 mg • Iodine (from potassium iodide) 150 mcg • Magnesium (from magnesium oxide) 200 mg • Zinc (from zinc oxide) 15 mg • Selenium (as proteinate) 50 mcg • Copper (from copper gluconate) 1 mg • Manganese (from manganese sulfate) 4 mg • Chromium (as chromium proteinate complex) 50 mcg • Molybdenum (as amino acid chelate) 50 mcg • Potassium (as potassium citrate) 99 mg • Lecithin 1.4 g • Fructooligosaccharides (FOS) 1 g • Lemon Bioflavonoid complex 400 mg • Inositol (from inositol and lecithin) 100 mg • Choline (from lecithin) 50 mg • Ginkgo Biloba powder 25 mg • Hesperidin complex 25 mg • PABA (para-aminobenzoic acid) 25 mg • Rutin (from buckwheat) Coenzyme Q10 20 mg • Reishi Mushroom extract 5 mg • Betaine HCl 2 mg • Papain (from papaya) 2 mg • Kelp 1.5 mg.

Aller-B - Progressive Labs
Each capsule contains: Thiamin (Vitamin B1) 50 mg • Riboflavin (Vitamin B2) 50 mg • Niacinamide 50 mg • Vitamin B6 50 mg • Folate (Folic Acid) 400 mcg • Vitamin B12 60 mcg • Biotin 50 mcg • Pantothenic Acid 100 mg • Choline Bitartrate 50 mg • Inositol 25 mg • PABA (Para Aminobenzioc Acid) 50 mg.

Aller-C Support Formula - The Vitamin Factory
Each tablet contains: Vitamin C (Calcium Ascorbate) 500 mg • Calcium (Ascorbate, Citrate, Pantothenate) 100 mg • Vitamin B5 (Calcium Pantothenate) 50 mg • Pycnogenol (Maritime Pine bark extract) 15 mg.

Aller-Cal - Atrium Inc.
Each tablet contains: Adrenal 80 mg • Pituitary 10 mg • Liver Substance 6 mg • Parathyroid 5 mg • Calcium 20.4 mg • Pantothenic Acid 26 mg • Folic Acid 130 mcg • Ammonium Chloride 30 mg • Choline Bitartrate 25 mg • Methionine 14 mg • Inositol 12 mg • Glutamic Acid HCL 12 mg • Betaine HCL 3.6 mg • Hydrolized Amino Acids 150 mg • Dulse 50 mg • Persic oil 36 mg • Linseed oil 12 mg.
See Editor's Note No. 14, page 1817.

AllerClear - Enzymatic Therapy
Active ingredient: Pseudophedrine HCl (from Ephedra sinensis) 60 mg. Other ingredients: Vitamin E (DL-Alpha Tocopherol) 75 IU • Vitamin C (Ascorbic Acid) 150 mg • Pantothenic Acid (D-Calcium Pantothenate) 150 mg • Choline (Bitartrate) 150 mg • Macrocystis pyrifera 150 mg • Lung extract 90 mg • Adrenal extract 80 mg •

Methionine 75 mg • Pancreatic Enzymes (3X) treated for enteric activity 65 mg • Ammonium Chloride 50 mg • Calcium Chloride 50 mg • Glutamic Acid HCL 50 mg • Betaine HCL 50 mg • Pepsin (1:10000) 49 mg • Magnesium Glycerophosphate 30 mg • Spleen extract 25 mg • Pancreas extract 15 mg • Thymus extract 15 mg • Niacinamide 10 mg • Liver Fractions 10 mg • Vitamin B6 (Pyridoxine HCl) 5 mg. Contains no sugar, salt, yeast, wheat, corn, soy, dairy products, coloring, flavoring or preservatives.
See Editor's Note No. 14, page 1817.

Aller-G Formula 25 - Olympian Labs
Two capsules contain: Vitamin C 200 mg • Histidine 60 mg • Citrus Aurantium extract 200 mg • Bee Pollen 75 mg • Propolis 25 mg • Pantothenic Acid 75 mg • Citrus Bioflavonoid Complex 30 mg • Niacin 20 mg • Goldenseal 25 mg • Echinacea 50 mg • Garlic 25 mg • Yerba Santa 50 mg • Nettle 80 mg • Mullein 40 mg • White Willow Bark 6 mg.

Allergia - HerbaSway
Bitter Orange • Ginger • Panax Ginseng • Blackberry • Kudzu • HerbaSwee (Cucurbitaceae fruit).

Allergy Essentials - Swanson
Three capsules contain: Vitamin C (as calcium ascorbate) 100 mg • Zinc (from zinc chelate and zinc gluconate) 15 mg • Ma Huang extract (6% ephedra) 250 mg • Bromelain (2400 GDU) 100 mg • Licorice root extract (1% glycyrrhizic acid) 100 mg • N-Acetyl-Cysteine 100 mg • Nettle extract (5:1) 100 mg • Quercetin 100 mg • White Willow Bark 100 mg • Cayenne pepper 100,000 HU 50 mg • Echinacea root extract (4% echinacosides) 50 mg • Goldenseal root 50 mg • Grapeseed extract (95% proanthocyanidins) 30 mg.

Allergy Relief - Futurebiotics
Three capsules contain: Vitamin A (as beta-carotene) 5000 IU • Vitamin C 1000 mg • Pantothenic Acid 100 mg • Zinc (as OptiZinc zinc monomethionine) 15 mg • MSM (methyl-sulfonyl-methane) 500 mg • Citrus Bioflavonoids 100 mg • Quercetin 25 mg • Rutin 25 mg • Bitter Orange (Citrus aurantium) peel powder extract (standardized for 4% synephrine, 4 mg) 100 mg • Grape Seed extract powder (standardized for 95% polyphenols, 29 mg) 30 mg • Stinging Nettle extract powder (leaf) (standardized for 2% plant silica, 2 mg) 100 mg • N-Acetyl-Cysteine (NAC) 100 mg • L-Histidine 200 mg. Other ingredients: Gelatin, Cellulose, Magnesium stearate, Water.

Allergy Support - Amazon Support
Each capsule contains: Nettles • Yerba Mate • Jatoba • Gervao • Pau d'arco • Picao Preto • Bitter Melon • Carqueja • Suma.

Allergy Support - Olympia Nutrition
Quercetin • Nettle • Licorice • Vitamin C.

AllergyCare - Nature's Way
Each capsule contains: Pseudoephedrine HCl 60 mg. Other Ingredients: Brigham Tea Herb, Elder Flowers, Eyebright (stem, leaf, flower), Ginger, Golden Rod Herb, Licorice Root.

Aller-Max - Biochem
Two capsules contain: Quercetin 250 mg • N-Acetyl Cysteine 200 mg • Bromelain 100 mg • L-Histidine 200 mg • Vitamin A (Palmitate) 2500 IU • Vitamin C (Calcium Ascorbate) 250 mg • Pantothenic Acid 200 mg • Zinc 10 mg • Grape seed extract 5 mg • Stinging Nettle 100 mg • Cayenne 20 mg.

AllerPlus - PhytoPharmica
Two capsules contain: Pseudoephedrine HCl (from Ephedra sinensis) 60 mg • Vitamin E (DL-Alpha Tocopherol) 75 IU • Vitamin C (Ascorbic Acid) 150 mg • Pantothenic Acid (D-Calcium Pantothenate) 150 mg • Choline (Bitartrate) 150 mg • Macrocystis Pyrifera 150 mg • Lung extract 90 mg • Adrenal extract 80 mg • Methionine 75 mg • Pancreatic Enzymes (3X) 65 mg (Treated for enteric activity) •

Ammonium Chloride 50 mg • Calcium Chloride 50 mg • Glutamic Acid HCL 50 mg • Betaine HCL 50 mg • Pepsin (1:10000) 49 mg • Magnesium Glycerophosphate 30 mg • Spleen extract 25 mg • Pancreas extract 15 mg • Thymus extract 15 mg • Niacinamide 10 mg • Liver Fractions 10 mg • Vitamin B6 (Pyridoxine HCl) 5 mg.
See Editor's Note No. 14, page 1817.

Aller-Response - Source Naturals
Three tablets contain: Quercetin 600 mg • Vitamin C (ascorbic acid and zinc ascorbate) 500 mg • Bitter orange standardized extract 500 mg • Bromelain (2000 GDU per g) 300 mg • Nettle root extract 100 mg • Ginkgo Biloba standardized leaf extract 75 mg • Licorice root extract 50 mg • Magnesium (amino acid chelate) 50 mg • Vitamin A (palmitate) 2500 IU • Vitamin B-6 (pyridoxine HCl) 5 mg • Vitamin B-12 (cyanocobalamin) 12 mcg • Zinc (ascorbate) 10 mg.

AllerZinc - Quantum Health
One drop contains: Zinc 9 mg • Ephedrine from Ephedra Extract 2 mg • Quercetin 80 mg • Lobelia 15 mg • Licorice 15 mg. Other Ingredients: Sugar, Corn Syrup, Natural Flavor.

Allicin Rich Garlic Powder - Jamieson
Each caplet contains: Garlic bulb powder (containing 750 mcg Allicin and 5000 mcg Alliin) 300 mg.

Alluna - SmithKline Beecham
Two tablets contain: Valerian root extract 500 mg • Hops extract 120 mg. Other ingredients: Microcrystalline Cellulose, Soy Polysaccharide, Hydrogenated Castor oil, Hydroxypropyl Methylcellulose, Titanium Dioxide (less than 20%), Propylene Glycol, Magnesium Stearate, Silica, Polyethylene Glycol (400, 6000, 20000), Blue 2 Lake, Artificial flavoring.

Aloe & E with Allantoin - Derma E
Aloe Vera gel • Vitamin E.

Aloe Vera - Leiner Health Products
Each softgel contains: Aloe Vera gel 25 mg. Other Ingredients: Vegetable Oil, Gelatin, Hydrogenated Soybean and Cottonseed Oil, White Beeswax.

Aloe Vera 200 - New Chapter, Inc.
Two tablets contain: Freeze dried Aloe Vera juice concentrate (200:1) 300 mg.

Aloe Vera Deep Skin Moisturizer Vitamin D Cell Refining Cream - Orjene
85% pure Aloe Vera • Bee Pollen • Vitamin F Complex • PABA-free sunblock.

Aloe Vera Gel - Puritan's Pride
Each softgel contains: Premium Concentrated Aloe Vera Gel 200:1 (Equivalent to 5000 mg or approximately one teaspoonful of 100% pure aloe vera inner leaf gel) 25 mg.

Aloe Vera Gel - Nature's Bounty
Each softgel contains: Aloe Vera Gel (200:1 extract: Equivalent to 5,000 mg or approximately one teaspoonful of 100% pure aloe vera inner leaf gel) 25 mg. Other Ingredients: Beeswax/Soybean Oil Mixture, Gelatin, Glycerin, Cottonseed Oil. Contains no yeast, wheat, gluten, milk or milk derivatives, lactose, sugar, preservatives, artificial color, artificial flavor, or sodium (less than 5 mg per serving).

Aloe Vital - Source Naturals
Each tablet contains: Organic whole leaf aloe vera powder (200:1 concentrate) 200 mg.

Alozone-M - T-Up Biosystems
Each teaspoon (5mL) contains: Proprietary Blend 670 mg: Aloe Vera •

Some Brand Name Natural Products - What they Contain
www.NaturalDatabase.com contains MANY more listings than appear here.

Iron • Boron • Lithium • Fluoride • Copper • Zinc • Selenium • Chromium • Valadium • Cobalt • Nickel • All Natural Ultra-Wide Mineral System.

Alpha betic - Abkit
Each caplet contains: Vitamin A 5000 IU • Vitamin C (as ascorbic acid) 120 mg • Vitamin D (as cholecalciferol) 400 IU • Vitamin E (d-alpha tocopheryl succinate) 60 IU • Thiamin (Vitamin B1) 1.5 mg • Riboflavin (Vitamin B2) 1.7 mg • Niacin (Vitamin B3) 20 mg • Vitamin B6 (as pyroxidine) 2 mg • Folic Acid 400 mcg • Vitamin B12 (as cyanocobalamin) 6 mcg • Biotin 150 mcg • Pantothenic Acid (as d-calcium pantothenate) 10 mg • Magnesium 200 mg • Zinc (as Zinc Citrate) 15 mg • Selenium (Selenite) 50 mcg • Copper (as Copper Gluconate) 2 mg • Manganese (Sulfate) 5 mg • Chromium (as Chromium Picolinate) 200 mcg • Potassium (as Potassium Chloride) 100 mg • Vanadium (as Vanadium Sulfate) 100 mcg • Alpha Lipoic Acid (Imported from Germany) 60 mg. Other Ingredients: Calcium Sulfate, Stearic Acid, Cellulose, Magnesium Stearate. Coating: Beta Carotene, Riboflavin (B2).

Alpha Lipoic Acid - Leiner Health Products
Each tablet contains: Alpha Lipoic Acid 50 mg. Other Ingredients: Cellulose, Calcium Carbonate, Croscarmellose Sodium, Stearic Acid, Magnesium Stearate, Silicon Dioxide, Hydroxypropyl Methylcellulose, Polyethylene Glycol, Hydroxypropyl Cellulose.

Alpha Lipoic Acid - Metabolic Response Modifiers
Each capsule contains: Alpha Lipoic acid 100 mg.

Alpha Lipoic Acid - Now
Each Vcap contains: Vitamin C (as ascorbic acid) 250 mg • Vitamin E (as d-alpha tocopheryl succinate) 30 IU • Alpha Lipoic Acid 100 mg. Other Ingredients: Rice Flour, Cellulose (capsule). Contains no yeast, wheat, gluten, corn, milk, egg, or animal products.

Alpha Lipoic Acid - Olympian Labs
Each capsule contains: Crystalline Alpha Lipoic Acid 100 mg.

Alpha Lipoic Acid - Swanson
Each capsule contains: Alpha Lipoic Acid 50 mg.

Alpha Lipoic Acid 100 mg - Puritan's Pride
Each capsule contains: Alpha Lipoic Acid 100 mg.

Alpha Lipoic Acid 200 mg - Puritan's Pride
Each capsule contains: Alpha Lipoic Acid 200 mg.

Alpha Lipoic Acid 30 mg - Puritan's Pride
Each capsule contains: Alpha Lipoic Acid 30 mg.

Alpha Lipoic Acid Extra Strength with MAT - Olympian Labs
Each capsule contains: Crystalline Alpha Lipoic Acid 200 mg. Other Ingredients: MAT (a proprietary blend of nutritional ingredients).

Alpha-Lipoic Acid - Source Naturals
Each tablet contains: Alpha-Lipoic acid 50 mg.

Alternecal-Rx - Alternecare Health Products
Each tablet contains: Tri- Calcium Phosphate 1000 mg • Magnesium 500 mg • Zinc 10 mg • Copper 3 mg • Oat Straw 25 mg • Boron 3 mg • Vitamin C 30 mg • Vitamin D 400 IU • Ashwagandha 25 mg • Silica 25 mg.

Alticort - PhytoPharmica
Contains: 1.8% Salicylic Acid. Other Ingredients: Purified Water • Organic Fatty Acid Complex (C11-C18), Glyceryl Stearate, Chamomile extract (0.5% Flavonoid Content) •

18-Beta-Glycyrrhetinic Acid (from Licorice root extract) • Allantoin 2.0% from Comfrey root extract • Dimethicone, Vitamin E (Antioxidant). Hypoallergenic Fragrance.

AM Menopause Formula - PhytoPharmica
Each tablet contains: Green Tea (Camellia sinesis) leaf extract (standardized to contain 14% caffeine) 250 mg • Panax Ginseng root phytosome (bound to phosphatidylcholine under patent) 50 mg • Black Cohosh (Cimicifuga racemosa) root and rhizome extract 20 mg.

AM Plus (Brain 111 Formula) - Alpha Zebra
AM Super capsule: Two capsules contain: Beta Carotene 25 IU • Thiamine HCl (Vitamin B1) 50 mg • Riboflavin (Vitamin B2) 50 mg • Niacin (Vitamin B3) 20 mg • Pantothenic Acid (Vitamin B5) 75 mg • Pyridoxine HCl (Vitamin B6) 50 mg • Cyanocobalamin concentrate (Vitamin B12/Sorbitol) 500 mcg • Vitamin C 55 mg • Bioflavonoids with Rose Hips 45 mg • Vitamin E Dry (dl-Alpha Tocopherol) 25 IU • Biotin 300 mcg • Choline Bitartrate (Phosphatidyl) 75 mg • Soya Lecithin(Phospholipids) 50 mg • Folic Acid 500 mcg • Inositol 50 mg • Inosine 40 mg • Para-Aminobenzoic Acid (PABA) 30 mg • Calcium Phosphate (Chelated) 40 mg • Chromium Picolinate (Chelated) 200 mcg • Copper (Oxide) (Chelated) 1 mg • Magnesium (Oxide) (Chelated) 25 mg • Manganese (Oxide) (Chelated) 45 mg • Phosphorus (Oxide) (Chelated)12 mg • Potassium (Oxide) (Chelated) 50 mg • Zinc (Oxide) (Chelated) 50 mg • Boron (Chelated) 1 mg • Molybdenum (Oxide) (Chelated) 100 mcg • Selenium (Oxide) (Chelated) 200 mcg • Silicon 400 mcg • L-Aspartic Acid 25 mg • L-Cysteine 15 mg • L-Glutamine 115 mg • L-Glycine 15 mg • L-Leucine 50 mg • L-Lysine 15 mg • L-Methionine 70 mg • L-Tyrosine 70 mg • L-Phenylalanine 100 mg • L-Serine 25 mg • A-Ketoglutaric Acid 15 mg • Adrenal Raw freeze dried concentrate 25 mg • Gamma Aminobutyric Acid - GABA 25 mg • Glutamic Acid 5 mg • RNA/DNA (Complex) 25 mg • Beta Hydrochloride 5 mg • Bromelain 3 mg • Pancreatin 10 mg • Papain 10 mg • Pepsin 10 mg • Protease Enzyme 3 mg • Bee Pollen 40 mg • Royal Jelly 35 mg • Ginkgo Biloba (50:1) (contains 24% Ginkgolides Heterosides) 50 mg • Ginkgo Biloba (8:1) contains 24% Ginkgolides 160 mg • Heterosides Gotu Kola 128 mg • Panax Korean Ginseng 88 mg • Ginger root 80 mg • Mexican Yam 80 mg • Echinacea augustifolia 76 mg • Spirulina algae 75 mg • Fo-Ti 60 mg • Oat Straw 60 mg • Siberian Ginseng 60 mg • Beet root powder 60 mg • Alfalfa 50 mg • Peppermint leaves 60 mg • Eyebright (Euphrasia herb) 60 mg • Licorice root (De-Glycyrrhiznated) 56 mg • Passionflower 48 mg • Capsicum 40 mg • Dandelion root 40 mg • Hawthorn berry 40 mg • Mexican Damiana leaves 32 mg • Kelp 28 mg • Aloe Vera 28 mg • Fennel 28 mg • Sarsaparilla 28 mg • Cabbage seed 24 mg • Sea Plant concentrate 20 mg • Saw Palmetto berry 20 mg • Burdock root 20 mg • Chamomile 20 mg • Slippery Elm 20 mg • Kava Kava 16 mg • Horseradish 16 mg • Suma 12 mg. Energizer Formula: Each capsule contains: Niacinamide (Vitamin B3) 40 mg • Pyridoxine HCl (Vitamin B6) 25 mg • Cyanocobalamin concentrate (Vitamin B12 w/ Sorbitol) 500 mcg • Bioflavonoids (including Rose Hips) 30 mg • L-Glutamine 50 mg • L-Phenylalanine 50 mg • L-Methionine 30 mg • L-Tyrosine 25 mg • L-Aspartic Acid 10 mg • L-Taurine 10 mg • L-Asparigne 10 mg • L-Alanine 10 mg • L-Glycine 10 mg • Pancreatin 20 mg • Gamma Aminobutyric Acid (GABA) 10 mg • Soy Lecithin (Phospholipids) 10 mg • Royal Jelly 25 mg • Beet root powder 80 mg • Cantaloupe 80 mg • Yucca 60 mg • American Cenuary 60 mg • Mexican Yam 60 mg • Bissy Nut 60 mg • Kava Kava root 56 mg • Fo-Ti 48 mg • Oat Straw 48 mg • Capsicum/Cayenne 44 mg • Bee Pollen 40 mg • Dandelion root 40 mg • Brigham Tea 40 mg • Artichoke 40 mg • Wild Lettuce 40 mg • Rosemary leaves 40 mg • Yerba Mate 32 mg • Peppermint leaves 32 mg • Sarsaparilla 25 mg • Ginger root 24 mg • Suma 24 mg • Hawthorn berry 16 mg • American Ginseng 16 mg • Cabbage seed 16 mg • Parsley 16 mg • Fenugreek 16 mg • Gotu Kola 16 mg • Muira Puama 12 mg • Spirulina algae 12 mg.

AmbroDerm Lotion - Mannatech
Water • Emu Oil • Sorbitol • Glycerin • Glycereth-26 • Polysorbate

Some Brand Name Natural Products - What they Contain

80 • Tocopherol acetate • Ambrotose Complex: naturally occurring plant polysaccharides including freeze-dried Aloe Vera inner leaf gel extract - Manapol powder • Carbomer • Germaben II (propylene glycol, Diazolidinyl urea, methylparaben, propylparaben) • Aminomethyl propanol • Fragrance • Retinyl palmitate • Allantoin.
See Editor's Note No. 17, page 1817.

AmbroStart beverage mix - Mannatech
Contains three grams of soluble fiber, Ambrotose Complex, Orange Flavor.
See Editor's Note No. 17, page 1817.

Ambrotose Complex - Mannatech
Ambrotose Complex: naturally occurring plant polysaccharides including freeze-dried Aloe Vera inner leaf gel extract - Manapol powder. Other Ingredients: Brown Rice Flour, Silicon dioxide, Magnesium stearate.
See Editor's Note No. 17, page 1817.

American Ginseng - Nature's Way
Two capsules contain: American Ginseng root 1.1 g. Other Ingredients: Gelatin, Magnesium stearate.

American Ginzing - Traditional Medicinals
Contains: American Ginseng root • Licorice root • Ginger rhizome • Cinnamon bark • Sarsaparilla root • Dong Quai root.

Amino 1000 - Puritan's Pride
Three tablets contain: Vitamin C (as ascorbyl palmitate) 30 mg • Hydrolyzed Protein 3,000 mg • L-Alanine 210 mg • L-Arginine 189 mg • L-Aspartic Acid 114 mg • L-Cysteine 9.9 mg • L-Glutamic Acid 114 mg • L-Glycine 588 mg • L-Histidine 23.4 mg • L-Hydroxyproline 378 mg • L-Isoleucine 40.8 mg • L-Leucine 66.6 mg • L-Lysine 99 mg • L-Methionine 22.8 mg • L-Phenylalanine 45 mg • L-Proline 303 mg • L-Serine 106.8 mg • L-Threonine 38.4 mg • L-Tyrosine 17.1 mg • L-Valine 57.3 mg.

Amino 1500 - Puritan's Pride
Six tablets contain: L-Ornithine HCl 161.1 mg • L-Lysine 836.2 mg • L-Histidine 198.6 mg • L-Arginine 329.2 mg • L-Aspartic Acid 861.3 mg • L-Threonine 376.3 mg • L-Serine 629.2 mg • L-Glutamic Acid 1259.7 mg • L-Proline 635.6 mg • L-Glycine 162.0 mg • L-Alanine 388.8 mg • L-Cystine 250.9 mg • L-Valine 445.3 mg • L-Methionine 203.8 mg • L-Isoleucine 543.5 mg • L-Leucine 977.4 mg • L-Tyrosine 339.7 mg • L-Phenylalanine 376.3 mg.

Amino 2000 - Puritan's Pride
Each tablet contains: L-Lysine 282.4 mg • L-Histidine 61.6 mg • L-Arginine 84.6 mg • L-Aspartic Acid 326.0 mg • L-Threonine 211.8 mg • L-Serine 164.6 mg • L-Proline 190.4 mg • L-Alanine 127.2 mg • L-Glycine 59.2 mg • L-Glutamic Acid 275.4 mg • L-Cysteine 80.4 mg • L-Valine 173.6 mg • L-Methionine 64.2 mg • L-Isoleucine 187.6 mg • L-Leucine 321.8 mg • L-Tyrosine 90.4 mg • L-Phenylalanine 97.6 mg • L-Tryptophan 52.2 mg • L-Carnitine 10.0 mg.

Amino 2222 Capsules - Optimum Nutrition
Two capsules contain: Pharmaceutical Grade 3Amino Acids2 (derived from Predigested Lactalbumen, Soy Protein Isolate & Whey Protein concentrate) 2222 mg • L-Ornithine • L-Carnitine.

Amino Acid 1000 mg - Nature's Life
Ten capsules contain: Casein Hydrolysate • Glycine • L-Proline • L-Arginine • L-Alanine • Pyridoxine HCl • L-Ornithine • L-Serine • L-Cystine • whole Egg powder. Ten capsules provide, based on a typical analysis: L-Alanine 663 mg • L-Arginine 665 mg • L-Aspartic Acid 447 mg • L-Cystine 4 mg • L-Glutamic Acid 1222 mg • Glycine 1806 mg • L-Histidine 157 mg • L-Isoleucine (Esssential Amino Acid) 313 mg • L-Leucine (Essential Amino Acid) 512 mg • L-Ornithine 250 mg • L-Lysine (Essential Amino Acid) 471 mg • L-Methionine

(Essential Amino Acid) 166 mg • L-Phenylalanine (Essential Amino Acid) 313 mg • L-Proline 1640 mg • L-Serine 505 mg • L-Threonine (Essential Amino Acid) 262 mg • L-Tryptophan (Essential Amino Acid) 70 mg • L-Tyrosine 200 mg • L-Valine (Essential Amino Acid) 408 mg.

Amino Athlete - Source Naturals
Each tablet contains: Vitamin B6 5 mg • Vitamin C (ascorbic acid) 15 mg.

Amino Blend - Progressive Labs
Three 750 mg capsules contain: L-Alanine 147 mg • L-Arginine 138 mg • L-Cysteine 23 mg • L-Cystine 26 mg • L-Glutamine 28 mg • Glycine 95 mg • L-Histidine 73 mg • L-Isoleucine 71 mg • L-Leucine 203 mg • L-Lysine 203 mg • L-Methionine 55 mg • L-Ornithine 23 mg • L-Proline 77 mg • L-Serine 95 mg • L-Threonine 91 mg • L-Tyrosine 77 mg • L-Valine 120 mg • Taurine 48 mg • L-Aspartic Acid 206 mg • L-Phenylalanine 102 mg • L-Glutamic Acid 349 mg.

Amino Complex - Puritan's Pride
Each tablet contains: L-Arginine 50 mg • L-Cysteine 50 mg • L-Histidine 50 mg • L-Isoleucine 50 mg • L-Leucine 50 mg • L-Lysine Hydrochloride 50 mg • L-Methionine 50 mg • L-Ornithine Hydrochloride 50 mg • L-Phenylalanine 50 mg • L-Threonine 50 mg • L-Tyrosine 50 mg • L-Valine 50 mg.

Amino Day - Source Naturals
Each tablet contains: Vitamin B6 5 mg • Vitamin C (ascorbic acdi) 15 mg.

Amino Fuel (Anabolic Amino Acid Drink) - TwinLab
Peptide Bonded & Free Amino Acids (derived from the natural Pancreatic digests of Whey Protein & Egg White Protein) 20 g • Protein-sparing Carbohydrates (predominantly from Glucose Polymers) 50 g. Other Ingredients: L-Carnitine, Branched Chain Amino Acids (L-Leucine, L-Isoleucine & L-Valine), Essential Vitamins & Minerals, Zinc Picolinate, Boron, GTF Chromium, Chromium Picolinate & Chromium Polynicotinate.

Amino Fuel (Mega Anabolic Chewable Wafers) 7500 mg - TwinLab
Two wafers contain: Peptide Bonded & Free Amino Acids 7500 mg (7.5 g). Each wafer contains: L-Carnitine • Branched Chain Amino Acids (L-Leucine, L-Isoleucine & L-Valine) • Pharmaceutical Grade Peptide Bonded & Free Amino Acids derived from the natural Pancreatic digests of Whey Protein (Lactalbumin) & Egg White (Albumin).

Amino Fuel (Peptide Bonded Amino Acid Liquid Concentrate) - TwinLab
L-Carnitine • Branched Chain Amino Acids (L-Leucine, L-Isoleucine & L-Valine) • Pharmaceutical Grade, Peptide Bonded & Free Amino Acids • Stress B Complex Vitamins • Lipotropic Factors: Choline & Inositol • Complex Carbohydrates (Glucose Polymers) • Pure Crystalline Fructose. Each serving contains: Peptide Bonded & Free Amino Acids [derived from the natural Pancreatic digests of Whey Protein (Lactalbumin), Egg Protein (Albumin), Liver Protein & other Animal Proteins] 15 g.

Amino Fuel (Peptide Bonded Amino Acid Tablets) - TwinLab
L-Carnitine • Branched Chain Amino Acids (L-Leucine, L-Isoleucine & L-Valine) • Peptide Bonded Amino Acids [derived from Pharmaceutical Grade Pancreatic (Enzymatic) digests of Whey Protein (Lactalbumin) & Egg White Protein (Albumin)].

Amino Fuel 1000 Tabs - TwinLab
L-Carnitine • Branched Chain Amino Acids (L-Leucine, L-Isoleucine

BRAND NAMES

& L-Valine) • Peptide Bonded Amino Acids [derived from Pharmaceutical Grade Pancreatic (Enzymatic) digests of Whey Protein (Albumin)].

Amino Fuel 1500 Tablets - TwinLab
Each tablet contains: Peptide Bonded Amino Acids & Branched Chain Amino Acids [derived from Pharmaceutical Grade Pancreatic digests of Whey Protein (Lactalbumin) & Egg White Protein (Albumin)] 1500 mg. No lower quality amino acid sources are present, such as soy or casein.

Amino Fuel 2000 (Extra Strength Amino Acid Tablets) - TwinLab
Each tablet contains: Protein (as Peptide Bonded Amino Acids) derived from Pharmaceutical Grade Pancreatic digests of Whey Protein (Lactalbumin) & Egg White Protein 2000 mg.

Amino Fuel Stack - TwinLab
Six capsules contain: HMB (B-Hydroxy B-Methylbutyrate Monohydrate) 3000 mg • L-Glutamine 2000 mg • Acetyl-L-Carnitine 1000 mg • Taurine 200 mg • N-Acetyl-Cysteine (NAC) 200 mg.

Amino Mass - Source Naturals
Four tablets contain: L-Arginine Pyroglutamate 1,000 mg • L-Lysine HCl 1,000 mg • ChromeMate Chromium GTF (Chromium Polynicotinate) 100 mcg.

Amino Night - Source Naturals
Four tablets contain: Arginine Pyroglutamate 816 mg • L-Lysine HCl 816 mg • L-Ornithine (from 469 mg of L-ornithine HCl) 368 mg.

Amino Strength - Source Naturals
Each tablet contains: Arginine Pyroglutamate 330 mg • l-Ornithine (from 382 mg of L-Ornithine HCl) 300 mg.

Amino-BC - ANS
Branched Chain Amino Acids.

AminoBuild: Chocolate Flavor - Pharmanex
Three scoops (45 g) contain: Vitamin A (as Vitamin A Palmitate) 1000 IU • Vitamin C (as Ascorbic Acid) 60 mg • Vitamin D (as Vitamin D3) (as Cholecalciferol) 40 IU • Vitamin E (as d-Alpha Tocopheryl Acetate) 30 IU • Thiamin (as Thiamin Mononitrate) 0.3 mg • Riboflavin (as Riboflavin) 0.34 mg • Niacin (as Niacinamide) 4 mg • Vitamin B6 (as Pyridoxine Hydrochloride) 0.4 mg • Folate (as Folic Acid) 80 mcg • Vitamin B12 (as Cyanocobalamin) 1.2 mcg • Biotin (as Biotin) 60 mcg • Pantothenic Acid (as d-Calcium Pantothenate) 2 mg • Calcium (as Dicalcium Phosphate) 540 mg • Phosphorus (as Dicalcium Phosphate) 400 mg • Iodine (as Calcium Iodate) 15 mcg • Magnesium (as Magnesium Citrate) 80 mg • Zinc (as Zinc Gluconate) 3 mg • Selenium (as Sodium Selenate) 14 mcg • Copper (as Copper Gluconate) 0.2 mg • Manganese (as Manganese Gluconate) 0.4 mg • Chromium (as Chromium Polynicotinate 24 mcg • Molybdenum (as Sodium Molybdate) 15 mcg • Sodium (as Sodium Chloride, Soy Protein Isolate) 250 mg • Potassium (from Soy Protein Isolate) 360 mg • Stevia (Stevia Rebaudiana) (Leaves) 50 mg. Other Ingredients: Protein Blend (Supro7 Soy Protein Isolate, Cross Flow Microfiltration Whey Protein Isolate, Whey Protein Hydrolysate), Crystalline Fructose, Natural Flavors, Alkalized Cocoa Powder, Magnesium Citrate, Sodium Chloride, Dicalcium Phosphate, Ascorbic Acid, dl-Alpha Tocopheryl Acetate, Stevia, Medium Chain Triglycerides, Zinc Gluconate, Chromium Polynicotinate, Biotin, Vitamin A Palmitate, Niacinamide, Manganese Gluconate, Copper Gluconate, d-Calcium Pantothenate, Pyridoxine Hydrochloride, Cholecalciferol, Riboflavin, Thiamin Mononitrate, Cyanocobalamin, Folic Acid, Calcium Iodate, Sodium Molybdate, Sodium Selenate.

AminoBuild: Vanilla Flavor - Pharmanex
Three scoops (45 g) contain: Vitamin A (as Vitamin A Palmitate)

1000 IU • Vitamin C (as Ascorbic Acid) 60 mg • Vitamin D3 (as Cholecalciferol) 40 IU • Vitamin E (as d-Alpha Tocopheryl Acetate) 30 IU • Thiamin (as Thiamin Mononitrate) 0.3 mg • Riboflavin (as Riboflavin) 0.34 mg • Niacin (as Niacinamide) 4 mg • Vitamin B6 (as Pyridoxine Hydrochloride) 0.4 mg • Folate (as Folic Acid) 80 mcg • Vitamin B12 (as Cyanocobalamin) 1.2 mcg • Biotin (as Biotin) 60 mcg • Pantothenic Acid (as d-Calcium Pantothenate) 2 mg • Calcium (as Dicalcium Phosphate) 540 mg • Phosphorus (as Dicalcium Phosphate) 400 mg • Iodine (as Calcium Iodate) 15 mcg • Magnesium (as Magnesium Citrate) 80 mg • Zinc (as Zinc Gluconate) 3 mg • Selenium (as Sodium Selenate) 14 mcg • Copper (as Copper Gluconate) 0.2 mg • Manganese (as Manganese Gluconate) 0.4 mg • Chromium (as Chromium Polynicotinate 24 mcg • Molybdenum (as Sodium Molybdate) 15 mcg • Sodium (as Sodium Chloride, Soy Protein Isolate) 250 mg • Potassium (from Soy Protein Isolate) 360 mg • Stevia (Stevia Rebaudiana) (Leaves) 50 mg. Other Ingredients: Protein Blend (Supro7 Soy Protein Isolate, Cross Flow Microfiltration Whey Protein Isolate, Whey Protein Hydrolysate), Crystalline Fructose, Natural Vanilla Flavors, Magnesium Citrate, Sodium Chloride, Dicalcium Phosphate, Ascorbic Acid, Stevia, Medium Chain Triglycerides, dl-Alpha Tocopheryl Acetate, Zinc Gluconate, Chromium Polynicotinate, Biotin, Vitamin A Palmitate, Niacinamide, Manganese Gluconate, Copper Gluconate, d-Calcium Pantothenate, Pyridoxine Hydrochloride, Cholecalciferol, Riboflavin, Thiamin Mononitrate, Cyanocobalamin, Folic Acid, Calcium Iodate, Sodium Molybdate, Sodium Selenate.

Amino-Cartilage - Nutri-Quest
Each tablet contains: Natural Hydrolyzed Protein 1000 mg (minimum 16% Nitrogen content, 92-97% Protein content). Six tablets contain: Natural Laevorotatory Amino Acids (L): Isoleucine 66 mg • Leucine 174 mg • Lysine 216 mg • Methionine 30 mg • Phenylalanine 126 mg • Threonine 120 mg • Valine 168 mg • Arginine 468 mg • Histidine 36 mg • Alanine 546 mg • Tyrosine 24 mg • Serine 198 mg • Aspartic Acid 336 mg • Glutamic Acid 582 mg • Glycine 1362 mg • Hydroxylysine 60 mg • Hydroxyproline 654 mg • Proline 834 mg.

Aminologic - PhysioLogics
Three capsules contain: L-Glutamine 185 mg • L-Aspartic Acid 107 mg • L-Tyrosine 103 mg • L-Leucine 97 mg • L-Valine 97 mg • Taurine 90 mg • L-Phenylalanine 88 mg • L-Proline 82 mg • L-Lysine 77 mg • L-Isoleucine 71 mg • L-Serine 71 mg • L-Alanine 60 mg • L-Threonine 59 mg • L-Methionine 55 mg • L-Arginine 54 mg • Papain NF 50 mg • Bromelain 50 mg • Glycine 48 mg • L-Histidine 41 mg • Pancreatin 4X 25 mg • L-Cystine 23 mg.
See Editor's Note No. 14, page 1817.

AminoZyme - Nature's Plus
Each capsule contains: AMINOGEN (Aspergillus niger & Aspergillus oryzae proteolytic complex) 250 mg • Vitamin B6 (Pyridoxine HCL) 10 mg • CoQ10 (Ubiquinone) 2.5 mg • Chromium (Polynicotinate) 25 mcg • Vanadium (Sulfate) 10 mcg. Contains no yeast, wheat, corn, soy, milk, salt, sugar or starch.

Amore Plus-Rx - H Enterprise
Vitamin E • Calcium • Arginine • Saw Palmetto • Damiana • Celery • Cinnamon (chinese) • Pygeum Africanum bark • Gotu Kola • Rice flour • Magnesium Stearate • Silica.

Anabolic Complex - The Kutting Edge
Two capsules contain: 10-Norandrosenedione 100 mg • 5-Andro-3B-17B Diol 100 mg • Androstenedione 100 mg • Phosphatidylserine 100 mg • Tribulus 150 mg • Chrysin 50 mg.

Anabolic Fuel - TwinLab
Four capsules contain: L-Leucine 2000 mg • L-Valine 500 mg • L-Isoleucine 500 mg.

Anabolic Max - Biochem
Four tablets contain: L-Glutamine 1000 mg • L-Arginine

(Pyroglutamate) 900 mg • Creatine Monohydrate 500 mg • L-Citrulline 300 mg • Taurine 300 mg • Betaine HCL 300 mg • Cinnamon extract 250 mg • Green Tea extract 100mg • DHA (Docosahaexaenoic Acid) 100 mg • Ginseng (Panax ginseng) 50 mg • PAK (Pyridoxine, Alpha-Ketoglutarate) 25 mg • Niacin 25 mg • Pantothenic Acid /Pantethine 90/10 25 mg.

Andro Heat - Substrate Solutions
Four capsules contain: Caffeine (naturally occuring in 2000 mg of Kola Nut herb) 200 mg • Ephedrine (naturally occuring in 250 mg of Ma Huang herb) 20 mg • 4-Androstenediol 100 mg.

Andro Stack - Substrate Solutions
Each capsule contains: 4-Androstenediol 100 mg • 4-Androstenedione 100 mg.

Andro Surge - Country Life
Each capsule contains: Tribulus Terrestris 100 mg • Moomiyo 50 mg • Dehydroepiandrosterone 50 mg • Vitamin E 25 IU.

Andro Surge - MRM
Each capsule contains: Androstenedione 100 mg.

Andro-6 - EAS
Four tablets contain: DHEA 50 mg • Androstenedione 100 mg • Tribulus terrestris 250 mg • Chrysin 150 mg • Saw Palmetto extract 180 mg • Indole-3-Carbinol 50 mg • Zinc Glycinate 8 mg.
See Editor's Note No. 22, page 1818.

Androbolic - ProLab
Each two tablets contain: 19-Norandrostenedione 100 mg • 4-Androstene-3,17 Diol 100 mg • 5-Androstene-3,17 Diol 50 mg • Tribulus Terrestris 250 mg • Saw Palmetto 180 mg • Chrysin 150 mg • Indole 3 Carbinol 50 mg.

Andro-Diol - New Hope Health Products
Each capsule contains: 4-androstene-3, 17-diol 100 mg.

Androdyne - Cytodyne Technologies
Three capsules contain: 19-Norandrostenedione 100 mg • 5-Androstene-3B, 17b-Diol 50 mg • 4-Androstene-3, 17-dione 50 mg • AA-t3 Anti-Aromatase Complex 100 mg (proprietary blend of Chrysin, Indole 3-Carbinol & 7-IsoPropoxyIsoflavone) • Zinc Gluconate 20 mg • B3 Nicotinic Acid 50 mg.

AndroPlex 700 - AST Sports Science
Two capsules contain: Tribulus Terrestris 500 mg • Androstenedione 100 mg • DHEA 100 mg.

Andro-Stack 850 - Optimum Nutrition
Two capsules contain: pharmaceutical grade Androstenedione (Delta-4-androstene-3-17-dione) 100 mg • pharmaceutical grade DHEA (Dehydroepiandrosterone) 100 mg • Tribulus terrestris 650 mg.

AndrosteDERM - MedLean
2 ml contain: 4-Androstenediol (Androdiol from Pat Arnold's LPJ Research) 90 mg • Androstenedione 30 mg.

Androstene Power - Olympian Labs
Each capsule contains: 4-Androstene 3, 17-dione 50 mg.

Androstenedione with Yohimbe - Puritan's Pride
Each capsule contains: Androstenedione 100 mg • Yohimbe bark extract (standardized for 8 mg Yohimbine) 400 mg.

Andro-Surge - New Hope Health Products
Each capsule contains: Androstenedione (4-androstene-3, 17-dione) 100 mg.

Andro-Surge - Metabolic Response Modifiers
Each capsule contains: Androstenedione (4-androstene-3, 17-dione) 100 mg.

ANDRO-Xtreme - New Hope Health Products
Each capsule contains: Dehydroepiandrosterone (DHEA) 100 mg • Androstenedione (4-androstene-3, 17-dione) 100 mg • 5-androstenediol (5-androstene-3, 17-diol) 50 mg • Tribulus terrestris 500 mg • Chrysin 250 mg.

Andro-Xtreme - Metabolic Response Modifiers
Two capsules contain: Dehydroepiandrosterone (DHEA) 100 mg • Androstenedione (4-androstene-3, 17-dione) 100 mg • 5-androstenediol (5-androstene 3, 17- diol) 50 mg • Tribulus terrestris 500 mg • Chrysin 250 mg.

Androzyme - Progressive Labs
Each capsule contains: Vitamin E (d-alpha tocopheryl succinate) 50 IU • Zinc (as zinc aspartate) 15 mg • Raw Orchic concentrate (bovine) 100 mg • Siberian Ginseng (Eleutherococcus senticosus) 100 mg • L-Carnitine 30 mg.
See Editor's Note No. 14, page 1817.

Animal Chews - Puritan's Pride
Two tablets contain: Vitamin A (as retinyl palmitate & beta carotene) 5,000 IU • Vitamin C (as calcium ascorbate) 120 mg • Vitamin D (as cholecalciferol) 400 IU • Vitamin E (as d-alpha tocopheryl acid succinate) 30 IU • Vitamin K (as phytonadione) 2 mcg • Thiamin (Vitamin B1; as thiamine mononitrate) 1.5 mg • Riboflavin (Vitamin B2) 1.7 mg • Niacin (as niacinamide) 20 mg • Vitamin B6 (as pyridoxine hydrochloride) 2 mg • Folic Acid 400 mcg • Vitamin B12 (as cyanocovalamin) 6 mcg • Biotin (as d-biotin) 300 mcg • Pantothenic Acid (as d-calcium pantothenate) 10 mg • Calcium (as calcium carbonate, calcium citrate, and calcium ascorbate) 250 mg • Iron (as ferrous fumarate) 4 mg • Iodine (as potassium iodide and kelp) 75 mcg • Magnesium (as magnesium ascorbate and magnesium oxide) 100 mg • Zinc (as zinc amino acid chelate) 7.5 mg • Selenium (as L-Selenomethionine) 15 mcg • Copper (as cupric gluconate) 1 mg • Manganese (as manganese gluconate) 1 mg • Chromium (as chromium polynicotinate) 15 mcg • Molybdenum (as sodium molybdate) 10 mcg • Boron (sodium borate) 10 mcg • Vanadium (as vanadyl sulfate) 5 mcg • Nickel (as nickelous sulfate) 2 mcg • Tin (as stannous chloride) 2 mcg • Choline Phosphatides (as lecithin) 2 mg • Inositol Phosphatides (as lecithin) 5 mg • Rutin 5 mg • Green Barley juice powder 3 mg • Chlorella powder 3 mg • Spirulina powder 5 mg • Alfalfa juice powder 5 mg • Rice Bran powder 10 mg • Carrot juice powder 5 mg • Natural Licorice root 4 mg.

Animal Chews with Calcium - Puritan's Pride
Two tablets contain: Vitamin A (50% as retinyl palmitate and 50% as beta-carotene) 5,000 IU • Vitamin C (as calcium ascorbate) 120 mg • Vitamin D (as cholecalciferol) 400 IU • Vitamin E (as d-alpha tocopheryl acid succinate) 30 IU • Thiamin (as thiamine mononitrate) 1.5 mg • Riboflavin 1.7 mg • Niacin (as niacinamide) 20 mg • Vitamin B6 (as pyridoxine hydrochloride) 2 mg • Folic Acid 0.4 mg • Vitamin B12 (as cyanocobalamin) 6 mcg • Biotin 100 mcg • Pantothenic Acid (as d-calcium pantothenate) 10 mg • Calcium (as calcium carbonate, calcium citrate, and calcium ascorbate) 250 mg. In a base containing Raspberry Juice Concentrate, Rose Hips, Acerola, Black Currant Juice, Fructose, Fruit Juice Solids, Dried Dates, Dried Apricots, and Dried Peaches.

Animal Joint Formula Dog & Cat Arthritis Formula - Puritan's Pride
Each capsule contains: Glucosamine Sulfate (Aminomonosaccharide) 333 mg • Sea Cucumber (Beche De-Mer) 333 mg • Shark Cartilage 166 mg.

Some Brand Name Natural Products - What they Contain

Anorex S-F - Klein-Becker
Contains: Calcium (amino acid chelate) 132 mg • Calcium phosphate • Commiphora mukul extract • Garcinia cambogia • L-Tyrosine • Acetylsalicylic acid 162.5 mg • Dipotassium phosphate • Sodium phosphate • Disodium phosphate • Phosphatidyl choline • Scutellaria • Bupleurum • Epimedium

Anotesten - Muscletech
Six capsules contain: 4-Androstenediol 150 mg • Androstenedione 250 mg • DHEA 100 mg • Tribulus Terrestris 1000 mg • Chrysin 150 mg • Indole-3-Carbinol (I3C) 50 mg • Saw Palmetto (standardized for 25% fatty acids) 320 mg.

Antacid - Progressive Labs
Each tablet contains: Calcium Carbonate 500 mg which supplies: Calcium (from calcium carbonate) 200 mg. Other Ingredients: Dextrose, Mannitol, Cellulose, Magnesium Stearate, Glycine and Spearmint oil. Free of Sodium & Aluminum.

Anthocyan - PhytoPharmica
Two capsules contain: Vitamin A (beta-carotene) 10,000 IU • Vitamin C (ascorbic acid) 200 mg • Riboflavin (vitamin B2) 10 mg • Bilberry (Vaccinium myrtillus fruit berry) extract (standardized to contain 25% anthocyanosides [40 mg per 2 capsules] calculated as anthocyanidins) 160 mg.

Anti-Aging Breakthrough - Jason
Six antioxidant Vitamin C.

Anti-Anxiety - PhytoPharmica
Twenty drops contain: Cicuta virosa 4x • Gaultheria 4x • Ignatia 4x • Staphysagria 4x • Asa foetida 3x • Corydalis formosa 3x • Hyoscyamus 3x • Sumbulus 3x • Valeriana officianalis 3x • Avena sativa 1x. In a base of 40% USP alcohol by volume.
See Editor's Note No. 1, page 1816.

Anti-Arthritis Glucosamine Chondroitin - Crystal Springs
Each tablet contains: Glucosamine (Sulfate) 600 mg • Chondroitin Sulfate 400 mg.
See Editor's Note No. 15, page 1817.

AntiBetic Pancreas Tonic - Gero Vita International
Each capsule contains: Pterocarpus marsupium (Indian Kino Tree) Fabaceae family 195 mg • Gymnema sylvestre (Gymnema) 175 mg • Momordica Charantia (Bitter Melon) 40 mg • Azadirachta indica (Neem) 20 mg • Tinospora cordifolia (Heart Leaved Moonseed) 30 mg • Aegle marmelose (Bael) 40 mg • Syzgium cumini (Jambolan) 50 mg • Cinnamonum tamala (Cinnamonleaf) 20 mg • Trigonella foenum-graecum (Fenugreek) 65 mg • Ficus racemosa (Cluster Fig) 15 mg.

AntiBio 1 - Dial Herbs
Echinacea • Goldenseal • Poke root • Cayenne.

AntiBio 2 - Dial Herbs
Echinacea • Myrrh • Poke root • Cayenne.

Anti-Catabolic Fuel - TwinLab
Four capsules contain: L-Leucine 1000 mg • L-Valine 225 mg • L-Isoleucine 225 mg • Ketoisocaproate (KIC) 100 mg • L-Ornithine, Alpha-Ketoglutarate 1000 mg • L-Glutamine 250 mg.

Anti-Depression Support - Amazon Support
Each capsule contains: Tayuya • Damiana • Muira Puama • Passion Flower • Chamomile.

Anti-Fatigue - PhytoPharmica
Twenty drops contain: Zincum muriaticum 8x • Gelsemium

sempervirens 6x • Picricum acidum 6x • Acidum phosphoricum 3x • Valeriana officinalis 1x. In a base of 45% USP alcohol by volume.
See Editor's Note No. 1, page 1816.

Anti-Fungal - The Herbalist
Thuja leaf • Usnea lichen • Spilanthes herb • Pau D'Arco inner bark • Echinacea root • Calendula flower • Cayenne pepper.

Anti-Fungal Salve - Blessed Herbs
Jewelweed • Black Walnut hulls • Pau d'Arco bark • Usnea lichen • Calendula flowers • Spilanthes • Echinacea Angustifolia root • Goldenseal root • Myrrh Gum • Organic Cold-Pressed Olive oil • Beeswax • Essential oils of Tea Tree & Thyme linalol.

Anti-Fungal Support - Amazon Support
Each capsule contains: Jatoba • Fedegosa • Brazilian Peppertree • Pau d'Arco.

Anti-Insom - Dial Herbs
Hops • Lobelia • Valerian • Cayenne.

Anti-Ox: Herbal Antioxidant - The Herbalist
Pau D'Arco inner bark • Astragalus root • Ginkgo leaf • Milk Thistle seed • Licorice root • Cayenne pepper.

Antioxidant 4000 Vitamins & Mineral - Nature's Bounty
Two softgels contain: Vitamin A (as Beta Carotene) 20000 IU • Vitamin C (as Ascorbic Acid) 400 mg • Vitamin E (as dl-Alpha Tocopheryl Acetate) 250 IU • Selenium (as Selenium Yeast) 50 mcg • Proprietary Blend: Carrot powder, Broccoli powder, Spinach powder 6 mg. Other Ingredients: Gelatin, Soy Lecithin, Glycerin, Vegetable Oil.

Antioxidant Caps - Now
Two capsules contain: Vitamin A (from 15 mg Beta-Carotene) 25000 IU • Vitamin C (from Calcium Ascorbate) 500 mg • Vitamin E (natural d-Alpha Succinate) 300 IU • Calcium (Ascorbate) 50 mg • Zinc (Picolinate) 5 mg • Selenium (L-Selenomethionine) 25 mcg • N-Acetyl-Cysteine 100 mg • L-Glutathione 25 mg • Alfalfa juice concentrate (Green Superfood) 250 mg • Wheat Sprout concentrate (Enzyme active) 100 mg.

Antioxidant Cocktail Custom Paks - The Vitamin Shoppe
Each packet contains: Vitamin A (as 100% beta-carotene) 15 mg (25000 IU) • Vitamin C (as ascorbic acid) 2000 mg • Vitamin E (as d-alpha, d-gamma, d-beta, d-delta tocopherol) 400 IU • Selenium (as selenomethionine) 200 mcg • Alpha-carotene 1 mg (833 IU) • Lycopene (LYC-O-MATO) 5 mg • Lutein 5 mg • Zeaxanthin 0.24 mg • Phytoene 0.055 mg • Phytofluene 0.026 mg • Citrus Bioflavonoids 1000 mg • Hesperidin 100 mg • Rutin 100 mg • Rose Hips (Rosa canina) fruit 160 mg • Acerola 20 mg.

Antioxidant Cocktail II - The Vitamin Shoppe
Two capsules contain: Pine bark extract (Pycnogenol) 30 mg • Grape Seed Extract (Vitis vinifera) (Activin) 50 mg • Alpha Lipoic Acid 50 mg • Green Tea leaves (Camellia sinensis) standardized to 75% polyphenols 50 mg.

Antioxidant Formula - Nature's Way
Two capsules contain: Beta Carotene 25,000 IU • Coenzyme Q10 (ubiquinone) 5 mg • Copper amino acid chelate 2 mg • Green Tea, polyphenol catechin extract 10 mg • L-Cysteine 100 mg • Quercetin (eucalyptus) 100 mg • Selenium (l-selenomethione) 200 mcg • Vitamin C 500 mg • Vitamin E (d-alpha tocopheryl) 400 IU • Zinc amino acid chelate 15 mg. Other Ingredients: Gelatin, Magnesium stearate, Maltodextrin, Silica.

Anti-Oxidant Formula #1 - Olympian Labs
Two capsules contain: Cat's Claw (uncaria tomentosa) 500 mg

• Ginkgo Biloba extract 60 mg • Crystalline CoQ10 30 mg • Grape Seed extract 50 mg.

Antioxidant Fuel - TwinLab
Three capsules contain: Beta-Carotene (pro-Vitamin A) 25000 IU • Vitamin C 1000 mg • Natural Vitamin E (Succinate) 800 IU • CoQ10 (Coenzyme Q10) 30 mg • N-Acetyl Cysteine (NAC) 200 mg • L-Glutathione 100 mg • Selenium (from Selenomethionine & Selenate 50/50 mixture) 100 mcg • Alpha-Lipoic Acid (reduced) 100 mcg.

Antioxidant Tablet - Leiner Health Products
Each tablet contains: Vitamin E (d-Alpha Tocopherol Acid Succinate and dl-Alpha Tocopheryl Acetate) 200 IU • Vitamin C (Ascorbic Acid) 250 mg • Selenium 70 mcg • Lutein 0.5 mg • Pine bark extract (Pycnogenol brand) 1 mg. Other Ingredients: Calcium Carbonate, Gelatin, Cellulose, Maltodextrin, Crospovidone, Croscarmellose Sodium, Silicon Dioxide, Spinach, Magnesium Stearate, Tricalcium Phosphate, Starch, Dicalcium Phosphate, Hydroxypropyl Methylcellulose, Pharmaceutical Glaze, Vegetable Oil, Ethylcellulose, Hydroxypropyl Cellulose, Sorbitol, Polysorbate 80, Ascorbyl Palmitate, Sodium Selenate, Polyethylene Glycol, Tocopherols, Zeaxanthin.

Anti-Parasite Support - Amazon Support
Each capsule contains: Macela • Graviola • Quinine Bark • Picao Preto • Carqueja • Papaya • Fedegosa • Simaruba • Epazote • Cat's Claw.

AntiSpasmodic - Dial Herbs
Scullcap • Skunk Cabbage • Black Cohosh • Myrrh • Lobelia • Cayenne

Anti-Stress Support - Amazon Support
Each capsule contains: Passion Flower • Chamomile • Manaca • Bitter Melon • Suma • Sarsaparilla • Tayuya • Damiana • Mulungu • Muira Puama.

Anti-Viral - Amazon Support
Each capsule contains: Bitter Melon • Brazilian Peppertree • Catuaba • Cha de Bugre • Chanca Piedra • Clavelilla • Macela • Vassourinha.

Anxiety Control - Pain & Stress Center
Four capsules contain: GABA 800 mg • Glycine 200 mg • Glutamine 280 mg • Magnesium 200 mg • Passion Flower 300 mg • Primula officinalis 300 mg • Vitamin B6 20 mg.

Anxiety-X - Olympian Labs
Two capsules contain: GABA (gamma aminobutyric acid) 150 mg • Niacinamide 150 mg • L-Tyrosine 40 mg • Glycine 40 mg • L-Glutamine 40 mg • Inositol 150 mg • Kava Kava 20 mg • Motherwort 20 mg • Wintergreen 30 mg.

Aorta-Glycan - Enzymatic Therapy
Each capsule contains: Aorta-Glycan (Mesoglycan) 50 mg, a mixture of highly-purified bovine-derived glycosaminoglycans (GAGs) naturally present in the aorta including: Dermatan Sulfate, Heparan Sulfate, Hyaluronic Acid, Chondroitin Sulfate, & related Hexosaminoglycans. Contains no sugar, salt, yeast, wheat, corn, soy, dairy products, coloring, flavoring or preservatives.
See Editor's Note No. 14, page 1817.

APM 60- Chocolate - Nutripeak
Each packet contains: Protein 60 g • Vitamin A (Retinyl Palmitate and Beta Carotene) 4500 IU • Vitamin C (Ascorbic Acid) 60 mg • Vitamin D (Cholecalciferol) 240 IU • Vitamin E (dl-Tocopheryl Acetate) 45 IU • Vitamin K (phytonadione) 40 mcg • Thiamin (Vitamin B1) 0.9 mcg • Riboflavin (Vitamin B2) 1 mg • Niacin (Niacinamide) 20 mg • Vitamin B-6 (Pyridoxine Hydrochloride) 1 mg • Folic Acid 400 mcg • Vitamin B-12 (Cyanocobalamin) 3 mcg • Biotin 180 mcg

• Pantothenic Acid (Calcium D-Pantothenate) 4 mg • Calcium Lactate 2 g • Iron (Ferrous Fumarate) 7.2 mg • Phosphorus (Tricalcium Phosphate and Dicalcium Phosphate) 1.3 mg • Iodine (Potassium Iodide) 52 mg • Magnesium (Trimagnesium Phosphate and Magnesium Oxide) 440 mg • Zinc Oxide 5.2 mg • Selenium (Sodium Molybdate) 31 mcg • Copper (Cupric Sulfate) 0.7 mg • Manganese Sulfate 1 mg • Chromium 48 mcg • Molybdenum (Sodium Molybdate) 60 mcg • Sodium 340 mg • Potassium Chloride and Citrate 1 g • ARS Proprietary Blend: L-Glutamine, Potassium Bicarbonate, Monosodium Orthophosphate, Sodium Citrate Dihydrate, L-Carnosine, Trans-Ferulic Acid 1.6 g • TNA Proprietary Blend: DL-Phenylalanine, L-Tyrosine, Taurine 800 mg • Proulin Proprietary Blend: Myo-Inositol, Alpha-Lipoic Acid, Vanadium, Chromium 201 mg. Other Ingredients: Metamyosyn Protein Blend: Milk Protein Concentrate, Calcium Sodium Caseinate, Whey Protein Concentrate, Dried Egg Albumen, Whey Protein Isolate, Bovine lactoferrin; Cocoa (processed with alkali); Xanthan Gum; Sodium Carboxymethylcellulose; Maltodextrin; Sucralose; Acesulfame Potassium; Natural and Artificial Flavors.

Appleheart Chondroitin Sulfate - Appleheart
Each capsule contains: Chondroitin Sulfate 300 mg.
Other Ingredients: Cellulose, Gelatin, Vegetable Stearate.
See Editor's Note No. 15, page 1817.

Appleheart Echinacea - Appleheart
Each capsule contains: standarized Echinacea Angustifolia and Echinacea Purpurea 250 mg • Rice Protein • Gelatin • Cellulose • Vegetable Stearate. Contains no Dairy, Yeast, Corn, Sugar, Starch, Soy, Preservatives, Hydrogenated Oils.

Appleheart Glucosamine Sulfate - Appleheart
Each capsule contains: Glucosamine Sulfate (from Glucosamine Sulfate Potassium) 500 mg • Potassium 65 mg. Other Ingredients: Gelatin, Cellulose, Vegetable Stearate.

Appleheart Melatonin - Appleheart
Each capsule contains: Melatonin 3mg.
See Editor's Note No. 16, page 1817.

Appleheart Saw Palmetto - Appleheart
Each capsule contains: Saw Palmetto berry 160 mg • Olive Oil • Water • Gelatin. Contains no dairy, yeast, corn, sugar, starch, soy, preservatives or hydrogenated oils.

Appleheart St. John's Wort - Appleheart
Each capsule contains: standardized St. John's Wort 250 mg • Gelatin • Rice Protein • Cellulose • Magnesium Stearate (Vegetable Source).

Apple-Honey Lactobacillus Acidophilus - Nature's Life
Two tablespoons (1 fl.oz or 29.6 ml) contain: Calories: 11 • Cholesterol: 0 • Fiber 0.1 g • Protein: 0.7 g • Fat: 0 • Carbohydrates: 2 g. Full disclosure ingredients: Unfiltered Apple juice, Purified Water, Pasteurized Honey, Soy Protein Isolate & Lactobacillus Acidophilus Culture.

AppSignal - Pharmanex
Two wafers contain: Sucrose • Cocoa Powder • Microcrystalline Cellulose • Protein Complex (Hydrolyzed Soy Protein, Soy Protein Isolate, Egg Albumin) • L-Tyrosine • AbsorbaLean Fiber Complex: Apple Pectin, Fructooligosaccharides, Locust Bean Gum, Carrageenan, Microcrystalline Cellulose • Stearic Acid • Lecithin Powder • Natural and Artificial Flavors • Sorbitol • L-Histidine Hydrochloride • Pyridoxine Hydrochloride • Magnesium Stearate • Folic Acid.

Aqua Ban - Thompson Medical Co
Each tablet contains: Active Ingredient: Pamabrom 50 mg (Diuretic). Other ingredients: Carnauba Wax • Croscarmellose Sodium • FD&C

Blue No. 1 Aluminum Lake • Hydroxypropyl Methylcellulose • Lactose • Magnesium Stearate • Microcrystalline Cellulose • Polyethylene Glycol • Polysorbate 80 • Starch • Titanium Dioxide.

Aqua Greens - Futurebiotics
Twelve tablets contain: Chlorella 1000 mg • Spirulina 2500 mg • Klamath Blue/Green Algae 500 mg • Kelp 250 mg • D. Salina 100 mg.

AquaActin - Nature's Plus
Two capsules contain: Chinese Green Tea [(Camellia sinensis leaf) decaffeinated, standardized 50% Polyphenols] 250 mg • Horsetail [(Equisetum arvense stem) standardized 10% Silicic Acid, 7% Silica] 150 mg • Uva Ursi [(Arctostaphylos uva-ursi leaf) standardized 20-25% Arbutin] 100 mg • Vitamin B6 (Pyridoxine HCI) 75 mg • Goldenseal [(Hydrastis canadensis root & rhizome) standardized 10% Alkaloids, 5% Hydrastine] 50 mg • Artichoke [(Cynara scolymus flower) standardized 2.5-5% Caffeylquinic Acids] 50 mg.

Aqua-Action - Nature's Plus
Each capsule contains: Buchu leaves 125 mg • Couchgrass 100 mg • Juniper berries 100 mg • Parsley leaves 100 mg • Corn Silk 75 mg • Uva Ursi leaves 50 mg • Celery seed 50 mg. Contains no yeast, wheat, soy, milk, salt, sugar or starch.

Aqua-Flow - Enzymatic Therapy
Two capsules contain: Potassium Citrate 200 mg • Magnesium (Oxide) 50 mg • Vitamin B6 (Pyridoxine HCL) 25 mg • Other ingredients: Bearberry extract (Uva Ursi) contains 10% Arbutin 200 mg • Lespedeza extract (Lespedeza capitatae) contains 8% Flavonoids 100 mg • Boldo extract (Peumus boldo) contains 1.52% essential oils 100 mg • Goldenrod extract (Solidago virgaurea) contains 5% flavonoids 100 mg. Contains no sugar, salt, yeast, wheat, corn, soy, dairy products, coloring, flavoring, or preservatives.

Aqua-Lim - Aspen Group, Inc.
Each tablet contains: Buchu leaves 70 mg • Couch Grass 70 mg • Hydrangea root 35 mg • Corn Silk 35 mg • Uva Ursi 10 mg • Hypothalamus 30 mg • Raw Kidney concentrate 30 mg • Vitamin B6 16 mg • Bladder Wrack 100 mg • Magnesium: Protein Chelated 50 mg.
See Editor's Note No. 14, page 1817.

Aquatone - PharmAssure
Two tablets contain: Vitamin B6 (as Pyridoxine Hydrochloride) 15 mg • Magnesium (as Magnesium Gluconate) 25 mg • Potassium (as Potassium Gluconate) 99 mg • Uva Ursi Extract (Arctostaphylos uva ursi;20% Arbutin=150 mg) 750 mg. Other ingredients: Cellulose, Calcium Carbonate.

Aqueous Liver Extract - PhytoPharmica
Two capsules contain: Vitamin B12 (cyanocobalamin) 200 mcg • Liquid Liver Fractions (predigested soluble concentrate) 1,100 mg.
See Editor's Note No. 14, page 1817.

Aqueous Liver Extract with Siberian Ginseng - PhytoPharmica
Two capsules contain: Vitamin B12 (cyanocobalamin) 200 mcg • Liquid Liver fractions (predigested soluble concentrate) 1,100 mg • Siberian Ginseng (Eleutherococcus senticosus) root extract 20:1 (standardized to contain greater than 0.5% eleutheroside E) 50 mg.
See Editor's Note No. 14, page 1817.

Arbu-Tone - PhytoPharmica
Two capsules contain: Potassium Citrate 200 mg • Magnesium (Oxide) 50 mg • Vitamin B6 (Pyridoxine HCL) 25 mg • Bearberry extract (Uva Ursi) standardized to contain 10% arbutin 200 mg • Lespedeza extract (Lespedeza capitatae) standardized to contain 8% flavonoids 100 mg • Boldo extract (Peumus boldo) standardized to

contain 1.52% essential oils 100 mg • Goldenrod extract (Solidago vigaurea) standardized to contain 5% flavonoids 100 mg . Contains no sugar, salt, yeast, wheat, corn, soy, dairy products, coloring, flavoring, or preservatives.

Arctic Root - Swedish Herbal Institute
Each tablet contains Rhodiola rosea, extract SHI-Rr5 180 mg.

Arginine & Ornithine - Olympian Labs
Each capsule contains: L-Arginine 500 mg • L-Ornithine 250 mg.

Arginine Pyroglutamate/Lysine - Ultimate Nutrition
Each capsule contains: L-Arginine Pyroglutamate 500 mg • L-Lysine 250 mg.

Arginine Ultra - FreeLife
Two caplets contain: Calcium as Calcium carbonate and Calcium hydrogen phosphate 100 mg • L-Arginine Hydrochloride 1500 mg. Other Ingredients: Galactomannan, Cellulose, Fractionated Vegetable oil, Fruit Pectin, Vita-Coat: vegetable resin, alpha-lipoic acid

Arginine-Ornithine 1500 - Puritan's Pride
Two capsules contain: L-Arginine 1000 mg • L-Ornithine 500 mg • Chromium picolinate 6.2 mcg.

ArginMax - Daily Wellness Co.
Six capsules contain: Vitamin A palmitate 5,000 IU • L-Arginine 3000 mg • Folate (as Folic Acid) 400 mcg • Biotin 300 mcg 90% • American Ginseng (Panax quinquefolius) standardized (5% Ginsenosides) 100 mg • Korean Ginseng (Panax Ginseng) standardized (30% ginsenosides) 100 mg • Selenium (Sodium Selenate) 70 mcg • Vitamin C (Ascorbic Acid) 60 mg • Ginkgo Biloba standardized (24% Flavone Glycosides, 6% Terpene Lactones) 50 mg • Vitamin E (as d-Alpha-Tocopheryl Acetate) 30 IU • Niacin (as Niacinamide) 20 mg • Zinc (Zinc Gluconate) 15 mg • Vitamin B5 (Pantothenic Acid) (as Calcium Pantothenate) 10 mg • Vitamin B12 (Cyanocobalamin) 6 mcg • Vitamin B6 (Pyridoxine HCl) 2 mg • Vitamin B2 (Riboflavin) • Vitamin B1 (Thiamin) (as Thiamin Mononitrate) 1.5 mg.

ArginMax for Men - Daily Wellness Co.
Six capsules contain: L-Arginine 3000 mg • American Ginseng 100 mg • Korean Ginseng 100 mg • Ginkgo Biloba 50 mg • Vitamin A 5000 IU • Vitamin C 60 mg • Vitamin E 30 IU • Thiamin 1.5 mg • Riboflavin 1.7 mg • Niacin 20 mg • Vitamin B6 2 mg • Folate 400 mcg • Vitamin B12 6 mcg • Biotin 300 mcg • Pantothenic Acid 10 mg • Zinc 15 mg • Selenium 70 mcg.

ArginMax for Men-GNC - GNC
Six tablets contain: Vitamin A (as retinyl palmitate) 5000 IU • Vitamin C (as ascorbic acid) 60 mg • Vitamin E (as d-alpha tocopherol succinate) 30 IU • Thiamin (as thiamin mononitrate) 1.5 mg • Riboflavin (B2) 1.7 mg • Niacin (as niacinamide) 20 mg • Vitamin B-6 (pyridoxine hydrochloride) 2 mg • Folic Acid 400 mcg • Vitamin B-12 (cyanocobalamin) 6 mcg • Biotin 300 mcg • Pantothenic Acid (as calcium d-pantothenate) 10 mg • Zinc (as zinc gluconate) 15 mg • Selenium 70 mcg • L-Arginine 3000 mg • Korean Ginseng extract aerial parts and roots 100 mg • American Ginseng root 100 mg • Ginkgo Biloba extract leaf 50 mg • Other Ingredients: Microcrystallin Cellulose, Magnesium Stearate, Hydroxypropyl Methylcellulose, Pharmaceutical Glaze, Silica, Titanium Dioxide, PEG, Polysorbate 80.

ArginMax for Women - Daily Wellness Co.
Six capsules contain: L-arginine 2500 mg • Korean Ginseng 100 mg • Ginkgo Biloba 50 mg • Damiana leaves 50 mg • Vitamin A 5000 IU • Vitamin C 60 mg • Vitamin E 30 IU • Thiamin 1.5 mg • Riboflavin 1.7 mg • Niacin 20 mg • Vitamin B6 2 mg • Folate 400 mcg • Vitamin B12 6 mcg • Biotin 300 mcg • Pantothenic Acid 10 mg • Calcium 500 mg • Iron 9 mg • Zinc 7.5 mg.

Some Brand Name Natural Products - What they Contain
www.NaturalDatabase.com contains MANY more listings than appear here.

ArginMax for Women-GNC - GNC
Six tablets contain: Vitamin A (as retinyl palmitate) 5000 IU • Vitamin C (as ascorbic acid) 60 mg • Vitamin E (as d-alpha tocopherol succinate) 30 IU • Thiamin (as thiamin mononitrate) 1.5 mg • Riboflavin (B2) 1.7 mg • Niacin (as niacinamide) 20 mg • Vitamin B-6 (pyridoxine hydrochloride) 2 mg • Folic Acid 400 mcg • Vitamin B-12 (cyanocobalamin) 6 mcg • Biotin 300 mcg • Pantothenic Acid (as calcium d-pantothenate) 10 mg • Calcium (as calcium carbonate) 500 mg • Iron (as ferrous gluconate) 9 mg • Zinc (as zinc gluconate) 7.5 mg • L-Arginine 2500 mg • Korean Ginseng extract aerial parts and roots 100 mg • Ginkgo Biloba extract leaf 50 mg • Damiana leaf 50 mg. Other Ingredients: Microcrystalline Cellulose, Hydroxypropyl Methylcellulose, Pharmaceutical Glaze, Silica, Titanium Dioxide, Magnesium Stearate, PEG, Polysorbate 80.

Arnica Oil - Blessed Herbs
Arnica flower & leaf • Organic Cold-Pressed Olive oil.

ArteClear - Pacific BioLogic
Rhubarb rhizome • Salvia root • Sea Weed • Polygonum root • Polygonatum rhizome • Cassia seeds • Aucklandia root • Hawthorn fruit • Pseudoginseng root.

Arth Rx - Symmetry
Each packet contains: Glucosamine • Chondroitin Sulfate • Hydrolyzed gelatin • Boswellia • Curcumin • Bilberry • Grape Seed extract • Grape Skin extract • Tumeric extract.
See Editor's Note No. 15, page 1817.

Arth-9 - Rx Vitamins
Four capsules contain: Glucosamine Sulfate (Aminomonosaccharide) 1000 mg • Vitamin C (Ascorbic Acid) 250 mg • Bromelain 250 mg • Calcium (Citrate) 250 mg • Boswellin 250 mg • Curcumin 100 mg • Zinc (L-Monomethionine) 30 mg • Chondroitin Sulfate A (CSA) 25 mg • Copper (Glycinate) 2 mg.
See Editor's Note No. 15, page 1817.

Artho-Health Formula - Youngevity
Cosamin (Glucosamine Sulfate 200 mg, Chondroitin Sulfate 160 mg) • Vitamin C 15 mg • Manganese 500 mcg • Vilcabamba Mineral Essence: Potassium, Calcium, Magnesium, Zinc, Chromium, Selenium, Iron, Copper, Molybdenum, Vanadium, Iodine, Cobalt, Manganese.
See Editor's Note No. 15, page 1817.

Artho-Therapy - PhytoPharmica
Each tablet contains: Capsaicin 0.025%. Other Ingredients: Purified water, Alcohol, Glycerin, Triethanolamine, Escin (Horse chestnut extract), Glory Lily, Methylparaben, Lavender essential oil.

Arthred-G - Richardson Labs
One rounded scoop contains: Arthred (enzymatically hydrolyzed collagen protein) 7 g • Glucosamine & Chondroitin complex: glucosamine HCL, glucosamine sulfate (potassium salt, sodium free), chondroitin sulfate.
See Editor's Note No. 15, page 1817.

Arth-Rid Us - The Herbalist
Devil's Claw root bark • Yucca root • Yerba Mansa root • Black Cohosh root • Wild Yam root.

Arthri-Gesic Liquid Glucosamine - Quantum Health
Each 10 mL dose contains: Glucosamine HCL 500 mg • White Willow Bark extract 50 mg • Devil's Claw extract 25 mg • Curcumin extract 500 mcg. Other Ingredients: Glycerin, Water, Potassium Sorbate, Stevia, Natural Beet Color, Tangerine Oil.

Arthrimin GS Glucosamine Sulfate 500 mg - Jamieson
Each capsule contains: Glucosamine Sulfate (from Potassium Chloride Complex) 500 mg. Other Ingredients: Peppermint Leaf, and Betaine Hydrochloride.

Arthritis Guardian - Clinician's Choice
Three tablets contain: Shark Cartilage 1500 mg • Glucosamine Sulfate 450 mg • Linoleic Acid, Gamma Linolenic Acid (sunflower oil, borage oil) 150 mg • Boswellia 30 mg • Cayenne Fruit 30 mg • Glycosaminoglycan 30 mg • White Willow Bark 30 mg • Proprietary blend: Carrot Powder, Citrus Bioflavonoids Complex, Grape Powder 9 mg.

Arthritis Remedy - PhytoPharmica
Each tablespoon contains: Aurum muriaticum natronatum 8x • Mercurius corrosivus 6x • Silicea 6x • Sulphur 4x • Bryonia 3x • Colchicum 3x • Natrum salicylicum 3x • Viscum album 3x • Dulcamara 2x • Kalium iodatum 2x • Betula 1x • Rubia tinctorum 1x. In a base of 20% USP alcohol by volume.
See Editor's Note No. 1, page 1816.

Arthro Herbal-Rx - Alternecare Health Products
Two capsules contain: Chondroitin Sulfate (Bovine Cartilage) 150 mg • Glucosamine Sulfate 350 mg • Cat's Claw 25 mg • Quercetin 50 mg • Bromelain 50 mg • Alfalfa 25 mg • Devil's Claw 10 mg • Yucca 20 mg • Pycnogenol 5 mg • Grape seed 5 mg • Suma 25 mg • Siberian Ginseng 25 mg • Lipoic Acid 25 mg.
See Editor's Note No. 15, page 1817.

Arthro-7 - Gero Vita
Each capsule contains: Chicken Collagen type II 400 mg • Methylsulfonylmethane (MSM) 50 mg • Cetyl Myristoleate (CMO) 50 mg • Bromelain (2400 GDU) 15 mg • Curcuma Longa Extract (root, 95% Curcumin) • Vitamin C (as Ascorbic Acid) 70 mg • Lipase (30 USP units) 50 mg.
See Editor's Note No. 14, page 1817.

Arthro-Glucosamine - Nutri-Quest
Each tablet supples: Glucosamine Sulfate 100 mg • N-Acetyl Glucosamine 50 mg • L-Glutathione 2 mg • N-Acetyl Cysteine 5 mg • L-Cysteine 50 mg • L-Glutamic Acid 50 mg • L-Glycine 50 mg • L-Taurine 25 mg • Vitamin C 50 mg • Vitamin E (Succinate) 25 IU • Pantothenic Acid 50 mg • Soluble Trachea (16% Chondroitin Sulfate-A) 25 mg • Silymarin 5 mg • Milk Thistle 100 mg • Green Lipped Mussel 25 mg (natural source of Mucopolysaccharides & Superoxide Dismutase).
See Editor's Note No. 15, page 1817.

Arthro-HCP - Met-Rx
Fourteen grams contain: Arthred (Hydrolyzed Collagen Protein) 10 g • Maltodextrin • Glucosamine Hydrochloride & Glucosamine Sulfate 1.5 g.
See Editor's Note No. 21, page 1818.

Artichoke Extract - PhytoPharmica
Two capsules contain: Artichoke (Cynara scolymus leaf extract 5:1) 320 mg.

Artichoke Extract - Nature's Way
Two capsules contain: Artichoke dried extract 600 mg • Milk Thistle seed 300 mg. Other Ingredients: Gelatin, Magnesium stearate, Maltodextrin, Silica.

As-Comp - Enzymatic Therapy
Each capsule contains: Active Ingredient: Ephedrine [From Ma Huang extract (Ephedra sinensis) 200 mg] 12 mg • Other ingredients: Ginger root extract 6.5:1 (Zingiber officinale) 65 mg • Licorice root extract (Glycyrrhiza glabra) standardized to contain 5% Glycyrrhizic acid) 50 mg • Marshmallow root extract 4:1 (Althaea officinalis) (Mucilage content 30-40%) 50 mg • Sundew Herb extract 4:1 (Drosera rotundifolia) 40 mg • Euphorbia Herb extract 4:1 (Euphorbia hirta)

40 mg • Senega root extract 4:1 (Polygala senega) 40 mg • Goldenseal root extract (Hydrastis canadensis) standardized to contain 5% total Alkaloids including Berberine, Hydrastine & Canadine 20 mg. Contains no sugar, salt, yeast, wheat, corn, soy, dairy products, coloring, flavoring, or preservatives.

Ascorbate-C - Atrium Inc.
Each teaspoon (5 gm) contains: Vitamin C (Calcium Ascorbate) 2000 mg • Rose Hips 1450 mg • Acerola 1000 mg • Lemon Bioflavonoids 500 mg • Rutin 25 mg • Hesperidin 25 mg • Calcium (from Calcium Ascorbate) 230 mg.

Asparagus Extract - PhytoPharmica
Each capsule contains: Asparagus (Asparagus officinalis) root (rhizome) extract (standardized to contain 4.0%-8.0% asparagosides) 170 mg.

Aspen - Body Booster with Power - Aspen Group, Inc.
Each tablet contains: Raw Testicular concentrate (not an extract) of Bovine sources 300 mg • Multiple Glans Raw Gland concentrate (not an extract) containing Raw Liver Duodenum, Pancreas (porcine sources) & Raw Heart , Pituitary, Kidney, Spleen, Thymus & Adrenal concentrates of Bovine sources 225 mg • Cayenne 25 mg • Gotu Kola 25 mg • Fo-Ti 25 mg • Damiana 32 mg • Guarana 50 mg.
See Editor's Note No. 14, page 1817.

Aspen - Candida - Aspen Group, Inc.
Each capsule contains: Pau D'Arco 4:1 extract 100 mg • Calcium Caprylate 100 mg • Goldenseal root extract 100 mg • Garlic extract (odorless) 50 mg • Licorice root extract 50 mg • Caprilic Acid 25 mg • Oregano 25 mg • Tea Tree oil 5 mg.

Aspen - Cardio- Health - Aspen Group, Inc.
Each caplet contains: Vitamin E (d-alpha tocopheryl acetate) 200 IU • Vitamin C 50 mg • Garlic extract (allium sativum) 300 mg • Hawthorn extract of leaf & flower (crategus laevigata) 50 mg • Co-Enzyme Q10 (ubiquinone) 5 mg.

Aspen - Daily Essentials - Aspen Group, Inc.
Three tablets contain: Vitamin E (d-alpha) 200 IU • Vitamin A 5000 IU • Beta Carotene 5000 IU • Vitamin D 400 IU • Vitamin C 400 mg • Folic Acid 400 mcg • Thiamine 1.5 mg • Riboflavin 1.7 mg • Niacin 20 mg • Vitamin B6 2 mg • Vitamin B12 6 mcg • Biotin 300 mcg • Pantothenic Acid 10 mg • Calcium (citrate) 600 mg • Phosphorus 450 mg • Iodine (kelp) 150 mcg • Magnesium (carbonate) 200 mg • Copper (gluconate) 2 mg • Zinc (gluconate) 15 mg • Vitamin K 100 mcg • Selenium (yeast) 75 mcg • Manganese (gluconate) 5 mg • Chromium (aspartate) 200 mcg • Molybdenum 150 mcg • Nickel 15 mcg • Tin 15 mcg • Vanadium 5 mg • Boron (citrate) 2 mg • Potassium (gluconate) 100 mg • Grape seed extract 10 mg • CoQ10 10 mg. Contains no sugar, starch, salt, wheat, corn, milk or soy derivatives.

Aspen - Flexile Plus - Aspen Group, Inc.
Three capsules contain: Glucosamine HCl 99% 1500 mg • Chondroitin Sulfate (purified chondroitin sulfate 95%, mixed glycosominoglycans 5%) 1200 mg • Manganese Ascorbate 240 mg • Bromelain 100 mg • Boswellia Serrata extract 100 mg.
See Editor's Note No. 15, page 1817.

Aspen - Imun- Comp - Aspen Group, Inc.
Two tablets contain: Vitamin C (Ascorbic Acid) 250 mg • Vitamin B1 (Thiamin HCl) 30 mg • Vitamin E (d-Alpha Tocopherol) 200 IU • Beta Carotene 5000 IU • Copper (Gluconate) 300 mcg • Selenium Chelate 25 mcg • Zinc (Gluconate) 15 mg • Bone Marrow 65 mg • Lymph 65 mg • Papain 50 mg • Pituitary Whole 15 mg • Spleen 130 mg • Thymus 550 mg • Bromelain 50 mg • Echinacea extract 300 mg • L-Lysine HCl 250 mg • Trypsin 1:75 25 mg • Blue Flag 130 mg • Fennel 70 mg • Goldenseal herb 70 mg.
See Editor's Note No. 14, page 1817.

Aspen - Maximal Sterol Complex - Aspen Group, Inc.
Six tablets contain: Fucosterol 6963 mcg • Beta Sitosterol 5148 mcg • Campestrol 3.069 mcg • Stigmatero 1749 mcg • Other Naturally Occuring Sterols 9174 mcg • (26103 mcg of Sterols) • Liver 2600 mg • Orchic 1000 mg • Thymus 200 mg • Heart 200 mg • Lung 200 mg • Kidney 200 mg • Adrenal 150 mg • Prostate 120 mg • Pituitary 150 mg • Hypothalamus 60 mg • Pancreas 120 mg • Bee pollen 1000 mg • Korean Ginseng 100 mg • Royal Jelly 30 mg • Calcium 200 mg • Magnesium 100 mg • Potassium 99 mg • Octacosanol 1650 mcg • RNA 60 mg • DNA 30 mg • Linoleic Acid 1040 mg • Oleic Acid 698 mg • Palmitic Acid 263 mg • Linolenic Acid 109 mg • Stearic Acid 56 mg • Lignoceric Acid 14 mg • Arachidonic Acid 13 mg • Elcoanoic Acid 11 mg • Behenic C Acid 6 mg • Myristic Acid 5 mg • Capsicum 100 mg • Alfalfa 100 mg • Dandelion root 100 mg • Garlic 100 mg • Yellow Dock 100 mg • Gota Kola 100 mg • Licorice root 100 mg • Arginine 1200 mg • Lysine 600 mg • Ornithine 600 mg • Leucine 40 mg • Valine 38 mg • Lysine 34 mg • Isoleucine 30 mg • Phenylalanine 30 mg • Theronine 24 mg • Methionine 20 mg • Tryptophan 8 mg • Trace Minerals.
See Editor's Note No. 14, page 1817.

Aspen - Mega Max - Aspen Group, Inc.
Each tablet contains: Vitamin C 250 mg • Vitamin E 150 IU • Vitamin A 25,000 USP Units • Vitamin D 1000 USP Units • Vitamin B1 75 mg • Vitamin B2 75 mg • Vitamin B6 75 mg • Vitamin B12 75 mg • Niacinamide 75 mg • Choline 75 mg • Inositol 75 mg • Para Aminobenzoic Acid 75 mg • Pantothenic Acid 75 mg • Biotin 75 mg • Folic Acid 400 mcg • Rutin 25 mg • Citrus bioflavonoids complex 25 mg • Hesperiden complex 5 mg • Betaine HCl 25 mg • Glutamic Acid 25 mg • Iodine .15 mg • Calcium 50 mg • Potassium 10 mg • Iron 10 mg • Magnesium 7.2 mg • Manganese 6.1 mg • Zinc 15 mg • Selenium 10 mcg • Amino Acids: Arginine, Aspartic Acid, Alanine, Cystine, Glutamic Acid, Glycine, Histidine, Isoleucine, Lucine, Lysine, Methionine, Ornithine, Phenylalanine, Proline, Serine, Threonine, Tyrosine, Tryptophan & Valine in a natural base of Alfalfa • Parsley • Golden Seal root • Buckthorne root • Rosemary • Watercress • Mandrake root • Spinach • Lovage • Kelp • Kale • Ginseng & Rhubarb root.

Aspen - Mid-Life Plus - Aspen Group, Inc.
Each caplet contains: Vitamin E (as natural d-alpha tocopherol succinate) 30 IU • Vitamin C 60 mg • Thiamin (as thiamin mononitrate) 2 mg • Riboflavin 2 mg • Niacin (niacinamide) 20 mg • Vitamin B6 (as pyridoxine HCl) 10 mg • Vitamin B12 (as cyanocobalamin) 6 mcg • Folate (as folic acid) 400 mcg • Calcium (from calcium carbonate) 150 mg • Selenium (from L-Selenomethionine) 70 mcg • Boron (chelate) 1.5 mg • Purified Isoflavones (from soybean & pueraria root) 50 mg • Kava Kava root standardized extract (30% kavalactones) 100 mg • Black Cohosh root 40 mg.

Aspen - Muscle Builder - Aspen Group, Inc.
Four tablets contain: Gamma Oryzanol 50 mg • Inosine 200 mg • Testicular Glan 600 mg • L-Ornithine 700 mg • Beta-Sitosterol 200 mg • Adrenal 400 mg • Thymus 400 mg.
See Editor's Note No. 14, page 1817.

Aspen - Osteo - Aspen Group, Inc.
Each tablet contains: Calcium Orotate 376 mg • Magnesium Orotate 200 mg • Calcium Aspartate 24 mg • Vitamin D 400 mg.

Aspen - Primrose - Aspen Group, Inc.
Each softgel contains: Evening Primrose oil 500 mg • Vitamin E (d-alpha tocopherol) 10 IU • Gamma Linolenic Acid 40 mg • Linoleic Acid 350 mg. Contains no sugar, starch, salt, wheat, corn, yeast or soy derivatives.

Aspen - Soy Special - Aspen Group, Inc.
Each tablet contains: Soy isoflavones 50 mg.

Some Brand Name Natural Products - What they Contain
www.NaturalDatabase.com contains MANY more listings than appear here.

Aspen - Super Max 1600 Weight Gain - Aspen Group, Inc.
Each flavor (vanilla or chocolate) contains: Vitamin C 332 mg • Rose Hips 6.8 mg • Vitamin E 400 IU • Vitamin A 13332 USP Units • Vitamin D 532 USP Units • Vitamin B1 20 mg • Vitamin B2 16 mg • Vitamin B6 68 mg • Vitamin B12 8 mcg • Niacin 56 mg • Choline 40 mg • Inositol 26.8 mg • Para Aminobenzoic Acid 1600 mg • Pantothenic 132 mg • Biotin 400 mcg • Folic Acid 532 mcg • Rutin 1700 mcg • Glutamic Acid 880 mg • Iodine 200 mcg • Calcium 1280 mg • Phosphorus 1200 mg • Potassium 10 mg • Iron 36 mg • Copper 2800 mg • Magnesium 13.2 mg • Manganese 3200 mg • Zinc 20 mg • Amino Acids Arginine 7883 mg • Aspartic Acid 220 mg • Alanine 880 mg • Cystine 1100 mg • Glutamic Acid 880 mg • Glycine 1980 mg • Histidine 2332 mg • Isoleucine 7152 mg • Lucine 4840 mg • Lysine 5060 mg • Methionine 1100 mg • Phenylalanine 944 mg • Proline 328 mg • Serine 4840 mg • Threonine 3300 mg • Tyrosine 220 mg • Tryptophan 880 mg • Valine 4840 mg.

AspirActin - Nature's Plus
Three capsules contain: White Willow bark [(Salix alba) standardized 7-9% Salicin] 500 mg • Kava Kava [(Piper methysticum root) standardized 29-31% Kavalactones] 50 mg • Inositol Hexanicotinate (Flush-Free Niacin) 50 mg • Cayenne [(Capsicum frutescens fruit) standardized 100000 STU] 25 mg • Ginkgo Biloba leaf (standardized 24% Ginkgo Flavone-Glycosides, 6% Terpene Lactones) 10 mg.

AstaZanthin - Source Naturals
Marine Algae (Haematococcus pluvialis) 10 mg. Natural concentrate (AstaZanthin) yielding Astaxanthin complex 1 mg.

Asthma & Allergy Remedy - PhytoPharmica
Twenty to fifty drops contain: Adrenalinum 6x • Stramonium 6x • Belladonna 4x • Ephedra vulgaris 4x • Ipecacuanha 4x • Lobelia 3x • Solidago virgaurea 3x • Yerba santa 3x • Sambucus 1x. In a base of 40% USP alcohol by volume.
See Editor's Note No. 1, pag 1816.

Asthma-X5 - Olympian Labs
Each capsule contains: Proprietary Blend: Schisandra Berries, Green Tea, Mormon Tea, Coleus Forskohlii, Lobelia, Feverfew, Skullcap, Licorice root, Ginger 500 mg.

Astragalus - Nature's Way
Three capsules contain: Astragalus root 1.41 g. Other Ingredients: Gelatin, Magnesium stearate.

Astragalus - Now
Two capsules contain: Total Carbohydrate 0.7 g • Dietary Fiber 0.5 g • Astragalus root powder (a. membranaceus) 1.0 g. Other Ingredients: Stearic Acid. Contains no milk, wheat, corn, yeast, sugar, salt, starch, soy, preservatives, or additives.

Astragalus - Pharmanex
Each capsule contains: Astragalus root extract(Astragalus membranaceus) (10:1) 250 mg. Other Ingredients: Rice Flour, Gelatin, Magnesium Stearate, Silicon Dioxide.

Astragalus Plus - The Herbalist
Astragalus root • Echinacea root • Lomatium root • Myrrh Gum • Poke root • Wild Indigo root • Yarrow flower • Cayenne pepper.

Astragalus-Shitake Virtue - Blessed Herbs
Astragalus root • Echinacea Angustifolia root • Licorice root • Shitake mycelium • Grain alcohol & Distilled Water.

A-Team: Adrenal Support - The Herbalist
Siberian Ginseng fresh-dried root (Eleuthero sent) • Oats fresh milky seed (Avena sativa) • Licorice fresh-dried root (Glycyrrhiza glabra) • Gotu Kola fresh herb (Hydrocotyle asiatica) • Cayenne fresh-dried pepper (Capsicum anuum).

Athero Chelate - PhytoPharmica
Six tablets contain: Vitamin C (ascorbic acid) 1,500 mg • Niacin/niacinamide 630 mg • Vitamin B6 (pyridoxine HCl) 150 mg • Calcium chloride 291 mg • Iodine (kelp) 600 mcg • Magnesium orotate 1,800 mg • Magnesium ascorbate 300 mg • Zinc ascorbate 45 mg • Selenium ascorbate (provides 300 mcg of selenium) 30 mg • Copper gluconate 750 mcg • Manganese ascorbate 30 mg • Sodium 18 mg • Potassium (orotate, aspartate, phosphate, chloride) 315 mg • Taurine 300 mg • Beta-sitosterol (rye germ) 450 mg • Mucopolysaccharide (soluble) 300 mg • Betaine HCl 300 mg • Ammonium chloride 291 mg • L-Methionine 195 mg • Bromelain (1,800 M.C.U.) enzymes derived from pineapple stems 150 mg.

Athero-Plus - Atrium Inc.
Two film coated tablets contain: Vitamin A Palmitate 3334 IU • Vitamin D (as Vitamin D3) (Fish oil) 67 IU • Vitamin B1 (Thiamine Mononitrate) 34 mg • Vitamin B2 (Riboflavin) 17 mg • Vitamin B6 (Pyridoxine HCL) 34 mg • Vitamin B12 (Cyanocobalamin) 34 mcg • Vitamin C (Ascorbic Acid, Sago Palm) 400 mg • Vitamin E Succinate 134 IU • Beta Carotene 5000 IU • Biotin 100 mcg • Niacin/Niacinamide 67 mg • D-Calcium Pantothenate 167 mg • Folic Acid 267 mcg • Calcium Orotate 170 mg • Chromium Aspartate 67 mcg • Copper Gluconate 0.67 mg • Iodine (Kelp) 40 mcg • Iron (Ferrous Fumerate) 6.67 mg • Magnesium Orotate 170 mg • Magnesium Aspartate 6.67 mg • Molybdenum (Kelp) 34 mcg • Potassium Orotate 34 mg • Selenium Aspartate 67 mcg • Zinc Orotate 6.67 mg • Bromelain 50 mg • Choline Bitartrate 34 mg • L-Methionine 20 mg • PABA 17 mg • Rutin 17 mg.

Athle-Peak - The Herbalist
Jamaican Sarsaparilla root • Siberian Ginseng root • American Ginseng root • Licorice root • Wild Yam root • Cinnamon bark • Cayenne pepper.

Athletic Support - Amazon Support
Each capsule contains: Suma • Sarsaparilla • Maca • Catuaba • Chuchuhuasi • Guarana • Muira Puama • Yerba Mate • Tayuya • Iporuru.

Athletica - HerbaSway
Bitter Orange • Kudzu • Panax Ginseng • Siberian Ginseng • Astragalus • Schisandra • Ginger • Knotweed • Blackberry • Licorice • HerbaSwee (Cucurbitaceae fruit).

Atkins Allergy - Atkins
Six tablets contain: Pantethine (co-enzyme A precursor) 360 mg • Bioperine (Piperine) 5 mg • Citrus Bioflavonoids 1000 mg • Grape seed extract (Activin) 60 mg • Vitamin B12 (Cyanocobalamin) 1000 mcg • Vitamin B6 (Pyridoxine) 50 mg • Vitamin C (buffered) 2000 mg • Vitamin A (Acetate) 10000 IU • Quercetin (Flavonoid) 840 mg • Calcium (3-Phosphate, Ascorbate) 700 mg • Magnesium (Carbonate) 200 mg.

Atkins Basic #3 - Atkins
Each tablet contains: Magnesium Oxide 8 mg • Copper Sulfate 200 mcg • Vitamin E (d Alpha Tocopherol) 20 IU • Cyanocobalamin (Vitamin B12) 30 mcg • Biotin 75 mcg • Folic Acid 100 mcg • Pyridoxine (HCL) (Vitamin B6) 20 mg • Pyridoxal 5-Phosphate 2 mg • Calcium Pantothenate (Vitamin B5) 25 mg • Pantethine (80%) 25 mg • Niacinamide 5 mg • Niacin (Vitamin B3) 2 mg • Vitamin C (Calcium Ascorbate) 120 mg • Riboflavin (Vitamin B2) 4 mg • Thiamine (HCL) (Vitamin B1) 5 mg • Vitamin D (as Vitamin D2) 15 IU • Beta Carotene 500 IU • Vitamin A 200 IU • L-Glutathione (reduced) 5 mg • N-Acetyl-L-Cysteine 20 mg • Octacosanol 150 mcg • Selenium 40 mcg • Vanadyl Sulfate 15 mcg • Molybdenum (Sodium) 10 mcg • Chromium (Polynicotinate) 50 mcg • Zinc (Chelate) 10 mg • Manganese (Chelate) 4 mg • PABA 100 mg • Inositol 80 mg • Choline Bitartrate 100 mg.

BRAND NAMES

Some Brand Name Natural Products - What they Contain
www.NaturalDatabase.com contains MANY more listings than appear here.

Atkins Blood Pressure - Atkins
Six tablets contain: Taurine 1500 mg • Bioperine (Piperine) 5 mg • Hawthorn (1.5% Vitexin conc.) 300 mg • Calcium (from Ascorbate) 75 mg • Magnesium (Carbonate, Glycinate) 600 mg • Vitamin C (buffered) 600 mg • Pantethine (co-enzyme A precursor) 35 mg • L-Arginine base 100 mg • Inositol 600 mg • N-Acetyl-L-Cysteine 150 mg • Chromium (Picolinate) 200 mcg • Garlic 600 mg • Vitamin B6 (Pyridoxine) 150 mg • Potassium (Citrate) 99 mg.

Atkins Blood Sugar Tablets - Atkins
Six tablets contain: Chromium (Picolinate) 500 mcg • Bioperine (Piperine) 5 mg • Folic Acid (Folate) 800 mcg • Vitamin E natural 150 IU • Manganese (Glycinate) 30 mg • Selenium (Selenomethionine) 120 mcg • Inositol 900 mg • Niacinamide 300 mg • Vitamin C (buffered) 1200 mg • Bis-Glycinato Oxovanadium Complex (BGOV) 15 mg • Biotin 4 mg • Taurine 600 mg • Alpha-Lipoic Acid 240 mg • Magnesium (Glycinate, Carbonate) 600 mg • Zinc (Monomethionine) 50 mg.

Atkins Cholesterol - Atkins
Three tablets contain: Calcium (as phosphate) approx. 200 mg • Phosphorus (as calcium phosphate) approx. 115 mg • Inositol Hexanicotinate 1600 mg • Guggul Lipids 100 mg • Beta-, Stigma-, Campa-Sterol 225 mg • Garlic 300 mg • Pantethine (as a co-enzyme A precursor) 100 mg • L-Arginine 100 mg • Absorb Best Tablet Base (an exclusive all natural digestion-supporting base) 345 mg. Other Ingredients: Cellulose, Lecithin extracts, Croscarmellose Sodium, Magnesium Stearate, Silica, Natural Food Glaze. Includes: Pantethine, Garlic, Arginine, DGL Licorice, Lactoferrin, Spirulina, Bromelain, Inulin, Bioperine, Acidophilus (lactal and bifido bacterium).

Atkins Cold & Flu - Atkins
Four tablets contain: natural Beta-Carotene 20000 IU • Bioperine (Piperine) 5 mg • Copper (Chelate) 4 mg • Vitamin B6 (Pyridoxine) 16 mg • Vitamin B3 (Niacinamide) 60 mg • Vitamin B2 (Riboflavin) 8 mg • Dimethylglycine (DMG) 80 mg • Folic Acid (Folate) 800 mcg • Garlic 640 mg • Magnesium (Ascorbate) 60 mg • Selenium (Selenate) 120 mcg • Citrus Bioflavonoids 320 mg • Calcium Pantothenate (Vitamin B5) 320 mg • Vitamin C buffered 2000 mg • Zinc (Monomethionine) 100 mg • Quercetin (Flavonoid) 320 mg • Vitamin A (Acetate) 13333 IU.

Atkins Dieters Advantage - Atkins
Four tablets contain: Citrin (55% Hydroxycitric Acid) 450 mg • Chromium (Polynicotinate) 200 mcg • Soy extract (containing active Saponins) 1500 mg • Methionine 250 mg • L-Carnitine Peptide Complex 500 mg • Vitamin B6 (Pyridoxine) 20 mg • Pantethine (Co-enzyme A precursor) 20 mg • Asparagus concentrate 50 mg • Parsley concentrate 50 mg • Kelp 20 mg • Spirulina 50 mg • Potassium (Citrate) 99 mg • Magnesium (Citrate/Carbonate) 60 mg • L-Glutamine 75 mg • DL-Phenylalanine 150 mg • L-Tyrosine 75 mg • Bioperine (Piperine) 5 mg.

Atkins Essential Oils - Atkins
Each capsule contains: Flaxseed oil 400 mg • Vitamin E 5 IU • Fish oil (50% Omega-3 potency) 400 mg • Borage seed oil 400 mg.

Atkins Heart Care - Atkins
Eight tablets contain: Magnesium (Glycinate, Carbonate) 400 mg • Bioperine (Piperine) 5 mg • Cayenne 500 mg • Bromelain (Proteolytic Enzyme) 500 mg • Vitamin B6 (Pyridoxine) 10 mg • Folic Acid (Folate) 800 mcg • Selenium (Methionate) 150 mcg • Hawthorn (1.5% Vitexin conc.) 100 mg • Ginkgo Biloba (6% Terpene conc.) 60 mg • natural Beta-Carotene (Dunaliella salina) 12000 IU • Chromium (Picolinate) 200 mcg • Vitamin C (buffered) 1000 mg • Vitamin E natural 400 IU • Taurine 500 mg • Calcium (3-Phosphate) 500 mg.

Atkins Memory - Atkins
Eight tablets contain: Phosphatidylserine (PS) 160 mg • Bioperine (Piperine) 5 mg • Folic Acid (Folate) 800 mcg • Vitamin B12 (Cyanocobalamin) 1000 mcg • Vitamin B1 (Thiamine) 100 mg • N-Acetyl-L-Cysteine 1000 mg • Octacosanol 6 mg • Ginkgo Biloba (6% Terpene lactone conc.) 60 mg.

Atkins Menopause - Atkins
Four tablets contain: Black Cohosh (Cimicifuga rademosal) (2.5% Triterpenes) 25 mg • Vitamin E (d-Alpha-Tocopheryl) 200 IU • Bioperine (Piperine) 5 mg • Vitamin K 50 mg • Folic Acid 800 mcg • Tocotrienols mixed 3 mg • Boron (Boroglutamate) 3 mg • Alpha Lipoic Acid 10 mg • Pantethine (co-enzyme A precursor) 25 mg • Vitamin B6 (Pyridoxine) 50 mg • Calcium (Sulfate) 65 mg • Magnesium (Sulfate) 70 mg • Beta-Sitosterol 50 mg • Gamma Oryzanol 150 mg • Garlic (PurGar) 250 mg • Soy Phosphatidylcholine 400 mg • PABA (Para Amino Benzoic Acid) 500 mg • Soy Isoflavones concentrate (23.6% Genistein/Genistin; 3.8% Daidzin/Daldzein) 100 mg.

Atkins Shake Mix - Cappuccino - Atkins
Cappuccino shake mix contains: Protein 23 g • Carbohydrates 2 g • Fat 8 g • Calories 175. Ingredients: Lipo-Pro Blend (special formulation containing: Calcium Caseinate, Milk Protein concentrate, Egg Whites, Glutamine Peptides, Hydrolyzed Whey Protein concentrate & Whey Protein Isolate) • High Oleic Sunflower oil • Lecithin • Enzyme Modified Soy Protein • Carmel Color • Guar Gum • Vitamins & Minerals • Natural & Artificial Flavors • Acesulfame Potassium • Beta-Carotene.

Atkins Shake Mix - Chocolate - Atkins
Chocolate shake mix contains: Protein 24 g • Carbohydrates 1 g • Fat 9 g • Calories 180. Ingredients: Lipo-Pro Blend (special formulation containing: Calcium Caseinate, Milk Protein concentrate, Egg Whites, Glutamine Peptides, Hydrolyzed Whey Protein concentrate & Whey Protein Isolate) • Dutch Cocoa • High Oleic Sunflower oil • Polydextrose • Lecithin • Guar Gum • Vitamins & Minerals • Vanillin • Acesulfame Potassium • Beta-Carotene.

Atkins Shake Mix - Vanilla - Atkins
Vanilla Shake Mix contains: Protein 23 g • Carbohydrates 1 g • Fat 8 g • Calories 170. Ingredients: Lipo-Pro Blend (special formulation containing: Calcium Caseinate, Milk Protein concentrate, Egg Whites, Glutamine Peptides, Hydrolyed Whey Protein concentrate & Whey Protein Isolate) • High Oleci Sunflower oil • Lecithin • Guar Gum • Vitamins & Minerals • Natural & Artificial Flavors • Acesulfame Potassium • Beta-Carotene.

ATP Fuel - TwinLab
Three capsules contain: Creatine Monohydrate & Creatine Pyruvate 3000 mg • Potassium Phosphate 300 mg • ATP (Adenosine Triphosphate) 60 mg.

ATP Plus - Progressive Labs
Six tablets contain: Magnesium (as magnesium hydroxide) 300 mg • Malic Acid 1200 mg.

Atri A.S.F - Atrium Inc.
Each tablet contains: Raw Tissue concentrates (not extracts) of Bovine source of the following 200 mg: Thymus 80 mg • Partoid 80 mg • Adrenal 20 mg • Spleen 20 mg.
See Editor's Note No. 14, page 1817.

Atri CU- Chelate - Atrium Inc.
Each tablet contains: Spleen 28.5 mg • Brain 7.5 mg • Liver 5 mg • Heart 3.5 mg • Kidney 3.5 mg • Thymus 2 mg • Adrenal 2 mg • Pituitary 1 mg • Pancreas 1 mg • Duodenum 1 mg • Copper (Protein Chelated) 2 mg.
See Editor's Note No. 14, page 1817.

Atri E-Derm - Atrium Inc.
Each gram contains: Natural Vitamin E (d-Alpha Tocopheryl Acetate)

30 IU. In an absorbent base containing unsaturated fatty acids from Flax & Beet Lipids, Natural Vitamin A & Lecithin.

Atri Flexile - Atrium Inc.

Each capsule contains: Glucosamine Sulfate 500 mg • Uncaria tomentosa 200 mg • Curcumin 50 mg • Bromelain 25 mg. Contains no sugar, starch, salt, wheat, corn, yeast or soy derivatives.

Atri Free Amino - Atrium Inc.

Each 600 mg capsule contains: Free form Amino Acids: L- Alanine • L-Arginine • L- Aspartic Acid • L- Citruline • L -Cystine • L-Glutamic Acid • L-Glutamine • L-Glysine • L-Histidine HCL • L-Hydroxproline • L-Isoleucine • L-Leucine • L-Lysine • L-Methionine • L-Phenylalanine • L-Proline • L-Serine • L-Threonine • L-Tyrosine • L-Valine • L-Taurine.

Atri K-Chelate - Atrium Inc.

Each tablet contains: As chelated proteinates (Amino Acid Chelated Minerals): Potassium 100 mg • Raw Tissue concentrate from the following: (Spleen 28.5 mg, Brain 7.5 mg, Liver 5 mg, Heart 3.5 mg, Kidney 3.5 mg, Thymus 2 mg, Adrenal 2 mg, Pituitary 1 mg, Pancreas 1 mg & Duodenum 1 mg) 55 mg.
See Editor's Note No. 14, page 1817.

Atri Multi-Hypo - Atrium Inc.

Three tablets contain: Vitamin A (from Fish Liver oil) 10000 IU • Vitamin D (as Vitamin D3) 400 IU • Vitamin B 10 mg • Vitamin B2 10 mg • Vitamin B6 10 mg • Vitamin B12 50 mcg • Niacinamide 100 mg • Pantothenic Acid 50 mg • Folic Acid 400 mcg • Vitamin C 120 mg • Vitamin E (d-Alpha Tocopherol Succinate) 15 mg • Biotin 30 mcg • Calcium 97 mg • Magnesium 72 mg • Manganese 15 mg • Potassium 53 mg • Zinc 15 mg • Iron (from Iron Sulfate) 18 mg • Iodine (from Kelp) 150 mcg • Choline Bitartrate 30 mg • Inositol 30 mg • PABA (Para Amino Benzoic Acid) 30 mg • Citrus Bioflavonoids 100 mg • Hesperidin 25 mg • Rutin 20 mg • Glutamic Acid 18 mg • L-Lysine (Monohydrochloride) 30 mg • L-Methionine 30 mg.

Atri- Stress-B+C - Atrium Inc.

Two tablets contain: Vitamin C (Ascorbic Acid) 500 mg • Vitamin B1 (Thiamine HCL) 100 mg • Vitamin B2 (Riboflavin) 100 mg • Vitamin B6 (Pyridoxine HCL) 100 mg • Vitamin B12 (Cyanocobalamin) 500 mcg • Niacinamide 100 mg • Pantothenic Acid 100 mg • Folic Acid 400 mcg • Biotin 100 mcg • Lemon Bioflavonoids 250 mg • Choline (Choline Bitartrate) 100 mg • Inositol 100 mg • PABA 50 mg.

Atri Zinc Plus - Atrium Inc.

Each tablet contains: Ascorbic Acid & Sodium Ascorbate 125 mg • Zinc Gluconate 25 mg • Rutin 25 mg.

Atri-770 - Atrium Inc.

Each capsule contains: Cold Pressed concentrated Wheat Germ oil 770 mg.

Atri-A + E Mulsion High concentrate - Atrium Inc.

Each drop contains: Emulsified Vitamin A Palmitate 15000 IU • Vitamin E (d-Alpha Tocopheryl Acetate) 10 IU.

Atri-A + E Mulsion Regular concentrate - Atrium Inc.

Each drop contains: Emulsified Vitamin A Palmitate 5000 IU • Vitamin E (d-Alpha Tocopheryl Acetate) 10 IU.

Atri-Acidic - Atrium Inc.

Each tablet contains: Raw Stomach concentrate (Bovine) 50 mg • Raw Duodenum concentrate (Bovine) 50 mg • Betaine HCL 460 mg • Glutamic Acid HCL 200 mg • Pepsin 1:20000 25 mg • Potassium Chloride 25 mg.
See Editor's Note No. 14, page 1817.

Atri-Aloe-Lax - Atrium Inc.

Each capsule contains: Aloe 450 mg. Contains no sugar, starch, salt, wheat, corn, yeast or soy derivatives.

Atri-Aloe-V - Atrium Inc.

Each capsule contains: Aloe ferox (Aloe Vera resin) 430 mg • Aloe barbadensis (Aloe Vera leaf) 100 mg.

Atri-Amino - Atrium Inc.

Six tablets contain: Isoleucine 90 mg • Leucine 216 mg • Lysine 270 mg • Methionine 54 mg • Phenylalanine 132 mg • Threonine 132 mg • Valine 156 mg • Arginine 528 mg • Histidine 48 mg • Alanine 660 mg • Tyrosine 18 mg • Serine 252 mg • Aspartic Acid 402 mg • Cystine 18 mg • Glutamic Acid 684 mg • Glycine 1650 mg • Hydroxylysine 54 mg • Hydroxyproline 846 mg • Proline 984 mg. All of the Amino Acids in this preparation are of the natural (L) form.

Atri-Arthritis Spray - Atrium Inc.

Four fluid ounces contains: Oil of Wintergreen (Methyl Salicylate) 15% • Menthol 6% • IPA Alcohol. In a specially formulated, non-greasy base.

Atri-Bio-C - Atrium Inc.

Each tablet contains: Calcium Ascorbate 500 mg • Bioflavonoids 500 mg • Acerola 10 mg • Hesperidin 10 mg • Rutin 10 mg.

Atri-BLP - Atrium Inc.

Each capsule contains: Cayenne 200 mg • Parsley 90 mg • Ginger root 50 mg • Goldenseal root 40 mg • Garlic 35 mg • Siberian Ginseng 30 mg. Contains no sugar, starch, salt, wheat, corn, yeast or soy derivatives. Professional Formula.

Atri-Cal Chelate - Atrium Inc.

Three tablets contain: As Chelated Proteinates (AminoAcid Chelated Minerals) Calcium 450 mg • Raw Tissue concentrate from: (Spleen 74.1 mg, Brain 19.5 mg, Liver 13 mg, Heart 9.1 mg, Kidney 9.1 mg, Thymus 2 mg, Adrenal 2 mg, Pituitary 1 mg, Pancreas 2.6 mg, Duodenum 2.6 mg) 135 mg.
See Editor's Note No. 14, page 1817.

Atri-C-Flu - Atrium Inc.

Each capsule contains: Garlic 300 mg • Parsley 60 mg • Rose Hips 60 mg • Rosemary 25 mg • Watercress 20 mg. Professional Formula. Contains no sugar, starch, salt, wheat, corn, yeast or soy derivatives.

Atri-Daily Essentials - Atrium Inc.

Three tablets contain: Vitamin E (d-Alpha) 200 IU • Beta Carotene 5000 IU • Vitamin D 400 IU • Folic Acid 400 mcg • Thiamine 1.5 mg • Riboflavin 1.7 mg • Niacin 20 mg • Vitamin B6 2 mg • Vitamin B12 6 mcg • Biotin 300 mcg • Pantothenic Acid 10 mg • Calcium Citrate 600 mg • Phosphorous 450 mg • Iodine (Kelp) 150 mcg • Magnesium (Carbonate) 200 mg • Copper (Gluconate) 2mg • Zinc (Gluconate) 15 mg • Vitamin K 100 mcg • Selenium (yeast) 75 mcg • Manganese (Gluconate) 5 mg • Chromium (Aspartate) 200 mcg • Molybdenum 150 mcg • Nickel 15 mcg • Tin 15 mcg • Vanadium 5 mg • Boron (Citrate) 2 mg • Potassium (Gluconate) 100 mg • Grape seed extract 10 mg • CoQ10 10 mg. Contains no sugar, starch, salt, wheat, corn, milk or soy derivatives.

Atri-Detox - Atrium Inc.

Each capsule contains: Red Clover Blossoms 150 mg • Chaparral 80 mg • Licorice root 50 mg • Peach bark 50 mg • Oregon Grape root 40 mg • Stillingia 35 mg • Cascara Sagrada bark 30 mg • Sarsaparilla root 30 mg • Burdock root 15 mg • Buckthorn bark 10 mg. Professional Formula. Contains no sugar, starch, salt, wheat, corn, yeast or soy derivatives.

Atri-Disco - Atrium Inc.

Each tablet contains: First Phase (in Stomach) Manganese Sulfate

BRAND NAMES

200 mg • Calcium Ascorbate 100 mg • Magnesium Aspartate 50 mg. Second Phase (in Duodenum) Alpha-Chymotrypsin 4 mg • Papain 100 mg • Bromelain 100 mg • Pancreatin 5x 50 mg.
See Editor's Note No. 14, page 1817.

Atri-DMG Plus - Atrium Inc.
Each tablet contains: NN Dimethyl Glycine 19.3 mg • Calcium Gluconate 30.7 mg • Glycine 25 mg • Lysine 25 mg.

Atri-EPA Plus - Atrium Inc.
Each capsule contains: Salmon oil [containing EPA Eicosapentaenoic Acid 180 mg & DHA Docosahexaenoic Acid 120 mg] 1000 mg • Vitamin A (Fish oil) 100 IU • Vitamin E (Fish oil) 5 IU.

Atri-F - Atrium Inc.
Each capsule contains: Cold Processed Persic oil (yielding the following Lipid Acids referred to as Vitamin F factors: Oleic 192 mg, Linoleic 109 mg, Palmitic 18 mg, Stearic 4 mg, Linolenic 701 mcg, Heptodecanoic 400 mcg, Arachadic 330 mcg, Arachidonic 111 mcg) 370 mg • Potassium 113 mcg • Sodium 14 mcg • Magnesium 7 mcg • Phosphorus 4 mg • Calcium 4 mcg • "trace amounts of: Manganese, Chromium, Zinc, Iron, Copper, Boron & Barium" • Palmitoleic 5 mg.

Atri-Fem-Reg - Atrium Inc.
Each capsule contains: Goldenseal root 120 mg • Blessed Thistle 100 mg • Cramp bark 80 mg • Uva Ursi leaves 70 mg • False Unicorn 50 mg • Raspberry leaves 30 mg • Squaw Vine 20 mg • Ginger root 10 mg. Professional Formula. Contains no sugar, starch, salt, wheat, corn, yeast or soy derivatives.

Atri-Flav-1000 - Atrium Inc.
Three tablets contain: Vitamin C 1000 mg • Citrus Bioflavonoids 1000 mg • Rutin 100 mg. Other Ingredients: Rose Hips & Acerola, in a base containing Raw Spleen concentrate 4 mg.
See Editor's Note No. 14, page 1817.

Atri-FM-H - Atrium Inc.
Each capsule contains: Black Cohosh 200 mg • Sarsaparilla root 150 mg • Siberian Ginseng 40 mg • Licorice root 35 mg • False Unicorn 30 mg • Blessed Thistle 25 mg • Squaw Vine 20 mg. Professional Formula. Contains no sugar, starch, salt, wheat, corn, yeast or soy derivatives.

Atri-Gastro - Atrium Inc.
Each capsule contains: Colloidal Silica 200 mg • Irish Moss 50 mg • Beef Duodenum 20 mg • Pepsin 20 mg • Stomach Mucosa 10 mg • Di-Sodium Phosphate 10 mg. Glandulars are processed by freeze drying method. Contains no sugar, starch, salt, wheat, corn, yeast or soy derivatives.
See Editor's Note No. 14, page 1817.

Atri-GE-132 - Atrium Inc.
Each capsule contains: Germanium Sesquioxide 150 mg.

Atri-GE-132 Sub - Atrium Inc.
Each tablet contains: Germanium Sesquioxide 25 mg.

Atri-Gesic - Atrium Inc.
Three ounces contain: Lanolin • Menthol • Methyl Salicylate • Oil of Cassia • Stearic Acid • Spermwax • GMS • Tea • Methyl Gluceth E 10 • Camphor • Methyl Nicotinate • Propyl Parasept • Deionized Water.

Atri-Glucomannan - Atrium Inc.
Each capsule contains: Glucomannan Dietary Fiber (Konjac root source) 500 mg.

Atri-Greens Plus - Atrium Inc.
Each tablet contains: Vitamin A (Palmitate) 5000 IU • Vitamin C (Ascorbic Acid) 240 mg • Vitamin E (Acetate) 45 mg • Beta Carotene 150 mg • Selenium (Yeast) 50 mcg • Spirulina 25 mg • Chlorophyll 2 mg. In a base of cruciferous vegetables: Broccoli, Brussels Sprouts, Cabbage, Carrot, Cauliflower, Kale, Mustard Greens, Pumpkin, Spinach & Turnip Greens.

Atri-Herb-CLS - Atrium Inc.
Each capsule contains: Gentian root 50 mg • Valerian root 50 mg • Catnip 40 mg • Goldenseal root 40 mg • Barberry bark 30 mg • Cascara Sagrada 30 mg • Irish Moss 30 mg • Fenugreek seed 30 mg • Bugleweed 25 mg • Yellow Dock root 25 mg • St. John's Wort 25 mg • Brigham Tea 25 mg • Red Clover Blossoms 25 mg • Chickweed 25 mg. Professional Formula. Contains no sugar, starch, salt, wheat, corn, yeast or soy derivatives.

Atri-IBC - Atrium Inc.
Each capsule contains: Eyebright 100 mg • Goldenseal root • Barberry bark 100 mg • Red Raspberry leaves 100 mg • Cayenne 100 mg. Professional Formula. Contains no sugar, starch, salt, wheat, corn, yeast or soy derivatives.

Atri-INF - Atrium Inc.
Each capsule contains: Plantain 200 mg • Black Walnut leaves 100 mg • Goldenseal root 60 mg • Marshmallow root 50 mg • Bugleweed 40 mg. Professional Formula. Contains no sugar, salt, wheat, corn, yeast or soy derivatives.

Atri-Kid-Uri - Atrium Inc.
Each capsule contains: Juniper berries 200 mg • Parsley 120 mg • Uva Ursi leaves 50 mg • Marshmallow root 45 mg • Ginger root 40 mg • Goldenseal root 20 mg. Professional Formula. Contains no sugar, starch, salt, wheat, corn, yeast or soy derivatives.

Atri-Lacto - Atrium Inc.
Each capsule contains: Lactobacillus Acidophilus & Bulgaras culture 400 mg. Contains a minimum two million total bacteria count.

Atri-Lax - Atrium Inc.
Each capsule contains: Psyllium husks 100 mg • Cascara Sagrada bark 100 mg • Prune concentrate 100 mg • Senna leaves 100 mg • Licorice root 45 mg • Chlorophyll 10 mg. Professional Formula. Contains no sugar, starch, salt, wheat, corn, yeast or soy derivatives.

Atri-LB-CLS - Atrium Inc.
Each capsule contains: Cascara Sagrada 150 mg • Bayberry root bark 75 mg • Cayenne 75 mg • Ginger root 50 mg • Goldenseal root 50 mg • Lobelia 30 mg • Red Raspberry leaves 30 mg • Turkey Rhubarb root 30 mg • Fennel seed 20 mg. Professional Formula. Contains no sugar, starch, salt, wheat, corn, yeast or soy derivatives.

Atri-Lipotropic - Atrium Inc.
Three capsules contain: Choline Bitartrate 1000 mg • Inositol 1000 mg • Methionine 300 mg.

Atri-Liv-GLB - Atrium Inc.
Each capsule contains: Barberry root bark 120 mg • Wild Yam 80 mg • Cramp bark 60 mg • Fennel seed 50 mg • Yellow Dock 40 mg • Ginger root 35 mg • Catnip 30 mg • Peppermint leaves 30 mg. Professional Formula. Contains no sugar, starch, salt, wheat, corn, yeast or soy derivatives.

Atri-Ly Poll - Atrium Inc.
Each tablet contains: Raw Bovine Tissue concentrate (not extracts) 20 mg: (Pituitary 5 mg • Adrenal 15 mg) • special blend of Bee Pollen 250 mg. In a base of L-Lysine 400 mg (an Amino Acid known to be essential in human nutrition).
See Editor's Note No. 14, page 1817.

Atri-Lym-Inf - Atrium Inc.
Each capsule contains: Cayenne 150 mg • Echinacea 120 mg • Myrrh

Gum 100 mg • Hawthorn berries 100 mg • Licorice root 30 mg. Professional Formula. Contains no sugar, starch, salt, wheat, corn, yeast or soy derivatives.

Atri-Mag Chelate Plus - Atrium Inc.
Each tablet contains: Amino Acid Chelated Minerals as: Magnesium 300 mg. Raw Tissue concentrates (Bovine source) from: Spleen 29 mg • Brain 8 mg • Liver 5 mg • Heart 4 mg • Kidney 4 mg • Thymus 2 mg • Adrenal 2 mg • Pituitary 1 mg • Duodenum 1 mg • Pancreas 1 mg.
See Editor's Note No. 14, page 1817.

Atri-Medicated Psoriasis Shampoo - Atrium Inc.
Eight fluid ounces contain: Active Ingredients: Coal Tar solution USP 5% • Colloidal Sulfur 2% • Salicylic Acid 2%. In a special base of Surface Active Cleansers, Wetting Agents & Lanolin.

Atri-Mega Plus - Atrium Inc.
Four tablets contain: Vitamin A Acetate 25000 IU • Vitamin D (as Vitamin D3) Cholecalciferol 1000 IU • Vitamin E Acetate 100 IU • Vitamin C (with Rose Hips) 500 mg • Folic Acid 0.1 mg • Thiamine (Vitamin B1) 50 mg • Riboflavin (Vitamin B2) 50 mg • Niacin 100 mg • Vitamin B6 50 mg • Vitamin B12 50 mcg • Biotin 50 mcg • Pantothenic Acid 50 mg • Choline Bitartrate 50 mg • Calcium (as Oyster Shell & Calcium Carbonate) 700 mg • Iodine (Kelp) 225 mcg • Iron (Ferrous Fumerate) 30 mg • Magnesium (as Oxide) 200 mg • Zinc (as Sulfate) 36 mg • Manganese (as Carbonate) 3mg • Potassium (Chloride & Kelp) 99 mg • Chromium (as Chelate) 20 mcg • Selenium (Yeast) 60 mcg • Betaine HCl 50 mg • Papain 200 mg • Para Aminobenzoic Acid 50 mg • Citrus Bioflavonoids 50 mg • Inositol 50 mg • Ribonucleic Acid (Yeast extract) 200 mg.

Atri-Mega-Lacto - Atrium Inc.
Each capsule contains: Lactobacillus Acidophilus with Bifidus Four Billion CFU (Colony Forming Units). Contains no preservatives or artificial color. Contains no wheat, sugar, corn or soy.

Atri-Min 74 - Atrium Inc.
Each tablet contains: Sea Bed Montmorillonite (also known as Mineral 74100 mg Volcanic Montmorillonite) 900 mg.

Atri-Multi - Atrium Inc.
Each tablet contains: Vitamin A (from Fish Liver oil) 3333 IU • Vitamin D (as Vitamin D3) 133 IU • Vitamin B1 4 mg • Vitamin B2 3 mg • Vitamin B6 3 mg • Vitamin B12 11 mcg • Niacinamide 34 mg • Pantothenic Acid 17 mg • Folic Acid 134 mcg • Vitamin C 40 mg • Vitamin E (d-Alpha Tocopherol) 5 mg • Biotin 10 mcg • Calcium 32 mg • Magnesium 24 mg • Manganese 5 mg • Potassium 18 mg • Zinc 5 mg • Iron (from Sulfate) 6 mg • Iodine (from Kelp) 50 mcg • Choline Bitartrate 10 mg • PABA 9 mg • Citrus Bioflavonoids 100 mg • Hesperidin 9 mg • Rutin 7 mg • Glutamic Acid 6 mg • L-Lysine 10 mg • L-Methionine 10 mg • RNA (from Yeast) 15 mg. In a base of Watercress, Kelp, Alfalfa, Parsley.

Atri-Nerv - Atrium Inc.
Each capsule contains: Black Cohosh 100 mg • Cayenne 100 mg • Hops Flowers 80 mg • Scullcap 70 mg • Wood Betony 50 mg • Passiflora 40 mg • Valerian root 20 mg • Ladys Slipper 10 mg. Professional Formula. Contains no sugar, starch, salt, wheat, corn, yeast or soy derivatives.

Atri-Neuro - Atrium Inc.
Each tablet contains: Choline (Choline Bitartrate) 200 mg • L-Histidine 50 mg • L-Phenylalanine 50 mg • GABA (Amino Buteric Acid) 50 mg • L-Tyrosine 50 mg • Raw Brain concentrate 25 mg • Niacin 15 mg • Pyridoxine HCI 50 mg.
See Editor's Note No. 14, page 1817.

Atri-NTL-CA - Atrium Inc.
Each capsule contains: Horsetail grass 300 mg • Oat Straw 100 mg. Professional Formula. Contains no sugar, starch, salt, wheat, corn, yeast or soy derivatives.

Atri-Ortho-Phos - Atrium Inc.
Each drop contains: Ortho Phosphoric Acid 13 mg • Inositol 0.57 mg • Choline Bitartrate 0.27 mg. Thirty drops contain: Ortho Phosphoic Acid 390 mg • Inositol 17 mg • Choline Bitartrate 8 mg.

Atri-Oxy - Atrium Inc.
Two tablets contain: Vitamin A (Beta Carotene) 25000 IU • Vitamin E (d-Alpha Tocopherol) 400 IU • Vitamin C 1000 mg • Bioflavonoid Complex 150 mg • Superoxide Dismutase 100 mg • Selenium 100 mcg • Zinc 25 mg • Copper 2 mg • Astragalus 50 mg • Rosemary 50 mg • Milk Thistle (Slymarin) 50 mg • Spirulina 100 mg • Chromium Picolinate 25 mcg • Grape seed extract 50 mg • CoEnzyme Q-10 10 mg • L-Glutathione 10 mg • L-Cysteine 100 mg • Reishi Mushroom 50 mg • Curcumin 50 mg.

Atri-PMS - Atrium Inc.
Three tablets contain: Vitamin A Acetate 5000 IU • Vitamin B6 (Pyridoxine HCL) 100 mg • Adrenal concentrate 50 mg • Hypothalamus concentrate 10 mg • Ovary concentrate 50 mg • Pituitary concentrate 10 mg • Passion Flower 75 mg • Dong Quai 50 mg • Cramp bark 50 mg • Chionanthus 50 mg • Valerian 75 mg • Magnesium (Oxide) 200 mg • Iron (Peptonate) 20 mg • Red Raspberry 50 mg.
See Editor's Note No. 14, page 1817.

Atri-Pros - Atrium Inc.
Each capsule contains: Cayenne 160 mg • Uva Ursi leaves 70 mg • Parsley 60 mg • Goldenseal root 50 mg • Gravel root 50 mg • Juniper berries 30 mg • Marshmallow root 25 mg • Ginger root 20 mg • Siberian Ginseng 15 mg. Professional Formula. Contains no sugar, starch, salt, wheat, corn, yeast or soy derivatives.

Atri-Psoriasis Ointment - Atrium Inc.
Four ounces contains: Sulfur ppt 1.5% • Salicylic Acid 1.5%, Coal Tar Solution USP 2%. In a specially formulated base designed to retain the skin's moisure.

Atri-Res - Atrium Inc.
Each capsule contains: Marshmallow root 200 mg • Mullein 120 mg • Comfrey leaves 100 mg • Chickweed 50 mg. Professional Formula. Contains no sugar, starch, salt, wheat, corn, yeast or soy derivatives.

Atri-RNA/DNA - Atrium Inc.
Each tablet contains: RiboNucleic Acid (RNA) 180 mg • DeoxyNucleic Acid (DNA) 40 mg.

Atri-SDT - Atrium Inc.
Each tablet contains: Trypsin 4 mg • Chymotrypsin 2 mg • Pancreatin 2 mg • Bromelain 3 mg • Papayotin 4 mg • Thymus concentrate (Bovine) 2 mg • Mannitol 13 mg. In a specially prepared natural spearmint flavored slow dissolving tablet base.
See Editor's Note No. 14, page 1817.

Atri-Selenium+E - Atrium Inc.
Each tablet contains: Vitamin C (Ascorbic Acid) 250 mg • Vitamin E (d-Alpha Tocopherol) 200 IU • Vitamin B1 (Thiamine HCL) 4 mg • Vitamin B2 (Riboflavin) 4 mg • Vitamin B6 (Pyridoxine HCL) 4 mg • Niacin 10 mg • Pantothenic Acid 50 mg • Selenium (Selenium Yeast) 50 mcg • Raw Heart concentrate 10 mg. In a base of Bone Meal.
See Editor's Note No. 14, page 1817.

Atri-S-G-V - Atrium Inc.
Each tablet contains: Selenium 50 mcg • Germanium 225 mcg • Vanadium 225 mcg, as Protein Chelates.

BRAND NAMES

Some Brand Name Natural Products - What they Contain
www.NaturalDatabase.com contains MANY more listings than appear here.

Atri-Statin - Atrium Inc.
Each tablet contains: Caprylic Acid 110 mg. Contains no sugar, starch, salt, wheat, corn, yeast or soy derivatives.

Atri-Thy-Kelp - Atrium Inc.
Each capsule contains: Mullein 140 mg • Parsley 90 mg • Watercress 80 mg • Kelp (Norwegian) 70 mg • Irish Moss 60 mg • Iceland Moss 40 mg. Professional Formula. Contains no sugar, starch, salt, wheat, corn, yeast or soy derivatives.

Atri-Trace - Atrium Inc.
Three tablets contain: Calcium (Egg & Oyster Shells) 250 mg • Magnesium (Gluconate) 50 mg • Manganese (Gluconate) 10 mg • Potassium (Gluconate) 50 mg • Zinc (Gluconate)15 mg • Vitamin D (as Vitamin D3) 133 IU • Vitamin B6 50 mg • Glutamic Acid HCL 325 mg.

Atri-V&M+Complete - Atrium Inc.
Six tablets contains: Vitamin A (Fish oil) 10000 IU • Vitamin D (Fish oil) 400 IU • Vitamin C (Calcium Ascorbate, Acerola, Rose Hips) 400 mg • Vitamin E 60 IU • Vitamin B1 • Vitamin B2 10 mg • Vitamin B6 10 mg • Vitamin B12 25 mcg • Niacin 60 mg • Calcium (Bone Meal & Calcium Carbonate) 750 mg • Magnesium (Oxide) 375 mg • Phosphorus (Bone Meal) 700 mg • Iron (Amino Acid Chelate) 20 mg • Iodine (Kelp) 150 mcg • Potassium (Proteinate) 20 mg • Zinc (Amino Acid Chelate) 20 mg • Manganese (Amino Acid Chelate) 15 mg • Choline (Bitartrate) 50 mg • Inositol 500 mg • Lecithin 50 mg • Pantothenic Acid 50 mg • Folic Acid 400 mcg • PABA 30 mg • RNA-DNA 15 mg • Betaine HCL 25 mg • Biotin 100 mcg. In a base of Alfalfa, Kelp, Rose Hips, Acerola, Fish Liver oils, Bone Meal, Citrus Bioflavonoids, Papaya, Bromelain Enzymes & Essential Amino Acids.

Atri-Vana - Atrium Inc.
Each capsule contains: Vanadyl Sulfate 25 mg. Contains no wheat, sugar, starch, salt, corn, yeast, milk or soy.

Atri-Verm - Atrium Inc.
Each capsule contains: Pumpkin seed 100 mg • Culver's root 70 mg • Violet leaves 60 mg • Cascara Sagrada bark 50 mg • Slippery Elm bark 45 mg • Witch Hazel bark 40 mg • Mullein 30 mg • Echinacea 20 mg. Professional Formula. Contains no sugar, starch, salt, wheat, corn, yeast or soy derivatives.

Atri-Yeast - Atrium Inc.
Four tablets contain: Protein from a Special Yeast 1200 mg • Niacin 66 mg • Pantothenic Acid 13 mg • Vitamin B1 13 mg • Vitamin B2 13 mg • Vitamin B6 3 mg • Chromium 25 mcg • Selenium 7.5 mcg.

Atri-Zinc Chelate Plus - Atrium Inc.
Each tablet contains: Amino Acid Chelated Minerals as: Zinc 29 mg. Raw Tissue concentrates (Bovine source) from: Spleen 29 mg • Brain 8 mg • Liver 5 mg • Heart 4 mg • Kidney 4 mg • Thymus 2 mg • Adrenal 2 mg • Pituitary 1 mg • Duodenum 1 mg.
See Editor's Note No. 14, page 1817.

Attention! - Olympia Nutrition
Contains DHA 250 mg • Phosphatidylserine 20 mg • DMAE 100 mg • Choline 100 mg • TMG. No yeast, wheat, corn, milk, egg, soy glutens, preservatives, or artificial colors.

Avena Sativa Complex - Puritan's Pride
Each capsule contains: Avena Sativa 300 mg • Siberian Ginseng 150 mg • Nettle 50 mg.

B Complex - Nature's Sunshine
Each capsule contains: Vitamin B1 (thiamine) 33 mg • Vitamin B2 (riboflavin) 33 mg • Niacinamide 33 mg • Vitamin B6 (pyridoxine HCl) 33 mg • Folic Acid 133 mcg • Vitamin B12 (cyanocobalamin) 33 mcg • Biotin 100 mcg • Pantothenic Acid (d-calcium pantothenate) 33 mg • Choline (bitartrate) 33 mg • Inositol 33 mg.

B/P Formula - Nature's Way
Two capsules contain: Proprietary Formula: Cayenne pepper fruit • Garlic bulb • Ginger • Goldenseal stem, leaf, flower • Parsley herb • Siberian Ginseng root. Other ingredients: Gelatin.

B-1 100 mg - Puritan's Pride
Each tablet contains: Vitamin B-1 (Thiamine Hydrochloride) 100 mg.

B-1 250 mg - Puritan's Pride
Each tablet contains: Vitamin B-1 (Thiamine Hydrochloride) 250 mg.

B100 Complex - Natrol
One tablet contains: Vitamin B1 (Thiamine) 100 mg • Vitamin B2 (Riboflavin) 100 mg • Vitamin B6 (Pyroxidoxine) 100 mg • Vitamin B12 (Cobalamin) 100 mcg • Niacinamide 100 mg • Folic Acid 400 mcg • Biotin 100 mcg • Pantothenic Acid 100 mg • Choline 100 mg • Inositol 100 mg • PABA 100 mg • ULTRAGREEN 150 mg. Other ingredients: Microcrystalline Cellulose, Calcium Carbonate, Croscarmellose Sodium, Stearic Acid, Silicon Dioxide, Magnesium Stearate.

B-100 Ultra B-Complex - Puritan's Pride
Each tablet contains: Thiamin (Vitamin B1; as thiamine mononitrate) 100 mg • Riboflavin (Vitamin B2) 100 mg • Niacin (as niacinamide) 100 mg • Vitamin B6 (as pyridoxine hydrochloride) 100 mg • Folic Acid 400 mcg • Vitamin B12 (as cyanocobalamin) 100 mcg • Biotin (as d-biotin) 100 mcg • Pantothenic Acid (as d-calcium pantothenate) 100 mg • Inositol 100 mg • PABA (para-aminobenzoic acid) 100 mg • Choline Bitartrate 100 mg • Proprietary Blend: Parsley leaves powder, Rice Bran, Defatted powder, Watercress leaves powder, Alfalfa leaves powder, Lecithin granules 5 mg.

B-12 100 mcg - Puritan's Pride
Each tablet contains: Vitamin B-12 (Cyanocobalamin) 100 mcg.

B-12 1000 mcg - Puritan's Pride
Each tablet contains: Vitamin B-12 (Cyanocobalamin) 1000 mcg.

B-12 1500 mcg - Puritan's Pride
Each tablet contains: Vitamin B-12 (Cobalamin concentrate) 1500 mcg.

B-12 250 mcg - Puritan's Pride
Each tablet contains: Vitamin B-12 (Cyanocobalamin) 250 mcg.

B-12 500 mcg - Puritan's Pride
Each tablet contains: Vitamin B-12 (Cyanocobalamin) 500 mcg.

B-12 Lingual - Progressive Labs
Each tablet contains: Vitamin B12 1000 mcg • Folate (folic acid) 400 mcg, in a base of Mannitol and Natural Cherry flavor.

B12-Active - PhytoPharmica
Each tablet contains: Vitamin B12 (methylcobalamin) 1,000 mcg.

B-150 - Puritan's Pride
Each tablet contains: Thiamin (Vitamin B1; as thiamine mononitrate) 150 mg • Riboflavin (Vitamin B2) 150 mg • Niacin (as niacinamide) 150 mg • Vitamin B6 (as pyridoxine hydrochloride) 150 mg • Folic Acid 150 mcg • Vitamin B12 (as cyanocobalamin) 150 mcg • Biotin (as d-biotin) 150 mcg • Pantothenic Acid (as d-calcium pantothenate) 150 mg • Choline Bitartrate 150 mg • PABA (para-aminobenzoic acid) 150 mg • Inositol 150 mg • Proprietary Blend: Alfalfa, Watercress, Parsley, Lecithin, and Rice Bran 7.5 mg.

B-2 - Puritan's Pride
Each tablet contains: Vitamin B-2 (Riboflavin) 100 mg.

B-50 Caps With C - Now
Each capsule contains: Vitamin B1 (Thiamine) 50 mg • Vitamin B2 (Riboflavin) 50 mg • Vitamin B3 (Niacinamide) 50 mg • Vitamin B6 (Pyridoxine) 50 mg • Vitamin B12 100 mcg • Biotin 100 mcg • Folic Acid 400 mcg • Pantothenic Acid 100 mg • Vitamin C (Ascorbic Acid) 250 mg • PABA 50 mg • Choline (Bitartrate) 50 mg • Inositol 50 mg.

B-50 Complex - Now
Each capsule contains: Vitamin B1 (Thiamine HCL) 50 mg • Vitamin B2 (Riboflavin) 50 mg • Vitamin B3 (Niacinamide) 50 mg • Vitamin B5 Pantothenic Acid 50 mg • Vitamin B6 (Pyridoxine HCL) 50 mg • Vitamin B12 (Cyanocobalamin) 50 mcg • Biotin 50 mcg • Folic Acid 400 mcg • PABA 50 mg • Choline (Bitartrate) 50 mg • Inositol 50 mg.

B-50 Vitamin B-Complex - Puritan's Pride
Each capsule contains: Thiamin (Vitamin B1; as thiamine mononitrate) 50 mg • Riboflavin (Vitamin B-2) 50 mg • Niacin (as niacinamide) 50 mg • Vitamin B6 (as pyridoxine hydrochloride) 50 mg • Folic Acid 100 mcg • Vitamin B12 (as cyanocobalamin) 50 mcg • Biotin (as d-biotin) 50 mcg • Pantothenic Acid (as d-calcium pantothenate) 50 mg • PABA (as para-aminobenzoic acid) 50 mg • Inositol 50 mg • Choline Bitartrate 50 mg.

B-6 100 mg - Puritan's Pride
Each tablet contains: Vitamin B-6 (Pyridoxine Hydrochloride) 100 mg.

B-6 200 mg - Puritan's Pride
Each tablet contains: Vitamin B-6 (Pyridoxine Hydrochloride) 200 mg.

B-6 50 mg - Puritan's Pride
Each tablet contains: Vitamin B-6 (Pyridoxine Hydrochloride) 50 mg.

B6 Min - Atrium Inc.
Each capsule contains: Vitamin B6 (Pyridoxine HCL) 200 mg • Magnesium Gluconate 120 mg • Potassium Gluconate 120 mg.

Back-Relief - Futurebiotics
Four capsules contain: Magnesium (as magnesium amino acid chelate) 300 mg • Alfalfa whole juice 225 mg • Yucca root powder 200 mg • Cayenne fruit powder extract 25 mg • Valerian root powder extract 12 mg • Pancreatin 4X quadruple strength (supplying 1600 USP units lipase, 10000 USP units amylase, 1000 USP protease) 125 mg • DL-Phenylalanine 250 mg. Other ingredients: Magnesium stearate, Gelatin, Water.
See Editor's Note No. 14, page 1817.

Barlean's Flax Oil - The Vitamin Shoppe
One teaspoon provides: Omega-3 7.7 g • Omega-6 2.3 g • Omega 9 2.2 g • VitaLox [a natural protectant blend of Ascorbic Acid and Rosemary extracts] 30 mg.

Barlean's Flax Oil High Lignin Formula - The Vitamin Shoppe
One tablespoon provides: Omega-3 6.1 g • Omega-6 1.8 g • Omega 9 1.7 g • Flaxseed Particles 2.6 g • VitaLox [a natural protectant blend of ascorbic acid and rosemary extracts] 30 mg.

Barlean's Vita-Flax - The Vitamin Shoppe
Certified Organic Flax Seed Powder containing: Protein (NX6.25) 34.7% • Fat 14.7% • Energy 435 Kcal/100 g. Vitamin E 0.01% • Dietary Fiber 34.2%. Total Fiber: Soluble Fiber 38%, Insoluble Fiber 62%.

B-Assure - The Vitamin Shoppe
Each capsule contains: 100 mg Champignon (Agaricus bisporus) stem and cap.

B-Complex - Nutri-Quest
Two tablets contain: Vitamin B1 100 mg • Vitamin B2 100 mg • Vitamin B6 50 mg • Niacinamide 100 mg • Pantothenic Acid 100 mg • Vitamin B12 100 mcg • Folic Acid 300 mcg • Biotin 100 mcg • Choline Bitartrate 100 mg • Inositol 100 mg • PABA 50 mg.

B-Complex - Health Smart Vitamins
Each caplet contains: Thiamin (as thiamin mononitrate) 100 mg • Riboflavin 100 mg • Niacin (as niacinamide) 100 mg • Vitamin B6 (as pyridoxine hydrochloride) 100 mg • Folate (folic acid) 400 mcg • Vitamin B12 (as cyanocobalamin) 100 mcg • Biotin 300 mcg • Pantothenic acid (as calcium pantothenate) 100 mg • Calcium (as dicalcium phosphate, calcium pantothenate, calcium stearate) 100 mg • Phosphorus (as dicalcium phosphate) 70 mg • Choline (as choline bitartrate) 100 mg • Inositol 100 mg • Para-aminobenzoic acid 100 mg.

B-Complex & B-12 - Puritan's Pride
Each tablet contains: Thiamin (Vitamin B1; as Thiamine Hydrochloride and Brewer's Yeast) 7 mg • Riboflavin (Vitamin B2) (as Riboflavin and Brewer's Yeast) 14 mg • Niacin (as Niacin and Brewer's Yeast) 4.5 mg • Vitamin B12 (as Cyanocobalamin and Brewer's Yeast) 25 mcg • Protease (as Papain Powder) 10 mg.

B-Complex 100 - The Vitamin Shoppe
Each capsule contains: Vitamin B1 100 mg • Vitamin B2 100 mg • Vitamin B6 100 mg • Vitamin B12 100 mcg • Niacinamide 100 mg • Folic Acid 400 mcg • Pantothenic Acid 100 mg • D-Biotin 100 mcg • Choline Bitartrate 100 mg • Inositol 100 mg • PABA 100 mg. No Yeast, Corn, Wheat, Soy, Salt, Sugar, Starch, Milk, Eggs, Preservatives, Artificial Colors or Flavors added.

B-Complex 50 mg - Nature's Life
Each tablet contains: Vitamin B1 (Thiamine HCl) 50 mg • Vitamin B2 (Riboflavin) 50 mg • Vitamin B6 (Pyridoxine HCl) 50 mg • Vitamin B12 (Cobalamin concentrate) 50 mcg • Niacinamide 50 mg • Pantothenic Acid (d-Calcium Pantothenate) 50 mg • Choline (Bitartrate) 50 mg • Inositol 50 mg • Biotin 50 mcg • Folic Acid 400 mcg • PABA (Para Aminobenzoic Acid) 50 mg • Lecithin 8 mg. In a natural base of Alfalfa, Parsley, Rice Bran & Watercress.

B-Complex Sublingual Liquid - Puritan's Pride
One dropper (1.0 cc) contains: Vitamin C (as Ascorbic Acid) 60 mg • Riboflavin (Vitamin B2; as Riboflavin 5-Phosphate Sodium) 1.7 mg • Niacin (as Niacinamide) 20 mg • Vitamin B6 (as Pyridoxine Hydrochloride) 2 mg • Vitamin B12 (as Cyanocobalamin) 1,200 mcg • Pantothenic Acid (as Dexpanthenol) 30 mg.

B-Complex Supplement - Leiner Health Products
Each tablet contains: Thiamin Mononitrate (Vitamin B1) 10 mg • Riboflavin (Vitamin B2) 10 mg • Vitamin B6 (Pyridoxine Hydrochloride) 10 mg • Niacin (Niacinamide) 10 mg • Biotin (USP Method 2) 10 mcg • Folate (Folic Acid) 100 mcg • Vitamin B12 (Cyanocobalamin - USP Method 2) 10 mcg • Pantothenic Acid 10 mg. Other Ingredients: Calcium Carbonate, Maltodextrin, Hydroxypropyl Methycellulose, d-Calcium Pantothenate, Cellulose, Starch, Para-Aminobenzoic Acid, Croscarmellose Sodium, Sodium Starch Glycolate, Silicon Dioxide, Hydroxypropyl Cellulose, Red 40 Lake, Polyethylene Glycol 3350, Magnesium Stearate, Resin, Dicalcium Phosphate, Polysorbate 80, Titanium Dioxide, Povidone, Pharmaceutical Glaze.

B-Complex with Folic Acid - Biodelivery Nutritional Systems
Two tablets contain: Choline Bitartrate 250 mg • D-Calcium Pantothenate 100 mg • Inositol 100 mg • Niacinamide 100 mg • PABA 50 mg • Riboflavin 50 mg • Thiamine HCL 50 mg • Pyridoxine HCL

BRAND NAMES

45 mg • Pantethine 25 mg • Pyridoxal -5-Phosphate 5 mg • Biotin 200 mcg • Folic Acid 800 mcg • Cyanocobalamin 200 mcg • NT Factor tablet base 355 mg.

Be Sure - Wakunaga of America
Two caplets contain: Aspergillus Enzyme Complex 300 mg. Other Ingredients: Cellulose, Silica, Magnesium Stearate (vegetable source).

beCalm'd - Neuro Health Products
Each capsule contains: Vitamin A (beta carotene) 1000 mg • Vitamin B as pyridoxine HCl 1 mg • d/ L-Phenylalanine 150 mg • L-Phenylalanine 75 mg • L-Glutamine 225 mg • Calcium (chelate, carbonate) 50 mg • Magnesium (chelate, oxide) 25 mg • Chromium picolinate 0.01 mg • Folic Acid 0.1 mg.

Bedwetting Tablets - Hyland's
Each tablet contains: Equisetum hyemale as Scouring Rush 3X HPUS • Rhus aromatica (Fragrant Sumac) 3X HPUS • Belladonna 3X HPUS (0.0003% Allkaloids). In a base of Lactose NF (Milk Sugar). See Editor's Note No. 1, page 1816.

Bee Complete - Futurebiotics
Two tablets contain: • Bee Pollen 1,000 mg • Royal Jelly 25 mg • Bee Propolis 500 mg.

Bee Pollen - Source Naturals
Each tablet contains: Whole nugget Bee Pollen 500 mg.

Bee Pollen Chewable - Atrium Inc.
Each tablet contains: Bee Pollen 300 mg. Contains no sugar, starch, salt, wheat, corn, yeast or soy derivatives.

Bee Pollen Complex - Puritan's Pride
Each tablet contains: Bee Pollen 1000 mg • Bee Propolis 10 mg • Royal Jelly 10 mg.

Beef Liver 1500 mg - Nature's Life
Six tablets contain: Argentine Beef Liver (Defatted, Desicated & Pesticide Free) 9000 mg • Vitamin B12 (Cobalamin concentrate) 1000 mcg • Vitamin B2 457 mcg • Vitamin B6 224 mcg • Vitamin B12 1 mg • Niacin 2.2 mg • Choline 94 mg • Calcium 2.7 mg • Copper 90 mcg • Iron 6.3 mg • Manganese 90 mcg • Potassium 94 mg • Sodium 28 mg • Zinc 1.3 mg. Amino Acids (naturally occurring): Alanine 747 mg • Arginine 297 mg • Aspartic Acid 99 mg • Cysteine 351 mg • Cystine 103 mg • Glutamic Acid 108 mg • Glycine 792 mg • Histidine (essential amino acid) 198 mg • Isoleucine (essential amino acid) 207 mg • Leucine (essential amino acid) 198 mg • Lysine (essential amino acid) 558 mg • Methionine (essential amino acid) 315 mg • Phenylalanine (essential amino acid) 369 mg • Proline 99 mg • Serine 441 mg • Threonine(essential amino acid) 306 mg • Tyrosine 396 mg • Tryptophan (essential amino acid) 36 mg • Valine (essential amino acid) 90 mg.
See Editor's Note No. 14, page 1817.

Beelith - Beach Pharmaceuticals
Each tablet contains: Magnesium Oxide (equivalent 362 mg of magnesium) 600 mg • Pyridoxine Hydrochloride (equivalent of Vitamin B6 20 mg).

Benecol - McNeil Consumer Healthcare
Three softgels contain: Plant Stanol Esters 1.5 g. Other Ingredients: Gelatin, Glycerin, Sunflower Oil, Titanium Dioxide, Soybean Oil, Annatto Extract, Red 40, Yellow 8, Blue 1, Yellow 5.

Benefin - LaneLabs
Shark Cartilage 750 mg.
See Editor's Note No. 28, page 1819.

Benejoint - LaneLabs
Capsaicin • Shark Cartilage • Aloe Vera • Essential Oils.

Berberine Complex - PhytoPharmica
Two capsules contain: Barberry (Berberis vulgaris) bark of root extract 6:1 400 mg • Oregon Grape (Berberis aquifolium) root extract 6:1 400 mg • Goldenseal (Hydrastis canadensis) root and rhizome extract 4:1 (standardized to contain 5% total alkaloids including berberine, hydrastine, and canadine) 100 mg.

Best Friends - Changes - TwinLab
One tablet contains: Vitamin A (as Alpha- and Beta-Carotene with mixed Carotenoids from D. Salina algae) 5000 IU • Vitamin C (as Ascorbic Acid with Sodium and Calcium Ascorbates) 100 mg • Vitamin D (as Cholecalciferol) 400 IU • Vitamin E (as mixed natural D-Alpha and DL-Alpha-Tocopherol Acetate) 80 IU • Thiamin (as Thiamin HCl) 1.5 mg • Riboflavin 1.7 mg • Niacin (as Niacinamide) 2 mg • Vitamin B6 (as Pyridoxine HCl) 2 mg • Folate (as Folic Acid) 400 mcg • Vitamin B12 (as Cyanocobalamin) 12 mcg • Biotin 75 mcg • Pantothenic Acid (as D-Calcium Pantothenate) 10 mg • Calcium (as Calcium Carbonate and Citrate) 125 mg • Iron (as Ferrous Fumarate) 5 mg • Iodine (as Potassium Iodide) 75 mcg • Magnesium (as Magnesium Oxide, Glycinate, and Citrate) 40 mg • Zinc (as Zinc Citrate and Glycinate) 5 mg • Selenium (as Selenomethionine) 25 mcg • Copper (as Copper Oxide, Citrate, Gluconate, and Glycinate) 2 mg • Manganese (as Manganese Sulfate, Citrate, Gluconate, and Glycinate) 1 mg • Chromium (as Chromium Dinicotinate Glycinate) 50 mcg • Molybdenum (as natural Molybdic Acid) 50 mcg • Fruit and vegetable phytonutrient concentrates 1500 mg: Dunaliela salina algae, Parsley, Tomato, Spinach, Kale, Yellow Squash, Turmeric, Orange, Cranberry, Lemon, Tangerine, Grapefruit, Red Grape, Strawberry, Cherry, Peach, Raspberry, Onion, Garlic, Leek, Broccoli, Cauliflower, Mustard Greens, Cabbage. Other Ingredients: Fructose, Sorbitol, Natural and Artificial flavors, Microcrystalline Cellulose, Stearic Acid, Carrageenan, Glycine, Maltodextrin, Citric Acid, Magnesium Stearate, Silica, Fractionated vegetable oil, Salt, and Carmine red.

Beta Carotene - Puritan's Pride
Each softgel contains: Beta Carotene (25,000 IU) 15 mg.

Beta Carotene - Olympian Labs
Each softgel contains: Beta Carotene 25000 IU.

Beta Carotene (Provitamin A) - Puritan's Pride
Each softgel contains: Beta Carotene (10000 IU) 6 mg.

Beta Carotene Provitamin A - Nature's Bounty
Each softgel contains: Vitamin A (as 100% Beta Carotene) 10000 IU. Other Ingredients: Soybean Oil, Gelatin, Beeswax, Glycerin, Lecithin.

Beta Carotene with Vitamin D - Puritan's Pride
Each softgel contains: Beta Carotene (25,000 IU) 15 mg • Vitamin D 400 IU.

Beta Fast GXR - Informulab
Gymnema Sylvestre (25% standardized extract) 400 mg.

Beta Glucan - Source Naturals
Each capsule contains: Purified beta-1, 3-glucan (derived from baker's yeast cell wall) 7.5 mg.

Beta Glucans - Natrol
Two capsules contain: Oat Bran extract Seed (Avena sativa) 1500 mg, supplying Beta Glucan 185 mg. Other ingredients: Oat Bran powder, Magnesium Stearate, Gelatin.

BETA-C - Pharmagel
Beta Hydroxy Acid • Stabilized Vitamin C.

Some Brand Name Natural Products - What they Contain

BetaGen - EAS
Each 6.6 gram serving contains: Ca HMB Monohydrate 1000 mg • Creatine Monohydrate 2000 mg • Potassium Phosphate 50 mg • L-Glutamine 400 mg • Taurine 200 mg. Ingredients: Dextrose, Phosphagen (HPCE pure Creatine Monohydrate) • Calcium b-Hydroxy b-Methylbutyrate Monohydrate • Citric Acid • L-Glutamine • Natural Flavors • Taurine • Potassium Phosphate • Aspartame • Beta-Carotene for color. Contains Phenylalanine.

Beta-mannan - Alotek Supplement Company
Two capsules contain: Vitamin E (as d-alpha-tocopherol) 100 IU • Proprietary blend of freeze-dried Aloe vera gel concentrates and extracts containing beta-mannans and beta-glucans 600 mg • IP6 (inositol hexaphosphate, derived from grains) 184 mg. Other Ingredients: defatted rice bran flour.

Beta-Sea 10,000 IU - Holista
Each capsule contains: Beta Carotene (from Dunaliella salina algea) 10000 IU. Other Ingredients: Carotenoids.

Beta-Sea 25,000 IU - Holista
Each capsule contains: Beta Carotene (from Dunaliella salina algea) 25000 IU. Other Ingredients: Carotenoids.

Better BodyEnergy for Life - HealthWatchers System
Ma Huang • Chromium Picolinate • Brindel Berry • White Willow Bark • Ginger Root • Hawthorn Berry • Licorice Root • Gotu Kola • Passion Flower • Siberian Ginseng • Guarana • Rhemannia Root • Bladderwrack • Reishi Mushroom • Astragalus.

Better Living Multi Vitamins - Health Center for Better Living
Each tablet contains: Vitamin A (Natural Fish Liver Oil) 10,000 IU• Beta Carotene (6 mg) 10000 mg • Vitamin B1 (Thiamine HCL) 75 mg • Vitamin B2 (Riboflavin) 75 mg • Vitamin B3 (Niacinamide) 75 mg • Vitamin B5 (Pantothenic) 75 mg • Vitamin B6 (as pyridoxine HCl) 75 mg • Vitamin B12 (as cyanocobalamin) 100 mcg • Biotin 100 mcg• Folic Acid 400 mcg • Vitamin C (Ascorbic Acid) 250 mg • Vitamin D (Natural FLO) 400 IU • Vitamin E (100% Natural d-alpha) 150 IU • Calcium (Ostershell) 100 mg • Magnesium (Oxide, amino acid chelate) 60 mg • Zinc (Amino acid chelate) 1 mg • Iodine (Kelp) 150 mcg • Iron (Amino acid chelate) • Chromium (Yeast Free GFT) 50 mcg • Boron (Amino acid chelate) 500 mcg • Molybdenum (Amino acid chelate) 50 mcg • Nucleic 50 mg.

BetterMan - Interceuticals
Each capsule contains: Proprietary Blend of Radix Ginseng, Rhizoma Dioscoreae, Radix Paeonie Alba, Herba Epimedii, Cornu Cervi Pantotrichum, Radix Astragali, Poria Cocos, Radix Morindae officinalis, Fructus Corni, Cortex Eucommiae, Radix Angelicae Sinensis, Fructus Lycii, Radix Rehmanniae, Rhizoma Chuanxiong, Fructus Schisandrae, Acanthopanax Senticosus, Cynomorium Songaricum Rupr, Cortex Cinnamomi.

Beyond Basics - Metabolic Response Modifiers
Three tablets contain: Vitamin A (as Beta-Carotene Palmitate) 15,000 IU • Vitamin C (as Ascorbic acid) 500 mg • Vitamin E (as d-Alpha Tocopherol Acetate) 200 IU • Vitamin B1 (as Thiamine HCl) 20 mg • Vitamin B2 (as Riboflavin) 30 mg • Vitamin D (as Cholecalciferol) 400 lU • Vitamin K1 (as Phylloquinine) 60 mcg • Niacin (Niacinamide 1:1) 30 mg • Pantothenic Acid (as Calcium d-Pantothenate) 25 mg • Vitamin B6 (as Pyridoxine HCl) 20 mg • Vitamin B12 (as Cyanocobalamin) 200 mcg • Biotin 75 mcg • Folic Acid 400 mcg • Calcium (as Calcium Carbonate Citrate 4:1) 200 mg • Magnesium (as Oxide Glycinate 4:1) 125 mg • Zinc (as Zinc Citrate) 10 mg • Copper (as Copper Citrate) 2 mg • Potassium (as Potassium Citrate) 75 mg • Molybdenum (as Molybdate) 100 mcg • Iodine (as Kelp) 150 mcg • Selenium (as l-Selenomethionine) 50 mcg • Chromium (as Chromium Chelate) 200 mcg • Boran (as Potassium

Borate) 3 mg • Silica (as Colloidal Silica) 10 mg • Organic Horsetail 275 mg • Vanadium (as Vanadyl Sulfate) 50 mcg • Choline (as Choline Bitartrate) 25 mg • Inositol 30 mg.

Beyond Calcium - KAL - Nutraceutical
Five tablets contain: Vitamin D (as Vitamin D3) (as natural Cholecalciferol) 400 IU • Calcium (as Calcium Citrate) 1000 mg • Magnesium (as Magnesium Citrate) 400 mg • Boron (as Boron Amino Acid Chelate) 6 mg • Horsetail 20 mg • Guaranteed Potency Soy Isoflavones (from NovaSoy supplying 25 mg (40%) Isoflavones and 12.5 mg (20%) Genistin) 62.5 • Ipriflavone (as 7-Isopropoxy - Isoflavone from Ostivone) 200 mg • ActiSorb Base 10 mg: Bioperine extract (Black Pepper - Piper longum), Cayenne (Capsicum frutecens), Turmeric (Curcuma longa), Rosemary (Rosmarinus officinalis), Ginger (Zingiber officinale). Other ingredients: Cellulose, Stearic Acid, Silica, and Magnesium Stearate.

Beyond Echinacea - Flora
Echinacea • Balsam root • Peruvian Cat's Claw bark.

BF & SC - MMS Pro
Each capsule contains: Calendula flowers • White Oak bark • Marshmallow root • Mullein leaves • Black Walnut hulls • Gravel root • Slippery Elm bark • Wormwood • Scullcap.

Bifidus Balance +FOS - Jarrow Formulas
Each capsule contains: FOS (Fructo-Oligo-Saccharides) 210 mg • Bifidobacterium Breve R070 40% 800 million • Bifidobacterium Longum R023 40% 800 million • Bifidobacterium Bifidum R071 15% 300 million • Bifidobacterium Infantis R033 5% 100 million. Other Ingredients: Maltodextrin, Magnesium Stearate, Ascorbic Acid.

Big Daddy - SNS - Sports Nutrition Source.com
A 225 gram serving contains: Sodium 50 mg • Potassium 145 mg • Protein 40 g.

Bilberry - Progressive Labs
Each all-vegetable capsule contains: Bilberry leaf powder (Vaccinum myrtillus) 370 mg • Bilberry extract (Vaccinum myrtillus) 80 mg • Anthocyanids (from above) 25 mg.

Bilberry - Leiner Health Products
Each caplet contains: Bilberry extract (Vaccinium myrtillus) berry 80 mg. Other Ingredients: Calcium Carbonate, Cellulose, Maltodextrin, Hydroxypropyl Methylcellulose, Silicon Dioxide, Polyethylene Glycol 3350, Croscarmellose Sodium, Hydroxypropyl Cellulose, Pharmaceutical Glaze, Yellow 5 Lake, Blue 1 Lake, Crospovidone, Magnesium Stearate, Polysorbate 80, Titanium Dioxide.

Bilberry - Solaray - Nutraceutical
Each capsule contains: Bilberry berry extract 60 mg. Other Ingredients: Cellulose, Gelatin, Magnesium Stearate.

Bilberry Extract - Source Naturals
Each tablet contains: Bilberry (Vaccinium myrtillus, standardized extract, yielding 18.5 mg Anthocyanosides) 50 mg.

Bilberry Extract - Nature's Way
Each capsule contains: Bilberry fruit (dried extract 25% anthocyanins) 80 mg • Elderberry 125 mg • Other Ingredients: Gelatin, Millet.

Bilberry Extract - PhytoPharmica
Two capsules contain: Bilberry (Vaccinium myrtillus fructus) berry extract (standardized to contain 25% anthocyanosides [40 mg] calculated as anthocyanidins) 160 mg.

Bilberry Extract - Swanson
Each capsule contains: Bilberry extract (25% anthocyanidins) 60 mg • Bilberry powder 360 mg • Citrus Bioflavonoids 50 mg.

Some Brand Name Natural Products - What they Contain
www.NaturalDatabase.com contains MANY more listings than appear here.

BRAND NAMES

Bilberry Formula - Quest
Each caplet contains: Bilberry (Vaccinium myrtillus) (provided by 50 mg P.E. 1:100 standardized to contain 25% anthocyanosides) 5000 mg • Citrus Bioflavonoids (providing Hesperidin 50 mg) 200 mg • Carrot powder (Daucus carota) 100 mg. Other Ingredients: Calcium Phosphate, Microcrystalline Cellulose, Vegetable Stearin, Croscarmellose Sodium, Magnesium Stearate (vegetable source).

Bilberry i sight - Nature's Life
Two capsules contain: Bilberry extract [(Viccinium myrtullus) standardized to 25% anthocyanosides] 360 mg • Vitamin C (Calcium Ascorbate) 300 mg • Vitamin B3 (Niacin) 40 mg • Vitamin B2 (Riboflavin) 3 mg • Vitamin E (d-Alpha Tocopheryl Succinate) 400 IU • Beta Carotene [(Dunaliella salina) equivalent to 15000 IU Vitamin A] 9 mg • Other naturally occurring carotenoids in D. salina: [Alpha Carotene 288 mcg, Cryptoxanthin 70 mcg, Zeaxanthin 58 mcg, Lutein 45 mcg].

Bilberry-Go! - Wakunaga of America
Each caplet contains: Bilberry Standardized Extract (fruit) 120 mg. Other Ingredients: Cellulose, Starch, Magnesium Stearate (vegetable source), Silica.

Bile-Gest - Atrium Inc.
Each tablet contains: Ox Bile concentrate 195 mg • Collinsonia root 310 mg • Glycine 50 mg • Pepsin 30 mg • Raw Liver concentrate 30 mg.
See Editor's Note No. 14, page 1817.

Binge Breaker - Enforma Natural Products
Two capsules contain: St. John's Wort (.2 -.3 Hypericin) • Kava Kava (70% Kavalactones) • Vitamin C (Ascorbic Acid) • Vitamin B1 (Thiamine) • Vitamin B2 (Riboflavin) • Vitamin B6 (Pyridoxine) • Vitamin B3 (Niacin).

Bio Berry Grape Seed Extract Plus - Flora
Grape Seed Extract 50 mg • Bilberry 10 mg. In a base of Cranberry powder.

Bio C Plus - Nutrilite
Each tablet contains: Vitamin C (30 mg from acerola cherries) 250 mg • Lemon Bioflavonoid concentrate (from lemon pulp and peel) 35 mg. Other Ingredients: Corn Starch, Microcrystalline Cellulose, Modified Cellulose Gum, Hydroxypropyl Methylcellulose, Magnesium Stearate, Acacia, Maltodextrin, Glycerin.
See Editor's Note No. 4, page 1816.

Bio C-Complex 1000 - The Vitamin Shoppe
Each capsule contains: Pure Crystalline Vitamin C (fortified with Rose Hips) 1000 mg • Citrus Bioflavonoids Complex 100 mg. No Yeast, Wheat, Corn, Dairy, Soy, Salt, Sugar, Starch, Milk, Eggs, Gluten, Preservatives, Artificial Colors or Flavors added.

Bio C-Complex 500 - The Vitamin Shoppe
Vitamin C (fortified with Rose Hips Conc.) 500 mg • Citrus Bioflavonoids Complex 250 mg. No Yeast, Wheat, Corn, Dairy, Soy, Salt, Sugar, Starch, Milk, Eggs, Gluten, Preservatives, Artificial Colors or Flavors added.

Bio Ginkgo 27/7 - Pharmanex
Each tablet contains: Ginkgo (50:1) leaf extract (Ginkgo Biloba) 60 mg. Other Ingredients: Lactose Anhydrous, Microcrystaline Cellulose, Corn Starch, Sodium Starch Glycolate, Opadry Colors (which contain the Lakes of Yellow 5 and Blue 1), Colloidal Silicon Dioxide, Magnesium Stearate.

Bio St. Johns - Pharmanex
Each capsule contains: CordyMax Cs-4 standardized to adenosine & mannitol content 375 mg • Hypericum extract standardized to 0.3% hypericin 225 mg.

Bio St. John's - Pharmanex
Two capsules contain: St. John's Wort flowering tops and leaves (5:1) extract (Hypericum perforatum) 450 mg • Cordyceps Cs-4 Mushroom Mycleia (Cordyceps sinensis [Berk.] Sacc.) 750 mg. Other Ingredient: Gelatin.

Bio Trim - Dial Herbs
Ma Huang • Kola Nut • Ginger • White Willow • Ginkgo Biloba • Bladderwrack • Fo-Ti • Hawthorn berries • Saw Palmetto • Beet Powder • Chromium Proteinate • Zinc Picolinate • Boron Proteinate • Chromium Picolinate • Kola Nut extract.

BioChoice Immune Support - Chocolate - Legacy for Life - A DCV Company
Each packet (27 g) contains: Sodium 160 mg • Potassium 55 mg • Protein 7 g • Vitamin A 5000 IU • Vitamin C 60 mg • Vitamin D (as Vitamin D3) 400 IU • Vitamin E 30 IU • Niacin 20 mg • Folic Acid 0.4 mg • Pantothenic Acid 10 mg • Vitamin B6 2 mg • Vitamin B2 (Riboflavin) 1.7 mg • Vitamin B1 (Thiamin) 1.5 mg • Vitamin B12 6 mcg • Biotin 0.3 mg • Calcium 100 mg • Copper 0.6 mg • Iodine 45 mcg • Iron 5.4 mg • Magnesium 10 mg • Phosphorus 120 mg • Zinc 4.5 mg • Vitamin K (as Vitamin K1) 80 mcg • Manganese 0.6 mg • Chromium 36 mcg. Other Ingredients: Protein blend (Egcel [egg powder], soy protein isolate, milk protein), Maltodextrin, Oat fiber, Cocoa, Natural Chocolate and Vanilla flavor, Soy lecithin, Guar Gum, Xanthan Gum.

BioChoice Immune Support - Strawberry - Legacy for Life - A DCV Company
Each packet (24 g) contains: Sodium 160 mg • Potassium 55 mg • Protein 7 g • Vitamin A 5000 IU • Vitamin C 60 mg • Vitamin D (as Vitamin D3) 400 IU • Vitamin E 30 IU • Niacin 20 mg • Folic Acid 0.4 mg • Pantothenic Acid 10 mg • Vitamin B6 2 mg • Vitamin B2 (Riboflavin) 1.7 mg • Vitamin B1 (Thiamin) 1.5 mg • Vitamin B12 6 mcg • Biotin 0.3 mg • Calcium 100 mg • Copper 0.6 mg • Iodine 45 mcg • Iron 5.4 mg • Magnesium 10 mg • Phosphorus 120 mg • Zinc 4.5 mg • Vitamin K (as Vitamin K1) 80 mcg • Manganese 0.6 mg • Chromium 36 mcg. Other Ingredients: Protein Blend (Egcel [egg powder], Soy protein isolate, milk protein), Maltodextrin, Oat fiber, artificial Strawberry flavor, Beet extract, Soy lecithin, Guar Gum, Xanthan Gum.

BioChoice Immune Support - Vanilla - Legacy for Life - A DCV Company
Each packet (24 g) contains: Vitamin A 5000 IU • Vitamin C 60 mg • Vitamin D (Vitamin D3) 400 IU • Vitamin E 30 IU • Niacin 20 mg • Folic Acid 0.4 mg • Pantothenic Acid 10 mg • Vitamin B6 2 mg • Vitamin B2 (Riboflavin) 1.7 mg • Vitamin B1 (Thiamin) 1.5 mg • Vitamin B12 6 mcg • Biotin 0.3 mg • Calcium 100 mg • Copper 0.6 mg • Iodine 45 mcg • Iron 5.4 mg • Magnesium 10 mg • Phosphorus 120 mg • Zinc 4.5 mg • Vitamin K (as Vitamin K1) 80 mcg • Manganese 0.6 mg • Chromium 36 mcg. Other Ingredients: Protein blend (Egcel [egg powder], soy protein isolate, milk protein), Maltodextrin, Oat fiber, Natural Vanilla flavor, Soy lecithin, Guar Gum, Xanthan Gum.

Biochol - Ketopharm USA
Each capsule contains: Fenugreek seed 305 mg • Garlic bulb 55 mg • Cloves 55 mg • Cinnamon bark 55 mg • Ginger root 55 mg • Costus root 55 mg. Contains no added sugars, starch, salt, milk products, yeast, artificial colors, flavors or preservatives.

Bio-EFA Borage Oil 90 - Health From The Sun
Each capsule contains: Cis- Linoleic Acid (Omega-6) 190 mg • Gamma Linolenic Acid (GLA) (Omega-6) 90 mg • Oleic Acids (Omega-9) 75 mg. Ingredients: 100% Pure Borage oil 500 mg. No sugar, starch, artificial preservatives, or colors.

Bioflora & Bioflora Powder - PhysioLogics
Each caplet contains: Fructooligosaccharides (FOS) 500 mg •
Lactobacillus acidophilus 180 mg • Lactobacillus Bulgaricus 30 mg •
Streptococcus Thermophilus 30 mg.

BioGinkgo 27/7 - Pharmanex
Ginkgo biloba leaf extract 50:1 concentration standardized to contain
27% ginkgo flavone glycosides and 7% terpene lactones 60 mg.

Biogra - Olympian Labs
Each capsule contains: DHEA 10 mg • Thymus Gland 20 mg
• Octacosanol 600 mg • Raw Orchic 20 mg • L-Tyrosine 250 mg
• Vitamin C 30 mg • Vitamin B-6 10 mg • Damiana 80 mg • Wild Yam
20 mg • Yohimbe Bark 20 mg • Gotu Kola 20 mg • Siberian Ginseng
20 mg • Licorice root powder 20 mg • Jamaican Ginger 20 mg • Dong
Quai 20 mg • Sarsaparilla 20 mg • Zinc Gluconate 20 mg.
See Editor's Note No. 14, page 1817.

Biogra for Women - Olympian Labs
Each capsule contains: Proprietary Blend: Damiana, Wild Yam, Gotu
Kola, Sarsaparilla, Saw Palmetto, Siberian Ginseng, Dong Quai, Kelp,
L-Tyrosine, L-Phenylalanine, Fo-Ti, Para-Aminobenzoic Acid, Bee
Propolis 685 mg.

BioGreens - The Vitamin Shoppe
Three teaspoons contain: Organically grown wheatgrass, alfalfa
1923 mg • Soy Lecithin (99% oil-free, 97% phosphatides) 1862 mg •
Royal Jelly, Bee Pollen, Honey Extract 1070 mg • Spirulina, Chlorella
700 mg • Vegetable Concentrate (carrot, spinach, bean sprout, celery,
tomato, daikon) 700 mg • High Pectin Fruit Fibers (apple, banana,
pineapple, papaya) 500 mg • Fructooligosaccharides from Chicory
root 400 mg • Dairy-Free Probiotic Cultures (Lactobacillus
acidophilus, L. bifidus, L. plantarum, L. rhamnosus, S. thermopilus)
360 mg • Wheat Germ Extract 350 mg • Vitamin E 120 IU • Acerola
Berry Powder 120 mg • Licorice Root Extract 120 mg • Brown Rice
112 mg • Red Beet Extract 90 mg • Lipase 0.5 units • Amylase
0.5 skb units • Protease 10 hut • Aloe Vera 50 mg • Green Tea extract
30 mg • Reishi Mushroom 30 mg • Cat's Claw Extract 30 mg • Yucca
Root Extract 30 mg • Ginger Root 30 mg • Ginkgo Biloba 20 mg •
Bilberry Extract (25% anthocyanidins) 20 mg • Garcinia Extract
20 mg • Konjac Yam extract 20 mg • Maltodextrin 900 mg. Plus
60 mg of the following herbal extracts: Milk Thistle, Siberian
Ginseng, Echinacea, American Ginseng.

Bio-Guard - Progressive Labs
Micellized antioxidant formula. Two mL contain: Vitamin A
10000 IU • Beta Carotene 2500 IU • Vitamin C 50 mg • Vitamin E
100 IU • Selenium (as selenomethionine) 50 mcg.

BioLax - Body Wise International, Inc.
Two caplets contain: Aloe Vera leaf extract 200:1 500 mg • Senna leaf
400 mg • Prune fruit 250 mg • Fig fruit 200 mg • Psyllium whole
husks 100 mg • Celery seed 100 mg • Green Barley Grass 100 mg •
Cruciferous Vegetables 100 mg • Lactobacillus Acidophilus 100 mg •
Anise Seed 20 mg.

BioPectin - Flora
Modified citrus pectin.

Bioperine - Source Naturals
Each tablet contains: Bioperine (95% pure piperine extracted from
black pepper) 10 mg.

Bio-Phoria - Olympian Labs
Two capsules contain: Proprietary Blend: St. John's Wort extract,
Phosphatidyl Serine, Acetyl L-Carnitine, Gotu Kola 700 mg.

BioPro - PhytoPharmica
Two capsules contain: Vitamin A (fish liver oil) 3,000 IU • Vitamin B6
(pyridoxine HCl) 20 mg • Zinc (chelate) 40 mg • Essential fatty acids

(unrefined vegetable lipids) 1,260 mg • Amino acid complex 300 mg
• Prostate extract (freeze-dried) 300 mg • Saw Palmetto berry extract
(4:1) 200 mg.

Biopure E 400 - Dial Herbs
Natural Vitamin E (soy-free d-alpha tocopherol) • Medium Chain
Triglycerides (coconut) • Oleic Acid (canola oil). Capsule Shell:
(gelatin, vegetable glycerine, water).

Biosorb Silymarin - Metabolic Response Modifiers
Each capsule contains: Biosorb Silymarin (yielding 80 mg silymarin)
250 mg.

Biotin - Nature's Bounty
Each tablet contains: Biotin 300 mcg. Other Ingredients: Dicalcium
Phosphate, Cellulose, Vegetable Stearic Acid, Vegetable Magnesium
Stearate.

Biovital Plus - Enzymatic Therapy
Vitamin A (Beta Carotene) non-toxic form of Vitamin A 40000 IU •
Vitamin A Fish Liver oil 25000 IU • Vitamin E (D-Tocopherol
Succinate) 800 IU • Vitamin D Fish Liver oil 600 IU • Vitamin C
(Ascorbic Acid/Rose Hips) 3000 mg • Calcium (Carbonate, Citrate,
Aspartate, Gluconate) 625 mg • Potassium Aspartate 375 mg •
Magnesium Aspartate 375 mg • Pantothenic Acid (D-Calcium
Pantothenate) 250 mg • Thiamine HCL (Vitamin B1) 250 mg • Niacin/
Niacinamide 250 mg • Manganese (Aspartate) 186 mg • Vitamin B6
(Pyridoxine HCL) 150 mg • Riboflavin (Vitamin B2/Liver) 100 mg •
Zinc (Aspartate) 92 mg • Iron (Aspartate) 60 mg • Copper (Aspartate)
2 mg • Biotin 1 mg • Folic Acid 800 mcg • Chromium Aspartate 428
mcg • Iodine (Kelp) 225 mcg • Selenium (Aspartate) 120 mcg •
Vitamin B12 /Liver (Cyanocobalamin)100 mcg • Other ingredients:
Choline Bitartrate /Liver 750 mg • Bromelain (600 MCU) 400 mg •
Pancreatic Enzymes (10X) 400 mg • PABA (Para Aminobenzoic
Acid) 250 mg • Citrus Bioflavonoids 250 mg • Lipase 200 mg •
L-Methionine 200 mg • Trace Mineral Complex "Containing 72 trace
minerals" 200 mg • Alfalfa juice concentrate 200 mg • Liver
concentrate (20X) 200 mg • Multi-Glandular concentrate 200 mg •
Adrenal extract freeze-dried 200 mg • Thymus extract freeze-dried
200 mg • Saw Palmetto Berry extract 4:1 (Serenoa repens) 125 mg •
Ma Huang extract (Ephedra sinensis) standardized to contain 6%
Ephedrine 125 mg • Sarsaparilla root 4:1 (Smilax officinalis) 125 mg •
Inositol 100 mg. Contains no sugar, salt, yeast, wheat, corn, dairy
products, coloring, flavoring, or preservatives.
See Editor's Note No. 14, page 1817.

Bio-Zyme - PhytoPharmica
Two tablets contain: Pancreatic enzymes (full strength, undiluted, and
uncut) USP units of activity: (Protease 81,250, Amylase 81,250,
Lipase 6,500) 3250 mg • Trypsin 75 mg • Papain 50 mg • Bromelain
(1,200 M.C.U.) 50 mg • Amylase 10 mg • Lipase 10 mg • Lysozyme
10 mg • Chymotrypsin 2 mg.
See Editor's Note No. 14, page 1817.

Bitters Virtue - Blessed Herbs
Aloe • Myrrh Gum • Senna • Camphor • Turkey Rhubarb root •
Zedoary root • Manna • Carline Thistle • Angelica root • Licorice root
• Fennel seed • Anise seed • Pomeranz peel • Gentian root • Galangal
root & Peach brandy.

Black Cohosh - Leiner Health Products
Each caplet contains: Black Cohosh extract powder (Cimicifuga
racemosa) root 40 mg • Lecithin 25 mg. Other Ingredients: Calcium
Carbonate, Dicalcium Phosphate, Cellulose, Maltodextrin, Stearic
Acid, Croscarmellose Sodium, Silicon Dioxide, Magnesium Stearate,
Dextrin, Hydroxypropyl Methylcellulose, Polyethylene Glycol 3350.

Black Cohosh - Nature's Way
Each capsule contains: Black Cohosh root 515 mg. Other Ingredients:
Gelatin, Magnesium stearate, Millet.

BRAND NAMES

Black Cohosh Extract - Nature's Way
Each tablet contains: Black Cohosh dried extract 40 mg. Other Ingredients: Cellulose, Maltodextrin, Modified Cellulose Gum, Silica, Stearic Acid.

Black Cohosh Root - Now
Two capsules contain: Black Cohosh (Cimicifuga Racemosa) root 1100 mg. Other Ingredients: Gelatin (capsule), Stearic Acid. Contains no yeast, wheat, gluten, corn, soy, milk, or preservatives.

Black Cohosh Standardized Extract - Now
Two capsules contain: Black Cohosh root & rhizome 160 mg • Cimicifuga racemosa (standardized to contain 2.5% total triterpene Glycosides, calculated as 27-Deoxyactein) 4 mg • Licorice root 250 mg • Dong Quai root (Angelica sinensis) 250 mg.

Black Cohosh-Blue Cohosh Virtue - Blessed Herbs
Black Cohosh root • Blue Cohosh root • Ginger root • Beth root • Grain alcohol & Distilled Water.

Black Cohosh-Source Naturals - Source Naturals
Each tablet contains: Black Cohosh standardized extract 2.5% (Cimicifuga racemosa roots and rhizome) (yielding 2 mg of Triterpene Glycosides) (containing 27-deoxyactein) 80 mg.

Black Currant 1000 - Health From The Sun
Each capsule contains: Alpha-Linolenic Acid (ALA) (Omega-3) 130 mg • Gamma Linolenic Acid (Omega-6) 170 mg • Linoleic Acid (Omega-6) 430 mg • Oleic Acid (Omega-9) 90 mg • Stearidonic Acid (Omega -3) 25 mg. Ingredients: Black Currant seed oil, Gelatin, Glycerine, Water.

Black Currant 500 - Health From The Sun
Each capsule contains: Alpha-Linolenic Acid (ALA) (Omega-3) 65 mg • Gamma Linolenic Acid (GLA) (Omega-6) 85 mg • Linoleic Acid (Omega-6) 215 mg • Oleic Acid (Omega-9) 45 mg • Stearidonic Acid (Omega-3) 12 mg. Ingredients: Black Currant seed oil, Gelatin, Glycerine, Water.

Black Currant Oil - Puritan's Pride
Each softgel contains: Black Currant oil 460 mg.

Black Currant seed oil - Nutri-Quest
Each capsule contains: Black Currant seed oil 250 mg • Fatty Acid composition %: Gamma Linolenic acid 16.9% • Linoleic 45.2% • Oleic 12.7% • Alpha Linolenic 11.7% • Palmitic 7.4% • Stearidonic 2.9% • Stearic 1.6% • Eicosenoic Acid 1.1%. Other Ingredients: Myristic, Arachidic, Behenic, Lignoceric, Palmitoleic Acids with nautral Vitamin E 5 IU.

Black Ointment - 1st Herb Source
Chaparral herb • Lobelia herb • Comfrey herb • Red Clover herb • Plantain root • Golden Seal root • Myrrh gum • Marshmallow root • Mullein herb • Chickweed herb. In a base of Olive oil, Beeswax, Pine Tar, Vitamin E oil.

Blackstrap Molasses with Iron - Swanson
Each tablet contains: Blackstrap Molasses with 29 mg of Iron.

Bladderwrack-Dandelion Virtue - Blessed Herbs
Ma Huang • Guarana seed • Dandelion blend of flower, leaf & root • Bladderwrack • Grain alcohol & Distilled Water.

BLF # Breathe Easy Without Stimulants - Health Center for Better Living
Two tablets contain: Siberian Ginseng root extract (0.8% eleutherosides) 250 mg • American Ginseng root 250 mg • Ginger root standardized extract (5% gingerols) • Peppermint leaf 75 mg • Chickweed herb (aerial parts) 50 mg • Myrrh resin 50 mg • Mullein leaf 50 mg • Yerba Mate leaf (20% alkaloids) • MSM (methyisul-foraimethan, 36% organic sulfur) 1,000 mg.

BLF #1 Clear Complexion - Health Center for Better Living
Each capsule contains: Burdock Root 84 mg • Dandelion Root 84 mg • Red Clover tops 84 mg • Echinacea root 56 mg • Yellow Dock root 56 mg • Capsicum 28 mg • Alfalfa Leaf 28 mg • Valerian Root 28 mg.

BLF #12 Cholest-A Ingredients - Health Center for Better Living
Each capsule contains: Hawthorn Berry 113 mg • Fenugreek Seed 75 mg • Capsicum 75 mg • Plantain Herb 75 mg • Red Clover Blossom 75 mg • Black Cohosh Root 38 mg.

BLF #125 Woman's Balance - Health Center for Better Living
Each capsule contains: Dong Quai Root 102 mg • Damiana Leaf 61 mg • Kelp Atlantic 61 mg • Sarsaparilla Root 61 mg • Saw Palmetto Berry 41 mg • Chickweed Herb 41 mg • Capsicum 41 mg • Black Cohosh Root 41 mg.

BLF #13 Body Circulation - Health Center for Better Living
Each capsule contains Capsicum 84 mg • Bayberry Bark 34 mg • Hyssop Leaf 17 mg • Skullcap 17 mg • Witch Hazel Bark 17 mg.

BLF #16 Colon Helper - Health Center for Better Living
Each capsule contains: Slippery Elm Bark 145 mg • Aloe 145 mg • White Oak Bark 73 mg • Blue Vervain Herb 73 mg • Gentain Root 36 mg • Goldenseal Herb 15 mg.

BLF #17 Regularity Ingredients - Health Center for Better Living
Each capsule contains: Buckthorn Bark 113 mg • Cascara Sagrada Bark 113 mg • Chickweed Herb 75 mg • Elder Flower 75 mg • Oregon Grape Root 38 mg • Mandrake Root 38 mg.

BLF #2 Allergy First Aid - Health Center for Better Living
Each caplet contains: Allergy Herbal Blend [Hyssop whole plant, Mullein leaves, Thyme whole plant, Chrysanthemum flower, Magnolia flower, Angelica root, Vitex fruit, Atractylodes Rhizome, Bellflower root, Field Mint, Immature Tangerine peel, Ledebouriella root, Moutan bark, Perilla leaf and Schizonepeta stem] 200 mg • Boswellia Gum resin (40% boswellic acid) 100 mg • Yerba Mate leaf (20% alkaloids) 50 mg • Meadowsweet 4:1 extract 50 mg • Eucalyptus leaf extract 25 mg • Fennel seed 25 mg.

BLF #21 Endless Energy - Health Center for Better Living
Each capsule contains: Ginseng Root 75 mg • Foti Root • Bee Pollen Granules 75 mg • Damiana Leaf 75 mg • Capsicum 50 mg • Kola Nut 50 mg • Echinacea Root 25 mg • Licorice Root 25 mg.

BLF #225 Man's Rejuvenator - Health Center for Better Living
Each capsule contains: Saw Palmetto Berry 75 mg • Cornsilk 75 mg • Gota Kola Herb 75 mg • Damiana Leaf 75 mg • Juniper Berry 38 mg • Kelp Atlantic 38 mg • Parsley Leaf 38 mg • Uva Ursi Leaf 38 mg.

BLF #23 Vision Booster - Health Center for Better Living
Vitamin A [as retinyl palmitate and 75% as beta-carotene with natural mixed carotenoids (alpha-carotene, beta-carotene, cryptoxanthin, zeaxanthin and lutein)] 10,000 IU • Vitamin C (as ascorbic acid) 250 mg • Vitamin E (as d-alpha-tocopheryl succinate and 50% as dl-alpha-tocopheryl acetate) 100 IU • Selenium (as selenomethionine) 100 mcg • Bilberry Herb blend [Bilberry leaf and Bilberry fruit standardized extract (25% anthocyanins)] 75 mg • Eyebright herb blend [Eyebright herb and eyebright herb 4:1 extract (whole plant)] 75 mg • Lutein (from marigold flower) 5 mg • L-Glutathione 5 mg • Taurine 5 mg • Quercetin dihydrate 75 mg • Lycium berry 5:1 extract 50 mg.

Some Brand Name Natural Products - What they Contain

BLF #24 Fresh Start - Health Center for Better Living
Alfalfa • Hyssop • Chamomile • Cornsilk • "Vitamins and minerals with antioxidant and diuretic qualities."

BLF #3 Love Formula - Health Center for Better Living
Two caplets contain: Tribulus terrestris extract (20% furanosterois) fruit and root 400 mg • Damiana leaf 125 mg • Fo-ti root 125 mg • Gota Kola leaf extract (10% total asiaticosides) 50 mg • Saw Palmetto berry extract (85-95% sterols and fatty acid) 150 mg • Korean Ginseng root extract (10% ginsenosides) 200 mg.

BLF #30 Head-X - Health Center for Better Living
Each capsule contains: Fenugreek Seed 107 mg • Feverfew Herb 107 mg • Passion Flower Herb 43 mg • Rosemary leaf 43 mg • Peppermint Leaf 43 mg • Thyme leaf 21 mg • Marjoram leaf 21 mg • Blue Violet leaf 21 mg • Wood Betony Herb 21 mg • Lobelia Herb 21 mg.

BLF #31 Healthy Heart - Health Center for Better Living
Each capsule contains: Angelica Root 45 mg • Blue Cohosh Root 45 mg • Borage Herb 45 mg • Capsicum 45 mg • Blue Vervain Herb 45 mg • Peppermint Leaf 45 mg • Wood Betony Herb 45 mg • Sheep Sorrel Herb 23 mg • Garlic Bulb 23 mg • Barberry Bark 23 mg • Goldenseal Root 23 mg • Motherwort Herb 23 mg • Scullcap Herb 23 mg.

BLF #35 Sleep Like a Baby - Health Center for Better Living
Each capsule contains: Hops flower 113 mg • Passion flower 113 mg • Scullcap Herb 75 mg • Catnip Leaf 38 mg • Peppermint Leaf 38 mg • Rosemary Leaf 38 mg • Mullein Leaf 38 mg.

BLF #38 Kidney Flush - Health Center for Better Living
Each caplet contains: Vitamin B6 (as pyridoxine HCl) 5 mg • Magnesium (as magnesium oxide) • Potassium (as potassium citrate) • Uva Ursi Leaf standardized extract (20% arbutin) 100 mg • Chokeberry fruit standardized extract (35% quinic acid) 100 mg • Cranberry juice 10:1 concentrate 50 mg • Dandelion root standardized extract (20% taraxasterol) 50 mg • Aloe Vera 200x gel (25 mg) • Herbal Blend [Couchgrass (whole plant), Buchu leaf, Uva Ursi leaf, Juniper berry, Hydrangea root, and Cornsilk stylus)] 200 mg.

BLF #41 Liver De-Tox - Health Center for Better Living
Each capsule contains: Fennel Seed 107 mg • Chicory Root 107 mg • Angelica Root 54 mg • Cleavers Herb 54 mg • Dandelion Root 27 mg • Gentian Root 27 mg • Hops Flower 27 mg • Elder Flower 27 mg • Wormwood Herb 11 mg • Lobelia Herb 11 mg.

BLF #42 Prime Lung - Health Center for Better Living
Each capsule contains: Mullein leaf 101 mg • Coltsfoot Herb 101 mg • Chickweed Herb 67 mg • Fenugreek Seed 34 mg • Pennyroyal Leaf 34 mg • Myrrh Gum 34 mg • Yarrow Flower 34 mg • Nettle Leaf 34 mg • Lobelia Herb 13 mg.

BLF #43 Bone & Nail Builder - Health Center for Better Living
Each Capsule contains: Bee Pollen Granules 87 mg • Horsetail 43 mg • Oatstraw 43 mg • Kelp Atlantic 43 mg • Ginseng root 43 mg • Foti root 43 mg • Chamomile flower 43 mg • Rose hips 43 mg • Red Clover blossom 43 mg • Lobelia Herb 17 mg.

BLF #44 Woman's Change - Health Center for Better Living
Two tablets contain: Black Cohosh root extract (2.5% triterpene glycosides) 160 mg • Dong Quai root extract (1% lingustilide) 200 mg • Chaste Tree berry extract (5% vitexi cacpin) 100 mg • Licorice Root extract (13% glycyrrhizin) 100 mg • Soybean and Kudzu root extract (20% total isoflavones) 150 mg • Damiana leaf 100 mg • Wild Yam root extract (5% diosgenin) 150 mg • Red Clover flowers 100 mg.

BLF #47 Rest Ease Ingredients - Health Center for Better Living
Each capsule contains: Valerian Root 101 mg • Wintergreen Leaf 67 mg • Peppermint Leaf 67 mg • Spearmint Leaf 67 mg • Sassafras Root Bark 34 mg • Capsicum 34 mg • Burdock root 34 mg • Buckthorn bark 34 mg • Lobelia Herb 13 mg.

BLF #48 Anti-Stress - Health Center for Better Living
Each capsule contains: Hops flower 99 mg • Valerian root 99 mg • Scullcap Herb 66 mg • Catnip leaf 66 mg • Passion Flower Herb 66 mg • Red Clover Herb 33 mg • Black Cohosh Root 20 mg.

BLF #49 Stable Sugar - Health Center for Better Living
Each capsule contains: Juniper Berries 94 mg • Uva Ursi Leaf 94 mg • Garlic Bulb 94 mg • Dandelion Root 47 mg • Capsicum 47 mg • Mullein Leaf 47 mg • Licorice Root 28 mg.

BLF #52 Fatigue Fighter - Health Center for Better Living
Prime Ingredients: Capsicum • Ginseng

BLF #53 Male Vigor - Health Center for Better Living
Two caplets contain: Yohimbe bark extract (2% yohimbe, 4% total alkaiods) 500 mg • Tribulus terrestris extract (20% furanosterols) fruit and root • Korean Ginseng root extract (10% ginsenosides) 200 mg • Yerba Mate leaf extract (20% total alkaloids) 125 mg • Saw Palmetto berry extract (85-95% sterols and fatty acid) 160 mg • Male support blend of Damiana leaf, Fo-ti root, Gota Kola leaf, and Pumpkin Seed concentrate 250 mg.

BLF #54 Sinus & Hayfever Ingredients - Health Center for Better Living
Each capsule contains: Myrrh Gum 148 mg • Echinacea Root 74 mg • Bayberry Bark 74 mg • Plantain Herb 74 mg • Saw Palmetto Berry 22 mg • Licorice Root 22 mg • Goldenseal Herb.

BLF #55 Pro Skin Enhancer - Health Center for Better Living
Each capsule contains: Red Clover Blossom 115 mg • Spikenard root 115 mg • Dandelion root 58 mg • Chickweed Herb 29 mg • Plantain Herb 29 mg • Blue Vervain Herb 29 mg • Sarsaparilla root 29 mg • Buckthorn bark 29 mg • Goldenseal root 17 mg.

BLF #57 Vein Vanish - Health Center for Better Living
Each capsule contains: White Oak Bark 87 mg • Witch Hazel Bark 87 mg • Bayberry Bark 87 mg • Capsicum 87 mg • Kelp Atlantic 43 mg • Goldenseal Root 43 mg • Lobelia Herb 17 mg.

BLF #59 Weight Loss - Health Center for Better Living
Each capsule contains: Nettle Leaf 139 mg • Chickweed Herb 93 mg • Seawrack 93 mg • Kelp Atlantic 35 mg • Fennel Seed 23 mg • Hawthorn Berry 23 mg • Dandelion Root 12 mg • Echinacea Root 12 mg • Burdock Root 12 mg • Licorice Root 5 mg • Chia Seed 5 mg.

BLF #6 Healthy Joints - Health Center for Better Living
Burdock • Alfalfa • Kelp • Vitamin C • Vitamin E • Vitamin B6.

BLF #61 P.M.S. Stop - Health Center for Better Living
Each capsule contains: Black Cohosh Root 82 mg • Dong Quai Root 82 mg • Red Raspberry Leaf 82 mg • Chaste Tree Berry 57 mg • Ginger Root 49 mg • Dandelion Root 41 mg • Motherwort Herb 33 mg • Valerian Root 25 mg.

BLF #75 Prostate Support - Health Center for Better Living
Two tablets contain: Zinc (as zinc glycinate) 15 mg • Saw Palmetto berry extract (85-95% sterols and fatty acid) 320 mg • Pygeum bark 4:1 extract 100 mg • Pumpkin seed 10:1 concentrate 100 mg • Tomato lycopene concentrate (10,000 lycopene) 100 mg • Urinary tract support blend [Chokeberry extract (35% quinic acid), Cranberry juice 10:1 concentrate, Uva-Ursi leaf extract (20% arbutin)].

BRAND NAMES

BLF #9: 120 Over 80 - Health Center for Better Living
Two tablets contain: Calcium (as calcium carbonate and calcium citratemalate-glycinate) 500 mg • Magnesium (as magnesium oxide and magnesium amino acid chelate) 200 mg • Potassium (as postassium citrate) • Ginger root extract (5% gingerols) 100 mg • Odor-controlled Garlic Extract (10,000 ppm allicin) 300 mg • Hawthorn berry extract (5% flavonoid glycosides) 250 mg • Capsicum pepper 50 mg • Panax Ginseng root extract (10% ginsenosides) 100 mg • Onion bulb 50 mg • Parsley leaf 50 mg.

Blood Formula - Dr. Morrow's Homeopathic Formula
Ten drops contain: Hamamelis virginica 3C • Pulsatilla nigricans 3C • Echinacea angustifolia 3C • Acidum hydrofluoricum 3C • Viburnum prunifolium 3C • Tussilago farfara 3C • Aesculus hippocastanum 3X. See Editor's Note No. 1, page 1816.

Blood Pressure - Nutrivention
Three tablets contain: Vitamin B6 100 mg • Calcium 50 mg • Potassium 45 mg • Magnesium 30 mg • Manganese 15 mg • Vitamin D 50 IU • Hawthorne berries 500 mg • Apple Pectin 500 mg • Garlic powder concentrate 500 mg • Cayenne pepper 500 mg • Black Cohosh 300 mg • Valerian root (Star root) 200 mg • Hops 200 mg • L-Taurine 100 mg.

Blood Sugar Balance - ProHerbs
Two tablets contain: Biotin 600 mcg • Magnesium (as Oxide) 200 mg • Zinc (as Sulfate) 30 mg • Gymnema Sylvestre leaves (standardized to 24% Gymnemic Acid) 300 mg • Bitter Melon powder (Momordica charantia fruit) 200 mg • Ginkgo Biloba leaf (standardized to 24% flavonoids glycosides & 6% terpene lactones) 120 mg • Chromium Picolinate 400 mcg • Alpha Lipoic Acid 150 mg • Quercetin 50 mg • Vanadium (as Vanadyl Pentoxide) 40 mcg. Other ingredients: Dicalcium Phosphate, Microcrystalline Cellulose, Croscarmellose Sodium, Hydroxypropylmethylcellulose, Magnesium Stearate, Mineral Oil, Polyethylene Glycol, Stearic Acid, Titanium Dioxide, Sodium Lauryl Sulfate, FD&C Yellow #6 Lake, Red #40 Lake, Iron Oxide.

Blood Sugar Blues - The Herbalist
Devil's Club root bark • Blueberry leaf • Dandelion root • Oregon Grape root • Uva Ursi leaf • Juniper berry • Licorice root • Elecampane root.

Blood Sugar Essentials - Swanson
Each tablet contains: Vitamin C (as calcium ascorbate) 100 mg • Vitamin E (as d-alpha tocopheryl succinate) 133.3 IU • Magnesium (from magnesium oxide) 66.7 mg • Biotin 333.3 mcg • Zinc (OptiZinc) 5 mg • Chromium (from Chromax chromium picolinate) 66.7 mcg • Gymnema Sylvestre powder 134 mg • Momordica Charantia (2.5%) 100 mg • Fenugreek seed powder 67 mg • Inositol 50 mg • Vanadyl Sulfate 4 mg.

Blood Sugar Formula - Nature's Way
Three capsules contain: Bilberry leaf 255 mg • Bitter Melon dried extract 150 mg • Caromix (Mixed Carotenoids) 30 mg • Chromium Polynicotinate 300 mcg • Fenugreek dried extract 210 mg • Gymnema sylvestre dried extract 66 mg • Prickly Pear leaf pad 420 mg. Other ingredients: Gelatin, Magnesium Stearate, Millet.

Bloussant - WellQuest International, Inc.
Each tablet contains: Saw Palmetto extract (Serenoa Repens) leaf 150 mg • Fennel Seed (Foeniculum Vulgare) fruit 50 mg • Dong Quai leaf 50 mg • Damiana (Tumera Diffusa) leaf 100 mg • Blessed Thistle (Cnicus Benedictus) leaf 40 mg • Dandelion (Taraxaci Herba) root 40 mg • Watercress (Nasturtium Officinale) leaf 40 mg • Black Cohosh (Cimicifuga Racemosa) root 50 mg • Wild Yam (Dioscorea Villosa) root 40 mg. Other Ingredients: Silicon Dioxide, Magnesium Stearate, Titanium Dioxide, Gelatin, and Water.

Blubberwack - The Herbalist
Bladderwrack • Gotu Kola herb • Kelp • Echinacea root • Kola Nut • Licorice root.

Blue Green Algae from Upper Klamath Lake - Futurebiotics
Blue-Green algae 500 mg.

Blue Green Micro Algae - Olympian Labs
Each capsule contains: Blue Green Micro Algae 380 mg.

Blue-Green Connection - HealthWatchers System
Spirulina • Chlorella • Klamath Lake Algae • Ginkgo Biloba • CoQ10 • Wheatgrass • Alfalfa • Chlorophyll

Body Ache Formula - Dr. Morrow's Homeopathic Formulas
Ten drops contain: Aconite 3C • Bryonia alba 3C • Eupatorium perfoliatum 3C • Ferrum Phosphate 6C • Apis mellifica 3C • Mercurius dulcis 6C • Arnica 3C. See Editor's Note No. 1, page 1816.

Body Guard - Jamieson
Chlorhexidine Gluconate • Glycerin • Nonoxynol-9 • Witch Hazel Herbal Extract.

Body Smoothing Lotion - Cellex-C
Ascorbic Acid • Vitamin E • Tomato extract • Evening Primrose oil • Tyrosine • Zinc • Glycine • Hyaluronic Acid • Aloe Vera extract • Chamomile extract • Allantoin • Bioflavonoids.

Body Solutions - Evening Formula - Mark Nutritionals, Inc.
Each tablespoon contains: Chromium (as chromium picolinate, chromium polynicotinate, and chromium cruciferate) 15 mcg • Proprietary Blend of Aloe Vera Gel, Collmark, Fosmark, Leanmark, Conjugated Linoleic Acid, Stevia 6 mL. Other Ingredients: Purified Water, Glycerin, Natural Kiwi Flavor, Natural Strawberry Flavor, Xanthan Gum, Sodium benzoate and Potassium sorbate as preservatives.

BodySynergy Meal Replacement Drink Mix - Vanilla - Rexall
Each packet contains: Sodium 100 mg • Protein 18 g • Potassium 340 mg • Vitamin A (Retinyl Palmitate) 1250 IU • Vitamin C (Ascorbic Acid) 15 g • Calcium 500 mg • Electrolytic Iron 4.5 mg • Vitamin D (Cholecalciferol) 100 IU • Vitamin E (dl-Alpha Tocopheryl Acetate) 7.5 IU • Thiamin Mononitrate .375 mg • Riboflavin .425 mg • Niacin (Niacinamide) 5 mg • Vitamin B6 (Pyrodoxine Hydrochloride) .5 mg • Folate (Folic Acid) 100 mcg • Vitamin B12 (Cyanocobalamin) 1.5 mcg • Biotin 75 mcg • Pantothenic Acid (Calcium D-Pantothenate) 2.5 mg • Phosphorus (Dicalcium Phosphate) 700 mg • Iodine (Potassium Iodide) 37.5 mcg • Magnesium 8 mg • Zinc Oxide 3.75 mg • Copper Gluconate .5 mg. Other Ingredients: Fructose, Maltodextrin, Soy Protein isolate, Whey Protein isolate, Whey Protein concentrate, Cocoa processed with alkali, Natural and Artificial Chocolate Flavor, Carrageenan, DiPotassium Phosphate, Natural Cream Flavor, Xanthan Gum, Stevia Extract.

BodySynergy Anti-Craving Formula - Rexall
Two tablets contain: Vitamin B-6 (from pyridoxine HCl and pyridoxal-5-phophate) 12 mg • Calcium 125 mg • Chromium (from chromium polynicotinate) 133 mcg • Sodium 10 mg • BodySynergy proprietary blend: DL-Phenylalanine, L-Tyrosine, Stinging Nettle leaf, L-Glutamine, L-Carnitine 1237 mg. Other Ingredients: Dicalcium Phosphate, Cellulose, Croscarmellose Sodium, Silica, Stearic Acid, Calcium Citrate, Hydroxypropyl Methylcellulose, Magnesium Stearate, PEG.

Some Brand Name Natural Products - What they Contain
www.NaturalDatabase.com contains MANY more listings than appear here.

BodySynergy Meal Replacement Drink Mix - Chocolate - Rexall
Each packet contains: Sodium 100 mg • Protein 18 g. Vitamin A (Retinyl Palmitate) 1250 IU • Vitamin C (Ascorbic Acid) 15 mg • Calcium 500 mg • Electrolytic Iron 4.5 mg • Vitamin D (Cholecalciferol) 100 IU • Vitamin E (dl-Alpha Tocopheryl Acetate) 7.5 IU • Thiamin Mononitrate 0.375 mg • Riboflavin 0.425 mg • Niacin (Niacinamide) 5 mg • Vitamin B6 (Pyridoxine Hydrochloride) 0.5 mg • Folate (Folic Acid) 100 mcg • Vitamin B12 (Cyanocobalamin) 1.5 mg • Biotin 75 mcg • Pantothenic Acid (Calicum D-Pantothenate) 2.5 mg • Phosphorous (Dicalcium Phosphate) 700 mg • Iodine (Potassium Iodide) 37.5 mcg • Magnesium 8 mg • Zinc Oxide 3.75 mg • Copper Gluconate 0.5 mg. Other Ingredients: Fructose, Maltodextrin, Soy Protein isolate, Whey Protein isolate, Whey Protein concentrate, Cocoa Processed with Alkali, Dicalcium Phosphate, Natural and Artificial Chocolate flavor, Carrageenan, Dipotassium Phosphate, Natural Cream flavor, Xanthan Gum, Stevia extract.

Bone & Joint Care - Natrol
Three capsules contain: Vitamin D (as cholecalciferol) 20 IU • Vitamin K (as Phytonadione) 10 mcg • Calcium (as calcium carbonate & calcium citrate) 250 mg • Magnesium (as Magnesium oxide) 125 mg • Zinc (as zinc citrate) 5 mg • Copper (as copper gluconate) 100 mcg • Glucosamine Sulfate 250 mg • MSM (Methyl Sulfonyl Methane) 250 mg • IpriFlavone 100 mg • Sea Cucumber • 100 mg Mucopolysaccarides (26%) 26 mg • Horsetail grass 100 mg • Silica (8%) 8 mg • Bamboo 100 mg • Salicylic Acid 10 mg • Boron 2 mg. Other ingredients: Silicon Dioxide, Magnesium Stearate, Gelatin.

Bone & Joint Defense System - Puritan's Pride
Each tablet contains: Vitamin A 208.34 IU • Vitamin C 8.33 mg • Vitamin D 66.67 IU • Vitamin E 8.33 IU • Vitamin K 8.33 mcg • Vitamin B-6 1.33 mg • Folic Acid 100 mcg • Vitamin B-12 8.33 mcg • Pantothenic Acid 8.33 mg • Calcium 333.33 mg • Magnesium 83.33 mg • Zinc 6 mg • Selenium 2 mcg • Copper 1 mg • Manganese 3.67 mg • Molybdenum 83.33 mcg • Potassium 33 mg • Silica 667 mcg • Boron 1.33 mg • Vanadium 66.67 mcg • Glucosamine Sulfate 41.67 mg • N-Acetyl Cysteine 4.3 mg • Pycnogenol Pine bark extract 80 mcg • Coenzyme Q-10 84 mcg • DL-Phenylalanine 4.33 mg • L-Proline 4.33 mg • Glycine 16.67 mg • S.O.D. 8.33 mcg • Mucopolysaccharide complex 21 mg • Hydrolyzed Collagen Protein 21 mg • Herbal Support Complex 36.67 mg. Other Ingredients: Milk Thistle, Alfalfa, Garlic, Young Barley Grass, Spirulina, Kelp, Devil's Claw, Hydrangea Root, Irish Moss, Yucca Root, White Willow Bark, Slippery Elm Bark.

Bone & Joints - ProHerbs - ProHerbs
Three tablets contain: Vitamin D (D3) 240 IU • Calcium (as Calcium Carbonate) 1005 mg • Isoflavones (as Soy standardized extract) 60 mg • Glucosamine Sulfate 510 mg • Chondroitin Sulfate 405 mg • Boron 4.5 mg. Other Ingredients: Croscarmellose Sodium, Hydroxypropylmethylcellulose, Magnesium Stearate, Mineral Oil, Polyethylene Glycol, Stearic Acid, Titanium Dioxide, Sodium Lauryl Sulfate, Iron Oxide.
See Editor's Note No. 15, page 1817.

Bone 350 Plus - Atrium Inc.
Each tablet contains: Raw Calf Bone concentrate 350 mg • Equisetum (Horsetail Rush) 150 mg.
See Editor's Note No. 14, page 1817.

Bone Builder - Schiff
Three tablets contain: Calcium (Carbonate, Chelate, Citrate-Malate) 1000 mg • Magnesium (Oxide, Chelate) 400 mg • Vitamin D (as Vitamin D3) (Cholecalciferol) 400 IU • Vitamin C (Ascorbic Acid) 150 mg • Vitamin K (Phytonadione) 25 mcg • Vitamin B6 (Pyridoxine, Coenzyme Pyridoxal-5-Phosphate) 10 mg • Vitamin B12 (Cyanocobalamin, Coenzyme Dibencozide) 25 mcg • Folic Acid (Folic Acid, Coenzyme Tetrahydrafolate) 200 mcg • Boron (Chelate)

1 mg • Zinc (Optizinc) 7.5 mg • Copper (Lysinate) 1 mg • Manganese (Glycinate) 10 mg • Molybdenum (Chelate) 50 mcg • Silica (Magnesium Trisillicate) 25mg • Strontium (Chloride) 100 mcg • Vanadium (Vanadyl Sulfate) 50 mcg • Sulphur (Vanadyl Sulfate) 30 mcg • Betaine HCI 50 mg • Glucose Polymers (Maltodextrin) 50 mcg • Citrus Bioflavonoids Complex 250 mg • Fennel (4:1 extract) 100 mg • Black Cohosh (4:1 extract) 100 mg • Blessed Thistle (4:1 extract) 100 mg. Natural base: Cellulose, Vegetable Sterates, Silica.

Bone Building Hair Teeth & Nails Formula - Youngevity
Calcium 250 mg • Magnesium 100 mg • Manganese 0.5 mg • Boron 240 mg • Vitamin D (as Vitamin D3) 150 IU • Horsetail grass 25 mg • Rose Hips 25 mg • Vilcabamba Mineral Essence: Potassium, Calcium, Magnesium, Zinc, Chromium, Selenium, Iron, Copper, Molybdenum, Vanadium, Iodine, Cobalt, Manganese.

Bone Calcium - Now
Four tablets contain: Calcium (from 4000 mg Microcrystalline Hydroxyapatite) 1000 mg • Magnesium (from 835 mg Magnesium Oxide) 500 mg • Phosphorus (Hydroxyapatite) 500 mg • Zinc (Amino Acid Chelate) 15 mg • Copper (Amino Acid Chelate) 2 mg • Vitamin D (Cholecalciferol) 200 IU • Manganese (Amino Acid Chelate) 7 mg • Boron (Amino Acid Chelate) 3 mg.

Bone Care - Puritan's Pride
Two tablets contain: Vitamin D (as Cholecalciferol) 800 IU • Vitamin K (as Phytonadione) 100 mcg • Calcium (as Calcium Carbonate and Calcium Gluconate) 1,200 mg • Magnesium (as Magnesium Oxide and Magnesium Gluconate) 300 mg. Other Ingredients: Cellulose (Plant Origin), Croscarmellose, Cellulose Coating, Vegetable Magnesium Stearate, Mannitol.

Bone Essentials - Swanson
Two capsules contain: Vitamin D (as cholecalciferol) 400 IU • Vitamin K (as phytonadione) 100 mcg • Calcium (from citrate/citrate maleate) 350 mg • Magnesium (from glycinate/oxide) 174 mg • Zinc (from zinc oxide) 30 mg • Copper (from copper gluconate) 2 mg • Manganese (from manganese gluconate) 3.6 mg • SoyLife Soy extract (3% soy isoflavones) 50 mg • Lactose 5 mg • L-Arginine 5 mg • L-Lysine (HCl) 5 mg • Silica (horsetail herb) 5 mg • Boron (from gluconate) 3 mg • Strontium Chloride 20 mcg.

Bone Formula - Pharmanex
Two capsules contain: Vitamin C (as Calcium Ascorbate Complex - Ester C) 60 mg • Vitamin D (as Vitamin D3) (as Cholecalciferol) 50 IU • Vitamin K (as Vitamin K1) (as Phytonadione) 20 mcg • Calcium (as Calcium Carbonate, Calcium Propionate) 250 mg • Magnesium (as Magnesium Asparate, Magnesium Oxide) 125 mg • Isoflavones (from Soy extract) 12.5 mg • Silicon (as Sodium Metasilicate) 5 mg • Boron (as Boron Citrate) 1.5 mg. Other Ingredients: Magnesium Stearate, Sodium Carboxymethylcellulose.

Bone Health - Centrum Focused Formulas
Two tablets contain: Supplement facts: Vitamin D 200 IU • Calcium (Citrate) 500 mg • Magnesium 40 mg • Zinc 7.5 mg • Copper 1 mg • Manganese 1.8 mg • Boron 250 mcg • Lycopene 1.5 mg • Saw Palmetto (Standardized lipophilic fruit extract, Serenoa repens) 160 mg. Ingredients: Calcium Citrate, Magnesium Oxide, Talc, Hydroxypropyl Methylcellulose, Sodium Starch Glycolate, Titanium Dioxide, Magnesium Stearate, Zinc Oxide, Mineral Oil, Manganese Sulfate Monohydrate, Vitamin D (Cholecalciferol), Polysorbate 80, Sodium Borate, Polyethlene Glycol, Cupric Oxide, Gelatin, Sucrose, Starch, Carnauba Wax, Vegetable Oil, DL-Alpha-Tocopherol

Bone Maximizer - Metabolic Response Modifiers
Six capsules contain: Hydroxyapatite (MCHC) 4,000 mg • Calcium (from MCHC) 1,000 mg • Protein (from MCHC) 1,000 mg • Phosphorus (from MCHC) 500 mg • Magnesium oxide glycinate 300 mg • Zinc (citrate) 18 mg • Boron (citrate) 2 mg • Vitamin D (as Vitamin D3 cholecalciferol) 480 IU • Vitamin K (as Vitamin K1,

BRAND NAMES

phylloquinone) 120 mcg • Vitamin C (ascorbic acid) 72 mg • MSM (methyl-sulfonyl-methane) 120 mg • Glucosamine (HCl) 120 mg • Horsetail extract (silica) 25 mg • Pregnenolone 10 mg.

Bone Maximizer II - Metabolic Response Modifiers
Six capsules contain: Hydroxyapatite (MCHC) 4,000 mg • Calcium (from MCHC) 1,000 mg • Protein (from MCHC) 1,000 mg • Phosphorus (from MCHC) 500 mg • Magnesium Glycinate 200 mg • Zinc (citrate) 18 mg • Boron (citrate) 2 mg • Vitamin D (as Vitamin D3 cholecalciferol) 480 IU • Vitamin K1 (phylloquinone) 120 mcg • Vitamin C (ascorbic acid) 72 mg • MSM (methyl-sulfonyl-methane) 120 mg • Glucosamine (HCl) 120 mg • Horsetail extract (silica) 25 mg.

Bone Meal with Natural Vitamin D - Puritan's Pride
Four tablets contain: Vitamin D (as Cholecalciferol) 400 IU • Calcium (as Bone Meal) 880 mg • Iron (as Ferrous Sulfate) 1.8 mg • Phosphorus (as Bone Meal) 400 mg • Magnesium (as Magnesium Gluconate) 3.7 mg • Zinc (as Zinc Gluconate) 0.080 mg • Copper (as Copper Gluconate) 0.013 mg • Manganese (as Manganese Gluconate) 0.011 mg • Red Beef Bone Marrow 15 mg.

Bone Protector with Ostivone - Natrol
Six capsules contain: Calcium (as calcium citrate) 1200 mg • 7-Isopropoxy-Isoflavone 600 mg. Other ingredients: Rice powder, Magnesium Stearate, Gelatin.

Bone Reinforcer with Hydroxyapatite - Puritan's Pride
Four tablets contain: Vitamin C 60 mg • Vitamin D 400 IU • Calcium 1200 mg • Magnesium 400 mg • Zinc 15 mg • Copper 2 mg • Manganese 2.5 mg • Boron 3 mg • Silica 20 mg • Betaine Hydrochloride 100 mg.

Bone Renew with Ostivone - Source Naturals
Four tablets contain: Calcium (as Calcium Citrate, Ethanolamine Phosphate and Malate) 800 mg • Ipriflavone (Ostivone) 600 mg.

Bone Review - Source Naturals
Four tablets contain: Calcium (as Calcium Citrate, Ethanolamine Phosphate and Malate) 800 mg • Ipriflavone (Ostivone) 600 mg.

Bone Support - TwinLab
Four tablets contain: Vitamin D (from Cholecalciferol) 800 IU • Calcium (from Calcium Citrate & Carbonate) 1500 mg • Magnesium (from Magnesium Aspartate & Oxide) 750 mg • Ostivone (Ipriflavone) (7-Isopropoxy Isoflavone) 600 mg • Novasoy Phytoestrogen extract (containing 40 mg of Soy Isoflavones) 100 mg • Boron (from Boron Citrate, Glycinate & Aspartate) 3 mg. Other Ingredients: Pharmaceutical Glaze, Cellulose, Stearic Acid Sodium Lauryl Sulfate, Magnesium Stearate, Colloidal Silicon Dioxide.

Bone Support Formula with Vitamin D - Health Smart Vitamins
Four caplets contain: Vitamin A (as beta-carotene) 25,000 IU • Vitamin D (cholecalciferol) 4 mg • Vitamin K (phytonadione) 0.08 mg • Calcium (as 50% calcium carbonate, 25% calcium citrate, 25% calcium glycinate) 1000 mg • Magnesium (as 75% magnesium oxide, 25% magnesium glycinate) 400 mg • Zinc (as zinc citrate) 15 mg • Copper (as copper asparate) 1.50 mg • Boron (as sodium borate) 1.50 mg.

Bones & Joints Body Benefits Pak - Leiner Health Products
Each packet contains: Magnesium 233 mg • Calcium Carbonate 498 mg • Iron 8 mg • Manganese 7.5 mg • Riboflavin (Vitamin B2) 5.1 mg • Thiamin (Vitamin B1) 4.5 mg • Vitamin B12 18 mcg • Vitamin B6 6 mg • Selenium 200 mcg • Molybdenum 208 mcg • Niacin 40 mg • Biotin 60 mcg • Chloride 72 mg • Potassium 80 mg • Copper 3.5 mg • Chromium 200 mcg • Vitamin E 460 IU • Vitamin A 7500 IU • Zinc 20 mg • Phosphorus 130 mg • Vitamin C 620 mg • Folate 400 mcg • Iodine 150 mcg • Pantothenic Acid 10 mg •

Vitamin D 400 IU • Vitamin K 80 mcg • Boron 200 mcg • Citrus Bioflavonoids complex 10 mg • Ginkgo Biloba leaf 25 mg • Grape Seed extract (Vitis vinefera) seed 1 mg • Hesperidin complex 5 mg • Kelp powder (Macrocystis pyrifera) frond 5 mg • Lecithin 10 mg • Mixed Carotenoids complex 10 mg • Nickel 6.5 mcg • Siberian Ginseng powder (Eleutherococcus senticosus) root 25 mg • Silicon Dioxide 2 mg • Tin 13 mcg • Tocotrienol complex 5 mg • Trace Mineral complex 10 mg • Vanadium 13 mcg. Other Ingredients: Glucosamine Sulfate, Glucosamine Hydrochloride, Cellulose, Methylcellulose, Maltodextrin, Hydroxypropyl Methylcellulose, Polyethylene Glycol 3350, Propylene Glycol, Starch, Crospovidone, Croscarmellose Sodium, Acacia.

Borage oil 240 - Health From The Sun
Each capsule contains: Gamma Linolenic Acid (GLA) (Omega-6) 240 mg • Linoleic Acid (Omega-6) 370 mg • Oleic Acid (Omega-9) 15 mg. Ingredients: Borage seed oil, Gelatin, Glycerine, Water.

Borage oil 300 - Health From The Sun
Each capsule contains: Gamma Linolenic Acid (GLA) (Omega-6) 300 mg • Linoleic Acid (Omega-6) 480 mg • Oleic Acid (Omega-9) 190 mg. Ingredients: Borage seed oil, Gelatin, Glycerine, Water.

Borage-Licorice Virtue - Blessed Herbs
Borage • Astragalus root • Licorice root • Siberian Ginseng root • Wild American Ginseng root • Suma root • Reishi mycelium • Ginger root • Grain alcohol & Distilled water.

Boron - Nature's Way
Each capsule contains: Boron amino acid chelate 3 mg. Other Ingredients: Cellulose, Gelatin, Maltodextrin, Millet.

Boron Complex Plus - The Vitamin Shoppe
Four capsules contain: Boron 3 mg • Calcium 1000 mg • Magnesium 500 mg • Vitamin D (as Vitamin D3) 400 IU • Zinc 15 mg • Manganese 5 mg • Copper 500 mcg • Betaine HCl 324 mg.

Boswellia Extract - Source Naturals
Three tablets contain: Boswellia serrata extract (yielding 788 mg of Boswellic Acids) 1,125 mg.

Boswellin - Now
Each capule contains: Boswellin (Boswellia serrata; extract of gum resins standardized to contain 65% [162 mg] Boswellic Acids) 250 mg • Curcumin extract (Curcuma longa; min 90% standardized extract of turmeric root powder) 100 mg • Turmeric root powder 150 mg. Other Ingredients: Rice Flour, Magnesium Stearate, Silica. Contains no sugar, salt, starch, yeast, wheat, corn, milk, or preservatives.

Botanaflor - Pharmanex
Each capsule contains: Jerusalem Artichoke with Fructooligosaccharides 100 mg • Cellulose Powder 100 mg • Citrus Pectin 98 mg • Apple Pectin Fiber 66 mg • Konjac Root (Glucomannan) 59 mg • Date Fiber 52 mg • Prune Fiber 48 mg • Soybean Fiber 43 mg • Papaya Powder with Papain 30 mg • Pineapple Powder with Bromelain 30 mg • Bifidobacterium Bifidum 30 mg • Lactobacillus Acidophilus.

Botaname - Pharmanex
Two capsules contain: Garcinia Cambogia 500 mg • Peppermint powder 104 mg • Brewer's Yeast 100 mg • Cinnamon Ramulus powder 86 mg • Lemon Verabanae powder 86 mg • Chamomile flower powder 69 mg • Ginger root powder 69 mg • Chinese Licorice root extract 35 mg • Sweet Citrus Peel 35 mg • Chicory powder 16 mg.

Bounty Bears Plus Extra C - Nature's Bounty
Each tablet contains: Vitamin A (as Retinyl Acetate and Beta Carotene) 2500 IU • Vitamin C (as Ascorbic Acid and Sodium

Ascorbate) 250 mg • Vitamin D (as Cholecalciferol) 400 IU • Vitamin E (as d-Alpha Tocopheryl Acetate) 15 IU • Thiamin (as Thiamine Mononitrate) 1.05 mg • Riboflavin (Vitamin B-2) 1.2 mg • Niacin (as Niacinamide) 13.5 mg • Vitamin B-6 (as Pyridoxine Hydrochloride) 1.05 mg • Folic Acid 300 mg • Vitamin B-12 (as Cyanocobalamin) 4.5 mcg. Other Ingredients: Sugar, Vegetable Stearic Acid, Natural Orange Flavor, Vegetable Magnesium Stearate, Silica, Mannitol, FD&C Red No. 40, FD&C Yellow No. 6, FD&C Blue No. 2.

Bovine Cartilage Plus - Atrium Inc.
Each capsule contains: Freeze Dried Bovine Cartilage 600 mg • Freeze Dried Soluble Trachea Substance 150 mg. Contains no sugar, starch, salt, wheat, corn or soy derivatives.
See Editor's Note No. 14, page 1817.

Bowel Support - Amazon Support
Each capsule contains: Cat's Claw • Macela • Jatoba • Jurubeba • Papaya • Carqueja.

BowelSoothe - Neopharmica
Each packet contains: Herbal Concentrate: White Peony Root,

Atractylodes Rhizome, Cardamon Seed, Paederia Scandens stem, Sonchus Brachyotus, Chinese Licorice root 10 g.

Brain Actives - VitaStore
Six tablets contain: Ginkgo Biloba (24% Flavoneglycosides, 6% Terpene Lactones) 100 mg • Phosphatidylserine 300 mg • L-Methionine 300 mg • OPC Complex (Pine Bark & Grapeseed Extracts) 100 mg • Vitamin B1 (Thiamine) 1.5 mg • Vitamin B2 (Riboflavin) 1.5 mg • Vitamin B3 (Niacin) 20 mg • Vitamin B5 (Pantothenic Acid) 10 mg • Vitamin B6 (Pyridoxine) 2 mg • Vitamin B12 6 mcg • Lecithin 1000 mcg • Acetyl L-Carnitine 500 mg • L-Glutamine 250 mg • Manganese 35 mg.

Brain Alert - Nutrapathic
Two tablets contain: Vitamin B1 10 mg • Vitamin B6 20 mg • Vitamin B12 40 mcg • Niacin 10 mg • Niacinamide 10 mg • Biotin 30 mcg • Choline Bitartrate 20 mg • Inositol 10 mg • PABA 20 mg • Vitamin F 4 mg • Calcium 20 mg • Chloride 4 mg • Copper 4 mg • Magnesium 10 mg • Manganese 6 mg • Phosphorus 10 mg • Potassium 10 mg • Selenium 10 mcg • Silica 4 mg • Zinc 20 mg. Other Ingredients: Brain, Egg Lecithin, Rye Green, Red Clover, Peppermint leaves, L-Tyrosine, L-Arginine, Lecithin granules, Barley Green, Bee Pollen, Gotu Kola, Ginkgo, Glutamic Acid, L-Phenylalanine, L-Glutamine, DNA, RNA, Hypothalamus, Pineal, Pituitary, Valerian, Ginseng, Spirulina, Wood Betony, Bupleurum root, Chondroitin Sulfate, CoQ10.
See Editor's Note No. 15, page 1817.

Brain Booster - Optimum Nutrition
Ginkgo Biloba • Siberian Ginseng.

Brain Care - Quantum
Two tablets contain: Vitamin E (d-Alpha Tocopherol) 100 IU • Phosphatidylserine complex 100 mg • Phosphatidyl Choline 95 mg • Ginkgo leaf (Ginkgo Biloba) (24% Ginkgo Flavone Glycosides) 60 mg • Alpha-Linolenic Acid (Borage Oil) 50 mg • Coenzyme Q10 30 mg • DHA (Docosahexaenoic Acid) 10 mg • EPA (Eicosahexaenoic Acid) 10 mg. In a base of Stearic acid, Guar Gum, Magnesium Stearate.

Brain Essentials - PhytoPharmica
Three tablets contain: Vitamin C (Ascorbic Acid) 300 mg • Magnesium Aspartate 100 mg • Potassium Aspartate 100 mg • Zinc Aspartate 30 mg • Manganese (Chelate) 15 mg • Folic Acid 800 mcg • Vitamin B12 (Cyanocobalamin) 500 mcg • L-Glutamine 300 mg • L-Phenylalanine 300 mg • Brain extract freeze-dried 300 mg • Choline (Bitartrate) 200 mg • Gamma-Aminobutyric Acid (GABA) 100 mg • Alpha-Ketoglutaric Acid 100 mg • Glycine 100 mg •

L-Tyrosine 100 mg • Pituitary extract freeze-dried 65 mg • L-Methionine 50 mg • RNA/DNA Complex 50 mg • L-Cysteine 50 mg • Pyridoxal Phosphate 15 mg. Contains no sugar, salt, yeast, wheat, corn, soy, dairy products, coloring, flavoring, or preservatives. All organs & glands derived from bovine sources.
See Editor's Note No. 14, page 1817.

Brain Essentials - Swanson
Each capsule contains: Vitamin E (as d-alpha tocopheryl succinate) 100 IU • Vitamin B-6 (as pyridoxine HCl) 25 mg • Vitamin B-12 (as cyanocobalamin) 250 mcg • Pantothenic Acid (as d-calcium pantothenate) 25 mg • Gotu Kola extract (10% asiaticosides) 150 mg • L-Glutamine 100 mg • L-Tyrosine 100 mg • Phosphatidylcholine (from lecithin) 100 mg • Ginkgo Biloba leaf extract (24% flavone glycosides, 6% terpene lactones) 60 mg • DHA (docosahexaenoic acid) 30 mg • Alpha Lipoic Acid 25 mg • DMAE Bitartrate 2 mg • Phosphatidylserine 1 mg.

Brain Fuel - Futurebiotics
Three tablets contain: Ginkgo Biloba (24% standardized extract) 45 mg • Korean Ginseng (7% ginsenoside extract) 15 mg • American Ginseng (7% ginsenoside extract) 10 mg • Gotu Kola extract (4:1 extract equivalent to) 150 mg • Ginkgo Biloba leaves 200 mg • Gotu Kola leaves 250 mg • Chinese Licorice extract (glycyrrhiza) 150 mg • Tyrosine 150 mg • Glutamine 275 mg • Phosphatidyl Choline (55% strength) 250 mg • Vitamin C 60 mg • Vitamin E (natural succinate) 5 IU • Vitamin B6 25 mg • Folic Acid 400 mcg • Vitamin B12 25 mcg • Vitamin B5 35 mg • Potassium 200 mg • Betaine HCl 50 mg • Bromelain 50 mg • Para Amino Benzoic Acid (PABA) 75 mg • L-Methionine 75 mg • Ribonucleic Acid (RNA) 50 mg.

Brain Fuel II - Futurebiotics
Two capsules contain: Vitamin E (as d-alpha tocopheryl acetate) 100 IU • Vitamin B6 (as pyridoxine hydrochloride) 25 mg • Vitamin B12 (as Cyanocobalamin) 25 mcg • Pantothenic acid (as calcium pantothenate) 25 mg • DHA (decosahexaenoic acid) 100 mg • Phosphatidylcholine (supplying 55% (110 g) choline) 200 mg • Alpha Lipoic Acid 100 mg • Ginkgo biloba leaf powder extract [standardized for 24% (11 g) ginkgo heterosides] 45 mg • Korean ginseng root powder extract [standardized for 7% (1 mg) ginsenosides] 15 mg • Gotu Kola leaf 4:1 powder extract 38 mg. Other ingredients: Gelatin, Water.

Brain Lightning - Future Dynamic Advantage
Three capsules contain: Vitamin E 100 IU • Vitamin B-1 (Thiamin) 25 mg • Vitamin B-3 (Niacin, non-flushing, as niacinamide) 10 mg • Vitamin B-5 (Pantothenic Acid) 25 mg • Vitamin B-6 (Pyridoxine 5- Phosphate) 25 mg • Vitamin B-12 (as Cyanocobalamin) 250 mcg • Magnesium 50 mg • Zinc (as Amino Acid Chelate) 10 mg • Manganese (as Manganese Chelate) 5 mg • Selenium (as Amino Acid Chelate) 200 mcg. Proprietary Synergistic Blend: [DMAE (dimethylaminoethanol), Pregnenolone, Trimethylglycine (TMG), L-Tyrosine, Huperzine A (pure molecular alkaloid), Vinpocetine, DL Phenylalanine (DLPA), GABA (gamma aminobutyric acid), Ginkgo Biloba] 1490 mg. Other Ingredients: Magnesium Silicate, Calcium Carbonate, Silicon Dioxide, Cellulose (non-reactive mixing agents).

Brain Link Complex - Pain & Stress Center
Five tablespoons contain: Vitamin A • Vitamin C • Calcium • Iron • Vitamin D • Vitamin E • Thiamin • Riboflavin • Niacin • Vitamin B6 • Folate • Vitamin B12 • Biotin • Pantothenic Acid • Iodine • Magnesium • Zinc • Selenium • Copper • Manganese • Chromium • Molybdenum. Amino Acid Profile: Alanine 290 mg • Arginine 149 mg • Aspartic Acid 573 mg • Cystine/Cysteine 167 mg • Glutamic Acid 837 mg • Glycine 2101 mg • Histidine 103 mg • Isoleucine 485 mg • Leucine 852 mg • Lysine 521 mg • Methionine 149 mg • Phenylalanine 335 mg • Proline 242 mg • Serine 202 mg • Threonine 252 mg • Tryptophan (from natural milk & egg protein) 111 mg • Tyrosine 898 mg • Valine 478 mg • Taurine 1500 mg • GABA 1500 mg • L-Glutamine 3000 mg • Inositol 50 mg • Choline 50 mg • PABA 2 mg.

Some Brand Name Natural Products - What they Contain
www.NaturalDatabase.com contains MANY more listings than appear here.

Brain Nutrition - Enzymatic Therapy
Three tablets contain: Vitamin C (Ascorbic Acid) 300 mg • Magnesium Aspartate 100 mg • Potassium Aspartate 100 mg • Zinc Aspartate 30 mg • Manganese (Chelate) 15 mg • Folic Acid 800 mcg • Vitamin B12 (Cyanocobalamin) 500 mcg • Other ingredients: L-Glutamine 300 mg • L-Phenylalanine 300 mg • Brain extract freeze-dried 300 mg • Choline (Bitatrate) 200 mg • Gamma-Aminobutyric Acid (GABA) 100 mg • Alpha-Ketoglutaric Acid 100 mg • Glycine 100 mg • L-Tyrosine 100 mg • Pituitary extract freeze-dried 65 mg • L-Methionine 50 mg • RNA-DNA Complex 50 mg • L-Cysteine 50 mg • Pyridoxal Phosphate 15 mg. Contains no sugar, salt, yeast, wheat, corn, soy, dairy products, coloring, flavoring or preservatives. All organs & glands derived from bovine sources. See Editor's Note No. 14, page 1817.

Brain Pep - Pep Products, Inc.
One capsule contains: Ginkgo Biloba • Kola Nut • Gotu Kola • Siberian Ginseng • Schizandra • Ginger • L-Glutamine 130 mg.

Brain Plus - Progressive Labs
Each capsule contains: Raw Porcine Brain concentrate 100 mg • Choline (bitartrate) 100 mg • Inositol 100 mg. This product contains naturally occuring RNA/DNA qualitatively from the brain concentrate.
See Editor's Note No. 14, page 1817.

BrainStorm - Allergy Research Group
Two tablets contain: Vitamin B6 15 mg • Pyridoxal-Phosphate 5 mg • Dibencoside 50 mcg • Biotin 100 mcg • Folic Acid 100 mcg • Chromium (Nicotinate) 50 mcg • Zinc (Citrate) 10 mg • Selenium 50 mcg • Molybdenum 50 mcg • Boron (Citrate) 500 mcg • L-Glutamine 250 mg • Bacosides 100 mg • L-Tyrosine 200 mg • Choline (Bitartrate) 80 mg • Inositol 50 mg • DMAE 80 mg • Acetyl-L-Carnitine 50 mg • Phosphatidyl Serine 20 mg • Vitamin E 10 IU • Vitamin C 10 mg • Ginkgo Biloba 30 mg • Siberian Ginseng 40 mg • Korean Ginseng 40 mg • Gota Kola 100 mg • Phosphatidyl Choline 250 mg • Copper Sebacate 1 mg • Beta Carotene 2000 IU • Vitamin B1 10 mg • Thiamine Tetrahydro-Furfuryl Disulfide 5 mg • Vitamin B2 (Riboflavin) 10 mg • B2 Activated (Riboflavin 5 Phosphate) 5 mg • Vitamin B3 (Niacin) 5 mg • Vitamin B3 (Niacinamide) 30 mg • Calcium Pantothenate 40 mg.

Brainwash Shampoo - Evergreen Research
Active Ingredients: Ginkgo Biloba • Grape Seed Extract. Other Ingredients: Peppermint Oil, Calendula Oil, Arnica.

Brave Hart Deer Velvet Capsules - Hart Products
Deer Velvet 300 mg.

Breast Care System-3 - Natrol
Calcium 24 mg • Calcium D-Glucarate 200 mg. Breast Care Formula: Selenium 50 mcg • Green Tea Extract 50 mg • Garlic 50 mg • Grape Seed Extract 20 mg. Ultra Green Breast Care Ingredients: Rice Powder, Silica, Magnesium Stearate, Gelatin.
See Editor's Note No. 21, page 1818.

Breast Essentials - Swanson
Two capsules contain: Calcium (from calcium d-glucarate) 24 mg • Selenium (as selenomethionine) 100 mcg • SoyLife Soy extract (3% soy isoflavones) 400 mg • Calcium D-Glucarate 200 mg • Green Tea extract (48% polyphenols) 200 mg • Rosemary leaf extract (6% rosemaric acid) 200 mg • Citrus Bioflavonoids (Citrus aurantium; 25% bioflavonoids) 100 mg • Boron (from boron aspartate) 3 mg.

Breast Health - ProHerbs
Two tablets contain: Vitamin C (as Ascorbic Acid) 200 mg • Selenium (as Selenomethionine) 200 mcg • Broccoli extract (20:1 extract) 170 mg • Curcumin root extract (Curcuma longa standardized to 2% curcuminoids) 600 mg • Genistein (Soy extract) 20 mg • Citrus

Bioflavonoids 100 mg • Flaxseed powder 400 mg. Other Ingredients: Dicalcium Phosphate, Microcrystalline Cellulose, Croscarmellose Sodium, Stearic Acid, Magnesium Stearate, Hydroxypropylmethylcellulose, Mineral Oil, Triacetin, Titanium Dioxide, FD&C Yellow #6 Lake.

Breast Health Formula - Great American Nutrition
Two capsules contain: Calcium (as calcium d-glucarate) 24 mg • Selenium (as selenomethionine, from SelenoMax) 100 mcg • Calcium D-Glucarate 200 mg • Green Tea leaf extract (Camellia sinensis, standardized to 48% polyphenols) 200 mg • Rosemary folia extract (Rosemarinus officialis, standardized to 6% rosemaric acid) 200 mg • Soy extract (standardized to 3% isoflavones) 400 mg • Citrus peel bioflavonoids (Citrus aurantium, standardized to 25% bioflavonoids) 100 mg • Boron Aspartate 3 mg. Other Ingredient: White Rice powder.

Breath Aid - D & E Pharmaceuticals
Each tablet contains: Ephedrine 12.5 mg • Guaifenesin 100 mg.

Breath Easy - Traditional Medicinals
Contains: Pseudoephedrine: 0.5 mg per cup as it naturally occurs in the whole Ma Huang herb (Ephedra sinisa) present in the blend. Other herbal ingredients: Peppermint leaf, Licorice root, Fennel seed, Eucalyptus leaf, Pleurisy root, Calendula flower, Ginger rhizome.

Breathe-Aid Formula - Nature's Way
Two capsules contain: Proprietary Formula: Chickweed leaf & stem • Ephedra HCL • Guafinesin • Lobelia herb • Marshmallow root • Mullein leaf. Other ingredients: Gelatin, Magnesium Stearate, Millet.

Breathe-Eze - Bio-Organics
Each capsule contains: Inula helenium (Elecampane) root & rhiz dry 500 mg • Grindelia robusta (Grindelia) herb fl. dry 400 mg • Thymus vulgaris (Thyme) herb fl. dry 300 mg • Glycyrrhiza glabra (Licorice) root & stolon dry 250 mg • Euphorbia hirta (Euphorbia) herb dry 40 mg.

BreatheSmart - Health Smart Vitamins
Each capsule contains: Vitamin C (ascorbic acid) 150 mg • Piper longum fruit (1.5% piperine, 1.5 mg) 100 mg • Picrorhiza kurroa root (4%-5% kutkin, 2 mg - 2.5 mg) 50 mg • Quercetin 50 mg • Ginkgo leaf (24% ginkgo flavonglycosides, 9.6 mg; 6% terpene lactones, 2.4 mg) 40 mg • Tylophora asthmatica leaf (0.1%- 0.25% tylophorine alkaloids, 0.03 mg - 0.075 mg) 30 mg • Serratiopeptidasse 7.5 mg.

Brewer's Yeast - Nature's Life
Twelve tablets contain, based on a typical analysis: Vitamin B1 1 mg • Vitamin B2 1 mg • Vitamin B6 240 mg • Choline 23 mg • Folic Acid 120 mcg • Niacin 3 mg • Inositol 23 mg • Pantothenic Acid 600 mcg • Calcium 360 mcg • Chromium 9 mcg • Copper 300 mcg • Iodine 18 mcg • Iron 2 mg • Magnesium 6 mg • Manganese 30 mcg • Phosphorus 8 mg • Potassium 10 mg • Selenium 12 mcg • Sodium 460 mcg • Zinc 600 mcg. Twelve tablets also supply 2.9 g of protein as follows: Alanine 216 mg • Arginine 155mg • Aspartic Acid 302 mg • Cysteine 72 mg • Glycine 148 mg • Glutamic Acid 402 mg • Histidine (essential amino acid) 78 mg • Isoleucine (essential amino acid) 140 mg • Leucine (essential amino acid) 222 mg • Lysine(essential amino acid) 234 mg • Methionine (essential amino acid) 43 mg • Phenylalanine (essential amino acid) 135 mg • Proline 140 mg • Serine 150 mg • Threonine (essential amino acid) 143 mg • Tryptophan (essential amino acid) 50 mg • Tyrosine 81 mg • Valine (essential amino acid) 179 mg • "plus all the remaining nutrients found in yeast."

Brewer's Yeast - The Vitamin Shoppe
Typical analysis per six tablets: Vitamin B1 48 mg • Vitamin B2 16 mg • Niacin 1.6 mg • Folic Acid 13 mcg • Vitamin B6 160 mcg •

BRAND NAMES

Choline 15 mg • Pantothenic Acid 200 mcg • Biotin 20 mcg • Inositol 15 mg. No Corn, Wheat, Soy, Salt, Sugar, Starch, Milk, Eggs, Fish or Animal Derivatives, Preservatives, Artificial Colors of Flavors added.

Brigham Tea - Nature's Way
Two capsules contain: Brigham Tea herb 830 mg. Other Ingredients: Gelatin, Magnesium stearate, Millet.

Brighten-Up - Changes - TwinLab
Two caplets contain: St. John's Wort standardized extract aerial parts (0.3% hypericin) 300 mg • Panax Ginseng root standardized extract (4% ginsenosides) 200 mg • Ashwagandha root (Withania somnifera) 200 mg • Green Tea leaf standardized extract (20% methylxanthines) 150 mg • Kava Kava root standardized extract (30% kavalactones) 50 mg • Siberian Ginseng root standardized extract (0.8% eleutherosides) 50 mg • Schizandra berry standardized extract (9% schizandrins) 50 mg. Other Ingredients: Dicalcium Phosphate, Vegetable Cellulose, Fractionated vegetable oil, Soy polysaccharides, Silica, and Vegetable resin glaze.

Bright-Eyes - Futurebiotics
Three tablets contain: Bilberry extract (standardized for 25% anthocyanidins) 10 mg • Eyebright (extract equivalent to) 500 mg • Chamomile (extract equivalent to) 250 mg • Rosemary (extract equivalent to) 200 mg • Beta Carotene 20,000 IU • Vitamin A 5000 IU • Quercetin 100 mg • Citrus bioflavonoids 100 mg • Vitamin C 1000 mg • Natural Vitamin E (d-alpha succinate) 200 IU • Vitamin B2 (riboflavin) 40 mg • Rutin 100 mg • Selenium (from selenomethionine) 100 mcg • Zinc (monomethionine) 15 mg • Vitamin B6 5 mg • Niacinamide 10 mg • Pantothenic Acid (B5) 40 mg • Chromium (GTF) 200 mcg • L-Cysteine 100 mg • L-Glutamine 75 mg. In a base of: Alfalfa, Carrot, Parsley & Dandelion.

Bromelain - Source Naturals
One tablet contains: Bromelain (2000 GDU per g) 500 mg.

Bromelain Complex - PhytoPharmica
Two capsules contain: Vitamin C (calcium ascorbate) 225 mg • Pantothenic Acid (calcium D-pantothenate) 125 mg • Bromelain (1,800 M.C.U.) enzymes derived from pineapple stems 750 mg.

Bromelain Forte - Ortho Molecular Products
Each capsule contains: Bromelain 1200 GDU • Papain 110 MCU.

Bromelain Joint-Ease - Nature's Life
Four capsules contain: Bromelain [an enzyme from Pineapple fruit (Ananassa sativa) activity of 1500 mg = 3000 GDU (4500 MCU)] 1500 mg • Quercetin (Dimorphandra pod) 400 mg • Vitamin C (Ascorbic Acid) 750 mg • Zinc (Picolinate, Gluconate, Citrate) 15 mg • Copper (Gluconate, Citrate) 1 mg • Manganese (Citrate, Aspartate) 3 mg.

Bromelain Plus - Enzymatic Therapy
Each tablet contains: Vitamin C (Calcium Ascorbate) 225 mg • Pantothenic Acid (D-Calcium Pantothenate) 125 mg. Other ingredients: Bromelain (1800 MCU) pineapple enzyme 750 mg. Contains no sugar, salt, yeast, wheat, corn, soy, dairy products, coloring, flavoring or preservatives.

Bromezyme - Progressive Labs
Each capsule contains: Bromelain 50 mg • Papain 20 mg • Raw Spleen concentrate 20 mg • Raw Calf Thymus 10 mg.
See Editor's Note No. 14, page 1817.

Bronchitis Remedy - PhytoPharmica
Twenty drops contain: Antimonium tartaricum 4x • Ipecacuanha 4x • Pimpinella saxifraga 2x • Cetraria islandica 1x • Eucalyptus globulus 1x. In a base of 45% USP alcohol by volume.
See Editor's Note No. 1, page 1816.

Bronchoril - PhytoPharmica
Each tablet contains: Glycerol Guaiacolate 200 mg • Fenugreek Seed Powder 4:1 (Trigonella foenum-graecum) 350 mg • Marshmallow Extract 4:1 (Althaea officinalis; Mucilage content 30%-40%) 125 mg • PABA (Para-Aminobenzoic Acid) 50 mg • Mullein Leaf (Verbascum nigrum) 50 mg.

B-Stress with Siberian Ginseng and Coenzymes - Nature's Way
Two capsules contain: Biotin (biotin triurate) 300 mcg • Calcium Pantethonate 150 mg • Choline Bitartrate 50 mg • Chromium Picolinate 200 mcg • Folic Acid (folate) 400 mcg • Inositol 100 mg • Niacin (Vitamin B3) 25 mg • Niacinamide 100 mg • PABA (para aminobenzoic acid) 50 mg • Pyridoxine HCl 100 mg • Riboflavin (Vitamin B2) 40 mg • Siberian Ginseng root 250 mg • Thiamine (Vitamin B1) 50 mg • Vitamin B12 (Cyanocobalamin) 100 mcg • Vitamin C (Ascorbic Acid) 500 mg.

Buckley's Mixture - W.K. Buckley Limited
Each teaspoonful (15 mL) contains: 12.5 mg of Dextromethorphan Hydrobromide in a sugar-free base.

Buckley's Mixture Cough Suppresant - W.K. Buckley
Each teaspoonful (5 mL) contains: Dextromethorphan Hydrobromide 12.5 mg • Ammonium Carbonate • Camphor • Canada Balsam • Carrageenan • Glycerine • Menthol • Pine Needle Oil • Sodium Butylparaben • Sodium Propylparaben • Sodium Saccharin • Tincture of Capsicum • Water.

Buffered C Powder 2000 mg - The Vitamin Shoppe
One teaspoon contains: Vitamin C (calcium ascorbate) 2000 mg • Rose Hips 1450 mg • Acerola 1000 mg • Lemon Bioflavonoids 500 mg • Rutin 25 mg • Hesperidin 25 mg • Calcium (ascorbate) 230 mg. No Yeast, Wheat, Corn, Soy, Salt, Sugar, Starch, Gluten, Dairy, Milk, Eggs, Fish Or Animal Derivatives, Preservatives, Artificial Colors or Flavors added.

Buffered TLC - Jarrow Formulas
Two teaspoons contain: Vitamin C 3000 mg • Calcium 450 mg • Magnesium 250 mg • Potassium 99 mg • L-Taurine 1,000 mg • L-Lysine 250 mg • L-Proline 250 mg • Bromelain (2,000 mcu) 300 mg. Other Ingredients: Ribose, Mannitol, L-Glycine, Natural Lime and Mandarin flavors.

Burdock - Nature's Way
Two capsules contain: Burdock root 1.08 g.
Other Ingredients: Gelatin, Magnesium stearate.

Burdock-Dandelion Formula - Quest
Each caplet contains: Burdock root powder (Arctium lappa) 90 mg • Dandelion root powder (Taraxacum officinale) 90 mg • Oregon Grape root powder (Mahonia aquifolium) 90 mg • Red Clover blossoms powder (Trifolium praetense) 90 mg • Echinacea angustifolia root powder (Echinacea angustifolia) 30 mg • Yellow Dock root powder (Rhumex) 30 mg • Cayenne powder (Capsicum) 20 mg • Kelp powder (Fucus vesiculosis) 20 mg • Licorice root powder (Glycirrhiza glabra) 5 mg. Other Ingredients: Calcium Phosphate, Microcrystalline Cellulose, Vegetable Stearin, Croscarmellose Sodium, Magnesium Stearate (vegetable source).

Burn It - ANS
Chromium Picolinate • Vitamin E • Selenium • Zinc.

Butchers Broom - Now
Two capsules contain: Butchers Broom 5:1 extract (rascus aculeatus) (root) 200 mg. Other Ingredients: Rice Flour. Contains no sugar, salt, yeast, wheat, corn, soy, egg, or milk.

BRAND NAMES

Butcher's Broom - Source Naturals
Each tablet contains: Butcher's Broom 500 mg.

Butcher's Broom - Nature's Way
Two capsules contain: Butchers Broom root 940 mg. Other Ingredients: Gelatin, Magnesium stearate.

C + Herbs - Jarrow Formulas
Each tablet contains: Silymarin (Silybum marianum) 30:1 Concentrate (standardized to 80% silybin) 75 mg • PicroLiv (3.5- 4% Kutkin from Picrorrhiza kurroa) 50 mg • Astragalus Root 6:1 Concentrate 150 mg • Schisandra 5:1 Concentrate 75 mg • Scutelluria root (Skullcap) 4:1 concentrate 150 mg • Vitamin C (Ascorbic Acid) 500 mg.
Other Ingredients: Magnesium Stearate. Contains no soy, yeast, corn, sugar, starch, or artificial color, flavor, preservatives, or other common allergen.

C Aspa Scorb - Progressive Labs
Each teaspoon (5100 mg) supplies: Vitamin C 4000 mg • Magnesium (from magnesium ascorbate and magnesium aspartate) 250 mg • Zinc (from zinc ascorbate) 30 mg • Selenium (from selenium ascorbate) 50 mcg • Manganese (from manganese ascorbate) 4.2 mg • Potassium (from potassium ascorbate and potassium aspartate) 96 mg.

C&F Formula - Dial Herbs
Vinegar • Glycerine • Honey • the Tinctures of Garlic, Comfrey, Wormwood, Marshmallow, White Oak bark, Black Walnut, Mullein, Scullcap, Uva Ursi, Lobelia.

C-1000 - Biodelivery Nutritional Systems
Each tablet contains: Vitamin C (Calcium Ascorbate-Niascorbate) 1000 mg • Bioflavonoids 100 mg • Pantethine 5 mg • NT Factor tablet base 50 mg.

C-1000-TR - Atrium Inc.
Each tablet contains: Vitamin C 1000 mg • Naturally Associated Bioflavonoid Complex 100 mg.

C-500 - Biodelivery Nutritional Systems
Each tablet contains: Vitamin C (Calcium Ascorbate-Niascorbate) 500 mg • Bioflavonoids 100 mg • Pantethine 5 mg • NT Factor tablet base 50 mg.

CAC Tabs - Dial Herbs
Cascara Sagrada • Buckthorn • Burdock • Chaparral • Dandelion • Licorice root • Barberry • Red Clover.

Cactus (Nopal) - Natural Dynamics
Each capsule contains: Nopal 650 mg.

Cactus Diet - Cactu-Life
Each capsule contains: Opuntia Streptacantha 500 mg.

Cal Burst - Nature Made
Each soft chew contains: Calcium Carbonate (providing Elemental Calcium 500 mg) 1250 mg • Vitamin D 200 IU. Other Ingredients: Corn Syrup, Calcium Carbonate, Sugar, Hydrogenated Coconut Oil, Cocoa (Chocolate Flavor only), Nonfat Dried Milk, Glycerin, Corn Starch, Salt, Lecithin, Natural and Artificial Flavors.
See Editor's Note No. 5, page 1816.

Cal/Mag Balance - Nutri-Quest
Each tablet contains: Calcium Aspartate 175 mg • Calcium Citrate 175 mg • Magnesium Aspartate 175 mg • Magnesium Glycinate 175 mg • Vitamin C 25 IU • Vitamin D 20 mg of HCL.

Cal-1000 Complete - Puritan's Pride
Two tablets contain: Vitamin A (as Retinyl Acetate) 5,000 IU • Vitamin C (as Ascorbic Acid) 60 mg • Vitamin C (as Cholecalciferol) 400 IU • Vitamin E (as dl-Alpha Tocopheryl Acetate) 30 IU • Thiamin (Vitamin B-1; as Thiamine Mononitrate) 1.5 mg • Riboflavin (Vitamin B-2) 1.7 mg • Niacin (as Niacinamide) 20 mg • Vitamin B-6 (as Pyridoxine Hydrochloride) 2 mg • Folic Acid 400 mcg • Vitamin B-12 (as Cyanocobalamin) 6 mcg • Biotin (as d-Biotin) 300 mcg • Pantothenic Acid (as d-Calcium Pantothenate) 10 mg • Calcium (as Calcium Carbonate) 1,000 mg • Iron (as Ferrous Fumarate) 18 mg.

Cal-Acid Complex - Atrium Inc.
Four tablets contain: Calcium (from Oyster Shell, Oyster Shell-Citrus Juice Complex, & Calcium Caseinate) 750 mg • Magnesium (from Magnesium Citrus Juice Complex & Oxide) 210 mg • Manganese (Manganese-Citrus Carbonate Juice Complex) 5 mg • Copper (as Gluconate) 0.1 mg • Vitamin D (Fish oil) 400 USP IU • Vitamin C with Rose Hips 40 mg • Vitamin E 10 IU • Betaine HCL & Glutamic Acid HCL sufficient to provide dilute HCL 10 min. Amino Acids, Peptids, & Polypetids from Hydrolized Soy Protein with Lecithin & Alfalfa juice concentrate. Contains no sugar, starch, salt, wheat or corn derivatives.

Cal-Acid Maxi - Atrium Inc.
Four tablets contain: Calcium (Calcium Citrate, Calcium Caseinate & Oyster Shell) 1500 mg • Magnesium (Magnesium Citrus Juice Complex & Oxide) 500 mg • Manganese (Manganese Citrus Carbonate Juice) 10 mg • Vitamin D (Fish oil) 500 IU • Vitamin C with Rose Hips 100 mg • Vitamin E (d-Alpha Tocopherol) 20 IU • Horsetail (Silica) 250 mg • Boron (Citrate) 3 mg. Betaine HCL & Glutamic Acid HCL sufficient to provide dilute HCL. Amino acids, peptids & polypeptids from hydrolyzed soy protein with Lecithin & Alfalfa juice concentrate. Contains no sugar, starch, salt, wheat, yeast or corn derivatives.

Calamacin - MMS Pros
Each capsule contains: Scullcap herb • Wood Betony • Black Cohosh root • Hops flowers • Valerian root • Cayenne.

Calcet Triple Calcium - Mission Pharmacal
Two tablets contain: Vitamin D (Vitamin D3; as cholecalciferol) 200 IU • Calcium (as calcium carbonate, calcium gluconate, calcium lactate) 300 mg. Other Ingredients: Polyethylene Glycol, HPMC, Croscarmellose Sodium, Color, Magnesium Stearate, FD & C Yellow 5 Lake, Magnesium Silicate, Carnauba Wax.

Cal-Chew Calcium 350 mg - Jamieson
Each tablet contains: Calcium (as Calcium Carbonate, Calcium Citrate, Calcium Malate, Calcium Succinate, Calcium Aspartate, Calcium Glutamate, Calcium Fumarate) 350 mg • Iron 0.4 mg.

Calcimate - GNC
Two tablets contain: Vitamin D (as cholecalciferol) 200 IU V Calcium (as calcium citrate malate) 500 mg • Magnesium (as magnesium oxide) 125 mg • Zinc (as zinc oxide) 8 mg • Copper (as cupric oxide) 1 mg • Boron (as boron citrate) 1 mg. Other Ingredients: Cellulose.

Calcimate Plus 800 - GNC
Vitamin D 200 IU • Calcimate (calcium citrate malate) 800 mg • Magnesium 100 mg • Potassium 99 mg.
See Editor's Note No. 5, page 1816.

Calcium - Natrol
Three tablets contain: Calcium 500 mg • Magnesium (Calcium & Magnesium are bound Krebs Cycle Carriers) 200 mg • Fruitbase 640 mg. Other ingredients: Mono- and Di-Glycerides, Croscarmellose Sodium, Silicon Dioxide, Stearic Acid, Magnesium Stearate.

Calcium - Animal Parade - Nature's Plus
Two tablets contain: Calcium (as aminoate complex) 250 mg • Magnesium (as aminoate complex) 50 mg.
See Editor's Note No. 5, page 1816.

BRAND NAMES

Some Brand Name Natural Products - What they Contain
www.NaturalDatabase.com contains MANY more listings than appear here.

Calcium & Magnesium - Source Naturals
Each tablet contains: Calcium (from 1,250 mg of Amino Acid Chelate) 250 mg • Magnesium (from 625 mg of Amino Acid Chelate) 125 mg • Vitamin D (Cholecalciferol) 500 IU.

Calcium & Magnesium - Nature's Way
Three capsules contain: Calcium (citrate, carbonate, malate) 500 mg • Magnesium (oxide, aspartate) 250 mg • Sodium 5 mg. Other Ingredients: Cellulose, Gelatin, Magnesium Stearate.

Calcium & Magnesium Complex - Health Smart Vitamins
Three caplets contain: Calcium (as 80% calcium citrate, 19% calcium carbonate, 1% calcium stearate) 503 mg • Magnesium (as 50% magnesium citrate, 50% magnesium glycinate) 250 mg.

Calcium + D, Natural Source - Leiner Health Products
Each tablet contains: Calcium Carbonate 600 mg • Vitamin D (Cholecalciferol) 200 IU. Other Ingredients: Maltodextrin, Hydroxypropyl Methylcellulose, Talc, Croscarmellose Sodium, Acacia, Hydroxypropyl Cellulose, Titanium Dioxide, Silicon Dioxide, Starch, Magnesium Stearate, Polysorbate 80, Polyethylene Glycol 3350, Sodium Citrate, Yellow 6 Lake.

Calcium and Magnesium with Zinc - Nature Made
Each tablet contains: Calcium Carbonate 333 mg • Magnesium Oxide 133 mg • Zinc Sulfate 5 mg. Other Ingredients: Maltodextrin, Croscarmellose Sodium, Silicon Dioxide, Magnesium Stearate, Hydroxypropyl Methylcellulose, Cellulose, Polyethylene Glycol. See Editor's Note No. 5, page 1816.

Calcium Ascorbate - Atrium Inc.
Each tablet contains: Vitamin C (Ascorbic Acid) 1000 mg.

Calcium Ascorbate C-Complex 1000 mg - The Vitamin Shoppe
Each 1000 mg capsule contains: Vitamin C as calcium ascorbate 750 mg • Citrus Bioflavonoids 100 mg • Hesperidin 50 mg • Rutin 25 mg • Calcium 75 mg. No Yeast, Wheat, Corn, Dairy, Soy, Salt, Sugar, Starch, Milk, Eggs, Gluten, Preservatives, Artificial Colors or Flavors added.

Calcium Ascorbate Crystals - Nature's Life
Each teaspoon contains: Vitamin C (Calcium Ascorbate) 3240 mg • Calcium (Calcium Ascorbate) 360 mg.

Calcium Citrate Plus Vitamin D - Progressive Labs
Four tablets contain: Calcium (as calcium citrate) 3240 mg • Calcium (Calcium Ascorbate) 360 mg.

Calcium Citrate with Zinc & Magnesium - Now
Two tablets contain: Vitamin D (Fish oil) 100 IU • Calcium (Citrate) 600 mg • Magnesium (Oxide, Aspartate) 300 mg • Zinc (Amino Acid Chelate) 15 mg • Manganese (Amino Acid Chelate) 5 mg • Copper (Amino Acid Chelate) 1 mg.

Calcium Effervescent - Progressive Labs
Two tablets contain: Calcium (from calcium carbonate) 1000 mg • Vitamin D (as cholecaciferol) 400 IU. Ingredients: Citric Acid, Calcium Carbonate, Sorbitol, Sodium Bicarbonate, Sodium Carbonate, Magnesium Carbonate, Aspartame, Mineral oil, Natural Orange flavor, Cholecalciferol. Contains Phenylalanine.

Calcium Lactate - Puritan's Pride
Three tablets contain: Calcium (as calcium lactate trihydrate) 250 mg.

Calcium Magnesium Phosphorus Superabsorbeze - Nature's Life
Each tablespoon contains: Calcium (Calcium Phosphate) 600 mg • Magnesium (Hydroxide, Carbonate) 300 mg • Vitamin D (as Vitamin D3) (Cholecalciferol) 200 IU. In a natural base of Purified Water, Citric Acid, Sorbital, natural Orange flavor & Cellulose.

Calcium Magnesium Superabsorbeze - Nature's Life
Each tablespoon contains: Calcium (Citrate, Lactate/Gluconate) 600 mg • Phosphorus (Calcium Phosphate) 600 mg • Magnesium (Hydroxide, Carbonate) 300 mg • Vitamin D (as Vitamin D3) (Cholecalciferol) 200 IU. In a natural base of Purified Water, Citric Acid, Fructose, natural Orange flavor, Cellulose & Ascorbic Acid.

Calcium Magnesium Zinc - Nature's Life
Three tablets contain: Calcium (Carbonate, Citrate/Malate) 1000 mg • Magnesium (Oxide, Citrate) 600 mg • Zinc (Picolinate, Citrate) 15 mg • Copper (Gluconate, Citrate) 1 mg • Silicon (Dioxide) 20 mg • Boron (Citrate) 100 mcg • Glutamic Acid HCl 100 mg. In a natural base of Springtime Horsetail Herb (Equisetum arvense).

Calcium Night - Source Naturals
Four tablets contain: Calcium (Citrate, Malate, Carbonate, Fumarate and Ascorbate) 600 mg • Magnesium (Oxide, Malate, Citrate, Fumarate and Ascorbate) 600 mg • Vitamin C (Magnesium and Calcium Ascorbate, Ascorbic Acid, and Manganese Ascorbate) 275 mg • Vitamin B-6 (Pyridoxine HCl) 20 mg • Vitamin D-3 (Cholecalciferol) 200 IU • Folic Acid 200 mcg • Silica (Horsetail Silica extract) 9 mg • Manganese (Ascorbate) 6 mg • Boron (Amino Acid Chelate) 3 mg • Copper Sebacate 1 mg.

Calcium Plus Vitamin D & Minerals - Leiner Health Products
Each tablet contains: Manganese Sulfate 1.8 mg • Calcium Carbonate 600 mg • Copper (Cupric Oxide) 1 mg • Vitamin D (Cholecalciferol) 200 IU • Zinc Oxide 7.5 mg • Magnesium Oxide 40 mg • Boron 250 mcg. Other Ingredients: Maltodextrin, Hydroxypropyl Methylcellulose, Titanium Dioxide, Magnesium Stearate, Sodium Borate, Red 40 Lake, Yellow 6 Lake, Blue 1 Lake, and may contain less than 2% of Cellulose, Talc, Starch, Mineral Oil, Croscarmellose Sodium, Hydroxypropyl Cellulose, Silicon Dioxide, Polyethylene Glycol 8000, Polysorbate 80, Sodium Lauryl Sulfate, Polyethylene Glycol 3350, Crospovidone, Gelatin, Stearic Acid.

Calcium Xtra - Puritan's Pride
Three tablets contain: Vitamin A (as Retinyl Acetate) 4,000 IU • Vitamin C (as Ascorbic Acid) 100 mg • Vitamin D (as Cholecalciferol) 400 IU • Calcium (as Calcium Carbonate) 1,000 mg • Iron (as Ferrous Gluconate) 10 mg • Magnesium (as Magnesium Oxide) 500 mg.

Calcium/Magnesium with Vitamin D - Jamieson
Each caplet contains: Vitamin D (as Cholecalciferol) 133 IU • Calcium (as Calcium Carbonate, Calcium Citrate, Calcium Succinate, Calcium Asparate, Calcium Glutamate, Calcium Furmarate) 333 mg • Magnesium (as Magnesium Oxide, Magnesium Citrate, Magnesium Malate, Magnesium Succiante, Magnesium Asparate, Magnesium Glutamate, Magnesium Fumarate) 167 mg.

Calcium-Magnesium - Biodelivery Nutritional Systems
Each tablet contains: Calcium (Citrate) 250 mg • Magnesium (Oxide) 250 mg • NT Factor tablet base 200 mg.

Calcium-Magnesium Complex - The Vitamin Shoppe
Four tablets provide: Calcium 1500 mg • Magnesium 420 mg • Vitamin D 1000 IU • Vitamin E 20 IU • Vitamin C 80 mg • Manganese 10 mg. Plus Betaine HCl and Glutamic Acid HCl. In a base containing: Hydrolyzed Soy Protein, Lecithin, and Alfalfa Powder.

Calcium-Magnesium for Children - The Vitamin Shoppe
Each tablet contains: Calcium 200 mg • Magnesium 100 mg.

BRAND NAMES

Calcium-Magnesium-Zinc - The Vitamin Shoppe
Three tablets contain: Elemental Calcium 1500 mg • Elemental Magnesium 750 mg • Elemental Zinc 45 mg.

CalciWise - Resource Wellness
One chew contains: Calories 20 • Calories from Fat 5 • Total Fat 0.5 g • Total Carbohydrate 4 g • Sugars 3 g • Vitamin A 1,000 IU • Vitamin D 200 IU • Vitamin K 40 mcg • Riboflavin 0.8 mg • Calcium 600 mg • Sodium 10 mg. Other Ingredients: Corn Syrup, High Fructose Corn Syrup, Sweetened Condensed Skim Milk, Sugar, Chocolate Liqueur, High Oleic Sunflower Oil, Cocoa (Processed with Alkali), Glycerol Monostearate, Salt, Artificial Flavor, Maltodexrin, Soy Lecithin.

Calendula Oil - Blessed Herbs
Calendula flower & Organic Cold-Pressed Olive oil.

Calendula Salve - Dial Herbs
Calendula • Chamomile • Mullein. In a base of Beeswax, Glycerine & Cold Pressed Olive oil.

Calgest - PhytoPharmica
Two capsules contain: Vitamin C (ascorbic acid/rose hips) 100 mg • Vitamin B6 (pyridoxine HCl) 50 mg • Calcium chloride 192 mg • Calcium phosphate 180 mg • Magnesium glycerophosphate 104 mg • Betaine HCl 192 mg • Ammonium chloride 192 mg • Kidney extract (freeze-dried) 60 mg • Mixed bioflavonoids (citrus) 60 mg. See Editor's Note No. 14, page 1817.

Calm Aid Formula - Nature's Way
Two capsules contain: Blue Vervain stem, leaf, flower, fruit 150 mg • Chamomile flower 75 mg • Kava (dried extract 30% Kavalactones) 350 mg • L-5 Hydroxytryptophan (Griffonia bean extract) 5 mg • Niacin (Vitamin B3) 6.66 mg • Passion flower stem, leaf, flower, fruit 75 mg • Riboflavin (Vitamin B2) 568 mcg • Scullcap herb 60 mg • Thiamine (Vitamin B1) 500 mcg • Vitamin B12 (Cyanocobalamin) 2 mcg • Vitamin B6 (Pyridoxine HCL) 660 mcg • Wood Betony stem, leaf, flower 100 mg. Other ingredients: Gelatin, Magnesium Stearate, Millet.

Calm Thoughts - Source Naturals
Three tablets contain: Kava root extract (Piper methysticum) (Standardized to 30% kavalactones yielding 105 mg of kavalactones) 350 mg • Siberian Ginseng root 200 mg • Bacopa Monniera leaf extract (Standardized to 20% bacosides yielding 20 mg of bacosides) 100 mg • Lemon Balm herb 100 mg • St. John's Wort extract (Hypericum perforatum) (50 mg Standardized to 0.3% hypericin and 50 mg 4:1 extract) 100 mg • Valerian root 60 mg • Ashwagandha root 50 mg • Ginger root 50 mg • Licorice root extract (4:1) 50 mg • Ginkgo Biloba leaf extract (50:1) (Standardized to 24% Ginkgo flavone glycosides and 6% terpene lactones) 30 mg • Schizandra fruit 30 mg • Vitamin C (as Ascorbic Acid) 100 mg • Vitamin B1 (Thiamin) 25 mg • Vitamin B2 (Riboflavin) 25 mg • Niacinamide 25 mg • Vitamin B6 (Pyridoxine HCl) 25 mg • Vitamin B12 (Cyanocobalamin) 25 mcg • Vitamin B5 (Pantothenic Acid) 50 mg • Calcium (as Calcium Citrate) 100 mg • Magnesium (275 mg Magnesium Oxide and 25 mg Magnesium Taurinate) 300 mg • Zinc (as Zinc Citrate) 15 mg • Manganese (as Manganese Citrate) 3 mg • GABA (Gamma Amino Butyric Acid) 500 mg • Taurine (as Magnesium Taurinate) 300 mg • L-Tyrosine (200 mg as L-Tyrosine and 50 mg N-Acetyl L-Tyrosine) 250 mg.

Calm Thoughts Kava - Source Naturals
Three tablets contain: Kava root extract (Piper methysticum) standardized to 30% Kavalactones, Yielding 105 mg to Kavalactones 350 mg • Siberian Ginseng root 200 mg • Bacopa monniera leaf extract, standardized to 20% Bacosides, Yielding 20 mg of Bacosides 100 mg • Lemon Balm herb 100 mg • St. John's wort extract (Hypericum perforatum) 50 mg standardized to 0.3 % Hypericin and 50 mg 4:1 extract 100 mg • Valerian root 60 mg • Ashwagandha root

50 mg • Ginger root 50 mg • Licorice root extract (4:1) 50 mg • Ginkgo Biloba leaf extract (50:1) standardized to 24% Ginkgo Flavone Glycosides and 6% Terpene Lactones 30 mg • Schizandra fruit 30 mg • Vitamin C (as Ascorbic Acid) 100 mg • Vitamin B1 (Thiamin) 25 mg • Vitamin B2 (Riboflavin) 25 mg • Niacinamide 25 mg • Vitamin B6 (Pyridoxine HCl) 25 mg • Vitamin B12 (Cyanocobalamin) 25 mcg • Vitamin B5 (Pantothenic Acid) 50 mg • Calcium (as Calcium Citrate) 100 mg • Magnesium (275 mg Magnesium Oxide and 25 mg Magnesium Taurinate) 300 mg • Zinc (as Zinc Citrate) 15 mg • Manganese (as Manganese Citrate) 3 mg • GABA (Gamma Amino Butyric Acid) 500 mg • Taurine (as Magnesium Taurinate) 300 mg • L-Tyrosine (200 mg as L-Tyrosine and 50 mg N-Acetyl-l-Tyrosine) 250 mg.

CAL-MAG - The Vitamin Shoppe
Each tablet contains: Calcium 500 mg • Magnesium 250 mg.

Cal-Mag Boron - Puritan's Pride
Three tablets contain: Calcium (as Calcium Carbonate, Calcium Citrate and Calcium Gluconate) 1,000 mg • Magnesium (as Magnesium Oxide, Magnesium Citrate, and Magnesium Gluconate) 400 mg • Boron (as Boron Citrate) 3 mg.

Cal-Mag Chewable - Quest
Each tablet contains: Elemental Calcium (Citrate, Phosphate) 300 mg • Elemental Magnesium (Citrate, Oxide) 150 mg • Vitamin D (as Vitamin D3) 100 IU. Other Ingredients: Sorbitol, Silicon Dioxide, Magnesium Stearate, Sucralose and Spearmint Flavor.

Cal-Mag Citrate - Puritan's Pride
Four tablets contain: Calcium (as Calcium Carbonate, Calcium Aspartate) 1,000 mg • Magnesium (as Magnesium Oxide and Magnesium Citrate) 500 mg.

Cal-Mag Potassium - Puritan's Pride
Two tablets contain: Calcium (carbonate, citrate, asparate) 500 mg • Magnesium (oxide, citrate, aspartate) 500 mg • Potassium (gluconate, aspartate, citrate) 99 mg.

CAL-MAG w/Zinc and Vitamin D - Dial Herbs
Vitamin D • Calcium from Gluconate & Lactate • Magnesium • Zinc • Aqueous Extracts from: Hibiscus, Chamomile, Fennel, Spinach • Fructose • Mango Juice • Orange Juice • Natural Flavor • Locust Seed Flour.

Cal-Mag-Zinc - Puritan's Pride
Three tablets contain: Calcium (as Calcium Carbonate and Calcium Gluconate) 1,000 mg • Magnesium (as Magnesium Oxide and Magnesium Gluconate) 400 mg • Zinc (as Zinc Gluconate and Zinc Citrate) 25 mg.

Cal-Mag-Zinc Liquid - Metabolic Response Modifiers
Each tablespoon contains: Vitamin D (as Vitamin D3 cholecalciferol) 400 IU • Calcium (tri-calcium phosphate citrate, gluconate, lactate) 600 mg • Magnesium (hydroxide, carbonate) 300 mg • Phosphate (tri-calcium phosphate) 300 mg • Zinc (citrate) 22.5 mg • Potassium (citrate) 50 mg.

Cal-Min - Progressive Labs
Each tablet contains: Calcium (as calcium proteinate) 300 mg. In a base of mixed vegetable concentrate from: Cultured Peas, Lentils, Buckwheat, Millet, and Chlorophyll, carefully dried to preserve their natural trace nutrient and enzyme content.

CalmingBlend - Rexall
Each capsule contains: Ashwaganda root extract (standardized to 1.5% withanolides, 3 mg; standardized to 1% alkaloids, 2 mg) 200 mg • Valerian root extract (standardized to 0.8% valerenic acid,

0.5 mg) 67 mg • Proprietary Blend: Kava Kava root, German Chamomile flower head, Hops (strobiles) 133 mg. Other Ingredients: Gelatin.

CalmTabs - Puritan's Pride
Four tablets contain: Valerian root 258 mg • Passiflora flower 258 mg • Celery seed 258 mg • Catnip leaf 258 mg • Hops flower 129 mg • Dried Orange Peel 129 mg.

Calorad - Essentially Yours Industries Corp.
Demineralized Water • Collagen Hydrolysat • Aloe Vera • Vegetal Glycerin • Potassium Sorbate • Citrus Extracts • Natural Peach Flavor.

Cal-Para - Atrium Inc.
Each tablet contains: Alkalinizing Calcium Lactate 325 mg • Calcium Aspartate (supplying Elemental Calcium 52) 80 mg • Magnesium Aspartate 75 mg • Magnesium Citrate (supplying Elemental Magnesium 21 mg) 70 mg.

Calsorb - PhysioLogics
Three caplets contain: Calcium (80% Citrate, 20% Carbonate) 500 mg • Magnesium (50% Citrate, 50% Glycinate) 250 mg.

Calsure - Rexall
Each tablet contains: Calcium 250 mg. Other Ingredients: Stearic Acid, Titanium Dioxide, Silica, Magnesium Stearate, Hydroxypropyl Methylcellulose, Microcrystalline Cellulose.

Cal-Sym - Atrium Inc.
Each tablet contains: Acidifying Calcium Phosphate 100 mg • Calcium Ascorbate 50 mg • Calcium Aspartate (supplies Elemental Calcium 34 mg compounded to insure acidic pH) 35 mg • Ammonium Chloride 100 mg • Betaine HCL 12 mg • Glutamic Acid HCL120 mg.

Caltrate 600 + Soy - Whitehall-Robbins Healthcare
Two tablets contain: Soy Isoflavones 50 mg • Calcium 1200 mg • Vitamin D 400 IU.

Caltrate Plus - Lederle Consumer Health Division
Each tablet contains: Vitamin D 200 IU • Calcium 600 mg • Magnesium 40 mg • Zinc 7.5 mg • Copper 1 mg • Manganese 1.8 mg • Boron 250 mcg. Other Ingredients: Maltodextrin, Cellulose, Mineral Oil, Hydroxypropyl Methylcellulose, Titanium Dioxide, Sodium Lauryl Sulfate, Cupric Oxide, FD&C Red No. 40, FD&C Yellow No. 6, FD&C Blue No. 1, Gelatin, Crospovidone, Stearic Acid, Magnesium Stearate.

Canadian Ginseng - Jamieson
Each capsule contains: Canadian Ginseng whole root (Panax quinquefolium) (Containing a minimum of 5% Ginsenosides 250 mg).

Candicidal - Source Naturals
Each capsule contains: Brevibacterium linens 2 billion cells • Vitamin B-6 (pyridoxine HCl) 10 mg • Methionine 200 mg.

Candid Care - Natrol
Two capsules contain: Zinc 9 mg • FOS 500 mg • Garlic 100 mg • Undecylenic Acid (as Zinc undecylenate acid) 50 mg • Citrus extract, dried powder from grapefruit Seed 25 mg. Other ingredients: Microcrystalline Cellulose, Silicon Dioxide, Magnesium Stearate, Gelatin

Candida Formula - Enzymatic Therapy
Each capsule contains: Oregano oil extract (Origanum vulgare) 0.1 ml • Thyme oil extract (Thymus vulgaris) 0.05 ml • Peppermint oil extract (Mentha piperita) 0.05 ml • Goldenseal root (Hydrastis canadensis) standardized to contain 5% total Alkaloids including: Berberine, Hydrastine, & Canadine 50 mg. Developed in accordance with the recommendations & safety standards set forth by the German Kommission E. Contains no sugar, salt, yeast, wheat, corn, dairy products, flavoring or preservatives.

Candida Forte - Nature's Plus
Two softgels contain: Safflower oil 1000 mg • Vitamin C (Ascorbate) 500 mg • L-Cysteine free form amino acid 100 mg • Zinc (Ascorbate) 50 mg • Pau D'Arco 50 mg • Vitamin B6 (Pyridoxine HCL) 50 mg • Acidophilus (Lactobacillus) supplying 80 million viable cells 20 mg • Vitamin A Fish Liver oil 10000 IU • Beta Carotene supplying 15000 IU Vitamin A activity 9 mg • Garlic equivalent to 500 mg of fresh garlic 1 mg • Biotin 100 mcg • Free Form Amino Acid Complex containing 198.08 mg: L-Glutamine 40.8 mg, L-Lysine 25 mg, L-Leucine 20.2 mg, L-Proline 16.2 mg, L-Valine 14 mg, L-Serine 12.6 mg, L-Isoleucine 11 mg, L-Phenylalanine 9.32 mg, L-Threonine 8.64 mg, L-Arginine 7.3 mg, L-Alanine 6.28 mg, L-Aspartic Acid 7 mg, L-Methionine 6.08 mg, L-Histidine 5.74 mg, L-Glycine 3.52 mg, L-Tyrosine 3 mg, L-Cysteine 1.4 mg. In a natural herbal base of black walnut. Contains no yeast, wheat, corn, soy, milk, salt, sugar or starch.

Candimyacin - PhytoPharmica
Each capsule contains: Oregano oil extract (Origanum vulgare) 0.1 ml • Thyme oil extract (Thymus vulgaris) 0.05 ml • Peppermint oil extract (Mentha piperita) 0.05 ml • Goldenseal root extract (Hydrastis canadensis) standardized to contain 5% total alkaloids including berberine, hydrastine, and canadine 50 mg.

Candistatin - PhysioLogics
Two capsules contain: Calcium (as Calcium Caprylate) 65 mg • Magnesium (as 92% Magnesium Caprylate, 8% Magnesium Stearate) 79 mg • Caprylic Acid (as 63% Magnesium Caprylate, 37% Calcium Caprylate) 800 mg • Goldthread root (10% Alkaloids, 10 mg) 100 mg • Pau D'Arco bark & stem (3% Napthoquinones 1.8 mg) 60 mg.

Candistroy - Nature's Secret
Two tablets contain: Zinc tannates • Barberry root extract • Goldenseal root • Pau d'Arco bark • Oregon Grape root • Peppermint oil • Orange peel • Licorice root • Cinnamon bark • Clove buds • Thyme leaf • Allicin.

Caprylate Complex - Progressive Labs
Three capsules contain: Caprylic Acid (as caprylate) 1290 mg • Calcium (as caprylate) 100 mg • Magnesium (as caprylate) 50 mg • Zinc (as caprylate) 5 mg.

CapsiCool Cayenne - Nature's Way
Two capsules contain: Proprietary Formula: Cayenne pepper fruit • Ginger • Glucomannan root. Other ingredients: Gelatin.

Carb Explosion - Orange - Rexall
Each scoop contains: Vitamin A 3000 IU • Vitamin C (Ascorbic Acid) 6 mg • Vitamin D (Cholecalciferol) 40 IU • Vitamin E (dl-Alpha Tocopheryl Acetate) 3 IU • Thiamin Mononitrate (Vitamin B-1) 0.15 mg • Riboflavin (Vitamin B-2) 0.17 mg • Niacin (Niacinamide) 2 mg • Vitamin B-6 (Pyridoxine HCl) 0.2 mg • Folic Acid 40 mcg • Vitamin B-12 (Cyanocobalamin) 0.6 mcg • Biotin 30 mcg • Pantothenic Acid (Calcium D-Pantothenate) 1 mg • Electrolytic Iron 1.8 mg • Phosphorus 50 mg • Iodine 0.15 mg • Magnesium Phosphate Dibasic 40 mg • Zinc Oxide 1.5 mg • Copper Gluconate 0.2 mg • Chromium Polynicotinate 90 mcg • Sodium Chloride 100 mg • Potassium Chloride 75 mg • Carb Explosion Enzyme Blend: Glucoamylase, Malt Diastase, Amylase, Phytase, Hemicellulase, Beta-Glucanase 250 mg. Other Ingredients: Crystalline Fructose, Maltodextrin, Dextrose, Natural and Artificial Orange Flavor, Citric Acid, Malic Acid, Dicalcium Phosphate, Beta-Carotene, Potassium Iodide.

BRAND NAMES

Carba-E-A-C - Atrium Inc.

Each rounded teaspoon contains approximately: Vitamin A Acetate 4000 IU • Vitamin C from Ascorbic Acid 100 mg • Vitamin E 33 IU. In a carrier of Carbamide (food grade).

Carbo Fuel (Complex Carbohydrate Peak Performance Energy Drink) - TwinLab

Each serving contains: Carbohydrates (from Glucose Polymers & Crystalline Pure Fructose) (no high fructose corn syrups are present) 80 grams. Other Ingredients: Vitamin B1 • Vitamin B2 • Vitamin B3 • Vitamin B6 • Pantothenic Acid • Biotin • Potassium • Magnesium • Yeast-Free GTF Chromium • Inosine • L-Carnitine • CoQ10 • Lipoic Acid • Pantetheine • Pyridoxine-Alpha-Ketoglutarate • Soluble Potassium (Phosphate & Succinates) • Citrates • Aspartates • Fumarates • Malates • Alpha-Ketoglutarates.

Carbo-Meta - Atrium Inc.

Each tablet contains: Pyridoxal-5-Phosphate 20 mg • Pyridoxine HCL 50 mg • Chromium Aspartate 500 mcg • Magnesium 50 mg • Manganese 5 mg • Zinc Aspartate 15 mg.

Cardio 150 - Atrium Inc.

Each tablet contains: Raw Heart concentrate (not an extract) of Bovine source 150 mg.
See Editor's Note No. 14, page 1817.

Cardio 20 - Futurebiotics

Six capsules supply: Beta-carotene 25,000 IU • Vitamin C (buffered ascorbate)1000 mg • Vitamin E (natural) 400 IU • Niacin (timed release, flush-free) 250 mg • Choline Bitartrate 150 mg • Inositol 75 mg • Calcium (ascorbate) 250 mg • Magnesium (oxide, chelate) 400 mg • Potassium (gluconate) 99 mg • Coenzyme Q10 15 mg • L-Carnitine 100 mg • Taurine 100 mg • Procyanidol 35 mg • Hawthorn berries (4:1 extract) 250 mg • Soy Isoflavone extract 100 mg • Cholestatin Beta-sitosterol complex 250 mg • Garlic (pure-gar 1500 deodorized concentrate) 400 mg • Cayenne 100 mg • Ginger 50 mg • Chlorella 250 mg. "Procyanidol is a concentrated, solvent-free, whole grape extract containing high levels of flavonoid polyphenols."

Cardio Chelate - Nutri-Quest

Six tablets contain: Vitamin A (Palmitate) 3000 IU • Beta Carotene 7500 IU • Vitamin D (as Vitamin D3) 100 IU • Vitamin C (Sago) 300 mg • Vitamin B1 30 mg • Vitamin B2 30 mg • Vitamin B6 75 mg • Vitamin B12 500 mcg • Biotin 200 mcg • Niacin 60 mg • D-Calcium Pantothenate (Pantothenic Acid) 150 mg • Folic Acid 300 mcg • Vitamin E (Succinate) 300 IU • Iodine (Kelp) 100 mcg • PABA 100 mg • Lecithin 120 mg • Choline Bitartrate 250 mg • Cysteine HCL 250 mg • L-Methionine 75 mg • L-Lysine 100 mg • Bromelaine 30 mg • Lemon Bioflavonoid 900 mg • Rutin 30 mg • Inositol 75 mg • Garlic 120 mg • Cayenne 30 mg • Hawthorne berries 100 mg • Pancreatin 6X 25 mg • Thymus 30 mg • Spleen 30 mg • Heart 30 mg • Adrenal (Nutritrophic) 30 mg • Whole Pituitary 30 mg • Papain 30 mg • L-Glycine 75 mg • Calcium Gluconate 37 mg • Manganese Chelate 2.5 mg • Copper Gluconate 7.8 mcg • Molybdenum Chelate 12 mcg • Chromium Chelate 102 mcg • Selenium Chelate 30 mcg • Calcium Ascorbate 100 mg • Calcium Aspartate 100 mg • Potassium Aspartate 25 mg • Magnesium Ascorbate 75 mg • Magnesium Aspartate 75 mg • Ferrous Gluconate 15 mg • Zinc Aspartate 15 mg. In a base containing: Calcium Phosphate, Magnesium Phosphate, Calcium Flouride, Ferric Phosphate, Kali Phosphate, Silica, Chiorinum, Peppermint leaves, Black Cohosh, Scullcap, Licorice root, Watercress, Siberian Ginseng, Red Beet root, Parsley.
See Editor's Note No. 14, page 1817.

Cardio Complex - Leiner Health Products

Each softgel contains: Vitamin E (dl-Alpha Tocopherol and d-Alpha Tocopherol) 400 IU • Folate (Folic Acid) 400 mcg • Vitamin B12

(Cyanocobalamin) 6 mcg • Vitamin B6 (Pyridoxine Hydrochloride) 2 mg. Other Ingredients: Gelatin, Vegetable Oil, Glycerin, Yellow Beeswax, Unbleached Lecithin, Titanium Dioxide, Dicalcium Phosphate, Red 40.

Cardio EDTA Chelate - Olympia Nutrition

EDTA 400 mg • MSM 100 mg • NAC 50 mg • Vitamin C 100 mg.

Cardio Flow - Progressive Labs

Six capsules contain: Vitamin A (retinyl palmitate) 10,000 IU • Vitamin C (ascorbic acid and zinc ascorbate) 640 mg • Elemental Potassium (from Potassium Aspartate 684 mg, from Potassium Orotate 300 mg) 210 mg • Elemental Magnesium (from Magnesium Aspartate 1400 mg, from Magnesium Orotate 714 mg) 330 mg • Elemental Zinc (from Zinc Ascorbate 168 mg) 25 mg • Elemental Selenium (Selenium Ascorbate 70 mg) 70 mcg • Sodium 28 mg • EDTA (Ethylenediamine tetra-acetic acid) 800 mg • Disodium EDTA 200 mg • L-Glutathione, reduced 20 mg • Bromelain (2000 GDU) 300 mg • Papain (525 TU/mg) 30 mg • Cilantro (coriander) 500 mg • Butcher's Broom 150 mg • Cardio Flow 600 mg: a proprietary blend of the following extracts: [Inula racemosa (root), Saussurea lappa (root), Terminalia arjuna (root), Desmodium gingatic (leaves), Commiphora mukul (resin), Bacopa monniera (leaves), Convolvulous pluricaulis (leaves)]. Other Ingredients: Rice flour, Magnesium Stearate.

Cardio Guardian - Clinician's Choice

Three tablets contain: Vitamin C (ascorbic acid) 180 mg • Vitamin E (dl-alpha tocopheryl acetate) 400 IU • Niacin (niacinamide) 300 mg • Niacin 100 mg • Vitamin B6 (pyridoxine hydrochloride) 23 mg • Folate (folic acid) 600 mcg • Vitamin B12 (cyanocobalmin) 150 mcg • Magnesium (glycinate) 15 mg • Zinc (gluconate) 15 mg • Selenium (aspartate) 120 mcg • RoseOx (patented, standardized process for an extract of Rosemary) 150 mg • Hawthorn 4:1 Extract 150 mg • Triphala Extract (Sstd. 40% tannin) 90 mg • White Willow Bark 60 mg • Motherwort 4:1 Extract 30 mg • L-Carnitine 30 mg • Seacol 30 mg • Linoleic Acid, Gamma Linolenic Acid (sunflower oil, borage oil) 30 mg • Proprietary blend: Grape Powder, Cayenne Fruit, Coenzyme Q10 45 mg.

Cardio Plus - Atrium Inc.

Three tablets contain: Vitamin E Acetate 300 IU • Vitamin C (with Rose Hips) 60 mg • Thiamine Mononitrate 15 mg • Vitamin B2 Riboflavin 2 mg • Niacin 100 mg • Vitamin B6 15 mg • Vitamin B12 2 mcg • Magnesium (as Citrus Juice Complex & Oxide) 100 mg • Zinc (as Gluconate) 5 mg • Potassium (as Citrus Juice Complex & Chloride) 99 mg • Chromium (amino acid complex) 10 mcg • Selenium (in yeast) 48 mcg • Choline Bitartrate 66 mg. In a base containing Lecithin 80 mg, Para Aminobenzoic Acid 30 mg, Inositol 4 mg, Cold Processed Heart Protein 90 mg.
See Editor's Note No. 14, page 1817.

Cardio ProtoChol - Fields of Nature

Each capsule contains: Vitamin E (as D-Alpha Tocopheryl Acid Succinate) 10 IU • Niacin Powder 3 mg • Soybean Isoflavones extract (Novasoy) (Isoflavones 13 mg) 33 mg • Garlic bulb extract (Allicin 333 mcg) 33 mg • Guggulipids Extract (Guggulsterones 0.8 mg) 33 mg • Red Rice Yeast Extract (Lovastain 134 mcg) 33 mg • Lemon Bioflavonoids Complex 10 mg • Chitosan Powder 50 mg. Other Ingredients: Calcium Carbonate, Hydroxymethyl Propylcellulose, Magnesium Stearate, Silicon Dioxide.

Cardio Q10 - PhysioLogics

Each capsule contains: Vitamin E (as d-Alpha Tocopherol) 200 IU • Calcium (as Dicalcium Phosphate) 2 mg • Selenium (as Selenomethionine) 25 mcg • Coenzyme Q10 30 mg.

Cardio Q10 - Health Smart Vitamins

Two capsules contain: Vitamin E (as d-alpha tocopheryl acetate)

542 IU • Calcium (as dicalcium phosphate) 3 mg • Selenium (as selenonmethionine) 50 mcg • Coenzyme Q10 60 mg.

Cardio Results - Changes - TwinLab
Two caplets contain: Vitamin B6 (as Pyridoxine HCl) 15 mg • Folate (as Folic acid) 400 mcg • Vitamin B12 (as Cyanocobalamin) 250 mcg • Red Yeast rice (from fermentation of Monascus pupureus Went) 600 mg • Purified Soy phytosterols (45-55% Beta-Sitosterol) 50 mg. Other ingredients: Dicalcium phosphate, Vegetable cellulose, Fractionated vegetable oil, Soy polysaccharides, Silica, and Vita-Lok vegetable resin glaze.

Cardio Support Formula - The Vitamin Factory
Each tablet contains: Vitamin E (d-Alpha Tocopheryl-Succinate) 100 IU • Folic Acid 100 mcg • White Willow bark extract 4:1 100 mg • Hawthorne berry extract 50 mg • Coenzyme Q10 30 mg • Oat Beta Glucan powder (min 18%) 25 mg • Pycnogenol (Maritime Pine bark extract) 15 mg.

Cardio Tonic - Puritan's Pride
Three caplets contain: Coenzyme Q10 20 mg • Vitamin E 100 IU • Vitamin C 300 mg • Folic Acid 400 mcg • Niacin (Vitamin B3) 20 mg • Vitamin B6 (pyridoxine) 50 mg • Calcium 100 mg • Magnesium 100 mg • Potassium 99 mg • Selenium Proteinate 150 mcg • L-Carnitine 50 mg • L-Taurine 300 mg • Garlic 100 mg • Hawthorn berry 5:1 50 mg • Lecithin 50 mg • Ginger 25 mg.

Cardio•Logic - Wakunaga of America Co., Ltd.
Each capsule contains: Vitamin E (d-alpha-tocopheryl acid succinate) 50 IU • Vitamin B6 5 mg • Folate (as folic acid) 200 mg • Vitamin B12 100 mg • Aged Garlic extract power (bulb) 200 mg • L-Carnitine 30 mg • Coenzyme Q10 30 mg • Alpha Lipoic Acid 30 mg. Other Ingredients: Cellulose, Colloidal Silica, and Magnesium Stearate (vegetable source).

Cardio-Basics - Rexall
Two tablets contain: Vitamin A (100% as beta-carotene) 2500 IU • Vitamin C (as ascorbyl palmitate and ascorbic acid) 300 mg • Vitamin D (as cholecalciferol) 200 IU • Vitamin E (as d-alpha-tocopheryl acid succinate) 200 IU • Thiamin (as thiamin mononitrate) 10 mg • Riboflavin (Vitamin B-2) 10 mg • Niacin (as niacinamide and niacin) 65 mg • Vitamin B-6 (as pyridoxine HCl) 15 mg • Folic Acid 130 mcg • Vitamin B-12 (as cyanocobalamin) 30 mcg • Biotin 100 mcg • Pantothenic Acid (as calcium d-pantothenate) 60 mg • Calcium 50 mg • Phosphorus 20 mg • Magnesium (as magnesium oxide) 60 mg • Zinc (as zinc oxide) 10 mg • Selenium (as sodium selenate) 30 mcg • Copper (as cupric oxide) 0.5 mg • Manganese (as manganese sulfate) 2 mg • Chromium (as chromium amino acid chelate) 15 mcg • Molybdenum (as molybdenum yeast chelate) 6 mcg • Sodium 5 mg • Potassium (as potassium chloride) 30 mg • L-Proline 150 mg • L-Lysine HCl 150 mg • L-Arginine HCl 50 mg • L-Carnitine Tartrate 50 mg • L-Cysteine HCl 50 mg • Inositol 50 mg • Coenzyme Q-10 10 mg • Pycnogenol Pine Bark extract 10 mg.
Other Ingredients: Cellulose, Tricalcium Phosphate, Croscarmellose Sodium, Stearic Acid, Povidone, Dicalcium Phosphate, Silica, Pharmaceutical Glaze, Magnesium Stearate, Hydroxypropyl Methylcellulose, Hydroxypropyl Cellulose, PEG.

Cardio-Chelate - Metabolic Response Modifiers
Each capsule contains: EDTA (Ethylenediamine-Tetra-Acetic acid) 400 mg • MSM (Methyl-Sulfonyl-Methane) 100 mg • NAC (N-Acetyl-Cysteine) 50 mg • Vitamin C (ascorbic acid) 100 mg.

Cardiogarl - Olympian Labs
Three capsules contain: Ginkgo Biloba leaf extract 120 mg • Garlic extract 600 mg • Bilberry extract 150 mg • Coenzyme Q10 60 mg • Hawthorn Berry extract 210 mg.

Cardio-Glycan - PhytoPharmica
Each capsule contains: Glycosaminoglycans (GAGs) Highly purified bovine-derived glycosaminoglycans 50 mg.
See Editor's Note No. 14, page 1817.

Cardiotrate - Progressive Labs
Each capsule contains: Raw Bovine heart concentrate 140 mg prepared by a special process which does not exceed physiological temperature (37º C). Guaranteed to be free of chemical pesticides and synthetic hormones.
See Editor's Note No. 14, page 1817.

Cardio-Vite - Atrium Inc.
Each tablet contains: Vitamin B1 2.2 mg • Vitamin B2 2.2 mg • Vitamin B6 50 mg • Pantothenic Acid 50 mg • Niacinamide 15 mg • Magnesium 50 mg • Potassium 50 mg.

Caribbean Tanning Secret - Futurebiotics
One tablet contains: Vitamin C 13 mg • Vitamin B 625 mg • Copper Gluconate 0.7 mg • Para Amino Benzoic Acid (PABA) 13 mg. In a base containing: L-tyrosine, Aloe Vera, Carrot powder, & Yucca powder.

Carni Fuel - TwinLab
Each capsule contains: Carni Fuel L-Carnitine Magnesium Citrate 500 mg • L-Carnitine 200 mg • Magnesium 30 mg.

Carni Fuel (L-Carnitine Liquid Concentrate) - TwinLab
Each tablespoonful (15 ml) contains: L-Carnitine 1000 mg.

Carni Lean - Sports Nutrition Source.com
Each capsule contains: L-Carnitine 1000 mg.

Carotenoid Complex - The Vitamin Shoppe
Each softgel contains: Phytofluene 0.033 mg • Lycopene (LYC-O-MATO) 5 mg • Lutein 5 mg • Beta-carotene (6251 IU Vitamin A) 3.75 mg • Alpha-carotene (1042 IU Vitamin A) 1.25 mg • Zeaxanthin 0.26 mg • Phytoene 0.098 mg. In a base of tomato and carrot concentrate.

Carpal-X - Olympian Labs
Two capsules contain: Vitamin C 120 mg • Vitamin B-6 (pyridoxine HCl) 100 mg • Vitamin B-2 (riboflavin) 10 mg • Zinc 5 mg • Copper 500 mcg • Proprietary Blend: Grape Seed extract, CoQ10, White Willow Bark extract, Horse Chestnut extract, Cayenne Pepper, Enzyme blend (protease, lipase, amylase), Sea Cucumber, Yucca, Devil's Claw, Boswellia Serrata extract, Curcumin extract 795 mg.

Cartilade - BioTherapies, Inc.
Shark Cartilage.

Cartilage Care - PhysioLogics
Each capsule contains: Vitamin C (as Ascorbic Acid) 60 mg • Manganese (as Manganese Glycinate) 2 mg • Glucosamine Sulfate 200 mg • Chondroitin Sulfate 100 mg • Glucosamine Hydrochloride 100 mg • Sea Cucumber 100 mg.
See Editor's Note No. 15, page 1817.

Cartilage Companion - PhysioLogics
Each capsule contains: Glucosamine Sulfate 200 mg • Chondroitin Sulfate 67 mg • Methylsulfonylmethane (MSM) 333 mg.
See Editor's Note No. 15, page 1817.

Cartilage Formula - Pharmanex
Two capsules contain: Vitamin C (Ascorbic Acid) 100 mg • Vitamin E (d-Alpha Tocopheryl Succinate, Beta, Delta, Gamma Tocopherols) 50 IU • Zinc (Zinc Propionate) 7.5 mg • Boron (Boron Citrate) 3 mg • Glucosamine (Glucosamine Sulfate, Glucosamine Hydrochloride) 750 mg • Boswellia Serrata extract (Min. 95% Boswellic Acids)

BRAND NAMES

BRAND NAMES

150 mg • Tumeric extract (Min. 95% Curcumin) 100 mg • Quercetin 25 mg • Rutin 25 mg. Other Ingredients: Silicon Dioxide, Magnesium Stearate.

Cata-Comp - Enzymatic Therapy
Two capsules contain: Vitamin A (Beta Carotene) non-toxic form of Vitamin A 10000 IU • Vitamin E (D-Alpha Tocopherol Succinate) 75 IU • Vitamin C (Ascorbic Acid) 500 mg • Zinc (Picolinate) 10 mg • Manganese (Picolinate) 2 mg • Riboflavin (Vitamin B2) 2 mg • Selenium selenomethionine 75 mcg • Other ingredients: Hachimijiogan Herbal Complex 200 mg • Curcuma root extract [(Curcuma longa) standardized to contain 97% Curcumin] 100 mg • L-Cysteine 50 mg • L-Glutamine 50 mg • L-Glycine 50 mg. Contains no sugar, salt, yeast, wheat, corn, dairy products, coloring, flavoring, or preservatives.

Catnip - Nature's Way - Nature's Way
Two capsules contain: Catnip (stem, leaf, flower) 760 mg. Other Ingredients: Gelatin.

Catnip and Fennel - Dial Herbs
Catnip • Peppermint • Fennel • Lobelia.

Catnip and Peppermint - Dial Herbs
Catnip • Peppermint • Lobelia.

Cat's Claw - Nature's Way
Three capsules contain: Cat's Claw bark 1.45 g. Other Ingredients: Gelatin, Magnesium stearate, Millet.

Cat's Claw - Olympian Labs
Each capsule contains: Cat's Claw (uncaria tomentosa) 500 mg.

Cat's Claw 5000 - Now
Each capsule contains: Cat's Claw (Uncaria tomentosa) (Inner bark) 15:1 standardized extract equivalent 333 mg. Other Ingredients: Stearic Acid. Contains no yeast, wheat, corn, soy, milk, or preservatives.

Cat's Claw Caplet - Leiner Health Products
Each caplet contains: Cat's Claw extract (Uncaria tomentosa) 250 mg. Other Ingredients: Calcium Carbonate, Cellulose, Maltodextrin, Hydroxypropyl Methylcellulose, Silicon Dioxide, Polyethylene Glycol 3350, Croscarmellose Sodium, Hyroxypropyl Cellulose, Pharmaceutical Glaze, Crospovidone, Magnesium Stearate, Yellow 5 Lake, Blue 1 Lake, Polysorbate 80, Titanium Dioxide.

Cat's Claw Defense Complex - Source Naturals
Four tablets contain: Cat's Claw inner bark (Uncaria Tomentosa) 2000 mg • Whole-Leaf Aloe Vera powder (200:1 Concentrate) 200 mg • Proanthodyn (from Grape Seed extract) 60 mg • Quercetin 400 mg • Green Tea extract 40 mg • Turmeric root extract (Yielding 95% Curcumin) 400 mg • Silymarin (Milk Thistle seed extract) 50 mg • Reishi Mycelia biomass 200 mg • Shiitake Mycelia biomass 200 mg • Maitake Mycelia biomass 150 mg • Astragalus root 200 mg • St. John's Wort herb extract 100 mg • St. John's Wort herb powder 100 mg • Siberian Ginseng root 100 mg • Siberian Ginseng root extract 100 mg • Schizandra berries 200 mg • Pau d'Arco bark 100 mg • Pau d'Arco bark extract 100 mg • Isatis leaf 150 mg • Vitamin A (Beta Carotene) 10000 IU • Vitamin C (Ascorbic Acid, Magnesium and Zinc Ascorbates) 350 mg • Magnesium (Ascorbate) 10 mg • Zinc (Ascorbate) 12 mg • N-Acetyl Cysteine 600 mg.

Cayenne - Leiner Health Products
Each softgel contains: Oleoresin Capsicum extract (Oleoresin capsicum) fruit 25 mg. Other Ingredients: Soybean Oil, Gelatin, Glycerin, Beeswax, Lecithin, Caramel, Titanium Dioxide, Red 40, Yellow 6, Blue 1.

Cayenne - Nature's Way
Each capsule contains: Cayenne pepper fruit 450 mg. Other Ingredients: Gelatin.

Cayenne - Now
Each capsule contains: Cayenne Pepper (Capsium Frutescens) 500 mg. Contains no sugar, yeast, wheat, corn, soy, or milk.

Cayenne - Pharmanex
Each capsule contains: Cayenne (Capisicum Annum) (Pepper) (40000 Heat Units) 450 mg. Other Ingredients: Gelatin, Magnesium Stearate, Silicon Dioxide.

Cayenne Extra Hot - Nature's Way
Each capsule contains: Proprietary Formula: Cayenne pepper fruit • Ginger • Hawthorne berry. Other ingredients: Gelatin.

Cayenne, Super - Swanson
Two capsules contain: Cayenne pepper (100,000 heating units) 450 mg • Ginger root powder 200 mg • Hawthorn berry powder 200 mg • Lecithin granules 50 mg.

CCM Calcium - Source Naturals
Each tablet contains: Calcium (from Calcium Citrate and Calcium Malate) 300 mg.

C-Complex 1000 - Puritan's Pride
Each tablet contains: Vitamin C (as Ascorbic Acid and Rose Hips) 1000 mg • Citrus Bioflavonoids 100 mg • Rutin 50 mg • Hesperidin complex 25 mg • Acerola powder 1 mg • Alfalfa leaf powder 1 mg • Barley grass powder 1 mg.

C-Complex 500 - Puritan's Pride
Each tablet contains: Vitamin C (with Rose Hips and other natural sources) 500 mg • Citrus Bioflavonoids 100 mg • Rutin (Buckwheat) 50 mg • Hesperidin complex 25 mg • Acerola 1.0 mg • Alfalfa leaf 1 mg • Barley Grass 1 mg. Other Ingredients: Vegetable Stearic Acid, Cellulose Coating, Silica, Vegetable Magnesium Stearate. See Editor's Note No. 4, page 1816.

C-Complex/ Bioflavonoids/ Rutin - Nature's Life
Each tablet contains: Vitamin C 500 mg • Lemon Bioflavonoids Complex (natural whole unaltered TESTLAB concentrate containing Hesperidin, Eriocitrin, Flavonols, & Flavones derived from freshly dejuiced Lemons.) 500 mg • Acerola (Malpighia glabra) 50 mg • Hesperidin 50 mg • Rutin (Saphora japonica) 50 mg • Calcium (naturally buffering Calcium Carbonate) 12 mg. In a natural base of Bell Peppers & Rose Hips powder.

CDT CoQ10 - Olympian Labs
Each capsule contains: Crystalline Coenzyme Q10 60 mg.

Celestial Seasonings - Saw Palmetto - Celestial Seasonings
Two capsules contain: Vitamin E (as d-alpha tocopherol acetate) 90 IU • Zinc (as gluconate) 15 mg • Proprietary Blend: Saw Palmetto berries, Saw Palmetto extract, Stinging Nettle root extract 1230 mg.

Celite-Complex 75 - Jamieson
Two capsules contain: Concentrated Citrus Bioflavonoids (Vitamin P) 100 mg • Ginkgo Biloba extract flavoglycoside-rich JGB24 250 mg • Bilberry extract anthocyanoside-rich JMF25 750 mg • Oil of Madagascar Cinnamon 20 mg • South Pacific Sea Kelp extract 25 mg • Bromelain Enzyme (from Pineapple) 100 mg • Kola Nut extract 250 mg. Other Ingredients: Soybean Oil, Vegetable Oil, Gelatin, Glycerin, Lecithin, Purified Water.

Celite-Complex 75-Firming Gel - Jamieson
Water • Glycerin • Butylene Glycol • Kola Nut (Cola acuminata) extract • Coneflower (Echinacea purpurea) extract • Propylene Glycol

• Butylene Glycol • Camellia oleifera extract • Arnica montana extract • Dimethylsilanol Hyaluronate • Jojoba Esters • Butcher's Broom (Rucus aculeatus) extract • Kelp (Macrocystis pyrifera) extract • Imidazolidinyl Urea • Triethanolamine • Carbomer • Methyl Paraben • Ethyl Paraben • Fragrance.

Cell Boost with IP-6 - Ultimate Nutrition
Two capsules contain: Calcium 101 mg • Phosphorous 195 mg • Calcium Magnesium Phytate (Inositol Hexaphosphate) 1000 mg.

Cell Forte with IP-6 - Enzymatic Therapy
Each capsule contains: IP-6 (inositol hexaphosphate, from rice) 400 mg • Inositol (from rice) 110 mg. Contains no sugar, salt, yeast, wheat, gluten, corn, soy, dairy products, coloring, flavoring or preservatives.

Cell Guard - Source Naturals
Three tablets contain: Vitamin A (beta carotene 15000 IU and palmitate 10000 IU) 25000 IU • Vitamin B-1 (thiamin) 10 mg • Vitamin B-2 (riboflavin) 10 mg • Niacin 30 mg • Vitamin B-5 (calcium D-Pantothenate) 50 mg • Vitamin B-6 (pyridoxine HCl) 30 mg • Vitamin B-12 (cyanocobalamin) 100 mcg • Vitamin C (ascorbic acid, magnesium and calcium ascorbates) 2000 mg • Vitamin E D-alpha Tocopheryl (natural) 400 IU • Folic acid 800 mcg • Calcium (ascorbate) 30 mg • Copper (sebacate) 1 mg • Magnesium (ascorbate, citrate, succinate and oxide) 120 mg • Selenium (from high-selenium yeast and sodium selenite) 200 mcg • Zinc (OptiZinc zinc monomethionine) 30 mg. Other ingredients: N-Acetyl Cysteine 300 mg, N,N-Dimethyl Glycine HCl 150 mg, Coenzyme Q10 (ubiquinone) 30 mg, Herbal blend (unique) 600 mg.

Cell Strength - Source Naturals
Each tablet contains: Calcium ethanolamine phosphate 600 mg.

Cell Strength - Source Naturals
Four tablets contain: Phosphorus 460 mg • Calcium 300 mg.

Cell U Less - Olympian Labs
Each capsule contains: Grape Seed extract 50 mg • Bladderwrack extract 100 mg • Gotu Kola extract 300 mg • Horse Chestnut extract 100 mg.

Cella Free - Bodyonics
Six tablets contain: Herbal BioModulators [From Evening Primrose Oil (contains Gamma Linolenic Acid (GLA)], Borage (Seed Oil), Bladderwreck Extract, Dried Fucus Vesiculosus Extract, Fish Oil [containing the Omega-3 polyunsaturated fatty acids EPA (eicosapentaenoic acid) and DHA (docosahezaenoic acid)], Grape Seed Extract, Bioflavonoids, Soya Lecithin, Fatty Acids, Dried Sweet Red Clover Extract (Mellotus Officinals) (Tri Folium pratense) (Standardized to 1% biochanina), Dried Ginkgo Biloba Extract (Standardized to contain flavonglycosides) 1000 mg • Protein/Fiber BioModulators (From a mixture of Bioactive Oligopeptides prepared from food grade proteins by means of Enzymatic Hydrolysis of Bovine Globin Proteins, Casein and Wheat Protein. Plus Fibrabind (Chitosan) a naturally occuring fiber extracted from shellfish with vegetable pupl and citrus pectin (grapefruit)) 1750 mg • Therma/ Fluid Balance BioModulators (From UVA URSI Standardized to contain 120 mg of Hydroxyquinone and Yerba Mate Standardized to contain 300 mg Methyl Xanthines) 1000 mg. Other Ingredients: Calcium Carbonate, Stearic Acid, Croscarmellose, Magnesium Stearate. See Editor's Note No. 14, page 1817.

Cellasene - Thompson Nutritional Products
Three softgels contain: Iodine 720 mcg • Cellasene Lipovascolen 702 mg • Cellasene support blend 1230 g. Other Ingredients: Bladderwrack extract, Grape seed extract, Sweet Clover extract, Ginko Biloba, Borage, Fish oil, Soya Lecithin.

Cell-FX - HerbTech
Each capsule contains: Shark Cartilage extract 200 mg.

Cell-FX (Bulk Powder) - HerbTech
Water-soluble concentrated Shark Cartilage 227 mg.

Cell-FX 500 mg - HerbTech
Each capsule contains: Shark Cartilage extract 500 mg.

CELL-Tech - Muscletech
Each serving contains: Creatine Monohydrate 10 g • Insulin-releasing Dextrose 75 g • Insulin-potentiating Lipoic Acid 200 mg • Chromium Picolinate 300 mcg • Potassium 150 mg • Phosphates 100 mg • Taurine • Magnesium.

Cellular Forte with IP-6 and Inositol - PhytoPharmica
Each capsule contains: IP-6 as Inositol hexaphosphate (rice) 400 mg • Inositol (rice) 110 mg. Contains no sugar, salt, wheat, gluten, corn, soy, dairy products, coloring, flavoring, or preservatives.

Cellular Forte with IP-6 and Inositol, Ultra Strength Powder - PhytoPharmica
Each scoop contains: Calories 10 • Carbohydrate 2 g • IP-6 (Inositol Hexaphosphate) from rice 3,200 mg • Inositol from rice 880 mg.

Cellu-Trim - Enforma Natural Products
Two capsules contain: White Willow bark • Vitamin C (Ascorbic Acid) • Hydragia (root) • Sida Cordifolia • Uva Ursi • Tinospora Cordifolia • Potassium (Chloride).

Cellu-Var Capsules - Enzymatic Therapy/PhytoPharmica
Each capsule contains: Butchers Broom extract (Ruscus aculeatus) standardized to contain 10% Saponins calculated as Ruscogenin 100 mg • Gotu Kola extract (Centella asiatica) standardized to contain 70% of selected Triterpenic Acids: Asiaticoside, Asiatic Acid, & Madecassic Acid from Centella 30 mg • Escin extract (Aesculus hippocastanum) 10 mg.

Cellu-Var Cream - Enzymatic Therapy
Contains: Deionized Water • Horse Chestnut (Escin) extract • Sea Ware extract • Cola vera extract • Rosemary extract in a base of Cholestanol (Dihydrocholesterol), a natural emulsifying agent. Contains no animal products.

Central-Vite Select Formula Plus - Leiner Health Products
Each tablet contains: Folate (Folic Acid) 200 mcg • Iron (Ferrous Fumarate) 9 mg • Phosphorus 48 mg • Vitamin B12 (Cyanocobalamin, USP Method 2) 25 mcg • Magnesium Oxide 100 mg • Molybdenum 160 mcg • Calcium Carbonate 200 mg • Chloride 72 mg • Potassium Chloride and Iodide 80 mg • Manganese Sulfate 3.5 mg • Vitamin A (Acetate) 7500 IU • Vitamin B6 (Pyridoxine Hydrochloride) 3 mg • Vitamin C (Ascorbic Acid) 90 mg • Vitamin E (dl-Alpha Tocopheryl Acetate) 45 IU • Zinc Oxide 22.5 mg • Vitamin K (Phytonadione) 10 mcg • Chromium Chloride 130 mcg • Copper Oxide 2 mg • Iodine 150 mcg • Niacin (Niacinamide) 20 mg • Pantothenic Acid 10 mg • Riboflavin (Vitamin B2) 1.7 mg • Selenium 70 mcg • Thiamin Mononitrate (Vitamin B1) 1.5 mg • Vitamin D 400 IU • Biotin (USP Method 2) 30 mcg • Boron 150 mcg • Nickel (Nickelous Sulfate) 5 mcg • Silicon Dioxide 10 mcg • Vanadium 10 mcg. Other Ingredients: Dicalcium Phosphate, Gelatin, Cellulose, Starch, Croscarmellose Sodium, Sodium Starch Glycolate, Hydroxypropyl Methylcellulose, Polyethylene Glycol 3350, Tricalcium Phosphate, Magnesium Stearate, Hydroxypropyl Cellulose, Resin, Beta Carotene, Polysorbate 80, Pharmaceutical Glaze, Sodium Metasilicate.

Centrum - Whitehall-Robbins Healthcare
Each tablet contains: Nickel (Nickelous Sulfate) 5.0 mcg • Vitamin A Acetate 5000.0 IU • Tin (Stannous Chloride) 10.0 mcg • Vitamin C (Ascorbic Acid) 60.0 mg • Vitamin D 400.0 IU • Vanadium (Sodium

BRAND NAMES

Metavanadate) 10.0 mcg • Silicon Dioxide 2.0 mg • Vitamin E (dl-Alpha Tocopheryl Acetate) 30.0 IU • Boron (Potassium Borate) 150.0 mcg • Vitamin K (Phytonadione) 25.0 mcg • Thiamin Mononitrate (Vitamin B1) 1.5 mg • Riboflavin (Vitamin B2) 1.7 mg • Niacin (Vitamin B3, Niacinamide) 20.0 mg • Vitamin B6 (Pyridoxine Hydrochloride) 2.0 mg • Folate (Folic Acid) 400.0 mcg • Vitamin B12 (Cyanocobalamin) 6.0 mcg • Biotin 30.0 mcg • Pantothenic Acid (Calcium Pantothenate) 10.0 mg • Calcium Carbonate 162.0 mg • Iron (Ferrous Fumarate) 18.0 mg • Phosphorus (Calcium Carbonate) 109.0 mg • Iodine 150.0 mcg • Magnesium Oxide 100.00 mg • Zinc Oxide 15.0 mg • Selenium (Sodium Selenate) 20.0 mcg • Copper (Cupric Acid) 2.0 mg • Manganese Sulfate 3.5 mg • Chromium 65.0 mcg • Molybdenum 160.0 mg • Chloride 72.0 mg • Potassium Chloride 80.0 mg. Other Ingredients: Microcrystalline Cellulose, Gelatin, Crospovidone, Hydroxypropyl Methylcellulose, Titanium Dioxide, Magnesium Stearate, Stearic Acid, Triethyl Citrate, Polysorbate 80, FD&C Yellow #6.

Centrum Kids - Whitehall-Robbins Healthcare
Each tablet contains: Vitamin A Acetate 5000.0 IU • Sodium 14.0 mg • Vitamin C (Ascorbic Acid and Sodium Ascorbate) 250.0 mg • Vitamin D 400.0 IU • Vitamin E (dl-Alpha Tocopheryl Acetate) 15.0 IU • Thiamin Mononitrate (Vitamin B1) 1.5 mg • Riboflavin (Vitamin B2) 1.7 mg • Niacin (Niacinamide, Vitamin B3) 13.5 mg • Vitamin B6 (Pyridoxine Hydrochloride) 1.0 mg • Folate (Folic Acid) 300.0 mcg • Vitamin B12 (Cyanocobalamin) 5.0 mcg • Calcium Carbonate 108.0 mg • Phosphorus (Calicum Phosphate) 50.0 mg • Zinc Oxide 4.0 mg • Copper (Cupric Oxide) 0.5 mg.
Other Ingredients: Sugar, Mannitol, Mono- and Diglycerides, Microcrystalline Cellulose, Modified Food Starch, Gelatin, Stearic Acid, FD&C Yellow #6 Lake, Food Starch, Aspartame, Carrageenan, Magnesium Stearate, Natural and Artificial Flavors, Guar Gum, FD&C Red #40 Lake, FD&C Blue #2 Lake, Silicon Dioxide, Partially Hydrogenated Coconut Oil, Dextrose, Beta Carotene, Lactose, Acacia.
See Editor's Note No. 4, page 1816.

Centrum Liquid Supplement - Whitehall-Robbins Healthcare
Each tablespoonful (15 mL) contains: Vitamin A Palmitate 2500.0 IU • Vitamin C (Ascorbic Acid) 60.0 mg • Vitamin D (as Vitamin D3) 400.0 IU • Vitamin E (dl-Alpha Tocopheryl Acetate) 30.0 IU • Thiamin Hydrochloride (Vitamin B1) 1.5 mg • Riboflavin 5-Phosphate Sodium (Vitamin B2) 1.7 mg • Niacin (Vitamin B3, Niacinamide) 20.0 mg • Vitamin B6 (Pyridoxine Hydrochloride) 2.0 mg • Vitamin B12 (Cyanocobalamin) 6.0 mcg • Biotin 300.0 mcg • Pantothenic Acid (D-Panthenol) 10.0 mg • Iron (Ferrous Gluconate) 9.0 mg • Iodine (Potassium Iodide) 150.0 mcg • Zinc Gluconate 3.0 mg • Manganese Chloride 2.0 mg • Chromium Chloride 25.0 mcg • Molybdenum (Sodium Molybdate) 25.0 mg. Other Ingredients: Water, Sucrose, Ethyl Alcohol 5.4% w/v, Glycerin, Polysorbate 80, Citric Acid, Sodium Benzoate, D-Panthenol, BHA, Natural and Artificial Flavor, Food Starch, Edetic Acid.

Centrum Performance - Whitehall-Robbins Healthcare
Each tablet contains: Ginseng root extract 50.0 mg • Vitamin A 5000.0 IU • Ginkgo root extract 60.0 mg • Vitamin C 120.0 mg • Vitamin D 400.0 IU • Boron 60.0 mg • Vitamin E 60.0 IU • Nickel 5.0 mcg • Silicon 4.0 mg • Vitamin K 25.0 mcg • Tin 10.0 mg • Thiamin (B1) 4.5 mg • Vanadium 10.0 mcg • Riboflavin (B2) 5.1 mg • Niacin (B3) 40.0 mg • Vitamin B6 6.0 mg • Folate (Folic Acid) 400.0 mcg • Vitamin B12 18.0 mcg • Biotin 40.0 mcg • Pantothenic Acid 10.0 mg • Calcium 100.0 mg • Iron 18.0 mg • Phosphorus 48.0 mg • Iodine 150.0 mcg • Magnesium 40.0 mg • Zinc 15.0 mg • Selenium 70.0 mcg • Copper 2.0 mg • Manganese 4.0 mg • Chromium 120.0 mcg • Molybdenum 75.0 mg • Chloride 72.0 mg • Potassium 80.0 mg.

Centrum Silver - Whitehall-Robbins Healthcare
Boron (Borates) 150.0 mcg • Vitamin E (dl-Alpha Tocopheryl Acetate) 45.0 IU • Vitamin K (Phytonadione) 10.0 mcg • Thiamin Mononitrate (Vitamin B1) 1.5 mg • Riboflavin (Vitamin B2) 1.7 mg •

Niacin (Niacinamide, Vitamin B3) 20.0 mg • Vitamin B6 (Pyridoxine Hydrochloride) 3.0 mg • Folate (Folic Acid) 400.0 mcg • Vitamin B12 (Cyanocobalamin) 25.0 mcg • Biotin 30.0 mcg • Pantothenic Acid (Calcium Pantothenate) 10.0 mg • Calcium Carbonate 200.0 mg • Phosphorus 48.0 mg • Iodine (Potassium Iodide) 150.0 mcg • Magnesium Oxide 100.0 mg • Zinc Oxide 15.0 mg • Selenium (Sodium Selenate) 20.0 mcg • Copper (Cupric Oxide) 2.0 mg • Manganese Sulfate 2.0 mg • Chromium Chloride 150.0 mcg • Molybdenum (Sodium Molybdate) 75.0 mg • Chloride 72.0 mg • Potassium Chloride 80.0 mg. Other Ingredients: Microcrystalline Cellulose, Gelatin, Starch, Crospovidone, Hydroxypropyl Methylcellulose, Titanium Dioxide, Sucrose, Magnesium Stearate, Triethyl Citrate, Lactose, Polysorbate 80, Beta Carotene, Lutein, Glucose, FD&C Yellow No. 6 Lake, FD&C Blue No. 2 Lake, FD&C Red No. 40 Lake.
See Editor's Note No. 3, page 1816.

Centrum with Lutein - Whitehall-Robbins Healthcare
Each tablet contains: Boron (Borates) 120.0 mcg • Vitamin A Acetate 5000.0 IU • Nickel (Nickelous Sulfate) 5.0 mcg • Vitamin C (Ascorbic Acid) 60.0 mg • Silicon Dioxide 2.0 mcg • Vitamin D 400.0 IU • Vitamin E (dl-Alpha Tocopheryl Acetate) 30.0 IU • Tin (Stannous Chloride) 10.0 mcg • Vanadium (Sodium Metavanadate) 10.0 mcg • Vitamin K (Phytonadione) 25.0 mcg • Lutein 250.0 mcg • Thiamin Mononitrate (Vitamin B1) 1.5 mg • Riboflavin (Vitamin B2) 1.7 mg • Niacin (Vitamin B3, Niacinamide) 20.0 mg • Vitamin B6 (Pyridoxine HCl) 2.0 mg • Folate (Folic Acid) 400.0 mcg • Vitamin B12 (Cyanocobalamin) 6.0 mcg • Biotin 30.0 mcg • Pantothenic Acid (Calcium Pantothenate) 10.0 mg • Calcium Carbonate 162.0 mg • Iron (Ferrous Fumarate) 18.0 mg • Phosphorus 109.0 mg • Iodine (Potassium Iodide) 150.0 mcg • Magnesium Oxide 100.0 mg • Zinc Oxide 15.0 mg • Selenium (Sodium Selenate) 20.0 mcg • Copper (Cupric Oxide) 2.0 mg • Manganese Sulfate 2.0 mg • Chromium Chloride 120.0 mcg • Molybdenum (Sodium Molybdate) 75.0 mg • Potassium Chloride 80.0 mg. Other Ingredients: Calcium Phosphate, Microcrystalline Cellulose, Gelatin, Crospovidone, Hydroxypropyl Methylcellulose, Starch, Titanium Dioxide, Sucrose, Magnesium Stearate, Triethyl Citrate, Lactose, Polysorbate 80, Beta Carotene, Glucose, FD&C Yellow #6 Lake.

Century Formula - Swanson
Each tablet contains: Vitamin A (as acetate) 5000 IU • Vitamin C USP (as ascorbic acid) 90 mg • Vitamin D USP (as cholecalciferol) 400 IU • Vitamin E (as d-alpha tocopheryl acetate) 30 IU • Vitamin K (as phytonadione) 25 mcg • Thiamin USP (as thiamin mononitrate; vitamin B-1) 2.25 mg • Riboflavin USP (vitamin B-2) 2.6 mg • Niacinamide 20 mg • Vitamin B-6 (pyridoxine HCl) 3 mg • Folic Acid 400 mcg • Vitamin B-12 (as cyanocobalamin) 9 mcg • Biotin 25 mcg • Pantothenic Acid (as d-calcium pantothenate) 10 mg • Calcium (from dicalcium phosphate) 162 mg • Iron (as ferrous fumarate) 27 mg • Iodine (as potassium iodide) 150 mcg • Magnesium (from magnesium oxide) 100 mg • Zinc (from zinc fultate) 15 mg • Selenium (as sodium selenate) 25 mcg • Copper (from copper gluconate) 2 mg • Manganese (from manganese sulfate) 5 mg • Chromium (as chromium chloride) 25 mcg • Molybdenum (sodium molybdate) 25 mcg • Potassium (as potassium chloride) 57.2 mg.

Cerebra - DHM, Inc.
Each tablet contains: Huperzine A (Chinese club moss) 50 mcg • Vitamin E.

Cernilton Flower Pollen - Cernitin America
Two tablets contain: Cernitin Flower Pollen (Rye Grass Pollen) Extract Water-Soluble Pollen Extract (T60) 120 mg • Cernitin Flower Pollen Extract Fat-Soluble Pollen Concentrate (GBX) 6 mg.
Other Ingredients: Cellulose (plant fiber), Magnesium Stearate (vegetable source).

Some Brand Name Natural Products - What they Contain

Cernilton T.S. Flower Pollen Triple Strength - Cernitin America
Two capsules contain: Cernitin Flower Pollen (Rye Grass Pollen) Extract Water-Soluble Pollen concentrate (T60) 360 mg • Cernitin Flower Pollen extract fat-soluble pollen concentrate (GBX) 18 mg. Other Ingredients: Cellulose (plant fiber), Magnesium Stearate (vegetable source).

CetylPure - Natrol
Two capsules contain: Cetyl Myristoleate proprietary blend (CetylPure) 1100 mg. Other Ingredients: Silica, Magnesium Stearate, Gelatin. Contains no yeast, wheat, milk, egg, soy, glutens, artificial colors or flavors, added sugar, starch, or preservatives.

Chamomile - Nature's Way
Two capsules contain: Chamomile flower 700 mg.
Other Ingredients: Gelatin.

Change-O-Life Formula - Nature's Way
Three capsules contain: Black Cohosh root • Blessed Thistle • False Unicorn root • Licorice root • Sarsaparilla root • Siberian Ginseng root • Squaw Vine vine, leaf, fruit. Other ingredients: Gelatin, Magnesium Stearate.

Changes Now - Changes - TwinLab
Two capsules contain: Vitamin C (Ascorbic acid) 50 mg • Lipase 300 LU • Calcium sulfate 100 mg • Multi-Source Fiber Complex 650 mg: Chitosan (Deacylated cellulose biopolymer), Glucomannan, Citrus Pectin, and Oat fiber. Other ingredients: Gelatin, Magnesium stearate, and Silica.

Changes Relief - Changes - TwinLab
Three caplets contain: Vitamin C (as Ascorbic Acid) 100 mg • Calcium (as Calcium Monohydrogen Phosphate) 300 mg • Phosphorus (as Calcium Monohydrogen Phosphate) 225 mg • Zinc (as Zinc Monomethionine) 13.75 mg • Copper (as Copper Gluconate) 500 mcg • Manganese (as Manganese Sulfate) 5 mg • Glucosamine Hydrochloride/Glucosamine Sulfate/N-Acetyl Glucosamine blend (with Chondroitin precursors) 750 mg • Turmeric rhizome standardized extract (12x) 300 mg • Boswellia serrata gum-resin 300 mg • Devil's Claw root standardized extract (5% harpagosides) 125 mg • Bromelain (80 GDU/g) 125 mg • White Willow bark 4:1 extract 150 mg • Ginger root standardized extract (5% gingerols) 125 mg • Alpine Snow Rose leaf (50% active polyphenolic proanthocyanidins) 213 mg. Other Ingredients: Vegetable cellulose, Fractionated vegetable oil, Soy polysaccharides, Silica, and Vegetable resin glaze.
See Editor's Note No. 15, page 1817.

Changing Times - Nature's Plus
Two tablets contain: Wild Brazilian SUMA (Pfaffia paniculata [Martius] Kuntze) 300 mg • Calcium amino acid chelate/complex 200 mg • Magnesium amino acid chelate/complex 100 mg • Vitamin B6 (Pyridoxine HCL) 100 mg • Pantothenic Acid 100 mg • Phosphatidylcholine 100 mg • Siberian Ginseng (Eleutherococcus senticosus) 100 mg • Niacinamide 25 mg • Vitamin E natural 200 IU • Vitamin B12 from Cobalamin 200 mcg • Selenium yeast free, amino acid complex 50 mcg. Yeast free. Sugar & starch free.

Chaparral and Red Clover - Dial Herbs
Chaparral • Red Clover • Echinacea • Buchu Leaves • Blood root.

Charcoal - Source Naturals
Each capsule contains: Charcoal 260 mg.

Charco-Zyme - Atrium Inc.
Each capsule contains: Papaya leaf 65 mg • Papain 32.5 mg • Mycozyme 32.5 mg • Rennin NF 3.75 mg • Activated Charcoal 130 mg. In a base of Alfalfa & Peppermint. Contains no sugar, salt, wheat, corn, yeast or soy derivatives.

Chaste Tree-Siberian Ginseng Virtue - Blessed Herbs
Chaste Tree berry • Siberian Ginseng root • Hawthorn berry, leaf & flower • Lavender flower • Wild Yam root • Licorice root • Grain alcohol & Distilled Water.

Chelated Calcium - Puritan's Pride
Six tablets contain: Calcium (as Calcium Amino Acid Chelate) 900 mg.

Chelated Calcium Magnesium Zinc - Nature's Bounty
Three tablets contain: Calcium (as Calcium Carbonate and Calcium Gluconate) 1000 mg • Magnesium (as Magnesium Oxide and Magnesium Gluconate) 400 mg • Zinc (as Zinc Gluconate and Zinc Citrate) 25 mg. Other Ingredients: Cellulose, Croscarmellose, Acacia Gum, Maltodextrin, Titanium Dioxide Color, Cellulose Coating, Vegetable Magnesium Stearate.

Chelated CAL-MAG - Puritan's Pride
Each tablet contains: Calcium 500 mg • Magnesium 250 mg.

Chelated Zinc 100 mg - Puritan's Pride
Each tablet contains: Zinc (from Zinc Gluconate) 100 mg.

Chelated Zinc 25 mg - Puritan's Pride
Each tablet contains: Zinc (from Zinc Gluconate) 25 mg.

Chelated Zinc 50 mg - Puritan's Pride
Each tablet contains: Zinc (from Zinc Gluconate) 50 mg.

Chem-Defense - Source Naturals
Each tablet contains: Molybdenum (aspartate, citrate) 120 mcg • Glutathione 50 mg • Coenzymated Vitamin B-2 (flavin mononucleotide) 2.25 mg.

Chem-Ex - Enzymatic Therapy
Two capsules contain: Pantothenic Acid (D-Calcium Pantothenate) 80 mg • Zinc (Chelate) 40 mg. Other ingredients: L-Cysteine 300 mg • L-Methionine 200 mg • Alpha-Ketoglutarate 60 mg • Taurine 50 mg • Glycine 40 mg. This exclusive formula also contains Licorice root extracts (Glycyrrhiza glabra). Contains no sugar, salt, yeast, wheat, corn, soy, dairy products, coloring, flavoring or preservatives.

Cherry Fruit Extract - PhytoPharmica
Two capsules contain: Cherry (Prunus avium) fruit extract 10:1 1,000 mg.

Chew Chew Vites Multiple - Nature's Life
Two tablets contain: Vitamin A (Fish Liver oil) 5000 IU • Vitamin D (as Vitamin D3) (Cholecalciferol) 400 IU • Vitamin E (d-Alpha Tocopheryl with Beta, Gamma, & Delta Tocopherols) 30 IU • Vitamin B1 (Thiamine HCI) 5 mg • Vitamin B2 (Riboflavin) 5 mg • Vitamin B6 Pyridoxine HCI) 5 mg • Vitamin B12 (Cyanocobalamin) 10 mcg • Niacinamide 10 mg • Pantothenic Acid (d-Calcium Pantothenate) 10 mg • Folic Acid 0.1 mg • Choline (Bitartrate) 25 mcg • Inositol 25 mcg • PABA (Para Aminobenzoic Acid) 300 mcg • Biotin 75 mcg • Vitamin C (with Rose Hips) 150 mg • Calcium (Carbonate, Gluconate, Citrate) 28 mg • Chromium (Picolinate Nutrition 21) 50 mcg • Copper (Full ranged Amino Acid Chelate) 0.1 mg • Iodine (Kelp) 0.1 mg • Iron (Full ranged Amino Acid Chelate) 5 mg • Magnesium (Full ranged Amino Acid Chelate)15 mg • Manganese (Full ranged Amino Acid Chelate) 0.3 mg • Phosphorus (Proteinate) 4 mg • Potassium (Proteinate) 11.5 mg • Silicon (Dioxide) 5 mg • Zinc (Picolinate) 2 mcg • Essential Fatty Acids 5 mg • Hawaiian Spirulina 10 mg • Chlorophyll, Alfalfa 10 mg • Chlorella algae 10 mg. In a natural base of low Glycemic pure Crystalline Fructose, pasteurized Honey powder, natural Lemon flavor, Vegetarian Acidophilus powder, natural Pineapple flavor, Rose Hips powder, Lecithin, Lemon Bioflavonoids, Barley Grass, Sunflower Seed powder, Rice Bran, Wheat Germ, Alfalfa leaf, Watercress & Parsley.

Chewable Acerola C Complex 500 mg - The Vitamin Shoppe
Each wafer contains: Vitamin C (fortified with Acerola extract & Rose Hips Concentrate) 500 mg • Bioflavonoid complex 50 mg. Sweetened exclusively with fructose, a naturally occurring sweetener found in fruit, and all-natural Acerola cherry flavoring. No yeast, corn, wheat, salt, starch, soy, dairy, sucrose, fish or animal derivatives, preservatives, artificial colors or flavors added.

Chewable C-500 mg with Rose Hips - Puritan's Pride
Each tablet contains: Vitamin C with Rose Hips 500 mg.

Chewable Calcium + D - Leiner Health Products
Each tablet contains: Total Carbohydrate 1 g • Calcium Carbonate 300 mg • Vitamin D (Ergocalciferol) 100 IU • Calories 5. Other Ingredients: Sorbitol, Stearic Acid, Cocoa, Magnesium Stearate, Maltodextrin, Silicon Dioixde, Natural Vanilla, Maltol, Gelatin.

Chewable Calcium with Vitamin D - Nature's Bounty
Four wafers contain: Vitamin D (as Ergocalciferol) 400 IU • Calcium (as Calcium Carbonate and Dicalcium Phosphate) 560 mg • Phosphorus (as Dicalcium Phosphate) 100 mg • Buckwheat (Fagopyrum esculentum) seed 10.4 mg • Corn Bran (Zea mays) seed 10.4 mg. Other Ingredients: Sucrose, Dextrose, Cellulose, Acacia Gum, Cottonseed Oil, Artificial Flavor, Silica, Vegetable Magnesium Stearate, Sodium Chloride.

Chewable E - Country Life
Each wafer contains: Vitamin E (D-alpha tocopheryl succinate) 450 IU. No yeast, corn, wheat, soy, milk, salt, starch, or artificial colors, sweeteners, flavors or preservatives.

Chewable Echinacea - Leiner Health Products
Two tablets contain: Vitamin C (Ascorbic Acid) 60 mg • Total Carbohydrates 2 g • Echinacea Purpurea root powder 25 mg. Other Ingredients: Dextrose, Natural Raspberry Flavor, Magnesium Stearate, Silicon Dioxide, Carmine.

Chewable Glucosamine Sulfate - Carlson
One tablet contains: Glucosamine Sulfate (providing Sulfur 4 g) 500 mg.

Chewable Orange Juice C 500 mg - The Vitamin Shoppe
Each chewable tablet contains: 500 mg Vitamin C, blend of natural Orange Juice concentrate, Orange Juice pulp, Orange peels, and natural fruit sugar. No Yeast, Wheat, Corn, Sucrose, Salt, Starch, Gluten, Milk, Eggs, Dairy, Fish or Animal Derivatives, Preservatives, Artificial Colors or Flavors added.

Chewable Vitamin C - Your Life - YourLife/Leiner Health Products
Each tablet contains: Vitamin C (Ascorbic Acid) 500 mg • Sodium 40 mg. Other Ingredients: Sucrose, Sodium Ascorbate, Stearic Acid, Starch, Natural flavor, Magnesium Stearate, Silicon Dioxide, Sorbitol, Yellow 6 Lake, Lactose, Ethylmaltol.

Chewable Vitamin C with Acerola - Leiner Health Products
Each wafer contains: Vitamin C 500 mg • Total carbohydrate 3 g • Calories 10 • Sugars 3 g. Other Ingredients: Sugar, Ascorbic Acid, Stearic Acid, Cellulose, Silicon Dioxide, Artificial Flavor, Acerola, Magnesium Stearate, Starch, Rose Hips, Lemon Bioflavonoids Complex, Hesperidin Complex, Buckwheat, Caramel, Rutin, Green Pepper Extract, Black Currant Extract.

CHI Chinese Herbal Bar - Nature's Plus
Each 1.5 oz. bar contains: Ancient Chinese Herbs: Huang-Ch'i (Astragalus root) 312 mg • Dang Shen (Relative root) 228 mg • Ling Zhi (Reishi mushroom) 192 mg • Bai Zhu (Attractylodes root) 144 mg • Ji Xue Teng (Millettia stem) 144 mg • Tu Si Zi (Dodder seed) 144 mg • Shan Yao (Chinese Yam root) 144 mg • Nu Zhen zi (Privet fruit) 144 mg • Di Huang (Rehmannia root) 138 mg • Bei Sha Shen (Sand root) 136 mg • Wu Wei Zi (Schisandra fruit) 114 mg • Jiang (Ginger root) 114 mg • Suan Zao Ren (Jujube seed) 114 mg • Chieh Keng (Balloon Flower root) 114 mg • Gan Cao (Licorice root) 108 mg • Bai Shoa (Peony root) 72 mg • Ju Luo (Tangerine peel) 72 mg.

Chickweed Formula - Quest
Each caplet contains: Chickweed powder (Stellaria media) 120 mg • Fennel seed powder (Foeniculum vulgare) 80 mg • Burdock root powder (Actium lappa) 80 mg • Chia seeds powder (Salvia columbariae) 70 mg • Bladderwrack powder (Fucus Vesiculosis) 30 mg • Kelp powder (Fucus Vesiculosis) 30 mg. Other Ingredients: Calcium Phosphate, Microcrystalline Cellulose, Vegetable Stearin, Croscarmellose Sodium, Magnesium Stearate (vegetable source).

Child Lax - Dial Herbs
Senna • Fennel • Rhubarb.

Children Immu-C - Nutri-Quest
Each tablet contains: Vitamin C (Sago Palm) 125 mg • Biotin 20 mcg • Folic Acid 10 mcg • Vitamin A (Palmitate) 1500 IU • Rutin 7.5 mg • Lemon Bioflavonoids 10 mg • Hesperidin Complex 7.5 mg • Propolis 1 mg • Lymph 1 mg • Thymus 1 mg • Spleen 1 mg. In a base of Fructose & Maltodextrin, with pleasant tasting Tropical Fruit Flavoring.
See Editor's Note No. 14, page 1817.

Children's Chewable Vita-Bear - The Vitamin Shoppe
Each tablet contains: Vitamin C 200 mg • Citrus Bioflavonoid Complex 20 mg. No Yeast, Wheat, Corn, Sucrose, Salt, Starch, Soy, Gluten, Milk, Eggs, Dairy, Fish or Animal Derivatives, Preservatives, Artificial Colors or Flavors added.

Children's Chewable Vitamin C - Health Smart Vitamins
Each tablet contains: Vitamin C (as ascorbic acid) 250 mg.

Children's Chewable Vitamins with Minerals - Schiff
Each tablet contains: Vitamin A (as palmitate) 5000 IU • Vitamin C (as ascorbic acid) 60 mg • Vitamin D (as cholecalciferol) 400 IU • Vitamin E (as d-alpha tocopheryl succinate) 30 IU • Thiamin (as mononitrate) 1.5 mg • Riboflavin 1.7 mg • Niacin (as niacinamide) 20 mg • Vitamin B-6 (as pyridoxine hydrochloride) 2 mg • Folic Acid 400 mcg • Vitamin B-12 (as cyanocobalamin) 6 mcg • Calcium (as calcium phosphate) 41 mg • Iron (as ferrous fumarate) 18 mg • Phosphorus (as calcium phosphate) 31 mg • Magnesium (as oxide) 6 mg • Zinc (as oxide) 2 mg. Other Ingredients: Fructose, Cellulose, Sorbitol, Stearic Acid, Natural Flavor, Silica, Magnesium Stearate, Citric Acid.

Children's Chewables - Swanson
Each tablet contains: Vitamin A (as acetate, beta-carotene) 2500 IU • Vitamin C USP (as ascorbic acid) 60 mg • Vitamin D (as cholecalciferol) 400 IU • Vitamin E (as d-alpha tocopheryl acetate) 15 IU • Thiamin USP (as thiamin HCl; vitamin B-1) 1.05 mg • Riboflavin USP (vitamin B-2) 1.2 mg • Niacinamide 13.5 mg • Vitamin B-6 (pyridoxine HCl) 1.05 mg • Folic Acid 300 mcg • Vitamin B-12 (cyanocobalamin) 4.5 mcg.

Children's Echinacea+C+Zinc Raspberry Flavor - LiFizz Effervescent Vitamins
Each tablet contains: Vitamin C 400 mg • Zinc (Zinc Oxide, Zinc Sulfate) 10 mg • Echinacea extract (Echinacea purpurea) 67 mg. Other ingredients: Citric Acid, Sodium Bicarbonate, Sorbitol, Mannitol, Red Beet Powder, Raspberry Flavor, Polyethylene Glycol 6000, Aspartame, Acesulfame Potassium, Wild Berry Powder, Magnesium Stearate, Silicon Dioxide.

Children's Multi-Vitamins - LiFizz Effervescent Vitamins
Each tablet contains: Vitamin A 2500 IU • Vitamin C 60 mg • Vitamin D 200 IU • Vitamin E 9 IU • Thiamin 1.05 mg • Riboflavin 1.19 mg •

Niacinamide 14 mg • Vitamin B6 1.4 mg • Folic Acid 280 mcg • Vitamin B12 4.2 mcg • Biotin 210 mcg • Pantothenic Acid 7.9 mg • Calcium 200 mg. Available in Grape, Bubblegum, Orange, and Fruit Punch flavors.

Child's Chewable Vitamins + Iron - Penwel
Each tablet contains: Vitamin A (Acetate & Beta Carotene) 2500 IU • Vitamin D (Ergocalciferol) 400 IU • Vitamin E (dl-Alpha tocopheryl Acetate) 15 IU • Vitamin C (Ascorbic Acid & Sodium Ascorbate) 60 mg • Folic Acid 0.3 mcg • Thiamine Mononitrate (Vitamin B1) 1.05 mg • Riboflavin (Vitamin B2) 1.2 mg • Niacin (Niacinamide) 13.5 mg • Vitamin B6 (Pyridoxine HCl) 1.05 mg • Vitamin B12 (Cyanocobalamin) 4.5 mcg • Iron (Ferrous Fumarate) 15 mg. Other Ingredients: Sugar, Corn Syrup Solids, Partially Hydrogenated Vegetable Oil, Stearic Acid, Maltodextrin, Natural and Artificial Flavorings, Starch, Tartaric Acid, Artificial Colors (Red #40, Blue #2, Yellow #6), Magnesium Stearate, and Gelatin.

Chill Out - Pacific BioLogic
Gotu Kola • Peony root • Polygoni vine • Valerian root • Passion flower • Skullcap • Lemon Balm • Sweetflag rhizome • Polygala root • Citrus peel (unripened) • Salvia root • Schizandra fruit.

Chill Pill - Futurebiotics
Three tablets contain: Vitamin B1 (thiamin) 5 mg • Vitamin B2 (riboflavin) 5 mg • Niacinamide 200 mg • Calcium: (carbonate, phosphate, amino acid chelate) 150 mg • Vitamin B6 5 mg. In a balanced formula of Herbal extracts & powders: Valerian root, Chamomile, Avena Sativa, Kava Kava, Hops, Skullcap, Spearmint, Nettles, Hawthorn, Fennel, Horsetail, Peppermint, Motherwort

China Chlorella 200 Mg - Natrol
Fifteen tablets contain: Protein 2 mg • Vitamin A 1665 mg • Vitamin C 500 mg • Thiamine (B1) 45 mcg • Riboflavin (B2) 140 mcg • Niacin 714 mcg • Calcium 6.2 mg • Iron 5 mg • Vitamin E 0.03 IU • Vitamin B6 51 mcg • Folic Acid 0.8 mcg • Vitamin B12 4 mcg • Phosphorus 30 mg • Iodine 18 mcg • Potassium 27.3 mg • Magnesium 10 mg • Zinc 2.2 mg • Copper 3 mcg • Biotin 6 mcg • Pantothenic Acid 40 mcg • Chlorophyll 90.1 mg • RNA 89.1 mg • DNA 8.5 mg • Germanium 76 ppm.

Chinac Digestive Health Formula - Metabolife
Each caplet contains: Amomum longiligulare (Chinese Amomum) • Oryza sativa (Rice) • Artemisia annua (Sweet Wormwood) • Crataegus cuneata (Chinese Hawthorn) • Armeniaca amarum (Apricot) • Xanthium sibiricum (Xanthium) • Wolfiporia cocos (Poria) • Coix Lacryma-jobi (Job's Tears).

Chinac Immune Health Formula - Metabolife
Each caplet contains: Forsythia suspensa (Forsythia) • Isatis tinctoria (Isatis) • Astragalus membranaceus (Astragalus) • Lonicera dasystyla (Honeysuckle) • Belamcanda chinensis (Blackberry Lily) • Paeonia veitchii (Chinese Peony).

Chinac Joint Health Formula - Metabolife
Each caplet contains: Achryanthes bidentata (Achyranthes) • Wenyujin concisa (Wen Curcuma) • Erythrina variegata (Coral Tree) • Atractylodes macrocephala (Bai-Zhu Atractylodes) • Notopterygium incisum (Notopterygium) • Angelica pubescens (Pubescent Angelica).

Chinac Menstrual Health Formula - Metabolife
Each caplet contains: Lindera aggregata (Lindera) • Leonurus japonicus (Chinese Motherwort) • Angelica sinensis (Dong Quai) • Cyperus rotundus (Cyperus) • Corydalis yanhusuo (Corydalis).

Chinac Stress and Tension Formula - Metabolife
Each caplet contains: Corydalis yanhusuo (Corydalis) • Angelica dahurica (Fragrant Angelica) • Ligusticum sinense (Sichuan Lovage) • Saposhnikovia divaricata (Siler) • Arctium lappa (Burdock).

Chinese Herbal Formula - Futurebiotics
Four tablets contain: Extracts &/or Powders [Siberian Ginseng, Foti, Astragalus, Schizandra, LEM, Shiitake-Ganoderma Mushroom complex, Chinese Licorice, Codonopsis, Echinacea] equivalent to a minimum of 7000 mg • Beta Carotene 10,000 IU • Vitamin E (mixed tocopherols) 100 IU • Vitamin C 1000 mg • Selenium 100 mcg.

Chitosan - The Vitamin Shoppe
Each capsule contains: Chitosan, minimum 90% Deacetylated Chitin 250 mg • Aloe Vera 50 mg.

Chitosan - Leiner Health Products
Two tablets contain: Chromium (Chromium picolinate) 100 mcg • Vitamin C 120 mg • Chitosan 1000 mg. Other Ingredients: Calcium Carbonate, Cellulose, Sodium Ascorbate, Maltodextrin, Acacia, Stearic Acid, Hydroxypropyl Methylcellulose, Magnesium Stearate, Hydroxypropyl Cellulose, Starch, Polysorbate 80, Polyethylene Glycol 3350.

Chitosan - Olympian Labs
Two capsules contain: Chitosan 1000 mg.

Chitosan - Puritan's Pride
Two tablets contain: Chitosan 1000 mg.

Chitosan - Swanson
Two capsules contain: LipoSan Ultra Chitosan (90%-93% deacetylated) 1 g.

Chitosan Plus - Progressive Labs
Each capsule contains: Chitosan (marine fiber concentrate) 250 mg • Citric Acid 75 mg • Lipase (3000 units) 25 mg.

Chitosan-C with Biozan - Richardson Labs
Four caplets contain: BioZan: [Purified Chitosan, Betaine HCl, Oat bran, Aloe & Beta Glucan] 2500 mg • Chromium (picolinate) 200 mcg.

Chit-O-Slim Plus - Aspen Group, Inc.
Each capsule contains: Chitosan 500 mg • Chromium (picolinate) 50 mcg.

Chitosol - Sheldon Marketing
Four capsules contain: Chitosan 2000 mg • Vitamin C 400 mg.

Chlorella - Source Naturals
Six tablets contain: Vitamin A (Beta Carotene) 1,665 IU • Vitamin B1 (Thiamin) 45 mcg • Vitamin B2 (Riboflavin) 140 mcg • Vitamin B3 (Niacin) 710 mcg • Vitamin B6 (Pyridoxine) 50 mcg • Vitamin B12 (Cyanocobalamin) 3.75 mcg • Biotin 5.7 mcg • Vitamin C (Ascorbic Acid) 460 mcg • Calcium 6 mg • Iodine 18 mcg • Iron 5 mg • Magnesium 9.45 mg • Phosphorus 29 mg • Zinc 2.1 mg • Chlorella Growth Factor (CGF) 60 mg • Chlorophyll 60 mg.

Chlorella Regularis - New Chapter, Inc.
Six capsules contain: Chlorella regularis 2340 mg.

Chlorophyll Concentrate - Puritan's Pride
Each softgel contains: Chlorophyllin Copper 50 mg.

Chlorophyll Liquid - Dial Herbs
Chlorophyllin Copper complex • Water • Oil of Mint • Glycerine, vegetable derived.

Chlorophyll Softgels - Dial Herbs
Chlorophyllin Copper complex • Water • Oil of Mint • Glycerine, vegetable derived.

Chloroplex - Progressive Labs
Each softgel contains: Chlorophyllin 50 mg.

Chloroplus - Atrium Inc.
Each capsule contains: Vitamin A 11000 IU • Vitamin D (as Vitamin D3) 250 IU • Chlorophyll (oil soluble) 10 mg • Vitamin E (d-Alpha Tocopherol) 3 IU • Lecithin (Raw Unbleached) 210 mg • Pumpkin seed oil 45 mg • Sesame seed oil 22 mg • Halibut Liver oil • Skip Jack Liver oil.

CholesFiber - Source Naturals
Three heaping scoops contain: Dietary Fiber 15 g • Soluble Fiber 15 g • Protein 15 g • Soy Isoflavones 60 mg. Other Ingredients: Soy Protein, Apple Pectin, Grapefruit Pectin, Mixed Gums: Guar Gum, Arabic Gum, Xanthan Gum.

Cholesta Balance - PhysioLogics
Each softgel contains: Pantethine (80% purity, 307 mg) 384 mg • Gamma Oryzanol (from Rice Bran) 100 mg.

Cholestaid - Omni Nutraceuticals
Two tablets contain: Esterin extract of Alfalfa 900 mg • Citric Acid 100 mg. Other ingredients: Microcrystalline, Croscarmellose Sodium, Stearic Acid, Silica.

Cholesta-Lo - Futurebiotics
Three tablets contain: Cholestatin 600 mg • Niacin (flush free) 200 mg • Chromium (polynicotinate) 100 mcg • Garlic (odorless) concentrate (2:1) 350 mg • Siberian Ginseng extract (10:1) 75 mg • Parsley 250 mg • Chickweed 200 mg • Hawthorn 150 mg • Ginger 200 mg • Cayenne 200 mg. ("75 mg of 10:1 Siberian Ginseng extract is equal to 750 mg of raw Siberian Ginseng. 350 mg of 2:1 Garlic is equal to 875 mg of raw Garlic.")

CholesTame - Jarrow Formulas
Four tablets contain: Red Yeast Rice Extract (Monascus purpureus) (Xie Zhi Kang) 4% Statins 2400 mg • Coenzyme Q10 (Ubiquinone) 30 mg • Artichoke Leaf Extract (Cynara scolymus) 2% cynarine 400 mg • Guggul (Commiphora mukul) 4% guggulsterones 500 mg • Alpha Lipoic Acid 100 mg • Grape Seed Extract (Vitis vinifera) 95% polyphenols 50 mg • Pantethine 200 mg • Lutein 10 mg • Taurine 250 mg.

Cholestatin - Futurebiotics
One tablet contains: Beta Sitosterol 200 mg • Campesterol 100 mg • Stigmasterol 80 mg. Other ingredients: Dicalcium phosphate, Cellulose, Magnesium Stearate, Silica.

Cholesterol Essentials - Swanson
Two tablets contain: Vitamin C (ascorbic acid) 500 mg • Thiamin (as thiamin HCl; vitamin B-1) 7 mg • Riboflavin (vitamin B-2) 7 mg • Niacin (100 mg as flush-free inositol hexanicotinate and 7 mg as niacinamide) 107 mg • Vitamin B-6 (as pyridoxine HCl) 7 mg • Folic Acid 200 mcg • Vitamin B-12 (as cyanocobalamin) 200 mcg • Biotin 6.24 mcg • Pantothenic Acid (as d-calcium pantothenate) 6.24 mg • Chromium (from Chromax® chromium picolinate) 200 mcg • Gugulipid® (Commiphora mukul, 2.5% guggulsterones) 500 mg • Lecithin 300 mg • Oat Bran fiber 300 mg • Phosphatidylcholine (from lecithin and phosphatidylcholine) 200 mg • Odor-Controlled Garlic bulb (PureGar® 10,000 ppm allicin potential) 150 mg • Beta Sitosterol 50 mg • Citrus Bioflavonoids 50 mg • Choline Bitartrate 6.4 mg • Inositol 6.4 mg • PABA (para-aminobenzoic acid) 6.4 mg.

Cholesterol Metabolism - Nutrivention
Six tablets contain: Choline 500 mg • Inositol 500 mg • Niacinamide 200 mg Unsaturated Fatty Acids (7% GAMA Linolenic Acid • 64% Linoleic Acid) 500 mg • Pantothenic Acid 200 mg • Magnesium 200 mg • Vitamin B6 100 mg • Vitamin D 600 IU • Lecithin 600 mg • Hawthorne berries 400 mg • Garlic powder concentrate 400 mg •

Apple Pectin 360 mg • L-Methionine 340 mg • Capsicum 200 mg • Ginger root 200 mg • Butcher's Broom 100 mg • Betaine HCL 100 mg.

Cholesterol Support - Amazon Support
Each capsule contains: Artichoke • Mullaca • Annatto • Suma • Cat's Claw • Bitter Melon • Yerba Mate • Sarsaparilla.

Cholestin - Pharmanex
Each capsule contains: Policosanol (Beeswax extract 5:1) 15 mg. Other Ingredients: Soybean Oil, Lecithin, Gelatin, Glycerin, Purified Water, Carmine (for color).

Cholestoril - Enzymatic Therapy
Each tablet contains: Pantethine 300 mg. Contains no sugar, salt, yeast, wheat, corn, soy, dairy products, coloring, flavoring or preservatives.

Cholestra - HerbaSway
Soy • Hawthorn berry • Green Tea • He Sho Wu • Cassia tora • Blackberry • HerbaSwee (Cucurbitaceae fruit).

Cholestrex - Source Naturals
Nine tablets contain: Niacin 480 mg • Vitamin C (Calcium Ascorbate, Ascorbic Acid and Zinc Ascorbate) 900 mg • Vitamin E (D-Alpha Tocopheryl)(Natural) 100 IU • Calcium (Calcium Ascorbate) 100 mg • Zinc (Zinc Ascorbate) 6 mg • Copper (Copper Sevacate) 2 mg • Chromium (ChromeMate GTF Chromium Polynicotinate) 300 mcg • Oats (bran and fiber) 2500 mg • Grapefruit Pectin 1400 mg • Psyllium seed husk 1100 mg • Lecithin (with 24% Phosphatidyl Choline) 900 mg • Alfalfa seed 600 mg • Beta Sitosterol 300 mg • L-Arginine 300 mg.

Cholest-Rite - Nu-Creations
Each capsule contains: Niacin 20 mg • Red Yeast 600 mg. Other Ingredients: Hawthorn extract, Artichoke extract, Gelatin, Magnesium Stearate.

Choline - Puritan's Pride
Each tablet contains: Choline (from Choline Bitartrate) 650 mg.

Choline - Nature's Bounty
Each tablet contains: Choline Bitartrate 650 mg. Other Ingredients: Cellulose, Vegetable Stearic Acid, Food Glaze, Silica, Vegetable Magnesium Stearate, Magnesium Silicate, Croscarmellose.

Choline & Inositol - Puritan's Pride
Each tablet contains: Choline Bitartrate 250 mg • Inositol 250 mg.

Chondroitin Complex - Puritan's Pride
Each capsule contains: Glucosamine Sulfate (2KCl) 250 mg • Chondroitin Sulfate 200 mg • Vitamin C (Ascorbic Acid) 100 mg • Manganese 1 mg.
See Editor's Note No. 15, page 1817.

Chondroitin Plus - Atrium Inc.
Two capsules contain: Calcium Ascorbate 60 mg • Magnesium Ascorbate 60 mg • Vitamin C Content 100 mg • Thiamine HCL 25 mg • Pyridoxine HCL 10 mg • Niacinamide 60 mg • Manganese (Sulfate) 65 mg • Potassium (Citrate) 25 mg • Zinc (Citrate) 25 mg • Chondroitin Sulfates 125 mg • Mocopoly Saccharides 65 mg • Bioflavonoid Complex 50 mg • Betaine HCL 15 mg • Rutin 10 g • Black Cohosh 75 mg • Passiflora 75 mg • Valerian root 75 mg • Equestium 65 mg. Contains no sugar, starch, salt, wheat, corn, yeast or soy derivatives.
See Editor's Note No. 15, page 1817.

Some Brand Name Natural Products - What they Contain
www.NaturalDatabase.com contains MANY more listings than appear here.

Chondroitin Sulfate - Leiner Health Products
Each tablet contains: Chondroitin Sulfate 600 mg. Other Ingredients: Cellulose, Dicalcium Phosphate, Stearic Acid, Croscarmellose Sodium, Magnesium Stearate, Silicon Dioxide, Titanium Dioxide, Hydroxypropyl Methylcellulose, Talc, Polyethylene Glycol 3350, Wax, Polysorbate 80.
See Editor's Note No. 15, page 1817.

Chondroitin Sulfate - Jamieson
Each caplet contains: Chondroitin Sulfate (Equivalent to 400 mg Sodium Chondroitin Sulfate) 360 mg.
See Editor's Note No. 15, page 1817.

Chondroitin Sulfate - Olympian Labs
Each capsule contains: Chondroitin Sulfate 400 mg.
See Editor's Note No. 15, page 1817.

Chondroitin Sulfate - Swanson
Each capsule contains: Chondroitin Sulfate 500 mg.
See Editor's Note No. 15, page 1817.

Chondroitin Sulfate/Glucosamine Sulfate - Metabolic Response Modifiers
Each capsule contains: Glucosamine sulfate KCl 500 mg • Chondroitin sulfate 400 mg.
See Editor's Note No. 15, page 1817.

Chondroytamine HCl - Olympian Labs
Each capsule contains: Chondroitin Sulfate 200 mg • Glucosamine HCl 250 mg.
See Editor's Note No. 15, page 1817.

Chondroytamine HCl (Double Strength) - Olympian Labs
Each capsule contains: Chondroitin Sulfate 400 mg • Glucosamine HCl 500 mg • Cat's Claw 30 mg • White Willow Bark 30 mg.
See Editor's Note No. 15, page 1817.

Chroma Slim for Men - Richardson Labs
Four caplets contain: Trace Mineral Blend: Chromium Picolinate 400 mcg, Vanadium 120 mcg, Manganese Picolinate 2.5 mg • Proprietary Lipotropic Blend 3000 mg: Choline Bitartrate, L-Carnitine, Inositol, L-Methionine • Essential Nutrient & Amino Acid Blend 500 mg: Ferulic Acid Esters, Taurine, L-Lysine HCl, L-Glutamic Acid, Base, Glycine USP, Cernitin flower pollen extract 500 mg • Vitamin Blend: Pantothenic Acid 10 mg, Vitamin B6 5 mg • Thermogenic Herbal Blend 424 mg: Panax Ginseng powdered extract • Cayenne • Mustard seed powder • Cinnamon powder • Ginger root powdered extract • Uva Ursi • Standardized White Willow bark powder. In a base of Natural Peppermint, Saw Palmetto berries, Juniper berries, Spirulina.

Chroma Slim Plus - Richardson Labs
Four caplets contain: Trace Mineral Blend: Chromium Picolinate 400 mcg, Vanadium 120 mcg, Manganese Picolinate 2.5 mg • Proprietary Lipotropic & Lipid Transport Blend 3000 mg: Choline Bitartrate, L-Carnitine, Inositol, L-Methionine • Essential Nutrient & Amino Acid Blend 500 mg: Ferulic Acid Esters, Taurine, L-Lysine HCl, L-Glutamic Acid, Base, Glycine USP, Cernitin flower pollen extract • Vitamin Blend: Potassium Chloride USP, Pantothenic Acid 10 mg, Vitamin B6 5 mg. In a base of natural Peppermint and Bromelain.

Chrom-Adyl Surge - Biochem
Each capsule contains: Chromium 500 mcg • BMOV (Bis-Maltol OXO Vandium) 5 mg • Vanadyl Sulfate 5 mg.

ChromaSlim Biozan - Richardson Labs
Four caplets contain: BioZan: [Purified Chitosan, Betaine HCl, Oat bran, Aloe, Beta Glucan] 2500 mg • Chromium (Picolinate) 250 mcg.

Chromemate - Natrol
One capsule contains: Chromium (Polynicotinate) 200 mcg • L-Arginine 50 mg • L-Lysine 50 mg • Vitamin B6 (Pyridoxine) 10 mg. Other ingredients: Microcrystalline Cellulose, Magnesium Stearate, Gelatin.

Chromic Fuel (Chromium Picolinate) - TwinLab
Pure Crystalline Chromium Picolinate (supplying of Trivalent Chromium 200 mcg) 1.67 mg.

Chromium - Source Naturals
Each tablet contains: Chromium (amino acid chelate) 200 mcg.

Chromium GTF - Nature's Sunshine
Each tablet contains: Calcium (di-calcium phosphate) 80 mg • Phosphorus (di-calcium phosphate) 61 mg • Chromium (chromium amino acid chelate, chromium nicotinate) 500 mcg • Proprietary Blend: Horsetail (Equisetum arvense), Red Clover tops (Trifolium pratense), Yarrow flower (Achillea millefolium) 60 mg.

Chromium GTF - Source Naturals
Each tablet contains: Chromium GTF (Polynicotinate) 200 mcg • Niacin (Polynicotinate) 1.8 mg.

Chromium HCA - PhysioLogics
Each capsule contains: Calcium (as Calcium Salt of Hydroxy Citric Acid) 79 mg • Chromium (as Chromium Picolinate) 100 mcg • Garcinia cambogia [50% (-)- Hydroxy Citric Acid (HCA) 250 mg] 500 mg.

Chromium Nicotinate Complex - Progressive Labs
Each capsule contains: Niacin (as polynicotinate) 1300 mcg • Chromium (as polynicotinate) 200 mcg • Glutathione 250 mcg • Glycine 50 mcg • Cysteine 100 mcg • Aspartic Acid 100 mcg.

Chromium Picolinate - The Vitamin Shoppe
Each softgel contains: Chromium Picolinate, a compound of yeast-free Trivalent Chromium and Picolinic Acid 200 mcg.

Chromium Picolinate - Great American Nutrition
One tablet contains: Chromium (Picolinate) 200 mcg. Other Ingredients: Calcium Carbonate, Cellulose, Magnesium Stearate. Contains no added Sugar, Salt, Starch, Preservatives, Artificial Flavors, or Colors. Free of Corn, Soy, Wheat, Yeast, & Dairy Products. Suitable for vegetarians. Contains no animal products.

Chromium Picolinate - Metabolic Response Modifiers
Each capsule contains: Chromium (picolinate) 200 mcg.

Chromium Picolinate - Olympian Labs
Each capsule contains: Chromium (picolinate) 200 mcg.

Chromium Picolinate - PhytoPharmica
Each capsule contains: Chromium (picolinate) 200 mcg.

Chromium Picolinate - Richardson Labs
Each tablet contains: Chromium (Picolinate), derived from 3.2 mg of pure crystalline Chromium Picolinate. Contains no added sugar, salt, starch, preservatives, artificial flavors, or colors. Free of corn, soy, wheat, yeast, and dairy. Suitable for vegetarians. Contains no animal products.

Chromium Picolinate - Swanson
Each capsule contains: Chromium (from Chromax® chromium picolinate) 200 mcg.

Chromium Picolinate - Source Naturals
Each tablet contains: Trivalent Chromium (from Chromax brand of yeast-free Chromium Picolinate) 200 mcg.

Chromium Picolinate GTF - Atrium Inc.
Each capsule contains: Chromium (Chromium Picolinate) 200 mcg. Contains no sugar, starch, salt, wheat, corn, yeast, or soy derivatives.

Chromium Picolinate Plus - Progressive Labs
Each capsule contains: Chromium 200 mcg (from 1640 mg of chromium picolinate) • Gamma Oryzanol 15 mg • Boron (as boron aspartate) 2 mg.

Chromium Plus with Oxidative Factors - The Vitamin Shoppe
Each tablet contains: Zinc 30 mg • Chromium 100 mcg • Selenium 100 mcg.

ChronFS-X - Olympian Labs
Each capsule contains: Raw Adrenal 50 mg • Licorice Rhizome 150 mg • Shitake Mushrooms 30 mg • Maitake Mushrooms 30 mg • Malic Acid 200 mg • Magnesium Glycinate 50 mg • Manganese Glycinate 10 mg • Potassium Gluconate 30 mg • Zinc Gluconate 20 mg.
See Editor's Note No. 14, page 1817.

Chrysin - ProLab
Each capsule contains: 5,7-Dihydroxyflanone (Chrysin) 250 mg.

Chrysin - Metabolic Response Modifiers
Each capsule contains: Chrysin (5,7-dihydroxyflavone) 500 mg.

Circulate Dietary Supplement Tablets - HealthWatchers System
Vitamin B6 • Vitamin B2 • Vitamin B12 • Vitamin B15 • Vitamin D • OrthoPhosphoric Acid • EDTA • Fenugreek Seed • Superoxide Dismutase • Rutin • Catalase • Beet Leaf • Phosphatidyl Choline • Alfalfa • Spanish Moss • Urea • Orchick Hyaluridase • Beta Carotene • Protomorphagens Pituitary • Heart • Liver • Kidney • Brain.
See Editor's Note No. 14, page 1817.

Circuleg - Puritan's Pride
Each tablet contains: Horse Chestnut Seed extract (aesculus hippocastanum: Standardized to 20% Aescin) 300 mg • Proprietary Herbal Blend: Butcher's Broom (Ruscus aculeatus) root, Bilberry (Vaccinium myrtillus) fruit, Cayenne (Capsicum annum) fruit, Ginger (Zingiber officinale) fruit, Ginkgo leaf extract (Ginkgo biloba) 200 mg.

Circulite Oil - The Herbalist
Oils of Sweet Almond, Eucalyptus, Camphor, St. John's Wort flower, Calendula flower, French Lavender, Peppermint, Sage & Extracts of Prickly Ash bark, Ginger root, Lobelia leaf.

Circuplex - Futurebiotics
Two tablets contain: Vitamin C 100 mg • Vitamin B1 (thiamin) 8 mg • Niacinamide 414 mg • Vitamin B2 (riboflavin) 8 mg • Niacin 20 mg • Vitamin B6 20 mg • Vitamin B12 10 mcg • Zinc (gluconate) 5 mg • Manganese (amino acid chelate) 5 mg. In a tablet base of: [Betaine HCl 20 mg, Citrus Bioflavonoids 50 mg, Alfalfa seed meal 200 mg, Oyster shell Calcium 50 mg, Cayenne 10 mg, Ginger 200 mg, Prickly Ash bark 200 mg & Peppermint] 100 mg.

Circutone - The Herbalist
Prickly Ash bark • Hawthorn berry, leaf & flower • Bayberry root bark • Ginger root • Yarrow flower • Cayenne pepper.

Citra Garcinia Cambogia - Olympian Labs
Each capsule contains: Garcinia- Hydroxycitrate 500 mg.

Citracal Calcium Citrate - Mission Pharmacal
Two tablets contain: Calcium (as Ultradense calcium citrate) 400 mg. Other Ingredients: Polyethylene Glycol, Croscarmellose Sodium, HPMC, Color, Magnesium Silicate, Magnesium Stearate.
See Editor's Note No. 5, page 1816.

Citracal Calcium Citrate 250 mg + D - Mission Pharmacal
Two tablets contain: Vitamin D (as vitamin D3; as cholecalciferol) 125 IU • Calcium (as Ultradense calcium citrate) 500 mg. Other Ingredients: Polyethylene Glycol, Citric Acid, Microcrystalline Cellulose, HPMC, Croscarmellose Sodium, Color, Magnesium Silicate, Magnesium Stearate.

Citracal Calcium Citrate Caplets + D - Mission Pharmacal
Two caplets contain: Vitamin D (as Vitamin D3; as cholecalciferol) 400 IU • Calcium (as Ultradense calcium citrate) 630 mg. Other Ingredients: Polyethylene Glycol, Croscarmellose Sodium, HPMC, Color, Magnesium Silicate, Magnesium Stearate.

Citracal Calcium Citrate Liquitab - Mission Pharmacal
Each dissolved tablet contains: Calcium (as calcium citrate) 500 mg. Other Ingredients: Citric Acid, Adipic Acid, Saccharin Sodium, Orange Flavor, Cellulose Gum, Aspartame. This Product contains Nutrasweet. Phenylketonurics: contains 6 mg Phenylalanine per tablet.

Citracal Plus - Mission Pharmacal
Two tablets contain: Vitamin D (as vitamin D3; as cholecalciferol) 250 IU • Vitamin B6 (as pyridoxine hydrochloride) 10 mg • Calcium (as Ultradense calcium citrate) 500 mg • Magnesium (as magnesium oxide) 80 mg • Zinc (as zinc oxide) 10 mg • Copper (as copper gluconate) 1 mg • Manganese (as manganese gluconate) 1 mg • Boron (as sodium borate) 1 mg. Other Ingredients: Polyethylene Glycol, Povidone, Croscarmellose Sodium, HPMS, Color, Magnesium Stearate, Magnesium Silicate, Maltodextrin, Carnauba Wax.

Citracal Prenatal Rx - Mission Pharmacal
Each tablet contains: Vitamin A (Vitamin A palmitate) 2700 IU • Vitamin C (Ascorbic acid) 120 mg • Calcium (Calcium citrate) 125 mg • Iron (Carbonyl iron, Ferrous gluconate) 27 mg • Vitamin D (as Vitamin D3) (Cholecalciferol) 400 IU • Vitamin E (dl Alpha Tocopheryl acetate) 30 IU • Thiamin (Vitamin B1) 3 mg • Riboflavin (Vitamin B2) 3.4 mg • Niacinamide (Vitamin B3) 20 mg • Vitamin B6 (Pyridoxine HCl) 20 mg • Folic Acid 1 mg • Iodine (Potassium iodide) 150 mcg • Zinc (Zinc oxide) 25 mg • Copper (Cupric oxide) 2 mg • Docusate Sodium 50 mg.

Citramannan - The Vitamin Shoppe
Each capsule contains: Citrimax (Hydroxy Citric Acid) 400 mg • Glucomannan (Konjac) root 400 mg.

Citratherm - MetPro
Citrus aurantium • Chromium Picolinate • Vitamin C • Niacin • St. John's Wort.

Citri-Caps - Progressive Labs
Each capsule contains: Malibar Tamarind [Garcinia cambogia, standardized to contain 50% (-) hydroxycitric acid] 333 mg • Atractylodes (Atractylodes lancea) 50 mg • Seville Orange flower (Citrus aurantii) 50 mg • Chromium (as chromium picolinate) 50 mcg • Chromium (as chromium arginate) 15 mcg.

Citri-Caps Plus - Progressive Labs
Each capsule contains: Malibar Tamarind [Garcinia cambogia, standardized to contain 50% (-) hydroxycitric acid] 333 mg • Ma Huang Extract (Ephedra sinica) 200 mg • Yerba Mate 75 mg • Atractylodes (Atractylodes lancea) 50 mg • Seville Orange flower (Citrus Aurantii) 50 mg • Chromium (as chromium picolinate) 50 mcg • Chromium (as chromium arginate) 15 mcg.

CitriChrome - Swanson
Each capsule contains: Chromium (from Chromax chromium picolinate) • CitriMax™ (Garcinia cambogia fruit extract) 500 mg, (-) Hydroxycitric Acid 250 mg.

CitriGenics - Roex
Six tablets contain: Citrimax Garcinia Cambogia 1500 mg • L-Carnitine 300 mg • Choline Bitartrate 100 mg • Inositol 100 mg • Betaine HCl 50 mg • Chromium 200 mcg • Green Tea extract 150 mg • Kola Nut extract 150 mg • Yerba Mate 100 mg • Ginger 100 mg • Spirulina 100 mg • Kelp with Trace Minerals 100 mg • Vitamin C 100 mg • Vitamin E 30 IU • Potassium 25 mg • Biotin 300 mcg • Niacinamide 50 mg • Vitamin A 5000 IU • Vitamin B6 20 mg • Vitamin B2 20 mg • Vitamin B12 6 mcg • Folic Acid 400 mcg • Iodine 150 mcg • Selenium 50 mcg.

CitriLean - Enzymatic Therapy
Each capsule contains: Garcinia cambogia extract (CitriMax) standardized to contain 50% (-) hydroxycitrate (125 mg/capsule) 250 mg • Ginger root extract 6.5:1 (Zingiber officinale) 50 mg • Fenugreek seed extract 4:1 (Trigonella foenum-graecum) 50 mg • Curcuma root extract (Curcuma longa) standardized to contain 4% curcumin 50 mg • Chromium Polynicotinate (ChromeMate) 25 mcg. Contains no sugar, salt, yeast, wheat, corn, soy, dairy products, coloring, flavoring, or preservatives.

Citrimate - Nature's Plus
Each tablet contains: Standardized Garcinia cambogia extract supplying 50% [-] Hydroxycitrate 500 mg • Chromium (Polynicotinate) 100 mcg. Contains no yeast, wheat, corn, soy, milk, salt, sugar or starch.

Citrimax - Nature's Plus
Each tablet contains: Standardized Garcinia cambogia extract supplying 50% [-] Hydroxycitrate 1000 mg. Contains no yeast, wheat, corn, soy, milk, salt, sugar or starch.

Citrimax Fat Burners - Optimum Nutrition
Citrimax (H.C.A).

CitrimaxPlus with ChromeMate - Natrol
One capsule contains: Chromium (Polynicotinate) 100 mcg • (-) Hydroxycitric Acid 250 mg • Uva Ursi 100 mg • Cascara Sagrada 75 mg. Other ingredients: Gelatin, Magnesium Stearate.

Citrin + Chromium - Olympia Nutrition
Hydroxycitrate (-) HCA + Chromium Picolinate.

CitriThin - PhytoPharmica
Two capsules contain: Garcinia Cambogia extract (CitriMax) 500 mg standardized to contain 50% (-)hydroxycitrate (125 mg per capsule) • Ginger root extract 6.5:1 (Zingiber officinale) 100 mg • Fenugreek seed extract 4:1 (Trigonella foenum-graecum) 100 mg • Curcuma root extract (Curcuma longa) 100 mg standardized to contain 4% curcumin • Chromium Polynicotinate (ChromeMate) 50 mcg. Contains no sugar, salt, yeast, wheat, corn, soy, dairy products, coloring, flavoring, or preservatives.

Citrus Slender - Nature's Way
Each 14 g scoop contains: Arabinogalactan 2 g • Chromium Polynicotinate 100 mcg • Citrin 1.5 g • L-Carnitine L-Tartrate 800 mg. Other ingredients: Citric Acid, Fructose, Lemon Crystals, Lemon/Lime Crystals, Lime Crystals, Sodium Chloride, Sorbitol, Stevia, dried extract.

CLA - EAS
Each capsule contains: 1000 mg Vegetable oil with 60% conjugated Linoleic Acid (CLA) & 40% other Monounsaturated & Saturated Fatty Acid • 0.02% TBHQ (antioxidant) has been added to preserve freshness.

CLA 1000 - Human Development Technologies
Each softgel capsule contains: Tonalin 1000 mg yielding Conjugated Linoleic Acid 700 mg.

Classic Perfor-Max - Changes - TwinLab
One capsule contains: Proanthocyanidin Blend (85% Proanthocyanidins) Grape seed extract and Pine Bark 4:1 extract 50 mg • Turmeric rhizome extract 25 mg. Other Ingredients: Maltodextrin, Calcium Sulfate, Gelatin, Cellulose, Magnesium Stearate, Silica, and Riboflavin color.

Classic Thermo-Lift (Classic ThermoLift) - Changes - TwinLab
Each capsule contains: Chromium (as Chromium picolinate) 200 mcg • MaHuang extract (aerial parts) (Standardized for 25 mg Ephedrine alkaloids) 310 mg • Proprietary herbal blend 260 mg: Guarana seed extract (39 mg Caffeine), White Willow bark, Siberian Ginseng root, Astragalus root, Bee Pollen, Bladderwrack kelp (Fucus vesiculosus), Ginger root, Gotu Kola leaf, Licorice root, Rehmannia root, and Reishi mushroom (fruiting body). Other ingredients: Gelatin, Maltodextrin, Magnesium stearate, Wheat Germ, Silica, and Turmeric extract.

CleanseSMART I - RenewLife
Artichoke leaf • Ashwaganda Root • Beet leaf (green rind) • Bupleurum root • Burdock root • Celandine • Chlorella • Corn silk • Dandelion root • Hawthorne berry • Larch gum • Milk Thistle seed • Mullein leaf • Red clover leaf and stem • Turmeric root.

CleanseSMART II - RenewLife
Magnesium Hydroxide • Cape aloe gel • Rhubarb • Slippery Elm bark • Marshmallow root • Fennel seed • Triphalia • Ginger root.

Cleansing Herbs - Youngevity
Vitamin B2 • Cascara sagrada • Fennel • Peppermint • Yucca root • Pau d'Arco • Yellow Dock root • Vilcabamba Mineral Essence: Potassium, Calcium, Magnesium, Zinc, Chromium, Selenium, Iron, Copper, Molybdenum, Vanadium, Iodine, Cobalt, Manganese.

Cleansing Laxative - Zand
Each tablet contains: Active Ingredient: Cascara Sagrada bark 150 mg. Other Ingredients include : Chinese Rhubarb root, Frangula bark, Gentian root, Goldenseal root, Fennel seed, Kaolin clay, Anise seed, Oregon Grape root.

Clear Skin - PhytoPharmica
Twenty drops contain: Cantharis 8x • Croton tiglium 8x • Arsenicum album 6x • Mercurius currosivus 6x • Pulsatilla 4x • Cistus canadensis 3x • Natrum phosphoricum 2x • Echinacea 1x • Juglans 1x • Viola tricolor 1x. In a base of 45% USP alcohol by volume.
See Editor's Note No. 1, page 1816.

Clear Thoughts - Rexall
Two capsules contain: Vitamin E (as dl-alpha-tocopheryl acetate and d-alpha-tocopheryl succinate) 30 IU • Niacin (as niacinamide) 20 mg • Folic Acid 400 mcg • Vitamin B-12 (as cyanocobalamin) 60 mcg • Zinc (as zinc amino acid chelate) 15 mg • Ginkgo Biloba extract (standardized to 24% ginkgo flavonol glycosides, 14.4 mg; standardized to 6% terpene lactones, 3.6 mg) 60 mg • Gotu Kola aerial parts 150 mg • L-Glutamine 200 mg • L-Tyrosine 100 mg • Choline (as choline bitartrate) 50 mg • Phosphatidylserine complex (standardized to 30% phosphatidylserine, 15 mg) 50 mg • Damiana leaf 50 mg. Other Ingredients: Gelatin, Maltodextrin, Silica, Talc, Magnesium Stearate.

Clensa-Herb - Dial Herbs
Red Clover • Burdock • Echinacea • Chaparral • Mullein • Uva Ursi • Parsley • Marshmallow • Cascara Sagrada.

BRAND NAMES

B R A N D   N A M E S

Clinical Nutrients Antioxidant - PhytoPharmica
Three capsules contain: Vitamin A (beta-carotene) 10,000 IU • Vitamin C (ascorbic acid) 500 mg • Vitamin E (d-alpha tocopheryl succinate) 200 IU • Riboflavin (vitamin B2) 6 mg • Zinc (picolinate) 15 mg • Selenium (L-selenomethionine) 200 mcg • Manganese (gluconate) 15 mg • N-Acetylcysteine 100 mg • Red Cabbage (Brassica oleracea) leaf extract 4:1 100 mg • Garlic (Allium sativum) bulb extract (deodorized) 100 mg • Ginger (Zingiber officinale) root (rhizome) extract 100 mg • Green Tea (Camellia sinensis) leaf extract 100 mg • Klamath Blue-Green Algae 100 mg • Curcuma (Curcuma longa) root extract (standardized to contain 85%-97% curcumin) 50 mg • Grape (Vitis vinifera) seed (PCO) extract (standardized to contain 95% procyanidolic oligomers [PCOs] 10 mg.

Clinical Nutrients Eye Formula - PhytoPharmica
Three tablets contain: Vitamin A (50% beta-carotene and 50% fish liver oil) 5,000 IU • Vitamin C (ascorbic acid) 600 mg • Vitamin E (D-alpha tocopheryl acetate) 60 IU • Riboflavin (vitamin B2) 1.5 mg • Zinc (picolinate) 9 mg • Selenium (L-selenomethionine) 50 mcg • Copper (picolinate) 1 mg • Hachimijiogan herbal complex: Rhemania glutinosa (root), Poria cocos sclerotium (whole plant), Dioscorea opposita (root), Cornus officinalis (aerial part), Astragalus membranaceus (root), Cinnamonum cassia (bark) 400 mg • Bilberry (Vaccinium myrtillus fructus) berry extract (standardized to contain 25% anthocyanosides calculated as anthocyanidins) 160 mg • Curcuma (Curcuma longa) root extract (standardized to contain 85%-97% curcumin) 50 mg • Grape (Vitis vinifera) seed (PCO) extract (standardized to contain 95% procyanidolic oligomers [PCOs]) 50 mg • Lutein (Marigold flower extract) 2 mg.

Clinical Nutrients Flax Oil - PhytoPharmica
Each tablespoon (14ml) contains: Calories 120 • Calories from Fat 120 • Total Fat 14 g • Saturated Fat 1 g • Flaxseed Oil 11 ml • Pumpkin Seed oil 2 ml • Borage seed oil 1 ml. Average analysis: Omega-3 (LNA) 5,250 mg • Omega-6 (LA) 2,625 mg • Omega-9 (Oleic) 2,600 mg • Gamma-Linolenic Acid (GLA) 325 mg.

Clinical Nutrients Flax Oil Capsules - PhytoPharmica
Seven capsules contain: Calories 60 • Calories from Fat 60 • Total Fat 7 g • Saturated Fat 0.5 g • Flaxseed Oil 5,250 mg • Pumpkin Seed Oil 1,050 mg • Borage Seed Oil 700 mg. Average analysis: Omega-3 (LNA) 2,625 mg • Omega-6 (LA) 1,313 mg • Omega-9 (Oleic) 1,300 mg • Gamma-Linolenic Acid (GLA) 163 mg.

Clinical Nutrients for 45-Plus Women - PhytoPharmica
Six tablets contain: Vitamin A (beta-carotene) 15,000 IU • Vitamin A (retinol) 2,500 IU • Vitamin C (ascorbic acid) 300 mg • Vitamin D (ergocalciferol) 400 IU • Vitamin E (d-alpha tocopheryl succinate) 200 IU • Vitamin K (phytonadione) 60 mcg • Thiamin (thiamin HCl; vitamin B1) 60 mg • Riboflavin (vitamin B2) 60 mg • Niacin/Niacinamide 45 mg • Vitamin B6 (pyridoxine HCl) 60 mg • Folic Acid 800 mcg • Vitamin B12 (cyanocobalamin) 800 mcg • Biotin 600 mcg • Pantothenic Acid (calcium D-pantothenate) 50 mg • Calcium (citrate, carbonate) 600 mg • Iodine (kelp) 300 mcg • Magnesium (aspartate) 300 mg • Zinc (picolinate) 15 mg • Selenium (L-selenomethionine) 100 mcg • Copper (gluconate) 1.5 mg • Manganese (citrate) 15 mg • Chromium (polynicotinate) 200 mcg • Molybdenum (sodium molybdate) 25 mcg • Sodium 18 mg • Potassium (aspartate) 99 mg • Mixed flavonoids (citrus) 100 mg • Alfalfa (Medicaga sativa) leaf and stem juice concentrate 100 mg • Dong Quai (Angelica sinensis) root extract 4:1 90 mg • Ginger (Zingiber officinale) root (rhizome) extract 60 mg • Fennel (Foeniculum vulgare) seed extract 4.4:1 30 mg • Green Tea (Camellia sinensis) leaf extract 30 mg • Choline Bitartrate 30 mg • Inositol 30 mg • Para-Aminobenzoic Acid (PABA) 30 mg • Betaine HCl 25 mg • L-Glutamic Acid HCl 25 mg • Bromelain 15 mg • Papain 15 mg • Protease (acid stable) 5 mg • Lipase 5 mg • Boron (sodium tetraborate decahydrate) 3 mg • Silica (sodium metasilicate) 1 mg • Vanadium (sulfate) 50 mcg.

Clinical Nutrients for 50-Plus Men - PhytoPharmica
Four tablets contain: Vitamin A (beta-carotene) 15,000 IU • Vitamin A (acetate) 2,500 IU • Vitamin C (ascorbic acid) 300 mg • Vitamin D (cholecalciferol) 100 IU • Vitamin E (d-alpha tocopheryl succinate) 200 IU • Vitamin K (phytonadione) 60 mcg • Thiamin (thiamin HCl; vitamin B1) 60 mg • Riboflavin (vitamin B2) 60 mg • Niacin/Niacinamide 120 mg • Vitamin B6 (pyridoxine HCl) 60 mg • Folic Acid 800 mcg • Vitamin B12 (cyanocobalamin) 800 mcg • Biotin 600 mcg • Pantothenic Acid (calcium D-pantothenate) 100 mg • Calcium (citrate, carbonate) 250 mg • Iodine (potassium iodide) 300 mcg • Magnesium (aspartate) 250 mg • Zinc (picolinate) 30 mg • Selenium (L-selenomethionine) 100 mcg • Copper (gluconate) 1.5 mg • Manganese (citrate) 15 mg • Chromium (polynicotinate) 200 mcg • Molybdenum (sodium molybdate) 25 mcg • Sodium 10 mg • Potassium (aspartate) 99 mg • Mixed flavonoids 50% (citrus) 100 mg • Saw Palmetto (Serenoa repens) berry extract 4:1 80 mg • Ginger (Zingiber officinale) root (rhizome) extract 60 mg • Alfalfa (Medicago sativa) leaf and stem juice concentrate 60 mg • Choline Bitartrate 30 mg • Inositol 30 mg • Para-Aminobenzoic Acid (PABA) 30 mg • Green Tea (Camellia sinensis) leaf extract 30 mg • Betaine HCl 25 mg • L-Glutamic Acid HCl 25 mg • Korean Ginseng (Panax ginseng) root extract (standardized to contain 7% ginsenosides) 15 mg • Bromelain 15 mg • Papain 15 mg • Protease (acid stable) 5 mg • Lipase 5 mg • Boron (sodium borate) 2 mg • Vanadium (sulfate) 50 mcg.

Clinical Nutrients for Bone Health - PhytoPharmica
Three tablets contain: Vitamin C (ascorbic acid) 100 mg • Vitamin D (fish liver oil) 300 IU • Vitamin K (phytonadione) 300 mcg • Folic Acid 800 mcg • Vitamin B12 (cyanocobalamin) 800 mcg • Calcium (Krebs cycle chlelate/carbonate) 600 mg • Magnesium (Krebs cycle chelate) 150 mg • Zinc (picolinate) 15 mg • Copper (picolinate) 1 mg • Sodium 5 mg • Mixed flavonoids (citrus) 100 mg • Betaine HCl 30 mg • Soy (Glycine Max.) bean extract 20 mg • Boron (sodium tetrahydroborate) 3 mg • Silicon (sodium metasilicate) 1 mg • Strontium (chloride) 500 mcg.

Clinical Nutrients for Diabetics - PhytoPharmica
Two tablets contain: Vitamin C (ascorbic acid) 300 mg • Vitamin E (mixed tocopherols) 100 IU • Vitamin B6 (pyridoxine HCl) 10 mg • Folic Acid 400 mcg • Vitamin B12 (cyanocobalamin) 400 mcg • Biotin 1,000 mcg • Magnesium (Krebs cycle chelate) 100 mg • Zinc (picolinate) 7.5 mg • Selenium (aspartate) 50 mcg • Copper (picolinate) 0.5 mg • Manganese (Krebs cycle chelate) 7.5 mg • Chromium (picolinate) 200 mcg • Sodium 5 mg • Gymnema Sylvestre leaf extract (standardized to contain 24% gymnemic acid) 200 mg • Bitter Melon (Momordica charantia) whole fruit extract 200 mg • Fenugreek (Trigonella feonum-graecum) seed extract 4:1 100 mg • Bilberry (Vaccinium myrtillus fructus) berry extract (standardized to contain 25% anthocyanosides calculated as anthocyanidins) 40 mg • Mixed bioflavonoids (citrus) 25 mg • Vanadyl sulfate 5 mg.

Clinical Nutrients for Heart Health - PhytoPharmica
Two tablets contain: Vitamin C (ascorbic acid) 100 mg • Vitamin E (D-alpha tocopheryl acetate) 100 IU • Niacin 100 mg • Vitamin B6 (pyridoxine HCl) 10 mg • Folic Acid 200 mcg • Vitamin B12 (cyanocobalamin) 200 mcg • Calcium pangamate 20 mg • Magnesium (oxide) 150 mg • Potassium (chloride) 75 mg • Hawthorn (Crataegus oxyacantha) leaf and flower extract (standardized to contain 1.8% vitexin-2-rhamnoside) 150 mg • Super seven complex mixture of herbs: Hydrangea (Hydrangea arborescens) root, Black Cohosh (Cimicifuga racemosa) root, (Rhizome) extract, Buchu (Barosma crenata) leaf extract, Couch Grass (Elytrigia repens) rhizome extract, Cornsilk (Zea mays) extract, Dandelion (Taraxacum officinale) leaf, Ginger (Zingiber officinale) root] 150 mg • Khella (ammi visnaga) fruit extract (standardized to contain a minimum of 10% pyrones calculated as khellin) 100 mg • L-Cysteine 100 mg • Carbamide 100 mg.

Clinical Nutrients for Joint Health - Capsules - PhytoPharmica

Four capsules contain: Vitamin C (ascorbic acid) 100 mg • Niacin/Niacinamide 330 mg • Vitamin B6 (pyridoxine HCl) 20 mg • Pantothenic Acid (calcium D-pantothenate) 100 mg • Magnesium (oxide) 100 mg • Zinc (picolinate) 3 mg • Copper (gluconate) 200 mcg • Manganese (chelate) 10 mg • Chloride (from glucosamine sulfate) 78 mg • Sodium 60 mg • Stabilized Glucosamine Sulfate 500 mg • Boswellia Serrata (gum resin) standardized to contain 65% boswellic acids 400 mg • Bio-Min T.R. 8 (a source of trace minerals) 100 mg • Chlorophyll 10 mg • Boron (sodium borate) 3 mg.

Clinical Nutrients for Joint Health - Tablets - PhytoPharmica

Two tablets contain: Vitamin C (ascorbic acid) 100 mg • Niacin/Niacinamide 330 mg • Vitamin B6 (pyridoxine HCl) 20 mg • Pantothenic Acid (calcium D-pantothenate) 100 mg • Magnesium (oxide) 100 mg • Zinc (picolinate) 3 mg • Copper (gluconate) 200 mcg • Manganese (chelate) 10 mg • Chloride (from glucosamine sulfate) 78 mg • Sodium 60 mg • Stabilized Glucosamine Sulfate 500 mg • Boswellia Serrata (gum resin) standardized to contain 65% boswellic acids 400 mg • Bio-Min T.R. 8 (a source of trace minerals) 100 mg • Chlorophyll 10 mg • Boron (sodium borate) 3 mg.

Clinical Nutrients for Men - PhytoPharmica

Three tablets contain: Vitamin A (beta-carotene) 15,000 IU • Vitamin A (retinol) 2,500 IU • Vitamin C (ascorbic acid) 300 mg • Vitamin D (cholecalciferol) 100 IU • Vitamin E (d-alpha tocopheryl succinate) 200 IU • Vitamin K (phytonadione) 60 mcg • Thiamin (thiamin HCl; vitamin B1) 60 mg • Riboflavin (vitamin B2) 60 mg • Niacin 90 mg • Vitamin B6 (pyridoxine HCl) 60 mg • Folic Acid 800 mcg • Vitamin B12 (cyanocobalamin) 800 mcg • Biotin 600 mcg • Pantothenic Acid (calcium D-pantothenate) 60 mg • Calcium (citrate, carbonate) 200 mg • Iodine (kelp) 300 mcg • Magnesium (aspartate, oxide, chloride) 400 mg • Zinc (picolinate) 30 mg • Selenium (selenomethionine) 200 mcg • Copper (gluconate) 1 mg • Manganese (citrate) 5 mg • Chromium (polynicotinate) 200 mcg • Molybdenum (sodium molybdate) 25 mcg • Sodium 10 mg • Potassium (aspartate) 99 mg • Mixed Flavonoids (citrus) 50 mg • Alfalfa (Medicago sativa) leaf and stem juice concentrate 50 mg • Choline Bitartrate 30 mg • Inositol 30 mg • Ginger (Zingiber officinale) root (rhizome) extract 30 mg • Green Tea (Camellia sinensis) leaf extract 30 mg • Muira Puama (Ptychopetalum olacoides) root extract 6:1 30 mg • Para-aminobenzoic Acid (PABA) 30 mg • Saw Palmetto (Serenoa repens) berry extract 4:1 30 mg • Korean Ginseng (Panax ginseng) root extract (standardized to contain 7% gensenosides) 15 mg • Mixed carotenes (from dunaliella salina; sea algae) 5 mg • Boron (sodium tetraborate decahydrate) 2 mg • Vanadium (sulfate) 50 mcg.

Clinical Nutrients for Senior Women - PhytoPharmica

Six tablets contain: Vitamin A (Beta Carotene) 15000 IU • Vitamin A (Retinol) 2500 IU • Vitamin E 200 IU • Calcium (Citrate, Carbonate) 600 mcg • Vitamin C 300 mg • Magnesium (Aspartate) 300mg • Potassium (Aspartate) 99 mg • Vitamin B6 60 mg • Vitamin B1 60 mg • Vitamin B2 60 mg • Pantothenic Acid 50 mg • Niacin/Niacinamide 45 mg • Zinc (Picolinate) 15 mg • Manganese (Citrate) 15 mg • Copper (Gluconate) 1.5 mg • Folic Acid 800 mcg • Vitamin B12 800 mcg • Biotin 600 mcg • Iodine (Kelp) 300 mcg • Chromium (Polynicotinate) 200 mcg • Selenium 100 mcg • Vitamin K 60 mcg • Molybdenum 25 mcg • Flavonoids 100 mg • Alfalfa Juice concentrate 100 mg • Dong Quai extract 90 mg • Ginger root extract 60 mg • Fennel seed extract 30 mg • Green Tea extract 30 mg • Choline Bitartrate 30 mg • Inositol 30 mg • PABA 30 mg • Betaine HCL 25 mg • Glutamic Acid HCL 25 mg • Bromelain 15 mg • Papain 15 mg • Protease acid stable 5 mg • Lipase 5 mg • Boron 3 mg • Silica 1 mg • Vanadium (Sulfate) 50 mcg.

Clinical Nutrients for Teens: Female Formula - PhytoPharmica

Four tablets contain: Vitamin A (88% beta-carotene and 12% retinol) 17,000 IU • Vitamin C (ascorbic acid) 300 mg • Vitamin D (ergocalciferol) 100 IU • Vitamin E (d-alpha tocopheryl succinate) 200 IU • Vitamin K (phytonadione) 60 mcg • Thiamin (thiamin HCl; vitamin B1) 30 mg • Riboflavin (vitamin B2) 30 mg • Niacin/Niacinamide 45 mg • Vitamin B6 (pyridoxine HCl) 90 mg • Folic Acid 800 mcg • Vitamin B12 (cyanocobalamin) 800 mcg • Biotin 300 mcg • Pantothenic Acid (calcium D-pantothenate) 30 mg • Calcium (citrate, carbonate) 500 mg • Iron (ferrous succinate) 30 mg • Iodine (kelp) 300 mcg • Magnesium (aspartate) 200 mg • Zinc (picolinate) 20 mg • Selenium (L-selenomethionine) 100 mcg • Copper (gluconate) 1.5 mg • Manganese (citrate) 15 mg • Chromium (polynicotinate) 200 mcg • Molybdenum (sodium molybdate) 25 mcg • Sodium 30 mg • Potassium (aspartate) 99 mg • Mixed flavonoids (citrus) 100 mg • Alfalfa (Medicago sativa) leaf and stem juice concentrate 60 mg • Choline Bitartrate 60 mg • Inositol 60 mg • Ginger (Zingiber officinale) root (rhizome) extract 60 mg • Dandelion (Taraxacum officinale) root extract 4:1 60 mg • Licorice (Glycyrrhiza glabra) root extract (standardized to contain 5% glycyrrhizic acid) 30 mg • Boron (sodium tetraborate decahydrate) 2 mg • Silica (sodium metasilicate) 1 mg • Vanadium (sulfate) 50 mcg.

Clinical Nutrients for Teens: Male Formula - PhytoPharmica

Four tablets contain: Vitamin A (86% beta-carotene and 14% retinol) 17,500 IU • Vitamin C (ascorbic acid) 300 mg • Vitamin D (ergocalciferol) 100 IU • Vitamin E (d-alpha tocopheryl succinate) 200 IU • Vitamin K (phytonadione) 60 mcg • Thiamin (thiamin HCl; vitamin B1) 30 mg • Riboflavin (vitamin B2) 30 mg • Niacin/Niacinamide 45 mg • Vitamin B6 (pyridoxine HCl) 30 mg • Folic Acid 800 mcg • Vitamin B12 (cyanocobalamin) 800 mcg • Biotin 300 mcg • Pantothenic Acid (calcium D-pantothenate) 30 mg • Calcium (citrate, carbonate) 400 mg • Iodine (kelp) 300 mcg • Magnesium (aspartate) 200 mg • Zinc (picolinate) 30 mg • Selenium (L-selenomethionine) 100 mcg • Copper (gluconate) 1.5 mg • Manganese (citrate) 15 mg • Chromium (polynicotinate) 200 mcg • Molybdenum (sodium molybdate) 25 mcg • Sodium 30 mg • Potassium (aspartate) 99 mg • Mixed flavonoids (citrus) 100 mg • Alfalfa (Medicago sativa) leaf and stem juice concentrate 60 mg • Dandelion (Taraxacum officinale) root extract 4:1 60 mg • Ginger (Zingiber officinale) root (rhizome) extract 60 mg • Sarsaparilla (Smilax officinalis) root extract 4:1 60 mg • Choline Bitartrate 30 mg • Inositol 30 mg • Boron (sodium tetraborate decahydrate) 2 mg • Vanadium (sulfate) 50 mcg.

Clinical Nutrients for Women - PhytoPharmica

Three tablets contain: Vitamin A (86% beta-carotene and 14% acetate) 17,500 IU • Vitamin C (as ascorbic acid) 300 mg • Vitamin D (as cholecalciferol) 100 IU • Vitamin E (as d-alpha tocopheryl succinate) 200 IU • Vitamin K (as phytonadione) 60 mcg • Thiamin (thiamin HCl; vitamin B1) 60 mg • Riboflavin (vitamin B2) 60 mg • Niacin (as niacinamide) 90 mg • Vitamin B6 (as pyridoxine HCl, and pyridoxal-5-phosphate) 95 mg • Folic Acid 800 mcg • Vitamin B12 (as cyanocobalamin) 800 mcg • Biotin 600 mcg • Pantothenic Acid (as calcium D-pantothenate) 30 mg • Calcium (as calcium carbonate and calcium citrate) 400 mg • Iron (as ferrous succinate) 18 mg • Iodine (kelp) 300 mcg • Magnesium (as magnesium citrate) 300 mg • Zinc (as zinc picolinate) 20 mg • Selenium (as L-selenomethionine) 200 mcg • Copper (as copper gluconate) 1 mg • Manganese (as citrate) 5 mg • Chromium (as chromium polynicotinate) 200 mcg • Molybdenum (as sodium molybdate) 25 mcg • Sodium 10 mg • Potassium (as potassium aspartate) 99 mg • Mixed flavonoids (citrus) 50 mg • Alfalfa (Medicago sativa) leaf and stem juice concentrate 50 mg • Choline Bitartrate 30 mg • Inositol 30 mg • Dong Quai (Angelica sinensis) root extract 4:1 30 mg • Ginger (Zingiber officinale) root (rhizome) extract 30 mg • Licorice (Glycyrrhiza glabra) root extract (standardized to contain 5% glycyrrhizic acid) 30 mg • Para-Aminobenzoic Acid (PABA) 30 mg • Chaste Tree (Vitex-agnus castus) berry extract (standardized to contain 0.5% agnuside) 15 mg • Fennel (Foeniculum vulgare) seed extract 4.4:1 15 mg • Carotenes 5 mg • Boron (as sodium tetraborate decahydrate) 3 mg • Silica (as magnesium metasilicate) 1 mg • Vanadium (as vanadyl sulfate) 50 mcg.

BRAND NAMES

Clinical Nutrients Prenatal Formula - PhytoPharmica

Four tablets contain: Vitamin A (Beta Carotene) 15000 IU • Vitamin E (D-Alpha Tocopherol Succinate) 200 IU • Vitamin D 100 IU • Calcium (Citrate, Carbonate) 800 mg • Magnesium (Citrate) 400 mg • Vitamin C (Ascorbic Acid) 300 mg • Vitamin B6 (Pyridoxine HCL) 120 mg • Pantothenic Acid (D-Calcium Pantothenate) 100 mg • Potassium (Aspartate) 99 mg • Thiamine HCL (Vitamin B1) 60 mg • Riboflavin (Vitamin B2) 60 mg • Niacin/Niacinamide 45 mg • Iron (Ferrous Succinate) 30 mg • Zinc (Picolinate) 30 mg • Manganese (Citrate) 15 mg • Copper (Gluconate) 1.5 mg • Folic Acid 800 mcg • Vitamin B12 (Cyanocobalamin) 800 mcg • Biotin 600 mcg • Vitamin K (Phytonandione) 500 mcg • Iodine (Kelp) 300 mcg • Chromium (Polynicotinate) 200 mcg • Selenium (L-Selenomethionine) 100 mcg • Molybdenum (Sodium Molybdate) 25 mcg • Ginger root extract 6.5:1 (Zingiber officinale) 150 mg • Flavonoids (Mixed) 90 mg • Choline Bitartrate 90 mg • Inositol 90 mg • Dandelion root extract 4:1 (Taraxacum officinale) 60 mg • Red Raspberry leaves 60 mg • Boron (Sodium Tetraborate Decahydrate) 1 mg • Silica (Sodium Metasilicate) 1 mg • Vanadium (Sulfate) 50 mcg.

Clinical Nutrients to Retain Healthy Cholesterol Levels - PhytoPharmica

Each capsule contains: Red Yeast (Monascus purpureus) rice 475 mg • Artichoke (Cynara scolymus) leaf extract (standardized to contain 13%-18% caffeylquinic acids calculated as chlorogenic acid) 50 mg • Ginger (Zingiber officinale) root (rhizome) extract 50 mg • Coenzyme Q10 (CoQ10) 8 mg.

CM Complex - Source Naturals

Three 500 mg softgels contain: Cetyl Myristoleate 180 mg • Cetyl Oleate (base of mixed fatty acid esters, olive oil and vitamin E) 375 mg.

CM Source - Now

Each 500 mg capsule contains : Cetyl Myristoleate 100 mg.

CM+ - Metabolic Response Modifiers

Each softgel contains: Cetylmyristoleate (CMO) complex (Yielding 100 mg CMO) 500 mg.

CMG - Natrol

Two capsules contain: Cetyl Myristoleate Proprietary Blend (CetylPure) 500 mg • MSM (Methyl Sulfonyl Methane) 500 mg • Glucosamine Sulfate 500 mg • Sea Cucumber 25 mg. Other Ingredients: Silica, Magnesium stearate, Gelatin. Contains no yeast, wheat, milk, egg, soy, glutens, artificial colors, or flavors, added sugar, or preservatives.

C-M-K Citrate - Progressive Labs

Each capsule contains: Calcium (as calcium citrate) 100 mg • Magnesium (as magnesium citrate) 100 mg • Potassium (as potassium citrate) 25 mg.

Co Q10 - Pharmanex - Pharmanex

Each softgel contains: Vitamin E (from Mixed Tocopherols) 30 IU • Coenzyme Q10 (Ubiquinone) 30 mg. Other Ingredients: Rice Bran Oil, Gelatin, Glycerin, Yellow Beeswax, Annatto Extract, Titanium Dioxide.

Coat and Skin (For Animal Use Only) - Puritan's Pride

Each serving contains: Linoleic & Linolenic acids (as the glycerides) 12.43 gm • Other unsaturated fatty acids: Arachidonic, Oleic, Palmitoleic, Clupanodonic (as the glycerides) 9.12 gm • Vitamin A 8100 IU • Vitamin D 540 IU • Vitamin E 162 IU.

Cod Liver Oil - Puritan's Pride

Each softgel contains: Natural Vitamin A 2,664 IU • Natural Vitamin D (from 1,000 mg of Cod Liver Oil) 200 IU. Provides a rich source of Omega 3 fatty acids, EPA and DHA.

Cod Liver Oil & Evening Primrose Oil - Puritan's Pride

Each softgel contains: Natural Vitamin A 2,664 IU • Natural Vitamin D (from 500 mg of Cod Liver Oil) 200 IU • Evening Primrose Oil 500 mg. Provides a rich source of Omega-3 fatty acids, EPA and DHA.

CoenZest - Holista

Each capsule contains: CoEnzyme Q10 (ubiquinone) 30 mg. Other Ingredients: Organic Flax Seed Oil.

Coenzymated B-1 - Source Naturals

Each tablet contains: Coenzyme Vitamin B1 (Cocarboxylase) (Yielding 16.25 mg of activated Vitamin B1) 25 mg. In a base of Mannitol, Sorbitol, Natural Peppermint, and Sodium Citrate.

Coenzyme Q10 - Source Naturals

Each sublingual tablet contains: Coenzyme Q10 30 mg. See Editor's Note No. 6, page 1816.

Coenzyme Q10 - YourLife/Leiner Health Products, Inc.

Each softgel contains: Coenzyme Q10 30 mg. Other Ingredients: Hydrogenated Vegetable Oil, Refined Soybean Oil, Gelatin, Glycerin, Lecithin, Titanium Dioxide, Red 40 Lake, d-Alpha Tocopherol, Yellow 6 Lake, Blue 1 Lake. See Editor's Note No. 6, page 1816.

Coenzyme Q10 - Leiner Health Products

Each softgel contains: Coenzyme Q10 30 mg. Other Ingredients: Hydrogenated Vegetable Oil, Refined Soybean Oil, Gelatin, Glycerin, Lecithin, Titanium Dioxide, Red 40 Lake, d-Alpha Tocopherol, Yellow 6 Lake, Blue 1 Lake.

Coenzyme Q10 - Leiner Health Products

Each capsule contains: Coenzyme Q10 100 mg. Other Ingredients: Maltodextrin, Gelatin, Magnesium Stearate.

Coenzyme Q-10 - GNC Preventive Nutrition

Each capsule contains: Coenzyme Q-10 30 mg. Other Ingredients: Dicalcium Phosphate, Cellulose, Gelatin, Stearic Acid. Contains no sugar, starch, artificial colors or flavors, sodium, corn, wheat, gluten, soy, dairy, or yeast. See Editor's Note No. 6, page 1816.

Coenzyme Q-10 - Natrol

Each capsule contains: CoEnzyme Q10 30 mg. Other Ingredients: Rice Powder, Magnesium Stearate, Gelatin. See Editor's Note No. 6, page 1816.

Coenzyme Q-10 - Puritan's Pride

Each softgel contains: Coenzyme Q-10 10 mg. Other Ingredients: Ricebran Oil, Gelatin, Glycerin, Yellow Beeswax. Contains no yeast, wheat, gluten, milk or milk derivatives, lactose, sugar, preservatives, soy, artificial color or flavor, sodium (less than 5 mg per serving). See Editor's Note No. 6, page 1816.

Coenzyme Q-10 - The Vitamin Shoppe

Each capsule contains: Co-Enzyme Q10 75 mg. Other Ingredients: Cellulose, Magnesium Stearate, Water. Contains no yeast, corn, wheat, soy, salt, gluten, sugar, starch, milk, eggs, dairy, fish, citrus, preservatives, artificial colors or flavors. See Editor's Note No. 6, page 1816.

Coenzyme Q-10 - Fields of Nature - Fields of Nature

Each capsule contains: Coenzyme Q-10 30 mg. Other Ingredients: Microcrystalline Cellulose, Gelatin, Magnesium Stearate. Contains no corn, soy, yeast, wheat, milk, egg, sugar, starch, salt, artificial colors or preservatives.

Some Brand Name Natural Products - What they Contain
www.NaturalDatabase.com contains MANY more listings than appear here.

Cognicine - Pacific BioLogic
DMAE • Bacopin • Ashwagandha extract • Black Pepper extract (bioperine).

CognoBlend - Rexall
Two capsules contain: Bacopa monniera leaf extract (standardized to 20% bacosides A&B, 30 mg) 150 mg • Ginkgo Biloba leaf extract (standardized to 24% ginkgo flavone glycosides, 14.4 mg; standardized to 6% terpene lactones, 3.6 mg) 60 mg • Proprietary Blend: Cat's Claw bark (Uncaria tomentosa), Gotu Kola leaf, Rosemary leaf 600 mg. Other Ingredients: Gelatin.

Cold & Flu (Cold and Flu) Capsules - Quantum Health
Three capsules contain: Vitamin C 25 mg • Echinacea angustifolia standardized to 4% phenolic compounds 100 mg • Elderberry (10:1 extract) 100 mg • Goldenseal root (3:1 extract) 25 mg. Other Ingredients: Vegetable Sterine, Magnesium stearate, Micro Crystalline Cellulose.

Cold & Flu (Cold and Flu) Liquid Extract - Quantum Health
Two ounces contain: Fresh undried Echinacea purpurea whole plant 30% • Goldenseal root 20% • Elderberry 40% • Echinacea angustifolia 10%. In a base of Alcohol (approximately 20%), Distilled Water.

Cold & Flu Remedy - PhytoPharmica
Twenty-five drops contain: Gelsemium sempervirens 6x • Aconitum napellus 4x • Arnica montana 4x • Belladonna 4x • Cinchona officinalis 4x • Bryonia 3x • Drosera rotundifolia 3x • Eupatorium 3x • Senega officinalis 3x • Eucalyptus globulus 1x. In a base of 50% USP alcohol by volume.
See Editor's Note No. 1, page 1816.

Cold & Flu Support - Amazon Support
Each capsule contains: Picao Preto • Fedegosa • Amor Seco • Guaco • Bitter Melon • Clavillia • Mullaca • Samambaia • Quinine Bark • Gervao • Pau d'Arco • Cat's Claw • Simaruba.

Cold Care P.M. - Traditional Medicinals
Contains: Menthol: 5 mg per cup as it naturally occurs in the Peppermint leaf (Mentha x piperia) present in the blend. Other herbal ingredients: Licorice root, Chamomile flower, Tilla Starflower, Yarrow flower, Passion flower herb, Eucalyptus leaf, Elder flower.

Cold Cayenne - Olympian Labs
Each capsule contains: Cayenne (40000 h.u.) 500 mg.

Cold Season Formula - Nature's Way
Three capsules contain: Echinacea purpurea (stem, leaf, flower) 450 mg • Ester-C (patented form of Vitamin C) 200 mg • Isatis 150 mg • Ligustrum fruits 70 mg • Sambucol (patented Black Elderberry extract) 100 mg • Siberian Ginseng root 150 mg • Usnea Barbata 100 mg • Vitamin A (retinol palmitate) 6,722 IU • Zinc amino acid chelate 25 mg. Other Ingredients: Cellulose, Gelatin, Magnesium stearate.

Cold Season Plus+ Zinc Lozenges - Quantum Health
Each lozenge contains: Zinc acetate 14 mg • Vitamin A acetate 500 IU • Slippery Elm bark (Ulmus fulva) 20 mg • Propolis 5 mg. In a base of Goldenseal, Sugar, Dextrose, Fructose.

Cold-Eeze - Quigley Co.
Each lozenge contains: Zinc Gluconate 11.5 mg.
Other ingredients: Glycine, corn syrup, sucrose, and natural flavors.

Cold-Eezer Plus - Quigley Co.
Each lozenge contains: Zinc Gluconate 14.5 mg.
Other ingredients: Glycerine, corn syrup, sucrose, and natural flavors.

Coldflua - HerbaSway
Bitter Orange • Kudzu • Ginger • Echinacea • Astragalus • Knotweed • Schisandra • Blackberry • Licorice • Skullcap • Cayenne pepper • HerbaSwee (Cucurbitaceae fruit).

Cold-FX - HerbTech - CV Technologies
Each capsule contains: Concentrated North American Ginseng (Panax quinquefolium) extract 200 mg.

Cold-X10 - Olympian Labs
Three capsules contain: Ester C 180 mg • Zinc Gluconate 15 mg • Garlic 500 mg • Cat's Claw 250 mg • Echinacea 500 mg • Gotu Kola 100 mg • Proteolytic Enzymes 100 mg.

Coleus Forskohlii extract - Enzymatic Therapy
One capsule contains: Coleus Forskohlii extract standardized to contain 18% Forskolin (9 mg per capsule) 50 mg. Contains no sugar, salt, yeast, wheat, corn, soy, dairy products, coloring, flavoring or preservatives.

Colic Tablets - Hyland's
Each tablet contains: Dioscorea as Wild Yam 2X HPUS • Chamomilla as Chamomile 3X HPUS • Colocynth as Bitter Apple 3X HPUS. In a base of Lactose NF (Milk Sugar).
See Editor's Note No. 1, page 1816.

Collagen Type II - Swanson
Six capsules contain: Hydrolyzed Type II Collagen (certified 100% chicken sternal cartilage) 3 g.
See Editor's Note No. 14, page 1817.

Colloidal Magnesium Plus - Progressive Labs
Each capsule contains: Colloidal Calcium 25 mg • Colloidal Magnesium 50 mg • Colloidal Zinc 1.5 mg • Colloidal Copper 1 mg • Colloidal Manganese 0.1 mg • Colloidal Chromium 0.03 mg • Colloidal Molybdenum 0.012 mg.

Colloidal Minerals - Progressive Labs
One half ounce contains: Calcium 109 mg • Iron 0.24 mg • Phosphorus 109 mg • Iodine 180 mcg • Magnesium 56.9 mg • Zinc 16.3 mg • Selenium 0.09 mcg • Copper 1.24 mg • Manganese 2.8 mg • Chromium 0.4 mcg • Molybdenum 0.01 mcg • Chloride 0.1 mg • Sodium 0.74 mg • Potassium 171 mg • Sulfur 0.08 mg • Aluminum 2.15 mg • Silicon 0.4 mg • Lanthanum 0.1 mg • Thallium 0.02 mg • Cesium 0.4 mcg • Strontium 5.8 mcg • Vanadium 5.4 mcg • Boron 4.62 mcg • Nickel 4.45 mcg • Scandium 3.3 mcg • Ruthenium 3.13 mcg • Lithium 2.15 mcg • Titanium 1.57 mcg • Neodynium 0.15 mcg • Antimony 1.3 mcg • Cobalt 1.06 mcg • Flouride 0.94 mcg • Bismuth 0.33 mcg • Thallium 0.28 mcg • Zirconium 0.23 mcg • Beryllium 0.2 mcg • Cerium 0.2 mcg • Erbium 0.2 mcg • Bromine 0.16 mcg • Indium 0.13 mcg • Rubidium 0.13 mcg • Silver 0.1 mcg • Tin 0.1 mcg • Yttrium 0.1 mcg • Gallium 0.08 mcg • Tellurium 0.07 mcg • Praseodymium 0.05 mcg • Samarium 0.05 mcg • Barium 0.02 mcg • Cadmium 0.02 mcg • Dysprosium 0.02 mcg • Germanium 0.01 mcg • Gold < 0.01 mcg • Europium < 0.01 mcg • Niobium < 0.01 mcg • Palladium < 0.01 mcg • Ytterbium < 0.01 mcg • Hafnium < 0.01 mcg • Iridium < 0.01 mcg • Rhodium < 0.01 mcg • Terbium < 0.01 mcg • Holmium < 0.01 mcg • Lutetium < 0.01 mcg • Rhenium < 0.01 mcg • Tantalum < 0.01 mcg • Thorium < 0.01 mcg • Tungsten < 0.01 mcg • Plantium < 0.01 mcg • Carbon 7.8%. Other ingredients: Water, Glycerine, Natural Flavor, Grapefruit seed extract, Stevia.

Colloidal Silver - Changes - TwinLab
Four droppers (4 mL) contain: Colloidal Silver 20 mcg. Other Ingredients: Demineralized water.

Colloidal Vitamins - Progressive Labs
One half ounce contains: Vitamin A (as beta carotene) 5000 IU • Vitamin C (ascorbic acid) 300 mg • Vitamin D 400 IU • Vitamin E

BRAND NAMES

BRAND NAMES

60 IU • Vitamin K 300 mcg • Thiamin (Vitamin B1) 3 mg • Riboflavin (Vitamin B2) 3.4 mg • Niacin (as niacinamide) 40 mg • Vitamin B6 4 mg • Folate (folic acid) 400 mcg • Vitamin B12 3 mcg • Biotin 300 mcg • Pantothenic Acid 20 mg • Choline Bitartrate 50 mg • Myonositol (inositol) 50 mg • Essential Fatty Acid complex 10 mg • Amino Acid complex 10 mg • Aloe powder 3 mg. Other Ingredients: Water, Glycerine, Natural Flavor, Grapefruit seed extract, Stevia.

Coloklysis - PhysioLogics
Each scoop contains: Psyllium seed & husk 10,000 mg • Oat fiber (Avena sativa) 1000 mg • Rice Bran 500 mg • Fructooligosaccharides (FOS) 250 mg • Alfalfa (Medicago sativa) 38 mg • Barley (Hordium vulgare) 38 mg • Apple Pectin (Malus sylvestris) 30 mg • Buckthorn bark (Rhamnus fangula) 38 mg • Papain (Carica papaya) 38 mg • Cascara sagrada (Rhamnus purshiana) 38 mg • Goldenseal (Hydrastis canadensis) 38 mg • Triphala 30 mg • natural Orange flavor 150 mg • Stevia extract 50 mg.

Coloklysis Daily - PhysioLogics
Each scoop contains: Psyllium 3400 mg • Oat fiber (Avena sativa) 2500 mg • Guar Gum 2500 mg • Acacia Gum 1200 mg • Apple Pectin 1000 mg • Rice Bran 500 mg • Fructooligosaccharides (FOS) 250 mg • L-Glutamine 100 mg • Aloe Vera 100 mg • Licorice 100 mg • Ginger 100 mg • Acesulfame Potassium 15 mg • Stevia 10 mg. Contains natural coloring and flavoring.

Colon Cleanse - Nature's Rx
Each capsule contains: Bentonita Clay • Micro-Crystalline Cellulose • Psyllium Seed • Senna Leaf • Citrus Pectin • Oat Bran • Nutra Flora FOS • Acidophilus Blend • Barley Grass • Golden Seal • Prune Concentrate • Slippery Elm Bark • Aloe Vera Leaf Extract • Bio-Perine • Cascara Sagrada.

Colon Cleanser Daily - Health Smart Vitamins
One scoop contains: Calories 7 • Total Carbohydrates 11g • Dietary Fiber 11 g • Blonde Psyllium (seed husks) 3 g • Oat Fiber 3 g • Guar Gum 3 g • Acacia Gum 1 mg • Apple Pectin 1 g • Rice Bran 500 mg • Fructooligosaccharides (FOS; from chicory root) 250 mg • Aloe Vera leaf 100 mg • Ginger root 100 mg • L-Glutamine 100 mg • Licorice root 100 mg • Stevia leaf 10 mg.

Colon Clear - Metabolic Response Modifiers
Each capsule contains: AG (Arabinogalactan) 200 mg • Cascara Sagrada bark 100 mg • Fennel seed 75 mg • Licorice root 50 mg • Ginger root 50 mg • Senna leaf 50 mg • Peppermint leaf 25 mg • Celery seed 25 mg • Triphala (Anala, Behada, Harada) 25 mg.

Colon Green - Futurebiotics
Six capsules contain: Psyllium seed husk powder 2490 mg • Alfalfa leaf powder 600 mg • Alfalfa juice powder 180 mg • Lactobacillus acidophilus (supplying 12 billion cells) 60 mg • Pau D'Arco bark powder 120 mg • Echinacea leaf powder extract 120 mg • Black Walnut hull powder extract 120 mg • Fenugreek seed powder 120 mg • Watercress powder 120 mg • Parsley leaf powder 120 mg • Rosemary leaf powder 120 mg • Clove flower powder 120 mg • Bayberry bark powder 120 mg • Cayenne fruit powder 120 mg • Lipase 114 LU* • Protease 1380 HUT* • Amylase 114 DU*. Other ingredients: LU are Lipase Units, HUT are Hemoglobin Units-Tyrosine basis, DU are Alpha-Amylase Dextrinizing Units.

Colostrum - Olympian Labs
Two capsules contain: Colostrum 1000 mg.

Colostrum Lozenges - Olympian Labs
Two lozenges contain: Colostrum 1000 mg.

Comfrey and Fenugreek - Dial Herbs
Comfrey • Fenugreek.

Comfrey/Aloe Capsules - Aloe Farms
Comfrey powder 100 mg, Aloe Vera powder 50 mg.

Commando 2000 - Nature's Plus
Two tablets contain: Commando Vitamin & Mineral Blend: Vitamin C corn free fortified with Rose Hips 1000 mg • Citrus Bioflavonoid Complex active flavonols, flavones, flavones & narigen - 44% 200 mg • Vitamin E natural 200 IU • Beta Carotene [carrot (Dunaliella salina) supplying 10000 IU Vitamin A activity] 60 mg • Zinc (Monomethionine) 20 mg • Selenium (Selenomethionine) 100 mcg. Commando Herbal Blend: Echinacea (Echinacea purpurea) 250 mg • Astragalus (Astragalus membranoceus) 150 mg • Garlic, odorless 70 mg • Ginkgo Biloba 50:1 standardized 24% ginkgo flavone-glycosides 5 mg. Commando Amino Acid Blend: NAC (N-Acetyl-Cysteine) 20 mg • L-Methionine free form amino acid 15 mg • L-Glutathione free form amino acid 10 mg. In a natural base of Pycnogenol (Pine bark extract), standardized 85-95% proanthocyanidins, antioxidant plant enzymes: catalase, glucose oxidase & peroxidase; & antioxidant vegetables : broccoli rich in sulforaphane, cabbage, cauliflower & tomato rich in lycopene. Contains no yeast, wheat, corn, soy, milk, salt, sugar or starch.

Compete - Mission Pharmacal
Each tablet contains: Vitamin A 5,000 IU • Vitamin C 90 mg • Vitamin D (as Vitamin D3) 400 IU • Vitamin E 43 IU • Thiamine 2 mg • Riboflavin 2.6 mg • Niacin 30 mg • Vitamin B6 20 mg • Folate 0.4 mg • Vitamin B12 9 mcg • Iron 27 mg • Zinc 25 mg. Other Ingredients: Microcrystalline Cellulose, Sugar, Calcium Carbonate, Color, Croscarmellose Sodium, Povidone, Food Glaze, Cyanocobalamin, Magnesium Stearate, Yellow 6 Lake, Carnauba Wax, White Beeswax, Sodium Benzoate.

Complete B - Puritan's Pride
Two tablets contain: Thiamin (Vitamin B1: as thiamine mononitrate) 10 mg • Riboflavin (Vitamin B2) 15 mg • Niacin (as niacinamide) 25 mg • Vitamin B6 (as pyridoxine hydrochloride) 10 mg • Folic Acid 400 mcg • Vitamin B12 (as cyancobalamin) 25 mcg • Biotin (as d-biotin) 100 mcg • Pantothenic Acid (as d-calcium pantothenate) 100 mg • PABA (para-aminobenzoic acid) 50 mg • Choline Bitartrate 250 mg • Inositol 250 mg.

Complete Cleanse - PhysioLogics
Each caplet contains: Calcium (from Dicalcium Phosphate) 260 mg • Phosphorus (from Dicalcium Phosphate) 200 mg. Rapid Release Layer: Enzyme Activated Herbal Digestive extract blend containing: [Cellulose, Beet fiber root, Fenugreek seed, Licorice root, Fennel seed, Lipase (from Aspargillus cryzae), Date fruit, Fig fruit, Ginger root, Prune fruit] 500 mg • Herbal Detox extract blend 250 mg containing: [Tea Green leaf, Grapefruit seed, Burdock root, Chickweed aerial parts, Gentian root, Milk Thistle seed, Red Clover blossom, Dandelion root, Marshmallow root, Rosemary leaf, Yarrow flower, Yellow Dock root] 500 mg. Extended Release Layer: Enzyme-Activated Cleansing Fiber & Herb Blend containing: [Butternut bark, Beet fiber root, Licorice root, Flax seed, Peppermint oil] 250 mg • Probiotic Flora Replenishment Complex containing: [Lactic Culture of B.Coagulins, Fructooligosaccharides & Inulides (from dahlia tuber & chicory root)] 75 million cells • Intestinal Tract Immune Complex containing: [Black Walnut leaf, Methylsulfonylmethane (MSM), Garlic bulb] 250 mg.

Complete Protein Diet - Optimum Nutrition
Each serving contains: Vanilla flavor Ingredients: Proprietary Protein Blend of Calcium Caseinate, Whey Protein Concentrate, Egg Albumen, Hydrolyzed Whey Peptides, Whey Protein Isolate, L-Glutamine • Canola oil • Artificial Flavor • Complete Vitamin Mineral Blend: di-Potassium Phosphate, Magnesium Oxide, Potassium Chloride, Ascorbic Acid, dl-Alpha Tocopherol Acetate, Niacinamide, Vitamin A Palmitate, Zinc Oxide, Potassium Iodide, Vitamin K, D-Calcium Pantothenate, Copper Sulfate, Manganese Sulfate, Vitamin D (as Vitamin D3), Pyridoxine Hydrochloride,

Thiamine Mononitrate, Riboflavin, Selenium Glycinate, Molybdenum Glycinate, Chromium Picolinate, Folic Acid, Biotin, Cyanocobalamin • Lecithin • Cellulose Gum • Xanthan Gum • Aspartame • Acesulfame Potassium • Salt • FD&C Yellow #5 • FD&C Yellow #6.

Complexion Perfect - Aspen Group, Inc.
Four tablets contain: Vitamin A 5000 IU • Beta Carotene 5000 IU • Vitamin B1 (thiamine) 25 mg • Vitamin B2 (riboflavin) 25 mg • Vitamin B3 (niacin) 50 mg • Vitamin B5 (pantothenic acid) 25 mg • Vitamin B6 (pyridoxine HCl) 50 mg • Biotin 300 mcg • Vitamin C (calcium ascorbate) 500 mg • Vitamin E (succinate) 400 IU • Magnesium Oxide 200 mg • Zinc (gluconate) 12 mg • Burdock root 600 mg • L-Lysine HCl 500 mg • L-Proline 500 mg • Yellow Dock 500 mg • Silica (derived from horsetail extract) 400 mg • Grape seed extract (proanthodyn) 50 mg • Selenomethionine 200 mcg • Chromium Picolinate 50 mcg • GTF Chromium 25 mcg. Contains no sugar, starch, salt, wheat, corn, yeast or soy derivatives.

Composition 1 - Dial Herbs
Bayberry • White Pine bark • Clove • Cinnamon • Ginger • Cayenne.

Concentrated Broccoli - Jamieson
Each caplet contains: Concentrated Broccoli florets (Equivalent to 25000 mg fresh Broccoli) 450 mg • Concentrated Kale leaf and Radish root (Standardized to Active Isothiocyanates 450 mcg) 10 mg.

Concentrated Garlic - Leiner Health Products
Two tablets contain: Garlic (Allium sativum) clove powder 300 mg. Other Ingredients: Dicalcium Phosphate, Cellulose, Starch, Silicon Dioxide, Vanilla Flavor, Magnesium Stearate, Ethylcellulose, may contain less than 2% of Croscarmellose Sodium.

Connect-All - Nature's Plus
Two tablets contain: Glucosamine Sulfate (Aminomonosaccharide) 300 mg • Bromelain, proteolytic enzyme 600 GDU/gram, 200 mg • Calcium (Aminoate) 200 mg • Vitamin C corn free 60 mg • Aloe Vera leaf naturally rich in Mucopolysaccharide 50 mg • Chondroitin Sulfate A (CSA) 50 mg • Zinc (Monomethionine) 15 mg • Chinese Sea Cucumber (Microchele nobilis) 10 mg • Copper (Aminoate) 1 mg . In a highly active base of Alfalfa, Chlorella, Spirulina & low temperature dried Barley Grass juice, supplying naturally occuring chlorophyll & trace minerals. Contains no yeast, wheat, corn, soy, milk, salt, sugar or starch.
See Editor's Note No. 15, page 1817.

Continence with Flowtrol - Solaray - Nutraceutical
Two capsules contain: Butterbur root extract (Petasites hybridus) (Guaranteed to contain 15 mg sesquiterpenes) 100 mg • Flowtrol Prorietary Blend 870 mg: Cranberry berry extract (Vaccinium macrocarpon as CranActin Cranberry AF Extract), Morinda root extract 5:1, Psoralea fruit extract 5:1, Raspberry fruit extract 5:1 (Rubus chingii), Alpinia oxyphylla fruit and seed extract 5:1, Lobelia (aerial). Other Ingredients: Gelatin (capsule), Cellulose, Maltodextrin, Magnesium Stearate, Silica, and Magnesium Hydroxide.

Controlled-Release Melatonin - Amni
Each tablet contains: Melatonin 2 mg.
See Editor's Note No. 16, page 1817.

Copper Sebacate - Source Naturals
Each tablet contains: Copper sebacate 22 mg.

CoQ10 - Nature's Way
Each capsule or softgel contains: Coenzyme Q10 (ubiquinone) 60 mg. Other Ingredients: Gelatin, Millet, Turmeric Root. Contains no soy, corn, yeast, wheat, milk, sugars, artificial color or preservatives.
See Editor's Note No. 6, page 1816.

CoQ10 - Now
Each capsule contains: Coenzyme Q10 30 mg. Other Ingredients: White Rice Powder. Contains no yeast, wheat, corn, milk, preservatives, or additives.
See Editor's Note No. 6, page 1816.

Co-Q10 - Carlson
Each softgel contains: Vitamin E (as d-Alpha Tocopherol) 1 IU • Co-Q10 (as Coenzyme Q10 50 mg).
See Editor's Note No. 6, page 1816.

CoQ-10 - Schiff
Each capsule contains: Coenzyme Q-10 30 mg. Other Ingredients: Rice Powder, Silica. Contains no sugar, starch, salt, soy, yeast, wheat, corn, milk, preservatives, artificial colors or flavors.
See Editor's Note No. 6, page 1816.

CoQ-10 - Solgar
Each capsule contains: CoEnzyme Q-10 (ubiquinone) 30 mg. Other Ingredients: Microcrystalline Cellulose, Gelatin, Vegetable Cellulose, Silica, Vegetable Magnesium Stearate, Water. Contains no corn, yeast, wheat, soy, dairy products, preservatives, artificial flavors or colors.
See Editor's Note No. 6, page 1816.

CoQ-10 - Metabolic Response Modifiers
Each capsule contains: Ubiquinone (Coenzyme Q-10) 30 mg.

CoQ10 - 100 mg - Nature's Way
Each capsule contains: Coenzyme Q10 (ubiquinone) 100 mg • Vitamin E (d-alpha tocopheryl) 5 IU. Other Ingredients: Annatto Oil, Gelatin, Glycerin, Rice Bran Oil, Titanium Dioxide, Water.

CoQ10 100 mg - PhytoPharmica
Each capsule contains: Coenzyme Q10 (CoQ10) verified by HPLC 100 mg.

COQ10 100 mg PLUS E - Progressive Labs
Each capsule contains: Co-Enzyme Q10 100 mg • Vitamin E (dl-alpha tocopheryl acetate) 100 IU.

CoQ10 30 mg - Swanson
Each capsule contains: Coenzyme Q10 30 mg.

CoQ10 30 mg - PhytoPharmica
Each capsule contains: Coenzyme Q10 (CoQ10) verified by HPLC 30 mg.

CoQ10 50 mg - PhytoPharmica
Each capsule contains: Coenzyme Q10 (CoQ10) verified by HPLC 50 mg.

CoQ10 Extra Strength - Olympian Labs
Each capsule contains: Crystalline Coenzyme Q10 150 mg.

CoQ10 Spray - Nature's Plus
Each spray contains: CoQ10 pharmaceutical grade Ubiquinone 30 mg. In a proprietary Liposomal Complex of Essential Metabolic Factors, Purified Water, Vegetable Glycerine, Purified Lecithin, Citrus seed extract (Citrus sinensis), Vitamin E & natural Mandarin Tangerine flavor.

Cordephrine XC - HealthDesigns
Each vegicap contains: Cordyceps Mycelia (Cordyceps sinensis) 450 mg. Other Ingredients: Pure plant cellulose (vegicaps). Does not contain ephedra or ephedrine.

Cordyceps - Metabolic Response Modifiers
Each capsule contains: Cordyceps mycelia (Cordyceps sinensis) 750 mg.

BRAND NAMES

***Cordyceps (Caterpillar Fungus)* - Olympia Nutrition**
Caterpillar fungus 500 mg.

***Cordyceps 500* - Pinnacle**
Each tablet contains: 100% Purified Chinese Herbs 500 mg (Dong Chong Zia Cao, Sha Shen, Wuwei Zi, Gan Jiang, Duhlulin). Free of yeast, corn, soy, wheat, lactose, citrus, milk, egg & fish products. No sugar, salt, starch, yeast, artificial coloring, flavoring, or preservatives.

***Cordyceps 520 mg* - Solaray**
Each capsule contains: Cordyceps 520 mg. Other Ingredients: Gelatin, Cellulose, & Magnesium stearate.

***Cordyceps Power 800 mg* - Planetary Formulations**
Two capsules contain: Cordyceps Proprietary Blend 1600 mg. Other Ingredients: Dibasic calcium phosphate, colloidal silicon dioxide, magnesium stearate, modified cellulose gum, & stearic acid.

***Cordyceps with Siberian Ginseng* - Natrol**
Each capsule contains: Cordyceps 300 mg • Siberian Ginseng 50 mg. Other Ingredients: Rice powder, silica, & gelatin. No yeast, wheat, corn, milk, egg, soy, glutens, artificial colors or flavors, added sugar, starch or preservatives.

***CordyMax Cs-4* - Pharmanex**
Two capsules contain: Cordyceps Cs-4 Mushroom Mycelia (Cordyceps sinensis [Berk.] Sacc.) 1050 mg. Other Ingredient: Gelatin.

***Coreplex* - Flora**
Hawthorn blossoms & leaves • Passion Flower Herb • Hibiscus flowers • Hawthorn berry extract (1:4).

***Coromega Orange Flavor* - European Reference Botanical Laboratorie**
Each packet contains: Vitamin C 45 mg • Vitamin E 7 IU • Folic Acid 100 mcg • Omega-3 fatty acids (EPA 350 mg, DHA 230 mg) 650 mg • Stevia Leaf extract 5 mg. Ingredients: Water, Egg Yolk, Natural Orange Flavor, Citric Acid, Sodium Benzoate, Vanillin, Beta Carotene, Potassium Sorbate, Menthol, Folic Acid.

***Cortistat-PS* - Champion Nutrition**
Four capsules contain: Phosphatidylserine 100 mg • Phosphatidylcholine 105 mg • Phosphatidylethanolamine 70 mg • Phosphatidylinositol 30 mg • Arginine Aspartate 576 mg • Potassium Succinate 576 mg • Quercetin 100 mg • Feverfew 100 mg.

***Coryza Forte* - Progressive Labs**
Each capsule contains: Vitamin A (as retinol & beta carotene) 4000 IU • Vitamin C (ascorbic acid) 300 mg • Vitamin B6 (pyridoxine HCl) 15 mg •Pantothenic Acid (as d-calcium pantothenate) 25 mg • Calcium (as calcium carbonate) 40 mg • Zinc (as zinc picolinate) 5 mg • Echinacea 50 mg • Citrus Bioflavonoid 5X complex (as undiluted hesperidin, naringin and rutin) 150 mg. Other ingredients: Pollen, Raw Bovine Trachea, Raw Bovine Thymus, Raw Bovine Adrenal, Raw Bovine Lymph, Raw Bovine Spleen, RNA, Rose Hips, Whey, Cellulose, Magnesium Stearate, Gelatin.
See Editor's Note No. 14, page 1817.

***Coryza-Comp* - Atrium Inc.**
Each tablet contains: Vitamin A (Fish oil) 2000 IU • Vitamin C Ascorbic Acid 300 mg • Vitamin B6 Pyridoxine HCL 15 mg • Pantothenic Acid 25 mg • Calcium (Aspartate) 10 mg • Magnesium (Aspartate) 10 mg • Zinc (Aspartate) 2 mg • Citrus Bioflavonoids 150 mg • High RNA Yeast 50 mg • Bee Pollen 10 mg • Raw Spleen concentrate (Bovine) 10 mg • Raw Thymus concentrate (Bovine) 10 mg • Raw Adrenal concentrate 5 mg • Raw Lymph concentrate (Bovine) 5 mg. In a base of Alfalfa & Rose Hips.
See Editor's Note No. 14, page 1817.

***Cosamin* - Nutramax Laboratories, Inc.**
Each capsule contains: Glucosamine HCl (99%) 250 mg • Sodium Chondroitin Sulfate (95%) with Mixed Glycosaminoglycans (5%) 200 mg • Ascorbate (as manganese ascorbate) 33 mg • Manganese (as manganese ascorbate) 5 mg.
See Editor's Note No. 33, page 1820.

***Cosamin ProTek* - Nutramax Laboratories, Inc.**
Each capsule contains: Sodium 30 mg • Vitamin C 359 mg • Vitamin D3 400 IU • Vitamin E (d-alpha tocopherol) 35 IU • Manganese 1 mg • Glucosamine HCl 200 mg • Sodium Chondroitin Sulfate 95% and Mixed Glycosaminoglycans 5% 400 mg.
See Editor's Note No. 33, page 1820.

***Cosamin ProTek Women's Formula* - Nutramax Laboratories, Inc.**
Each capsule contains: Sodium 30 mg • Vitamin C 9 mg • Vitamin D3 400 IU • Calcium 115 mg • Manganese 1 mg • Glucosamine HCl 200 mg • Sodium Chondroitin Sulfate 95% and Mixed Glycosaminoglycans 5% 400 mg.
See Editor's Note No. 33, page 1820.

***CosaminDS* - Nutramax Laboratories, Inc.**
Each capsule contains: Glucosamine HCl (99%) 500 mg • Sodium Chondroitin Sulfate (95%) with Mixed Glycosaminoglycans (5%) 400 mg • Ascorbate (as manganese ascorbate) 66 mg • Manganese (as manganese ascorbate) 10 mg.
See Editor's Note No. 33, page 1820.

***Cosamine 500 mg* - Kripps Pharmacy**
Each capsule contains: Chondroitin Sulfate & Glucosamine powder (1:1 ratio) 500 mg.
See Editor's Note No. 15, page 1817.

***Cough Syrup* - Progressive Labs**
Each 10 ml contains: Dextromethorphan Hydrobromide 10 mg • Guaifenesin 100 mg • Potassium Citrate 85 mg • Citric Acid 35 mg. Contains no sugar, alcohol, sodium, or antihistamine.

***Cough Syrup with Honey* - Hyland's**
Ipecacuanha as Ipecac 6X HPUS • Aconitum napellus as Aconite 6X HPUS • Spongia tosta as Sponge 6X HPUS • Antimonium tartaricum as Potassium antimonium tartrate 6X HPUS. In simple syrup with Honey.
See Editor's Note No. 1, page 1816.

***Cough-Eze Syrup* - The Herbalist**
Herbs of Marshmallow root, Slippery Elm bark, Elecampane root, Wild Cherry bark, Mullein leaf, Horehound leaf, Licorice root, Cubeb berry, Orange peel, Cinnamon bark & Ginger root • Extracts of Skunk Cabbage root & Lobelia leaf • Honey • Vegetable Glycerine & Peppermint Oil.

***C-Plus Cold Tablets* - Hyland's**
Each tablet contains: Eupatorium perforliatum as Boneset 3X HPUS • Euphrasia officinalis as Eyebright 2X HPUS • Gelsemium sempervirens as Yellow Jasmine 3X HPUS • Kali iodatum as Potassium Iodide 3X HPUS. In a base of Lactose NF (Milk Sugar).
See Editor's Note No. 1, page 1816.

***C-Plus-Citrus* - Atrium Inc.**
Each level teaspoon (3300 mg approx. wt.) contains: Vitamin C from: (Ascorbic Acid 900 mg & Sodium Ascorbate 625 mg) 1500 mg • Mannitol 1395 mg • Lemon Bioflavonoids 150 mg • Rose Hips 100 mg • Hesperidin Complex 50 mg • Rutin 30 mg. Contains natural Orange Juice flavor.

***Cramp Bark-Catnip Virtue* - Blessed Herbs**
Cramp bark • Catnip flower & herb • Motherwort • Scullcap • Yarrow flower & herb • Grain alcohol & Distilled Water.

Some Brand Name Natural Products - What they Contain
www.NaturalDatabase.com contains MANY more listings than appear here.

Cramp Free - Health Center for Better Living
Calcium • Magnesium • Potassium • other herbs.

Cran Support - Natrol
One capsule contains: Guaranteed Potency Cranberry extract supplying 90% solids 30-40% organic acids 400 mg • Uva Ursi leaves 115 mg • Vitamin C (Ascorbic Acid) 100 mg • FOS (Fruiti-Vin FructoOgligoSaccharides) 100 mg • Cat's Claw root 50 mg • Corn Silk 30 mg • Kava Kava root 8.5 mg. Other ingredients: Silica, Magnesium Stearate, Annatto, Gelatin.

Cran-Aid - Traditional Medicinals
Roselle Hibiscus flower • Cranberry Fruit concentrate • German Chamomile flower • Rose Hip • Uva Ursi leaf • Cleavers herb • Althea root • Peppermint leaf • Stevia leaf.

Cranberry - Aspen Group, Inc.
Each tablet contains: Cranberry extract (25:1 extract) 250 mg • Vitamin C 60 mg • Echinacea (4:1 extract) 30 mg • Buchu (4:1 extract) 15 mg • Juniper berry (4:1 extract) 15 mg • Uva Ursi (4:1 extract) 15 mg. Contains no sugar, starch, salt, wheat, corn, yeast or soy derivatives.

Cranberry - Leiner Health Products
Two caplets contain: Cranberry extract (Vaccinium macrocarpon) berry 600 mg. Other Ingredients: Calcium Carbonate, Cellulose, Maltodextrin, Croscarmellose Sodium, Talc, Silicon Dioxide, Polyethylene Glycol 3350, Crospovidone, Hyroxypropyl Methylcellulose, Magnesium Stearate, Hydroxypropyl Cellulose, Polysorbate 80.

Cranberry - Pharmanex
Each capsule contains: Cranberry fruit (15:1) concentrate (Vaccinium macrocarpon) 500 mg. Other Ingredients: Gelatin and Titanium Dioxide.

Cranberry + - PhysioLogics
Four tablets contain: Vitamin C (Ascorbic Acid) 300 mg • Cranberry extract (30% natural organic acids, 600 mg; 5% Anthocyanidins, 100 mg) 2000 mg • Goldenseal root (5% total Alkaloids, 10 mg) 200 mg.

Cranberry Concentrate - Now
Two capsules contain: Calories 5 • Total Carbohydrate 1.1 g • Dietary Fiber 560 mg • Sugars 630 mg • Vitamin C (as Ascorbic Acid) 20 mg • Cranberry concentrate fruit (1400 mg of 8:1 concentrate) 1.4 g. Other Ingredients: Magnesium Stearate. Contains no salt, sugar, yeast, corn, wheat, milk, or preservatives.

Cranberry Juice Concentrate 1000 mg - Jamieson
Each capsule contains: Vitamin C (as Ascorbic Acid) 10 mg • Cranberry juice concentrate 1000 mg.

Cranberry Plus - Futurebiotics
Cranberry Extract (25:1 extract) 250 mg • Vitamin C 50 mg • Echinacea (4:1 extract equivalent to) 25 mg • Buchu (4:1 extract equivalent to) 12.5 mg • Juniper Berry (4:1 extract equivalent to) 12.5 mg • Uva Ursi (4:1 extract equivalent to) 12.5 mg.

Cran-C - Holista
Each capsule contains: Vitamin C 100 mg • Concentrated Cranberries (Vaccinum macrocarpon) of 25:1 extract (equivalent to 1132 mg of fresh cranberry juice) 45.3 mg.

Cran-Caps - Progressive Labs
Three softgels contain: Vitamin C 30 mg • Cranberry juice concentrate 3000 mg • Phosphatide complex 90 mg. Free of sugar and artificial sweeteners.

CranExtra - Enzymatic Therapy
Each capsule contains: Vitamin C (Ascorbic Acid) 1000 mg. Other ingredients: Cranberry extract (Vaccinium macrocarpon) standardized to contain 5% Anthocyanidins & 30% Organic Acids: Quinic, Malic, Citric & Hippuric Acid 100 mg • Uva Ursi (Arctostaphylos uva ursi) standardized to contain 20% Arbutin 100 mg. Contains no sugar, salt, yeast, wheat, corn, soy, dairy products, coloring, flavoring or preservatives.

CranGuard - PhytoPharmica
Two capsules contain: Vitamin C (ascorbic Acid) 100 mg • Cranberry extract (Vaccinium macrocarpon) standardized to contain 5% anthocyanidins & 30% organic acids (quinic, malic, citric & hippuric acid) 100 mg • Uva Ursi (Arctostaphylos uva ursi) standardized to contain 20% arbutin 100 mg. Contains no sugar, salt, yeast, wheat, corn, soy, dairy products, coloring, flavoring, or preservatives.

Cravex - Natrol
Two tablets contain: Calcium 230 mg • Iodine (as Potassium Iodine) 150 mcg • Chromium (as Chromium Picolinate) 200 mcg • Gymnema Sylvestre powdered extract leaves 300 mg • Licorice root 250 mg Deglycyrrhizinated Licorice • powdered extract Glycerinic Acid (1%) 2.5 mg • L-Glutamine 250 mg • DL-Phenylalanine 250 mg • 5-Hydroxytryptophan (5-HTP) 10 mg. Other ingredients: Calcium Sulfate Dihydrate, Mono & Di-Glycerides, Microcrystalline Cellulose, Croscarmellose Sodium, Stearic Acid, Silicon Dioxide, Magnesium Stearate.

CreActiv - Metabolic Response Modifiers
Two scoops (95.5 g) contains: Creatine monohydrate 12 g • L-Glutamine 5 g • BCAA blend 2 g • Alpha Lipoic Acid 300 mg • Dextrose 70 g • L-Taurine 1 g • L-Arginine 500 mg • Vitamin C 250 mg • Calcium 21 mg • Potassium 101 mg • Sodium 85 mg • Magnesium 100 mg • Phosphorus 160 mg • Chloride 122 mg • RNA 200 mg.

Creage - ANS
Creatine Monohydrate.

Creagen Plus - ANS
Creatine Monohydrate • Dextrose • Taurine.

Creatine - Source Naturals
Each tablet contains: Creatine monohydrate 1,000 mg.

Creatine 6000-ES - Muscletech
Each teaspoon contains: Creatine Monohydrate 6000 mg • Proprietary blend: Creatine Monohydrate, L-Methionine, L-Arginine, L-Glycine 500 mg.
See Editor's Note No. 7, page 1816.

Creatine Blast - Pharmanex
Each scoop (42 g) contains: Phosphorus (as Dimagnesium Phosphate) 60 mg • Magnesium (as Dimagnesium Phosphate) 50 mg • Creatine Monohydrate 4 g • Taurine 1000 mg. Other Ingredients: Dextrose, Citric Acid, Natural Grape Flavor, Grape Skin Extract (color).

Creatine Chewable with FOS - Natural Sport Supplements - Nutraceutica
Two wafers contain: Creatine Monohydrate 3 g • Proprietary FOS Fiber Blend (BeFlora) (265 mg Fructo-oligosaccharides) 530 mg. Other Ingredients: Guar gum, Cellulose, Natural Tangerine flavor, Citric acid, Stearic acid, Maltose, Natural Orange flavor, Silica, and Magnesium Stearate.

Creatine Fuel - TwinLab
Each capsule contains: Creatine Monohydrate 700 mg. Each teaspoonful of powder contains: Creatine Monohydrate 5 g (5000 mg).

BRAND NAMES

BRAND NAMES

Creatine Fuel Loading Drink - TwinLab
HPLC Pure Creatine Monohydrate with added Dextrose (a high glycemic carbohydrate) • Chromium • Taurine • Magnesium • Alpha Lipoic Acid. Other Ingredients: L-Glutamine 2 g.

Creatine Fuel Plus - TwinLab
Creatine (Creatine Monohydrate) 7 g. It also contains muscle cell volumizers, insulin potentiators & anti-catabolic, lean body mass stimulators. Fat free.

Creatine Fuel Stack - TwinLab
Six capsules contain: Creatine Monohydrate 5000 mg • L-Glutamine 2000 mg • Taurine 200 mg.

Creatine Fuelchews - TwinLab
Each chew contains: Pure Creatine Monohydrate 1 g • Dextrose 3 g. No sucrose or fructose is present.

Creatine Monohydrate Powder - ProLab
Each teaspoon contains: Creatine Monohydrate 5 g.
See Editor's Note No. 7, page 1816.

Creatine Now - Wild Cherry - Rexall
Each packet contains: Vitamin C (Ascorbic Acid) 1000 mg • Thiamin Hydrochloride (Vitamin B-1) 15 mg • Riboflavin USP (Vitamin B-2) 20 mg • Niacin (Niacinamide) 50 mg • Vitamin B-6 (Pyridoxine Hydrochloride) 8.3 mg • Vitamin B-12 (Cyanocobalamin) 10 mcg • Biotin 150 mcg • Pantothenic Acid (Calcium D-Pantothenate) 25 mg • Calcium Citrate 175 mg • Sodium Bicarbonate 200 mg • Potassium Bicarbonate 180 mg • Creatine Citrate 5 g • Stevia extract 26 mg. Other Ingredients: Dextrose, Citric Acid, Natural and Artificial Cherry flavor, Cochineal extract.

Creatine Powder - Olympian Labs
Each teaspoon contains: Creatine Monohydrate 5000 mg.

Creatine Sport Gel - Metabolic Response Modifiers
Contains: Creatine monohydrate 6,000 mg • L-Glutamine 1,000 mg • L-Taurine 500 mg • Dextrose 25 g.

CreaVATE - ProLab
Each capsule contains: Creatine Pyruvate 750 mg.

Creavescent - GEN
Each serving contains: L-Glutamine 2 g • TCT TM (Total Creatine Transport) proprietary blend of: (Creatine Monohydrate) 5 g. Ingredients: Creatine Monohydrate • Fructose • L-Glutamine • Mono Poly-Saccharide • 2-Hydroxy-1, 2, 3-Propanetricarboxylic Acid • Sodium Hydrogen Carbonate • Orange Solids • Calcium Phosphate • Vitamin A • Vitamin D • Riboflavin.

CreaVol ATP - SportPharma
Each 41 g serving contains: 99% pure microfine Crystalline Creatine 5 g • Adenine Mucleotides including ATP • Vanadyl Sulfate • Taurine • Disodium & Potassium Phosphate • Dextrose (about 35 g per serving).

C-Time 1000 with Rose Hips - Puritan's Pride
Each tablet contains: Vitamin C with Rose Hips 1000 mg.

C-Time 1500 with Rose Hips - Puritan's Pride
Each tablet contains: Vitamin C with Rose Hips 1500 mg.

C-Time 500 with Rose Hips - Puritan's Pride
Each tablet contains: Vitamin C with Rose Hips 500 mg.

CTR Support - PhysioLogics
Each capsule contains: Turmeric (95% Curcumin) 250 mg • Boswellia (60% Boswellic Acids) 166.67 mg • Bromelain (2400 GDU)83.33 mg • Ginger (5% Gingerols) 33.33 mg • Yucca (14% Saponins) 16.67 mg • Devils Claw (3.5% Harpagosides) 16.67 mg • Quercetin (98% bioflavonoids) 16.67 mg.

Culturelle with Lactobacillus GG - Klaire Laboratories
Each capsule contains: Lactobacillus GG.

Curazyme - Enzymatic Therapy
Each capsule contains: Vitamin C (Ascorbic Acid) 50 mg • Pantothenic Acid (D-Calcium Pantothenate) 25 mg • Magnesium (Oxide) 25 mg • Curcuma root extract (Curcuma longa) standardized to contain 97% Curcumin 200 mg • Bromelain (2000 MCU) 200 mg • Butchers Broom extract (Ruscus aculeatus) standardized to contain 10% Saponins calculated as Ruscogenin 100 mg • Pancreatic Enzymes (10X) 50 mg • L-Cysteine 25 mg. Contains no sugar, salt, yeast, wheat, corn, soy, dairy products, coloring, flavoring, or preservatives.
See Editor's Note No. 14, page 1817.

CurcuMax - PhytoPharmica
Each capsule contains: Vitamin C (ascorbic acid) 50 mg • Pantothenic Acid (calcium D-pantothenate) 25 mg • Magnesium (oxide) 25 mg • Curcuma (Curcuma longa) root (rhizome) extract (standardized to contain 85%-97% curcumin) 200 mg • Bromelain (2,000 M.C.U.) enzymes derived from pineapple stems 200 mg • Butcher's Broom (Ruscus aculeatus) root and rhizome extract (standardized to contain 10% saponins calculated as ruscogenin) 100 mg • Pancreatic enzymes (10X) 50 mg • L-Cysteine 25 mg.
See Editor's Note No. 14, page 1817.

CV-10 (Cardiovascular Nutritional Support) - Rx Vitamins
Six capsules contain: L-Taurine 500 mg • L-Carnitine 500 mg • Magnesium (Taurate) 400 mg • Hawthorne berry 100 mg • Potassium (Citrate) 99 mg • CoQ10 30 mg • Vitamin B3 (Niacin) 25 mg • Vitamin B6 (Pyridoxine) 25 mg • Folic Acid 400 mcg • Vitamin E 200 IU.

CVS Echinacea - CVS
Three capsules contain: Echinacea 1140 mg. Other Ingredients: Echinacea Purpurea Herb powder, Gelatin, Maltodextrin, Cellulose, Calcium Carbonate, Magnesium Stearate, Silicon Dioxide, Dicalcium Phosphate, Microcrystalline Cellulose, Stearic Acid, Croscarmellose Sodium, Hydroxypropyl Methylcellulose, Hydroxypropyl Cellulose, Polyethylene Glycol.

CVS Saw Palmetto - CVS
Two capsules contain: Maltodextrin • Cellulose • Gelatin • Saw Palmetto extract • Calcium carbonate • Magnesium stearate • Silicon Dioxide.
See Editor's Note No. 20, page 1818.

CVS Saw Palmetto Softgels - CVS
Each softgel contains: Saw Palmetto extract (serenoa repens) fruit 160 mg. Other Ingredients: Olive Oil, Gelatin, Purified Water, Glycerin, FD & C Red #40, FD & C Yellow #6.
See Editor's Note No. 2, page 1816.

Cycla-Action - Nature's Plus
Each capsule contains: Blue Cohosh root 150 mg • Black Currant seed 125 mg • Mustard seed 75 mg • Red Raspberry leaves 75 mg • Cramp bark 75 mg • Squaw Vine 50 mg • False Unicorn 50 mg. Contains no yeast, wheat, corn, soy, milk, salt, sugar or starch.

Cycl-A-Vites - Nature's Plus
Two tablets contain: whole Black Currant seeds naturally supplying GLA 300 mg • Magnesium amino acid chelate/complex 250 mg • Vitamin B6 (Pyridoxine HCL) 200 mg • Bromelain natural pineapple 150 mg • Calcium amino acid chelate/complex 125 mg • Iron amino

Some Brand Name Natural Products - What they Contain
www.NaturalDatabase.com contains MANY more listings than appear here.

acid chelate/complex 18 mg. In a natural base of Red Raspberry leaves, Strawberry Leaves, Dong Quai, Uva Ursi, & Peppermint. Yeast free. Sugar & starch free.

Cyclo 3 Fort - Unknown
One capsule contains: Ruscus aculeatus root extract 150 mg • Trimethylhesperidin-chalcon 150 mg • Ascorbic acid 100 mg.

CycloDiol-4 (Sports One Cycloplex Pro-Hormone) - Sports One
Each lozenge contains: 4-Androstenediol Cycloplex (cyclodextrin complex) 25 mg.

CycloDiol-5 (Sports One Cycloplex Pro-Hormone) - Sports One
Each lozenge contains: 5-Androstenediol Cycloplex (cyclodextrin complex) 25 mg.

CycloDiol-XS (Sports One Cycloplex Pro-Hormone) - Sports One
Each lozenge contains: Nor-4-Androstenediol Cycloplex (cyclodextrin complex) 10 mg & 4-Androstenediol Cycloplex (cyclodextrin complex) 15 mg.

Cyclovar - Warner Laboratories
Proprietary Blend 250 mg, containing: L-Arginine, Cnidium Monnier extract, Xanthoparmelia extract, ZMA, Gamma Amino Butyric acid, Narigen, Quebracho extract, Microcrystalline Cellulose, Lactose Solutab, Magnesium Stearate.

Cynara-SL Artichoke - Lichtwer Pharma
One capsule contains: Artichoke extract (Dried leaf extract) 320 mg. Other Ingredients: Gelatin, Magnesium Stearate, Silicon Dioxide, Talc, Titanium Dioxide, Sodium Lauryl Sulphate, FD&C Blue No. 1, FD&C Yellow No. 5.

Cytodrene - Weightlosscontrol
Each capsule contains: Propietary Blend 700 mg: Sida cordifolia extract, Kola Nut extract, Green Tea extract, Yohimbe bark extract, White Willow bark, Chromium picolinate, Guggulsterones.

Cytodyne - Cytodyne Technologies
Six capsules contain: Acetyl L-Carnitine 1100 mg • Phosphatidylserine 175 mg • L-Alanine 200 mg • Alpha Ketoglutaric Acid 150 mg • L-Glutamine 2150 mg • Taurine 1050 mg • Ketoisocaporate 50 mg • Inositol 50 mg.

Cytolog - Allergy Research Group
Colostrum.

Cytomax - Champion Nutrition
Each 25 gram serving contains: Apple: Alpha-L-Polyactate • Energy 90 Kcal • Total Fat 0g • Sodium 100 mg • Potassium 120 mg • Total Carbohydrate 22 g • Sugars 10 g • Protein 0 g. Citrus: Energy 90 Kcal • Total Fat 0g • Sodium 100 mg • Potassium 120 mg • Total Carbohydrate 22 g • Sugars 10 g • Protein 0 g. Tangy-Orange: Energy 90 Kcal • Total Fat 0g • Sodium 100 mg • Potassium 120 mg • Total Carbohydrate 21 g • Sugars 11 g • Protein 0. Tropical: Energy 90 Kcal • Total Fat 0g • Sodium 100 mg • Potassium 100 mg • Total Carbohydrate 22 g • Sugars 11 g • Protein 0. Ingredients: Fructose • Alpha-L-Polyactate: our non-acidic patented L-Lactate formula combined with Sodium L-Lactate & Potassium L-Lactate • Metacarb (Champion Nutrition's original complex carbohydrate blend including Amylopectin Starches & Maltodextrins from Corn Hybrids) • Glucose • Citric Acid • Succinate ETF Our Exclusive Succinate Compound containing: Potassium Succinate, L-Glutamic Acid, Inosine, Magnesium Succinate, Calcium Succinate • Natural Flavoring • Malic Acid • L-Alanine • L-Glutamine • Ascorbic Acid • Natural Caramel Coloring • Potassium Citrate • Xanthan Gum • Sunett (Acesulfame-K) • Chromium Polynicotinate (Chromemate - GTF).

CytoPro - Cytodyne Technologies
Each rounded scoop contains: Cross Flow Micro/Ultra Filtered 100% pure Whey Protein Isolate (Beta Lactoglobulin 19100 MW/50% Alpha Lactoalbumin 14700 MW/20%, Glycomacropeptides 16200 MW/20%, Glutamine Peptides 6700 MW/5%, Immunoglobulin 95000 MW/3%, Bovine Serum Albumin 65000 MW/2%, Protease Peptone). CytoPro WPI (typical Amino Acid profile): L-Alanine 1071 mg • L-Arginine 538 mg • L-Aspartic Acid 2303 mg • L-Cysteine 276 mg • L-Glutamic Acid 3870 mg • L-Glutamine 548 mg • L-Glycine 522 mg • L-Histidine 393 mg • L-Isoleucine 1433 mg • L-Leucine 2341 mg • L-Lysine 1999 mg • L-Methionine 409 mg • L-Phenylalanine 768 mg • L-Proline 1553 mg • L-Serine 1184 mg • L-Taurine 1000 mg • L-Threonine 1409 mg • L-Tryptophan 464 mg • L-Tyrosine 567 mg • L-Valine 1328 mg. Total amino profile in milligrams: 23976 mg.

CytoVol - EAS
Each 15 gram serving contains: L-Glutamine 2500 mg • Taurine 2000 mg • Manganese 50 mcg • Calcium AKG 1500 mg • Inositol 500 mg • Glycine 500 mg • RNA 250 mg • L-Alanine 2000 mg. Ingredients: Dextrose • L-Glutamine • Taurine • L-Alanine • Calcium Alpha-Ketoglutarate (AKG) • Citric Acid • Natural Flavors • Inositol • Glycine • Sodium Ribonucleic Acid (RNA) • Sodium Phosphate • Turmeric mixed with Maltodextrin for color • Aspartame • Manganese Glycinate. Contains Phenylalanine.

Daily 3 Complete - The Vitamin Shoppe
Each tablet contains: Vitamin D 400 IU • Vitamin A Activity 25000 IU • Vitamin C 500 mg • Vitamin E 400 IU • Vitamin B1 50 mg • Vitamin B2 50 mg • Vitamin B6 50 mg • Vitamin B12 500 mcg • Niacinamide 50 mg • PABA 50 mg • Pantothenic Acid 50 mg • Choline Bitartrate 50 mg • Inositol 50 mg • Biotin 50 mcg • Folic Acid 800 mcg • Vitamin K 30 mcg • Selenium 50 mcg • Green Tea extract 50 mg • CoQ10 100 mcg • L-Glutathione 10 mg • Pycnogenol 100 mcg • N-Acetyl Cysteine 15 mg • Molybdenum 50 mcg • Calcium 100 mg • Magnesium 50 mg • Potassium 50 mg • Zinc 15 mg • Iodine 150 mcg • Iron 10 mg • Manganese 5 mg • Chromium 100 mcg • Boron 3 mg • Apple pectin 50 mg • Papain 25 mg • Lipase 10 mcg • Probiotics 10 mg • Betaine HCl 25 mg • Pepsin 25 mg • Protease 10 mcg • Glutamic Acid 25 mg • Amylase 10 mcg • Chlorophyll 10 mg • Spirulina 45 mg • Bee Pollen 45 mg • Echinacea/Golden Seal 50 mg • Shiitake/Reishi mushrooms 45 mg • Barley grass 45 mg • Royal Jelly 15 mg • Alfalfa concentrate 45 mg • Siberian Ginseng 45 mg • Chlorella 45 mg • RNA/DNA 45 mg. A concentrated blend of: broccoli, tomato, garlic, onions, cauliflower, brussel sprouts, carrots, parsley, watercress. Pure dry, cold-pressed borage, flaxseed, safflower oils providing the essential fatty acids, Omega 3-6-9.

Daily 3 with Antioxidant Factors - Puritan's Pride
Three capsules contain: Vitamin A (as Beta-Carotene) 25,000 IU • Vitamin C (as Calcium Ascorbate) 500 mg • Vitamin D (as Cholecalcifeol) 400 IU • Vitamin E (as d-Alpha Tocopherol Succinate) 400 IU • Vitamin K (as Phytonadione) 30 mcg • Thiamin (Vitamin B-1; as Thiamine Hydrochloride) 50 mg • Riboflavin (Vitamin B-2) 50 mg • Niacin (as Niacinamide) 50 mg • Vitamin B-6 (as Pyridoxine Hydrochloride) 50 mg • Folic Acid 800 mcg • Vitamin B-12 (as Coenzyme B-12) 500 mcg • Biotin 50 mcg • Pantothenic Acid (as d-Calcium Pantothenate) 50 mg • Calcium (as Calcium Carbonate) 100 mg • Iron (as Carbonyl Iron) 10 mg • Iodine (as Kelp) 150 mcg • Magnesium (as Magnesium Oxide) 50 mg • Zinc (as Zinc Picolinate) 15 mg • Selenium (as Selenomethionate) 50 mcg • Manganese (as Manganese Carbonate) 5 mg • Chromium (as GTF Chromium Yeast) 100 mcg • Potassium (as Potassium Chloride) 50 mg • Green Tea (Camellia sinensis) leaf 50 mg • N-Acetyl Cysteine 15 mg • L-Glutathione 10 mg • Coenzyme Q10 100 mcg • Pine bark extract (Pycnogenol®) 100 mcg • Choline Bitartrate 50 mg • Inositol 50 mg • PABA (Para-Aminobenzoic Acid) 50 mg • Boron (as Boron Citrate) 3 mg • Spirulina (Spirulina plantensis) plant 20 mg • Chinese Chlorella (Chlorella pyrenoidosa) 20 mg • Barley Grass (plant) 20 mg • Alfalfa juice concentrate 20 mg • Octacosanol 100 mcg • Siberian Ginseng (Eleutherococcus senticosus) root 20 mg • Bee Pollen 20 mg

• Citrus Bioflavonoids 20 mg • Rutin 20 mg • Echinacea/Goldenseal (Echinacea purpurea/Hydrastis canadensis) root 20 mg • Royal Jelly 15 mg • Reishi Mushroom (Ganoderma lucidum) aerial 15 mg • Shiitake Mushroom (Lentinus edodes) aerial 15 mg • Shark Cartilage 45 mg • Apple Pectin 20 mg • Betaine Hydrochloride 20 mg • L-Glutamic Acid 20 mg • Papain (Papaya) 20 mg • Pepsin Enzyme 20 mg • Lipase 10 mg • Amylase 10 mg • Chlorophyll (as Sodium Copper Chlorophyllin) 10 mg • Proprietary Blend: Broccoli, Tomato, Orange, Lemon, Blueberry, Cranberry, Garlic, Onion, Cauliflower, and Brussels Sprout Concentrates 20 mg.

Daily Antioxidant Packs - Puritan's Pride
Each pack (2 softgels, 3 tablets) contains: Beta Carotene 25,000 IU • Multi-Vitamin: Providing Vitamin A (as beta carotene), Vitamin D, and B-Complex Vitamins • Vitamin E 400 IU • Vitamin C with Rose Hips 500 mg • Multi-Mineral: A full accompaniment of major and trace minerals including Chromium, Calcium, Zinc, and the antioxidant Selenium.

Daily Basics - Original - Rexall
Each packet contains: Vitamin A (100% as Beta-Carotene) 1,000 IU • Vitamin C (Ascorbic Acid) 60 mg • Vitamin E (dl-Alpha Tocopheryl Acetate) 30 IU • Niacin (Niacinamide) 36 mg • Vitamin B12 (Cyanocobalamin) 10.8 mcg • Selenium Chelate (Sodium Selenite) 4 mcg • Calcium Carbonate 100 mg • Thiamin HCl 2.7 mg • Vitamin B6 (Pyridoxine HCl) 3.6 mg • Biotin 29 mcg • Chromium Polynicotinate (ChromeMate) 52 mcg • Riboflavin 3 mg • Folate (Folic Acid) 120 mcg • Zinc Gluconate 0.9 mg. Other Ingredients: Guar Gum, Locust Bean Gum, Pectins, Oat Fiber, Maltodextrin, Gum Arabic, Natural and Artifical Orange Flavor, Aspartame, Artifical Vanilla Flavor.

Daily Detox - M.D. Labs
Sarsaparilla • Milk Thistle • Red Clover • Dandelion • Yellow Dock • Burdock • Hibiscus • Echinacea • Fenugreek • Ginger • Cascara Sagrada. Other Ingredients: All Natural Fruit & Spice extracts.

Daily Enzyme Complex - Futurebiotics
Pancreas* 235 mg • Ox bile 35 mg • Duodenum 20 mg • Papaya enzyme 125 mg • Betaine 20 mg • Liver 20 mg • Vitamin B1 (thiamin) 3 mg • Bromelain 50 mg • Niacinamide 10 mg • Vitamin B2 (riboflavin) 3 mg • Peppermint 25 mg • Anise 25 mg • Chamomile 25 mg. *Whole dried pancreas, a source of Pancreatin, Trypsin, Amylase, Lipase, Lisotozyme, Diatase & Chymosin.
See Editor's Note No. 14, page 1817.

Daily Essentials - Aspen Group, Inc.
Each three tablets contain: Vitamin E (d-alpha) 200 IU • Vitamin A 5000 IU • Beta Carotene 5000 IU • Vitamin D 400 IU • Vitamin C 400 mg • Folic Acid 400 mcg • Thiamine 1.5 mg • Riboflavin 1.7 mg • Niacin 20 mg • Vitamin B6 2 mg • Vitamin B12 6 mcg • Biotin 300 mcg • Pantothenic Acid 10 mg • Calcium (citrate) 600 mg • Phosphorus 450 mg • Iodine (kelp) 150 mcg • Magnesium (carbonate) 200 mg • Copper (gluconate) 2 mg • Zinc (gluconate) 15 mg • Vitamin K 100 mcg • Selenium (yeast) 75 mcg • Manganese (gluconate) 5 mg • Chromium (aspartate) 200 mcg • Molybdenum 150 mcg • Nickel 15 mcg • Tin 15 mcg • Vanadium 5 mg • Boron (citrate) 2 mg • Potassium (gluconate) 100 mg • Grape seed extract 10 mg • CO Q10 10 mg. Contains no sugar, starch, salt, wheat, corn, milk or soy derivatives.

Daily Essentials for Men - Health Smart Vitamins
Two caplets contain: Vitamin A (as 83% beta-carotene, 17% palmitate) 15,000 IU • Vitamin C (ascorbic acid) 250 mg • Vitamin D (as cholecalciferol) 400 IU • Vitamin E (as d-alpha tocopheryl) 200 IU • Vitamin K (as phytonadione) 25 mcg • Thiamin (as thiamin mononitrate) 25 mg • Riboflavin 25 mg • Niacin (as 50% nicotinic acid, 50% niacinamide) 50 mg • Vitamin B6 (as pyridoxine HCl) 25 mg • Folate (folic acid) 400 mcg • Vitamin B12 (as cyanocobalamin) 50 mcg • Biotin 300 mcg • Pantothenic acid

(as calcium pantothenate) 25 mg • Calcium (as 87% calcium carbonate, 13% mixed calcium complexes) 258 mg • Iron (as iron sulfate) 6 mg • Iodine (as potassium iodide) 150 mcg • Magnesium (as 80% magnesium oxide, 10% magnesium citrate, 10% mangesium glycinate) 125 mg • Zinc (as zinc ascorbate) 30 mg • Selenium (as selenomethionine) 75 mcg • Copper (as copper citrate) 3 mg • Manganese (as manganese gluconate) 2 mg • Chromium (as chromium polynicotinate) 100 mcg • Molybdenum (as molybdenum amino acid chelate) 50 mcg • Oriental Ginseng root (Panax ginseng) 75 mg • Pumpkin seed 75 mg • Saw Palmetto berry 75 mg • Betaine HCl 25 mg • Citrus bioflavonoids 25 mg • Choline (as bitartrate) 25 mg • Insitol 25 mg • Lecithin (from soybean) 25 mg • Bromelain (from pineapple 6,000 PU/g, 120 PU) 20 mg • Lipase (from fermentation of Aspergillus niger) 10 mg • Papain (from latex of fruit) 10 mg • Para-aminobenzoic acid (PABA) 10 mg • Boron (as boron aspartate) 2 mg • Silicon (as silicon dioxide) 2 mg • Vanadium (as vanadium amino acid chelate) 10 mcg.

Daily Essentials for Women - Health Smart Vitamins
Two caplets contain: Vitamin A (as 83% beta-carotene, 17% palmitate) 15000 IU • Vitamin C (ascorbic acid) 250 mg • Vitamin D (as cholecalciferol) 400 IU • Vitamin E (as d-alpha-tocopherol) 200 IU • Vitamin K (as phytonadione) 25 mcg • Thiamin (as thiamin mononitrate) 25 mg • Riboflavin 25 mg • Niacin 50 mg • Vitamin B-6 (as pyridoxine HCl) 25 mg • Folate (folic acid) 400 mcg • Vitamin B-12 (cyanocobalamin) 100 mcg • Biotin 300 mcg • Pantothenic Acid (as calcium pantothenate) 25 mg • Calcium 507 mg • Iron (as iron glycinate) 18 mg • Magnesium 200 mg • Iodine (as potassium iodide) 150 mcg • Zinc (as zinc ascorbate) 15 mg • Selenium (as seleno-methione) 75 mcg • Copper (as copper citrate) 2 mg • Manganese (as manganese gluconate) 2 mg • Chromium (as chromium polynicotinate) 100 mcg • Molybdenum 50 mcg • Dong Quai root 50 mg • Royal Jelly from bees 50 mg • Betaine HCl 25 mg • Bioflavonoids (from citrus) 25 mg • Choline (as choline bitartrate) 25 mg • Inositol 25 mg • Lecithin (from soybean) 25 mg • Bromelain 20 mg • Lipase 10 mg • Papain 10 mg • PABA (Para-Amino Benzoic Acid) 10 mg • Rutin 5 mg • Boron (as boron aspartate) 2 mg • Silicon (as silicon dioxide) 2 mg • Vanadium 10 mcg.

Daily Multi-Vitamin & Mineral - Swanson
Each capsule contains: Vitamin A (from fish liver oil) 10000 • Vitamin C (Ester-C®, as calcium ascorbate) 200 mg • Vitamin D (from fish liver oil) 400 IU • Vitamin E (as d-alpha tocopheryl succinate) 15 IU • Thiamin (as thiamin mononitrate; vitamin B-1) 10 mg • Riboflavin USP (vitamin B-2) 10 mg • Niacinamide 100 mg • Vitamin B-6 (as pyridoxine HCl) 5 mg • Folic Acid 400 mcg • Vitamin B-12 (as cyanocobalamin) 5 mcg • Pantothenic Acid (as d-calcium pantothenate) 20 mg • Calcium (from bone meal and dolomite) 125 mg • Iron (from ferrous sulfate) 12 mg • Iodine (from kelp) 150 mcg • Magnesium (from magnesium oxide) 32.5 mg • Zinc (from zinc sulfate) 15 mg • Copper (from copper sulfate) 2 mg • Manganese (from manganese sulfate) 1 mg.

Daily Pak Maximum - Leiner Health Products
Each packet contains: Zinc 12.5 mg • Biotin 25 mg • Copper 1.5 mg • Iodine 112.5 mg • Manganese 1.5 mg • Vitamin D 200 IU • Vitamin B12 25 mg • Chromium 425 mcg • Vitamin E (dl-Alpha Tocopheryl Acetate) 900 IU • Pantothenic Acid 25 mg • Iron 4.1 mg • Vitamin C (Ascorbic Acid) 1200 mg • Selenium 12.5 mcg • Thiamin (Vitamin B1) 25 mg • Riboflavin (Vitamin B2) 25 mg • Calcium Carbonate 130 mg • Vitamin B6 25 mg • Niacin 25 mg • Magnesium • Folate 400 mg • Vitamin A 5000 IU • Molybdenum 7.5 mcg • Phosphorus 100 mg • Ginseng 250 mg • Inositol 5 mg • PABA 2.5 mg. Other Ingredients: Dicalcium Phosphate, Gelatin, Siberian Ginseng, Glycerin, Cellulose, Hydroxypropyl Methylcellulose, Hydrogenated Vegetable Oil, Magnesium Oxide, Starch, Silicon Dioxide, Stearic Acid, Maltodextrin.

Daily Therapy 7-Vitamin Foaming Cleansing Gel - Orjene
Vitamin-packed antioxidant formula with Sea Minerals.

Daily Vits One-A-Day Multiple - Now
Each tablet contains: Vitamin A (100% as Beta Carotene) 5000 IU • Vitamin B1 (Thiamine HCL) 1.5 mg • Vitamin B2 (Riboflavin) 1.7 mg • Vitamin B3 (Niacinamide) 20 mg • Vitamin B5 (Pantothenic Acid) 10 mg • Vitamin B6 (Pyridoxine HCL) 3 mg • Vitamin B12 (Cyanocobalamin) 9 mcg • Biotin 300 mcg • Folic Acid 400 mcg • Vitamin C (Ascorbic Acid) 90 mg • Vitamin D (Calciferol) 400 IU • Vitamin E (natural d-Alpha Tocopherol) 30 IU • Calcium (Carbonate, Phosphate) 100 mg • Magnesium (Oxide) 80 mg • Zinc (Amino Acid Chelate) 15 mg • Iron (Ferrochel Bisglycinate) 9 mg • Copper (Amino Acid Chelate) 1 mg • Iodine (Kelp) 150 mcg • Potassium (Chloride) 50 mg • Manganese (Amino Acid Chelate) 2 mg • Selenium (Amino Acid Chelate) 70 mcg • Chromium (Chelavite Chelate) 120 mcg • Molybdenum (Amino Acid Chelate) 50 mcg • Choline (Bitartrate) 10 mg • Inositol 10 mg • PABA 10 mg • Boron (Amino Acid Chelate) 500 mcg • Vanadium (Amino Acid Chelate) 50 mcg • Panax ginseng (5% Ginsenosides) 100 mg.

Daily VM Caps - The Vitamin Shoppe
Each capsule contains: Vitamin A 10000 IU • Vitamin D 400 IU • Vitamin C 250 mg • Thiamin 8 mg • Riboflavin 8 mg • Niacin 25 mg • Vitamin B6 10 mg • Vitamin B12 25 mcg • Vitamin E 100 IU • Pantothenic Acid 25 mg • Biotin 300 mcg • Folate 400 mcg • Calcium 100 mg • Magnesium 50 mg • Iron 10 mg • Manganese 2 mg • Zinc 7 mg • Selenium 70 mcg • Chromium 50 mcg • Iodine 125 mcg • Citrus Bioflavonoids 25 mg • Para Aminobenzoic Acid 10 mg • Choline 10 mg • Inositol 10 mg • Potassium 10 mg • Betaine HCl 10 mg • Pepsin 10 mg • Papain 10 mg • Pancreatin 10 mg.
See Editor's Note No. 14, page 1817.

Damiana/Ginseng Formula - Nature's Way
Two capsules contain: Proprietary Formula: Damiana leaves • Fo-Ti root • Gotu Kola stem, leaf • Licorice root • Sarsaparilla root • Saw Palmetto berry • Siberian Ginseng root • Wild Yam root • Other ingredients: Gelatin.

Damiana-Sarsaparilla Formula - Quest
Each caplet contains: Damiana leaf powder (Tunera aphrodisiaca) 120 mg • Sarsaparilla root powder (Smilax officinalis) 90 mg • Saw Palmetto berry powder (Serenoa serrulata) 90 mg • Siberian Ginseng root powder (Eleutherococcus senticosus) 90 mg • Licorice root powder (Glycyrrhiza glabra) 60 mg • Kelp powder (Fucus versiculosis) 50 mg. Other Ingredients: Calcium Phosphate, Microcrystalline Cellulose, Vegetable Stearin, Croscarmellose Sodium, Magnesium Stearate (vegetable source).

Dandelion - Nature's Way
Three capsules contain: Dandelion root 1.62 g.
Other Ingredients: Gelatin.

Dandelion Root - Now
Two capsules contain: Total Carbohydrate 0.7 g • Dandelion root (Taraxacom Officinale) 1.0 g.
Other Ingredients: Magnesium Stearate. Contains no sugar, wheat, yeast, corn, starch, egg, soy, milk, or additives.

Dandelion-Milk Thistle Virtue - Blessed Herbs
Dandelion blend of flower, leaf & root • Milk Thistle seed • Bladderwrack • Reishi mycelium • Scullcap • Licorice root • Prickly Ash bark • Grain alcohol & Distilled Water.

Deep Pore Cleanser - Jason
Vitamin C Complex • Alpha Lipoic Acid.

Defender - Health Factor
Each tablet contains: Beta Carotene 5000 IU • Vitamin C (Ascorbic Acid) 60 mg • Vitamin E (d-Alpha Tocopheryl) 30 IU • Zinc (Amino Acid Chelate) 20 mg • Copper (Citrate) 2 mg • Selenium (Amino Acid Chelate) 100 mcg • Manganese (Citrate) 2 mg • Chromium (Nicotinate) 100 mcg • Boron (Citrate) 100 mcg • Vanadium (Citrate) 50 mcg • Molybdenum (Citrate) 50 mcg • Silicon (Citrate) 20 mcg • Grape seed (95% Polyphenols) 20 mg • Bilberry (25% Anthocyanidins) 5 mg.

Defender BVM - PhysioLogics
Two caplets contain: Vitamin A (as Beta Carotene) 5000 IU • Vitamin C (as Ascorbic Acid) 100 mg • Vitamin E (as d-Alpha Tocopherol Succinate) 240 IU • Selenium (as Selenomethionine) 400 mcg • Manganese (as Manganese Glycinate) 1.75 mg • Tea Green leaf (50% Polyphenols, 75 mg) 150 mg • N-Acetyl L-Cysteine 50 mg • Resveratrol (8% Resveratrol, 4 mg) 50 mg • Alpha Lipoic Acid 25 mg.

Deferol - IDIST Laboratories, LLC
Each capsule contains: Pyridoxine HCl 50 mg • Folic Acid 0.4 mg • Proprietary Blend: Passiflora Coerulea leaf extract, Griffonia seed extract, Pyridoxyl 5-phosphate 125 mg.
Other Ingredients: Magnesium Stearate, Rice Powder, Gelatin.

Defy Your Age - Pharmagel
10% Alpha Hydroxy Acids • Stabilized Oxygen.

Dental-Aid - Futurebiotics
Three capsules contain: Vitamin C (as ascorbic acid) 1000 mg • Calcium (as calcium citrate) 250 mg • MSM (methyl-sulfonyl methane) 200 mg • Citrus Bioflavonoids 110 mg • Hesperidin 55 mg • Rutin 55 mg • Quercetin 50 mg • CoEnzyme Q-10 15 mg • Ginger root powder 110 mg • Chamomile flower powder 35 mg • Prickly Ash bark powder 50 mg • Barberry fruit powder 35 mg • Cloves 17 mg • Lemon Grass 15 mg • Sage 12 mg • Angelica root 12 mg.
Other ingredients: Magnesium stearate, Gelatin, Water.

Dentalgel - NutriBiotic
Contains 0.4% Grapefruit extract.

Dentaplex - Collagenex Pharmaceuticals
Each tablet contains: Vitamin A (20% [1000 IU] as Beta Carotene, 80% [4000 IU] as Vitamin A Acetate) 5000 IU • Vitamin C (as Ascorbic Acid) 300 mg • Vitamin D 200 IU • Vitamin E (as dl-Alpha Tocopheryl Acetate) 30 IU • Thiamin (Vitamin B1) 7.5 mg • Riboflavin (Vitamin B2) 8.5 mg • Vitamin B6 (as Pyridoxine Hydrochloride) 10 mg • Folic Acid 400 mcg • Vitamin B12 (as Cyanocobalamin) 30 mcg • Calcium (as Calcium Carbonate) 333 mg • Magnesium (as Magnesium Oxide) 40 mg • Zinc (as Zinc Oxide) 20 mg • Selenium (as Sodium Selenate) 15 mcg • Copper (as Cupric Oxide) 2 mg • Molybdenum (as Sodium Molybdate) 25 mcg • Vanadium (as Sodium Metavanadate) 10 mcg.

Depremin - FreeLife
Each tablet contains: St. John's Wort extract (Hypericum perforatum) patented St. John's Wort extract EV.EXT 119 300 mg.
Other Ingredients: Calcium Hydrogen Phosphate, Potato Starch, Hydrous Magnesium Silicate, Silica Dioxide, Microcrystalline Cellulose, Magnesium Stearate.

Depress-X - Olympian Labs
Each capsule contains: 5-HTP 10 mg • Ginkgo Biloba extract 40 mg • Vitamin B-6 50 mg • Magnesium 120 mg • Vitamin B-3 (niacinamide) 20 mg.

Derma Care - PhytoPharmica
Two capsules contain: Vitamin A (fish liver oil) 3,332 IU • Vitamin C (ascorbic acid) 200 mg • Vitamin D (fish liver oil) 666 IU • Vitamin E (d-alpha tocopherol) 66 IU • Riboflavin (vitamin B2) 3.4 mg • Niacin/Niacinamide 66 mg • Vitamin B6 (pyridoxine HCl) 20 mg • Folic Acid 66 mcg • Biotin 666 mcg • Pantothenic Acid (calcium D-pantothenate) 17 mg • Zinc (chelate) 30 mg • Unsaturated free fatty acids (linoleic, arachidonic, and linolenic from unrefined germ oil and

safflower seed oil) 600 mg • Lecithin (soy) 400 mg • Choline Bitartrate 100 mg • Intrinsic glandular lipids 100 mg • Inositol 66 mg.

Derma Q-Gel - Tishcon Corp.
Active Ingredients: Coenzyme Q10 • Vitamin E • Vitamin C • Vitamin A (Retinyl palmitate) • Alpha-Lipoic Acid (Thioctic Acid) • Vitamin K (as Vitamin K1) • Vitamin D • Biotin • Panthenol • Grape Seed extract • Green Tea extract • Chamomile extract • GLA from Borage Oil, Evening Primrose Oil • Aloe Vera gel • Squalane • Kikui Nut oil • Jojoba oil • Sweet Almond oil • Wheat Germ oil • Avocado oil.

Derma Teen - Futurebiotics
MSM, combination of vitamins, minerals, and horsetail.

Derma-Klear Akne Treatment Cream - Enzymatic Therapy
Contains: Sulfur 2.5%. Other ingredients: Purified Water, Zinc, Sage extract, Silymarin Phytosome, Hawthorne extract, Chamomile extract, 18-Beta-Glycyrrhetinic Acid, Essential Oil of Rosemary, Urea & Vitamin E (Tocopherol). Fragrance is natural & hypoallergenic. Contains no Benzoyl Peroxide.

DermaSlim TD - Alvin Last
Abies Canadensis • Ammonium Bromatum • Ammonium Carbonicum • Antimonium Crudem • Argentum Metallicum • Argentum Nitircum • Calcarea Carbonica • Capsicum Annuum • Cinchona Officinalis • Fucus Vesiculosus • Graphites • Kali Bichromicum • Kali Carbonicum • Kali Phosphoricum • Lycopodium Clavatum • Natrum Muriaticum • Phosphorus • Pulsatilla • Silicea • Spongia Tosta • Staphsagria • Sulphur • Thyroidunum • Veratrum Album.

DermaVite Dietary Supplement - Stiefel Laboratories
Each tablet contains: Vitamin A (29% as beta carotene) 3500 IU • Vitamin C 120 mg • Vitamin E 60 IU • Riboflavin 8.5 mg • Vitamin B-6 10 mg • Folate 400 mcg • Biotin 600 mcg • Calcium 270 mg • Zinc 45 mg • Selenium 50 mcg • Copper 2 mg • Manganese 5 mg • Chromium 200 mcg • Lycopene 5 mg • Silicon 20 mg.

Desiccated Liver Tablets with B-12 and B-Complex - Puritan's Pride
Each tablet contains: Thiamin (Vitamin B-1; Thiamine Hydrochloride) 1 mg • Vitamin B-12 (as Cyanocobalamin) 1 mcg • Desiccated Liver 680 mg.

Dessert Avert - Enforma Natural Products
Each lozenge contains: Gymnema Sylvestre • Clove oil (or Clove powder) • Fructose.

Detox - The Herbalist
Oregon Grape root • Yellow Dock root • Dandelion root • Burdock root • Fennel seed.

Detox Formula - Gary Nulls
Each capsule contains: Apple Pectin 25 mg • Buckthorn bark 25 mg • Burdock root 25 mg • Cascara Sagrada bark 25 mg • Chrysanthemum 25 mg • Dandelion root 25 mg • Fennel seed 25 mg • Fiber 75 mg • Garlic 25 mg • Ginger root 25 mg • Goldenseal root 50 mg • Hibiscus 25 mg • Kelp 25 mg • Licorice root 25 mg • Marshmallow 25 mg • Orange peel 25 mg • Oregon Grape root 25 mg • Peppermint 25 mg • Prickly Ash bark 25 mg • Psyllium 50 mg • Red Clover 25 mg • Rose Hips 25 mg • Sarsaparilla root 25 mg • Stillingia 25 mg • Yellow Dock 25 mg.

Detox Support - Amazon Support
Each capsule contains: Graviola • Carquija • Erva Tostao • Fedegosa • Tayuya • Artichoke • Mutmaba • Espinheira Santa • Boldo • Chanca Piedra • Samambaia • Brazilian Peppertree • Sarsaparilla • Pau d'arco • Cat's Claw.

Detox Support - Now
Each capsule contains: Milk Thistle • Sodium Alginate • Chlorella • MSM as central ingredients.

Detoxene - Health Smart Vitamins
Two capsules contain: Vitamin C (as ascorbic acid) 50 mg • Vitamin E (as d-alpha tocopheryl acetate) 10 IU • Pectin (from citrus) 120 mg • Chlorella 60 mg • Algin (as alginic acid) 50 mg • Burdock root 50 mg • Red Clover flower 50 mg • Sarsaparilla root 50 mg • Cornsilk style and stigma 30 mg • Bromelain (from pineapple) 20 mg • Garlic bulb 20 mg • Goldenseal (whole herb) 20 mg • Juniper berry 20 mg • Kelp 20 mg • Turmeric root (95% curcumin; 19 mg) 20 mg • Dandelion root 10 mg • Milk Thistle seed (80% silymarin; 8 mg) 10 mg.

Detoxinal - PhysioLogics
Two capsules contain: Vitamin C (Ascorbic Acid) 200 mg • Chlorella 200 mg • Garlic 100 mg • Milk Thistle (80% Silymarin, 80 mg) 100 mg • Burdock root 50 mg • Cascara sagrada 50 mg • Dandelion root 50 mg • Red Clover 50 mg • Algin 50 mg • Pectin 50 mg • Bromelain 50 mg.

Detoxygen - Nature's Plus
Two tablets contain: Botanical Blend: Hibiscus (Hibiscus sabdariffa) 250 mg • Red Clover (Trifolium pratense) 200 mg • Dandelion (Taraxacum officinale) 200 mg • Chinese Mushroom Complex 200 mg: Shiitake (Lentinus edodes) 150 mg • Reishi (Ganoderma lucidum) 50 mg • Echinacea (Echinacea purpurea) 100 mg • Cayenne (Capsicum frutescens) 75 mg • Yellow Dock (Rumex crispus) 50 mg • Milk Thistle (standardized 80% Silymarin) 50 mg • Celery Seed (Apium graveolens) 25 mg • Ginger root (Zingiber officinale) 25 mg • Juniper berries (Juniperus communis) 20 mg • Essential Cofactor blend: Creatine Monohydrate Energy Precursor 100 mg • Co-Enzyme Q10 (Ubiquinone) 10 mg • Vitamin B12 (Cobalamin concentrate) 250 mcg. Contains no yeast, wheat, corn, soy, milk, salt, sugar or starch.

Devil's Claw Complex - PhytoPharmica
Two capsules contain: Devil's Claw (Harpagophytum procumbens) root extract (standardized to contain 1.8%-2.2% harpagoside) 500 mg • Nettle leaf (Urticae dioica) leaf extract (standardized to contain 1% silicic acid) 500 mg • Ginger (Zingiber officinale) root extract (standardized to contain a minimum of 4.5% pungent compounds) 200 mg.

Devil's Club-Bilberry Virtue - Blessed Herbs
Devil's Club Root bark • Bilberry leaf • Reishi mycelium • Siberian Ginseng root • Grain alcohol & Distilled Water.

Dexatrim - Chattem, Inc.
Each gelcap contains: Active Ingredient: Phenylpropanolamine HCl 75 mg. Inactive Ingredients: Carnauba wax, D&C Yellow No. 10 Aluminum Lake, FD&C Yellow No. 6. Aluminum Lake, Hydroxypropyl Methylcellulose, Iron Oxide, Magnesium Stearate, Microcrystalline Cellulose, Polyethylene Glycol, Polysorbate 80, Povidone, Silicon Dioxide, Stearic Acid, Titanium Dioxide.

Dexatrim Natural Ephedrine - Free Formula - Chattem, Inc.
Each caplet contains: Calcium 23 mg • Chromium (as Chromium Dinicotinate Glycinate) 83 mcg • Bitter Orange Peel powder extract 120 mg • Proprietary Blend: Siberian Ginseng extract, Green Tea leaf with added Caffeine, Fenugreed seed extract, Guarana seed extract with added Caffeine, Kola Nut extract with added Caffeine, Ginger root, Licorice root and Vanadium amino acid chelate 340 mg. Other Ingredients: Microcrystalline Cellulose, Maltodextrin, Dicalcium Phosphate, Croscarmellose Sodium, Stearic Acid, Silicon Dioxide, Hydroxypropyl Methylcellulose, Polyethylene Glycol.

Some Brand Name Natural Products - What they Contain
www.NaturalDatabase.com contains MANY more listings than appear here.

Dexatrim Natural Green Tea Formula - Chattem, Inc.
Each caplet contains: Calcium 70 mg • Iodine (from Kelp) 30 mcg •
Chromium (as Chromium Dinicotinate Glycinate) 250 mcg
• Vanadium (as Vanadium Amino Acid Chelate) 100 mcg
• Standardized Green Tea extract (leaf, 40 mg Caffeine) 200 mg •
Heartleaf extract (Sida cordifolia, 12 mg Ephedrine Alkaloids) 120 mg
• Herbal Blend: Standardized Panax Ginseng extract root, Licorice
root, Cinnamon bark, Ginger root, Sarsaparilla root, and Kelp 150 mg.
Other Ingredients: Dicalcium Phosphate, Microcrystalline Cellulose,
Croscarmellose Sodium, Stearic Acid, Silica, Magnesium Stearate,
Hydroxypropyl Methylcellulose, Hydroxypropyl Cellulose,
Polywthylene Glycol, Titanium Dioxide, Riboflavin, Caramel.

Dexatrim Natural No Caffeine Formula - Chattem, Inc.
Each caplet contains: Chromium (as chromium dinicotinate glycinate)
250 mcg • Vanadium (as vanadium amino acid chelate) 100 mcg •
Heartleaf Standardized Extract (Sida cordifolia, 12 mg naturally
occurring ephedrine) 120 mg • Thermonutrient Blend
100 mg: Steatite, Atractylodes rhizome, Baikal Skullcap root,
Balloon-Flower root, Licorice root, Terra Alba, Da Huang root,
Mirabilite, Dong Quai root, Field Mint leaf, Forsythia fruit, Gardenia
fruit, Ginger root, Lovage root, Schizonepeta stem, Siler root, White
Peony root. Other Ingredients: Dicalcium Phosphate,
Microchrystalline Cellulose, Croscarmellose Sodium, Stearic Acid,
Hydroxypropyl Cellulose, Polyethylene glycol.

Dexatrim No Caffeine - Chattem, Inc.
Each gelcap contains: Active Ingredient: Phenylpropanolamine HCl
75 mg. Inactive Ingredients: Carnauba wax, D&C Yellow No. 10
Aluminum Lake, Edetate Disodium, FD&C Blue No. 1., FD&C Red
No. 40 Aluminum Lake, FD&C Yellow No. 6 Aluminum Lake,
Gelatin, Glycerin, Hydroxypropyl Methylcellulose, Magnesium
Stearate, Microcrystalline Cellulose, Pharmaceutical Glaze,
Polyethylene Glycol, Polysorbate 80, Povidone, Propylene Glycol,
Silicon Dioxide, Stearic Acid, Titanium Dioxide.

DGL - Enzymatic Therapy
Each chewable tablet contains: Licorice root extract 4:1
Deglycrrhizinated (Glycyrrhiza glabra) 380 mg • Glycine (Amino
Acid) 50 mg. In a base of Fructose. Contains no sugar, salt, yeast,
wheat, corn, soy, dairy products, coloring, flavoring or preservatives.

DGL Chewable Licorice - Puritan's Pride
Each tablet contains: Deglycyrrihizinated Licorice root (Glycyrrihiza
glabra) extract (4:1) 380 mg • Glycine (Amino Acid) 50 mg.

DGL Plus - Progressive Labs
Two capsules contain: Licorice root (Glycyrrhiza glabra):
Deglycyrrhizinated Licorice extract 400 mg • NAG (N-Acetyl
Glucosamine) 60 mg • Parotid Gland 10 mg • Gamma Oryzanol
50 mg • Glycine 50 mg.

DHA - Brain Support Complex - Leiner Health Products
Each softgel contains: DHA (Docosahexaenoic Acid) 100 mg. Other
Ingredients: High Oleic Sunflower Oil, Algal Oil, Gelatin, Glycerin,
Vanillin, Ascorbyl Pamitate, Mixed Natural Tocopherols.

DHA Neuromins - Source Naturals
Each softgel contains: Docosahexaenoic acid 100 mg.

DHEA - Leiner Health Products
Each tablet contains: DHEA (Dehydroepiandrosterone) 25 mg. Other
Ingredients: Dicalcium Phosphate, Cellulose, Stearic Acid, Silicon
Dioxide, Magnesium Stearate, Polyethylene Glycol 3350,
Crospovidone, Croscarmellose Sodium, Hydroxypropyl
Methylcellulose, Hydroxypropyl Cellulose, Polysorbate 80.

DHEA - Body Wise International, Inc.
Each capsule contains: DHEA (Dehydroepiandrosterone) 25 mg •
Calcium (from Dicalcium Phosphate) 6 mg.

DHEA - Olympian Labs
Each capsule contains: DHEA (dehydroepiandrosterone) 25 mg.

DHEA - Swanson
Each capsule contains: DHEA (dehydroepiandrosterone) 25 mg.

DHEA (50 mg) - Olympian Labs
Each capsule contains: DHEA (dehydroepiandrosterone) 50 mg.

DHEA -25- X-TRA - Progressive Labs
Each capsule contains: DHEA (dehydroepiandrosterone) 25 mg •
Herbal Base: [Green Tea leaf extract (Camellia sinensis) - 35%
polyphenols, Schizandra berry (Schizandra chinensis), Soybean
extract (Glycine max) - 1% isoflavones (hypoallergenic), Ginkgo
Biloba leaf extract (24% ginkgoflavonglycosides), Grape seed extract
(Vitis vinifera) - 40% proanthocyanidins] 250 mg.

DHEA Ultra - FreeLife
Each tablet contains: DHEA (micronized dehydroepiandrosterone -
100% pharmaceutical grade) 25 mg • Metabolic Activation System
(an exclusive coenzyme complex of Nicotinamide, Pyridoxal-5'-
phosphate, Riboflavin-5'-phosphate, Pantothenic Acid, Thiamine)
10 mg • Bioavailability Enhancing System (ancient herbal tricatu
blend - 2.5 mg of Bioperine [Piper nigrum fruit standardized 95%
1-piperoylpiperidine], Piper longum fruit, Zingiber officinalis root)
12.5 mg.

DHEA X-TRA - Progressive Labs
Each capsule contains: DHEA (dehydroepiandrosterone) 50 mg •
Herbal Base: [Green Tea leaf extract (Camellia sinensis) - 35%
polyphelols, Schizandra berry (Schizandra chinensis), Soybean extract
(Glycine max) - 1% isoflavones (hypoallergenic), Ginkgo Biloba leaf
extract (24% ginkgoflavonglycosides), Grape seed extract (Vitis
vinifera) - 40% proanthocyanidins] 250 mg.

DHEA-25 - PhytoPharmica
Each capsule contains: DHEA (Dehydroepiandrosterone)
pharmaceutical grade 25 mg.

DHEA-5 - PhytoPharmica
Each capsule contains: DHEA (Dehydroepiandrosterone)
pharmaceutical grade 5 mg.

DHEAX - HealthWatchers System
Dioscorea Villosa • Alpha Ketoglutaric Acid • Phosphatidyl Serine •
Pantothenic Acid • Gotu Kola Powder • Ginkgo Biloba Powder •
Siberian Ginseng Powder • L-Glutamine • L-Tyrosine • L-Glycine •
L-Arginine-HCl • L-Ornithine • L-Lysine • Pantathine • Beta
Sitosterol.

Diabest - PhysioLogics
Three tablets contain: Vitamin A (Palmitate) 2500 IU • Vitamin E
(d-Alpha Tocopherol) 300 IU • Vitamin C (Ascorbic Acid) 300 mg
• Magnesium (Glycinate) 300 mg • Niacin 150 mg • Zinc (Glycinate)
23 mg • Vitamin B6 (Pyridoxine HCI) 15 mg • Copper (Glycinate)
3 mg • Biotin 900 mcg • Chromium (Niacin/Glycine Chelate)
200 mcg • Selenium (as Selenomethionine) 50 mcg • Quercetin
150 mg • Ginkgo leaf (24% Ginkgo flavonglycosides 75 mg,
6% terpene lactones 4.5 mg) 75 mg • Vanadyl Sulfate 750 mcg.

Diabest 2 - PhysioLogics
Each capsule contains: Chromium (33% Niacin/Glycine Chelate, 67%
Picolinate) 300 mcg • Gymnema sylvestre (24% Gymnemic Acid 48
mg) 200 mg • Mormodica charantia 4:1 extract 100 mg • Bis
(Glycinato) Oxovanadium (BGOV) 10 mg • Vanadyl Sulfate 10 mg.

Diabetic Support Formula - Nutrition Warehouse
Each tablet contains: Vitamin C (as Ascorbic Acid) 100 mg • Vitamin
E (as dl-Alpha Tocopheryl Acetate) 30 IU • Biotin 350 mcg • Calcium

(as Dicalcium Phosphate) 85 mg • Magnesium (as Magnesium Oxide) 250 mg • Zinc (as Zinc Oxide) 7.5 mg • Selenium (as Sodium Selenate) 70 mcg • Manganese (as Manganese Sulfate) 2 mg • Chromium (as Chromium Picolinate) 500 mcg • Lipoic Acid 30 mg • Vanadyl Sulfate 10 mg • Ginkgo Biloba (24% flavone glycosides) 20 mg • Coenzyme Q-10 5 mg • Taurine 50 mg • L-Carnitine 125 mg.

Diabetic Support Formula - Puritan's Pride
Each tablet contains: Vitamin C (as Ascorbic Acid) 100 mg • Vitamin E (as dl-Alpha Tocopheryl Acetate) 30 IU • Biotin 350 mcg • Calcium (as Dicalcium Phosphate) 85 mg • Magnesium (as Magnesium Oxide) 250 mg • Zinc (as Zinc Oxide) 7.5 mg • Selenium (as Sodium Selenate) 70 mcg • Manganese (as Manganese Sulfate) 2 mg • Chromium (as Chromium Picolinate) 500 mcg • Lipoic Acid 30 mg • Vanadyl Sulfate 10 mg • Ginkgo Biloba (24% flavone glycosides) 20 mg • Coenzyme Q-10 5 mg • Taurine 50 mg • L-Carnitine 125 mg.

Diabetica Tea - HerbaSway
Panax Ginseng • Siberian Ginseng • Astragalus • Kudzu • Blackberry • Licorice • HerbaSwee (Cucurbitaceae fruit).

Dia-B-Tea - Amazon Support
One rounded teaspoon contains: Pata de Vaca • Pedra Hume Caa • Bitter Melon • Chanca Piedra • Stevia.

Di-Acid Dim - Atrium Inc.
Each tablet contains: First Phase (in Stomach): Glycine 32 mg • Pepsin 100 mg • Papain 50 mg. Second Phase (in Duodenum): Pancreatin 100 mg • Pancrelipase 50 mg • Amylase 30 mg • Bromelain 30 mg • Ox Bile extract 65 mg.
See Editor's Note No. 14, page 1817.

Di-Acid Stim - Atrium Inc.
Each tablet contains: First Phase (in Stomach): Betaine HCL 100 mg • Glutamic Acid HCL 110 mg • Pepsin 100 mg • Papain 50 mg. Second Phase (in Duodenum): Pancreatin 100 mg • Pancrelipase 50 mg. Amylase 30 mg • Bromelain 40 mg • Ox Bile extract 60 mg.
See Editor's Note No. 14, page 1817.

Dia-Comp - Enzymatic Therapy
Two capsules contain: Vitamin E (Mixed Tocopherols) 50 IU • Magnesium (Chelate) 100 mg • Vitamin C (Ascorbic Acid) 100 mg • Vitamin B6 (Pyridoxine HCL) 10 mg • Manganese (Chelate) 10 mg • Zinc (Picolinate) 5 mg • Biotin 1000 mcg • Vitamin B12 (Cyanocobalamin) 250 mcg • Chromium (Picolinate) 50 mcg • Selenium (Aspartate) 40 mcg • Other ingredients: Blueberry extract 4:1 (Vaccinium myrtillus fructus) 300 mg • Gymnema sylvestre extract standardized to contain 24% Gymnemic Acid 150 mg • Bitter Melon extract (Momordica charanita) 100 mg • Fenugreek seed extract (4:1) (Trigonella foenum-Ggaecum) 100 mg.

Dibencozide - Source Naturals
Each tablet contains: Dibencozide (Coenzyme Vitamin B12) 10,000 mcg.

Diene-O-Lean - Pharmanex
Two capsules contain: Sunflower Oil 2000 mg • Conjugated Linoleic Acid 1200 mg • Capsaicin 100 mg.

Diet Chitosan - Source Naturals
Each capsule contains: Chitosan (minimum 80% Deacetylated Chitin) 250 mg.

Diet CitriMax - Source Naturals
Each tablet contains: Garcinia cambogia extract [yielding 500 mg of (-) Hydroxycitric Acid as Calcium Hydroxycitrate] 1,000 mg • Chromium (60 mcg ChromeMate Chromium Polynicotinate and 60 mcg of Chromium Picolinate) 120 mcg.

Diet CitriMax Complex - Source Naturals
Three tablets contain: Garcinia cambogia extract [yielding 1,000 mg of (-) Hydroxycitric Acid as Calcium Hydroxycitrate] 2,000 mg • L-Phenylalanine 200 mg • Chromium (200 mcg ChromeMate Chromium Polynicotinate and 200 mcg Chromium Picolinate) 400 mcg.

Diet Fuel - TwinLab
Three capsules contain: Chromium 200 mcg • Citrimax: Garcinia cambogia, Hydroxycitrate extract 500 mg • Guarana extract 909 mg • L-Carnitine 100 mg • Ma Huang extract 334 mg • Potassium & Magnesium Phosphate 100 mg.

Diet Fuel With Chitosan Formula - TwinLab
Two capsules contain: Chitosan (fiber) 1000 mg. Other Ingredients: Cellulose, Gelatin, Purified Water, Magnesium Stearate, MCT.

Diet Metabo-7 - Source Naturals
Each tablet contains: Vitamin C (as Ascorbic Acid) 80 mg • Niacinamide 30 mg • Vitamin B6 (as Pyridoxine HCl) 30 mg • Pantothenic Acid (as calcium-d-pantothenate) 80 mg • Chromium (as Picolinate & Polynicotinate) 400 mcg • Potassium (as Potassium Citrate) 20 mg • Iodine (from Kelp) 100 mcg • GABA (Gamma-Aminobutyric Acid) 500 mg • Phenylalanine (as L-& DL-Phenylalanine) 500 mg • Sida cordifolia extract 6% yielding 30 mg ephedrine alkaloids 500 mg • Gymnema sylveste extract (GS4) 400 mg • Green Tea leaf extract 20% yielding 60 mg of caffeine 300 mg • Glutamine 200 mg • Yogaraj Guggul Gum Resin 200 mg • Kola Nut extract 20% yielding 30 mg of caffeine 150 mg • Yerba Mate extract 8% yielding 10 mg of caffeine 125 mg • Dandelion leaf 100 mg • Bupleurum root 100 mg • L-Tryosine 100 mg • Horse Chestnut extract yielding 14 mg Aescin 70 mg • Dandelion root extract (4:1) 50 mg • Bladderwrack extract 30 mg • Ginkgo Biloba leaf extract (50:1) 30 mg • Ginger root 30 mg • N-Acetyl-Cysteine 30 mg • Black Pepper Fruit extract (Bioperine) 3 mg.

Diet Support Formula - Now
Two capsules contain: Vitamin B6 (pyridoxine HCL) 10 mg • Chromium (chelavite chelate) 300 mcg • Iodine (kelp extract) 300 mcg • Bitter Orange extract (Citrus aurantium) containing 6% synepherine 350 mg • L-Carnitine (from 365 mg l-carnitine tartrate) 250 mg • Super Citrimax as Garcinia cambogia extract containing 225 mg (-)hydroxycitric acid 375 mg • Uva Ursi (Uvae ursi folium) 4:1 extract 50 mg • Green Tea extract (Carmellia sinenis) 30% calechins 200 mg.

Diet System 6 - Applied Nutrition
Six capsules contain: Super Citrimax : Garcinia extract 1500 mg. Energizing Herbs (Thermogenic Herbs): Kola nut extract 550 mg, Guarana extract 100 mg, Ginger 100 mg. Three Lipotropics including: Choline Bitartrate 100 mg, Inositol 100 mg, Betaine HCL 25 mg. Chromium (Chromium Picolinate 150 mcg, ChromeMate 150 mcg). L-Carnitine (L-Carnitine Complex) 300 mg. Vitamins & Minerals: "72 Trace Mineral Complex" 100 mg: Vitamin B3 20 mg, Vitamin B6 2 mg, Vitamin B12 6 mcg, Vitamin B2 1.7 mg, Vitamin E 15 IU, Folic Acid 400 mcg, Selenium 50 mcg , Vitamin C 60 mg, Potassium 25 mg, Iodine 150 mcg.

Diet Ultra III - The Vitamin Shoppe
Three tablets contain: Vitamin A (as acetate, beta-carotene) 10000 IU • Vitamin C (as ascorbic acid) 100 mg • Vitamin D (cholecalciferol) 400 IU • Vitamin E (as d-alpha tocopherol) 50 IU • Vitamin B1 (as thiamin hydrochloride) 25 mg • Vitamin B2 (as riboflavin) 25 mg • Vitamin B12 (as cobalamin) 25 mcg • Niacin (as nicotinic acid) 25 mg • Folic Acid 100 mcg • Biotin 100 mcg • Pantothenic Acid (as d-calcium pantothenate) 20 mg • Iron (as chelate) 10 mg • Calcium (as citrate) 100 mg • Iodine (from kelp) 150 mcg • Magnesium (as citrate) 50 mg • Zinc (as chelate) 15 mg • Selenium (as chelate)

25 mcg • Chromium (as chelate) 300 mcg • Gotu Kola (Centella asiatica) 50 mg • Siberian Ginseng (Eleutherococcus senticosus) root 50 mg • L-Carnitine 50 mg • Choline 150 mg • Inositol 150 mg • Omega-3 (fish) 15 mg.

Diet-Metabo-7 - Source Naturals
Three tablets contain: Vitamin C (as Ascorbic Acid) 80 mg • Niacinamide 30 mg • Vitamin B6 (as Pyridoxine HCl) 30 mg • Pantothenic Acid (as Calcium-D-Pantothenate) 80 mg • Calcium 20 mg • Chromium (200 mcg Chromium 400 mcg Picolinate 200 mcg chromium polynicatinate) • Potassium (as Potassium Citrate) 20 mg • GABA (Gamma-Aminobutyric Acid) 500 mg • Phenylalanine (as L- & DL-Phenylalanine) 500 mg • Sida cordifolia extract (6% yielding 30 mg ephedrine alkaloids) 500 mg • Gymnema sylvestre extract (GS4) 400 mg • Green Tea leaf extract (20% yielding 60 mg of caffeine) 300 mg • Glutamine 200 mg • Guggul Yogaraj Gum Resin 200 mg • Kola Nut extract 20% yielding 30 mg of caffeine) 150 mg • Dandelion extract 4:1 (root & herb) 150 mg • Yerba Mate extract (8% yielding 10 mg of caffeine) 125 mg • Bupleurum root 100 mg • L-Tyrosine 100 mg • Horse Chestnut extract (Yielding 14 mg Aescin) 70 mg • Bladderwrack extract 30 mg • Ginkgo Biloba leaf extract (50:1) 30 mg • Ginger root 30 mg • N-Acetyl Cysteine 30 mg • Black Pepper fruit extract (Bioperine) 3 mg • Iodine (from Kelp) 100 mcg.

Diet-Phen - Source Naturals
Three tablets contain: St. John's Wort extract (Hypericum perforatum standardized extract 0.3% yielding 2.7 mg of hypericin) 900 mg • L-Phenylalanine 750 mg • Green Tea 300 mg • Cayenne 100 mg • Mustard seed 100 mg • Ginger root 100 mg • Piper nigrum 100 mg • Acetyl L-Carnitine 50 mg • Niacinamide 25 mg • Vitamin B6 (Pyridoxine HCl) 25 mg • Chromium (100 mcg ChromeMate Polynicotinate, 100 mcg Chromium Picolinate) 200 mcg.

Diet-Phen For Men - Source Naturals
Three tablets contain: St. John's Wort extract (Hypericum perforatum standardized extract 0.3% yielding 2.7 mg of hypericin) 900 mg • Creatine Monohydrate 500 mg • L-Glutamine 200 mg • L-Phenylalanine 500 mg • Ma Huang standardized extract 8% (Yielding 18 mg of Ephedra alkaloids) 225 mg • Panax Ginseng root extract (Standardized to 8% ginsenosides) 100 mg • L-Carnitine L-Tartrate 50 mg • Niacinamide 25 mg • Vitamin B6 (Pyridoxine HCl) 25 mg • Chromium (300 mcg ChromeMate Polynicotinate and 100 mcg Chromium Picolinate) 400 mcg.

Digest RC - Cxresearch Inc.
Each tablet contains: Black Radish 75 mg • Charcoal 75 • Artichoke 47 mg • Calcium Phospate 45 mg • Cholic Acid 40 mg • Peppermint 15 mg.

Digest Support - Natrol
Two capsules contain: Proteolytic Enzymes: Protease I (20000 HUT) 200 mg • Protease II (16600 FCC) 8 mg • Amylolytic Enzymes: Amylase (10200 DU) 408 mg • Cellulase (410 CMC) 100 mg • Lactase (200 LAC) 20 mg • Lipolytic Enzymes: Lipase (300 LU) 100 mg • Maltase (90 DU) 90 mg • Sucrase (200 SU) 20 mg • Anti Gas Factor: Alpha Galactosidase (54 GAL) 54 mg. Other ingredients: TriCalcium Phosphate, Silica, Magnesium Stearate, Gelatin.

Digestabs - Puritan's Pride
Two tablets contain: Pancreatin 600 mg • Amylase 260 mg • Pepsin 130 mg • Papain 130 mg • Ox Bile 130 mg • Betaine HCl 130 mg • Duodenal substance 60 mg.
See Editor's Note No. 14, page 1817.

DigestEase - Pacific BioLogic
Ginger • Rhubarb • Elecampane • Gentian • Long Pepper • Tropical Almond • Emblic Myrobalan • Beleric Myrobalan • Glauber's Salt • Kaolin.

Di-Gest-Eze - Nutri-Quest
Each two-phase tablet contains: Phase One (Stomach): Betaine HCL 155 mg • L-Glutamic Acid HCL 100 mg • Pepsin 105 mg • Papain 50 mg. Phase Two (Duodenum): Pancreatin 100 mg • Pancrelipase 50 mg • Amylase 30 mg • Bromelain 30 mg • Ox Bile 65 mg • Parotid 2 mg.
See Editor's Note No. 14, page 1817.

Digestion Formula - Dr. Morrow's Homeopathic Formulas
Ten drops contain: Nux vomica 3C • Bryonia alba 3C • Argentum nitricum 3C • Condurango 3C • Abies nigra 3C • Robinia pseudacacia 3C • Solidago 3X.
See Editor's Note No. 1, page 1816.

Digestion Formula - Nature's Way
Two capsules contain: Angelica root 90 mg • Barberry bark 135 mg • Beet root 100 mg • Cayenne pepper fruit 25 mg • Dandelion root 315 mg • Fizyme enzyme formula 100 mg • Gentian root 135 mg.
Other Ingredients: Gelatin, Magnesium stearate, Millet.

Digestion Support - Amazon Support
Each capsule contains: Boldo • Carqueja • Espinheira Santa • Sarsaparilla • Jurubeba • Gervao • Cat's Claw.

Digestive Enzyme Complex - Nutrilite
Each capsule contains: Lipase 31 mg • Lactase 40 mg • Amylase 20 mg • Alpha-Galactosidase 10 mg • Ginger Root Extract 150 mg • NUTRILITE Parsley Concentrate with Phytofactors Plant Compounds.

Diol Stack - Substrate Solutions
Each tablet contains: Nor-4-Androstenediol 100 mg • 4-Androstenediol 100 mg.

Diurex Long Acting Water Capsules - Alva-Amco Pharmacal Cos., Inc.
Each capsule contains: Active Ingredients: Caffeine Anhydrous • Acetaminophen • Potassium Salicylate. Other Ingredients: Non-Pariell seeds, Magnesium Oxide, Titanium Dioxide, plus other coloring & coating ingredients.

Diurex Water Caplets - Alva-Amco Pharmacal Cos., Inc.
Each caplet contains: Active Ingredient: Pamabrom 50 mg. Other Ingredients: Dicalcium Phosphate, FD&C Blue #1, Hydroxypropyl Methylcellulose, Magnesium Stearate, Polyethylene Glycol, Potassium Gluconate, Riboflavin, Stearic Acid, Titanium Dioxide. May also contain: Calcium Sulfate, Croscarmellose Sodium, Microcrystalline Cellulose, Mineral Oil, Polysorbate, Silicon Dioxide, Sodium Lauryl Sulfate.

Diurex Water Pills - Alva-Amco Pharmacal Cos., Inc.
Each pill contains: Active Ingredients: Potassium Salicylate • Caffeine Anhydrous • Salicylamide. Other Ingredients: Calcium Sulfate, Dicalcium Phosphate, Magnesium Trisilicate, Microcrystalline Cellulose, Starch, Magnesium Stearate, Stearic Acid, plus other fillers, coloring & coating ingredients.

Diutrate - Atrium Inc.
Each tablet contains: Buchu leaves 70 mg • Couch grass 70 mg • Hydrangea root 35 mg • Corn Silk 35 mg • Uva Ursi 10 mg • Hypothalamus 30 mg • Raw Kidney concentrate 60 mg • Vitamin B6 16 mg • Magnesium (Protein Chelated) 50 mg.
See Editor's Note No. 14, page 1817.

DMG-B15-Plus - Enzymatic Therapy
Each capsule contains: Potassium Aspartate 125 mg • Magnesium Aspartate 125 mg • Calcium Gluconate 31 mg. Other ingredients: Trimethylglycine (TMG) 100 mg • N,N-Dimethylglycine 100 mg • Glycine 25 mg. Contains no sugar, salt, yeast, wheat, corn, soy, dairy products, coloring, flavoring or preservatives.

BRAND NAMES

BRAND NAMES

D-MNS - Dial Herbs
Mistletoe • Blessed Thistle • Witch Hazel • Nettle • Shepherd's Purse • Red Raspberry • Cayenne.

DN-24 Hydracreme - Pharmagel
Vitamin Retinyl-A 25000 IU.

DNE Ephedrana 12.5 - D & E Pharmaceuticals
Each tablet contains: Ephedrine HCL 12.5 mg. In a proprietary herbal base of Ephedra, Guarana, Chromium.

Doctor's Choice Antioxidant - Enzymatic Therapy
Three capsules contain: Vitamin A (Beta Carotene) non-toxic form of Vitamin A 10000 IU • Vitamin E (D-Alpha Tocopherol) 200 IU • Vitamin C (Ascorbic Acid) 500 mg • Zinc (Picolinate) 15 mg • Manganese (Gluconate) 15 mg • Riboflavin (Vitamin B2) 6 mg • Selenium (L-Selenomethionine) 200 mcg • N-Acetylcysteine 100 mg • Cabbage extract (Brassica oleracea) 100 mg • Garlic extract, deodorized 100 mg • Ginger root extract 6.5:1 (Zingiber officinale) 100 mg • Green Tea extract (Camellia sinensis) 100 mg • Klamath Blue-Green Algae 100 mg • Curcuma root extract (Curcuma longa) standardized to contain 97% Curcumin 50 mg • Grape seed (PCO) extract (Procyanidolic oligomers (PCO) from grape seed extract) 10 mg. Other ingredients: Cellulose, Calcium Silicate, Silicon Dioxide, & Gelatin Capsule. Contains no sugar, salt, yeast, wheat, corn, dairy products, artificial coloring, artificial flavoring or preservatives.

Doctor's Choice Eye Formula - Enzymatic Therapy
Three tablets contain: Vitamin A (Fish Liver oil) 2500 IU • Vitamin A (Beta Carotene) non-toxic form of Vitamin A 2500 IU • Vitamin C (Ascorbic Acid) 600 mg • Vitamin E (D-Alpha Tocopheryl Acetate) 60 IU • Vitamin B2 (Riboflavin) 1.5 mg • Zinc (Picolinate) 9 mg • Selenium (L Selenomethionine) 50 mcg • Copper (Picolinate) 1 mg • Hachimijiogan Herbal Complex 400 mg • Bilberry (Vaccinium myrtillus fructus) Berry extract standardized to contain 25% Anthocyanosides (calculated as Anthocyanidins) 160 mg • Curcuma (Curcuma Longa) root extract standardized to contain 85-97% Curcumin) 50 mg • Grape (Vitis vinifera) seed (PCO) extract standardized to contain 95% Procyanidolic Oligomers (PCOs) 50 mg • Lutein (Marigold flower extract) 2 mg. Other ingredients: Cellulose, Calcium Carbonate, Cellulose Gum, Stearic Acid, Silicon Dioxide & Magnesium Stearate. Contains no sugar, salt, yeast, wheat, gluten, corn, dairy products, artificial coloring, artificial flavoring or preservatives.

Doctor's Choice Flax oil fortified with Borage & Pumpkin - Enzymatic Therapy
Flaxseed oil • Pumpkin seed oil • Borage seed oil • Rosemary Antioxidant S-327 • Average analysis per tablespoon: Omega-3 (LNA) 5250 mg • Omega-6 (LA) 2625 mg • Omega-9 (Oleic) 2600 mg • Gamma-Linolenic Acid (GLA) 325 mg. Contains no sugar, salt, yeast, wheat, corn, soy, dairy products, artificial coloring, artificial flavoring or preservatives.

Doctor's Choice for 45-Plus Women - Enzymatic Therapy
Six tablets contain: Vitamin A (Beta Carotene) 15000 IU • Vitamin A (Retinol) 2500 IU • Vitamin D 400 IU • Vitamin E (D-Alpha Tocopherol Succinate) 200 IU • Vitamin D 400 IU • Calcium (Citrate, Carbonate) 600 mg • Vitamin C (Ascorbic Acid) 300 mg • Magnesium (Aspartate) 300 mg • Potassium (Aspartate) 99 mg • Vitamin B6 (Pyridoxine HCL) 60 mg • Thiamine HCL (Vitamin B1) 60 mg • Riboflavin (Vitamin B2) 60 mg • Pantothenic Acid (D-Calcium Pantothenate) 50 mg • Niacin/Niacinamide 45 mg • Zinc (Picolinate) 15 mg • Manganese (Citrate) 15 mg • Copper (Gluconate) 1.5 mg • Folic Acid 800 mcg • Vitamin B12 (Cyanocobalamin) 800 mcg • Biotin 600 mcg • Vitamin K (Phytonadione) 60 mcg • Iodine (Kelp) 300 mcg • Chromium (Polynicotinate) 200 mcg • Selenium (L-Selenomet hionine) 100 mcg • Molybdenum (Sodium Molybdate)

25 mcg • Flavonoids mixed 100 mg • Alfalfa juice concentrate 100 mg • Dong Quai extract 4:1 (Angelica sinensis) 90 mg • Ginger root extract 6.5:1 (Zingiber officinale) 15 mg • Green Tea extract (Camellia sinensis) 30 mg • Choline Bitartrate 30 mg • Fennel seed extract 6:1 (Foeniculum vulgare) 30 mg • Inositol 30 mg • PABA (Para-Aminobenzoic Acid) 30 mg • Betaine HCL 25 mg • Glutamic Acid HCL 25 mg • Bromelain 15 mg • Papain 15 mg • Protease acid stable 5 mg • Lipase 5 mg • Boron (Sodium Tetraborate Decahydrate 3 mg • Silica (Sodium Metasilicate) 1 mg • Vanadium (Sulfate) 50 mcg. Other ingredients: Cellulose, Cellulose Gum, Stearic Acid, Silicon Dioxide & Magnesium Stearate. Contains no sugar, salt, yeast, wheat, corn, dairy products, artificial coloring, artificial flavoring, or preservatives.

Doctor's Choice for 50-Plus Men - Enzymatic Therapy
Four tablets contain: Vitamin A (Beta Carotene) 15000 IU • Vitamin A (Retinol) 2500 IU • Vitamin E (d-Alpha Tocopherol Succinate) 200 IU • Vitamin D (Ergocalciferol) 100 IU • Vitamin C (Ascorbic Acid) 300 mg • Magnesium (Aspartate) 250 mg • Calcium (Citrate • Carbonate) 250 mg • Niacin/Niacinamide 120 mg • Pantothenic Acid (D-Calcium Pantothenate) 100 mg • Potassium (Aspartate) 99 mg • Thiamine HCL (Vitamin B1) 60 mg • Riboflavin (Vitamin B2) 60 mg • Vitamin B6 (Pyridoxine HCL) 60 mg • Zinc (Picolinate) 30 mg • Manganese (Citrate) 15 mg • Copper (Gluconate) 1.5 mg • Folic Acid 800 mcg • Vitamin B12 (Cyanocobalamin) 800 mcg • Biotin 600 mcg • Iodine (Kelp) 300 mcg • Chromium (Polynicotinate) 200 mcg • Selenium (L-Selenomethionine) 100 mcg • Vitamin K (Phytonadione) 60 mcg • Molybdenum (Sodium Molybdate) 25 mcg • Mixed Flavonoids citrus 100 mg • Saw Palmetto Berry extract 4:1 (Serenoa repens) 80 mg • Ginger root extract 6.5:1 (Zingiber officinale) 60 mg • Alfalfa juice concentrate 60 mg • Choline Bitartrate 30 mg • Inositol 30 mg • PABA (Para-Aminobenzoic Acid) 30 mg • Green Tea extract (Camellia sinensis) 30 mg • Betaine HCL 25 mg • Glutamic Acid HCL 25 mg • Korean Ginseng root extract (Panax ginseng) standardized to contain 7% Saponins (calculated as Rg1) 15 mg • Bromelain 15 mg • Papain 15 mg • Protease acid stable 5 mg • Lipase 5 mg • Boron (Sodium Tetraborate Decahydrate) 2 mg • Vanadium (Sulfate) 50 mcg. Other ingredients: Cellulose, Stearic Acid, Cellulose Gum, Silicon Dioxide, & Magnesium Stearate. Contains no sugar, salt, yeast, wheat, corn, dairy products, artificial coloring, artificial flavoring or preservatives.

Doctor's Choice for Arthritics - Enzymatic Therapy
Two tablets contain: Niacin/Niacinamide 330 mg • Pantothenic Acid (D-Calcium Pantothenate) 100 mg • Magnesium (Oxide) 100 mg • Calcium Chloride 32 mg • Vitamin C (Ascorbic Acid) 30 mg • Zinc (Picolinate) 3 mg • Manganese (Chelate) 3 mg • Glucosamine Sulfate 500 mg • PABA (Para-Aminobenzoic Acid) 400 mg • Bio-Min TR8 a source of trace minerals 100 mg • Glutamic Acid HCL 40 mg • Ammonium Chloride 32 mg • Betaine HCL 20 mg • Chlorophyll 10 mg • Boron (Sodium Tetraborate Decahydrate) 3 mg. Other ingredients: Cellulose, Cellulose Gum, Stearic Acid, Silicon Dioxide, Magnesium Stearate, Alfalfa (Medicago sativa) leaves & stems juice concentrate, Black Cohosh (Cimicituga racemosa) root, Licorice (Glycyrrhiza glabra) root extract & Scullcap (Scutellaria baicalensis) whole plant. Contains no sugar, salt, yeast, wheat, corn, soy, dairy products, artificial coloring, artificial flavoring or preservatives.

Doctor's Choice for Bone Health - Enzymatic Therapy
Three tablets contain: Vitamin C (Ascorbic Acid) 100 mg • Vitamin D (Fish Liver oil) 300 IU • Vitamin K (Phytonadione) 300 mcg • Folic Acid 800 mcg • Vitamin B12 (Cyanocobalamin) 800 mcg • Calcium (Krebs Cycle Chelate) 600 mg • Magnesium (Krebs Cycle Chelate) 150 mg • Vitamin C (Ascorbic Acid) 100 mg • Zinc (Picolinate) 15 mg • Sodium 6 mg • Copper (Picolinate) 1 mg • Mixed Flavonoids (Citrus) 100 mg • Betaine HCL 30 mg • Soy Bean extract standardized to contain 25% Saponins & 13-17% Isoflavones calculated as Genistein 20 mg • Boron (Sodium Tetrahydroborate) 3 mg • Silicon (Sodium Metasilicate) 1 mg • Strontium (Chloride) 500 mcg. Other ingredients: Cellulose, Cellulose Gum, Stearic Acid, Silicon Dioxide, & Magnesium Stearate.

Doctor's Choice for Diabetics - Enzymatic Therapy
Two tablets contain: Vitamin E (Mixed Tocopherols) 100 IU • Vitamin C (Ascorbic Acid) 300 mg • Magnesium (Krebs Cycle Chelate) 100 mg • Vitamin B6 (Pyridoxine HCL) 10 mg • Manganese (Krebs Cycle Chelate) 7.5 mg • Zinc (Picolinate) 7.5 mg • Copper (Picolinate) 0.5 mg • Biotin 1000 mcg • Folic Acid 400 mcg • Vitamin B12 (Cyanocobalamin) 400 mcg • Chromium (Picolinate) 200 mcg • Selenium (Aspartate) 50 mcg • Gymnema sylvestre leaves extract standardized to contain 25% Gymnemic Acid 200 mg • Bitter Melon extract (Momordica charantia) 200 mg • Fenugreek seed extract (4:1) (Trigonella foenum-graecum) 100 mg • Bilberry extract (Vaccinium myrtillus fructus) standardized to contain 25% Anthocyanosides calculated as Anthocyanidins 40 mg • Mixed Bioflavonoids (Citrus) 25 mg • Vanadyl Sulfate 5 mg. Other ingredients: Calcium Carbonate, Cellulose, Cellulose Gum, Silicon Dioxide, Dicalcium Phosphate, Magnesium Stearate & Calcium Silicate. Contains no sugar, salt, yeast, wheat, gluten, corn, dairy products, artificial coloring, artificial flavoring or preservatives.

Doctor's Choice for Female Teens - Enzymatic Therapy
Four tablets contain: Vitamin A (Beta Carotene) 15000 IU • Vitamin A (Retinol) 2500 IU • Vitamin E (D-Alpha Tocopherol Succinate) 200 IU • Vitamin D (Ergocalciferol) 100 IU • Calcium (Citrate, Carbonate) 500 mg • Vitamin C (Ascorbic Acid) 300 mg • Magnesium (Aspartate) 200 mg • Potassium (Aspartate) 99 mg • Vitamin B6 (Pyridoxine HCL) 90 mg • Niacin/Niacinamide 45 mg • Iron (Ferrous Succinate) 30 mg • Pantothenic Acid (D-Calcium Pantothenate) 30 mg • Thiamine HCL (Vitamin B1) 30 mg • Riboflavin (Vitamin B2) 30 mg • Zinc (Picolinate) 20 mg • Manganese (Citrate) 15 mg • Copper (Gluconate) 1.5 mg • Folic Acid 800 mcg • Vitamin B12 (Cyanocobalamin) 800 mcg • Biotin 300 mcg • Iodine (Kelp) 300 mcg • Chromium (Polynicotinate) 200 mcg • Selenium (L-Selenomethionine) 100 mcg • Vitamin K (Phytonadione) 60 mcg • Molybdenum (Sodium molybdate) 25 mcg • Mixed Flavonoids (Citrus) 100 mg • Alfalfa juice concentrate 60 mg • Choline Bitartrate 60 mg • Inositol 60 mg • Ginger root extract 6.5:1 (Zingiber officinale) 60 mg • 8 Dandelion root extract 4:1 (Taraxacum officinale) 60 mg • Licorice root extract (Glycyrrhiza glabra) standardized to contain 5% Glycyrrhizic Acid 30 mg • Boron (Sodium Tetraborate Decahydrate) 2 mg • Silica (Sodium Metasilicate) 1 mg • Vanadium (Sulfate) 50 mcg. Other ingredients: Cellulose, Cellulose Gum, Stearic Acid, Magnesium Stearate & Silicon Dioxide. Contains no sugar, salt, yeast, wheat, corn, dairy products, coloring, flavoring, or preservatives.

Doctor's Choice for Healthy Cholesterol Levels - Enzymatic Therapy
Each capsule contains: Red Yeast Rice (Standardized to contain 1% Mevinolin) 475 mg • Artichoke (Cynara scolymus) leaf extract 50 mg • Ginger (Zingiber officinale) root extract 50 mg • Coenzyme Q10 (CoQ10) 8 mg. Other ingredients: Soybean oil, Vegetable oil, Beeswax, Lecithin, and Gelatin capsule.

Doctor's Choice for Heart Health - Enzymatic Therapy
Two tablets contain: Vitamin E (D-Alpha Tocopherol) 100 IU • Magnesium (Oxide) 150 mg • Niacin 100 mg • Vitamin C (Ascorbic Acid) 100 mg • Potassium (Chloride) 75 mg • Calcium Pangamate 20 mg • Vitamin B6 (Pyridoxine HCL) 10 mg • Sodium 6 mg • Folic Acid 200 mcg • Vitamin B12 (Cyanocobalamin) 200 mcg • Hawthorne berry extract (Crataegus oxyacantha) standardized to contain 1.8% Vitexin-2'-Rhamnoside 150 mg • Super Seven Complex Mixture of Herbs: Hydrangea, Black Cohosh (Cimicifuga racemosa), Buchu leaves, Couch Grass, Corn Silk, Dandelion leaf (Taraxacum officinale) & Ginger root (Zingiber officinale) 150 mg • Khella extract (Ammi visnaga) standardized to contain a minimum of 10% Pyrones calculated as Khellin 100 mg • L-Cysteine 100 mg • Carbamide 100 mg. Other ingredients: Cellulose, Cellulose Gum, Stearic Acid, Sodium Starch, Glycolate, Silicon Dioxide, Magnesium Stearate & Vanillin.

Doctor's Choice for Male Teens - Enzymatic Therapy
Four tablets contain: Vitamin A (Beta Carotene) 15000 IU • Vitamin A (Retinol) 2500 IU • Vitamin E (D-Alpha Tocopherol Succinate) 200 IU • Vitamin D (Ergocalciferol) 100 IU • Calcium (Citrate, Carbonate) 400 mg • Vitamin C (Ascorbic Acid) 300 mg • Magnesium (Aspartate) 200 mg • Potassium (Aspartate) 99 mg • Niacin/Niacinamide 45 mg • Pantothenic Acid (D-Calcium Pantothenate) 30 mg • Vitamin B6 (Pyridoxine HCL) 30 mg • Thiamine HCL (Vitamin B1) 30 mg • Riboflavin (Vitamin B2) 30 mg • Zinc (Picolinate) 30 mg • Manganese (Citrate) 15 mg • Copper (Gluconate) 1.5 mg • Folic Acid 800 mcg • Vitamin B12 (Cyanocobalamin) 800 mcg • Iodine (Kelp) 300 mcg • Chromium (Polynicotinate) 200 mcg • Selenium (L-Selenomethionine) 100 mcg • Vitamin K (Phytonadione) 60 mcg • Molybdenum (sodium Molybdate) 25 mcg • Biotin 300 mcg • Mixed Flavonoids (Citrus) 100 mg • Alfalfa juice concentrate 60 mg • Dandelion root extract 4:1 (Taraxacum officinale) 60 mg • Ginger root extract 6.5:1 (Zingiber officinale) 60 mg • Sarsaparilla root extract 4:1 (Similax officinalis) 60 mg • Choline Bitartrate 30 mg • Inositol 30 mg • Boron (Sodium Tetraborate Decahydrate) 2 mg • Vanadium (Sulfate) 50 mcg.

Doctor's Choice for Men - Enzymatic Therapy
Three tablets contain: Vitamin A (Beta Carotene) non-toxic form of Vitamin A 15000 IU • Vitamin A (Retinol) 2500 IU • Vitamin E (D-Alpha Tocopherol Succinate) 200 IU • Vitamin D 100 IU • Magnesium (Aspartate, Chloride) 400 mg • Vitamin C (Ascorbic Acid) 300 mg • Calcium (Citrate, Carbonate) 200 mg • Potassium (Aspartate) 99 mg • Niacin 90 mg • Thiamine HCL (Vitamin B1) 60 mg • Riboflavin (Vitamin B2) 60 mg • Vitamin B6 (Pyridoxine HCL) 60 mg • Pantothenic Acid (D-Calcium Pantothenate) 60 mg • Zinc (Picolinate) 30 mg • Manganese (Citrate) 5 mg • Copper (Gluconate) 1 mg • Folic Acid 800 mcg • Vitamin B12 (Cyanocobalamin) 800 mcg • Biotin 600 mcg • Iodine (Kelp) 300 mcg • Chromium (Polynicotinate) 200 mcg • Selenium (Selenomethionine) 200 mcg • Vitamin K (Phytonadione) 60 mcg • Molybdenum (Sodium Molybdate) 25 mcg • Flavonoids mixed 50 mg • Alfalfa juice concentrate 50 mg • Choline Bitartrate 30 mg • Inositol 30 mg • Ginger root extract 6.5:1 (Zingiber officinale) 30 mg • Green Tea extract (Camellia sinensis) standardized to contain 70% Polyphenols 30 mg • Muira Puama extract 6:1 (Ptychopetalum olacoides) 30 mg • PABA (Para-Aminobenzoic Acid) 30 mg • Saw Palmetto Berry extract 4:1 (Serenoa repens) 30 mg • Korean Ginseng root extract (Panax ginseng) standardized to contain 7% Saponins (calculated as Ginsenoside Rg1) 15 mg • Carotenes from natural sources 5 mg • Boron (Sodium Tetraborate Decahydrate) 2 mg • Vanadium (Sulfate) 50 mcg. Other ingredients: Cellulose, Cellulose Gum, Stearic Acid, Silicon Dioxide & Magnesium Stearate. Contains no sugar, salt, yeast, wheat, corn, dairy products, artificial coloring, artificial flavoring, or preservatives.

Doctor's Choice for Women - Enzymatic Therapy
Four tablets contain: Vitamin A (Beta Carotene) non-toxic form of Vitamin A 15000 IU • Vitamin A (Retinol) 2500 IU • Vitamin E (D-Alpha Tocopherol Succinate) 200 IU • Vitamin D 100 IU • Calcium (Citrate, Carbonate) 400 mg • Vitamin C (Ascorbic Acid) 300 mg • Magnesium (Aspartate, Chloride) 300 mg • Potassium (Aspartate) 99 mg • Vitamin B6 (Pyridoxine HCL) 90 mg • Niacin/Niacinamide 90 mg • Thiamine HCL (Vitamin B1) 60 mg • Riboflavin (Vitamin B2) 60 mg • Pantothenic Acid (D-Calcium Pantothenate) 30 mg • Zinc (Picolinate) 20 mg • Iron (Ferrous Succinate) 18 mg • Manganese (Citrate) 5 mg • Vitamin B6 (Pyridoxal-5-Phosphate) 5 mg • Copper (Gluconate) 1 mg • Folic Acid 800 mcg • Vitamin B12 (Cyanocobalamin) 800 mcg • Biotin 600 mcg • Iodine (Kelp) 300 mcg • Chromium (Polynicotinate) 200 mcg • Selenium (Selenomethionine) 200 mcg • Vitamin K (Phytonadione) 60 mcg • Molybdenum (Sodium molybdate) 25 mcg • Flavonoids, mixed 50 mg • Alfalfa juice concentrate 50 mg • Choline Bitartrate 30 mg • Inositol 30 mg • Dong Quai extract 4:1 (Angelica sinensis) 30 mg • Ginger root extract (6.5:1) (Zingiber officinale) 30 mg • Licorice root extract (Glycyrrhiza glabra) standardized to contain 5% Glycyrrhizic Acid 30 mg • PABA

BRAND NAMES

(Para-Aminobenzoic Acid) 30 mg • Chaste Tree Berry extract 5:1 (Vitex agnus-castus) 15 mg • Fennel seed extract 6:1 (Foeniculum vulgare) 15 mg • Carotenes from natural sources 5 mg • Boron (Sodium Tetraborate Decahydrate) 3 mg • Silica (Sodium Metasilicate) 1 mg • Vanadium (Sulfate) 50 mcg. Other Ingredients: Cellulose, Cellulose Gum, Magnesium Stearate, Stearic Acid, & Silicon Dioxide. Contains no sugar, salt, yeast, wheat, corn, dairy products, artificial coloring, artificial flavoring or preservatives.

Doctor's Choice Prenatal Supplement - Enzymatic Therapy
Four tablets contain: Vitamin A (Beta Carotene) 15000 IU • Vitamin E (D-Alpha Tocopherol Succinate) 200 IU • Vitamin D (Ergocalciferol) 100 IU • Calcium (Citrate, Carbonate) 800 mg • Magnesium (Citrate) 400 mg • Vitamin C (Ascorbic Acid) 300 mg • Vitamin B6 (Pyridoxine HCL) 120 mg • Pantothenic Acid (D-Calcium Pantothenate) 100 mg • Potassium (Aspartate) 99 mg • Thiamine HCL (Vitamin B1) 60 mg • Riboflavin (Vitamin B2) 60 mg • Niacin/Niacinamide 45 mg • Iron (Ferrous succinate) 30 mg • Zinc (Picolinate) 30 mg • Manganese (Citrate) 15 mg • Copper (Gluconate) 1.5 mg • Folic Acid 800 mcg • Vitamin B12 (Cyanocobalamin) 800 mcg • Biotin 600 mcg • Vitamin K (Phytonadione) 500 mcg • Iodine (Kelp) 300 mcg • Chromium (Polynicotinate) 200 mcg • Selenium (L-Selenomethionine) 100 mcg • Molybdenum (Sodium Molybdate) 25 mcg • Ginger root extract 6.5:1 (Zingiber officinale) 150 mg • Mixed Flavonoids (Citrus) 90 mg • Choline Bitartrate 90 mg • Inositol 90 mg • Dandelion root extract 4:1 (Taraxacum officinale) 60 mg • Red Raspberry leaves 60 mg • Boron (Sodium Tetraborate Decahydrate) 1 mg • Silica (Sodium Metasilicate) 1 mg • Vanadium (Sulfate) 50 mcg. Other ingredients: Cellulose, Cellulose Gum, Stearic Acid, Silicon Dioxide & Magnesium Stearate.

Dolomite - The Vitamin Shoppe
Four tablets supply: Calcium 520 mg • Magnesium 312 mg.

Dolomite - Puritan's Pride
One tablet contains: Calcium (as Dolomite) 130 mg • Magnesium (as Dolomite) 78 mg.

Dona Glucosamine Sulfate - Rotta Pharmaceuticals
Each packet contains: Crystalline Glucosamine Sulfate 1500 mg.

Dong Quai - Fingerprint Botanicals
Each capsule contains: Dong Quai 500 mg.

Dong Quai - Leiner Health Products
Each caplet contains: Dong Quai extract (Angelica sinensis) root 200 mg • Ligustilides (Dong Quai extract) 2 mg. Other Ingredients: Cellulose, Calcium Carbonate, Stearic Acid, Croscarmellose Sodium, Silicon Dioxide, Magnesium Stearate.

Dong Quai - Nature's Way
Two capsules contain: Dong Quai root 1110 mg. Other Ingredients: Gelatin, Magnesium stearate.

Dong Quai - Olympian Labs
Each capsule contains: Dong Quai 500 mg.

Dong Quai & Royal Jelly - Puritan's Pride
Each capsule contains: Dong Quai root powder 200 mg • Royal Jelly powder (from Royal Jelly 2:1 150 mg) 300 mg.

Dong Quai and Royal Jelly - GNC
Each capsule contains: Dong Quai 300 mg • Agnus Castus berry 50 mg • Royal Jelly 50 mg • Wild Yam root 50 mg.

Dong Quai Extract - Montana Big Sky
Each capsule contains: Dong Quai 200 mg.

Dong Quai Extract in Vegetable Glycerin - Nature's Herbs
Each drop contains: Dong Quai 565 mg.

Dong Quai Root - Herbal Plus
Each capsule contains: Dong Quai 250 mg.

DopaBean 333 mg - Solaray - Nutraceutical
One capsule contains: Velvet Bean seed extract (Mucuna pruriens) 333 mg • Catecholamines 66 mg • L-dopa 50 mg. Other Ingredients: Gelatin (capsule), Rice Flour, Maltodextrin, Magnesium Stearate, Silica, Alpha Galactosidase.

Down Size - Dial Herbs
Purified Water • Hydrolyzed Collagen • Glycerine • Natural Flavors • Aloe concentrate • Acesulfame Potassium • Citric Acid • Potassium Sorbate • Sodium Benzoate • Potassium Iodide.

Dr. Powers Liquid Colloidal Mineral Source with Trace Minerals - Puritan's Pride
Each 1 fl oz (30 ml) contains: Vitamin B12 1100 mcg • Biotin 200 mcg • Calcium 25 mg • Magnesium 100 mg • Zinc 10 mg • Selenium 50 mcg • Manganese 5 mg • Chromium 50 mcg • Potassium 10 mg • Silica 1000 mcg.

Dream Sleep - The Herbalist
Hops blossom • Passionflower herb • Skullcap herb • Valerian root.

Dream Time - Health Smart Vitamins
Two capsules contain: Calcium (as calcium stearate) 1 mg • Valerian root (0.8% valernic acids, 3 mg) 380 mg • German Chamomile flowers 180 mg • Peppermint leaf 180 mg • Bee Propolis extract 90 mg • Passionflower aerial parts 90 mg • American Ginseng root 80 mg.

Dry Vitamin D - Nature's Way
Each capsule contains: Vitamin D (as Vitamin D3) cholecalciferol 400 IU. Other Ingredients: Cellulose, Gelatin, Maltodextrin, Millet.

D-Snore - Quest
Sweet Almond Oil • Sesame Oil • Sunflower Oil • Olive Oil • Grape Seed Oil • Lecithin • Orange Seed Extract in a base of glycerin • Purified de-ionized Water • Natural Peppermint extract.

Dymetadrine 25 - AST Sports Science
Each tablet contains: Ephedrine HCL 25 mg • Guaifenesin 200 mg.

Dymetadrine Xtrem - AST Sports Science
Two capsules contain: Ephedra extract 8% 600 mg • L-Phenylalanine 300 mg • L-Tyrosine 300 mg • Caffeine 200 mg • Willow Bark extract 100 mg.

E.T.-(Essiac Tonic) - The Herbalist
Burdock root • Sheep Sorrel leaf • Slippery Elm bark • Turkey Rhubarb root.

E-400 Caps - TwinLab
Each capsule contains: Vitamin E 400 IU. Other Ingredients: Cellulose, Magnesium, Silicate, Croscarmellose, Sodium, Gelatin, Crospovidone, Purified Water, Silica, Magnesium Stearate, MCT.

E-400 Plus Selenium - The Vitamin Shoppe
Each softgel contains: Vitamin E (d-alpha, d-beta, d-delta tocopheryls) 400 IU • Selenium (Selenomethionine) 50 mcg.

E-400 Sesame - Progressive Labs
Each softgel capsule contains: Vitamin E (d-alpha tocopherol) 400 IU • Sesame oil 200 mg. With Natural, Unesterified Mixed Tocopherols.

Ear Drops - NutriBiotic
Contains 0.1% grapefruit extract in a base of tea tree oil and vegetable glycerin.

Ear Oil - Blessed Herbs
Calendula flower • St. John's Wort flower • Mullein flower • Garlic & Organic Cold-Pressed Olive oil.

Earache Tablets - Hyland's
Each tablet contains: Pulsatilla as Passion Flower 30C HPUS • Chamomilla as Chamomile 30C HPUS • Sulphur 30C HPUS • Calcarea carbonica as Carbonate of Lime 30C HPUS • Belladonna 30C HPUS (3x10-60% Alkaloids) • Lycopodium as Club Moss 30C HPUS. In a base of Lactose NF (Milk Sugar).
See Editor's Note No. 1, page 1816.

Earthmends Breast Health Program - Cancer Wellness Institute
One packet (containing one softgel and four capsules) contains: Vitamin A (as natural beta-carotene and mixed carotenes from natural antioxidant blend) 9000 IU • Vitamin E (as natural vitamin E succiante and d-alpha tocopherol) 200 IU • Selenium (from selenium yeast) 150 mcg. Energizing Complex - Yellow: Glutamine (as L-glutamine polypeptides) 100 mg • Propolis 75 mg • Bee Pollen 75 mg • Ginger extract (root) (3.75 mg gingerols/shoagols) 75 mg • Turmeric extract (root) (71.25 mg curcumins) 75 mg • Oriental Ginseng extract (root) (3.5 mg ginsenosides) 50 mg • Garlic concentrate (bulb) 50 mg. Mushroom Complex - Speckled: Chinese Skullcap (aerial) 75 mg • Maitake Mushroom (aerial) 50 mg • Reishi Mushroom (mycelia) 50 mg • Shitake Mushroom (aerial) 50 mg • Agaricus Mushroom (aerial) 50 mg • Panax Pseudoginseng Wal. (root) 50 mg • Rabdosia Rubescens (Hemsl.) Hara. (aerial) 35 mg • Dyer's Woad (aerial) 35 mg • Licorice (root) 25 mg • Chrysanthemum (flower) 25 mg • Agaricus Mushroom extract (aerial) 25 mg • Maitaki Mushroom extract (6.25 mg polysaccharides) 25 mg • Shitake Mushroom Lenode extract mycelia (aerial) (0.375 mg) 25 mg • Reishi Mushroom extract (aerial) (3.125 mg polysaccharides) 25 mg. Antioxidant Complex - Burgundy: Broccoli concentrate (with natural sulforophanes) (aerial) 200 mg • Colostrum 200 mg • Green Tea extract (leaf) (50 mg polyphenols) 100 mg • Grape Seed Extract (45 mg gallic acid equivalent) (40 mg polyphenols) 100 mg • Quercetin (flavonoid) 50 mg • Indole-3-Carbinol 40 mg. Red Clover Complex - Brown: Red Clover extract (flower) (20 mg isoflavones) 200 mg • Black Cohosh extract (root) (2.83 mg triterpeneglycosides) 113 mg • Dong Quai extract (root) (0.042 mg ferulic acids) 83 mg • Tocotrienols 43 mg. Flax Seed Oil Complex - Red: Flax Oil (seed) 200 mg • Natural Antioxidant Blend 100 mg from Carrot oil (root), Palm (fruit), Marigold (flower), Tomato (fruit), supplying Lutein, Lycopene, Phytoene, Phytofluene, Tocotrienols/Tocopherols, Zeaxanthin • Beta Sitosterol Complex (90 mg free sterols) 100 mg • Natural Lycopene (from Tomato fruit) 5 mg • Astaxanthin 2 mg. Other Ingredients: Gelatin, Soybean oil, Lecithin, Glycerin, Rice flour, Magnesium stearate, Silicon dioxide, Natural Beeswax. No sugar or starch added.

Earthmends Prostate Health Program - Cancer Wellness Institute
One packet (containing two softgels and three capsules) contains: Vitamin A (as natural beta-carotene and mixed carotenes from natural antioxidant blend) 9000 IU • Vitamin E (as natural vitamin E succiante and d-alpha-tocopherol) 200 IU • Zinc (as zinc amino acid chelate) 15 mg • Selenium (from selenium yeast) 150 mcg. Energizing Complex - Yellow: Glutamine (as L-glutamine polypeptides) 100 mg • Propolis 75 mg • Bee Pollen 75 mg • Ginger extract (root) (3.75 mg gingerols/shoagols) 75 mg • Turmeric extract (root) (71.25 mg curcumins) 75 mg • Oriental Ginseng extract (root) (3.5 mg ginsenosides) 50 mg • Garlic concentrate (bulb) 50 mg. Mushroom Complex - Speckled: Chinese Skullcap (aerial) 75 mg • Maitake Mushroom (aerial) 50 mg • Reishi Mushroom (mycelia) 50 mg • Shitake Mushroom (aerial) 50 mg • Agaricus Mushroom (aerial) 50 mg • Panax Pseudoginseng Wall. (root) 50 mg • Rabdosia Rubescens (Hemsl.) Hara. (aerial) 50 mg • Dyer's Woad (aerial) 35 mg • Licorice (root) 25 mg • Chrysanthemum (flower) 25 mg • Agaricus Mushroom extract (aerial) 25 mg • Maitaki Mushroom

extract (6.25 mg polysaccharides) 25 mg • Shitake Mushroom Lenode extract mycelia (aerial) (0.375 mg) 25 mg • Reishi Mushroom extract (aerial)(3.125 mg polysaccharides) 25 mg. Antioxidant Complex - Burgundy: Broccoli concentrate (with natural sulforophanes) (aerial) 200 mg • Colostrum 200 mg • Green Tea extract (leaf) (50 mg polyphenols) 100 mg • Grape Seed extract (45 mg gallic acid equivalent) (40 mg polyphenols) 100 mg • Quercetin (flavonoid) 50 mg • Indole-3-Carbinol 40 mg. Saw Palmetto Complex - Brown: Red Clover (flower) 200 mg • Saw Palmetto berry extract (seed) (136 mg free fatty acids) 160 mg • Stinging Nettle extract (root) (0.96 mg beta sitosterol) 120 mg • Pygeum extract (Pygeum africanum) (bark) (6.5 mg sterols) 50 mg • Beta Sitosterol complex (45 mg free sterols) 50 mg. Flax Seed Complex - Red: Flax Oil (seed) 200 mg • Natural Antioxidant Blend [(from Carrot oil (root)), Palm (fruit), Marigold (flower), Tomato (fruit), supplying Lutein, Lycopene, Phytoene, Phytofluene, Tocotrienols/Tocopherols, Zeaxanthin] 150 mg • Beta Sitosterol complex (90 mg free sterols) 100 mg • Natural Lycopene (from Tomato fruit) 5 mg • Astaxanthin 2 mg. Other Ingredients: Gelatin, Soybean oil, Lecithin, Glycerin, Magnesium stearate, Silicon dioxide, Natural Beeswax. No sugar or starch added.

Earthmends Total Health Program - Cancer Wellness Institute
Five capsules contain: Fruit extract blend 900 mg: Banana (fruit), New Jersey Tomato (fruit), Delicious Apple (fruit), Strawberry (fruit), Kiwi (fruit), Peach (fruit), Whole Red Wine Grape (fruit), Wild Blueberry (fruit), Mango (fruit), Cantaloupe Melon (fruit), Hawaiian Pineapple (fruit), Cranberry (fruit), Bing Cherry (fruit), Plum (fruit), Elderberry (fruit), Apricot (fruit), Red Raspberry (fruit), Red Pepper (fruit), Eggplant (fruit) • Root Vegetable Extract Blend 450 mg: Carrot (root), Ginger (root), Beet (root), Onion (bulb), Sweet Potato (root), Potato (root) • Cruciferous Vegetable Extract Blend 375 mg: Broccoli (aerial), Spinach (leaf), Kale (leaf), Brussel Sprout (bud), Cabbage (leaf) • Citrus Fruit Extract Blend 350 mg: Orange (fruit), Grapefruit (fruit), Lemon (fruit), Lime (fruit) • Micro-Algae Blend 250 mg: Spirulina (Spirulina planatensis whole cell), Broken Cell Wall Chlorella (Chlorella spp. broken cells) • Soy isolate protein extract (Soybeans)(seed) 250 mg • Whole Cereal Grains and Grass Extract Blend 100 mg: Alfalfa (aerial), Barley (whole plant), Wheat (whole plant), Rye (whole plant) • Vegetable Extract Blend 75 mg: Cauliflower (florets), Corn (seed). Other Ingredients: Malarin, Collagen, Silicon Dioxide, Magnesium Stearate.

Earthrise Chlorella - Earthrise
Fifteen tablets contain: Sodium 3 mg • Vitamin A (100% Beta Carotene) 1500 IU • Calcium 4 mg • Iron 2 mg • Niacin 0.75 mg • Riboflavin 0.15 mg • Protein 1.8 g • Total Carb. 0.4 g • Potassium 35 mg • Vitamin C 4 mg • Vitamin E 0.7 IU • Magnesium 8.0 mg • Thiamin 0.05 mg • Vitamin B6 0.05 mg • Vitamin B12 0.12 mcg • Chlorophyll 80 mg • Mixed Carotenoids 8 mg.

Earthrise NutraGreens - Earthrise
Twenty tablets contain: Vitamin A 5000 IU • Vitamin C 90 mg • Vitamin D 80 IU • Vitamin E (d-alpha-tocopherol acetate) 30 IU • Thiamin (Vitamin B-1) 1.5 mg • Riboflavin (Vitamin B-12) 1.7 mg • Niacin (Vitamin B-3) 20 mg • Vitamin B6 2 mg • Folic Acid 400 mcg • Vitamin B12 7.2 mcg • Biotin 300 mcg • Pantothenic Acid 10 mg • Calcium (Citrate) 24 mg • Iron (Gluconate) 2.7 mg • Iodine (Kelp) 30 mcg • Magnesium (Citrate) 18 mg • Zinc (Methionine) 10 mg • Selenium (Aminoate) 18 mcg • Copper (Gluconate) 1 mg • Manganese (Gluconate) 2 mg • Chromium (Aminoate) 50 mcg • Potassium (Spirulina & Asparatate) 25 mg • Proprietary Blend: Earthrise Spirulina, Lecithin, Natural Apple Concentrate, Prune Powder, Boron (Aminoate), Licorice extract (DGL), Sarsaparilla root, Siberian Ginseng extract (35:1, root), Ginkgo Biloba extract (24% Flavone Glycosides, 6% Terpene Lactones), Milk Thistle extract (80% Silymarin), Royal Jelly, Kelp, Dulse, Astragalus root, Stevia leaf, Ginger root extract (5%), Green Tea extract (50% Polyphenols),

B R A N D

N A M E S

BRAND NAMES

Broccoli Powder, Carrot Powder, Beet Powder, Celery Powder, Grape Seed extract (95% OPC), Octacosanol, Pine Bark extract (50% OPC), Cayenne Pepper fruit, Coenzyme Q-10 4242 mg • Proprietary Digestive Complex: Gum Arabic, Lactobacillus acidophilus DDS, Bifidobacterium longum, Aloe Vera, Amylase, Cellulase 253 mg.

Earthrise Spirulina - Earthrise
Six tablets contain: Sodium 35 mg • Vitamin A (100% Beta Carotene) 4,000 IU • Calcium 7 mg • Iron 2 mg • Riboflavin 0.06 mg • Niacin 0.35 mg • Potassium 50 mg • Total Carb. 0.5 g • Protein 2 g • Magnesium 7 mg • Thiamin 0.03 mg • Vitamin B12 4.2 mcg • Vitamin K 17 mcg • Phycocyanin 330 mg • Chlorophyll 30 mg • Mixed Carotenoids 8 mg • Gamma Linolenic Acid 30 mg • Sulfolipids 30 mg • Polysaccharides 140 mg.

Earthrise Spirulina Bio - Earthrise
Six tablets contain: Sodium 35 mg • Vitamin A (100% Beta Carotene) 4,000 IU • Calcium 7 mg • Iron 2 mg • Riboflavin 0.06 mg • Niacin 0.35 mg • Potassium 50 mg • Total Carb. 0.5 g • Protein 2 g • Magnesium 7 mg • Thiamin 0.03 mg • Vitamin B12 4.2 mcg • Vitamin K 17 mcg • Phycocyanin 330 mg • Chlorophyll 30 mg • Mixed Carotenoids 8 mg • Gamma Linolenic Acid 30 mg • Sulfolipids 30 mg • Polysaccharides 140 mg.

Earthrise Spirulina Bio Powder - Earthrise
Three grams contain: Sodium 60 mg • Vitamin A (100% Beta Carotene) 8300 IU • Calcium 12 mg • Iron 3.3 mg • Riboflavin 0.1 mg • Niacin 0.6 mg • Potassium 80 mg • Total Carb. .8 g • Protein 3 g • Magnesium 11 mg • Thiamin 0.05 mg • Vitamin B12 7 mcg • Vitamin K 29 mcg • Phycocyanin 550 mg • Chlorophyll 50 mg • Mixed Carotenoids 17 mg • Gamma Linolenic Acid 50 mg • Sulfolipids 50 mg • Polysaccharides 230 mg.

Earthrise Spirulina Gold - Earthrise
Twelve tablets contain: Sodium 35 mg • Vitamin A (100% Beta Carotene) 5,000 IU • Calcium 7 mg • Iron 2 mg • Riboflavin 0.306 mg • Niacin 0.35 mg • Zinc 3 mg • Potassium 50 mg • Total Carb. 0.5 g • Protein 2 g • Vitamin C 1.2 mg • Magnesium 7 mg • Thiamin 0.03 mg • Vitamin B12 4.2 mcg • Vitamin K 17 mcg • Phycocyanin 330 mg • Chlorophyll 30 mg • Mixed Carotenoids 10 mg • Gamma Linolenic Acid 30 mg • Sulfolipids 50 mg • Polysaccharides 140 mg.

Earthrise Spirulina Gold Powder - Earthrise
Three grams contain: Sodium 80 mg • Vitamin A (100% Beta Carotene) 10000 IU • Calcium 12 mg • Iron 3.3 mg • Riboflavin 0.1 mg • Niacin 0.6 mg • Zinc 5 mg • Potassium 80 mg • Total Carb. 0.8 mg • Protein 3 g • Vitamin C 2 mg • Magnesium 11 mg • Thiamin 0.05 mg • Vitamin B12 7 mcg • Vitamin K 29 mcg • Phycocyanin 550 mg • Chlorophyll 60 mg • Mixed Carotenoids 18.5 mg • Gamma Linolenic Acid 50 mg • Sulfolipids 50 mg • Polysaccharides 230 mg,

Earthrise Spirulina Powder - Earthrise
Three grams contain: Sodium 60 mg • Vitamin A (100% Beta Carotene) 8,300 IU • Calcium 12 mg • Iron 3.3 mg • Riboflavin 0.1 mg • Niacin 0.6 mg • Potassium 80 mg • Total Carb. .8 g • Protein 3 g • Magnesium 11 mg • Thiamin 0.05 mg • Vitamin B12 7 mcg • Vitamin K 29 mcg • Phycocyanin 550 mg • Chlorophyll 50 mg • Mixed Carotenoids 17 mg • Gamma Linolenic Acid 50 mg • Sulfolipids 50 mg • Polysaccharides 230 mg.

Earthrise Spirulina- Vegi-Capsules - Earthrise
Seven Vegi-Capsules Contain: Sodium 35 mg • Vitamin A (100% Beta Carotene) 4,000 IU • Calcium 7 mg • Iron 2 mg • Riboflavin 0.06 mg • Niacin 0.35 mg • Potassium 50 mg • Total Carb. 0.5 mg • Protein 2 g • Magnesium 7 mg • Thiamin 0.03 mg • Vitamin B12 4.2 mcg • Vitamin K 17 mcg • Phycocyanin 330 mg • Chlorophyll 30 mg • Mixed Carotenoids 8 mg • Gamma Linolenic Acid 30 mg • Sulfolipids 30 mg • Polysaccharides 140 mg.

Earthrise Spirulina+Chlorella - Earthrise
Eight tablets contain: Sodium 20 mg • Vitamin A (100% Beta Carotene) 2900 IU • Calcium 6 mg • Iron 2 mg • Vitamin E 0.51 IU • Riboflavin 0.1 mg • Niacin 0.35 mg • Protein 2 g • Total Carb. 0.5 g • Potassium 45 mg • Vitamin C 30 mg • Magnesium 8.0 mg • Thiamin 0.04 mg • Vitamin B6 0.05 mg • Vitamin B12 2 mcg • Vitamin K 17 mcg • Phycocyanin 176 mg • Chlorophyll 60 mg • Mixed Carotenoids 8 mg • Gamma Linolenic Acid 16 mg • Sulfolipids 16 mg • Polysaccharides 75 mg.

Easy Iron - Puritan's Pride
Each capsule contains: Iron (as Ferrous Bis-Glycinate) 28 mg • Vitamin C (as Ascorbic Acid) 60 mg • Folate (as Folic Acid) 400 mcg • Vitamin B12 (as Cyanocobalamin) 8 mcg.

Easy Now - Traditional Medicinals
Contains: Peppermint leaf • Spearmint leaf • Passion flower herb • Valerian root • Licorice root • Catnip leaf • Chamomile flower • Rosemary leaf • Lavender flower • natural flavors.

Eater's Digest - Traditional Medicinals
Peppermint leaf • Ginger rhizome • Fennel seed • Rose Hip • Papaya leaf • Alfalfa Herb • Cinnamon bark.

EB5 Age Spot Formula - Pharmacist Heldfond's eb5 Formulas for Y
Hydroquinone 2% • Deionized Water • Mineral Oil • Cetearyl Alcohol • Cetearyl Phosphate • Glycerin • Petroleum • Steareth-2 • Stearyl Alcohol • Steareth-10 • Bilberry Extract • Sugar Cane Extract • Sugar Maple Extract • Orange Extract • Lemon Extract • Octyl Methoxcinnamate • Benzophenone-3 • Sodium Sulfite • Sodium Meta Bisulfite • Citric Acid • Propylene Glycol • Diazolidinyl Urea • Methylparaben • Propylparaben.

EB5 Body Formula - Pharmacist Heldfond's eb5 Formulas for Y
Purified Water • Methylsilanol Mannuronate • Mate Extract • Gotu Kola Extract • Thea Sinensis Extract • Butylene Glycol • Glyeryl Stearate • Stearic Acid • Cyclomehticome • Octyl Palmitate • Myristy Myristate • Dimethicone • Sunflower Oil • Isopropyl Lanolate • Soy Serol • Cetareth 20 • Tocopheryl Acetate • Choleth-24 • Ceteth 24 • Panthenol • Ivy Extract • Horsetail Extract • Kelp Extract • Algae Extract • Ginkgo Extract • Arnica Extract • Triethanolamine • Carbomer • Hydroxykpropyl • Methycellulose • Disodium EDTA • Methylparaben • Propylparaben • Imadazolidinyl Urea • Fragrance.

EB5 Body Lotion - Pharmacist Heldfond's eb5 Formulas for Y
Water • Tocopheryl Acetate • Stearic Acid • Propylene Glycol • Dicaprylate/Dicaprate • Mineral Oil • Butylene glycol • Clyeryl Stearate SE • Sorbitan Stearate • Polysorbate-60 • Squalane • Soy Sterol • Panthenol • Oat Flour • Lanolin Alcohol • Retinyl Palmitate • Ergocalciferol • Dimenthicone • Imidazolidinyl Urea • Disodium EDTA • Carbomer-940 • Polyamino Sugar • Condensate • Urea • Methylparaben • Propylparaben • Triethanolamine • Fragrance.

EB5 Cleansing Formula - Pharmacist Heldfond's eb5 Formulas for Y
Purified Water • Cycerin • Caprylic/Capric Triglyceride • Stearic Acid • Peg 8 • Glycol Distearate • Cetyl Alcohol • Triethanolamine • Tocopheryl Acetate • Lactic Acid • Polyquatemium-7 • Panthenol • Peg-10 • Soya Sterol • Oat Flour • Cetearyl Alcohol • Peg-40 Castor Oil • Sodium Cetearyl Sulfate • Cocamide DEA • Carbomer • Disodium • EDTA • BHA • Methylparaben • Propylparaben • Quantemium-15 • fragrance.

EB5 Facial Creme - Pharmacist Heldfond's eb5 Formulas for Y

Water • Propylene Glycol • Tocopheryl Acetate • Stearic Acid • Mineral Oil • Cetyl Alcohol • Oat Flour • Retinyl Palmitate • Ergocalciferol • Propylparaben • Triethanolamine • Methylparaben • Potassium Sorbate • Allantoin • Imidazolidinyl • Urea • Panthenol • Cobomer-940 • Soluble Animal Collagen.

EB5 Footcare Formula - Pharmacist Heldfond's eb5 Formulas for Y

Deionized Water • Mineral Oil • Propylene Glycol • Stearic Acid • Microcrystalline Wax • Cetyl Alcohol • PEG-100 Stearate • vitamin E Acetate • Oat Protein • Triethanolamine • Menthol • Eucalyptus Oil • Fragrance • DL Panthenol • Allantoin • Imidazolidiny Urea • Methylparaben • Propylparaben • Potassium Sorbate • Chamomile • Comfrey • Tea Tree Oil • White Lily Extract • Corn Flower Extract • Sandalwood Extract • Sunflower Extract • Basil Extract • Sage Extract • Jasmine Extract • Sugar Cane Extract • Maple Extract • Citrus Extract • Apple Extract • Vitamin A • Vitamin D (as Vitamin D3) • Dipotassium • Glycyrrhzinate • Soluble Collagen • FD&C Blue #1 • FD&C Yellow #5.

EB5 Men's Facial Formula - Pharmacist Heldfond's eb5 Formulas for Y

Water • Propylene Glycol • Tocopheryl Acetate • Stearic Acid • Mineral Oil • Cetyl Alcohol • Oat Flour • Sodium PCA • Retinyl Palmiate • Ergocalciferol • Allantoin • Panthenol • Soluble Animal Collagen • Propylparaben • Triethanolamine • Methylparaben • Potassium Sorbate • Imidazolidinyl Urea • Carbomer-940 • Fragrance • FD&C Blue No. 1 and D&C Red No. 33.

EB5 Toning Formula - Pharmacist Heldfond's eb5 Formulas for Y

Purified Water • Hydrolyzed Wheat Protein • Arnica Extract • Barley Extract • Triethanolamine • Lactic Acid • Polysorbate 20 • Sodium PCA • Vitamin E Acetate • Allantoin • Panthenol • Witch Hazel Distillate • Sage Extract • Birch Leaf Extract • Comfrey Extract • Sambucus Extract • Blackberry Extract • Horsetail Extract • Tetrasodium EDTA • Methylparaben • Imidazolidinyl Uera • Quantemium-15 • Fragrance.

EB-C - MMS Pro

Each capsule contains: Eyebright • Golden Seal root • Bayberry root bark • Red Raspberry • Cayenne.

ECA Stack - Nutra Sport

Two capsules contain: Ephedrine alkaloids (from whole ma huang plant extract) 20 mg • Caffeine (32.2 mg from bissey nut) 200 mg • Acetylsalicylic Acid 324 mg. Other Ingredients: Rice flour.

EchinaCare Capsules - PhytoPharmica

Each capsule contains: Echinacea purpurea (aerial part) concentrate 50:1 50 mg.

EchinaCare Liquid - PhytoPharmica

Fourty to sixty drops contain: Echinacea purpurea (fresh-pressed juice from stems, leaves, and flowers) 1.5 ml.

Echinacea - Nature's Way

Three capsules contain: Echinacea Purpurea stem, leaf, flower 1.20 g. Other ingredients: Gelatin.

Echinacea - Centrum Herbals

One capsule contains: Echinacea extract flower and root (Echinacea purpurea) 100 mg. Standardized to contain (based on extract weight): Total Phenols (marker) 3.0%, Cichoric Acid (natural active), Isobutyl Alkylamides (natural active), Activity Measure 15-lipoxygenase enzymatic assay. Other Ingredients: Dibasic Calcium Phosphate, Cellulose, Lactose Monohydrate, Hydroxypropyl Cellulose, Ethylcellulose, Castor Oil, Gelatin, Silicon Dioxide, Sodium Lauryl Sulfate, Propylene Glycol, Titanium Dioxide.

Echinacea - Gaia Herbs

Echinacea standardized for 1% isobutylamides and 4% phenolic compounds. Standardized Full Spectrum 90 mg of extract per capsule. Guaranteed Potency 45 mg of extract per capsule.

Echinacea - Leiner Health Products

Each caplet contains: Echinacea extract (Echinacea angustifolia & Echinacea purpurea) root 125 mg. Other Ingredients: Calcium Carbonate, Cellulose, Maltodextrin, Hydroxypropyl Methylcellulose, Silicon Dioxide, Polyethylene Glycol 3350, Croscarmellose Sodium, Hydroxypropyl Cellulose, Red 40 Lake, Blue 2 Lake, Pharmaceutical Glaze, Crospovidone, Magnesium Stearate, Polysorbate 80, Titanium Dioxide.

Echinacea - Nature's Bounty

Each capsule contains: Echinacea (Echinacea purpurea) root 400 mg. Other Ingredients: Gelatin, Vegetable Stearic Acid. Contain no yeast, wheat, gluten, milk or milk derivatives, lactose, sugar, preservatives, soy, artifical color, artificial flavor, sodium (less than 5 mg per serving).

Echinacea - Nature's Way

Three capsules contain: Echinacea Purpurea stem, leaf, flower 1.20 g. Other Ingredients: Gelatin.

Echinacea - Now

Two capsules contain: Total Carbohydrate 620 mg • Echinacea purpurea powder root 800 mg. Other Ingredients: Stearic Acid. Contains no sugar, salt, preservatives, yeast, wheat, corn, soy, or milk.

Echinacea - Pharmanex

Each capsule contains: Echinacea purpurea root 6:1 extract 225 mg. Other Ingredients: Rice Flour, Gelatin.

Echinacea - Puritan's Pride

Each capsule contains: Echinacea (Echinacea purpurea) root 400 mg. Other Ingredients: Gelatin, Vegetable Stearic Acid.

Echinacea & Elderberry - Leiner Health Products

Each softgel contains: Zinc Gluconate 8 mg • Echinacea extract (Echinacea angustifolia, Echinacea purpurea) root and aerial parts 150 mg • Elderberry extract (Sambucus nigra) fruit 100 mg • Golden Seal extract (Hydrastis canadensis) root 100 mg. Other Ingredients: Flaxseed Oil, Gelatin, Lecithin, Wax, Yellow Turmeric, Caramel Powder, Titanium Dioxide.

Echinacea & Golden Seal Combo - Optimum Nutrition

Each capsule contains: Horse Chestnut extract (Aesculus hippocastanum) root 250 mg • Butcher's Broom powdered root 145 mg • Ginger powdered root 145 mg. Other Ingredients: Gelatin, Magnesium Stearate.

Echinacea & Goldenseal - Leiner Health Products

Each caplet contains: Echinacea extract (Echinacea angustifolia & Echinacea purpurea) root 75 mg • Golden Seal extract (Hydrastis canadensis) root 100 mg • Hesperidin 40 mg • Quercetin 20 mg • Rutin 40 mg. Other Ingredients: Calcium Carbonate, Cellulose, Maltodextrin, Hydroxypropyl Methylcellulose, Stearic Acid, Silicon Dioxide, Polyethylene Glycol 3350, Croscarmellose Sodium, Talc, Magnesium Stearate, Hydroxypropyl Cellulose, Pharmaceutical Glaze, Crospovidone, Yellow 5 Lake, Red 40 Lake, Blue 2 Lake, Titanium Dioxide, Polysorbate 80.

BRAND NAMES

Some Brand Name Natural Products - What they Contain

B R A N D   N A M E S

Echinacea & Goldenseal Combination - Atrium Inc.
Two fluid ounces contains: Echinacea • Goldenseal. In a synergistic base of Red Clover, Burdock, Parsley, Fennel, Ginger, Chamomile, Barberry & Cayenne. Contains 16-18% Grain Alcohol.

Echinacea & Goldenseal Root - Now
Two capsules contain: Total Carbohydrate 710 mg • Echinacea purpurea root powder 450 mg • Goldenseal root powder (Hydrastis canadensis) 450 mg. Contains no sugar, salt, starch, yeast, wheat, soy, milk, corn, or fillers.

Echinacea 150 mg - Jamieson
Each capsule contains: Echinacea (Echinacea purpurea, powdered extract 1:3) 150 mg • Panax Ginseng (Standardized to 4% ginsenosides) 250 mg.

Echinacea 300 mg - Jamieson
Each capsule contains: Echinacea herb (Echinacea Purpurea, powdered 1:3) 300 mg • Allicin Rich Garlic bulb powder 300 mg • Ginger root (Zingiber Officinale, powdered Extract 1:6) 300 mg.

Echinacea and Golden Seal - Optimum Nutrition
Echinacea Angustifolia extract • Goldenseal powder.

Echinacea and Goldenseal - Dial Herbs
Echinacea • Goldenseal • Cayenne.

Echinacea Angustifolia - Now
One and one half droppersful contains: Echinacea Angustifolia root extract 1.2 ml. Other Ingredients: Grain Alcohol, Water.

Echinacea Angustifolia - Optimum Nutrition
Each capsule contains: Echinacea Angustifolia extract (Echinacea angustifoliae) (root) (standardized to 4% echinacosides) 125 mg • Echinacea Angustifola, powered (root) 225 mg • Echinacea Purpurea aerial 10 mg. Other Ingredients: Gelatin, Magnesium Stearate.

Echinacea Angustifolia, Extract - Nature's Way
Each capsule contains: Echinacea Angustifolia, dried extract 250 mg • Echinacea Purpurea stem, leaf, flower 190 mg. Other Ingredients: Gelatin, Millet.

Echinacea Balance - HerbaSway
Echinacea • Green Tea • Ginger • Blackberry • HerbaSwee (Cucurbitaceae fruit).

Echinacea Complete Care - Celestial Seasonings
Two capsules contain: Vitamin C (as ascorbic acid) 180 mg • Zinc (as gluconate) 15 mg • Proprietary Blend, 1000 mg: Echinacea (root, stem, leaf, flower), Echinacea (standardized extract), Arabinogalactan. Other ingredients: May contain one or more of the following: Dicalcium phosphate, gelatin, rice flour, stearic acid, magnesium stearate and silicon dioxide. This product contains no artificial colors, flavors, or preservatives. One serving size is equivalent to: Echinacea 500 mg standardized to 4% phenols.

Echinacea Extract - Progressive Labs
Each capsule contains: Echinacea 250 mg • Polysaccharides (from Echinacea) 37.5 mg • Phenolic compounds (from Echinacea) 10 mg.

Echinacea Extract - Jamieson
Each capsule contains: Echinacea herb (Echinacea purpurea 1:3 powdered extract) 350 mg. Other Ingredients: Dicalcium Phosphate, Micorcrystalline Cellulose, Magnesium Stearate, Silicon Dioxide.

Echinacea Extract - Ortho Molecular Products
Each capsule contains: Echinacea Angustifolia extract 200 mg • Echinacea Purpurea 200 mg.

Echinacea Goldenseal - Jamieson
Each capsule contains: Calcium (as Calcium Sulfate) 30 mg • Echinacea root extract 4:1 (Echinacea purpurea Moench.) (4% Phenolic Compounds) 185 mg • Goldenseal root extract 2:1 (Hydrastis canadensis L.) (5% Alkaloids and Hydrastine Compounds) 45 mg.

Echinacea Plus - Traditional Medicinals
Echinacea purpurea herb • Lemongrass leaf • Spearmint leaf • Echinacea angustifolia herb • concentrated extract of E. Purpurea root.

Echinacea Root Complex - Nature's Way
Two capsules contain: Echinacea Angustifolia root • Echinacea Purpurea stem, leaf, flower • Proprietary Blend 900 mg. Other ingredients: Gelatin, Magnesium Stearate.

Echinacea Tincture - Jamieson
Each 2 ml (40 drops) contains: Echinacea angustifolia 1000 mg (1:2 pure tincture in 45% Ethanol) Derived from alcohol maceration of fresh plants (aerial parts).

Echinacea with Goldenseal Liquid Extract - Quantum Health
Two ounces contain: Fresh undried Echinacea purpurea whole plant 70% • Echinacea angustifolia 10% • Goldenseal root 20% • Alcohol 50%.

Echinacea with Zinc - Aspen Group, Inc.
Each capsule contains: Echinacea Purpurea 380 mg • Zinc (citrate) 3 mg. Contains no sugar, starch, salt, wheat, yeast, corn or soy derivatives.

Echinacea, Propolis & Ester C - Futurebiotics
Two capsules contain: Vitamin C (as Ester-C ascorbate) 500 mg • Calcium (as calcium ascorbate) 59 mg • Echinacea angustifolia leaf powder extract (standardized for 4% (5 mg) echinacosides) 125 mg • Echinacea angustifolia leaf powder 150 mg • Echinacea purpurea leaf powder 150 mg • Citrus bioflavonoid peel powder 250 mg • Bee Propolis powder 100 mg • Acerola berry (Rose Hips) powder 50 mg. Other ingredients: Magnesium stearate, Gelatin, Water.

Echinacea/Astragalus/Reishi Formula - Nature's Way
Three capsules contain: Proprietary Formula: Astragalus root • Echinacea Purpurea stem, leaf, flower • Reishi (dried extract 10% Polysaccharides). Other ingredients: Gelatin.

Echinacea/Ester-C Formula - Nature's Way
Two capsules contain: Calcium 27 mg • Echinacea Purpurea stem, leaf, flower 722 mg • Ester-C (Patented form of Vitamin C) 207 mg. Other ingredients: Gelatin.

Echinacea/Ginseng Formula - Nature's Way
Two capsules contain: Proprietary Formula: Echinacea Angustifolia root • Echinacea Purpurea stem, leaf, flower • Siberian Ginseng root . Other ingredients: Gelatin, Magnesium Stearate, Millet.

Echinacea/Goldenseal - Gaia Herbs
Echinacea and Goldenseal standardized for 1% isobutylamides and 15% total alkaloids. Standardized Full Spectrum 100 mg of extract per capsule. Guaranteed Potency 50 mg of extract per capsule.

Echinacea/GSR Formula - Nature's Way
Three capsules contain: Proprietary Formula: Burdock root • Cayenne pepper fruit • Echinacea Angustifolia root • Echinacea Purpurea stem, leaf, flower • Gentain root • Goldenseal stem, leaf, flower • Wood Betony stem, leaf, flower. Other ingredients: Gelatin.

Some Brand Name Natural Products - What they Contain
www.NaturalDatabase.com contains MANY more listings than appear here.

Echinacea-Go! - Wakunaga of America
Each capsule contains: Echinacea Standardized Extract (angustifolia & purpurea blend) leaf/root, standardized to 4% Phenolic Compounds. Other Ingredients: Cellulose, Colloidal Silica, Magnesium Stearate (vegetable source).

Echinacea-Goldenseal Formula - Quest
Each caplet contains: Echinacea angustifolia powder (provided by 100 mg P.E. 1:7 standardized to contain 4% echinacosides) 700 mg • Goldenseal root powder (Hydrastis canadensis) (provided by 50 mg P.E. 1:6 standardized to contain 5% hydrastine) 300 mg • Echinacea purpurea powder (Provided by 50 mg P.E. 1:5 standardized to contain 0.7% flavonoids) 250 mg • Astragalus root powder (Astragalus membranaceus) 100 mg. Other Ingredients: Calcium Phosphate, Microcrystalline Cellulose, Vegetable Stearin, Croscarmellose Sodium, Magnesium Stearate (vegetable source).

Echinacea-Reishi Virtue - Blessed Herbs
Astragalus root • Echinacea Angustifolia root • Pau d'Arco bark • Suma root • Siberian Ginseng root • Reishi mycelium • Licorice root • German Chamomile flower • Calendula flower • Grain alcohol & Distilled Water.

EchinaFresh - Enzymatic Therapy
Each capsule contains: Echinacea purpurea 50:1 concentration of powder from the fresh-pressed juice of stems, leaves, & flowers of organically grown Echinacea purpurea 50 mg.

EchinaGuard - Nature's Way
Each capsule contains: Echinacea purpurea (stem, leaf, flower) 250 mg • EchinaGuard (Echinacea purpurea dried extract) 85 mg. Other Ingredients: Gelatin, Silica.

EchinaGuard Flexitabs - Nature's Way
Each flexitab contains: EchinaGuard (Echinacea Purpurea dried extract) 88 mg. Other Ingredients: Cherry Flavor, Citric Acid, Corn Starch, Fructose, Gelatin, Glycerol, Guar Gum, Lecithin.

Echinex - Chattem, Inc.
Each tablet contains: Standardized extract of Echinacea purpurea root & herb (4% total phenolic compounds) 250 mg • Standardized extract of Siberian Ginseng root (0.8% eleutherosides) 100 mg • Standardized extract of Ginger root (5% gingerols) 100 mg. Other ingredients: Cellulose, Croscarmellose Sodium, Stearic Acid, Magnesium Stearate, Silicon Dioxide, Hydroxypropyl Methylcellulose (aqueous film coating). Contains no sugar, starch, yeast, sodium, dairy or preservatives.

EchinKids - Health Smart Vitamins
Two drops contains: Zinc (as zinc glycinate) 4 mg • Copper (as copper glycinate) 0.50 mg • Echinacea (root, aerial parts) 150 mg.

EchinSeal - Health Smart Vitamins
Two capsules contain: Goldenseal root 800 mg • Echinacea purpurea aerial parts 400 mg.

Eco-Green Multi - Now
Two tablets contain: Vitamin A (Beta Carotene) (15 mg) 25000 IU • Vitamin B1 (Thiamine HCL) 50 mg • Vitamin B2 (Riboflavin) 50 mg • Vitamin B3 (Niacinamide) 50 mg • Vitamin B5 (Pantothenic Acid) 50 mg • Vitamin B6 (Pyridoxine HCL) 50 mg • Vitamin B12 (Cyanocobalamin) 200 mcg • Biotin 100 mcg • Folic Acid 800 mcg • Vitamin C (Calcium Ascorbate) 500 mg • Vitamin D (Calciferol) 200 IU • Vitamin E (d-Alpha Succinate) 200 IU • Vitamin K (from green foods) 70 mcg • Calcium (Ascorbate, Citrate, Carbonate) 100 mg • Magnesium (50% Citrate, 50% Oxide) 100 mg • Zinc (Picolinate) 15 mg • Copper (Amino Acid Chelate) 500 mcg • Iodine (Kelp) 150 mcg • Potassium (Chloride) 25 mg • Manganese (Amino Acid Chelate) 5 mg • Selenium (L-Selenomethionine) 50 mcg •

Chromium (Picolinate) 100 mcg • Molybdenum (Amino Acid Chelate) 50 mcg • Spirulina US grown 250 mg • Barley grass organically grown 250 mg • Chlorella (broken cell wall) 100 mg • Wheat grass organically grown 100 mg • Alfalfa juice concentrate 100 mg • Green Tea extract (40% Catechins) 50 mg • Choline (Bitartrate) 50 mg • Inositol 50 mg • PABA 30 mg • Trace Mineral concentrate 100 mg • Boron (Amino Acid Chelate) 1 mg • Vanadium (Amino Acid Chelate) 50 mcg • Panax ginseng (5% Ginsenosides) 100 mg • Bioflavonoids (40%) 50 mg • Rutin 25 mg • Bromelain (2000 GDU from pineapple) 50 mg • Papain (140 MCU from papaya) 25 mg • Pepsin Enzymes (NF 1:10000) 25 mg • Lipase (3400 Usp Units) 25 mg • Amylase (20000 USP Units) 10 mg • Chlorophyll from green foods 8 mg • Amino Acids from green foods 350 mg. Vegetarian formula base ingredients contain: Di-Calcium Phosphate, Cellulose, Stearic Acid, Magnesium Stearate & Silica. Contains no yeast, soy, milk, corn, gluten or preservatives.

EFA Attention Formula - Health From The Sun
Each capsule contains: Vitamin E (as d-Alpha Tocopherol) 5 IU • Magnesium from Magnesium Oxide 55 mg • Zinc from Zinc Sulfate 0.5 mg • High DHA Fish oil (70 mg Omega-3 DHA) 175 mg • Arachidonic Acid (from Fish oil) 3 mg • Borage oil (16 mg Omega-6 GLA) 80 mg • Lecithin 50 mg • Ashwagandha root extract 25 mg • Bacopa Monnieri Whole Plant extract 25 mg. Other Ingredients: Gelatin, Glycerine, Beeswax (emulsifier), Water, Carob powder.

EFA Complex - PhysioLogics
Two soft gels contain: Vitamin E (as d-Alpha Tocopherol) 20 IU • Eicosapentaenoic Acid (from Marine Lipids) 120 mg • Docosahexaenoic Acid (from Marine Lipids) 80 mg • Gamma-linolenic Acid (from Borage oil) 30 mg.

EFA Derma-Skin Formula - Health From The Sun
Each capsule contains: Vitamin A from Palmitate 3000 IU • Vitamin C from Ascorbic Acid 60 mg • Vitamin D as Cholecalciferol 100 IU • Vitamin E as d-Alpha Tocopherol 40 IU • Zinc from Zinc Sulfate 10 mg • Organic Flax seed oil (450 mg Omega-3 ALA) 800 mg • Borage seed oil (120 mg Omega-6 GLA) 600 mg • Burdock root extract 4:1 50 mg • Yellow Dock root extract 4:1 50 mg. Other Ingredients: Gelatin, Glycerine, Beeswax (emulsifier), Water, Carob powder, Lecithin.

EFA Heart Formula - Health From The Sun
Three capsules contain: Borage oil (180 mg GLA) 900 mg • Fish oil (18% EPA, 12% DHA) 1200 mg • Flax seed oil, organic 300 mg • Folic Acid 300 mcg • Garlic extract (0.8% Allicin) 300 mg • Gugulipid (10% Gugulsterone) 300 mg • Hawthorne extract (2% Vitexin) 105 mg • Tocopherols, mixed 3.9 mg • Tocotrienols 11 mg • Vitamin B6 from Pyridoxine Hydrochloride 1.2 mg. No sugar, starch, artificial preservatives, or colors.

EFA Joint Formula - Health From The Sun
Three capsules contain: Protein 1 g • Vitamin C as Ascorbic Acid 75 mg • Vitamin D (as Vitamin D3) as Cholecalciferol 100 IU • Vitamin E as d-Alpha Tocopherol 30 IU • Zinc from Zinc Sulfate 15 mg • Manganese from Manganese Gluconate 330 mcg • Borage seed oil 300 mg GLA 1500 mg • Glucosamine Sulfate 1200 mg • Organic Flax seed oil (250 mg ALA) 450 mg • Boswellic Acid from Boswellia Resin extract 100 mg. Ingredients: Gelatin, Glycerine, Beeswax (emulsifer), Water, Carob powder, Soy Lecithin.

Efalex - Efamol
Two capsules contain: Efamol Pure Evening Primrose Oil 280 mg • DHA 120 mg • GLA 24 mg • Arachidonic Acid 10.5 mg • Thyme Oil 2 mg • Vitamin E 15 IU. Other Ingredients: Tuna Oil, Gelatin, Glycerin.

Efalex Liquid - Efamol
Four teaspoons contain: Efamol Pure Evening Primrose Oil 1200 mg • DHA 480 mg • GLA 96 mg • Arachidonic Acid 42 mg • Thyme Oil 8 mg • Vitamin E 15 IU. Other Ingredients: Sunflower Oil, Tuna Oil, Flavoring: lemon oil, lime oil.

Efamol Fortify - Efamol
Two capsules contain: Efamol Pure Evening Primrose Oil 800 mg • EPA 14 mg • GLA 64 mg • Vitamin E 30 IU • Calcium 200 mg. Other Ingredients: Calcium Carbonate, Gelatin, Glycerin, Marine Fish Oil, Glyceryl Monostearate, Titanium Dioxide Color.

Efamol PMS Control - Efamol
Two capsules contain: Efamol Pure Evening Primrose Oil 500 mg • GLA 40 mg • Vitamin C 60 mg • Vitamin E 30 IU • Niacin 12 mg • Vitamin B6 40 mg • Biotin 80 mcg • Magnesium 40 mg • Zinc 4 mg. Other Ingredients: Gelatin, Sorbitol Syrup, Glyceryl Monostearate, Glycerin, Ascorbic Acid, Heavy Magnesium Oxide, Pyridoxine HCl, Lecithin, Nicotinamide, Zinc Sulphate Monohydrate, d-Biotin.

Efamol Pure Evening Primrose Oil - Efamol
Two capsules contain: Efamol Pure Evening Primrose Oil 1000 mg • Linoleic Acid 330 mg • Gamma Linolenic Acid 80 mg . Other Ingredients: Gelatin, Glycerin.

Efanatal - Efamol
Two capsules contain: Efamol Pure Evening Primrose Oil 500 mg • DHA (Docosahexaenoic Acid) 107 mg • Arachidonic Acid 9.4 mg • GLA 40 mg • Vitamin E 15 IU. Other Ingredients: Fish Oil, Gelatin, Glycerol, Carmine Color, Titanium Dioxide Color, Ammonium Phosphatide, Ascorbyl Palmitate.

E-Gems - Carlson
Each softgel contains: Vitamin E (as d-alpha tocopheryl acetate) 400 IU.

Egg Fuel - TwinLab
Each serving contains: Calories 110 • Protein 25 g. Ingredient: Pure egg white protein. Fat free, sugar free, & lactose free.

Elan Vital Multiple - Source Naturals
Six tablets contain: Pro-Vitamin A (beta carotene) 25000 IU • Vitamin A (palmitate) 10000 IU • Total Vitamin A activity 35000 IU • Vitamin B-1 (thiamin nitrate) 100 mg • Vitamin B-2 (riboflavin) 100 mg • Inositol Hexanicotinate, Niacinamide and Niacin 200 mg • Vitamin B-5 (calcium D-pantothenate) 100 mg • Vitamin B-6 (pyridoxine HCl) 100 mg • Vitamin B-12 (cyanocobalamin) 200 mcg • Biotin 500 mcg • Folic acid 800 mcg • Vitamin C (magnesium, manganese and zinc ascorbates) 1800 mg • Fat-Soluble Vitamin C (from 476 mg of ascorbyl palmitate) 200 mg • Total Vitamin C activity 2000 mg • Vitamin D-3 (cholecalciferol) 400 IU • Vitamin E D-alpha Tocopheryl (natural) 600 IU • Boron (amino acid chelate) 2 mg • Calcium (succinate, carbonate, malate) 200 mg • Chromium (ChromeMate yeast-free polynicotinate 150 mcg and yeast-free picolinate 150 mcg) 300 mcg • Copper (sebacate) 1 mg • Iodine (from kelp) 150 mcg • Magnesium (ascorbate, oxide, succinate) 300 mg • Manganese (ascorbate) 10 mg • Molybdenum (amino acid chelate) 300 mcg • Potassium (succinate, alpha-ketoglutarate) 99 mg • Selenium (L-selenomethionine and sodium selenite) 250 mcg • Zinc (OptiZinc zinc monomethionine and ascorbate) 30 mg. Other Ingredients: N-Acetyl Cysteine 600 mg, Succinic Acid (free form) 300 mg, Choline (bitartrate) 100 mg, Inositol (hexanicotinate and inositol) 100 mg, N-A-G (N-acetyl glucosamine) 200 mg, DMAE (bitartrate) 40 mg, N-Acetyl L-Tyrosine 80 mg, Coenzyme Q10 (ubiquinone) 40 mg, alpha-Lipoic acid (thioctic acid) 40 mg, Quercetin 300 mg, Silymarin (milk thistle seed extract) 200 mg, Proanthodyn (from grape seed extract) 100 mg, Ginkgo Biloba 24% (50:1 extract) 40 mg, Bilberry extract (37% anthocyanosides) 20 mg.

Ela-Vites L-Phenylalanine Complex - Nature's Plus
Two tablets contain: L-Phenylalanine free form amino acid 600 mg • Vitamin C with Rose Hips 400 mg • L-Tyrosine free form amino acid 200 mg • Vitamin B6 (Pyridoxine HCl) 100 mg. In a natural herbal base containing Ginseng, Gotu Kola & Fo-Ti. Contains no yeast, wheat, corn, soy, milk, salt, sugar or starch.

Elderberry - Natrol
One lozenge contains: Vitamin C (as Calcium Ascorbate) 50 mg • Zinc (as Zinc Gluconate) 7.5 mg • Echinacea angustfolia entire plant 10 mg • Bee Propolis 10 mg • Slippery Elm Bark 10 mg • Elderberry 10 mg • Bee Pollen 10 mg. Other ingredients: Hydrogenated Starch, Hydrolysate, natural Elderberry flavor, Grape skin for color.

Elderberry - Extra Strength - Jamieson
Each capsule contains: Elderberry fruit (Sambucus Nigra L. 40 mg powdered extract 1:50) 2000 mg.

Elderberry Lozenges - Quantum Health
Each lozenge contains: Elderberry extract standardized to 5% total flavonoids (Sambucus nigra) 200 mg • Vitamin C (ascorbic acid) 100 mg • Marshmallow Althea powder 50 mg • Echinacea angustifolia standardized powder extract 4% phenolic compounds 25 mg • Mullein powder 10 mg. Other Ingredients: Menthol Crystals, Eucalyptus Oil, Peppermint Oil, Stevia Leaves and Stevioside, Sorbitol, Raspberry Flavoring.

Elder-Zinc Lozenges - Now
Two lozenges contain: Vitamin C (Ascorbic Acid • Sodium Ascorbate) 300 mg • Zinc (as Zinc Gluconate) 24 mg • Elderberry (Sambucus nigra) 10:1 extract 200 mg • Echinacea purpurea root 50 mg • Bee Propolis 50 mg • Slippery Elm bark (Ulmus fulva) 50 mg.

Electrolyte Balance - The Vitamin Shoppe
Two tablets provide: Potassium 99 mg • Magnesium 500 mg • Calcium 250 mg • Boron 3 mg • Vitamin D 100 IU.

Elemax - Naturodoc
Each capsule contains: L-Glycine 200 mg • L-Tyrosine 150 mg • St. John's Wort (hypericum perforatum extract, .3% Hypericin) 150 mg • Niacin (Niacinol) 100 mg • 5-HTP (5-hydroxytryptophan) 25 mg • Siberian Ginseng (eleutherococcus senticosus, 1.2% eleutherosides) 25 mg • Ginkgo Biloba Extract (24% Ginkgo Extract) 25 mg • Colecus Forskohlii Extract (5-10% Forskolin) 25 mg • Coenzyme B6 (pyridoxal-5-phosphate) 5 mg • Folic Acid 500 mcg.

Elo-Plex - Progressive Labs
Each capsule contains: Vitamin C 100 mg • Vitamin B6 10 mg • Pantothenic Acid 50 mg • Zinc (as zinc proteinate) 3.3 mg • Copper (as copper proteinate) 0.3 mg • L-Tyrosine 150 mg • DL-Phenylalanine 80 mg • Adrenal 10 mg • Hypothalamus 15 mg. See Editor's Note No. 14, page 1817.

Elusan Prostate - Plantes & Medecines Inc.
Each capsule contains: Serenoa Repens Lipidosterolic extract 160 mg.

E-mergen-C - Alacer
Each packet contains: Vitamin C 1000 mg • Vitamin B1 (Thiamine HCl) 0.38 mg • Vitamin B2 (Riboflavin) 0.43 mg • Special Niacin Complexes 5 mg • Vitamin B6 (Pyridoxine HCl) 10 mg • Folic Acid 12.5 mcg • Vitamin B12 (Cyanocobalamin) 25 mcg • Pantothenic Acid 2.5 mg • Calcium 50 mg • Magnesium 20 mg • Zinc 2 mg • Sodium 60 mg • Potassium 200 mg • Manganese 1.5 mg • Chromium (Ascorbate) 10 mg. Sweetened with Fructose. All nutrients in a base of Citric, Tartaric, Aspartic, & Malic (Apple) Acids. Naturally flavored with concentrates of Lemon & Lime.

Emerita - Transitions of Health
Aloe Vera gel • Distilled Water • D-Alpha Tocopherol • Mixed Tocopherols • Cetyl Alcohol • Almond oil • Octyl Palmitate • Panthenol • Peg 8 Stearate • Glycerine • Progesterone • Polysorbate 60 • Hyaluronic Acid, Oil of Lemon, Keratin, Carbomer 940 • Grapefruit seed extract.

Emerita Hot Flash Formula - Transitions for Health, Inc.
One capsule contains: Vitamin C (sodium ascorbate) 400 mg • Vitamin E (as d-alpha tocopheryl succinate) 100 mg • Bioflavonoids (as citrus bioflavonoid complex) 200 mg • Para-aminobenzoic acid 20 mg • Pantothenic acid (as calcium pantothenate) 20 mg • Adrenal Complex 5 mg. Other Ingredients: Rice Bran, Gelatin, Water, and Glycerin.

Emerita Libido Formula - Transitions for Health, Inc.
Three capsules contain: Damiana leaf and stem 200 mg • Siberian Ginseng root 150 mg • Black Cohosh root 100 mg • Motherwort leaf 100 mg • Wild Oats leaf and stem 100 mg • Ginkgo Biloba leaf 60 mg • Wild Lettuce leaf 50 mg. Other Ingredients: Rice Bran, Gelatin, Water, and Glycerin.

Emerita Sleep Formula - Transitions for Health, Inc.
One capsule contains: Valerian root 100 mg • Scullcap leaf and flower 100 mg • Wild Lettuce leaves 50 mg • Lavender flowers 50 mg • Oat Straw tops 50 mg • Lady's Mantle leaves 50 mg. Other Ingredients: Rice Bran, Gelatin, Water, and Glycerin.

Em-Pact - Mannatech
Energy Complex: Fructose, Medium chain triglycerides, Creatine monohydrate, Calcium citrate, Magnesium aspartate, Magnesium succinate, Potassium aspartate, Potassium succinate, Choline bitartrate, L-carnitine, Lecithin • Ambrotose Complex: naturally occurring plant polysaccharides including freeze-dried Aloe Vera inner leaf gel extract - Manapol powder. Other Ingredients: Citric Acid, Natural Flavors.
See Editor's Note No. 17, page 1817.

Emulsified A Complex - Nature's Life
Each capsule contains: Vitamin A (Fish Liver oil) 7500 IU • Beta Carotene (Vitamin A equivalent to 7500 IU) 4.5 mg.

Emulsified Vitamin A Complex with Vitamin D - Puritan's Pride
Each softgel contains: Vitamin A 10,000 IU • Vitamin D 400 IU • Apple Pectin.

ENADA NADH - Menuco
Each micro tab provides: NADH 5.0 mg • Baking Soda (sodium bicarbonate) 3.0 mg • Vitamin C (sodium ascorbate) 0.3 mg. Other Ingredients: D-Mannitol, Microcrystalline Cellulose, Magnesium Stearate.

ENADAlert (e-NAD-alert) - Menuco Corp.
Each tablet contains: NADH 10 mg. Other Ingredients: D-Mannitol, Sodium Bicarbonate, Microcrystalline Cellulose, Natural Flavoring, Magnesium Stearate.

EnadaNADH 2.5 Mg - Natrol
One micro tab contains: NADH (reduced 5-nicotinamide adenine dinucleotide) 2.5 mg • Baking Soda (Sodium Bicarbonate) 0.3 mg • Vitamin C (Sodium Ascorbate) 0.3 mg. Other ingredients: D-Mannitol, Microcrystalline Cellulose, Magnesium Stearate.

EnadaNADH 5 Mg - Natrol
One microtab contains: NADH (reduced 5-nicotinamide adenine dinucleotide) 5 mg • Baking Soda (Sodium Bicarbonate) 0.3 mg • Vitamin C (Sodium Ascorbate) 0.3 mg. Other ingredients: D-Mannitol, Microcrystalline Cellulose, Magnesium Stearate.

Endorphin+ - PhysioLogics
Each capsule contains: DL-Phenylalanine 450 mg • White Willow bark (7.5% Salicin, 1.9 mg) 25 mg • Feverfew flower, leaf (1.2% Parthenolide, 0.3 mg) 25 mg • Ginger root (5% Gingerols, 1.25 mg) 25 mg.

Endurox - PacificHealth Labs
Two Caplets Contains: Ciwujia root extract 800 mg • Calcium (sulfate) 130 mg. Other Ingredients: Microcrystalline Cellulose, Stearic Acid, Hydroxypropyl Cellulose, Magnesium Stearate, Titanium Dioxide, P.E.G., Caramel Color, Beet juice powder & Annatto extract.

Endurox Excel - Pacific Health Labs
Two caplets contain: Endurox (standardized root extract of the herb ciwujia) 1200 mg • Vitamin E 60 IU.

Endurox R4 - Pacific Health Labs
Two scoops contain: Vitamin C 470 mg • Vitamin E 400 IU • Calcium 100 mg • Iron 1.8 mg • Magnesium 250 mg • Chloride 270 mg • Sodium 230 mg • Potassium 140 mg • Ciwujia (Endurox) 600 mg • L-Glutamine 420 mg • L-Arginine 1420 mg. Other Ingredients: Complex Carbohydrates, Glucose, Whey Protein concentrate, Crystalline Fructose, L-Arginine, Vitamin E Acetate, Ciwujia, Ascorbic Acid, Sodium Chloride, Citric Acid, L-Glutamine, Magnesium Oxide, Artificial Flavor, Potassium Phosphate, FD&C Red #40.

Enerblast - Nature's Plus
Each tablet contains: Potassium Glycero-Phosphate 250 mg • Pyridoxal Alpha Ketoglutarate (PAK) 50 mg • Trimethylglycine (TMG) 25 mg • Inosine (HXR-Hypoxanthine Riboside) 25 mg • Creatine Phosphate 50 mcg. Contains no yeast, wheat, corn, soy, milk, salt, sugar or starch.

Energiza - HerbaSway
Bitter Orange • Panax Ginseng • Siberian Ginseng • Schisandra • Astragalus • Ginger • Kudzu • Blackberry • Licorice • HerbaSwee (Cucurbitaceae fruit).

Energizer Formula - Nature's Way
Two capsules contain: Proprietary Formula: Bee Pollen • Cayenne pepper fruit • Coenzyme Q10 (Ubiquinone) • Magnesium Stearate • Siberian Ginseng root • Spirulina • Thiamine (Vitamin B1) • Vitamin B12 (Cyanocobalamin). Other ingredients: Gelatin, Millet.

Energy - Nutrivention
Each tablet contains: Pantothenic Acid 100 mg • Vitamin B12 300 mcg • Folic Acid 200 mcg • Aspartic Acid 100 mg • Gotu Kola 100 mg • Licorice root 100 mg • Siberian Ginseng 100 mg.

Energy - Whitehall-Robbins Healthcare
One tablet contains: Supplement facts: Thiamin (B1) 3 mg • Riboflavin (B2) 0.85 mg • Niacin (B3) 10 mg • Vitamin B6 1 mg • Vitamin B12 3 mcg • Biotin 15 mcg • Pantothenic Acid 5 mg • Taurine 100 mg • Panax Ginseng standardized extract (root) 62.5 mg. Other Ingredients: Dibasic Calcium Phosphate, Taurine, Ginseng standardized root extract (Panax Ginseng), Microcrystalline Cellulose, Crospovidone, Maltodextrin, Hydroxypropyl Methylcellulose, Niacinamide, Calcium Pantothenate, Magnesium Stearate, Titanium Dioxide, Polyethylene Glycol, Thiamin Mononitrate, Polysorbate 80, FD&C Yellow #6 Aluminum Lake, Pyridoxine Hydrochloride, Riboflavin, Starch, Biotin, Citric Acid, Sodium Citrate, Silicon Dioxide, Cyanocobalamin, Sodium Benzoate, Sorbic Acid.

Energy - Now
Two capsules contain: Vitamin E (as d-alpha tocopheryl succinate) 15 IU • Vitamin B1 (from Thiamine HCL) 10 mg • Riboflavin

B R A N D   N A M E S

(Vitamin B2) 10 mg • Niacin (Vitamin B3) 25 mg • Vitamin B6 (from Pyridoxine HCL) 10 mg • Vitamin B12 (as Cyanocobalamin) 100 mg • Vitamin B5 (from Calcium Pantothenate) 10 mg • Iodine (from Kelp) 225 mg • Chromium (as Chromium Chelavite) 200 mcg • Potassium (from Potassium Aspartate) 55 mg • Guarana standardized extract (Paullinia Cupane, seed extract contains 42 mg caffeine) 280 mg • Green Tea extract (Camellia Sinensis, leaf extract contains 8 mg caffeine) 200 mg • Bitter Orange extract (Citrus Aurantium) fruit (min. 3% Synephrine) 150 mg • Panax Ginseng (5% Ginsenosides) root 150 mg • Siberian Ginseng (Eleutherococcus Senticosus) root 150 mg • Licorice (Glycyrrhiza Glabra) root 100 mg • Gotu Kola (Centella Asiatica) whole plant 100 mg • Cayenne (Capsicum annuum: 40,000 SHU) fruit 50 mg • Alpha Lipoic Acid 25 mg • COQ10 10 mg • Octacosanol (Spinach) 30 mcg. Other Ingredients: Gelatin (capsule), Magnesium Stearate. Contains no sugar, yeast, corn, soy, wheat, gluten, milk, or preservatives.

Energy - ProHerbs
One tablet contains: Thiamin HCl (B1) 25 mg • Riboflavin (B2) 25 mg • Vitamin B6 (Pyridoxine HCl) 25 mg • Vitamin B12 (Cyanocobalamin) 50 mcg • Folic Acid 400 mcg • Korean Ginseng root (Panax Ginseng standardized to 10% ginsenosides) 100 mg • Kola Nut (3:1 extract) (Cola acuminata) 500 mg • Guarana root (Paullina cupana 3:1 extract) 200 mg • Royal Jelly 50 mg. Other Ingredients: Dicalcium Phosphate, Microcrystalline Cellulose, Croscarmellose Sodium, Hydroxypropylmethylcellulose, Magnesium Stearate, Mineral Oil, Stearic Acid, Titanium Dioxide, Triacetin, FD&C Yellow #6 Lake.

Energy Body Benefits Pak - Leiner Health Products
Each packet contains: Thiamin Mononitrate (Vitamin B1) 100 mg • Riboflavin (Vitamin B2) 100 mg • Vitamin B6 (Pyridoxine Hydrochloride) 100 mg • Niacin (Niacinamide) 100 mg • Biotin 100 mcg • Vitamin B12 100 mcg • Pantothenic Acid (d-Calcium Pantothenate)100 mg • Folate 400 mcg • American Ginseng extract (Panax quinquefolius) root 70 mg • Chinese Panax Ginseng extract (Panax ginseng) root 60 mg • Damiana (Turnera diffusa) leaf 2 mg • Fo-Ti (Polygonum multiflorum) root 2 mg • Gotu Kola (Centella asiatica) leaf 78 mg • Green Tea extract (Camellia sinensis) leaf (50% catechins) 2 mg • Guarana extract (Paullinia cupana) seed 78 mg • Jamaican Ginger (Zingiber officinalis) rhizome 2 mg • Korean Ginseng extract (Panax ginseng) root 70 mg • Siberian Ginseng (Eleutherococcus senticosus) root 500 mg • Yerba Mate extract (Ilex paraguariensis) leaf 575 mg. Other Ingredients: Dicalcium Phosphate, Calcium Carbonate, Croscarmellose Sodium, Hydrogenated Vegetable Oil, Cellulose.

Energy Elxir - Nature's Plus
Each serving contains: Royal Jelly lyophilized 3X-4.2% 10-HDA 250 mg • Guarana seed 125 mg • Spanish Bee Pollen 125 mg • Korean Ginseng 50 mg • Siberian Ginseng 50 mg • American Ginseng 12.5 mg. In a natural base of Purified Water, Wild Clover Honey, Citric Acid & Potassium Sorbate added to maintain freshness.

Energy Reserve - Clinician's Choice
Two tablets contain: Thiamin (mononitrate) 20 mg • Riboflavin 20 mg • Vitamin B12 (cyanocobalamin) 20 mcg • Siberian Ginseng Root 400 mg • Panax Ginseng Leaves 400 mg • Brazilian Guarana Seeds 200 mg • Green Tea Leaves 200 mg • Wild American Ginseng Root 100 mg • Red Chinese Ginseng Root 100 mg • Tienchi Ginseng Root 100 mg • Cayenne Fruit 20 mg • Proprietary blend 6 mg: Bee Pollen, Citrus Bioflavonoids, Soy Isoflavones.

Energy Support - Amazon Support
Each capsule contains: Jatoba • Guarana Extract • Yerba Mate Extract • Maca • Suma.

Ener-T - Atrium Inc.
Each tablet contains: Primary Yeast 705 mg. Specially grown & formulated because of its content of an accessory factor known as Termitin, Complex-T or Vitamin T. This yeast also typically contains 50% Protein, trace amounts of many B-Complex Vitamins & Inositol as well as trace amounts of many minerals.

EnerX - Quest
Niacin • Zinc • Yohimbe • Tribulus Terrestris • Panax Ginseng • Guarana • Ashwagandha • Arginine • Damiana • Muira Puama • Potent Herbal Blend.

EnVigor - Resource Wellness
One caplet contains: Vitamin C 60 mg • Vitamin E 30 IU • Thiamin 1.5 mg • Riboflavin 1.7 mg • Niacin 20 mg • Vitamin B6 2 mg • Vitamin B12 6 mcg • Biotin 300 mcg • Pantothenic Acid 10 mg • Calcium 260 mg • Standardized Ginkgo Biloba extract leaves 120 mg • Standardized Panax Ginseng extract root 200 mg. Other Ingredients: Dicalcium Phosphate, Microcrystalline Cellulose, Croscarmellose Sodium, Calcium Silicate, Stearic Acid, Magnesium Stearate, Methylcellulose, Hydroxypropyl Cellulose, Polyethylene Glycol.

Enviro-Gard - Aspen Group, Inc.
Four tablets contain: Vitamin A Palmitate 8000 IU • Beta Carotene 16,000 IU • Vitamin C 800 mg • Vitamin E 320 IU • Quercetin 160 mg • Zinc (gluconate) 12 mg • Copper Gluconate 0.1 mg • Yellow Dock 364 mg • Bupleurum 192 mg • Poria Cocos 192 mg • Gentian root 192 mg • Goldenseal 192 mg • Myrrh Gum 192 mg • Echinacea extract 192 mg • Milk Thistle extract (83% silymarin) 192 mg • N-Acetyl Cysteine 160 mg • Rosemary extract 160 mg • Hawthorn Berry extract 80 mg • Wild Yam root 80 mg • Wild Yam extract 77 mg • Marshmallow root 58 mg • Magnesium Ascorbate 24 mg • Grape seed extract 20 mg • Ginkgo Biloba 4 mg • Manganese Ascorbate 4 mg • Selenomethionine 80 mcg. Contains no sugar, starch, salt, wheat, yeast, corn or soy derivatives.

ENZOGENOL - Pharmacy Express Ltd.
Each tablet contains: Enzogenol (Pinus radiata bark extract) 50 mg • Citrus Bioflavonoids 100 mg • Beta carotene (ProVitA) 5 mg • Natural Vitamin E (80 IU) 66.7 mg • Ester C 250 mg • Selenium (from selenomethionine) 75 ug • Zinc (from OptiZinc) 7.5 mg • Pyridoxine Hydrochloride (Vitamin B6) 25 mg • Cysteine 50 mg • Methionine 50 mg • Folic Acid 100 ug. Contains no added yeast, gluten, artificial colors or preservatives.

Enzolen - Enzo Nutraceuticals Ltd.
Each capsule contains: Shiitake mushroom extract 250 mg • Vitamin C 120 mg.

Enzy-Derm - Atrium Inc.
Each gram contains: Pancreatin 12 mg • Papayotin 7 mg • Bromelain 6 mg • Trypsin 4 mg • Lipase 1.5 mg • Amylase 1.5 mg • Chymotrypsin 0.15 mg. In a base containing Vitamin A & Vitamin E. See Editor's Note No. 14, page 1817.

Enzygen - Rexall
Each tablet contains: Calcium 100 mg • Enzyme Blend: Lipase 2400 LU, Cellulase 250 CAU, Amylase 750 SKBU, Lactose 350 LacU, Protease 100 SAPU 200 mg. Other Ingredients: Dicalcium Phosphate, Croscarmellose Sodium, Magnesium Stearate.

Enzyme Aid Digestive Support - Nature's Life
Each tablet contains: Pancreatin (concentrate 4X NF) containing: (Protease activity 50000 USP IU; Amylase activity 50000 USP IU, Lipase activity 4000 USP IU) 500 mg • Glutamic Acid Hydrochloride 200 mg • Ox Bile extract 200 mg • Pepsin (NF 10000X) 200 mg • Lipase (activity 425 USP IU) 50 mg • Cellulase (activity 10 CMC-ASE IU) 10 mg.
See Editor's Note No. 14, page 1817.

Enzyme Digestant - Natural Brand
One tablet contains: Pancreatin 400 mg • Alpha Amylase 130 mg • Betaine hydrochloride 65 mg • Pepsin 65 mg • Papain 65 mg • Ox Bile Extract (8:1) 8.1 mg. Other ingredients: Dicalcium Phosphate, Cellulose, Food Glaze.
See Editor's Note No. 14, page 1817.

Enzymes - Nutrivention
Each capsule contains: Pancreatin 100 mg • Papain 60 mg • Anise (Pimpinella anisum) 50 mg • Fennel (Foeniculum vulgare) 50 mg • Rutin 50 mg • Bromelain (natural Pineapple Enzyme) 45 mg • Trypsin 24 mg • Amylase 10 mg • Lipase 10 mg • L-Chymotrypsin 1 mg.
See Editor's Note No. 14, page 1817.

EPA Natural Fish Oil - Puritan's Pride
Each softgel contains: EPA (Eicosapentaenoic Acid) 180 mg • DHA (Docosahexaenoic Acid) 120 mg.

EPA with Garlic - Puritan's Pride
Each softgel contains: Marine Lipid Concentrate 1000 mg • EPA (Eicosapentaenoic Acid) 180 mg • DHA (Docosahexaenoic Acid) 120 mg • Odorless Garlic powder 50 mg • Vitamin E (d-Alpha Tocopherol) 10 IU.

EPA-1000 - PhysioLogics
Each softgel contains: Vitamin E (d-Alpha Tocopherol) 10 IU • Marine Lipid concentrate (18% EPA, 12% DHA) 1000 mg.

EPAForte - Nature's Plus
Each softgel contains: Marine Lipid concentrate 900 mg supplying: Eicosapentaenoic Acid (EPA) 162 mg, Docosahexaenoic Acid (DHA) 108 mg, total Omega-3 Fatty Acids 270 mg • Magnesium Aspartate equivalent to 60 mg of elemental Magnesium 300 mg • Vitamin E natural 50 IU • Vitamin B6 (Pyridoxine HCL) 10 mg • Garlic equivalent to 500 mg of fresh garlic 1 mg • Selenium, Biotron yeast-free amino acid complex 25 mcg. Contains no yeast, wheat, corn, soy, milk, salt, sugar or starch.

EPH-833 - AST Sports Science
Each capsule contains: standardized 8% Ephedra extract 750 mg.

Ephedra Plus - PhytoPharmica
Each capsule contains: Ephedrine from 200 mg of Ma Huang extract (Ephedra sinensis) 12 mg • Ginger root extract 6.5:1 (Zingiber officinale) 65 mg • Licorice root extract (Glycyrrhiza glabra) standardized to contain 5% glycyrrhizic acid 50 mg • Marshmallow root extract 4:1 (Althaea officinalis; Mucilage content of 30-40%) 50 mg • Sundew Herb extract 4:1 (Drosera rotundifolia) 40 mg • Euphorbia Herb extract 4:1 (Euphorbia hirta) 40 mg • Senega root extract 4:1 (Polygala senega) 40 mg • Goldenseal root extract (Hydrastis canadensis) standardized to contain 5% total alkaloids, including berberine, hydrastine, & canadine 20 mg.

Ephedra Super Cap - D & E Pharmaceuticals
Each capsule contains: 883 mg of pure Ephedra extract.

Ephedrine Formula 100 - D & E Pharmaceuticals
Each tablet contains: Ephedrine HCL 25 mg • Guaifenesin 100 mg.

Ephedrine Formula 200 - D & E Pharmaceuticals
Each tablet contains: Ephedrine HCL 25 mg • Guaifenesin 200 mg.

Ephedrine HCL 25 mg - D & E Pharmaceuticals
Each tablet contains: Ephedrine HCL 25 mg.

Ephedrine Sulphate 25 mg - D & E Pharmaceuticals
Each tablet contains: Ephedrine Sulphate 25 mg.

Epresat Multivitamin - Flora
Each tablet contains: Vitamin A • Vitamin B1 • Vitamin B2 • Vitamin B6 • Vitamin C • Vitamin D • Vitamin E • Niacinamide

E-Prime - USANA Nutritionals
Each capsule contains: Vitamin E (as d-alpha tocopherol) 200 IU • D-Gamma Tocotrienol 7 mg • Mixed Tocopherols 3.4 mg.
Other Ingredients: Medium Chain Glycerides, Gelatin, Purified Water, Lecithin.

Equal Ratio CAL-MAG - Quest
Each tablet contains: Calcium (HVP Chelate) 100 mg • Magnesium (HVP Chelate) 100 mg • Vitamin D (as Vitamin D3) 200 IU.
Other Ingredients: Croscarmellose Sodium, Magnesium Stearate (vegetable source), Microcrystalline Cellulose, Vegetable Stearin.

Erotikava - Pacific Sensuals
Each 1 oz. serving contains: Vanuatu Kava Kava • Honey • Ginger • Lycium • Epimedium • Polygala • Liquid Amber • Saigon Cinnamon bark • Licorice • Vegetable Glycerine • Cnidium seed.

Esberitox - Enzymatic Therapy/PhytoPharmica
Each tablet contains: Baptista tinctoria root extract (Wild Indigo root) 10 mg • Echinacea purpurea & pallida 1:1 root extract (Purple Coneflower root) 7.5 mg • Thuja occidentalis leaf extract (White Cedar leaf) 2 mg. Contains no salt, yeast, wheat, gluten, corn, soy, dairy products (except lactose), coloring, flavoring, or preservatives.

Escalation - Enzymatic Therapy
Each capsule contains: Cola Nut extract (Cola nitida) (contains Caffeine 35 mg) 250 mg • Green Tea extract (Camellia sinensis) (contains Caffeine 15 mg) 250 mg • Ma Huang extract (Ephedra sinensis) (contains Ephedrine 15 mg) 250 mg.
Contains no sugar, salt, yeast, wheat, corn, soy, dairy products, coloring, flavoring, or preservatives.

Escalert - Enzymatic Therapy
Two capsules contain: Cola Nut extract (Cola nitida) (Contains 35 mg of Caffeine) 250 mg • Green Tea extract (Camellia sinensis) (contains 15 mg of Caffeine) 250 mg • Oat Straw extract 10:1 (Avena sativa) 50 mg • Schisandra extract standardized to contain 9% Schizandrin 50 mg • Siberian Ginseng extract (Eleutherococcus senticosus) standardized to contain greater than 1% Eleutherosides E 50 mg • Ginger root extract 6.5:1 (Zingiber officinale) 25 mg • Korean Ginseng root extract (Panax ginseng) standardized to contain 7% Saponins calculated as Ginsenoside Rg1 10 mg • Chromium (Polynicotinate) 100 mcg. Contains no sugar, salt, yeast, wheat, corn, soy, dairy products, coloring, flavoring or preservatives.

Esiak Caps - Now
Each capsule contains: 450 mg Proprietary Blend: Burdock (Articum Lappa) root (4:1 extract) • Sheep Sorrel (Rumex Acetosella) leaf (4:1 extract) • Slippery Elm bark (Ulmus fulva) bark (4:1 extract) • Turkey Rhubarb (Rheum palmatum) root (4:1 extract).
Other Ingredients: Maltodextrin, Magnesium Stearate. Contains no yeast, wheat, corn, milk, soy, or preservatives.

Especially for "Women" - The Vitamin Shoppe
Three capsules contain: Vitamin A Activity 10000 IU • Vitamin E 200 IU • Vitamin D 200 IU • Vitamin C 250 mg • Selenium 50 mcg • Vitamin B1 25 mg • Vitamin B2 25 mg • Niacinamide 25 mg • Vitamin B6 25 mg • Vitamin B12 250 mcg • Pantothenic Acid 25 mg • Citrus Bioflavonoids 100 mg • Biotin 100 mcg • Folic Acid 400 mcg • Choline Bitartrate 25 mg • Inositol 25 mg • PABA 25 mg • Calcium 200 mg • Magnesium 100 mg • Potassium 25 mg • Phosphorus 50 mg • Manganese 15 mg • Zinc 15 mg • Iron 18 mg • Chromium 50 mcg • Iodine 225 mcg • Boron 3 mg • Silica 5 mg • Black Currant 100 mg • Dong Quai 50 mg • Royal Jelly 100 mg.

BRAND NAMES

BRAND NAMES

Especially for MEN - The Vitamin Shoppe
Two capsules contain: Vitamin A 5000 IU • Vitamin C 30 mg • Vitamin D 200 IU • Vitamin E 100 IU • Vitamin K 75 mcg • Niacin 30 mg • Vitamin B1 30 mg • Vitamin B2 30 mg • Vitamin B6 30 mg • Folic Acid 400 mcg • Vitamin B12 30 mcg • Biotin 250 mcg • Pantothenic Acid 30 mg • Calcium 200 mg • Iodine 150 mcg • Magnesium 100 mg • Zinc 25 mg • Selenium 100 mcg • Copper 2 mg • Manganese 5 mg • Chromium 50 mcg • Chloride 28 mg • Beta-carotene 3 mg • Potassium 30 mg • Silica 10 mcg • Choline 10 mg • Inositol 10 mg • PABA 10 mg • Citrus Bioflavonoids 25 mg • Korean Ginseng 70 mg • Damiana leaf 70 mg • Oat Straw 50 mg • Garlic 50 mg • Oyster extract 50 mg • Prostate Glandular 50 mg • Saw Palmetto 50 mg • L-Cysteine 50 mg • Nettles leaf 30 mg • Pumpkin seed 30 mg • L-Methionine 10 mg • Alpha Lipoic Acid 5 mg • Lycopene 1 mg.

Essential B Complete - Rexall
Each tablet contains: Thiamin (as thiamin mononitrate) 1.5 mg • Riboflavin (Vitamin B-2) 1.7 mg • Niacin (as niacinamide) 20 mg • Vitamin B-6 (as pyridoxine HCl) 2 mg • Folic Acid 400 mcg • Vitamin B-12 (as cyanocobalamin) 6 mcg • Calcium 35 mg. Other Ingredients: Dicalcium Phosphate, Cellulose, Croscarmellose Sodium, Hydroxypropyl Methylcellulose, Magnesium Stearate, Triethyl Citrate.

Essential Bodyguard - Rexall
Two tablets contain: Vitamin A (from retinyl acetate and 25% as beta-carotene) 4000 IU • Vitamin C 600 mg • Vitamin D (from cholecalciferol) 160 IU • Vitamin E (from dl-alpha-tocopheryl acetate and d-alpha-tocopheryl acid succinate) 120 IU • Thiamin (from thiamin HCl) 4 mg • Riboflavin (Vitamin B2) 8 mg • Niacin (as niacinamide) 4 mg • Vitamin B-6 (from pyridoxine HCl) 40 mg • Folic Acid 160 mcg • Vitamin B-12 (as cyanocobalamin) 100 mcg • Biotin 100 mcg • Pantothenic Acid (from calcium d-pantothenate) 40 mg • Calcium 20 mg • Iron (from ferrous fumarate) 4 mg • Magnesium (from magnesium oxide) 80 mg • Zinc (from zinc gluconate) 20 mg • Selenium (from selenium amino acid chelate) 80 mcg • Copper (from copper gluconate) 0.8 mg • Manganese (from manganese gluconate) 2 mg • Sodium 5 mg • Whey Protein Concentrate 200 mg • Echinacea Purpurea root 120 mg • Rutin 30 mg • Choline Bitartrate 40 mg • Goldenseal aerial parts 24 mg • Garlic extract 15:1 bulb 8 mg. Other Ingredients: Croscarmellose Sodium, Cellulose, Stearic Acid, Sodium Starch Glycolate, Magnesium Stearate, Silica, Hydroxypropyl Methylcellulose, Hydroxypropyl Cellulose, PEG.

Essential E - PhysioLogics
Each softgel contains: Vitamin E (d-Alpha Tocopheryl Acetate) 400 IU.

Essential Enzymes - Source Naturals
Each capsule contains: Vegetal analog of Pancreatin with acid-stable Protease (28652 FCC) 298 mg • Lipase (375 FCC) 125 mg • Alpha Amylase (630 FCC) 52 mg • Amyloglucosidase (2 FCC) 12.5 mg • Cellulase (100 FCC) 5 mg • Hemicellulase (650 FCC) 3 mg • Lactase (40 FCC) 5 mg.
See Editor's Note No. 14, page 1817.

Essential Fatty Acid Complex - Health Smart Vitamins
Three softgels contain: Vitamin E (as d-alpha tocopherol) 30 IU • Eicosapentaenoic Acid (EPA: from marine lipids) 180 mg • Docosahexaenoic Acid (DHA: from marine lipids) 120 mg • Gamma Linolenic Acid (GLA: from borage oil) 45 mg.

Essential Fatty Acids - Nutri-Quest
Each capsule contains: Cod Liver 500 mg • Flaxseed oil 135 mg • Extra Virgin Olive oil 135 mg • Vitamin A 1190 IU • Vitamin D 124 IU. Also contains: Oleic, Linoleic, Palmitic, Arachidic & Linolenic, Eicosapentaenoic, & Docosahexaenoic.

Essential Fish Oil Concentrate - Rexall
Three softgels contain: Vitamin E (as dl-alpha-tocopheryl acetate) 300 IU • Fish Oil (Eicosapentaenoic Acid 540 mg, Docosahexaenoic Acid 360 mg) 3 g. Other Ingredients: Gelatin, Glycerin, Water.

Essential Meal - Gary Nulls
Fortified with branched chain amino acids.

Essential Minerals - Futurebiotics
Four tablets provide: Calcium: (carbonate, aspartate, citrate) 1000 mg • Magnesium: (oxide, aspartate, citrate) 800 mg • Vitamin D 200 IU • Boron (citrate) 3 mg • Iron (gluconate) 9 mg • Manganese (amino acid chelate) 5 mg • Copper (gluconate) 1.5 mg • Zinc (gluconate) 15 mg • Betaine HCl 250 mg • Potassium (chloride, proteinate) 75 mg.

Essential Nutrients - Progressive Labs
Six capsules contain: Vitamin A (retinyl palmitate) 10,000 IU • Vitamin A (beta carotene) 15,000 IU • Vitamin C (ascorbic acid) 1000 mg • Vitamin D (cholecalciferol) 80 IU • Vitamin E (d-alpha tocopheryl succinate) 400 IU • Thiamin (Vitamin B1) 50 mg • Riboflavin-5-Phosphate (Vitamin B2) 20 mg • Niacin 25 mg • Niacinamide 125 mg • Vitamin B6 (pyridoxine HCl with pyridoxal-5'-phosphate) 20 mg • Folate (folic acid) 800 mcg • Vitamin B12 (cyanocobalamin with adenosylocobalamin) 500 mcg • Biotin 800 mcg • Pantothenic Acid (d-calcium pantothenate) 500 mg • Calcium (aspartate & carbonate) 500 mg • Iodine (potassium iodide) 225 mcg • Magnesium (aspartate and oxide) 500 mg • Zinc (picolinate) 25 mg • Selenium (selenomethionine) 200 mcg • Copper (glycinate & oxide) 2 mg • Manganese (aspartate & sulfate) 20 mg • Chromium (as chromium picolinate) 200 mcg • Molybdenum (sodium molybdate) 100 mcg • Potassium (aspartate and chloride) 99 mg • Boron (chelate) 3 mg • Vanadium (vanadyl sulfate) 100 mcg • Choline Citrate 250 mg.

Essential Oils - Puritan's Pride
Each softgel contains: Flaxseed oil 400 mg • Borage oil 400 mg • Super EPA 400 mg • Oleic Acid (Omega 9) 152 mg • Linoleic Acid (Omega 6) 180 mg • Gamma/Alpha Linolenic Acid (Omega 3) 260 mg • Eicosapentaenoic Acid (EPA) 120 mg • Docosahexaenoic Acid (DHA) 80 mg • Vitamin E (d-alpha tocopherol) 5 IU.

Essiac - Dial Herbs
Burdock • Sheep Sorrel • Rhubarb • Slippery Elm.

Ester C - Derma E
Each tablet contains: Vitamin C • Vitamin E •Antioxidants and Skin Rejuvenators.

Ester C 1000 mg - The Vitamin Shoppe
Each tablet contains: Vitamin C (Calcium Ascorbate) 1000 mg • Calcium (as Ascorbate, Threonate) 125 mg. No yeast, corn, wheat, sugar, salt, starch, soy, citrus, milk, eggs, fish or animal derivatives, preservatives, artificial colors or flavors added.

Ester C 1000 mg with Bioflavonoids - The Vitamin Shoppe
Each tablet contains: Vitamin C (Calcium Ascorbate) (from 1250 mg Ester C) 1000 mg, plus Bioflavonoids Complex. No yeast, corn, wheat, sugar, salt, starch, soy, gluten, dairy, milk, eggs, fish or animal derivatives, preservatives, artificial colors or flavors added.

Ester C 500 mg - The Vitamin Shoppe
Each tablet contains: Vitamin C (Calcium Ascorbate) 500 mg • Calcium (as Ascorbate, Threonate) 60 mg. No yeast, corn, wheat, sugar, salt, starch, soy, citrus, milk, eggs, fish or animal derivatives, preservatives, artificial colors or flavors added.

Some Brand Name Natural Products - What they Contain

www.NaturalDatabase.com contains MANY more listings than appear here.

Ester C 500 mg with Bioflavonoids - The Vitamin Shoppe
Each tablet contains: Vitamin C (Calcium Ascorbate) (from 625 mg Ester C) 500 mg, plus Bioflavonoids Complex. No yeast, corn, wheat, sugar, salt, starch, soy, gluten, dairy, milk, eggs, fish or animal derivatives, preservatives, artificial colors or flavors added.

Ester C Caps - Progressive Labs
Each capsule contains: Vitamin C (as calcium polyascorbate) 500 mg • Calcium (as calcium polyascorbate) 50 mg.

Ester C Plus Bioflavonoids and Pycnogenol 500 mg - The Vitamin Shoppe
Each capsule contains: Vitamin C (Calcium Ascorbate) (from 625 mg Ester C) 500 mg • Calcium (Calcium Ascorbate) 60 mg • Quercetin 25 mg • Pycnogenol 2.5 mg • Citrus Bioflavonoid Complex with Hesperidin and Rutin 200 mg. No yeast, corn, wheat, sugar, salt, starch, soy, dairy, preservatives, artificial colors or flavors added.

Ester C Powder 2000 mg with Bioflavonoids - The Vitamin Shoppe
Each teaspoon contains: Vitamin C (Calcium Ascorbate) 2000 mg, plus Bioflavonoids Complex. No yeast, corn, wheat, sugar, salt, starch, soy, gluten, dairy, milk, eggs, fish or animal derivatives, preservatives, artificial colors or flavors added.

Ester C with Bioflavonoids, Vitamin C - Leiner Health Products
Each tablet contains: Vitamin C 500 mg • Citrus Bioflavonoids complex 200 mg. Other Ingredients: Ester-C Calcium Ascorbate, Calcium Carbonate, Cellulose, Croscarmellose Sodium, Crospovidone, Silicon Dioxide, Maltodextrin, Polyethylene Glycol 3350, Talc, Magnesium Stearate, Hydroxypropyl Methylcellulose, Hydroxypropyl Cellulose, Polysorbate 80.

Ester-C 1000 Mg with Bioflavonoids - Natrol
Each tablet contains: Vitamin C (as calcium ascorbate) 1000 mg • Calcium (as calcium ascorbate) 100 mg • Lemon Bioflavonoid Complex consisting of extracts from lemon 200 mg. Other ingredients: Mono & Di-Glycerides, Stearic Acid, Croscarmellose Sodium, Silicon Dioxide, Magnesium Stearate.

Ester-C 250 Mg with Bioflavonoids - Natrol
Each tablet contains: Vitamin C (as calcium ascorbate) 250 mg • Calcium (as calcium ascorbate) 25 mg • Lemon Bioflavonoid Complex consisting of extracts from lemon 100 mg. Other ingredients: Microcrystalline Cellulose, Stearic Acid, Croscarmellose Sodium, Silicon Dioxide, Magnesium Stearate.

Ester-C 500 Mg with Bioflavonoids - Natrol
Each tablet contains: Vitamin C (as calcium ascorbate) 500 mg • Calcium (as calcium ascorbate) 50 mg • Lemon Bioflavonoid Complex consisting of extracts from lemon 200 mg. Other ingredients: Mono & Di-Glycerides, Stearic Acid, Croscarmellose Sodium, Silicon Dioxide, Magnesium Stearate.

Ester-C 1000 - Now
Each tablet contains: Vitamin C 1000 mg • Citrus Bioflavonoids (40%) 200 mg • Acerola powder 25 mg • Rose Hips powder 25 mg • Rutin 20 mg • Calcium 125 mg.

Ester-C 250 Mg - Natrol
Each tablet contains: Vitamin C (as calcium ascorbate) 250 mg • Calcium (as calcium ascorbate) 25 mg. Other ingredients: Microcrystalline Cellulose, Stearic Acid, Mono & Di-Glycerides, Croscarmellose Sodium, Magnesium Stearate.
See Editor's Note No. 4, page 1816.

Ester-C 250 Mg Chewable - Natrol
Each wafer contains: Vitamin C (as calcium ascorbate) 250 mg • Calcium (as calcium ascorbate) 25 mg. Other ingredients: Fructose, Glycine, Mono & Di-Glycerides, Stearic Acid, natural Orange flavor, Citric Acid, Silicon Dioxide, Microcrystalline Cellulose, Gum Acacia, Magnesium Stearate.

Ester-C 500 Mg capsule - Natrol
Each capsule contains: Vitamin C (as calcium ascorbate) 500 mg • Calcium (as calcium ascorbate) 50 mg. Other ingredients: Magnesium Stearate, Microcrystalline Cellulose, Gelatin.

Ester-C 500 Mg tablets - Natrol
Each tablet contains: Vitamin C (as calcium ascorbate) 500 mg • Calcium (as calcium ascorbate) 50 mg. Other ingredients: Microcrystalline Cellulose, Stearic Acid, Croscarmellose Sodium, Magnesium Stearate, Silicon Dioxide.

Ester-C 500 Mg with Bioflavonoids Vegetarian capsules - Natrol
Each capsule contains: Vitamin C (as calcium ascorbate) 500 mg • Calcium (as calcium ascorbate) 50 mg • Citrus Bioflavonoid Complex consisting of extracts from: lemon, orange, grapefruit, lime, & tangerine 200 mg. Other ingredients: Magnesium Stearate, Silicon Dioxide, Vegetable Carbohydrate Gum, Glycerine.

Ester-C 500 Mg with Echinacea - Natrol
Each tablet contains: Vitamin C (as calcium ascorbate) 500 mg • Calcium (as calcium ascorbate) 50 mg • Echinacea extract (Phenolic compounds 4%) 50 mg • Echinacea (angustifolia) leaf powder 80 mg • Echinacea (Purpurea) leaf powder 80 mg • Echinacea (angustifolia) root powder 20 mg • Echinacea (Purpurea) root powder 20 mg. Other ingredients: Calcium Carbonate, Mono & Di-Glycerides, Croscarmellose Sodium, Stearic Acid, Silicon Dioxide, Magnesium Stearate.

Ester-C 500 Mg with Pycnogenol & Proanthocyanidis capsules - Natrol
Each capsule contains: Vitamin C (as calcium ascorbate) 500 mg • Calcium (as calcium ascorbate) 50 mg • Grape skin powder 50 mg • Rutin 50 mg • Hesperidin Complex 50 mg • Quercetin 25 mg • Pycnogenol (pine bark extract) 5 mg. Other ingredients: Silicon Dioxide, Magnesium Stearate, Gelatin.

Ester-C 500 Mg with Pycnogenol & Proanthocyanidis tablets - Natrol
Each tablet contains: Vitamin C (as calcium ascorbate) 500 mg • Calcium (as calcium ascorbate-carbonate) 70 mg • Grape skin powder 50 mg • Rutin 50 mg • Hesperidin 50 mg • Quercetin 25 mg • Pycnogenol (pine bark extract) 5 mg. Other ingredients: Mono & Di-Glycerides, Calcium Carbonate, Croscarmellose Sodium, Silicon Dioxide, Stearic Acid & Magnesium Stearate.

Ester-C Antioxidant - Natrol
Two tablets contain: Vitamin A (as d-Salina beta carotene) 5000 IU • Vitamin C (as calcium ascorbate) 500 mg • Vitamin E (as d-alpha tocopheryl succinate with mixed tocopherols) 200 IU • Calcium (as ascorbate) 50 mg • Lemon Bioflavonoid Complex consisting of extracts from lemon 25 mg • a-Lipoic Acid 25 mg. Other ingredients: TriCalcium Phosphate, Microcrystalline Cellulose, Stearic Acid, Silicon Dioxide, Croscarmellose Sodium, Magnesium Stearate.

Ester-C Cold Season - Natrol
Two capsules contain: Vitamin C (as calcium ascorbate) 500 mg • Calcium (as calcium ascorbate) 50 mg • Zinc (chelate) 10 mg • Reishi/ Shiitake/ Maitake Blend, powdered extract (mushrooms) 150 mg •

B R A N D   N A M E S

Echinacea 50:50 (purpurea & angustifolia), powdered extract supplying Phenolic compounds (4%) 75 mg • Citrus Bioflavonoid Complex extracts of: lemon, orange, grapefruit, lime & tangerine 50 mg • Black Elderberry extract, powdered 30 mg • Garlic, powdered extract bulb 30 mg • Licorice root extract supplying 25 % Glycerenic Acid 25 mg • Astragalus 25 mg • Cayenne supplying 40000 SCU 10 mg • Beta Glucans, oats 5 mg. Other ingredients: Silica, Magnesium Stearate, Rice powder, Gelatin.

Ester-C Complex - Olympian Labs
Each capsule contains: Vitamin C (Ester C) 500 mg • Citrus Bioflavonoid Complex 200 mg.

Ester-C Complex Extra Strength - Olympian Labs
Each tablet contains: Ester C (Vitamin C) 1000 mg • Calcium (from Ester-C) 80 mg • Citrus Bioflavonoid Complex 50 mg • Grape Skin extract 50 mg • Rose Hips 50 mg.

Ester-C Complex Plus Calcium - Olympian Labs
Each capsule contains: Ester C (Vitamin C) 500 mg • Calcium (from Ester-C) 40 mg • Citrus Bioflavonoid Complex 200 mg.

Ester-C For Kids - Natrol
Each wafer contains: Vitamin C (as calcium ascrobate) 100 mg • Calcium (as calcium ascorbate) 10 mg • Citrus Bioflavonoids consisting of extracts from lemon 25 mg. Other ingredients: Fructose, Mono & Di-Glycerides, Glycine, Cellulose, natural Tropical fruit flavor, Stearic Acid, Silica, Magnesium Stearate, Guar Gum, Citric Acid.

Ester-C Nightime Formula - Natrol
Each tablet contains: Vitamin C (as calcium ascrobate) 500 mg • Calcium (as calcium ascorbate) 50 mg • Kava Kava root supplying 30% Kavalactones 100 mg • Valerian root supplying 0.8% Valerenic Acid 100 mg • Melatonin 1 mg. Other ingredients: TriCalcium Phosphate, Cellulose, Stearic Acid, Silica, Magnesium Stearate. See Editor's Note No. 16, page 1817.

Ester-C Powder - Natrol
Each teaspoon contains: Vitamin C (as calcium ascorbate) 3200 mg • Calcium (as calcium ascorbate) 320 mg.

Ester-C Powder with Bioflavonoids - Natrol
Each teaspoon contains: Vitamin C (as calcium ascorbate) 3000 mg • Calcium (as calcium ascorbate) 300 mg • Citrus Bioflavonoid Complex consisting of extracts from: lemon, orange, grapefruit, lime, & tangerine 300 mg.

Ester-C with Bioflavonoids - Natrol
Each capsule contains: Vitamin C (as calcium ascorbate) 500 mg • Calcium (as calcium ascorbate) 50 mg • Citrus Bioflavonoid Complex consisting of extracts from: lemon, orange, grapefruit, lime & tangerine 200 mg. Other ingredients: Magnesium Stearate, Gelatin.

Ester-C with Echinacea - Natrol
One capsule contains: Vitamin C (as calcium ascorbate) 500 mg • Calcium (as calcium ascorbate) 50 mg Echinacea extract (Phenolic compounds 4%) 50 mg • Echinacea (angustifolia) leaf powder 80 mg • Echinacea (Purpurea) leaf powder 80 mg • Echinacea (angustifolia) root powder 20 mg • Echinacea (Purpurea) root powder 20 mg. Other ingredients: Silicon Dioxide, Magnesium Stearate, Gelatin.

Ester-C with Echinacea & Goldenseal Root - Puritan's Pride
Each capsule contains: Ester C (Polysascorbate) 500 mg • Echinacea (Eachinacea angustifolia) 100 mg • Goldenseal root (Hydrastis canadensis) 50 mg.

Ester-C Zinc Lozenges - Natrol
Each lozenge contains: Vitamin C (as calcium ascorbate) 150 mg • Calcium (as calcium ascorbate) 15 mg • Citrus Bioflavonoids consisting of extracts from lemon 25 mg • Zinc (Gluconate) 4.5 mg. Other ingredients: Fructose, Mono & Di-Glycerides, Glycine, Cellulose, natural fruit flavors, Stearic Acid, Silica, Magnesium Stearate, Guar Gum, Citric Acid.

EstrAttune - Health Smart Vitamins
Each capsule contains: Vitamin E (as d-alpha tocopheryl acetate) 50 IU • Vitamin B6 (as pyridoxine HCl) 25 mg • Folate (folic acid) 200 mcg • Magnesium (as magnesium oxide) 100 mg • Zinc (as zinc amino acid chelate) 3.75 mg • Copper (as copper amino acid chelate) 0.5 mg • Black Cohosh root 100 mg • Chastetree berry (5% flavonoids) 100 mg • Dong Quai root (>= 0.8% ligustilides, >= 0.8 mg) 100 mg • Soy bean (5% isoflavones, 2.5 mg) 50 mg • Kava Kava root (30% kavalactones, 7.5 mg) 25 mg.

Estro Balance - Puritan's Pride
Each tablet contains: Vitamin E 30 IU • Thiamin (Vitamin B1) 2 mg • Riboflavin (Vitamin B2) 2 mg • Niacin 20 mg • Vitamin B6 10 mg • Calcium 150 mg • Selenium 150 mg • Boron 1.5 mg • Soy Isoflavones 50 mg • Kava Kava root extract (30% kavalactones) 100 mg • Black Cohosh root (cimicifuga racemosa) 40 mg.

EstroGentle - Pinnacle
Contains Black Cohosh • Soy germ • Red Clover leaf extract • Licorice root • Wild Yam • Chaste Tree berry • Other botanicals.

EstroSoy - Nature's Way
Two capsules contain: Fermented Soy extract 890 mg • Red Clover blossoms 100 mg.

Estrotone - New Chapter, Inc.
Two softgels contain: Dong Quai (Angelica sinensis) root, extract (1%lingustilide- .80 mg) 80 mg • Schizandra (wu-wei-zi) berry extract (2% schizandrins- 1.6 mg) 80 mg • Ginger rhizome, certified organic, extract (minimum 20% pungent compounds- 10 mg, 5% ziniberene- 2.5 mg) 50 mg • Black Cohosh root and rhizome, extract (8% triterpene glycoside- 3.2 mg) 40 mg • Chaste Tree berry, exract (0.6% aucubin- 2.4mg, % 0.5 agnuside- 20 mg) 40 mg • Rosemary leaf and essential oil, extract (23% total phenolic anitoxidants - 2.3 mg) 10 mg. Other Ingredients: Evening primrose oil, Olive Oil, Yellow Beeswax, Gelatin, Vegetable glycerin, Purified Water, Carob.

Estroven - Amerifit
Each caplet contains: Vitamin E (as natural d-alpha tocopherol succinate) 30 IU • Thiamin (as thiamin mononitrate) 2 mg • Riboflavin 2 mg • Niacin (niacinamide) 20 mg • Vitamin B6 (as pyridoxine HCl) 10 mg • Vitamin B12 (as cyanocobalamin) 6 mcg • Folate (as folic acid) 400 mcg • Calcium (from calcium carbonate) 150 mg • Selenium (from l-selenomethionine) 70 mcg • Boron (chelate) 1.5 mg • Purified Isoflavones (from soybean & pueraria root) 50 mg • Kava Kava root standardized extract (30% kavalactones) 100 mg • Black Cohosh root 40 mg. Other Ingredients: Cellulose • Cellulose Gum • Fractionated Vegetable oil • Silica • Titanium Dioxide (natural mineral source) & Caramel Color.

Estroven Memory - Amerifit
Each tablet contains: Zinc 7.5 mg • Ginkgo Biloba leaf standardized extract 60 mg • Panax Ginseng root standardized extract 125 mg • Green Tea leaf standardized extract 250 mg • Isoflavones 10 mg • Grape skin standardized extract 75 mg.

E-TOCO 400 - Progressive Labs
Each softgel contains: Vitamin E (mixed tocopherols) 400 IU • Sesame seed oil 200 mg • Nutriene 100 mg • Mixed Tocotrienols from Nutriene 15 mg. Two softgels will supply 800 IU of Mixed Tocopherols and 30 mg of Tocotrienols.

Some Brand Name Natural Products - What they Contain
www.NaturalDatabase.com contains MANY more listings than appear here.

Eucalyptus Salve - Dial Herbs
Eucalyptus • Camphor • Mint. In a base of Beeswax , Glycerine & Cold Pressed Olive oil.

European Grape Seed Extract 50 mg - Jamieson
Each caplet contains: Calcium 30 mg • Grape Seed 60:1 extract (Vitis vinifera) (Standardized to 95% Oligomeric Procyanidins) 50 mg.

Evening Primrose Deluxe - Health From The Sun
Each capsule contains: Gamma Linolenic Acid (GLA) (Omega-6) 130 mg • Linoleic Acid (Omega-6) 950 mg • Oleic Acid (Omega-9) 80 mg. Ingredients: Evening Primrose seed oil, Gelatin, Glycerine, Water.

Evening Primrose Oil - Health From The Sun
Two capsules contain: Gamma-Linolenic Acid (GLA) (Omega-6) 100 mg • Linoleic Acid (Omega-6) 730 mg • Oleic Acid (Omega-9) 60 mg. Ingredients: Evening Primrose seed oil, Gelatin, Glycerine, Water.

Evening Primrose Oil - Jamieson
Each capsule contains: Vitamin E (as D-Alpha Tocopheryl Acetate) 13.6 IU • Gamma Linolenic Acid (GLA) 50 mg.

Evening Primrose Oil - Leiner Health Products
Each softgel contains: Evening Primrose Oil (Oenothera biennis) seed 500 mg. Other Ingredients: Gelatin, Glycerin, Purified Water.

Evening Primrose Oil - Olympian Labs
Each softgel contains: Evening Primrose Oil 500 mg.

Evening Primrose Oil 1300 mg - Nature's Way
Each capsule contains: Evening Primrose oil, cold pressed 1.3 g • Vitamin E d-alpha tocopheryl 6 IU. Other Ingredients: Gelatin, Glycerin, Water.

Evening Primrose Oil 500 mg - Nature's Way
Each softgel contains: Evening Primrose Oil (cold pressed) 500 mg • Vitamin E (d-alpha tocopheryl) 6 IU. Other Ingredients: Gelatin, Glycerin, Water.

Evening Primrose Oil Extra Strength - Olympian Labs
Each softgel contains: Evening Primrose Oil 1300 mg.

EverCLR - Herpes Relief, Ltd.
Each capsule contains: Burdock root • Ashwaganda root • Echinacea Angustifolia root • Echinacea Purpurea root • Hydrangea root.

Everyday Detox - Traditional Medicinals
Contains: Sweet Tea Vine herb (Gynostemma pentaphyllum) • Schisandra fruit dried aqueous extract • Licorice root • Ginger rhizome • Star Anise fruit • Lycium fruit dried aqueous extract • Schisandra fruit • Kukicha twig (Camellia sinensis).

Exandra Lean - The Kutting Edge
Two capsules contain: Citrus Aurantium 125 mg • Nor-Ephedrine 23 mg • L-Phenylalanine 300 mg • Citri Max 500 mg • Acetyl L-Carnitine 100 mg • L-Tyrosine 80 mg • Ginger Root 50 mg • Vitamin B5 40 mg.

Exec-U-Stress - Nature's Plus
Three tablets contain: Vitamin C with Rose Hips 600 mg • Niacinamide (Vitamin B3) 300 mg • Pantothenic Acid (Vitamin B5) 300 mg • L-Cysteine free form amino acid 200 mg • L-Glycine free form amino acid 200 mg • Vitamin B1 (Thiamine) 200 mg • Vitamin E natural 200 IU • Vitamin B6 (Pyridoxine HCL) 100 mg • Inositol 100 mg • PABA (Para-aminobenzoic acid) 75 mg • Zinc amino acid chelate/complex 50 mg • Vitamin B2 (Riboflavin) 50 mg • Choline (Bitartrate) 32 mg • Beta Carotene supplying 15000 IU Vitamin A activity 9 mg • Folic Acid 400 mcg • Vitamin B12 from Cobalamin 200 mcg • Selenium amino acid complex 100 mcg • Biotin 100 mcg. B-Complex vitamins in a fortified rice bran base. In a special base which provides for the gradual release of ingredients over a prolonged period of time for 40% better absorption & utilization. Sugar & starch free.

Exercise In A Bottle - Enforma Natural Products
Two capsules contain: Calcium Pyruvate 300 mg • CitriMax [Providing 40 mg of (-)Hydroxycitric Acid] 60 mg • Chromium Picolinate 25 mcg • Ginkgo Biloba 10 mg.

Expectorant - Dial Herbs
Garlic • Bayberry • Mullein • Blood root • Cayenne • Lobelia.

Ex-Stress Formula - Nature's Way
Two capsules contain: Proprietary Formula: Black Cohosh root • Cayenne pepper fruit • Hops flower • Scullcap herb • Valerian root • Wood Betony stem, leaf, flower. Other ingredients: Gelatin.

Ex-Tox - Progressive Labs
Three capsules contain: Vitamin C 600 mg • Bentonite 300 mg • L-Lysine 60 mg • DL-Methionine 600 mg • Sodium Alginate 450 mg • Chlorophyll 60 mg • Fruit pectin 150 mg • Garlic powder 30 mg.

Extra Strength Glucosamine Chondroitin - Source Naturals
Two tablets contain: Glucosamine (as glucosamine sulfate) 1.5 g • Chondroitin (as chondroitin sulfate) 1.2 g.
See Editor's Note No. 15, page 1817.

Extra Strength Joint Maintenance - Puritan's Pride
Three tablets contain: Glucosamine Sulfate 1500 mg • Chondroitin Sulfate 1200 mg • Vitamin C (ascorbic acid) 500 mg • Manganese 5 mg.
See Editor's Note No. 15, page 1817.

Extra Strength Joint Maintenance Gels - Puritan's Pride
Three softgels contain: Glucosamine Sulfate 1500 mg • Chondroitin Sulfate 1200 mg • Citrus Bioflavonoids 45 mg • Manganese (as manganese aspartate) 1.02 mg.
See Editor's Note No. 15, page 1817.

Extra Strength Prosta-Metto - Puritan's Pride
Each softgel contains: Saw Palmetto extract (Serenoa repens: standardized to contain 85-95% fatty acids and biologically active sterol compounds) 160 mg • Pumpkin Seed oil extract (Cucurbita pepo) 40 mg • Pygeum Africanum extract 10 mg • Bearberry extract (Uva Ursi) 5 mg • Zinc (as Zinc Gluconate) 15 mg • Vitamin B6 5 mg.

Extra Strength Water Pill - Puritan's Pride
One tablet contains: Potassium (as Potassium Gluconate) 40 mg • Buchu (Barosma betulina) leaf (25 mg of 4:1 extract) 100 mg • Uva Ursi (Arctostaphylos uva-ursi) leaf (33.3 mg of 3:1 extract) 100 mg • Juniper (Juniperus communis) berry 20 mg • Parsley (Petroselinum crispum) leaf 100 mg.

Extreme Cordyceps - Natural Sport Supplements - Nutraceutica
One capsule contains: Cordyceps CS-4 mycelial biomass (Cordyceps sinensis) (Minimum 36 mg Cordycepic acid) 525 mg • Cordyceps mycelial biomass (Cordyceps sinensis) (Minimum 10 mg Cordydepic acid, Minimum 1 mg Cordycepin) 100 mg • Reishi mushroom (Ganoderma lucidum) 75 mg • Maitake mushroom (Grifolia fondosa) 75 mg. Other Ingredients: Gelatin, Magnesium Stearate, Silica, Brown Rice.

BRAND NAMES

Some Brand Name Natural Products - What they Contain
www.NaturalDatabase.com contains MANY more listings than appear here.

Extreme Power Plus - Dutch International Products
Green Tea • Kola Nut • 72 Trace Mineral Complex • Siberian
Ginseng • Royal Jelly • White Willow bark • Ginger • Fo-Ti •
Hawthorn berries • Saw Palmetto • Beet root powder • Chromium
Picolinate • Guarana • Ma Huang • Zi Chi • Kelp • Citrimax • Calcium
Carbonate • Magnesium Carbonate • Korean Ginseng • American
Ginseng • Yerba Mate • Vitamin B12 • Bee Pollen.

Eye Beaute Pads - Pharmagel
Chamomile • Cucumber • Cornflower • Rosemary • Yarrow • Birch
leaf • Sage • Nettle • Clover blossom.

Eye Care Complex - Leiner Health Products
Each tablet contains: Selenium 40 mcg • Vitamin A (Acetate)
2500 IU • Vitamin C (Ascorbic Acid) 30 mg • Bilberry 30 mg •
Lutein 8 mg • Spinach 70 mg • Zeaxanthin 640 mcg.
Other Ingredients: Calcium Carbonate, Gelatin, Glycerol, Starch,
Cellulose, Maltodextrin Hydroxypropyl Methylcellulose,
Croscarmellose Sodium, Crospovidone, Silicon Dioxide, Ascorbyl
Palmitate, Dicalcium Phosphate, Polyethylene Glycol 3350,
Tocopherols, Hydroxypropyl Cellulose, Magnesium Stearate,
Pharmaceutical Glaze, Riboflavin, Blue 1 Lake, Titanium Dioxide,
Polysorbate 80, Sodium Selenate.

Eye Contour Cream Plus - Cellex-C
Ascorbic Acid • Tyrosine • Zinc • Bioflavonoids • Vitamin E • Sodium
Hyaluronate • Evening Primrose Oil • Glycine • Tomato oil • Aloe
barbadensis gel • Chamomile extract • Allantoin.

Eye Contour Gel - Cellex-C
Ascorbic Acid • Tyrosine • Zinc • Bioflavonoids • Sodium
Hyaluronate.

Eye Firming Gel - Pharmagel
Ginseng and plant extracts.

Eye Formula - Pharmanex
Each capsule contains: Beta-Carotene (Dunaliella Salina) 2500 IU •
Vitamin C (Calcium Ascorbate, Ascorbic Acid) 150 mg • Vitamin E
(d-Alpha Tocopheryl Succinate, Beta, Delta, Gamma Tocopherols)
75 IU • Zinc (Zinc Propionate) 2.5 mg • Selenium
(L-Selenomethionine) 35 mcg • N-Acetyl-L-Cysteine 100 mg •
Taurine 100 mg • Tumeric extract (Min. 95% Curcumin) 50 mg •
Ginkgo Biloba extract (Min. 95% Flavonglycosides, Min. 6% Terpene
Lactones) 30 mg • Alpha-Lipoic Acid 10 mg • Lutein (from Marigold
flower extract) 2.5 mg. Other Ingredients: Calcium Carbonate,
Sodium Carboxymethylcellulose, Magnesium Stearate, Talc.

Eye Guard Plus - Nutrition Warehouse
Four capsules contain: Beta Carotene (pro-vitamin A) 40,000 IU •
Natural Vitamin E (succinate) 400 IU • Vitamin C 1500 mg • Citrus
Bioflavonoid Complex 250 mg • Quercetin (bioflavonoid) 100 mg •
Bilberry extract (standardized 25%) 10 mg • Rutin 100 mg • Zinc
(picolinate) 25 mg • Selenium (selenomethionine) 100 mcg • Taurine
200 mg • N-Acetyl Cysteine 200 mg • L-Glutathione 10 mg • Vitamin
B2 (riboflavin) 50 mg • Chromium (GTF) 200 mcg • Lutein 20 mg.

Eye Guard Plus - Puritan's Pride
Four capsules contain: Beta Carotene (pro-vitamin A) 40,000 IU •
Natural Vitamin E (succinate) 400 IU • Vitamin C 1,500 mg • Citrus
Bioflavonoids Complex 250 mg • Quercetin (bioflavonoid) 100 mg •
Bilberry extract (standardized 25%) 10 mg • Rutin 100 mg • Zinc
(picolinate) 25 mg • Selenium (selenomethionine) 100 mcg • Taurine
200 mg • N-Acetyl-Cysteine 200 mg • L-Glutathione 10 mg
• Vitamin B2 (Riboflavin) 50 mg • Chromium (GTF) 200 mcg •
Lutein 20 mg.

Eye Support - Now
Three capsules contain: Vitamin A (natural Beta Carotene • D. salina)
15 mg/25 000 IU • Vitamin C (as Ascorbic Acid) 300 mg • Vitamin E
(as d-Alpha-Tocopheryl Succinate) 200 IU • Riboflavin (Vitamin B2)
20 mg • Zinc (as L-OptiZinc) 25 mg • Selenium 100 mcg • Bilberry
standardized extract (Vaccinum myrtillus) (25% Anthocyanidins)
100 mg • Lutein 10 mg • Green Tea extract (Camellia sinensis)
(40% Catechins) 150 mg • N-Acetyl-Cysteine (NAC) 100 mg • Rutin
100 mg.

Eye Treatment - Jason
Complete Vitamin C Complex • Vitamin E • Aloe Vera gel • Rose
Hips.

Eyebright Formula - Nature's Way
Two capsules contain: Proprietary Formula: Bayberry bark • Cayenne
pepper fruit • Eyebright stem, leaf, flower • Goldenseal root • Red
Raspberry leaves. Other ingredients: Gelatin.

Eyebright Herb - Now
Two capsules contain: Total Carbohydrate 650 mg • Eyebright herb
(Euphrasia Officinalis) leaves and stems 940 mg. Other Ingredients:
Stearic Acid. Contains no sugar, salt, yeast, wheat, corn, soy, or milk.

Eye-Vites - Nature's Bounty
Each tablet contains: Vitamin A (as Beta Carotene) 5000 IU • Vitamin
C (as Ascorbic Acid) 60 mg • Vitamin E (as dl-Alpha Tocopheryl
Acetate) 30 IU • Zinc (as Zinc Oxide) 40 mg • Selenium (as Sodium
Selenate) 40 mcg • Copper (as Cupric Oxide) 2 mg. Other Ingredients:
Whey, Calcium Carbonate, Cellulose, Gelatin, Dicalcium Phosphate,
Vegetable Stearic Acid, Croscarmellose, Cellulose Coating,
Crospovidone, Vegetable Magnesium Stearate.

E-Z Vite Multiple - Nature's Life
Two tablets contain: Vitamin A (Fish Liver oil) 10000 IU • Vitamin D
(as Vitamin D3) (Cholecalciferol) 400 IU • Vitamin B1 (Thiamine
HCl) 10 mg • Vitamin B2 (Riboflavin) 10 mg • Vitamin B6
Pyridoxine HCl) 10 mg • Vitamin B12 (Cobalamin) 100 mcg • Niacin
30 mg • Pantothenic Acid (d-Calcium Pantothenate) 20 mg • Folic
Acid 400 mcg • PABA (Para Aminobenzoic Acid) 30 mg • Biotin
(d-Biotin) 3.5 mcg • Choline (Choline Bitartrate) 3 mg • Inositol
50 mg • Vitamin E (d-Alpha tocopherol, with Beta, Gamma & Delta
Tocopherols) 10 IU • Vitamin C 100 mg • Lemon Bioflavonoids
(TESTLAB) 30 mg • Rutin (Saphora japonica) 20 mg • Hesperidin
Complex 5 mg • Calcium (Bone Meal) 40 mg • Copper (Gluconate)
100 mcg • Phosphorus (Bone Meal) 25 mg • Iodine (Icelandic Kelp)
100 mcg • Iron (Ferrous Fumarate) 10 mg • Magnesium (Oxide)
10 mg • Zinc (Gluconate) 2 mg • Potassium (Chloride) 10 mg •
Manganese (Gluconate) 2 mg • Betaine HCl 25 mg • Liver (Defatted
& Desiccated) 100 mg • RNA powder (Torula Yeast) 25 mg •
Pancreatin (4 X N.F.) 25 mg. In a natural base of Raw Pancreas,
Sodium Alginate, Torula B Yeast, Rose Hips & Acerola berries.
See Editor's Note No. 14, page 1817.

Fade Away Gel For Sun And Age Spots - Cellex-C
Glucosamine • Ascorbic Acid • Tyrosine • Zinc • Green Tea extract •
Sodium Hyaluronate • Cucumber extract • Thyme extract.

Fade-Out Creme - Pharmagel
Vitamin C • Licorice Extract • PABA-free sunblock.

False Unicorn-Squaw Vine Virtue - Blessed Herbs
False Unicorn root • Squaw vine • Black Haw bark • Grain alcohol &
Distilled Water.

Fast Food - Sports Nutrition Source.com
Two scoops contain: Sodium 300 mg • Potassium 600 mg • Protein
38 g • Vitamin A 2500 IU • Vitamin C 30 mg • Calcium 500 mg • Iron
9 mg • Vitamin D 200 IU • Vitamin E 15 IU • Vitamin K 35 mcg

• Vitamin B-1 75 mg • Vitamin B-2 85 mg • Vitamin B-3 10 mg • Vitamin B-6 1 mg • Vitamin B-12 3 mcg • Biotin 125 mcg • Zinc 7.5 mcg • Copper 1 mg.

Fast-Acting Zinaxin - FreeLife
Each softgel contains: Patented Extract EV.EXT 77 [highly standardized extracts of rhizomes of Ginger (Zungiber officinale and Alpinia galanga)] 255 mg. Other Ingredients: Sunflower Seed oil, Gelatin, Beeswax, Lecithin, Vegetable Glycerin, Purified Water, Natural Chlorophyll Complex, Titanium Dioxide (natural mineral color).

Fat Binding Diet System 6 - Applied Nutrition
Two capsules contain: Vitamin C (ascorbic acid) 14 mg • Vitamin E (dl-alpha tocopheryl acetate) 4 IU • Riboflavin 0.5 mg • Niacin (niacinamide) 5 mg • Vitamin B6 (pyridoxine hydrochloride) 0.54 mg • Folic Acid 107 mcg • Vitamin B12 (cyanocobalamin) 2 mcg • Iodine (potassium iodine) 40 mcg • Selenium (sodium selenite) 14 mcg • Chromium (picolinate & 50% as polynicotinate) ChromeMate 80 mcg • Potassium (chloride) 6 mg • Garcinia Cambogia fruit (Super CitriMax, 60% Hydroxycitric acid extract) 460 mg • Chitosan (82% Deacetylated) 190 mg • Kola nut seed kernel extract (10% caffeine) 146 mg • Guarana seed extract (15% guaranine) 26 mg • Choline (bitartrate) 26 mg • Inositol 26 mg • Carnitine (L-Carnitine fumarate) 20 mg • Betaine (hydrochloride) 7 mg • Proprietary blend: [Ginger root, "72 Trace Minerals", Bioperine fruit (Piper nigrum extract, 95% Piperine)] 60 mg. Other Ingredients: Gelatin, montnirollinite, silica & magnesium stearate.

Fat Burner - Swanson
Three tablets contain: Vitamin B-6 (as pyridoxine HCl) 50 mg • Chromium (from Chromax® chromium picolinate) 200 mcg • CitriMax™ (Garcinia cambogia fruit extract) 1 g, (-) Hydroxycitric Acid 500 mg • Choline Bitartrate 500 mg • Inositol 250 mg • L-Methionine 200 mg • Cider Vinegar powder 100 mg • Grapefruit powder 100 mg • Lecithin 100 mg • Taurine 100 mg.

Fat Burners - Amerifit
Two caplets contain: Vitamin B6 (as pyridoxine HCl) 10 mg • Iron (as ferrous fumarate) 4 mg • Chromium (chromium picolinate) 50 mcg • Choline complex: (Choline Citrate, Buchu leaves, Uva Ursi root & fiber) 1000 mg • Inositol 250 mg • L-Carnitine (as carnitine tartrate, carnitine HCl) 50 mg • L-Lysine 100 mg • Methionine 200 mg • Lecithin (from glycine max) 100 mg • Betaine HCl 200 mg • Essential Fatty Acids: (Linoleic, Oleic) 100 mg. Other Ingredients: Dicalcium Phosphate, Microcrystalline Cellulose, Magnesium Stearate, Croscarmellose Sodium• Stearic Acid & Vegetable glaze.

Fat Busters - Nature's Plus
Two softgels contain: Plant Phytosterols 500 mg, supplying: Beta Sitosterol 200 mg • Campesterol 86 mg • Stigmasterol 80 mg • Safflower oil supplying 190 mg of free unsaturated fatty acids 240 mg • Lemon Grass oil 100 mg • Brindall berry extract 60 mg with naturally occuring [-] hydroxycitrate. Yeast free, sugar & starch free, no preservatives.

Fat Free Gainers Fuel 1000 - TwinLab
Each serving contains: Chromium (from Chromic Fuel Chromium Picolinate) 400 mcg. Other Ingredients: Branched Chain Amino Acids (L-Leucine, L-Isoleucine, L-Valine), Milk & Egg White Proteins, L-Carnitine & Kreb's Cycle Mineral Complexes (including Citrates, Aspartates, Succinates & Alpha-Ketoglutarates). Fat free with no added sugar.

Fat Free Gainers Fuel 2500 - TwinLab
Chromium (from patented Chromic Fuel Chromium Picolinate) 400 mcg • Kreb's Cycle Mineral Complexes (including Citrates, Aspartates, Succinates & Alpha-Ketoglutarates) • Milk & Egg White Proteins • Branched Chain Amino Acids (L-Leucine, L-Isoleucine & L-Valine), L-Carnitine. Fat free with no added sugar. Each serving supplies 2500 calories.

Fat Metabolizer 2000 - Youngevity
Cat's Claw • Siberian Ginseng • Bee Pollen • Kelp • Ephedra Sinica herb • White Willow bark • Licorice root • Hops flowers • Valerian root • Pantothenic Acid • Chromium Chelavite • Manganese Chelazome • Vilcabamba Mineral Essence: Potassium, Calcium, Magnesium, Zinc, Chromium, Selenium, Iron, Copper, Molybdenum, Vanadium, Iodine, Cobalt, Manganese.

Fat Metabolizer 2001+ - Youngevity
Cat's Claw • Ephedra Sinica herb • White Willow bark • Caffeine • Kelp • Pantothenic Acid • Chromium Chelavite • Manganese Chelazome • Vilcabamba Mineral Essence: Potassium, Calcium, Magnesium, Zinc, Chromium, Selenium, Iron, Copper, Molybdenum, Vanadium, Iodine, Cobalt, Manganese.

Fat Predator - Fat Predator Weight Loss Company, Inc.
Each capsule contains: Ephedra extract • Cola Nut extract • White Willow bark

Fat Snatcher - Youngevity
Chitosan • Aloe Vera leaf • Citric Acid • Iso-Ascorbic Acid (Vitamin C).

Fat Stopper Formula - Dr. Bussan's
Two capsules contain: Chitosan 250 mg • TAT Metabolite (a proprietary process of Dews Research Laboratories) 100 mg • Bile Salts Extract NF 50 mg • Vitamin C (polyascorbic acid) 50 mg • Acetyl Pyruvate Bile 12 mg • Niacin 5 mg • Chromium Picolinate 25 mcg. Other Ingredients: Magnesium trisilicate, Magnesium stearate, trace F.D.& C. Yellow #5 and natural Gelatin capsules.

Fat Trap - Sports Nutrition Source.com
Each capsule contains: Chitosan shellfish 500 mg • Fiber 500 mg.

Fat Trapper - Enforma Natural Products
Two capsules contain: Psyllium seed husk 420 mg • Chitin 80 mg.

Fat Trapper Plus - Enforma Natural Products
Two capsules contain: Psyllium seed husk 420 mg • Chitin 80 mg. Other ingredients: Gelatin, Magnesium Stearate, Vegetable Stearine, Glycerin.

FatFree - Starlight International
Two tablets contain: Maitake Mushroom extract, 4:1 (Grifola frondosa, plant) 50 mg • Platycodon grandiflorum extract 5:1 (root) 140 mg • Glucomannan (Amorphophalius konjac, root) 1000 mg • Gymnema sylvestre leaf 100 mg. Other Ingredients: Dicalcium Phosphate, Microcrystalline Cellulose, Stearic Acid Croscarmellose Sodium, Magnesium Stearate, Silicon Dioxide, Food Glaze, Ethylcellulose, Dextrin, Dextrose, Lecithin, Sodium Citrate.

Fatigue-Aid - Futurebiotics
Two capsules contain: Vitamin C (as buffered calcium ascorbate) 120 mg • Thiamin (as thiamin HCl) 25 mg • Riboflavin 25 mg • Niacin (as niacinamide) 25 mg • Vitamin B6 (as pyridoxine hydrochloride) 25 mg • Vitamin B12 (as cyanocobalamin) 250 mcg • Folic Acid 400 mcg • Pantothenic Acid 25 mg • Selenium (as amino acid chelate) 100 mcg • Citrus Bioflavonoids 250 mg • MSM (methyl-sulfonyl-methane) 200 mg • St. John's Wort powder extract (standardized for 0.3% (0.75 mg) hypericin) 250 mg • Astragalus root powder 200 mg • Pancreatin 4x (quadruple strength) (supplying 1600 USP units Lipase, 10000 USP units Amylase, 10000 USP units Protease) 125 mg

BRAND NAMES

BRAND NAMES

• Spirulina 100 mg • Blackstrap Molasses powder 25 mg • Red Beet powder 25 mg • Licorice root powder 25 mg • Siberian Ginseng (50:1) root powder 25 mg. Other ingredients: Gelatin, Water. See Editor's Note No. 14, page 1817.

FATmelt - with Gymnema Sylvestre - Slimming and Nutrition Consultancy
Each capsule contains: L-Carnitine • Gymnema Sylvestre • Chromium Picolinate • Forskolii (4:1 extract) • Bioperine. In a Maltodextrin and Magnesium stearate base.

Fem Balance - The Vitamin Shoppe
Each capsule contains: Black Cohosh 20 mg.

Fem Fit - Sports Nutrition Source.com
Two scoops contain: Sodium 200 mg • Potassium 400 mg • Protein 26 g • Vitamin A 1675 IU • Vitamin C 20 mg • Calcium 335 mg • Iron 6 mg • Vitamin D 134 IU • Vitamin E 10 IU • Vitamin K 23 mcg • Vitamin B-1 50 mg • Vitamin B-2 57 mg • Vitamin B-3 6.7 mg • Vitamin B-6 670 mcg • Vitamin B-12 3 mcg • Biotin 64 mcg • Zinc 5 mcg • Copper 670 mcg.

FemActin - Nature's Plus
Three capsules contain: Dong Quai [(Angelica sinensis root) standardized 0.9% Ligustilide] 100 mg • Evening Primrose [(Oenothera biennis seed) standardized 4% Gamma-Linolenic Acid] 100 mg • Uva Ursi [(Arctostaphylos uva-ursi leaf) standardized 20-25% Arbutin] 75 mg • Suma [(Pfaffia paniculata root) standardized 5% Beta-Ecdysterone] 50 mg • Butcher's Broom [(Ruscus aculeatus L. rhizome) standardized 10% Saponin Glycosides] 50 mg • Nettle [(Urtica dioica leaf) standardized 1-2% Plant Silica] 50 mg • Goldenseal [(Hydrastis canadensis root & rhizome) standardized 10% Alkaloids, 5% Hydrastine]50 mg • Chasteberry [(Vitex agnus-castus fruit) standardized 0.5% Agnuside, 0.6% Aucubin] 50 mg • Vitamin B6 (Pyridoxine HCI) 25 mg • Iron (Amino Acid Chelate) 12 mg.

Female Advantage - Body Wise International, Inc.
Three capsules contain: Genestein (Soy Protein) 150 mg • Daidzein (Soy Protein) 80 mg • Black Cohosh root 50 mg • Bromelain substance 50 mg • Dong Quai 200 mg • Echinacea Purpurea root 20 mg • Evening Primrose oil 50 mg • Korean Ginseng 75 mg • Siberian Ginseng 75 mg • Goldenseal root 50 mg • Gotu Kola 50 mg • Alpha-Ketoglutaric Acid 200 mg • Lady Slipper 25 mg • Licorice root 10 mg • Magnesium (Krebs Cycle Chelate) 15 mg • Passion Flower 50 mg • Suma root 50 mg • Valerian root 400 mg • Mexican Yam 100 mg • Zinc (Krebs Cycle Chelate) 10 mg • Flax Seed 100 mg • Kava Kava 250 mg.

Female Balance - Enzymatic Therapy
Three capsules contain: Vitamin A (Beta Carotene) (Non-toxic form of Vitamin A) 16665 IU • Vitamin E (D-Alpha Tocopherol Succinate) 200 IU • Vitamin C (Ascorbic Acid) 200 mg • Magnesium L-Aspartate 150 mg • Pantothenic Acid (D-Calcium Pantothenate) 100 mg • Thiamine HCL (Vitamin B1) 50 mg • Riboflavin (Vitamin B2) 50 mg • Calcium Citrate 50 mg • Iron (Ferrous Succinate) 18 mg • Zinc (Gluconate) 15 mg • Chromium (Polynicotinate) 250 mcg • Folic Acid 100 mcg • Vitamin B12 (Cyanocobalamin concentrate) 50 mcg • Selenium (L-Selenomethionine) 50 mcg • Other ingredients: Dong Quai extract (4:1) (Angelica sinensis) 75 mg • Licorice root extract (Glycyrrhiza glabra) standardized to contain 5% Glycyrrhizic acid) 60 mg • Milk Thistle extract (Silybum Marianum) standardized to contain 70% Silymarin calculated as Silybin) 50 mg • Black Cohosh extract (4:1) (Cimicifuga racemosa) 30 mg • Chaste Berry extract (5:1) (Vitex agnus-castus) 20 mg • Pyridoxal-5'-Phosphate 10 mg. Contains no sugar, salt, yeast, wheat, corn, dairy products, coloring, flavoring or preservatives.

Female Balance - Now
Three capsules contain: Vitamin B6 50 mg • Folic Acid 400 mcg • Borage oil powder (45 mg GLA) 325 mg • Wild Yam root extract (6% Diosgenin) 225 mg • Dong Quai root extract 5:1 150 mg • Vitex Agnus castus extract 10:1 150 mg.

Female Balance - Olympia Nutrition
Borage Oil powder • Wild Yam root • Dong Quai • Vitex Agnus • Vitamin B6.

Female Fertility Blend - Daily Wellness Co.
Three capsules contain: Vitamin E (as d-alpha tocopherol) 150 mg • Vitamin B6 (as pyridoxine hydrochloride) 6 mg • Vitamin B12 (as cyanocobalamin) 12 mcg • Folate (as folic acid) 400 mcg • Iron (as gluconate) 18 mg • Magnesium (as oxide) 400 mg • Zinc (as gluconate) • Selenium (as sodium selenate) 70 mcg • Proprietary Blend 1080 mg: Chasteberry (Vitex agnus castus standardized to .5% agnusides), Green Tea (Camellia sinensis standardized to 50% phenols), L-arginine. Other Ingredients: Rice Flour Powder, Magnesium Stearate, Silica.

Female Multi Vitamin - Health Center for Better Living
Each tablet contains: Vitamin A (as retinyl palmitate and 50% from beta-carotene) 3000 IU • Vitamin C (as ascorbic acid) 100 mg • Vitamin D (as cholecalciferol) 200 IU • Vitamin E (as dl-alpha-tocopheryl acetate) 25 IU • Thiamin (as thiamin HCl) 7 mg • Riboflavin 7 mg • Niacin (as niacinarnide) 25 mg • Vitamin B6 (as pyridoxine HCl) 25 mg • Folate (as folic acid) 200 mcg • Vitamin B12 (as cyanocobalamin) 50 mcg • Biotin 35 mcg • Pantothenic Acid (as D-calcium patothenate) 25 mg • Calcium (as dicalcium phosphate) 75 mg • Iron (as ferrous fumarate) 18 mg • Iodine (from Kelp) 25 mcg • Magnesium (as magnesium oxide) 75 mg • Zinc (as zinc citrate) 5 mg • Copper (as copper gluconate) 250 mcg • Manganese (as manganese gluconate) 1 mg • Chromium (as chromium dinicotinate glycinate) 50 mcg • Inositol 10 mg • Choline bitartrate 10 mg • Bioflavonoids complex: Citrus bioflavonoids, Hesperidin, Rutin, and Quercetin trace.

Female Sage - Traditional Medicinals
Sage leaf • Chaste berry dry extract • Blue Vervain leaf • Oatstraw herb • Lemongrass leaf • Fennel seed • Rosemary leaf • Blessed Thistle leaf • Stevia leaf.

Female Toner - Traditional Medicinals
Spearmint leaf • Rose Hip • Red Raspberry leaf • Licorice root • Strawberry Leaf • Lemongrass leaf • Lemon Verbena leaf • Nettle leaf • Ginger rhizome • Chamomile flower • Angelica root • Blessed Thistle herb • Cramp bark.

Femaprin - Nature's Way
Each capsule contains: Chaste Tree (vitex dried extract standardized to 6% agnusides) 3.85 mg. Other Ingredients: Lactose.

Femdiol - PhytoPharmica
Each capsule contains: Vitamin E (D-Alpha Tocopherol) 150 IU • Barlean's Flaxseed oil 300 mg • Gamma-Oryzanol 100 mg • Pumpkin seed oil (Curcurbita pepo) 50 mg • Soy extract 20 mg.

FEMFOCUS - Solgar
Three tablets contain: Protein 1 g • Vitamin A (as palmitate 5000 IU, 75% as natural beta-carotene from D.salina) 20000 IU • Vitamin C (as L-ascorbic acid) 400 mg • Vitamin D (as cholecalciferol) 400 IU • Vitamin E (as D-alpha tocopheryl succinate) 400 IU • Vitamin K (as phytonadione) 20 mcg • Thiamin (as thiamin mononitrate) 50 mg • Riboflavin 50 mg • Niacin (as niacinamide) 60 mg • Vitamin B-6 (as pyridoxine HCl) 50 mg • Folic Acid 800 mcg • Vitamin B-12 (as cobalamin) 200 mcg • Biotin (as D-biotin) 300 mcg • Pantothenic Acid (as D-ca pantothenate) 80 mg • Calcium (as calcium carbonate, glycinate, citrate) 400 mg • Iron (as iron bisglycinate) 18 mg • Iodine

(as kelp) 150 mcg • Magnesium (as magnesium oxide, glycinate, citrate) 400 mg • Zinc (as zinc glycinate, histidinate) 30 mg • Selenium (as L-selenomethionine) 200 mcg • Copper (as copper glycinate) 1.5 mg • Manganese (as manganese glycinate) 2 mg • Chromium (as chromium nicotinoglycinate) 200 mcg • Molybdenum (as molybdenum glycinate) 50 mcg • Sodium 25 mg • Potassium (as potassium glycinate complex) 99 mg • Citrus Bioflavonoids 100 mg • Choline (as choline bitartrate) 100 mg • Inositol 100 mg • Pantethine 7 mg • Cocarboxylase 6 mg • Pyridoxal-5-Phosphate 6 mg • Riboflavin-5-Phosphate 6 mg • Dibencozide 21 mcg • Boron (as boron glycinate complex) 500 mcg • Dong Quai extract root (angelica sinensis) 25 mg • Uva Ursi extract leaf (arcostaphylos uva ursi) 25 mg • Chaste berry extract (vitex agnus-castus) 25 mg • American Ginseng extract root 25 mg • Milk Thistle extract aerial (silybum marianum) 25 mg • Black Cohosh extract root (cimicifuga racemosa) 25 mg • Soy Isoflavone extract seed 25 mg • Carotenoid Mix (alpha carotene, lutein, zeaxanthin, cryptoxanthin) 172 mcg. Other Ingredients: Microcrystalline Cellulose, Vegetable Cellulose, Vegetable Stearic Acid, Red Beet Powder, Titanium Dioxide, Vegetable Glycerin, Silica, Vegetable Magnesium Stearate.

FEMFOCUS - Black Cohosh - Solgar
Each vegicap contains: Black Cohosh extract root (triterpine glycosides 5 mg as 27-deoxyactein) 200 mg • Raw Black Cohosh powder root 200 mg • Soy Isoflavone concentrate seed (isoflavone 6 mg) 200 mg. Other Ingredients: Microcrystalline Cellulose; Vegetable Cellulose; Vegetable Magnesium Stearate; Vegetable Glycerin; Phyt02X Blend: Vitamin E, Beta Carotene and other Carotenoids, Rosemary extract aerial, Vitamin C (L-Ascorbic Acid), Water.

FEMFOCUS - Bone Support - Solgar
Four tablets contain: Vitamin D (as cholecalciferol) 600 IU • Vitamin K (as phytonadione) 80 mcg • Calcium (as calcium carbonate, glycinate, citrate) 800 mg • Iron 0.7 mg • Magnesium (as magnesium glycinate, citrate, oxide) 400 mg • Zinc (as zinc glycinate, histidinate) 10 mg • Copper (as copper lysinate) 0.5 mg • Sodium 20 mg • Ipriflavone (as 7-isopropoxyisoflavone) 600 mg • Soy Isoflavone Concentrate seed 400 mg • Boron (as boron glycinate complex) 1.5 mg. Other Ingredients: Microcrystalline Cellulose; Vegetable Cellulose; Methacrylic Acid; Vegetable Magnesium Stearate; Vegetable Stearic Acid; Glyceryl Triacetate; Vegetable Glycerin; PhytO2X Blend: Vitamin E, Beta-Carotene and other Carotenoids, Rosemary extract aerial, Vitamin C (L-Ascorbic Acid), Annatto, Grapeskin.

FEMFOCUS - Calcium Citrate - Solgar
Four tablets contain: Vitamin D (as cholecalciferol) 600 IU • Calcium (as calcium citrate) 1000 mg. Other Ingredients: Microcrystalline Cellulose, Silica, Vegetable Magnesium Stearate, Titanium Dioxide, Vegetable Cellulose, Vegetable Glycerin.

FEMFOCUS - Cranberry Berry Extract - Solgar
Each vegicap contains: Cranberry extract berry (organic acids 30 mg) 100 mg • Cranberry concentrate powder berry 300 mg. Other Ingredients: Vegetable Cellulose; Microcrystalline Cellulose; Silica; Vegetable Magnesium Stearate; Vegetable Glycerin; PhytO2X Blend: Vitamin E, Beta-Carotene and other Carotenoids, Rosemary extract aerial, Vitamin C, Water.

FEMFOCUS - Cranberry Extract with Vitamin C - Solgar
Each vegicap contains: Vitamin C (as L-ascorbic acid) 60 mg • Cranberry extract berry 400 mg. Other Ingredients: Vegetable Cellulose, Silica, Vegetable Magnesium Stearate, Vegetable Glycerin, Water.

FEMFOCUS - Dong Quai - Solgar
Each vegicap contains: Dong Quai extract root 150 mg • Raw Dong Quai powder root 300 mg. Other Ingredients: Microcrystalline

Cellulose; Vegetable Cellulose; Vegetable Magnesium Stearate; Vegetable Glycerin; Phyt02X Blend: Vitamin E, Beta Carotene and other Carotenoids, Rosemary extract aerial, Vitamin C (L-Ascorbic Acid), Water.

FEMFOCUS - Ester-C Plus - Solgar
Each vegicaps contain: Vitamin C (as Ester-C calcium ascorbate) 500 mg • Calcium (as calcium ascorbate) 62 mg • Citrus Bioflavonoids 25 mg • Acerola 10 mg • Rose Hips fruit 10 mg • Rutin 5 mg. Other Ingredients: Vegetable Cellulose, Vegetable Magnesium Stearate, Silica, L-Threonic Acid, Vegetable Glycerin, Water.

FEMFOCUS - Evening Primrose Oil - Solgar
Each softgel contains: Vitamin E (as D-alpha tocopheryl acetate) 14 IU • Linoleic Acid 360 mg • Gamma-Linolenic Acid 50 mg • Oleic Acid 50 mg • Other Fatty Acids 40 mg. Other Ingredients: Evening Primrose Oil, Gelatin, Glycerin, Water.

FEMFOCUS - Flaxseed Oil - Solgar
Two softgels contain: Linolenic Acid 1425 mg • Oleic Acid 450 mg • Linoleic Acid 400 mg • Palmitic Acid 150 mg • Stearic Acid 75 mg. Other Ingredients: Flaxseed Oil, Gelatin, Glycerin, Carob Flavor, Water.

FEMFOCUS - Folic Acid - Solgar
Each tablet contains: Folic Acid 400 mcg • Calcium (as dicalcium phosphate) 70 mg. Other Ingredients: Vegetable Stearic Acid, Silica, Vegetable Cellulose.

FEMFOCUS - Gentle Iron - Solgar
Each vegicap contains: Iron (as iron bisglycinate) 25 mg. Other Ingredients: Microcrystalline Cellulose, Vegetable Cellulose, Vegetable Magnesium Stearate, Vegetable Glycerin, Water.

FEMFOCUS - Herbal Female Complex - Solgar
Each vegicap contains: Iron 1 mg • Standardized Chaste berry extract 75 mg • Dong Quai extract root 75 mg • Soy Isoflavone extract seed 100 mg • Milk Thistle extract aerial, seed (silymarin 40 mg) 50 mg • Black Cohosh extract root 100 mg • Motherwort extract aerial 75 mg • Raw Astragalus powder root 75 mg • Raw Korean Ginseng powder root 50 mg • Raw Dong Quai powder root 50 mg. Other Ingredients: Microcrystalline Cellulose; Vegetable Cellulose; Vegetable Stearic Acid; Vegetable Magnesium Stearate; Vegetable Glycerin; Phyt02X Blend: Vitamin E, Beta-Carotene and other Carotenoids, Rosemary extract aerial, Vitamin C (L-Ascorbic Acid), Water.

FEMFOCUS - Ipriflavone - Solgar
Each vegicap contains: Ipriflavone (as 7-isopropoxyisoflavone) 200 mg. Other Ingredients: Microcrystalline Cellulose, Vegetable Cellulose, Vegetable Magnesium Stearate, Vegetable Glycerin, Water.

FEMFOCUS - Non-GMO Isoflavones - Solgar
Each tablet contains: Total Soy Isoflavones seed (from soy isoflavone extract) 38 mg. Other Ingredients: Microcrystalline Cellulose, Vegetable Cellulose, Silica, Vegetable Magnesium Stearate, Caramel, Titanium Dioxide, Vegetable Glycerin.

FEMFOCUS - Oceanic Silica - Solgar
Each vegicap contains: Calcium 30 mg • Silica (from red algae powder, 25 mg elemental silicon) 54 mg. Other Ingredients: Vegetable Cellulose, Microcrystalline Cellulose, Vegetable Magnesium Stearate, Vegetable Glycerin, Water.

FEMFOCUS - Prenatal Tablets - Solgar
Four tablets contain: Vitamin A (as palmitate 3000 IU, 63% as natural beta-carotene from D.salina) 8000 IU • Vitamin C (as L-ascorbic acid) 100 mg • Vitamin D (as cholecalciferol) 400 IU • Vitamin E (as D-alpha tocopheryl succinate) 30 IU • Thiamin (as thiamin mononitrate)

1.7 mg • Riboflavin 2 mg • Niacin (as niacinamide) 20 mg • Vitamin B-6 (as pyridoxine HCl) 2.5 mg • Folic Acid 800 mcg • Vitamin B-12 (as cobalamin) 8 mcg • Biotin 300 mcg • Pantothenic Acid (as D-ca pantothenate) 10 mg • Calcium (as calcium carbonate, calcium citrate) 1300 mg • Iron (as iron bisglycinate) 27 mg • Iodine (as kelp) 150 mcg • Magnesium (as magnesium oxide, magnesium citrate) 450 mg • Zinc (as zinc chelate, zinc oxide) 15 mg • Copper (as copper chelate, copper gluconate) 2 mg • Selenium (as L-selenomethionine) 25 mcg • Manganese (as manganese chelate, manganese gluconate) 2 mg • Chromium (as chromium picolinate) 25 mcg • Potassium (from potassium amino acid complex, potassium gluconate) 50 mg • Inositol 10 mg • Choline (as choline bitartrate) 4 mg • PABA (as para aminobenzoic acid) 2 mg • Alpha Carotene 114 mcg • Cryptoxanthin 28 mcg • Zeaxanthin 23 mcg • Lutein 18 mcg • Soy Protein Isolate/ Amino Acid Blend: L-Glutamic Acid, L-Aspartic Acid, L-Leucine, L-Arginine, L-Lysine, L-Phenylalanine, L-Serine, L-Proline, L-Valine, L-Isoleucine, L-Alanine, Glycine, L-Threonine, L-Tyrosine, L-Histidine, L-Cysteine, L-Methionine, L-Ornithine, Taurine 160 mg. Other Ingredients: Microcrystalline Cellulose, Vegetable Cellulose, Vegetable Stearic Acid, Grapeskin, Titanium Dioxide, Silica, Vegetable Magnesium Stearate, Vegetable Glycerin.

FEMFOCUS - Red Clover - Solgar
Each vegicap contains: Standardized Red Clover extract leaf (biochanin A 3 mg) 250 mg • Raw Red Clover powder leaf 225 mg. Other Ingredients: Vegetable Cellulose; Vegetable Magnesium Stearate; Vegetable Glycerin; PhytO2X Blend: Vitamin E, Beta-Carotene and other Carotenoids, Rosemary extract aerial, Vitamin C (L-absorbic acid), Water.

FEMFOCUS - Super GLA - Solgar
Each softgel contains: Linoleic Acid 498 mg • Gamma-Linolenic Acid 300 mg • Other Fatty Acids 296 mg • Oleic Acid 206 mg • Borage Oil 1300 mg. Other Ingredients: Gelatin, Glycerin, Water.

FEMFOCUS - Vitamin B12 - Solgar
Each nugget contains: Vitamin B-12 (as cobalamin) 1000 mcg. Other Ingredients: Mannitol, Vegetable Magnesium Stearate, Vegetable Stearic Acid, Natural Cherry Flavor.

FEMFOCUS - Vitamin B-6 - Solgar
Each tablet contains: Vitamin B-6 (as pyridoxine HCl) 50 mg • Calcium (as dicalcium phosphate) 50 mg. Other Ingredients: Dicalcium Phosphate, Vegetable Stearic Acid, Vegetable Magnesium Stearate, Vegetable Cellulose.

FEMFOCUS - Vitamin K - Solgar
Each tablet contains: Calcium (as dicalcium phosphate) 90 mg • Vitamin K (as phytonadione) 100 mcg. Other Ingredients: Vegetable Cellulose, Vegetable Stearic Acid, Vegetable Magnesium Stearate.

Fem-Gest - Progressive Labs
Ingredients: Stabilized Aloe Vera gel • Mexican Yam extract • Chamomile extract • Chaste Tree berry • Tocopheryl Acetate • Lavender extract • Jojoba oil • Safflower oil • Progesterone 950 mg • Carbomer 940 • Glyceryl Stearate (and) PEG-100 Stearate • C12-15 Alkyl Benzoate • Stearic Acid • Octyl Palmitate • Triethanolamine • Cetyl Alcohol • Methylparaben • Tetrasodium EDTA • Dimethicone • Propylparaben • Diazolidyl Urea.

FEM-H - MMS Pros
Each capsule contains: Black Cohosh root • Sarsaparilla root • Siberian Ginseng root • Licorice root • Blessed Thistle herb • Squaw Vine • False Unicorn root.

FeminEstra - Pacific BioLogic
Poria Plant Fungus (hoelen) • Polygonum root (thin) • Moutan Root bark • Chinese Yam • Cherry (cornelian asiatic) • Rehmannia root (fresh) • Rehmannia root (cooked in wine) • Curculigo rhizome • Alisma (water plantain rhizome) • Pearl – No Concentration.

Femme Advantage Creatine Serum - Muscle Marketing USA
Each serving comtains: Creatine Monohydrate • Vitamin B12 • Ginseng • Royal Jelly • Vitamin B5 • Soluable Bioflavonoids • Ginkgo extract • Wild Yam extract • Papain extract.

Fem-Mend Formula - Nature's Way
Two capsules contain: Proprietary Formula: Blessed Thistle • Cayenne pepper fruit • Cramp bark • False Unicorn root • Ginger • Goldenseal stem, leaf, flower • Red Raspberry leaves • Squaw Vine vine, leaf, fruit • Uva Ursi leaves. Other ingredients: Gelatin.

FemTone - PhytoPharmica
Two capsules contain: Vitamin C (Ascorbic Acid) 100 mg • Dong Quai extract 4:1 (Angelica sinensis) 250 mg • Hesperidin Complex standardized to contain 50% bioflavonoids 200 mg • Licorice root extract (Glycyrrhiza glabra) standardized to contain 5% glycyrrhizic acid 50 mg • Chaste Tree berry extract 5:1 (Vitex agnus-castus) 50 mg • Black Cohosh extract 4:1 (Cimicifuga racemosa) 50 mg • False Unicorn root extract 4:1 (Helonias opulus) 50 mg • Fennel seed extract 6:1 (Foeniculum vulgare) 25 mg.

Femtrol - Enzymatic Therapy
Two capsules contain: Vitamin C (Ascorbic Acid) 100 mg. Other ingredients: Dong Quai extract 4:1 (Angelica sinensis) 250 mg • Hesperidin Complex standardized to contain 50% Bioflavonoids 200 mg • Licorice root extract (Glycyrrhiza glabra) standardized to contain 5% Glycyrrhizic Acid 50 mg • Chaste Tree Berry extract 5:1 (Vitex agnus-castus) 50 mg • Black Cohosh root extract 4:1 (Cimicifuga racemosa) 50 mg • False Unicorn root extract 4:1 (Helonias opulus) 50 mg • Fennel seed extract 6:1 (Foeniculum vulgare) 25 mg. Contains no sugar, salt, yeast, wheat, corn, soy, dairy products, coloring, flavoring or preservatives.

Fennel-Yam - Atrium Inc.
Each capsule contains: Fennel 250 mg • Wild Yam 250 mg. Contains no sugar, starch, salt, wheat, corn, yeast or soy derivatives.

Fen-Tastic - The Vitamin Shoppe
Two tablets contain: St. John's Wort root standardized for 3% hypericin 400 mg • Citrus Aurantium fruit 600 mg • 5-HTP 150 mg • Yerba Santa • Mate leaves standardized 20% methylzanthine 250 mg • White Willow bark 400 mg.

Fenugreek - Nature's Way
Two capsules contain: Fenugreek seed 1.22 g. Other Ingredients: Gelatin.

Fenu-Thyme Formula - Nature's Way
Two capsules contain: Proprietary Formula: Fenugreek seed • Thyme leaf. Other ingredients: Gelatin.

FerroComp - PhytoPharmica
Each capsule contains: Vitamin C (Ascorbic Acid) 60 mg • Iron (Ferrous Succinate) 25 mg • Folic Acid 200 mcg • Vitamin B12 (Cyanocobalamin) 100 mcg • Liquid Liver Fractions (predigested soluble concentrate) 250 mg • Chlorophyll (Fat-Soluble) 5 mg. Contains no sugar, salt, yeast, wheat, corn, dairy products, flavoring or preservatives. All organs & glands derived from bovine sources. See Editor's Note No. 14, page 1817.

Fevera - HerbaSway
Cassia tora • Kudzu • Skullcap • Knotweed • Licorice • Blackberry • HerbaSwee (Cucurbitaceae fruit).

Feverfew - Now
Each capsule contains: Feverfew 0.9% 400 mg.

Feverfew - Leiner Health Products

Each caplet contains: Feverfew extract (Tanacetum parhenium) leaf 100 mg • Feverfew leaf (Tanacetum parthenium) 20 mg. Other Ingredients: Calcium Carbonate, Cellulose, Maltodextrin, Mannitol, Hydroxypropyl Methylcellulose, Silicon Dioxide, Polyethylene Glycol 3350, Croscarmellose Sodium, Titanium Dioxide, Hydroxypropyl Cellulose, Pharmaceutical Glaze, Crospovidone, Magnesium Stearate, Polysorbate 80, Blue 1 Lake, Yellow 6 Lake.

Feverfew - Pharmanex

Each capsule contains: Feverfew leaves and flowers (12:1) extract (Tanacetum parthenium) 125 mg. Other Ingredients: Rice Flour, Gelatin.

Feverfew (Nomigraine) Caplets - Life Brand

Dried Feverfew leaf (Tanacetum parthenium) 125 mg. This product is guaranteed to contain a minimum of 0.2% Parthenolide. Excipients: Dicalcium Phosphate, Microcrystalline Cellulose, Silicon Dioxide, Magnesium Stearate (plant source), Stearic Acid (plant source).

Feverfew-Source Naturals - Source Naturals

Each tablet contains: Feverfew extract 200 mg • Feverfew whole herb 50 mg • Magnesium (Oxide) 70 mg • Calcium (Carbonate) 35 mg • Vitamin C (Ascorbic Acid) 10 mg.

Fiber Clense - Nutri-Quest

Three tablets contain: Vitamin C 300 mg • Apple Pectin 150 mg • Garlic 150 mg • Rice Bran 600 mg • Sodium Alginate 300 mg • L-Cysteine 200 mg • DL-Methionine 100 mg • L-Lysine 30 mg • Chlorophyll 10 mg • Oat Bran 600 mg • Red Beet root 100 mg.

Fiber Soy-Pro - The Vitamin Shoppe

SUPRO Soy Protein Isolate and BeneFiber Soluble Fiber. Orange citrus natural flavor. No yeast, corn, wheat, salt, starch, milk, gluten, eggs, fish or animal derivatives, preservatives, artificial colors or flavors added.

Fiberific - Nature's Plus

Each 1.4 oz. bar contains: Calories 120 • Calories from Fat 18 • Total Fat 2 g Saturated Fat 0 g • Cholesterol 0 mg • Total Carbohydrate 23 g • Complex Carbohydrate 14 g • Sugars 9 g • Dietary Fiber 8 g • Soluble Fiber 3.6 g • Insoluble Fiber 4.4 g • Protein 3 g • Sodium 43 mg • Potassium 196 mg. Ingredients include: Rolled Oats, Wheat Germ, Brown Rice, Apples, Prunes & Oat Bran. Naturally flavored with Fruit Juice & Honey. No tropical oils.

FiberPlus - PhytoPharmica

Two capsules contain: FiberPlus Proprietary Blend: [Psyllium hydrophilic muciloid, Grapefruit pectin, Oat (Avena sativa) fiber, Beet fiber, Carrot fiber, Fructooligosaccharides (FOS; from Jerusalem artichoke), Prune fiber, Ginger (Zingiber officinale) root and rhizome extract, Fenugreek (Trigonella foenum-graecum) seed extract 4:1, Goldenseal (Hydrastis canadensis) root and rhizome extract (standardized to contain 5% total alkaloids including berberine, hydrastine, and canadine), Chamomile (Matricaria recutita) root extract, Marshmallow (Althaea officinalis) root extract 4.25:1, Aloe Vera (Aloe barbadensis) leaf extract, and Cascara sagrada (Rhamnus purshiana) bark, trunk, and branch extract] 1,000 mg.

Fibersol - TwinLab

Each rounded teaspoonful contains: Fiber Blend Concentrate [from Psyllium Seed Husks, Guar Gum, Apple Pectin] 4 g • Vitamin C 100 mg.

Fiber-Time - Atrium Inc.

Twelve ounces contain: Bran Fiber • Cascara Sagrada bark • Citrus Fiber • Karaya Gum • Apple Pectin • Prune powder • Psyllium Plantago Ovata Blond • Rhubarb root • Rice Fiber • Sweet Whey.

FibreNet - Pharmanex

Four capsules contain: Chitosan (from shellfish) PolmerPlex 1000 mg. Other Ingredients: Calcium Carbonate, Magnesium Stearate.

FibreNet Plus - Pharmanex

Each scoop contains: Vitamin A (85% Beta-Carotene) 6877 IU • Vitamin C 12 mg • Vitamin D 80 IU • Vitamin E 4 IU • Thiamin 0.30 mg • Riboflavin 0.34 mg • Niacin 4 mg • Vitamin B6 0.40 mg • Folate 80 mcg • Vitamin B12 1.2 mg • Biotin 60 mcg • Pantothenic Acid 2 mg • Calcium 187 mg • Iron 3.8 mg • Phosphorus 100 mg • Iodine 30 mcg • Magnesium 60 mg • Zinc 3 mg • Copper 0.40 mg • Sodium 60 mg • Potassium 190 mg • PolmerPlex 1000 mg. Ingredients: Crystalline Fructose, Oat Bran, Stabilized Rice Bran, Gum Arabic, Natural and Artificial Flavors, PolmerPlex, High Oleic Sunflower Oil, Corn Syrup Solids, Tricalcium Phosphate, Citric Acid, Beta-Carotene, Dipotassium Phosphate Cellulose Gum, Sugar Beet Fiber, Potassium Citrate, Sodium Caseinate, Magnesium Oxide, Soy Fiber, Salt, Pea Fiber, Xanthan Gum, Ground Psyllium Husks, Ascorbic Acid, dl-Alpha Tocopheryl Acetate, Dicalcium Phosphate, Soy Lecithin, Vitamin A Palmitate, Niacinamide, Zinc Oxide, Electric Iron, Copper Gluconate, d-Calcium Pantothenate, Cholecalciferol, Pyridoxine Hydrochloride, Riboflavin, Thiamine Mononitrate, Cyanocobalamin, Folic Acid, Biotin, Potassium Iodide.

Fibro Plus - Aspen Group, Inc.

Two capsules contain: Elemental Magnesium 200 mg • Malic Acid 300 mg • Glyciante 50 mg.

FibroLeve - PharmAssure

Four tablets contain: Vitamin B6 (as Pyridoxine Hydrochloride) 15 mg • Magnesium (as Magnesium Oxide) 400 mg • Manganese (as Manganese Sulfate) 10 mg • Malic Acid 1200 mg • Boswellin serrata Resin Extract (65% Boswellic Acid=75 mg) 115 mg. Other ingredients: Cellulose.

Fibromyalgin - Olympia Nutrition

Glucosamine, Collagen, Mag. Malate.

Fibro-X - Olympian Labs

Two capsules contain: Malic Acid 600 mg • Shark Cartilage 600 mg • White Willow Bark 50 mg • Valerian root 20 mg • Grape Seed extract 40 mg • Magnesium Glycinate 100 mg • Manganese Glycinate 5 mg.

Firm Lotion - Mannatech

Water • Parrafin • Caprylic/capric triglycerides C12-15 • Alkyl Benzoate • Cetyl Alcohol • Propylene Glycol • Dimethicone • Germanben II (propylene glycol, diazolidinyl urea, methylparaben, propylparaben) • Aminomethyl propanol • Ambrotose Complex: naturally occurring plant polysaccharides including freeze-dried Aloe Vera inner leaf gel extract - Manapol powder • Lactic Acid • Niacinamide • Emu Oil • Stearic Acid • Cholesterol • Lavender Oil • Carbomer • Herbal Complex: barley extract, clover extract, ivy extract, butcherbroom extract, camellia oleifera extract, lady's thistle extract • Wild Yam extract.
See Editor's Note No. 17, page 1817.

Fish Body Oil - Health Center for Better Living

Each softgel contains: EPA 180 mg • DHA 120 mg • Vitamin E 5 IU.

Flash Fighters - Puritan's Pride

Three tablets contain: Soy concentrate (yielding 65 mg total Isoflavones) 2,100 mg • Black Cohosh extract (Cimicifuga racemosa) root (2.5% triterpene glycosides) 160 mg • Dong Quai (Angelica sinensis) root 150 mg • Licorice (Glycyrrhiza glabra) root 150 mg • Vitex extract (Vitex agnus-castus) fruit 100 mg.

BRAND NAMES

B R A N D   N A M E S

Flax Borage Combo - Health From The Sun
Three capsules contain: Alpha-Linolenic Acid (ALA) (Omega-3) 825 mg • Gamma-Linolenic Acid (Omega-6) 72 mg • Linoleic Acid (Omega-6) 320 mg • Oleic Acid (Omega-9) 260 mg. Ingredients: Certified Organic Flax seed oil, Borage seed oil, Gelatin, Glycerine, Water, Carob powder.

Flax Lignan Gold - Health From The Sun
One tablespoon contains: 100% Certified Organic Flax seed oil & Particulate with Rosemary extract • Mixed Tocopherols (Vitamin E) • Ascorbyl Palmitate (Vitamin C) • Citric Acid to protect freshness.

Flax Liquid Gold - Health From The Sun
One tablespoon contains: 100% Certified Organic Flax seed oil with Rosemary extract • Mixed Tocopherols (Vitamin E) • Ascorbyl Palmitate (Vitamin C) • Citric Acid to protect freshness.

Flax Oil - Swanson
Each softgel contains: Calories 10 • Calories from Fat 9 • Total Fat 1 g • Organic Flax Oil 1 g.

Flax Oil - Metabolic Response Modifiers
Each softgel contains: Flax oil 1,000 mg • Linolenic acid (Omega-3) 550 mg • Linoleic acid (Omega-6) 170 mg • Oleic acid (Omega-9) 170 mg • Mixed short chain fatty acids 110 mg.

Flax Seed Oil 1000 mg - Jamieson
Each capsule contains: Alpha Linolenic Acid (ALA) (from Flax seed oil) 500 mg.

Flax-O-Mega - Flora
Cold pressed Flax Seed oil 1000 mg.

Flaxseed & Cod Liver Oil - Puritan's Pride
Each softgel contains: Cold-Pressed Linseed oil 500 mg • Vitamin A (from Cod Liver Oil) 1250 IU • Vitamin D (from Cod Liver Oil) 135 IU.

Flexa-Herb - Dial Herbs
Kava Kava • Cramp bark • Cayenne • Ginger • Lobelia • Lady Slipper • Red Clover.

Flex-A-Min - Puritan's Pride
Three capsules contain: Glucosamine Sulfate 500 mg • Vitamin C 250 mg • Bromelain (2400 GDU per gram) 250 mg • Boswellin (Boswellia Serrata) 250 mg • Curcumin (Curcuma Longa) 50 mg • Zinc (Amino Acid Chelate) 10 mg • Chondroitin Sulfate A 10 mg • White Willow Bark 100 mg • Shark Cartilage 500 mg • Vervain 100 mg.
See Editor's Note No. 15, page 1817.

FlexAnew - Natrol
Two tablets contain: Calcium (as Calcium Carbonate) 330 mg • Glucosamine Sulfate 750 mg • Chondroitin Sulfate 300 mg • Nexrutine (Phellodendron Amurense bark extract) 250 mg.
See Editor's Note No. 15, page 1817.

Flexaplex - Progressive Labs
Three capsules contain: Vitamin A 3000 IU • Vitamin B6 150 mg • Vitamin B12 300 mcg • Magnesium 300 mg • Copper 3 mg • Potassium 25 mg • Adrenal (Bovine) 30 mg • Valerian root 150 mg • Slippery Elm 30 mg • Gentian root 30 mg • Cape Aloes 30 mg • Skullcap 30 mg • Rue powder 30 mg.
See Editor's Note No. 14, page 1817.

FlexTend - Nature's Way
Three caplets contain: Vitamin C (Ascorbic Acid) 180 mg • Vitamin E Acetate 60 IU • Iron 0.78 mg • Sodium 160 mg • Glucosamine Sulfate (sodium salt) 1.5 g. Other Ingredients: Microcrystalline Cellulose,

Maltodextrin, Croscarmellose Sodium, Stearic Acid, Magnesium Stearate, Silicon Dioxide, Hydroxypropyl Methylcellulose, Titanium Dioxide, Polyethylene Glycol, Caramel, Polysorbate 80.

Flintstones Plus Iron Children's Multivitamin - Bayer
Each chewable tablet contains: Vitamin A 2500 IU • Vitamin C 60 mg • Vitamin D 400 IU • Vitamin E 15 IU • Thiamin 1.05 mg • Riboflavin 1.2 mg • Niacin 13.5 mg • Vitamin B-6 1.05 mg • Folic Acid 300 mcg • Vitamin B-12 4.5 mcg • Iron 15 mg.

Flor*Essence - Flora
Burdock root • Sheep Sorrel • Slippery Elm • Turkish Rhubarb • Watercress • Kelp • Blessed Thistle • Red Clover.

Flora Vision - Flora
Bilberry extract 250mg • Blueberry.

Floradix Iron and Herbs - Dial Herbs
Vitamin B1 • Vitamin B2 • Vitamin B6 • Folic Acid • Vitamin B12 • Vitamin C • Iron • Aqueous Extract from Carrot • Nettle Worth • Spinach • Quitch roots • Angelica roots • Fennel • Ocean Kelp • African Allow blossom • Orange peel • Juice concentrates: Pear, Red Grape, Blackcurrant, Orange, Blackberry, Cherry, Beetroot • Yeast (Saccharomyces cerevisiae) Extract • Honey • Rose Hip extract • Wheat Germ Extract • Natural Flavor.

Flush Free Niacin - Puritan's Pride
Each capsule contains: Niacin 400 mg • Inositol 100 mg.

Flush-Free HexaNiacin - Enzymatic Therapy
Each capsule contains: Niacin (Inositol hexaniacinate) contains 500 mg elemental Niacin 650 mg. Contains no sugar, salt, yeast, wheat, corn, soy, dairy products, coloring, flavoring, or preservatives.

Flush-Free Niacin - PhytoPharmica
Each capsule contains: Niacin (flush-free Inositol hexaniacinate) 590 mg.

Flush-free Niacin 500 mg - Nature's Life
Each tablet contains: Niacin (Inositol, Hexaniacinate) 500 mg.

Focus Child - Source Naturals
Two tablets contain: Magnesium (from Magnesium Aspartate and Oxide) 100 mg • Zinc (as Zinc Picolinate) 2 mg • L-Aspartate (from Magnesium Aspartate) 310 mg • DMAE (as DMAE Bitartrate) 100 mg • Standardized Soybean Lecithin (LECI-PS) 50 mg • Yielding 40% Phosphatidylserine 20 mg • Phosphatidylcholine 6 mg • Phosphatidylethanolamine 3.5 mg • Phosphatidylinositol 1 mg • DHA (Docosahexaenoic Acid (Neuromins)) 15 mg • Grape Seed extract 15 mg.

Focus DHA - Source Naturals
One softgel contains: Docosahexaenoic Acid (DHA) (from Alga Oil [Neuromins]) 100 mg.

Focus Factor - Vital Basics, Inc.
Four tablets contain: Vitamin A (from natural beta-carotene and mixed carotenoids) 4,000 IU • Vitamin C (as ascorbic acid, sodium ascorbate, calcium ascorbate, potassium ascorbate, zinc ascorbate, and ascorbyl palmitate) 250 mg • Vitamin D (as cholecalciferol) 100 IU • Vitamin E (as natural d-alpha- tocopheryl succinate) 30 IU • Thiamin (as thiamin mononitrate) 3mg • Riboflavin 1.7 mg • Niacin (from inositol hexanicotinate and 50% as niacinamide) 25 mg • Vitamin B6 (as pyridoxal-alpha-ketoglutarate, pyridoxal 5-phosphate) 15 mg • Folate (as folic acid) 400 mcg • Vitamin B12 (as cyanocobalamin) 20 mcg • Biotin 300 mcg • Pantothenic acid (as D-calcium pantothenate) 12 mg • Calcium (as calcium citrate, calcium succinate

and calcium ascorbate) 50 mg • Iron (as Ferronly carbonyl Iron) 5 mg • Iodine (as potassium iodide and kelp (Ascophyllum nodosum)) 15 mcg • Magnesium (as magnesium citrate, magnesium malate and magnesium taurinate) 100 mg • Zinc (as zinc citrate and zinc ascorbate) 10 mg • Selenium (as selenomethionine) 20 mcg • Copper (as copper citrate and copper Chelazome) 0.4 mg • Manganese (as manganese citrate) 2 mg • Chromium (as chromium polynicotinate) 100 mcg • Molybdenum (as molybdenum amino acid chelate) 10 mcg • Potassium (as potassium citrate, potassium aspartate, and potassium ascorbate) 50 mg • Synergistic and proprietary formulation, L-Glutamine, DMAE (as DMAE bitartrate), L-pyroglutamic acid, phosphatidylserine, DHA concentrate (15% DHA from fish body oil), choline (as choline bitartrate), inositol, pyridoxal-alpha-ketoglutarate, N-acetyltyrosine, Bacopin (Bacopa monnieri extract) (leaf), bilberry fruit standardized extract (25% anthocyansides), GABA, pine bark and Activin (grape seed extract), vinpocetine, Trace-Lyte Electrolyte concentrate, Huperzine (extract of Huperzia serrata) (whole plant), boron (as boron chelate), vanadium (as vanadyl sulfate) 471 mg. Other Ingredients: Dicalcium Phosphate, Microcrystalline Cellulose, Croscarmellose Sodium, Stearic Acid, Silica, Magnesium Stearate and Pharmaceutical Glaze.

Focus Factor - Children's Chewable - Vital Basics, Inc.
Four Wafers contain: Vitamin A (from natural beta-carotene and mixed carotenoids) 4,000 UI • Vitamin C (as ascorbic acid, sodium ascorbate and zinc ascorbate) 250 mg • Vitamin D (as cholecalciferol) 100 UI • Vitamin E (as natural d-alpha-tocopheryl succinate) 30 UI • Thiamin (as thiamin mononitrate) 3 mg • Riboflavin 1.7 mg • Niacin (from inositol hexanicotinate and 50% as niacinamide) 25 mg • Vitamin B6 (as pyridoxal alpha ketoglutarate) 5 mg • Folate (as folic acid) 40 mcg • Vitamin B12 (as cyanocobalamin) 20 mcg • Biotin 300 mcg • Pantothenic Acid (as D-calcium pantothenate) 12 mg • Calcium (as calcium citrate, calcium ascorbate, calcium malate and calcium succinate) 100 mg • Iron (as ferrous glycinate) 10 mg • Iodine (as potassium iodide and kelp) 15 mcg • Magnesium (as magnesium citrate, magnesium malate and magnesium taurinate) 100 mg • Zinc (as zinc aspartate and zinc ascorbate) 10 mg • Selenium (as selenomathionine) 20 mcg • Copper (as copper citrate and copper Chelazome) 400 mcg • Manganese (as manganese citrate) 2 mg • Chromium (as chromium polynicotinate) 100 mcg • Potassium (as potassium citrate, potassium ascorbate and potassium aspartate) 50 mg • Synergistic and proprietary formulation, Phosphatidyl serine / soya lecithin complex, DMAE (as DMAE birartrate), Neuromins (Martex Docosahexaenoic acid concentrate), L-glutamine, L-pyroglutamic acid, pyridoxial alpha ketoglutarate, trace mineral complex, N-acetyl-tyrosine, GABA, Inositol, Bilberry (from 100:1 concentrate), Proanthocyanidin blend from Pine Bark and Activin (grape seed extract), Bacopin (Bacopa monnieri extract), Coenzyme Q-10, Huperzine (extract of huperzia serrata), Boron (as boron citrate), Vanadium (as vanadyl sulfate) 640 mg. Other Ingredients: Simple and Complex Carbohydrates from corn, Organic Sucanat with honey, Mixed Fruit, and Cherry Crystals, Cellulose, Magnesium Stearate and Silica.

Folgard - Upsher-Smith Laboratories
Each tablet contains: Folic Acid 800 mcg • Vitamin B-6 10 mg • Vitamin B-12 115 mcg.

Folic Acid - Leiner Health Products
Each tablet contains: Folate (Folic Acid) 400 mcg. Other Ingredients: Dicalcium Phosphate, Cellulose, Stearic Acid, Croscarmellose Sodium, Magnesium Stearate.

Folic Acid - Nature's Bounty
Each tablet contains: Folic Acid 400 mcg. Other Ingredients: Dicalcium Phosphate, Vegetable Stearic Acid, Croscarmellose, Silica, Vegetable Magnesium Stearate.

Folic Acid 400 mcg - Jamieson
Each tablet contains: Folate (as Folic Acid) 400 mcg.

Folic Acid Dophilus Plus B-12 - Dial Herbs
Two wafers contain: Folic Acid 800 mcg • Vitamin B12 400 mcg • Lactobacillus acidophilus • Lactobacillus plantarum • Lactobacillus bulgaricus • Lactobacillus casei 200 mcg.

For Men Only - Doctor's Best
Each tablet contains: L-Glycine 135 mg • L-Alanine 135 mg • L-Glutamic Acid 135 mg • Raw Prostate concentrate 100 mg • Saw Palmetto 100 mg • Golden Rod 50 mg • Pumpkin seed concentrate 10 mg • Vitamin E 10 IU • Zinc 5 mg • Flax Seed Oil 3 mg. See Editor's Note No. 14, page 1817.

Formula 100 - Puritan's Pride
Each tablet contains: Vitamin A (as retinyl palmitate and 20% as beta carotene) 10,000 IU • Vitamin C (as ascorbic acid and rose hips) 250 mg • Vitamin D (as cholecalciferol) 400 IU • Vitamin E (as d-alpha tocopheryl acid succinate) 150 IU • Thiamin (Vitamin B1; as thiamine mononitrate) 100 mg • Riboflavin (Vitamin B2) 100 mg • Niacin (as niacinamide) 100 mg • Vitamin B6 (as pyridoxine hydrochloride) 100 mg • Folic Acid 300 mcg • Vitamin B12 (as cyanocobalamin) 100 mcg • Biotin 100 mcg • Pantothenic Acid (as d-calcium pantothenate) 100 mg • Calcium (as calcium carbonate) 100 mg • Iron (as ferrous fumarate) 18 mg • Iodine (as kelp) 150 mcg • Magnesium (as magnesium oxide) 50 mg • Zinc (as zinc oxide) 15 mg • Selenium (as sodium selenate) 25 mcg • Copper (as cupric oxide) 0.5 mg • Manganese (as manganese sulfate) 6.1 mg • Chromium (as GTF chromium yeast) 200 mcg • Potassium (as potassium citrate) 10 mg • PABA (para-aminobenzoic acid) 100 mg • Choline Bitartrate 100 mg • Inositol 100 mg • Rutin 25 mg • Lemon Bioflavonoids 50 mg • Hesperidin 12.5 mg • Betaine Hydrochloride 30 mg • Octacosanol 50 mcg • Proprietary Blend: Alfalfa Leaf, Watercress, Parsley Leaf, Rice Bran, and Lecithin 5 mg.

Formula 560 - Immunity Today, LLC.
Each capsule contains: Vitamin C 30 mg • Coenzyme Q10 5 mg • Proprietary Blend of Transfer Factor derived from Bovine Colostrum 165 mg.

Formula 600 Plus for Men - Nature's Life
Two capsules contain: Saw Palmetto berry (Serenoa repens B.) 600 mg • Active Aminos (l-Glutamic Acid, Glycine & L-Alanine) 170 mg • Zinc (Picolinate) 15 mg • Pumpkin seed (Curcurbita pepo) 50 mg • Pygeum africanum H. bark extract [(150:1) equivalent to 300 mg whole herb] 2 mg • Burdock root (Arctium lappa L.) 5 mg • Cayenne fruit (Capsicum annuum L. var. annuum) 5 mg • Goldenseal root (Hydrastis canadensis L.) 5 mg • Gravel root (Eupatorium purpureum L.) 5 mg • Juniper berry (Juniperus oxycedrus L.) 5 mg • Marshmallow root (Althaea officinalis L.) 5 mg • Parsley leaf (Petroselinum crispum(Mill) Nym.ex. A.W. Hill) 5 mg • White Pond Lily root (Nymphaea odorata) 5 mg • Vitamin B6 (Pyridoxine HCI) 5 mg • Copper (Gluconate) 1 mg • Nature's Life Active Aminos is an exclusive free-form blend of l-Glutamic Acid, l-Alanine & Glycine.

Formula 75 - Futurebiotics
Vitamin C (Rose hips) 250 mg • Vitamin A (palmitate 10,000 IU, beta carotene 7500 IU) 17,500 IU • Vitamin E (natural) 150 IU • Vitamin D (cholecalciferol) 400 IU • Riboflavin 75 mg • Thiamin 75 mg • Vitamin B6 (pyridoxine HCl) 75 mg • Niacinamide 75 mg • Vitamin B12 (cyanocobalamin) 75 mcg • Folic Acid 400 mcg • Pantothenic Acid 75 mg • Biotin 75 mcg • Iron (chelate) 1.3 mg • Calcium (chelate) 20 mg • Magnesium (chelate) 10 mg • Iodine (kelp) 150 mcg • Selenium (chelate) 25 mcg • Zinc (chelate) 10 mg • Manganese (chelate) 1 mg • Copper (chelate) 1 mg • Molybdenum (chelate) 25 mcg • Chromium (picolinate) 25 mcg • Boron (chelate

complex) 0.5 mg • Potassium (chelate complex) 1.8 mg • Inositol 75 mg • Choline (bitartrate) 31 mg • Rutin 25 mg • Para Amino Benzoic Acid (PABA) 75 mg • Hesperidin complex 5 mg • Citrus bioflavonoid complex 25 mg • Betaine HCl 25 mg. In a Green Foods base of: Alfalfa, Barley & Chlorella.

ForSight - Resource Wellness
Three caplets contain: Vitamin A (89% as Beta Carotene) 15,000 IU • Vitamin C (Ascorbis Acid) 300 mg • Vitamin E Acetate 400 IU • Calcium 650 mg • Iron 0.74 mg • Sodium 10 mg • Lutein/Zeaxanthin 6 mg • Alpha Carotene 2 mg • Grape Seed extract 50 mg. Other Ingredients: Dicalcium Phosphate, Microcrystalline Cellulose, Croscramellose Sodium, Calcium Silicate, Magnesium Stearate, Stearic Acid, Hydroxypropyl Methylcellulose, Propylene Glycol, Polyethylene Glycol, Titanium Dioxide, FD&C Yellow No. 6 Lake, FD&C Red No. 40 Lake, FD&C Blue No. 2 Lake.

Forskolin Extract - PhytoPharmica
Each capsule contains: Coleus Forskohlii extract (standardized to contain 18% forskolin [9 mg per capsule]) 50 mg.

Forten-Zyme 550 - Atrium Inc.
Each tablet contains: Maxistrength Pancreatin 550 mg (which has been prepared by the lyophilization method to insure the preservation & concentration of natural occuring factors such as Amylase, Lipase & Protease enzyme activity. Proteolytic activity is ensured as specific Chymotrypsin & Trypsin content.). This formula is compounded in a buffered base of Amino Acids for maximum stability.
See Editor's Note No. 14, page 1817.

Fortified Pycnogenol - Puritan's Pride
Three tablets contain: Vitamin A (100% as Beta-Carotene) 25,000 IU • Calcium 340 mg • Selenium (from Selenium Yeast Chelate) 100 mcg • Pine bark extract (Pinus maritmus) 25 mg • Coenzyme Q-10 10 mg • Grape Seed extract (Vitis vinifera) 100 mcg • Whole Food Phytonutrient Blend: Broccoli (entire plant), Carrot (root), Spinach (leaf), Tomato (fruit) 120 mg.

FOS Daily - Health Smart Vitamins
Each caplet contains: Fructooligosaccharides (FOS) 500 mg • Lactobacillus acidophilus 180 mg • Lactobacillus bulgaricus 30 mg • Streptococcus thermophilus 30 mg.

Fosfree - Mission Pharmacal
Two tablets contain: Vitamin A 3,000 IU • Vitamin C 100 mg • Vitamin D (as Vitamin D3) 300 IU • Thiamine 9 mg • Riboflavin 4 mg • Niacin 21 mg • Vitamin B6 5 mg • Vitamin B12 4 mcg • Pantothenic Acid 2 mg • Calcium 351 mg • Iron 29 mg. Other Ingredients: Sugar, Polyethylene Glycol, Color, Croscarmellose Sodium, Povidone, Food Glaze, Cyanocobalamin, Magnesium Stearate, Yellow 5 Lake, Carnauba Wax, White Beeswax, Sodium Benzoate.

Four-In-One - Changes - TwinLab
Each capsule contains: Vitamin C (as Calcium Ascorbate) 120 mg • Aloe 200:1 concentrate leaf gel 200 mg • Wild Yam root (Mexican Yam) 50 mg • Cat's Claw root bark (Uncaria tomentosa) 300 mg • DHEA (Dehydroepiandrosterone) 5 mg. Other Ingredients: Gelatin, Magnesium Stearate, Calcium Stearate, and Silica.

Free Amino - Atrium Inc.
Full Spectrum - Composed of 22 Free Form Pure Amino Acids.

Free-B - Atrium Inc.
Each tablet contains: Vitamin B1 (Thiamine HCL) 100 mg • Vitamin B2 (Riboflavin) 50 mg • Vitamin B6 (Pyridoxine HCL) 50 mg • Vitamin B12 (Cyanocobalamin) 100 mcg • Niacinamide 150 mg • Pantothenic Acid 100 mg • Biotin 150 mcg • Calcium (Dicalcium Phosphate) 20 mg • Copper (Gluconate) 1 mg • Phosphorus

(Dicalcium Phosphate) 20 mg • Zinc (Aspartate) 30 mg.
In a base specially formulated to complement metabolic type concepts containing trace minerals in specific proportions. This product is completely yeast free & contains no sugar, starch, salt, corn, wheat or soy derivatives.

Fresh Green Black Walnut Wormwood Complex - Now
Two droppersful (16 ml) contain: Proprietary blend: Green Black Walnut hulls (Juglans species) 1.6 ml • Wormwood herb (Artemisia absinthium) • Clove buds (Carophyllus species) extracts. Other Ingredients: Grain Alcohol, Distilled Water.

Fresh Nettle Leaf - Gaia Herbs
Nettle leaf (2% caffeic acids and derivatives). Standardized Full Spectrum 100 mg of extract per capsule. Guaranteed Potency 50 mg of extract per capsule.

Friendly Flora - Nutri-Quest
Each capsule contains: Jerusalem Artichoke (rich source of Fructooligosaccharides) 200 mg • Cellulase 1200 CU • Lactobacillus Acidophilus 400 million • Acerola extract 25 mg • Rose Hips 25 mg • Bifidobacterium Bifidum 200 million • Bifidobacterium Longum 200 million • Protease 7500 HUT • Lipase 52 LU • Lactobacillus Casei 100 million • Lactobacillus Plantarum 100 million • Lactobacillus Rueteri 100 million • Lactobacillus Salicarius 100 million • Amylase 275 DU • EDS Mineral Mix: Kelp, Calcium Ascorbate, Magnesium Citrate, Zinc Gluconate, Manganese Gluconate. In a base of pure plant fiber.

From The Earth - The Vitamin Shoppe
Three tablets contain: Vitamin A 15000 IU • Vitamin D 400 IU • Vitamin E 200 IU • Vitamin C 1000 mg • Vitamin B1 25 mg • Vitamin B2 25 mg • Vitamin B6 25 mg • Vitamin B12 500 mcg • Vitamin B3 25 mg • Inositol 25 mg • Choline 50 mg • PABA 25 mg • Pantothenic Acid 25 mg • Biotin 50 mcg • Folic Acid 400 mcg • Citrus Bioflavonoids Complex 125 mg • Rutin 25 mg • Quercetin 25 mg • Hesperidin 25 mg • Calcium 200 mg • Magnesium 100 mg • Potassium 99 mg • Zinc 15 mg • Manganese 5 mg • Molybdenum 50 mcg • Iodine 150 mcg • Copper 500 mcg • Selenium 50 mcg • Chromium 200 mcg • Boron 1 mg • Silica 5 mg • RNA 35 mg • DNA 10 mg • Carotenoids 4 mg • Chlorophyll 4 mg • Borage, Flax Seed, and Sunflower Oils 200 mg • L-Glutathione 5 mg • Spirulina 1000 mg • Wheat Grass 100 mg • Barley Grass 100 mg • Chlorella 100 mg • Bee Pollen 100 mg • Korean Ginseng root 50 mg • Garlic 10 mg • Bee Propolis extract 10 mg • Royal Jelly 5 mg • Bromelain 50 mg • Betaine HCl 50 mg • Papain 50 mg • Amylase 5 mg • Lipase 5 mg • Cellulase 5 mg • Lactobacillus Acidophilus, B. bifidum, L-bulgaricus (dairy free) 50 mg • Oat Bran 50 mg • Apple Pectin 50 mg • A unique blend of: Echinacea, Milk Thistle, Goldenseal, Ginger root, Ginkgo Biloba, Capsicum 50 mg.

From The Sea - Nutrition Warehouse
Three capsules contain: Glucosamine Sulfate (Aminomonosaccharide) 1000 mg • Sea Cucumber (Beche De-Mer) 1000 mg • Shark Cartilage 500 mg.

From The Sea - Puritan's Pride
Three capsules contain: Glucosamine Sulfate (Aminomonosaccharide) 1000 mg • Sea Cucumber (Beche De-Mer) 1000 mg • Shark Cartilage 500 mg.

Fruit Max - Swanson
Two tablets contain: Apple fruit powder 80 mg • Apricot fruit powder 80 mg • Cherry fruit powder 80 mg • Lemon peel powder 80 mg • Orange peel powder 80 mg • Papaya powder 80 mg • Peach fruit powder 80 mg • Strawberry fruit powder 80 mg • Freeze-Dried Grape juice 50 mg • Freeze-Dried Orange juice 50 mg • Freeze-Dried Pineapple juice 50 mg • Prune juice powder 40 mg • Cranberry juice concentrate 20 mg.

Fruit4Life - Swanson
Two tablets contain: Apple fruit powder 80 mg • Apricot fruit powder 80 mg • Cherry fruit powder 80 mg • Lemon peel powder 80 mg • Orange peel powder 80 mg • Papaya powder 80 mg • Peach fruit powder 80 mg • Strawberry fruit powder 80 mg • Freeze-Dried Grape juice 50 mg • Freeze-Dried Orange juice 50 mg • Freeze-Dried Pineapple juice 50 mg • Prune juice powder 40 mg • Cranberry juice concentrate 20 mg.

Fruit-Easy - Progressive Labs
Two tablets contain: A blend of the following 1400 mg: Apples • Cranberry powder • Orange juice powder • Pineapple juice powder • Siberian Ginseng • Ginkgo Biloba • Peaches • Dates • Bromelain • Papain • Lipase • Amylase • Protease • Cellulase • Powdered Cellulose • Apple pectin • Citris pectin • Prune powder • Glucomannan • Lactobacillus Acidophilus • Calcium Gluconate & Green Tea

Fruitplex - HealthWatchers System
Apple • Lemon • Strawberry • Blueberry • Plum • Cantaloupe • Pear • Cherry • Grapefruit • Raspberry • Grape • Orange • Peach • Watermelon • Pineapple • Papaya

Fuel for Thought Neuro Nutrition - Nature's Plus
Two tablets contain: L-Glutamine free form amino acid 250 mg • Lecithin (Soya) 250 mg • RNA (Ribonucleic acid) 200 mg • L-Tyrosine free form amino acid 200 mg • L-Phenylalanine free form amino acid 100 mg • Phosphatidylcholine 100 mg • Raw Pituitary concentrate 25 mg • Vitamin B6 (Pyridoxine HCL) 10 mg. Sugar & starch free.
See Editor's Note No. 14, page 1817.

Full Spectrum Mineral Caps - Now
Four capsules contain: Vitamin D (as Cholecalciferol) 4000 IU • Calcium (from Hydroxapatite) 500 mg • Phosphorus (from Hydroxapatite) 193 mg • Iodine (from Kelp) 225 mcg • Magnesium (as Magnesium Oxide and Citrate) 500 mg • Zinc (as Amino Acid Chelate) 15 mg • Selenium (as l-Selenomethionine) 100 mcg • Copper (as Amino Acid Chelate) 2 mg • Manganese (as Amino Acid Chelate) 5 mg • Chromium (as Chromium Chelavite) 200 mcg • Molybdenum (as Amino Acid Chelate) 100 mcg • Potassium (as Amino Acid Chelate) 99 mg • Boron (as Amino Acid Chelate) 3 mg • Vanadium (as Amino Acid Chelate) 50 mcg. Other Ingredients: Gelatin (capsule), Rice Flour, Magnesium Stearate. Contains no sugar, yeast, corn, soy, wheat, gluten, milk, or preservatives.

Full Spectrum Minerals - Now
Each tablet contains: Calcium (Carbonate, Amino Acid Chelate, Citrate) 1000 mg • Magnesium (Oxide, Amino Acid Chelate, Citrate) 500 mg • Zinc (Amino Acid Chelate) 22.5 mg • Iron (Amino Acid Chelate) 20 mg • Copper (Amino Acid Chelate) 1 mg • Potassium (Proteinate) 99 mg • Manganese (Amino Acid Chelate) 5 mg • Selenium (L-Selenium Methionine) 50 mcg • Chromium (yeast-free, Proteinate) 100 mcg • Molybdenum (Amino Acid Chelate) 59 mcg • Vanadium (Amino Acid Chelate) 50 mcg • Iodine (Kelp) 150 mcg • L-Glutamic Acid (HCL) 50mg • Vitamin D (Cholecalciferol) 200 IU • Boron 3 mg.

FX-Chrysin - GEN
Each capsule contains: Chrysin 250 mg • LPC (Lysophosphatidyl Choline) 200 mg.

G.I. Gel: Gastro-Intestinal Tonic - The Herbalist
Slippery Elm bark• Marshmallow root.

G.I. Support - Now
Three capsules contain: Vitamin A (as Retinol Palmitate) 5000 IU • Vitamin B3 (as Niacinamide) 40 mg • Vitamin B5 (as Calcium Pantothenate) 50 mg • Biotin 1000 mcg • Folic Acid (Folate) 400 mcg • Zinc (as Zn Monomethionine) 15 mg • Selenium

(as Selenomethionine) 140 mcg • L-Glutamine 500 mg • Apple Pectin 300 mg • N-Acetyl Glucosamine (NAG) 250 mg • Methylsulfonylmethane (MSM) 250 mg • Deglycyrrhizinated Licorice (DGL) 100 mg • Licorice extract 4:1 root 100 mg • Cat's Claw extract 15:1 bark 100 mg • Ginger powder root 100 mg • Aloe Vera concentrate 200:1 leaf (equivalent to 5000 mg fresh Aloe Vera) 25 mg • Pepsin Enzymes NF 1:10000) 50 mg • Pepsin (2000 USP papaya) 50 mg.

G/C 1000 - Progressive Labs
Each capsule contains: Vitamin C (from manganese ascorbate) 60 mg • Manganese (from manganese ascorbate) 15 mg • Glucosamine Hydrochloride 750 mg • Chondroitin Sulfate 250 mg.
See Editor's Note No. 15, page 1817.

GABA - Source Naturals
Each tablet contains: GABA (Gamma amino butyric acid) 750 mg.

GABA - PhytoPharmica
Each capsule contains: Gamma-aminobutyric acid (GABA) 250 mg.

GABA Calm - Source Naturals
Each tablet contains: GABA (Gamma Amino Butyric Acid) 100 mg • Glycine 50 mg • Magnesium Taurinate (Yielding 3 mg of Elemental Magnesium) 40 mg • N-Acetyl-L-Tyrosine 25 mg.

GABA Complex - Puritan's Pride
Each capsule contains: GABA 500 mg • Inositol 3000 mg • Niacinamide 1000 mg.

GABA-Val - Progressive Labs
Each capsule contains: Gamma Amino Butyric Acid (GABA) 50 mg • Valerian root extract (Valeriana officinalis) 300 mg • Thiamine HCl (Vitamin B1) 25 mg • Niacinamide 25 mg • Magnesium (amino acid chelate) 25 mg • Inositol 175 mg • Lupulin (hops pollen) 50 mg • Passion flower (Passiflora incarnata) 25 mg • Glutamic Acid 25 mg • Brain tissue 25 mg.
See Editor's Note No. 14, page 1817.

Gainers Fuel (Anabolic Weight Gain Formula) - TwinLab
Each serving contains: Calories 531. Each serving also contains Branched Chain Amino Acids (including Peptide Bonded & Free Amino Acids) 21 g, Essential Vitamins, Minerals, Trace Elements, Key Metabolic Optimizers & Lipotropic Factors.

Gainers Fuel 1000 (Super Anabolic Weight Gain Formula) - TwinLab
Each serving contains: Calories 1000 • Predigested Proteins & Amino Acids (Complex Carbohydrates, Anabolic Branched Chain Amino Acids) • Vitamins & Minerals • Pharmaceutical Grade Pancreatic digests of Whey Protein (Lactalbumin) & Egg White Protein (Albumin) • Chromium 400 mcg • Boron • L-Carnitine • Beta-Carotene • Kreb's Cycle Mineral Complexes (including Citrates, Aspartates, Succinates & Alpha-Ketoglutarates).

Gainers Fuel 2500 - TwinLab
Whey & Egg White Proteins • Branched Chain Amino Acids (L-Leucine, L-Isoleucine & L-Valine) • Essential Vitamins & Minerals • Chromium Picolinate & L-Carnitine (100% predigested). Low in fat without high levels of medium chain triglycerides that may cause gastrointestinal upset.

Gall & Liver Tablets - Life Brand
Agrimony herb 100.1 mg • Goose Grass 100.1 mg • Horehound herb 72.8 mg • Senna leaf 18.2 mg • Woodruff herb 81.25 mg • Wormwood herb 18.2 mg • Yarrow 81.9 mg. Excipients: Corn Starch, Sodium Bicarbonate, Silicon Dioxide, Magnesium Stearate, Methyl Paraben, Propyl Paraben.

BRAND NAMES

Gallbladder Support - Amazon Support
Each capsule contains: Chanca Piedra • Boldo • Artichoke 4:1 Extract • Erva Tostao • Carqueja • Jurubeba.

Gallexier Herbal Bitters - Flora
Artichoke • Dandelion • "other bitter herbs."

Gamma Oryzanol - Source Naturals
Each tablet contains: Gamma Oryzanol 30 mg.

GammaFrac - Source Naturals
Each tablet contains: Famma Oryzanol 25 mg • FRAC (Ferulic Acid Complex) 50 mg.

Garcinia 1000 - Source Naturals
Two tablets contain: Citrin Garcinia cambogia extract [yielding 1,000 mg of (-) Hydroxycitric Acid as Calcium Hydroxycitrate] 2,000 mg • Chromium (150 mcg from ChromeMate GTF Yeast-Free Polynicotinate and 150 mcg from Yeast-Free Chromium Picolinate) 300 mcg.

Garcinia Cambogia Plus - Atrium Inc.
Each capsule contains: Garcinia cambogia (standardized to contain 50% Hydroxycitric Acid) 340 mg • Atractylodes 80 mg • Citrus aurantii 80 mg • Chromium Picolinate 500 mcg • Chromium Arginate 160 mcg. Contains no sugar, starch, salt, wheat, corn or soy derivatives.

Garlic - Centrum Focused Formulas
One capsule contains: Garlic powder (bulb) Allium sativum 300 mg • Allin (marker) allicin potential 45% 1300 mcg. Standardized to contain: Gamma Glytamyl-S allyl-cysteine (natural active) • Gamma Glytamyl-S-trans-1-propenyl-cysteine (natural active) • Gamma glutamyl-phenylalanine (natural active) • Activity Measure Angiotensin converting enzyme assay.

Garlic - Olympian Labs
Each capsule contains: Garlic 500 mg.

Garlic - Pharmanex
Each caplet contains: Garlic clove powder (Allium sativum) 650 mg. Other Ingredients: Excipients, Binders, Caplet Coating.

Garlic - Plus - Aspen Group, Inc.
Each tablet contains: High Potency Garlic (standardized to contain 2500 mcg of allicin) 300 mg • Enzyme Complex 60 mg • Rice Protein-Calcium complex 40 mg.

Garlic & Golden Seal - Nutrivention
Two fl oz contains: Garlic oil • Goldenseal root • Safflower oil • cold-pressed Olive oil • Tocopherol (natural Vitamin E).

Garlic (Allicin-Rich) - Life Brand
Garlic extract powder 500 mg (equivalent to 1500 mg of fresh Garlic cloves). Contains Allicin potential yield of 1.5 mg/g; Thiosulphonates 1.6 mg/g; Allicin 10 mg/g; Gamma Glutamylcysteines 20 mg/g. Excipients: Cellulose, Calcium Phosphate, Stearic Acid, Magnesium Stearate, aqueous base film coat.

Garlic Echinacea Goldenseal+ - Futurebiotics
Two tablets contain: Echinacea angustifolia leaf powder extract (standardized for 4% (5 mg) echinacosides) 125 mg • Echinacea purpurea leaf powder 80 mg • Echinacea angustifolia leaf powder 20 mg • Goldenseal root powder 225 mg • Garlic bulb powder extract (odorless) 200 mg • Chinese Cinnamon root powder 30 mg • Black Pepper bud powder 20 mg • Clove flower powder 50 mg • Astragalus root powder 50 mg • Ginger root powder 50 mg • Peppermint leaf powder 10 mg • Parsley leaf powder 100 mg • Chamomile flower powder 100 mg • Bayberry bark powder 100 mg • Cayenne fruit powder 25 mg • Barberry bark powder 50 mg • Myrrh resin powder 50 mg. Other ingredients: Dicalcium phosphate, Cellulose, Stearic acid, Magnesium stearate, Silica.

Garlic HP - PhysioLogics
Each tablet contains: Garlic bulb (10000 mcg Allicin/gram) 400 mg.

Garlic/Parsley Formula - Nature's Way
Two capsules contain: Proprietary Formula: Garlic bulb • Parsley herb. Other ingredients: Gelatin.

Garlic-Go! - Wakunaga of America
Each caplet contains: Aged Garlic Extract Powder (bulb) 1000 mg. Other Ingredients: Cellulose, Silica, Magnesium Stearate (vegetable source).

Garlic-Gold - Olympian Labs
Each caplet contains: Garlic extract (alium satium) 600 mg • Allicin 7200 mcg.

Garlicin - Nature's Way
Each tablet contains: Garlicin (alliinaise-rich garlic powder) 300 mg. Other Ingredients: Aqueous Coating Solution, Cellulose, Modified Cellulose Gum, Silica, Stearic Acid, Xylitol.

Garlicin HC - Nature's Way
One tablet contains: Calcium 26 mg • Cayenne pepper fruit 15 mg • Garlic bulb 259 mg • Hawthorn dried extract (19% oligomeric procyanidins) 25 mg • Rutin 12 mg • Vitamin E (d-alpha tocopheryl) 15 IU. Other Ingredients: Aqueous Coating Solution, Cellulose, Maltodextrin, Modified Cellulose Gum, Silica, Stearic Acid.

Garlinase 4000 - Enzymatic Therapy
Each tablet contains: Garlic extract, equal to 4000 mg of fresh garlic, standardized to contain a minimum of 3.4% (11000 mcg) of Allicin per tablet by a unique patented process to assure maximum Allicin production in your body 320 mg. Contains no sugar, salt, yeast, wheat, corn, soy, dairy products, coloring, flavoring, or preservatives.

GarliPure Daily Formula - Natrol
One vegetarian capsule contains: Garlic (Allium sativum) powdered extract bulb 600 mg containing: Gamma Glutamylcysteines 12000 mcg • Allicin 6000 mcg • Sulfur 4800 mcg • Thiosulfinates 1200 mcg • Allicin Yield 1200 mcg. Other ingredients: 100% Vegetarian capsule Shell made of Kosher Vegetable Cellulose & Water, Magnesium Stearate.

GarliPure Formula 500 - Natrol
Two tablets contain: Garlic (Allium sativum) powdered extract bulb 1000 mg containing: Gamma Glutamylcysteines 20000 mcg • Allicin 10000 mcg • Sulfur 8000 mcg • Thiosulfinates 1600 mcg • Allicin Yield 1500 mcg. Other ingredients: Dicalcium Phosphate, Microcrystalline Cellulose, Stearic Acid, Magnesium Stearate, aqueous base film coat.

GarliPure Maximum Allicin Formula - Natrol
One caplet contains: Garlic (Allium sativum) powdered extract bulb 600 mg containing: Gamma Glutamylcysteines 12000 mcg • Allicin 4800 mcg • Sulfur 3900 mcg • Thiosulfinates 3800 mcg • Allicin Yield 3600 mcg. Other ingredients: Microcrystalline Cellulose, Stearic Acid, Dicalcium Phosphate, Magnesium Stearate Silicon Dioxide, aqueous base film coat.

GarliPure Once Daily Potency - Natrol
One tablet contains: Garlic (Allium sativum) 600 mg Powdered extract bulb containing: Allicin 13800 mcg • Thiosulfinates 6060 mcg • Allicin Yield 6000 mcg • Gamma Glutamylcysteines

4800 mcg • Sulfur 3900 mcg. Other ingredients: Dicalcium Phosphate, Microcrystalline Cellulose, Croscarmellose Sodium, Silicon Dioxide, Stearic Acid, Magnesium Stearate.

GarliPure Organic Formula - Natrol
Two capsules contain: Garlic (Alium sativum), organically grown powdered extract bulb 1000 mg containing: Gamma Glutamylcysteines 15000 mcg • Allicin 10000 mcg • Sulfur 7000 mcg • Thiosulfinates 1600 mcg • Allicin Yield 1500 mcg. Other ingredients: 100% Vegetarian capsule Shell made of Kosher Vegetable Cellulose & Water, Silicon Dioxide, Magnesium Stearate.

GarliPure Selenium Plus Formula - Natrol
Each capsule contains: Selenium 67 mcg • Garlic (Allium sativum) powdered extract bulb 400 mg containing: Gamma Glutamylcysteines 8000 mcg • Allicin 4400 mcg • Sulfur 3200 mcg • Thiosulfinates 2040 mcg • Allicin Yield 2000 mcg. Other ingredients: Gelatin.

GarliPure Selenium Plus Formulas - Natrol
One capsule contains: Selenium 67 mcg • Garlic (Allium sativum) powdered extract bulb 400 mg containing: Gamma Glutamylcysteines 8000 mcg • Allicin 4400 mcg • Sulfur 3200 mcg • Thiosulfinates 2040 mcg • Allicin Yield 2000 mcg. Other ingredients:Gelatin.

Garlique - SunSource/Chattem Inc.
Each tablet contains: Garlic bulb powder (not less than 500 mcg of allicin yield) 400 mg. Other Ingredients: Dicalcium Phosphate, Microcrystalline Cellulose, Croscarmellose Sodium, Stearic Acid, Magnesium Stearate, Sodium Lauryl Sulfate, Colloidal Silicon Dioxide, Hydroxypropyl Methylcellulose Phthalate, Talc, Titanium Dioxide, Triacetin, Pharmaceutical glaze, (214-112). Contains no sugar, starch, yeast, caffeine, dairy or preservatives.

Garlite - Nature's Plus
Each Vegicap contains: Deodorized Garlic equivalent to a minimum of 2.5 times its weight in fresh garlic 500 mg. Contains no yeast, wheat, corn, soy, milk, salt, sugar or starch.

Garlitrin 4000 - PhytoPharmica
Each tablet contains: Garlic extract (Allium sativum) bulb extract (standardized to contain a minimum of 3.4% [11,000 mcg] of alliin per tablet) 320 mg.

Gastritix Formula - Nature's Way
Two capsules contain: Chamomile flower 62.5 mg • Fennel seed 237.5 mg • Ginger 237.5 mg • Marshmallow root 50 mg • Slippery Elm bark 125 mg • Wild Yam root 237.5 mg.
Other ingredients: Gelatin, Magnesium Stearate, Maltodextrin.

Gastro-Relief - PhytoPharmica
Each chewable tablet contains: Calcium Carbonate 250 mg • Deglycyrrhizinated Licorice (DGL) root extract (Glycyrrhiza glabra) 380 mg • Glycine (Amino Acid) 50 mg.
No added sugar or fructose. Contains no sugar, salt, yeast, wheat, corn, soy, dairy products, coloring, flavoring, or preservatives.

GastroSoothe - Enzymatic Therapy
Each tablet contains: Active ingredient: Calcium Carbonate 250 mg. Other ingredients: Deglycyrrhizinated Licorice (DGL) root extract (Glycyrrhiza glabra) 380 mg • Glycine (Amino Acid) 50 mg. No added sugar or fructose. Contains no sugar, salt, yeast, wheat, corn, soy, dairy products, coloring, flavoring or preservatives.

GastroSoothe Chocolate-Mint - Enzymatic Therapy
Each tablet contains: Active ingredient: Calcium Carbonate 250 mg • Deglycyrrhizinated Licorice (DGL) root extract (Glycyrrhiza glabra) 380 mg • Glycine (Amino Acid) 50 mg. No added sugar or fructose. Flavored with Dutch Cocoa powder, Creme Flavor, & Peppermint.

GBLVR - Nutri-Quest
Proprietary blend 500 mg: Bayberry • Red Beet root • Yellow Dock • Dandelion root • Fennel seeds • Peppermint • Ginger root • Wild Yam • Blessed Thistle • Garlic 500 mg. In a base of 6X tissue salts: Calc Fluor.

GEN Andro*Gen - GEN
Each capsule contains: Androstenedione 100 mg.

GEN CM Relief - GEN
Each capsule contains: CMO (Cetyl-Myristoleate) 500 mg.

GEN Multi*GenX - GEN
Each six capsules contain: Antioxidants:Vitamin C (Ascorbic Acid) 1000 mg • Vitamin E (natural d-Alpha Tocopherol) 40 IU • Propanthocyanidins (Grape seed extract) 25 mg • Citrus bioflavonoids 100 mg • Lipoic Acid 50 mg. Vitamins: Vitamin A (Retinol Palmitate) 5000 IU • Vitamin A (Beta Carotene) 20000 IU • Vitamin D (as Vitamin D3)(Cholecalciferol) 400 IU • Vitamin B1 (Thiamine HCL) 50 mg • Vitamin B2 (Riboflavin) 50 mg • Vitamin B3 (Niacinamide) 50 mg • Vitamin B5 (Calcium d-Pantothenate) 50 mg • Vitamin B6 (Pyroxine HCL) 50 mg • Vitamin B12 (Cyanocobalamin) 40 mcg • Folic Acid 400 mcg • Biotin 300 mcg. Minerals: Calcium (from Citrate) 400 mg • Magnesium (from Citrate) 200 mg • Iron (from Fe glycinate) 9 mg • Potassium (from Chloride) 150 mg • Zinc (from Monomethionate-OptiZinc) 15 mg • Manganese (from Citrate) 10 mg • Iodine (from Kelp) 100 mcg • Copper (from Co Gluconate) 270 mcg • Chromium (from Cr Nicotinate/Glycinate) 200 mcg • Molybdenum (from Sodium Molybdate) 150 mcg • Selenium (from Amino Acid Chelate) 200 mcg. Lean Muscle Enhancement: RNA (Sodium Ribonucleic Acid) 150 mg • Inositol 40 mg • L-Carnitine 35 mg • Taurine (HCL) 75 mg • L-Glutamine 25 mg • MSM (Methyl Sulfonylmethane) 100 mg • Coenzyme Q10 (Ubiquinone) 30 mg.

GEN Pyruvate Burn - GEN
Each capsule contains: MED-PRO licensed Pyruvate, from a Pyruvic Acid Complex with Dihydroxyacetone 500 mg. Pyruvic Acid is stabalized with Calcium, Sodium, Potassium or Magnesium to form Pyruvate.

GEN Thermogen - GEN
Two capsules contain: Ma Huang extract standardized at 6%: 334 (334 x .06 = 20 mg) • Caffeine 200 mg • Naringin 40 mg • White Willow bark extract 75 mg • Potassium (Phosphate) 50 mg • Cayenne 35 mg.

Genistein - Source Naturals
Four tablets contain: Soybean powder 4000 mg • Genistein 11.6 mg • Daidzein 42.4 mg • Glycitein 32 mg • Total Isoflavones 86 mg.

Geritol Complete - SmithKline Beecham
Each tablet contains: Vitamin A 6000 IU • Vitamin C 60 mg • Vitamin D (Vitamin D3, Cyanocobalamin) 400 IU • Vitamin E Acetate 30 IU • Vitamin K (Vitamin K1) 25 mcg • Thiamin Mononitrate (Vitamin B1) 1.5 mg • Riboflavin (Vitamin B2) 1.7 mg • Niacin (Vitamin B3, Niacinamide Ascorbate) 20 mg • Vitamin B6 (Pyridoxine HCl) 2 mg • Folate (Folic Acid, Folacin) 0.4 mg • Vitamin B12 6 mcg • Biotin 0.045 mcg • Pantothenic Acid (Calcium D-Pantothenate) 10 mg • Calcium 162 mg • Carbonyl Iron 18 mg • Phosphorus (Dicalcium Phosphate) 125 mg • Iodine (Potassium Iodide) 174 mcg • Magnesium Oxide 100 mg • Zinc Oxide 15 mg • Selenium (Sodium Selenate) 15 mg • Copper (Cupric Oxide) 2 mg • Manganese Sulfate 2.5 mg • Chromium Chloride 15 mcg • Molybdenum (Sodium Molybdate) 15 mg • Chloride 35 mg • Potassium Chloride 40 mg • Nickel (Nickelous Sulfate) 5 mcg • Tin (Stannous Chloride)10 mcg • Silicon Yeast 80 mg • Vanadium (Sodium Chloride) 10 mcg. Other Ingredients: Microcrystalline Cellulose, Gelatin, Hydrolized Protein,

B R A N D   N A M E S

Beta Carotene, Stearic Acid, Crospovidone, Hydroxypopyl Methylcellulose, Hydroxypropyl Cellulose, Glycerides of Stearic and Palmitic Acid, Polyethylene Glycol, Magnesium Stearate, Silica, Titanium Dioxide, FD&C Blue #2, FD&C Red #40, FD&C Yellow #6.
See Editor's Note No. 3, page 1816.

Gest-Tonic - The Herbalist
Angelica root • Gentian root • Oregon Grape root • Bayberry root bark • Fennel seed • Prickly Ash bark • Ginger root.

GH Fuel - TwinLab
Six capsules contain: L-Ornithine Alpha-Ketoglutarate 3000 mg • Ma Huang extract (standardized for 6% Ephedrine) 334 mg • Kola extract (standardized for 12% Caffeine) 1000 mg • L-Carnitine 100 mg • Chromium (from Chromic Fuel patented Chromium Picolinate) 400 mcg.

GH Fuel Cocktail - TwinLab
Two tablespoonfuls contain: L-Arginine 6 g • L-Ornithine 1 g • Taurine 250 mg • L-Carnitine 200 mg • Beta-Carotene 10000 IU • Vitamin D 100 IU • Vitamin C 1000 mg • Natural Vitamin E 400 IU • Vitamin B1 1.5 mg • Vitamin B2 1.9 mg • Vitamin B6 2 mg • Niacinamide 20 mg • Vitamin B12 12 mcg • Pantothenic Acid 500 mg • Folic Acid 400 mcg • Biotin 300 mcg • Choline 700 mg • Inositol 250 mg • Calcium (from KrebMins Calcium) 250 mg • Magnesium (from KrebMins Magnesium) 100 mg • Potassium (from KrebMins Potassium) 325 mg • Zinc (from Zinc Picolinate & KrebMins Zinc) 15 mg • Manganese (from KrebMins Manganese) 2 mg • Copper (from KrebMins Copper) 1 mg • Iodine (from Kelp) 10 mcg • Molybdenum (from KrebMins Molybdenum) 50 mcg • Chromium (from Chromium Picolinate) 100 mcg • Selenium (from KrebMins Selenium) 50 mcg • Boron (from Tri-Boron citrate, Aspartate & Glycinate) 1.5 mg. Natural orange flavor 100%.

GH Release - Nature's Plus
Two capsules contain: L-Ornithine free form amino acid 500 mg • L-Arginine free form amino acid 150 mg • Raw Pituitary concentrate 100 mg • Vitamin B6 (Pyridoxine HCL) 50 mg. Contains no yeast, wheat, corn, soy, milk, salt, sugar or starch.
See Editor's Note No. 14, page 1817.

GH3 (GH-3, GH 3) - Gero Vita
Each tablet contains: Hypericum perforatum extract (0.3% hypericin) 400 mg • 2-Dimethyl Aminoethanol Bitartrate (DMAE) 100 mg • Calcium Carbonate 100 mg • Para-aminobenzoic Acid (PABA) 50 mg • Thiamine Mononitrate 50 mg • Riboflavin 50 mg • Acorbyl Palmitate 50 mg • Ginkgo Biloba 50 mg • Pyridoxine HCL 25 mg • Niacin 10 mg • Zinc Picolinate 3 mg • L-Glutathione 2 mg • Chromium Polynicotinate 0.1 mg • Folic Acid 400 mcg • Selenium (amino acid chelated) 50 mcg • Cobalamin 10 mcg • Beta-Carotene 2000 IU • Vitamin E 100 IU.

GH3XL - HealthWatchers System
L-Glutamic Acid • L-Tyrosine • L-Taurine • Glucosamine HCL • Choline Bitartrate "needed to form the neurotransmitter acetylcholine" • Magnesium • Vitamin B6 • Vitamin Bee pollen • Kelp • Dulse • Irish Moss • Ginseng • Nettles • Alfalfa • Fo-Ti • Pau d'Arco • Fennel Seed • Schizandra • Barley Grass • Acacia Gum • Saussurea • Cat's Claw • Ginger • Licorice.

Ginger - Leiner Health Products
Each softgel contains: Ginger extract (Zingiber officinale) root 125 mg. Other Ingredients: Canola Oil, Gelatin, Glycerin, Yellow Beeswax, Lecithin, Caramel, Turmeric, Titanium Dioxide, Red 40, Annatto, Blue 1.

Ginger - Nature's Way
Two capsules contain: Ginger 1.1 g. Other Ingredients: Gelatin.

Ginger - Pharmanex
Each capsule contains: Ginger (Zingiber officinalis) (root extract) (20:1) 125 mg. Other Ingredients: Soybean Oil, Gelatin, Purified Water, Glycerin, Beeswax, Carob.

Ginger & Curcumin Joint-Ease - Nature's Life
Four capsules contain: Ginger root (Zingiber officinale) 1300 mg • Curcumin [from Turmeric root (Curcuma longa) providing 90-95% Curcuminoids] 1300 mg.

Ginger Aid - Traditional Medicinals
Ginger rhizome • Blackberry leaf • Stevia leaf • natural Lemon flavor.

Gingerall - Enzymatic Therapy
Each capsule contains: Ginger root extract (Zingiber officinale) standardized to contain 20% pungent compounds calculated as 6-Gingerol & 6-Shogaol 100 mg. Contains no sugar, salt, yeast, wheat, corn, dairy products, flavoring, or preservatives.

GingerMax - PhytoPharmica
Each capsule contains: Ginger (Zingiber officinale) root extract (standardized to contain 20% pungent compounds calculated as 6-Gingerol and 6-Shogaol) 100 mg.

Ginkai - Lichtwer Pharma
Each tablet contains: LI 1370 Ginkgo Biloba leaf extract, standardized to 25% ginkgo flavonoids & 6% terpenoids 50 mg.
See Editor's Note No. 8, page 1816.

Ginkgo- 24 - Source Naturals
Each tablet contains: Ginkgo Biloba leaf extract (50:1) (Yielding 24% Ginkgo Flavone Glycosides and 6% Terpene Lactones from 2,000 mg of Ginkgo biloba leaf) 40 mg.

Ginkgo 5 - Pharmline
Active Ingredients: Ginkgo Biloba extract 24/6, standardized to not less than 24% total Ginkgo flavone glycosides & not less than 6% total terpene lactones.

Ginkgo Alert Formula - PhysioLogics
Each capsule contains: Niacin 5 mg • Vitamin B6 (Pyridoxine HCI) 5mg • Vitamin B12 (Cyanocobalamin) 250 mcg • DMAE 150 mg • L-Glutamine 150 mg • L-Pyroglutamic Acid 100 mg • L-Tyrosine 100 mg • Choline (Bitartrate) 50 mg • Ginkgo leaf (24% Ginkgo Flavonglycosides, 9.6 mg/ 6% Terpene Lactones, 2.4 mg) 40 mg • Panax ginseng (14% Ginsenosides, 3.5 mg) 25 mg.

Ginkgo B - Metabolic Response Modifiers
Each capsule contains: Ginkgo biloba extract (100:1) 60 mg.

Ginkgo Biloba - Centrum Herbals
One capsule contains: Ginkgo Biloba leaf extract 60 mg. Standardized to contain (based on extract weight): Ginkgo Flavone glycosides (marker) 24%, Terpene Lactones (marker) 6%, ginkgolide A (natural active), Ginkgolide B (natural active), Amentoflavone (natural active). Activity measure: GABA Central binding assay. Other Ingredients: Sucrose, Cellulose, Lactose, Monohydrate, Dibasic Calcium Phosphate, Hydroxypropyl Cellulose, Ethylcellulose, Castor Oil, Flavor Extractives of St. John's Bread, Glucose, Caramel color, Silicon Dioxide, Sodium Lauryl Sulfate, Propylene Glycol, Tianium Dioxide.
See Editor's Note No. 8, page 1816.

Ginkgo Biloba - Nature's Resource
Each capsule contains: Ginkgo Biloba leaf extract standardized to 24% Ginkgo flavone glycosides 60 mg. Other Ingredients: Rice Flour, Gelatin, and Water. No artifical colors, flavors, or preservatives.
See Editor's Note No. 8, page 1816.

Ginkgo Biloba - Sundown Vitamins
Two capsules contain: Ginkgo Biloba extract leaf 40.0 mg • Ginkgo Biloba leaf 400.0 mg.
See Editor's Note No. 8, page 1816.

Ginkgo Biloba - Celestial Seasonings
Two capsules contain: Proprietary Blend, 1700 mg: Ginkgo Biloba (leaves), Ginkgo Biloba (standardized extract). Other ingredients: May contain one or more of the following: Dicalcium phosphate, gelatin, rice flour, stearic acid, magnesium stearate, and silicon dioxide. One serving size is equivalent to: Ginkgo Biloba 120 mg standardized to 24% ginkgoflavonone glycosides and 6% ginkgolides.

Ginkgo Biloba - CVS
Each softgel contains: Ginkgo Biloba extract (standardized to 24% Flavone Glyosides; 6% Terpene Lactones) 60 mg. Other Ingredients: Soybean Oil, Gelatin, Purified Water, Glycerin, Yellow Beeswax, Lecithin, Annatto, Titanium Dioxide, FD&C Yellow #5, FD&C Blue #1, FD&C Red #40.

Ginkgo Biloba - Herbal Harvest, Inc.
Each tablet contains: Ginkgo Biloba extract (Standardized for a minimum of 24% Ginkgo Flavone Glycosides and 6% terpenes) 30 mg.

Ginkgo Biloba - Jamieson
Each tablet contains: Ginkgo extract (50:1) (Ginkgo biloba) (leaf) (24% flavoglycosides) 40 mg.

Ginkgo Biloba - Natrol
Each capsule contains: Ginkgo Biloba leaf 50:1 extract (24% Ginkgo Flavonglycosides) (6% Terpene Lactone) 120 mg.

Ginkgo Biloba - Nature's Bounty
Each tablet contains: Ginkgo Biloba extract 30 mg. Other Ingredients: Dicalcium Phosphate, Cellulose, Vegetable Stearic Acid, Cellulose Coating, Silica, Vegetable Magnesium Stearate.

Ginkgo Biloba - Now
Each Vcaps contains: Ginkgo Biloba extract (50:1 standardized extract containing 24% ginkgoflavonglycosides) 120 mg • Gotu Kola (Centella asiatica) (leaf) 200 mg • Siberian Ginseng (Eleutherococcus senticosus) (root) 150 mg. Contains no yeast, wheat, soy, milk, sugar, salt, preservatives, caffeine.

Ginkgo Biloba - Olympian Labs
Each capsule contains: Ginkgo Biloba extract 120 mg.

Ginkgo Biloba - Puritan's Pride
Each tablet contains: Ginkgo Biloba Extract (standardized for a minumum of 24% Ginkgo Flavone Glycosides and 6% terpenes) 60 mg. Other Ingredients: Dicalcium Phosphate, Cellulose (Plant Origin), Vegetable Stearic Acid, Cellulose Coating, Croscarmellose, Silica, Vegetable Magnesium Stearate. Contains no yeast, wheat, gluten, milk or milk derivatives, lactose, sugar, preservatives, soy, artificial color or flavor, sodium (less than 5 mg per serving).

Ginkgo Biloba (50:1 extract) - Atrium Inc.
Each capsule contains: Ginkgo Biloba, 50:1 extract (24% Ginkgocides) 60 mg. Contains no sugar, starch, salt, wheat, corn, milk, yeast or soy.

Ginkgo Biloba 24% - Swanson
Each capsule contains: Ginkgo Biloba leaf extract (24% flavone glycosides, 6% terpene lactones) 60 mg.

Ginkgo Biloba 24% Standardized Extract - Now
Each capsule contains: Ginkgo Biloba leaf powder 300 mg • Ginkgo Biloba extract (50:1 standardized extract containing 24% ginkgoflavonglycosides) 60 mg. Other Ingredients: Stearic Acid.

Ginkgo Biloba 40 mg - Leiner Health Products
Each tablet contains: Ginkgo Biloba extract (Ginkgo biloba) leaf 40 mg. Other Ingredients: Calcium Carbonate, Maltodextrin, Cellulose, Hydroxypropyl Methylcellulose, Polyethylene Glycol 3350, Crospovidone, Silicon Dioxide, Hydroxypropyl Cellulose, Titanium Dioxide, Magnesium Stearate, Yellow 5 Lake, Polysorbate 80, Yellow 6 Lake, Blue 2 Lake, Sodium Citrate.
See Editor's Note No. 8, page 1816.

Ginkgo Biloba 60 mg - Leiner Health Products
Each caplet contains: Ginkgo Biloba extract (Ginkgo biloba) leaf 60 mg. Other Ingredients: Calcium Carbonate, Cellulose, Maltodextrin, Hydroxypropyl Methylcellulose, Silicon Dioxide, Polyethylene Glycol 3350, Croscarmellose Sodium, Hydroxypropyl Cellulose, Yellow 5 Lake, Blue 1 Lake, Pharmaceutical Glaze, Crospovidone, Magnesium Stearate, Polysorbate 80, Titanium Dioxide.

Ginkgo Biloba 60 mg - Puritan's Pride
Each tablet contains: Ginkgo Biloba extract (Standardized for a minimum of 24% Ginkgo Flavone Glycosides and 6% terpenes) 60 mg. Other Ingredients: Dicalcium Phosphate, Cellulose (Plant Origin), Vegetable Stearic Acid, Cellulose Coating, Croscarmellose, Silica, Vegetable Magnesium Stearate.

Ginkgo Biloba Double Strength - Now
Each Vcap contain: Ginkgo Biloba extract leaf (50:1 standardized extract containing 24% ginkgoflaconglycosides) 120 mg • Gotu Kola (Centella Asiatica) leaf 200 mg • Siberian Ginseng (Eleutherococcus Senticoscus) root 150 mg. Other Ingredients: Stearic Acid. Contains no yeast, wheat, corn, soy, milk, sugar, salt, preservatives, or caffeine.

Ginkgo Biloba Extract - MotherNature.com
Each capsule contains: Ginkgo Biloba extract 50:1 (Standardized to 24% [14.4 mg] Flavonglycosides, 6% [3.6 mg] Terpene Lactones and 0.8% [0.48] Ginkgolide B) 60 mg. Other Ingredients: Gelatin, Rice Powder, Magnesium Stearate, and Silica.
See Editor's Note No. 8, page 1816.

Ginkgo Biloba Extract - Nature's Bounty
Each tablet contains: Ginkgo Biloba extract (Standardized for a minimum of 24% Ginkgo Flavone Glycosides and 6% terpenes) 30 mg. Other Ingredients: Dicalcium Phosphate, Cellulose (Plant Origin), Vegetable Stearic Acid, Cellulose Coating, Silica, Vegetable Magnesium Stearate.
See Editor's Note No. 8, page 1816.

Ginkgo Biloba Extract - The Vitamin Shoppe
Each capsule contains: Ginkgo Biloba leaf standardized to 24% ginkgoflavoglycosides and 6% ginkgolides-bilobalides.

Ginkgo Biloba Extract - Now
Each dropperful (0.8 ml) contains: Ginkgo Biloba extract 0.8 ml. Other Ingredients: Gotu Kola (Centella Asiatica); Siberian Ginseng (Eleutherococcus Senticosus); in a base of Distilled Water, Vegetable Glycerine, and Grain Alcohol.

Ginkgo Biloba Plus - Wakunaga of America
Each capsule contains: Aged Garlic Extract powder (bulb) 200 mg • Siberian Ginseng Extract 5:1 (root) 80 mg • Ginkgo Biloba Extract 50:1 (leaf) standardized to 24% ginkgoflavonglycosides & 6% terpene lactones 40 mg. Other Ingredients: Cellulose, Magnesium Stearate (vegetable source).
See Editor's Note No. 8, page 1816.

Ginkgo Biloba/Gotu Kola - Futurebiotics
One capsule contains: Ginkgo Biloba leaf powder extract (standardized for 24% (29 mg) ginkgo heterosides) 120 mg • Gotu Kola leaf powder extract (standardized for 16% (32 mg) triterpenes) 200 mg. Other ingredients: Gelatin, Water.

Ginkgo Biloba-24% - Enzymatic Therapy
Each capsule contains: Ginkgo Biloba Leaves Extract (Ginkgo biloba folia) standardized to contain 24% ginkgoflavonglycosides, 6% terpene lactones, and 2% bilobalide. Contains no sugar, salt, yeast, wheat, corn, soy, dairy products, coloring, flavoring or preservatives. See Editor's Note No. 8, page 1816.

Ginkgo Booster - Puritan's Pride
Two tablets contain: Ginkgo Biloba extract (24%) 60 mg • L-Glutamine 100 mg • Lecithin 100 mg • L-Tyrosine 50 mg • Choline (Bitartrate) 100 mg • DMAE (2-Di Methylaminothanol) 40 mg • Vitamin B1 (Thiamine HCl) 20 mg • Vitamin B2 (Riboflavin) 20 mg • Vitamin B12 (Sobalamin/Dibencozide) 50 mcg • Niacin 10 mg • Niacinamide 40 mg • Pantothenic Acid (Calcium d-Pantothenate) 50 mg • Folic Acid 200 mcg • Biotin 50 mcg • Inositol 20 mg • Vitamin C (Ascorbic Acid) 50 mg • Iodine 50 mcg • Betaine HCl 20 mg. In a base of Fo-Ti and Siberian Ginseng.

Ginkgo DHA Mind - The Vitamin Shoppe
Each capsule contains: Ginkgo Biloba leaf 24% ginkgoflavoglycosides 6% terpene 60 mg • DHA 50 mg.

Ginkgo Energizer - The Vitamin Shoppe
Each capsule contains: Ginkgo Biloba leaf standardized to 24% ginkgoflavoglycosides 6% ginkgolides-bilobalides 60 mg • CoQ10 30 mg.

Ginkgo Neuro-Mind - The Vitamin Shoppe
Each tablet contains: Vitamin B12 (as cyanocobalamin) 0.25 mcg • Vitamin B6 (as pyridoxine HCl) 10 mg • Ginkgo Biloba (Ginkgo biloba) leaf standardized to 24% ginkgoflavoglycosides 6% terpene lactones 50 mg • Phosphatidylserine (LECI-PS) 50 mg • DHA (Docosahexaenoic acid) (Neuromins) 50 mg. No yeast, corn, wheat, sugar, salt, starch, gluten, soy, milk, dairy, eggs, fish, citrus, preservatives, artificial colors or flavors added.

Ginkgo Phytosome - PhytoPharmica
Each capsule contains: Ginkgo Phytosome 80 mg.

Ginkgo Sharp - Celestial Seasonings
Two capsules contain: Vitamin B3 (as niacinamide) 40 mg • Proprietary Blend, 930 mg: Ginkgo Biloba (leaf), Ginkgo Biloba (standardized extract), DHA (50 mg as docohexaenoic acid). Other Ingredients: May contain one or more of the following: Dicalcium phosphate, gelatin, rice flour, stearic acid, magnesium stearate, and silicon dioxide. This product contains no artificial colors, flavors, or preservatives. One serving size is equivalent to: Ginkgo Biloba 120 mg standardized to 24% ginkgoflavonone glycosides and 6% ginkgolides.

Ginkgo/Gotu Kola - Gaia Herbs
Ginkgo and Gotu Kola standardized for 12% flavonoid glycosides & 2.5% triterpenoids. Standardized Full Spectrum 100 mg of extract per capsule. Guaranteed Potency 50 mg of extract per capsule.

Ginkgo-Combo Ginkgo Biloba Complex in Vegetarian Capsules - Nature's Plus
Two vegicaps contain: Ginkgo Biloba (8:1 extract Ginkgoaceae) 240 mg • Capsicum fruit 160 mg • Gotu Kola root 160 mg • Vitamin E natural 100 IU. Naturally rich in the flavonoids & bioflavonoids Quercetin, Kaempferol, Ginkgetin, Bilobetin, Isoginkgetin & Isorhamnetin. Contains no yeast, wheat, corn, soy, milk, salt, sugar or starch.

Ginkgo-Go! - Wakunaga of America
Each caplet contains: Ginkgo Biloba Standardized Extract 50:1 (leaf) standardized with 24% Ginkgo flavonglycosides & 6% Terpene lactones 120 mg. Other Ingredients: Cellulose, Vegetable Starch, Magnesium Stearate (vegetable source), Silica. See Editor's Note No. 8, page 1816.

Ginkgold - Nature's Way
Each tablet contains: Egb 761 Ginkgo Biloba leaf extract; standardized to 24% Ginkgo flavone glycosides & 6% terpene lactones 60 mg. See Editor's Note No. 8, page 1816.

Ginkgolidin - PhytoPharmica
Each capsule contains: Ginkgo Biloba leaves extract (Ginkgo biloba folia; standardized to contain 24% ginkgoflavonglycosides, 6% terpene lactones & 2% bilobalide) 40 mg. See Editor's Note No. 8, page 1816.

Ginko Biloba - HealthWatchers System
Two capsules contain: Standard Ginkgo Biloba 120 mg • Ginko Biloba Powder equivalent to 6000 mg.

Ginkoba - Pharmaton
Each tablet contains: Standardized Ginkgo Biloba leaf extract (50:1) 40 mg. Other Ingredients: Hydroxypropyl Methylcellulose, Lactose, Talc, Polyethylene Glycol, Magnesium Stearate, Titanium Dioxide, Synthetic Iron Oxides. Contains no sugar, caffeine, or artificial stimulants. See Editor's Note No. 8, page 1816.

Ginkoba M/E - Pharmaton
Each capsule contains: Panax Ginseng Extract (standardized G115) 100 mg • Ginkgo Biloba Extract (standarized GK501) 60 mg. Other Ingredients: Mannitol, Gelatin, Sicon dioxide, Magnesium Stearate.

Ginsana - Pharmaton
Each capsule contains: Standardized G115 Ginseng root extract (Panax Ginseng, C.A. Meyer) 100 mg. Other Ingredients: Sunflower oil, gelatin, glycerin, lecithin, beeswax, chlorophyll. Contains no sugar, caffeine, or artificial stimulants. See Editor's Note No. 9, page 1817.

Ginsana Chewy Squares - Pharmaton
Each chewy square contains: Vitamin C • Standardized G115 Ginseng root extract (Panax Ginseng, C.A. Meyer) 50 mg. Other Ingredients: Sucrose, Glucose, Palm kernel oil, Gelatin, Citric Acid, Ascorbic Acid, Lecithin, Natural Flavoring & Coloring.

GinsanaSport - Boehringer Ingelheim Pharmaceuticals, In
Each capsule contains: Standardized G-115 Panax Ginseng Extract (Panax Ginseng, C.A. Meyer) (root) 200 mg. Other Ingredients: Sunflower oil, gelatin, glycerin, beeswax, lecithin, turmeric, titanium dioxide, FD&C Green No. 3. Contains no sugar, caffeine, or atificial stimulants.

Ginseng - Celestial Seasonings
Two capsules contain: Proprietary Blend, 180 mg: Panax Ginseng (root), Panax Ginseng (standardized extract). Other ingredients: May contain one or more of the following: Dicalcium phosphate, gelatin, rice flour, stearic acid, magnesium stearate and silicon dioxide. This product contains no artificial colors, flavors or preservatives. One serving size is equivalent to: Panax Ginseng 200 mg standardized to 7% ginsenosides. See Editor's Note No. 9, page 1817.

Ginseng - Centrum Herbals
One capsule contains: Ginseng root extract 100 mg. Standardized to contain (based on extract weight): Total Ginenosides (marker) 7.0%, Ginsenoside Rb1 (natural active), Ginsenoside Rg1 (natural active). Activity measure: Phospholipase A2 enzymatic assay. Other ingredients: Dibasic Calcium Phosphate, Cellulose, Lactose, Monohydrate, Hydroxypropyl Cellulose, Ethylcellulose, Castor Oil, Gelatin, Silicon Dioxide, Sodium Lauryl Sulfate, Propylene Glycol, Titanium Dioxide. See Editor's Note No. 9, page 1817.

Some Brand Name Natural Products - What they Contain
www.NaturalDatabase.com contains MANY more listings than appear here.

Ginseng - Leiner Health Products
Each softgel contains: Ginseng extract (Panax ginseng) root 100 mg. Other Ingredients: Gelatin, Soybean Oil, Vegetable Oil, Lecithin, Palm Oil, Glycerin, Sorbitol, Yellow Beeswax, Hydrogenated Coconut Oil, Titanium Dioxide, Yellow 5, Blue 1, Red 40, Green 3, Chlorophyll.

Ginseng Complex - Puritan's Pride
Each capsule contains: American Panax Ginseng 200 mg • Korean Panax Ginseng 200 mg • Red Chinese Panax Ginseng 200 mg • Siberian Ginseng 200 mg • Royal Jelly 200 mg.

Ginseng Energy - Celestial Seasonings
Two capsules contain: Vitamin E (as d-alpha tocopherol acetate) 10 IU • Vitamin B12 (as cyanocobalamin) 30 mcg • Proprietary Blend, 1590 mg: Siberian Ginseng (root), Siberian Ginseng (standardized extract), Panax Ginseng (root), Panax Ginseng (standardized extract), Coenzyme Q10 (as ubiquinone) 10 mg. Other ingredients: May contain one or more of the following: Dicalcium phosphate, gelatin, rice flour, stearic acid, magnesium stearate, and silicon dioxide. This product contains no artificial colors, flavors or preservatives. One serving size is equivalent to: Panax Ginseng 200 mg standardized to 7% ginsenosides, Siberian Ginseng 250 mg standardized to 0.8% eleutherosides.

Ginseng Extract - The Vitamin Shoppe
Each softgel contains: 100 mg Panax Ginseng extract standardized for 8% ginsenosides.

Ginseng Phytosome - PhytoPharmica
Each capsule contains: Panax Ginseng root phytosome (bound to phosphatidylcholine under patent) 50 mg.

Ginseng/Aloe Capsules - Aloe Farms
Siberian Ginseng powder 150 mg, Aloe Vera powder 100 mg.

Ginseng/Collagen Firming Creme - Derma E
Ginseng • Collagen (contains 22 amino acids).

Ginseng-Go! - Wakunaga of America
Each capsule contains: Korean Ginseng Extract Powder (root) 300 mg. Other Ingredients: Cellulose, Magnesium Stearate (vegetable source).

Ginseng-Source Naturals - Source Naturals
Each tablet contains: Panax Ginseng root 648 mg.

Ginseven - Leiner Health Products
Each caplet contains: American Ginseng extract (Panax quinquefolius) root 75 mg • Ashwagandha extract (Withania somnifera) root 50 mg • Notoginseng extract (Panax notoginseng) root 50 mg • Panax Ginseng extract (Panax ginseng) root 100 mg • Schisandra extract (Schisandra chinensis) fruit 75 mg • Siberian Ginseng extract (Eleutherococcus senticosus) root 75 mg • Suma extract (Pfaffia paniculata) root 100 mg. Other Ingredients: Cellulose, Dicalcium Phosphate, Stearic Acid, Magnesium Stearate, Silicon Dioxide, Sodium Starch Glycolate, Polyethylene Glycol 3350.

GinSting - Futurebiotics
Two tablets contain: Korean Ginseng 1000 mg • Bee Pollen 500 mg.

GinSwee Tea - HerbaSway
Ginger • Panax Ginseng • Blackberry • HerbaSwee (Cucurbitaceae fruit).

GKG - EAS
Each capsule contains: Alpha-Ketoglutaric Acid 250 mg • L-Glutamine 275 mg • Taurine 150 mg • Calcium 63 mg • Potassium 25 mg • Magnesium 25 mg • RNA 9.5 mg • Manganese 400 mcg.

GLA Forte - Nature's Plus
Two softgels contain: GLA (Gamma Linolenic Acid) from Borage & Black Currant Seed oils, 100 mg • Vitamin E (d-Alpha Tocopherol) 200 IU • Vitamin C corn free 100 mg • Vitamin B6 (Pyridoxine HCL) 50 mg • Niacinamide 25 mg • Zinc (Gluconate) 5 mg. In a base containing safflower oil, octacosanol, lecithin & rapeseed.

GLA Mega-260 - Progressive Labs
Each softgel contains: Borage oil 1300 mg which supplies no less than Gamma Linolenic Acid (GLA) 260 mg and Vitamin E 1.5 IU: Fatty Acid Composition: Gamma Linolenic Acid 260 mg • Linoleic Acid 494 mg • Oleic Acid 221 mg.

Glan-Fem Plus - Atrium Inc.
Each tablet contains: Ovary 80 mg • Adrenal 20 mg • Thyroid (Thyroxin Free) 20 mg • Pituitary 10 mg • Vitamin B1 15 mg • Vitamin B2 17 mg • Vitamin B6 16 mg • Vitamin C 120 mg • Niacinamide 60 mg • Folic Acid 200 mcg • Vitamin E (d-Alpha Tocopherol) 60 IU • Manganese (Protein Chelated) 5 mg • Selenium 20 mcg.
See Editor's Note No. 14, page 1817.

Glan-Male Plus - Atrium Inc.
Each tablet contains: Orchic 80 mg • Adrenal 20 mg • Pituitary 10 mg • Vitamin B1 15 mg • Vitamin B2 17 mg • Vitamin B6 16 mg • Vitamin C 120 mg • Niacinamide 60 mg • Folic Acid 200 mcg • Vitamin E (d-Alpha Tocopherol) 60 IU • Manganese (Protein Chelated) 5 mg • Selenium 20 mcg.
See Editor's Note No. 14, page 1817.

Gla-Plus - Atrium Inc.
Each capsule contains: Gamma Linolenic Acid (from Black Currant) 40 mg • Vitamin E (d-Alpha Tocopheryl Acetate) 10 IU.

Global Source No-Jet-Lag - Vitamin Express
One tablet contains: Arnica Montana (Leopard's Bane) 30 C • Bellis Perennis (Daisy) 30 C • Chamomilla (Wild Chamomile) 30 C • Ipecacuanha (Ipecac) 30 C • Lycopodium (Clubmoss) 30 C.
See Editor's Note No. 1, page 1816.

Gluca-Herb - Dial Herbs
Cedar berries • Uva Ursi • Licorice • Mullein • Cayenne.

Glucogen Ace - ANS
Glucose • Vitamin A • Vitamin C • Vitamin E.

Glucogen Sport - ANS
"Vitamins & Minerals enriched Glucose Drink for Sports people."

GlucoLean - Nutripeak
Two tablets contain: Selenium (as selenium amino acid chelate) 50 mcg • Chromium (as chromium polynicotinate) 200 mcg • Guggul extract 1000 mg • Gymnema Sylvestre leaf 150 mg • Coleus Forskohlii extract 130 mg • Alpha-Lipoic Acid 100 mg • D-Pinitol 25 mg • Bitter Melon extract fruit, seed 18.8 mg. Other Ingredients: Cellulose, Stearic Acid, Magnesium Stearate, Silica.

Glucomannan 500 Mg - Natrol
Two capsules contain: Hemicellulose 913 mg • Cellulose 61 mg • Pectin Substance 25 mg • Lignin 1 mg. From Amorphophallus Konjac root.

Glucomannan+ - Swanson
Three capsules contain: Chromium (50% from Chromax chromium picolinate, 50% from chromium polynicotinate) 150 mcg • Psyllium husk fiber 600 mg • Konjac Glucomannan 450 mg • Apple Pectin •

BRAND NAMES

300 mg • Chitosan (93% deacetylated) 300 mg • Guar Gum 300 mg • Oat Bran fiber 300 mg • Gymnema sylvestre extract (25% gymnemic acids) 75 mg • L-Carnitine (as tartrate) 30 mg.

Glucomine - Body Wise International, Inc.
Three capsules contain: Glucosamine Sulfate 1500 mg • Chondroitin Sulfate 150 mg • Boswellia Gum Std. Extract (Boswellia serrata) 25 mg • White Willow Bark (Salix alba) 25 mg • Devils Claw-Inner Bark (Harpagophytum procumbens) 25 mg • Tea Tree Oil (Melaleuca alternifolia) 25 mg • Una de Gato (Uncaria tomentosa) 25 mg
See Editor's Note No. 15, page 1817.

Gluco-Pro 900 - Thompson Nutritional Products
Each tablet contains: Glucosamine HCl 500 mg • Chondroitin Sulfate 400 mg.
See Editor's Note No. 15, page 1817.

Glucoril - PhytoPharmica
Two capsules contain: Vitamin C (ascorbic acid) 100 mg • Vitamin E (mixed tocopherols) 50 IU • Vitamin B6 (pyridoxine HCl) 10 mg • Vitamin B12 (cyanocobalamin) 250 mcg • Biotin 1,000 mcg • Magnesium (Krebs chelate) 100 mg • Zinc (picolinate) 5 mg • Selenium (L-selenomethionine) 40 mcg • Manganese (Krebs chelate) 10 mg • Chromium (picolinate) 50 mcg • Blueberry (Vaccinium myrtillus fructus) extract 5:1 300 mg • Gymnema Sylvestre leaf extract 6:1 (standardized to contain 24% gymnemic acid) 150 mg • Bitter Melon (Momordica charantia) whole fruit extract 100 mg • Fenugreek (Trigonella foenum-graecum) seed extract 4:1 100 mg.

Glucosalage SO4 - Olympian Labs
Each capsule contains: Shark Cartilage 200 mg • Cat's Claw (uncaria tomentosa) 200 mg • Glucosamine Sulfate 2 KCl 200 mg.

Glucosalage SO4 (Extra Strength) - Olympian Labs
Two capsules contain: Shark Cartilage 400 mg • Cat's Claw 400 mg • Glucosamine Sulfate 400 mg • Proprietary Blend: Protease, Amylase, Lipase 100 mg. In a base of White Willow Bark, Valerian Root, Devil's Claw, and Black Willow.

Glucosamine & Chondroitin 500/400 - Now
Each capsule contains: Sodium 40 mg • Potassium (as Potassium Chloride) 60 mg • Glucosamine Sulfate (from 500 mg Glusocamine Potassium Sulfate complex) 375 mg • Chondroitin Sulfate (min. 90%) (Bovine Source) 400 mg • MSM 100 mg.
See Editor's Note No. 15, page 1817.

Glucosamine & Chondroitin Combo - Swanson
Each capsule contains: Glucosamine Sulfate (2KCl) 500 mg • Chondroitin Sulfate 250 mg.
See Editor's Note No. 15, page 1817.

Glucosamine & MSM Complex - Puritan's Pride
Three tablets contain: Glucosamine Sulfate 1500 mg • MSM 1000 mg • Ginger (Standardized 4% Volatile Oil) 100 mg • Vitamin C (Ascorbic Acid) 60 mg • Manganese 5 mg • White Willow 100 mg.

Glucosamine Chondroitin Complex with MSM - Source Naturals
Three tablets contain: Vitamin C (as ascorbic acid) 250 mg • Molybdenum (as molybdenum chelate) 320 mcg • Glucosamine Sulfate 1,500 mg • Chondroitin Sulfate 1,200 mg • MSM (methylsulfonylmethane) 800 mg.
See Editor's Note No. 15, page 1817.

Glucosamine Chondroitin Sulfate - HealthWatchers System
Glucosamine Sulfate • Chondroitin Sulfate • Vitamin C.
See Editor's Note No. 15, page 1817.

Glucosamine Complex - Natrol
One capsule contains: Glucosamine Sulfate 100 mg • Glucosamine HCl 300 mg • Glucosamine N-Acetyl 100 mg. Other ingredients: Rice powder, Silicon Dioxide, Magnesium Stearate, Gelatin.

Glucosamine Formula - Symmetry
Each packet contains: Glucosamine • Chondroitin Sulfate • Hydrolyzed gelatin • Boswellia • Curcumin • Bilberry • Grape Seed extract • Grape Skin extract • Tumeric extract.
See Editor's Note No. 15, page 1817.

Glucosamine Fuel - TwinLab
Two tablets contain: Glucosamine Sulfate (Pure Pharmaceutical Grade) 1500mg • Chondroitin Sulfate (Pure Pharmaceutical Grade) 1200 mg • Glycerol Fuel (contains 99.7% Pure Pharmaceutical Grade Glycerol).
See Editor's Note No. 15, page 1817.

Glucosamine HCl, Chondroitin & MSM - Swanson
Three tablets contain: Glucosamine HCl 750 mg • Chondroitin Sulfate 600 mg • OptiMSM (methylsulfonylmethane) 450 mg.
See Editor's Note No. 15, page 1817.

Glucosamine Plus Dietary Supplement - Dr. Art Ulene's Prescriptive Formulas
Two tablets contain: Niacin (B3) 100 mg • Curcumin 100 mg • Glucosamine Hydrochloride 730 mg • Frankincense Extract (boswellia serrata, roxb. excolabr, gum resin) 300 mg • Glucosamine Sulfate 50 mg • Quercetin 100 mg • Turmeric (Curcuma longa, rhizome powder) 100 mg.

Glucosamine Sulfate - PhytoPharmica
Each capsule contains: Glucosamine Sulfate 500 mg.
Contains no sugar, yeast, wheat, corn, soy, dairy products, coloring, flavoring or preservatives. Each capsule contains 60 mg of sodium.

Glucosamine Sulfate - Olympian Labs
Each capsule contains: Glucosamine Sulfate (yielding Glucosamine Sulfate 500 mg and Potassium Chloride 170 mg) 670 mg.

Glucosamine Sulfate - Swanson
Each capsule contains: Glucosamine Sulfate (2KCl) 500 mg.

Glucosamine Sulfate - Capsules - PhytoPharmica
Three capsules contain: Stabilized Glucosamine Sulfate 1,500 mg • Chloride (from glucosamine sulfate) 234 mg • Sodium (from glucosamine sulfate) 150 mg.

Glucosamine Sulfate - Packets - PhytoPharmica
Each packet contains: Stabilized Glucosamine Sulfate (equivalent to three, 500 mg capsules) 1,500 mg • Carbohydrate <1 gm • Chloride (from glucosamine sulfate) 234 mg • Sodium (from glucosamine sulfate) 150 mg.

Glucosamine Sulfate - Packets, Orange-flavored - PhytoPharmica
Each packet contains: Carbohydrate <1 gm • Chloride (from glucosamine sulfate) 234 mg • Sodium (from glucosamine sulfate) 150 mg • Stabilized Glucosamine Sulfate (equivalent to three, 500 mg capsules) 1,500 mg.

Glucosamine Sulfate & Shark Cartilage - Swanson
Each tablet contains: Glucosamine Sulfate (2KCl) 500 mg • Shark Cartilage 250 mg.

Some Brand Name Natural Products - What they Contain
www.NaturalDatabase.com contains MANY more listings than appear here.

Glucosamine Sulfate Chondroitin Sulfate - Progressive Natural Products
One tablespoon contains: Glucosamine Sulfate 500 mg • Vitamin C 500 mg • Chondroitin Sulfate 150 mg • Shark Cartilage 50 mg • CMO 25 mg • Cherry extract 25 mg • Sea Cucumber 25 mg • Manganese Aspartate 5 mg • Zinc Citrate 5 mg • Boron Citrate 1 mg.
See Editor's Note No. 15, page 1817.

Glucosamine Sulfate Complex - PhytoPharmica
Three capsules contain: Vitamin C (ascorbic acid) 1,000 mg • Chloride (from glucosamine sulfate) 156 mg • Sodium 100 mg • Stabilized Glucosamine Sulfate 1,000 mg • L-Tyrosine 500 mg.

Glucosamine, Chondroitin & MSM - Swanson
Each tablet contains: Glucosamine Sulfate (2KCl) 500 mg • Chondroitin Sulfate 400 mg • OptiMSM (methylsulfonylmethane) 200 mg.
See Editor's Note No. 15, page 1817.

Glucosa-Plex - Progressive Labs
Each capsule contains: Vitamin C 50 mg • Vitamin E (succinate) 25 IU • Pantothenic Acid 50 mg • Glucosamine Sulfate 100 mg • N-Acetyl Glucosamine 50 mg • L-Glutathione 2 mg • N-Acetyl Cysteine 5 mg • L-Cysteine 50 mg • L-Glutamic Acid 50 mg • L-Glycine 50 mg • L-Taurine 25 mg • Soluble Trachea (16% pure chondroitin sulfate-A) 25 mg • Milk Thistle (Silybum marianum) 100 mg • Silymarin 5 mg • Green Lipped Mussel 25 mg (natural source of mucopolysaccharides and superoxide dismutase).
See Editor's Note No. 15, page 1817.

Glucos-Bal - Nutri-Quest
Each tablet contains: Vanadyl Sulfate 3 mg • Chromium (Picolinate) 200 mcg • Vitamin B1 10 mg • Vitamin B2 5 mg • Vitamin B6 5 mg • Vitamin B12 10 mcg • Folic Acid 200 mcg • Biotin 500 mcg • Pantothenic Acid (D-Calcium Pantothenate) 20 mg • Niacinamide 20 mg • Niacin 6 mg • Magnesium Aspartate 100 mg • Calcium Ascorbate 100 mg • Manganese Aspartate 4 mg • Zinc (Picolinate) 1 mg • Selenium (Chelate) 30 mcg.

Glucotize - MRI
Each tablet contains: a-Lipoic Acid (thioctic acid) 300 mg. Inactive Ingredients: Calcium Phosphate, Cellulose ethers & composites, Magnesium Stearate. Contains no yeast, corn, wheat, soy, sugar or sweeteners, artificial flavors, colors or preservatives.

Glucovite - TheraNutria
Six tablets provide: Vitamin A (67% as Beta-Carotene, 33% as Vitamin A Palmitate) 7500 IU • Vitamin C (Calcium Ascorbate) 1000 mg • Vitamin D (as Vitamin D3) 400 IU • Vitamin E (natural d-alpha,d-beta, d-gamma, d-delta-tocopherols) 100 IU • Vitamin K (as Vitamin K1) (Phylloquinone) 40 mcg • Thiamine (Mononitrate) 4.5 mg • Riboflavin 3.4 mg • Niacin (50% Niacin, 50% Niacinamide) 40 mg • Vitamin B6 (Pyridoxine HCI) 10 mg • Folic Acid 600 mcg • Vitamin B12 (Cyanocobalamin) 60 mcg • Biotin 200 mcg • Pantothenic Acid (D-Calcium Pantothenate) 20 mg • Calcium (Ascorbate, Propionate, Carbonate) 300 mg • Magnesium (Amino Acid Chelate) 200 mg • Iron (Amino Acid Chelate) 3.6 mg • Iodine (Potassium Iodide) 150 mcg • Zinc (Amino Acid Chelate) 15 mg • Copper (Amino Acid Chelate) 2 mg • Manganese (Amino Acid Chelate) 2 mg • Selenium (50% L-Selenomethionine, 50% Sodium Selenite) 140 mcg • Chromium (Glycine-Niacin Chelate) 600 mcg • Molybdenum (Amino Acid Chelate) 75 mcg • Boron (Citrate) 3 mg • Silicon (Sodium Metasilicate) 3 mg • Vanadium (Vanadyl Sulfate) 100 mcg • Citrus Bioflavonoids 10 mg • Quercetin 10 mcg • Glucosol Banaba leaf extract (L. speciosa L., min. 1% corosolic acid) 2 • Alpha-Lipoic acid (Thioctic acid). Other ingredients: modified cellulose gum, cellulose, vegetable stearine, silicon dioxide, magnesium stearate, hydroxymethyl propylcellulose, titanium dioxide, chlorophyll. Contains no yeast, corn, wheat, dairy, sugar or other sweeteners, artificial colors, flavors or preservatives.

Glutagen - ANS
Pure Glutamine.

Glutamine Capsules - Universal Nutrition
Each capsule contains: L-Glutamine 750 mg • Manganese Sulfate 400 mcg • Potassium Phosphate 30 mg.

Glutamine Flora - Nutri-Quest
Each tablet contains: Combined stabalized microencapsulated freeze-dried Lactobacillus Acidophilus, Bulgaricus & Bifidus 4.5 million IU • L-Glutamine 500 mg • Chlorophyll 20 mg • natural Vitamin E Succinate 5 IU.

Glutamine Fuel Capsules - TwinLab
Two capsules contain: L-Glutamine 1500 mg.

Glutamine Fuel Powder - TwinLab
Each teaspoonful contains: L-Glutamine 4500 mg (4.5 g).

Glutathione Plus - Atrium Inc.
Each capsule contains: L-Glutathione 50 mg • L-Glutamine 200 mg.

GLYCO-8 - Pharmagel
Glycolic Acid • Alpha Hydroxy Acids • Antioxidants.

Glyco-B - Atrium Inc.
Each tablet contains: Vitamin B1 35 mg • Vitamin B2 35 mg • Vitamin B6 35 mg • Vitamin B12 35 mcg • Vitamin C 180 mg • Pantothenic Acid 80 mg • Niacinamide 180 mg • Folic Acid 135 mcg • Choline Bitartrate 25 mg • Inositol 10 mg • Biotin 10 mcg • L-Lysine HCL 10 mg • Brewer's Yeast 50 mg • Pancrelipase 20 mg • Selenium 2 mcg • Adrenal 4 mg • Brain 4 mg • Liver 7 mg • Pancreas 2 mg.
See Editor's Note No. 14, page 1817.

Glycobar: Chocolate Chip - Pharmanex
Each bar contains: Honey • Peanut Butter: Peanuts, Salt • Semi Sweet Chocolate Chips: Sugar, Chocolate Liquor, Cocoa Butter, Soy Lecithin, Vanilla • Brown Sugar • Date Puree • Prune Puree • Rolled Oats • Sugar Beet Fiber • Brown Crisp Rice: Rice Flour, Rice Bran, Rosemary Extract • Modified Guar Gum • Oat Bran • Peanuts • Barley Flakes • Rye Flakes • Soybean Oil • Soy Lecithin • Whey Powder.

Glycobar: Peanut Butter and Jelly - Pharmanex
Each bar contains: Honey • Peanut Butter: Peanuts, Salt • Brown Sugar • Date Puree • Prune Puree • Rolled Oats • Strawberry and Blueberry Fruit Chips: Sugar, Strawberries, Blueberries, Glucose, Pectin, Citric Acid, Sodium Citrate, Natural Flavor • Brown Crisp Rice: Rice Flour, Rice Bran, Rosemary Extract • Modified Guar Gum • Oat Bran • Peanuts • Yogurt Chips: Sugar, Hydrogenated Palm Kernel Oil, Milk Solids, Color (Titanium Dioxide), Soy Lecithin, Vanilla • Barley Flakes • Rye Flakes • Soybean Oil • Soy Lecithin • Whey Powder.

GlycoLean Accelerator - Mannatech
Country Mallow (contains ephedrine) • Proprietary Blend of antioxidants, digestive enzymes, and nutrients.
See Editor's Note No. 17, page 1817.

GlycoLean Catalyst - Mannatech
Multiple vitamin, mineral and herbal tablet.
See Editor's Note No. 17, page 1817.

GlycoLean Fiber Full - Mannatech
Ambrotose FiberMax • Whole Aloe Gel • Magnesium.
See Editor's Note No. 17, page 1817.

GlycoLean Manager - Mannatech
Bitter Orange (contains synephrine) • Proprietary Blend of antioxidants, digestive enzymes, and nutrients.
See Editor's Note No. 17, page 1817.

BRAND NAMES

Glycoplex - Progressive Labs
Three capsules provide: Vitamin C 500 mg • Thiamin (Vitamin B1) 100 mg • Riboflavin (Vitamin B2) 100 mg • Niacinamide 500 mg • Vitamin B6 100 mg • Folate (folic acid) 300 mcg • Vitamin B12 50 mcg • Biotin 15 mcg • Pantothenic Acid (calcium pantothenate) 250 mcg • Chromium (chromium picolinate) 200 mcg • Inositol 50 mg • Pancrelipase 50 mg • Choline Bitartrate 50 mg • Pyloric substance 45 mg • Para Amino Benzoic Acid (PABA) 60 mg • L-Lysine Monohydrochloride 30 mg. Other ingredients: Raw Adrenal, Raw Pancreas, Raw Brain and Raw Liver concentrates.
See Editor's Note No. 14, page 1817.

GlycoSlim Meal Replacement Shake - Mannatech
No ingredients listed. Chocolate, strawberry and vanilla flavors.
See Editor's Note No. 17, page 1817.

GlyMordica - Amazing Herbs
Bitter Melon (Momordica Charantia).

GNC Herbal Plus Standardized Saw Palmetto - GNC
Each capsule contains: Saw Palmetto berries extract (Serenoa repens; 85% Fatty Acids=136 mg; 0.2% Sterols=0.32 mg) 160 mg. Other Ingredients: Olive Oil, Gelatin, Glycerin, Caramel Color, Titanium Dioxide (natural mineral whitener).
See Editor's Note No. 20, page 1818.

GNC SAMe 100mg - GNC
Each tablet contains: S-Adenosyl-Methionine (SAMe) 100 mg. Other Ingredients: Microcrystalline Cellulose, Magnesium Stearate, Talc, Metacrylic Copolymer.
See Editor's Note No. 10, page 1817.

Golden Flax Meal - Nature's Life
Two tablespoons (17 g) contain: Low fat Omegaflo Flax seed meal (certified organic by Farm Verified Organic). Naturally occuring fatty acids: Alpha Linolenic Acid (Omega-3) 1710 mg • Linoleic Acid (Omega-6) 480 mg • Oleic Acid (Omega-9) 50 mg • Lignin Fiber 1003 mg • Lignan 13.6 mg.

Golden Flax Oil - Nature's Life
One tablespoon contains: Lipid profile, based on a typical analysis of: Omega-3 as Alpha-Linolenic Acid EFA 8.6 g • Omega-6 as Alpha- Linoleic Acid EFA 2.7 g • Omega-9 as Oleic (Monounsaturated Fatty Acid) 2.4 g.

Golden Flax Oil 1000 mg - Nature's Life
Each capsule contains: 100% pure Flax oil (Certified Organically Grown) (Omegaflo Process fresh, unrefined, unfiltered, unbleached, virgin seed oil; Organically grown & processed according to California Organic Foods Act of 1990; Farm Verified Organic). Lipid profile based on a typical analysis: Omega-3 EFA as Alpha-Lenolic Acid 570 mg • Omega-6 EFA as Linoleic Acid 180 mg • Omega-9 as Oleic Acid 160 mg • Vitamin A (from naturally occuring Beta Carotene) 286 IU • Vitamin E (from naturally occuring Tocopherols) 1 IU.

Golden Spleen 500 - Enzymatic Therapy
Each capsule contains: Spleen Polypeptides 375 mg: A mixture of highly purified bovine-derived spleen polypeptides naturally present in the spleen, including: Tuftsin, Splenopentin, Splenin, & Leukokinin • Goldenseal root extract 125 mg: (Hydrastis canadensis) standardized to contain 5% total Alkaloids including: Berberine, Hydrastine, & Canadine. Contains no sugar, salt, yeast, wheat, corn, dairy products, flavoring, or preservatives.
See Editor's Note No. 14, page 1817.

Goldenseal - Leiner Health Products
Each caplet contains: Golden Seal extract (Hydrastis canadensis) root 100 mg. Other Ingredients: Calcium Carbonate, Cellulose, Maltodextrin, Hydroxypropyl Methylcellulose, Silicon Dioxide, Polyethylene Glycol 3350, Croscarmellose Sodium, Hydroxypropyl Cellulose, Pharmaceutical Glaze, Crospovidone, Magnesium Stearate, Yellow 5 Lake, Red 40 Lake, Blue 2 Lake, Titanium Dioxide, Polysorbate 80.

Goldenseal - Olympian Labs
Each capsule contains: Goldenseal root 500 mg.

Goldenseal - Pharmanex
Each capsule contains: Goldenseal root extract (Hydrastis canadensis) (4:1) 250 mg. Other Ingredients: Rice Flour, Gelatin, Magnesium Stearate, Silicon Dioxide.

Goldenseal & Echinacea - Olympian Labs
Each capsule contains: Goldenseal 225 mg • Echinacea 225 mg.

Goldenseal and Myrrh - Dial Herbs
Goldenseal • Myrrh.

Goldenseal Root - Now
Two capsules contain: Goldenseal root powder (hydrastis canadensis) 1000 mg. Contains no milk, wheat, corn, yeast, sugar, salt, or soy.

Goldenseal Salve - Dial Herbs
Goldenseal • Myrrh • Shavegrass • Echinacea • Comfrey • Slippery Elm • Lobelia. In a base of Bees Wax , Glycerine & Cold Pressed Olive oil.

Goldenseal-Myrrh Virtue - Blessed Herbs
Goldenseal root • Myrrh Gum • Propolis • Grain alcohol & Distilled Water.

GO-lite/am (Appetite Manager) - Enviro- Tech Nutritionals
Griffonia simplicifolia (Containing 5-hydroxytryptophan) • St. John's Wort.

GO-lite/fm (Fat Metabolizer) - Enviro- Tech Nutritionals
Chitosan • Vitamin C • Iodine • Chromium • Thermal Herbal Blend: Sida Cordifolia and bitter orange peel • Yerba mate leaf • Chitosan.

Good-Nite - Changes - TwinLab
Each caplet contains: Melatonin 3 mg • Kava Kava root standardized extract (30% kavalactones) 250 mg • Herbal Extract Blend 275 mg: Valerian root standardized extract (0.8% valerenic acids), Catnip aerial parts, Chamomile flower, Hops stobile, Passion flower aerial parts, Skullcap root. Other Ingredients: Dicalcium Phosphate, Vegetable cellulose, Fractionated vegetable oil, Silica, Soy polysaccharides, and Vegetable resin glaze.
See Editor's Note No. 16, page 1817.

Gotu Kola - Nature's Way
Two capsules contain: Gotu Kola (stem, leaf) 870 mg.

Gotu Kola - Now
Two capsules contain: Sodium 10 mg • Total Carbohydrate 540 mg • Gotu Kola leaf (Centella Asiatica) 900 mg. Other Ingredients: Stearic Acid. Contains no salt, yeast, wheat, sugar, corn, milk, or preservatives.

Gotu Kola - Olympian Labs
Each capsule contains: Gotu Kola 450 mg.

GP Cordyceps - Solaray - Nutraceutical
Two capsules contain: Cordyceps (Cordyceps sinensis) 520 mg • Other Ingredients: Gelatin (capsule), Cellulose, Magnesium.

Gram-Two Vitamin C - The Vitamin Shoppe
Two tablets contain: Vitamin C [as ascorbic acid and as mineral ascorbates of calcium, magnesium, zinc, and manganese] 2000 mg • Bioflavonoids [Hesperidin, Rose Hips, Acerola Cherry, Pectin, Orange, Grapefruit, Lemon, Rutin] 250 mg. No Yeast, Corn, Wheat, Sugar, Salt, Soy, Starch, Dairy, Milk, Eggs, gluten, Fish Or Animal Derivatives, Preservatives, Artificial Colors or Flavors added.

Grape Seed - Pharmanex
Each capsule contains: Grape seed extract (Vitis vinifera) (100:1) 75 mg. Other Ingredients: Rice Flour, Gelatin, Magnesium Stearate, Silicon Dioxide.

Grape Seed (PCO) Extract - PhytoPharmica
Each capsule contains: Grape Seed (PCO) extract (standardized to contain 95% procyanidolic oligomers [PCOs] 50 mg.

Grape Seed (PCO) Phytosome - PhytoPharmica
Each capsule contains: Grape (Vitis vinifera) seed (PCO) phytosome (standardized to contain 95% procyanidolic oligomers [PCOs] from Grape seed extract bound to Phosphatidylcholine under patent) 50 mg.

Grape Seed (PCO) Phytosome - 100 - PhytoPharmica
Each capsule contains: Grape (Vitis vinifera) seed (PCO) phytosome (standardized to contain 95% procyanidolic oligomers [PCOs] from Grape seed extract bound to Phosphatidylcholine under patent) 100 mg.

Grape Seed Antioxidant - Now
Each capsule contains: Grape seed extract (95%) 60 mg • Citrus Bioflavonoids (40%) 300 mg.

Grape Seed Extract - Leiner Health Products
Each tablet contains: Grape seed extract (Vitis vinifera) seed 100 mg. Other Ingredients: Calcium Carbonate, Maltodextrin, Cellulose, Silicon Dioxide, Polyethylene Glycol 3350, Croscarmellose Sodium, Crospovidone, Magnesium Stearate, Hydroxypropyl Methylcellulose, Hydroxypropyl Cellulose, Polysorbate 80.

Grape Seed Extract - Metabolic Response Modifiers
Each capsule contains: Grape Seed extract (85-95% OPC's - offering a minimum 100 mg of OPC's with 20 mg of other vital flavonoids) 120 mg.

Grape Seed Extract - Olympian Labs
Each capsule contains: Grape Seed extract (120:1, consists of 85% Oligomeric Procyanidins) 100 mg.

Grape Seed Extract Extra Strength with MAT - Olympian Labs
Each capsule contains: Grape Seed extract (120:1, consists of 85% Oligomeric Procyanidins) 200 mg. Other Ingredients: MAT (proprietary blend of nutritional ingredients).

Grape Seed Extract Formula - Quest
Each caplet contains: Grape Seed powder (Vitis vinffera) (Provided by 25 mg P.E. 1:100 standardized to contain not less than 95% leucoanthocyanins) 2500 mg • Citrus Bioflavonoids 200 mg providing Hesperidin 50 mg • Rutin powder 25 mg. Other Ingredients: Calcium Phosphate, Microcrystalline Cellulose, Vegetable Stearin, Croscarmellose Sodium, Magnesium Stearate (vegetable source).

Grape Seed Extract Plus - Atrium Inc.
Each capsule contains: Grape seed extract (Leucocyanidins) 50 mg • Bioflavonoids 200 mg.

Grapefruit Concentrate With Fiber & Herbs - Natrol
Two capsules contain: Grapefruit concentrate 10:1 300 mg • Psyllium Husk fiber 100 mg • Rice Bran fiber 100 mg • Oat Bran fiber 100 mg • Licorice root 100 mg • Uva Ursi 100 mg • Apple Cider vinegar 50 mg • Deep Ocean Kelp 50 mg • Lecithin 50 mg • Spirulina 50 mg • Vitamin B6 (Pyridoxine HCL) 25 mg • L-Phenylalanine 25 mg • Cascara Sagrada 20 mg. This is a 10 time concentration of the equivalent of 3000 mg of Whole Grapefruit. Other ingredients: Silicon Dioxide, Magnesium Stearate, Gelatin, Microcrystalline Cellulose.

Grapefruit Extract - NutriBiotic
Grapefruit extract.

Grapeseed Extract - Swanson
Each capsule contains: Grapeseed extract (95% proanthocyanidins) 50 mg.

Grapeseed Extract 100 mg - Puritan's Pride
Each capsule contains: Grapeseed extract 100 mg • Citrus Bioflavonoids 300 mg.

Grapeseed Extract 50 mg - Puritan's Pride
Each capsule contains: Grapeseed extract 50 mg • Citrus Bioflavonoids 500 mg.

Green Black Walnut Wormwood Complex - Now
Two droppersful (16ml) contains: 1.6 ml proprietary blend of Green Black Walnut hulls (Juglans species) • Wormwood herb (Artemisia absinthium) • Clove buds (Carophyllus species) extracts. Other Ingredients: Grain Alcohol, Distilled Water.

Green Max Powder - Swanson
Each tablespoon (8.5 grams) contains: Vitamin A (as beta-carotene 40 mg) 66,666 IU • Soy Lecithin 2,142 g • Spirulina powder 1,356 g • Apple Fiber 1.35 g • Wheat Grass powder 445 mg • Alfalfa leaf powder 435 mg • Barley bran powder 435 mg • Brown Rice powder 350 mg • Chlorella (broken cell wall) 350 mg • Soy sprout powder 350 mg • Beet powder 335 mg • Lactobacillus probiotic culture 200 mg • Bee Pollen powder 150 mg • Royal Jelly powder 150 mg • Acerola cherry powder 115 mg • Barley grass powder 97 mg • Licorice root powder 60 mg • Dulse Thallus powder 20 mg • Ginkgo Biloba leaf powder 20 mg • Grape Seed extract (90% proanthocyanidins) 20 mg • Green Tea extract (50% polyphenols) 20 mg • Milk Thistle seed extract (80% silymarin) 20 mg • Astragalus root powder 10 mg • Bilberry powder 10 mg • Echinacea root powder 10 mg • Siberian Ginseng root powder 10 mg.

Green Multi - Nature's Life
Three tablets contain: Beta Carotene (equivalent to 25000 IU Vitamin A) 15 mg • Vitamin C 1000 mg • Vitamin E (d-Alpha Tocopheryl Succinate) 300 IU • Vitamin B1 (Thiamine Mononitrate) 25 mg • Vitamin B2 (Riboflavin, Riboflavin 5'-Phosphate) 25 mg • Vitamin B3 (Niacin) 25 mg • Pantothenic Acid (Calcium Pantothenate, Pantetheine-5' -Phosphate) 25 mg • Vitamin B6 (Pyridoxine HCl, Pyridoxal-5'-Phosphate) 25 mg • Folic Acid (Folacin) 400 mcg • Vitamin B12 100 mcg • Biotin (d-Biotin) 60 mcg • Choline (Bitartrate) 14 mg • Inositol (Niacinate) 20 mg • PABA (Para Aminobenzoic Acid) 25 mg • Boron (Citrate, Nature's Life Greens) 100 mg • Calcium (Carbonate, Citrate/Malate) 250 mg • Chromium (Picolinate, Polynicotinate) 100 mcg • Copper (Citrate, Gluconate) 1 mg • Iodine (Potassium Iodine, Nature's Life Greens) 75 mcg • Iron (Glycinate, Nature's Life Greens) 10 mg • Magnesium (Oxide, Nature's Life Greens) 125 mg • Manganese (Gluconate, Citrate) 6 mg • Molybdenum (Molybdate, Nature's Life Greens) 50mcg • Potassium (Gluconate, Iodide, Nature's Life Greens) 90 mg • Selenium (Selenite, Cysteine) 100 mcg • Vanadium (Vanadyl Sulfate) 25 mcg • Zinc (Picoliante, Monomethionine) 15 mg • Lemon Bioflavonoids

B R A N D N A M E S

Complex (50% active) 100 mg • Quercetin (Saphora japonica) 25 mg • Rutin (Sapora japonica) 25 mg • Hesperidin (Citrus fruit peel) 25 mg • Bromelain from Pineapple (2000 GDU/g) 25 mg • Papain from Papaya (2000 USP units/g) 25 mg • Betaine HCL, beets 25 mg • Amylase (30000 SKB IU/g) 6 mg • Lipase 10000 Usp IU/g) 6 mg • Cellulase (10000 USP IU/g) 6 mg • Nature's Life Greens powder 1000 mg.

Green Phytofoods - Now
Each nine gram serving contains: Lecithin fine powder 2000 mg • Spirulina (Hawaiian) 1000 mg • Alfalfa juice concentrate 700 mg • Wheat grass powder organic 500 mg • Barley grass powder organic 500 mg • Carrot powder 500 mg • Barley Malt powder 400 mg • Broccoli powder 350 mg • Brown Rice Bran 350 mg • Apple fiber 350 mg • Apple Pectin 300 mg • Oat Bran 300 mg • Chlorella powder 300 mg • Red Beet powder 300 mg • Panax ginseng root powder (min 5% Ginsenosides) 250 mg • Siberian Ginseng root powder (Eleutherococcus senticosus) 100 mg • Peppermint powder 150 mg • Green Tea extract (Camellia sinensis) (40% Catechins) 100 mg • Royal Jelly powder (min 5% 10-HDA) 100 mg • Fructo Oligo Saccharides (NutraFlora FOS) 100 mg • Trace Mineral concentrate 100 mg • Milk Thistle extract (80% Silymarin) 80 mg • Kelp powder 50 mg • Ginkgo Biloba extract (24% Ginkgo Flavonglycosides) 20 mg • Grape seed extract (95% Polyphenols) 20 mg • Bilberry extract (25% Anthocyanidins) 20 mg • Plant Based Enzymes 100 mg: Protease 12500 HUT, Lipase 200 LU, Lactase 200 LAC, Bromelain 5000 FCC, Amylase 2500 DU, Cellulase 500 CMC, Papain 6000 PU • Coenzyme Q10 10 mg • Alpha Lipoic Acid 10 mg • Stevia extract 10 mg.

Green Source - Puritan's Pride
Three tablets contain: Vitamin A (100% as Beta Carotene) 15,000 IU • Vitamin C 1,000 mg • Vitamin D 400 IU • Vitamin E 250 IU • Thiamin (Vitamin B-1) 25 mg • Riboflavin (Vitamin B-2) 25 mg • Niacin 25 mg • Vitamin B-6 25 mg • Folic Acid 400 mcg • Vitamin B-12 25 mcg • Biotin 50 mcg • Pantothenic Acid 25 mg • Calcium 250 mg • Iron 15 mg • Iodine 150 mcg • Magnesium 125 mg • Zinc 15 mg • Selenium 25 mcg • Copper 500 mcg • Manganese 4 mg • Chromium 100 mcg • Molybdenum 50 mcg • Potassium 50 mg • Boron 1 mg • Choline Bitartrate 50 mg • Inositol 25 mg • PABA (Para-Aminobenzoic Acid) 25 mg • Citrus Bioflavonoids complex (Orange) 100 mg • Quercetin 25 mg • Rutin 25 mg • Hesperidin (Orange) 10 mg • Bromelain (Pineapple-2000 GDU/gm) 20 mg • Betaine Hydrochloride 20 mg • Papain (Papaya) 20 mg • Amylase 5 mg • Lipase 5 mg • Protease 1.0 mg • Cellulase 2.5 mg • Proprietary Lactobacilus blend: L. Acidophilus, L. Bifidus, L. Bulgaricus (Milk-Free: minimum 1 billion viable micro-organisms per gram) 25 mg • Oat Bran 25 mg • Pectin (Apple) 25 mg • RNA 35 mg • DNA 10 mg • Carotenoids 10 mg • Chlorophyll 4 mg • Vegetable Oil: Borage and Sunflower (dry, cold-pressed - providing Essential Fatty Acids, GLA) 100 mg • L-Glutathione 5 mg • Spirulina 1,000 mg • Wheat grass juice (dry) 100 mg • Sprouted Barley juice (dry) 100 mg • Flaxseed Oil (dry) 100 mg • Chlorella (broken cell wall) 100 mg • Bee Pollen 100 mg • Siberian Ginseng (Eleutherococcus senticosus) root 50 mg • Dehydrated Garlic (allium sativum) bulb 10 mg • Proprietary herbal blend: Echinacea (Echinacea purpurea) arial, Milk Thistle (Silybum marianum) seed, Goldenseal (Hydrastis canadensis) root, Ginger Root (Zingiber officinale) root, Ginkgo Biloba (Ginkgo biloba) leaf, Cayenne Pepper (Capsicum annuum) fruit 60 mg.

Green Stuff - Gary Nulls
Contains a Green Mix [Green Kamut juice, Wheat Grass juice, Barley Green Juice, Alfalfa Leaf, Oat Grass Juice, Broccoli, Parsley, Kale], Flaxseed, Raw Brown Rice, Fruit Juice Mix [Pineapple, Lemon, Lime], Carrot juice, Earthrise Farms Spirulina, Yucca root, and Black Licorice root extract.

Green Tea Complex - Leiner Health Products
Each tablet contains: Vitamin C (Ascorbic Acid) 120 mg • Green Tea extract (Camellia sinensis) leaf 100 mg. Other Ingredients: Calcium Carbonate, Cellulose, Hesperidin Complex, Rutin, Maltodextrin, Quercetin, Silicon Dioxide, Polyethylene Glycol 3350, Croscarmellose Sodium, Starch, Crospovidone, Magnesium Stearate, Hydroxypropyl Methylcellulose, Hydroxypropyl Cellulose, Polysorbate 80.

Green Tea Diet - Schiff
Each tablet contains: Green Tea extract 225 mg • EGCG 90 mg • Caffeine 50 mg.

Green Tea Extract - HealthWatchers System
Green Tea Extract • Green Tea Powder. Each capsule is the equivalent of 700 mg. of Green Tea Powder.

Green Tea Extract - Nature's Way
Each capsule contains: Green Tea dried extract 170 mg • Red Clover blossoms 315 mg. Other Ingredients: Gelatin.

Green Tea Extract - Olympian Labs
Each capsule contains: Green Tea extract 500 mg.

Green Tea Extract - PhytoPharmica
Each capsule contains: Green Tea (camellia sinensis) leaf extract (standardized to contain 47%-52% polyphenols [catechin, epicatechin, epicatechin gallate, and epigallocatechin gallate] and 5%-10% Caffeine) 250 mg.

Green Tea Phytosome - PhytoPharmica
Each capsule contains: Green Tea (Camellia sinensis) leaf phytosome (bound to Phosphatidylcholine using a unique patented process) 100 mg.

Green Tea Remedy - Puritan's Pride
Each caplet contains: Green Tea extract 200 mg • Reishi mushroom 25 mg • Maitake mushroom 25 mg • Shiitake mushroom 25 mg • Astragalus 100 mg • Ligustrum 50 mg • Cat's Claw 100 mg • Vitamin C 60 mg • Selenium 50 mcg • Zinc 6 mg • Spirulina 50 mcg • Super-Oxide Dismutase 10 mg • N-acetyl Cysteine 25 mg.

Gro Pro - Universal Nutrition
Ten capsules contain: Creatine Monohydrate 5000 mg • L-Glutamine 2000 mg • Acetyl L-Carnitine 500 mg • L-Leucine (BCAA) 250 mg • L-Isoleucine (BCAA) 250 mg • L-Valine (BCAA) 250 mg • N-Acetyl-Cysteine (NAC) 200 mg • Tribulus Terrestris L. 250 mg • DHEA 50 mg • Zinc 15 mg.

Growth Fuel - TwinLab
Nine capsules contain: B-Hydroxy B-Methylbutyrate Monohydrate (HMB) 3000 mg • L-Glutamine 2000 mg • Creatine Monohydrate 5000 mg • N-Acetyl-Cysteine (NAC) 200 mg • Acetyl-L-Carnitine 50 mg • Zinc (from Zinc Picolinate) 30 mg • DHEA (Dehydroepiandrosterone) 50 mg.

GSC (Glandular Stress Complex) - Progressive Labs
Each capsule contains: Vitamin B12 24 mcg • Raw Bovine Adrenal 15 mg • Raw Bovine Liver 15 mg • Raw Bovine Thymus 60 mg • Raw Bovine Spleen 15 mg • Raw Bovine Stomach 15 mg. See Editor's Note No. 14, page 1817.

Guar Gum - Atrium Inc.
Each tablet contains: Pure Guar Gum 1000 mg.

Guarana Chai - Traditional Medicinals
Assam Black leaf Tea • Cardamom seed Ginger rhizome • Roasted Chicory root • Nutmeg seed • Organic Black Peppercorn • Guarana seed dry extract • Stevia leaf • Vanilla Bean dry extract • Clove stem • Rose petal • Cinnamon bark oil.

B R A N D   N A M E S

Guarana Energizer - Source Naturals
Each tablet contains: Guarana 900 mg.

Guarana-Gotu Kola Virtue - Blessed Herbs
Ma Huang • Siberian Ginseng root • Guarana seed • Gotu Kola • Licorice root • Grain alcohol & Distilled Water.

Guggulbolic - Syntrax Innovations
Each capsule contains: Guggulsterones 30 mg.

GugulPlex - PhytoPharmica
Each tablet contains: Niacin 250 mg • Vitamin C 100 mg • Chromium 50 mcg • Guggul extract 250 mg • Ginger root extract 200 mg.

GugulPlus - Enzymatic Therapy
Each tablet contains: Niacin (Inositol hexaniacinate) 250 mg • Vitamin C (Potassium Ascorbate) 100 mg • Chromium (Chromium Polynicotinate) (ChromeMate brand of patented Niacin-bound GTF Chromium) 50 mcg • Other ingredients: Guggul extract (Commiphora Mukul) standardized to contain Guggulsterones 25 mg/gram) 250 mg • Ginger root extract 6.5:1 (Zingiber officinale) 200 mg. Contains no sugar, salt, yeast, wheat, corn, soy, dairy products, flavoring, or preservatives.

Gum Weed Salve - Dial Herbs
Gum Weed • Licorice • Myrrh • Goldenseal • Arnica • Strawberry • Lobelia • Cayenne. In a base of Bees Wax, Glycerine & Cold Pressed Olive oil.

Gum-Ease - The Herbalist
Echinacea root • Myrrh Gum • Blood root • Bayberry root bark • Essential oils of Peppermint, Cinnamon, Clove.

Gymnema Sylvestre - Puritan's Pride
Each tablet contains: Gymnema Sylvestre 400 mg • Citrus Fiber 200 mg.

Gynecrine - Progressive Labs
Each capsule contains: Vitamin A 1000 IU • Vitamin C 100 mg • Vitamin E (dl-alpha tocopherol) 50 IU • Thiamin (Vitamin B1) 10 mg • Riboflavin (Vitamin B2) 10 mg • Vitamin B6 (pyridoxine) 18 mg • Iodine (as potassium iodide) 150 mcg • Magnesium (as magnesium oxide) 100 mg • Manganese (as manganese gluconate) 10 mg • Ovary concentrate (bovine) 20 mg • Mammary concentrate 10 mg • Pancreas concentrate 10 mg • Adrenal concentrate 10 mg • Pituitary concentrate 10 mg • Lecithin 10 mg • Flax seed oil 10 mg.
See Editor's Note No. 14, page 1817.

Gypsy Cold Care - Traditional Medicinals
Contains: Menthol: 5 mg per cup as it naturally occurs in the Peppermint leaf (Mentha x piperia) present in the blend. Other herbal ingredients: Rose Hip, Cinnamon bark, Yarrow flower, Ginger rhizome, Elder flower, Safflower petal, Clover stem, Hyssop herb, Licorice root dry extract.

Hair & Skin Formula - Nature's Way
Four capsules contain: Biotin (Biotin Triurate) 1.6 mg • Calcium 50 mg • Cayenne pepper fruit 160 mg • Fizyme Enzyme Formula 100 mg • Fo-Ti root 160 mg • Glucosamine HCL 400 mg • Horsetail grass 160 mg • Kelp (whole Thallus) 160 mg • MSM (Methyl Sulfonyl Methane) 600 mg • Nettle herb 160 mg • Oatstraw stem, leaf 160 mg • Rosemary herb 160 mg. Other ingredients: Gelatin, Magnesium Stearate, Millet.

Hair & Skin Nutrition - Enzymatic Therapy
Each capsule contains: Vitamin A (Fish Liver oil) 1666 IU • Vitamin D (Fish Liver oil) 333 IU • Vitamin E (D-Alpha Tocopherol) 33 IU • Vitamin C (Ascorbic Acid) 100 mg • Niacin/Niacinamide 33 mg • Zinc (Chelate) 15 mg • Vitamin B6 (Pyridoxine HCL) 10 mg •

Pantothenic Acid (D-Calcium Pantothenate) 8.3 mg • Riboflavin (Vitamin B2) 1.7 mg • Biotin 333 mcg • Folic Acid 33 mcg • Other ingredients: Unsaturated Free Fatty Acids (Linoleic, Arachidonic & Linolenic from Unrefined Germ oil & Safflower seed oil) 300 mg • Lecithin (Soy) 200 mg • Choline Bitartrate 50 mg • Intrinsic Glandular Lipids 50 mg • Inositol 33 mg. In a base of L-Cysteine as a natural amino acid synergistic component. Contains no sugar, salt, yeast, corn, dairy products, flavoring or preservatives. All organs & glands derived from bovine sources.
See Editor's Note No. 14, page 1817.

Hair Clean 1-2-3 Lice Remover - Quantum Health
Each one or two oz. tube contains: Coconut Oil • Anise Oil • Ylang Ylang Oil • Isopropyl Alcohol.

Hair Formula - Pharmanex
Each capsule contains: Vitamin E (as D-Alpha Tocopheryl Acetate) 3 IU • Riboflavin (as Riboflavin-5-Phosphate) 0.75 mg • Vitamin B6 (as Pyridoxine Hydrochloride) 3 IU • Biotin (as Biotin) 200 mcg • Pantothenic Acid (as Calcium Pantothenate) 25 mg • DL-Methionine 200 mg • L-Cysteine 105 mg • Lactalbumin Hydrolysate 25 mg • Millet Extract 20 mg. Other Ingredients: Gelatin, Maltodextrin, Starch, Vanillin, Stearic Acid (Vegetable Derived), Silicon Dioxide.

Hair Genesis - Crawford Co.
Each softgel contains: Beta Sitosterol 50 mg • Saw Palmetto Berry extract (85/95% liposterolic standardized) 200 mg • Lecithin 50 mg • Inositol 100 mg • Phosphatidyl Choline 25 mg • Niacin 15 mg • Biotin 100 mcg. Other Ingredients: Alcohol SDA-40, Propylene Glycol, Deionized Water, Polysorbate-80, Isoceteth-20, Hydrolyzed Mucopolysaccharides, Beta-Sitosterol, Biotin, and Citric Acid.

Hair Nutrients - Biotech
Three tablets contain: Shen Min [a proprietary blend of 12:1 standardized He Shou Wu (Fo Ti) root extract and He Shou Wu root powder] 1755 mg • BioPerine Black Pepper extract 3 mg.

Hair Support - Amazon Support
Each capsule contains: Nettles • Mutamba • Muira Puama • Sarsaparilla • Avenca • Gervao • Catuaba.

Hair Support for Men - Futurebiotics
Two capsules contain: Vitamin A (5000 IU as fish liver oil, 5000 IU as beta carotene) 10000 IU • Vitamin C (ascorbic acid) 250 mg • Vitamin D (ergocalciferol) 200 IU • Vitamin E (d-alpha tocopherol succinate) 30 IU • Vitamin B1 (thiamine HCl) 10 mg • Vitamin B2 (riboflavin) 10 mg • Vitamin B6 (pyridoxine HCl) 10 mg • Vitamin B12 (cyanocobalamin) 16 mcg • Folic Acid 400 mcg • Biotin (d-biotin) 500 mcg • Pantothenic Acid (calcium pantothenate) 100 mg • Zinc (amino acid chelate) 25 mg • Selenium (amino acid chelate) 100 mcg • Para Aminobenzoic Acid (PABA) 30 mg • Boron (amino acid chelate) 3 mg • MSM (methyl-sulfonyl-methane) 500 mg • Horsetail leaf powder extract (4:1) 50 mg • Saw Palmetto berry extract (4:1) powder 50 mg • Hair Support Herbal Base, 200 mg: Citrus Bioflavonoids, Saw Palmetto berry powder, Schizandra berry extract powder, Horsetail leaf powder. Other ingredients: Gelatin, Water.

Hair, Skin & Nails - Health Factor
Each capsule contains: Choline Bitartrate 100 mg • DL Methionine 100 mg • Borage Seed 150 mg • Flax Seed 150 mg • Gelatin 150 mg • Lecithin 100 mg.

Hair, Skin & Nails for Men - Futurebiotics
Three tablets contain: • Beta Carotene 10,000 IU • Vitamin C 120 mg • Vitamin B2 (Riboflavin) 10 mg • Vitamin B1 (Thiamin) 10 mg • Calcium 600 mg • Iron (Amino Acid Chelate) 6 mg • Vitamin D (Fish Liver Oil) 200 IU • Vitamin E (Natural Mixed Tocopherols) 30 IU • Vitamin B6 (Pyridoxine) 10 mg • Folic Acid 400 mcg • Vitamin B12 16 mcg • Phosphorus 300 mg • Iodine (Kelp) 225 mcg • Magnesium

BRAND NAMES

(Oxide) 200 mg • Zinc (Gluconate) 25 mg • Biotin 400 mcg • Pantothenic Acid (Calcium Salt) 30 mg • Choline (Bitartrate) 150 mg • Inositol 60 mg • Para Amino Benzoic Acid (PABA) 50 mg • Selenium (Amino Acid Chelate) 25 mcg • Manganese (Amino Acid Chelate) 10 mg • Niacinamide 50 mg • In a special potentiating base containing: Gelatin, Cysteine, Methionine, Ribonucleic Acid (RNA), Bioflavonoids, Betaine HCl, Oat Straw, Horsetail Extract, Saw Palmetto Berry, Smilax Extract, Siberian Ginseng Extract, Standardized Panax Ginseng Extract & Rutin.

Hair, Skin & Nails for Women - Futurebiotics
Three tablets contain: Vitamin A (Beta Carotene) 10,000 IU • Vitamin C 120 mg • Thiamin (B1) 10 mg • Riboflavin 10 mg • Niacinamide 50 mg • Calcium 600 mg • Iron (Amino Acid Chelate) 6 mg • Vitamin D (Fish Liver Oil) 200 IU • Vitamin E (Natural Mixed Tocopherols) 30 IU • Vitamin B6 (Pyridoxine) 10 mg • Folic Acid 400 mcg • Vitamin B12 16 mcg • Phosphorus 300 mg • Iodine (Kelp) 225 mcg • Magnesium (Oxide) 200 mg • Zinc (Gluconate) 15 mg • Biotin 400 mcg • Pantothenic Acid (Calcium Salt) 30 mg • Choline (Bitartrate) 150 mg • Inositol 60 mg • Para Amino Benzoic Acid (PABA) 50 mg • Selenium (Amino Acid Chelate) 25 mcg • Manganese (Amino Acid Chelate) 10 mg • Ribonucleic Acid (RNA) 60 mg • Bioflavonoids 50 mg • Rutin 25 mg • Betaine HCl 50 mg • In a base containing L-Cysteine, L-Methionine, Gelatin, Papain, Oat Straw, Echinacea, Horsetail, Asparagus.

Hair, Skin, & Nails - Health Smart Vitamins
Each capsule contains: Vitamin A (as beta carotene) 5,000 IU • MSM (methylsulfonylmethane) 233 mg • Tea green leaf (50% polyphenols, 60 mg) 120 mg • Horsetail stem (7% silica, 3.15 mg) 45 mg • Gotu Kola whole plant (10% triterpenes, 4 mg) 40 mg • Blueberry fruit (5% anthocyanins, 1.5 mg) 30 mg • Dandelion root 10 mg.

Hangover Relief - Hangover Solutions Inc.
Each tablet contains: Sodium (carbonates) 333 mg • Magnesium (oxide) 20 mg • Vitamin C (ascorbic acid) 200 mg • Vitamin B-1 4.5 mg • Vitamin B-2 5.1 mg • Niacinamide 60 mg • Pantothenic Acid (d-calcium pantothenate) 30 mg • Vitamin B-6 (pyridoxine) 6 mg • Vitamin B-12 18 mcg • Biotin 200 mcg • Folic Acid 400 mcg • Choline (bitartrate) 100 mg • Inositol 1 mg • PABA 1 mg • Acerola Cherry extract 50 mg • Ginger extract 50 mg • White Willow Bark 100 mg • L-Glutamine 600 mg • Yerba Mate 50 mg. Other Ingredients: Citric Acid, Sorbitol, Natural Orange Flavor, Acosulfame Potassium, Canola Oil, Docusate Sodium.

Happy Camper - Natural Balance
Two capsules contain: Proprietary blend 840 mg: Passion Flower • Kava Kava • Siberian Ginseng • Gotu Kola • Schisandra • Wood Betony • Lavender.

Harmonex - Chattem, Inc.
Each caplet contains: Standardized St. John's Wort flower extract (0.3% hypericin) 450 mg • Standardized Siberian Ginseng root extract (0.8% eleutherosides) 90 mg. Other Ingredients: Microcrystalline Cellulose, Croscarmellose Sodium, Hydroxypropyl Methylcellulose, Sodium Carboxymethyl Cellulose, Magnesium Stearate, Dextrin, Dextrose, Mineral oil, Polyethylene Glycol, Caramel, Polysorbate 80, Propylene Glycol, Riboflavin, Silicon Dioxide, Sodium Citrate, Titanium Dioxide.

HAS Original Formula - Nature's Way
Two capsules contain: Proprietary Formula: Brigham Tea herb • Burdock root • Cayenne pepper fruit • Cleavers herb • Elecampane • Goldenseal root • Marshmallow root • Parsley herb • Rosemary herb. Other ingredients: Gelatin.

Hawaiian Noni Juice - Youngevity
Purified Water • Morinda citrifolia • Lecithin • Potassium Sorbate • Artificial Flavoring • Vilcabamba Mineral Essence: Potassium, Calcium, Magnesium, Zinc, Chromium, Selenium, Iron, Copper, Molybdenum, Vanadium, Iodine, Cobalt, Manganese.

Hawthorn - Leiner Health Products
Each caplet contains: Hawthorn extract (Crataegus spp.) leaves and flowers 250 mg. Other Ingredients: Calcium Carbonate, Glucose, Cellulose, Maltodextrin, Silicon Dioxide, Hydroxypropyl Methylcellulose, Polyethylene Glycol 3350, Croscarmellose Sodium, Pharmaceutical Glaze, Crospovidone, Magnesium Stearate, Hydroxypropyl Cellulose, Red 40 Lake, Polysorbate 80, Titanium Dioxide, Povidone.

Hawthorn - Pharmanex
Each capsule contains: Hawthorn flowers & leaves (5.5:1) extract (Crategus oxyacantha) 125 mg. Other Ingredients: Rice Flour, Gelatin.

Hawthorn Phytosome - PhytoPharmica
Two capsules contain: Hawthorn (Crataegus oxyacantha) branch and flower phytosome (bound to phosphatidylcholine using a unique patented process) 200 mg.

Hay Relief - Rainbow Light
Each caplet contains: Nettle tops 260 mg • Golden seal rhizome and root powder 40 mg • Licorice root 40 mg • Lemon thyme herb 30 mg • Dong Quai root 20 mg • Eyebright herb 8 mg. Other ingredients: Cellulose or gum arabic, vegetable stearin, and silica.

H-Complex - Progressive Labs
Each capsule contains: Vitamin E 15 IU • Stone root (Collinsonia canadensis) 400 mg • Comfrey root (Symphytum officinale) 50 mg • Bayberry bark (Myrica cerifera) 50 mg • Goldenseal root (Hydrastis canadensis) 40 mg • Green Beet leaf powder 25 mg • Betony (Betonica officinalis) 10 mg.

HDT Andros-D 100 - Human Development Technologies
Each capsule contains: Androstenedione 100 mg • Zinc 15 mg • Bioperine 2.5 mg.

HDT GLX-37.5 - Human Development Technologies
Each capsule contains: Vanadyl Sulfate (yielding 7.5 mg elemental Vanadium) 37.5 mg • Taurine 600 mg • Magnesium 200 mg • Selenium 33 mcg • Ginger 20 mg • Cinnamon 20 mg • Chromium Picolinate 200 mcg.

Head Relief - Now
Two capsules contain: Feverfew leaf (Tanacetum parthenium) (min. 0.9% Parthenolide) 400 mg • Kava root extract (Piper methysticum) (30% Kavalactones) 100 mg • Ginger root extract (Zingiber officinale) 5% standardized 50 mg • Proprietary Blend of extracts 50 mg containing: Purple Willow Bark (Salix purpurea), Meadow Sweet (Filipendula ulmaria), Wintergreen (Gaultheria procumbens) to 25% standardized Salicin content.

Headacha - HerbaSway
Ginkgo Biloba • Dong Quai • Ginger • Kudzu • Bupleurum • Coptis • Blackberry • HerbaSwee (Cucurbitaceae fruit).

Headache Relief - New Chapter, Inc.
Each capsule contains: Feverfew stem, leaf & flower, supercritical extract (1% parthenolide- 1.25 mg) 125 mg • Green Tea leaf extract (50% polyphenols- 50 mg) (7% caffeine) 100 mg • Wintergreen leaf extract, salicylic acid derivatives 75 mg • Ginger (rhizome) certified organic (minimum 20% pungent compounds- 10 mg, 4% zingiberene- 2 mg) 50 mg • Meadowsweet herb, extract, salicylic acid derivatives 38 mg • Purple Willow bark (Salix purpurea) extract salicylic acid derivatives 38 mg • California Poppy whole plant, extract 5:1(leaf & essential oil), supercritical extract (23% total phenolic antioxidants - 2.3 mg) 20 mg • Rosemary leaf & essential oil, supercritical extract (23% total phenolic antioxidants - 2.3 mg) 10 mg • Ginger rhizome, certified organic (post - supercritical ethanolic extract) (3% pungent compounds - 0.3 mg) 10 mg • Lavender flower, supercritical extract (25% linalool - 2.5 mg) 10 mg • Hops strobiles, supercritical extract

(35% humulones - 1.7 mg) (12% lupulones - 0.6 mg) 5 mg • Valerian root (Valeriana officinalis & Valerians mexicanus) supercritical extract (60% valepotrates - 3 mg) 5 mg. Other Ingredients: Olive Oil certified organic, Yellow Beeswax, Gelatin, Vegetable Glycerine, Purified Water, Carob.

Headache Remedy - Lehning Laboratories
Ruta graveolens 8X • Argentum nitricum 6X • Digitalis purpurea 6X • Cimicifuga racemosa 4X • Gelsemium sempervirens 4X • Sanguinaria canadensis 4X • Chelidonium majus 3X • Cyclamen europaeum 3X • Iris versicolor 3X • Melilotus 3X. In a base of 40% USP alcohol by volume.
See Editor's Note No. 1, page 1816.

Headache Remedy - PhytoPharmica
Twenty drops contain: Ruta graveolens 8x • Argentum nitricum 6x • Digitalis purpurea 6x • Cimicifuga racemosa 4x • Gelsemium sempervirens 4x • Sanguinaria canadensis 4x • Chelidonium majus 3x • Cyclamen europaeum 3x • Iris versicolor 3x • Melilotus 3x. In a base of 40% USP alcohol by volume.
See Editor's Note No. 1, page 1816.

Heal-All Salve - Blessed Herbs
Goldenseal root • Heal-All • Comfrey root • German Chamomile flower • Plantain leaf • Echinacea Angustifolia root • Yarrow flower • Gotu Kola • St. John's Wort flower • Calendula flower • Organic Cold-Pressed Olive oil & Essential oil of Lavender.

HealthSmiles - Health Smart Vitamins
Two tablets contain: Vitamin A (as beta-carotene) 5,000 IU • Vitamin C (as ascorbic acid) 60 mg • Vitamin D (as ergocalciferol) 400 IU • Vitamin E (d-alpha tocopheryl acetate) 30 IU • Thiamin (as thiamin HCl) 1.5 mg • Riboflavin 1.7 mg • Niacin (as niacinamide) 20 mg • Vitamin B6 (as pyridoxine HCl) 2 mg • Folate (as folic acid) 10 mcg • Vitamin B12 (cyanocobalamin) 6 mcg • Biotin 50 mcg • Pantothenic acid (as calcium pantothenate) 10 mg • Calcium (as calcium amino acid chelate) 20 mg • Iron (as iron amino acid chelate) 5 mg • Iodine (from kelp) 100 mcg • Magnesium (as magnesium amino acid chelate) 10 mg • Zinc (as zinc amino acid chelate) 3 mg • Copper (as copper amino acid chelate) 50 mcg • Manganese (as maganese amino acid chelate) 50 mcg • Potassium (as potassium amino acid chelate) 1 mg • Apple fruit 50 mg • Papaya fruit 50 mg • Pineapple fruit 50 mg • Lemon Bioflavonoids 20 mg • Spirulina 20 mg • Sunflower oil seed 20 mg • Rice bran 10 mg • Beet Greens leaf 5 mg • Broccoli aerial parts 5 mg • Brown rice 5 mg • Carrot root 5 mg • Dog Rose (rose hips) 5 mg • Mango fruit 5 mg • Spinach leaf 5 mg • West Indian Cherry (fruit, Malpighia pruncifolia) 5 mg • Para-aminobenzoic acid (PABA) 400 mcg • Choline (as choline bitartrate) 10 mcg • Inositol 10 mcg.

Healthy Antioxidants - Health Smart Vitamins
Three tablets contain: Vitamin A (as beta-carotene) 20,000 IU • Vitamin C (ascorbic acid) 60 mg • Vitamin E (as d-alpha tocopheryl acetate) 30 IU • Calcium (as dicalcium phosphate) 3.5 mg • Selenium (as selenomethionine) 60 mcg • Garlic bulb (>=10,000 mcg allicin/g, >=4 mg) 400 mg • Tomato fruit (1% lycopene, 3 mg) 300 mg • Oregano leaf 150 mg • Rosemary leaf (>=6% carnosic acid, >=9 mg) 150 mg.

Healthy Cells Breast - PhytoPharmica
Each tablet contains: Folic Acid 200 mcg • Vitamin B12 (cyanocobalamin) 500 mcg • Calcium D-Glucarate 200 mg • Protein-bound Iodine (from Casein iodide) 212.5 mcg • Broccoli (Brassica oleracea) floret and stalk concentrate standardized to contain a minimum of 125 mcg sulforaphane 125 mg • Green Tea (Camellia sinensis) leaf extract (decaffeinated; standardized to contain a minimum of 70% polyphenols) 50 mg • Maitake (Grifola frondosa) mushroom powder 50 mg • Maitake (Grifola frondosa) mushroom extract (standardized to contain a minimum of 28% D-fraction compound) 5 mg.

Healthy Cells Prostate - PhytoPharmica
Each tablet contains: Calcium D-Glucarate 200 mg • Selenium (L-selenomethionine) 200 mcg • Broccoli (Brassica oleracea) floret and stalk concentrate (standardized to contain a minimum of 125 mcg of sulforaphane) 125 mg • Green Tea (Camillia sinensis) leaf extract (decaffeinated) 50 mg • Maitake (Grifola frondosa) mushroom powder 50 mg • Maitake (Grifola frondosa) mushroom extract (standardized to contain a minimum of 28% D-fraction compound) 5 mg • Lycopene 2.5 mg.

Healthy Digestion - Health Smart Vitamins
Each capsule contains: Digestive Enzyme Blend: Ox Bile, Protease, Amylase, Lipase, Cellulase, Bromelain, Papain 138 mg • Plant Fiber Base: Sugar Beet Fiber, Rice Bran, Beech cellulose, Spruce cellulose 77 mg.
See Editor's Note No. 14, page 1817.

Healthy Eyes - Health Smart Vitamins
Each capsule contains: Vitamin A (as beta-carotene) 6,000 IU • Vitamin E (as dl-alpha-tocopheryl acetate) 50 IU • Zinc (as zinc citrate) 25 mg • Selenium (as selenomethionine) 40 mcg • Copper (as copper citrate) 2 mg • Bilberry fruit (36% anthocyanosides, 21.6 mg) 60 mg.

Healthy Hair, Skin, & Nails (60) - Rainbow Light
Each capsule contains: Beta-Carotene 5000 IU • Vitamin E natural 100 IU • Tomato Paste concentrate (Lycopene)300 mg • Vitamin C (Zinc & Copper Ascorbates) 180 mg • Rice Bran 150 mg • Inositol 150 mg • Horsetail herb 4:1 extract 150 mg • Nettles tops 4:1 extract 120 mg • Ginger rhizome 4:1 extract 120 mg • L-Cysteine 100 mg • Spirulina 100 mg • PABA (Para Aminobenzioc Acid) 75 mg • Red Pepper fruit 60 mg • Pantothenic Acid (Vitamn B5) 60 mg • Rosemary leaf 4:1 extract 50 mg • Maidenhair Fern 40 mg • Marine Mineral Complex 25 mg • Niacin (Vitamin B3) 20 mg • Zinc (Ascorbate)15 mg • Rosemary oil 3 mg • Pyridoxine (Vitamin B6) 2 mg • Biotin 1800 mcg • Copper (Ascorbate) 1500 mcg • Folic Acid 400 mcg • Cyanocobalamin (Vitamin B12) 6 mcg.

Healthy Hearing - Health Smart Vitamins
Each capsule contains: Vitamin B12 (as cyanocobalamin) 100 mcg • Magnesium (as magnesium aspartate) 50 mg • Black Cohosh root 50 mg • Ginkgo leaf 2(4% ginkgo flavonglycosides, 7.2 mg; 6% terpene lactones, 1.8 mg) 30 mg • Vinpocetine 5 mg.

Healthy Heart with Folic Acid and B6 - Discount, Inc.
Each tablet contains: Vitamin B6 5 mg • Pyridoxal 5 Phosphate 0.5 mg • Folic Acid 600 mcg • Folinic Acid 1 mcg.

Healthy Immunity - Health Smart Vitamins
Each capsule contains: Astragalus root (70% polysaccharides, 70 mg) 100 mg • Elderberry (European elder berry - 10% anthocyanins, 10 mg) 100 mg • Tea green leaf (90% polyphenols, 90 mg) 100 mg • Shiitake (Mycelia extract, LEM, fruiting body) 60 mg • Reishi mycelica 30 mg • Grifola frondosa (maitake mushroom, fruiting body) 25 mg.

Healthy Joints - Health Smart Vitamins
Each capsule contains: Vitamin C (ascorbic acid) 60 mg • Manganese (as manganese glycinate) 2 mg • Glucosamine Sulfate 200 mg • Chondroitin Sulfate 100 mg • Glucosamine Hydrochloride 100 mg • Sea Cucumber 100 mg.
See Editor's Note No. 15, page 1817.

Healthy Legs Horse Chestnut Seed Extract - Leiner Health Products
Each caplet contains: Citrus Bioflavonoids complex 15 mg • Ginger powder (Zingiber officinale) root 100 mg • Gotu Kola (Centella asiatica) leaf 33 mg • Grape Seed extract (Vitis vinifera) seed 2 mg •

BRAND NAMES

Horse Chestnut extract (Aesculus hippocastanum) seed 300 mg. Other Ingredients: Dicalcium Phosphate, Hydroxypropyl Methylcellulose, Stearic Acid, Dextrin, Titanium Dioxide, Magnesium Stearate, Polyethylene Glycol 8000, Lecithin.

Healthy Mood Body Benefits Pak - Leiner Health Products
Each packet contains: Kava Kava extract (Piper methysticum) root 200 mg • Lecithin 45 mg • Licorice extract (Glycyrrhiza glabra) root 60 mg • Siberian Ginseng extract (Eleutherococcus senticosus) root 150 mg • Siberian Ginseng powder (Eleutherococcus senticosus) root 45 mg • St. John's Wort extract (Hypericum perforatum) aerial parts 900 mg. Other Ingredients: Cellulose, Dicalcium Phosphate, Calcium Carbonate, Croscarmellose Sodium, Silicon Dioxide, Stearic Acid, Maltodextrin, Magnesium.

Healthy Prostate - Health Smart Vitamins
Each softgel contains: Saw Palmetto berry (85-95% fatty acids and sterols, 136-152 mg)160 mg • Pygeum africanum bark (>13% total sterols, >6.5 mg) 50 mg • Pumpkin seed oil 40 mg.

Healthy Soy Chocolate - Nature's Life
Each scoop (35 g) contains: Supro Soy Protein Isolate (with less than 2% Lecithin) • Rice Syrup Solids • Fructose • Cocoa powder (with less than 2% Lecithin) • Fructooligosaccharides • Magnesium Citrate • Calcium Carbonate • Glycine • Apple Pectin • Ascorbic Acid • d-Alpha Tocopherol Acetate • Zinc Citrate • Niacinamide • Copper Gluconate • d-Calcium Pantothenate • Manganese Gluconate • Vitamin A Palmitate • l-Selenomethionine • Cholecalciferol • Chromium Niacinate • Pyridoxine HCl • Thiamine Mononitrate • Riboflavin • Folic Acid • Biotin • Potassium Iodide • Sodium Selenite • Sodium Molybdate • Cyanocobalamin.

Healthy Soy Formula - Health Smart Vitamins
Each capsule contains: Soy bean (10% isoflavones, 30 mg) 300 mg • Red Clover aerial parts (8% isoflavones, 16 mg) 200 mg.

Healthy Soy Vanilla - Nature's Life
Each scoop (33 g) contains: Supro Soy Protein Isolate (with less than 2% lecithin) • Maltodextrin • Rice Syrup Solids • Fructose • Fructooligosaccharides • Magnesium Citrate • Calcium Carbonate • Glycine • Apple Pectin • natural Flavors • Ascorbic Acid • d-Alpha Tocopherol Acetate • Zinc Citrate • Niacinamide • Copper Gluconate • d-Calcium Pantothenate • Manganese Gluconate • Vitamin A Palmitate • l-Selenomethionine • Cholecalciferol • Chromium Niacinate • Pyridoxine HCl • Thiamine Mononitrate • Riboflavin • Folic Acid • Biotin • Potassium Iodide • Sodium Selenite • Sodium Molybdate • Cyanocobalamin.

Healthy Vein Support - Health Smart Vitamins
Each capsule contains: Vitamin C (ascorbic acid) 50 mg • Horse Chestnut aerial parts (15% escin, 33.75 mg) 225 mg • Butcher's Broom root (10% ruscogennis, 16.7 mg) 167 mg • Rutin 90 mg • Hesperidin (35% bioflavonoids, 26.25 mg) 75 mg.

Healthy Weight - Health Smart Vitamins
Two capsules contain: Calcium (as calcium salt of hydroxy citric acid) 79 mg • Chromium (as chromium picolinate) 100 mcg • Garcinia cambogia fruit (50% (-) hydroxy citric acid [HCA], 250 mg) 500 mg • L-carnitine (as L-carnitine tartrate) 166 mg.

Healthy Whey - Nature's Life
Three tablespoons or one rounded scoop (23 g) contain: Whey Protein concentrate • natural Flavor composed of Di, Tri, Oligo & Polypeptides (providing 58% B-lactoglobulin, 22% A-Lactalbumin, 10% Immunoglobulin, 10% Minor Proteins & Lactoferrin).

Healthy Woman Soy Menopause - Personal Products
Each tablet contains Soy Standardized extract 320 mg • Includes Isoflavones 55 mg.

Heart - Centrum - Whitehall-Robbins Healthcare
One tablet contains: Supplement facts: Vitamin E 200 IU • Vitamin B6 5 mg • Folate, Folic Acid, Folacin 200 mcg • Vitamin B12 200 mcg • Selenium 25 mcg • Manganese 1 mg • Garlic Powder (bulb) (Allium sativum) 300 mg • Taurine 33 mg • Coenzyme Q10 4 mg. Other Ingredients: DL-Alpha Tocopherol Acetate, Garlic powder (Bulb, Alium sativum), Microcrystalline Cellulose, Dibasic Calcium Phosphate, Calcium Silicate, Taurine, Croscarmellose sodium, Sodium Selenate, Gelatin, Hydroxypropyl methylcellulose, Silicon Dioxide, Magnesium Stearate, Pyridoxine Hydrochloride, Ubidecarenone, Titanium Dioxide, Polyethylene Glycol, Polysorbate 80, Magnesium Sulfate Monohydrate, FD&C Red #40 Aluminum Lake, FD&C Blue #2 Aluminum Lake, Folic Acid, Cyanocobalamin, Citric Acid, Starch, Sodium Citrate, Sodium Benzoate, Sorbic Acid.

Heart Actives - VitaStore
Six tablets contain: Coenzyme Q-10 5 mg • Chitosan 500 mg • Hawthorne 200 mg • Chromium 100 mcg • Green Tea Extract 200 mg • Fiber Complex (Oat Bran & Psyllium) 1000 mg • Lecithin 500 mg • Vitamin B3 (Niacin) 50 mg • Calcium 500 mg • L-Carnitine 250 mg • Ginger 200 mg • EFA Complex (Essential Fatty Acids) 500 mg • Selenium 150 mcg • Vitamin B1 (Thiamine) 1.5 mg.

Heart Essentials - Health Smart Vitamins
Two caplets contain: Vitamin A (as 83% beta-carotene, 17% palmitate) 15,000 IU • Vitamin C (as ascorbic acid) 250 mg • Vitamin D (as cholecalciferol) 400 IU • Vitamin E (as d-alpha tocopheryl) 400 IU • Thiamin (as thiamin mononitrate) 25 mg • Riboflavin 25 mg • Niacin (as 50% nicotinic acid, 50% niacinamide) 50 mg • Vitamin B6 (as pyridoxine HCl) 25 mg • Folate (folic acid) 400 mcg • Vitamin B12 (as cyanocobalamin) 100 mcg • Biotin 300 mcg • Pantothenic Acid (as calcium pantothenate) 25 mg • Calcium (as 71% calcium carbonate, 24% dicalcium phosphate, 5% mixed calcium complexes) 269 mg • Phosphorus (as dicalcium phosphate) 10 mg • Iodine (as potassium iodide) 150 mcg • Magnesium (as 90% magnesium oxide, 5% magnesium citrate, 5% magnesium glycinate) 100 mg • Zinc (as zinc ascorbate) 15 mg • Selenium (as selenomethionine) 100 mcg • Copper (as copper citrate) 2 mg • Manganese (as manganese gluconate) 2 mg • Chromium (as chromium polynicotinate) 200 mcg • Molybdenum (as molybdenum amino acid chelate) 50 mcg • Potassium (as potassium citrate) 99 mg • Chondroitin Sulfate 50 mg • Betaine HCl 25 mg • Bioflavonoids 25 mg • Choline (as bitartrate) 25 mg • Garlic bulb (250 mcg allicin) 25 mg • Hawthorn leaf, flower (1.8% vitexin - 2" - rhamnoside) 0.45 mg • Inositol 25 mg • L-Carnitine 25 mg • Lecithin (from soybean) 25 mg • Bromelain (from pineapple, 6,000 PU/g, 120 PU) 20 mg • Coenzyme Q10 10 mg • Lipase (from fermentation of Aspergillus niger) 10 mg • Alpha Lipoic acid 10 mg • Papain (from latex of fruit) 10 mg • Para-aminobenzoic acid (PABA) 10 mg • Rutin 5 mg • Boron (as boron asparate) 2 mg • Silicon (as silicon dioxide) 2 mg • Vanadium (as vanadium amino acid chelate) 10 mcg.
See Editor's Note No. 15, page 1817.

Heart Essentials - Swanson
Each tablet contains: Vitamin C (as ascorbic acid) 100 mg • Vitamin E (as d-alpha tocopheryl succinate) 33.3 IU • Niacin 9 mg • Vitamin B-6 (as pyridoxine HCl) 17 mg • Folic Acid 135 mcg • Vitamin B-12 (as cyanocobalamin) 33.3 mcg • Calcium (from amino acid chelate) 33.3 mg • Magnesium (from amino acid chelate) 33.3 mg • Selenium (as selenomethionine) 50 mcg • Chromium (ChromeMate) 33 mcg • Potassium (from amino acid chelate) 33 mg • Taurine 100 mg • Trimethylglycine 84 mg • Odor-Controlled Garlic bulb (PureGar 10,000 ppm allicin potential) 34 mg • Hawthorn berry extract (1.8% vitexin-2' rhamnosides) 17 mg • L-Carnitine 17 mg • Lecithin 17 mg • Coenzyme Q10 10 mg • Ginger root extract (5% gingerols) 8.4 mg.

Heart Formula - Nature's Way
Two capsules contain: Betaine Anhydrous 200 mg • Coenzyme Q10 (Ubiquinone) 15 mg • Folic Acid (Folate) 300 mc • Hawthorne dried

extract (1.8%-2.2% Vitexin) 350 mg • Niacin (Vitamin B3) 20 mg • Potassium (Aspartate, Chloride) 20 mg • Pyridoxine HCL 50 mg • Reishi dried extract (10% Polysaccharides) 25 mg • Siberian Ginseng root 250 mg • Vitamin B12 (Cyanocobalamin) 400 mcg • Vitamin E (d-Alpha Tocopheryl) 50 IU. Other ingredients: Gelatin, Magnesium Stearate, Millet.

Heart Science - Source Naturals
Six tablets contain: Vitamin A (Beta Carotene) 45000 IU • Vitamin B1 (Thiamin) 50 mg • Inositol Hexanicotinate 500 mg • Vitamin B6 (Pyridoxine HCl) 25 mg • Coenzymated B6 (Pyridoxal-5'-Phosphate)(Yielding 16.9 mg of Vitamin B6) 25 mg • Vitamin B12 (Cyanocobalamin) 500 mcg • Folic Acid 800 mcg • Vitamin C (Magnesium Ascorbate) 1500 mg • Vitamin E (D-Alpha Tocopheryl) (Natural) 400 IU • Chromium (ChromeMate Polynicotinate 150 mcg and Chromium Picolinate 150 mcg) 300 mcg • Copper (Sebacate) 750 mcg • Magnesium (Ascorbate, Taurinate and Oxide) 300 mg • Potassium (Citrate) 99 mg • Selenium (L-Selenomethionine) 200 mcg • Silica (from 400 mg of Horsetail Extract) 28 mg • Coenzyme Q10 (Ubiquinone) 60 mg • L-Carnitine L-Tartrate 500 mg • Hawthorn berry extract 400 mg • Proanthodyn (grape seed extract)(with a Proanthocyanidolic Value of 95) 100 mg • L-Proline 500 mg • L-Lysine (HCl) 500 mg • N-A-G (N-Acetyl Glucosamine) 500 mg • Bromelain (2000 GDU per g) 1200 mg • Taurine (Magnesium Taurinate) 500 mg • Inositol (Hexanicotinate) 50 mg.

Heart Support - Nutri-Quest
Each tablet contains: Heart 100 mg • Spleen 40 mg • Co-Enzyme Q-10 2 mg • Vitamin C (Sago Palm) 100 mg • Vitamin E (Succinate) 100 IU • L-Carnitine HCL 20 mg.
See Editor's Note No. 14, page 1817.

Heart Support - Amazon Support
Each capsule contains: Abuta • Hawthorn • Bitter Melon • Chanca Piedra • Periwinkle • Mulungu • Artichoke.

Heart Support - Now
Three tablets contain: Vitamin B1 (Thiamine HCL) 50 mg • Vitamin B6 (Pyridoxine HCL) 50 mg • Vitamin B12 (Cyanocobalamin) 1000 mcg • Folic Acid 800 mcg • Magnesium (Oxide/Aspartate) 200 mg • Potassium (Chloride/Aspartate) 200 mg • Iodine (Kelp extract) 300 mcg • Selenium (Selenomethionine) 140 mcg • Coenzyme Q10, pure 30 mg • L-Carnitine 400 mg • Pure-Gar Garlic 1000 mg • Hawthorne berry extract (standardized to contain 1.25% Vitexin-4' Rhamnoside) 150 mg • Alpha Lipoic Acid 20 mg • Ginger root 250 mg • Cayenne pepper (40000 Heat units) 150 mg.

Heart Support - Olympia Nutrition
CoQ10 • Alpha Lipoic Acid • Garlic • Hawthorn • Cayenne • Magnesium.

HeartCare - Nature's Way
Each tablet contains: Hawthorn dried extract (19% oligomeric procyanidins) 80 mg.

Heart's Ease - The Herbalist
Hawthorn berry, leaf & flower • Dandelion root, leaf & flower • Skullcap herb • Yarrow flower • Horsetail herb • Lemon Balm herb • Prickly Ash bark • Cayenne pepper.

Heat - Sports Nutrition Source.com
Each capsule contains: Ma Huang Concentrate aerial parts 24 mg • Caffeine USP 80 mg • Guarana Concentrate seed 75 mg • White Willow Bark Concentrate 75 mg • Cayenne fruit 60 mg • Ginger root 40 mg.

Heavenly Skin & Hair Care - Gary Nulls
Whole leaf Aloe Vera concentrate, Jojoba oil, Licorice and Grape seed extracts, Tri-Silica complex, MSM, Antioxidant Botanical extracts, Liposomal Vitamins, Oat Bran glucan, Tissue Respiratory Factor, and more.

Heavyweight Gainer 900 - Champion Nutrition
Each serving contains: Metacarb-III (branching complex carbohydrates extracted from Corn Hybrids including Maltodextrins) • Peptol-III: pre-digested highly efficient protein blend consisting of Whey Protein Concentrate, Fat-Free, Cholesterol-Free, Red-Muscle Protein Complex, Debitterized Enzyme Digest of Lactalbumin, & Egg White Protein • extra grade Whey • Fructose • low-fat Cocoa powder • MCT's • Metavite-III [Champion Nutrition's advanced Vitamin/ Mineral formula consisting of di-Calcium Pantothenate, Potassium, Citrate, Magnesium Gluconate, Potassium Chloride, Choline Bitartrate, Inositol, Ascorbic Acid, D-Calcium Pantothenate, Niacin, Zinc Gluconate, d-Alpha Tocopherol Succinate, Molybdenum Aspartate, Selenium Aspartate, Manganese Gluconate, Chromemate-GTF (Chromium Polynicotinate), Copper Gluconate, Pyridoxal-5-Phosphate, Thiamine HCL, D-Biotin, Potassium Iodid, Ergocalciferol, Folic Acid, Cyanocobalamin] • Cellulose Gum • Xanthan • Natural & Artificial Flavors • Lecithin • Sunnette Brand of Acesulfame-K • Carrageenan • Aspartame. Contains Phenylalanine.

Hemaplex - Progressive Labs
Each capsule contains: Iron (from 200 mg iron peptonate) 32 mg • Vitamin C (ascorbic acid) 200 mg • Thiamin HCl (Vitamin B1) 2 mg • Riboflavin (Vitamin B2) 2 mg • Niacin 13 mg • Niacinamide 15 mg • Vitamin B6 (pyridoxine HCl) 2 mg • Folate (folic acid) 400 mcg • Vitamin B12 (cyanocobalamin) 50 mcg • Base: [Raw Duodenum, Raw Liver, Raw Stomach, Red Bone Marrow, Beef Peptone, Citrus pectin, Betaine HCl, Bile Salts, Rose Hips, Alfalfa & Wheat germ] 50 mg.
See Editor's Note No. 14, page 1817.

Hem-Care - PhytoPharmica
Two capsules contain: Vitamin C (ascorbic acid) 100 mg • Vitamin E (d-alpha tocopheryl succinate) 30 IU • Calcium lactate 130 mg • Phosphorus (tricalcium phosphate) 25 mg • Collinsonia Canadensis (stoneroot) 500 mg • Choline Bitartrate 150 mg • Butcher's Broom (Ruscus aculeatus) root and rhizome extract (standardized to contain 10% saponins calculated as ruscogenin) 100 mg • Rutin (Buckwheat) flower buds 100 mg • Glycosaminoglycans (GAGs) Highly purified bovine-derived glycosaminoglycans 25 mg.
See Editor's Note No. 14, page 1817.

Hem-Mend: Hemorrhoid Support - The Herbalist
Stone root fresh dried (Collinsonia canadensis) • Celandine fresh-flowering herb (Chaelidonium majus) • Witch Hazel fresh-dried leaf (Hamamelis virginiana) • Horse chestnut fresh nut (Aesculus hippocastanum).

Hemo-Plus - Atrium Inc.
Each tablet contains: Vitamin C 300 mg • Vitamin B1 10 mg • Vitamin B2 10 mg • Vitamin B6 10 mg • Vitamin B12 250 mcg • Folic Acid 800 mcg • Niacinamide 20 mg • Iron Peptonate 113 mg • Manganese (Proteinate Chelated) 5 mg • Liver 75 mg.
See Editor's Note No. 14, page 1817.

Hemorrhoid Remedy - PhytoPharmica
Twenty drops contain: Aloe socotrina 4x • Sulphur 4x • Collinsonia canadensis 3x • Narum nitricum 3x • Nux vomica 3x • Paeonia officinalis 3x • Teucrium scorodonia 3x • Verbascum thapsus 2x • Aesculus hippocastanum 1x • Boldo 1x • Hamamelis virginiana 1x. In a base of 45% USP alcohol by volume.
See Editor's Note No. 1, page 1816.

Hem-Tone - Enzymatic Therapy
Two capsules contain: Vitamin E (D-Alpha Tocopherol Succinate) 30 IU • Calcium Lactate 130 mg • Vitamin C (Ascorbic Acid) 100 mg • Phosphorus (Tricalcium Phosphate) 25 mg • Other ingredients: Colinsonia root (Stone root) 500 mg • Choline Bitartrate 150 mg • Butchers Broom extract (Ruscus aculeatus) standardized to contain

BRAND NAMES

BRAND NAMES

10% Saponins (calculated as Ruscogenin) 100 mg • Rutin (Buckwheat) 100 mg • Glycosaminoglycans 25 mg: A mixture of highly purified bovine-derived Glycosaminoglycans naturally present in the aorta including: Dermatan Sulfate, Heparan Sulfate, Hyaluronic Acid, Chondroitin Sulfate, & related Hexosaminoglycans. Contains no sugar, salt, yeast, wheat, corn, dairy products, coloring, flavoring, or preservatives. All organs & glands derived from bovine sources. See Editor's Note No. 15, page 1817.

Hepato-C - Pacific BioLogic
Salvia root • Heydyotis • Scutellaria (barbat skullcap) • Peony root (red) • Codonopsis root (natural) • Lycium fruit • Dryopteris rhizome • Rhodiole Sachelanensi root • Polygonum root (thin) • Magnolia bark • Knotweed rhizome (bushy) • Astragalus root (Grade 1) • Capillaris shoots & leaves • Bitter Orange (ripened fruit) • Polyporus Sclerotium.

Hepato-Detox - Pacific BioLogic
Salvia root • Codonopsis root (natural) • Lycium fruit • Polygonatum rhizome • Astragalus root (Grade 1) • Reishi Mushroom • Privet fruit (ligustrum) • Ginseng root (red ji lin) • Cherry (cornelian asiatic).

Hepatox - PhytoPharmica
Three tablets contain: Vitamin A (Fish Liver oil) 4500 IU • Niacin 40 mg • Vitamin C (Ascorbic Acid/Rose Hips) 25 mg • Biotin 200 mcg • Vitamin B12 (Cyanocobalamin) 3 mcg • Choline Bitartrate 850 mg • Dehydrated Green Beet leaf juice powder 300 mg • L-Methionine 250 mg • Barberry Bark of root 4:1 (Berberis vulgaris) 150 mg • Boldo extract (peumus boldo) 150 mg standardized to contain 1.52% essential oils • Greater Celandine extract (Chelidonium majus) 135 mg • Fringe Tree (Cheonanthus) 135 mg • Ox Bile extract 90 mg • Betaine HCL 75 mg • Inositol 50 mg • Liver (Desiccated) 40 mg • Unsaturated Free Fatty Acids 30 mg. Chlorophyll is used in this product as a natural coloring agent. Contains no sugar, salt, yeast, wheat, corn, soy, dairy products, flavorings or preservatives. All organs & glands derived from bovine sources. See Editor's Note No. 14, page 1817.

Herba Fuel - TwinLab
Three capsules contain: Ma Huang extract (standardized for 6% Ephedrine) 334 mg • Chinese Green Tea extract (standardized for 7% Caffeine & 20% Polyphenols) 1500 mg. In a natural base of Siberian Ginseng (Eleutherococcus senticosus).

Herbal Cold - Puritan's Pride
Each tablet contains: Vitamin C (calcium ascorbate) 500 mg • Calcium (calcium ascorbate) 50 mg • Poplar Bud extract 25 mg • Senega extract 10 mg • Oil of Thyme 5 mg • Oil of Eucalyptus 5 mg • Hore Hound powdered 10 mg • Coltsfoot powdered 10 mg • Licorice root powdered 15 mg • Capsicum powdered 10 mg • Cubeb powdered 10 mg • Slippery Elm bark powdered 10 mg • Fennel powdered 10 mg • Jamaican Ginger powdered 10 mg • Honey 10 mg • Lemon Juice 1 mg • Rutin 10 mg • Bee Pollen 10 mg • Bee Propolis 50 mg.

Herbal Cold Relief - Jamieson
Each capsule contains: Ephedra stem extract (Ephedra since)(equivalent to 10.2 mg of ephedrine) 62.5 mg • Grindelia aerial parts 1:4 extract (Grindelia Camporum) 0.5 mg • Eucalyptus oil (Eucalypyus Globulus) 0.05 mg • Echinacea Root (Echinacea purpurea) 100 mg.

Herbal Cold Season Defense - Quantum Health
Three capsules contain: Vitamin C 250 mg • Echinacea angustifolia standardized to 4% phenolic compounds 100 mg • Elderberry (10:1) extract 100 mg • Goldenseal root (3:1) extract 25 mg. Other Ingredients: Vegetable Sterine, Magnesium Stearate, Micro Crystalline Cellulose.

Herbal Decongestant Expectorant Capsules - Life Brand
Ma Huang (Ephedra) 50 mg as a standardized extract 1:10 (equivalent to 500 mg Ma Huang) with 4 mg of total Ephedrines • Wild Horehound leaf 150 mg • Thyme herb extract (1:4) 100 mg (equivalent to 400 mg of Thyme) • Coltsfoot leaf 50 mg • Mullein leaf 50 mg • Cayenne 1.125 mg • Marshmallow root 9 mg • Slippery Elm bark 9 mg. Excipients: Gelatin & water.

Herbal Diuretic - Progressive Labs
Each capsule contains: Active Ingredients: Proprietary blend 120 mg: Buchu leaves (Barsoma crenata) • Couch Grass root (Triticum repens). Other Herbs: Proprietary blend 330 mg: [Hydrangea root (Hydrangea arborescens), Corn Silk (Stigmata maidis), Juniper berry (Juniperus communis), Burdock root (Arctium lappa), Uva Ursi leaf (Arctostaphylos Uva-Ursi), Ginger root (Zingiber officinale) Parsley (Petroselium sativum), Marshmallow root (Althaea officinalis)].

Herbal Diuretic Formula - Quest
Each caplet contains: Uva Ursi leaf (Arctostaphylos uva-ursi) (Provided by 50 mg P.E. 1:4) 200 mg • Juniper berry extract (Junuperus communis) (Provided by 80 mg P.E. 1:4) 320 mg • Parsley root (Petroselinum crispum) (Provided by 40 mg P.E. 1:4) 160 mg. Other Ingredients: Buchu leaves, Cayenne, Corn Silk, Kelp, Parsley leaf, Pumpkin seed, Saw Palmetto berries, Calcium Phosphate, Vegetable Stearin, Croscarmellose Sodium, Magnesium Stearate (vegetable source).

Herbal Diuretic Tablets - Life Brand
Buchu leaf extract (1:4) 25 mg (equivalent to 100 mg Buchu leaf) • Uva Ursi leaf extract (1:3) 33.3 mg (equivalent to 100 mg Uva Ursi leaf) • Juniper berry extract (1:2) 50 mg (equivalent to 100 mg of Juniper berries) • Celery seed 75 mg • Parsley root 75 mg. Excipients: Microcrystalline Cellulose, Tricalcium Phosphate, Corn Starch, Magnesium Stearate.

Herbal Douche - Dial Herbs
Mineral Water • Aloe Vera • White Oak bark • Slippery Elm • Uva Ursi • Cayenne.

Herbal Ecstacy - Global World Media
Each pill contains: Ephedra • Ma Huang • Guarana • Gingko biloba • Cola Nut • Gotu-Kola • Fo-Ti-Tient (Fo-Ti) • Green Tea • Rou Gui (Chinese Nutmeg).
See Editor's Note No. 32, page 1820.

Herbal Expector-Aid - Quantum Health
Each softgel contains: Vitamin C (ascorbic acid) 200 mg • Elderberry extract berry standardized to 5% flavonoids 200 mg • Fenugreek powder seed (4:1) extract 100 mg • Horehound powder flower, leaf, stem (4:1) extract 100 mg • Anise seed (4:1) extract 100 mg • Marshmallow root (4:1) extract 60 mg • Anise seed oil 40 mg • Echinacea extract flower, leaf (4:1 PE) 40 mg • Menthol Crystals 20 mg • Eucalyptus Oil 10 mg. Other Ingredients: Gelatin Shell: Gelatin, Glycerin, St. John's Bread, Titanium Dioxide; Liquid Fill: Sunflower Seed Oil, Beeswax, Lecithin.

Herbal Fem - Nutri-Quest
Golden Seal root, Dong Quai, Blessed Thistle, Red Raspberry leaves, Squaw Vine, Scullcap, Cayenne, Blue Cohosh, Licorice root, Wild Yam root, Passion Flower 408 mg. In a base of 6X tissue salts: Calc Fluor, Calc Phos, Calc Sulph, Kali Mur, Kali Phos, Kali Sulph, Mag Phos, Nat Mur, Nat Phos, Nat Sulph, Silica.

Herbal Gargle - Dial Herbs
Sage • Myrrh • Goldenseal • Bayberry • Cayenne • Ginger • pure Apple cider vinegar aged in wood.

Herbal GI - PhysioLogics
Each capsule contains: Glucosamine (HCl) 150 mg • Gamma

Oryzanol 200 mg • Chamomile (1.2% Apigenin, 1.8 mg; 0.5% Essential oil, 0.75 mg) 150 mg • Aloe Vera 100 mg • Wild Yam (6% total Saponins, 4.5 mg) 75 mg.

Herbal Gold Cigarettes - Alternative Cigarettes Inc
Each cigarette contains: Marshmallow • Yerba Santa • Damiana • Passion Flower • Jasmine • Ginseng. Regular, menthol, vanilla, and cherry are available.
See Editor's Note No. 31, page 1820.

Herbal Grobust - HomeCure, Inc.
Sabal • Damiana • Dong Quai • Blessed Thistle • Kava Kava • Dandelion root • Oat Bran • Wild Yam • Mother's Wort.

Herbal Immune Complex - Solgar
Standardized Astragalus root (glucosides 0.5 mg [0.5%], polysaccharides 70 mg [70%]) 100 mg • Standardized Cat's Claw extract inner bark (mitraphylline 3 mg [3%], polyphenols 15 mg [15%]) 100 mg • Standardized Echinacea purpurea extract root, leaf (echinacosides 4 mg [4%], polysaccharides 15 mg [15%]) 100 mg • Standardized Deglycyrrhized Licorice extract root (glycyrrhizin<1 mg [1%]) 100 mg • Standardized Elderberry extract berry (polyphenols 30 mg [30%]) 100 mg • Standardized Olive Leaf extract leaf (oleuropein 6 mg [6%]) 100 mg • Raw Elderberry powder flower 20 mg • Raw Echinacea powder root, leaf 20 mg • Raw Licorice powder root 20 mg • Raw Olive Leaf powder 20 mg • Raw Astragalus powder root 20 mg. Other Ingredients: Vegetable Cellulose, Vegetable Stearic Acid, Vegetable Magnesium Stearate, Vegetable Glycerin, PhytO2X Blend containing: Natural Vitamin E (mixed tocopherols), Natural Beta Carotene and other Carotenoids, Rosemary extract aerial, Vitamin C (L-ascorbic-acid), Water.

Herbal Insomnia Tablets - Life Brand
Valerian root extract (1:4) 50 mg (equivalent to 200 mg Valerian root) • Passion Flower herb 80 mg • Chamomile flower extract (1:4) 15 mg (equivalent to 60 mg Chamomile flowers) • Mistletoe herb 50 mg • Hops flower 50 mg • Wild Lettuce leaf 40 mg. Excipients: Tricalcium Phosphate, Corn Starch, Silicon dioxide, Magnesium Stearate.

Herbal Klenz - Progressive Labs
Each capsule contains: Vitamin A 3500 IU • Echinacea (Echinacea angustifolia) 200 mg • Golden Seal (Hydrastis canadensis) 125 mg • Irish Moss (Chondrus crispus) 40 mg • Ginger root (Zingiber officinale) 35 mg • Burdock root (Arctium lappa) 35 mg • Peony root (Paeonia officinalis) 35 mg • Peony root skin (Paeonia officinalis) 35 mg • Licorice root (Glycyrrhiza glabra) 25 mg • Red Clover flower (Trifolium pratense) 20 mg.

Herbal Laxative - Holista
Each capsule contains: Cascara Sagrada extract 200 mg • Senna leaves 250 mg.

Herbal Laxative (Stomach-Ease) Tablets - Life Brand
Senna leaves 240 mg • Cascara Sagrada bark 150 mg • Licorice root 30 mg • Juniper berries 8 mg • Rhubarb root 8 mg • Gentian root 8 mg • Buchu leaves 4 mg. Excipients: Corn Starch, Sodium Bicarbonate, Silicon Dioxide, Magnesium Stearate, oil of Peppermint.

Herbal Laxative Formula - Quest
Each caplet contains: Cascara Sagrada bark (Rhamnus purshiana) (Provided by 50 mg P.E. 7:1) 350 mg • Rhubarb root (Rheum officinale L.) (Provided by 30 mg P.E. 1:4) 120 mg. Other Ingredients: Cayenne, Ginger root, Licorice root, Marshmallow root, Calcium Phosphate, Croscarmellose Sodium, Microcrystalline Cellulose, Magnesium Stearate (vegetable source), Vegetable Stearin.

Herbal Lite - BioTreasures
Each caplet contains: Calcium Pyruvate 1050 mg • L-Phenylalanine 116 mg • Manganese Chelate 6 mcg • Chromium Polynicotinate

500 mcg • Proprietary Herbal Blend 1830 mg: Citrus Aurantium • Garcinia Cambogia • St. John's Wort • Green Tea • Gotu Kola • Siberian Ginseng • Stevia.

Herbal Liver Complex - Solgar
Each vegicap contains: Standardized Milk Thistle extract aerial, seed (silymarin 80 mg [80%]) 100 mg • Standardized Dandelion extract whole plant (vitexin 3 mg [3%]) 100 mg • Standardized Turmeric extract root (curcuminoids 71 mg [95%]) 75 mg • Standardized Schisandra extract fruit (schisandrins 0.5 mg [1%]) 50 mg • Standardized Picrorizha kurroavv extract Picroliv (kutkin 3 mg [3.5%]) 75 mg • Standardized Phyllanthus amarus extract leaf (sesquiterpenes>2 mg [4%]) 50 mg • Phosphatidylcholine 100 mg • Raw Milk Thistle powder aerial 75 mg • Raw Dandelion powder root 75 mg. Other Ingredients: Microcrystalline Cellulose; Vegetable Cellulose; Vegetable Stearic Acid; Vegetable Magnesium Stearate; Vegetable Glycerin; PhytO2X Blend containing: Natural Vitamin E (mixed tocopherols), Natural Beta Carotene and other Carotenoids, Rosemary extract aerial, Vitamin C (L-ascorbic acid), Water.

Herbal Male Complex - Solgar
Each vegicap contains: Standardized Saw Palmetto extract berry (FFA 34 mg-38 mg [45%-50%]) 75 mg • Standardized Nettles extract leaf (silic acid 0.75 mg [1%]) 75 mg • Standardized Astragalus extract root (glucosides 0.38 mg [0.5%], polysaccharides 53 mg [70%]) 75 mg • Standardized Korean Panax Ginseng extract root (eleutherosides 0.6 mg [0.8%]) 75 mg • Soy Isoflavone extract seed 75 mg • Raw Astragalus powder root 50 mg • Raw Korean Ginseng powder root 25 mg • Raw Siberian Ginseng powder root 25 mg • Raw Nettles powder leaf 25 mg. Other Ingredients: Microcrystalline Cellulose; Vegetable Cellulose; Vegetable Stearic Acid; Vegetable Magnesium Stearate; Vegetable Glycerin; PhtO2X blend containing Natural Vitamin E (mixed tocopherols), Natural Beta Carotene and Other Carotenoids, Rosemary extract aerial, Vitamin C (L-ascorbic acid), Water.

Herbal Migraine Formula - Quest
Each caplet contains: Feverfew powder (Tanacetum parthenium) (contains no less than 0.2% parthenolides) 125 mg. Other Ingredients: Calcium Phosphate, Croscarmellose Sodium, Microcrystalline Cellulose, Vegetable Stearin, Magnesium Stearate (vegetable source).

Herbal Nerve Tablets - Life Brand
Valerian root extract (1:4) 50 mg (equivalent to 200 mg Valerian root) • Skullcap herb 100 mg • Hops flowers 50 mg. Excipients: Tricalcium Phosphate, Corn Starch, Magnesium Stearate, Silicon Dioxide.

Herbal Niagra - Young Again Nutrients
Three capsules contain: Bulgarian Tribulus Terrestris 750 mg • Ginseng Panax 500 mg • Yohimbe Bark 300 mg • Saw Palmetto (25%) 100 mg • Vitamin B3 (Niacinamide) 50 mg.

Herbal Nightcap - Trader Joe's
Passion flower 150 mg • Chamomile 4 mg • Hops 60 mg.

Herbal Pain and Fever Relief - Holista
Each capsule contains: White Willow bark powder 300 mg • Meadowsweet extract 250 mg.

Herbal Pain Relief Formula - Quest
Each caplet contains: White Willow bark (Salix alba) (Provided by 250 mg P.E. 1:12 standardized to contain 11% Salicin) 3000 mg. Other Ingredients: Blue Vervain, Kelp, Red Raspberry leaf, Skullcap and Wood Betony. Calcium Phosphate, Magnesium Stearate (vegetable source), Microcrystalline Cellulose, Vegetable Stearin.

Herbal Phen Fen Stage 2 - HPF L.L.C.
Two tablets contain: St. John's Wort 400 mg • Ma Huang 250 mg • Green Tea leaf extract 450 mg. Other Ingredients: Dicalcium

Phosphate, Microcrystalline Cellulose, Croscarmellose Sodium, Stearic Acid, Silica, Magnesium Stearate, Pharmaceutical glaze.

Herbal Regulator - VitaStore
Two tablets contain: Potassium (as gluconate) 25 mg • Hydrangea root 100 mg • Graminis Rhizoma root 50 mg • Cornsilk 50 mg • Parsley whole herb 25 mg • Uva Ursi leaves 75 mg.

Herbal Relaxant Formula - Quest
Each caplet contains: Valerian root (Valeriana officinalis) (Provided by 100 mg P.E. 1:5 standardized to contain 0.8% Valerenic Acid) 500 mg • Chamomile flower (Chamomilla recutita L.) (Provided by 50 mg P.E. 1:4 standardized to contain 1% Apigenin) 200 mg. Other Ingredients: Ginger root, Hops, Marshmallow root, Skullcap, Calcium Phosphate, Croscarmellose Sodium, Magnesium Stearate (vegetable source), Microcrystalline Cellulose, Vegetable Stearin.

Herbal Seltzer - Dial Herbs
Sodium • White Willow bark • Fever Few • Ginger • Mint • Stevia • Potassium Bicarbonate • Sodium Bicarbonate • Citric Acid. Flavored & sweetened with natural orange flavorings, natural fruit flavors & dextrose.

Herbal Slim - Nature's Way
Four capsules contain: Proprietary formula: Black Walnut hulls • Burdock root • Chickweed leaf & stem • Echinacea Purpurea stem, leaf, flower • Fennel seed • Hawthorne berry • Kelp (whole Thallus) • Licorice root • Papaya leaves • Parsley herb • Safflower flower. Other ingredients: Gelatin.

Herbal Tranquility - Optimum Nutrition
Valerian Root • Passionflower extract.

Herbal Tranquility Complex - Solgar
Each vegicap contains: Standardized Kava Kava extract root (kavalactones 30 mg [30%]) 100 mg • Standardized Valerian extract root (valernic acid 0.8 mg [0.8%]) 100 mg • Standardized Passionflower extract aerial (isovitexin 2mg-3mg [3%-4%]) 75 mg • Standardized Schisandra extract fruit (schisandrins 0.75 mg [1%]) 75 mg • Standardized St. John's Wort extract aerial (hypericin 0.23 mg [0.3%]) 75 mg • Standardized American Ginseng extract root (ginsenosides 5 mg [10%]) 50 mg • Raw Kava Kava powder root 50 mg • Raw St. John's Wort powder aerial 50 mg • Raw Valerian powder root 50 mg. Other Ingredients: Microcrystalline Cellulose; Vegetable Cellulose; Vegetable Stearic Acid; Vegetable Magnesium Stearate; Vegetable Glycerin; PhytO2X Blend containing: Natural Vitamin E (mixed tocopherols), Natural Beta Carotene and other Carotenoids, Rosemary extract aerial, Vitamin C (L-ascorbic acid), Water.

Herbal Treasures - BioTreasures
Each caplet contains: Kelp 40 mg • Reishi Mushroom 40 mg • Papain (from Papaya) 40 mg • Alfalfa 200 mg • Vitamin A (Beta Carotene) 5000 IU • Vitamin C (Ester-C Calcium Ascorbate) 75 mg • Vitamin E (D-Alpha Tocopheryl Acetate) 30 IU • Vitamin B1 (Thiamine) 1.5 mg • Vitamin B2 (Riboflavin) 1.7 mg • Vitamin B3 (Niacin) 20 mg • Vitamin B5 (Pantothenic Acid) 10 mg • Vitamin B6 (Pyridoxine) 2 mg • Vitamin B12 (Cyanocobalamin) 6 mcg • Folic Acid 400 mcg • Calcium (Calcium Chelate) 400 mg • Magnesium (Ascorbate) 150 mg • Zinc (Zinc Chelate) 74 mg • Chromium (Chromium Polynicotate) 1000 mcg • Proprietary Herbal Blend 610 mg: Grape Seed extract, Garlic extract, Ginkgo biloba extract, Green Tea extract, Siberian Ginseng, Silymarin (Milk Thistle extract), Astragalus extract, Hawthorne berries extract, Horsetail extract, Ashwaganda extract, Stevia extract.

Herbal Up Formula - Nature's Way
Two capsules contain: Bee Pollen • Cayenne pepper fruit • Gotu Kola stem, leaf • Proprietary Blend (840 mg) • Siberian Ginseng root. Other ingredients: Gelatin.

Herbal UR-Kidney - Nutri-Quest
Proprietary blend 430 mg: Juniper Berries • Parsley • Uva Ursi, Marshmallow • Ginger • Golden Seal root • Corn Silk • Cleavers root. In a base of 6X tissue salts: Mag Phos, Nat Sulph, Calc Phos, Calc Sulph.

Herbal V - Ultra-V
Two tablets contain: Yohimbe extract 2% 250 mg • Avena Sativa extract 10:1 150 mg • Androstenedione 90 mg • Saw Palmetto extract 4:1 100 mg • Guarana extract 22% 300 mg • Taurine 200 mg • Siberian Ginseng extract 35:1 30 mg • Tribulus Terrestris extract 40% 50 mg. Other ingredients: Dicalcium Phosphate, Microcrystalline Cellulose, Magnesium Sterate, Stearic Acid.

Herbal V: Women's Formula - VitaZip, Inc.
Avena Sativa 10:1 Extract • Kava Kava 30% • Muira Puama 4:1 Extract • St. John's Wort .3% • Ginkgo Biloba 24%/6%.

Herbal Water Control - Jamieson
Two capsules contain: Calcium (as Calcium Sulfate) 54 mg • Uva Ursi leaf (Arctostaghylos uva-ursi (L) Spreng) 400 mg • Buchu leaf (Barosma Betulina Bartl. Et Wendl.) 200 mg.

Herbal Women's Formula - Quest
Each caplet contains: White Willow bark powder (Salix alba) (Provided by 85 mg P.E. 1:12 standardized to contain 11% Salicin) 1000 mg • Valerian root (Valeriana officinalis) (Provided by 40 mg P.E. 1:5 standardized to contain 0.8% Valerenic Acid) 200 mg • Chamomile flower (Chamomilla recutita L.) (Provided by 20 mg P.E. 1:4 standardized to contain 1% Apigenin) 80 mg • Uva Ursi leaf (Arctostaphylos uva-ursi) (Provided by 50 P.E. 1:4 standardized to contain 10% Arbutin) 200 mg • Juniper berry (Juniperus communis) (Provided by 80 mg P.E. 1:4) 320 mg • Parsley root (Petroselinum crispum) (Provided by 40 mg P.E. 1:4) 160 mg. Other Ingredients: Calcium Phosphate, Croscarmellose Sodium, Magnesium Stearate (vegetable source), Microcrystalline Cellulose, Silicon Dioxide.

Herbalax - Health Factor
Each capsule contains: Cascara Sagrada (Rhamnus purshiana) 260 mg • Peppermint (Menta piperita) 90 mg.

Herbal-Biotic - The Herbalist
Oregon Grape Root • Golden Seal root • Yerba Mansa root.

Herbal-F - Progressive Labs
Each capsule contains: Vitamin B6 (as pyridoxine HCl) 20 mg • Magnesium (as magnesium oxide/soy protein complex) 15 mg • Damiana leaf (Turnera aphrodisiaca) 60 mg • Passion flower (Passiflora incarnata) 40 mg • Black Cohosh root (Cimicifuga racemosa) 20 mg • Blue Cohosh root (Caulophyllum thalictroides) 20 mg • Ginger root (Zingiber officinale) 60 mg • Cramp bark (Viburnum opulus) 75 mg • Wild Yam root (Dioscorea villosa) 40 mg • False Unicorn root (Chamaelirium luteum) 40 mg • Squaw vine (Mitchella repens) 40 mg • Blackhaw bark (Viburnum punifolium) 40 mg • Prickly Ash bark (Zanthoxylum americanum) 40 mg • White Birch bark (Betula alba) 40 mg • Ovarian substance 10 mg. See Editor's Note No. 14, page 1817.

Herbalife - Activated Fiber Tablets - Herbalife
Each tablet contains: Sodium Choleate • L-Carnitine.

Herbalife - Aminogen - Herbalife
Each tablet contains: Aminogen 250 mg.

Herbalife - Body Contouring Cream - Herbalife
Water • Cetyl Esters • Isopropyl Myristate • Stearyl Alcohol • Hydrogenated Coco-glycerides • Steareth-20 • Caffeine • Propylene Glycol • Lecithin • Aminophylline • Imidazolidinyl • Urea

• Methylparaben • Carbomer • Propylparaben • Triethanolamine • Algae • Magnolia Bark Extract • Fragrance • Horsetail Extract • Rose Hips Extract • Mate.

Herbalife - Cell-U-Loss - Herbalife
Each tablet contains: Vitamin C 250 mg • Potassium 297 mg • Iron 9 mg • Exclusive Combination [Buchu, Couch Grass, Cornsilk, Hydrangea, Juniper Berry, & Uva Ursi] 1000 mg • Lecithin 50 mg • Kelp 100 mg • Cider Vinegar 100 mg.

Herbalife - Herbal Aloe Drink - Herbalife
Water • Aloe Vera Juice • Sodium Citrate • Citric Acid • Potassium Sorbate • Chamomile • Sodium Benzoate.

Herbalife - NRG-Nature's Raw Guarana Instant Tea - Herbalife
Maltodextrins • Roasted Guarana Seed Extract • Pekoe Tea Extract • Lemon Peel Extract • Citric Acid.

Herbalife - NRG-Nature's Raw Guarana Tablets - Herbalife
Each tablet contains: Guarana powder (contains 4% naturally occuring caffeine) 800 mg.

Herbalife - Thermo Bond - Herbalife
Each tablet contains: Sodium Choleate • Fiber Blend: natural fibers from apple, grains, citrus, & cellulose.

Herbalife - Thermojetics Beige - Herbalife
Each tablet contains: English Hawthorn Berry fruit 80 mg • Alfalfa leaves 70 mg • Parsley leaves 60 mg • Marshmallow root 55 mg • Uva Ursi leaves 50 mg • Corn cornsilk 50 mg • Magnolia Bark bark 30 mg • Fennel seed 25 mg • Astragalus root 20 mg • Pfaffia root 20 mg • Pau d'Arco bark 20 mg • European Goldenrod leaves 15 mg • Licorice root 15 mg. Other Ingredients: Microcrystalene cellulose, tapioca & corn starches, stearic acid, cross-linked sodium carboxymethylcellulose, sodium starch glyconate, silicon dioxide, magnesium stearate, food grade shellac, hydroxypropyl methylcellulose, titianium dioxide, & caramel.

Herbalife - Thermojetics Green Refresh - Herbalife
Each tablet contains: Balu • Yerba Mate Extract • Bladderwrack • Meadowsweet • Garcinia Cambogia • Valerian Root • Green Tea Extract • Fumitory Herb • Honeysuckle • FD&C Blue No. 1 Lake.

Herbalife - Thermojetics Herbal Concentrate - Herbalife
Each serving contains: Camellia sinensis (Green Tea & Orange Pekoe Tea) Extract • Maltodextrin • Fructose • Malva Sylvestris Extract • Cardamom Extract • Hibiscus Extract • Lemon Peel Extract.

Herbalife - Thermojetics Original Green - Herbalife
Each tablet contains: Calcium (as calcium carbonate) 58 mg • Iodine (from bladderwrack) 30 mg • Chinese Ephedra leaf 140 mg • Yerba Mate leaf 115 mg • Dried MaHuang Extract whole 70 mg • Bladderwrack whole 40 mg • Valerian root 40 mg • Fumaria Officinalis whole 30 mg • Dried Salix purpurea Extract bark 30 mg • Chondrus crispus whole 5 mg. Other Ingredients: Stearic acid, tapioca starch, microcrystalline cellulose, papain, cross-linked sodium carboxymethylcellulose, silicon dioxide, sodium starch glyconate, magnesium stearate, sodium laurel sulfate, food grade shellac, titanium dioxide, polyethylene glycol, riboflavin, & blue #1.

Herbalife - Thermojetics Yellow - Herbalife
Each tablet contains: Garcinia (Garcinia Cambogia Extract) 400 mg • GTF Chromium (Chomium Polynicotinate) 400 mg.

Herbalist's Choice - The Herbalist
Gotu Kola herb • Guarana seed • Kola Nut • American Ginseng root • Licorice root • Damiana leaf • Echinacea root • Osha root • Cinnamon bark • Ginger root • Cayenne pepper.

Herbal-M - Progressive Labs
Each capsule contains: Vitamin E 30 IU • Zinc (as zinc oxide) 15 mg • Damiana leaf (Turnera aphrodesiaca) 60 mg • Siberian Ginseng/ Korean Ginseng blend (Eleutherococcus senticosus & Panax ginseng) • Cayenne (Capsicum annuum) 50 mg • Dong Quai (Angelica sinensis) 25 mg • Yohimbe (Pausinystalia johimbe) 10 mg • Muira Puama (Pytchopetalum olacoides) 10 mg • Goldenrod (Solidago virguarea) 10 mg • Orchic Substance 10 mg.
See Editor's Note No. 14, page 1817.

Herbaretic - Suddenly Slender
Each tablet contains: Alfalfa 50 mg • Buchu 50 mg • Uva Ursi 50 mg • Couch Grass 50 mg • Parsley 50 mg • Juniper berries 50 mg • Asparagus 50 mg • Watermelon seed powder 50 mg • Cubebs 50 mg • Shave Grass 50 mg • Corn Silk 50 mg • Golden Rod 50 mg • Cranberries 50 mg.

HerbaSlim - HerbaSway
St. John's Wort • Bitter Orange • Green Tea • Cassia tora • Panax Ginseng • Kudzu • Knotweed • Lycium • Cayenne pepper • Blackberry • HerbaSwee (Cucurbitaceae fruit).

Herbs & Prunes Formula - Nature's Life
Each tablet contains: Senna leaf (Senna alexandrina) 400 mg • Rhubarb root (Rheum officinale) 10 mg • Chinese Asparagus root (Tian dong, Asparagus cochinchinensis) 5 mg • Beet leaf (Beta vulgaris rubra) 5 mg • Buckthorn bark (Rhamnus frangula) 5 mg • Cabbage leaf (Brassica oleracea capitata) 5 mg • Cascara Sagrada (Rhamnus purshiana) 5 mg • Celery leaf (Apium graveolens) 5 mg • Cranberry (Vaccinium macrocarpon) 5 mg • Culvers root (Leptandra virginica) 5 mg • Dried Prune (Prunus aractus) 5 mg • Parsley leaf (Petroselinum crispum) 5 mg • Spinach leaf (Spinacia oleracea) 5 mg.

Herpalieve - PhytoPharmica
Contains: Allantoin 1% Other Ingredients: Melissa extract (Lemon balm) 70:1, and white soft paraffin with benzyl alcohol.

Herpanacine - Diamond Formulas
Six capsules contain: L-Lysine 1500 mg • A-Beta-Carotene 25000 IU • L-Tyrosine 500 mg • E-D-Alpha 200 IU • Selenium 100 mcg • Dandelion leaf • Sarsaparilla • Astragalus • Ligustrum • Echinacea.

Herp-Eeze - Olympian Labs
Each capsule contains: Larreastat 50 mg • Ascorbic Acid 250 mg.

Herpilyn - Enzymatic Therapy
Each 0.18 oz tube contains: Active ingredient: Allantoin 1%. Other ingredients: Melissa extract (Lemon Balm) 70:1 • White Soft Paraffin with Benzyl Alcohol.

Hi Energy Multi for Men - Futurebiotics
Three tablets contain: Beta Carotene 25,000 IU • Vitamin C • (Ascorbic Acid, Palmitate) 250 mg • Vitamin D 200 IU • Vitamin E 60 IU • Vitamin B1 (Thiamin) 25 mg • Vitamin B2 (Riboflavin) 25 mg • Niacinamide 50 mg • Pantothenic Acid 25 mg • Vitamin B6 25 mg • Vitamin B12 100 mcg • Biotin 300 mcg • Folic Acid 400 mcg • Phosphatidyl Choline 100 mg • Inositol 75 mg • Ribonucleic Acid (RNA) 75 mg • Para Amino Benzoic Acid (PABA) 75 mg • Zinc (Monomethionine) 30 mg • Calcium (Phosphate, Citrate, Amino Acid Chelate) 200 mg • Magnesium (Citrate, Amino Acid Chelate) 200 mg • Iron (Gluconate) 6 mg • Potassium (Citrate) 99 mg • Chromium (Polynicotinate) 200 mcg • Copper (Gluconate) 2 mg • Iodine (Kelp) 200 mcg • Manganese (Proteinate) 5 mg • Molybdenum (Amino Acid Chelate) 25 mcg • Selenium (Selenomethionine) 200 mcg. In a base of herbal extracts, powders & nutritional concentrates equivalent to 2,000 mg: Active Ginsenosides (from Standardized Ginseng Extract), Saw Palmetto, Avena Sativa, Ginseng, Hawthorn, Garlic (Odorless Extract), Bee Pollen, Foti, Adrenal Concentrate, Octacosanol (Wheat Free), Alfalfa Juice Concentrate & Spirulina.
See Editor's Note No. 14, page 1817.

BRAND NAMES

Some Brand Name Natural Products - What they Contain
www.NaturalDatabase.com contains MANY more listings than appear here.

Hi-B 100 B-Complex - Nature's Life
Each tablet contains: Vitamin B1 (Thiamine Hydrochloride) 100 mg • Vitamin B2 (Riboflavin) 100 mg • Vitamin B6 (Pyridoxine Hydrochloride) 100 mg • Vitamin B12 (Cobalamin concentrate) 100 mcg • Folic Acid 400 mcg • Biotin 100 mcg • Niacinamide 100 mg • Pantothenic Acid (d-Calcium Pantothenate) 100 mg • Choline (Bitartrate) 100 mg • PABA (Para Aminobenzoic Acid) 100 mg • Inositol 100 mg. In a natural base of Alfalfa, Parsley, Rice Bran & Watercress.

Hi-B-100 Complex - Nature's Life
Each capsule contains: Vitamin B1 (Thiamine HCl) 100 mg • Vitamin B2 (Riboflavin) 100 mg • Vitamin B6 (Pyridoxine HCl) 100 mg • Vitamin B12 (Cobalamin concentrate) 100 mcg • Niacinamide 100 mg • Pantothenic Acid (d-Calcium Pantothenate) 100 mg • Choline (Bitartrate) 100 mg • Inositol 100 mg • Biotin 100 mcg • Folic Acid 400 mcg • PABA (Para-Aminobenzioc Acid) 100 mg. In a natural base of Rice Bran.

High Five - Pharmanex
Each tablet contains: Boswellia Serrata Extract (stem) 125 mg • Fungal Protease (Aspergillus Oryzae) 100 mg • Bromelain (from Pineapple extract) 50 mg • Quercetin 25 mg • Papain (from Papaya extract) 10 mg. Other Ingredients: Dicalcium Phosphate, Microcrystalline Cellulose, Cellulose Powder, Silica, Magnesium Stearate.

High Performance Creatine - Puritan's Pride
Each serving contains: Creatine Monohydrate 5.25 g • Taurine 1000 mg.

High Potency B-Complex with Vitamin C - Puritan's Pride
Each caplet contains: Vitamin C (as ascorbic acid) 300 mg • Thiamin (Vitamin B1; as thiamine mononitrate) 15 mg • Riboflavin (Vitamin B2) 10.2 mg • Niacin (as niacinamide) 50 mg • Vitamin B6 (as pyridoxine hydrochloride) 5 mg • Pantothenic Acid (as d-calcium pantothenate) 10 mg. Other Ingredients: Dicalcium Phosphate, Cellulose (Plant Origin), Cellulose Coating, Croscarmellose, Vegetable Magnesium Stearate, Silica, FD&C Yellow No.5 Aluminum Lake, Titanium Dioxide Color, Vegetable Stearic Acid, Guar Gum.

High Potency Cal-Mag Plus - Quest
Each tablet contains: Calcium (Citrate) 250 mg • Magnesium (Oxide) 250 mg • Vitamin C (Ascorbic Acid) 150 mg • Vitamin D (as Vitamin D3) 100 IU • Zinc (Citrate) 10 mg. Other Ingredients: Croscarmellose Sodium, Magnesium Stearate (vegetable source), Microcrystalline Cellulose, Silicon Dioxide, Vegetable Stearin.

High Potency Iron from Ferrous Sulfate - Leiner Health Products
Each tablet contains: Iron (Ferrous Sulfate) 27 mg. Other Ingredients: Calcium Carbonate, Starch, Maltodextrin, Cellulose, Croscarmellose Sodium, Tricalcium Phosphate, Hydroxypropyl Methylcellulose, Polyethylene Glycol 3350, Silicon Dioxide, Talc, Magnesium Stearate, Hydroxypropyl Cellulose, Red 40 Lake, Polysorbate 80, Titanium Dioxide, Povidone.

High Potency Soft Multiple - Swanson
Each softgel contains: Calories 10 • Calories from Fat 10 • Total Fat 1 g • Vitamin A (as beta-carotene) 5000 IU • Vitamin C USP (as ascorbic acid) 150 mg • Vitamin D (as cholecalciferol) 200 IU • Vitamin E (as d-alpha tocopherol) 100 IU • Thiamin USP (as thiamin mononitrate; vitamin B-1) 25 mg • Riboflavin USP (vitamin B-2) 25 mg • Niacin (as niacin 5 mg; as niacinamide 25 mg) 30 mg • Vitamin B-6 (as pyridoxine HCl) 25 mg • Folic Acid 200 mcg • Vitamin B-12 (as cyanocobalamin) 25 mcg • Biotin 25 mcg • Pantothenic Acid (as d-calcium pantothenate) 25 mg • Calcium (from calcium carbonate) 100 mg • Iron (as ferrous fumarate) 7.5 mg • Iodine (as potassium iodide) 75 mcg • Magnesium (from magnesium oxide) 50 mg • Zinc (from zinc oxide) 7.5 mg • Selenium (from selenomethionine) 12.5 mcg • Copper (from copper gluconate) 0.5 mg • Manganese (from manganese sulfate) 5 mg • Chromium (from Chromax® chromium picolinate) 12.5 mcg • Molybdenum (sodium molybdate) 12.5 mcg. Lecithin 40 mg • Choline (as choline bitartrate) 25 mg • Inositol 25 mg • PABA (para-aminobenzoic acid) 25 mg, Boron (from calcium borogluconate) 0.5 mg • Silica (from silicon dioxide) 0.25 mg • Vanadium (from vanadyl sulfate) 5 mcg.

High Strength Cod Liver Oil - Nature's Bounty
Each softgel contains: Vitamin A (as Cod Liver Oil and Retinyl Palmitate) 2664 IU • Vitamin D (as Cod Liver Oil and Cholecalciferol) 200 IU • Cod Liver Oil 1000 mg • Eicosapentaenoic Acid 110 mg • Docosahexaenoic Acid 100 mg. Other Ingredients: Gelatin, Glycerin.

Higher Mind - Source Naturals
Four tablets contain: Phosphatidyl Serine (Leci-PS) 150 mg • Vitamin B1 (Thiamin) 100 mg • Vitamin B2 (Riboflavin) 25 mg • Vitamin B3 (Inositol Hexanicotinate 100 mg and Niacin 50 mg) 150 mg • Vitamin B5 (Pantothenic Acid) 50 mg • Vitamin B6 (PAK and Pyridoxine HCl) 100 mg • Vitamin B12 50 mcg • Folic Acid 800 mcg • Biotin 50 mcg • Vitamin C (Calcium and Zinc Ascorbates) 200 mg • Calcium (Ascorbate, Carbonate, Malate, Succinate) 100 mg • Magnesium (Malate, Succinate, Taurinate, Oxide) 200 mg • Zinc (Ascorbate) 10 mg • Manganese (Citrate) 5 mg • L-Pyroglutamic Acid 750 mg • L-Glutamine 500 mg • Acetyl L-Carnitine 300 mg • DMAE (Bitartrate) 100 mg • Taurine (Magnesium Taurinate) 200 mg • DLPA (DL-Phenylalanine) 200 mg • Phosphatidyl Choline 157.5 mg • Phosphatidyl Ethanolamine 105 mg • N-Acetyl L-Tyrosine 100 mg • GABA (Gamma Amino Butyric Acid) 100 mg • PAK (Pyridoxine Alpha-Ketoglutarate) 100 mg • Ginkgo Biloba extract 24% (50:1) 50 mg • Phosphatidyl Inositol 45 mg • Alpha-Lipoic Acid (Thioctic Acid) 20 mg • Coenzyme Q10 (Ubiquinone) 10 mg • Inositol 10 mg.

High-Potency Serum - Cellex-C
Ascorbic Acid • Tyrosine • Zinc • Sodium Hyaluronate • Bioflavonoids.

Hi-Potent-C (powdered) - Nutri-Quest
Each level teaspoonful contains: Vitamin C 1500 mg • Mannitol 1355 mg • Rose Hips 250 mg • Lemon Bioflavinoids 130 mg • Hesperidin Complex 50 mg • Rutin 35 mg • Acerola concentrate 35 mg • natural Flavor.

Hives, Allergies, Poison Ivy, Poison Oak Formula - Dr. Morrow's Homeopathic Formulas
Ten drops contain: Ammonium carbonate 12X • Apis mellifica 30X • Arsinucum album 30X • Gridelia robusta 30X • Echinacea 6X • Crotalus horridus 20X.
See Editor's Note No. 1, page 1816.

HMB - EAS
Each 4 capsule serving contains: HMB 1000 mg • Potassium Phosphate 200 mg.

Holista Echinacea - Holista
Each capsule contains: Echinacea angustifolia/purpurea (root) (16:1 extract) 500 mg.

Holista Echinacea Tincture - Holista
Each mL contains: Echinacea angustifolia dried root 1:1 standardized extract in alcohol 45% 200 mg.

Holista Evening Primrose Oil 1000 mg - Holista
Each capsule contains: Evening Primrose Oil 1000 mg, containing 10% gamma-linolenic acid and 70% linoleic acid.

Holista Evening Primrose Oil 500 mg - Holista
Each capsule contains: Evening Primrose Oil (not less than 50 mg of gamma-linolenic acid and 350 mg of lenoleic acid) standardized to 10% GLA 500 mg.

Holista Feverfew - Holista
Each capsule contains: Feverfew (Tanacetum parthenium) standardized to a minimum of 0.2% parthenolide 125 mg.

Holista Lactase enzyme - Holista
Each capsule contains: Food Chemical Codex Lactase 3000 units.

Holista Milk Thistle - Holista
Each capsule contains: Milk Thistle (Silybum marianum) standardized to silymarin 80% 150 mg.

Holista Milk Thistle Tincture - Holista
Each mL contains: Milk Thistle seed from 1:1 fluid extract in 65% alcohol 0.2 mg.

Holista Saw Palmetto - Holista
Each caplet contains: Saw Palmetto (Serenoa repens) extract from berries 10:1 160 mg.

Holista Saw Palmetto Tincture - Holista
Each mL contains: Saw Palmetto dried berries of Seronoa repens 1:1 in 45% alcohol 0.2 mg.

Holista Tea Tree Oil 20% Lotion - Holista
Tea Tree oil (Melaleuca alternifolia) 0.2 mL.
Other Ingredients: Water, Alcohol.

Holista Valerian - Holista
Each capsule contains: Valerian Root Extract standardized to 0.8% Valerenic Acid 500 mg.

Holista Valerian Tincture - Holista
Each mL contains: Valerian Root from the rhizome and roots of Valeriana officianalis 1:1 in 60% alcohol 0.2 mg.

Holista Zinc Lozenges - Holista
Each lozenge contains: Zinc (citrate) 5 mg • Echinacea 50 mg • Vitamin C 50 mg.

Homocysteine Control - Nature's Way
Each capsule contains: Betaine Anhydrous 500 mg • Folic Acid (folate) 800 mcg • Pyridoxine HCl 20 mg • Vitamin B-12 (cyanocobalamin) 400 mcg. Other Ingredients: Cellulose, Gelatin, Magnesium stearate, Millet.

Homocysteine De-Crease - Nutri-Quest
Each tablet contains: Trimethylglycine 300 mg • Pyridoxal 5 Phosphate 5 mg (enteric coated) • Vitamin B12 200 mcg • Dimethyl Gluyine 25 mg • Niacinamide 20 mg • Cysteine 15 mg • Molybdenum Chelate 30 mcg • Selenium Chelate 15 mcg • Vitamin B6 15 mg (enertic coated) • Folic Acid 275 mg • Vitamin E Succinate 10 IU • Red Beet root 25 mg • Choline Bitartrate 10 mg • Magnesium Chelate 100 mg • Zinc Chelate 10 mg.

Homocysteine Formula - Nature's Life
Each capsule contains: Vitamin B6 (Pyridoxine HCl) 10 mg • Folic Acid 800 mcg • Vitamin B12 400 mcg • Choline (Bitartrate) 50 mg • Betaine HCl 50 mg.

Homocysteine Regulators - Now
Each Vcap contains: Vitamin B6 (as Coenzyme Pyridoxyl-5-Phosphate) 20 mg • Vitamin B12 (as Cyanocobalamin) 250 mcg • Folic Acid 800 mcg • Trimethylglycine (Betaine) 400 mg.

HomocystexPlus with TMG & TroxeRutin - Natrol
One capsule contains: Riboflavin (Vitamin B2) 25 mg • Vitamin B6 (as pyridoxine HCl) 25 mg • Folic Acid 800 mcg • Vitamin B12 (as cobalamin) 500 mcg • Betaine TMG (as betaine trimethylglycine) 500 mg • TroxeRutin 100 mg • Choline (as choline bitartrate) 25 mg. Other ingredients: Silicon Dioxide, Magnesium Stearate, Gelatin.

Honey Apple Double Ginseng - Traditional Medicinals
Asian Ginseng root (Panax ginseng) • American Ginseng root (Panax quinquefolius) • Siberian Ginseng root (Eleutherococcus senticosus) • Chamomile flower • Licorice root • Orange peel • dried Apples • Prince Ginseng rootlets (Pseudostellada heterophylla) • Natural Honey & Apple flavors.

Honey C Chews Chewable C 100 mg - Nature's Life
Each wafer contains: Vitamin C (Buffered) 100 mg • Rose Hips powder (Rosa canina) 50 mg • Acerola berry powder (Malpighia glabra) 25 mg.

Honey C Chews Chewable C 300 mg - Nature's Life
Each wafer contains: Vitamin C (Buffered) 300 mg • Rose Hips powder (Rosa canina) 50 mg • Acerola berry powder (Malpighia glabra) 25 mg.

Hops, Valerian & Scullcap - Dial Herbs
Hops • Valerian • Scullcap.

Hormogen - Atrium Inc.
Each capsule contains: Lecithin 200 mg • Safflower oil 200 mg • Wheat Germ oil (Cold Pressed) 66.667 mg • Rice Bran oil 66.667 mg • Soybean oil 66.667 mg. Contains no sugar, starch, salt, wheat, corn, yeast, or soy derivatives.

Hormone Nutrients - Wellness for Women
Each capsule contains: Vitamin B-6 (as pyridoxine HCl) 50 mg • Magnesium (from amino acid chelate) 75 mg • Motherwort (5:1 concentrate) 100 mg • Vitex Chasteberry extract (0.5% agnusides) 100 mg • Dong Quai extract (1% ligustilides) 75 mg • SoyLife Soy protein extract (1% soy isoflavones) 75 mg • Black Cohosh extract (2.5% triterpene-glycosides) 50 mg.

Horse Chestnut Extract - PhytoPharmica
Each capsule contains: Horse Chestnut (Aesculus hippocastanum) seed extract (standardized to contain 20%-22% saponins calculated as escin) 250 mg.

Horse Chestnut Herbal Balm - Nature's Life
Deionized Water • Horse Chestnut seed extract [(Aesculus hippocastanum L.) standardized to 2% aescin] • Phospholipids from Safflower & Sunflower seed oil • Caprylic/Capric Triglyceride • Apricot Kernel oil • Soy Lecithin • Glycerine (Vegetable) • Tocopherol (natural Vitamin E) • Arnica extract • Panthenol • Saccharide Isomerate • Xanthan Gum • Carrageenan (Irish Moss) • Dimethicone • Lauroyl Lysine • Natural Fragrant Essential Oils Blend • Sodium Hydroxymethylglycinate.

Horsetail Extract Formula - Quest
Each caplet contains: Horsetail powder (Equisetum arvense) (provided by 125 mg 1:4 Aqueous Extract) 500 mg • Rosehips powder (Rose canina) 50 mg • Burdock root powder (Arctium lappa) 30 mg • Marshmallow root powder (Althaea officinalis) 30 mg • Parsley leaf powder (Plantago major) 30 mg • Slippery Elm bark powder (Ulmus fulva) 30 mg. Other Ingredients: Calcium Phosphate, Microcrystalline Cellulose, Croscarmellose Sodium, Magnesium Stearate (vegetable source), Vegetable Stearin.

Horsetail Plus Fo-Ti - The Herbalist
Horsetail fresh-dried herb (Equisetum arvense) • Fo-Ti fresh-dried

BRAND NAMES

root (Polygonum multiforum) • Nettles fresh-dried leaf (Urtica dioica) • Red Clover fresh-dried blossom (Trifolium pratense) • Burdock fresh-dried root (Arctium lappa).

Hot Flash - Source Naturals
Three tablets contain: Soy concentrate, yielding 65 mg Isoflavones 2100 mg • Black Cohosh 160 mg • Dong Quai extract 150 mg • Licorice root extract 150 mg • Vitex extract 100 mg.

Hot Flashex - Natrol
One tablet contains: Vitamin E (as d-alpha tocopherol) 50 IU • Calcium (as tri-calcium phosphate) 70 mg • Licorice 100 mg • Black Cohosh root 60 mg, Triterpenes (2.5%) 15 mg • Chamomile extract 50 mg • Kava Kava root 30 mg, Kavalactones (30%) 9 mg. Other ingredients: Mono & Di-Glycerides, Croscarmellose Sodium, Silicon Dioxide, Stearic Acid, Magnesium Stearate.

Hoxsey Formula - The Herbalist
Red Clover fresh-dried blossoms (Trifolium pratense) • Chaparral fresh-dried leaf (Larrea tridentata) • Licorice fresh-dried root (Glycyrrhiza glabra) • Oregon Grape fresh-dried root (Berberis nervosa) • Burdock fresh-dried root (Arcticum lappa) • Sarsaparilla fresh-dried root (Smilax ornata) • Echinacea fresh root (Echinacea angustifolia) • Prickly Ash fresh-dried bark (Zanthoxylum americanum).

Human Growth Hormone (HGH) - Youngevity
Each capsule contains: L-Lysine HCL • L-Arginine • L-Ornithine • L-Glutamine • L-Tyrosine • Vilcabamba Mineral Essence: Potassium, Calcium, Magnesium, Zinc, Chromium, Selenium, Iron, Copper, Molybdenum, Vanadium, Iodine, Cobalt, Manganese.

Huperzine A Complex - Puritan's Pride
Each tablet contains: Folic Acid 200 mcg • Vitamin B12 (as cyanocobalamin) 6 mcg • DMAE (from DMAE bitartrate) (dimethylaminoethanol) 50 mg • Panax ginseng (root standardized extract: provides 5 mg ginsenosides) 125 mg • Huperzine A (from standardized Huperiza serrata) leaf extract 50 mcg • L-Tyrosine 75 mg • Bioperine (from standardized piperine) 2.5 mg.

Huperzine A Ginkgo/Ginseng - Nutrapharm, Inc.
Each capsule contains: Huperzine A 50 mcg • Ginkgo biloba extract 60 mg • Panax ginseng extract 150 mg. Other Ingredients: Malto dextrin, magnesium stearate, microcrystalline cellulose, & silica. Free of sugar, yeast, milk, artificial colors, flavors & dyes.

Huperzine A w/Ginkgo - Nutrapharm, Inc.
Each capsule contains: Huperzine A 50 mcg • Ginkgo biloba extract 60 mg. Other Ingredients: Malto dextrin, magnesium stearate, microcrystalline cellulose, & silica. Free of sugar, yeast, corn, milk, artificial colors, flavors & dyes.

Huperzine A w/Ginseng - Nutrapharm, Inc.
Each capsule contains: Huperzine A 50 mcg • Panax ginseng extract (standardized to 8% ginsenosides) 150 mg. Other Ingredients: Malto dextrin, magnesium stearate, microcrystalline cellulose, & silica. Free of sugar, yeast, corn, milk products, artificial colors, flavors & dyes.

Huperzine A w/Vitamin E - Nutrapharm, Inc.
Each capsule contains: Huperzine A 50 mcg • Vitamin E (D-alpha tocopheryl acetate) 100 IU. Other Ingredients: Malto dextrin, magnesium stearate, & silica. Free of sugar, yeast, corn, milk, artificial colors, flavors & dyes.

HVP - Nature's Sunshine
Each capsule contains: Proprietary Blend 390 mg: Valerian root • Skullcap herb • Hops flowers.

HY 2 - Pacific BioLogic
St. John's Wort.

Hydra Cleanse - Pharmagel
Aloe Vera • a complex of marine-based extracts of Seaweed, Algae, and Spirulina • Oat extract • Beta Glucan • Panthenol.

Hydra Fuel (The Ultimate Fluid Replacement Sports Drink) - TwinLab
Glucose Polymers & Glucose (approximately 5%) • Fructose (about 2%). Replenishes important Electrolytes & Minerals: Sodium, Potassium, Magnesium, Chloride, Chromium & Phosphorus.

Hydroxy Ripped - Puritan's Pride
Four capsules contain: Chromium 300 mcg • Hydroripped 2000 (Garcinia cambogia) fruit rind (containing 1,000 of HCA) 1,667 mg • Guarana extract (Paullina cupana) seed (standardized for 22% caffeine) 1,000 mg • Ma Huang extract (Ephedra sinica) aerial (standardized for 21 mg of ephedra alkaloids) 360 mg • Salicin complex (from White Willow Bark) Salix alba (containing 15% salicin) 150 mg • L-Carnitine 150 mg.

Hydroxycut - Muscletech
Four capsules contain: Hydroxagen (supplying 100 mg of Hydroxycitric Acid) 2000 mg • MaHuang extract 334 mg • Guarana extract 910 mg • Willow bark extract 100 mg • L-Carnitine 100 mg • Chromium Picolinate 300 mcg.

Hy-Gear - Met-Rx
Each 40 g serving contains: Creatine Monohydrate 5 g, Carbohydrate 34 g, Ingredients: Citrus Mist flavor: CeraSport (Rice Syrup Solids, Sodium Chloride, Potassium Chloride & Trisodium Citrate) • Fructose • Creatine Monohydrate • Glucose • Natural & Artificial Flavors • Citric Acid • Malic Acid • Beta Carotene & Beet juice powder for color. Strazzyberry Flavor: CeraSport (Rice Syrup Solids, Sodium Chloride, Potassium Chloride & Trisodium Citrate) • Fructose • Creatine Monohydrate • Glucose • Natural & Artificial Flavors • Beet juice powder for color.

HyperiCalm - Enzymatic Therapy
Each capsule contains: St. John's Wort (Hypericum perforatum) extract standardized to 0.3% hypericins (900 mcg) & 4% hyperforin (12 mg), verified by HPLC 300 mg. Contains no sugar, salt, yeast, wheat, corn, soy, dairy products, coloring, flavoring, or preservatives.

HyperiMed - PhytoPharmica
Each capsule contains: St. John's Wort (Hypericum perforatum) extract standardized to 0.3% hypericins (900 mcg) & 4% hyperforin (12 mg), verified by HPLC 300 mg. Contains no sugar, salt, yeast, wheat, corn, soy, dairy products, coloring, flavoring, or preservatives.

Hypertension Support - Amazon Support
Each capsule contains: Abuta • Artichoke • Bitter Melon • Chanca Piedra • Graviola • Jurubeba • Mullaca • Suma • Periwinkle • Stevia • Pedra hume caa.

Hypo-Ade - Enzymatic Therapy
Two tablets contain: Vitamin A (Fish Liver oil) 5000 IU • Vitamin C (Ascorbic Acid) 200 mg • Niacin/Niacinamide 115 mg • Potassium Chloride 100 mg • Pantothenic Acid (D-Calcium Pantothenate) 100 mg • Thiamine HCL (Vitamin B1) 25 mg • Riboflavin (Vitamin B2) 25 mg • Vitamin B6 (Pyridoxine HCL) 25 mg • Zinc (Oxide) 10 mg • Manganese (Gluconate) 10 mg • Chromium (Polynicotinate) 267 mcg • Vitamin B12 (Cyanocobalamin) 25 mcg • Other ingredients: Inositol 200 mg • Pancreas extract 150 mg • Choline Bitartrate 100 mg • L-Methionine 100 mg • Green Beet leaf powder 100 mg • Adrenal extract 65 mg • Betaine HCL 50 mg • Wild Yam 50 mg • Pituitary extract 40 mg • Barberry, Bark of root extract (4:1) (Berberis vulgaris) 30 mg. This exclusive formulation also contains

Dandelion (Taraxacum officinale), Goldenseal (Hydrastis canadensis), Raw Liver, Raw Lung, Raw Pancreas, Raw Heart, Raw Kidney, Raw Spleen, & Raw Brain. Contains no sugar, salt, yeast, wheat, corn, soy, dairy products, coloring, flavoring or preservatives. See Editor's Note No. 14, page 1817.

Hyporil - PhytoPharmica
Two tablets contain: Vitamin A (Fish Liver oil) 5000 IU • Vitamin C (Ascorbic Acid) 200 mg • Niacin/Niacinamide 115 mg • Potassium Chloride 100 mg • Pantothenic Acid (D-Calcium Pantothenate) 100 mg • Thiamine HCL (Vitamin B1) 25 mg • Riboflavin (Vitamin B2) 25 mg • Vitamin B6 (Pyridoxine HCL) 25 mg • Zinc (Oxide) 10 mg • Manganese (Gluconate) 10 mg • Chromium (Polynicotinate) 267 mcg • Vitamin B12 (Cyanocobalamin) 25 mcg • Inositol 200 mg • Pancreas extract 150 mg • Choline Bitartrate 100 mg • L-Methionine 100 mg • Green Beet leaf powder 100 mg • Adrenal extract 65 mg • Betaine HCL 50 mg • Wild Yam 50 mg • Pituitary extract 40 mg • Barberry bark of root extract 4:1 (Berberis vulgaris) 30 mg. This exclusive formulation also contains Dandelion (Taraxacum officinale), Goldenseal (Hydrastis canadensis), Raw Liver, Raw Lung, Raw Pancreas, Raw Heart, Raw Kidney, Raw Spleen, and Raw Brain. Contains no sugar, salt, yeast, wheat, corn, soy, dairy products, coloring, flavoring, or preservatives. See Editor's Note No. 14, page 1817.

Iberogast - PhytoPharmica
20 drops (1ml) contains: Proprietary Blend: Clown's Mustard Plant (Iberis amara), Chamomile flower (Matricariae flos), Angelica root (Angelicae radix), Caraway fruit (Carvi fructus), Milk Thistle fruit (Cardui mariae fructus), Melissa leaf (Melissae folium), Celandine herbs (Chelidonii herba), Licorice root (Liquiritiae radix), Peppermint leaf (Menthae pipertae folium) 1 ml. Other Ingredients: Water, Alcohol (31%).

Ideas - Starlight International
Four tablets contain: St. John's Wort, 0.3% (Hypericum perforatum, flowering parts) 400 mg • Gingko biloba extract, 4:1 (leaf) 100 mg • Basil / Tulsi extract, 4:1 (Ocimum sanctum, leaf) 150 mg • Lemon Balm (Melissa officinalis, leaf) 150 mg • Siberian Ginseng extract, 4:1 (Eleutherococcus senticosus, root) 200 mg • Gotu Kola extract, 4:1 (Cantella asiatica, plant) 150 mg • Water Hyssop extract, 4:1 (Bacopa monneria, plant) 150 mg • Spirulina 5 mg • Rosemary (Rosmarinus officinalis, leaf) 5 mg • English Lavender (Lavandula officinalis, flower) 5 mg. Other Ingredients: Dicalcium Phosphate, Microcrystalline Cellulose, Stearic Acid, Croscarmellose Sodium, Magnesium Stearate, Silicon Dioxide, Dextrin, Dextrose, Lecithin, Carboxymethylcellulose Sodium, Sodium Citrate.

IGF Fuel - TwinLab
Two capsules contain: DHEA (dehydroepiandrosterone) 50 mg • Zinc (from zinc picolinate) 50 mg • L-Glutamine 2000 mg.

Immortale for Men - Roex
Each tablet contains: Tribulus Terrestris 250 mg • Panax ginseng 50 mg • Damiana 50 mg • Avena sativa 100 mg • Sarsaparilla 50 mg.

Immortale for Women - Roex
Each tablet contains: Tribulus Terrestris 250 mg • Panax ginseng 50 mg • Damiana 50 mg • Avena sativa 100 mg • Dong Quai 50 mg.

IMMU-C - Nutri-Quest
Each tablet contains: Vitamin C (Sago Palm) 500 mg • Rutin 15 mg • Lemon Bioflavonoids 15 mg • Hesperidin Complex 15 mg • Tissue concentrates (not extracts) of Bovine Source from Lymph, Thymus, Spleen • 5X Propolis 2 mg. See Editor's Note No. 14, page 1817.

Immuguard - Optimum Nutrition
Echinacea Angustifolia extract • Goldenseal root.

Immumax-Rx - Alternecare Health Products
Each tablet contains: Bee Propolis 50 mg • Shiitake Mushroom 50 mg • Reishi Mushroom 50 mg • Garlic 25 mg • Suma 25 mg • Red Clover 25 mg • Pau d'Arco 25 mg • Milk Thistle 25 mg • Shark Cartilage 15 mg • Golden Seal 25 mg • Siberian Ginseng 25 mg • Echinacea 25 mg • Astragalus 25 mg • N-Acetyl Cysteine 15 mg • Zinc 15 mg • L-Glutathione 15 mg • CO Q10 5 mg.

ImmunACE - Nature's Plus
Two tablets contain: Vitamin C corn free 1000 mg • Vitamin E natural 400 IU • Beta Carotene pro-vitamin A, supplying Vitamin A 20000 IU • Zinc Amino Acid Chelate 300 mg, supplying Elemental Zinc 30 mg • L-Cysteine free form amino acid 200 mg • Iron Amino Acid Chelate 180 mg, supplying Elemental Iron 18 m • Selenium Amino Acid Complex 100 mg, supplying Elemental Selenium 200 mcg • Folic Acid 200 mcg. In a natural base of Pau D'Arco, Chlorophyll, Echinacea, Thyme, Juniper berry, Korean Ginseng, Irish Moss & Rosemary. Yeast free. Sugar & starch free.

ImmunActin Throat Spray - Nature's Plus
Purified Water • Exclusive Liposomal Herbal Complex [Olivir (Olea europa leaf extract) (supplying purified Calcium Elenolate), Kava Kava extract (Piper methysticum root) (standardized 4% Kavalactones), Echinacea extract (Echinacea angustifolia root & rhizome) (standardized 4% Echinacosides), Elderberry extract (Sambucus canadensis fruit) (standardized 30% Flavonoids), Ginger (Zingiber officinale root) (standardized 4% Volatile oils)] • Wild Clover Honey • Oil of Peppermint.

ImmunActin Throat Syrup - Nature's Plus
Vegetable Glycerine • Exclusive Liposomal Herbal Complex [Elderberry extract (Sambucus canadensis fruit) (standardized 30% Falvonoids), Echinacea extract (Echinacea angustifolia root & rhizome) (standardized 4% Echinacosides), Slippery Elm (Ulmus rubra bark) (naturally rich in Phytosterols, Sesquitepenes & Mucilage), Goldenseal extract (Hydrastis canadensis root) (standardized 10% Alkaloids, 5% Hydrastine), White Willow extract (Salix alba bark) (standardized 7-9% Salicin), Astragalus extract (Astragalus membranaceus root) (standardized 0.4% 4'-Hydroxy-3'-Methoxyisoflavone 7-Sug), Schisandra extract (Schisandra chinensis fruit) (standardized 9% schisandrins), Zinc Gluconate] • Wild Clover • Honey • Methol • natural Cherry flavor.

ImmunActinB - Nature's Plus
Two capsules contain: Vitamin C corn free 300 mg • Vitamin E natural 100 IU • Echinacea [(Echinacea angustifolia root & rhizome) standardized 4% Echinacosides] 50 mg • Astragalus [(Astragalus membranaceus root) standardized 0.4% 4'-Hydroxy-3'-Methoxyisoflavone 7-Sug] 50 mg • Chinese Green Tea [(Camellia sinensis leaf) decaffeinated, standardized 20% Polyphelols] 50 mg • Tumeric [(Curcuma longa rhizome) standardized 95% Curcumin] 50 mg • Garlic odor-modified [(Allium sativum clove) standardized 0.35% Allicin, 0.65% Allicin, 0.40% Thiosulfinates, 0.085% Allyl Mercaptan] 50 mg • Schisandra [(Schisandra chinensis fruit) standardized 9% Schisandrins] 25 mg • Pau D'Arco [(Tabebuia impetiginosa bark) standardized 3% Naphthoquinones] 25 mg • Goldenseal [(Hydrastis canadensis root & rhizome) standardized 10% Alkaloids, 5% Hydrastine] 25 mg • Shiitake Mushroom [(Lentinus edodes mycelia) standardized 3.2% KS-2 Polysaccharides (peptidomannan)] 15 mg • Zinc (Monomethionine) 15 mg • Beta Carotene (supplying 10000 IU of Vitamin A activity) 6 mg • Grape seed [(Vitis vinifera) standardized 95% Proanthocyanidins] 5 mg • Bioperine [(Piper nigrum fruit) standardized 95% 1-Piperoylpiperidine] 5 mg.

Immune Actives - VitaStore
Each tablet contains: Echinacea 500 mg • Goldenseal 250 mg • Beta Carotene (Vitamin A) 2500 IU • Zinc Gluconate 30 mg • Vitamin C 120 mg • Licorice 150 mg • Astragalus 145 mg • Grape Seed extract 50 mg • Green Tea 200 mg • Garlic 300 mg • L-Lysine 500 mg.

BRAND NAMES

Some Brand Name Natural Products - What they Contain
www.NaturalDatabase.com contains MANY more listings than appear here.

BRAND NAMES

Immune Booster Body Benefits Pak - Leiner Health Products
Each packet contains: Zinc Gluconate 50 mg • Vitamin C 740 mg • Echinacea extract (Echinacea augustifolia, Echinacea purpurea) root 200 mg • Garlic (Allium sativum) clove 200 mg • Propolis 100 mg. Other Ingredients: Ascorbic Acid, Dicalcium Phosphate, Starch, Hydroxypropyl Methylcellulose, Maltodextrin, Croscarmellose Sodium, Silicon Dioxide, Cellulose, Stearic Acid, Rose Hips, Sodium Starch Glycolate, Magnesium.

Immune Builder - JHSPRO.com
Each capsule contains: Coriolus Versicolor extract 75 mg • Reishi fruit body extract 75 mg • Maitake fruit body extract 75 mg • Shiitake (lentinula edodes) extract 75 mg • Cordyceps Sinensis Cs-4 Mycelial extract 75 mg.

Immune Defense - ProHerbs
Two tablets contain: Vitamin C (Ascorbic Acid) 500 mg • Vitamin E (DI-Alpha Tocopherol Acetate) 400 IU • Zinc (as Sulfate) 15 mg • Selenium (as Selenomethionine) 200 mcg • ActiVin Grape Seed extract (Vitis vinifera seeds standardized to 95% polyphenols) 100 mg • Echinacea root (Echinacea purpurea) 100 mg • Alpha Lipoic Acid (standardized to 4% phenolic compounds) 50 mg. Other Ingredients: Dicalcium Phosphate, Croscarmellose Sodium, Hydroxypropylmethylcellulose, Magnesium Stearate, Microcrystalline Cellulose, Mineral Oil, Polyethylene Glycol, Silicon Dioxide, Stearic Acid, Titanium Dioxide, Sodium Lauryl Sulfate, FD&C Yellow, #6 Lake, Yellow #10 Lake.

Immune Formula - Nature's Life
Three tablets contain: Antioxidant Vitamins: Beta Carotene [(Dunaliella salina) equivalent to 25000 IU Vitamin A] 15 mg • Other naturally occurring carotenoids in D. salina: Alpha Carotene (equivalent to 393 IU Vitamin A) 473 mcg • Cryptoxanthin (equivalent to 96 IU Vitamin A) 116 mcg • Zeaxanthin 95 mcg • Lutein 74 mcg • Vitamin C (Calcium Ascorbate) 1000 mg • Vitamin E (d-Alpha Tocopheryl Succinate) 200 IU. Other Nutrients: Vitamin A (Retinyl Palmitate) 8000 IU • Vitamin B6 (Pyridoxine HCl) 50 mg • Vitamin B12 (Cobalamin) 100 mcg • Folic Acid 400 mcg • Selenium (l-Selenomethionine) 100 mcg • Zinc (Citrate) 25 mg • Copper (Citrate) 2 mg • Medical Herbs: Echinacea purpurea root (Trout Lake Farm Certified Organically Grown) 500 mg • Korean Ginseng root extract [(Panax ginseng) standardized to 10% ginsenosides] 100 mg • Natural Base: Lemon Bioflavonoid Complex (50% active flavonols) 100 mg.

Immune Guardian - Clinician's Choice
Three tablets contain: Vitamin C (ascorbic acid, calcium ascorbate) 150 mg • Vitamin E (dl-alpha tocopheryl acetate) 90 IU • Zinc (amino acid chelate) 90 IU • Selenium (selenomethionine) 150 mcg • Echinacea Angustifolia 450 mg • Echinacea Purpurea Root 300 mg • Golden Seal Root 150 mg • Kudzu Root 150 mg • Odor Modified Garlic Bulb 150 mg • Bee Pollen 150 mg • RoseOx (patented, standardized process for an extract of Rosemary) 90 mg • Ascorbyl Palmitate 75 mg • Schizandra Fruit 75 mg • Proprietary blend 15 mg: Beta-Carotene, Reishi Mushroom, Shiitake Mushroom, Cinnamon Bark, Grape Powder.

Immune Support - Amazon Support
Each capsule contains: Cat's Claw • Suma • Avenca • Samambaia • Simauba • Chanca Piedra • Mullaca • Macela • Pau d'arco • Yerba Mate.

Immune System - Nutrivention
Each tablet contains: Vitamin A 5000 IU • Pantothenic Acid 25 mg • Vitamin B6 25 mg • Vitamin C 20 mg • Vitamin B1 18 mg • Vitamin B2 18 mg • Vitamin E 15 IU • Inositol 15 mg • Choline 8 mg • Magnesium 5 mg • Zinc 5 mg • Folic Acid 400 mcg • Selenium 50 mcg • Echinacea 100 mg • Astragalus 100 mg • L-Cysteine 100 mg • Suma 100 mg • Codonopsis 75 mg • Rei-Shi Mushroom 75 mg •

White Astractylodes 50 mg • Schizandra berries 50 mg • Privet berries 50 mg • Watercress 50 mg • Shiitake Mushroom 50 mg • Juniper berries 50 mg.

Immune System Booster Formula - Cambridge Nutraceuticals
Each serving contains: Glutamine 10 g • Vitamin A (as mixed carotenoids) 6500 IU • Vitamin C 200 mg • Vitamin E 125 IU • Selenium 70 mcg • N-Acetyl-Cysteine 600 mg. Available in 650 g jar or single dose packets.

Immune-Action - Nature's Plus
Each capsule contains: Astragalus root 200 mg • Ligustrum berries 100 mg • Schisandra berries 100 mg • Shiitake Mushrooms 100 mg • Echinacea root 100 mg • Young Barley leaves 50 mg • Pau D'Arco bark 50 mg. Contains no yeast, wheat, corn, soy, milk, salt, sugar or starch.

Immunectar - Nature's Plus
Two tablespoons contain: Egg Yolk Lecithin 2000 mg & Phosphatidylcholine 250 mg, The above combination supplies: Neutral Lipids 60%, Phosphatidylcholine 20%, Phosphatidylethanolamine 3% • Colostrum Whey, naturally rich in immunoglobulins, nucleotides, gamma interferon, enzymes & vitamins 150 mg • SUMA (Pfaffia paniculata [Martius] Kuntze root) 150 mg • Chlorella 150 mg • Astragalus (Astragalus membranaceus root) 75 mg • Ligustrum (Ligustrum lucidum berries) 75 mg • Echinacea (Echinacea angustifolia root) 75 mg • Schisandra (Schisandra chinensis berries) 75 mg • Shiitake (Lentinus edodes mushrooms) 75 mg • Coenzyme Q10 15 mg.

Immun-Eeze - Allergy Limited
Each capsule and lozenge together contain: Vitamin C (as ascorbic acid) 250 mg • Thiamin (as thiamine mononitrate) 25 mg • Riboflavin 25 mg • Niacin (as niacinamide) 20 mg • Vitamin B6 (as pyridoxine HCL) 25 mg • Vitamin B12 (as cyanocobalamin) 3 mg • Manganese (as manganese citrate) 6 mg. Other ingredients: Maltodextrin, sucrose, gelatin, vegetable derived magnesium stearate, croscarmellose sodium, silicon dioxide.

Immunene - PhysioLogics
Each capsule contains: Cats Claw inner bark (Una de Gato) (2% Oxindole Alkaloids, 2 mg) 100 mg • Astragalus (70% Polysaccharides, 70 mg) 100 mg • Reishi (4% Triterpenes, 2 mg; 10% Polysaccharides, 5mg) 50 mg • Shiitake 50 mg • Shiitake extract (3.2% KS-2, 3.2 mg) 10 mg • Maitake 10 mg.

Immuno Support Complex - Nutrition Dynamics Inc.
Each capsule contains: Vitamin C 200 mg • Pantothenic Acid 10 mg • Vitamin A 10,000 IU • Vitamin B12 10 mcg • Calcium Chelate 60 mg • Zinc Chelate • RNA 60 mg • Thymus 50 mg • Lemon Bioflavonoids 40 mg • Lymph 25 mg • Spleen 25 mg • Bromelain 20 mg. Other Ingredients: Bee pollen, dehydrated pineapple. See Editor's Note No. 14, page 1817.

ImmunoBlend - Rexall
Each capsule contains: Turmeric Rhizome extract (standardized to 95% curcuminoids, 95 mg) 100 mg • Echinacea Purpurea extract (standardized to 4% phenolic compounds, 4 mg) 100 mg • Immuno Proprietary Blend: Garlic bulb, Astragalus root, Reishi Mushroom, Cat's Claw Bark 175 mg. Other Ingredients: Gelatin.

Immunoboost - Shawnee Moon
Peony root • Gotu Kola • Chrysanthemum • Astragalus • Licorice • Kelp • Suma • Pau d'arco • Red Clover.

Immunocal - Immunotec
100% Milk Whey Protein.

1682 • © Copyright 2002, Natural Medicines Comprehensive Database (209) 472-2244. For updated data, go to www.NaturalDatabase.com.

ImmunoFin - LaneLabs
G-E Lipids 50 mg • Shark Liver Oil 250 mg.

Immunogarl-1 - Olympian Labs
Three capsules contain: Garlic extract 600 mg • Ginkgo Biloba leaf extract 120 mg • Proprietary Blend: Amylase, Protease, Lipase 600 mg • Ascorbic Acid 240 mg • L-Glutamine 450 mg • Maitake Mushroom 30 mg.

Immuplex - Standard Process
Two capsules contain: Proprietary Blend 565 mg: Bovine Liver (PMG) extract, Veal Bone extract, Nutritional Yeast, Bovine Spleen (PMG) extract, Bovine Thymus (PMG) extract, Bovine Thymus (Cytosol) extract, Bovine Liver, Bovine Spleen, Ovine Spleen, Calcium Lactate. Other Ingredients: Gelatin, Zinc Liver Chelate, Ascorbic Acid, Iron Liver Chelate, Water, Chromium Yeast, Copper Liver Chleate, Selenium Yeast, Mixed Tocopherols, Natural Colors, Pyridoxine hydrochloride, Calcium stearate, Vitamin A palmitate, Folic Acid, Cyanocobalamin.
See Editor's Note No. 14, page 1817.

IMMU-Power - Nutri-Quest
Each tablet contains: Tissue concentrate (not an extract) from Thymus 60 mg • Vitamin A (Palmitate) 300 IU • Vitamin B6 15 mg • Niacin 10 mg • Pantothenic Acid 55.5 mg • Vitamin B12 200 mcg • Folic Acid 150 mcg • Vitamin C (Sago Palm) 150 mg • Natural Vitamin E (Succinate) 70 IU • Suma 7 mg • ISB Complex 107 mg includes: Magnesium, Selenium, SOD Type G, Zinc, Echinacea purpurea, Goldenseal, L-Cysteine HCL, L-Ornithine, Ferric Phosphate, Garlic & L-Aspartic Acid & natural Flavor.
See Editor's Note No. 14, page 1817.

Immutol - Immunocorp
Each capsule contains: Beta Glucan 375 mg.

I-MNS - Dial Herbs
Black Cohosh • Blue Cohosh • Red Raspberry • Catnip • Wild Yam • Wild Carrot • Motherwort • Pennyroyal • St. John's Wort.

Imperial Green Tea - Jamieson
Each tea bag contains: Chinese Green Tea leaf (Camellia sinensis) • Ginger root (Singiber officinale) • Leechee fruit (Litchi chinensis).

Imumax - FreeLife
Each tablet contains: Patented EV.EXT 10 standardized American Feverfew (Parthenium integrifolium) root 75 mg • standardized Echinacea (Echinacea purpurea) root 25 mg. Other Ingredients: Calcium Hydrogen Phosphate, Microcrystalline Cellulose, Silica Dioxide, Hydrous Magnesium Silicate, Magnesium Stearate, Zein, Alginates.

Indigestion Remedy - PhytoPharmica
Twenty drops contain: Podophyllum peltatum 4x • Carduus marianus 3x • Dolichos pruriens 3x • Leptandra virginica 3x • Lycopodium clavatum 3x • Nux vomica 3x • Boldo 1x • Chelidonium majus 1x. In a base of 50% USP alcohol by volume.
See Editor's Note No. 1, page 1816.

Indole-3-Carbinol - Solaray
Each capsule contains: Vitamin C (as ascorbic acid) 200 mg • Broccoli 50 mg • Brussel Sprouts 50 mg • Cabbage 50 mg • Cauliflower 50 mg • Kale 50 mg • Indole-3-Carbinol (I3C) 25 mg. Other Ingredients: Gelatin (capsule), Magnesium stearate.

Indolplex - PhytoPharmica
Each tablet contains: Diindolylmethane (DIM) from Indolplex 30 mg.

InflamActin - Nature's Plus
Two capsules contain: Boswellin [(Boswellia serrata gum resin) (standardized 65% Boswellic Acids)] 250 mg • Bromelain (standardized 90 Gelatin Digesting Units) 150 mg • DLPA (dl-Phenylalanine) (Free Form Amino Acid) 100 mg • Turmeric [(Curcuma longa rhizome) standardized 95% Curcumin) 75 mg • Vitamin C corn free 60 mg • St. John's Wort [(Hypericum perforatum flower) (standardized 0.3-0.5% Hypericin)] 50 mg • Chamomile [(Matricaria recutita flower) standardized 1% Apigenin, 0.5% Essential oil] 50 mg • Feverfew [(Tanacetum parthenium leaf) standardized 0.7% Parthenolide] 50 mg • Goldenseal [(Hydrastis canadensis root & rhizome) standardized 10% Alkaloids, 5% Hydrastine] 25 mg • Ginger [(Zingiber officinale root) standardized 4% Volatile oils] 25 mg.

InflamActin Cream - Nature's Plus
Active ingredient: Methyl Salicylate 18%.
Other Ingredients: Exclusive Liposomal Herbal Complex [Boswellin (Boswellia serrata gum resin extract) (standardized 65% Boswellic Acids), Tumeric rhizome extract (Curcuma longa) (standardized 95% Curcumin), Gorgonian extract (Pseudopterogoria elisbethae leaf) (standardized 4% Pseudopterosin), & natural Vitamin E] in a vanishing Liposomal Cream Base.

Inflamase - Progressive Labs
Each capsule contains: Enteric release phase: Pancreatin 100 mg • Lipase 10 mg • Amylase 10 mg • Trypsin 200 mg • Alpha Chymotrypsin 2 mg. Gastric release phase: Bromelain 100 mg • Catalase 25 mcg • Superoxide Dismutase 25 mcg. The two phase pH sensitive release of the ingredients in this product is due to its exclusive enteric matrix formulation.
See Editor's Note No. 14, page 1817.

Inflamzyme - PhytoPharmica
Each tablet contains: Vitamin C (ascorbic acid) 100 mg • Magnesium (carbonate) 25 mg • Bromelain pineapple whole fruit (1,800 M.C.U.) 125 mg • Quercetin 125 mg • Mixed bioflavonoids complex (50% concentrate) citrus 100 mg • L-Cysteine (HCl) 75 mg.

Inholtra - Omni Nutraceuticals
Two Quicksorb gels contain: Vitamin C (as Ascorbyl Palmitate) 1 mg • Vitamin E (as D-Alpha Tocopherol) 7 IU • Manganese (as Manganese Aspartate) 0.60 mg • Omega-3 fatty acid (Eicosapentainoic Acid 400 mg and Docosahexaenoic Acid 300 mg) 465 mg • D-Glucosamine Sulfate 335 mg • N-Acetyl D-Glucosamine 335 mg • Omega-6 fatty acid (as Gamma-Linolenic Acid) 135 mg. Other Ingredients: Vegetable Oil, Fish Oil, Gelatin, Glycerin, Carob, Water.
See Editor's Note No. 15, page 1817.

Inholtra Natural Pain Relief Formula - Omni Nutraceuticals
Three quicksorb gels contain: Glucosamine Sulfate 500 mg • N-Acetyl D-Glucosamine 500 mg • Chondroitin Sulfate (as Chondroitin Sulfates A & B) 200 mg • EPA 400 mg • DHA 300 mg • GLA 300 mg • Vitamin E 10 IU • Ascorbyl Palmitate 5 mg • Manganese 1 mg.
See Editor's Note No. 15, page 1817.

Inositol - Puritan's Pride
Each tablet contains: Inositol 650 mg.

Inositol - Nature's Bounty
Each tablet contains: Inositol 650 mg. Other Ingredients: Cellulose, Vegetable Stearic Acid, Food Glaze, Talc, Magnesium Silicate, Vegetable Magnesium Stearate.

Inositol Hexaphosphate - Olympian Labs
Two capsules contain: Inositol Hexaphosphate 1000 mg • Kelp 100 mg • Wheat grass 60 mg.

BRAND NAMES

Some Brand Name Natural Products - What they Contain
www.NaturalDatabase.com contains MANY more listings than appear here.

Inositol Powder - Puritan's Pride
Each 1/4 teaspoon contains: Inositol powder 600 mg.

Insomnia Formula - Dr. Morrow's Homeopathic Formulas
Ten drops contain: Passiflora 3X • Ignatia 4C • Coffee cruda 5C • Tellurium 6C • Acid phosphorica 7C • Palladium 6C • Magnesia phosphorica 6C.
See Editor's Note No. 1, page 1816.

Instant Soy'n Whey - Next Nutrition
One serving contains: Water-Extracted Soy Protein concentrate • Non-Denatured Whey Protein concentrate • Fructose • Natural Vanilla flavoring • Lecithin • Modified Food starch • Malic acid • Cellulose gum • Kudzu extract • Momordica extract • Stevia • Vitamin E.

Intact Colostrum - GNC
Each packet (20.4 grams) contains: Bovine Colostrum powder (standardized for minumum 15% IgG content).
Other Ingredients: Artificial Vanilla Flavoring, Acesulfame Potassium.

Intensive Therapy Support - Amazon Support
Each capsule contains: Graviola • Cat's Claw (3% standardized extract) • Pau d'arco (4:1 extract) • Suma (5% standardized extract) • Bitter Melon (4:1 extract) • Espinheira Santa (leaf & bark) • Mullaca • Mutamba • Vassourinha.

IntestaLife - Holista
Each capsule contains: 4 billion active cells specially cultured strains of Lactobacillus Rhamnosus • Lactobacillus acidophilus • Bifido longum.

Intestamend - Health From The Sun
Three capsules contain: Protein 1 g • Calcium 24 mg • Glutamine 200 mg • Lysine 132 mg • Leucine 103 mg • Methionine 49 mg • Threonine 59 mg • Valine 69 mg • Trypophane 11 mg • Isoleucine 60 mg • Phenylalanine 48 mg. Ingredients: Deep-Ocean White Fish, Gelatin, Glycerine, Water, natural Rosemary flavor.

Intestinal Fortitude - Nutri-Quest
Each tablet contains: L-Glutamine 150 mg • Buffered Vitamin C (Sago) 25 mg • N-Acetyl Glucosamine 75 mg • Vitamin E Succinate 10 IU • Lipoic Acid 2 mg • Ginkgo Biloba extract 2 mg • Deglycerrized Licorice 50 mg • Slippery Elm 100 mg • Lactobacillus Acidophilus 1 million IU • Cats Claw 15 mg • Ginkgo Biloba herb 50 mg • Jerusalem Artichoke 25 mg • Zinc Chelate 5 mg • Lactobacillus Bifidus 1 million IU.

Intestinal Rescue - The Herbalist
Psyllium seed & husk • Guar gum • Ginger root • Medical Grade Pectin • Bentonite clay • Rhubarb root • Cinnamon bark.

Intlecs Huperzine A - Intlecs
Each tablet contains: Huperzine A (Chinese club moss, Huperzia serrata) 50 mcg.

Intrasound Cleanse Formula - TriStar Online
Each scoop contains: Maltodextrin • Calcium Citrate • Natural Flavors • Magnesium Citrate • Gum • Citric Acid • Beta Carotene Gum • Stevia • Rebaudiana Extract • Soy Lecithin • Beet Powder • Lactobacillus Acidophilus • Lactobacillus Bifidus • Fructooligosaccharides • Papaya Powder • Prune Powder • Ascorbic Acid • Barley Sprout Powder • Wheat Sprout Powder • Oat Sprout Powder • Fenugreek. Fiber blend: Oat Fiber, Cellulose Gel/Cellulose, Purified Cellulose, Partially Hydrolyzed Soy Fiber, Psyllium Husk, Rice Bran, Citrus Pectin.

Intrasound Energy Drink - TriStar Online
Whole leaf aloe • Purified water • Natural Flavor • Fructose • Kaolin Clay • Trace Minerals • Citric Acid • Stevia • Xanthan Gum • Fiber •

Ginseng Extract • Sage Extract • Dandelion Extract • Potassium Gluconate • Sodium Benzoate • Potassium Sorbate.

Intrasound Enzyme Formulas - TriStar Online
Each capsule contains: Amylase • Lipase • Protease • Cellulase • Intervase or Sucrase • Lactase • Malt Diastase • Calcium Citrate • Kaolin Clay • Beef Gelatin Capsule.

Intrasound Gel - TriStar Online
Generic Conductive Gel • Kaolin Clay.

Intrasound Herbal Accelerator - TriStar Online
Each capsule contains: Lipase • Cellulase • Amylase • Protease • Chromium Picolinate • Chromium Polynicotinate • Garcinia Cambogia Extract • Sida Cordifolia Herb • Yerba Mate • Kola Nut • Bladderwrack Algae • Cayenne Pepper • Siberian Ginseng Root.

Intrasound Mouth Rinse - TriStar Online
Whole leaf aloe • Purified Water • Natural Flavor • Kaolin Clay • Chlorophyll • Stevia • Sodium Benzoate.

Intrasound Powder - TriStar Online
Kaolin Clay.

Intrasound Tooth Gel - TriStar Online
Whole Leaf Aloe • Purified Water • Glycerin • Carrageenan (seaweed) • Hydrated Silica • Sodium Lauroyl Sarcosinate • Chlorophyll • Kaolin Clay • Natural Flavor • Stevia • Potassium Sorbate.

Intrinsic Plus - Progressive Labs
Each capsule contains: Vitamin B12 (cyanocobalamin) 500 mcg • Folate (folic acid) 800 mcg • Pancreatic enzyme concentrate 50 mg • Porcine Stomach 250 mg • Pyloric Substance 60 mg.
See Editor's Note No. 14, page 1817.

IP6 Capsule - Jarrow Formulas
Each capsule contains: Calcium-Magnesium Inositol Hexaphosphate 615 mg • IP6 50 mg • Calcium 85 mg • Magnesium 30 mg.
Other Ingredients: Rice powder, Magnesium Stearate.

IP6 Powder - Jarrow Formulas
Each scoop contains: Calcium-Magnesium Inositol Hexaphosophate 1230 mg • IP6 (extracted from rice bran) 1000 mg • Calcium 170 mg • Magnesium 60 mg.

IpriBone - GNC Preventive Nutrition
Two tablets contain: Vitamin D (as Cholecalciferol) 400 IU • Calcium (as Calcimate Calcium Citrate Malate) 200 mg • 7-Isopropoxy Isoflavone (Ostivone) 600 mg.

Iromin-G - Mission Pharmacal
Each tablet contains: Vitamin A 4000 IU • Vitamin C 100 mg • Vitamin D (as Vitamin D3; Cholecalciferol) 400 IU • Vitamin B1 4.8 mg • Vitamin B2 (Cyanocobalamin) 2 mg • Vitamin B3 10 mg • Vitamin B6 20 mg • Folate 0.8 mg • Vitamin B12 2 mcg • Vitamin B5 1 mg • Calcium 57 mg • Iron 29.5 mg. Other Ingredients: Sugar, Microcrystalline Cellulose, Color, Croscarmellose Sodium, Magnesium Stearate, Povidone, Red 40 Lake, Food Glaze, Carnauba Wax, Sodium Benzoate, White Beeswax, Yellow 6 Lake.

Iron - Source Naturals
Each tablet contains: Iron (from 250 mg of Iron Amino Acid Chelate) 25 mg.

Iron Complex - PhytoPharmica
Two capsules contain: Vitamin C (ascorbic acid) 120 mg • Folic Acid 400 mcg • Vitamin B12 (cyanocobalamin) 200 mcg • Iron (ferrous succinate) 50 mg • Liquid Liver fractions (predigested soluble concentrate) 500 mg • Chlorophyll (fat-soluble) 1 mg.
See Editor's Note No. 14, page 1817 .

Iron Complex - Nature's Life
Each capsule contains: Iron (Peptonate) 25 mg • Vitamin C 20 mg •
Niacinamide 10 mg • Vitamin B1 (Thiamine HCl) 1 mg • Vitamin B2
(Riboflavin) 1 mg • Vitamin B6 (Pyridoxine HCl) 1 mg • Folic Acid
30 mcg • Vitamin B12 (Cobalamin concentrate) 15 mcg • Copper
(Gluconate) 100 mcg • Manganese (Gluconate) 1 mg • Betaine HCl
15 mg. In a natural base of Rose Hips concentrate.

Iron Plex - PhysioLogics
Each capsule contains: Iron (from Ferrous Bisglycinate) 28 mg • Folic
Acid 400 mcg • Dibencozide 250 mcg • Intrinsic Factor 20 mg.

Iron Plus - Nutri-Quest
Each tablet contains: Iron (Ferrous Fumarate) 50 mg • Vitamin C
100 mg • L-Glycine 100 mg • Niacinamide 15 mg • Betaine HCL
15 mg • Vitamin E (Succinate) 15 IU • D-Calcium Pantothenate
(Pantothenic Acid) 13 mg • Vitamin B2 4 mg • Vitamin B1 3 mg •
Vitamin B6 2 mg • Folic Acid 200 mcg • Vitamin B12 25 mcg •
Choline Bitartrate 12.5 mg.

Iron Woman - Traditional Medicinals
Yellow Dock root • Burdock root • Dandelion root • Licorice root •
Nettle leaf • Prune fruit • Astragalus root • Stevia leaf.

Iron-All - Puritan's Pride
Three tablets contain: Vitamin C (as Ascorbic Acid with Rose Hips)
100 mg • Thiamin (as Thiamine Hydrochloride) 2.25 mg • Riboflavin
4.5 mg • Niacin 0.75 mg • Vitamin B6 (as Pyridoxine Hydrochloride)
0.026 mg • Folate (as Folic Acid) 16.5 mg • Vitamin B12 (as
Cyanocobalamin) 12.5 mg • Biotin 0.00075 mg • Pantothenic Acid
(as D-Calcium Pantothenate) 0.0675 mg • Iron (Ferrous Gluconate)
57.5 mg • Desiccated Liver 100 mg • L-Lysine 30 mg • Inositol 3 mg •
Choline Bitartrate 2.25 mg • PABA 15 mcg.
See Editor's Note No. 14, page 1817.

Iron-Folic Plus - Nutrilite
Each tablet contains: Folic Acid 33% DV • Ferrous Fumarate •
Ferrous Gluconate • Nutrilite Spinach concentrate with phytofactors
plant compounds.

Iron-Free MultiLogics - PhysioLogics
Each tablet contains: Vitamin A (Beta-Carotene) 12500 IU • Vitamin
A (Palmitate) 2500 IU • Thiamine 75 mg • Riboflavin 75 mg • Niacin
75 mg • Pantothenic Acid 75 mg • Vitamin B6 (Pyridoxine HCl)
75 mg • Vitamin B12 (Cyanocobalamin) 75 mcg • Folic Acid 400 mcg
• Biotin 300 mcg • Vitamin C (Ascorbic Acid) 250 mg • Vitamin D
(Cholecalciferol) 400 IU • Vitamin E (d-Alpha Tocopherol) 150 IU •
Calcium (Amino Acid Chelate) 20 mg • Magnesium (Amino Acid
Chelate) 10 mg • Zinc (Amino Acid Chelate) 10 mg • Copper (Amino
Acid Chelate) 1 mg • Manganese (Amino Acid Chelate) 1 mg •
Chromium (Niacin/Glycine Chelate) 25 mcg • Iodine (Potassium
Iodide) 150 mcg • Selenium (Amino Acid Chelate) 25 mcg •
Molybdenum (Amino Acid Chelate) 25 mcg • Boron (Amino Acid
Chelate) 500 mcg • Potassium (Amino Acid Complex) 1.8 mg •
Bioflavonoids lemon 25 mg • Rutin 25 mg • Betaine (HCl) 25 mg •
Choline (Bitartrate) 31 mg • Inositol 75 mg • PABA 75 mg •
Hesperidin 5 mg.

IsoPure - Nature's Best
Each serving contains: Creamy Vanilla Ingredients: Ion Exchanged
Whey Protein Isolate, Maltodextrin, Vitamin, Mineral & Amino Acid
Blend, Natural & Artificial Flavor, Xanthan Gum, Aspartame,
Acesulfame K. Dutch Chocolate Ingredients: Ion Exchange Whey
Protein Isolate, Maltodextrin, Vitamin, Mineral & Amino Acid Blend,
Cocoa, Xanthan Gum, Natural & Artificial Flavor, Aspartame,
Acesulfame K. Orange Creamsicle Ingredients: Ion Exchange Whey
Protein Isolate, Maltodextrin, Vitamin, Mineral & Amino Acid Blend,
Natural & Artificial Flavor, Xanthan Gum, Aspartame, Acesulfame
K, Artificial Color (Yellow #6). Strawberries & Cream Ingredients:

Ion Exchange Whey Protein Isolate, Maltodextrin, Vitamin, Mineral
& Amino Acid Blend, Natural & Artificial Flavor, Freeze-Dried
Strawberry Crystals, Xanthan Gum, Aspartame, Acesulfame K,
Artificial Color (Red #3). Chocolate Peanut Butter Swirl Ingredients:
Ion Exchange Whey Protein Isolate, Maltodextrin, Vitamin, Mineral
& Amino Acid Blend, Cocoa, Natural & Artificial Flavor, Xanthan
Gum, Aspartame, Acesulfame K.

Isotonix OPC-3 - Isotonix
Grape Seed extract 25 mg • Red Wine extract 25 mg • Pine Bark
extract 25 mg • Bilberry extract 25 mg • Bioflavonoids 25 mg.
In a base of citric acid, fructose, dextrose, maltodextrin, apple pectin,
silica, calcium sulfate, and potassium.

Ivy Extract - PhytoPharmica
Two tablets contain: Ivy (Hedera helix) leaf extract 5-7.5:1 (Contains
glycosidic saponins) 50 mg.

Jarro-Dophilus + Colostrum - Jarrow Formulas
Each capsule contains: Lactobacillus Rhamnosus R049 20% 672
million • Lactobacillus Casei R215 20 % 672 million • Lactobacillus
Plantarum R202 20% 672 million • Lactobacillus Acidophilus R052
10% 336 million • Bifidobacterium Longum R023 20% 672 million •
Bifidobacterium Breve R070 10% 336 million • Colostrum 500 mg.
Other Ingredients: Ascorbic Acid, Magnesium Stearate.

Jarro-Dophilus +FOS - Jarrow Formulas
Each capsule Contains: FOS (Fructo-Oligo-Saccharides) 210 mg •
Lactobacillus Rhamnosus R049 20% 672 million • Lactobacillus
Casei R215 20 % 672 million • Lactobacillus Plantarum R202 20%
672 million • Lactobacillus Acidophilus R052 10% 336 million •
Bifidobacterium Longum R023 672 million • Bifidobacterium breve
R070 10% 336 million • Vitamin C 1 mg. Other Ingredients:
Maltodextrin, Magnesium Stearate.

Jarro-Dophilus +FOS Powder - Jarrow Formulas
Each capsule Contains: FOS (Fructo-Oligo-Saccharides) 4000 mg •
Lactobacillus Rhamnosus R049 20% 2.4 billion • Lactobacillus Casei
R215 20 % 2.4 billion • Lactobacillus Plantarum R202 20% 2.4
billion • Lactobacillus Acidophilus R052 10% 1.2 billion •
Bifidobacterium Longum R023 2.4 billion • Bifidobacterium Breve
R070 10% 1.2 billion • Vitamin C 1 mg. Other Ingredients:
Maltodextrin, Magnesium Stearate.

Jarro-Dophilus +Lactoferrin - Jarrow Formulas
Each capsule Contains: Lactobacillus Rhamnosus R049 20% 672
million • Lactobacillis Casei R215 20 % 672 million • Lactobacillus
Plantarum R202 20% 672 million • Lactobacillus Acidophilus R052
10% 336 million • Bifidobacterium Longum R023 20% 672 million •
Bifidobacterium Breve R070 10% 336 million • Lactoferrin 200 mg.
Other Ingredients: Ascorbic Acid, Magnesium Stearate.

Jarsin 300 - Lichtwer Pharma
Each tablet contains: Dry St. John's Wort extract 300 mg.
Other Ingredients: Lactose Monohydrate, Silicon Dioxide, Cellulose
powder, Magnesium Stearate, Vanillin, Dimeticon Emulsion,
Hypromellose, Macrogol 4000, Saccharin Sodium, Talcum, Titanium
Dioxide, Iron Oxide Hydrate.

Joint Actives - VitaStore
Six tablets contain: Glucosamine HCl 1500 mg • Shark Cartilage
500 mg • Salix Alba 200 mg • Boswellia 250 mg • Green-Lipped
Mussel 250 mg • Quercetin 300 mg • Manganese 5 mg •
L-Methionine 100 mg • Zinc Gluconate 25 mg • Turmeric 250 mg •
Bromelain 200 mg • Vitamin C 300 mg • Vitamin E 90 IU.

Joint Complex - Puritan's Pride
Three capsules contain: Glucosamine Sulfate 500 mg • Vitamin C 250
mg • Bromelain (2400 GDU per gram) 250 mg • Boswellin

BRAND NAMES

(Boswellia Serrata) 250 mg • Curcumin (Curcuma Longa) 50 mg • Zinc (Amino Acid Chelate) 10 mg • Chondroitin Sulfate A 10 mg • White Willow Bark 100 mg • Shark Cartilage 500 mg • Vervain 100 mg.
See Editor's Note No. 15, page 1817.

Joint Cream - The Vitamin Shoppe
Glucosamine • Boswellin • Capsaicin.

Joint Essentials - Swanson
Three capsules contain: Vitamin C (as ascorbic acid) 250 mg • Zinc (from amino acid chelate) 15 mg • Manganese 5 mg • Glucosamine Sulfate (2KCl) 500 mg • Boswellian Boswellia Serrata Resin (65% boswellic acid) 250 mg • Bromelain (2400 GDU) 250 mg • Chondroitin Sulfate 200 mg • OptiMSM (methylsulfonylmethane) 100 mg • White Willow Bark 100 mg • Curcumin 50 mg • Devil's Claw powder 25 mg • Quercetin 25 mg • Sea Cucumber 25 mg • Yucca root extract 25 mg.
See Editor's Note No. 15, page 1817.

Joint Fitness - Celestial Seasonings
Two capsules contain: Vitamin C (as ascorbic acid) 225 mg • Pantothenic Acid (as calcium pantothenate) 15 mg • Glucosamine Sulfate/HCL 150 mg • Flax Seeds 225 mg • Turmeric extract 185 mg. Other ingredients: May contain one or more of the following: Dicalcium phosphate, gelatin, rice flour, stearic acid, magnesium stearate, and silicon dioxide. This product contains no artificial colors, flavors, or preservatives. One serving size is equivalent to: Turmeric 185 mg standardized to 95% curcuminoids.

Joint Formula - PharmAssure
Two tablets contain: Sodium 140 mg • Vitamin C (as Ascorbic Acid) 60mg • Selenium (as Selenium Chelate) 100 mcg • D-Glucosamine Sulfate 750 mg • .2NaCl Chondroitin Sulfate, Sodium 600 mg • Boswellin serrate Resin Extract (65% Boswellic Acid=200 mg) 308 mg • Bromelain 200 GDU. Other ingredients: Cellulose, Croscarmellose sodium, Dicalcium Phosphate
See Editor's Note No. 15, page 1817.

Joint Fuel - TwinLab
Six capsules contain: Glucosamine Sulfate 1500 mg • Chondroitin Sulfate A (CSA) 100 mg • Zinc (from Chelated Zinc Picolinate) 30 mg • Manganese (from Chelated Manganese Gluconate) 5 mg • Vitamin C 1000 mg • Natural Vitamin E (Succinate) 800 IU • Selenium (from Selenomethionine) 200 mcg • Turmeric extract (Curcuma longa) (standardized for 95% Curcumin) 1300 mg • Quercetin (Bioflavonoid) 100 mg • Bromelain 200 mg.
See Editor's Note No. 15, page 1817.

Joint Fuel Liquid Concentrate - TwinLab
Each tablespoonful contains: Glucosamine HCl 500 mg • Chondroitin Sulfate 400 mg • Betaine 166 mg • Hydrolyzed Collagen 33 mg • Chicken Type II Collagen 33 mg • Vitamin B6 3.3 mg • Folic Acid 400 mcg • Vitamin B12 166 mcg.
See Editor's Note No. 15, page 1817.

Joint Performance - Metabolic Response Modifiers
Four capsules contain: Glucosamine Sulfate 1000 mg • MSM (Methyl-Sulfonyl-Methane) 500 mg • Noto-Gin (Panax Ginseng 45% saponins) 100 mg • Chondroitin complex 280 mg • Collagen complex 200 mg • Sea Cucumber 100 mg • CMO (25%) 100 mg • Boswellia 200 mg • Bromelain (2400 GDU) 100 mg • White Willow bark (0.1% salicylates) 80 mg • Tumeric (95% curcuminoids) 75 mg • Manganese (citrate) 8 mg.
See Editor's Note No. 15, page 1817.

Joint Rejuvenator - BioTreasures
Each caplet contains: Glucosamine Sulfate 1500 mg • Chondroitin Sulfate 750 mg • Turmeric 750 mg • Devil's Claw 400 mg • Bromelain 100 mg.
See Editor's Note No. 15, page 1817.

Joint Rescue - TwinLab
Three softgels contain: Vitamin E (from d-Alpha Tocopherols) 400 IU • Glucosamine HCl & Glucosamine Sulfate 750 mg • Chondroitin Sulfate 50 mg • Turmeric powder extract (standardized for 95% Curcumin) 650 mg • Boswellin (Boswellia serrata extract) (standardized for 65% Boswellic Acids) 13 mg • Ginger root extract 50 mg • EPA 750 mg • DHA 750 mg • Borage Oil 100 mg.
See Editor's Note No. 15, page 1817.

Joint Rescue Formula with Glucosamine+ - Dr. Bussan's
Each capsule contains: Glucosamine sulfate 500 mg • Herbal Extract Complex 125 mg: Wild Yam, Licorice root, Aloe Vera, Pfaffia root, Red Poppy flower, Tumeric, White Peony root, Yucca, Corydalis rhizome, Super Dioxide Dismutase (SOD), Catalase Oxidants • Methionine 75 mg • Malic Acid 50 mg • Polyascorbic Acid (vitamin c) 25 mg • Niacinamide 10 mg • Pantothenic Acid (vitamin B5) 5 mg • Manganese Gluconate Chelate 5 mg.

Joint Support - Futurebiotics
Four tablets contain: Devil's Claw 400 mg • Yucca 300 mg • Horsetail 200 mg • Ginger 200 mg • Alfalfa juice concentrate 200 mg • Chinese Cinnamon 250 mg • Magnesium: (oxide, chloride, ascorbate) 400 mg • Beta Carotene 250 mg • Vitamin C (ascorbic acid, Rose hips) 120 mg • Niacin 8 mg • Niacinamide 250 mg • Vitamin D (Fish oils) 200 IU • Vitamin E (natural) 25 IU • Vitamin B6 (pyridoxine HCl) 8 mg • Vitamin B12 (cyanocobalamin) 12 mcg • Zinc (sulfate) 15 mg • Copper (gluconate) 750 mcg • Biotin 80 mcg • Pantothenic Acid 35 mg • Selenium (methionate) 120 mcg • Glutamic Acid HCl 100 mg • Lecithin 100 mg • Betaine HCl 75 mg • Para Amino Benzoic Acid (PABA) 25 mg • Potassium (sulfate) 20 mg.

Joint Support - Now
Three capsules contain: Vitamin B3 (Niacinamide) 100mg • Vitamin B5 (Pantothenic Acid) 100 mg • Vitamin B6 (Pyridoxine HCl) 50 mg • Vitamin C (Ascorbic Acid) 100 mg • Magnesium (Oxide) 200 mg • Zinc (Picolinate) 15 mg • Manganese (Amino Acid Chelate) 7 mg • Copper (Amino Acid Chelate) 3 mg • Glucosamine HCL 1000 mg • Boswellin standardized herbal extract of Boswellia serrata 300 mg • Sea Cucumber 300 mg • Bromelain (2000 GDU activity from pineapple) 150 mg • PABA (Para-Aminobenzoic Acid) 10 mg • Devil's Claw (Harpagophytum procumbens) 100 mg.

Joint Support - Olympia Nutrition
Glucosamine, Boswellin, Sea Cucumber, Bromelain, Yucca, Alfalfa.

Joint Support Formula - Health Smart Vitamins
Each capsule contains: Methylsulfonylmethane (MSM) 333 mg • Glucosamine Sulfate 200 mg • Chondroitin Sulfate 67 mg.
See Editor's Note No. 15, page 1817.

Joint Synergy - Olympia Nutrition
Glucosamine Sulfate • Sea Cucumber • MSM • Hydrolyzed Cartilage.

Joint Synergy + - Metabolic Response Modifiers
Four capsules contain: Glucosamine Sulfate (KCl) 1000 mg • MSM (methyl-sulfonyl-methane) 500 mg • Noto-Panax Ginseng (50-60% Saponins supplying 45% Ginsenosides) 100 mg • Chondroitin complex 280 mg • Collagen complex 200 mg • Sea Cucumber (25% mucopolysaccharides) 100 mg • CMO (25%) 100 mg • Boswellia serrata 200 mg • Bromelain (2400 GDU) 100 mg • White Willow bark (0.1% salicylates) 80 mg • Tumeric (95% curcuminoids) 75 mg • Manganese (citrate) 8 mg.
See Editor's Note No. 15, page 1817.

Joint/Arthritis Support - Amazon Support
Each capsule contains: Amor Seco • Cat's Claw Extract • Chuchuhuasi • Tayuya • Iporuru • Pucao Preto • Mullaca • Sarsaparilla.

Some Brand Name Natural Products - What they Contain

JointFlex - Eden Laboratories, Inc.
Active Ingredient: Camphor (3.1%). Inactive Ingredients: Acetylated lanolin, acrylates/C10-30, alkyl acrylate, crosspolymer, aloe vera, C12-15 alkyl benzoate, chondroitin sulfate, purified water, diazolidnyl urea, dimethicone, dimethiconol stearate, disodium EDTA, dl panthenol, glucosamine sulfate, glycerin, glycerol stearate, glycosaminoglycans, hydroxylated lanolin, hydroxypropylene methylcellulose, lodopropynyl, butylcarbomate, methyl gluceth-20, methyl glucose, sesquistearate, peppermint oil, polysorbate 20, potassium carbomer, tocopheryl acetate.
See Editor's Note No. 15, page 1817.

JointPower - Trimedica
Six capsules contain: Glucosamine Sulfate 1500 mg • Vitamin C 1000 mg • natural Vitamin E (Succinate) 800 IU • Manganese (Chelated Manganese Gluconate) 5 mg • Zinc (Chelated Zinc Picolinate) 15 mg • Copper (Chelated Copper Gluconate) 1.5 mg • Tumeric (Curcuma longa) extract (standardized for 95% Curcumin) 1300 mg • Boswellia serrata extract (standardized for 60-65 Boswellic Acids) 100 mg • Bromelain 100 mg • Selenium (from Selenomethionine) 200 mcg.

Joints Formula - Nature's Way
Three capsules contain: Alfalfa concentrate 125 mg • Boswellia dried extract 300 mg • Copper (Amino Acid Chelate) 1 mg • Glucosamine HCL 750 mg • Grape seed dried extract 48 mg • Manganese Amino Acid Chelate 5 mg • Nettle root 250 mg • Wild Yam root 75 mg • Zinc Amino Acid Chelate 7.5 mg. Other ingredients: Gelatin, Magnesium Stearate, Millet.

Jojoba & E Skin Oil - Derma E
90% Jojoba • 10% Vitamin E oil.

Juice Plus Garden Blend - Juice Plus+
Two capsules contain: Carrots • Barley • Parsley • Beets- Folic Acid, Iron, Calcium, Potassium • Kale • Broccoli- Beta Carotene, Indoles, Sulforaphane, Vitamin C, Calcium, Chromium • Cabbage • Oats • Spinach- Lutein, Zeaxanthin • Tomatoes- Lycopene, Coumarine • Soluble and Insoluble Fibers- Beet Fiber, Oat Bran, Barley Bran, Cabbage Fiber, Plant Cellulose, Glucomannan • Enzymes- Lipase, Amylase, Protease, Cellulase • Food Actives- Allicin, Lycopene, Acidophilus, Polyphenol Catechins, Indole Carbinols, d-Calcium Glucarate • Vitamins & Minerals- Vitamin C, Beta Carotene, Vitamin E, Vitamin B, Calcium, Magnesium.

Juice Plus Orchard Blend - Juice Plus+
Two capsules contain: Apples- Boron • Oranges- Vitamin C, Beta Carotene • Pineapples- Bromelain • Cranberries • Peaches- Boron • Acerola Cherries- Vitamin C, Iron • Papaya- Vitamin C, Papain, Carpaine • Soluble and Insoluble Fibers- Apple and Citrus Pectin, Date Fiber, Prune powder, Dried Plant Fiber, Glucomannan • Enzymes- Bromelain, Papain, Lipase, Amylase, Protease, Cellulase • Food Actives- Citrus Bioflavonoids, Acidophilus Polyphenol Catechins, d-Calcium Glucarate, Indole Carbinols • Vitamins & Minerals- Vitamin C, Beta Carotene, Vitamin E, Vitamin B Complex, Calcium, Magnesium.

Just-Whey - SportPharma
Each serving contains: Calories 110 • Protein 23 g • Carbohydrates 2.5 g • Fat 1 g.

K & MG Aspartate - Atrium Inc.
Each tablet contains: Potassium Aspartate (which yields Potassium 78 mg & L-Aspartic Acid 209 mg) 261 mg • Magnesium Aspartate (which yields Magnesium 28 mg & L-Aspartic Acid 242 mg) 278 mg.

K & U - MMS Pros
Each capsule contains: Juniper berries • Parsley herb • Ginger root • Uva Ursi leaves • Marshmallow root • Cramp bark • Golden Seal root.

Kalm-Assure - Nature's Plus
Each tablet contains: Rapid Release Layer: Pantothenic Acid (Vitamin B5) 50 mg • GABA (Gamma Aminobutyric Acid) 25 mg • Magnesium (Citrate) 25 mg • Pyridoxal-5-Phosphate (P5P) 5 mg. Sustained Release Layer: Kava (Piper methysticum root) standardized 30% kavalactones 100 mg • Passion Flower (Passiflora incarnata) standardized 4% Isovitexin 75 mg • Hops fruit (Humulus lupulus) standardized 5.2% bitter acids 10 mg • Siberian Ginseng (Eleutherococcus senticosus) standardized 0.8% Eleutherosides 25 mg • Chamomile (Matricaria recutita flower) standardized 1% Apigenin 25 mg. Contains no yeast, wheat, corn, soy, milk, salt or starch.

Kan Jang (Kanjang) - Swedish Herbal Institute
Each tablet contains: Standardized Andrographis paniculata root extract (4% Andrographolides) 300 mg. Other ingredients: Mycrocrystalline, Sodium Starch Glyconate, Magnesium Stearate, Zien.

Kava 30% - Nature's Way
Each capsule contains: Kava Dried Extract (30% kavalactones) 350 mg • Passion Flower stem, leaf, fruit & flower 500 mg.

Kava Kava - Leiner Health Products
Each caplet contains: Kava Kava extract (Piper methysticum) root 200 mg. Other Ingredients: Calcium Carbonate, Cellulose, Maltodextrin, Hydroxypropyl Methylcellulose, Silicon Dioxide, Polyethylene Glycol 3350, Croscarmellose Sodium, Hydroxypropyl Cellulose, Crospovidone, Magnesium Stearate, Yellow 6 Lake, Red 40 Lake, Blue 2 Lake, Pharmaceutical Glaze, Polysorbate 80, Titanium Dioxide.

Kava Kava - Gaia Herbs
Kava Kava standardized for 5% kavalactones. Standardized Full Spectrum 136 mg of extract per capsule. Guaranteed Potency 68 mg of extract per capsule.

Kava Kava - Olympian Labs
Each capsule contains: Kava extract 500 mg.

Kava Kava - Pharmanex
Each softgel contains: Kava Kava root (11:1) extract (Piper methysticum) 175 mg. Other Ingredients: Soybean Oil, Gelatin, Glycerin, Maltodextrin, Beeswax, Lecithin, Carob.

Kava Kava - Puritan's Pride
Each capsule contains: Kava Kava root (in a millet grain base) 300 mg.

Kava Kava 3000 mg - Jamieson
Each capsule contains: Kava Kava root (Piper methysticum, 250 mg powdered extract 1:12) 3000 mg. Other Ingredients: Gelatin, Calcium Sulfate, Maltodextrin, Cellulose, Magnesium Stearate, Silica.

Kava Kava Plus - The Herbalist
Kava Kava root • Siberian Ginseng root • St. John's Wort flowering tops • Oat seed • Skullcap herb.

Kava Kava Root Extract - Source Naturals
Each softgel contains: Kava Kava root extract (Piper methysticum) (standardized to 40% Kavalactones, yielding 70 mg of Kavalactones) 175 mg. In a base of Soybean Oil, Lecithin and Beeswax.

Kava Kava-Valerian Virtue - Blessed Herbs
Kava Kava root • Scullcap • Valerian root • St. John's Wort flower • Lobelia • Arnica flower & herb • Grain alcohol & Distilled Water.

B R A N D   N A M E S

Some Brand Name Natural Products - What they Contain
www.NaturalDatabase.com contains MANY more listings than appear here.

B R A N D   N A M E S

Kava Oasis - New Chapter, Inc.
One softgel contains: Kava root, supercritical extract, (60% kavapyrones- 75 mg) 125 mg• Valerian root, (Valeriana officinalis & Valeriana mexicanus) supercritical extract, (60% valepotriates- 3 mg) 5 mg • Lavender flower, supercritical extract (25% Linalool- 1.2 mg) 5 mg • Passion Flower herb, extract, (3% vitexin- 0.15 mg) 5 mg • Chastetree berry, extract (0.6% aucubin- 0.03 mg) (0.5% agnuside- 0.025 mg) 5 mg • Gotu Kola leaf, extract, (10% asiaticoside- 0.5 mg) (3.% triterpenes- 1.5 mg) 5 mg • Ginger supercritical broad spectrum complex (rhizome), certified organic, (minimum 20% pungent compounds- 1 mg, 4% zingiberene- 0.2 mg) 5 mg • Chamomile flower, supercritical extract (minimum 25% alpha-bisabolol- 1.2 mg) 5 mg. Other Ingredients: Olive Oil -certified organic, Yellow Beeswax.

Kava-30 - PhytoPharmica
Each capsule contains: Kava (Piper methysticum) root and rhizome extract (standardized to contain 30% kavalactones [75 mg of kavalactones]) 250 mg.

Kava-55 - PhytoPharmica
Each capsule contains: Kava (Piper methysticum) root (rhizome) extract (standardized to contain 55% kavalactones [82.5 mg kavalactones]) 150 mg.

Kava-77 - Source Naturals
Each softgel contains: Kava Kava root extract (Piper methysticum) (standardized to 55% Kavalactones yielding 75 mg of Kavalactones) 140 mg. In a base of Rice Bran Oil, Lecithin, Silicon Dioxide and Beeswax.

Kavacin - PhytoPharmica
Each capsule contains: Kava root extract (Piper methysticum) 200 mg standardized to contain 30% kavalactones (60 mg per capsule) • Oat Straw extract 10:1 (Avena sativa) 100 mg • Pyridoxine-Alpha-Ketoglutarate (PAK) 50 mg • Pantothenic Acid 50 mg • Nicotinamide 50 mg • Thiamine HCL (Vitamin B1) 25 mg. Contains no sugar, salt, yeast, wheat, corn, soy, dairy products, coloring, flavoring or preservatives.

KaValerian Caplet - Leiner Health Products
Each caplet contains: Magnesium Citrate 10 mg • Chamomile extract (Matricaria recutita) flower 50 mg • Kava Kava extract (Piper methysticum) root 75 mg • Lecithin 15 mg • Valerian extract (Valeriana officinalis) root 200 mg. Other Ingredients: Dicalcium Phosphate, Cellulose, Stearic Acid, Magnesium Stearate, Dextrin, Silicon Dioxide, Dextrose, Sodium Carboxymethylcellulose, Sodium Citrate.

Kavatime - Bodyonics
Each tablet contains: Kava Kava Root (Piper Methysticum) 350 mg • Kava Kava Powdered Extract 150 mg • Herbolics Support Complex [Derived from barley Malt Flour, Brewers Yeast (saccharomyces cerevisiae), Hops (humulus lupulus), and Ginger Root Extract (zingiber officinale)] 50 mg. Other Ingredients: Calcium Phosphate, Magnesium Stearate, Gelatin.

KavaTone - Enzymatic Therapy
Each capsule contains: Kava Root Extract (Piper methysticum) (standardized to contain 30% Kavalactones 60 mg per capsule) 200 mg • Oat Straw Extract 10:1 (Avena sativa) 100 mg • Pyridoxine-Alpha-Ketoglutarate (PAK) 50 mg • Pantothenic Acid 50 mg, Nicotinamide 50 mg • Thiamin HCL (Vitamin B1) 25 mg. Contains no sugar, salt, yeast, wheat, corn, soy, dairy products, coloring, flavoring, or preservatives.

Kavatrol - Capsule - Natrol
One capsule contains: Kava root extract (30% Kavalactones) 200 mg • In an exclusive base of complementary herbs: Passion flower, Chamomile flower, Hops flower, Schizandra fruit. Other ingredients: Magnesium Stearate, Silicon Dioxide, Gelatin.

Keto Pro - Met-Rx
Metamyosyn V.4 (unique blend of Milk Protein Isolates, Caseinate, Whey Protein Concentrate, Glutamine, Calcium-B-Hydroxy B-Methylbutyrate Monhydrate, Lactoferrin) • Medium Chain Triglycerides • Natural & Artifical Flavor • Cellulose Gum • Maltodextrin • Dipotassium Phosphate • Potassium Chloride • Potassium Citrate • Carrageenan • Salt • Sodium Citrate • Sucralose.

Key-E - Carlson
Each tablet contains: Vitamin E (as d-alpha tocopheryl succinate) 200 IU.

KIC Fuel - TwinLab
Each capsule contains: KIC 500 mg.

Kid Vits - Now
Two tablets contain: Beta-Carotene 4000 IU • Vitamin A (as Palmitate) 1000 IU • Vitamin B1 (Thiamine HCL) 3 mg • Vitamin B2 (Riboflavin) 3.4 mg • Vitamin B3 (Niacinamide) 20 mg • Vitamin B5 (Pantothenic Acid) 15 mg • Vitamin B6 (Pyridoxine HCL) 4 mg • Vitamin B12 (Cyanocobalamin) 10 mcg • Biotin 100 mcg • Folic Acid 400 mcg • Vitamin C (Ascorbic Acid, Calcium Ascorbate) 120 mg • Vitamin D (Cholecalciferol) 200 IU • Vitamin E (d-Alpha Tocopheryl Succinate) 30 IU • Calcium (Carbonate, Ascorbate) 30 mg • Magnesium (Oxide, Amino Acid Chelate) 20 mg • Zinc (Amino Acid Chelate) 5 mg • Iron (Ferrochel Iron Bisglycinate) 5 mg • Copper (Amino Acid Chelate) 0.2 mg • Iodine (Kelp) 75 mcg • Manganese (Amino Acid Chelate) 1 mg • Selenium (Amino Acid Chelate) 10 mcg • Chromium (Chelavite) 60 mcg • Molybdenum (Amino Acid Chelate) 15 mcg • Acerola 25 mg • Bioflavonoids (40 % Hesperidin) 25 mg • Choline 10 mg • Inositol 10 mg • PABA 4 mg.

Kid-Alert - The Herbalist
Ginkgo fresh leaf (Ginkgo biloba) • Gotu Kola fresh herb (Hydrocotyle asiatica) • Lemon Balm fresh leaf (Melissa officinalis) • St. John's Wort fresh flower tops (Hypericum perf.) • Siberian Ginseng fresh-dried root (Eleuthero sent.) in a base of kosher glycerine and distilled water • grapefruit seed extract.

KidCalm St. John's Wort Complex - Enzymatic Therapy
Two capsules contain: Magnesium (Krebs Cycle Chelate) 50 mg • Vitamin B6 (Pyridoxal-5-Phosphate) 15 mg • Zinc (Krebs Cycle chelate) 15 mg. Other ingredients: St. John's Wort extract (Hypericum perforatum) standardized to contain 0.3% Hypericin, verified by HPLC 100 mg • Valerian root extract (Valerian officinalis) standardized to contain a minimum of 0.8% Valeric acids 100 mg • GABA (Gamma-Aminobutyric Acid) 100 mg • L-Tyrosine 100 mg • Kava root extract (Piper methysticum) standardized to contain 30% Kavalactones 50 mg • Melissa extract (Melissa officinalis) standardized to contain a minimum of 5% Rosmarinic Acid 50 mg • Grape seed (PCO) extract standardized to contain 95% Procyanidolic Oligomers (PCOs) 20 mg. Contains no sugar, salt, yeast, wheat, gluten, corn, soy, dairy products, coloring, flavoring, or preservatives.

Kid-Ease - The Herbalist
Lemon Balm fresh leaf (Melissa officinalis) Valerian fresh root (Valeriana officinalis) • St. John's Wort fresh flower tops (Hypericum perf.) In a base of kosher glycerine and grapefruit seed extract.

Kidney Bladder Formula - Nature's Way
Two capsules contain: Proprietary formula: Cramp bark • Ginger • Goldenseal root • Juniper berries • Marshmallow root • Parsley herb • Uva Ursi leaves. Other ingredients: Gelatin.

Kidney Blend - The Herbalist
Dandelion root • Burdock seed • Uva Ursi leaf • Corn Silk • Echinacea root • St. John's Wort flower • Yarrow flower • Cayenne pepper.

Kidney Plus - The Herbalist
Uva Ursi leaf • Juniper berry • Buchu leaf • Echinacea root • Pipsissewa leaf • St. John's Wort flower • Yarrow flower • Cayenne pepper.

Kidney Support - Amazon Support
Each capsule contains: Chanca Piedra • Boldo • Cipo Cabeludo • Erva Tostao • Abuta • Jatoba.

Kidney Tea: Soothing Diuretic Tea - The Herbalist
Marshmallow root• Juniper berry• Plantain leaf• Dandelion root• Parsley root• Mullein leaf• Horsetail herb• Nettles leaf• Rosehips.

Kidneycare - PhysioLogics
Two capsules contain: Potassium 50 mg • Dandelion root 300 mg • Astragalus root (70% Polysaccharides, 175 mg) 250 mg • Corn silk 150 mg • Yarrow 150 mg.

Kidney-Liver Complex - Enzymatic Therapy
Two capsules contain: Kidney-Liver Complex (Predigested Soluble concentrate*) 500 mg • Artichoke extract (Cynara solymus) standardized to contain 15% Caffeylquinic Acids 100 mg • Multi-Glandular Complex: Raw Liver, Raw Lung, Raw Pancreas, Raw Heart, Raw Kidney, Raw Spleen & Raw Brain 100 mg. *Free-form concentrate predigested by enzymatic action, creating a highly absorbable form of glandular concentrate containing all the natural principles with a standardized content. Contains no sugar, salt, yeast, wheat, corn, soy, dairy products, coloring, flavoring, or preservatives.
See Editor's Note No. 14, page 1817.

Kids Be Well - The Herbalist
Astragalus fresh root (Astragalus membranaceous)• Echinacea fresh root (Echinacea angustifolia)• Lemon Balm fresh leaf (Melissa officinalis)• St. John's Wort fresh flower tops (Hypericum perf.)• Ginkgo fresh leaf (Ginkgo biloba)• in a base of kosher glycerine• and grapefruit seed extract.

Kid's Choice: Versatile Herbal for Children - The Herbalist
Echinacea root • Lemon Balm leaf • Goldenseal root.

KidSoothe - PhytoPharmica
Two capsules contain: Vitamin B6 (pyridoxal-5-phosphate) 15 mg • Magnesium (Krebs cycle chelate) 50 mg • Zinc (Krebs cycle chelate) 15 mg • St. John's Wort (Hypericum perforatum) flower head extract (standardized to contain a minimum of 0.3% hypericin and 4% hyperforin) 100 mg • Valerian (Valeriana officinalis) root extract (standardized to contain a minimum of 0.8% valerinic acids) 100 mg • GABA (Gamma-aminobutyric acid) 100 mg • L-Tyrosine 100 mg • Kava (Piper methysticum) root extract (standardized to contain 30% kavalactones) 50 mg • Melissa (Melissa officinalis) leaf extract (standardized to contain a minimum of 5% rosmarinic acid) 50 mg • Grape Seed (PCO) extract (standardized to contain 95% procyanidolic oligomers [PCOs]) 20 mg.

Kinder Love Children's Multivitamin - Dial Herbs
Vitamin A • Vitamin C • Vitamin B from Yeast extract • Vitamin E • Thiamin • Niacin • Vitamin B6 • Calcium • Phosphorus • Magnesium • Aqueous extract from: Carrots, Anise, Licorice root, Milfoil herb, Horsetail herb, Chamomile flowers, Peppermint Leaves, Watercress, Wheat Germ, Coriander seeds, Nettles, Spinach, Orange peel • Orange juice • Pear juice concentrate • Malt extract • Yeast extract • Maple Syrup • Honey • Rose Hip extract • Wheat Germ extract • Natural Flavor.

Kindervital - Flora
Vitamin A • Vitamin B Complex • Vitamin C • Vitamin D • Vitamin E.

Kinder-Vites - Atrium Inc.
Two chewable tablets contain: Vitamins: Vitamin A (Palmitate) 2500 IU • Vitamin D (as Vitamin D3) 200 IU • Vitamin E 10 IU • Vitamin K 10 mcg • Vitamin B1 3.2 mg • Vitamin B2 3 mg • Vitamin B6 3.2 mg • Vitamin B12 10 mcg • Vitamin C 100 mg • Niacinamide 13.5 mg • Folic Acid 200 mcg • Pantothenic Acid 5 mg • Biotin 60 mcg. Minerals: Calcium 12 mg • Magnesium 3.2 mg • Manganese 2.5 mg • Copper 100 mcg • Zinc 8 mg • Iron 12 mg • Iodine 100 mcg • Selenium 10 mcg • Chromium 10 mcg • Molybdenum 5 mcg • Vanadium 5 mcg. Associated Nutritional Factors: Citrus Bioflavonoids, Rutin, & Hesperidin 60 mg • Choline 10 mg • Inositol 2 mg • PABA 10 mg. Formulated in a base of pleasant tasting, natural source flavoring & excipients.

Kira - Lichtwer Pharma US
Each tablet contains: St. John's Wort (Hypericum perforatum, extract LI 160, standardized to contain 0.3% hypericin) 300 mg. Other Ingredients: Sucrose, Lactose, Talc, Powdered Cellulose, Hydroxypropyl Methylcellulose, Polyethylene Glycol, Castor Oil, Magnesium Stearate, Polyvinylpyrrolidone (pvp), Silicon Dioxide, Gelatin, Titanium Dioxide, Carnauba Wax.

Kirkland Signature Daily Multi-Vitamin - CWC, Inc
Each tablet contains: Vitamin A (25% as beta carotene) 10000 IU • Vitamin C 120 mg • Vitamin D 400 IU • Vitamin E 60 IU • Vitamin K 25 mcg • Thiamin 1.5 mg • Riboflavin 1.7 mg • Niacin 20 mg • Vitamin B-6 2 mg • Folic Acid 400 mcg • Vitamin B-12 6 mcg • Biotin 30 mcg • Pantothenic Acid 10 mg • Calcium 162 mg • Iron 9 mg • Phosphorus 109 mg • Iodine 150 mcg • Magnesium 100 mg • Zinc 22.5 mg • Selenium 45 mcg • Copper 3 mg • Manganese 2.5 mg • Chromium 100 mcg • Molybdenum 25 mcg • Chloride 36.3 mg • Potassium 40 mg • Nickel 5 mcg • Tin 10 mcg • Silicon 2 mg • Vanadium 10 mcg • Boron 150 mcg.

KLB6 Grapefruit Diet - Puritan's Pride
Four tablets contain: Grapefruit extract 800 mg • Glucomannan 800 mg • Vitamin B6 20 mg • Lecithin 200 mg • Kelp 75 mg • Cider Vinegar 100 mg • Uva Ursi 25 mg • L-Phenylalanine 25 mg.

K-Mag Aspartate - Source Naturals
Each tablet contains: Potassium (from 565.7 mg of Potassium Aspartate HCl) 99 mg • Magnesium (from 1,027.4 mg of Magnesium Aspartate HCl) 75 mg.

K-Mag C - Source Naturals
Each tablet contains: Potassium (Citrate and Ascorbate) 99 mg • Magnesium (Malate and Ascorbate) 75 mg • Vitamin C (Magnesium and Potassium Ascorbates) 500 mg.

K-Mag KG - Source Naturals
Each tablet contains: Potassium (from 285 mg Potassium alpha-Ketoglutarate) 99 mg • Magnesium (from 715 mg Magnesium alpha-Ketoglutarate) 100 mg.

Knock Out - Schiff
Each caplet contains: Vitamin B6 (Pyroxidal-5-Phosphate) 0.5 mg • Magnesium (as Glycinate) 10 mg • Melatonin synthetic 3 mg • Kava Kava 2:1 extract 100 mg • Valerian extract (0.89% Valeric Acid) 100 mg • Gamma Aminobutyric Acid GABA 100 mg • Glycine 40 mg.
See Editor's Note No. 16, page 1817.

Korean Ginseng - Basic Nutrition
Each capsule contains: Korean Ginseng root powder 648 mg. Other Ingredients: Gelatin.

BRAND NAMES

Some Brand Name Natural Products - What they Contain

BRAND NAMES

Korean Red Ginseng - Jamieson
Each caplet contains: Calcium 65 mg • Korean Red Ginseng root (Panax Ginseng) 4% ginsenosides saponins 250 mg.

Korean White Ginseng - Nature's Way
Two capsules contain: Korean Ginseng root 1.02 g. Other Ingredients: Gelatin, Magnesium stearate.

Krebs Calcium-Magnesium Chelate - PhytoPharmica
Each tablet contains: Calcium 200 mg • Magnesium 120 mg • Sodium 5 mg.

Krebs Ionized Calcium - PhytoPharmica
Two tablets contain: Calcium 250 mg.

Krebs Ionized Chelates - PhytoPharmica
Four tablets contain: Calcium 600 mg • Iron 5 mg • Iodine (marine organic minerals) 100 mcg • Magnesium 400 mg • Zinc 15 mg • Selenium 75 mcg • Copper 1 mg • Manganese 2 mg • Chromium 100 mcg • Molybdenum 25 mcg • Sodium 10 mg • Potassium 99 mg • Boron 4 mg • Vanadium 50 mcg.

Krebs Ionized Zinc - PhytoPharmica
Each tablet contains: Zinc 15 mg.

Krebs Magnesium-Potassium Chelates - PhytoPharmica
Each tablet contains: Magnesium 250 mg • Potassium 99 mg.

Kudja - HerbaSway
Kudzu • Ginkgo Biloba • Blackberry • Green Tea • HerbaSwee (Cucurbitaceae fruit).

Kwai Heart Fit - Lichtwer Pharma
Each tablet contains: Garlic powder sucrose 300 mg • Vitamin C (Ascorbic Acid Sorbitol) 80 mg • Vitamin E (Tocopherol Acetate) 20 IU • Vitamin A (Acetate) 2640 IU. Other Ingredients: Talc, Corn Starch, Hydroxypropylmethylcellulose, Polivinylpyrrolidone, Silicon Dioxide, Stearic Acid, Castor oil, Magnesium Stearate, Powdered Cellulose, Glucose Syrup, Titanium Dioxide, Carnauba Wax/Bees Wax, Riboflavin, Beta-Carotene.

Kwai Odor-Free Garlic - Lichtwer Pharma
Each tablet contains: Dried Garlic clove powder 150 mg. Other Ingredients: Hydroxypropylmethylcellulose, Silicon Dioxide, Maltitol, Magnesium Stearate, Magnesium Silicate, Carnauba Wax, Powdered Cellulose, Castor Oil, Gum Arabic.

Kwik Size XXXL - Labrada Bodybuilding Nutrition
Each serving contains: Kwik Carb (Unique blend of Maltodextrin & Polydextrose) • Kwik Pro (Unique blend of cross flow ultrafiltered Whey Protein Concentrate, Calcium Caseinate, Specially Extracted & Spray-Dried Soy Protein Concentrate) • Cocoa powder (dutch processed) • Natural & Artificial flavors • Vitamin & Mineral Blend • Xanthan Gum • Dipotassium Phosphate • Aspartame • Peptigen (proprietary blend of Alpha Amylase, Malt Diatase, Protease, Lactase) • Medium Chain Triglycerides.

Kyo-Chlorella - Wakunaga of America
Six tablets contain: 100% pure broken cell wall Chlorella powder 3 g.

Kyo-Chrome Aged Garlic Extract Cholesterol Formula - Wakunaga of America
Two capsules contain: Aged Garlic extract powder 400 mg • Niacin 20 mg • Chromium (as Chromium Picolinate) 200 mcg. Other Ingredients: Microcrystalline Cellulose, Magnesium Stearate (vegetable source).

Kyo-Dophilus L. Acidophilus; B. Bifidum; B. Longum - Wakunaga of America
Each capsule contains: L. Acidophilus [Lactobacillus Acidophilus], B. Bifidum [Bifidobacterium Bifidum], and B. Longum [Bifidobacterium Longum] 1.5 billion cells. Other Ingredients: Vegetable Starch Complex.

Kyo-Green - Wakunaga of America
Each teaspoon contains: Kyo-Green Proprietary Blend 2.5 g • Barley Grass Powder • Cooked Brown Rice • Wheat Grass Powder • Bulgarian Chlorella • Pacific Kelp.

Kyolic - Wakunaga Consumer Products
Each caplet contains: Aged Garlic extract powder 600 mg • Microcrystalline Cellulose • Magnesium Stearate • Silicon Dioxide. Kyolic is free of dairy, sodium & yeast.

Kyolic Aged Garlic Extract Enriched with Vitamin B1 and B12 - Wakunaga of America
Each capsule contains: Vitamin B1 (Thiamine hydrochloride) 8 mg • Vitamin B12 (cyanocobalamin) 1 mcg. Other Ingredients: Aged Garlic Extract, Liver Extract, Water, Residual Alcohol from extraction.
See Editor's Note No. 14, page 1817.

Kyolic Aged Garlic Extract Garlic Plus - Wakunaga of America
Two capsules or tablets contain: Aged Garlic extract powder 540 mg • Brewer's Yeast 54 mg • Kelp 18 mg. Other Ingredients: Whey, Brewer's Yeast, Alginic Acid (seaweed), Kelp, Collodial Silica, Magnesium Stearate (vegetable source).

Kyolic Aged Garlic Extract Kyolic HI-PO - Wakunaga of America
Two capsules or tablets contain: Aged Garlic extract powder (bulb) 600 mg. Other Ingredients: Whey, Alginic Acid (seaweed), Silica, Cellulose, Magnesium Stearate (vegetable source).

Kyolic Aged Garlic Extract Plus Enzyme - Wakunaga of America
Two tablets contain: Aged Garlic powder 700 mg • KYOLIC Enzyme Complex (Amylase, Protease, Cellulose, and Lipase from Aspergillus oryzae and A. niger) 60 mg • Rice Protein-Calcium Complex 40 mg. Other Ingredients: Alginic Acid (seaweed), Colloidal Silica, and Magnesium Stearate (vegetable source).

Kyolic Aged Garlic Extract Plus Lecithin - Wakunaga of America
Two capsules contain: Aged Garlic extract powder (bulb) 600 mg • Lecithin 380 mg. Other Ingredients: Silica, Magnesium Stearate (vegetable source).

Kyolic Aged Garlic Extract Vitamin A, C, E, Selenium - Wakunaga of America
Two capsules contain: Vitamin A (from 12 mg of Beta-Carotene) 20000 IU • Vitamin C (Calcium ascorbate) 240 mg • Vitamin E (d-alpha-Tocopheryl succinate) 120 IU • Selenium (L-Selenomethionine) 50 mcg • Aged Garlic Extract Powder (bulb) 400 mg • Green Tea Powder (leaf) 89 mg. Other Ingredients: Silica, Magnesium Stearate (vegetable source).

Kyolic Aged Garlic Extract Vitamin C, Astragalus - Wakunaga of America
Two capsules contain: Vitamin C (Ester C) 210 mg • Calcium (Citrate Polyascorbate) 46 mg • Aged Garlic extract powder (bulb) 440 mg • Astragalus extract powder (root) 200 mg. Other Ingredients: Calcium Citrate, Magnesium Stearate (vegetable source).

Some Brand Name Natural Products - What they Contain
www.NaturalDatabase.com contains MANY more listings than appear here.

Kyolic Aged Garlic Extract Vitamin E, Cayenne, Hawthorn Berry - Wakunaga of America
Two capsules contain: Vitamin E (d-alpha-tocopheryl Succinate) 200 IU • Aged Garlic Extract Powder (bulb) 600 mg • Hawthorn Berry (fruit) 100 mg • Cayenne Pepper (fruit) 20 mg. Other Ingredients: Cellulose, Magnesium Stearate (vegetable source), Silica.

Kyolic Cardio Logic - Wakunaga of America
Each capsule contains: Vitamin E (as D-Alpha-Tocopheryl Acid Succinate) 50 IU • Vitamin B6 5 mg • Folate (as Folic acid) 200 mcg • Vitamin B12 100 mcg • Aged Garlic bulb extract powder 200 mg • L-Carnitine 30 mg • Coenzyme Q10 30 mg • Alpha-Lipoic Acid 30 mg. Other Ingredients: Cellulose, Colloidal Silica, Magnesium Stearate (vegetable source).

Kyolic Echinacea Aged Garlic Extract - Wakunaga of America
Two capsules contain: Aged Garlic powder (bulb) 600 mg • Echinacea extract powder (root) 100 mg. Other Ingredients: Cellulose (pine), Magnesium Stearate (vegetable source).

Kyolic Estro Logic - Wakunaga of America
Each capsule contains: Black Cohosh root extract (standardized to 2.5% triterpene glycosides) 100 mg • Soybean Isoflavones (seed) (Standardized to 40% isoflavones) 50 mg • Wild Yam root extract (Standardized to 6% total saponins) 33.3 mg • Sage leaf extract 25 mg • Chaste Tree berry extract 12.5 mg • Vervain leaf extract 12.5 mg • Astragalus root extract 12.5 mg • Motherwort leaf extract 12.5 mg. Other Ingredients: Cellulose, Silica, Magnesium Stearate (vegetable source).

Kyolic Liquid Aged Garlic Extract - Wakunaga of America
1/4 teaspoon contains: Aged Garlic extract (bulb) 1 ml. Other Ingredients: Water and Residual Alcohol from Extraction.

Kyolic Neuro Logic - Wakunaga Consumer Products
Two capsules contain: Folate (as Folic acid) 200 mcg • Vitamin B12 100 mcg • Aged Garlic bulb powder 400 mg • Lecithin 200 mg • Ginkgo Biloba leaf extract 60 mg • Phosphatidylserine (30%) 50 mg • Acetyl-L-Carnitine 25 mg. Other Ingredients: Cellulose, Colloidal Silica, Magnesium Stearate (vegetable source).

Kyolic Prosta Logic - Wakunaga of America
Each capsule contains: Zinc (as Zinc Picolinate) 7.5 mg • Saw Palmetto berry extract 160 mg • Aged Garlic bulb extract powder 100 mg • Pumpkin seed oil extract 50 mg • Pygeum Africanum bark extract 50 mg • Lycopene (as tomato oleoresin) 2.5 mg. Other Ingredients: Wheat Germ Oil, Beeswax, Soft Gelatin Capsule.

Kyolic Reserve Aged Garlic Extract - Wakunaga of America
Each capsule contains: Aged Garlic Extract powder (bulb) 600 mg. Other Ingredients: Vegetable Protein, Magnesium Stearate (vegetable source), Silica.

Kyolic-EPA Aged Garlic Extract - Wakunaga of America
Two capsules contain: EPA (Eicosapentaenoic Acid) 560 mg • DHA (Docosahexaenoic Acid) 240 mg • Aged Garlic powder 240 mg • Vitamin E mixed Tocopherol 10 mg. Other Ingredients: Glycerin, Soft gelatin capsule.

L & V Formula - Dial Herbs
Wild Lettuce • Valerian • Wood Betony.

L.B.T. Caps: Lower Bowel Tonic - The Herbalist
Cascara Sagrada fresh-dried bark (Rhamnus purshiana) • Barberry root bark (Berberis vulgaris) • Fennel fresh-dried seed (Foeniculum vulgare) • Bayberry fresh-dried root bark (Myrica cerifera) • Ginger fresh root (Zingiber officinale) • Turkey Rhubarb fresh-dried root

(Rheum palmatum) • Lobelia fresh-dried herb (Lobelia inflata) • Cayenne fresh-dried pepper (Capsicum annum).

Lactase Enzyme - Nature's Way
Three capsules contain: Lactase enzyme 690 mg.
Other Ingredients: Gelatin, Magnesium stearate, Maltodextrin.

Lactobacillus Acidophilus Milk-Base - Nature's Life
Each capsule contains: Lactobacillus species (Combined L. Acidophilus, L. Bulgaricus & L. Caucasious) 250 mg.

Lactobacillus Acidophilus Milk-Free - Nature's Life
Each capsule contains: Lactobacillus acidophilus 500 mg.

Lactoferrin with Colostrum - The Vitamin Shoppe
Each capsule contains: Lactoferrin (from whey) 100 mg • Colostrum (from bovine) providing 20% immunoglobulins 250 mg • Lysozyme (from whey) 5 mg. No yeast, corn, wheat, sugar, salt, starch, gluten, soy, eggs, fish or animal derivatives, citrus, preservatives, artificial colors or flavors added.

Lady V - Ultra-V
Three capsules contain: Vitamin D (as Cholecalciferol) 21 IU • Niacin (as Niacinamide) 20 mg • Vitamin B6 (as Pyridoxine HCl) 2.4 mg • Folic Acid (as Folacin) 6.4 mg • Vitamin B12 (as Cyancolalamine) 6 mg • Avena Sativa extract 10:1 150 mg • Kava Kava 10 mg • Guarana 300 mg • White Willow bark 10 mg • Muira Puama 4:1 20 mg • St. John's Wort 250 mg • Siberian Ginseng 35:1 30 mg • Ginkgo Biloba 40 mg • Cordyceps 100 mg • Damiana 20 mg • L-Taurine 200 mg.

Lava - Universal Nutrition
Each 83 g serving contains: Creatine Monohydrate 5.5 g • Chromium 75 mcg • Glutamine 2.5 g • Taurine 1.2 g • Sodium 180 mg • Potassium 360 mg. Ingredients: Ultra & Micro-Filtrated Whey Protein Concentrate (Containing Whey Peptide-Rich Lactoglobulins, Lactalbumin, Immunoglobulins & Lactoferrin) • GlycoCarb Complex (Dextrose & Glucose Polymers) • Maltodextrin • 100% Pure Creatine Monohydrate • Glutamine • Taurine • Magnesium Oxide • Disodium Phosphate • Potassium Phosphate • Fruit Flavor • Lecithin • Ascorbic Acid • Vitamin E Succinate • Niacin • Citric Acid • Aspartame • Carmine (for color) • Chromium (GTF).

Laxaco - Jamieson
Each capsule contains: Calcium (as Calcium Sulfate) 25 mg • Senna leaf (Cassia senna L.) 240 mg • Cascara Sagrada bark (Rhamnus purshiana DC) 150 mg.

LaxActin - Nature's Plus
Each capsule contains: Cascara Sagrada (Rhamnus purshiana bark) (standardized 25-30% Hydroxyanthracene derivatives - HAD) 100 mg • Passion Flower [(Passiflora incarnata flower) standardized 3.5-4% Flavonoids] 100 mg • Senna [(Cassia senna leaf) standardized 5% Sennosides] 50 mg.

Laxaherb - Dial Herbs
Cascara Sagrada • Buckthorn • Ginger • Bayberry • Goldenseal • Raspberry • Fennel • Lobelia • Rhubarb.

L-Carnitine - New Hope Health Products
Each capsule contains: L-Carnitine 500 mg • Vitamin B5 15 mg • Vitamin B6 5 mg.

L-Carnitine - Metabolic Response Modifiers
Each capsule contains: L-Carnitine 500 mg • Vitamin B5 15 mg • Vitamin B6 5 mg.

L-Carnitine - Olympian Labs
Two capsules contain: L-Carnitine Fumarate 1000 mg.

BRAND NAMES

Some Brand Name Natural Products - What they Contain
www.NaturalDatabase.com contains MANY more listings than appear here.

L-Carnitine - Source Naturals
Each capsule contains: L-Carnitine 250 mg.

L-Carnitine - Swanson
Two capsules contain: L-Carnitine (from tartrate and free-form) 500 mg.

LDL-RX - Athletic Technologies Inc.
Two capsules contain: Red Yeast Rice 1000 mg • Niacin 50 mg • Guggulipids 50 mg • Beta-Sisterol 50 mg • Capiscum 50 mg • Garlic 50 mg • Lecithin 200 mg.

Lean & Clean - Sports Nutrition Source.com
Each capsule contains: Proprietary Blend: Papaya fruit, Echinacea root, Black Walnut leaves, Fennel seeds, Parsley plant, Norwegian Kelp plant, Safflower flowers, Burdock root, Chickweed herb, Hawthorn berries, Cayenne fruit 470 mg.

Lean "4" - The Vitamin Shoppe
Each six tablets contain: Lecithin 1200 mg • Vitamin B6 (pyridoxine HCl) 50 mg • Iodine (kelp) 210 mcg • Cider Vinegar Powder 240 mg • Grapefruit Powder 300 mg.

Lean Body - Labrada Bodybuilding Nutrition
Each 45 g serving contains: Vanilla: Calories 300 • Protein 45 g • Carbohydrates 28 g • Fat 1.5 g. Ingredients: Lean Pro unique blend of ProPlex (cross flow ultrafiltered Whey Protein Concentrate, Ion Exchange Whey Protein Isolate, Cross Flow Microfiltered Whey Protein Isolate, Hydrolyzed Whey Protein Isolate Peptides) • Milk Protein Isolate • Caseinate • L-Glutamine • Taurine • Magnesium • Alpha Ketoglutarate • Maltodextrin • Vitamin & Mineral Blend • Polydextrose • Natural Flavors • Soy Lecithin • Xanthan Gum • Cellulose Fiber • Aspartame • L-Carnitine • Beta-Carotene for color. Chocolate Peanut Butter: Calories 300 • Protein 45 g • Carbohydrates 28 g • Fat 1.5 g. Ingredients: Lean Pro [Unique Blend of Proplete (Cross Flow Ultrafiltered Whey Protein concentrate, Ion Exchange Whey Protein Isolate, Cross Flow Microfiltered Whey Protein Isolate, Hydrolyzed Whey Protein Isolate Peptides), Caseinate, Milk Protein Isolate, L-Glutamine, Taurine, Magnesium Alpha Keto Glutarate] • Maltodextrin • Natural & Artificial Flavors including Hershey's Cocoa • Polydextrose • Cocoa (Dutch Processed) • Vitamin & Mineral Blend [Diacalcium Phosphate, Potassium Chloride, Magnesium Oxide, Vitamin C (Ascorbic Acid), Vitamin E (Alpha Tocopherol Acetate), Ferrous Fumarate, Beta Carotene, Vitamin B3 (Niacinamide), Zinc Oxide, Manganese Sulfate, Calcium Pantothenate, Vitamin A Palmitate, Zinc Picolinate, Copper Sulfate, Vitamin B6 (Pyridoxine Hydrochloride), Chromium Polynicotinate, Vitamin B2 (Riboflavin), Vitamin B1 (Thiamine Hydrochloride), Vitamin B12 (Cyanocobalamin), Vitamin D3 (Cholecalciferol), Folic Acid, Sodium Molybdate, Chromium Chloride, Biotin, Potassium Iodide, Sodium Selenite] • Xanthan Gum • Soy Lecithin • Aspartame • Salt • Cellulose Fiber. Wildberry: Calories 305 • Protein 45 g • Carbohydrates 28 g • Fat 1.5 g. Ingredients: Lean Pro [Unique Blend of Proplex+ (Cross Flow Ultrafiltered Whey Protein concentrate, Ion Exchange Whey Protein Isolate, Cross Flow Microfiltered Whey Protein Isolate, Hydrolyzed Whey Protein Isolate Peptides), Milk Protein Isolate, Caseinate, L-Glutamine, Taurine, Magnesium Alpha Keto Glutarate], Maltodextrin, Vitamin & Mineral Blend (Diacalcium Phosphate, Magnesium Oxide, Ascorbic Acid, Vitamin E Acetate, Niacinamide, Electrolytic Iron, Riboflavin, Folic Acid, Biotin, Manganese Sulfate, Potassium Iodide, Chromium Picolinate, Cholecalciferol, Sodium Molybdate, Cyanocobalamin, Sodium Selenite) • Natural & Artificial flavors • Polydextrose • Medium Chain Triglycerides • Xanthan Gum • Cellulose Gum • Aspartame. Peanut Butter: Calories 300 • Protein 45 g • Carbohydrates 28 g, Fat 1.5 g.

Lean Dreams - Sports Nutrition Source.com
Each tablet contains: Vitamin B-6 (Pyridoxine) 15 mg • Niacin (niacinamide) 50 mg • L-Ornithine 500 mg • L-Glycine 667 mg • Valerian root extract 150 mg • Hops powder 20 mg.

Lean Gainer - Champion Nutrition
Each serving contains: Protein 50 g • Carbohydrates 12 g • Fat 4.5 g • Calories 280. Ingredients: Peptol-C: Whey Protein Concentrate, Creatine Monohydrate, Amino Acids, L-Leucine, L-Glutamine • Metabarb-V (blend of Simple & Complex Carbohydrates containing Glucose Polymers & Whey) • Low Fat Cocoa powder • Natural & Artificial Flavors • Metavite IV (Vitamin-Mineral Complex) • FIBR3: Cellulose, Oat Fiber, Psyllium husks • Aspartame • Succinate ETF: Potassium Succinate, L-Glutamic Acid, Inosine, Magnesium Succinate, Calcium Succinate • Bromelain • Papain • Defatted Peanut Flour • Sunette (Brand of Acesulfame-K) • Vanadyl Polynicotinate. Contains Phenylalanine. No added sucrose or fructose.

Lean Machine - Sports Nutrition Source.com
Two scoops contain: Sodium 85 mg • Potassium 85 mg • Protein 37 g • Creatine Monohydrate 3000 mg • L-Glutamine 2000 mg • Methylsulfonylmethane 1000 mg • Glucosamine Sulfate 500 mg • Chondroitin Sulfate 350 mg • White Willow Bark extract 75 mg • Ascorbic Acid 100 mg • Bromelain 100 mg.
See Editor's Note No. 15, page 1817.

Leci-Plus - Atrium Inc.
Each capsule contains: Raw Unbleached Lecithin 650 mg • Choline Bitartrate 50 mg • Inositol 50 mg • Biotin 60 mcg • Niacinamide 30 mg • Vitamin B6 2 mg • Magnesium Glycero Phosphate 100 mg • Magnesium 12 mg • Phosphorus 16 mg.

Lecithin - Health Center for Better Living
"Rich source of choline, a B-complex nutrient," HCBL Lecithin. (Derived from soybeans).

Leci-Thin - Nature's Plus
Each wafer contains: Lecithin 1500 mg derived from natural Soybean, rich in Choline, Inositol & Phosphorus • Wheat Bran 500 mg • Vegetable Cellulose 200 mg • Protein, vegetable soy & peanut 150 mg. Made from the finest quality Lecithin, containing 95% Soy Phosphatides. In an all natural base of carob, coconut & vanilla bean. Each wafer contains approximatly 16 calories. Yeast free; sweetened with VitaSweet.

Lecithin & Milk powder - Nature's Life
Two heaping tablespoons contain: Lipids: Linoleic Acid (Omega-6) 3681 mg • Linolenic Acid (Omega-3) 438 mg • Oleic Acid (Omega-9) 575 mg • Palmitic Acid 1269 mg • Stearic Acid 288 mg. Phospholipids: Phosphatidyl choline 2.8g • Phosphatidyl ethanolamine 2.5 g • Phosphatidyl inositol 1.8 g. Vitamins: Choline 378 mg • Inositol 275 mg. Minerals: Calcium 132 mg • Iron 1 mg • Magnesium 11 mg • Phosphorus 471 mg • Potassium 276 mg • Sodium 57 mg. Amino Acids: Alanine 103 mg • Arginine 137 mg • Aspartic Acid 213 mg • Cysteine 11 mg • Glutamic Acid 779 mg • Glycine 68 mg • Histidine (essential amino acid) 99 mg • Isoleucine (essential amino acid) 216 mg • Leucine (essential amino acid) 334 mg • Lysine (essential amino acid) 270 mg • Methionine (essential amino acid) 110 mg • Phenylalanine (essential amino acid) 190 mg • Proline 407 mg • Serine 209 mg • Threonine (essential amino acid) 148 mg • Tryptophan (essential amino acid) 49 mg • Tyrosine 209 mg • Valine (essential amino acid) 243 mg.

Lecithin-E - Nutrilite - Nutrilite
Each tablet contains: Lecithin (from Soybean Oil) 290 mg • Vitamin E 30 IU.

Leg Vein & Circulation - ProHerbs
Two tablets contain: Vitamin C 240 mg • Green Tea leaves (Camellia sinensis standardized to 50% catechins) 100 mg • Horse Chestnut seed (Aesculus hippocastanum standardized to 18-20% total saponins) 300 mg • Butcher's Broom root (Ruscus aculeatus standardized to 10% saponins) 200 mg • Citrus Bioflavonoid complex 200 mg. Other Ingredients: Dicalcium Phosphate, Croscarmellose Sodium, Mineral

Oil, Hydroxypropylmethylcellulose, Magnesium Stearate, Microcrystalline Cellulose, Polyethylene Glycol, Silicon Dioxide, Stearic Acid, Titanium Dioxide, FD&C Red #27 Lake and FD&C Blue #1 Lake.

Leg Vein Essentials - Swanson
Two time-release capsules contain: Vitamin C (as calcium ascorbate) 120 mg • Horse Chestnut extract (22% escin) 400 mg • Butcher's Broom extract (10% saponins calculated as ruscogenin) 150 mg • Gotu Kola extract (10% asiaticosides) 100 mg • Hesperidin (40% bioflavonoids) 100 mg • Bilberry extract (25% anthocyanidins) 20 mg • Grapeseed extract (90%-95% proanthocyanidins) 20 mg • Hawthorn berry extract (2% vitexin-2' rhamnosides) 20 mg.

Leg Veins Formula - Nature's Way
Two capsules contain: Butcher's Broom root 200 mg • Cayenne pepper fruit 50 mg • Dandelion leaf 250 mg • Grape seed dried extract 37.5 mg • Horse chestnut dried extract 200 mg • Prickly Ash bark 100 mg • Vitamin C (Ascorbic Acid) 30 mg.
Other ingredients: Gelatin, Magnesium Stearate, Millet.

Leg-Aid - Futurebiotics
Two capsules contain: Niacin (as flush free niacin) 20 mg • MSM (methyl-sulfonyl-methane) 400 mg • Citrus Bioflavonoids 220 mg • Glucosamine sulfate 400 mg • Grape Seed powder extract (standardized for 95% (24 mg) proanthocyanidins) 25 mg • Horse Chestnut (standardized at 18-22% (50-62 mg) aescin) 280 mg • Butcher's Broom root powder 200 mg • Prickly Ash bark powder 125 mg • Ginkgo Biloba leaf powder 30 mg.
Other ingredients: Magnesium stearate, Gelatin, Water.

Lemon-Lime Multi-Vitamin For Adults - LiFizz Effervescent Vitamins
Each tablet contains: Magnesium 80 mg • Calcium 200 mg • Zinc 5 mg • Iron 6 mg • Vitamin A 5000 IU • Vitamin E 15 IU • Vitamin C 60 mg • Vitamin B2 (Riboflavin) 1.7 mg • Vitamin B6 (Pyridoxine) 2 mg • Vitamin B12 (Cyanocobalamin) 6 mcg • Vitamin B1 (Thiamin) 1.5 mg • Niacin (Vitamin PP or B3) 20 mg • Pantothenic Acid 10 mg • Free Folic Acid 400 mcg • Biotin 300 mcg • Vitamin D 400 IU.

L-Glutamine Plus - Atrium Inc.
Each tablet contains: L-Glutamine (an essential amino acid) 300 mg • L-Tryosine (an essential amino acid) 100 mg • Raw Bovine Adrenal concentrate 50 mg • Calcium Ascorbate (Vitamin C) 100 mg.
See Editor's Note No. 14, page 1817.

Lice Treatment & Prevention: Herbal Hair Oil - The Herbalist
Pure essential oils of Rosemary• Lavender • Bay • Sage • Formulated with botanical extracts of Nettles leaf • Burdock root • Red Clover blossom • Chaparral leaf • in a base of cold-pressed oils of Sweet Almond and Jojoba.

Licorice - Nature's Way
Three capsules contain: Licorice root 1.35 g.
Other Ingredients: Gelatin.

Licorice Garlic - Atrium Inc.
Each capsule contains: Licorice root 250 mg • Garlic 260 mg.
Contains no sugar, starch, salt, wheat, corn, yeast or soy derivatives.

Life Essentials Dietary Supplement - Pharmanex
Each capsule contains: Vitamin A (as vitamin A palmitate, 29% as beta carotene from dunaliella salina) 3500 IU • Vitamin C (as ascorbic acid, acerola cherry extract) 70 mg • Vitamin D (as cholecalciferol) 200 IU • Vitamin E (as d-alpha tocopheryl succinate, beta, gamma, delta tocopherols) 30 IU • Thiamin (as thiamine mononitrate) 0.75 mg • Riboflavin 0.85 mg • Niacin (as niacinamide) 10 mg • Vitamin B-6 (as pyridoxine hydrochloride, pyridoxal-5-phosphate) 1 mg • Folic

Acid 200 mcg • Vitamin B-12 (as cyanocobalamin) 3 mcg • Biotin 75 mcg • Pantothenic Acid (as D-calcium pantothenate) 5 mg • Calcium (as calcium carbonate, calcium chelate) 100 mg • Iron (as iron chelate) 1.5 mg • Iodine (as potassium iodide) 37.5 mcg • Magnesium (as magnesium chelate, magnesium citrate, magnesium oxide) 50 mg • Zinc (as zinc chelate) 7.5 mg • Selenium (as L-selenomethionine) 17.5 mcg • Copper (as copper chelate) 1 mg • Manganese (as manganese chelate) 1.75 mg • Chromium (as chromium chelate) 60 mcg • Molybdenum (as molybdenum chelate) 37.5 mcg • Potassium (as potassium chloride) 40 mg • Boron (as boron citrate) 0.5 mg • Horsetail extract 75 mg.

Life Extension Mix - Olympia Nutrition
Multiple Vitamin, Mineral Enzyme, Antioxidant Flavonoid formula.

Life Force Multiple - Source Naturals
Two tablets contain: Vitamin A (beta carotene) 7500 IU • Vitamin A (palmitate) 5000 IU • Total Vitamin A activity 12500 IU • Vitamin B-1 (thiamin) 50 mg • Vitamin B-2 (riboflavin) 50 mg • Niacinamide 35 mg • Niacin 15 mg • Vitamin B-5 (pantothenic acid) 50 mg • Vitamin B-6 (pyridoxine HCl) 50 mg • Vitamin B-12 (cyanocobalamin) 100 mcg • Biotin 150 mcg • Folic Acid 400 mcg • Vitamin C (ascorbic acid crystals, ascorbyl palmitate) 500 mg • Vitamin D-3 (cholecalciferol) 200 IU • Vitamin E D-alpha Tocopheryl (natural) 200 IU • Boron (amino acid chelate) 2 mg • Calcium (chelate, citrate, malate) 100 mg • Chromium (ChromeMate yeast-free polynicotinate) 100 mcg • Copper (sebacate) 1 mg • Iodine (from kelp) 100 mcg • Iron (fumarate) 6 mg • Magnesium (chelate, citrate, oxide) 100 mg • Manganese (citrate) 3 mg • Molybdenum (amino acid chelate) 100 mcg • Potassium (citrate) 50 mg • Selenium (L-Selenomethionine and sodium selenite) 100 mcg • Zinc (citrate and OptiZinc monomethionine) 15 mg. Other Ingredients: Coenzyme Q10 (ubiquinone) 20mg, Alpha-Lipoic Acid (thioctic acid) 25 mg, N-Acetyl Cysteine 100 mg, DMAE (bitartrate) 30 mg, Silymarin (milk thistle seed extract) 60 mg, Ginkgo Biloba 24% (50:1 extract) 20 mg, Choline (bitartrate) 50 mg, Inositol 50mg , Hawthorn berry 75 mg, Turmeric root 75 mg, Bilberry fruit extract standardized to 25% anthocyanidins 10 mg, Proanthodyn (grape seed extract) 25 mg, L-Tyrosine 50 mg, Methylsulfonylmethane 25 mg, Bioperine 3 mg.

Life Force Multiple No Iron - Source Naturals
Two tablets contain: Vitamin A (beta carotene) 7500 IU • Vitamin A (palmitate) 5000 IU • Total Vitamin A activity 12500 IU • Vitamin B-1 (thiamin) 50 mg • Vitamin B-2 (riboflavin) 50 mg • Niacinamide 35 mg • Niacin 15 mg • Vitamin B-5 (pantothenic acid) 50 mg • Vitamin B-6 (pyridoxine HCl) 50 mg • Vitamin B-12 (cyanocobalamin) 100 mcg • Biotin 150 mcg • Folic acid 400 mcg • Vitamin C (ascorbic acid crystals, ascorbyl palmitate) 500 mg • Vitamin D-3 (cholecalciferol) 200 IU • Vitamin E D-alpha Tocopheryl (natural) 200 IU • Boron (amino acid chelate) 2 mg • Calcium (chelate, citrate, malate) 100 mg • Chromium (ChromeMate yeast-free polynicotinate) 100 mcg • Copper (sebacate) 1 mg • Iodine (from kelp) 100 mcg • Magnesium (chelate, citrate, oxide) 100 mg • Manganese (citrate) 3 mg • Molybdenum (amino acid chelate) 100 mcg • Potassium (citrate) 50 mg • Selenium (L-Selenomethionine and sodium selenite) 100 mcg • Zinc (citrate and OptiZinc monomethionine) 15 mg. Other Ingredients: Coenzyme Q10 (ubiquinone) 20mg, Alpha-Lipoic Acid (thioctic acid) 25 mg, N-Acetyl Cysteine 100 mg, DMAE (bitartrate) 30 mg, Silymarin (milk thistle seed extract) 60 mg, Ginkgo Biloba 24% (50:1 extract) 20 mg, Choline (bitartrate) 50 mg, Inositol 50mg , Hawthorn berry 75 mg, Turmeric root 75 mg, Bilberry fruit extract standardized to 25% anthocyanidins 10 mg, Proanthodyn (grape seed extract) 25 mg, L-Tyrosine 50 mg, Methylsulfonylmethane 25 mg, Bioperine 3 mg.

Life Minerals - Source Naturals
Four tablets contain: Calcium (Citrate, Fumarate, Malate, Succinate and alpha-Ketoglutarate) 480 mg • Magnesium (Citrate, Fumarate, Malate, Succinate and alpha-Ketoglutarate) 480 mg • Potassium (Citrate, Malate, Fumarate, Succinate, and alpha-Ketoglutarate)

BRAND NAMES

99 mg • Zinc (OptiZinc Zinc Monomethionine 20 mg and Ascorbate 10 mg) 30mg • Chromium (ChromeMate GTF Chromium Polynicotinate) 300 mcg • Selenium (Selenomethionine and Sodium Selenite) 200 mcg • Iron (Fumarate, Citrate and Succinate) 15 mg • Boron(Amino Acid Chelate) 3 mg • Silica (Horsetail Silica extract) 4.5 mg • Iodine (from Kelp) 150 mcg • Copper (Sebacate) 2 mg • Molybdenum (Chelate) 300 mcg • Vitamin B-6 (Pyridoxine HCl) 10 mg • Vitamin C (Zinc and Manganese Ascorbates) 78 mg • Vitamin D-3 (Cholecalciferol) 200 IU.

Life Minerals-No Iron - Source Naturals
Four tablets contain: Calcium (Citrate, Fumarate, Malate, Succinate and alpha-Ketoglutarate) 480 mg • Magnesium (Citrate, Fumarate, Malate, Succinate and alpha-Ketoglutarate) 480 mg • Potassium (Citrate, Malate, Fumarate, Succinate, and alpha-Ketoglutarate) 99 mg • Zinc (OptiZinc Zinc Monomethionine 20 mg and Ascorbate 10 mg) 30mg • Chromium (ChromeMate GTF Chromium Polynicotinate) 300 mcg • Selenium (Selenomethionine and Sodium Selenite) 200 mcg • Boron (Amino Acid Chelate) 3 mg • Silica (Horsetail Silica extract) 4.5 mg • Iodine (from Kelp) 150 mcg • Copper (Sebacate) 2 mg • Molybdenum (Chelate) 300 mcg • Vitamin B-6 (Pyridoxine HCl) 10 mg • Vitamin C (Zinc and Manganese Ascorbates) 78 mg • Vitamin D-3 (Cholecalciferol) 200 IU.

Life Spark - Source Naturals
Four tablets contain: Vitamin B1 (Thiamin) 30 mg • Vitamin B2 (Riboflavin) 30 mg • Vitamin B3 (Niacin 25 mg and Niacinamide 125 mg) 150 mg • Vitamin B5 (Pantothenic Acid) 100 mg • Vitamin B6 (Pyridoxine HCl) 25 mg • Vitamin B12 (Cyanocobalamin) 100 mcg • Vitamin E (D-Alpha Tocopheryl) (Natural) 150 IU • Magnesium (Oxide, Citrate) 250 mg • Potassium (Citrate) 99 mg • Glycine 500 mg • Tyrosine 250 mg • Coenzyme Q10 (Ubiquinone) 50 mg • Alpha-Lipoic Acid 25 mg • Herbal Blend 1170 mg: Siberian Ginseng, Panax Ginseng, Polygonum Multiflori (Fo Ti), Cyperus, Panax Ginseng extract, Tien Chi, and Siberian Ginseng extract.

LifeGuard Advanced Antioxidant - Starlight International
Two tablets contain: Vitamin A (as beta carotene) 5000 IU • Vitamin C (as asorbic acid) 300 mg • Vitamin E (as d-alpha tocopheryl succintate) 30 IU • Zinc (as zinc picolinate) 50 mg • Selenium (as sodium selenite) 60 mcg • Bilberry extract 4:1 (vaccinium myrtillus, fruit) 400 mg • Green Tea extract 4:1 (carmellia sinensis, leaf) 150 mg • Turmeric (curcuma longa, rhizome) 150 mg • Pine Bark extract (pinus strobus, bark) 40 mg • Ginkgo Biloba extract (leaf) 24% Ginkgo flavone glycosides, 6% terpene lactones 20 mg • Garlic (allim salivum, root) deodorized 10 mg • Echinacea purpurea (plant) 10 mg • Goldenseal (hydrastis caradensis, plant) 2 mg. Other Ingredients: Croscarmellose Sodium, Dicalcium Phosphate, Hydroxpropylcellulose, Stearic Acid, Magnesium Stearate, Microcrystalline Cellulose, Calcium Carbonate, Calcium Sulfate, Silicon Dioxide, Dextrin, Dextrose, Lecithin, Sodium Citrate.

LifeGuard Cholesterol Control - Starlight International
Two tablets contain: Red Rice Yeast (Monascus purpureus, Plant) 800 mg • Fo-Ti (Polygonum multiforum, Plant) 50 mg • Soy 80 mg • Beta Sitosterol 100 mg • English Hawthorn (Crataegus laevigata, Fruit) 30 mg. Other Ingredients: Calcium Carbonate, Microcrystalline Cellulose, Stearic Acid, Croscarmellose Sodium, Magnesium Stearate, Silicon Dioxide, Hydroxypropylcellulose, Dextrin, Dextrose, Lecithin, Sodium Citrate.

LifeGuard Joint Formula - Starlight International
Three tablets contain: Manganese (as Manganese Ascorbate) 6 mg • Glucosamine HCl 750 mg • Chondroitin Sulfate, 95% 250 mg • MSM (Methyl-Sulfonyl-Methane) 100 mg • Sulfate (Sodium-Sulfate) 30 mg • Turmeric, 90% curcumin (Curcuma Longa, root) 25 mg • Boswell Serrata extract, 65% (Boswellic Acid, trunk) 25 mg. Other Ingredients: Dicalcium Phosphate, Microcrystalline Cellulose,

Stearic Acid, Croscarmellose Sodium, Silicon Dioxide, Magnesium Stearate, Dextrin, Dextrose, Lecithin, Sodium Carboxymethylcellulose, Sodium Citrate.
See Editor's Note No. 15, page 1817.

LifeGuard Junior - Starlight International
Two tablets contain: Vitamin A (as beta carotene) 1000 IU • Vitamin C (as sodium ascorbate) 100 mg • Vitamin E (as d-alpha tocopheryl acetate) 20 IU • Bilberry extract 4:1 (vaccinium myrtillus, fruit) 100 mg • Vegetable complex (tomato, carrot, cabbage, broccoli, and green pepper powder) 100 mg • Acerola (malpighia glabra, fruit) 75 mg • Rosehips powder (rosa canina, fruit) 25 mg • Grape Seed extract, 95% flavanols (vitis vinifera seed) 2 mg.

Life's Greens - Puritan's Pride
One scoop (8.8 g) contains: Green Organic Gluten-Free Grasses: Wheat Grass powder 350 mg • Barley grass powder 350 mg • Alfalfa grass powder 350 mg • Oat grass powder 350 mg. Blue-Green And Sea Algae: Spirulina 1,000 mg • Chlorella (cracked-cell) 350 mg • Dunaliella salina 40 mg • Nova Scotia Dulse 30 mg. Adapogenic And Support Herbs: Licorice root 100 mg • Siberian Ginseng (Eleuthrococcus senticosus) 60 mg • Suma (Pfaffia paniculata) 60 mg • Astragalus membraneceus 60 mg • Echinacea purpurea 60 mg • Powdered Ginger root 5 mg. Nutrient-Rich Superfoods: Lecithin 99% oil-free 2,000 mg • Wheat sprout powder 350 mg • Acerola berry juice powder 200 mg • Beet juice powder 200 mg • Spinach octacosanol 150 mg • Royal Jelly (5% 10-HDA) 150 mg • Bee Pollen 150 mg • Vitamin E (d'alpha tocopheryl succinate) 100 IU. Dairy-Free Probiotic Cultures (Total count, Non-dairy culture: 5.0 billion): Lactoacillus group (L. rhamnosus A, L. rhamnosus B, L. acidophilus, L. casei, L. delbrueckii subsp. bulgaricus) 3.5 billion • Bifidobacterium group (B. longum, B. breve) 1.0 billion • Streptococcus salivarius subsp. thermophilus 500 million. Natural Fibers: Flaxseed meal 500 mg • Apple Pectin and fiber 500 mg • Fructooligosaccharides (FOS) 500 mg. Standardized Bioflavonoid Extracts: Milk Thistle extract (silybum marianum: standardized for 80% silymarin) 60 mg • Ginkgo Biloba extract (standardized for 6% terpene: lactones & 24 % ginkgo flavoglycosides) 20 mg • Green Tea catechins (standadized for 60% catechins) 20 mg • Grape pip extract (92% proanthocyanidins) 20 mg • Bilberry extract (standardized to 25% anthocyanidins) 20 mg.

Liga-Pane - Nutri-Quest
Each tablet contains: Shark Cartilage 50 mg • N-Acetyl Glucosamine 10 mg • Bromelain 10 mg • Valerian 50 mg • Feverfew 150 mg • Passion Flower 50 mg • Scullcap 25 mg • White Willow 100 mg • Magnesium Citrate 150 mg • Calcium Lactate 100 mg • Kava Kava 15 mg • Tumeric 10 mg • Vitamin B6 10 mg • Oregano 10 mg • Marjoram 10 mg • Thyme 10 mg • Basil powder 10 mg • Ginger 10 mg • Suma 10 mg • Manganese Chelate 15 mg • Molybdenum Chelate 50 mcg.

Line Assist Creme - Aspen Group, Inc.
Each gram contains: Tocopheryl Acetate 1% • Panthenol 1% • Ascorbyl Palmitate .3% • Water • Diisopropyl Adipate • Cetearyl Alcohol • Potassium Cetyl Phosphate • Retinyl Palmitate • Palmitate • Tocopherol • Dimethicone • Carbomer • Ammonium Hydroxide • Quaternium-15 • Disodium EDTA.

Liniment Virtue - Blessed Herbs
St. John's Wort flower • Comfrey root • Angelica root • Valerian root • Lobelia herb • Ginger root • Calendula flower • Arnica flower & herb • Cayenne pepper • Essential oils of Myrrh, Hyssop, Rosemary, Lavender & German Chamomile • Grain alcohol & Distilled Water.

Lipo Trim - Now
Three tablets contain: Choline 1000 mg • Inositol 1000 mg • L-Methionine 500 mg • Taurine 250 mg • L-Carnitine 100 mg • Pyridoxine (B6) 10 mg • Chromium Picolinate 200 mcg.

BRAND NAMES

Some Brand Name Natural Products - What they Contain
www.NaturalDatabase.com contains MANY more listings than appear here.

Lipo-Complex - Progressive Labs
Each capsule contains: Pancreatic enzyme concentrate 400 mg (equivalent in enzymatic activity to 4X USP) • Pepsin 1:3000 (from Pepsin 1:10,000) 100 mg • Green Beet leaf powder 100 mg • Raw Liver concentrate 10 mg • Ox bile 10 mg.
See Editor's Note No. 14, page 1817.

Lipoicare - PhysioLogics
Each capsule contains: Taurine 200 mg • Alpha-Lipoic Acid 25 mg • Calendula flower, Marigold (5% Lutein 3 mg; > 0.22% Zeaxanthin, 0.13 mg) 60 mg.

Lipokinetix - Syntrax Innovations
Norephedrine • Caffeine • Yohimbine • Diiodothyronine • Sodium usniate.

Lipotrope - Progressive Labs
Each capsule contains: Vitamin C 50 mg • Vitamin B6 5 mg • Folate (folic acid) 200 mcg • Vitamin B12 200 mcg • Pantothenic Acid 60 mg • Magnesium Aspartate 25 mg • Milk Thistle (Silybum marianum) 100 mg • Choline Bitartrate 150 mg • Inositol 75 mg • Betaine HCl 60 mg • DL-Methionine 50 mg • Black Radish (Raphanus nigra) 50 mg • Green Beet leaf powder 50 mg • Celandine (Chelidonium majus) 15 mg • Chionanthus (Chionanthus virginica) 15 mg • PABA 25 mg.

Lipotropic Action - Puritan's Pride
Each capsule contains: Iodine (as Potassium Iodide) 25 mcg • Magnesium (as Magnesium Amino Acid Chelate) 8.3 mg • Selenium (as Selenomethionine) 0.33 mcg • Manganese (as Manganese Amino Acid Chelate) 1.6 mg • Molybdenum (as Molybdenum Amino Acid Chelate) 8.33 mg • Potassium (as Potassium Amino Acid Chelate) 16.5 mg • Boron (as Boron Chelate) 0.33 mcg • Vanadium (as Vanadium Amino Acid Chelate) 0.33 mcg • Choline Bitartrate 35.46 mg • Inositol 25 mg • Ginger (Zingiber officinale) root 25 mg • L-Methionine 16.67 mg • L-Carnitine (as L-Carnitine Fumarate) 16.67 mg • Beta Sitosterol 16.67 mg • Dandelion (Taraxacum officinale) root 12.5 mg • Barberry (Berberis vulgaris) root 12.5 mg • Turmeric (Curcuma longa) root 12.5 mg • Milk Thistle (Silybum marianum) seed 12.5 mg • Cinnamon (Cinnamonum verum) bark 12.5 mg • Siberian Ginseng (Eleutherococcus senticosus) root 8.33 mg • Gotu Kola (Centella asiatica) aerial 8.33 mg • Fo-Ti (Polygonum multiflorum) root 8.33 mg • Cayenne pepper (Capsicum annuum) fruit 4.16 mg • DigeZyme enzyme complex: Anylase (1:2,000), Neutral Protease, Cellulase, Galactohydrolase Lactase, Lipase 50 mg.

Lipotropic Complex - Nature's Life
Three tablets contain: L-Methionine (Free-Form Amino Acid) 1000 mg • Choline (from 2040 mg Choline Bitartrate) 1000 mg • Inositol 1000 mg • Betaine HCl (Sugar Beets) 250 mg • Milk Thistle (Silybum marianum) 50 mg • Vitamin B6 (Pyridoxine Hydrochloride) 10 mg • L-Carnitine (Free-Form Amino Acid) 10 mg • L-Taurine (Free-Form Amino Acid) 10 mg • Lecithin (Soy) (61% Phosphatides) 10 mg • Beet root powder (Beta vulgaris rubra) 5 mg • Dandelion root powder (Taraxacum officinale) 5 mg • Culvers root powder (Leptandra virginica) 5 mg • Apple Cider Vinegar 5 mg • Barberry root bark (Berberis vulgaris) 5 mg • Chromium (Nutrition 21 Picolinate) 25 mcg.

Lipotropic Fuel - TwinLab
Five capsules contain: Choline 500 mg • Inositol 250 mg • L-Methionine 100 mg • Vitamin B12 100 mcg • Betaine 100 mg • L-Carnitine 100 mg • Milk Thistle extract (standardized for 80% Silymarin) 500 mg • Natural Vitamin E (Succinate) 400 IU • Vitamin C 1000 mg • Vitamin B1 25 mg • N-Acetyl Cysteine (NAC) 250 mg • L-Glutathione 100 mg • Vitamin B2 25 mg • Selenium (from Selenomethionine) 150 mcg • Zinc (from Zinc Mono-Methionine) 15 mg.

Lipotropic Plus - Vitamin Express
Three tablets contain: Niacin (as nicotinic acid) 100 mg • Vitamin B12 (as cobalamin) 50 mcg • Betaine HCL 50 mg • Choline (as choline bitartrate) 450 mg • Clove 90 mg • DL-Methionine 1000 mg • Hawthorn Berry 30 mg • Inositol 1000 mg • Liver (from desiccated whole liver) 6 mg • Yucca 30 mg. Other Ingredients: Calcium Phosphate, Calcium Stearate, Cellulose, Lecithin, Silica, Stearic Acid. Contains NO sugar, starch, artificial colors, flavors, preservatives, corn, yeast, wheat, grain, egg or milk products.
See Editor's Note No. 14, page 1817.

Liquid Aminos - Puritan's Pride
Each softgel contains: L-Alanine 30 mg • L-Arginine 54 mg • L-Aspartic Acid 83 mg • L-Cysteine 10 mg • L-Glutamic Acid 145 mg • L-Glycine 33 mg • L-Histidine 20 mg • L-Isoleucine 35 mg • L-Leucine 60 mg • L-Lysine 59 mg • L-Methionine 9 mg • L-Phenylalanine 41 mg • L-Proline 38 mg • L-Serine 39 mg • L-Threonine 32 mg • L-Tryptophan 7 mg • L-Tyrosine 22 mg • L-Valine 33 mg.

Liquid Anti-Oxidant - Natrol
Two teaspoons (10 ml) contain: Anti-Oxidant Vitamins & Trace Minerals: Vitamin A (beta carotene) 10000 IU • Vitamin C (Calcium ascorbate) 500 mg • Vitamin E (acetate) 200 IU • Selenium (monomethionine) 90 mcg • Advanced Flavonoids: GP Complex+ 80 mg • Rutin, Quercetin, & Hesperidin 10 mg • Tropical fruit extracts from: Acerola, Cashew fruit, Passion fruit, Orange, Lime & Mango in a specially formulated base of: Purified Water, Brown Rice Syrup, Honey & Citric Acid.

Liquid Calcium - Nature's Bounty
Three softgels contain: Vitamin A (as Retinyl Palmitate) 825 IU • Vitamin D (as Cholecalciferol) 180 IU • Calcium (as Calcium Carbonate) 600 mg. Other Ingredients: Soybean Oil, Gelatin, Glycerin, Lecithin, Titanium Dioxide Color.

Liquid Calcium Magnesium Citrate - Puritan's Pride
Each teaspoon (15 ml) contains: Calcium (Citrate, Lactate, Gluconate) 600 mg • Magnesium (Citrate) 300 mg • Vitamin D (Cholecalciferol) 400 IU.

Liquid Children's Multiple - Natrol
Two teaspoons contain: Essential Vitamins: Vitamin A (beta carotene) 2,500 IU • Vitamin C (calcium ascorbate & ascorbic acid) 100 mg • Vitamin D (as Vitamin D3)(calciferol) 400 IU • Vitamin E (Acetate) 30 IU • Thiamine (Vitamin B1) 1 mg • Riboflavin(Vitamin B2) 1 mg • Niacin (Niacinamide) 12 mg • Vitamin B6 (pyridoxine HCl) 1.4 mg • Vitamin B12 (cyanocobalamin) 2.5 mcg • Pantothenic Acid (calcium d-pantothenate) 6 mg • Folic Acid 100 mcg • Biotin 20 mcg • Flavonoid: Hesperidin, Acerola, Cashew fruit, Passion fruit, Orange & Lime 10 mg • Tropical fruit extracts from: Lemon, Orange, Lime, Mango • Other extracts from: natural Vanilla Bean extract • Herbal extracts: Anise Seed, Licorice root, Millefolium plant, Horsetail Grass plant, Chamomile leaf & flowers, Peppermint leaf, Nettles plant, Spinach leaf & Sodium Benzoate (0.1% added to help protect flavor). In a base of Purified Water, Brown Rice Syrup, Glycerine & Citric Acid.

Liquid Children's Multi-Vitamin - Natrol
Two teaspoons (10 ml) contain: Essential Vitamins: Vitamin A (beta carotene) 2500 IU • Vitamin C (calcium ascorbate & ascorbic acid) 100 mg • Vitamin D (as Vitamin D3)(calciferol) 400 IU • Vitamin E (Acetate) 30 IU • Vitamin B1 (Thiamine) 1 mg • Vitamin B2 (Riboflavin) 1 mg • Niacin (Niacinamide) Vitamin B3 12 mg • Vitamin B6 (pyridoxine HCl) 1.4 mg • Vitamin B12 (cyanocobalamin) 2.5 mcg • Pantothenic Acid (calcium d-pantothenate) 6 mg • Folic Acid 100 mcg • Biotin 20 mcg • Flavonoid: Hesperidin 10 mg • Tropical fruit extracts from: Lemon,

B R A N D   N A M E S

Orange, Lime, Mango • Other extracts from: natural Vanilla Bean extract • Herbal extracts: Anise Seed, Licorice root, Millefolium plant, Plantain root, Horsetail Grass plant, Chamomile leaf & flowers, Peppermint leaf, Nettles plant, Spinach leaf & Sodium Benzoate (0.1% added to help protect Flavor). In a base of: Purified Water, Brown Rice Syrup, Glycerine & Citric Acid.

Liquid Ester-C - Natrol
Two teaspoons (10 ml) contain: Vitamin C (from Ester-C calcium ascorbate) 250 mg • Calcium (from Ester-C calcium ascorbate) 25 mg • Pure Bioflavonoids containing: Rutin, Quercetin, & Hesperidin 10 mg • Tropical fruit extracts from: Acerola, Cashew fruit, Passion fruit, Orange, Lime & Mango. In a specially formulated base of: Purified Water, Brown Rice Syrup, Honey, natural Vanilla Bean extract, Citric Acid & Sodium Benzoate (0.1% added to help protect flavor). Ester-C is a unique ascorbate complex bound with calcium carbonate. It is naturally processed in purified water without the use of alcohol or acetone solvents.

Liquid Iron Ferrochel - Natrol
Four teaspoons (20 mL) contain: Iron & Vitamins: Iron (Ferrochel chelate) 14.5 mg • Vitamin C (Calcium Ascorbate) 100 mg • Vitamin B1 (Thiamine) 1 mg • Vitamin B6 (Pyridoxine HCl) 2 mg • Vitamin B12 (Cyanocobalamin) 3 mcg • Niacinamide 13 mg • Herbal extracts: Nettles, Kelp, Spinach, Yarrow, Angelica, Horsetail Grass, Siberian Ginseng, Yellow Dock, Burdock root, Pau D'Arco, Rose Hips & Alfalfa • Tropical fruit extracts from: Acerola, Pineapple, Cashew fruit, Passion fruit, Lime & Mango. In a specially formulated base of: Purified Water, Brown Rice Syrup, Honey & natural fruit flavors.

Liquid Kalm With Kava Kava root extract - Natrol
Two teaspoons (10 ml) contain: Guaranteed Potency Herbal extracts: Kava Kava root extract standardized to contain 30% Kavalactones 25 mg • Passion flower Herb extract standardized to Contain 3.5% Isovitexin 20 mg • Chamomile flower extract standardized to Contain 0.5% Apigenin 25 mg • Hops Cone extract standardized to Contain 0.35% Flavonoids 25 mg • Vitamin: Vitamin B6 2 mg • Herbal extract blend: Lemon Balm leaf, Oat Straw, Marjoram leaf, Cowslip herb, Rosemary leaf, Scullcap herb. Other ingredients: Honey & Brown Rice Syrup, natural Lemon & Ginger flavor, Cashew fruit & Passion fruit powder, Citric Acid, Sodium Benzoate (0.1% added to protect flavor).

Liquid Multi-Vitamin - Natrol
Two teaspoons (10 ml) contain: Vitamins & Minerals: Vitamin A (beta carotene) 10000 IU • Vitamin C (Calcium Ascorbate) 200 mg • Vitamin D (cholecalciferol) 400 IU • Vitamin E (Acetate) 100 IU • Vitamin B1 (Thiamine) 7.5 mg • Vitamin B2 (Riboflavin) 8.5 mg • Niacin (Niacinamide) Vitamin B3 20 mg • Vitamin B6 (Pyridoxine HCl) 17 mg • Vitamin B12 (cyanocobalamin) 50 mcg • Pantothenic Acid (calcium d-pantothenate) 50 mg • Inositol 25 mg • Folic Acid 400 mcg • Biotin 300 mcg. Advanced Flavonoids: GP Flavonoids Complex+ 50 mg • Rutin, Quercetin, & Hesperidin 10 mg • Herbal extracts: Nettles, Kelp, Parsley, Ginger, Oats, Alfalfa, Hops, Peppermint, Rose Hips, Spinach & Echinacea, Natural Vanilla Bean flavor, natural Ginger flavor • Tropical fruit extracts from: Acerola, Pineapple, Cashew fruit, Passion fruit, Mango, Orange, Lime & Lemon. In a Specially Formulated Base of: Purified Water, Brown Rice Syrup, Honey, Glycerine, Citric Acid, Sodium Benzoate to help protect flavor, Milk Thistle & Citrus fruits.

Liquid Multi-Vitamin - Puritan's Pride
Each tablespoonful (15 ml) contains: Vitamin A (as Retinyl Palmitate) 5,000 IU • Vitamin C (as Ascorbic Acid) 250 mg • Vitamin D (as Cholecalciferol) 400 IU • Vitamin E (as d-Alpha Tocopheryl plus Mixed Tocopherols) 125 IU • Thiamin (Vitamin B1; as Thiamine Mononitrate) 25 mg • Riboflavin (Vitamin B2; as Riboflavin-5'-Phosphate Sodium) 25 mg • Niacin (as Niacinamide) 150 mg • Vitamin B-6 (as Pyridoxine Hydrochloride) 50 mg • Folic Acid

400 mcg • Vitamin B-12 (as Cyanocobalamin) 50 mcg • Biotin (as D-Biotin) 50 mcg • Pantothenic Acid (as Dexpanthenol) 150 mg • PABA (Para-Aminobenzoic Acid) 25 mg • Choline Bitartrate 200 mg • Inositol 100 mg.

Liquid NewBust (Liquid New Bust) - Tiger-One.com
Water • Saw Palmetto • Extra Virgin Olive Oil • Dong Quai • Damiana • Glycerin • Foenugreek seed • Blessed Thistle • Violet • Wild Yam • Fennel Seed • Althea root • Cumin seed • Hops.
See Editor's Note No. 17, page 1817.

Lithinase - Progressive Labs
Each capsule contains: Lithium Amino Acid Chelate 25 mg • Elemental Lithium 50 mcg • Pea powder 25 mg • Buckwheat 25 mg • Millet flour 25 mg • Lentil powder 25 mg (carefully dried to preserve their natural nutrient content).

Little One Children's Multiple - Metabolic Products
One tablet contains: Vitamin A (Palmitate) 2500 IU • Vitamin A (Natural Mixed Carotenoids) 2500 IU • Vitamin C (Hypoallergenic from Beet sugar and Ascorbyl Palmitate) 100 mg • Vitamin E (D-Alpha, Natural) 60 IU • Vitamin B1 (Thiamin Mononitrate) 5 mg • Vitamin B2 (Riboflavin) 5 mg • Vitamin B3 (Niacinamide) 25 mg • Vitamin B5 (D-Calcium Pantothenate) 25 mg • Vitamin B6 (Pyridoxine) 5 mg • Vitamin B12 (Cyanocobalamin) 10 mcg • Folic Acid 400 mcg • Biotin 300 mcg • Vitamin D (Cholecalciferol) 400 IU • Iron (Carbonyl) 9 mg • Iodine (K-Iodine) 100 mcg • Copper (Gluconate) 2 mg • Manganese (Gluconate) 1 mg • Zinc (Citrate) 15 mg • Molybdenum (Sodium Molybdate) 25 mcg • Chromium (GTF-Polynicotinate) 100 mcg • Selenium (L-Selenomethionine, Sodium Selenite) 100 mcg.

Liv-A-Tox - Enzymatic Therapy
Three tablets contain: Vitamin A (Fish Liver oil) 4500 IU • Niacin 40 mg • Vitamin C (Ascorbic Acid/Rose Hips) 25 mg • Biotin 200 mcg • Vitamin B12 (Cyanocobalamin) 3 mcg • Other ingredients: Choline Bitartrate 850 mg • Dehydrated Green Beet leaf juice powder 300 mg • L-Methionine 250 mg • Barberry • bark of root 4:1 (Berberis vulgaris) 150 mg • Boldo extract (Peumus boldo) standardized to contain 1.52% essential oils 150 mg • Greater Celandine extract (Chelidonium majus) 135 mg • Fringetree (Cheonanthus) 135 mg • Ox Bile extract 90 mg • Betaine HCL 75 mg • Inositol 50 mg • Liver, desiccated 40 mg • Unsaturated Free Fatty Acids 30 mg. Chlorophyll is used in this product as a natural coloring agent. All organs & glands derived from bovine sources.
See Editor's Note No. 14, page 1817.

Live Calm Sleep Deep - Cocoon Nutrition
Each capsule contains: L-Tetrahydropalmatine (Rotundine) 30 mg • Magnesium Chloride 12.6 mg. Other Ingredients: Microcrystalline Cellulose.

Liver - Nutrivention
Each tablet contains: Inositol 100 mg • Choline Bitartrate 100 mg • Vitamin E 50 IU • Vitamin B1 10 mg • Niacin 10 mg • Pantothenic Acid 10 mg • Vitamin A (Beta Carotene) 500 IU • Vitamin B12 100 mcg • Vitamin K 15 mcg • Lecithin 300 mg • Milk Thistle (Cardus marianus) 200 mg • Dandelion root 200 mg • Burdock root 50 mg • L-Methionine 50 mg • L-Theronine 30 mg • Yellow Dock 25 mg • Butternut root bark 25 mg.

Liver Chelate - Atrium Inc.
Each tablet contains: Ferrous Fumarate as Chelated Proteinates 55 mg • Copper 1 mg • Folic Acid 40 mcg • Vitamin B12 20 mcg • Raw Liver concentrate (not an extract) of Bovine source 190 mg.
See Editor's Note No. 14, page 1817.

Some Brand Name Natural Products - What they Contain

Liver Essentials - Swanson

Two capsules contain: Milk Thistle seed extract (85% silymarin) 350 mg • Dandelion root 170 mg • Burdock root 120 mg • Parsley root 120 mg • Picroliv® (Picrorhiza kurroa) 100 mg • Black Radish root 70 mg • N-Acetyl Cysteine 50 mg • Trimethylglycine (as betaine anhydrous) 50 mg • Alpha Lipoic Acid 20 mg.

Liver Formula - Dr. Morrow's Homeopathic Formulas

Ten drops contain: Chelidonium 3X • Taraxacum 3X • Carduus marianus 3X • Solidago 3X • Hydrastis 3C • Magnesia muriatica 3C • Cinchona 3C.
See Editor's Note No. 1, page 1816.

Liver Guard - Source Naturals

Two tablets contain: Vitamin B1 (Thiamin) 7.5 mg • Vitamin B2 (Riboflavin) 7.5 mg • Niacinamide and Niacin 50 mg • Vitamin B5 (Pantothenic Acid) 15 mg • Vitamin B6 (Pyridoxine HCl) 10 mg • Vitamin B12 (Cyanocobalamin) 25 mcg • Folic Acid 200 mcg • Vitamin C (Ascorbic Acid and Zinc Ascorbate) 527 mg • Fat-Soluble Vitamin C (from 238 mg of Ascorbyl Palmitate) 100 mg • Vitamin E (D-Alpha Tocopheryl) (Natural) 75 IU • Magnesium (Oxide, Malate) 60 mg • Potassium (Citrate) 49.5 mg • Selenium (as L-Selenomethionine) 50 mcg • Zinc (OptiZinc Zinc Monomethionine 10 mg and Zinc Ascorbate 5 mg) 15 mg • Silymarin (from Milk Thistle seed extract) 200 mg • N-Acetyl Cysteine 200 mg • Dandelion root extract 125 mg • Dandelion root 125 mg • Turmeric extract (95% Curcumin) 76 mg • Choline (Bitartrate) 50 mg • Inositol 50 mg • Alpha-Lipoic Acid (Thioctic acid) 25 mg • Coenzyme Q10 (Ubiquinone) 12.5 mg.

Liver Maintenance Formula - PhysioLogics

Each capsule contains: Milk Thistle (80% Silymarin, 80 mg) 100 mg • Dandelion (20% Taraxasterol, 20 mg; 3% Choline, 3 mg) 100 mg • Picrorhiza kurroa (4% Kutkin, 4 mg) 100 mg • Artichoke (5% Cynarin, 2.5 mg) 50 mg • Phylannthus amarus (4% Sesquiterpenes, 2 mg) 50 mg • Boldo (0.2% Boldine, 500 mcg) 25 mg • Black Radish 25 mg • Alpha Lipoic Acid 25 mg.

Liver Performance - Metabolic Response Modifiers

Each capsule contains: N-Acetyl-Cysteine (NAC) 400 mg • Alpha Lipoic Acid 100 mg • Choline bitartrate 100 mg • Silymarin (32 mg of milk thistle extract standardized to 80% silymarin) 100 mg • Picrorhiza kurroa 25 mg • Andographis paniculata 25 mg • Vitamin E 40 IU • Vitamin B12 (methylcobalamin) 20 mcg.

Liver Support - Amazon Support

Each capsule contains: Carqueja • Picao Preto • Erva Tostao • Tayuya • Tumeric • Artichoke • Mutamba • Boldo • Chanca Piedra • Sarsaparilla • Jurubeba • Gervao.

Liver-Enhancer - HerbaSway

Reishi • Poria • Cordyceps • Maitake • Shiitake • Hericium • Schisandra • Lycium • Milk Thistle • Blackberry • HerbaSwee (Cucurbitaceae fruit).

LiveRx - Metabolic Response Modifiers

Each capsule contains: N-Acetyl-Cysteine (NAC) 400 mg • Alpha Lipoic Acid 100 mg • Choline 100 mg • Silymarin 100 mg • Picrorhiza kurroa 25 mg • Andographis paniculata 25 mg • Vitamin E 40 IU • Vitamin B12 (methylcobalamin) 20 mcg.

Living Energy - Futurebiotics

Four tablets contain: Chlorella 500 mg • Bee Pollen 1000 mg • Ginseng 4:1 extract equivalent to 250 mg • Royal Jelly (freeze dried) 25 mg • Schizandra 4:1 extract equivalent to 250 mg • Astragalus 4:1 extract equivalent to 250 mg • Spirulina 500 mg • Alfalfa juice concentrate 1200 mg.

Livr D-Tox - Nutri-Quest

Each tablet contains: Glucuronic Acid 10 mg • Liver 5 mg • Vitamin A 1000 IU • Vitamin C 25 mg • Vitamin B1 5 mg • Vitamin E 10 IU • Black Currant seed oil 5 mg • Cellulase 50 mg • Amylase 50 mg • Lipase 50 mg • Protease 50 mg • Lipoic Acid 2 mg • Phosphatidyl Choline 5.75 mg • Choline Bitartrate 15 mg • DL-Methionine 5 mg • Calcium Chelate 50 mg • Magnesium 50 mg • Zinc Chelate 5 mg • Selenium Chelate 25 mcg • Manganese 1 mg • Milk Thistle 100 mg • Silymarin 5 mg • Garlic 50 mg • Beet root 25 mg • Beet leaf 25 mg.
See Editor's Note No. 14, page 1817.

Liv-R-Actin Milk Thistle Blend in Vegetarian Capsules - Nature's Plus

Two Vegicaps contain: Herbal Blend containing: Dandelion, Barberry, Goldenseal, Wild Oregon Grape & Celery seed 600 mg • Milk Thistle extract, providing 70%, 98 mg of the active flavonoid Silymarin 140 mg. Contains no yeast, wheat, corn, soy, milk, salt, sugar or starch.

Livral - AIE Pharmaceuticals

Each capsule contains: Proprietary Blend 750 mg: Milk Thistle extract • Phyllanthus amarus • Dandelion root (Taraxacum officinale) • Grape seed extract (Vitis vinifera) • Artichoke • Choline • Inositol.

Livral Complex - AIE Pharmaceuticals

Each capsule contains: Proprietary Blend 750 mg: Milk Thistle extract • Phyllanthus Amarus • Dandelion root (Taraxacum officinale) • Cat's Claw bark • Licorice root • Tribulus terrestris • Culver's root • Oregon Grape root • Yellow Dock • Burdock root • Echinacea root • Grape seed extract (Vitis vinifera) • Artichoke • Catechin.

L-Lysine Plus - Atrium Inc.

Each tablet contains: L-Lysine HCL (an essential amino acid) 500 mg • Ascorbic Acid (Vitamin C) 100 mg.

Lobelia - Nature's Way

Each capsule contains: Lobelia 425 mg. Other Ingredients: Gelatin, Magnesium Stearate.

Lobelia and Cayenne - Dial Herbs

Lobelia • Cayenne.

Lomatium-Goldenseal Virtue - Blessed Herbs

Lomatium root • Astragalus root • Osha root • Echinacea Angustifolia root • Goldenseal root • Siberian Ginseng root • Licorice root • Reishi mycelium • Shitake mycelium • Grain alcohol & Distilled Water.

Longest Living Acidophilus - Futurebiotics

Each capsule contains: Acidophilus fortified with Rhamnosus, encapsulated in a base of Rice powder & Beet fiber. 1 billion Live Organisms per capsule.

Longe-Vit-E - Holista

Each capsule contains: Vitamin C (Ester-C) 250 mg • Beta Carotene 10000 IU • Vitamin E (d-alpha tocopherol) 200 IU • Selenium 50 mcg • Vitamin B6 25 mg • Magnesium 50 mg • Manganese 1.5 mg • Copper 1.0 mg.

Love-Berries - Nature's Plus

Each pill contains: Cranberry concentrate 45X 200 mg • Vitamin C corn free 60 mg. Sweetened with VitaSweet. Contains no yeast, wheat, corn, soy, milk, salt.

LPC - OSMO Therapy

Each capsule contains: Lysophosphatidyl Choline 300 mg.

BRAND NAMES

LPC Serum - The Vitamin Factory
One ounce of serum contains: Pycnogenol • Liquid Vitamin C
Applied topically to the face. Using a highly stable derivative of
Vitamin C called Magnesium Ascorbyl Phosphate (Mega-C), the
Vitamin C and Pycnogenol are released into the skin by a liposomal
delivery system which protects the ingredients.

L-Pyroglutamic Acid - Source Naturals
Each tablet contains: L-Pyroglutamic acid 1,000 mg.

Lullaby Nighttime Formula - Starlight International
Two tablets contain: Niacin (Niacinamide) 50 mg • Vitamin B6
(Pyridoxine HCl) 20 mg • Calcium (as Calcium Lactate) 10 mg •
Magnesium (as Magnesium Oxide) 114 mg • Kava Kava extract, 4:1
(Piper methysticum, root) 200 mg • Valerian extract, 4:1 (Valeriana
officinalis, root) 150 mg • Lemon Balm (Melissa officinalis, leaf)
150 mg • Passion Flower (Passiflora incarnata, plant) 150 mg •
Melatonin 5 mg. Other Ingredients: Dicalcium Phosphate,
Microcrystalline Cellulose, Stearic Acid, Gum Acacia, Croscarmellose
Sodium, Silicon Dioxide, Magnesium Stearate, Pharmaceutical Glaze,
Ethylcellulose, Dextrin, Dextrose, Lecithin, Sodium Citrate.

Lung Support Formula - Gero Vita
Astragalus membranaceus • Cordyceps sinensis • Ophiopogon
japonicus.

Lung-Mend - The Herbalist
Elecampane root • Grindelia herb • Pleurisy root • Butterbur root •
Marshmallow root • Usnea lichen • Yerba Santa leaf • Lobelia leaf •
Yerba Mansa root.

Luprinol - Klein-Becker
Two capsules contain: Ephedrine alkaloids (from standardized whole
plant Ma Huang extract 200 mg) 20 mg • Caffeine (34 mg from
standardized Kola nut 280 mg) 200 mg • Acetylsalicylic acid 324 mg •
DHEA 8.4 mg • Schizonepeta (spica) 250 mg. Other Ingredients: Rice
Flour.

Lustre - Source Naturals
Six tablets contain: Vitamin A (Beta Carotene) 15000 IU • Vitamin A
(Palmitate) 5000 IU • Vitamin B1 (Thiamin) 10 mg • Vitamin B2
(Riboflavin) 10 mg • Niacinamide 30 mg • Vitamin B5 (Calcium
D-Pantothenate) 50 mg • Vitamin B6 (Pyridoxine HCl) 20 mg •
Vitamin B12 (Cyanocobalamin) 30 mcg • Biotin 2000 mcg • Folic
Acid 800 mcg • Vitamin C (Magnesium, Zinc and Manganese
Ascorbates) 1000 mg • Vitamin E (D-Alpha Tocopheryl)(Natural)
200 IU • Copper (Sebacate) 1.5 mg • Magnesium (Ascorbate) 59 mg •
Silica (Horsetail Silica Extract) 36 mg • Manganese (Ascorbate) 6 mg
• Selenium (as L-Selenomethionine and Sodium Selenite) 200 mcg •
L-Proline 600 mg • Inositol 500 mg • L-Cysteine (HCl) 400 mg •
Choline (Bitartrate) 100 mg • L-Methionine 100 mg • N-Acetyl
Cysteine 100 mg • PABA (Para Amino Benzoic Acid) 100 mg.

Lutein i care - Nature's Life
Each capsule contains: Lutein (FloraGLO) [from Marigold petals
(Tagetes erecta)] 5 mg • Beta Carotene [(Dunaliella salina) equivalent
to 5000 IU Vitamin A] 3 mg • Other naturally occurring carotenoids in
D. salina: Zeaxanthin (T. erecta, D. salina) 370 mcg • Alpha Carotene
106 mcg • Cryptoxanthin 20 mcg • Zinc (Gluconate) 5 mg • Copper
(Gluconate) 2.5 mg.

Lutein Plus - Nutrition Warehouse
Each capsule contains: Lutein (with 240-600 mcg Zeaxanthin) 6 mg •
In a 330 mg base of: Spinach, Blueberry Powder and Bilberry extract.

Lycopene - Nature's Life
Each capsule contains: Lycopene 6 mg • Carrot Carotenoids 2 mg
providing: Beta Carotene (Vitamin A equivalent 2500 IU) 1500 mcg,
Alpha Carotene (Vitamin A equivalent 417 IU) 500 mcg, Phytoene
39 mcg, Phytofluene 13 mcg.

Lycopene - Olympian Labs
Two capsules contain: Tomato Lycopene 300 mg • Vegetable Enzymes
(amylase, lipase, protease) 100 mg.

Lycopene 10 mg - Puritan's Pride
Each softgel contains: Lycopene 10 mg.

Lycopene 5 mg - Puritan's Pride
Each softgel contains: Lycopene 5 mg.

Lycosoy - TwinLab
Two softgels contain: Vitamin D 400 IU • Vitamin E 200 IU •
Selenium 200 mcg • Omega-3 Fish Oil conc. 460 mcg • Soy Bean
extract 150 mg • Lycopene 5 mg • Green Tea leaf extract 2 mg.

Lymphatone - The Herbalist
Echinacea root • Red root • Cleavers herb • Yellow Dock root •
Burdock root • Wild Indigo root • Poke root.

Lympho-Clear - Enzymatic Therapy
Each capsule contains: Red Clover extract 4:1 (Trifolium pratense)
200 mg • Burdock root extract 4:1 (Arctium lappa) 200 mg • Oregon
Grape root extract 6:1 (Berberis aquifolium) 100 mg • Licorice root
extract (Glycyrrhiza glabra) standardized to contain 5% Glycyrrhizic
Acid 50 mg • Goldenseal root extract (Hydrastis canadensis)
standardized to contain 5% total Alkaloids including: Berberine,
Hydrastine & Canadine 50 mg. Contains no sugar, salt, yeast, wheat,
corn, soy, dairy products, coloring, flavoring, or preservatives.

Lymph-Spleen Soluble Fractions - PhytoPharmica
Each capsule contains: Lymph-Spleen Complex (predigested soluble
concentrate) 250 mg • Multi-Glandular Complex : Raw Liver, Raw
Lung, Raw Pancreas, Raw Heart, Raw Kidney, Raw Spleen & Raw
Brain 100 mg. All organs and glands derived from bovine sources
except raw pancreas (porcine).
See Editor's Note No. 14, page 1817.

Lysozyme Plus - Atrium Inc.
Each tablet contains: Pancreatin (maximum strength) 200 mg • Papain
100 mg • Bromelain 75 mg • Rutin 60 mg • Trypsin 35 mg • Thymus
35 mg • Amylase 15 mg • Lipase 15 mg • Lysozyme 10 mg • Cellulase
2 mg • Zinc Gluconate 4 mg • a-Chymotrypsin 1 mg.
See Editor's Note No. 14, page 1817.

M.C.H.C. Capsules - Progressive Labs
Each capsule contains: Calcium 250 mg, from 500 mg M.C.H.C.
125 mg, from 500 mg Calcium Citrate 125 mg • Iron (from M.C.H.C.)
0.3 mg • Vitamin K 20 mcg • Phosphorus (from M.C.H.C.) 65 mg •
Magnesium (from M.C.H.C.) 4 mg • Zinc (from M.C.H.C.) 0.075 mg
• Copper (from M.C.H.C.) 0.01 mg • Manganese (from M.C.H.C.)
0.045 mg • Potassium (from M.C.H.C.) 0.035 mg • Protein (from
M.C.H.C. as collagen glycosaminoglycans) 125 mg • Boron (as boron
aspartate) 0.75 mg • Fluorapatite (from M.C.H.C.) 31 mcg • Silicon
(from M.C.H.C.) 19 mcg • Strontium (from M.C.H.C.) 10 mcg.

M.C.H.C. Tablets - Progressive Labs
Each tablet contains: Calcium (elemental) 250 mg, from 500 mg
M.C.H.C. 125 mg, from 500 mg. Calcium Citrate 125 mg • Iron (from
M.C.H.C.) 0.3 mg • Vitamin K 20 mcg • Phosphorum (from
M.C.H.C.) 65 mg • Magnesium (from M.C.H.C.) 4 mg • Zinc (from
M.C.H.C.) 0.075 mg • Copper (from M.C.H.C.) 0.01 mg • Manganese
(from M.C.H.C.) 0.045 mg • Potassium (from M.C.H.C.) 0.035 mg •
Protein (from M.C.H.C. as collagen glycosaminoglycans) 125 mg •
Boron (as aspartate) 750 mcg • Fluorapatite (from M.C.H.C.) 31 mcg
• Silicon (from M.C.H.C.) 19 mcg • Strontium (from M.C.H.C.)
10 mcg.

M.V. Teen - Futurebiotics
100% or more of the USRDA for 16 vitamins and minerals, 100 mcg of chromium and selenium.

Maca - Source Naturals
Three tablets contain: Maca root extract (MacaPure) (Lepidium meyenii) Standardized to 0.6% macamides and macaenes yielding 4.5 mg macamides and macaenes 750 mg

MacroForce Plus C - ImmuDyne, Inc.
Each capsule contains: Vitamin C (as Calcium Ascorbate) 394 mg • Calcium (as Calcium Carbonate) 44 mg • Beta-1,3-D-glucan (from cell walls of yeast, Saccharomyces cerevisiae) 7.5 mg.

Macro-Min - Atrium Inc.
Each tablet contains: Calcium Aspartate 600 mg • Magnesium Gluconate 300 mg • Potassium Aspartate 88.3 mg • Manganese Aspartate 50 mg • Vitamin D (as Vitamin D3) 250 IU.

Macular Guardian - Clinician's Choice
Two tablets contain: Vitamin A (as retinyl acetate) 2000 IU • Vitamin C (as ascorbic acid) 120 mg • Vitamin E (as dl-alpha tocopheryl acetate) 200 IU • Riboflavin 6 mg • Selenium (as selenomethionine) 40 mcg • Manganese (as amino acid chelate) 10 mg • Eyebright Herb 200 mg • RoseOx (patented, standardized process for an extract of Rosemary) 100 mg • Ascorbyl Palmitate 20 mg • L-Lysine HCl 20 mg • Lutein 12 mg • L-Glutathione 10 mg • Lycopene 10 mg • Beta-Carotene 6 mg • Proprietary blend 8 mg: Cruciferex, Carrot Powder, Citrus Bioflavonoid Complex, Bilberry, Zeaxanthin.

MacuVision - Health Smart Vitamins
Two capsules contain: Taurine 400 mg • Calendula (5% Lutein, 6 mg; >0.22% Zeaxanthin, 264 mcg) 120 mg • Alpha-Lipoic Acid 50 mg.

Mag Link - Pain & Stress Center
Two tablets contain: Calcium (Calcium Carbonate) 225 mg • Magnesium (Magnesium Chloride Hexahydrate) 130 mg • Chloride 375 mg.

Magic Cigarettes - Alternative Cigarettes Inc
Each cigarette contains: Marshmallow • Yerba Santa • Damiana • Passion Flower • Jasmine • Ginseng. Regular and menthol are available.
See Editor's Note No. 31, page 1820.

Magna Pac Daily Basics - Swanson
Each packet (three softgels, five tablets) contains: Calories 15 • Calories from Fat 15 • Total Fat 1.5 g • Vitamin A (as beta-carotene) 25000 IU • Vitamin C USP (as ascorbic acid) 1 g • Vitamin D (from fish liver oil) 400 IU • Vitamin E (as d-alpha tocopheryl acetate) 400 IU • Thiamin (as thiamin HCl; vitamin B-1) 50 mg • Riboflavin (vitamin B-2) 50 mg • Niacin (as niacinamide) 50 mg • Vitamin B-6 (as pyridoxine HCl) 50 mg • Folic Acid USP 40 mcg • Vitamin B-12 (as Cyanocobalamin) 50 mcg • Biotin USP 50 mcg • Pantothenic Acid (as d-calcium pantothenate) 50 mg • Calcium (500 mg from oyster shell, 500 mg from carbonate, aspartate, citrate) 1 g • Iron (from Albion amino acid chelate) 18 mg • Iodine (from kelp) 150 mcg • Magnesium (from magnesium oxide) 250 mg • Zinc 50 mg • Selenium (from selenomethionine) 50 mcg • Copper 2 mg • Manganese 10 mg • Chromium 50 mcg • Potassium (from potassium proteinate) 99 mg • Lecithin 1.2 g • 72 Trace Mineral compound 72 mg • Betaine HCl 50 mg • Choline (as choline bitartrate) 50 mg • Inositol FCC 50 mg • PABA (para-aminobenzoic acid) 50 mg • Rose Hips (from concentrate) 50 mg.

Magna Pac for Cardio - Swanson
Each packet (four capsules, three softgels) contains: Calories 16 • Calories from Fat 16 • Total Fat 1.5 g • Vitamin E (as d-alpha tocopherol from mixed tocopherols) 400 IU • Thiamin (as thiamin HCl; vitamin B-1) 100 mg • Riboflavin (vitamin B-2) 100 mg • Niacinamide USP 100 mg • Vitamin B-6 USP (as pyridoxine HCl) 100 mg • Folic Acid 400 mcg • Vitamin B-12 USP (as cyanocobalamin) 100 mcg • Biotin USP 100 mcg • Pantothenic Acid (as d-calcium pantothenate) 100 mg • Flaxseed Oil 1 g • Trimethylglycine (as betaine anhydrous) 1 g • Standardized Hawthorn berry extract (1.8% vitexin-2' rhamnosides) 250 mg • Hawthorn berry powder 250 mg • Choline (as choline bitartrate) 100 mg • Inositol 100 mg • PABA (para-aminobenzoic acid) 100 mg • Coenzyme Q10 30 mg • Garlic (500:1 concentrate equal to 500 mg of fresh garlic) 1 mg.

Magna Pac for Joints - Swanson
Each packet (seven capsules, one softgel) contains: Calories 10.6 • Calories from Fat 9 • Total Fat 1 g • Saturated Fat 119 mg • Polyunsaturated Fat 211 mg • Monounsaturated Fat 610 mg • Manganese (Albion® amino acid chelate) 40 mg • Glucosamine Sulfate (2KCl) 1.5 g • Borage Oil (24% GLA) 1 g • Chondroitin Sulfate 1 g • OptiMSM (methylsulfonylmethane) 1 g • Boswellia Serrata powder 300 mg • Boswellia Serrata (65% boswellic acid) 200 mg • Optimum Abzorption™ Complex Proprietary Blend: Ginger (root), Piper longum, Piper nigrum 45 mg.
See Editor's Note No. 15, page 1817.

Magna Pac for Menopause - Swanson
Each packet (six capsules, two softgels) contains: Calories 11.8 • Calories from Fat 10.2 • Total Fat 1.1 g • Saturated Fat 119 mg • Polyunsaturated Fat 343 mg • Monounsaturated Fat 610 mg • Vitamin C (ascorbic acid) 1 g • Vitamin E (as d-alpha tocopherol from mixed tocopherols) 400 IU • Borage Oil (24% GLA) 1 g • Black Cohosh powder 860 mg • SoyLife® Soy extract (3% soy isoflavones) 750 mg • Dong Quai herb powder 300 mg • Licorice root extract (15% glycyrrhizic acid) 300 mg • Dong Quai extract (1% ligustilides) 200 mg • Licorice root powder 170 mg • Rose Hips (from concentrate) 60 mg • Black Cohosh (5% triterpene glycosides calculated as 27-deoxyactein) 40 mg.

Magna Pac for Prostate - Swanson
Each packet (five capsules, one tablet) contains: Calories 14 • Calories from Fat 14 • Total Fat 1.5 g • Saturated Fat 0.3 g • Polyunsaturated Fat 0.9 g • Monounsaturated Fat 0.3 g • Vitamin E (as d-alpha tocopherol from mixed tocopherols) 400 IU • Zinc (from zinc gluconate) 50 mg • Selenium (L-selenomethionine) 50 mcg • Pumpkin Seed oil 1 g • Saw Palmetto (25% fatty acids) 1 g • Pygeum powder 400 mg • Beta Sitosterol (Cholestatin™) 120 mg • Pygeum extract (6.5% phytosterols) 100 mg • Lycopene (Lyc-O-Mato) 5 mg.

MagnaCal - Holista
Each capsule contains: Calcium from citrate (equivalent to 625 mg) 125 mg • Magnesium from oxide (equivalent to 206 mg) 125 mg • Vitamin D (as Vitamin D3) 100 IU.

Magnesium - Source Naturals
Each tablet contains: Magnesium (from 500 mg of magnesium amino acid chelate) 100 mg.

Magnesium Complex - Klaire Laboratories
Each capsule contains: Magnesium Glycinate (Amino Acid Chelate) 100 mg.

Magnesium Malate - Source Naturals
Each tablet contains: Magnesium Malate 1000mg • Malic Acid 825 mg • Magnesium 152 mg.

Magnesium Multi-Min - Nutri-Quest
Each tablet contains: As an Aspartic Acid Chelate (Amino Acid Chelate): Phosphorus 10 mg • Calcium 100 mg • Magnesium 500 mg • Iron 5 mg • Potassium 200 mg • Zinc 30 mg • Copper 250 mcg •

BRAND NAMES

B R A N D   N A M E S

Manganese 30 mg • Chromium 500 mcg • Molybdenum 10 mcg • Selenium 25 mcg • Vanadium 60 mcg • Silicon 0.33 mcg • Lithium 0.05 mcg.

Magnesium-Potassium Aspartate - The Vitamin Shoppe
Magnesium 100 mg • Potassium 100 mg.

Maharishi Amrit Kalash Ambrosia - Maharishi Ayurveda Products
Meda Milkweed • Black Musale • Heart-Leaved Moonseed • East Indian Globe Thistle • Butterfly Pea • Licorice • Vanda Orchid • Elephant Creeper • Indian Wild Pepper.

Maharishi Amrit Kalash Nectar - Maharishi Ayurveda Products
Whole Cane Sugar • Indian Gooseberry • Indian Gallnut • Ghee • Honey • Cardamom • Cinnamon • Dried Catkins • Indian Pennywort • Cyperus • Nutgrass • White Sandalwood • Aloeweed • Butterfly Pea • Shoe Flower • Licorice • Turmeric. Processed in the aqueous extract of: Castor root • Country Mallow • Thatch Grass • Eragrostis cynosuroides • Sugar Cane • Indian Asparagus • Spreading Hogweed • Giant Potato • Winter Cherry • Indian Kudju • Trumpet flower • Premna Integrifolia • Desmodium gangeticum • Uraria picta • Yellow-berried Night Shade • Small Caltrops • Phaseolus trilobus • Teramnus labialis • Bengal Quince • Cashmere bark.

Maharishi Amrit Kalash Sugar-Free Nectar - Maharishi Ayurveda Products
Indian Gooseberry • Indian Gallnut • Cardamom • Cinnamon • Dried Catkins • Indian Pennywort • Cyperus • Nutgrass • White Sandalwood • Aloeweed • Butterfly Pea • Shoe Flower • Licorice • Turmeric. Processed in the aqueous extract of: Castor root • Country Mallow • Thatch Grass • Eragrostis cynosuroides • Sugar Cane • Indian Asparagus • Spreading Hogweed • Giant Potato • Winter Cherry • Indian Kudju • Trumpet flower • Premna Integrifolia • Desmodium gangeticum • Uraria picta • Yellow-berried Night Shade • Small Caltrops • Phaseolus trilobus • Teramnus labialis • Bengal Quince • Cashmere bark.

Male Activator - Sports Nutrition Source.com
Two capsules contain: Niacin 20 mg • Wild Oats extract 200 mg • Yohimbe bark 250 mg • Damiana leaves 150 mg • Siberian Ginseng root 100 mg • Bee Pollen 100 mg • Cordyceps Mushroom 50 mg • Cayenne 50 mg.

Male Advantage - Body Wise International
Three capsules contain: Zinc (Krebs Cycle Chelate) 15 mg • Saw Palmetto berry fruit extract 4:1 (Equivalent to 1000 mg Saw Palmetto) 250 mg • Kava Kava root 250 mg • Alpha-Ketoglutaric Acid 200 mg • Flaxseed 100 mg • Pumpkin seed 75 mg • Korean Ginseng root 75 mg • Siberian Ginseng root 75 mg • Turmeric root extract (95% Curcumin) 50 mg • Damiana leaf 50 mg • L-Alanine 50 mg • L-Glutamic Acid 50 mg • Glycine 50 mg • Pygeum Africana Bark wet extract 150:1 50 mg • Gotu Kola whole plant 50 mg • Bromelain 50 mg.

Male Drive - Dial Herbs
Vitamin E • Yohimbe • Green Oats • Zinc • Siberian Ginseng • l-Histidine. In a base of Velvet Antler, Rehmanniae, Cormus Wolfberries, Astragalus seed, Epimedii, Vaccriae, Cyperi.

Male Ferility Blend - Daily Wellness Co.
Two capsules contain: Vitamin C as ascorbic acid 120 mg • Vitamin E as d-alpha tocopherol 150 mg • Vitamin B6 as pyridoxine hydrochloride 2 mg • Vitamin B12 as cyanocobalamin 6 mcg • Folate as folic acid 400 mcg • Zinc as gluconate 15 mg • Selenium as sodium selenate 70 mcg • Proprietary Blend 610 mg: L-Carnitine as tartrate, Dong quai (standardized to .1% ferulic acid), Coenzyme Q10. Other Ingredients: Rice Flour Powder, Magnesium Stearate, Silica.

Male Fuel - TwinLab
Six capsules contain: Yohimbe bark extract (standardized for Yohimbine) 800 mg • L-Arginine HCl 2800 mg • Ginkgo Biloba extract (standardized for 24% flavonoid glycosides) 60 mg • Natural Vitamin E 400 IU • Zinc (from Zinc Picolinate) 30 mg • L-Tyrosine 100 mg • Vitamin B6 50 mg • Choline Bitartrate 200 mg • Vitamin B5 (Pantothenic Acid) 100 mg • Saw Palmetto (Serenoa repens) extract 120 mg • Phytosterol Complex (providing Beta-Sitosterol 60 mg) 120 mg.

Male Multi Vitamins - Health Center for Better Living
Each tablet contains: Vitamin A (as retinyl palmitate and 50% from beta-carotene) 5,000 IU • Vitamin C (as ascorbic acid) 150 mg • Vitamin D (as cholecalciferol) 100 IU • Vitamin E (as dl-alpha-tocopheryl acetate) 50 IU • Vitamin K (as phytonadione) 10 mcg • Thiamin (as thiamin HCl) 10 mg • Riboflavin 10 mg • Niacin (as niacinarnide) 30 mg • Vitamin B6 (as pyridoxine HCl) 5 mg • Folate (as folic acid) 100 mcg • Vitamin B12 (as cyanocobalamin) 10 mcg • Biotin 100 mcg• Pantothenic Acid (as D-calcium patothenate) 5 mg • Calcium (as calcium carbonate and dicalcium phosphate) 150 mg • Iodine (from Kelp) 50 mcg • Magnesium (as magnesium oxide) 25 mg • Zinc (as zinc citrate) 5 mg • Selenium (as selenomethionine) 100 mcg • Copper (as copper oxide) 1 mg • Manganese (as manganese sulfate) 1 mg • Chromium (as chromium dinicotinate glycinate) 100 mcg • Molybdenum (as sodium molybdate) 20 mcg • Boron (as boron chelate) 300 mcg • Grape seed extract (40% proanthocyanidins) 10 mg • Citrus bioflavonoids complex 15 mg • Rutin 10 mg • Silica (from horsetail herb) 5 mg • Montmorillonite (source of 72 trace minerals) 25 mg • Octacosanol (from rice bran) 2 mg • Saw palmetto berry 50 mg.

Male Performax - PhysioLogics
Each capsule contains: Muira Puama root 500 mg • Oriental Ginseng root (Panax ginseng) (14% Ginsenosides, 3.5 mg) 25 mg • Ginkgo leaf (24% Ginkgo Flavonglycosides, 3.2 mg; 6% Terpene Lactones, 0.8 mg) 13 mg.

Male Potential - Health Smart Vitamins
Each capsule contains: Muira Puama bark 500 mg • Oriental Ginseng (root, Panax ginseng; 14% ginsenosides, 3.5 mg) 25 mg • Ginkgo leaf (24 % ginkgo glavonglycosides 3.2 mg; 6% terpene lactones, 0.8 mg) 13 mg.

Male Power - Futurebiotics
Panax Ginseng (Active Standardized Ginsenosides) 5 mg • Siberian Ginseng (50:1 extract from) 750 mg • Avena Sativa (Wild Oats, extract from) 200 mg • Smilax (Sarsaparilla) 200 mg • Saw Palmetto (extract from) 200 mg • Mexican Yam (extract from) 200 mg • Polygonum Multiflorum (extract from) 250 mg • Astragalus (extract from) 250 mg • Schizandra (extract from) 250 mg • Alfalfa 500 mg • Licorice Root (extract from) 500 mg • Muira Puama 150 mg • Deer Antler 50 mg • Kelp 150 mg • Spirulina 100 mg • Black Cohosh 100 mg • Mullein 100 mg • Ginger 35 mg • Bee Pollen 500 mg • Royal Jelly 30 mg • Vitamin B12 500 mcg • Zinc (Citrate) 25 mg • Glandulars: • Pancreas 100 mg • Orchic 90 mg • Thymus 90 mg • Adrenal 80 mg • Heart 75 mg • Lymph 35 mg • Prostate 35 mg • Spleen 20 mg • Pituitary 15 mg.
See Editor's Note No. 14, page 1817.

Male Response - Source Naturals
Three tablets contain: Vitamin E (as Natural D-Alpha Tocopheryl) 100 IU • Vitamin B6 (Pyridoxine HCl) 25 mg • Pantothenic Acid (Vitamin B5) 50 mg • Zinc (as OptiZinc Monomethionine) 15 mg • Selenium (as L-Selenomethionine and Selenium Chelate) 150 mcg • Copper (as Copper Sebacate) 1 mg • Tribulus leaf, stem and flower (Yielding 200 mg of Furostanol Saponins) 500 mg • Maca root extract (Lepidium Meyenii) 300 mg • Yohimbe bark standardized extract 4% (Yielding 9 mg of Yohimbine) 225 mg • Muira Puama stem extract 200 mg • Oat Straw leaf extract (Avena sativa) 200 mg •

Siberian Ginseng root 200 mg • Damiana leaf and stem 200 mg • Saw Palmetto berry 200 mg • Mexican Sarsaparilla root 200 mg • Ashwagandha root 150 mg • Panax Ginseng root standardized extract 8% (Yielding 8 mg of Ginsenosides) 100 mg • Ginkgo Biloba leaf extract (50:1) (Yielding 14 mg of Ginkgo Flaconglycosides) 60 mg • Stinging Nettle root extract (16:1) 60 mg • Ginger root 60 mg.

Malic Acid Plus - Pain & Stress Center
Two capsules contain: Malic Acid 800 mg • Boswellia 300 mg • Magnesium 100 mg • Chromium Picolinate 50 mcg • Vitamin C 10 mg • Vitamin B6 5 mg.

Malic Acid+ - PhysioLogics
Each capsule contains: Magnesium (Oxide, Aspartate) 100 mg • Potassium (Aspartate) 10 mg • Malic Acid 250 mg • Coenzyme Q10 15 mg.

Maltsupex - Wallace Laboratories
Each level scoop contains: Malt Soup Extract derived from natural barley malt 8 g.

Man-Aloe (Ambrotose with Lecithin) - Mannatech
Ambrotose Complex: naturally occurring plant polysaccharides including freeze-dried Aloe Vera inner leaf gel extract - Manapol powder. Other Ingredients: Calcium carbonate, Dibasic calcium phosphate, Brown rice flour, Cellulose, Silicon dioxide, Magnesium stearate.
See Editor's Note No. 17, page 1817.

Manganese - Source Naturals
Each tablet contains: Manganese (from 150 mg of manganese amino acid chelate) 15 mg.

Manganese Extra - Olympian Labs
Each capsule contains: Manganese Chelate 30 mg • Huckleberry 100 mg • Blueberry 100 mg • Lady Slipper 50 mg • Black Walnut 50 mg.

Mangaplex - Progressive Labs
Each tablet contains: Vitamin C (ascorbic acid) 80 mg • Vitamin D (as Vitamin D3) (cholecalciferol) 50 IU • Vitamin E (d-alpha tocopheryl succinate) 10 IU • Thiamin HCl (Vitamin B1) 5 mg • Vitamin B6 (pyridoxine HCl) 10 mg • Vitamin B12 (cyanocobalamin) 10 mcg • Calcium (calcium lactate 175 mg) 26 mg • Manganese (manganese sulfate 200 mg) 73 mg • Choline Bitartrate 30 mg • Bioflavonoids 20 mg • Horsetail 100 mg • Rose Hips 5 mg • Green Pea concentrate 200 mg • Raw Liver concentrate 10 mg.
See Editor's Note No. 14, page 1817.

MannaBar - Mannatech
Solnuts (Soybeans, Soya, Toasted Soya Pieces) • Roasted Cashew Butter wtih Safflower Oil • Rice Syrup (partially polished Brown Rice, Kojl, Water) • Isolated Soy Protein • Dried Apricots • Dried Cranberries sweetened with Apple juice • Date Paste • Natural Vegetable Glycerine • Raspberry Flavor • Energy Smart (Fruit Juice, Natural Grain Dextrins) • Honey Granola (Quick Oats, Canola Oil, Honey, Lecithin) • Supro Plus Nuggets (Isolated Soy Protein, Rice Flour, Malt, Salt) • Pear Juice concentrate • Nonfat Dry Milk Solids • Rolled Oats • Flax Seed • Whey Protein Concentrate • Wheat Bran • Calcium Caseinate • Ambrotose Complex: naturally occurring plant polysaccharides including freeze-dried Aloe Vera inner leaf gel extract - Manapol powder • Phytosterols from Wild Yam root • PhytAloe Complex Flash dried: Broccoli, Brussels Sprout, Cabbage, Carrot, Cauliflower, Garlic, Kale, Onion, Tomato, Turnip, Papaya, Pineapple. Other Ingredients: Citric Acid, Natural Flavoring.
See Editor's Note No. 17, page 1817.

Manna-C - Mannatech
Vitamin C from Acerola fruit • Ambrotose Complex: naturally occurring plant polysaccharides including freeze-dried Aloe Vera inner leaf gel extract - Manapol powder • Herbal Blend: Boneset aerial part, Lemon Verbena leaves, Sage leaves, Catnip aerial part, Peppermint leaves, Yarrow flowers, Horehound aerial part. Other Ingredients: Sodium starch glycolate, Stearic acid.
See Editor's Note No. 17, page 1817.

Manna-Cleanse - Mannatech
I. Essential Fibers Blend: Whole Oat fiber (Avena sativa), Black Currant seed fiber (Ribes nigrum), Psyllium seed husk fiber (Plantago ovata), Flax seed fiber (Linum usitatissimum), Irish Moss, Carrageenan (Chondrus crispus), Konjac Glucomannan (Amorphophallus konjac). II. Essential Oils and Botanicals Blend: Fenugreek seed (Trigonella foenum-graecum), Fennel seed (Foeniculum vulgare), Ginger root (Zingiber officinale), Rosemary leaf (Rosmarinus officinalis), Neroli Orange blossom (Citrus neroli), Peppermint leaf (Mentha piperita). III. Essential Enteric Ecology and Flora Growth Promotants Blend: Dahlulin (Inulin and Fructo-oligosaccharides), Mannan-oligosaccharides, Beta-glucans Ambrotose Complex. IV. Essential Fatty Acids Blend: Caprylic Acid, Rice Bran concentrate, Linoleic and oleic soy phosphatides, Omega 6 concentrate (from borage seed meal), Omega 3 concentrate (from flax seed meal). V. Essential Live Probiotics Flora Blend: Lactobacillus sporogenes, Lactobacillus acidophilus, Lactobacillus plantarum, Lactobacillus rhamnosus, Lactobacillus casei, Bifidobacterium bifidum. VI. Essential Plant Enzymes Blend: Amylase, Lipase, Cellulase, Protease, Saccharase, Lactase. Other Ingredients: Calcium Monohydrogen phosphate, Plant cellulose, Fractional vegetable oil, Silica.
See Editor's Note No. 17, page 1817.

Mannatonin - Mannatech
Melatonin • Ambrotose Complex: naturally occurring plant polysaccharides including freeze-dried Aloe Vera inner leaf gel extract - Manapol powder • Valerian root • Lecithin. Other Ingredients: Dibasic calcium phosphate, Microcrystalline cellulose tribasic calcium phosphate, Molasses, Wheat germ, Croscarmellose sodium, Magnesium stearate, Silicon dioxide, Calcium silicate, and coating.
See Editor's Note No. 25, page 1818.

Marine Beta Carotene - Jarrow Formulas
Each softgel contains: Beta Carotene (from Dunaliella salina) (Equivalent to 25000 IU of pro Vitamin A) activity 15 mg • Vitamin E 5 IU. Other Ingredients: Soybean Oil, Lecithin.

Marine Beta Carotene 25000 IU - Nature's Life
Each capsule contains: Beta Carotene (Dunaliella salina) (Vitamin A equivalent 25000 IU) (Other natural Carotenoids occuring in D. Salina) 15 mg • Alpha Carotene 500 mcg • Cryptoxanthin 130 mcg • Zeaxanthin 100 mcg • Lutein 86 mcg. Added as a naturally protective antioxidant: Vitamin E (d-Alpha Tocopherol) 1.5 IU.

Marine Carotene - The Vitamin Shoppe
Each softgel contains: 15 mg Natural Beta-carotene equivalent to 25000 IU Vitamin A activity along with other naturally occurring Carotenoids; Alpha-carotene, Lutein, Cryptoxanthin, and Zeaxanthin. No Yeast, Corn, Wheat, Fish, Dairy, Milk, Eggs, Salt, Sugar, Starch, Preservatives, Artificial Colors or Flavors added.

Marshmallow - Nature's Way
Two capsules contain: Marshmallow root 910 mg. Other Ingredients: Gelatin.

Martrim - VitaStore
Cayenne • Ginseng (Siberian) • Guarana (Paullinia Cupana) • Gymnema Sylvestre • Kelp • Phenylalanine • Pullulan • Sidacordifilia

BRAND NAMES

Extract • Zingiber • Vitamin A • Vitamin B1 • Vitamin B6 • Vitamin B12 • Vitamin C • Vitamin D • Vitamin E (d-alpha tocopherol) • Folic Acid • Iodine (Kelp) • Niacin • d-Biotin • Pantothenic Acid • Potassium Gluconate.

Masculex - Enzymatic Therapy
Two capsules contain: Vitamin E (D-Alpha Tocopherol) 100 IU. Other ingredients: Muira Puama Powdered extract 6:1 (Ptychopetalum olacoides) 250 mg • Liquid Liver Fractions (predigested soluble concentrate) 250 mg • Wheat Germ oil concentrate 100 mg • Beta-Sitosterol 100 mg • Mexican Damiana leaves extract (Tunera diffusa) 100 mg • Saw Palmetto Berry extract (Serenoa repens) standardized to contain 85%-95% fatty acids & biologically active sterols 40 mg • Cola Nut extract (Cola nitida) (contains 4.8 mg Caffeine) 40 mg • Panax ginseng extract standardized to contain 7% Saponins (calculated as Ginsenoside Rg1) 40 mg • Ginkgo Biloba leaves extract (Ginkgo biloba folia) standardized to contain 24% ginkgoflavonglycosides 20 mg. Contains no sugar, salt, yeast, corn, dairy products, flavoring or preservatives.
See Editor's Note No. 14, page 1817.

MascuPlex - PhytoPharmica
Two capsules contain: Vitamin E (D-Alpha Tocopherol)100 IU • Muira Puama powdered extract 6:1 (Ptychopetalum olacoides) 250 mg • Liquid Liver Fractions, predigested soluble concentrate 250 mg • Wheat Germ oil concentrate 100 mg • Beta-Sitosterol 100 mg • Mexican Damiana leaves extract (Turnera diffusa) 100 mg • Saw Palmetto berry extract (Serenoa repens) standardized to contain 85%-95% fatty acids & biologically active sterols 40 mg • Cola Nut extract (Cola nitida) contains 4.8 g caffeine 40 mg • Panax Ginseng extract 40 mg • Ginkgo Biloba leaves extract (Ginkgo biloba folia) 20 mg.
See Editor's Note No. 14, page 1817.

Mass Action - Met-Rx
Each serving contains: Micronized Creatine 5 g • HMB 1.5 g • Trimethylglycine (TMG) 500 mg • Improved Nutrient Uptake. Ingredients: Glucose • Creatine Monohydrate • HMB • Trimethylglycine • Natural & Artificial Flavors • Beta Carotene & Beet juice powder for colors • Xanthan Gum • Aspartame.

Mass Fuel - TwinLab
High Biological-Quality Milk & Egg Proteins • Branched Chain Amino Acids (L-Leucine, L-Isoleucine & L-Valine) • L-Glutamine • Alpha-Ketoglutarates • Keto-Isocaproate (KIC) • L-Ornithine Alpha-Ketoglutarate • L-Carnitine • Creatine Monohydrate • High Potencies Of Vitamins & Minerals • Potassium 2000 mg • Chromium 300 mcg (from patented Chromic Fuel Chromium Picolinate). Mass Fuel is rich in complex carbohydrates. Contains no simple sugars & is fat free.

Masters - Pharmanex
Two capsules contain: Vitamin A (100% as Beta-Carotene)(Beta-Carotene, Dunaliella Salina) 3750 IU • Vitamin C (as Ascorbic Acid) 150 mg • Vitamin D (as Vitamin D3)(as Cholecalciferol) 200 IU • Vitamin E (as d-Alpha Tocopheryl Succinate) 150 IU • Riboflavin (as Riboflavin) 0.85 mg • Vitamin B6 (as Pyridoxine Hydrochloride) 1 mg • Folate (as Folic Acid) 200 mcg • Vitamin B12 (as Cyanocobalamin) 3 mcg • Calcium (Calcium Carbonate, Calcium Chelate, Calcium Citrate) 250 mg • Magnesium (Magnesium Oxide, Magnesium Chelate) 100 mg • Zinc (Zinc Chelate) 7.5 mg • Chromium (Chromium Chelate, Chromium Picolinate) 100 mcg • Korean Panax Ginseng with Ginsenosides 25 mcg • Siberian Ginseng extract with Eleutherosides 25 mg • Ginkgo Biloba Powder with Ginkgoflavonglycosides 20 mg • Echinacea Purpurea Powder with Echinacosides 20 mg • Cranberry Concentrate with Quinnic Acid 12.5 mg • Bilberry Powder with Anthocyanosides 10 mg.

Max GLA - PhysioLogics
Each softgel contains: Linolenic Acid 375 mg • Gamma-Linolenic

Acid (GLA) 229 mg • Oleic Acid 190 mg • Palmitic Acid 114 mg • Stearic Acid 41 mg • Palmitoleic Acid 3 mg.

Maxativa - Futurebiotics
Two tablets contain: Oat extract (4:1) 300 mg • Nettles extract (4:1) 150 mg • Glycine 100 mg • Vitamin C 100 mg • Smilax-Ginseng-Damiana Complex 400 mg • Bee Pollen (Lyophilized) 350 mg • Zinc (Oxide, Gluconate) 15 mg • Royal Jelly (Lyophilized) 45 mg • Niacinamide 15 mg.

MaxEPA - Puritan's Pride
Each softgel contains: Eicosapentaenoic Acid (EPA) 180 mg • Docosahexaenoic Acid (DHA) 120 mg. Contains not less than 30% Omega-3 polyunsaturates.

MaxEPA 1000 mg - Nature's Life
Each capsule contains: MaxEPA 1000 mg providing the following naturally occuring essential nutrients: EPA (Eicosapentaneoic Acid) 180 mg • DHA (Docosahexaenoic Acid) 180 mg • Vitamin E (d-Alpha Tocopherol) 30 IU. In a natural base of certified organic Safflower oil.

Maxi-Complete - Atrium Inc.
Each tablet contains: Vitamin A Palmitate 10000 IU • Vitamin D (as Vitamin D2 Fish oil) 400 IU • Vitamin B1 Thiamine HCL 10 mg • Vitamin B2 Riboflavin 10 mg • Vitamin B6 Pyridoxine HCL 10 mg • Vitamin B12 Cyanocobalamin 15 mcg • Vitamin C Ascorbic Acid 150 mg • Vitamin E Acetate 60 IU • Biotin 6 mcg • Niacin-Niacinamide 50 mg • Pantothenic Acid 25 mg • Folic Acid 400 mcg • Calcium Amino Acid Chelate 30 mg • Iodine 100 mcg • Iron Amino Acid Chelate 50 mg • Magnesium Amino Acid Chelate 20 mg • Manganese Amino Acid Chelate 6 mg • Phosphorus 20 mg • Zinc Amino Acid Chelate 5 mg • Choline Bitartrate 100 mg • Inositol 100 mg • PABA 30 mg • Rutin 25 mg. In a base of Alfalfa, Bone Meal, Bromelain, Kelp, Papaya, Rose Hips.

Maximum Anti-Oxidant Formula - Nature's Bounty
Two tablets contain: Vitamin A (as Beta Carotene) 15000 IU • Vitamin C (as Calcium Ascorbate and Ascorbyl Palmitate) 500 mg • Vitamin E (as d-Alpha Tocopheryl Succinate) 400 IU • Zinc (as Zinc Picolinate) 7.5 mg • Selenium (as L-Selenomethionine) 50 mcg • Copper (as Copper Lysinate) 1 mg • Manganese (as Manganese Arginate) 2.5 mg • Coenzyme Q-10 1000 mcg • Pycnogenol 3000 mcg • Quercetin 15 mg • Citrus Bioflavonoid Complex 50 mg • L-Glutathione 1000 mcg • N-Acetyl Cysteine 5000 mcg • L-Cysteine Hydrochloride 50 mg • Green Tea extract aerial 500 mcg • Echinacea root 25 mg • Bilberry leaf 25 mg • Schizandra berry 25 mg • Barley Juice powder 2 mg • Broccoli powder 2.5 mg • Spirulina 2 mg • Chlorella 2.5 mg • Citrus Fiber 50 mg.
Other Ingredients: Cellulose, Dicalcium Phosphate, Vegetable Stearic Acid, Food Glaze, Magnesium Silicate, Vegetable Magnesium Stearate, Silica, Croscarmellose.

Maximum Anti-Oxidant Formula - Vegetarian - Puritan's Pride
Two tablets contain: Vitamin A (as beta carotene) 15,000 IU • Vitamin C (as calcium ascorbate & ascorbyl palmitate) 500 mg • Vitamin E (as d-alpha tocopheryl succinate) 400 IU • Selenium (as l-selenomethionine) 50 mcg • Coenzyme Q10 1000 mcg • Pycnogenol 3000 mg • Quercetin 15 mg • Citrus Bioflavonoids Complex 50 mg • L-Glutathione 1000 mcg • N-Acetyl-Cysteine 5000 mcg • L-Cysteine HCl 50 mg • Copper (as copper lysinate) 1 mg • Manganese (as manganese arginate) 2.5 mg • Zinc (as zinc picolinate) 7.5 mg • Green Tea extract 500 mcg • Echinacea 25 mg • Bilberry 25 mg • Schizandra 25 mg. In a natural base of Broccoli powder 2.5 mg, Spirulina 2 mg, Chlorella 2.5 mg, Barley juice powder 2 mg, and Citrus fiber 50 mg.

Some Brand Name Natural Products - What they Contain

www.NaturalDatabase.com contains MANY more listings than appear here.

Maximum Fat Burners - Optimum Nutrition
Citrimax 500 mg • L-Carnitine • Choline • Inositol • Methionine.

Maximum Strength Flex-A-Min - Arthritis Research Corp.
Three tablets contain: Glucosamine Sulfate 1,500 mg • Chondroitin Sulfate 1,200 mg • MSM 500 mg.
See Editor's Note No. 15, page 1817.

Maximum Strength Glucosamine Chondroitin - Puritan's Pride
Three tablets contain: Glucosamine Hydrochloride 1500 mg • Chondroitin Sulfate 1200 mg.
See Editor's Note No. 15, page 1817.

MBX (Meta-Burn Xtreme) - Metabolic Response Modifiers
Each capsule contains: Caffeine (USP) 90 mg • 1R, 2S-norephedrine (HCl) 25 mg • Coleus Forskohlii (20% forskolin) 25 mg • Naringin 5 mg • Yohimbine (HCl) 2.75 mg.

MCH-Cal - Natrol
Two capsules contain: Vitamin D (as Cholecalciferol) 200 IU • Calcium (as calcium hydroxyapatite) 125 mg • Magnesium (as Magnesium oxide) 300 mg. Other ingredients: Magnesium Stearate, Silicon Dioxide, Gelatin.

MCT Fuel (Emulsified Medium-Chain Triglycerides) - TwinLab
Emulsified Medium Chain Triglycerides (MCTs) • Emulsified Vitamin E. Contains: 100% natural Orange flavor & small amounts of Lecithin & Apple Pectin. MCT Fuel's formula contains no chemical emulsifiers.

Medphen - Olympian Labs
Six capsules contain: Proprietary Blend: Green Tea extract, Garcinia Cambogia, Ginger, Mustard Seed, Cayenne, Astragalus, White Willow Bark, Uva Ursi, Siberian Ginseng, Gotu Kola 3000 mg.

Medroid - Sports One
19-Nor-4-Androstenediol • 19-Norandrostenedione • Androstenedione • 4-Androstenediol • 5-Androstenediol • Tribulus Terrestris • Acetyl-L-Carnitine • Thermogenic Formula using a proprietary half-life enzymatic conversion excelerator. Capsule 1: (Tribulus Terrestris 250 mg, 5-Androstene-3B,17B-Diol 50 mg). Capsule 2: (Androstenedione 100 mg, Acetyl L-Carnitine 100 mg, 4-Androstene-3, 17-Diol 100 mg). Capsule 3 (Proprietary half-life excelerator): (Ma Huang herb 10:1 extract, Green Tea leaf 10:1 extract, White Willow bark, Secret Half Life Enzymatic Conversion Excelerator). Capsule 4: (5-Androstene-3B,17B-Diol 50 mg, 19-Nor-4-Androstene-3B, 17B-Diol 50 mg, 19-Norandrostenedione 100 mg).

Mega B-125 - The Vitamin Shoppe
Each sustained-release tablet contains: Vitamin B1 (Thiamin) 125 mg • Vitamin B2 (Riboflavin) 125 mg • Vitamin B6 (Pyridoxine Hcl) 125 mg • Vitamin B12 (Cobalamin Concentrate) 125 mcg • Niacinamide 125 mg • Folic Acid 400 mcg • Pantothenic Acid (d-Calcium Pantothenate) 125 mg • D-Biotin 125 mcg • Choline Bitartrate 125 mg • Inositol 125 mg • PABA 125 mg. In a base of Alfalfa, Watercress, Parsley, and Rice Concentrate. No Yeast, Corn, Wheat, Soy, Salt, Sugar, Starch, Milk, Eggs, Dairy, Fish or Animal Derivatives, Preservative, Artificial Colors of Flavors added.

Mega C-Complex 1000 - The Vitamin Shoppe
Each tablet contains: Vitamin C (fortified with Rose Hips) 1000 mg • Citrus Bioflavonoids 500 mg • Hesperidin Complex 50 mg • Rutin 50 mg • Acerola 10 mg. No Yeast, Wheat, Corn, Dairy, Milk, Eggs, Fish or Animal Derivatives, Soy, Salt, Sugar, Starch, Preservatives, Artificial Colors or Flavors added.

Mega Chromic Fuel (Chromium Picolinate) 500 mcg - TwinLab
Each capsule contains: Trivalent Chromium (from Pure Crystalline Chromium Picolinate) 500 mcg.

Mega Chromium Picolinate - Source Naturals
Each tablet contains: Trivalent Chromium (from Chromax brand of yeast-free Chromium Picolinate) 300 mcg.

Mega CoQ10 - TwinLab
Each capsule contains: Coenzyme Q10 30 mg. Contains no tablet binders, coatings, or colorings. Free of the most common allergens such as corn, soy, yeast, rice, barley, wheat, lactose (milk sugar), and all milk, citrus, fish, and egg products. No added flavorings, sugars, salt, artificial sweeteners, colorings, preservatives, or salicylates.

Mega Creatine Fuel - TwinLab
Each capsule contains: University-Tested Pure Creatine Monohydrate 1200 mg.

Mega Diet Caps - Puritan's Pride
Three capsules contain: Ma Huang extract (standardized for 6% Ephedra) 334 mg • Guarana extract (standardized for 22% caffeine) 910 mg • Citrimax (Garcinia Cambogia-Hydroxycitrate) 500 mg • Chromium (Picolinate) 200 mcg • L-Carnitine 100 mg • Potassium Phosphate 50 mg • Magnesium Phosphate 50 mg • Green Tea 10 mg • Citrus Bioflavonoids 10 mg • Ginger root 10 mg • Cayenne 10 mg.

Mega Glucosamine 750 - Swanson
Each capsule contains: Glucosamine Sulfate (2KCI) 750 mg.

Mega Manna 500 mg - Nature's Life
Each capsule contains: Glucomannan (Amorphophallus konjac) 500 mg.

Mega Mind - Source Naturals
Four tablets contain: Vitamin B1 (Thiamin) 500 mg • Vitamin B2 (Riboflavin) 50 mg • Vitamin B3 (150 mg Niacinamide and 50 mg Niacin) 200 mg • Vitamin B5 (Pantothenic Acid) 50 mg • Vitamin B6 (Pyridoxine HCl) 50 mg • Vitamin B12 (Cyanocobalamin) 50 mcg • Folic Acid 800 mcg • Biotin 500 mcg • Vitamin C (Calcium and Zinc Ascorbates) 197 mg • Calcium (Ascorbate, Carbonate, Malate, Succinate) 100 mg • Magnesium (Malate, Succinate, Taurinate, Oxide) 200 mg • Zinc (Ascorbate) 10 mg • Manganese (Citrate) 5 mg • L-Pyroglutamic Acid 1000 mg • L-Glutamine 500 mg • DMAE (Bitartrate) 160 mg • Acetyl L-Carnitine 400 mg • N-Acetyl L-Tyrosine 300 mg • Taurine (Magnesium Taurinate) 198 mg • Ginkgo Biloba 24% with a Proanthocyanidolic value of 95 (50:1 Extract) 120 mg • Proanthodyn (from Grape Seed extract) 100 mg • GABA (Gamma Amino Butyric Acid) 100 mg • Coenzyme Q10 (Ubiquinone) 15 mg • Alpha-Lipoic Acid (Thioctic Acid) 15 mg.

Mega Minerals - Nature's Life
Four capsules contain: Boron (Citrate) 1 mg • Calcium (Carbonate, Citrate/Malate) 1000 mg • Chromium (Picolinate {US Patent #33988}, Polynicotinate) 200 mcg • Copper (Glyconate, Citrate) 1 mg • Iodine (Kelp) 25 mcg • Iron (Fumerate, Peptonate) 15 mg • Magnesium (Oxide, Citrate) 500 mg • Manganese (Citrate) 10 mg • Molybdenum (Sodium Molybdate) 20 mcg • Potassium (Citrate) 99 mg • Selenium (l-Selenomethionine) 100 mcg • Silicon Dioxide 20 mg • Vanadium (Vanadyl Sulfate) 20 mcg • Zinc (Picolinate, Citrate) 15 mg • Vitamin D (as Vitamin D3)(Cholecalciferol) 200 IU • Betaine HCl 100 mg • Glutamic Acid 100 mg.

Mega N-R-G Thirty - Progressive Labs
Four tablets contain: Vitamin A (50% as beta carotene) 15000 IU • Vitamin C 600 mg • Vitamin D (as Vitamin D3) 100 IU • Vitamin E 200 IU • Thiamin (Vitamin B1) 25 mg • Riboflavin (Vitamin B2) 15 mg • Niacin (Vitamin B3) 50 mg • Niacinamide (Vitamin B3)

BRAND NAMES

100 mg • Vitamin B6 25 mg • Folate (folic acid) 400 mcg • Vitamin B12 100 mcg • Biotin 300 mcg • Pantothenic Acid (as calcium pantothenate) 250 mg • Calcium (as aspartate) 120 mg • Iodine (from kelp) 150 mcg • Magnesium (as aspartate) 120 mg • Zinc Gluconate 15 mg • Selenium (as aspartate) 200 mcg • Manganese (as aspartate) 2 mg • Chromium (as aspartate) 200 mcg • Potassium (as aspartate) 9.9 mg • Choline 100 mg • Inositol 100 mg • Bioflavonoids 300 mg • PABA 100 mg • L-Methionine 75 mg • L-Lysine 75 mg.

Mega Once-A-Day - Progressive Labs

Each tablet supplies: Vitamin A (as palmitate and beta carotene) 25000 IU • Vitamin C 250 mg • Vitamin D 500 IU • Vitamin E 150 IU • Thiamin (Vitamin B1) 75 mg • Riboflavin (Vitamin B2) 75 mg • Niacinamide 75 mg • Vitamin B6 (pyridoxine) 75 mg • Folate (folic acid) 400 mcg • Vitamin B12 (cyanocobalamin) 75 mcg • Biotin 75 mcg • Pantothenic Acid 75 mg • Calcium (amino acid chelate) 50 mg • Iron (amino acid chelate) 10 mg • Iodine (from kelp) 225 mcg • Magnesium (amino acid chelate) 7 mg • Zinc (amino acid chelate) 15 mg • Selenium (amino acid chelate) 15 mcg • Copper (amino acid chelate) 25 mcg • Manganese (amino acid chelate) 6 mg • Silicon (amino acid chelate) 15 mg • Chromium (amino acid chelate) 10 mg • Molybdenum (amino acid chelate) 5 mcg • Potassium 10 mg • Boron (as boron gluconate) 750 mcg • Choline Bitartrate 75 mg • Inositol 75 mg • Para Amino Benzoic Acid (PABA) 75 mg • Betaine HCl 25 mg • Glutamic Acid HCl 25 mg • Rutin 25 mg • Lemon bioflavonoid complex 25 mg • Hesperidin complex 25 mg. Natural base of: Oat fiber, Alfalfa, Lecithin, Parsley, Bee Pollen, Royal Jelly, and Albumin.

Mega Pak Multiple - Nature's Life

Each packet of nine capsules contains: Vitamin A (Fish Liver oil) 7500 IU • Beta Carotene (equivalent to 7500 IU Vitamin A) 4.5 mg • Vitamin B1 (Thiamine HCl) 100 mg • Vitamin B2 (Riboflavin) 100 mg • Vitamin B6 (Pyridoxine HCl) 100 mg • Vitamin B12 (Cobalamin) 100 mcg • Folic Acid 400 mcg • Niacinamide 100 mg • Pantothenic Acid (d-Calcium Pantothenate) 100 mg • Choline (Bitartrate) 100 mg • Inositol 100 mg • Biotin (d-Biotin) 100 mg • PABA (Para Aminobenzoic Acid) 100 mg • Vitamin C 1000 mg • Lemon Bioflavonoids Complex (TESTLAB) 25 mg • Rose Hips (Rosa canina) 15 mg • Acerola (Malpighia glabra) 5 mg • Hesperidin Conplex (Citrus) 5 mg • Rutin (Saphora japonica) 5 mg • Vitamin E (d-Alpha Tocopherol, Beta, Delta & Gamma Tocopherols) 400 IU • Boron (Citrate) 1 mg • Calcium (Carbonate, Citrate/Malate) 1000 mg • Chromium (Picolinate, Polynicotinate) 200 mcg • Copper (Gluconate, Citrate) 1 mg • Iodine (Kelp) 25 mcg • Iron (Fumerate, Peptonate) 15 mg • Magnesium (Oxide, Citrate) 500 mg • Manganese (Citrate) 10 mg • Molybdenum (Sodium Molybdate) 20 mcg • Potassium (Citrate) 99 mg • Selenium (l-Selenomethionine) 100 mcg • Silicon Dioxide 20 mg • Vanadium (Vanadyl Sulfate) 20 mcg • Zinc (Picolinate • Citrate) 15 mg • Vitamin D (as Vitamin D3) (Cholecalciferol) 200 IU • Betaine HCI 100 mg • Glutamic Acid HCI 100 mg • Bromelain (Proteolytic Enzyme from Pineapple, activity: 225 MCU) 250 mg • Papain (Proteolytic Enzyme from Papaya, acivity 17.5 MCU) 250 mg. In a natural base of Lecithin, Rice Bran & Soy oil.

Mega Plus - Swanson

Each tablet contains: Vitamin A (from fish liver oil) 10,000 IU • Vitamin C USP (as ascorbic acid) 250 mg • Vitamin D (from fish liver oil) 400 IU • Vitamin E (as d-alpha tocopheryl succinate) 100 IU • Thiamin USP (as thiamin HCl; vitamin B-1) 75 mg • Riboflavin USP (vitamin B-2) 75 mg • Niacinamide 100 mg • Vitamin B-6 (as pyridoxine HCl) 75 mg • Folic Acid USP 400 mcg • Vitamin B-12 (as cyanocobalamin) 250 mcg • Biotin 150 mcg • Pantothenic Acid (as d-calcium pantothenate) 100 mg • Calcium (from bone meal) 150 mg • Iron (as ferrous fumarate) 18 mg • Phosphorus (from bone meal) 72 mg • Iodine (from kelp) 225 mcg • Magnesium (from magnesium oxide) 75 mg • Zinc (from zinc gluconate) 10 mg • Selenium (from amino acid chelate) 50 mcg • Copper (from copper gluconate) 2 mg • Manganese (from manganese carbonate sulfate) 7 mg • Chromium (from amino acid chelate) 20 mcg • Choline (as choline bitartrate) 100 mg.

Mega Potency Fat Burner - Optimum Nutrition

L-Carnitine • Citrimax Chromium Picolinate • Chromium Polynicotinate.

Mega Vita Gel - Puritan's Pride

Two softgels contain: Vitamin A (as fish liver oil and 40% beta carotene) 10,000 IU • Vitamin C (as ascorbic acid and rose hips) 300 mg • Vitamin D (as fish liver oil) 400 IU • Vitamin E (as mixed tocopherols) 300 IU • Thiamin (Vitamin B1; as thiamine mononitrate) 50 mg • Riboflavin (Vitamin B2) 50 mg • Niacin (as niacinamide) 50 mg • Vitamin B6 (as pyridoxine hydrochloride) 50 mg • Folic Acid 400 mcg • Vitamin B12 (as cyanocobalamin) 50 mcg • Biotin (as d-biotin) 50 mcg • Pantothenic Acid (as d-calcium pantothenate) 50 mg • Calcium (as calcium carbonate and dicalcium phosphate) 200 mg • Iron (as ferrous fumarate) 15 mg • Phosphorus (as dicalcium phosphate) 50 mg • Iodine (as kelp) 150 mcg • Magnesium (as magnesium oxide) 50 mg • Zinc (as zinc citrate) 15 mg • Selenium (as selenium yeast) 25 mcg • Copper (as copper gluconate) 2 mg • Manganese (as manganese carbonate) 10 mg • Chromium (as chromium picolinate) 3.1 mcg • Potassium (as potassium citrate) 30 mg • Boron (as boron amino acid chelate) 1 mg • Rutin 10 mg • Citrus Bioflavonoids 30 mg • PABA 50 mg • Royal Jelly 5 mg • Choline Bitartrate 50 mg • Inositol 50 mcg • Garlic oil 135 mg • Lecithin 80 mg • Octacosanol 10 mcg • RNA 2 mg • DNA 2 mg • Coenzyme Q10 100 mcg.

Mega Vita Liquid - Puritan's Pride

Each 15ml tablespoonful contains: Vitamin A (as retinyl palmitate) 5,000 IU • Vitamin C (as ascorbic acid) 250 mg • Vitamin D (as cholecaliferol) 400 IU • Vitamin E (as d-alpha tocopherol plus mixed tocopherols) 125 IU • Thiamin (Vitamin B1) (as thiamine mononitrate) 25 mg • Riboflavin (Vitamin B2) (as Riboflavin 5'-Phosphate Sodium) 25 mg • Niacin (as niacinamide) 150 mg • Vitamin B6 (as pyridoxine hydrochloride) 50 mg • Folic Acid 400 mcg • Vitamin B12 (as cyanocobalamin) 50 mcg • Biotin (as d-biotin) 50 mcg • Pantothenic Acid (as dexpanthenol) 150 mg • PABA (para-aminobenzoic acid) 25 mg • Choline Bitartrate 200 mg • Inositol 100 mg.

Mega Vita Min for Teens - Puritan's Pride

Three tablets contain: Vitamin A (100% as beta carotene) 5, 000 IU • Vitamin C (as ascorbic acid) 350 mg • Vitamin D (as cholecalciferol) 400 IU • Vitamin E (as d-alpha tocopheryl succinate) 30 IU • Vitamin K (as phytonadione) 10 mcg • Thiamin (Vitamin B1; as thiamine mononitrate) 4.5 mg • Riboflavin (Vitamin B2) 5.1 mg • Niacin (as niacinamide) 20 mg • Vitamin B6 (as pyridoxine hydrochloride) 6 mg • Folic Acid 400 mcg • Vitamin B12 (as cyanocobalamin) 1 mcg • Biotin (as d-biotin) 45 mcg • Pantothenic Acid (as d-calcium pantothenate) 10 mg • Calcium (as dicalcium phosphate and calcium citrate) 100 mg • Iron (as ferrous fumarate) 18 mg • Phosphorus (as dicalicum phosphate) 20 mg • Iodine (as potassium iodide) 150 mcg • Magnesium (as Magnesium oxide) 50 mg • Zinc (as zinc oxide) 15 mg • Selenium (as selenium yeast) 5 mcg • Copper (as copper sulfate) 2 mg • Manganese (as manganese sulfate) 2 mg • Chromium (as GTF chromium yeast) 20 mcg • Molybdenum (as molybdenum yeast) 20 mcg • Choline (as choline bitartrate) 50 mcg • Inositol 50 mcg. Other Ingredients: Cellulose (Plant Origin), Vegetable Stearic Acid, Cellulose Coating, Croscarmellose, Silica, Guar Gum, Mannitol.

Mega Vita Min for Women - Puritan's Pride

Two tablets contain: Vitamin A (as retinyl palmitate and beta carotene) 10,000 IU • Vitamin C (as ascorbic acid and rose hips) 250 mg • Vitamin D (as cholecalciferol) 400 IU • Vitamin E (as d-alpha tocopheryl acetate) 125 IU • Thiamin (Vitamin B1) 80 mg • Riboflavin (Vitamin B2) 80 mg • Niacin 80 mg • Vitamin B6 80 mg • Folic Acid 400 mcg • Vitamin B12 80 mcg • Biotin 300 mcg • Pantothenic Acid 80 mg • Calcium (as calcium carbonate and calcium phosphate) 500 mg • Iron 15 mg • Phosphorus 225 mg • Iodine

150 mcg • Magnesium 200 mg • Zinc 15 mg • Selenium 100 mcg • Copper 2 mg • Manganese 2 mg • Chromium 100 mcg • Molybdenum 25 mcg • Chloride 10 mg • Potassium 10 mg • Boron 2 mg • Silica 2 mg • Cranberry 25 mg • Deodorized Garlic (Allium sativum) bulb 25 mg • Dong Quai (Angelica sinensis) root 25 mg • Black Cohosh (Cimicifuga racemosa) root 25 mg • Red Clover (Trifolium pratense) blossom 25 mg • Wild Yam (Discorea villosa) root 25 mg • Vitex extract (Vitex agnus castus) fruit 25 mg • Chamomile (Matricaria chamomilla) flower 25 mg • Soy isoflavones 25 mg • Ipriflavone 25 mg • Bee Pollen 25 mg • Royal Jelly 5 mg • Barley Grass 5 mg • Choline 10 mg • Inositol 10 mg • Para Aminobenzoic acid 10 mg • Rutin 25 mg • Citrus Bioflavonoids Complex 25 mg • Hesperine Complex 5 mg • Betaine Hydrochloride 25 mg • Coenzyme Q10 500 mcg • Pycnogenol (Pinus maritima) bark 500 mcg.

Mega-16 Permathene Maximum Strength - CCA Industries, Inc.
Each tablet contains: Active Ingredient: Phenylpropanolamine HCl 75 mg. Other Ingredients: Croscarmellose, D&C Yellow #10, Dicalcium Phosphate, FD&C Blue #1, FD&C Yellow #6, Lactose, Magnesium Stearate, Methylcellulose , Microcrystalline Cellulose, Stearic Acid, Titanium Dioxide.

Mega-Cal Calcium 650 mg - Jamieson
Each caplet contains: Vitamin D (as Cholecalciferol) 200 IU • Calcium (as Calcium Carbonate, Calcium Citrate, Calcium Fumarate, Calcium Malate, Calcium Succinate, Calcium Glutamate) 650 mg.

Mega-Energy - Puritan's Pride
Two tablets contain: Total Carbohydrate 1 g • Calcium 67 mg • Sodium 10 mg • Guarana extract 8:1 seed 225 mg • Kola Nut extract 8:1 seed 200 mg • Royal Jelly 65 mg • Korean Ginseng extract 15:1 root 64 mg • Gotu Kola extract 6:1 aerial parts 23 mg • Alfalfa Parsley blend (Alfalfa aerial parts, Parsley leaf) 16 mg • Barley Grass aerial parts 16 mg • Bee Pollen 16 mg • Disodium Inosinate 16 mg • Suma root 16 mg • Wheat Grass aerial parts 16 mg • Beta-Sitosterol 8.8 mg • Stigmasterol 4 mg • Campesterol 3.2 mg • Octacosanol 1 mg.

Mega-Kid Multiple - Source Naturals
Two tablets contain: Vitamin A (beta-carotene) 6000 IU • Vitamin B-1 (thiamin) 3 mg • Vitamin B-2 (riboflavin) 3 mg • Niacinamide 10 mg • Vitamin B-5 (calcium D-Pantothenate) 8 mg • Vitamin B-6 (pyridoxine HCl) 3 mg • Vitamin B-12 (cyanocobalamin) 10 mcg • Biotin 100 mcg • Folic acid 200 mcg • Vitamin C (calcium and manganese ascorbates) 200 mg • Vitamin D-3 (cholecalciferol) 400 IU • Vitamin E (natural D-alpha) 30 IU • Vitamin K (phytonadione) 20 mcg • Calcium (ascorbate) 21.28 mg • Chromium (ChromeMate yeast-free polynicotinate) 10 mcg •

MegaMind - Source Naturals
DMAE • Acetyl L-Carnitine • GABA • Pyroglutamic • Ginkgo • Lipoic • CoQ10.

MegaMuscle - Life Extension
L-Arginine 5000 mg • L-Ornithine 2500 mg • Vitamin B6 • Vitamin C.

Mega-Stress Complex - Nature's Plus
Each tablet contains: Vitamin C with Rose Hips 500 mg • Pantothenic Acid 200 mg • Niacinamide 125 mg • Inositol 100 mg • Vitamin B6 (Pyridoxine HCL) 100 mg • Calcium amino acid chelate/complex 100 mg • Vitamin B1 (Thiamine) 60 mg • Vitamin B2 (Riboflavin) 60 mg • Valerian root 50 mg • Magnesium amino acid chelate/complex 50 mg • Choline (Bitartrate) 32 mg • PABA (Para-aminobenzoic acid) 30 mg • Chamomile 25 mg • Zinc amino acid chelate/complex 25 mg • Folic Acid 400 mcg • Vitamin B12

from Cobalamin 250 mcg • Biotin 75 mcg. B-Complex Vitamins in a fortified rice bran base. Yeast, sugar, & starch free. In a special base which provides for the gradual release of ingredients over a prolonged period of time for 40% better absorption & utilization.

Mega-Vim 75 - Jamieson
Each caplet contains: Vitamin A (from Acetate) 8500 IU • Beta-Carotene (Provitamin A) 1500 IU • Vitamin D 400 IU • Vitamin C (Ascorbic Acid) 250 mg • Vitamin E (from Succinate) 150 IU • Vitamin B1 (Thiamin Mononitrate) 75 mg • Vitamin B2 (Riboflavin) 75 mg • Vitamin B6 (Pyridoxine HCl) 75 mg • Vitamin B12 (Cyanocobalamin) 75 mcg • Niacinamide 75 mg • Vitamin B5 (Pantothenic Acid from Calcium D-Pantothenate) 75 mg • Biotin (D-Biotin) 75 mcg • Folic Acid 0.4 mg • Chelated Calcium, Calcium (Carbonate) 130 mg • Chelated Iron 4 mg • Chelated Copper 1 mg • Iodine (from Kelp) 0.15 mg • Chelated Magnesium, Magnesium (Oxide) 50 mg • Chelated Manganese 0.61 mg • Chelated Zinc 1.5 mg • Chelated Potassium 2 mg • Chelated Chromium 10 mcg • Chelated Selenium 10 mcg • Choline Bitartrate 75 mg • Inositol 75 mg.

Megavital Forte - Futurebiotics
One tablet contains: Vitamin C 60 mg • Vitamin B1 (thiamin HCl) 10 mg • Vitamin B2 (riboflavin) 10 mg • Niacinamide 25 mg • Vitamin E 15 IU • Vitamin B6 (pyridoxine Hcl) 10 mg • Folic Acid 400 mcg • Vitamin B12 (cyanocobalamin) 50 mcg • Magnesium (oxide, gluconate) 25 mg • Zinc (gluconate) 15 mg • Biotin 201 mcg • Pantothenic Acid 20 mg • Choline Bitartrate 100 mg • Inositol 40 mg • Iodine (potassium iodide) 180 mcg • Sodium Phosphate 500 mcg • Phosphatidylcholine (55% strength) 50 mg • Papain 15 mg • Lecithin 25 mg • Selenium (yeast) 100 mcg • Chromium (polynicotinate) 25 mcg • Betaine HCl 25 mg. In a biological base containing a special blend of: Selenium Rich Yeast, Soy protein, Power Green complex (Barley grass, Chlorella, Alfalfa juice concentrate) & Para Amino Benzoic Acid (PABA).

Mega-Vita-Min - Puritan's Pride
Each tablet contains: Vitamin A (as Retinyl Palmitate) 8,000 IU • Vitamin C (as Ascorbic Acid) 250 mg • Vitamin D (as Cholecalciferol) 400 IU • Vitamin E (as d-Alpha Tocopheryl Acetate) 125 IU • Thiamin (Vitamin B-1; as Thiamine Mononitrate) 80 mg • Riboflavin (Vitamin B-2) 80 mg • Niacin (as Niacinamide) 80 mg • Vitamin B-6 (as Pyridoxine Hydrochloride) 80 mg • Folic Acid 400 mcg • Vitamin B-12 (as Cyanoccobalamin) 80 mcg • Biotin 80 mcg • Pantothenic Acid (as-d-Calcium Panothenate) 80 mg • Calcium (as Calcium Carbonate) 8 mg • Iron (as Ferrous Gluconate) 2 mg • Iodine (as Kelp) 150 mcg • Magnesium (as Magnesium Oxide) 6 mg • Zinc (as Zinc Gluconate) 1.4 mg • Selenium (as Sodium Selenate) 25 mcg • Copper (as Copper Gluconate) 0.07 mg • Manganese (as Manganese Gluconate) 0.12 mg • Chromium (as Chromium Picolinate) 25 mcg • Molybdenum (as Sodium Molybdate) 25 mcg • Potassium (as Potassium Gluconate) 1.6 mg • Boron (as Sodium Borate) 0.5 mg • Choline Bitartrate 80 mg • Inositol 80 mg • PABA 80 mg • Rutin 30 mg • Citrus Bioflavonoid Complex 25 mg • Hesperidin Complex 5 mg • Betaine Hydrochloride 25 mg • Coenzyme Q-10 500 mcg • Deodorized Garlic 1 mg • Korean Ginseng 1 mg • Pycnogenol 500 mcg.

Mega-Vita-Min Multiple - Nature's Life
Each tablet contains: Beta Carotene (Vitamin A equivalent to 5000 IU) 3 mg • Vitamin B1 (Thiamine HCI) 10 mg • Vitamin B2 (Riboflavin) 10 mg • Vitamin B6 (Pyridoxine HCI) 10 mg • Vitamin B12 (Cobalamin concentrate) 100 mcg • Niacin 10 mg • Pantothenic Acid (D-Calcium Pantothenate) 20 mg • Folic Acid 400 mcg • Choline (Bitartrate) 90 mg • Inositol 90 mg • Biotin (D-Biotin) 50 mcg • PABA (Para Aminobenzoic Acid) 20 mg • Lemon Bioflavonoids Complex (Testlab) 15mg • Vitamin C 100 mg • Vitamin E (d-Alpha Tocopherol mixed with Tocopherols) 10 IU • Boron (Full-Ranged Amino Acid Chelated) 25 mg • Calcium (Full-Ranged Amino Acid Chelated) 50 mg • Chromium (Nutrition 21 Picolinate) 50 mcg •

Copper (Full-Ranged Amino Acid Chelated) 200 mcg • Iodine (Icelandic Kelp) 225 mcg • Magnesium (Full-Ranged Amino Acid Chelated) 50 mg • Manganese (Full-Ranged Amino Acid Chelated) 2 mg • Molybdenum (Proteinate) 25 mcg • Phosphorus (Full-Ranged Amino Acid Chelated & Complexed) 19 mg • Potassium (Proteinate) 15 mg • Selenium (Nutrition 21 Selenomethionine) 25 mcg • Silicon (Dioxide) 25 mcg • Vanadium (Full-Ranged Amino Acid Chelated) 25 mcg • Zinc (Nutrition 21 Picolinate) 2 mg • Betaine HCl 30 mg • Nucleic Acids (RNA & DNA from Yeast) 30 mg • CoQ10 (Co-Enzyme Ubiquione) 500 mcg, Essential Fatty Acids (Soy, Spirulina) 25 mg • Super Green Pro 96 (Soy Protein Super Food) 330 Mg. In a natural base containing: Rose Hips concentrate, Acerola, Rutin, Hesperidin, Lecithin, Milk-Free Lactobacillus Acidophilus, Alfalfa leaf, Watercress, Parsley, "72 Trace Minerals", Rice Bran, Spirulina, Barley Green, Psyllium, Apple Pectin, Oat Bran, Bromelain, Papain, Chlorella & Chlorophyll.

Mega-Vite 85 Multiple - Source Naturals
Each tablet contains: Vitamin A (palmitate 10000 IU, beta carotene 2000 IU) 12000 IU • Vitamin C (calcium, zinc and manganese ascorbates) 250 mg • Vitamin B-1 (thiamin) 85 mg • Vitamin B-2 (riboflavin) 85 mg • Niacinamide 85 mg • Vitamin B-6 (pyridoxine HCl) 85 mg • Folic acid 420 mcg • Vitamin B-12 (cyanocobalamin) 85 mcg • Biotin 85 mcg • Vitamin B-5 (calcium D-Pantothenate) 85 mg • Vitamin D-3 (cholecalciferol) 400 IU • Vitamin E (D-alpha tocopheryl) 100 IU • Calcium (ascorbate, citrate) 30 mg • Iron (fumarate) 12 mg • Iodine (from kelp) 150 mcg • Magnesium (citrate, oxide) 20 mg • Zinc (ascorbate) 15 mg • Copper (sebacate) 1 mg • Potassium (citrate) 10 mg • Manganese (ascorbate) 6 mg • Chromium (amino acid chelate) 100 mcg • Selenium (amino acid chelate) 50 mcg • Molybdenum (amino acid chelate) 100 mcg • Boron (amino acid chelate) 1 mg. Other ingredients: PABA (para amino benzoic acid) 85 mg, Choline Bitartrate 85 mg, Inositol 85 mg, Bioflavonoid complex 25 mg, Rutin 20 mg, Hesperidin complex 5 mg.

Mega-Vites 75 - The Vitamin Shoppe
Each tablet contains: Vitamin D 400 IU • Vitamin A Activity 10000 IU • Vitamin C 250 mg • Vitamin E 150 IU • Vitamin B1 75 mg • Vitamin B2 75 mg • Vitamin B6 75 mg • Vitamin B12 75 mcg • Niacinamide 75 mg • PABA 75 mg • Pantothenic Acid 75 mg • Choline Bitartrate 75 mg • Inositol 75 mg • D-Biotin 75 mcg • Folic Acid 400 mcg • Rutin 25 mg • Citrus Bioflavonoid Complex 5 mg • Hesperidin 5 mg • Betaine Hydrochloride 25 mg • L-Glutamic Acid 25 mg • Iodine 150 mcg • Calcium 50 mg • Potassium 10 mg • Iron 10 mg • Magnesium 10 mg • Manganese 6.1 mg • Zinc 15 mg • Chromium 10 mcg • Selenium 10 mcg.

Mega-Zyme - Enzymatic Therapy
Two tablets contain: Pancreatic Enzymes 10X full strength, undiluted & uncut 325 mg: Units of Activity: Protease 96580, Amylase 98780, Lipase 24496 • Trypsin 75 mg • Papain 50 mg • Bromelain (1200 MCU) 50 mg • Amylase 10 mg • Lipase 10 mg • Lysozyme 10 mg • Chymotrypsin 2 mg. Potency levels found at time of manufacturing. In a base of other proteolytic enzymes in a special Bicarbonate Complex. Bicarbonates are key factors in triggering the release of Pancreatic Enzymes. Contains no sugar, salt, yeast, wheat, corn, soy, dairy products, coloring, flavoring or preservatives. See Editor's Note No. 14, page 1817.

Melatonex - Chattem, Inc.
Each tablet contains: Vitamin B6 (as pyridoxine hydrochloride) 10 mg • Melatonin 3 mg. Other Ingredients: Dicalcium phosphate (binder and hardening agent), microcrystalline cellulose (binder and disintegrant), glyceryl monostearate (binder and disintegration retardant), magnesium stearate (lubricant). See Editor's Note No. 16, page 1817.

Melatonin - BioDynamax
Each capsule contains: Melatonin 3 mg. See Editor's Note No. 16, page 1817.

Melatonin - Metabolic Response Modifiers
Each capsule contains: Melatonin (5-methoxy-tryptamine) 3 mg. See Editor's Note No. 16, page 1817.

Melatonin - New Hope Health Products
Each capsule contains: Melatonin (5-Methoxy-tryptamine) 3 mg. See Editor's Note No. 16, page 1817.

Melatonin - Olympian Labs
Each capsule contains: Melatonin 3 mg. See Editor's Note No. 16, page 1817.

Melatonin - Optimum Nutrition
Each tablet contains: Melatonin 3 mg. See Editor's Note No. 16, page 1817.

Melatonin 3 mg - TwinLab
Each tablet contains: Melatonin 3 mg. See Editor's Note No. 16, page 1817.

Melatonin 500 mcg - Nature's Way
Each lozenge contains: Melatonin 500 mcg. Other Ingredients: Magnesium Stearate, Sorbitol. See Editor's Note No. 16, page 1817.

Melatonin Controlled Release 2 mg - TwinLab
Each tablet contains: Melatonin 2 mg. See Editor's Note No. 16, page 1817.

Melatonin Forte - PhytoPharmica
Two capsules contain: Kava (Piper methysticum) root extract (standardized to contain 30% kavalactones) 210 mg • Valerian (Valeriana officinalis) root extract (standardized to contain a minimum of 0.8% valerenic acids) 150 mg • Melatonin 500 mcg.

Melatonin PM Complex - Anabolic Laboratories
Each tablet contains: Melatonin 1 mg • Vitamin B6 (pyridoxine HCl) 5 mg • Vitamin B2 (riboflavin) 3 mg • Vitamin B3 (niacinamide) 10 mg • Vitamin B12 (ion-exchange resin) 12.5 mcg • Calcium (lactate) 40 mg • Magnesium (oxide) 30 mg • Chinese Herbal Complex 195 mg: Valerian Root extract, Zizyphus Spinosa seed, Salviae Miltiorrhiza root, Succinum (Amber), Biotae Orientalis seed, Coptis Chiensis rhizome, Chamomile flower, Hops Strobile, Passion Flower, Skullcap herb. Other Ingredients: Cellulose, Stearic Acid, Magnesium Stearate, Vanillin, Vegetable Oil, Silica. See Editor's Note No. 16, page 1817.

Melatonin Spray - Nature's Plus
Each spray contains: Melatonin (N-Acetyl-5-Methoxytryptamine) 1.5 mg • GABA (Gamma Aminobutyric Acid) 2500 mcg • Pyridoxal-5-Phosphate (P5P) 2500 mcg. In a proprietary liposomal complex of Essential Metabolic Factors, Purified Water, Vegetable Glycerine, Purified Lecithin, Citrus seed extract (Citrus sinensis), Vitamin E & natural Peppermint flavor. See Editor's Note No. 16, page 1817.

Melatonin Tablets, Accurate Release, 1 mg - Nature's Bounty
Each tablet contains: Melatonin (n-Acetyl-5 Methoxytryptamine) 1 mg. Inactive Ingredients: Dicalcium Phosphate, Microcrystalline, Cellulose, Vegetable Magnesium Stearate, Croscarmellose Sodium. See Editor's Note No. 16, page 1817.

Melatonin Tablets, Accurate Release, 200 mcg - Nature's Bounty
Each tablet contains: Pure Melatonin 200 mcg. See Editor's Note No. 16, page 1817.

Melatonin Time Release - 1 mg - Natrol
Each tablet contains: Calcium (as Dicalcium Phosphate) 40 mg • Melatonin 1 mg. Other Ingredients: Time Release Agent (Hydrogenated Vegetable Oil), stearic acid, silica, magnesium stearate.
See Editor's Note No. 16, page 1817.

Melatonin Time Release - 3 mg - Natrol
Each tablet contains: Calcium (as Calcium Carbonate) 63 mg • Melatonin 3 mg. Other Ingredients: Cellulose, silica, stearic acid, cellulose gum, magnesium stearate.
See Editor's Note No. 16, page 1817.

MemorAble - Resource Wellness
Two softgels contain: Vitamin B6 (Pyridoxine HCl) 2 mg • Vitamin B12 (cyanocobalamin) 6 mcg • Ginkgo Biloba extract (leaves) 120 mg • Lecithin 1200 mg. Other Ingredients: Gelatin, Soybean Oil, Glycerin, Beeswax, Titanium Dioxide, FD&C Yellow No. 6, FD&C Red No. 40, FD&C Blue No. 1.

MemorActin - Nature's Plus
Two capsules contain: Phosphatidylcholine 250 mg • Inositol 125 mg • Ginkgo Biloba leaf (standardized 24% Ginkgo Flavone-Glycosides, 6% Terpene Lactones) 100 mg • Vitamin C corn free 100 mg • Pantothenic Acid (Calcium Pantothenate) 50 mg • Phosphatidylserine 25 mg • Bilberry [(Vaccinium myrtillus fruit) standardized 25% Anthocyanosides] 10 mg • Beta Carotene pro-Vitamin A (supplying 10000 IU of Vitamin A activity) 6 mg • Coenzyme Q10 (Ubiquinone) 2.5 mg.

Memorall - PharmAssure
One softgel contains: Vitamin E 50 IU • Huperzine A 50 mcg. Other Ingredients: Soybean Oil, Gelatin, Glycerin, Caramel Color, Titanium Dioxide as a natural mineral whitener.

Memory - ProHerbs
One tablet contains: Thiamin HCI (B1) 25 mg • Niacin (as Niacinamide) 10 mg • Vitamin B6 (Pyridoxine HCI) 25 mg • Vitamin B12 (Cyanocobalamin) 25 mcg • Ginkgo Biloba extract (Ginkgo biloba leaves standardized to 24% ginkgo flavonoid glycosides & 6% terpene lactones) 120 mg • Memorzine (Huperzia serrata moss extract) 25 mcg • Korean Ginseng (Panax Ginseng root standardized to 4% ginsenosides) 100 mg. Other Ingredients: Dicalcium Phosphate, Microcrystalline Cellulose, Croscarmellose Sodium, Hydroxypropylmethylcellulose, Magnesium Stearate, Mineral Oil, Polyethylene Glycol, Stearic Acid, Titanium Dioxide, Sodium Lauryl Sulfate, FD&C Yellow #10 Lake, FD&C Blue #1 Lake and FD&C Blue #2 Lake.

Memory 2000 - Natural Balance
Two tablets contain: Niacin 40 mg • Ginkgo leaf standardized extract 120 mg • Phosphatidylserine 100 mg • DMAE 100 mg • Acetyl-L-Carnitine 20 mg • Vinpocetine 5 mg.

Memory Formula - Youngevity
Ginkgo biloba leaf • Gotu Kola herb • Cayenne pepper • Siberian Ginseng • Magnesium • Lecithin • L-Glutamine • L-Tyrosine • Vitamin B6 • Vitamin B3 • Vilcabamba Mineral Essence: Potassium, Calcium, Magnesium, Zinc, Chromium, Selenium, Iron, Copper, Molybdenum, Vanadium, Iodine, Cobalt, Manganese.

Memory Power - The Vitamin Shoppe
Two tablets contain: Ginkgo Biloba extract standardized to contain 24% ginkgoflavonglycosides • L-Phenylalanine • L-Glutamine • RNA • Choline • Gotu Kola • Lecithin • Ginkgo Biloba leaf powder.

Memory Support Complex - Leiner Health Products
Each caplet contains: Vitamin B12 (Cyanocobalamin) 6 mcg • Ginkgo Biloba extract (Ginkgo biloba) leaf 60 mg • Gotu Kola extract

(Centella asiatica) leaf 10 mg • Phosphatidylserine 25 mg • Phosphatidylserine complex 83 mg. Other Ingredients: Caclium Carbonate, Maltodextrin, Cellulose, Silicon Dioxide, Polyethylene Glycol 3350, Croscarmellose Sodium, Tricalcium Phosphate, Crospovidone, Magnesium Stearate, Hydroxypropyl Methycellulose, Resin, Hydroxypropyl Cellulose, Polysorbate 80.

Memorya - HerbaSway
Ginkgo Biloba • Dong Quai • Kudzu • Rehmannia • Panax Ginseng • Schisandra • Knotweed • Blackberry • HerbaSwee (Cucurbitaceae fruit).

Men Plus Ester C - Nutrivention
Two tablets contain: Vitamin C 300 mg • Vitamin E 200 IU • Choline Bitartrate 150 mg • Inositol 150 mg • Niacinamide 150 mg • Pantothenic Acid 150 mg • Essential Fatty Acids 100mg • Vitamin A 1500 IU • Vitamin B6 75 mg • Vitamin B2 75 mg • Vitamin B1 75 mg • Vitamin D 1000 IU • Biotin 500 mcg • Vitamin B12 500 mcg • Folic Acid 400 mcg • Iodine (Kelp) 150 mcg • Saw Palmetto berry 200 mg • Sarsaparilla 200 mg • Bioflavonoids 150 mg.

Men-Applause - The Herbalist
Dong Quai root • Black Cohosh root • Chaste Tree berry • Siberian Ginseng root • Oat seed • Wild Yam root.

MenoEase - Wellness for Women
Each capsule contains: Black Cohosh (5% triterpene glycosides calculated as 27-deoxyactein) 20 mg • Black Cohosh powder 430 mg.

Menoflash - Olympian Labs
Two capsules contain: Black Cohosh extract 100 mg.
In a base of Dong Quai, Siberian Ginseng, and Passion Flower.

Menopausal Formula - Nature's Herbs
Each capsule contains: Dong Quai 75 mg • Siberian Ginseng 100 mg.

Menopause - Nutrivention
Each tablet contains: Pantothenic Acid 50 mg • Vitamin B6 50 mg • Vitamin C 50 mg • Vitamin E 100 IU • PABA 50 mg • Calcium 50 mg • Iodine (Kelp) 150mcg • Borage GLA concentrate 150 mg • Mexican Wild Yam root 150 mg • Chaste Tree berry 150 mg • Dong Quai root 150 mg • Licorice root 100 mg • Unicorn root 100 mg • Black Cohosh root 50 mg • Passion flower 50 mg.

Menopause Formula - Pharmanex
Each capsule contains: Isoflavones (from Soy extract) 25 mg • Kava Lactones (from Kava Kava root extract) 25.5 mg • Black Cohosh root powder 50 mg. Other Ingredients: Calcium Carbonate, Maltodextrin, Magnesium Stearate, Silicon Dioxide.

Menopause Formula - Natrol
Three capsules contain: Calcium (as calcium carbonate) 250 mg • Magnesium (as magnesium oxide) 125 mg • Soy Isoflavones 100 mg Genistein (10%) 10 mg • Kava Kava 100 mg Kavalactones (30%) 30 mg • Red Raspberry 100 mg • Mexican Wild Yam 50 mg • Licorice root 50 mg • Red Clover 50 mg • Horse Chestnut 50 mg • Dong Quai 50 mg • Black Cohosh root 40 mg • Damiana 30 mg • Vitex (agnus-castus) 25 mg • Gingko Biloba 24:6 25 mg • Gotu Kola 25 mg • Gamma Oryzanol 20 mg. Other Ingredients: Rice powder, Silicon Dioxide, Magnesium Stearate, Gelatin.

Menopause Formula - Nature's Life
Four capsules contain: Black Cohosh root extract (Cimicifuga racemosa) (standardized to provide 2.5% or 4 mg Triterpene Glycosides as 27-Deoxyactein) 160 mg • Vitamin C (Calcium Ascorbate) 1200 mg • Vitamin E (d-Alpha Tocopheryl Succinate) 200 IU • Hesperidin (plant source flavonols) 1200 mg • Women's Phyto-Estrogen Blend (Soy bean, Wild Yam, Rice Flour, Flax seed & Amaranth) 100 mg.

B R A N D   N A M E S

Menopause Multiple - Source Naturals

Six tablets contain: SoyLife genistein-rich Soy concentrate (Yielding 62 mg of Isoflavones: Daidzein 34 mg, Glycitein 20 mg, Genistein 8 mg) • CimiPure Black Cohosh standardized extract 2.5% (Yielding 4 mg Triterpene Glycosides) (Containing 27-Deoxyactein) 160 mg • Vitex extract (Vitex Agnus-Castus) 150 mg • Dong Quai extract (Angelica sinensis) 100 mg • Licorice root extract (Glycyrrhiza glabra) 15 mg • Taurine (Magnesium taurinate) 455 mg • N-Acetyl Cysteine 100 mg • Silymarin (Milk Thistle seed extract) 60 mg • Alpha-Lipoic Acid (Thioctic Acid) 30 mg • Ginkgo Biloba 24% (50:1 Extract) 20 mg • Coenzyme Q10 (Ubiquinone) 15 mg • Vitamin A (Beta Carotene) 13000 IU • Vitamin A (Palmitate) 7000 IU • Vitamin B1 (Thiamin) 50 mg • Vitamin B2 (Riboflavin) 50 mg • Niacinamide 50 mg • Vitamin B5 (Calcium D-Pantothenate) 70 mg • Vitamin B6 (Pyridoxine HCI) 50 mg • Vitamin B12 (Cyanocobalamin) 50 mcg • Biotin 200 mcg • Folic Acid 600 mcg • Vitamin C (Ascorbic Acid, Calcium and Magnesium Ascorbates) 1000 mg • Vitamin D (as Vitamin D3)(Cholecalciferol) 400 IU • Vitamin E (D-Alpha Tocopheryl)(Natural) 400 IU • Boron (Chelate) 3 mg • Calcium (Carbonate, Citrate and Ascorbate) 300 mg • Chromium (ChromeMate Polynicotinate 100 mcg and Chromium Picolinate 100 mcg) 200 mcg • Magnesium (Oxide, Taurinate, Malate, and Ascorbate) 400 mg • Manganese (Citrate) 2 mg • Selenium (L-Selenomethionine) 200 mcg • Zinc (OptiZinc Monomethionine) 12 mg.

Menopause Nutritional System 1 - Schiff

Four caplets contain: Vitamin A (as 50% Acetate & 50% Beta Carotene) 5000 IU • Vitamin C (as Ascorbic Acid) 500 mg • Vitamin D (as Cholecalciferol) 200 IU • Vitamin E (as d-Alpha Tocopheryl Succinate) 400 IU • Thiamin (as Thiamin Hydrochloride) 25 mg • Riboflavin 25 mg • Niacin (Niacinamide) 25 mg • Vitamin B6 (as Pyridoxine Hydrochloride) 15 mg • Folate (as Folic Acid) • Vitamin B12 (as Cyanocobalamin) 25 mcg • Biotin 100 mcg • Pantothenic Acid (as d-Calcium Pantothenate) 25 mg • Calcium (as Citrate) 500 mg • Iron (as Ferrous Fumerate) 7.5 mg • Iodine (from Kelp) 75 mcg • Magnesium (as Oxide) 250 mg • Zinc (as Gluconate) 7.5 mg • Selenium (as L-Selenomethionine) 12.5 mg • Copper (as Gluconate) 1 mg • Manganese (as Gluconate) 5 mg • Chromium (as Polynicotinate) 50 mcg. Potassium (as Gluconate) 50 mg • Choline (as Bitartrate) 25 mg • Inositol 25 mg • PABA (Para AminoBenzioc Acid) 25 mg • Boron (as Amino Acid Chelate) 1.5 mg • Bromelain 50 mg • Papain 32.5 mg • Bioflavonoids (from citrus) 400 mg • Rutin 100 mg. Other Ingredients: Cellulose, Maltodextrin, Stearic Acid, Sillica, Magnesium Sterate, Plyethylene Glycol.

Menopause Nutritional System 2 - Schiff

Four caplets contain: Fennel (Foeniculum vulgare) fruit 100 mg • Black Cohosh (Cimicifuga racemosa) root 100 mg • Anise (Pimpinella anisum) seed 100 mg • Blessed Thistle (Cnicus benedictus) whole herb 100 mg.

Menopause Support - Amazon Support

Each capsule contains: Abuta • Chuchuhuasi • Muira Puama • Suma • Damiana • Maca • Wild Yam • Dong Quai • Mutamba • Licorice Root • Black Cohosh.

Menophase - Futurebiotics

Complex of 4:1 extracts & powders (equivalent to 1700 mg of raw herbs) 450 mg containing: Foti, Peony Root, Withania Somnifera, Dong Quai, Chinese Sage & Carlina Ancalis • Pantothenic Acid (Vitamin B5) 75 mg • Ribonucleic Acid (RNA) 40 mg • Pyridoxine (Vitamin B6) 15 mg • Zinc (from gluconate) 7.5 mg.

Menopryn - Rx Vitamins

Black Cohosh (standardized) 50 mg • Isoflavone complex.

Men's AM Multi - Clinician's Choice

Two tablets contain: Vitamin A (retinyl acetate & 26% as beta-carotene) 3900 IU • Vitamin C (ascorbic acid) 250 mg • Vitamin D (cholecalciferol) 400 IU • Vitamin E (dl-alpha tocopheryl acetate) 150 IU • Thiamin (mononitrate) 1 mg • Riboflavin 1 mg • Niacin (niacinamide) 10 mg • Vitamin B6 (pyridoxine hydrochloride) 1 mg • Folate (folic acid) 200 mcg • Vitamin B12 (cyanocobalamin) 4 mcg • Biotin 210 mcg • Pantothenic Acid (d-calcium pantothenate) 5 mg • Iodine (potassium iodide) 76 mcg • Calcium (amino acid chelate) 4 mg • Magnesium (oxide, amnio acid chelate) 9 mg • Potassium (chloride, amino acid chelate) 12 mg • Zinc (amino acid chelate, gluconate) 2 mg • Selenium (selenomethionine) 100 mcg • Copper (amino acid chelate) 1 mg • Manganese (amino acid chelate) 3 mg • Chromium (nicotinate, amino acid chelate, chelavite, picolinate) 40 mcg • Molybdenum (amino acid chelate) 4 mcg • RoseOx (patented, standardized process for an extract of Rosemary) 50 mg • Citrus Bioflavonoid Complex 10 mg • Saw Palmetto Berries 10 mg • Whole Oats 10 mg • Panax Ginseng Extract 4 mg • Proprietary blend 12 mg: Gingko Biloba Leaf, Echinacea Angustifolia, Panax Ginseng Root, Bee Pollen, Cruciferex, Grape Powder.

Men's Formula - Rexall

Two capsules contain: Vitamin A (100% as beta-carotene, 20% of which is from Dunaliella salina algae) 5000 IU • Vitamin D (as cholecalciferol) 40 IU • Vitamin E (as dl-alpha-tocopheryl acetate and d-alpha-tocopheryl succinate) 60 IU • Niacin (as niacinamide) 10 mg • Vitamin B-6 (as pyridoxine HCl and pyridoxal 5-phosphate) 2 mg • Folic Acid 200 mcg • Vitamin B-12 (as cyanocobalamin) 12 mcg • Biotin 50 mcg • Pantothenic Acid (as calcium d-pantothenate) 20 mg • Calcium (as calcium carbonate, calcium malate, calcium citrate, and hydroxyapatite) 100 mg • Magnesium (as magnesium oxide, magnesium citrate and magnesium chelate) 150 mg • Zinc (as zinc chelate, zinc gluconate and zinc citrate) 7.5 mg • Selenium (as L-selenomethionine and sodium selenate) 50 mcg • Copper (as copper chelate, copper citrate, and copper aspartate) 1 mg • Manganese (as manganese chelate and manganese aspartate) 1 mg • Chromium (as chromium chelate, chromium glutathionate and chromium nicotinate) 100 mcg • Molybdenum (as molybdenum aspartate and molybdenum chelate) 25 mcg • Potassium (as potassium chloride, potassium aspartate and potassium citrate) 50 mcg • Saw Palmetto fruit 200 mg • Dry Fish Oil (omega-3 fatty acids) 50 mg • L-Arginine 50 mg • Bromelain 25 mg • L-Carnitine 25 mg • L-Glutamine 25 mg • Papain 25 mg • Taurine 25 mg • Coenzyme Q-10 2.5 mg • Glutathione 2.5 mg • Vanadium (as vanadium aspartate and vanadium chelate) 10 mcg • Men's Formula Blend: Nettle aerial parts, Oats, Pumpkin Seed (curcubita pepo), Tomato, Alfalfa Juice Concentrate aerial parts, Spirulina pacifica blue-green algae, Grape Seed extract, Lycopene, Alpha-Lipoic Acid, Lutein 205 mg. Other Ingredients: Gelatin, Maltodextrin, Magnesium Stearate.

Men's Formula 800+ Prostate Support - Nature's Life

Two capsules contain: Saw Palmetto berry extract (Serenoa repens B. standardized to 85% Liposterolic Acids equivalent to 1600 mg whole herb) 160 mg • Stinging Nettle plant (Urtica dioica L.) 150 mg • Pygeum africanum H. bark extract (concentrated 130:1; equivalent to 6500 mg whole herb) 50 mg • Beta Sitosterol (Soy oil) 10 mg • Zinc (Gluconate, Citrate, Picolinate) 15 mg • Copper (Gluconate, Citrate) 1 mg • Flax seed oil (Linum usitatissimum L.) 235 mg • (Omegaflo Process Certified Organically Grown) Providing naturally occuring Omega 3 Essential Fatty Acid: Alpha Linolenic Acid 133 mg.

Men's Formula Plus - Swanson

Two softgels contain: Zinc (from zinc gluconate) 15 mg • Saw Palmetto extract (85% free fatty acids) 320 mg • Pumpkin Seed oil 80 mg • Lycopene (tomato) 10 mg.

Men's Mood-Enhancer - HerbaSway

St. John's Wort • Ginkgo biloba • He Sho Wu • Horny Goat Weed • Schisandra • Knotweed • Astragalus • Lycium • Skullcap • Blackberry • Bupleurum • HerbaSwee (Cucurbitaceae fruit).

Some Brand Name Natural Products - What they Contain
www.NaturalDatabase.com contains MANY more listings than appear here.

Men's PM Multi - Clinician's Choice
Two tablets contain: Vitamin A (retinyl acetate & 20% as beta-carotene) 1250 IU • Vitamin C (ascorbic acid) 450 mg • Vitamin D (cholecalciferol) 60 IU • Vitamin E (dl-alpha tocopheryl acetate) 150 IU • Thiamin (mononitrate) 0.5 mg • Riboflavin 0.7 mg • Niacin (niacinamide) 10 mg • Vitamin B6 (pyridoxine hydrochloride) 1 mg • Folate (folic acid) 200 mcg • Vitamin B12 (cyanocobalamin) 2 mcg • Biotin 90 mcg • Pantothenic Acid (d-calcium pantothenate) 5 mg • Calcium (carbonate, amino acid chelate) 84 mg • Iodine (potassium iodide) 74 mcg • Magnesium (oxide, amino acid chelate) 20 mg • Potassium (chloride, amino acid chelate) 16 mg • Zinc (oxide, amino acid chelate, gluconate) 32 mg • Selenium (selenomethionine) 100 mcg • Copper (amino acid chelate) 1 mg • Manganese (amino acid chelate) 1 mg • Chromium (nicotinate, picolinate, chelavite, amino acid chelate) 10 mcg • Molybdenum (amino acid chelate) 2 mcg • RoseOx (patented, standardized process for an extract of Rosemary) 50 mg • Citrus Bioflavonoid Complex 10 mg • Chamomile Flowers 10 mg • Passion Flower 10 mg • Valerian Root 10 mg • Mint Leaves 10 mg • Saw Palmetto Berries 10 mg • Whole Oats 10 mg • Hesperidin Complex 4 mg • Proprietary blend 8 mg: Reishi Mushroom, Shiitake Mushroom, Cruciferex, Grape Powder.

Men's Prime Multi - Swanson
Each tablet contains: Vitamin A (as beta-carotene) 3000 IU • Vitamin C (as ascorbic acid) 100 mg • Vitamin D (as cholecalciferol) 50 IU • Vitamin E (as d-alpha tocopheryl succinate) 60 IU • Thiamin (as thiamin HCl; vitamin B-1) 5 mg • Riboflavin (vitamin B-2) 5 mg • Vitamin B-6 (as pyridoxine HCl) 5 mg • Folic Acid 200 mcg • Vitamin B-12 (as cyanocobalamin) 5 mcg • Biotin 5 mcg • Pantothenic Acid (as d-calcium pantothenate) 5 mg • Iron (from Albion® amino acid chelate) 5 mg • Iodine (from kelp) 50 mcg • Magnesium (from magnesium oxide) 50 mg • Zinc (from Albion amino acid chelate) 15 mg • Selenium (from Albion amino acid chelate) 100 mcg • Chromium (from Albion amino acid chelate) 25 mcg • Green Tea powder 50 mg • Pygeum powder 50 mg • Saw Palmetto Extract (5% fatty acids) 50 mg • Rutin 25 mg • Muira Puama 20 mg • Tribulus Terrestris (20% saponins) 20 mg • Yohimbe powder (4:1) 20 mg • Korean Ginseng powder (5% ginsenosides) 15 mg • Nettle Concentrate (4:1) 15 mg • Pumpkin Seed powder 15 mg • Inositol 10 mg, Bilberry powder (25% anthocyanidins) 5 mg • Choline (as choline bitartrate) 5 mg • Ginkgo Biloba leaf extract (24% flavone glycosides, 6% terpene lactones) 5 mg • PABA (para-aminobenzoic acid) 5 mg • Coenzyme Q10 2 mg • Lycopene Complex 100 mcg.

Men's Support - Rainbow Light
Each tablet provides: Sarsaparilla root 50 mg • Wild Oat green tops 100 mg • Damiana oxide 100 mg • Kava Kava rhizome 75 mg • Saw Palmetto fruit 50 mg • Pumpkin seed 25 mg • Ginseng 25 mg • Selenium 25 mg • Wood Betony 50 mg • Blue Vervain 50 mg • Ginger rhizome 100 mg • Vitamin A 1000 IU • Vitamin E 25 IU • Zinc 5 mg.

Men's Virility Power - Now
Two capsules contain: Epimedium extract 375 mg • Muira Puama 100 mg • Maca 100 mg • Tribulus extract 75 mg • Panax Ginseng 50 mg • Damiana 50 mg • Ginkgo Biloba 30 mg • Cayenne 25 mg. Other Ingredients: Cellulose, Stearic Acid, Silica, Magnesium Stearate.

MenstraCalm - Jarrow Formulas
Four capsules contain: Vitamin C (calcium acsorbate) 100 mg • Vitamin D 100 IU • Vitamin E (natural d-alpha- tocopheryl succinate) 100 IU • Vitamin B6 (pyridoxine HCl) 25 mg • Folic Acid 200 mcg • Calcium (as calcium citrate) 132 mg • Magnesium (as magnesium oxide) 60 mg • Potassium (as potassium chloride) 99 mg • Dong Quai Root Extract 5:1 (Angelicae sinensis) 500 mg • Xiang Fu Tuber Extract 5:1 (Cyperus rotundus) 500 mg • Shu Di Huang 5:1 (Rehmannia glutinosa) 400 mg • Lindera 5:1 (Lindera strychnifolin) 200 mg • Chaste Tree Fruit Extract 5:1 (vitex agnus-castus) 300 mg • Dandelion Root (Taraxacum officinale) 200 mg.

Menstrual Support - Amazon Support
Each capsule contains: Abuta • Jatoba • Suma • Chuchuhuasi • Sarsaparilla • Picao Preto • Tayuya • Iporuru • Cramp Bark.

Menstru-Care - Natrol
Two tablets contain: Vitamin B12 (as cobalamin) 75 mcg • Folic Acid 100 mcg • Calcium (as calcium carbonate) 299 mg • Iron (as iron glycinate) 30 mg • Chasteberry 75 mg • CrampBark 4:1 (Viburnum opulus) 75 mg • Dong Quai 75 mg, Ferulic Acid (1%) 750 mcg • Uva Ursi 50 mg • Kava Kava 50 mg, Kavalactones (30%) 15 mg • Squaw Vine 50 mg • Black Cohosh 20 mg, Triterpenes (2.5%) 0.5 mg. Other ingredients: Mono & Di-Glycerides, Stearic Acid, Croscarmellose Sodium, Silicon Dioxide, Magnesium Stearate.

Menta-FX - HerbTech
St. John's Wort 200 mg • HT-1001 (extract of American Ginseng) 100 mg • Ginkgo Biloba 25 mg.

Mental Advantage + Ginkgo - PhytoPharmica
Each chewable tablet contains: Plumbum metallicum 8x • Ambra grisea 5x • Kali phosphoricum 5x • Ginkgo 1x • Magnesia muriatica 1x • Magnesia phosphorica 1x.
See Editor's Note No. 1, page 1816.

Mental Clarity - Centrum - Whitehall-Robbins Healthcare
One tablet contains: Supplement Facts: Vitamin E 20 IU • Thiamin (B1) 0.55 mg • Riboflavin (B2) 0.85 mg • Niacin (B3) 10 mg • Vitamin B6 1 mg • Folate, Folic Acid, Folacin 200 mcg • Vitamin B12 3 mcg • Biotin 5 mcg • Pantothenic Acid 7.5 mg • Ginkgo Biloba standardized leaf extract 60 mg • Choline 8 mg. Other Ingredients: Dibasic Calcium Phosphate, Microcrystalline Cellulose, Ginkgo Biloba standardized extract, Dl-alpha Tocopheryl Acetate, Choline Bitartrate, Hydroxypropyl methylcellulose Crospovidone, maltodextrin, Niacinamide, Zinc Oxide, Calcium Pantothenate, Calcium Silicate, Magnesium Stearate, Titanium Dioxide, Gelatin, Polyethylene Glycol, Polysorbate 80, Silicon Dioxide, FD&C Blue #2 Aluminum Lake, FD&C Red #40 Aluminum Lake, FD&C Yellow #6 Aluminum Lake, Pyridoxine Hydrochloride, Riboflavin, Thiamine Mononitrate, Folic Acid, Starch, Citric Acid, Sodium Citrate, Cyanocobalamin, Sodium Benzoate, Sorbic Acid.

Mental Edge - Source Naturals
Four tablets contain: Phosphatidyl Choline 350 mg • Choline (Bitartrate) 100 mg • DMAE (Bitartrate) 160 mg • Ginkgo Biloba leaf extract (50:1) 20 mg • Vitamin B1 (Thiamin) 50 mg • Vitamin B2 (Riboflavin) 20 mg • Vitamin B3 (80 mg Niacinamide and 40 mg Niacin) 120 mg • Vitamin B5 (Calcium D-Pantothenate) 120 mg • Vitamin B6 (Pyridoxine HCl) 25 mg • Vitamin B12 (Cyanocobalamin) 50 mcg • Folic Acid 400 mcg • Biotin 50 mcg • Inositol 30 mg • Vitamin C (Ascorbic Acid, Zinc and Magnesium Ascorbates) 150 mg • Calcium (Citrate) 60 mg • Magnesium (Oxide, Citrate) 120 mg • Potassium (Citrate) 99 mg • Zinc (Ascorbate) 10 mg • Manganese (Ascorbate) 5 mg • L-Pyroglutamic Acid 500 mg • L-Glutamine 500 mg • L-Tyrosine 275 mg • L-Phenylalanine 125 mg • Taurine 100 mg • Herbal Formula 595 mg: Siberian Ginseng 225 mg, Gotu Kola 150 mg, Schizandra 80 mg, Ginger root 80 mg, Cayenne 60 mg.

Mentharil - PhytoPharmica
Two softgels contain: Peppermint (Mentha peperita) leaf oil extract 0.4 mL • Rosemary (Rosmarinus officinalis) leaf and stem oil extract 0.04 mL • Thyme (Thymus vulgaris) whole plant oil extract 0.04 mL. Contains no sugar, salt, yeast, wheat, gluten, corn, soy, dairy products, artificial flavoring, or preservatives.

MESO-Tech - Muscletech
Each packet contains: MesoPro (Whey Protein concentrate, specially filtered & new Ion-Exchanged Whey Protein) • Maltodextrin • Glutamine Blend • natural & artificial Flavors • Cellulose Gums •

Some Brand Name Natural Products - What they Contain
www.NaturalDatabase.com contains MANY more listings than appear here.

Vitamin & Mineral Blend • Phenylalanine • Taurine • Guar Gum • Xanthan Gum • Acesulfame Potassium • Aspartame • Carrageenan • Essential Fatty Acid Blend (EFA's): Borage oil, Lecithin, Flax seed oil. Phenylketonurics: Contains Phenylalanine.

Metabolean - Premier Marketing
Each caplet contains: Ginger • Magnesium • Vitamin E • Zinc • Mahuang • Astragalus • Guarana • Bee Pollen • Chromium Picolinate • Siberian Ginseng • Sarsaparilla • Goldenseal • Nettles • Gotu Kola • Lecithin • Damiana • Royal Jelly • Bladderwrack • Blue Green Algae • Licorice.

Metabolic Action - Puritan's Pride
Each capsule contains: Vitamin B6 (as Pyridoxine Hydrochloride) 10 mg • Vitamin B12 (as Cyanocoballamin) 6.67 mcg • Chromium (as Chromium Picolinate) 66 mcg • PABA (Para-Aminobenzoic Acid) 16.67 mg • Licorice (Glycyrrhiza glabra) root 116.67 mg • Siberian Ginseng (Eleuterococcus senticosus) root 66.67 mg • Bee Pollen 66.67 mg • L-Glutamine 33.33 mg • L-Tyrosine 33.33 mg • DMAE (as Dimethylaminoethanol Bitartrate) 33.33 mg • L-Taurine 33.33 mg • Korean Ginseng (Panax ginseng) root 33.33 mg • Suma (Pfaffia paniculata) root 33.33 mg • Schizandra (Schisandra chinensis) fruit 33.33 mg • Chlorella plant 33.33 mg • Gymnema (Gymnema Sylvestre) leaf 33.33 mg • American Ginseng (Panax quinquefolius) root 16.67 mg.

Metabolic Fat Loss - Olympian Labs
Two capsules contain: Chromium Picolinate 100 mcg • L-Carnitine Fumarate 150 mg • Garcinia Cambogia 500 mg • Uva Ursi 150 mg • Vitamin B6 25 mg • White Willow Bark 20 mg.
In a natural base of Guarana.

Metabolic Thyrolean - ProLab
Each capsule contains: Phosphatidyl Choline 12.5 mg • Calcium Phosphate 125 mg • Dipotassium Phosphate 75 mg • Sodium Phosphate 37.5 mg • Disodium Phosphate 37.5 mg • Gum Guggul extract (Guggelsterone) 125 mg • Garcinia cambogia 125 mg • L-Tyrosine 125 mg.

Metabolife 356 - Metabolife
Each tablet contains: Vitamin E 6 IU • Magnesium (as magnesium chelate) 75 mg • Zinc (as zinc chelate) 5 mg • Chromium (as chromium picolinate) 75 mcg • Proprietary Blend: Guarana Concentrate seed (40 mg naturally- occurring caffeine), Ma Huang concentrate aerial part (12 mg naturally- occurring ephedrines), Bee Pollen, Ginseng root, Ginger root, lecithin, Bovine Complex, Damiana leaf, Sarsaparilla root, Golden Seal aerial part, Nettles leaf, Gotu Kola aerial part, Spirulina Algae, Royal Jelly 728 mg.
Other Ingredients: Methocel, Silica, Croscarmellose Sodium, Magnesium Stearate.
See Editor's Note No. 14, page 1817.

Metabolift - TwinLab
Two capsules contain: Ma Huang extract 334 mg • Guarana extract (standardized for 22% Caffeine) 910 mg • Chromium (from Chromic Fuel patented Chromium Picolinate) 200 mg. In a concentrated herbal base of White Willow bark extract & Cayenne.

Metab-O-Lite (Metabolite) - Man-Richardson Labs
One tablet contains: Vitamin E 6 IU • Magnesium (as Magnesium chelate) 75 mg • Zinc (as Zinc chelate) 5 mg • Chromium (as Chromium Picolinate) 75 mcg • Proprietary Blend 728 mg: Ephedra (Ma Huang) concentrate (aerial part) (12 mg naturally-occurring ephedrines) • Bee Pollen • Siberian Ginseng root • Ginger root • Lecithin • Bovine Cartilage • Damiana leaf • Sarsaparilla root • Goldenseal aerial part • Nettles leaf • Gotu Kola aerial part • Spirulina Algae • Royal Jelly. Other Ingredients: Cellulose, Croscarmellose Sodium, Hydroxypropyl Cellulose, Silica, Hydroxypropyl Methylcellulose, DL-Alpha-Tocopheryl Acetate, Magnesium Stearate, Maltodextrin, PEG.

Metabolol II - Champion Nutrition
Each serving contains: Chocolate: Calories 260 • Carbohydrates 40 g • Protein 18 g • Plain flavor: Calories 260 • Carbohydrates 39 g, Protein 21 g • Fat 2.5 g. Ingredients: Metacarb Plus (Champion Nutrition's new longer lasting blend of complex carbohydrates from corn hybrids) • Peptol PER4 + Our scientifically balanced, highest bio-availability protein formulation containing: Enzyme Modified Egg Albumin, Whey Protein Concentrate, Potassium Caseinate, Peptides from Enzyme Modified Lactalbumin, & Pharmaceutical Grade Amino Acids: L-Leucine, L-Isoleucine, L-Valine, L-Cystine, L-Phenylalanine, L-Methionine, L-Threonine, L-Lysine, L-Glutamic Acid • Polylactate (Our revolutionary new liver energy source) • Medium Chain Triglycerides • Metavite Our uniquely balanced, highest bioactive vitamin mineral formula containing: Calcium Carbonate, Pyridoxine Alpha-Ketoglutarate (PAK), Choline Bitartrate, Inositol, Di-Calcium Phosphate, Calcium Lactate, Calcium Citrate, Magnesium Oxide, Magnesium Citrate, Zinc Picolinate, Ester-C, (Esterified Calcium Polyascorbate), Potassium Phosphate, D-Alpha Tocopherol Succinate Esterified Zinc Polyascorbate, Molybdenum Aspartate, Iron Succinate, Manganese Citrate, Niacin, Calcium Pantothenate, Copper Glycinate, Chromium-Polynicotinate • Pyridoxal-5-Phosphate • Retinyl Palmitote, Riboflavin-5-Phosphate • Thiamine HCL • D-Biotin • Potassium Iodide • Ergocalciferol • Folic Acid • Cyanocobalamin • Intrinsic Factor Complex • Succinate ETF Complex Our exclusive Succinate Compound including: Potassium Succinate, Magnesium Succinate, Calcium Succinate, L-Glutamic Acid, Inosine, & Pyridoxine Alpha-Ketoglutarate (PAK) Inosine, Lecithin, Natural Flavors, L-Carnitine, Lipoic Acid, Selenium Aspartate.

Metaboloss - Metaboloss
Ginger • Magnesium • Vitamin E • Zinc • Ma Huang • Astragalus • Bee Pollen • Chromium Picolinate • Siberian Ginseng • Sarsaparilla • Goldenseal • Nettles • Gotu Kola • Lecithin • Damiana • Royal Jelly • Bladderwrack • Blue Green Algae • Licorice.

MetaboMax - Nature's Sunshine
Each tablet contains: Chinese Ephedra (12 mg total ephedra alkaloids) • Bee Pollen • Siberian Ginseng • Ginger • Lecithin • Cordyceps • Kelp • Damiana • Sarsaparilla • Golden Seal • Nettle • Gotu Kola • Spirulina • Royal Jelly.

Meta-Booster - Nu-Creations
Each capsule contains: Vitamin E 6 IU • Magnesium 75 mg • Zinc 5 mg • Chromium Picolinate 75 mcg • Meta-Booster Proprietary Blend 803 mg: Guarana, Ma Huang concentrate, Bee Pollen, Siberian Ginseng, Ginger, Lecithin, Bovine Complex, Damiana, Sarsaparilla, Goldenseal, Canadensis, Nettle, Gotu Kola, Spirulina, Royal Jelly.
Other Ingredients: Dicalcium Phosphate, Pharmaceutical Glaze, Magnesium Stearate.
See Editor's Note No. 14, page 1817.

Metabosurge - Puritan's Pride
Each tablet contains: Vitamin C (as Ascorbic Acid) 20 mg • Vitamin E (as dl-Alpha Tocopheryl Acetate) 6 IU • Magnesium (as Magnesium Oxide) 75 mg • Zinc (as Zinc Oxide) 5 mg • Chromium (as Chromium Picoline) 75 mcg • Proprietary Blend: Ma Huang (Ephedra sinica) aerial (standardized for 12 mg ephedra alkaloids), Guarana extract, Citrus Aurantium, Bee Pollen, Korean Ginseng, Ginger, Lecithin, White Willow, Damiana, Sarsaparilla, Golden Seal, Nettles, Gotu Kola, Spirulina, Green Tea extract, Bladderwrack extract 750 mg.

MetaboTrim - VitaStore
Each tablet contains: Vitamin E 6 IU • Magnesium (as Magnesium Chelate) 75 mg • Zinc (as Zinc Chelate) 5 mg • Chromium (as Chromium Picolinate) 75 mcg. Blended Formula 728 mg: Guarana Concentrate (seed) (40 mg Naturally-occurring caffeine), Ma Huang Concentrate (herb: aerial part) (12 mg naturally-occurring ephedrine),

Bee Pollen, Ginseng (root), Lecithin (vitamin), Bovine Complex, Damiana (leaf), Sarsaparilla (root), Goldenseal (aerial part), Nettles (leaf), Gotu Kola (aerial part), Spirulina Algae, Royal Jelly. Other Ingredients: Methocel, Silica, Croscarmellose Sodium, Magnesium Stearate.
See Editor's Note No. 14, page 1817.

Metabotrim - Pharmanex
Each capsule contains: Vitamin C (Calcium Ascorbate) 75 mg • Niacin (Niacinamide) 10 mg • Vitamin B6 (Pyridoxine Hydrochloride, Pycodoxal-5-Phosphate) 3 mg • Vitamin B12 (Cyanocobalamin, Dibencozide) 6 mcg • Magnesium (Magnesium Asparate, Magnesium Citrate, Magnesium Chelate) 20 mg • Chromium (Chromium Chelate, Chromium Picolinate) 100 mcg • Potassium (Potassium Asparate, Potassium Citrate) 20 mg • Carnitine (L-Carnitine L-Tartrate) 100 mg. Other Ingredients: Cellulose, Magnesium Stearate, Vanillin, Silicon Dioxide.

Meta-Burn - Metabolic Response Modifiers
Two capsules contain: Garcinia cambogia (50%) HCA 500 mg • Ma Huang (8% ephedra) 225 mg • Green Tea (50% caffeine) 100 mg • Caffeine (anhydrous) 100 mg • White Willow bark (2%salicylates) 60 mg • Naringin 20 mg • L-Tyrosine 50 mg • Choline bitartrate 100 mg • Chromium (chelate 10%) 200 mcg • Vanadium (sulfate) 3 mg • Alpha Lipoic Acid 50 mg • Vitamin B5 (pantothenic acid) 50 mg • Potassium (phosphate) 74 mg • Iodine (as potassium iodide) 750 mcg • Cayenne Pepper 10 mg.

Meta-Burn EF - Metabolic Response Modifiers
Four capsules contain: Garcinia cambogia (50%) HCA 2000 mg • Citrus aurantium (6% synephrine) 350 mg • Green Tea (40% caffeine) 225 mg • Phosphate (potassium phosphate) 124 mg • White Willow bark (1% salicylates) 60 mg • Coleus Forskohlii (10% Forskolin) 50 mg • Naringin 20 mg • Alpha Lipoic Acid 25 mg • Cayenne Pepper 20 mg • Potassium (potassium phosphate) 101 mg • Iodine (Iodine USP) 750 mcg • Chromium (as chelate) 300 mcg.

Meta-Dream - Meta-Sure Health
Two caplets contain: Potassium (as potassium phosphate) 160 mg • Calcium (as calcium phosphate) 30 mg • Cellulex Blend: Borage extract seed, Bladderwrack extract, Sweet Clover extract, Grape Seed extract, Lecithin (soy), Ginkgo Biloba extract 250 mg • L-Carnitine 25 mg • L-Tyrosine 70 mg • Collagen Complex 120 mg • Valerian powder root 15 mg • Skullcap powder root 10 mg • Passion Flower powder leaf 10 mg • 5-HTP seed 750 mcg • Melatonin 250 mcg.
See Editor's Note No. 16, page 1817.

Metalogic - PhysioLogics
Each capsule contains: Vitamin C (Ascorbic Acid) 250 mg • Zinc 15 mg • Copper (Glycinate) 500 mcg • N-Acetyl cysteine 200 mg • L-Methionine 30 mg • Alpha-Lipoic Acid 25 mg • L-Glutathione 5 mg • Selenium (Selenomethionine) 75 mcg.

Meta-Sure Metagizer - Meta-Sure Health
One caplet contains: Vitamin E (as d-alpha Tocopheryl) 7 IU • Niacin 5 mg • Vitamin B6 5 mg • Folic Acid 50 mcg • Vitamin B12 10 mcg • Magnesium (as Magnesium Chelate, Magnesium Salicylate) 11 mg • Zinc (as Zinc Chelate) 3 mg • Chromium (as Chromium Aspartate, Chromium Picolinate) 75 mcg • Sure Plex Blend: Guarana concentrate seed (contains 46 mg naturally occuring caffeine), Ma Huang concentrate aerial part (contains 12 mg naturally occuring ephedrines), Taurine, Potassium Citrate, Siberian Ginseng root, Spirulina algae, Ginger root, Green Tea concentrate leaf (contains 2 mg naturally occuring caffeine), Lecithin, Farcinia Cambogia concentrate fruit, Bladderwrack leaf, Inositol, Nettle leaf, Royal leaf, Sarsaparilla root, Cayenne fruit, White Willow bark, Naringen fruit, Hawthorne fruit, L-Methionine, Ginkgo Biloba leaf, Gotu Kola (aerial part) 700 mg. Other Ingredients: Croscarmellose Sodium, Magnesium Stearate, Methocel, Microcrystalline Cellulose, Silica.

Meta-Thin - New Hope Health Products
Two capsules contain: Garcinia cambogia (50%) HCA 750 mg • Ma Huang (8% ephedra) 225 mg • Green Tea (50% caffeine) 125 mg • Caffeine (anhydrous) 100 mg • White Willow bark (2% salicylates) 60 mg • Naringin 20 mg • L-Tyrosine 50 mg • Choline bitartrate 100 mg • Chromium (chelate 10%) 200 mcg • Vanadium (sulfate) 3 mg • Alpha-lipoic acid 50 mg • Vitamin B-5 (Pantothenic acid) 50 mg • Potassium (Phosphate) 74 mg • Iodine (as Potassium iodide) 750 mcg • Cayenne Pepper 10 mg.

MetaTox Oral - PhysioLogics
Each capsule contains: Vitamin C (Ascorbic Acid) 250 mg • N-Acetylcysteine 200 mg • L-Methionine (Zn/Se Monomethionine) 52.5 mg • Alpha-Lipoic Acid (USP) 5 mg • L-Glutathione (USP) 5 mg • Zinc (as Zinc Monomethionine) 15 mg • Copper (Glycinate) 0.5 mg • Selenium (Methionine) 75 mcg.

Methoxy-7 - BioTest
Two teaspoons contain: 5-Methyl-7-Methoxy-Isoflavone 400 mg • Cholesterol 520 mg. Other Ingredients: Purified Water, Fatty-Acid Ethyl Esters, Polysorbate 60, Lecithin, Natural and Artificial Flavors, Potassium Sorbate, Methyl Paraben, Disodium EDTA, Butylated Hydroxyanisole, Sucralose, Vegetable Gum.

MethOxyvone - Metabolic Response Modifiers
Each capsule contains: 5-methyl-7-methoxyisoflavone 150 mg • 7-isopropoxyisoflavone (ipriflavone) 40 mg • Lysophosphatidylcholine 40 mg.

MET-Rx Meal Replacement For The Best Shape Of Your Life - Met-Rx
Each powdered packet contains: Extreme Chocolate: Glutamine 6 g • Calories 240 • Protein 38 g • Carbohydrates 19 g • Fat 2.5 g. Ingredients: METAMYOSYN: Unique blend of Milk Protein Isolates, Caseinate, Glutamine, Whey Protein Concentrate, Egg White • Maltodextrin • Dutch Cocoa (alkali processed) • Vitamins & Minerals [Dicalcium Phosphate, Potassium Chloride, Dipotassium Phosphate, Potassium Citrate, Salt, Sodium Citrate, Magnesium Oxide, Choline Bitartrate, Ascorbic Acid, d- Alpha Tocopheryl Acetate, Ferrous Fumarate, Niacinamide, Vitamin A Palmitate, Zinc Oxide, Calcium Pantothenate, Vitamin K, Manganese Sulfate, Vitamin D (as Vitamin D3), Copper Sulfate, Pyridoxine Hydrochloride, Riboflavin, Thiamine Hydrochloride, Chromium Picolinate, Cobalamin Concentrate (Vitamin B12), Folic Acid, Biotin, Sodium Molybdate, Sodium Selenite, Potassium Iodide] • Natural & Artificial Flavors • Partially Hydrogenated Coconut oil • Corn Syrup Solids • Cellulose Gum • Xanthan Gum • Aspartame • Carrageenan • Beta Carotene • Acesulfame Potassium • Lecithin • Mono & Diglycerides. Original: Calories 260 • Protein 37 g, • Carbohydrates 24 g • Fat 2 g. Ingredients: METAMYOSYN: Unique blend of Milk Protein Isolates, Caseinate, Glutamine, Whey Protein Concentrate, Egg White, Maltodextrin • Vitamins & Minerals [Dicalcium Phosphate, Potassium Chloride, Dipotassium Phosphate, Potassium Citrate, Salt, Sodium Citrate, Magnesium Oxide, Choline Bitartrate, Ascorbic Acid, d-Alpha Tocopheryl Acetate, Ferrous Fumarate, Niacinamide, Vitamin A Palmitate, Zinc Oxide, Calcium Pantothenate, Vitamin K, Manganese Sulfate, Vitamin D (as Vitamin D3), Copper Sulfate, Pyridoxine Hydrochloride, Riboflavin, Thiamine Hydrochloride, Chromium Picolinate, Cobalamin Concentrate (Vitamin B12), Folic Acid, Biotin, Sodium Molybdate, Sodium Selenite, Potassium Iodide] • Natural & Atrificial Flavors • Corn Syrup Solids • Cellulose Gum • Xanthan Gum • Aspartame • Carrageenan • Beta Carotene • Acesulfame Potassium • Lecithin • Mono & Diglycerides. White Chocolate Mocha: Calories 250 • Protein 37 g • Carbohydrates 22 g • Fat 2 g. Ingredients: METAMYOSYN: Unique blend of Milk Protein Isolates, Caseinate, Glutamine, Whey Protein Concentrate, Egg White, Maltodextrin • Vitamins & Minerals [Dicalcium Phosphate, Potassium Chloride, Dipotassium Phosphate, Potassium Citrate, Salt, Sodium Citrate, Magnesium Oxide, Choline Bitartrate, Ascorbic Acid,

d-Alpha Tocopheryl Acetate, Ferrous Fumarate, Niacinamide, Vitamin A Palmitate, Zinc Oxide, Calcium Pantothenate, Vitamin K, Manganese Sulfate, Vitamin D (as Vitamin D3), Copper Sulfate, Pyridoxine Hydrochloride, Riboflavin, Thiamine Hydrochloride, Chromium Picolinate, Cobalamin Concentrate (Vitamin B12), Folic Acid, Biotin, Sodium Molybdate, Sodium Selenite, Potassium Iodide] • Natural & Artificial Flavors • Soluble Coffee • Dutch Cocoa (alkali processed) • Partially Hydrogenated Coconut oil • Corn Syrup Solids • Cellulose Gum • Xanthan Gum • Aspartame • Carrageenan • Beta Carotene • Acesulfame Potassium • Lecithin • Mono & Diglycerides.

MGN3 (MGN-3, MGN 3) - LaneLabs
Two capsules contain: MGN-3 proprietary blend 500 mg: Rice Bran, Hyphomycetes Mycelia extract, Beet Root Fiber, Calcium Phosphate, Silica, Magnesium Stearate, Gelatin, Water, Glycerin.

Microhydrin - Royal BodyCare
Each capsule contains: Silica hydride powder 250 mg • Flanaga Microclusters (Silica, Potassium Carbonate, Magnesium Sulfate) • Rice flour • Rice Bran oil.

Mid-Life - Aspen Group, Inc.
Each tablet contains: The compounds Triterpine Glycosides, standardized at 1 mg - derived from approximately 40 mg of Cimicufuga Racemosa root & rhizome. MID-LIFE contains natural plant extracts from Cimicufuga Racemosa.

Midlife Care - Health Factor
Each capsule contains: Oat Straw extract (10:1) (Avena sativa) 250 mg • Dong Quai extract (4:1) (Angelica sinensis) 100 mg • Black Cohosh extract (4:1) (Cimicifuga racemosa) 80 mg • Licorice extract (4:1) (Glycyrrhiza glabra) 70 mg • Chasteberry (Vitex agnus-castus) 50 mg • Pomegranate (Punica granatum) 39.5 mg.

Mid-Life Creme - Aspen Group, Inc.
Aloe Vera gel in Distilled Water with Catalyst Altered Normalizer • d-Alpha-Tocopherol & mixed Tocopherols • Cetyl Alcohol • Almond oil • Ociyl Palmitate • Panthenol • Peg 8 Stearate • Hydrogenated Vegetable oil • Glycerine • extract of Wild Yam • Micronized Progesterone • Polysorbate 60 • Propylene Glycol • Hyaluronic Acid • oil of Lemon • Keratin • Carbomer 940 • Grapefruit seed extract.

MigraActin - Nature's Plus
Two capsules contain: Feverfew [(Tanacetum parthenium leaf) standardized 1.2% Parthenolide] 700 mg • Pantothenic Acid 50 mg • Ginkgo Biloba leaf (standardized 24% Ginkgo Flavone-Glycosides, 6% Terpene Lactones) 10 mg • Bioperine [(Piper nigrum fruit) standardized 95% 1-Piperoylpiperidine] 5 mg • Trimethylglycine (TMG) 5 mg.

Migraban Feverfew - Jamieson
Each tablet contains: Dried Feverfew leaf (Tanacetum parthenium L.) (Equivalent to 250 mcg of Parthenolide with a complete active sesquiterpene lactone complex) 125 mg.

Migracare - Enzymatic Therapy
Each capsule contains: Feverfew extract (Tanacetum parthenium) standardized to contain 0.6% Parthenolide 100 mg.

MigraDaily - NatureWell Inc.
Each tablet contains: Magnesium (as magnesium oxide) 180 mg • Vitamin B-2 (riboflavin) 200 mg • Vitamin B-1 (thiamin) 15 mg • Feverfew powder 25 mg • White Willow Bark powder 15 mg.

Migra-Ease - Optimum Nutrition
Feverfew • White Willow.

Migra-Lieve - Natural Science Corp. of America
Two caplets contain: Feverfew Extract (Tanacetum parthenium, standardized to 0.7% Parthenolide) 100 mg • Magnesium (Citrate/Oxide 1:1) 300 mg • Riboflavin (Vitamin B2) 400 mg. Contains no yeast, milk, corn, wheat, gluten, soy sodium, salt, sugar, flavorings, preservatives, artificial colors.

Migraplex - PharmAssure
Two tablets contain: Riboflavin (B2) 50mg • Magnesium (as Magnesium stearate) 200 mg • Ginger Root Extract (Zingiber officinale) 150 mg • Feverfew Leaves Extract (Tanacetum parthenium; 0.5% Parthenolide=0.75mg) 150 mg. Other ingredients: Dicalcium Phosphate, Cellulose.

Migraway - PhysioLogics
Each capsule contains: Riboflavin (Vitamin B2) 100 mg • Vitamin B6 (as Pyridoxine Hydrochloride) 20 mg • Ginger root (5% Gingerols, 7.5 mg) 150 mg • Feverfew leaf (1.2% Parthenolides, 0.6 mg) 50 mg • White Willow bark (7.5% Salicin, 3.75 mg) 50 mg • Ginkgo leaf (24% Ginkgoflavonglycosides, 9.6 mg; 6% Terpene Lactones, 2.4 mg) 40 mg.

Migra-X - Olympian Labs
Two capsules contain: Feverfew extract 600 mg. In a 300 mg natural base of Ginkgo Biloba extract, Gotu Kola, and White Willow Bark.

Migrelief - Quantum
Each capsule contains: DHEA (Dehydroepiandrosterone) 25 mg • White Willow extract (4:1) (Salix alba) 125 mg • Meadowsweet extract (4:1) (Filipendula ulmaria) 125 mg • Feverfew (4:1) extract (Tanacetum parthenium) 75 mg. Standardized 4% Parthenolide I in a base of Vegetable Sterine & Magnesium Stearate.

Milagro For Men - Changes - TwinLab
Four caplets contain: Zinc (from Zinc Citrate) 30 mg • L-Arginine Hydrochloride 2800 mg • African Yohimbe bark standardized extract (2% yohimbine) (Pausinystalia johimbe) 800 mg • DHEA (Dehydroepiandrosterone) 50 mg • Global Male Herbal Blend 300 mg: Damiana leaf (Turnera aphrodisiaca), Muira Puama bark (Ptychopetalum olacoides), Jamaica Ginger root (Zingiber officinale), Mucuna pruriens seed, Withania somnifera root, Tinospora cordifolia leaf, Licorice root (Glycyrrhiza uralensis), Tribulus terrestris root, Nutmeg fruit (Myristica fragans), Korean Ginseng (Panax ginseng), Siberian Ginseng (Acanthopanax senticosus), Chinese Red Panax Ginseng (Panax ginseng), Manchurian Tienchi Ginseng (Panax notoginseng), Oat Straw (Avena sativa), Stinging Nettle (Urtica dioica). Other Ingredients: Calcium Phosphate, Vegetable Cellulose, Fractionated Vegetable Oil, Silica, and Vita-Lok Vegetable Resin Glaze.

Milagro For Women - Changes - TwinLab
Four caplets contain: Vitamin E (as natural D-Alpha Tocopheral Succinate) 400 IU • Soy phytoestrogens concentrate (providing 80 mg isoflavones as daidzin and daidzein, genistin and genistein, glycitin and glycetein) 2670 mg • DHEA (Dehydroepiandrosterone) 50 mg • Global Female Herbal Blend 500 mg: Wild Yam (Discorea villosa), Red Clover blossom (Trifolium pratense), Damiana leaf (Turnera aphrodisiaca), Squaw Vine (Mitchella repens), Jamaica Ginger root (Zingiber officinale), Tribulus terrestris root, Licorice root (Glycyrrhiza uralensis), Fennel seed (Foeniculum vulgare), Magnolia bark (Magnolia officinalis), Korean Ginseng root (Panax ginseng), Siberian Ginseng root (Acanthopanax ginseng), Chinese Red Panax Ginseng root (Panax ginseng), Manchurian Tienchi Ginseng (Panax notoginseng), Black Cohosh root (Cimicifuaga racemosa), Oat Straw (Avena sativa), Stinging Nettle (Urtica dioica). Other ingredients: Dicalcium Phosphate, Vegatable cellulose, Fractionated vegetable oil, Silica, and Vita-Lok.

Mild Child - The Herbalist
Catnip leaf • Fennel seed • Chamomile flower • Lemon Balm leaf.

Milk Thistle - BioDynamax
Each tablet contains: Milk Thistle 175 mg.

Milk Thistle - Leiner Health Products
Each softgel contains: Milk Thistle extract (Silybum marianum) fruit 150 mg. Other Ingredients: Soybean Oil, Gelatin, Glycerin, Yellow Beeswax, Lecithin, Polysorbate 80, Caramel, Titanium Dioxide, Red 40, Blue 1.

Milk Thistle - Pharmanex
Each capsule contains: Milk Thistle seed extract (Silybum marianum) (30:1) 175 mg. Other Ingredients: Rice Flour, Gelatin, Magnesium Stearate, Silicon Dioxide.

Milk Thistle Combination - Swanson
Each capsule contains: Milk Thistle seed extract (standardized to 80% silymarin) 175 mg • Dandelion root 85 mg • Black Radish root 60 mg • Burdock root 60 mg • Ginger root 60 mg • Parsley root 35 mg.

Milk Thistle Formula - Quest
Each caplet contains: Milk Thistle seed powder (Silybum marianum) (provided by 60 mg of P.E. 1:8) 480 mg • Butternut bark of root powder (Juglans cineraria) 155 mg • Dandelion root powder (Taraxacum oficinale) 155 mg • Licorice root powder (Glycyrrhiza glabra) 40 mg • Wild Yam root powder (Dioscorea villosa) 10 mg. Other Ingredients: Calcium Phosphate, Microcrystalline Cellulose, Vegetable Stearin, Croscarmellose Sodium, Magnesium Stearate (vegetable source).

Milk Thistle Seed - Gaia Herbs
Milk Thistle seed (Standardized for 80% silymarins) Standardized Full Spectrum 150 mg of extract per capsule. Guaranteed Potency 75 mg of extract per capsule.

Milk-Based Soy-Free Lactobacillus Acidophilus - Nature's Life
Two tablespoons (1 fl.oz or 29.6 ml) contain: Purified Water • Non-fat Milk powder • viable Lactobacillus Acidophilus Culture.

Milk-Zyme - Atrium Inc.
Each capsule contains: Lactase 30 mg • Rennin 10 mg.

Min-Chex - Standard Process
Each capsule contains: Bovine Orchic Cytosol extract 95 mg • Niacinamide 25 mg • Vitamin B6 5 mg. Other Ingredients: Calcium lactate, Kelp powder, Vacuum Dried Bovine and Ovine Spleen, Magnesium citrate, Manganese lactate, Bone Liver powder, Vacuum Dried Porcine Stomach, Processed Soy Bean powder, Potassium Para-Aminobenzoate, Pyridoxine Hydrochloride, Defatted Wheat Germ, Vacuum Dried Bovine Brain, and Ascorbic acid.
See Editor's Note No. 14, page 1817.

Mind & Memory - Health Factor
Each capsule contains: Ginkgo Biloba extract (4:1) (standardized extract to 24% Gingkoflavonglycosides) 160 mg • Gotu Kola extract (4:1) (Hydrocotyle asaitica) 150 mg • Rosemary (Rosmarinus officinalis) 150 mg.

Minerogen - ANS
Each capsule contains: Calcium 200 mg • Magnesium 75 mg • Copper 250 mcg • Chromium 25 mcg • Manganese 100 mcg • Molybdenum 50 mcg • Selenium 25 mcg • Potassium 100 mg • Vanadium 25 mcg • Boron 1 mg • Zinc 7.5 mg.

Mintacin - Enzymatic Therapy
Each capsule contains: Active ingredient: Simethicone 25 mg. Other ingredients: Peppermint oil extract (Mentha piperita) 0.2 mL. Contains no sugar, salt, yeast, wheat, corn, soy, dairy products, coloring, flavoring or preservatives. Chlorophyll is used as a nautral coloring agent.

Mission Prenatal - Mission Pharmacal
Each tablet contains: Vitamin A 4000 IU • Vitamin C 100 mg • Vitamin D (as Vitamin D3) 400 IU • Vitamin B1 4.7 mg • Vitamin B2 2 mg • Vitamin B3 10 mg • Vitamin B6 2.8 mg • Folate 0.4 mg • Vitamin B12 2 mcg • Vitamin B5 1 mg • Calcium 50 mg • Iron 29.5 mg. Other Ingredients: Sugar, Microcrystalline Cellulose, Color, Povidone, Croscarmellose Sodium, Magnesium Stearate, FD & C Red 40 Lake, Food Glaze, Carnauba Wax, Cholecalciferol, White Beeswax, Sodium Benzoate, Cyanocobalamin.

Mission Prenatal FA - Mission Pharmacal
Each tablet contains: Vitamin A 4000 IU • Vitamin C 100 mg • Vitamin D (as Vitamin D3) 400 IU • Vitamin B1 4.7 mg • Vitamin B2 2 mg • Vitamin B3 10 mg • Vitamin B6 10 mg • Folate 0.8 mg • Vitamin B12 2 mcg • Vitamin B5 1 mg • Calcium 50 mg • Iron 29.5 mg • Zinc 15 mg. Other Ingredients: Sugar, Microsrystalline Cellulose, Color, Magnesium Stearate, Croscarmellose Sodium, Povidone, Food Glaze, Blue 1 Lake, Carnauba Wax, Sodium Benzoate, White Beeswax, Cholecalciferol, Cyanocobalamin.

Mission Prenatal HP - Mission Pharmacal
Each tablet contains: Vitamin A 4000 IU • Vitamin C 100 mg • Vitamin D (Vitamin D3; Cholecalciferol) 400 IU • Vitamin B1 4 mg • Vitamin B2 2 mg • Vitamin B3 10 mg • Vitamin B6 20 mg • Folate 0.8 mg • Vitamin B12 (Cyanocobalamin) 2 mcg • Vitamin B5 1 mg • Calcium 50 mg • Iron 29.5 mg. Other Ingredients: Sugar, Microcrystalline Cellulose, Color, Magnesium Stearate, Croscarmellose Sodium, Povidone, FD & C Yellow 5 Lake, Food Glaze, FD & C Blue 1 Lake, Sodium Benzoate, Carnauba Wax, FD & C Yellow 6 Lake, White Beeswax.

MI-T-Cell - Progressive Labs
Each capsule contains: Vitamin C (ascorbyl palmitate) 50 mg • Vitamin E Succinate 30 mg • Thiamin HCl (Vitamin B1) 5 mg • Riboflavin (Vitamin B2) 5 mg • Magnesium (as magnesium malate) 50 mg • L-Glutathione 50 mg • N-Acetyl-Carnitine 30 mg • N-Acetyl Cysteine 50 mg • CoEnzyme Q10 10 mg • Lipoic Acid 50 mg • L-Isoleucine 225 mcg • Red Grape skin (Vitis vinifera) 2% polyphenols 50 mg.

Mixed Greens - Health Smart Vitamins
Each capsule contains: Broccoli aerial parts (2% glucosinolates, 2 mg) 100 mg • Tea green, leaf (50% polyphenols, 50 mg) 100 mg • Tomato fruit (1% lycopene, 0.5 mg) 50 mg • Calendula flower (5% lutein, 1.9 mg) 38 mg • Garlic bulb (10,000 mcg allicin/g, 250 mg) 25 mg • Ginger root (5% gingerols, 1.25 mg) 25 mg • Milk Thistle seed (80% silymarin, 20 mg) 25 mg • Red Grape (Vitis vinifera, skin; 30% anthocyanidins, 7.5 mg) 25 mg • Soy Isoflavones bean (5% isoflavones, 1.25 mg) 25 mg • Turmeric root (95% curcumin, 23.75 mg) 25 mg.

Mixed Vegetable Phytonutrients - Leiner Health Products
Two tablets contain: Lutein 3000 mcg • Lycopene 1000 mcg • Sulforaphane 33 mcg • Zeaxanthin 150 mcg. Other Ingredients: Calcium Carbonate, Broccoli, Carrot, Spinach, Tomato, Cellulose, Maltodextrin, Gelatin, Lutein/Lycopene Suspension, Sucrose, Starch, Hydroxypropyl Methylcellulose, Titanium Dioxide, Hydroxypropyl Cellulose, Crospovidone, Silicon Dioxide, Pharmaceutical Glaze, Polyethylene Glycol 3350, Ascorbyl Palmitate, Tocopherols, Magnesium Stearate, Polysorbate 80, Yellow 6 Lake, Blue 2 Lake.

Mixed Vegetables - Nature's Plus
Three tablets contain: Broccoli floret (Brassica oleracea) naturally rich in sulorophane & indole-3-carbinol equivalent to 10000 mg fresh broccoli 1000 mg • Spinach leaf (Spinacia oleracea) naturally rich in monoterpenes equivalent to 1000 mg fresh Spinach 100 mg • Carrot root (Daucus carota) naturally rich in carotenoids, coumarins & Polyacetylenes equivalent to 1000 mg fresh Carrot 100 mg • Cabbage leaf (Brassica chinensis) naturally rich in Sterols, Phenolic Acids &

BRAND NAMES

Indoles equivalent to 1000 mg. fresh Cabbage 100 mg. Contains no yeast, wheat, corn, soy, milk, salt, sugar or starch.

Modrenal GF - PhysioLogics
Three caplets contain: Vitamin B1 (Thiamine HCI) 40 mg • Vitamin B2 (Riboflavin) 30 mg • Vitamin B5 (Calcium Pantothenate) 150 mg • Vitamin B6 (Pyridoxine HCI) 25 mg • Vitamin B12 (Cyanocobalamin) 30 mcg • Vitamin C (Ascorbic Acid) 200 mg • Vitamin E (D-Alpha Tocopherol) 100 IU • Vitamin B3 (Niacinamide) 50 mg • Iron (Ferrous Succinate) 10 mg • Magnesium (Citrate) 200 mg • Calcium (Citrate) 250 mg • Folic Acid 100 mcg • Biotin 20 mcg • Siberian Ginseng (Eleutherococcus senticosus; GPH: 0.3% eleutherosides b & e) 75 mg • Lemon Bioflavonoids 50 mg • Passion Flower 50 mg • Chamomile 50 mg • Skullcap 50 mg • Choline 40 mg • PABA 10 mg • Inositol 10 mg • Chromium GTF (Nicotinate) 250 mcg.

Moducare Sterinol - Dynapro
Each capsule contains: Plant Sterols 20 mg • Plant Sterolins 200 mcg. Other Ingredients: White Rice Flour, Magnesium Silicate, Gel Cap.

Moisturizing Cleansing Creme - Aspen Group, Inc.
Each gram contains: Tocopheryl Acetate 1% • Panthenol 1% • Water • Mineral Oil • Steareth-2 • PPG-15 • Stearyl Ether • Tocopheryl Acetate • Octyl Palmitate • Isoceteth-20 • Cetearyl Octanoate • Carbomer • Dimethicone • Ammonium Hydroxide • Propylene Glycol • Diazolidinyl Urea • Methylparaben • Propylparaben.

Molymin - Progressive Labs
Each capsule contains: Molybdenum (amino acid chelate) 50 mcg • Pea powder 150 mg • Lentil powder 75 mg • Buckwheat 75 mg • Millet flour 75 mg. Carefully dried to preserve their natural trace nutrient content.

Monolaurin (Coconut Extract) - Olympia Nutrition
Coconut extract 300 mg.

Monthly Comfort - Source Naturals
Six tablets contain: Vitamin A (Palmitate) 6000 IU • Vitamin C (Ascorbic Acid and Zinc Ascorbate) 600 mg • Vitamin E (D-Alpha Tocopheryl) (Natural) 150 IU • Vitamin B1 (Thiamin) 20 mg • Vitamin B2 (Riboflavin) 20 mg • Niacinamide 100 mg • Vitamin B5 (Calcium D-Pantothenate) 30 mg • Vitamin B6 (Pyridoxine HCl) 150 mg • Vitamin B12 (Cyanocobalamin) 30 mcg • Folic Acid 800 mcg • Calcium (Carbonate, Citrate) 200 mg • Chromium (ChromeMate GTF Yeast-Free Polynicotinate) 300 mcg • Magnesium (Oxide, Citrate) 450 mg • Zinc (Ascorbate) 20 mg • Taurine 500 mg • N-Acetyl Cysteine 300 mg • DLPA (DL-Phenylalanine) 250 mg • Choline (Bitartrate) 100 mg • Inositol 100 mg • Herbal Formula 1350 mg • Chasteberry 400 mgl • Dong Quai root 200 mg • Black Cohosh root 175 mg • Blue Cohosh root 175 mg • Silymarin (Milk Thistle seed extract) 100 mg • Cyperus rhizome 100 mg • Dong Quai root extract 100 mg • Dandelion root extract 100 mg.

Mood Actives - VitaStore
Four tablets contain: St. John's Wort (0.3% Hypericin) 450 mg • Kava Kava 325 mg • Ginseng 200 mg • Valerian 200 mg • Licorice Root 150 mg • L-Methionine 100 mg • L-Phenylalanine 200 mg • L-Tyrosine 500 mg • L-Taurine 500 mg • Folic Acid 0.4 mg • Vitamin C 300 mg • Vitamin B6 (Pyridoxine) 4 mg • Vitamin B12 12 mcg • Zinc 50 mg.

Mood Aid Formula - Nature's Way
Each capsule contains: Korean Ginseng dried extract 33.3 mg • L-5 Hydroxytryptophan (Griffonia bean extract) 3.33 mg • Niacin (Vitamin B3) 3.33 mg • Riboflavin (Vitamin B2) 284 mcg • Scullcap herb 100 mg • St. John's Wort dried extract (0.3% Dianthrones measures as Hypercin) 300 mg • Thiamine (Vitamin B1) 350 mcg • Vitamin B12 (Cyanocobalamin) 1 mcg • Vitamin B6 (Pyridoxine HCL) 330 mcg. Other ingredients: Gelatin, Magnesium Stearate, Millet.

Mood Enhancer - Clinician's Choice
Three tablets contain: Valerian Root 300 mg • St. John's Wort Extract (std. 0.3% hypericin) 300 mg • Chamomile Flowers 300 mg • L-Tyrosine 30 mg • Proprietary blend 15 mg: Passion Flower, Sage Leaves, Isoflavones, Grape Powder, Acetyl-L-Carnitine.

Mood Mender - Celestial Seasonings
Two capsules contain: Vitamin B6 (as pyridoxine HCL) 6 mg • Folic Acid 200 mcg • Vitamin B12 (as cyanocobalamin) 12 mcg • Selenium (as methionine chelate) 140 mcg • Chromium (as polynicotinate) 120 mcg • Proprietary Blend, 1930 mg: St. John's Wort (leaf,stem, flower), St. John's Wort (standardized extract), Siberian Ginseng (root), Siberian Ginseng (standardized extract). Other ingredients: May contain one or more of the following: Dicalcium phosphate, gelatin, rice flour, stearic acid, magnesium stearate, and silicon dioxide. This product contains no artificial colors, flavors or preservatives. One serving size is equivalent to St. John's Wort 900 mg, standardized to .3% hypericin, Siberian Ginseng 200 mg standardized to 0.8% eleutherosides.

Mood Support with St. John's Wort - Natrol
One capsule contains: Guaranteed Potency St. John's Wort supplying 0.3% Hypericin 300 mg • Ginseng supplying 8% Ginsenosides 100 mg • L-Tyrosine 50 mg • Lemon Balm 25 mg • DMAE (Di Methyl Amino Ethanol Bitartrate) 25 mg • Vitamin E (d-Alpha Tocopheryl Acetate) 30 IU • Folic Acid 400 mcg • Vitamin B12 (Cyanocobalamin) 50 mcg • Selenium (l-Selenomethionine) 25 mcg. Other ingredients: Silica, Magnesium Stearate, Gelatin.

Mood Sync - Pain & Stress Center
Each capsule contains: St. John's Wort 175 mg • GABA 125 mg • Taurine 100 mg • Glutamine 75 mg • 5-HTP 25 mg • Vitamin B6 (Pyridoxine HCl) 5 mg.

MoodPlex - PharmAssure
Three capsules contain: St. John's Wort with Flowers Extract (Hypericum perforatum;0.3% Hypericin=2.7mg) 900 mg • Griffonia Simplicifolia Seed Extract (20% 5-Hydroxy-Tryptopan=20 mg) 100 mg • D,L-Phenylalanine 100 mg. Other ingredients: Cellulose, Gelatin, Calcium Carbonate.

Mor-Andro 200 - OSMO Therapy
Each capsule contains: 4-Androstene-3Beta,17Beta-Diol (androdiol) 100 mg • 4-Androstene 3, 17-Dione (androstenedione) 100 mg • Elemental Zinc Gluconate 5 mg • Niacin (nicotinic acid) 20 mg.

More - Puritan's Pride
Six tablets contain: Vitamins: Vitamin A 10,000 IU • Vitamin C (w/Rose Hips) 500 mg • Vitamin D 400 IU • Vitamin E 100 IU • Thiamine (B-1) 10 mg • Riboflavin (B-2) 15 mg • Niacinamide (B-3) 100 mg • Vitamin B-6 10 mg • Vitamin B-12 25 mcg • Biotin 150 mcg • Choline Bitartrate 250 mg • Folic Acid 400 mcg • Inositol 25 mg • PABA 30 mg • Pantothenic Acid 100 mg. Minerals: Calcium 750 mg • Copper 2 mg • Iodine 0.15 mg • Iron 30 mg • Magnesium 40 mg • Manganese 5 mg • Phosphorus 350 mg • Potassium 50 mg • Sodium 0.3 mg • Zinc 30 mg • Trace amounts of chlorine, flourine, sulphur, silicon, molybdenum, boron, etc. Amino Acids (from yeast and liver): Arginine 6.6 mg • Cysteine 2.8 mg • Glutamic Acid 8 mg • Histidine 3.2 mg • Isoleucine 11 mg • Leucine 12.4 mg • Lysine 13 mg • Methionine 4.2 mg • Phenylalanine 7.4 mg • Threonine 2.25 mg • Tyrosine 9.2 mg • Valine 8.8 mg. Additional Ingredients: Algin 150 mg • Bee Pollen 10 mg • Desiccated Liver 100 mg • Hesperidin 25 mg • Lemon Bioflavonoid complex 50 mg • Red Bone Marrow 60 mg • Rutin 40 mg • Yeast 100 mg. Formulated in a natural food base of vegetable concentrate of watercress, tomato, onion, celery, celery seeds and garlic. Plus lecithin, papain, pepsin, chlorophyll, EFA's, and many others.
See Editor's Note No. 14, page 1817.

More than a Diet - American Health

Three duotabs contain: Chromium Factors: (Chromium Picolinate, Chromium Polynicotinate) 100 mg • Lipoactive Factors: L-Carnitine, Inositol, Choline L-Methionine, Lecithin, Phosphatidyl Choline (pc), Phosphatidyl Serine (ps), Taurine, Betaine HCl, Vanadium, Vanadyl Sulfate Amino Factors 333mg • Herbal Thermal Factors 350 mg • Capsicum, Ginger, Licorice, Mustard seed, Green Tea, American Ginseng, Cinnamon, Korean Ginseng, Siberian Ginseng, Piper Longum, Gugulipid, Suma, Schizandra, Astragalus, Hawthorne, Kola Nut, Guarana 232 mg • Fiber Factors: Oat Bran Fiber, Citrus Pectin Fiber, Pulp Cellulose, Vegetable Cellulose, Beet Fiber 500 mg • Herbal Fluid Factors: Uva Ursi, Buchu Leaves, Couch Grass, Corn Silk, Hydrangea, Juniper berries 190 mg • Essential Fatty Acid Factors: Gotu Kola, Milk Thistle (Silymarin), Chickweed, Borage oil, Black Currant oil, Primrose oil, Flaxseed oil (cla), Dandelion 80 mg • Appetite Factors : Citrimax (hca from Garnicia cambogia), Chitosan (Shellfish Fiber), OP's (Wheat Oligio Peptides), Gymnema, Sylvestre, Apple Cider Vinegar 450 mg • Green Super Food Factors: Spirulina, Chlorella, Barley Grass, Wheat Grass, Kelp 500 mg • Alfalfa Enzyme Factors: Bromelain, Bipase, Protease, Cellulase, Aspergillus niger, Aspergillus oryzae, FOS 215 mg • Pancreatin Fruit Extract Factors: Apple, Apricot, Banana, Cranberry, Orange, Lemon, Lime, Papaya, Pineapple, Strawberry, Watermelon, Grapeseed (opc), Grapefruit 67.5 mg • Vegetable extract Factors: Cabbage, Celery, Broccoli, Brussels Sprouts, Yams, Carrots, Kale, Collard Greens, Spinach, Cauliflower 50 mg • Youth Factors: DHEA (does not contain more than 2 mg per tablet of DHEA), CoEnzyme Q10, Phaseolus vulgaris 109 mg.

MotherNature Saw Palmetto Berry Extract - MotherNature.com

Each softgel contains: Saw Palmetto extract (serenoa repens) 160 mg. Other Ingredients: Olive Oil, Gelatin, Glycerin, Water.
See Editor's Note No. 2, page 1816.

Mother's Milk - Traditional Medicinals

Contains: Fennel seed • Anise seed • Coriander seed • Spearmint leaf • Lemongrass leaf • Lemon Verbena leaf • Althea root • Blessed Thistle leaf • Fenugreek seed.

Motion Mate - Nature's Way

Two capsules contain: Ginger • Hyssop herb • Meadowsweet herb • Peppermint leaves • Red Raspberry leaves. Other Ingredients: Gelatin, Magnesium Stearate, Millet.

Motion Sickness Formula - Dr. Morrow's Homeopathic Formulas

Ten drops contain: Tabacum 3C • Cocculus indicus 3C • Arnica montana 3C • Petroleum 3C • Belladonna 3C • Ipecac 3C • Ignatia 3C.
See Editor's Note No. 1, page 1816.

Motion Sickness Remedy - PhytoPharmica

Twenty drops contain: Cocculus indicus 8x • Plumbum aceticum 8x • Argentum nitricum 6x • Glonoinum 6x • Zincum valerianicum 6x • Belladonna 4x • Nux vomica 4x • Pulsatilla 4x • Vinca minor 3x • Artemesia vulgaris 1x. In a base of 45% USP alcohol by volume.
See Editor's Note No. 1, page 1816.

Mouth-Mend - The Herbalist

Echinacea root • Golden Seal root • Myrrh Gum • Propolis • Spilanthes herb • Yerba Mansa root.

Movana - Pharmaton

Each tablet contains: St. John's Wort flower & leaves extract WS-5572 (Stabalized minimum hyperforin content 3%, Standardized Hypericin content 0.3%) 300 mg. Other Ingredients: Microcrystalline Cellulose • Corn Starch • Croscarmellose Sodium • Hydroxypropyl Methylcellulose, PEG-4000 • Magnesium Stearate • Silicon Dioxide • Ascorbic Acid • Synthetic Iron Oxide • Titanium Dioxide • Talc • Vanillin. Contains no artificial stimulants, caffeine, or sugar.

Move Free- formerly called Pain Free - Schiff

One caplet contains: Glucosamine Complex [Includes: Glucosamine Hydrochloride, N-Acetyl D-Glucosamine, and Glucosamine Sulfate] 500 mg • Chondroitin Sulfate (Bovine Cartilage Sources) 400 mg. Other ingredients: Cellulose, Coating (Titanium Dioxide, Dextrose, Hydroxypropyl methylcellulose, Polyethelyne Glycol, Sodium Carboxymethyl Cellulose, Mineral Oil, Sodium Citrate, Polysorbate 80, Dextrin), Copolyvidone, Silicon Dioxide, Magnesium Stearate.
See Editor's Note No. 15, page 1817.

MPF - Progressive Labs

Six capsules contain: Vitamin A 25000 IU • Vitamin E 180 IU • Folic Acid 780 mcg • Zinc Picolinate 60 mg • L-Glutamine 1500 mg • N-Acetyl Glucosamine 1050 mg • Gamma Oryzanol 360 mg • Cat's Claw (Uncaria tomentosa) 450 mg.

MRP-44 - Human Development Technologies

Each serving contains: Calories 297 • Protein 44 g • Total Carbohydrate 26 g • Sugar 5 g • Total Fat 1.5 g • Saturated Fat 1 g • L-Glutamine 2 g • Taurine 1 g. Ingredients: MRP1000 (Micro Ultra Filtered Whey Protein concentrate • Egg Albumen • Micro Ultra Filtered Whey Protein Isolate, Ion Exchanged Whey Protein Isolate) • Maltodextrin • natural & artificial flavorings • L-Glutamine • Di-Calcium Phosphate • Taurine • Inulin • Cellulose Gum • Xanthan Gum • Magnesium Oxide • Lecithin • Fructose • Stevia • Acesulfame Potassium • Ascorbic Acid • Vitamin A Acetate • Vitamin E Acetate • Niacinamide • Iron Electrolytic • Zinc Oxide • D-Calcium Pantothenate • Ergocalciferol • Pyridoxine HCL • Copper Gluconate • Riboflavin • Thiamine Mononitrate • Folic Acid • Biotin • Potassium Ionide • Cyanocobalamin.

MSM - Trimedica

Each capsule contains: Methylsulfonylmethane 99.9% • Water 0.1%.

MSM - CVS

Each tablet contains: MSM (methylsulfonylmethane) 1000 mg. Other Ingredients: Cellulose, Stearic Acid, Magnesium Stearate, Silicon Dioxide.

MSM - Metabolic Response Modifiers

Each capsule contains: MSM (methyl-sulfonyl-methane) 750 mg.

MSM - Natural Balance

Each tablet contains: MSM (methylsulfonylmethane) 1000 mg. Other Ingredients: Cellulose, Silicon Dioxide, Stearic Acid, Magnesium Stearate.

MSM - Nature's Bounty

Each capsule contains: Methylsulfonylmethane (255 mg organic sulfur) 750 mg. Other Ingredients: Dicalcium Phosphate, Gelatin, Vegetable Magnesium Stearate, Silica.

MSM - Now

Two capsules contain: Lignisul MSM (methylsulphonylmethane) 2 g. Other Ingredients: Magnesium Stearate, Stearic Acid.

MSM - Olympian Labs

Each capsule contains: MSM (methylsulfonylmethane) 500 mg.

MSM - PhytoPharmica

Each tablet contains: MSM (methylsulfonylmethane) 1,000 mg.

MSM - Swanson

Two capsules contain: OptiMSM (methylsulfonylmethane) 1 g.

MSM 1000 - Aspen Group, Inc.

Each capsule contains: 100% pure MSM (Methyl Sulfonyl Methane) 1000 mg. Contains no sugar, starch, salt, wheat, corn, yeast or soy derivatives.

BRAND NAMES

BRAND NAMES

MSM 1000 - Jarrow Formulas
Each capsule contains: Methylsulfonylmethane 1000 mg.
Other Ingredients: Magnesium Stearate, Gelatin.

MSM Extra Strength - Olympian Labs
Each tablet contains: MSM (methylsulfonylmethane) 1300 mg.

MSM Formula with White Willow - Health Smart Vitamins
Two capsules contain: Vitamin C (as ascorbyl palmitate) 30 mg •
MSM (methylsulfonylmethane) 500 mg • Chondroitin Sulfate 300 mg
• White Willow bark (3% salicins, 1.5 mg) 50 mg.
See Editor's Note No. 15, page 1817.

MSM Plex - PharmAssure
Each capsule contains: MSM (methyl-sulfonyl-methane) 500 mg •
Glucosamine Sulfate 500 mg.

MSM Plus - Progressive Labs
Each capsule contains: Vitamin C (as magnesium ascorbate) 100 mg •
Magnesium (as magnesium ascorbate) 7 mg • Methyl Sulfonyl
Methane (MSM) 800 mg.

MSM Rejuvenator - Progressive Labs
Ingredients: Stabilized Aloe Vera gel • Methylsulfonyl Methane •
Glycerine • Caprylic/Capric Triglycerides • Jojoba oil •
Polyquanterium-32 (colloidal polymers) • Evening Primrose oil •
Cetyl Alcohol • Steryl Alcohol • Tetrahexyldecyl Ascorbate (lipid
soluble Vitamin C) • Tocopheryl Acetate (Vitamin E) • Ginseng
extract • Chamomile extract. Extracts of: Grape seed, Willow bark,
Calendula, White Lily, Japanese Green Tea, Gum Mint, Cucumber,
Soapbark, Balm of Gilead, Bee Propolis: Betaglucans. Essential oils
of: Lemongrass, Rosemary, Sage, Cedarwood, Tetrasodium EDTA,
Methylparaben, Propylparben, Diazolidiny Lurea.

MSM with Glucosamine Sulfate - PhytoPharmica
Each capsule contains: Chloride (from glucosamine sulfate)
78 mg • Sodium (from glucosamine sulfate) 50 mg • Stabilized
Glucosamine Sulfate 500 mg • MSM (methylsulfonylmethane)
250 mg.

Mucho Mate - Traditional Medicinals
Green & Roasted Yerba Mate leaf • Ginger rhizome • Lemon peel •
natural Lemon flavor • Stevia leaf.

Mucoplex - Progressive Labs
Each capsule contains: Comfrey root (Symphytum officinale) 225 mg
• Pepsin (1:3000) 65 mg • Bromelain 50 mg • Raw Duodenum 10 mg.
See Editor's Note No. 14, page 1817.

Muco-Plex - Enzymatic Therapy
Two tablets contain: Niacin 30 mg • Vitamin B6 (Pyridoxine HCl)
10 mg • Iodine (Potassium Iodide) 75 mcg. Other Ingredients:
Marshmallow extract 8:1 (Althea officinalis) mucilage content
30-40% 450 mg • Raw Duodenum Tissue 450 mg • Pancreatic
Enzymes 3X 100 mg • L-Methionine 100 mg • Gastric Mucin powder
100 mg • Pepsin 1:10000 65 mg • Pituitary extract 15 mg.
In a base of Crude Licorice extract (Glycyrrhiza glabra) & derivatives
with an organically bound Allantoin-Methionine (Comfrey) Complex,
Acidophilus, & Aloe Vera. Contains no sugar, salt, yeast, wheat, corn,
soy, dairy products, coloring, flavoring or preservatives.
See Editor's Note No. 14, page 1817.

Mullein Lobelia - Atrium Inc.
Each capsule contains: Mullein leaves 375 mg • Lobelia 125 mg.
Professional Formula. Contains no sugar, starch, salt, wheat, corn,
yeast or soy derivatives.

Multi Caps - Progressive Labs
Three capsules contain: Vitamin A 10000 IU • Vitamin C 120 mg •
Vitamin D (as Vitamin D3) 400 IU • Vitamin E 15 IU • Thiamin
(Vitamin B1) 10 mg • Riboflavin (Vitamin B2) 10 mg • Niacinamide
100 mg • Vitamin B6 10 mg • Folate (folic acid) 400 mcg • Vitamin
B12 50 mcg • Biotin 25 mcg • Pantothenic Acid 40 mg • Calcium
200 mg • Iron 15 mg • Magnesium 100 mg • Zinc 15 mg • Selenium
25 mcg • Manganese 20 mg • Iodine 150 mcg • Chromium 20 mcg •
Potassium 99 mg • Choline 75 mg • Inositol 75 mg • PABA 30 mg •
Citrus bioflavonoids 100 mg • Rutin 25 mg • Hesperidin 25 mg •
Glutamic Acid 30 mg • L-Lysine 50 mg • DL-Methionine 50 mg •
Pancreatin 60 mg • Bile Salts 5 mg • RNA (Brain) 50 mg •
Unsaturated Fatty Acids 50 mg. Other ingredients: Rose Hips,
Ginseng, Goldenseal, Fo Ti Teng, Gotu Kola, Sarsaparilla, Watercress,
Kelp, Green Cabbage, Rice polishings, Raw Stomach substance (not
an extract), Alfalfa, Parsley, Papaya.
See Editor's Note No. 14, page 1817.

Multi Carotene - Puritan's Pride
Each softgel contains: Beta Carotene (Pro-Vitamin A Activity)
25,000 IU • Alpha-Carotene 1 mg • Lycopene 5 mg • Lutein 6 mg •
Zeaxanthin 0.3 mg.

Multi Chelate - Progressive Labs
Six capsules contain: Calcium 500 mg • Iron 15 mg • Magnesium
250 mg • Zinc 10 mg • Iodine 150 mcg • Selenium 25 mcg • Copper
1 mg • Manganese 10 mg • Chromium 50 mcg • Molybdenum
150 mcg • Potassium 99 mg • Vanadium 150 mcg • Silicone 2 mg •
Raw Glandular concentrate 200 mg. The raw glandular materal in this
product is prepared by a special process which does not exceed
physiological temperature (37 Celcius). Guaranteed free of chemical
pesticides and synthetic hormones.
See Editor's Note No. 14, page 1817.

Multi fiber Complex - Natrol
One capsule contains: Psyllium Seed husk 400 mg • Guar Gum
50 mg • Slippery Elm Bark 50 mg • Licorice root 50 mg • Apple
Pectin 50 mg • Grapefruit Pectin 50 mg • Glucomannan 50 mg.
Other ingredients: Magnesium Stearate, Silicon Dioxide, Gelatin.

Multi for Seniors - Health Center for Better Living
Each tablet contains: Vitamin A (as retinyl acetate and beta-carotene)
6,000 IU • Vitamin C (as ascorbic acid) 60 mg • Vitamin D (as
cholecalciferol) 400 IU • Vitamin E (as dl-alpha-tocopheryl acetate)
45 IU • Vitamin K (as phytonadione) 10 mcg • Vitamin B1 (as thiamin
mononitrate) 1.5 mg • Vitamin B2 (as riboflavin) 1.7 mg • Niacin (as
niacinarnide) 20 mg • Vitamin B6 (as pyridoxine HCl) 3 mg • Folate
(as folic acid) 200 mcg • Vitamin B12 (as cyanocobalamin) 25 mcg •
Biotin 30 mcg • Pantothenic Acid (as D-calcium patothenate) 10 mg •
Calcium (as calcium carbonate and dicalcium phosphate) 200 mg •
Iron (as ferrous fumarate) 9 mcg • Phosphorus (as dicalcium
phosphate) 48 mcg • Iodine (as potassium iodide) 150 mcg •
Magnesium (as magnesium oxide) 100 mg • Zinc (as zinc oxide)
15 mg • Selenium (as sodium selenate) 25 mcg • Copper (as cupric
oxide) 2 mg • Manganese (as manganese sulfate (2.5 mg) • Chromium
(as chromium amino acid chelate) 100 mcg • Molybdenum (as sodium
molybdate) 25 mcg • Potassium (as postassium chloride)80 mg •
Nickel (as nickelous sulfate) 5 mcg • Silicon (as sodium metasilicate)
10 mcg • Vanadium (as sodium metavanadate) 10 mcg.

Multi Mineral Citrate Complete - Puritan's Pride
Four capsules contain: Calcium (Citrate, Carbonate, Aspartate)
1000 mg • Magnesium (Citrate, Oxide, Aspartate) 500 mg • Potassium
99 mg • Zinc 50 mg • Iron (Fumarate) 10 mg • Manganese 10 mg •
Copper (Gluconate) 2 mg • Selenium (Chelate) 100 mcg • Chromium
(Chelate) 200 mcg • Molybdenum (Chelate) 100 mcg • Silica
(Chelate) 10 mcg • Boron 3 mg.

Multi Minerals with Boron - Nutrition Warehouse
Three tablets contain: Calcium (Carbonate, Citrate) 1000 mg •
Magnesium (Oxide, Citrate) 500 mg • Zinc 22.5 mg • Iron 20 mg •

Copper 1 mg • Potassium 99 mg • Manganese 5 mg • Selenium 50 mcg • Chromium (yeast-free) 100 mcg • Molybdenum 50 mcg • Vanadium 50 mcg • Iodine (Kelp) 150 mcg • L-Glutamic Acid (HCL) 50 mg • Vitamin D (Cholecalciferol) 200 IU • Boron Citrate 3 mg.

Multi Vitamin Energy Plus for Women - Futurebiotics
Two tablets contain: Beta Carotene 8500 IU • Vitamin C (Acerola, Ascorbic Acid) 225 mg • Thiamin 12.5 mg • Riboflavin 12.5 mg • Niacinamide 50 mg • Calcium (Phosphate, Carbonate) 625 mg • Iron (Amino Acid Chelate) 8 mg • Vitamin D 400 IU • Vitamin E (Natural Mixed Tocopherols) 30 IU • Vitamin B6 15 mg • Folic Acid 400 mcg • Vitamin B12 30 mcg • Biotin 300 mcg • Pantothenic Acid 25 mg • Para Amino Benzoic Acid (PABA) 85 mg • Choline 150 mg • Inositol 30 mg • Iodine (Kelp) 150 mcg • Magnesium (Oxide, Ascorbate) 150 mg • Zinc (Amino Acid Chelate) 15 mg • Ribonucleic Acid (RNA) 50 mg • Chromium (Polynicotinate) 60 mcg • Potassium (Amino Acid Chelate) 90 mg • Selenium (Selenomethionine) • In a base of Peony Root, Dong Quai, Aloe Vera, Methionine, Chamomile, Rosemary, American Ginseng, Chlorella, Bee Pollen, Sea Vegetable, Dandelion Root, Betaine HCl, Chinese Licorice & Raw Alfalfa Juice Concentrate.

MultiBite Plus Iron - GNC
Each tablet contains: Vitamin A (14% as Beta Carotene, 86% as Retinyl Acetate) 2500 IU • Vitamin C (as sodium ascorbate) 60 mg • Vitamin D (as cholecaliferol) 400 IU • Vitamin E (as d-alpha tocopheryl acetate) 15 IU • Thiamin (as thiamin mononitrate) 1.05 mg • Riboflavin 1.2 mg • Niacin (as niacinamide) 13.5 mg • Vitamin B-6 (as pyridoxine hydrochloride) 1.05 mg • Folic Acid 300 mcg • Vitamin B-12 (as cyanocobalamin) 4.5 mcg • Iron (as carbonyl iron) 15 mg. Other Ingredients: Fructose, Sorbitol, Natural Flavors, Carmine Color.

Multi-Carotene - PhysioLogics
Each softgel contains: Carotenoids 306 mg • Beta Carotene (30000 IU) 18 mg • Alpha Carotene 10.8 mg • Gamma Carotene 0.9 mg • Lycopene 0.9 mg • Vitamin E (D-Alpha Tocopherol) 1 IU.

Multi-Carotene Antioxidant - Nature's Way
Each softgel contains: Alpha Carotene 9900 mcg • Beta Carotene 18600 mcg • Gamma Carotene 1200 mcg • Lycopene 30 mcg.

Multi-Enzyme Formula - Puritan's Pride
Each tablet contains: Betaine 200 mg • Pepsin 50 mg • Bromelain 50 mg • Amylase 100 mg • Lipase 25 mg • Cellulase 10 mg • Papain 50 mg • Protease 100 mg • Ox Bile 30 mg • Pancrease Substance 200 mg.
See Editor's Note No. 14, page 1817.

Multiglan Chelate - Atrium Inc.
Six tablets contain: Calcium 500 mg • Magnesium 250 mg • Potassium 99 mg • Manganese 10 mg • Iron 18 mg • Silicon 2 mg • Zinc 15 mg • Iodine (Kelp) 150 mcg • Chromium 200 mcg • Selenium 25 mcg • Molybdenum 150 mcg • Vanadium 150 mcg • As Chelated Proteinates, together in a base of Raw Tissue concentrates (not extracts) from: [Spleen 144 mg, Brain 30 mg, Liver 20 mg, Heart 14 mg, Thymus 4 mg, Adrenal 4 mg, Pancreas 4 mg, Duodenum 4 mg, Pituitary 2 mg] 240 mg.
See Editor's Note No. 14, page 1817.

MultiLogics - PhysioLogics
Each tablet contains: Vitamin A (Beta-Carotene) 12500 IU • Vitamin A (Palmitate) 2500 IU • Thiamine 75 mg • Riboflavin 75 mg • Niacin 75 mg • Pantothenic Acid 75 mg • Vitamin B6 (Pyridoxine HCl) 75 mg • Vitamin B12 (Cyanocobalamin) 75 mcg • Folic Acid 400 mcg • Biotin 300 mcg • Vitamin C (Ascorbic Acid) 250 mg • Vitamin D (Cholecalciferol) 400 IU • Vitamin E (d-Alpha Tocopherol) 150 IU • Calcium (Amino Acid Chelate) 20 mg • Iron (Bisglycinate) 1.3 mg • Magnesium (Amino Acid Chelate) 10 mg • Zinc (Amino Acid Chelate) 10 mg • Copper (Amino Acid Chelate) 1 mg • Manganese (Amino Acid Chelate) 1 mg • Chromium (Niacin/Glycine Chelate) 25 mcg • Iodine (Potassium Iodide) 150 mcg • Selenium (Amino Acid Chelate) 25 mcg • Molybdenum (Amino Acid Chelate) 25 mcg • Boron (Amino Acid Chelate) 500 mcg • Potassium (Amino Acid Complex) 1.8 mg • Bioflavonoids lemon 25 mg • Rutin 25 mg • Betaine (HCl) 25 mg • Choline (Bitartrate) 31 mg • Inositol 75 mg • PABA 75 mg • Hesperidin 5 mg.

MultiLogics for Children - PhysioLogics
Two tablets contain: Vitamin A (as 67% Beta-Carotene, 33% Fish Liver oil) 7500 IU • Vitamin C (as Ascorbic Acid) 180 mg • Vitamin D (as Vitamin D3) (from Fish Liver oil) 200 IU • Vitamin E (as d-Alpha Tocopherol Succinate) 90 IU • Vitamin K (as Phytonadione) 30 mcg • Thiamine (as Thiamine Mononitrate) 3 mg • Riboflavin (Vitamin B2) 3.4 mg • Niacin (as Niacinamide) 20 mg • Vitamin B6 (as Pyridoxine HCl) 4 mg • Folic Acid 400 mcg • Vitamin B12 12 mcg • Biotin 300 mcg • Pantothenic Acid (as d-Calcium Panthothenate) 20 mg • Calcium (as Calcium Citrate-Aspartate Complex) 100 mg • Iron (as Iron Carbonyl) 4.5 mg • Iodine (as Potassium Iodide, Kelp) 75 mcg • Magnesium (as Magnesium Citrate-Aspartate Complex) 100 mg • Zinc (as Amino Acid Zinc Chelate) 5 mg • Selenium (as Amino Acid Selenium Complex) 50 mcg • Copper (as Copper Gluconate) 400 mcg • Manganese (as Amino Acid Manganese Chelate) 1 mg • Chromium (as Chromium Polynicotinate) 50 mcg • Molybdenum (as Amino Acid Molybdenum Chelate) 50 mcg • Black Currant seed 5 mg • Choline (Bitartate) 5 mg • Boron (Aspartate-Citrate) 1 mg.

MultiLogics for Men - PhysioLogics
Three tablets contain: Vitamin E (d-Alpha Tocopherol Acetate) 250 IU • Calcium (Aquamins, Carbonate) 530 mg • Magnesium (Amino Acid Chelate/Oxide) 140 mg • Zinc (Amino Acid Chelate) 15 mg • Iron (Ferrous Bisglycinate) 5 mg • Copper (Amino Acid Chelate) 1 mg • Chromium (Amino Acid Chelate) 175 mcg • Selenium (Amino Acid Complex) 175 mcg • Tomato extract (1% Lycopene, 1.6 mg) 160 mg • Saw Palmetto berry (20-25% fatty acids & Lipid Sterols 15-18.75 mg) 75 mg • Bioflavonoids lemon 50 mg • Rutin 50 mg • Hesperidin 50 mg • Green Tea leaf (45% Polyphenols, 22.5 mg) 50 mg • Betaine HCl 50 mg • Ginkgo Biloba leaf (24% Ginkgo Flavonglycosides, 9.6 mg; 6% Terpene Lactones, 24 mg) 40 mg • Nettles (1-2% Silica, 300-600 mcg) 30 mg • Beta Sitosterol 30 mg • Black Cohosh root (Cimicifuga racemosa) 25 mg • Whole Grape/Wine Complex (45% Polyphenols, 11.25 mg) 25 mg • Bioperine (95% Piperine, 4.75 mg) 5 mg • Calendula flower Marigold (5% Lutein, 150 mg) 3 mg • Potassium (Amino Acid Chelate) 3.6 mg • Boron (Amino Acid Chelate) 500 mcg • Calendula flower Marigold (0.25% Zeaxanthin, 3.75 mcg) 150 mcg.

MultiLogics for Women - PhysioLogics
Three tablets contain: Vitamin E (d-Alpha Tocopherol Acetate) 250 IU • Calcium (Aquamins, Carbonate) 530 mg • Magnesium (Amino Acid Chelate/Oxide) 140 mg • Zinc (Amino Acid Chelate) 15 mg • Iron (Ferrous Bisglycinate) 5 mg • Copper (Amino Acid Chelate) 1 mg • Chromium (Amino Acid Chelate) 175 mcg • Selenium (Amino Acid Complex) 175 mcg • Tomato extract (1% Lycopene, 1.6 mg) 160 mg • Bioflavonoids lemon 50 mg • Rutin 50 mg • Hesperidin 50 mg • Green Tea leaf (45% Polyphenols, 22.5 mg) 50 mg • Betaine HCl 50 mg • Ginkgo Biloba leaf (24% Ginkgo Flavonglycosides. 9.6 mg; 6% Terpene Lactones, 24 mg) 40 mg • Black Cohosh root 25 mg • Whole Grape/Wine Complex (45% Polyphenols, 11.25 mg) 25 mg • Dong Quai (1% Ligustilides, 250 mcg) 25 mg • Chasteberry (0.5% Isoflavones, 125 mcg) 25 mg • Choline (Bitartate) 20 mg • Daidzein 13 mg • Bioperine (95% Piperine, 4.75 mg) 5 mg • Calendula flower Marigold (5% Lutein, 150 mg) 3 mg • Potassium (Amino Acid Chelate) 3.6 mg • Boron (Amino Acid Chelate) 500 mcg • Calendula flower Marigold (0.25% Zeaxanthin, 3.75 mcg) 150 mcg.

BRAND NAMES

Multi-Mega Minerals - Puritan's Pride
Two tablets contain: Calcium 1,000 mg • Magnesium 500 mg • Iron 30 mg • Manganese 10 mg • Potassium 95 mg • Chromium 100 mcg • Vitamin D 400 IU • Iodine 150 mcg • Copper 3 mg • Zinc 22.5 mg. Other Components: Betaine Hydrochloride 100 mg • Glutamic Acid Hydrochloride 100 mg • Chloride 90 mg.

Multi-Mineral Citrate Complete - The Vitamin Shoppe
Eight capsules contain: Calcium 1000 mg • Magnesium 500 mg • Potassium 99 mg • Zinc 50 mg • Boron 3 mg • Copper 2 mg • Selenium 100 mcg • Chromium 200 mcg • Molybdenum 100 mcg • Iron 10 mg • Manganese 10 mg.

Multi-Minerals - The Vitamin Shoppe
Three tablets provide: Calcium 1000 mg • Zinc 22.5 • Copper 1 mg • Selenium 50 mcg • Chromium 100 mcg • Vanadium 50 mcg • Glutamic Acid 50 mg • Magnesium 500 mg • Iron 20 mg • Potassium 99 mg • Manganese 5 mg • Boron 3 mg • Molybdenum 50 mcg • Iodine 150 mcg • Vitamin D 200 IU.

Multi-Quest - Nutri-Quest
Three tablets contain: Vitamin A (Palmitate) 2000 IU • Vitamin D (as Vitamin D3) 400 IU • Vitamin E (Succinate) 200 IU • Vitamin C (Sago Palm) 1000 mg • Lemon Bioflavonoids 100 mg • Rutin 25 mg • Hesperidin Complex 50 mg • Vitamin B6 25 mg • Vitamin B1 13 mg • Vitamin B2 10 mg • Niacin 45 mg • Vitamin B12 30 mcg • Pantothenic Acid (Calcium Pantothenate) 50 mg • Folic Acid 200 mcg • Choline Bitartrate 100 mg • Inositol 100 mg • Biotin 400 mcg • PABA 50 mg • L-Glycine 9.66 mg • Calcium Gluconate 15.36 mg • Vitamin F 5 mg • Chlorophyll 16 mg • Calcium Aspartate 500 mg • Magnesium Aspartate 250 mg • Phosphorus Chelate 200 mg • Potassium Proteinate 30 mg • Copper Chelate 1 mg • Zinc Aspartate 5 mg • Manganese Aspartate 15 mg • Molybdenum Chelate 50 mcg • Chromium Chelate 25 mcg • Selenium Chelate 30 mcg • Iodine (kelp) 50 mcg • Sodium Proteinate 30 mcg • Rubidium Chelate 15 mcg • Lithium Chelate 8 mcg • L-Phenylalanine 13 mg • L-Histidine 6 mg • L-Tyrosine 9 mg • L-Lysine 13 mg • L-Valine 15 mg • DL-Methionine 9 mg • L-Isoleucine 13 mg • L-Leucine 18 mg • L-Threonine 9 mg • L-Glutamic Acid 2 mg • Goldenseal root 45 mg • Siberian Ginseng 45 mg • Garlic 40 mg • Tillandsia 30 mg • Rice Bran 176 mg • Almond Meal 150 mg.

Multi-Scorb - Progressive Labs
Each tablet contains: Vitamin C (as mineral ascorbates) 1000 mg • Calcium (ascorbate) 50 mg • Magnesium (ascorbate) 30 mg • Zinc (ascorbate) 3 mg • Manganese (ascorbate) 3 mg • Potassium (ascorbate) 60 mg • Citrus BioFlavonoid 5X complex 125 mg (as undiluted hesperidin, naringin and rutin).

Munit-E - Holista
Each capsule contains: Beta Carotene 10000 IU • Vitamin A 5000 IU • Vitamin C 500 mg • Vitamin B6 25 mg • Zinc 20 mg • Echinacea (angustifolia/purpurea) 300 mg • Bioflavonoids 100 mg • Garlic 50 mg • Ginger 50 mg.

Muscle - Gary Nulls
Composed of plant sources. Fortified with Methionine, Leucine, Valine, Isoleucine, and Lysine.

Muscle Dynamo - Source Naturals
Four tablets contain: Vitamin B1 (Thiamin) 30 mg • Vitamin B2 (Riboflavin) 30 mg • Niacinamide (125 mg) and Niacin (25 mg) 150 mg • Vitamin B5 (Calcium D-Pantothenate) 100 mg • Vitamin B6 (Pyridoxine HCl) 25 mg • Vitamin B12 (Cyanocobalamin) 100 mcg • Folic Acid 400 mcg • Vitamin E D-Alpha Tocopheryl (Natural) 100 IU • Magnesium (Citrate and Succinate) 181 mg • Potassium (Succinate) 99 mg • Calciium (Succinate) 89 mg • Succinate Complex (Magnesium/Calcium/Potassium Succinates) 1,300 mg • Inosine 500 mg • PAK (Pyridoxine alpha-Ketoglutarate) 100 mg • Coenzyme

Q10 (Ubiquinone) 30 mg • Alpha-Lipoic Acid (Thioctic Acid) 25 mg • l-Isoleucine 120 mg • L-Leucine 360 mg • L-Valine 120 mg • Glycine 500 mg • L-Tyrosine 150 mg • Korean Ginseng root 250 mg • Siberian Ginseng root extract 100 mg.

Muscle Dynamo II - Source Naturals
One oz contains: Vitamin A 1,250 IU • Vitamin C (Ascorbic Acid) 30 mg • Thiamin (Vitamin B1) 380 mcg • Riboflavin (Vitamin B2) 430 mcg • Niacin 20 mg • Calcium 150 mg • Iron 1 mg • Vitamin D 100 IU • Vitamin E 15 IU • Vitamin B6 500 mcg • Folic Acid 100 mcg • Vitamin B12 3 mcg • Phosphorus 150 mg • Iodine 25 mcg • Magnesium 50 mg • Zinc 7.5 mg • Copper 250 mcg • Biotin 75 mcg • Pantothenic Acid 2.5 mg • Potassium 300 mg • Manganese 2 mg • Chromium 150 mcg • Molybdenum 50 mcg • Selenium 30 mcg.

Muscle Mass - Source Naturals
Two tablets contain: Vitamin C (Ascorbic Acid) 50 mg • Vitamin B5 (Calcium D-Pantothenate) 20 mg • Vitamin B6 (Pyridoxine HCl) 20 mg • Iodine (from kelp) 56 mcg. Other Ingredients: Arginine Pyroglutamate 718 mg, L-Lysine HCl 718 mg, L-Ornithine (Ornithine HCl) 200 mg, Branched Chain Amino Acids (BCAAs) 174 mg (L-Leucine 100 mg, L-Isoleucine 30 mg and L-Valine 44 mg), Lipotropic Factors 360 mg (Choline Bitartrate 200 mg, Inositol 100 mg, L-Methionine 30 mg and Betaine HCI 30 mg), Glycine 50 mg, Trans-Ferulic Acid 50 mg, L-Carnitine (L-Carnitine L-Tartrate) 10 mg, Special Herbal Blend 590 mg: Saw Palmetto, Sarsaparilla, Wild Yam Root, Astragalus, Kelp, Ginseng, Pueraria, Licorice Root.

Muscle Mass - Source Naturals
Two tablets contain: Vitamin C (Ascorbic Acid) 50 mg • Vitamin B5 (Calcium D-Pantothenate) 20 mg • Vitamin b6 (Pyridoxine HCl) 20 mg • Iodine (from Kelp) 56 mcg • Arginine Pyroglutamate 718 mg • L-Lysine HCl 718 mg • L-Ornithine (Ornithine HCl) 200 mg • Branched-Chain Amino Acids (BCAA's), L-Leucine 100 mg, L-Isoleucine 30 mg and L-Valine 44 mg 174 mg • Lipotropic Factors: Choline Bitartrate 200 mg, Inositol 100 mg, L-Methionine 30 mg and Betaine HCl 30 mg 360 mg • Glycine 60 mg • trans-Ferulic Acid 50 mg • L-Carnitine (L-Carnitine, L-Tartrate) 10 mg • Herbal Blend: Saw Palmetto, Sarsaparilla, Wild Yam Root, Astragalus, Kelp, Ginseng, Pueraria and Licorice Root 590 mg.

Musclease - PhysioLogics
Two capsules contain: Magnesium (Aspartate) 100 mg • Calcium (Citrate) 50 mg • Valerian (0.8% Valernic Acids, 800 mcg) 100 mg • Kava Kava root (30% Kavalactones, 30 mg) 100 mg • Passion flower (3.5% Flavonoids, 3.5 mg) 100 mg.

MuscleSoothe - Neopharmica
Two tablets contain: Proprietary Blend: San-Qi Ginseng root, Dong-Quai root, Sichuan teasel rhizome, Safflower Flower, Astilbe Chinensis plant 2000 mg.

MuscleTech - Muscletech
Six capsules contain: Acetyl-L-Carnitine 1000 mg • Glutamine 2000 mg • L-Leucine 1000 mg • L-Valine 250 mg • L-Isoleucine 250 mg • OKG 100 mg • Zinc 60 mg • Taurine 1000 mg.

Mustard Salve - Dial Herbs
Mustard • Wintergreen • Comfrey • Arnica • Camphor • Cayenne. In a base of Beeswax , Glycerine & Cold Pressed Olive oil.

Mutiglan Plus - Atrium Inc.
Each tablet contains: Spleen 256.5 mg • Brain 67.5 mg • Liver 45 mg • Heart 31.5 mg • Kidney 31.5 mg • Thymus 8 mg • Adrenal 8 mg • Pituitary 2 mg • Pancreas 9 mg • Duodenum 9 mg. See Editor's Note No. 14, page 1817.

Some Brand Name Natural Products - What they Contain
www.NaturalDatabase.com contains MANY more listings than appear here.

MVP - Mannatech

Wild Yam root standardized for phytosterols • Kola Nut seed • Country Mallow (Sida cortifolia aerial) • Atlantic Kelp whole plant • Cayenne Pepper fruit • Ambrotose Complex: naturally occurring plant polysaccharides including freeze-dried Aloe Vera inner leaf gel extract - Manapol powder. Other Ingredients: Cellulose, Calcium carbonate, Silicon dioxide, Hydroxypropyl methylcellulose, Coscarmellose sodium, Stearic acid, Magnesium stearate. Each caplet contains 10 mg of Ephedrine from Country Mallow and 40 mg of Caffeine from Kola Nut.
See Editor's Note No. 17, page 1817.

My Favorite Multiple Original - Capsules - Natrol

Six capsules contain: Vitamin A (as beta carotene & Vitamin A palmitate) 10000 IU • Vitamin C (as calcium ascorbate) 250 mg • Vitamin D (as cholecalciferol) 400 IU • Vitamin E (as d-alpha tocopheryl succinate) 400 IU • Thiamine (as thiamin HCI) (Vitamin B1) 50 mg • Riboflavin (Vitamin B2) 50 mg • Niacin (as niacin & niacinamide) 50 mg • Vitamin B6 (as pyridoxine HCI) 50 mg • Folic Acid 400 mcg • Vitamin B12 (as cyanocobalamin) 50 mcg • Biotin 300 mcg • Pantothenic Acid (as d-calcium pantothenate) 50 mg • Calcium (as calcium carbonate & calcium citrate) 1 g • Iron (as iron glycinate) 18 mg • Iodine (from kelp) 150 mcg • Magnesium (as magnesium citrate & magnesium oxide) 400 mg • Zinc 25 mg • Selenium 200 mcg • Copper 2 mg • Manganese (as manganese gluconate) 2 mg • Chromium 200 mcg • Molybdenum 50 mcg • Potassium (as potassium chloride) 99 mg • Betaine (as betaine TMG trimethylglycine) 300 mg • MultiEnzyme Blend: Amylase, Papain, Protease, Bromelain, Lipase 110 mg • GP Flavonoid Complex + 100 mg extracted from: Rose Hips fruit, Tumeric root, Acerola berries, Bilberry berries, Hawthorne berries, Grape skin, Milk Thistle seed, & Citrus fruit • PABA (as para amino benzoic acid) 50 mg • Choline (as choline bitartrate) 50 mg • Inositol 50 mg • Hesperidin 25 mg • Rutin 25 mg • Siberian Ginseng 4:1 extract root 1 mg • Boron 200 mcg. Other ingredients: Silicon Dioxide, Magnesium Stearate, Gelatin.

My Favorite Multiple Original - tablets - Natrol

Four tablets contain: Vitamin A (as d-Salina beta carotene & Vitamin A palmitate) 10000 IU • Vitamin C (as calcium ascorbate) 250 mg • Vitamin D (as cholecalciferol) 400 IU • Vitamin E (as d-alpha tocopheryl succinate) 400 IU • Thiamine (asThiamine HCI) (Vitamin B1) 50 mg • Riboflavin (Vitamin B2) 50 mg • Niacin (as Niacin & Niacinamide) 50 mg • Vitamin B6 (as pyridoxine HCI) 50 mg • Folic Acid 400 mcg • Vitamin B12 (as cyanocobalamin) 50 mcg • Biotin 300 mcg • Pantothenic Acid (as d-calcium pantothenate) 50 mg • Calcium (as calcium carbonate & calcium citrate) 1 g • Iron (as iron glycinate) 18 mg • Iodine (from kelp) 150 mcg • Magnesium (as magnesium citrate & magnesium oxide) 400 mg • Zinc 25 mg • Selenium 200 mcg • Copper 2 mg • Manganese (as manganese gluconate) 2 mg • Chromium 200 mcg • Molybdenum 50 mcg • Potassium (as potassium chloride) 99 mg • Betaine (as betaine TMG trimethylglycine) 300 mg • Multi Enzyme Blend consisting of: amylase, papain, protease, bromelain, lipase 110 mg • GP Flavonoid Complex 100 mg extracted from: Rose Hips fruit, Tumeric root, Acerola berries, Bilberry berries, Hawthorne berries, Grape skin, Milk Thistle Seed, & citrus fruit • PABA (as para amino benzoic acid) 50 mg • Choline (as choline bitartrate) 50 mg • Inositol 50 mg • Hesperidin 25 mg • Rutin 25 mg • Siberian Ginseng 4:1 extract root 15 mg • Boron 200 mcg. Other ingredients: Microcrystalline Cellulose, Mono & Di-Glycerides, Silicon Dioxide, Magnesium Stearate, Stearic Acid, Croscarmellose Sodium.

My Favorite Multiple Take One - Natrol

One tablet contains: Vitamin A (as beta carotene) 10000 IU • Vitamin C (as calcium ascorbate)100 mg • Vitamin D (as cholecalciferol) 400 IU • Vitamin E (as d-alpha tocopheryl succinate) 100 IU • Thiamine (as thiamin HCI) (Vitamin B1) 15 mg • Riboflavin (Vitamin B2) 17 mg • Niacin 20 mg • Vitamin B6 (as pyridoxine HCI) 17 mg • Folic Acid 400 mcg • Vitamin B12 (as cyanocobalamin) 50 mcg •

Biotin 300 mcg • Pantothenic Acid (as d-calcium pantothenate) 50 mg • Calcium 25 mg • Iron 18 mg • Iodine 150 mcg • Magnesium 10 mg • Zinc 15 mg • Selenium 200 mcg • Copper 2 mg • Manganese 5 mg • Chromium 200 mcg • Molybdenum 50 mcg • Potassium 5 mg • Silica 10 mg • Vanadium 10 mcg • Boron 3 mg • GP Flavonoid Complex + 100 mg, extracted from: Rose Hips fruit, Tumeric root, Acerola berries, Bilberry berries, Hawthorne berries, Grape skin, Milk Thistle Seed & Citrus fruit • UltraGreen Blend concentrate extract 100 mg from: Alfalfa juice leaf, barley grass, spirulina algae, parsley leaf, spinach leaf, peppermint leaf, & spearmint leaf • Lecithin 50 mg • Choline (as choline bitartrate) 50 mg • PABA (as para amino benzoic acid) 25 mg • Inositol 25 mg. Other ingredients: Mono & Di-Glycerides, Silicon Dioxide, Stearic Acid, Croscarmellose Sodium, Magnesium Stearate.

My Favorite Multiple Take One Without Iron - Tablets - Natrol

Each tablet contains: Vitamin A (as beta carotene) 10000 IU • Vitamin C (as calcium ascorbate) 100 mg • Vitamin D (as cholecalciferol) 400 IU • Vitamin E (as d-alpha tocopheryl succinate) 100 IU • Thiamine (as thiamin HCI) (Vitamin B1) 15 mg • Riboflavin (Vitamin B2) 17 mg • Niacin 20 mg • Vitamin B6 (as pyridoxine HCI) 17 mg • Folic Acid 400 mcg • Vitamin B12 (as cyanocobalamin) 50 mcg • Biotin 300 mcg • Pantothenic Acid (as d-calcium pantothenate) 50 mg • Calcium 25 mg • Iodine 150 mcg • Magnesium 10 mg • Zinc 15 mg • Selenium 200 mcg • Copper 2 mg • Manganese 5 mg • Chromium 200 mcg • Molybdenum 50 mcg • Potassium 5 mg • Silica 10 mg • Vanadium 10 mcg • Boron 3 mg • GP Flavonoids 100 mg, extracted from: Rose Hips fruit, Tumeric root, Acerola berries, Bilberry berries, Hawthorne berries, Grape skin, Milk Thistle seed, & Citrus fruit • UltraGreen Blend 100 mg concentrate extract from: Alfalfa juice leaf, Barley grass, Spirulina algae, Parsley leaf, Spinach leaf, Peppermint leaf, & Spearmint leaf • Lecithin 50 mg • Choline (as choline bitartrate) 50 mg • PABA (as para amino benzoic acid) 25 mg • Inositol 25 mg. Other ingredients: Mono & Di-Glycerides, Silicon Dioxide, Stearic Acid, Croscarmellose Sodium, Magnesium Stearate.

My Favorite Multiple Without Iron – Capsules - Natrol

Six capsules contain: Vitamin A (as beta carotene & Vitamin A palmitate) 10000 IU • Vitamin C (as calcium ascorbate) 250 mg • Vitamin D (as cholecalciferol) 400 IU • Vitamin E (as d-alpha tocopheryl succinate) 400 IU • Thiamine (as thiamin HCl) (Vitamin B1) 50 mg • Riboflavin (Vitamin B2) 50 mg • Niacin (as niacin & niacinamide) 50 mg • Vitamin B6 (as pyridoxine HCl) 50 mg • Folic Acid 400 mcg • Vitamin B12 (as cyanocobalamin) 50 mcg • Biotin 300 mcg • Pantothenic Acid (as d-calcium pantothenate) 50 mg • Calcium (as calcium carbonate & calcium citrate) 1 g • Iodine (from kelp) 150 mcg • Magnesium (as magnesium citrate & magnesium, oxide) 400 mg • Zinc 25 mg • Selenium 200 mcg • Copper 2 mg • Manganese (as manganese gluconate) 2 mg • Chromium 200 mcg • Molybdenum 50 mcg • Potassium(as potassium chloride) 99 mg • Betaine (as betaine TMG trimethylglycine) 300 mg • MultiEnzyme Blend 110 mg: amylase, papain, protease, bromelain & lipase • GP Flavonoid Complex + 100 mg extracted from: Rose Hips fruit, Tumeric root, Acerola berries, Bilberry berries, Hawthorne berries, Grape skin, Milk Thistle Seed & Citrus fruit • PABA (as para amino benzoic acid) 50 mg • Choline (as choline bitartrate) 50 mg • Inositol 50 mg • Hesperidin 25 mg • Rutin 25 mg • Siberian Ginseng 4:1 extract root 15 mg • Boron 200 mcg. Other ingredients: Silicon Dioxide, Magnesium Stearate, Gelatin.

My Favorite Multiple Without Iron - Tablets - Natrol

Four tablets contain: Vitamin A (as d-Salina beta carotene & Vitamin A palmitate) 10000 IU • Vitamin C (as calcium ascorbate) 250 mg • Vitamin D (as cholecalciferol) 400 IU • Vitamin E (as d-alpha tocopheryl succinate) 400 IU • Thiamine (as Thiamine HCl) (Vitamin B1) 50 mg • Riboflavin (Vitamin B2) 50 mg • Niacin (as Niacin & Niacinamide) 50 mg • Vitamin B6 (as pyridoxine HCl) 50 mg • Folic Acid 400 mcg • Vitamin B12 (as cyanocobalamin) 50 mcg • Biotin

B R A N D   N A M E S

300 mcg • Pantothenic Acid (as d-calcium pantothenate) 50 mg • Calcium (as calcium carbonate & calcium citrate) 1 g • Iodine (from kelp) 150 mcg • Magnesium (as magnesium citrate & magnesium oxide) 400 mg • Zinc 25 mg • Selenium 200 mcg • Copper 2 mg • Manganese (as manganese gluconate) 2 mg • Chromium 200 mcg • Molybdenum 50 mcg • Potassium (as potassium chloride) 99 mg • Betaine (as betaine TMG trimethylglycine) 300 mg • MultiEnzyme Blend 110 mg consisting of: Amylase, Papain, Protease, Bromelain & Lipase • GP Flavonoid Complex 100 mg extracted from: Rose Hips fruit, Tumeric root, Acerola berries, Bilberry berries, Hawthorne berries, Grape skin, Milk Thistle seed & Citrus fruit • PABA (as para amino benzoic acid) 50 mg • Choline (as choline bitartrate) 50 mg • Inositol 50 mg • Hesperidin 25 mg • Rutin 25 mg • Siberian Ginseng 4:1 extract root 15 mg • Boron 200 mcg. Other ingredients: Microcrystalline Cellulose, Mono & Di-Glycerides, Silicon Dioxide, Magnesium Stearate, Stearic Acid, Croscarmellose Sodium.

Mycelin3 - Allergy Research Group
Each capsule contains: Reishi (ganoderma lucidum) 300 mg • Shiitake (lentinus edodes) 300 mg • Cordyceps Sinensis 150 mg • Ascorbic Acid (vitamin C) 40 mg.

Myelin-MS - Olympia Nutrition
Spingomyelin- pharmaceutical grade.

MygraFew Standardized Feverfew Extract - Nature's Way
Each tablet contains: Dried Feverfew Extract (leaf, standardized Feverfew Extract delivering 600 mcg parthenolide, 5% parthenolide) 12 mg.

MygraFree - PhytoPharmica
Each capsule contains: Feverfew extract (standardized to contain 0.6% Parthenolide) 100 mg.

MygrAid Formula - Nature's Way
Each capsule contains: Feverfew leaves 100 mg • Feverfew dried extract 33.3 mg • Lavender flower 50 mg • Linden leaf & flower 70 mg • Magnesium Amino Acid Chelate 33.3 mg. Other ingredients: Gelatin, Magnesium Stearate, Millet.

Mylanta Calci Tabs - Ultra Strength - Johnson & Johnson
Two tablets contain: Calcium Carbonate 1000 mg. Other Ingredients: Dextrose, Maltodextrin, Microcrystalline Cellulose, Magnesium Stearate, Starch, Cellulose, Citric and Fumaric Acids, Natural and Artificial Flavors, Mineral Oil, Sucrose, FD&C Yellow #6, FD&C Yellow #5, FD&C Blue #1, FD&C Red #27, Ethylmaltol, Crospovidone, Hydroxypropyl Methylcellulose, Stearic Acid.

Mylanta Calci Tabs-Extra Strength - Johnson & Johnson
Two tablets contain: Calcium 600 mg. Other ingredients: Dextrose, Maltodextrin, Microcrystalline Cellulose, Magnesium Stearate, Starch, Cellulose, Citric and Fumaric Acids, Natural and Artificial Flavors, Mineral Oil, Sucrose, FD & C Yellow #6, FD & C Yellow #5, FD & C Blue #1, D & C Red #27, Ethylmaltol, Crospovidone, Hydroxypropyl Methylcellulose and Stearic Acid.
See Editor's Note No. 5, page 1816.

Myo-Comp - PhytoPharmica
Two tablets contain: Vitamin C (ascorbic acid) 120 mg • Vitamin D (fish liver oil) 266 IU • Vitamin E (d-alpha tocopheryl succinate) 20 IU • Thiamin (thiamin HCl; vitamin B1) 10 mg • Riboflavin (vitamin B2) 10 mg • Niacin 10 mg • Vitamin B6 (pyridoxine HCl) 12 mg • Vitamin B12 (cyanocobalamin) 20 mcg • Calcium (bone meal) 360 mg • Magnesium (chelate) 60 mg • Manganese (chelate) 3.3 mg • Sodium 10 mg • Potassium chloride 100 mg • Choline Bitartrate 100 mg • Muscle extract 100 mg • Inositol 100 mg • Betaine HCl 60 mg • Ammonium chloride 60 mg • RNA powder 6 mg.
See Editor's Note No. 14, page 1817.

Myoplex Low Carb-Chocolate Cream - Nutripeak
Each packet contains: Protein 50 g • Vitamin A Palmitate (35% as Beta Carotene) 7500 IU • Vitamin D (Cholecalciferol) 400 mg • Niacin (Niacinamide) 10 mg • Biotin 150 mcg • Magnesium Oxide 240 mg • Manganese Sulfate 2 mg • Vitamin C (Ascorbic Acid) 90 mg • Vitamin E (dl-Alpha Tocopheryl Acetate) 45 IU • Vitamin B6 (Pyridoxine Hydrochloride) 1 mg • Pantothenic Acid (D-Calcium Pantothenate) 5 mg • Zinc Oxide 7.5 mg • Chromium Citrate 96 mcg • Calcium (Tricalcium Phosphate and Dipotassium Phosphate) 0.5 mg • Thiamin Hydrochloride 0.75 mcg • Folic Acid 200 mcg • Phosphorus 0.35 g • Selenium Amino Acid Chelate 32 mcg • Molybdenum Amino Acid Chelate 52.5 mcg • Iron (Ferrous Fumarate) 9 mg • Riboflavin .83 mg • Vitamin B12 (Cyanocobalamin) 3 mcg • Iodine (Potassium Iodide) 74 mg • Copper Sulfate 1 mg. Other Ingredients: Protein Blend: Calcium Caseinate, Whey Protein Concentrate, Milk Protein Isolate, Whey Protein Isolate, Sodium Caseinate, Dutch Processed Cocoa, Partially Hydrogenated Canola Oil, Corn Syrup Solids, Natural and Artificial Flavors, Fibersol (Maltodextrin), Salt, Soy Lecithin, Aspartame, Xanthan Gum, Cellulose Gum, Medium Chain Triglycerides, Carrageenan, Mono & Diglycerides.

Myoplex Plus - EAS
Each 76 gram Vanilla Serving contains: Calories 280 • Protein 42 g • Carbohydrates 24 g • Fat 2 g • Cholesterol 15 mg • Sodium 330 mg • Potassium 550 mg • Fiber < 1 g. Ingredients: Myopro [A unique blend of Whey Protein Isolate from specially filtered & ion-exchanged Whey Protein, Calcium Caseinate, Milk Protein Isolate, Taurine, L-Glutamine, Sodium Caseinate, Egg Albumin, & Calcium Alpha-Ketoglutarate (AKG)] • Maltodextrin • Corn Syrup Solids • Vitamin & Mineral Blend [Potassium Chloride, Disodium Phosphate, Calcium Phosphate, Magnesium Oxide, Potassium Citrate, Potassium Phosphate, Choline Bitartrate, Beta-Carotene, Ascorbic Acid, Dl-Alpha Tocopheryl Acetate, Ferrous Fumarate, Molybdenum Amino Acid Chelate, Boron Proteinate, Manganese Gluconate, Selenium Amino Acid Chelate, Niacinamide, Zinc Oxide, Calcium Pantothenate, Chromium Citrate, Copper Sulfate, Vitamin A Palmitate, Pyridoxine Hydrochloride, Riboflavin, Thiamine Hydrochloride, Vitamin D (as Vitamin D3), Folic Acid, Biotin, Potassium Iodide, & Cyanocobalamin] • Natural & Artificial Flavor • Partially Hydrogenated Canola oil • Aspartame • Citrimax (Garcinia cambogia), Salt • Medium-Chain Triglycerides • Xanthan Gum • Soy Lecithin • Cellulose Gum • Mono & Diglycerides • Borage oil. Contains Phenylalanine.

Myoplex Plus Deluxe - EAS
Each 83 gram Vanilla serving contains: Calories 300 • Protein 42 g • Carbohydrates 25 g • Fat 2 g • Cholesterol 5 mg • Sodium 450 mg • Potassium 550 mg • Fiber 1 g • Choline 100 mg • Molybdenum 50 mcg • Boron 1 mcg • Manganese 400 mcg • Selenium 33 mcg • Chromium 100 mcg • Vanadyl Sulfate 10 mg • Conjugated Linoleic Acid 1000 mg • Sodium RNA 9.5 mg. Ingredients: MyoPro: A proprietary protein blend containing Whey Protein Isolate from ion-exchanged Whey, Milk Protein Isolate, Calcium Caseinate, Sodium Caseinate, & Egg Albumin • Maltodextrin GKG [A proprietary blend containing L-Glutamine, Calcium Alpha-Ketoglutarate (AKG), Taurine, Potassium Chloride, Potassium Phosphate, Magnesium Phosphate, Magnesium Oxide, Sodium RNA, & Manganese Glycinate] • CLA (Calcium Conjugated Linoleic Acid from Sunflower oil) • Natural & Artificial Flavors • Partially Hydrogenated Canola oil • Xanthan Gum • V2G: A proprietary blend containing Taurine, Vanadyl Sulfate, & Sodium Selenate • Vitamin & Mineral Blend [Choline Bitartrate, Beta-Carotene, Ascorbic Acid, Dl-Alpha Tocopheryl Acetate, Ferrous Fumarate, Molybdenum Amino Acid Chelate, Boron Proteinate, Niacinamide, Zinc Oxide, Calcium Pantothenate, Chromium Citrate, Copper Sulfate, Vitamin A Palmitate, Pyridoxine Hydrochloride, Riboflavin, Thiamine Hydrochloride, Vitamin D (as Vitamin D3), Folic Acid, Biotin, Potassium Iodide, & Cyanocobalamin] • Corn Syrup Solids • Salt • Soy Lecithin •

Some Brand Name Natural Products - What they Contain

Asparatame • Cellulose Gum • Carrageenan • Citrimax (Garcinia cambogia) • Medium-Chain Triglycerides • Mono & Diglycerides • Borage oil. Contains Phenylalanine.

Myoplex Plus Deluxe Bar - EAS
Gral & Artificial Flavors • Nonfat Milk • Milk • Cocoa • Unsweetened Chocolate • GKG [A proprietary blend containing L-Glutamine, Calcium Alpha-Ketoglutarate (AKG), Taurine, Potassium Chloride, Potassium Phosphate, Magnesium Oxide, Magnesium Phosphate, Sodium RNA, & Manganese Glycinate] • V2G: A proprietary blend containing Taurine, Vanadyl Sulfate, Sodium Selenate • Vitamin & Mineral Blend [Dicalcium Phosphate, Sodium Ascorbate, Ferric Orthophosphate, Dl-Alpha Tocopherol Acetate, Niacinamide, Zinc Oxide, Copper Gluconate, Calcium Pantothenate, Chromium Citrate, Vitamin A Palmitate, Pyridoxine Hydrochloride, Riboflavin, Thiamine Mononitrate, Folic Acid, Chromium Chloride, Sodium Molybdate, Biotin, Potassium Iodide, Phylloquinone, Cholecalciferol, & Cyanocobalamin] • CLA (Calcium Conjugated Linoleic Acid from Sunflower oil) • Lecithin.

Myo-Tone - Enzymatic Therapy
Each tablet contains: Vitamin D (Fish Liver oil) 133 IU • Vitamin E succinate/Wheat Germ) 10 IU • Calcium (Bone Meal) 180 mg • Manganese (Chelate) 63 mg • Vitamin C (Ascorbic Acid/Rose Hips) 60 mg • Potassium Chloride 50 mg • Magnesium (Chelate) 30 mg • Vitamin B6 (Pyridoxine HCL) 6 mg • Thiamine HCL (Vitamin B1) 5 mg • Niacin 5 mg • Riboflavin (Vitamin B2) 5 mg • Vitamin B12 (Cyanocobalamin) 10 mcg • Other ingredients: Choline Bitartrate 50 mg • Muscle extract 50 mg • Inositol 50 mg • Betaine HCL 30 mg • Ammonium Chloride 30 mg, RNA Powder 3 mg. Contains no sugar, salt, yeast, corn, dairy products, coloring, flavoring or preservatives. All organs & glands derived from bovine sources.
See Editor's Note No. 14, page 1817.

MyoVive - Nutricia
One pack (4 fl oz) contains: Vitamin A 1113 IU • Vitamin C 125 mg • Vitamin D 100 IU • Vitamin E 400 IU • Thiamin (Vitamin B1) 13 mg • Riboflavin (Vitamin B2) 1.5 mg • Niacin (Vitamin B3) 10 mg • Vitamin B6 3 mg • Folic Acid 300 mcg • Vitamin B12 1.5 mcg • Biotin 50 mcg • Pantothenic Acid (Vitamin B5) 2 mg • Calcium 126 mg • Iron 0.4 mg • Phosphorus 74 mg • Iodine 40 mcg • Magnesium 9 mg • Zinc 6 mg • Selenium 20 mcg • Copper 0.6 mg • Manganese 1.2 mg • Chromium 13 mcg • Molybdenum 20 mcg • Chloride 81 mg • Sodium 50 mg • Potassium 300 mg • Cysteine 115 mg • Choline 40 mg • Coenzyme Q10 68 mg • L-Carnitine 1.4 g • Creatine 875 mg • Taurine 1.4 g • Fluoride 0.4 mg.

Myrrh Salve - Dial Herbs
Myrrh • White Poplar • Balsam Fir • Black Walnut • Cayenne. In a base of Beeswax, Glycerine & Cold Pressed Olive oil.

Myrrh-Goldenseal Plus Formula - Nature's Way
Two capsules contain: Proprietary formula: Cayenne pepper fruit • Goldenseal root • Myrrh Gum (Oleo-Gum Resin from stems). Other ingredients: Gelatin.

Myrrh-Prickly Ash Bark Virtue - Blessed Herbs
Echinacea Angustifolia root • Goldenseal root • Myrrh Gum • Propolis • Prickly Ash bark • Grain alcohol & Distilled Water.

NAC Fuel - TwinLab
Each capsule contains: Highest Quality Pharmaceutical Grade NAC (N-Acetyl-Cysteine) 600 mg.

N-A-C Sustain - Jarrow Formulas
Each tablet contains: N-Acetyl-L-Cysteine 600 mg. Other Ingredients: Cellulose, Calcium Phosphate, Magnesium Stearate, Silicon Dioxide.

Nasal Spray - NutriBiotic
Contains 0.1% Grapefruit extract, combined with Sodium Ascorbate (buffered Vitamin C).

Natrol High Nutrition - Natrol
Each capsule contains: Vitamin C (as Ascorbic Acid) 60 mg • Niacin (as Niacinamide) (Vitamin B3) 2 mg • Vitamin B6 (as Pyridoxine HCI) 2 mg, Thiamine (Vitamin B1) 1.5 mg • In a specially formulated base containing: Winter Berry root 4:1 • Country Malva leaf 5:1, Siberian Ginseng root, Ginger root, Licorice root. Other ingredients: Silicon Dioxide, Magnesium Stearate, Gelatin.

Naturafed - Pacific BioLogic
Angelica root (dahurica) • Peppermint (field mint) • Bupleurum root (natural) • Ligusticum root (cnidium) • Ligusticum root (Chinese) • Astragalus root (Grade 1) • Scute root • Platycodon root • Honeysuckle flower • Schizonepta stem • Gentian root (Chinese) • Ephedra Herba (aerial) • Jasmine fruit (cape) • Magnolia flower • Houtuynia.

Natural B-12 with Liver - Leiner Health Products
Each tablet contains: Vitamin B12 (Cyanocobalamin) 1000 mcg. Other Ingredients: Dicalcium Phosphate, Stearic Acid, Liver, Croscarmellose Sodium, Yeast, Silicon Dioxide, Magnesium Stearate.

Natural Balance B-100 Complex - Leiner Health Products
Each tablet contains: Thiamin Mononitrate (Vitamin B1) 100 mg • Riboflavin (Vitamin B2) 100 mg • Vitamin B6 (Pyridoxine Hydrochloride) 100 mg • Niacin 100 mg • Biotin 100 mcg • Vitamin B12 100 mcg • Pantothenic Acid 100 mg • Folate 400 mcg. Other Ingredients: Calcium Carbonate, Cellulose, Maltodextrin, Croscarmellose Sodium, Silicon Dioxide, Polyethylene Glycol 3350, Dicalcium Phosphate, Crospovidone, Tricalcium Phosphate.

Natural Balance B-50 Complex - Leiner Health Products
Each tablet contains: Vitamin B12 50 mcg • Pantothenic Acid (d-Calcium Pantothenate) 50 mg • Thiamin Mononitrate (Vitamin B1) 50 mg • Riboflavin (Vitamin B2) 50 mg • Vitamin B6 (Pyridoxine Hydrochloride) 50 mg • Niacin (Niacinamide) 50 mg • Folate 100 mcg • Biotin 50 mcg. Other Ingredients: Calcium Carbonate, Cellulose, Maltodextrin, Croscarmellose Sodium, Sodium Starch Glycolate, Silicon Dioxide, Polyethylene Glycol 3350, Tricalcium Phosphate.

Natural Balanced B Complex + C - Leiner Health Products
One tablet contains: Vitamin B12 50 mcg • Vitamin C (Ascorbic Acid) 500 mg • Pantothenic Acid (d-Calcium Pantothenate) 50 mg • Thiamin Mononitrate (Vitamin B1) 50 mg • Riboflavin (Vitamin B2) 50 mg • Vitamin B6 (Pyridoxine Hydrochloride) 50 mg • Niacin 50 mg • Biotin 50 mcg • Folate 400 mcg. Other Ingredients: Calcium Carbonate, Yeast, Cellulose, Croscarmellose Sodium, Sodium Starch Glycolate, Silicon Dioxide, Rose Hips, Polyethylene Glycol 3350, Cyanocobalamin.

Natural Bee Pollen - Lichtwer Pharma US
Each tablet contains: Bee Pollen 500 mg. Other Ingredients: Sorbitol, Calcium Carbonate, Sodium Starch Glycolate, Silicon Dioxide, Maltodextrin, Crospovidone, Hydroxypropyl Methylcellulose, Stearic Acid, Hydroxypropyl Cellulose, Magnesium Stearate, Polysorbate 80, Polyethylene Glycol 3350.

Natural Beta Carotene - Leiner Health Products
Each softgel contains: Vitamin A 25000 IU. Other Ingredients: Soybean Oil, Gelatin, Glycerin, Vegetable Oil (Partially Hydrogenated Cottonseed and Soybean oils), Yellow Beeswax, Beta Carotene, Carrot Oil.

BRAND NAMES

Some Brand Name Natural Products - What they Contain
www.NaturalDatabase.com contains MANY more listings than appear here.

B R A N D   N A M E S

Natural Brewer's Yeast - Leiner Health Products
Two tablets contain: Vitamin B1 0.12 mg • Vitamin B2 0.04 mg • Niacin 0.30 mg • Vitamin B6 0.02 mg. Other Ingredients: Brewer's Yeast, Cellulose, Guar Gum, Silicon Dioxide.

Natural Bronchial Syrup - Tom's of Maine
Each teaspoon (5 ml) contains: Thyme extract (Thymus vulgaris L) 190 mg • Pine extract (Pinus strobus L) 125 mg • Marshmallow aqueous extract (Althaea officinalis L) 103 mg • Licorice extract (Glycyrrhiza glabra L) 75 mg. Other ingredients: Honey, Natural Black Cherry extract, Natural Almond extract, Xanthan Gum, or Natural Benzoic Acid.

Natural Calcium & Magnesium - Leiner Health Products
Each tablet contains: Magnesium Oxide 167 mg • Calcium 334 mg. Other Ingredients: Oyster Shell, Maltodextrin, Cellulose, Talc, may contain less than 2% of Mineral Oil, Soy Fiber, Croscarmellose Sodium, Sodium Starch Glycolate, Crospovidone, Magnesium Stearate, Stearic Acid.

Natural Calcium Magnesium & Zinc - Leiner Health Products
Each tablet contains: Calcium Carbonate 333 mg • Magnesium Oxide 133 mg • Zinc Sulfate 5 mg. Other Ingredients: Maltodextrin, Starch, Cellulose, Croscarmellose Sodium, Tricalcium Phosphate, Talc, Sodium Starch Glyolate, Hydroxypropyl Methylcellulose, Silicon Dioxide, Magnesium Stearate, Hydroxypropyl Cellulose, Egg.

Natural Coenzyme Q10 - Nature's Bounty
Each softgel contains: Coenzyme Q-10 30 mg.
Other Ingredients: Rice Bran Oil, Gelatin, Glycerin, Beeswax, Soybean Oil Mixture, Lecithin.
See Editor's Note No. 6, page 1816.

Natural Dolomite with Bone Meal - Puritan's Pride
Six tablets contain: Calcium (from Dolomite and Bone Meal) 1,287 mg • Magnesium (from Dolomite) 303 mg • Phosphorus (from Bone Meal) 294 mg.

Natural Fast Release Lysine - Leiner Health Products
Each tablet contains: L-Lysine Monohydrochloride 500 mg.
Other Ingredients: Dicalcium Phosphate, Cellulose, Croscarmellose Sodium, Stearic Acid, Silicon Dioxide, Magnesium Stearate.

Natural Fish Oil Concentrate - Leiner Health Products
Two softgels contain: Total Fat 2 g • Saturated Fat 0.5 g • Natural Fish Oil concentrate 2000 mg • Calories 20 • Calories form Fat 20 • Containing EPA (Eicosapentaenoic acid) 360 mg • DHA (Docosahexaenoic acid) 240 mg • Protein less than 1 g. Other Ingredients: Fish Oil Concentrate, Gelatin, Glycerin, d-Alpha Tocopherol.

Natural Garlic Oil - Leiner Health Products
Each softgel contains: Garlic oil 3 mg.
Other Ingredients: Vegetable Oil, Gelatin, Glycerin.

Natural Herbal Energizer Caps - Leiner Health Products
Each caplet contains: Ginseng concentrate (American Ginseng, Korean Ginseng, Chinese Panax Ginseng) 200 mg • Herbal Blend 740 mg. Other Ingredients: Yerba Mate Extract, Croscarmellose Sodium, Gotu Kola, Guarana Extract, Dicalcium Phosphate, Stearic Acid, Magnesium Stearate, Silicon Dioxide, Cellulose, Hydroxypropyl Methylcellulose, Polyethylene Glycol 3350, Hydroxypropyl Cellulose, Damiana, Fo-Ti, Green Tea Extract, Jamaican Ginger.

Natural High Potency Iron - Leiner Health Products
Each softgel contains: Iron (Ferrous Fumarate) 27 mg.
Other Ingredients: Vegetable Oil, Gelatin, Vegetable Shortening (Partially hydrogenated Soybean and Palm Oils), Glycerin, Blackstrap Molasses, Yellow Beeswax, Hydrogenated Soybean Oil, Lecithin, Polysorbate 80, Caramel Color, Titanium Dioxide.

Natural High Potency Multivitamin/Mineral - Leiner Health Products
Each tablet contains: Thiamin (Vitamin B1) 10 mg • Riboflavin (Vitamin B2) 10 mg • Phosphorus 40 mg • Biotin 10 mcg • Magnesium Oxide 100 mg • Vitamin B12 12 mcg • Vitamin C (Ascorbic Acid) 100 mg • Calcium Carbonate 62 mg • Iron (Ferrous Fumarate) 27 mg • Vitamin A 7500 IU • Vitamin B6 3 mg • Selenium 10 mcg • Copper 2 mg • Folate 400 mcg • Iodine 150 mcg • Niacin (Niacinamide) 20 mg • Pantothenic Acid 10 mg • Vitamin D 400 IU • Vitamin E (dl-Alpha Tocopheryl Acetate) 30 IU • Zinc Sulfate 15 mg. Other Ingredients: Dicalcium Phosphate, Cellulose, Gelatin, Starch, Maltodextrin, Croscarmellose Sodium, Sodium Starch Glycolate, Kelp, Silicon Dioxide.

Natural Imperial Ginseng - Leiner Health Products
Each tablet contains: Ginseng (Siberian) root 250 mg.
\Other Ingredients: Dicalcium Phosphate, Hydrogenated Vegetable Oil, Croscarmellose Sodium, Silicon Dioxide, Magnesium Stearate, Hydroxopropyl Methylcellulose, Hydroxypropyl Cellulose, Pharmaceutical Glaze, Polysorbate 80, Polyethylene Glycol 3350.

Natural Iron-Free Multivitamin/Mineral Formula - Leiner Health Products
Each tablet contains: Molybdenum (Sodium Molybdate) 25 mcg • Vitamin K (Phytonadione) 25 mcg • Selenium (Sodium Selenate) 20 mcg • Magnesium Oxide 100 mg • Chromium Chloride 25 mcg • Calcium Carbonate 162 mg • Manganese Sulfate 2.5 mg • Phosphorus 109 mg • Copper (Cupric Oxide) 2 mg • Folate (Folic Acid) 400 mcg • Iodine (Potassium Iodide) 150 mcg • Niacin (Niacinamide) 20 mg • Pantothenic Acid (d-Calcium Pantothenate) 10 mg • Riboflavin (Vitamin B2) 1.7 mg • Thiamin Mononitrate (Vitamin B1) 1.5 mg • Vitamin A Acetate 5000 IU • Vitamin B12 (Cyanocobalamin - USP Method 2) 6 mcg • Vitamin B6 (Pyridoxine Hydrochloride) 2 mg • Vitamin C (Ascorbic Acid) 60 mg • Vitamin D (Ergocalciferol) 400 IU • Vitamin E (dl-Alpha Tocopheryl Acetate) 30 IU • Zinc Oxide 15 mg • Biotin (USP Method 2) 30 mcg • Chloride 36.3 mg • Potassium Chloride 40 mg • Nickel (Nickelous Sulfate) 5 mcg • Silicon 2 mg • Tin (Stannous Chloride) 10 mcg • Vanadium (Sodium Metavanadate) 10 mcg. Other Ingredients: Dicalcium Phosphate, Gelatin, Cellulose, Croscarmellose Sodium, Sodium Starch Glycolate, Hydroxypropyl Methylcellulose, Starch, Sodium Metasilicates & Oxides, Pharmaceutical Glaze, Polyethylene Glycol 3350, Magnesium Stearate, Maltodextrin, Hydroxypropyl Cellulose, Mannitol, Sodium & Potassium Borates, Polysorbate 80, Beta Carotene, Resin.

Natural KLB6 - Puritan's Pride
Two softgels contain: Vitamin B6 (Pyridoxine HCl) 7 mg • Lecithin 200 mg • Kelp 50 mg • Cider Vinegar 80 mg.

Natural L-Formula Lysine - Leiner Health Products
Each tablet contains: L-Lysine Monohydrochloride 500 mg.
Other Ingredients: Cellulose, Polyethylene Glycol 3350, Croscarmellose Sodium, Silicon Dioxide, Magnesium Stearate.

Natural Magnesium - Leiner Health Products
Each tablet contains: Magnesium Oxide 250 mg.
Other Ingredients: Cellulose, Talc, Sodium Starch Glycolate, Starch, Silicon Dioxide, Croscarmellose Sodium, Polyethylene Glycol, Kelp, Magnesium Stearate.

Natural Oyster Shell Calcium - Leiner Health Products
Each tablet contains: Calcium 500 mg.
Other Ingredients: Oyster Shell, Maltodextrin, Acacia Gum, Croscarmellose Sodium, Tricalcium Phosphate, Magnesium Stearate.

Some Brand Name Natural Products - What they Contain

Natural Oyster Shell Calcium with D - Leiner Health Products
Each tablet contains: Vitamin D 200 IU • Calcium 500 mg.
Other Ingredients: Oyster Shell, Maltodextrin, Acacia, may contain less than 2% of Cellulose, Mineral Oil, Croscarmellose Sodium, Tricalcium Phosphate, Soy Fiber, Magnesium Stearate, Ergocalciferol, Crospovidone, Stearic Acid.

Natural Potassium Gluconate - Leiner Health Products
Each tablet contains: Potassium Gluconate 90 mg. Other Ingredients: Cellulose, Croscarmellose Sodium, Sodium Starch Glycolate, Starch, Polyethylene Glycol 3350, Silicon Dioxide, Magnesium Stearate.

Natural Quit - JBS Natural Products
Denicotizing Formula: Alfalfa leaf • Barberry bark • Buckthorn bark • Burdock root • Cascara Sagrada • Chaparral • Dandelion root • Goldenseal root • Hyssop • Kelp • Oregon Grape root • Pau D'Arco • Prickly Ash • Yellow Dock root • Yucca root. Anti-Addiction Formula: Anise seed • Barberry bark • Bee Pollen • Blue Cohosh root • Catnip herb • Cayenne 40M • Chamomile • Echinacea angustifolia herb • Eleutherococcus • Fennel seed • Gentian root • Gotu Kola • Hops flower • Lemongrass • Licorice root • Lobelia herb • Myrrh gum • Passionflower • Peppermint leaf • Safflower • Sarsaparilla • Skullcap herb • Slippery Elm bark • Valerian root • Wood Betony . Aromatherapy Formula: Camphor • Eucalyptus • Denatured Alcohol 40 • Peppermint • Rosemary • Ylang Ylang.

Natural Source Calcium & Magnesium - Leiner Health Products
Each tablet contains: Magnesium Oxide 167 mg • Calcium Carbonate 333 mg. Other Ingredients: Maltodextrin, Cellulose, Talc, Croscarmellose Sodium, Mineral Oil, Hydroxypropyl Methylcellulose, Soy Polysaccharide, Citric Acid, Starch Silicon Dioxide, Polyethylene Glycol, Magnesium Stearate, Crospovidone, Gum Arabic Stearic Acid.

Natural Source Calcium + Vitamin D - Leiner Health Products
Each tablet contains: Vitamin D (Cholecalciferol) 125 IU • Calcium Carbonate 250 mg. Other Ingredients: Maltodextrin, Talc, Pregelatinized Starch, Croscarmellose Sodium, Acacia, Silicon Dioxide, Magnesium Stearate.

Natural Source Calcium + Vitamin D - Pharmaceutical Grade - Leiner Health Products
Each tablet contains: Calcium Carbonate 500 mg • Vitamin D (Cholecalciferol) 125 IU.
Other Ingredients: Maltodextrin, Talc, Pregelatinized Starch, Croscarmellose Sodium, Acacia, Hydroxypropyl Methylcellulose, Silicon Dioxide, Magnesium Stearate, Hydroxypropyl Cellulose, Polysorbate 80, Polyethylene Glycol 3350.

Natural Source Calcium Pharmaceutical Grade - Leiner Health Products
Each tablet contains: Calcium Carbonate 500 mg. Other Ingredients: Maltodextrin, Acacia, Starch, Croscarmellose Sodium, Cellulose, Hydroxypropyl Methylcellulose, Talc, Silicon Dioxide, Mineral Oil, Soy Polysaccharide, Magnesium Stearate, Polyethylene Glycol 3350, Hydroxypropyl Cellulose, Polysorbate 80, Crospovidone, Stearic Acid.

Natural Source Calcium, Magnesium, & Zinc - Leiner Health Products
Each tablet contains: Calcium Carbonate 333 mg • Magnesium Oxide 133 mg • Zinc Sulfate 5 mg. Other ingredients: Maltodextrin, Cellulose, Croscarmellose Sodium, Talc, Hydroxypropyl Methylcellulose, Acacia, Soy Polysaccharide, Mineral Oil, Silicon Dioxide, Starch, Magnesium Stearate, Stearic Acid, Citric Acid, Sodium Starch Glycolate, Polyethylene Glycol, Hydroxypropyl Cellulose, Polysorbate 80, Crospovidone.

Natural Soya Lecithin - Leiner Health Products
Each softgel contains: Total Fat 1 g • Calories 10 • Calories from Fat 10 • Soya Lecithin 1200 mg. Other Ingredients: Gelatin, Glycerin.

Natural Sterol Complex - Universal Nutrition
Two tablets contain: Mexican Wild Yam root 1000 mg • Smilax officinalis extract 1000 mg • Muira puama 1000 mg • Gotu Kola 515 mg • Boron 3 mg • Gamma Oryzanol 500 mg • Fucosterol 7959 mcg • Beta Sitosterol 5663 mcg • Campesterol 3376 mcg • Stigmasterol 1924 mcg • "other Sterols" 1009 mcg • Bee Pollen 1000 mg • Guarana 500 mg • Korean Ginseng 100 mg • Cytochrome C 100 mg • Dimethylglycine 100 mg • Inosine 100 mg • Royal Jelly 30 mg • Kola Nut 25 mg • Calcium 200 mg • Magnesium 100 mg • Potassium 99 mg • Linoleic Acid 1040 mg • Oleic Acid 698 mg • Palmitic Acid 263 mg • Linoleic Acid 109 mg • Stearic Acid 56 mg • Lignoceric Acid 14 mg • Arachidonic Acid 13 mg • Behenic Acid 6 mg • Myristic Acid 5 mg • Octacosanol 1650 mcg • RNA 60 mg • DNA 30 mg • Capsicum 100 mg • Alfalfa 100 mg • Dandelion root 100 mg • Garlic 100 mg • Yellow Dock 100 mg • Licorice root 100 mg • Hops 100 mg • Milk Thistle 10 mg.

Natural Time Release B-12 - Leiner Health Products
Each tablet contains: Vitamin B12 (Cyanocobalamin) 1000 mcg. Other Ingredients: Dicalcium Phosphate, Hydrogenated Vegetable Oil, Cellulose, Magnesium Stearate, Silicon Dioxide.

Natural Time Release B-6 - Leiner Health Products
Each tablet contains: Vitamin B6 (Pyridoxine Hydrochloride) 200 mg. Other Ingredients: Dicalcium Phosphate, Hydrogenated Vegetable Oil, Silicon Dioxide, Stearic Acid, Magnesium Stearate, Yeast, Rose Hips, Watercress.

Natural Time Release Balanced B-100 - Leiner Health Products
Each tablet contains: Thiamin Mononitrate (Vitamin B1) 100 mg • Riboflavin (Vitamin B2) 100 mg • Vitamin B6 (Pyridoxine Hydrochloride) 100 mg • Niacin (Niacinamide) 100 mg • Biotin 100 mcg • Vitamin B12 100 mcg • Pantothenic Acid 100 mg • Folate 400 mcg. Other Ingredients: Dicalcium Phosphate, Hydrogenated Vegetable Oil, Stearic Acid, Silicon Dioxide, Magnesium Stearate, Resin, Gum Acacia, Wheat Bran, Cellulose, Para Aminobenzoic Acid.

Natural Time Release Balanced B-50 - Leiner Health Products
Each tablet contains: Vitamin B12 50 mcg • Pantothenic Acid (d-Calcium Pantothenate) 50 mg • Thiamin Mononitrate (Vitamin B1) 50 mg • Riboflavin (Vitamin B2) 50 mg • Vitamin B6 (Pyridoxine Hydrochloride) 50 mg • Niacin (Niacinamide) 50 mg • Biotin 50 mcg • Folate 400 mcg. Other Ingredients: Dicalcium Phosphate, Hydrogenated Vegetable Oil, Stearic Acid, Cellulose, Magnesium Stearate, Silicon Dioxide, Resin, Gum Acacia, Hydroxypropyl Cellulose.

Natural Time Release Complete Multivitamin/Mineral - Leiner Health Products
Each tablet contains: Selenium 5 mcg • Calcium 62.5 mg • Magnesium 25 mg • Molybdenum 5 mcg • Vitamin B12 35 mcg • Copper 1 mg • Vitamin C (Ascorbic Acid) 250 mg • Chromium 5 mcg • Pantothenic Acid (d-Calcium Pantothenate) 30 mg • Manganese 5 mg • Thiamin Mononitrate (Vitamin B1) 35 mg • Riboflavin (Vitamin B2) 35 mg • Potassium Chloride 99 mg • Vitamin B6 (Pyridoxine Hydrochloride) 35 mg • Niacin 35 mg • Iodine 225 mcg • Vitamin A 7500 IU • Folate 400 mcg • Iron (Ferrous Sulfate) 18 mg • Vitamin D 400 IU • Vitamin E 30 IU • Zinc 15 mg • Biotin 5 mcg. Other Ingredients: Dicalcium Phosphate, Hydrogenated Vegetable Oil, Cellulose, Stearic Acid, Gelatin, Silicon Dioxide, Magnesium Oxide.

BRAND NAMES

Some Brand Name Natural Products - What they Contain
www.NaturalDatabase.com contains MANY more listings than appear here.

BRAND NAMES

Natural Time Release Maximum Choice - Leiner Health Products
Two tablets contain: Chloride 18 mg • Potassium 20 mg • Vitamin B12 50 mcg • Vitamin C (Ascorbic Acid) 400 mg • Vitamin E (d-Alpha Tocopheryl Acid Succinate) 200 IU • Pantothenic Acid (d-Calcium Pantothenate) 50 mg • Iron 8.2 mg • Chromium 50 mcg • Selenium 25 mcg • Thiamin Mononitrate (Vitamin B1) 50 mg • Riboflavin (Vitamin B2) 50 mg • Calcium 260 mg • Vitamin B6 (Pyridoxine Hydrochloride) 50 mg • Niacin (Niacinamide) 50 mg • Magnesium Oxide 100 mg • Vitamin A 10000 IU • Molybdenum 15 mcg • Phosphorus 200 mg • Zinc Sulfate 25 mg • Biotin 50 mcg • Copper 3 mg • Iodine 225 mcg • Manganese 3 mg • Folate 400 mcg • Vitamin D 400 IU. Other Ingredients: Dicalcium Phosphate,Hydrogenated Vegetable Oil, Beta Carotene, Stearic Acid.

Natural Time Release Vitamin C with Rose Hips - Leiner Health Products
Each tablet contains: Vitamin C 500 mg. Other Ingredients: Dicalcium Phosphate, Hydrogenated Vegetable Oil, Stearic Acid, Rose Hips, Silicon Dioxide, Magnesium Stearate, Starch, Ethylcellulose.

Natural Vitamin A - Leiner Health Products
Each softgel contains: Vitamin A 8000 IU.
Other Ingredients: Vegetable Oil, Gelatin, Glycerin, Fish Liver Oil.

Natural Vitamin A & D (Cod Liver Oil) USP - Leiner Health Products
Each softgel contains: Vitamin D 135 IU • Vitamin A 1250 IU. Other Ingredients: Cod Liver Oil, Gelatin, Glycerin, and may contain Water.

Natural Vitamin C with Rose Hips - Leiner Health Products
Each tablet contains: Vitamin C 250 mg. Other Ingredients: Ascorbic Acid, Calcium Carbonate, Cellulose, Rose Hips, Silicon Dioxide, Talc, Polyethylene Glycol 3350, Tricalcium Phosphate, Crospovidone, Magnesium Stearate.

Natural Vitamin E - Biodelivery Nutritional Systems
Each tablet contains: Vitamin E 200 IU • Pantethine (Coenzyme A Precursor) 25 mg • Selenium 12.5 mg • NT Factor tablet base 47.5 mg.

Natural Vitamin E - Puritan's Pride
Each softgel contains: Vitamin E (as d-alpha tocopheryl acetate) 400 IU. Other Ingredients: Gelatin, Glycerin, Soybean Oil.

Natural Vitamin E - Leiner Health Products
Each softgel contains: Vitamin E (dl-Alpha Tocopheryl Acetate and d-Alpha Tocopherol) 200 IU. Other Ingedients: Gelatin, Glycerin, Vegetable Oil.

Natural Vitamin E - Swanson
Eash softgel contains: Natural Vitamin E (as d-alpha tocopheryl acetate) 400 IU.

Natural Vitamin E 400 I.U. - Leiner Health Products
Each softgel contains: Vitamin E (dl-Alpha Tocopheryl Acetate and d-Alpha Tocopherol) 400 IU. Other Ingredients: Gelatin, Glycerin, Vegetable Oil.

Natural Vitamin E d-Alpha - Leiner Health Products
Each softgel contains: Vitamin E (d-Alpha Tocopheryl Acetate) 400 IU. Other Ingredients: Vegetable Oil, Gelatin, Glycerin, and may contain Water.

Natural Zinc Gluconate - Leiner Health Products
Each tablet contains: Zinc Gluconate 50 mg. Other Ingredients: Starch, Croscarmellose Sodium, Sodium Starch Glycolate, Magnesium Stearate.

Naturally Herbal Phen - Optimum Nutrition
St. John's Wort • Bitter Orange.

Naturally Kids' Calcees Chewable Calcium + D - Naturally Vitamins
Each tablet contains: Calcium 300 mg • Vitamin D (cholecalciferol) 50 IU. Other Ingredients: Fruit concentrate, Vanilla powder. See Editor's Note No. 5, page 1816.

Naturally Phen - Optimum Nutrition
DL-Phenylalanine L-5-Hydroxytryptophan Tyrosine.

Naturally Ripped - Optimum Nutrition
Ma Huang • Guarana • L-Carnitine • Chromium Picolinate.

Naturatussin 1 - Pacific BioLogic
Platycodon root (balloon flower) • Licorice root • Cynanchum root • Red Date (Chinese jujube) • Sophora root • Burdock fruit (great) • Fritillaria bulb (tendrilled) • Peppermint (field mint) • Ephedra Herba (aerial) • Apricot kernal (northern) • Aster root (purple).

Naturatussin 2 - Pacific BioLogic
Houttuynia Herba • Platycodon root (balloon flower) • Hogfennel root (peucedanum) • Aster root (purple) • Honeysuckle flower • Cynanchum root • Trichosanthes fruit peel • Peach kernal • Momordica Fruit (arhat) • Fritillaria bulb (tendrilled) • Burdock fruit (great).

Natura-UR - Pacific BioLogic
Angelica root (dahurica) • Citrus peel (tangerine) • Andrographis • Isatis leaves • Licorice root • Scute root • Platycodon root • Honey Suckle flower • Chrysanthemum flower • Forsynthia fruit • Burdock fruit • Notopterygium root & rhizome.

Nature Cleanse BotaniCleanse - Nature's Plus
Each tablet contains: Botanical Complex containing a proprietary blend of: [Butternut bark (Juglans cinera), Yellow Dock root (Rumex crispus), Blessed Thistle flower (Cnicus benedictus), Red Clover leaf (Trifolium pratense), Clove bud (Eugenia caryophyllata), Milk Thistle seed (Silybum marianum), Uva Ursi leaf (Arctostaphylos uva-ursi), Cranberry fruit (Vaccinium macrocarpon), Ginger root (Zingiber officinale), Cascara Sagrada bark (Rhamnus purshiana) Hibiscus flower (Hibiscus abelmoschus), Juniper berry (Juniperus oxycedrus), Senna leaf (Cassia senna), Slippery Elm bark (Ulmus rubra), Fennel seed (Foeniculum vulgare), Cayenne fruit (Capsicum frutescens), Dandelion root (Taraxacum officinale), Parsley leaf (Petroselinum crispum), Alfalfa leaf (Medicago sativa), Fenugreek seed (Trigonella foenum-graecum), Aloe Vera & Apple Cider Vinegar • Green Food Complex 100 mg, a proprietary blend of Chlorophyll & trace mineral rich foods: Chlorella broken cell Blue-Green Micro-Algae, Spirulina Algae (Spirulina platensis), Irish Moss (Chondrus crispus), Barley grass juice (Hordeum vulgare), Pacific Kelp (Laminaria)] 500 mg • Vitamin C corn free 100 mg.

Nature Cleanse Fiber Diet - Nature's Plus
Nine capsules contain: Oat Bran (87% Fiber) 1912.5 mg • Psyllium husks (80% Fiber) 1912.5 mg • Apple pectin (84% Fiber) 180 mg • Vitamin C 157.5 mg • Butcher's Broom (15% Fiber) 135 mg • Bentonite U.S.P. grade 90 mg • Cellulose (100% Fiber) 90 mg • Lactobacillus acidophilus 90 million viable cells 22.5 mg. Contains no yeast, wheat, corn, soy, salt, sugar or starch.

Nature Cleanse PuriFiber Internal Cleansing & Revitalizing Powder - Nature's Plus
Each teaspoon (3.75g) contains: Fiber Complex 3500 mg containing a proprietary blend of fiber rich concentrates: Psyllium husks (Plantago ovata), Apple pectin (Malus sylvestris), Butcher's Broom rhizome (Ruscus aceleatus), Bentonite, modified citrus pectin, Cellulose, Rice fiber (Oryza sativa), Slippery Elm bark (Ulmus rubra), Oat bran

(Avena sativa), Beet juice & fiber (Beta vulgaris), Prune fiber (Prunus) • Chitosan, vegetarian 50 mg • FOS (Fructooligosaccharides) Lactic flora growth accelerant 50 mg • Lipase fat-digesting enzyme 50 mg • Peptide FM bioactive oligopeptide 25 mg • Lactospor micro-encapsulated pure culture of B. Coagulans, provides 1 million viable cells 1.7 mg.

Nature Derm - Skin Care System Nutritional Supplement -
PhytoPharmica

Two capsules contain: Vitamin A (acetate) 10,000 IU • Vitamin C (ascorbic acid) 200 mg • Niacin 10 mg • Vitamin B6 (pyridoxine HCl) 8 mg • Vitamin B12 (cyanocobalamin) 3 mcg • Pantothenic Acid (calcium D-pantothenate) 10 mg • Calcium lactate 60 mg • Magnesium oxide 120 mg • Zinc (chelate) 30 mg • Potassium chloride 200 mg • Sublimed Sulfur 200 mg • Bromelain (1,200 M.C.U.) 200 mg • Thymus extract 25 mg • RNA powder 20 mg • Burdock (Arctium lappa) root extract 10 mg.
See Editor's Note No. 14, page 1817.

Nature Derm Skin Care System Acne Cream -
PhytoPharmica

Each application contains: Sulfur 3%. Other ingredients: Purified Water, Zinc, Sage Extract, Silymarin Phytosome, Hawthorne Extract, Chamomile Extract, 18-Beta-Glycyrrhetinic Acid, Essential Oil of Rosemary, Urea, and Vitamin E (Tocopherol).

Nature Force - Rexall
Two tablets contain: Vitamin A (100% beta-carotene) 10000 IU • Vitamin C 300 mg • Vitamin E (dl-alpha-tocopheryl acid succinate) 90 IU • Calcium 255 mg • Selenium (from selenium amino acid chelate) 50 mcg • Sodium 5 mg • Nature Force Proprietary Blend: Mixed Berry Skin extract, Alfalfa aerial parts, Tomato, European Wine Grape concentrate (vitis vinifera), Plant Enzymes (glucose oxidase, peroxidase, catalase), Cruciferous Vegetable concentrate (cabbage head, cauliflower flower head, broccoli flower head), Green Tea leaf extract, Garlic, Rose Hips, and Seeds extract (rosa canina), Freeze-Dried Carrot root juice 188 mg. Other ingredients: Dicalcium Phosphate, Croscarmellose Sodium, Silica, Magnesium Stearate.

Nature's Cure Two-Part Acne Treatment System for Females - Nature's Cure
This is a 2 component product that includes tablets and a cream. Each tablet contains: Juglans regia (walnut) 6x • Antimonium Crudum (antimonius sulfide) 12x • Candida albicans (yeast) 12x, 30x, 60x, 200x • Echinacea angustifolia (cone flower) 12x • Kali Bromatum (potassium bromide) 12x • Ledum palustre (wild rosemary) 12x • Oophorunum (glandular) 12x • Hepar Sulfuris Calcareum (calcium sulfide) 24x • Carbo Vegetabilis (vegetable carbon) • Cimicifuga racemosa (black cohosh) 30x • Cistus canadensis (frost weed) 30 x • Graphites (graphite) 30x. Other Ingredients: Lactose. The cream contains: Benzoyl Peroxide (5%). Other Ingredients: Purified Water, Carbomer 940, Alantoin, Aloe Vera concentrate, Diazolidinyl Urea, Disodium Edetate, Dioctyl Sodium Sulfosuccinate, Sodium Hydroxide.
See Editor's Note No. 1, page 1816.

Nature's Cure Two-Part Acne Treatment System for Males - Nature's Cure
This is a 2 component product that includes tablets and a cream. Each tablet contains: Calendula officinalis (marigold) 6x • Hydrastis canadensis (golden seal) 6x • Juglans regia (walnut) 6x • Antimonium crudum (antimonius sulfide) 12x • Echinacea angustifolia (cone flower) 12x • Ledum palustre (wild rosemary) 12x • Orchitimun (glandular) 12x • Sarsaparilla (wild licorice) 12x • Hepar Sulfuris Calcareum (calcium sulfide) 24x • Carbo Vegetabilis (vegetable carbon) 30x. Other Ingredients: Lactose. The cream contains: Benzoyl Peroxide (5%). Other Ingredients: Purified Water, Carbomer 940, Allantoin, Aloe Vera concentrate, Diazolidinyl Urea, Disodium Edetate, Dioctyl Sodium Sulfosuccinate, Sodium Hydroxide.
See Editor's Note No. 1, page 1816.

Nature's Fingerprint - Fingerprint Botanicals
Each capsule contains: Wild Yam root 150 mg • Evening Primrose 90 mg • Chaste Tree berry 50 mg.

Nature's Life Greens - Capsule - Nature's Life
Each 500 mg capsule contains: Green Peas (Pisum sativum) • Celery (Apium graveolens) Cabbage (Brassica oleracea capitata) • Cauliflower (Brassica oleracea botrutis) • Broccoli (Brassica oleracea italica) • Spinach (Spinacia oleracea) • Green Bell Peppers (Capsicum frutescens) • Green Onions (Allium cepa) • Hawaiian grown Spirulina plantesis • Parsley (Petroselinum crispum) • Green Chili Peppers (Capsicum annum) • Green Garlic sprouts (Allium sativum) • Jalepeno Peppers (Capsicum annum) • Green Tea leaves (Camellia sinensis) • Alfalfa (Medicago sativa) • Barley Grass (Hordeum vulgare) • Dunaliella salina • Chlorella • Pacific Alaria (Alaria marginata) • Kelp (Laminaria species) • Pacific Nori (Porphyra tenera) Dulse (Phodymenia palmata) • Kombu (Laminaria setchellii) • Sea Lettuce (Ulva lactuca) • Sea Palm (Pastelsi palmaeformis).

Nature's Life Greens - Powder - Nature's Life
Five grams of powder contain: Green Peas (Pisum sativum) • Celery (Apium graveolens) Cabbage (Brassica oleracea capitata) • Cauliflower (Brassica oleracea botrutis) • Broccoli (Brassica oleracea italica) • Spinach (Spinacia oleracea) • Green Bell Peppers (Capsicum frutescens) • Green Onions (Allium cepa) • Hawaiian grown Spirulina plantesis • Parsley (Petroselinum crispum) • Green Chili Peppers (Capsicum annum) • Green Garlic sprouts (Allium sativum) • Jalepeno Peppers (Capsicum annum) • Green Tea leaves (Camellia sinensis) • Alfalfa (Medicago sativa) • Barley Grass (Hordeum vulgare) • Dunaliella salina • Chlorella • Pacific Alaria (Alaria marginata) • Kelp (Laminaria species) • Pacific Nori (Porphyra tenera) Dulse (Phodymenia palmata) • Kombu (Laminaria setchellii) • Sea Lettuce (Ulva lactuca) • Sea Palm (Pastelsi palmaeformis).

Nature's Way Digestion Formula - Nature's Way
Two capsules contain: Angelica root 90 mg • Barberry bark 135 mg • Beet root 100 mg • Cayenne pepper fruit 25 mg • Dandelion root 315 mg • Fizyme Enzyme Formula 100 mg • Gentian root 135 mg. Other ingredients: Gelatin, Magnesium Stearate, Millet.

Nature's Way Lycopene - Nature's Way
Each softgel capsule contains: Tomato seed oil standardized to (Lycopene) 5000 mcg • Canola oil • Beeswax • Lecithin • natural Vitamin E (d-Alpha Tocopheryl).

Nature's White Cross - D & E Pharmaceuticals
Each tablet contains: pure Ephedra extract 400 mg.

Naturex Multi II - Swanson
Each capsule contains: Vitamin A (as palmitate) 5000 IU • Vitamin C USP (as ascorbic acid) 150 mg • Vitamin D (as cholecalciferol) 200 IU • Vitamin E (as d-alpha tocopheryl succinate) 75 IU • Thiamin USP (as thiamin HCl; vitamin B-1) 50 mg • Riboflavin (vitamin B-2) 50 mg • Niacinamide 50 mg • Vitamin B-6 (as pyridoxine HCl) 50 mg • Folic Acid 200 mcg • Vitamin B-12 (as cyanocobalamin) 20 mcg • Biotin 25 mcg • Pantothenic Acid (as d-calcium pantothenate) 50 mg • Iron (from ferrous gluconate) 0.5 mg • Iodine (from potassium iodide) 75 mcg • Zinc (from zinc gluconate) 1.5 mg • Selenium (as selenomethionine) 5 mcg • Copper (from copper gluconate) 0.5 mg • Manganese (from manganese gluconate) 0.5 mg • Chromium (from amino acid chelate) 50 mcg • Choline (as choline bitartrate) 25 mg • Inositol 25 mg • PABA (para-aminobenzoic acid) 25 mg • Betaine HCl 12.5 mg • Lemon Bioflavonoid Complex 12.5 mg • L-Glutamic Acid 12.5 mg • Rutin (from buckwheat) 12.5 mg • Hesperidin Complex 2.5 mg.

Natur-Leaf - Lifeline, Inc.
Each caspule contains: Blend of sprout phytochemicals 300 mg: Wild African Potato root • Lupins sprouts • Fenugreek sprouts • Barley

BRAND NAMES

B R A N D N A M E S

sprouts • Wheat sprouts • Soybean sprouts • African Sunflower sprouts. Blend of enzymes 50 mg: Enzyme Mineral blend • Protease • Amylase • Lipase • Cellulase • Sucrase • Maltase • Lactase • Bromelain • Ionic Mineral blend.

NeoProstate B-300 - BCN
Each caplet contains: Beta-sitosterol 300 mg • Zinc Citrate 15 mg. Ingredients: Mixed Sterols including Beta-sitosterol (at least 50%), Stig-masterol, Campesterol, Lupeol, Cycloartenon, Famesol, Phytol and Zinc.

Nerve Guard - Flora
St. John's Wort.

Nettle - Nature's Way
Two capsules contain: Nettle herb 870 mg. Other Ingredients: Gelatin.

Nettle & Pygeum with Pumpkin - Enzymatic Therapy
Each capsule contains: Nettle root extract 16:1 (Urticae dioica radix) 300 mg • Pumpkin seed oil (Cucurbita pepo) 175 mg • Pygeum africanum extract standardized to contain 13% total sterols 25 mg.

Nettle-Pygeum Complex - PhytoPharmica
Each capsule contains: Nettle (Urtica dioica) root extract 16:1 300 mg • Pumpkin (Cucurbita pepo) seed oil 175 mg • Pygeum africanum (Prunus africana) bark extract (standardized to contain 13% total sterols) 25 mg.

Nettle-Reishi Virtue - Blessed Herbs
Nettle • Reishi mycelium • Chinese Ephedra • Yerba Santa leaf • Propolis • Ginkgo leaf • Licorice root • Grain alcohol & Distilled Water.

Neural Support Formula - The Vitamin Factory
Each tablet contains: Vitamin E (d-Alpha Tocopheryl-Succinate) 100 IU • Neuromins (13% DHA powder) 100 mg • Phosphatidylserine Complex 20% 50 mg • Ginkgo Biloba Leaf extract (24/6) 40 mg • Bacopin extract (Bacopa monniera, min. 20% Bacosides) 25 mg • Pycnogenol (Maritime Pine bark extract) 15 mg.

NeuRecover-DA (Depressant Abuse) - Natural Distributors International, Inc.
Six capsules contain: Vitamin A 2000 IU • Vitamin C 600 mg • Vitamin B1 14.5 mg • Vitamin B2 5 mg • Niacin (Niacinamide Ascorbate) 200 mg • Calcium (Chelate) 150 mg • Iron 9 mg • Vitamin E 30 IU • Vitamin B6 18 mg • Folic Acid 0.4 mg • Vitamin B12 0.03 mg • Magnesium 150 mg • Zinc 15 mg • Biotin 0.3 mg • Pantothenic Acid 90 mg • Chromium (Picolinate) 0.06 mg • DL-Phenylalanine 2760 mg • L-Glutamine 150 mg.

NeuRecover-SA (Stimulant Abuse) - Natural Distributors International, Inc.
Six capsules contain: Vitamin C (Ascorbate) 600 mg • Vitamin B1 10 mg • Vitamin B2 15 mg • Niacin (Niacinamide) 100 mg • Calcium (Chelate) 150 mg • Iron 9 mg • Vitamin B6 (Pyridoxal-5-Phosphate) 20 mg • Folic Acid 0.4 mg • Vitamin B12 0.03 mg • Magnesium (Oxide) 150 mg • Zinc (Chelate) 30 mg • Pantothenic Acid 90 mg • Chromium (Picolinate) 0.06 mg • DL-Phenylalanine 1500 mg • L-Tyrosine 900 mg • L-Glutamine 300 mg.

Neuro Care-Rx - Alternecare Health Products
Each capsule contains: Cayenne 125 mg • Ginger 125 mg • St. John's Wort 125 mg • Ginko Biloba 40 mg • Malic Acid 100 mg • Vitamin B3 100 mg • Vitamin C 60 mg • Manganese 10 mg • Copper 1 mg • Vitamin B6 50 mg.

Neuro Guardian - Clinician's Choice
Two tablets contain: Vitamin E (as dl-alpha tocopheryl acetate) 200 IU • Thiamin (as mononitrate) 10 mg • Riboflavin 10 mg • Niacin

(as niacinamide) 50 mg • Pantothenic Acid (d-calcium pantothenate) 10 mg • Zinc (as amino acid chelate) 10 mg • Selenium (selenomethionine) 50 mcg • Chromium (as nicotinate, chelavite, picolinate) 100 mcg • Ginkgo Biloba Leaf Extract 4:1 150 mg • Lecithin 100 mg • Natural Beta Carotene 40 mg • Acetyl-L-Carnitine 30 mg • RoseOx (patented, standardized process for an extract of Rosemary) 30 mg • Lecithin (standardized to 30% phosphatidyl serine) 30 mg • Aminogen 20 mg • Cayenne Fruit Powder 200 mg • Choline (as choline bitartrate) 20 mg • L-Tyrosine 20 mg • Proprietary blend 8 mg: Astragalus, Carrot Powder, Pacific Kelp, Piper Longum Fruit Powder.

Neuro Optimizer - Jarrow Formulas
Four capsules contain: Cytidine 5'-diphoscholine (CDP Choline) 300 mg • Phosphatidyl Serine (PS) 100 mg • Acetyl L-Carnitine 500 mg • L-Glutamine 500 mg • Alpha Lipoic Acid 50 mg • Taurine 500 mg • Phosphatidylcholine 135 mg. Other Ingredients: Tricalcium Phosphate, Silicon Dioxide.

Neuro-Boost Spray - Nature's Plus
Each spray contains: Phosphatidylserine-rich purified Lecithin concentrate supplying Activated Phosphatides: [Phosphatidylserine (PS) 10 mg, Phosphatidylcholine (PC) 10 mg, Cephalin (Phosphatidylethanolamine) 6 mg, Phosphoinositides 3 mg] 50 mg • DMAE (2-Dimethylaminoethanol Bitartrate) 12.5 mg • N-Acetyl-Tyrosine pharmaceutical grade free form amino acid 5 mg • Pantothenic Acid 5 mg • Korean Ginseng root (Panax ginseng CA Meyer) standardized 15% ginsenosides 5 mg • Chinese Green Tea leaf (Camellia sinensis) standardized 50% polyphenols 5 mg • Chinese Green Tea leaf standardized 24% ginkgo flavone glycosides, 6% terpene lactones 1000 mcg. In a proprietary Liposomal Complex of Essential Metabolic Factors , Purified Water, Vegetable Glycerine, Purified Lecithin, Citrus seed extract (Citrus sinensis), Vitamin E & (natural Root Beer) Sarsaparilla flavor.

Neuro-DHA - Metabolic Response Modifiers
Each sofgel contains: Fish Oil concentrate 500 mg • Min. 50% DHA 250 mg • Max. 20% EPA 100 mg • 20% Mixed fatty acids 100 mg • 10% stearidonic acid 50 mg • Vitamin C (Ascorbyl palmitate) 2 mg • Vitamin E (mixed-tocopherols) 4 mg.

NeuroGenic - Nature's Plus
Two tablets contain: Phosphatidyl Choline 250 mg • L-Glutamine free form amino acid 200 mg • Vitamin C corn free 150 mg • Pantothenic Acid 100 mg • L-Phenylalanine free form amino acid 100 mg • Ginkgo Biloba standardized 24% Ginkgo flavone-glycosides, 6% terpene lactones 60 mg • Ashwagandha (Withania somnifera) standardized 1.5% withanols 50 mg • Chinese Green Tea (Camellian sinensis) standardized 20% polyphenols 20 mg • Standardized Bilberry (Swedish Vaccinium myrtillus) standardized 25% Anthocyanosides 15 mg • PAK (Pyridoxal Alpha-Ketoglutarate) 10 mg • Co-Enzyme Q10 (Ubiquinone) 5mg. Contains no yeast, wheat, corn, soy, milk, salt, sugar or starch.

Neuro-Max - Metabolic Response Modifiers
Two capsules contain: Phospholipid Complex 500 mg • Ashwaganda extract 100 mg • Ginkgo Biloba extract 40 mg • Pregnenolone 50 mg.

Neuro-Max - New Hope Health Products
Two capsules contain: Phospholipid Complex [containing 100 mg Phosphatidylserine] 500 mg • Ashwagandha Extract 80 mg • Bacopa Monniera Extract 80 mg • Ginkgo Biloba Extract (28/11) 60 mg • Cytidine diphosphate choline 12 mg • Vinpocetine 5 mg • Niacin 10 mg.

Neuro-Max - Olympia Nutrition
Phosphatidylserine 50 mg • Ashwaganda 50 mg • Ginkgo 20 mg • Pregnenolone 25 mg.

Neuro-Max II - Metabolic Response Modifiers
Each capsule contains: Phospholipid complex (containing 100 mg Phosphatidlyserine) 500 mg • Ashwagandha extract 80 mg • Ginkgo Biloba extract (28/11) 60 mg • Cytidine diphosphate choline 12 mg • Vinpocetine 5 mg • Niacin 10 mg.

Neuromins DHA - Source Naturals
Each softgel contains: Docosahexaenoic Acid (DHA) (Derived rom algal oil (oceanic phytophankton), in a base of high-oleic sunflower oil, vitamin C (ascorbyl palmitate) and vitamin E (mixed tocopherols) as antioxidants) 100 mg.

Neuromins DHA - Nature's Way
Each softgel contains: Neruomins DHA 100 mg.
Other Ingredients: Gelatin, Glycerin, Sunflower Oil, Vitamin C, Vitamin E d-alpha tocopheryl, Water.

NeuroSyn - PharmAssure
Two softgel capsules contain: Vitamin E (as Natural d-alpha tocopheryl Acetate) 30 IU • High Choline Soy Lecithin (35% Phosphatidylcholine=175mg) 500 mg • DHA (Docosahaenioc Acid;as Marine Microalgae Oil) 100 mg • Ginkgo Biloba Leaves Extract (24% Ginkgo Flavonglycosides=28.8mg, 6% Terpene Lactones=7.2mg) 120 mg • Vinpocetine 5 mg. Other ingredients: Gelatin, Soybean Oil, Glycerin, Caramel Color, Titanium Dioxide (Natural Mineral Whitener).

Neurozyme - New Chapter, Inc.
One softgel contains: DHA (Docosahexaenoic acid), supercritical extract (from Arctic fish oil- 100 mg) (DPA min. 10%- 10 mg, EPA min. 5%- 5 mg) 50 mg • Rosemary leaf, supercritical extract (23% total phenolic antioxidants- 7 mg) 30 mg • Ginger (rhizome), certified organic, supercritical extract (minimum 20% pungent compounds-6 mg, 5% zingiberence- 1.5 mg) 30 mg • Sage leaf, supercritical extract (38%- 42% total phenolic antioxidants- 6 mg) 15 mg • Chamomile flower, supercritical extract (25% alpha-bisabolol 3.8 mg) 15 mg • Clove bud, supercritical extract, (65% euaenol 6.5 mg) 10 mg • Potency Assured Extracts, Ginkgo leaf (12% flavone glycosides- 14 mg) 120 mg • Gotu Kola leaf (10% asiaticoside 12 mg, 30% triterpenes- 36 mg) 120 mg • Club Moss, Chinese Huperzia serrata (0.5% Huperzine A -0.3 mg) 60 mg • Ashwaganda root (extract 4:1) 60 mg • Cat's Claw root (extract 4:1) (3% alkaloids-1.5 mg) 50 mg • Lemon Balm, Melissa officinalis leaf (5% rosemarininc acid- 1.5 mg) 30 mg • Bacopin, Bacopa monniera (Brahil), (leaf), (extract), (Bacosides A and B = 20.65%- 6.2 mg), (0.6% alkaloids- 0.2 mg) 30 mg • Paeonia, Eurpoean (extract 5:1) 20 mg • Holy Basil, Ocimum sanctum, (leaf) (2.5% ursalic acid-0.5 mg) 20 mg • Turmeric (rhizome), (7-9% curcumin- 1.6 mg) 20 mg • Red Wine, (30% total polyphenols- 6 mg) 20 mg • Chamomile flower (extract 5:1) 15 mg • Vitamin E 2 UI. Other Ingredients: Olive Oil - certified organic, Yellow Beeswax.

Neutra-Gas - PhytoPharmica
Each capsule contains: Simethicone 25 mg • Peppermint oil extract (Mentha piperita) 0.2 ml. Chlorophyll is used as a natural coloring agent.

New Choice - The Herbalist
Gingko leaf • Gotu Kola herb • Guarana seed • American Ginseng root • Siberian Ginseng root • Jamaican Sarsaparilla root • Kola Nut • Licorice root • Cinnamon bark • Ginger root • Cayenne pepper.

New Life Colostrum - Symbiotics
100% Bovine Colostrum

New Life Colostrum Capsules - Symbiotics
Two capsules contain: 100% Bovine Colostrum from New Zealand cows 960 mg • Vitamin A 336 IU • Vitamin C 2.8 mg • Iron 1.4 mg • Calcium 10 mg.

New Life Colostrum High-IG - Symbiotics
Two capsules contain: 100% Bovine Colostrum 960 mg • Vitamin A 504 IU • Vitamin C 4.2 mg • Iron 2.1 mg • Calcium 15 mg • Immunoglobulin 288 mg.

New Life Colostrum Powder - Symbiotics
One teaspoon contains: 100% Bovine Colostrum from New Zealand cows 1440 mg • Vitamin A 504 IU • Vitamin C 4.2 mg • Iron 2.1 mg • Calcium 15 mg • Immunoglobulin 246 mg.

New Man Tea - The Herbalist
Damiana leaf • Fo-ti root • Sassafras bark • Licorice root • Cinnamon bark • Saw Palmetto berry • Sarsaparilla bark • Parsley root • Marshmallow root • Orange peel.

New Woman Tonic - The Herbalist
Chaste Tree berry • Black Cohosh root • Black Haw bark • Motherwort herb • Cramp bark • Skullcap herb • Ginger root.

NewBust (New Bust) - Tiger-One.com
Saw Palmetto • Dong Quai • Damiana • Fenugreek seed • Blessed Thistle • Violet • Wild Yam • Fennel seed • Althea root • Cumin seed • Hops.
See Editor's Note No. 17, page 1817.

NewBust Lotion (New Bust Lotion) - Tiger-One.com
Water • Saw Palmetto • Extra Virgin Olive Oil • Dong Quai • Damiana • Glycerin • Foenugreek seed • Blessed Thistle • Violet • Wild Yam • Fennel seed • Althea root • Cumin seed • Hops.
See Editor's Note No. 17, page 1817.

NewPhase - New Phase - Chattem
Each caplet contains: Multi-herbal blend 410 mg: Soy Protein Concentrate, Standardized Kudzu extract root, Standardized Red Clover Extract leaf • Standardized Chastetree Extract berry 75 mg • Standardized Black Cohosh Extract root 40 mg.

Nexcite - Nordic Drinks
Each 100 mL serving contains: Carbonated Water 93 g • Sugar 8.5 g • Citric Acid 0.2 g • Damiana -extract 59 mg • Schizandra -extract 58 mg • Mate -extract 57 mg • Guarana -extract 56 mg • Caffeine 30 mg • Flavoring 23 mg • Ginseng -extract 18 mg • Sodium benzoate (E211) 15 mg • Colour (E133) 65 pg.

NFA-500 - Human Development Technologies
Each capsule contains: L-Tyrosine 500 mg • Acetylcholine 25 mg • DMAE 25 mg • St. John's Wort 60 mg. Additional Ingredients: DLPA • Ginkgo Biloba • Vitamin B12 • Vitamin B6 • Vitamin B1 • Vitamin C • Copper Sulfate • Folic Acid • Phosphorus • Zinc • Bioperine.

N-FLAM Plus - Nutri-Quest
Each enteric coated tablet contains: Pancreatin 170 mg • Papain 100 mg • Bromelain 80 mg • Trypsin 40 mg (Chymotrypsin 8 mg) • Lipase 15 mg • Amylase 17 mg • Rutin 85 mg • Calf Thymus 45 mg • Zinc Gluconate 4 mg • Partoid concentrate 1 mg.
See Editor's Note No. 14, page 1817.

Niacin - Leiner Health Products
Each tablet contains: Niacin (Nicotinic acid) 100 mg.
Other Ingredients: Lactose, Starch, Stearic Acid, Silicon Dioxide, Magnesium Stearate.

Niacin - Nature's Bounty
Each tablet contains: Niacin 100 mg. Other Ingredients: Cellulose, Dicalcium Phosphate, Vegetable Stearic Acid, Povidone, Vegetable Magnesium Stearate, Silica.

BRAND NAMES

Niacin - Flush Free - Nature's Bounty
Each capsule contains: Niacin (as Inositol Hexanicotinate) 400 mg
• Inositol (as Inositol Hexanicotinate) 100 mg. Other Ingredients:
Gelatin, Dicalcium Phosphate, Vegetable Magnesium Stearate, Silica.

Niacin Time Release - Puritan's Pride
Each capsule contains: Niacin 250 mg.

Niacin with Cholestatin - Futurebiotics
Each tablet contains: Niacin 400 mg • Cholestatin 400 mg.

Niacin+ - PhysioLogics
Each capsule contains: Niacin (Inositol Hexanicotinate) 400 mg
• Vitamin C (Magnesium Ascorbate) 100 mg • Chromium
(Niacinamide/Glycinate) 66 mcg.

Niacinamide - Nature's Bounty
Each tablet contains: Niacin (as Niacinamide) 500 mg.
Other Ingredients: Cellulose, Dicalcium Phosphate, Vegetable Stearic
Acid, Silica, Vegetable Magnesium Stearate.

Nico-End - PhytoPharmica
Each tablet contains: Nux vomica 8x • Lobelia 6x • Staphysagria 6x •
Tabacum 6x.
See Editor's Note No. 1, page 1816.

Night Time Formulation - Olympian Labs
Each capsule contains: Valerian root 200 mg • Passion Flower 200 mg
• Skullcap 50 mg • L-Tyrosine 25 mg • Parsley 50 mg • Peppermint
75 mg • Calcium Citrate 80 mg • Pantothenic Acid 20 mg.

NightRest - Source Naturals
Two tablets contain: Melatonin 4 mg • Magnesium (Magnesium
Glycinate and Magnesium Taurinate) 200 mg • Glycine (Magnesium
Glycinate and Glycine) 502 mg • Taurine (Magnesium Taurinate)
435 mg • Passionflower 120 mg • GABA (Gamma Amino Butyric
Acid) 100 mg • Skullcap 70 mg • Chamomile extract (4:1) 60 mg.
See Editor's Note No. 16, page 1817.

NightTime Complex with Melotonin - Pharmanex
Each capsule contains: Valerian root extract 75 mg • Passion Flower
extract 37.5 mg • Kava Lactones (from Kava Kava root extract)
7.5 mg • Hops Strobile powder (fruit) 25 mg • Chamomile flower
powder 25 mg • Melissa officinalis powder (leaf & flower) 25 mg •
Mixed Tocopherols 0.5 mg • Melatonin 0.5 mg. Other Ingredients:
Maltodextrin, Magnesium, Silicon Dioxide.
See Editor's Note No. 16, page 1817.

Nighty Night - Traditional Medicinals
Contains: Passionflower • Spearmint leaf • Chamomile herb • Lemon
Verbena leaf • Licorice root • Lilia Star flower • Lemon peel •
Lemongrass leaf • Catnip leaf • Hop Strobile.

Nitro Fuel (Ion Exchange Whey Protein Powder) - TwinLab
Each serving contains: Pure Protein 25 g.

Nitro Fuel (The Ultimate Anti-Catabolic Amino Acid Drink) - TwinLab
Protein (Amino Acids) & Carbohydrates • Whey Protein Concentrate
[a source of Branched Chain Amino Acids (L-Leucine, L-Isoleucine,
L-Valine)] • Chromium Picolinate • Alpha-Ketoglutarates. No
preservatives or artificial flavors.

No. 1 GARLIC PLUS ESTER-C & FOS - Dial Herbs
Two capsules contain: Pure-Gar deodorized Garlic concentrate
300 mg • FOS Micro Flora Growth concentrate 300 mg • Vitamin C
from Ester-C 200 mg.

No. 56 K KIDNEY - Systemic Formulas
Rose Hips • RNA/DNA Kidney Factors • Gelatin • Magnesium
Sulfate • Vitamin C • Ch de Bugre • Fish Liver Oil (Source of
Vitamins A and D) • Sete Sangrias • Calcium Carbonate • RNA/DNA
Adrenal Factors • Hesperidin • Serine • RNA/DNA Thalamus Factors
• Tyrosine • Spearmint Oil • Rose Petal Essence • Aloe Vera.
See Editor's Note No. 14, page 1817.

Noni - Source Naturals
Each capsule contains: Hawaiian Noni (Morinda citrifolia) 375 mg.

Nopal (Opuntia S.P.) - Concord
Each capsule contains: Nopal 500 mg.

Nopal Strepta (Prickly Pear Cactus) - Cactu-Life
Each capsule contains: 100% Opuntia Streptacantha 450 mg.

Nor Stack - Substrate Solutions
Each tablet contains: 19-Nor-4-Androstenediol 100 mg •
19-Nor-4-Androstenedione 100 mg.

NorCycloDiol-4 (Sports One Cycloplex Pro-Hormone) - Sports One
Each lozenge contains: Nor-4-Androstenediol Cycloplex (cyclodextrin
complex) 10 mg.

NorCycloDione (Sports One Cycloplex Pro-Hormone) - Sports One
Each lozenge contains: 19-Nor-4-Androstenedione Cycloplex
(cyclodextrin complex) 25 mg.

Nordisk of Denmark Propolis - Health From The Sun
Each capsule contains: 50% Propolis • 50% Bee Pollen in a natural
mineral base of Calcium Phosphate. No sugar added. No
preservatives. No artificial coloring or flavoring.

Norwegian Cod Liver Oil - Puritan's Pride
Each softgel contains: Natural Vitamin A 1,250 IU •
Natural Vitamin D (from Cod Liver Oil) 135 IU.

Norwegian Cod Liver Oil - Nature's Bounty
Each softgel contains: Vitamin A (from Cod Liver Oil) 1250 IU
• Vitamin D (from Cod Liver Oil) 135 IU. Other Ingredients: Cod
Liver Oil, Soybean Oil, Gelatin, Glycerin.

N-R-G Protein Powder - Naturade
Each 1 oz serving contains: Isolated Soy Protein • Calcium Caseinate
• Sweet Dairy whey • Carrageenan • Soy Lecithin • Enzymatically
Predigested Lactalbumin • Egg albumin • Papain & Natural Vanilla
flavor.

N-TENSE - Raintree Nutrition
Each capsule contains: Graviola • Mullaca • Vassournha • Espinheira
Santa • Mutamba • Bitter Melon • Suma • Cat's Claw.
See Editor's Note No. 17, page 1817.

Nu Knees - Sports Nutrition Source.com
Three capsules contain: Glucosamine Sulfate 1000 mg • Chondroitin
Sulfate 750 mg • MSM 750 mg • White Willow Bark 150 mg •
Bromelain 100 mg • Vitamin C 90 mg.
See Editor's Note No. 15, page 1817.

NuBiotic - PhytoPharmica
Each tablet contains: Vitamin A (fish liver oil) 10,000 IU • Vitamin C
(ascorbic acid) 200 mg • Vitamin D (fish liver oil) 35 IU • Vitamin
B12 (cyanocobalamin) 2.5 mcg • Pantothenic Acid (calcium
D-pantothenate) 25 mg • Calcium (lactate) 41 mg • Magnesium
(citrate) 6.7 mg • Zinc (gluconate) 10.5 mg • RNA powder 60 mg •

Alfalfa (Medicago sativa) leaf and stem juice powder 50 mg • Lemon Bioflavonoids 30 mg • Spleen extract 30 mg • Thymus extract 25 mg • Trace Mineral Concentrate (kelp) 25 mg • Unsaturated free fatty acids (oil of evening primrose) 15 mg • Lung extract 10 mg.
See Editor's Note No. 14, page 1817.

Nucleic Acid with RNA and DNA - Quest
Each tablet contains: RNA (Ribonucleic Acid) 200 mg • DNA (Deoxyribonucleic Acid) 60 mg • Brewer's Yeast 190 mg. Other Ingredients: Dibasic Calcium Phosphate, Microcrystalline Cellulose, Vegetable Stearin, Magnesium Stearate (vegetable source), Silicon Dioxide.

NutraFloraFOS - Natrol
One capsule contains: FOS (Fructooligosaccharides) 500 mg.
Other ingredients: Magnesium Stearate, Gelatin.

NutraLife - SAMe - NutraLife
Each tablet contains: S-Adenosyl-Methionine Tosylate Disulfate 200 mg.

Nutramin Body System - Informulab
One Capsule contains: Vitamin A (Beta Carotene) 1562 IU • Vitamin C 125 mg • Vitamin E 25 IU • Vitamin B-1 (Thiamine Mononitrate) 2.5 mg • Vitamin B2 (Riboflavin) 2.5 mg • Vitamin B6 (Pyridoxine HCl) 2.5 mg • Vitamin B12 (Cyanocobalamin) 2.5 mcg • Vitamin B3 (Niacinimide) 5 mg • Vitamin B5 (Pantothenic Acid) 10 mg • Vitamin B8 (Folic Acid) 50 mcg • Biotin (Water soluble Vit. B) 12.5 mcg • Vitamin D 50 IU • Calcium (Amino acid chelate) 62.5 mg • Phosphorus (Di-calcium phosphate) 6.25 mg • Magnesium (Amino acid chelate) 37.5 mg • Iron (Amino acid chelate) 2.25 mg • Zinc (Amino acid chelate) 1.875 mg • Manganese (Amino acid chelate) 0.625 mg • Copper (Amino acid chelate) 0.25 mg • Chromium Chelavite 18.75 mcg • Selenium (Amino acid chelate) 0.625 mcg • Potassium (Amino acid chelate) 3.125 mg • Iodine (as Potassium iodine) 18.75 mcg • Horsetail Herb 3.125 mg • White Willow Bark 3.125 mg • Bee Pollen 3.125 mg • Hops Flower 3.125 mg • Licorice Root 3.125 mg • Skullcap 3.125 mg • Valerian 3.125 mg • Garlic (Bulb-odorless) 3.125 mg • Citrus Bioflavonoids 3.125 mg • Rosehips 3.125 mg • Rutin 3.125 mg • Ginseng Root (Siberian) 3.125 mg • Alfalfa Herb 3.125 mg • Ginkgo Leaf 3.125 mg • Hawthorne Berry 3.125 mg • Beet Root 3.125 mg • Cayenne Fruit 3.125 mg • L-Lysine 3.125 mg • L-Proline 3.125 mg • L-Glutamine 3.125 mg • Live Food Enzyme Blend (vegetable source Protease, Lipase and Amylase) 6.25 mg • Pycnogenol 0.25 mg.

Nutramine - Calwood Nutritionals
Each scoop contains: L-Histidine 280 mg • L-Isoleucine 360 mg • L-Leucine 560 mg • L-Lysine 410 mg • L-Methionine 560 mg • L-Phenylalanine 560 mg • L-Threonine 250 mg • L-Tryptophan 130 mg • L-Valine 410 mg.

Nutramine T - Calwood Nutritionals
Two scoops contain: L-Histidine 220 mg • L-Isoleucine 290 mg • L-Leucine 440 mg • L-Lysine 310 mg • L-Methionine 440 mg • L-Phenylalanine 340 mg • L-Threonine 320 mg • L-Tryptophan 120 mg • L-Valine 360 mg • L-Tyrosine 660 mg.

NutraSleep - Source Naturals
Four tablets contain: Niacinamide 10 mg • Vitamin B6 (Pyridoxine HCl) 2 mg • Calcium (citrate and carbonate) 250 mg • Magnesium (citrate, oxide and taurinate) 450 mg • Taurine (Magnesium taurinate) 1000 mg • Inositol 700 mg • GABA (Gamma Amino Butyric Acid) 600 mg • Skullcap 250 mg • Passionflower 200 mg • Valerian root 200 mg • Chamomile extract 100 mg.

NutraSpray Quercetin - Source Naturals
Each spray contains: Quercetin 50 mg.

Nutri Fiber - Progressive Labs
One tablespoon contains: Calcium 10.2 mg • Iron 0.35% • Thiamin (Vitamin B1) 0.36 mg • Riboflavin (Vitamin B2) 0.18 mg • Niacin 1.89 mg • Vitamin B6 1.66 mg • Pantothenic Acid 044 mg • Phosphorus 11.5 mg • Magnesium 31.8 mg • Zinc 2.42 mg • Copper 0.26 mg • Manganese 0.13 mg • Sodium 0.6% • Potassium 34.2 mg • Linolenic Acid (omega 3) 1.36 g.

Nutri Plex - Sports Nutrition Source.com
One and a half scoops contain: Sodium 200 mg • Potassium 680 mg • Protein 25 g • Vitamin A 2500 IU • Vitamin C 30 mg • Calcium 800 mg • Iron 9 mg • Vitamin D 200 IU • Vitamin E 15 IU • Pantothenic Acid 5 mg • Vitamin B-1 75 mg • Vitamin B-2 85 mg • Vitamin B-3 10 mg • Vitamin B-6 1 mg • Vitamin B-12 3 mcg • Biotin 125 mcg • Zinc 7.5 mcg • Copper 1 mg • Magnesium 200 mg • Manganese 2 mg • Iodine 75 mcg • Phosphorus 160 mg • Selenium 32 mcg • Molybdenum 60 mcg • Chromium 78 mcg.

Nutri-1000 - The Vitamin Shoppe
Each tablet contains: Vitamin D 400 IU • Vitamin A 25000 IU • Vitamin C 100 mg • Vitamin E 100 IU • Vitamin B1 100 mg • Vitamin B2 100 mg • Vitamin B6 100 mg • Vitamin B12 100 mcg • Niacinamide 100 mg • PABA 100 mg • Pantothenic Acid 100 mg • Choline 100 mg • Inositol 100 mg • Biotin 100 mcg • Folic Acid 400 mcg • Rutin 25 mg • Citrus Bioflavonoid Complex 25 mg • Hesperidin Complex 5 mg • Betaine Hydrochloride 25 mg • Glutamic Acid 25 mg • Iodine 150 mcg • Calcium 50 mg • Potassium 15 mg • Iron 25 mg • Magnesium 20 mg Manganese 6.1 mg • Zinc 20 mg • Chromium 15 mcg • Selenium 10 mcg. In a whole-food base of rice concentrate, parsley, kelp, alfalfa, green cabbage, acerola, sarsaparilla, watercress, and golden seal.

Nutri-All Multiple Powder - Nature's Life
Each scoop (about 15 g) contains: Vitamin A (Beta Carotene) 20000 IU • Vitamin E (d-Alpha Tocopheryl Acetate) 390 IU • Vitamin B1 (Thiamine Mononitrate) 30 mg • Vitamin B2 (Riboflavin) 30 mg • Vitamin B3 (Niacinamide) 110 mg • Vitamin B6 (Pyridoxine HCI) 30 mg • Vitamin B12 (Cobalamin concentrate) 30 mcg • Folic Acid 400 mcg • Biotin 30 mcg • Pantothenic Acid (d-Calcium Pantothenate) 110 mg • Inositol 110 mg • Choline (Citrate) 110 mg • Vitamin C 510 mg • Lemon Bioflavonoids (TESTLAB 50% Flavonoids) 100 mg • Rutin 30 mg • Boron (Proteinate) 25 mcg • Calcium (Carbonate , Ascorbate, Citrate/Malate) 800 mg • Chromium (Polinicotinate, Aspartate) 60 mcg • Copper (Citrate) 1 mg • Iodine (Kelp) 22.5 mg • Iron (Fumerate) 8 mg • Magnesium (Oxide, Citrate) 400 mg • Manganese (Citrate) 4 mg • Molybdenum (Molybdate) 60 mcg • Potassium (Gluconate) 99 mg • Selenium (Selenomethionine) 60 mcg • Silicone (Dioxide) 10 mg • Zinc (Picolinate) 20 mg. In a natural base of Protein powder, Oat Fiber, Rice Syrup solids, Psyllium husks & natural Orange flavor. Contains 10 mg of naturally occurring Sodium.

Nutri-All Multiple Softgel - Nature's Life
Six softgel capsules contain: Beta Carotene (Vitamin A equivalent 10000 IU) 6 mg • Vitamin A (Fish Liver oil) 10000 IU • Vitamin D (as Vitamin D3) (Cholecalciferol) 400 IU • Vitamin B1 (Thiamine Mononitrate) 80 mg • Vitamin B2 (Riboflavin) 80 mg • Vitamin B3 (Niacinamide) 80 mg • Vitamin B6 (Pyridoxine HCI) 80 mg • Folic Acid 400 mcg • Vitamin B12 (Trituration of concentrate) 100 mcg • Biotin 50 mcg • Pantothenic Acid (d-Calcium Pantothenate) 80 mg • Choline Bitartrate 50 mg • Inositol 50 mg • Vitamin E (d-Alpha Tocopherol) 400 IU • Vitamin C (Ascorbic Acid & Rose Hips) 500 mg • Lemon Bioflavonoids (50% TESTLAB) 50 mg • Rutin Complex (Dimorphandra mollis) 25 mg • Hesperidin Complex (Citrus) 25 mg • Calcium (Carbonate) 1000 mg • Chromium (Picolinate, Nutrition 21) 200 mcg • Copper (Gluconate) 1 mg • Iodine (Potassium Iodide) 225 mcg • Magnesium (Oxide) 600 mg • Manganese (Citrate) 10 mg • Molybdenum (Molybdate) 20 mcg • Potassium (Citrate) 50 mg • Selenium (l-Selenomethionine) 50 mcg • Vanadium (Vanadyl Sulfate)

BRAND NAMES

20 mcg • Zinc (Citrate) 15 mg • Betaine HCl 25 mg • CoEnzyme Q10 5 mg • Chlorophyll (oil-soluble) 100 mg.
In a natural base of Safflower oil, Lecithin & Soy.

NutriBiotic Capsules Plus - NutriBiotic
Grapefruit extract • Echinacea extract • Artemisa annua extract.

NutriBiotic Tablets - NutriBiotic
Grapefruit extract 100 mg.

Nutri-Cleanse - Nu-Creations
Each tablet contains: Aloe Vera resin 430 mg • Aloe Vera leaf 200 mg. Other Ingredients: Anise, Fennel, Psyllium, Rhubarb, Kelp, Flax, Dicalcium Phosphate, Pharmaceutical Glaze, Magnesium Stearate.

Nutri-Fast Trim - Nu-Creations
Three tablets contain: Chromium 400 mcg. Other Ingredients: Guar Gum, Gum Karaya, American Desert Herb, Guarana, Korean Ginseng, Bee Pollen, White Willow, Bladderwrack, Gotu Kola, Licorice, Reishi Mushroom, Chickweed, Mate, Gymnema Sylvestis, Fennel, Astragalus, Ginger, Rehmannia, Dicalcium Phosphate, Pharmaceutical Glaze, Magnesium Stearate.

NutriFi - Pharmanex
Each teaspoon contains: Oat Fiber • Maltodextrin • Dextrose (Glucose) • Cellulose • Citrus Pectin • Psyllium Fiber • Gum Arabic.

Nutrilite Antioxidant Complex with Pycnogenol - Nutrilite
Each capsule contains: Pycnogenol 60 mg • Grape Seed extract 30 mg • Green Tea extract (Decaffeinated) 300 mg • Alpha-Lipoic Acid 45 mg • Glutathione 60 mg • Turmeric extract 75 mg.

Nutrilite Bilberry with Lutein - Nutrilite
Each softgel contains: Bilberry extract • Lutein • Zeaxanthin • DHA.

Nutrilite Black Cohosh and Soy - Nutrilite
Each tablet contains: Black Cohosh extract 120 mg • Soy Protein 300 mg • Isoflavones 49.8 mg • Acerola Cherry Concentrate 30 mg • Calcium 60 mg.

Nutrilite Calcium Magnesium Plus - Nutrilite
Each tablet contains: Calcium 651 mg • Magnesium 324 mg • Zinc 10 mg • Copper 2 mg • Manganese 2.5 mg • NUTRILITE Alfalfa Concentrate with Phytofactors Plant Compounds.
See Editor's Note No. 5, page 1816.

Nutrilite ChromPic Extra - Nutrilite
Each capsule contains: Chromium 300 mcg (providing Chromium picolinate 2400 mcg) • Vanadium 220 mcg • Gymnema sylvestre 100 mcg.

Nutrilite CoEnzyme Q10 Complex - Nutrilite
Each capsule contains: CoEnzyme Q10 30 mg • L-Carnitine 100 mg • Taurine 125 mg • Bioflavonoids 25 mg.

Nutrilite Daily Multivitamin and Multimineral - Nutrilite
Each tablet contains: Vitamin A (20% as beta carotene) 5000 IU • Vitamin C 90 mg • Vitamin D 400 IU • Vitamin E 30 IU • Vitamin K 80 mcg • Thiamin 2.3 mg • Riboflavin 2.6 mg • Niacin 20 mg • Vitamin B-6 2 mg • Folic Acid 400 mcg • Vitamin B-12 9 mcg • Biotin 300 mcg • Pantothenic Acid 10 mg • Calcium 200 mg • Iron 6 mg • Phosphorus 45 mg • Iodine 150 mcg • Magnesium 100 mg • Zinc 15 mg • Selenium 70 mcg • Copper 2 mg • Manganese 2 mg • Chromium 120 mcg • Molybdenum 75 mcg • Nutrilite concentrate 518 mg.

Nutrilite Double X - Nutrilite
Each tablet contains: Vitamin A (75% as beta carotene) 5000 IU • Vitamin C (from ascorbic acid, acerola powder) 250 mg • Vitamin D

200 IU • Vitamin E (d-alpha tocopheryl succinate) 150 IU • Vitamin K (from phytonadione) 40 mcg • Thiamin 12.5 mg • Riboflavin 12.5 mg • Niacin 35 mg • Vitamin B-6 25 mg • Folic Acid 400 mcg • Vitamin B-12 50 mcg • Biotin (from d-biotin) 150 mcg • Pantothenic Acid 25 mg • Calcium (from calcium carbonate) 450 mg • Phosphorous (from calcium phosphate) 10 mg • Iodine 75 mcg • Magnesium (from magnesium oxide) 225 mg • Zinc (from zinc gluconate) 10 mg • Selenium (from sodium selenite) 50 mcg • Copper (from copper gluconate) 1 mg • Manganese (from manganese gluconate) 2.5 mg • Chromium (from chromium chloride) 60 mcg • Molybdenum (from sodium molybdate) 37.5 mcg • Potassium (from potassium chloride) 40 mg • Alpha Lipoic Acid 5 mg • MSM (methylsulfonyl methane) 30 mg • Lycopene 0.5 mg • Lutein 0.5 mg • Quercetin 50 mg • Spirulina 25 mg • Boron (from boron aspartate) 500 mcg • Vanadium (from vanadyl sulfate) 10 mcg. Other Ingredients: Alfalfa extract, Parsley Dehydrate, Acerola concentrate, Citrus Bioflavonoid concentrate, Quercetin, Methylsulfonyl Methane, Brassica concentrate, Horseradish root, Mixed Tocopheryls, Calcium Pantothenate, Pyridoxine Hydrochloride, Niacinamide, Spirulina algae, Thiamine Mononitrate.

Nutrilite Echinacea with Astragalus - Nutrilite
Each tablet contains: Echinacea extract 200.1 mg • Astragalus extract 50.1 mg • Chlorella powder 50.1 mg.

Nutrilite Garlic & Licorice - Nutrilite
Each tablet contains: Pure concentrated Garlic 1000 mg • Licorice extract 21 mg.

Nutrilite Ginkgo Biloba and DHA - Nutrilite
Each softgel contains: Standardized Ginkgo Biloba extract 160 mg • DHA 180 mg • Gotu Kola 68 mg.

Nutrilite Glucosamine HCl with Boswellia - Nutrilite
Four tablets contain: Glucosamine HCL 1500 mg • Boswellia 75.2 mg • Bromelain 160 mg • NUTRILITE Acerola concentrate • Lemon Bioflavonoid concentrate with specific Phytofactors plant compounds.

Nutrilite LeadingEdge Heart Pack - Nutrilite
Each packet contains: CoEnzyme Q10 • Garlic • Licorice • Omega 3 Complex • Natural B Complex.

Nutrilite Milk Thistle and Dandelion - Nutrilite
Each tablet contains: Milk Thistle extract (Silybin Extract 228 mg) 468 mg • Dandelion root extract 375 mg • Turmeric extract 225 mg • Lemon Bioflavonoids • Acerola Cherry Concentrate.

Nutrilite Passionflower with Chamomile - Nutrilite
Each tablet contains: Passionflower 129.9 mg • Chamomile 81.3 mg • Hops 18.75 mg.

Nutrilite Saw Palmetto with Nettle Root - Nutrilite
Each softgel contains: Saw Palmetto 318 mg • Pumpkin Seed Oil 480 mg • Nettle Root 240 mg.
See Editor's Note No. 2, page 1816.

Nutrilite Siberian Ginseng with Ginkgo Biloba - Nutrilite
Each capsule contains: Siberian Ginseng extract 200 mg • Ginkgo Biloba extract 133.6 mg • NUTRILITE Acerola Cherry and Citrus Bioflavonoid Concentrates.

Nutrilite St. John's Wort with Lemon Balm - Nutrilite
Each capsule contains: St. John's Wort (0.3% Hypericin) 900 mg • Lemon Balm 78 mg • Lemon Bioflavonoid Concentrate 72 mg • Vitamin C (from Acerola Cherry Concentrate) 10 mg.

Nutrilite Women's GLA Blend with Evening Primrose Oil - Nutrilite
Each softgel contains: Evening Primrose • Borage Oil • Black Currant Oil • Chasteberry • Dong Quai • Ginger Extract.

Nutri-Plex - Nu-Creations
Three tablets contain: Vitamin A 5000 IU • Vitamin C 180 mg • Vitamin D 400 IU • Vitamin E 50 IU • Vitamin K 80 mcg • Vitamin B1 1.5 mg • Vitamin B2 1.7 mg • Niacin 20 mg • Vitamin B6 2 mg • Folic Acid 400 mcg • Vitamin B12 6 mcg • Biotin 300 mcg • Pantothenic Acid 10 mg • Calcium 100 mg • Phosphorus 100 mg • Iodine 100 mcg • Magnesium 150 mcg • Zinc 50 mg • Selenium 15 mg • Copper 70 mcg • Manganese 2 mg • Chromium 2 mg • Molybdenum 400 mcg • Vanadium 75 mcg • Boron 1 mcg • Potassium 79 mg • Choline 10 mg • Inositol 10 mg • Garcinia cambogia 300 mg • Korean Ginseng 100 mg • Siberian Ginseng 200 mg.
Other Ingredients: Anise, Fennel, Psyllium, Rhubarb, Kelp, Flax, Dicalcium Phosphate, Pharmaceutical Glaze, Magnesium Stearate.

Nutri-Shield - Nu-Creations
Two capsules contain: Vitamin A 25,000 mg • Vitamin C 1000 mg • Vitamin E 400 mg • Vitamin B6 25 mg • Zinc 25 mg • Selenium 100 mg • Copper 2 mg • Chromium 25 mg • Bioflavonoid Complex 150 mg • Rutin 40 mg • Quercetin 10 mg • Superoxide 100 mg • Astragalus 50 mg • Ginkgo biloba 15 mg • Rosemary 50 mg • Alpha Lipoic Acid 20 mg • Silymarin 50 mg • Lutein 6 mg • Spirulina 100 mg • Grape Seed extract 25 mg • Pine Bark extract 25 mg • Coenzyme Q-10 20 mg • L-Glutathione 10 mg • L-Glycerine 100 mg • Siberian Ginseng 50 mg • Reishi Mushroom 50 mg • Curcumin 50 mg. Other Ingredients: Dicalcium Phosphate, Pharmaceutical Glaze, Magnesium Stearate.

Nutrition Warehouse Boron Complex Plus - Nutrition Warehouse
Four capsules contain: Boron 3 mg • MCHA (microcrystalline hydroxyapatite) 2000 mg • Calcium (from MCHA) 520 mg • Phosphorous (from MCHA) 260 mg • Magnesium carbonate elemental 160 mg • Magnesium aspartate elemental 40 mg • Vitamin D (as Vitamin D3) 260 IU • Vitamin K 120 mcg • Manganese 10 mg • Silica 100 mg. Other Ingredients: Magnesium, Potassium, Zinc, Selenium, Manganese, Iron, Collagen, Glycosaminoglycans, substituent Amino Acids.

Nutri-Vit - Progressive Labs
One tablespoon (15 ml) contains: Vitamin A 3750 IU • Vitamin C 60 mg • Vitamin D 600 IU • Vitamin E 15 IU • Thiamin (B1) 1.05 mg • Riboflavin (B2) 1.2 mg • Niacin 13.5 mg • Vitamin B6 1.05 mg • Folate (folic acid) 300 mcg • Vitamin B12 4.5 mcg • Biotin 225 mcg • Pantothenic Acid 7.5 mg • Iron 15 mg • Zinc 12 mg.

NxTrim - Nova Pharmaceutical, Inc.
Two tablets contain: Vitamin C (ascorbic acid) 200 mg • Niacin 10 mg • Vitamin B6 (as pyridoxine hydrochloride) 4 mg • Vitamin B12 (as cyanocobalamin) 166 mcg • Calcium (as dibasic calcium phosphate) 55 mg • Chromium (as chromium polynicotinate) 100 mcg • Phenylalanine (as L-phenylalanine hydrochloride) 300 mg • Glutamine (as L-glutamine hydrochloride) 50 mg • Tyrosine (as L-tyrosine hydrochloride)100 mg • St. John's Wort extract 50 mg • L-Carnitine 20 mg • Korean Ginseng powdered root 70 mg • Uva Ursi powdered leaves 50 mg. Other ingredients: Whey , Stearic Acid , Magnesium Stearate, Pharmaceutical Glaze.

Nytol - Block Drug Company
Each capsule contains: Diphenhydramine Hydrochloride 25 mg. Other Ingredients: Corn Starch, Lactose, Microcrystalline Cellulose, Silica, Stearic Acid.

O.U.T. (Ovarian Uterine Tonic) - The Herbalist
Chaparral leaf • Pipsissewa leaf • False Unicorn root • Prickly Ash bark • Cramp bark • Licorice root • Saw Palmetto berry • Red Clover blossom.

Oats-Scullcap Virtue - Blessed Herbs
Oats in milk stage • Scullcap • St. John's Wort flower • Lemon Balm • Lavender flower • Rosemary & Blackberry brandy.

Occuplex - Puritan's Pride
Eight capsules contain: Vitamin A 32,800 IU • Vitamin C (Ascorbic Acid) 500 mg • Vitamin E (as dl-Alpha Tocopheryl Acetate) 400 IU • Thiamin 20 mg • Riboflavin 25 mg • Niacin (as Niacinamide and Niacin) 60 mg • Vitamin B6 30 mg • Folic Acid 800 mcg • Vitamin B12 50 mcg • Pantothenic Acid 100 mg • Calcium 100 mg • Magnesium 250 mg • Zinc 30 mg • Selenium 200 mcg • Copper 3 mg • Lutein 10 mg • N-Acetyl-Cysteine 250 mg • Bilberry leaf 40 mg • Ginkgo Biloba 24% extract 60 mg • Quercetin 300 mg • L-Taurine 500 mg • L-Methionine 200 mg • Glutamic acid 50 mg • L-Glycine 50 mg.

OcuActin - Nature's Plus
Two capsules contain: Vitamin C corn free 100 mg • Citrus Bioflavonoid Complex 100 mg • Vitamin E natural 50 IU • Zinc (Monomethionine) 30 mg • Bilberry [(Vaccinium myrtillus fruit) standardized 25% Anthocyanosides] 25 mg • Goldenseal [(Hydrastis canadensis root & rhizome) standardized 10% Alkaloids, 5% Hydrastine] 25 mg • Echinacea [(Echinacea angustifolia root & rhizome) standardized 4% Echinacosides] 25 mg • Chinese Green Tea [(Camellia sinensis leaf) decaffeinated, standardized 50% Polyphenols] 25 mg • Grape Seed [(Vitis vinifera) standardized 95% Proanthocyanidins] 10 mg Glutathione (pharmaceutical grade Free Form Amino Acid) 10 mg • Beta Carotene (supplying 15000 IU of Vitamin A activity) 9 mg • Lutein (active Carotenoid from Marigold flower extract) 6 mg • Coenzyme Q10 (Ubiquinone) 5 mg • Copper (Glycinate) 2 mg • Zeaxanthin (active Carotenoid from Marigold flower extract) 263 mcg • Vitamin A (Retinol) 5000 IU • Selenium (Selenomethionine) 50 mcg.

Ocu-Care - Nature's Plus
Two tablets contain: Strengthening Nutrients: Bilberry standardized 25% Anthocyanosides 30 mg • Citrus Bioflavonoid Complex supplying: (Active Flavonones with Hesperidin & Eriocitrin 24%, Active Flavonols & Flavones, Pectin, Cellulose & Narigen 20%) 250 mg • Rutin (Saphora japonica) 100 mg. Protectant Nutrients: Pantothenic Acid 100 mg • L-Lysine free form amino acid 50 mg. Antioxidant Nutrients: Beta Carotene pro-Vitamin A, supplying 20000 IU Vitamin A activity • Vitamin A Fish Liver oil 5000 IU • Vitamin E natural 200 IU • NAC (N-Acetyl-Cysteine) 50 mg • Zinc (Monomethionine) 20 mg.

Ocular Defense - PhysioLogics
Two capsules contain: Vitamin A (Beta-Carotene) 10000 IU • Vitamin A (Palmitate) 2500 IU • Vitamin E (d-Alpha Tocopherol) 100 IU • Vitamin B2 (Riboflavin) 10 mg • Vitamin B6 (Pyridoxine HCl) 10 mg • Zinc (Glycinate) 15 mg • Copper (Glycinate) 2 mg • Chromium (Niacin/Glycine Chelate) 100 mcg • Selenium (Selenomethionine) 50 mcg • Taurine 200 mg • Bilberry fruit (36% Anthocyanosides, 36 mg) 100 mg • N-Acetylcysteine 100 mg • Quercetin (98% Bioflavonoids, 49 mg) 50 mg • Glutathione 25 mg.

Ocu-Plus - Aspen Group, Inc.
Two tablets contain: Beta-Carotene 25,000 IU • Vitamin E (d-alpha tocopherol) 400 IU • Vitamin C 1000 mg • Citrus bioflavonoid complex 250 mg • Quercetin 100 mg • Bilberry extract (25% anthocyanosides) 80 mg • Rutin 100 mg • Zinc (gluconate) 50 mg • Copper (gluconate) 2 mg • Selenium (selenomethionine) 50 mcg • N-Acetyl L-Cysteine (glutathione precursor) 200 mg • L-Glutathione 10 mg • Eyebright 50 mg • Alpha-Lipoic Acid 50 mg • Chromium Picolinate 200 mcg • Lutein (containing zeaxanthin) 6 mg • Ginkgo Biloba 25 mg.

Ocuvite - Bausch & Lomb
Each tablet contains: Vitamin A (100% as beta carotene) 5000 IU • Vitamin C (ascorbic acid) 60 mg • Vitamin E (dl-alpha tocopherol acetate) 30 IU • Zinc (from zinc oxide) 40 mg • Selenium (from sodium selenate) 40 mcg • Copper (from cupric oxide) 2 mg. Inactive Ingredients: Dibasic Calcium Phosphate, Microcrystalline Cellulose,

BRAND NAMES

Calcium Carbonate, Crospovidone, Hydroxypropyl Methylcellulose, Titanium Dioxide, Silica Gel, Magnesium Stearate, Stearic Acid, FD&C Yellow No. 6, Triethyl Citrate, Polysorbate 80, and Sodium Lauryl Sulfate.

Ocuvite Extra - Bausch & Lomb
Each tablet contains: Vitamin A (100% as beta carotene) 6000 IU • Vitamin C (ascorbic acid) 200 mg • Vitamin E (dl-alpha tocopherol acetate) 50 IU • Riboflavin (Vitamin B2) 3 mg • Niacinamide (Vitamin B3) 40 mg • Zinc (from zinc oxide) 40 mg • Selenium (from sodium selenate) 40 mcg • Copper (from cupric oxide) 2 mg • Manganese 5 mg • L-Glutathione 5 mg. Inactive Ingredients: Dibasic Calcium Phosphate, Microcrystalline Cellulose, Calcium Carbonate, Crospovidone, Hydroxypropyl Methylcellulose, Titanium Dioxide, Silica Gel, Magnesium Stearate, Stearic Acid, FD&C Yellow No. 6, Triethyl Citrate, Polysorbate 80, & Sodium Lauryl Sulfate.

Ocuvite PreserVision - Bausch & Lomb
Each tablet contains: Vitamin C 500 mg • Vitamin E 400 mg • Beta-carotene 15 mg • Zinc (zinc oxide) 80 mg • Copper (copper oxide) 2 mg.

OKG Fuel Capsules OKG (L-Ornithine Alphaketoglutarate) - TwinLab
Each capsule contians: OKG 650 mg.

OKG Fuel Powder - TwinLab
Each teaspoonful contains: OKG 3.5 grams (3500 mg).

Olimmune - PhysioLogics
Three capsules contain: Licorice DGL (1% Glycyrrhizin, 7.6 mg) 760 mg • Astragalus (70% Polysaccharides, 140 mg) 200 mg • Ligusticum 200 mg • N-Acetyl-Cysteine (NAC) 135 mg • Olive leaf extract (17% Oleuropein, 17 mg) 100 mg.

Olive Leaf Extract - Swanson
Each capsule contains: Olive leaf extract (15% oleuropein) 500 mg.

Olive Leaf Extract - Olympian Labs
Each capsule contains: Olive Leaf extract 500 mg.

Olive Leaf Extract with Hawthorn - PhytoPharmica
Two capsules contain: Olive (Olea europaea) leaf extract (standardized to contain 17%-23% oleuropein) 500 mg • Hawthorn (Crataegus oxyacantha) leaf and flower extract (standardized to contain 1.8% vitexin-2'-rhamnoside) 300 mg.

Olive Leaf Plus - Health Smart Vitamins
Four capsules contain: Echinacea Blend: Echinacea purpurea root, leaf, Echinacea angustifolia root (4% total phenolic compounds, 10 mg) 1000 mg • Olive leaf, (Olea europaea: 17% oleuropein, 136 mg) 800 mg • Una de Gato inner bark, (Uncaria tomentosa; 2% oxindole alkaloids 1.3 mg) 80 mg.

Olympian Energy - Olympian Labs
Each capsule contains: Siberian Ginseng 100 mg • Gotu Kola 100 mg • Guarana 100 mg • Kola Nut 100 mg • Ma Huang 100 mg • Cayenne 10 mg • Vitamin B-6 (pyridoxine HCl) 5 mg.

Oly-Zymes - Olympian Labs
Each capsule contains: Proprietary Blend: Amylase, Protease, Lipase 200 mg.

Omega 3 Fatty Acids - Trader Joe's
EPA (eicosapentaenoic acid) 300 mg • DHA (docosahexaenoic acid) 200 mg • Calories 10. Contains no vitamin A, D, or cholesterol.

Omega 3 Fish Oils - Olympian Labs
Each softgel contains: Marine Lipid concentrate 1000 mg • EPA (eicosapentaenoic acid) 180 mg • DHA (docasahexaenoic acid) 120 mg • Vitamin E (d-alpha tocopherol) 1 mg.

Omega 3-6-9 - The Vitamin Shoppe
Two softgels contain the Omega 3-6-9 essential fatty acids from 100% pure cold-pressed vegetable seed oils of: Borage 500 mg • Flaxseed 150 mg • Safflower 50 mg • Canola 200 mg • Olive 100 mg. Plus 150 mg of Omega-3 components (EPA-DHA) naturally present in Salmon Oil, providing the following: A/Gamma Linolenic Acid (Omega-3) 220 mg • Linoleic Acid (Omega-6) 290 mg • Oleic Acid (Omega-9) 306 mg.

Omega III Essential Fatty Acids - Nature's Life
Three capsules contain: Eicosapentaenoic Acid (EPA) (Fish Body oils) 540 mg • Docosahexaenoic Acid (DHA) (Fish Body oils) 360 mg • Garlic extract (1000:1) (Allium sativum) 150 mg • Vitamin C (Ascorbate Palmitate) 10 mg • Vitamin E (d-Alpha Tocopherol) 30 IU. In a natural base of certified organic Safflower oil.

Omega-3 - Natrol
Two softgels contain: Fish Oil concentrate 2 g • EPA (Eiicosapentaenoic Acid) (18%) 360 mg • DHA (Docosahexaenoic Acid) (12%) 240 mg • Total Omega-3; Fatty Acids (36%) 720 mg. Other Ingredients: Gelatin, Mixed Natural Tocopherols.

OmegaTru™ Organic Flaxseed Oil - Swanson
Each tablespoon (1/2 oz) contains: Calories 126 • Calories from Fat 125 • Total Fat 14 g • Saturated Fat 1.5 g • Polyunsaturated Fat 9.7 g • Monounsaturated Fat 2.8 g • Cholesterol 0.6 mg • Sodium 0 mg • Total Carbohydrate 0 g • Protein 0 g • Alpha Linolenic Acid 7 g • Linoleic Acid 2 g • Oleic Acid 2.8 g.

Oncotax - American Metabolic Institute
Unknown
See Editor's Note No. 19, page 1818.

Oncovite - Mission Pharmacal
Each tablet contains: Vitamin A 9,000 IU • Vitamin C 500 mg • Vitamin D (as Vitamin D3) 400 IU • Vitamin E 100 IU • Thiamine 0.34 mg • Riboflavin 0.5 mg • Niacin 5 mg • Vitamin B6 25 mg • Folate 0.4 mg • Vitamin B12 1.6 mcg • Pantothenic Acid 2.3 mg • Zinc 7.5 mg. Other ingredients: Microcrystalline Cellulose, Color, Acrylic Resin, Croscarmellose Sodium, Magnesium Silicate, Magnesium Stearate, Ethylcellulose, Silicon Dioxide, Polyethylene Glycol, Food Glaze, Ethyl Vanallin, Cholecalciferol, Cyanocobalamin.

One A Day - Maximum Formula - Bayer
Each tablet contains: Vitamin A Acetate 5000 IU • Vitamin C (Ascorbic Acid) 60 mg • Vitamin D 400 IU • Vitamin E Acetate 30 IU • Vitamin K (Phytonadione) 25 mcg • Thiamin Mononitrate 1.5 mg • Riboflavin (Vitamin B2) 1.7 mg • Niacin (Vitamin B3) 20 mg • Vitamin B6 (Pyridoxine Hydrochloride) 2 mg • Folate (Folic Acid, Folacin) 400 mcg • Vitamin B12 6 mcg • Biotin 30 mcg • Pantothenic Acid (Calcium Pantothenate) 10 mg • Calcium Carbonate 162 mg • Iron (Ferrous Fumarate) 18 mg • Phosphorus 109 mg • Iodine (Potassium Iodide) 150 mcg • Magnesium Hydroxide 100 mg • Zinc Sulfate 15 mg • Selenium (Sodium Selenate) 20 mcg • Copper (Cupric Sulfate) 2 mg • Manganese 3.5 mg • Chromium Chloride 65 mcg • Molybdenum (Sodium Molybdate) 160 mcg • Chloride 72 mg • Potassium Chloride 80 mg • Nickel (Nickelous Sulfate) 5 mcg • Tin (Stannous Chloride)10 mcg • Silicon (Sodium Metasilicate) 2 mg • Vanadium (Sodium Metavanadate) 10 mcg • Boron (Disodium Borate) 150 mcg. Other Ingredients: Dicalcium Phosphate, Cellulose, Modified Cellulose Gum, Gelatin, Citric Acid, Hydroxypropyl Methylcellulose, Calcium Pantothenate, Magnesium Stearate, Artificial Color, Cupric Sulfate, Silicon Dioxide, Disodium Borate, Beta Carotene.
See Editor's Note No. 3, page 1816.

Some Brand Name Natural Products - What they Contain
www.NaturalDatabase.com contains MANY more listings than appear here.

One Daily - The Vitamin Shoppe
Each tablet contains: Vitamin A 10000 IU • Vitamin D (as Vitamin D3) 400 IU • Vitamin C 100 mg • Citrus Bioflavonoids 25 mg • Rutin 5 mg • Hesperidin Complex 5 mg • Vitamin E 150 IU • Vitamin B1 25 mg • Vitamin B2 25 mg • Vitamin B6 25 mg • Vitamin B12 100 mcg • Calcium Pangamate 25 mg • Pantothenic Acid 25 mg • Biotin 50 mcg • Folic Acid 400 mcg • Niacinamide 25 mg • Inositol 25 mg • Choline 25 mg • PABA 25 mg • Calcium 100 mg • Magnesium 50 mg • Potassium 25 mg • Manganese 5 mg • Zinc 15 mg • Iron 18 mg • Selenium 50 mcg • GTF Chromium 50 mcg • Iodine 150 mcg • Copper 2 mg • Molybdenum 100 mcg • Vitamin K 25 mcg • SOD 25 mcg • Octacosanol 100 mcg • L-Carnitine 5 mg • CoQ10 10 mcg • GLA 5 mg • Korean Ginseng 10 mg • Bee Pollen 10 mg • Royal Jelly 5 mg • Betaine HCl 10 mg • Pepsin 10 mg • Bromelain 10 mg • Papain 10 mg • Lecithin 25 mg • L-Glutathione 5 mg • L-Cysteine 5 mg • L-Methionine 5 mg • EPA & DHA 50 mg.

One Daily - Leiner Health Products
Each tablet contains: Folate (Folic Acid) 400 mcg • Niacin (Niacinamide) 20 mg • Pantothenic Acid (d-Calcium Pantothenate) 10 mg • Riboflavin (Vitamin B2) 1.7 mg • Thiamin Mononitrate (Vitamin B1) 1.5 mg • Vitamin A Acetate 5000 IU • Vitamin B12 (Cyanocobalamin - USP Mehtod 2) 6 mcg • Vitamin B6 (Pyridoxine Hydrochloride) 2 mg • Vitamin C (Ascorbic Acid) 60 mg • Vitamin D (Ergocalciferol) 400 IU • Vitamin E (dl-Alpha Tocopheryl Acetate) 30 IU. Other Ingredients: Calcium Carbonate, Gelatin, Maltodextrin, Hydroxypropyl Methylcellulose, Starch, Cellulose, Croscarmellose Sodium, Sodium Starch Glycolate, Silicon Dioxide, Hydroypropyl Cellulose, Red 40 Lake, Polyethylene Glycol 3350, Pharmaceutical Glaze, Magnesium Stearate, Polysorbate 80, Resin, Titanium Dioxide, Povidone, Beta Carotene.

One Daily + Minerals - Leiner Health Products
Each tablet contains: Chromium Yeast 10 mcg • Magnesium Hydroxide100 mg • Selenium Yeast 10 mcg • Calcium 130 mg • Molybdenum Yeast 10 mcg • Manganese Sulfate 2.5 mg • Copper (Cupric Sulfate) 2 mg • Folate (Folic Acid) 400 mcg • Iodine (Potassium Iodide) 150 mcg • Iron (Ferrous Fumarate) 18 mg • Niacin (Niacinamide) 20 mg • Pantothenic Acid (d-Calcium Pantothenate) 10 mg • Riboflavin (Vitamin B2) 1.7 mg • Thiamin Mononitrate (Vitamin B1) 1.5 mg • Vitamin A Acetate 5000 IU • Vitamin B12 (Cyanocobalamin - USP Method 2) 6 mcg • Vitamin B6 (Pyridoxine Hydrochloride) 2 mg • Vitamin C (Ascorbic Acid) 60 mg • Vitamin D (Ergocalciferol) 400 IU • Vitamin E (dl-Alpha Tocopheryl Acetate) 30 IU • Zinc Sulfate 15 mg • Biotin (USP Method 2) 30 mcg • Phosphorus 100 mg • Chloride 34 mg • Potassium Chloride 37.5 mg. Other Ingredients: Dicalcium Phosphate, Gelatin, Pregelatinized Starch, Cellulose, Sodium Starch Glycolate, Hydroxypropyl Methylcellulose, Croscarmellose Sodium, Silicon Dioxide, Tricalcium Phosphate, Red 40 Lake, Polyethylene Glycol 3350, Hydroxypropyl Cellulose, Pharmaceutical Glaze, Magnesium Stearate, Crospovidone, Polysorbate 80, Titanium Dioxide, Beta Carotene, Resin, Povidone.

One Daily 50+ - Leiner Health Products
Each tablet contains: Vitamin B12 (Cyanocobalamin - USP Method 2) 30 mcg • Thiamin Mononitrate (Vitamin B1) 4.5 mg • Vitamin B6 (Pyridoxine Hydrochloride) 6 mg • Magnesium Hydroxide 100 mg • Vitamin K (Phytonadione) 20 mcg • Manganese Sulfate 4 mg • Riboflavin (Vitamin B2) 3.4 mg • Vitamin C (Ascorbic Acid) 120 mg • Vitamin E (dl-Alpha Tocopheryl Acetate) 60 IU • Chromium Chloride 180 mcg • Pantothenic Acid (d-Calcium Pantothenate) 15 mg • Selenium (Sodium Molybdate) 105 mcg • Zinc Sulfate 22.5 mg • Molybdenum (Sodium Molybdate) 93.75 mcg • Calcium Carbonate 120 mg • Copper (Cupric Sulfate) 2 mg • Folate (Folic Acid) 400 mcg • Iodine (Potassium Iodide)150 mcg • Niacin (Niacinamide Ascorbate) 20 mg • Vitamin A Acetate 5000 IU • Vitamin D (Cholecalciferol) 400 IU • Biotin (USP Method 2) 30 mcg • Chloride 34 mg • Potassium Chloride 37.5 mg. Other Ingredients: Starch, Cellulose, Dicalcium Phosphate, Maltodextrin, Hydroxypropyl Methylcellulose, Croscarmellose Sodium, Gelatin, Titanium Dioxide, Calcium Silicate, Crospovidone, Pharmaceutical Glaze, Magnesium Stearate, Hydroxypropyl Cellulose, Resin, Mannitol, Polyethylene Glycol 3350, Polysorbate 80, Yellow 6 Lake, Blue 2 Lake, Beta Carotene.

One Daily Men's Formula - Leiner Health Products
Each tablet contains: Magnesium Hydroxide 100 mg • Manganese Sulfate 3.5 mg • Riboflavin (Vitamin B2) 2.55 mg • Thiamin Mononitrate (Vitamin B1) 2.25 mg • Vitamin B12 (Cyanocobalamin - USP Mehtod 2) 9 mcg • Vitamin B6 (Pyridoxine Hyrochloride) 3 mg • Vitamin C (Ascorbic Acid) 90 mg • Vitamin E (dl-Alpha Tocopheryl Acetate) 45 IU • Chromium Chloride 150 mcg • Selenium (Sodium Selenate) 87.5 mcg • Copper (Cupric Sulfate) 2 mg • Folate (Folic Acid) 400 mcg • Iodine (Potassium Iodide) 150 mcg • Molybdenum (Sodium Molybdate) 75 mcg • Niacin (Niacinamide Ascorbate) 20 mg • Pantothenic Acid (d-Calcium Pantothenate) 10 mg • Vitamin A 5000 IU • Vitamin D (Cholecalciferol) 400 IU • Zinc Sulfate 15 mg • Chloride 34 mg • Potassium Chloride 37.5 mg. Other Ingredients: Starch, Cellulose, Dicalcium Phosphate, Gelatin, Croscarmellose Sodium, Hydroxypropyl Methylcellulose, Calcium Silicate, Crospovidone, Hydroxypropyl Cellulose, Pharmaceutical Glaze, Polyethylene Glycol 3350, Yellow 6 Lake, Titanium Dioxide, Resin, Beta Carotene, Polysorbate 80.

One Daily Multiple - Nature's Life
Each capsule contains: Beta Carotene (Vitamin A equivalent to 10000 IU) 6 mg • Vitamin D (as Vitamin D3) (Cholecalciferol) 200 IU • Vitamin E (d-Alpha Tocopheryl Succinate) 100 IU • Vitamin B1 (Thiamine Mononitrate) 25 mg • Vitamin B2 (Riboflavin & Riboflavin 5'-Phosphate) 25 mg • Vitamin B6 Pyridoxine HCl & Pyridoxine 5'-Phosphate) 25 mg • Niacinamide 50 mg • Vitamin B12 (Cyancobalamin) 100 mcg • Folic Acid 400 mcg • Pantothenic Acid (d-Calcium Pantothenate) 50 mg • Biotin (d-Biotin) 300 mcg • Choline (Bitartrate) 25 mg • Inositol 25 mg • PABA (Para Aminobenzoic Acid) 25 mg • Vitamin C 100 mg • Boron (Citrate) 50 mcg • Calcium (Carbonate, Citrate/ Malate) 50 mg • Chromium (Picolinate) 100 mcg • Copper (Gluconate, Citrate) 1 mg • Magnesium (Oxide,Citrate) 10 mg • Manganese (Gluconate) 5 mg • Molybdenum (Sodium Molybdate) 150 mcg • Potassium (Chloride) 5 mg • Selenium (Selenomethionine) 100 mcg • Silicon (Dioxide) 10 mg • Vanadium(Vandyl Sulfate) 25 mcg • Zinc (Picolinate) 15 mg.

One Daily with Calcium, Iron, & Zinc - Leiner Health Products
Each tablet contains: Calcium Carbonate 45 mg • Iron (Ferrous Fumarate) 27 mg • Folate (Folic Acid) 400 mcg • Niacin (Niacinamide) 20 mg • Pantothenic Acid (d-Calcium Pantothenate) 10 mg • Riboflavin (Vitamin B2) 1.7 mg • Thiamin Mononitrate (Vitamin B1) 1.5 mg • Vitamin A Acetate 5000 IU • Vitamin B12 (Cyanocobalamin - USP Method 2) 6 mcg • Vitamin B6 (Pyridoxine Hydrochloride) 2 mg • Vitamin C (Ascorbic Acid) 60 mg • Vitamin D (Cholecalciferol) 400 IU • Vitamin E (dl-Alpha Tocopheryl Acetate) 30 IU • Zinc Oxide 15 mg. Other Ingredients: Maltodextrin, Gelatin, Hydroxypropyl Methylcellulose, Croscarmellose Silicon Dioxide, Propylene Glycol, Titanium Dioxide, Hydroxypropyl Cellulose, Polyethylene Glycol 3350, Pharmaceutical Glaze, Starch, Magnesium Stearate, Yellow 5 Lake, Yellow 6 Lake, Polysorbate 80, Beta Carotene, Povidone, Resin.

One Daily without Iron - The Vitamin Shoppe
Each tablet contains: Vitamin A 10000 IU • Vitamin D (as Vitamin D3) 400 IU • Vitamin C 100 mg • Citrus Bioflavonoids 25 mg • Rutin 5 mg • Hesperidin Complex 5 mg • Vitamin E 150 IU • Vitamin B1 25 mg • Vitamin B2 25 mg • Vitamin B6 25 mg • Vitamin B12 100 mcg • Calcium Pangamate 25 mg • Pantothenic Acid 25 mg • Biotin 50 mcg • Folic Acid 400 mcg • Niacinamide 25 mg • Inositol 25 mg • Choline 25 mg • PABA 25 mg • Calcium 100 mg • Magnesium 50 mg • Potassium 25 mg • Manganese 5 mg • Zinc 15 mg • Selenium 50 mcg • GTF Chromium 50 mcg • Iodine 150 mcg • Copper 2 mg • Molybdenum 100 mcg • Vitamin D 25 mcg • SOD 25 mcg •

B
R
A
N
D

N
A
M
E
S

BRAND NAMES

Octacosanol 100 mcg • L-Carnitine 5 mg • CoQ10 10 mcg • GLA 5 mg • Korean Ginseng 10 mg • Bee Pollen 10 mg • Royal Jelly 5 mg • Betaine HCl 10 mg • Pepsin 10 mg • Bromelain 10 mg • Papain 10 mg • Lecithin 25 mg • L-Glutathione 5 mg • L-Cysteine 5 mg • L-Methionine 5 mg • EPA & DHA 50 mg.

One Step - Progressive Labs
One level scoop (approx. 31 g.) contains: Calories 120 • Calories from fat 27 • Total Fat 3 g • Saturated Fat 0.625 g • Cholesterol 0 g • Sodium 28 mg • Potassium 419 mg • Total Carbohydrate 12 g • Dietary Fiber 6 g • Sugars 1 g • Protein 11 g • Vitamin A 5000 IU • Vitamin C 177 mg • Vitamin D 200 IU • Vitamin E 70 IU • Vitamin K 40 mcg • Thiamin (B1) 3 mg • Riboflavin (B2) 3 mg • Niacinamide (B3) 13 mg • Vitamin B6 30 mg • Folate (folic acid) 446 mcg • Vitamin B12 250 mcg • Biotin 150 mcg • Pantothenic Acid 23 mg • Calcium 326 mg • Iron 3 mg • Phosphorus 266 mg • Iodine 38 mcg • Magnesium 255 mg • Zinc (as ascorbate) 8 mg • Selenium 40 mcg • Copper (as amino acid chelate) 2 mg • Manganese (as ascorbate) 6 mg • Chromium (as nicotinate) 100 mcg • Molybdenum 13 mg • Chloride 175 mg. Amino acids from Soy Protein & Rice Bran: Aspartic Acid 1583 mg, Threonine 551 mg, Serine 696 mg, Glutamic Acid 2491 mg, Proline 755 mg, Glycine 630 mg, Alanine 637 mg, Cysteine 378 mg, Valine 740 mg, Methionine 202 mg, Isoleucine 691 mg, Leucine 1109 mg, Tyrosine 499 mg, Phenylalanine 723 mg, Histidine 371 mg, Lysine 888 mg, Arginine 1028 mg, Tryptophan 173 mg. Ingredients: Arcon VF Hypoallergenic, Predigested Soy Protein concentrate, Rice bran, Lecithin, Colloidal Magnesium, Glucosamine HCl, Nopal (detoxifier and sugar regulator), Colloidal Calcium, MSM (methyl sulfonyl methane), Beta 1,3 Glucans, Inulin, Gamma Oryzanol, L-Glutamine, L-Ornithine, L-Taurine, Vitamin E Succinate, CitriMax, Globulin Protein, Ester C, Ascorbic Acid, Trimethylglycine, Citrus Bioflavonoid 5X complex, Aloe Isolate, Zinc Ascorbate, Pantothenic Acid, Pyridoxine HCl, Inositol, Creatine Pyruvate, Siberian Ginseng extract, Betatene (lycopene and mixed carotenoids), Alpha Lipoic Acid, Manganese Ascorbate, Borage Oil, NovaSoy (soy isoflavones), Gugulipid Extract, Leci-PS (phosphatidyl serine), Beta Carotene, Niacinamide, L-Glutathione, Quercetin, Copper Amino Acid Chelate, Seleno-L-Methionine, Atlantic Sea Kelp, Lutein, Pyridoxal-5-Phosphate, Ginkgo Biloba leaf extract, Grape seed extract, Grape skin extract, Bioperine (black pepper extract), Mixed Tocotrienols, Coenzyme Q10, Pycnogenol, Boron, Natural Vanilla and other Natural Flavors, Stevia.

One-A-Day Bedtime & Rest - Bayer
Two tablets contain: Calcium 450 mg • Magnesium 80 mg • Lecithin 20 mg • Kava Kava Standardized extract (Piper methysticum) root 100 mg • Valerian Standardized extract (Valeriana officinalis) root 200 mg • Rosemary Standardized extract (Rosmannus officinalis) leaf 10 mg.

One-A-Day Bone Strength - Bayer
Each tablet contains: Vitamin D 100 IU • Calcium (precipitated) 500 mg • Soy Standardized extract (Glycine max or spp.) bean 28 mg.

One-A-Day Cholesterol Health - Bayer
Two tablets contain: Vitamin E 200 IU • Lecithin 100 mg • Garlic (Allium sativum) freeze dried/bulb 30 mg • Soy Standardized extract (Glycine max or spp.) bean 140 mg.

One-A-Day Cold Season - Bayer
Each tablet contains: Vitamin C 500 mg • Zinc 7.5 mg • Echinacea Standardized extract (Echinacea purpurea) whole plant/root 50 mg.
See Editor's Note No. 4, page 1816.

One-A-Day Energy Formula - Bayer
Each tablet contains: Thiamin (B1) 2.25 mg • Niacin 20 mg • Vitamin B6 3 mg • Folic Acid 200 mcg • Pantothenic Acid 10 mg • Chromium (as Picolinate) 100 mcg • Ginseng Standardized extract (Panax ginseng) root 200 mg.
See Editor's Note No. 9, page 1817.

One-A-Day Joint Health - Bayer
Each tablet contains: Vitamin C 30 mg • Vitamin E 30 IU • Manganese 1.5 mg • Lecithin 10 mg • Glucosamine Sulfate powder (includes Dipotassium CI 125 mg) 500 mg • Devil's Claw Standardized extract (Harpagophytum procumbens) root 134 mg.

One-A-Day Memory & Concentration - Bayer
Each tablet contains: Vitamin B6 1 mg • Vitamin B12 3 mcg • Choline 60 mg • Ginkgo Standardized extract (Ginkgo biloba) leaf 60 mg.
See Editor's Note No. 8, page 1816.

One-A-Day Menopause Health - Bayer
Each tablet contains: Vitamin E 15 IU • Calcium (precipitated) 250 mg • Lecithin 15 mg • Black Cohosh Standardized extract (Cimicifuga racemosa) root 10 mg • Soy Standardized extract (Glycine max or spp.) bean 42 mg.

One-A-Day Prostate Health - Bayer
Two softgels contain: Zinc Gluconate 15 mg • Pumpkin Seed Oil Standardized extract 80 mg • Saw Palmetto Standardized extract (Serenoa repens) berry 320 mg. Other Ingredients: Gelatin, Glycerin, Vegetable Oil, Beeswax, Lecithin, Titanium Dioxide, FD&C Red #40 (Tartrazine), FD&C Yellow #6, FD&C Blue #1, FD&C Yellow #5 (Tartrazine).
See Editor's Note No. 20, page 1818.

One-A-Day Tension & Mood - Bayer
Each tablet contains: Vitamin C 60 mg • Thiamin (B1) 1.125 mg • Niacin 10 mg • Folic Acid 100 mcg • Pantothenic Acid 5 mg • Lecithin 15 mg • Kava Kava Standardized extract (Piper methysticum) rhizome/root 100 mg • St. John's Wort Standardized extract (Hypericum perforatum) leaves/flowers 225 mg.

One-A-Day Women's Formula - Bayer
Each tablet contains: Vitamin A 5000 IU • Vitamin C 60 mg • Vitamin D 400 IU • Vitamin E 30 IU • Thiamin (Vitamin B1) 1.5 mg • Riboflavin (Vitamin B2) 1.7 mg • Niacin 20 mg • Vitamin B-6 2 mg • Folic Acid 400 mcg • Vitamin B-12 6 mcg • Pantothenic Acid 10 mg • Calcium 450 mg • Iron 27 mg • Zinc 15 mg.

OneSource - Health Smart Vitamins
Each caplet contains: Vitamin D (as cholecalciferol) 400 IU • Vitamin A (as 60% retinyl acetate, 40% beta-carotene) 5,000 IU • Vitamin C (as ascorbic acid) 60 mg • Vitamin E (as dl-alpha-tocopheryl acetate) 30 IU • Vitamin K (phytonadione) 25 mcg • Thiamin (as thiamin mononitrate) 1.5 mg • Riboflavin 1.7 mg • Niacin (as niacinamide) 20 mg • Vitamin B6 (as pyridoxine HCl) 2 mg • Folate (as folic acid) 400 mcg • Vitamin B12 (as cyanocobalamin) 6 mcg • Biotin 30 mcg • Pantothenic Acid (as D-calcium pantothenate) 10 mg • Calcium (dicalcium phosphate) 162 mg • Iron (as ferrous fumarate) 18 mg • Phosphorus (as dicalcium phosphate) 125 mg • Iodine (as potassium iodide) 150 mcg • Magnesium (as 90% magnesium oxide, 10% magnesium amino acid chelate) 100 mg • Zinc (as zinc amino acid chelate) 15 mg • Selenium (as selenomethionine) 20 mcg • Copper (as copper sulfate) 2 mg • Manganese (as maganese sulfate) 2.5 mg • Chromium (as chromium picolinate) 25 mcg • Molybdenum (as sodium molybdenate) 25 mcg • Chloride (as potassium chloride) 36 mg • Potassium (as potassium chloride) 40 mg • Silica (as silica dioxide) 2 mg • Boron (as sodium borate) 150 mcg • Tin (as stannous chloride) 10 mcg • Vanadium (as vanadium amino acid chelate) 10 mcg • Nickel (as nickel sulfate) 5 mcg.

Ophthaplus - Atrium Inc.
Each tablet contains: Raw Eye concentrate 120 mg • Raw Brain concentrate 20 mg • Eyebright 150 mg • Rutin 125 mg • Hesperidin Complex 20 mg.
See Editor's Note No. 14, page 1817.

Optein - Solgar

Each level scoop (35 grams) contains: Vitamin A (3600 IU palmitate 18%, 1400 IU as natural beta carotene from Dunaliella salina) 5000 IU • Vitamin C (as L-ascorbic-acid) 45 mg • Vitamin D (as cholecalciferol) 300 IU • Vitamin E (as D-alpha tocopheryl acetate) 23 IU • Thiamin (as thiamin mononitrate) 1.1 mg • Riboflavin 1.3 mg • Niacin (as niacinamide) 15 mg • Vitamin B6 (as pyridoxine hydrochloride) 1.5 mg • Folic Acid 300 mcg • Vitamin B12 (as cyanocobalamin) 5 mcg • Biotin (as D-biotin) 200 mcg • Pantothenic Acid (as D-calcium pantothenate) 7.5 mg • Calcium (as calcium carbonate, calcium from proteinate) 200 mg • Iron (as reduced iron, iron from proteinate) 9 mg • Iodine (as potassium iodide, brown seaweed extract) 115 mcg • Magnesium (as magnesium oxide, magnesium from proteinate) 100 mg • Zinc (as zinc oxide) 11 mg • Selenium (selenium from proteinate) 14 mcg • Copper (as copper gluconate) 1.5 mg • Manganese (as manganese from proteinate) 0.4 mg • Chromium (as chromium polynicotinate) 24 mcg • Molybdenum (molybdenum from proteinate) 15 mcg • Sodium 120 mg • Potassium (from malted oat cereal solids) 70 mg • Lecithin (from lecithin oil) 500 mg • Dried Red Beet powder 50 mg • Dried Broccoli powder (Brassica aleracea) aerial 50 mg • Dried Carrot powder (Daucus carota) root 40 mg • Spirulina powder 50 mg • Alfalfa Sprouts powder (Medicago sativa) aerial 50 mg • Kamut Grass powder (triticum durham egyptum) aerial 50 mg • Wheat Grass powder (Tritizum vulgare) aerial 50 mg • Barley Grass powder (Hordeum vulgare) aerial 50 mg • Reishi Mushroom extract (Ganoderma lucidum) 20 mg • Maitake Mushroom extract (Gifola frondosa) 20 mg • Shiitake Mushroom powder (Lentinus edodes) 20 mg • Brown Seaweed Extract 30 mg • Isoflavones (from soy concentrate) 20 mg • Octacosanol (from wheat germ oil) 250 mcg • Lactoferrins 10 mg • Glutamine Peptides 100 mg • Astragalus extract (Astragalus membranaceus) root 20 mg • Schisandra extract (Schizandra chinensis) fruit 20 mg • American Ginseng extract (Panax quinquefolium) root 20 mg • Siberian Ginseng extract (Acanthopanax seticosus) root 20 mg • Korean Ginseng extract (Panax ginseng) root 20 mg • Rhodiola extract (Rhodiola rosea) root 20 mg • Elderberry extract (Sambucus nigra, canadensis) berry 20 mg • Fruit Polyphenols (from apple, apricot, nectarine, cherry, prune, pomegranate) 20 mg • Beta Glucan (from oat fiber) 25 mg • Dried Colostrum powder 50 mg • Cytidine Monophosphate 5 mg • Adenosine Monophosphate 5 mg • Uridine Monophosphate 5 mg • Guanosine Monophosphate 5 mg • Phosphatidylcholine (from lecithin oil) 100 mg • Phosphatidylinositol (from lecithin oil) 20 mg. Other Ingredients: Malted Oat Cereal Solids, Crystalline Fructose, Soy Protein Isolate, Whey Protein Isolate, Whey Protein Concentrate, Dried Malt, Oat Fiber, Natural Chocolate Flavor, Dutch Cocoa, Soy Concentrate, Apple Fiber, Gum Arabic, Apple Pectin, Dried Cream, Black Currant Fiber, Lemon Fiber, Rice Fiber Concentrate, Fruit Concentrate.

Opti Fuel (The Ultimate Metabolic Optimizer) - TwinLab

Each serving contains: Pharmaceutical Grade Pep-Tide Bonded & Free Amino Acids [derived from the natural Pancreatic digests of Whey Protein (Lactalbumin) & Egg White Protein (Albumin)] 15 g • Branched Chain Amino Acids (L-Leucine, L-Isoleucine & L-Valine) • Carbohydrates & Medium Chain Triglycerides (MCTs) • High Potency Metabolic Activator Vitamins & Minerals • Electro-Lytes • Antioxidants • Stress B Complex • Lipotropic Factors • Methyl Donors • TMG (Trimethylglycine) • Siberian Ginseng • Octacosanol • Gamma-Oryzanol & Synergistic Metabolic Optimizers (such as Inosine) • L-Carnitine • CoQ10 • Lipoic Acid • Pantetheine • Pyridoxine-Alpha-Ketoglutarate • Soluble Potassium Phosphate & Mineral Succinates • Aspartates • Citrates • Fumarates • Malates • Alpha-Ketoglutarates.

Opti Fuel 2 - TwinLab

Each serving contains: Carbohydrates (derived primarily from Glucose Polymers & Glucose with small amounts of 100% Pure Crystalline Fructose) 100 g • Predigested Whey Protein • Extra Branched Chain Amino Acids (L-Leucine, L-Isoleucine, L-Valine) • Vitamin C • Vitamin E • Beta-Carotene • Other Important Antioxidant

Nutrients such as: Selenium, Coenzyme Q10 & Alpha Lipoic Acid, High Potency B Complex Vitamins, Calcium, Magnesium, Potassium, Zinc & Chromium Picolinate • Carni Fuel, (L-Carnitine Magnesium Citrate). All predigested for easier digestion & assimilation.

Opti-Lean - Optimum Nutrition

Citrimax™ 500 mg • High Quality Protien 20 g • Carbohydrates 20 g.

Optimal Performance - Rexall

Each tablet contains: Zinc (as zinc gluconate) 7.5 mg • Spirulina (spirulina pacifica) 125 mg • Bee Pollen 100 mg • Royal Jelly 100 mg • Siberian Ginseng root 75 mg • Octacosanol 0.5 mg.
Other Ingredients: Corn Syrup solids, Croscarmellose Sodium, Alfalfa leaf, Hydrogenated Vegetable Oil, Silica, Magnesium Stearate.

OptimEyes - Body Wise International, Inc.

Three tablets contain: Beta Carotene (Dunaliella salina algae) 9 mg (Equivalent to Vitamin A 15000 IU) • Vitamin C (as Ascorbic Acid) 1000 mg • Vitamin E (as D-Alpha Tocopheryl Succinate and Mixed Tocopherols-Alpha, Beta, Gamma and Delta) 100 IU • Zinc (Krebs Cycle Chelate) 20 mg • Selenium (as L-Selenomethionine) 250 mcg • Copper (Krebs Cycle Chelate) 2 mg • Taurine 500 mg • N-Acetyl-L-Cysteine 200 mg • Bilberry fruit extract 100:1 (25% Anthocyanidins) 80 mg • Ginkgo Biloba leaf extract 50:1 (24% Flavonglycosides) 60 mg • Alpha Lipoic Acid 25 mg • Lutein 6 mg.

Optimum Nutrition - Optimum Nutrition

Hawthorn Berry • Garlic Extract.

Optimum Omega - Pharmanex

Each capsule contains: Vitamin E (as d-Alpha Tocopheryl Acetate) 5 IU • Marine Lipid Concentrate 1000 mg (Omega 3 Fatty Acids: EPA 180 mg, DHA 120 mg, Other Omega 3 Fatty Acids 50 mg) • Deodorized Garlic Oil 1 mg. Other Ingredients: Gelatin, Glycerin, Purified Water.

Optimune - Rx Vitamins

Pharmaceutical Grade Arabinogalactan 250 mg • Phosphoric Nucleotides 4000 mcg.

OptiVision - PhysioLogics

Two capsules contain: Vitamin A (Beta-Carotene) 10000 IU • Vitamin A (Palmitate) 2500 IU • Taurine 200 mg • Bilberry (GPH: 36% anthocyanosides) 100 mg • Vitamin E (D-Alpha Tocopherol) 100 IU • N-Acetylcysteine 100 mg • Quercetin (GPH: 98% Bioflavonoids) 50 mg • Glutathione 25 mg • Vitamin B2 (Riboflavin) 10 mg • Vitamin B6 (Pyridoxine HCI) 10 mg • Zinc (Glycinate) 15 mg • Copper (Glycinate) 2 mg • Chromium (Niacin/Glycine Chelate) 100 mcg • Selenium (Selenomethionine) 50 mcg.

OptiVision Forte - Similasan

Four caplets contain: Vitamin A (45% (1,650 IU) as Beta Carotene) 3,650 IU • Vitamin C 150 mg • Vitamin D (cholecalciferol) 200 IU • Vitamin E (d-alpha tocopheryl acetate) 75 IU • Thiamin (Vitamin B-1) 25 mg • Riboflavin (Vitamin B-2) 38 mg • Niacin 20 mg • Vitamin B6 (from 25 mg pyridoxyl-5 phosphate) 17 mg • Folic Acid 400 mcg • Vitamin B12 (dibencozide) 84 mcg • Biotin 100 mcg • Pantothenic Acid (from d-calcium panthothenate) 25 mg • Calcium (rice protein chelate) 75 mg • Magnesium (rice protein chelate) 75 mg • Zinc (rice protein chelate) 19 mg • Selenium (rice protein chelate) 50 mcg • Manganese (rice protein chelate) 10 mg • Chromium (rice protein chelate) 25 mcg • Bioflavinoids (citrus) 75 mg • Alpha-Lipoic Acid 30 mg • Lutein (from Calendula officinalis flowers) 5,065 mcg • Coenzyme Q-10 (emulsified) 2.5 mg • Alpha-Carotene 415 mcg • Zeaxanthine 333 mcg • Lycopene 300 mcg • Cryptoxanthine 100 mcg • Proprietary Blend: Eye Bright Herb, Taurine, L-Cysteine, L-Arginine, Cayenne, Garlic Bulb, Ginger Root, Ginkgo Biloba leaf, L-Glutamine, Glycine, Bilberry 5:1 extract, Inositol, L-Histidine, Raw

Eye Concentrate, L-Glutathione, Lecithin, and SuperOxide Dismutase (SOD) 1,130 mg. Other Ingredients: Special Plant Cellulose, Vegtable Stearates, Acacia, Gum Tragacanth, Natural Silica, and Magnesium Stearate. This forumulation contains NO corn, soy, yeast, wheat, milk & egg products, sugar, starch, or preservatives.
See Editor's Note No. 14, page 1817.

Opti-Vue - The Vitamin Shoppe
Two capsules contain: Vitamin A 10000 IU • Vitamin C 200 mg • Vitamin E 50 IU • Potassium 100 mg • Niacin 30 mg • Zinc 5 mg • Riboflavin 3 mg • Selenium 50 mcg • Lutein 6 mg • Zeaxanthin 240-600 mcg • Eyebright Extract 200 mg • Raw Eye Tissue 160 mg • Raw Muscle Tissue 100 mg • Inositol 100 mg • Alfalfa concentrate 50 mg • Citrus Bioflavonoids 50 mg • Quercetin 200 mg • Rutin 25 mg • Bilberry extract 40 mg • Glutathione 5 mg • N-Acetyl Cysteine 50 mg. In a special food base of rice carrot parsley, and spinach concentrates.
See Editor's Note No. 14, page 1817.

Optizinc - Natrol
One capsule contains: Zinc (Monomethionine) 30 mg. Other ingredients: Microcrystalline Cellulose, Magnesium Stearate, Gelatin.

OptiZinc - Source Naturals
Each tablet contains: Zinc (from 150 mg of OptiZinc zinc monomethionine) 30 mg • Copper (sebacate) 300 mcg.

Opti-Zyme - Changes - TwinLab
One caplet contains: Calcium (from 500 mg Calcium Carbonate) 180 mg • Amylase 4250 DU • Protease 10255 HUT • Cellulase 630 CU • Lactase 350 Lac U • Lipase 65 LU • Invertase 0.6 IAU • Glucoamylase 15 AG • Multi-algae blend: Spirulina algae, Bladderwrack kelp, Klamath Lake algae, Canary Island algae, Chlorella algae, Maine coast kelp, and Sargassi seaweed • Supporting herbal blend: Turmeric rhizome, Fennel seed, Ginger root, and Soy sprouts. Other Ingredients: Vegetable cellulose, Fractionated vegetable oil, Soy polysaccherides, Silica, and Vegetable resin glaze.

Opti-Zyme Pro - Changes - TwinLab
One capsule contains: Amylase 3400 SKB • Lipase 2250 LU • Cellulase 5400 C-ase • Protease 10200 HUT • Amyloglucosidase 22 AG • Acid stable protease 340 APU • Invertase 102 Sumner U • Lactase 351 LAU • Lactobacillus acidophilus 100 million CFU • Bifidobacterium bifidum 50 million CFU • Dulse algae 50 mg • Trace mineral complex (Montmorillonite) 100 mg • Spirulina blue-green algae 50 mg • Bromelain 50 mg. Other Ingredients: Gelatin, Calcium Sulfate, Magnesium Stearate, and Silica.

Organic Flax 1000 - Health From The Sun
Two capsules contain: Alpha-Linolenic Acid (ALA) (Omega-3) 1.1 g • Linoleic Acid (Omega-6) 280 mg • Oleic Acid (Omega-9) 290 mg. Ingredients: Certified Organic Flax seed oil, Gelatin, Glycerine, Water, Carob powder.

OS-Cal - SmithKline Beecham
Each tablet contains: Calcium Carbonate 500 mg. Other Ingredients: Dextrose Monohydrate, Maltodextrin, Microcrystalline Cellulose, Magnesium Stearate, Artificial Flavors, Sodium Chloride.
See Editor's Note No. 5, page 1816.

Oscillococcinum - Boiron
Each tube contains: Active Ingredients: Anas barbariae hepatis et cordis extractum HPUS 200 CK. Inactive Ingredients: Sucrose 0.85 g, Lactose 0.15 g.

Osha-Lomatium Virtue - Blessed Herbs
Osha root • Lomatium root • Pau d'Arco bark • Propolis • Shitake mycelium • Echinacea Angustifolia root • Goldenseal root • Licorice root • Grain alcohol & Distilled Water.

Osteo Bi-Flex - Rexall
Three caplets contain: Sodium 105 mg • Vitamin C 60 mg • Vitamin D 400 IU • Calcium 500 mg • Glucosamine HCl 1500 mg • Chondroitin Sulfate 1200 mg. Other Ingredients: Red Beet Juice powder, Crospovidone, Magnesium Stearate, Croscarmellose Sodium, Silica.
See Editor's Note No. 15, page 1817.

Osteo Bi-Flex: Double Strength Caplets - Rexall
Three caplets contain: Sodium 100 mg • Glucosamine HCl 1500 mg • Chondroitin Sulfate 1200 mg. Other Ingredients: Red Beet Juice powder, Crospovidone, Magnesium Stearate, Croscarmellose Sodium, Silica.
See Editor's Note No. 15, page 1817.

Osteo Bi-Flex: Double Strength Softgels - Rexall
Three softgels contain: Sodium 100 mg • Glucosamine HCl 1500 mg • Chondroitin Sulfate 1200 mg. Other Ingredients: Red Beet Juice powder, Crospovidone, Magnesium Stearate, Croscarmellose Sodium, Silica.
See Editor's Note No. 15, page 1817.

Osteo Formula - Quest
Each tablet contains: Calcium (HVP Chelate) 125 mg • Magnesium (HVP Chelate) 125 mg • Vitamin C 50 mg • Vitamin D (as Vitamin D3) 50 IU • Silicon (HVP Chelate) 125 mcg • N-Acetyl Glucosamine (NAG) 125 mg • Betaine HCl 25 mg. Other Ingredients: Croscarmellose Sodium, Magnesium Stearate (vegetable source), Microcrystalline Cellulose, Vegetable Stearin.

Osteo Guard - Clinician's Choice
Four tablets contain: Vitamin C (ascorbic acid) 120 mg • Vitamin D (cholecalciferol) 400 IU • Calcium (carbonate, glycinate, gluconate, citrate, succinate, amino acid chelate, aspartate) 1000 mg • Magnesium (oxide, carbonate, citrate, amino acid chelate) 480 mg • Zinc (amino acid chelate) 10 mg • Manganese (amino acid chelate) 1 mg • L-Glutamic Acid 20 mg • Betaine Hydrochloride 20 mg • Proprietary blend 20 mg: Piper Longum Fruit, Pacific Kelp, Carrot Powder, Astragalus Membranaceus, Silica (horsetail herb), Boron (boron aspartate).

Osteo Plex - Olympian Labs
Four capsules contain: Calcium Citrate 800 mg • Magnesium (oxide) 400 mg • Boron (proteinate) 400 mcg • Zinc (amino acid chelate) 10 mg.

Osteo Protector - The Vitamin Shoppe
Each tablet contains: Vitamin D (as cholecalciferol) 100 IU • Calcium (as carbonate, hydroxyapatite) 500 mg • Magnesium (as oxide, citrate) 250 mg • Ipriflavone (7-Isopropoxy Isoflavone (Ostivone)) 200 mg. No yeast, corn, wheat, sugar, salt, starch, milk, gluten, soy, eggs, dairy, fish, citrus, preservatives, artificial colors or flavors added.

Osteo-Aid - Futurebiotics
Six capsules contain: Vitamin D 400 IU • Calcium (as calcium citrate) 1000 mg • Magnesium (as magnesium amino acid chelate) 400 mg • Boron (as amino acid chelate) 1.5 mg • Ostivone Ipriflavone (7-isopropoxy isoflavone) 100 mg • Soy Isoflavone extract powder (standardized for 10% (5 mg) phytoestrogen isoflavones) 50 mg. Other ingredients: Gelatin, Water.

Osteocare - Vitabiotics
Two tablets contain: Calcium 800 mg • Magnesium 300 mg • Zinc 10 mg • Vitamin D 5 UG. Ingredients: Calcium Carbonate, Magnesium Hydroxide, Maize Starch, Starch Glyconate, Zinc Sulphate, Vitamin D (as cholecaciferol prep), Carboxymethylcellulose prep, Magnesium Stearate.

Osteocare - Puritan's Pride

Two capsules contain: Vitamin D (as cholecalciferol) 133 IU • Calcium (as calcium citrate) 400 mg • Ipriflavone (as 7-isopropoxy isoflavone) 200 mg.

Osteo-Joint - Leiner Health Products

Each caplet contains: Deoiled Lecithin (Glycine max) bean 25 mg • Devil's Claw extract 40 mg • Glucosamine Sulfate powder 500 mg • Methylsulfonylmethane 25 mg • Rice Starch (Oryza sativa) 25 mg. Other Ingredients: Calcium Carbonate, Cellulose, Methylcellulose, Maltodextrin, Deoiled Lecithin, Rice Starch, Silicon Dioxide, Croscarmellose Sodium, Stearic Acid, Dextrin, Crospovidone, Magnesium Stearate.

Osteologic - PhysioLogics

Four tablets contain: Vitamin D (as Cholecalciferol) 400 IU • Vitamin K (as Phytonadione) 80 mcg • Vitamin B6 (as Pyridoxine HCl) 2 mg • Folate (Folic Acid) 400 mcg • Pantothenic Acid (as D-Calcium Pantothenate) 10 mg • Calcium (as Calcium Carbonate) 1000 mg • Iodine (from Kelp) 471 mcg • Magnesium (as 58% Magnesium Oxide, 25% Magnesium Glycinate, 17% Magnesium Carbonate) 400 mg • Zinc (as Zinc Citrate) 15 mg • Selenium (from natural salts) 3 mcg • Copper (as Copper Aspartate) 2 mg • Manganese (as mixed Manganese salts) 378 mcg • Chromium (from natural salts) 38 mcg • Molybdenum (from natural salts) 115 mcg • Silicon (as Silicon Dioxide) 20 mg • Boron (as 98% Boron Aspartate, 2% natural salts) 3 mg.

Osteo-Max - Metabolic Response Modifiers

Each capsule contains: Ipriflavone 200 mg • MCHC (yielding 167 mg elemental calcium) 667 mg.

Osteo-Plus - Nutri-Quest

Each tablet contains: Boron (special organic complex) 1 mg • Magnesium Chelate 400 mg • Calcium Chelate 100 mg • Calcium Aspartate 100 mg • Calcium Giuconate 50 mg • Calcium (Hydroxyapatite) 156 mg • Calcium (Veal Bone) 39 mg • Red Bone Marrow 10 mg • Calcium Citrate 50 mg • Vitamin C 25 mg • Vitamin D 50 IU • L-Glutamic Acid HCL 15 mg • Betaine HCL 15 mg • Salmiac 10 mg • Parathyroid 2 mg. In a base containing Horsetail Rush (Shave grass), Source of Natural Silicon 15 mg, Calcium Fluoride (Cell Salt) Safflower herb 25 mg. See Editor's Note No. 14, page 1817.

Osteoporosis Formula - Nature's Life

Each four capsules contain: Calcium (Citrate/Malate, Carbonate) 1000 mg • Magnesium (Oxide, Citrate) 500 mg • Vitamin C (Ascorbic Acid) 40 mg • Betaine HCl 40 mg • Zinc (Picolinate) 15 mg • Manganese (Gluconate) 5 mg • Boron (Citrate) 2 mg • Vitamin K (as Vitamin K1) mg • Copper (Gluconate) 1 mg • Silicon (Dioxide) 1 mg • Vitamin D (as Vitamin D3) (Cholecalciferol) 400 IU. In a natural base of Springtime Horsetail herb (Equisetum arvernse).

OsteoPrime - Enzymatic Therapy

Four tablets contain: Vitamin D 200 IU • Calcium (Aspartate, Citrate, Succinate, Fumarate, Carbonate, Lactate, Malate) 600 mg • Magnesium (Aspartate, Oxide) 250 mg • Vitamin C (Ascorbic Acid) 100 mg • Vitamin B6 (Pyridoxine) 25 mg • Niacinamide 20 mg • Zinc (Picolinate) 15 mg • Manganese (Aspartate) 15 mg • Thiamine HCL (Vitamin B1) 10 mg • Riboflavin (Vitamin B2) 10 mg • Pantothenic Acid (D-Calcium Pantothenate) 10 mg • Copper (Gluconate) 1.5 mg • Folic Acid 400 mcg • Vitamin K (Phytonadione) 150 mcg • Chromium (Aspartate) 100 mcg • Selenium sodium Selenite) 100 mcg • Molybdenum (Sodium Molybdate) 50 mcg • Vitamin B12 (Cyanocobalamin) 10 mcg. Other ingredients: Betaine HCL 20 mg • Silicon sodium Metasilicate) 1 mg • Boron (Chelated) 750 mcg • Strontium (Nonradioactice) 500 mcg. Contains no sugar, yeast, wheat, corn, soy, dairy products, coloring or preservatives.

OsteoPrime Forte - PhytoPharmica

Four tablets contain: Vitamin D 200 IU • Calcium (aspartate, citrate, succinate, fumarate, carbonate, lactate, malate) 600 mg • Magnesium (aspartate, oxide) 250 mg • Vitamin C (ascorbic acid) 100 mg • Niacinamide 50 mg • Vitamin B6 (pyridoxine) 25 mg • Zinc (picolinate) 20 mg • Manganese (aspartate) 20 mg • Thiamine HCL (Vitamin B1) 20 mg • Riboflavin (Vitamin B2) 20 mg • Pantothenic Acid (D-Calcium pantothenate) 20mg • Copper (gluconate) 2 mg • Folic Acid 800 mcg • Vitamin K (phytonadione) 300 mcg • Chromium (aspartate) 100 mcg • Selenium (sodium selenite) 100 mcg • Molybdenum (sodium molybdate) 50 mcg • Vitamin B12 (cyanocobalamin) 20 mcg • Betaine HCL 20 mg • Boron (chelated) 2 mg • Silicon (sodium metasilicate) 1 mg • Strontium (nonradioactive) 500 mcg.

Osteosupport - Health Factor

Four tablets contain: Calcium (Citrate/Hydroxylapatite) 850 mg • Vitamin D (as Vitamin D3) (Cholecalciferol) 100 IU • Iodine (Kelp) 100 mcg • Magnesium (Citrate) 650 mg • Boron (Citrate) 2 mg • Silicon (Citrate) 500 mcg • Vanadium (Pentoxide) 75 mcg • Betaine HCl 65 mg • Glutamic Acid 65 mg.

Osteo-Support - The Vitamin Shoppe

Two tablets provide: Calcium 500 mg • Magnesium 250 mg • Vitamin D 100 IU.

OstiBone - NaturalMax - Nutraceutical

One capsule contains: Calcium (as Calcium Carbonate) 120 mg • Ostivone (as Isoproproxy Isoflavone) 200 mg. Other ingredients: Gelatin, Cellulose, Magnesium Stearate

Ostivone - Enzymatic Therapy

Each capsule contains: Ostivone(tm) (Ipriflavone) 200 mg. Contains no sugar, salt, yeast, wheat, gluten, corn, soy, dairy products, coloring, flavoring or preservatives.

Ostivone - Anabolic Laboratories

Each tablet contains: Ipriflavone (Ostivone 7-Isopropoxy Isoflavone) 200 mg.

Ostivone - PhytoPharmica

Each capsule contains: Ipriflavone (Ostivone brand) 200 mg.

Ostivone - Source Naturals

One tablet contains: Ipriflavone (Ostivone) 300 mg.

Ostivone 100 mg - Natrol

Each capsule contains: 7-Isopropoxy-Isoflavone 100 mg. Other ingredients: Rice Powder, Magnesium Stearate, Gelatin.

Otrthoflex - Pacific BioLogic

Siberian Ginseng • Angelica root (Chinese) • Angelica root (pubescent) • Eucommia bark • Siler root • Cinnamon Twig • Astragalus root (Grade 1) • Homalomena rhizome • Notopterygium root & rhizome • Gentiana root • Pseudoginseng root (whole) • Teasal root • Ginger (Chinese Wild).

Ouch Ointment - Earth Science

Each 100 mL tube contains: Water • Tea Tree oil • Glyceryl Stearate • Capric Caprylic Triglycerides • Echinacea extract • Witch Hazel extract • Steareth-20 • Glycerine • Calendula extract • Saccharomyces Lysate • St. John's Wort • Dimethicone • Plantain extract • Potassium Sorbate • Sodium Carbomer 940 • Peppermint oil • Mont-Morillonite Clay • Grape extract.

Ovary-Uterus Complex - Enzymatic Therapy

Each capsule contains: Ovary-Uterus Complex (Predigested Soluble concentrate*) 250 mg • Multi-Glandular Complex: Raw Liver, Raw

Lung, Raw Pancreas, Raw Heart, Raw Kidney, Raw Spleen, & Raw Brain 100 mg. *Free-form concentrate predigested by enzymatic action, creating a highly absorbable form of glandular concentrate containing all the natural principles with a standardized content. Contains no sugar, salt, yeast, wheat, corn, soy, dairy products, coloring, flavoring or preservatives.
See Editor's Note No. 14, page 1817.

Overdrive - Pharmanex
Each capsule contains: Vitamin A (100% as Beta-Carotene from Dunaliella Salina, Beta-Carotene) 2500 IU • Vitamin C (as Ascorbic Acid) 300 mg • Vitamin E (d-Alpha Tocopheryl Succinate) 75 IU • Thiamin (as Thiamine Mononitrate) 0.75 mg • Riboflavin (as Riboflavin) 0.85 mg • Vitamin B6 (as Pyridoxine Hydrochloride) 1 mg • Folate (as Folic Acid) 100 mcg • Vitamin B12 (as Cyanocobalamin) 3 mcg • Pantothenic Acid (as d-Calcium Pantothenate) 5 mg • Magnesium (as Magnesium Asparate, Magnesium Oxide) 60 mg • Selenium (as L-Selenomethionine) 35 mcg • Chromium (as Chromium Chelate, Chromium Picolinate) 100 mcg • Bromelain (from Pineapple extract) 50 mg • Papain (from Papaya extract) 50 mg • Citrus Bioflavonoid Complex 50 mg • Hydromins (from Sea Salt extract) 50 mg • N-Acetyl-L-Cysteine 20 mg • Quercetin 12.5 mg • Grape Seed Extract with Leucoanthocyanin 2.5 mg.

Overexertion Formula - Dr. Morrow's Homeopathic Formulas
Ten drops contain: Phosphoric Acid 3C • Kali phosphoricum 6C • Anacardium 3C • Arnica 3C • Gelsemium 3C • Selenium 6C • Argentum nitricum 3C • Avena sativa 3X.
See Editor's Note No. 1, page 1816.

Oxy Shield - Futurebiotics
Three tablets contain: Vitamin E (natural d-alpha tocopherol) 400 IU • Beta Carotene 25,000 IU • Vitamin C 1000 mg • N-Acetyl Cysteine 125 mg • Cysteine 125 mg • Zinc (citrate, gluconate) 25 mg • Copper 1 mg • Selenium (selenomethionine) 150 mcg • Garlic (pure-gar) 400 mg • Green Tea 400 mg • Licorice (extract from) 700 mg • Astragalus (extract from) 350 mg • Tricosanthes (extract from) 150 mg • Siberian Ginseng (extract from) 750 mg • Pau D'Arco 50 mg • Cayenne 30 mg • Methionine 50 mg • Red Clover flowers 100 mg • Barley grass powder 100 mg • Chamomile 100 mg • Ribonucleic Acid (RNA) 50 mg • Kelp 100 mg • Iodine (kelp) 150 mcg • Molybdenum 20 mcg.

Oxy-G2 - Body Wise International, Inc.
Two capsules contain: Beta Carotene (Vitamin A 6250 IU) 3.75 mg • Vitamin C 75 mg • Vitamin E (as d-alpha Tocopheryl Succinate) 30 IU • Pantothenic Acid (from Calcium Pantothenate) 50 mg • Selenium (as L-Selenomethionine) 100 mcg • Molybdenum (Krebs Cycle Chelate) 100 mcg • Organic Germanium 100 mg • Ginkgo Biloba Leaf 100 mg • Milk Thistle Seed Std. Extract (80% Silymarin) 50 mg • Echinacea Purpurea Root 50 mg • Cytochrome C Oxidase 50 mg • Krebs Cycle Chelated Replenished Factors 50 mg • L-Glutathione 50 mg • Ascorbyl Palmitate 50 mg • L-Cysteine 25 mg • L-Tyrosine 25 mg • Pau D'Arco (Taheebo Tea Bark) 25 mg • Chlorophyll 20 mg.

Oxy-Pro - Progressive Labs
Each capsule contains: Vitamin A (as beta carotene) 12500 IU • Vitamin C 150 mg • Vitamin E (d-alpha tocopheryl succinate) 100 IU • Riboflavin (B2) 12.5 mg • Niacinamide 12.5 mg • Vitamin B6 10 mg • Zinc (as zinc glycinate) 7.5 mg • Selenium (as selenomethionine) 100 mcg • Copper (as copper lysinate) 0.5 mg • Manganese (as manganese glycinate) 4 mg • Molybdenum (as sodium molybdate) 5 mcg • Quercetin 50 mg • N-Acetyl Cysteine 50 mg • Glutathione 2.5 mg.

Oyster Calcium - Puritan's Pride
Each tablet contains: Vitamin A (as Retinyl Acetate) 1600 IU • Vitamin D (as Cholecalciferol) 400 IU • Calcium (as Oyster Shell) 750 mg.

Oyster Calcium - Nature's Bounty
Two tablets contain: Vitamin A (as Retinyl Acetate) 1600 IU • Vitamin D (as Cholecalciferol) 400 IU • Calcium (as Oyster Shell) 750 mg. Other Ingredients: Maltodextrin, Acacia, Cellulose, Croscarmellose, Cellulose Coating, Vegetable Magnesium Stearate.

Oyster Shell Calcium - Nature's Bounty
Each tablet contains: Calcium (as Oyster Shell Powder) 500 mg. Other Ingredients: Maltodextrin, Acacia Gum, Cellulose, Croscarmellose, Cellulose Coating, Vegetable Magnesium Stearate.

Oystercal 500 - Puritan's Pride
Each tablet contains: Calcium (as Calcium Carbonate from Oyster Shell) 500 mg.

Oystercal 500 + D - Puritan's Pride
Each tablet contains: Vitamin D (as Ergocalciferol) 125 IU • Calcium (as Oyster Shell) 500 mg.

Pacific Kelp - Quest
Each tablet contains: Pacific Kelp 650 mg. Other Ingredients: Calcium Carbonate, Silicon Dioxide, Magnesium Stearate (vegetable source).

Padma 28 - Padma A.G.
Each tablet contains: Saussuria 40 mg • Iceland Moss 40 mg • Margosa 35 mg • Myrobalan 30 mg • Red Sandalwood 30 mg • Cardamom 30 mg • Allspice 25 mg • Bengal Quince 20 mg • Potentilla 15 mg • Golden Seal 15 mg • Licorice 15 mg • Ribwort 15 mg • Columbine 15 mg • Knot grass 15 mg • Cloves 12 mg • Gingerlily 10 mg • Heartleaved Sida 10 mg • Valerian 10 mg • Wild Lettuce 6 mg • Marigold 5 mg • Camphor 4 mg • Aconite 1 mg • Calcium sulfate 20 mg • Sorbitol 73 mg • Cilicum dioxide 12 mg.

Pain Relief Support - Amazon Support
Each capsule contains: Iporuru • Tayuya • Picao Preto.

Pain Stop - Flora
Willow bark.

Pain-Less - The Herbalist
White Willow bark • Feverfew herb • Jamaican Dogwood root bark • Black Cohosh root • Passionflower herb • Butterbur root • St. John's Wort flower.

Pain-Less Rub - The Herbalist
Oils of Sweet Almond, Aloe Vera, St. John's Wort flower, Calendula flower & Arnica flower • Essential oils of French Lavender, Peppermint, Lemon Grass, Wintergreen, Nutmeg, Bergamot & Camphor • Extracts of Comfrey root, Echinacea root, White Willow bark & Cayenne pepper.

Palmitol - Flora
Saw Palmetto berries • Zinc 50 mg • Vitamin B6 120 mg.

Palmvitee - LaneLabs
Two capsules contain: Vitamin E 350 IU (as gamma tocotrienol, alpha tocotrienol, delta tocotrienol, & d-alpha tocopherol). Other Ingredients: Gelatin, water, & glycerin. Free of corn, yeast, wheat, & dairy products and contains no sugar, salt, starch, preservatives, artificial flavors or colors.

Panax Ginseng - Pharmanex
Each capsule contains: Ginseng Panax root (5:1) extract (Panax Ginseng C.A. Meyer) 100 mg. Other Ingredients: Rice Flour, Gelatin.

Some Brand Name Natural Products - What they Contain
www.NaturalDatabase.com contains MANY more listings than appear here.

Panaxin - PhytoPharmica
Each capsule contains: Korean Ginseng (Panax ginseng) root extract (standardized to contain 7% ginsenosides) 100 mg.

Pancreas Chelate Plus - Atrium Inc.
Each tablet contains: Zinc (Protein Chelated) 15 mg • Chromium (Protein Chelated) 200 mcg • Pancreas Substance (from total maxi strength Pancreatin 75 mg, Raw Pancreas concentrate 75 mg) 150 mg. To insure the naturally occuring factors as well as the concentrated forms of Lipase & Amylase Enzymes.
See Editor's Note No. 14, page 1817.

Pancreas Plus - Nutri-Quest
Each tablet contains: Pancreatin 270 mg • Pancreas 130 mg [Tissue concentrate (not extract) of Bovine Source]. Natural occuring factors as well as concentrated forms of Protease, Lipase, & Amylase enzymes.
See Editor's Note No. 14, page 1817.

Pantethine - Puritan's Pride
Each tablet contains: Pantethine 165 mg.

Pantethine - PhytoPharmica
Each tablet contains: Pantethine 300 mg.

Pantethine Complex - The Vitamin Shoppe
Each tablet contains 300 mg of Pantethine Complex supplying: Pantethine (coenzyme A precursor) 150 mg • Pantothenic Acid (d-calcium pantothenate) 150 mg. No Yeast, Corn, Wheat, Salt, Sugar, Starch, Soy, Gluten, Milk, Eggs, Dairy, Fish or Animal Derivatives, Preservatives, Artificial Colors or Flavors added.

Pantothenic Acid - Nature's Bounty
Each tablet contains: Pantothenic Acid (as d-Calcium Pantothenate) 200 mg. Other Ingredients: Cellulose, Vegetable Stearic Acid, Starch, Croscarmellose, Silica, Vegetable Magnesium Stearate.

Pantothenic Acid 100 mg - Puritan's Pride
Each tablet contains: Calcium Pantothenate 109 mg.

Pantothenic Acid 200 mg - Puritan's Pride
Each tablet contains: Calcium Pantothenate 218 mg.

Papaya - Leiner Health Products
Each tablet contains: Total Carbohydrate 1 g • Papain 10 mg • Papaya fruit powder 250 mg • Pineapple juice solid powder 150 mg. Other Ingredients: Compressible Sugar, Stearic Acid, Mannitol, Cellulose, Magnesium Stearate, Silicon Dioxide, Artificial Pineapple Flavor.

Para Thyrolate - Progressive Labs
Each capsule contains: Calcium 100 mg • Iodine 225 mcg • Phosphorus 40 mg • Parathyroid concentrate 500 mcg • Thyroid concentrate (thyroxin-free) 25 mg. Other Ingredients: Dicalcium Phosphate, Cellulose, Protein Conjugate, Pacific Sea Kelp, Calcium Carbonate, Papain, Guar Gum, Stearic Acid, Gelatin. The glandular material in this product is prepared by a special process which does not exceed physiological temperature (37° C). Guaranteed free of chemical pesticides and synthetic hormones.
See Editor's Note No. 14, page 1817.

Para-Cid - Atrium Inc.
Each tablet contains: Betaine HCL 250 mg • Pepsin 20 mg. In a slow release matrix.

Paraclear - PhysioLogics
Two capsules contain: Sweet Annie leaf, stem 400 mg • Garlic bulb (10000 mcg Allicin/g • 2 mg) 200 mg • Pau D'Arco bark, stem (3% Napthoquinone 6 mg) 200 mg • Goldthread root (10% Alkaloids, 15 mg) 150 mg • Black Walnut husk 100 mg • Ficin (from fig) 10 mg.

Para-Clens - Nutri-Quest
Each tablet contains: Artemisia Annua 50 mg • Garlic powder 50 mg • Black Walnut 50 mg • Pumpkin seed 50 mg • Oregano oil 1 mg • Tea Tree 2 mg • Grapefruit seed extract 50 mg • Bromelain 50 mg • Papain 50 mg.

Parasillan - Olympian Labs
Each capsule contains: Proprietary Blend: Plaintain, Barberry Bark, Chaparral, Citrus Bioflavonoids, Lobelia, Black Walnut, Wormwood, Psyllium Hull, Cayenne Pepper 700 mg.

Parathyroid - Atrium Inc.
Each tablet contains: Parathyroid (Bovine) 10 mg • Thyroid (Thyroxin free) 30 mg • Stomach (Bovine) 32 mg • Dulse 300 mg • Calcium 50 mg • Phosphorus 22 mg • Vitamin D (as Vitamin D3) 100 IU • Vitamin B12 20 mcg • Folic Acid 440 mcg • Beet 50 mg • Carrot 50 mg. Calcium & Phosphorus from Bone Meal, Beet & Carrot powders, Iodine from Dulse powder.
See Editor's Note No. 14, page 1817.

Parselenium-E - Nutrilite
Each tablet contains: Vitamin E (d-alpha tocopheryl acid succinate) 400 IU • Selenium 10 mcg. Other Ingredients: Parsley concentrate, Selenium yeast, Tri-calcium Phosphate.

PatentLEAN - Patent Health, LLC
Each capsule contains: 3-acetyl-7-oxo-dehdyroepiandrosterone 100 mg. Contains no sugar, salt, yeast, wheat, gluten, corn, soy, dairy products, artificial coloring, artificial flavoring, or preservatives.

Pau D'Arco - Source Naturals
Each tablet contains: Pau d'Arco extract (Tabebuia altissima) 500 mg • Pau d'Arco (Inner Bark) 25 mg • Vitamin C (Ascorbic Acid) 10 mg • Pro- Vitamin A (Beta Carotene) 500 IU.

Pau d'Arco-Black Walnut Virtue - Blessed Herbs
Pau d'Arco bark • Usnea lichen • Calendula flower • Echinacea Angustifolia root • Black Walnut hull • Goldenseal root • Myrrh Gum • Grain alcohol & Distilled Water.

PC-SPES (PCSPES, PC SPES) - BotanicLab, Inc
Each capsule contains: Proprietary Blend: Da Qing Ye (Isatis indigotica), Licorice (Glycyrrhiza glabra, Glycyrrhiza uralensis), San Qi (Panax Pseudoginseng), Reishi Mushroom (Ganoderma lucidum), Baikal Skullcap (Scutellaria baicalensis), Chrysanthemum (Dendranthema morifolium), Rabdosia Rubescens, Saw Palmetto (Serenoa repens) 320 mg.
See Editor's Note No. 30, page 1819.

Pedi-Active A.D.D. Chewables - Nature's Plus
Two tablets contain: LECI-PS (Phosphatidylserine-rich purified Lecithin concentrate) 100 mg • DMAE (2-dimethylaminoethanol bitartrate) 100 mg.

Pedi-Active Spray - Nature's Plus
Each spray contains: DMAE (2-Dimethylaminoethanol Bitartrate) 50 mg • LECI-PS Phosphatidylserine-rich purified Lecithin concentrate supplying Activated Phosphatides: [Phosphatidylserine 10 mg, Phosphatidylcholine 10 mg, Cephalin (Phosphati-dylethanolamine) 6 mg, Phosphoinositides 3 mg] 50 mg. In a proprietary liposomal complex of Essential Metabolic Factors , Purified Water, Vegetable Glycerine, Purified Lecithin, Citrus seed extract (Citrus sinensis), Vitamin E & natural Wild Berry flavor.

Pedi-ADD - Aspen Group, Inc.
Each chewable tablet contains: Phosphatidylserine - Purified Lecithin concentrate supplying Activated Phosphatides 50 mg: Phosphatidylserine 10 mg • Phosphatidylcholine 10 mg • Cephalin (phosphatidylethanolamine) 6 mg • Phosphoinositides 5 mg • DMAE (2-dimethylaminoethanol bitartrate) 50 mg.

BRAND NAMES

Some Brand Name Natural Products - What they Contain

Pediatric Chewable - Clinician's Choice
One tablet contains: Vitamin A (as retinyl acetate & 50% as betacarotene) 2500 IU • Vitamin C (as ascorbic acid & sodium ascorbate) 60 mg • Vitamin D (as cholecalciferol) 200 IU • Vitamin E (as dl-alpha tocopheryl acetate) 15 IU • Thiamin (as mononitrate) 0.75 mg • Riboflavin 0.9 mg • Niacin (as niacinamide) 10 mg • Vitamin B6 (as pyridoxine hydrochloride) 1 mg • Folate (as folic acid) 200 mcg • Vitamin B12 (as cyanocobalamin) 3 mcg • Biotin 30 mcg • Pantothenic Acid (as d-calcium pantothenate) 5 mg • Calcium (as carbonate & gluconate) 85 mg • Iodine (as potassium Iodide) 75 mcg • Magnesium (as oxide) 15 mg • Zinc (as oxide) 7.5 mg • Copper (as cupric oxide) 1 mg • Manganese (as citrate) 0.5 mg • Chromium (as nicotinate) 10 mcg • Molybdenum (sodium molybdate) 5 mcg • Proprietary blend: Acerola powdered extract 4:1 • Carrot Powder, Spinach Powder 6 mg.

Pedia-Vit - Progressive Labs
Two teaspoons (10 ml) contain: Vitamin A 2500 IU • Vitamin C 40 mg • Vitamin D 400 IU • Vitamin E 10 IU • Thiamin (B1) 0.7 mg • Riboflavin (B2) 0.8 mg • Niacin (B3) 9 mg • Vitamin B6 0.7 mg • Folate (folic acid) 200 mcg • Vitamin B12 3 mcg • Biotin 150 mcg • Pantothenic Acid 5 mg • Iron 10 mg • Zinc 8 mg.

Pedi-Vites Multiple - Aspen Group, Inc.
Each tablet contains: Vitamin A Palmitate 180 IU • Vitamin D (as Vitamin D3) 150 IU • Vitamin E 10 IU • Vitamin B1 2 mg • Vitamin B2 2 mg • Vitamin B6 2 mg • Vitamin B12 6 mcg • Vitamin C 60 mg • Niacinamide 5 mg • Folic Acid 100 mcg • Pantothenic Acid 3 mg • Biotin 30 mcg • Calcium (carbonate) 10 mg • Magnesium (gluconate) 2 mg • Manganese (gluconate) 1 mg • Selenium (selenium aspartate) 5 mcg • Chromium (chromium ACP) 5 mcg • Molybdenum (sodium molybdate) 2 mcg • Vanadium (vanadium sulfate) 2 mcg • Chlorophyll 1 mg • Boron (boron citrate) 50 mcg.

Peppermint Plus - Enzymatic Therapy
Each enteric-coated capsule contains: Peppermint oil extract (Mentha piperita) 0.2 ml • Rosemary oil extract (Rosemarinus officinalis) 0.02 ml • Thyme oil extract (Thymus vulgaris) 0.02 ml.
Contains no sugar, salt, yeast, wheat, corn, dairy products, flavoring or preservatives.

Perfect Cal - Futurebiotics
Four tablets contain: Calcium (from Hydroxyappatite crystal) 400 mg • Calcium Complex (Citrate, Carbonate) 600 mg • Magnesium (Citrate, Oxide, Hydroxyappatite) 600 mg • Vitamin D 200 IU • Boron 1.5 mg • Horsetail (from extract) 750 mg.

PerfectRx - Nature's Best
Chocolate flavor contains: Protein 37 g • Carbohydrates 24 g • Fat 2 g. Vanilla flavor contains: Protein 37 g • Carbohydrates 26 g • Fat 0 g • Calories 260. Vanilla Perfect Rx Ingredients: Perfect Unique Protein Blend (Milk Protein Isolate, Calcium Caseinate, Whey Protein Concentrates, Egg Albumin), Maltodextrin, Potassium Chloride, Potassium Citrate, Sodium Chloride, Sodium Citrate, Dipotassium Phosphate, Natural & Artificial Flavors, Aspartame, Magnesium Oxide, Choline Bitartrate, Cellulose, Ascorbic Acid, d-Alpha Tocopheryl Acetate, Ferrous Fumarate, Niacin, Biotin, Xanthan Gum, Vitamin A Palmitate, Zinc, Oxide, D-Calcium Pantothenate, Vitamin K, Manganese Sulfate, Beta-Carotene, Copper Sulfate, Pyridoxine HCL, Riboflavin, Thiamine HCL, L-Glutamine, Chromium Picolinate, Cobalamin Concentrate (vitamin B12), Vitamin D (as Vitamin D3), Folic Acid, Sodium Molybdate, Potassium Iodide, Sodium Selenite.

Performance Enhancer Creatine Fuel - TwinLab
Each capsule contains: Creatine Monohydrate 700 mg.
See Editor's Note No. 7, page 1816.

Perfor-Max - Changes - TwinLab
One caplet contains: Grape seed extract (vitis vinifera) 25 mg • Pine bark extract (Pinus pinaster) 25 mg • Turmeric rhisome extract 25 mg • Botanical Blend 50 mg: Green Tea leaf standardized extract (36% catechin & polyphenols), Hawthorn berry standardized extract (5% flavonoid glycosides), and Rosemary leaf extract. Other Ingredients: Dicalcium Phosphate, Vegetable cellulose, Fractionated vegetable oil, Soy polysaccharides, Silica, and Vegetable resin glaze.

Peridin-C - Beutlich Pharmaceuticals
Each tablet contains: Ascorbic Acid (Vitamin C) 200 mg • Hesperidin Complex (Bioflavonoid) 150 mg • Hesperidin Methyl Chalcone (Bioflavonoid) 50 mg.

Perika St. John's Wort - Nature's Way
Each tablet contains: Perika (WS 5572) dried St. John's Wort extract 300 mg.

Permathene-16 Maximum Strength Caffeine Free - CCA Industries, Inc.
Each tablet contains: Active Ingredient: Phenylpropanolamine HCl 75 mg. Other Ingredients: Croscarmellose, D&C Yellow #10, Dicalcium Phosphate, FD&C Blue #1, FD&C Yellow #6, Lactose, Magnesium Stearate, Methylcellulose, Microcrystalline Cellulose, Stearic Acid, Titanium Dioxide.

Persic-GLA - Atrium Inc.
Each capsule contains: Borage oil 100 mg • Cold Processed Persic oil yielding to the following Lipid Acids: Referred to as Vitamin F Factors, (Oleic 192 mg, Linoleic 109 mg, Gamma Linolenic 30 mg, Palmitic 18 mg, Palmitoleic 5 mg, Stearic 4mg, Linolenic 701 mcg, Heptodecanoic 409 mcg, Arachadic 330 mcg, Arachidonic 111 mcg) 370 mg • Potassium 113 mcg • Sodium 14 mcg • Magnesium 7 mcg • Phosphorus 4 mg • Calcium 4 mcg • "trace amounts of Manganese, Chromium, Zinc, Iron, Copper, Baron, Barium". Contains no sugar, starch, salt, wheat, corn, yeast or soy derivatives.

Personal Lubricant with Aloe Vera, Calendula and Vitamin E - Transitions for Health, Inc.
Deionized Water • Glycerin • Carbomer • Aloe Vera Gel • Butylene Glycol • Hydroxpropyl Methylcellulose • Calendula Extract • Black Walnut Leaf Extract • Imidazolidinyl Urea • Methylparaben • Allantoin • Citric Acid • Tocopheryl Acetate • Retinyl Palmitate • Squalene.

Petadolex - Weber
Each capsule contains: Petasites hybridus extract (Butterbur root, 30:1) 50 mg • Petasin and Isopetasin 7.5 mg. Contains all natural coloring: Carmine, Glycerole, Gelatin, Titanoxide.

PhenCal 106 - Great American Nutrition
Six tablets contain: Vitamin B6 (as pyridoxal-5-phosphate) 30 mg • Chromium (as picolinate) 200 mcg • DL-Phenylalanine 2700 mg • L-Tyrosine 300 mg • L-Glutamine 150 mg • L-5-Hydroxytryptophan 15 mg • L-Carnitine 60 mg.

Phen-Free - EAS
Four capsules contain: Caffeine 99 mg • Citrus aurantium 300 mg (Bitter Orange peel standardized to 6% Synephrine) • Yohimbe 100 mg • Cordyceps 500 mg (standardized to 7% Cordyceptic Acid) • L-Tyrosine 500 mg • St. John's Wort 200 Mg (standardized to 0.3% Hypericin) • Cayenne Pepper powder 30 mg.

PhenSafe - Applied Nutrition
Three capsules contain: St. John's Wort (.3% hypericin) 300 mg • L-Glutamic Acid HCl 100 mg • B6 Pyridoxine HCl 20 mg • Niacinamide (B3) 10 mg • Zinc 8 mg • Folic Acid 200 mcg • ChromeMate 125 mcg • B12 100 mcg • Selenium 75 mcg. Each

serving of the above nutrients is formulated with a special mixture containing these natural ingredients: [Advantra Z (citrus aurantium), Licorice root powder, Ginger root powder, Cayenne powder, Mustard seed powder, Green Tea extract, Fennel seed powder, BioPerine] 640 mg.

Phoenaz - Dazzle, Inc.
Three tablets contain: Vitamin E 60 mg · Vitamin B6 · Calcium carbonate granularV Proprietary Blend 3012 mg: Rye Flour, Malt powder diastatic, Barley Grass, Wheat Grass powder, Blessed Thistle, Wild Yam extract, Corn powder, Damiana leaf powder, Saw Palmetto extract, Soy Isoflavones, European Hops.

Phos Fuel - TwinLab
Four capsules contain: Sodium Phosphate (Dibasic) 4000 mg • Potassium Bicarbonate 816 mg • L-Carnosine 50 mg • Lipoic Acid 100 mcg • Vitamin B1 1.5 mg • Vitamin B2 1.9 mg • Vitamin B3 (Niacinamide) 20 mg • Vitamin B6 2 mg • Pantothenic Acid 10 mg • Biotin 300 mcg.

Phosphagain 2 - EAS
Each 59 gram Vanilla serving contains: Calories 180 • Protein 25 g • Carbohydrates 13 g • Fat 1.5 g • Cholesterol 10 mg • Sodium 380 mg • Potassium 730 mg • Chromium 50 mcg • Selenium 30 mcg • Manganese 1 mg • Vitamin K 40 mcg • Molybdenum 60 mcg • Choline 80 mg. Ingredients: Nitrogenin 2 proprietary Protein/Nitrogen reinforcing matrix [Milk Protein Isolate, Calcium Caseinate, L-Glutamine, Taurine, Calcium Alpha-Ketoglutarate (AKG) & Egg Albumin] • Phosphagen (HPCE Pure Creatine Monohydrate) • Maltodextrin, Dextrose • Vitamin & Mineral Blend: Potassium Phosphate, Potassium Citrate, Salt, Magnesium Oxide, Choline Bitartrate, Disodium Phosphate, Beta-Carotene, Ascorbic Acid, Dl-Alpha Tocopheryl Acetate, Ferrous Fumarate, Niacin, Zinc Oxide, D-Calcium Pantothenate, Copper Sulfate,Vitamin A Palmitate, Manganese Sulfate, Chromium Citrate, Pyridoxine Hydrochloride, Riboflavin, Thiamine Hydrochloride, Sodium Molybdate, Vitamin D (as Vitamin D3), Folic Acid, Biotin, Potassium Iodide, Sodium Selenate, Vitamin K, & Cyanocobalamin • Corn Syrup Solids • Partially Hydrogenated Canola oil • Xanthan Gum • Natural & Artificial Flavors • Sodium RNA • Soy Lecithin • Aspartame • Carrageenan, Phenylalanine.

PhosphaGems - EAS
Each 42 gram serving contains: Calories 135 • Carbohydrates 35 g • Sodium 100 mg • Phosphagen (HPCE pure Creatine Monohydrate) 5.2 g. Ingredients: TriCarb Complex (Sucrose, High-Dextrose Corn Syrup & Dextrose) • Phosphagen (HPCE pure Creatine Monohydrate) • Modified Starch • Natural & Artificial Flavor • Disodium Phosphate • Malic Acid • colored with Cochineal extracts.

Phosphagen - EAS
Each 5 gram serving contains: Phosphagen 5 g.

Phosphagen HP - EAS
Each 43 gram Fruit Punch serving contains: Calories 140 • Carbohydrates 34 g • Sodium 95 mg • Potassium 80 mg • Phosphagen 5.25 g • Taurine 1000 mg. Ingredients: Dextrose • Phosphagen (HPCE pure Creatine Monohydrate), Taurine • Natural & Artificial Flavor • Citric Acid • Beet Powder for color • Magnesium Phosphate • Disodium Phosphate • Potassium Phosphate.

Phosphatide I-C-E - Progressive Labs
Each softgel contains: Phosphatidylcholine 420 mg • Phosphatidylethanolamine 210 mg • Phosphatidylinositol 120 mg • Total Phosphatides 750 mg. All phosphatides extracted from soybeans. This product contains the highest known concentration of naturally occuring phosphatides.

Phosphatidyl Choline - Source Naturals
Each softgel contains: Soy lecithin 1,200 mg • Phosphatidyl Choline 420 mg.

Phosphatidyl Choline Complex - Nature's Life
Each capsule contains: Phosphatidyl Choline Complex (Soy) 120 mg. Nutrient profile based on a typical analysis: Phosphatides: Phosphatidyl Choline (contains 65 mg Choline) 420 mg • Phosphatidyl Ethanolamine 108 mg • Phosphatidyl Inositol (contains 6 mg Inositol) 24 mg • Phosphatidic Acid 36 mg. Lipids: Linoleic Acid (Omega-6) 313 mg • Linolenic Acid (Omega-3) 24 mg • Oleic Acid (Omega-9) 73 mg • Palmitic Acid 78 mg • Stearic Acid 24 mg.

Phosphatidyl Serine - Progressive Labs
Each softgel contains: Phospholipids: Phosphatidylserine (soy phospholipid) 100 mg • Phosphatidylcholine (soy phospholipid) 45 mg • Phosphatidylethanolamine (soy phospholipid) 10 mg • Phosphatidylinositol (soy phospholipid) 10 mg. Fatty Acids: Linoleic Acid 113 mg • Linolenic Acid 11 mg • Oleic Acid 12 mg • Stearic Acid 1 mg • Palmitic Acid 24 mg • Capric Acid 49 mg • Caprylic Acid 130 mg. Minerals: Phosphorus 8 mg • Potassium 3 mg.

Phosphatidylserine - PhysioLogics
Two capsules contain: Phosphatidylserine Complex 500 mg. Phospholipids: Phosphatidylserine 100 mg • Phosphatidylcholine 100 mg • Phosphatidylethanolamine 60 mg • Phosphatidylinositol 30 mg. Fatty Acids: Linoleic Acid 135 mg • Linolenic Acid 30 mg • Oleic Acid 25 mg • Stearic Acid 15 mg • Palmitic Acid 45 mg. Minerals: Phosphorus 15 mg • Potassium 5 mg.

Phosphatidylserine Complex - The Vitamin Shoppe
Each softgel contains: 500 mg Phospholipids providing 100 mg of Phosphatidylserine and 400 mg other Phospholipids. No Yeast, Wheat, Salt, Sugar, Starch, Corn, Milk, Dairy, Eggs, Preservatives, Artificial Colors or Flavors added.

Phospholoba Q10 - Olympian Labs
Two capsules contain: Phophatidylserine Complex 500 mg • Ginkgo Biloba 30 mg • Coenzyme Q10 15 mg • Fatty Acids & Minerals 270 mg.

Phyt-Aloe - Mannatech
Each capsule contains: PhytoAloe Complex: broccoli, brussels sprout, cabbage, carrot, cauliflower, garlic, kale, onion, tomato, turnip, papaya, pineapple • Ambrotose Complex: naturally occurring plant polysaccharides including freeze-dried Aloe Vera inner leaf gel extract - Manapol powder. Other Ingredients: Magnesium stearate. See Editor's Note No. 17, page 1817.

Phyto Estrogen Power - Nature's Herbs
Four capsules contain: Soy Germ Isoflavone concentrate 1400 mg • Kudzu root extract 100 mg • Certified Potency Korean Ginseng extract 100 mg • Certified Potency Dong Quai extract 100 mg • Mexican Wild Yam extract 100 mg • Boron 3 mg • Natural Vitamin E 800 IU. In a base of Chasteberry powder and Arrowroot.

Phyto Flavonoids - Olympia Nutrition
Contains the extracts of Silymarin, Curcumin, Green Tea, Quercetin, Rosemary, Bilberry, Hawthorn, Ginger, Ginkgo Biloba, Bromelain, Cranberry.

Phyto Surge - PhytoPharmica
One tablespoon contains: Arsenicum album 6x • Nux vomica 3x • Podophyllum peltatum 3x • Cinchona officinalis 2x • Rhamnus frangula 2x • Artemisia vulgaris 1x • Avena sativa 1x • Cinnamomum 1x • Gentiana lutea 1x • Sterculia acuminata 1x. In a base of 20% USP alcohol by volume. See Editor's Note No. 1, page 1816.

BRAND NAMES

Phyto-Bears - Mannatech
Each Phyto-Bear contains: PhytoAloe Complex: broccoli, brussels sprout, cabbage, carrot, cauliflower, garlic, kale, onion, tomato, turnip, papaya, pineapple • Ambrotose Complex: naturally occurring plant polysaccharides including freeze-dried Aloe Vera inner leaf gel extract - Manapol powder. Other Ingredients: Corn syrup, Sucrose water, Gelatin, Citric acid, Grape juice concentrate, Natural flavors, Natural colors, Olive oil, Beeswax.
See Editor's Note No. 17, page 1817.

Phyto-Biotic - Enzymatic Therapy
Each capsule contains: Barberry Bark of root extract 6:1 (Berberis vulgaris) 200 mg • Oregon Grape root extract 6:1 (Berberis aquifolium) 200 mg • Goldenseal root extract (Hydrastis canadensis) standardized to contain 5% total Alkaloids including Berberine, Hydrastine & Canadine 50 mg. Contains no sugar, salt, yeast, wheat, corn, soy, dairy products, coloring, flavoring, or preservatives.

Phytodolor - PhytoPharmica
Active Ingredients: Common ash (Fraxinus excelsior) bark (4.5:1) 0.20 ml • Aspen (Populus tremula) leaves & bark (4.5:1) 0.60 ml • Goldenrod (Solidago virgaurea) aerial (4.8:1) 0.20 ml. Other Ingredients: Water, Alcohol (45.6%). This patented liquid formula is standardized to contain: Salicin-0.75 mg/ml, Salicylic alcohol-0.042 mg/ml, Isofraxidin-0.015 mg/ml, and Rutin-0.06 mg/ml.

Phytoestrin - USANA Nutritionals
Each tablet contains: Soy Isoflavones (Glycine Max) seed 14.0 mg • Black Cohosh extract (Cimicifuga Racemosa) root 50.0 mg • Chasteberry powder (Vitex Agnus-Castus) fruit 50.0 mg • Licorice root extract (Glycyrrhiza Glabrera) 30.0 mg • Dong Quai extract (Angelica Sinensis) root 15.0 mg. Other Ingredients: Dextrose, Ascorbyl Palmitate, Croscarmellose Sodium, Dextrin (Modified Food Starch), Collodial Silicon Dioxide.

Phytoestrogen Body Cream - Transitions for Health, Inc.
Deionized Water • Carbomer • Jojoba Oil • Caprylic / Caprice Triglycerides • Cetyl Ester • Glyceryl Stearate • Ginseng Extract • Glycerin • Peg-100 Stearate • Stearic Acid • Aloe Vera Gel • Hydrolyzed Glycosaminoglycans • Black Walnut Leaf Extract • Black Cohosh Extract • Licorice Root Extract • Chaste Tree Berry Extract • Evening Primrose Oil • Tocopheryl Acetate • Triethanolamine • Imidazolidinyl Urea • Methylparaben • Xanthan Gum • Grape Seed Extract • Red Clover Blossom Extract • Propylparaben • Butylene Glycol • Orange Oil.

Phyto-Flavonoids - Futurebiotics
Two capsules contain: Procyanidol • Whole Grape extract* 50 mg • Green Tea powder concentrate 150 mg • Citrus bioflavonoids 500 mg • Rutin 75 mg • Quercetin 150 mg • Soy isoflavone extract 500 mg • Berry blend (Raspberry, Blackberry, Blueberry) 200 mg • Cruciferous Vegetable powder blend 200 mg. *Procyanidol is a concentrated solvent-free grape extract containing high levels of flavonoid polyphenols.

Phyto-Fruit - Olympia Nutrition
Guava, Papaya, Mango, Raspberry, Blueberry, Grapefruit, Grape, Ginseng.

PhytoFruit Concentrates - Now
Two V Caps contain: Grape seed extract (95% Polyphenols) 20 mg • Concentrated fruit extract powders: Acerola Cherry 50 mg, Cranberry 50 mg, Guava 50 mg, Papaya 50 mg, Raspberry 50 mg, Blueberry 50 mg, Grapefruit 50 mg, Mango 50 mg, Pineapple 50 mg, Strawberry 50 mg • Panax ginseng (5% Ginsenosides) 50 mg • Bromelain (2000 GDU from pineapple) 50 mg • Protease (100 SAP Units) 50 mg • Amylase (3000 DU Units) 50 mg • Lipase (100 LU Units) 50 mg • Cellulase (500 CMC Units) 50 mg.

PhytoMax - PhytoPharmica
Two capsules contain: St. John's Wort (Hypericum perforatum) flower head extract (standardized to contain 0.3% hypericin and 4% hyperforin) 500 mg • Valerian (Valeriana officinalis) root extract (standardized to contain a minimum of 0.8% valerenic acids) 30 mg • Passion Flower (Passiflora incarnata) dried aerial part extract 4:1 30 mg.

Phytosterol Complex - Progressive Labs
Each capsule contains: Niacin (vitamin B3) 20 mg • Beta-Sitosterol 106 mg • Campesterol 52 mg • Stigmasterol 42 mg.

Phytotality - PhysioLogics
Each capsule contains: Broccoli extract (2% Glucosinolates, 2 mg) 100 mg • TeaGreen leaf (50 % Polyphenols, 50 mg) 100 mg • Tomato extract (1% Lycopene, 500 mcg) 50 mg • Calendula flower Marigold (5% Lutein, 150 mcg) 3 mg • Soy Isoflavones extract (5 % Isoflavones, 1.25 mg) 25 mg • Red Grape skin extract (30% Anthocyanidins, 7.5 mg) 25 mg • Garlic bulb (10000 mcg Allicin/g, 250 mcg) 25 mg • Turmeric (95% Curcumin, 1.9 mg) 2 mg • Ginger root (5% Gingerols, 100 mcg) 2 mg • Milk Thistle seed (80% Silymarin, 20 mg) 25 mg • Onion 2 mg • Carrot 2 mg • Beet root 2 mg • Celery 2 mg • Leek 2 mg • Garlic 2 mg • Cauliflower 2 mg • Asparagus 2 mg • Broccoli 2 mg • Cabbage 2 mg.

PhytoxyActin - Nature's Plus
Two capsules contain: Vitamin C corn free 250 mg • Broccoli [(Brassica oleracea floret) standardized 0.035% Lutein, 0.004% B-Cryptoxanthin, 0.0025% Lycopene, 0.0025% Alpha Carotene, 0.0025% Beta Carotene, 0.004% Sulforaphane] 100 mg • Carrot [(Daucus carota root) standardized 0.003% Lutein, 0.0010% Lycopene, 0.0063% Alpha Carotene, 0.0075% Beta Carotene] 100 mg • Vitamin E natural 100 IU • Spinach [(Spinacia oleracea leaf) standardized 0.0043% Lutein, 0.0024% Lycopene, 0.0043% Beta Carotene, 0.0038% B-Cryptoxanthin] 75 mg • Tomato [(Lycopersicon esculentum fruit) standardized 0.0075% Lutein, 0.0155% Lycopene, 0.0015% Beta Carotene] 75 mg • Echinacea [(Echinacea angustifolia root) standardized 4% Echinacosides] 75 mg • Astragalus [(Astragalus membranaceus root) standardized 0.4% 4'-Hydroxy-3'-Methoxyisoflavone 7-sug] 50 mg • Green Tea [(Camellia sinensis leaf) standardized 50% Polyphenols] 50 mg • Red Wine concentrate alcohol free [(Vitis vinifera fruit) standardized 20% Polyphenols] 50 mg • Turmeric [(Cuizome) standardized 95% Curcumin] 50 mg • Garlic odor-modified [(Allium sativum clove) standardized 0.35% Allicin, 0.65% Allicin, 0.40% Thiosulfinates, 0.085% Allyl Mercaptan] 50 mg • Shiitake Mushroom [(Lentinus edodes mycelia) standardized 3.2% KS-2 Polysaccharides] 25 mg • Grape seed extract [(Vitis vinifera) standardized 95% Proanthocyanidins] 25 mg • Beta Carotene pro-Vitamin A (naturally supplying 25000 IU of Vitamin A activity) 15 mg.

Pile Formula - Dr. Morrow's Homeopathic Formulas
Ten drops contain: Aesculus hippocastanum 10X • Hamamelis canadensis 10X • Hydrastis canadensis 10X • Viburnum prunifolium 10X.
See Editor's Note No. 1, page 1816.

Pineal Concentrate - Progressive Labs
Each capsule contains: Veal bone concentrate 100 mg • Flaxseed oil 20 mg • Pineal concentrate 7 mg • Pituitary concentrate 3 mg. The glandular concentrate in this product is prepared by a special process which does not exceed physiological temperature (37° C). Guaranteed free of chemical pesticides and synthetic hormones.
See Editor's Note No. 14, page 1817.

Pineal Plus - Atrium Inc.
Each tablet contains: Raw Pineal Tissue concentrate (Bovine) 8 mg • Raw Whole Pituitary concentrate (Bovine) 20 mg • Raw Calf Bone concentrate (Bovine) 150 mg • Cold Pressed Flaxseed oil 10 mg.
See Editor's Note No. 14, page 1817.

Pinna-Cal - Changes - TwinLab

Six caplets contain: Vitamin D (as Cholecalciferol) 125 IU • Vitamin K (as Phytonadione) 80 mcg • Calcium (as purified Calcite, Hydroxyapatite, Calcium Citrate, and Calcium Lactate) 1000 mg • Magnesium (as Magnesium Citrate and Oxide) 400 mg • Boron (as Boron Citrate) 2 mg • Ipriflavone 600 mg.
Other Ingredients: Vegetable cellulose, Fractionated vegetable oil, Silica, Soy polysaccharides, and Vita-Lok vegetable resin glaze.

Pinnacle 5-HTP Tryptobol - Bodyonics

Two capsules contain: Griffonia Simplicifolia (providing 10% (100 mg) 5-HTP (5-Hydroxy-L-Tryptophan)) 1000 mg • Herbolics Support Complex (from Jatoba, Maca, Para Todo, Yerba Mate) 100 mg. Other Ingredients: Calcium Phosphate, Microcrystalline Cellulose, Magnesium Stearate, Gelatin.

Pinnacle Androstat 100 - Bodyonics

Each tablet contains Androstenedione 100 mg.
Other Ingredients: Calcium Phosphate, Lecithin, Xanthan Gum, Stearic Acid, Magnesium Stearate.

Pinnacle Androstat Pro Six - Bodyonics

Each tablet contains balanced andro complex: 4-androstene-3, 17-diol (4-androstenediol) 125 mg • 4-androstenedione-3, 17-dione (4-androstenedione) 5 mg • 5-androstene-3, 17-dione (5-androstenedione) 5 mg • 5-androstene-3, 17-diol (5-androstenediol) 5 mg • 19-nor-5-androstene-3, 17-diol (19-nor 5-androstendiol) 5 mg.
Other Ingredients: Calcium Phosphate, Lecithin, Xanthan Gum, Stearic Acid, Magnesium Stearate. Inulinized in a bioactive complex of Phosephorolytic Dahlin.

Pinnacle Androstat100 Poppers Cool Mint Flavor - Bodyonics

Two tablets contain balanced andro complex: 4-androstene-3, 17-diol (4-androstenediol) 83.33 mg • 4-androstenedione-3, 17-dione (4-androstenedione) 3.33 mg • 5-androstene-3, 17-dione (5-androstenedione) 3.33 mg • 5-androstene-3, 17-diol (5-androstenediol) 3.33 mg • 19-nor-5-androstene-3, 17-diol (19-nor 5-androstendiol) 3.33 mg. Other Ingredients: Fructose, Sorbitol, Natural Flavor, Stearic Acid, Magnesium Stearate, Cellulose, Croscarmellose, Sucralose.

Pinnacle Androstat100 poppers Licorice Flavor - Bodyonics

Two tablets contain balanced andro complex: 4-androstene-3, 17-diol (4-androstenediol) 83.33 mg • 4-androstenedione-3, 17-dione (4-androstenedione) 3.33 mg • 5-androstene-3, 17-dione (5-androstenedione) 3.33 mg • 5-androstene-3, 17-diol (5-androstenediol) 3.33 mg • 19-nor-5-androstene-3, 17-diol (19-nor 5-androstendiol) 3.33 mg. Other Ingredients: Fructose, Sorbitol, Natural Flavor, Stearic Acid, Magnesium Stearate, Cellulose, Croscarmellose, Sucralose.

Pinnacle Androstat100 Poppers Wild Berry Flavor - Bodyonics

Two tablets contain balanced andro complex: 4-androstene-3, 17-diol (4-androstenediol) 83.33 mg • 4-androstenedione-3, 17-dione (4-androstenedione) 3.33 mg • 5-androstene-3, 17-dione (5-androstenedione) 3.33 mg • 5-androstene-3, 17-diol (5-androstenediol) 3.33 mg • 19-nor-5-androstene-3, 17-diol (19-nor 5-androstendiol) 3.33 mg. Other Ingredients: Fructose, Sorbitol, Natural Flavor, Stearic Acid, Magnesium Stearate, Cellulose, Croscarmellose, Sucralose.

Pinnacle Androstat6 - Bodyonics

Two tablet contains balanced andro complex: 4-androstene-3, 17-diol (4-androstenediol) 125 mg • 4-androstenedione-3, 17-dione (4-androstenedione) 5 mg • 5-androstene-3, 17-dione (5-androstenedione) 5 mg • 5-androstene-3, 17-diol (5-androstenediol) 5 mg • 19-nor-5-androstene-3, 17-diol (19-nor 5-androstendiol) 5 mg.

Other Ingredients: Fructose, Sorbitol, Natural Licorice Flavor, Stearic Acid, Magnesium, Stearate and 100% Natural Beta Cyclodextrins.

Pinnacle Beta Activated Protein with HMB - Bodyonics

Twelve tablets contain: Calcium B-Hydroxy B-Methylbutyrate Monohydrate (HMB) 3 g • Beta Peptide (a proprietary blend of very distinct cosein, whey and aligopeptides) 12 g • Alanine 392 mg •Arginine 419 mg • Aspartic Acid 713 mg • Cystine 74 mg • Glutamic Acid 2806 mg • Glycine 232 mg • Isoleucine (BCAA) 635 mg • Leucine (BCAA) 1044 mg • Lysine 906 mg • Methionine 307 mg • Phenylalanine 556 mg • Proline 1178 mg • Serine 617 mg • Threonine 494 mg • Tryptophan 142 mg • Tyrosine 461 mg • Valine (BCAA) 732 mg. Other Ingredients: Calcium Phosphate, Stearic Acid, Magnesium Stearate, Croscarmellose, Silica.

Pinnacle BHP-5 - Bodyonics

Each tablet contains: Hydrolyzed BHP5 (Pregnenolone) 15 mg.
Other Ingredients: Calcium Phosphate, Stearic Acid, Magnesium Stearate, Croscarmellose.

Pinnacle Chrysinex 250 - Bodyonics

Each tablet contains: Chrysin Complex [Derived from a customized blend of 98% pure 5,7-Dihydroxyflavone and natural powered extract poplar bud (Populus candicans)] 250 mg • Cruciferous Vegetable Concentrate (Standardized to contain 10% Indole 3-Carbinol) 25 mg. Other Ingredients: Calcium Phosphate, Stearic Acid, Magnesium Stearate, Lecithin, Xanthan Gum.

Pinnacle Cordyceps 500 - Bodyonics

Each tablet contains: Dong Chong Zia Cao (Cordyceps sinensis-winter bug, summer herb) • Sha Shen (Adenophora tetraphylla) • WuWei Zi (Schisandra chinensis) • Gan Jiang (Zingiber officinale) • Dahlulin (Dahlia inulin juice concentrate).
Other ingredients: Dicalcium Phosphate, Croscarmellose, Magnesium Stearate, Stearic Acid.

Pinnacle Crea Glutide 2400 - Bodyonics

Each tablet contains: Crea-Glutide 2400 mg • Creatine Monohydrate 2 g • Glutamine Peptide 400 mg. Other Ingredients: Calcium Phosphate, Stearic Acid, Magnesium Stearate, Croscarmellose.

Pinnacle Crea-Glutide - Bodyonics

Two tablespoons contains: Dextrose • BioReacted Crea-Glutide Complex • Complex Carbohydrate • Dahlulin (Dry Dahlia Inulin Juice Complex) • Citric Acid • Natural Cranberry Flavor • Xanthan Gum • Stevia Extract • Beet Extract.

Pinnacle CreaRibose ATP Kichers - Bodyonics

Six tablets contain: Creatine Monohydrate 5 grams • D-Ribose 3 grams. Other Ingredients: Magnesium Stearate, Cellulose, Calcium Phosphate, Stearic Acid.

Pinnacle Fractionized CCK 100 - Bodyonics

Each tablet contains: Cholecystokinin (CCK) (Derived from a purified blend of edible bovine tissuse fractions, providing 1000 picomotes of standardized Cholecystokinin (CCK) a bioactive substance) 100 mg. Other ingredients: Calcium Phosphate, Microcrystalline Cellulose, Stearic Acid, Magnesium Stearate, Croscarmellose Silica.
See Editor's Note No. 14, page 1817.

Pinnacle Gro Tropin - Bodyonics

Three capsules contains: Alpha GPC (Alpha-Glycerylphosarylcholine) 500 mg • AminoGlutein Peptide (standardized to provide 30% Glutamine Peptide) 500 mg • Colostrum (Colostral Isoform Extract) (standardized to provide 1300 nanograms of platelet derived growth factor) 500 mg • Tribulus Terrestris (standardized to provide 40% Furostanol Saponins) 500 mg •

BRAND NAMES

B R A N D   N A M E S

Phosphatidyl Serine 500 mcg • Chrysin (98% pure 5,7 Dehydroxyflavone) 750 mcg. Other Ingredients: Magnesium Strearate, Gelatin.

Pinnacle Horny Goat Weed - Bodyonics
Two capsules contain: Horny Goat Weed (Epimedium grandiflorum) standardized 10% Icariin 500 mg • Maca Pure (Lepidium meyenii)standardized to contain 0.6% macamides and macaenes 250 mg • Mucuna pruriens standardized 15% L-Dopa (L-dihydroxyphenylalanine) 33.3 mg • Polypodium vulgare standardized 8% 20-hydroxyecdysone 25 mg. Other Ingredients: Calcium Phosphate, Magnesium Stearate, Gelatin.

Pinnacle P-ALC 500 - Bodyonics
Each tablet contains: Phosphorolytic Acetyl L-Carnitine (PALC) (Including Inulin and Succunates) 500 mg. Other Ingredients: Calcium Phosphate, Stearic Acid, Magnesium Stearate, Silica, Croscarmellose.

Pinnacle PS Complex 500 - Bodyonics
Each tablet contains: Cephalized PS (Phosphatidyl Serine Complex) (BioActivated Phospholipid fractions standardized to 55% cephalins phosphatidyl serine, choline, inositol and ethanolamine) 500 mg. Other Ingredients: Microcrystalline Cellulose, Calcium Phosphate, Stearic Acid, Magnesium Stearate, Croscarmellose, Silica.

Pinnacle PYRUVATE 1000 - Bodyonics
Each tablet contains: Sodium 60 mg • Potassium 40 mg • Calcium 100 mg • Stabilized Trimin Pyruvate Complex 1000 mg (From Calcium, Potassium, and Sodium salts of Pyruvic Acid, plus Dihydroxyacetone. Inulinized in a bioactive complex of Phosphorolytic Dahlia Inulin providing a long chain carbohydrate molecule). Other Ingredients: Calcium Phosphate, Stearic Acid, Magnesium Stearate, Silica, Croscarmellose.

Pinnacle PYRUVATE 500 - Bodyonics
Each tablet contains: Sodium 30 mg • Potassium 20 mg • Calcium 50 mg • Stabilized Trimin Pyruvate Complex 500 mg (From Calcium, Potassium, and Sodium salts of Pyruvic Acid, plus Dihydroxyacetone. Inulinized in a bioactive complex of Phosphorolytic Dahlia Inulin providing a long chain carbohydrate molecule). Other Ingredients: Calcium Phosphate, Stearic Acid, Magnesium Stearate, Silica, Croscarmellose.

Pinnacle Super Crea Glutide A-DS - Bodyonics
One scoop contains: Creatine Monohydrate 6 g • Glutamine Peptide 2 g • Taurine 2 g • Dahlulin (Dry Dahlia Inulin Juice Complex) 500 mg • Complex Carbohydrate • Natural Flavor • Xanthan Gum • Stevia Extract • Beta Carotene.

Pinnacle Thermophen - Bodyonics
Two tablets contain: St. John's Wort (0.3% hypericin) 150 mg • Citrus Aurantium (Bitter Orange peel) (1.5- 3% synephrine) 200 mg • Kava Kava (40% Kavalactones) 100 mg • Yerba Mate (20% Methylxanthines) 200 mg. Other Ingredients: Calcium Phosphate, Microcrystalline Cellulose, Stearic Acid, Magnesium Stearate, Croscarmellose.

Pinnacle Tribestrol 250 - Bodyonics
Two captabs contain: Tribulus Terrestris (providing 40% (100 mg) Furostanol Saponins) 250 mg • Herbolics Support Complex (from Catuaga, Muira Puama, Chachuhuasu, Iporuru) 100 mg. Other Ingredients: Calcium Phosphate, Stearic Acid, Magnesium Stearate, Croscarmellose.

Pinnacle Ultra Strength Volumax Chocolate Flavor - Bodyonics
Two scoops contain: Whey Protein Concentrate (Ion Exchange) • complex Carbohydrate (Maliodextrin) • Creatine Monohydrate •

Dutch Cocoa Powder • Soy Fiber • Oat Fiber • Nat. & Art. Vanilla Flavor • Glutamine Peptide • Dahluin (Dry Dahlia Inulin Juice Complex) • Whey Protein Hydrolysate • Tourine • Potassium Phosphate • Calcium Phosphate • Magnesium Oxide • Potassium Chloride • Xanthan Gum • Aspartame • Psyllium, Monosodium Phosphate • Ascorbic Acid • Beta Carotene • dl-Alpha • Tocopheryl Acetate • ferrous Fumarate • Niacinamide • Zinc Oxide • Vitamin A Palmitate • D-Calcium Pantothenate • Manganese Sulfate • RNA Powder • Soy Lecithin • Vitamin K (as Vitamin K1) • Copper Sulfate • Pyridoxine Hydrochloride • Riboflavin • Thiamine Hydrochloride • Cyanocobalamin • Vitamin D (as Vitamin D3) • Folic Acid • Chromium Chloride • Biotin • Selenomethionine • Chromium Picolinate • Sodium Molybdate • Potassium Iodide • Sodium Selenate.

Pinnacle Ultra Strength Volumax Vanilla Flavored - Bodyonics
Two scoops contain: Whey Protein Concentrate (Ion Exchange) • complex Carbohydrate (Maliodextrin) • Creatine Monohydrate • Soy Fiber • Oat Fiber • Nat. & Art. Vanilla Flavor • Glutamine Peptide • Dahluin (Dry Dahlia Inulin Juice Complex) • Whey Protein Hydrolysate • Taurine • Potassium Phosphate • Calcium Phosphate • Magnesium Oxide • Potassium Chloride • Xanthan Gum • Aspartame • Psyllium, Monosodium Phosphate • Ascorbic Acid • Beta Carotene • dl-Alpha • Tocopheryl Acetate • ferrous Fumarate • Niacinamide • Zinc Oxide • Vitamin A • Palmitate • D-Calcium Pantothenate • Manganese Sulfate • RNA Powder • Soy Lecithin • Vitamin K (as Vitamin K1) • Copper Sulfate • Pyridoxine Hydrochloride • Riboflavin • Thiamine Hydrochloride • Cyanocobalamin • Vitamin D (as Vitamin D3) • Folic Acid • Chromium Chloride • Biotin • Selenomethionine • Chromium Picolinate • Sodium Molybdate • Potassium Iodide • Sodium Selenate.

Pinnacle Whey Ahead Chocolate Flavor - Bodyonics
One scoop contains: Whey Ahead Complex (a blend of Whey Protein Concentrates and Whey Protein Isolates, and Partially Pre-digested Ion Exchanged Whey Protein Hydrolysates) • Creatine Monohydrate • Glutamin Peptide • Dutch Cocoa Powder • Natural and Artifical Vanilla Flavor • Tourine • Dahlulin (Dry Dahlia Inulin Juice Complex) • Xanthan Gum • Beta Carotene • Aspartame.

Pinnacle Whey Ahead Vanilla Flavored - Bodyonics
One scoop contains: Whey Ahead Complex a blend of Whey Protein Concentrates and Whey Protein Isolates and partially Pre-digested Ion Exchanged Whey Protein Hydrolysates • Creatine Monohydrate • Glutamine Peptide • Natural and Artifical Vanilla Flavor • Tourine • Dahlulin (Dry Dahlia Inulin Juice Complex) • Xanthan Gum • Beta Carotene • Aspartame.

Pizazz - Nature's Plus
Each tablespoon contains: L-Phenylalanine free form amino acid 250 mg • Pantothenic Acid 75 mg • Inositol 50 mg • Niacinamide 40 mg • Vitamin B1 (Thiamine) 30 mg • Vitamin B2 (Riboflavin) 30 mg • Vitamin B6 (Pyridoxine HCL) 30 mg • Choline (Bitartrate) 21 mg • Vitamin B12 (from Cobalamin) 100 mcg • Biotin 30 mcg. In a natural high-energy base of Bee Pollen, Ginseng, Gotu Kola, & Fo-Ti. Sweetened with Honey & Blackstrap Molasses. Contains no yeast, wheat, corn, soy, milk or salt.

Plant Enzimase - Nutri-Quest
Each 360 mg capsule contains: Amylase 4500 DU • Protease 15000 HUT • Lipase 65 IU • Invertase 0.25 IAU • Malt Diastase 150 DPI • Lactase 200 LacU • Cellulase 60 CU. In a base of pure Beet root Fiber.

Plantain Salve - Dial Herbs
Plantain • Chickweed • Mint • Comfrey • Oat Straw. In a base of Bees Wax, Glycerine & Cold Pressed Olive oil.

Plus - Mannatech
Wild Yam root standardized for phytosterols • L-Glutamic Acid • L-Glycine • L-Lysine • L-Arginine • Beta Sitosterol • Ambrotose Complex: naturally occurring plant polysaccharides including freeze-dried Aloe Vera inner leaf gel extract - Manapol powder. Other Ingredients: Microcrystalline cellulose, Cellulose Silicon dioxide, Polyvinylpyrrolidone, Croscarmellose sodium, Magnesium stearate. See Editor's Note No. 17, page 1817.

PM Menopause formula - PhytoPharmica
Each tablet contains: Valerian (Valeriana officinalis) root extract (standardized to contain a minimum of 0.8% valerenic acids) 200 mg • Kava (Piper methysticum) root extract (standardized to contain 30% kavalactones) 200 mg • Hops (Humulus lupulus) flower extract 7.5:1 100 mg • Black Cohosh (Cimicifuga racemosa) root and rhizome extract (standardized to contain 2.5% triterpene glycosides [calculated as 27-deoxyactein]) 20 mg.

PMS Escape - PMS Escape
One packet (50 g) contains: Calories 188 • Total Carbohydrates 47 g • Vitamin C 60 mg • Vitamin B6 05 mg • Calcium 50 mg • Magnesium 20 mg. Other Ingredients: Natural and Artificial Flavor, FD&C Red #40.

PMS Formula - Puritan's Pride
Three tablets contain: Vitamin B-6 354 mg • Folic Acid 400 mcg • Calcium 125 mg • Magnesium 250 mg • Potassium 99 mg • Evening Primrose oil 500 mg • Proprietary Herbal Complex Blend: derived from Dong Quai, Black Cohosh, Fo-Ti, Dandelion, Watercress, Parsley, and Yellow Dock 150 mg.

PMS Formula - Nature's Way
Three capsules contain: Black Cohosh root 150 mg • Cramp bark 250 mg • Dandelion leaf 150 mg • L-5 Hydroxytryptophan (griffonia bean extract) 5 mg • Lobelia herb 150 mg • Magnesium amino acid chelate 50 mg • Niacin (Vitamin B3) 10 mg • Pyridoxine HCl 76 mg • Riboflavin (Vitamin B2) 852 mcg • Thiamine (Vitamin B1) 750 mcg • Vitamin B12 (Cyanacobalamin) 3 mcg. Other Ingredients: Gelatin, Millet.

PMS Formula - Nature's Way
Three capsules contain: Black Cohosh root 150 mg • Cramp bark 250 mg • Dandelion leaf 150 mg • L-5 Hydroxytryptophan (Griffonia bean extract) 5 mg • Lobelia herb 150 mg • Magnesium Amino Acid Chelate 50 mg • Niacin (Vitamin B3) 10 mg • Pyridoxine HCL 76 mg • Riboflavin (Vitamin B2) 852 mcg • Thiamine (Vitamin B1) 750 mcg • Vitamin B12 (Cyanocobalamin) 3 mcg. Other ingredients: Gelatin, Millet.

PMS Formula - The Vitamin Shoppe
Each capsule contains: Vitamin B12 25 mcg • Vitamin B6 10 mg • St. John's Wort 150 mg • Siberian Ginseng 100 mg • Korean Ginseng root 50 mg • Chamomile 100 mg.

PMS Formula with Indolplex - PhytoPharmica
Two tablets contain: Vitamin D (as cholecalciferol) 250 IU • Calcium (as calcium citrate and calcium carbonate) 200 mg • Iodine (as potassium iodide) 80 mcg • Magnesium (as magnesium aspartate) 100 mg • Chaste Tree (Vitex-agnus castus) berry extract (standardized to contain a minimum of 0.5% agnuside) 20 mg • Diindolylmethane (DIM) as Indolplex blend 14 mg.

PMS Forte - Futurebiotics
Two tablets contain: Thiamin HCl (B1) 12 mg • Riboflavin (B2) 12 mg • Pyridoxine HCl (B6) 65 mg • Niacinamide 50 mg • Vitamin C (Ascorbic Acid) 60 mg • Dong Quai (extract equal to) 300 mg • Choline Bitartrate 75 mg • Para Amino Benzoic Acid (PABA) 85 mg • Methionine 60 mg • Inositol 50 mg • Iron (Ferrous Fumarate) 8 mg •

Potassium (Citrate, Gluconate) 60 mg • Magnesium (Oxide, Amino Acid Chelate) 350 mg • Vitamin B12 40 mcg • Iodine (Potassium, Iodide) 150 mcg • Zinc (Gluconate) 15 mg • Pantothenic Acid 60 mg • Folic Acid 400 mcg • Calcium (Carbonate, Phosphate) 300 mg • Vitamin E 30 IU • Ribonucleic Acid (RNA) 40 mg • Biotin 300 mcg • In a base containing Vitex (Agnus Castus), Uva Ursi, Royal Jelly, Raw Alfalfa Juice Concentrate, Cramp Bark, Betaine HCl, Chamomile, Squawvine, American Ginseng Extract, Chinese Licorice, Melissa, Marjoram, Polygonum Multiflorum.

PMS Nutritional Systems Part I - Schiff
Eight softgels contain: Beta Carotene (Vitamin A activity) 15000 IU • Vitamin D 100 IU • Vitamin E (d-Alpha Tocopheryl Acetate) 600 IU • Vitamin C (Ascorbic Acid) 1000 mg • Folic Acid 200 mcg • Thiamine Mononitrate (Vitamin B2) 50 mg • Riboflavin (Vitamin B2) 50 mg • Niacinamide 50 mg • Vitamin B6 (Pyridoxine HCl) 200 mg • Biotin 30 mcg • Pantothenic Acid (d-Calcium Pantothenate) 50 mg • Calcium (Calcium Chlelate) 150 mg • Magnesium (Magnesium Oxide) 300 mg • Iodine (Potassium Iodide) 150 mcg • Iron (Ferrous Chelate) 15 mg • Copper (Cupric Oxide) 0.5 • Zinc (Zinc Gluconate) 25 mg • Choline Bitartrate 500 mg • Manganese (Gluconate) 10 mg • Potassium (Potassuim Chloride) 100 mg • Selenium (Selenium Chelate) 100 mcg • Chromium (Chromium Chelate) 500 mg • Inositol 500 mg • Para Aminobenzoic Acid 50 mg.

PMS Nutritional Sytems Part II - Schiff
Each softgel contains: Sarsaparilla root 210 mg • Burdock root 210 mg • Ginger root 70 mg.

PMS Tea - Traditional Medicinals
One tea bag contains: Dandelion root (Tanaxacum officinale): 500 mg. Other herbal ingredients: Roasted Carob pod, Roasted Barley, Roasted Chicory root, Parsley leaf, Oat Straw herb, Nettle leaf, Chickweed herb, Uva Ursi leaf, Cramp bark, Cornsilk style & stigma.

PMSOS - Nature's Herbs
Four capsules contain: Vitamin B6 500 mg • natural Vitamin E (d-Alpha Tocopherol Succinate) 400 IU • Uva Ursi extract (concentrated standardized for 10% Arbutin equivalent to 1200 of dried herb) 400 mg • Valerian root extract (standardized for .72-.88% valernic acid = to 1600 mg of dried herb) 400mg • White Willow bark extract (standardized for 15% salicin - White Willow extract 5:1= to 1600 mg of dried herb) 200 mg • Chasteberry extract (Vitex agnus castus - standardized for 11k ppm Glycosides equivalent to 600 mg of dried herb) 100 mg • Ginger root 305 mg • Dong Quai root 200 mg.

Pneumotrate - Progressive Labs
Each capsule contains: Vitamin A 2500 IU • Beta Carotene 2500 IU • Vitamin C 90 mg • Bovine lung concentrate 200 mg.
See Editor's Note No. 14, page 1817.

PoisePlus - Atrium Inc.
Six tablets contain: Vitamin A 15000 IU • Vitamin E 140 IU • Vitamin C 1050 mg • Bioflavonoids 300 mg • Chlorophyll (oil) 60 mg • Along with the following Amino Acid chelated minerals: Calcium 500 mg • Magnesium 250 mg • Potassium 99 mg • Manganese 10 mg • Iron 15 mg • Zinc 10 mg • Copper 2 mg • Iodine 150 mcg • Chromium 200 mcg • Selenium 25 mcg • Molybdenum 150 mcg • Vanadium 150 mcg • Silicon 2 mcg. In a base of Raw Bovine Tissue concentrates (not extracts) from the following: (Spleen 150 mg, Brain 30 mg, Liver 25 mg, Heart 15 mg, Kidney 15 mg, Thymus 10 mg, Adrenal 10 mg, Pituitary 10 mg, Pancreas 10 mg, Duodenus 10 mg) 285 mg.
See Editor's Note No. 14, page 1817.

Polysorbate 80 - The Vitamin Shoppe
Contains 100% pharmaceutical-grade Polysorbate 80.

BRAND NAMES

B R A N D   N A M E S

Poly-Vi-Sol Chewable Vitamins - Mead Johnson Nutritionals
Each chewable tablet contains: Vitamin A Acetate 2500 IU • Vitamin C (Ascorbic Acid) 60 mg • Vitamin D (Vitamin D3) 400 IU • Vitamin E Acetate 15 IU • Thiamin Mononitrate 1.05 mg • Riboflavin 1.2 mg • Niacin (Niacinamide) 13.5 mg • Vitamin B-6 Hydrochloride 1.05 mg • Folate (Folic Acid) 0.3 mg • Vitamin B-12 4.5 mcg • Iron (Ferrous Fumarate)12 mg • Zinc Oxide 8 mg • Copper (Cupric Oxide) 0.8 mg. Other Ingredients: Dextrates, Sugar, Sodium Ascorbate, Magnesium Stearate, Stearic Acid, Silicon Dioxide, Artificial Flavor and Color (Red 40 Lake), Salt.
See Editor's Note No. 3, page 1816.

Positive Thoughts - Source Naturals
Three tablets contain: St. John's Wort (Hypericum Perforatum) 900 mg (Yielding 0.3% Hypericin 2.7 mg) • Valerian root extract (Valeriana officinalis) 100 mg (Yielding 0.8% Valerenic Acids 800 mcg) • Kava Root Extract (Piper methysticum) 85 mg (Yielding 30% Kavalactones 25 mg) • Lemon Balm (Melissa officinalis) 100 mg • GABA (Gamma Amino Butyric Acid) 300 mg • Taurine (Magnesium Taurinate) 200 mg • Magnesium (oxide, taurinate) 200 mg • L-Tyrosine 200 mg • N-Acetyl L-Tyrosine 50 mg • L-Phenylalanine 100 mg • DMAE (Dimethylaminoethanol bitartrate) 60 mg • Vitamin C (Zinc ascorbate) 50 mg • Vitamin B1 (Thiamin) 25 mg • Vitamin B2 (Riboflavin) 25 mg • Niacinamide 50 mg • Vitamin B5 (Pantothenic Acid) 25 mg • Vitamin B6 (Pyridoxine HCl) 50 mg • Vitamin B12 (Cyanocobalamin) 25 mg • Biotin 300 mcg • Folic Acid 400 mcg • Manganese (citrate) 3 mg • Zinc (Zinc ascorbate) 10 mg.

Posture-D - Inverness Medical, Inc.
Each tablet contains: Vitamin D (as cholecalciferol) 125 IU • Calcium (as tribasic) 600 mg. Other Ingredients: Maltodextrin, Croscarmellose Sodium, Cellulose, Hydroxypropyl Methylcellulose, Citric Acid, Starch, Silicon Dioxide, Magnesium Stearate, Titanium Dioxide, Mineral Oil, Polysorbate 80, Sodium Lauryl Sulfate.
See Editor's Note No. 5, page 1816.

Posture-D - S.C.P.I.
Two tablets contain: Calcium (as tribasic calcium phosphate) 1200 mg • Vitamin D (as cholecalciferol) 250 IU. Other Ingredients: Dextrose, Carboxymethylcellulose Sodium, Magnesium Stearate, Adipic Acid, Natural & Artificial Flavors, FD&C Red #40 Aluminum Lake, FD&C Blue #2 Aluminum Lake, FD&C Yellow #6 Aluminum Lake.

Potassium - Source Naturals
Each tablet contains: Potassium (from 495 mg of potassium amino acid chelate) 99 mg.

Potassium 50 mg - Jamieson
Each tablet contains: Potassium (as Potassium Gluconate) 50 mg.

Potassium Fuel - TwinLab
Two capsules contain: Potassium Alpha-Ketoglutarate (supplying Elemental Potassium 99 mg) 325 mg • Magnesium Alpha-Ketoglutarate (supplying Elemental Magnesium 100 mg) 700 mg.

Potassium Gluconate with Folic Acid - Quest
Each tablet contains: Potassium Gluconate 650 mg • Folic Acid 400 mcg. Other Ingredients: Croscarmellose Sodium, Calcium phosphate, Magnesium Stearate (vegetable source), Microcrystalline Cellulose, Vegetable Stearin.

Potassium Plus - Enzymatic Therapy
Each tablet contains: Potassium (Chloride/Citrate) 99 mg • Magnesium Citrate 10 mg • Magnesium Sulfate 5 mg • Pantothenic Acid (D-Calcium Pantothenate) 5 mg • Vitamin B6 (Pyroxidine HCL) 1 mg. Other ingredients: Colloidal Alkaline Ash Mineral concentrate: Alfalfa juice concentrate, Sea Plant extract, Bio-Min TR8 (Enzymatic Tract Mineral concentrate), Orange juice concentrate, Banana concentrate, & Sugar Cane juice concentrate (no sugar) 855 mg,

Yucca 25 mg. Contains no sugar, salt, yeast, wheat, corn, soy, dairy products, coloring, flavoring or preservatives.

Potassium Plus - Olympian Labs
Each capsule contains: Potassium Gluconate 99 mg • Dandelion 100 mg • Barley Grass 100 mg • Red Clover 50 mg • Basil 50 mg • Mulberry leaf 100 mg • Blessed Thistle 50 mg.

Potassium Plus - PhytoPharmica
Each tablet contains: Vitamin B6 (pyridoxine HCl) 1 mg • Pantothenic Acid (calcium D-pantothenate) 5 mg • Magnesium citrate (provides 0.9 mg of magnesium) 10 mg • Magnesium sulfate (provides 0.9 mg of magnesium) 5 mg • Potassium (chloride/citrate) 99 mg • Colloidal Alkaline Ash Mineral Concentrate: Alfalfa stem and leaf juice, Sea Plant extract, Bio-Min T.R. 8 enzymatic trace mineral concentrate, Orange fruit juice, Banana fruit concentrate, Molasses (glucose), no sucrose or fructose 855 mg • Yucca (Yucca filamentosa) root 25 mg.

Power Fuel (Exercise & Recovery Drink) - TwinLab
Each serving contains: Carbohydrates (derived from Glucose Polymers & Glucose with small amounts of Fructose) 100 g • Anticatabolic Branched Chain Amino Acids (L-Leucine, L-Isoleucine, L-Valine) • L-Glutamine & Alpha-Ketoglutarates • Antioxidant Nutrients: Vitamin E, Vitamin C, & Beta-Carotene • B Vitamins • Chromium (from patented Chromic Fuel Chromium Picolinate) • Coenzyme Q10 • L-Carnitine • Potassium • Magnesium • Phosphate & Creatine • Carni Fuel (a preferred form of L-Carnitine & Magnesium).

Power Generation - Rexall
Three capsules contain: L-Tyrosine 750 mg • DMAE (as 2-dimethylaminoethanol L-bitartrate) 200 mg • Korean Ginseng extract root (standardized to 7% ginsenosides, 10 mg) 143 mg • Caffeine (as caffeine citrate) 50 mg • Ginkgo Biloba extract leaf (standardized to 24% ginkgo flavone glycosides, 9.6 mg; standardized to 6% terpene lactones, 2.4 mg) 40 mg • Cayenne fruit 30 mg. Other Ingredients: Gelatin, Citric Acid, Maltodextrin, Magnesium Stearate.

Power Herbs Migracin - Quantum
Two capsules contain: DHEA (Dehydroepiandrosterone) 25 mg • Feverfew extract 4:1 (equal to 200 mg of fresh Feverfew) 50 mg • White Willow bark extract: standardized for 15% Salicin 30 mg • extract 5:1 & powder of White Willow bark (equal to 1700 fresh Willow) 500 mg • DLPA (DL-Phenylalanine) 250 mg.

Power Nutrient - Changes - Changes - TwinLab
Two tablespoons (1 oz/30 ml) contain: Vitamin A (as 37% Beta-Carotene, 63% Retinyl palmitate) • Vitamin C (as Ascorbic acid) 60 mg • Vitamin D (as Cholecalciferol) 400 IU • Vitamin E (as DL-tocopherol) 30 IU • Thiamin (as Thiamine mononitrate) 1.5 mg • Riboflavin (as Riboflavin monophosphate) 1.7 mg • Niacin (as Niacinamide) 20 mg • Vitamin B6 (as Pyrodoxine HCL) 2 mg • Folate (as Folic acid) 400 mcg • Vitamin B12 (as Cyanocobalamin) 6 mcg • Biotin 300 mcg • Pantothenic acid (Vitamin B5) (as D-calcium pantothenate) 10 mg • Calcium (as Calcium lactate-gluconate) 40 mg • Iron 6 mg. Other ingredients: Purified water, Fructose, Citric acid, Colloidal mineral blend, Natural Cranberry flavor, Sodium benzoate, Potassium sorbate and Maltodextrin.

Power Nutrient Plus - Changes - TwinLab
One tablespoonful (15 ml) contains: Vitamin A (as 100% Beta-Carotene) 5000 IU • Vitamin C (Ascorbic acid) 60 mg • Vitamin D (as Cholecalciferol) 400 IU • Thiamin (as Thiamin HCI) 1.5 mg • Riboflavin (as Riboflavin-5-phosphate) 1.7 mg • Niacin (as Niacinamide) 5 mg • Vitamin B6 (as Pyridoxine HCl) 2 mg • Folate (Folic acid) 400 mcg • Vitamin B12 (as Cyanocobalamin) 6 mcg • Biotin 300 mcg • Pantothenic acid (as D-calcium pantothenate) 10 mg • Calcium (as Calcium lactate-gluconate) 40 mg • Korean Ginseng root extract 50 mg. Other ingredients: Purified water,

Fructose, Citric acid, Natural flavors, Aloe vera gel, Poly-colloidal organic minerals, Electrolyte complex (Potassium chloride, Magnesium citrate and Sodium citrate), Cellulose gum, Potassium sorbate, and Sodium benzoate.

Power Thin - Gold Star Nutrition
Ma Huang • Guarana • Magnesium • Chromium • Ginseng • Bladderwrack • Kola Nut • White Willow Bark • Fo-Ti • Ginger root • Gotu Kola • Licorice root • Hawthorne Berries • Saw Palmetto • Ginkgo Biloba • Boron • Spirulina • Potassium Citrate • Vitamin B12 • Folic Acid.

Power Vitamins for Men - Jamieson
Three caplets contain: Vitamin B1 (Thiamine Mononitrate) 20 mg • Vitamin B2 (Riboflavin) 20 mg • Vitamin B6 (Pyrodixine HCl) 20 mg • Niacinamide 150 mg • Vitamin B12 (Cyanocobalamin) 50 mcg • Pantothenic Acid (Calcium D-Panthenate) 30 mg • Folic Acid 0.2 mg • Vitamin A (Acetate) 7500 IU • Beta Carotene (Pro-Vitamin A) 1500 IU • Vitamin D 200 IU • Vitamin E (D-Alpha Tocopheryl Succinate) 30 IU • Vitamin C (Ascorbic Acid) 200 mg • Calcium (Carbonate) 250 mg • Magnesium (Oxide) 100 mg • Potassium 50 mg • Zinc 5 mg • Iodine (Kelp) 15 mg • Selenium 10 mcg • Chromium 10 mcg • Siberian Ginseng root (PE 1:8) 100 mg • Astragalus root (PE 1:4) 50 mg • Codonopsis root 50 mg • Damiana leaves (PE 1:6.5) 50 mg • Licorice root (PE 1:2) 50 mg • Fo-Ti root (PE 1:8) 50 mg • Grape Seed (PE 1:5) 50 mg • Citrus Bioflavonoids 50 mg • European Garlic 80 mg • Spirulina 80 mg • Chlorella 80 mg • Wheat Grass 80 mg • Borage 50 mg • Sunflower Oil 50 mg • Coenzyme Q10 (Ubiquinone) 10 mg • Seed Source Protein (Amaranth, Sunflower, Bean, Quinoa, Diu, Radish) 80 mg • Inositol 20 mg • Dl-Methionine 2.2 mg • Bromelain 48.5 mg • Papain 36.4 mg • Amylase 6.1 mg • Lipase 6.1 mg • Cellulase 3.0 mg.

PowerActin - Nature's Plus
Two capsules contain: Korean Ginseng [(Panax ginseng root) standardized 15% Ginsenosides] 250 mg • Siberian Ginseng [(Eleutherococcus senticosus root) standardized 0.8% Eleutherosides] 150 mg • Cayenne [(Capsicum frutescens fruit) standardized 100000 STU] 150 mg • Ashwagandha ([Withania somnifera root) standardized 1.5% Withanolids] 50 mg • Schisandra [(Schisandra chinensis fruit) standardized 9% Schisandrins] 50 mg • Coenzyme Q10 (Ubiquinone) 5 mg • Vitamin B12 (from Cobalamin) 500 mcg.

PoweRelief - Pain & Stress Center
Two capsules contain: DLPA (DL-Phenylalanine) 500 mg • GABA 200 mg • Boswellia 300 mg • Passion Flower 150 mg • Magnesium 10 mg • Vitamin B6 4 mg.

Pre. - Pacific BioLogic
Patrina • Peony root (white) • Bupleurum root (natural) • Ligusticum root • Jack-in-the-Pulpit rhizome • Angelica root (Chinese) • Hornet Nest • Vaccaria seeds • Argimony • Cyperus rhizome • Motherwort (Chinese) • Tumeric tuber • Bitter Orange ripened fruit.

PreCare Conceive - KV Pharmaceutical Co.
Each tablet contains: Vitamin C (as Ester-C1) 60 mg • Calcium (as Calcium Carbonate) 200 mg • Iron (as Ferrous Fumarate and Carbonyl Iron) 30 mg • Vitamin E (as dl-Alpha-Tocopheryl Acetate) 30 IU • Thiamine (as Thiamine Mononitrate) 3 mg • Riboflavin, USP 3.4 mg • Niacin (as Niacinamide, USP) 20 mg • Pyridoxine (as Pyridoxine HCl, USP) 50 mg • Folic Acid, USP 1 mg • Magnesium (as Magnesium Oxide) 100 mg • Cyanocobalamin 12 mcg • Zinc (as Zinc Oxide) 15 mg • Copper (as Cupric Oxide) 2 mg. Inactive Ingredients: Cellulose Polymers, Flow Agents, Pigment Natural Wax, FD&C yellow #10 aluminum lake, FD&C yellow #6 aluminum lake, Lactose, and other ingredients.

Pregnancy Tea - Traditional Medicinals
Spearmint leaf • Red Raspberry leaf • Lemongrass leaf • Strawberry Leaf • Fennel seed • Nettle leaf • Rose Hip • Alfalfa herb • Lemon Verbena leaf.

Pregnancy-6 Formula (Pregnancy 6) - Nature's Way
Each capsule contains a proprietary formula, 425 mg: Black Cohosh root • Blessed Thistle • False Unicorn root • Penny Royal flowering top • Red Raspberry leaves • Squaw Vine vine, leaf, fruit. Other ingredients: Gelatin.
See Editor's Note No. 29, page 1819.

Pregnenolone - Metabolic Response Modifiers
Each capsule contains: Pregnenolone 10 mg.

Pregnenolone-15 - PhytoPharmica
Each capsule contains: Pregnenolone 15 mg.

Prelieve PMS - Boehringer Ingelheim Pharmaceuticals, In
One mini-tablet contains: Standardized Vitex Agnus-Castus Extract (2:1) (fruit) 20 mg. Other Ingredients: Lactose, magnesium stearate, polyvidone, talc, PEG-100, polymethacrylic acid derivatives, FD&C blue #2, titanium dioxide, synthetic iron oxide.

Premenstra - HerbaSway
Dong Quai • Wild Yam • Knotweed • Ginger • Licorice • Blackberry • HerbaSwee (Cucurbitaceae fruit).

Premium Echinacea - Holista
Each capsule contains: Echinacea angustifolia (root) from standardized 6.5:1 extract (4% echinacoside) 500 mg.

Premium Echinacea - Olympian Labs
Each capsule contains: Premium Echinacea 400 mg.

Premium Korean Ginseng - Olympian Labs
Each capsule contains: Korean Ginseng 650 mg.

Premium Soy Protein Isolate Powder - Puritan's Pride
Each serving approximately contains: Total Isoflavones 60 mg • Genistein 36 mg • Daidzein 21 mg • Glycitein 3 mg.

Pre-Natal - Aspen Group, Inc.
Each tablet contains: Vitamin A (from vitamin A acetate & beta carotene) 4000 IU • Vitamin D (cholecalciferol) 400 IU • Vitamin E (d2-alpha tocopherol acetate) 11 mg • Vitamin C (ascorbic acid) 100 mg • Folic acid 0.8 mg • Vitamin B1 (thiamine mononitrate) 1.84 mg • Vitamin B2 (riboflavin) 1.7 mg • Niacinamide 18 mg • Vitamin B6 (pyridoxine hydrochloride) 2.6 mg • Vitamin B12 (cyanocobalamin) 4 mcg • Calcium (calcium sulfate) 200 mg • Iron (ferrous fumerate) 20 mg • Zinc (zinc oxide) 25 mg.

Pre-Natal Caps - Now
Four capsules contain: Vitamin A (Beta Carotene) 10000 IU • Vitamin B1 (Thiamine HCL) 5 mg • Vitamin B2 (Riboflavin) 5 mg • Vitamin B3 (Niacinamide) 20 mg • Vitamin B5 (Pantothenic Acid) 20 mg • Vitamin B6 (Pyridoxine HCL) 5 mg • Vitamin B12 (Cyanocobalamin) 20 mcg • Biotin 300 mcg • Folic Acid 800 mcg • Vitamin C (Calcium Ascorbate) 120 mg • Vitamin D (Fish Liver oil) 400 IU • Vitamin E (d-Alpha Tocopheryl Succinate) 150 IU • Vitamin K 80 mcg • Calcium (Carbonate • Ascorbate) 1200 mg • Magnesium (Oxide) 500 mg • Zinc (Amino Acid Chelate) 15 mg • Iron (Bisglycinate) 36 mg • Copper (Amino Acid Chelate) 1 mg • Iodine (Kelp) 150 mcg • Manganese (Amino Acid Chelate) 3.5 mg • Selenium (L-Selenomethionine) 50 mcg • Chromium (Picolinate) 100 mcg • Molybdenum (Amino Acid Chelate) 80 mcg • Potassium (Chloride) 50 mg • Vanadium (Amino Acid Chelate) 25 mcg • Choline 10 mg • Inositol 10 mg • PABA 4 mg.

PreNatal Care - Natrol
Three tablets contain: Vitamin A (as Vitamin A palmitate & d-Salina beta carotene) 5000 IU • Vitamin C (calcium ascorbate) 100 mg • Vitamin D (as cholecalciferol) 200 IU • Vitamin E (as d-alpha tocopherol) 100 IU • Vitamin K 25 mcg • Thiamine (Vitamin B1)

BRAND NAMES

(as Thiamine HCl) 25 mg • Riboflavin (Vitamin B2) 25 mg • Niacinamide 25 mg • Vitamin B6 (pyridoxine HCl) 25 mg • Folic Acid 800 mcg• Vitamin B12 (as cobalamin) 50 mcg • Biotin 100 mcg • Pantothenic Acid (as calcium pantothenate) 50 mg • Calcium (as calcium carbonate) 250 mg • Iron 25 mg • Iodine (from kelp) 150 mcg • Magnesium (as magnesium oxide) 125 mg • Zinc (as zinc gluconate) 15 mg • Selenium (as l-Selenomethionine) 100 mcg • Copper (copper gluconate) 2 mg • Manganese (as manganese gluconate) 50 mcg • Potassium (as potassium proteinate) 99 mg • DHA (docosahexanoic acid) 100 mg • Choline (as choline bitartrate) 50 mg • Betaine (as betaine HCl) 50 mg • Ginger root extract 50 mg • Inositol 25 mg • PABA (para amino benzoic acid) 25 mg • Red Raspberry extract leaf 15 mg • Rosemary extract leaf 15 mg • Squaw Vine powdered aerial part 15 mg. Other ingredients: Mono & Di-Glycerides, Microcrystalline Cellulose, Stearic Acid, Silicon Dioxide, Magnesium Stearate.

Pre-Natal Complex - Puritan's Pride
Four capsules contain: Vitamin A (as retinyl acetate) 8,000 IU • Vitamin C (as ascorbic acid) 120 mg • Vitamin D (as cholecalciferol) 400 IU • Vitamin E (as d-alpha tocopheryl acid succinate) 30 IU • Thiamin (Vitamin B1; as thiamine mononitrate) 1.7 mg • Riboflavin (Vitamin B2) 2.0 mg • Niacin (as niacinamide) 20 mg • Vitamin B6 (as pyridoxine hydrochloride) 2.5 mg • Folate (as folic acid) 800 mcg • Vitamin B12 (as cyanocobalamin) 8 mcg • Biotin 300 mcg • Pantothenic Acid (as d-calcium pantothenate) 10 mg • Calcium (as calcium carbonate and calcium citrate) 1,300 mg • Iron (as ferrous fumarate) 28 mg • Iodine (as potassium iodide) 150 mcg • Magnesium (as magnesium oxide) 450 mg • Zinc (as zinc citrate) 15 mg • Selenium (as sodium selenate) 70 mcg • Copper (as cupric gluconate) 2 mg • Manganese (as manganese gluconate) 2 mg • Chromium (as chromium picolinate) 120 mcg • Molybdenum (as sodium molybdate) 75 mcg • Potassium (as potassium chloride and potassium citrate) 10 mg • Choline (as choline bitartrate) 20 mg • Inositol 20 mg • PABA (as Para-Aminobenzoic acid) 2 mg • Cranberry fruit 60 mg • Peppermint Oil 20 mg • Ginger root 20 mg.

Prenatal Daily - Health Factor
Three capsules contain: Beta Carotene (pro Vitamin A) 2500 IU • Vitamin A (Acetate) 4000 IU • Vitamin B1 (Thiamine HCl) 10 mg • Vitamin B2 (Riboflavin & R5'P) 10 mg • Vitamin B3 (Niacinamide) 20 mg • Calcium (Ascorbate & Carbonate) 250 mg • Iron (Feronyl) 40 mg • Vitamin D (Ergocalciferol) 400 IU • Vitamin E (d-Alpha Tocopheryl) 100 IU • Vitamin B6 (Pyridoxine HCl & P5'P) 30 mg • Folic Acid 800 mcg • Vitamin B12 (Cobalamin) 100 mcg • Iodine (Potassium Iodide) 150 mcg • Magnesium (Oxide) 125 mg • Zinc (Picolinate) 20 mg • Copper (Citrate) 2 mg • Biotin 300 mcg • Vitamin B5 (Pantothenic Acid) 25 mg • Vitamin B10 (PABA) 25 mg • Vitamin K (Phytonadione) 15 mcg • Choline (Bitartrate) 12.5 mg • Inositol 12.5 mg • Chromium (Nichrome-3) 200 mcg • Manganese (Citrate) 7 mg • Selenium (Amino Acid Chelate) 100 mcg • Lemon Bioflavonoids 25 mg • Rutin 5 mg • Hesperidin 5 mg • Lactobacillus Acidophilus (3 billion/gm) 20 mg.

Prenatal Formulation - Olympian Labs
Four tablets contain: Beta Carotene 5000 IU • Vitamin B-1 (thiamine HCl) 1.5 mg • Vitamin B-2 (riboflavin) 1.6 mg • Vitamin B-3 (inositol hexanicotinate) 17 mg • Vitamin B-5 (calcium pantothenate) 10 mg • Vitamin B-6 (pyridoxine HCl) 2.2 mg • Vitamin B-9 (folic Acid) 600 mcg • Vitamin B-12 (cyanocobalamin) 6 mcg • Vitamin C (ascorbic acid) 70 mg • Vitamin D (cholecalciferol) 400 IU • Vitamin E (d-alpha-tocopherol acetate) 30 IU • d-Biotin 300 mcg • Inositol 10 mg • PABA 2 mg • Choline Bitartrate 10 mg • Chromium 25 mcg • Calcium 1200 mg • Copper 2 mg • Iron 30 mg • Magnesium 320 mg • Manganese 2 mg • Potassium 50 mg • Selenium 65 mcg • Zinc 15 mg • Phosphorus 130 mg • Iodine (kelp) 150 mcg.

Prenatal Multiple - Nature's Life
Six capsules contain: Beta Carotene (Vitamin A equivalent to 15000 IU) 9 mg • Vitamin D (Cholecalciferol) 200 IU • Vitamin B1 (Thiamine HCl) 50 mg • Vitamin B2 (Riboflavin) 50 mg • Vitamin B3

(Niacinamide) 50 mg • Vitamin B6 (Pyridoxine HCl) 75 mg • Vitamin B12 (Cyancobalamin concentrate) 50 mcg • Folic Acid 800 mcg • Pantothenic Acid (d-Calcium Pantothenate) 50 mg • Biotin (d-Biotin) 800 mcg • Inositol 50 mg • Choline (Bitartrate) 50 mg • PABA (Para Aminobenzoic Acid) 25 mg • Vitamin C 300 mg • Lemon Bioflavonoids Complex (TESTLAB 50%, Flavonoids, Flavones, Naringen & Eriocitrin) 50 mg • Rutin (Saphora japonica) 25 mg • Vitamin E (d-Alpha Tocopheryl Succinate) 200 IU • Vitamin K (Phylloquinone) 5 mg • Boron (Citrate) 50 mcg • Calcium (Carbonate, Citrate/ Malate) 1000 mg • Chromium (Picolinate, Nutrition 21, US Patent #33988) 200 mcg • Copper (Gluconate, Citrate) 1.5 mg • Iodine (Potassium Iodide) 25 mcg • Iron (Fumarate, Peptonate) 18 mg • Magnesium (Oxide, Citrate) 500 mg • Manganese (Citrate) 10 mg • Molybdenum (Molybdate) 20 mcg • Potassium (Citrate, Iodide) 99 mg • Selenium (l- Selenomethionine) 100 mcg • Silicon (Dioxide) 20 mcg • Vanadium (Vanadyl Sulfate) 20 mcg • Zinc (Picolinate, Methionine) 15 mg • Red Raspberry leaf (Rubus idaeus) 100 mg • Betaine HCl 50 mg.

Prenatal Plus Optizinc - Nutrivention
Four tablets contain: Calcium (Chelate) 1200 mg • Magnesium (Chelate) 300 mg • Vitamin C 300 mg • Phosphorus (Chelate) 150 mg • Niacinamide 100 mg • Vitamin E 100 IU • Potassium 99 mg • Vitamin A 1500 IU • Pantothenic Acid 60 mg • Choline Bitartrate 60 mg • Inositol 50 mg • Vitamin B1 50 mg • Iron (Amino Acid Chelate) 45 mg • Vitamin B1 25 mg • Vitamin B2 25 mg • Zinc 25 mg • Manganese (Amino Acid Chelate) 10 mg • Vitamin D 400 IU • Copper 1 mg • Folic Acid 800 mcg • Biotin 300 mcg • Iodine (Kelp) 150 mcg • Chromium 100 mcg • Selenium 100 mcg • Vitamin B12 100 mcg • Vitamin K 100 mcg • Pumpkin seeds 200 mg • Yellow Dock 200 mg • Alfalfa 100 mg • Bioflavonoids 100 mg • Beet tops 100 mg • Horsetail grass 100 mg • Hesperidin 50 mg • PABA 30 mg • Rutin 25 mg.

Prenatal Tablets - Leiner Health Products
Each tablet contains: Niacin (Niacinamide) 18 mg • Riboflavin (Vitamin B2) 1.7 mg • Vitamin A Acetate 4000 IU • Vitamin B12 (Cyanocobalamin - USP Method 2) 4 mcg • Vitamin E (dl-Alpha Tocopheryl Acetate) 11 IU • Vitamin C (Ascorbic Acid) 100 mg • Zinc Oxide 25 mg • Iron (Ferrous Fumarate) 27 mg • Calcium Sulfate 200 mg • Thiamin Mononitrate (Vitamin B1) 1.84 mg • Vitamin B6 (Pyridoxine Hydrochloride) 2.6 mg • Folate (Folic Acid) 800 mcg • Vitamin D (Ergocalciferol) 400 IU. Other Ingredients: Cellulose, Maltodextrin, Starch, Hydroxypropyl Methylcellulose, Croscarmellose Sodium, Sodium Starch Glycolate, Gelatin, Silicon Dioxide, Tricalcium Phosphate, Polyethylene Glycol 3350, Hydroxypropyl Cellulose, Titanium Dioxide, Magnesium Stearate, Phamaceutical Glaze, Polysorbate 80, Lactose, Yellow 6 Lake, Red 40 Lake, Blue 1 Lake, Beta Carotene, Resin.

Prenatal Vitamins - Nature's Bounty
Each tablet contains: Vitamin A (as Retinyl Acetate and Beta Carotene) 4000 IU • Vitamin C (as Ascorbic Acid) 100 mg • Vitamin D (as Cholecalciferol) 400 IU • Vitamin E (as dl-Alpha Tocopheryl Acetate) 11 IU • Thiamin (as Thiamine Mononitrate) 1.84 mg • Riboflavin (Vitamin B-2) 1.7 mg • Niacin (as Niacinamide) 18 mg • Vitamin B-6 (Pyridoxine Hydrochloride) 2.6 mg • Folic Acid 800 mcg • Vitamin B-12 (as Cyanocobalamin) 4 mcg • Calcium (as Calcium Sulfate) 200 mg • Iron (as Ferrous Fumarate) 27 mg • Zinc (as Zinc Oxide) 25 mg. Other Ingredients: Cellulose, Vegetable Stearic Acid, Croscarmellose, Cellulose Coating, Vegetable Magnesium Stearate, Titanium Dioxide, FD&C Yellow No. 6 Aluminum Lake, FD&C Red No. 40 Aluminum Lake, FD&C Blue No. 1 Aluminum Lake.

Pre-Nate Oil - The Herbalist
Herbal oils of Sweet Almond, Safflower, Aloe Vera, Vitamin E, St. John's Wort flower, Calendula flower • Essential oils of French Lavender & Lemon.

Pressure-FX - HerbTech
Each capsule contains: Shark Cartilage 180 mg • Cordyceps extract 20 mg.

Pressur-Lo - Futurebiotics
Six tablets contain: Vitamin A (as beta-carotene) 6,000 IU • Vitamin C (as ascorbic acid) 360 mg • Vitamin D (as ergocalciferol) 150 IU • Thiamin 12 mg • Riboflavin 12 mg • Niacin (as niacinamide) 180 mg • Vitamin B6 (as pyridoxine hydrochloride) 12 mg • Vitamin B12 (as cyanocobalamin) 30 mcg • Pantothenic Acid (as calcium pantothenate) 120 mg • Calcium (as calcium carbonate, ascorbate) 480 mg • Magnesium (as magnesium oxide, chloride, citrate) 360 mg • Zinc (as zinc gluconate) 18 mg • Selenium (as selenomethionine) 120 mcg • Manganese (as manganese amino acid chelate) 24 mg • Chromium (as chromium polynicotinate) 180 mcg • Potassium (as potassium chloride, citrate) 330 mg • Garlic bulb powder concentrate 480 mg • Hawthorn berry powder extract (4:1) 282 mg • Horsetail leaf powder 180 mg • Juniper berry powder 180 mg • Valerian root powder 180 mg • Cayenne fruit powder 150 mg • Beta-sitosterol complex 210 mg • Rutin 150 mg • Betaine hydrochloride 150 mg • Taurine 480 mg. Other Ingredients: Cellulose, Stearic Acid, Magnesium Stearate, and Silica.

Prevalin - VitaStore
Bee Pollen • Brindal Berry (Hydroxycitric Acid, HCA) • Chromium Picolinate • Ginger • Ginseng • Carnitine • White Willow Bark • Vitamin A • Vitamin B1 • Vitamin B6 • Vitamin B12 • Vitamin C • Vitamin D • Vitamin E (D-Alpha Tocopherol) • Folic Acid • Iodine (Kelp) • Niacin • d-Biotin • Pantothenic Acid • Potassium Gluconate.

Preventa Tea - HerbaSway
Soy • Green Tea • Ginger • Blackberry • HerbaSwee (Cucurbitaceae fruit).

Prevent-X - Cambridge Nutraceuticals
Each serving contains: L-Glutamine 10 g • N-Acetyl-Cysteine 4 g • Vitamin A (as mixed carotenoids) 4000 IU • Vitamin C 2000 mg • Vitamin E 700 IU • Folate 300 mcg • Magnesium 300 mg • Selenium 70 mcg • Zinc 10 mg • Copper 0.5 mg.

Pre-Vites - Puritan's Pride
Each tablet contains: Vitamin A 2500 IU • Vitamin C 60 mg • Vitamin D 400 IU • Vitamin E 15 IU • Thiamin 1.05 mg • Riboflavin 1.2 mg • Niacin 13.5 mg • Vitamin B6 1.05 mg • Folic Acid 0.3 mg • Vitamin B12 4.5 mcg.

Pre-Vites - Nature's Bounty
Each tablet contains: Vitamin A (as Retinyl Acetate) 2500 IU • Vitamin C (as Ascorbic Acid) 60 mg • Vitamin D (as Cholecalciferol) 400 IU • Vitamin E (as d-Alpha Tocopheryl Acetate) 15 IU • Thiamin Mononitrate (Vitamin B1) 1.05 mg • Riboflavin (Vitamin B2) 1.2 mg • Niacin (as Niacinamide) 13.5 mg • Vitamin B-6 (as Pyridoxine Hydrochloride) 1.05 mg • Folic Acid 0.3 mg • Vitamin B-12 (as Cyanocobalamin) 4.5 mcg. Other Ingredients: Sugar, Vegetable Stearic Acid, Natural Orange Flavor, Vegetable Magnesium Stearate, Silica, Mannitol.

Pre-Vites with Iron - Nature's Bounty
Each tablet contains: Vitamin A (as Retinyl Acetate) 2500 IU • Vitamin C (as Ascorbic Acid) 60 mg • Vitamin D (as Cholecalciferol) 400 IU • Vitamin E (as d-Alpha Tocopheryl Acetate) 15 IU • Thiamin Mononitrate (Vitamin B1) 0.05 mg • Riboflavin (Vitamin B2) 1.2 mg • Niacin (as Niacinamide) 13.5 mg • Vitamin B6 (as Pyridoxine Hydrochloride) 1.05 mg • Folic Acid 0.3 mg • Vitamin B12 (as Cyanocobalamin) 4.5 mcg • Iron (as Ferrous Fumarate) 7.5 mg. Other Ingredients: Sugar, Vegetable Stearic Acid, Natural Orange Flavor, Vegetable Magnesium Stearate, Silica, Mannitol.

Prima-C - PhysioLogics
Each capsule contains: Vitamin C (as Calcium Ascorbate) 500 mg • Calcium (as Calcium Ascorbate) 57 mg • Bioflavonoids (from citrus) 7 mg • Hesperidin 10 mg • Rutin 10 mg.

Primaderm - Prime Pharmaceutical Corp. (Canadian)
Active Ingredient: Mahonia Aquifolium.

Primavar - Unknown
Each capsule contains: 19-Norandrostenedione 100 mg • 4-Androstenediol 100 mg.

Primavar II - Unknown
Each capsule contains: Bolandiol (Norandrostenediol) 100 mg • 4-Androstenediol 100 mg.

Prime Advantage Creatine Serum - Muscle Marketing USA
Each serving contains: Damiana • Yohimbe • Pygeum africanum • Glucosamine • Vitamin B12.

Primrose Oil - Atrium Inc.
Each capsule contains: Oil of Evening Primrose 500 mg • Vitamin E (d-Alpha Tocopheryl Acetate) 10 IU • Gamma Linolenic Acid 40 mg • Lenoleic Acid 350 mg.

Pro Blend 55 - Human Development Technologies
Two scoops contain: Protein Blend of Micro Ultra Filtered Whey Protein concentrate, Egg Albumen, Calcium Caseinate, Micro Ultra Filtered Whey Protein Isolate, Ion Exchanged Whey Protein Isolate, Hydrolyzed Whey Protein Isolate • Natural & artificial Chocolate Flavorings • Acesulfame Potassium • Stevia.

Pro Fuel (Milk & Egg Protein Drink) - TwinLab
Each serving contains: Pure Milk & Egg Protein 40 g • Extra Branched Chain Amino Acids (L-Leucine, L-Isoleucine, L-Valine) • L-Glutamine • All Essential Vitamins & Minerals including B Complex Vitamins plus Antioxidant Vitamin C & Vitamin E, Calcium & Magnesium. Patented Chromic Fuel Chromium Picolinate including Potassium, Zinc & Chromium.

Pro Lite - Optimum Nutrition
L-Carnitine • Choline • Inositol.

Pro-50 - Enzymatic Therapy
Each capsule contains: Vitamin A (Fish Liver oil) 1500 IU • Zinc (Chelate) 20 mg • Vitamin B6 (Pyridoxine HCL) 10 mg • Other ingredients: EFA (unrefined Vegetable Lipids) 630 mg • Amino Acid Complex 150 mg • Prostate extract freeze-dried 150 mg • Saw Palmetto Berry extract 4:1 100 mg. Contains no sugar, salt, yeast, corn, dairy products, flavoring or preservatives. All organs & glands derived from bovine sources.
See Editor's Note No. 14, page 1817.

Pro-Antho Forte - Progressive Labs
Each capsule contains: Pycnogenol 10 mg • Grape seed extract (Vitis vinifera) (5:1 concentrate) 50 mg • Ginkgo leaf extract (Ginkgo biloba) (50:1 concentrate) 20 mg • Green Tea leaf extract (Camellia sinensis) (65% standardized extract) 75 mg • Quercetin 100 mg • Milk Thistle (Silibum marianum) (80% standardized extract) 10 mg. Pycnogenol is the registered trademark of Horphag Research Ltd. Pycnogenol is an extract of the bark of French Coastal Pine (Pinus maritime). Contains no animal products.

Probiata - Wakunaga of America
Each tablet contains: Lactobacillus acidophilus 1 billion live cells in a vegetable starch complex.

BRAND NAMES

Probiotic A.Y. - Futurebiotics
Lactobacillus acidophilus 3 billion cells at formulation NutraFlora FOS (Fructooligosaccharides) 600 mg • Inulin FOS 200 mg • Garlic (Pure-Gar 1500TM deodorized concentrate) 75 mg • Pau D'Arco 25 mg • Licorice (4:1 extract) 25 mg • Caprylic Acid (MCT) 100 mg • Echinacea (4:1 extract) 25 mg.

Probiotica - McNeil Consumer Healthcare
Each tablet contains: Lactobacillus reuteri 100 million cells. Other Ingredients: Mannitol, Xylitol, Lactulose, Mono- and Diglycerides, Malic Acid, Lemon Flavor, Zein (corn protein), Riboflavin Phosphate (for color).

Pro-Brom - Atrium Inc.
Each tablet contains: Bromelain 100 mg • Papayotin 30 mg.

Pro-DMG-B15 - PhytoPharmica
Each capsule contains: Calcium Gluconate 31 mg • Magnesium Aspartate 125 mg • Potassium Aspartate 125 mg • Trimethylglycine (TMG) 100 mg • N,N-Dimethylglycine HCl 100 mg • Glycine 25 mg.

Pro-Enz 99+ - Country Road Naturals
Ephedra stem (Ephedrine) 8 mg • Bladderwrack herb 15 mg • Astragalus root 15 mg • Rehmannia root 10 mg • White Willow bark 10 mg • Siberian Ginseng 10 mg • Kola Nut 85 mg • Reishi Mushroom 5 mg • Dandelion root 5 mg • Ginger root 5 mg • Black Pepper extract 2.5 mg. In a base of Green Tea 85 mg, Bee Pollen 10 mg, Chromium (Chloride) 100 mcg, Niacin 1 mg.

Proenzi 99 + - Abundance Marketing
Ephedra stem (Ephedrine) 8 mg • Bladderwrack herb 15 mg • Astragalus root 15 mg • Rehmannia root 10 mg • White Willow bark 10 mg • Siberian Ginseng 10 mg • Kola nut 85 mg • Reishi Mushroom 5 mg • Dandelion root 5 mg • Ginger root 5 mg • Black Pepper extract 2.5 mg. In a base of Green Tea 85 mg • Bee Pollen 10 mg • Chromium (Chloride) 100 mcg • Niacin 1 mg.

Pro-Essence - Flora
Burdock root • Juniper Berry • Prickley Ash bark • Slippery Elm bark • Uva Ursi.

Pro-F Complex - PhytoPharmica
Two tablets contain: Vitamin A (Fish Liver oil) 3000 IU • Vitamin D (Fish Liver oil) 100 IU • Calcium (Lactate) 82 mg • Zinc (Chelate) 20 mg • Magnesium (Citrate) 13 mg • Pacific Sea Kelp 200 mg • Ovarian extract 90 mg • Whole Pituitary extract 60 mg • Adrenal extract 60 mg • Uterus extract 60 mg • RNA powder 60 mg. All organs and glands derived from bovine sources.
See Editor's Note No. 14, page 1817.

Profile 1 - Mannatech
Three tablets contain: Vitamin A 2500 IU • Vitamin B1 27 mg • Vitamin B12 18 mcg • Vitamin B2 24 mg • Vitamin B6 26 mg • Beta Carotene 100 IU • Bioflavonoids 95 mg • Biotin 36 mcg • Vitamin C 187 mg • Choline 19 mg • Vitamin D 400 IU • Vitamin E 30 IU • Folic Acid 400 mcg • Inositol 90 mcg • Vitamin K 90 mcg • Niacinamide 30 mg • PABA 5 mg • Pantothenic Acid 5 mg • Boron 150 mcg • Calcium 10 mg • Copper 20 mcg • GTF Chromium 150 mcg • Iodine 3 mcg • Iron 5 mg • Magnesium 50 mg • Manganese 12 mg • Molybdenum 70 mcg • Potassium 75 mg • Selenium 15 mcg • Silicon 500 mcg • Vanadium 10 mcg • Zinc 7 mg • Ambrotose Complex (naturally occurring plant polysaccharides including freeze-dried Aloe Vera inner leaf gel extract - Manapol powder) 25 mg.
See Editor's Note No. 17, page 1817.

Profile 2 - Mannatech
Three tablets contain: Vitamin A 15000 IU • Vitamin B1 2 mg • Vitamin B12 125 mcg • Vitamin B2 5 mg • Vitamin B6 2 mg • Beta Carotene 5000 IU • Bioflavonoids 56 mg • Biotin 57 mcg • Vitamin C 130 mg • Choline 55 mg • Vitamin D 170 IU • Vitamin E 62 IU • Folic Acid 200 mcg • Inositol 25 mg • Vitamin K 50 mcg • Niacinamide 38 mg • PABA 7 mg • Pantothenic Acid 29 mg • Boron 500 mcg • Calcium 75 mg • Copper 700 mcg • GTF Chromium 50 mcg • Iodine 100 mcg • Iron 2 mg • Magnesium 10 mg • Manganese 2 mg • Molybdenum 70 mcg • Potassium 7 mg • Selenium 15 mcg • Silicon 2.5 mcg • Vanadium 10 mcg • Zinc 15 mg • Ambrotose Complex (naturally occurring plant polysaccharides including freeze-dried aloe Vera inner leaf gel extract - Manapol powder) 25 mg.
See Editor's Note No. 17, page 1817.

Profile 3 - Mannatech
Three tablets contain: Vitamin A 7500 IU • Vitamin B1 7 mg • Vitamin B12 68 mcg • Vitamin B2 8 mg • Vitamin B6 10 mg • Beta Carotene 2500 IU • Bioflavonoids 75 mg • Biotin 52 mcg • Vitamin C 170 mg • Choline 40 mg • Vitamin D 210 IU • Vitamin E 50 IU • Folic Acid 300 mcg • Inositol 20 mcg • Vitamin K 90 mcg • Niacinamide 32 mg • PABA 6 mg • Pantothenic Acid 23 mg • Boron 300 mcg • Calcium 60 mg • Copper 300 mcg • GTF Chromium 80 mcg • Iodine 30 mcg • Iron 3.5 mg • Magnesium 25 mg • Manganese 8 mg • Molybdenum 70 mcg • Potassium 12 mg • Selenium 15 mcg • Silicon 2 mg • Vanadium 10 mcg • Zinc 10 mg • Ambrotose Complex (naturally occurring plant polysaccharides including freeze-dried Aloe Vera inner leaf gel extract - Manapol powder) 25 mg.
See Editor's Note No. 17, page 1817.

Pro-Gain - Nature's Life
Two scoops (28.35 g) contain: SUPRO brand soy protein isolate containing Lecithin • Whey • Fructose • Non-fat Dry Milk • natural Vanilla Flavor • Yeast • Egg Albumin • Eggshell powder • Kelp • natural Papain Enzyme concentrate • Cobalamin concentrate (B12). Pro-Gain also contains 34 mg of naturally occuring Isoflavones, including 21 mg Genistein & 10 mg Daidzen.

Progensa - Life-Flo
Each ounce contains: Natural Progesterone USP Grade 480 mg. Other Ingredients: Grape seed extract, aloe vera, vitamin E, & primrose.

Pro-Gest - PhytoPharmica
Two tablets contain: Niacinamide 20 mg • Betaine HCl 310 mg • L-Glutamic Acid HCl 310 mg • Bromelain (pineapple whole fruit) 10:1 200 mg • Papain 200 mg • Mylase (lipase) 200 mg • Mycozyme (Fungal amylase) 50 mg • Ox Bile extract 32 mg • Pancreas extract 32 mg.
See Editor's Note No. 14, page 1817.

Pro-Gest Body Cream - Transitions for Health, Inc.
Aloe Vera Gel in Distilled Water • D-Alpha Tocopherol and Mixed Tocopherols • Cetyl Alcohol • Almond Oil • Octyl Palmitate • Panthenol • Peg 8 Stearate • Glycerin • USP Progesterone • Polysorbate 60 • Hyaluronic Acid • Oil of Lemon • Keratin • Carbomer 940 • Grapefruit Seed Extract.

Pro-Gest Progesterone Body Cream/ Original Formula - Transitions for Health, Inc.
Deionized Water • Aloe Vera Gel • D-Alpha Tocopherol • Mixed Tocopherols (Vit. E) • Cetyl Alcohol • Almond Oil • Octyl Palmitate • Panthenol • PEG-8 Stearate • USP Progesterone • Glycerin • Polysorbate 60 • Hyaluronic Acid • Oil of Lemon (Oleum Limonis) • Keratin • Carbomer 940 • Grapefruit Seed Extract (Citrus Grandis).

ProgestaCare - Life-Flo
Aloe Vera gel • Caprylic/Capric Triglyceride • natural Progesterone derived from the Mexican Wild Yam root • Evening Primrose oil (Oenothera biennis) • Vitamin E Acetate • Isostearic Acid • Glyceryl Stearate • Siberian Ginseng • Burdock root • Black Cohosh • MSM • Chamomile • Glycerin • Allantoin • Grape seed extract.

Some Brand Name Natural Products - What they Contain

Pro-Gest-Ade - Enzymatic Therapy
Each tablet contains: Niacinamide 10 mg. Other ingredients: Betaine HCL 155 mg • Glutamic Acid HCL 155 mg • Bromelain (600 MCU) 100 mg • Papain 100 mg • Mylase (Lipase) 100 mg • Mycozyme (Fungal amylase) 25 mg • Ox Bile extract 16 mg • Pancreas extract 16 mg. Contains no sugar, salt, yeast, wheat, corn, soy, dairy products, coloring, flavoring or preservatives.
See Editor's Note No. 14, page 1817.

Progesterone Plus Creme - Nutri-Quest
Water • Stearic Acid • Cetyl Alcohol • Sesame oil • Progesterone USP (Homeopathic) • Triethanolame • Arnica oil • Evening Primrose oil • Zinc • Copper • Magnesium • Glyconucleopeptides • Peg 10 Soya Sterol • Hydroxyethycellulose • Disodium EDTA • Cetyl Ricinoleate • Canola oil • Wild Yam • Dex-Panthenol (Vitamin B5) • Progesterone USP • Honey • Lecithin • NaPCA • Silicon • Iron • Peg 7 Glycerol Cocoate • Carrot oil • Carbomer • Phenyldimethicone • Sodium Hydroxymethylglycinate.

ProGram16: Chocolate - Pharmanex
One bar contains: High Fructose Corn Syrup • Whey Protein Isolate • Soy Protein Isolate • Sugar • Milk Protein Isolate • Cocoa Butter • Unsweetened Chocolate • Lowfat Cocoa (Processed with Alkali) • Milk • Creatine Monohydrate 1 g • Glycerin • Maltodextrin • Dicalcium Phosphate • Natural and Artificial Flavors • Taurine 250 mg • Magnesium Carbonate • Potassium Chloride • Potassium Citrate • Egg Whites • Ascorbic Acid • Lecithin • d-Alpha Tocopherol Acetate • Beta-Carotene • Niacinamide • Calcium Pantothenate • Zinc Oxide • Chromium Chelate • Carbonyl Iron • Copper Gluconate • Manganese Sulfate • Pyridoxine Hydrochloride • Riboflavin • Thiamine Mononitrate • Folate (Folic Acid) • Biotin • Potassium Iodide • Sodium Molybdate • Sodium Selenite • Phytonadine • Cholecalciferol • Cyanocobalamin.

ProGram16: Coconut - Pharmanex
Each bar contains: High Fructose Corn Syrup • Whey Protein Isolate • Soy Protein Isolate • Sugar • Partially Defatted Peanut Flour • Milk Protein Isolate • Cocoa Butter • Unsweetened Chocolate • Milk • Creatine Monohydrate 1 g • Glycerin • Natural and Artificial Flavors • Maltodextrin • Dicalcium Phosphate • Potassium Chloride • Taurine 250 mg • Magnesium Carbonate • Egg Whites • Ascorbic Acid • Lecithin • Salt • d-Alpha Tocopherol Acetate • Beta-Carotene • Niacinamide • Calcium Pantothenate • Zinc Oxide • Chromium Chelate • Carbonyl Iron • Copper Gluconate • Manganese Sulfate • Pyridoxine Hydrochloride • Riboflavin • Thiamine Mononitrate • Folate (Folic Acid) • Biotin • Potassium Iodide • Sodium Molybdate • Sodium Selenite • Phytonadine • Cholecalciferol • Cyanocobalamin.

ProGram16: Peanut Butter - Pharmanex
Each bar contains: High Fructose Corn Syrup • Whey Protein Isolate • Soy Protein Isolate • Sugar • Partially Defatted Peanut Flour • Milk Protein Isolate • Cocoa Butter • Unsweetened Chocolate • Milk • Creatine Monohydrate 1 g • Glycerin • Maltodextrin • Dicalcium Phosphate • Natural and Artificial Flavors • Taurine 250 mg • Magnesium Carbonate • Potassium Chloride • Egg Whites • Ascorbic Acid • Lecithin • Salt • d-Alpha Tocopherol Acetate • Beta-Carotene • Niacinamide • Calcium Pantothenate • Zinc Oxide • Chromium Chelate • Carbonyl Iron • Copper Gluconate • Manganese Sulfate • Pyridoxine Hydrochloride • Riboflavin • Thiamine Mononitrate • Folate (Folic Acid) • Biotin • Potassium Iodide • Sodium Molybdate • Sodium Selenite • Phytonadine • Cholecalciferol • Cyanocobalamin.

Pro-Guard - Man-Nutra-Life Health and Fitness
Each tablet contains: Saw Palmetto Fruit 500 mg • Hydrangea Root and Rhiz. 100 mg • Golden Rod Herb 50 mg • Couch Grass Root 200 mg • Horsetail Herb 100 mg • Panax Ginseng Root 100 mg • Zinc Gluconate (Providing 15 mg zinc) 112.5 mg • Magnesium Amino Acid Chelate (Providing magnesium 15 mg) 75 mg • Calcium Ascorbate 250 mg • Pyridoxine Hydrocholoride (Vitamin B6) 15 mg •

Glutamine 100 mg • Glycine 100 mg • Alanine 100 mg. No added sugar, yeast, artificial colours, gluten or animal products.

ProhGH Symbiotropin - Nutraceutics Co.
Two tablets contain: Glycoamino Acid Complex 4200 mg • Aminotrope-7 Anterior Pituitary Peptides Polyose Complex 2300 mg. Other Ingredients: Citric Acid, Potassium Bicarbonate, Glucose, L-Glutamine, L-Arginine, L-Pyroglutamate, Sodium Bicarbonate, L-Lysine Monohydrochloride, Gamma Aminobutyric Acid, Glycine, Sodium Carbonate, Polyethlene Glycol, Mixed Berry Flavor, Magnesium Stearate, Sodium Benzoate powder.
See Editor's Note No. 14, page 1817.

PRO-hGH Symbiotropin Growth Hormone Releasing Complex - Nutraceutics Co.
Two tablets contain: Anterior Pituitary Peptides • Aminotrope-7 (a sequenced glycoamino acid complex) 4200 mg • Novel Polyose complex (pharmaceutical mono, poly & oligo saccharides) 2230 mg. All in a base of: L-Glutamine, L-Arginine, L-Pyroglutamate, GABA, L-Glycine, L-Lysine, L-Tyrosine & Vicia Faba Major. Naturally sweetened & flavored.
See Editor's Note No. 14, page 1817.

Prolab CarbPRO - ProLab
Granulated Medium Length Complex Carbohydrates (Maltodextrin) extracted from grains.

ProLab GlutaMASS - ProLab
Each capsule contains: L-Glutamine 275 mg • Alpha-Ketoglutaric Acid 250 mg • Taurine 150 mg • Calcium (AKG) 63 mg • Magnesium (oxide) 25 mg • Potassium (citrate) 25 mg • RNA 9.5 mg • Manganese 400 mcg.

ProLab Lean Rx - ProLab
Each 72 g packet contains: Protein Blend of Milk Protein Isolates • Caseinates • Whey Protein Concentrates & Egg Whites • Maltodextrin • Cocoa • Natural Flavors • Dicalcium Phosphate • Potassium Chloride • Dipotassium Phosphate • Potassium Citrate • Sodium Chloride • Sodium Citrate • Magnesium Oxide • Medium Chain Triglycerides • Choline Bitartrate • Vegetable Gum • Aspartame • Lecithin • Betaine • Beta Carotene • Manganese Sulfate • Canola oil • Glutamine • Inositol • Vitamin E Acetate • Vitamin B12 • Vitamin A Palmitate • Thiamine • Riboflavin • Vitamin D • Niacin • Pyridoxine HCL • Calcium Pantothenate • Potassium Iodide • Ferrous Gluconate • Copper Gluconate • Zinc Oxide • Biotin • Folic Acid • Selenium Chelate • Molybdenium Yeast • Vitamin K • Paba • Chromium Picolinate.

ProLab MSM - ProLab
Each capsule contains: MSM (Methyl-Sulfonyl-Methane) 1000 mg.

ProLab N-Large 2 - ProLab
Each serving (153 g) contains: Maltodextrin • Cross-Flow Micro-Filtered Cold Processed Ion Exchanged Whey • Fructose • Natural Flavoring.

ProLab Stoked - ProLab
Each rounded scoop contains: Caffeine 200 mg • Ephedra alkaloids 20 mg • Guarana 10 mg • Green Tea extract 10 mg • White Willow 75 mg. In a base of Yohimbe bark, Quercetin & Citrus aurantium.

Pro-Life Soy Protein - Nature's Life
Two scoops (28.35 g) contain: SUPRO brand soy protein isolate containing Lecithin • natural Vanilla Flavor • natural Papain Enzyme concentrate • Cobalamin concentrate.

Pro-Lite Soy Protein - Nature's Life
Two scoops (28.35 g) contain: SUPRO brand soy protein isolate containing Lecithin • natural Vanilla Flavor • natural Papain Enzyme concentrate • Cobalamin concentrate.

BRAND NAMES

Some Brand Name Natural Products - What they Contain
www.NaturalDatabase.com contains MANY more listings than appear here.

Promend - The Herbalist
Saw Palmetto berry • Goldenrod flower tops • Echinacea root • Horsetail herb • Plantain herb • Ginger root.

Promensil - Novogen
Each tablet contains: Isoflavone Phytoestrogens (as Red Clover leaf extract) 40 mg. Other Ingredients: Dicalcium phosphate, Microcrystalline cellulose, Hydroxypropyl methylcellulose, Magnesium stearate, Mixed tocopherols, Silica, Soy polysaccharide, Titanium dioxide, Polyethylene glycol, & Organic coloring containing: Red 40, Yellow 6, Yellow 5, Blue 1.
See Editor's Note No. 11, page 1817.

ProOmega - Nordic Naturals
Each gelcap contains: EPA 173 mg • DHA 123 mg • Other Omega-3 49 mg.

Propalmex - Chattem, Inc.
Each softgel contains: Zinc (chelated from zinc gluconate) 75 mg • Standardized Saw Palmetto berry extract (85%-95% free fatty acids & phytosterols) 160 mg • Standardized Pumpkin seed oil extract (85%-95% free fatty acids) 40 mg.

Propalmex Saw Palmetto - SunSource/Chattem Inc.
Each softgel contains: Zinc (as zinc gluconate) 75 mg • Saw Palmetto berry extract 160 mg • Pumpkin Seed Oil extract 40 mg • Lycopene (from Lyc-O-Mato tomato extract) 1.5 mg.
See Editor's Note No. 2, page 1816.

Propax - Nutritional Therapeutics
Each multipack contains: Vitamin A (as acetate) 4375 IU • Vitamin A (as natural beta-carotene) 3750 IU • Vitamin C (as calcium ascorbate) 150 mg • Vitamin D (as Vitamin D3 cholecalciferol) 32 IU • Vitamin E (as d-alpha tocopherol) 145 IU • Vitamin K (as phytonadione) 2.5 mcg • Vitamin B1 6.25 mg • Vitamin B2 30 mg • Vitamin B3 (as niacinamide) 60 mg • Vitamin B6 (as pyridoxine/P-5-P) 40 mg • Folic Acid (as folate) 200 mcg • Vitamin B12 25 mcg • Biotin 25 mcg • Pantothenic Acid (as d-calcium) 25 mg • Calcium (as phosphate, ascorbate, citrate, sulfate, borogluconate) 360 mg • Iodine (as kelp) 18.75 mcg • Magnesium (as carbonate, oxide, glycinate, sulfate) 160 mg • Zinc (as methionate) 12.5 mg • Selenium (as selenomethionate) 75 mcg • Copper (as tyrosinate) 300 mcg • Manganese (as glycinate) 2.5 mg • Chromium (as nicotinate) 50 mcg • Molybdenum (as glycinate) 20 mcg • Potassium (as citrate) 12.8 mg • DHA (as Docosahexaenoic Acid) 120 mg • EPA (as Eicosopentaenoic Acid) 180 mg • Bioflavonoids (as citrus, rutin, rosehips, quercetin) 165 mg • Boron (as calcium borogluconate) 500 mcg • CoEnzyme Q10 4 mg • Grape Seed Extract 5 mg • Inositol 24 mg • Pantethine (as coenzyme A precursor) 70 mg • Phosphoglycolipids 160 mg • Vanadium (as vanadyl sulfate) 12.5 mcg • Creatine (Monohydrate, Phosphate) 122.5 mg • Alpha-Keto Glutarate 125 mg • Glutathione (as reduced) 5 mg • L-Tyrosine 60 mg • N-Acetyl-L-Cysteine 25 mg • Taurine 110 mg • Green Tea Extract 50 mg • Horsetail (as silica) 12.5 mg • Lactoferrin 4 mg • NT Factor (as tablet base) proprietary blend 1400 mg: defatted rice bran, arginine, beet root fiber, black strap molasses, glycine, magnesium sulfate, enriched polyunsaturated phosphatidyl choline (phospholipids), saponin (glycolipids), para-amino benzoate, leek, pantethine (bifidus growth factor), taurine, garlic, calcium borogluconate, omega-6 essential fatty acids, omega-3 essential fatty acids, artichoke, barley malt, potassium citrate, calcium sulfate, spirulina, bromelain, natural vitamin E, calcium ascorbate, alpha-lipoic acid, oligosaccharides, B-6, niacinamide, tocotrienols, riboflavin, inositol, niacin, calcium pantothenate, thiamin, B-12, bifidus, acidophilus, folic acid, chromium picolinate. Other Ingredients: Gelatin (soft gel capsules), microcrystalline cellulose, croscarmellose sodium, vegetable magnesium stearate, silica, water & glycerin.

Prophet 3H (Prophet3H) - Prophet 3H
Unknown.
See Editor's Note No. 24, page 1818.

Propo-Mune - Atrium Inc.
Each tablet contains: Propolis 5X 92 mg • Thymus 67 mg • Lymph 30 mg • Spleen 25 mg • Brain 25 mg • Folic Acid 400 mcg.
See Editor's Note No. 14, page 1817.

ProPortion Bars - Chocolate Peanut Butter - Rexall
Each bar contains: Protein 12 g • Vitamin A 2250 IU • Vitamin C 27 mg • Calcium 100 mg • Iron 9 mg • Vitamin D 180 IU • Vitamin E 13.5 IU • Thiamin 0.675 mg • Riboflavin 0.765 mg • Niacin 9 mg • Vitamin B6 0.9 mg • Folate 200 mcg • Vitamin B12 2.7 mcg • Biotin 135 mcg • Pantothenic Acid 4.5 mg • Phosphorus 150 mg • Iodine 67.5 mcg • Magnesium 80 mg • Zinc 6.75 mg • Copper 1 mg • Chromium 52.5 mcg.

Prosplex - Olympian Labs
Two capsules contain: Inositol Hexaphosphate 400 mg • Quercetin 200 mg • Saw Palmetto 320 mg • Tomato Lycopene 200 mg • Zinc (gluconate) 10 mg • Pumpkin Seed 10 mg • Pygeum Aficanum 20 mg.

Prosta Glan - Progressive Labs
Each capsule contains: Magnesium (as magnesium gluconate) 10 mg • Zinc (as zinc glycinate) 3.3 mg • Raw Bovine prostate concentrate 80 mg • Saw Palmetto 4:1 extract Lipoic Sterolic (Serenoa repens) 100 mg • Pygeum (Prunus africanum) 25 mg • Glutamic Acid 135 mg • Alanine 135 mg • Glycine 135 mg • Uva Ursi leaf (Arctostaphylos uva-ursi) 10 mg • Unsaturated Fatty Acids 10 mg • Pumpkin seed concentrate (Curcurbita pepo) 10 mg • Pollen 5 mg. The glandular concentrate in this product is prepared by a special process which does not exceed physiological temperature (37° C). Guaranteed free of chemical pesticides and synthetic hormones.
See Editor's Note No. 14, page 1817.

Prosta Kit - Flora
Formula 1: Palmitol Saw Palmetto berries • Zinc 50 mg • Vitamin B6 120 mg. Formula 2: Flax-O-Mega cold pressed flax seed oil 1000 mg. Formula 3: Pro-Essence Burdock root • Juniper Berry • Prickly Ash bark • Slippery Elm bark • Uva Ursi.

Prosta Support - Nutri-Quest
Each tablet contains: Vitamin C 10 mg • Vitamin B6 10 mg • Vitamin E (Succinate) 5 IU • Zinc Chelate 10 mg • L-Glycine 120 mg • L-Alanine 120 mg • L-Glutamic Acid 120 mg • Saw Palmetto 106 mg • Pygeum africanus extract 10 mg • Pygeum africanus herb 20 mg • Pumpkin seed 200 mg • Stinging Nettle leaves 75 mg • Echinacea 25 mg • Ginkgo Biloba 20 mg • Wild Yam 20 mg • Uva Ursi 10 mg.

Prostabs Plus - Futurebiotics
Three tablets contain: Glutamic Acid 390 mg • Glycine 390 mg • Raw Prostate Concentrate 150 mg • Alanine 390 mg • Vitamin B6 7.5 mg • Vitamin C (Ascorbate) 15 mg • Zinc (Gluconate) 30 mg • Magnesium (Oxide) 105 mg • Saw Palmetto Berry Extract (4:1 extract equivalent to) 300 mg.
See Editor's Note No. 14, page 1817.

Prosta-Comp - Atrium Inc.
Each tablet contains: Saw Palmetto berry extract 100 mg • Pumpkin seed oil extract 50 mg • Pygeum africanum extract 25 mg • Uva Ursi 50 mg • Zinc Gluconate 25 mg • Hydrangea extract 150 mg • Panax ginseng extract 100 mg. Contains no sugar, starch, salt, wheat, corn, milk, yeast or soy derivatives.

ProstActin - Nature's Plus
Two softgels contain: Pygeum [(Prunus africanum bark) standardized 12-13% Phytosterols] 200 mg • Saw Palmetto [(Serenoa repens fruit)

standardized 95% Fatty Acids] 80 mg • Glycine (Free form Amino Acid) 50 mg • Alanine (Free Form Amino Acid) 50 mg • Glutamine (Free Form Amino Acid) 50 mg • Turmeric [(Curcuma longa rhizome) standardized 95% Curcumin] 50 mg • Pumpkin Seed oil [(Curcurbita maxima seed) standardized 7% Alpha-Linolenic Acid] 50 mg • Zinc (Zinc Monomethionine) 30 mg • Vitamin E natural 200 IU.

Prost-Actin - Nature's Plus
Each tablet contains: Saw Palmetto berries 250 mg • Raw Prostate concentrate 140 mg • Zinc (Monomethionine) 50 mg • Vitamin A (Beta Carotene) 10000 IU • Vitamin E natural 200 IU. Contains no yeast, wheat, corn, soy, milk, salt, sugar or starch.
See Editor's Note No. 14, page 1817.

Prostactive Plus Saw Palmetto - Nature's Way
Each softgel contains: Concentrated 12:1 Saw Palmetto Berry Extract 160 mg • Concentrated 10:1 Nettle Root Extract 120 mg.

ProstaMed - Enzymatic Therapy
Each capsule contains: Saw Palmetto Berry extract 160 mg standardized to contain 85%-95% fatty acids & sterols: 0.15% - 0.3% fatty alcohols, 0.2%-0.4% total sterols, 0.1%-0.3% beta-sitosterol. Contains no sugar, salt, yeast, wheat, corn, dairy products, flavoring or preservatives.

Prosta-Metto - The Vitamin Shoppe
Each softgel contains: Saw Palmetto extract 160 mg • Pumpkin seed oil 40 mg • Pygeum Africanum extract 10 mg • Bearberry extract 10 mg • Zinc 15 mg • Vitamin B6 5 mg.

Prosta-Metto Saw Palmetto Complex - Puritan's Pride
Each softgel contains: Saw Palmetto berry extract (Serenoa repens: Standardized to contain 85%-95% fatty acids and biologically active sterol compounds) 80 mg • Pumpkin Seed oil extract (Curburbita pepo) 40 mg • Pygeum Africanum extract 10 mg • Bearberry extract (Uva Ursi) 5 mg.

Prostaprime - Puritan's Pride
Each tablet contains: Raw Prostate concentrate 100 mg • Saw Palmetto 100 mg • Pygeum extract 75 mg. Other Ingredients: Golden Rod, Pumpkin Seed Concentrate, Flaxseed Oil, Glycine, Glutamic Acid, and Alanine.
See Editor's Note No. 14, page 1817.

ProstaPro - PhytoPharmica
Each capsule contains: Saw Palmetto Berry extract 160 mg.
See Editor's Note No. 2, page 1816.

Prosta-Q - Farr Laboratories, LLC
Each capsule contains: Zinc (from zinc gluconate) 5 mg • Proprietary Blend [Quercetin, Cranberry (berry), Saw Palmetto (berry), Bromelain, Papain] 540 mg.

Prostata - Gero Vita
Urtica Dioica extract 16:1 150 mg • Serenoa Serrulata extract 106 mg • Apis Mellifica 83.33 mg • L-Alanine 66.67 mg • Glycine 66.67 mg • L-Glutamic Acid 66.67 mg • Pygeum Africanum extract 50 mg • Vitamin B6 15 mg • Panax Ginseng extract 8.33 mg • Zinc Arginate 7.5 mg • Hydrangea extract 5 mg • Copper 0.5 mg • Beta Carotene 8333 IU.

Prostate - Centrum Focused Formulas
One softgel contains: Vitamin A as Beta-carotene 5000 IU • Lycopene 1.5 mg • Saw Palmetto standardized Lipophilic fruit extract (Serenoa repens) 160 mg.

Prostate - ProHerbs
Two softgels contain: Vitamin E (Dl-Alpha Tocopheryl Acetate) 30 IU • Zinc (as Sulfate) 15 mg • Selenium (as Selenomethionine) 200 mcg •

LycoPure (equivalent to 5 mg Lycopene) 71 mg • Saw Palmetto berries (Serenoa repens standardized to 85%-95% free fatty acids) 320 mg • Stinging Nettle root (Urtica dioca L. 2% minimum plant silica) 200 mg • Pumpkin Seed Oil (Cucurbita pepo seeds) 30 mg. Other Ingredients: Soybean Oil, Beeswax, Gelatin, Glycerin, Water, Chlorophyllin, Sodium, Copper, Titanium Dioxide.

Prostate 5LX - New Chapter, Inc.
Two softgels contain: Saw Palmetto berry, extract (85-95% total fatty acids- 272-304 mg) 320 mg • Green Tea leaf, extract (45% polyphenols- 45 mg) 100 mg • Pumpkin Seed Oil 96 mg • Ginger rhizome, certified organic, extract (minimum 20% pungent compounds- 16 mg 5% zingiberene- 4 mg) 80 mg • Urtica root extract (Nettle) hydroalcoholic, 10:1 50 mg • Urtica root extract (Nettle) aqueous, 5:1 50 mg • Selenium, bio-grown 50 mcg • Rosemary leaf and essential oil, extract (23% total phenolic antioxidants- 2.3 mg) 10 mg. Other Ingredients: Olive Oil, Yellow Beeswax, Gelatin, Vegetable Glycerin, Purified Water, Carob.

Prostate Essentials - Swanson
Each capsule contains: Zinc (as zinc picolinate) 15 mg • Saw Palmetto extract (20% free fatty acids) 160 mg • Stinging Nettle concentrate 120 mg • Korean Ginseng root 50 mg • Pygeum extract (3% sterols) 50 mg • Pumpkin Seed concentrate 40 mg • Glycine 25 mg • L-Alanine 25 mg • L-Glutamic Acid 25 mg • Beta Sitosterol 20 mg.

Prostate Formula - Nature's Way
Two capsules contain: Beta Glucan 2.2 mg • Calcium 26 mg • Dandelion leaf 230 mg • Lycopene 2.4 mg • Saw Palmetto dried extract 360 mg • Soy Isoflavone dried extract 25 mg • Zinc (Amino Acid Chelate) 7 mg. Other ingredients: Gelatin, Magnesium Stearate, Millet, Silica.

Prostate Formula - Youngevity
Saw Palmetto 400 mg • Pygeum bark 80 mg • Pumpkin seed 80 mg • Atractylodes herb • Licorice root 40 mg • Bupleurum root 40 mg • Vitamin E 100 IU • Vitamin C 60 mg • Vitamin B6 4 mg • Vilcabamba Mineral Essence: Potassium, Calcium, Magnesium, Zinc, Chromium, Selenium, Iron, Copper, Molybdenum, Vanadium, Iodine, Cobalt, Manganese.

Prostate Guardian - Clinician's Choice
Three tablets contain: Vitamin E (dl-alpha tocopheryl acetate) 150 IU • Zinc (glycinate) 15 mg • Niacin (niacinamide) 15 mg • Pygeum Bark Powder 30 mg • Saw Palmetto Berries 450 mg • Kudzu Root 450 mg • Pumpkin Seeds 360 mg • Panax Ginseng Root 150 mg • Siberian Ginseng Root 150 mg • Oat Straw Extract (10:1) 150 mg • Horny Goat Weed 90 mg • RoseOx (patented, standardized process for an extract of Rosemary) 75 mg • Cayenne Fruit • Proprietary blend 12 mg: Lycopene 1%, Citrus Bioflavonoid Complex, Horsetail Herb, Isoflavones.

Prostate Health - Celestial Seasonings
Two capsules contain: Vitamin E (as d-alpha tocopherol acetate) 90 IU • Zinc (as gluconate) 15 mg • Proprietary Blend: Saw Palmetto (berries), Saw Palmetto (standardized extract), Stinging Nettle root (standardized extract) 1230 mg. Other Ingredients: (May contain one or more of the following) Dicalcium Phosphate, Gelatin, Rice Flour, Stearic Acid, Magnesium Stearate, and Silicon Dioxide. One servings size is equivalent to: Saw Palmetto 320 mg standardized to 95% fatty acids.
See Editor's Note No. 2, page 1816.

Prostate Health - Doctor's A-Z
Each capsule contains: Zinc (as zinc picolinate) 15 mg • Saw Palmetto extract (20% fatty acids) 160 mg • Stinging Nettle concentrate 120 mg • Korean Ginseng root 50 mg • Pygeum extract (3% sterols) 50 mg • Pumpkin Seed concentrate 40 mg • Glycine 25 mg • L-Alanine 25 mg • L-Glutamic Acid 25 mg • Beta Sitosterol 20 mg.

BRAND NAMES

BRAND NAMES

Prostate Support - Amazon Support
Each capsule contains: Mutamba • Brazilian Peppertree • Jatoba • Nettles • Pau D'Arco • Chanca Piedra • Cipo Cabeludo • Sarsaparilla.

Prostate Support - Now
Each gelcap contains: Saw Palmetto • Pygeum • Stinging Nettle • Lycopene. Other ingredients: Pumpkin seed oil, Zinc & Vitamin B6.

Prostate Support Formula - PhysioLogics
Two capsules contain: Zinc (Glycinate) 15 mg • Copper (Glycinate) 2 mg • Vitamin B6 (Pyridoxine HCL) 100 mg • Beta Sitosterol 60 mg • Pygeum (2.5% Phytosterols 2.5 mg) 100 mg • Pumpkin seed powder 100 mg • Nettles (1-2% Plant Silica, 4-8 mg) 400 mg.

Prostate-Duo - Uronat Nutrition Company, Inc.
Each softgel contains: Saw Palmetto extract (minimun 85% free fatty acids & 5% sterols) 160 mg • Pygeum africanum extract (minimum 13% sterols) 50 mg. Other Ingredients: Gelatin, Glycerin, Pumpkin seed oil, Water, Carob. Free from sugar, salt, starch, artificial colors, preservatives, yeast, wheat, corn & milk.

Prostatonin - Pharmaton
Each capsule contains: Pygeum africanum 25 mg • Nettle Root 300 mg. Other Ingredients: Grape oil, gelatin, triglycerides, glycerol, sorbitol, soya lecithin, synthetic iron oxides, & titanium dioxide.

Prostex - Metabolic Products
Two capsules contain: Proprietary Amino Acid blend: Glutamic Acid, Alanine, Aminoacetic Acid (glycine) 810 mg. Other Ingredients: Gelatin, Polyethylene glycol 8000.

ProstGard - Holista
Each capsule contains: Zinc (from gluconate) 15 mg • Vitamin B6 (pyridoxine HCl) 5 mg • Saw Palmetto (Serenoa repens) extract of berries (10:1) 80 mg • Pumpkin Seed Oil 500 mg.

Prostoid - HealthWatchers System
Vitamin C • Vitamin A • Vitamin E • Vitamin B6 • Serenoa Senulata • Pygeum Africanum Extract • Hydrangea Extract • Bee Pollen • Siberian Ginseng Extract • Glutamic Acid • L-Glycine • L-Alanine • Silica • Solidago Fragrans Extract • Zinc • Damiana • Dong Quai • Gotu Kola • Juniper • Copper

Protagest - PhytoPharmica
Three tablets contain: Niacinamide 30 mg • Vitamin B6 (pyridoxine HCl) 1,500 mcg • Potassium Chloride 96 mg • Betaine HCl 975 mg • Glutamic Acid HCl 585 mg • Pepsin (1:10,000) 291 mg • Ammonium Chloride 96 mg • Papain (6X) 90 mg • Ox Bile extract 45 mg • Pancreatic enzymes (4X) 30 mg.
See Editor's Note No. 14, page 1817.

Protazyme - Enzymatic Therapy
Each tablet contains: Potassium Chloride 32 mg • Niacinamide 10 mg • Vitamin B6 (Pyridoxine HCL) 500 mcg • Other Ingredients: Betaine HCL 325 mg • Glutamic Acid HCL 195 mg • Pepsin 1:10000 97 mg • Ammonium Chloride 32 mg • Papain 6X 30 mg • Ox Bile extract 15 mg • Pancreatic Enzymes 4X 10 mg. Contains no sugar, salt, yeast, wheat, corn, soy, dairy products, coloring, flavoring or preservatives.
See Editor's Note No. 14, page 1817.

Protector Caps - The Vitamin Shoppe
Three capsules contain: Vitamin A (Beta-carotene) 10000 IU • Vitamin E (d-alpha tocopheryl succinate) 200 IU • Ester C 500 mg • Pycnogenol 10 mg • Selenium (L-Selenomethionine) 50 mcg • CoQ10 10 mg • Green Tea extract (30% Polyphenols) 25 mg • Quercetin 25 mg.

Protector SPF 15 - Jason
Vitamin C Complex • Beta Hydroxy Acid.

Protein 95 Soy Protein - Nature's Life
Two 2 scoops (28.35 g) contain: SUPRO brand Soy Protein Isolate containing Lecithin • natural Vanilla Flavor • natural Papain Enzyme concentrate.

Protein Boost - Nutri-Quest
Two tablespoons contain: Alanine 646 mg • Arginine 1190 mg • Aspartic Acid 1853 mg • Cystine 187 mg • Glutamic Acid 3060 mg • Glycine 680 mg • Histidine 408 mg • Isoleucine 765 mg • Leucine 1275 mg • Lysine 986 mg • Methionine 221 mg • Phenylalanine 850 mg • Proline 901 mg • Serine 833 mg • Threonine 612 mg • Tyrosine 629 mg • Valine 782 mg. Ingredients: Isolated Soy Protein, Calcium & Sodium Caseinate, Tri Calcium Phosphate, Lecithin, Soybean oil, Magnesium Oxide, Papain, Ascorbic Acid, Ferrous Fumarate, Kelp, Niacin, Calcium Pantothenate, Vitamin A, Pyridoxine HCL, Thiamine HCL, Riboflavin, Vitamin D & natural Vanilla Flavor. All acids of (L) form.

ProtoChol Chewables - Fields of Nature
Each tablet contains: Phytosterol Concentrate 400 mg (as Beta-Sitosterol 172 mg, Campesterol 100 mg, Stigmasterol 44 mg). Other Ingredients: Dextrose, Magnesium Stearate, Adipic Acid, Aspartame, Natural and artificial flavors, Artificial colors (FD&C Red No. 40 Lake).

Protykin/ Resveratrol - Natrol
Two capsules contain: Polygonum cuspidatum extract root 50 mg • Trans-Resveratrol 10 mg Total Reservatrols 12 mg • Emodin 5 mg. Other ingredients: Rice powder, Magnesium Stearate, Gelatin.

Provol - Upsher-Smith Laboratories
Pygeum africanum bark extract 50 mg.

ProXeed. - Sigma-Tau Pharmaceuticals, Inc.
Each packet contains: Active Ingredients: L-Carnitine Fumarate 1 g • Fructose • Acetyl L-Carnitine HCL .5 g • Citric Acid. Inactive Ingredients: Mannitol, polyethylene glycol, artificial flavorings, povidone, & silicone dioxide.

Proxylon - Syntrax Innovations
Each capsule contains: 7-Isopropoxyisoflavone 250 mg.

PS (Phosphatidylserine) - Metabolic Response Modifiers
Each softgel contains: Phosphatidylserine 100 mg • Other Phospholipids 380 mg • Soy oil 200 mg • Vitamin C 10 mg.

PS Memory Care - Sundown Vitamins
Each softgel contains: Phosphatidylserine complex 500 mg Standardized to: Phosphatidylserine 100 mg • Phosphatidylcholine 45 mg • Phosphatidylethanolamine 10 mg • Phosphatidylinositol 5 mg. Other Ingredients: Soya Lecithin, Gelatin, Glycerine, Soybean Oil, Water.

Pseudo Ephedrine 30 mg - D & E Pharmaceuticals
Each tablet contains: Psuedo Ephedrine 30 mg.

Pseudo Ephedrine 60 mg - D & E Pharmaceuticals
Each tablet contains: Psuedo Ephedrine 60 mg.

Psoriasis Support - Amazon Support
Each capsule contains: Samambaia • Cat's Claw • Suma • Sarsaparilla • Bitter Melon • Chanca Piedra • Fedegosa • Gervao • Boldo.

Psyllium - Metabolic Response Modifiers
Each tablespoon contains: Psyllium husk (4 g dietary fiber) 5 g.

Some Brand Name Natural Products - What they Contain

Psyllium (Secrets of the Psyllium & Orange Flavored Psyllium Powder) - Trader Joe's
Psyllium husk fiber • Secrets of the Psyllium 85%: Fiber (per heaping tablespoon) 6 g • Orange flavored Psyllium powder 35%: Fiber (per heaping tablespoon) 3 g.

PTE Support - PhysioLogics
Two capsules contain: Bromelain (2400 GDU) 500 mg • Serratiopeptidase 10 mg.

Pumpkin Seed Extract - PhytoPharmica
Each capsule contains: Pumpkin (Cocurbita pepo) seed extract 20:1 300 mg.

Pure C Crystals - Nature's Life
Each 1/4 teaspoon contains: Vitamin C (Ascorbic Acid) 1250 mg.

Pure Citrimax - Natrol
One capsule contains: (-) Hydroxycitric Acid 250 mg.
Other ingredients: Gelatin, Magnesium Stearate.

Pure CoQ-10 - Solaray
Each capsule contains: Coenzyme Q-10 30 mg.
Other Ingredients: Cellulose, Gelatin (capsule).

Pure CoQ10-30 - Solaray
Each capsule contains: Coenzyme Q-10 30 mg.
Other Ingredients: Cellulose, Gelatin.

Pure Energy - Montana Big Sky
Each 800 mg caplet contains: Bee Pollen (Apis pollenus) • Dibaxic Calcium Phosphate • Gotu Kola (Centella asiatica) • Siberian Ginseng (Eleutherococcus senticosus) • Gotu Kola standardized extract • Royal Jelly • Siberian Ginseng standardized extract.

Pure Soy Protein Powder - Puritan's Pride
Each scoop (28 g) contains: Calories 110 • Protein 25 g • Fat 1 g • L-Alanine 1064 mg • L-Arginine 1876 mg • L-Aspartic Acid 2856 mg • L-Cysteine 308 mg • L-Glutamic Acid 4704 mg • L-Glycine 1036 mg • L-Histidine 644 mg • L-Isoleucine 1204 mg • L-Lysine 1540 mg • L-Methionine 336 mg • L-Phenylalanine 1288 mg • L-Proline 1260 mg • L-Serine 1288 mg • L-Threonine 924 mg • L-Tryptophan 308 mg • L-Tyrosine 924 mg • L-Valine 1232 mg.

Pur-Gar - Now
Each tablet contains: Pur-Gar 600 mg.

Puritan's Pride One - Puritan's Pride
Each tablet contains: Vitamin A (as Retinyl Palmitate and Beta Carotene) 10,000 IU • Vitamin C (as Ascorbic Acid with Rose Hips) 250 mg • Vitamin D (as Cholecalciferol) 400 IU • Vitamin E (as d-Alpha Tocopheryl Acetate) 30 IU • Thiamin (Vitamin B-1; as Thiamine Hydrochloride) 25 mg • Riboflavin (Vitamin B-2) 25 mg • Niacin (as Niacinamide) 50 mg • Vitamin B-6 (as Pyridoxine Hydrochloride) 50 mg • Folic Acid 400 mcg • Vitamin B-12 (as Cyanocobalamin) 50 mcg • Biotin (as D-Biotin) 50 mcg • Pantothenic Acid (as D-Calcium Pantothenate) 50 mg • Calcium (as Bone Meal) 50 mg • Iron (as Ferrous Fumarate) 10 mg • Phosphorus (as Bone Meal) 23 mg • Iodine (as Potassium Iodide) 150 mcg • Magnesium (as Magnesium Oxide) 100 mg • Zinc (as Zinc Sulfate) 15 mg • Selenium (as Selenium Yeast) 25 mcg • Copper (as Copper Sulfate) 2 mg • Manganese (as Manganese Sulfate) 5 mg • Chromium (as Chromium Chloride) 100 mcg • Molybdenum (as Sodium Molybdate) 15 mcg • Chloride (as Potassium Chloride) 1 mg • Potassium (as Potassium Chloride) 1 mg • PABA (Para-Aminobenzoic Acid) 50 mg • Inositol 15 mg • Choline Bitartrate 15 mg. In a natural base of Bioflavonoids, Rutin, Rose Hips, Yeast, Kelp, and Dolomite.

Puritron - Puritan's Pride
Six tablets contain: Vitamin A (as Fish Liver Oil) 10,000 IU • Vitamin C (as Ascorbic Acid) 300 mg • Vitamin D (as Cholecalciferol) 400 IU • Vitamin E (as d-Alpha Tocopheryl Acetate) 100 IU • Thiamin (Vitamin B-1; as Thiamine Mononitrate) 25 mg • Riboflavin (Vitamin B-2) 25 mg • Niacin (as Niacinamide) 25 mg • Vitamin B-6 (as Pyridoxine Hydrochloride) 25 mg • Folic Acid 400 mcg • Vitamin B-12 (as Cyanocobalamin) 25 mcg • Biotin 150 mcg • Pantothenic Acid (as D-Calcium Pantothenate) 25 mg • Calcium (as Bone Meal) 800 mg • Iron (as Ferrous Gluconate) 30 mg • Phosphorus (as Bone Meal) 400 mg • Iodine (as Kelp) 150 mcg • Magnesium (as Magnesium Oxide) 100 mg • Zinc (as Zinc Gluconate) 30 mg • Selenium (as Selenium Yeast) 25 mcg • Copper (as Copper Gluconate) 1 mg • Manganese (as Manganese Gluconate) 0.07 mg • Potassium (as Potassium Gluconate) 40 mg • Brewer's Yeast 600 mg • Choline Bitartrate 24 mg • Inositol 36 mcg • PABA (Para-Aminobenzoic Acid) 40 mcg • Rutin 30 mg • Citrus Bioflavonoid complex 30 mg • Hesperidin complex 25 mg • Nucleic Acid 40 mg • Desiccated Liver 100 mg • Red Bone Marrow 60 mg • Lecithin 60 mg • Wheat Germ Oil 20 mg • Papain 20 mg • Rose Hips 1 mg. Brewer's Yeast and Desiccated Liver provide the following Amino Acids per 6 tablets: Alanine 19.3 mg, Arginine 8.1 mg, Aspartic Acid 20.0 mg, Cysteine 2.7 mg, Glutamic Acid 32.8 mg, Glycine 12.8 mg, Histidine 8.0 mg, Isoleucine 13.1 mg, Leucine 21.1 mg, Lysine 21.9 mg, Methionine 5.4 mg, Phenylalanine 12.5 mg, Proline 11.9 mg, Serine 13.6 mg, Threonine 13.2 mg, Tryptophan 3.8 mg, Tyrosine 8.9 mg, Valine 12.6 mg.
See Editor's Note No. 14, page 1817.

Pycnogenol - Now
Each capsule contains: European Pine bark.

Pycnogenol - Leiner Health Products
Each tablet contains: Pycnogenol 50 mg. Other Ingredients: Calcium Carbonate, Maltodextrin, Cellulose, Tricalcium Phosphate, Talc, Polyethylene Glycol 3350, Silicon Dioxide, Crospovidone, Croscarmellose Sodium, Magnesium Stearate.

Pycnogenol 25 Mg - Natrol
One capsule contains: Pine Bark extract 25 mg. Other ingredients: Microcrystalline Cellulose, Magnesium Stearate, Gelatin.

Pycnogenol 50 Mg - Natrol
One capsule contains: Pine Bark extract 50 mg. Other ingredients: Microcrystalline Cellulose, Magnesium Stearate, Gelatin.

Pycnogenol Plus - Aspen Group, Inc.
Each capsule contains: Bioflavonoids 200 mg • Grape Seed extract 25 mg • Pycnogenol 25 mg.

Pycnogenol with Vitamins C, E, & A - Derma E
Pycnogenol • Vitamin C • Vitamin E • Vitamin A.

Pycno-Plus Protection - HealthWatchers System
Grape Seed Extract • Pine Bark Pwder Plus • Beta Carotene • Vitamin C • Cat's Claw Powder • Bioflavonoids • Rutin • Acerola.

Pygeum - Nature's Way
Each capsule contains: Pygeum bark extract concentrate (standardized to 13% sterols 6.5 mg) 50 mg • B6 (Pyridoxine HCl) 12.5 mg • Zinc (Citrate) 15 mg • Copper (Citrate) 1.5 mg • Selenium 50 mcg. In a base of Pumpkin seed oil.

Pygeum and Saw Palmetto - Solaray
Six capsules contain: Vitamin B-6 (as pyridoxine HCl) 20 mg • Zinc (as optizinc) 15 mg • Cranberry extract 800 mg • Saw Palmetto berry oil 320 mg • Pygeum bark extract 100 mg. Other Ingredients: Gelatin, Cellulose, Pumpkin Seed, L-Glycerine, Glutamic Acid, L-Alanine, Magnesium Stearate.

BRAND NAMES

Pyridoxal 5-Phosphate Plus - Klaire Laboratories
Each capsule contains: Pyridoxal 5-Phosphate 50 mg • Magnesium (as Magnesium Glycinate Chelate) 100 mg.

Pyruvate - Aspen Group, Inc.
Each capsule contains: Calcium Pyruvate 750 mg. Contains no sugar, starch, salt, wheat, yeast, corn, milk or soy derivatives.

Pyruvate 1000 - Pinnacle
Each tablet provides 1000 mg of Pyruvate 1000 from calcium and sodium salts of Pyruvic Acid, plus Dihydroxyacetone. Inulized in a bioactive complex of Phosphorolytic Dahlia Inulin providing a long chain carbohydrate molecule.

Pyruvate Fuel - TwinLab
Each capsule contains: Calcium Pyruvate Monohydrate 750 mg.

Pyruvate Powder - Source Naturals
Each capsule contains: Calcium Pyruvate Monohydrate 750 mg.

Pyruvate Power - Swanson
Two capsules contain: Calcium (as calcium pyruvate) 244 mg • Pyruvate (as calcium pyruvate) 1.05 g • Cayenne 100 mg.

Pyruvate-C - Richardson Labs
Four caplets contain: Pyruvate: (Potassium Pyruvate, Calcium Pyruvate) 2 g • Chromium (picolinate) 400 mcg.

Python - Swedish Herbal Institute
One tablet contains: Damiana 100 mg • Gotu Kola 30 mg • Green Oat Straw seeds 100 mg • Muira Puama 100 mg • Saw Palmetto 100 mg • Ginkgo Biloba 30 mg • Siberian Ginseng 200 mg • Korean Ginseng root 200 mg • Guarana seeds 50 mg • Schisandra fruit/seed 100 mg • Stinging Nettle leaf 200 mg • Tribulus Terrestris 250 mg.

Pytodolor - Enzymatic Therapy
Each drop contains: Common Ash bark 0.20 ml • Aspen leaves and bark 0.60 ml • Goldenrod aerial 0.20 ml. Other ingredients: Water, Alcohol 45.6%.

Q-Gel 15 mg - Tishcon
One softsule contains: Vitamin E 3 IU • Coenzyme Q-10 15 mg. Other ingredients: Gelatin, Glycerin, Purified water, Titanium dioxide, Annatto seed extract, Proprietary Biosolv (Polysorbate 80, Lecithin, Sorbitan monoleate, Medium Chain Triglycerides).

Q-Gel Forte 30 mg - Tishcon
One softsule contains: Vitamin E 6 IU • Coenzyme Q-10 30 mg. Other ingredients: Gelatin, Glycerin, Purified water, Titanium dioxide, Annatto seed extract, Proprietary Biosolv (Polysorbate 80, Lecithin, Sorbitan monoleate, Medium Chain Triglycerides).

Q-Gel Ultra - Tishcon - Tishcon
Each softgel capsule contains: Coenzyme Q-10 60 mg • Vitamin E 150 IU.

Q-Sorb Coenzyme Q-10 - Nature's Bounty
Each softgel contains: Coenzyme Q-10 50 mg. Other Ingredients: Rice Bran Oil, Gelatin, Glycerin, Mixture of Beeswax and Soybean Oil, Lecithin, Titanium Dioxide Color.
See Editor's Note No. 6, page 1816.

Q-Sorb Coenzyme Q-10 (120 mg) - VitaStore
Each softgel capsule contains: Coenzyme Q-10 120 mg. Other Ingredients: Rice Bran Oil, Gelatin, Glycerin, Mixture of Beeswax and Soybean Oil, Lecithin, Titanium Dioxide Color. Contains no yeast, wheat, gluten, milk or milk derivatives, lactose, sugar, preservatives, artificial flavor, sodium (less than 5 mg per serving).

Q-Sorb Coenzyme Q-10 (75 mg) - Vitamin World
Each softgel capsule contains: Coenzyme Q-10 75 mg. Other Ingredients: Rice Bran Oil, Gelatin, Glycerin, Mixture of Beeswax and Soybean Oil, Lecithin, Titanium Dioxide Color. Contains no yeast, wheat, gluten, milk or milk derivatives, lactose, sugar, preservatives, artificial flavor, sodium (less than 5 mg per serving)

Quanterra Emotional Balance - Warner-Lambert
Each tablet contains: LI 160 WS (hyperforin stabilized) St. John's Wort standardized extract 300 mg.

Quanterra Mental Sharpness, Ginkgo Biloba - Warner-Lambert
Each tablet contain: Egb 761 Ginkgo Biloba leaf extract; standardized to 24% Ginkgo flavone glycosides & 6% terpene lactones) 60 mg. Other Ingredients: Lactose, microcrystalline cellulose, maize starch, hydroxypropyl methylcellulose, croscarmellose sodium, polyethylene glycol, magnesium stearate, silicon dioxide, artificial color, talc, ferric oxide, & dimethicone.
See Editor's Note No. 21, page 1818.

Quanterra Prostate, Saw Palmetto - Warner-Lambert
Each softgel contains: Saw Palmetto Berry dried extract (Seronoa repens, berry, dried extract) 160 mg. Other Ingredients: Gelatin, Glycerol, & Ferric Oxide.
See Editor's Note No. 20, page 1818.

Quanterra Sinus Defense, Sinupret - Warner-Lambert
Each tablet contains: Gentian Root (Gentian lutea) 9 mg • Elder Flower (Sambucus nigra) 29 mg • European Vervain Aerial Parts (Verbena) 29 mg • Primrose Flower (Primula veris) 29 mg • Sorrel Aerial Parts (Rumex acesota) 29 mg. Other Ingredients: Sucrose, talc, lactose monohydrate, calcium carbonate, potato starch, maize starch, maize swell-starch flour, colloidal anhydrous silica, stearic palmitic acid, titanium dioxide, glucose syrup, gelatin, shellac, magnesium oxide, sorbitol, eudragit E 12.5, montan glycol wax, povidone, & castor oil.
See Editor's Note No. 21, page 1818.

Quanterra Sleep Valerian - Warner-Lambert
Three tablets contain: Valerian (Valeriana officinalis) root, dried extract 300 mg • Lemon Balm (Melissa officinalis) leaf, dried extract 150 mg. Other Ingredients: Sucrose, Castor Oil, Talc, Methylhydroxypropyl Cellulose, Microcrystalline Cellulose, Crospovidone, Silicon Dioxide, Calcium Carbonate, Polyethylene Glycol, Titanium Dioxide, Eudragit L 30 D, Glucose Syrup, Carmellose Sodium, FD&C Blue No. 2 Aluminum Lake, Magnesium Stearate, Polyvidon, Carnauba Wax, Polysorbate 80.

Quanterra Stomach Comfort, Ginger - Warner-Lambert
Two capsules contain: Ginger (Zingiber Officinale, root) 500 mg. Other Ingredients: Gelatin, colloidal anhydrous silica, & sodium laurel sulfate.

QueaseEase - Pacific BioLogic
Pinellia rhizome • Citrus peel • Fritillaria bulb • Poria Plant Fungus (hoelen) • Licorice root • Ginger rhizome • Chrysanthemum flower • Astragalus seed • Gastrodia rhizome • Bamboo shavings • Perilla leaf • Peppermint.

Quercetin - Metabolic Response Modifiers
Each capsule contains: Quercetin 500 mg.

Quercetin + C - Puritan's Pride
Two capsules contain: Quercetin 500 mg • Vitamin C 1400 mg.

Quercetin-Bromelain - Doctor's Best
Each capsule contains: Quercetin 250 mg • Bromelain 125 mg.

Quercezyme-Plus - Enzymatic Therapy
Each capsule contain: Vitamin C (Ascorbic Acid) 100 mg • Magnesium (Carbonate) 25 mg • Other ingredients: Bromelain (1800 MCU) 125 mg • Quercetin 125 mg • Mixed Bioflavonoids Complex 50% concentrate 100 mg • L-Cysteine (HCL) 75 mg. Contains no sugar, salt, yeast, wheat, corn, soy, dairy products, coloring, flavoring or preservatives.

Quest Chromium GTF - Quest
Each capsule contains: Chromium (HVP Chelate) 200 mcg. Other Ingredients: Microcrystalline Cellulose, Magnesium Stearate (vegetable source).

Quest Ginkgo Biloba Extract - Quest
Each caplet contains: Ginkgo Biloba leaf extract (Ginkgo biloba) (provided by 60 mg P.E. 1:50 standardized to contain 24% Ginkgosides) 3000 mg • Citrus Bioflavonoids 200 mg providing Hesperidin 50 mg. Other Ingredients: Calcium Phosphate, Microcrystalline Cellulose, Croscarmellose Sodium, Vegetable Stearin, Magnesium Stearate (vegetable source).

Quest Green-Lipped Mussel - Quest
Each capsule contains: Freeze-Dried Green Lipped Mussel (Perna canaliculus) 625 mg.

Quest Kava Kava - Quest
Each capsule contains: Kava Kava (provided by 150 mg P.E. 1:12 standardized to 30% Kavalactones) 1800 mg. Other Ingredients: Microcrystalline Cellulose, Magnesium Stearate (vegetable source).

Quest Lycopene - Quest
Each capsule contains: Lyc-o-Mato brand Lycopene 5000 mcg. Other Ingredients: Rice Bran Oil, Sunflower Oil, Vegetable Stearin, Beeswax, Lecithin.

Quest MSM - Quest
Each caplet contains: Lignisul brand MSM 1000 mg. Other Ingredients: Croscarmellose Sodium, Silicon Dioxide, and Magnesium Stearate.

Quest SAM-e - Quest
Each caplet contains: S-adenosyl-methionine tosylate (providing 50 mg S-adenosyl-methionine) 100 mg. Other Ingredients: Croscarmellose Sodium, Microcrystalline Cellulose, Calcium Phosphate, Vegetable Stearin, Magnesium Stearate (vegetable source).

Quest Siberian Ginseng - Quest
Each capsule contains: Siberian Ginseng 500 mg.

Quick Dissolve Maalox - Novartis Consumer Health
Each tablet contains: Calcium Carbonate 600 mg. Other Ingredients: Aspartame, Colloidal Silicon Dioxide, Croscarmellose Sodium, Dextrose, Flavors, Magnesium Stearate, Maltodextrin, Mannitol, Pregelatinized Starch, Red #30 Lake.

Quick Dissolve Maalox - Maximum Strength - Novartis Consumer Health
Each tablet contains: Calcium Carbonate 1000 mg • Sodium 2 mg. Other Ingredients: Aspartame, Corn Starch, Croscarmellose Sodium, Dextrose, Flavors, Magnesium Stearate, Maltodextrin, Mannitol, Pregelatinized Starch, Silica, Sodium Chloride, Red #30 Lake. See Editor's Note No. 5, page 1816.

Quick Trim - Cybergenics America Co.
Each caplet contains: Complex 1: Guarana seed extract • L-Tyrosine • L-Phenylalanine • Garcinia Cambogia (Citrimax) • Griffonia extract • Kola Nut powder • Chinese Ginseng • Cayenne pepper • Phenalgin • Astragalus root • Cinnamon bark • Green Tea • Pacific Kelp. Complex 2: Lecithin • Ginger • Cascara Sagrada • Buchu leaf extract • Uva Ursi leaf • Juniper berry extract • Choline Bitartrate • Inositol • L-Methionine • Chickweed herb • Red Clover powder • Dandelion root extract • Senna leaf extract • Cynarin complex. Complex 3: Chamomile flower • Valerian root extract • Hawthorne extract • Kava Kava root • Immature Orange peel • Lemon Verbena • Skullcap. Complex 4: Enzyme blend • Magnesium Oxide • Calcium Chelate • Selenium Yeast • Zinccitrata • Zinc Picolinate • Ascorbic Acid • Beta Carotene • Niacin • D Alpha Tocopheryl Acetate • Pyridoxine HCl • Riboflavin • Thiamin HCl • Potassium Iodide • Folic Acid • Cyanocobalamin • Chromium Picolinate • Phytonadione • Cholecalciferol.

Radical Raiders - Puritan's Pride
Three capsules contain: Vitamin A (beta carotene) 25,000 IU • Vitamin E (d-alpha tocopheryl) 400 IU • Vitamin C (Ester C) 500 mg • Selenium (l-selenomethionine) 50 mcg • Zinc (picolinate) 50 mg • Calcium (Ester C) 50 mg • Coenzyme Q10 3,000 mcg • Pycnogenol 3,000 mcg • Citrus Bioflavonoids complex 50 mg • Quercetin 30 mg • L-Glutathione 1,000 mcg • N-Acetyl-Cysteine 100 mg • Green Tea extract 3,000 mcg • Bilberry extract 30 mg.

Raspberry - Natrol
Each single serving contains: Vitamin C (Ascorbic Acid) 250 mg • Acerola berry extract 20 mg • Echinacea (Purpurea extract 16:1) 12.5 mg • White Willow bark 100 mg • Slippery Elm bark 75 mg • Stevia powder 20 mg. Other ingredients: Lemon Juice powder, Fructose, natural Raspberry flavor, Honey powder, Citric Acid, Natural Elderberry flavor, Calcium Carbonate.

Raw Adrenal - Enzymatic Therapy
Each two capsules contain: Vitamin C (Ascorbic Acid/Rose Hips) 250 mg • Pantothenic Acid (D-Calcium Pantothenate) 100 mg • Vitamin B6 (Pyridoxine HCL) 50 mg • Other ingredients: L-Tyrosine 250 mg • Betaine 250 mg • Pituitary extract freeze-dried 120 mg • Adrenal extract (Predigested Soluble concentrate*) 400 mg • Adrenal Cortex extract 33 mg. *Free-form concentrate predigested by enzymatic action, creating a highly absorbable form of glandular concentrate containing all the natural principles with a standardized content. All organs & glands derived from bovine sources. See Editor's Note No. 14, page 1817.

Raw Adrenal II - Enzymatic Therapy
Two tablets contain: Vitamin C (Ascorbic Acid/Rose Hips) 250 mg • Pantothenic Acid (D-Calcium Pantothenate) 250 mg • Vitamin B6 (Pyridoxine HCL) 50 mg • Other ingredients: L-Tyrosine 500 mg • Betaine 250 mg • Pituitary extract freeze-dried 120 mg • Adrenal extract (Predigested Soluble concentrate*) 100 mg • Ginger root extract 6.5:1 (Zingiber officinale) 100 mg • Adrenal Cortex extract 33 mg. *Free-form concentrate predigested by enzymatic action, creating a highly absorbable form of glandular concentrate containing all the natural principles with a standardized content. All organs & glands derived from bovine sources. See Editor's Note No. 14, page 1817.

RealSJW - Indena
Each tablet contains: St. John's Wort (0.03% Hypericin, 4% min. Hyperforin) 300 mg • LeucoSelect 1 mg. Other Ingredients: Calcium Phosphate, Dipacic Microcrystalline Cellulose, Vegetable Oil, Croscarmellose Sodium, Magnesium Stearate, Silicon Dioxide.

Recall Support - The Vitamin Shoppe
Two tablets contain: Ginkgo Biloba Extract 24% ginkgoflavoglycosides 25 mg • Phosphatidylserine 10 mg • L-Phenylalanine 250 mg • L-Glutamine 250 mg • Choline 250 mg • Gotu Kola 200 mg • RNA/DNA 100 mg • Magnesium (citrate, gluconate) 50 mg • Ginseng Extract (Panax Ginseng) 50 mg • B6 10 mg. In a base of Lecithin and Rice concentrate.

BRAND NAMES

Some Brand Name Natural Products - What they Contain

BRAND NAMES *(side margin)*

Red Clover - Nature's Way
Each capsule contains: Red Clover blossoms 430 mg.
Other Ingredients: Gelatin.

Red Clover Combination - Nature's Way
Each capsule contains: Barberry bark • Buckthorn bark • Burdock root • Cascara Sagrada bark • Echinacea Purpurea stem, leaf, flower • Licorice root • Peach bark • Prickly Ash bark • Red Clover blossoms • Rosemary herb • Sarsaparilla root • Sheep Sorrell. Other ingredients: Gelatin.

Red Clover Support Complex - Puritan's Pride
Each tablet contains: Vitamin E 10 IU • Red Clover extract (Trifolium pratense) aerial (dried weight equivalent) standardized for 40 mg of isoflavone phytoestrogens (naturally contains: genistein, biochanin A, daidzein, formononetin) 200 mg • Soy Isoflavones 40 mg • Black Cohosh extract (Cimicifuga racemosa) root (standarized to contain 2.5% Triterpene) 50 mg • Wild Yam (Dioscorea villosa) root 50 mg • Horse Chestnut extract (Aesculus hippocastanum) seed (standardized to contain 2.5% aescin) 25 mg • Rosemary extract (Rosmarinus officinalis) leaf 15 mg • Silica 25 mg.

Red Dragon Cold & Flu Relief - Jamieson
Each capsule contains: Honeysuckle flower (Lonicera japonica Thunb. PE 1:2) 149.3 mg • Forsythia fruit (Forsythia suspensa Thunb. PE 1:2) 149.3 mg • White Mulberry Leaf (Morus Alba L.PE 1:2) 119.4 mg • Chrysanthemum flower (Chrysanthemum morifolium Ramat PE 1:2) 89.6 mg • Adenophora root (Adenophora Tetraphylla Thunb PE 1:2) 89.6 mg • Schizonepata stem (Schizonepata tenifolia Briq PE 1:2) 89.6 mg • Ningpo Figwort root (Scrophularia ninpoensis Hemsl PE 1:2) 74.6 mg • Great Burdock fruit (Arctium Lappa L PE 1:2) 74.6 mg • Hogfennel root (Peucedanum praeruptorum Dunn PE 1:2) 74.6 mg • Field Mint leaf (Mentha haplocalyx Briq PE 1:2) 44.8 mg • Licorice root (Glycyrrhiza uralensis Fischer PE 1:2) 44.8 mg. (PE = Powdered Extract).

Red Dragon Imperial Ginseng - Jamieson
Each caplet contains: Panax Ginseng (derived from Shiu Chu, Tien Chi and Red Kirin) • 500 mg Roots of: Prince Adenophorae, Salvia, Scrophulara, Codonopsis and Polygonum Ginsengs, Radix Astragail, Canodermae Lucidum, Fructus Lycii Berry.

Red Dragon Imperial Ginseng and Garlic - Jamieson
Each capsule contains: Panax Ginseng (derived from Shiu Chu, Tien Chi and Red Kirin) • Roots of: Prince Adenophorae, Salvia, Scrophulara, Codonopsis and Polygonum Ginseng, Radix Astragail, Canodermae Lucidum, Fructus Lycii Berry 250 mg • Tibetan Plateau Garlic 250 mg.

Red Dragon Imperial Ginseng and Royal Jelly - Jamieson
Each caplet contains: Panax Ginseng (derived from Shiu Chu, Tien Chi and Red Kirin) • Roots of: Prince Adenophorae, Salvia, Scrophulara, Codonopsis and Polygonum Ginseng, Radix Astragail, Canodermae Lucidum, Fructus Lycii Berry 500 mg • Fresh Royal Jelly 250 mg.

Red Dragon Imperial Royal Jelly - Jamieson
Each capsule contains: Pure Royal Jelly concentrate equivalent to fresh Royal Jelly 500 mg.

Red Root-Cleavers Virtue - Blessed Herbs
Nettle • Horsetail Grass • Red Root • Cleavers • Sage leaf • Mullein leaf • Goldenseal root • Poke root • Ginger root • Grain alcohol & Distilled Water.

Red Stuff - Gary Nulls
Contains a fruit mix including Cranberries, Cherries, Pears, Watermelons, Pink Grapefruit, Lecithin, Apple Pectin, Papayas, and Peaches.

Red Wine Formula - Health Smart Vitamins
Each capsule contains: Tea (green, leaf: 90% polyphenols, 180 mg) 200 mg • Vitis vinifera (grape seed: 95% proanthocyanidins, 95 mg or >260 Porter Value Units)100 mg • Resveratrol (from Polygonum cuspidatum) 4 mg.

Reduced L-Glutathione 150 mg - Klaire Laboratories
Reduced L-Glutathione 150 mg.

Reduced L-Glutathione 75 mg - Klaire Laboratories
Reduced L-Glutathione 75 mg.

Regal Pro-Meal - Nature's Life
Two scoops (28.35 g) contain: Supro brand Soy Protein Isolate containing Lecithin • Whey • Fructose • Non-fat Dry Milk • natural Vanilla Flavor • Yeast • Egg Albumin • Eggshell powder • Kelp • natural Papain Enzyme concentrate & Cobalamin concentrate (B12). Regal Pro-Meal also contains 34 mg of naturally occuring Isoflavones including 21 mg Genistein & 10 mg Daidzein.

Rehab Forte - Progressive Labs
Two capsules contain: Vitamin C (ascorbic acid) 500 mg • Niacinamide 200 mg • Vitamin B6 (pyridoxine HCl) 50 mg • Calcium (amino acid chelate) 200 mg • Elemental Calcium 40 mg • Magnesium (amino acid chelate) 100 mg • Elemental Magnesium 20 mg • Zinc (amino acid chelate) 30 mg • Elemental Zinc 7.6 mg • Manganese (amino acid chelate) 50 mg • Elemental Manganese 5 mg • Copper (amino acid chelate) 2 mg • Elemental Copper 0.01 mg • Potassium Sulfate 200 mg • Elemental Potassium 90 mg • Chondroitin Sulfate 50 mg • Lemon bioflavonoids 500 mg • Rutin 50 mg. See Editor's Note No. 15, page 1817.

Reishi 5 - New Chapter, Inc.
Two capsules contain: Vitamin C 60 mg • Ginger extract (rhizome) 5% pungent compounds 50 mg • Mushroom Mycelia Reishi (mycelia), certified organic 200 mg • Shiitake (mycelia), certified organic mushroom extract 200 mg • Reishi (mushroom) minimum 4% triterpenes, 12.5% polysaccharides 40 mg • Maitake (mushroom) minimum 25% total polysaccharides 40 mg • Shiitake (mycelia) LEM, freeze dried, minimum EP3 1.5% PPT1 6% 40 mg • Cordyceps (mycelia) (dong-chong-zia-cao) 4:1 20 mg • Coriolus (mushroom) 8:1 20 mg. Other Ingredients: Vegetable Cellulose.

Reishi Defense - Traditional Medicinals
Red Reishi Mushroom (Ganoderma lucidum) Mycclium & Fruit Body • Ginger rhizome • Astragalus root • Roasted Barley grain • Licorice root • Stevia leaf.

Reishi Extract - Nature's Way
Two capsules contain: Reishi dried extract 376 mg. Other Ingredients: Gelatin, Millet.

Rejoyn Veromax - American MedTech
Two capsules contain: L-Arginine 200 mg • Zizyphi fructus 200 mg • Siberian Ginseng 200 mg • Saw Palmetto 200 mg • Ginkgo Biloba 75 mg • L-Alanine 75 mg • Glutamic Acid 75 mg • L-Lysine 75 mg. Other Ingredients: Pvp, Dicalcium Phosphate, Cellulose, Croscarmellose Sodium, Vegetable sterine, Magnesium stearate, Silicon dioxide and Pharmaceutical glaze.

Rejuveinate - PhysioLogics
Each capsule contains: Vitamin C (Ascorbic Acid) 60 mg • Horse Chestnut seed extract (15% Escin, 22.5 mg) 150 mg • Butcher's Broom (10% Ruscogenins, 10 mg) 100 mg • Gotu Kola (20% Terpenes, 12 mg) 60 mg • Hesperidin (35% Bioflavonoids, 14 mg) 40 mg • Bilberry fruit (36% Anthocyanosides, 7.2 mg) 20 mg.

Some Brand Name Natural Products - What they Contain
www.NaturalDatabase.com contains MANY more listings than appear here.

Rejuvex - Chattem, Inc.
Each caplet contains: Vitamin E (as dl-alpha tocopherol acetate) 30 IU • Thiamin HCl (Vitamin B1) 2 mg • Riboflavin (Vitamin B2) 2 mg • Niacin 10 mg • Vitamin B6 (as pyridoxine hydrochloride) 10 mg • Pantothenic Acid (as d-calcium pantothenate) 10 mg • Magnesium (as magnesium oxide) 500 mg • Selenium (as sodium selenate) 25 mcg • Manganese (as manganese sulfate) 2 mg • Standardized Dong Quai root extract 200 mg • Mammary gland powder 25 mg • Ovary gland powder 19 mg • Uterus gland powder 10 mg • Adrenal gland powder 10 mg • Pituitary gland powder 5 mg • Boron (chelated with citrate & aspartate) 3 mg. Other Ingredients: Microcrystalline Cellulose, Stearic Acid, Silicon Dioxide, Croscarmellose Sodium, Hydroxypropyl Methylcellulose, Magnesium Stearate, Polyethylene Glycol, Mineral oil, Shellac, & Talc. See Editor's Note No. 14, page 1817.

Rejuvine - Metabolic Response Modifiers
Two teaspoons contain: DHEA 25 mg • Pregnenolone 25 mg.

Relax & Ease Tension - ProHerbs
Two tablets contain: Thiamine HCl (B1) 50 mg • Riboflavin (B2) 50 mg • Vitamin B6 (Pyridoxine HCl) 50 mg • Vitamin B12 (Cyanocobalamin) 100 mcg • Kava Kava root (Piper methysticum standardized to 30% kavalactones) 300 mg • Passion Flower (Passiflora incarnata standardized to 4% flavonoids) 100 mg • Chamomile flower (Matricaria chamomilla standardized to greater than 1% apigenin) 100 mg. Other Ingredients: Dicalcium Phosphate, Microcrystalline Cellulose, Croscarmellose Sodium, Hydroxypropylmethylcellulose, Magnesium Stearate, Mineral Oil, Polyethylene Glycol, Stearic Acid, Titanium Dioxide, Sodium Lauryl Sulfate, Yellow #6 Lake, FD&C Blue #1 Lake, FD&C Red #40 Lake, FD&C Blue #2 Lake.

Relax & Sleep - Futurebiotics
Two tablets contain: Calcium (as calcium carbonate, phosphate, amino acid chelate) 150 mg • Magnesium (as magnesium oxide, amino acid chelate) 150 mg • Relax & Sleep Blend, 860 mg: Valerian root powder, Chamomile flower powder, Hawthorn berry powder, Fennel seed powder, Passion flower powder, Skullcap leaf powder, Hops flower powder, Lemon Balm herb powder, Oat Straw leaf/stem powder, Red Clover herb powder, Catnip leaf powder, Spearmint leaf powder, Vanilla bean powder. Other ingredients: Dicalcium phosphate, Stearic acid, Magnesium stearate, Silica.

Relax & Sleep Formula 2 - Futurebiotics
Two tablets contain: Valerian root - A balanced blend of extract & powder equivalent to dried root 500 mg. • Chamomile - A balanced blend of extract & powder equivalent to dried blossoms 250 mg • Magnesium (oxide, amino acid chelate) 150 mg • Calcium (carbonate, phosphate, amino acid chelate) 150 mg. Specially formulated in a base of natural, time-tested herbs (in the form of extracts & powders) including: Hawthorn berry, Fennel, Passion flower, Scullcap, Hops, Lemon Balm, Avena Sativa, Red Clover, Catnip, Spearmint leaves & Vanilla.

Relax Now - Health Factor
Each capsule contains: Kava Kava 100 mg • Valerian 100 mg • Scutellaria 100 mg • Passion flower (2:1 extract) 75 mg • Hops 25 mg • Chamomilla 6X • Lady Slipper 3X.

Relax-O-Comp - PhytoPharmica
Each tablet contains: Vitamin D (Fish Liver oil) 50 IU • Calcium Citrate 162 mg • Niacin/Niacinamide 65 mg • Magnesium Gluconate 50 mg • Magnesium (Oxide) 50 mg • Vitamin B6 (Pyridoxine HCL) 10 mg • Zinc (Chelate) 10 mg • Other Ingredients: Valerian extract Extra Strength (Valeriana officinalis) 75 mg • Chamomile extract (Matricaria chamomilla) 75 mg • Passion flower extract (Passiflora) 30 mg • Hops extract (Humulus lupulus) 30 mg • Unsaturated Free Fatty Acids 10 mg. In a base of Raw Crude Licorice extract, Peppermint & Anise seeds. Contains no sugar, salt, yeast, wheat, corn, soy, dairy products, flavoring, or preservatives.

Relax-U - The Herbalist
Valerian root • Skullcap herb • Passionflower herb.

Relief Plus - Health Factor
Each capsule contains: Goldenseal extract (4:1)(Hydrastis canadensis) 125 mg • Chamomile (Matricaria chamomilla) 100 mg • Valerian (Valeriana officinalis) 85 mg • Feverfew (Tanacetum parthenium) 590 mg • Cayenne Pepper 50 mg.

Reliv Arthaffect - Reliv International
Each scoop (8.5 g) contains: Arthred (hydrolyzed collagen) • Glucosamine Sulfate • Ginkgo Biloba • Borage Oil Powder • Turmeric • Boswellia Serrata • Ashwagandha • Cat's Claw • Sarsaparilla Root • Licorice Root • Kelp • Burdock Root • Alfalfa • Barley Grass • Echinacea Root • Yucca Extract • Devil's Claw Extract • Bilberry Extract • Celery Seed • Capsicum • Aloe Vera • Bioperine (Piper nigrum extract) • Soy Lecithin.

Reliv Celleboost - Reliv International
Two capsules contain: (-)Hydroxycitric Acid 375 mg • Oatrim (Hydrolyzed Oat Flour) 360 mg • Chromium 50 mcg.

Reliv Cellebrate - Reliv International
Each scoop contains: (-) Hydroxycitric Acid 375 mg • L-Carnitine 75 mg • Chromium 50 mcg • Choline 50 mg • Inositol 50 mg • Gamma-Linolenic Acid (as Borage Oil Powder) 50 mg • Ginkgo Biloba Leaves 33 mg • Coenzyme Q10 15 mg. Other Ingredients: Maltodextrin, Soy Lecithin, & Quaker Oatrim (Hydrolyzed Oat Flour).

Reliv Classic - Reliv International
Each scoop (16 g) contains: Soy Protein Isolate • Soy Flour • Brewer's Yeast • Lecithin • Psyllium Fiber • Dicalcium Phosphate • Ascorbic Acid • Methionine • Potassium Chloride • Magnesium Phosphate • Natural Flavor • Licorice Root • Garlic Rhubarb Root • Rose Hips • Cayenne • Kelp • OptiZinc Brand of Zinc Momomethionine • Ferrous Fumarate • Calcium Pantothenate • Niacinamide • Vitamin E Acetate • Vitamin A Palmitate • Vitamin D • Copper • Gluconate • Papain • Bromelain • Thiamin HCL • Riboflavin • Beta Carotene • Pyridoxine HCL • Biotin • Folic Acid • Potassium Iodine • Vitamin B12 • Soldium Selenite • ChromeMate Brand of Niacin Bound Chromium Polynicotinate.

Reliv FibRestore - Reliv International
Each scoop (30 g) contains: Fructose • Fiber Blend: Oat Fiber, Corn Bran, Apple Fiber, Soy Fiber, Pea Fiber, Citrus Fiber, Carrageenan Gum, Guar Gum, Xanthan Gum, Gum Arabic • Maltodextrin • Natural Flavor • Herbal Blend: Oriental Ginseng, Garlic, Cayenne, Licorice Root, Kelp, Rhubarb Root, Hibiscus, Irish Moss, Siberian Ginseng, Aloe Vera Powder, Chicory Root, Dandelion Root, Chamomile Powder, Alfalfa Powder, Pearl Barley, Ginger Root, Celery Seed, Sarsaparilla, Passion Flower, Capsicum Fruit Powder, Fenugreek • Lecithin • Ascorbic Acid • Citric Acid • Beta Carotene • Alpha Tocopheryl Acetate • Pepsin • Papain • Bromelain.

Reliv Innergize! - Reliv International
Each scoop (19 g) contains: Fructose • Maltodextrin • Citric Acid • Potassium Citrate • Natural Flavor • Tricalcium Phosphate • Sodium Chloride • Magnesium Oxide • Ascorbic Acid • Beta Carotene • OptiZinc Brand of Zinc Monomethionine • ChromeMate Brand of Niacin Bound Chromium Polynicotinate.

Reliv Now - Reliv International
Each scoop (15 g) contains: Whey • Soy Protein Isolate • Fructose • Dicalcium Phosphate • Magnesium Phosphate • Calcium Caseinate • Calcium Carbonate • Natural Flavor • Ascorbic Acid • Potassium Chloride • Lecithin • PABA (para-aminobenzoic acid) • Kelp • OptiZinc Brand of Zinc Monomethionine • Ferrous Fumarate • Calcium Pantothenate • Beta Carotene • Vitamin A Palmitate •

BRAND NAMES

Vitamin D (as Vitamin D3) • Thiamin HCL • Riboflavin • Niacinamide • Vitamin E Acetate • Pyridoxine HCL • Folic Acid • Vitamin B12 • Potassium Iodide • Copper Gluconate • Biotin • Sodium Selenite • ChromeMate Brand of Niacin Bound Chromium Polynicotinate • Sodium Molybdate • Vitamin K • Manganese Sulfate • Rutin • Garlic • Cayenne • Butternut Bark • Rhubarb Root • Blue Vervain • Licorice Root • Irish Moss.

Reliv ProVantage - Reliv International
Each scoop (26 g) contains: Soy Protein Isolate • Fructose • Medium Chain Triglycerides • Creatine Monohydrate • Tonalin (Conjugated Linoleic Acid-CLA) • Lecithin • L-Arginine • L-Glutamine • L-Leucine • L-Lysine • L-Carnitine • L-Alanine • Glycine • Ornithine Alpha Ketoglutarate • Coenzyme Q10 • Activin (Grape Seed extract) • Phosphatidylserine & Phosphatidylcholine (as Phosphatidylserine/Phosphatidylcholine Complex) • Bioperine (Piper nigrum extract) • Natural & Artificial Flavors • Alpha-Lipoic Acid

Reliv SoySentials - Reliv International
Each scoop (22 g) contains: Soy Protein Isolate • Fructose • Inulin • Dehydrated Cranberries • Calcium Carbonate • Dicalcium Phosphate • Lactobacillus Acidophilus • Lecithin • Natural & Artifical Flavors • Activin (Grape seed extract) • Protykin (Resveratrol) • Ipriflavone • Black Cohosh Root • Dong Quai Root • Wild Yam • Panax Ginseng • Green Tea Extract • Chasteberry • Horse Chestnut • Nettle Root • Hops • Licorice Root • Coenzyme Q10 • Folic Acid • Ascorbic Acid • Pyridoxine HCL • Alpha Tocopheryl Acetate • Beet Powder • Stevia Extract • Acesulfame Potassium • Alpha Lipoic Acid.

Reliv Ultrim-Plus - Reliv International
Each scoop (28 g) contains: Soy Protein Isolate • Whey • Fructose • Milk Protein • Nonfat Dry Milk • Xanthan Gum • Dicalcium Phosphate • Magnesium Phosphate • Calcium Carbonate • Natural & Artificial Flavor • Ascorbic Acid • Potassium Chloride • Lecithin • Aspartame • PABA (Para-aminobenzoic acid) • Kelp • OptiZinc Brand of Zinc Monomethionine • Ferrous Fumarate • Calcium Pantothenate • Vitamin A Palmitate • Vitamin D (as Vitamin D3) • Thiamin HCL • Riboflavin • Niacinamide • Vitamin E Acetate • Pyridoxine HCL • Folic Acid • Vitamin B12 • Potassium Iodide • Copper Gluconate • Biotin • Sodium Selenite • ChromeMate Brand of Niacin Bound Chromium Polynicotinate • Sodium Molybdate • Vitamin K • Manganese Sulfate • Rutin • Garlic • Cayenne • Butternut Bark • Rhubarb Root • Blue Vervain • Licorice Root • Irish Moss.

Remember-FX - HerbTech
North American Ginseng (Panax quinquefolium) 100 mg.

Remifemin - SmithKline Beecham
Each tablet contains: Black Cohosh (Cimicifuga racemosa) & rhizome extract (standardized to contain 1 mg of triterpene glycosides calculated as 27-Deoxyacetin) 20 mg. Other Ingredients: Lactose, Cellulose, Potato Starch, Magnesium Stearate, Natural Peppermint Flavor.

Remifemin - PhytoPharmica
Each tablet contains: Black Cohosh (Cimicifuga racemosa) root and rhizome extract (standardized to contain triterpene glycosides [calculated as 27-deoxyactein]) 20 mg.

Remifemin Plus - Enzymatic Therapy/PhytoPharmica
Each tablet contains: Standardized Cimicifuga racemosa (Black Cohosh) root & rhizome extract (standardized for triterpene glycosides content, calculated as 27-Deoxyactein) 20 mg • St. John's Wort extract standardized to contain hypericin 250 mcg. Contains no sugar, salt, yeast, wheat, gluten, corn, soy, dairy products (except lactose), coloring, flavoring, or preservatives.

Remotiv - Zeller
Each tablet contains: Hypericum extract Ze 117, standardized to a daily amount of 1 mg hypericin (St. John's Wort) 250 mg.

Renatrate - Progressive Labs
Each capsule contains: Vitamin A 5000 IU • Vitamin C 90 mg • Bovine kidney concentrate 300 mg. The glandular concentrate in this product is prepared by a special process which does not exceed physiological temperature (37° C). Guaranteed free of chemical pesticides and synthetic hormones. See Editor's Note No. 14, page 1817.

Renew-U - The Herbalist
Milk Thistle seed • Echinacea root • Oregon Grape root • Dandelion herb • Burdock root • Yellow Dock root • Cleavers herb • Wild Indigo root • Ginger root • Fennel seed.

Repagene Emulsion - Atrium Inc.
Each teaspoon contains: Squalene 1 1/2 g in an Emulsified form. Contains no sugar or artificial flavor.

Repose - Chattem
One caplet contains: Vitamin C (as Calcium Ascorbate) 100 mg • Vitamin B6 (as Pyridoxine HCl) 14 mg • Pantothenic Acid (as D-Calcium Pantothenate) 17 mg • Magnesium (as Magnesium Oxide) 70 mg • Standardized Kava root extract (30% kavalactones) 200 mg • Standardized Siberian Ginseng root extract (0.8% eleutherosides) 65 mg. Contains no starch, yeast, caffeine, dairy or preservatives.

Resist - Pacific BioLogic
Astragalus root (Grade 1) • Ganoderma Fungus • Codonopsis root • Jujube fruit • Atractylodes (white) rhizome • Peony root (white) • Citrus peel (tangerine) • Cuscuta seeds • Dioscorea root • Schizandra fruit • Licorice root • Milletta root • Platycodon root • Ligustrum fruit • Glehnia root • Rehmannia root (prep.) • Ginger rhizome (fresh).

Resist 2 - Pacific BioLogic
Bitter Melon • St. John's Wort • Red Marine Algae • Echinacea Angustifolia • Tumeric rhizome • Licorice root (honey-baked) • Ligustrum root (Chinese) • Citrus peel (tangerine) • Viola (whole plant) • Prunella (selfheal spike) • Trichosanthis root • Knotweed rhizome (bushy) • Aucklandia root.

Respa-Herb - Dial Herbs
Ma Huang • Mullein • Goldenseal • Colts Foot • Comfrey • Marshmallow • Lobelia • Cayenne.

Resphora - PhysioLogics
Each capsule contains: Tylophora (GPH: 0.1% tylophorine alkaloids) 30 mg • Piper longum (GPH: 2% piperine) • Picrorhiza kurroa (GPH: 4% kutkin) 50 mg.

Respi-Oil - The Herbalist
Essential oils of Eucalyptus, Rosemary, Sage, Tea Tree & Nutmeg in a Sweet Almond oil base.

Respir-all - Now
Three tablets contain: Vitamin B5 (Pantothenic Acid) 100 mg • Vitamin B6 (Pyridoxine HCL) 20 mg • Vitamin C (as Magnesium Ascorbate) 500 mg • Magnesium (as Magnesium Ascorbate) 40 mg • Zinc (as L-OptiZinc Monomethionine) 10 mg • Quercetin 800 mg • Nettle root extract (Urtica dioica) (standardized 30 ppm Scopoletin) 500 mg • Bromelain (2000 GDU) 500 mg • Licorice root (Glycyrrhiza glabra) 4:1 extract 200 mg.

Respiratory Support - Amazon Support
Each capsule contains: Amor Seco • Embauba • Samambaia • Espinheira Santa • Fedegosa • Mullaca • Mutamba • Sarsaparilla • Jatoba • Vassourinha.

Respiratory Support Formula - PhysioLogics
Two capsules contain: Vitamin C (Ascorbic Acid) 130 mg • Ephedra root, stem (6% total Ephedrine Alkaloids, 12 mg) 200 mg • Lemon

Bioflavonoids citrus 66 mg • Pleurisy root 45 mg • Mullein leaf 38 mg • Slippery Elm bark 38 mg • Licorice root 35 mg • Red Clover tops 35 mg • Ginkgo leaf (24% Ginkgo Flavonglycosides, 7.2 mg; 6 % Terpene Lactones, 1.8 mg) 30 mg.

Respiratory Support Formula - Health Smart Vitamins
Two capsules contain: Vitamin C (as ascorbic acid) 130 mg • Ma Huang stem (6% total ephedrine alkaloids 12 mg) 200 mg • Citrus Bioflavonoids 66 mg • Pleurisy Root 45 mg • Mullein leaf 38 mg • Slippery Elm bark 38 mg • Licorice root 35 mg • Red Clover flower 35 mg • Ginkgo leaf (24% ginkgo flavonglycosides, 7.2 mg; 6% terpene lactones 1.8 mg) 30 mg.

Respi-Tea - The Herbalist
Wild Cherry bark • Slippery Elm bark • Coltsfoot leaf • Marshmallow root • Licorice root • Cinnamon bark • Yarrow blossom • Ginger root.

Respitonic - The Herbalist
Echinacea root • Golden Seal root • Osha root • Yerba Santa leaf • Horseradish root • Yarrow blossom • Cayenne pepper.

Restful - BioDynamax
Two capsules contain: Kava Kava root extract 300 mg • Chamomile 100 mg • Passion flower 100 mg • Calcium 100 mg • Magnesium 50 mg.

Restore-X - Cambridge Nutraceuticals
Each serving contains: L-Glutamine 10 g • N-Acetyl-Cysteine 600 mg • L-Arginine (from Zinc Arginate) 140 mg • Vitamin A (as mixed carotenoids) 5000 IU • Vitamin C 500 mg • Vitamin E 200 IU • Thiamin 6 mg • Riboflavin 6.8 mg • Niacin 80 mg • Vitamin B6 8 mg • Pantothenic Acid 40 mg • Magnesium 200 mg • Zinc 20 mg • Selenium 100 mcg • Copper 0.75 mg • Folate 400 mcg • Vitamin B12 50 mcg.

Resveratone - Metabolic Response Modifiers
Each capsule contains: Polygonum cuspidatum (yielding 16 mg Resveratrol) 200 mg.

Revenge - Champion Nutrition
Each 29 g serving contains: Vitamin C 60 mg • Vitamin E 60 IU • Thiamine 5 mg • Riboflavin 3 mg • Vitamin B6 5 mg • Pantothenic Acid 10 mg • Magnesium 12 mg • Chromium 240 mcg • Potassium 160 mg. Tropical Mango Blast Ingredients: Metacarb VII (proprietary carbohydrate blend which contains Amylopectin Food Starch Modified, Glucose Polymer [Maltodextrin]) • Fructose • Peptol-7 (proprietary Protein-Amino Acid Blend which contains: Whey Protein Concentrate, L-Leucine, Glycine, L-Glutamine, Taurine, L-Isoleucine & L-Valine) • Lactate Blend (Sodium Potassium Lactate, Creatine Lactate, Glycerol Stearate, Magnesium Lactate, Glycerol Lactate) • Glucose (Dextrose) • Natural & Artificial Flavoring • Cellulose • Malic Acid • Trutina Dulcem (Natural Kiwi extract) • Phosphatidylcholine • D-Ribose • Vitamin E Acetate • Talc • Ginseng Root extract • Proteoglycan Support (proprietary blend which includes Glucosamine Hcl & Glucosamine Ascorbate) • Creatine Alpha-Ketoglutarate • Citric Acid • Potassium Phosphate • Guarana seed extract (standardized to 50% Caffeine) • Potassium Citrate • Ascorbic Acid • Quercetin • Willow Bark extract (standardized to 50% Salycin) • Sunett (Acesulfame-K) • Sodium Citrate • Omega-3 Fatty Acids (Fish oil) • Xanthan Gum • Feverfew extract • Vitamin B Blend (Vitamin B1, Vitamin B2, Vitamin B3, Vitamin B5, Vitamin B6, Pantethine) • Curcumin • N-Acetylcysteine • Periwinkle standardized extract • Coenzyme Q10 • Lipoic Acid • Chromium Polynicotinate • Annatto & Carmine (natural colors).

ReVitalize - Rx Vitamins
Three purecaps contain: Mixed Carotenoid complex (alpha, beta & gamma carotenes) 25000 IU • Vitamin C (ascorbic acid) 200 mg • Pantothenic Acid (calcium pantothenate) 100 mg • Calcium (amino

acid chelate/complex) 50 mg • Magnesium (amino acid chelate/complex) 50 mg • Vitamin B1 (thiamine) 50 mg • Vitamin B2 (riboflavin) 50 mg • Vitamin B3 (niacin) 50 mg • Vitamin B6 (pyridoxine HCl) 50 mg • Citrus Flavonoid complex (active flavonols, flavonones, flavones & naringen-44%) 50 mg • Choline (bitartrate) 50 mg • Inositol 50 mg • Potassium (glycero-phosphate) 25 mg • Zinc (amino acid chelate/complex) 15 mg • Manganese (amino acid chelate/complex) 5 mg • Iron (amino acid chelate/complex) 4.5 mg • Copper (glycinate) 1 mg • Vanadium (as vanadyl sulfate) 1 mg • Vitamin D (calciferol) 400 IU • Vitamin E (d-alpha tocopherol) 200 IU • Folic Acid 400 mcg • Biotin 300 mcg • Iodine (kelp) 150 mcg • Vitamin B12 (cyanocobalamin) 100 mcg • Chromium (polynicotinate) 50 mcg • Selenium (amino acid complex) 50 mcg • Molybdenum (amino acid complex) 20 mcg • Korean Ginseng (Panax ginseng, standardized 5% ginsenosides) 50 mg • Chinese Green Tea extract (Camilla sinensis, standardized 40% polyphenols) 25 mg • Ginkgo Biloba (standardized 24% ginkgoflavoneglycosides, 6% terpene lactones) 10 mg • Bilberry (Vaccinium myrtillus, standardized 25% anthocyanosides) 5 mg • Wild Grape seed extract (Mahonia aquifolia, standardized 95-100% leucoanthocyanins) 5 mg • Oleoresin Turmeric (Curcuma longa, standardized 90-95% curcuminoids) 5 mg • Milk Thistle (Silybum marianum, standardized 80% Silymarin) 75 mg • Parsley Leaves (Petroselinum crispum, naturally rich in apiin & luteolin-7-apiolglucoside) 75 mg • Juniper Berries (juniperus communis, naturally rich in glucuronic acid) 50 mg • Celery seed 4x (Aplum graveolens, naturally rich in limonene) 50 mg • Cayenne (Capsicum frutescens, naturally rich in capsaicin) 50 mg • Glucosamine Sulfate (aminomonosaccharide) 30 mg • Borage Seed Oil (Borago officinalis, standardized 25% gamma linolenic acid) 25 mg.

Rezyme - Nature's Secret
Vegetarian Enzyme that contains a proprietary blend of Amylase, Glucoamylase, Cellulase, Lipase, Lactase, Alpha Galactosidase, Bromelain, Papain, Betaine HCl, Gentian, Licorice, and Ginger root. Enzyme Rebuilder, which contains Bitters, Lecithin, L-Glutamine, and Piper longum fruit.

Rhino Acidophilus - Dial Herbs
Lactobacillus acidophilus • Bifidobacterium bifidum • Bifidobacterium infantis • FOS, in a base of rice powder & natural flavors • Vitamin C from Ester-C. Flavored & sweetened with all-natural raspberry fruit juice crystals, dextrose & fructose.

Rhino Actalin Bars - Nutrition Now
Soy Protein Isolate, Calcium Sodium Caseinate, Whey Protein Concentrate, Glucose, High Fructose Glucose Syrup, Fractionated Vegetable Oils, Turbinado Sugar, Non-Fat Dry Milk, Yogurt Solids, Vanilla, Lecithin, Raisins, Apple Paste, Natural Flavors, Apple Fiber, Graham Flour, and Cinnamon.

Rhino Actalin Dietary Supplement - Nutrition Now
Each tablet contains: Magnesium 20 mg • Inosine 50 mg • Phosphatidylserine 50 mg • Amino Acid Blend 50 mg.
See Editor's Note No. 21, page 1818.

Rhino Chewy Vites - Dial Herbs
Vitamin A • Vitamin C • Vitamin D • Vitamin E • Vitamin B6 • Vitamin B12 • Calcium • Thiamin • Riboflavin • Folic Acid • Biotin • Pantothenic Acid • Iodine • Magnesium • Zinc • Choline • Inositol • Fruitrim: (Fruit juice, Natural grain dextrins) • Evaporated Cane juice (natural milled sugar) • Gelatin • Lactate • Gluconate • Ascorbic Acid • d-Alpha Tocopheryl Acetate • Citrate Palmitate • Betartrate • Citric Acid • Lactic Acid • Natural Flavors • Natural Colors added including Annatto, Turmeric, Carmine & Grape skin liquid • Lightly polished with Fractionated Vegetable oil (Coconut origin) to prevent sticking • Beeswax.

BRAND NAMES

Some Brand Name Natural Products - What they Contain

B R A N D   N A M E S

Rhino Daily Pack - Nutrition Now
Each packet contains two Rhino Vites- 100% natural daily multi-vitamin, two Rhino Calcium, one Rhino Ester-C (Vitamin C).

Rhino Echinacea - Dial Herbs
Two tablets contain: Echinacea 100 mg • Vitamin C 60 mg. Flavored & sweetened with all natural raspberry fruit juice crystals, dextrose & fructose.

Rhino Ester-C - Dial Herbs
Vitamin C from Ester-C • Calcium. Flavored & sweetened with all-natural cherry flavorings, natural fruit flavors, fructose, dextrose & bilberry.

Rhino Pops Box - Dial Herbs
Each lollipop contains: Isomalt • Maltitol • Citric Acid • Ascorbic Acid 50 mg • Natural Flavor • Color from Beet liquid • Echinacea • Goldenseal • Phosphorus 6x • Drosera 6x • Kali Carbonicum 6x • Belladonna 6x • Rumex Crispus 6x • Hydrastis 6x.
See Editor's Note No. 1, page 1816.

Rhino Support Pack - Nutrition Now
Each packet contains: Two Rhino Echinacea, two Rhino Acidophilus, one Rhino Ester-C (Vitamin C).

Rhizinate - PhytoPharmica
Two tablets contain: Licorice root extract (deglycyrrhizinated; Glycyrhiza glabra) 760 mg • Glycine (amino acid) in a base of fructose 100 mg.

Rhizinate - Chocolate-Mint - PhytoPharmica
Two tablets contain: Licorice (Glycyrhiza glabra) root extract 4:1 (deglycyrrhizinated) 760 mg • Glycine (amino acid) in a base of fructose 100 mg. Flavored with Dutch Cocoa Powder, Creme Flavor, and Peppermint.

Riboflavin - PhytoPharmica
Each tablet contains: Riboflavin (vitamin B2) 400 mg.

Rice Bran Oil - Progressive Labs
Each tablespoon contains: Rice bran oil 14 g.

Rich's MSM Eye and Ear Drops - Rich Distributing
Methylsulfonylmethane • Sterilized Activated Water.
See Editor's Note No. 27, page 1819.

Ripped Fuel - TwinLab
Ma Huang 20 mg • Guarana 200 mg • Chromium 200 mcg • L-Carnitine 100 mg.

Ripped Fuel (Metabolic Enhancer) - TwinLab
Two capsules contain: Ma Huang extract (standardized for 6% Ephedrine) 334 mg • Guarana extract (standardized for 22% Caffeine) 910 mg • L-Carnitine 100 mg • Chromium (Chromium Picolinate) 200 mcg.

RNA/DNA - Puritan's Pride
Each tablet contains: RNA (Ribonucleic Acid) 100 mg • DNA (Deoxyribonucleic Acid) 100 mg. In a base containing 400 mg of Dried Debittered Brewer's Yeast.

Robert's Complex - Enzymatic Therapy
Each capsule contains: Niacinamide 5 m. Other ingredients: American Cranesbill (Geranium maculatum) 100 mg • Cabbage extract (Braccica oleracea) 100 mg • Marshmallow extract 4:1 (Althaea officinalis) mucilage content 30-40%)75 mg • Okra (Hibiscus esculentis) 75 mg • Slippery Elm (Ulma fulva) 75 mg • Duodenal Substance 75 mg • Echinacea root extract (Echinacea angustifolia)

standardized to contain greater than 3.5% Echinacosides & 0.65% essential oils 25 mg • Goldenseal root extract (Hydrastis canadensis) standardized to contain 5% total Alkaloids including: Berberine, Hydrastine, & Canadine 25 mg • Pancreatic Enzymes 25 mg. Contains no sugar, salt, yeast, wheat, corn, soy, dairy products, coloring, flavoring or preservatives.
See Editor's Note No. 14, page 1817.

Robert's Formula - PhytoPharmica
Two capsules contain: Niacinamide 10 mg • American Cranesbill (Geranium maculatum) root 200 mg • Cabbage (Brassica oleracea) leaf extract 4:1 200 mg • Marshmallow (althaea officinalis) root extract 4.25:1 150 mg • Okra (Abelmoschus esculentis) whole plant 150 mg • Slippery Elm (Ulma fulva) bark 150 mg • Duodenal substance 50 mg • Echinacea (Echinacea angustifolia) root extract (standardized to contain greater than 4% echinacosides) 50 mg • Goldenseal (Hydrastis canadensis) root and rhizome extract 4:1 (standardized to contain 5% total alkaloids including berberine, hydrastine, and canadine) 50 mg • Pancreatic enzymes 50 mg.
See Editor's Note No. 14, page 1817.

Rolaids - Extra Strength - Pfizer Inc
Each tablet contains: Calcium Carbonate (providing Calcium 271 mg) 675 mg • Magnesium Hydroxide (providing Magnesium 56 mg) 135 mg • Calcium Carbonate 675 mg • Magnesium Hydroxide 135 mg. Other ingredients: Dextrose, Magnesium Stearate, Polyethylene Glycol, Pregelatinized Starch, Sucrose.
See Editor's Note No. 5, page 1816.

Rosemary - Nature's Way
Two capsules contain: Rosemary herb 800 mg. Other Ingredients: Gelatin, Magnesium Stearate.

RoseOx - Natrol
One capsule contains: Rosemary dried powdered extract leaf 250 mg. Other ingredients: Rice powder, Magnesium Stearate, Gelatin.

Royal Bee Power - Nature's Plus
Two tablets contain: Bee Pollen 500 mg • Propolis from extract 500 mg Royal Jelly 50 mg. In a high energy natural base containing Gotu Kola, Ginseng & Fo-Ti. Contains no yeast, wheat, corn, soy, milk or salt.

Royal Jelly 2000 - Premier One - Nutraceutical
One capsule contains: Royal Jelly 3.5x (equivalent to 2000 mg) 572 mg.

RTD 40 Advanced Mega Protein Shake - Nutripeak
Each can contains: Protein 40 g • Vitamin A (Retinyl Palmitate) 5000 IU • Vitamin C (Ascorbic Acid) 24 mg • Calcium Caseinate 24 mg • Iron (Ferrous Fumarate) 2.7 mg • Vitamin D (Cholecalciferol) 60 IU • Vitamin E (dl-Alpha Tocopheryl Acetate) 51 IU • Vitamin K (Phytonadione) 8 mcg • Thiamin Mononitrate .225 mg • Riboflavin .225 mg • Niacin (Niacinamide) 5 mg • Vitamin B6 (Pyridoxine Hydrochloride) .3 mg • Folic Acid 100 mcg • Vitamin B12 (Cyanocobalamin) .6 mcg • Biotin 45 mcg • Pantothenic Acid (Calcium D-Pantothenate) 1 mg • Phosphorus (Dipotassium Phosphorus and Potassium Triphosphate) 700 mg • Iodine (Potassium Iodide) 15 mcg • Magnesium Oxide 140 mg • Zinc Oxide 4.5 mg • Selenium (Sodium Selenate) 7 mcg • Copper (Cupric Sulfate) .2 mg • Manganese Sulfate .2 mg • Chromium Picolinate 12 mcg • Molybdenum (Sodium Molybdate) 15 mcg. Other Ingredients: Water Metamyosyn V4 Protein Blend: Milk Protein Concentrate, Milk Protein Isolate, Calcium Sodium Casseinate, Hydrolyzed Wheat Protein (Gluten), Maltodextrin, High Fat Cocoa (processed with alkali); Sodium Phosphate; Sodium Citrate; Sodium Polyphosphate; Beta Carotene; Natural and Artificial Flavors; Microcrystalline.

Rubus-Ginger Tea - HerbaSway
Ginger • Green Tea • Blackberry • HerbaSwee (Cucurbitaceae fruit).

Runners' Shield - Source Naturals
Two tablets contain: Vitamin A (Beta Carotene 12,500 IU and Palmitate 5,000 IU) 17,500 IU • Vitamin C (Magnesium Ascorbate, Ascorbic Acid and Manganese Ascorbate) 500 mg • Fat-Soluble Vitamin C (from 186 mg of Ascorbyl Palmitate) 80 mg • Vitamin E (Natural d-alpha) 200 IU • Magnesium (Ascorbate) 30 mg • Zinc (OptiZinc Monomethionine) 15 mg • Manganese (Ascorbate) 5 mg • Copper (Sebacate) 750 mcg • Selenium (Selenomethionine) 100 mcg • Quercetin 200 mg • N-Acetyl-Cysteine 100 mg • Silymarin (Milk Thistle Seed Extract) 50 mg • Ginkgo Biloba extract 24% (50:1) 5 mg • Hawthorn Berry extract (4:1) 150 mg • Rosemary 150 mg • Schizandra 125 mg • Marshmallow root 85 mg • Astragalus 60 mg.

Runny Nose formula - Dr. Morrow's Homeopathic Formulas
Ten drops contain: Allium cepa 3C • Belladonna 3C • Euphrasia 3C • Mercurius dulcis 6C • Hydrastis 3C • Kali bichromicum 3C • Sambucus nigra 3C.
See Editor's Note No. 1, page 1816.

Rx for Life Cellular Essentials Pack (Bio-C) - Rexall
Each tablet contains: Vitamin C (from ascorbyl palmitate, calcium ascorbate, magnesium ascorbate and ascorbic acid) 300 mg • Citrus Bioflavonoids 75 mg. Other Ingredients: Cellulose, Stearic Acid, Crospovidone, Croscarmellose Sodium, Silica, Magnesium Stearate.

Rx Fuel Bio-Designed Food Formula - TwinLab
Two servings contain: Branched Chain Amino Acids (L-Leucine, L-Isoleucine, & L-Valine) • L-Glutamine 1000 mg • L-Carnitine 100 mg • Chromium (from Chromic Fuel Chromium Picolinate) 200 mcg. No added sugar, fructose, corn syrup solids, artificial colors, artificial flavors, mono- & diglycerides, or salt. This unique formulation is rich in potassium, yet has only 200 mg of sodium per serving.

Rx-Bone Ostivone - Nutritional Dynamics
Two tablets contain: Vitamin D 100 IU • Calcium 1000 mg • Ostivone 200 mg. Other ingredients: Dicalcium Phosphate, Microcrystalline Cellulose, Silica, Stearic Acid, Pharmaceutical glaze.

SAF for Kids - Natrol
Six capsules contain: Vitamin C (Ester-C brand) 60 mg • Calcium 100 mg • Vitamin B6 (pyridoxine HCl) 50 mg • Magnesium 50 mg • Additional ingredients: GABA 800 mg • Glycine 800 mg • Passion flower extract 6:1 500 mg • L-Taurine 500 mg • Other ingredients: Microcrystalline Cellulose, Magnesium Stearate, Gelatin. SAF Patent #1,540,075.

SAF The Stress Formula - Natrol
Four capsules contain: Vitamin C (Ester-C Brand) 100 mg • Thiamine (Vitamin B1) 3 mg • Riboflavin (Vitamin B2) 3.1 mg • Niacin (Niacinamide) 50 mg • Vitamin B6 (Pyridoxine HCl) 4 mg • Magnesium 100 mg • GABA 650 mg • L-Tyrosine 650 mg • Siberian Ginseng 100 mg • Inositol 100 mg, Patent #4,973,467. Other ingredients: Calcium Carbonate, Magnesium Stearate, Microcrystalline Cellulose, Gelatin.

Safeway Select Women's One Tablet Multivitamin - Safeway, Inc.
Each tablet contains: Vitamin A (50% as beta carotene) 5000 IU • Vitamin C 60 mg • Vitamin D 400 IU • Vitamin E 30 IU • Thiamin 1.5 mg • Riboflavin 1.7 mg • Niacin 20 mg • Vitamin B-6 2 mg • Folate 400 mcg • Vitamin B-12 6 mcg • Pantothenic Acid 10 mg • Calcium 450 mg • Iron 27 mg • Zinc 15 mg.
See Editor's Note No. 3, page 1816.

Salad-Tabs - Wakunaga Consumer Products
Two tablets contain: Vitamin A (as Palmitate and Beta-Carotene) 5000 IU • Vitamin C (as Asorbic Acid) 60 mg • Vitamin D (as Cholecalciferol) 400 IU • Vitamin E (as D-Alpha-Tocopherol Acid Succinate) 30 IU • Thiamine (Vitamin B1) 1.5 mg • Riboflavin (Vitamin B2) 1.7 mg • Niacin 20 mg • Vitamin B6 (as Pyridoxine Hydrochloride) 2 mg • Folate (as Folic Acid) 400 mcg • Vitamin B12 (as Cyanocobalamin) 6 mcg • Biotin 300 mcg • Pantothenic Acid (as Calcium Pantothenate) 10 mg • Iron (as Ferrous Fumarate) 18 mg • Iodine (as Potassium Iodide) 150 mcg • Zinc (as Zinc Oxide) 15 mg • Copper (as Copper Gluconate) 2 mg • Manganese (as Manganese sulfate) 2 mg • Young Barley and Wheat Grass powder 600 mg • Chlorella 180 mg. Other Ingredients: Cellulose, Silica, Magnesium Stearate (vegetable source).

Salmon Oil - Puritan's Pride
Two softgels contain: EPA 240 mg • DHA 160 mg.

Salmon Oil 1000 mg - Jamieson
Each capsule contains: EPA (Eicosapentaenoic Acid) 180 mg • DHA (Docosahexaenoic Acid) 120 mg.

Salonpas - Hisamitsu Pharmaceutical Co., Inc.
Active Ingredients: Methyl Salicylate 132 mg • l-Menthol 120 mg • dl-Camphor 26 mg • Tocopherol Acetate 21 mg.

Salusan Herbal Rest - Flora
St. John's Wort • Passion Flower • Valerian "& other calming herbs."

Sambu - Flora
Elderberry.

Sambu Guard - Flora
Wildgrown elder fruit & flower • Echinacea • Acerola Cherry fruit powder) & Vitamin C.

Sambucol - Black Elderberry Extract - Nature's Way
Two teaspoons contain: Elderberry extract 3.8 g. Other Ingredients: Glucose Syrup, Rasberry extract, Honey, Citric Acid, Natural Flavor.

Sambucol Black Elder - Jb Harris
Each lozenge contains: Vitamin C (as ascorbic acid) 100 mg • Elderberry dried extract (berries) 130 mg. Other Ingredients: Sorbitol, Peppermint extract.

Sambucol Immune System - Jb Harris
Two teaspoons (10 mL) contain: Zinc 10 mg • Vitamin C 100 mg • Proprietary blend 4 g: Elderberry extract (berries), Propolis, Echinacea angustifolia (root), Echinacea purpurea (stems, leaves, flowers). Other Ingredients: Glucose syrup, raspberry extract (berries), honey, citric acid, & natural flavors.

Sambucol Lozenge - Nature's Way
Each lozenge contains: Sambucol (Black Elderberry extract) 130 mg • Vitamin C 100 mg. Other Ingredients: Peppermint extract, Sorbitol.

Sambucol Original - Jb Harris
Each lozenge contains: Black Elder Tree extract (sambucus nigra).

Sambucol-D (Sugar Free) - Jb Harris
Each tablespoon contains: Elderberry juice (Black Elder tree, sambucus nigra 1). Other Ingredients: Liquid sorbitol, water, citric acid, natural flavor, & raspberry.

SAMe - Natrol
Two tablets contain: S-Adenosyl-Methionine (SAMe) (as S-Adenosyl-Methionine Disulfate Ditosylate) 400 mg. Other Ingredients: Cellulose, Mannitol, Hydroxypropyl Methylcellulose Phthalate, Citric Acid, Sodium Starch Glycolate, Glyceryl Triacetate, Croscarmellose Sodium, Stearic Acid, Silica.
See Editor's Note No. 10, page 1817.

Some Brand Name Natural Products - What they Contain

SAMe - Pinnacle
Each tablet contains SAM-e 200 mg • Vitamin B12 50 mcg • Folic Acid 100 mcg.

SAMe - Olympian Labs
Each tablet contains: SAMe (S-adenosyl-L-methionine-tosylate-disulfate) 200 mg.

SAM-e - Nature Made Nutritional Products
Two tablets contain: S-adenosylmethionine 400 mg • 4-butanedisulfonate • Cellulose • Sodium Starch Glycolate • Methacrylic Acid Copolymer • Talc • Polyethylene Glycol • Silica • Magnesium Stearate • Polysorbate 80 • Sodium Hydroxide • Iron Oxide • Simethicone.
See Editor's Note No. 10, page 1817.

SAM-e - The Vitamin Shoppe
Two tablets contain: S-Adenosyl-L-Methionine 400 mg. Other Ingredients: Colloidal Silica, Microcrystalline Cellulose, Sodium Starch Glycolate, Magnesium Stearate, Methacrylic Acid Copolymer, Polyethylene Glycol, Simethicone, Polysorbate 80, Sodium Hydroxide, Magnesium Silicate, Iron Oxide.
See Editor's Note No. 10, page 1817.

SAM-e - TwinLab
Two tablets contain: SAMe (S-adenosylmethionine tosylate) 400 mg. Other Ingredients: Cellulose, Mannitol, Hydroxypropyl Methylcellulose, Citric Acid, Sodium Starch, Glycolate, Glyceryl Triacetate, Croscarmellose Sodium, Stearic Acid.
See Editor's Note No. 10, page 1817.

SAMe Extra Strength Super Size - Olympian Labs
Each tablet contains: SAMe (S-adenosyl-L-methionine-tosylate-disulfate) 400 mg.

SAMe Supersize - Olympian Labs
Each tablet contains: SAMe (s-adenosyl-l-methionine-tosylate-disulfate) 200 mg.

SAMe-Source Naturals - Source Naturals
Two tablets contain: SAMe (S-Adenosyl-L-Methionine) from 800 mg of SAMe Disulfate Tosylate 400 mg.
See Editor's Note No. 10, page 1817.

Sandal Turmeric (soap) - Auromere Ayurvedic Soaps
Coconut oil • Palmyra oil • Rice Bran oil • Alkali • Water • Hydnocarpus (Cactus) oil • Castor oil • Neem oil • Indian Beech oil • Mohwa (Madhuca Indica) oil • Sesame oil • Sandalwood oil • Neem Bark • Dhub Grass (Cynodon Dactylon) • Indian Gooseberry (Amla) • Turmeric • Peepal (Bodhi Tree) • Licorice • Celastrus seed • Tulsi (Holy Basil) • Corallacarpus epigaeus • Nutgrass • Zedoary • Indian Madder Root • Costus • Mung Bean • Fenugreek.

Sandelios Beauty Caps - Health From The Sun
Each capsule contains: Wheat Germ oil 150 mg • Yeast 50 mg • Vitamin E (d-Alpha Tocopherol) 10 mg • Nicotinamide 10 mg • Vitamin B2 1 mg • Calcium D-Pantothenate 6.5 mg • Vitamin B1 1.2 mg • Vitamin B6 1 mg • Carotin 0.8mg • D-Biotin 20 mcg • Vitamin B12 2 mcg. No sugar, preservatives, artificial coloring or flavoring.

Sandelios Garlic Caps - Health From The Sun
Each capsule contains: Garlic oil with Allicin 270 mg. No sugar, preservatives, artificial coloring or flavoring.

Sanhelios Circu Caps with Butcher's Broom - Health From The Sun
Each capsule contains: natural Rusci aculeati (Butcher's Broom) extract 75 mg • Rosemary oil 2 mg. No sugar. No preservatives. No artificial coloring or flavoring.

Sanhelios Devil's Claw Caps - Health From The Sun
Each capsule contains: natural Devil's Claw extract 120 mg. No sugar, preservatives, artificial coloring or flavoring.

Sanhelios Garlic Forte - Health From The Sun
Each gelcap contains: Garlic oil, Maceration 2-3:1 280 mg. No sugar, starch, salt, preservatives, coloring, or flavoring.

Sanhelios Kalm Caps - Health From The Sun
Each capsule contains: Valerian root extract 4:1 150 mg. No sugar, preservatives, artificial coloring or flavoring.

Sanhelios Onion Caps - Health From The Sun
Each capsule contains: natural etherial Onion oil from Allium Cepa Linne 1.5 mg. No sugar, preservatives, artificial coloring or flavoring.

Sanhelios Propolentum Capsules - Health From The Sun
Each capsule contains: Propolis 250 mg.

Sanhelios Propolentum Throat Lozenges - Health From The Sun
Each lozenge contains: Isomalt 1465 mg • Menthol Crystals 3 mg • Propolis powder 30 mg • Peppermint oil 2 mg.

Sanhelios Prosta Caps - Health From The Sun
Each capsule contains: Pumpkin seed oil with Cucurbitin 150 mg • Alpha-Tocopherolacetate equalling 40.8 IU • Vitamin E 30 mg. No sugar, preservatives, artificial coloring or flavoring.

Sanhelios Water Caps - Health From The Sun
Each capsule contains: natural Juniper berry oil 20 mg. No sugar, preservatives, artificial coloring or flavoring.

Satietrol - PacificHealth Laboratories
Each (18 g) packet contains: Casein from Whey Protein Isolate enriched with glycomacropeptides • Potato Fiber • Sunflower Oil • Corn Syrup Solids • Natural & Artificial Flavors • Konjac Flour • Maltodextrin • Guar Gum • Calcium Lactate • Sodium Caseinate • Soy Lecithin • Alfalfa Powder • Monoglycerides • Diglycerides • Dipotassium Phosphate • Sodium Silicoaluminate • Aspartame.

Saventaro - PhytoPharmica
Each capsule contains: Saventaro (Uncaria tomentosa) pentacylic chemotype standardized to contain a minimum of 1.3% pentacyclic oxindole alkaloids (POAs) and to be free of tetracyclic oxindole alkaloids (TOAs) 20 mg. Other Ingredients: Cellulose, Calcium Carbonate, Magnesium Stearate, Silicon Dioxide, Gelatin Capsule.

Saw Palmetto - Centrum Herbals
One softgel contains: Saw Palmetto berry extract (Serenoa repens) 160 mg. Total Fatty Acids (marker) 80% (Standardized to contain- based on extract weight): Linolenic Acid (natural active) • Lauric Acid, Ethyl Ester (natural active) • Linoleic Acid, Ethyl Ester (natural active) • Activity measure: Adrenergic alpha 1B binding assay. Other ingredients: Corn oil, Yellow Wax, Gelatin, Propylene Glycol, Hydroxypropyl Methylcellulose, Titanium Dioxide, Carmine.
See Editor's Note No. 2, page 1816.

Saw Palmetto - Natrol
Each softgel contains: Saw Palmetto extract berries (serenoa repens) 160 mg. Other Ingredients: Olive Oil, Glycerin, Gelatin.
See Editor's Note No. 2, page 1816.

Saw Palmetto - Leiner Health Products
Two softgels contain: Saw Palmetto extract (Serenoa repens) berry 160 mg. Other Ingredients: Soybean Oil, Gelatin, Glycerin, Caramel, Titanium Dioxide, Red 40, Blue 1.

Some Brand Name Natural Products - What they Contain
www.NaturalDatabase.com contains MANY more listings than appear here.

Saw Palmetto - Gaia Herbs
Saw Palmetto standardized for 90% fatty acids. Standardized Full Spectrum 150 mg of extract per capsule. Guaranteed Potency 75 mg of extract per capsule.

Saw Palmetto - Metabolic Response Modifiers
Each capsule contains: Saw Palmetto oil (Serenoa repens, containing 85-95% saponins) 160 mg.

Saw Palmetto - Pharmanex
Each softgel contains: Saw Palmetto berries (10:1) extract (Serenoa repens) 160 mg. Other Ingredients: Olive Oil, Gelatin, Glycerin, Carob.

Saw Palmetto - Puritan's Pride
Each softgel contains: Saw Palmetto extract berry (serenoa repens) 320 mg. Other Ingredients: Gelatin, Glycerin.

Saw Palmetto - Smart Basics
Each softgel contains: Saw Palmetto extract berry (Serenoa Repens) 160 mg. Other Ingredients: Olive Oil, Gelatin, Glycerin.

Saw Palmetto - Swanson
Each capsule contains: Saw Palmetto berries powder 540 mg.

Saw Palmetto - Suma Virtue - Blessed Herbs
Saw Palmetto berry • Siberian Ginseng root • Jamaican Sarsaparilla root • Suma root • Astragalus root • Damiana • Grain alcohol & Distilled Water.

Saw Palmetto Complex - Enzymatic Therapy
Each capsule contains: Saw Palmetto Berry extract standardized to contain 85% to 95% fatty acids & sterols 80 mg • Pumpkin seed oil extract (Cucurbita pepo) 40 mg • Pygeum africanum extract standardized to contain 13% total sterols 10 mg • Bearberry extract (Uva Ursi) standardized to contain 10% Arbutin 5 mg. Contains no sugar, salt, yeast, wheat, corn, dairy products, flavoring or preservatives.

Saw Palmetto Complex - Leiner Health Products
Each softgel contains: Zinc Gluconate 7.5 mg • Pumpkin Seed oil extract (Cucurbita pepeo) 40 mg • Saw Palmetto berry extract (serenoa repens) 160 mg. Other Ingredients: Gelatin, Glycerin, Vegetable Oil, Beeswax, Lecithin, Titanium Dioxide, Red 40, Yellow 6, Blue 1, Yellow 5.

Saw Palmetto Complex - PhytoPharmica
Saw Palmetto (Serenoa repens) berry extract (standardized to contain 85%-95% fatty acids and sterols) 160 mg • Pumpkin (Curcubita pepo) seed oil extract 80 mg • Pygeum africanum (Prunus africana) bark extract (standardized to contain 13% total sterols) 20 mg • Bearberry (Uva ursi) leaf extract (standardized to contain 10% arbutin) 10 mg.

Saw Palmetto Extract - Jamieson
Each capsule contains: Pumpkin seed oil (Curcubita pepo) 100 mg • Saw Palmetto berry 4:1 extract (Serenoa repens) 50 mg • Pygeum bark 150:1 extract (Pygeum africanum) 50 mg • Cranberry fruit 25:1 extract (Viccinum macrocarpon) 10 mg.

Saw Palmetto Formula - Quest
Each caplet contains: Saw Palmetto berry powder (Serenoa serrulate/repens) 110 mg • Corn Silk powder (Zea mays) 110 mg • Pumpkin Seed powder 90 mg • Parsley leaf powder (Petroselinum crispu) 55 mg • Buchu leaf powder (Barosma betulina) 35 mg • Cayenne powder (Capsicum) 35 mg • Kelp powder (Fucus vesiculosis) 35 mg. Other Ingredients: Calcium Phosphate, Microcrystalline Cellulose, Vegetable Stearin, Croscarmellose Sodium, Magnesium Stearate (vegetable source).

Saw Palmetto Male Toner - Traditional Medicinals
Hibiscus flower • Saw Palmetto berry • Nettle root • Uva Ursi leaf • Ginger rhizome • Saw Palmetto berry dry extract • Althea root • Rose Hip • natural Lemon flavor • Stevia leaf.

Saw Palmetto Plus - Atrium Inc.
Each capsule contains: Saw Palmetto oil (50:1 extract) 160 mg • Olive oil 90 mg. Contains no wheat, sugar, starch, corn, salt, yeast, milk or soy.

Saw Palmetto with Lycopene - Health Smart Vitamins
Each soft gel contains: Saw Palmetto berry (85-95% fatty acids, 272 mg-304 mg) 320 mg • Lycopene (from tomato) 5 mg.

Say Yes to Beans - Nature's Plus
Each Vegicap contains: Legumase (Saccharamyces cerevisae & Aspergillus enzyme complex) 125 mg • Licorice root (Glycyrrhiza glabra) standardized < 2% Glycyrrhizinic acid 75 mg • Ginger root (Zingiber officinale) standardized 5% gingerols 25 mg • Parsley seed (Petroselinum crispum) 20 mg. Contains no yeast, wheat, corn, soy, milk, salt, sugar or starch.

SB Normal Stool Formula - Shaman Botanicals
Each tablet contains: Croton lechleri extract (sap) (standardized to contain 250 mg of SP-303). Other Ingredients: Microcrystalline Cellulose, Coating [Methacrylic Acid Copolymer, Magnesium Silicate, Triethyl Citrate], Glyceryl Monostearate, Sodium Starch Glycolate, Silicon Dioxide.

Schisandra - Pharmanex - Pharmanex
Each capsule contains: Schisandra berry extract (Schisandra chinensis) (10:1) 200 mg. Other Ingredients: Rice Flour, Gelatin, Magnesium Stearate, Silicon Dioxide.

Sea & Earth - The Vitamin Shoppe
Sea-life protein • Vitamin C • Zinc • Silica • Green Tea extract • Red Wine extract • Red Cabbage extract • Grape Juice extract • Pine Bark extract • Citrus Bioflavonoids • Carotene.

Sea Cal Oyster Shell Calcium - Nature's Life
Two tablets contain: Calcium (Oyster Shell) 500 mg • Vitamin D (as Vitamin D3) (Cholecaciferol) 250 IU.

Sea Cucumber - Futurebiotics
Sea Cucumber 500 mg.

Sea Mussel - Futurebiotics
New Zealand Greenshell Mussel 500 mg.

Seaweed Virtue - Blessed Herbs
Kelp • Bladderwrack • Dulse & "Other Seaweeds as Available" • Grain alcohol & Distilled Water.

Secretagogue-One - MHP
Each packet contains: Anterior Pituitary Substance 25 mg • Glycoamino Acid-Glucose Complex 4200 mg • Novel polyose complex 2230 mg • Amino Acid Blend 500 mg • Broad Bean 10 mg. See Editor's Note No. 14, page 1817.

See - Quantum Health
Three tablets contain: Bilberry extract 10 mg • Omega-3 Flax Meal (partially defatted) 500 mg • Beta-Carotene (Pro Vitamin A) 25000 IU • Vitamin A (Palmitate) 5000 IU • Vitamin C (Ascorbic Acid) 1000 mg • Natural Vitamin E (D-Alpha Succinate) 200 IU • Citrus Bioflavonoid 250 mg • Vitamin B2 (Riboflavin) 40 mg • Rutin NF (Bioflavonoid) 100 mg • Selenium (Selenomethionine) 100 mcg • Pantothenic Acid (d-Calcium Pantothenate) 40 mg • Chromium (GTF) 200 mcg • Zinc (Citrate) 25 mg • Lutein 5 mg.

Some Brand Name Natural Products - What they Contain
www.NaturalDatabase.com contains MANY more listings than appear here.

BRAND NAMES

Selenium - Source Naturals
Each tablet contains: Selenium (yeast free, from 40 mg of L-Selonomethionine) 200 mcg.

Selenium 200 - Leiner Health Products
Each tablet contains: Selenium (High Selenium yeast) 200 mcg. Other Ingredients: Calcium Carbonate, Maltodectrin, Cellulose, Croscarmellose Sodium, Tricalcium Phosphate, Crospovidone, Polyethylene Glycol 3350, Silicon Dioxide, Magnesium Stearate, Hydroxypropyl Methylcellulose, Hydroxypropyl Cellulose, Polysorbate 80.

Selenium 50 mcg - Jamieson
Each caplet contains: Selenium (Proteinate) 50 mcg • Beta-Carotene (Provitamin A) 5000 IU • Vitamin C (Ascorbic Acid) 60 mg • Vitamin E (Natural D-Alpha Tocopheryl Acetate) 10 IU.

Selenium Tablets - Leiner Health Products
Each tablet contains: Selenium Yeast 50 mcg. Other Ingredients: Brewer's Yeast, Dicalcium Phosphate, Cellulose, Stearic Acid, Croscarmellose Sodium, Silicon Dioxide.

Selenomax - Source Naturals
Each tablet contains: Selenium (from 100 selenomax high selenium yeast) 100 mcg.

Selenomax Selenium 200 Mcg - Nature's Life
Each tablet contains: Selenium (natural food yeast-based) (Nutrition 21 Selenomax) 200 mcg.

Senescegarl - Olympian Labs
Three capsules contain: Ginkgo Biloba leaf extract 120 mg • Garlic extract 600 mg • Coenzyme Q10 60 mg • Ascorbic Acid 300 mg • Grape Seed extract 90 mg • Vitamin B-6 (pyridoxine HCl) 30 mg • Zinc (gluconate) 15 mg • Copper (cupric oxide) 1800 mcg • Manganese (manganese sulfate) 1800 mcg.

Senior Moment - Nutramax Laboratories, Inc.
Each capsule contains: Cerebral Phospholipids including: Phosphatidylserine, Phosphatidylethanolamine, and Phosphatidylinositol, 50 mg • Docosahexaenoic acid 40mg. Other Ingredients: Sunflower Oil, Gelatin, Water, Ascorbyl Palmitate, Tocopherols, Titanium dioxide color, FD&C Red #3, Sodium Lauryl sulfate, FD&C Yellow #5, FD&C Blue #1.

Senior-Vites Plus - The Vitamin Shoppe
Three tablets contain: Vitamin A Activity 20000 IU • Vitamin D 400 IU • Vitamin C 150 mg • Vitamin E 200 IU • Vitamin B1 35 mg • Vitamin B2 35 mg • Niacinamide 50 mg • Vitamin B6 35 mg • Vitamin B12 50 mcg • Pantothenic Acid 75 mg • Folic Acid 400 mcg • Biotin 300 mcg • PABA 35 mg • Inositol 100 mg • Choline 100 mg • Citrus Bioflavonoids 25 mg • Rutin 25 mg • Glutamine 100 mg • Taurine 100 mg • Glutamic Acid 50 mg • Pancreatin 25 mg • Ox Bile 10 mg • Calcium 100 mg • Magnesium 50 mg • Iron 18 mg • Zinc 15 mg • Manganese 6 mg • Potassium 45 mg • Iodine 225 mcg • Selenium 50 mcg • Chromium 25 mcg • Fo-Ti 50 mg • Gotu Kola 50 mg • Avena Sativa 25 mg • Siberian Ginseng 25 mg • Nettles extract 10 mg.
See Editor's Note No. 14, page 1817.

Senna Leaves - Now
Each capsule contains: Senna leaves (Cassia Angustifolia) 470 mg. Other Ingredients: Gelatin (capsule), Magnesium Stearate. Contains no yeast, wheat, gluten, corn, soy, milk, or preservatives.

Sentinel Multi Vitamin - Health Center for Better Living
Each tablet contains: Vitamin A (as retinyl acetate and beta-carotene) 5000 IU• Vitamin C (as ascorbic acid) 60 mg • Vitamin D (as

cholecalciferol) 400 IU • Vitamin E (as dl-alpha-tocopheryl acetate) 30 IU • Vitamin K (as phytonadione) 25 mcg • Thiamin (as thiamin mononitrate) 1.5 mg • Riboflavin 1.7 mg • Niacin (as niacinamide) 20 mg • Vitamin B6 (as pyridoxine HCl) 2 mg • Folate (as folic acid) 400 mcg • Vitamin B12 (as cyancobalamin) 6 mcg • Biotin 30 mcg • Pantothenic acid (as D-calcium pantothenate) 10 mg • Calcium (as dicalcium phosphate) 162 mg • Iron (as ferrous fumarate) 18 mg • Phosphorus (as dicalcium phosphate) 125 mg • Iodine (as potassium iodide) 150 mcg • Magnesium (as magnesium oxide) 100 mg • Zinc (as zinc oxide) 15 mg • Selenium (as sodium selenate) 25 mcg • Copper (as cupric oxide) 2 mg • Manganese (as manganese sulfate) 2.5 mcg • Chromium (as chromium chloride)• Molybdenum (as sodium moybdate) 25 mcg • Chloride (as potassium choride) 36.3 mg Potassium (as potassium choride) 40 mg • Vanadium (as sodium metavandate) 10 mcg • Tin (as stannous chloride) 10 mcg • Silicon (as sodium metasilicate) 10 mcg • Nickel (as nickelous sulfate) 5 mcg.

SerenAid - Klaire Laboratories
Each capsule contains: Multi-Enzyme Complex (proprietary blend) 317 mg: L-Lysine, Peptidase FP, Papain (sulfite free), Protease, Acid-stable Protease, Lactase. Contains no gluten, casein, soy, corn, sugars, flavors, fragrances, preservatives, salicylates, artificial colors or other common allergenic substances.

Serenoa Repens - Progressive Labs
Each softgel contains: Saw Palmetto purified extract (95% free fatty acids) 160 mg • Olive oil 160 mg.

Serrapeptase (Serraflazyme) - Olympia Nutrition
Silk worm enzyme.

Serum For Sensitive Skin - Cellex-C
Ascorbic Acid • Tyrosine • Zinc • Sodium Hyaluronate • Pine Bark extract.

Seven Day Souper Cabbage Diet - Puritan's Pride
Three capsules contain: 3 Green Onions (organo-sulfurs) • 1 Green Pepper (flavonoids) • 1 small stalk of Celery (polyacetylenes) • 1 whole Tomato (lycopene) • 2 large Carrots (carotenoids) • 1 Zucchini Squash (sulforaphane) • 1 small head of Cabbage (Indole 3 Carbinol: I-3C).

Shake and Bake - The Herbalist
Oils of Sweet Almond, Aloe Vera, Safflower, St. John's Wort flower, Calendula flower, & Vitamin E • Extracts of St. John's Wort flower, Calendula flower & Chamomile flower • Essential oils of Sandalwood, Lite Musk, French Vanilla.

Shark / Glucosamine Formula - Health Smart Vitamins
Three capsules contain: Protein 0.675 g • Calcium (from shark cartilage) 210 mg • Phosphorus (from shark cartilage) 135 mg • Potassium (from glucosamine sulfate) 98 mg • Shark Cartilage 1500 mg • Glucosamine Sulfate 750 mg.

Shark Cartilage - Leiner Health Products
Each capsule contains: Shark Cartilage 500 mg. Other Ingredients: Gelatin, Maltodextrin, Magnesium Stearate, Calcium Carbonate, Sodium Starch Glycolate.

Shark Cartilage - Olympian Labs
Each capsule contains: Shark Cartilage 750 mg.

Shark Cartilage - Swanson
Three capsules contain: Shark Cartilage 2.25 g.

Shark Oil - Futurebiotics
Shark liver oil 460 mg.

Some Brand Name Natural Products - What they Contain
www.NaturalDatabase.com contains MANY more listings than appear here.

Sharp Thinking - Changes - TwinLab
Two caplets contain: Ginkgo Biloba leaf standardized extract (24% flavonglycosides, 6% terpene lactones) 120 mg • Huperzine A (from Huperzia serrata extract whole plant) 50 mcg • Green Tea leaf standardized extract (30% polyphenols, 20% methylxanthines) 500 mg • Panax Ginseng root standardized extract (4% ginsenosides) 200 mg • Brahmi leaf standardized extract (10% asiaticosides) (Centella asiatica) 100 mg • Citrus aurantium fruit standardized extract (5-7% alkaloids) 50 mg. Other Ingredients: Dicalcium Phosphate, Vegetable Cellulose, Fractionated vegetable oil, Soy polysaccharides, Silica, and Vegetable resin glaze.

Shen Min - Biotech
Three tablets contain: Shen Min: a proprietary blend of 12:1 standardized He Shou Wu (Fo Ti) root extract and He Shou Wu root powder providing a synergistic complex of chrysophanics and resveratrol 1775 mg • Bioperine Black Pepper (Piper nigrum) 3.0 mg. Other ingredients: Dicalcium phosphate, Microcrystalline Cellulose, Croscarmellose Sodium, Stearic Acid, Magnesium Stearate, Pharmaceutical glaze.

Shen Min - Puritan's Pride
Three tablets contain: Shen Min (a proprietary blend of 12:1 standardized He Shou Wu (Fo Ti) root powder providing a synergistic complex of chrysophanics and resveratrol) 1,775 mg • BioPerine black pepper extract (Piper nigrum) 3.0 mg. Other Ingredients: Dicalcium Phosphate, Microcrystalline Cellulose, Croscarmellose Sodium, Stearic Acid, Magnesium Stearate, Pharmaceutical Glaze.

Shiitake/Maitake Extract - Nature's Way
Each capsule contains: Maitake dried extract 100 mg • Oat grain 200 mg • Shiitake dried extract 100 mg. Other Ingredients: Gelatin, Magnesium stearate, Millet.

Ship-Assure - Nature's Plus
Two tablets contain: Ginger root [(Zingiber officinale) standardized 4% Volatile oils] 350 mg • Kava [(Piper methysticum) standardized 29-31% kavalactones] 50 mg • Chamomile flower [(Matricaria recutita) standardized 1% apigenin, 0.5% essential oil] 50 mg • Hops fruit [(Humulus lupulus) standardized 5.2% bitter acids, 4% flavonoids] 50 mg • Siberian Ginseng root [(Eleutherococcus senticosus) standardized 0.8% Eleutherosides] 50 mg • Passion Flower [(Passiflora incarnata) standardized 3.5-4% flavonoids, calculated as isovitexin] 50 mg • Wild Cherry (Prunus virginlana fruit) 50 mg. Contains no yeast, wheat, corn, soy, milk, salt, or starch.

SHN Skin-Hair-Nails - The Vitamin Shoppe
Three tablets contain: Vitamin A (beta carotene) 10,000 IU • Vitamin C 120 mg • Vitamin B1 10 mg • Vitamin B2 10 mg • Niacinamide 50 mg • Calcium 600 mg • Iron 6 mg • Vitamin D 200 IU • Vitamin E 30 IU • Vitamin B6 10 mg • Folic Acid 400 mcg • Vitamin B12 16 mcg • Phosphorus 300 mg • Iodine (kelp) 225 mcg • Magnesium 200 mg • Zinc 15 mg • Biotin 400 mcg • Pantothenic Acid 30 mg • Choline 150 mcg • Inositol 60 mg • PABA 50 mg • Selenium 25 mcg • Manganese 10 mg • RNA 60 mg • Bioflavonoids 50 mg • Rutin 25 mg • Betaine Hydrochloride 50 mg. In a base of L-Cysteine, Methionine, Gelatin, Papain, Oat Straw, Echinacea, Horse Tail, and Asparagus.

Siberian Ginseng - Gaia Herbs
Siberian Ginseng standardized for 0.8% eleutherosides B & E. Standardized Full Spectrum 200 mg of extract per capsule. Guaranteed Potency 100 mg of extract per capsule.

Siberian Ginseng - Nature's Way
Three capsules contain: Siberian Ginseng root 1.23 g. Other Ingredients: Gelatin, Magnesium stearate.

Siberian Ginseng - Olympian Labs
Each capsule contains: Siberian Ginseng 500 mg.

Siberian Ginseng - Pharmanex
Each capsule contains: Ginseng, Siberian root extract (Eleutherococcus senticosus Max) (10:1) 150 mg. Other Ingredients: Rice Flour, Gelatin, Magnesium Stearate, Silicon Dioxide.

Siberian Ginseng Extract - PhytoPharmica
Each capsule contains: Siberian Ginseng (Eleutherococcus senticosus) root extract 10:1 (standardized to contain greater than 0.5% eleutheroside E) 200 mg.

Sil-150 - PhytoPharmica
Each capsule contains: Milk Thistle extract (Silybum marianum) standardized to contain 70% silymarin (105 mg per capsule) calculated as silybin 150 mg. Contains no sugar, salt, yeast, wheat, corn, soy, dairy products, flavorings, or preservatives.

Silent Night Formula - Nature's Way
Four capsules contain: Proprietary Formula: Hops flower • Scullcap herb • Valerian root. Other ingredients: Gelatin.

Silica 10 mg - Jamieson
Each caplet contains: Standardized Silica from pure spring Horsetail herb 3080 mg (Equisetum arvense L 770 mg powdered extract 1:4) 10 mg. With natural occurring flavonoids, saponins and minerals.

Silica Complex - Puritan's Pride
Each tablet contains: Calcium (as calcium carbonate and calcium citrate) 200 mg • Magnesium (as magnesium oxide and magnesium citrate) 150 mg • Zinc (as zinc gluconate and zinc citrate) 15 mg • Boron (as Boron Citrate, Boron Glycinate, and Boron Aspartate) 1.5 mg • Betaine (as Betaine Hydrochloride) 38 mg • Horsetail extract (Euisetum arvense) arial (standardized to contain 7% Silica) 500 mg.

SiliCare - Holista
Each capsule contains Silicon (dioxide) derived from 410 mg 2.9% Spring Horsetail Equisetum arvense extract 5 mg.

Silybin Phytosome - PhytoPharmica
Each capsule contains: Silybin Phytosome (milk thistle extract) bound to phosphatidylcholine under patent 120 mg. Contains no sugar, salt, yeast, wheat, gluten, corn, dairy products, coloring, flavorings, or preservatives.

Silymarin - Aspen Group, Inc.
Each capsule contains: Silymarin (Milk Thistle, standardized at 80%) 150 mg.

Silymarin Plus - Futurebiotics
Three tablets contain: Milk Thistle seed powder extract (standardized for 80% (420 mg) silymarin) 525 mg • Inositol 240 mg • Choline (as choline bitartrate) 240 mg • Dandelion root powder 300 mg • Alfalfa leaf powder extract 300 mg • Black Radish root powder 300 mg • Beet root powder 300 mg. Other ingredients: Dicalcium phosphate, Magnesium stearate, Vegetable stearate, Silica, Cellulose.

Silymarin Plus - Source Naturals
Each tablet contains: Silymarin (from Milk Thistle Seed extract) 140 mg • Vitamin C (Ascorbic Acid) 100 mg • Choline (Bitartrate) 50 mg • Inositol 50 mg • Vitamin E (d-alpha tocopheryl natural) 25 IU.

Simicort - Enzymatic Therapy
Active ingredient: Salicylic Acid 1.8%. Other ingredients: Purified Water, Organic Fatty Acid Complex (C11-C18), Glyceryl Stearate, Chamomile extract (0.5% Flavonoid Content), 18-Beta-Glycyrrhetinic Acid from Licorice root extract, Allantoin 2.0% from Comfrey root extract, Dimethicone, Vitamin E antioxidant, & Hypoallergenic Fragrance.

Sino-Lung Res-Q - Nutri-Quest
Each tablet contains: Lung 35 mg • Thymus 35 mg • Spleen 35 mg •

BRAND NAMES

Vitamin C 75 mg • Beta Carotene 12600 IU • Lemon Bioflavonoids 125 mg • Rutin 20 mg • Hesperidin Complex 75 mg • N-Acetyl Cysteine 35 mg • Propolis 20 mg • Cranberry 36 mg • Echinacea 30 mg • Goldenseal 35 mg • Elderberry 10 mg • Scullcap 35 mg. See Editor's Note No. 14, page 1817.

SinuCheck - Enzymatic Therapy
Each capsule contains: Active ingredient: Pseudoephedrine HCl (from Ephedra sinensis) 30 mg • Other ingredients: Scullcap extract 4:1 (Scutellaria baicalensis) 100 mg • Chinese Thoroughwax extract (Bupleurum falcatum) 100 mg • Chinese Peony extract 4:1 (Paeonia Lactiflora) 100 mg • Dong Quai extract (4:1) (Angelica sinensis) 100 mg • Licorice root extract (Glycyrrhiza glabra) standardized to contain 5% Glycyrrhizic Acid 40 mg • Curcuma root extract (Curcuma longa) standardized to contain 4% Curcumin 20 mg • Ginger root extract 6.5:1 (Zingiber officinale) 20 mg. Contains no sugar, salt, yeast, wheat, corn, soy, dairy products, coloring, flavoring or preservatives.

SinuClear - PhytoPharmica
Each capsule contains: Pseudoephedrine HCL 30 mg (from Ephedra sinensis) • Scullcap extract 4:1 (Scutellaria baicalensis) 100 mg • Chinese Thoroughwax extract (Bupleurum falcatum) 100 mg • Chinese Peony extract 4:1 (Paeonia lactiflora) 100 mg • Dong Quai extract 4:1 (Angelica sinensis) 100 mg • Licorice root extract (Glycyrrhiza glabra) 40 mg standardized to contain 5% glycyrrhizic acid • Curcuma root extract (Curcuma longa) 20 mg standardized to contain 2.5% curcumin • Ginger root extract 6.5:1 (Zingiber officinale) 20 mg. Contains no sugar, salt, yeast, wheat, corn, soy, dairy products, coloring, flavoring, or preservatives.

SinuComp - PhytoPharmica
Each tablet contains: Cowslip flowers (Primula veris) 36 mg • Sour Dock (Rumex acetosa) 36 mg • Elder flowers (Sambucus nigra) 36 mg • Verbena (Verbena officinalis) 36 mg • Gentian root (Gentiana lutea) 12 mg. Product contains no sugar, salt, yeast, wheat, gluten, corn, soy, dairy products, coloring, flavoring, or preservatives.

SinuGuard - Enzymatic Therapy
Each tablet contains: Cowslip flower (Primula veris) 36 mg • Sour Dock (Rumex acetosa) 36 mg • Elder flower (Sambucus nigra) 36 mg • Verbena (Verbena officinalis) 36 mg • Gentian root (Gentiana lutea) 12 mg. Contains no sugar, salt, yeast, wheat, gluten, corn, soy, dairy products, coloring, flavoring or preservatives.

Sinus Ease - Nature's Life
Three capsules contain: Bromelain [an enzyme from Pineapple fruit (Ananassa sativa) activity of 1200 mg = 2,880 GDU (4320 MCU)] 1200 mg • Quercetin (a flavonoid from Pilocarpus gaborandi) 300 mg • Vitamin C (Buffered, as Calcium Ascorbic) 133 mg.

Sinus Essentials - Swanson
Three capsules contain: Ma Huang (8% ephedra) 252 mg • Fenugreek seed powder 100 mg • Slippery Elm bark 100 mg • Cayenne Pepper 100,000 HU 60 mg • Eucalyptus leaves powder 50 mg • Goldenseal root 50 mg • Aloe Vera leaf powder 25 mg.

Sinus Remedy - PhytoPharmica
Two chewable tablets contain: Kalium bichromicum 5x • Silicea 5x • Mercurius sulphuratus ruber 4x • Kali sulphuricum 4x • Belladonna 3x • Calcarea carbonica 3x • Calcarea fluorica 3x • Hepar sulphuris calcareum 3x • Hydrastis canadensis 3x • Manganum sulphuricum 3x • Sabadilla 3x • Thuja 2x.
See Editor's Note No. 1, page 1816.

SinusHealth - Neopharmica
Two tablets contain: Proprietary Blend: Baikal Skullcap root, Schizonpeta Tenuifolia, Angelica root, Cinnamon twig, Xanthium Strumarium, Astragalus root 2500 mg.

Sinutone - The Herbalist
Eyebright herb • Golden Seal root • Bayberry root bark • Osha root • Yarrow flower • Horseradish root • Cayenne pepper.

Sinu-X - Olympian Labs
Two capsules contain: Proteolytic Enzymes 150 mg • Spearmint 50 mg • Clove 10 mg • Sea Mussel 50 mg • Zinc Gluconate 20 mg • Echinacea 40 mg • Red Clover 20 mg • Goldenseal 30 mg • Citrus Aurantium 30 mg • Green Tea extract 20 mg.

Sitol - PharmaGen
Each capsule contains: Serenoa repens extract (standardized) 320 mg.

Sitol PA - PharmaGen
Each capsule contains: Serenoa repens extract (standardized) 320 mg • Pygeum africanum extract (standardized) 100 mg.

Skin Clear - The Herbalist
Echinacea root • Yellow Dock root • Oregon Grape root • Burdock root • Red Clover blossom • Jamaican Sarsaparilla root.

Skin Firming Cream Plus - Cellex-C
Ascorbic Acid • Tyrosine • Vitamin E • Zinc • Bioflavonoids • Sodium Hyaluronate • Evening Primrose oil • Glycine • Tomato extract • Aloe barbadensis gel • Chamomile extract • Allantoin.

Skin Formula - Dr. Morrow's Homeopathic Formulas
Ten drops contain: Saponaria officinalis 3X • Fumaria officinalis 3X • Sarsaparilla 3X • Hydrocotyle asiatica 3X • Viola tricolor 3X • Rhus venenata 3C • Lappa major 3C • Berberis vulgaris 3C.
See Editor's Note No. 1, page 1816.

Skin Support for Women - Futurebiotics
Two capsules contain: Vitamin A (5000 IU beta carotene, 5000 IU fish liver oil) 10000 IU • Vitamin C (ascorbic acid) 250 mg • Vitamin D (ergocalciferol) 200 IU • Vitamin E (d-alpha tocopherol succinate) 30 IU • Zinc (amino acid chelate) 30 mg • Selenium (amino acid chelate) 100 mcg • Boron (amino acid chelate) 3 mg • MSM (methyl-sulfonyl-methane) 500 mg • Collagen 500 mg • Glucosamine Sulfate 100 mg • Skin Support Herbal Base, 200 mg: Citrus Bioflavonoids, Grape Seed extract, Horsetail leaf powder, Papain, Chamomile flower powder, Aloe Vera leaf powder. Other ingredients: Gelatin, Water.

Skin Tone Balancer - Jason
10% Complete Vitamin C Complex with Kojic Ester, beta Hydroxy Acids, and Barberry extract. Super Oxide Dismutase liposome.

Skin, Hair & Nails Formula - Puritan's Pride
Three tablets contain: Vitamin A (as Retinyl Palmitate) 5000 IU • Vitamin C (as Ascorbic Acid) 60 mg • Vitamin D (as Cholecalciferol) 100 IU • Vitamin E (as d-Alpha Tocopheryl Acetate) 15 IU • Thiamin (Vitamin B-1; as Thiamine Hydrochloride) 5 mg • Riboflavin (Vitamin B-2) 5 mg • Niacin (as Niacinamide) 25 mg • Vitamin B-6 (as Pyridoxine Hydrochloride) 5 mg • Folic Acid 200 mcg • Vitamin B-12 (as Cyanocobalamin) 8 mcg • Biotin (as D-Biotin) 200 mcg • Pantothenic Acid (as D-Calcium Pantothentate) 15 mg • Calcium (as Dicalcium Phosphate and Calcium Carbonate) 834 mg • Iron (as Ferrous Gluconate) 3 mg • Phosphorus (as Dicalcium Phosphate) 331 mg • Iodine (as Potassium Iodide) 112.5 mcg • Magnesium (as Magnesium Oxide) 100 mg • Zinc (as Zinc Gluconate) 7.5 mg • Selenium (as L-Selenomethionine) 12.5 mg • Manganese (as Manganese Gluconate) 5 mg • Para-Aminobenzoic Acid 25 mg • Choline Bitartrate 75 mg • Inositol 30 mg • RNA 30 mg • Citrus Bioflavonoid 25 mg • Rutin 12.5 mg • Betaine Hydrochloride 25 mg • Rose Hips 60 mg.

Skin, Hair and Nails - Aspen Group, Inc.
Three tablets contain: Vitamin A 5000 IU • Vitamin C 60 mg • Vitamin B1 5 mg • Riboflavin 5 mg • Niacinamide 25 mg • Calcium 300 mg • Iron 3 mg • Vitamin D 100 IU • Vitamin E 15 IU • Vitamin

B6 5 mg • Folic Acid 200 mcg • Vitamin B12 8 mcg • Phosphorus 150 mg • Iodine 112.5 mg • Magnesium 100 mg • Zinc 7.5 mg • Biotin 200 mcg • Pantothenic Acid 15 mg • Choline 75 mg • Inositol 30 mg • PABA 25 mg • Selenium 12.5 mcg • Manganese 5 mg • RNA 30 mg • Bioflavonoids 25 mg • Rutin 12.5 mg • Betaine HCl 25 mg • Horsetail Silica 50 mg. Contains no sugar, starch, salt, wheat, corn, yeast or soy derivatives.

Skin, Hair, Nails - Natrol
Two capsules contain: Vitamin A (as Vitamin A palmitate) 5000 mg • Vitamin C (ascorbic acid) 100 mg • Vitamin E (as d-alpha tocopherol succinate) 50 IU • Thiamine (Vitamin B1) (as Thiamine HCl) 10 mg • Riboflavin (Vitamin B2) 10 mg • Vitamin B6 (pyridoxine HCl) 20 mg • Vitamin B12 (as cobalamin) 50 mcg • Biotin 500 mcg • Zinc (as zinc oxide) 8 mg • Copper (as amino acid chelate) 2 mg • Manganese (as manganese carbonate) 2 mg • MSM (methyl sulfonyl methane) 250 mg • Trace Mineral Complex 100 mg • Cysteine (as L-cysteine hydrochloride) 75 mg • PABA (para amino benzoic acid) 50 mg • Burdock root 50 mg • Choline (as choline bitartrate) 25 mg • Inositol 25 mg • Silicon (as colloidal silicon) 20 mg • Glutathione (as L-glutathione reduced) 2 mg. Other ingredients: Rice powder, Magnesium Stearate, Gelatin.

Sleep Ease - PhytoPharmica
Twenty drops contain: Secale cornutum 4x • Belladonna 3x • Avena sativa 1x • Passiflora incarnata 1x • Valeriana officinalis 1x. In a base of 40% USP alcohol by volume.
See Editor's Note No. 1, page 1816.

Sleep Formula - Preventive Nutrition
One capsule contains: Kava Kava Root Extract (Piper methysticum; 55% Kavalactones=49.5 mg) 90 mg • Griffonia Seed Extract (20% 5-Hydroxyl-L-Tryptophan=10mg) 50 mg • Melatonin (n-acetyl-5-Methoxytryptamine) 2 mg. Other ingredients: Polyethylene Glycol, Gelatin, Glycerin, Chlorophyll, Titanium Dioxide (Natural Mineral Whitener).
See Editor's Note No. 16, page 1817.

Sleep-Assure - Nature's Plus
Each tablet contains: Rapid Release Layer: Melatonin (N-Acetyl-5-Methoxytryptamine) 1.5 mg • GABA (Gamma Aminobutyric Acid) 10 mg • Pyridoxal-5-Phosphate (P5P) 10 mg. Sustained Release Layer: Melatonin (N-Acetyl-5-Methoxytryptamine) 1.5 mg • Herbal Blend containing equal proportions of: [Kava Kava root extract (Piper methysticum) standardized 29-31% kavalactones], Passion Flower extract (Passiflora incarnata) standardized 3.5-4% flavonoids calculated as isovitexin, Valerian root extract (Valeriana officinalis) standardized 1% Valerenic Acid, Chamomile flower (Matricaria recutita) standardized 1% Apigenin 0.5% essential oil] 25 mg. Contains no yeast, wheat, corn, soy, milk, salt, sugar or starch.
See Editor's Note No. 16, page 1817.

Sleepytime Extra - Celestial Seasonings
Two capsules contain: Calcium (as carbonate, citrate, and malate) 200 mg • Magnesium (as oxide) 100 mg • Proprietary Blend 800 mg: Valerian (root), Valerian (standardized extract), Kava Kava (root), Kava Kava (standardized extract). Other ingredients: May contain one or more of the following: Dicalcium phosphate, gelatin, rice flour, stearic acid, spearmint extract, magnesium stearate, and silicon dioxide. This product contains no artificial colors, flavors or preservatives. One serving size is equivalent to: Valerian 375 mg standardized to .8% valerenic acid, Kava Kava 100 mg standardized to 30% kavalactones.

Slender Shaper - Pharmagel
E-L-A Complex.

Slender-Mist - KareMor International
Vitamin B6 • Pantothenic Acid • Chromium • Hydroxy-Citric Acid • L-Carnitine. Available in Arctic Mint, Berry Supreme, chocolate Fudge, and Tropical Delite.

Slim 7 - Swanson
Two tablets contain: Vitamin A (as retinyl palmitate) 1667 IU • Vitamin C (as ascorbic acid) 20 mg • Vitamin E (as d-alpha tocopheryl succinate) 10 IU • Riboflavin (vitamin B-2) 0.6 mg • Niacin 6.6 mg • Vitamin B-6 (as pyridoxine HCl) 0.66 mg • Folic Acid 133.3 mcg • Vitamin B-12 (as cyanocobalamin) 2 mcg • Biotin 100 mcg • Iodine (from kelp) 50 mcg • Selenium (as selenomethionine) 16.6 mcg • Chromium (from Chromax® chromium picolinate) 375 mcg • Chromium (from chromium polynicotinate) 375 mcg • CitriMax™ (Garcinia cambogia fruit extract) 500 mg, (-) Hydroxycitric Acid 250 mg • Proprietary blend of 72 Trace Minerals 200 mg • L-Carnitine (as tartrate) 100 mg • Choline (as choline bitartrate) 67 mg • Green Tea extract (20% polyphenols) 50 mg • Kola Nut extract 50 mg • Capsicum 33.3 mg • Chitosan 33.3 mg • Ginger 33.3 mg • Inositol 33.3 mg • Spirulina 33.3 mg • Betaine HCl 8 mg.

Slim Down GTF Chromium 200 mcg - Jamieson
Each tablet contains: Chromium (from brewer's yeast) 200 mcg.

Slim Smart - Health Center for Better Living
Chromium Picolinate 200 mcg, other herbs.

Slim Trim - Life Extension
L-Arginine 500 mg L-Ornithine 250 mg.

Slimmer - Dr. Roopas
Each capsule contains: Propietary Formula 250 mg: Powder of Cassia Angustifolia, Cinnamomum Tamala, Garcinia Cambogia, Balsamodendron Mukul.

Slimming Formula - PhytoPharmica
One tablet contains: Thyroidinum 8x • Antimonium crudum 3x • Calcarea acetica 2x • Fucus vesiculosus 2x.
See Editor's Note No. 1, page 1816.

Slow-Mag - Roberts
Two tablets contain: Calcium (from calcium carbonate) 212 mg • Magnesium 128 mg & Chloride 373 mg (from magnesium chloride hexahydrate) • Cellulose Acetate Phthalate • Pregelatinized Starch • Povidone • Diethylphthalate • Talc • Titanium Dioxide • Magnesium Stearate & FD&C Blue No. 2 Lake.

Slumber - Nutrivention
Two tablets contain: Calcium (Amino Acid Chelate) 500 mg • Magnesium (Amino Acid Chelate) 500 mg • Inositol 200 mg • Niacinamide 20 mg • Biotin 100 mcg • Passion flower 200 mg • Blue Vervain 200 mg • Hops 100 mg • Valerian root (Star root) 100 mg • Wild Lettuce 100 mg.

SlumberActin - Nature's Plus
Three capsules contain: Chamomile [(Matricaria recutita root) standardized 1% Apigenin, 0.5% Essential oil] 200 mg • Valerian [(Valeriana officinalis root) standardized 1% Valernic Acids] 100 mg • Passion Flower [(Passiflora incarnata flower) standardized 3.5-4% Flavonoids] 75 mg • Hops [(Humulus lupulus fruit) standardized 5.2% Bitter Acids, 4% Flavonoids] 75 mg • Kava Kava [(Piper methysticum root) standardized 29-31% Kavalactones] 50 mg • English Hawthorne [(Crataegus laevigata berry) standardized 3.2% Vitexin] 50 mg • Magnesium (Amino Acid Chelate) 50 mg • Calcium (Amino Acid Chelate) 25 mg.

Smart Coffee w/ Ginkgo Biloba - Nature's Plus
Each 3 g serving contains: Instant herbal coffee blend: naturally decaffeinated Brazilian coffee (coffea) • Ginkgo Biloba (standardized 24% ginkgo flavone-glycosides, 6% terpene lactones) • Rosemary (Rosmarinus officinalis) • Fo-Ti (Polygonum multiflorum) • Wild Grape (Mahonia aquifolia) standardized 95-100% leucoanthocyanidins • Chinese Apricot (Prunus armeniaca). Contains no yeast, wheat, corn, soy, milk, salt, or starch.

BRAND NAMES

Some Brand Name Natural Products - What they Contain

Smart Pill - Only Natural, Inc.
Two tablets contain: Ginkgo Biloba leaf extract 10:1 250 mg • Gotu Kola 250 mg • Ginseng 100 mg • Capsicum 50 mg • L-Phenylalanine 200 mg • L-Glutamine 500 mg • L-Tyrosine 200 mg • GABA 300 mg • Vitamin B1 50 mg • Vitamin B3 50 mg • Vitamin B5 100 mg • Vitamin B6 50 mg • Vitamin B12 500 mcg • Folic Acid 200 mcg • Inositol 100 mg • Phosphatidylcholine 500 mg • RNA 100 mg • TMG 50 mg.

Smart Vitamins - Jamieson
Each capsule contains: Choline Bitartrate • Molasses cone • L-Glutamine • Brewers Yeast (a natural source of the B complex vitamin family) • Acerola (a natural source of Vitamin C) • Taurine • Kola Nut • Korean Ginseng • Vegetable Magnesium Stearate • Wheat Germ Powder • Silica • Chromium Yeast • Turnera (Damiana aphrodesiaca) • Capsicum (Cayenne) • Ginkgo Biloba • Fo-Ti (Polygonum multiflorum).

Smoke-Less - The Herbalist
Lobelia leaf • Milk Thistle seed • Oat seed • Siberian Ginseng root • Licorice root.

Smooth Food 2 - New Chapter, Inc.
Three capsules contain: Okra fruit 201 mg • Slippery Elm bark 201 mg • Psyllium husk 159 mg • Licorice root 159 mg • Ginger (rhizome) 159 mg • Marshmallow root 120 mg • Wheat Grass 21 mg • Bio Flora (tm) (100 million probiotic live cells per teaspoon) 21 mg • Chlorella regularis 6 mg • Cayenne fruit 3 mg. Other Ingredients: Vegetable cellulose.

Smooth Move - Traditional Medicinals
Sennosides A & B: 20 mg per cup as they naturally occur in Senna leaf (Casala angustifolia) present in the blend. Other herbal ingredients: Licorice root, Fennel seed, Orange peel, Cinnamon bark, Coriander seed, Ginger rhizome, natural Orange flavor.

Snooze - Pacific BioLogic
Valerian root • Dragon Bone (fossilized) • Oyster Shell (untreated) • Mimosa Tree flower • Chamomile • Gotu Kola • Hops • Polygala root • Jujube seed (sour) • Passion flower • Scullcap • Melatonin 1.5 mg per capsule.
See Editor's Note No. 16, page 1817.

Snoreless - Nutrition for Life International
Three sprays (approx. 3 mL) contains: Vitamin C 4.5 mg • Vitamin E 7.5 mg • Vitamin B6 3 mg • Olive Oil 210 mg • Sunflower Oil 90 mg • Peppermint Oil 60 mg • Almond Oil 37.5 mg • Sesame Oil 30 mg. Other Ingredients: Purified Water, Glycerine.

Snorenz - MedGen, Inc.
Peppermint Oil • Sunflower Oil • Sesame Oil • Olive Oil • Almond Oil.

SnoreStop - The Green Pharmacy
Each tablet contains: Nux vomica 4X • Nux vomica 6X • Belladonna 6X • Ephedra vulgaris 6X • Hydrastis canadensis 6X • Kali bichromicum 6X • Teucrium marum 6X • Histaminum hydrochloricum 12X.
See Editor's Note No. 1, page 1816.

Soft Gelatin Multiple - Nature's Life
Two capsules contain: Beta Carotene (Vitamin A equivalent 15000 IU) 9 mg • Vitamin A (Fish Liver oil) 10000 IU • Vitamin D (as Vitamin D3) (Cholecalciferol) 400 IU • Vitamin E (d-Alpha Tocopherol) 400 IU • Vitamin C 300 mg • Rose Hips 20 mg • Folic Acid 400 mcg • Vitamin B1 (Thiamine Mononitrate) 50 mg • Vitamin B2 (Riboflavin) 50 mg • Niacinamide 50 mg • Vitamin B6 (Pyridoxine HCl) 50 mg • Vitamin B12 (Cyanocobalamin) 100 mcg • Biotin (d-Biotin) 300 mcg • Pantothenic Acid(d-Calcium Pantothenate) 50 mg • Choline (Bitartrate) 25 mg • Inositol 25 mg •

PABA (Para Aminobenzoic Acid) 25 mg • Boron (Calcium Boron Gluconate) 25 mcg • Calcium (Carbonate, Citrate, Aspartate) 200 mg • Chromium (Nutrition 21 Picolinate) 25 mcg • Copper (Gluconate) 2 mg • Iodine (Potassium Iodide) 150 mcg • Iron (Peptonate) 10 mg • Magnesium (Magnesium Oxide) 100 mg • Manganese (Amino Acid Chelate) 15 mg • Molybdenum (Free-Form Amino Acid Chelate) 25 mcg • Potassium (Phosphate & Iodide) 15 mg • Selenium (l-Selenomethionine, yeast-free) 15 mcg • Silicon Dioxide 20 mg • Vanadium (Vanadyl Sulfate) 25 mcg • Zinc (Citrate, Gluconate, Picolinate) 15 mg • Essential Fatty Acids (Safflower oil) 540 mg.

Solovites - Puritan's Pride
Each tablet contains: Vitamin A 10,000 IU • Vitamin C 200 mg • Vitamin D 400 IU • Vitamin E 30 IU • Thiamin 30 mg • Riboflavin 30 mg • Niacin 30 mg • Vitamin B-6 30 mg • Folic Acid 400 mcg • Vitamin B-12 30 mcg • Biotin 30 mcg • Pantothenic Acid 30 mg • Calcium 60 mg • Iron 18 mg • Phosphorus 30 mg • Iodine 150 mcg • Magnesium 30 mg • Zinc 30 mg • Selenium 25 mcg • Copper 0.5 mg • Manganese 0.6 mg • Chromium 25 mcg • Molybdenum 25 mcg • Potassium 11 mg • PABA (Para-Aminobenzoic Acid) 30 mg • Choline Bitartrate 30 mg • Inositol 30 mcg • Citrus Bioflavonoid complex 25 mg • Betaine Hydrochloride 25 mg. In a base of Alfalfa, Parsley, Oyster Shell, Watercress, Kelp, and Lecithin.

Soluble Enzyme Caps - Atrium Inc.
Each capsule contains: Papayotin 110 mg • Pancreatin (Bovine) 90 mg • Calf Thymus (Bovine) 50 mg • Bromelain 50 mg • Lipase 10 mg • Chymotrypsin 15 mg. Lemon flavor.
See Editor's Note No. 14, page 1817.

Solu-Min - Aspen Group, Inc.
Calcium • Phosphorus • Magnesium • Potassium • Sulfur • Iron • Iodine • Copper • Cobalt • Zinc • Chromium • Manganese • Molybdenum • Selenium • Aluminum • Antimony • Barium • Bismuth • Cadmium • Sodium • Cesium • Carbon • Lithium • Nickel • Platinum • Rubidium • Silver • Strontium • Silicon • Tungsten • Tin • Titanium • Tantalum • Thorium • Vanadium • Zirconium • Yttrium. Plus up to 30 other randomly occurring trace minerals in natural combinations.

Sore Muscle Formula - Dr. Morrow's Homeopathic Formulas
Ten drops contain: Rhus toxicodendron 3C • Urtica urens 3C • Benzoic Acid 3C • Formic Acid 3C • Berberis vulgaris 3C • Ranunculus bulbosus 3C • Lithium carbonate 3C.
See Editor's Note No. 1, paeg 1816.

Sore Throat Lozenge - Jamieson
Each lozenge contains: Slippery Elm bark 50 mg • White Horehound leaves 50 mg • Parsley root 20 mg • Thyme leaves 10 mg • Menthol 5 mg. Other Ingredients: Camphor 50 mcg, Acerola Cherry 40 mg, Sugar, Glucose, Honey, Anise Oil, and natural flavors.

Source of Life Oxygenic - Nature's Plus
Three tablets contain: Mixed Wild berry extract containing: [European Red Wine Grape, Bilberry, Blackberry, Black Raspberry, & Red Raspberry (standardized 20% Polyphenols, 4% Anthocyanosides)] 300 mg • Chinese Green Tea extract (standardized 20% Polyphenols) 300 mg • Horseradish concentrate naturally rich in Peroxidase & Catalase 250 mg • Vitamin C fortified with Rose Hips, Mango, Guava & West Indian Cherry 100 mg • Beta Carotene (Dunaliella salina, Carrot) 2500 IU • Wild Grape seed extract standardized 95-100% Leucoanthocyanins 10 mg • Pycnogenol (Pine bark extract) standardized 85-95% Proanthocyanidins 5 mg. In a whole food base of Broccoli, Spinach, Cauliflower & Beet Greens. Contains no yeast, wheat, corn, soy, milk, salt, sugar or starch.

Source of Life Vibra-Gest - Nature's Plus
Each vegicap contains: Brown rice fermentation: Amylase, 30000 units/gram 50 mg • Lactase, 1000 units/gram 50 mg • Lipase, 5000 units/gram 50 mg • Cellulase, 5000 units/gram 30 mg • Protease, 100000 units/gram 20 mg • Oxidase, 5000 units/gram 10 mg

- Barley malt: Diastase, 1000 units/gram 10 mg • Maltase, 1000 units/gram 10 mg • Sweet potato: Phosphatase, 4000 units/gram 5 mg • Pineapple: Bromelain, 600 GDU/gram 35 mg • Papaya: Papain, 2 million units/gram 30 mg • Carrot powder: Lactobacillus acidophilus 4 billion viable cells/gram 100 mg • Natural cultures: Bifidobacterium longum 1 billion viable cells/gram 50 mg • Lactobacillus bulgaricus 1 billion viable cells/gram 50 mg. Contains no yeast, wheat, corn, soy, milk, salt, sugar or starch.

Soy Defense - Changes - TwinLab
Two caplets contain: Vitamin E (as D-Alpha-Tocopheryl Succinate and Dl-Alpha-Tocopheryl Acetate) 200 IU • Mixed Soy phytosterols 50 mg • Tri-source isoflavone concentrate [defatted Soy Germ, Red Clover flower, and Kudzu root (providing 40 mg total isoflavones)] 1333 mg • Soy polysaccharides 150 mg. Other Ingredients: Dicalcium Phosphate, Vegetable Cellulose, Fractionated vegetable oil, Silica, Calcium Sulfate, and Vegetable resin glaze.

Soy Essentials - Health From The Sun
Four tablets contain: Genistein (Aglycone) 2.88 mg • Daidzein (Aglycone) 2.20 mg • Beta Glucans 7.87 mg. Ingredients: Certified GMO-Free Fermented Soymeal (Soynatto), Microcrystalline Cellulose, Stearic Acid, HPC (cellulose), Croscarmellose Sodium, Magnesium Stearate, Silicon Dioxide, Pharmaceutical Glaze.

Soy Extract - PhytoPharmica
Each capsule contains: Soy (Glycine Max.) bean extract (standardized to contain 15% isoflavones calculated as their glycoside forms, genistin and daidzin) 100 mg.

Soy Force Rx - Biotech
Two tablets contain: Soy Isoflavones 80 mg • Soy Protein Concentrate 500 mg • OPTiSOY Blend 300 mg.

Soy Isoflavone - Natrol
One capsule contains: Soy Isoflavone extract 100 mg containing: Isoflavones (10%) 10 mg • Daidzin & Daidzein (2%) 2 mg • Genistin & Genistein (9%) 9 mg • Glycitin & Glycitein (0.1%) 0.1 mg. Other ingredients: Rice powder, Magnesium Stearate, Gelatin.

Soy Isoflavones - Olympian Labs
Each capsule contains: Soy Isoflavone dried extract 100 mg.

Soy Isoflavones 50 mg - Nature Made
Each tablet contains: Soy Isoflavones 50 mg. Other Ingredients: Dibasic Calcium Phosphate, Cellulose, Soy Extract, Croscarmellose Sodium, Magnesium Stearate, Silicon Dioxide.

Soy Isoflavones Concentrate Caplet - Leiner Health Products
Each caplet contains: Isoflavones (Soy extract) 50 mg • Lecithin 15 mg. Other Ingredients: Dicalcium Phosphate, Cellulose, Stearic Acid, Silicon Dioxide, Croscarmellose Sodium, Magnesium Stearate, Dextrin, Dextrose, Sodium Carboxymethylcellulose, Sodium Citrate.

Soy Preventive - GNC
Two capsules contain: Vitamin A (100% as Acetate) 5000 IU • Vitamin C (as Ascorbic Acid) 200 mg • Vitamin E (as d-alpha Tocopheryl Succinate) 100 IU • Selenium (as Selenium Yeast) 100 mcg • Soy Isoflavone Concentrate (34% Isoflavones = 8.5 mg) 25 mg. Other Ingredients: Cellulose, Calcium Carbonate, Gelatin.

Soy-Based Milk-Free Lactobacillus Acidophilus powder - Nature's Life
Each level tablespoon (6 g) contains: A freeze-dried blend of unrefined Apple Juice, Maltodextrin NF, SUPRO brand Soy Protein, pure Crystalline Fructose & our uniquely cultured probiotics Lactobacillus Acidophilus (95%), L. Bulgaricus (3%) & Bifidobacteria Bifidus (2%).

Soygenol 100 - FreeLife
Each tablet contains: Soygenol 100 [soy-phosphatide-bonded premium Grape Seed OPCs (2:1)] 100 mg • Green Tea leaf standardized extract (30% polyphenols) 100 mg • Ultra Soy Delivery System (Soy polysaccharides and plant enzymes) 5000 Units. Other Ingredients: Calcium Hydrogen Phosphate, Cellulose, Cellulose Gum, Vegetable Stearic Acid, Silica, Vegetable Magnesium Stearate, Calcium Silicate, Vita-Coat (vegetable resin, alpha-lipoic acid).

SoySwee Tea - HerbaSway
Soy • Ginger • Panax Ginseng • Siberian Ginseng • Blackberry • HerbaSwee (Cucurbitaceae fruit).

SP-500 - PhytoPharmica
Each capsule contains: Spleen Polypeptides (a mixture of highly purified bovine-derived spleen polypeptides naturally present in the spleen, including tuftsin, splenopentin, splenin and leukokinin) 375 mg • Goldenseal root extract (Hydrastis canadensis) standardized to contain 5% total alkaloids including Berberine, Hydrastine and Canadine 125 mg. Contains no sugar, salt, yeast, wheat, corn, dairy products, flavoring, or preservatives. All organs and glands derived from bovine sources.
See Editor's Note No. 14, page 1817.

Speak Easy Throat Spray - The Herbalist
Yerba Mansa root • Echinacea root • Marshmallow root • Propolis • Myrrh Gum • Licorice root in a base of Vegetable Glycerine.

Special B-Complex 50 mg - Nature's Life
Each capsule contains: Vitamin C 50 mg • Vitamin B1 (Thiamine HCl) 50 mg • Vitamin B2 (Riboflavin) 50 mg • Niacinamide 50 mg • Vitamin B6 (Pyridoxine HCl) 50 mg • Folic Acid 800 mcg • Vitamin B12 (Cobalamin concentrate) 50 mcg • Biotin 50 mcg • Pantothenic Acid (d-Calcium Pantothenate) 50 mg • Choline (Choline Bitartrate) 50 mg • Inositol 50 mg • PABA (Para-Aminobenzioc Acid) 50 mg. In a natural base of Rice Bran, Alfalfa, Parsley, Watercress, Rose Hips & Acerola.

Special Two - Now
Two tablets contain: Vitamin A (Beta Carotene) (6 mg) 10000 IU • Vitamin B1 (Thiamine HCL) 50 mg • Vitamin B2 (Riboflavin) 50 mg • Vitamin B3 (Niacinamide) 50 mg • Vitamin B5 (Pantothenic Acid) 50 mg • Vitamin B6 (Pyridoxine HCL) 50 mg • Vitamin B12 (Cyanocobalamin) 100 mcg • Biotin 100 mcg • Folic Acid 400 mcg • Vitamin C (Calcium Ascorbate) 500 mg • Vitamin D (Calciferol) 200 IU • Vitamin E (d-Alpha Succinate) 200 IU • Vitamin K (from green foods) 70 mcg • Calcium (Ascorbate, Carbonate) 100 mg • Magnesium (Oxide , Amino Acid Chelate) 50 mg • Zinc (Amino Acid Chelate) 15 mg • Iron (Amino Acid Chelate) 10 mg • Copper (Amino Acid Chelate) 1 mg • Iodine (Kelp) 150 mcg • Potassium 50 mg • Manganese (Amino Acid Chelate) 5 mg • Selenium (Amino Acid Chelate) 50 mcg • Chromium (Yeast-free GTF) 100 mcg • Molybdenum (Amino Acid Chelate) 50 mcg • Boron (Amino Acid Chelate) 1 mg • Vanadium (Amino Acid Chelate) 50 mcg • Choline (Bitartrate) 50 mg • Inositol 50 mg • PABA 30 mg • Spirulina 250 mg • Chlorella (broken cell wall) 250 mg • Barley grass organic 250 mg • Alfalfa juice concentrate 100 mg • Octacosanol wheat-free 100 mcg • Siberian Ginseng 50 mg • Bioflavonoids (40%) 50 mg • Rutin 25 mg • Psyllium husk fiber 50 mg • Echinacea 50 mg • Apple Pectin 25 mg • Betaine Hydrochloride 25 mg • Glutamic Acid 25 mg • Papain (Papaya) 25 mg • Lipase 10 mg • Amylase 10 mg • Chlorophyll 9 mg • 17 Amino Acids 380 mg derived from Spirulina, Chlorella , Barley grass & Alfalfa juice concentrate. Natural base includes Alfalfa, Rose Hips, Di-Calcium Phosphate, Cellulose, Stearic Acid & natural vegetable protein coating.

Spectro 3 - Solaray - Nutraceutical
Three tablets contain: Vitamin A (from Retinyl Palmitate, and 60% as natural Beta Carotene [Dunaliella salina algae]) 25000 IU • Vitamin C (as natural Ascorbic acid, Rose Hips, Acerola cherry) 1000 mg •

BRAND NAMES

BRAND NAMES

Vitamin D (as Cholecalciferol D-3) 400 IU • Vitamin E (as natural d-Alpha Tocopheryl Succinate, d-Alpha Tocopheryl Acetate) 400 IU • Vitamin K 50 mcg • Thiamin (as Thiamine Mononitrate) (Vitamin B1) 25 mg • Riboflavin (Vitamin B2)25 mg • Niacin (as Niacinamide) 125 mg • Vitamin B6 (as Pyridoxine HCl) 50 mg • Folic Acid 400 mcg • Vitamin B12 (as Cyanocobalamin) 100 mcg • Biotin 300 mcg • Pantothenic Acid (as d-Calcium Pantothenate) 125 mg • Calcium (as Calcium Carbonate, Calcium Amino Acid Chelate) 500 mg • Iron (as Iron Fumarate, Iron Amino Acid Chelate) 18 mg • Phosphorous (as Potassium Phosphate) 23 mg • Iodine (from Kelp) 225 mcg • Magnesium (Magnesium Oxide, Magnesium Amino Acid Chelate) 250 mg • Zinc (as Zinc Citrate, Zinc Picolinate, Zinc Amino Acid Chelate) 15 mg • Selenium (as yeast free I-Selenomethionine) 100 mcg • Copper (as Copper Amino Acid Chelate) 0.5 mg • Potassium (as Potassium Phosphate, Potassium Chloride) 88 mg • Choline Bitartrate 50 mg • Inositol 50 mg • PABA (Para-Aminobenzoic Acid) 30 mg • Lecithin 50 mg • Bioflavonoid concentrate (from Citrus) 150 mg • Rutin concentrate 50 mg • Hesperidin concentrate 50 mg • Pectin 25 mg • Boron (as Tetra-Boron: Boron Citrate, Boron Glycinate, Boron Aspartate, Boron Lysinate) 1.5 mg • Spirulina (Spirulina platensis) 50 mg • Alfalfa juice (aerial) 125 mg • Carrot and Yam concentrate 100 mg • Barley Grass juice concentrate 75 mg • Rosemary leaf extract 25 mg • Aloe Vera gel concentrate 200x (equivalent to 400 mg) 2 mg • Parsley leaf 50 mg • Pancreatin 4x (equivalent to 120 mg) 30 mg • Diatase 20 mg • Papain (from Papaya) 50 mg • Ox Bile extract 20 mg • Glutamic Acid HCl 50 mg • Propolis 2x (equivalent to 50 mg) 25 mg • Royal Jelly 3.5x (equivalent to 14 mg) 4 mg • Bee Pollen. Other ingredients: Cellulose, Stearic Acid, Silica, Siberian Ginseng root, Calcium Phosphate, Whole Rice concentrate, Alfalfa herb, Montmorillonite Clay, Maltodextrin, Natural flavors and Natural food glazed coating. See Editor's Note No. 14, page 1817.

SPES - BotanicLab, Inc
Each capsule contains: Proprietary Blend: Pyrola (pyrola rotundifolia L), Agrimony (Agrimonia pilosa Ledeb), Corydalis (Corydalis yanhusuo W.T. Wang), Reishi (Ganoderma lucidum Karst), Rubescens (Rabdosia rubescens Hara), Stephania (Stephania delavayi Diels), Stephania (Stephania sinica Diels), Lycoris (Lycoris radiata Herb), Partinia (Partrinia heterophylla Bunga), Oriental Ginseng (Panax ginseng C.A. Meyer), Pollen (Pollen), Prickly Ash (Zanthoxylum nitidum DC), Chinese Licorice (Glycyrrhiza uralensis Fisch), Cervus (Cervus nippon Temmiinck), Broomrape (Cistanche deserticola Y.C. Ma) 300 mg.

Spirulina - Quest
Each capsule contains: Spirulina 500 mg.

Spirulina - Source Naturals
Six tablets contain: Vitamin A (Beta Carotene) 14,000 IU • Vitamin B1 (Thiamin) 100 mcg • Vitamin B2 (Riboflavin) 99 mcg • Niacin 620 mcg • Vitamin B12 (Cobalamin) 6.6 mg • Boron 30 mcg • Iron 3.2 mg • Magnesium 14 mg • Phosphorus 31 mg • Protein 1,800 mg • Phycocyanin 333 mg • Linoleic Acid 33 mg • Gamma-Linoleic Acid (GLA) 30 mg • Omega-3 Fatty Acids 87 mcg • Chlorophyll 23.7 mg • Total Carotenoids 16.2 mg • Superoxide Dismutase (SOD) 1.2 mg.

Spirulina Blue Green Algae - Leiner Health Products
Each capsule contains: Spirulina Blue Green Algae (Spirulina pacifica) cell 250 mg. Other Ingredients: Maltodextrin, Gelatin, Cellulose, Magnesium Stearate, Croscarmellose Sodium.

Spirulina Multiple - Source Naturals
Two tablets contain: Spirulina Plankton (Spirulina platensis) 200 mg • Rose Hips 25 mg • Beta Carotene (Pro-Vitamin A) 10,000 IU • Vitamin B1 (Thiamin Mononitrate) 25 mg • Vitamin B2 (Riboflavin) 25 mg • Niacin 25 mg • Vitamin B6 (Pyridoxine HCl) 25 mg • Vitamin B12 (Cobalamin) 100 mcg • Folic Acid 100 mcg • Vitamin C (Ascoribic Acid) 250 mg • Vitamin D (as Vitamin D3)

(Cholecalciferol) 400 IU • Vitamin E d-alpha tocopheryl 60 IU • Calcium (Carbonate) 99 mg • Iodine (from Kelp) 150 mcg • Iron (Fumarate) 18 mg • Magnesium (Oxide) 33 mg • Potassium (Chelate) 7.5 mg • Zinc (Citrate) 5 mg.

Spirulina Powder - Source Naturals
Each teaspoon contains: Vitamin A (Beta Carotene) 42,000 IU • Vitamin B1 (Thiamin) 300 mcg • Vitamin B2 (Riboflavin) 300 mcg • Niacin 2 mg • Vitamin B12 (Cobalamin) 20 mg • Boron 90 mcg • Iron 9.5 mg • Magnesium 43 mg • Phosphorus 93 mg • Protein 5,400 mg • Phycocyanin 1,000 mg • Linoleic Acid 99 mg • Gamma-Linolenic Acid (GLA) 90 mg • Omega-3 Fatty Acids 261 mcg • Chlorophyll 71 mg • Total Carotenoids 48.6 mg • Superoxide Dismutase (SOD) 3.6 mg.

SPL and PAN - Dial Herbs
Chamomile • Dandelion • Goldenseal • Parsley • Uva Ursi • Yellow Dock • Cayenne • Yarrow.

Sport - Mannatech
Chromium Picolinate • Sterol Complex: bovine testes extract, wild yam root standardized for phytosterols, Mexican Sarsaparilla root • Boron Citrate • Ambrotose Complex: naturally occurring plant polysaccharides including freeze-dried Aloe Vera inner leaf gel extract - Manapol powder. Other Ingredients: Brown Rice Flour, Silicon Dioxide, Magnesium Stearate. See Editor's Note No. 26, page 1818.

Sport Fuel - TwinLab
Six capsules contain: Beta-Carotene (pro-Vitamin A) 25000 IU • Vitamin D (from natural Vitamin D3) 400 IU • Vitamin C 1000 mg • Natural Vitamin E (Succinate) 800 IU • CoQ10 (Coenzyme Q10) 30 mg • L-Glutathione 100 mg • N-Acetyl Cysteine (NAC) 200 mg • Alpha Lipoic Acid 100 mg • Vitamin B1 (Thiamine) 50 mg • Vitamin B2 (Riboflavin) 50 mg • Vitamin B6 (Pyridoxine) 50 mg • Vitamin B12 (Cobalamin) 100 mg • Folic Acid 400 mcg • Niacinamide 150 mg • Pantothenic Acid 250 mg • Biotin 300 mcg • PABA (Para-Aminobenzoic Acid) 25 mg • Choline Bitartrate 100 mg • Inositol 100 mg • L-Carnitine (from Carni Fuel L-Carnitine Magnesium Citrate) 100 mg • Magnesium (from L-Carnitine Magnesium Citrate, Aspartate, Alpha-Ketoglutarate & Oxide) 600 mg • Potassium (from Potassium Aspartate, Alpha-Ketoglutarate & Citrate) 100 mg • Zinc (from Zinc Picolinate) 30 mg • Manganese (from Manganese Gluconate) 5 mg • Copper (from Copper Gluconate) 2 mg • Iron (from Ferrous Fumarate) 10 mg • Iodine (from Potassium Iodide) 150 mcg • Selenium (from Selenomethionine & Selenate 50/50 mixture) 200 mcg • Chromium (from Chromic Fuel Chromium Picolinate) 400 mcg • Molybdenum (from natural Molybdic Acid) 150 mcg.

Sport Fuel With Iron - TwinLab
Six capsules contain: Beta-Carotene (pro-Vitamin A) 25000 IU • Vitamin D (from natural form Vitamin D3) 400 IU • Vitamin C 1000 mg • Natural Vitamin E (Succinate) 800 IU • CoQ10 (Coenzyme Q10) 30 mg • L-Glutathione 100 mg • N-Acetyl Cysteine (NAC) 200 mg • Alpha Lipoic Acid 100 mcg • Vitamin B1 (Thiamine) 50 mg • Vitamin B2 (Riboflavin) 50 mg • Vitamin B6 (Pyridoxine) 50 mg • Vitamin B12 (Cobalamin) 100 mcg • Folic Acid 400 mcg • Niacinamide 150 mg • Pantothenic Acid 250 mg • Biotin 300 mcg • PABA (Para-Aminobenzoic Acid) 25 mg • Choline Bitartrate 100 mg • Inositol 100 mg • L-Carnitine (from Carni Fuel L-Carnitine Magnesium Citrate) 100 mg • Calcium (from Calcium Citrate, Carbonate) 25 mg • Magnesium (from L-Carnitine Magnesium Citrate, Aspartate, Alpha-Ketoglutarate & Oxide) 600 mg • Potassium (from Potassium Aspartate, Alpha-Ketoglutarate & Citrate) 100 mg • Zinc (from Zinc Picolinate) 30 mg • Manganese (from Manganese Gluconate) 5 mg • Copper (from Copper Gluconate) 2 mg • Iron (from

Ferrous Fumarate) 10 mg • Iodine (from Potassium Iodide) 150 mcg • Selenium (from Selenomethionine & Selenate‹50/50 mixture) 200 mcg • Chromium (from Chromic Fuel Chromium Picolinate) 400 mcg • Molybdenum (from natural Molybdic Acid) 150 mcg.

Sport Fuel Without Iron - TwinLab
Six capsules contain: Beta-Carotene (pro-Vitamin A) 25000 IU • Vitamin D (from natural form Vitamin D3) 400 IU • Vitamin C 1000 mg • Natural Vitamin E (Succinate) 800 IU • CoQ10 (Coenzyme Q10) 30 mg • L-Glutathione 100 mg • N-Acetyl Cysteine (NAC) 200 mg • Alpha Lipoic Acid 100 mcg • Vitamin B1 (Thiamine) 50 mg • Vitamin B2 (Riboflavin) 50 mg • Vitamin B6 (Pyridoxine) 50 mg • Vitamin B12 (Cobalamin) 100 mcg • Folic Acid 400 mcg • Niacinamide 150 mg • Pantothenic Acid 250 mg • Biotin 300 mcg • PABA (Para-Aminobenzoic Acid) 25 mg • Choline Bitartrate 100 mg • Inositol 100 mg • L-Carnitine (from Carni Fuel L-Carnitine Magnesium Citrate) 100 mg • Calcium (from Calcium Citrate, Carbonate) 25 mg • Magnesium (from L-Carnitine Magnesium Citrate, Aspartate, Alpha-Ketoglutarate & Oxide) 600 mg • Potassium (from Potassium Aspartate, Alpha-Ketoglutarate & Citrate) 100 mg • Zinc (from Zinc Picolinate) 30 mg • Manganese (from Manganese Gluconate) 5 mg • Copper (from Copper Gluconate) 2 mg • Iodine (from Potassium Iodide) 150 mcg • Selenium (from Selenomethionine & Selenate‹50/50 mixture) 200 mcg • Chromium (from Chromic Fuel Chromium Picolinate) 400 mcg • Molybdenum (from natural Molybdic Acid) 150 mcg.

Sportalyte - Pharmanex
Twenty grams Contain: Glucose • Fructose • Maltodextrin • Citric Acid • Natural Flavor • Sodium Chloride • Silicon Dioxide • Sodium Citrate • Magnesium Carbonate • Tricalcium Phosphate • Potassium Citrate • Magnesium Oxide • Ascorbic Acid • d- Alpha Tocopheryl Acetate • Potassium Chloride • Hydromins • Taurine • Fructooligosaccharides.

Sports One DIOL XS - Sports One
Each capsule contains: 4-Androstenediol 100 mg • Nor-4-Androstenediol 100 mg.

Spring Valley Children's Chewables Complete - Leiner Health Products
Each tablet contains: Vitamin A Acetate (as Acetate and Beta Carotene) 5000 IU • Vitamin C (Ascorbic Acid) 60 mg • Vitamin D (Ergocalciferol) 400 IU • Vitamin E (dl-Alpha Tocopheryl Acetate) 30 IU • Thiamin Mononitrate (Vitamin B1) 1.5 mg • Riboflavin (Vitamin B2) 1.7 mg • Niacin (Niacinamide) 20 mg • Vitamin B-6 (Pyridoxine Hydrochloride) 2 mg • Folic Acid 400 mcg • Vitamin B-12 (Cyanocobalamin) 6 mcg • Biotin (USP Method 2) 40 mcg • Pantothenic Acid (d-Calcium Pantothenate) 10 mg • Calcium 100 mg • Iron (Ferrous Fumarate) 18 mg • Phosphorus 100 mg • Iodine (Potassium Iodide) 150 mcg • Magnesium Oxide 20 mg • Zinc Oxide 15 mg • Copper (Cupric Oxide) 2 mg. Other Ingredients: Sorbitol, Dicalcium Phosphate, Magnesium Phosphate, Fructose, Stearic Acid, Mono- & Diglycerides, Xylitol, Gelatin, Sodium Ascorbate, Carrageenan, Aspartame, Citric Acid, Red 40 Lake, Yellow 6 Lake, Starch, Silicon Dioxide, Magnesium Stearate, Blue 2 Lake, Hydroxypropyl Methylcellulose, Resin, Hydroxypropyl Cellulose, Lactose, Polyvinyl Pyrrolidone.
See Editor's Note No. 3, page 1816.

Spring Valley Vitamin C with Rose Hips - Leiner Health Products
Each tablet contains: Vitamin C 500 mg. Other Ingredients: Ascorbic Acid, Starch, Cellulose, Rose Hips, Stearic Acid, Silicon Croscarmellose Sodium.

SS Cream (SS-Cream) - Cheil Jedang Corporation
70% ethanol extract of Bufonis venenum 10 mg • 100 mg extract of Angelicae gigantic radix, Cistanchis caulis, Torilidis semen, Ginseng radix alba, Zanthoxylli fructos • 10 mg extract of Asiasari radix, Caryophilli flos, Cinnamomi cortex.
See Editor's Note No. 23, page 1818

St. John's Complex - Body Wise International, Inc.
Each tablet contains: St. John's Wort extract (0.3% Hypericin) 300 mg • Chamomile flowers (Anthemis flores) 25 mg • Passion Flower (Passiflora incarnata) 25 mg.

St. John's Formula - Health Smart Vitamins
Each capsule contains: Vitamin B6 (as pyridoxine hydrochloride) 10 mg • Folate (folic acid) 200 mcg • Vitamin B12 (as cyanocobalamin) 50 mcg • Magnesium (as magnesium oxide) 100 mg • St. John's Wort aerial parts (0.3% hypercins, 0.9 mg) 300 mg • Kava Kava root (30% kavalactones, 22.5 mg) 75 mg • Ginkgo leaf (24% ginkgo flavonglycosides, 9.6 mg; 6% terpene lactone, 2.4 mg) 40 mg.

St. John's Good Mood - Traditional Medicinals
Contains: St. John's Wort herb & dry extract • Lemon Balm leaf (Melissa) • Oatstraw herb • Damiana herb • Lavender flower • Berganot herb • Sage leaf • Spearmint leaf • Lemongrass leaf • Licorice root • Rose petals • Stevia leaf.

St. John's Plus - Nutri-Quest
Each tablet contains: St. John's Wort herb 400 mg • Pyridoxal-5-Phosphate 5 mg • Riboflavin (as Riboflavin-5-Phosphate) 5 mg • Folic Acid 100 mcg • Vitamin B1 10 mg • Vitamin B12 250 mcg • Ginkgo Biloba extract 5 mg • Damiana herb 25 mg • Ginkgo Biloba herb 30 mg • Blue Vervain 25 mg • Kava Kava herb 10 mg • Hyssop herb 15 mg • Siberian Ginseng 10 mg • Niacinamide 50 mg • Calcium Citrate 100 mg • Magnesium Citrate 100 mg.

St. John's Plus - Rx Vitamins
Each caplet provides: St. John's Wort flower (Hypericum perforatum, standardized 0.3-0.5 hypericin) 300 mg • Kava root (Piper methylsticum, standardized 29-31% kavalactones) 50 mg • Siberian ginseng root (Eleutherococcus senticosis, standardized 0.8% eleutherosides) 50 mg • Feverfew leaf (Tanacetum parthenium, standardized 0.7% parthenolide) 25 mg • L-Tyrosine (pharmaceutical grade, free form amino acid) 25 mg • Zinc (l-monomethionine) 10 mg • Vitamin B6 (pyridoxine HCl) 5 mg • Vitamin B12 (cyanocobalamin) 10 mcg.

St. John's Plus Kava Kava - Progressive Labs
Each capsule contains: Vitamin B6 (pyridoxine HCl) 25 mg • St. John's Wort 0.3% Hypericin 200 mg • Kava Kava 100 mg.

St. John's Solution - Quantum
One softgel contains: St. John's Wort (Hypericum perforatum) (Standardized .3% hypericin) 300 mg.

St. John's Wort - Leiner Health Products
Each caplet contains: St. John's Wort extract (Hypericum perforatum) herb 330 mg. Other Ingredients: Cellulose, Dicalcium Phosphate, Croscarmellose Sodium, Stearic Acid, Hydroxypropyl Methycellulose, Magnesium Stearate, Silicon Dioxide, Hydroxypropyl Cellulose, Red 40 Lake, Blue 2 Lake, Pharmaceutical Glaze, Polyethylene Glycol 3350, Polysorbate 80, Titanium Dioxide.

St. John's Wort - Centrum Herbals
One capsule contains: St. John's Wort (Hypericum perforatum) flower and leaves 300 mg. Standardized to contain (based on extract weight): Total Hypericin compounds (marker) 0.3%, Hyperforin (marker), Quercetin (natural active), Amentoflavone (natural active), Gaba & Proline (natural actives). Activity measure: Muscarinic M1 binding assay. Other ingredients: Dibasic Calcium Phosphate, Maltodextrin, Cellulose, Lactose Monohydrate, Silicon Dioxide, Hydroxypropyl Cellulose, Ethycellulose, Castor Oil, Gelatin, Sodium Lauryl Sulfate, Propylene Glycol, Titanium Dioxide.

BRAND NAMES

St. John's Wort - Gaia Herbs
St. John's Wort standardized for 0.5% hypericins. Standardized Full Spectrum 180 mg of extract per capsule. Guaranteed Potency 90 mg of extract per capsule.

St. John's Wort - Jamieson
Each tablet contains: Vitamin C 2.5 mg • St. John's Wort 4.4:1 extract (Hypericum perforatum L.) (Aerial parts of flower, stamen and leaf) (Containing 0.3% hypericin) 225 mg.

St. John's Wort - Nature's Way
Two capsules contain: St. John's Wort stem, leaf, flower 600 mg • St. John's Wort (dried extract 0.3% Dianthrones measures as Hypericin) 300 mg. Other ingredients: Gelatin, Magnesium Stearate, Millet.

St. John's Wort - Pharmanex
Each capsule contains: St. John's Wort flower tops/leaves (Hypericum perforatum) (5:1) 300 mg. Other Ingredients: Rice Flour, Gelatin, Magnesium Stearate, Silicon Dioxide.

St. John's Wort - Quest
Each caplet contains: St. John's Wort (Hypericum perfortum) (provided by 300 mg P.E. 1:5 standardized to contain 0.3% Hypercin) 1500 mg. Other Ingredients: Microcrystalline Cellulose, Calcium phosphate, Croscarmellose Sodium Dioxide, Vegetable Stearin, Magnesium Stearate.

St. John's Wort - Swanson
Each capsule contains: St. John's Wort powder 375 mg.

St. John's Wort - Celestial Seasonings - Celestial Seasonings
Three capsules contain: Proprietary Blend, 1800 mg: St. John's Wort (leaves,stems, flowers), St. John's Wort (standardized extract). Other ingredients: May contain one or more of the following: Dicalcium phosphate, gelatin, rice flour, stearic acid, magnesium stearate, and silicon dioxide. This product contains no artificial colors, flavors, or preservatives. One serving size is equivalent to: St. John's Wort 900 mg standardized to 0.3% hypericin.

St. John's Wort + Ginseng Caplet - Leiner Health Products
Each caplet contains: Lecithin 15 mg • Licorice extract (Glycyrrhiza glabra) root 20 mg • Siberian Ginseng extract (Eleutheroxoxxus senticosus) root 50 mg • Siberian Ginseng powder (Eleuterococcus senticosus) root 15 mg • St. John's Wort extract (Hypericum perforatum) aerial parts 300 mg. Other Ingredients: Cellulose, Dicalcium Phosphate, Croscarmellose Sodium, Silicon Dioxide, Stearic Acid, Magnesium Stearate, Hydroxypropyl Methylcellulose, Dextrin.

St. John's Wort + Kava Kava - Leiner Health Products
Each caplet contains: Kava Kava extract (Piper methysticum) root 60 mg • St. John's Wort extract (Hypericum perforatum) aerial parts 300 mg. Other Ingredients: Cellulose, Dicalcium Phosphate, Croscarmellose Sodium, Silicon Dioxide, Stearic Acid, Magnesium Stearate, Dextrin, Dextrose, Lecithin, Sodium Carboxymethylcellulose, Sodium Citrate.

St. John's Wort Blend - VitaStore
Each capsule contains: St. John's Wort (standardized for 0.3% Hypericin) • Kava Kava • Ginkgo Biloba.

St. John's Wort Complete - Futurebiotics
Two capsules contain: Vitamin C (as ascorbic acid) 300 mg • Thiamin 25 mg • Riboflavin 25 mg • Niacin (as niacinamide) 25 mg • Vitamin B6 (as pyridoxine hydrochloride) 25 mg • Folic Acid 400 mcg • Vitamin B12 (as cyanocobalamin) 250 mcg • Biotin 300 mcg • Pantothenic Acid (as calcium pantothenate) 25 mg • St. John's Wort

flower powder extract (standardized for 0.3% (0.8 mg) hypericin) 250 mg • Choline (as choline bitartrate) 25 mg • Inositol 25 mg • Para-Aminobenzoic Acid 25 mg • L-Tyrosine 50 mg • L-Phenylalanine 100 mg. Other ingredients: Gelatin, Water.

St. John's Wort Forte with Kava - PhytoPharmica
Each capsule contains: St. John's Wort (Hypericum peroratum) flower head extract (standardized to contain a minimum of 0.3% hypericin and 4% hyperforin) 300 mg • Valerian (Valeriana officinalis) root extract (standardized to contain a minimum of 0.8% valerenic acids) 100 mg • Kava (Piper methysticum) root extract (standardized to contain 30% kavalactones) 100 mg.

St. John's Wort Modifiers - Metabolic Response Modifiers
Each capsule contains: Hypericum perforatum (0.3% Hypericin) 450 mg.

St. John's Wort NutraSpray - Source Naturals
Each spray contains: St. John's Wort standardized extract (Hypericum perforatum) 2.7 mg.

St. John's Wort Oil - Blessed Herbs
St. John's Wort flowering tops • organic cold-pressed Olive oil.

St. John's Wort Plus - Aspen Group, Inc.
Each capsule contains: St. John's Wort herb extract standardized to 0.3% Hypericin 300 mg • Kava Kava 100 mg • Vitamin B6 25 mg • Standardized extract St. John's Wort herb extract Hypericum Perforatum. No artificial colors, flavors or preservatives.

St. John's Wort Supreme - Gaia Herbs
St. John's Wort and Kava Kava standardized for 0.5% hypericins and 55% kavalactones. Standardized Full Spectrum 150 mg of extract per capsule. Guaranteed Potency 75 mg of extract per capsule.

St. John's Wort-Go! - Wakunaga of America
Each caplet contains: St. John's Wort Standardized Extract (herb with flower) standardized to 0.3% Hypericin 600 mg. Other Ingredients: Cellulose, Magnesium Stearate (vegetable source), Silica.

St. John's Wort-Kava Kava - Futurebiotics
St. John's Wort flower powder extract (standardized for 0.3% (0.8 mg) hypericin) 250 mg • Kava Kava root powder extract (standardized for 30% (30 mg) kavalactones) 100 mg. Other ingredients: Gelatin, Water.

Stabilium - Smart Basics
Each capsule contains: Predigested Garum Armoricum 105 mg • Virgin Sunflower Oil 83 mg • Soya Lecithin Oil 12 mg.

Stabilized Acidophilus Three Billion - Now
Each tablet contains: Lactobacillus Acidophilus 3 billion. Other Ingredients: Anhydrous Dicalcium Phosphate, Microcrystalline Cellulose, Silica, Modified Cellulose Gum, Magnesium Stearate. Contains no sugar, yeast, corn, soy, wheat, gluten, or preservatives.

Stamina - HerbaSway
Horny Goat Weed • Yohimbe • Dong Quai • Knotweed • Panax Ginseng • Licorice • Blackberry • HerbaSwee (Cucurbitaceae fruit).

Stamina 100 - Jamieson
Three caplets contain: Vitamin A (as Retinyl Acetate) 7500 IU • Vitamin C (as Ascorbic Acid) 125 mg • Vitamin D (as Cholecalciferol) 200 IU • Vitamin E (as Dl-Alpha Tocopheryl Acetate) 25 IU • Thiamin (as Thiamine Mononitrate) 12.5 mg • Riboflavin (Vitamin B2) 12.5 mg • Niacin (as Nicacinamide) 190 mg • Vitamin B6 (as Pyridoxine Hydrochloride) 12.5 mg • Folate (as Folic Acid) 200 mcg • Vitamin B12 (as Cyanocobalamin) 50 mcg • Pantothenic

Acid (as Calcium D-Pantothenate) 30 mg • Calcium (as Calcium Carbonate) 600 mg • Iron (as Ferrous Fumarate) 10 mg • Iodine (as Potassium Iodide) 150 mcg • Magnesium (as Magnesium Oxide) 100 mg • Zinc (as Zinc Gluconate) 5 mg • Selenium (as Seleium Brown Rice Protein Chelate) 12.5 mcg • Manganese (as Manganese Gluconate) 3.5 • Chromium (as Chromium Brown Rice Protein Chelate) 10 mcg • Potassium (as Potassium Gluconate) 50 mg.

Stamina Beverage - Jamieson
Each bottle contains: Purified Water • Canadian Maple Syrup • Glucose • Natural Lemon and Orange Flavor (Tocopherols, Soybean Oil) • Canadian Ginseng root (Panax Quinquegolium) • Citric Acid • Sodium Benzoate • Xanthan Gum • Caramel (natural color) • Potassium Sorbate.

Standardized Cider Vinegar with Apple Pectin - The Vitamin Shoppe
Each tablet has been standardized to provide 27 mg of acetic acid and 27 mg of apple pectin.

Standardized Feverfew Extract - Nature's Way
Each capsule contains: Feverfew leaves (standardized 0.7% Parthenolide) 370 mg.

Standardized Ginkgo Extract - Nature's Way
Each capsule contains: Ginkgo Biloba leaf extract; standardized to 24% Ginkgo flavone glycosides & 6% terpene lactones) 60 mg • Gotu Kola stem & leaf 400 mg. Other Ingredients: Gelatin & Millet.

Standardized Kava Extract - Nature's Way
Each softgel contains: Concentrated 10:1 Kava Extract (rhizome, standardized to 55% kavalactones) 128 mg.

Standardized Lutein & Bilberry - Swanson
Each softgel contains: Bilberry extract (25% anthocyanidins) 20 mg • FloraGLO® Lutein extract (from marigold) 6 mg.

Standardized Saw Palmetto Extract - Nature's Way
Each softgel contains: Saw Palmetto extract (berry, standardized to 85-95% Fatty Acids) 160 mg.
See Editor's Note No. 2, page 1816.

StayCalm - Resource Wellness
Each caplet contains: Vitamin C (Ascorbic Acid) 10 mg • Thiamin Mononitrate 0.25 mg • Vitamin B6 (Pyridoxine HCl) 0.33 mg • Vitamin B12 (Cyanocobalamin) 1 mcg • Calcium 190 mg • St. John's Wort extract aerial parts 300 mg • Valerian root extract (root) 50 mg. Other Ingredients: Dicalcium Phosphate, Microcrystalline Cellulose, Croscarmellose Sodium, Magnesium Stearate, Stearic Acid, Maltodextrin, Silicon Dioxide, Hydroxypropyl Methylcellulose, Hydroxypropyl Cellulose, Polyethylene Glycol.

StimuMax for Men - Natrol
Proprietary Blend 2.02 g: Maca 4:1 root extract (Lepidium meyenii), Muira Puama 5:1 root extract (Ptychopetalum olacoides), Wild Oats 10:1 extract (Avena sativa), Guarana seed extract (Paullinia Cupana) (20% Caffeine), Korean ginseng root extract (Panax Ginseng), Ginkgo Biloba leaf extract, Epimedium 10% aerial extract (Epimedium grandiflorum). Other Ingredients: Rice powder, Silica, Magnesium Stearate, Gelatin.

StimuMax for Women - Natrol
Proprietary Blend 1.90g: Maca 4:1 root extract (Lepidium meyenii), Muira Puama 5:1 root extract (Ptychopetalum olacoides), Wild Oats 10:1 extract (Avena sativa), Kava Kava standardized root extract (Piper methsyticum), Dong Quai standardized extract (Angelica sinensis), Damiana 4:1 leaf extract (Turnera diffusa), Korean Ginseng root extract (Panax). Other ingredients: Rice Powder, Silica, Magnesium Stearate, Gelatin.

Stinging Nettle Leaf Extract - PhytoPharmica
Two capsules contain: Stinging Nettle (Urtica dioica) leaf extract (standardized to contain 1% silicic acid) 600 mg.

Stomach Plus - Atrium Inc.
Each tablet contains: Raw Stomach concentrate Bovine 323 mg • Folic Acid 100 mcg • Vitamin B12 50 mcg • Glycine 32 mg.
See Editor's Note No. 14, page 1817.

Stomach-Aid - Futurebiotics
Two capsules contain: Calcium (carbonate) 200 mg • MSM (methyl-sulfonyl-methane) 300 mg • Ginger (root powder) 400 mg • Peppermint (leaf powder) 100 mg • Bromelain (600 GDU) 100 mg • Pancreatin 4X (Supplying 1600 USP units lipase, 10000 USP units amylase, 10000 USP units protease) 100 mg • Aloe Vera (leaf powder) 50 mg • Papain 50 mg • Stomach Aid Herbal Base, 200 mg: Chamomile (flower powder), Catnip (leaf powder), Parsley (leaf powder), Fennel (seed powder). Other ingredients: Gelatin, Cellulose, Magnesium stearate, Water.
See Editor's Note No. 14, page 1817.

StomachEase - Neopharmica
Two tablets contain: Proprietary Concentrate: Corydalis Tuber, Astragalus root, San-Qi Ginseng root, Chekiang Fritillary bulb, Chinese Licorice root, Gambir leaf and stem, Brown's Lilly bulb, Bletilla Striata, Sepia Esculenta shell 1500 mg.

Stone Root-Corn Silk Virtue - Blessed Herbs
Stone root • Gravel root • Hydrangea root • Goldenrod • Corn Silk • Nettle • Grain alcohol & Distilled Water.

Stop Cough Formula - Dr. Morrow's Homeopathic Formulas
Ten drops contain: Drosera 3C • Arnica 3C • Belladonna 3C • Cina 3C • Coccus cacti 3C • Corallium rubrum 6C • Cuprum metallicum 6C • Ferrum Phosphate 6C • Ipecac 3C • Solidago 1C.
See Editor's Note No. 1, page 1816.

Strawberry-Apple Lactobacillus Acidophilus - Nature's Life
Two tablespoons (1 fl.oz or 29.6 ml) contain: Purified Water • Strawberry concentrate • Unfiltered Apple Juice • Pasteurized Honey • Soy Protein Isolate • Lactobacillus Acidophilus Culture.

ST-Res-Q - Nutri-Quest
Each tablet contains: Adrenal 25 mg • Thymus 70 mg • Spleen 20 mg • Stomach 10 mg • Parotid 80 mg (All bovine source).• Vitamin C 175 mg • Vitamin B2 15 mg • Vitamin B6 10 mg • Niacinamide 15 mg • Pantothenic Acid (D-Calcium Pantothenate) 105 mg • Grape seed extract 1 mg • Lemon Bioflavonoids 225 mg • L-Tyrosine 175 mg • Magnesium Oxide 75 mg • Zinc Chelate 5 mg • Chromium Chelate 50 mcg • Potassium Chelate 10 mg • Chlorella 50 mg.
See Editor's Note No. 14, page 1817.

Stress - Centrum - Centrum Focused Formulas
One tablet contains: Vitamin C 150 mg • Vitamin E 22.5 IU • Thiamin (B1) 15 mg • Riboflavin (B2) 4.8 mg • Niacin (B3) 50 mg • Vitamin B6 5 mg • Folate, Folic Acid, Folacin 200 mcg • Vitamin B12 12.5 mcg • Biotin 15 mcg • Pantothenic Acid 12.5 mg • Zinc 7.5 mg • Copper 1 mg • Ginseng standardized root extract (Panax ginseng) 62.5 mg

Stress Action - Nature's Plus
Two tablets contain: Vitamin C as Mineral Ascorbate 1000 mg • Desiccated Beef Liver 500 mg • Pantothenic Acid (Calcium Pantothenate) 125 mg • Vitamin B1 (Thiamine) 100 mg • Vitamin B2 (Riboflavin) 100 mg • Vitamin B6 (Pyridoxine HCL) 100 mg • Niacinamide 100 mg • Vitamin E natural 100 IU • Choline (Bitartrate) 75 mg • Inositol 75 mg • PABA (Para-aminobenzoic acid) 50 mg • Bee Pollen 50 mg • Ginseng Korean 50 mg • Calcium ascorbate

BRAND NAMES

B R A N D   N A M E S

50 mg • Zinc Ascorbate 25 mg • Magnesium Ascorbate 25 mg • L-Phenylalanine free form amino acid 20 mg • Iron (Gluconate) 20 mg • Potassium (Citrate) 15 mg • L-Cysteine free form amino acid 15 mg • L-Methionine free form amino acid 15 mg • Folic Acid 400 mcg • Vitamin B12 from Cobalamin 250 mcg • Biotin 100 mcg • Octacosanol 50 mcg • Chromium amino acid chelate 20 mcg • Selenium amino acid complex 10 mcg . In a natural rice bran base. In a special base which provides for the gradual release of ingredients over a prolonged period of time for 40% better absorption & utilization. Sugar & starch free.
See Editor's Note No. 14, page 1817.

Stress Away - Futurebiotics
Two tablets contain: Vitamin C (ascorbic acid/ascorbyl palmitate) 250 mg • Vitamin A (beta carotene) 5000 IU • Vitamin B1 (thiamin) 25 mg • Vitamin B2 (riboflavin) 25 mg • Niacinamide 200 mg • Calcium (phosphate, aspartate) 100 mg • Vitamin B6 5 mg • Folic Acid 400 mcg • Vitamin B12 50 mcg • Iodine (kelp) 75 mg • Magnesium (oxide, amino acid chelate) 100 mg • Zinc (oxide, picolinate) 15 mg • Biotin 300 mcg • Pantothenic Acid 50 mg • Inositol 50 mg • Choline Bitartrate 100 mg • Manganese (amino acid chelate) 3 mg • Chromium (amino acid chelate, polynicotinate) 40 mcg • Para Amino Benzoic Acid (PABA) 50 mg • Valerian 200 mg • Chamomile 100 mg • Skullcap 50 mg • Passion flower 50 mg • Methionine 50 mg • Ribonucleic Acid (RNA) 50 mg.

Stress B with C - Nature's Life
Two capsules contain: Vitamin B1 (Thiamine Mononitrate) 50 mg • Vitamin B2 (Riboflavin and Riboflavin 5'-Phosphate) 50 mg • Vitamin B6 (Pyridoxine HCl & Pyridoxal 5'-Phosphate) 50 mg • Vitamin B12 (Cobalamin concentrate) 250 mcg • Niacinamide 100 mg • Folic Acid 400 mcg • Pantothenic Acid (d-Calcium Pantothenate) 250 mg • Biotin (d-Biotin)100 mcg • PABA (Para Aminobenzoic Acid) 50 mg • Choline (Bitartrate) 100 mg • Vitamin C 1000 mg.

Stress Essentials - PhytoPharmica
Each capsule contains: Vitamin C (Ascorbic Acid & Rose Hips) 100 mg • Calcium (Oyster Shell) 50 mg • Magnesium (Oxide) 30 mg • Potassium (Citrate) 25 mg • Pantothenic Acid (D-Calcium Pantothenate) 20 mg • Vitamin B6 (Pyridoxine HCL) 15 mg • Thiamine HCL (Vitamin B1) 12.5 mg • Riboflavin (Vitamin B2) 12.5 mg • Niacin 10 mg • Manganese (Chelate) 5 mg • Zinc (Chelate) 1.5 mg • Biotin 100 mcg • Folic Acid 75 mcg • Vitamin B12 (Cyanocobalamin) 25 mcg • Inositol 50 mg • Siberian Ginseng extract 5:1 (Eleutherococcus senticosus) 50 mg • Valerian extract (Valeriana officinalis; standardized to contain 0.2% to 0.8% valerenic acids) 50 mg • L-Tyrosine 50 mg • Skullcap extract 4:1 (Scutellaria baicalensis) 50 mg • Passion flower extract (Passiflora) 50 mg • Hops extract (Humulus lupulus) 50 mg • PABA (Para-Aminobenzoic Acid) 5 mg. Contains no sugar, salt, yeast, wheat, corn, soy, dairy products, coloring, flavoring, or preservatives.

Stress Fighter - Puritan's Pride
Each tablet contains: Vitamin B1 20 mg • Vitamin B2 15 mg • Vitamin B6 10 mg • Vitamin B12 25 mcg • Folic Acid 400 mcg • Niacinamide 100 mg • Pantothenic Acid 25 mg • Vitamin C 600 mg • Vitamin E 45 IU. Plus valuable minerals such as Zinc, Iron, and Copper.

Stress Formula Calcet Plus - Mission Pharmacal
Each tablet contains: Vitamin A 5000 IU • Vitamin C 500 mg • Vitamin D (as Vitamin D3) 400 IU • Vitamin E 30 IU • Vitamin B1 2.25 mg • Vitamin B2 2.55 mg • Vitamin B3 30 mg • Vitamin B6 3 mg • Folate 0.8 mg • Vitamin B12 9 mcg • Vitamin B5 15 mg • Calcium 160 mg • Iron 18 mg • Zinc 15 mg. Other Ingredients: Sugar, Povidone, Magnesium Stearate, Color, Croscarmellose Sodium, Food Glaze, Carnauba Wax, White Beeswax, Sodium Benzoate, Cyanocobalamin.

Stress Plex - Nature's Plus
Two tablets contain: Vitamin C with Rose Hips 500 mg • Pantothenic Acid (Calcium pantothenate) 100 mg • Niacinamide 100 mg • Choline (Bitartrate) 100 mg • Inositol 100 mg • PABA (Para-aminobenzoic acid) 30 mg • Vitamin B1 (Thiamine) 10 mg • Vitamin B2 (Riboflavin) 10 mg • Vitamin B6 (Pyridoxine HCL) 10 mg • Folic Acid 100 mcg • Vitamin B12 (from Cobalamin) 25 mcg • Biotin   25 mcg. B-Complex vitamins in a fortified rice bran base. Contains no yeast, wheat, corn, soy, milk, salt, sugar or starch.

Stress Plus - Now
Each tablet contains: Vitamin B1 (Thiamine) 30 mg • Vitamin B2 (Riboflavin) 30 mg • Vitamin B3 (Niacinamide) 150 mg • Vitamin B6 (Pyridoxine) 30 mg • Vitamin B12 50 mcg • Pantothenic Acid 150 mg • Vitamin C (Ascorbic Acid) 500 mg • Biotin 300 mcg • Folic Acid 400 mcg • Magnesium (Oxide) 100 mg • PABA 40 mg • Choline (Bitartrate) 150 mg • Inositol 150 mg • Valerian root (50 mg of 4:1 extract) 200 mg.

Stress Tab B - Nature's Life
Two tablets contain: Vitamin B1 (Thiamine HCl) 60 mg • Vitamin B2 (Riboflavin) 60 mg • Vitamin B6 (Pyridoxine HCl) 60 mg • Vitamin B12 (Cobalamin concentrate) 60 mcg • Vitamin C 600 mg • Niacin 30 mg • Niacinamide 30 mg • Folic Acid 600 mcg • Pantothenic Acid (d-Calcium Pantothenate) 600 mg • Biotin (d-Biotin) 600 mcg • Choline (Bitartrate) 60 mg • Inositol 60 mg • PABA (Para Aminobenzoic Acid) 60 mg.

Stressease - Jamieson
Each caplet contains: Thiamin (as Thiamine Mononitrate) 50 mg • Riboflavin (Vitamin B2) 50 mg • Niacin (as Niacinamide) 50 mg • Vitamin B6 (as Pyridoxine Hydrochloride) 50 mg • Folate (as Folic Acid) 400 mcg • Vitamin B12 (as Cyanocobalamin) 50 mg • Biotin 50 mg • Pantothenic Acid (as Calcium D-Pantothenate) 50 mg • Choline Bitartrate 50 mg • Inositol 50 mg.

Stress-End - Enzymatic Therapy
Each capsule contains: Vitamin C (Ascorbic Acid/Rose Hips) 100 mg • Calcium (Oyster Shell) 50 mg • Magnesium (Oxide) 30 mg • Potassium (Citrate) 25 mg • Pantothenic Acid (D-Calcium Pantothenate) 20 mg • Vitamin B6 (Pyridoxine HCL) 15 mg • Thiamine HCL (Vitamin B1) 12.5 mg • Riboflavin (Vitamin B2) 12.5 mg • Niacin 10 mg • Manganese (Chelate) 5 mg • Zinc (Chelate) 1.5 mg • Biotin 100 mcg • Folic Acid 75 mcg • Vitamin B12 (Cyanocobalamin) 25 mcg • Other ingredients: Inositol 50 mg • Siberian Ginseng extract 5:1 (Eleutherococcus senticosus) 50 mg • Valerian extract (Valeriana officinalis) standardized to contain 0.2% to 0.8% Valerenic Acids 50 mg • L-Tyrosine 50 mg • Skullcap extract 4:1 (Scutellaria baicalensis) 50 mg • Passion flower extract (Passiflora) 50 mg • Hops extract (Humulus lupulus) 50 mg • PABA (Para-Aminobenzoic Acid) 5 mg. Contains no sugar, salt, yeast, wheat, corn, soy, dairy products, coloring, flavoring, or preservatives.

Stresstabs - Unknown
Each tablet contains: Vitamin C 500 mg • Vitamin E 30 IU • Thiamin 10 mg • Riboflavin 10 mg • Niacinamide 100 mg • Vitamin B6 5 mg • Folic Acid 400 mcg • Vitamin B12 12 mcg • Biotin 45 mcg • Pantothenic Acid 20 mg. Ingredients: Ascorbic Acid • Calcium Carbonate • Cellulose • Niacinamide • dl-Alpha Tocopheryl Acetate (Vitamin E) • Starch • d-Calcium Pantothenate • Hydroxypropyl Methylcellulose • Riboflavin (Vitamin B2) • Thiamine Mononitrate (Vitamin B1) • Dicalcium Phosphate • Pyridoxine Hydrochloride (Vitamin B6) • Silicon Dioxide • Magnesium Stearate • Triethyl Citrate • Stearic Acid • Mineral oil • Folic Acid • Titanium Dioxide • FD&C Yellow #6 Aluminum Lake • Biotin • Cyanocobalamin (Vitamin B12).

Stresstabs + Zinc - Unknown
Each tablet contains: Vitamin C 500 mg • Vitamin E 30 IU • Thiamin 10 mg • Riboflavin 10 mg • Niacinamide 100 mg • Vitamin B6 5 mg •

Folic Acid 400 mcg • Vitamin B12 12 mcg • Biotin 45 mcg • Pantothenic Acid 20 mg • Zinc 23.9 mg • Copper 3 mg. Ingredients: Ascorbic Acid • Calcium Carbonate • Cellulose • Niacinamide • dl-Alpha Tocopheryl Acetate (Vitamin E) • Starch • Zinc Oxide • d-Calcium Pantothenate • Hydroxypropyl Methylcellulose • Riboflavin (Vitamin B2) • Thiamine Mononitrate (Vitamin B1) • Dicalcium Phosphate • Pyridoxine Hydrochloride (Vitamin B6) • Silicon Dioxide • Triethyl Stearate • Stearic Acid • Magnesium Stearate • Cupric Oxide • Crospovidone • Providone • Mineral oil • Folic Acid • Titanium Dioxide • FD&C Yellow #6 Aluminum Lake • Biotin • Cyanocobalamin (Vitamin B12).

Stuart Prenatal Multivitamin/Multimineral Supplement - Integrity Pharmaceutical Corp.
Each tablet contains: Vitamin A Acetate (25% as Beta Carotene) 4000 IU • Vitamin C (Ascorbic Acid) 100 mg • Vitamin D (Cholecalciferol) 400 IU • Vitamin E (dl-Alpha Tocopheryl Acetate) 11 IU • Thiamin Mononitrate (Vitamin B1) 1.8 mg • Riboflavin (Vitamin B2) 1.7 mg • Niacin (Vitamin B3, Niacinamide) 18 mg • Vitamin B6 (Pyridoxine Hydrochloride) 2.6 mg • Folate (Folic Acid, Folacin) 0.8 mcg • Vitamin B12 (Cyanocobalamin) 4 mcg • Calcium Sulfate 200 mg • Iron (Ferrous Fumarate) 27 mg • Zinc Oxide 25 mg. Other Ingredients: Beta Carotene, Croscarmellose Sodium, Hydroxypropyl Methylcellulose, Microcrystalline Cellulose, Pregelatinized Starch, Red Iron Oxide, Titanium Dioxide.

Sublingual B-12 Lozenge Tablets 2500 mcg - Puritan's Pride
Each lozenge contains: Vitamin B-12 2500 mcg.

Sublingual B-12 Lozenge Tablets 500 mcg - Puritan's Pride
Each lozenge contains: Vitamin B-12 500 mcg.

Sublingual B-12 Lozenge Tablets 5000 mcg - Puritan's Pride
Each lozenge contains: Vitamin B-12 5000 mcg.

Substrate Solutions Di-Indolin - Substrate Solutions
Three tablets contain: Di-Indolin [proprietary blend of Diindolymethane, Vitamin E (as d-Alpha Tocopheryl Succinate), Phosphatidylcholine] 300 mg. Other Ingredients: Calcium Carbonate, Cellulose, Food Grade Starch, Magnesium Sterate, Tocophersolan, Silica.

Sugar Free Zinc Drops - Quantum Health
Each drop contains: Vitamin A acetate 500 IU • Elemental Zinc (Zinc acetate) 14 mg • Slippery Elm bark (Ulmus fulva) 20 mg • Bee Propolis extract powder (5:1) 5 mg • Goldenseal 2 mg. Other Ingredients: HSH (Hydrogenated Starch Hydrolysate), Natural and Artificial Flavors, Aspartame. Phenylketonurics- contains Phenylalanine.

Sugar Stopper - Sports Nutrition Source.com
Each capsule contains: Gymnena Sylvestre 300 mg • Chitosan shellfish 100 mg • Garcinia Cambogia 100 mg • Vitamin C 50 mg.

Sun Pollen - Futurebiotics
Cracked Flower Pollen & Pollen Extract.

Sundown Pokemon Children's Multiple Vitamin - Sundown Vitamins
Each chewable tablet contains: Vitamin A 5000 IU • Vitamin C (as sodium ascorbate and ascorbic acid) 60 mg • Vitamin D (as cholecalciferol) 400 IU • Vitamin E (as dl-alpha tocopheryl acetate) 30 IU • Thiamin (as thiamin mononitrate) 1.5 mg • Riboflavin 1.7 mg • Niacin (as niacinamide) 20 mg • Vitamin B-6 (as pyridoxine HCl) 2 mg • Folic Acid 400 mcg • Vitamin B-12 (as cyanocobalamin) 6 mcg • Biotin 40 mcg • Pantothenic Acid (as calcium d-pantothenate) 10 mg • Calcium 150 mg • Iron (as ferrous sulfate) 18 mg • Phosphorous 80 mg • Iodine (as potassium iodide) 150 mcg

• Magnesium (as magnesium oxide) 20 mg • Zinc (as zinc oxide) 15 mg • Copper (as cupric oxide) 2 mg. See Editor's Note No. 3, page 1816.

Super All-Day Nutricom - Puritan's Pride
Each scoop contains: Vitamin A 10,000 IU • Vitamin C 1,000 mg • Vitamin D 500 IU • Vitamin E 400 IU • Vitamin K 5 mcg • Thiamin 25 mg • Riboflavin 25 mg • Niacin 100 mg • Vitamin B-6 25 mg • Biotin 25 mcg • Pantothenic Acid 100 mg • Calcium 500 mg • Iron 18 mg • Phosphorus 200 mg • Iodine 150 mcg • Magnesium 200 mg • Zinc 50 mg • Selenium 50 mcg • Copper 0.2 mg • Manganese 4 mg • Chromium 50 mcg • Molybdenum 50 mcg • Potassium 99 mg • Inositol 100 mg • Choline 100 mg • Para-Aminobenzoic Acid (PABA) 25 mg • Rutin 25 mg • Citrus Bioflavonoids 25 mg • Hesperidin complex 25 mg • Lecithin 350 mg. Typical Amino Acid content per 15 g serving: Alanine 235 mg, Arginine 285 mg, Aspartic Acid 518 mg, Cysteine 27 mg, Glutamic Acid 1,614 mg, Glycine 139 mg, Histidine 212 mg, Isoleucine 458 mg, Leucine 703 mg, Lysine 561 mg, Methionine 216 mg, Phenylalanine 377 mg, Proline 822 mg, Serine 469 mg, Threonine 300 mg, Tryptophan 93 mg, Tyrosine 407 mg, Valine 517 mg.

Super Anti-OX - Nutri-Quest
Each tablet contains: Grape seed extract 20 mg (92-95% Proanthocyanidins) • Zinc (as Ester-C 2 mg) 14 mg • Vitamin C 100 mg • Vitamin E (Succinate) 50 IU • L-Glutathione 2 mg • N-Acetyl Cysteine 5 mg • Magnesium Aspartate 5 mg • Manganese Chelate 1 mg • Selenium Chelate 50 mcg • Chromium Chelate 50 mcg • Milk Thistle 150 mg • Silymarin 5 mg.

Super Antioxidant - Health Center for Better Living
Vitamin C 500 mg • Vitamin E 300 IU.

Super Antioxidant Capsules - The Vitamin Shoppe
Two capsules contain: Vitamin A (beta carotene and mixed carotenoids) 10,000 IU • Vitamin E 200 IU • Vitamin C (Calcium ascorbate) 60 mg • Vitamin B1 25 mg • Vitamin B2 25 mg • Vitamin B3 25 mg • Vitamin B5 25 mg • Vitamin B6 25 mg • Vitamin B12 250 mcg • N-Acetyl Cysteine 50 mg • Glutathione 50 mg • Selenium 75 mcg • Zinc 15 mg • Green Tea Extract (30% Polyphenols) 25 mg • CoQ10 10 mg • Quercetin 25 mg • Alpha Lipoic Acid 10 mg • Garlic (odorless) 100 mg • Grape Seed Extract (minimum 85%-95% proanthocyanidins) 10 mg • Manganese (Gluconate/Citrate) 15 mg

Super Anti-Oxidant Complex - Nature's Plus
Two tablets contain: Vitamin C with Rose Hips 500 mg • Vitamin E natural 200 IU • Vitamin A (Beta Carotene) 10000 IU • Selenium amino acid complex 200 mcg • Chromium amino acid chelate 200 mcg. In a natural base of Carrots, Broccoli, Spinach & Beet Greens. In a special base which provides for the gradual release of ingredients over a prolonged period of time for 40% better absorption & utilization. Sugar & starch free.

Super Antioxidant Formula - Puritan's Pride
Each softgel contains: Vitamin E 400 IU • Beta Carotene 25,000 IU • Vitamin C 500 mg • Selenium 50 mcg.

Super Antioxidant Formula - High Potency - Nature's Bounty
Each softgel contains: Vitamin A 25000 IU • Vitamin C (as Ascorbic Acid) 500 mg • Vitamin E (as d-Alpha Tocopherol) 400 IU • Selenium (as Selenium Yeast) 50 mcg. Other Ingredients: Gelatin, Glycerin, Soybean Oil, Soy Lecithin, Beeswax, St. John's Bread extract, Caramel Color.

Super Antioxidant Tablets - Clinician's Choice
Two tablets contain: Vitamin C (as ascorbic acid) 120 mg • Vitamin E (as dl-alpha tocopheryl acetate) 200 IU • Zinc (as amino acid chelate) 4 mg • Selenium (selenomethionine) 100 mcg • RoseOx (patented,

BRAND NAMES

standardized process for an extract of Rosemary) 200 mg • Schizandra Fruit Powder 100 mg • Grape Powder 60 mg • Ascorbyl Palmitate 20 mg • Proprietary blend 10 mg: Astragalus, Beta Carotene, Carrot Powder, Coenzyme Q10, Cruciferex, Pycnogenol.

Super Antioxidants - Now
Two Vcaps contain: Green Tea extract (Camellia sinensis) (40% Catechins) 200 mg • Milk Thistle extract (Silybum marianum) (80% Silymarin) 100 mg • Curcumin extract (Curcuma longa) (min. 90% extract) 100 mg • Quercetin 100 mg • Bromelain from pineapple (2000 GDU) 100 mg • Cranberry powder extract 100 mg • Rosemary extract (Rosmarinus officinalis) 100 mg • Grape seed extract (95% Polyphenols) 30 mg • Ginkgo Biloba extract (24% Ginkgoflavoglycosides) 30 mg • Ginger root (Zingiber officinalis) 30 mg • Hawthorne berry extract (Crataegus oxyacantha) (1.8% Vitexin-4"-Rhamnoside) 30 mg • Bilberry extract (Vaccimum myrtillus) (25% Anthocyanidins) 20 mg.

Super B Complex 100 - The Vitamin Shoppe
Each tablet contains: Vitamin B1 (Thiamin) 100 mg • Vitamin B2 (Riboflavin) 100 mg • Vitamin B6 (Pyridoxine HCl) 100 mg • Vitamin B12 (Cobalamin Concentrate) 100 mcg • Niacinamide 100 mg • Folic Acid 400 mcg • D-Biotin 100 mcg • Choline Bitartrate 100 mg • Inositol 100 mg • Pantothenic Acid (d-calcium pantothenate) 100 mg • PABA 100 mg. In a base of Alfalfa, Watercress, Parsley, Lecithin, and Rice Concentrate. No Yeast, Corn, Wheat, Soy, Salt, Sugar, Starch, Milk, Eggs, Fish or Animal Derivatives, Preservatives, Artificial Colors or Flavors added.

Super Blue Stuff Gel - Natural Relief Marketing
4 oz contains: MSM • Emu Oil • Whole leaf Aloe Vera • Purified Water • Carbomer 940 • Willow Bark extract • SD-alcohol-40 • Sorbitol • Triethanolamine • Capsicum oleoresin • Witch Hazel extract • Menthol • Coriander Oil • Grape Seed extract • Fragrance • FD&C Blue #2 • Extracts of: Blue Bottle, Roman Chamomile, Feverfew, St. John's Wort, Marigold, and Lime Tree.

Super Calcium 1200 - Schiff
Two softgels contain: Vitamin D (as cholecalciferol) 400 IU • Calcium (as calcium carbonate) 1200 mg. Other Ingredients: Vegetable Oil, Gelatin, Glycerin, Lecithin, and Titanium Dioxide.
See Editor's Note No. 5, page 1816.

Super Cal-Mag - Nature's Life
Two tablets contain: Calcium (Chelated) (Carbonate, Aspartate, Aminoate, Citrate Complex) 1000 mg • Magnesium (Chelated) (Oxide, Aspartate, Aminoate, Citrate Complex) 500 mg.

Super Cayenne - Swanson
Two capsules contain: Cayenne pepper (100,000 heating units) 450 mg • Ginger root powder 200 mg • Hawthorn berry powder 200 mg • Lecithin granules 50 mg.

Super C-Complex 500 - The Vitamin Shoppe
Each tablet contains: Vitamin C (with Rose Hips) 500 mg • Citrus Bioflavonoid Complex 100 mg • Hesperidin Complex 25 mg • Rutin 50 mg • Acerola 1 mg. No Yeast, Corn, Wheat, Dairy, Soy, Salt, Starch, Sugar, Gluten, Milk, Eggs, Fish or Animal Derivatives, Preservatives, Artificial Colors or Flavors added.

Super Chelated Multi-Mineral - Puritan's Pride
Three tablets contain: Calcium 750 mg • Phosphorus 300 mg • Magnesium 375 mg • Potassium 99 mg • Manganese 15 mg • Iron 15 mg • Zinc 15 mg • Copper 375 mcg • Iodine 225 mcg • Chromium 30 mcg • Selenium 38 mcg.

Super Coenzyme Q-10 - Gary Nulls
Each tablet contains: Coenzyme Q10 100 mg. Other Ingredients: Di-calcium Phosphate, Cellulose and Modified Cellulose, Stearic

Acid, Magnesium Stearate, Silicon Dioxide, Pharmaceutical Glaze. See Editor's Note No. 6, page 1816.

Super Complete Capsules - Ultimate Nutrition
Nine capsules contain: Vitamin A 10000 IU • Vitamin D 400 IU • Vitamin E 400 IU • Vitamin B1 100 mg • Vitamin B2 100 mg • Vitamin B6 100 mg • Vitamin B12 100 mcg • Niacinamide 100 mg • Pantothenic Acid 100 mg • Folic Acid 400 mcg • Biotin 300 mcg • Choline 100 mg • Inositol 100 mg • PABA 100 mg • Vitamin C 1500 mg • Bioflavonoids 250 mg • Rutin 50 mg • Rose Hips powder 20 mg • Hesperidin 20 mg • Acerola Cherry 10 mg • Glutamic Acid HCL 100 mg • Betaine HCl 100 mg • Calcium 1000 mg • Magnesium 500 mg • Iodine 150 mcg • Potassium 95 mg • Iron 30 mg • Zinc 22.5 mg • Manganese 10 mg • Copper 3 mg • Boron 3 mg • Chromium 200 mcg • Selenium 50 mcg.

Super Cranberry Concentrate - Wellness for Women
Each softgel contains: Vitamin C USP (as ascorbic acid) 100 mg • Vitamin E (as dl-alpha tocopheryl acetate) 3 IU • Cranberry juice concentrate, 10:1 (equivalent to 800 mg) 80 mg.

Super Energy Oil - Puritan's Pride
Each softgel contains: Soybean oil 650 mg • Rice Bran oil 228 mg • Wheat Germ oil (cold pressed) 228 mg • Vitamin E (d-alpha tocopherol) 5 IU.

Super Energy Up - The Vitamin Shoppe
Each capsule contains: Standardized Panax Ginseng extract, Fo-Ti root, Sukday, Licorice, Lycii Berries, and Damiana leaves in a base of Royal Jelly, Bee Pollen, Vitamin B12, and Octacosanol.

Super Enzymes - Now
Each tablet contains: Betaine HCL (from beet molasses) 200 mg • Bromelain (2000 GDU from pineapple) 50 mg • Papain (140 MCU uncoated from papaya) 50 mg • Pancreatin 4x (equivalent to 800 mg) 200 mg supplying: Amylase (20000 USP Units) 100 mg, Protease [Chymotrypsin & Trypsin (20000 USP Units)] 100 mg, Lipase (3400 USP Units) 25 mg • Pepsin Enzymes NF 1:10000 50 mg • Cellulase 10 mg • Ox Bile extract 100 mg • Papaya Enzymes 45 mg • Pineapple Enzymes 45 mg.
See Editor's Note No. 14, page 1817.

Super EPA DHA 500 mg - The Vitamin Shoppe
Each softgel contains: Vitamin E (as d-alpha tocopherol) 5 IU • EPA Eicosapentaenoic Acid (as marine fish oil) 300 mg • DHA Docosahexaenoic Acid (as marine fish oil) 200 mg.

Super Food - Youngevity
Phosphorus • Sulfur • Chloride • Sodium • Vitamin A • Vitamin B1 • Vitamin B2 • Vitamin B3 • Vitamin B5 • Vitamin B6 • Vitamin B12 • Vitamin C • Vitamin D • Vitamin E • Vitamin K • Folic Acid • Biotin • Soy Protein • Soybean Oil • Soy Lecithin • Lactobacillus Acidophilus • FOS • Papaya • Protease • Bromelain • Amylase • Lipase • Cellulase • Soy • Rice • Barley • Oats • Prunes • Citrus • Alfalfa • Capsicum fruit • Chlorella • Garcinia fruit • Licorice.

Super Gainers Fuel - TwinLab
Each serving contains: Calories 3000 • Milk & Egg Proteins 100 g • High Levels of Complex Carbohydrates • Branched Chain Amino Acids (L-Leucine, L-Isoleucine & L-Valine) • L-Glutamine • L-Carnitine • Alpha-Ketoglutarate • Creatine Monohydrate • High Potencies of Vitamins & Minerals including Potassium 2000 mcg & Chromium 600 mcg • Fat 29 g [from Medium Chain Triglycerides (MCTs)]. MCTs are lipids composed of Medium Chain Fatty Acids.

Super Ginseng - Dial Herbs
Siberian Ginseng • Korean Ginseng • Brazilian Ginseng • Chinese Ginseng • American Ginseng.

Some Brand Name Natural Products - What they Contain
www.NaturalDatabase.com contains MANY more listings than appear here.

Super Growth Enhancer - Optimum Nutrition
L-Arginine L-Ornithine Vitamin B6 20 mg • Vitamin C 200 mg.

Super Herbal V - MD Healthline
Two capsules contain: Yohimbe Bark 250 mg • Damiana Extract 50 mg • Bilberry Powder 100 mg • Gingko Biloba Extract (24%) 60 mg • Siberian Ginseng Extract 100 mg • Schisandra Extract 200 mg • Avena Sativa Extract 10:1 250 mg • Saw Palmetto (30%) 100 mg.

Super Immuno-Comp - Enzymatic Therapy
Two capsules contain: Vitamin A (Beta Carotene) non-toxic form of Vitamin A 5000 IU • Vitamin C (Ascorbic Acid/Rose Hips) 100 mg • Vitamin B6 (Pyridoxine HCL) 5 mg • Zinc (Picolinate) 3 mg • Other ingredients: Astragalus extract (Astragalus membranaceus) 150 mg • Echinacea extract (Echinacea angustifolia) standardized to contain greater than 3.5% Echinacosides & 0.65% essential oils 150 mg • Goldenseal extract (Hydrastis canadensis) standardized to contain 5% total Alkaloids including: Berberine, Hydrastine & Canadine 150 mg • KS-2 (Peptidomannan Complex) Shiitake Mushroom, a purified extract of Lentinus Edodes 50 mg • Licorice root extract (Glycyrrhiza glabra) standardized to contain 5% Glycyrrhizic Acid 50 mg. Contains no sugar, salt, yeast, wheat, corn, soy, dairy products, coloring, flavoring, or preservatives.

Super Immuno-Tone - PhytoPharmica
Two capsules contain: Vitamin A 5000 IU • Vitamin C 100 mg • Vitamin B6 5 mg • Zinc 3 mg • Astragalus extract 150 mg • Echinacea extract 150 mg • Goldenseal extract 150 mg • Shiitake Mushroom (KS-2) 50 mg • Licorice root extract 50 mg.

Super Leci-Thins - Nature's Life
Three tablets contain: Lecithin (Soy) 1300 mg • Cider Vinegar 255 mg • Kelp 150 mg • Vitamin B6 (Pyridoxine HCI) 50 mg.

Super Liquid Absorbable Calcium - Puritan's Pride
Two softgels contain: Vitamin D (as Cholecalciferol) 100 IU • Calcium (as Calcium Carbonate) 1,000 mg.

Super Lysine Plus+ Cream - Quantum Health
L-lysine • Lithium Carbonate 3X • Propolis extract • Calendula Flower extract • Echinacea Flower extract • Zinc Oxide • Goldenseal extract • Vitamin A • Vitamin D • Vitamin E • Cajeput Oil • Tea Tree Oil • Gum Benzoin Tincture. Prepared in a Beeswax and Olive Base.

Super Lysine Plus+ Tablets - Quantum Health
Three tablets contain: L-lysine 1500 mg • Vitamin C (ascorbic acid) 100 mg • Garlic (odorless) 200 mg • Echinacea extract (4:1 PE) 100 mg • Propolis 50 mg • Licorice extract (4:1 PE) 15 mg • Goldenseal root USP (Hydrastis) 15 mg.

Super Male Plex - The Vitamin Shoppe
Two tablets contain: Yohimbe extract 10 mg • Raw Testicular 250 mg • Damiana 250 mg • Ginseng (Korean/Siberian) 500 mg • Octacosanol 250 mcg • Vitamin E 250 IU • Histidine 200 mg • Sarsaparilla 100 mg • Saw Palmetto 100 mg • Raw Prostate 100 mg • Bee Pollen 100 mg • Zinc 100 mg • Oyster extract 50 mg • Cayenne 50 mg • Gotu Kola 50 mg • Selenium 50 mcg • Niacin 15 mg • Royal Jelly 5 mg
See Editor's Note No. 14, page 1817.

Super Male-Plex - Puritan's Pride
Two tablets contain: Raw Testicular 250 mg • Damiana 250 mg • Siberian Ginseng 250 mg • Korean Ginseng 250 mg • Octacosanol 250 mcg • Vitamin E 250 IU • Histidine 200 mg • Sarsaparilla 100 mg • Saw Palmetto 100 mg • Raw Prostate 100 mg • Bee Pollen 100 mg • Zinc 30 mg • Oyster extract 50 mg • Cayenne 50 mg • Gotu Kola 50 mg • Selenium 50 mcg • Niacin 15 mg • Royal Jelly 5 mg • Oatstraw 50 mg.
See Editor's Note No. 14, page 1817.

Super Malic - Optimox
Six tablets contain: Magnesium (Hydroxide) 300 mg • Malic Acid 1200 mg.

Super Mega Vite II Multiple - Nature's Life
Each tablet contains: Beta Carotene (Vitamin A equivalent to 10000 IU) 6 mg • Vitamin B1 (Thiamine HCI) 50 mg • Vitamin B2 (Riboflavin) 50 mg • Niacinamide 75 mg • Pantothenic Acid (Calcium Pantothenate) 75 mg • Vitamin B6 Pyridoxine HCI) 50 mg • Vitamin B12 (Cobalamin concentrate) 250 mcg • Folic Acid 400 mcg • Biotin (d-Biotin) 50 mcg • Choline (Bitartrate) 50 mg • Inositol 50mg • l-Methionine (free form) 25 mg • Vitamin E (d-Alpha Tocopherol plus mixed Tocopherols) 100 IU • Vitamin C 250 mg • Rutin 5 mg • Lemon Bioflavonoids Complex (TESTLAB 50%) 25 mg • Hesperidin Complex 5 mg • Calcium (Carbonate) 100 mg • Chromium (Chelate) 25 mcg • Copper (Chelate) 200 mcg • Iodine (Postassium Idodine) 100 mg • Iron (Chelate) 10 mg • Magnesium (Oxide) 40 mg • Manganese (Chelate) 7 mg • Phosporus (Potassium Phosphate) 45 mg • Potassium (Phosphate, Chloride, Iodide) 67 mg • Selenium (Nutrition 21) (l-Selenomethionine) 10 mcg • Silicon (Dioxide) 20 mg • Zinc (Chelate) 10 mg • Coenzyme Q-10 (Ubiquinone) 500 mcg • Betaine HCl 25 mg • Glutamic Acid HCL 25 mg. In a natural base of "72 Trace Minerals" from an ancient sedimentary sea bed, Chamomile, Rice Bran & Rose Hips.

Super Mega Vite Multiple - Nature's Life
Each tablet contains: Vitamin A (Fish Liver oil) 25000 IU • Vitamin D (as Vitamin D3) (Cholecalciferol) 400 IU • Vitamin B1 (Thiamine HCI) 30 mg • Vitamin B2 (Riboflavin) 30 mg • Niacinamide 100 mg • Pantothenic Acid (d-Calcium Pantothenate) 100 mg • Vitamin B6 Pyridoxine HCI) 30 mg • Vitamin B12 (Cyanocobalamin) 250 mcg • Folic Acid 400 mcg • PABA (Para Aminobenzoic Acid) 60 mg • Biotin (d-Biotin) 50 mcg • Choline (Choline Bitartrate) 100 mg • Inositol 100 mg • Vitamin E (d-Alpha Tocopheryl Succinate) 100 IU • Vitamin C 250 mg • Lemon Bioflavonoids Complex (50% Total Flavanones) 25 mg • Rutin 25 mg • Hesperidin Complex (50% Total Flavanones) 5 mg • Calcium (Bone Meal) 82.5 mg • Chromium (Chelate) 25 mcg • Copper (Gluconate) 200 mcg • Iodine (Potassium Iodide) 100 mcg • Iron (Ferrous Fumarate) 10 mg • Magnesium (Oxide) 40 mg • Manganese (Gluconate) 7 mg • Phosphorus (Bone Meal) 37.5 mg • Potassium (Iodide) 10 mg • Selenium (Nutrition 21 l-Selenomethionine) 10 mcg • Zinc (Gluconate) 10 mg • Super Oxide Dismutase 30 IU • Betaine HCl 25 mg • Glutamic Acid HCI 25 mg • Methionine 50 mg. In a natural base of Lecithin, Alfalfa, Watercress, Parsley, Duodenal Substance, Rose Hips powder, Chamomile, Molasses, Kale, Cabbage, Goldenseal, Sarsaparilla, "72 Trace Minerals", Pepsin & Kelp.

Super Milk Thistle X - PhytoPharmica
Each capsule contains: Milk Thistle (Silybum marianum) fruit extract bound to phosphatidylcholine under patent 100 mg • Dandelion (Taraxacum officinale) root extract 4:1 10 mg • Artichoke (Cynara scolymus) leaf extract (standardized to contain 13%-18% caffeylquinic acids calculated as chlorogenic acid) 10 mg • Licorice (Glycyrrhiza glabra) root extract (standardized to contain 5% glycyrrhizic acid) 10 mg.

Super Multi with Herbs - Leiner Health Products
Each tablet contains: Iron (Ferrous Fumarate) 9 mg • Magnesium (Magnesium Oxide) 100 mg • Calcium (Calcium Carbonate) 225 mg • Vitamin B12 (Cyanocobalamin) 12 mcg • Vitamin C (Ascorbic Acid) 120 mg • Vitamin E (dl-Tocopheryl Acetate) 60 IU • Chromium (Chromium Picolinate, Chromium Chloride) 120 mcg • Copper (Cupric Oxide) 2 mg • Folate (Folic Acid) 400 mcg • Iodine (Potassium Iodide) 150 mcg • Manganese (Manganese Sulfate) 2 mg • Molybdenum (Sodium Molybdate) 75 mcg • Niacin (Niacinamide) 20 mg • Pantothenic Acid (d-Calcium Pantothenate) 10 mg • Riboflavin (Vitamin B2) 1.7 mg • Selenium (Sodium Selenate) 70 mcg • Thiamin (Vitamin B1) 1.5 mg • Vitamin A (40% as Beta

BRAND NAMES

Carotene) 5000 IU • Vitamin B6 (Pyridoxine Hydrochloride) 2 mg • Vitamin D (Ergocalciferol) 400 IU • Vitamin K (Phytonadione) 80 mcg • Zinc (Zinc Oxide) 15 mg • Biotin (d-Biotin) 30 mcg • Boron (Boron Citrate) 150 mcg • Ginkgo Biloba (Ginkgo biloba) leaf 25 mg • Herbal Complex Blend 25 mg • Siberian Ginseng (Eleutherococcus senticosus) root 25 mg. Other Ingredients: Gelatin, Maltodextrin, Starch, Cellulose, Dicalcium Phosphate, Croscarmellose Sodium, Silicon Dioxide, Polyethylene Glycol 3350, Crospovidone, Tricalcium Phosphate, Hydroxypropyl Methylcellulose, Mannitol, Magnesium Stearate, Pharmaceutical Glaze, Hydroxypropyl Cellulose, Resin, Polysorbate 80.

Super Nails - Puritan's Pride
Three tablets contain: Vitamin A (as Fish Liver Oil) 10,000 IU • Vitamin D (as Fish Liver Oil and Cholecalciferol) 400 IU • Riboflavin (Vitamin B2) 50 mg • Folic Acid 200 mcg • Vitamin B12 (as Cyanocobalamin) 100 mcg • Calcium (as Calcium Amino Acid Chelate and Dicalcium Phosphate) 730 mg • Iron (as Iron Amino Acid Chelate) 5 mg • Phosphorus (as Phosphorus Amino Acid Chelate and Dicalcium Phosphate) 372 mg • Magnesium (as Magnesium Amino Acid Chelate) 25 mg • Gelatin 260 mg • Horsetail (Equisetum arvense) stem 250 mg • L-Cysteine 100 mg • DL-Methionine 100 mg • Sulfur (as Potassium Sulfate and from amino acids) 25 mg • Oat Straw (Avena sativa) stem 25 mg • Rice Bran powder 12 mg.

Super Nutrition Power - Mascot Enterprise
Deer Velvet • Shark Cartilage • Fish Oil (Salmon) • Royal Jelly • Oyster Extract • Orchic Substance • Siberian Ginseng extract 5:1 • Cinnamon • Garlic • Noni • Muira Puama • Guarana extract 4:1 • Smilax • Avena Sativa 10:1 • Damiana leaf extract 4:1 • Vitamin E • Vitamin C • Vitamin B6 • Boron (Citrate) • Zinc (Sulfate) • Niacinamide.
See Editor's Note No. 14, page 1817.

Super Octacosanol - The Vitamin Shoppe
Each softgel contains: Octacosanol 3000 mcg • Wheat Germ Oil 235 mg • Lecithin 9 mg.

Super Odorless Garlic - Now
Each capsule contains: odorless Garlic extract 100:1 concentrate (equivalent to 5000 mg fresh Garlic) 50 mg • Hawthorne berry extract (standardized to contain 1.8% Vitexin-2"-Rhamnoside) 100 mg • Hawthorne berry powder 250 mg • Cayenne pepper (40,000 Heat units) 100 mg.

Super Omega 3 - Nutri-Quest
Each capsule contains: Natural marine lipid concentrate 1 g • Omega-3 Fatty Acids 110 mg/1 g of Eicosapentaenoic Acid (EPA) • Omega-3 90 mg/1 g of Docosahexaenoic Acid (DHA).

Super Phos 30 - Dew Research
Ninety drops contain: Phosphorus 360 mg • Inositol 51 mg • Choline Bitartrate 18 mg.

Super Salve - The Herbalist
Oils of Sweet Almond, St. John's Wort flower, Plantain herb, Calendula flower, & Beeswax • Extracts of Poplar bud, Golden Seal root, Echinacea root, Plantain herb, Comfrey root, Marshmallow root, Yarrow flower.

Super Saw Palmetto - Enzymatic Therapy
Each softgel contains: Saw Palmetto berry extract (serenoa repens) 160 mg.
See Editor's Note No. 2, page 1816.

Super Silica Complex - Futurebiotics
One tablet contains: Calcium (as calcium carbonate, citrate) 200 mg • Magnesium (as magnesium oxide, citrate) 150 mg • Zinc (as zinc

gluconate) 15 mg • Betaine hydrochloride 50 mg • Boron 1.5 mg • Horsetail leaf powder extract 275 mg. Other ingredients: Dicalcium phosphate, Cellulose, Stearic acid, Magnesium stearate.

Super Snooze with Melatonin - Puritan's Pride
Each capsule contains: Valerian root 100 mg • Hops 75 mg • Scullcap 75 mg • Chamomile 75 mg • Passion Flower 50 mg • Calcium carbonate 100 mg • Magnesium oxide 50 mg • Inositol 50 mg • L-Taurine 50 mg • Melatonin 3 mg.
See Editor's Note No. 16, page 1817.

Super Stress Formula - The Vitamin Shoppe
Two capsules contain: Vitamin C 1000 mg • Vitamin B1 (Thiamin) 50 mg • Vitamin B2 (Riboflavin) 50 mg • Vitamin B6 (Pyridoxine Hcl) 50 mg • Vitamin B12 (Cobalamin) 400 mcg • Niacinamide 100 mg • Folic Acid 400 mcg • Pantothenic Acid 250 mg • Biotin 100 mcg • Choline Bitartrate 100 mg • Inositol 100 mg • PABA 50 mg. No Yeast, Corn, Wheat, Soy, Salt, Sugar, Starch, Gluten, Milk, Eggs, Dairy, Preservatives, Artificial Colors or Flavors added.

Super Suppositories - The Herbalist
Tea Tree Oil • Herbal extracts of Usnea & Calendula in a base of Cocoa Butter & Purified Bees Wax.

Super Vanadyl Fuel - TwinLab
Four capsules contain: Vanadyl Sulfate (supplying elemental Vanadium IV 4.87 mg) 25 mg • BMOV [Bis (maltolato) Oxovanadium] (supplying elemental Vanadium IV 320 mcg) 2 mg • Chromium (from Chromic Fuel Chromium Picolinate) 300 mcg • Chromium (from ChromeMate Chromium Nicotinate) 300 mcg • Natural Vitamin E 900 IU • Taurine 1000 mg • Selenium (from Sodium Selenate) 150 mcg • Zinc (from Zinc Picolinate) 30 mg • Manganese (from Manganese Gluconate) 5 mg • Magnesium (from Magnesium Oxide & Aspartate) 400 mg • Biotin 1000 mcg • Niacinamide 100 mg.

Super Vitamin E Creme - Aspen Group, Inc.
Each gram contains: Tocopheryl Acetate 25% • Panthenol 1% • Water • Glyceryl Stearate SE • Octyl Palmitate • Isopropyl Palmitate • Propylene Glycol • Cetearyl Alcohol • Cetyl Phosphate • Decyl Oleate • Aminomethyl Propanol • Carbomer • Allantoin • Diazolidinyl Urea • Methylparaben • Propylparaben.

Super Vita-Vim with Beta Carotene - Jamieson
Each caplet contains: Vitamin A (as Tetinyl Acetate and 15% [1500] IU as Beta-Carotene) 10000 IU • Vitamin C (as Ascorbic Acid) 200 mg • Vitamin D (as Cholecalciferol) 400 IU • Vitamin E (as Dl-Alpha Tocopheryl Acetate) 60 IU • Thiamin (as Thiamine Mononitrate) 30 mg • Riboflavin (Vitamin B2) 30 mg • Niacin (as Niacin and Niacinamide) 60 mg • Vitamin B6 (as Pyridoxine Hydrochloride) 30 mg • Folate (as Folic Acid) 400 mcg • Vitamin B12 (as Cyanocobalamin) 60 mcg • Biotin 30 mg • Pantothenic Acid (as Calcium D-Pantothenate) 30 mg • Calcium (as Calcium Carbonate) 140 mg • Iron (as reduced Iron) 4 mg • Iodine (from kelp) 100 mcg • Magnesium (as Magnesium Oxide) 100 mg • Zinc (as Zinc Gluconate) 10 mg • Selenium (from yeast) 10 mcg • Copper (as Copper Gluconate) 1 mg • Chromium (as Chromium Rice Protein Chelate) 50 mcg • Potassium (as Potassium Gluconate) 30 mg • Choline Bitartrate 30 mg • Inositol 30 mg • Dl-Methionine 2.2 mg.

Super VM - Puritan's Pride
Each tablet contains: Vitamin A (as Retinyl Palmitate) 10,000 IU • Vitamin C (as Ascorbic Acid and Rose Hips) 250 mg • Vitamin D (as Ergocalciferol) 400 IU • Vitamin E (as d-Alpha Tocopheryl Acetate) 150 IU • Thiamin (Vitamin B-1) 60.8 mg • Riboflavin (Vitamin B-2) 75 mg • Niacin (as Niacinamide) 75 mg • Vitamin B-6 (as Pyridoxine Hydrochloride) 61.5 mg • Folic Acid 400 mcg • Vitamin B-12 (as Cyanocobalamin) 75 mcg • Biotin (as D-Biotin) 75 mcg • Pantothenic Acid (as d-Calcium Pantothenate) 75 mg • Calcium (as Calcium Amino Acid Chelate) 50 mg • Iron (as Iron Amino Acid Chelate)

B R A N D   N A M E S

10 mg • Iodine (as Kelp) 150 mcg • Magnesium (as Magnesium Amino Acid Chelate) 25 mg • Zinc (as Zinc Amino Acid Chelate) 15 mg • Selenium (as Sodium Selenate) 10 mcg • Copper (as Cupric Amino Acid Chelate) 0.25 mg • Manganese (as Manganese Amino Acid Chelate) 6.1 mg • Potassium (as Potassium Amino Acid Chelate) 10 mg • PABA (Para-Aminobenzoic Acid) 75 mg • Choline Bitartrate 75 mg • Inositol 75 mg • Rutin 25 mg • Citrus Bioflavonoids 25 mg • Hesperidin 5 mg • Betaine Hydrochloride 25 mg • L-Glutamic Acid 25 mg • Proprietary Blend: Alfalfa (leaf), Watercress (plant), Parsley (leaf) 3 mg.

Super Whey Fuel - TwinLab
Blend of Three key Whey Proteins: Micro-Filtered & Ion-Exchange Whey Protein Isolate, Modified Molecular Weight & Partially Pre-Digested Whey Protein, & Whey Protein Concentrate enriched with Glutamine, Taurine, Arginine, Leucine, Isoleucine, Valine, Carnitine & Carnosine. Contains no added sugar, is low in lactose & contains Whey Protein 17 g per serving.

SuperCitriMax - Now
Each capsule contains: Calcium (from Citrimax) 90 mg • ChromeMate brand of Chromium (Chromium Polynicotinate) 100 mcg • Iodine (from Kelp) 150 mcg • CitriMax Garcinia cambogia extract 750 mg • Panax ginseng root powder 100 mg.

Super-Green Pro-96 Soy Protein - Nature's Life
Two scoops (28.35 g) contain: Full disclosure ingredients: SUPRO brand Soy Protein Isolate (including Lecithin) • Hawaiian Spirulina • natural Vanilla Flavor • Barley Grass • Psyllium seed husks • Apple Pectin • Oat Fiber • Chlorophyll • Lemon Bioflavonoids Complex • Bromelain • Papain • Kelp • Milk-free Lactobacillus acidophilus • Pyridoxine Hydrochloride (Vitamin B6).

Superior One Plus - Swanson
Each tablet contains: Vitamin A (as beta-carotene) 25000 IU • Vitamin C USP (as ascorbic acid) 300 mg • Vitamin D (as cholecalciferol) 400 IU • Vitamin E USP (as d-alpha tocopheryl succinate) 15- IU • Thiamin USP (as thiamin HCl; vitamin B-1) 125 mg • Riboflavin (vitamin B-2) 125 mg • Niacinamide 125 mg • Vitamin B-6 USP (as pyridoxine HCl) 125 mg • Folic Acid USP 400 mcg • Vitamin B-12 USP (as cyanocobalamin) 125 mcg • Biotin 125 mcg • Pantothenic Acid USP (as d-calcium pantothenate) 125 mg • Calcium (from calcium carbonate) 75 mg • Iron USP (from ferrous fumarate) 18 mg • Iodine (from kelp) 225 mcg • Magnesium USP (from magnesium oxide) 40 mg • Zinc (from zinc gluconate) 20 mg • Selenium (from yeast) 100 mcg • Manganese USP (from manganese sulfate) 7 mg • Chromium (from yeast) 225 mcg • Inositol 125 mg • Choline (as choline bitartrate) 100 mg • Lemon Bioflavonoid Complex 50 mg • Betaine HCl 30 mg • PABA (para-aminobenzoic acid) 30 mg • Rutin 30 mg, Glutamic Acid HCl 25 mg, Hesperidin Complex 25 mg.

Support Tonic For Men - Amazon Support
Each capsule contains: Muira Puama • Catuaba • Chuchuhuasi • Suma • Maca • Simaruba • Sarsaparilla • Jurubeba • Carqueja • Jatoba.

Support Tonic For Women - Amazon Support
Each capsule contains: Abuta • Catuaba • Suma • Maca • Simaruba • Sarsaparilla • Wild Yam • Chuchuhuasi • Espinheira Santa • Gervao • Jurubeba • Damiana.

Supra Renal 220 - Atrium Inc.
Each tablet contains: Raw Tissue concentrate from Bovine Sources (not extracts): (Adrenal 220 mg & Pituitary 15 mg) 235 mg • Vitamin C 175 mg • Bioflavonoid Complex 45 mg • Pantothenic Acid 70 mg • Methionine 60 mg • Choline 60 mg • Vitamin B1 25 mg • Vitamin B2 25 mg • Vitamin B6 25 mg • Niacinamide 50 mg • Magnesium 100 mg • Folic Acid 400 mcg • RNA 25 mg.
See Editor's Note No. 14, page 1817.

Supraene Creme - Atrium Inc.
Two ounces contains: Squalene 30 mg • Triethanolamine 5 mg • Ceresin Wax 5 mg • Glucam F-20 4 mg • Amerchol L-101 2.5 mg • Solulan 16 2.5 mg • Steral 2.5 mg • Cetyl Alcohol 2.5 mg • Carbopol 934 0.5 mg • Methyl Paraben 10 mg • Propyl Paraben 0.05 mg • Distilled Water 45.35 mg.

Suprema C Powder - Gary Nulls
One teaspoon contains: Vitamin C 2500 mg • Selenium 65 mcg • Bioflavonoids 150 mg.

Suprema C Tablets - Gary Nulls
Each tablet contains Vitamin C 500 mg • Selenium 6 mcg • Bioflavonoids 10 mg.

Swiss Herbal - The Vitamin Shoppe
Each tablet contains: Senna (Cassia senna) leaves standardized to 3% sennosides 100 mg • Strawberry (Fragaria vesca) leaves 50 mg • Peach (Prunus persica) leaves 50 mg • Anise (Pimpinella anisum) fruit and seeds 50 mg • Cranberry (Vaccinium macrocarpon) fruit 50 mg • Calendula (Calendula officinalis) flower and leaves 25 mg. No yeast, corn, wheat, sugar, salt, starch, milk, gluten, soy, eggs, dairy, fish or animal derivatives, citrus, preservatives, artificial colors or flavors added.

Swiss Kriss Tabs - Swiss Kriss
Each tablet contains: Active Ingredient: Finely powdered sun dried Senna leaves. Also contains the following natural herbs: Finely powdered Strawberry Leaves • Peach Leaves • Anise seed • Caraway seed • Hibiscus & Calendula flowers for their flavoring & carminative principals.

Symbiotropin hGH - ASN
Each two tablets contain: Anterior Pituitary Peptides Aminotrope-7 (a sequenced glycoamino acid complex) 4200 mg • Novel Polyose Complex (pharmaceutical mono, poly & oligo saccharides) 2230 mg. In a base of L-Glutamine, L-Arginine, L-Pyroglutamate, GABA, L-Glycine, L-Lysine, L-Tyrosine & Vica faba major, all naturally sweetened & flavored.

Sympt-X Plus - Cambridge Nutraceuticals
Each serving contains: Glutamine 10 g • Vitamin A (as mixed carotenoids) 6500 IU • Vitamin C 330 mg • Vitamin E 100 IU • Selenium 50 mcg. Available in 650 g jar and Single Dose Packets.

Synadrene - Metaphysics - Pro-Soma Enterprises
One capsule contains: Citrus Aurantium (Bitter Orange Peel) 350 mg • Chromium Picolinate 400 mcg.

Synergistic Iron - Quest
Each capsule contains: Iron (HVP Chelate) 25 mg • Copper (HVP Chelate) 2 mg • Molybdenum (HVP Chelate) 50 mcg • Vitamin C (Ascorbic Acid) 100 mg • Niacin 10 mg • Vitamin B1 (Thiamine HCl) 5 mg • Vitamin B6 (Pyridoxine HCl) 5 mg • Vitamin B2 (Riboflavin) 2 mg • Pantothenic Acid (d-Calcium Pantothenate) 10 mg • Folic Acid 0.2 mg • Vitamin B12 (Cobalamin) 20 mcg • Biotin 50 mcg. Other Ingredients: Magnesium Stearate (vegetable source), Microcrystalline Cellulose.

Synergistic Magnesium - Quest
Each tablet contains: Magnesium (HVP Chelate) 150 mg • Calcium (HVP Chelate) 30 mg • Phosphorus (HVP Complex) 15 mg • Vitamin B6 (Pyridoxine HCl) 20 mg. Other Ingredients: Croscarmellose Sodium, Magnesium Stearate (vegetable source), Microcrystalline Cellulose, Vegetable Stearin.

Synergistic Manganese - Quest
Each capsule contains: Manganese (HVP Chelate) 50 mg • Vitamin B1 (Thiamine HCl) 20 mg • Vitamin C 100 mg. Other Ingredients: Magnesium Stearate (vegetable source), Microcrystalline Cellulose.

Some Brand Name Natural Products - What they Contain

B R A N D   N A M E S

Synergistic Multiple Mineral - Quest
Each tablet contains: Calcium (HVP Chelate) 100 mg • Magnesium (HVP Chelate) 100 mg • Potassium (HVP Chelate) 33 mg • Iron (HVP Chelate) 5 mg • Manganese (HVP Chelate) 5 mg • Zinc (HVP Chelate) 5 mg • Copper (HVP Chelate) 1 mg • Iodine (Potassium Iodide) 50 mcg • Molybdenum (HVP Chelate) 50 mcg • Chromium (HVP Chelate) 10 mcg • Selenium (HVP Complex) 10 mcg. Other Ingredients: Croscarmellose Sodium, Magnesium Stearate (vegetable source), Mircocrystalline Cellulose, Vegetable Stearin.

Synergistic Selenium - Quest
Each capsule contains: Selenium (HVP Chelate) 200 mcg • Vitamin E (d-Alpha Tocopheryl Acetate) 25 IU • Vitamin C (Ascorbic Acid) 100 mg. Other Ingredients: Magnesium Stearate (vegetable source), Microcrystalline Cellulose.

Synergistic Zinc - Quest
Each tablet contains: Vitamin A (Palmitate) 5000 IU • Zinc (HVP Chelate) 20 mg • Copper (HVP Chelate) 1 mg. Other Ingredients: Calcium Phosphate, Croscarmellose Sodium, Magnesium Stearate (vegetable source), Microcrystalline Cellulose, Vegetable Stearin.

Synerpro Multiple Vitamins & Minerals - Nature's Sunshine
Each tablet contains: Vitamin A (beta-carotene) 2,500 IU • Vitamin C 30 mg • Vitamin D 200 IU • Vitamin E (d-alpha tocopherol) 15 IU • Thiamine (Vitamin 1) 0.75 mg • Riboflavin (Vitamin B2) 0.85 mg • Niacin (as nicotinic acid) 10 mg • Vitamin B6 (pyridoxine HCl) 1 mg • Folate (folic acid) 200 mcg • Vitamin B12 (cyanocobalamin) 3 mcg • Biotin 150 mcg • Pantothenic acid (d-calcium pantothenate) 5 mg • Calcium (d-calcium pantothenate and dicalcium phosphate) 125 mg • Iron (ferrous fumarate) 9 mg • Phosphorus (dicalcium phosphate) 90 mg • Iodine (potassium iodide) 75 mcg • Magnesium (magnesium oxide) 50 mg • Zinc (zinc oxide) 7.5 • Selenium (amino acid chelate) 25 mcg • Copper (copper gluconate) 1 mg • Manganese (amino acid chelate) 0.5 mg • Chromium (amino acid chelate) 50 mcg • Molybdenum (amino acid chelate) 38 mcg. Other Ingredients: Broccoli flowers (Brassica oleracera), Turmeric root (Curcuma longa), Red Beet root (Beta vulgaris), Rosemary leaves (Rosmarinus officinalis), Carrot root (Daucus carota), Tomato fruit (Solanum lycopersicum), Chinese Cabbage leaves (Brassica rapa), Cabbage leaves (Brassica oleracea, Orange Bioflavonoids, Grapefruit Bioflavonoids, Hesperidin, cellulose (plant fiber), Stearic Acid, and Silicon Dioxide (powdered silica).

System D-Tox - Nutri-Quest
Six capsules contain: Vitamin A Palmitate 2000 IU • Vitamin C 750 mg • Vitamin B1 20 mg • Niacin 25 mg • Vitamin B12 50 mcg • Folic Acid 300 mcg • Calcium Aspartate 75 mg • Magnesium Glycinate 200 mg • Magnesium Aspartate 100 mg • Chromium Picolinate 50 mcg • Zinc Picolinate 20 mg • N-Acetyl Cysteine 30 mg • L-Glutamine 200 mg • Silymarin extract 5 mg • Quercetin 25 mg • L-Taurine 50 mg • L-Ornithine 20 mg • L-Glutamic Acid 20 mg • L-Carnitine 20 mg • Choline 50 mg • Propolis 20 mg • Yellow Dock 25 mg • Beta Carotene 7500 IU • Vitamin E Succinate Natural 200 IU • Vitamin B2 20 mg • Pyridoxal 5 Phosphate 20 mg • Pantothenic Acid 50 mg • Biotin 200 mcg • Calcium Gluconate 75 mg • Magnesium Citrate 100 mg • Selenomethionine 150 mcg • Manganese Aspartate 5 mg • Molybdenum Citrate 50 mcg • Reduced Glutathione 20 mg • Milk Thistle 50 mg • Beet root 50 mg • Glucaronic Acid 5 mg • L-Glycine 50 mg • L-Methionine 50 mg • L-Arginine 20 mg • L-Tyrosine 20 mg • Inositol 50 mg • Curcumin 5 mg • Chlorophyll 10 mg • Asparagus 15 mg • Dandelion root 25 mg • Siberian Ginseng 30 mg • Broccoli 15 mg • Mullein 25 mg • Co-Enzyme Q-10 1 mg.

Syste-Max (SysteMax) - Changes - TwinLab
One heaping teaspoonful (6.8 g) contains: Vitamin A 668 IU • Vitamin C 100 mg • Vitamin E 60 IU • Psyllium seed husk 4000 mg • Soy Germ flour (providing 15 mg of isoflavones) 500 mg • Chitosan 100 mg • Phytosterol complex (providing 43 mg of beta-sitosterol) 100 mg • Oat flour 100 mg.

T-5W - Dial Herbs
Red Raspberry • Blue Cohosh • Bayberry • Squaw Vine • Blessed Thistle • Ginger • Motherwort • False Unicorn • Wild Yam • Lobelia • Cayenne.

T-ACN - Dial Herbs
Black Walnut • Burdock • Chaparral • Yellow Dock • Sassafras • Valerian.

Tadenan - European; Not available in the US.
Pygeum africanum extract standardized to contain 14% triterpenes and 0.5% n-docosanol usually in dosages of 100 - 200 mg.

T-AFT - Dial Herbs
Wild Lettuce • St. John's Wort • Valerian • Cayenne.

T-AIS - Dial Herbs
Rose Hips • Sage • Yarrow • Burdock • Echinacea • Goldenseal • Yellow Dock • Garlic • Nettle • Lemon Grass • White Oak bark • Black Cohosh • Fenugreek • Juniper berry • Oregon Grape • Plantain • Thyme.

T-AKE - Dial Herbs
Clove Oil • Oat Straw • Lobelia • Cayenne.

Take Control - Lipton
Water • Liquid Canola Oil • Vegetable Oil Sterol Esters • Liquid Sunflower Oil • Partially Hydrogenated Soybean Oil • Salt • Whey • Vegetable Mono- and Diglycerides • Potassium Sorbate • Lactic Acid • Calcium Disodium EDTA • Soy Lecithin • Artificial Flavor • Beta Carotene • Vitamin A (Palmitate).

T-ALER - Dial Herbs
Bayberry • Echinacea • Yarrow • Wild Cherry bark • Cayenne • Goldenseal.

T-ANEM - Dial Herbs
Comfrey root • Dandelion • Barberry • Parsley • Yellow Dock • Myrrh • Kelp.

Taraxatone - Cytodyne Technologies
Six capsules contain: Vitamin B6 24 mg • Magnesium 8.4 mg • Dandelion leaf powder 1500 mg • Uva Ursi leaf extract 900 mg • Guarana extract 600 mg • Taurine 115 mg.

T-ARTH - Dial Herbs
Yucca • Alfalfa • Buckthorn • Burdock • Parsley • Slippery Elm • Yarrow • Cayenne.

T-ASMA - Dial Herbs
Blood root • St. John's Wort • Mullein • Comfrey • Saw Palmetto • Wild Cherry bark • Goldenseal • Lobelia • Cayenne.

T-BB - Dial Herbs
Buckthorn • Yellow Dock • Garlic • Cayenne • Dandelion • Poke root.

T-BC - Dial Herbs
White Oak bark • Comfrey • Black Walnut • Marshmallow root • Mullein • Gravel root • Wormwood • Lobelia • Scullcap • Glycerine.

T-BDW - Dial Herbs
Corn Silk • Plantain • St. John's Wort • Sanicle • Mullein • Sarsaparilla • Cubeb berries • Watermelon seeds • Cayenne.

T-BF - Dial Herbs
Oat Straw • Shavegrass • Comfrey • Slippery Elm • Burdock • Lobelia.

Some Brand Name Natural Products - What they Contain
www.NaturalDatabase.com contains MANY more listings than appear here.

T-CAC - Dial Herbs
Buckthorn • Burdock • Chaparral • Dandelion • Cascara Sagrada • Licorice • Red Clover • Barberry.

T-CIRC - Dial Herbs
Witch Hazel • Garlic • Ginger • Cayenne.

T-CS - Dial Herbs
Bayberry • Myrrh • Echinacea • Goldenseal • Cayenne.

T-DI - Dial Herbs
Hyssop • Garlic • Hydrangea • Catnip • Peppermint • Cayenne.

T-DIA - Dial Herbs
Yarrow • Juniper berries • Huckleberry • Cayenne • Goldenseal.

T-DREA - Dial Herbs
Witch Hazel • Slippery Elm • Ginger • Shepherd's Purse • Raspberry.

T-DRY - Dial Herbs
Sage • Yarrow.

T-DTX - Dial Herbs
Echinacea • Yellow Dock • Garlic • Lobelia • Cayenne.

Tea Tree Oil - Holista - Holista
Tea Tree oil (Melaleuca alternifolia) 100% pure.

T-EC - Dial Herbs
Eyebright • Bayberry • Passion flower • Goldenseal • Cayenne.

Teen Advantage Creatine Serum - Muscle Marketing USA
Each serving contains: Creatine Monohydrate • Glucosamine • Vitamin B12 • L-Glutamine • Sodium Pyruvate • Royal Jelly • Ginseng • Honey • Natural Glycerine • Natural Flavor • Distilled Water.

Teen Essentials - Rexall
Two tablets contain: Vitamin A (from retinyl palmitate) 10000 IU • Vitamin C 400 mg • Vitamin D (as cholecalciferol) 400 IU • Vitamin E (as d-alpha-tocopheryl acid succinate and dl-alpha-tocopheryl acetate) 100 IU • Thiamin (as thiamin HCl) 50 mg • Riboflavin (Vitamin B2) 50 mg • Niacin (as niacinamide) 100 mg • Vitamin B-6 (from pyridoxine HCl) 50 mg • Folic Acid 400 mcg • Vitamin B-12 (as cyanocobalamin) 50 mcg • Biotin 150 mcg • Pantothenic Acid (from calcium d-pantothenate) 100 mg • Calcium 200 mg • Iron (from ferrous fumarate) 9 mg • Phosphorus 154 mg • Iodine (from potassium iodide) 75 mg • Magnesium (from magnesium oxide) 100 mg • Zinc (from zinc gluconate) 22 mg • Manganese (from manganese gluconate) 3 mg • Potassium (from potassium gluconate) 90 mg • Choline Bitartrate 100 mg • Para-Aminobenzoic Acid 30 mg • Inositol 10 mg. Other Ingredients: Dicalcium Phosphate, Cellulose, Stearic Acid, Croscarmellose Sodium, Silica, Magnesium Stearate, Hydroxypropyl Methylcellulose, PEG.

Teen Link - Pain & Stress Center
Each capsule contains: 5-HTP 25 mg • St. John's Wort 165 mg • GABA 120 mg • Glutamine 100 mg • Taurine 110 mg • Vitamin B6 5 mg.

Teething Gel - Hyland's
Calcarea phosphorica as Calcium phosphate 12X HPUS • Chamomilla as Chamomile 6X HPUS • Coffea cruda as Coffee 6X HPUS • Belladonna (Alkaloids 0.0000003%) 6X HPUS. In a base of Deionized Water, Vegetable Glycerin, Hydroxyethyl Cellulose, Methyl Paraben, Propyl Paraben.
See Editor's Note No. 1, page 1816.

Teething Tablets - Hyland's
Each tablet contains: Calcarea phosphorica as Calcium Phosphate 3X HPUS • Chamomilla as Chamomile 3X HPUS • Coffea cruda as Coffee 3X HPUS • Belladonna as Alkaloids 0.0003% 3X HPUS. In a base of Lactose NF (Milk Sugar).
See Editor's Note No. 1, page 1816.

Tegreen 97 - Pharmanex
Each 250 mg capsule contains a 15:1 extract of Green Tea extract that is standardized to contain a minimum of 97% pure polyphenols including >160 mg of catechins of which >100 mg is EGC.

Ten Mushroom Combination - Smart Basics
Each capsule contains: Cordyceps • Reishi • Maitake • Shiitake • Coriolus • Umbellatus Polyporus • Wood Ear • Tremella • Poria • Hericium.

T-ENDO - Dial Herbs
Chaparral • Pipsissewa • Licorice • Prickly Ash • Cramp bark • False Unicorn • Saw Palmetto • Red Clover.

Tension Tamer Extra - Celestial Seasonings
Two capsules contain: Vitamin B6 (as pyridoxine HCL) 6 mg • Vitamin B12 (as cyanocobalamin) 12 mcg • Magnesium (as ascorbate and oxide) 60 mg • Proprietary Blend, 1180 mg: Kava Kava (root), Kava Kava (standardized extract), Chamomile (standardized extract). Other ingredients: May contain one or more of the following: Dicalcium phosphate, gelatin, rice flour, stearic acid, magnesium stearate, and silicon dioxide. This product contains no artificial colors, flavors or preservatives. One serving size is equivalent to: Kava Kava 330 mg standardized to 30% kavalactones.

T-ER - Dial Herbs
Eyebright • Bayberry • Passion flower • Goldenseal • Cayenne • Mineral Water • Honey.

Testatropinol - ASN
Each tablet contains: Testatropinol is a 100% natural, non-herbal, non-glandular, synergistic, homeopathic compound, consisting of: Testosterone • Growth Hormone • Adrenalinum • Adrenocorticotropic Hormone • Lutenizing Hormone • Follicle Stimulating Hormone • Thyroid Stimulating Hormone • Progesterone • Estrone.
See Editor's Note No. 1, page 1816.

Testosterone Fuel Booster - TwinLab
Two capsules contain: Natural Testosterone Boosters DHEA (Dehydroepiandrosterone) (Pure Pharmaceutical Grade) 50 mg • Zinc (from Zinc Picolinate) 50 mg • Natural LH Boosters Acetyl-L-Carnitine 500 mg • Tribulus Terrestris extract 150 mg • Natural Aromatase Inhibitor (anti-estrogen) • Novasoy Purified Soy extract (providing 40% isoflavones) (providing isoflavones 80 mg including: Genistein 39 mg, Daidzein 34 mg & Glycitein 7 mg) 200 mg • Natural DHT Inhibitors • Saw Palmetto (Serenoa repens) extract 120 mg • Phytosterol Complex (providing 130 mg of Beta-Sitosterol) 250 mg.

T-FC1 - Dial Herbs
Red Raspberry • Black Cohosh • Lady Slipper • Blessed Thistle • Damiana.

T-FC2 - Dial Herbs
Black Cohosh • Licorice root • Sarsaparilla • Ginseng • Goldenseal.

T-FC3 - Dial Herbs
Black Cohosh • Wood Betony • Blessed Thistle • Chamomile • Fennel • Ginger • Cayenne.

T-FC4 - Dial Herbs
Wood Betony • Sarsaparilla • Valerian • Blessed Thistle • Dandelion • Garlic • Chamomile.

BRAND NAMES

Some Brand Name Natural Products - What they Contain
www.NaturalDatabase.com contains MANY more listings than appear here.

B R A N D N A M E S

T-FLO - Dial Herbs
Sanicle • Marshmallow • Fennel • Blessed Thistle • Ginger.

T-FVR - Dial Herbs
Peppermint • Garlic • Valerian • Yarrow • Echinacea • Goldenseal • Cayenne • Lobelia.

_T-GB_ - Dial Herbs
Dandelion • Oregon Grape • Rhubarb • Bayberry • Yellow Dock • Lobelia.

_T-GS_ - Dial Herbs
Catnip • Peppermint • Fennel • Cayenne • Lobelia.

_T-H_ - Dial Herbs
White Willow bark • Valerian • Scullcap • Wood Betony.

T-HBP - Dial Herbs
Black Cohosh • Blue Cohosh • Wild Cherry bark.

T-HBRN - Dial Herbs
Sarsaparilla • Thyme • Valerian • Wood Betony • Peppermint • Catnip • White Willow bark.

The Antioxidant Formula - Rx Vitamins
Three capsules contain: Vitamin C (Ascorbate) 500 mg • Beta Carotene 25000 IU • Phytonutrient Blend (Broccoli, Spinach, Tomato) 150 mg • Citrus Bioflavonoid Complex 50 mg • Vitamin E 200 IU • Selenium 50 mcg • Zinc 15 mg • NAC (N-Acetyl-Cysteine) 15 mg • Bilberry 10 mg • L-Glutathione 10 mg • Wild Grape seed extract 10 mg.

The Antioxidant Phyters - The Vitamin Shoppe
Each tablet contains: Green and Red Wine 100 mg • Licorice 100 mg • Pine bark and Grape seed 30 mg • Bilberry 50 mg • Ginkgo Biloba 50 mg • Marigold, Sunflowers 60 mg.

The AstaFactor - Aquasearch
Two softgels contain: Natural Astaxanthin (6 mg total carotenoids) 5 mg. Ingredients: Algal meal (Haematococcus pluvialis), Rice Bran Oil, Natural Gelatin, Beeswax, Natural Vitamin E, Vegetal Glycerin.

The B-Total Solution with Extra B12 - Dial Herbs
Vitamin C • Vitamin B2 • Vitamin B3 • Vitamin B6 • Vitamin B12 • Pantothenic Acid. In a base of Distilled Water, Glycerine, Sorbitol, Sodium Bicarbonate, Citric Acid, Fruit flavors & Sodium Benzoate.

The Fat Metabolizer - The Vitamin Shoppe
Three tablets contain: Elemental Choline (from Choline Bitartrate) 1000 mg • Inositol 100 mg • L-Methionine 500 mg • Taurine 500 mg • Vitamin B6 (Pyridoxine HCl) 30 mg • Betaine HCl 150 mg • Barberry Extract (Berberis vulgaris) 100 mg.

The Fruit Phyters - The Vitamin Shoppe
Two tablets contain: Tomato, Red Grapefruit, Apricot, Watermelon 100 mg • Walnut, Berries, Grape, Apple, Tea • Orange, Lemon, Lime, Grapefruit, Tangerine, Cherry, Tomato, Strawberry 400 mg • Apricot, Cantaloupe, Citrus Fruit 150 mg • Citrus Fruit 100 mg • Papaya, Kiwi, Pineapple 50 mg • Mango, Citrus Fruit 100 mg.

The Green Phyters - The Vitamin Shoppe
Two tablets contain: Spirulina 200 mg • Chlorella 200 mg • Barley Juice 200 mg • Wheat Grass 200 mg • Alfalfa Leaf 200 mg • Chlorophyll 200 mg.

The Missing Link: Master Nutrient Formula - Designing Health, Inc.
Each tablespoon contains: Vitamin A (90% as beta carotene) 55 IU • Thiamine (Vitamin B1) 0.1 mg • Calcium 22 mg • Iron 0.7 mg • Omega-3 1000 mg • Omega-6 450 mg • Omega-9 400 mg • Hesperidin 80 mg • Spirulina 8 mg • Kelp (macrocystis pyrifuri) 6 mg. Other Ingredients: Flax Seed, Blackstrap Molasses, Rice Bran, Nutritional Yeast, Sunflower Seed, Alfalfa, Carrot, Apple, Sesame Seed, Licorice Root, Broccoli, Cherry, Parsely, Sprouted Green Barley, Nettle, Vanilla Bean, Ginger Root, Sage, Rosemary, Garlic, and Yucca Schidigera Extract.

The Natural Choice Hepol - Allergon AB
Each tablet contains: Botanical Glutathione Yeast extract YH 85 mg • Aloe Vera extract 45 mg • Polbax extract 40 mg. Other Ingredients: Lacrose Alfa, Microcrystalline Cellulose, Magnesium Stearate, Colloidal Silicon Dioxide, Talc, Natural Resin.

The Natural Choice Probacillus Plus - Allergon AB
Each tablet contans: proprietary blend [Lactobacillus Acidophilus • Bifidobacterium Bifidum] 4 Billion Cells. Other Ingredients: Inositol, Monoatril Glutamas, Ascorbate, Yeast extract, Polysaccharides, Skim Milk Powder, stearate, Dextrose.

The Natural Choice Profemme - Allergon AB
Each tablet contains: Flower Pollen extract WSI 72 mg • Flower Pollen extract LS1 4 mg. Other Ingredients: Microcrystalline Cellulose, Lactose, Magnesium stearate, Silicon Dioxide, Natural Resin, Polyethylene Glycol, Talc.

The Natural Choice Prostat - Allergon AB
Each tablet contains: Standardized extract of Graminae Pollen 70 mg • Fat soluble Gramanie extract EA 10 4 mg. Other Ingredients: Microcrystalline Cellulose, Lactose, Magnesium Stearate, Colloidal Silicon Dioxide, Natural Resin, Talc, Propylene Glycol.

The Ocular Formula - Rx Vitamins
Three capsules contain: Vitamin C (Ascorbate) 200 mg • Citrus Flavonoid Complex 100 mg • Vitamin E 100 IU • Zinc 30 mg • Glutathione 10 mg • Beta Carotene 9 mg • Vitamin A (Retinol) 5000 IU • Selenium 50 mcg • Lutein 6 mg • Zeaxanthin 260 mcg • Bilberry 100 mg • Grape seed 10 mg • Essential Cofactors: CoQ10 5 mg, Copper 3 mg.

The One-Minute Facial - Jason
Seven different Vitamin Cs • Alpha Lipoic Acid.

The Prostate Formula - Real Health Laboratories
Three tablets contain: Vitamin D 200.0 IU • Saw Palmetto powder 320.0 mg • Pygeum powder 300.0 mg • Vitamin E 100.0 IU • Stinging Nettle powder 100.0 mg • Vitamin B6 50.00 mg • Pumpkin seed powder 100.0 mg • Zinc 15.0 mg • L-Lysine HCl 250.0 mg • L- Glutamic acid 250.0 mg • Glycine 250.0 mg. Other Ingredients: Dicalcium Phosphate, Hydroxyproplyl Methylcellulose, Microcrystalline Cellulose, Croscarmellose Sodium, Stearic Acid, Polyethylene Glycos, Silica, Titanium Dioxide, Magnesium Stearate, Peppermint oil, Polysorbate 80.

The Total EFA - Health From The Sun
Three capsules contain: Calories 35 • Calories from Fat 30 • Total Fat 3.5 g • Saturated Fat 0.5 g • Cholesterol 5 mg • Protein 1 g • Vitamin E 30 IU • Alpha-Linolenic Acid (ALA) (Omega-3) 699 mg • Docosahexaenoic Acid (DHA) (Omega-3) 138 mg • Eicosapentaenoic Acid (EPA) (Omega-3) 216 mg • Gamma Linolenic Acid (GLA) (Omega-6) 288 mg • Lenoleic Acid (Omega-6) 620 mg • Oleic Acid (Omega-9) 520 mg. Ingredients: Certified Organic Flax seed oil, Borage seed oil, Fish oil, Gelatin, Glycerine, Water, Mixed Tocopherols.

Some Brand Name Natural Products - What they Contain
www.NaturalDatabase.com contains MANY more listings than appear here.

The Ultimate Anti-Oxidant Formula - Natrol
Two capsules contain: Vitamin A (Beta Carotene from d-Salina) 10000 IU • Vitamin E (d-alpha tocopheryl) 200 IU • Vitamin C (Ester-C Brand) 250 mg • Niacinamide 40 mg • Zinc (Krebs Cycle) 25 mg • Copper (Krebs Cycle) 2 mg • Selenium (Selenomethionine) 125 mcg • Flavonoids, Herbs, & other selected ingredients: Spirulina 300 mg GP Flavonoids Complex+ 200 mg, a 30% guaranteed potency extract of mixed flavonoids extracted from: Rose Hips, Turmeric, Acerola berry, Bilberry, Hawthorne berry, Grape skin, Milk Thistle, & Citrus fruits • Calendula 50 mg • Artichoke extract 10 mg. Other ingredients: Silicon Dioxide, Magnesium Stearate, Gelatin.

The Ultimate Calcium Formula - Roex
Six tablets contain: Calcium (Chelate, Citrate, Hydroxyapatite, Aspartate, Lactate) 1000 mg • Magnesium (Chelate, Oxide, Aspartate) 500 mg • Zinc (Gluconate , Citrate, Aspartate) 15 mg • Manganese 5 mg • Copper 2 mg • Vitamin D (Cholecalciferol) 400 IU • Boron 3 mg • Trace Minerals 25 mg • Silica 150 mg • Selenium 50 mcg • Chromium 50 mcg • Molybdenum 10 mcg.

The Ultimate Weight Loss & Nutrition System - Nature's Secret
Three tablets provide: Vitamin B6 30 mg • Garcinia cambogia extract 600 mg • Pantothenic Acid 100 mg • Magnesium (aspartate) 25 mg • Chromium 300 mcg • Potassium (citrate) 128 mg • L-Carnitine 250 mg • Betaine HCl 100 mg • Lipotropic factors 800 mg • Choline, L-Methionine, Inositol, Lecithin, Triphala powder, Echinacea angustifolia, Cascara sagrada • Astragalus. Thermogenic support factors 757 mg: N-Acetyl Glucosamine, Uva Ursi leaf, Gotu Kola, Siberian Ginseng, L-Glutamine, Parsley leaf, Ginger root, Borage oil, Shave Grass herb, Piper longum, Licorice root. L-Phenylalanine, Corn Silk, Gugulipid, Pacific Kelp, L-Tyrosine, Atractylodes, Bladderwrack, Dulse, Chickweed herb, Dandelion root, Capsicum fruit, Lipase, Mustard seed, Protease, Cellulase.

The Vegi Phyters - The Vitamin Shoppe
Two tablets contain: Red, Yellow, and Dark vegetable, Carrots, Kale, Parsley, Spinach, Sweet Potatoes, Turnip Greens, Winter Squash, and Yams 300 mg • Cruciferous Vegetable 300 mg • Horseradish 100 mg • Chili Peppers 100 mg • Cabbage, Brussel Sprouts, Kale, Collard Greens, Broccoli, Mustard Greens 200 mg.

The Vitamin Shoppe Flax Seed Oil 1000 mg - The Vitamin Shoppe
Each softgel contains: 1000 mg of 100% pure, organically grown cold-pressed, unrefined virgin flax oil providing the following approximate essential fatty acids: Alpha-Linolenic Acid 550 mg • Linoleic Acid 150 mg • Oleic Acid 190 mg • natural Vitamin E 1 IU.

Thera Zinc Lozenges-Menthol - Natrol
One lozenge contains: Vitamin C (as Calcium Ascorbate) 50 mg • Zinc (as Zinc Gluconate) 7.5 mg • Echinacea angustifolia entire plant 10 mg • Bee Propolis 10 mg • Slippery Elm Bark 10 mg • Elderberry 10 mg • Bee Pollen 10 mg. Other ingredients: Hydrogenated Starch, Hydrolysate, natural Menthol Eucalyptus flavor.

Thera-C 3 Grams Lemon - Natrol
One single serving contains: Vitamin C (Ascorbic Acid) 250 mg • Acerola berry extract 20 mg • Echinacea (Purpurea extract 16:1) 12.5 mg • White Willow bark 100 mg • Slippery Elm bark 75 mg • Stevia powder 20 mg. Other ingredients: Lemon Juice powder, Citric Acid, Menthol from Peppermint, Honey powder, Fructose, Calcium Carbonate.

Theragran Heart Right - Bristol-Myers Squibb Co.
Two caplets contain: Vitamin A (8% as Beta-carotene, 2% as Alpha-carotene, Lutein, Lypcopene, Zeaxanthin, Cryptoxanthin 10 mcg) 5000 IU • Vitamin C 120 mg • Vitamin D 400 IU • Vitamin E 400 IU • Vitamin K 14 mcg • Thiamin (B1) 3 mg • Riboflavin (B2) 3.4 mg •

Niacin (B3) 20 mg • Vitamin B6 16 mg • Folate, Folic Acid, Folacin 600 mcg • Vitamin B12 30 mcg • Biotin 30 mcg • Pantothenic acid 10 mg • Calcium 55 mg • Iron 4 mg • Iodine 150 mcg • Magnesium 150 mg • Zinc 15 mg • Selenium 70 mcg • Copper 1.5 mg • Manganese 2 mg • Chromium 50 mcg • Molybdenum 75 mcg • Proprietary Blend, 10 mg: Beta Carotene, Alpha Carotene, Lutein, Lycopene, Zeaxanthin, Cryptoxanthin.

Theragran-M Advanced - Bristol-Myers Squibb Co.
Each caplet contains: Vitamin A Acetate (20% as Beta Carotene) 5000 IU • Vitamin C (Ascorbic Acid) 90 mg • Vitamin D (Vitamin D3) 400 IU • Vitamin E (dl-Alpha Tocopheryl) 60 IU • Vitamin K (Phytonadione) 28 mcg • Thiamin Mononitrate (Vitamin B1) 3 mg • Riboflavin (Vitamin B2) 3.4 mg • Niacin (Vitamin B3, Niacinamide) 20 mg • Vitamin B6 (Pyridoxine Hydrochloride) 6 mg • Folate (Folic acid, Folacin) 400 mcg • Vitamin B12 (Cyanocobalamin) 12 mcg • Biotin 30 mcg • Pantothenic Acid (Calcium Pantothenate) 10 mg • Calcium 40 mg • Iron (Ferrous Fumarate) 9 mg • Phosphorus (Calcium Phosphate) 31 mg • Iodine (Potassium Iodide) 150 mcg • Magnesium Oxide 100 mg • Zinc Oxide 15 mg • Selenium (Sodium Selenate) 70 mcg • Copper (Cupic Sulfate) 2 mg • Manganese Sulfate 2 mg • Chromium Chloride 50 mcg • Molybdenum (Sodium Molybdate) 75 mcg • Chloride 7.5 mg • Potassium Chloride 7.5 mg • Nickel Sulfate 5 mcg • Tin (Stannous Chloride) 10 mcg • Silicon 2 mg • Vanadium (Sodium Metavanadate) 10 mcg • Boron (Sodium Borate) 150 mcg. Other Ingredients: Beta Carotene, Carnauba Wax, Crospovidone, FD&C Blue No.2 Aluminum Lake, FD&C Red No. 40 Aluminum Lake, Flavor, Gelatin, Hydroxypropyl Cellulose, Hydroxypropyl Methylcellulose, Lactose, Magnesium Stearate, Maltodextrin, Microcrystaline Cellulose, Polyethylene Glycol, Polysorbate 80, Potassium Citrate, Povidone, Silica Gel, Stearic Acid, Titanium Dioxide, Triacetin.
See Editor's Note No. 3, page 1816.

Theravim-M - Puritan's Pride
Each tablet contains: Vitamin A (as retinyl acetate and beta carotene) 5,000 IU • Vitamin C (as ascorbic acid) 90 mg • Vitamin D (as cholecalciferol) 400 IU • Vitamin E (as dl-alpha tocopheryl acetate) 30 IU • Thiamin (Vitamin B1: as thiamine hydrochloride) 3 mg • Riboflavin (Vitamin B2) 3.4 mg • Niacin (as niacinamide) 20 mg • Vitamin B6 (as pyridoxine hydrochloride) 3 mg • Folic Acid 400 mcg • Vitamin B12 (as cyancobalamin) 9 mcg • Biotin (as d-biotin) 30 mcg • Pantothenic Acid (as d-calcium pantothenate) 10 mg • Calcium (as dicalcium phosphate) 40 mg • Iron (ferrous fumarate) 27 mg • Phosphorus (as dicalcium phosphate) 31 mg • Iodine (as potassium iodide) 150 mcg • Magnesium (as magnesium oxide) 100 mg • Zinc (as zinc oxide) 15 mg • Selenium (as sodium selenate) 10 mcg • Copper (as copper sulfate) 2 mg • Manganese (as manganese sulfate) 5 mg • Chromium (as chromium chloride) 15 mcg • Molybdenum (as sodium molybdate) 15 mcg • Chloride (as potassium chloride) 7.5 mg • Potassium (as potassium chloride) 7.5 mg.

Thermadrene - SportPharma
Each capsule contains: Ephedra Standardized extract 300 mg (equals 24 mg of Ephedrine) • USP Caffeine 80 mg • Guarana extract 150 mg (equals 15 mg of Caffeine) • Willow Bark extract 75 mg (natural Aspirin; equals less than 5 mg of Aspirin) • Cayenne 60 mg • Ginger root 40 mg.

Thermic Blast - Human Development Technologies
Four sprays contain: Caffeine 100 mg • Ephedra extract 8% aerial (Ephedrine 8 mg) 100 mg • Stevia extract 80% leaf (Steviosides 32 mg) 40 mg • White Willow bark 1% bark (Salicin 200 mcg) 20 mg • Green Tea extract 30% leaf (Polyphenols 6 mg) 20 mg • Guarana extract 10% seed (Caffeine 2 mg) 20 mg • Chromium Picolinate 400 mcg. Other Ingredients: Purified Water, Propylene Glycol, natural Cherry & Vanilla Flavors, Polysorbate 20, Benzyl Alcohol, Hydrochloric Acid Lecithin.

BRAND NAMES

Some Brand Name Natural Products - What they Contain
www.NaturalDatabase.com contains MANY more listings than appear here.

Thermicore - Met-Rx
Three capsules contain: Ma Huang extract 250 mg • Caffeine 200 mg • Bitter Orange extract 400 mg. Other Ingredients: Cellulose, Polyvinylpyrrolidone & Gelatin.

Thermo Cuts - Optimum Nutrition
Four capsules contain: Citrimax 2000 mg • MaHuang extract 334 mg • Guarana extract 910 mg • Willow bark extract 100 mg • L-Carnitine 100 mg • Chromium Picolinate 300 mcg.

Thermo Trim - Swanson
Three capsules contain: Chromium (from Chromax® chromium picolinate) 200 mcg • Guarana extract (standardized to 22% caffeine) 909 mg • Citrin® (Garcinia cambogia extract, 50% hydroxycitrate acid) 500 mg • Ma Huang extract (standardized to 20 mg ephedra alkaloids) 334 mg • L-Carnitine (tartrate) 100 mg.

Thermo-Actives - Natrol
One capsule contains: Ginger extract roots (5% Gingerols) 150 mg • Sida cordifolia extract (0.8% Ephedrine) 100 mg • Mucuna pruriens 5:1 extract 100 mg • Cayenne Guaranteed Potency extract (90000 SHU) 50 mg • Mustard extract Seed (50% Saponins) 15 mg • Bioperine 4:1 extract 15 mg. Other ingredients: Rice powder, Silicon Dioxide, Magnesium Stearate, Gelatin.

ThermoDiet for Men - Futurebiotics
Two tablets contain: Spirulina 100 mg • MaHuang (Standardized Extract) 200 mg • Mustard Seed Powder 100 mg • Vitamin C 100 mg • Potassium (Citrate) 99 mg • Magnesium (Aspartate) 50 mg • Chromium (Picolinate) 200 mcg • Kelp 150 mg • Chinese Licorice 250 mg • Smilax.

ThermoDiet For Women - Futurebiotics
Two tablets contain: Spirulina 100 mg • MaHuang (Standardized Extract) 200 mg • Mustard Seed Powder 100 mg • Vitamin C 100 mg • Potassium (Citrate) 99 mg • Magnesium (Aspartate) 50 mg • Chromium (Picolinate) 200 mcg • Kelp 150 mg • Peony 250 mg • Fo-Ti 250 mg • Dong Quai 250 mg.

Thermogenic Herbal Complex - Starlight International
Each capsule contains: Chromium (as chromium picolinate) 6 mcg • Ma Huang (Ephedra Sinica, plant) 275 mg (Total Ephedrine Alkaloids) 22mg • Cascara Sagrada (Rhamnus purshiana, bark) 35 mg • Bladderwrack (Focus vesiculosus, plant) 35 mg • Uva Ursi extract, 4:1 (Arctostaphylos uva ursi, leaf) 25 mg • Parsley leaf extract, 4:1 (Petroselinum crispum, leaf) 10 mg • Calcium Gluconate 5 mg • Corn Silk Pistils (Zea mays, flower) 7 mg • Goldenrod (Solidago odora, leaf) 6 mg • Fumitory Herb (Fumaria officinalis, aerial parts) 6 mg • Magnesium Gluconate 7 mg • English Hawthorn (Crategus laevigata, fruit) 5 mg • Licorice root (Glycymhiza glabra, root) 5 mg • Marshmallow root (Athea officinalis, root) 5 mg • Apple Pectin 5 mg. Other Ingredients: Magnesium Stearate, Silicon Dioxide, Dicalcium Phosphate, Calcium Sulfate.

Thermogenics Original Formula - Silver Sage
Each capsule contains: Ephedrine alkaloids (from standardized Ma Huang plant extract 310 mg) 25 mg • Caffeine (16.8 mg from standardized Bissy Nut 140 mg) 50 mg • Acetylsalicylic Acid (Aspirin) 110 mg • Proprietary Blend of synergistic ingredients 249 mg: Siberian Ginseng root, Schizonepeta spica extract 5:1, Forsythia fruit extract 5:1, Green Tea leaf extract standardized for polyphenols/catechins content, Cayenne fruit, Ginger root • Vitamin C 50 mg • Pantothenic Acid 25 mg • Zinc amino acid chelate 7 mg • Selenium amino acid chelate 1 mcg • Manganese amino acid chelate 2.5 mg.

ThermoGenics Plus - Silver Sage
Each capsule contains: Ephedrine (in standardized whole Ma Huang extract) 14 mg • Caffeine (in standardized Bissy Nut) • Acetylsalicylic Acid • In a base of Vitamin C, Siberian Ginseng, Green Tea extract (standardized to 50% polyphenols/catechins), Schizonepeta spica extract (5:1), Forsythia fruit extract (5:1), White Willow bark, Cayenne, Pantothenic Acid, Ginger root, Zinc (Amino Acid Chelate), Manganese (Amino Acid Chelate), Selenium (Amino Acid Chelate).

Thermogenics Quick Start - Silver Sage
Each capsule contains: Ephedrine alkaloids (from standardized Ma Huang plant extract 250 mg) 20 mg • Caffeine (26 mg from standardized Bissy Nut 106 mg) 200 mg • Acetylsalicylic Acid (Aspirin) 324 mg • Proprietary Blend of synergistic ingredients 198 mg: Siberian Ginseng root, Schizonepeta spica extract 5:1, Forsythia fruit extract 5:1, Cayenne fruit, Ginger root • Vitamin C 40 mg • Pantothenic Acid 23 mg • Zinc amino acid chelate 14 mg • Selenium amino acid chelate 167 mcg • Manganese amino acid chelate 5 mg.

Thermo-Lift (ThermoLift) - Changes - TwinLab
One caplet contains: Chromium (Chromium dinicotinate glycinate, Chromium picolinate, and Niacin bound Chromium) 200 mcg • Vanadium (as bis(maltoalto)oxovanadium(iv)) 100 mcg • Mahuang stem standardized extract (Supplying 25 mg Ephedrine alkaloids) 310 mg • Thermogenic herbal blend 325 mg: Guarana seed standardized extract (20%) (Supplying 43 mg Caffeine), Citrus Peel standardized extract (5-7% alkaloids) (Citrus aurantium), White Willow bark, Siberian Ginseng root, Astragalus root, Bee Pollen, Bladderwrack kelp, Ginger root, Gotu Kola leaf, Licorice root, Rehmannia root, Reishi mushroom (Fruiting body). Other ingredients: Dicalcium phosphate, Vegetable cellulose, Fractionated Vegetable oil, Soy polysaccharides, Silica, and Vegetable resin glaze.

Thermo-Lift II (ThermoLift II) - Changes - TwinLab
Each caplet contains: Niacin 10 mg • Chromium (as Chromium dinicotinate glycinate, Chromium polynicotinate and chromium picolinate) 100 mcg • Vanadium (as Vanadyl sulfate) 50 mcg • Panax Ginseng root standardized extract (8% ginsenosides) 100 mg • Guarana seed standardized extract (20% Caffeine) 225 mg • Yerba Mate leaf standardized extract 100 mg • L-Tyrosine 100 mg • Thermogenic herbal blend 75 mg: Standardized Citrus Peel extract (5% phenethylamines) (Citrus aurantium), Cayenne pepper, Cinnamon bark standardized extract, Ginger root, and White Willow bark • Supporting herbal blend 50 mg: Astragalus root, Bladderwrack kelp, Licorice root, Siberian Ginseng root, and Arctic root (Rhodiola rosea) standardized extract. Other ingredients: Dicalcium phosphate, Vegetable cellulose, Fractionated Vegetable oil, Soy polysaccharides, Silica, and Vegetable resin glaze.

ThermoSculpt - For Your Health
Four softgels contain: Citrus Aurantium 1000 mg • Glucosol TM 48 mg • Corosolic Acid 480 mg • Vitamin B-5 (pantothenic acid) 60 mg • Chromium 400 mg • Vanadium 200 mg • Zinc Oxide 40 mg.

ThermoSyn - PharmAssure
One tablet contains: Chromium (as Chromium Picolinate) 400 mcg • MaHuang Extract (Ephedra sinica; 6% Ephedrine=20mcg) 333 mg • Guarana Seed Extract (Paullinia cupana; 365 Caffeine=90mg) 250 mg • Citrus aurantium Fruit Extract (4% Synephrine=6mg) 150 mg • White Willow Bark Extract (Salix alba; 15% Salicin=15mg) 100 mg. Other ingredients: Dicalcium Phosphate, Croscarmellose Sodium, Cellulose.

THERMOthin - Slimming and Nutrition Consultancy
Each capsule contains: Citrus aurantium • Citrin (HCA) • Guarana • Caffeine • White Willow bark • Chromium • Liquorice extract • Cayenne extract • Siberian Ginseng • Vitamin B6 • Iodine • Betaine HCL.

T-HFV - Dial Herbs
Bayberry • Cayenne • Mullein • Lobelia.

B R A N D   N A M E S

Some Brand Name Natural Products - What they Contain
www.NaturalDatabase.com contains MANY more listings than appear here.

ThiaMind - Source Naturals
Each tablet contains: Vitamin B1 (Thiamin Mononitrate) 500 mg • Magnesium (Citrate, Malate, Succinate and Oxide) 100 mg.

Think Sharp - Health Smart Vitamins
Three capsules contain: Vitamin C (ascorbic acid) 250 mg • Thiamin (as thiamin mononitrate) 10 mg • Riboflavin 10 mg • Niacin (as 50% niacinamide, 50% nicotinic acid) 20 mg • Vitamin B6 (as pyridoxine HCl) 10 mg • Folic Acid 400 mcg • Vitamin B12 (as cyanocobalamin) 100 mcg • Biotin 300 mcg • Pantothenic Acid (as calcium pantothenate) 10 mg • Dimethylaminoethanol (DMAE; as Dimethylaminoethanol bitartrate) 500 mg • L-Glutamine 250 mg • L-Pyroglutamic Acid 100 mg • Acetyl-L-carnitine (as Acetyl-L-carnitine HCl) 50 mg.

Think-O2 - Traditional Medicinals
Contains: Peppermint leaf • Ginkgo leaf and Ginkgo dry leaf extract • Gotu Kola leaf • Sage leaf • Siberian Ginseng root • Lemon Balm leaf • Rosemary leaf • natural Lemon flavor • Stevia leaf.

Thinz Back-To-Nature - Alva-Amco Pharmacal Cos., Inc.
One tablet contains: Active Ingredient: Phenylpropanolamine HCl 75 mg. Other Ingredients: Apple powder • Brown Lake color blend • Dicalcium Phosphate • D&C Yellow #10 • FD&C Yellow #6 • Hydroxypropyl Methylcellulose • Magnesium Stearate • Mineral oil • Oat bran • Polyethylene Glycol • Titanium Dioxide • Wheat bran.

Thinz-Span - Alva-Amco Pharmacal Cos., Inc.
Each capsule contains: Phenylpropanolamine HCl 75 mg.

Thiodox - Allergy Research Group
Glutathione • N-Acetyl Cysteine • Lipoic Acid.

Thisilyn - Nature's Way
Each capsule contains: Milk thistle extract (standardized for a flavanoid content of 140 mg silymarin [80%], which includes silybinin, silychristin, and 85 mg of lactose) 175 mg.

ThistleComp - PhytoPharmica
Each capsule contains: Artichoke leaves extract (Cynara scolymus) 250 mg • Curcuma root extract (Curcuma longa) 150 mg • Boldo extract (Peumus boldo) 100 mg • Milk Thistle extract (Silybum marianum) (56 mg) calculated as silybin 70 mg. Contains no sugar, salt, yeast, wheat, corn, soy, dairy products, coloring, flavoring, or preservatives.

ThistlePlex - Enzymatic Therapy
Each capsule contains: Artichoke leaves extract (Cynara scolymus) standardized to contain 3% Caffeylquinic Acids 250 mg • Curcuma root extract (Curcuma longa) standardized to contain 2.5% Curcumin) 150 mg • Boldo extract (Peumus boldo) standardized to contain 1.52% essential oils) 100 mg • Milk Thistle extract (Silybum marianum) standardized to contain 80% Silymarin (56 mg) calculated as Silybin 70 mg. Contains no sugar, salt, yeast, wheat, corn, soy, dairy products, coloring, flavoring, or preservatives.

ThistleRex - PhytoPharmica
Each capsule contains: Milk Thistle extract standardized to contain 80% silymarin (120 mg) calculated as silybin 150 mg• Dandelion root extract 4:1 (Taraxacum officinale) 10 mg • Artichoke leaves extract (Cynara scolymus) 10 mg • Licorice root extract (Glycyrrhiza glabra) 10 mg.

Thistlezyme - Olympian Labs
Two capsules contain: Milk Thistle extract (standardized to contain at least 80% Silymarin) 200 mg.

Thorene - Thorene Research Inc.
Each capsule contains: Tylophora asthmatica 30 mg • Boswellia serrata extract (60% Boswellin) 150 mg • Piper longa 100 mg • Hesperidin Methyl Chalcone 100 mg.

Three-In-One - Changes - TwinLab
Each capsule contains: Vitamin C (as Calcium Ascorbate) 120 mg • Aloe Vera leaf gel 200:1 concentrate 200 mg • Mexican Yam root 4:1 (equivalent to 150 mg) 37.5 mg. Other Ingredients: Gelatin, Maltodextrin, Calcium Sulfate, Magnesium Stearate, and Silica.

Throat Coat - Traditional Medicinals
Contains: Slippery Elm bark (Ulmus rubra). Other herbal ingredients: Licorice root, Wild Cherry bark, Fennel seed, Cinnamon bark, Orange peel, Althea root.

T-HRT - Dial Herbs
Hawthorne • Lecithin • Tansy • Fenugreek • Garlic • Cayenne.

T-HS - Dial Herbs
Ginseng • Damiana • Gotu Kola • Sarsaparilla • Sassafras • Saw Palmetto.

Thyme and Myrrh - Dial Herbs
Thyme • Myrrh.

Thymex - Standard Process
Each tablet contains: Proprietary Blend 195 mg: Bovine Thymus extract (Cytosol), Magnesium citrate. Other Ingredients: Calcium lactate, Cellulose, Calcium stearate, Ascorbic Acid.
See Editor's Note No. 14, page 1817.

Thymucin - PhytoPharmica
Two capsules contain: Enzymatic Polypeptide Fractions (Thymus fractions) 750 mg • Astragalus (Astragalus membranaceus) root extract 4-6:1 (standardized to contain 0.5% minimum of the isoflavone 4' hydroxy 3' methoxy isoflavone 7-SUG [GHMIF]) 250 mg.

Thymuril Capsules - PhytoPharmica
Four capsules contain: Vitamin A (beta-carotene) 25,000 IU • Vitamin C (ascorbic acid) 250 mg • Vitamin E (d-alpha tocopheryl acetate) 200 IU • Zinc (Krebs chelate) 15 mg • Selenium (L-selenomethionine) chelate 25 mcg • Polypeptide Fractions Thymus Complex (Predigested, concentrated soluble extract standardized for peptides and polypeptides with molecular weight less than 10,000 daltons) 945 mg • Echinacea (Echinacea purpurea) root 300 mg • L-Lysine (HCl) 250 mg • Blue Flag (Iris versicolor) extract 130 mg • Goldenseal (Hydrastis canadensis) root extract 64 mg.
See Editor's Note No. 14, page 1817.

Thymuril Tablets - PhytoPharmica
Two tablets contain: Vitamin A (Beta Carotene) 25000 IU • Vitamin E 200 IU • Vitamin C (Ascorbate) 250 mg • Zinc (Chelate) 15 mg • Selenium (Chelate) 25 mcg • Enzymatic Polypeptide fractions 750 mg.

Thymus Cream - Atrium Inc.
Three fluid ounces contain: Extract of Thymus (Viobin) • Glycerin Hexadecenol • Sodium Laureth Sulfate • Stearic Acid • Methylparaben • Sodium Sulfate • Propylparaben • Natural Fragrance.
See Editor's Note No. 14, page 1817.

T-HYPO - Dial Herbs
Licorice • Juniper berry • Wild Yam • Dandelion • Ginger.

B R A N D   N A M E S

B R A N D   N A M E S

Thyro Complex - Progressive Labs

Each capsule contains: Raw Thyroid concentrate (thyroxin free) 60 mg • Raw Adrenal concentrate 30 mg • Raw Pituitary concentrate 10 mg • Raw Spleen concentrate 10 mg • Kelp 300 mg. This natural product is prepared by a special process which does not exceed physiological temperature (37° C). Guaranteed to be free of chemical pesticides and synthetic hormones.
See Editor's Note No. 14, page 1817.

Thyroid & L-Tyrosine Complex - Enzymatic Therapy

Each capsule contains: Magnesium (Oxide) 100 mg • Manganese (Chelate) 3 mg • Zinc (Chelate) 3 mg • Copper (Chelate) 150 mcg • Iodine (Kelp) 100 mcg • Molybdenum (Chelate) 50 mcg • Vitamin B12 (Cyanocobalamin) 50 mcg • Other ingredients: L-Tyrosine 124 mg • Multi-Glandular Complex: Raw Liver, Raw Lung, Raw Pancreas, Raw Heart, Raw Kidney, Raw Spleen, & Raw Brain 35 mg • Thyroid Substance (thyroxin-free) 4X. Contains no sugar, salt, yeast, wheat, corn, soy, dairy products, coloring, flavoring or preservatives.
See Editor's Note No. 14, page 1817.

Thyroid Complex - The Vitamin Shoppe

Each capsule contains: Thiamine (Vitamin B1) 10 mg • Riboflavin (Vitamin B2) 10 mg • Vitamin B6 (as pyridoxine HCl) 10 mg • Vitamin B12 (as cyanocobalamin) 25 mcg • Iodine (from kelp) 150 mcg • Magnesium (as magnesium oxide) 100 mg • Zinc (as zinc chelate) 3 mg • Selenium (as selenium chelate) 70 mcg • Copper (as copper chelate) 150 mcg • Manganese (as manganese chelate) 3 mg • Molybdenum (as molybdenum chelate) 150 mcg • L-Tyrosine 150 mg • Multi Gland Complex (from Bovine Liver, Lung, Pancreas, Heart, Kidney, Spleen, Brain) 35 mg. No yeast, corn, wheat, sugar, salt, starch, milk, gluten, eggs, fish, citrus, preservatives, artificial colors or flavors added.
See Editor's Note No. 14, page 1817.

Thyroid Essentials - Swanson

Each capsule contains: Thiamin USP (as thiamin HCl; vitamin B-1) 25 mg • Riboflavin USP (vitamin B-2) 25 mg • Niacinamide 25 mg • Vitamin B6 (as pyridoxine HCl) 25 mg • Folic Acid 25 mcg • Vitamin B12 (as cyanocobalamin) 25 mcg • Pantothenic Acid (as d-calcium pantothenate) 25 mg • Iodine (from kelp) 100 mcg • Magnesium (from magnesium oxide) 25 mg • Zinc (from zinc oxide) 25 mg • Selenium (as L-selenomethionine) 50 mcg • Copper (from copper gluconate) 2 mg • L-Tyrosine 150 mg • Coleus Forskohlii (18% forskolin) 50 mg.

Thyroid Support Formula - PhysioLogics

Each capsule contains: Riboflavin 20 mg • Niacin (as Niacinamide) 20 mg • Vitamin B6 (as Pyridoxine Hydrochloride) 1 mg • Iodine (from Kelp) 110 mcg • Zinc (as Zinc Gluconate) 5 mg • Copper (as Copper Glycinate) 300 mcg • Chromium (as Chromium Chelavite) 80 mcg • L-Tyrosine 300 mg • Coleus Forskohlii leaf (18% Forskolin, 9 mg) 50 mg.

Thyrosine Complex - PhytoPharmica

Each capsule contains: Magnesium (Oxide) 100 mg • Manganese (Chelate) 3 mg • Zinc (Chelate) 3 mg • Copper (Chelate) 150 mcg • Iodine (Kelp) 100 mcg • Molybdenum (Chelate) 50 mcg • Vitamin B12 (Cyanocobalamin) 50 mcg • L-Tyrosine 124 mg • Multi-Glandular Complex containing: Raw Liver, Raw Lung, Raw Pancreas, Raw Heart, Raw Kidney, Raw Spleen, and Raw Brain 35 mg • Thyroid Substance (Thyroxin-free) 4X. Contains no sugar, salt, yeast, wheat, corn, soy, dairy products, coloring, flavoring, or preservatives. All organs & glands are derived from bovine sources except raw pancreas (porcine).
See Editor's Note No. 14, page 1817.

ThyroStart - Silver Sage

Two capsules contain: Kelp meal 500 mg • Vitamin C 20 mg • Magnesium 20 mg • L-Tryosine 20 mg • Vitamin B3 20 mg • Vitamin B2 10 mg • Zinc 10 mg • Vitamin B5 10 mg • Horsetail grass 5 mg •

Gentian root 5 mg • Blue Flag 5 mg • Nettle leaf herb 5 mg • Radish extract 4:1 5 mg • Parathyroid substance 5 mg • Thymus substance 2.5 mg • Adrenal substance 2.5 mg • Pancreas substance 2.5 mg • Vitamin B6 2 mg • Vitamin B1 1.5 mg • Manganese 1 mg • Copper 0.02 mg • Vitamin A 2000 IU • Beta Carotene 2000 IU • Vitamin E 50 IU • Biotin 50 mcg • Folic Acid 50 mcg • Vitamin B12 10 mcg • Selenium 10 mcg • Molybdenum 10 mcg.
See Editor's Note No. 14, page 1817.

Tiger Vites - Body Wise International, Inc.

Two caplets contain: Beta Carotene (Dunaliella Salina Algae) (Equivalent to Vitamin A 5000 IU) 3 mg • Vitamin D (as Vitamin D3) (Cholecalciferol) 200 IU • Vitamin E (d-Alpha Tocopherol Acid Succinate and Mixed Tocopherols Beta, Gamma and Delta) 30 IU • Vitamin C 60 mg • Folic Acid 400 mcg • Vitamin B1 1.5 mg • Vitamin B2 1.7 mg • Vitamin B6 2 mg • Niacin (Niacinamide) 20 mg • Vitamin B12 6 mcg • Pantothenic Acid (d-Calcium Pantothenate) 5 mg • Biotin 150 mcg • Choline (Choline Bitartrate) 10 mcg • Inositol 10 mcg • Calcium (Krebs Cycle Chelate) 50 mg • Magnesium 40 mg • Copper 1 mg • Zinc 7.5 mg • Molybdenum 37.5 mcg • Iodine (Kelp) 75 mcg • Chromium 120 mcg • Selenium (L-Seleno-methionine) 17.5 mcg • Manganese 0.5 mg • Potassium 0.5 mg • Iron 1.8 mg • PhytoNutrient Garden Blend* 25 mg • PhytoNutrient Orchard Blend 25 mg • Pineapple 12.5 mg • Papaya 12.5 mg • Citrus Bioflavonoids 12.5 mg. Other Ingredients: Spirulina, Whole Brown Rice, Spinach, Beet Leaf, Cherry, Rose Hips, Mango.

Tigra Pill - Universal Products, Performance Industri

Each tablet contains: Hydrolyzed protein rich in Arginine • D-Alpha-Tocopherol • Aromatic plant extract (Diamiana aphrodisiaca, Dioscorea villosa, Panax Ginseng, Smilax officinalis) • Choline sulfate • Vitamin B3 • Vitamin B1 • Zinc sulfate • Grape Seed extract • Essential oils of Peppermint • Savory • Clove • Magnesium stearate • Carboxymethylcellulosis • Magnesium silicate.

Time Fighters For Men - Changes - TwinLab

Four caplets contain: Vitamin A (as Beta-Carotene and mixed carotenoids from D. salina algae) 25000 IU • Vitamin C (as Ascorbic Acid) 500 mg • Vitamin D (as Cholecalciferol) 400 IU • Vitamin E (as Dl-Alpha-Tocopheryl and D-Alpha Tocopheryl Succinate) 200 IU • Vitamin B1 (as Thiamin HCl) 50 mg • Vitamin B2 (as Riboflavin) 50 mg • Niacin (as Niacinamide) 125 mg • Vitamin B6 (as Pyridoxine HCl) 50 mg • Folate (as Folic Acid) 800 mcg • Vitamin B12 (as Cyanocobalamin) 500 mcg • Biotin 300 mcg • Pantothenic acid (as D-Calcium Pantothenate) 50 mg • Calcium (as Calcium Carbonate and Citrate) 400 mg • Iodine (as Potassium Iodide) 150 mcg • Magnesium (as Magnesium Oxide and Aspartate) 500 mg • Zinc (as Zinc Citrate and Picolinate) 50 mg • Selenium (as Selenomethionine) 200 mcg • Copper (as Copper Gluconate) 2 mg • Manganese (as Manganese Gluconate) 2 mg • Chromium (as Chromium Dinicotinate Glycinate) 200 mcg • Molybdenum (as Sodium Molybdate) 150 mcg • Potassium (as Potassium Citrate and Chloride) 10 mg • Life Enhancement Men's Herbal Blend 360 mg: Soybean phytosterol complex (120 mg Beta-Sitosterol), Saw Palmetto berry 4:1 extract, Panax Ginseng extract (4% ginsenosides) • Marigold flower concentrate (2% Lutein) 50 mg • Tomato fruit concentrate (2% Lycopene) 50 mg • Choline Bitartrate 25 mg • Inositol 25 mg • PABA 10 mg • Whole Food Phytonutrient Concentrates 500 mg: Parsley, Dunaliela salina algae, Kale, Spinach, Cantoloupe, Carrot, Papaya, Red Peppers, Tomato, Yellow Squash, Turmeric, Cranberry, Tangerine, Grapefruit, Lemon, Orange, Pineapple, Leek, Onion, Garlic, Raspberry, Green Tea, Alfalfa, Soybean, Cherry, Peach, Pear, Red Grape, Strawberry, Asparagus, Broccoli, Bruessels Sprout, Cabbage, Cauliflower, Mustard Greens. Other Ingredients: Microcrystaline Cellulose, Croscarmellose Sodium, Stearic Acid, Silica, Caramel color, Magnesium Stearate, Vanillin, Pharmaceutical Glaze.

Some Brand Name Natural Products - What they Contain
www.NaturalDatabase.com contains MANY more listings than appear here.

Time Fighters For Women With Iron - Changes - TwinLab
Four caplets contain: Vitamin A (as Beta-Carotene and mixed carotenoids from D. salina algae) 25000 IU • Vitamin C (as Ascorbic Acid) 500 mg • Vitamin D (as Cholecalciferol) 800 IU • Vitamin E (as Dl-Alpha-Tocopheryl Acetate and D-Alpha Tocopheryl Succinate) 200 IU • Thiamin (as Thiamin HCl) 25 mg • Riboflavin 25 mg • Niacin (as Niacinamide) 100 mg • Vitamin B6 (as Pyridoxine HCl) 25 mg • Folate (as Folic Acid) 800 mcg • Vitamin B12 (as Cyanocobalamin) 250 mcg • Biotin 300 mcg • Pantothenic Acid (as D-Calcium Pantothenate) 50 mg • Calcium (as Calcium Carbonate and Citrate) 500 mg • Iron (as Ferrous Fumarate) 18 mg • Iodine (as Potassium Iodide) 150 mcg • Magnesium (as Magnesium Oxide and Aspartate) 400 mg • Zinc (as Zinc Citrate and Picolinate) 30 mg • Selenium (as Selenomethionine) 200 mcg • Copper (as Copper Gluconate) 2 mg • Manganese (as Manganese Gluconate) 2 mg • Chromium (as Chromium Dinicotinate Glycinate) 200 mcg • Molybdenum (as Sodium Molybdate) 150 mcg • Potassium (as Potassium Citrate and Chloride) 10 mg • Boron (from Boron Citrate) 3 mg • Marigold flower concentrate (2% Lutein) 50 mg • Tomato fruit concentrate (2% Lycopene) 50 mg • Choline Bitartrate 25 mg • Inositol 25 mg • PABA 10 mg • Life Enhancement Women's Herbal Blend 200 mg : Panax Ginseng root extract, Black Cohosh root, Chaste Tree fruit • Whole Food Phytonutrient Concentrates 500 mg: Parsley, Dunaliela Salina Algae, Kale, Spinach, Cantaloupe, Carrot, Papaya, Tomato, Yellow Squash, Turmeric rhizome, Tangerine, Grapefruit, Lemon, Orange, Red Pepper, Alfalfa, Soybean, Cranberry, Green Tea, Raspberry, Cherry, Peach, Pear, Pineapple, Red Grape, Strawberry, Asparagus spear, Brussesl sprouts, Garlic, Leek, Onion, Broccoli, Cauliflower, Cabbage, Mustard Greens. Other Ingredients: Microcrystalline Cellulose, Croscarmellose Sodium, Stearic Acid, Silica, Magnesium Stearate, Vanillin, and Pharmaceutical Glaze.

Time Fighters For Women Without Iron - Changes - TwinLab
Four caplets contain: Vitamin A (as Beta-Carotene and mixed carotenoids from D. salina algae) 25000 IU • Vitamin C (as Ascorbic Acid) 500 mg • Vitamin D (as Cholecalciferol) 800 IU • Vitamin E (as Dl-Alpha-Tocopheryl Acetate and D-Alpha Tocopheryl Succinate) 200 IU • Thiamin (as Thiamin HCl) 25 mg • Riboflavin 25 mg • Niacin (as Niacinamide) 100 mg • Vitamin B6 (as Pyridoxine HCl) 25 mg • Folate (as Folic Acid) 800 mcg • Vitamin B12 (as Cyanocobalamin) 250 mcg • Biotin 300 mcg • Pantothenic Acid (as D-Calcium Pantothenate) 50 mg • Calcium (as Calcium Carbonate and Citrate) 500 mg • Iodine (as Potassium Iodide) 150 mcg • Magnesium (as Magnesium Oxide and Aspartate) 400 mg • Zinc (as Zinc Citrate and Picolinate) 30 mg • Selenium (as Selenomethionine) 200 mcg • Copper (as Copper Gluconate) 2 mg • Manganese (as Manganese Gluconate) 2 mg • Chromium (as Chromium Dinicotinate Glycinate) 200 mcg • Molybdenum (as Sodium Molybdate) 150 mcg • Potassium (as Potassium Citrate and Chloride) 10 mg • Boron (from Boron Citrate) 3 mg • Marigold flower concentrate (2% Lutein) 50 mg • Tomato fruit concentrate (2% Lycopene) 50 mg • Choline Bitartrate 25 mg • Inositol 25 mg • PABA 10 mg • Life Enhancement Women's Herbal Blend 200 mg: Panax Ginseng root extract, Black Cohosh root, Chaste Tree fruit • Whole Food Phytonutrient Concentrates 500 mg: Parsley, Dunaliela Salina Algae, Kale, Spinach, Cantaloupe, Carrot, Papaya, Tomato, Yellow Squash, Turmeric rhizome, Tangerine, Grapefruit, Lemon, Orange, Red Pepper, Alfalfa, Soybean, Cranberry, Green Tea, Raspberry, Cherry, Peach, Pear, Pineapple, Red Grape, Strawberry, Asparagus spear, Brussel sprouts, Garlic, Leek, Onion, Broccoli, Cauliflower, Cabbage, Mustard Greens. Other ingredients: Microcrystalline Cellulose, Croscarmellose Sodium, Stearic Acid, Silica, Magnesium Stearate, Vanillin, and Pharmaceutical Glaze.

Time Release Athletes Formula - Puritan's Pride
Two caplets contain: Vitamin A 10,000 IU • Vitamin C 300 mg • Vitamin D 800 IU • Vitamin E 100 IU • Thiamin (Vitamin B1) 22.25 mg • Riboflavin (Vitamin B2) 25 mg • Niacin 100 mg • Vitamin B6 20.5 mg • Folic Acid 400 mcg • Vitamin B12 100 mcg • Biotin

50 mcg • Pantothenic Acid 25 mg • Calcium 250 mg • Iron 25 mg • Iodine 225 mcg • Magnesium 20 mg • Zinc 50 mg • Selenium (as Yeast) 25 mcg • Copper 0.05 mg • Manganese 5 mg • Chromium 50 mcg • Chloride 240 mg • Sodium 100 mg • Potassium 99 mg • Choline 25 mg • Inositol 25 mg • Lecithin 100 mg • RNA - DNA 25 mg • PABA 25 mg • Bee Pollen 50 mg • Rose Hips 20 mg • Isoleucine 389 mcg • Leucine 610 mcg • Lysine 632 mcg • Methionine 122 mcg • Phenylalanine 337 mcg • Threonine 390 mcg • Valine 500 mcg.

Time Release B-100 Ultra B-Complex - Puritan's Pride
Each tablet contains: Thiamin (Vitamin B1; as thiamine mononitrate) 100 mg • Riboflavin (Vitamin B2) 100 mg • Niacin (as niacinamide) 100 mg • Vitamin B6 (as pyridoxine hydrochloride) 100 mg • Folic Acid 100 mcg • Vitamin B12 (as cyanocobalamin) 100 mcg • Biotin (as D-Biotin) 100 mcg • Pantothenic Acid (as D-Calcium Pantothenate) 100 mg • Proprietary Blend: Choline Bitartrate, Inositol, PABA (Para-Aminobenzoic Acid), Alfalfa, Watercress, Parsley, Lecithin, and Rice Bran 100 mg.

Time Release B-50 Vitamin B-Complex - Puritan's Pride
Each tablet contains: Thiamin (Vitamin B1; as thiamine mononitrate) 50 mg • Riboflavin (Vitamin B2) 50 mg • Niacin (as niacinamide) 50 mg • Vitamin B6 (as pyridoxine hydrochloride) 50 mg • Folic Acid 100 mcg • Vitamin B12 (as cyanocobalamin) 50 mcg • Biotin (as d-biotin) 50 mcg • Pantothenic Acid (as d-calcium pantothenate) 50 mg • Proprietary Blend: Choline Bitartrate, Inositol, PABA (Para-Aminobenzoic Acid), Alfalfa, Watercress, Parsley, Lecithin, and Rice Bran 50 mg.

Time Release B-Complex + C - Puritan's Pride
Each tablet contains: Vitamin C (as Ascorbic Acid and Rose Hips) 200 mg • Thiamin (Vitamin B1; as Thiamine Mononitrate) 10 mg • Riboflavin (Vitamin B2) 10 mg • Niacin (as Niacinamide) 50 mg • Vitamin B6 (as Pyridoxine Hydrochloride) 5 mg • Vitamin B12 (as Cyanocobalamin) 10 mcg • Pantothenic Acid (as D-Calcium Pantothenate) 10 mg.

Time Release Mega Vitamins for the Hair - Puritan's Pride
Three tablets contain: Vitamin A (as 100% Beta Carotene) 10,000 IU • Vitamin C (as Ascorbic Acid) 1,000 mg • Thiamin (Vitamin B1; as Thiamine Hydrochloride) 89 mg • Riboflavin (Vitamin B2) 100 mg • Niacin (as niacinamide) 100 mg • Vitamin B6 (as Pyridoxine Hydrochloride) 82 mg • Folic Acid 400 mcg • Vitamin B12 (as Cyanocobalamin) 100 mcg • Biotin 2,000 mcg • Zinc (as Zinc Amino Acid Chelate) 5 mg • Copper (Cupric Sulfate) 2 mg • Choline Bitartrate 500 mg • Inositol 500 mg • PABA (Para-Aminobenzoic Acid) 100 mg • L-Cysteine (as L-Cysteine Hydrochloride) 334 mg.

Time Release Stress B with 500 mg Vitamin C - Puritan's Pride
Each tablet contains: Vitamin C (as ascorbic acid) 500 mg • Vitamin B1 (as thiamine hydrochloride) 100 mg • Vitamin B2 (riboflavin) 100 mg • Niacin (as niacinamide) 100 mg • Vitamin B6 (as pyridoxine hydrochloride) 100 mg • Folic Acid 400 mcg • Vitamin B12 (as cyanocobalamin) 500 mcg • Biotin (as D-Biotin) 50 mcg • Pantothenic Acid (as d-calcium pantothenate) 100 mg • Choline Bitartrate 50 mg • Inositol 50 mg • PABA (para-aminobenzoic acid) 50 mg • Citrus Bioflavonoids 50 mg.

Time Release Ultra Man - Puritan's Pride
Two tablets contain: Vitamin A (Acetate) 5,000 IU • Vitamin E (d alpha Tocopheryl Acetate) 100 IU • Vitamin C (Ascorbic Acid) 300 mg • Selenium (Selenite) 25 mcg • Citrus Bioflavonoids 25 mg • Superoxide Dismutase (SOD) 10 mcg • Pycnogenol 1 mcg • Biotin 300 mcg • Silica 20 mcg • Inositol 10 mg • L-Cysteine 100 mg • Yohimbe extract 50 mg • Korean Ginseng root 50 mg • Swiss Avena Sativa (Oat Straw) 50 mg • Damiana leaves 50 mg • Muira Puama 50 mg • Nettles leaves 30 mg • Oyster Extract 25 mg • Saw Palmetto

BRAND NAMES

berries 50 mg • Prostate glandular 50 mg • Pumpkin Seed 30 mg • Pygeum 25 mg • Golden Seal herb 25 mg • Zinc (Oxide) 2 mg • Vitamin B1 (Thiamine Mononitrate) 30 mg • Vitamin B2 (Riboflavin) 30 mg • Vitamin B3 (Niacin) 30 mg • Vitamin B6 (Pyridoxine Hydrochloride) 30 mg • Vitamin B12 (Cyanocobalamin) 30 mcg • Folic Acid 400 mcg • Pantothenic Acid (Calcium d-Pantothenate) 30 mg • Choline (Choline Bitartrate) 10 mg • PABA (Para Aminobenzoic Acid) 10 mg • Vitamin D (Cholecalciferol) 200 IU • Calcium (Dicalcium Phosphate) 275 mg • Phosphorus (Dicalcium Phosphate) 210 mg • Iodine (Potassium Iodide) 150 mcg • Magnesium (Oxide) 100 mg • Manganese (Gluconate) 5 mg • Potassium (Chloride) 30 mg • Chromium (Picolinate) 50 mcg • Vitamin K (Phytonadione) 25 mcg. In a base of Garlic, Oat Bran, Spirulina, Alfalfa, Parsley, Lecithin, Watercress, Smilax (Sarsaparilla), and Cayenne.
See Editor's Note No. 14, page 1817.

T-ING - Dial Herbs
Valerian root • Chamomile • Lobelia • Arnica • Cayenne.

T-JAUN - Dial Herbs
Barberry • Chamomile • Dandelion • Horehound • St. John's Wort • Tansy • Wood Betony • Yellow Dock.

T-KB - Dial Herbs
Peach bark • Marshmallow • Buchu Leaves • Corn Silk • Echinacea.

T-LB - Dial Herbs
Barberry • Cascara Sagrada • Licorice root • Senna Leaves • Red Raspberry • Lobelia • Cayenne.

T-LS - Dial Herbs
Prickly Ash • Sarsaparilla • Poke root • Stillingia • Red Clover • Burdock • Barberry • Peach bark • Licorice root • Chaparral • Echinacea • Cayenne.

T-MEM - Dial Herbs
Lady Slipper • Rosemary • Gotu Kola • Borage • Siberian Ginseng • Licorice • Lobelia.

TMG Plus - Progressive Labs
Each tablet contains: Trimethylglycine (anhydrous) 500 mg • Vitamin B6 (pyridoxine HCl) 37.5 mg • Vitamin B6 (pyridoxine-5'-phosphate) 7.5 mg • Folate (folic acid) 450 mcg • Vitamin B12 375 mcg • Selenium (from seleno-L-methionine) 7.5 mcg.

T-MISS - Dial Herbs
Wild Yam • Ginger • Red Raspberry • Catnip • False Unicorn • Squaw vine.

T-MSLE - Dial Herbs
Cleavers • Pleurisy root • Saffron • Valerian root • Yarrow • Bistort • Catnip • Cayenne • Lobelia.

T-MUSCL - Dial Herbs
Sarsaparilla • Saw Palmetto • Strawberry.

T-NAUS - Dial Herbs
Catnip • Peppermint • Cinnamon • Ginger • Alfalfa • Lobelia.

T-NRV - Dial Herbs
Black Cohosh • Blue Cohosh • Blue Vervain • Scullcap • Lobelia.

T-NSU - Dial Herbs
Cranesbill • Goldenseal • Marshmallow • Poke root • Echinacea.

Tocotrien-All - Natrol
One softgel contains: Tocotrienol Complex 50 mg containing alpha-tocopherols 30 IU • gamma-tocotrienols 45 mg • alpha-tocopherols 4 mg • delta-tocotrienols 1 mg. Other ingredients: Gelatin, Nutriene (Rice oil).

Tocotrienols plus E-100 I.U. - The Vitamin Shoppe
Each softgel contains: Vitamin E (as d-alpha, d-gamma, d-beta, d-delta tocopherols) 100 IU • Tocotrienols (NuTriene) (as d-alpha, d-gamma, d-beta, d-delta tocopherols) 35 mg.

Tomentosin Plus - Atrium Inc.
Each capsule contains: Uncaris tomentosa 400 mg • Bromelain 100 mg • Salix alba 50 mg • Curcuma longa 40 mg.

Tonalin CLA 1000 Mg - Natrol
One softgel contains: Tonalin supplies 60-70% Conjugated Linoleic Acid from Sunflower oil 1000 mg. Other ingredients: Lecithin, Beeswax, Soybean oil, Gelatin.

Tonalin CLA 750 Mg - Natrol
One softgel contains: Tonalin supplies 60-70% Conjugated Linoleic Acid from Sunflower oil 750 mg • Chromium (Picolinate) 75 mcg • ThermoActives Capsicum (200 SCU) 100 mcg • Ginger root 100 mg. Other ingredients: Lecithin, Beeswax, Soybean oil, Gelatin.

Tonalin CLA for Men - Natrol
One capsule contains: Chromium (as Chromium Picolinate) 50 mcg • Sunflower oil 75 mg • CLA • Conjugated Linoleic Acid 150 mg • Alpha Lipoic Acid 8 mg • Vanadyl Sulfate 2 mg • Siberian Ginseng extract root 50 mg • Leucine (as L-Leucine Hydrochloride) 50 mg • Arginine (as L-Arginine Hydrochloride) 50 mg • Isoleucine (as L-Isoleucine Hydrochloride) 12 mg • Valine (as L-Valine Hydrochloride) 25 mg. Other ingredients: Silicon Dioxide, Magnesium Stearate, Gelatin.

Tone 'N' Trim - Optimum Nutrition
Citrimax • L-Carnitine • Chromium Picolinate.

Tot Tonic - The Herbalist
Echinacea root • Golden Seal root • Lemon Balm herb • Yarrow flower • Yerba Santa leaf.

Total Greens - Solar Green/Nutraceutical
Four tablets contains: Barley Grass Juice powder (Hordeum vulgare) 600 mg • Wheat Grass (Triticum aestivum) 600 mg • Alfalfa leaf (medicago sativa) 600 mg. Other Ingredients: Cellulose, Stearic Acid, Silica and Magnesium Stearate, Chlorella Broken Cell Algae (chlorella pyrenoidosa), Spirulina (algae pratensis), Norwegian Kelp (fucus vesiculosis).

Total Immune - Allergy Research Group
Each serving scoop (20 g) provides: Co-Enzyme Q10 75 mg • Grape seed extract (95%) 250 mg • Alpha Carotene 5 mg • Beta Carotene (from mixed carotenoids) 7500 IU • Lycopene 1.5 mg • Vitamin E (mixed tocopherols) 200 IU • Vitamin C 1175 mg • Folic Acid 400 mcg • Vitamin A 2500 IU • Vitamin B1 23 mg • Vitamin B2 23 mg • Vitamin B3 (niacinamide) 150 mg • Vitamin B3 (niacin) 10 mg • Vitamin B5 150 mg • Vitamin B6 25 mg • Vitamin B12 200 mcg • Biotin 200 mcg • Inositol hexaphosphate 175 mg • Choline 63 mg • Germanium Sesquioxide 50 mg • N-Acetyl Cysteine 375 mg • Glutathione 175 mg • L-Carnitine 100 mg • Calcium (carbonate, glycinate) 50 mg • Magnesium (carbonate, glycinate) 75 mg • Vitamin D (as Vitamin D3) 200 IU • Zinc (arginate) 15 mg • Copper (glycinate) 1 mg • Potassium (ascorbate) 50 mg • Chromium (picolinate) 100 mcg • Molybdenum 125 mcg • Manganese 1.25 mg • Selenium 100 mcg • EPA 500 mg • Iron (aspartate) 1.5 mg • Iodine 75 mcg • MSM 100 mg • Borage oil 150 mg • Genistein (soy isolate) 5 mg • Tocotrienol 25 mg • Biofavonoid complex 50 mg • Trimethyl

Some Brand Name Natural Products - What they Contain
www.NaturalDatabase.com contains MANY more listings than appear here.

Glycine 250 mg • Sulforaphane (broccoli) 50 mg • Beta Glucan (1-3) 25 mg • Green Tea extract 50 mg • Mushroom extract 1500 mg • Bromelain 163 mg • Turmeric 100 mg • Panax Ginseng 50 mg • Astragalus 50 mg • Taurine 250 mg • Lactoferrin 50 mg • In a base of Wheat bran, Hydrolized Whey protein, Oat bran, Rice bran, Psyllium bran, Apple fiber, Lemon flavor, Stevia, Lemon oil & Lime oil.

Total Life Care Nutrition System for Men - Rexall
One packet contains: Vitamin A 5000 IU • Vitamin C (as ascorbic acid) 210 mg • Vitamin D (as cholecalciferol) 400 IU • Vitamin E (as dl-alpha-tocopheryl acetate and d-alpha-tocopherol) 100 IU • Thiamin (vitamin B1; as thiamin mononitrate) 1.5 mg • Riboflavin (vitamin B2) 1.7 mg • Niacin (as niacinamide) 20 mg • Vitamin B-6 (as pyridoxine HCl) 11 mg • Folic Acid 1 mg • Vitamin B-12 (as cyanocobalamin) 101 mcg • Pantothenic Acid (as calcium d-pantothenate) 1 mg • Calcium 100 mg • Magnesium (as magnesium oxide) 200 mg • Zinc (as zinc oxide) 5 mg • Selenium (as selenium amino acid chelate) 200 mcg • Fish Oil (EPA [eicosapentaenoic acid] 180 mg, DHA [docosahexaenoic acid] 120 mg) • L-Arginine (L-arginine and L-arginine HCl) 800 mg • Saw Palmetto fruit 450 mg • Calcium D-Glucarate 400 mg • Grape seed extract (vitis vinifera) 60 mg • Nettle root 50 mg • Pygeum (pygeum africanum) 50 mg • Coenzyme Q-10 20 mg. Other Ingredients: Gelatin, Cellulose, Dicalcium Phosphate, Glycerin, White Rice Powder, Croscarmellose Sodium, Calcium Silicate, Water, Hydroxypropyl Methylcellulose, Magnesium Stearate, PEG, Red 40 lake, Retinyl Acetate, Yellow 6 lake, Titanium Dioxide, Polysorbate 80, Blue 2 lake, Beta-carotene.

Total Life Care Nutrition System for Women - Rexall
One packet contains: Vitamin A 5000 IU • Vitamin C (as ascorbic acid) 410 mg • Vitamin D (as cholecalciferol) 400 IU • Vitamin E (as dl-alpha-tocopheryl acetate and d-alpha-tocopherol) 100 IU • Thiamin (vitamin B1); (as thiamin mononitrate) 1.5 mg • Riboflavin (vitamin B2) 1.7 mg • Niacin (as niacinamide) 20 mg • Vitamin B-6 (as pyridoxine HCl) 11 mg • Folic Acid 1 mg • Vitamin B-12 (as cyanocobalamin) 101 mcg • Pantothenic Acid (as calcium d-pantothenate) 1 mg • Calcium 100 mg • Magnesium (as magnesium oxide) 200 mg • Selenium (as selenium amino acid chelate) 200 mcg • Fish Oil (Eicosapentaenoic Acid [EPA] 180 mg, Docosahexaenoic acid [DHA] 120 mg) 1000 mg • L-Arginine (L-arginine and L-arginine HCl) 800 mg • Calcium D-Glucarate 400 mg • Cranberry fruit juice concentrate 140 mg • Grape seed extract (vitis vinifera) 60 mg • Coenzyme Q-10 20 mg. Other Ingredients: Gelatin, Cellulose, Soybean oil, Glycerin, Dicalcium Phosphate, White Rice Powder, Partially Hydrogenated Soybean Oil, Water, Croscarmellose Sodium, Calcium Silicate, Hydrogenated Soybean Oil, Yellow Beeswax, Hydroxypropyl Methylcellulose, Soy Lecithin, Magnesium Stearate, PEG, Red 40 lake, Retinyl acetate, Silica, Yellow 6 lake, Titanium Dioxide, Polysorbate 80, Blue 2 lake, Beta-carotene.

Total Woman Formula - Youngevity
Damiana leaf (Turnera aphrodisiaca) • Dong Quai root (Angelica sinensis) • Saw Palmetto (Serenoa repens) • Fennel seed (Foeniculum vulgare) • Oat Bran (Avena sativa) • Vilcabamba Mineral Essence: Potassium, Calcium, Magnesium, Zinc, Chromium, Selenium, Iron, Copper, Molybdenum, Vanadium, Iodine, Cobalt, Manganese.

Toxoid OTC's Toxoid First Aid - HealthWatchers System
Zinc (as Zincboracyl crystals) • Menthol • Denatured Ethyl Alcohol 60%.

Toxoid OTC's Toxoid Pain - HealthWatchers System
Zinc (as Zincboracyl crystals) • Menthol • Camphor • Fang Fang Extract • Dong Quai Extract • Ling Man Zhin • Qin Jiu Extract.

Toxoid OTC's Toxoid Relief - HealthWatchers System
Trace Minerals • Zinc (as Zincboracyl crystals) • Red Cabbage Extract • Aluminum Acetate.

Toxoid OTC's Toxoid Skin - HealthWatchers System
Salicylic Acid • Zinc (as Zincoracyl crystals) • Purified Water.

T-PARA - Dial Herbs
Wormwood • Black Walnut • Senna • Wild Carrot.

T-PEP - Dial Herbs
Gotu Kola • Kelp • Alfalfa • Dandelion • Brigham Tea • Hydrangea • Saffron • Parsley.

T-PERSP - Dial Herbs
Pennyroyal • Cayenne • Catnip • Ginger • Chamomile • Mustard.

T-PNF - Dial Herbs
Wild Lettuce • Valerian • Scullcap • Blue Vervain • Arnica • Lobelia • Cayenne.

T-PR - Dial Herbs
Strawberry • Sassafras • Sarsaparilla • Echinacea • Garlic.

Trace-Min Plus - Progressive Labs
Three capsules contain: Vitamin B6 (pyridoxine HCl) 50 mg • Vitamin D (cholecalciferol) 50 IU • Calcium (as calcium carbonate and calcium citrate) 300 mg • Magnesium (as magnesium oxide and magnesium gluconate) 150 mg • Zinc (as zinc gluconate) 15 mg • Manganese (as manganese gluconate) 10 mg • Potassium (as potassium gluconate) 99 mg • Glutamic Acid HCl 325 mg.

Tranquility - Nature's Plus
Each tablet contains: Valerian root 200 mg • Magnesium amino acid chelate/complex 200 mg • Calcium Caseinate, amino acid chelate/complex 100 mg • Chamomile 50 mg. In a base of milk protein concentrate (750 mg), containing 10 mg of naturally occuring L-Tryptophan. Yeast free. Sugar & starch free.

Transfer Factor Plus - 4 Life
Two capsules contain: Zinc Monomethionine 10 mg • Transfer Factor XF (concentrated transfer factor from bovine colostrum) 300 mg • Proprietary blend: ThyRx (Thymus complex containing liposterolics, thymic T factor proteins and other proteinaceous compounds), Cordyvant polysaccharide complex (Inositol hexaphate IP6, Cordyceps sinensis (whole herb containing 7% cordyceptic acid), Beta glucan from Brewers Yeast, Saacharomyces cerevisiae (whole plant), Mannans from Aloe Vera leaf, Shiitake mushroom (Lentinus edodes whole plant 5:1 extract), Maitake mushroom (Grifola frondosa whole plant with concentrated D-fraction) 580 mg.

T-RHU - Dial Herbs
Buchu Leaves • Oregon Grape • Cayenne • Black Cohosh • Buckthorn • Burdock • Hydrangea • Lobelia • Nettle • Scullcap • Wild Yam • White Willow bark • Yellow Dock • Arnica.

Tri-40 - Progressive Labs
Each capsule contains: Iodine (from kelp) 150 mcg • Thyroid concentrate (thyroxin free) 40 mg • Spleen concentrate 40 mg • Thymus concentrate 40 mg • Pacific Sea Kelp 100 mg. The glandular concentrate in this product is prepared by a special process which does not exceed physiological temperature (37° C). Guaranteed free of chemical pesticides and synthetic hormones.
See Editor's Note No. 14, page 1817.

Tri-Amino Supplement - Puritan's Pride
Four tablets contain: L-Arginine Hydrochloride 1447 mg • L-Ornithine Hydrochloride 900 mg • L-Lysine Hydrochloride 1200 mg.

Triax - Syntrax Innovations
Each capsule contains: Tiratricol 1 mg. Other ingredients: Barley flour, gelatin, titanium dioxide, red #40, blue #1.

Some Brand Name Natural Products - What they Contain
www.NaturalDatabase.com contains MANY more listings than appear here.

TRIBEST - New Hope Health Products
Each capsule contains: Tribulus terrestris (containing Furostanol and Protodioscin) 750 mg.

Tribest - Metabolic Response Modifiers - Metabolic Response Modifiers
Each capsule contains: Tribulus terrestris (containing Furostanol and Protodioscin) 750 mg.

Tribestan - Sopharma
Each tablet contains: Tribestan from Tribulus Terrestris herb.

Tribestrone II - ASN
Each tablet contains: Tribulus Terrestris L. extract 450 mg • Ashwaganda extract 100 mg • Mucuna extract 100 mg • Bioperine standardized extract 1.5 mg.

Tribulus - The Vitamin Shoppe
Each capsule contains: Tribulus terrestris (fruit) standardized to 20% saponins 625 mg. No yeast, corn, wheat, sugar, salt, starch, milk, gluten, soy, eggs, dairy, fish, citrus, preservatives, artificial colors or flavors added.

Tribulus Fuel - TwinLab
Each capsule contains: Tribulus Terrestris extract (standardized for 20-29% steroidal saponins) 625 mg.

Tribulus Fuel Stack - TwinLab
Two capsules contain: Tribulus Terrestris extract 1250 mg • DHEA (dehydroepiandrosterone) 50 mg.

Trilean - VitaStore
Guarana (Paullinia Cupana) • Glutamine • Fennel • Choline • Spirulina • Hawthorne • Inositol • Bladderwrack • Vitamin A • Vitamin C • Vitamin D • Vitamin E • Vitamin B1 • Vitamin B2 • Vitamin B6 • Vitamin B12 • Folic Acid • Niacin • d-Biotin • Pantothenic Acid • Potassium • Calcium.

Trim Fit - Quest
Six caplets contain: Advantra-Z (Citrus aurantium) (Bitter Orange peel standardized to 4% Synephrine) 1050 mg • Green Tea extract (Camellia sinesis) (P.E. 1:6) 1050 mg • Tonalin (source of conjugated Linoleic Acid) 900 mg • Kelp (Fucus vesiculosus) 300 mg • St. John's Wort extract (Hypericum perforatum) (P.E. 1:5, Standardized to 0.3% Hypericin) 150 mg • Trim-zyme enzyme blend (Protease, Lipase, Amylase, Cellulase) 150 mg • Lipoic Acid 30 mg. Other Ingredients: Silicon Dioxide, Magnesium Stearate (vegetable source).

Trim Lite - Health Smart Vitamins
Three capsules contain: Vitamin C (ascorbic acid) 250 mg • Vitamin E (d-alpha tocopheryl succinate) 150 IU • Vitamin B6 (pyridoxine HCl) 7 mg • Chromium (as chromium nicotinate) 150 mcg • Cola Nut (14% caffeine, 70 mg) 500 mg • Ma Huang root (6% total ephedrine alkaloids, 6 mg) 100 mg • DL-Phenylalanine 75 mg • English Hawthorn leaf & flower (1.8% vitexin, 0.9 mg) 50 mg • l-Carnitine (as L-carnitine tartrate) 30 mg.

Trimax - Enzymatic Therapy
Each capsule contains: St. John's Wort extract (Hypericum perforatum) standardized to contain 0.15% Hypericins, verified by HPLC 500 mg • Valerian extract (Valeriana officinalis) standardized to contain a minimum of 0.8%, 15 mg • Passionflower extract (Passiflora) 15 mg. Contains no sugar, salt, yeast, wheat, corn, soy, dairy products, coloring, flavoring, or preservatives.

TrimFast (Trim Fast) - Preferred Price Plus
Each capsule contains: Natural Ephedra • White Willow bark • Chromium Polynicotinate.

Trim-Plex - Nature's Plus
Three softgels contain: Lecithin (Soya) 600 mg • Kelp 300 mg • Apple Cider Vinegar 240 mg • Vitamin B6 (Pyridoxine HCL) 50 mg. In a natural blend of Vegetable (soy) oil & Chlorophyll. Sugar & starch free.

Trinovin - Novogen
Each tablet contains: Natural Isoflavones 40mg. Trinovin is made from red clover, which contains isoflavones (genistein, biochanin, daidzein, formononetin) with a high biochanin content. Other Ingredients: Dicalcium phosphate, Microcrystalline cellulose, Hydroxypropyl methylcellulose, Magnesium stearate, Mixed tocopherols, Silica, Soy polysaccharide, & Natural caramel color.

Trioxalon 500 - AST Sports Science
Each capsule contains: Tribulus Terrestris extract 500 mg.

Triple Defense - Olympian Labs
Two capsules contain: Soy Isoflavone dried extract 100 mg • D-Glucarate 400 mg • Lycopene extract (5% Standardized Yielding 30 mg of pure Lycopene) 600 mg • Citrus Bioflavonoids 40 mg.

Triple Stack - Crystal Springs
Each tablet contains: Tribulis 250 mg • DHEA 50 mg • Androstenedione 50 mg • Saw Palmetto 200mg • Pygeum 100 mg.

Triple Whey Fuel - TwinLab
Blend of three key Whey Proteins: Micro-Filtered & Ion-Exchange Whey Protein Isolate (with ~57% Beta-Lactoglobulin, ~24% Alpha-Lactalbumin, ~12% Immunoglobulins, ~7% Minor Peptones & Lactoferrin) • modified molecular weight & partially predigested (hydrolyzed) Whey Protein (providing di-, tri-, oligo- & poly-peptides) • Whey Protein Concentrate enriched with Glutamine. Contains no added sugar, is low in lactose & contains 20 g of whey protein per serving.

Tropical Noni - NutraMed
Morinda citrifolia.

Trym Tone 1200 - Futurebiotics
Four tablets contain: L-Arginine HCl 2100 mg • L-Glycine 1800 mg • L-Lysine HCl 300 mg • Vitamin C 30 mg • Pyridoxine HCl 15 mg • Chromium (polynicotinate) 75 mcg.

T-SEPT - Dial Herbs
Bayberry • Goldenseal • Myrrh • Mineral Water.

T-SHK - Dial Herbs
Lobelia • Cayenne • Mineral Water.

T-SKT - Dial Herbs
Myrrh • White Poplar bark • Balsam.

T-SLC - Dial Herbs
Comfrey • Mullein • Peppermint • Chickweed • Lobelia • Cayenne.

T-SS - Dial Herbs
Damiana • Licorice • Ginseng • Passion flower • Cayenne.

T-THD - Dial Herbs
Kelp • Parsley • Irish Moss • Cayenne • Licorice • Dulse • Bayberry • Bugleweed.

T-ULC - Dial Herbs
Goldenseal • Cayenne • Myrrh • Ginger • Comfrey • Poke root • Yellow Dock.

Some Brand Name Natural Products - What they Contain
www.NaturalDatabase.com contains MANY more listings than appear here.

Tulsi-Neem (soap) - Auromere Ayurvedic Soaps
Coconut oil • Palmyra oil • Rice Bran oil • Alkali • Water • Neem oil • Hydnocarpus (cactus) oil • Castor Oil • Tulsi (Holy Basil) • Rose Petals • Zedoary • Turmeric • Fenugreek • Psoralea corlifolia (Babchi Seed) • Peepal (Bodhi Tree) • Alangium salviifolium • Costus • Indian Sarsaparilla • Shiva Neem (variety of Neem) • Hibiscus.

Tum-Ease - The Herbalist
Catnip leaf • Fennel seed • Angelica root • Gentian root • Oregon Grape root • Ginger root.

Tumeric Extract - Nature's Way
Each capsule contains: Tumeric root 50 mg • Tumeric dried extract 450 mg. Other Ingredients: Cellulose, Gelatin, Silica.

Tums Calcium for Life Bone Health Calcium Supplement - Glaxo Smith Kline
Each tablet contains: Calories 10 • Sugars 2 g • Calcium Carbonate 500 mg. Other Ingredients: Sucrose, Corn Starch, Talc, Mineral Oil, Natural and Artificial Flavors, Adipic Acid, Sodium Polyphosphate, Red 40 Lake, Yellow 6 Lake, Yellow 5 Lake, Blue 1 Lake.
See Editor's Note No. 5, page 1816.

TurboTrim Plus - Trim International
Each tablet contains: MaHuang • Guarana • Chromium Picolinate • Chitosan • Gymnema Sylvestre • Garcinia Cambogia • Vitamin E • Magnesium Chelate • Zinc Chelate • Proprietary Blend: Bee Pollen, Ginseng root, Ginger root, Lecithin, Bovine complex, Damiana herb, Sarsaparilla root, Goldenseal herb, Nettle leaf, Gotu Kola herb, Spirulina, Royal Jelly. Other Ingredients: Di-Calcium Phosphate, Magnesium Stearate, Stearic Acid. Contains no yeast, sugar, or artificial colors or preservatives.
See Editor's Note No. 14, page 1817.

T-VV - Dial Herbs
Oat Straw • Buckthorn • Yarrow • Brigham Tea • Witch Hazel • St. John's Wort • Cayenne.

T-WRT - Dial Herbs
Garlic • Celandine • Mullein • Buckthorn.

Ty-Glute - Atrium Inc.
Each tablet contains: L-Glutamine 255 mg • L-Tyrosine 155 mg • Vitamin C 150 mg • Adrenal concentrate 45 mg.
See Editor's Note No. 14, page 1817.

T-YI - Dial Herbs
Echinacea • Goldenseal • Bayberry • Myrrh • Plantain • Slippery Elm • Wild Carrot.

Udo's Choice Beyond Greens - Flora
One tablespoon (8 g) contains: Udo's Choice perfected seed blend: (Certified Organic Flax seed & Defatted Flax, Certified Organic Sunflower seed & Defatted Sunflower seed, Certified Organic Sesame seed & Defatted Sesame seed, Rice germ & Bran powder, Oat germ & Bran powder) • Pines Barley Grass powder • Cracked Golden Flax seed • Pumpkin seed • Pines Alfalfa Grass powder • Rice bran • Dried Cane juice • Carrot • Soyforce Sprouted Soybeans • Tomato • Pines Oat Grass • Pines Rye Grass • Red Beet • Cinnamon • Peppermint • Ginger • Bilberry leaf • Spirulina • Bee pollen • Dulse • Chlorella • Broccoli • Parsley • Kelp • Hawthorne berry • Milk Thistle • Burdock root • Red Clover • Kale • Licorice root • Chrysanthemum • Yucca • Natural Almond flavor • Lemon Grass • Udo's Choice Digestive Enzyme blend: (Protease, Lipase, Amylase, Cellulase, Maltase, Glucoamylase, Invertase, Pectinase, with Phytase, Lactase) • Beet juice • American Ginseng • Ginkgo extract • Psyllium • Slippery Elm • Stevia leaf • Artichoke • Dandeloin root • Dandelion leaf • Rosemary • Thyme • Sage • Standardized Grape seed extract.

Udo's Choice Fast Food Blend - Flora
Certified Organic Flax • Sunflower & Sesame seeds • Pines Organic Cereal Grasses • Soyforce Powdered Sprouted Soybeans & "much more."

Udo's Choice Oil Blend - Flora
Flax oil • Sunflower oil • Sesame oil • Medium Chain Triglycerides • Evening Primrose oil (12.6 mg GLA per tablespoon) • Rice germ & Bran oil • Soy Lecithin • d-Alpha Tocopheral (natural Vitamin E) • Oat germ & Bran oil. One tablespoon LIQUID FORM contains: Calories 135 • Total Fat 14.5 g • Saturated Fat 1.5 g • Polyunsaturated Fat: (Omega-3 Fatty Acids 6.4 g, Omega-6 Fatty Acids 3.2 g) 10 g • Monounsaturated Fat (Omega-9 fatty acids 3 g) 3 g • Medium Chain Triglycerides 231 mg. Two CAPSULES contain: Calories 20 • Total Fat 2 g • Saturated Fat .2 g • Polyunsaturated Fat : (Omega-3 Fatty Acids 920 mg, Omega-6 Fatty Acids 460 mg) 1.4 g • Monounsaturated Fat (Omega-9 fatty acids 400 mg) .4g • Medium Chain Triglycerides 38 mg.

Udo's Choice Perfect Oil Blend - Flora
Flax oil • sesame seed oil • Sunflower oil & other unrefined oils • medium triglycerides • lecithin & d-alpha tocopherol.

Udo's Choice Super 5 - Flora
Each tablet contains: 1 billion plus viable organisms of Lactobacillus acidophilus DDS-1 • B. bifidum • L. bulgaricus • S. thermophilus & L. salivarius in a base of: (Maltodextrin, Fructose & Ascorbic Acid).

Ultimate Antioxidant II - Gary Nulls
Three capsules contain: Citrus Bioflavonoid Complex 300 mg • Rutin 25 mg • Bilberry extract 25 mg • Red Wine Concentrate 25 mg • Grape Skin extract 200 mg • China Green Tea 200 mg • Beta Carotene 10000 IU • L-Glutathione 5 mg • L-Cysteine 200 mg • Vitamin C 500 mg • Vitamin E 200 IU • Selenium 10 mcg • Zinc Picolinate 25 mg • CoQ10 10 mg • NAC 25 mg • Alpha Lipoic Acid 100 mg • Ascorbyl Palmitate 100 mg • SOD 25 mg • Vitamin B6 10 mg • Copper Lysinate 2 mg • Taurine 50 mg • Quercetin 50 mg • Pycnogenol 5 mg • Licorice 25 mg • Broccoli 25 mg • Lutein 25 mg • Cabbage 25 mg • Carrot powder 25 mg • Milk Thistle 25 mg.

Ultimate Athlete's Pain Formula - Biochem
Three softgel capsules contain: Boswellia serrata extract 500 mg • Omega-3 Fish oil concentrate 400 mg • Glucosamine HCL 250 mg • Glucosamine Sulfate 250 mg • Chondroitin Sulfate 200 mg • PolyNAG (N-Acetyl Glucosamine) 50 mg • Vitamin C (Ascorbyl Palmitate) 50 mg • Green-lipped Mussel extract 50 mg • CMO (Cetyl Myristoleate) 50 mg • Gamma-Lenolenic Acid (Borage seed oil) 50 mg • Vitamin E (d-Alpha Tocopheryl Acetate) 25 IU • Manganese (Sulfate) 5 mg • Boron (Borogluconate) 1.5 mg.
See Editor's Note No. 15, page 1817.

Ultimate Balance - Antioxidant Formula - Bioadvantex Pharma
Two caplets contain: N-Acetyl Cysteine (NAC) 700 mg • Alpha-Lipoic Acid 200 mg • Milk Thistle seed extract 200 mg

Ultimate Cleanse - Nature's Secret
Each tablet contains: Multi-Herb: Alfalfa Leaf • Fenugreek Seed • Ginger Root • Dandelion Root • Fennel Seed • Yarrow Flower • Hawthorne Berries • Horsetail Herb • Licorice Root • Marshmallow Root • Peppermint Leaf • Red Clover Tops • Red Raspberry Leaf • Safflower Oil • Scullcap Herb • Burdock Root • Chickweed Herb • Mullein Leaf • Papaya Leaf • Black Cohosh Root • Cayenne Fruit • Irish Moss • Pacific Kelp • Slippery Elm Bark • Yellow Dock Root • Plantain Herb • Echinacea Angustifolia Extract • Ginkgo Biloba Leaf Extract • Milk Thistle Extract. Multi-Fiber: Cascara Sagrada Bark • Fennel Seed • Psyllium Seed • Ginger Root • Acacia Gum • Alfalfa

BRAND NAMES

Leaf • Apple Pectin • Apple Powder • Barley Rice Fiber • Beet Root • Glucomannan • Karaya Gum • Peppermint Leaf • Lemon Peel • Oat Bran • Red Raspberry Leaf • Slippery Elm Bark • Shattered Cell Wall Chlorella • Lactobacillus Acidophilus (dairy free) • Guar Gum.

Ultimate Eye Formula - Purity Products
Three capsules contain: Vitamin C (magnesium ascorbate) 360 mg • Vitamin E 50 IU • Vitamin B-6 10 mg • Vitamin B-12 500 mcg • Alpha-Lipoic Acid 150 mg • L-Taurine 250 mg • Bilberry fruit extract 120 mg • Lutein 10 mg • Wolfberry fruit powder 25 mg • Pomegranate fruit 50 mg • IP6 (inositol hexaphosphate) 150 mg • Soy Isoflavones 200 mg • Gamma Oryzanol 100 mg.

Ultimate Fat Metabolizer - Biochem
Three tablets contain: Choline Bitartrate 500 mg • Inositol 500 mg • L-Carnitine 500 mg • L-Methionine 500 mg • Taurine 500 mg • Phosphatidyl Choline 200 mg • Betaine HCL 200 mg • Dandelion 100 mg • Milk Thistle 100 mg • Barberry 100 mg • Artichoke extract 50 mg • Vitamin B6 (Pyridoxine • Alpha-Ketoglutarate/Pyridoxal-5-Phosphate) 10 mg • Chromium 400 mcg.

Ultimate Fiber - Nature's Secret
Psyllium husks, Slippery Elm bark, Acidophilus powder, Fructooligosaccharides.

Ultimate Green - Nature's Secret
Each packet contain: Shattered Cell Wall Chlorella • Hawaiian Blue-Green Algae • Barley Grass • Wheat Grass • Alfalfa • Spinach.

Ultimate Libido Formula for Women - MD Healthline
Two capsules contain: Niacin 40 mg • Yohimbe Bark 500 mg • Dong Quai 150 mg • Sativari (Asparagus racemosus) 150 mg • Ashwagandha 100 mg • L-Tyrosine 100 mg • L-Histidine 66 mg • Tree Peony 4:1 Extract 50 mg • Royal Jelly 50 mg • Wild Yam 10:1 Extract 40 mg • Quebracho Bark 20 mg • Ginger Root 5:1 Extract 20 mg • Sundew 20 mg • Guarana 20 mg • Damiana 20 mg • DHEA 10 mg.

Ultimate Men's Peak Performance - Swanson
Each tablet contains: Vitamin E (as d-alpha tocopheryl succinate) 50 IU • Niacin 25 mg • Zinc (from zinc amino acid chelate) 7.5 mg • Yohimbe extract (2% yohimbine alkaloids) 250 mg • Tribulus Terrestris extract (40% steroidal saponins) 125 mg • Avena Sativa wild oats (5:1 extract) 50 mg • Cayenne Pepper 50 mg • Damiana leaf powder 50 mg • Ginger root powder 50 mg • Ginkgo Biloba leaf powder 50 mg • Ginseng extract (5% ginsenosides) 50 mg • Guarana extract (12.5% alkaloids) 50 mg • Hawthorn berry powder 50 mg • L-Arginine HCl 50 mg • Oyster extract 50 mg • Saw Palmetto berry powder 50 mg • Rhodiola Rosea extract (1% rosevin) 25 mg.

Ultimate Multi Plus - Nature's Secret
Contains over 90 vitamins, minerals, amino acids, antioxidants, herbs, superfoods, digestive enzymes and Herbalgest.

Ultimate Oil - Nature's Secret
Blend of oils that offer a mixture of the essential fatty acids, Omega 3 and Omega 6.

Ultimate Orange Powercaps - Next Nutrition
Three softgels contain: Magnesium 9.7 mg • L-Tyrosine 500 mg • Ma Huang whole plant 313 mg • Guarana seed 227 mg • Caffeine 200 mg • Proprietary Blend: Sida Cordifolia root, Korean Ginseng root, Green Tea leaf, Coleus Forskohlii root, Orange Peel Bioflavonoids, Grapefruit extract, Cayenne Pepper 100 mg. Other Ingredients: Soybean Oil, Gelatin, Glycerin Water, Titanium Dioxide, FD&C Yellow 6, FD&C Red 40.

Ultimate Performance Max Protein Bar - Vanilla Almond - Rexall
Each bar contains: Protein 18 g • Vitamin A (as retinyl palmitate) 2500 IU • Vitamin C 30 mg • Vitamin D (as cholecalciferol) 200 IU • Vitamin E (as dl-alpha-tocopheryl acetate) 15 IU • Thiamin (as thiamine HCl) 0.75 mg • Riboflavin (Vitamin B-2) 0.85 mg • Niacin (as niacinamide) 10 mg • Vitamin B-6 (as pyridoxine HCl) 1 mg • Folic Acid 200 mcg • Vitamin B-12 (as cyanocobalamin) 3 mcg • Biotin 150 mcg • Pantothenic Acid (as calcium d-pantothenate) 5 mg • Calcium 500 mg • Iron (as ferrous fumarate) 9 mg • Phosphorus 700 mg • Iodine (as potassium iodide) 75 mcg • Magnesium (as magnesium oxide) 200 mg • Zinc (as zinc oxide) 7.5 mg • Copper (as copper gluconate) 1 mg • Chromium (as chromium picolinate) 5 mcg • Sodium 110 mg. Other Ingredients: Brown Rice Syrup, Cocoa Coating (sugar, fractionated palm kernel oil, cocoa powder, whey powder, nonfat dry milk powder, soy lecithin, natural vanilla flavor), Whey Protein Isolate, High Fructose Corn Syrup, Whey Protein Concentrate, Crystaline Fructose, Almond Butter, Natural flavor, Oat Fiber, Dicalcium Phosphate, L-Glutamine, Taurine.

Ultimate Plenamins - Rexall
Each tablet contains: Vitamin A (from retinyl acetate) 5000 IU • Vitamin C (as niacinamide ascorbate and ascorbic acid) 120 mg • Vitamin D (as cholecalciferol) 400 IU • Vitamin E (as dl-alpha-tocopheryl acetate and d-alpha-tocopheryl acid succinate) 30 IU • Vitamin K (as phytonadione) 25 mcg • Thiamin (as thiamin HCl) 3 mg • Riboflavin (vitamin B-2) 3.4 mg • Niacin (from niacinamide ascorbate) 20 mg • Vitamin B-6 (from pyridoxine HCl) 4 mg • Folic Acid 400 mcg • Vitamin B-12 (as cyanocobalamin) 25 mcg • Biotin 50 mcg • Pantothenic Acid (from d-calcium pantothenate) 10 mg • Calcium (from dicalcium phosphate and calcium carbonate) 200 mg • Iron (from ferrous fumarate) 18 mg • Phosphorus (as dicalcium phosphate) 125 mg • Iodine (from potassium iodide) 150 mcg • Magnesium (from magnesium oxide) 100 mg • Zinc (from zinc sulfate) 15 mg • Selenium (from sodium selenate) 25 mcg • Copper (from cupric oxide) 2 mg • Manganese (from manganese sulfate) 5 mg • Chromium (from chromium chloride) 15 mcg • Molybdenum (from sodium molybdate) 25 mcg • Potassium (from potassium chloride) 30 mg • Vanadium (from vanadium aspartate) 10 mcg • Silicon (from silicon dioxide) 10 mcg • Nickel (from nickel sulfate) 5 mcg • PABA (para-aminobenzoic acid) 1 mg • Choline Bitartrate 1 mg • Inositol 100 mcg • Bee Pollen 25 mg • Siberian Ginseng root 25 mg • Fish Oil (EPA [eicosapentaenoic acid] 18 mg, DHA [docosahexaenoic acid] 12 mg) 100 mg • Plenamin nutritional catalyst base: Rose Hips and seed extract, Kelp, Soy Lecithin, Soy protein isolate, Wheat Germ, Hesperidin, Rutin, Acerola fruit extract, Citrus Bioflavonoids 3.5 mg. Other Ingredients: Cellulose, Croscarmellose sodium, Hydroxypropyl methylcellulose, Magnesium stearate, PEG, Red 40 lake, Blue 2 lake, Titanium dioxide, Polysorbate 80, Beta-carotene.

Ultimate Prostate Formula - Purity Products
Three capsules contain: Vitamin E 60 IU • Vitamin B-6 50 mg • Zinc (zinc citrate) 15 mg • Selenium (selenomethionine) 50 mcg • Saw Palmetto extract 575 mg • Pygeum extract 310 mg • Nettle root extract 300 mg • Lycopene 7 mg • L-Alanine 400 mg • Glutamic Acid 400 mg • Glycine 400 mg • Quercetin 100 mg.

Ultimate Sleep System - Rainbow Light
Two tablets contain: Valerian rhizome (standardized to 0.8% valernic acid) 160 mg • Kava Kava root(standardized to 30% kavalactones) 40 mg • Spirulina 100 mg • 4:1 Custom Herbal extracts: [Valerian rhizome, Hops strobiles, Kava Kava root, Orange oil, Passion flower herb, Valerian oil, Reishi fruiting body (providing 3200 mg herbal powder equivalent)] 800 mg. Nutritional Cofactors: N-Acetyl-L-Carnitine (NAC) 10 mg • Niacin/Niacinamide (Vitamin B3)115 mg • Magnesium (Oxide, Pyroglutamate) 47.3 mg • Chromium (Polynicotinate) 30 mcg.

Ultimate Sports Multiple - Biochem

Four tablets contain: Vitamin A (Carotene Complex) 5000 IU • Vitamin D (Ergocalciferol) 200 IU • Vitamin E (d-Alpha Tocopheryl Succinate) 400 IU • Vitamin C (Ascorbic Acid) 1000 mg • Grape seed extract/Grape skin 100 mg • Vitamin B1 (Thiamine HCL/Thiamine Cocarboxylase) 100 mg • Vitamin B2 (Riboflavin/Riboflavin 5 Phosphate) 100 mg • Vitamin B3 (Niacin/Niacinamide) 200 mg • Vitamin B5 (d-Calcium Pantothenate/Pantethine) 200 mg • Vitamin B6 (Pyridoxine HCL/Pyridoxal 5 Phosphate) 100 mg • Folic Acid 400mcg • Vitamin B12 (Cyanocobalamine/Didencozide) 200 mcg • d-Biotin 300 mcg • PABA 200 mcg • Selenium 100 mcg • Molybdenum 10 mcg • Choline Bitartrate 200 mg • Inositol 100 mg • Bromelain 100 mg • Betaine HCL 200 mg • L-Methionine 50 mg • Taurine 50 mg.

Ultimate Wild Yam - Swanson

Four tablets contain: Yam extract 12 mg • Avena sativa 2 mg • Camellia sinensis 2 mg • Crataegus oxyacantha 2 mg • Dioscorea Quat 2 mg • Extracts of Barbasco 2 mg • Lactase 2 mg • Licorice root 2 mg • Medicago sativa 2 mg • Prunus SPP 2 mg • Smilax aristolochiaefolia 2 mg • Soy extracts 2 mg.

Ultimate Women's Intimate Performance - Swanson

Each tablet contains: Niacin 8.3 mg • Ginseng extract (6% ginsenosides) 100 mg • Avena Sativa oats (5:1 extract) 33.3 mg • Cayenne pepper 33.3 mg • Damiana leaf powder 33.3 mg • Dong Quai extract (1% ligustilides) 33.3 mg • Ginger root powder 33.3 mg • Guarana extract (12.5% alkaloids) 33.3 mg • L-Arginine HCl 33.3 mg • Licorice extract (12% glycyrrhizic acid) 33.3 mg • Muira Puama root 33.3 mg • Agnus Castus (chasteberry) extract (0.5% agnusides) 8.3 mg • Black Cohosh extract (2.5% triterpene glycosides) 8.3 mg • Ovary extract 8.3 mg.
See Editor's Note No. 14, page 1817.

Ultimate Zinc-C Lozenges - Now

Each lozenge contains: Vitamin A (from Fish Liver oil) 1000 IU • Vitamin C (as Ascorbic Acid) 150 mg • Zinc (as Zinc Gluconate) 24 mg • Echinacea root powder 100 mg • Bee Propolis 100 mg • Slippery Elm bark powder (Ulmus fulva) 25 mg.

Ultra 30/20 Fish oil - Health From The Sun

Two capsules contain: Vitamin E 4 IU • Omega-3 Fatty Acids 1.2 g [EPA (600 mg) DHA (400 mg)]. Ingredients: All natural Fish Body oil concentrate, Gelatin, Glycerine, Mixed Tocopherols.

Ultra Beauty Formula - Leiner Health Products

Two tablets contain: Biotin 266 mcg • Folate 266 mcg • Vitamin E (Mixed Tocopherols) 20 IU • Zinc Gluconate 10 mg • Thiamin (Vitamin B1) 6.6 mg • Calcium Carbonate 400 mg • Riboflavin (Vitamin B2) 6.6 mg • Manganese Oxide 6.6 mg • Vitamin B6 6.6 mg • Magnesium Oxide 133 mg • Vitamin D 133 IU • Iron 4 mg • Selenium 16 mcg • Pantothenic Acid 20 mg • Phosphorus 200 mg • Vitamin B12 10 mcg • Niacin 33 mg • Vitamin A 6666 IU • Vitamin C (Ascorbic Acid) 80 mg • Iodine 150 mcg • Betaine 33 mg • Bioflavonoids 33 mg • Choline Bitartrate 100 mg • Inositol 40 mg • L-Cysteine 680 mcg • PABA 33 mg • Ribonucleic Acid 40 mg • Rutin 16 mg. Other Ingredients: Dicalcium Phosphate, Cellulose, Stearic Acid, Croscarmellose Sodium, Sodium Starch Glycolate. In a base containing: Asparagus, Echinacea, Horsetail, L-Methionine, Gelatin, Oat Straw, and Papain.

Ultra Bone Balance - Source Naturals

Four tablets contain: Vitamin C (as Calcium, Magnesium, Manganese Ascorbates) 52 mg • Vitamin D (as Cholecalciferol) 300 IU • Vitamin B6 (as Pyridoxine HCl) 20 mg • Folate (as Folic Acid) 200 mcg • Calcium (as Calcium Carbonate, Citrate, Ethanolamine Phosphate, Malate, Ascorbate) 1200 mg • Magnesium (as Magnesium Oxide, Citrate, Fumarate, Malate, Ascorbate) 600 mg • Zinc (as Zinc Chelate) 7.5 mg • Copper (as Copper Sebacate) 1 mg • Manganese (as Manganese Ascorbate) 6 mg • Ipriflavone (Ostivone) 600 mg • Genistein Rich Soy concentrate (Yielding 50 mg total isoflavones) 125 mg • Silica (from Horsetail silica extract) 10 mg • Boron (as Boron Chelate) 3 mg.

Ultra Carotenoid Complex - The Vitamin Shoppe

Each softgel contains: Phytofluene 0.026 mg • Lycopene (LYC-O-MATO) 5 mg • Lutein 5 mg • Beta-carotene (25000 IU Vitamin A) 15 mg • Alpha-carotene (833 IU Vitamin A) 1 mg • Zeaxanthin 0.24 mg • Phytoene 0.055 mg.

Ultra Cee 500 mg - Puritan's Pride

Each capsule contains: Vitamin C 500 mg.

Ultra Chondroitin 600 - Nature's Plus

Each protein coated tablet contains: Chondroitin Sulfate A - CSA (Glucuronic, N-Acetyl-D-Galactosamine 4-Sulfate) 600 mg • Bioperine bioavailability enhancing thermonutrient, (95% 1-piperoylpiperdine) 2.5 mg. Contains no yeast, wheat, corn, soy, milk, salt, sugar or starch.
See Editor's Note No. 15, page 1817.

Ultra Chroma Slim Plan with Biotrol - Richardson Labs

Three caplets contain: Manganese (as manganese picolinate) 1.25 mg • Chromium (as chromium picolinate) 200 mcg • Blood Sugar Support blend: [Manganese Picolinate, Chromium Picolinate, Vanadium (as vanadyl sulfate) 60 mcg] 10.4 mg • Lipotropic & Metabolic Support blend: [Choline Bitartrate, L-Carnitine Tartrate] 1.1 g • Appetite Control & Neurotransmitter Support blend: [Inulin, L-Phenylalanine, St. John's Wort extract leaves & flowers standardized to 0.3% hypercin, Capsicum fruit extract 10:1, Peppermint oil] 1.6 g • Energy Support blend: [Siberian Ginseng root, Calcium Pyruvate] 252 mg. Other Ingredients: Cellulose, Modified Cellulose Gum, Stearic Acid, Silica, Hydroxypropyl Methylcellulose, Magnesium Stearate, Peppermint leaves.

Ultra Chromium GTF - Source Naturals

Each tablet contains: Chromium GTF (100 mcg of ChromeMate Chromium Polynicotinate and 100 mcg of Chromium Picolinate) 200 mcg • Niacin (Polynicotinate) .9 mg.

Ultra Chromium Picolinate - The Vitamin Shoppe

Each capsule contains: Chromium Picolinate, a compound of yeast-free trivalent chromium and picolinic acid 500 mcg.

Ultra Chromium Picolinate 500 - Source Naturals

Each tablet contains: Trivalent Chromium (from Chromax brand of yeast-free chromium picolinate) 500 mcg.

Ultra Colloidal Silver - Olympia Nutrition

Deionized Water • Silver (10 ppm). Contains no animal proteins or artificial additives.

Ultra CoQ10 - Nature's Plus

Each softgel contains: Coenzyme Q10 (ubiquinone) 100 mg.

Ultra Cranberry 1000 - Nature's Plus

Each protein coated tablet contains: Cranberry concentrate 45X 1000 mg • Vitamin C corn free 100 mg. In a highly active herbal base of Juniper berries (Juniperus communis), Parsley (Petroselinum crispum), Uva Ursi (Arctostaphylos uva ursi) & Red Clover (Trifolium pratense). Contains no yeast, wheat, corn, soy, milk, salt, sugar or starch.

Ultra DHA 50 - Health From The Sun

Two capsules contain: Vitamin E 4 IU • Omega-3 Fatty Acids 700 mg [DHA (425 mg) EPA (200 mg)]. Ingredients: All natural Fish Body oil concentrate, Gelatin, Glycerine, Mixed Tocopherols.

BRAND NAMES

Some Brand Name Natural Products - What they Contain

Ultra Diet Pep - Natural Balance

Two tablets contain an herbal blend of Kola Nut, Ma Huang, Siberian Ginseng, Green Tea extract, Dandelion, Ginger, Passion Flower, Kelp, Gymnema Sylvestre, Pullulan and Fennel • Vitamin B6 15 mg • Vitamin B12 6 mcg • Pantothenic Acid 25 mg • Inositol 100 mg • DynaChrome Chromium 200 mcg • Bromelain 100 mg • Potassium 99 mg.

Ultra Diet-Phen - Source Naturals

Two tablets contain: St. John's Wort (Hypericum perforatum) standardized extract 0.3 %, yielding 1.2 of Hypericin 400 mg • Bitter Orange peel standardized extract, yielding 24 mg of Synepherine 570 mg • Green Tea standardized extract, yieildng 40 mg of Polypheols and 10 mg of Caffeine 100 mg • L-Phenylalanine 500 mg • Cayenne fruit 150 mg • Piper nigrum seed 150 mg • Mustard Seed 150 mg • Ginger root 150 mg • Dandelion Leaf 100 mg • Dandelion Root 100 mg • Chromium (300 mcg ChromeMate Polynicotinate and 100 mcg Chromium Picolinate) 400 mcg.

Ultra Fuel (The Ultimate Carbohydrate Energy & Recovery Drink) - TwinLab

Each 16 ounce serving contains: Carbohydrates 100 g • Carbohydrate & Energy Metabolizers including Chromium • Stress B Vitamins • Vitamin C. No added preservatives or sodium.

Ultra Garlite - Nature's Plus

Each tablet contains: Deodorized Garlic equivalent to a minimum of 2.5 times its weight in fresh garlic 1000 mg. In a special base which provides for the gradual release of ingredients over a prolonged period of time, for 40% better absorption & utilization. Contains no yeast, wheat, corn, soy, milk, salt, sugar or starch.

Ultra Hair - Nature's Plus

Two tablets contain: Vitamin C with Rose Hips 500 mg • Pantothenic Acid 500 mg • Inositol 500 mg • Choline (Bitartrate) 210 mg • L-Cysteine free form amino acid 100 mg • Vitamin B6 (Pyridoxine HCL) 100 mg • Vitamin B2 (Riboflavin) 100 mg • PABA (Para-aminobenzoic acid) 100 mg • Vitamin B1 (Thiamine) 30 mg • Niacinamide 30 mg • Zinc (Amino Acid Chelate) 5 mg • Vitamin A (Beta Carotene) 10000 IU • Biotin 2000 mcg • Folic Acid 400 mcg. In a natural base of unsaturated fatty acids from safflower oil, rice bran & spirulina, naturally rich in RNA, DNA, amino acids & trace minerals. Yeast free. Sugar & starch free.

Ultra High Carb - Sports Nutrition Source.com

Four level scoops contain: Biotin 300 mcg • Chromium 200 mcg • Vitamin B-1 1.5 mg • Vitamin B-2 1.7 mg • Vitamin B-3 20 mg • Vitamin B-6 2 mg • Pantothenic Acid 100 mg • Vitamin C 60 mg • Potassium (from soluble potassium phosphate) 99 mg • Magnesium (from magnesium succinate) 25 mg.

Ultra Inosine - Source Naturals

Two tablets contain: Vitamin C (Potassium and Sodium Ascorbates) 350 mg • Calcium (Carbonate) 100 mg • Vitamin B6 (Pyridoxine HCl) 10 mg • Magnesium (Oxide, Aspartate) 100 mg • Vitamin B5 (Pantothenic Acid) 50 mg • Potassium (Citrate, Ascorbate and Aspartate) 99 mg • Sodium (Ascorbate) 20 mg • Inosine (Pure Crystalline) 1000 mg • Aspartic Acid (Potassium and Magnesium Aspartates and L-Aspartic Acid) 200 mg • Branched Chain Amino Acids (BCAAs) (L-Leucine 100 mg, L-Isoleucine 30 mg, L-Valine 44 mg) 174 mg • L-Carnitine L-Tartrate 20 mg • L-Lysine (HCl) 60 mg • Glycine 60 mg • Bee Pollen 200 mg • Octacosanol 4000 mcg • Spirulina 70 mg • Siberian Ginseng 100 mg • Tienchi Ginseng 100 mg.

Ultra Joint Response - Source Naturals

Three tablets contain: Vitamin A 5000 IU • Vitamin C 250 mg • Niacinamide 50 mg • Vitamin B6 12.5 mg • Zinc 15 mg • Selenium 100 mcg • Copper 1 mg • Manganese 10 mg • Molybdenum 130 mcg

• MSM 1125 mg • Glucosamine Sulfate 900 mg • Boswellia serrata extract 321 mg • Quercetin 150 mg • Horse Chestnut extract 100 mg • Turmeric root extract 50 mg • Stinging Nettle leaf extract 50 mg • Ashwagandha root extract 50 mg • N-Acetyl Cysteine 50 mg • Sea Cucumber 40 mg • Grape Seed extract 25 mg • Aloe Vera whole leaf concentrate 25 mg • Black Pepper fruit extract 1 mg.

Ultra KLB6 - Puritan's Pride

Three tablets contain: Lecithin 1200 mg • Vitamin B6 (Pyridoxine HCl) 50 mg • Kelp powder 100 mg • Cider Vinegar 240 mg.

Ultra Lean - Schiff

Two tablets contains: Garcinia cambogia extract (min. 50% HCA) 500 mg • Dandelion Root 4:1 extract (Taraxacum officinate) 100 mg • Horsetail standardized extract (10% silicic acid, 6.3% organic silica - from Springtime Equisetum arvense) 50 mg • Juniper Berries 4:1 extract (Juniper communis) 50 mg • Cayenne (oleoresin capsium 6:1 extract from capsicum frutescens) 25 mg • Betaine HCl 50 mg • Iodine (Norwegian kelp) 150 mcg • Potassium (glycerophosphate) 25 mg • Magnesium (glycinate) 40 mg • Chromium (picolinate) 200 mcg.

Ultra Lipo-Plex - Nature's Plus

Two tablets contain: Choline Bitartrate equivalent to 1000 mg of choline 2381 mg • Inositol 1000 mg • L-Methionine free form amino acid 500 mg • Vitamin B6 (Pyridoxine HCL) 100 mg. In a natural herbal base containing Dandelion root, Fennel seed, Barberry bark, Parsley, Capsicum & Ginger. In a special base which provides for the gradual release of ingredients over a prolonged period of time, for 40% better absorption & utilization. Contains no yeast, wheat, corn, soy, milk, salt, sugar or starch.

Ultra Max 46 - Puritan's Pride

Each tablet contains: Vitamin A (13% as beta-carotene) 7,500 IU • Vitamin D 400 IU • Vitamin K 10 mcg • Thiamine (Vitamin B-1) 50 mg • Riboflavin (Vitamin B-2) 50 mg • Niacin 50 mg • Vitamin B-6 50 mg • Folic Acid 400 mcg • Vitamin B-12 50 mcg • Biotin 300 mcg • Pantothenic Acid 50 mg • Calcium 106 mg • Iron 9 mg • Iodine 150 mcg • Magnesium 100 mg • Zinc 50 mg • Selenium 50 mcg • Copper 1 mg • Manganese 5 mg • Chromium 50 mcg • Sodium 5 mg • Potassium 50 mg • Choline Bitartrate 50 mg • PABA (para-aminobenzoic acid) 25 mg • Inositol 10 mg.

Ultra Mega Vite Multiple - Nature's Life

Each tablet contains: Vitamin A (Fish Liver oil) 10000 IU • Vitamin D (as Vitamin D3) (Cholecalciferol) 400 IU • Vitamin E (d-Alpha Tocopherol) 200 IU • Vitamin B1 (Thiamine Mononitrate) 100 mg • Vitamin B2 100 mg • Vitamin B3 (Niacinamide) 100 mg • Vitamin B6 (Pyridoxine HCl • Pyridoxal 5'-Phosphate) 100 mg • Vitamin B12 (Cobalamin concentrate) 100 mg • Folic Acid 400 mcg • Biotin 300 mcg • Pantothenic Acid (d-Calcium Pantothenate) 100 mg • Inositol 10 mg • Choline (Bitartrate) 10 mg • PABA (Para Aminobenzoic Acid) 10 mg • Vitamin C 300 mg • Lemon Bioflavonoids (TESTLAB 50% Flavonoids) 50 mg • Rutin 25 mg • Hesperidin Complex (10% Flavonoids) 25 mg • Boron (Citrate) 25 mcg • Calcium (Carbonate, Citrate/Malate) 100 mg • Chromium (Amino-Nicotinate) 100 mcg • Copper (Gluconate, Citrate) 1 mg • Iodine (Potassium) 25 mcg • Iron (Fumerate, Peptonate) 10 mg • Magnesium (Oxide, Citrate) 60 mg • Manganese (Citrate, Gluconate) 5 mg • Molybdenum (Molybdate) 25 mcg • Potassium (Citrate) 15 mg • Selenium (Yeast) 50 mcg • Silicon (Dioxide) 10 mg • Vanadium (Sulfate) 25 mcg • Zinc (Citrate) 20 mg • Chlorophyll 5 mg • Betaine HCl 30 mg • Glutamic Acid HCl 30 mg • Nature's Life Greens 20 mg.

Ultra Multiple - Source Naturals

Six tablets contain: Vitamin A (palmitate 10000 IU and beta carotene 3000 IU) 13000 IU • Vitamin B-1 (thiamin) 100 mg • Vitamin B-2 (riboflavin) 75 mg • Niacinamide 75 mg and Niacin 25 mg 100mg • Vitamin B-5 (calcium D-Pantothenate) 150 mg • Vitamin B-6 (pyridoxine HCl) 125 mg • Vitamin B-12 (cyanocobalamin) 300 mcg

• Biotin 150 mcg • Folic acid 420 mcg • Vitamin C (calcium, magnesium and manganese ascorbates) 500 mg • Vitamin D-3 (cholecalciferol) 402 IU • Vitamin E (natural D-alpha succinate) 200 IU • Magnesium (ascorbate, oxide, citrate) 125 mg • Potassium (citrate) 10 mg • Iron (fumarate) 12 mg • Calcium (ascorbate, carbonate, citrate) 125 mg • Zinc (citrate) 15 mg • Manganese (ascorbate) 6 mg • Chromium (ChromeMate polynicotinate) 50 mcg • Copper (sebacate) 250 mcg • Selenium (sodium selenite) 100 mcg • Iodine (from kelp) 225 mcg.

Ultra Nails - Nature's Plus
Two tablets contain: Calcium amino acid chelate/complex 500 mg • Gelatin 260 mg • Horsetail supplying natural silica 250 mg • Phosphorus amino acid complex 200 mg • L-Cysteine free form amino acid 100 mg • L-Methionine free form amino acid 100 mg • Vitamin B2 (Riboflavin) 50 mg • Sulphur from Sulphur containing amino acids 25 mg • Oat straw 25 mg • Magnesium amino acid chelate/complex 25 mg • Iron (Amino Acid Chelate) 5 mg • Vitamin A Fish Liver oil 10000 IU • Folic Acid 200 mcg • Vitamin B12 from Cobalamin 100 mcg • Vitamin D Fish Liver oil 400 IU. In a natural rice bran base, supplying a complete balance of B-Complex vitamins & trace minerals. Yeast free. Sugar & starch free.

Ultra Omega-3 Fish oil - Health From The Sun
Two capsules contain: Omega-3 Fatty Acids 600 mg [EPA (360) DHA (240 mg)]. Ingredients: All natural Fish Body Oil, Gelatin, Glycerine, Water, Carob powder, Mixed Tocopherols (Vitamin E).

Ultra Potassium - Source Naturals
Each tablet contains: Potassium (citrate, malate, ketoglutarate, fumarate, succinate, asparate, glycinate, and ascorbate) 99 mg.

Ultra Power Nutrient - Changes - TwinLab
One packet (6g) contains: Vitamin A (as Retinyl palmitate with Lemongrass and Beta Carotene) 5000 IU • Vitamin C (as buffered mineral ascorbates) 60 mg • Vitamin D (as Cholecalciferol) 400 IU • Thiamin (Vitamin B1 as Thiamine hydrochloride) 1.5 mg • Riboflavin (Vitamin B2) 1.7 mg • Vitamin B6 (as Pyridoxine hydrochloride) 2 mg • Folate (as Folic acid) 400 mcg • Vitamin B12 (as Cyanocobalamin) 6 mcg • Biotin 300 mcg • Pantothenic acid (Vitamin B5) (as Calcium pantothenate) 10 mg • Calcium (as Calcium citrate ascorbate) 40 mg • Magnesium (as Magnesium citrate ascorbate) 20 mg • Sodium (as Sodium citrate ascorbate) 60 mg • Potassium (as Potassium citrate ascorbate) 200 mg • Sea minerals from Celtic marine algae 10 mg. Other ingredients: Crystalline fructose, Maltodextrin, Natural citrus flavors, Non-nutritive sweetener.

Ultra Prosta-Metto - The Vitamin Shoppe
Each softgel contains: Vitamin E 50 IU • Vitamin B6 5 mg • Zinc 15 mg • Saw Palmetto berries 160 mg • Pumpkin seed 40 mg • Pygeum Africanum bark 10 mg • Stinging Nettle leaf 50 mg • Lycopene 2.5 mg.

Ultra Skin - Nature's Plus
Two tablets contain: Unsaturated Fatty Acids from natural Safflower oil 500 mg • Vitamin C with Rose Hips 200 mg • Vitamin B2 (Riboflavin) 200 mg • Vitamin B6 (Pyridoxine HCL) 200 mg • Vitamin E natural 200 IU • Niacinamide 150 mg • PABA (Para-Aminobenzoic Acid) 150 mg • Pantothenic Acid 150 mg • Vitamin B1 (Thiamine) 100 mg • Zinc amino acid chelate/complex 50 mg • Vitamin A (Beta Carotene) 25000 IU • Biotin 400 mcg • Folic Acid 100 mcg • Vitamin B12 (from Cobalamin) 100 mcg • Vitamin D (Calciferol) 1000 IU. In a natural base of rice bran & spirulina (naturally rich in RNA, DNA, amino acids & trace minerals). In a special base which provides for the gradual release of ingredients over a prolonged period of time for 40% better absorption & utilization. Yeast free. Sugar & starch free.

Ultra Stress with Iron - Nature's Plus
Each tablet contains: Vitamin C with Rose Hips 500 mg • Pantothenic Acid 200 mg • Vitamin B1 (Thiamine) 125 mg • Vitamin B2 (Riboflavin) 125 mg • Vitamin B6 (Pyridoxine HCL) 125 mg • Niacinamide 125 mg •Inositol 75 mg • PABA (Para-aminobenzoic acid) 50 mg • Choline (Bitartrate) 32 mg • Iron amino acid chelate/complex 20 mg • Vitamin B12 from Cobalamin 500 mcg • Folic Acid 400 mcg • Biotin 125 mcg. B-Complex vitamins in a fortified rice bran base. In a special base which provides for the gradual release of ingredients over a prolonged period of time for 40% better absorption & utilization.

Ultra Sugar Control - Nature's Plus
Two tablets contain: CITRIMAX (Garcinia cambogia fruit) standardized 50% [-] hydroxycitrate 500 mg • Rehmannia Glutinosa root [naturally rich in Beta-Sitosterol, Catalpol & Aucubin] 400 mg • L-Glutamine pharmaceutical grade free form amino acid 250 mg • L-Alanine pharmaceutical grade free form amino acid 250 mg • Gymnema Sylvestre leaf standardized 75% Gymnemic acids 200 mg • Chromium (Polynicotinate) 500 mcg. Contains no yeast, wheat, corn, soy, milk, salt, sugar or starch.

Ultra Virile-Actin - Nature's Plus
Two protein coated tablets contain: Vitamin E natural 200 IU • Korean Ginseng [(Panax ginseng root) standardized 15% Ginsenosides] 100 mg • Siberian Ginseng [Eleutherococcus senticosus root) standardized 0.8% Eleutherosides] 100 mg • Bee Pollen, Spanish 75 mg • Saw Palmetto [(Serenoa repens berry) standardized 35%-45% free fatty acids] 60 mg • Brazilian Muirapuama (Phychopetalum olacoides root & rhizome) 50 mg • L-Histidine, pharmaceutical grade free form amino acid 50 mg • Zinc (Monomethionine) 50 mg • Cayenne [(Capsicum frutescens fruit) standardized 125000 STU/gram] 50 mg • L-Phenylalanine pharmaceutical grade free form amino acid 50 mg • St. John's Wort [(Hypericum perforatum flower) 0.3%-0.5% Hypericin) 50 mg • Royal Jelly 25 mg • L-Carnitine (L-Carnitine-L-Tartrate) 25 mg • Pacific Oyster extract [(Crassostreagis thunberg) naturally rich in trace elements & amino acids] 10 mg • Vitamin B6 (Pyridoxine HCL) 5 mg • Coenzyme Q10 (Ubiquinone) 2500 mcg. Contains no yeast, wheat, corn, soy, milk, salt, sugar or starch.

Ultra Vita-Min - Puritan's Pride
Each tablet contains: Vitamin A (as retinyl palmitate and beta carotene) 10,000 IU • Vitamin C (as ascorbic acid) 150 mg • Vitamin D (as cholecalciferol) 400 IU • Vitamin E (as d-alpha tocopheryl succinate) 12.5 IU • Thiamin (Vitamin B-1; as thiamine hydrochloride) 25 mg • Riboflavin (Vitamin B-2) 25 mg • Niacin (as niacinamide) 50 mg • Vitamin B6 (pyridoxine hydrochloride) 15 mg • Folic Acid 400 mcg • Vitamin B12 (as cyanocobalamin) 50 mcg • Biotin 1 mcg • Pantothenic Acid (as d-calcium pantothenate) 12.5 mg • Calcium (as oyster shell and bone meal) 60 mg • Iron (as ferrous gluconate) 6.26 mg • Phosphorus (as bone meal) 24.3 mg • Iodine (as potassium iodide) 100 mcg • Magnesium (as magnesium gluconate) 0.42 mg • Zinc (as zinc gluconate) 0.72 mg • Selenium (as sodium selenate) 10 mcg • Copper (as cupric gluconate) 0.035 mg • Manganese (as manganese gluconate) 0.76 mg • Chromium (as chromium picolinate) 2.35 mg • Molybdenum (as sodium molybdate) 10 mcg • Potassium (as potassium gluconate) 0.5 mg • PABA 15 mg • Choline Bitartrate 25 mg • Inositol 25 mg • Boron (as sodium borate) 500 mcg • Betaine Hydrochloride 25 mg • Rose Hips powder 10 mg • Rutin 5 mg • Citrus Bioflavonoids complex 15 mg • Royal Jelly 5 mg • Bee Propolis powder 5 mg • Coenzyme Q10 30 mcg • Octacosanol 50 mcg • Deodorized Garlic powder 10 mg • Ginseng root 15 mg • RNA 2 mg • DNA 2 mg.

UltraAC - Great American Nutrition
Four capsules contain: Potassium (as potassium glycerophosphate) 112 mg • Chromium (as chromium picolinate) 200 mcg • Potassium Glycerophosphate 450 mg • DL-Phenylalanine 1000 mg • Zhi Shi

BRAND NAMES

BRAND NAMES

fruit (Citrus aurantium (Bitter Orange peel) containing 10 mg synephrine from a 4% standardized extract) 250 mg • Kola Nut nut (Cola acuminata, containing 50 mg caffeine from a 10% standardized extract) 500 mg • Ginger root (Zingiber officinale) 100 mg. Other Ingredients: Rice powder, Magnesium Silicate & Magnesium Stearate.

UltraAP Activated Pyruvate - Great American Nutrition
Four capsules contain: Potassium (as potassium glycerophosphate) 125 mg • Potassium Glycerophosphate 500 mg • Caffeine (from caffeine citrate & Kola nut) 150 mg • Zhi Shi fruit (Citrus aurantium (Bitter Orange peel), synephrine from a 4% standardized extract 10 mg) 250 mg • Kola Nut nut (Cola acuminata) 500 mg • Siberian Ginseng root (Eleutherococcus senticosus) 200 mg • Quercetin 100 mg • Jing jie leaves(Schizonepeta divaricata, 5:1 extract) 10 mg • Fang feng leaves (Ledebouriella tenuifolia, 5:1 extract) 10 mg. Other Ingredients: Rice powder, Maltodextrin, Magnesium Silicate and Magnesium Stearate.

Ultra-Cal Night - Source Naturals
Four tablets contain: Calcium (Citrate, Carbonate, Malate, Fumarate, Ethanolamine Phosphate, and Ascorbate) 600 mg • Magnesium (Oxide, Citrate, Fumarate, Malate, and Ascorbate) 600 mg • SoyLife Genistein Rich Soy Concentrate (Daidzein 13 mg, Glycitein 9 mg, Genistein 3 mg, total Isoflavones 25 mg) 830 mg • Vitamin C (Magnesium and Calcium Ascorbates, Ascorbic Acid and Manganese Ascorbate) 285 mg • Vitamin B6 (Pyridoxine HCl) 20 mg • Vitamin D (as Vitamin D3) (Cholecalciferol) 200 IU • Folic Acid 200 mcg • L-Lysine (HCl) 60 mg • Silica (Horsetail Silica Extract) 10 mg • Zinc (Chelate) 7.5 mg • Manganese (Ascorbate) 6 mg • Boron (Amino Acid Chelate) 3 mg • Copper (Sebacate) 1 mg.

Ultra-Eyebright - Nutri-Quest
Each tablet contains: Eyebright 100 mg • Bilberry extract 6 mg • Ginkgo Biloba 6 mg • Siberian Ginseng 15 mg • Gymnema sylvestre 100 mg • Tumeric 25 mg • Quercetin 10 mg • Lemon Bioflavonoids 40 mg • Bromelain 30 mg • Pancreatin 30 mg • Papain 30 mg • Trypsin 40 mg (Chymotrypsin 8 mg) • Pancreolipase 15 mg • Amylase-Diastase 15 mg • Ox Bile 30 mg • Betaine HCL 10 mg • Rutin 50 mg • L-Glutathione 2.5 mg • L-Taurine 15 mg • N-Acetyl Cysteine 10 mg • Selenium Chelate 10 mcg • Zinc Chelate 15 mg • Chromium Aspartate 1 mg • Parotid 1 mg • Beta Carotene 1000 IU • Vitamin C 75 mg • Vitamin D 200 IU • Vitamin E (Succinate) 20 IU • Vitamin B2 20 mg • Vitamin B6 10 mg • Folic Acid 50 mcg. See Editor's Note No. 14, page 1817.

Ultra-Mag - Source Naturals
Two tablets contain: Magnesium (citrate, taurinate, glycinate, malate and succinate) 400 mg • Vitamin B-6 (pyridoxine HCl) 50 mg.

Ultramet - Vanilla Flavor - Champion Nutrition
Each packet of Vanilla flavor contains: Peptol-EX protein 42 grams including Ion-Exchange Whey Protein Isolate, Calcium Caseinate, Milk Protein Isolate, Potassium Caseinate, Egg Albumen, Whey Protein Concentrate, Sodium Caseinate, L-Glutamine, Taurine, Calcium Alpha-Ketoglutarate & L-Arginine • Carbohydrates 24 g (1.5 g Fiber) • Fat 2 g • Calories 280.

Ultra-Pro Training Pak - Sports Nutrition Source.com
One packet of eight tablets contains: Vitamin A 20000 IU • Vitamin C 1000 mg • Vitamin D 200 IU • Vitamin E 400 IU • Thiamin (B-1) 100 mg • Riboflavin (B-2) 120 mg • Niacin 125 mg • Vitamin B-6 100 mg • Biotin 300 mcg • Pantothenic Acid 200 mg • Folic Acid 400 mcg • Vitamin B-12 200 mcg • Calcium 1000 mg • Iron 25 mg • Iodine 150 mcg • Magnesium 600 mg • Zinc 25 mg • Selenium 200 mcg • Copper 500 mcg • Manganese 15 mg • Chromium 100 mcg • Molybdenum 20 mcg • Potassium 99 mg • Rutin 100 mg • Bioflavonoids 100 mg • Gamma Oryzanol 40 mg • Inosine 10 mg • Coenzyme Q10 5 mg • Germanium 100 mcg • PABA 25 mcg • Choline 200 mg • Inositol 100 mg • Bromelain 25 mg • Papain

25 mg • Beta Sisterol 20 mg • L-Carnitine 10 mg • Cayenne 20 mg • Gotu Kola 10 mg • Sarsaparilla 10 mg • Siberian Ginseng 10 mg • L-Leucine 78 mg • L-Isoleucine 48 mg • L-Valine 60 mg • L-Alanine 47 mg • L-Arginine 84 mg • L-Aspartic Acid 77 mg • L-Cystine 14 mg • L-Glutamic Acid 193 mg • L-Glycine 50 mg • L-Histidine 15 mg • L-Lysine 47 mg • L-Methionine 50 mg • L-Ornithine 46 mg • L-Phenylalanine 58 mg • L-Proline 35 mg • L-Serine 47 mg • L-Taurine 50 mg • L-Threonine 35 mg • L-Typtophan 13 mg • L-Tyrosine 53 mg.

Ultra-Zyme - Nature's Plus
Two tablets contain: Pancreatin 4X quadruple strength 325 mg, supplying: Amylase 32500 USP Units, Protease (Trypsin & Chymotrypsin) 32500 USP Units, Lipase (Pancreatic lipase) 2600 USP Units • Glutamic Acid HCL 200 mg • Acidophilus (Lactobacillus, Bulgaricus, Bifidus) 150 mg • Ox Bile 120 mg • Bromelain, 1:10, pineapple, 100 mg • Pepsin NF 1:15000 65 mg • Malt Diastase 65 mg • Cellulase • Hemicellulase • 5 mg • Lactase 5 mg. In a natural herbal base of Peppermint, Fennel seed, Ginger & Rosemary. Contains no yeast, wheat, corn, soy, milk, salt, sugar or starch. See Editor's Note No. 14, page 1817.

Una De Gato-Go! Cat's Claw Extract - Wakunaga of America
Each capsule contains: Cat's Claw standardized extract (Una De Gato) (bark) 250 mg. Other Ingredients: Cellulose, Colloidal Silica, Magnesium Stearate (vegetable source).

UnDo - Lindsey Duncan's Home Nutrition
Blended Fiber Formula: Each tablet contains: Proprietary blend 495 mg: Fiber blend: [Apple pectin, Beet fiber, Barley fiber, Psyllium husk, Karaya Gum, Oat Bran] • Fennel seed • Buckthorn bark • Cascara Sagrada bark • Kava Kava root • Red Raspberry leaf • Ginger root • Capsicum Fruit. Blended Herb Formula: Each tablet contains: Proprietary blend 368 mg: Panax Ginseng root • Ginkgo Biloba leaf extract (50:1) • Garlic bulb • Milk Thistle extract (80% Silymarin) • Echinacea Angustifolia leaf extract (6:1) • Cat's Claw bark • Uva Ursi leaf • Alfalfa leaf • Hawthorn berries • Licorice root • Ginger root • Rosemary leaf • Oregon Grape root • Turmeric root • Dandelion leaf • Burdock root • Yellow Dock root • Mullein leaf • Fenugreek seed • Horsetail herb • Safflower flower • Butcher's Broom root • Red root • Capsicum fruit • Schizandra fruit.

Up Your Gas - National Health Products
Each tablet contains 1200 mg blend of the following ingredients: Guarana seed (Paullinia cupana) • Ma Huang herb (Ephedra sinica) (Standardized 6% extract) 285 mg • Korean Ginseng root (Panax ginseng) • Bee Pollen • Vitamin E (D-Alpha-Tocopheryl Acetate) • Spirulina Blue-Green Algae (Spirulina pratensis) • Gotu Kola (Centella asiatica) • Inosine • Octacosanol • Pyridoxal-Alpha-Ketoglutarate • Wheat Grass (Triticum aestivum) • Cayenne pepper (Capsicum frutescens) • Lipoic Acid • Cytochrome C. In a base of Calcium, Magnesium, Potassium Succinates.

Upper Di-GST - Nutri-Quest
Each tablet contains: L-Glutamine 50 mg • Okra 25 mg • Stomach 125 mg • Folic Acid 250 mcg • Vitamin A 1500 IU • Parotid 10 mg • Aloe Vera 5 mg • N-Acetyl Glucosamine 50 mg • Bromelain 25 mg • Duodenum 125 mg • Deglycerrized Licorice root 156 mg • Cabigen extract (Vitamin U) 20 mg • Slippery Elm 25 mg • Magnesium Chelate 75 mg. See Editor's Note No. 15, page 1817.

UpTime Herbal - Uptime Sports Nutrition
Three caplets contain: Vitamin A (beta-carotene) (10% DV) 501 IU • Vitamin C (150% DV) 90 mg • Thiamin (thiamin mononitrate) (100% DV) 1.5 mg • Riboflavin (100% DV) 1.71 mg • Niacin (niacinamide) (225% DV) 45 mg • Vitamin B6 (pyridoxine hydrochloride) (300% DV) 6 mg • Folate (folic acid) (98% DV) 390 mcg • Vitamin B12

(cyanocabalamin) (300% DV) 18 mcg • Pantothenic Acid (Calcium pantothenate) (300% DV) 30 mg • Chromium (aspartate) (250% DV) 300 mcg • Molybdenum (amino acid chelate) (300% DV) 225 mcg • Vanadium (vanadyl sulfate) 2.85 mcg • Herbal Powder Base: Green Tea leaf, Dong Quai, Schisandra berry, Kola Nut seed, Ashwaganda leaf, Organic Bee Pollen, Yerba Mate leaf, Siberian Ginseng root, Papain (from papaya), Long Pepper fruit, Jujube fruit, Gamma Oryzanol, Wild Yam root, White Ginseng root, Fo-ti root, Ligustrum fruit, Astragalus root, Ginger root 1014 mg.

UpTime Nutritional Fitness - Uptime Sports Nutrition
Three caplets contain: Vitamin C (as ascorbic acid) (1500% DV) 900 mg • Calcium (as Calcium carbonate) (70% DV) 700 mg • Chromium (as picolinate) (8% DV) 10 mcg • Uptime Power Base: Spirulina Blue Green Algae, Wheat Grass, Alfalfa leaf, Caffeine, Papaya fruit, Silica, Cayenne fruit, Siberian Ginseng extract, Echinacea herb, Ginkgo Biloba extract, Carnitine (tartrate), Coenzyme Q10, Chromium (picolinate) 750 mg.

Urban Air Defense - Source Naturals
Two tablets contain: Vitamin A (Beta Carotene 12500 IU and Palmitate 5000 IU) 17500 IU • Vitamin C (Magnesium Ascorbate, Vitamin C and Manganese Ascorbate) 500 mg • Fat-Soluble Vitamin C (from 186 mg of Ascorbyl Palmitate) 80 mg • Vitamin E (D-Alpha Tocopheryl)(Natural) 200 IU • Magnesium (Ascorbate) 30 mg • Zinc (OptiZinc Monomethionine) 15 mg • Manganese (Ascorbate) 5 mg • Copper (Sebacate) 750 mcg • Selenium (as L-Selenomethionine) 100 mcg • Quercetin 200 mg • N-Acetyl Cysteine 100 mg • Silymarin (Milk Thistle seed extract) 50 mg • Ginkgo Biloba extract 24% (50:1) 5 mg • Hawthorn berry 150 mg • Rosemary 150 mg • Schizandra 125 mg • Marshmallow root 85 mg • Astragalus 60 mg.

Urinary & Kidney Care - Wellness for Women
Each capsule contains: Vitamin C (as ascorbic acid) 50 mg • Thiamin USP (as thiamin HCl; vitamin B-1) 12.5 mg • Riboflavin (vitamin B-2) 12.5 mg • Niacinamide 12.5 mg • Vitamin B-6 (as pyridoxine HCl) 12.5 mg • Folic Acid 100 mcg • Vitamin B-12 (as cyanocobalamin) 100 mcg • Biotin 12.5 mcg • Pantothenic Acid (as d-calcium pantothenate) 12.5 mg • Potassium (from potassium gluconate and potassium chloride) 99 mg • Cranberry extract (10:1 concentrate) 200 mg • Juniper berry powder 50 mg • Corn Silk 25 mg • Uva Ursi 25 mg • Choline (as choline bitartrate) 12.5 mg • Inositol 12.5 mg • PABA (para-aminobenzoic acid) 12.5 mg.

Urinary Formula - Nature's Way
Three capsules contain: Cleavers herb 180 mg • Corn Silk 150 mg • Cranberry concentrate fruit 600 mg • Dandelion leaf 180 mg • Goldenseal stem, leaf, flower 60 mg • Marshmallow root 180 mg. Other ingredients: Gelatin, Magnesium Stearate, Millet.

Urinary Support - Amazon Support
Each capsule contains: Chanca Piedra • Boldo • Cipo Cabeludo • Anamu • Jatoba • Brazilian Peppertree • Cha de Bugre.

Uriphron - PhytoPharmica
Each tablet contains: Goldenrod extract 5.9:1 (Solidago virgaurea) 136 mg • Birch leaf extract 5.5:1 (Betula pendula) 109 mg • Orthosiphon leaf extract 6.2:1 (O. aristata) 97 mg. Contains no sugar, salt, yeast, wheat, gluten, corn, soy, dairy products, coloring, flavoring, or preservatives.

Uriplex - Enzymatic Therapy
Each tablet contains: Goldenrod extract 5.9:1 (Solidago virgaurea) 136 mg • Birch Leaf extract 5.5:1 (Betula pendula) 109 mg • Orthosiphon Leaf extract 6.2:1 (O. aristata) 97 mg. Contains no sugar, salt, yeast, wheat, gluten, corn, soy, dairy products, coloring, flavoring, or preservatives.

Usnea-Propolis Virtue - Blessed Herbs
Usnea lichen • Pau d'Arco bark • Echinacea Angustifolia root • Propolis • Goldenseal root • Myrrh Gum • Grain alcohol & Distilled Water.

Utrophin PMG - Standard Process
Each tablet contains: Proprietary Blend 192 mg: Bovine uterus (PMG) extract, Magnesium citrate. Other Ingredients: Calcium Lactate, Cellulose, Calcium stearate.
See Editor's Note No. 14, page 1817.

Uva Ursi Formula - Quest - Quest
Each caplet contains: Uva Ursi leaf powder (Arctostaphylos uva-ursi) 85 mg • Dandelion root powder (Taraxacum officinale) 60 mg • Gentian root powder (Gentiana lutea) 55 mg • Huckleberry leaf powder (Vaccinium Myrtillus) 55 mg • Parsley leaf powder (Petroselinum crispum) 45 mg • Buchu leaf powder (Barosma betulina) 35 mg • Kelp powder (Fucus vesiculosis) 35 mg • Raspberry leaf powder (Rubus idaeus) 35 mg • Saw Palmetto berry powder (Serenoa serrulata/repens) 35 mg • Bladderwrack powder (Fuccus vesiculosis) 20 mg. Other Ingredients: Calcium Phosphate, Microcrystalline Cellulose, Vegetable Stearin, Croscarmellose Sodium, Magnesium Stearate (vegetable source).

U-Viva Vitamin E (Chewable) - Uviva
Each tablet contains: Vitamin E (d-alpha tocopheryl succinate) 400 IU. Other Ingredients: Sucrose, Wheat Starch, Talc Purified, Kaolin, CL 75470, Gelatin. No synthetic vitamin E, yeast, salt, preservatives, gluten, glucose, artifical colors & flavors.

V2G - EAS
Each capsule contains: Vanadyl Sulfate 7.5 mg • Taurine 800 mg • Selenium (Sodium Selenate) 33 mcg.

Vag-Mend - The Herbalist
Golden Seal root • Thuja leaf • Usnea lichen • Bayberry root bark • Echinacea root • Red Raspberry leaf.

Valer-A-Somn - PhytoPharmica
Each capsule contains: Valerian extract (Valeriana officinalis) - (standardized to contain 0.2%-0.8% valerenic acids) 150 mg.

Valerian - Pharmanex
Each capsule contains: Valerian root extract (6:1) (Valerian officinalis) 350 mg. Other Ingredients: Gelatin, Rice Flour, Magnesium Stearate, Silicon Dioxide.
See Editor's Note No. 12, page 1817.

Valerian - Leiner Health Products
Two caplets contain: Valerian extract (Valeriana officinalis) root 200 mg. Other Ingredients: Calcium Carbonate, Cellulose, Maltodextrin, Hydroxypropyl Methylcellulose, Silicon Dioxide, Polyethylene Glycol 3350, Croscarmellose Sodium, Hydroxypropyl Cellulose, Pharmaceutical Glaze, Crospovidone, Magnesium Stearate, Blue 1 Lake, Polysorbate 80, Titanium Dioxide, Sodium Citrate.

Valerian Extract - Nature's Way
Two capsules contain: Calcium 30 mg • Valerian Nighttime (dried valerian extract) 220 mg • Valerian root 800 mg. Other Ingredients: Gelatin.

Valerian Nighttime - Nature's Way
Each tablet contains: Lemon Balm dried extract 80 mg • Valerian Nighttime (dried valerian extract) 160 mg.

Valerian Plus - PhysioLogics
Each capsule contains: Valerian (0.8% Valerenic Acids, 1.52 mg) 190 mg • Chamomile 90 mg • Peppermint 90 mg • Propolis 45 mg • Passion flower 45 mg • American Ginseng 40 mg.

B R A N D   N A M E S

Some Brand Name Natural Products - What they Contain

B R A N D   N A M E S

Valerian Root - Gaia Herbs
Each capsule contains: Valerian root (standardized for 0.8% valerenic acid, and full spectrum up to 100 mg of extract per capsule) 50 mg

Valerian Root - Olympian Labs
Each capsule contains: Valerian root 500 mg.

Valerian-400 - PhytoPharmica
Two capsules contain: Valerian (Valeriana officinalis) root extract (standardized to contain a minimum of 0.8% valerenic acids) 800 mg.

Valerian-Primrose Virtue - Blessed Herbs
Valerian root • Primrose flower & leaf • California Poppy flower & leaf • Hops strobile • Wild Lettuce • Passion flower • Scullcap • Grain alcohol & Distilled Water.

Val-Tran - Atrium Inc.
Each tablet contains: Valerian (standardized extract) 100 mg • Vitamin B6 5 mg • Magnesium Gluconate 50 mg • Magnesium Oxide 50 mg. In a base containing Chamomile, Anise & Peppermint.

Vanadyl Factors - Olympia Nutrition
Vanadyl Sulfate + 800 mg Taurine.

Vanadyl pH - SportPharma
Each capsule contains: Vanadyl Sulfate 7.5 mg.

Vanadyl Plus with Chromium - Olympian Labs
Each capsule contains: Chromium Picolinate 200 mcg • Vanadyl Sulfate 10 mg • Niacin 20 mg.

Vanadyl Sulfate - Ultimate Nutrition
Each tablet contains: Vanadyl Sulfate 10 mg.

Vanadyl Sulfate with Niacin - Olympian Labs
Each capsule contains: Vanadyl Sulfate 20 mg • Niacin 25 mg.

Vancol (Cholesterol Lowering Plan) - Omnicron International
Two chewable tablets contain: Beta Sitosterol 10 mg • Psyllium 200 mg • Chromium from Picolinate 50 mcg with natural Quinone Antioxidants. In a base of Calcium Carbonate & Magnesium Stearate.

VariCare - Enzymatic Therapy
Each tablet contains: Butcher's Broom extract (Ruscus aculeatus) standardized to contain 9 - 11% Saponins calculated as Ruscogenin 150 mg • Horse Chestnut extract (Aesculus hippocastanum) standardized to contain 20 - 22% Saponins calculated as Escin 125 mg • Gotu Kola Phytosome (Centella asiatica) standardized to contain 30 - 35% Centella Triterpenes 15 mg.

Varicosin - PhytoPharmica
Each tablet contains: Butcher's Broom extract 150 mg • Horse Chestnut extract 125 mg • Gotu Kola Phytosome 15 mg.

Vascular Complete - Rexall
Each tablet contains: Vitamin C 33.3 mg • Calcium 260 mg • Sodium 10 mg • Chondroitin Sulfate 66.7 mg • Alpha-Ketoglutaric Acid (from calcium alpha-ketoglutarate) 33.3 mg • Citric Acid 33.3 mg • L-Arginine (from L-arginine HCl) 33.3 mg • L-Lysine (from L-lysine HCl) 33.3 mg • L-Proline 33.3 mg • L-Ornithine (from L-ornithine HCl) 16.7 mg • Choline (from choline bitartrate) 16.7 mg • Silica 7 mg • Vascular Complete base blend: Rose Hips and seeds extract (Rosa canina), Citrus Bioflavonoids, rutin, Hesperidin, Acerola Fruit extract (malpighia punicifolia) 7 mg. Other Ingredients: Calcium Carbonate, Cellulose, Croscarmellose Sodium, Hydroxypropyl Methylcellulose, Talc, Magnesium Stearate, Riboflavin (colorant), Titanium Dioxide, Calcium Sulfate, Polysaccharides.

Vascular Support Formula - The Vitamin Factory
Each tablet contains: Vitamin C (Ascorbic Acid) 500 mg • Pycnogenol (Maritime Pine bark extract) 100 mg.

VasoRect - Real Health Laboratories
Each capsule contains: L-Arginine 625 mg • Calcium 12.5 mg.

Vege Fuel - TwinLab
Pure Isolated Soy (All-Vegetable) Protein 100%. Contains no sugar, artificial sweeteners or flavors. It is fat free, cholesterol free & lactose free.

Vege Fuel (Aspartame Free) - TwinLab
Pure Isolated Soy (All-Vegetable) Protein 100%. Contains no sugar, artificial sweeteners or flavors. It is fat free, cholesterol free & lactose free.

Veg-Easy - Progressive Labs
Two tablets contain: Blend 1400 mg: Broccoli powder • Spirulina • Wheat Grass • Alfalfa powder • Spinach powder • Cabbage powder • Green Tea • Carrot • Barley grass • Parsley • Beet root powder • Kale • Oat fiber medium • Brussels Sprouts • Lipase • Amylase • Protease • Cellulase • Powdered Cellulose • Beet leaf powder • Barley fiber • Oat bran • Lactobacillus Acidophilus • Glucomannan & Calcium Gluconate.

Veg-Enzyme - Atrium Inc.
Each capsule contains: Protease Enzymes 150 mg • Amylase Enzymes 140 mg • Lipase Enzymes 25 mg • Cellulase Enzymes 10 mg.

VegeSil - Flora
Silica extract • Spring Horsetail.

Vegetarian Enzyme Complex - Futurebiotics
Protease 6500 HUT • Amylase 2000 DU • Cellulase 20 CU • Lipase 14.5 LU • Papaya enzyme (papain) 50 mg • Lactase 100 LacU • Alfalfa powder 50 mg • Pineapple enzyme (bromelain) 50 mg • Betaine HCl 3 mg. Enzyme activity is determined & reported according to Standard Food Chemical Codex procedures accepted by the FDA.

Vegetarian Enzyme Complex 50 Plus - Futurebiotics
Protease 8000 HUT* • Amylase 4000 DU* • Cellulase 100 CU* • Lipase 40 LU* • Invertase 0.2 IAU* • Lactase 240 LacU* • Papain 10 mg • Maltase 15 AGU* • Gentian root 100 mg • Bromelain 10 mg • Fennel seed 50 mg. *Enzyme activity is determined & reported according to Standard Food Chemical Codex procedures accepted by the FDA.

Vegetarian Mega Minerals - Nature's Life
Two tablets contain: Boron (Citrate) 1 mg • Calcium (Carbonate, Citrate/Malate) 1000 mg • Chromium (Picolinate {US Patent #33,988}, Polynicotinate) 200 mcg • Copper (Glyconate, Citrate) 1 mg • Iodine (Kelp) 25 mcg • Iron (Fumerate, Peptonate) 15 mg • Magnesium (Oxide, Citrate) 500 mg • Manganese (Citrate) 10 mg • Molybdenum (Sodium Molybdate) 20 mcg • Potassium (Citrate) 99 mg • Selenium (l-Selenomethionine) 100 mcg • Silicon Dioxide 20 mg • Vanadium (Vanadyl Sulfate) 20 mcg • Zinc (Picolinate, Citrate) 15 mg • Betaine HCl 100 mg • Glutamic Acid HCl 100 mg.

Vegetarian Super Multi - Futurebiotics
Three tablets contain: Vitamin C 500 mg • Beta Carotene 15,000 IU • Vitamin B1 (thiamin) 20 mg • Vitamin B2 (riboflavin) 20 mg • Niacinamide 75 mg • Vitamin D 200 IU • Vitamin E (natural succinate) 100 IU • Vitamin B6 20 mg • Folic Acid 400 mcg • Vitamin B12 100 mcg • Biotin 300 mcg • Pantothenic Acid 50 mg • Inositol 50 mg. Minerals: Calcium: (carbonate, phosphate, ascorbate) 200 mg • Iron (gluconate) 8 mg • Phosphorus 100 mg • Iodine (kelp) 150 mcg • Magnesium: (oxide, ascorbate, amino acid chelate) 25 mcg • Zinc

(gluconate, oxide) 25 mg • Copper (gluconate) 1 mg • Selenium (amino acid chelate) 200 mcg • Chromium (amino acid chelate) 200 mcg • Manganese (proteinate) 5 mg • Molybdenum (amino acid chelate) 25 mcg. Other ingredients: Choline 150 mg • Para Amino Benzoic Acid (PABA) 75 mg • Bioflavonoid complex 100 mg • Sodium Phosphate 1 mg • Methionine 75 mg • Betaine HCl 75 mg • Bromelain 75 mg • RNA/DNA (chlorella) 50 mg • Chlorella 400 mg. In a base of: [Sea Vegetable, Ginkgo Biloba, Milk Thistle, Goldenseal, Dandelion, Burdock root, Alfalfa & Horsetail] 500 mg.

Veggie Carotenoids - Now
Two VCaps contain: natural Beta-Carotene (D. salina) 12 mg/20000 IU • Alpha Carotene (D. salina) 400 mcg containing additional Carotenoids from D. salina algae: Xeaxanthin, Cryptoxanthin, Lycopene & Lutein • Lutein Floraglo Marigolds 3 mg • Lycopene natural source 3 mg • Broccoli concentrate (250 mcg Sulforaphane) 250 mg • Spinach concentrate (75 mcg Lutein) 100 mg • Tomato concentrate (140 mcg Lycopene) 100 mg • Kale powder 50 mg • Cabbage powder 50 mg • Brussels Sprouts powder 50 mg.

Veggies4Life - Swanson
Two tablets contain: Alfalfa leaf powder 100 mg • Beet powder 100 mg • Broccoli powder 100 mg • Carrot powder 100 mg • Odor-Controlled Garlic bulb (PureGar® 10,000 ppm allicin potential) 100 mg • Parsley powder 100 mg • Spinach powder 100 mg • Tomato powder 100 mg • Barley Grass powder 50 mg • Cabbage powder 50 mg • Celery Seed powder 50 mg • Kale powder 50 mg • Kelp powder 50 mg • Wheat Grass powder 50 mg • Oregano powder 40 mg.

Vegie-Tabs One - Dial Herbs
Parsley • Garlic • Black Walnut hulls • Red Beet • Kelp • Dulse • Wheat bran • Wheat germ • Oat straw • Honey • Spinach • Cabbage • Carrots • Squash • Onion • Broccoli • Yellow Dock • Chickweed • Echinacea • Ginger • Cloves • Alfalfa • Alfalfa seeds • Papaya seeds • Rice Bran Capsicum • Sweet Potato.

Vegie-Tabs Two - Dial Herbs
Parsley • Hawthorne • Black Walnut hulls • Red Beet • Kelp • Dulse • Millet • Oat Straw • Honey • Spinach • Cabbage • Carrots • Squash • Onion • Broccoli • Yellow Dock • Chickweed • Echinacea • Alfalfa • Alfalfa seeds • Papaya seeds • Rice Bran • Capsicum • Ginger • Cloves.

Vegiplex - HealthWatchers System
Brocolli • Kale • Sprouts • Spinach • Radish • Carrot • Beet • Tomato • Celery • Onion • Leek • Cauliflower • Brussel Sprouts. (all ingredients are whole and powdered.)

Vegzyme - Progressive Labs
Each 500 mg capsule contains: Protease 10000 NP Units • Lipase 3600 NL Units • Amylase 4000 NA Units • Cellulase 30 NC Units • Papaya leaf powder 25 mg. Other Ingredients: Plant fiber. All-vegetable source from cultures of Aspergillus Oryzae & Niger & Papaya. Naturally occurring Invertase, Maltase, Beta-Amylase, Hemicellulase, Phosphatase, Peroxidase, Catalase & Hydrolase are also present.

Vein Formula - Pharmanex
Each tablet contains: Vitamin C (as Calcium Ascorbate) 60 mg • Grape Seed Extract (as Masquelier's Original OPC's) 75 mg. Other Ingredients: Gelatin, Maltodextrin, Microcrystalline Cellulose, Magnesium stearate, Silicon dioxide.

Vein Support Formula - Baywood International
Each tablet contains: Proprietary Flavonoid Blend: Diosmin • Hesperidin 500 mg. Other ingredients: Microcrystalline Cellulose, Maize Starch, Opadry II Orange, Povidone.

Veinish - Quest
Sesame Oil • Emulsifying Wax • Stearic Acid • Marine Algae •

Propylene Glycol • Cetyl Alcohol • Canola Oil • Calendula Oil • Marigold Extract • Chickweed Extract • Lecithin • Essence of Lemon.

VeinTain - Resource Wellness
Each caplet contains: Vitamin A 250 IU • Vitamin C 30 mg • Calcium 175 mg • Grape Seed extract 25 mg • Horse Chestnut extract 250 mg. Other Ingredients: Dicalcium Phosphate, Microcrystalline Cellulose, Croscarmellose Sodium, Stearic Acid, Magnesium Stearate, Silicon Dioxide, Hydroxypropyl Methylcellulose, Hydroxypropyl Cellulose, Polyethylene Glycol.

VeinTrain - Resource Wellness
One caplet contains: Vitamin A 250 IU • Vitamin C 30 mg • Calcium 175 mg • Standardized Grape Seed extract 25 mg • Standardized Horse Chestnut extract 250 mg. Other Ingredients: Dicalcium Phosphate, Microcrystalline Cellulose, Ascorbic Acid (Vitamin C), Croscarmellose Sodium, Stearic Acid, Magnesium Stearate, Silicon Dioxide, Hydroxypropyl Methylcellulose, Hydroxypropyl Cellulose, Polyethylene Glycol, Vitamin A Acetate.

VelvaMax - Gold Mountain
Ginseng (Panax Ginseng) • Reishi (Ganoderma lucidum) • Tienchi (Radix Pseudoginseng) • Astragalus (Astragalus membranaceus) • Licorice (Radix glycyrrhizae uralensis).

Venastat - Pharmaton
Each Supro Cap contains: Sustained Release Pellets of Standardized Horse Chestnut seed extract as Triterpene glycosides calculated as Escin (16%) 300 mg. Other Ingredients: Dextrin, Gelatin, Copolyvidone, Talc, Polymethacrylic Acid Derivatives, Titanium Dioxide, Dibutyl Phthalate, Synthetic Iron Oxide.

Venix - Pharmanex
Two capsules contain: Triacin, a proprietary blend of 1325 mg: Cs-4 Mushroom Mycelia Cordyceps Sinensis ([Berk.]Sacc.), L-Arginine (as L-Arginine HCL), Ginkgo Biloba leaf extract (50:1). Other Ingredients: Gelatin, Magnesium Stearate, Silicon Dioxide.

Veromax for Men - Veromax International
Each tablet contains: Jujube Dates (Zizyphi fructus) fruit 100 mg • 213 mg Proprietary Amino Blend of L-Arginine • L-Alanine • Glutamic Acid • Lysine (L-Lysine hydrochloride) • 238 mg Proprietary Herbal Blend of Korean Ginseng root powder • Ginkgo Biloba leaf powder • Saw Palmetto berry powder. Other ingredients: Calcium Carbonate, Microcrystalline Cellulose, Croscarmellose Sodium, Stearic Acid, Silica, Magnesium Stearate, Hydroxypropyl Methylcellulose.

Veromax for Women - Veromax International
Each tablet contains: Jujube Dates (Zizyphi fructus) fruit 100 mg • Proprietary Amino Blend: Arginine (L-Arginine Hydrochloride), Alanine, Glutamic Acid, Lysine (L-Lysine Hydrochloride) 175 mg. Proprietary Herbal Blend: Siberian Ginseng root powder, Ginkgo Biloba leaf powder, Isoflavones (Kidzo root extract) 177.5 mg. Other Ingredients: Calcium Carbonate, Microcrystalline Cellulose, Croscarmellose Sodium, Stearic Acid, Silica, Magnesium Stearate, Hydroxypropyl Methylcellulose.

Vertigoheel - Heel Biotherapeutics
50 ml contains: Cocculus (Indian berries) 4X 35 ml • Conium (Spotted Hemlock) 3x • Ambra (Amber) 6X • Petroleum (Mineral Oil) 8X 5 mg. Contains 35 Vol.% alcohol.
See Editor's Note No. 1, page 1816.

Vertigoheel Tablets - Heel Biotherapeutics
One tablet contains: Cocculus (Indian berries) 4X 210 mg • Conium (Spotted Hemlock) 3X • Ambra (Amber) 6X • Petroleum (Mineral Oil) 8X ana 30 mg.
See Editor's Note No. 1, page 1816.

BRAND NAMES

VHandC Tabs - Dial Herbs
Vinegar • Honey • Cayenne.

Viactiv Soft Calcium Chews - Mead Johnson Nutritionals
Each chew contains: Calcium (as calcium carbonate) 500 mg •
Vitamin D 100 IU • Vitamin K 40 mcg • Potassium 15 mg •
Phosphorus 8 mg • Lactose 0.5 mg • Caffeine 1.14 mg. Other
Ingredients: Corn syrup, calcium carbonate, sugar, chocolate, nonfat
milk, cocoa butter, salt, soy lecithin, glyceryl monostearate, artificial
flavor, carrageenan, & sodium phosphate.
See Editor's Note No. 5, page 1816.

Vigorex Femme - New Hope Health Products
Each tablet contains: Sabal Serrulata (Saw Palmetto) • Avena Sativa
(Common Oats).

Vigorex forte - Doc Johnson Enterprises
Active Ingredient: Avena sativa 1X. In a base of lactose.
See Editor's Note No. 1, page 1816.

Vigorex Forte - New Hope Health Products
Each capsule contains: Avena Sativa Extract 300 mg.

Vigrex - Puritan's Pride
Each tablet contains: Yohimbe 500 mg • Tribulus Terrestris herb
225 mg • Maca root 200 mg • Muira Puama root 200 mg • Panax
Ginseng 150 mg • Ginger extract 100 mg • Citrus Aurantium extract
(Bitter Orange) 50 mg • Fructooligosaccharides (FOS) 50 mg • Saw
Palmetto (Standardized for 30% fatty acids) 15 mg. Other Ingredients:
Dicalcium Phosphate, Cellulose, Magnesium Stearate, Silica, Stearic
Acid.

Vincamine - Source Naturals
Each tablet contains: Vincamine 30 mg.

Vincazine - Smart Basics
Each capsule contains: Vinpocetine 10 mg • (-) Huperzine A 50 mcg.

Vinpocetine - Amerifit
Each tablet contains: Vinpocetine 5 mg • Green Tea standardized
extract 200 mg. Other Ingredients: Dicalcium phosphate,
croscarmellose sodium, microcrystalline cellulose, magnesium
stearate, silica stearic acid, & pharmaceutical glaze.

Vinpocetine - Nature Made
Each tablet contains: Vinpocetine 5 mg.

Vinpocetine - PhysioLogics
Each capsule contains: Vinpocetine 10 mg.

Vinpo-Zine - Smart Nutrition
Each capsule contains: Vinpocetine 10 mg • Huperzine A 50 mcg.

Viper - Puritan's Pride
Each capsule contains: Kola Nut 175 mg • Oatstraw 150 mg • Nettles
100 mg • Yohimbe 2% extract 50 mg • Siberian Ginseng 50 mg •
Horny Goat Weed 20 mg • Catuaba 10 mg • Muira Puama 10 mg •
Korean Ginseng 10 mg • Turnera Aphrodisiaca 10 mg • Saw Palmetto
10 mg.

ViraMax - Solaray
Two capsules contain: Catuaba 500 mg • Yohimbe bark extract
(supplying 10 mg of yohimbine) 500 mg • Muira Puama root 250 mg
• Peruvian Maca root extract (4:1) 100 mg.

ViraPlex - Enzymatic Therapy
Each tablet contains: Vitamin A (Fish Liver oil) 10000 IU • Vitamin D
(Fish Liver oil) 35 IU • Vitamin C (Ascorbic Acid/Rose Hips) 200 mg
• Calcium (Lactate) 41 mg • Pantothenic Acid (D-Calcium

Pantothenate) 25 mg • Zinc (Gluconate) 10.5 mg • Magnesium
(Citrate) 6.7 mg • Vitamin B12 (Cyanocobalamin) 2.5 mcg • Other
ingredients: RNA Powder 60 mg • Alfalfa juice powder 50 mg •
Lemon Bioflavonoids 30 mg • Spleen extract 30 mg • Thymus extract
25 mg • Trace Mineral concentrate (Kelp) 25 mg • Unsaturated Free
Fatty Acids 15 mg • Lung extract 10 mg. In a base of Chlorophyll,
Lymph, & Fermentation extract. Contains no sugar, salt, yeast, wheat,
gluten, corn, soy, dairy products, flavoring or preservatives.
Chlorophyll is used in this product as a natural coloring agent. All
organs & glands derived from bovine sources.
See Editor's Note No. 14, page 1817.

Virile V for Him - USA Pharmacal Sales
Two tablets contain: Niacin 10 mg • Yohimbe 250 mg • Avena Sativa
150 mg • Androstenedione 100 mg • Saw Palmetto 100 mg • Guarana
300 mg • Taurine 200 mg • Siberian Ginseng 30 mg • Panax Ginseng
30 mg • Tribulus Terrestris 50 mg • Rhodiola Roseo 10 mg • Wild
Yam 250 mg • Maca 100 mg • Arginine 100 mg.

Virility Support Formula - The Vitamin Factory
Each tablet contains: Niacin 10 mg • L-Arginine 250 mg •
Muirapuama root & bark extract 10:1 100 mg • Yohimbe bark extract
(min 1% Yohimbe) 100 mg • Quebracho Branco bark extract
(Aspidosperma • min. 6% Quebrachine) 25 mg • Catuaba bark extract
4:1 50 mg • Pycnogenol (Maritime Pine bark extract) 10 mg.

Virility-V - Aspen Group, Inc.
Two tablets contain: Yohimbe extract 2% 500 mg • Avena Sativa
extract 10.1 150 mg • Androstenedione 90 mg • Saw Palmetto extract
4.1 100 mg • Guarana extract 22% 300 mg • Taurine 200 mg •
Siberian Ginseng extract 35.1 30 mg • Tribulus Terrestris extract 40%
50 mg. Inactive ingredients: Dicalcium Phosphate, Microcrystaline
Cellulose, Magnesium Stearte, Stearic Acid.

Virility-V Female - Aspen Group, Inc.
Three tablets contain: Vitamin D (as colecalciferol) 21 IU • Niacin (as
Niacinamide) 20 mg • Vitamin B6 (as pyridoxine hydrochloride)
2.4 mg • Folic Acid (as folacin) 6.4 mg • Vitamin B12 (as
cyanocobalamin) 6 mg. Other Ingredients: Avena Sativa (10:1)
150 mg, Kava Kava (30%) 10 mg, Muira Puama (4:1) 20 mg,
St. John's Wort (0.3%) 250 mg, Siberian Ginseng (35:1) 30 mg,
Gingko Biloba (24%) 40 mg, Cordyceps 100 mg, Damiana 20 mg,
L-Taurine 200 mg.

Virilogarl - Olympian Labs
Three capsules contain: Ginkgo Biloba leaf extract 120 mg • Garlic
extract 600 mg • L-Arginine 390 mg • Bilberry extract 150 mg
• Grape Seed extract 75 mg • Green Tea leaf extract 225 mg.

Virx - Nutri-Quest
Each tablet contains: Olive leaf 100 mg • L-Lysine 100 mg • Vitamin
C 25 mg • Zinc Chelate 10 mg • Elderberry extract 100 mg • Selenium
Chelate 50 mcg • Olive leaf extract 5 mg • Vitamin A 3333.33 IU •
Echinacea 100 mg • Goldenseal 50 mg • Astragalus 100 mg • natural
Beta Carotene 3333.33 IU.

Vision Complete - Rexall
Two capsules contain: Vitamin A (100% as beta-carotene, 60% of
which is from dunaliella salina algae) 5000 IU • Vitamin C (as
ascorbic acid and ascorbyl palmitate) 60 mg • Vitamin E (as
dl-alpha-tocopheryl acetate and d-alpha-tocopheryl succinate) 30 IU •
Riboflavin (Vitamin B2) 3.4 mg • Vitamin B-6 (as pyridoxine HCl)
2 mg • Lutein (from marigold flower extract) 5 mg • Bilberry leaf
10 mg • Piperine (from black pepper fruit extract) 4.75 mg •
Alpha-Lipoic Acid 10 mg • Glutathione 5 mg • Spinach leaf 20 mg.
Other Ingredients: Maltodextrin, Gelatin, Water, Magnesium Stearate.

Vision Essentials - Enzymatic Therapy
Each capsule contains: Vitamin A (Beta Carotene) non-toxic form of
Vitamin A 5000 IU • Vitamin C (Ascorbic Acid) 100 mg • Riboflavin

(Vitamin B2) 5 mg • Other ingredients: Bilberry extract (Vaccinium myrtillus Fructus) standardized to contain 25% Anthocyanosides (20 mg per capsule) calculated as Anthocyanidins 80 mg. Contains no sugar, salt, yeast, wheat, corn, soy, dairy products, coloring, flavoring, or preservatives.

Vision Formula - Nature's Way
Two capsules contain: Bilberry fruit (dried extract 25% Anthocyanins) 50 mg • Biotin (Biotin Triurate) 40 mcg • Cayenne pepper fruit 100 mg • Citrus Bioflavonoids 150 mg • Copper (Amino Acid Chelate) 1 mg • Lutein 6 mg • Niacin (Vitamin B3) 20 mg • Riboflavin (Vitamin B2) 8 mg • Siberian Ginseng root 50 mg • Taurine 150 mg • Tru-OPCs (dried Grape seed extract) 20 mg • Vitamin A (Retinol Palmitate) 2000 IU • Vitamin E (d-Alpha Tocopheryl) 80 IU • Zinc (Amino Acid Chelate) 16 mg. Other ingredients: Gelatin, Magnesium Stearate, Millet.

Vision Health - ProHerbs
Two tablets contain: Vitamin A (100% Beta Carotene) 2500 IU • Zinc (as Sulfate) 15 mg • Selenium (as Selenomethionine) 200 mcg • Copper (as Cupric Oxide) 2 mg • Bilberry extract (Vaccinium myrtillus fruit standardized to 25% anthocyanidins) 160 mg • Lutein 6 mg • Lycopene 5 mg. Other Ingredients: Dicalcium Phosphate, Microcrystalline Cellulose, Croscarmellose Sodium, Hydroxypropylmethylcellulose, Magnesium Stearate, Mineral Oil, Polyethylene Glycol, Stearic Acid, Titanium Dioxide, Sodium lauryl Sulfate, FD&C Red #40 Lake, FD&C Blue #1 Lake, FD&C Blue #2 Lake.

Vision Nutrients - Puritan's Pride
Each tablet contains: Pro-Vitamin A (Beta Carotene) 5,000 IU • Vitamin E (dl-alpha Tocopheryl) 30 IU • Vitamin C (Ascorbic Acid) 60 mg • Zinc (Zinc Oxide) 40 mg • Copper (Cupric Oxide) 2 mg • Selenium 40 mcg.

Visionace - Vitabiotics
Each capsule contains: Vitamin A 300 mcg • Vitamin D (as Vitamin D3) 2.5 mcg • Vitamin E 60 mg • Vitamin C 150 mg • Vitamin B1 (Thiamin) 7.5 mg • Vitamin B2 (Riboflavin) 5 mg • Vitamin B3 (Niacin) 9 mg • Vitamin B6 4.5 mg • Folic Acid 250 mcg • Vitamin B12 4.5 mcg • Pantothenic Acid 10 mg • Vitamin K 45 mcg • Iron 3 mg • Magnesium 50 mg • Zinc 7.5 mg • Iodine 100 mcg • Copper 1 mg • Manganese 2 mg • Selenium 100 mcg • Chromium 50 mcg • Natural Mixed Carotenoids 3 mg • Citrus Bioflavonoids 15 mg • Bilberry extract 60 mg.

Visioplex - Progressive Labs
Each capsule contains: Vitamin A (acetate) 937 IU • Vitamin A (beta carotene) 3125 IU • Vitamin C 62.5 mg • Calcium (as calcium citrate) 12.5 mg • Vitamin E (dl-alpha tocopherol) 50 IU • Thiamin (vitamin B1) 2.5 mg • Riboflavin (vitamin B2) 3.1 mg • Niacin 1.25 mg • Niacinamide 6.25 mg • Vitamin B6 (pyridoxine HCl) 3.75 mg • Folate (folic acid) 100 mcg • Vitamin B12 6.25 mcg • Pantothenic Acid 12.5 mg • Magnesium (as magnesium citrate) 31.25 mg • Zinc (as zinc picolinate) 6.25 mg • Selenium (selenomethionine) 25 mcg • Copper (amino acid chelate) 0.375 mg • Raw Eye concentrate 8.75 mg • Eyebright (Euphrasia officinalis) 18.75 mg • Bilberry powder (Vaccinium myrtillis) 5 mg • Ginkgo extract (Ginkgo biloba) 7.5 mg • N-Acetyl-Cysteine (NAC) 31.25 • Quercetin 37.5 mg • Taurine 62.5 mg • L-Methionine 25 mg • Glutamic Acid 6.25 mg • Glycine 6.25 mg.
See Editor's Note No. 14, page 1817.

Visual Eyes - Source Naturals
Four tablets contain: Vitamin A (Beta Carotene) 25000 IU • Vitamin A (Palmitate) 7500 IU • Vitamin B2 50 mg • Inositol Hexanicotinate 100 mg • Vitamin C (Magnesium Ascorbate) 1500 mg • Vitamin E (D-Alpha Tocopheryl Succinate) 400 IU • Chromium (ChromeMate Polynicotinate 125 mcg and Chromium Picolinate 125 mcg)

250 mcg • Copper (Sebacate) 1 mg • Magnesium (Ascorbate, Taurinate) 164 mg • Selenium (L-Selenomethionine) 200 mcg • Zinc (Monomethionine) 30 mg • Bilberry extract (Yielding 37 mg of Anthocyanosides)100 mg • Lutein 10 mg • Alpha-Lipoic Acid 25 mg • Ginkgo Biloba 24% (50:1 Extract) 45 mg • Grape Seed extract (Proanthodyn with a Proanthocyanidolic Value of 95) 45 mg • Quercetin 320 mg • N-Acetyl Cysteine 400 mg • Taurine (Magnesium Taurinate) 500 mg • Inositol (Hexanicotinate) 10 mg.

Vita Fuel With Iron - TwinLab
Nine capsules contain: Beta-Carotene (pro-Vitamin A) 25000 IU • Vitamin D (from natural form Vitamin D3) 400 IU • Vitamin C 2000 mg • Natural Vitamin E (Succinate) 800 IU • CoQ10 (Coenzyme Q10) 30 mg • L-Glutathione 100 mg • N-Acetyl Cysteine (NAC) 200 mg • Alpha-Lipoic Acid 100 mcg • Vitamin B1 (Thiamine) 50 mg • Vitamin B2 (Riboflavin) 50 mg • Vitamin B6 (Pyridoxine) 50 mg • Vitamin B12 (Cobalamin) 100 mcg • Niacinamide 75 mg • Pantothenic Acid 100 mg • Folic Acid 800 mcg • Biotin 600 mcg • PABA 10 mg • Choline Bitartrate 100 mg • Inositol 100 mg • L-Carnitine (from Carni Fuel L-Carnitine Magnesium Citrate) 100 mg • Creatine (Monohydrate) 1000 mg • Calcium (from Calcium Citrate & Carbonate) 500 mg • Magnesium (from L-Carnitine Magnesium Citrate, Aspartate, Alpha-Ketoglutarate & Oxide) 500 mg • Potassium (from Potassium Alpha-Ketoglutarate, Citrate & Aspartate) 500 mg • Zinc (from Zinc Picolinate) 50 mg • Manganese (from Manganese Gluconate) 10 mg • Iron (from Ferrous Fumarate) 10 mg • Copper (from Copper Gluconate) 2 mg • Iodine (from Potassium Iodide) 150 mcg • Selenium (from Selenomethionine & Selenate‹50/50 mixture) 200 mcg • Chromium (from Chromic Fuel patented Chromium Picolinate) 400 mcg • Molybdenum (from natural Molybdic Acid) 150 mcg.

Vita Fuel Without Iron - TwinLab
Nine capsules contain: Beta-Carotene (pro-Vitamin A) 25000 IU • Vitamin D (from natural form Vitamin D3) 400 IU • Vitamin C 2000 mg • Natural Vitamin E (Succinate) 800 IU • CoQ10 (Coenzyme Q10) 30 mg • L-Glutathione 100 mg • N-Acetyl Cysteine (NAC) 200 mg • Alpha-Lipoic Acid 100 mcg • Vitamin B1 (Thiamine) 50 mg • Vitamin B2 (Riboflavin) 50 mg • Vitamin B6 (Pyridoxine) 50 mg • Vitamin B12 (Cobalamin) 100 mcg • Niacinamide 75 mg • Pantothenic Acid 100 mg • Folic Acid 800 mcg • Biotin 600 mcg • PABA 10 mg • Choline Bitartrate 100 mg • Inositol 100 mg • L-Carnitine (from Carni Fuel L-Carnitine Magnesium Citrate) 100 mg • Creatine (Monohydrate) 1000 mg • Calcium (from Calcium Citrate & Carbonate) 500 mg • Magnesium (from L-Carnitine Magnesium Citrate, Aspartate, Alpha-Ketoglutarate & Oxide) 500 mg • Potassium (from Potassium Alpha-Ketoglutarate, Citrate & Aspartate) 500 mg • Zinc (from Zinc Picolinate) 50 mg • Manganese (from Manganese Gluconate) 10 mg • Copper (from Copper Gluconate) 2 mg • Iodine (from Potassium Iodide) 150 mcg • Selenium (from Selenomethionine & Selenate‹50/50 mixture) 200 mcg • Chromium (from Chromic Fuel patented Chromium Picolinate) 400 mcg • Molybdenum (from natural Molybdic Acid) 150 mcg.

Vita Male - Nutri-Quest
Each tablet contains: Yohimbe bark 250 mg • Damiana 40 mg • Gotu Kola 25 mg • Hawthorne berries 25 mg • Beet root.

Vita-Bear Children's Chewables - The Vitamin Shoppe
Each tablet contains: Vitamin C 200 mg • Citrus Bioflavonoid Complex 20 mg. Naturally flavored with freeze-dried fruit juices. No yeast, corn, wheat, sucrose, salt, starch, soy, gluten, milk, eggs, dairy, fish or animal derivatives, preservatives, artificial colors or flavors added.

VitaCardia - PhysioLogics
Three capsules contain: Vitamin B6 (as Pyridoxine HCl) 10 mg • Folic Acid 810 mcg • Vitamin B12 (as Cyanocobalamin) 510 mcg • Magnesium (as Magnesium Glycinate) 50 mg • Potassium (as

Potassium Chloride) 100 mg • Hawthorne flower, leaf (1.8% Vitexin, 10.8 mg) 600 mg • Cordyceps (7% Cordyceptic Acid, 28 mg; 0.2% Adenosine, 800 mcg) 400 mg • Taurine 200 mg.

Vitacor Plus - Matthias Rath, Inc.
Each tablet contains: Ascorbic Acid 230 mg • Ascorbyl Palmitate 170 mg • Calcium Ascorbate 100 mg • Magnesium Ascorbate 100 mg • Vitamin E (d-Alpha-Tocopherol) 130 IU • Vitamin A (Beta-Carotene) 1665 IU • Vitamin B1 (Thiamine) 7 mg • Vitamin B2 (Riboflavin) 7 mg • Niacin 10 mg • Niacinamide 35 mg • Pantothenic Acid (d-Calcium Pantothenate) 40 mg • Vitamin B6 (Pyridoxal Phosphate) 10 mg • Vitamin B12 (Cyanocobalamin) 20 mcg • Vitamin D (as Vitamin D3) (Cholecalciferol) 130 IU • Folic Acid 90 mcg • Biotin 65 mcg • L-Proline 110 mg • L-Lysine 110 mg • L-Carnitine 35 mg • L-Arginine 40 mg • L-Cysteine 35 mg • Calcium (Glycinate, Ascorbate) 35 mg • Magnesium (Glycinate, Ascorbate) 40 mg • Potassium (Chelate) 20 mg • Zinc (Glycinate) 7 mg • Manganese (Chelate) 1.3 mg • Copper (Glycinate) 330 mcg • Selenium (L-Seleno Methionine) 20 mcg • Chromium (Glycinate) 10 mcg • Molybdenum (Glycinate) 4 mcg • Inositol 35 mg • Coenzyme Q10 7 mg • Phosphorous (Dicalcium Phosphate) 15 mg • Pycnogenol 7 mg • Citrus Bioflavonoids 100 mg • Vitamin E (Beta, Gamma & Delta Tocopherols) 22 mg • Carotenoids [Alpha-Carotene, Lutein, Zeaxanthin, & Cryptoxanthin] 50 mcg.

Vital Green - Futurebiotics
Ten tablets contain: Alfalfa leaf juice powder concentrate 1350 mg • Barley grass juice powder concentrate 100 mg • Wheat Grass juice powder concentrate 250 mg • Spirulina powder 150 mg • Chlorella powder (broken cell) 150 mg. Other ingredients: Dicalcium phosphate, Cellulose, Magnesium stearate, Vegetable stearate, Silica.

Vital K + Ginseng Capsules - Futurebiotics
Potassium • Calcium • Magnesium • 16 Herbal extracts Plus the Triple Ginseng Action of Korean, Siberian & American Ginseng.

Vital K + Ginseng Extra - Futurebiotics
Siberian, Korean, & American Ginseng • "16 Invigorating Herbal extracts" • Potassium • Calcium & Iron found in the Original Vital K.

Vital K Original with Magnesium - Futurebiotics
Potassium • Magnesium • Calcium • Iron & "17 Herbal extracts," including the major Chinese adaptogenic herbs: (Ginseng, Astragalus, Schizandra & Dong Quai).

Vital Vein - Puritan's Pride
Three capsules contain: Vitamin A 10,000 IU • Vitamin C 250 mg • Vitamin E 100 IU • Magnesium 100 mg • Zinc 3 mg • Selenium 0.42 mcg • Grape Seed extract 15 mg • Gotu Kola herb (centella asiatica) 800 mg • Lecithin 200 mg • Butchers' Broom herb (Ruscus aculeatus) 400 mg • Rutin 125 mg • Spirulina 100 mg • White Oak Bark (Quercus alba) 75 mg • Ginkgo Biloba leaf (Ginkgo biloba) 100 mg • Kelp 100 mg • Bromelain 50 mg • Ginger root (Zingiber officinate) 50 mg • Hawthorn berry (Crataegus laevigata) 50 mg.

Vitaline CoQ10 - 100 mg - Chocolate Flavor - PhytoPharmica
Each chewable wafer contains: Vitamin E (as dl-alpha tocopheryl acetate, d-alpha tocopheryl acetate, and mixed tocopherals) 300 IU • Coenzyme Q10 (CoQ10; Ubiquinone) certified by Assay 100 mg.

Vitaline CoQ10 - 100 mg - Maple Nut Flavor - PhytoPharmica
Each chewable wafer contains: Vitamin E (as dl-alpha tocopheryl acetate, d-alpha tocopheryl acetate, and mixed tocopherols) 300 IU • Coenzyme Q10 (CoQ10; Ubiquinone) certified by Assay 100 mg.

Vitaline CoQ10 - 200 mg - Chocolate Flavor - PhytoPharmica
Each chewable wafer contains: Vitamin E (as dl-alpha tocopheryl acetate, d-alpha tocopheryl acetate, and mixed tocopherols) 400 IU • Coenzyme Q10 (CoQ10; Ubiquinone) certified by Assay 200 mg.

Vitaline CoQ10 - 200 mg - Maple Nut Flavor - PhytoPharmica
Each chewable wafer contains: Vitamin E (as dl-alpha tocopheryl acetate, d-alpha tocopheryl acetate, and mixed tocopherols) 400 IU • Coenzyme Q10 (CoQ10; Ubiquinone) certified by Assay 200 mg.

Vitaline CoQ10 - 60 mg - Chocolate Flavor - PhytoPharmica
Each chewable wafer contains: Vitamin E (as dl-alpha tocopheryl acetate, d-alpha tocopheryl acetate, and mixed tocopherols) 180 IU • Coenzyme Q10 (CoQ10; Ubiquinone) certified by Assay 60 mg.

Vitaline CoQ10 - 60 mg - Maple Nut Flavor - PhytoPharmica
Each chewable wafer contains: Vitamin E (as dl-alpha tocopheryl acetate, d-alpha tocopheryl acetate, and mixed tocopherols) 180 IU • Coenzyme Q10 (CoQ10; Ubiquinone) certified by Assay 60 mg.

Vitaliza - HerbaSway
Horny Goat Weed • Dong Quai • He Sho Wu • Panax Ginseng • Knotweed • Schisandra • Blackberry • HerbaSwee (Cucurbitaceae fruit).

Vita-Min - Puritan's Pride
Six tablets contain: Vitamin A (as Retinyl Acetate and Beta Carotene) 7,650 IU • Vitamin D (as Cholecalciferol) 200 IU • Vitamin C (as Ascorbic Acid) 200 mg • Vitamin E (as d-Alpha Tocopheryl Acid Succinate) 10 IU • Thiamin (Vitamin B-1; as Thiamine Hydrochloride) 6 mg • Riboflavin (Vitamin B-2) 12 mg • Niacin 3 mg • Vitamin B-6 (as Pyridoxine Hydrochloride) 2 mg • Folic Acid 400 mcg • Vitamin B-12 (as Cyanocobalamin) 5 mcg • Biotin (as D-Biotin) 5 mcg • Pantothenic Acid (as D-Calcium Pantothenate) 0.12 mg • Calcium (as Dicalcium Phosphate) 800 mg • Iron (as Ferrous Gluconate) 14 mg • Phosphorus (as Dicalcium Phosphate) 600 mg • Iodine (as Potassium Iodide) 100 mcg • Magnesium (as Magnesium Oxide) 50 mg • Zinc (as Zinc Sulfate) 0.022 mg • Selenium (as Sodium Selenate) 70 mcg • Copper (as Copper Sulfate) 0.022 mg • Manganese (as Manganese Sulfate) 0.0042 mg • Potassium (as Potassium Chloride and Potassium Iodide) 0.0574 mg • Silicon (as Silicon Dioxide) 0.097 mcg • Boron (as Sodium Borate Decahydrate) 300 mcg • PABA (Para-Aminobenzoic Acid) 37.5 mg • Choline Bitartrate 5.25 mg • Inositol 10 mg • Alfalfa 40 mg • L-Lysine 10 mg • Methionine 1.25 mg • Leucine 4.5 mg • Cysteine 1.25 mg • Isoleucine 4.5 mg • Phenylalanine 2.6 mg • Arginine 1.93 mg • Histidine 1.09 mg • Threonine 2.08 mg • Valine 3.16 mg • Wheat Germ powder 60 mg • Papain 20 mg • Chlorophyll 10 mg • Citrus Bioflavonoid 30 mg • Wheat Germ oil 20 mg • Peppermint leaves 20 mg • Ginkgo Biloba leaf 30 mg • Coenzyme Q-10 30 mcg • Ginseng 12 mg • Deodorized Garlic 12 mg • Echinacea Purpurea 24 mg • Spirulina 12 mg • Chlorella 12 mg • Klamath Lake Blue Green Algae 12 mg • Grapeseed extract complex 200 mcg. In a natural base of Watercress, Parsley, Kelp, and Lecithin.

Vitamin & Aloe Mosturizing Creme - Aspen Group, Inc.
Each gram contains: Tocopheryl Acetate 1% • Panthenol 1% • Water • Hydrogenated Polyisobutane • Octyl Methoxycinnamate • Mineral Oil • Ceteraryl Alcohol • Cetyl Phosphate • Dimethicone • Aloe Vera Gel • Aminomethyl Propanol • Fragrance • Carbomer • Propylene Glycol • Diazolidinyl Urea • Methylparaben • Propylparaben.

Vitamin A - Puritan's Pride
Each softgel contains: Vitamin A (as derived from fish liver oils) 10,000 IU.

Vitamin A - Jamieson
Each capsule contains: Vitamin A (from Halibut liver oil) 10000 IU.

Vitamin A - Nature's Bounty
Each softgel contains: Vitamin A (from Fish Liver Oils) 10000 IU.
Other Ingredients: Soybean Oil, Gelatin, Glycerin.

Vitamin A - Nature's Way
Each softgel contains: Vitamin A (cod liver oil) 10,000 IU. Other Ingredients: Gelatin, Glycerin, Soybean Oil, Water.

Vitamin A - In Water Soluble Base - Nature's Bounty
Each softgel contains: Vitamin A (as Retinyl Palmitate) 10000 IU. Other Ingredients: Polysorbate 80, Gelatin, Glycerin, Propylene Glycol.

Vitamin A & D - Health Smart Vitamins
Each softgel contains: Vitamin A (from cod liver oil) 10,000 IU • Vitamin D (from cod liver oil) 400 IU.

Vitamin A & D - Nature's Bounty
Each tablet contains: Vitamin A (as Retinyl Palmitate) 10000 IU • Vitamin D (as Cholecalciferol) 400 IU. Other Ingredients: Dicalcium Phosphate, Cellulose, Calcium Sulfate, Vegetable Stearic Acid, Cellulose Coating, Vegetable Magnesium Stearate, Silica.

Vitamin A Retinyl Palmitate Wrinkle Treatment - Derma E
Vitamin A 10000 IU/100 gm, Vitamin E, Vitamin D, Allantoin.

Vitamin B 100 Complex - Jamieson
Each caplet contains: Thiamin (as Thiamine Mononitrate) 100 mg • Riboflavin (Vitamin B2) 100 mg • Niacin (as Niacinamide) 100 mg • Vitamin B6 (as Pyridoxine Hydrochloride) 100 mg • Folate (as Folic Acid) 400 mcg • Vitamin B12 (as Cyanocobalamin) 100 mcg • Biotin 100 mcg • Pantothenic Acid (as Calcium D-Pantothenate) 100 mg • Calcium 555 mg • Choline Bitartrate 100 mg • Inositol 100 mg.

Vitamin B-1 - Nature's Bounty
Each tablet contains: Thiamin (as Thiamine Hydrochloride) 100 mg. Other Ingredients: Dicalcium Phosphate, Cellulose, Vegetable Stearic Acid, Silica, Vegetable Magnesium Stearate.

Vitamin B12 - Jamieson
Each tablet contains: Vitamin B12 (as Cyanocobalamin) 1200 mcg • Calcium 80 mg.

Vitamin B-12 - Leiner Health Products
Each tablet contains: Vitamin B12 (Cyanocobalamin) 100 mcg. Other Ingredients: Lactose, Starch, Dicalcium Phosphate, Magnesium Stearate, Red 40 Lake.

Vitamin B-12 - Nature's Bounty
Each tablet contains: Vitamin B-12 (as Cyanocobalamin) 100 mcg. Other Ingredients: Dicalcium Phosphate, Cellulose, Vegetable Stearic Acid, Mannitol, Silica, Vegetable Magnesium Stearate.

Vitamin B12 100 mcg - Jamieson
Each tablet contains: Vitamin B12 (Cyanocobalamin) 100 mcg.

Vitamin B-2 - Nature's Bounty
Each tablet contains: Riboflavin 100 mg. Other Ingredients: Dicalcium Phosphate, Cellulose, Vegetable Stearic Acid, Guar Gum, Croscarmellose, Silica.

Vitamin B6 - Jamieson
Each tablet contains: Vitamin B6 (as Pyridoxine Hydrochloride) 100 mg.

Vitamin B-6 - Leiner Health Products
Each tablet contains: Vitamin B6 (Pyridoxine Hydrochloride) 100 mg. Other Ingredients: Dicalcium Phosphate, Cellulose, Starch, Croscarmellose Sodium, Polyethylene Glycol 3350, Silicon Dioxide, Magnesium Stearate.

Vitamin B-6 - Nature's Bounty
Each tablet contains: Vitamin B-6 (Pyridoxine Hydrochloride) 50 mg. Other Ingredients: Dicalcium Phosphate, Cellulose, Vegetable Stearic Acid, Croscarmellose, Vegetable Magnesium Stearate, Silica.

Vitamin B-Complex - PhysioLogics
Each capsule contains: Thiamine (as Thiamine Mononitrate) 50 mg • Riboflavin 50 mg • Niacin 55 mg • Pantothenic Acid (as Calcium Pantothenate) 100 mg • Vitamin B6 (as Pyridoxine HCl) 50 mg • Vitamin B12 (as Cyanocobalamin) 50 mcg • Folic Acid 400 mcg • Biotin 300 mcg • Inositol 50 mg • Choline (Bitartrate) 50 mg • PABA 50 mg.

Vitamin C - Leiner Health Products
Each tablet contains: Vitamin C (Ascorbic Acid) 250 mg. Other Ingredients: Calcium Carbonate, Maltodextrin, Cellulose, Starch, Silicon Dioxide, Stearic Acid, Magnesium Stearate, Sodium Starch Glycolate, Croscarmellose Sodium.

Vitamin C - 1000 - Nature Made
Each tablet contains: Vitamin C 1000 mg. Other Ingredients: Ascorbic Acid, Corn Starch, Cellulose, Magnesium Stearate, Stearic Acid, Silica Gel.
See Editor's Note No. 4, page 1816.

Vitamin C - 1000 - Nature's Bounty
Each tablet contains: Vitamin C (as ascorbic acid) 1000 mg. Other ingredients: Cellulose Plant Origin, Vegetable Magnesium Stearate, Vegetable Stearic Acid, Silica.
See Editor's Note No. 4, page 1816.

Vitamin C - 1000 - PhysioLogics
Each tablet contains: Vitamin C (Ascorbic Acid) 1000 mg • Bioflavonoids lemon 30 mg.

Vitamin C - 1000 mg Capsules with Bioflavonoids - Puritan's Pride
Each capsule contains: Vitamin C 1000 mg • Bioflavonoids 30 mg.

Vitamin C - 1500 mg Tablets with Rose Hips - Puritan's Pride
Each tablet contains: Vitamin C with Rose Hips 1500 mg.

Vitamin C - 500 with Rose Hips - Windmill Health Products
Each tablet contains: Vitamin C 500 mg • Ascorbic Acid 500 mg • Rose Hips 30 mg.
See Editor's Note No. 4, page 1816.

Vitamin C - CVS - CVS
Each tablet contains: Vitamin C 500 mg. Other Ingredients: Ascorbic Acid, Starch, Cellulose, Stearic Acid, Croscarmellose Sodium, Lactose, Magnesium Stearate, Silicon Dioxide.
See Editor's Note No. 4, page 1816.

Vitamin C & Zinc Lozenges - Puritan's Pride
Each lozenge contains: Vitamin C (as Ascorbic Acid and Rose Hips) 300 mg • Zinc (as Zinc Citrate) 7 mg • Natural Food Base: Rutin, Hesperidin, Acerola, Citrus Bioflavonoids, Black Currant 15 mg.

Vitamin C + Echinacea - Leiner Health Products
Each tablet contains: Vitamin C (Ascorbic Acid) 500 mg • Echinacea (Echinacea angustifolia) herb 35 mg • Echinacea (Echinacea

BRAND NAMES

angustifolia) root 15 mg • Echinacea (Echinacea purpurea) herb 50 mg. Other Ingredients: Cellulose, Hydroxypropyl Methylcellulose, Croscarmellose Sodium, Magnesium Stearate, Silicon Dioxide, Lemon Bioflavonoids, Rose Hips, Acerola, Hesperidin, Orange Peel, Quercetin, Rutin, Polyethylene Glycol 3350.

Vitamin C 1000 - Olympian Labs
Each capsule contains: Vitamin C 1000 mg • Rose Hips 50 mg • Citrus Bioflavonoids 100 mg.

Vitamin C 1000 mg Timed Release - Jamieson
Each caplet contains: Vitamin C (as Ascorbic Acid) 1000. Other Ingredients: Rutin, Hesperidin, Lemon Bioflavonoids, Acerola, Rosehips.

Vitamin C 1000 with Rose Hips - Nature's Way
Each capsule contains: Vitamin C 1000 mg. Other Ingredients: Cellulose, Gelatin, Magnesium Stearate, Rose Hips.
See Editor's Note No. 4, page 1816.

Vitamin C 200 mg - The Vitamin Shoppe
Each tablet contains: Vitamin C 200 mg • Citrus Bioflavonoid Complex 20 mg.

Vitamin C 500 mg - Jamieson
Each tablet contains: Vitamin C (as Ascorbic Acid and Sodium Ascorbate) 500 mg • Sodium (as Sodium Ascorbate) 35 mg. Available in Chewable Orange, Grape Juice-Chewable, and Chewable Tropical Fruit flavors.

Vitamin C 500 with Bioflavonoids - Nature's Way
Two capsules contain: Citrus Bioflavonoids 600 mg • Vitamin C (ascorbic acid) 1000 mg.

Vitamin C Chewable - Leiner Health Products
Each tablet contains: Vitamin C (Ascorbic Acid) 500 mg • Sodium 40 mg • Total Carbohydrate less than 1 g • Sugars less than 1 g. Other Ingredients: Sucrose, Sodium Ascorbate, Stearic Acid, Starch, Natural Flavor, Magnesium Stearate, Silicon Dioxide, Sorbitol, Yellow 6 Lake, Lactose, Ethylmaltol.

Vitamin C Citrus Complex - Sunkist
Each tablet contains: Vitamin C 250 mg. Other Ingredients: Fructose, Sorbitol, Sucrose, Sodium Ascorbate, Ascorbic Acid, Hydrogenated Soybean Oil, Maltodextrin, Magnesium Stearate, Corn Starch, Hydrogenated Castor oil, Colloidal Silicon Dioxide, Lactose, Natural Flavors, Bioflavonoids.

Vitamin C Crystals - Puritan's Pride
Each teaspoon contains: Vitamin C 5000 mg.

Vitamin C Plex - Olympian Labs
Each capsule contains: Vitamin C (calcium ascorbate) 500 mg • Calcium (ascorbate) 55 mg • Citrus Bioflavonoid Complex 50 mg • Hesperidin 25 mg • Rutin 20 mg • Ascorbyl Palmitate 10 mg.

Vitamin C Skin Supplement Cream - Orjene
Antioxidants • Vitamin C • Ginkgo Biloba • Germanium • Chamomile.

Vitamin C Solution - Dial Herbs
Vitamin C • Vitamin B3 • Citrus bioflavonoids extract. In a base of Distilled Water, Fructose, Sorbitol, Vegetable Glycerine (kosher), Fruit flavors, Sodium Benzoate & Caramel color. Contains no fillers, binders, yeast, wheat, gluten, soy, dairy, artificial colors, or starch.

Vitamin C with Echinacea - Holista
Each tablet contains: Vitamin C 500 mg • Echinacea 100 mg.

Vitamin C, 500 mg (special) - Nature's Life
Vitamin C (Ascorbic Acid), 500 mg. In a natural base of Rose Hips Powder. Excipients: Cellulose, Magnesium stearate and Micro-Cellulose (tm) coating.

Vitamin C, Hesperidin & Mineral Powder - Wonder Foods
Two grams of powder contain: Ascorbic Acid 800 mg • Calcium Ascorbate 200 mg • Hesperidin 190 mg • Calcium Phosphate 100 mg • Magnesium Phosphate 190 mg • Zinc Sulfate Monohydrate 2.9 mg.

Vitamin C-1000 mg Tablets with Rose Hips - Puritan's Pride
Each tablet contains: Vitamin C with Rose Hips 1000 mg.

Vitamin C-500 mg Softgels with Rose Hips - Puritan's Pride
Each softgel contains: Vitamin C with Rose Hips 500 mg. Other Ingredients: Soybean Oil, Gelatin, Lecithin, Beeswax, St. John's Bread extract, Caramel Color.

Vitamin C-500 mg Tablets with Rose Hips - Puritan's Pride
Each tablet contains: Vitamin C with Rose Hips 500 mg.

Vitamin D - Puritan's Pride
Each tablet contains: Vitamin D 400 IU.

Vitamin D 1000 IU - Jamieson
Each tablet contains: Vitamin D (as Cholecaliciferol) 1000 IU • Calcium (as Dicalcium Phosphate) 20 mg • Peanut oil.

Vitamin E - Nature's Way
Each softgel contains: Vitamin E (d-alpha tocopheryl) 400 IU. Other Ingredients: Gelatin.
See Editor's Note No. 13, page 1817.

Vitamin E - drugstore.com
Each softgel contains: Vitamin E (dl-Alpha Tocopheryl Acetate) 400 IU. Other Ingredients: Gelatin, Glycerin, Vegetable Oil.

Vitamin E - Health Smart Vitamins
Each softgel contains: Vitamin E (as 50% d-alpha tocopherol, 50% dl-alpha tocopheryl acetate) 1,000 IU.

Vitamin E - Nature Made
Each softgel contains: Vitamin E 400 IU. Other Ingredients: dl-Alpha Tocopheryl Acetate, Gelatin, Glycerin, Water.

Vitamin E - Olympian Labs
Each capsule contains: Vitamin E (d-alpha tocopherol) 400 IU. In a base of Soybean Oil or Safflower Oil.

Vitamin E - Vitamins.com
Each softgel contains: Vitamin E Complex 400 IU. Other Ingredients: Glycerin, Gelatin.

Vitamin E - 400 - PhytoPharmica
Each capsule contains: Vitamin E (natural d-alpha tocopheryl acetate) 400 IU.

Vitamin E - A&D Cream - Atrium Inc.
Three ounces contain: Vitamin E 1500 IU • Vitamin A 750 IU • Vitamin D 300 IU. In a Silicone Cream Base: Stearic Acid, Glycerol, Cetyl Alcohol, Beeswax, Apricot Kernel oil, Triethanolamine, Borax, Allantoin, Methyl Parasept.

Vitamin E & Selenium - Swanson
Each softgel contains: Vitamin E (as d-alpha tocopherol) 400 IU • Selenium (as selenomethionine) 50 mcg.

Some Brand Name Natural Products - What they Contain
www.NaturalDatabase.com contains MANY more listings than appear here.

Vitamin E 200 I.U. - Leiner Health Products
Each softgel contains: Vitamin E (dl-Alpha Tocopheryl Acetate) 200 IU. Other Ingredients: Gelatin, Glycerin, Vegetable Oil.

Vitamin E 200 IU Supplement - Jamieson
Each tablet contains: Vitamin E (as Dl-Alpha Tocopheryl Acetate) 200 IU.

Vitamin E 400IU 294mg - Nature's Sunshine
Each capsule contains: Vitamin E (d-alpha tocopherol) 294 mg (400 IU).

Vitamin E 800 I.U. - Leiner Health Products
Each softgel contains: Vitamin E (dl-Alpha Tocopheryl Acetate) 800 IU. Other ingredients: Gelatin, Glycerin.

Vitamin E Complex - Schiff
Each softgel contains: Vitamin E 400 IU.

Vitamin E Essential Skin Cream - Orjene
Vitamin E 6000 IU • Vitamin A 20000 USP units • Vitamin D 5000 USP units.

Vitamin E Oil - Orjene
6000 IU of Vitamin E and Vitamin A and Vitamin D.

Vitamin E Succinate - Life Extension
Each capsule contains: Vitamin E (as d-alpha-tocopheryl succinate) 400 IU. Other Ingredients: Magnesium Stearate, Rice Flour, Gelatin, Water.

Vitamin E Water Dispersible - Leiner Health Products
Each softgel contains: Vitamin E (dl-Alpha Tocopheryl Acetate) 400 IU. Other Ingredients: Gelatin, Polysorbate 80, Glycerin, Soybean Oil.

Vitamin for the Hair - Puritan's Pride
Each tablet contains: Calcium Pantothenate 100 mg • Choline Bitartrate 125 mg • Inositol 50 mg • Niacin (Nicotinic Acid) 35 mg • Para-Aminobenzoic Acid 30 mg • Folic Acid 0.4 mg • Cobalamin (Vitamin B12) 6 mcg • Iron (Ferrous Sulfate) 18 mg • Copper (Copper Gluconate) 2 mg • Iodine (Kelp) 0.15 mg • Manganese (Manganese Gluconate) 5 mg • Protein (from Soy Protein) 100 mg • Zinc (Zinc Gluconate) 15 mg.

Vitamin Foundation Creme - Aspen Group, Inc.
Each gram contains: Tocopheryl Acetate • Panthenol • Water • Octyldodecyl Neopetanoate • Octyl Methoxycinnmate • Cetearyl Alcohol • Cetyl Phosphate • Dimethicone • Beeswax • Carbomer • Aminomethyl Propanol • Propylene Glycol • Diazolidinyl Urea • Methylparaben • Propylparaben.

Vitamin O - R-Garden Internationale
Stabilized Oxygen in a solution of distilled water, Sodium Chloride, and trace minerals.

Vitasana - Boehringer Ingelheim Pharmaceuticals, In
Two gelcaps contain: Vitamin A (as beta carotene) 4000 IU • Vitamin C (as ascorbic acid) 120 mg • Vitamin D (as cholecalciferol) 400 IU • Vitamin E (as dl-alpha tocopheryl acetate) 30 IU • Vitamin B1 (as thiamine mononitrate) 2.4 mg • Vitamin B2 (riboflavin) 3.4 mg • Vitamin B3 (niacinamide) 30 mg • Vitamin B6 (as pyridoxine HCl) 4 mg • Folic Acid 400 mcg • Vitamin B12 (as cobalamin conc.) 2 mcg • Calcium (as calcium phosphate) 200 mg • Iron (as ferrous sulfate) 18 mg • Phosphorus (as calcium phosphate) 160 mg • Magnesium (as magnesium oxide) 20 mg • Zinc (as zinc sulfate) 2 mg • Copper (as copper sulfate) 2 mg • Manganese (as manganese sulfate) 2 mg • Standardized G115 Ginseng Extract (from Panax Ginseng, C.A. Meyer) (root) 80 mg.

Vita-Smart High Potency Vitamins and Minerals - K-mart
Each tablet contains: Vitamin A 8000 IU • Vitamin C 120 mg • Vitamin D 400 IU • Vitamin E 30 IU • Thiamin 5 mg • Riboflavin 5 mg • Niacin 30 mg • Vitamin B-6 5 mg • Folic Acid 400 mcg • Vitamin B-12 10 mcg • Biotin 10 mcg • Pantothenic Acid 10 mg • Calcium 100 mg • Iron 18 mg • Phosphorous 78 mg • Iodine 150 mcg • Magnesium 100 mg • Zinc 15 mg • Copper 2 mg • Chloride 15 mg • Potassium 15 mg.

Vita-Vim - Jamieson
Each caplet contains: Vitamin A (as Retinyl Acetate) 10000 IU • Vitamin C (as Ascorbic Acid) 150 mg • Vitamin D (as Cholecalciferol) 400 IU • Vitamin E (as Dl-Alpha Tocopheryl Acetate) 15 IU • Thiamin (as Thiamine Mononitrate) 4.5 mg • Riboflavin (Vitamin B2) 7.5 mg • Niacin (as Niacin and Nicacinamide) 65 mg • Vitamin B6 (as Pyridoxine Hydrochloride) 3 mg • Folate (as Folic Acid) 400 mcg • Vitamin B12 (as Cyanocobalamin) 14 mcg • Biotin 10 mcg • Pantothenic Acid (as Calcium D-Pantothenate) 15 mg • Calcium (as Calcium Carbonate) 130 mg • Iron (as reduced Iron) 4 mg • Iodine (as from Kelp) 100 mcg • Magnesium (as Magnesium Oxide) 100 mg • Zinc (as Zinc Gluconate) 10 mg • Selenium (from yeast) 15 mcg • Copper (as Copper Gluconate) 1 mg • Choline Bitartrate 20 mg • Inositol 20 mg • Dl-Methionine 2.2 mg.

Vita-Vitamin - Olympian Labs
Two tablets contain: Vitamin A (palmitate) 5000 IU • Vitamin B-1 (thiamine HCl) 50 mg • Vitamin B-2 (riboflavin) 80 mg • Vitamin B-3 (inositol hexanicotinate) 80 mg • Vitamin B-5 (calcium pantothenate) 80 mg • Vitamin B-6 (pyridoxine HCl) 80 mg • Vitamin B-9 (folic acid) 400 mcg • Vitamin B-12 (cyanocobalamin) 60 mcg • Vitamin C (ascorbic acid) 300 mg • Vitamin D (cholecalciferol) 400 IU • Vitamin E (d-alpha-tocopherol acetate) 100 IU • Alpha Lipoic Acid 10 mg • Betaine HCl 30 mg • Boron 100 mcg • Calcium (citrate and phosphate) 120 mg • Choline Bitartrate 50 mg • Chromium 120 mcg • Citrus Bioflavonoid Complex 30 mg • Coenzyme Q10 10 mg • d-Biotin 300 mcg • Grape Skin extract 50 mg • Hesperidin 5 mg • Inositol 50 mg • Iodine (Kelp) 150 mcg • Lutein/Zeaxanthin 3 mg • Lycopene (100 mg Yielding 5 mg Pure Lycopene) 5 mg • Magnesium (Citrate and Magnesium Oxide) 40 mg • Manganese (Amino Acid Chelate) 2 mg • Molybdenum (Amino Acid Chelate) 75 mcg • PABA 50 mg • Potassium (Amino Acid Chelate) 7 mg • Rutin 30 mg • Selenium (L-Selenomethionine) 50 mcg • Vanadium (Amino Acid Chelate) 5 mcg • Zinc (Amino Acid Chelate) 20 mg. In a Proprietary Base: Barley Grass, Echinacea purpurea, Goldenseal root, Lecithin, Parsley, Pau d' Arco, Rice Bran and Watercress.

Vitex - Puritan's Pride
Each capsule contains: Vitex (Chastetree fruit powder: Vitex agnus-castus) 400 mg.

Vitex - Pharmanex
Each capsule contains: Vitex fruit 20:1 extract 175 mg. Other Ingredients: Rice flour, Gelatin.

Vitex Extract - PhytoPharmica
Each capsule contains: Chaste Tree (Vitex agnus-castus) berry extract (standardized to contain a minimum of 0.5% agnuside [1,130 mcg per capsule]) 225 mg.

Vit-Min 100+ - Now
Each tablet contains: Vitamin A (6 mg Beta-Carotene) 10000 IU • Vitamin A (Acetate) 10000 IU • Vitamin B1 (Thiamine HCL) 100 mg • Vitamin B2 (Riboflavin) 100 mg • Vitamin B3 (Niacinamide) 100 mg • Vitamin B5 (Pantothenic Acid) 100 mg • Vitamin B6 (Pyridoxine HCL) 100 mg • Vitamin B12 (Cyanocobalamin) 100 mcg • Biotin 100 mcg • Folic Acid 400 mcg • Vitamin C (Calcium Ascorbate) 250 mg • Vitamin D (Calciferol) 400 IU • Vitamin E (d-Alpha Tocopheryl Succinate) 150 IU • Calcium (Ascorbate,

BRAND NAMES

BRAND NAMES

Carbonate) 50 mg • Magnesium (Oxide • Amino Acid Chelate) 30 mg • Zinc (Amino Acid Chelate) 15 mg • Copper (Amino Acid Chelate) 500 mcg • Iodine (Kelp) 150 mcg • Iron (Amino Acid Chelate) 10 mg • Potassium 10 mg • Manganese (Amino Acid Chelate) 5 mg • Selenium (Amino Acid Chelate) 25 mcg • Chromium (Yeast-free GTF) 100 mcg • Molybdenum (Amino Acid Chelate) 50 mcg • Boron (Amino Acid Chelate) 500 mcg • Vanadium (Amino Acid Chelate) 50 mcg • Choline (Bitartrate) 100 mg • Inositol 100 mg • PABA 50 mg • Rutin 25 mg • Betaine (HCL) 25 mg • Glutamic Acid 25 mg • Spirulina 50 mg • Barley grass organic 50 mg • Citrus Bioflavonoids (40% Hesperidin) 25 mg • Psyllium husk fiber 25 mg. This timed release multiple is formulated in a base of 72 Trace Minerals, Dicalcium Phosphate, Cellulose, Stearic Acid, Silica & natural vegetable protein coating.

Vit-Min 75+ - Now
Each tablet contains: Vitamin A (natural Fish Liver oil) 10000 IU • Beta-Carotene (6 mg) 10000 IU • Vitamin B1 (Thiamine HCL) 75 mg • Vitamin B2 (Riboflavin) 75 mg • Vitamin B3 (Niacinamide) 75 mg • Vitamin B5 (Pantothenic Acid) 75 mg • Vitamin B6 (Pyridoxine HCL) 75 mg • Vitamin B12 (Cyanocobalamin) 100 mcg • Biotin 100 mcg • Folic Acid 400 mcg • Vitamin C (Ascorbic Acid) 250 mg • Vitamin D (natural Fish Liver oil) 400 IU • Vitamin E (100% d-Alpha) 150 IU • Calcium (Amino Acid Chelate, Oystershell) 100 mg • Magnesium (Oxide, Amino Acid Chelate) 60 mg • Zinc (Amino Acid Chelate) 15 mg • Copper (Amino Acid Chelate) 1 mg • Iodine (Kelp) 150 mcg • Iron (Amino Acid Chelate) 10 mg • Choline (Bitartrate) 100 mg • Inositol 75 mg • PABA 30 mg • Rutin 25 mg • Citrus Bioflavonoids (40%) 100 mg • Betaine (HCL) 25 mg • Glutamic Acid 25 mg • Potassium (Amino Acid Chelate) 10 mg • Manganese (Amino Acid Chelate) 5 mg • Selenium (Amino Acid Chelate) 25 mcg • Chromium (Yeast-free GTF) 50 mcg • Boron (Amino Acid Chelate) 500 mcg • Molybdenum (Amino Acid Chelate) 50 mcg • Nucleic Acid 50 mg. In a natural base containing Alfalfa, Parsley, Rice polishings, Lecithin & Rose Hips, Dicalcium Phosphate, Cellulose, Stearic Acid & Silica. Contains no sugar, salt, starch, yeast, wheat, corn, soy, milk or preservatives.

Vitox - Pharmanex
Two capsules contain: Vitamin A (Vitamin A Palmitate) 3750 IU • Beta-Carotene (Beta-Carotene, Spirulina Pacifica) 6250 IU • Vitamin C (Calcium Ascorbate Complex-Ester-C, Acorbyl Palmitate) 250 mg • Vitamin D (as Vitamin D3) (Cholecalciferol) 200 IU • Vitamin E (d-Alpha Tocopheryl Succinate, Beta, Gamma, Delta Tocopherols) 150 IU • Vitamin K (Phylloquinone) 35 mcg • Thiamin (Thiamine Mononitrate) 1.5 mg • Riboflavin (Riboflavin, Riboflavin-5-Phosphate) 1.7 mg • Niacin (Niacinamide Ascorbate) 20 mg • Vitamin B6 (Pyridoxine Hydrochloride, Pyridoxal-5-Phosphate) 2 mg • Folate (Folic Acid) 200 mcg • Vitamin B12 (Cyanocobalamin, Dibencozide) 6 mg • Biotin (Biotin) 150 mcg • Pantothenic Acid (d-Calcium Pantothenate) 25 mg • Calcium (Calcium Carbonate, Calcium Citrate, Calcium Chelate) 250 mg • Iron (Iron Chelate) 3 mg • Magnesium (Magnesium Oxide, Magnesium Citrate, Magnesium Chelate) 100 mg • Zinc (Zinc Chelate) 7.5 mg • Selenium (L-Selenomethionine) 50 mcg • Copper (Copper Chelate) 2.5 mg • Manganese (Manganese Chelate) 2.5 mg • Chromium (Chromium Chelate, Chromium Picolinate) 50 mcg • Boron (Boron) 0.5 mg • Reduced Glutathione 0.5 mg • Leucoanthocyanin (Grape Seed extract) 0.5 mg.

Vivace - Veromax International
Each tablet contains: Siberian Ginseng root 100 mg • Ginkgo Biloba leaf 37.5 mg • Jujube Dates (Zizyphi fructus) 100 mg • Isoflavones 40 mg • Proprietary Blend: Glutamic acid, L-lysine HCL, L-Alanine 175 mg. Other Ingredients: Dicalcium Phosphate, Microcrystalline Cellulose, Croscarmellose Sodium, Stearic Acid, Magnesium Stearate, Silicon Dioxide.

Vivarin - Glaxo Smith Kline
Each tablet contains: Caffeine 200 mg. Other Ingredients: Carnauba Wax, Colloidal Silicon Dioxide, FD&C Yellow #10 Lake, Dextrose,

FD&C Yellow #6 Lake, Hydroxypropyl Methylcellulose, Magnesium Stearate, Microcrystalline Cellulose, Polyethylene Glycol, Polysorbate 80, Starch, Titanium Dioxide.

Volumax - Pinnacle
Includes Colostrum 1000 mg, Super Crea-Glutide A-DS. Super Crea-Glutide tri-bonds pure Creatine Monohydrate with Glutamine Peptide and Taurine.

VP2 - AST Sports Science
Each serving contains: Calories 100 • Protein 24 g • Carbohydrates 1g • Fat 0.5 g. Ingredients: 100% Hydrolyzed "Oligopeptide" Isolated Whey Protein Fractions consisting of precision engineered Whey Protein Isolate Fractions (Beta-Lactoglobulin, Alpha-Lacalbumin, Immunoglobulin, Proteose-Peptone, Glycomacropeptides (GMP), Bovine Serum Albumin, Lactoferrin, Lactoperoxidase. Lysozyme, Relaxin, Lactollin, & Beta-Microglobulin), natural & artificial Flavors & Aspartame.

VPS Coriolus versicolor - JHS Natural Products
Each capsule contains: Coriolus extract 625 mg.

VS-10 Vanadyl Sulfate - Optimum Nutrition
Each tablet contains: Vanadyl Sulfate 10 mg.

VyoPro - AST Sports Science
Each serving contains: Fat-Free Whey Protein (L-Glutamine & B Vitamins) 18 g • Calories 82 • Protein 18 g • Carbohydrates 3 g • Fat per serving 1 g. Ingredients: 100% cool processed, (partially digested) "amino-specific" controlled Chymotrypsin/ Trypsin Hydrolyzed CCTH (Tryptic Hydrolysate) Oligopeptide Whey Protein from "Micro Filtered" & "Stirred-Bed Reactor" Ion-Exchange Whey Protein providing the highest percentage of Oligopeptides along with Di-, Tri-, & Poly-Peptides (multi-spectrum short & long amino acid chains) with specifically tailored & precision engineered molecular weight profiles [isolate fractions 53% Beta-Lactalbumin (molecular weight - MW 18,400 - 36,800D), 24% Alpha-Lactalbumin (MW 14,200) 17% Immunoglobulin (MW 16,000-160,000D) 6% Minor Peptones {lactoferrin, lactoperoxidase, lysozyme, relaxin, lactollin, & Beta-microglobulin (MW 4,000 - 40,000D)}] • Dual Stage Glutamine Composite, consisting of low molecular weight Whey Glutamine Peptides (MW 500 - 10,000) & Microencapsulated Pure Crystalline L-Glutamine • Protein Absorption Enhancing Matrix (Cyanocobalamin, Pyridoxine HCL, Thiamin, Riboflavin, & Calcium Pantothenate) • natural Flavors • Aspartame.

Walgreens Multiple Vitamins - Walgreens
Each tablet contains: Vitamin A 5000 IU • Vitamin C 60 mg • Vitamin D 400 IU • Vitamin E 30 IU • Thiamin 1.5 mg • Riboflavin 1.7 mg • Niacin 20 mg • Vitamin B-6 2 mg • Folic Acid 400 mcg • Vitamin B-12 6 mcg • Pantothenic Acid 10 mg • Iron 18 mg.

Warm Cream - Strategic Science & Technology
Water • Choline chloride • L-Arginine • Sodium chloride • Mineral oil • Glyceryl stearate SE • Squalane • Cetyl alcohol • Magnesium chloride • Propylene glycol stearate SE • Wheat germ oil • Glyceryl stearate • Isopropyl myristate • Stearyl stearate • Polysorbate-60 • Propylene gylcol • Oleic acid • Tocopherol acetate • Collagen • Sorbitan stearate • Vitamin A • Vitamin D • Triethanolamine • O capsic • Methylparaben • Aloe vera extract • Imidazolidinyl urea • Propylparaben • BHA.

Water Balance - Nutrivention
Three tablets contain: Vitamin B6 (Pyridoxine) 150 mg • Potassium (Amino Acid Complex) 149 mg • Corn Silk (Stigmata maidis) 900 mg • Buchu (Barosma betulina) 600 mg • Elder flowers (Sambuccua canadensis nigra) 300 mg • Hydrangea (Hydrangea arborescens) 300 mg • Uva Ursi (Arctostaphylos uva ursi) 300 mg • Parsley (Petroselinum sativum) 150 mg • Samphire (Crithmum maritimum) 150 mg • Watermelon seed (Citrullus vulgaris) 150 mg.

Some Brand Name Natural Products - What they Contain
www.NaturalDatabase.com contains MANY more listings than appear here.

Water Garden Pycnogenol Skin Lotion - Quantum Health
Purified Water • Aloe Vera gel • Propylene Glycol • Hybrid Safflower Oil • Glyceryl Stearate • Stearic Acid • Octyl Palmitate • Sorbitol • Cetyl Alcohol • Tocopherol Acetate (vitamin E) • Panthenol • Allantoin • Sodium PCA • Jojoba Oil • Shea Butter • Kelp extract • Chamomile extract • Calendula extract • Lecithin • Tocopherol • Dimethicone • Triethanolamine • Methylparaben • Propylparaben • Vitamin A • Vitamin D (as Vitamin D3) • Diazolidinyl Urea • Pycnogenol • Super Oxide Dismutase.

Water Garden Pycnogenol Wrinkle Therapy Cream - Quantum Health
Deionized Water • Aloe Vera gel • Dioctyl Dodecyl Dodecane Dioate • Propylene Glycol • Dimethicone • Toccopheryl Acetate (vitamin E) • Stearic Acid • Emulsifying Wax • Cetyl Alcohol • Jojoba Oil • Pycnogenol • Lecithin • Panthenol • Allantoin • Extracts of Ginkgo Biloba • Echinacea • Chamomile • Super Oxide Dismutase SOD • Lipoderm • Glyceryl Stearate • Xanthan Gum • Triethanolamine • Methylparaben • Propylparaben • Diazolidinyl Urea • Tocopherol (Vitamin E).

Water Garden Pycnogenol+ - Quantum Health
Each tablet contains: Pycnogenol Atlantic Pine Bark extract (Pinus maritma) 30 mg • Grape Seed extract standardized 85% proanthocyanidins (Vinus vinifera) 20 mg.

Water Pill - Natrol
Two tablets contain: Vitamin B6 (as Pyridoxine HCI) 150 mg • Potassium (as Potassium Gluconate) 99 mg • Buchu extract leaf 4:1 100 mg • Parsley extract leaf 4:1 100 mg • Uva Ursi extract leaf 4:1 100 mg • Juniper extract berry 4:1 20 mg. Other ingredients: Calcium Carbonate, Mono & Di-Glycerides, Stearic Acid, Croscarmellose Sodium, Silicon Dioxide, Magnesium Stearate.

Water Pill - Puritan's Pride
Two tablets contain: Potassium (as Potassium Gluconate) 40 mg • Buchu (Barosma betulina) leaf (25 mg of Buchu leaves 4:1 extract) 100 mg • Uva Ursi (Arctostaphylos uva-ursi) leaf (33.4 mg of Uva Ursi 3:1 extract) 100 mg • Juniper (Juniperus communis) berry 20 mg • Parsley (Petroselinum crispum) leaf 100 mg.

Weight Loss Support - Amazon Support
Each capsule contains: Cha de Bugre • Carqueja • Guarana • Jurubeba • Mutamba • Picao Preto • Yerba Mate • Annatto.

Weightless Cinnamon-Spice - Traditional Medicinals
Cinnamon bark • Fennel seed • Roasted Chicory root • Uva Ursi leaf • Cleavers Herb • Flax seed • Licorice root • Red Clover Top • Clove stem • Star Anise seed • Hibiscus flower • Buchu leaf • natural flavors.

Weightless Cranberry - Traditional Medicinals
Contains: Hibiscus flower • Roasted Chicory root • Fennel seed • Red Clover top • Uva Ursi leaf • Parsley leaf • Cleavers herb • Cranberry • Other natural flavors.

Weightless Tea - Traditional Medicinals
Contains: Fennel seed • Hibiscus flower • Lemongrass leaf • Uva Ursi leaf • Lemon Verbena leaf • Flax seed • Spearmint leaf • Cleavers herb • Red Clover top • Parsley leaf • Buchu leaf • Natural flavors.

Welah Mide - Shawnee Moon
Buchu leaf • Red Clover • Saw Palmetto • Uva Ursi.

Wellness Cell Response - Source Naturals
Each capsule contains: Polyvalent Transfer Factor (as colostral fraction with minimum 20 potency units) 5 mg.

Wellness Formulas - Source Naturals
Three tablets contain: Vitamin A (Palmitate 4000 IU, Beta Carotene 1000 IU) 5000 IU • Vitamin C (Ascorbic Acid, and Zinc, Calcium, and Magnesium Ascorbates) 1075 mg • Calcium (Ascorbate) 7.5 mg • Copper (Sebacate) 300 mcg • Magnesium (Ascorbate) 3.8 mg • Selenium (Sodium Selenite) 25 mcg • Zinc (Ascorbate) 23 mg • Propolis 324 mg • Propolis extract 126 mg • Garlic clove 360 mg • Boneset leaf 328 mg • Polygonum Odoratum 200 mg • Echinacea root 196 mg • Echinacea extract 164 mg • Isatis (root and leaf) 159 mg • Horehound stems 150 mg • Bioflavonoids 120 mg • Astragalus root 90 mg • Angelica Archangelica root 87 mg • Mullein leaf 80 mg • Goldenseal root 75 mg • Siberian Ginseng root 66 mg • Hawthorn berry 55 mg • Oregon Grape root 55 mg • Siberian Ginseng extract 54 mg • Pau d'Arco extract 36 mg • Cayenne fruit 30 mg.

Wellness Source - HealthWatchers System
Vitamin A • Vitamin D • Vitamin E • Vitamin C • Vitamin B6 • Vitamin B2 • Vitamin B1 • Vitamin B12 • Vitamin U • Bioflavonoids • Choline Bitartrate • Niacin-Niacinamide • Pantothenic Acid • Inositol • Rutin • Papain • PABA • Lecithin • Quercetin • RNA • Hesperidin • DNA • CoQ10 • Folic Acid • Octacosanol • Biotin • Magnesium • Calcium • Zinc • Boron • Potassium • Manganese • Copper • Iodine (Kelp) • Selenium • Chromium.

Wellness Source Booster - HealthWatchers System
Beta Carotene • Vitamin E • Vitamin C • Calcium • Magnesium • Choline • Potassium • Silica • Niacinamide.

Wheat Grass - Pines International
Seven tablets (or 1 teaspoon of powder) contain: Protein 860 mg • Chlorophyl 18.5 mg • Biotin 4 mcg • Choline 5 mg • Lutein 1 mg • Lycopene 29 mcg • Vitamin A (beta-carotene) 1668 IU • Vitamin B-1 (thiamine) 11 mcg • Vitamin B-2 (riboflavin) 260 mcg • Vitamin B-3 (niacin) 252 mcg • Vitamin B-5 (pantothenic acid) 36 mcg • Vitamin B-6 (pyridoxine) 39 mcg • Vitamin B-8 (folic acid) 21 mcg • Vitamin B-12 (cobalamin) .05 mcg • Vitamin C 7.5 mg • Vitamin E 320 mcg • Vitamin K 35 mcg • Zeaxanthin 279 mcg • Calcium 15 mg • Cobalt 1.7 mcg • Copper 17 mcg • Iodine 8 mcg • Iron 870 mcg • Magnesium 3.9 mcg • Manganese 240 mcg • Phosphorus 14 mg • Potassium 137 mg • Selenium 3.5 mcg • Sodium 1 mg • Sulfur 10.5 mg • Zinc 62 mcg • Alanine 69 mg • Arginine 66 mg • Aspartic Acid 50 mg • Cystine 11 mg • Glutamic Acid 76 mg • Glycine 49 mg • Histidine 18 mg • Isoleucine 35 mg • Leucine 72 mg • Lysine 38 mg • Methionine 18 mg • Phenylalanine 36 mg • Proline 46 mg • Serine 31 mg • Threonine 42 mg • Tryptophan 6 mg • Tyrosine 33 mg • Valine 48 mg.

Whey Protein - Sports Nutrition Source.com
Each scoop contains: Sodium 50 mg • Potassium 75 mg • Protein 16 g.

White Willow Bark Extract - Nature's Way
Each capsule contains: White Willow Bark 250 mg • White Willow Bark, dried extract 200 mg. Other Ingredients: Gelatin.

Wild Brazilian SUMA-750 - Nature's Plus
Each capsule contains: Wild Brazilian SUMA (Pfaffia paniculata [Martius] Kuntze) 750 mg. Naturally rich in the 6 Saponins, Pfaffosides A,B,C,D,E & F - average 6%; 100% pure. Contains no yeast, wheat, corn, soy, milk, salt, sugar or starch.

Wild Cherry Syrup - Dial Herbs
Wild Cherry bark • Cubeb berry • Mullein • Skunk Cabbage • Lobelia • Honey • Clove.

Wild Cherry Virtue - Blessed Herbs
Wild Cherry bark • Plantain leaf • Mullein leaf • Mullein flower • Licorice root • Black Cherry concentrate.

BRAND NAMES

Some Brand Name Natural Products - What they Contain
www.NaturalDatabase.com contains MANY more listings than appear here.

***Wild Cherry-Slippery Elm Bark Formula* - Quest**
Each caplet contains: Wild Cherry bark powder (Prunus serotina) 60 mg • Slippery Elm bark powder (Ulmus fulva) 60 mg • Pleurisy Root powder (Asclepias tuberosa) 60 mg • Chickweed powder (Stellaria media) 40 mg • Horehound powder (Marrubium vulgare) 40 mg • Kelp powder (Fucus vesiculosus) 40 mg • Licorice root powder (Glycyrrhiza glabra) 40 mg • Mullein leaf powder (Verbascum thapsus) 40 mg • Cayenne powder (Capsicum minimum) 35 mg • Saw Palmetto berry powder (Serenoa serrulata) 15 mg. Other Ingredients: Calcium Phosphate, Microcrystalline Cellulose, Vegetable Stearin, Croscarmellose Sodium, Magnesium Stearate (vegetable source).

***Wild Rose Nerve Formula* - Dial Herbs**
Valerian root • Mistletoe • Scullcap • Hops • Lady Slipper • Passion flower.

***Wild Vites* - Nature's Life**
Each tablet contains: Vitamin A (Acetate) 5000 IU • Vitamin D3 (Cholecalciferol) 400 IU • Vitamin E (d-Alpha Tocopheryl acetate) 30 IU • Vitamin C (Ascorbic Acid) 60 mg • Vitamin B1 (Thiamine Monoitrate) 1.5 mg • Vitamin B2 (Riboflavin) 1.7 mg • Vitamin B3 (Niacinamide) 20 mg • Vitamin B5 (Pantothenic Acid) 10 mg • Vitamin B6 Pyridoxine HCI) 2 mg • Vitamin B12 (Cobalamin) 6 mcg • Folic Acid 400 mcg • Biotin 300 mg. In a natural base of low-Glycemic pure Crystalline Fructose & Sorbitol.

***Wild Yam* - Alvin Last**
Wild Yam extract • Aloe Vera gel • Soybean Oil • Stearic Acid • Cetyl Alcohol • Triethanolamine • Tocopheryl Acetate • Glycerin • Methylparaben • Propylparaben.

***Wild Yam Cream* - Youngevity**
Wild Yam root extract (Dioscorea villosa) • Aloe Vera gel • Natural Emollients and Moisturizers • Avocado oil • Oat oil • Key Lime fragrance • Chamomile (Matricaria chamomilla) • Burdock root (Arctium lappa) • Black Cohosh (Cimicifuga racemosa) • Siberian Ginseng (Eleutherococcus senticosus) • D-Alpha Tocopherol Acetate • Methylparaben • Propylparaben.

***Wild Yam Extract* - PhytoPharmica**
Two capsules contain: Wild (Mexican) Yam (Dioscorea villosa) root extract 10:1 (standardized to contain 10% diosgenin) 480 mg • Adrenal extract (freeze-dried) 200 mg • Beta-sitosterol 42 mg.

***Wild Yam Root* - Nature's Bounty**
Two capsules contain: Wild Yam root (Dioscorea Villosa) 810 mg. Other Ingredients: Cellulose, Gelatin, Vegetable Magnesium Stearate, Silica.

***Wild Yam/Dong Quai Formula* - PhysioLogics**
Each capsule contains: Wild Yam extract (6% Diosgenin, 12 mg) 200 mg • Dong Quai (1% Ligustilides, 2 mg) 200 mg • Soy bean (5% Isoflavones, 5 mg) 100 mg.

***Wild Yam-False Unicorn Virtue* - Blessed Herbs**
False Unicorn root • Black Haw bark • Wild Yam root • Lobelia • Grain alcohol & Distilled Water.

***Winter Wellness* - Now**
Two tablets contain: Vitamin A 5000 IU • Vitamin C 500 mg • Potassium 20 mg • Zinc 15 mg • Bee Propolis 200 mg • Deodorized Garlic Extract 200 mg • Ginger root 200 mg • Oregon Grape root 150 mg • Peptizyme 125 mg • Echinacea angustifolia root extract 100 mg • Elderberry extract 100 mg • Olive leaf extract 100 mg • Quercetin 100 mg • Shitake mushroom extract 100 mg • Reishi mushroom 100 mg • American Ginseng root 100 mg • Licorice root extract 100 mg • Goldenseal root 75 mg • Cayenne pepper 50 mg.

***Wobenzym N (Wobenzym-N)* - Mucos Pharma GMBH & Co**
Each tablet contains: Pancreatin 100 mg • Trypsin 24 mg • Chymotrypsin 1 mg • Bromelain 45 mg • Papain 60 mg • Rutosid 50 mg.
See Editor's Notes No. 14 and No. 18, page1817.

***Woman's Choice* - PhytoPharmica**
Three capsules contain: Vitamin A (Beta Carotene) - (Non-toxic form of Vitamin A) 16665 IU • Vitamin E (D-Alpha Tocopherol Succinate) 200 IU • Vitamin C (Ascorbic Acid) 200 mg • Magnesium L-Aspartate 150 mg • Pantothenic Acid (D-Calcium Pantothenate) 100 mg • Thiamine HCL (Vitamin B1) 50 mg • Riboflavin (Vitamin B2) 50 mg • Calcium Citrate 50 mg • Iron (Ferrous Succinate) 18 mg • Zinc (Gluconate) 15 mg • Chromium (Polynicotinate) 250 mcg • Folic Acid 100 mcg • Vitamin B12 (Cyanocobalamin) 50 mcg • Selenium (L-Selenomethionine) 50 mcg • Dong Quai extract 4:1 (Angelica sinensis) 75 mg • Licorice root extract (Glycyrrhiza glabra) 60 mg • Milk Thistle extract 50 mg (Silybum marianum) • Black Cohosh extract 4:1 (Cimicifuga racemosa) 30 mg • Chaste Tree berry extract (Vitex agnus-castus) 20 mg • Pyridoxal-5'-Phosphate 10 mg.

***Women's AM Multi* - Clinician's Choice**
Two tablets contain: Vitamin A (retinyl acetate & 26% as beta-carotene) 3900 IU • Vitamin C (ascorbic acid) 250 mg • Vitamin D (cholecalciferol) 400 IU • Vitamin E (dl-alpha tocopheryl acetate) 150 IU • Thiamin (mononitrate) 1 mg • Riboflavin 1 mg • Niacin (nianicamide) 10 mg • Vitamin B6 (pyridoxine hydrochloride) 2 mg • Folate (folic acid) 250 mg • Vitamin B12 (cyanocobalamin) 4 mcg • Biotin 200 mcg • Pantothenic Acid (d-calcium pantothenate) 5 mg • Calcium (carbonate, amino acid chelate, ascorbate, aspartate, citrate, gluconate) 220 mg • Iron (amino acid chelate) 12 mg • Iodine (potassium iodide) 76 mcg • Magnesium (oxide, amino acid chelate) 9 mg • Zinc (oxide, amino acid chelate, gluconate) 8 mg • Selenium (selenomethionine) 100 mcg • Copper (amino acid chelate) 1 mg • Manganese (amino acid chelate) 3 mg • Potassium (chloride, amino acid chelate) 12 mg • Chromium (nicotrate, picolinate, chelavite, amino acid chelate) 40 mcg • Molybdenum (amino acid chelate) 4 mcg • RoseOx (patented, standardized process for an extract of Rosemary) 60 mg • Citrus Bioflavonoid Complex 10 mg • Dong Quai 10 mg • Wild Yam 10 mg • Black Currant 10 mg • Red Raspberry Leaf 10 mg • Proprietary blend 12 mg: Panax Ginseng Extract, Schizandra Fruit, Echinacea Angustifolia, Grape Powder, Bee Pollen, Cruciferex.

***Women's Cycle Multivitamins* - Leiner Health Products**
Each caplet contains: Iron (Ferrous Fumarate) 15 mg • Vitamin K (Phytonadione) 65 mcg • Folate (Folic Acid) 300 mcg • Biotin 200 mcg • Molybdenum (Sodium Molybdate) 38 mcg • Niacin (Niacinamide) 8.5 mg • Calcium 160 mg • Vitamin B6 (Pyrodoxine Hydrochloride) 3 mg • Vitamin E (dl-Alpha Tocopheryl Acetate) 45 IU • Riboflavin (Vitamin B2) 2.5 mg • Selenium 100 mcg • Thiamin Mononitrate(Vitamin B1) 2 mg • Magnesium Oxide 50 mg • Phosphorus 124 mg • Chromium Chloride 120 mcg • Copper (Cupric Oxide) 2 mg • Iodine 10 mcg • Manganese Sulfate 2 mg • Pantothenic Acid (d-Calcium Pantothenate)10 mg • Vitamin A Acetate 5000 IU • Vitamin B12 (Cyanocobalamin - USP Mehtod 2) 6 mcg • Vitamin C (Ascorbic Acid) 60 mg • Vitamin D (Ergocalciferol) 400 IU • Zinc Oxide 15 mg • Borage Oil complex (Borage officinalis) (seed) (Standardized to 10% GLA) 25 mg • Chloride 18 mg • Isoflavones (Soy extract) 5 mg • Kelp (Macrocystis pyrifera) (frond) 5 mg • Lecithin powder (Glycine max) (bean) 20 mg • Nickel (Nickelous Sulfate) 5 mcg • Potassium Chloride 20 mg • Silicon Dioxide 2 mg • Tin (Stannous Chloride) 10 mcg • Trace Mineral complex 5 mg • Vanadium (Sodium Metavandate) 10 mcg. Other Ingredients: Dicalcium Phosphate, Cellulose, Gelatin, Stearic Acid, Croscarmellose Sodium, Hydroxypropyl Methylcellulose, Titanium Dioxide, Red Raspberry Powder, Dextrin, Maltodextrin, Mannitol, Hydroxypropyl Cellulose, Polyethylene Glycol, Kelp Powder, Trace Mineral Complex, Starch, Polysorbate 80, Chromium Chloride, Blue 1 Lake, Red 40 Lake, Dextrose.

Women's Daily Pack - YourLife/Leiner Health Products

Each packet contains: Vitamin A (Acetate) 2500 IU • Vitamin A (Beta Carotene) 5000 IU • Vitamin C (Ascorbic Acid) 120 mg • Vitamin D (Ergocalciferol) 200 IU • Vitamin E (dl-Alpha Tocopheryl Acetate) 230 IU • Vitamin K (Phytonadione) 10 mcg • Vitamin B1 (Thiamine Mononitrate) 2 mg • Vitamin B2 (Riboflavin) 3 mg • Niacin (Niacinamide) 20 mg • Vitamin B6 (Pyridoxine HCl) 2 mg • Folate (Folic Acid) 400 mcg • Vitamin B12 (Cyanocobalamin) 3 mcg • Biotin (d-Biotin) 30 mcg • Pantothenic Acid (d-Calcium Pantothenate) 10 mg • Calcium (Oyster Shell, Calcium Carbonate, Calcium Phosphate) 725 mg • Iron (Ferrous Fumarate) 4 mg • Phosphorus (Calcium Phosphate) 50 mg • Iodine (Potassium Iodide) 100 mcg • Magnesium (Magnesium Oxide) 100 mg • Zinc (Zinc Oxide) 20 mg • Selenium (Selenium Amino Acid Chelate) 30 mcg • Copper (Copper Oxide) 3 mg • Manganese (Manganese Sulfate) 4 mg • Chromium (Chromium Amino Acid Chelate) 20 mcg • Molybdenum (Molybdenum Amino Acid Chelate) 25 mcg • Chloride (Potassium Chloride) 36 mg • Evening Primrose oil (Evening Primrose Seed) 500 mg. 7 day iron strip contains: Iron (Ferrous Sulfate) 18 mg. Contains no added yeast. Contains colors: Titanium Dioxide, Yellow 6 Lake, Red 40 Lake, Blue 2 Lake.

Women's Exclusive Formula - Puritan's Pride

Two tablets contain: Vitamin A 5,000 IU • Vitamin C 60 mg • Vitamin D 400 IU • Vitamin E (as d-Alpha Tocopheryl Acetate) 30 IU • Thiamin (Vitamin B-1) 26.7 mg • Riboflavin (Vitamin B-2) 30 mg • Niacin 30 mg • Vitamin B-6 24.6 mg • Folic Acid 400 mcg • Vitamin B-12 100 mcg • Biotin 30 mcg • Pantothenic Acid 30 mg • Calcium 500 mg • Iron 15 mg • Phosphorus 30 mg • Iodine 150 mcg • Magnesium 250 mg • Zinc 15 mg • Selenium 25 mcg • Copper 0.5 mg • Manganese 5 mg • Chromium 25 mcg • Molybdenum 25 mcg • Potassium 11.5 mg • Inositol 30 mg • Choline Bitartrate 30 mg • PABA (Para-Aminobenzoic Acid) 30 mg • Citrus Bioflavonoids 25 mg • Betaine Hydrochloride 25 mg • L-Cysteine 50 mg • Dong Quai 50 mg • Rose Hips 6 mg.

Women's Formula 1 - Rexall

Two tablets contain: Vitamin C 67 mg • Vitamin D (as cholecalciferol) 67 IU • Vitamin B-6 (as pyridoxine HCl) 3.3 mg • Folic Acid 100 mcg • Vitamin B-12 (as cyanocobalamin) 3.3 mcg • Calcium (as calcium carbonate, calcium citrate and calcium gluconate) 333 mg • Iron (as carbonyl iron) 3 mg • Magnesium (as magnesium gluconate and magnesium oxide) 133 mg • Zinc (as zinc gluconate) 3.3 mg • Selenium (as sodium selenate) 16.7 mcg • Copper (as copper gluconate) 0.17 mg • Manganese (as manganese sulfate) 5 mg • Molybdenum (as sodium molybdate) 16.7 mcg • Potassium (as potassium chloride) 35 mg • Boron (as potassium borate and sodium borate) 16.7 mcg • Silica 7 mg • Phytonutrient Vegetable Blend (Broccoli, Carrot, Spinach, Tomato) 40 mg. Other Ingredients: Cellulose, Croscarmellose Sodium, Hydroxypropyl Methylcellulose, Magnesium Stearate, PEG.

Women's Formula 2 - Rexall

Two tablets contain: Vitamin C 33 mg • Vitamin D (as cholecalciferol) 67 IU • Vitamin K (as phytonadione) 3.3 mcg • Vitamin B-6 (as pyridoxine HCl) 3.3 mg • Folic Acid 33.3 mcg • Vitamin B-12 (as cyanocobalamin) 6.7 mcg • Calcium (as calcium carbonate, calcium citrate and calcium gluconate) 400 mg • Iodine (as potassium iodide) 16.7 mcg • Magnesium (as magnesium gluconate and magnesium oxide) 150 mg • Zinc (as zinc gluconate) 1.7 mg • Selenium (as sodium selenate) 16.7 mcg • Copper (as copper gluconate) 0.1 mg • Manganese (as manganese sulfate) 5 mg • Molybdenum (as sodium molybdate) 16.7 mcg • Potassium (as potassium chloride) 35 mg • Boron (as potassium borate and sodium borate) 16.7 mcg • Betaine (as betaine HCl) 33.3 mg • Silica 6.9 mg • Phytonutrient Vegetable Blend (Broccoli, Carrot, Spinach, Tomato) 40 mg. Other Ingredients: Cellulose, Croscarmellose Sodium, Magnesium Stearate, Hydroxypropyl Methylcellulose, PEG.

Women's Formula Plus - Rexall

Two caplets contain: Calcium 518 mg • Calcium D-Glucarate 400 mg • Women's Nutritional Blend: Flaxseed, Citrus Bioflavonoids, Red Clover (flower head), Soybean (standardized to 3.5% Isoflavones) 176 mg. Other Ingredients: Calcium Carbonate, Cellulose, Croscarmellose Sodium, Stearic Acid, Magnesium Stearate.

Women's Group Formulas Vaginal Lubricant - Transitions for Health, Inc.

Deionized Water • Glycerin • Butylene Glycol • Aloe Vera Gel • Citric Acid • Black Cohosh (Cimicifuga racemosa) Extract • Marigold (Calendula officinalis) Extract • Chamomile (Matricaria chamomilla) Extract • Ginseng (Panax ginseng) Extract • Black Walnut (Juglans nigra) Extract • d-alpha Tocopherol and Mixed Tocopherols (Vit. E) • Retinyl Palmitate • Evening Primrose (Oenothera biennis) Oil

Women's Guardian - Clinician's Choice

Two tablets contain: Vitamin B6 (pyridoxine HCl) 2 mg • Pantothenic Acid (calcium pantothenate) 50 mg • Beta-Sitosterol 300 mg • Dong Quai Herb 200 mg • Red Raspberry Leaf 160 mg • Kudzu Root 100 mg • Wild Yam 100 mg • Squaw Vine 50 mg • L-Isoleucine 40 mg • L-Leucine 40 mg • L-Valine 40 mg • Aminogen 20 mg • Black Cohosh Root 20 mg • Evening Primrose 20 mg • Lycopene (1%) 20 mg • Proprietary blend 12 mg: Lutein (5%), Chamomile Flowers, Passion Flower, Sage Leaves, Isoflavones, Grape Powder.

Women's Liberty - Traditional Medicinals

Licorice root • Orange peel • Wild Yam root • Ginger rhizome • Cinnamon bark • Dong Quai root • Clove stem • Fo Ti root • Angelica root.

Women's Mood-Enhancer - HerbaSway

St. John's Wort • Dong Quai • Rehmannia • Schisandra • Coptis • Ginkgo biloba • Cassia tora • Astragalus • Blackberry • HerbaSwee (Cucurbitaceae fruit).

Women's Nutritional System - Rainbow Light

Six tablets contain: Beta Carotene 10000 IU • Vitamin D 400 IU • Vitamin E natural 120 IU • Vitamin K 30 mcg • Thiamin (Vitamin B1) 36 mg • Riboflavin (Vitamin B2) 41 mg • Niacinamide 80 mg • Pantothenic Acid 80 mg • Pyridoxine (Vitamin B6) 48 mg • Folic Acid 800 mcg • Biotin (d-Biotin) 300 mcg • Cyanocobalamin (Vitamin B12) 144 mcg • Vitamin C 500 mg • Calcium (Amino Acid Chelate, Citrate) 200 mg • Magnesium (Amino Acid Chelate, Ascorbate, Oxide) 400 mg • Potassium (Aspartate, Chloride) 99 mg • Manganese (Amino Acid Chelate) 2.5 mg • Iron (Amino Chelate) 22.5 mg • Zinc (Picolinate) 15 mg • Copper (Amino Acid Chelate) 1 mg • GTF Chromium (Polynicotinate) 30 mcg • Selenium (l-Selenomethionine) 40 mcg • Iodine (Kelp) 150 mcg • Molybdenum (Aspartate) 50 mcg • Choline (Bitartrate) 40 mg • Inositol 40 mg • PABA (Para Aminobenzoic Acid) 30 mg • Octacosanol (Spinach) 300 mcg • Black Currant (seed) 30 mg • Bioflavonoids 250 mg • Rutin 20 mg • L-Tyrosine 20 mg • Hesperidin Complex 15 mg • Protease 3600 HUT • Amylase 282 DU • Lipase 3 LU • Cellulase 3.2 CU. Superfood & Herbal Ingredients: Bee Pollen • Spirulina • Lemon juice powder • Wheatgrass • Dong Quai • Barley Grass • Echinacea agustifolia • Reishi (Ling Chi) • Rosemary oil • Blue Cohosh 4:1) 530 mg. Custom Herbal extracts: Vitex • Red Raspberry • Mulberry • Fo-Ti • Bladderwrack • Tumeric • Peony Cistanche • Cynomorium 270 mg.

Women's PM Multi - Clinician's Choice

Two tablets provide: Vitamin A (retinyl acetate & 20% as beta-carotene) 1250 IU • Vitamin C (ascorbic acid) 250 mg • Vitamin D (cholecalciferol) 60 IU • Vitamin E (dl-alpha tocopheryl acetate) 150 IU • Thiamin (mononitrate) 0.5 mg • Riboflavin 0.7 mg • Niacin (niacinamide) 10 mg • Folate (folic acid) 200 mcg • Vitamin B12 (cyanocobalamin) 2 mcg • Biotin 150 mcg • Pantothenic Acid (d-calcium pantothenate) 5 mg • Calcium (amino acid chelate, aspartate, citrate, gluconate) 16 mg • Iron (glycinate) 6 mg • Iodine (potassium iodide) 76 mcg • Magnesium (oxide, amino acid chelate) 20 mg • Potassium (chloride, amino acid chelate, gluconate) 16 mg • Zinc (oxide, amino acid chelate, gluconate) 12 mg • Selenium (selenomethionine) 100 mcg • Copper (amino acid chelate) 1 mg • Manganese (amino acid chelate) 1 mg • Chromium (nicotinate, picolinate, chelavite, amino acid chelate) 10 mcg • Molybdenum (amino acid chelate) 2 mcg • RoseOx (patented, standardized process for an extract of Rosemary) 50 mg • Citrus Bioflavonoid Complex 10 mg • Chamomile Flower 10 mg • Passion Flower 10 mg • Valerian Root 10 mg • Mint Leaves 10 mg • Dong Quai 10 mg • Wild Yam 10 mg • Black Currant 10 mg • Red Raspberry Leaf 10 mg • Hesperidin 4 mg • Proprietary blend: Isoflavones, Echinacea, Milk Thistle Fruit, Cruciferex, Grape Powder 10 mg.

Women's Prime Multi - Swanson
Each tablet contains: Vitamin A (as beta-carotene) 3000 IU • Vitamin C (as ascorbic acid) 100 mg • Vitamin D (as cholecalciferol) 60 IU • Vitamin E (as d-alpha tocopheryl succinate) 60 IU • Thiamin USP (as thiamin HCl; Vitamin B-1) 5 mg • Riboflavin USP (Vitamin B-2) 5 mg • Niacin (as niacinamide) 5 mg • Vitamin B-6 (as pyridoxine HCl) 5 mg • Folic Acid 200 mcg • Vitamin B-12 (as cyanocobalamin) 50 mcg • Biotin 5 mcg • Pantothenic Acid (as d-calcium pantothenate) 5 mg • Calcium (50 mg from calcium citrate, 12 mg from calcium glucarate, 4 mg from calcium phytate) 66 mg • Iron (from Albion amino acid chelate) 5 mg • Iodine (from kelp) 50 mcg • Magnesium (from magnesium oxide) 30 mg • Zinc (from Albion amino acid chelate) 7.5 mg • Selenium (from Albion amino acid chelate) 100 mcg • Manganese (from Albion® amino acid chelate) 2 mg • Chromium (from Albion amino acid chelate) 25 mcg • Dong Quai powder 50 mg • Green Tea powder 50 mg • Soy powder 50 mg • IP-6 (inositol hexaphosphate)-(from calcium phytate) 25 mg • Korean Ginseng powder (5% ginsenosides) 15 mg • Black Cohosh (2.5% triterpenoids) 10 mg • Choline (as choline bitartrate) 10 mg • GLA (gamma-linolenic acid from borage) 10 mg • Inositol 10 mg • Bilberry powder (25% anthocyanidins) 5 mg • Ginkgo Biloba leaf extract (24% flavon glycosides, 6% terpene lactones) 5 mg • PABA (para-aminobenzoic acid) 5 mg • Rutin (from buckwheat) 5 mg • Coenzyme Q10 2 mg • Boron 1 mg.

Women's Stress System - Rainbow Light
Two tablets contain: Vitamin A (Beta Carotene) 250 IU • Vitamin E (d-Alpa Tocopheryl Acetate) 30 IU • Vitamin C (Ascorbic Acid) 120 mg • Magnesium (Citrate) 60 mg • Potassium (Chloride) 40 mg • Niacin-Niacinamide (Vitamin B3) 40 mg • Pantothenic Acid (Vitamin B5) 20 mg • Pyridoxine (Vitamin B6) 10 mg • Zinc (Glycinate) 8 mg • Riboflavin (Vitamin B2) 3 mg • Thiamin (Vitamin B1) 3 mcg • Copper (Glycinate) 750 mcg • Folic Acid 400 mcg • Biotin 300 mcg • Cyanocobalamin (Vitamin B12) 12 mcg • Soy extract 150 mg • Hawaiian Spirulina 70 mg • standardized to 1.5% Isoflavoids Citrus Bioflavonoids 50 mg • Wheat Grass 80 mg • 4:1 Custom Herbal extracts containing: [Siberian Ginseng (Eleuthero root), St. John's Wort herb, Kava root, Codonopsis root, Vitex berry, Lavender oil] 302 mg. Other Nutritional Ingredients: L-Glutamine 50 mg, L-Taurine 20 mg, Alpha-Lipoic Acid 25 mg, L-Methionine 15 mg, L-Tyrosine 25 mg.

Women's Support Formula - PhysioLogics
Each capsule contains: Vitamin E (as d-Alpha Tocopheryl Acetate) 50 IU • Vitamin B6 (as Pyridoxine HCl) 25 mg • Folate (Folic Acid) 200 mcg • Magnesium (as Magnesium Oxide) 100 mg • Zinc (as Zinc Glycinate) 3.75 mg • Copper (as Copper Glycinate) 0.5 mg • Black Cohosh root 100 mg • Chastetree berry (5% Vitexicarpin, 5 mg) 100 mg • Dong Quai root (0.8% Ligustilides, 0.8 mg) 100 mg • Soy bean (5% Isoflavones, 2.5 mg) 50 mg • Kava Kava root (30% Kavalactones, 7.5 mg) 25 mg.

Xenadrine RFA-1 - Cytodyne Technologies
Two capsules contain: Citrus aurantium (Bitter Orange peel standardized for 4% Synephrine) 125 mg • MaHuang (standardized for 6% Ephedrine) 335 mg • Guarana extract (standardized for 22% Caffeine) 910 mg • White Willow bark extract (standardized for 15% Salicin) 105 mg • Acetyl L-Carnitine 100 mg • L-Tyrosine 80 mg • Ginger root 50 mg • Vitamin B5 (Pathothenic Acid) 40 mg.

Xomatropin hGH Spray - ASN
Each two part formula contains: Part One: Secreatagoges • GH & IGF-1 Peptides. Part Two: Anti-Soatosatin called Revosatin (a power suppressor of an antagonistic hormone called somatosatin responsible for what is called the negative feedback loop for GH).

XTEND-LIFE Prostate - Xtend-Life Nutraceuticals Inc.
Each capsule contains: Saw Palmetto extract 160 mg • Pygeum extract 50 mg • Pumpkin Seed extract 40 mg.

XTEND-LIFE Total Balance - Xtend-Life Nutraceuticals Inc.
Each tablet contains: Amino Acid Blend: L-Arginine, Aspartic Acid, L-Glutamic Acid, L-Lysine, Glycine, Tryptophan, L-Phenylalanine, L-Serine, L-Methionine, L-Leucine, L-Isoleucine, L-Alanine, L-Proline, L-Threonine, L-Histidine 200 mg • N-Acetyl L-Tyrosine 20 mg • L-Carnitine 20 mg • L-Glutathione 20 mg • N-Acetyl Cysteine 20 mg • L-Taurine 20 mg • Bromelain 2000 GUI 10 mg • Lipase 10 mg • Catalase 10 mg • Betaine HCl 10 mg • Citrus Bioflavonoids 30 mg • Hesperidin 10 mg • Quercetin 10 mg • Trimethylglycine 15 mg • Inositol 20 mg • N-Acetyl Glucosamine 20 mg • Chondroitin Sulfate 20 mg • MSM (Methyl Sulfonyl Methane) 20 mg • DMAE (Bitartrate) 20 mg • Lutein 2 mg • Lycopene 2 mg • Alpha-Lipoic Acid 10 mg • Rutin 10 mg • Phosphatidyl Choline 25 mg • Choline (Bitartrate) 25 mg • Octacosanol 5 mg • 1,3-Beta Glucan 10 mg • Hawthorne berry extract 25 mg • Grape Seed extract 25 mg • Ginkgo Biloba 40 mg • Bilberry extract 20 mg • Whole Leaf Aloe Vera extract 20 mg • Turmeric extract 20 mg • Green Tea extract 60 mg • Silymarin (Milk Thistle Seed extract) 20 mg • Ginger root extract 25 mg • Barley Grass Juice powder 80 mg • Artichoke powder 50 mg • Green Oat Juice powder 50 mg • Beet Juice powder 50 mg • Vitamin A (Beta Carotene) 2500 IU • Vitamin A (Palmitate) 1000 IU • Vitamin B-1 (Thiamin Nitrate) 2 mg • Vitamin B-2 (Riboflavin) 2 mg • Vitamin B-3 (Niacinamide) 12 mg • Vitamin B-5 (d-Pantothenate) 12 mg • Vitamin B-6 (Pyridoxine HCl) 6 mg • Vitamin B-12 (Cyanocobalamin) 24 mcg • Biotin 100 mcg • Folic Acid 200 mcg • Vitamin C 20 mg • Vitamin D (Cholecalciferol) 100 IU • Vitamin E (d-Alpha Tocopheryl) 25 mg • Vitamin K (Phytonadione) 20 mcg • PABA 10 mg • Boron (Chelate) 1 mg • Calcium (Citrate) 50 mg • Chromium (Polynicotinate) 120 mcg • Copper (Gluconate) 150 mcg • Iodine (from Kelp) 50 mcg • Magnesium (Aspartate) 50 mg • Manganese (Chelate) 1.5 mg • Molybdenum 75 mcg • Potassium (Aspartate) 20 mg • Selenium 70 mcg • Vanadium 25 mcg • Zinc (Gluconate) 10 mg. Other Ingredients: Cellulose Powder, Hydroxypropylcellulose, Magnesium Stearate, Silicon Dioxide. See Editor's Note No. 15, page 1817.

Xtra Advantage Creatine Serum - Muscle Marketing USA
Each 5 mL serving contains: Creatine Monohydrate • Glucosamine • L-Glutamine • L-Taurine • L-Carnitine • Magnesium • Zinc • Calcium • Vitamin B12 • Royal Jelly • Ginseng • Honey • Natural Glycerine • Natural Flavor • Distilled Water.

Xtra Fuel - TwinLab
Three capsules contain: Guarana extract (standardized for 22% Caffeine) 910 mg • Citrus aurantium extract (Bitter Orange peel standardized for 4% Synephrine) 325 mg • L-Tyrosine 500 mg • Vitamin C 250 mg • Vitamin B6 10 mg • Ginkgo Biloba extract (standardized for 24% flavonoid glycoside) 60 mg • DMAE (2-Dimethylaminoethanol) 100 mg • Vitamin B5 (Pantothenic Acid) 100 mg.

Xtra-Mineral - The Herbalist
Yellow Dock root • Red Raspberry leaf • Nettles leaf • Dandelion root.

Some Brand Name Natural Products - What they Contain
www.NaturalDatabase.com contains MANY more listings than appear here.

Xtreme Trim - Puritan's Pride
Two capsules contain: Pantothenic Acid (as d-Calcium Pantothenate) 10 mg • Citrus Aurantium extract fruit (standardized for 4% synephrine) 125 mg • Ma Huang extract (Ephedra sinica) leaf (standardized for 6% ephedrine) 335 mg • Guarana extract (Paullinia cupana) seed (standardized for 22% caffeine) 910 mg • White Willow extract (Salix alba) bark (standardized for 15% silicin) 105 mg • Acetyl-L-Carnitine Hydrochloride 50 mg • L-Tyrosine 40 mg • Ginger (Zingiber officinale) root 25 mg.

Yam Extract Plus 30 - Aspen Group, Inc.
Each capsule contains: Mexican Yam extract 500 mg • Adrenal substance (freeze dried) 200 mg.
See Editor's Note No. 14, page 1817.

Yam Extract Plus 30 - Atrium Inc.
Each capsule contains: Mexican Yam extract 500 mg • Adrenal Substance (freeze dried) 200 mg.
See Editor's Note No. 14, page 1817.

Yarrow-Pipsissewa Virtue - Blessed Herbs
Echinacea Angustifolia root • Yarrow flower • Pipsissewa • Oregon Grape root • Corn Silk • Kava Kava root • Hydrangea root • Grain alcohol & Distilled Water.

Yeast Raiders - Puritan's Pride
Five capsules contain: Vitamin C 60 mg • Biotin 900 mcg • Zinc 10 mg • Selenium 50 mcg • Freeze Dried Lactobacillus Acidophilus 1,000 mg • Concentrated Odorless Garlic extract (equivalent to 1,500 mg of fresh Garlic) 100 mg • Natural Caprylic Acid 100 mg • Fiber Blend: Psyllium seed husks (Plantago ovata), Guar Gum, Apple Pectin 3,000 mg • Barberry (Berberis vulgaris) root 100 mg • Ginger (Zingiber officinale) root 10 mg • Thyme (Thymus vulgaris) herb 10 mg • Cinnamon (Cinnamomum verum) bark 10 mg • Proprietary Blend: Pau D'Arco, Onion powder, Black Walnut, Echinacea, Goldenseal root 50 mg.

Yellow Dock - Nature's Way
Two capsules contain: Yellow Dock root 1 g. Other Ingredients: Gelatin.

Yerba Manza-Eyebright Virtue - Blessed Herbs
Yerba Manza root • Yerba Santa leaf • Usnea lichen • Osha root • Eyebright • Propolis • Goldenseal root • Myrrh Gum • Licorice root • Grain alcohol & Distilled Water.

Yerba Santa-Echinacea Virtue - Blessed Herbs
Yerba Santa leaf • Osha root • Usnea lichen • Lomatium root • Pau d'Arco bark • Echinacea Angustifolia root • Goldenseal root • Myrrh Gum • Shitake mycelium • Propolis • Licorice root • Grain alcohol & Distilled Water.

Yin-Yang Athletic Tone - Flora
Chinese Red Ginseng • American Ginseng • Astragalus • Reishi Mushroom • Schisandra • Noto Ginseng • He Shou Wu • Codonopsis • Lycii berries • Licorice • Rehmania • Du Zhong • Prince Ginseng • Dodder Seed • Asparagus root.

Yin-Yang Beautiful Lady - Flora
Peony • Schisandra • Lycii berries • Licorice • He Shou Wu • Asparagus root • Noto Ginseng • Dang Gui • Codonopsis • Atractylodes • Poria.

Yin-Yang Crystal Clear Vision - Flora
Rehmania • Dodder Seed • Lycii berries • Chrysanthemum • He Shou Wu • Poria • Ligusticum • Acorus • Plantago Seeds.

Yin-Yang Golden Passage - Flora
Curculigo • Epimedii • Morinda root • Dang Gui • Phellodendron bark • Anemarrhena • Schisandra • Lycii berries • He Shou Wu • Licorice.

Yin-Yang Premenstrual Harmony - Flora
Bupleurum • Dang Gui • Peony • Poria • Atractylodes • Ginger • Licorice • Peppermint • Peony root bark • Cyperus berries • Ligusticum • Citrus Peel.

Yin-Yang Secret of Longevity - Flora
Chinese Red Ginseng • Astragalus • Noto Ginseng • Reishi Mushroom • Dang gui • Lycii berries • Asparagus root • Licorice • Poria • Prince Ginseng • Rehmania • Ligustrum Fruit • Schisandra • He Shou Wu.

Yin-Yang Tranquil Spirit - Flora
Zizyphus Jujube seed • Poria • Biota Seed • Anemarrhena • Licorice • Schisandra • Dang Gui.

YoHIMbe - HVL
Two capsules contain: Yohimbe 500 mg (Ultra Strength extract 4:1 equivalent to 2000 mg of Yohimbe) • Cellulose • Gelatin • Silica and Magnesium Stearate (vegetable source).

Yohimbe B-12 - Puritan's Pride
Each 1 ml serving contains: Yohimbe extract (Pausinystalia yohimbe) bark (dried weight equivalent) 1,000 mg • Co-Enzyme B-12 (as Dibencozide) 5,000 mcg.

Yohimbe Fuel - TwinLab
Yohimbine (the active component in Yohimbe bark) 8 mg.

Young Again - Aspen Group, Inc.
Four tablets contain: Vitamin A Palmitate 500,000 IU/GR 8000 IU • Niacinamide 80 mg • Vitamin B6 20 mg • Vitamin C (magnesium ascorbate) 400 mg • Vitamin E (succinate) 100 IU • N-Acetyl Glucosamine 160 mg • L-Proline 360 mg • L-Lysine 320 mg • Glucosamine Sulfate 560 mg • Chondroitin Sulfate 160 mg • N-Acetyl Cysteine 120 mg • Quercetin Powder 80 mg • Grape seed extract (proanthodyn) 30 mg • Zinc (gluconate) 12 mg • Manganese Ascorbate 12 mg • Copper (gluconate) 0.5 mg • Selenomethionine 80 mcg. Contains no sugar, starch, salt, wheat, corn, yeast or soy derivatives.
See Editor's Note No. 15, page 1817.

Youth-Assure - Nature's Plus
Two tablets contain: Rapid Release Layer: Melatonin (N-Acetyl-5-Methoxytryptamine) 3 mg. Sustained Release Layer: Pregnenolone pharmaceutical grade 50 mg • DHEA pharmaceutical grade Dehydroepiandrosterone 25 mg • LECI-PS, Phosphatidylserine-rich purified Lecithin concentrate supplying Activated Phosphatides: [Phosphatidylserine (PS) 5 mg, Phosphatidylcholine (PC) 5 mg, Cephalin (Phosphatidylethanolamine) 3 mg, Phosphoinositides 1.5 mg] 25 mg. Contains no yeast, wheat, corn, soy, milk, salt, or starch.
See Editor's Note No. 16, page 1817.

YST-RES-Q - Nutri-Quest
Two tablets contain: Lacto Bacillus 1 million IU • Caprylic Acid 50 mg • Grapefruit seed extract 100 mg • Garlic 25 mg • Berberis aquifolium 100 mg • Aloe Vera 25 mg • Undecenoic Acid 50 mg.

Yucca-AR Formula - Nature's Way
Two capsules contain: Proprietary Formula: Black Cohosh root • Black Walnut hulls • Brigham Tea herb • Burdock root • Cayenne pepper fruit • Hydrangea root • Rosemary herb • Sarsaparilla root • Valerian root • Wild Lettuce leaves • Wild Yam root • Yucca stalk. Other ingredients: Gelatin.

BRAND NAMES

Some Brand Name Natural Products - What they Contain

Zallnex Male Formula - Nutranex
Two capsules contain: Vitamin B6 (pyridoxine HCl) 3 mg • Magnesium (magnesium aspartate) 8.5 mg • Zinc (zinc aspartate) 1.6 mg • Zallouh root (Ferula harmonis L.) 250 mg • Muira Puama bark (pxchopetalum olecosides L.) 250 mg • Arginine HCl 200 mg • Tribulis terrestris L. fruit 100 mg. Other Ingredients: Gelatin (capsules), Rice Flour.

Zamoreve Female Formula - Nutranex
Two capsules contain: Vitamin B6 (pyridoxine HCl) 3 mg • Magnesium (magnesium aspartate) 8.5 mg • Zinc (zinc aspartate) 1.6 mg • Zallouh root (Ferula harmonis L) 200 mg • Tribulis terrestris L. fruit 100 mg • Avena sativa L. fruit 100 mg • Nettle root 100 mg. Other Ingredients: Gelatin (capsules), Rice Flour.

Zenibolin - Syntrax Innovations
Each .25 mL contains: 19-Nor (5) Androstenediol • Isotonic Saline • Carboxymethylcellulose • Benzyl Alcohol.

Zicam Cold Remedy Nasal Spray - Gel Tech
Active Ingredients: Zincum Gluconium (Zinc) 2%. Inactive Ingredients: Benzalkonium chloride, glycerine, hydroxyethylcellulose, purified water, sodium chloride, & sodium hydroxide.

Zinaxin - FreeLife - FreeLife
Each softgel contains: Patented Ginger extract EV.EXT 33 (Zingiber officinale) root 255 mg. Other Ingredients: Soybean oil, Silicon Dioxide, Lecithin, Gelatine, Glycerin, Sorbitol, Water, Natural Chlorophyll Complex, Titanium Dioxide (natural mineral color).

Zinaxin (HMP-33) - Eurovita A/S, Denmark
Each capsule contains: Zingiber Officinale Roscoe Extract (HMP-33 Extract) 255 mg. Recommended dosage is 2 capsules per day, in divided doses with liquid for the first month.

Zinaxin Rapid - Eurovita A/S, Denmark
Each capsule contains: Ginger Extract EV.EXT 77 (255 mg is equivalent to approximately 3000 mg of dried ginger rhizome and 1500 mg of dried galanga rhizome) • Sunflower Seed Oil • Gelatin • Glycerol • Beeswax Yellow • Lecithin • Titanium Dioxide • Copper Chlorophyllins. Recommended dosage is 2 capsules daily. Results should become noticeable within 2-4 weeks.

Zinc - Source Naturals
Each tablet contains: Zinc (from 500 mg of zinc amino acid chelate) 50 mg • Copper (from 3.57 mg of copper sebacate) 500 mcg.

Zinc Chewable - Aspen Group, Inc.
Each tablet contains: Amino Acid Chelated Minerals as Zinc 29 mg • Raw Tissue concentrates (bovine source) from: Spleen 29 mg, Brain 8 mg, Liver 5 mg, Heart 4 mg, Kidney 4 mg, Thymus 2 mg, Adrenal 2 mg, Pituitary 1 mg, Duodenum 1 mg.
See Editor's Note No. 14, page 1817.

Zinc Citrate - Quest
Each tablet contains: Zinc (Citrate) 50 mg. Other Ingredients: Croscarmellose Sodium, Calcium Phosphate, Magnesium Stearate (vegetable source), Microcrystalline Cellulose, Silicon Dioxide, Vegetable Stearin.

Zinc for Acne - Puritan's Pride
Two tablets contain: Vitamin A (as Retinyl Palmitate) 1,000 IU • Vitamin C (as Ascorbic Acid and Rose Hips) 150 mg • Vitamin E (as dl-alpha tocopheryl acetate) 50 IU • Vitamin B6 (Pyridoxine Hydrochloride) 20 mg • Zinc (as Zinc Gluconate) 50 mg.

Zinc Lozenge - Nutri-Quest
Each lozenge contains: Zinc Gluconate 75 mg.

Zinc Lozenge - Nature's Way
Each lozenge contains: Echinacea Purpurea (stem, leaf, flower) 20 mg • Stevia dried extract 3 mg • Vitamin C (ascorbic acid) 100 mg • Zinc Citrate 23 mg. Other Ingredients: French Vanilla flavor, Fructose, Magnesium stearate, Mannitol, Sodium, Sorbitol, Wild Berry flavor.

Zinc Lozenges - Nature's Life
Each lozenge contains: Zinc (Gluconate) 10 mg • Vitamin C 100 mg • Beta Carotene (equivalent to 500 IU Vitamin A) 300 mcg • Purple Cone Flower root (Echinacea purpurea) 25 mg. In a natural base of low-Glycemic, pure Crystalline Fructose, pasteurized Honey powder, Hydrogenated Vegetable oil, natural Peppermint flavor, Eucalyptus leaf (Eucalyptus globulus) Licorice root (Glycyrrhiza glabra), Goldenseal root (Hydrastis canadensis), Slippery Elm bark (Ulmus ruba), & Fenugreek seed (Trigonella foenum-graecum).

Zinc Lozenges - Futurebiotics
One lozenge contains: Vitamin C (from ascorbic acid) 60 mg • Zinc (as zinc citrate) 15 mg • Herbal Lozenge Blend, 8 mg: Echinacea leaf powder 4:1 extract, Goldenseal root powder 4:1 extract, Elderberry flower powder, Bee Propolis powder, Peppermint leaf powder, Kava Kava root powder. Other ingredients: Orange crystals, Orange flavor, Magnesium stearate, Stearic acid, Mannitol, Fructose, Cane sugar.

Zinc Lozenges - Jamieson
Each lozenge contains: Vitamin C (as Ascorbic Acid) 50 mg • Zinc (as Zinc Gluconate) 5 mg. Other Ingredients: Eucalyptus, Anise Oil, Menthol, Camphor, Lemon.

Zinc Lozenges Cherry with Vitamin C and B-6 - Leiner Health Products
Each lozenge contains: Vitamin B6 (Pyridoxine Hydrochloride) 5 mg • Vitamin C 60 mg • Zinc 15 mg • Total carbohydrate 1 g • Calories 5 • Sugars 1 g. Other Ingredients: Sugar, Zinc Aspartate, Stearic Acid, Sodium Ascorbate, Maltodextrin, Ascorbic Acid, Mono- and Diglycerides, Magnesium Stearate, Silicon Dioxide, Aspartame, Red 40 Lake, Artificial Cherry Flavor, Starch. Phenylketonurics: Contains Phenylalanine.

Zinc Lozenges Plus - The Vitamin Shoppe
Each lozenge contains: Zinc 24 mg • Echinacea 100 mg • Vitamin C 150 mg • Propolis 100 mg • Vitamin A 1000 IU • Slippery Elm 25 mg. In a base of Golden Seal, Acerola, Fructose Cellulose, with Vanilla and Orange flavor.

Zinc Magnesium Aspartate - Substrate Solutions
Three capsules contain: Zinc (as L-OptiZinc & Aspartate) 30 mg • Magnesium (as Aspartate) 450 mg • Vitamin B6 (Pyridoxine Hydrochloride) 10.5 mg. Other Ingredients: Cellulose, Magnesium Stearate, Gelatin.

Zinc Plex - PhysioLogics
Each capsule contains: Zinc (as 50% Arginate, 25% Histidinate, 25% Glycinate) 30 mg • Copper (as 50% Glycinate, 50% Lysinate) 2 mg.

Zinc Plus - Olympian Labs
Each capsule contains: Zinc Chelate 30 mg. In a base of Pumpkin Seeds, Kelp, and Dulse.

ZincEchinacea Drops - Quantum Health
Each drop contains: Vitamin A acetate 500 IU • Elemental Zinc (Zinc acetate) 14 mg • Echinacea purpurea extract (4:1) 20 mg • Slippery Elm bark (Ulmus fulva) 20 mg • Bee Propolis extract powder (5:1) 5 mg • Goldenseal 2 mg. Other Ingredients: Sugar, Corn Syrup, Natural and Artificial Flavors.

ZincEchinacea Lozenges - Quantum Health
Each lozenge contains: Zinc acetate 14 mg • Vitamin A acetate 500 IU • Slippery Elm bark (Ulmus fulva) 20 mg • Echinacea (4:1) 20 mg • Propolis 5 mg. In a base of Goldenseal, Sugar, Dextrose, Fructose.

ZincEchinacea Pops - Quantum Health
Each pop contains: Vitamin A acetate 167 IU • Elemental Zinc (Zinc acetate) 5 mg • Echinacea purpurea extract (4:1) 7 mg • Slippery Elm bark 7 mg • Bee Propolis extract powder (5:1) 2 mg • Goldenseal 1 mg. Other Ingredients: Sugar, Corn Syrup, Natural Flavor.

Zing! - Health Center for Better Living
Each capsule contains: Siberian Ginseng Root 106 mg.• Ginkgo Biloba Leaf 79 mg.• Gota Kola Herb 79 mg.• Kola Nut 79 mg.• Bee Pollen 53 mg.• Foti Root 26 mg.• Rehmannia Root 26 mg.• Spirulina 26 mg.

Zingiforce - New Chapter, Inc.
One softgel contains: Ginger (rhizome), certified organic, supercritical extract (minimum 20% pungent compounds- 20 mg, 4% zingiberene- 4 mg) 100 mg • Rosemary leaf & essential oil, supercritical extract (23% total phenolic antioxidants [TPA] -1.15 mg) 5 mg. Other Ingredients: Olive Oil - certified organic, Yellow Beeswax, Gelatin, Vegetable Glycerin, Purified Water, Carob.

ZMA - SNAC (Balco Labs)
Each capsule contains: Zinc (Monomethionine/ Asparate) 10 mg • Magnesium (Aspartate) 150 mg • Vitamin B6 3.5 mg.

ZMA Rx-Strength - Advanced Therapeutics - Nature's Plus
Three capsules contain: Vitamin B6 (as Pyridoxine HCl) 0.5 mg • Magnesium (as Aspartate) 450 mg • Zinc (As Aspartate/ Monomethionine) 30 mg • ZMA (Proprietary Anabolic Support Factor) 2424 mg.

ZonePerfect Fish Oil Capsules - ZonePerfect
Each capsule contains: Molecularly Distilled Fish oil • Natural Vitamin E 20 IU • EPA 160 mg • DHA 107 mg.

Z-Plex - PharmAssure
One softgel capsule contains: Kava Kava Root Extract (Piper methysticum; 55% Kavalactones=55mg) 100 mg • Griffonia Seed Extract (Griffonia simplicifolia; 20% 5-Hydroxy-L-Tryptophan =10mg) 50 mg • Melatonin (N-Acetyl-5-Methoxytryptamine) 2 mg. Other ingredients: Polyethylene Glycol, Gelatin, Glycerin, Chlorophyll, Titanium Dioxide (Natural Mineral Whitener). See Editor's Note No. 16, page 1817.

Zyflamend - New Chapter, Inc.
Two softgels contain: Holy Basil leaf extract 100 mg • Turmeric rhizome extract 100 mg • Ginger rhizome, certified, organic, supercritical extract 100 mg • Green Tea leaf extract 100 mg • Rosemary leaf/essential oil supercritical extract 100 mg • Hu Zhang (polygonum cuspidatum) root extract, radix/rhizome 80 mg • Rosemary leaf extract 5:1 50 mg • Chinese Goldenthread root extract 40 mg • Barberry root extract 40 mg • Oregano leaf, supercritical extract 40 mg • Scutellariae baicalensis root extract 5:1 20 mg. Other Ingredients: Olive oil- certified organic, yellow beeswax.

Zyflamend PM - New Chapter, Inc.
Two softgels contain: Holy Basil leaf, extract (2% ursolic acid- mg) 150 mg • Melissa leaf, extract (1% essential oil- 0.85 mg) (including neral and geranial) 85 mg • Tumeric (rhizome) extract (7% curcumin- 7 mg) 100 mg • Scutellaria baicalensis root, extract 5:1 100 mg • Ginger (rhizome) certified organic (post-ethanolic extract) (3% pungent compunds- 1.5 mg) 50 mg • Ginger, SBSC (rhizome), certified organic (minimum 20% pungent compounds 5 mg, 4% zingiberene-1 mg) 25 mg • Chamomile flower, extract

(25% alpha-bisabolol- 12.5 mg) 50 mg • Hops (strobiles) ethanolic extract (1.5% xanthohumol- 0.37 mg) 25 mg • Chamomile flower, extract (3% apigeninglycosides- 0.75 mg) 25 mg • Mexican Valerian and Valerian root, extract 30:1 20 mg. Other Ingredients: Olive oil - certified organic, Yellow Beeswax.

Zygest - PhysioLogics
Two capsules contain: Acid Protease (100 FCC/gm) 100 mg • Papain (6000 USP/mg) 100 mg • Protease (5000 FCC/gm) 80 mg • Amylase (5000 FCC/gm) 80 mg • Bromelain (2400 GDU/gm) 50 mg • Lipase (1000 LU/gm) 60 mg • Lactase (1000 FCC/gm) 20 mg • Cellulase (1000 FCC/gm) 10 mg • Hemicellulase (1000 FCC/gm) 10 mg.

Zymax - HealthWatchers System
Pancreatin • Papain • Rutin • Bromelain • Pancrelipase • Peppermint • Trypsin • Lipase • Amylase • Lysozyme • Cellulase • Chymotrypsin. See Editor's Note No. 14, page 1817.

Zypan - Standard Process
Two tablets contain: Proprietary Blend 700 mg: Betaine hydrochloride, Pancreas extract (Cytosol), Pancreatin (3X), Fatty Acid, Pepsin (1:10,000), Ammonium chloride, Bovine Spleen, Ovine Spleen. Other Ingredients: Cellulose, Lactose, Calcium stearate. See Editor's Note No. 14, page 1817.

BRAND NAMES

BRAND NAMES

Editor's Note No. 1

This is a homeopathic product. It is so extremely diluted that its activity can not be explained by conventional scientific methods. Therefore this product can not be rated by the scientific criteria used in this Database. A patient receiving the extreme dilution of this product will not receive many, if any, molecules of the original active ingredient. Therefore, there are no harmful pharmacologic effects, and any beneficial effects are controversial and not due to a direct biochemical action of the ingredient on the body. Homeopathic products are allowed for sale in the U.S. due to legislation passed in the 19th century sponsored by a homeopathic physician who was also a Senator. The law still requires that the FDA allow the sale of products listed in this Homeopathic Pharmacopea of the United States.

Editor's Note No. 2

This brand product might be an acceptable choice for patients interested in taking saw palmetto. It has been tested by an independent laboratory and found to contain what is stated on the label (5655). Although these findings are promising, they are not conclusive. These findings have not yet been verified by a second independent lab. Furthermore, these findings only pertain to one bottle of product, manufactured at a particular time. These findings do not guarantee that this product will continue to maintain the same level of quality.
References:
5655. Anon. Product Review: Saw Palmetto. ConsumerLab.com 2001. www.consumerlab.com/results/sawpalmetto.asp (accessed 7/16/01).

Editor's Note No. 3

This brand name product might be an acceptable choice for patients interested in taking multivitamins/multiminerals. It has been tested by an independent laboratory and found to contain what is stated on the label (6207). Although these findings are promising, they are not conclusive. These findings have not yet been verified by a second independent lab. Furthermore, these findings only pertain to one bottle of product, manufactured at a particular time. These findings do not guarantee that this product will continue to maintain the same level of quality.
References:
6207. Anon. Product Review: Multivitamins/Multiminerals. ConsumerLab.com 2001. www.consumerlab.com/results/multivit.asp (Accessed 7/18/01).

Editor's Note No. 4

This brand name product might be an acceptable choice for patients interested in taking vitamin C. It has been tested by an independent laboratory and found to contain what is stated on the label (6205). Although these findings are promising, they are not conclusive. These findings have not yet been verified by a second independent lab. Furthermore, these findings only pertain to one bottle of product, manufactured at a particular time. These findings do not guarantee that this product will continue to maintain the same level of quality.
References:
6205. Anon. Product Review: Vitamin C. Consumerlab.com 2001. www.consumerlab.com/results/vitaminc.asp (Accessed 7/18/01).

Editor's Note No. 5

This brand name product might be an acceptable choice for patients interested in taking calcium. It has been tested by an independent laboratory and found to contain what is stated on the label (6209). Although these findings are promising, they are not conclusive. These findings have not yet been verified by a second independent lab. Furthermore, these findings only pertain to one bottle of product, manufactured at a particular time. These findings do not guarantee that this product will continue to maintain the same level of quality.
References:
6209. Anon. Product Review: Calcium. ConsumerLab.com 2001. www.consumerlab.com/results/calcium.asp (Accessed 7/18/01).

Editor's Note No. 6

This brand name product might be an acceptable choice for patients interested in taking coenzyme Q10. It has been tested by an independent laboratory and found to contain what is stated on the label (7001). Although these findings are promising, they are not conclusive. These findings only pertain to one bottle of product, manufactured at a particular time. These findings do not guarantee that this product will continue to maintain the same level of quality.
References:
7001. Anon. Product Review: Coenzyme Q10. ConsumerLab.com 2001. www.consumerlabs.com/results/CoQ10.asp (accessed 7/18/01).

Editor's Note No. 7

This brand name product might be an acceptable choice for patients interested in taking creatine. It has been tested by an independent laboratory and found to contain what is stated on the label (7201). Although these findings are promising, they are not conclusive. These findings have not yet been verified by a second independent lab. Furthermore, these findings only pertain to one bottle of product, manufactured at a particular time. These findings do not guarantee that this product will continue to maintain the same level of quality.
References:
7201. Anon. Product Review: Creatine. ConsumerLab.com 2001. www.consumerlab.com/results/creatine.asp (Accessed 7/18/01).

Editor's Note No. 8

This brand name product might be an acceptable choice for patients interested in taking ginkgo biloba. It has been tested by an independent laboratory and found to contain what is stated on the label (5838). Although these findings are promising, they are not conclusive. These findings have not yet been verified by a second independent lab. Futhermore, these findings only pertain to one bottle of product, manufactured at a particular time. These findings do not guarantee that this product will continue to maintain the same level of quality.
References:
5838. Anon. Product Review: Ginkgo Biloba. ConsumerLab.com 2001. www.consumerlab.com/results/ginkgobiloba.asp (accessed 7/18/01).

Editor's Note No. 9

This brand name product might be an acceptable choice for patients interested in taking ginseng. It has been tested by an independent laboratory and found to contain what is stated on the label (1902). Although these findings are promising, they are not conclusive. These findings have not yet been verified by a second independent lab. Furthermore, these findings only pertain to one bottle of product, manufactured at a particular time. These findings do not guarantee that this product will continue to maintain the same level of quality.

References:

1902. Anon. Product Review:Ginseng. ConsumerLab.com 2001. www.consumerlab.com/results/ginseng.asp (accessed 7/18/01).

Editor's Note No. 10

This brand name product might be an acceptable choice for patients interested in taking SAMe. It has been tested by an independent laboratory and found to contain what is stated on the label (6210). Although these findings are promising, they are not conclusive. These findings have not yet been verified by a second independent lab. Furthermore, these findings only pertain to one bottle of product, manufactured at a particular time. These findings do not guarantee that this product will continue to maintain the same level of quality.

References:

6210. Anon. Product Review: SAMe. ConsumerLab.com 2001. www.consumerlab.com/results/same.asp (Accessed 7/18/01).

Editor's Note No. 11

This brand name product might be an acceptable choice for patients interested in taking soy and red clover isoflavones. It has been tested by an independent laboratory and found to contain what is stated on the label (4017). Although these findings are promising, they are not conclusive. These findings have not yet been verified by a second independent lab. Furthermore, these findings only pertain to one bottle of product, manufactured at a particular time. These findings do not guarantee that this product wil continue to maintain the same level of quality.

References:

4017. Anon. Product Review: Soy and Red Clover Isoflavones. ConsumerLab.com 2001. www.consumerlab.com/results/phytoestrogens2.asp. (Accessed 8/16/01).

Editor's Note No. 12

This brand name product might be an acceptable choice for patients interested in taking valerian. It has been tested by an independent labortory and found to contain what is stated on the label (5809). Although these findings are promising, they are not conclusive. These findings have not yet been verified by a second independent lab. Furthermore, these findings only pertain to one bottle of product, manufactured at a particular time. These findings do not guarantee that this product will continue to maintain the same level of quality.

References:

5809. Anon. Product Review: Valerian. ConsumerLab.com 2001. www.consumerlab.com/results/valerian.asp (accessed 7/11/01).

Editor's Note No. 13

This brand name product might be an acceptable choice for patients interested in taking vitamin E. It has been tested by an independent laboratory and found to contain what is stated on the label (6203). Although these findings are promising, they are not conclusive. These findings have not yet been verified by a second independent lab. Furthermore, these findings only pertain to one bottle of product, manufactured at a particular time. These findings do not guarantee that this product will continue to maintain the same level of quality.

References:

6203. Anon. Product Review: Vitamin E. ConsumerLab.com 2001. www.consumerlab.com/results/vitamine.asp (Accessed 7/18/01).

Editor's Note No. 14

There is some concern about the safety of this product because it contains glandular or organ material derived from animals. The concern is that animal materials might be obtained from diseased animals, including those harboring bovine spongiform encephalopathy (BSE, mad cow disease). There are no reports of BSE or other disease transmission to humans from dietary supplements containing glandular or organ material and the risk of potential disease transmission is thought to be low. However, until more is known about the safety of these products, tell patients to avoid this and other supplements containing glandular or organ materials.

Editor's Note No. 15

The potential risk of transmission of bovine spongiform encephalopathy (BSE, mad cow disease) is raising patients' concerns about products containing chondroitin. Chondroitin is produced from bovine trachea. Although bovine trachea tissue does not seem to carry a high risk of BSE disease infectivity, in some cases manufacturing methods might lead to contamination with other diseased animal tissues. So far there are no reports of BSE or other disease transmission to humans from dietary supplements containing animal materials and the risk of potential disease transmission is thought to be low. However, until more is known about the quality of manufacturing practices, tell patients to avoid this product.

Editor's Note No. 16

The potential risk of transmission of bovine spongiform encephalopathy (BSE, mad cow disease) is raising patients' concerns about products containing melatonin. Melatonin is a hormone sometimes harvested from the pineal gland of animals. However, some melatonin products are made synthetically and are free of this potential risk. The manufacturer of this product has not disclosed its source of melatonin. Until more is known, tell patients to avoid this product.

Editor's Note No. 17

The manufacturer of this product refuses to disclose specific details about the ingredients. Because the exact amounts of ingredients are unknown, tell patients to avoid this product.

Editor's Note No. 18

Wobenzym N is promoted for reducing inflammation and edema, and speeding recovery from certain injuries. Often it is used by individuals with arthritis and by athletes, including

some professional and Olympic athletes. Enzymes in this product are thought to activate macrophages that attack inflammation-causing circulating immune complexes. Rutoside, an additional ingredient, acts as an antioxidant. To date there is no convincing clinical evidence that Wobenzym is effective for these uses. Because these enzymes do not affect prostaglandin synthesis, Wobenzym N is also promoted to be free of many of the side effects associated with non-steroidal anti-inflammatory drugs (NSAIDS). Adverse reactions reported after oral administration include loose stools, increased gas, and skin reactions. Wobenzym N contains enzymes with fibrinolytic activity and might affect coagulation. It should be used cautiously by people on anticoagulant medications such as aspirin, clopidogrel (Plavix), dalteparin (Fragmin), enoxaparin (Lovenox), heparin, ticlopidine (Ticlid), warfarin (Coumadin), and others (6060).
References:
6060. Wobenzym N media kit. Naturally Vitamins (Marlyn Nutraceuticals, Inc.): Scottsdale, AZ.

Editor's Note No. 19
This product is utilized at the Mexican cancer clinic American Metabolic Institute and promoted by Geronimo Rubio, MD, the clinic's medical director. However, the clinic does not disclose the ingredients of this preparation. Tell patients to avoid this and other products that do not disclose ingredients.

Editor's Note No. 20
This product is a good choice for patients interested in using saw palmetto for benign prostatic hyperplasia (BPH). Independent laboratories have found that this product reliably contains the contents stated on the label (6467,6468). This product also provides the amount of saw palmetto extract found in clinical studies to be beneficial for reducing symptoms of BPH.
References:
6467. Anon. Product Review: Saw Palmetto. ConsumerLab.com 2000. www.consumerlab.com/results/sawpalmetto.html (Accessed 8/31/00).
6468. Anon. Herbal Rx for prostate problems. Consumer Reports 2000;Sep: 60-2.

Editor's Note No. 21
This product has been discontinued by the manufacturer.

Editor's Note No. 22
This product and others similar to it have been marketed as an alternative to anabolic steroids for increasing testosterone levels and improving muscle size and strength. So far, evidence indicates that Andro-6 does not increase testosterone levels or significantly improve muscle strength (6795). However, this product, like other products containing androstenedione, has been shown to significantly increase levels of estrogens (6795) and might be associated with estrogenic side effects in men, including acne, behavior changes, testicular atrophy, and gynecomastia (674,6000).
References:
674. Anon. Creatine and androstenedione-two "dietary supplements." Med Lett Drugs Ther 1998;40(1039):105-6.
6000. King DS, et al. Effect of oral androstenedione on serum testosterone and adaptations to resistance training in young

men. A randomized controlled trial JAMA 1999; 281(21): 2020-8.
6795. Brown GA, Vukovich MD, Reifenrath TA, et al. Effects of Anabolic Precursors on Serum Testosterone Concentrations and Adaptations to Resistance Training in Young Men. Int J Sport Nutr Exerc Metab 2000;10:340-359.

Editor's Note No. 23
There is some evidence that SS Cream can be helpful for premature ejaculation. Applying SS Cream to the glans penis one hour prior to intercourse and washing off immediately before intercourse seems to significantly delay ejaculation compared to placebo. A single application of SS Cream seems to be safe. However, the safety of SS Cream with repeated application is not known. SS Cream seems to be well tolerated, but can sometimes cause sporadic erectile dysfunction, excessively delayed ejaculation, mild pain, and local irritation and burning.
References:
2537. Choi HK, Jung GW, Moon KH, et al. Clinical study of SS-Cream in patients with lifelong premature ejaculation. Urology 2000;55(2):257-61.

Editor's Note No. 24
The manufacturer refuses to disclose the ingredients of this product. Anecdotal evidence suggests that this product may have induced a seizure in one patient. Patients should be strongly encouraged to avoid using this product until more is known about its contents and safety.

Editor's Note No. 25
The manufacturer of this product refuses to disclose specific details about the ingredients. Because the exact amounts of ingredients are unknown, tell patients to avoid this product. The potential risk of transmission of bovine spongiform encephalopathy (BSE, mad cow disease) is raising patients' concerns about products containing melatonin. Melatonin is a hormone sometimes harvested from the pineal gland of animals. However, some melatonin products are made synthetically and are free of this potential risk. The manufacturer of this product has not disclosed its source of melatonin. Until more is known, tell patients to avoid this product.

Editor's Note No. 26
The manufacturer of this product refuses to disclose specific details about the ingredients. Because the exact amounts of ingredients are unknown, tell patients to avoid this product. There is some concern about the safety of this product because it contains glandular or organ material derived from animals. The concern is that animal materials might be obtained from diseased animals, including those harboring bovine spongiform encephalopathy (BSE, mad cow disease). There are no reports of BSE or other disease transmission to humans from dietary supplements containing glandular or organ material and the risk of potential disease transmission is thought to be low. However, until more is known about the safety of these products, tell patients to avoid this and other supplements containing glandular or organ materials.

Editor's Note No. 27

The manufacturer has voluntarily recalled this product after FDA laboratories found contamination problems. It might be contaminated with yeast and Pseudomonas fluorescens. Use of this contaminated product might result in severe eye injury and loss of sight. This product should not be used. People who have used this product should contact their physician or other health care professional.

Editor's Note No. 28

The FDA is seeking a permanent injunction against this product due to charges that BeneFin is an unapproved drug promoted as a treatment for cancer and other diseases. The action against the BeneFin brand of shark cartilage does not affect brands of shark cartilage that are not intended for use in the treatment of disease and that are otherwise lawfully marketed as dietary supplements (387). In June 2000, the manufacturer of BeneFin agreed to settle Federal Trade Commission charges of making unsubstantiated claims for a one million dollar judgement (6999). Part of the settlement will be used to help fund a placebo-controlled study of shark cartilage to be conducted by the National Cancer Institute (6999).

References:
387. FDA Talk Paper: FDA Takes Action Against Firm Marketing Unapproved Drugs. FDA website. URL: www.fda.gov/bbs/topics/ANSWERS/ANS00988.html (Accessed 14 December 1999).
6999. Federal Trade Commission. "FTC Action against Lane Laboratories" website: http://www.ftc.gov/opa/2000/06/lanelabs.htm (Accessed 10 August 2000).

Editor's Note No. 29

The FDA has recently declared this product as adulterated and misbranded. It is adulterated because it is promoted for use during the last 6 weeks of pregnancy, but contains ingredients that should not be used during any stage of pregnancy. These include black cohosh, blessed thistle, false unicorn root, and pennyroyal. It also contains raspberry leaf which should be avoided during pregnancy unless used under the guidance of a health professional. It is misbranded because its labeling does not state that it should not be used by pregnant women.

Editor's Note No. 30

PC-SPES is a combination product containing 8 Chinese herbs that has been available commercially since 1996. It is used therapeutically for prostate cancer. "PC" stands for prostate cancer and "spes" is Latin for hope (5548). So far, studies look promising. Preliminary clinical evidence from several small uncontrolled studies and anecdotal reports show that PC-SPES can benefit patients with both hormone-sensitive and hormone-insensitive or refractory prostate cancers. In both groups of patients, PC-SPES can significantly decrease serum prostate-specific antigen (PSA) levels (3576,5122,5548,6284,6286,6483). In patients with hormone-senstive prostate cancer, PC-SPES can decrease PSA levels by at least 50% in 78-100% of patients (3576,3577,5548,6483,6484). In 56-80% of patients PSA levels become undetectable after approximately 6 months (3576,3577,6484). PC-SPES also seems to signficantly decrease PSA in patients with hormone-insensitive prostate cancer. PSA levels decrease more than 50% in about 50-90% of patients after 6 months of treatment (3576,3577,6286,6483,6484). PC-SPES also seems to cause clinically significant reductions in serum testosterone (5548,6484), improve quality of life, and reduce pain and analgesic use (6286) in patients with prostate cancer. There is also some evidence that PC-SPES in combination with conventional hormonal therapy for 5 months can improve quality of life, reduce PSA levels, and reduce pain in patients with metastatic prostate cancer (6286). Although PC-SPES does not contain estrogen, the licorice and Panax-pseudoginseng constituents have estrogenic activity. The saw palmetto constituent also inhibits 5-alpha reductase, an enzyme involved in conversion of testosterone to the more biologically active dihydrotestosterone (5548). Laboratory studies on prostate cancer cell lines show PC-SPES might decrease tumor cell proliferation and might induce apoptosis in both hormone sensitive and insensitive cancer cells (6284,6285,6483). However, PC-SPES seems to reduce tumor cell proliferation more in hormone sensitive prostate cancer (6483). Although PC-SPES is generally well-tolerated, some side effects are relatively common. Most side effects can be attributed to the estrogenic effects of PC-SPES. One of the most common side effects is nipple and breast tenderness and breast enlargement. This seems to occur in up to approximately 90% of patients (3577,6483). Other frequently reported side effects include leg cramps, nausea, decreased libido, erectile dysfunction, and hot flashes. Other side effects that might occur are reduction in overall body hair, pitting edema, significant drop in lipoprotein a, hypertriglyceridemia, and venous and pulmonary thrombosis (5122,5548,6287,6483,6484). There is a lot of concern about the potential for thrombosis formation in patients taking PC-SPES. So far, it seems to occur in about 2-4% of patients (3577,6483). Since PC-SPES has estrogenic effects, there is also some concern that it might interfere with conventional hormone therapies for prostate cancer if used concurrently. Because of these risks patients should avoid using PC-SPES without the supervision of a health care provider. Tell patients not to attempt to self-treat prostate cancer with PC-SPES. Although PC-SPES might be helpful for some patients, it should only be used in conjunction with a comprehensive treatment plan developed between the patient and oncologist. Clinical trials have used 6-9 capsules daily. Each capsule contains 320 mg of the herbal combination. In some studies patients started with one capsule three times daily during the first week and 2 capsules three times daily during the second week. Then, if this dose was tolerated, it was increased to 3 capsules three times daily. PC-SPES should be taken on an empty stomach and should not be administered concurrently with antacids or other medicines (3577). Depending on the dose required, cost is estimated to range from $162-$486/month (5233).

References:
3576. Ault A. Chinese herbal remedy holds promise for prostate cancer. Reuters Health May 23,2000. URL: http://www.medscape.com/reuters/prof/2000/05/05.23/20000523clin013.html (Accessed 2 June 2000).
3577. Anon. PC-SPES. UCSF Cancer Center Communications 2000. URL: http://cc.ucsf.edu/clinical/uro_pc-spes.html (Accessed 2 June 2000).
5122. Moyad MA, Pienta KJ, Montie JE. Use of PC-SPES, a commercially available supplement for prostate cancer, in a patient with hormone-naive disease. Urology 54(2):319-328.

BRAND NAMES

BRAND NAMES

5233. Moyad MA. Alternative therapies for advanced prostate cancer. What should I tell my patients? Urologic Clinics of North America 1999;26:413-17.

5548. DiPaola RS, Zhang H, Lambert GH, et al. Clinical and biologic activity of an estrogenic herbal combination (PC-SPES) in Prostate Cancer. NEJM 1998;785-91.

6284. de la Taille A, Hayek OR, Buttyan R, et al. Effects of a phytotherapeutic agent, PC-SPES, on prostate cancer: a preliminary investigation on human cell lines and patients. BJU Int 1999;84:845-850.

6285. Kubota T, Hisatake J, Hisatake Y, et al. PC-SPES: a unique inhibitor of proliferation of prostate cancer cells in vitro and in vivo. Prostate 2000;42:163-171.

6286. Pfeifer BL, Pirani JF, Hamann SR, Klippel KF. PC-SPES, a dietary supplement for the treatment of hormone-refractory prostate cancer. BJU Int 2000;85:481-5.

6287. Porterfield H. Survey of UsToo Members and Other Prostate Cancer Patients to Evaluate the Efficacy and Safety of PC-SPES. Mol Urol 1999;3(3):333-336.

6483. De La Taille A, Buttyan R, Hayek O, et al. Herbal therapy PC-SPES: In vitro effects and evaluation of its efficacy in 69 patients with prostate cancer. J Urol 2000;164:1229-34.

6484. Small EJ, Frohlich MW, Bok R, et al. Prospective trial of the herbal supplement, PC-SPES, in patients with pregressive prostate cancer. J Clin Oncol 2000;18:3595-603.

Editor's Note No. 31

In April 2000, the Federal Trade Commission filed a complaint against manufacturers of natural or herbal cigarettes for making claims that these products were safer than conventional cigarettes. The labeling on these products is now required to state "Herbal cigarettes are dangerous to your health. They produce tar and carbon monoxide." If they use the term "No additives" they must also state "No additives in our tobacco does NOT mean a safer cigarette."

Editor's Note No. 32

Herbal Ecstacy is no longer being produced under an agreement with the FDA. Global World Media now produces Organic Ecstacy which they claim to be ephedra free. The ingredients of Organic Ecstacy are currently unknown.

Editor's Note No. 33

The potential risk of transmission of bovine spongiform encephalopathy (BSE, mad cow disease) is raising patients' concerns about products containing chondroitin. Chondroitin is produced from bovine trachea. Although bovine trachea tissue does not seem to carry a high risk of BSE disease infectivity, in some cases manufacturing methods might lead to contamination with other diseased animal tissues. So far there are no reports of BSE, or other disease transmission to humans from dietary supplements containing animal materials and the risk of potential disease transmission is thought to be low. The manufacturer of this product reports taking extensive steps to ensure that their chondroitin is not contaminated.

Therapeutic Efficacy

For more information on any of the natural medicines identified in this list, review the listing for that monograph in the database. Just because a product has a positive effectiveness rating does not mean it is appropriate for all patients. In some cases natural medicines that are rated effective might be unsafe for certain patients due to contraindications, drug interactions, or other reasons.

Abdominal Bloating
(see Dyspepsia)

Abdominal Pain
(see Dyspepsia)

Abscesses
Possibly Effective
Maggots

Absence Seizures
(see Epilepsy)

Acetaminophen Overdose/Poisoning
Effective
N-Acetyl Cysteine
Possibly Effective
Methionine

Achlorhydria
None

Acne
(see also Nodulocystic Acne)
Possibly Effective
Alpha Hydroxy Acids
Bovine Cartilage
Brewer's Yeast (Hansen CBS 5926)
Chasteberry
Guggul
Tea Tree Oil
Vitamin A
Zinc

Acrodermatitis Enteropathica
Possibly Effective
Zinc

Acrylonitrile Poisoning
Effective
N-Acetyl Cysteine

Actinic Keratoses
Possibly Effective
Vitamin D

Acute Alcohol Withdrawal
(see Alcohol Withdrawal)

Acute Bronchitis
(see Bronchitis)

Adenitis
None

Adnexitis
None

Adrenal Insufficiency
Possibly Effective
DHEA

Adrenoleukodystrophy
Likely Ineffective
Lorenzo's Oil

Adrenomyeloneuropathy
Likely Ineffective
Lorenzo's Oil

Age Spots
None

Age-Related Macular Degeneration (ARMD)
Possibly Effective
Beta-Carotene
Ginkgo leaf
Lutein
Vitamin C
Vitamin E
Zinc (Treatment)
Possibly Ineffective
Zinc (Prevention)

Age-Related Memory Impairment
Possibly Effective
Ginkgo leaf

Aging
None

Aging Skin
None

AIDS
(see HIV/AIDS)

Alcohol Dependence
Possibly Effective
Gamma Hydroxybutyrate (GHB)

Alcohol Intoxication
None

Alcohol Poisoning
None

Alcohol Withdrawal
Possibly Effective
Gamma-Hydroxybutyrate (GHB)

Alcoholism
None

Allergy
Possibly Effective
EPA (Eicosapentaenoic Acid)
Whey Protein

Alopecia Areata
Possibly Effective
Cedarwood oil
Lavender
Rosemary
Thyme
Zinc

Alopecia Totalis
None

Altitude Sickness
Possibly Effective
Ginkgo leaf

Alzheimer's Disease
(see also Dementia)
Possibly Effective
Acetyl-L-Carnitine
Ginkgo leaf
Phosphatidylserine
Huperzine A
Possibly Ineffective
Inositol
Vitamin C
Vitamin E
Likely Ineffective
Choline
Deanol
Lecithin

Amanita Mushroom Poisoning
Possibly Effective
Milk Thistle

Amenorrhea
Likely Effective
Progesterone

Amyloidosis
Possibly Effective
Dimethylsulfoxide (DMSO)

Amyotrophic Lateral Sclerosis (ALS, Lou Gehrig's Disease)
Possibly Ineffective
N-Acetyl Cysteine
Likely Ineffective
Branched-Chain Amino Acids
Octacosanol

Anal Fissures
None

Anal Pruritus
(see Pruritus Ani)

Anemia
Effective
Iron
Pyridoxine
Vitamin B12
Likely Effective
Copper
Possibly Effective
Chitosan
Vitamin E
Possibly Ineffective
Histidine

CHARTS

Angina
Possibly Effective
- Coenzyme Q10
- L-Arginine
- L-Carnitine
- Magnesium
- N-Acetyl Cysteine
- Propionyl-L-Carnitine
- Terminalia

Possibly Ineffective
- Vitamin E

Angina Pectoris
(see Angina)

Anhydrosis
Possibly Effective
- N-Acetyl Cysteine

Ankylosing Spondylitis
None

Anorexia
(see Anorexia Nervosa)

Anorexia Nervosa
Possibly Effective
- Zinc

Anthrax
None

Anticonvulsant-Induced Osteomalacia
Possibly Effective
- Vitamin D

Anxiety
Likely Effective
- Kava

Possibly Effective
- 5-HTP
- Valerian
- Wine

Aphthous Ulcers
Possibly Ineffective
- Zinc

Appendicitis
None

Ariboflavinosis
Effective
- Riboflavin

ARMD
(see Age-Related Macular Degeneration)

Arrhythmia
Possibly Effective
- Magnesium

Asthma
Possibly Effective
- Beta-Carotene
- Caffeine
- Choline
- Ephedra
- Forskolin
- Thymus Extract
- Vitamin C

Asthma (Cont.)
Possibly Ineffective
- EPA (Eicosapentaenoic Acid)
- Magnesium
- Yogurt

Atherosclerosis
Possibly Effective
- Black Tea
- Garlic
- Niacin and Niacinamide

Possibly Ineffective
- Fish Oils

Athlete's Foot
(see Tinea Pedis)

Athletic Performance, Improving
Possibly Ineffective
- Bee Pollen
- Branched-Chain Amino Acids
- Ginseng, Panax
- L-Tryptophan
- Ornithine
- Ornithine Ketoglutarate

Likely Ineffective
- Dimethylglycine
- Inosine
- L-Carnitine

Atonia of the Uterus
Possibly Effective
- Ergot

Atopic Dermatitis
Possibly Effective
- Borage Seed Oil
- Rice Bran

Possibly Ineffective
- Fish Oils

Attention Deficit Disorder
Possibly Ineffective
- Inositol
- Tyrosine

Attention Deficit Hyperactivity Disorder (ADHD)
Possibly Effective
- Magnesium
- Pyridoxine

Possibly Ineffective
- Evening Primrose Oil

Autism
Possibly Effective
- Pyridoxine

Possibly Ineffective
- Dimethylglycine
- Inositol
- Pyridoxine

Likely Ineffective
- Secretin

Backache
None

Bacteremia
None

Bacterial Prostatitis
None

Bacterial Vaginosis
Possibly Effective
- Yogurt

Possibly Ineffective
- Lactobacillus

Bed Sores
Possibly Effective
- Peru Balsam

Bedwetting
(see Enuresis)

Bee Stings
Likely Effective
- Bee Venom

Behcet's Disease
None

Bell's Palsy
None

Benign Prostatic Hyperplasia (BPH)
Likely Effective
- Beta-Sitosterol
- Pygeum
- Saw Palmetto

Possibly Effective
- Pumpkin
- Red Clover
- Stinging Nettle root

Benzodiazepine Withdrawal
Possibly Effective
- Melatonin

Beriberi
Effective
- Thiamine

Beta-Thalassemia
Possibly Effective
- Vitamin E

Biliary Stones
None

Binge Eating
None

Biotin Deficiency
Likely Effective
- Biotin

Bipolar Disorder
Possibly Effective
- Fish Oils

Bladder Cancer
Possibly Effective
- Green Tea

Possibly Ineffective
- Lycopene

Likely Ineffective
- Beta-Carotene

Bladder Extrophy
None

Blepharitis
None

Boils
Possibly Effective
- Magnesium

Bowel Obstruction
  Effective
        N-Acetyl Cysteine
Brachial Plexus Neuralgia
  None
Bradycardia
  None
Brain Cancer
  Possibly Ineffective
        Shark Cartilage
  Likely Ineffective
        Beta-Carotene
Breast Cancer
  Possibly Effective
        Beta-Carotene
        Lentinan
        Olive Oil
        Melatonin
        Vitamin A
  Possibly Ineffective
        Beer
        Garlic
        Shark Cartilage
  Likely Ineffective
        Vitamin E
Breast Pain (Mastalgia)
  Possibly Effective
        Bugleweed
        Chasteberry
        Progesterone
        Pyridoxine
Breast Tenderness
  Possibly Effective
        Ginkgo leaf
        Pyridoxine
Bright's Disease
  None
Brittle Nails
  Possibly Effective
        Biotin
Bronchitis
  Possibly Effective
        Beta-Carotene
        English Ivy
        Ephedra
        Ginseng, Siberian
        Great Plantain
        N-Acetyl Cysteine
        Thyme flower, leaf
Bruises
  Possibly Effective
        Peru Balsam
Bruxism
  Possibly Ineffective
        L-Tryptophan
Bubonic Plague
  None
Buerger's Disease
  None
Bunions
  None

Burning Feet Syndrome
  None
Burns
  Possibly Effective
        Aloe gel
        Camphor
        Chymotrypsin
        Honey
        Maggots
        Peru Balsam
        Zinc
Bursitis
  None
Cachexia
  None
Calluses
  None
Cancer
  (see specific Cancers)
Candidiasis
  (see also Yeast Infection)
  Possibly Effective
        Yogurt
Canker Sores
  None
Carbuncles
  Possibly Effective
        Maggots
        Magnesium
Cardiac Arrhythmia
  (see Arrhythmia)
Cardiac Failure
  (see Congestive Heart Failure)
Cardiac Glycoside-Induced Arrhythmias
  Likely Effective
        EDTA
Cardiomyopathy
  None
Cardiotoxicity Associated With Doxorubicin Chemotherapy
  Possibly Effective
        Coenzyme Q10
Carpal Tunnel Syndrome (CTS)
  None
Cataracts
  Possibly Effective
        Lutein
        Niacin and Niacinamide
        Riboflavin
        Thiamine
        Vitamin A
  Possibly Ineffective
        Vitamin E
Celiac Disease
  Possibly Effective
        Magnesium
Cellulitis
  None

Cerebellar Ataxia
  Possibly Effective
        5-HTP
  Possibly Ineffective
        Choline
Cerebral Hemorrhage
  (see Stroke)
Cerebral Insufficiency
  (see also Dementia)
  Possibly Effective
        Acetyl-L-Carnitine
Cerebral Ischemia
  (see also Stroke)
  Possibly Effective
        Acetyl-L-Carnitine
Cerebrovascular Disease
  Possibly Effective
        Mesoglycan
        Vinpocetine
Cervical Cancer
  Likely Ineffective
        Beta-Carotene
Cervical Dysplasia
  Possibly Effective
        Indole-3-Carbinol
Cervical Lymphadenitis
  None
Chancre
  None
Chapped Lips
  None
Chapped Skin
  None
Chemotherapy-Induced Nausea And Vomiting
  None
Chemotherapy-Induced Mucositis
  Possibly Effective
        Glutamine
Chemotherapy-Induced Nausea
  Possibly Effective
        Ginger
Chest Pain
  (see Angina)
CHF
  (see Congestive Heart Failure)
Chicken Pox
  None
Chilblains
  None
Cholecystitis
  None
Cholera
  None
Cholestasis of Pregnancy
  Possibly Effective
        Activated Charcoal
Chorea
  None

CHARTS

Chronic Brain Syndrome
None
Chronic Bronchitis
(see Bronchitis)
Chronic Fatigue Syndrome
None
Chronic Hepatic Encephalopathy
Possibly Effective
Branched-Chain Amino Acids
Chronic Lead Poisoning
Effective
EDTA
Chronic Low Back Pain
Possibly Ineffective
Phenylalanine
Chronic Obstructive Pulmonary Disease (COPD)
Possibly Effective
Magnesium
Possibly Ineffective
Beta-Carotene
Chronic Venous Insufficiency
Likely Effective
Horse Chestnut seed
Possibly Effective
Butcher's Broom
Gotu Kola
Grape leaf
Grape seed
Mesoglycan
Pycnogenol
Sweet Clover
Ciguatera Fish Poisoning
None
Circadian Rhythm Sleep Disorders
Likely Effective
Melatonin
Possibly Ineffective
Vitamin B12
Cirrhosis
(see Liver Cirrhosis)
Climacteric
(see Menopausal Symptoms)
Clostridium Difficile Infection
Possibly Effective
Lactobacillus
Possibly Ineffective
Saccharomyces Boulardii
Cluster Headache
Possibly Effective
Magnesium
Melatonin
Coccidiomycosis
None
Cognitive Impairment
Possibly Effective
Acetyl-L-Carnitine
Cold Sores
(see also Fever Blisters)
Possibly Effective

Cold Sores (Cont.)
Camphor
Lemon Balm
Possibly Ineffective
Tannic Acid
Colon/Colorectal Cancer
Possibly Effective
Barley
Calcium
Folic Acid
Garlic
Lutein
Melatonin
Oats
Olive Oil
Pyridoxine
Selenium
Vitamin C
Vitamin E
Possibly Ineffective
Hydrazine Sulfate
Shark Cartilage
Wheat Bran
Likely Ineffective
Beta-Carotene
Oat Bran
Common Cold (Cold)
Possibly Effective
Andrographis
Echinacea (Treatment)
Ginseng, Panax
Great Plantain
Peppermint Oil
White Horehound
Vitamin C (Treatment)
Zinc
Possibly Ineffective
Vitamin C (Prevention)
Echinacea (Prevention)
Complex Partial Seizures
(see Epilepsy)
Complex Regional Pain Syndromes
None
Condyloma Acuminata (HPV, Human Papilloma Virus)
Likely Effective
Podophyllum
Congestive Heart Failure (CHF)
Likely Effective
Digitalis
Hawthorn
Possibly Effective
Coenzyme Q10
Creatine
Ginseng, Panax
L-Arginine
L-Carnitine
Propionyl-L-Carnitine
Taurine
Terminalia
Conjunctivitis
None

Contact Dermatitis
None
Copper Deficiency
Likely Effective
Copper
Cor Pulmonale
None
Corns
None
Coronary Heart Disease
Effective
Oat Bran
Possibly Effective
Alpha-Linolenic Acid
Beer (Prevention)
Ginseng, Siberian
Propionyl-L-Carnitine
Vitamin E
Wine
Possibly Ineffective
Beer (Treatment)
L-Arginine
Wine
Likely Ineffective
Beta-Carotene
EDTA
Corticosteroid-Induced Hyperglycemia
None
Corticosteroid-Induced Osteopenia
Effective
Vitamin D
Cough
Possibly Effective
Marshmallow
Mullein
Peppermint Oil
White Horehound
Possibly Ineffective
EPA (Eicosapentaenoic Acid)
Crohn's Disease
None
Croup
None
Cutaneous Sporotrichosis
Effective
Iodine
Cystic Fibrosis
Effective
N-Acetyl Cysteine
Possibly Ineffective
EPA (Eicosapentaenoic Acid)
Pancreatin
Cystitis
(see Urinary Tract Infection)
Dandruff
None
Decubitus Ulcers
Possibly Effective
Peru Balsam

CHARTS

Deep Vein Thrombosis (DVT)
Possibly Ineffective
  Mesoglycan
Dementia
  (see also Alzheimer's Disease)
Possibly Effective
  Acetyl-L-Carnitine
  Ginkgo leaf
  Huperzine A
  Phosphatidylserine
  Vitamin C
  Vitamin E
Likely Ineffective
  Choline
  Lecithin
Dengue Fever
  None
Dental Caries
  None
Depression
Likely Effective
  SAMe
  St. John's Wort
Possibly Effective
  5-HTP
  Acetyl-L-Carnitine
  DHEA
  Inositol
  L-Tryptophan
  Phenylalanine
Possibly Ineffective
  Tyrosine
Likely Ineffective
  Melatonin
Dermatitis
  (see also Atopic Dermatitis or
  Seborrheic Dermatitis)
Likely Effective
  Lecithin
Dermatitis Herpetiformis
  None
Dermatomyositis
  None
Diabetes
Possibly Effective
  Beer
  Blond Psyllium
  Chromium
  Fenugreek
  Ginseng, Panax
  Ginseng, Siberian
  Glucomannan
  Gymnema
  Niacin and Niacinamide
  Oat Bran
  Oats
  Prickly Pear Cactus
  Vanadium
  Wheat Bran
  Wine
  Xanthan Gum
Possibly Ineffective
  Alpha-Lipoic Acid

Diabetes (Cont.)
  Coenzyme Q10
  Garlic
  Magnesium
Diabetes Insipidus
  None
Diabetes Mellitus
  (see Diabetes)
Diabetic Foot Ulcers
Possibly Effective
  Iodine
  Maggots
Diabetic Neuropathy
Effective
  Capsicum
Possibly Effective
  Alpha-Lipoic Acid
  Gamma Linolenic Acid
  Thiamine
Likely Ineffective
  Inositol
  Pyridoxine
Diabetic Retinopathy
Possibly Effective
  Ginkgo leaf
Diarrhea
Effective
  Pectin
Likely Effective
  Apple
  Lactobacillus
  Zinc
Possibly Effective
  Betony
  Bifidobacteria
  Black Tea
  Blond Psyllium
  Bovine Colostrum
  Brewer's Yeast
  Calcium
  Cherokee Rosehip
  Green Tea
  Kaolin
  Lactobacillus
  Oak bark
  Rhubarb
  Saccharomyces Boulardii
  Soy
  Tormentil
Diphtheria
  None
Diverticulitis
  None
Diverticulosis
  None
Dizziness
  (see also Vertigo)
Possibly Effective
  Fish Oils
  Ginkgo leaf
Down Syndrome
  None

Dropsy
  None
Dry Skin
Likely Effective
  Alpha Hydroxy Acids
  Lecithin
Dysentery
  None
Dysmenorrhea
  None
Dyspepsia
Possibly Effective
  Artichoke
  Bitter Orange
  Peppermint Oil
  Sage
  Sandy Everlasting
Dyspnea
Likely Effective
  Coenzyme Q10
Possibly Effective
  Beta-Carotene
Dysuria
Possibly Effective
  Pumpkin
Eczema
Possibly Effective
  Bifidobacteria
  Bittersweet Nightshade
  Lactobacillus
Possibly Ineffective
  Zinc
Edema
Likely Effective
  Digitalis
  Horse Chestnut seed
Possibly Effective
  Chasteberry
  Chymotrypsin
  Grape leaf
  Horsetail
  Pycnogenol
Emphysema
  None
Empyema
Possibly Effective
  Maggots
Endometrial Hyperplasia
Possibly Effective
  Progesterone
Endometriosis
  None
Enteritis
Possibly Effective
  Cherokee Rosehip
Enuresis
  None
Epididymis
  None
Epilepsy
Possibly Ineffective
  Dimethylglycine

CHARTS

Epistaxis
None
Erectile Dysfunction
Possibly Effective
DHEA
L-Arginine
Melanotan II
Yohimbe
Erysipelas
None
Erythropoietic Protoporphyria (EPP)
Likely Effective
Beta-Carotene
Canthaxanthin
Erythrodysesthesia
Possibly Effective
Pyridoxine
Esophageal Cancer
(see also Gastroesophageal Cancer)
Possibly Effective
Green Tea
Vitamin C
Exfoliative Glossitis
None
External Hemorrhoids
Possibly Effective
Poplar
External Otitis
None
Facial Neuralgia
None
Facial Pain
Possibly Effective
Betony
Facial Paralysis
None
Fanconi Syndrome
None
Febrile Convulsions
None
Fever
Possibly Effective
Willowbark
Fever Blisters
(see also Cold Sores)
Possibly Ineffective
Tannic Acid
Fibrocystic Breast Disease
Possibly Effective
Iodine
Fibromyalgia
Possibly Effective
5-HTP
Alpha Hydroxy Acids
Capsicum
Gamma-Hydroxybutyrate (GHB)
Magnesium
SAMe

Fibrositis
None
Flatulence
Possibly Effective
Artichoke
Caraway Oil
Chlorophyllin
Fennel Oil
Japanese Mint
Sage
White Horehound
Ineffective
Pancreatin
Flu
(see Influenza & Influenza-Like-Infections)
Foehn Illness
None
Food Allergies
Possibly Effective
Thymus Extract
Fragile-X Syndrome
Likely Ineffective
Folic Acid
Frost Bite
Possibly Effective
Peru Balsam
Furuncles
Possibly Effective
Larch Turpentine
Gallstones
Possibly Effective
Apple
Likely Ineffective
Beta-Sitosterol
Gangrene
None
Gas
(see Flatulence)
Gastric and Duodenal Ulcers
(see Peptic Ulcers)
Gastric/Stomach Cancer
(see also Gastroesophageal Cancer)
Possibly Effective
Beta-Carotene
Garlic
Lentinan
Melatonin
Vitamin C
Possibly Ineffective
Green Tea
Gastric Hyperacidity
Effective
Magnesium
Gastroesophageal Cancer
(see also Gastric Cancer and Esophageal Cancer)
Possibly Effective
Vitamin E
Generalized Seizure
(see Epilepsy)

Genital Herpes
Possibly Effective
Zinc
Possibly Ineffective
Echinacea
Genital Tumors
None
Genital Ulcers
None
Gingival Hyperplasia
Possibly Effective
Folic Acid
Possibly Ineffective
Folic Acid
Gingivitis
Possibly Effective
Folic Acid
Possibly Ineffective
Fish Oils
Glaucoma
Possibly Effective
Marijuana
Glioblastoma
Possibly Effective
Melatonin
Glomerulonephritis
None
Glomerulosclerosis
Possibly Effective
Vitamin E
Glossitis
None
Glucose-6-Phosphate Dehydrogenase (G6PD) Deficiency
Possibly Effective
Vitamin E
Glutamate Toxicity
None
Glycine Encephalopathy
None
Goiter
Effective
Iodine
Gonorrhea
None
Gout
Possibly Effective
Autumn Crocus
Granuloma Annulare
Possibly Effective
Vitamin E
Gray Hair
None
Grinding Teeth during Sleep
(see Bruxism)
Gyrate Atrophy of the Chorid and Retina
Possibly Effective
Creatine

CHARTS

Hangover
None
Hansen's Disease
Possibly Effective
Zinc
Hayfever
(see Allergy)
Head and Neck Cancer
Likely Ineffective
Vitamin A
Headache
Likely Effective
Caffeine
Possibly Effective
Betony
Guarana
Mate
Willowbark
Heart Attack
(see Myocardial Infarction)
Heart Disease
(see Coronary Heart Disease)
Heart Failure
(see Congestive Heart Failure)
Hemophilia
None
Hemoptysis
None
Hemorrhoids
Possibly Effective
Bovine Cartilage
Butcher's Broom
Camphor
Diosmin
Hesperidin
Peru Balsam
Poplar
Wheat Bran
Hepatic Osteodystrophy
Effective
Vitamin E
Hepatitis
Possibly Effective
Danshen
Milk Thistle fruit, seed
Schisandra
Yin Chen
Hepatitis A
Possibly Ineffective
Phosphatidylcholine
Hepatitis B
Possibly Effective
Cordyceps
Possibly Ineffective
Chanca Piedra
Phosphatidylcholine
Hepatitis C
Possibly Effective
Phosphatidylcholine

Hepatomegaly
None
Hepatorenal Syndrome
None
Hernia
None
Herpes Labialis
Possibly Effective
Lemon Balm
Lysine
Herpes Simplex
Possibly Effective
Ginseng, Siberian
Propolis
Sangre de Grado
Zinc
Herpes Zoster
Possibly Effective
Dimethylsulfoxide (DMSO)
Papain
Herpetic Genital Lesions
Possibly Effective
Propolis
Hiccups
None
High Blood Pressure
(see Hypertension)
High Cholesterol
(see Hypercholesterolemia)
HIV/AIDS
Possibly Effective
Coenzyme Q10
HIV/AIDS-Related Anorexia
Effective
Marijuana
HIV/AIDS-Related Dementia
Possibly Ineffective
Alpha-Lipoic Acid
HIV/AIDS-Related Diarrhea
Possibly Effective
Saccharomyces Boulardii
Bovine Colostrum
Sangre de Grado
Possibly Ineffective
Zinc
HIV/AIDS-Related Myelopathy
Possibly Effective
SAMe
**HIV/AIDS-Related
Peripheral Neuropathy**
Possibly Ineffective
Capsicum
HIV/AIDS-Related Wasting
Possibly Effective
Glutamine
L-Arginine
Possibly Ineffective
Zinc

Homocystinuria
Effective
Betaine Anhydrous
Pyridoxine
Hot Flashes
Possibly Effective
Black Cohosh
Progesterone
Soy
**Hot Flashes associated with Breast
Cancer**
Possibly Ineffective
Black Cohosh
Soy
Vitamin E
Huntington's Chorea
None
Hurler Syndrome
None
Hyperacidity
(see Gastric Hyperacidity)
Hyperactivity
(see Attention Deficit Hyperactivity
Disorder)
Hypercalcemia
Likely Effective
EDTA
Phosphate Salts
Hypercalciuria
Likely Effective
Potassium
Possibly Effective
Phosphate Salts
Rice Bran
Hypercholesterolemia
(see also Hyperlipidemia)
Likely Effective
Beta-Sitosterol
Blond Psyllium
Flaxseed
Sitostanol
Possibly Effective
Chitosan
Hydroxymethylbutyrate
(HMB)
Magnesium
Olive Oil
Policosanol
Possibly Effective
Rice Bran
Yucca
Possibly Ineffective
Garlic
Lecithin
Red Clover
Likely Ineffective
Pyridoxine
Hyperglycemia
None
Hyperhidrosis
None

CHARTs

Hyperhomocysteinemia
Likely Effective
Folic Acid
Pyridoxine
Vitamin B12

Hyperkalemia
None

Hyperkinesis
None

Hyperlipidemia
(see also Hypercholesterolemia)
Effective
Niacin and Niacinamide
Likely Effective
Soy
Possibly Effective
Artichoke
Fish Oils
Garlic
Guggul
Inositol Nicotinate
Yogurt

Hyperparathyroidism
Likely Effective
Calcium
Possibly Effective
Vitamin D

Hyperpigmentation
None

Hypersensitive Teeth
None

Hypertension
Possibly Effective
Calcium
Coenzyme Q10
Fish Oils
Garlic
Ginseng, Siberian
Hydroxymethylbutyrate
(HMB)
Magnesium
Olive leaf
Olive Oil
Potassium
Sweet Orange
Vitamin C
Vitamin E
Yucca
Possibly Ineffective
EPA (Eicosapentaenoic Acid)

Hyperthyroidism
Effective
Iodine

Hypertriglyceridemia
Likely Effective
Fish Oils
Possibly Effective
Mesoglycan

Hypocalcemia
Effective
Calcium
Vitamin D

Hypochondria
None

Hypoglycemia
Possibly Effective
Chromium

Hypokalemia
Effective
Potassium

Hypomagnesemia
Effective
Magnesium

Hypotension
Possibly Effective
Caffeine
Ginseng, Siberian
Guarana
Mate

Hypothyroidism
Possibly Effective
Tiratricol

Idiopathic Congestive Myopathy
Possibly Effective
Forskolin

Idiopathic Methemoglobinemia
None

Idiopathic Thrombocytopenia Purpura (ITP)
None

Impetigo
None

Impotence
Possibly Effective
Yohimbe

Infertility
Likely Effective
Progesterone
Possibly Effective
Chasteberry
Vitamin E

Inflammatory Bowel Disease (IBD)
Possibly Ineffective
Zinc

Influenza and Influenza-Like Infections
Possibly Effective
Echinacea
Elderberry
Ginseng, Panax
N-Acetyl Cysteine
Possibly Ineffective
Zinc

Insomnia
Possibly Effective
Lavender
Melatonin
Passionflower
Valerian

Intention Myoclonus
None

Intermittent Claudication
Possibly Effective
Ginkgo leaf

Intermittent Claudication (Cont.)
Inositol Nicotinate
L-Arginine
Policosanol
Propionyl-L-Carnitine
Possibly Ineffective
Vitamin E

Interstitial Cystitis
Possibly Effective
L-Arginine
Superoxide Dismutase

Irritable Bowel Syndrome (IBS)
Possibly Effective
Artichoke
Blond Psyllium
Evening Primrose Oil
Peppermint Oil
Possibly Ineffective
Lactobacillus

Ischemic Stroke
(see also Stroke)
Possibly Effective
Beer
Calcium

Itching
(see also Pruritis)
Possibly Effective
Bittersweet Nightshade
Camphor
Witch Hazel

Jaundice
(see also Hepatitis)
Possibly Effective
Yin Chen

Jet Lag
Possibly Effective
Melatonin

Juvenile Rheumatoid Arthritis
None

Kearns-Sayre Syndrome
None

Keloids
Possibly Effective
Gotu Kola

Keratosis Follicularis
None

Kidney Cancer
Possibly Effective
Melatonin
Possibly Ineffective
European Mistletoe

Kidney Stones
Possibly Effective
Black Tea
Magnesium
Phosphate Salts
Pyridoxine

Laryngeal Papillomatosis
None

Laryngeal Spasm
None

Laryngismus Stridulus
None
Laryngitis
None
Leg Cramps
Possibly Effective
Magnesium
Leg Ulcers
Possibly Effective
Alkanna
Mesoglycan
Zinc
Leishmaniasis
None
Leprosy
None
Leukemia
None
Leukoplakia
(see Oral Leukoplakia)
Leukorrhea
None
Lice
Effective
Pyrethrum
Possibly Effective
Quassia
Lichen Planus Pigmentosus
None
Lithuria
None
Liver Cancer
Possibly Effective
Ginseng, Panax
Liver Cirrhosis
Possibly Effective
Milk Thistle fruit, seed
SAMe (Early Cirrhosis)
Possibly Ineffective
SAMe (Advanced Cirrhosis)
Low Back Pain
Possibly Effective
Willowbark
Possibly Ineffective
Phenylalanine
Low Blood Pressure
(see Hypotension)
Lung Cancer
Possibly Effective
Apple
Ginseng, Panax
Lycopene
Melatonin
Selenium
Vitamin C
Possibly Ineffective
Garlic
Shark Cartilage
Vitamin E
Likely Ineffective
Beta-Carotene

Lung Cancer (Cont.)
Hydrazine Sulfate
Vitamin A
Lupus Erythematosus
[see Systemic Lupus Erythematosus, (SLE)]
Lupus Nephritis
[see Systemic Lupus Erythematosus (SLE)]
Lupus Vulgaris
None
Lyme Disease
None
Lymphadenitis
None
Lymphadenoid Goiter
None
Lymphangitis
None
Lymphedema
None
Macroglossia
None
Macular Degeneration
(see Age-Related Macular Degeneration)
Malaria
Effective
Sweet Annie
Possibly Effective
Vitamin A
Male Climacteric
None
Male Impotence
(see Impotence)
Mammary Dysplasia
Likely Ineffective
Vitamin E
Mandibular Alveolitis
Possibly Effective
Bovine Cartilage
Mania
None
Manic-Depressive Disorder
(see Bipolar Disorder)
Mastitis
None
Mastodynia
Possibly Effective
Progesterone
Mastoiditis
Possibly Effective
Maggots
McArdle's Disease
Likely Ineffective
Ribose
Measles
None
Meconium Ileus
Possibly Effective
N-Acetyl Cysteine

Mediterranean Fever
Likely Effective
Autumn Crocus
Meniere's Syndrome
None
Meningitis
None
Menopausal Symptoms
(see also Hot Flashes)
Possibly Effective
Black Cohosh
Possibly Ineffective
Dong Quai
Menorrhagia
Possibly Effective
Chasteberry
Ergot
Menstrual Cramps
None
Menstrual Irregularities
None
Menstrual Pain
(see Dysmenorrhea)
Mental Retardation
None
Metrorrhagia
Possibly Effective
Ergot
Microcytic Anemia
None
Migraine
Likely Effective
Caffeine
Possibly Effective
Feverfew (Prevention)
Fish Oils
L-Arginine
Magnesium
Olive Oil
Riboflavin (Prevention)
Possibly Ineffective
Feverfew (Treatment)
Riboflavin (Treatment)
Mitral Valve Prolapse
Possibly Effective
Magnesium
Mononucleosis
None
Morning Sickness
(Pregnancy Related Nausea)
Possibly Effective
Ginger
Pyridoxine
Motion Sickness
Possibly Effective
Ginger
Ginseng, Siberian
Mouth Cancer
Possibly Effective
Vitamin C
Mouth Sores
None

CHARTS

Mouth Ulcers
None
Mucous Colitis
None
Multiple Sclerosis
Possibly Ineffective
Vitamin D
Mumps
None
Muscle Cramps
Possibly Effective
Zinc
Muscular Dystrophy
Possibly Effective
Coenzyme Q10
Creatine
Vitamin E
Myalgia
Possibly Effective
Horseradish
Japanese Mint
Peppermint Oil
Possibly Ineffective
Glutamine
Myasthenia Gravis
None
Myelodysplastic Syndrome
Possibly Effective
Vitamin D
Myelopathy
(see HIV/AIDS-Related
Myelopathy)
Myocardial Infarction
Possibly Effective
Alpha-Linolenic Acid
Beer
Black Tea
Fish Oils
L-Carnitine
Magnesium
Niacin and Niacinamide
Terminalia
Possibly Ineffective
Vitamin E
Likely Ineffective
Beta-Carotene
Superoxide Dismutase
Myocardial Ischemia
Possibly Effective
Propionyl-L-Carnitine
Myocarditis
Possibly Effective
L-Carnitine
Myoclonus Epilepsy
Possibly Effective
N-Acetyl Cysteine
Myofascial Pain
Possibly Ineffective
L-Tryptophan
Myopathy
Possibly Effective
Vitamin D

Myositis Ossificans Generalis
None
Myxedema
None
Nasal Polyps
None
Nasopharyngeal Carcinoma
None
Nematodes
Possibly Effective
Costus root
Neonatal Apnea
Possibly Effective
Caffeine
Nephritis
(see Systemic Lupus Erythematosus
Nephritis)
Nerve Pain
(see Neuropathy)
Nervousness
(see Anxiety)
Neuralgia
Effective
Capsicum
Possibly Effective
Peppermint Oil
Neurasthenia
None
Neuritis
(see Peripheral Neuritis)
Neurodermatitis
None
Neuropathy
(see Diabetic Neuropathy and
Polyneuropathy)
Niacin Deficiency
(Vitamin B3 Deficiency)
Effective
Niacin and Niacinamide
Nicotine Withdrawal
Possibly Effective
Melatonin
Night Blindness
Effective
Vitamin A
Possibly Effective
Beta-Carotene
Nocturia
Likely Effective
Saw Palmetto
Possibly Effective
Rye Grass
Nocturnal Enuresis
(see Enuresis)
Nodulocystic Acne
(see also Acne)
Possibly Effective
Guggul
Non-Hodgkins Lymphoma
Possibly Ineffective
Shark Cartilage

Obesity
(see also Weight Loss)
Possibly Effective
5-HTP
Ephedra
Obstructive Jaundice
(see Jaundice)
Ocular Stress
Possibly Effective
Grape seed
Oligomenorrhea
Possibly Effective
Chasteberry
Oliguria
None
Onychomycosis
Possibly Effective
Tea Tree Oil
Oohyoideus Myofascial Pain Syndrome
None
Oral Leukoplakia
Possibly Effective
Beta-Carotene
Blue-Green Algae
Green Tea
Oral Mucoceles
None
Orchitis
None
Osgood-Schlatter Disease
None
Osteoarthritis
Effective
Capsicum
Likely Effective
Chondroitin Sulfate
Glucosamine Sulfate
SAMe
Possibly Effective
Beta-Carotene
Boron
Bovine Cartilage
Bromelain
Devil's Claw
DMSO (Dimethylsulfoxide)
Glucosamine Hydrochloride
Niacin and Niacinamide
Rutin
Stinging Nettle
above ground parts
Superoxide Dismutase
Trypsin
Vitamin C
Vitamin E
Possibly Ineffective
Cod Liver Oil
Osteogenesis Imperfecta
Possibly Effective
Vitamin D

Osteomalacia
Effective
Vitamin D
Osteomyelitis
Possibly Effective
Maggots
Osteoporosis
Likely Effective
Calcium
Ipriflavone
Possibly Effective
Magnesium
Manganese
Red Clover
Soy
Vitamin D
Osteosarcoma
None
Otitis Media
Possibly Effective
Xylitol
Ovarian Cancer
Possibly Effective
Ginseng, Panax
Likely Ineffective
Beta-Carotene
Pancreatic Cancer
Possibly Effective
Fish Oils
Green Tea
Melatonin
Possibly Ineffective
European Mistletoe
Vitamin E
Likely Ineffective
Beta-Carotene
Painful Menses
(see Dysmenorrhea)
Pancreatitis
Effective
Pancreatin
Possibly Effective
Chlorophyll
Panic Disorder
(see also Anxiety)
Possibly Effective
Inositol
Paralysis
Possibly Effective
Scullcap
Parkinson's Disease
Possibly Effective
Caffeine
Phenylalanine
(L-Phenylalanine)
Possibly Ineffective
Phenylalanine
(DL-Phenylalanine)
Peptic Ulcer Disease (PUD)
(see Peptic Ulcers)

Peptic Ulcers
Possibly Effective
Carrageenan
Licorice
Zinc
Peripheral Neuritis
Effective
Thiamine
Peripheral Neuropathy
Possibly Effective
Alpha-Lipoic Acid
Possibly Ineffective
Capsicum
Peripheral Vascular Disease
Possibly Effective
Inositol Nicotinate
Propionyl-L-Carnitine
Likely Ineffective
Propionyl-L-Carnitine
Pertussis
Possibly Effective
Thyme flower, leaf
Pharyngitis
Possibly Effective
Papain
Pharyngotonsillitis
Possibly Effective
Andrographis
Photo-Aged Skin
Possibly Effective
Vitamin C
Pimples
(see Acne)
Pleurisy
None
PMS
(see Premenstrual Syndrome)
Pneumocystis Carinii Pneumonia
None
Pneumonia
Likely Ineffective
Vitamin A
Poison Oak and Poison Ivy Dermatitis
Possibly Effective
Bovine Cartilage
Polyneuropathy
Possibly Effective
St. John's Wort
Porphyria
[see Erythropoietic Protoporphyria (EPP)]
Post-Anoxia Myoclonus
None
Post-Operative Nausea and Vomiting
Possibly Effective
Ginger (Absence of Narcotic Analgesia)
Peppermint Oil

Post-Operative Nausea and Vomiting (Cont.)
Possibly Ineffective
Ginger (Presence of Narcotic Analgesia)
Post-Partum Diarrhea
Possibly Effective
Beta-Carotene
Post-Partum Hemorrhage
None
Postherpetic Neuralgia
Possibly Effective
Dimethylsulfoxide (DMSO)
Postirradiation Dermatitis
None
Postpartum Depression
None
Pre-Eclampsia
Likely Effective
Magnesium
Possibly Effective
Calcium
Vitamin C
Vitamin E
Likely Ineffective
Evening Primrose Oil
Fish Oils
Premature Ejaculation
Possibly Effective
Angelica root
Cinnamon bark
Clove dried flowerbud
Ginseng, Panax
Premenstrual Syndrome (PMS)
Likely Effective
Calcium
Possibly Effective
Chasteberry
Ginkgo leaf
L-Tryptophan
Magnesium
Manganese
Potentilla
Pyridoxine
Vitamin E
Possibly Ineffective
Evening Primrose Oil
Progesterone
Preoperative Anxiety
Possibly Effective
Melatonin
Priapism
None
Primary L-Carnitine Deficiency
Effective
L-Carnitine
Proctitis
None
Progressive Systemic Sclerosis
None

CHARTS

Prostate Cancer
Possibly Effective
Baikal Skullcap
Beta-Carotene
Chrysanthemum
Da Qing Ye
Garlic
Lentinan
Licorice
Lycopene
Panax Pseudoginseng
Reishi Mushroom
Saw Palmetto
Selenium
Soy
Tomato
Vitamin E
Possibly Ineffective
Shark Cartilage
Prostate Enlargement
[see Benign Prostatic Hyperplasia (BPH)]
Prostatitis
Possibly Effective
Quercetin
Rye Grass
Protozoal Infections
None
Pruritus
(see Itching)
Pruritus Ani
Possibly Effective
Bovine Cartilage
Pseudotumor Cerebri
None
Psoriasis
Effective
Vitamin D
Possibly Effective
Aloe gel
Bovine Cartilage
Fish Oils
Folic Acid
Gotu Kola
Possibly Ineffective
Zinc
Pulmonary Tuberculosis
(see also Tuberculosis)
Possibly Effective
Ginseng, Siberian
Purpura Fulminans
None
Pyelonephritis
Possibly Effective
Ginseng, Siberian
Pyodermia
None
Pyorrhea
None
Rabies
None

Radiation Burns
None
Radiation Sickness
None
Ramsey-Hunt Syndrome
Possibly Effective
5-HTP
Raynaud's Disease
Possibly Effective
Inositol Nicotinate
Red Blood Cell Aplasia
None
Reiter's Syndrome
None
Renal Calculus
(see Kidney Stones)
Renal Gravel
(see Kidney Stones)
Renal Insufficiency
None
Renal Osteodystrophy
Effective
Vitamin D
Possibly Effective
Ipriflavone
Restenosis after Angioplasty
Likely Ineffective
Fish Oils
Restless Leg Syndrome
None
Retinal Hemorrhage
None
Retinitis Pigmentosa
Possibly Ineffective
Vitamin E
Rett Syndrome
None
Reye's Syndrome
None
Rheumatoid Arthritis
Effective
Capsicum
Likely Effective
Folic Acid
Possibly Effective
Borage Seed Oil
Bovine Cartilage
Dimethylsulfoxide (DMSO)
Evening Primrose Oil
Fish Oils
Gamma Linolenic Acid
Olive Oil
Superoxide Dismutase
Thunder God Vine
Vitamin E
Possibly Ineffective
Creatine
Feverfew
Flaxseed Oil
Histidine
Zinc

Rheumatoid Arthritis (Cont.)
Likely Ineffective
New Zealand Green-Lipped Mussel
Rhinitis
Possibly Effective
Thymus Extract
Rickets
Effective
Vitamin D
Ringing in the Ears
(see Tinnitus)
Ringworm
None
Roemheld's Syndrome
None
Rosacea
None
Scabies
Possibly Effective
Peru Balsam
Ineffective
Pyrethrum
Scarlet Fever
None
Schistosomiasis
Possibly Effective
Gotu Kola
Schizophrenia
Possibly Effective
Eicosapentaenoic Acid (EPA)
Possibly Ineffective
Inositol
Niacin and Niacinamide
Likely Ineffective
Choline
Sciatica
None
Scleroderma
Possibly Effective
Vitamin E
Possibly Ineffective
Dimethylsulfoxide (DMSO)
EDTA
PABA
Scurvy
Effective
Vitamin C
Possibly Effective
Acerola
Seasickness
(see Motion Sickness)
Seborrheic Dermatitis
Possibly Effective
Biotin
Secondary Amenorrhea
Likely Effective
Progesterone
Possibly Effective
Chasteberry

Secondary L-Carnitine Deficiencies in People with Inborn Errors of Metabolism
Effective
L-Carnitine
Seizure Disorders
(see Epilepsy)
Septicemia
None
Sexual Dysfunction in Men
Possibly Effective
DHEA
Sexual Dysfunction in Women
None
Sexual Dysfunction - SSRI-Induced
Possibly Effective
Yohimbe
Shin Splints
None
Shingles
None
Shock
None
Short Bowel Syndrome
Possibly Effective
Glutamine
Sickle Cell Anemia
None
Silicone Breast Disease
None
Sinusitis
Possibly Effective
Cowslip
Elderflower
Gentian
Sorrel
Verbena
Sjogren's Syndrome
Possibly Effective
Xanthan Gum
Skin Cancer
Possibly Effective
Ginseng, Panax
Likely Ineffective
Beta-Carotene
Skin Ulcerations
Possibly Effective
Aloe gel
Honey
Skin Wounds
Possibly Effective
Echinacea
Maggots
Smallpox
None
Snake Bites
None
Snoring
None

Sore Throat
Possibly Effective
Mullein
Slippery Elm
Spermatorrhea
None
Spider Bites
None
Splenomegaly
None
Sprue
None
Steatorrhea
Effective
Medium Chain Triglycerides (MCT)
Stomach Cancer
Possibly Effective
Garlic
Vitamin E
Stomatitis
Possibly Effective
Glutamine
Thyme flower, leaf
Striae Gravidarum
None
Stroke
Possibly Effective
Acetyl-L-Carnitine
Scullcap
Possibly Ineffective
Vinpocetine
Vitamin E
Likely Ineffective
Glycerol
Stroke Prevention
Possibly Ineffective
Beta-Carotene
Potassium
Sweet Orange
Vitamin C
Wine
Sunburn
Possibly Effective
Beta-Carotene
Melatonin
Poplar
Vitamin C
Vitamin E
Possibly Ineffective
Tannic Acid
Sulcoplasty
Possibly Effective
Propolis
Sunstroke
None
Sydenham's Chorea and Acute Cystitis
None
Syphilis
None

Systemic Lupus Erythematosus (SLE)
Possibly Effective
DHEA
Flaxseed
Possibly Ineffective
Fish Oils
Systemic Sclerosis
Possibly Ineffective
Gamma Linolenic Acid
Tachycardia
Possibly Effective
Magnesium
Tapeworm Infestation
Possibly Effective
Male Fern
Tardive Dyskinesia
Possibly Effective
Vitamin E
Possibly Ineffective
Phosphatidylcholine
Likely Ineffective
Deanol
Telangiectasias
None
Temporomandibular Joint Disease (TMJ)
Possibly Effective
Glucosamine Sulfate
Tendonitis
None
Tenesmus
None
Tenosynovitis
None
Tension Headaches
(see also Headaches)
Possibly Effective
Peppermint Oil
Possibly Ineffective
5-HTP
Tetanus
Possibly Effective
Magnesium
Thalassemia
(see Beta-Thalassemia)
Thallium Poisoning
None
Thrombocytopenia
Possibly Effective
Melatonin
Thrombophlebitis
Possibly Effective
Mesoglycan
Thrombosis
Possibly Effective
Scullcap
Thrush
None
Thumb-Sucking
None

C H A R T S

Thyroid Cancer
Possibly Effective
    Tiratricol
Likely Ineffective
    Beta-Carotene
Tic Doloreaux
  None
Tinea Corporis
Possibly Effective
    Bitter Orange
    Garlic
Tinea Cruris
Possibly Effective
    Bitter Orange
    Garlic
Tinea Pedis (Athlete's Foot)
Possibly Effective
    Bitter Orange
    Tea Tree Oil
Tinnitus
Possibly Ineffective
    Ginkgo leaf
    Zinc
Tonsillitis
  (see Pharyngotonsillitis)
Tooth Decay
  None
Toothache
  None
Tourette's Syndrome
  None
Tracheitis
  None
Travel Sickness
  (see Motion Sickness)
Traveler's Diarrhea
Possibly Effective
    Bifidobacteria
    Lactobacillus
    Sangre de Grado
Tremors
  None
Trench Foot
  None
Trigeminal Neuralgia
  None
Tuberculosis
  (see also Pulmonary Tuberculosis)
Possibly Ineffective
    Beta-Sitosterol
Typhoid Fever
  None
Typhus
  None
Ulcerative Colitis
Possibly Effective
    Bifidobacteria
    Indian Frankincense

Ulcus Cruris
Possibly Effective
    Peru Balsam
Ulcus Ventriculi
  None
Upset Stomach
  (see Dyspepsia)
Ureteritis
  None
Urethritis
  None
Urinary Calculi
  (see Kidney Stones)
Urinary Incontinence
Possibly Effective
    Magnesium
Urinary Retention
  None
Urinary Stones
  (see Kidney Stones)
Urinary Tract Infection (UTI)
Possibly Effective
    Cranberry
    Dandelion entire plant
    Uva Ursi
Possibly Ineffective
    Yogurt
Uterine Cancer
Likely Ineffective
    Beta-Carotene
Uterine Fibroids
  None
UTI
  (see Urinary Tract Infection)
Vaginal Candidiasis
  (see Yeast Infection)
Vaginitis
  None
Varicella
  None
Varicose Veins
  (see also Chronic Venous
  Insufficiency)
Possibly Effective
    Mesoglycan
    Sweet Clover
    Witch Hazel
Vasculitis
  None
Venereal Disease
  (see specific conditions)
Venereal Warts
  (Human Papilloma Virus)
Likely Effective
    Podophyllum
Venous Insufficiency
  (see Chronic Venous Insufficiency)
Venous Stasis
Possibly Effective
    Maggots

Vertigo
  (see also Dizziness)
Possibly Effective
    Gingko leaf
Vitamin A Deficiency
Effective
    Vitamin A
Vitamin B12 Deficiency
Effective
    Vitamin B12
Vitamin B3 Deficiency
  (see Niacin Deficiency)
Vitamin B6 Deficiency
Effective
    Pyridoxine
Vitamin C Deficiency
Effective
    Vitamin C
Possibly Ineffective
    Rose Hips
Vitamin D Deficiency
Possibly Effective
    Vitamin D
Vitamin E Deficiency
Effective
    Vitamin E
Vitiligo
Possibly Effective
    Folic Acid
    Phenylalanine
    Vitamin D
Vomiting
Possibly Effective
    Pyridoxine
Vulval Leukoplakias
  None
Vulval Lichen Sclerosis
Possibly Ineffective
    Progesterone
Warts
Likely Ineffective
    Camphor
    Podophyllum
Wasp Stings
  None
Weight Loss
  (see also Obesity)
Possibly Effective
    Caffeine
    Fish Oils
    Glucomannan
    Guarana
    Mate
    Pyruvate
Possibly Ineffective
    Blue-Green Algae
    Chromium
    Garcinia
    Glycerol
Likely Ineffective
    Chitosan
    Tiratricol

CHARTS

Whooping Cough
　　None
Wilson's Disease
　　None
Wiskott-Aldrich Syndrome
　　None
Wound Healing
　　Possibly Effective
　　　　Alkanna
　　　　Aloe gel
　　　　Gotu Kola
　　　　Magnesium
　　　　Ornithine Ketoglutarate
　　　　Trypsin
Wrinkles
　　Possibly Effective
　　　　Vitamin C
Yeast Infection
　　(see also Candidiasis)
　　Possibly Effective
　　　　Echinacea
Yellow Fever
　　None
Yuppie Flu
　　(see Chronic Fatigue Syndrome)
Zollinger-Ellison Syndrome
　　Likely Effective
　　　　Secretin

CHARTS

Potential Interactions Between Drugs and Natural Medicines

For details on possible interactions between natural medicines and drugs, see the listing for the specific natural medicine in the body of this database. This chart does not contain all theoretical or unknown interactions.

Drug	Natural Medicine
5-HT1 AGONISTS (Triptans) Some drugs in this category include: Eletriptan (*Relpax*) • Naratriptan (*Amerge*) • Rizatriptan (*Maxalt*) • Sumatriptan (*Imitrex*) • Zolmitriptan (*Zomig*)	St. John's Wort
5-HT2 ANTAGONISTS	Hawaiian Baby Woodrose
ACARBOSE (*Precose*)	Pancreatin
ACE INHIBITORS (ACEIs) Some drugs in this category include: Captopril (*Capoten*) • Enalapril (*Vasotec*) • Lisinopril (*Prinivil, Zestril*) • Fosinopril (*Monopril*) • Moexipril (*Univasc*) • Perindopril (*Aceon*) • Quinapril (*Accupril*) • Ramipril (*Altace*) • Spirapril (*Renormax*) • Trandolapril (*Mavik*)	Capsicum • L-Arginine • Laminaria • Potassium
ACENOCOUMAROL	L-Carnitine
ACETAMINOPHEN (*Tylenol*)	Black Tea • Cabbage • Caffeine • Cocoa • Coffee • Cola Nut • Coriolus Mushroom • Green Tea • Guarana • Leech • Mate • Methionine • Smokeless Tobacco • Vitamin C (Ascorbic Acid)
ACID-INHIBITING DRUGS Some drugs in this category include: H2-blockers: Famotidine (*Pepcid*) • Ranitidine (*Zantac*) • Nizatidine (*Axid*) • Cimetidine (*Tagamet*) Proton Pump Inhibitors: Omeprazole (*Prilosec*) • Lansoprazole (*Prevacid*) • Esomeprazole (*Nexium*) • Rabeprazole (*Aciphex*) • Pantoprazole (*Protonix*)	Aletris • Alpinia • Angelica herb, seed • Angelica root • Aristolochia • Bitter Orange • Black Mustard oil • Black Mustard seed • Blessed Thistle • Calamus • Capsicum • Cinchona • Cinnamon bark • Coffee • Colombo • Cubebs • Dandelion entire plant • Devil's Claw • Dibencozide • Gentian • Ginger • Goldenseal • Goldthread • Pancreatin • Peppermint Oil • Northern Prickly Ash • Southern Prickly Ash • Quassia • Wormwood above ground parts • Yarrow
ACID-SENSITIVE DRUGS **ACIDIC OR BASIC DRUGS** Some drugs in this category include: Cefpodoxime (*Vantin*) • Ampicillin (*Omnipen*) • Theophylline (*TheoDur*)	Kombucha Tea • Acerola
ACTIVATED CHARCOAL	N-Acetyl Cysteine
ADENOSINE (*Adenocard*)	Black Tea • Green Tea • Smokeless Tobacco
ALCOHOL	Acacia • Alpha-Lipoic Acid • Baikal Skullcap • Butanediol (BD) • Caffeine • Calcium D-Glucarate • Cetyl Myristoleate • Coca • Gamma Butyrolactone (GBL) • Gamma-Hydroxybutyrate (GHB) • Ginseng, Siberian • Hops • Indian Snakeroot • Peyote • Red Yeast • Tansy • Valerian • Vitamin A
ALENDRONATE (*Fosamax*)	Coffee
ALLOPURINOL (*Zyloprim*)	Inosine
ALPHA 2-ADRENERGIC-BLOCKING DRUGS Some drugs in this category include: Phenoxybenzamine (*Dibenzyline*) • Phentolamine (*Regitine*) • Tamsulosin (*Flomax*) • Terazosin (*Hytrin*) • Prazosin (*Minipress*) • Doxazosin (*Cardura*)	Yohimbe
ALPRAZOLAM (*Xanax*)	Kava
ALUMINUM-CONTAINING ANTACIDS (*Maalox, Mylanta, Amphojel*)	Rose Hip • Vitamin C (Ascorbic Acid)

Potential Interactions: Drug/Natural Medicine   For additional data, refer to the database.

Drug	Natural Medicine
AMANTADINE (*Symmetrel*)	Scopolia
AMINOGLYCOSIDES Some drugs in this category include: Gentamicin (*Garamycin*) • Amikacin (*Amikin*) • Tobramycin (*Tobrex*)	Cordyceps • Dibencozide
AMINOPHYLLINE (*Slo-bid, Theo-Dur, Theolair, Uni-Dur, Uniphyl*)	L-Arginine
AMINOSALICYLIC ACID (*Paser, Teebacin, Tubasal*)	Dibencozide • Para-Aminobenzoic Acid (PABA) • Procaine
AMIODARONE (*Cordarone*)	Pyridoxine (Vitamin B6)
AMITRIPTYLINE (*Elavil*)	Country Mallow • Ephedra • St. John's Wort
AMOBARBITOL (*Amytal*)	Smokeless Tobacco
AMPHETAMINE	Ashwaganda • Butanediol (BD) • Gamma Butyrolactone (GBL) • Gamma-Hydroxybutyrate (GHB)
ANALEPTICS	Boxwood • Ignatius Bean • Nux Vomica
ANDROGENIC DRUGS Some drugs in this category include: Danazol (*Danocrine*) • Methyltestosterone (*Android-10*) • Nadrolone Decanoate (*Androlone-D*) • Testosterone (*Andro, Testoderm*)	Androstenediol
ANESTHESIA Some drugs in this category include: Thiopental Sodium (*Pentothal*) • Methohexital Sodium (*Brevital*) • Etomidate (*Amidate*) • Ketamine (*Ketalar*) • Propofol (*Diprivan*) • Nitrous Oxide • Enflurane (*Ethrane*) • Halothane (*Fluothane*) • Methoxyflurane (*Penthrane*) • Sevoflurane (*Ultane*) • Isoflurane (*Forane*) • Desflurane (*Suprane*)	Borage Seed Oil • Cowhage • Evening Primrose Oil • Feverfew
ANTACIDS (*Tums, Maalox, Mylanta*)	Colombo • Iron • Peppermint Oil • Phosphate Salts
ANTIARRHYTHMIC DRUGS Some drugs in this category include: Moricizine (*Ethmozine*) • Ibutilide Fumarate (*Corvert*) • Quinidine Sulfate (*Quinidex*) • Quinidine Gluconate (*Quinaglute*) • Procainamide (*Pronestyl*) • Adenosine (*Adenocard*) • Digoxin (*Lanoxin*) • Lidocaine (*Xylocaine*) • Tocainide (*Tonocard*) • Flecainide (*Tambocor*) • Disopyramide (*Norpace*) • Mexiletine (*Mexitil*) • Propafenone (*Rythmol*) • Bretylium Tosylate • Amiodarone (*Cordarone*)	Aloe dried juice from leaf, latex • Butternut • Rhubarb
ANTIBIOTICS Some drugs in this category include: Fluoroquinolones: Ciprofloxacin (*Cipro*) • Levofloxacin (*Levaquin*) • Norfloxacin (*Noroxin*) • Ofloxacin (*Floxin*) • Enoxacin (*Penetrax*) • Lomefloxacin (*Maxaquin*) • Trovafloxacin;Alatrofloxacin (*Trovan*) Penicillins: Penicillin (*Bicillin, Veetids*) • Nafcillin (*Unipen*) • Oxacillin (*Bactocill*) • Dicloxacillin (*Dynapen*) • Cloxacillin (*Cloxapen*) • Ampicillin (*Principen*) • Amoxicillin (*Amoxil*) • Amoxicillin;Potassium Clavulanate (*Augmentin*) • Ticarcillin (*Ticar*) • Ticarcillin;Clavulanate (*Timentin*) • Mezlocillin (*Mezlin*) • Piperacillin (*Pipracil*) • Piperacillin;Tazobactam (*Zosyn*) • Carbenicillin (*Geocillin*) Macrolides: Clarithromycin (*Biaxin*) • Azithromycin (*Zithromax*) • Dirithromycin (*Dynabac*) • Erythromycin Base (*E-Mycin, Ery-Tab*) • Erythromycin Ethylsuccinate (*E.E.S.*) Vancomycin (*Vancocin*) Clindamycin (*Cleocin*) Aminoglycosides: Tobramycin (*Nebcin*) • Amikacin (*Amikin*) • Kanamycin (*Kantrex*) • Gentamicin (*Garamycin*) Metronidazole (*Flagyl*)	Lactobacillus • Saccharomyces Boulardii

C
H
A
R
T
S

Drug	Natural Medicine
ANTIBIOTICS (Cont.) Sulfadiazine • Sulfasoxazole • Sulfamethoxazole (*Gantanol*) • Sulfamethoxazole;Trimethoprim (*Bactrim*) Nitrofurantoin (*Macrodantin*) Tetracycline (*Sumycin*) • Doxycycline (*Vibramycin*) • Minocycline (*Minocin*) Cefpodoxime (*Vantin*) • Cefaclor (*Ceclor*) • Cephalexin (*Keflex*) • Cefadroxil (*Duricef*) • Cephradine (*Velosef*) • Loracarbef (*Lorabid*) • Cefprozil (*Cefzil*) • Ceftibuten (*Cedax*) • Cefdinir (*Omnicef*) • Cephapirin (*Cefadyl*) • Cefazolin (*Ancef*) • Cefoxitin (*Mefoxin*) • Cefuroxime (*Ceftin*) • Cefonicid (*Monocid*) • Ceftriaxone (*Rocephin*) • Cefixime (*Suprax*) • Cefoperazone (*Cefobid*) • Cefotaxime (*Claforan*) • Cefotetan (*Cefotan*) • Ceftazidime (*Fortaz*) • Cefamandole (*Mandol*) • Imipenem;Cilastatin (*Primaxin*) • Aztreonam (*Azactam*)	
ANTICHOLINERGIC DRUGS Some drugs in this category include: Diphenhydramine (*Bendryl*) • Cyproheptadine (*Periactin*) • Amantadine (*Symmetrel*) • Atropine;Belladonna;Scopolamine (*Donnatal*) • Clozapine (*Clozaril*) • Procholperazine (*Compazine*) • Amitriptyline (*Elavil*)	Angel's Trumpet • Areca • Belladonna • Calabar Bean • Chinese Club Moss • Deanol • European Mandrake • Henbane • Huperzine A • Iboga • Jimson Weed • Scopolia • Secretin
ANTICHOLINESTERASE DRUGS Some drugs in this category include: Donepezil (*Aricept*) • Galantamine (*Reminyl*) • Rivastigmine (*Exelon*) • Tacrine (*Cognex*)	Pantothenic Acid (Vitamin B5) • Procaine
ANTICOAGULANT AND ANTIPLATELET DRUGS Some drugs in this category include: Ardeparin (*Normiflo*) • Dalteparin (*Fragmin*) • Enoxaparin (*Lovenox*) • Danaparoid (*Organan*) Heparin Antithrombin III (*Thrombate III*) Lepirudin (*Refludan*) Warfarin (*Coumadin*) • Dicumarol • Clopidogel (*Plavix*) • Cilostazol (*Pletal*) • Dipyridamole (*Persantine*) • Ticlopidine (*Ticlid*) • Tirofiban (*Aggrastat*) • Eptifibatide (*Integrilin*) • Abciximab (*ReoPro*) • Anagrelide (*Agrylin*)	Agrimony • Alfalfa • Allspice • Andorgraphis • Angelica herb, seed • Angelica root • Arnica • Asafoetida • Bladderwrack • Bishop's Weed • Bogbean • Borage Seed Oil • Bromelain • Buchu • Capsicum • Celery • Cinchona • Chlorella • Chondroitin Sulfate • Clove dried flowerbud, leaf, stem • Clove Oil • Cod Liver Oil • Corn Silk • Danshen • Deertongue • DHA (Docosahexanenoic Acid) • Dong Quai • Emu Oil • EPA (Eicosapentoenoic Acid) • Fenugreek • Feverfew • Fish Oils • Flaxseed • Flaxseed Oil • Gamma Linolenic Acid • Garlic • German Chamomile • Ginger • Ginkgo leaf (Ginkgo leaf extract) • Ginseng, Panax • Ginseng, Siberian • Green Tea • Horse Chestnut branch • Horse Chestnut leaf • Horse Chestnut seed • Inositol Nicotinate • IP-6 • Jiaogulan • Kudzu • Mesoglycan • Northern Prickly Ash • Onion • Papain • Parsley leaf, root • Pau D'Arco • Policosanol • Poplar • Quassia • Red Clover • Reishi Mushroom • Resveratrol • Roman Chamomile • Safflower • Spinach • Stinging Nettle above ground parts • Sweet Clover • Sweet Vernal Grass • Tiratricol • Tonka Bean • Turmeric • Vanadium • Vinpocetine • Vitamin E • Willow Bark • Yarrow
ANTICONVULSANTS Some drugs in this category include: Carbamazepine (*Tegretol*) • Clonazepam (*Klonopin*) • Ethosuximide (*Zarontin*) • Gabapentin (*Neurontin*) • Lamotrigine (*Lamictal*) • Levetiracetam (*Keppra*) • Methsuximide (*Celontin*) • Oxcarbazepine (*Trileptal*) • Tiagabine (*Gabitril*) • Topiramate (*Topamax*) • Valproic Acid (*Depakote*) • Zonisamide (*Zonegran*)	Butanediol (BD) • Cedar leaf • Cedar leaf oil • Dibencozide • Gamma Butyrolactone (GBL) • Gamma-Hydroxybutyrate (GHB) • Ginkgo seed • Sage • Wormwood above ground parts
ANTIDEPRESSANTS Some drugs in this category include: Bupropion (*Wellbutrin*) Nefazodone (*Serzone*) Tetracylic: Maprotiline (*Ludiomil*) • Mirtazapine (*Remeron*) Trazodone (*Desyrel*)	Pleurisy Root • SAMe • St. John's Wort

C
H
A
R
T
S

Drug	Natural Medicine

ANTIDEPRESSANTS (Cont.)

<u>Monoamine Oxidase Inhibitors</u>: Phenelzine (*Nardil*) • Tranylcypromine (*Parnate*) • Isocarboxazid (*Marplan*)

<u>Selective Serotonin Reuptake Inhibitors</u>: Citalopram (*Celexa*) • Fluoxetine (*Prozac*) • Fluvoxamine (*Luvox*) • Paroxetine (*Paxil*) • Sertraline (*Zoloft*) • Venlafaxine (*Effexor*)

<u>Tricylic</u>: Amitriptyline (*Elavil*) • Clomipramine (*Anafranil*) • Amoxapine (*Asendin*) • Desipramine (*Norpramin*) • Doxepin (*Sinequan*) • Imipramine (*Tofranil*) • Nortriptyline (*Pamelor*)

ANTIDIABETES DRUGS

Some drugs in this category include:

Insulin (*Humulin, Novolin, Lantus, Humalog, Novolog*)

<u>Biguanides</u>: Metformin (*Glucophage*)

<u>Meglitinides</u>: Repaglinide (*Prandin*) • Nateglinide (*Starlix*)

<u>Alpha-Glucosidase Inhibitors</u>: Acarbose (*Precose*) • Miglitol (*Glyset*)

<u>Sulfonylureas</u>: Chlorpropamide (*Diabinese*) • Glimepiride (*Amaryl*) • Glipizide (*Glucotrol*) • Glyburide (*DiaBeta, Glynase, Micronase*) • Tolbutamide (*Orinase*)

<u>Thiazolidinediones</u>: Pioglitazone (*Actos*) • Rosiglitazone (*Avandia*)

Natural Medicine: Ackee • Agrimony • Aloe gel • Alpha-Lipoic Acid • Annatto • Baikal Skullcap • Barley • Bean Pod • Beer • Bilberry leaf • Bitter Melon • Black Mulberry • Black Psyllium • Blond Psyllium • Blue Cohosh • Blueberry • Bugleweed • Burdock • Caffeine • Cassia • Chanca Piedra • Chinese Cucumber root • Cocoa • Coffee • Cola Nut • Corn Silk • Country Mallow • Cowhage • Cumin • Damiana • Dandelion entire plant • Devil's Claw • Devil's Club • Elecampane • Ephedra • Eucalyptus dried leaf • Eucalyptus Oil • Fenugreek • Fish Oils • Fo-Ti • Garlic • Ginger • Ginseng, American • Ginseng, Panax • Ginseng, Siberian • Glucomannan • Glucosamine Hydrochloride • Glucosamine Sulfate • Goat's Rue • Gotu Kola • Guar Gum • Guarana • Gymnema • Horse Chestnut branch bark • Horse Chestnut seed • Inositol Nicotinate • Juniper • Kudzu • Lycium • Madagascar Periwinkle • Maitake Mushroom • Marshmallow • Mate • Myrrh • N-Acetyl Glucosamine • Niacin and Niacinamide (Vitamin B3) • Olive Oil • Onion • Potato • Ribose • Sage • Solomon's Seal • Spinach • Stevia • Stinging Nettle above ground parts • Tansy • Tiratricol • Vanadium • Wine • Yohimbe • Xanthan Gum

---

ANTIFUNGALS

Some drugs in this category include: Ciclopirox (*Loprox*) • Griseofulvin (*Grisactin, Gris-PEG*) • Terbinafine (*Lamisil*) • Clotrimazole (*Lotrimin, Mycelex*) • Fluconazole (*Diflucan*) • Itraconazole (*Sporanox*) • Ketoconazole (*Nizoral*) • Miconazole (*Desenex, Monistat*) • Terconazole (*Terazol*) • Amphotericin B (*Amphotec*) • Nystatin (*Mycostatin*)

Natural Medicine: Brewer's Yeast • Brewer's Yeast (Hansen CBS 5926) • Saccharomyces Boulardii

---

ANTIGOUT AGENTS

Some drugs in this category include:
Allopurinol (*Zyloprim*) • Probenicid (*Benemid*) • Colchicine

Natural Medicine: Alpine Cranberry

ANTIHYPERTENSIVE DRUGS

Some drugs in this category include:

<u>Beta-Adrenergic Blockers</u>: Atenolol (*Tenormin*) • Labetalol (*Normodyne*) • Metoprolol (*Lopressor*) • Nadolol (*Corgard*) • Propranolol (*Inderal*)

<u>Calcium Channel Blockers</u>: Amlodipine (*Norvasc*) • Diltiazem (*Cardizem*) • Felodipine (*Plendil*) • Nifedipine (*Adalat, Procardia*) • Verapamil (*Calan*)

<u>Antiadrenergic Agents</u>: Reserpine • Methyldopa (*Aldomet*) • Clonidine (*Catapres*) • Guanfacine (*Tenex*) • Guanabenz (*Wytensin*)

<u>Alpha-1 Adrenergic Blockers</u>: Doxazosin (*Cardura*) • Prazosin (*Minipress*) • Terazocin (*Hytrin*)

<u>Angiotensin II Receptor Antagonists</u>: Irbesartan (*Avapro*) • Losartan (*Cozaar*) • Valsartan (*Diovan*)

<u>Angiotensin-Converting Enzyme Inhibitors</u>: Benazepril (*Lotensin*) •

Natural Medicine: Agrimony • Andographis • Asafoetida • Betony • Capsicum • Cassia • Cat's Claw • Coenzyme Q10 • Coltsfoot • Corn Silk • Cowslip • Devil's Claw • Elecampane • European Mistletoe • Mistletoe • Fish Oils • Ginger • Goldenseal • Indian Snakeroot • L-Arginine • Licorice • Lycium • Periwinkle • Reishi Mushroom • Shepherd's Purse • Stinging Nettle above ground parts • Verbena • Vinpocetine • Wallflower • Wild Carrot • Yarrow • Yohimbe

C
H
A
R
T
S

Drug	Natural Medicine
ANTIHYPERTENSIVE DRUGS (Cont.) Captopril (*Capoten*) • Enalapril (*Vasotec*) • Fosinopril (*Monopril*) • Lisinopril (*Prinivil*) • Quinapril (*Accupril*) • Ramipril (*Altace*)	
ANTIHYPOTENSIVE DRUGS Fludrocortisone (*Florinef*) • Desmopressin (*DDAVP*) • Midodrine (*ProAmatine*) • Norepinephrine (*Levophed*)	Agrimony • Asafoetida • Cowslip • Elecampane • Periwinkle • Shepherd's Purse • Verbena • Yarrow
ANTIPSYCHOTIC DRUGS Some drugs in this category include: <u>Benzisoxazoles</u>: Risperidone (*Risperdal*) <u>Dibenzapines</u>: Clozapine (*Clozaril*) • Loxapine (*Loxitane*) • Olanzapine (*Zyprexa*) • Quetiapine (*Seroquel*) • Ziprasidone (*Geodon*) <u>Thioanthenes</u>: Thiothixene (*Navane*) <u>Phenylbutylpiperadines</u>: Haloperidol (*Haldol*) <u>Phenothiazines</u>: Chlorpromazine (*Thorazine*) • Fluphenazine (*Prolixin*) • Mesoridazine (*Serentil*) • Perphenazine (*Trilafon*) • Thioridazine (*Mellaril*) • Trifluoperazine (*Stelazine*)	Black Tea • Butanediol (BD) • Chasteberry • Cowhage • Gamma Butyrolactone (GBL) • Gamma-Hydroxybutyrate (GHB) • Ginseng, American • Ginseng, Panax • Ginseng, Siberian • Green Tea • Indian Snakeroot • Olive leaf • Phenylalanine
ANTITHYROID DRUGS Some drugs in this category include: Methimazole (*Tapazole*) • Potassium Iodide (*SSKI, Pima*) • Propylthiouracil, PTU	Iodine
APOMORPHINE (*Uprima*)	Acacia • Oak bark
ARRHYTHMOGENIC AGENTS Some drugs in this category include: Theophylline (*Theolair, TheoDur*) • Pseudophedrine (*Sudafed*) • Fenfluramine (*Pondimin*) • Phentermine (*Fastin*) • Dextroamphetamine (*Dexadrine*) • Epinephrine (*Adrenalin, EpiPen*)	Squill
ARTEMETHER (*Artenam, Paluther*)	Grapefruit • Grapefruit seed extract
ASPIRIN AND OTHER SALICYLATES Some drugs in this category include: Diflunisal (*Dolobid*) • Magnesium Salicylate (*Doan's*) • Salsalate (*Disalcid*)	Black Tea • Beer • Caffeine • Capsicum • Cherokee Rosehip • Cocoa • Coffee • Cola Nut • Emu Oil • Gelesemium • Green Tea • Guarana • Horse Chestnut branch bark • Horse Chestnut leaf • Kudzu • Leech • Licorice • Mate • Meadowsweet • Milk Thistle • Onion • Parsley leaf, root • Riboflavin (Vitamin B2) • Ribose • Rose Hip • Vitamin C (Ascorbic Acid) • Willowbark • Wine • Wintergreen Oil
ATROPINE	Acacia • Oak bark
BARBITURATES Some drugs in this category include: Pentobarbital (*Nembutal*) • Phenobarbital • Primidone (*Mysoline*) • Secobarbital (*Seconal*)	Ashwaganda • Beer • Black Tea • Calendula • California Poppy • Capsicum • Catnip • Cedarwood bark, berry, leaf, seed, twig • Cocoa • Cumin • Ginger • Ginseng, Siberian • Goldenseal • Green Tea • Hops • Indian Snakeroot • Jiaogulan • Lavender • Lemon Balm • Marijuana • Passion flower • Sassafras • St. John's Wort • Valerian • Wine • Yarrow • Yerba Mansa
BENZODIAZEPINES Some drugs in this category include: Alprazolam (*Xanax*) • Lorazepam (*Ativan*) • Clonazepam (*Klonopin*) • Clorazepate (*Tranxene*) • Chlordiazepoxide (*Librium*) • Diazepam (*Valium*) • Estazolam (*Prosom*) • Flurazepam (*Dalmane*) • Midazolam (*Versed*) • Oxazepam (*Serax*) • Quazepam (*Doral*) • Triazolam (*Halcion*) • Temazepam (*Restoril*)	Ashwaganda • Baikal Skullcap • Beer • Black Tea • Butanediol (BD) • Caffeine • Coffee • Cola Nut • Gamma Butyrolactone (GBL) • Gamma-Hydroxybutyrate (GHB) • German Chamomile • Grapefruit • Grapefruit seed extract • Green Tea • Guarana • Lavender • L-Tryptophan • Mate • Melatonin • Smokeless Tobacco • Valerian • Wine
BETA-ADRENERGIC AGONISTS Some drugs in this category include: Albuterol (*Ventolin*) • Metaproterenol (*Alupent*) • Terbutaline (*Brethine*) • Isoproterenol (*Isuprel*)	Black Tea • Caffeine • Cocoa • Coffee • Cola Nut • Green Tea • Guarana • Mate

C
H
A
R
T
S

Potential Interactions: Drug/Natural Medicine   For additional data, refer to the database.

Drug	Natural Medicine
BETA-BLOCKERS (BETA-ADRENERGIC ANTAGONISTS) Some drugs in this category include: Acebutolol (*Sectral*) • Atenolol (*Tenormin*) • Betaxolol (*Betoptic*) • Bisoprolol (*Zebeta*) • Carvedilol (*Coreg*) • Esmolol (*Brevibloc*) • Labetalol (*Normodyne*) • Levobunolol (*Betagan*) • Metoprolol (*Lopressor*) • Nadolol (*Corgard*) • Pindolol (*Visken*) • Propranolol (*Inderal*) • Sotalol (*Betapace*) • Timolol (*Timoptic*)	Black Tea • Chromium • Melatonin • Riboflavin (Vitamin B2) • Smokeless Tobacco • Yohimbe
BILE ACID SEQUESTRANTS Some drugs in this category include: Cholestyramine (*Questran*) • Colesevelam (*WelChol*) • Colestipol (*Colestid*)	Niacin and Niacinamide (Vitamin B3)
BISPHOSPHONATES Some drugs in this category include: Alendronate (*Fosamax*) • Etidronate (*Didronel*) • Pamidronate (*Aredia*) • Risedronate (*Actonel*) • Tiludronate (*Skelid*)	Calcium
BUSPIRONE (*Buspar*)	Grapefruit • Grapefruit seed extract
CAFFEINE (*NoDoz, Stay Alert, Vivarin*)	Country Mallow • Ephedra • Ginseng, Panax • Grapefruit • Grapefruit seed extract • Smokeless Tobacco
CALCITONIN (*Miacalcin*)	Ipriflavone
CALCIUM (*Citracal, Caltrate, Os-cal, Titralac*)	Lily-Of-The-Valley • Lysine • Oleander • Pheasant's Eye • Squill • Strophanthus • Wallflower • Zinc
CALCIUM CHANNEL BLOCKERS Some drugs in this category include: Amlodipine (*Norvasc*) • Diltiazem (*Cardizem*) • Felodipine (*Plendil*) • Isradipine (*DynaCirc*) • Nicardipine (*Cardene*) • Nifedipine (*Procardia, Adalat*) • Nisoldipine (*Sular*) • Verapamil (*Calan*)	Grapefruit • Grapefruit seed extract
CARBAMAZEPINE (*Tegretol*)	Biotin • Black Psyllium • Blond Psyllium • Cinchona • Grapefruit • Grapefruit seed extract • N-Acetyl Cysteine • Niacin And Niacinamide (Vitamin B3) • St. John's Wort
CARBIDOPA (*Lodosyn*)	5-HTP • Octacosanol
CARDIOVASCULAR DRUGS	Apple Cider Vinegar • Black Hellebore • Blue Cohosh • Chrysanthemum • Coltsfoot • Devil's Claw • Digitalis • European Mistletoe • Ginger • Hawthorn • Hedge Mustard • Kudzu • Lily-Of-The-Valley • Oleander • Panax Psuedoginseng • Quassia • Strophanthus • Swamp Milkweed • Wahoo • Wallflower • Wild Carrot • Uzara
CARVEDILOL (*Coreg*)	Grapefruit • Grapefruit seed extract
CHEMOTHERAPEUTIC AGENTS Some drugs in this category include: <u>Alkyl Sulfonates:</u> Busulfan (*Myleran*) <u>Triazines:</u> Dacarbazine (*DTIC-Dome*) <u>Nitrogen Mustards:</u> Chlorambucil (*Leukeran*) • Cyclophosphamide (*Cytoxan*) • Ifosfamide (*Ifex*) • Melphalan (*Alkeran*) <u>Nitrosoureas:</u> Carmustine, BCNU (*Gliadel*) • Lomustine (*CeeNu*) • Streptozocin (*Zanosar*) <u>Platinum Coordination Complex:</u> Carboplatin (*Paraplatin*) • Cisplatin (*Zanosar*) Hydroxyurea (*Hydrea*) <u>Folic Acid Analogs:</u> Methotrexate (*Rheumatrex*) <u>Pyrimidine Analogs:</u> Cytarabine ARA-C (*Cytosar-U*) • Fluorouracil, 5-FU (*Efudex*) • Gemcitabine (*Gemzar*)	Alpha-Lipoic Acid • Coenzyme Q10 • Vitamin A • Vitamin E

Potential Interactions: Drug/Natural Medicine   For additional data, refer to the database.

Drug	Natural Medicine
CHEMOTHERAPEUTIC AGENTS (Cont.) Purine Analogs: Cladribine (*Leustatin*) • Fludarabine (*Fludara*) • Mercaptopurine (*Purinethol*) • Pentostatin (*Nipent*) • Thioguanine Vinca Alkaloids: Vinblastine (*Velban*) • Vincristine (*Oncovin*) Taxoids: Paclitaxel (*Taxol*) • Docetaxel (*Taxotere*) Anthracyclines: Daunorubicin (*DaunoXome*) • Doxorubicin (*Adriamycin*) • Idarubicin (*Idamycin*) • Valrubicin (*Valstar*)	
CHLORAL HYDRATE (*Aquachloral*)	Ashwaganda • Clary Sage • Lavender
CHLORAMPHENICOL (*Chloromycetin*)	Dibencozide • Folic Acid • Iron • Vitamin B12
CHLORPROMAZINE (*Thorazine*)	Alfalfa • Black Tea • Green Tea • Yerba Mansa
CHLORPROPAMIDE (*Diabinese*)	Bitter Melon • Prickly Pear Cactus • Solomon's Seal
CHLORTHALIDONE (*Hygroton*)	Zinc
CHLORZOXAZONE (*Paraflex, Parafon Forte*)	Watercress
CHOLESTEROL-REDUCING DRUGS Some drugs in this category include: Niacin (*Nicobid, Niaspan*) Bile Acid Sequestrants: Cholestyramine (*Questran*) • Colesevelam (*WelChol*) • Colestipol (*Colestid*) Fibric Acid Derivatives: Clofibrate (*Atromid-S*) • Fenofibrate (*Tri-Cor*) • Gemfibrozil (*Lopid*) HMG-CoA Reductase Inhibitors: Atorvastatin (*Lipitor*) • Fluvastatin (*Lescol*) • Lovastatin (*Mevacor*) • Pravastatin (*Pravachol*) • Simvastatin (*Zocor*)	Gotu Kola
CHOLESTYRAMINE (*Questran*)	Folic Acid • Tiratricol
CHOLINERGIC DRUGS Some drugs in this category include: Bethanechol (*Urecholine*) • Echothiophate (*Phospholine Iodide*) • Neostigmine (*Prostigmin*) • Physostigmine (*Antilirium*) • Pyridostigmine (*Mestinon*) • Succinylcholine (*Anectine*)	Areca • Chinese Club Moss • Huperzine A • Iboga • Procaine
CIMETIDINE (*Tagamet*)	Black Tea • Caffeine • Cocoa • Green Tea • Licorice • Smokeless Tobacco
CIPROFLOXACIN (*Cipro*)	Fennel fruit, seed • Yogurt
CISAPRIDE (*Propulsid*)	Beer • Grapefruit • Grapefruit seed extract • Wine
CISPLATIN (*Platinol-AQ*)	Glutathione • Milk Thistle • Selenium • Squalamine • Zinc
CLOMIPRAMINE (*Anafranil*)	Grapefruit • Grapefruit seed extract
CLONIDINE (*Catapres*)	Yohimbe
CLOZAPINE (*Clozaril*)	Black Tea • Caffeine • Cocoa • Coffee • Cola Nut • Green Tea • Guarana • Mate
CNS DEPRESSANTS Some drugs in this category include: Secobarbital (*Seconal*) • Pentobarbital (*Nembutal*) • Clonazepam (*Klonopin*) • Diazepam (*Valium*) • Midazolam (*Versed*) • Zolpidem (*Ambien*) • Zaleplon (*Sonata*) • Hydroxyzine (*Atarax*)	Beer • Bitter Almond • Black Tea • Butanediol (BD) • Calamus • Hawthorn • Hydrazine Sulfate • Kava • Lavender • Marsh Tea • Melatonin • Motherwort • Wine
CNS STIMULANTS Some drugs in this category include: Pemoline (*Cylert*) • Methylphenidate (*Ritalin*) • Fenfluramine (*Pondimin*) • Dextroamphetamine (*Dexedrine*) • Dexfenfluramine (*Redux*) • Caffeine (*NoDoz*)	Bitter Orange • Caffeine • Coffee • Cola Nut • Ephedra Guarana • Ginseng, American • Ginseng, Panax • Mate

Potential Interactions: Drug/Natural Medicine
For additional data, refer to the database.

Drug	Natural Medicine
COCAINE	Acacia • Capsicum • Oak bark
COLCHICINE	Autumn Crocus • Dibencozide
COLESTIPOL (*Colestid*)	Folic Acid • Phosphate Salts
CONJUGATED EQUINE ESTROGENS (*Premarin*)	Progesterone
CORONARY VASODILATORS Some drugs in this category include: Theophylline (*Theolair*, *TheoDur*) • Caffeine (*NoDoz*) • Papaverine (*Pavabid*) • Sodium Nitrate • Adenosine (*Adenocard*) • Epinephrine (*Adrenalin*, *EpiPen*)	Hawthorn
CORTICOSTEROIDS Some drugs in this category include: Beclomethasone (*Beclovent*) • Betamethasone (*Valisone*) • Budesonide (*Rhinocort*) • Cortisone (*Cortone*) • Dexamethasone (*Decadron*) • Fludrocortisone (*Florinef*) • Flunisolide (*Aerobid*) • Fluocinonide (*Lidex*) • Fluticasone (*Flovent*) • Hydrocortisone (*Cortef*) • Methylprednisolone (*Medrol*) • Prednisolone (*Prelone*) • Prednisone (*Orasone*,*Deltasone*) • Triamcinolone (*Kenalog*)	Alder Buckthorn • Aloe dried juice from leaf, latex • Butternut • Cascara • Castor Oil • Chromium • Fenugreek • Fo-Ti • Licorice • Pheasant's Eye • Rhubarb • Squill • Vitamin D
CYCLOPHOSPHAMIDE (*Cytoxan*)	Astragalus • Cordyceps
CYCLOSPORINE (*Neoral*, *Sandimmune*)	Astragalus • Cordyceps • Fish Oils • Garlic • Grapefruit • Grapefruit seed extract • L-Arginine • Red Yeast • St. John's Wort • Wine
CYTOCHROME P450 1A2 (CYP1A2) SUBSTRATES Some drugs in this category include: Clozapine (*Clozaril*) • Cyclobenzaprine (*Flexeril*) • Fluvoxamine (*Luvox*) • Haloperidol (*Haldol*) • Imipramine (*Tofranil*) • Mexiletine (*Mexitil*) • Olanzapine (*Zyprexa*) • Pentazocine (*Talwin*) • Propranolol (*Inderal*) • Tacrine (*Cognex*) • Theophylline (*TheoDur*) • Zileuton (*Zyflo*) • Zolmitriptan (*Zomig*)	Cabbage • Ginkgo leaf (Ginkgo leaf extract) • Grape fruit, skin • Indole-3-Carbinol • Ipriflavone • Nutmeg and Mace
CYTOCHROME P450 2C9 (CYP2C9) SUBSTRATES Some drugs in this category include: Amitriptyline (*Elavil*) • Clopidogrel (*Plavix*) • Clozapine (*Clozaril*) • Diazepam (*Valium*) • Estradiol (*Estrace*) • Grepafloxacin (*Raxar*) • Mirtazepine (*Remeron*) • Ondansetron (*Zofran*) • Tacrine (*Cognex*) • Verapamil (*Calan*) • Warfarin (*Coumadin*) • Zileuton (*Zyflo*)	Ipriflavone • St. John's Wort
CYTOCHROME P450 2D6 (CYP2D6) SUBSTRATES Some drugs in this category include: Amitriptyline (*Elavil*) • Clozapine (*Clozaril*) • Codeine • Desipramine (*Norpramin*) • Donepezil (*Aricept*) • Fentanyl (*Duragesic*,*others*) • Flecainide (*Tambocor*) • Fluoxetine (*Prozac*) • Meperidine (*Demerol*) • Methadone (*Dolophine*) • Metoprolol (*Lopressor*, *Toprol XL*) • Olanzapine (*Zyprexa*) • Ondansetron (*Zofran*) • Tramadol (*Ultram*) • Trazodone (*Desyrel*)	Ginkgo leaf (Ginkgo leaf extract) • Ginseng, Panax • St. John's Wort
CYTOCHROME P450 3A4 (CYP3A4) SUBSTRATES Some drugs in this category include: Alfentanil (*Alfenta*) • Alprazolam (*Xanax*) • Amitriptyline (*Elavil*) • Amlodipine (*Norvasc*) • Amiodarone (*Cordarone*) • Astemizole (*Hismanal*) • Atorvastatin (*Lipitor*) • Bepridil (*Vascor*) • Buspirone (*Wellbutrin*) • Carbamazepine (*Tegretol*) • Chlorpheniramine (*Chlor-Trimeton*, others) • Clarithromycin (*Biaxin*) • Clindamycin (*Cleocin*) • Clomipramine (*Anafranil*) • Clonazepam (*Klonopin*) • Cyclobenzaprine (*Flexeril*) • Cyclophosphamide (*Cytoxan*) • Cyclosporine (*Neoral*, *Sandimmune*) • Delavirdine (*Rescriptor*) • Dexamethasone (*Decadron*, others) • Dextromethorphan • Diazepam (*Valium*) • Diltiazem (*Cardizem*) • Donepezil (*Aricept*) • Doxorubicin	American Elder • Bishop's Weed • Bitter Orange • Cat's Claw • DHEA • Echinacea • Garlic • German Chamomile • Ginkgo leaf (Ginkgo leaf extract) • Goldenseal • Licorice • Milk Thistle • Red Clover • Red Yeast • St. John's Wort • Valerian

CHARTS

Drug	Natural Medicine
CYTOCHROME P450 3A4 (CYP3A4) SUBSTRATES (Cont.) (*Adriamycin*) • Erythromycin • Estrogens, oral contraceptives • Ethinyl estradiol • Etoposide (*Toposar*) • Felodipine (*Plendil*) • Fentanyl (*Duragesic*, others) • Fexofenadine (*Allegra*) • Finasteride (*Proscar, Propecia*) • Fluvastatin (*Lescol*) • Haloperidol (*Haldol*) • Hydrocortisone • Ifosfamide (*Ifex*) • Imipramine (*Tofranil*) • Indinavir (*Crixivan*) • Itraconazole (*Sporanox*) • Ketoconazole (*Nizoral*) • Lansoprazole (*Prevacid*) • Loratadine (*Claritin*) • Losartan (*Cozaar*) • Lovastatin (*Mevacor*) • Midazolam (*Versed*) • Mirtazapine (*Remeron*)	
DAPSONE (*Avlosulfon*)	Para-Aminobenzoic Acid (PABA)
DEXAMETHASONE (*Decadron*)	Country Mallow • Ephedra • Marshmallow
DICOUMAROL	Cedarwood bark, berry, leaf, seed, twig
DIDANOSINE (ddI, *Videx*)	Lentinan
DIFLUNISAL (*Dolobid*)	Smokeless Tobacco
DIGITOXIN (*Crystodigin*)	Khella
DIGOXIN (*Lanoxin*)	Alder Buckthorn • Aloe dried juice from leaf, latex • Black Hellebore • Black Psyllium • Black Root • Blue Flag • Butternut • Calotropis • Canadian Hemp • Cascara • Castor Oil • Cereus • Colocynth • Country Mallow • Digitalis • Ephedra • European Buckthorn • Fo-Ti • Gamboge • Ginseng, Siberian • Greater Bindweed • Gossypol • Hawthorn • Hedge Mustard • Horsetail • Indian Snakeroot • Jalap • Khella • Laminaria • Licorice • Lily-Of-The-Valley • Manna • Mexican Scammony Root • Oleander • Pangamic Acid • Pectin • Pheasant's Eye • Pleurisy Root • Procaine • Rhubarb • Rice Bran • Sarsaparilla •Senna • Squill • St. John's Wort • Strophanthus • Swamp Milkweed • Uzara • Vanadium • Vitamin D • Wahoo • Wallflower • Wheat Bran • Yellow Dock
DILTIAZEM (*Cardizem*)	Guggul
DISULFIRAM (*Antabuse*)	Beet • Bilberry leaf • Black Tea • Caffeine • Cocoa • Coffee • Cola Nut • Green Tea • Guarana • Kombucha Tea • Marijuana • Mate • Wine
DIURETICS Some drugs in this category include: Thiazides: Indapamide (*Lozol*) • Chlorothiazide (*Diuril*) • Hydrochlorothiazide (*Esidrix, Hydrodiuril*, others) • Chlorthalidone (*Hygroton*) •Metolazone (*Zaroxolyn*) Loop Diuretics: Bumetanide (*Bumex*) • Ethacrynic Acid (*Edecrin*) • Furosemide (*Lasix*) • Torsemide (*Demadex*) Potassium-Sparing: Amiloride (*Midamor*) • Triamterene (*Dyrenium*) • Spironolactone (*Aldacton*)	Aloe dried juice from leaf, latex • Birch • Bladderwrack • Cowslip • Dandelion entire plant • EDTA • European Buckthorn • Goldenrod • Indian Snakeroot • Juniper • Lovage • Parsley leaf, root • Parsley seed • Stone Root
DOPAMINE AGONISTS Some drugs in this category include: Bromocriptine (*Parlodel*) • Carbidopa (*Lodosyn*) • Carbidopa;Levodopa (*Sinemet*) • Pergolide (*Permax*) • Pramipexole (*Mirapex*) • Ropinirole (*Requip*)	Black Horehound
DOPAMINE ANTAGONISTS Some drugs in this category include: Metoclopramide (*Reglan*) • Chlorpromazine (*Thorazine*) • Thiothixene (*Navane*) • Clozapine (*Clozaril*)	Chasteberry
DOXYCYCLINE (*Vibramycin*)	Cowslip • Elderflower • Gentian • Sorrel • Verbena
ECONAZOLE NITRATE (*Spectazole*)	Echinacea

C H A R T S

Potential Interactions: Drug/Natural Medicine   For additional data, refer to the database.

Drug	Natural Medicine
EPHEDRINE	Caffeine • Coffee • Cola Nut • Green Tea • Guarana • Indian Snakeroot • Mate
ERGOT A LKALOIDS Some drugs in this category include: Bromocriptine (*Parlodel*) • Caffeine;Ergotamine (*Cafergot*) • Dihydroergotamine (D.H.E.) • Ergotamine (*Ergostat*) • Methylergonovine (*Methergine*) • Methysergide (*Sansert*)	Ergot
ERGOTAMINE (*Ergostat*)	Black Tea • Caffeine • Cocoa • Coffee • Cola Nut • Ephedra • Green Tea • Guarana • Mate
ERYTHROMYCIN (*E.E.S., E-Mycin, PCE*)	Beer • Wine • Yogurt
ESTROGEN (*Estratest, Estrace, Ogen, Menogen*) See also **CONJUGATED EQUINE ESTROGENS**	Acerola • Alfalfa • Androdenedione • Androstenediol • Boron • Caffeine • Calcium • Chasteberry • Cherokee Rosehip • Coffee • Cola Nut • Dolomite • Fenugreek • Ginseng, American • Ginseng, Siberian • Grapefruit • Grapefruit seed extract • Guarana • Ipriflavone • L-Arginine • Licorice • Mate • Pleurisy Root • Red Clover • Saw Palmetto • Smokeless Tobacco • Soy • Verbena • Wild Carrot
ETHACRYNIC ACID (*Edecrin*)	Licorice
ETHYL ALCOHOL	Acacia
ETRETINATE (*Tegison*)	EPA (Eicosapentaenoic Acid) • Fish Oils
FELODIPINE (*Plendil*)	Bitter Orange
FENFLURAMINE (*Pondimin*)	St. John's Wort
FEXOFENADINE (*Allegra*)	Apple • Grapefruit • Sweet Orange
FLUCONAZOLE (*Diflucan*)	Cocoa
FLUOROQUINOLONES Some drugs in this category include: Ciprofloxacin (*Cipro*) • Gatifloxacin (*Tequin*) • Levofloxacin (*Levaquin*) • Moxifloxacin (*Avelox*) • Norfloxacin (*Noroxin*) • Ofloxacin (*Floxin*) • Trovafloxacin (*Trovan*)	Calcium • Iron • Magnesium • Manganese • Zinc
FLUOXETINE (*Prozac*)	Marijuana • Melatonin
FLUPHENAZINE (*Prolixin*)	Acerola • Cherokee Rosehip
FLUVOXAMINE (*Luvox*)	Caffeine • Melatonin
FOSPHENYTOIN (*Cerebyx*)	Folic Acid
FUROSEMIDE (*Lasix*)	Germanium • Ginseng, Panax • Smokeless Tobacco • Licorice
GANGLIONIC BLOCKING DRUGS Trimethaphan	Inositol Nicotinate • Niacin and Niacinamide (Vitamin B3)
GEMFIBROZIL (*Lopid*)	Red Yeast
GLAUCOMA DRUGS Some drugs in this category include: Timolol (*Timoptic*) • Betaxolol (*Betoptic*) • Levobunonol (*Betagan*) • Pilocarpine (*Pilocar*) • Dipivefrin (*Propine*) • Lantanoprost (*Xalatan*) • Acetazolamide (*Diamox*)	Greater Celandine dried above ground parts
GLUCOCORTICOIDS Some drugs in this category include: Hydrocortisone (*Cortef*) • Triamcinolone (*Kenalog*) • Betamethasone (*Celestone*)	Dolomite • Lily-Of-The-Valley • Strophanthus • Wallflower
GLUTETHIMIDE (*Cytadren*)	Smokeless Tobacco
GLYBURIDE (*DiaBeta, Micronase, Glynase*)	Aloe gel
GUANABENZ (*Wytensin*)	Yohimbe
GUANETHIDINE (*Ismelin*)	Cowhage

CHARTS

Potential Interactions: Drug/Natural Medicine   For additional data, refer to the database.

Drug	Natural Medicine
H2-BLOCKERS Some drugs in this category include: • Famotidine (*Pepcid*) • Ranitidine (*Zantac*) • Nizatidine (*Axid*) • Cimetidine (*Tagamet*)	Beet • Colombo • Iron • Pancreatin • Peppermint Oil • Wine
HALOPERIDOL (*Haldol*)	Butanediol (BD) • Gamma Butyrolactone (GBL) • Gamma-Hydroxybutyrate (GHB) • Smokeless Tobacco • Peyote
HEPARIN	Goldenseal • L-Carnitine • Smokeless Tobacco • Vitamin C (Ascorbic Acid)
HEPATOTOXIC DRUGS Some drugs in this category include: • Amphotericin B (*Fungizone*) • Azathioprine (*Imuran*) • Carbamazepine (*Tegretol*) • Disulfiram (*Antabuse*) • Felbamate (*Felbatol*) • Flutamide (*Eulexin*) • Hydroxychloroquine (*Plaquenil*) • Indinavir (*Crixivan*) • Interferon (*Roferon, Intron, Wellferon*) • Itraconazole (*Sporanox*) • Leflunomide (*Arava*) • Methotrexate (*Rheumatrex*) • Procainamide (*Procan*) • Rosiglitazone (*Avandia*) • Stavudine, d4T (*Zerit*) • Tacrine (*Cognex*) • Terbinafine (*Lamisil*) • Ticlopidine (*Ticlid*) • Tolcapone (*Tasmar*) • Zalcitabine, ddC (*Hivid*)	Beer • Bishop's Weed • Kava • Khella • Sweet Clover • Wine
HEXOBARBITAL	Greek Sage
HEXOBARBITONE	Angelica herb, seed • Clary Sage
HIGHLY PROTEIN BOUND DRUGS Some drugs in this category include: Digoxin (*Lanoxin*) • Phenytoin (*Dilantin*)	Goldenseal
HMG-CoA REDUCTASE INHIBITORS ("Statins") Some drugs in this category include: Atorvastatin (*Lipitor*) • Fluvastatin (*Lescol*) • Lovastatin (*Mevacor*) • Pravastatin (*Pravachol*) • Simvastatin (*Zocor*)	Grapefruit • Grapefruit seed extract • Inositol Nicotinate • Lavender • Niacin and Niacinamide (Vitamin B3) • Red Yeast • Sitostanol
HOMATROPINE (*Homapin*)	Acacia • Oak bark
HORMONE REPLACEMENT THERAPY Some drugs in this category include: Conjugated Estrogens (*Premarin, Premphase, Prempro*) • Esterified Estrogens (*Estratest*)	Alfalfa • Chasteberry • Saw Palmetto
HYALURONIC ACID	Chondroitin Sulfate
HYDROCORTISONE (*Cortef*)	Aloe gel • Bee Venom
IMMUNOSUPPRESSANTS Some drugs in this category include: Azathioprine (*Imuran*) • Basiliximab (*Simulect*) • Cyclosporine (*Neoral, Sandimmune*) • Daclizumab(*Zenapax*) • Muromonab-CD3 (*OKT3*) • Mycophenolate (*CellCept*) • Tacrolimus (*FK506, Prograf*) • Sirolimus (*Rapamune*) • Prednisone (*Orasone, Deltasone*)	Andrographis • Astragalus • Cat's Claw • Echinacea • European Mistletoe • Ginseng, Panax • Ipriflavone • Larch Arabinogalactan • Melatonin • Pycnogenol • Thunder God Vine • Thymus Extract
INDOMETHACIN (*Indocin*)	Turmeric
INSULIN (*Humulin, Humalog, Novolin, Lantus, Novolog*)	Apple Cider Vinegar • Bitter Melon • Black Psyllium • Burdock • Chromium • Coenzyme Q10 • EDTA • Fenugreek • Garlic • Ginkgo leaf (Ginkgo leaf extract) • Ginseng, Panax • Ginseng, Siberian • Guar Gum • Licorice • Peyote • Ribose • Smokeless Tobacco • Solomon's Seal
INTERFERON	Licorice • Zinc
IRON (*Feosol, Slow FE*)	Acacia • Acerola • Cherokee Rosehip • Gymnema • Liver Extract • Oak bark • Rose Hip • Vitamin C (Ascorbic Acid)
ISONIAZID (*INH, Laniazid*)	Melatonin • Niacin and Niacinamide (Vitamin B3)
ITRACONAZOLE (*Sporanox*)	Grapefruit
KANAMYCIN (*Kantrex*)	Calcium D-Glucarate • Ginseng, Siberian

CHARTS

Potential Interactions: Drug/Natural Medicine

For additional data, refer to the database.

Drug	Natural Medicine
LAMIVUDINE (*3TC, Epivir*), **STAVUDINE** (*d4T*, Zerit), **ZIDOVUDINE** (*AZT, Retrovir*)	Riboflavin (Vitamin B2)
LAXATIVES Some drugs in this category include: Bisacodyl (*Dulcolax*) • Lactulose (*Chronulac*) • Methylcellulose (*Citrucel*) • Polyethylene Glycol (*Miralax*) • Psyllium (*Metamucil*) • Senna (*Senokot*)	Butternut • Cascara • Castor Oil • Fo-Ti • Gamboge • Rhubarb • Strophanthus • Wallflower
LEVODOPA (*Larodopa*)	Branched-Chain Amino Acids • Indian Snakeroot • Kava • Octacosanol • Phenylalanine • Pyridoxine (Vitamin B6) • Tyrosine • Verbena • Whey Protein
LEVOTHYROXINE (*Synthroid, Levothroid, Levoxyl*)	Bladderwrack • Bugleweed • Calcium • Guggul • Horseradish • Lemon Balm • Red Yeast • Shepherd's Purse • Tiratricol • Tyrosin
LITHIUM (*Eskalith, Lithobid*)	Black Psyllium • Black Tea • Bladderwrack • Blond Psyllium • Caffeine • Cocoa • Coffee • Cola Nut • Dandelion entire plant • Green Tea • Guarana • Iodine • Mate
LOSARTAN (*Cozaar*)	Grapefruit
LOVASTATIN (*Mevacor*)	Pectin
MACROLIDE ANTIBIOTICS Some drugs in this category include: Azithromycin (*Zithromax*) • Clarithromycin (*Biaxin*) • Dirithromycin (*Dynabec*) • Erthromycin (*E-Mycin, E.E.S., Ery-Tab*)	Black Hellebore • Digitalis • Hedge Mustard • Lily-Of-The-Valley • Oleander • Swamp Milkweed • Uzara • Wahoo
MAGNESIUM (*Slo-Mag, Mag-Ox*)	Alpha Hydroxy Acids
MEDROXYPROGESTERONE (*Provera*)	L-Arginine
METFORMIN (*Gucophage*)	Beer • Quillaia • Water Avens • Wine • Raspberry leaf
METHADONE (*Dolophine*)	Peyote
METHOTREXATE (*MTX, Rheumatrex*)	Cetyl Myristoleate • Folic Acid
METHYLDOPA (*Aldomet*)	Colloidal Silver • Cowhage
METHYLPREDNISOLONE (*Adlone, A-Methapred, depMedalone, Depoject, Medrol, Solu-Medrol*)	Grapefruit
METHYLXANTHINES Some drugs in this category include: Caffeine (*NoDoz, Vivarin*) • Theophylline (*Theo-Dur, Slo-bid, Theolair*)	Country Mallow
METHYSERGIDE (*Sansert*)	Peyote
MEXILETINE (*Mexitil*)	Caffeine • Cocoa • Coffee • Cola Nut • Green Tea • Guarana • Mate
MIDAZOLAM (*Versed*)	Bitter Orange
MINOCYCLINE (*Minocin*)	Vitamin A
MONOAMINE OXIDASE INHIBITORS (MAOIs) Some drugs in this category include: Phenelzine (*Nardil*) • Tranylcypromine (*Parnate*)	Black Tea • Bitter Orange • Brewer's Yeast • Brewer's Yeast (Hansen CBS 5926) • Caffeine • Calamus • California Poppy • Capsicum • Cereus • Chaparral • Cocoa • Coffee • Cola Nut • Country Mallow • Cowhage • Ephedra • Fenugreek • Ginkgo leaf (Ginkgo leaf extract) • Ginseng, American • Ginseng, Panax • Guarana • Green Tea • Hydrazine Sulfate • Indian Snakeroot • L-Tryptophan • Licorice • Mate • Nutmeg and Mace • Parsley leaf, root • Parsley Seed • Passionflower • Phenylalanine • Ribose • SAMe • Scotch Broom, flower • Scotch Broom herb • St. John's Wort • Wine • Yohimbe
MORPHINE (*Roxanol, Oramorph, MS Contin, MSIR, Kadian*)	Acacia • Deer Velvet • Oak bark • Oat above ground parts • Oats

CHARTS

Potential Interactions: Drug/Natural Medicine   For additional data, refer to the database.

Drug	Natural Medicine
NALOXONE (*Narcan*)	Butanediol (BD) • Fever Bark • Gamma Butyrolactone (GBL) • Gamma-Hydroxybutyrate (GHB) • Yohimbe
NARCOTIC ANALGESICS Some drugs in this category include: Acetaminophen;Oxycodone (*Percocet*) • Acetaminophen;Propoxyphene (*Darvocet*) • Aspirin;Oxycodone (*Percodan*) • Fentanyl (*Duragesic*) • Hydromorphone (*Dilaudid*) • Meperidine (*Demerol*) • Methadone (*Methadose, Dolophine*) • Morphine (*MS Contin, Roxanol*) • Oxycodone (*OxyContin*) • Propoxyphene (*Darvon*) • Sufentanil (*Sufenta*)	Beer • Beet • Butanediol (BD) • Gamma Butyrolactone (GBL) • Gamma-Hydroxybutyrate (GHB) • Meadowsweet • St. John's Wort • Sweet Bay • Wine
NEFAZODONE (*Serzone*)	St. John's Wort
NEOMYCIN (*Neo-Fradin*)	Vitamin A
NEPHROTOXIC DRUGS Some drugs in this category include: Carbamazepine (*Tegretol*) • Diclofenac (*Voltaren*) • Diflunisal (*Dolobid*) • Ganciclovir (*Cytovene*) • Gatifloxacin (*Tequin*) • Interferon • Meloxicam (*Mobic*) • Spironolactone (*Aldactone*) • Tacrolimus (*Prograf*) • Valacyclovir (*Valtrex*) • Amphotericin B (*Fungizone*) • Cisplatin (*Platinol*) • Cyclosporine (*Neoral*) • Enalapril (*Vasotec*) • Nafcillin (*Unipen*) • Tobramycin (*Nebcin*)	Creatine
NEUROMUSCULAR BLOCKING AGENTS Some drugs in this category include: Pancuronium (*Pavulon*) • Succinylcholine (*Anectine*)	Thiamine (Vitamin B1)
NIACIN (*Niacor, Niaspan, Nicobid, Slo-Niacin*)	Red Yeast
NICOTINE (*Nicotrol, Habitrol, Nicorette, Nicoderm, Prostep*)	Blue Cohosh • Inositol Nicotinate • Niacin and Niacinamide (Vitamin B3) • Oat above ground parts • Oats
NICOTINIC ACID	Chromium
NIFEDIPINE (*Adalat, Procardia*)	Coca • Magnesium • Melatonin
NITRATES Some drugs in this category include: Isosorbide Dinitrate (*Isordil*) • Isosorbide Mononitrate (*Imdur*) • Nitroglycerin (*Nitrostat*)	L-Arginine • Vitamin E
NITROGLYCERIN (*Nitrostat, Minitran, Nitrek*)	N-Acetyl Cysteine
NONNUCLEOSIDE REVERSE TRANSCRIPTASE INHIBITORS (NNRTIs) Some drugs in this category include: Nevirapine (*Viramune*) • Delavirdine (*Rescriptor*) • Efavirenz (*Sustiva*)	Garlic • St. John's Wort
NONSTEROIDAL ANTI-INFLAMMATORY DRUGS (NSAIDs) Some drugs in this category include: Diclofenac (*Voltaren*) • Etodolac (*Lodine*) • Flurbiprofen (*Ansaid*) • Ibuprofen (*Motrin*) • Indomethacin (*Indocin*) • Ketoprofen (*Orudis*) • Ketoralac (*Toradol*) • Meclofenamate, Mefenamic Acid (*Ponstel*) • Nabumetone (*Relafen*) • Naproxen (*Naprosyn*) • Oxaprozine (*Daypro*) • Piroxicam (*Feldene*) • Sulindac (*Clinoril*)	Beer • Beeswax • Feverfew • Gossypol • Leech • Licorice • Veronica • Wine
NORETHINDRONE (*Aygestin*)	L-Arginine
NORFLOXACIN (*Noroxin*)	Colloidal Silver
NORTRIPTYLINE (*Pamelor, Aventyl*)	St. John's Wort
OFLOXACIN (*Ocuflox, Floxin*)	Colloidal Silver
ORAL CONTRACEPTIVES Some drugs in this category include: Ethinyl Estradiol;Ethynodiol Diacetate (*Demulen*) • Ethinyl Estradiol;Levonorgestrel (*Triphasil*) • Ethinyl Estradiol;Norethindrone (*Ortho-Novum*) •	Alfalfa • Black Tea • Caffeine • Chasteberry • Cocoa • Coffee • Cola Nut • Fenugreek • Garlic • Ginseng, American • Ginseng, Siberian • Green Tea • Guarana • L-Arginine • Licorice • Mate • Pleurisy Root • Red Clover • Saw Palmetto •

Drug	Natural Medicine
ORAL CONTRACEPTIVES (Cont.) Ethinyl Estradiol;Norethindrone Acetate (*Loestrin*) • Ethinyl Estradiol;Norgestimate (*Ortho-Cyclen*)	Smokeless Tobacco • St. John's Wort • Wild Carrot • Verbena
ORAL DRUGS	Acacia • Activated Charcoal • Agar • Alder Buckthorn • Algin • Aloe dried juice from leaf, latex • American Chestnut • Bistort • Black Psyllium • Black Walnut • Blond Psyllium • Butternut • Cascara • Castor Oil • Coffee Charcoal • European Buckthorn • European Chestnut • European Mandrake • Fenugreek • Flaxseed • Glucomannan • Guar Gum • Iceland Moss • Ipecac • Kaolin • Karaya Gum • Larch Arabinogalactan • Marshmallow • Mormon Tea • Oats • Pectin • Pinus Bark •Pomegranate • Quillaia • Raspberry leaf • Rhatany • Rhubarb • Rice Bran • Sarsaparilla • Slippery Elm • Sorrel • Tannic Acid • Tragacanth • Water Avens • Willow Bark
OXAZEPAM (*Serax*)	Cabbage
OXYTOCIN (*Pitocin*)	Aletris • Country Mallow • Ephedra
PANCREATIC ENZYMES (*Pancreatin*)	Folic Acid
PARASYMPATHOMIMETICS Neostigmine (*Prostigmin*)	Pantothenic Acid (Vitamin B5)
PAROXETINE (*Paxil*)	St. John's Wort
PENICILLAMINE (*Cuprimine*)	Colloidal Silver • Copper • Zinc
PENTAZOCINE (*Talwin*)	Smokeless Tobacco
PHENACETIN	Gelsemium • Grape fruit, skin
PHENOBARBITAL	Biotin • Cinchona • Folic Acid • Nutmeg and Mace • Pyridoxine (Vitamin B6) • Vitamin D
PHENOTHIAZINES Some drugs in this category include: Thioridazine (*Mellaril*) • Mesoridazine (*Serentil*) • Trifluoperazine (*Stelazine*) • Chlorpromazine (*Thorazine*) • Fluphenazine (*Prolixin*)	Borage flower, dried above ground parts • Borage Seed Oil • Boxwood • Brahmi • Chastberry • Evening Primrose Oil • Fever Bark • Ignatius Bean • L-Tryptophan • Nux Vomica • Smokeless Tobacco • Yohimbe
PHENYLBUTAZONE	Smokeless Tobacco
PHENYLPROPANOLAMINE (*Acutrim*)	Black Tea • Caffeine • Cocoa • Coffee • Cola Nut • Green Tea • Guarana • Mate
PHENYTOIN (*Dilantin*)	Beer • Biotin • Black Pepper and White Pepper • Black Tea • Folic Acid • Green Tea • Indian Long Pepper • Pyridoxine (Vitamin B6) • Vitamin D • Wine
PHOTOSENSITIZING DRUGS Some drugs in this category include: Acyclovir (*Zovirax*) • Amitriptyline (*Elavil*) • Azithromycin (*Zithromax*) • Captopril (*Capoten*) • Carbamazepine (*Tegretol*) • Chloroquine (*Arelan*) • Chlorthiazide (*Diuril*) • Chlorpromazine (*Thorazine*) • Ciprofloxacin (*Cipro*) • Dantrolene (*Dantrium*) • Dapsone • Divalproex (*Depakote*) • Oral Contraceptives • Felbamate (*Felbatol*) • Fluorouracil (*Efudex, Carac*) • Flutamide (*Eulexin*) • Furosemide (*Lasix*) • Glipizide (*Glucotrol*) • Glyburide (*Micronase*) • Hydroxychloroquine (*Plaquenil*) • Isotretinoin (*Accutane*) • Methoxsalen (*Oxsoralen*) • Minocycline (*Minocin*) • Phenobarbital • Promethazine (*Phenergan*) • Quinidine (*Quinidex*) • Sulfamethoxale;Trimethotrim (*Bactrim, Septra*) • Tacrolimus (*Prograf*) • Tolbutamide (*Orinase*) • Trazodone (*Desyrel*) • Tretinoin (*Retin A*) • Valproic Acid (*Depakene*)	Angelica root • Bergamot Oil • Bishop's Weed • Chlorophyll • Khella • St. John's Wort
PHYSOSTIGMINE (*Antilirium*)	Acacia • Oak bark • Peyote
POTASSIUM DEPLETING DIURETICS Some drugs in this category include: Furosemide (*Lasix*) • Bumetanide(*Bumex*) • Chlorothiazide (*Diuril*) • Chlorthalidone	Agropyron • Alder Buckthorn • Apple Cider Vinegar • Butternut • Calatropis • Cascara • Castor Oil • Corn Silk • Couch Grass • Fo-Ti • Gamboge

CHARTS

Potential Interactions: Drug/Natural Medicine

For additional data, refer to the database.

Drug	Natural Medicine
POTASSIUM DEPLETING DIURETICS (Cont.) (*Hygroton*) • Indapamide (*Lozol*) • Torsemide (*Demadex*)	Lily-Of-The-Valley • Oleander • Pheasant's Eye • Quassia • Rhubarb • Squill • Strophanthus • Swamp Milkweed • Uzara • Wahoo • Wallflower
POTASSIUM (*K-Dur, K-Lyte, Micro-K*)	Dibencozide • Laminaria
POTASSIUM INCREASING DRUGS Some drugs in this category include: Potassium supplements (*K-Dur, K-Lyte, Micro-K*) • Enalapril (*Vasotec*) • Lisinopril (*Prinivil, Zestril*) • Quinapril (*Accupril*) • Ramipril (*Altace*) • Moexipril (*Univasc*) • Spironolactone (*Aldactone*) • Triamterene (*Dyrenium*)	L-Arginine • Laminaria • Morinda • Potassium
POTASSIUM IODIDE (*Pima, SSKI*)	Iodine
POTASSIUM-SPARING DIURETICS Some drugs in this category include: Spironolactone (*Aldactone*) • Triamterene (*Dyrenium*)	L-Arginine • Laminaria • Morinda • Potassium • Zinc
PRAVASTATIN (*Pravachol*)	Beta-Sitosterol
PREDNISOLONE (*Pediapred*)	Cordyceps
PRIMIDONE (*Mysoline*)	Biotin • Cinchona • Folic Acid
PROBENECID (*Benemid*)	Inosine
PROCYCLIDINE (*Kemadrin*)	Areca
PROPOXYPHENE (*Darvon*)	Smokeless Tobacco
PROPRANOLOL (*Inderal*)	Black Pepper and White Pepper • Guggul • Indian Long Pepper • Indian Snakeroot
PROTEASE INHIBITORS (PIs) Some drugs in this category include: Indinavir (*Crixivan*) • Nelfinavir (*Viracept*) • Saquinavir (*Invirase*)	St. John's Wort
PROTEIN-BINDING DRUGS Some drugs in this category include: • Phenytoin (*Dilantin*) • Digoxin (*Lanoxin*)	Horse Chestnut seed
PROTON PUMP INHIBITORS Some drugs in this category include: Esomeprazole (*Nexium*) • Lansoprazole (*Prevacid*) • Omeprazole (*Prilosec*) • Pantoprazole (*Protonix*) • Rabeprazole (*Aciphex*)	Cranberry • Pancreatin • Peppermint Oil
PSEUDOCHOLINESTERASE INHIBITORS	Cocoa
PSORALENS Some drugs in this category include: • Methoxsalen (*Oxsoralen*) • Trioxsalen (*Trisoralen*)	Arrach • Lime oil • Masterwort • Wild Carrot
PUVA	Celery • Rue
PYRIMETHAMINE (*Daraprim*)	Folic Acid
QUINIDINE (*Quinidex*)	Cinchona • Grapefruit • Grapefruit seed extract • Pheasant's Eye • Scopolia • Squill
QUININE	Black Hellebore • Cinchona • Hedge Mustard • Lily-Of-The-Valley • Oleander • Smokeless Tobacco • Swamp Milkweed • Uzara • Wahoo
QUINOLONES Some drugs in this category include: Ciprofloxacin (*Cipro*) • Gatifloxacin (*Tequin*) • Levofloxacin (*Levaquin*) • Moxifloxacin (*Avelox*) • Norfloxacin (*Noroxin*) • Ofloxacin (*Floxin*) • Trovafloxacin (*Trovan*)	Black Tea • Caffeine • Cocoa • Coffee • Cola Nut • Green Tea • Guarana • Mate • Quercetin
RANITIDINE (*Zantac*)	Smokeless Tobacco
RESERPINE	Country Mallow • Ephedra • St. John's Wort • Turmeric
RILUZOLE (*Rilutek*)	Caffeine • Coffee • Cola Nut • Guarana • Mate

C H A R T S

•

Potential Interactions: Drug/Natural Medicine   For additional data, refer to the database.

Drug	Natural Medicine
RITONAVIR (*Norvir*)	Gamma-Hydroxybutyrate (GHB)
SAQUINAVIR (*Fortovase, Invirase*)	Bitter Orange • Gamma-Hydroxybutyrate (GHB) • Garlic • Grapefruit • Grapefruit seed extract • St. John's Wort
SCOPOLAMINE (*Transderm Scop*)	Acacia • Oak bark
SECALE ALKALOID DERIVATIVES (*Ergot*)	Country Mallow
SEDATIVE DRUGS Some drugs in this category include: Zolpidem (*Ambien*) • Zaleplon (*Sonata*) • Temazepam (*Restoril*) • Flurazepam (*Dalmane*) • Triazolam (*Halcion*) • Lorazepam (*Ativan*) • Estazolam (*Prosom*) • Secobarbital (*Seconal*) • Phenobarbital	Baikal Skullcap • Beer • Bitter Almond • Black Tea • Butanediol (BD) • Calamus • Calendula • California Poppy • Catnip • Celery • Couch Grass • Cowslip • Elecampane • Gamma Butyrolactone (GBL) • Gamma-Hydroxybutyrate (GHB) • German Chamomile • Ginseng, Siberian • Goldenseal • Gotu Kola • Hawthorn • Hops • Hydrazine Sulfate • Jamaican Dogwood • Kava • L-Tryptophan • Lavender • Lemon Balm • Marsh Tea • Melatonin • Motherwort • Passionflower • Sage • Sarsaparilla • Sassafras • Shepherd's Purse • Stinging Nettle above ground parts • Sweet Bay • Valerian • Wild Lettuce • Wine • Yerba Mansa
SELECTIVE SEROTONIN REUPTAKE INHIBITORS (SSRIs) Some drugs in this category include: Citalopram (*Celexa*) • Fluoxetine (*Prozac*) • Fluvoxamine (*Luvox*) • Paroxetine (*Paxil*) • Sertraline (*Zoloft*) • Venlafaxine (*Effexor*)	Hawaiian Baby Woodrose • L-Tryptophan • SAMe • St. John's Wort
SELEGILINE (*Eldepryl*)	Phenylalanine
SEROTONIN AGONISTS Some drugs in this category include: Citalopram (*Celexa*) • Fluoxetine (*Prozac*) • Fluvoxamine (*Luvox*) • Paroxetine (*Paxil*) • Sertraline (*Zoloft*) • Venlafaxine (*Effexor*) • Phenelizine (*Nardil*) • Tranycypromine (*Parnate*) • Amitriptyline (*Elavil*) • Nortriptyline (*Pamelor*)	5-HTP • L-tryptophan • SAMe • St. John's Wort
SEROTONIN ANTAGONISTS Some drugs in this category include: Methylsergide • Cyproheptadine (*Periactin*)	5-HTP
SERTRALINE (*Zoloft*)	St. John's Wort
SILDENAFIL (*Viagra*)	L-Arginine
SKELETAL MUSCLE RELAXANTS Some drugs in this category include: • Baclofen (*Lioresal*) • Botulinum Toxin Type A (*Botox*) • Chlorzoxazone (*Parafon Forte*) • Cyclobenzaprine (*Flexeril*) • Dantrolene (*Dantrium*) • Metaxalone (*Skelaxin*) • Orphenadrine (*Norflex*)	Butanediol (BD) • Gamma Butyrolactone (GBL) • Gamma-Hydroxybutyrate (GHB) • Magnesium
STIMULANT LAXATIVES Some drugs in this category include: Senna (*Senokot*) • Bisacodyl (*Dulcolax*)	Black Hellebore • Calatropis • Digitalis • Gossypol • Hedge Mustard • Lily-Of-The-Valley • Oleander • Pheasant's Eye • Squill • Swamp Milkweed • Uzara • Wahoo
SUCCINYLCHOLINE (*Quelicin*)	Procaine
SULFASALAZINE (*Azulfidine*)	Folic Acid
SULFONAMIDE ANTIBIOTICS Some drugs in this category include: Sulfamethoxazole;Trimethoprim (*Bactrim*) • Sulfacetamide (*Sodium Sulamyd*) • Sulfisoxazole (*Gantrisin*)	Para-Aminobenzoic Acid (PABA) • Procaine
SULINDAC (*Clinoril*)	DMSO (Dimethylsulfoxide)
SYMPATHOMIMETICS Pseudophedrine (*Sudafed*)	Barley • Ergot • Fever Bark • Indian Snakeroot • Tiratricol • Yohimbe
SYRUP OF IPECAC	Activated Charcoal
TACRINE (*Cognex*)	Smokeless Tobacco

CHARTS

Potential Interactions: Drug/Natural Medicine

For additional data, refer to the database.

Drug	Natural Medicine
TERBINAFINE (*Lamisil*)	Caffeine • Coffee • Cola Nut • Guarana • Mate
TERFENADINE (*Seldane*)	Grapefruit • Grapefruit seed extract
TETRACYCLINE (*Sumycin*)	Black Hellebore • Bromelain • Calcium • Colloidal Silver • Digitalis • Hedge Mustard • Iron • Lily-Of-The-Valley • Manganese • Oleander • Pectin • Swamp Milkweed • Uzara • Wahoo • Yogurt • Zinc
THEOPHYLLINE (*Theo-Dur*)	Black Pepper and White Pepper • Black Tea • Caffeine • Capsicum • Cocoa • Coffee • Cola Nut • Country Mallow • Ephedra • Green Tea • Guarana • Indian Long Pepper • Ipriflavone • Marijuana • Mate • Smokeless Tobacco • St. John's Wort
THIAZIDE DIURETICS Some drugs in this category include: Chlorothiazide (*Diuril*) • Chlorthalidone (*Hygroton*) • Hydrochlorothiazide (*Esidrix*) • Metolazone (*Zaroxolyn*)	Calcium • Dolomite • Ginkgo leaf (Ginkgo leaf extract) • Pangamic Acid • Vitamin D • Zinc
THIOTHIXENE (*Navane*)	Smokeless Tobacco
THROMBOLYTICS (*tPA, Alterplase*)	Mesoglycan • Potato
THYROXINE	Colloidal Silver
TRAZODONE (*Desyrel*)	Ginkgo leaf (Ginkgo leaf extract) • L-Tryptophan
TRIAZOLAM (*Halcion*)	DHEA
TRICYCLIC ANTIDEPRESSANTS (TCAs) Some drugs in this category include: Amitriptyline (*Elavil*) • Clomipramine (*Anafranil*) • Desipramine (*Norpramin*) • Doxepin (*Sinequan*) • Imipramine (*Tofranil*) • Nortriptyline (*Pamelor*) • Protriptyline (*Vivactil*)	Black Tea • Cowhage • Scopolia • Smokeless Tobacco • Yohimbe
URINARY ACIDIFIERS Ammonium Chloride	Country Mallow • Ephedra • Uva Ursi
URINARY ALKALINIZERS Potassium Citrate (*Polycitra-K*)	Country Mallow • Ephedra • Uva Ursi
VALPROIC ACID (*Depakene*)	L-Carnitine
VERAPAMIL (*Calan, Covera, Isoptin, Verelan*)	Black Tea • Caffeine • Calcium • Cocoa • Coffee • Cola Nut • Guarana • Green Tea • Mate • Melatonin • Pangamic Acid • Peyote • Stevia
VITAMIN B12 (*Cobex*)	Smokeless Tobacco
VITAMIN C	Dibencozide • Smokeless Tobacco
VITAMIN K (*Mephyton*)	Tiratricol
WARFARIN (*Coumadin*)	Acerola • Avocado • Beer • Black Psyllium • Blond Psyllium • Cabbage • Cherokee Rosehip • Coenzyme Q-10 • Danshen • Devil's Claw • Dong Quai • EDTA • Ginkgo leaf (Ginkgo leaf extract) • Ginseng, American • Ginseng, Panax • Grape Seed • Grapefruit • Grapefruit seed extract • Great Plantain • Green Tea • Leech • Lycium • Papaya • Rose Hip • Smartweed • St. John's Wort • Vinpocetine • Vitamin C (Ascorbic Acid) • Vitamin E • Vitamin K • Watercress • Wheatgrass • Wine • Wintergreen Oil
XYLITOL	L-Arginine
ZOLPIDEM (*Ambien*)	Smokeless Tobacco

C
H
A
R
T
S

•

Potential Interactions Between
Natural Medicines and Drugs

For details on possible interactions between natural medicines and drugs, see the listing for the specific natural medicine in the body of this database. This chart does not contain all theoretical or unknown interactions.

Natural Medicine	Drug
5-HTP	Carbidopa (*Lodosyn*) • Serotonin Agonists • Serotonin Antagonists
Acacia	Alcohol • Apomorphine (*Uprima*) • Atropine • Cocaine • Ethyl Alcohol • Homatropine (*Homapin*) • Iron (*Feosol, Slow Fe*) • Morphine (*Roxanol, Oramorph, MS Contin, MSIR, Kadian*) • Oral Drugs • Physostigmine (*Antilirium*) • Scopolamine (*Transderm Scop*)
Acerola	Acid-Sensitive Drugs • Acidic or Basic Drugs • Estrogen (*Estratest, Estrace, Ogen, Menogen*) • Fluphenazine (*Prolixin*) • Iron (*Feosol, Slow Fe*) • Warfarin (*Coumadin*)
Ackee	Antidiabetes Drugs
Activated Charcoal	Oral Drugs • Syrup of Ipecac
Agar	Oral Drugs
Agrimony	Anticoagulant and Antiplatelet Drugs • Antidiabetes Drugs • Antihypertensive Drugs • Antihypotensive Drugs
Agropyron	Potassium Depleting Diuretics
Alder Buckthorn	Corticosteroids • Digoxin (*Lanoxin*) • Oral Drugs • Potassium Depleting Diuretics
Aletris	Acid-Inhibiting Drugs • Oxytocin (*Pitocin*)
Alfalfa	Anticoagulant and Antiplatelet Drugs • Chlorpromazine (*Thorazine*) • Estrogen (*Estratest, Estrace, Ogen, Menogen*) • Hormone Replacement Therapy • Oral Contraceptives
Algin	Oral Drugs
Allspice	Anticoagulant and Antiplatelet Drugs
Aloe dried juice from leaf, latex	Antiarrhythmic Drugs • Corticosteroids • Digoxin (*Lanoxin*) • Diuretics • Oral Drugs
Aloe gel	Antidiabetes Drugs • Glyburide (*Diabeta, Micronase, Glynase*) • Hydrocortisone (*Cortef*)
Alpha Hydroxy Acids	Magnesium (*Slo-Mag, Mag-Ox*)
Alpha-Lipoic Acid	Alcohol • Antidiabetes Drugs • Chemotherapeutic Agents
Alpine Cranberry	Antigout Agents
Alpinia	Acid-Inhibiting Drugs
American Chestnut	Oral Drugs
American Elder	Cytochrome P450 3A4 (CYP3A4) Substrates
Andorgraphis	Anticoagulant and Antiplatelet Drugs • Antihypertensive Drugs • Immunosuppressants
Androdenedione	Estrogen (*Estratest, Estrace, Ogen, Menogen*)
Androstenediol	Androgenic Drugs • Estrogen (*Estratest, Estrace, Ogen, Menogen*)
Angelica herb, seed	Acid-Inhibiting Drugs • Anticoagulant and Antiplatelet Drugs • Hexobarbiton
Angelica root	Acid-Inhibiting Drugs • Anticoagulant and Antiplatelet Drugs • Photosensitizing Drugs

CHARTS

Potential Interactions: Natural Medicine/Drug   For additional data, refer to the database.

Natural Medicine	Drug
Angel's Trumpet	Anticholinergic Drugs
Annatto	Antidiabetes Drugs
Apple	Fexofenadine (*Allegra*)
Apple Cider Vinegar	Cardiovascular Drugs • Insulin (*Humulin, Humalog, Novolin, Lantus*) • Potassium Depleting Diuretics
Areca	Anticholinergic Drugs • Cholinergic Drugs • Procyclidine (*Kemadrin*)
Aristolochia	Acid-Inhibiting Drugs
Arnica	Anticoagulant and Antiplatelet Drugs
Arrach	Psoralens
Asafoetida	Anticoagulant and Antiplatelet Drugs • Antihypertensive Drugs • Antihypotensive Drugs
Ashwaganda	Amphetamines • Barbiturates • Benzodiazepines • Chloral Hydrate (*Aquachloral*)
Astragalus	Cyclophosphamide (*Cytoxan*) • Cyclosporine (*Neoral, Sandimmune*) • Immunosuppressants
Autumn Crocus	Colchicine
Avocado	Warfarin (*Coumadin*)
Baikal Skullcap	Alcohol • Antidiabetes Drugs • Benzodiazepines • Sedative Drugs
Barley	Antidiabetes Drugs • Sympathomimetics
Bean Pod	Antidiabetes Drugs
Bee Venom	Hydrocortisone (*Cortef*)
Beer	Antidiabetes Drugs • Aspirin and other Salicylates • Barbiturates • Benzodiazepines • Cisapride (*Propulsid*) • CNS Depressants • Erythromycin (*E.E.S., E-Mycin, PCE*) • Hepatotoxic Drugs • Metformin (*Gucophage*) • Narcotic Analgesics • Nonsteroidal Anti-Inflammatory Drugs (NSAIDS) • Phenytoin (*Dilantin*) • Sedative Drugs • Warfarin (*Coumadin*)
Beeswax	Nonsteroidal Anti-Inflammatory Drugs (NSAIDS)
Beet	Disulfiram (*Antabuse*) • H2-Blockers • Narcotic Analgesics
Belladonna	Anticholinergic Drugs
Bergamot Oil	Photosensitizing Drugs
Beta-Sitosterol	Pravastatin (*Pravachol*)
Betony	Antihypertensive Drugs
Bilberry leaf	Antidiabetes Drugs • Disulfiram (*Antabuse*)
Biotin	Carbamazepine (*Tegretol*) • Phenobarbital • Phenytoin (*Dilantin*) • Primidone (*Mysoline*)
Birch	Diuretics
Bishop's Weed	Anticoagulant and Antiplatelet Drugs • Cytochrome P450 3A4 (CYP3A4) Substrates • Hepatotoxic Drugs • Photosensitizing Drugs
Bistort	Oral Drugs
Bitter Almond	CNS Depressants • Sedative Drugs
Bitter Melon	Antidiabetes Drugs • Chlorpropamide (*Diabinese*) • Insulin (*Humulin, Humalog, Novolin, Lantus*)

C H A R T S

•

Potential Interactions: Natural Medicine/Drug
For additional data, refer to the database.

Natural Medicine	Drug
Bitter Orange	Acid-Inhibiting Drugs • CNS Stimulants • Cytochrome P450 3A4 (CYP3A4) Substrates • Felodipine (*Plendil*) • Midazolam (*Versed*) • Monoamine Oxidase Inhibitors (MAOIs) • Saquinavir (*Fortovase, Invirase*)
Black Hellebore	Cardiovascular Drugs • Digoxin (*Lanoxin*) • Macrolide Antibiotics • Quinine • Stimulant Laxatives • Tetracyclines (*Sumycin*)
Black Horehound	Dopamine Agonists
Black Mulberry	Antidiabetes Drugs
Black Mustard oil	Acid-Inhibiting Drugs
Black Mustard seed	Acid-Inhibiting Drugs
Black Pepper and White Pepper	Phenytoin (*Dilantin*) • Propranolol (*Inderal*) • Theophylline (*Theo-Dur, Slo-Bid, Theolair*)
Black Psyllium	Antidiabetes Drugs • Carbamazepine (*Tegretol*) • Digoxin (*Lanoxin*) • Insulin (*Humulin, Humalog, Novolin, Lantus*) • Lithium (*Eskalith, Lithobid*) • Oral Drugs • Warfarin (*Coumadin*)
Black Root	Digoxin (*Lanoxin*)
Black Tea	Acetaminophen (*Tylenol*) • Adenosine (*Adenocard*) • Antipsychotic Drugs • Aspirin and other Salicylates • Barbiturates • Benzodiazepines • Beta-Adrenergic Agonists • Beta-Blockers • Chlorpromazine (*Thorazine*) • Cimetidine (*Tagamet*) • Clozapine (*Clozaril*) • CNS Depressants • Disulfiram (*Antabuse*) • Ergotamine (*Ergostat*) • Lithium (*Eskalith, Lithobid*) • Monoamine Oxidase Inhibitors (MAOIs) • Oral Contraceptives • Phenylpropanolamine (*Acutrim*) • Phenytoin (*Dilantin*) • Quinolones • Sedative Drugs • Theophylline (*Theo-Dur, Slo-Bid, Theolair*) • Tricyclic Antidepressants (TCAs) • Verapamil (*Calan, Covera, Isoptin, Verelan*)
Black Walnut	Oral Drugs
Bladderwrack	Anticoagulant and Antiplatelet Drugs • Diuretics • Levothyroxine (*Synthroid, Levothroid, Levoxyl*) • Lithium (*Eskalith, Lithobid*)
Blessed Thistle	Acid-Inhibiting Drugs
Blond Psyllium	Antidiabetes Drugs • Carbamazepine (*Tegretol*) • Lithium (*Eskalith, Lithobid*) • Oral Drugs • Warfarin (*Coumadin*)
Blue Cohosh	Antidiabetes Drugs • Cardiovascular Drugs • Nicotine (*Nicotrol, Habitrol, Nicorette, Nicoderm, Prostep*)
Blue Flag	Digoxin (*Lanoxin*)
Blueberry	Antidiabetes Drugs
Bogbean	Anticoagulant and Antiplatelet Drugs
Borage flower, dried above ground parts	Phenothiazines
Borage Seed Oil	Anesthesia • Anticoagulant and Antiplatelet Drugs • Phenothiazines
Boron	Estrogen (*Estratest, Estrace, Ogen, Menogen*)
Boxwood	Analeptics • Phenothiazines
Brahmi	Phenothiazines
Branched-Chain Amino Acids	Levodopa (*Larodopa*)
Brewer's Yeast	Antifungals • Monoamine Oxidase Inhibitors (MAOIs)
Brewer's Yeast (Hansen CBS 5926)	Antifungals • Monoamine Oxidase Inhibitors (MAOIs)
Bromelain	Anticoagulant and Antiplatelet Drugs • Tetracyclines (*Sumycin*)
Buchu	Anticoagulant and Antiplatelet Drugs

CHARTS

Natural Medicine	Drug
Bugleweed	Antidiabetes Drugs • Levothyroxine (*Synthroid, Levothroid, Levoxyl*)
Burdock	Antidiabetes Drugs • Insulin (*Humulin, Humalog, Novolin, Lantus*)
Butanediol (BD)	Alcohol • Amphetamines • Anticonvulsants • Antipsychotic Drugs • Benzodiazepines • CNS Depressants • Haloperidol (*Haldol*) • Naloxone (*Narcan*) • Narcotic Analgesics • Sedative Drugs • Skeletal Muscle Relaxants
Butternut	Antiarrhythmic Drugs • Corticosteroids • Digoxin (*Lanoxin*) • Laxatives • Oral Drugs • Potassium Depleting Diuretics
Cabbage	Acetaminophen (*Tylenol*) • Cytochrome P450 1A2 (CYP1A2) Substrates • Oxazepam (*Serax*) • Warfarin (*Coumadin*)
Caffeine	Acetaminophen (*Tylenol*) • Alcohol • Antidiabetes Drugs • Aspirin and other Salicylates • Benzodiazepines • Beta-Adrenergic Agonists • Cimetidine (*Tagamet*) • Clozapine (*Clozaril*) • CNS Stimulants • Disulfiram (*Antabuse*) • Ephedrine • Ergotamine (*Ergostat*) • Estrogen (*Estratest, Estrace, Ogen, Menogen*) • Fluvoxamine (*Luvox*) • Lithium (*Eskalith, Lithobid*) • Mexiletine (*Mexitil*) • Monoamine Oxidase Inhibitors (MAOIs) • Oral Contraceptives • Phenylpropanolamine (*Acutrim*) • Quinolones • Riluzole (*Rilutek*) • Terbinafine (*Lamisil*) • Theophylline (*Theo-Dur, Slo-Bid, Theolair*) • Verapamil (*Calan, Covera, Isoptin, Verelan*)
Calabar Bean	Anticholinergic Drugs
Calamus	Acid-Inhibiting Drugs • CNS Depressants • Monoamine Oxidase Inhibitors (MAOIs) • Sedative Drugs
Calcium	Bisphosphonates • Estrogen (*Estratest, Estrace, Ogen, Menogen*) • Fluoroquinolones • Levothyroxine (*Synthroid, Levothroid, Levoxyl*) • Tetracyclines (*Sumycin*) • Thiazide Diuretics • Verapamil (*Calan, Covera, Isoptin, Verelan*)
Calcium D-Glucarate	Alcohol • Kanamycin (*Kantrex*)
Calendula	Barbiturates • Sedative Drugs
California Poppy	Barbiturates • Monoamine Oxidase Inhibitors (MAOIs) • Sedative Drugs
Calotropis	Digoxin (*Lanoxin*) • Potassium Depleting Diuretics • Stimulant Laxatives
Canadian Hemp	Digoxin (*Lanoxin*)
Capsicum	Ace Inhibitors (ACEIs) • Acid-Inhibiting Drugs • Anticoagulant and Antiplatelet Drugs • Antihypertensive Drugs • Aspirin and other Salicylates • Barbiturates • Cocaine • Monoamine Oxidase Inhibitors (MAOIs) • Theophylline (*Theo-Dur, Slo-Bid, Theolair*)
Cascara	Corticosteroids • Digoxin (*Lanoxin*) • Laxatives • Oral Drugs • Potassium Depleting Diuretics
Cassia	Antidiabetes Drugs • Antihypertensive Drugs
Castor Oil	Corticosteroids • Digoxin (*Lanoxin*) • Laxatives • Oral Drugs • Potassium Depleting Diuretics
Cat's Claw	Antihypertensive Drugs • Cytochrome P450 3A4 (CYP3A4) Substrates • Immunosuppressants
Catnip	Barbiturates • Sedative Drugs
Cedar leaf	Anticonvulsants
Cedar leaf oil	Anticonvulsants
Cedarwood bark, berry, leaf, seed, twig	Barbiturates • Dicoumarol
Celery	Anticoagulant and Antiplatelet Drugs • PUVA • Sedative Drugs
Cereus	Digoxin (*Lanoxin*) • Monoamine Oxidase Inhibitors (MAOIs)
Cetyl Myristoleate	Alcohol • Methotrexate (*MTX, Rheumatrex*)
Chanca Piedra	Antidiabetes Drugs

Potential Interactions: Natural Medicine/Drug	For additional data, refer to the database.
Natural Medicine	**Drug**
Chaparral	Monoamine Oxidase Inhibitors (MAOIs)
Chasteberry	Antipsychotic Drugs • Dopamine Antagonists • Estrogen (*Estratest, Estrace, Ogen, Menogen*) • Hormone Replacement Therapy • Oral Contraceptives • Phenothiazines
Cherokee Rosehip	Aspirin and other Salicylates • Estrogen (*Estratest, Estrace, Ogen, Menogen*) • Fluphenazine (*Prolixin*) • Iron (*Feosol, Slow Fe*) • Warfarin (*Coumadin*)
Chinese Club Moss	Anticholinergic Drugs • Cholinergic Drugs
Chinese Cucumber Root	Antidiabetes Drugs
Chlorella	Anticoagulant and Antiplatelet Drugs
Chlorophyll	Photosensitizing Drugs
Chondroitin Sulfate	Anticoagulant and Antiplatelet Drugs • Hyaluronic Acid
Chromium	Beta-Blockers (*Beta-Adrenergic Antagonists*) • Corticosteroids • Insulin (*Humulin, Humalog, Novolin, Lantus*) • Nicotinic Acid
Chrysanthemum	Cardiovascular Drugs
Cinchona	Acid-Inhibiting Drugs • Anticoagulant and Antiplatelet Drugs • Carbamazepine (*Tegretol*) • Phenobarbital • Primidone (*Mysoline*) • Quinidine (*Quinidex*) • Quinine
Cinnamon bark	Acid-Inhibiting Drugs
Clary Sage	Chloral Hydrate (*Aquachloral*) • Hexobarbitone
Clove dried flowerbud, leaf, stem	Anticoagulant and Antiplatelet Drugs
Clove oil	Anticoagulant and Antiplatelet Drugs
Cocoa	Acetaminophen (*Tylenol*) • Alcohol • Antidiabetes Drugs • Aspirin and other Salicylates • Barbiturates • Beta-Adrenergic Agonists • Cimetidine (*Tagamet*) • Clozapine (*Clozaril*) • Disulfiram (*Antabuse*) • Ergotamine (*Ergostat*) • Fluconazole (*Diflucan*) • Lithium (*Eskalith, Lithobid*) • Mexiletine (*Mexitil*) • Monoamine Oxidase Inhibitors (MAOIs) • Nifedipine (*Adalat, Procardia*) • Oral Contraceptives • Phenylpropanolamine (*Acutrim*) • Pseudocholinesterase Inhibitors • Quinolones • Theophylline (*Theo-Dur, Slo-Bid, Theolair*) • Verapamil (*Calan, Covera, Isoptin, Verelan*)
Coenzyme Q10	Antihypertensive Drugs • Chemotherapeutic Agents • Insulin (*Humulin, Humalog, Novolin, Lantus*) • Warfarin (*Coumadin*)
Coffee	Acetaminophen (*Tylenol*) • Acid-Inhibiting Drugs • Alendronate (*Fosamax*) • Antidiabetes Drugs • Aspirin and other Salicylates • Benzodiazepines • Beta-Adrenergic Agonists • Clozapine (*Clozaril*) • CNS Stimulants • Disulfiram (*Antabuse*) • Ephedrine • Ergotamine (*Ergostat*) • Estrogen (*Estratest, Estrace, Ogen, Menogen*) • Lithium (*Eskalith, Lithobid*) • Mexiletine (*Mexitil*) • Monoamine Oxidase Inhibitors (MAOIs) • Oral Contraceptives • Phenylpropanolamine (*Acutrim*) • Quinolones • Riluzole (*Rilutek*) • Terbinafine (*Lamisil*) • Theophylline (*Theo-Dur, Slo-Bid, Theolair*) • Verapamil (*Calan, Covera, Isoptin, Verelan*)
Coffee Charcoal	Oral Drugs
Cola Nut	Acetaminophen (*Tylenol*) • Antidiabetes Drugs • Aspirin and other Salicylates • Benzodiazepines • Beta-Adrenergic Agonists • Clozapine (*Clozaril*) • CNS Stimulants • Disulfiram (*Antabuse*) • Ephedrine • Ergotamine (*Ergostat*) • Estrogen (*Estratest, Estrace, Ogen, Menogen*) • Lithium (*Eskalith, Lithobid*) • Mexiletine (*Mexitil*) • Monoamine Oxidase Inhibitors (MAOIs) • Oral Contraceptives • Phenylpropanolamine (*Acutrim*) • Quinolones • Riluzole (*Rilutek*) • Terbinafine (*Lamisil*) • Theophylline (*Theo-Dur, Slo-Bid, Theolair*) • Verapamil (*Calan, Covera, Isoptin, Verelan*)
Colloidal Silver	Methyldopa (*Aldomet*) • Norfloxacin (*Noroxin*) • Ofloxacin (*Ocuflox, Floxin*) • Penicillamine (*Cuprimine*) • Tetracyclines (*Sumycin*) • Thyroxine
Colocynth	Digoxin (*Lanoxin*)
Colombo	Acid-Inhibiting Drugs • Antacids (*Tums, Maalox, Mylanta*) • H2-Blockers

CHARTS

Potential Interactions: Natural Medicine/Drug	For additional data, refer to the database.
Natural Medicine	**Drug**
Coltsfoot	Antihypertensive Drugs • Cardiovascular Drugs
Copper	Penicillamine (*Cuprimine*)
Cordyceps	Aminoglycosides • Cyclophosphamide (*Cytoxan*) • Cyclosporine (*Neoral, Sandimmune*) • Prednisolone (*Pediapred*)
Coriolus Mushroom	Acetaminophen (*Tylenol*)
Cornsilk	Anticoagulant and Antiplatelet Drugs • Antidiabetes Drugs • Antihypertensives Drugs • Potassium Depleting Diuretics
Couch Grass	Potassium Depleting Diuretics • Sedative Drugs
Country Mallow	Amitriptyline (*Elavil*) • Antidiabetes Drugs • Caffeine (*NoDoz, Stay Alert, Vivarin*) • Dexamethasone (*Decadron*) • Digoxin (*Lanoxin*) • Monoamine Oxidase Inhibitors (MAOIs) • Oxytocin (*Pitocin*) • Reserpine • Secale Alkaloid Derivatives (*Ergot*) • Theophylline (*Theo-Dur, Slo-Bid, Theolair*) • Urinary Acidifiers • Urinary Alkalinizers
Cowhage	Anesthesia • Antidiabetes Drugs • Antipsychotic Drugs • Guanethidine (*Ismelin*) • Methyldopa (*Aldomet*) • Monoamine Oxidase Inhibitors (MAOIs) • Tricyclic Antidepressants (TCAs)
Cowslip	Antihypertensive Drugs • Antihypotensive Drugs • Diuretics • Doxycycline (*Vibramycin*) • Sedative Drugs
Cranberry	Proton Pump Inhibitors
Creatine	Nephrotoxic Drugs
Cubebs	Acid-Inhibiting Drugs
Cumin	Antidiabetes Drugs • Barbiturates
Damiana	Antidiabetes Drugs
Dandelion entire plant	Acid-Inhibiting Drugs • Antidiabetes Drugs • Diuretics • Lithium (*Eskalith, Lithobid*)
Danshen	Anticoagulant and Antiplatelet Drugs • Warfarin (*Coumadin*)
Deanol	Anticholinergic Drugs
Deer Velvet	Morphine (*Roxanol, Oramorph, MS Contin, MSIR, Kadian*)
Deertongue	Anticoagulant and Antiplatelet Drugs
Devil's Club	Antidiabetes Drugs
Devil's Claw	Acid-Inhibiting Drugs • Antidiabetes Drugs • Antihypertensive Drugs • Cardiovascular Drugs • Warfarin (*Coumadin*)
DHA (Docosahexanenoic Acid)	Anticoagulant and Antiplatelet Drugs
DHEA	Cytochrome P450 3A4 (CYP3A4) Substrates • Triazolam (*Halcion*)
Dibencozide	Acid-Inhibiting Drugs • Aminoglycosides • Aminosalicylic Acid (*Paser, Teebacin, Tubasal*) • Anticonvulsants • Chloramphenicol (*Chloromycetin*) • Colchicine • Potassium (*K-Dur, K-Lyte, Micro-K*) • Vitamin C
Digitalis	Cardiovascular Drugs • Digoxin (*Lanoxin*) • Macrolide Antibiotics • Stimulant Laxatives • Tetracyclines (*Sumycin*)
DMSO (Dimethylsulfoxide)	Sulindac (*Clinoril*)
Dolomite	Estrogen (*Estratest, Estrace, Ogen, Menogen*) • Glucocorticoids • Thiazide Diuretics
Dong Quai	Anticoagulant and Antiplatelet Drugs • Warfarin (*Coumadin*)
Echinacea	Cytochrome P450 3A4 (CYP3A4) Substrates • Econazole Nitrate (*Spectazole*) • Immunosuppressants
EDTA	Diuretics • Insulin (*Humulin, Humalog, Novolin, Lantus*) • Warfarin (*Coumadin*)

CHARTS

Potential Interactions: Natural Medicine/Drug
For additional data, refer to the database.

Natural Medicine	Drug
Elderflower	Doxycycline (*Vibramycin*)
Elecampane	Antidiabetes Drugs • Antihypertensive Drugs • Antihypotensive Drugs • Sedative Drugs
Emu Oil	Anticoagulant and Antiplatelet Drugs • Aspirin and other Salicylates
EPA (Eicosapentoenoic Acid)	Anticoagulant and Antiplatelet Drugs • Etretinate (*Tegison*)
Ephedra	Amitriptyline (*Elavil*) • Antidiabetes Drugs • Caffeine (*NoDoz, Stay Alert, Vivarin*) • Dexamethasone (*Decadron*) • Digoxin (*Lanoxin*) • Ergotamine (*Ergostat*) • Monoamine Oxidase Inhibitors (MAOIs) • Oxytocin (*Pitocin*) • Reserpine • Theophylline (*Theo-Dur, Slo-Bid, Theolair*) • Urinary Acidifiers • Urinary Alkalinizers
Ergot	Ergot Alkaloids • Sympathomimetics
Eucalyptus dried leaf	Antidiabetes Drugs
Eucalyptus oil	Antidiabetes Drugs
European Buckthorn	Digoxin (*Lanoxin*) • Diuretics • Oral Drugs
European Chestnut	Oral Drugs
European Mandrake	Anticholinergic Drugs • Oral Drugs
European Mistletoe	Antihypertensive Drugs • Cardiovascular Drugs • Immunosuppressants
Evening Primrose Oil	Anesthesia • Phenothiazines
Fennel fruit, seed	Ciprofloxacin (*Cipro*)
Fenugreek	Anticoagulant and Antiplatelet Drugs • Antidiabetes Drugs • Corticosteroids • Estrogen (*Estratest, Estrace, Ogen, Menogen*) • Insulin (*Humulin, Humalog, Novolin, Lantus*) • Monoamine Oxidase Inhibitors (MAOIs) • Oral Contraceptives • Oral Drugs
Fever Bark	Naloxone (*Narcan*) • Phenothiazines • Sympathomimetics
Feverfew	Anesthesia • Anticoagulant and Antiplatelet Drugs • Nonsteroidal Anti-Inflammatory Drugs (NSAIDs)
Fish Oils	Anticoagulant and Antiplatelet Drugs • Antidiabetes Drugs • Antihypertensive Drugs • Cyclosporine (*Neoral, Sandimmune*) • Etretinate (*Tegison*)
Flaxseed	Anticoagulant and Antiplatelet Drugs • Oral Drugs
Flaxseed Oil	Anticoagulant and Antiplatelet Drugs
Folic Acid	Chloramphenicol (*Chloromycetin*) • Cholestyramine (*Questran*) • Colestipol (*Colestid*) • Fosphenytoin (*Cerebyx*) • Methotrexate (*MTX, Rheumatrex*) • Pancreatic Enzymes (*Pancreatin*) • Phenobarbital • Phenytoin (*Dilantin*) • Primidone (*Mysoline*) • Pyrimethamine (*Daraprim*) • Sulfasalazine (*Azulfidine*)
Fo-Ti	Antidiabetes Drugs • Corticosteroids • Digoxin (*Lanoxin*) • Laxatives • Potassium Depleting Diuretics
Gamboge	Digoxin (*Lanoxin*) • Laxatives • Potassium Depleting Diuretics
Gamma Butyrolactone (GBL)	Alcohol • Amphetamines • Anticonvulsants • Antipsychotic Drugs • Benzodiazepines • Haloperidol (*Haldol*) • Naloxone (*Narcan*) • Narcotic Analgesics • Sedative Drugs • Skeletal Muscle Relaxants
Gamma Linolenic Acid	Anticoagulant and Antiplatelet Drugs
Gamma-Hydroxybutyrate (GHB)	Alcohol • Amphetamines • Anticonvulsants • Antipsychotic Drugs • Benzodiazepines • Haloperidol (*Haldol*) • Naloxone (*Narcan*) • Narcotic Analgesics • Ritonavir (*Norvir*) • Saquinavir (*Fortovase, Invirase*) • Sedative Drugs • Skeletal Muscle Relaxants
Garlic	Anticoagulant and Antiplatelet Drugs • Antidiabetes Drugs • Cyclosporine (Neoral, Sandimmune) • Cytochrome P450 3A4 (CYP3A4) Substrates • Insulin (*Humulin, Humalog, Novolin, Lantus*) • Nonnucleoside Reverse Transcriptase Inhibitors (NNRTIs) • Oral Contraceptives • Saquinavir (*Fortovase, Invirase*)

CHARTS

Potential Interactions: Natural Medicine/Drug	For additional data, refer to the database.
Natural Medicine	**Drug**
Gelesemium	Aspirin and other Salicylates • Phenacetin
Gentian	Acid-Inhibiting Drugs • Doxycycline (*Vibramycin*)
German Chamomile	Anticoagulant and Antiplatelet Drugs • Benzodiazepines • Cytochrome P450 3A4 (CYP3A4) Substrates • Sedative Drugs
Germanium	Furosemide (*Lasix*)
Ginger	Acid-Inhibiting Drugs • Anticoagulant and Antiplatelet Drugs • Antidiabetes Drugs • Antihypertensive Drugs • Barbiturates • Cardiovascular Drugs
Ginkgo leaf (Ginkgo Leaf Extract)	Anticoagulant and Antiplatelet Drugs • Cytochrome P450 1A2 (CYP1A2) Substrates • Cytochrome P450 2D6 (CYP2D6) Substrates • Cytochrome P450 3A4 (CYP3A4) Substrates • Insulin (*Humulin, Humalog, Novolin, Lantus*) • Monoamine Oxidase Inhibitors (*MAOIs*) • Thiazide Diuretics • Trazodone (*Desyrel*) • Warfarin (*Coumadin*)
Ginkgo seed	Anticonvulsants
Ginseng, American	Antidiabetes Drugs • Antipsychotic Drugs • CNS Stimulants • Estrogen (*Estratest, Estrace, Ogen, Menogen*) • Monoamine Oxidase Inhibitors (MAOIs) • Oral Contraceptives • Warfarin (*Coumadin*)
Ginseng, Panax	Anticoagulant and Antiplatelet Drugs • Antidiabetes Drugs • Antipsychotic Drugs • Caffeine (*NoDoz, Stay Alert, Vivarin*) • CNS Stimulants • Cytochrome P450 2D6 (CYP2D6) Substrates • Furosemide (*Lasix*) • Immunosuppressants • Insulin (*Humulin, Humalog, Novolin, Lantus*) • Monoamine Oxidase Inhibitors (MAOIs) • Warfarin (*Coumadin*)
Ginseng, Siberian	Alcohol • Anticoagulant and Antiplatelet Drugs • Antidiabetes Drugs • Antipsychotic Drugs • Barbiturates • Digoxin (*Lanoxin*) • Estrogen (*Estratest, Estrace, Ogen, Menogen*) • Insulin (*Humulin, Humalog, Novolin, Lantus*) • Kanamycin (*Kantrex*) • Oral Contraceptives • Sedative Drugs
Glucomannan	Antidiabetes Drugs • Oral Drugs
Glucosamine Hydrochloride	Antidiabetes Drugs
Glucosamine Sulfate	Antidiabetes Drugs
Glutathione	Cisplatin (*Platinol-AQ*)
Goat's Rue	Antidiabetes Drugs
Goldenrod	Diuretics
Goldenseal	Acid-Inhibiting Drugs • Antihypertensive Drugs • Barbiturates • Cytochrome P450 3A4 (*CYP3A4*) Substrates • Heparin • Highly Protein Bound Drugs • Sedative Drugs
Goldthread	Acid-Inhibiting Drugs
Gossypol	Digoxin (*Lanoxin*) • Nonsteroidal Anti-Inflammatory Drugs (NSAIDs) • Potassium Depleting Diuretics • Stimulant Laxatives
Gotu Kola	Antidiabetes Drugs • Cholesterol-Reducing Drugs • Sedative Drugs
Grape fruit, skin	Cytochrome P450 1A2 (CYP1A2) Substrates • Phenacetin
Grape seed	Warfarin (*Coumadin*)
Grapefruit	Artemether (*Artenam, Paluther*) • Benzodiazepines • Buspirone (*Buspar*) • Caffeine (*NoDoz, Stay Alert, Vivarin*) • Calcium Channel Blockers • Carbamazepine (*Tegretol*) • Carvedilol (*Coreg*) • Cisapride (*Propulsid*) • Clomipramine (*Anafranil*) • Cyclosporine (*Neoral, Sandimmune*) • Estrogen (*Estratest, Estrace, Ogen, Menogen*) • Fexofenadine (*Allegra*) • HMG-CoA Reductase Inhibitors (*"Statins"*) • Itraconazole (*Sporanox*) • Losartan (*Cozaar*) • Methylprednisolone (*Adlone, A-Methapred, Depmedalone, Depoject, Medrol, Solu-Medrol*) • Quinidine (*Quinidex*) • Saquinavir (*Fortovase, Invirase*) • Terfenadine (Seldane) • Warfarin (*Coumadin*)
Grapefruit seed extract	Artemether (*Artenam, Paluther*) • Benzodiazepines • Buspirone (*Buspar*) • Caffeine (*NoDoz, Stay Alert, Vivarin*) • Calcium Channel Blockers • Carbamazepine (*Tegretol*)

C
H
A
R
T
S

Potential Interactions: Natural Medicine/Drug	For additional data, refer to the database.
Natural Medicine	**Drug**
Grapefruit seed extract (Cont.)	Carvedilol (*Coreg*) • Cisapride (*Propulsid*) • Clomipramine (*Anafranil*) • Cyclosporine (*Neoral, Sandimmune*) • Estrogen (*Estratest, Estrace, Ogen, Menogen*) • HMG-CoA Reductase Inhibitors (*"Statins"*) • Quinidine (*Quinidex*) • Saquinavir (*Fortovase, Invirase*) • Terfenadine (*Seldane*) • Warfarin (*Coumadin*)
Great Plantain	Warfarin (*Coumadin*)
Greater Bindweed	Digoxin (*Lanoxin*)
Greater Celandine dried above ground parts	Glaucoma Drugs
Greek Sage	Hexobarbital
Green Tea	Acetaminophen (*Tylenol*) • Adenosine (*Adenocard*) • Anticoagulant and Antiplatelet Drugs • Antipsychotic Drugs • Aspirin and other Salicylates • Barbiturates • Benzodiazepines • Beta-Adrenergic Agonists • Chlorpromazine (*Thorazine*) • Cimetidine (*Tagamet*) • Clozapine (*Clozaril*) • Disulfiram (*Antabuse*) • Ephedrine • Ergotamine (*Ergostat*) • Lithium (*Eskalith, Lithobid*) • Mexiletine (*Mexitil*) • Monoamine Oxidase Inhibitors (MAOIs) • Oral Contraceptives • Phenylpropanolamine (*Acutrim*) • Phenytoin (*Dilantin*) • Quinolones • Theophylline (*Theo-Dur, Slo-Bid, Theolair*) • Verapamil (*Calan, Covera, Isoptin, Verelan*) • Warfarin (*Coumadin*)
Guar Gum	Antidiabetes Drugs • Insulin (*Humulin, Humalog, Novolin, Lantus*) • Oral Drugs
Guarana	Acetaminophen (*Tylenol*) • Antidiabetes Drugs • Aspirin and other Salicylates • Benzodiazepines • Beta-Adrenergic Agonists • Clozapine (*Clozaril*) • CNS Stimulants • Disulfiram (*Antabuse*) • Ephedrine • Ergotamine (*Ergostat*) • Estrogen (*Estratest, Estrace, Ogen, Menogen*) • Lithium (*Eskalith, Lithobid*) • Mexiletine (*Mexitil*) • Monoamine Oxidase Inhibitors (MAOIs) • Oral Contraceptives • Phenylpropanolamine (*Acutrim*) • Quinolones • Riluzole (*Rilutek*) • Terbinafine (*Lamisil*) • Theophylline (*Theo-Dur, Slo-Bid, Theolair*) • Verapamil (*Calan, Covera, Isoptin, Verelan*)
Guggul	Diltiazem (*Cardizem*) • Levothyroxine (*Synthroid, Levothroid, Levoxyl*) • Propranolol (*Inderal*)
Gymnema	Antidiabetes Drugs • Iron (*Feosol, Slow Fe*)
Hawaiian Baby Woodrose	5-HT2 Antagonists • Selective Serotonin Reuptake Inhibitors (SSRIs)
Hawthorn	Cardiovascular Drugs • CNS Depressants • Coronary Vasodilators • Digoxin (*Lanoxin*) • Sedative Drugs
Hedge Mustard	Cardiovascular Drugs • Digoxin (*Lanoxin*) • Macrolide Antibiotics • Potassium Depleting Diuretics • Quinine • Stimulant Laxatives • Tetracyclines (*Sumycin*)
Henbane	Anticholinergic Drugs
Hops	Alcohol • Barbiturates • Sedative Drugs
Horse Chestnut branch bark	Anticoagulant and Antiplatelet Drugs • Antidiabetes Drugs • Aspirin and other Salicylates
Horse Chestnut leaf	Anticoagulant and Antiplatelet Drugs • Aspirin and other Salicylates
Horse Chestnut seed	Anticoagulant and Antiplatelet Drugs • Antidiabetes Drugs • Protein-Binding Drugs
Horseradish	Levothyroxine (*Synthroid, Levothroid, Levoxyl*)
Horsetail	Digoxin (*Lanoxin*) • Potassium Depleting Diuretics
Huperzine A	Anticholinergic Drugs • Cholinergic Drugs
Hydrazine Sulfate	CNS Depressants • Monoamine Oxidase Inhibitors (MAOIs) • Sedative Drugs
Iboga	Anticholinergic Drugs • Cholinergic Drugs
Iceland Moss	Oral Drugs
Ignatius Bean	Analeptics • Phenothiazines

Potential Interactions: Natural Medicine/Drug   For additional data, refer to the database.

Natural Medicine	Drug
Indian Long Pepper	Phenytoin (*Dilantin*) • Propranolol (*Inderal*) • Theophylline (*Theo-Dur, Slo-Bid, Theolair*)
Indian Snakeroot	Alcohol • Antihypertensive Drugs • Antipsychotic Drugs • Barbiturates • Digoxin (*Lanoxin*) • Diuretics • Ephedrine • Levodopa (*Larodopa*) • Monoamine Oxidase Inhibitors (MAOIs) • Propranolol (*Inderal*) • Sympathomimetics
Indole-3-Carbinol	Cytochrome P450 1A2 (CYP1A2) Substrates
Inosine	Allopurinol (*Zyloprim*) • Probenecid (*Benemid*)
Inositol Nicotinate	Anticoagulant and Antiplatelet Drugs • Antidiabetes Drugs • Ganglionic Blocking Drugs • HMG-CoA Reductase Inhibitors ("*Statins*") • Nicotine (*Nicotrol, Habitrol, Nicorette, Nicoderm, Prostep*)
Iodine	Antithyroid Drugs • Lithium (*Eskalith, Lithobid*) • Potassium Iodide (*Pima, SSKI*)
IP-6	Anticoagulant and Antiplatelet Drugs
Ipecac	Oral Drugs
Ipriflavone	Calcitonin (*Miacalcin*) • Cytochrome P450 1A2 (CYP1A2) Substrates • Cytochrome P450 2C9 (CYP2C9) Substrates • Estrogen (*Estratest, Estrace, Ogen, Menogen*) • Immunosuppressants • Theophylline (*Theo-Dur*)
Iron	Antacids (*Tums, Maalox, Mylanta*) • Chloramphenicol (*Chloromycetin*) • Fluoroquinolones • H2-Blockers • Tetracyclines (*Sumycin*)
Jalap	Digoxin (*Lanoxin*)
Jamaican Dogwood	Sedative Drugs
Jiaogulan	Anticoagulant and Antiplatelet Drugs • Barbiturates
Jimson Weed	Anticholinergic Drugs
Juniper	Antidiabetes Drugs • Diuretics
Kaolin	Oral Drugs
Karaya Gum	Oral Drugs
Kava	Alprazolam (*Xanax*) • CNS Depressants • Hepatotoxic Drugs • Levodopa (*Larodopa*) • Sedative Drugs
Khella	Digitoxin (*Crystodigin*) • Digoxin (*Lanoxin*) • Hepatotoxic Drugs • Photosensitizing Drugs
Kombucha Tea	Acid-Sensitive Drugs • Acidic or Basic Drugs • Disulfiram (*Antabuse*)
Kudzu	Anticoagulant and Antiplatelet Drugs • Antidiabetes Drugs • Aspirin and other Salicylates • Cardiovascular Drugs
Lactobacillus	Antibiotics
Laminaria	Ace Inhibitors (ACEIs) • Digoxin (*Lanoxin*) • Potassium (*K-Dur, K-Lyte, Micro-K*) • Potassium-Sparing Diuretics
Larch Arabinogalactan	Immunosuppressants • Oral Drugs
L-Arginine	Ace Inhibitors (ACEIs) • Aminophylline (*Slo-Bid, Theo-Dur, Theolair, Uni-Dur, Uniphyl*) • Antihypertensive Drugs • Cyclosporine (*Neoral, Sandimmune*) • Estrogen (*Estratest, Estrace, Ogen, Menogen*) • Medroxyprogesterone (*Provera*) • Nitrates • Norethindrone (*Aygestin*) • Oral Contraceptives • Potassium Increasing Drugs • Potassium-Sparing Diuretics • Sildenafil (*Viagra*) • Xylitol
Lavender	Barbiturates • Benzodiazepines • Chloral Hydrate (*Aquachloral*) • CNS Depressants • HMG-CoA Reductase Inhibitors ("*Statins*") • Sedative Drugs
L-Carnitine	Acenocoumarol • Heparin • Valproic Acid (*Depakote*)
Leech	Acetaminophen (*Tylenol*) • Aspirin and other Salicylates • Nonsteroidal Anti-Inflammatory Drugs (NSAIDs) • Warfarin (*Coumadin*)

C
H
A
R
T
S

Potential Interactions: Natural Medicine/Drug

For additional data, refer to the database.

Natural Medicine	Drug
Lemon Balm	Barbiturates • Levothyroxine (*Synthroid, Levothroid, Levoxyl*) • Sedative Drugs
Lentinan	Didanosine (*ddI, Videx*)
Licorice	Antihypertensive Drugs • Aspirin and other Salicylates • Cimetidine (*Tagamet*) • Corticosteroids • Cytochrome P450 3A4 (CYP3A4) Substrates • Digoxin (*Lanoxin*) • Estrogen (*Estratest, Estrace, Ogen, Menogen*) • Ethacrynic Acid (*Edecrin*) • Furosemide (*Lasix*) • Insulin (*Humulin, Humalog, Novolin, Lantus*) • Interferon • Monoamine Oxidase Inhibitors (MAOIs) • Nonsteroidal Anti-Inflammatory Drugs (NSAIDs) • Oral Contraceptives • Potassium Depleting Diuretics
Lily-Of-The-Valley	Calcium (*Citracal, Caltrate, Os-Cal, Titralac*) • Cardiovascular Drugs • Digoxin (*Lanoxin*) • Glucocorticoids • Macrolide Antibiotics • Potasium Depleting Diuretics • Quinine • Stimulant Laxatives • Tetracyclines (*Sumycin*)
Lime oil	Psoralens
Liver extract	Iron (*Feosol, Slow Fe*)
Lovage	Diuretics
L-Tryptophan	Benzodiazepines • Monoamine Oxidase Inhibitors (MAOIs) • Phenothiazines • Sedative Drugs • Selective Serotonin Reuptake Inhibitors (SSRIs) • Trazodone (*Desyrel*)
Lycium	Antidiabetes Drugs • Antihypertensive Drugs • Warfarin (*Coumadin*)
Lysine	Calcium (*Citracal, Caltrate, Os-Cal, Titralac*)
Madagascar Periwinkle	Antidiabetes Drugs
Magnesium	Fluoroquinolones • Nifedipine (*Adalat, Procardia*) • Skeletal Muscle Relaxants
Maitake Mushroom	Antidiabetes Drugs
Manganese	Fluoroquinolones • Tetracyclines (*Sumycin*)
Manna	Digoxin (*Lanoxin*)
Marijuana	Barbiturates • Disulfiram (*Antabuse*) • Fluoxetine (*Prozac*) • Theophylline (*Theo-Dur, Slo-Bid, Theolair*)
Marsh Tea	CNS Depressants • Sedative Drugs
Marshmallow	Antidiabetes Drugs • Dexamethasone (*Decadron*) • Oral Drugs
Masterwort	Psoralens
Mate	Acetaminophen (*Tylenol*) • Antidiabetes Drugs • Aspirin and other Salicylates • Benzodiazepines • Beta-Adrenergic Agonists • Clozapine (*Clozaril*) • CNS Stimulants • Disulfiram (*Antabuse*) • Ephedrine • Ergotamine (*Ergostat*) • Estrogen (*Estratest, Estrace, Ogen, Menogen*) • Lithium (*Eskalith, Lithobid*) • Mexiletine (*Mexitil*) • Monoamine Oxidase Inhibitors (MAOIs) • Oral Contraceptives • Phenylpropanolamine (*Acutrim*) • Quinolones • Riluzole (*Rilutek*) • Terbinafine (*Lamisil*) • Theophylline (*Theo-Dur, Slo-Bid, Theolair*) • Verapamil (*Calan, Covera, Isoptin, Verelan*)
Meadowsweet	Aspirin and other Salicylates • Narcotic Analgesics
Melatonin	Benzodiazepines • Beta-Blockers (*Beta-Adrenergic Antagonists*) • CNS Depressants • Fluoxetine (*Prozac*) • Fluvoxamine (*Luvox*) • Immunosuppressants • Isoniazid (*INH, Laniazid*) • Nifedipine (*Adalat, Procardia*) • Sedative Drugs • Verapamil (*Calan, Covera, Isoptin, Verelan*)
Mesoglycan	Anticoagulant and Antiplatelet Drugs • Thrombolytics (*tPA, Alteplase*)
Methionine	Acetaminophen (*Tylenol*)
Mexican Scammony Root	Digoxin (*Lanoxin*)
Milk Thistle fruit, seed	Aspirin and other Salicylates • Cisplatin (*Platinol-AQ*) • Cytochrome P450 3A4 (CYP3A4) Substrates • Hepatotoxic Drugs

CHARTS

Potential Interactions: Natural Medicine/Drug For additional data, refer to the database.

Natural Medicine	Drug
Morinda	Potassium-Sparing Diuretics
Mormon Tea	Oral Drugs
Motherwort	CNS Depressants • Sedative Drugs
Myrrh	Antidiabetes Drugs
N-Acetyl Cysteine	Activated Charcoal • Carbamazepine (*Tegretol*) • Nitroglycerin (*Nitrostat, Minitran, Nitrek*)
N-Acetyl Glucosamine	Antidiabetes Drugs
Niacin And Niacinamide (Vitamin B3)	Antidiabetes Drugs • Bile Acid Sequestrants • Carbamazepine (*Tegretol*) • Ganglionic Blocking Drugs • HMG-CoA Reductase Inhibitors (*"Statins"*) • Isoniazid (*INH, Laniazid*) • Nicotine (*Nicotrol, Habitrol, Nicorette, Nicoderm, Prostep*)
Northern Prickly Ash	Acid-Inhibiting Drugs • Anticoagulant and Antiplatelet Drugs
Nutmeg And Mace	Cytochrome P450 1A2 (CYP1A2) Substrates • Monoamine Oxidase Inhibitors (MAOIs) • Phenobarbital
Nux Vomica	Analeptics • Phenothiazines
Oak bark	Apomorphine (*Uprima*) • Atropine • Cocaine • Homatropine (*Homapin*) • Iron (*Feosol, Slow Fe*) • Morphine (*Roxanol, Oramorph, MS Contin, MSIR, Kadian*) • Physostigmine (*Antilirium*) • Scopolamine (*Transderm Scop*)
Oat above ground parts	Morphine (*Roxanol, Oramorph, MS Contin, MSIR, Kadian*) • Nicotine (*Nicotrol, Habitrol, Nicorette, Nicoderm, Prostep*)
Oats	Morphine (*Roxanol, Oramorph, MS Contin, MSIR, Kadian*) • Nicotine (*Nicotrol, Habitrol, Nicorette, Nicoderm, Prostep*) • Oral Drugs
Octacosanol	Carbidopa (*Lodosyn*) • Levodopa (*Larodopa*)
Oleander	Calcium (*Citracal, Caltrate, Os-Cal, Titralac*) • Cardiovascular Drugs • Digoxin (*Lanoxin*) • Macrolide Antibiotics • Potasium Depleting Diuretics • Quinine • Stimulant Laxatives • Tetracyclines (*Sumycin*)
Olive leaf	Antipsychotic Drugs
Olive oil	Antidiabetes Drugs
Onion	Anticoagulant and Antiplatelet Drugs • Antidiabetes Drugs • Aspirin and other Salicylates
Panax Psuedoginseng	Cardiovascular Drugs
Pancreatin	Acarbose (*Precose*) • Acid-Inhibiting Drugs • H2-Blockers • Proton Pump Inhibitors
Pangamic Acid	Digoxin (*Lanoxin*) • Thiazide Diuretics • Verapamil (*Calan, Covera, Isoptin, Verelan*)
Pantothenic Acid (Vitamin B5)	Anticholinesterase Drugs • Parasympathomimetics
Papain	Anticoagulant and Antiplatelet Drugs
Papaya	Warfarin (*Coumadin*)
Para-Aminobenzoic Acid (PABA)	Aminosalicylic Acid (*Paser, Teebacin, Tubasal*) • Dapsone (*Avlosulfon*) • Sulfonamide Antibiotics
Parsley leaf, root	Anticoagulant and Antiplatelet Drugs • Aspirin and other Salicylates • Diuretics • Monoamine Oxidase Inhibitors (MAOIs)
Parsley seed	Diuretics • Monoamine Oxidase Inhibitors (MAOIs)
Passionflower	Barbiturates • Monoamine Oxidase Inhibitors (MAOIs) • Sedative Drugs
Pau D'Arco	Anticoagulant and Antiplatelet Drugs
Pectin	Digoxin (*Lanoxin*) • Lovastatin (*Mevacor*) • Oral Drugs • Tetracyclines (*Sumycin*)
Peppermint Oil	Acid-Inhibiting Drugs • Antacids (*Tums, Maalox, Mylanta*) • H2-Blockers • Proton Pump Inhibitors

CHARTS

Potential Interactions: Natural Medicine/Drug For additional data, refer to the database.

Natural Medicine	Drug
Periwinkle	Antihypertensive Drugs • Antihypotensive Drugs
Peyote	Alcohol • Haloperidol (*Haldol*) • Insulin (*Humulin, Humalog, Novolin, Lantus*) • Methadone (*Dolophine*) • Methysergide (*Sansert*) • Physostigmine (*Antilirium*) • Verapamil (*Calan, Covera, Isoptin, Verelan*)
Pheasant's Eye	Calcium (*Citracal, Caltrate, Os-Cal, Titralac*) • Corticosteroids • Digoxin (*Lanoxin*) • Potassium Depleting Diuretics • Quinidine (*Quinidex*) • Stimulant Laxatives
Phenylalanine	Antipsychotic Drugs • Levodopa (*Larodopa*) • Monoamine Oxidase Inhibitors (MAOIs) • Selegiline (*Eldepryl*)
Phosphate Salts	Antacids (*Tums, Maalox, Mylanta*) • Colestipol (Colestid)
Pinus Bark	Oral Drugs
Pleurisy Root	Antidepressants • Digoxin (*Lanoxin*) • Estrogen (*Estratest, Estrace, Ogen, Menogen*) • Oral Contraceptives
Policosanol	Anticoagulant and Antiplatelet Drugs
Pomegranate	Oral Drugs
Poplar	Anticoagulant and Antiplatelet Drugs
Potassium	Ace Inhibitors (ACEIs) • Potassium-Sparing Diuretics
Potato	Antidiabetes Drugs • Thrombolytics (*tPA, Alteplase*)
Prickly Pear Cactus	Chlorpropamide (*Diabinese*)
Procaine	Aminosalicylic Acid (*Paser, Teebacin, Tubasal*) • Anticholinesterase Drugs • Cholinergic Drugs • Digoxin (*Lanoxin*) • Succinylcholine (*Quelicin*) • Sulfonamides
Progesterone	Conjugated Equine Estrogens (*Premarin*)
Pycnogenol	Immunosuppressants
Pyridoxine (Vitamin B6)	Amiodarone (*Cordarone*) • Levodopa (*Larodopa*) • Phenobarbital • Phenytoin (*Dilantin*)
Quassia	Ace Inhibitors (ACEIs) • Acid-Inhibiting Drugs • Anticoagulant and Antiplatelet Drugs • Cardiovascular Drugs • Potassium Depleting Diuretics
Quercetin	Quinolones
Quillaia	Metformin (*Glucophage*) • Oral Drugs
Raspberry leaf	Metformin (*Glucophage*) • Oral Drugs
Red Clover	Anticoagulant and Antiplatelet Drugs • Cytochrome P450 3A4 (CYP3A4) Substrates • Estrogen (*Estratest, Estrace, Ogen, Menogen*) • Oral Contraceptives
Red Yeast	Alcohol • Cyclosporine (*Neoral, Sandimmune*) • Cytochrome P450 3A4 (CYP3A4) Substrates • Gemfibrozil (*Lopid*) • HMG-CoA Reductase Inhibitors (*"Statins"*) • Levothyroxine (*Synthroid, Levothroid, Levoxyl*) • Niacin (*Niacor, Niaspan, Nicobid, Slo-Niacin*)
Reishi Mushroom	Anticoagulant and Antiplatelet Drugs • Antihypertensive Drugs
Resveratrol	Anticoagulant and Antiplatelet Drugs
Rhatany	Oral Drugs
Rhubarb	Antiarrhythmic Drugs • Corticosteroids • Digoxin (*Lanoxin*) • Laxatives • Oral Drugs • Potassium Depleting Diuretics
Riboflavin (Vitamin B2)	Aspirin and other Salicylates • Beta-Blockers (*Beta-Adrenergic Antagonists*) • Lamivudine (*3TC, Epivir*), Stavudine (*D4T, Zerit*), Zidovudine (*AZT, Retrovir*)
Ribose	Antidiabetes Drugs • Aspirin and other Salicylates • Insulin (*Humulin, Humalog, Novolin, Lantus*) • Monoamine Oxidase Inhibitors (MAOIs)
Rice Bran	Digoxin (*Lanoxin*) • Oral Drugs
Roman Chamomile	Anticoagulant and Antiplatelet Drugs

CHARTS

Potential Interactions: Natural Medicine/Drug   For additional data, refer to the database.

Natural Medicine	Drug
Rose Hip	Aluminum-Containing Antacids (*Maalox, Mylanta, Amphojel*) • Aspirin and other Salicylates • Iron (*Feosol, Slow Fe*) • Warfarin (*Coumadin*)
Rue	PUVA
Saccharomyces Boulardii	Acid-Sensitive Drugs • Acidic or Basic Drugs • Antibiotics • Antifungals
Safflower	Anticoagulant and Antiplatelet Drugs
Sage	Anticonvulsants • Antidiabetes Drugs • Sedative Drugs
SAMe	Antidepressants • Hepatotoxic Drugs • Monoamine Oxidase Inhibitors (MAOIs)
Sarsaparilla	Digoxin (*Lanoxin*) • Oral Drugs • Sedative Drugs
Sassafras	Barbiturates • Sedative Drugs
Saw Palmetto	Estrogen (*Estratest, Estrace, Ogen, Menogen*) • Hormone Replacement Therapy • Oral Contraceptives
Scopolia	Amantadine (*Symmetrel*) • Antibiotics • Anticholinergic Drugs Quinidine (*Quinidex*) • Tricyclic Antidepressants (TCAs)
Scotch Broom herb	Monoamine Oxidase Inhibitors (MAOIs)
Scotch Broom, flower	Monoamine Oxidase Inhibitors (MAOIs)
Secretin	Anticholinergic Drugs
Selenium	Cisplatin (*Platinol-AQ*)
Senna	Digoxin (*Lanoxin*)
Shepherd's Purse	Antihypertensive Drugs • Antihypotensive Drugs • Levothyroxine (*Synthroid, Levothroid, Levoxyl*) • Sedative Drugs
Sitostanol	HMG-CoA Reductase Inhibitors ("*Statins*")
Slippery Elm	Oral Drugs
Smartweed	Warfarin (*Coumadin*)
Smokeless Tobacco	Acetaminophen (*Tylenol*) • Adenosine (*Adenocard*) • Amobarbitol (*Amytal*) • Benzodiazepines • Beta-Blockers (*Beta-Adrenergic Antagonists*) • Caffeine (*NoDoz, Stay Alert, Vivarin*) • Cimetidine (*Tagamet*) • Diflunisal (*Dolobid*) • Estrogen (*Estratest, Estrace, Ogen, Menogen*) • Furosemide (*Lasix*) • Glutethimide (*Cytadren*) • Haloperidol (*Haldol*) • Heparin • Insulin (*Humulin, Humalog, Novolin, Lantus*) • Oral Contraceptives • Pentazocine (*Talwin*) • Phenothiazines • Phenylbutazone • Propoxyphene (*Darvon*) • Quinine • Ranitidine (*Zantac*) • Tacrine (*Cognex*) • Theophylline (*Theo-Dur, Slo-Bid, Theolair*) • Thiothixene (*Navane*) • Tricyclic Antidepressants (TCAs) • Vitamin B12 (*Cobex*) • Vitamin C • Zolpidem (*Ambien*)
Solomon's Seal	Antidiabetes Drugs • Chlorpropamide (*Diabinese*) • Insulin (*Humulin, Humalog, Novolin, Lantus*)
Sorrel	Doxycycline (*Vibramycin*) • Oral Drugs
Southern Prickly Ash	Acid-Inhibiting Drugs
Soy	Estrogen (*Estratest, Estrace, Ogen, Menogen*)
Spinach	Anticoagulant and Antiplatelet Drugs • Antidiabetes Drugs
Squalamine	Cisplatin (*Platinol-AQ*)
Squill	Arrhythmogenic Agents • Calcium (*Citracal, Caltrate, Os-Cal, Titralac*) • Corticosteroids • Digoxin (*Lanoxin*) • Potassium Depleting Diuretics • Quinidine (*Quinidex*) • Stimulant Laxatives
St. John's Wort	5-HT1 Agonists (*Triptans*) • Amitriptyline (*Elavil*) • Antidepressants • Barbiturates • Carbamazepine (*Tegretol*) • Cyclosporine (*Neoral, Sandimmune*) • Cytochrome P450 2C9 (CYP2C9) Substrates • Cytochrome P450 2D6 (CYP2D6) Substrates • Cytochrome P450 3A4 (CYP3A4) Substrates • Digoxin (*Lanoxin*) • Fenfluramine (*Pondimin*) • Monoamine Oxidase Inhibitors (MAOIs) • Narcotic Analgesics •

Potential Interactions: Natural Medicine/Drug
For additional data, refer to the database.

Natural Medicine	Drug
St. John's Wort (Cont.)	Nefazodone (*Serzone*) • Nonnucleoside Reverse Transcriptase Inhibitors (NNRTIs) • Nortriptyline (*Pamelor, Aventyl*) • Oral Contraceptives • Paroxetine (*Paxil*) • Photosensitizing Drugs • Protease Inhibitors (PIs) • Reserpine • Sertraline (*Zoloft*) • Theophylline (*Theo-Dur, Slo-Bid, Theolair*) • Warfarin (*Coumadin*)
Stevia	Antidiabetes Drugs • Verapamil (*Calan, Covera, Isoptin, Verelan*)
Stinging Nettle above ground parts	Anticoagulant and Antiplatelet Drugs • Antidiabetes Drugs • Antihypertensive Drugs • Sedative Drugs
Stone Root	Diuretics
Strophanthus	Calcium (*Citracal, Caltrate, Os-Cal, Titralac*) • Cardiovascular Drugs • Digoxin (*Lanoxin*) • Glucocorticoids • Laxatives • Potassium Depleting Diuretics
Swamp Milkweed	Cardiovascular Drugs • Digoxin (*Lanoxin*) • Macrolide Antibiotics • Potassium Depleting Diuretics • Quinine • Stimulant Laxatives • Tetracyclines (*Sumycin*)
Sweet Bay	Narcotic Analgesics • Sedative Drugs
Sweet Clover	Anticoagulant and Antiplatelet Drugs • Hepatotoxic Drugs
Sweet Orange	Fexofenadine (*Allegra*)
Sweet Vernal Grass	Anticoagulant and Antiplatelet Drugs
Tannic Acid	Oral Drugs
Tansy	Alcohol • Antidiabetes Drugs
Thiamine (Vitamin B1)	Neuromuscular Blocking Agents
Thunder God Vine	Immunosuppressants
Thymus Extract	Immunosuppressants
Tiratricol	Anticoagulant and Antiplatelet Drugs • Antidiabetes Drugs • Cholestyramine (*Questran*) • Levothyroxine (*Synthroid, Levothroid, Levoxyl*) • Sympathomimetics • Vitamin K (*Mephyton*)
Tonka Bean	Anticoagulant and Antiplatelet Drugs
Tragacanth	Oral Drugs
Turmeric	Anticoagulant and Antiplatelet Drugs • Indomethacin (*Indocin*) • Reserpine
Tyrosine	Levodopa (*Larodopa*) • Levothyroxine (*Synthroid, Levothroid, Levoxyl*)
Uva Ursi	Urinary Acidifiers • Urinary Alkalinizers
Uzara	Cardiovascular Drugs • Digoxin (*Lanoxin*) • Macrolide Antibiotics • Potassium Depleting Diuretics • Quinine • Stimulant Laxatives • Tetracyclines (*Sumycin*)
Valerian	Alcohol • Barbiturates • Benzodiazepines • Cytochrome P450 3A4 (CYP3A4) Substrates • Sedative Drugs
Vanadium	Anticoagulant and Antiplatelet Drugs • Antidiabetes Drugs • Digoxin (*Lanoxin*)
Verbena	Antihypertensives Drugs • Antihypotensive Drugs • Doxycycline (*Vibramycin*) • Estrogen (*Estratest, Estrace, Ogen, Menogen*) • Levodopa (*Larodopa*) • Oral Contraceptives
Veronica	Nonsteroidal Anti-Inflammatory Drugs (NSAIDs)
Vinpocetine	Anticoagulant and Antiplatelet Drugs • Antihypertensive Drugs • Warfarin (*Coumadin*)
Vitamin A	Alcohol • Chemotherapeutic Agents • Minocycline (*Minocin*) • Neomycin (*Neo-Fradin*)
Vitamin B12	Chloramphenicol (*Chloromycetin*)
Vitamin C (Ascorbic Acid)	Acetaminophen (*Tylenol*) • Aluminum-Containing Antacids (*Maalox, Mylanta, Amphojel*) • Aspirin and other Salicylates • Heparin • Iron (*Feosol, Slow Fe*) • Warfarin (*Coumadin*)
Vitamin D	Corticosteroids • Digoxin (*Lanoxin*) • Phenobarbital • Phenytoin (*Dilantin*) • Thiazide Diuretics

CHARTS

Potential Interactions: Natural Medicine/Drug
For additional data, refer to the database.

Natural Medicine	Drug
Vitamin E	Anticoagulant and Antiplatelet Drugs • Chemotherapeutic Agents • Nitrates • Warfarin (*Coumadin*)
Vitamin K	Warfarin (*Coumadin*)
Wahoo	Cardiovascular Drugs • Digoxin (*Lanoxin*) • Macrolide Antibiotics • Potassium Depleting Diuretics • Quinine • Stimulant Laxatives • Tetracyclines (*Sumycin*)
Wallflower	Antihypertensive Drugs • Calcium (*Citracal, Caltrate, Os-Cal, Titralac*) • Cardiovascular Drugs • Digoxin (*Lanoxin*) • Glucocorticoids • Laxatives • Potassium Depleting Diuretics
Water Avens	Metformin (*Glucophage*) • Oral Drugs
Watercress	Chlorzoxazone (*Paraflex, Parafon Forte*) • Warfarin (*Coumadin*)
Wheat Bran	Digoxin (*Lanoxin*)
Wheatgrass	Warfarin (*Coumadin*)
Whey Protein	Levodopa (*Larodopa*)
Wild Carrot	Antihypertensive Drugs • Cardiovascular Drugs • Estrogen (*Estratest, Estrace, Ogen, Menogen*) • Oral Contraceptives • Psoralens
Wild Lettuce	Sedative Drugs
Willow Bark	Anticoagulant and Antiplatelet Drugs • Aspirin and other Salicylates • Oral Drugs
Wine	Antidiabetes Drugs • Aspirin and other Salicylates • Barbiturates • Benzodiazepines • Cisapride (*Propulsid*) • CNS Depressants • Cyclosporine (*Neoral, Sandimmune*) • Disulfiram (*Antabuse*) • Erythromycin (*E.E.S., E-Mycin, PCE*) • H2-Blockers • Hepatotoxic Drugs • Metformin (*Gucophage*) • Monoamine Oxidase Inhibitors (MAOIs) • Narcotic Analgesics • Nonsteroidal Anti-Inflammatory Drugs (NSAIDs) • Phenytoin (*Dilantin*) • Sedative Drugs • Warfarin (*Coumadin*)
Wintergreen oil	Aspirin and other Salicylates • Warfarin (*Coumadin*)
Wormwood above ground parts	Acid-Inhibiting Drugs • Anticonvulsants
Xanthan Gum	Antidiabetes Drugs
Yarrow	Acid-Inhibiting Drugs • Anticoagulant and Antiplatelet Drugs • Antihypertensive Drugs • Antihypotensive Drugs • Barbiturates
Yellow Dock	Digoxin (*Lanoxin*)
Yerba Mansa	Barbiturates • Chlorpromazine (*Thorazine*) • Sedative Drugs
Yogurt	Ciprofloxacin (*Cipro*) • Erythromycin (*E.E.S., E-Mycin, PCE*) • Tetracyclines (*Sumycin*)
Yohimbe	Alpha 2-Adrenergic-Blocking Drugs • Antidiabetes Drugs • Antihypertensive Drugs • Beta-Blockers • Clonidine (*Catapres*) • Guanabenz (*Wytensin*) • Monoamine Oxidase Inhibitors (MAOIs) • Naloxone (*Narcan*) • Phenothiazines • Sympathomimetics • Tricyclic Antidepressants (TCAs)
Zinc	Calcium (*Citracal, Caltrate, Os-Cal, Titralac*) • Chlorthalidone (*Hygroton*) • Cisplatin (*Platinol-AQ*) • Fluoroquinolones • Interferon ALFA-2B (*Intron A*) • Penicillamine (*Cuprimine*) • Potassium-Sparing Diuretics • Tetracyclines (*Sumycin*) • Thiazide Diuretics

C
H
A
R
T
S

•

Drug Influences on Nutrient Levels and Depletion

Some medications can affect the levels of certain nutrients in the body. There is considerable interest in using nutritional supplements to counteract these possible drug-induced "nutrient depletions." The chart below shows the current scientific understanding of these relationships, and suggested actions.

DRUGS (includes some representative U.S. and Canadian Brand Names.)	NUTRIENT DEPLETED	POSSIBLE MECHANISM	COMMENTS & REFERENCES
ANTI-INFECTIVES			
Antibiotics: Cephalosporins, Fluoroquinolones, Isoniazid, Macrolides, Penicillins, Sulfonamides, Tetracyclines, Trimethoprim/Sulfamethoxazole	Intestinal Micro Flora (B Vitamins, Vitamin K)	Destruction of normal intestinal microflora leads to decreased production of various B vitamins and vitamin K.	Various beneficial intestinal microflora are eliminated when antibiotics are taken. Some proponents of probiotics recommend taking them for 2-3 weeks during and after a course of antibiotics. Colonic bacteria are responsible for the production of various B vitamins and vitamin K. The nutritional importance of the quantity of vitamins produced by these organisms may not be clinically significant. Give supplements of these vitamins only if clinical judgment warrants it. [4434-4443]
Antiretrovirals: Zidovudine (AZT, Combivir, Retrovir)	Vitamin B12	Some HIV patients taking AZT have subnormal Vitamin B12 levels.	Give vitamin B12 supplements if clinical judgment warrants it. [30]
Cycloserine (*Seromycin*)	Folic Acid	Folate antagonism. (Decreases the availability of substrates required for nucleic acid biosynthesis.)	Although the depletion of folic acid can be documented, it may or may not be clinically significant. Give supplements of this nutrient only if clinical judgment warrants it. [4531]
Fluoroquinolones (Also See Antibiotics): Ciprofloxacin (*Cipro*), Enoxacin (*Penetrex*), Gatifloxacin (*Tequin*), Levofloxacin (*Levaquin*), Lomefloxacin (*Maxaquin*), Moxifloxacin (*Avelox*), Norfloxacin (*Noroxin*), Ofloxacin (*Floxin*), Sparfloxacin (*Zagam*), Trovafloxacin (*Trovan*)	Zinc	Decreases dietary zinc absorption.	The clinical significance is yet to be determined, and the need for supplementation has not been adequately studied. Give supplements of this vitamin only if clinical judgment warrants it. [506,828,2682]

CHARTS

Drug Influences on Nutrient Levels and Depletion

Some medications can affect the levels of certain nutrients in the body. There is considerable interest in using nutritional supplements to counteract these possible drug-induced "nutrient depletions." The chart below shows the current scientific understanding of these relationships, and suggested actions.

DRUGS (includes some representative U.S. and Canadian Brand Names.)	NUTRIENT DEPLETED	POSSIBLE MECHANISM	COMMENTS & REFERENCES
Isoniazid (*Laniazid*) (Also See Antibiotics)	Vitamin B6	Interferes with vitamin B6 metabolism.	Patients receiving > 10 mg/kg/day of INH should be supplemented with 50 - 100 mg of pyridoxine per day. [4481,4482]
Pentamidine (*NebuPent, Pentacarinat, Pentam 300*)	Folic Acid	Impairs folate absorption.	The need for supplementation has not been adequately studied. Give supplements of this vitamin only if clinical judgment warrants it. [4531]
Pyrimethamine (*Daraprim*)	Folic Acid	Folate antagonism. (Binds to dihydrofolate reductase)	At lower pyrimethamine doses, the need for supplementation has not been adequately studied. Give supplements of this vitamin only if clinical judgment warrants it. At larger pyrimethamine doses (those required to treat toxoplasmosis), if signs of folate deficiency develop, folinic acid (*Leucovorin*) should be administered in a dosage of 5 – 15 mg/day (orally, IV, or IM) until normal hematopoiesis is restored. [4425,4532]
Rifampin (*Rifadin, Rimactane, Rofact*)	Vitamin D	Inhibition of enzymes necessary for the formation of the most active metabolite of vitamin D (1,25-dihydroxyvitamin D).	There is no consensus that vitamin D supplementation is always required. Give supplements of this vitamin only if clinical judgment warrants it. [4514]
Tetracyclines (Also See Antibiotics): Tetracycline (*Achromycin V, Panmycin, Robitet, Robicaps, Sumycin, Teline, Tetracap, Tetracyn, Tetralan*), Demeclocycline (*Declomycin*), Doxycycline (*Bio-Tab, Doryx, Doxy Caps, Doxychel, Doxychel Hyclate, Monodox, Periostat, Vibra-Tabs, Vibramycin*), Minocycline (*Dynacinn, Vectrin*), Oxytetracycline (*Terramycin, Uri-Tet*)	Calcium Iron Zinc	Tetracyclines may form complexes with calcium, iron and zinc in the GI tract and thus prevent absorption of adequate amounts of these elements. Doxycycline does not reduce zinc absorption.	Tetracycline doses should be staggered 2 hrs before or 2 hrs after calcium-containing foods or calcium, iron, or zinc supplements to avoid this interaction. Consider giving supplemental calcium doses of 0.8 - 1.5 g/day. Give supplements of these nutrients only if clinical judgment warrants it. [506,4412,4453,4531,4549-4550]
Trimethoprim (*Proloprim, Trimpex*)	Folic Acid	Folate antagonism. (Binds to dihydrofolate reductase.)	Mild folate deficiency may develop in patients on long-term or high-dose therapy. The need for supplementation has not been adequately studied. Give supplements of this vitamin only if clinical judgment warrants it. [4468,4531]

CHARTS

Drug Influences on Nutrient Levels and Depletion

Some medications can affect the levels of certain nutrients in the body. There is considerable interest in using nutritional supplements to counteract these possible drug-induced "nutrient depletions." The chart below shows the current scientific understanding of these relationships, and suggested actions.

DRUGS (includes some representative U.S. and Canadian Brand Names.)	NUTRIENT DEPLETED	POSSIBLE MECHANISM	COMMENTS & REFERENCES
Trimethoprim/Sulfamethoxazole (Also See Antibiotics): (*Bactrim, Cotrim, Septra, Sulfatrim*)	Folic Acid	Folate antagonism. (Binds to dihydrofolate reductase.)	Mild folate deficiency may develop in patients on long-term or high-dose therapy (trimethoprim component). The need for supplementation has not been adequately studied. Give supplements of this vitamin only if clinical judgment warrants it. [4468,4531]
ANTIGOUT/ANTIRHEUMATIC			
Colchicine	Vitamin B12	Decreases intestinal absorption of vitamin B12.	There is evidence that patients on colchicine may have slightly lower levels of vitamin B12, but this does not represent a scientific consensus. Give supplements of this vitamin only if clinical judgment warrants it. [4543-4545]
Methotrexate (*Rheumatrex*)	Folic Acid	Folate antagonism. (Binds to dihydrofolate reductase.)	Recommend supplementation in patients receiving MTX for psoriasis, RA, and other indications requiring prolonged MTX therapy. Common but less serious toxicities of MTX include mucositis, mild alopecia, and GI disturbances, which may be caused by folate depletion. These toxicities are often treated or prevented with the use of folate supplementation. Folic acid at a dosage of 1 mg per day or 7 mg once a week is less expensive and less complicated than the use of folinic acid. Neither low-dose folate (1 mg per day) nor folinic acid ($\leq$ 5 mg per week) interferes with the beneficial effect of MTX. [1716,1719,4493-4494]
Penicillamine (*Cuprimine, Depen*)	Copper Magnesium Vitamin B6 Zinc	Vitamin B6 - Formation of a complex between penicillamine and the reactive coenzyme PLP (pyridoxal-5'-phosphate). This leads to an inactivation of PLP. PLP is an enzyme necessary for the formation of vitamin B6. Copper, Magnesium, Zinc – Forms chelation complexes in the GI tract. Decreases absorption of these elements.	The need for supplementation has not been adequately studied. Give supplements of these nutrients only if clinical judgment warrants it. [4453,4531,4534-4535]

CHARTS

Drug Influences on Nutrient Levels and Depletion

Some medications can affect the levels of certain nutrients in the body. There is considerable interest in using nutritional supplements to counteract these possible drug-induced "nutrient depletions." The chart below shows the current scientific understanding of these relationships, and suggested actions.

DRUGS (includes some representative U.S. and Canadian Brand Names.)	NUTRIENT DEPLETED	POSSIBLE MECHANISM	COMMENTS & REFERENCES
CARDIOVASCULAR			
ANTIHYPERTENSIVES			
Beta-Blockers: Atenolol (*Tenormin*) Metoprolol (*Lopressor, Toprol*) Nadolol (*Corgard*) Propranolol (*Inderal*)	Coenzyme Q10	Beta blockers seem to inhibit mitochandrial coenzyme Q10 enzymes.	The clinical significance is yet to be determined, and the need for supplementation has not been adequately studied.[3368,3369,3370]
Hydralazine (*Apresoline*)	Vitamin B6	Formation of a complex between hydralazine and the reactive coenzyme PLP (pyridoxal-5'-phosphate). This leads to an inactivation of PLP. PLP is an enzyme necessary for the formation of vitamin B6.	The need for supplementation has not been adequately studied. Give supplements of this mineral only if clinical judgement warrants it.[4453,4531,4533]
Captopril (*Capoten*)	Zinc	Captotril increases urinary elimination.	Clinical significance is unknown.[25,26,6543]
CARDIAC GLYCOSIDES			
Digoxin (*Lanoxicaps, Lanoxin*)	Magnesium	Limits reabsorption of magnesium in the renal tubule, leading to magnesium excretion.	The need for supplementation has not been adequately studied. Give supplements of this mineral only if clinical judgment warrants it.[4556]
CHOLESTEROL-REDUCING DRUGS			
HMG CoA Reductase Inhibitors ("Statins"): Atorvastatin (*Lipitor*), Cerivastatin (*Baycol*), Fluvastatin (*Lescol*), Pravastatin (*Pravacol*), Simvastatin (*Zocor*)	Coenzyme Q10	The enzyme HMG CoA reductase is also involved in the biosynthesis of coenzyme Q10. Inhibition of this enzyme leads to a decreased production of coenzyme Q10.	Clinical significance yet to be determined. Postulated potential decrease in cardiac function and possible contributor to liver dysfunction seen with HMG CoA reductase inhibitors.[4404-4410]
Cholestyramine (*LoCHOLEST, Prevalite, Questran*)	Beta-Carotene Folic Acid Vitamins A, B12, D, E, K	All nutrients – Reduces gastrointestinal absorption, lowering of serum cholesterol and triglyceride levels.	It is likely that cholestyramine does bind with some of these nutrients but there has never been clinical proof that supplements are necessary. Supplementation may be valuable in some patients.[4454-4459,4551-4553]
Colestipol (*Colestid*)	Beta-Carotene Folic Acid Vitamins A, B12, D, E, K	All nutrients – Reduces gastrointestinal absorption, lowering of serum cholesterol and triglyceride levels.	It is possible that supplementation with folic acid and vitamin D may be appropriate. In some cases it may be appropriate to supplement all nutrients depleted by colestipol.[4460-4461]
Gemfibrozil (*Lopid*)	Vitamin E	Gemfibrozil can decrease vitamin E serum levels.	The clinical significance is unknown.[4096]

CHARTS

Drug Influences on Nutrient Levels and Depletion

Some medications can affect the levels of certain nutrients in the body. There is considerable interest in using nutritional supplements to counteract these possible drug-induced "nutrient depletions." The chart below shows the current scientific understanding of these relationships, and suggested actions.

DRUGS (includes some representative U.S. and Canadian Brand Names.)	NUTRIENT DEPLETED	POSSIBLE MECHANISM	COMMENTS & REFERENCES
DIURETICS			
Loop Diuretics: Bumetanide (*Bumex, Burinex*), Ethacrynic acid (*Edecrin*), Furosemide (*Lasix*), Torsemide (*Demadex*)	Calcium Folic Acid Magnesium Potassium Sodium Vitamin B1 Zinc	Increased urinary excretion.	Electrolyte disturbances more likely with higher doses or when used in combination with diuretics of another class. Hypokalemia and hypomagnesemia are most commonly clinically encountered. Supplementation may be appropriate in certain patients.[4412,4425,4449] Thiamine depletion might contribute to impaired heart function in some patients with congestive heart failure (CHF) treated with long-term furosemide. Supplementation with 200 mg thiamine (orally or intravenously) per day can replete thiamine, and in some cases, improve left ventricular function in these patients. Consider thiamine supplementation in patients using loop diuretics, especially long-term.[1282-1286] The need for folic acid supplementation has not been adequately studied.[1891,1892,1893,1899]
Thiazide and Thiazide Derivatives: Bendroflumethiazide (Naturetin), Benzthiazide (*Exna*), Chlorothiazide (*Diuril*), Chlorthalidone (*Hygroton, Thalitone*), Hydrochlorothiazide (*Esidrix, Hydrodiuril, Oretic*), Hydroflumethiazide (*Diucardin, Saluron*), Indapamide (*Lozide, Lozol*), Methyclothiazide (*Aquatensen, Enduron*), Metolazone (*Mykrox, Zaroxolyn*), Polythiazide (*Renese*), Quinethazone (*Hydromox*), Trichlormethiazide (*Diurese, Metahydrin, Naqua*)	Folic Acid Magnesium Potassium Sodium Zinc	Increased urinary excretion.	Electrolyte disturbances more likely with higher doses or when used in combination with diuretics of another class. Hypokalemia and hypomagnesemia are most commonly clinically encountered. Supplementation may be appropriate in certain patients.[4412,4425,4453] The need for folic acid supplementation has not been adequately studied.[1891,1892,1893,1899]
Potassium Sparing: Triamterene (*Dyrenium*)	Folic Acid	Folate antagonism. (Binds to dihydrofolate reductase.)	The need for supplementation has not been adequately studied. Give supplements of this vitamin only if clinical judgment warrants it.[4425,4536-4537]

Drug Influences on Nutrient Levels and Depletion

Some medications can affect the levels of certain nutrients in the body. There is considerable interest in using nutritional supplements to counteract these possible drug-induced "nutrient depletions." The chart below shows the current scientific understanding of these relationships, and suggested actions.

DRUGS (includes some representative U.S. and Canadian Brand Names.)	NUTRIENT DEPLETED	POSSIBLE MECHANISM	COMMENTS & REFERENCES
CENTRAL NERVOUS SYSTEM			
ANTICONVULSANTS			
Carbamazepine (*Atretol, Epitol, Tegretol*)	Folic Acid Vitamin D (Ultimately may lead to decreases in serum calcium and potential bone loss.)	Folic Acid – Two mechanisms have been proposed: Induction of hepatic microsomal enzymes leading to increased folic acid metabolism and decreased intestinal absorption. Vitamin D – Increases the rate of vitamin D metabolism leading to decreased levels of various forms of vitamin D.	Studies of anticonvulsants in general demonstrate lower folic acid levels in treated patients. The necessity for supplementation to prevent peripheral neuropathies or red cell dyscrasias has not been adequately studied. The necessity for supplementation with vitamin D to potentially prevent osteomalacia has not been adequately studied. Give supplements of these vitamins only if clinical judgment warrants it. [4426-4431]
Phenytoin (*Dilantin*), Fosphenytoin (*Cerebyx*)	Folic Acid Vitamin D (Ultimately may lead to decreases in serum calcium and potential bone loss.)	Folic Acid - Several mechanisms have been proposed to explain the ability of phenytoin to deplete body folate. It appears to be more related to metabolic and distributional changes than decreases in dietary absorption. Vitamin D – Increases the rate of vitamin D metabolism leading to decreased levels of various forms of vitamin D. Phenytoin may also increase the renal excretion of polar vitamin D metabolites.	Based on patient specific circumstances, consider giving folic acid supplementation with the initial dose of phenytoin to prevent folate deficiency. Note that folic acid supplementation may alter phenytoin pharmacokinetics leading to lower serum concentrations and possible seizure breakthrough. [4471-4474, 4477-4531] Consider giving 400 – 800 IU/day of vitamin D to patients receiving long-term phenytoin therapy. Also recommend a diet rich in calcium. [4475]
Phenobarbital (*Luminal, Solfoton*)	Folic Acid Vitamin D (Ultimately may lead to decreases in serum calcium and potential bone loss.)	Folic Acid - Induces hepatic microsomal enzymes leading to an increase in folic acid metabolism. Vitamin D – Increases the rate of vitamin D metabolism leading to decreased levels of various forms of vitamin D.	The need for supplementation with folic acid has not been adequately studied. Give supplements of this vitamin only if clinical judgment warrants it. Consider giving 400 – 800 IU daily of vitamin D to patients receiving long-term phenobarbital therapy. Suggest a diet rich in calcium. Monitor vitamin D. Only give supplementation if deficiencies are noted. [4453,4530-4531]
Primidone (*Mysoline*)	Folic Acid	Folic Acid – Induces hepatic microsomal enzymes leading to an increase in folic acid metabolism.	The need for supplementation has not been adequately studied. Give supplements of this vitamin only if clinical judgment warrants it. [4453,4530-4531]
Valproic Acid (*Depakene, Depakote*)	L-Carnitine	Inhibits the biosynthesis of L-carnitine and possibly decreases the tissue uptake of L-carnitine.	Recommend oral L-carnitine supplementation in special subgroups of patients. See footnote at the end of the chart. [4523-4529,5798]

CHARTS

Drug Influences on Nutrient Levels and Depletion

Some medications can affect the levels of certain nutrients in the body. There is considerable interest in using nutritional supplements to counteract these possible drug-induced "nutrient depletions." The chart below shows the current scientific understanding of these relationships, and suggested actions.

DRUGS (includes some representative U.S. and Canadian Brand Names.)	NUTRIENT DEPLETED	POSSIBLE MECHANISM	COMMENTS & REFERENCES
PHENOTHIAZINES			
Phenothiazines: Chlorpromazine (*Thorazine*), Promazine (*Sparine*), Triflupromazine (*Vesprin*), Fluphenazine (*Moditen HCl, Permitil, Prolixin*), Perphenazine (*Trilafon*), Prochlorperazine (*Compazine, Stemetil*), Trifluoperazine (*Stelazine*), Mesoridazine (*Serentil*), Thioridazine (*Mellaril*), Thiothixene (*Navane*)	Vitamin B2	Increases renal excretion and possibly inhibits synthesis.	Give 2 - 5 mg/day of riboflavin to patients on phenothiazines if clinical judgment warrants it. [4425]
DIABETES			
Glyburide (*Diabeta, Euglucon, Glynase, Micronase*), Acetohexamide (*Dymelor*), Tolazamide (*Tolinase*)	Coenzyme Q10	Inhibits NADH-oxidase, an enzyme necessary in the formation of coenzyme Q10.	Clinical significance is yet to be determined. Postulated potential decrease in cardiac function and possible impairment of insulin production and/or secretion. Give supplements of this nutrient only if clinical judgment warrants it. [4479]
Metformin (*Glucophage*)	Folic Acid Vitamin B12	Causes malabsorption of dietary vitamin B12 and folic acid.	The *Glucophage* package insert recommends obtaining hematological parameters annually and obtaining B12 at 2-3 year intervals in patients at increased risk for B12 deficiency. Give supplements of this vitamin only if clinical judgment warrants it. [32,4487-4491]
GASTROINTESTINALS			
ANTACIDS			
Aluminum Salts (*Amphojel, Alternajel, Gaviscon, Maalox, Riopan*)	Calcium Phosphorus	Binds calcium and phosphate in the gastrointestinal tract.	Prolonged administration of large doses may lead to hypocalcemia and/or hypophosphatemia. Avoid prolonged administration of large doses. [4400]
Magnesium Salts (*Di-gel, Gelusil, Maalox, Mag-Ox, Milk of Magnesia, Mylanta, Riopan*)	Calcium Phosphorus	Binds calcium and phospate in the gastrointestinal tract.	Prolonged administration of large doses may lead to hypocalcemia and/or hypophosphatemia. Avoid prolonged administration of large doses. [4400]
GI ANTI-INFLAMMATORIES			
p-Aminosalicylic Acid [aminosalicylic acid, PAS]	Folic Acid Vitamin B12	Inhibits absorption in the gastrointestinal tract.	The need for supplementation has not been adequately studied. Give supplements of these vitamins only if clinical judgment warrants it. [4557-4560]

CHARTS

Drug Influences on Nutrient Levels and Depletion

Some medications can affect the levels of certain nutrients in the body. There is considerable interest in using nutritional supplements to counteract these possible drug-induced "nutrient depletions." The chart below shows the current scientific understanding of these relationships, and suggested actions.

DRUGS (includes some representative U.S. and Canadian Brand Names.)	NUTRIENT DEPLETED	POSSIBLE MECHANISM	COMMENTS & REFERENCES
Sulfasalazine (*Azulfidine, Salazopyrin*)	Folic Acid	Inhibits folate absorption in the gastrointestinal tract.	Folate depletion is proposed to be involved in the various blood dyscrasias seen with sulfasalazine. Foods high in folic acid rather than folic acid supplements are recommended. Give supplements of this vitamin only if clinical judgment warrants it, and adequate amounts cannot be maintained by diet. [4515-4517]
HISTAMINE-2 BLOCKERS			
H2 Blockers: Cimetidine (*Tagamet*), Famotidine (*Pepcid*), Nizatidine (*Axid*), Ranitidine (*Zantac*)	Iron Vitamin B12	Decreases iron and vitamin B12 absorption from the gastrointestinal tract.	The need for iron and vitamin B12 supplementation has not been adequately studied. B12 depletion may be particularly important in patients with inadequate diet, poor stores of the vitamin, and in patients receiving continuous therapy of more than two years. Give supplements of this vitamin if clinical judgment warrants it. [4539-4541]
LAXATIVES			
Bisacodyl (*Bisacodyl Uniserts, Bisco-Lax, Correctol, Dulcagen, Dulcolax, Feen-a-mint, Fleet Laxative*)	Potassium	Increases gastrointestinal losses of potassium.	Reported in patients undergoing bowel-cleansing regimens. Use caution in patients who may be predisposed to hypokalemia (i.e. aggressive diuretic therapy). Give supplements of this mineral if clinical judgment warrants it. [4411-4412]
Mineral Oil	Beta-Carotene Calcium Vitamins A,D,E, K	Decreases gastrointestinal absorption.	May be avoided by limiting duration of use. [4495-4496]
Stimulant Laxatives: Cascara (*Various...*) Senna (*Senexon, Senolax, Senokot , Senna-Gen, Senokotxtra, Black-Draught, Gentlax, Dr. Caldwell Senna, Fletcher's Castoria, Dosalax*), Bisacodyl Tablets (*Bisacodyl Uniserts, Bisco-Lax, Correctol, Dulcagen, Dulcolax, Feen-a-mint, Fleet Laxative*)	Calcium Potassium Sodium Vitamin D	Calcium and Vitamin D - Decreases gastrointestinal absorption. Sodium and Potassium – Increases gastrointestinal losses.	Excessive use of stimulant laxatives may result in depletion of these essential elements and vitamin D. Limit to short-term use. [4411-4412,4425,4453]
PROKINETIC AGENTS			
Metoclopramide (*Maxeran, Reglan*)	Vitamin B2	Decreases dietary vitamin B2 absorption from the gastrointestinal tract.	The need for supplementation has not been adequately studied. Give supplements of this vitamin only if clinical judgment warrants it. [4561]

CHARTS

Drug Influences on Nutrient Levels and Depletion

Some medications can affect the levels of certain nutrients in the body. There is considerable interest in using nutritional supplements to counteract these possible drug-induced "nutrient depletions." The chart below shows the current scientific understanding of these relationships, and suggested actions.

DRUGS (includes some representative U.S. and Canadian Brand Names.)	NUTRIENT DEPLETED	POSSIBLE MECHANISM	COMMENTS & REFERENCES
PROTON PUMP INHIBITORS			
Proton Pump Inhibitors: Lansoprazole (*Prevacid*), Omeprazole (*Losec, Prilosec*), Rabeprazole (*Aciphex*), Pantoprazole (*Pantoloc, Protonix*)	Beta-Carotene Iron Vitamin B12	Decreases beta carotene, iron and vitamin B12 absorption from the gastrointestinal tract.	The need for supplementation has not been adequately studied. Give supplementation of these vitamins only if clinical judgment warrants it. 31,4483-4486,4539-4541
HORMONES			
Corticosteroids [Glucocorticoids]: **Short-acting** Cortisone (*Cortone*), Hydrocortisone [Cortisol] (*Cortef, Hydrocortone*) **Intermediate-acting** Prednisone (*Deltasone, Meticorten, Orasone, Panasol-S*), Prednisolone (*Delta-Cortef, Prelone, Pediapred*), Triamcinolone (*Aristocort, Atolone, Kenacort*), Methylprednisolone (*Medrol*) **Long-acting** Dexamethasone (*Decadron, Dexameth, Dexone*), Betamethasone (*Celestone*)	Calcium (Indirectly – Vitamin D) Chromium	Calcium – Increases renal calcium excretion and decreases intestinal calcium absorption. Vitamin D - Depletion of calcium by steroids creates a greater need for vitamin D, which is necessary for appropriate GI absorption of calcium. Chromium - Increases renal excretion of chromium, possibly leading to chromium deficiency or hyperglycemia.	Steroid induced osteoporosis is a well-recognized consequence of long-term steroid administration. Supplement with calcium and vitamin D (calcitriol). Emerging data indicate that bisphosphonates may also be helpful. Depletion of calcium by steroids creates a greater need for vitamin D, which is necessary for appropriate GI absorption of calcium. It may be prudent to supplement these nutrients before, during, and after long-term and/or high-dose corticosteroids. 4462-4467 Consider chromium supplements based on clinical judgement. 5039
Estrogens: (*Cenestin, Estrace, Estratab, Ogen, Premarin, Premphase, Prempro*)	Magnesium Vitamin B6 Vitamin C	Magnesium – Proposed shift of magnesium from plasma to other tissues. Vitamin B6 – Disturbance of tryptophan and vitamin B6 metabolism. Vitamin C – Estrogens seem to increase elimination of vitamin C.	Although there has been much talk about giving vitamin B6 to people on estrogens, the need for supplementation has not been proven. Give supplements of these nutrients only if clinical judgment warrants it. 4470,4498
Oral Contraceptives [Containing Estrogen]	Folic Acid Magnesium Vitamin B2 Vitamin B6 Vitamin B12 Vitamin C	Folic Acid – Interferes with metabolism. Magnesium – Proposed shift of magnesium from plasma to other tissues. Vitamins B2, B6 – Interferes with metabolism. Vitamin B12 – Possibly due to increased metabolism and decreased B12 binding capacity. Vitamin C – Estrogens seem to increase elimination of vitamin C.	Although there has been much talk about giving vitamin B6 to people on oral contraceptives, the need for supplementation has not been proven. Give supplements of these nutrients only if clinical judgment warrants it. 4459,4470,4498,4547-4548
Thyroid Hormones	Calcium	Might increase urinary loss of calcium	There is not yet any proof that calcium supplementa-tion is either helpful or necessary. 27,28,29

CHARTS

Drug Influences on Nutrient Levels and Depletion

Some medications can affect the levels of certain nutrients in the body. There is considerable interest in using nutritional supplements to counteract these possible drug-induced "nutrient depletions." The chart below shows the current scientific understanding of these relationships, and suggested actions.

DRUGS (includes some representative U.S. and Canadian Brand Names.)	NUTRIENT DEPLETED	POSSIBLE MECHANISM	COMMENTS & REFERENCES
MISCELLANEOUS			
Orlistat (*Xenical*)	Beta-Carotene Vitamin A Vitamin D Vitamin E Vitamin K	Beta-Carotene - Decreases the absorption of beta-carotene supplements from the gastrointestinal tract. Vitamin E - Decreases the absorption of vitamin E supplements by 60%. Vitamin A, vitamin D, and vitamin K - Possibly decreases the absorption from the gastrointestinal tract.	Separate administration of orlistat and beta-carotene, vitamin A, vitamin D, vitamin E, and vitamin K supplements by 2-hours to avoid this interaction. The effect of orlistat on the absorption of nutritionally derived vitamins is unknown. The need for supplementation has not been adequately studied. Give supplements of these vitamins only if clinical judgment warrants it. [1725-1727,1730, 6001]
Potassium Chloride (Extended Release) (*K-Dur, Micro K, Slow K*)	Vitamin B12	Malabsorption of dietary vitamin B12.	The need for supplementation has not been adequately studied. Give supplements of this vitamin only if clinical judgment warrants it. [4511-4512]
RESPIRATORY			
Theophylline (*Slobid, Theo-24, Theo-Dur, Theolair*)	Vitamin B6	Inhibits pyridoxal kinase leading to decreases in vitamin B6 levels.	There have been several studies looking at the possible depletion of vitamin B6 due to theophylline. There is no consensus yet. Give supplements of this vitamin only if clinical judgment warrants it. [4522,7066]

Footnote: Oral L-carnitine supplementation is indicated for primary plasmalemmal carnitine transporter defect. In addition, oral L-carnitine supplementation is strongly suggested for the following groups: patients with certain secondary carnitine deficiency syndromes; symptomatic VPA-associated hyperammonemia; multiple risk factors for VPA-associated hepatotoxicity, or renal associated syndromes; infants and young children taking VPA; patients with epilepsy using the ketogenic diet who have hypocarnitinemia; patients on dialysis; and premature infants receiving TPN. An oral L-carnitine dosage of 100 mg/kg/day, up to a maximum of 2 g/day has been recommended.

GENERAL INDEX

(1S)-1,2,4/3,5,6-inositol .... see INOSITOL
(1S)-inositol .... see INOSITOL
(3 beta)-3-hydroxypregn-5-en-20-one
.... see PREGNENOLONE
(3-carboxy2-hydroxypropyl)trimethylammonium hydroxide
    inner salt ....see L-CARNITINE
(3-carboxy-2-hydroxy-propyl)trimethylammonium
    hydroxide inner salt acetate
    .... see ACETYL-L-CARNITINE
(beta-hydroxyethyl) trimethylammonium hydroxide
    .... see CHOLINE
(Dimethylamino)acetic Acid ..... see DIMETHYLGLYCINE
(R)-(3-carboxy-2-hydroxypropyl) trimethylammonium
    hydroxide ....see L-CARNITINE
(R)-3-hydroxy-4-trimethylammonio-butyrate
    ....see L-CARNITINE
(Z,Z,Z)-Octadeca-6,9,12-trienoic acid
    .... see GAMMA LINOLENIC ACID
1,2,3,4,5,6-Cyclohexanehexol .... see INOSITOL
1,2,3-propanetriol .... see GLYCEROL
1,2,5/3,4,6-inositol .... see INOSITOL
1,25-dihydroxycholecalciferol .... see VITAMIN D
1,2-Butanolide .... see GAMMA BUTYROLACTONE
1,2-dithiolane-3-pentanoic acid
    .... see ALPHA-LIPOIC ACID
1,2-dithiolane-3-valeric acid ...... see ALPHA-LIPOIC ACID
1,3,7-trimethylxanthine .... see CAFFEINE
1,4-BD .... see BUTANEDIOL
1,4-butanediol .... see BUTANEDIOL
1,4-butylene glycol .... see BUTANEDIOL
1,4-dihydroxybutane .... see BUTANEDIOL
1,4-tetramethylene glycol .... see BUTANEDIOL
1-3,1-6-beta-glucan .... see BETA GLUCANS
13-Docosenoic acid (erucic acid) .... see LORENZO'S OIL
17 beta-(1-ketoethyl)- delta 5-androsten-3 beta-ol
    .... see PREGNENOLONE
1-Octacosanol .... see OCTACOSANOL
2(3H) furanone dihydro
    .... see GAMMA BUTYROLACTONE
2(3H)-Furanone di-dihydro .... see BUTANEDIOL
2(3H)-Furanone Dihydro
    .... see GAMMA BUTYROLACTONE
2-(acetyloxy)-3-carboxy-N,N,N-trimethyl-1-propanaminium
    inner salt .... see ACETYL-L-CARNITINE
2,3 dihydro furanone ... see GAMMA BUTYROLACTONE
2,3-Diphosphoglycerate .... see INOSINE
20-Dione ....see PROGESTERONE
22,23-dihydrostigmasterol .... see BETA-SITOSTEROL
24-alpha-ethylcholestanol .... see SITOSTANOL
24-beta-ethyl-delta-5-cholesten-3beta-ol
    .... see BETA-SITOSTEROL
24-ethyl-cholesterol .... see BETA-SITOSTEROL
25-HCC .... see VITAMIN D
25-hydroxycholecalciferol .... see VITAMIN D
25-hydroxyvitamin D3 .... see VITAMIN D
25-OHCC .... see VITAMIN D
25-OHD3 .... see VITAMIN D
2-acetamido-2-deoxyglucose
    .... see N-ACETYL GLUCOSAMINE
2-amino-2-deoxy-beta-D-glucopyranose
    .... see GLUCOSAMINE HYDROCHLORIDE

2-amino-2-deoxyglucose hydrochloride
    .... see GLUCOSAMINE HYDROCHLORIDE
2-amino-2-deoxyglucose sulfate
    .... see GLUCOSAMINE SULFATE
2-amino-3-(4-hydroxyphenyl)propionic acid
    .... see TYROSINE
2-amino-3-methylbutanoic acid
    .... see BRANCHED-CHAIN AMINO ACIDS
2-amino-3-methylvaleric acid
    .... see BRANCHED-CHAIN AMINO ACIDS
2-amino-4-methylvaleric acid
    .... see BRANCHED-CHAIN AMINO ACIDS
2-Amino-5-guanidinopentanoic acid .... see L-ARGININE
2-Aminoethane sulfonic acid .... see TAURINE
2-Dietylaminoethyl p-aminobenzoate monohydrochloride
    .... see PROCAINE
2-Dimethyl Aminoethanol .... see DEANOL
2-Dimethylaminoethanol .... see DEANOL
2-hydroxypropionic acid (Lactic acid)
    .... see ALPHA HYDROXY ACIDS
2-Methyl-3-Phytyl-1,4-Naphthoquinone .... see VITAMIN K
2-Oxoglutaric acid .... see ALPHA-KETOGLUTARATE
2-Oxopentanedoicic acid
    .... see ALPHA-KETOGLUTARATE
2-Oxopropanoate (pyruvate) .... see PYRUVATE
2-oxopropanoic acid (pyruvic acid) .... see PYRUVATE
2-Oxypropanoic Acid .... see PYRUVATE
3 (hydroxymethyl) Indole .... see INDOLE-3-CARBINOL
3 Hydroxymethyl Indole .... see INDOLE-3-CARBINOL
3-(hydroxymethyl) .... see INDOLE-3-CARBINOL
3,3',4'5,7-Penthydroxyflavone .... see QUERCETIN
3,3',5-triiodothyroacetic acid .... see TIRATRICOL
3,3'-dihydroxy-4,4'-diketo-beta-carotene
    .... see MICROALGAE
3,4',5-stilbenetriol .... see RESVERATROL
3,4',5-trihydroxystilbene .... see RESVERATROL
3,5,4' -trihydroxystilbene .... see RESVERATROL
31-diol .... see LUTEIN
32-C .... see POLICOSANOL
3-acetyl-7-oxo-dehydroepiandrosterone
    .... see 7-KETO-DHEA
3-beta,5-alpha-stigmastan-3-ol .... see SITOSTANOL
3beta-acetoxy-androst-5-ene-7,17-dione
    .... see 7-KETO-DHEA
3-beta-stigmast-5-en-3-ol .... see BETA-SITOSTEROL
3-carboxy-2-hydroxy-N,N,N-trimethyl-1-propanaminium
    inner salt ....see L-CARNITINE
3-Dehydroretinol .... see VITAMIN A
3-hydroxy-4-N-trimethylaminobutyrate
    ....see L-CARNITINE
3-Hydroxybutyric Acid Lactone
    .... see GAMMA BUTYROLACTONE
3-Hydroxymethyl Indole .... see INDOLE-3-CARBINOL
3-Pyridine Carboxamide
    .... see NIACIN AND NIACINAMIDE
3R .... see MICROALGAE
3R,3'S-astaxanthin .... see MICROALGAE
3'R-astaxanthin .... see MICROALGAE
3S .... see MICROALGAE
3'S-astaxanthin .... see MICROALGAE
4,4-diketo-beta-carotene .... see CANTHAXANTHIN

4-AD .... see ANDROSTENEDIOL
4-amino-2-methyl-1-naphthol (K5) .... see VITAMIN K
4-Aminobenzoic Acid

         .... see PARA-AMINOBENZOIC ACID
4-androstene-3,17-dione .... see ANDROSTENEDIONE
4-androstene-3beta,17beta-diol

         .... see ANDROSTENEDIOL
4-Butanolide .... see GAMMA BUTYROLACTONE
4-Butyrolactone .... see GAMMA BUTYROLACTONE
4-Hydroxy Butyrate

         .... see GAMMA-HYDROXYBUTYRATE
4-Hydroxybutanoic Acid Lactone

         .... see GAMMA BUTYROLACTONE
4-hydroxybutyric acid

         .... see GAMMA-HYDROXYBUTYRATE
4-Pregnene-3 .... see PROGESTERONE
5-(1,2-dithiolan-3-yl) valeric acid

         .... see ALPHA-LIPOIC ACID
5-androsten-3-beta-17-one-DHEA .... see 7-KETO-DHEA
5-androstene-3beta,17beta-diol

         .... see ANDROSTENEDIOL
5-HTP .... see 5-HTP
5-Hydroxytryptophan .... see 5-HTP
6,8-dithiooctanoic acid .... see ALPHA-LIPOIC ACID
6,8-thioctic acid .... see ALPHA-LIPOIC ACID
6,9-Dihydro-9-B-D-ribofuranosyl-1H-puin-6-one

         .... see INOSINE
6-furfurylaminopurine .... see KINETIN
7 Keto Dhea .... see 7-KETO-DHEA
7-Isopropoxyisoflavone .... see IPRIFLAVONE
7-Keto .... see 7-KETO-DHEA
7-keto dehydroepiandrosterone .... see 7-KETO-DHEA
7-ketodehydroepiandrostenedione .... see 7-KETO-DHEA
7-KETO-DHEA .... see 7-KETO-DHEA
7-Oda .... see 7-KETO-DHEA
7-oxo-dehydroepiandrosterone-3-acetate

         .... see 7-KETO-DHEA
7-oxo-DHEA .... see 7-KETO-DHEA
7-oxo-DHEA-acetate .... see 7-KETO-DHEA
9-B-D-ribofuranosylhypoxanthine .... see INOSINE
Aamalaki .... see INDIAN GOOSEBERRY
Aaron's Rod

         .... see GOLDENROD, HOUSELEEK, MULLEIN
Abelmoschus moschatus .... see AMBRETTE
Abelmosk .... see AMBRETTE
A-Beta-Carotene .... see BETA-CAROTENE
Abies alba .... see FIR, FIR NEEDLE OIL
Abies balsamea .... see CANADA BALSAM
Abies excelsa .... see HEMLOCK SPRUCE
Abies pectinata .... see FIR
Abies sachalinensis .... see FIR NEEDLE OIL
Abies sibirica .... see FIR NEEDLE OIL
Abrojos .... see PUNCTURE VINE
Abrus pecatorius .... see PRECATORY BEAN
ABSCESS ROOT .... see ABSCESS ROOT
Absinth .... see WORMWOOD above ground parts
Absinthe .... see WORMWOOD above ground parts
Absinthii Herba ...... see WORMWOOD above ground parts
Absinthites .... see WORMWOOD above ground parts
Absinthium .... see WORMWOOD above ground parts
ABUTA .... see ABUTA
Abyssinian Myrrh .... see MYRRH
Abyssinian Tea .... see KHAT
ACACIA .... see ACACIA

Acacia farnesiana .... see CASSIE ABSOLUTE
Acacia senegal .... see ACACIA
Acanthopanax senticosus .... see GINSENG, SIBERIAN
Ace .... see ADRENAL EXTRACT
Acedera Común .... see SORREL
Acer rubrum .... see RED MAPLE
ACEROLA .... see ACEROLA
Acetate Replacing Factor .... see ALPHA-LIPOIC ACID
Acetyl Carnitine .... see ACETYL-L-CARNITINE
Acetyl Cysteine .... see N-ACETYL CYSTEINE
ACETYL-L-CARNITINE ..... see ACETYL-L-CARNITINE
Acetyl-Levocarnitine .... see ACETYL-L-CARNITINE
Acetylformic Acid .... see PYRUVATE
Acetylglucosamine .... see N-ACETYL GLUCOSAMINE
Ache des Marais .... see CELERY
Achilee .... see YARROW
Achillea .... see YARROW
Achillea millefolium .... see YARROW
Achillea ptarmica .... see SNEEZEWORT
Achiote .... see ANNATTO
Achiotillo .... see ANNATTO
Achras sapota .... see CHICLE
Achras zapotilla .... see CHICLE
Achweed .... see GOUTWEED
Acidophilus .... see LACTOBACILLUS
Acidophilus Milk .... see YOGURT
ACKEE .... see ACKEE
Ackerkraut .... see AGRIMONY
ACONITE .... see ACONITE
Aconiti Tuber .... see ACONITE
Aconitum Napellus .... see ACONITE
Aconitum species .... see ACONITE
Acorus calamus .... see CALAMUS
Acrid Crowfoot .... see BUTTERCUP
Acrid Lettuce .... see WILD LETTUCE
Actaea alba .... see WHITE COHOSH
Actaea macrotys .... see BLACK COHOSH
Actaea pachypoda .... see WHITE COHOSH
Actaea racemosa .... see BLACK COHOSH
Actaea rubra .... see WHITE COHOSH
Actinidia chinensis .... see KIWI
ACTIVATED CHARCOAL

         .... see ACTIVATED CHARCOAL
Activin .... see GRAPE seed
Acuilee .... see YARROW
Adam's Apple .... see LIME fruit, peel, LIME oil
Adam's Flannel .... see MULLEIN
ADAM'S NEEDLE .... see ADAM'S NEEDLE
Adam's Needle .... see YUCCA
Adaptogen .... see JIAOGULAN
Adder's Eyes .... see SCARLET PIMPERNEL
Adder's Root .... see ARUM
Adderwort .... see BISTORT
Ademetionine .... see SAMe
Adenosylcobalamin .... see DIBENCOZIDE
Adenosylmethionine .... see SAMe
Adermine Hydrochloride

         .... see PYRIDOXINE (VITAMIN B6)
Adiantifolia .... see GINKGO leaf (GINKGO leaf extract)
Adiantum capillus-veneris .... see MAIDENHAIR FERN
Adiantum pedatum .... see MAIDENHAIR FERN
Adiptam .... see BURNING BUSH leaf,
                            BURNING BUSH root
Adonis herba .... see PHEASANT'S EYE

Adonis vernalis .... see PHEASANT'S EYE
Adrenal .... see ADRENAL EXTRACT
Adrenal Complex .... see ADRENAL EXTRACT
Adrenal Concentrate
.... see ADRENAL EXTRACT
Adrenal Cortex Extract .... see ADRENAL EXTRACT
ADRENAL EXTRACT .... see ADRENAL EXTRACT
Adrenal Factors .... see ADRENAL EXTRACT
Adrenal Substance .... see ADRENAL EXTRACT
ADRUE .... see ADRUE
Adulsa .... see MALABAR NUT
AE-941 .... see SHARK CARTILAGE
Aegle marmelos .... see BAEL
Aegopodium podagraria .... see GOUTWEED
Aesculus Hippocastanum
.... see HORSE CHESTNUT branch bark,
HORSE CHESTNUT flower,
HORSE CHESTNUT leaf,
HORSE CHESTNUT seed
Aetheroleum Pelargonii .... see ROSE GERANIUM
Aethusa cynapium .... see FOOL'S PARSLEY
AFA .... see BLUE-GREEN ALGAE
Aframomum melegueta .... see GRAINS OF PARADISE
African Chillies .... see CAPSICUM
African Civet .... see CIVET
African Civet: Viverra civetta .... see CIVET
African Coffee Tree .... see CASTOR OIL
African Coffee Tree .... see CASTOR seed
African Cucumber .... see BITTER MELON
African Ginger .... see GINGER
African Marigold .... see TAGETES
African Myrrh .... see MYRRH
African Pepper .... see CAPSICUM
African Plum Tree .... see PYGEUM
African Potato .... see AFRICAN WILD POTATO
AFRICAN WILD POTATO
.... see AFRICAN WILD POTATO
AG .... see LARCH ARABINOGALACTAN
AGA .... see AGA
AGAR .... see AGAR
Agar-Agar .... see AGAR
Agarweed .... see AGAR
Agathosma betulina .... see BUCHU
Aged Garlic Extract .... see GARLIC
Agnolyt .... see CHASTEBERRY
Agnus Castus .... see CHASTEBERRY
Agracejo .... see EUROPEAN BARBERRY
Agrião .... see WATERCRESS
Agrimonia eupatoria .... see AGRIMONY
Agrimonia procera .... see AGRIMONY
Agrimoniae herba .... see AGRIMONY
AGRIMONY .... see AGRIMONY
Agromonia .... see AGRIMONY
AGROPYRON .... see AGROPYRON
Agropyron repens .... see AGROPYRON,
COUCH GRASS,
WHEATGRASS
Agrostemma githago .... see CORN COCKLE
Ague Grass .... see ALETRIS
Ague Root .... see ALETRIS
Ague Tree .... see SASSAFRAS
Agueweed .... see BONESET
AHA .... see ALPHA HYDROXY ACIDS
Ahuacate ....see AVOCADO

Ail .... see GARLIC
Ailanthus altissima .... see TREE OF HEAVEN
Ailanthus Glandulosa .... see TREE OF HEAVEN
Ailanto .... see TREE OF HEAVEN
Airelle .... see BILBERRY dried ripe fruit,
BILBERRY leaf
Ajagandha .... see ASHWAGANDHA
Ajava Seeds .... see BISHOP'S WEED
Ajenjo .... see WORMWOOD above ground parts
Ajenuz.................................. see BLACK SEED
Ajo .... see GARLIC
Ajowan .... see BISHOP'S WEED
Ajowan Caraway .... see BISHOP'S WEED
Ajowan Seed .... see BISHOP'S WEED
Ajowanj .... see BISHOP'S WEED
Ajuga chamaepitys .... see GROUND PINE
Ajuga reptans .... see BUGLE
Akee .... see ACKEE
A-KetoGlutaric Acid
.... see ALPHA-KETOGLUTARATE
AKG .... see ALPHA-KETOGLUTARATE
Aki .... see ACKEE
ALA .... see ALPHA-LINOLENIC ACID
ALPHA-LIPOIC ACID
Alant .... see ELECAMPANE
A-Lan-Thus .... see TREE OF HEAVEN
ALC .... see ACETYL-L-CARNITINE
Alcachofa .... see ARTICHOKE
Alcacuz.................................... see LICORICE
Alcanna .... see HENNA
Alcar .... see ACETYL-L-CARNITINE
Alcaucil .... see ARTICHOKE
Alcazuz.................................... see LICORICE
Alcea rosea .... see HOLLYHOCK
ALCHEMILLA .... see ALCHEMILLA
Alchemilla alpina .... see ALPINE LADY'S MANTLE
Alchemilla vulgaris .... see ALCHEMILLA
Alchemilla xanthochlora .... see ALCHEMILLA
Alchemillae alpinae herba
.... see ALPINE LADY'S MANTLE
Alchornea castaneifolia .... see IPORURU
ALDER BUCKTHORN .... see ALDER BUCKTHORN
Alder Dogwood .... see ALDER BUCKTHORN
Alehoof.................................. see GROUND IVY
ALETRIS .... see ALETRIS
Aletris farinosa .... see ALETRIS
Aleurites cordata .... see TUNG SEED
Aleurites moluccana .... see TUNG SEED
Alexandrian Senna ....see SENNA
Alexandrian-laurel .... see LAURELWOOD
Alexandrinische Senna .... see SENNA
Alexandrinischer Lorbeer .... see LAURELWOOD
Alfacalcidol .... see VITAMIN D
ALFALFA .... see ALFALFA
Algerian Geranium Oil .... see ROSE GERANIUM
ALGIN ....see ALGIN
Alginates ....see ALGIN
Alhucema .... see LAVENDER
A-Lipoic Acid .... see ALPHA-LIPOIC ACID
Alisma plantago-aquatica .... see WATER PLANTAIN
Alkanet .... see ALKANNA
ALKANNA .... see ALKANNA
Alkanna Radix .... see ALKANNA
Alkanna tinctoria .... see ALKANNA

INDEX

All-Heal .... see EUROPEAN MISTLETOE,
                                    SELF-HEAL, VALERIAN
All Rac-Alpha-Tocopherol .... see VITAMIN E
Alligator Pear .... see AVOCADO
Allii cepae bulbus .... see ONION
Allii Sativi Bulbus .... see GARLIC
Allium .... see GARLIC
Allium cepa .... see ONION
Allium sativum .... see GARLIC
Allium schoenoprasum .... see CHIVE
Allium ursinum .... see BEAR'S GARLIC
Allseed Nine-Joints .... see KNOTWEED HERB
ALLSPICE .... see ALLSPICE
All-Trans Lycopene .... see LYCOPENE
Almond .... see SWEET ALMOND
Almond Oil .... see SWEET ALMOND
Alnus glutinosa .... see BLACK ALDER
Alnus serrulata .... see SMOOTH ALDER
Aloe .... see ALOE dried juice from leaf, latex,
                                          ALOE gel
Aloe africana .... see ALOE dried juice from leaf, latex,
                                          ALOE gel
Aloe arborescens natalenis
       .... see ALOE dried juice from leaf, latex, ALOE gel
Aloe Barbadensis
       .... see ALOE dried juice from leaf, latex, ALOE gel
Aloe Capensis .... see ALOE gel
ALOE dried juice from leaf, latex
       .... see ALOE dried juice from leaf, latex
Aloe Ferox .... see ALOE dried juice from leaf, latex,
                                          ALOE gel
ALOE gel .... see ALOE gel
Aloe Juice .... see ALOE dried juice from leaf, latex
Aloe Latex .... see ALOE dried juice from leaf, latex
Aloe Leaf Gel .... see ALOE gel
Aloe perfoliata
       .... see ALOE dried juice from leaf, latex, ALOE gel
Aloe perryi
       .... see ALOE dried juice from leaf, latex, ALOE gel
Aloe spicata
       .... see ALOE dried juice from leaf, latex, ALOE gel
Aloe vera
       .... see ALOE dried juice from leaf, latex, ALOE gel
Aloe Yucca .... see YUCCA
Aloerot .... see ALETRIS
Alopecurus species .... see HAY FLOWER
Aloysia citriodora .... see LEMON VERBENA
Aloysia triphylla .... see LEMON VERBENA
Alpenkraut .... see HEMP AGRIMONY
Alpha-amino-4-imidazole propanoic acid ... see HISTIDINE
Alpha-aminohydrocinnamic acid
       .... see PHENYLALANINE
Alpha-Chymotrypsin .... see CHYMOTRYPSIN
ALPHA HYDROXY ACIDS
       .... see ALPHA HYDROXY ACIDS
Alpha-hydroxyethanoic Acid
       .... see ALPHA HYDROXY ACIDS
Alpha Keto Glutarate .... see ALPHA-KETOGLUTARATE
ALPHA-KETOGLUTARATE
       .... see ALPHA-KETOGLUTARATE
Alpha-Ketoglutarates .... see ALPHA-KETOGLUTARATE
Alpha Ketoglutaric Acid
       .... see ALPHA-KETOGLUTARATE
Alpha-Ketopropionic Acid .... see PYRUVATE

Alpha KG .... see ALPHA-KETOGLUTARATE
ALPHA-LINOLENIC ACID
       .... see ALPHA-LINOLENIC ACID
ALPHA-LIPOIC ACID .... see ALPHA-LIPOIC ACID
Alpha-Lipoic Acid Extract .... see ALPHA-LIPOIC ACID
Alpha-Tocopherol .... see VITAMIN E
Alpha tocotrienol .... see VITAMIN E
ALPINE CRANBERRY .... see ALPINE CRANBERRY
ALPINE LADY'S MANTLE
       .... see ALPINE LADY'S MANTLE
ALPINE RAGWORT .... see ALPINE RAGWORT
Alpine Strawberry .... see STRAWBERRY
ALPINIA .... see ALPINIA
Alpinia officinarum .... see ALPINIA
Alquitran de Enebro .... see CADE OIL
Alraunwurzel .... see EUROPEAN MANDRAKE
Alstonia Bark .... see FEVER BARK
Alstonia constricta .... see FEVER BARK
Altamisa .... see FEVERFEW
Alteia .... see MARSHMALLOW
Althaea officinalis .... see MARSHMALLOW
Althaea rosea .... see HOLLYHOCK
Althaeae folium .... see MARSHMALLOW
Althaeae radi .... see MARSHMALLOW
Althea .... see MARSHMALLOW
Althea Rose .... see HOLLYHOCK
Aluminum phosphate .... see PHOSPHATE SALTS
Amachazuru .... see JIAOGULAN
Amalaki .... see INDIAN GOOSEBERRY
Amangura .... see ASHWAGANDHA
Amanita muscaria .... see AGA
Amantilla .... see VALERIAN
AMARANTH .... see AMARANTH
Amaranthus hypochondriacus .... see AMARANTH
Amargo .... see QUASSIA
Amber .... see ST. JOHN'S WORT
Amber Touch-and-Heal .... see ST. JOHN'S WORT
Amblabaum .... see INDIAN GOOSEBERRY
Ambreine .... see LABDANUM
Ambretta .... see AMBRETTE
AMBRETTE .... see AMBRETTE
Ambroise .... see WOOD SAGE
AMERICAN ADDER'S TONGUE
       .... see AMERICAN ADDER'S TONGUE
American Arborvitae .... see CEDAR leaf,
                                          CEDAR LEAF OIL
American Aspidium .... see MALE FERN
AMERICAN BITTERSWEET
       .... see AMERICAN BITTERSWEET
AMERICAN CHESTNUT ... see AMERICAN CHESTNUT
American Cone Flower .... see ECHINACEA
American Cranberry .... see CRANBERRY
American Dill .... see DILL seed,
                                    DILL above ground parts
AMERICAN DOGWOOD ... see AMERICAN DOGWOOD
American Dwarf Palm Tree .... see SAW PALMETTO
AMERICAN ELDER .... see AMERICAN ELDER
American Elderberry .... see AMERICAN ELDER
AMERICAN GINSENG .... see GINSENG, AMERICAN
American Greek Valerian .... see ABSCESS ROOT
AMERICAN HELLEBORE
       .... see AMERICAN HELLEBORE
American Indigo .... see WILD INDIGO
American Ipecacuanha .... see INDIAN PHYSIC

AMERICAN IVY .... see AMERICAN IVY
American Liverleaf .... see LIVERWORT
American Mandrake .... see PODOPHYLLUM
AMERICAN MISTLETOE
.... see AMERICAN MISTLETOE
American Mullein .... see MULLEIN
American Nightshade .... see POKEWEED berry,
                                                        POKEWEED root
AMERICAN PAWPAW .... see AMERICAN PAWPAW
American Pennyroyal .... see PENNYROYAL leaf,
                                                        PENNYROYAL oil
American Saffron .... see SAFFLOWER
AMERICAN SPIKENARD
.... see AMERICAN SPIKENARD
American Spinach .... see POKEWEED berry,
                                                        POKEWEED root
American Storax .... see STORAX
American Valerian .... see NERVE ROOT
American Veratrum .... see AMERICAN HELLEBORE
American White Hellebore
.... see AMERICAN HELLEBORE
AMERICAN WHITE POND LILY
.... see AMERICAN WHITE POND LILY
American Woodbine .... see AMERICAN IVY
American Wormgrass .... see PINK ROOT
Aminobenzoate Potassium
.... see PARA-AMINOBENZOIC ACID (PABA)
Aminobenzoic Acid
.... see PARA-AMINOBENZOIC ACID (PABA)
Aminoethanesulfonate .... see TAURINE
Amla .... see INDIAN GOOSEBERRY
Ammi .... see KHELLA
Ammi daucoides .... see KHELLA
Ammi majus .... see BISHOP'S WEED
Ammi visnaga .... see KHELLA
Ammocallis rosea ...... see MADAGASCAR PERIWINKLE
Amomum cardamomum .... see CARDAMOM
Amomum melegueta .... see GRAINS OF PARADISE
Amoraciae Rusticanae Radix .... see HORSERADISH
Amorphophallus konjac .... see GLUCOMANNAN
Amukkirag .... see ASHWAGANDHA
Amygdala Amara .... see BITTER ALMOND
Amygdala Dulcis .... see SWEET ALMOND
Amygdaloside .... see APRICOT
Anabaena species .... see BLUE-GREEN ALGAE
Anacardium occidentale .... see CASHEW
Anacyclus pyrethrum .... see PELLITORY
Anagallis arvensis .... see SCARLET PIMPERNEL
Anamirta cocculus .... see LEVANT BERRY
Anamirta paniculata .... see LEVANT BERRY
Ananas sativus .... see BROMELAIN
Anashca .... see MARIJUANA
Anchi Ginseng .... see GINSENG, AMERICAN
Anchusa .... see ALKANNA
Andira araroba ....see GOA POWDER
ANDIROBA .... see ANDIROBA
Andiroba-Saruba .... see ANDIROBA
ANDRACHNE .... see ANDRACHNE
Andrachne aspera .... see ANDRACHNE
Andrachne cordifolia .... see ANDRACHNE
Andrachne phyllanthoides .... see ANDRACHNE
Andro .... see ANDROSTENEDIONE
ANDROGRAPHIS .... see ANDROGRAPHIS
Andrographis paniculata .... see ANDROGRAPHIS

Andrographolide .... see ANDROGRAPHIS
Andropogon citratus .... see LEMONGRASS
Andropogon nardus .... see CITRONELLA OIL
Androst-4-ene-3,17-dione .... see ANDROSTENEDIONE
Androstene .... see ANDROSTENEDIONE
ANDROSTENEDIOL .... see ANDROSTENEDIOL
ANDROSTENEDIONE .... see ANDROSTENEDIONE
Anémone à Lobes Aigus .... see LIVERWORT
Anemone acutiloba .... see LIVERWORT
Anemone americana .... see LIVERWORT
Anémone d'Amérique .... see LIVERWORT
Anemone hepatica .... see LIVERWORT
Anemone nemorosa .... see WOOD ANEMONE
Anemone nigricans .... see PULSATILLA
Anemone pratensis .... see PULSATILLA
Anemone pulsatilla .... see PULSATILLA
Anemopsis californica .... see YERBA MANSA
Anetheum graveolens .... see DILL seed,
                                                        DILL above ground parts
Anethi fructus .... see DILL seed
Anethi herba .... see DILL above ground parts
Anethum foeniculum .... see FENNEL fruit, seed,
                                                        FENNEL OIL
Aneurine Hydrochloride .... see THIAMINE (VITAMIN B1)
Angel Tulip .... see JIMSON WEED
Angelica .... see ANGELICA herb, seed,
                                                        ANGELICA root
Angelica archangelica .... see ANGELICA herb, seed,
                                                        ANGELICA root
Angelica atropurpurea .... see ANGELICA root
Angelica curtisi .... see ANGELICA root
ANGELICA herb, seed .... see ANGELICA herb, seed
Angelica levisticum .... see LOVAGE
Angelica polymorpha sinensis .... see DONG QUAI
Angelica pubescens .... see ANGELICA root
ANGELICA root .... see ANGELICA root
Angelica rosaefolia .... see ANGELICA root
Angelica sinensis .... see DONG QUAI
Angelica sylvestris .... see ANGELICA root
Angelica Tree .... see NORTHERN PRICKLY ASH
Angelicae ....see ANGELICA herb, seed
Angelicae Fructus .... see ANGELICA herb, seed
Angelicae Herba .... see ANGELICA herb, seed
Angelicin .... see BETA-SITOSTEROL
ANGEL'S TRUMPET .... see ANGEL'S TRUMPET
Angled Loofah .... see LUFFA
ANGOSTURA .... see ANGOSTURA
Angustura .... see ANGOSTURA
Anhydrous aluminum silicates
.... see COLLOIDAL MINERALS
Anhydrous Caffeine .... see CAFFEINE
Aniba rosaeodora ....see BOIS DE ROSE OIL
Animal Charcoal .... see ACTIVATED CHARCOAL
Anis des Vosges .... see CARAWAY dried fruit, seed
ANISE .... see ANISE
Aniseed .... see ANISE
Aniseed Stars .... see STAR ANISE
Anisi Fructus .... see ANISE
Anisi stellati fructus .... see STAR ANISE
ANNATTO .... see ANNATTO
Annotta .... see ANNATTO
Annual Mugwort .... see SWEET ANNIE
Annual Wormwood .... see SWEET ANNIE
Antennaria dioica .... see CAT'S FOOT

INDEX

Antennariase Dioicae Flos .... see CAT'S FOOT
Anthemis grandiflorum .... see CHRYSANTHEMUM
Anthemis stipulacea .... see CHRYSANTHEMUM
Anthoxanthum odoratum .... see SWEET VERNAL GRASS,
HAY FLOWER
Anthriscus cerefolium .... see CHERVIL
Anthriscus longirostris .... see CHERVIL
Antialopecia Factor .... see INOSITOL
Antiberiberi Factor .... see THIAMINE (VITAMIN B1)
Antiberiberi Vitamin .... see THIAMINE (VITAMIN B1)
Anti-Blacktongue Factor
.... see NIACIN AND NIACINAMIDE (VITAMIN B3)
Antineuritic Factor .... see THIAMINE (VITAMIN B1)
Antineuritic Vitamin .... see THIAMINE (VITAMIN B1)
Antipellagra Factor ...... see NIACIN AND NIACINAMIDE
Antiscorbutic Vitamin .... see VITAMIN C
Antitumor Angiogenesis Factor (anti-TAF)
.... see BOVINE CARTILAGE
Antixerophthalmic Vitamin .... see VITAMIN A
Anurine .... see THIAMINE (VITAMIN B1)
Aonla .... see INDIAN GOOSEBERRY
Aortic GAGs .... see MESOGLYCAN
Aortic Glycosaminoglycans .... see MESOGLYCAN
Aphanes arvensis .... see PARSLEY PIERT
Aphanizomenon flos-aquae ..... see BLUE-GREEN ALGAE
Apii Fructus .... see CELERY
Apis cerana .... see BEESWAX
Apis mellifera .... see BEESWAX,
ROYAL JELLY
Apis mellifera (honey bee) .... see BEE VENOM,
HONEY
Apis Venenum Purum .... see BEE VENOM
Apitoxin .... see BEE VENOM
Apium carvi .... see CARAWAY dried fruit, seed,
CARAWAY OIL
Apium graveolens .... see CELERY
Apium petroselinum .... see PARSLEY leaf, root,
PARSLEY seed
Apocynum cannabinum .... see CANADIAN HEMP
APPLE .... see APPLE
Apple Acid .... see ALPHA HYDROXY ACIDS
APPLE CIDER VINEGAR
.... see APPLE CIDER VINEGAR
APRICOT .... see APRICOT
Apricot Vine .... see PASSIONFLOWER
Aqua Pimentae .... see ALLSPICE
Aqueous Liver Extract .... see LIVER EXTRACT
Aquilegia vulgaris .... see COLUMBINE
Ara-6 .... see LARCH ARABINOGALACTAN
Arabian Myrrh .... see MYRRH
Arabinogalactan .... see LARCH ARABINOGALACTAN
Arachis .... see PEANUT OIL
Arachis hypogaea .... see PEANUT OIL
Aralia racemosa .... see AMERICAN SPIKENARD
Arandano Americano .... see CRANBERRY
Arandano Trepador .... see CRANBERRY
Arañuel .... see BLACK SEED
Araoba .... see GOA POWDER
Arberry .... see UVA URSI
Arborvitae .... see CEDAR leaf,
CEDAR LEAF OIL
Arbre Fricasse .... see ACKEE
Arbutus uva-ursi .... see UVA URSI
Archangel .... see WHITE DEAD NETTLE FLOWER

Archangelica officinalis .... see ANGELICA root
Archangle .... see BUGLEWEED
Arcostaphylos .... see UVA URSI
Arctic Root .... see ROSEROOT
Arctium .... see BURDOCK
Arctium lappa .... see BURDOCK
Arctium minus .... see BURDOCK
Arctium tomentosum .... see BURDOCK
Arctostaphylos uva-ursi .... see UVA URSI
ARECA .... see ARECA
Areca catechu .... see ARECA
Areca Nut .... see ARECA
ARENARIA RUBRA .... see ARENARIA RUBRA
Arg .... see L-ARGININE
Argasse .... see SEA BUCKTHORN
Argilla .... see KAOLIN
Arginine .... see L-ARGININE
Arginine Hydrochloride .... see L-ARGININE
Argousier .... see SEA BUCKTHORN
Argyreia nervosa ...... see HAWAIIAN BABY WOODROSE
Argyreia speciosa .... see HAWAIIAN BABY WOODROSE
ARISTOLOCHIA .... see ARISTOLOCHIA
Aristolochia auricularia .... see ARISTOLOCHIA
Aristolochia clematitis .... see ARISTOLOCHIA
Aristolochia fangchi .... see ARISTOLOCHIA
Aristolochia heterophylla .... see ARISTOLOCHIA
Aristolochia kwangsiensis .... see ARISTOLOCHIA
Aristolochia moupinensis .... see ARISTOLOCHIA
Aristolochia reticulata .... see ARISTOLOCHIA
Aristolochia serpentaria .... see ARISTOLOCHIA
Arjuna .... see TERMINALIA
Armeniaca .... see APRICOT
Armoise .... see WORMWOOD above ground parts
Armoise Capillaire .... see YIN CHEN
Armoise Commune .... see MUGWORT
Armoracia lopathifolia .... see HORSERADISH
Armoracia rusticana .... see HORSERADISH
Armstrong .... see KNOTWEED HERB
ARNICA .... see ARNICA
Arnica cordifolia .... see ARNICA
Arnica Flos .... see ARNICA
Arnica Flower .... see ARNICA
Arnica fulgens .... see ARNICA
Arnica latifolia .... see ARNICA
Arnica Montana .... see ARNICA
Arnica sororia .... see ARNICA
Arnikablüten .... see ARNICA
Arnotta .... see ANNATTO
ARRACH .... see ARRACH
Arrow Wood .... see ALDER BUCKTHORN
ARROWROOT .... see ARROWROOT
Arrowwood .... see WAHOO
Arruda Bravam .... see JABORANDI
Arruda Do Mato .... see JABORANDI
Arryan .... see CHEKEN
Arsesmart .... see SMARTWEED
Artemisia .... see MUGWORT,
WORMWOOD above ground parts,
WORMWOOD oil
Artemisia absinthium
.... see WORMWOOD above ground parts,
WORMWOOD oil
Artemisia annua .... see SWEET ANNIE
Artemisia capillaris .... see YIN CHEN

Artemisia cina .... see WORMSEED
Artemisia dracunculus .... see TARRAGON
Artemisia scoparia .... see YIN CHEN
Artemisia vulgaris .... see MUGWORT
Artemisiae vulgaris herba .... see MUGWORT
Artemisiae vulgaris radix .... see MUGWORT
Artemisinin .... see SWEET ANNIE
Artesian Absinthium
.... see WORMWOOD above ground parts
Arthritica .... see COWSLIP
Artichaut Commun .... see ARTICHOKE
ARTICHOKE .... see ARTICHOKE
Artischocke .... see ARTICHOKE
ARUM .... see ARUM
Arum maculatum .... see ARUM
Arundinaria japonica .... see BAMBOO
Arusa .... see MALABAR NUT
Asa Foetida .... see ASAFOETIDA
Asafetida .... see ASAFOETIDA
ASAFOETIDA .... see ASAFOETIDA
Asan .... see ASHWAGANDHA
ASARABACCA .... see ASARABACCA
Asaroun .... see ASARABACCA
Asarum .... see ASARABACCA
Asarum europaeum .... see ASARABACCA
Asclepias geminate .... see GYMNEMA
Asclepias incarnata .... see SWAMP MILKWEED
Asclepias tuberosa .... see PLEURISY ROOT
Ascophyllum nodosum .... see ALGIN
Ascophyllum nodosum .... see BLADDERWRACK
Ascorbate .... see VITAMIN C (ASCORBIC ACID)
Ascorbic Acid .... see VITAMIN C (ASCORBIC ACID)
Asgand .... see ASHWAGANDHA
Asgandh .... see ASHWAGANDHA
Asgandha .... see ASHWAGANDHA
ASH .... see ASH
Ashagandha .... see ASHWAGANDHA
Ashangee .... see BUGLEWEED
Ashe Juniper
.... see CEDARWOOD bark, berry, leaf, seed, twig
Ashvagandha .... see ASHWAGANDHA
Ashwaganda .... see ASHWAGANDHA
ASHWAGANDHA .... see ASHWAGANDHA
Ashweed .... see GOUTWEED
Asian Ginseng .... see GINSENG, PANAX
Asiatic Ginseng .... see GINSENG, PANAX
Asimina triloba .... see AMERICAN PAWPAW
Asoda .... see ASHWAGANDHA
Aspalathus contaminata .... see RED BUSH TEA
Aspalathus linearis .... see RED BUSH TEA
Asparagi Rhizoma Root .... see ASPARAGUS
ASPARAGUS .... see ASPARAGUS
Asparagus officinalis .... see ASPARAGUS
Aspartate Chelated Minerals .... see ASPARTATES
Aspartate Mineral Chelates .... see ASPARTATES
ASPARTATES .... see ASPARTATES
ASPEN .... see ASPEN
Asperge .... see ASPARAGUS
Asperula odorata .... see SWEET WOODRUFF
Aspidosperma quebracho-blanco .... see QUEBRACHO
Ass Ear .... see COMFREY
Assant .... see ASAFOETIDA
Ass's Foot .... see COLTSFOOT
Astaxanthin .... see MICROALGAE

Aster helenium .... see ELECAMPANE
Aster officinalis .... see ELECAMPANE
Asthma Weed .... see LOBELIA
Astragali .... see ASTRAGALUS
ASTRAGALUS .... see ASTRAGALUS
Astragalus gummifera .... see TRAGACANTH
Astragalus Membranaceus .... see ASTRAGALUS
Astragalus mongholicus .... see ASTRAGALUS
Asundha .... see ASHWAGANDHA
Asvagandha .... see ASHWAGANDHA
Aswagandha .... see ASHWAGANDHA
Athemis nobilis .... see ROMAN CHAMOMILE
Athyrium filix-femina .... see LADY FERN
Atlantic Yam .... see WILD YAM
Atmagupta .... see COWHAGE
Atomic number 5 .... see BORON
Atomic number 12 .... see MAGNESIUM
Atomic number 19 .... see POTASSIUM
Atomic number 20 .... see CALCIUM
Atomic number 23 .... see VANADIUM
Atomic number 24 .... see CHROMIUM
Atomic number 25 .... see MANGANESE
Atomic number 26 .... see IRON
Atomic number 29 .... see COPPER
Atomic number 30 .... see ZINC
Atomic number 32 .... see GERMANIUM
Atomic number 34 .... see SELENIUM
Atomic number 53 .... see IODINE
Atropa belladonna .... see BELLADONNA
Atropa belladonna acuminata .... see BELLADONNA
Aubepine .... see HAWTHORN
Auckland Costus .... see COSTUS OIL,
                                           COSTUS root
Aucklandia costus .... see COSTUS OIL,
                                           COSTUS root
Augentrostkraut .... see EYEBRIGHT
August Flower .... see GUMWEED
Aurantii Pericarpium .... see BITTER ORANGE
Australian Febrifuge .... see FEVER BARK
Australian Fever Bush .... see FEVER BARK
Australian Quinine .... see FEVER BARK
Australian Tea Tree Oil .... see TEA TREE OIL
AUTUMN CROCUS
.... see AUTUMN CROCUS
Autumn Crocus .... see SAFFRON
Autumn Monkshood .... see ACONITE
Ava .... see KAVA
Ava Pepper .... see KAVA
Avarada .... see ASHWAGANDHA
Aveleira .... see HAZELNUT
Avelinier .... see HAZELNUT
Avellano .... see HAZELNUT
Avena Fructus .... see OATS
Avena Sativa .... see OAT above ground parts,
                          OAT BRAN, OAT STRAW, OATS
Avenae herba .... see OAT above ground parts
Avenae stramentum .... see OAT STRAW
AVENS .... see AVENS
AVOCADO .... see AVOCADO
Avocato .... see AVOCADO
Awa .... see KAVA
Axerophtholum .... see VITAMIN A
Axjun Argun .... see TERMINALIA
AY-27255 .... see VINPOCETINE

Ayak Chichira .... see MACA
Ayegreen .... see HOUSELEEK
Ayron .... see HOUSELEEK
Ayuk Willku .... see MACA
Ayurvedic Ginseng .... see ASHWAGANDHA
Azadirachta indica .... see NEEM
Azafron .... see SAFFRON
Azarum .... see ASARABACCA
Azeda-Brava .... see SORREL
Aztec Marigold .... see TAGETES
Azucacaa .... see STEVIA
B .... see BORON
B Complex Vitamin .... see FOLIC ACID,
NIACIN AND NIACINAMIDE (VITAMIN B3) ,
PANTOTHENIC ACID (VITAMIN B6),
PYRIDOXINE (VITAMIN B6),
RIBOFLAVIN (VITAMIN B2),
THIAMINE (VITAMIN B1),
VITAMIN B12
B(t) Factor .... see L-CARNITINE
BA JI TIAN .... see BA JI TIAN
Baby Hawaiian Woodrose
.... see HAWAIIAN BABY WOODROSE
Baby Wood-rose ...... see HAWAIIAN BABY WOODROSE
Bac Ngu Vi Tu .... see SCHISANDRA
Baccae .... see ELDERBERRY
Bachelor's Button .... see FEVERFEW
Backache Root .... see MARSH BLAZING STAR
Bacopa monniera .... see BRAHMI
Bacopa monnieri .... see BRAHMI
Badiana .... see STAR ANISE
BAEL .... see BAEL
Bahama Cascarilla .... see CASCARILLA
Bahera .... see TERMINALIA
Bahia Powder .... see GOA POWDER
Bahira .... see TERMINALIA
Bai Dou Kou .... see CARDAMOM
Bai Guo Ye .... see GINKGO leaf (GINKGO leaf extract)
Bai Qu Cai
...... see GREATER CELANDINE dried above ground parts
Baiguo .... see GINKGO seed
BAIKAL SKULLCAP .... see BAIKAL SKULLCAP
Baikal Skullcap Root .... see BAIKAL SKULLCAP
Baises De Sureau .... see ELDERBERRY
Bal .... see MYRRH
Bala .... see COUNTRY MALLOW
Bala Harade .... see TERMINALIA
B-alanyl histidine .... see CARNOSINE
B-alanyl-L-histidine .... see CARNOSINE
Bald-faced Hornet .... see BEE VENOM
Baldrian .... see VALERIAN
Baldrianwurzel .... see VALERIAN
Balera .... see TERMINALIA
Ballota .... see BLACK HOREHOUND
Ballota nigra .... see BLACK HOREHOUND
Balm .... see LEMON BALM
Balm of Gilead .... see CANADA BALSAM, POPLAR
Balm of Gilead Fir .... see HEMLOCK SPRUCE
Balmony .... see TURTLE HEAD
Balsam .... see CANADA BALSAM,
COPAIBA BALSAM, OREGON FIR BALSAM,
PERU BALSAM, TOLU BALSAM
Balsam Apple .... see BITTER MELON
Balsam Canada .... see CANADA BALSAM
Balsam Fir .... see CANADA BALSAM

HEMLOCK SPRUCE
Balsam Fir Canada .... see CANADA BALSAM
Balsam Fir Oregon .... see OREGON FIR BALSAM
Balsam of Fir .... see CANADA BALSAM
Balsam of Peru .... see PERU BALSAM
Balsam of Tolu .... see TOLU BALSAM
Balsam Oregon .... see OREGON FIR BALSAM
Balsam Pear .... see BITTER MELON
Balsam Peru .... see PERU BALSAM
Balsam Poplar Buds .... see POPLAR
Balsam Styracis .... see STORAX
Balsam Tolu .... see TOLU BALSAM
Balsam Weed .... see JEWELWEED
Balsambirne .... see BITTER MELON
Balsamo .... see BITTER MELON
Balsamodendron Myrrha .... see MYRRH
Balsamum Peruvianum .... see PERU BALSAM
Balsamum Styrax Liquidus .... see STORAX
Balsamum Tolutanum .... see TOLU BALSAM
Balucanat .... see TUNG SEED
BAMBOO .... see BAMBOO
Band Man's Plaything .... see YARROW
Baneberry .... see BLACK COHOSH, WHITE COHOSH
Banji .... see MARIJUANA
Bannal .... see SCOTCH BROOM flower,
SCOTCH BROOM herb
Bantu Tulip .... see AFRICAN WILD POTATO
Baptista tinctoria .... see WILD INDIGO
Baraka .... see BLACK SEED
Barbados Cherry .... see ACEROLA
Barbasco .... see WILD YAM
Barberry .... see OREGON GRAPE
Barber's Brush .... see TEAZLE
Bardana .... see BURDOCK
Bardanae Radix .... see BURDOCK
Bardane .... see BURDOCK
Bariar .... see COUNTRY MALLOW
BARLEY .... see BARLEY
Barosma betulina .... see BUCHU
Barosma crenulata .... see BUCHU
Barosmae Folium .... see BUCHU
Barrenwort .... see EPIMEDIUM
Barweed .... see CLIVERS
Basam .... see SCOTCH BROOM herb
BASIL .... see BASIL
Basil Thyme .... see CALAMINT
Basilici Herba .... see BASIL
Basket Willow .... see WILLOW BARK
Basking Shark Liver Oil .... see SHARK LIVER OIL
Bassora Tragacanth .... see KARAYA GUM
Basswood
.... see LINDEN CHARCOAL, LINDEN dried flower,
LINDEN dried leaf, LINDEN dried sapwood
Bastard Cinnamon .... see CASSIA
Bastard Ginseng .... see CODONOPSIS
Bastard Mahogany .... see ANDIROBA
Bastard Saffron .... see SAFFLOWER
Batavia Cassia .... see CINNAMON bark
Batavia Cinnamon .... see CINNAMON bark
Batchelor's Buttons ..... see BUTTERCUP, CORNFLOWER
Bauchweh .... see YARROW
Baurenlilien .... see WHITE LILY
Bay .... see SWEET BAY
Bay Laurel .... see SWEET BAY
Bay Leaf .... see SWEET BAY

Bay Tree ....see SWEET BAY
Bay Willow ....see WILLOW BARK
BAYBERRY .... see BAYBERRY
Bayberry .... SWEET GALE
BCAA .... see BRANCHED-CHAIN AMINO ACIDS
B-Complex Vitamin .... see FOLIC ACID
BC PS .... see PHOSPHATIDYLSERINE
BD .... see BUTANEDIOL (BD)
Bdellium .... see MYRRH
BDO .... see BUTANEDIOL (BD)
B-DPNH .... see NADH
Bead Tree ....see NEEM
Bead Vine .... see PRECATORY BEAN
Bean Herb .... see SUMMER SAVORY
BEAN POD .... see BEAN POD
Bean Trifoil .... see LABURNUM
Bear Grass .... see YUCCA
Bear Root .... see OSHA
Bearberry .... see UVA URSI
Bearbind ....see GREATER BINDWEED
Beard Moss .... see USNEA
Bearded Darnel .... see TAUMELLOOLCH
Beargrape .... see UVA URSI
Bear's-Bind ....see GREATER BINDWEED
BEAR'S GARLIC .... see BEAR'S GARLIC
Bear's Grape............................... see POKEWEED berry,
                                          POKEWEED root, UVA URSI
Bear's Paw .... see MALE FERN
Bear's Weed .... see YERBA SANTA
Bearsgrape .... see UVA URSI
Beaumont Root .... see BLACK ROOT
Beaver Poison .... see WATER HEMLOCK
Beaver Tree .... see MAGNOLIA bark
Beccabunga............................... see BROOKLIME
Bedstraw .... see CLIVERS
Bedumil .... see VITAMIN B12
BEE VENOM .... see BEE VENOM
Bee Balm .... see OSWEGO TEA
Bee Glue .... see PROPOLIS
Bee Nettle .... see WHITE DEAD NETTLE FLOWER
Bee Plant .... see BORAGE flower, dried above ground parts
BEE POLLEN .... see BEE POLLEN
Bee Pollen Extract .... see BEE POLLEN
Bee Propolis .... see PROPOLIS
Bee saliva .... see ROYAL JELLY
Bee spit .... see ROYAL JELLY
Bee Sting Venom .... see BEE VENOM
Beebread ... see BORAGE flower, dried above ground parts,
                                                      RED CLOVER
Beeflower .... see WALLFLOWER
Beefsteak Plant .... see PERILLA
BEER .... see BEER
Bees Wax .... see BEESWAX
Beesnest Plant.......................... see WILD CARROT
BEESWAX .... see BEESWAX
BEET .... see BEET
Beets .... see BEET
Beg Kei .... see ASTRAGALUS
Beggar's Blanket .... see MULLEIN
Beggar's Buttons .... see BURDOCK
Beggarweed .... see DODDER, KNOTWEED HERB
Beggary .... see FUMITORY
Behada .... see TERMINALIA
Bei Chai Hu .... see BUPLEURUM

Bei Qi.................................... see ASTRAGALUS
Bei Wu Wei Zi .... see SCHISANDRA
Bejunco de Cerca .... see ABUTA
Bel .... see BAEL
Beleric Myrobalan .... see TERMINALIA
Belgium Valerian .... see VALERIAN
BELLADONNA .... see BELLADONNA
Belladonna .... see SCOPOLIA
Belladonna Scopola .... see SCOPOLIA
Bellflower .... see CODONOPSIS
Bellis perennis .... see WILD DAISY
Benedict's Herb .... see AVENS
Bengal Quince .... see BAEL
Bennet's Root .... see AVENS
Benzoe .... see BENZOIN
BENZOIN .... see BENZOIN
Berberidis cortex .... see EUROPEAN BARBERRY
Berberidis fructus .... see EUROPEAN BARBERRY
Berberidis radicis cortex ...... see EUROPEAN BARBERRY
Berberidis radix .... see EUROPEAN BARBERRY
Berberis AQuifolium .... see OREGON GRAPE
Berberis nervosa .... see OREGON GRAPE
Berberis repens .... see OREGON GRAPE
Berberis sonnei .... see OREGON GRAPE
Berberis Vulgaris .... see EUROPEAN BARBERRY
Berberitze .... see EUROPEAN BARBERRY
Berberry .... see EUROPEAN BARBERRY
Berbis .... see EUROPEAN BARBERRY
Bergamot .... see BERGAMOT OIL, OSWEGO TEA
BERGAMOT OIL .... see BERGAMOT OIL
Bergamot Orange .... see BERGAMOT OIL
Bergamota .... see BERGAMOT OIL
Bergamotier .... see BERGAMOT OIL
Bergamoto .... see BERGAMOT OIL
Bergamotte .... see BERGAMOT OIL
Bergamotto Bigarade Orange .... see BERGAMOT OIL
Bergwohlverleih .... see ARNICA
Berro .... see WATERCRESS
Berro Di Agua .... see WATERCRESS
Besenginaterkraut .... see SCOTCH BROOM flower
Besom .... see SCOTCH BROOM herb
Beta-1,3-D-glucan .... see BETA GLUCANS
Beta-1-6,1,3-beta-glucan .... see BETA GLUCANS
Beta-alanyl-L-histidine .... see CARNOSINE
Beta,beta-carotene-4,4-dione .... see CANTHAXANTHIN
BETA-CAROTENE .... see BETA-CAROTENE
Beta-D-fructofuranosidase
.... see FRUCTO-OLIGOSACCHARIDES
Beta-D-ribofuranose .... see RIBOSE
Beta-galactosidase .... see LACTASE
BETA GLUCANS .... see BETA GLUCANS
Beta Glycans .... see BETA GLUCANS
Beta-hydroxy-beta-methylbutyrate
.... see HYDROXYMETHYLBUTYRATE (HMB)
Beta-Hydroxy Beta-Methylbutyric Acid
.... see HYDROXYMETHYLBUTYRATE (HMB)
Beta-hydroxy-gamma-trimethylammonium butyrate
.... see L-CARNITINE
Beta-phenyl-alanine .... see PHENYLALANINE
Beta-sitostanol .... see SITOSTANOL
Beta sitosterin .... see BETA-SITOSTEROL
BETA-SITOSTEROL .... see BETA-SITOSTEROL
Beta-sitosterol glucoside .... see BETA-SITOSTEROL

INDEX

Beta-sitosterol glycoside .... see BETA-SITOSTEROL
Beta-tocopherol .... see VITAMIN E
Beta tocotrienol .... see VITAMIN E
Beta vulgaris .... see BEET
Betaine .... see BETAINE ANHYDROUS,
                                        BETAINE HYDROCHLORIDE
BETAINE ANHYDROUS ... see BETAINE ANHYDROUS
BETAINE HCL .... see BETAINE HYDROCHLORIDE
BETAINE HYDROCHLORIDE
            .... see BETAINE HYDROCHLORIDE
Betel Nut .... see ARECA
Betel Quid .... see ARECA
BETH ROOT .... see BETH ROOT
Betonica officinalis .... see BETONY
BETONY .... see BETONY
Betula .... see BIRCH
Betula Alnus .... see BLACK ALDER
Betula pendula .... see BIRCH
Betula pubescens .... see BIRCH
Betula verrucosa .... see BIRCH
Betulae folium .... see BIRCH
BGA .... see BLUE-GREEN ALGAE
Bhang .... see MARIJUANA
B-Hydroxy B-Mthylbutyrate Monohydrate
            .... see HYDROXYMETHYLBUTYRATE (HMB)
B-hydroxy-N-trimethyl aminobutyric acid
            .... see L-CARNITINE
Bianco spino .... see HAWTHORN
Bibernellkraut .... see PIMPINELLA above ground parts
Bible Frankincense .... see FRANKINCENSE
Bidara .... see ANDROGRAPHIS
Bidens tripartitia .... see BURR MARIGOLD
Bifido .... see BIFIDOBACTERIA
BIFIDOBACTERIA .... see BIFIDOBACTERIA
Bifidobacteria Bifidus .... see BIFIDOBACTERIA
Bifidobacterium .... see BIFIDOBACTERIA
Bifidobacterium adolescentis .... see BIFIDOBACTERIA
Bifidobacterium Bifidum .... see BIFIDOBACTERIA
Bifidobacterium Breve .... see BIFIDOBACTERIA
Bifidobacterium Infantis .... see BIFIDOBACTERIA
Bifidobacterium lactis .... see BIFIDOBACTERIA
Bifidobacterium Longum .... see BIFIDOBACTERIA
Bifidum .... see BIFIDOBACTERIA
Big Marigold .... see TAGETES
Bignonia sempervirens .... see GELSEMIUM
Bihara .... see TERMINALIA
Bilberry .... see BILBERRY dried ripe fruit,
                                                           BILBERRY leaf
BILBERRY dried ripe fruit
            .... see BILBERRY dried ripe fruit
BILBERRY leaf .... see BILBERRY leaf
Biletan .... see ALPHA-LIPOIC ACID
Biobran .... see MGN-3
Bioelectrical Minerals .... see COLLOIDAL MINERALS
Bioflavonoid Concentrate
            .... see GRAPEFRUIT SEED EXTRACT
Biota orientalis .... see ORIENTAL ARBORVITAE
BIOTIN .... see BIOTIN
Biowater .... see WILLARD WATER
Birangasifa .... see YARROW
BIRCH .... see BIRCH
Birch Sugar .... see XYLITOL
Bird Bread .... see COMMON STONECROP
Bird Pepper .... see CAPSICUM

Birdlime Mistletoe .... see EUROPEAN MISTLETOE
Bird's Eye Maple .... see RED MAPLE
Bird's Foot .... see FENUGREEK
Bird's Nest Root .... see WILD CARROT
Bird's Tongue .... see ASH, KNOTWEED HERB
Birdweed .... see KNOTWEED HERB
Birthroot .... see BETH ROOT
Birthwort .... see ARISTOLOCHIA
Bis-Carboxyethyl Germanium Sesquioxide
            .... see GERMANIUM
Bischofskrautfruchte .... see KHELLA
Biscuits .... see TORMENTIL
Bishop Wort .... see BETONY
Bishop's Elder .... see GOUTWEED
Bishop's Flower .... see BISHOP'S WEED
BISHOP'S WEED .... see BISHOP'S WEED
Bishop's Weed .... see KHELLA
Bishop's Weed Fruit .... see KHELLA
Bishopsweed .... see GOUTWEED
Bishopswort .... see BETONY, GOUTWEED
Bissy Nut .... see COLA NUT
BISTORT .... see BISTORT
BITTER ALMOND .... see BITTER ALMOND
Bitter Almond Oil .... see BITTER ALMOND
Bitter Apple .... see BITTER MELON, COLOCYNTH
Bitter Ash .... see QUASSIA, WAHOO
Bitter Bark .... see CASCARA
Bitter Buttons .... see TANSY
Bitter Candy Tuft .... see CLOWN'S MUSTARD PLANT
Bitter Candytuft .... see CLOWN'S MUSTARD PLANT
Bitter Cucumber ...... see BITTER MELON, COLOCYNTH
Bitter Damson .... see SIMARUBA
Bitter Fennel .... see FENNEL fruit, seed
Bitter Gourd .... see BITTER MELON
Bitter Herb .... see CENTAURY, TURTLE HEAD
Bitter Lettuce .... see WILD LETTUCE
BITTER MELON .... see BITTER MELON
BITTER MILKWORT .... see BITTER MILKWORT
Bitter Nightshade .... see BITTERSWEET NIGHTSHADE
BITTER ORANGE .... see BITTER ORANGE
Bitter Orange Flower .... see BITTER ORANGE
Bitter Orange Peel .... see BITTER ORANGE
Bitter Redberry .... see AMERICAN DOGWOOD
Bitter Root .... see GENTIAN
Bitter Stick .... see CHIRATA
Bitter Winter .... see PIPSISSEWA
Bitter Wintergreen .... see PIPSISSEWA
Bitter Wood .... see QUASSIA
Bittergurke .... see BITTER MELON
Bitterroot .... see CANADIAN HEMP
Bitterstick .... see CHIRATA
Bittersweet .... see BITTERSWEET NIGHTSHADE
BITTERSWEET NIGHTSHADE
            .... see BITTERSWEET NIGHTSHADE
Bitterwood .... see QUASSIA
Bitterwort .... see GENTIAN
Bixa orellana .... see ANNATTO
Bizzom .... see SCOTCH BROOM herb
BLACK ALDER .... see BLACK ALDER
Black Balsam .... see PERU BALSAM
Black Berry .... see BLACKBERRY leaf,
                                              BLACKBERRY root
Black-Berried Alder............................ see ELDERBERRY,
                                                           ELDERFLOWER

INDEX

BLACK BRYONY .... see BLACK BRYONY
Black Caraway .... see BLACK SEED
Black catechu: Acacia catechu .... see CATECHU
Black Catechu: Acacia Catechu Heartwood Extract
.... see CATECHU
Black Cherry .... see WILD CHERRY
Black Choke .... see WILD CHERRY
BLACK COHOSH .... see BLACK COHOSH
Black Cumin .... see BLACK SEED
Black Currant .... see BLACK CURRANT berry,
                                               BLACK CURRANT dried leaf
BLACK CURRANT berry ... see BLACK CURRANT berry
BLACK CURRANT dried leaf
.... see BLACK CURRANT dried leaf
BLACK CURRANT SEED OIL
.... see BLACK CURRANT SEED OIL
Black Cutch .... see CATECHU
Black Date .... see JUJUBE
Black Dogwood .... see ALDER BUCKTHORN
Black Elder .... see ELDERBERRY, ELDERFLOWER
Black Elderberry .... see ELDERBERRY
Black Ginger .... see GINGER
Black Grape Raisins .... see GRAPE fruit, skin
BLACK HAW .... see BLACK HAW
BLACK HELLEBORE .... see BLACK HELLEBORE
BLACK HOREHOUND .... see BLACK HOREHOUND
Black Leaf Tea ....see BLACK TEA
BLACK MULBERRY .... see BLACK MULBERRY
Black Mustard .... see BLACK MUSTARD oil,
                                               BLACK MUSTARD seed
BLACK MUSTARD oil .... see BLACK MUSTARD oil
BLACK MUSTARD seed ..... see BLACK MUSTARD seed
BLACK NIGHTSHADE ....see BLACK NIGHTSHADE
Black Pepper
.... see BLACK PEPPER AND WHITE PEPPER
BLACK PEPPER AND WHITE PEPPER
.... see BLACK PEPPER AND WHITE PEPPER
BLACK PSYLLIUM .... see BLACK PSYLLIUM
Black Root .... see BLACK ROOT, COMFREY
Black Sampson .... see ECHINACEA
BLACK SEED .... see BLACK SEED
Black Snakeroot .... see BLACK COHOSH
Black Stinking Horehound ...... see BLACK HOREHOUND
Black Susans .... see ECHINACEA
Black Tang .... see BLADDERWRACK
BLACK TEA .... see BLACK TEA
BLACK WALNUT .... see BLACK WALNUT
Black Whortles .... see BILBERRY dried ripe fruit,
                                               BILBERRY leaf
Blackberry .... see BLACKBERRY leaf,
                                               BLACKBERRY root
BLACKBERRY leaf...................... see BLACKBERRY leaf
BLACKBERRY root .... see BLACKBERRY root
Blackcurrant .... see BLACK CURRANT berry
Blackeye Root .... see BLACK BRYONY
Black-Eyed Susan .... see PRECATORY BEAN
Blackhaw .... see BLACK HAW
Blackthorn .... see BLACKTHORN berry,
                                               BLACKTHORN flower
BLACKTHORN berry .... see BLACKTHORN berry
BLACKTHORN flower .... see BLACKTHORN flower
Blackthorn Fruit........................... see BLACKTHORN berry
Blackwort .... see COMFREY
Bladder Fucus .... see BLADDERWRACK

Bladder Wrack .... see BLADDERWRACK
Bladderpod .... see LOBELIA
BLADDERWORT .... see BLADDERWORT
BLADDERWRACK .... see BLADDERWRACK
Blanc Poivre
.... see BLACK PEPPER AND WHITE PEPPER
Blanket Herb .... see MULLEIN
Blanket Leaf .... see MULLEIN
Blasentang .... see BLADDERWRACK
Blatterdock .... see BUTTERBUR
Blazing Star .... see ALETRIS,
                                               FALSE UNICORN
                                               MARSH BLAZING STAR
Bleaberry .... see BILBERRY dried ripe fruit,
                                               BILBERRY leaf
Bleached Beeswax .... see BEESWAX
Bleeding Heart .... see NERVE ROOT,
                                               TURKEY CORN, WAHOO
BLESSED THISTLE .... see BLESSED THISTLE
Blighia sapida .... see ACKEE
Blind Nettle .... see WHITE DEAD NETTLE FLOWER
Blind Weed .... see SHEPHERD'S PURSE
Blisterweed .... see BUTTERCUP
Blond Plantago .... see BLOND PSYLLIUM
BLOND PSYLLIUM .... see BLOND PSYLLIUM
Blonde Psyllium .... see BLOND PSYLLIUM
Blood Elder .... see DWARF ELDER
Blood Hilder .... see DWARF ELDER
Blood of the Dragon .... see SANGRE DE GRADO
Blood Root .... see BLOODROOT
Blood Vine ....see FIREWEED
BLOODROOT .... see BLOODROOT
Bloodroot .... see TORMENTIL
Bloodwood .... see LOGWOOD
Bloodwort ....see YARROW
Blooming Sally ....see FIREWEED,
                                               PURPLE LOOSESTRIFE
Blowball .... see DANDELION above ground parts,
                                               DANDELION entire plant
Blue Balm .... see OSWEGO TEA
Blue Barberry .... see OREGON GRAPE
Blue Bells .... see ABSCESS ROOT
Blue Cap .... see CORNFLOWER
Blue Centaury .... see CORNFLOWER
BLUE COHOSH .... see BLUE COHOSH
Blue Curls ....see SELF-HEAL
BLUE FLAG .... see BLUE FLAG
Blue Flag .... see ORRIS
Blue Ginseng .... see BLUE COHOSH
Blue Green Algae .... see BLUE-GREEN ALGAE
Blue Gum .... see EUCALYPTUS dried leaf
Blue Mallow .... see MALLOW leaf
Blue Mallow Flower .... see MALLOW flower
Blue Monkshood Root....................................see ACONITE
Blue Nightshade .... see BITTERSWEET NIGHTSHADE
Blue Pimpernel .... see SCULLCAP
Blue Sailors .... see CHICORY
Blue Vervain .... see VERBENA
Blueberries .... see BLUEBERRY
Blueberry .... see BILBERRY dried ripe fruit,
                                               BILBERRY leaf
BLUEBERRY .... see BLUEBERRY
Bluebonnet .... see CORNFLOWER
Bluebottle .... see CORNFLOWER

INDEX

Bluebow .... see CORNFLOWER
BLUE-GREEN ALGAE .... see BLUE-GREEN ALGAE
Blue-Green Micro-Algae .... see BLUE-GREEN ALGAE
Bnadh .... see NADH
Bobbins .... see ARUM
Bockshornsame .... see FENUGREEK
Bofareira .... see CASTOR OIL, CASTOR seed
BOG BILBERRY .... see BOG BILBERRY
Bog Myrtle .... see SWEET GALE
Bog Rhubarb .... see BUTTERBUR
BOGBEAN .... see BOGBEAN
Bogshorns .... see BUTTERBUR
Bohnenkraut .... see SUMMER SAVORY
BOIS DE ROSE OIL .... see BOIS DE ROSE OIL
Bois Douleur .... see MORINDA
Bol .... see MYRRH
Bola .... see MYRRH
Boldine .... see BOLDO
BOLDO .... see BOLDO
Boldo Folium .... see BOLDO
Boldoak Boldea .... see BOLDO
Boldus .... see BOLDO
Boldus Boldus .... see BOLDO
Boletus Versicolor .... see CORIOLUS MUSHROOM
Bolivian Coca .... see COCA
Bolus Alba .... see KAOLIN
Bombus terrestris (Bumblebee) .... see BEE VENOM
Bone Meal .... see CALCIUM
BONESET .... see BONESET
Bonnet Bellflower .... see CODONOPSIS
Bookoo .... see BUCHU
Boor Tree .... see ELDERBERRY,
                                                ELDERFLOWER
Borage .... see BORAGE flower, dried above ground parts
BORAGE flower, dried above ground parts
.... see BORAGE flower, dried above ground parts
Borage Oil .... see BORAGE SEED OIL
BORAGE SEED OIL .... see BORAGE SEED OIL
Borago .... see BORAGE flower, dried above ground parts
Borago officinalis
.... see BORAGE flower, dried above ground parts
Borago officinalis .... see BORAGE SEED OIL
Borate .... see BORON
Borates .... see BORON
Borbonia pinfolia .... see RED BUSH TEA
Borforsin .... see FORSKOLIN
Boric Acid .... see BORON
Boric Anhydride .... see BORON
Boric Tartate .... see BORON
Borneo-mahogany .... see LAURELWOOD
BORON .... see BORON
Boswellia .... see INDIAN FRANKINCENSE
Boswellia carteri .... see FRANKINCENSE
Boswellia Serrata .... see INDIAN FRANKINCENSE
Boswellin .... see INDIAN FRANKINCENSE
Boswellin Serrata Resin .... see INDIAN FRANKINCENSE
Botfly Maggot .... see MAGGOTS
Bottle Brush .... see HORSETAIL
Bouncing Bess .... see RED-SPUR VALERIAN
Bouncing-Bet .... see RED SOAPWORT
Bountry .... see ELDERBERRY,
                                                ELDERFLOWER
Bourbon Geranium Oil .... see ROSE GERANIUM
Bourbon Vanilla .... see VANILLA

Bouillon Blanc .... see MULLEIN
BOVINE CARTILAGE .... see BOVINE CARTILAGE
BOVINE COLOSTRUM .... see BOVINE COLOSTRUM
Bovine Cortex Phosphatidylserine
.... see PHOSPHATIDYLSERINE
Bovine Dialyzable Leukocyte Extract
.... see TRANSFER FACTOR
Bovine Dialyzable Transfer Factor
.... see TRANSFER FACTOR
Bovine Immunoglobulin .... see BOVINE COLOSTRUM
Bovine lactoferrin .... see LACTOFERRIN
Bovine Orchic Extract .... see ORCHIC EXTRACT
Bovine Phosphatidylserine
.... see PHOSPHATIDYLSERINE
Bovine Spleen .... see SPLEEN EXTRACT
Bovine Testicle Extract .... see ORCHIC EXTRACT
Bovine Tracheal Cartilage (BTC)
.... see BOVINE CARTILAGE
Bovine Transfer Factor .... see TRANSFER FACTOR
Bovine Whey Protein Concentrate .... see WHEY PROTEIN
Bovis and Soldier .... see RED-SPUR VALERIAN
Bovista .... see PUFF BALL
Bowman's Root .... see BLACK ROOT, INDIAN PHYSIC
Box Holly .... see BUTCHER'S BROOM
Box Tree .... see AMERICAN DOGWOOD
Boxberry .... see WINTERGREEN leaf,
                                                WINTERGREEN oil
Boxwood .... see AMERICAN DOGWOOD
BOXWOOD .... see BOXWOOD
Boxwood Extract .... see BOXWOOD
Brahma-Buti .... see GOTU KOLA
Brahma-Manduki .... see GOTU KOLA
BRAHMI .... see BRAHMI
Brake Root .... see LADY FERN
Bramble .... see BLACKBERRY leaf,
                                                BLACKBERRY root
Bran .... see WHEAT BRAN
BRANCHED-CHAIN AMINO ACIDS
.... see BRANCHED-CHAIN AMINO ACIDS
Branching Phytolacca .... see POKEWEED berry
                                                POKEWEED root
Brandlattich .... see COLTSFOOT
Brandy Mint .... see PEPPERMINT leaf
Brassica alba .... see WHITE MUSTARD
Brassica nigra .... see BLACK MUSTARD oil,
                                                BLACK MUSTARD seed
Brassica oleracea .... see CABBAGE
Brauneria Angustifolia .... see ECHINACEA
Brauneria Pallida .... see ECHINACEA
Brayera anthelmintica .... see KOUSSO
Brazil Powder .... see GOA POWDER
Brazil Root .... see IPECAC
Brazilian Cocoa .... see GUARANA
Brazilian Ginseng .... see SUMA
Brazilian Ipecac .... see IPECAC
Brazilian Mahogany .... see ANDIROBA
Brazilian Rhatany .... see RHATANY
Brechnusssamen .... see NUX VOMICA
Breeam .... see SCOTCH BROOM herb
Breiapfelbaum .... see CHICLE
Brewers Yeast .... see BREWER'S YEAST
BREWER'S YEAST .... see BREWER'S YEAST
BREWER'S YEAST (HANSEN CBS 5926)
.... see BREWER'S YEAST (HANSEN CBS 5926)

Brideweed .... see YELLOW TOADFLAX
Bridewort .... see MEADOWSWEET
Brigham Tea .... see MORMON TEA
Brindal Berry .... see GARCINIA
Brindall Berry .... see GARCINIA
Brindle Berry .... see GARCINIA
British Indian Lemongrass .... see LEMONGRASS
British Myrrh .... see SWEET CICELY
British Tobacco .... see COLTSFOOT
Brittle Willow .... see WILLOW BARK
Broad-Leafed Laurel .... see MOUNTAIN LAUREL
Broad-Leaved Dock .... see YELLOW DOCK
Broad-leaved Garlic .... see BEAR'S GARLIC
BROMELAIN .... see BROMELAIN
Bromelains .... see BROMELAIN
Bromelainum .... see BROMELAIN
Bromelin .... see BROMELAIN
Bromus hordeaceus .... see HAY FLOWER
Brook mint .... see JAPANESE MINT
BROOKLIME .... see BROOKLIME
Brook-Tongue .... see WATER HEMLOCK
Broom .... see SCOTCH BROOM herb
BROOM CORN .... see BROOM CORN
Broom Flower .... see DYER'S BROOM
Broom Tops .... see SCOTCH BROOM flower
Browme .... see SCOTCH BROOM herb
Brown Algae .... see LAMINARIA
Brown Psyllium .... see BLACK PSYLLIUM
Brownwort .... see SELF-HEAL
Bruchkraut .... see RUPTUREWORT
Bruisewort .... see COMFREY, WILD DAISY
Brum .... see SCOTCH BROOM herb
Brunfelsia hopeana .... see MANACA
Brunnenkresse .... see WATERCRESS
Brushes and Combs .... see TEAZLE
BRYONIA .... see BRYONIA
Bryonia Alba .... see BRYONIA
Bryonia cretica .... see BRYONIA
Bryoniae Radix .... see BRYONIA
B-sitosterol 3-B-D-glucoside .... see BETA-SITOSTEROL
B-sitosterolin .... see BETA-SITOSTEROL
Bucco .... see BUCHU
BUCHU .... see BUCHU
Buck Qi .... see ASTRAGALUS
Buckbean .... see BOGBEAN
Buckels .... see COWSLIP
Buckeye .... see HORSE CHESTNUT branch bark,
                                HORSE CHESTNUT flower,
                                HORSE CHESTNUT leaf
Buckhorn .... see BUCKHORN PLANTAIN
BUCKHORN PLANTAIN ... see BUCKHORN PLANTAIN
Buckthorn .... see ALDER BUCKTHORN,
                        CASCARA, EUROPEAN BUCKTHORN,
                                        SEA BUCKTHORN
Buckthorn Bark .... see ALDER BUCKTHORN
Buckthorn Berry .... see EUROPEAN BUCKTHORN
Bucku .... see BUCHU
BUCKWHEAT .... see BUCKWHEAT
Buckwheat Pollen .... see BEE POLLEN
Buddhist Rosary Bead .... see PRECATORY BEAN
Budwood .... see AMERICAN DOGWOOD
Bugbane .... see AMERICAN HELLEBORE,
                                        BLACK COHOSH
BUGLE .... see BUGLE

Bugle .... see GROUND PINE
Bugle Weed .... see BUGLEWEED
BUGLEWEED .... see BUGLEWEED
Bugloss .... see BORAGE SEED OIL
Bugula .... see BUGLE
Bugwort .... see BLACK COHOSH
BULBOUS BUTTERCUP ... see BULBOUS BUTTERCUP
Bulgarian Yogurt .... see YOGURT
Bull Balls Extract .... see ORCHIC EXTRACT
Bullock's Eye .... see HOUSELEEK
Bull's Eyes .... see MARSH MARIGOLD
Bullsfoot .... see COLTSFOOT
Bullwort .... see BISHOP'S WEED
Bulnesia sarmienti .... see GUAIAC WOOD OIL
Bumblebee Venom .... see BEE VENOM
BUPLEURUM .... see BUPLEURUM
Bupleurum chinense .... see BUPLEURUM
Bupleurum exaltatum .... see BUPLEURUM
Bupleurum falcatum .... see BUPLEURUM
Bupleurum fruticosum .... see BUPLEURUM
Bupleurum longifolium .... see BUPLEURUM
Bupleurum multinerve .... see BUPLEURUM
Bupleurum octoradiatum .... see BUPLEURUM
Bupleurum rotundifolium .... see BUPLEURUM
Bupleurum scorzonerifolium .... see BUPLEURUM
Burage .... see BORAGE SEED OIL
BURDOCK .... see BURDOCK
Burn Plant .... see ALOE dried juice from leaf, latex
Burnet Saxifrage ...... see PIMPINELLA above ground parts,
                                        PIMPINELLA root
Burning Bush .... see BURNING BUSH leaf,
                                BURNING BUSH root, WAHOO
BURNING BUSH leaf .... see BURNING BUSH leaf
BURNING BUSH root .... see BURNING BUSH root
BURR MARIGOLD .... see BURR MARIGOLD
Burr Seed .... see BURDOCK
Burrage ..... see BORAGE flower, dried above ground parts,
                                        BORAGE SEED OIL
Burren Myrtle .... see BILBERRY dried ripe fruit,
                                        BILBERRY leaf
Burrwort .... see BUTTERCUP
Bursae Pastoris Herba .... see SHEPHERD'S PURSE
Bursting Heart .... see WAHOO
Bush Tree .... see BOXWOOD
Butane-1,4-diol .... see BUTANEDIOL (BD)
BUTANEDIOL (BD) .... see BUTANEDIOL (BD)
Butcherbroom .... see BUTCHER'S BROOM
BUTCHER'S BROOM .... see BUTCHER'S BROOM
Butcher's-Broom .... see SCOTCH BROOM flower
Butter and Eggs .... see YELLOW TOADFLAX
Butter Bur .... see BUTTERBUR
Butter Daisy .... see OX-EYE DAISY
Butter-Dock .... see BUTTERBUR
Butter Rose .... see COWSLIP
BUTTERBUR .... see BUTTERBUR
Butterburr .... see BUTTERBUR
BUTTERCUP .... see BUTTERCUP
Buttered Hayhocks .... see YELLOW TOADFLAX
Butterfly Dock .... see BUTTERBUR
Butterfly Weed .... see PLEURISY ROOT
Butternussbaum .... see BUTTERNUT
BUTTERNUT .... see BUTTERNUT
Button Snakeroot .... see MARSH BLAZING STAR
Buttonhole .... see HARTSTONGUE

INDEX

Buttons .... see TANSY
Butua .... see ABUTA
Butylene Glycol .... see BUTANEDIOL (BD)
Butyrolactone
.... see GAMMA BUTYROLACTONE (GBL)
Butyrolactone Gamma
.... see GAMMA BUTYROLACTONE (GBL)
Buxus .... see BOXWOOD
Buxus chinensis .... see JOJOBA
Buxus sempervirens .... see BOXWOOD
Ca .... see CALCIUM
Caa-He-É .... see STEVIA
Ca-A-Jhei .... see STEVIA
Ca-A-Yupi .... see STEVIA
CABBAGE .... see CABBAGE
Cabbage Palm .... see SAW PALMETTO
Cabernet Franc .... see GRAPE fruit, skin
Cabernet Sauvignon .... see GRAPE fruit, skin
Cacao .... see COCOA
Cachou .... see CATECHU
Cactus Flowers .... see PRICKLY PEAR CACTUS
Cactus Grandiflorus .... see CEREUS
CADE OIL .... see CADE OIL
Caesalpinia bonducella .... see DIVI-DIVI
Cafe .... see COFFEE
Caffea .... see COFFEE
CAFFEINE .... see CAFFEINE
Caffeine and Sodium Benzoate .... see CAFFEINE
Caffeine Citrate .... see CAFFEINE
Caje Oil .... see NIAULI OIL
CAJEPUT OIL .... see CAJEPUT OIL
Cajeputi Aetheroleum .... see CAJEPUT OIL
Cajuput .... see CAJEPUT OIL
CALABAR BEAN .... see CALABAR BEAN
CALAMINT .... see CALAMINT
Calamintha ascendens .... see CALAMINT
Calamintha hortensis .... see SUMMER SAVORY
Calamintha montana .... see WINTER SAVORY
CALAMUS .... see CALAMUS
Calamus draco .... see DRAGON'S BLOOD
Calanolide .... see LAURELWOOD
Calcifediol .... see VITAMIN D
Calcii Pantothenas
.... see PANTOTHENIC ACID (VITAMIN B5)
Calcipotriene .... see VITAMIN D
Calcitriol .... see VITAMIN D
CALCIUM .... see CALCIUM
Calcium Acetate .... see CALCIUM
Calcium Ascorbate .... see VITAMIN C (ASCORBIC ACID)
Calcium Aspartate .... see CALCIUM
Calcium Carbonate .... see CALCIUM
Calcium Carbonate Matrix .... see CORAL
Calcium Chelate .... see CALCIUM
Calcium Chloride .... see CALCIUM, PANGAMIC ACID
Calcium Citrate .... see CALCIUM
Calcium Citrate Malate .... see CALCIUM
CALCIUM D-GLUCARATE
.... see CALCIUM D-GLUCARATE
Calcium Disodium Edathamil .... see EDTA
Calcium Disodium Edetate .... see EDTA
Calcium Disodium EDTA .... see EDTA
Calcium Disodium Versenate .... see EDTA
Calcium Edetate .... see EDTA
Calcium EDTA .... see EDTA

Calcium Glucarate .... see CALCIUM D-GLUCARATE,
CALCIUM, PANGAMIC ACID
Calcium Lactate .... see CALCIUM
Calcium Lactogluconate .... see CALCIUM
Calcium Orotate .... see CALCIUM
Calcium Pangamate .... see PANGAMIC ACID
Calcium Pantothenate
.... see PANTOTHENIC ACID (VITAMIN B5)
Calcium Phosphate .... see CALCIUM,
PHOSPHATE SALTS
Calcium Pyruvate .... see PYRUVATE
CALENDULA .... see CALENDULA
Calendula officinalis .... see CALENDULA
Caley Pea .... see LATHYRUS
Calico Bush .... see MOUNTAIN LAUREL
California Buckthorn .... see CASCARA
California Fern .... see HEMLOCK
California Poppies .... see CALIFORNIA POPPY
CALIFORNIA POPPY .... see CALIFORNIA POPPY
Calluna vulgaris .... see HEATHER
Calluna vulgaris flos .... see HEATHER
Callunae vulgaris herba .... see HEATHER
Calomba Root .... see COLOMBO
Calophyllum inophyllum .... see LAURELWOOD
CALOTROPIS .... see CALOTROPIS
Calotropis procera .... see CALOTROPIS
Caltha palustris .... see MARSH MARIGOLD
Caltrop .... see PUNCTURE VINE
Calumba .... see COLOMBO
Calumbo Root .... see COLOMBO
Calves' Snout .... see YELLOW TOADFLAX
Calystegia sepium .... see GREATER BINDWEED
Calzin .... see GRAPE fruit, skin
Camboge .... see GAMBOGE
Camellia Sinensis .... see BLACK TEA, GREEN TEA
Camellia thea .... see BLACK TEA, GREEN TEA
Camellia theifera .... see BLACK TEA, GREEN TEA
Cammock .... see SPINY RESTHARROW
Camolea .... see MEZEREON
Camomilla .... see GERMAN CHAMOMILE
Camomille Allemande .... see GERMAN CHAMOMILE
CAMPHOR .... see CAMPHOR
Camphor of the Poor .... see GARLIC
Camphor Tree .... see CAMPHOR
Camphora .... see CAMPHOR
Canada Balsam .... see CANADA BALSAM,
HEMLOCK SPRUCE
Canada Pitch .... see PINUS BARK
Canada Root .... see PLEURISY ROOT
Canada Tea .... see WINTERGREEN leaf,
WINTERGREEN oil
Canada Turpentine .... see CANADA BALSAM
Canadian Balsam .... see CANADA BALSAM
Canadian Beaver .... see CASTOREUM
CANADIAN FLEABANE ... see CANADIAN FLEABANE
Canadian Ginseng .... see GINSENG, AMERICAN
Canadian Hemlock .... see PINUS BARK
CANADIAN HEMP .... see CANADIAN HEMP
Canadian Trailing Arbutus .... see CANADIAN FLEABANE
Canagnium odoratum macrophylla ..... see CANANGA OIL
CANAIGRE .... see CANAIGRE
CANANGA OIL .... see CANANGA OIL
Canangium odoratum genuina .... see YLANG YLANG OIL

INDEX

Canarium commune .... see ELEMI
Canarium luzonicum .... see ELEMI
Cancer Jalap .... see POKEWEED berry,
POKEWEED root
Candleberry .... see BAYBERRY
Candle-berry .... see TUNG SEED
Candleberry Tree .... see TUNG SEED
Candleflower .... see MULLEIN
Candlenut .... see TUNG SEED
Candlewick .... see MULLEIN
Candytuft .... see CLOWN'S MUSTARD PLANT
CANELLA .... see CANELLA
Canella alba .... see CANELLA
Cangana odorata genuina .... see YLANG YLANG OIL
Cangana odorata macrophylla .... see CANANGA OIL
Cankerroot .... see GOLDTHREAD
Cankerwort .... see DANDELION above ground parts,
DANDELION entire plant,
TANSY RAGWORT
Cannabis .... see MARIJUANA
Cannabis sativa .... see MARIJUANA
CANTHAXANTHIN .... see CANTHAXANTHIN
Canthaxanthine .... see CANTHAXANTHIN
Canton Cassia .... see CASSIA
Cao Mahuang .... see EPHEDRA
Capdockin .... see BUTTERBUR
Cape Gooseberry .... see WINTER CHERRY
Cape Periwinkle .... see MADAGASCAR PERIWINKLE
CAPERS .... see CAPERS
Capillary Wormwood .... see YIN CHEN
Capim-Cidrao .... see LEMONGRASS
Capim Doce .... see STEVIA
Capparis spinosa .... see CAPERS
Cappero .... see CAPERS
Capsaicin .... see CAPSICUM
Capsella .... see SHEPHERD'S PURSE
Capsella bursa-pastoris .... see SHEPHERD'S PURSE
CAPSICUM .... see CAPSICUM
Capsicum annuum .... see CAPSICUM
Capsicum baccatum .... see CAPSICUM
Capsicum chinense .... see CAPSICUM
Capsicum Fruit .... see CAPSICUM
Capsicum frutescens .... see CAPSICUM
Capsicum pubescens .... see CAPSICUM
Caramel .... see CARAMEL COLOR
CARAMEL COLOR .... see CARAMEL COLOR
Caramuru .... see CATUABA
Carapa .... see ANDIROBA
Carapa guianensis .... see ANDIROBA
Caraway .... see CARAWAY dried fruit, seed
CARAWAY dried fruit, seed
.... see CARAWAY dried fruit, seed
CARAWAY OIL .... see CARAWAY OIL
Carbenia benedicta .... see BLESSED THISTLE
Carbon .... see ACTIVATED CHARCOAL
Carbonaceous Activated Water .... see WILLARD WATER
Carboxyethylgermanium Sesquioxide .... see GERMANIUM
Card Thistle .... see TEAZLE
CARDAMOM .... see CARDAMOM
Cardamon .... see CARDAMOM
Cardo .... see ARTICHOKE
Cardo de Comer .... see ARTICHOKE
Cardo Santo .... see BLESSED THISTLE
Cardomomi Fructus .... see CARDAMOM

Cardon d'Espagne .... see ARTICHOKE
Cardoon .... see ARTICHOKE
Cardui mariae fructus .... see MILK THISTLE
Cardui mariae herba .... see MILK THISTLE
Carduus .... see BLESSED THISTLE
Carduus benedictus .... see BLESSED THISTLE
Carduus marianum .... see MILK THISTLE
Carduus Marianus .... see MILK THISTLE
Carex arenaria .... see GERMAN SARSAPARILLA
Carica papaya .... see PAPAIN, PAPAYA
Caricae Fructus .... see FIG
Caricae papayae folium .... see PAPAYA
Caricis rhizoma .... see GERMAN SARSAPARILLA
Carilla Gourd .... see BITTER MELON
CARLINA .... see CARLINA
Carlina acaulis .... see CARLINA
Carlinae Radix .... see CARLINA
Carline Thistle .... see MUGWORT
Carmantina .... see ANDROGRAPHIS
Carnitine .... see L-CARNITINE
Carnitine Acetyl Ester .... see ACETYL-L-CARNITINE
Carnitor .... see L-CARNITINE
CARNOSINE .... see CARNOSINE
CAROB .... see CAROB
Carolina Pink .... see PINK ROOT
Carolina Vanilla .... see DEERTONGUE
Caroline Jasmine .... see GELSEMIUM
Carony Bark .... see ANGOSTURA
Carophyll Red .... see CANTHAXANTHIN
Carosella .... see FENNEL fruit, seed
Carotte a Moreau .... see WATER HEMLOCK
Carpenter's Herb .... see BUGLE, SELF-HEAL
Carpenter's Square .... see FIGWORT
Carpenter's Weed .... see SELF-HEAL, YARROW
Carphephorus odoratissimus .... see DEERTONGUE
CARRAGEENAN .... see CARRAGEENAN
Carrageenin .... see CARRAGEENAN
Carragheenan .... see CARRAGEENAN
Carrot Weed .... see HEMLOCK
Cartagena Ipecac .... see IPECAC
Carthamus tinctorius .... see SAFFLOWER
Carum .... see BISHOP'S WEED
Carum carvi .... see CARAWAY dried fruit, seed,
CARAWAY OIL
Carum petroselinum .... see PARSLEY leaf, root,
PARSLEY seed
Carvacrol .... see OREGANO
Carvacrol-rich Origanum species
.... see SPANISH ORIGANUM OIL
Carvi Fructus .... see CARAWAY dried fruit, seed
Caryophylli .... see CLOVE dried flowerbud, leaf, stem
Caryophyllum .... see CLOVE OIL
Caryophyllus .... see CLOVE dried flower bud, leaf, stem,
CLOVE OIL
Caryophyllus aromaticus
.... see CLOVE dried flowerbud, leaf, stem,
CLOVE OIL
CASCARA .... see CASCARA
Cascara Sagrada .... see CASCARA
CASCARILLA .... see CASCARILLA
Caseweed .... see SHEPHERD'S PURSE
CASHEW .... see CASHEW
Cashou .... see CATECHU
Casis .... see BLACK CURRANT SEED OIL

Casse .... see SENNA
CASSIA .... see CASSIA
Cassia acutifolia .... see SENNA
Cassia Angustifolia .... see SENNA
Cassia Aromaticum .... see CASSIA
Cassia Bark .... see CASSIA
Cassia Cinnamon .... see CASSIA
Cassia Lignea .... see CASSIA
Cassia senna .... see SENNA
CASSIE ABSOLUTE .... see CASSIE ABSOLUTE
Cassis .... see BLACK CURRANT berry,
                                       BLACK CURRANT SEED OIL
Castanea americana .... see AMERICAN CHESTNUT
Castanea dentata .... see AMERICAN CHESTNUT
Castanea sativa .... see EUROPEAN CHESTNUT
Castanea vesca .... see EUROPEAN CHESTNUT
Castanea vulgaris .... see EUROPEAN CHESTNUT
Castaneae Folium .... see EUROPEAN CHESTNUT
Castor .... see CASTOR OIL CASTOR seed
Castor Bean .... see CASTOR seed
Castor canadensis .... see CASTOREUM
Castor fiber .... see CASTOREUM
CASTOR OIL .... see CASTOR OIL
Castor Oil Plant .... see CASTOR OIL
CASTOR seed .... see CASTOR seed
CASTOREUM .... see CASTOREUM
Catalonina Jasmine .... see JASMINE
Catalyst Altered Water .... see WILLARD WATER
Catarrh Root .... see ALPINIA
Catchfly .... see CANADIAN HEMP
Catchweed .... see CLIVERS
CATECHU .... see CATECHU
Catechu nigrum .... see CATECHU
Caterpillar Fungus .... see CORDYCEPS
Catha edulis .... see KHAT
Catharanthus .... see MADAGASCAR PERIWINKLE
Catharanthus roseus ... see MADAGASCAR PERIWINKLE
Catmint .... see CATNIP
Catnep .... see CATNIP
CATNIP .... see CATNIP
Catrix .... see BOVINE CARTILAGE
Catrix-S .... see BOVINE CARTILAGE
CAT'S CLAW .... see CAT'S CLAW
Cat's Ear Flower .... see CAT'S FOOT
Cats Foot .... see GROUND IVY
CAT'S FOOT .... see CAT'S FOOT
Cat's-Head .... see PUNCTURE VINE
Cat's-Paw .... see GROUND IVY
Cat's Tails .... see HAY FLOWER
Catswort .... see CATNIP
CATUABA .... see CATUABA
Catuaba Casca .... see CATUABA
Caulophyllum .... see BLUE COHOSH
Caulophyllum thalictroides .... see BLUE COHOSH
Caulophyllum Tree .... see LAURELWOOD
Cavinton .... see VINPOCETINE
Cayenne .... see CAPSICUM
Cayenne Rosewood Oil .... see BOIS DE ROSE OIL
CDS .... see CHONDROITIN SULFATE
Ceanothus americanus .... see NEW JERSEY TEA
Cedar .... see CEDAR leaf,
                           CEDARWOOD bark, berry, leaf, seed, twig
CEDAR leaf .... see CEDAR leaf
CEDAR LEAF OIL .... see CEDAR LEAF OIL

Cedarwood
.... see CEDARWOOD bark, berry, leaf, seed, twig
CEDARWOOD bark, berry, leaf, seed, twig
.... see CEDARWOOD bark, berry, leaf, seed, twig
CEDARWOOD OIL .... see CEDARWOOD OIL
Cedoaria .... see ZEDOARY
Cedro .... see ANDIROBA
Celandine
...... see GREATER CELANDINE dried above ground parts
Celandine Herb
...... see GREATER CELANDINE dried above ground parts
Celandine Root
.... see GREATER CELANDINE rhizome, root
Celastrus scandens .... see AMERICAN BITTERSWEET
CELERY .... see CELERY
Celery Fruit .... see CELERY
Celery-Leafed Crowfoot ... see POISONOUS BUTTERCUP
Celery Seed .... see CELERY
Cemphire .... see CAMPHOR
Centaurea cyanus .... see CORNFLOWER
Centaurium erythraea .... see CENTAURY
Centaurium minus .... see CENTAURY
Centaurium umbellatum .... see CENTAURY
CENTAURY .... see CENTAURY
Centella .... see GOTU KOLA
Centella asiatica .... see GOTU KOLA
Centella coriacea .... see GOTU KOLA
Centellase .... see GOTU KOLA
Centinode .... see KNOTWEED HERB
Centranthus ruber .... see RED-SPUR VALERIAN
Centraria .... see ICELAND MOSS
Centroporus squamosus .... see SHARK LIVER OIL
Cephaelis acuminata .... see IPECAC
Cephaelis ipecacuanha .... see IPECAC
Cephalin .... see PHOSPHATIDYLSERINE
Cerasomal-cis-9-cetylmyristoleate
.... see CETYL MYRISTOLEATE
Cerasus vulgaris .... see SOUR CHERRY
Ceratonia siliqua .... see CAROB
CEREUS .... see CEREUS
Cereus grandiflorus .... see CEREUS
Cerezo Acido .... see SOUR CHERRY
Cerisier Acide .... see SOUR CHERRY
Cervus elaphus .... see DEER VELVET
Cervus nippon .... see DEER VELVET
Cetoal .... see ZEDOARY
Cetorhinus maximus .... see SHARK LIVER OIL
Cetraria Islandica .... see ICELAND MOSS
CETYL MYRISTOLEATE
.... see CETYL MYRISTOLEATE
Cetylmyristoleate .... see CETYL MYRISTOLEATE
Cevitamic Acid .... see VITAMIN C (ASCORBIC ACID)
Ceylon Cinnamon .... see CINNAMON bark
Ceylon Citronella Grass .... see LEMONGRASS
Ch'ih Shen .... see DANSHEN
Chaat .... see KHAT
Chamaelirium carolianum .... see FALSE UNICORN
Chamaelirium luteum .... see FALSE UNICORN
Chamaemelum nobile .... see ROMAN CHAMOMILE
Chamomile .... see GERMAN CHAMOMILE,
                                          ROMAN CHAMOMILE
Chamomilla .... see GERMAN CHAMOMILE,
                                          ROMAN CHAMOMILE
Chamomilla recutita .... see GERMAN CHAMOMILE

Chamomillae ramane flos .... see ROMAN CHAMOMILE
Champaca Wood Oil .... see GUAIAC WOOD OIL
Champagne Of Life .... see KOMBUCHA TEA
CHANCA PIEDRA .... see CHANCA PIEDRA
Chancapiedra .... see CHANCA PIEDRA
Chanca-Piedra Blanca .... see CHANCA PIEDRA
Chandrika .... see INDIAN SNAKEROOT
Chanvrin .... see HEMP AGRIMONY
CHAPARRAL .... see CHAPARRAL
Charas .... see MARIJUANA
Charcoal .... see ACTIVATED CHARCOAL
Chardonnay .... see GRAPE fruit, skin
Charity .... see JACOB'S LADDER
Charnuska .... see BLACK SEED
Chaste Berry .... see CHASTEBERRY
Chaste Tree .... see CHASTEBERRY
Chaste Tree Berry .... see CHASTEBERRY
CHASTEBERRY .... see CHASTEBERRY
Chastetree .... see CHASTEBERRY
CHAULMOOGRA .... see CHAULMOOGRA
Chaw .... see SMOKELESS TOBACCO
Cheat .... see TAUMELLOOLCH
Chebulic Myrobalan .... see TERMINALIA
Checkerberry .... see SQUAWVINE,
                                            WINTERGREEN leaf,
                                            WINTERGREEN oil
Cheese Rennet .... see LADY'S BEDSTRAW
Cheese Renning .... see LADY'S BEDSTRAW
Cheeseflower .... see MALLOW flower
Cheiranthus cheiri .... see WALLFLOWER
Chekan ....see CHEKEN
CHEKEN ....see CHEKEN
Chelated Boron .... see CHELATED MINERALS
Chelated Calcium .... see CHELATED MINERALS
Chelated Chromium .... see CHELATED MINERALS
Chelated Cobalt .... see CHELATED MINERALS
Chelated Copper .... see CHELATED MINERALS
Chelated Iron .... see CHELATED MINERALS
Chelated Magnesium .... see CHELATED MINERALS
Chelated Magnesium .... see MAGNESIUM
Chelated Manganese .... see CHELATED MINERALS
CHELATED MINERALS ..... see CHELATED MINERALS
Chelated Molybdenum .... see CHELATED MINERALS
Chelated Potassium .... see CHELATED MINERALS
Chelated Selenium .... see CHELATED MINERALS
Chelated Trace Minerals .... see CHELATED MINERALS
Chelated Vanadium .... see CHELATED MINERALS
Chelated Zinc........................ see CHELATED MINERALS
Chelidonii
...... see GREATER CELANDINE dried above ground parts
Chelidonii Herba
...... see GREATER CELANDINE dried above ground parts
Chelidonium Majus
...... see GREATER CELANDINE dried above ground parts
              see GREATER CELANDINE rhizome, root
Chelone ....see TURTLE HEAD
Chelone glabra .... see TURTLE HEAD
Chenopodium ambrosioides .... see CHENOPODIUM OIL
Chenopodium ambrosioides anthelminticum
                .... see CHENOPODIUM OIL
CHENOPODIUM OIL .... see CHENOPODIUM OIL
Chenopodium vulvaria .... see ARRACH
CHEROKEE ROSEHIP .... see CHEROKEE ROSEHIP
CHERRY LAUREL WATER
              .... see CHERRY LAUREL WATER

CHERVIL .... see CHERVIL
Chestnut .... see HORSE CHESTNUT seed
Chew .... see SMOKELESS TOBACCO
Chewing Tobacco .... see SMOKELESS TOBACCO
Chi Hu .... see BUPLEURUM
CHICKEN COLLAGEN .... see CHICKEN COLLAGEN
Chicken Collagen Type II ....see CHICKEN COLLAGEN
Chicken Toe .... see CORAL ROOT
Chicken Type II Collagen .... see CHICKEN COLLAGEN
Chickling Vetch .... see LATHYRUS
Chick-Pea .... see LATHYRUS
CHICKWEED .... see CHICKWEED
CHICLE .... see CHICLE
Chico Sapote .... see CHICLE
CHICORY .... see CHICORY
Chiendent Odorant .... see VETIVER
Child Pick-a-Back .... see CHANCA PIEDRA
Children's Bane .... see WATER HEMLOCK
Chili Pepper .... see CAPSICUM
Chimaphila .... see PIPSISSEWA
Chimaphila corymbosa .... see PIPSISSEWA
Chimaphila umbellata .... see PIPSISSEWA
Chimney-Sweeps .... see BUCKHORN PLANTAIN
Chin Cups .... see CUPMOSS
China Bark .... see QUILLAIA
China Clay ....see KAOLIN
China Gooseberry ....see KIWI
China Root .... see ALPINIA, WILD YAM
Chinarinde .... see CINCHONA
China-Wood Oil .... see TUNG SEED
Chinchilla Enana .... see TAGETES
Chinese Almond .... see APRICOT
Chinese Angelica .... see DONG QUAI
Chinese Anise .... see STAR ANISE
Chinese Arborvitae .... see ORIENTAL ARBORVITAE
Chinese Cinnamon....................................see CASSIA
CHINESE CLUB MOSS .... see CHINESE CLUB MOSS
Chinese Cornbind .... see FO-TI
Chinese Cucumber ....see CHINESE CUCUMBER fruit,
                        CHINESE CUCUMBER root,
                        CHINESE CUCUMBER seed
CHINESE CUCUMBER fruit
              ....see CHINESE CUCUMBER fruit
CHINESE CUCUMBER root
              ....see CHINESE CUCUMBER root
CHINESE CUCUMBER seed
              .... see CHINESE CUCUMBER seed
Chinese Gelatin .... see AGAR
Chinese Ginger .... see ALPINIA
Chinese Ginseng .... see GINSENG, PANAX
Chinese Goldthread .... see GOLDTHREAD
Chinese Gooseberry ....see KIWI
Chinese Jujube .... see JUJUBE
Chinese Knotweed .... see FO-TI
Chinese Licorice .... see LICORICE
Chinese Mint Oil .... see JAPANESE MINT
Chinese Parsley ....see CORIANDER
Chinese Privet .... see GLOSSY PRIVET
Chinese Rhubarb ....see RHUBARB
Chinese Rosehip .... see CHEROKEE ROSEHIP
Chinese Senega .... see SENEGA
Chinese Snake Gourd ..... see CHINESE CUCUMBER fruit,
                        CHINESE CUCUMBER root,
                        CHINESE CUCUMBER seed

INDEX

Chinese Star Anise .... see STAR ANISE
Chinese Sumach .... see TREE OF HEAVEN
Chinese Tea .... see BLACK TEA, GREEN TEA
Chinese Thoroughwax .... see BUPLEURUM
Chinese Wolfberry .... see LYCIUM
Chinese Wormwood .... see SWEET ANNIE
Chinesischer Limonenbaum .... see SCHISANDRA
Ching-hao .... see SWEET ANNIE
Chinli-Chih .... see BITTER MELON
Chinwood .... see YEW
Chionanthus .... see FRINGETREE
Chionanthus virginicus .... see FRINGETREE
CHIRATA .... see CHIRATA
Chirayta .... see CHIRATA
Chiretta .... see ANDROGRAPHIS, CHIRATA
CHITOSAN .... see CHITOSAN
Chitosan Ascorbate .... see CHITOSAN
Chittem Bark .... see CASCARA
Chiu .... see YIN CHEN
CHIVE .... see CHIVE
Chives .... see CHIVE
CHLORELLA .... see CHLORELLA
Chlorella pyrenoidosa .... see CHLORELLA
Chlorella Vulgaris .... see CHLORELLA
CHLOROPHYLL .... see CHLOROPHYLL
Chlorophyll a .... see CHLOROPHYLL
Chlorophyll b .... see CHLOROPHYLL
Chlorophyll c .... see CHLOROPHYLL
Chlorophyll d .... see CHLOROPHYLL
CHLOROPHYLLIN .... see CHLOROPHYLLIN
Chocola .... see COCOA
Chocolate Root .... see WATER AVENS
Choke Cherry .... see WILD CHERRY
Cholecalciferol .... see VITAMIN D
CHOLINE .... see CHOLINE
Choline Bitartrate .... see CHOLINE
Choline Chloride .... see CHOLINE
Chondrodendron tomentosum .... see PAREIRA
chondroitin 4- and 6-sulfate
.... see CHONDROITIN SULFATE
Chondroitin 4-sulfate .... see CHONDROITIN SULFATE
CHONDROITIN SULFATE
.... see CHONDROITIN SULFATE
Chondroitin Sulfate A .... see CHONDROITIN SULFATE
Chondroitin Sulfate B .... see CHONDROITIN SULFATE
Chondroitin Sulfate C .... see CHONDROITIN SULFATE
Chondroitin Sulfates .... see CHONDROITIN SULFATE
Chondroitin Sulphate A Sodium
.... see CHONDROITIN SULFATE
Chondrus Crispus .... see CARRAGEENAN
Chondrus Extract .... see CARRAGEENAN
Chongras .... see POKEWEED berry,
                                      POKEWEED root
Chop Nut .... see CALABAR BEAN
Chosen-Gomischi .... see SCHISANDRA
Chota-Chand .... see INDIAN SNAKEROOT
Christe Herbe .... see BLACK HELLEBORE
Christmas Flower .... see POINSETTIA
Christmas Rose .... see BLACK HELLEBORE
Christmas Rose Plant .... see BLACK HELLEBORE
Christ's Spear .... see ENGLISH ADDER'S TONGUE
Christ's Thorn .... see HOLLY
Chromic Chloride .... see CHROMIUM
CHROMIUM .... see CHROMIUM

Chromium (III) .... see CHROMIUM
Chromium 3 .... see CHROMIUM
Chromium 3+ .... see CHROMIUM
Chromium Acetate .... see CHROMIUM
Chromium Chloride .... see CHROMIUM
Chromium III .... see CHROMIUM
Chromium III Picolinate .... see CHROMIUM
Chromium Nicotinate .... see CHROMIUM
Chromium Picolinate .... see CHROMIUM
Chromium Polynicotinate .... see CHROMIUM
Chromium Trichloride .... see CHROMIUM
Chromium Tripicolinate .... see CHROMIUM
Chrysanthemi vulgaris flos .... see TANSY
Chrysanthemi vulgaris herba .... see TANSY
CHRYSANTHEMUM .... see CHRYSANTHEMUM
Chrysanthemum cinerariifolium .... see PYRETHRUM
Chrysanthemum leucanthemum .... see OX-EYE DAISY
Chrysanthemum morifolium ...... see CHRYSANTHEMUM
Chrysanthemum parthenium .... see FEVERFEW
Chrysanthemum sinense .... see CHRYSANTHEMUM
Chrysanthemum stipulaceum ..... see CHRYSANTHEMUM
Chrysanthemum vulgare .... see TANSY
Chrysatobine .... see GOA POWDER
Chuan Xin Lian .... see ANDROGRAPHIS
Chuan Xin Lin .... see ANDROGRAPHIS
Chuan-wu .... see ACONITE
Chuchuhuasha .... see CATUABA
Chuchupate .... see OSHA
Church Broom .... see TEAZLE
Church-Flower .... see MADAGASCAR PERIWINKLE
Churnstaff .... see YELLOW TOADFLAX
CHYMOTRYPSIN .... see CHYMOTRYPSIN
Chymotrypsin A .... see CHYMOTRYPSIN
Chymotrypsin B .... see CHYMOTRYPSIN
Chymotrypsinum .... see CHYMOTRYPSIN
CI Food Orange 8 .... see CANTHAXANTHIN
Ci Wu Jia .... see GINSENG, SIBERIAN
Cichorii Herba .... see CHICORY
Cichorii Radix .... see CHICORY
Cichorium intybus .... see CHICORY
Cicuta bulbifera .... see WATER HEMLOCK
Cicuta douglasii .... see WATER HEMLOCK
Cicuta maculata .... see WATER HEMLOCK
Cicuta occidentalis .... see WATER HEMLOCK
Cicuta vagans .... see WATER HEMLOCK
Cicuta Virosa .... see WATER HEMLOCK
Cider Vinegar .... see APPLE CIDER VINEGAR
CIGUATERA .... see CIGUATERA
Ciguatera Poisoning .... see CIGUATERA
Cilantro .... see CORIANDER
Cimicifuga .... see BLACK COHOSH
Cimicifuga Racemosa .... see BLACK COHOSH
Cinchol .... see BETA-SITOSTEROL
CINCHONA .... see CINCHONA
Cinchona calisaya .... see CINCHONA
Cinchona ledgeriana .... see CINCHONA
Cinchona pubescens .... see CINCHONA
Cinchona succirubra .... see CINCHONA
Cineraria maritima .... see DUSTY MILLER
Cinnamomi cassiae cortex .... see CASSIA
Cinnamomum aromaticum .... see CASSIA,
                                      CINNAMON flower
Cinnamomum camphora .... see CAMPHOR
Cinnamomum cassia .... see CASSIA,
                                      CINNAMON flower

INDEX

Cinnamomum verum .... see CINNAMON bark
Cinnamomum zeylanicum .... see CINNAMON bark
Cinnamon .... see CINNAMON bark,
CINNAMON flower
CINNAMON bark .... see CINNAMON bark
Cinnamon Flos .... see CINNAMON flower
CINNAMON flower .... see CINNAMON flower
Cinnamon Sedge .... see CALAMUS
Cinnamon Wood .... see SASSAFRAS
Cinnamonum .... see CINNAMON bark,
CINNAMON flower
Cinquefoil .... see EUROPEAN FIVE-FINGER G RASS,
TORMENTIL
Cique Vireuse .... see WATER HEMLOCK
cis-1,2,3,5-trans-4,6-Cyclohexanehexol .... see INOSITOL
cis-12 conjugated linoleic acid
.... see CONJUGATED LINOLEIC ACID
Cis-9 .... see CONJUGATED LINOLEIC ACID
Cis-9-cetylmyristoleate .... see CETYL MYRISTOLEATE
Cis-9-Octadecenoic acid (oleic acid) .. see LORENZO'S OIL
Cis-hexahydro-2-oxo-1H-thieno[3,4-d]-imidazole-4-valeric
acid .... see BIOTIN
Cis-Resveratrol .... see RESVERATROL
Cissampelos pareira ....see ABUTA
Ciste .... see LABDANUM
Cistus incanus .... see LABDANUM
Cistus ladanifer .... see LABDANUM
Cistus ladaniferus .... see LABDANUM
Cistus polymorphus .... see LABDANUM
Cistus villosus .... see LABDANUM
Citrated Caffeine .... see CAFFEINE
Citri Sinensis .... see SWEET ORANGE
Citric Acid .... see ALPHA HYDROXY ACIDS
Citronella .... see LEMONGRASS, STONE ROOT
CITRONELLA OIL .... see CITRONELLA OIL
Citrullus colocynthis .... see COLOCYNTH
Citrus aurantifolia .... see LIME fruit, peel, LIME oil
Citrus Aurantium .... see BITTER ORANGE
Citrus aurantium amara .... see BITTER ORANGE
Citrus aurantium bergamia .... see BERGAMOT OIL
Citrus aurantium dulcis .... see SWEET ORANGE
Citrus aurantium sinensis .... see SWEET ORANGE
Citrus bergamia .... see BERGAMOT OIL,
BITTER ORANGE
Citrus bigaradia .... see BITTER ORANGE
Citrus Bioflavonoid .... see DIOSMIN,
HESPERIDIN,
QUERCETIN, RUTIN
Citrus Bioflavonoids .... see DIOSMIN,
HESPERIDIN,
QUERCETIN, RUTIN
Citrus decumana .... see GRAPEFRUIT OIL
Citrus Grandis Extract
.... see GRAPEFRUIT SEED EXTRACT
Citrus limon .... see LEMON
Citrus maxima .... see GRAPEFRUIT OIL
Citrus medica var. acida .... see LIME oil
Citrus paradisi .... see GRAPEFRUIT,
GRAPEFRUIT SEED EXTRACT
Citrus racemosa .... see GRAPEFRUIT OIL
Citrus Seed Extract ... see GRAPEFRUIT SEED EXTRACT
Citrus Sinensis .... see SWEET ORANGE
Citrus vulgaris .... see BITTER ORANGE

Citrus X paradisi .... see GRAPEFRUIT OIL
Civan Percemi .... see YARROW
Cives .... see CHIVE
CIVET .... see CIVET
Civettictis civetta .... see CIVET
Ciwujia .... see GINSENG, SIBERIAN
CLA .... see CONJUGATED LINOLEIC ACID
Cladonia pyxidata .... see CUPMOSS
Clarified Honey .... see HONEY
Clary .... see CLARY SAGE
CLARY SAGE .... see CLARY SAGE
Clary Wort .... see CLARY SAGE
Claviceps purpurea ....see ERGOT
Clay Suspension Products ... see COLLOIDAL MINERALS
Clear Eye .... see CLARY SAGE
Cleavers .... see CLIVERS
Cleaverwort .... see CLIVERS
Clematis .... see CLEMATIS, WOODBINE
Clematis recta .... see CLEMATIS
Clematis virginiana .... see WOODBINE
Clematis vitalba .... see TRAVELER'S JOY
Climbing Knotweed ....see FO-TI
CLIVERS .... see CLIVERS
Clot Bur .... see BURDOCK, MULLEIN
Clous de Girolfe ... see CLOVE dried flowerbud, leaf, stem,
CLOVE OIL
Clove .... see CLOVE dried flowerbud, leaf, stem
CLOVE dried flowerbud, leaf, stem
.... see CLOVE dried flowerbud, leaf, stem
Clove Garlic .... see GARLIC
CLOVE OIL .... see CLOVE OIL
Clove Pepper .... see ALLSPICE
Cloves .... see CLOVE dried flowerbud, leaf, stem
Clown's Lungwort .... see MULLEIN
CLOWN'S MUSTARD PLANT
.... see CLOWN'S MUSTARD PLANT
CLUB MOSS .... see CLUB MOSS
Clustered Win7tercherry .... see ASHWAGANDHA
CM .... see CETYL MYRISTOLEATE
CMO .... see CETYL MYRISTOLEATE
Cnici Benedicti Herba .... see BLESSED THISTLE
Cnicus .... see BLESSED THISTLE
Cnicus benedictus .... see BLESSED THISTLE
Co Enzyme Q 10 .... see COENZYME Q-10
CO Q10 .... see COENZYME Q-10
Coachweed .... see CLIVERS
Coakum .... see POKEWEED berry, POKEWEED root
Coakum-Chorngras .... see POKEWEED berry,
POKEWEED root
Coastal Douglas Fir .... see OREGON FIR BALSAM
Cobalamin .... see VITAMIN B12
Cobalamin Enzyme .... see DIBENCOZIDE
Cobalamins .... see VITAMIN B12
Cobamamide .... see DIBENCOZIDE
Cobamin .... see VITAMIN B12
Cobnut ....see HAZELNUT
COCA .... see COCA
Cocaine Plant .... see COCA
Cocash Weed .... see GOLDEN RAGWORT
Cocculus .... see LEVANT BERRY
Cocculus Indicus .... see LEVANT BERRY
Cocculus lacunosus .... see LEVANT BERRY
Cocculus suberosus .... see LEVANT BERRY

I
N
D
E
X

Cochin Ginger .... see GINGER
Cochin Lemongrass .... see LEMONGRASS
Cochlearia armoracia .... see HORSERADISH
Cochlearia officinalis .... see SCURVY GRASS
COCILLANA .... see COCILLANA
Cockle .... see CORN COCKLE
Cockle Buttons .... see BURDOCK
Cocklebur .... see AGRIMONY, BURDOCK
Cockspur Rye .... see ERGOT
Cockup Hat .... see QUEEN'S DELIGHT
Cocky Baby .... see ARUM
COCOA .... see COCOA
Cocoa Bean .... see COCOA
Cocoa Oleum .... see COCOA
Cocoa Seed .... see COCOA
Cocoa Semen .... see COCOA
Cocoa Testae .... see COCOA
Cocowort .... see SHEPHERD'S PURSE
Coculus Fructus .... see LEVANT BERRY
Cod Liver Oil .... see COD LIVER OIL, FISH OILS
Cod Oil .... see COD LIVER OIL
CODONOPSIS .... see CODONOPSIS
Codonopsis pilosula .... see CODONOPSIS
Codonopsis pilosula modesta .... see CODONOPSIS
Codonopsis tangsheng .... see CODONOPSIS
Codonopsis tubulosa .... see CODONOPSIS
Coenzyme 1 .... see NADH
Coenzyme B-12 .... see DIBENCOZIDE
COENZYME Q-10 .... see COENZYME Q-10
Coenzyme R .... see BIOTIN
Coffea arabica .... see COFFEE,
                                        COFFEE CHARCOAL
Coffea canephora .... see COFFEE,
                                        COFFEE CHARCOAL
Coffea liberica .... see COFFEE,
                                        COFFEE CHARCOAL
Coffea robusta .... see COFFEE
COFFEE .... see COFFEE
COFFEE CHARCOAL .... see COFFEE CHARCOAL
Cokan .... see POKEWEED berry,
                                        POKEWEED root
Cola acuminata .... see COLA NUT
Cola nitida .... see COLA NUT
COLA NUT .... see COLA NUT
Cola Seed .... see COLA NUT
Colchicum .... see AUTUMN CROCUS
Colchicum autumnale .... see AUTUMN CROCUS
Colchicum speciosum .... see AUTUMN CROCUS
Colchicum vernum .... see AUTUMN CROCUS
Cold-Pressed Grapefruit Oil .... see GRAPEFRUIT OIL
Colecus forskohlii .... see FORSKOLIN
Coleus Forskohlii .... see FORSKOLIN
Coleus forskolii .... see FORSKOLIN
Colewort .... see AVENS, CABBAGE
Colforsin .... see FORSKOLIN
Colic Root .... see ALETRIS, ALPINIA
                                MARSH BLAZING STAR,
                                        WILD YAM
Colinsonia .... see STONE ROOT
Colius forskolii .... see FORSKOLIN
Colle du Japon .... see AGAR
Collinsonia canadensis .... see STONE ROOT
COLLOIDAL MINERALS
.... see COLLOIDAL MINERALS

COLLOIDAL SILVER .... see COLLOIDAL SILVER
Colloidal Silver Protein .... see COLLOIDAL SILVER
Colloidal Trace Minerals ..... see COLLOIDAL MINERALS
COLOCYNTH .... see COLOCYNTH
Colocynth Pulp .... see COLOCYNTH
Colocynthidis Fructus .... see COLOCYNTH
COLOMBO .... see COLOMBO
Colorado Cough Root .... see OSHA
Colostrum .... see BOVINE COLOSTRUM
Colour Index No. 40850 .... see CANTHAXANTHIN
Colts Foot .... see COLTSFOOT
COLTSFOOT .... see COLTSFOOT
Coltstail .... see CANADIAN FLEABANE
COLUMBINE .... see COLUMBINE
Comb Flower .... see ECHINACEA
Combretum .... see OPIUM ANTIDOTE
Combretum micranthum .... see OPIUM ANTIDOTE
Combucha Tea .... see KOMBUCHA TEA
COMFREY .... see COMFREY
Cominho Negro .... see BLACK SEED
Commiphora .... see MYRRH
Commiphora abyssinica .... see MYRRH
Commiphora erythraea .... see MYRRH
Commiphora madagascariensis .... see MYRRH
Commiphora molmol .... see MYRRH
Commiphora Mukul .... see GUGGUL
Commiphora myrrha .... see MYRRH
Common Alder .... see BLACK ALDER
Common Ash .... see ASH
Common Barberry .... see EUROPEAN BARBERRY
Common Basil .... see BASIL
Common Bean .... see BEAN POD
Common Bearberry .... see UVA URSI
Common Borage
.... see BORAGE flower, dried above ground parts
Common Bugloss
.... see BORAGE flower, dried above ground parts
Common Centaury .... see CENTAURY
Common Cherry Laurel .... see CHERRY LAUREL WATER
Common Chicory Root .... see CHICORY
Common Comfrey .... see COMFREY
Common Couch .... see HAY FLOWER
Common Dandelion
.... see DANDELION above ground parts,
                                DANDELION entire plant
Common Dubbletjie .... see PUNCTURE VINE
Common Elder .... see ELDERFLOWER
Common Elderberry .... see AMERICAN ELDER
Common Fennel .... see FENNEL fruit, seed
Common Figwort .... see FIGWORT
Common Groundsel .... see GROUNDSEL
Common Guelder-Rose .... see CRAMP BARK
Common Hoarhound .... see WHITE HOREHOUND
Common Hops .... see HOPS
Common Jasmine .... see JASMINE
Common Juniper Berry .... see JUNIPER
Common Lavender .... see LAVENDER
Common Melilot .... see SWEET CLOVER
Common Nettle
.... see STINGING NETTLE above ground parts,
                                STINGING NETTLE root
Common Nightshade
.... see BITTERSWEET NIGHTSHADE
Common Oak .... see OAK bark

Common Oleander .... see OLEANDER
Common Parsley .... see PARSLEY leaf, root, PARSLEY seed
Common Periwinkle .... see PERIWINKLE
Common Plantain .... see GREAT PLANTAIN
Common Polypod ....see LADY FERN
Common Ragwort .... see TANSY RAGWORT
Common Rue .... see RUE
Common Sage .... see SAGE
Common Sandspurry .... see ARENARIA RUBRA
Common Sassafras .... see SASSAFRAS
Common Shrubby Everlasting .... see IMMORTELLE, SANDY EVERLASTING
Common Sorrel .... see WOOD SORREL
COMMON STONECROP ... see COMMON STONECROP
Common Thyme .... see THYME flower, leaf, THYME OIL
Common Valerian .... see VALERIAN
Common Vanilla .... see VANILLA
Common Verbena .... see VERBENA
Common Vervain .... see VERBENA
Common Wormwood
.... see WORMWOOD above ground parts
Common Yarrow .... see YARROW
Common Yew .... see YEW
Compass Plant .... see ROSEMARY
Compass Weed................. see ROSINWEED, ROSEMARY
Compound Q .... see CHINESE CUCUMBER fruit, CHINESE CUCUMBER root, CHINESE CUCUMBER seed
Condensed Tannins .... see PYCNOGENOL
Condroitin .... see CHONDROITIN SULFATE
CONDURANGO .... see CONDURANGO
Condurango Cortex .... see CONDURANGO
Coneflower .... see ECHINACEA
Conium .... see HEMLOCK
Conium maculata .... see HEMLOCK
Conium maculatum .... see HEMLOCK
CONJUGATED LINOLEIC ACID
.... see CONJUGATED LINOLEIC ACID
Consolidae Radix ....see COMFREY
Consound ....see COMFREY
Constancy .... see LILY-OF-THE-VALLEY
Consumptive's Weed............................ see YERBA SANTA
Continental Tea .... see LABRADOR TEA
CONTRAYERVA .... see CONTRAYERVA
Convallaria .... see LILY-OF-THE-VALLEY
Convallaria herba.................... see LILY-OF-THE-VALLEY
Convallaria majalis .... see LILY-OF-THE-VALLEY
Convall-Lily .... see LILY-OF-THE-VALLEY
Convolvulus nervosus
.... see HAWAIIAN BABY WOODROSE
Convolvulus purga .... see JALAP
Convolvulus speciosus
.... see HAWAIIAN BABY WOODROSE
Cool Tankard
.... see BORAGE flower, dried above ground parts
COOLWORT .... see COOLWORT
Coon Root... see BLOODROOT
Copaiba .... see COPAIBA BALSAM
COPAIBA BALSAM .... see COPAIBA BALSAM
Copaiba Oleoresin .... see COPAIBA BALSAM
Copaifera langsdorfii .... see COPAIBA BALSAM
Copaifera officinalis .... see COPAIBA BALSAM

Copaifera reticulata .... see COPAIBA BALSAM
Copaiva .... see COPAIBA BALSAM
Copal Tree .... see TREE OF HEAVEN
Copalm .... see STORAX
COPPER .... see COPPER
Copperose .... see CORN POPPY
Coptide .... see GOLDTHREAD
Coptis .... see GOLDTHREAD
Coptis chinensis .... see GOLDTHREAD
Coptis chinesis .... see GOLDTHREAD
Coptis deltoidea .... see GOLDTHREAD
Coptis groenlandica .... see GOLDTHREAD
Coptis teetoides .... see GOLDTHREAD
Coptis trifolia .... see GOLDTHREAD
CoQ .... see COENZYME Q-10
Co-Q10 .... see COENZYME Q-10
Coqueret .... see WINTER CHERRY
CORAL .... see CORAL
CORAL ROOT .... see CORAL ROOT
Coralberry .... see WHITE COHOSH
Corallorhiza odontorihiza .... see CORAL ROOT
CORDYCEPS .... see CORDYCEPS
Cordyceps Sinensis .... see CORDYCEPS
CORIANDER .... see CORIANDER
Coriandri Fructus .... see CORIANDER
Coriandrum sativum .... see CORIANDER
Coridothymus capitatus .... see SPANISH ORIGANUM OIL
Coriolus .... see CORIOLUS MUSHROOM
CORIOLUS MUSHROOM
.... see CORIOLUS MUSHROOM
Coriolus versicolor .... see CORIOLUS MUSHROOM
CORKWOOD TREE .... see CORKWOOD TREE
Corn Campion .... see CORN COCKLE
CORN COCKLE .... see CORN COCKLE
Corn Flower .... see CORNFLOWER
Corn Horsetail .... see HORSETAIL
CORN POPPY .... see CORN POPPY
Corn Rose .... see CORN COCKLE, CORN POPPY
CORN SILK .... see CORN SILK
Corn Sugar Gum .... see XANTHAN GUM
Cornel .... see AMERICAN DOGWOOD
Cornelian tree .... see AMERICAN DOGWOOD
CORNFLOWER .... see CORNFLOWER
Cornmint Oil .... see JAPANESE MINT
CORN SILK .... see CORN SILK
Cornu Cervi Parvum .... see DEER VELVET
Cornus florida .... see AMERICAN DOGWOOD
Corona De Cristo .... see PASSIONFLOWER
Corona Solis .... see SUNFLOWER OIL
Corpus Luteum Hormone .... see PROGESTERONE
Cortex Cinnamomi ....see CASSIA
CORYDALIS .... see CORYDALIS
Corydalis........................... see TURKEY CORN
Corydalis cava .... see CORYDALIS
Corylus avellana .... see HAZELNUT
Corylus heterophylla .... see HAZELNUT
Corynanthe johimbi .... see YOHIMBE
Corynanthe yohimbi .... see YOHIMBE
Cossoo .... see KOUSSO
Costus .... see COSTUS root
COSTUS OIL .... see COSTUS OIL
COSTUS root .... see COSTUS root
COTTON .... see COTTON
Cotton Dawes .... see CUDWEED

INDEX

Cotton Root .... see COTTON
Cotton Weed .... see CUDWEED
Cottonseed Oil .... see GOSSYPOL
COUCH GRASS .... see COUCH GRASS
Couch Grass.. see AGROPYRON, WHEATGRASS
Coudrier .... see HAZELNUT
Coughroot .... see BETH ROOT
Coughweed .... see GOLDEN RAGWORT
Coughwort .... see COLTSFOOT
Couhage .... see COWHAGE
Coumarouna Odorata .... see TONKA BEAN
COUNTRY MALLOW .... see COUNTRY MALLOW
Country Walnut .... see TUNG SEED
Covanamilpori .... see INDIAN SNAKEROOT
Cow Cabbage .... see AMERICAN WHITE POND LILY, MASTERWORT
Cow Clover .... see RED CLOVER
Cow Grass .... see KNOTWEED HERB
Cow Milk Colostrum .... see BOVINE COLOSTRUM
Cow Parsnip .... see MASTERWORT
Cowbane .... see WATER HEMLOCK
Cowberry .... see ALPINE CRANBERRY
COWHAGE .... see COWHAGE
Cowitch .... see COWHAGE
COWSLIP .... see COWSLIP
Cowslip .... see MARSH MARIGOLD
Cr .... see CHROMIUM, CREATINE
Cr III .... see CHROMIUM
Cr-3 .... see CHROMIUM
Cr3+ .... see CHROMIUM
Crab's Eye .... see PRECATORY BEAN
Crabwood .... see ANDIROBA
Crack Willow .... see WILLOW BARK
CRAMP BARK .... see CRAMP BARK
Crampbark .... see CRAMP BARK
Crampweed .... see POTENTILLA
Cranberries .... see CRANBERRY
CRANBERRY .... see CRANBERRY
Crataegi Flos .... see HAWTHORN
Crataegi Folium .... see HAWTHORN
Crataegi Folium Cum Flore .... see HAWTHORN
Crataegi Fructus .... see HAWTHORN
Crataegus Cuneata .... see HAWTHORN
Crataegus laevigata .... see HAWTHORN
Crataegus monogyna .... see HAWTHORN
Crataegus oxyacantha .... see HAWTHORN
Crataegus pinnatifida .... see HAWTHORN
Crawley .... see CORAL ROOT
Crawley Root .... see CORAL ROOT
Crawlgrass .... see KNOTWEED HERB
Creat .... see ANDROGRAPHIS
CREATINE .... see CREATINE
Creatine Monohydrate .... see CREATINE
Creeper .... see AMERICAN IVY
Creeping Barberry .... see OREGON GRAPE
Creeping Charlie .... see GROUND IVY
Creeping Jenny .... see MONEYWORT
Creeping Joan .... see MONEYWORT
Creeping Tom .... see COMMON STONECROP
Creosote Bush .... see CHAPARRAL
Crescione Di Fonte .... see WATERCRESS
Cresson au Poulet .... see WATERCRESS
Cresson De Fontaine .... see WATERCRESS

Cresson D'eau .... see WATERCRESS
Crest Marine .... see SAMPHIRE
Crewel .... see COWSLIP
Crithum maritimum .... see SAMPHIRE
Croci stigma .... see SAFFRON
Crocus .... see AUTUMN CROCUS
Crocus sativus .... see SAFFRON
Crosswort .... see BONESET
Croton .... see CROTON SEEDS
Croton eleuteria .... see CASCARILLA
Croton lechleri .... see SANGRE DE GRADO
CROTON SEEDS .... see CROTON SEEDS
Croton tiglium .... see CROTON SEEDS
Crow Corn .... see ALETRIS
Crowberry .... see POKEWEED berry, POKEWEED root
Crowfoot .... see BULBOUS BUTTERCUP, WOOD ANEMONE
Crown-of-the-Field .... see CORN COCKLE
Crude Chrysarobin .... see GOA POWDER
Crystalline DMSO
.... see MSM (METHYLSULFONYLMETHANE)
Cs-4 .... see CORDYCEPS
CSA .... see CHONDROITIN SULFATE
CSC .... see CHONDROITIN SULFATE
CSE .... see GRAPEFRUIT SEED EXTRACT
Cu .... see COPPER
Cubeb .... see CUBEBS
Cubeb Berries .... see CUBEBS
Cubeba .... see CUBEBS
Cubeba officinaliz .... see CUBEBS
CUBEBS .... see CUBEBS
Cuckoo Bread .... see WOOD SORREL
Cuckoo Buds .... see BULBOUS BUTTERCUP
Cuckoo Flower .... see SALEP
Cuckoo Pint .... see ARUM
Cuckowes Meat .... see WOOD SORREL
Cucurbita Pepo .... see PUMPKIN
Cucurbitea peponis semen .... see PUMPKIN
Cuddy's Lungs .... see MULLEIN
Cudweed .... see CAT'S FOOT
CUDWEED .... see CUDWEED
Cuivre .... see COPPER
Cukilanarpak .... see DEVIL'S CLUB
Culveris Root .... see BLACK ROOT
Culvers .... see BLACK ROOT
Culver's Physic .... see BLACK ROOT
Culver's Root .... see BLACK ROOT
Culverwort .... see COLUMBINE
Cumaru .... see TONKA BEAN
CUMIN .... see CUMIN
Cumin des Pres .... see CARAWAY dried fruit, seed
Cuminum cyminum .... see CUMIN
Cuminum odorum .... see CUMIN
Cummin .... see CUMIN
Cundeamor .... see BITTER MELON
CUP PLANT .... see CUP PLANT
Cup-Puppy .... see CORN POPPY
CUPMOSS .... see CUPMOSS
Cupreol .... see BETA-SITOSTEROL
Cupressus sempervirens .... see CYPRESS
Curcuma .... see JAVANESE TURMERIC, TURMERIC
Curcuma aromatica .... see TURMERIC

INDEX

Curcuma domestica .... see TURMERIC
Curcuma Longa .... see TURMERIC
Curcuma xanthorrhiza .... see JAVANESE TURMERIC
Curcuma zedoaria .... see ZEDOARY
Curcumae longae rhizoma .... see TURMERIC
Curcumae xanthorrhizae rhizoma
.... see JAVANESE TURMERIC
Curcumin .... see TURMERIC
Curdwort .... see LADY'S BEDSTRAW
Cure All .... see WATER AVENS, LEMON BALM
Curled Dock .... see YELLOW DOCK
Curled Mint .... see SPEARMINT
Curly Dock .... see YELLOW DOCK
Cursed Crowfoot .... see POISONOUS BUTTERCUP
Cuscus .... see VETIVER
Cuscus Grass .... see VETIVER
Cuscuta chinensis .... see DODDER
Cuscuta epithymum .... see DODDER
Cuscutae .... see DODDER
Cusparia .... see ANGOSTURA
Cusparia Bark .... see ANGOSTURA
Custard Apple .... see AMERICAN PAWPAW
Cutch .... see AGROPYRON, CATECHU,
                                                            COUCH GRASS
Cutweed .... see BLADDERWRACK
Cyamopsis psoralioides .... see GUAR GUM
Cyamopsis tetragonolobus .... see GUAR GUM
Cyani Blossoms .... see CORNFLOWER
Cyani Flos .... see CORNFLOWER
Cyani Flower .... see CORNFLOWER
Cyani Petals .... see CORNFLOWER
Cyanobacteria .... see BLUE-GREEN ALGAE
Cyancobalamin .... see VITAMIN B12
Cyanocobalaminum .... see VITAMIN B12
CYCLAMEN .... see CYCLAMEN
Cyclamen Europaeum .... see CYCLAMEN
Cyclohexitol .... see INOSITOL
Cycobemin .... see VITAMIN B12
Cydonia oblongata .... see QUINCE
Cymbopogon citratus .... see LEMONGRASS
Cymbopogon flexuosus .... see LEMONGRASS
Cymbopogon nardis .... see LEMONGRASS
Cymbopogon nardus .... see CITRONELLA OIL
Cymbopogon winterianus .... see CITRONELLA OIL
Cynanchum vincetoxicum .... see GERMAN IPECAC
Cynara cardunculus .... see ARTICHOKE
Cynara scolymus .... see ARTICHOKE
Cynoglossi herba .... see HOUND'S TONGUE
Cynoglossi radix .... see HOUND'S TONGUE
Cynoglossum officinale .... see HOUND'S TONGUE
Cynosbatos .... see ROSE HIP
Cyperus articulatus .... see ADRUE
CYPRESS .... see CYPRESS
Cypress Powder .... see ARUM
CYPRESS SPURGE .... see CYPRESS SPURGE
Cypripedium .... see NERVE ROOT
Cypripedium calceolus .... see NERVE ROOT
Cypripedium pubescens .... see NERVE ROOT
Cystadane .... see BETAINE ANHYDROUS
Cyste .... see LABDANUM
Cystisi scoparii flos .... see SCOTCH BROOM flower
Cytisi scoparii herba .... see SCOTCH BROOM herb
Cytisus laburnum .... see LABURNUM
Cytisus scoparius .... see SCOTCH BROOM flower,
                                                         SCOTCH BROOM herb

Da Huang .... see RHUBARB
DA QING YE .... see DA QING YE
Da Zao .... see JUJUBE
Dactylis species .... see HAY FLOWER
Daemonorops draco .... see DRAGON'S BLOOD
DAFFODIL .... see DAFFODIL
Dage of Jerusalem .... see LUNGWORT
Dagger Plant .... see YUCCA
Daggers .... see ORRIS
Daidzein .... see KUDZU, RED CLOVER, SOY
Daisy .... see TANSY
Dalmatian Sage .... see SAGE
Dalmation Insect Flowers .... see PYRETHRUM
Dalmation Pellitory .... see PYRETHRUM
D-Alpha-Tocopherol .... see VITAMIN E
d-Alpha-Tocopheryl .... see VITAMIN E
d-Alpha-Tocopheryl Acetate .... see VITAMIN E
d-Alpha-Tocopheryl Succinate .... see VITAMIN E
Dambrose .... see INOSITOL
DAMIANA ....see DAMIANA
Damiana aphrodisiaca ....see DAMIANA
Damiana Herb ....see DAMIANA
Damiana Leaf ....see DAMIANA
Dan Shen .... see DANSHEN
Dancing Mushroom .... see MAITAKE MUSHROOM
Dandelion .... see DANDELION above ground parts,
                                             DANDELION entire plant
DANDELION above ground parts
.... see DANDELION above ground parts
DANDELION entire plant ... see DANDELION entire plant
Dandelion Herb .... see DANDELION above ground parts
Danewort .... see DWARF ELDER
Dang Gui .... see DONG QUAI
Danggui .... see DONG QUAI
Dangshen ....see CODONOPSIS
DANSHEN .... see DANSHEN
Daphne .... see MEZEREON, SWEET BAY
Daphne mezereum .... see MEZEREON
Daphne Willow .... see WILLOW BARK
Dark Catechu .... see CATECHU
Darnel .... see TAUMELLOOLCH
Darri .... see BROOM CORN
DATE PALM .... see DATE PALM
Datura .... see JIMSON WEED
Datura sauveolens .... see ANGEL'S TRUMPET
Datura stramonium .... see JIMSON WEED
Daucus .... see WILD CARROT
Daucus carota L. subspecies carota ..... see WILD CARROT
Daucus visagna .... see KHELLA
d-Beta-Tocopherol .... see VITAMIN E
D-Biotin .... see BIOTIN
D-Calcium Pantothenate
.... see PANTOTHENIC ACID (VITAMIN B5)
D-Carnitine .... see L-CARNITINE
D-chiro-inositol .... see INOSITOL
D-chiro-inositol, synonym (+)-chiroinositol
.... see INOSITOL
d-Delta-Tocopherol .... see VITAMIN E
Dead Man's Bells .... see DIGITALIS
Dead Tongue .... see HEMLOCK WATER DROPWORT
Deadly Nightshade ....see BELLADONNA,
                                             BITTERSWEET NIGHTSHADE
Deaf Nettle .... see WHITE DEAD NETTLE FLOWER

INDEX

DEANOL .... see DEANOL
Deanol aceglumate .... see DEANOL
Deanol acetamidobenzoate .... see DEANOL
Deanol benzilate .... see DEANOL
Deanol bisorcate .... see DEANOL
Deanol cyclohexylpropionate .... see DEANOL
Deanol hemisuccinate .... see DEANOL
Deanol pidolate .... see DEANOL
Deanol tartrate .... see DEANOL
Death-of-Man .... see WATER HEMLOCK
Deep Sea Shark Liver Oil .... see SHARK LIVER OIL
Deer Antler Velvet .... see DEER VELVET
Deer Balls .... see PUFF BALL
Deer Musk .... see MUSK
DEER VELVET .... see DEER VELVET
Deerberry .... see SQUAWVINE,
 WINTERGREEN leaf, WINTERGREEN oil
Deernut .... see JOJOBA
Deer's Tongue .... see DEERTONGUE
DEERTONGUE .... see DEERTONGUE
Dehydroepiandrosterone .... see DHEA
Dehydroretinol .... see VITAMIN A
Delicate Bess .... see RED-SPUR VALERIAN
Delphinii Flos .... see DELPHINIUM
DELPHINIUM .... see DELPHINIUM
Delphinium consolida .... see DELPHINIUM,
 LARKSPUR
Delphinium staphisagria .... see STAVESACRE
delta 5-pregnen-3 beta-ol-20-one .... see PREGNENOLONE
delta tocotrienol .... see VITAMIN E
delta-tocopherol .... see VITAMIN E
Demon Chaser .... see ST. JOHN'S WORT
Dendranthema morifolium .... see CHRYSANTHEMUM
Deoxynucleic Acid .... see RNA AND DNA
Deoxyribonucleic Acid .... see RNA AND DNA
Derriere Dos .... see CHANCA PIEDRA
Des Dos .... see CHANCA PIEDRA
Desert Herb .... see EPHEDRA
Desert Tea .... see MORMON TEA
Devil Tree .... see FEVER BARK
Devil's Apple .... see JIMSON WEED,
 PODOPHYLLUM
Devil's Bit .... see ALETRIS, FEVER BARK,
 PREMORSE
Devil's Bite .... see AMERICAN HELLEBORE
Devil's Bite Prairie-Pine ...... see MARSH BLAZING STAR
Devil's Bones .... see WILD YAM
Devil's Bush .... see GINSENG, SIBERIAN
Devil's Cherries .... see BELLADONNA
DEVIL'S CLAW .... see DEVIL'S CLAW
Devil's Claw Root .... see DEVIL'S CLAW
DEVIL'S CLUB .... see DEVIL'S CLUB
Devil's Darning-Needle .... see WOODBINE
Devil's Dung .... see ASAFOETIDA
Devil's Eye .... see HENBANE
Devil's Fuge .... see EUROPEAN MISTLETOE
Devil's Guts .... see DODDER
Devil's Head .... see YELLOW TOADFLAX
Devil's Herb .... see BELLADONNA
Devil's Nettle .... see YARROW
Devil's Plaything .... see YARROW
Devil's Ribbon .... see YELLOW TOADFLAX
Devil's Root .... see PEYOTE

Devil's Shrub .... see GINSENG, SIBERIAN
Devil's Thorn .... see PUNCTURE VINE
Devil's Trumpet .... see ANGEL'S TRUMPET,
 JIMSON WEED
Devil's Turnip .... see BRYONIA
Devil's Vine .... see GREATER BINDWEED
Devil's Weed .... see PUNCTURE VINE
Dew Plant .... see SUNDEW
Dewberry .... see BLACKBERRY leaf,
 BLACKBERRY root
Dexpanthenol
 see PANTOTHENIC ACID (VITAMIN B5)
Dexpanthenolum
 see PANTOTHENIC ACID (VITAMIN B5)
d-Gamma-Tocopherol .... see VITAMIN E
D-Glucarate (GA) .... see CALCIUM D-GLUCARATE
D-glucaro-1,4-lactone (1,4 GL)
 see CALCIUM D-GLUCARATE
D-Glucosamine .... see GLUCOSAMINE SULFATE
DHA .... see DHA (DOCOSAHEXAENOIC ACID)
DHA (DOCOSAHEXAENOIC ACID)
 see DHA (DOCOSAHEXAENOIC ACID)
Dhanburua .... see INDIAN SNAKEROOT
Dhar-Bu .... see SEA BUCKTHORN
DHEA .... see DHEA
Di Gu Pi .... see LYCIUM
Dialyzable Leukocyte Extract .... see TRANSFER FACTOR
Dialyzable Transfer Factor .... see TRANSFER FACTOR
DIBENCOZIDE .... see DIBENCOZIDE
Dicalcium Phosphate
 see CALCIUM, PANGAMIC ACID
Dicentra cucullaria .... see TURKEY CORN
Dictamnus albus
 see BURNING BUSH leaf, BURNING BUSH root
Didin .... see MYRRH
Didthin .... see MYRRH
Dietary Fiber .... see BARLEY, BLACK PSYLLIUM
 BLOND PSYLLIUM, GUAR GUM,
 LARCH ARABINOGALACTAN
 OAT BRAN, OATS, RICE BRAN,
 WHEAT BRAN
DIGITALIS .... see DIGITALIS
Digitalis lanata .... see DIGITALIS
Digitalis Purpurea .... see DIGITALIS
Digupi .... see LYCIUM
Dihe .... see BLUE-GREEN ALGAE
Dihydro-2(3H)-Furanone
 see GAMMA BUTYROLACTONE (GBL)
Dihydro-beta-sitosterol .... see SITOSTANOL
dihydrotachysterol .... see VITAMIN D
Dihydroxysuccinic Acid ... see ALPHA HYDROXY ACIDS
Dihydroxysuccinic acid (Tartaric acid)
 see ALPHA HYDROXY ACIDS
Di-isopropylamine Dichloroacetate
 see PANGAMIC ACID
Dill .... see DILL seed,
 DILL above ground parts
DILL above ground parts .... see DILL above ground parts
DILL seed .... see DILL seed
Dill Herb .... see DILL above ground parts
Dill Weed .... see DILL above ground parts
Dillweed .... see DILL above ground parts
Dilly .... see DILL seed, DILL above ground parts

INDEX

Dimethyl Glycine
.... see DIMETHYLGLYCINE, PANGAMIC ACID
Dimethyl Sulfone
.... see MSM (METHYLSULFONYLMETHANE)
Dimethyl Sulfoxide
................see DMSO (DIMETHYLSULFOXIDE)
Dimethyl Sulphoxide
................see DMSO (DIMETHYLSULFOXIDE)
Dimethylaminoethanol .... see DEANOL
Dimethylethanolamine .... see DEANOL
DIMETHYLGLYCINE .... see DIMETHYLGLYCINE
Dimethylglycine .... see PANGAMIC ACID
Dimethylis sulfoxidum
............................see DMSO (DIMETHYLSULFOXIDE)
Dimethylsulfone
.... see MSM (METHYLSULFONYLMETHANE)
Dimethylsulfoxide
............................see DMSO (DIMETHYLSULFOXIDE)
Dioscorea .... see WILD YAM
Dioscorea macrostachya .... see WILD YAM
Dioscoreae .... see WILD YAM
Diosma .... see BUCHU
Diosmetin .... see DIOSMIN
DIOSMIN .... see DIOSMIN
Dip ....see SMOKELESS TOBACCO
Dipsacus silvestris .... see TEAZLE
Dipteryx odorata .... see TONKA BEAN
Discorea composita .... see WILD YAM
Discorea floribunda .... see WILD YAM
Discorea mexicana.................................. see WILD YAM
Discorea villosa .... see WILD YAM
Dishcloth Sponge .... see LUFFA
Disodium Edathamil .... see EDTA
Disodium Edetate .... see EDTA
Disodium EDTA .... see EDTA
Disodium ethylenediamine tetraacetic acid .... see EDTA
Disodium Tetraacetate .... see EDTA
Distilled Oil from Aniba Rosaeodora Wood
....see BOIS DE ROSE OIL
Dita Bark .... see FEVER BARK
Dittany .... see BURNING BUSH leaf,
BURNING BUSH root
Divale ....see BELLADONNA
DIVI-DIVI .... see DIVI-DIVI
Divine Mexican Mint .... see DIVINER'S SAGE
Diviner's Mint .... see DIVINER'S SAGE
Diviners Sage................................ see DIVINER'S SAGE
DIVINER'S SAGE .... see DIVINER'S SAGE
Divinorin.................................... see DIVINER'S SAGE
Divinorin A .... see DIVINER'S SAGE
dl-Alpha-Tocopherol .... see VITAMIN E
dl-Alpha-Tocopheryl .... see VITAMIN E
dl-Alpha-Tocopheryl Acetate .... see VITAMIN E
DL-Carnitine...see L-CARNITINE
DLE .... see TRANSFER FACTOR
DL-Methionine .... see METHIONINE
DLPA .... see PHENYLALANINE
Dl-phenylalanine .... see PHENYLALANINE
dl-Tocopherol.................................. see VITAMIN E
DMAE .... see DEANOL
DMG .... see DIMETHYLGLYCINE, PANGAMIC ACID
DMSO (DIMETHYLSULFOXIDE)
...........................see DMSO (DIMETHYLSULFOXIDE)
DMSO2 ...... see MSM (METHYLSULFONYLMETHANE)

DNA .... see RNA AND DNA
Docosahexaenoic
.... see DHA (DOCOSAHEXAENOIC ACID)
Docosahexanoic Acid
.... see DHA (DOCOSAHEXAENOIC ACID)
Doctor Oje .... see FICIN
DODDER .... see DODDER
Dodder Of Thyme .... see DODDER
Dog-Bur .... see HOUND'S TONGUE
Dog Fish Liver Oil .... see SHARK LIVER OIL
Dog Grass .... see AGROPYRON,
COUCH GRASS
Dog Parsley .... see FOOL'S PARSLEY
Dog Poison .... see FOOL'S PARSLEY
Dog Rose .... see ROSE HIP
Dog Standard .... see TANSY RAGWORT
Dog-Tree .... see AMERICAN DOGWOOD
Dog Wood .... see ALDER BUCKTHORN
Dogbane .... see CANADIAN HEMP
Doggies .... see YELLOW TOADFLAX
Doggrass .... see AGROPYRON,
COUCH GRASS,
WHEATGRASS
Dog's Arrach .... see ARRACH
Dog's Tongue .... see HOUND'S TONGUE
Dog's Tooth Violet ... see AMERICAN ADDER'S TONGUE
Dogwood .... see AMERICAN DOGWOOD
Dogwood Bark .... see CASCARA
Dolichos lobatus .... see KUDZU
Dolloff .... see MEADOWSWEET
Doll's Eye ....see WHITE COHOSH
DOLOMITE .... see DOLOMITE
Dolomitic Limestone .... see DOLOMITE
Dong Chong Xia Cao .... see CORDYCEPS
Dong Chong Zia Cao .... see CORDYCEPS
Dong Qua .... see DONG QUAI
DONG QUAI.................................... see DONG QUAI
Dongqingzi .... see GLOSSY PRIVET
Donnerkraut .... see HEMP AGRIMONY
Doorweed ....see KNOTWEED HERB
Dorstenia contrayerva .... see CONTRAYERVA
Dostenkraut....................see HEMP AGRIMONY,
OREGANO
Dotriacontanol .... see POLICOSANOL
Douglas Fir .... see OREGON FIR BALSAM
Douglas Spruce .... see OREGON FIR BALSAM
Downy Birch ....see BIRCH
D-Panthenol .... see PANTOTHENIC ACID (VITAMIN B5)
D-pantothenic acid
.... see PANTOTHENIC ACID (VITAMIN B5)
D-Pantothenyl Alcohol
.... see PANTOTHENIC ACID (VITAMIN B5)
D-Phenylalanine .... see PHENYLALANINE
Dr. Sklenar's Kombucha Mushroom Infusion
.... see KOMBUCHA TEA
Drachenkraut .... see HEMP AGRIMONY
Draconis Resina .... see DRAGON'S BLOOD
Dracontium .... see SKUNK CABBAGE
Dracontium foetidum................... see SKUNK CABBAGE
Dracorubin .... see DRAGON'S BLOOD
Drago .... see SANGRE DE GRADO
Dragon-Bushes .... see YELLOW TOADFLAX
Dragon Root .... see ARUM

INDEX

Dragon's Blood .... see DRAGON'S BLOOD, HERB ROBERT, SANGRE DE GRADO
Dragon's-Blood Palm .... see DRAGON'S BLOOD
Dragonwort .... see BISTORT
Drake .... see TAUMELLOOLCH
D-Ribose .... see RIBOSE
Drimia indica .... see SQUILL
Drimia maritima .... see SQUILL
Drimys winteri .... see WINTER'S BARK
Dromiceius nova-hollandiae .... see EMU OIL
Dropberry .... see SOLOMON'S SEAL
Dropsy Plant .... see LEMON BALM
Dropwort .... see MEADOWSWEET
Drosera .... see SUNDEW
Drosera intermedia .... see SUNDEW
Drosera longifolia .... see SUNDEW
Drosera ramentacea .... see SUNDEW
Drosera rotundifolia .... see SUNDEW
Drudenfuss .... see EUROPEAN MISTLETOE
Drug Centaurium .... see CENTAURY
Drunken Sailor .... see RED-SPUR VALERIAN
Dry Ground Cranberry .... see ALPINE CRANBERRY
Dryopteris Filix-Mas .... see MALE FERN
d-Tocopherol .... see VITAMIN E
Duboisia myoporoides .... see CORKWOOD TREE
Duck's Foot .... see PODOPHYLLUM
DUCKWEED .... see DUCKWEED
Dudgeon .... see BOXWOOD
Duffle .... see MULLEIN
Dukong Anak .... see CHANCA PIEDRA
Dulcarara .... see BITTERSWEET NIGHTSHADE
Dumb Nettle .... see WHITE DEAD NETTLE FLOWER
Dumpling Cactus .... see PEYOTE
Dun Daisy .... see OX-EYE DAISY
Dungkulcha .... see JIAOGULAN
Durfa Grass .... see AGROPYRON, COUCH GRASS
Durmast Oak .... see OAK bark
Durri .... see BROOM CORN
DUSTY MILLER .... see DUSTY MILLER
Dutch Agrimony .... see HEMP AGRIMONY
Dutch Eupatoire Commune .... see HEMP AGRIMONY
Dutch Myrtle .... see SWEET GALE
Dutch Rushes .... see HORSETAIL
Dutch Tonka .... see TONKA BEAN
Dutchman's Breeches .... see TURKEY CORN
Dwale .... see BELLADONNA
Dwarf Bay .... see MEZEREON
Dwarf Bilberry .... see BILBERRY dried ripe fruit, BILBERRY leaf
Dwarf Carline .... see CARLINA
DWARF ELDER .... see DWARF ELDER
Dwarf Flax .... see MOUNTAIN FLAX
Dwarf Mallow .... see MALLOW leaf
Dwarf Marigold .... see TAGETES
Dwarf-Pine .... see PINE
DWARF PINE NEEDLE .... see DWARF PINE NEEDLE
Dwayberry .... see BELLADONNA
Dyeberry .... see BILBERRY dried ripe fruit, BILBERRY leaf
DYER'S BROOM .... see DYER'S BROOM
Dyer's Bugloss .... see ALKANNA
Dyer's Greenwood .... see DYER'S BROOM
Dyer's Madder .... see MADDER
Dyer's Saffron .... see SAFFLOWER

Dyer's Weed .... see DYER'S BROOM
Dyer's Whin .... see DYER'S BROOM
Dysentery Bark .... see SIMARUBA
Dysentery Weed .... see CUDWEED
E Zhu .... see ZEDOARY
E161 .... see CANTHAXANTHIN
E967 .... see XYLITOL
Eagle-Vine Bark .... see CONDURANGO
Early Fumitory .... see CORYDALIS
Earlyflowering .... see PERIWINKLE
Earth Gall .... see AMERICAN HELLEBORE
Earth-Nut .... see PEANUT OIL
Earth Smoke .... see FUMITORY
Earthbank .... see TORMENTIL
East India Catarrh Root .... see ALPINIA
East India Root .... see ALPINIA
East Indian Almond .... see CASHEW
East Indian Balmony .... see CHIRATA
East Indian Lemongrass .... see LEMONGRASS
East Indian Sandalwood
.... see WHITE SANDALWOOD wood
East Indian Sandalwood Oil
.... see WHITE SANDALWOOD oil
Easter Flower .... see POINSETTIA, PULSATILLA
Easter Giant .... see BISTORT
Easter Mangiant .... see BISTORT
Eastern Arborvitae .... see CEDAR leaf, CEDAR LEAF OIL
Eastern Burning Bush .... see WAHOO
Eastern Fir .... see CANADA BALSAM
Eastern Hemlock .... see PINUS BARK
Eastern Red Cedar
.... see CEDARWOOD bark, berry, leaf, seed, twig
Eastern White Cedar .... see CEDAR leaf, CEDAR LEAF OIL
Eberesche .... see MOUNTAIN ASH
Ebereschenbeeren .... see MOUNTAIN ASH
Eberwurz .... see CARLINA
Eburnamenine-14-carboxylic acid .... see VINPOCETINE
ECHINACEA .... see ECHINACEA
Echinacea Angustifolia .... see ECHINACEA
Echinacea pallida .... see ECHINACEA
Echinacea Purpurea .... see ECHINACEA
Echinaceawurzel .... see ECHINACEA
Echiopanax horridum .... see DEVIL'S CLUB
Echte Kamille .... see GERMAN CHAMOMILE
Ecorce de Quina .... see CINCHONA
Ecuadorian Sarsaparilla .... see SARSAPARILLA
Edamame .... see SOY
Edible Burdock .... see BURDOCK
EDTA .... see EDTA
Egg Lecithin .... see LECITHIN
Eggs and Bacon .... see YELLOW TOADFLAX
Eggs and Collops .... see YELLOW TOADFLAX
Egyptian Alcee .... see AMBRETTE
Egyptian Privet .... see HENNA
Ehrenpreiskraut .... see VERONICA
Eichenrinde .... see OAK bark
Eicosapentaenoic
.... see EPA (EICOSAPENTAENOIC ACID)
Eicosapentaenoic Acid
.... see EPA (EICOSAPENTAENOIC ACID)
Eight Horns .... see STAR ANISE
Eight-Horned Anise .... see STAR ANISE
Einbeere .... see HERB PARIS

INDEX

Eira-Caa .... see STEVIA
Eisenkraut .... see VERBENA
Elder .... see ELDERBERRY
Elder Flower .... see AMERICAN ELDER
Elderberry .... see AMERICAN ELDER
ELDERBERRY .... see ELDERBERRY
ELDERFLOWER .... see ELDERFLOWER
Eldrin .... see RUTIN
ELECAMPANE .... see ELECAMPANE
Elemental Copper .... see COPPER
Elemental Iron .... see IRON
ELEMI .... see ELEMI
Elemi Oleoresin .... see ELEMI
Elemi Resin .... see ELEMI
Elephant-Climber .... see HAWAIIAN BABY WOODROSE
Elephant Creeper ..... see HAWAIIAN BABY WOODROSE
Elephant's Gall .... see ALOE dried juice from leaf, latex
Elettaria cardamomum .... see CARDAMOM
Eleuthera .... see GINSENG, SIBERIAN
Eleuthero .... see GINSENG, SIBERIAN
Eleuthero Ginseng .... see GINSENG, SIBERIAN
Eleutherococ .... see GINSENG, SIBERIAN
Eleutherococci radix .... see GINSENG, SIBERIAN
Eleutherococcus .... see GINSENG, SIBERIAN
Eleutherococcus senticosus .... see GINSENG, SIBERIAN
Elfdock .... see ELECAMPANE
Elfwort .... see ELECAMPANE
Ellanwood .... see ELDERBERRY,
ELDERFLOWER
Ellhorn .... see ELDERBERRY,
ELDERFLOWER
ELM BARK .... see ELM BARK
Eltroot .... see GOUTWEED
Elymus repens .... see AGROPYRON,
COUCH GRASS, HAY FLOWER
Elytrigia repens .... see AGROPYRON,
COUCH GRASS, WHEATGRASS
Emblic .... see INDIAN GOOSEBERRY
Emblic Myrobalan .... see INDIAN GOOSEBERRY
Emblica .... see INDIAN GOOSEBERRY
Emblica officinalis .... see INDIAN GOOSEBERRY
Emetic Herb .... see LOBELIA
Emperor .... see GRAPE fruit, skin
Emu .... see EMU OIL
EMU OIL .... see EMU OIL
Enada .... see NADH
Enchanter's Plant .... see VERBENA
Enebro .... see JUNIPER
ENGLISH ADDER'S TONGUE
.... see ENGLISH ADDER'S TONGUE
English Alder .... see BLACK ALDER
English Chamomile .... see ROMAN CHAMOMILE
English Cowslip .... see COWSLIP
English Goatweed .... see GOUTWEED
English Green Valerian .... see JACOB'S LADDER
English Hawthorn .... see HAWTHORN
ENGLISH HORSEMINT ...... see ENGLISH HORSEMINT
ENGLISH IVY .... see ENGLISH IVY
English Lavender .... see LAVENDER
English Mandrake .... see BRYONIA
English Morello .... see SOUR CHERRY
English Oak .... see OAK bark
English Plantain .... see BUCKHORN PLANTAIN
English Sarsaparilla .... see TORMENTIL

English Tonka .... see TONKA BEAN
ENGLISH WALNUT .... see ENGLISH WALNUT
English Watercress .... see HEDGE MUSTARD
English Yew .... see YEW
Englishman's Foot .... see BLOND PSYLLIUM
Enocianina .... see GRAPE fruit, skin
EPA .... see EPA (EICOSAPENTAENOIC ACID)
EPA (EICOSAPENTAENOIC ACID)
.... see EPA (EICOSAPENTAENOIC ACID)
Epazote .... see CHENOPODIUM OIL
EPHEDRA .... see EPHEDRA
Ephedra distachya .... see EPHEDRA
Ephedra equisetina .... see EPHEDRA
Ephedra gerardiana .... see EPHEDRA
Ephedra intermedia .... see EPHEDRA
Ephedra nevadensis .... see MORMON TEA
Ephedra shennungiana .... see EPHEDRA
Ephedra Sinensis .... see EPHEDRA
Ephedra sinica .... see EPHEDRA
Ephedrae herba .... see EPHEDRA
Epigaea repens .... see TRAILING ARBUTUS
Epilobium angustifolium .... see FIREWEED
EPIMEDIUM .... see EPIMEDIUM
Epimedium acuminatum .... see EPIMEDIUM
Epimedium brevicornum .... see EPIMEDIUM
Epimedium grandiflorum .... see EPIMEDIUM
Epimedium koreanum .... see EPIMEDIUM
Epimedium pubescens .... see EPIMEDIUM
Epimedium sagittatum .... see EPIMEDIUM
Epimedium wushanese .... see EPIMEDIUM
Épine Blanche .... see HAWTHORN
Épine de Mai .... see HAWTHORN
Épine-Vinette .... see EUROPEAN BARBERRY
EPO .... see EVENING PRIMROSE OIL
Epsilon-Carotene-3 .... see LUTEIN
Epsom salts .... see MAGNESIUM
Equisetum .... see HORSETAIL
Equisetum arvense .... see HORSETAIL
Equisetum telmateia .... see HORSETAIL
Erba Da Cartentieri .... see YARROW
Erba Da Falegname .... see YARROW
Ergocalciferol .... see VITAMIN D
ERGOT .... see ERGOT
Eriffe .... see CLIVERS
Erigeron canadensis .... see CANADIAN FLEABANE
Eringo
.... see ERYNGO above ground parts, ERYNGO root
Eriodictyon .... see YERBA SANTA
Eriodictyon californicum .... see YERBA SANTA
Eriodictyon glutinosum .... see YERBA SANTA
Erva Doce .... see STEVIA
Eryngii Herba .... see ERYNGO above ground parts
Eryngii Radix .... see ERYNGO root
Eryngium campestre
.... see ERYNGO above ground parts, ERYNGO root
Eryngium maritinum
.... see ERYNGO above ground parts, ERYNGO root
Eryngium yuccifolium
.... see ERYNGO above ground parts, ERYNGO root
Eryngo
.... see ERYNGO above ground parts, ERYNGO root
ERYNGO above ground parts
.... see ERYNGO above ground parts
ERYNGO root .... see ERYNGO root

Eryngo-leaved Liverwort .... see ICELAND MOSS
Erysimum .... see HEDGE MUSTARD
Erysimum officinale .... see HEDGE MUSTARD
Erythraea centaurium .... see CENTAURY
Erythronium .... see AMERICAN ADDER'S TONGUE
Erythronium americanum
.... see AMERICAN ADDER'S TONGUE
Erythroxylon coca .... see COCA
Erythroxylum catuaba .... see CATUABA
Erythroxylum coca .... see COCA
Erythroxylum novogranatense .... see COCA
Eschscholzia californica .... see CALIFORNIA POPPY
Escine .... see HORSE CHESTNUT seed
Esere Nut .... see CALABAR BEAN
Espigón .... see PUNCTURE VINE
Espino Armarillo .... see SEA BUCKTHORN
Espino Cambrón .... see EUROPEAN BARBERRY
Espino Falso .... see SEA BUCKTHORN
Espresso .... see COFFEE
Esrar .... see MARIJUANA
Essential Fatty Acid .... see ALPHA-LINOLENIC ACID
Estoraque Liquido .... see STORAX
Estragon .... see TARRAGON
Eternal Flower
.... see IMMORTELLE, SANDY EVERLASTING
Ethyl Apovincaminate .... see VINPOCETINE
Ethyl Dihydroxypropyl Aminobenzoate
.... see PARA-AMINOBENZOIC ACID (PABA)
Ethyl Ester .... see VINPOCETINE
Ethylapovincaminoate .... see VINPOCETINE
Ethylenediamine Tetraacetic Acid .... see EDTA
Eucalypti Folium .... see EUCALYPTUS dried leaf
Eucalyptus .... see EUCALYPTUS dried leaf
EUCALYPTUS dried leaf ..... see EUCALYPTUS dried leaf
Eucalyptus fructicetorum ...... see EUCALYPTUS dried leaf,
EUCALYPTUS OIL
Eucalyptus Globulus .... see EUCALYPTUS dried leaf,
EUCALYPTUS OIL
EUCALYPTUS OIL .... see EUCALYPTUS OIL
Eucalyptus polybractea .... see EUCALYPTUS dried leaf,
EUCALYPTUS OIL
Eucalyptus smithii .... see EUCALYPTUS dried leaf,
EUCALYPTUS OIL
Eucalyptusblatter .... see EUCALYPTUS dried leaf
Euchema species .... see CARRAGEENAN
Eugenia aromatica
.... see CLOVE dried flowerbud, leaf, stem, CLOVE OIL
Eugenia caryophyllata
.... see CLOVE dried flowerbud, leaf, stem, CLOVE OIL
Eugenia caryophyllus
.... see CLOVE dried flowerbud, leaf, stem, CLOVE OIL
Eugenia chequen (dried leaf) ....see CHEKEN
Eugenia pimenta .... see ALLSPICE
Euonymus atropurpureus .... see WAHOO
Eupatorium .... see HEMP AGRIMONY
Eupatorium cannabinum .... see HEMP AGRIMONY
Eupatorium perfoliatum .... see BONESET
Eupatorium purpureum .... see GRAVEL ROOT
EUPHORBIA .... see EUPHORBIA
Euphorbia capitata .... see EUPHORBIA
Euphorbia cyparissias .... see CYPRESS SPURGE
Euphorbia hirta .... see EUPHORBIA
Euphorbia pilulifera .... see EUPHORBIA
Euphorbia poinsettia .... see POINSETTIA
Euphorbia pulcherrima .... see POINSETTIA

Euphraisia Eye Bright .... see EYEBRIGHT
Euphrasia officinalis .... see EYEBRIGHT
Euphrasiae herba .... see EYEBRIGHT
Eurixor .... see EUROPEAN MISTLETOE
European Alder .... see BLACK ALDER,
ELDERBERRY,
ELDERFLOWER
European Angelica .... see ANGELICA root
European Ash .... see ASH
European Aspidium .... see MALE FERN
EUROPEAN BARBERRY
.... see EUROPEAN BARBERRY
European Beaver .... see CASTOREUM
European Bitter Polygala .... see BITTER MILKWORT
European Black Alder .... see BLACK ALDER
European Black Currant
.... see BLACK CURRANT SEED OIL
European Blackcurrant
.... see BLACK CURRANT SEED OIL
EUROPEAN BUCKTHORN
.... see EUROPEAN BUCKTHORN
EUROPEAN CHESTNUT
.... see EUROPEAN CHESTNUT
European Cranberry .... see CRANBERRY
European Cranberry-Bush .... see CRAMP BARK
European Dill .... see DILL seed,
DILL above ground parts
European Elder Flower .... see ELDERFLOWER
European Elder Fruit .... see ELDERBERRY
European Elderberry .... see ELDERBERRY
European Filbert .... see HAZELNUT
EUROPEAN FIVE-FINGER GRASS
.... see EUROPEAN FIVE-FINGER GRASS
European Goldenrod .... see GOLDENROD
European Hazel .... see HAZELNUT
European Hellebore .... see WHITE HELLEBORE
European Hops .... see HOPS
European Linden .... see LINDEN CHARCOAL,
LINDEN dried flower, LINDEN dried leaf,
LINDEN dried sapwood
EUROPEAN MANDRAKE
.... see EUROPEAN MANDRAKE
EUROPEAN MISTLETOE
.... see EUROPEAN MISTLETOE
European Mountain-Ash .... see MOUNTAIN ASH
European Mullein .... see MULLEIN
European Oregano .... see OREGANO
European Pasqueflower .... see PULSATILLA
European Pennyroyal .... see PENNYROYAL leaf,
PENNYROYAL oil
European Peony .... see PEONY flower,
PEONY root
European Ragwort .... see TANSY RAGWORT
European Sanicle .... see SANICLE
European Senega .... see BITTER MILKWORT
European Squill .... see SQUILL
European Vervain .... see VERBENA
European Water Hemlock .... see WATER HEMLOCK
European White Hellebore .... see WHITE HELLEBORE
European Wild Pansy .... see HEART'S EASE
Eurphrasia rostkoviana .... see EYEBRIGHT
Evening Primrose .... see EVENING PRIMROSE OIL
EVENING PRIMROSE OIL
.... see EVENING PRIMROSE OIL

Evening Trumpet Flower .... see GELSEMIUM
Evergreen .... see PERIWINKLE
Evergreen Snakeroot .... see BITTER MILKWORT
Everlasting .... see CUDWEED,
                                                              SANDY EVERLASTING
Everlasting Friendship .... see CLIVERS
Everlasting Pea .... see LATHYRUS
Evernia prunastri .... see OAK MOSS
Eve's Cups .... see PITCHER PLANT
Ewe Daisy .... see TORMENTIL
Exogonium purga .... see JALAP
Expressed Almond Oil .... see SWEET ALMOND
Expressed Grapefruit Oil .... see GRAPEFRUIT OIL
Extrait De Pepins De Raisin .... see GRAPE seed
Eye Balm .... see GOLDENSEAL
Eye Bright .... see EYEBRIGHT
Eye Root .... see GOLDENSEAL
Eyebright .... see CLARY SAGE
EYEBRIGHT .... see EYEBRIGHT
Eyrnigium planum .... see ERYNGO above ground parts,
                                                              ERYNGO root
E-Zhu .... see ZEDOARY
Fa Tha Lai Jone .... see ANDROGRAPHIS
Faba Calabarica .... see CALABAR BEAN
Faex Medicinalis .... see BREWER'S YEAST
Fagopyrum esculentum .... see BUCKWHEAT
Fairy Bells .... see WOOD SORREL
Fairy Cap .... see DIGITALIS
Fairy Caps .... see COWSLIP
Fairy Finger .... see DIGITALIS
Fairy Flax .... see MOUNTAIN FLAX
Fairy Herb .... see JIAOGULAN
Fairywand .... see FALSE UNICORN
Fake Saffron .... see SAFFLOWER
Fall Crocus .... see AUTUMN CROCUS
False Bittersweet .... see AMERICAN BITTERSWEET
False Box .... see AMERICAN DOGWOOD
False Cinnamon .... see CASSIA
False Coltsfoot .... see ASARABACCA
False Grapes .... see AMERICAN IVY
False Hellebore .... see AMERICAN HELLEBORE,
                                                              PHEASANT'S EYE
False Indigo .... see WILD INDIGO
False Jacob's Ladder .... see ABSCESS ROOT
False Jasmin .... see GELSEMIUM
False Pareira .... see ABUTA
False Parsley .... see WATER HEMLOCK
False Saffron .... see SAFFLOWER
FALSE UNICORN .... see FALSE UNICORN
False Valerian .... see GOLDEN RAGWORT
Farberrote .... see MADDER
Farfarae Folium Leaf .... see COLTSFOOT
Farmer's Lily .... see WHITE LILY
Fa-Tha-Lai-Jone .... see ANDROGRAPHIS
Fatsia .... see DEVIL'S CLUB
Fe .... see IRON
Featerfoiul .... see FEVERFEW
Featherfew .... see FEVERFEW
Featherfoil .... see FEVERFEW
Feigen .... see FIG
Feijoa macaco .... see COWHAGE
Feldkamille .... see GERMAN CHAMOMILE
Fellen .... see BITTERSWEET NIGHTSHADE

Fellonwood .... see BITTERSWEET NIGHTSHADE
Felon Herb .... see MUGWORT
Felonwort .... see BITTERSWEET NIGHTSHADE
Feltwort .... see MULLEIN
Female Regulator .... see GOLDEN RAGWORT
Fen Ke .... see KUDZU
Fenge .... see KUDZU
Fennel .... see FENNEL fruit, seed
Fennel Flower .... see BLACK SEED
FENNEL fruit, seed .... see FENNEL fruit, seed
FENNEL OIL .... see FENNEL OIL
FENUGREEK .... see FENUGREEK
Fer .... see IRON
Ferrous Carbonate Anhydrous .... see IRON
Ferrous Fumarate .... see IRON
Ferrous Gluconate .... see IRON
Ferrous Pyrophosphate .... see IRON
Ferrous Sulfate .... see IRON
Ferrula .... see SUMBUL
Ferula assa-foetida .... see ASAFOETIDA
Ferula foetida .... see ASAFOETIDA
Ferula gummosa .... see GALBANUM
Ferula rubricaulis .... see ASAFOETIDA
Ferula sumbul .... see SUMBUL
Festuca pratensis .... see HAY FLOWER
Fetid Nightshade .... see HENBANE
Feuille De Luzerne .... see ALFALFA
Feuilles d'Alchemille .... see ALCHEMILLA
Feuilles la Fievre .... see CHANCA PIEDRA
FEVER BARK .... see FEVER BARK
Fever Few .... see FEVERFEW
Fever Grass .... see LEMONGRASS
Fever Plant .... see EVENING PRIMROSE OIL
Fever Root .... see CORAL ROOT,
                                                              WATER HEMLOCK
Fever Tree .... see EUCALYPTUS dried leaf
Fever Twig .... see BITTERSWEET NIGHTSHADE
FEVERFEW .... see FEVERFEW
Fevertree .... see EUCALYPTUS dried leaf
Feverwort .... see BONESET
Ficaria .... see LESSER CELANDINE
Fichtennadelöl .... see FIR NEEDLE OIL
FICIN .... see FICIN
Ficin anthelmintica .... see FICIN
Ficin glabrata .... see FICIN
Ficus carica .... see FIG
Ficus insipida .... see FICIN
Fieberbaumblatter .... see EUCALYPTUS dried leaf
Fieberrinde .... see CINCHONA
Field Balm .... see CATNIP
Field Horsetail .... see HORSETAIL
Field Lady's Mantle .... see PARSLEY PIERT
Field Melilot .... see SWEET CLOVER
Field Mint Oil .... see JAPANESE MINT
Field Pansy .... see HEART'S EASE
Field Pumpkin .... see PUMPKIN
FIELD SCABIOUS .... see FIELD SCABIOUS
Field Seven .... see PANAX PSEUDOGINSENG
Field Sorrel .... see YELLOW DOCK
Fieldhove .... see COLTSFOOT
FIG .... see FIG
FIGWORT .... see FIGWORT
Figwort .... see LESSER CELANDINE

INDEX

Filipendula .... see MEADOWSWEET
Filipendula ulmaria .... see MEADOWSWEET
Filuis Ante Patrem .... see COLTSFOOT
Finbar .... see SEA BUCKTHORN
Finnochio .... see FENNEL fruit, seed
FIR .... see FIR
FIR NEEDLE OIL .... see FIR NEEDLE OIL
Fir Tree .... see FIR, HEMLOCK SPRUCE
FIREWEED .... see FIREWEED
Fish Berries .... see LEVANT BERRY
Fish Body Oil .... see FISH OILS
Fish Killer .... see LEVANT BERRY
Fish Liver Oil .... see FISH OILS
Fish Liver Oils .... see FISH OILS
Fish Mint .... see SPEARMINT
Fish Oil .... see COD LIVER OIL,
FISH OILS

Fish Oil Fatty Acid
.... see DHA (DOCOSAHEXAENOIC ACID),
EPA (EICOSAPENTAENOIC ACID)
Fish Oil Fatty Acids .... see FISH OILS
FISH OILS .... see FISH OILS
Fish Poison Bark .... see JAMAICAN DOGWOOD
Fish-Poison Tree .... see JAMAICAN DOGWOOD
Fish Wood .... see WAHOO
Fishfudle .... see JAMAICAN DOGWOOD
Fitch .... see BLACK SEED
Fitolaca .... see POKEWEED berry,
POKEWEED root

Five-Finger Blossom
.... see EUROPEAN FIVE-FINGER GRASS
Five-Finger Fern .... see MAIDENHAIR FERN

Five-Fingered Root
.... see HEMLOCK WATER DROPWORT
Five Fingers .... see EUROPEAN FIVE-FINGER GRASS
Five-Flavor-Fruit .... see SCHISANDRA
Five-Flavor-Seed .... see SCHISANDRA
Five Leaves .... see AMERICAN IVY
Fixed Almond Oil .... see SWEET ALMOND
FL-113 .... see IPRIFLAVONE
Flag .... see ORRIS
Flag Lily .... see ORRIS
Flaggon .... see ORRIS
Flake Manna .... see MANNA
Flame Seedless .... see GRAPE fruit, skin
Flannelflower .... see MULLEIN
Flapperdock .... see BUTTERBUR
Flat-Podded Vetch .... see LATHYRUS
Flavin .... see RIBOFLAVIN (VITAMIN B2)
Flavine .... see RIBOFLAVIN (VITAMIN B2)
Flax .... see SENEGA
Flax Oil .... see FLAXSEED OIL
Flax Seed .... see FLAXSEED
Flax Seed Oil .... see FLAXSEED OIL
Flax weed .... see RUPTUREWORT
FLAXSEED .... see FLAXSEED
FLAXSEED OIL .... see FLAXSEED OIL
Flaxweed .... see YELLOW TOADFLAX
Flea Wort .... see CANADIAN FLEABANE
Fleaseed .... see BLACK PSYLLIUM
Fleawort .... see BLACK PSYLLIUM
Fleischfarbige .... see PASSIONFLOWER
Flesh and Blood .... see TORMENTIL
Fleur de Camomile .... see GERMAN CHAMOMILE

Fleur De Camomille Romaine
.... see ROMAN CHAMOMILE
Fleur De La Passion .... see PASSIONFLOWER
Fleur de Pied de Chat .... see SANDY EVERLASTING
Fleurs d'Arnica .... see ARNICA
Fliggers .... see ORRIS
Flirtwort Midsummer Daisy .... see FEVERFEW
Flor De Passion .... see PASSIONFLOWER
Florence Fennel .... see FENNEL fruit, seed
Florentine Iris .... see ORRIS
Flores Anthemidis .... see ROMAN CHAMOMILE
Flores Caryophylli .... see CLOVE OIL

Flores Caryophyllum
.... see CLOVE dried flowerbud, leaf, stem
Florist's Chrysanthemum .... see CHRYSANTHEMUM
Flos Magnoliae .... see MAGNOLIA flower bud
Flower Velure .... see COLTSFOOT
Flowering Ammi .... see BISHOP'S WEED
Flowering Ash .... see MANNA
Flowering Sally .... see PURPLE LOOSESTRIFE
Flowering Willow .... see FIREWEED
Flowering Wintergreen .... see BITTER MILKWORT
Flowery Knotweed .... see FO-TI
Fluelli .... see YELLOW TOADFLAX
Fluffweed .... see MULLEIN
Flux Root .... see PLEURISY ROOT
Fly Agaric .... see AGA
Fly-Catcher .... see PITCHER PLANT
Fly Larva .... see MAGGOTS
Fly-Trap .... see CANADIAN HEMP,
PITCHER PLANT
Fo Ti .... see FO-TI
Foal's Foot .... see COLTSFOOT
Foalswort .... see COLTSFOOT
Foam Flower .... see COOLWORT
Fodder Beet .... see BEET
Foeniculi antheroleum .... see FENNEL OIL
Foeniculum capillaceum .... see FENNEL fruit, seed,
FENNEL OIL
Foeniculum officinale .... see FENNEL fruit, seed,
FENNEL OIL
Foeniculum vulgare .... see FENNEL fruit, seed,
FENNEL OIL
Foenugraeci Semen .... see FENUGREEK
Foenugreek .... see FENUGREEK
Folacin .... see FOLIC ACID
Folate .... see FOLIC ACID
Folia Vitis Viniferae .... see GRAPE leaf
FOLIC ACID .... see FOLIC ACID
Food of the Gods .... see ASAFOETIDA
Fool's-Cicely .... see FOOL'S PARSLEY
FOOL'S PARSLEY .... see FOOL'S PARSLEY
Forest Mushroom .... see SHIITAKE MUSHROOM
FORGET-ME-NOT .... see FORGET-ME-NOT
Forscolin .... see FORSKOLIN
FORSKOLIN .... see FORSKOLIN
FOS .... see FRUCTO-OLIGOSACCHARIDES
Fossil Tree .... see GINKGO leaf (GINKGO leaf extract),
GINKGO seed
FO-TI .... see FO-TI
Fo-Ti-Tient .... see FO-TI
Foxberry .... see ALPINE CRANBERRY
Foxglove .... see DIGITALIS
Fox's Clote .... see BURDOCK

Foxtails .... see HAY FLOWER
Fragaria vesca .... see STRAWBERRY
Fragaria virginiana .... see STRAWBERRY
Fragaria viridis .... see STRAWBERRY
Fragariae folium .... see STRAWBERRY
Fragrant Agrimony .... see AGRIMONY
Fragrant Valerian .... see VALERIAN
Framboise .... see RASPBERRY leaf
Frangula .... see ALDER BUCKTHORN
Frangula alnus .... see ALDER BUCKTHORN
Frangula Bark .... see ALDER BUCKTHORN
Frangula purshiana .... see CASCARA
Frangulae Cortex .... see ALDER BUCKTHORN
FRANKINCENSE .... see FRANKINCENSE
Frauenmantelkraut .... see ALCHEMILLA
Fraxinella .... see BURNING BUSH leaf,
                                      BURNING BUSH root
Fraxinus americana .... see ASH
Fraxinus excelsior .... see ASH
Fraxinus ornus .... see MANNA
French Honeysuckle .... see GOAT'S RUE
French Lavender .... see LAVENDER
French Lilac .... see GOAT'S RUE
French Marigold .... see TAGETES
French Marine Pine Bark Extract .... see PYCNOGENOL
French Maritime Pine Bark Extract ...... see PYCNOGENOL
French Psyllium .... see BLACK PSYLLIUM
French Thyme .... see THYME flower, leaf
French Willow .... see FIREWEED
Fresh Water Leech .... see LEECH
Friar's Cowl .... see ARUM
Frijol de Soya .... see SOY
Fringe Tree .... see FRINGETREE
FRINGETREE .... see FRINGETREE
Frogsfoot .... see BULBOUS BUTTERCUP
Frogwort .... see BULBOUS BUTTERCUP
Frost Plant .... see FROSTWORT
Frostweed .... see FROSTWORT
FROSTWORT .... see FROSTWORT
Fructo Oligo Saccharides
    ....see FRUCTO-OLIGOSACCHARIDES
FRUCTO-OLIGOSACCHARIDES
    ....see FRUCTO-OLIGOSACCHARIDES
Fructus Cortex .... see ENGLISH WALNUT
Fructus Lycii .... see LYCIUM
Fructus Lycii Berry .... see LYCIUM
Fructus Rosae Laevigatae .... see CHEROKEE ROSEHIP
Fruit de Celeri .... see CELERY
Fruits De Khella .... see KHELLA
Fu Ling .... see PORIA MUSHROOM
Fucostanol .... see SITOSTANOL
Fucus .... see BLADDERWRACK
Fucus vesiculosis .... see BLADDERWRACK
Fuga Daemonum .... see ST. JOHN'S WORT
Fum .... see ASAFOETIDA
Fumaria Officinalis .... see FUMITORY
Fumiterry .... see FUMITORY
FUMITORY .... see FUMITORY
Fumus .... see FUMITORY
Funffing .... see AGRIMONY
Funffingerkraut .... see AGRIMONY
Fungus Japonicus .... see KOMBUCHA TEA
Furze .... see DYER'S BROOM

Fusanum .... see WAHOO
FuShen .... see PORIA MUSHROOM
Fusoria .... see WAHOO
Fytic Acid .... see IP-6
GABA .... see GABA (GAMMA-AMINOBUTYRIC ACID)
GABA (GAMMA-AMINOBUTYRIC ACID)
    .... see GABA (GAMMA-AMINOBUTYRIC ACID)
Gadrose .... see WAHOO
Gag .... see CHONDROITIN SULFATE
Gaga .... see MARIJUANA
Gaglee .... see ARUM
Gagroot .... see LOBELIA
Galactosaminoglucuronoglycan Sulfate
    .... see CHONDROITIN SULFATE
Galanga .... see ALPINIA
Galangal .... see ALPINIA
Galbanum .... see GALBANUM
Galbanum Gum .... see GALBANUM
Galbanum Gum Resin .... see GALBANUM
Galbanum Oleogum Resin .... see GALBANUM
Galbanum Oleoresin .... see GALBANUM
Galbanum Resin .... see GALBANUM
Galega officinalis .... see GOAT'S RUE
Galegae officinalis herba .... see GOAT'S RUE
Galeopsidis Herba .... see HEMPNETTLE
Galeopsis ochroleuca .... see HEMPNETTLE
Galeopsis segetum .... see HEMPNETTLE
Galii odorati herba .... see SWEET WOODRUFF
Galipea officinalis .... see ANGOSTURA
Galium aparine .... see CLIVERS
Galium odorata .... see SWEET WOODRUFF
Galium verum .... see LADY'S BEDSTRAW
Gall Weed .... see GENTIAN
Gallium .... see CLIVERS
Gallwort .... see YELLOW TOADFLAX
Gambierdiscus toxicus .... see CIGUATERA
Gambodia .... see GAMBOGE
GAMBOGE .... see GAMBOGE
Gamma Amino Butyric Acid
    .... see GABA (GAMMA-AMINOBUTYRIC ACID)
Gamma Aminobutyric Acid
    .... see GABA (GAMMA-AMINOBUTYRIC ACID)
Gamma Butyrolactone
    ....see GAMMA BUTYROLACTONE (GBL)
GAMMA BUTYROLACTONE (GBL)
    ....see GAMMA BUTYROLACTONE (GBL)
Gamma-Glutamylcysteinylglycine ...... see GLUTATHIONE
Gamma Hydrate
    .... see GAMMA-HYDROXYBUTYRATE (GHB)
GAMMA-HYDROXYBUTYRATE (GHB)
    .... see GAMMA-HYDROXYBUTYRATE (GHB)
Gamma Hydroxybutyrate Sodium
    .... see GAMMA-HYDROXYBUTYRATE (GHB)
Gamma Hydroxybutyric Acid
    .... see GAMMA-HYDROXYBUTYRATE (GHB)
Gamma Hydroxybutyric Acid Lactone
    .... see GAMMA BUTYROLACTONE (GBL)
Gamma-L-Glutamyl-L-cysteinylglycine
    .... see GLUTATHIONE
GAMMA LINOLENIC ACID
    .... see GAMMA LINOLENIC ACID
Gamma-OH
    .... see GAMMA-HYDROXYBUTYRATE (GHB)
GAMMA ORYZANOL .... see GAMMA ORYZANOL

INDEX

Gamma-OZ .... see GAMMA ORYZANOL
Gamma-tocopherol .... see VITAMIN E
Gamma tocotrienol .... see VITAMIN E
Gamma-Trimethyl-Beta-Acetylbutyrobetaine
.... see ACETYL-L-CARNITINE
Gamolenic Acid .... see GAMMA LINOLENIC ACID
Gan Cao .... see LICORICE
Gan Zao .... see LICORICE
Ganga .... see MARIJUANA
Gange .... see KUDZU
Ganoderma lucidum .... see REISHI MUSHROOM
Garacilaria confervoides .... see AGAR
Garance .... see MADDER
GARCINIA .... see GARCINIA
Garcinia Cambogi .... see GARCINIA
Garcinia Cambogia .... see GARCINIA
Garcinia hanburyi .... see GAMBOGE
Garden Angelica .... see ANGELICA root
Garden Artichoke .... see ARTICHOKE
Garden Asparagus .... see ASPARAGUS
Garden Balsam .... see JEWELWEED
Garden Basil .... see BASIL
Garden Beet .... see BEET
Garden Burnet .... see GREATER BURNET
Garden Chamomile .... see ROMAN CHAMOMILE
Garden Chervil .... see CHERVIL
GARDEN CRESS .... see GARDEN CRESS
Garden Fennel .... see FENNEL fruit, seed
Garden Heliotrope .... see VALERIAN
Garden Lavender .... see LAVENDER
Garden Marigold .... see CALENDULA
Garden Marjoram .... see MARJORAM
Garden Mint .... see SPEARMINT
Garden Nightshade .... see BLACK NIGHTSHADE
Garden Parsley .... see PARSLEY leaf, root,
                                          PARSLEY seed
Garden Pepper .... see CAPSICUM
Garden Rhubarb .... see RHUBARB
Garden Rue .... see RUE
Garden Sage .... see SAGE
Garden Sorrel .... see SORREL
Garden Thyme .... see THYME flower, leaf
Garden Valerian .... see VALERIAN
Garden Violet .... see GARDEN VIOLET,
                                          SWEET VIOLET
Gargaut .... see ALPINIA
Garget .... see POKEWEED berry,
                                          POKEWEED root
GARLIC .... see GARLIC
Garlic Clove .... see GARLIC
Garlic Sage .... see WOOD SAGE
Gartenmajoran .... see MARJORAM
Gas Black .... see ACTIVATED CHARCOAL
Gas Plant .... see BURNING BUSH leaf,
                                          BURNING BUSH root
Gat .... see KHAT
Gatten .... see WAHOO
Gatter .... see WAHOO
Gattilier .... see CHASTEBERRY
Gaultheria Oil .... see WINTERGREEN oil
Gaultheria procumbens .... see WINTERGREEN leaf,
                                          WINTERGREEN oil
Gay Feather .... see MARSH BLAZING STAR
GBL .... see GAMMA BUTYROLACTONE (GBL)

Ge .... see GERMANIUM
Ge-132 .... see GERMANIUM
Ge Gen .... see KUDZU
Gegen .... see KUDZU
Geissrautenkraut .... see GOAT'S RUE
Gelatin .... see AGAR
Gelidiella acerosa .... see AGAR
Gelidium amanasii .... see AGAR
Gelidium cartilagineum .... see AGAR
Gelidium crinale .... see AGAR
Gelidium divaricatum .... see AGAR
Gelidium pacificum .... see AGAR
Gelidium vagum .... see AGAR
Gelosa .... see AGAR
Gelosae .... see AGAR
Gelsemii Rhizoma .... see GELSEMIUM
Gelsemin .... see GELSEMIUM
GELSEMIUM .... see GELSEMIUM
Gelsemium nitidum .... see GELSEMIUM
Gelsemium Sempervirens .... see GELSEMIUM
Gelsemiumwurzelstock Jessamine .... see GELSEMIUM
Gemeine Schafgarbe .... see YARROW
Gemeiner Beifuss .... see MUGWORT
Gemeiner Wasswedost .... see HEMP AGRIMONY
Gemnema melicida .... see GYMNEMA
Gemuseartischocke .... see ARTICHOKE
General Plantain .... see GREAT PLANTAIN
Genet .... see SPANISH BROOM
Genet a Balais .... see SCOTCH BROOM flower
Geniévre .... see JUNIPER
Genista juncea .... see SPANISH BROOM
Genista tinctoria .... see DYER'S BROOM
Genistein .... see RED CLOVER, SOY
GENTIAN .... see GENTIAN
Gentiana .... see GENTIAN
Gentiana acaulis .... see GENTIAN
Gentiana Lutea .... see GENTIAN
Gentianae radix .... see GENTIAN
Ge-Oxy 132 .... see GERMANIUM
Geranium robertianum .... see HERB ROBERT
GERMAN CHAMOMILE ... see GERMAN CHAMOMILE
GERMAN IPECAC .... see GERMAN IPECAC
German Lactucarium .... see WILD LETTUCE
German Rue .... see RUE
GERMAN SARSAPARILLA
.... see GERMAN SARSAPARILLA
GERMANDER .... see GERMANDER
GERMANIUM .... see GERMANIUM
Germanium Lactate Citrate .... see GERMANIUM
Gero-Vita .... see PROCAINE
Gerovital .... see PROCAINE
Gerovital-H3 .... see PROCAINE
Geum .... see AVENS
Geum rivale .... see WATER AVENS
Geum urbanum .... see AVENS
Gewurznelken Nagelein
.... see CLOVE dried flowerbud, leaf, stem, CLOVE OIL
GH-3 .... see PROCAINE
GHB .... see GAMMA-HYDROXYBUTYRATE (GHB)
Ghoda Asoda .... see ASHWAGANDHA
Giant Fennel .... see ASAFOETIDA
Gifolan (GRN) .... see BETA GLUCANS
Gigartina mamillosa and other Gigartina species
.... see CARRAGEENAN

Gillenia .... see INDIAN PHYSIC
Gillenia trifoliata .... see INDIAN PHYSIC
Gill-Go-By-The-Hedge .... see GROUND IVY
Gill-Go-Over-The-Ground .... see GROUND IVY
Gillyflower .... see WALLFLOWER
Ginepro .... see JUNIPER
Gingembre .... see GINGER
GINGER .... see GINGER
Ginger Root .... see GINGER
Gingko .... see GINKGO leaf (GINKGO leaf extract),
GINKGO seed
Gingko Biloba .... see GINKGO leaf (GINKGO leaf extract)
Ginjeira .... see SOUR CHERRY
Ginkgo .... see GINKGO leaf (GINKGO leaf extract),
GINKGO seed
Ginkgo Biloba ... see GINKGO leaf (GINKGO leaf extract),
GINKGO seed
Ginkgo Folium .... see GINKGO leaf (GINKGO leaf extract)
Ginkgo leaf .... see GINKGO leaf (GINKGO leaf extract)
GINKGO leaf (GINKGO leaf extract)
.... see GINKGO leaf (GINKGO leaf extract)
Ginkgo Leaf Extract
.... see GINKGO leaf (GINKGO leaf extract)
GINKGO seed .... see GINKGO seed
Ginko Biloba ...... see GINKGO leaf (GINKGO leaf extract)
Ginkyo .... see GINKGO leaf (GINKGO leaf extract),
GINKGO seed
Ginseng .... see GINSENG, AMERICAN,
GINSENG, PANAX,
GINSENG, SIBERIAN
Ginseng Asiatique .... see GINSENG, PANAX
Ginseng Radix .... see GINSENG, PANAX
Ginseng Root .... see GINSENG, PANAX
GINSENG, AMERICAN .... see GINSENG, AMERICAN
GINSENG, PANAX .... see GINSENG, PANAX
GINSENG, SIBERIAN .... see GINSENG, SIBERIAN
Ginsterkraut .... see SCOTCH BROOM flower
Giroflier .... see WALLFLOWER
GL701 .... see DHEA
GLA .... see GAMMA LINOLENIC ACID
Gladdon .... see CALAMUS
Gladyne .... see ORRIS
Glandular .... see ADRENAL EXTRACT
Glechoma hederacea .... see GROUND IVY
Glicerol .... see GLYCEROL
GLN .... see GLUTAMINE
Globe Amaranth .... see BUTTERCUP
Globe Artichoke .... see ARTICHOKE
Globe Crowfoot .... see GLOBE FLOWER
GLOBE FLOWER .... see GLOBE FLOWER
Globe Ranunculus .... see GLOBE FLOWER
Globe Trollius .... see GLOBE FLOWER
Glockenbilsenkraut .... see SCOPOLIA
Glossy Buckthorn .... see ALDER BUCKTHORN
GLOSSY PRIVET .... see GLOSSY PRIVET
Glucerite .... see GLYCEROL
GLUCOMANNAN .... see GLUCOMANNAN
Gluconic Acid .... see PANGAMIC ACID
Gluconolactone .... see ALPHA HYDROXY ACIDS
Glucosamine
.... see GLUCOSAMINE HYDROCHLORIDE,
GLUCOSAMINE SULFATE
Glucosamine HCL
.... see GLUCOSAMINE HYDROCHLORIDE

GLUCOSAMINE HYDROCHLORIDE
.... see GLUCOSAMINE HYDROCHLORIDE
Glucosamine N-Acetyl
.... see N-ACETYL GLUCOSAMINE
GLUCOSAMINE SULFATE
.... see GLUCOSAMINE SULFATE
Glucosamine Sulphate ...... see GLUCOSAMINE SULFATE
Glucose Tolerance Factor .... see CHROMIUM
Glucose Tolerance Factor-Cr .... see CHROMIUM
Glutamate .... see GLUTAMINE
Glutamic Acid .... see GLUTAMINE
Glutaminate .... see GLUTAMINE
GLUTAMINE .... see GLUTAMINE
GLUTATHIONE .... see GLUTATHIONE
Glycerin .... see GLYCEROL
GLYCEROL .... see GLYCEROL
Glycerol Trierucate Oil .... see LORENZO'S OIL
Glycerol Trioleate Oil .... see LORENZO'S OIL
Glycerolum .... see GLYCEROL
Glyceryl Alcohol .... see GLYCEROL
Glyceryl Paraaminobenzoate
.... see PARA-AMINOBENZOIC ACID (PABA)
Glycine .... see PANGAMIC ACID
Glycine max .... see SOY
Glycine soja .... see SOY, SOYBEAN OIL
Glycolic Acid .... see ALPHA HYDROXY ACIDS
Glycosaminoglycans .... see MESOGLYCAN
Glycyrrhiza .... see LICORICE
Glycyrrhiza glabra .... see LICORICE
Glycyrrhiza glabra glandulifera .... see LICORICE
Glycyrrhiza glabra typica .... see LICORICE
Glycyrrhiza glabra violacea .... see LICORICE
Glycyrrhiza uralensis .... see LICORICE
Gnaphalium uliginosum .... see CUDWEED
GOA POWDER .... see GOA POWDER
Goathead .... see PUNCTURE VINE
Goatnut .... see JOJOBA
Goat's Arrach .... see ARRACH
Goat's Leaf .... see HONEYSUCKLE
Goat's Pod .... see CAPSICUM
GOAT'S RUE .... see GOAT'S RUE
Goat's Rue Herb .... see GOAT'S RUE
Goat's Thorn .... see TRAGACANTH
Goatweed .... see ST. JOHN'S WORT
God's-Hair .... see HARTSTONGUE
Gokhru .... see PUNCTURE VINE
Gold-Bloom .... see CALENDULA
Gold Chain .... see COMMON STONECROP
Gold Cup .... see BUTTERCUP
Gold Thread .... see GOLDTHREAD
Goldcup .... see BULBOUS BUTTERCUP
Golden Chain .... see LABURNUM
Golden Daisy .... see OX-EYE DAISY
Golden Groundsel .... see GOLDEN RAGWORT
Golden Moss .... see COMMON STONECROP
GOLDEN RAGWORT .... see GOLDEN RAGWORT
Golden Rod .... see GOLDENROD, MULLEIN
Golden Root .... see ROSEROOT
Golden Seal .... see GOLDENSEAL
Golden Senecio .... see GOLDEN RAGWORT
Golden Trumpet .... see CATUABA
GOLDENROD .... see GOLDENROD
Goldenroot .... see GOLDENSEAL
GOLDENSEAL .... see GOLDENSEAL

INDEX

Goldenseal .... see OX-EYE DAISY
Goldenthread .... see GOLDTHREAD
Goldilocks .... see IMMORTELLE,
SANDY EVERLASTING
Goldsiegel .... see GOLDENSEAL
GOLDTHREAD .... see GOLDTHREAD
Gomishi .... see SCHISANDRA
Gomme Arabique .... see ACACIA
Gomme de Senegal .... see ACACIA
Gommelaque .... see SHELLAC
Goniopora species .... see CORAL
Gonolobus condurango .... see CONDURANGO
Goose bill .... see CLIVERS
Goose Grass .... see CLIVERS
Goose Tansy .... see POTENTILLA
Goosefoot .... see ARRACH
Goosegrass .... see CLIVERS, POTENTILLA
Goosewort .... see POTENTILLA
Gorikapuli .... see GARCINIA
Gosling Weed .... see CLIVERS
Gossypium herbaceum .... see COTTON, GOSSYPOL
Gossypium hirsutum .... see COTTON, GOSSYPOL
GOSSYPOL .... see GOSSYPOL
Gotu Cola .... see GOTU KOLA
GOTU KOLA .... see GOTU KOLA
Gou Qi Zi .... see LYCIUM
Goudron de Cade .... see CADE OIL
Gouqizi .... see LYCIUM
Gout Herb .... see GOUTWEED
Goutberry .... see BLACKBERRY leaf,
BLACKBERRY root
GOUTWEED .... see GOUTWEED
Goutwort .... see GOUTWEED
Gracemere-Pear .... see PRICKLY PEAR CACTUS
Graine De Lin .... see FLAXSEED,
FLAXSEED OIL
Grains of Paradise .... see CAPSICUM
GRAINS OF PARADISE .... see GRAINS OF PARADISE
Graminis Flos .... see HAY FLOWER
Graminis Rhizoma .... see AGROPYRON
Granada .... see POMEGRANATE
Grape .... see GRAPE fruit, skin,
GRAPE leaf, GRAPE seed
Grape Bark .... see COCILLANA
Grape Fruit .... see GRAPE fruit, skin
Grape Fruit Skin .... see GRAPE fruit, skin
GRAPE fruit, skin .... see GRAPE fruit, skin
Grape Juice .... see GRAPE fruit, skin
GRAPE leaf .... see GRAPE leaf
Grape Leaf Extract .... see GRAPE leaf
GRAPE seed .... see GRAPE seed
Grape Seed Extract .... see GRAPE seed
Grape Seed Oil .... see GRAPE seed
Grape Skin .... see GRAPE fruit, skin
Grape Skin Extract .... see GRAPE fruit, skin
GRAPEFRUIT .... see GRAPEFRUIT
Grapefruit Extract ..... see GRAPEFRUIT SEED EXTRACT
GRAPEFRUIT OIL .... see GRAPEFRUIT OIL
GRAPEFRUIT SEED EXTRACT
.... see GRAPEFRUIT SEED EXTRACT
Grapefruit Seed Glycerate
.... see GRAPEFRUIT SEED EXTRACT
Grapes .... see GRAPE fruit, skin
Grapeseed .... see GRAPE seed

Grapple Plant .... see DEVIL'S CLAW
Grass .... see MARIJUANA,
SWEET VERNAL GRASS
Grass Flower .... see HAY FLOWER
Grass Myrtle .... see CALAMUS
Grass Pollen .... see RYE GRASS
Grass Pollen Extract .... see RYE GRASS
Gratiola .... see HEDGE-HYSSOP
Gratiola officinalis .... see HEDGE-HYSSOP
Gravel Plant .... see TRAILING ARBUTUS
GRAVEL ROOT .... see GRAVEL ROOT
Gray Beard Tree .... see FRINGETREE
Greasewood .... see CHAPARRAL
Great Bur .... see BURDOCK
Great Burdocks .... see BURDOCK
Great Morel .... see BELLADONNA
Great Ox-Eye .... see OX-EYE DAISY
GREAT PLANTAIN .... see GREAT PLANTAIN
Great Raifort .... see HORSERADISH
Great Stinging Nettle
.... see STINGING NETTLE above ground parts,
STINGING NETTLE root
Great Willowherb .... see FIREWEED
GREATER BINDWEED .... see GREATER BINDWEED
GREATER BURNET .... see GREATER BURNET
Greater Burnet-Saxifrage .... see PIMPINELLA root
Greater Celandine
..... see GREATER CELANDINE dried above ground parts,
GREATER CELANDINE rhizome, root
GREATER CELANDINE dried above ground parts
...... see GREATER CELANDINE dried above ground parts
GREATER CELANDINE rhizome, root
.... see GREATER CELANDINE rhizome, root
Greater Plantain .... see GREAT PLANTAIN
Grecian Laurel .... see SWEET BAY
Greek Hay .... see FENUGREEK
Greek Hay Seed .... see FENUGREEK
GREEK SAGE .... see GREEK SAGE
Green Arrow .... see YARROW
Green Bean .... see BEAN POD
Green Bell Pepper .... see CAPSICUM
Green Broom .... see DYER'S BROOM
Green Chili Pepper .... see CAPSICUM
Green Dragon .... see TRAGACANTH
Green Endive .... see WILD LETTUCE
Green Ginger .... see WORMWOOD above ground parts
Green Hellebore .... see AMERICAN HELLEBORE
Green Mint .... see SPEARMINT
Green Oil of Charity .... see ENGLISH ADDER'S TONGUE
Green Onion .... see ONION
Green Orange .... see BITTER ORANGE
Green Ozier .... see AMERICAN DOGWOOD
Green Sauce .... see WOOD SORREL
GREEN TEA .... see GREEN TEA
Green Veratrum .... see AMERICAN HELLEBORE
Green Wolf's Foot .... see BUGLEWEED
Greenweed .... see DYER'S BROOM
Grenadier .... see POMEGRANATE
Griffe Du Chat .... see CAT'S CLAW
Griffe Du Diable .... see DEVIL'S CLAW
Grifola .... see MAITAKE MUSHROOM
Grifola frondosa .... see MAITAKE MUSHROOM
Grindelia .... see GUMWEED
Grindelia robusta .... see GUMWEED

I
N
D
E
X

Grindelia squarrosa .... see GUMWEED
Grindeliae herba .... see GUMWEED
Griottier .... see SOUR CHERRY
Grip Grass .... see CLIVERS
Grisset .... see SEA BUCKTHORN
Groats .... see OATS
Groseillier de Ceylan .... see INDIAN GOOSEBERRY
Grosse Kamille .... see ROMAN CHAMOMILE
Grosse Moosbeere .... see CRANBERRY
Ground Apple .... see ROMAN CHAMOMILE
Ground Berry .... see WINTERGREEN leaf,
WINTERGREEN oil
Ground Elder .... see GOUTWEED
Ground Furze .... see SPINY RESTHARROW
Ground Glutton .... see GROUNDSEL
Ground Holly .... see PIPSISSEWA
GROUND IVY .... see GROUND IVY
Ground Laurel .... see TRAILING ARBUTUS
Ground Lemon .... see PODOPHYLLUM
Ground Lily .... see BETH ROOT
GROUND PINE .... see GROUND PINE
Ground Raspberry .... see GOLDENSEAL
Ground Thistle .... see CARLINA
Groundbread .... see CYCLAMEN
Groundnuts .... see PEANUT OIL
GROUNDSEL .... see GROUNDSEL
Grub .... see MAGGOTS
Grundy Swallow .... see GOLDEN RAGWORT,
GROUNDSEL
GSE .... see GRAPEFRUIT SEED EXTRACT
GSH .... see GLUTATHIONE
GTF .... see CHROMIUM
GTF Cr .... see CHROMIUM
Gua Lou .... see CHINESE CUCUMBER fruit
Gua Luo Ren .... see CHINESE CUCUMBER seed
Guaiac .... see GUAIAC WOOD resin, wood
Guaiac Heartwood .... see GUAIAC WOOD resin, wood
Guaiac Wood .... see GUAIAC WOOD resin, wood
GUAIAC WOOD OIL .... see GUAIAC WOOD OIL
GUAIAC WOOD resin, wood
.... see GUAIAC WOOD resin, wood
Guaiacum .... see GUAIAC WOOD resin, wood
Guaiacum officinale .... see GUAIAC WOOD resin, wood
Guaiacum sanctum .... see GUAIAC WOOD resin, wood
Guajaci Lignum .... see GUAIAC WOOD resin, wood
Gua-Lou .... see CHINESE CUCUMBER fruit
Gua-Luo-Ren .... see CHINESE CUCUMBER seed
Guapi .... see COCILLANA
Guar Flour .... see GUAR GUM
GUAR GUM .... see GUAR GUM
GUARANA .... see GUARANA
Guarana Bread .... see GUARANA
Guarana Gum .... see GUARANA
Guarana Seed Paste .... see GUARANA
Guarea rusbyi .... see COCILLANA
Guarea spiciflora .... see COCILLANA
Guarea tricholoides .... see COCILLANA
Guatemala Lemongrass .... see LEMONGRASS
GUAYULE .... see GUAYULE
Guelder Rose .... see CRAMP BARK
Guflatich .... see COLTSFOOT
Guggal .... see GUGGUL
Guggal Gum and Resin .... see MYRRH
GUGGUL .... see GUGGUL

Guggulu .... see GUGGUL
Guindo .... see SOUR CHERRY
Guinea Corn .... see BROOM CORN
Guinea Grains .... see GRAINS OF PARADISE
Guinea Rush .... see ADRUE
Guinea Sorrel .... see HIBISCUS
Gum Acacia .... see ACACIA
Gum Arabic .... see ACACIA
Gum Benjamin .... see BENZOIN
Gum Benzoin .... see BENZOIN
Gum Bush .... see YERBA SANTA
Gum Camphor .... see CAMPHOR
Gum Dragon .... see TRAGACANTH
Gum Guggal .... see GUGGUL
Gum Guggulu .... see GUGGUL
Gum Ivy .... see ENGLISH IVY
Gum Myrrh .... see MYRRH
Gum Plant .... see COMFREY, YERBA SANTA
Gum Senegal .... see ACACIA
Gum Tragacanth .... see TRAGACANTH
Gum Tree .... see EUCALYPTUS dried leaf,
STORAX
Gum Weed .... see GUMWEED
Gummae Mimosae .... see ACACIA
Gummi Tragacanthae .... see TRAGACANTH
Gummigutta .... see GAMBOGE
GUMWEED .... see GUMWEED
Gumweed Herb .... see GUMWEED
Gur Mar .... see GYMNEMA
Gurmarbooti .... see GYMNEMA
Guru Nut .... see COLA NUT
Gutta Cambodia .... see GAMBOGE
Gutta Gamba .... see GAMBOGE
GYMNEMA .... see GYMNEMA
Gymnema Sylvestre .... see GYMNEMA
Gynocardia Oil .... see CHAULMOOGRA
Gynostemma pedatum .... see JIAOGULAN
Gynostemma pentaphyllum .... see JIAOGULAN
Gypsophila paniculata and other Gypsophila species
.... see WHITE SOAPWORT
Gypsophilae radix .... see WHITE SOAPWORT
Gypsy Flower .... see HOUND'S TONGUE
Gypsy Weed .... see BUGLEWEED
Gypsyweed .... see VERONICA
Gypsywort .... see BUGLEWEED
Haagdorn .... see HAWTHORN
Haba Soya .... see SOY
Hackmatack .... see CEDAR leaf,
CEDAR LEAF OIL
Haematoxylon campechianum .... see LOGWOOD
Haematoxylon lignum .... see LOGWOOD
Hagedorn .... see HAWTHORN
Hagenia abyssinica .... see KOUSSO
Hag's Taper .... see MULLEIN
Hair of Venus .... see MAIDENHAIR FERN
Hairy Mint .... see WILD MINT
Hallelujah .... see WOOD SORREL
Hallfoot .... see COLTSFOOT
Hamamelis .... see WITCH HAZEL
Hamamelis virginiana .... see WITCH HAZEL
Hamburg Parsley .... see PARSLEY leaf, root
Handflower .... see WALLFLOWER
Happy Major .... see BURDOCK
Hara .... see TERMINALIA

INDEX

Harada .... see TERMINALIA
Hardback .... see STONE ROOT
Hardhack .... see STONE ROOT
Hardhay .... see ST. JOHN'S WORT
Hardock .... see BURDOCK
Harebur .... see BURDOCK
Hare's Beard .... see MULLEIN
Hare's Ear Root .... see BUPLEURUM
Haritaki .... see TERMINALIA
Harnblumen .... see SANDY EVERLASTING
HARONGA .... see HARONGA
Haronga madagascariensis .... see HARONGA
Harongablädder leaf .... see HARONGA
Harongarinde bark .... see HARONGA
Harpagophyti Radix .... see DEVIL'S CLAW
Harpagophytum .... see DEVIL'S CLAW
Harpagophytum procumbens .... see DEVIL'S CLAW
Harthorne .... see HAWTHORN
Hart's Tree .... see SWEET CLOVER
Hart's Truffle .... see PUFF BALL
Hartshorn .... see EUROPEAN BUCKTHORN
HARTSTONGUE .... see HARTSTONGUE
Harunganae madagascariensis cortex bark .. see HARONGA
Harunganae madagascariensis folium leaf .. see HARONGA
Haselnuss .... see HAZELNUT
Haselstrauch .... see HAZELNUT
Hash .... see MARIJUANA
Hashish .... see MARIJUANA
Hauhechelwurzel .... see SPINY RESTHARROW
Haw .... see HAWTHORN
HAWAIIAN BABY WOODROSE
.... see HAWAIIAN BABY WOODROSE
HAWTHORN .... see HAWTHORN
Hawthorn Extract .... see HAWTHORN
Hawthorn Flower .... see HAWTHORN
Hawthorn Fruit .... see HAWTHORN
Hawthorn Leaf .... see HAWTHORN
Hawthorne .... see HAWTHORN
Hay Flower .... see HAY FLOWER,
SWEET CLOVER
Hay Sack .... see HAY FLOWER
Hayflower .... see HAY FLOWER
Haymaids .... see GROUND IVY
Hayriffe .... see CLIVERS
Hayruff .... see CLIVERS
Hazel .... see HAZELNUT,
WITCH HAZEL
Hazel Alder .... see SMOOTH ALDER
Hazel Nut .... see HAZELNUT
HAZELNUT .... see HAZELNUT
Hazelwort .... see ASARABACCA
HCA .... see GARCINIA
He Shou Wu .... see FO-TI
He Zi .... see TERMINALIA
Headache .... see CORN POPPY
Headsman .... see BUCKHORN PLANTAIN
Headwark .... see CORN POPPY
Heal-All .... see FIGWORT,
SELF-HEAL,
STONE ROOT
Healing Herb .... see COMFREY
Heart of the Earth .... see SELF-HEAL
Heartleaf .... see COUNTRY MALLOW
HEART'S EASE .... see HEART'S EASE

Heartsease .... see HEART'S EASE
Heated Oyster Shell-Seaweed Calcium .... see CALCIUM
HEATHER .... see HEATHER
Heaven Tree .... see TREE OF HEAVEN
Heavy Kaolin .... see KAOLIN
Hedeoma pulegioides .... see PENNYROYAL leaf,
PENNYROYAL oil
Hedera helix .... see ENGLISH IVY
Hederae helicis folium .... see ENGLISH IVY
Hedge Bindweed .... see GREATER BINDWEED
Hedge-Burs .... see CLIVERS
Hedge Convolvulus .... see GREATER BINDWEED
Hedge Fumitory .... see FUMITORY
HEDGE-HYSSOP .... see HEDGE-HYSSOP
Hedge Lily .... see GREATER BINDWEED
HEDGE MUSTARD .... see HEDGE MUSTARD
Hedge Nettles .... see BETONY
Hedge Taper .... see MULLEIN
Hedgeheriff .... see CLIVERS
Hedgehog .... see ECHINACEA
Hedgemaids .... see GROUND IVY
Hedgethorn .... see HAWTHORN
Hediondilla .... see CHAPARRAL
Heeng .... see ASAFOETIDA
Heerabol .... see MYRRH
Hei Zao .... see JUJUBE
Helenium grandiflorum .... see ELECAMPANE
Helianthemum canadense .... see FROSTWORT
Helianthi Annui Oleum .... see SUNFLOWER OIL
Helianthus annuus .... see SUNFLOWER OIL
Helichrysum .... see SANDY EVERLASTING
Helichrysum arenarium .... see IMMORTELLE
Helichrysum augustifolium ... see SANDY EVERLASTING
Helichrysum italicum .... see SANDY EVERLASTING
Helichrysum oriental .... see SANDY EVERLASTING
Helichrysum stoechas .... see SANDY EVERLASTING
Helixor .... see EUROPEAN MISTLETOE
Helleborus niger .... see BLACK HELLEBORE
Hellweed .... see DODDER
Helmet Flower .... see SCULLCAP
Helonias .... see FALSE UNICORN
Helonias dioica .... see FALSE UNICORN
Helonias lutea .... see FALSE UNICORN
Hemicellulose Complex with Arabinoxylane ..... see MGN-3
HEMLOCK .... see HEMLOCK
Hemlock Bark .... see PINUS BARK
Hemlock Gum .... see PINUS BARK
HEMLOCK SPRUCE .... see HEMLOCK SPRUCE
Hemlock Spruce .... see PINUS BARK
HEMLOCK WATER DROPWORT
.... see HEMLOCK WATER DROPWORT
Hemlocktanne .... see PINUS BARK
Hemp .... see MARIJUANA
HEMP AGRIMONY .... see HEMP AGRIMONY
Hemp Tree .... see CHASTEBERRY
HEMPNETTLE .... see HEMPNETTLE
Hen Bell .... see HENBANE
Hen Of The Woods .... see MAITAKE MUSHROOM
HENBANE .... see HENBANE
Hendibeh .... see CHICORY
Henna .... see ALKANNA, HENNA
Hennae folium .... see HENNA
Henne .... see HENNA
Hens and Chickens .... see HOUSELEEK

Heparinoid Fraction .... see MESOGLYCAN
Heparinoids .... see MESOGLYCAN
Hepatica nobilis var. acuta .... see LIVERWORT
Hepatica nobilis var. obtusa .... see LIVERWORT
Hepatici noblis herba .... see LIVERWORT
Hépatique à Lobes Aigus .... see LIVERWORT
Hépatique d'Amérique .... see LIVERWORT
Heps .... see ROSE HIP
Heptacosanol .... see POLICOSANOL
Heracleum lanatum .... see MASTERWORT
Heracleum sphondylium .... see MASTERWORT
Herb Bennet .... see AVENS
Herb Gerard .... see GOUTWEED
Herb Louisa .... see LEMON VERBENA
Herb Margaret .... see OX-EYE DAISY
Herb of Grace .... see VERBENA
Herb of the Cross .... see VERBENA
HERB PARIS .... see HERB PARIS
Herb Perter .... see COWSLIP
HERB ROBERT .... see HERB ROBERT
Herb Trinity .... see LIVERWORT
Herb Two-Pence .... see MONEYWORT
Herba .... see SWEET VIOLET
Herba de la Pastora .... see DAMIANA
Herba de María .... see DIVINER'S SAGE
Herba Dictamni Herba .... see BURNING BUSH leaf,
                                                  BURNING BUSH root
Herba Epimedii .... see EPIMEDIUM
Herba eupatoriae .... see AGRIMONY
Herba fumariae .... see FUMITORY
Herba Malvae .... see MARSHMALLOW
Herbal Ecstasy .... see EPHEDRA
Herbe Aux Charpentiers .... see YARROW
Herbe d'Absinthe .... see WORMWOOD above ground parts
Herbe d'Aigremoine .... see AGRIMONY
Herbe de Hogweed .... see SCOTCH BROOM flower
Herbe de Sainte Cunegonde .... see HEMP AGRIMONY
Herbe de Saint-Guillaume .... see AGRIMONY
Herbed' Euphraise .... see EYEBRIGHT
Herb-of-Grace .... see RUE
Herb-of-the-Virgin .... see DIVINER'S SAGE
Herb-Paris .... see HERB PARIS
Herbygrass .... see RUE
Hercules Woundwort .... see SELF-HEAL
Herniaria glabra .... see RUPTUREWORT
Herniaria hirsuta .... see RUPTUREWORT
Herniariae herba .... see RUPTUREWORT
Herniary .... see RUPTUREWORT
Herpestis monniera .... see BRAHMI
Hervea .... see MATE
He Shou Wu .... see FO-TI
HESPERIDIN .... see HESPERIDIN
Hexacosanol .... see POLICOSANOL
Hexacosanol (26-C) .... see OCTACOSANOL
Hexahydroxycyclohexane .... see INOSITOL
Hexanicotinoyl Inositol .... see INOSITOL NICOTINATE
Hexanicotinyl cis-1,2,3-5-trans-4,6-cyclohexane
                   .... see INOSITOL NICOTINATE
Hexenbesen .... see EUROPEAN MISTLETOE
HIBISCUS .... see HIBISCUS
Hibiscus abelmoschus .... see AMBRETTE
Hibiscus sabdariffa .... see HIBISCUS
Hierba Carmín .... see POKEWEED berry,
                                                  POKEWEED root

Hierba de la Virgen .... see DIVINER'S SAGE
Hierba de San Juan .... see MUGWORT
Hierba Santa .... see YERBA SANTA
High Balm .... see OSWEGO TEA
High Mallow .... see MALLOW flower,
                                                     MALLOW leaf
Highbush Blueberry .... see BLUEBERRY
High-Bush Cranberry .... see CRAMP BARK
Highwaythorn .... see EUROPEAN BUCKTHORN
Higtaper .... see MULLEIN
Hilberry .... see WINTERGREEN leaf,
                                                 WINTERGREEN oil
Hillside Blueberry .... see BLUEBERRY
Himalayan Mayapple .... see PODOPHYLLUM
Himalayan Rhubarb .... see RHUBARB
Hind Heal .... see WOOD SAGE
Hindheal .... see TANSY
Hind's Tongue .... see HARTSTONGUE
Hing Hua .... see SAFFLOWER
Hini .... see BLACK ROOT
Hip .... see ROSE HIP
Hip Fruit .... see ROSE HIP
Hip Sweet .... see ROSE HIP
Hipberry .... see ROSE HIP
Hippocastani Cortex
         .... see HORSE CHESTNUT branch bark
Hippocastani Flos .... see HORSE CHESTNUT flower
Hippocastani folium .... see HORSE CHESTNUT leaf
Hippocastani Semen
         .... see HORSE CHESTNUT branch bark
Hippocastani Semen .... see HORSE CHESTNUT seed
Hippophae rhamnoides .... see SEA BUCKTHORN
Hipposelinum levisticum .... see LOVAGE
Hirala .... see TERMINALIA
Hirshklee .... see HEMP AGRIMONY
Hirudo medicinalis .... see LEECH
HISTIDINE .... see HISTIDINE
Hive Dross .... see PROPOLIS
Hive Vine .... see SQUAWVINE
HL-362 .... see FORSKOLIN
HMB .... see HYDROXYMETHYLBUTYRATE (HMB)
Ho Shou Wu .... see FO-TI
Hoarhound .... see BUGLEWEED,
                                          WHITE HOREHOUND
Hoary Plantain .... see BUCKHORN PLANTAIN
Hock-Heal .... see SELF-HEAL
Hockle Elderberry .... see LEVANT BERRY
Hoelen .... see PORIA MUSHROOM
Hog Apple .... see MORINDA,
                                             PODOPHYLLUM
Hog Bean .... see HENBANE
Hog Gum .... see TRAGACANTH
Hogberry .... see UVA URSI
Hogweed .... see KNOTWEED HERB,
                                          MASTERWORT,
                                    SCOTCH BROOM flower,
                                      SCOTCH BROOM herb
Hojas de la Pastora .... see DIVINER'S SAGE
Hoku-Gomishi .... see SCHISANDRA
Holligold .... see CALENDULA
HOLLY .... see HOLLY
Holly .... see PIPSISSEWA
Holly Barberry .... see OREGON GRAPE
Holly Bay .... see MAGNOLIA bark

INDEX

Holly Mahonia .... see OREGON GRAPE
HOLLYHOCK .... see HOLLYHOCK
Hollyhock Flower .... see HOLLYHOCK
Holly-Leaved Berberis .... see OREGON GRAPE
Holm .... see HOLLY
Holme Chase .... see HOLLY
Holunderbeeren .... see ELDERBERRY
Holy Basil .... see BASIL
Holy Herb .... see YERBA SANTA
Holy Rope .... see HEMP AGRIMONY
Holy Thistle .... see BLESSED THISTLE,
                                                    MILK THISTLE
Holy Tree .... see HOLLY, NEEM
Holy Weed .... see YERBA SANTA
Holywort .... see VERBENA
Honduras Sarsaparilla .... see SARSAPARILLA
HONEY .... see HONEY
Honey Bee Pollen .... see BEE POLLEN
Honey Bee's Milk .... see ROYAL JELLY
Honey Plant .... see LEMON BALM
Honey Suckle .... see HONEYSUCKLE
Honeybee Pollen .... see BEE POLLEN
Honeybee Venom .... see BEE VENOM
Honeybloom .... see CANADIAN HEMP
HONEYSUCKLE .... see HONEYSUCKLE
Hong Qu .... see RED YEAST
Hong Zao .... see JUJUBE
Honghua .... see SAFFLOWER
Honig .... see HONEY
Hoodwort .... see SCULLCAP
Hop Fruit .... see ROSE HIP
Hop Strobile .... see HOPS
Hop Strobiles .... see HOPS
Hopfenzapfen .... see HOPS
HOPS .... see HOPS
Hordeum .... see BARLEY
Hordeum distychum .... see BARLEY
Hordeum vulgare .... see BARLEY
Horehound .... see WHITE HOREHOUND
Horns of Gold .... see DEER VELVET
Hornseed .... see ERGOT
Horny Goat Weed .... see EPIMEDIUM
Horse Balm .... see STONE ROOT
Horse Blobs .... see MARSH MARIGOLD
Horse Chestnut .... see HORSE CHESTNUT branch bark,
                                    HORSE CHESTNUT flower,
                                    HORSE CHESTNUT leaf,
                                    HORSE CHESTNUT seed
HORSE CHESTNUT branch bark
        .... see HORSE CHESTNUT branch bark
HORSE CHESTNUT flower
        .... see HORSE CHESTNUT flower
HORSE CHESTNUT leaf ..... see HORSE CHESTNUT leaf
HORSE CHESTNUT seed ... see HORSE CHESTNUT seed
Horse Daisy .... see OX-EYE DAISY
Horse-Elder .... see ELECAMPANE
Horse Gowan .... see OX-EYE DAISY
Horse Tail .... see HORSETAIL
Horse Tongue .... see HARTSTONGUE
Horse Willow .... see HORSETAIL
Horsebane .... see HEMLOCK WATER DROPWORT,
                                    WATER FENNEL
Horsefly Weed .... see WILD INDIGO
Horsefoot .... see COLTSFOOT

Horseheal .... see ELECAMPANE
Horsehoof .... see COLTSFOOT
HORSEMINT .... see HORSEMINT
HORSERADISH .... see HORSERADISH
HORSETAIL .... see HORSETAIL
Horsetail .... see LAMINARIA
Horsetail Grass .... see HORSETAIL
Horsetail Rush .... see HORSETAIL
Horseweed .... see STONE ROOT
Horsewood .... see CANADIAN FLEABANE
Ho Shou Wu .... see FO-TI
Hot Pepper .... see CAPSICUM
Hou Po .... see MAGNOLIA bark,
                                    MAGNOLIA flower bud
Houblon .... see HOPS
Hound's Tongue .... see DEERTONGUE
HOUND'S TONGUE .... see HOUND'S TONGUE
Houndsbane .... see WHITE HOREHOUND
Houndsberry .... see BLACK NIGHTSHADE
HOUSELEEK .... see HOUSELEEK
HP 200 .... see COWHAGE
Hsia Ts'Ao Tung Ch'Ung .... see CORDYCEPS
Hsiang-Dan .... see ALOE dried juice from leaf, latex
Hu Lu Ba .... see FENUGREEK
Hua Gu .... see SHIITAKE MUSHROOM
Huacatay .... see TAGETES
Huang Ken .... see DANSHEN
Huang Lian .... see GOLDTHREAD
Huang Qi .... see ASTRAGALUS
Huang Qin .... see BAIKAL SKULLCAP
Huangquin .... see BAIKAL SKULLCAP
Huang-T'eng Ken .... see THUNDER GOD VINE
Huanuco Coca .... see COCA
Huckleberry .... see BILBERRY dried ripe fruit,
                                    BILBERRY leaf
Huile D'Onagre .... see EVENING PRIMROSE OIL
Huile De Bourrache .... see BORAGE SEED OIL
Huisache .... see CASSIE ABSOLUTE
Hulm .... see HOLLY
Hulver Bush .... see HOLLY
Hulver Tree .... see HOLLY
Humic Shale .... see COLLOIDAL MINERALS
Hummingbird Tree .... see TURTLE HEAD
Humulus lupulus .... see HOPS
Hungarian Chamomile .... see GERMAN CHAMOMILE
Hungarian Pepper .... see CAPSICUM
Huntsman's Cup .... see PITCHER PLANT
Huo xiang .... see PATCHOULY OIL
HupA .... see HUPERZINE A
Huperazon .... see CHINESE CLUB MOSS
Huperzia Serrata .... see CHINESE CLUB MOSS
Huperzine .... see HUPERZINE A
HUPERZINE A .... see HUPERZINE A
Hurtleberry .... see BILBERRY dried ripe fruit,
                                    BILBERRY leaf
Hurtsickle .... see CORNFLOWER
Husked Nut .... see EUROPEAN CHESTNUT
Hwanggi .... see ASTRAGALUS
Hwanggum .... see BAIKAL SKULLCAP
hybrid species .... see STINGING NETTLE root
Hydnocarp .... see CHAULMOOGRA
Hydnocarpus .... see CHAULMOOGRA
Hydnocarpus species .... see CHAULMOOGRA
HYDRANGEA .... see HYDRANGEA

Hydrangea arborescens ....see HYDRANGEA
Hydrastis .... see GOLDENSEAL
Hydrastis Canadensis......................... see GOLDENSEAL
Hydrated aluminum silicate ....see KAOLIN
Hydrazine ....see HYDRAZINE SULFATE
HYDRAZINE SULFATE .... see HYDRAZINE SULFATE
Hydrocotyle .... see GOTU KOLA
Hydrocotyle Asiatica ....see GOTU KOLA
Hydrocotyle Asiatique ....see GOTU KOLA
Hydrolyzed Liver Extract .... see LIVER EXTRACT
Hydrolyzed Soy Protein .... see SOY
Hydrolyzed Spleen Extract .... see SPLEEN EXTRACT
Hydroxocobalamin .... see VITAMIN B12
Hydroxocobalaminum .... see VITAMIN B12
Hydroxocobemine .... see VITAMIN B12
Hydroxyacetic acid (Glycolic acid)
.... see ALPHA HYDROXY ACIDS
Hydroxyapatite .... see CALCIUM
Hydroxycaprylic Acid ...... see ALPHA HYDROXY ACIDS
Hydroxycitrate .... see GARCINIA
Hydroxycitric Acid .... see GARCINIA
Hydroxymethyl Butyrate
.... see HYDROXYMETHYLBUTYRATE (HMB)
HYDROXYMETHYLBUTYRATE (HMB)
.... see HYDROXYMETHYLBUTYRATE (HMB)
Hydroxypropionic Acid .... see ALPHA HYDROXY ACIDS
Hydroxysuccinic Acid ...... see ALPHA HYDROXY ACIDS
Hyoscyami Folium .... see HENBANE
Hyoscyamus niger .... see HENBANE
Hypereikon .... see ST. JOHN'S WORT
Hyperici Herba .... see ST. JOHN'S WORT
Hypericum .... see ST. JOHN'S WORT
Hypericum perforatum .... see ST. JOHN'S WORT
Hyperimmune Bovine Colostrum
.... see BOVINE COLOSTRUM
Hypoxanthine Riboside .... see INOSINE
Hypoxanthosine .... see INOSINE
Hypoxis Plant .... see AFRICAN WILD POTATO
Hypoxis rooperi .... see AFRICAN WILD POTATO
HYSSOP .... see HYSSOP
Hyssopus officinalis .... see HYSSOP
I .... see IODINE
I3C .... see INDOLE-3-CARBINOL
Iandirova .... see ANDIROBA
Iberis amara .... see CLOWN'S MUSTARD PLANT
IBOGA .... see IBOGA
Ice Vine .... see PAREIRA
Iceland Lichen .... see ICELAND MOSS
ICELAND MOSS .... see ICELAND MOSS
Ichthyomethia piscipula .... see JAMAICAN DOGWOOD
Ici Fructus .... see CAPSICUM
Idrocotyle .... see GOTU KOLA
Idrossocobalamina .... see VITAMIN B12
Igelkopfwurzel .... see ECHINACEA
IGNATIUS BEAN .... see IGNATIUS BEAN
Ilex .... see MATE
Ilex aquifolium .... see HOLLY
Ilex opaca .... see HOLLY
Ilex paraguariensis .... see MATE
Ilex vomitoria .... see HOLLY
Illicium .... see STAR ANISE
Illicium verum .... see STAR ANISE
Imlee .... see TAMARIND
Immortality Herb .... see JIAOGULAN

IMMORTELLE .... see IMMORTELLE
Impatiens balsamina .... see JEWELWEED
Impatiens biflora .... see JEWELWEED
Impatiens capensis .... see JEWELWEED
Impatiens pallida .... see JEWELWEED
In Chen .... see YIN CHEN
Inchinko .... see YIN CHEN
Inchin-Ko-To .... see YIN CHEN
India Root .... see ALPINIA
Indian Almond .... see TERMINALIA
Indian Apple ....see PODOPHYLLUM
Indian Arrowroot .... see WAHOO, ZEDOARY
Indian Arrowwood .... see WAHOO
Indian Bael.. see BAEL
Indian Balm ....see BETH ROOT
Indian Balsam .... see PERU BALSAM
Indian Bark .... see MAGNOLIA bark
Indian Bdellium-Tree .... see GUGGUL
Indian Bead .... see PRECATORY BEAN
Indian Berry .... see LEVANT BERRY
Indian Bolonong .... see CHIRATA
Indian Bread .... see PORIA MUSHROOM
Indian Chocolate .... see WATER AVENS
Indian Corn .... see CORN SILK
Indian Cress .... see NASTURTIUM,
WATERCRESS
Indian Dye .... see GOLDENSEAL
Indian Echinacea .... see ANDROGRAPHIS
Indian Elm .... see SLIPPERY ELM
INDIAN FRANKINCENSE
.... see INDIAN FRANKINCENSE
Indian Gentian .... see CHIRATA
Indian Ginseng .... see ASHWAGANDHA
INDIAN GOOSEBERRY ..... see INDIAN GOOSEBERRY
Indian Gum .... see CUP PLANT
Indian Head .... see ECHINACEA
Indian-Hemp .... see CANADIAN HEMP
Indian Hippo .... see INDIAN PHYSIC
Indian-laurel .... see LAURELWOOD
Indian Lilac .... see NEEM
INDIAN LONG PEPPER ...... see INDIAN LONG PEPPER
Indian Mulberry .... see MORINDA
Indian Olibanum .... see INDIAN FRANKINCENSE
Indian Parsley .... see OSHA
Indian Pennywort.................... see GOTU KOLA
Indian Physic .... see CANADIAN HEMP
INDIAN PHYSIC .... see INDIAN PHYSIC
Indian Pink....................... see PINK ROOT
Indian Plant .... see BLOODROOT,
GOLDENSEAL
Indian Plantago .... see BLOND PSYLLIUM
Indian Podophyllum ....see PODOPHYLLUM
Indian Poke .... see AMERICAN HELLEBORE
Indian Red Paint .... see BLOODROOT
Indian Rhubarb .... see RHUBARB
Indian Root .... see AMERICAN SPIKENARD
Indian Saffron .... see SAFFRON, TURMERIC
Indian Sage .... see BONESET
Indian Senna .... see SENNA
Indian Shamrock ....see BETH ROOT
INDIAN SNAKEROOT .... see INDIAN SNAKEROOT
Indian Squill .... see SQUILL
Indian Tobacco .... see LOBELIA
Indian Tragacanth .... see KARAYA GUM

INDEX

Indian Tumeric .... see GOLDENSEAL
Indian Valerian .... see VALERIAN
Indian Walnut .... see TUNG SEED
Indian Water Navelwort .... see GOTU KOLA
Indigo Broom .... see WILD INDIGO
Indischer Wassernabel .... see GOTU KOLA
INDOLE-3-CARBINOL .... see INDOLE-3-CARBINOL
Indole-3-methanol .... see INDOLE-3-CARBINOL
Inkberry .... see POKEWEED berry,
                                            POKEWEED root
Inorganic Germanium .... see GERMANIUM
Inose .... see INOSITOL
INOSINE .... see INOSINE
Inosite .... see INOSITOL
INOSITOL .... see INOSITOL
Inositol Hexaniacinate .... see INOSITOL NICOTINATE
Inositol Hexanicotinate .... see INOSITOL NICOTINATE
Inositol Hexaphosphate .... see IP-6
Inositol Monophosphate .... see INOSITOL
Inositol Niacinate .... see INOSITOL NICOTINATE
INOSITOL NICOTINATE ... see INOSITOL NICOTINATE
Intoxicating Pepper .... see KAVA
Intrachol .... see CHOLINE
Intralipid .... see SOYBEAN OIL
Inula .... see ELECAMPANE
Inula helenium .... see ELECAMPANE
IODINE .... see IODINE
IP-6 .... see IP-6
Ipe Roxo .... see PAU D'ARCO
IPECAC .... see IPECAC
Ipecacuanha .... see IPECAC
Ipes .... see PAU D'ARCO
Ipomoea .... see MEXICAN SCAMMONY ROOT
Ipomoea orizabensis
        .... see MEXICAN SCAMMONY ROOT
Ipomoea purga .... see JALAP
Iporoni .... see IPORURU
Iporuro .... see IPORURU
IPORURU .... see IPORURU
IPRIFLAVONE .... see IPRIFLAVONE
Ipurosa .... see IPORURU
Ipururo .... see IPORURU
Iris .... see BLUE FLAG, ORRIS
Iris caroliniana .... see BLUE FLAG
Iris florentina .... see ORRIS
Iris germanica .... see ORRIS
Iris Versicolor .... see BLUE FLAG
Iris virginica .... see BLUE FLAG
Iris x germanica var. florentina .... see ORRIS
Irish Broom .... see SCOTCH BROOM herb
Irish Broom Tops .... see SCOTCH BROOM flower
Irish Moss Extract .... see CARRAGEENAN
Irish Potato .... see POTATO
IRON .... see IRON
Iron Edta .... see EDTA
Isatis indigota .... see DA QING YE
Iscador .... see EUROPEAN MISTLETOE
Iso-Ascorbic Acid ..... see VITAMIN C (ASCORBIC ACID)
Isoflavone .... see KUDZU, LICORICE,
                                            RED CLOVER, SOY
Isoflavones .... see KUDZU, LICORICE
                                            RED CLOVER, SOY
Isoleucine .... see BRANCHED-CHAIN AMINO ACIDS
Isorel .... see EUROPEAN MISTLETOE

Ispaghula .... see BLOND PSYLLIUM
Ispagol .... see BLOND PSYLLIUM
Italian Fitch .... see GOAT'S RUE
Italian Jasmine .... see JASMINE
Italian Limetta .... see LIME fruit, peel, LIME oil
Itchweed .... see AMERICAN HELLEBORE
Ivy .... see AMERICAN IVY,
                                            ENGLISH IVY
Ivy-Leafed Cyclamen .... see CYCLAMEN
JABORANDI .... see JABORANDI
Jaborandi Pepper .... see INDIAN LONG PEPPER
Jack-Jump-About .... see GOUTWEED
Jack-of-the-Buttery .... see COMMON STONECROP
JACOB'S LADDER .... see JACOB'S LADDER
Jacob's Ladder .... see LILY-OF-THE-VALLEY
Jacob's Staff .... see MULLEIN
Jacob's Sword .... see ORRIS
Jaffa Orange .... see SWEET ORANGE
Jaguar Gum .... see GUAR GUM
Jalanimba .... see BRAHMI
JALAP .... see JALAP
Jalap .... see POKEWEED berry,
                                            POKEWEED root
Jalapa .... see JALAP
Jalape .... see JALAP
Jalnaveri .... see BRAHMI
Jamaica Dogwood .... see JAMAICAN DOGWOOD
Jamaica Ginger .... see GINGER
Jamaica Mignonette .... see HENNA
Jamaica Pepper .... see ALLSPICE
Jamaica Sorrel .... see HIBISCUS
JAMAICAN DOGWOOD ... see JAMAICAN DOGWOOD
Jamaican Quassia .... see QUASSIA
Jamaican Sarsaparilla .... see SARSAPARILLA
Jambolan .... see JAMBOLAN bark,
                                            JAMBOLAN seed
JAMBOLAN bark .... see JAMBOLAN bark
JAMBOLAN seed .... see JAMBOLAN seed
Jambul .... see JAMBOLAN bark,
                                            JAMBOLAN seed
James' Tea .... see MARSH TEA
Jamestown Weed .... see JIMSON WEED
Jamguarandi .... see JABORANDI
Jamum .... see JAMBOLAN bark,
                                            JAMBOLAN seed
Japanese Arrowroot .... see KUDZU
Japanese Belladonna .... see SCOPOLIA
Japanese Epimedium .... see EPIMEDIUM
Japanese Ginseng .... see GINSENG, PANAX
Japanese Isinglas .... see AGAR
JAPANESE MINT .... see JAPANESE MINT
Japanese Silver Apricot
        .... see GINKGO leaf (GINKGO leaf extract),
                                            GINKGO seed
JASMINE .... see JASMINE
Jasminium grandiflorum .... see JASMINE
Jasminium officinale .... see JASMINE
Jateorhiza palmata .... see COLOMBO
Jaundice Berry .... see EUROPEAN BARBERRY
Jaundice Root .... see GOLDENSEAL
Java .... see COFFEE
Java Coca .... see COCA
Java Pepper .... see CUBEBS
Java Plum .... see JAMBOLAN bark,
                                            JAMBOLAN seed

JAVA TEA .... see JAVA TEA
JAVANESE TURMERIC .... see JAVANESE TURMERIC
Jequirity Bean .... see PRECATORY BEAN
Jequirity Seed .... see PRECATORY BEAN
Jersey Tea .... see NEW JERSEY TEA
Jesuit Tea .... see CHENOPODIUM OIL
Jesuit's Balsam .... see COPAIBA BALSAM
Jesuit's Bark .... see CINCHONA
Jesuit's Brazil Tea .... see MATE
Jesuit's Tea .... see MATE
Jewel Balsam Weed .... see JEWELWEED
Jewel Weed .... see JEWELWEED
JEWELWEED .... see JEWELWEED
Jew's Harp Plant .... see BETH ROOT
Jew's Myrtle .... see BUTCHER'S BROOM
JIAOGULAN .... see JIAOGULAN
JIMSON WEED .... see JIMSON WEED
Jintsam .... see GINSENG, PANAX
Jinyingzi .... see CHEROKEE ROSEHIP
Jinyinhua .... see HONEYSUCKLE
Joe Pye .... see GRAVEL ROOT
Joe-Pye Weed .... see GRAVEL ROOT
Johimbi .... see YOHIMBE
Johnny-Jump-Up .... see HEART'S EASE
Johns Wort .... see ST. JOHN'S WORT
Joint Fir .... see EPHEDRA
Joint-Podded Charlock .... see WILD RADISH
JOJOBA .... see JOJOBA
Joshua Tree .... see YUCCA
Ju Hua .... see CHRYSANTHEMUM
Juarandi .... see JABORANDI
Juglandis .... see ENGLISH WALNUT
Juglandis Folium .... see ENGLISH WALNUT
Juglans .... see ENGLISH WALNUT
Juglans cinerea .... see BUTTERNUT
Juglans nigra .... see BLACK WALNUT
Juglans regia .... see ENGLISH WALNUT
JUJUBE .... see JUJUBE
Jujube Plum .... see JUJUBE
Jujubi .... see JUJUBE
Jumbul .... see JAMBOLAN bark,
                                  JAMBOLAN seed
Jungle Weed .... see OPIUM ANTIDOTE
JUNIPER .... see JUNIPER
Juniper Tar .... see CADE OIL
Juniper Tar Oil .... see CADE OIL
Juniperi fructus .... see JUNIPER
Juniperus communis .... see JUNIPER
Juniperus mexicana (Cedarwood Oil Texas)
            .... see CEDARWOOD OIL
Juniperus oxycedrus .... see CADE OIL
Juniperus sabina .... see SAVIN TOPS
Juniperus virginiana
     .... see CEDARWOOD bark, berry, leaf, seed, twig
Juniperus virginiana (Cedarwood Oil Virginia)
            .... see CEDARWOOD OIL
Juno's Tears .... see VERBENA
Jupiter's Bean .... see HENBANE
Jupiter's Beard .... see HOUSELEEK
Jupiter's Eye .... see HOUSELEEK
Jupiter's Nut .... see EUROPEAN CHESTNUT
Justicia Adhatoda .... see MALABAR NUT
Justicia paniculata .... see ANDROGRAPHIS
Ju-Zhong .... see SAW PALMETTO

K .... see POTASSIUM
Kaa Jhee .... see STEVIA
Kadaya .... see KARAYA GUM
Kadeol .... see CADE OIL
Kadira .... see KARAYA GUM
Kaffree Tea .... see RED BUSH TEA
Kalmegh .... see ANDROGRAPHIS
Kalmia latifolia .... see MOUNTAIN LAUREL
KAMALA .... see KAMALA
Kamani Punna .... see LAURELWOOD
Kamcela .... see KAMALA
Kameela .... see KAMALA
Kamillen .... see GERMAN CHAMOMILE
Kanaje Hindi .... see ASHWAGANDHA
Kansas Snakeroot .... see ECHINACEA
KAOLIN .... see KAOLIN
Karaya .... see KARAYA GUM
KARAYA GUM .... see KARAYA GUM
Kardone .... see ARTICHOKE
Karela .... see BITTER MELON
Kargasok Tea .... see KOMBUCHA TEA
Kariyat .... see ANDROGRAPHIS
Karkade .... see HIBISCUS
Kastanienblaetter .... see EUROPEAN CHESTNUT
Kat .... see KHAT
Katila .... see KARAYA GUM
Katsenpfotchenbluten .... see CAT'S FOOT
Katzenkrat .... see YARROW
Katzenpfotchenbluten .... see SANDY EVERLASTING
Kaugummibaum .... see CHICLE
Kaunch .... see COWHAGE
KAVA .... see KAVA
Kava Kava .... see KAVA
Kava Pepper .... see KAVA
Kava Root .... see KAVA
Kawa .... see KAVA
Kawa-Kawa .... see KAVA
Kawanch .... see COWHAGE
Kawaratake .... see CORIOLUS MUSHROOM
Kawara-Yomogi .... see YIN CHEN
Keiri .... see WALLFLOWER
Kelp .... see BLADDERWRACK,
                                  LAMINARIA
Kelp Ware .... see BLADDERWRACK
Kephalin .... see PHOSPHATIDYLSERINE
Kermesbeere .... see POKEWEED berry,
                                  POKEWEED root
Kew .... see KAVA
Kew Tree .... see GINKGO leaf (GINKGO leaf extract),
                                  GINKGO seed
Key Flower .... see COWSLIP
Key Lime .... see LIME oil
Key of Heaven .... see COWSLIP
KH-3 .... see PROCAINE
Khareti .... see COUNTRY MALLOW
Khartoum Senna .... see SENNA
Khas-khas .... see VETIVER
KHAT .... see KHAT
KHELLA .... see KHELLA
Khella Fruit .... see KHELLA
Khellin .... see KHELLA
Kher .... see ACACIA
Khus Khus .... see VETIVER
Khus-khus Grass .... see VETIVER

INDEX

Kidney Bean .... see BEAN POD
Kidney Root .... see GRAVEL ROOT
Kidney Wort .... see LIVERWORT
Kif .... see MARIJUANA
Kijitsu .... see BITTER ORANGE
Kiln-Dried Allspice .... see ALLSPICE
Kinerase .... see KINETIN
Kinetase .... see KINETIN
KINETIN .... see KINETIN
King Cups .... see MARSH MARIGOLD
King of Bitters .... see ANDROGRAPHIS
King of Mushrooms .... see MAITAKE MUSHROOM
Kings And Queens .... see ARUM
King's Clover .... see SWEET CLOVER
King's Crown .... see ROSEROOT
King's Cup .... see BULBOUS BUTTERCUP
King's Cure .... see PIPSISSEWA
King's Cureall
.... see EVENING PRIMROSE OIL, PIPSISSEWA
Kinnikinnik .... see UVA URSI
Kirta .... see ANDROGRAPHIS
Kita-Gomishi .... see SCHISANDRA
Kiwach .... see COWHAGE
KIWI .... see KIWI
Kiwi Fruit .... see KIWI
Klamath Blue/Green Algae
.... see BLUE-GREEN ALGAE
Klamath Weed .... see ST. JOHN'S WORT
Klapperschlangen .... see SENEGA
Kleine Kamille .... see GERMAN CHAMOMILE
Knackweide .... see WILLOW BARK
Knautia arvensis .... see FIELD SCABIOUS
Knee Holly .... see BUTCHER'S BROOM
Kneeholm .... see BUTCHER'S BROOM
Kniepp Hay Sack .... see HAY FLOWER
Knight's Spur .... see DELPHINIUM,
                                      LARKSPUR
Knitback .... see COMFREY
Knitbone .... see COMFREY
Knob Grass .... see STONE ROOT
Knob Root .... see STONE ROOT
Knobweed .... see STONE ROOT
Knot Grass .... see KNOTWEED HERB
Knotgrass .... see KNOTWEED HERB
Knotted Marjoram .... see MARJORAM
Knotted Wrack .... see BLADDERWRACK
Knotty Brake .... see MALE FERN
Knotweed .... see KNOTWEED HERB
KNOTWEED HERB .... see KNOTWEED HERB
Kojo-Kon .... see RESVERATROL
Kola Nut .... see COLA NUT
Koloquinthen .... see COLOCYNTH
Kombe .... see STROPHANTHUS
Kombe-Strophanthus Seeds ...... see STROPHANTHUS
Kombu .... see LAMINARIA
Kombucha Mushroom Tea .... see KOMBUCHA TEA
KOMBUCHA TEA .... see KOMBUCHA TEA
Konjac .... see GLUCOMANNAN
Konjac Mannan .... see GLUCOMANNAN
Kooso .... see KOUSSO
Korean Ginseng .... see GINSENG, PANAX
Korean Panax Ginseng .... see GINSENG, PANAX
Korean Red Ginseng .... see GINSENG, PANAX
Koriander .... see CORIANDER

Kosho .... see BLACK PEPPER AND WHITE PEPPER
Kosso .... see KOUSSO
KOUSSO .... see KOUSSO
Kraftwurz .... see ARNICA
Krameria .... see RHATANY
Krameria argentea .... see RHATANY
Krameria triandra .... see RHATANY
Kranbeere .... see CRANBERRY
Krestin .... see CORIOLUS MUSHROOM
Kreuzdornbeeren .... see EUROPEAN BUCKTHORN
Kua .... see ZEDOARY
Kuandong Hua .... see COLTSFOOT
Kudsu .... see KUDZU
KUDZU .... see KUDZU
Kudzu Vine .... see KUDZU
Kuguazi .... see BITTER MELON
K'u-Kua .... see BITTER MELON
Kukui .... see TUNG SEED
Kullo .... see KARAYA GUM
Kummel .... see CARAWAY dried fruit, seed
Kummich .... see CARAWAY dried fruit, seed
Kunigundendraut .... see HEMP AGRIMONY
Kuntze Saloop .... see SASSAFRAS
Kus es Salahin .... see KHAT
Kuthmithi .... see ASHWAGANDHA
Kwaao Khruea .... see KUDZU
Kwassan .... see KOMBUCHA TEA
Kydney Root .... see GRAVEL ROOT
Kyunchinho .... see YIN CHEN
L Arginine .... see L-ARGININE
L-(+)-2-Aminoglutaramic acid .... see GLUTAMINE
L(+)-ornithine alpha-ketoglutarate
.... see ORNITHINE KETOGLUTARATE
L. Acidophilus .... see LACTOBACILLUS
L. johnsonii LC-1 .... see LACTOBACILLUS
L-2,5-diaminovaleric acid .... see ORNITHINE
L-2,6-diaminohexanoic acid .... see LYSINE
L-2-Amino-3-(1H-imidazol-4-yl) propionic acid
.... see HISTIDINE
L-2-amino-3-(indole-3-yl) propionic acid
.... see L-TRYPTOPHAN
L-2-amino-4-(methylthio)butyric acid ... see METHIONINE
L-3-hydroxy-4-(trimethylammonium)-butyrate
.... see L-CARNITINE
L-5 HTP .... see 5-HTP
L-5 HYDROXYTRYPTOPHAN .... see 5-HTP
L-5-aminorvaline .... see ORNITHINE
L-75-1362B .... see FORSKOLIN
La Hembra .... see DIVINER'S SAGE
LABDANUM .... see LABDANUM
LABRADOR TEA .... see LABRADOR TEA
Labrador Tea .... see MARSH TEA
LABURNUM .... see LABURNUM
Lac .... see SHELLAC
Lacca .... see SHELLAC
Laccifer .... see SHELLAC
L-acetylcarnitine .... see ACETYL-L-CARNITINE
Laciniaria spicata .... see MARSH BLAZING STAR
LACTASE .... see LACTASE
Lactic Acid .... see ALPHA HYDROXY ACIDS
Lacto Bacillus .... see LACTOBACILLUS
Lactobacilli .... see LACTOBACILLUS
LACTOBACILLUS .... see LACTOBACILLUS
Lactobacillus Acidophilus .... see LACTOBACILLUS

Lactobacillus brevis .... see LACTOBACILLUS
Lactobacillus Bulgaricus .... see LACTOBACILLUS
Lactobacillus casei sp. rhamnosus .. see LACTOBACILLUS
Lactobacillus delbrueckii............... see LACTOBACILLUS
Lactobacillus fermentum .... see LACTOBACILLUS
Lactobacillus GG .... see LACTOBACILLUS
Lactobacillus johnsonii .... see LACTOBACILLUS
Lactobacillus Plantarum .... see LACTOBACILLUS
Lactobacillus Rhamnosus .... see LACTOBACILLUS
Lactobacillus rhamnosus GG .... see LACTOBACILLUS
LACTOFERRIN .... see LACTOFERRIN
lactoferrins .... see LACTOFERRIN
Lactoflavin .... see RIBOFLAVIN (VITAMIN B2)
Lactuca virosa .... see WILD LETTUCE
Lactucarium .... see WILD LETTUCE
Ladder-To-Heaven .... see LILY-OF-THE-VALLEY
Ladies' Delight .... see HEART'S EASE
Ladies' Seal .... see BRYONIA
Lady Bleeding .... see AMARANTH
LADY FERN .... see LADY FERN
Lady Of The Meadow .... see MEADOWSWEET
LADY'S BEDSTRAW .... see LADY'S BEDSTRAW
Lady's Mantle .... see ALCHEMILLA
Lady's Nightcap .... see GREATER BINDWEED
Lady's Purse .... see SHEPHERD'S PURSE
Lady's Seals .... see SOLOMON'S SEAL
Lady's Slipper .... see NERVE ROOT
Lady's Thimble .... see DIGITALIS
Lady's Thistle .... see MILK THISTLE
Ladysmock .... see ARUM
Laetrile .... see APRICOT
Lai Margose .... see BITTER MELON
Lakritze .... see LICORICE
Lamb Mint .... see PEPPERMINT leaf, SPEARMINT
Lambkill .... see MOUNTAIN LAUREL
Lamb's Quarters .... see BETH ROOT
Lamb's Tongue .... see AMERICAN ADDER'S TONGUE
Lamii Albi Flos ..... see WHITE DEAD NETTLE FLOWER
LAMINARIA .... see LAMINARIA
Laminaria digitata .... see ALGIN, LAMINARIA
Laminaria japonica .... see LAMINARIA
Lamiumalbum .... see WHITE DEAD NETTLE FLOWER
Lamp Black .... see ACTIVATED CHARCOAL
Land Whin .... see SPINY RESTHARROW
Langer Pfeffer .... see INDIAN LONG PEPPER
Langwort .... see BUTTERBUR,
                                                    WHITE HELLEBORE
Lan-Hiqui .... see SANGRE DE GRADO
Laniqui .... see SANGRE DE GRADO
Lapacho .... see PAU D'ARCO
Lapacho Colorado .... see PAU D'ARCO
Lapacho Morado .... see PAU D'ARCO
Lappa .... see BURDOCK
Larch .... see LARCH ARABINOGALACTAN
LARCH ARABINOGALACTAN
.... see LARCH ARABINOGALACTAN
Larch Gum .... see LARCH ARABINOGALACTAN
LARCH TURPENTINE .... see LARCH TURPENTINE
Large Cranberry .... see CRANBERRY
Large Fennel .... see FENNEL fruit, seed
Large Indian Civet .... see CIVET
Large-Leaved Germander .... see WOOD SAGE
L-ARGININE .... see L-ARGININE
L-Arginine HCl.. see L-ARGININE

L-Arginine Hydrochloride .... see L-ARGININE
Larix .... see LARCH ARABINOGALACTAN
Larix dahurica .... see LARCH ARABINOGALACTAN
Larix decidua .... see LARCH TURPENTINE
Larix occidentalis ...... see LARCH ARABINOGALACTAN
Lark Heel .... see DELPHINIUM, LARKSPUR
Lark's Claw .... see DELPHINIUM, LARKSPUR
Lark's Toe .... see DELPHINIUM, LARKSPUR
Larkspur .... see DELPHINIUM
LARKSPUR .... see LARKSPUR
Larkspur Lion's Mouth .... see YELLOW TOADFLAX
Larrea divaricata .... see CHAPARRAL
Larrea tridentata .... see CHAPARRAL
LATHYRUS .... see LATHYRUS
Lathyrus cicera .... see LATHYRUS
Lathyrus clymenu .... see LATHYRUS
Lathyrus hirsutus .... see LATHYRUS
Lathyrus incanus .... see LATHYRUS
Lathyrus odoratus .... see LATHYRUS
Lathyrus pusillus .... see LATHYRUS
Lathyrus sativus .... see LATHYRUS
Lathyrus sylvestris .... see LATHYRUS
Laurel .... see MOUNTAIN LAUREL,
                                                           SWEET BAY
Laurel Camphor .... see CAMPHOR
Laurel Willow .... see WILLOW BARK
LAURELWOOD .... see LAURELWOOD
Laurocerasus Leaves .... see CHERRY LAUREL WATER
Laurocerasus officinalis .... see CHERRY LAUREL WATER
Laurus Cinnamomum .... see CINNAMON bark
Laurus nobilis .... see SWEET BAY
Laurus persea .... see AVOCADO
Lavandula angustifolia .... see LAVENDER
Lavandula dentata .... see LAVENDER
Lavandula latifolia .... see LAVENDER
Lavandula officinalis .... see LAVENDER
Lavandula pubescens .... see LAVENDER
Lavandula spica .... see LAVENDER
Lavandula stoechas .... see LAVENDER
Lavandula vera .... see LAVENDER
LAVENDER .... see LAVENDER
LAVENDER COTTON .... see LAVENDER COTTON
Lavose... see LOVAGE
Lawsonia alba .... see HENNA
Lawsonia inermis .... see HENNA
Layor Carang .... see AGAR
LC-1 L. johnsonii .... see LACTOBACILLUS
L-CARNITINE .... see L-CARNITINE
L-carnitine Propionyl ...... see PROPIONYL-L-CARNITINE
L-Carnosine .... see CARNOSINE
L-Cysteine .... see N-ACETYL CYSTEINE
Leaves of the Virgin Shepherdess .... see DIVINER'S SAGE
Leberbluemchenkraut .... see LIVERWORT
Leberkraut .... see HEMP AGRIMONY
Leche de Higueron .... see FICIN
Leche de Oje .... see FICIN
Leci PS .... see PHOSPHATIDYLSERINE
LECITHIN .... see LECITHIN
Lecithin Phosphatidylserine
.... see PHOSPHATIDYLSERINE
Ledi palustris herba .... see MARSH TEA
Ledum groenlandicum .... see LABRADOR TEA
Ledum latifolium .... see LABRADOR TEA
Ledum palustre .... see LABRADOR TEA,
                                                           MARSH TEA

LEECH .... see LEECH
Leeches .... see LEECH
Legalon .... see MILK THISTLE
Legume .... see BEAN POD, CALABAR BEAN,
             LABURNUM, PRECATORY BEAN,
             SOY, SOYBEAN OIL, TONKA BEAN
Lei Gong Teng .... see THUNDER GOD VINE
Lei-Kung T'eng .... see THUNDER GOD VINE
Leimmistel .... see EUROPEAN MISTLETOE
Leinsamen .... see FLAXSEED
LEMON .... see LEMON
LEMON BALM .... see LEMON BALM
Lemon Grass .... see LEMONGRASS
Lemon-Scented Verbena .... see LEMON VERBENA
LEMON VERBENA .... see LEMON VERBENA
Lemon Walnut .... see BUTTERNUT
LEMONGRASS .... see LEMONGRASS
Lent Lily .... see DAFFODIL
Lenticus edodes .... see LENTINAN,
             SHIITAKE MUSHROOM
Lentinan .... see BETA GLUCANS
LENTINAN .... see LENTINAN
Lentinan edodes .... see LENTINAN,
             SHIITAKE MUSHROOM
Lentinula .... see SHIITAKE MUSHROOM
Lentinula edodes .... see LENTINAN,
             SHIITAKE MUSHROOM
Lentinus edodes .... see SHIITAKE MUSHROOM
Lentisk .... see MASTIC
Leontodon taracum ... see DANDELION above ground parts
Leontodon taraxacum .... see DANDELION entire plant
Leontopodium .... see ALCHEMILLA
Leonuri cardiacae herba .... see MOTHERWORT
Leonurus .... see MOTHERWORT
Leonurus cardiaca and other Leonurus species
             .... see MOTHERWORT
Leopard's Bane .... see ARNICA
Leopard's Foot .... see MARSH MARIGOLD
Lepidium meyenii .... see MACA
Lepidium sativum .... see GARDEN CRESS
Leptandra virginica .... see BLACK ROOT
LESSER CELANDINE .... see LESSER CELANDINE
Lesser Centauru .... see CENTAURY
Lesser Dodder .... see DODDER
Lesser Hemlock .... see FOOL'S PARSLEY
Lesser Periwinkle .... see PERIWINKLE
Lettsomia nervosa .... see HAWAIIAN BABY WOODROSE
Lettuce Opium .... see WILD LETTUCE
Leucanthemum parthenium .... see FEVERFEW
Leucine .... see BRANCHED-CHAIN AMINO ACIDS
Leucoanthocyanidins .... see PYCNOGENOL
Leucoanthocyanin .... see GRAPE seed
Levacecarnine .... see ACETYL-L-CARNITINE
Levant .... see WORMSEED
LEVANT BERRY .... see LEVANT BERRY
Levant Nut .... see LEVANT BERRY
Levant Salep .... see SALEP
Levant Storax .... see STORAX
Levistici radix .... see LOVAGE
Levisticum officinale .... see LOVAGE
Levocarnitine .... see L-CARNITINE
Levoglutamide .... see GLUTAMINE
Levoglutamine .... see GLUTAMINE
Levo-Histidine .... see HISTIDINE

Levure De Biere .... see BREWER'S YEAST
L-Glutamic Acid .... see GLUTAMINE
L-Glutamic Acid 5-Amide .... see GLUTAMINE
L-Glutamine .... see GLUTAMINE
L-Glutathione .... see GLUTATHIONE
L-Histidine .... see HISTIDINE
LI 132 .... see HAWTHORN
Lian Fang .... see LOTUS flower
Lian Xu .... see LOTUS flower
Lian Zi .... see LOTUS seed
Liatris .... see DEERTONGUE
Liatris callilepis .... see MARSH BLAZING STAR
Liatris odoratis .... see DEERTONGUE
Liatris spicata .... see MARSH BLAZING STAR
Lichen Islandicus .... see ICELAND MOSS
Lichen Oak Moss .... see OAK MOSS
Lichwort .... see PELLITORY-OF-THE-WALL
LICORICE .... see LICORICE
Licorice Root .... see LICORICE
Life Everlasting .... see CAT'S FOOT
Life-giving Vine of Peru .... see CAT'S CLAW
Life of Man .... see AMERICAN SPIKENARD
Life Root .... see ALPINE RAGWORT,
             GOLDEN RAGWORT
Liferoot .... see ALPINE RAGWORT,
             GOLDEN RAGWORT
Light Kaolin .... see KAOLIN
Lignum rhodium .... see ROSEROOT
Ligusticum levisticum .... see LOVAGE
Ligusticum porteri .... see OSHA
Ligustilides .... see DONG QUAI
Ligustro .... see GLOSSY PRIVET
Ligustrum .... see GLOSSY PRIVET
Ligustrum Fruit .... see GLOSSY PRIVET
Ligustrum lucidum .... see GLOSSY PRIVET
Lilium candidium .... see WHITE LILY
Lilium martagon .... see MARTAGON
Lily .... see LILY-OF-THE-VALLEY
Lily of the Desert .... see ALOE dried juice from leaf, latex
LILY-OF-THE-VALLEY .... see LILY-OF-THE-VALLEY
Lime .... see LIME fruit, peel, LIME oil
Lime Blossom .... see LINDEN dried flower
Lime Flower .... see LINDEN dried flower
LIME fruit, peel .... see LIME fruit, peel
LIME oil .... see LIME oil
Lime Tree .... see LINDEN CHARCOAL,
             LINDEN dried flower, LINDEN dried leaf,
             LINDEN dried sapwood
Limette .... see LIME fruit, peel, LIME oil
Limon .... see LEMON
Limonnik Kitajskij .... see SCHISANDRA
Linaria vulgaris .... see YELLOW TOADFLAX
Linden .... see LINDEN dried flower,
             LINDEN dried leaf,
             LINDEN dried sapwood
LINDEN CHARCOAL .... see LINDEN CHARCOAL
LINDEN dried flower .... see LINDEN dried flower
LINDEN dried leaf .... see LINDEN dried leaf
LINDEN dried sapwood .... see LINDEN dried sapwood
Linden Tree .... see LINDEN dried flower
Linden Wood .... see LINDEN dried sapwood
Ling .... see HEATHER
Ling Chih .... see REISHI MUSHROOM
Ling Zhi .... see REISHI MUSHROOM

Lingen .... see ALPINE CRANBERRY
Lingenberry .... see ALPINE CRANBERRY
Lingon .... see ALPINE CRANBERRY
Lingonberry .... see ALPINE CRANBERRY
Lingum Vitae .... see GUAIAC WOOD resin, wood
Lini Semen .... see FLAXSEED
Linoleic .... see CONJUGATED LINOLEIC ACID
Linoleic Acid .... see FLAXSEED OIL
Linseed .... see FLAXSEED
Linseed Oil .... see FLAXSEED OIL
Lint Bells .... see FLAXSEED
Linum .... see FLAXSEED
Linum catharticum .... see MOUNTAIN FLAX
Linum usitatissimum .... see FLAXSEED,
                                                    FLAXSEED OIL
Lion's Ear .... see MOTHERWORT
Lion's Foot .... see ALCHEMILLA
Lion's Mouth .... see DIGITALIS
Lion's Tail .... see MOTHERWORT
Lion's Tooth .... see DANDELION above ground parts
                                  DANDELION entire plant
LIPASE .... see LIPASE
Lipoic Acid .... see ALPHA-LIPOIC ACID
Lipoicin .... see ALPHA-LIPOIC ACID
Lipositol .... see INOSITOL
Lipotropic Factor .... see CHOLINE
Lippia citriodora .... see LEMON VERBENA
Liquid Amber .... see STORAX
Liquid Liver Extract .... see LIVER EXTRACT
Liquid Oxygen .... see VITAMIN O
Liquid Storax .... see STORAX
Liquidambar styraciflua .... see STORAX
Liquidamber orientalis .... see STORAX
Liquiritiae radix .... see LICORICE
Liquirizia .... see LICORICE
Liquorice .... see LICORICE
L-Isoleucine ...... see BRANCHED-CHAIN AMINO ACIDS
Little Dragon .... see TARRAGON
Little Pollom .... see BITTER MILKWORT
Live Culture Yogurt .... see YOGURT
Liveforever .... see HOUSELEEK
Liver .... see LIVER EXTRACT
Liver Concentrate .... see LIVER EXTRACT
LIVER EXTRACT .... see LIVER EXTRACT
Liver Factors .... see LIVER EXTRACT
Liver Fractions .... see LIVER EXTRACT
Liver Hydrolysate .... see LIVER EXTRACT
Liver Lily .... see ORRIS
Liver Oil .... see COD LIVER OIL
Liver Substance .... see LIVER EXTRACT
Liverleaf .... see LIVERWORT
Liverweed .... see LIVERWORT
Liverwort .... see AGRIMONY
LIVERWORT .... see LIVERWORT
Liverwort-Leaf .... see LIVERWORT
Living Antiseptic .... see MAGGOTS
Lizard's Tail .... see YERBA MANSA
Lizzy-Run-Up-The-Hedge .... see GROUND IVY
L-Leucine .... see BRANCHED-CHAIN AMINO ACIDS
L-Lysine .... see LYSINE
L-Methionine .... see METHIONINE
LNA .... see ALPHA-LINOLENIC ACID
Lobaria pulmonaria .... see LUNGMOSS
LOBELIA .... see LOBELIA

Lobelia inflata .... see LOBELIA
Lobster Flower Plant .... see POINSETTIA
Lobsterplant .... see POINSETTIA
Lochnera rosea .... see MADAGASCAR PERIWINKLE
Locoweed .... see JIMSON WEED
Locust Bean .... see CAROB
Locust Pods .... see CAROB
LOGWOOD .... see LOGWOOD
Lolium perenne .... see HAY FLOWER
Lolium temulentum .... see TAUMELLOOLCH
Long Birthwort .... see ARISTOLOCHIA
Long Pepper .... see INDIAN LONG PEPPER
Long Purples .... see PURPLE LOOSESTRIFE
Longwort .... see MULLEIN
Lonicera .... see HONEYSUCKLE
Lonicera caprifolium .... see HONEYSUCKLE
Lonicera japonica .... see HONEYSUCKLE
Loofa .... see LUFFA
Loofah .... see LUFFA
Loosestrife .... see LOOSESTRIFE,
                                  PURPLE LOOSESTRIFE
Lop Grass .... see HAY FLOWER
Lophophora williamsii .... see PEYOTE
Lorbeerweide .... see WILLOW BARK
Lords and Ladies .... see ARUM
LORENZO'S OIL .... see LORENZO'S OIL
L-Ornithine .... see ORNITHINE
L-Ornithine Alpha-Ketoglutarate
.... see ORNITHINE KETOGLUTARATE
Lotus .... see LOTUS flower, LOTUS seed
LOTUS flower .... see LOTUS flower
LOTUS seed .... see LOTUS seed
Louisa .... see LEMON VERBENA
Louisiana Long Pepper .... see CAPSICUM
Louisiana Sport Pepper .... see CAPSICUM
Louseberry .... see LEVANT BERRY
Lousewort .... see STAVESACRE
LOVAGE .... see LOVAGE
Love Apple .... see TOMATO
Love Bean .... see PRECATORY BEAN
Love in a Mist .... see BLACK SEED
Love in Winter .... see PIPSISSEWA
Love Leaves .... see BURDOCK
Love-Lies-Bleeding .... see AMARANTH
Love-Man .... see CLIVERS
Love Parsley .... see LOVAGE
Lovely Bleeding .... see AMARANTH
Low Balm .... see OSWEGO TEA
Low Chamomile .... see ROMAN CHAMOMILE
Lowbush Blueberry .... see BLUEBERRY
Lowbush Cranberry .... see ALPINE CRANBERRY
LPC .... see PROPIONYL-L-CARNITINE
L-Phenylalanine .... see PHENYLALANINE
L-Selenomethionine .... see SELENIUM
L-Taurine .... see TAURINE
L-Trypt .... see L-TRYPTOPHAN
L-TRYPTOPHAN .... see L-TRYPTOPHAN
L-Tyrosine .... see TYROSINE
Lu Rong .... see DEER VELVET
Lucerne .... see ALFALFA
Lucilia sericata .... see MAGGOTS
Lucky Bean .... see PRECATORY BEAN
Luei Gong Gen .... see GOTU KOLA
LUFFA .... see LUFFA

INDEX

Luffa acutangula .... see LUFFA
Luffa aegyptiaca .... see LUFFA
Luffa cylindrica .... see LUFFA
Luffaschwamm .... see LUFFA
Lu-Hui .... see ALOE dried juice from leaf, latex
Lungenkraut .... see LUNGWORT
LUNGMOSS .... see LUNGMOSS
Lungwort .... see LUNGMOSS
LUNGWORT .... see LUNGWORT
Lupinus luteus .... see YELLOW LUPIN
Lupuli Strobulus .... see HOPS
Lurk-In-The-Ditch .... see PENNYROYAL leaf, PENNYROYAL oil
Lustwort .... see SUNDEW
Luteal Hormone .... see PROGESTERONE
LUTEIN .... see LUTEIN
Luteohormone .... see PROGESTERONE
Lutine .... see PROGESTERONE
L-Valine .... see BRANCHED-CHAIN AMINO ACIDS
Lycii Berries .... see LYCIUM
LYCIUM .... see LYCIUM
Lycium barbarum .... see LYCIUM
Lycium chinense .... see LYCIUM
LYCOPENE .... see LYCOPENE
Lycoperdon spp .... see PUFF BALL
Lycopersicon esculentum .... see TOMATO
Lycopi Herba .... see BUGLEWEED
Lycopodium .... see CLUB MOSS
Lycopodium clavatum .... see CLUB MOSS
Lycopus americanus .... see BUGLEWEED
Lycopus europaeus .... see BUGLEWEED
Lycopus virginicus .... see BUGLEWEED
Lyngbya wollei .... see BLUE-GREEN ALGAE
Lys .... see LYSINE
Lysimachia nummularia .... see MONEYWORT
Lysimachia vulgaris .... see LOOSESTRIFE
LYSINE .... see LYSINE
Lysine Hydrochloride .... see LYSINE
Lysine Monohydrochloride .... see LYSINE
Lythrum .... see PURPLE LOOSESTRIFE
Lythrum salicaria .... see PURPLE LOOSESTRIFE
M Mei Gee .... see SCHISANDRA
M. viridis .... see SPEARMINT
Ma Huang .... see EPHEDRA
MACA .... see MACA
Maca Maca .... see MACA
Mace .... see NUTMEG AND MACE
Macis .... see NUTMEG AND MACE
Mackerel Mint .... see SPEARMINT
Macochihua .... see IPORURU
Macrocystis Pyrifera .... see ALGIN
Mad-apple .... see JIMSON WEED
Mad-dog Herb .... see SCULLCAP
Mad-dog Weed .... see SCULLCAP, WATER PLANTAIN
Mad Weed .... see SCULLCAP
Madagascar Lemongrass .... see LEMONGRASS
MADAGASCAR PERIWINKLE
.... see MADAGASCAR PERIWINKLE
Madagascar Vanilla .... see VANILLA
MADDER .... see MADDER
Madecassol .... see GOTU KOLA
Madelonitrile .... see APRICOT
Madnep .... see MASTERWORT

Madonna Lily .... see WHITE LILY
Madre Selva .... see PASSIONFLOWER
Magdalena .... see MADAGASCAR PERIWINKLE
Maggi Plant .... see LOVAGE
MAGGOTS .... see MAGGOTS
Magnesia .... see MAGNESIUM
MAGNESIUM .... see MAGNESIUM
Magnesium Aspartate .... see MAGNESIUM
Magnesium Carbonate .... see MAGNESIUM
Magnesium Chloride .... see MAGNESIUM
Magnesium Citrate .... see MAGNESIUM
Magnesium Gluconate .... see MAGNESIUM
Magnesium Hydroxide .... see MAGNESIUM
Magnesium Lactate .... see MAGNESIUM
Magnesium Orotate .... see MAGNESIUM
Magnesium Oxide .... see MAGNESIUM
Magnesium Pyruvate .... see PYRUVATE
Magnesium Sulfate .... see MAGNESIUM
Magnesium Trisilicate .... see MAGNESIUM
Magnolia .... see MAGNOLIA bark, MAGNOLIA flower bud
MAGNOLIA bark .... see MAGNOLIA bark
Magnolia biondii .... see MAGNOLIA bark, MAGNOLIA flower bud
Magnolia denudata .... see MAGNOLIA bark, MAGNOLIA flower bud
Magnolia emargenata .... see MAGNOLIA bark, MAGNOLIA flower bud
Magnolia fargesii .... see MAGNOLIA bark, MAGNOLIA flower bud
MAGNOLIA flower bud .... see MAGNOLIA flower bud
Magnolia glauca .... see MAGNOLIA bark, MAGNOLIA flower bud
Magnolia heptaperta .... see MAGNOLIA bark, MAGNOLIA flower bud
Magnolia officinalis .... see MAGNOLIA bark, MAGNOLIA flower bud
Magnolia salicifolia .... see MAGNOLIA bark, MAGNOLIA flower bud
Magnolia sargentiana .... see MAGNOLIA bark, MAGNOLIA flower bud
Magnolia sprengeri .... see MAGNOLIA bark, MAGNOLIA flower bud
Magnolia Vine .... see SCHISANDRA
Magnolia wilsonii .... see MAGNOLIA bark, MAGNOLIA flower bud
Mahogany .... see LAURELWOOD
Mahongany .... see ANDIROBA
Mahonia Aquifolium .... see OREGON GRAPE
Mahonia nervosa .... see OREGON GRAPE
Mahonia repens .... see OREGON GRAPE
Ma Huang .... see EPHEDRA
Mahuanggen (ma huang root) .... see EPHEDRA
Mai Ya .... see BARLEY
Maiden Fern .... see MAIDENHAIR FERN
MAIDENHAIR FERN .... see MAIDENHAIR FERN
Maidenhair Tree
.... see GINKGO leaf (GINKGO leaf extract), GINKGO seed
Maidis Stigma .... see CORN SILK
Maid's Hair .... see LADY'S BEDSTRAW
Maino .... see MACA
Maitake .... see MAITAKE MUSHROOM
MAITAKE MUSHROOM ... see MAITAKE MUSHROOM

Maize Pollen .... see BEE POLLEN
Maize Silk .... see CORN SILK
Majoran .... see MARJORAM
Majorana aetheroleum oil .... see MARJORAM
Majorana herb .... see MARJORAM
Majorana hortensis .... see MARJORAM
Maka .... see MACA
Makombu Thallus .... see LAMINARIA
MALABAR NUT .... see MALABAR NUT
Malabar Tamarind .... see GARCINIA
MALE FERN .... see MALE FERN
Malic Acid .... see ALPHA HYDROXY ACIDS
Mallaguetta Pepper .... see GRAINS OF PARADISE
Mallards .... see MARSHMALLOW
Mallotus philippinensis .... see KAMALA
Mallow .... see MALLOW flower,
                                          MALLOW leaf
MALLOW flower .... see MALLOW flower
MALLOW leaf .... see MALLOW leaf
Malpidnia glabra .... see ACEROLA
Malpidnia punicifolia .... see ACEROLA
Malus sylvestris .... see APPLE
Malva .... see HOLLYHOCK
Malva Flower .... see HOLLYHOCK
Malva neglecta .... see MALLOW leaf
Malva Sylvestris .... see MALLOW flower,
                                          MALLOW leaf
Malvae arboreae flos .... see HOLLYHOCK
Malvae flos .... see MALLOW flower
Malvae folium .... see MALLOW leaf
Mamaerie .... see PAPAYA
MANACA .... see MANACA
Manchurian Fungus .... see KOMBUCHA TEA
Manchurian Mushroom Tea ...... see KOMBUCHA TEA
Mandragora .... see EUROPEAN MANDRAKE
Mandragora officinarum .... see EUROPEAN MANDRAKE
Mandragora vernalis .... see EUROPEAN MANDRAKE
Mandragore .... see EUROPEAN MANDRAKE
Mandrake .... see EUROPEAN MANDRAKE,
                                          PODOPHYLLUM
MANGANESE .... see MANGANESE
Manganese Amino Acid Chelate .... see MANGANESE
Manganese Aminoate .... see MANGANESE
Manganese Ascorbate .... see MANGANESE
Manganese Aspartate Complex .... see MANGANESE
Manganese Chloride .... see MANGANESE
Manganese Chloridetetrahydrate .... see MANGANESE
Manganese Dioxide .... see MANGANESE
Manganese Gluconate .... see MANGANESE
Manganese Sulfate .... see MANGANESE
Manganese Sulfate Monohydrate .... see MANGANESE
Manganese Sulfate Tetrahydrate .... see MANGANESE
Manganum .... see MANGANESE
Mangel .... see BEET
Mangold .... see BEET
Manila Elemi .... see ELEMI
Manilkara achras .... see CHICLE
Manilkara zapota .... see CHICLE
Manilkara zapotilla .... see CHICLE
MANNA .... see MANNA
Manna Ash .... see MANNA
Mannentake .... see REISHI MUSHROOM
Manzanilla .... see GERMAN CHAMOMILE,
                                          ROMAN CHAMOMILE

Manzanita .... see UVA URSI
Mapato .... see RHATANY
Maranhao Jaborandi .... see JABORANDI
Maranta .... see ARROWROOT
Maranta arundinaceae .... see ARROWROOT
Marcory .... see QUEEN'S DELIGHT
Marginal Fern .... see MALE FERN
Margosa .... see NEEM
Marguerite .... see OX-EYE DAISY
Marian Thistle .... see MILK THISTLE
Mariendistel .... see MILK THISTLE
Marienmantel .... see ALCHEMILLA
Marigold .... see CALENDULA
Marigold of Peru .... see SUNFLOWER OIL
Mariguana .... see MARIJUANA
Marihuana .... see MARIJUANA
MARIJUANA .... see MARIJUANA
Marine Oils .... see FISH OILS
Marjolaine .... see MARJORAM
MARJORAM .... see MARJORAM
Markweed .... see POISON IVY
Marron Europeen ..... see HORSE CHESTNUT branch bark,
                                  HORSE CHESTNUT flower,
                                  HORSE CHESTNUT leaf,
                                  HORSE CHESTNUT seed
Marrubii herba .... see WHITE HOREHOUND
Marrubium .... see WHITE HOREHOUND
Marrubium vulgare .... see WHITE HOREHOUND
Marsdenia condurango .... see CONDURANGO
MARSH BLAZING STAR
.... see MARSH BLAZING STAR
Marsh Citrus .... see MARSH TEA
MARSH MARIGOLD .... see MARSH MARIGOLD
Marsh Mint .... see WILD MINT
Marsh Penny .... see GOTU KOLA
Marsh Rosemary .... see LABRADOR TEA
Marsh Tea .... see LABRADOR TEA
MARSH TEA .... see MARSH TEA
Marsh Trefoil .... see BOGBEAN
MARSHMALLOW .... see MARSHMALLOW
MARTAGON .... see MARTAGON
Mary Thistle .... see MILK THISTLE
Marybud .... see CALENDULA
Maryland Pink .... see PINK ROOT
Master of the Wood .... see SWEET WOODRUFF
Masterwort .... see GOUTWEED, MASTERWORT
MASTIC .... see MASTIC
Mastich .... see MASTIC
Mastix .... see MASTIC
Mastranzo .... see WHITE HOREHOUND
MATE .... see MATE
Mate de Coca .... see COCA
Maté Folium .... see MATE
Matricaire .... see GERMAN CHAMOMILE
Matricaria chamomilla .... see GERMAN CHAMOMILE
Matricaria morifolia .... see CHRYSANTHEMUM
Matricaria recutita .... see GERMAN CHAMOMILE
Matricariae Flos .... see GERMAN CHAMOMILE
Matrimony Vine .... see LYCIUM
Matsbouza .... see SCHISANDRA
Matsuhodo .... see PORIA MUSHROOM
Matteucccia struthiopteris .... see OSTRICH FERN
Matto Grosso Ipecac .... see IPECAC
Maudlin Daisy .... see OX-EYE DAISY

INDEX

Maudlinwort .... see OX-EYE DAISY
Mauls .... see MALLOW flower
May .... see HAWTHORN
May Bells .... see LILY-OF-THE-VALLEY
May Lily .... see LILY-OF-THE-VALLEY
Mayapple .... see PODOPHYLLUM
Maybush .... see HAWTHORN
Mayflower .... see COWSLIP
Maypop .... see PASSIONFLOWER
Maypop Passion Flower .... see PASSIONFLOWER
Maythorn .... see HAWTHORN
MCT ..... see MEDIUM CHAIN TRIGLYCERIDES (MCT)
MCT's ... see MEDIUM CHAIN TRIGLYCERIDES (MCT)
Meadow Anenome .... see PULSATILLA
Meadow Cabbage .... see SKUNK CABBAGE
Meadow Clover .... see RED CLOVER
Meadow Fescue .... see HAY FLOWER
Meadow Lily .... see WHITE LILY
Meadow Queen .... see MEADOWSWEET
Meadow Routs .... see MARSH MARIGOLD
Meadow Runagates .... see MONEYWORT
Meadow Saffran .... see AUTUMN CROCUS
Meadow Saffron .... see AUTUMN CROCUS
Meadow Sage .... see SAGE
Meadow Sweet .... see MEADOWSWEET
Meadow Windflower .... see PULSATILLA
Meadowbloom .... see BULBOUS BUTTERCUP,
BUTTERCUP
MEADOWSWEET .... see MEADOWSWEET
Meadow-Wart .... see MEADOWSWEET
Mealy Kudzu .... see KUDZU
Mechoacán .... see JALAP
Medicago .... see ALFALFA
Medicago sativa .... see ALFALFA
Medicinal Charcoal .... see ACTIVATED CHARCOAL
Medicinal Leech .... see LEECH
Medicinal Rhubarb .... see RHUBARB
Medicinal Yeast .... see BREWER'S YEAST
Mediterranean Bay .... see SWEET BAY
Mediterranean Oregano .... see OREGANO
Mediterranean Squill .... see SQUILL
MEDIUM CHAIN TRIGLYCERIDES (MCT)
.... see MEDIUM CHAIN TRIGLYCERIDES (MCT)
Meerdorn .... see SEA BUCKTHORN
Meereiche .... see BLADDERWRACK
Meerrettich .... see HORSERADISH
Mehlbeebaum .... see HAWTHORN
Mehndi .... see HENNA
Meidorn .... see HAWTHORN
Mejorana .... see MARJORAM
Mel .... see HONEY, MELATONIN
Melaleuca alternifolia .... see TEA TREE OIL
Melaleuca leucodendra .... see CAJEPUT OIL
Melaleuca leucodendron .... see CAJEPUT OIL
Melaleuca Oil .... see TEA TREE OIL
Melaleuca quinquenervia .... see CAJEPUT OIL
Melaleuca viridiflora .... see NIAULI OIL
Melampode .... see BLACK HELLEBORE
MELANOTAN-II .... see MELANOTAN-II
MELATONIN .... see MELATONIN
Melegueta Pepper .... see GRAINS OF PARADISE
Meletin .... see QUERCETIN
Melilot .... see SWEET CLOVER
Meliloti herba .... see SWEET CLOVER

Melilotus .... see SWEET CLOVER
Melilotus altissimus .... see SWEET CLOVER
Melilotus officinalis .... see SWEET CLOVER
Melissa .... see LEMON BALM
Melissa officinalis .... see LEMON BALM
Melissa pulegioides
.... see PENNYROYAL leaf, PENNYROYAL oil
Melissae folium .... see LEMON BALM
Melissenblatt .... see LEMON BALM
Melon Tree .... see PAPAYA
Melonenbaumblaetter .... see PAPAYA
Membranous Milk Vetch .... see ASTRAGALUS
Memeniran .... see CHANCA PIEDRA
Menadiol acetate (K4) .... see VITAMIN K
Menadione (K3) .... see VITAMIN K
Menaquinone (K2) .... see VITAMIN K
Mendee .... see HENNA
Mengkudu .... see MORINDA
Menhaden Oil .... see FISH OILS
Meniran .... see CHANCA PIEDRA
Menispermum cocculus .... see LEVANT BERRY
Menispermum Lacunosum .... see LEVANT BERRY
Menkoedoe .... see MORINDA
Mentha aquatica .... see WILD MINT
Mentha arvensis aetheroleum .... see JAPANESE MINT
Mentha arvensis var. piperascens ..... see JAPANESE MINT
Mentha canadensis .... see JAPANESE MINT
Mentha longifolia .... see ENGLISH HORSEMINT
Mentha piperita .... see PEPPERMINT leaf,
PEPPERMINT OIL
Mentha pulegium .... see PENNYROYAL leaf,
PENNYROYAL oil
Mentha spicata .... see SPEARMINT
Menthae piperitae Aetheroleum ...... see PEPPERMINT OIL
Menthae piperitae folium .... see PEPPERMINT leaf
Menthe poivree .... see PEPPERMINT leaf,
PEPPERMINT OIL
MENTZELIA .... see MENTZELIA
Mentzelia cordifolia .... see MENTZELIA
Menyanthes .... see BOGBEAN
Menyanthes trifoliata .... see BOGBEAN
Merasingi .... see GYMNEMA
Mercurialis annua .... see MERCURY HERB
MERCURY HERB .... see MERCURY HERB
Merlot .... see GRAPE fruit, skin
Mescal Buttons .... see PEYOTE
Mescaline .... see PEYOTE
Meshashringi .... see GYMNEMA
MESOGLYCAN .... see MESOGLYCAN
Meso-inositol .... see INOSITOL
Meso-Inositol Hexanicotinate
.... see INOSITOL NICOTINATE
Meso-Xylitol .... see XYLITOL
Metavanadate .... see VANADIUM
Methi .... see FENUGREEK
METHIONINE .... see METHIONINE
Methyl Sulfonyl Methane
.... see MSM (METHYLSULFONYLMETHANE)
Methyl sulphoxide
.... see DMSO (DIMETHYLSULFOXIDE)
Methylcobalamin .... see VITAMIN B12
Methylsulfonyl Methane
.... see MSM (METHYLSULFONYLMETHANE)

Methylsulfonylmethane
.... see MSM (METHYLSULFONYLMETHANE)
Mexican Chilies .... see CAPSICUM
Mexican Damiana .... see DAMIANA
Mexican Flame Leaf .... see POINSETTIA
Mexican Flameleaf .... see POINSETTIA
Mexican Marigold .... see TAGETES
Mexican Sage .... see DIVINER'S SAGE
Mexican Sage Incense .... see DIVINER'S SAGE
Mexican Sarsaparilla .... see SARSAPARILLA
MEXICAN SCAMMONY ROOT
.... see MEXICAN SCAMMONY ROOT
Mexican Tea .... see CHENOPODIUM OIL
Mexican Valerian .... see VALERIAN
Mexican Vanilla .... see VANILLA
Mexican Yam .... see WILD YAM
Mexico Weed .... see CASTOR OIL, CASTOR seed
MEZEREON .... see MEZEREON
Mg .... see MAGNESIUM
MGN-3 .... see MGN-3
MICROALGAE .... see MICROALGAE
Microcystis aeruginosa .... see BLUE-GREEN ALGAE
Microcystis wesenbergii .... see BLUE-GREEN ALGAE
Middle Comfrey .... see BUGLE
Middle Confound .... see BUGLE
Miel Blanc .... see HONEY
Mignonette Tree .... see HENNA
Milefolio .... see YARROW
Milfoil .... see YARROW
Milk Ipecac .... see BETH ROOT,
                                                         CANADIAN HEMP
Milk of Magnesia .... see MAGNESIUM
MILK THISTLE .... see MILK THISTLE
Milk Thistle above ground parts .... see MILK THISTLE
Milk Thistle Fruit .... see MILK THISTLE
Milk Thistle Seed .... see MILK THISTLE
Milk Vetch .... see ASTRAGALUS
Milk Willow-Herb .... see PURPLE LOOSESTRIFE
Milkweed .... see CANADIAN HEMP
Milkwort .... see SENEGA
Mill Mint .... see CALAMINT
Mill Mountain .... see MOUNTAIN FLAX
Millefeuille .... see YARROW
Millefolii flos .... see YARROW
Millefolii herba .... see YARROW
Millefolium .... see YARROW
Millegoglie .... see YARROW
Millepertuis .... see ST. JOHN'S WORT
Mimosa farnesiana .... see CASSIE ABSOLUTE
Mineral-amino acid complex
.... see CHELATED MINERALS
Mineral Aspartates .... see ASPARTATES
Minor Centaury .... see CENTAURY
Mint Oil .... see JAPANESE MINT
Minzol .... see JAPANESE MINT
Miracle Grass .... see JIAOGULAN
Miracle Plant .... see ALOE dried juice from leaf, latex
Mirobalano .... see INDIAN GOOSEBERRY
Mirobalanus embilica .... see INDIAN GOOSEBERRY
Miso .... see SOY
Mistlekraut .... see EUROPEAN MISTLETOE
Mistletein .... see EUROPEAN MISTLETOE
Mistletoe .... see AMERICAN MISTLETOE,
                                               EUROPEAN MISTLETOE

Mitchella repens .... see SQUAWVINE
Mitoquinone .... see COENZYME Q-10
Mitrewort .... see COOLWORT
Mixed Fruit Acid .... see ALPHA HYDROXY ACIDS
Mixed Tocopherols .... see VITAMIN E
Mixed Vespids .... see BEE VENOM
Mizibcoc .... see DAMIANA
Mizu-Garashi .... see WATERCRESS
MLT .... see MELATONIN
Mn .... see MANGANESE
Moccasin Flower .... see NERVE ROOT
Mocha .... see COFFEE
Mockeel Root .... see WATER HEMLOCK
Mohave Yucca .... see YUCCA
Mokko .... see COSTUS OIL, COSTUS root
Mokkou .... see COSTUS root
Momordica charantia .... see BITTER MELON
Momordica murcata .... see BITTER MELON
Momordique .... see BITTER MELON
Monarda .... see OSWEGO TEA
Monarda didyma .... see OSWEGO TEA
Monarda Lutea .... see HORSEMINT
Monarda punctata .... see HORSEMINT
Monascus .... see RED YEAST
Monascus purpureus Went .... see RED YEAST
MONEYWORT .... see MONEYWORT
Mongolian Larch .... see LARCH ARABINOGALACTAN
Mongolian Larchwood
.... see LARCH ARABINOGALACTAN
Mongolian Milk .... see ASTRAGALUS
Moniera cuneifolia .... see BRAHMI
Monkey Flower .... see NERVE ROOT,
                                                  YELLOW TOADFLAX
Monkey Nuts .... see PEANUT OIL
Monkey's Bench .... see MAITAKE MUSHROOM
Monk's Pepper .... see CHASTEBERRY
Monkshood .... see ACONITE
Monkshood Tuber .... see ACONITE
Monohydroxysuccinic Acid
.... see ALPHA HYDROXY ACIDS
Monohydroxysuccinic acid (Malic acid)
.... see ALPHA HYDROXY ACIDS
Mono-Sulfated Saccharide
.... see GLUCOSAMINE SULFATE
Monounsaturated Fatty Acid .... see OLIVE OIL
Montmorency Cherry .... see SOUR CHERRY
Moon Daisy .... see OX-EYE DAISY
Moon Flower .... see OX-EYE DAISY
Moon Penny .... see OX-EYE DAISY
Moor Grass .... see POTENTILLA
Moose Elm .... see SLIPPERY ELM
Moosebeere .... see CRANBERRY
Mora De La India .... see MORINDA
Morello Cherry .... see SOUR CHERRY
Morinda .... see BA JI TIAN
MORINDA .... see MORINDA
Morinda Citrifolia .... see MORINDA
Morinda officinalis .... see BA JI TIAN
Morinda Root .... see BA JI TIAN
Morindae Officinalis .... see BA JI TIAN
Morindae radix .... see BA JI TIAN
MORMON TEA .... see MORMON TEA
Moroccan Geranium Oil .... see ROSE GERANIUM
Mortal .... see BITTERSWEET NIGHTSHADE

INDEX

Mortification Root .... see MARSHMALLOW
Morus nigra .... see BLACK MULBERRY
Moschus moschiferus .... see MUSK
Mosquito Plant .... see PENNYROYAL leaf,
                                     PENNYROYAL oil
Moss Cranberry .... see ALPINE CRANBERRY
Mossberry .... see CRANBERRY
Moth Herb .... see MARSH TEA
Mother of Rye .... see ERGOT
Mother of Thyme .... see WILD THYME
Mother's-Heart .... see SHEPHERD'S PURSE
MOTHERWORT .... see MOTHERWORT
MOUNTAIN ASH .... see MOUNTAIN ASH
Mountain Balm .... see CALAMINT,
                                    OSWEGO TEA,
                                    YERBA SANTA
Mountain Box .... see UVA URSI
Mountain Cranberry .... see UVA URSI
Mountain Damson .... see SIMARUBA
Mountain Everlasting .... see CAT'S FOOT
MOUNTAIN FLAX .... see MOUNTAIN FLAX
Mountain Grape .... see EUROPEAN BARBERRY,
                                    OREGON GRAPE
Mountain Hydrangea .... see HYDRANGEA
Mountain Ivy .... see MOUNTAIN LAUREL
MOUNTAIN LAUREL .... see MOUNTAIN LAUREL
Mountain Lovage .... see OSHA
Mountain Mint .... see CALAMINT,
                                    OREGANO,
                                    OSWEGO TEA
Mountain Pink .... see TRAILING ARBUTUS
Mountain Polygala .... see SENEGA
Mountain Radish .... see HORSERADISH
Mountain Sorrel .... see WOOD SORREL
Mountain Strawberry .... see STRAWBERRY
Mountain-Sweet .... see NEW JERSEY TEA
Mountain Tea .... see WINTERGREEN leaf,
                                  WINTERGREEN oil
Mountain Tobacco .... see ARNICA
Mouse Antialopecia Factor .... see INOSITOL
Mouse Ear .... see CUDWEED
MOUSE EAR .... see MOUSE EAR
Mousetail .... see COMMON STONECROP
Mousse D'Irlande .... see CARRAGEENAN
Mouth Root .... see GOLDTHREAD
Mouth-Smart .... see BROOKLIME
MSI-1256F .... see SHARK CARTILAGE
MSM .... see MSM (METHYLSULFONYLMETHANE)
MSM (METHYLSULFONYLMETHANE)
         .... see MSM (METHYLSULFONYLMETHANE)
MT-II .... see MELANOTAN-II
Mu Xiang .... see COSTUS OIL, COSTUS root
Mucara .... see KARAYA GUM
Mucopolysaccharide .... see MESOGLYCAN
Mucuna .... see COWHAGE
Mucuna Pruriens .... see COWHAGE
Mucuna prurient .... see COWHAGE
Mudar Bark .... see CALOTROPIS
Muder Yercum .... see CALOTROPIS
Muguet .... see LILY-OF-THE-VALLEY
MUGWORT .... see MUGWORT
Mugwort .... see TARRAGON
MUIRA PUAMA .... see MUIRA PUAMA
Mulberry .... see BLACK MULBERRY,
                                  MORINDA

MULLEIN .... see MULLEIN
Multiflora Preparata .... see FO-TI
Mum .... see CHRYSANTHEMUM
Murillo Bark .... see QUILLAIA
Muscadier .... see NUTMEG AND MACE
Muscatel Sage .... see CLARY SAGE
Mushroom Of Immortality .... see REISHI MUSHROOM
Mushroom of Spiritual Potency
                            see REISHI MUSHROOM
MUSK .... see MUSK
Musk Root .... see SUMBUL
Musk Seed .... see AMBRETTE
Muskat .... see GRAPE seed
Muskatbuam .... see NUTMEG AND MACE
Muskatnuss .... see NUTMEG AND MACE
Muskmallow .... see AMBRETTE
Muskrat Weed .... see WATER HEMLOCK
Musquash Root .... see WATER HEMLOCK
Mustard .... see BLACK MUSTARD seed
Mustard Oil .... see BLACK MUSTARD oil
Muster John Henry .... see TAGETES
Mutton Chops .... see CLIVERS
Muzei Mahuang .... see EPHEDRA
Myo-inositol .... see INOSITOL
Myo-inositol hexa-3-pyridine-carboxylate
                            see INOSITOL NICOTINATE
Myosotis arvensis .... see FORGET-ME-NOT
Myrica .... see BAYBERRY
Myrica cerifera .... see BAYBERRY
Myrica gale .... see SWEET GALE
Myrica pensylvanica .... see BAYBERRY
Myristica .... see NUTMEG AND MACE
Myristica fragrans .... see NUTMEG AND MACE
Myristica officinalis .... see NUTMEG AND MACE
Myristicae Aril .... see NUTMEG AND MACE
Myristicae Semen .... see NUTMEG AND MACE
Myrobalan .... see TERMINALIA
Myrobalan Emblic .... see INDIAN GOOSEBERRY
Myroxylan balsamum .... see TOLU BALSAM
Myroxylan toluiferum .... see TOLU BALSAM
Myroxylon balsamum .... see TOLU BALSAM
Myroxylon balsamum genuinum .... see TOLU BALSAM
Myroxylon balsamum pereirae .... see PERU BALSAM
Myroxylon pereirae .... see PERU BALSAM
MYRRH .... see MYRRH
Myrrhis odorata .... see SWEET CICELY
Myrti aetherolum .... see MYRTLE
Myrti folium .... see MYRTLE
Myrtilli Fructus .... see BILBERRY dried ripe fruit,
                                BILBERRY leaf
Myrtle .... see MADAGASCAR PERIWINKLE,
                                PERIWINKLE
MYRTLE .... see MYRTLE
Myrtle Flag .... see CALAMUS
Myrtle Flower .... see ORRIS
Myrtle Sedge .... see CALAMUS
Myrtus .... see CHEKEN
Myrtus communis .... see MYRTLE
Mysteria .... see AUTUMN CROCUS
Mystyldene .... see EUROPEAN MISTLETOE
N-(2-furanylmethyl)-1H-purin-6-amine .... see KINETIN
N(6)furfuryladenine .... see KINETIN
N-(aminoiminomethyl)-N methyl glycine .... see CREATINE
N-(N-L-gamma-Glutamyl-L-cysteinyl)glycine
                                see GLUTATHIONE

N,N-dimethylaminoacetic Acid
.... see DIMETHYLGLYCINE
N,N-dimethylglycine .... see DIMETHYLGLYCINE
N-3 Fatty Acid .... see ALPHA-LINOLENIC ACID,
DHA (DOCOSAHEXAENOIC ACID),
EPA (EICOSAPENTAENOIC ACID)
N-3 Fatty Acids .... see COD LIVER OIL, FISH OILS
N-3 Polyunsaturated Fatty Acid
.... see ALPHA-LINOLENIC ACID
N3-polyunsaturated Fatty Acids .... see FISH OILS
N-6 .... see OMEGA-6 FATTY ACIDS
N-6 EFAs .... see OMEGA-6 FATTY ACIDS
N-6 Essential Fatty Acids .... see OMEGA-6 FATTY ACIDS
N-9 Fatty Acid .... see OLIVE OIL
Nabin Chanvandi .... see ANDROGRAPHIS
NAC .... see N-ACETYL CYSTEINE
N-acetyl-5-methoxytryptamine .... see MELATONIN
N-Acetyl-B-Cysteine .... see N-ACETYL CYSTEINE
N-Acetyl-Carnitine .... see ACETYL-L-CARNITINE
N-ACETYL CYSTEINE .... see N-ACETYL CYSTEINE
N-Acetyl D-Glucosamine
.... see N-ACETYL GLUCOSAMINE
N-ACETYL GLUCOSAMINE
.... see N-ACETYL GLUCOSAMINE
N-Acetyl-L-Carnitine .... see ACETYL-L-CARNITINE
N-Acetyl L-Cysteine .... see N-ACETYL CYSTEINE
Nad .... see NADH
NADH .... see NADH
NAG .... see N-ACETYL GLUCOSAMINE
Naked Ladies .... see AUTUMN CROCUS
N-amidinosarcosine .... see CREATINE
Nan Shanzha .... see HAWTHORN
Nanwuweizi .... see SCHISANDRA
Narcissus pseudonarcissus .... see DAFFODIL
Narrow Dock .... see YELLOW DOCK
Narrow-leaved Purple Cone Flower .... see ECHINACEA
Naseberry .... see CHICLE
Nasilord .... see WATERCRESS
Nasturtii herba .... see WATERCRESS
NASTURTIUM .... see NASTURTIUM
Nasturtium armoracia .... see HORSERADISH
Nasturtium officinale .... see WATERCRESS
Natto .... see SOY
Natural DHEA .... see WILD YAM
Nature's Viagra .... see PUNCTURE VINE
Naughty Man's Cherries ....see BELLADONNA
Navel Orange .... see SWEET ORANGE
Navy Bean .... see BEAN POD
N-Carboxybutyl Chitosan .... see CHITOSAN
Nebraska Fern .... see HEMLOCK
Neckweed .... see BROOKLIME
Nectar of the Gods .... see GARLIC
NEEM .... see NEEM
Nees .... see CASSIA
Neli .... see INDIAN GOOSEBERRY
Nelumbo nucifera .... see LOTUS flower, LOTUS seed
Nepeta cataria .... see CATNIP
Nepeta hederacea .... see GROUND IVY
Nerium oleander .... see OLEANDER
Neroli Oil .... see BITTER ORANGE
NERVE ROOT .... see NERVE ROOT
Netchweed .... see ARRACH
Nettle .... see STINGING NETTLE above ground parts,
STINGING NETTLE root

Nettles .... see STINGING NETTLE above ground parts,
STINGING NETTLE root
Neuromins .... see DHA (DOCOSAHEXAENOIC ACID)
NEW JERSEY TEA .... see NEW JERSEY TEA
New Zealand Green Lipped Mussel
.... see NEW ZEALAND GREEN-LIPPED MUSSEL
NEW ZEALAND GREEN-LIPPED MUSSEL
.... see NEW ZEALAND GREEN-LIPPED MUSSEL
Ngu Mei Gee .... see SCHISANDRA
Nhau .... see MORINDA
Niacin
.... see NIACIN AND NIACINAMIDE (VITAMIN B3)
NIACIN AND NIACINAMIDE (VITAMIN B3)
.... see NIACIN AND NIACINAMIDE (VITAMIN B3)
Niacin/Niacinamide
.... see NIACIN AND NIACINAMIDE (VITAMIN B3)
Niacinamide
.... see NIACIN AND NIACINAMIDE (VITAMIN B3)
Niacin-Niacinamide
.... see NIACIN AND NIACINAMIDE (VITAMIN B3)
Niando .... see IPORURU
Niauli Aetheroleum .... see NIAULI OIL
NIAULI OIL .... see NIAULI OIL
Nicamid
.... see NIACIN AND NIACINAMIDE (VITAMIN B3)
Nicaragua Ipecac .... see IPECAC
Nichol Seeds .... see DIVI-DIVI
Nicosedine
.... see NIACIN AND NIACINAMIDE (VITAMIN B3)
Nicotiana tabacum .... see SMOKELESS TOBACCO
Nicotinamide
.... see NIACIN AND NIACINAMIDE (VITAMIN B3)
Nicotinic Acid
.... see NIACIN AND NIACINAMIDE (VITAMIN B3)
Nicotinic Acid Amide
.... see NIACIN AND NIACINAMIDE (VITAMIN B3)
Nicotylamidum
.... see NIACIN AND NIACINAMIDE (VITAMIN B3)
Nigella sativa .... see BLACK SEED
Nigelle de Crète .... see BLACK SEED
Night Blooming Cereus .... see CEREUS
Night Willow-Herb .... see EVENING PRIMROSE OIL
Nightshade .... see JIMSON WEED
Nikkar Nuts .... see DIVI-DIVI
Nim ....see NEEM
Nimba .... see NEEM
Nine Hooks .... see ALCHEMILLA
Ninety-Knot ....see KNOTWEED HERB
Ninjin .... see GINSENG, PANAX
Niruri .... see CHANCA PIEDRA
Níspero .... see CHICLE
N-methylsarcosine .... see DIMETHYLGLYCINE
Noah's Ark .... see NERVE ROOT
Noble Laurel .... see SWEET BAY
Noble Yarrow .... see YARROW
N-octacosanol .... see OCTACOSANOL
No-Flush Niacin .... see INOSITOL NICOTINATE
Nogal Americano .... see BLACK WALNUT
Nogal Ceniciento .... see BUTTERNUT
Nogueira-preta .... see BLACK WALNUT
Noisetier ....see HAZELNUT
Noix Muscade .... see NUTMEG AND MACE
Nokyong .... see DEER VELVET

INDEX

Nonacosanol .... see POLICOSANOL
Noni .... see MORINDA
Nono .... see MORINDA
Nonu .... see MORINDA
Noon Kie Oo Nah Yeah .... see SQUAWVINE
Nopal .... see PRICKLY PEAR CACTUS
Nopol .... see PRICKLY PEAR CACTUS
North American Ginseng .... see GINSENG, AMERICAN
NORTHERN PRICKLY ASH
.... see NORTHERN PRICKLY ASH
Northern Schisandra .... see SCHISANDRA
Northern White Cedar .... see CEDAR leaf,
CEDAR LEAF OIL
Norway Pine .... see HEMLOCK SPRUCE
Norway Spruce .... see FIR, HEMLOCK SPRUCE
Nosebleed .... see YARROW
Noyer Cerdré .... see BUTTERNUT
Noyer Noir .... see BLACK WALNUT
NSC-763 .... see DMSO (DIMETHYLSULFOXIDE)
NSC-9704 .... see PROGESTERONE
Nu Zhen .... see GLOSSY PRIVET
Nu Zhen Zi .... see GLOSSY PRIVET
Nuclei Acids .... see RNA AND DNA
Nucleic .... see RNA AND DNA
Nucleic Acid .... see RNA AND DNA
Nucleic Acids .... see RNA AND DNA
Nucleotides .... see RNA AND DNA
Nuez Moscada .... see NUTMEG AND MACE
Nutmeg .... see NUTMEG AND MACE
NUTMEG AND MACE .... see NUTMEG AND MACE
Nutmeg Flower .... see BLACK SEED
Nux Moschata .... see NUTMEG AND MACE
NUX VOMICA .... see NUX VOMICA
Nuzhenzi .... see GLOSSY PRIVET
Nymphaea odorata
.... see AMERICAN WHITE POND LILY
NZGLM
.... see NEW ZEALAND GREEN-LIPPED MUSSEL
Oak .... see OAK bark
OAK bark .... see OAK bark
Oak Fern .... see LADY FERN
Oak Lungs .... see LUNGMOSS
OAK MOSS .... see OAK MOSS
Oat .... see OAT above ground parts
OAT above ground parts .... see OAT above ground parts
OAT BRAN .... see OAT BRAN
Oat Fruit .... see OATS
Oat Grain .... see OATS
Oat Herb .... see OAT above ground parts
OAT STRAW .... see OAT STRAW
Oatmeal .... see OATS
OATS .... see OATS
Oatstraw .... see OAT STRAW
Oblepikha .... see SEA BUCKTHORN
Ocimum basilicum .... see BASIL
OCTACOSANOL .... see OCTACOSANOL
Octacosanol .... see POLICOSANOL
Octacosyl alcohol .... see OCTACOSANOL
Octyl Diemthyl PABA
.... see PARA-AMINOBENZOIC ACID (PABA)
Oderwort .... see BISTORT
Oenanthe aquatica .... see WATER FENNEL
Oenanthe crocata .... see HEMLOCK WATER DROPWORT

Oenothera biennis and other Oenothera species
.... see EVENING PRIMROSE OIL
Ofbit .... see PREMORSE
Ogi .... see ASTRAGALUS
Ogon .... see BAIKAL SKULLCAP
Oil Nut .... see BUTTERNUT
Oil of Cade .... see CADE OIL
Oil of Clove .... see CLOVE OIL
Oil of Juniper Tar .... see CADE OIL
Oil of Melaleuca .... see TEA TREE OIL
Oil of Oregano .... see OREGANO
Oje .... see FICIN
Ojo De Pajaro .... see PRECATORY BEAN
OKG .... see ORNITHINE KETOGLUTARATE
Okra .... see AMBRETTE
Old Maid .... see MADAGASCAR PERIWINKLE
Old Man .... see ROSEMARY
Old Man's Beard
.... see FRINGETREE, USNEA, WOODBINE
Old Man's Night Cap .... see GREATER BINDWEED
Old Man's Pepper .... see YARROW
Old Man's Root .... see AMERICAN SPIKENARD
Old Woman's Broom .... see DAMIANA
Olea europaea .... see OLIVE leaf, OLIVE OIL
Oleae folium .... see OLIVE leaf
OLEANDER .... see OLEANDER
Oleanderblatter .... see OLEANDER
Oleandri folium .... see OLEANDER
Oleovitamin A .... see VITAMIN A
Oleum Bergamotte .... see BERGAMOT OIL
Oleum Cadinum .... see CADE OIL
Oleum Chaulmoograe .... see CHAULMOOGRA
Oleum Geranii .... see ROSE GERANIUM
Oleum Juniperi Empyreumaticum .... see CADE OIL
Oleum Melaleucae .... see TEA TREE OIL
Olibanum .... see FRANKINCENSE
Oligofructose .... see FRUCTO-OLIGOSACCHARIDES
Oligomeric Proanthocyanidins .... see GRAPE seed,
PYCNOGENOL
Oligomeric Procyanidins .... see GRAPE seed
Olivae oleum .... see OLIVE OIL
Olive .... see OLIVE leaf
OLIVE Leaf .... see OLIVE leaf
OLIVE OIL .... see OLIVE OIL
Olivier .... see OLIVE leaf
Omega 3 Fatty Acids
.... see ALPHA-LINOLENIC ACID, COD LIVER OIL
DHA (DOCOSAHEXAENOIC ACID),
EPA (EICOSAPENTAENOIC ACID),
FISH OILS
Omega-3 Polyunsaturated Fatty Acid
.... see ALPHA-LINOLENIC ACID
OMEGA-6 FATTY ACIDS
.... see OMEGA-6 FATTY ACIDS
Omega-6 Oils .... see OMEGA-6 FATTY ACIDS
Omega-6 polyunsaturated fatty acids
.... see OMEGA-6 FATTY ACIDS
Omega-9 Fatty Acid .... see OLIVE OIL
Omega Fatty Acids
.... see DHA (DOCOSAHEXAENOIC ACID),
EPA (EICOSAPENTAENOIC ACID),
FISH OILS
Omicha .... see SCHISANDRA

Omum .... see BISHOP'S WEED
One Berry .... see HERB PARIS, SQUAWVINE
Oneseed Hawthorn .... see HAWTHORN
ONION .... see ONION
Onions.. see ONION
Ononidis radix .... see SPINY RESTHARROW
Ononis spinosa........................ see SPINY RESTHARROW
Onopordum acanthium .... see SCOTCH THISTLE
Ontario Ginseng..................... see GINSENG, AMERICAN
OPCs .... see GRAPE seed, PYCNOGENOL
Ophioglossum vulgatum
    .... see ENGLISH ADDER'S TONGUE
OPIUM ANTIDOTE .... see OPIUM ANTIDOTE
Oplopanax horridus .... see DEVIL'S CLUB
Opobalsam .... see TOLU BALSAM
Opopanax .... see MYRRH
Opossum Tree .... see STORAX
Optimsm ....see MSM (METHYLSULFONYLMETHANE)
Opuntia .... see PRICKLY PEAR CACTUS
Opuntia ficus indica .... see PRICKLY PEAR CACTUS
Opuntia hyptiacantha .... see PRICKLY PEAR CACTUS
Opuntia lasciacantha .... see PRICKLY PEAR CACTUS
Opuntia macrocentra .... see PRICKLY PEAR CACTUS
Opuntia megacantha .... see PRICKLY PEAR CACTUS
Opuntia puberula .... see PRICKLY PEAR CACTUS
Opuntia streptacantha .... see PRICKLY PEAR CACTUS
Opuntia velutina .... see PRICKLY PEAR CACTUS
Oraches .... see ARRACH
Oranda-Garashi .... see WATERCRESS
Orange Milkweed .... see PLEURISY ROOT
Orange Mullein................................... see MULLEIN
Orange Root .... see GOLDENSEAL
Orange Swallow-Wort .... see PLEURISY ROOT
Orchanet .... see ALKANNA
Orchic .... see ORCHIC EXTRACT
Oirchic Concentrate .... see ORCHIC EXTRACT
ORCHIC EXTRACT .... see ORCHIC EXTRACT
Orchic Factors .... see ORCHIC EXTRACT
Orchic Substance .... see ORCHIC EXTRACT
Orchid ....see SALEP
Orchis morio ....see SALEP
Ordeal Bean .... see CALABAR BEAN
OREGANO .... see OREGANO
Oregano Oil .... see OREGANO
Oregon Balsam .... see OREGON FIR BALSAM
Oregon Barberry .... see OREGON GRAPE
OREGON FIR BALSAM ...... see OREGON FIR BALSAM
Oregon Grape .... see EUROPEAN BARBERRY
OREGON GRAPE .... see OREGON GRAPE
Oregon Grape-Holly .... see OREGON GRAPE
Organic Germanium .... see GERMANIUM
Organy .... see OREGANO
Orgotein .... see SUPEROXIDE DISMUTASE
ORIENTAL ARBORVITAE
    .... see ORIENTAL ARBORVITAE
Oriental Ginseng.......................... see GINSENG, PANAX
Origan De Marais .... see HEMP AGRIMONY
Origani vulgaris herba .... see OREGANO
Origano .... see OREGANO
Origanum .... see OREGANO
Origanum majorana .... see MARJORAM
Origanum Oil .... see SPANISH ORIGANUM OIL
Origanum vulgare .... see OREGANO
Orizaba Jalap .... see MEXICAN SCAMMONY ROOT

Ornicetil .... see ORNITHINE KETOGLUTARATE
ORNITHINE .... see ORNITHINE
Ornithine Alpha Ketoglutarate
    .... see ORNITHINE KETOGLUTARATE
Ornithine Alphaketoglutarate
    .... see ORNITHINE KETOGLUTARATE
ORNITHINE KETOGLUTARATE
    .... see ORNITHINE KETOGLUTARATE
Orozuz .... see LICORICE
ORRIS .... see ORRIS
Orthosiphon .... see JAVA TEA
Orthosiphon spicatus .... see JAVA TEA
Orthosiphon stamineus .... see JAVA TEA
Orthosiphonis folium .... see JAVA TEA
Orthovanadate .... see VANADIUM
Ortie .... see STINGING NETTLE above ground parts
Oryza Sativa .... see RICE BRAN
Oryzanol .... see GAMMA ORYZANOL
OSHA .... see OSHA
Osier .... see AMERICAN DOGWOOD
Osier Rouge .... see WILLOW BARK
Osterick .... see BISTORT
OSTRICH FERN .... see OSTRICH FERN
O-Sulfated Chitosan .... see CHITOSAN
O-Sulfated N-Acetylchitosan .... see CHITOSAN
OSWEGO TEA .... see OSWEGO TEA
Otaheite Walnut .... see TUNG SEED
Our Lady's Flannel .... see MULLEIN
Our Lady's Keys .... see COWSLIP
Our Lady's Mint.................................. see SPEARMINT
Our Lady's Tears .... see LILY-OF-THE-VALLEY
Our Lady's Thistle .... see MILK THISTLE
Our-Lord's-Candle .... see YUCCA
Ovolecithin .... see LECITHIN
Owler .... see BLACK ALDER
Oxadoddy .... see BLACK ROOT
Oxalis acetosella .... see WOOD SORREL
Oxerutin .... see RUTIN
Oxeye .... see PHEASANT'S EYE
OX-EYE DAISY .... see OX-EYE DAISY
Oxitriptan .... see 5-HTP
Ox's Tongue
    .... see BORAGE flower, dried above ground parts
Oxycoccus hagerupii .... see CRANBERRY
Oxycoccus macrocarpos .... see CRANBERRY
Oxycoccus microcarpus .... see CRANBERRY
Oxycoccus palustris .... see CRANBERRY
Oxycoccus quadripetalus .... see CRANBERRY
Oxykrinin .... see SECRETIN
Oyster Shell Calcium .... see CALCIUM
PABA .... see PARA-AMINOBENZOIC ACID (PABA)
Pacific Valerian .... see VALERIAN
Pacific Yew .... see YEW
Padamate O ... see PARA-AMINOBENZOIC ACID (PABA)
Padang-Cassia .... see CINNAMON bark
Paddock-Pipes .... see HORSETAIL
Paeonia .... see PEONY flower, PEONY root
Paeonia mascula .... see PEONY flower, PEONY root
Paeonia officinalis .... see PEONY flower, PEONY root
Paeoniae flos .... see PEONY flower
Paeoniae Radix .... see PEONY root
Pagla-Ka-Dawa .... see INDIAN SNAKEROOT
PAGODA TREE .... see PAGODA TREE

Paigle .... see COWSLIP
Paigle Peggle .... see COWSLIP
Paintedleaf .... see POINSETTIA
Pale Coneflower .... see ECHINACEA
Pale Gentian .... see GENTIAN
Pale Mara .... see FEVER BARK
Pale Psyllium .... see BLOND PSYLLIUM
Pali-Mara .... see FEVER BARK
Palma Christi .... see CASTOR OIL, CASTOR seed
Palmier Nain .... see SAW PALMETTO
Palo de Santa Maria .... see LAURELWOOD
Palo Maria .... see LAURELWOOD
Palsy Root .... see MARSH MARIGOLD
Palsywort .... see COWSLIP
P-Aminobenzoic Acid
   .... see PARA-AMINOBENZOIC ACID (PABA)
Panama Bark .... see QUILLAIA
Panama Ipecac .... see IPECAC
Panang Cinnamon .... see CINNAMON bark
Panax Ginseng .... see GINSENG, PANAX
Panax horridum .... see DEVIL'S CLUB
Panax notoginseng .... see PANAX PSEUDOGINSENG
Panax pseudoginseng .... see PANAX PSEUDOGINSENG
PANAX PSEUDOGINSENG
   .... see PANAX PSEUDOGINSENG
Panax quinquefolius .... see GINSENG, AMERICAN
Panax schinseng .... see GINSENG, PANAX
Panax zingiberensis .... see PANAX PSEUDOGINSENG
PANCREATIN .... see PANCREATIN
Pancreatinum .... see PANCREATIN
Pancreatis pulvis .... see PANCREATIN
Pangamate .... see PANGAMIC ACID
PANGAMIC ACID .... see PANGAMIC ACID
Pansy .... see HEART'S EASE
Pantothenic ..... see PANTOTHENIC ACID (VITAMIN B5)
Pantothenic Acid
   .... see PANTOTHENIC ACID (VITAMIN B5)
PANTOTHENIC ACID (VITAMIN B5)
   .... see PANTOTHENIC ACID (VITAMIN B5)
Pantothenol ..... see PANTOTHENIC ACID (VITAMIN B5)
Pantothenylol
   .... see PANTOTHENIC ACID (VITAMIN B5)
Papagallo .... see POINSETTIA
PAPAIN .... see PAPAIN
Papainum Crudum .... see PAPAIN
Papaver rhoeas .... see CORN POPPY
Papaw .... see PAPAYA
PAPAYA .... see PAPAYA
Papayas .... see PAPAYA
Paperbark Tree Oil .... see CAJEPUT OIL
Papoose Root .... see BLUE COHOSH
Pappelknospen ....see POPLAR
Paprika .... see CAPSICUM
Para Amino Benzoic Acid
   .... see PARA-AMINOBENZOIC ACID (PABA)
PARA-AMINOBENZOIC ACID (PABA)
   .... see PARA-AMINOBENZOIC ACID (PABA)
Paradisapfel .... see GRAPEFRUIT
Paradise Tree .... see TREE OF HEAVEN
Paraguay Tea .... see MATE
Paraguayan Sweet Herb .... see STEVIA
Pareira .... see ABUTA, PAREIRA
Paricalcitol .... see VITAMIN D
Parietaria officinalis .... see PELLITORY-OF-THE-WALL

Paris quadrifolia .... see HERB PARIS
Pariswort .... see BETH ROOT
Parsley .... see PARSLEY leaf, root,
                                           PARSLEY seed
Parsley Breakstone .... see PARSLEY PIERT
Parsley Fern .... see TANSY
Parsley Fruit .... see PARSLEY seed
PARSLEY leaf, root .... see PARSLEY leaf, root
Parsley Piercestone .... see PARSLEY PIERT
PARSLEY PIERT .... see PARSLEY PIERT
PARSLEY seed .... see PARSLEY seed
Parsnip .... see PARSNIP above ground parts,
                                           PARSNIP root
PARSNIP above ground parts
   .... see PARSNIP above ground parts
PARSNIP root .... see PARSNIP root
Parson and Clerk .... see ARUM
Parthenium argentatum .... see GUAYULE
Parthenocissus quinquefolia .... see AMERICAN IVY
Partridge Berry .... see WINTERGREEN leaf,
                                           WINTERGREEN oil
Partridgeberry .... see ALPINE CRANBERRY,
                                           SQUAWVINE
Pas d'Ane .... see COLTSFOOT
Pas Diane .... see COLTSFOOT
Pasania Fungus .... see SHIITAKE MUSHROOM
Pasque Flower .... see PULSATILLA
Pasqueflower .... see PULSATILLA
Passe Flower .... see PULSATILLA
Passiflora .... see PASSIONFLOWER
Passiflora incarnata .... see PASSIONFLOWER
Passiflorae herba .... see PASSIONFLOWER
Passiflore .... see PASSIONFLOWER
Passiflorina .... see PASSIONFLOWER
Passion Flower .... see PASSIONFLOWER
Passion Vine .... see PASSIONFLOWER
Passionaria .... see PASSIONFLOWER
Passionblume .... see PASSIONFLOWER
PASSIONFLOWER .... see PASSIONFLOWER
Passionflower Herb .... see PASSIONFLOWER
Passionsblumenkraut .... see PASSIONFLOWER
Password .... see COWSLIP
Pastinaca sativa .... see PARSNIP above ground parts,
                                           PARSNIP root
Pastinacae herba .... see PARSNIP above ground parts
Pastinacae Radix .... see PARSNIP root
Patacon .... see ABUTA
Patalagandhi .... see INDIAN SNAKEROOT
Patchouli .... see PATCHOULY OIL
Patchouly .... see PATCHOULY OIL
PATCHOULY OIL .... see PATCHOULY OIL
Patience Dock .... see BISTORT
Pattens and Clogs .... see YELLOW TOADFLAX
Pau Darco .... see PAU D'ARCO
PAU D'ARCO .... see PAU D'ARCO
Pau de Arco .... see PAU D'ARCO
Pau De Reposta .... see CATUABA
Pau-Azeitona .... see MORINDA
Paullinia .... see GUARANA
Paullinia cupana .... see GUARANA
Paullinia sorbilis .... see GUARANA
Paul's Betony .... see BUGLEWEED
Pausinystalia johimbe .... see YOHIMBE
Pausinystalia yohimbe .... see YOHIMBE

Pauson .... see BLOODROOT
PCO .... see GRAPE seed, PYCNOGENOL
Pea Tree .... see LABURNUM
Peachwood .... see LOGWOOD
Peagle .... see COWSLIP
Peagles .... see COWSLIP
PEANUT OIL .... see PEANUT OIL
PEAR .... see PEAR
Pearl Barley .... see BARLEY
Pears .... see PEAR
PECTIN .... see PECTIN
Pectinic Acid .... see PECTIN
Pedlar's Basket .... see YELLOW TOADFLAX
Pedunculate Oak .... see OAK bark
Pegu Catechu .... see CATECHU
Pegwood .... see WAHOO
Pelargonium graveolens .... see ROSE GERANIUM
Pelargonium Oil .... see ROSE GERANIUM
Pelican Flower .... see ARISTOLOCHIA
Pellagra Preventing Factor
.... see NIACIN AND NIACINAMIDE (VITAMIN B3)
PELLITORY .... see PELLITORY
PELLITORY-OF-THE-WALL
.... see PELLITORY-OF-THE-WALL
Pellote .... see PEYOTE
Penny Royal .... see PENNYROYAL leaf,
                                                 PENNYROYAL oil
Pennyroyal .... see PENNYROYAL leaf,
                                                 PENNYROYAL oil
PENNYROYAL leaf .... see PENNYROYAL leaf
PENNYROYAL oil .... see PENNYROYAL oil
Pennywort .... see YELLOW TOADFLAX
Pensee Sauvage .... see HEART'S EASE
Penta Tea .... see JIAOGULAN
Peony .... see PEONY flower, PEONY root
PEONY flower .... see PEONY flower
PEONY root .... see PEONY root
Pepe .... see BLACK PEPPER AND WHITE PEPPER
Pepino Montero .... see BITTER MELON
Pepo .... see PUMPKIN
Pepper .... see BLACK PEPPER AND WHITE PEPPER
Pepper-And-Salt .... see SHEPHERD'S PURSE
Pepper Bark .... see WINTER'S BARK
Pepper Extract
.... see BLACK PEPPER AND WHITE PEPPER
Pepper Plant
.... see BLACK PEPPER AND WHITE PEPPER
Pepper Wood .... see NORTHERN PRICKLY ASH
Peppercorn .... see BLACK PEPPER AND WHITE PEPPER
Peppermint .... see PEPPERMINT leaf
PEPPERMINT leaf .... see PEPPERMINT leaf
PEPPERMINT OIL .... see PEPPERMINT OIL
Pepperrot .... see HORSERADISH
Pereira Brava .... see PAREIRA
Perennial Rye-Grass .... see HAY FLOWER
Pericarpium .... see SWEET ORANGE
PERILLA .... see PERILLA
Perilla frutescens .... see PERILLA
Periploca sylvestris .... see GYMNEMA
Periwinkle .... see MADAGASCAR PERIWINKLE
PERIWINKLE .... see PERIWINKLE
Perna canaliculus
.... see NEW ZEALAND GREEN-LIPPED MUSSEL

Persea americana .... see AVOCADO
Persea gratissima .... see AVOCADO
Persely .... see PARSLEY leaf, root
Persian Lilac .... see NEEM
Persian Willow .... see FIREWEED
Persil .... see PARSLEY leaf, root,
                                                                 PARSLEY seed
Personata .... see BURDOCK
Peru-Apple .... see JIMSON WEED
PERU BALSAM .... see PERU BALSAM
Peruvian Balsam .... see PERU BALSAM
Peruvian Bark .... see CINCHONA
Peruvian Coca .... see COCA
Peruvian Ginseng .... see MACA
Peruvian Rhatany .... see RHATANY
Petasites .... see BUTTERBUR
Petasites Flower .... see BUTTERBUR
Petasites hybridus .... see BUTTERBUR
Petasites Leaf .... see BUTTERBUR
Petasites officinalis .... see BUTTERBUR
Petasites Rhizome .... see BUTTERBUR
Petasites Root .... see BUTTERBUR
Petasitidis folium (flower) .... see BUTTERBUR
Petasitidis hybridus .... see BUTTERBUR
Petasitidis rhizoma (rhizome) .... see BUTTERBUR
Peter's Cress .... see SAMPHIRE
Petersylinge .... see PARSLEY leaf, root
Petite Sirah .... see GRAPE fruit, skin
Petroselini fructus .... see PARSLEY seed
Petroselini herba .... see PARSLEY leaf, root
Petroselinum crispum .... see PARSLEY leaf, root,
                                                                 PARSLEY seed
Petroselinum hortense .... see PARSLEY leaf, root,
                                                                 PARSLEY seed
Petroselinum sativum .... see PARSLEY leaf, root,
                                                                 PARSLEY seed
Petrosilini radix .... see PARSLEY leaf, root
Pettigree .... see BUTCHER'S BROOM
Petty Morel .... see BLACK NIGHTSHADE
Petty Mugget .... see LADY'S BEDSTRAW
Petty Mulleins .... see COWSLIP
Petty Whin .... see SPINY RESTHARROW
Pettymorell .... see AMERICAN SPIKENARD
Peumus boldus .... see BOLDO
Pewterwort .... see HORSETAIL
PEYOTE .... see PEYOTE
Pfaffia .... see SUMA
Pfaffia paniculata .... see SUMA
Pfeffer .... see BLACK PEPPER AND WHITE PEPPER
Pferdefut .... see COLTSFOOT
PGG-Glucan .... see BETA GLUCANS
Phaseoli fructus .... see BEAN POD
Phaseolus vulgaris varieties .... see BEAN POD
PHEASANT'S EYE .... see PHEASANT'S EYE
PHENYLALANINE .... see PHENYLALANINE
Philanthropium .... see BURDOCK
Phleum species .... see HAY FLOWER
Phoenix dactylifera .... see DATE PALM
Phoradendron flavescens ..... see AMERICAN MISTLETOE
Phoradendron leucarpum ..... see AMERICAN MISTLETOE
Phoradendron macrophyllum
.... see AMERICAN MISTLETOE
Phoradendron serontium ...... see AMERICAN MISTLETOE

Phoradendron tomentosum
.................................see AMERICAN MISTLETOE
Phormia regina .... see MAGGOTS
PHOSPHATE SALTS .... see PHOSPHATE SALTS
Phosphatidyl Choline .... see PHOSPHATIDYLCHOLINE
Phosphatidyl Serine
.... see PHOSPHATIDYLSERINE
PHOSPHATIDYLCHOLINE
.... see PHOSPHATIDYLCHOLINE
PHOSPHATIDYLSERINE
.... see PHOSPHATIDYLSERINE
Phragmites communis .... see REED HERB
Phyllanthus emblica .... see INDIAN GOOSEBERRY
Phyllanthus niruri .... see CHANCA PIEDRA
Phylloquinone .... see VITAMIN K
Physalis alkekengi .... see WINTER CHERRY
Physic Root .... see BLACK ROOT
Physostigma venenosum .... see CALABAR BEAN
Physotigma .... see CALABAR BEAN
Phytic Acid .... see IP-6
Phytoestrogen .... see ALFALFA, ANISE,
BLACK COHOSH, DONG QUAI,
FENNEL fruit, seed, FENNEL OIL,
FLAXSEED, GINSENG, SIBERIAN,
LICORICE, RED CLOVER,
RESVERATROL, SCARLET PIMPERNEL,
SOY, WILD YAM
Phytoestrogens .... see RED CLOVER
Phytolacca americana .... see POKEWEED berry,
POKEWEED root
Phytolacca Berry .... see POKEWEED berry,
POKEWEED root
Phytolacca decandra .... see POKEWEED berry,
POKEWEED root
Phytomenadione .... see VITAMIN K
Phytonadione .... see VITAMIN K
Phytonadione (K1) .... see VITAMIN K
Phytoprogestin .... see OREGANO
Phytostanol .... see SITOSTANOL
Phytosterols .... see BETA-SITOSTEROL
Pica-Pica .... see COWHAGE
Picea abies .... see FIR, FIR NEEDLE OIL,
HEMLOCK SPRUCE
Picea aetheroleum .... see HEMLOCK SPRUCE
Picea excelsa .... see FIR, FIR NEEDLE OIL,
HEMLOCK SPRUCE
Picea turiones recentes .... see HEMLOCK SPRUCE
Piceae aetheroleum .... see FIR NEEDLE OIL
Piceae turiones recentes .... see FIR
Pickaway Anise .... see WAFER ASH
Pick-Pocket .... see SHEPHERD'S PURSE
Picrasma .... see QUASSIA
Picrasma excelsa .... see QUASSIA
Pie Cherry .... see SOUR CHERRY
Pierce-Stone .... see SAMPHIRE
Pigeonberry .... see POKEWEED berry,
POKEWEED root
Pigeon's Grass .... see VERBENA
Pigeonweed .... see VERBENA
Pignut .... see JOJOBA
Pigrush .... see KNOTWEED HERB
Pigweed .... see GOUTWEED,
KNOTWEED HERB
Pigwood .... see WAHOO

Pilewort .... see AMARANTH,
BULBOUS BUTTERCUP,
LESSER CELANDINE
Piliolerial .... see PENNYROYAL leaf,
PENNYROYAL oil
Pillbearing Spurge .... see EUPHORBIA
Pilocarpus microphyllus .... see JABORANDI
Pilosella officinarum .... see MOUSE EAR
Pilot Plant .... see CUP PLANT
Pilot Weed .... see ROSINWEED
Pimenta .... see ALLSPICE,
BLACK PEPPER AND WHITE PEPPER
Pimenta dioica .... see ALLSPICE
Pimenta-Longa .... see INDIAN LONG PEPPER
Pimenta officinalis .... see ALLSPICE
Pimento .... see ALLSPICE, CAPSICUM
Pimento Oil .... see ALLSPICE
Pimento Water .... see ALLSPICE
Pimienta .... see BLACK PEPPER AND WHITE PEPPER
Pimpernell .... see PIMPINELLA above ground parts,
PIMPINELLA root
Pimpinella .... see PIMPINELLA above ground parts,
PIMPINELLA root
PIMPINELLA above ground parts
.... see PIMPINELLA above ground parts
Pimpinella anisum .... see ANISE
Pimpinella major ..... see PIMPINELLA above ground parts,
PIMPINELLA root
PIMPINELLA root .... see PIMPINELLA root
Pimpinella Saxifraga
.... see PIMPINELLA above ground parts,
PIMPINELLA root
Pimpinellae herba ..... see PIMPINELLA above ground parts
Pimpinellae radix .... see PIMPINELLA root
Pin Heads .... see GERMAN CHAMOMILE
Pinag .... see ARECA
PINE .... see PINE
Pine Bark .... see PYCNOGENOL
Pine Bark Extract .... see PYCNOGENOL
Pine Needle Oil .... see BUTANEDIOL (BD)
Pine Oils .... see SCOTCH PINE NEEDLE
Pine Pollen .... see BEE POLLEN
Pineal Hormone .... see MELATONIN
Pineapple: Ananas comosus .... see BROMELAIN
Piney .... see PEONY flower,
PEONY root
Pini Atheroleum .... see SCOTCH PINE NEEDLE
Pini Turiones .... see PINE
PINK ROOT .... see PINK ROOT
Pinkroot .... see PINK ROOT
Pinlag .... see ARECA
Pin-Ma Ts'ao .... see DANSHEN
Pinto Bean .... see BEAN POD
Pinus australis .... see TURPENTINE OIL
PINUS BARK .... see PINUS BARK
Pinus Maritima .... see PYCNOGENOL
Pinus marittima .... see PYCNOGENOL
Pinus montana .... see DWARF PINE NEEDLE
Pinus mugo .... see DWARF PINE NEEDLE
Pinus mugo pumilio .... see DWARF PINE NEEDLE
Pinus palustris .... see TURPENTINE OIL
Pinus Pinaster .... see PYCNOGENOL,
TURPENTINE OIL
Pinus pumilio .... see DWARF PINE NEEDLE

Pinus sylvestris .... see PINE, SCOTCH PINE NEEDLE
Piper .... see BLACK PEPPER AND WHITE PEPPER
Piper cubeba .... see CUBEBS
Piper Longum .... see INDIAN LONG PEPPER
Piper methysticum .... see KAVA
Piper Nigrum
.... see BLACK PEPPER AND WHITE PEPPER
Pipiltzintzintli .... see DIVINER'S SAGE
Pipperidge .... see EUROPEAN BARBERRY
Piprage .... see EUROPEAN BARBERRY
PIPSISSEWA .... see PIPSISSEWA
Piratancara .... see CATUABA
Piscidia communis .... see JAMAICAN DOGWOOD
Piscidia erythrina .... see JAMAICAN DOGWOOD
Piscidia piscipula .... see JAMAICAN DOGWOOD
Pissenlit .... see DANDELION above ground parts,
DANDELION entire plant
Pistacia lentiscus .... see MASTIC
PITCHER PLANT .... see PITCHER PLANT
Pitirishi .... see CHANCA PIEDRA
Pituri .... see CORKWOOD TREE
Pix Cadi .... see CADE OIL
Pix Juniper .... see CADE OIL
Pix Liquida .... see PINE
Pix Oxycedri .... see CADE OIL
Plant Estrogen .... see SOY
Plant of Immortality
.... see ALOE dried juice from leaf, latex
Plant Protease Concentrate .... see BROMELAIN,
PAPAIN
Plant Stanol .... see SITOSTANOL
Plant Sterols .... see BETA-SITOSTEROL
Plantaginis lanceolatae herba
.... see BUCKHORN PLANTAIN
Plantaginis ovatae semen .... see BLOND PSYLLIUM
Plantaginis ovatae testa .... see BLOND PSYLLIUM
Plantago decumbens .... see BLOND PSYLLIUM
Plantago isphagula .... see BLOND PSYLLIUM
Plantago lanceolata .... see BUCKHORN PLANTAIN
Plantago major .... see GREAT PLANTAIN
Plantago Ovata.............................. see BLOND PSYLLIUM
Plantago psyllium .... see BLACK PSYLLIUM
Plantain .... see BLACK PSYLLIUM,
BUCKHORN PLANTAIN
Plant-Derived Liquid Minerals
.... see COLLOIDAL MINERALS
Platycladus orientalis .... see ORIENTAL ARBORVITAE
PLC .... see PROPIONYL-L-CARNITINE
Pleurisy .... see PLEURISY ROOT
PLEURISY ROOT .... see PLEURISY ROOT
Plumrocks .... see COWSLIP
Pocan .... see POKEWEED berry
Pocan .... see POKEWEED root
Pockwood .... see GUAIAC WOOD resin, wood
Podophylli pelati rhizoma/resina .... see PODOPHYLLUM
PODOPHYLLUM ....see PODOPHYLLUM
Podophyllum emodi ....see PODOPHYLLUM
Podophyllum hexandrum ....see PODOPHYLLUM
Podophyllum Peltatum ....see PODOPHYLLUM
Poet's Jessamine .... see JASMINE
Pogostemon cablin........................... see PATCHOULY OIL
Pogostemon heyneanus .... see PATCHOULY OIL
Pogostemon patchouly...................... see PATCHOULY OIL
Pohl... see MANACA

POINSETTIA .... see POINSETTIA
Poinsettia pulcherrima .... see POINSETTIA
Poison Ash .... see FRINGETREE
Poison Black Cherries .... see BELLADONNA
Poison Flag .... see ORRIS
Poison Fool's Parsley .... see HEMLOCK
POISON IVY .... see POISON IVY
Poison Lettuce .... see WILD LETTUCE
Poison Nut .... see NUX VOMICA
Poison Parsnip .... see WATER HEMLOCK
Poison Tobacco .... see HENBANE
Poison Vine .... see POISON IVY
Poisonberry ....see BLACK NIGHTSHADE,
LEVANT BERRY
Poison-Hemlock .... see HEMLOCK
POISONOUS BUTTERCUP
.... see POISONOUS BUTTERCUP
Poivre .... see BLACK PEPPER AND WHITE PEPPER
Poivre Long .... see INDIAN LONG PEPPER
Poivre Noir ... see BLACK PEPPER AND WHITE PEPPER
Poke .... see POKEWEED berry,
POKEWEED root
Poke Root .... see POKEWEED root
Pokeberry .... see POKEWEED berry,
POKEWEED root
Pokeweed .... see POKEWEED berry,
POKEWEED root
POKEWEED berry .... see POKEWEED berry
POKEWEED root .... see POKEWEED root
Polar Plant .... see CUP PLANT,
ROSEMARY,
ROSINWEED
Polecatweed .... see SKUNK CABBAGE
Polemonium coeruleum .... see JACOB'S LADDER
Polemonium reptans .... see ABSCESS ROOT
Poleo .... see JAPANESE MINT
POLICOSANOL .... see POLICOSANOL
Pollen .... see BEE POLLEN
Pollen D'Abeille .... see BEE POLLEN
Poly-[1-6]-Beta-D-Glucopyranosyl-[1-3]-Beta-D-
Glucopyranose .... see BETA GLUCANS
Polygala amara .... see BITTER MILKWORT
Polygala glomerata .... see SENEGA
Polygala japonica .... see SENEGA
Polygala reinii .... see SENEGA
Polygala senega .... see SENEGA
Polygala senega latifolia .... see SENEGA
Polygala tenuifolia .... see SENEGA
Polygalae radix .... see SENEGA
Polygonatum multiflorum .... see SOLOMON'S SEAL
Polygoni Avicularis Herba .... see KNOTWEED HERB
Polygonum .... see FO-TI
Polygonum aviculare .... see KNOTWEED HERB
Polygonum bistorta .... see BISTORT
Polygonum hydropiper .... see SMARTWEED
Polygonum Multiflorum .... see FO-TI
Poly-NAG .... see N-ACETYL GLUCOSAMINE
Polyporus .... see PORIA MUSHROOM
Polyporus Versicolor........... see CORIOLUS MUSHROOM
Polysaccharide derived from Lentinus edodes
.... see LENTINAN
Polysaccharide Peptide .... see CORIOLUS MUSHROOM
Polysaccharide-K .... see CORIOLUS MUSHROOM
Polystictus Versicolor .... see CORIOLUS MUSHROOM

Polyunsaturated Fatty Acids .... see COD LIVER OIL, OMEGA-6 FATTY ACIDS
POMEGRANATE .... see POMEGRANATE
Pomelo .... see GRAPEFRUIT
Poolroot .... see SANICLE
Poor Man's Parmacettie .... see SHEPHERD'S PURSE
Poor Man's Treacle .... see GARLIC
Poor Man's Weatherglass .... see SCARLET PIMPERNEL
Popinac Absolute .... see CASSIE ABSOLUTE
POPLAR .... see POPLAR
Popotillo .... see EPHEDRA, MORMON TEA
Poppy California .... see CALIFORNIA POPPY
Populi cortex .... see ASPEN
Populi folium .... see ASPEN
Populi Gemma .... see POPLAR
Populus balsamifera .... see POPLAR
Populus candicans .... see POPLAR
Populus tacamahacca .... see POPLAR
Populus tremula .... see ASPEN
Populus tremuloides .... see ASPEN
Porcelain Clay .... see KAOLIN
Poria .... see PORIA MUSHROOM
Poria Cocos .... see PORIA MUSHROOM
PORIA MUSHROOM .... see PORIA MUSHROOM
Porites species .... see CORAL
Porter's Licorice Root .... see OSHA
Portland Arrowroot .... see ARUM
Pot .... see MARIJUANA
Pot Barley .... see BARLEY
Pot Marigold .... see CALENDULA
POTASSIUM .... see POTASSIUM
Potassium Acetate .... see POTASSIUM
Potassium Bicarbonate .... see POTASSIUM
Potassium Chloride .... see POTASSIUM
Potassium Citrate .... see POTASSIUM
Potassium Gluconate .... see POTASSIUM
Potassium Iodide .... see IODINE
Potassium Phosphate .... see PHOSPHATE SALTS, POTASSIUM
Potassium Pyruvate .... see PYRUVATE
POTATO .... see POTATO
Potency Wood .... see MUIRA PUAMA
POTENTILLA .... see POTENTILLA
Potentilla .... see TORMENTIL
Potentilla anserina .... see POTENTILLA
Potentilla erecta .... see TORMENTIL
Potentilla reptans
.... see EUROPEAN FIVE-FINGER GRASS
Poverty Weed .... see OX-EYE DAISY
Povidone Iodine .... see IODINE
Prairie Dock .... see CUP PLANT
Prairie Grub .... see WAFER ASH
Prasterone .... see DHEA
Prayer Beads .... see PRECATORY BEAN
Prayer Head .... see PRECATORY BEAN
PRECATORY BEAN .... see PRECATORY BEAN
Predigested Spleen Extract .... see SPLEEN EXTRACT
Predigested Thymus Extract .... see THYMUS EXTRACT
Pregnancy Hormone .... see PROGESTERONE
Pregnanedione .... see PROGESTERONE
PREGNENOLONE .... see PREGNENOLONE
Prele .... see HORSETAIL
PREMORSE .... see PREMORSE

Premorse Scaboius .... see PREMORSE
Pretty Betsy .... see RED-SPUR VALERIAN
Prick Madam .... see COMMON STONECROP
Prickly Ash .... see NORTHERN PRICKLY ASH, SOUTHERN PRICKLY ASH
Prickly Pear .... see PRICKLY PEAR CACTUS
PRICKLY PEAR CACTUS
.... see PRICKLY PEAR CACTUS
Prickly Yellow Wood ...... see SOUTHERN PRICKLY ASH
Prickwood .... see WAHOO
Pride of China .... see NEEM
Prideweed .... see CANADIAN FLEABANE
Priest's Crown .... see DANDELION entire plant, DANDELION above ground parts
Primrose .... see COWSLIP, EVENING PRIMROSE OIL
Primula .... see COWSLIP
Primula elatier .... see COWSLIP
Primula Officinalis .... see COWSLIP
Primula veris .... see COWSLIP
Prince's Feather .... see AMARANTH
Prince's Feathers .... see POTENTILLA
Prince's Pine .... see PIPSISSEWA
Privet .... see GLOSSY PRIVET
Proacemic Acid .... see PYRUVATE
Proanthodyn .... see GRAPE seed
Probiotics .... see BIFIDOBACTERIA, BREWER'S YEAST (HANSEN CBS 5926), LACTOBACILLUS, SACCHAROMYCES BOULARDII, YOGURT
PROCAINE .... see PROCAINE
Procaine Hydrochloride .... see PROCAINE
Processed Bovine Cartilage ...... see BOVINE CARTILAGE
Procyandiol Oligomers .... see PYCNOGENOL
Procyanidolic Oligomers .... see GRAPE seed
Procyanodolic Oligomers .... see PYCNOGENOL
Progestational Hormone .... see PROGESTERONE
PROGESTERONE .... see PROGESTERONE
Progesteronum .... see PROGESTERONE
PROPIONYL-L-CARNITINE
.... see PROPIONYL-L-CARNITINE
PROPOLIS .... see PROPOLIS
Propolis Balsam .... see PROPOLIS
Propolis Resin .... see PROPOLIS
Propolis Wax .... see PROPOLIS
Proteinase .... see TRYPSIN
Proteolytic Enzyme .... see TRYPSIN
Protykin .... see RESVERATROL
Provitamin A .... see BETA-CAROTENE
Pruche de l'Est .... see PINUS BARK
Prunella .... see SELF-HEAL
Prunella vulgaris .... see SELF-HEAL
Pruni Spinosae Fructus .... see BLACKTHORN berry
Pruni Spinosae Llos .... see BLACKTHORN flower
Prunus africana .... see PYGEUM
Prunus amygdalus amara .... see BITTER ALMOND
Prunus amygdalus dulcis .... see SWEET ALMOND
Prunus armeniaca .... see APRICOT
Prunus Cerasus .... see SOUR CHERRY
Prunus dulcis amara .... see BITTER ALMOND
Prunus laurocerasus .... see CHERRY LAUREL WATER
Prunus serotina .... see WILD CHERRY
Prunus spinosa .... see BLACKTHORN berry, BLACKTHORN flower

Prunus virginiana .... see WILD CHERRY
Prunus vulgaris .... see SOUR CHERRY
PS .... see PHOSPHATIDYLSERINE
Pseudoginseng Root .... see PANAX PSEUDOGINSENG
Pseudotsuga douglasii .... see OREGON FIR BALSAM
Pseudotsuga menziesii .... see OREGON FIR BALSAM
Pseudotsuga mucronata .... see OREGON FIR BALSAM
Pseudotsuga taxifolia .... see OREGON FIR BALSAM
Psi-Psi-Carotene .... see LYCOPENE
PSK .... see CORIOLUS MUSHROOM
Psoralea linearis .... see RED BUSH TEA
Psoriacin .... see BOVINE CARTILAGE
Psoriacin-T .... see BOVINE CARTILAGE
PSP .... see CORIOLUS MUSHROOM
Psychotria ipecacuanha .... see IPECAC
Psyllion .... see BLACK PSYLLIUM
Psyllios .... see BLACK PSYLLIUM
Psyllium .... see BLOND PSYLLIUM
Psyllium afra .... see BLACK PSYLLIUM
Psyllium arenaria .... see BLACK PSYLLIUM
Psyllium indica .... see BLACK PSYLLIUM
Psyllium Seed .... see BLACK PSYLLIUM
Ptarmigan Berry .... see UVA URSI
PtdSer .... see PHOSPHATIDYLSERINE
Ptelea trifoliata .... see WAFER ASH
Pterocarpus santalinus .... see RED SANDALWOOD
Pteroylglutamic acid .... see FOLIC ACID
Pteroylmonoglutamic acid .... see FOLIC ACID
Pteroylpolyglutamate .... see FOLIC ACID
Ptychopetali lignum .... see MUIRA PUAMA
Ptychopetalum olacoides .... see MUIRA PUAMA
Ptychopetalum unicatum .... see MUIRA PUAMA
Public House Plant .... see ASARABACCA
Pudding Grass .... see PENNYROYAL leaf,
                                                           PENNYROYAL oil
Pueraria .... see KUDZU
Pueraria lobata .... see KUDZU
Pueraria mirifica .... see KUDZU
Pueraria montana var. lobata .... see KUDZU
Pueraria montana var. thomsonii .... see KUDZU
Pueraria pseudohirsuta .... see KUDZU
Pueraria Root .... see KUDZU
Pueraria thomsonii .... see KUDZU
Pueraria thunbergiana .... see KUDZU
Pueraria tuberosa .... see KUDZU
Puerto Rican Cherry .... see ACEROLA
Pufa .... see FISH OILS
Pufas .... see OMEGA-6 FATTY ACIDS
PUFF BALL .... see PUFF BALL
Pukeweed .... see LOBELIA
Pulegium .... see PENNYROYAL leaf,
                                                           PENNYROYAL oil
Pulegium vulgare .... see PENNYROYAL leaf,
                                                           PENNYROYAL oil
Pulmonaria officinalis .... see LUNGWORT
Pulmonariae herba .... see LUNGWORT
PULSATILLA .... see PULSATILLA
Pulsatilla Nigricans .... see PULSATILLA
Pulsatilla pratensis .... see PULSATILLA
Pulsatilla vulgaris .... see PULSATILLA
Pumacuchu .... see RHATANY
Pumilio Pine .... see PINE
PUMPKIN .... see PUMPKIN
Pumpkin Seed .... see PUMPKIN

PUNCTURE VINE .... see PUNCTURE VINE
Puncturevine .... see PUNCTURE VINE
Punica granatum .... see POMEGRANATE
Punk Tree .... see CAJEPUT OIL
Punnanga .... see LAURELWOOD
Pupurweide .... see WILLOW BARK
Pure Bee Venom .... see BEE VENOM
Pure Thymic Extract .... see THYMUS EXTRACT
Purging Flax .... see MOUNTAIN FLAX
Purging Thorn .... see SEA BUCKTHORN
Purified Honey .... see HONEY
Purified Turpentine Oil .... see TURPENTINE OIL
Purines .... see RNA AND DNA
Purple Boneset .... see GRAVEL ROOT
Purple Clover .... see RED CLOVER
Purple Cockle .... see CORN COCKLE
Purple Cone Flower .... see ECHINACEA
Purple Foxglove .... see DIGITALIS
Purple Lapacho .... see PAU D'ARCO
Purple Leptandra .... see BLACK ROOT
PURPLE LOOSESTRIFE ..... see PURPLE LOOSESTRIFE
Purple Medick .... see ALFALFA
Purple Mulberry .... see BLACK MULBERRY
Purple Osier .... see WILLOW BARK
Purple Osier Willow .... see WILLOW BARK
Purple Passion Flower .... see PASSIONFLOWER
Purple Pitcher Plant .... see PITCHER PLANT
Purple Rocket .... see FIREWEED
Purple Side-Saddle Flower .... see PITCHER PLANT
Purple Turk's Cap Lily .... see MARTAGON
Purple Willow-Herb .... see PURPLE LOOSESTRIFE
Purpursonnenhutkraut .... see ECHINACEA
Purpursonnenhutwurzel .... see ECHINACEA
Purshiana Bark .... see CASCARA
P'u-T'ao .... see BITTER MELON
Putcha-Pat .... see PATCHOULY OIL
PYCNOGENOL .... see PYCNOGENOL
Pygenol .... see PYCNOGENOL
PYGEUM .... see PYGEUM
PYRETHRUM .... see PYRETHRUM
Pyrethrum parthenium .... see FEVERFEW
Pyridoxal .... see PYRIDOXINE (VITAMIN B6)
Pyridoxamine .... see PYRIDOXINE (VITAMIN B6)
Pyridoxine .... see PYRIDOXINE (VITAMIN B6)
PYRIDOXINE (VITAMIN B6)
.... see PYRIDOXINE (VITAMIN B6)
Pyridoxine Hydrochloride
.... see PYRIDOXINE (VITAMIN B6)
Pyrimidines .... see RNA AND DNA
Pyroleum Juniperi .... see CADE OIL
Pyroleum Oxycedri .... see CADE OIL
Pyrus communis .... see PEAR
PYRUVATE .... see PYRUVATE
Q .... see GLUTAMINE
Q10 .... see COENZYME Q-10
Qian Ceng Ta .... see CHINESE CLUB MOSS
Qing Hao .... see SWEET ANNIE
Qinghao .... see SWEET ANNIE
Qinghaosu .... see SWEET ANNIE
Quack Grass .... see AGROPYRON,
                                                           COUCH GRASS
Quackgrass .... see AGROPYRON,
                                                           COUCH GRASS,
                                                           WHEATGRASS

INDEX

Quaker .... see ARUM
Quaker Bonnet .... see SCULLCAP
Quaker Buttons .... see NUX VOMICA
QUASSIA .... see QUASSIA
Quassia amara .... see QUASSIA
Quassia Bark .... see QUASSIA
Quebra Pedra .... see CHANCA PIEDRA
QUEBRACHO .... see QUEBRACHO
Quebracho Blanco .... see QUEBRACHO
Quebrachol .... see BETA-SITOSTEROL
Quebrapedra .... see CHANCA PIEDRA
Queen Anne's Lace .... see WILD CARROT
Queen Of The Meadow .... see GRAVEL ROOT,
                                                 MEADOWSWEET
QUEEN'S DELIGHT .... see QUEEN'S DELIGHT
Queen's Root .... see QUEEN'S DELIGHT
QUERCETIN .... see QUERCETIN
Quercetin-3-rhamnoglucoside .... see RUTIN
Quercetin-3-rutinoside .... see RUTIN
Quercus alba .... see OAK bark
Quercus cortex .... see OAK bark
Quercus Marina .... see BLADDERWRACK
Quercus petraea .... see OAK bark
Quercus robur .... see OAK bark
Quickbeam .... see MOUNTAIN ASH
Quick-In-The-Hand .... see JEWELWEED
QUILLAIA .... see QUILLAIA
Quillaja .... see QUILLAIA
Quillaja saponaria .... see QUILLAIA
Quimotripsina .... see CHYMOTRYPSIN
QUINCE .... see QUINCE
Quing Dai .... see DA QING YE
Quinina Criolla .... see CHANCA PIEDRA
Quinine .... see CINCHONA
Quinine Créole .... see CHANCA PIEDRA
Quitch Grass .... see AGROPYRON
Qut .... see KHAT
Rabbiteye blueberry .... see BLUEBERRY
Rabbits .... see YELLOW TOADFLAX
Raccoon Berry .... see PODOPHYLLUM
Race Ginger .... see GINGER
Racine de Carline Acaule .... see CARLINA
Racine De Guimauve .... see MARSHMALLOW
Racine d'echininacea .... see ECHINACEA
Radis .... see RADISH
RADISH .... see RADISH
Radix Anchusae .... see ALKANNA
Radix Cardopatiae .... see CARLINA
Radix Chamaeleontis Albae .... see CARLINA
Radix Codonopsis .... see CODONOPSIS
Radix Peurariae .... see KUDZU
Radix Pimpinelle Franconiae .... see MASTERWORT
Radix Polygoni Multiflori .... see FO-TI
Radix Polygoni Shen Min .... see FO-TI
Rag Paper .... see MULLEIN
Ragged Cup .... see CUP PLANT
Ragweed .... see TANSY RAGWORT
Ragwort .... see GOLDEN RAGWORT,
                                           TANSY RAGWORT
Rainbow Weed .... see PURPLE LOOSESTRIFE
Raisin d'Amérique .... see POKEWEED berry,
                                             POKEWEED root
Raisin D'Ours .... see UVA URSI
Raisins .... see GRAPE fruit, skin

Raiz Para Los Dientes .... see RHATANY
Ram-Goat Rose .... see MADAGASCAR PERIWINKLE
Rami Buah .... see CHANCA PIEDRA
Ramp .... see ARUM
Ramsons .... see BEAR'S GARLIC
Ramsted .... see YELLOW TOADFLAX
Ramsthorn .... see EUROPEAN BUCKTHORN
Ranunculus .... see LESSER CELANDINE
Ranunculus acris .... see BUTTERCUP
Ranunculus Bulbosus ..... see BULBOUS BUTTERCUP
Ranunculus ficaria .... see LESSER CELANDINE
Ranunculus sceleratus ...... see POISONOUS BUTTERCUP
Raphani sativi radix .... see RADISH
Raphanus raphanistrum .... see WILD RADISH
Raphanus sativus .... see RADISH
Raspberry .... see RASPBERRY leaf
RASPBERRY leaf .... see RASPBERRY leaf
Ratanhiae radix .... see RHATANY
Ratanhiawurzel .... see RHATANY
Rattle Pouches .... see SHEPHERD'S PURSE
Rattle Root .... see BLACK COHOSH
Rattle Snakeroot .... see BLACK COHOSH
Rattlebush .... see WILD INDIGO
Rattlesnake Root .... see BETH ROOT,
                                       BLACK COHOSH, SENEGA
Rattlesnake Violet .... see AMERICAN ADDER'S TONGUE
Rattleweed .... see BLACK COHOSH
Rauschpfeffer .... see KAVA
Raute .... see RUE
Rauvolfia serpentina .... see INDIAN SNAKEROOT
Rauwolfae radix .... see INDIAN SNAKEROOT
Rauwolfia .... see INDIAN SNAKEROOT
Rauwolfia Serpentina .... see INDIAN SNAKEROOT
Rauwolfiawurzel .... see INDIAN SNAKEROOT
Raw Liver .... see LIVER EXTRACT
Raw Spleen .... see SPLEEN EXTRACT
Ray-Grass .... see TAUMELLOOLCH
Red .... see DANSHEN
Red American Ginseng .... see CANAIGRE
Red Bay .... see MAGNOLIA bark
Red Bearberry .... see UVA URSI
Red Beet .... see BEET
Red Berry .... see GINSENG, AMERICAN
Red Bilberry .... see ALPINE CRANBERRY
Red Bush .... see RED BUSH TEA
RED BUSH TEA .... see RED BUSH TEA
Red Cedarwood
.... see CEDARWOOD bark, berry, leaf, seed, twig
Red Cherry .... see SOUR CHERRY
Red Chickweed .... see SCARLET PIMPERNEL
Red Cinchona Bark .... see CINCHONA
RED CLOVER .... see RED CLOVER
Red Cockscomb .... see AMARANTH
Red Cole .... see HORSERADISH
Red Couchgrass .... see GERMAN SARSAPARILLA
Red Date .... see JUJUBE
Red Elm .... see SLIPPERY ELM
Red Fir .... see OREGON FIR BALSAM
Red Ginseng .... see GINSENG, PANAX
Red Globe .... see GRAPE fruit, skin
Red Gum .... see EUCALYPTUS dried leaf,
                                                 STORAX
Red Indian Paint .... see BLOODROOT
Red-Ink Plant .... see POKEWEED berry,
                                             POKEWEED root

Red Juniper
.... see CEDARWOOD bark, berry, leaf, seed, twig
Red Lapacho .... see PAU D'ARCO
Red Legs .... see BISTORT
Red Malaga .... see GRAPE fruit, skin
RED MAPLE .... see RED MAPLE
Red Morocco .... see PHEASANT'S EYE
Red Pepper .... see CAPSICUM
Red Periwinkle .... see MADAGASCAR PERIWINKLE
Red Pimpernel .... see SCARLET PIMPERNEL
Red Plant .... see POKEWEED berry,
POKEWEED root
Red Poppy .... see CORN POPPY
Red Puccoon .... see BLOODROOT
Red Raspberry .... see RASPBERRY leaf
Red Rhatany .... see RHATANY
Red Rice Yeast .... see RED YEAST
Red River Snakeroot .... see ARISTOLOCHIA
Red Robin .... see KNOTWEED HERB
Red Root .... see BLOODROOT,
NEW JERSEY TEA
Red Rot .... see SUNDEW
Red Sage .... see DANSHEN,
GERMAN SARSAPARILLA
RED SANDALWOOD .... see RED SANDALWOOD
Red Sanderswood .... see RED SANDALWOOD
Red Saunders .... see RED SANDALWOOD
RED SOAPWORT .... see RED SOAPWORT
RED-SPUR VALERIAN .... see RED-SPUR VALERIAN
Red Squill .... see SQUILL
Red Sunflower .... see ECHINACEA
Red Tea .... see HIBISCUS
Red Thyme Oil .... see THYME OIL
Red Vine Leaf AS 195 .... see GRAPE leaf
Red Vine Leaf Extract .... see GRAPE leaf
Red Weed .... see POKEWEED berry,
POKEWEED root
Red Whortleberry .... see ALPINE CRANBERRY
RED YEAST .... see RED YEAST
Red Yeast Rice .... see RED YEAST
Redberries .... see ALPINE CRANBERRY
Redberry .... see UVA URSI
Redroot .... see NEW JERSEY TEA
Reduced DPN .... see NADH
Reduced Nicotinamide Adenine Dinucleotide .... see NADH
Reed .... see REED HERB
REED HERB .... see REED HERB
Reglisse .... see LICORICE
Regliz .... see LICORICE
Reifweide .... see WILLOW BARK
Rei Shi .... see REISHI MUSHROOM
REISHI MUSHROOM .... see REISHI MUSHROOM
Ren Shen .... see GINSENG, AMERICAN
GINSENG, PANAX
Requia .... see ANDIROBA
Reseda .... see HENNA
Resin Tolu .... see TOLU BALSAM
Resina Tolutana .... see TOLU BALSAM
Restharrow .... see SPINY RESTHARROW
RESVERATROL .... see RESVERATROL
Resveratrols .... see RESVERATROL
Retinoids .... see VITAMIN A
Retinol .... see VITAMIN A
Retinol Acetate .... see VITAMIN A

Retinol Palmitate .... see VITAMIN A
Retinyl Acetate .... see VITAMIN A
Retinyl Palmitate .... see VITAMIN A
Réunion Vanilla .... see VANILLA
RGH-4405 .... see VINPOCETINE
Rhamni cathartica fructus
.... see EUROPEAN BUCKTHORN
Rhamni Purshianae Cortex .... see CASCARA
Rhamnol .... see BETA-SITOSTEROL
Rhamnus catharticus .... see EUROPEAN BUCKTHORN
Rhamnus Frangula .... see ALDER BUCKTHORN
Rhamnus purshiana .... see CASCARA
Rhatanhia .... see RHATANY
Rhatania .... see RHATANY
RHATANY .... see RHATANY
Rhei .... see RHUBARB
Rhei radix .... see RHUBARB
Rheum australe .... see RHUBARB
Rheum emodi .... see RHUBARB
Rheum officinale .... see RHUBARB
Rheum palmatum .... see RHUBARB
Rheum rhabarbarum .... see RHUBARB
Rheum tanguticum .... see RHUBARB
Rheum x cultorum .... see RHUBARB
Rheumatism Root .... see WILD YAM
Rheumatism Weed .... see PIPSISSEWA
Rhizoma iridis .... see ORRIS
Rhizome Galangae .... see ALPINIA
Rhodiola Rosea .... see ROSEROOT
Rhododendri Ferruginei Folium
.... see RUSTY-LEAVED RHODODENDRON
Rhododendron ferrugineum
.... see RUSTY-LEAVED RHODODENDRON
Rhoeados Flos .... see CORN POPPY
RHUBARB .... see RHUBARB
Rhus aromatica .... see SWEET SUMACH
Rhus Toxicodendron (Rhus radicans) .... see POISON IVY
Ribes Nero .... see BLACK CURRANT SEED OIL
Ribes nigri folium .... see BLACK CURRANT dried leaf
Ribes nigrum .... see BLACK CURRANT berry,
BLACK CURRANT dried leaf,
BLACK CURRANT SEED OIL
Ribgrass .... see BUCKHORN PLANTAIN
Riboflavin .... see RIBOFLAVIN (VITAMIN B2)
RIBOFLAVIN (VITAMIN B2)
.... see RIBOFLAVIN (VITAMIN B2)
Riboflavine .... see RIBOFLAVIN (VITAMIN B2)
Ribonucleic Acid .... see RNA AND DNA
RIBOSE .... see RIBOSE
Ribwort .... see BUCKHORN PLANTAIN
Ribwort Plantain .... see BUCKHORN PLANTAIN
RICE BRAN .... see RICE BRAN
Rice Bran Oil .... see RICE BRAN
Ricebran Oil .... see RICE BRAN
Rich Weed .... see STONE ROOT
Richleaf .... see STONE ROOT
Richmond .... see SOUR CHERRY
Ricinus communis .... see CASTOR OIL, CASTOR seed
Ricinus sanguines .... see CASTOR OIL, CASTOR seed
Ringworm Powder .... see GOA POWDER
Rio Ipecac .... see IPECAC
Ripplegrass .... see BUCKHORN PLANTAIN
Ritterspornblüten .... see DELPHINIUM
RNA .... see RNA AND DNA

RNA AND DNA .... see RNA AND DNA
RNA/DNA .... see RNA AND DNA
RNA-DNA .... see RNA AND DNA
Robbia .... see MADDER
Robin-Run-in-the-Grass .... see CLIVERS
Robin-Run-In-The-Hedge .... see GROUND IVY
Rock Brake .... see LADY FERN
Rock Cranberry .... see ALPINE CRANBERRY
Rock Fern .... see MAIDENHAIR FERN
Rock of Polypody .... see LADY FERN
Rock Parsley .... see PARSLEY leaf, root
Rockberry .... see UVA URSI
Rockrose .... see FROSTWORT, LABDANUM
Rock's-Foot .... see HAY FLOWER
Rock-Up-Hat .... see ECHINACEA
Rockweed .... see BLADDERWRACK
Rockwrack .... see BLADDERWRACK
Rodia riza .... see ROSEROOT
Roga Mari .... see YARROW
Rokitnik .... see SEA BUCKTHORN
Rokujo .... see DEER VELVET
ROMAN CHAMOMILE .... see ROMAN CHAMOMILE
Roman-Coriander .... see BLACK SEED
Roman Cumin .... see CARAWAY OIL
Roman Laurel .... see SWEET BAY
Roman Motherwort .... see MOTHERWORT
Romarin Sauvage .... see MARSH TEA
Römische Kamille .... see ROMAN CHAMOMILE
Ronce d'Amerique .... see CRANBERRY
Rooibos Tea .... see RED BUSH TEA
Root of the Holy Ghost .... see ANGELICA root
Rooted Sage .... see DANSHEN
Roripa armoracia .... see HORSERADISH
Rosa camellia .... see CHEROKEE ROSEHIP
Rosa canina .... see ROSE HIP
Rosa centifolia .... see ROSE HIP
Rosa cherokensis .... see CHEROKEE ROSEHIP
Rosa damascena .... see ROSE HIP
Rosa de castillo .... see ROSE HIP
Rosa gallica .... see ROSE HIP
Rosa laevigata .... see CHEROKEE ROSEHIP
Rosa nivea .... see CHEROKEE ROSEHIP
Rosa pomifera .... see ROSE HIP
Rosa rugosa .... see ROSE HIP
Rosa sinica .... see CHEROKEE ROSEHIP
Rosa ternata .... see CHEROKEE ROSEHIP
Rosa villosa .... see ROSE HIP
Rosae pseudofructus cum semen .... see ROSE HIP
Rosary Pea .... see PRECATORY BEAN
Rose Apple .... see JAMBOLAN bark,
                                                            JAMBOLAN seed
Rose-A-Rubie .... see PHEASANT'S EYE
Rose Bay .... see OLEANDER
Rose Bay Willow .... see FIREWEED
ROSE GERANIUM .... see ROSE GERANIUM
ROSE HIP .... see ROSE HIP
Rose Hip With Seed .... see ROSE HIP
Rose Hips .... see ROSE HIP
Rose Laurel .... see MOUNTAIN LAUREL,
                                                                    OLEANDER
Rose Mallow .... see HOLLYHOCK
Rose Root .... see ROSEROOT
Rose Root Extract .... see ROSEROOT
Rose Willow .... see AMERICAN DOGWOOD

Rosebay .... see RUSTY-LEAVED RHODODENDRON
Rosebay Willow .... see FIREWEED
Rosehips .... see ROSE HIP
Roselle .... see HIBISCUS
Rosemary .... see DAMIANA
ROSEMARY .... see ROSEMARY
Rosenoble .... see FIGWORT
Rosenroot .... see ROSEROOT
ROSEROOT .... see ROSEROOT
Rosewood Oil .... see BOIS DE ROSE OIL
Rosin Rose .... see ST. JOHN'S WORT
Rosin Weed .... see GUMWEED
Rosinweed .... see CUP PLANT
ROSINWEED .... see ROSINWEED
Rosmarinus officinalis .... see ROSEMARY
Roter Sonnenhut .... see ECHINACEA
Roter Wasserhanf .... see GRAVEL ROOT
Rottlera Tinctoria .... see KAMALA
Rou Gui .... see CASSIA
Round Buchu .... see BUCHU
Round-Leafed Sundew .... see SUNDEW
Round-Leaved Hepatica .... see LIVERWORT
Round-Lobe Hepatica .... see LIVERWORT
Rowan Tree .... see MOUNTAIN ASH
Roxanthin Red 10 .... see CANTHAXANTHIN
Royal Jasmine .... see JASMINE
ROYAL JELLY .... see ROYAL JELLY
RRR-Alpha-Tocopherol .... see VITAMIN E
Rubbed Thyme .... see THYME flower, leaf
Rubi Fruticosi Folium .... see BLACKBERRY leaf
Rubi Fruticosi Radix .... see BLACKBERRY root
Rubi idaei folium .... see RASPBERRY leaf
Rubia .... see MADDER
Rubia tinctorum .... see MADDER
Rubiae tinctorum radix .... see MADDER
Rubus .... see RASPBERRY leaf
Rubus fruticosus .... see BLACKBERRY leaf,
                                                             BLACKBERRY root
Rubus idaeus .... see RASPBERRY leaf
Rubus strigosus .... see RASPBERRY leaf
Rubywood .... see RED SANDALWOOD
Ruda .... see QUASSIA, RUE
RUE .... see RUE
Rue Officinale .... see RUE
Ruibarbo Caribe .... see MORINDA
Rum Cherry Bark .... see WILD CHERRY
Rumalon .... see BOVINE CARTILAGE
Rumex .... see YELLOW DOCK
Rumex acetosa .... see SORREL
Rumex aquaticus .... see WATER DOCK
Rumex crispus .... see YELLOW DOCK
Rumex hymenosepalus .... see CANAIGRE
Rumex obtusifolius .... see YELLOW DOCK
Rumput Roman .... see YIN CHEN
Run-By-The-Ground .... see PENNYROYAL leaf
                                                             PENNYROYAL oil
Running Box .... see SQUAWVINE
Running Jenny .... see MONEYWORT
RUPTUREWORT .... see RUPTUREWORT
Rusciaculeati .... see BUTCHER'S BROOM
Rusci Aculeati Rhizoma .... see BUTCHER'S BROOM
Ruscus Aculeatus .... see BUTCHER'S BROOM
Russian Formula .... see PANGAMIC ACID
Russian Krainer Tollkraut .... see SCOPOLIA

Russian Licorice .... see LICORICE
Russion Penicillin .... see PROPOLIS
Rust Treacle .... see GARLIC
Rust-Red Rhododendron
.... see RUSTY-LEAVED RHODODENDRON
RUSTY-LEAVED RHODODENDRON
.... see RUSTY-LEAVED RHODODENDRON
Ruta Graveolens .... see RUE
Rutae folium .... see RUE
Rutae herba .... see RUE
RUTIN .... see RUTIN
Rutine .... see RUTIN
Rutinum .... see RUTIN
Rutland Beauty .... see GREATER BINDWEED
Rutosid .... see RUTIN
Rutoside .... see RUTIN
Rutosidum .... see RUTIN
Rye .... see RYE GRASS
RYE GRASS .... see RYE GRASS
Rye Grass Pollen .... see RYE GRASS
Rye Grass Pollen Extract .... see RYE GRASS
Rye Pollen Extract .... see RYE GRASS
S. boulardii .... see SACCHAROMYCES BOULARDII
S.O.D. .... see SUPEROXIDE DISMUTASE
Sabal .... see SAW PALMETTO
Sabal Fructus .... see SAW PALMETTO
Sabal serrulata .... see SAW PALMETTO
Sabina .... see SAVIN TOPS
Sabline Rouge .... see ARENARIA RUBRA
Sabojira .... see CHICLE
Saccharomyces ..... see SACCHAROMYCES BOULARDII
SACCHAROMYCES BOULARDII
.... see SACCHAROMYCES BOULARDII
Saccharomyces Cerevisiae .... see BREWER'S YEAST
Saccharomyces cerevisiae Hansen CBS 5926
.... see BREWER'S YEAST (HANSEN CBS 5926)
Sacha Foster .... see CHANCA PIEDRA
Sacred Bark .... see CASCARA
Sacred Herb .... see YERBA SANTA
Sacred Mushroom .... see PEYOTE
S-Adenosyl Methionine .... see SAMe
S-Adenosyl-L-Methionine .... see SAMe
Sadi .... see DIVINER'S SAGE
Sadilata .... see ANDROGRAPHIS
SAFFLOWER .... see SAFFLOWER
SAFFRON .... see SAFFRON
Saffron Crocus .... see SAFFRON
Saffron Marigold .... see TAGETES
Safran .... see SAFFRON
Sagackhomi .... see UVA URSI
SAGE .... see SAGE
Sage of Bethlehem .... see SPEARMINT
Sage of the Seers .... see DIVINER'S SAGE
Sagrada Bark .... see CASCARA
Sahlep .... see SALEP
Saigon Cassia .... see CINNAMON bark
Saigon Cinnamon .... see CINNAMON bark
Sailor's Tobacco .... see MUGWORT
Saint John's Wort .... see ST. JOHN'S WORT
Sakau .... see KAVA
Salad Chervil .... see CHERVIL
Salad Oil .... see OLIVE OIL
Salai Guggal .... see INDIAN FRANKINCENSE
SALEP .... see SALEP

Salicare .... see PURPLE LOOSESTRIFE
Salicis cortex .... see WILLOW BARK
Salisburia .... see GINKGO leaf (GINKGO leaf extract)
Salisburia Adiantifolia
.... see GINKGO leaf (GINKGO leaf extract)
Salix Alba .... see WILLOW BARK
Salix daphnoides .... see WILLOW BARK
Salix fragilis .... see WILLOW BARK
Salix pentandra .... see WILLOW BARK
Salix Purpurea .... see WILLOW BARK
Sallow Thorn .... see SEA BUCKTHORN
Saloop .... see SALEP
Salsaparilha .... see SARSAPARILLA
Salsepareille .... see SARSAPARILLA
Salsify .... see COMFREY
Salt-Rheum Weed .... see TURTLE HEAD
Salvia .... see ALOE gel, DIVINER'S SAGE
Salvia bowelyana .... see DIVINER'S SAGE
Salvia divinorum .... see DIVINER'S SAGE
Salvia lavandulaefolia .... see SAGE
Salvia miltiorrhiza .... see DANSHEN
Salvia officinalis .... see SAGE
Salvia przewalskii .... see DANSHEN
Salvia przewalskii mandarinorum .... see DANSHEN
Salvia Root .... see DANSHEN
Salvia sclarea .... see CLARY SAGE
Salvia triloba .... see GREEK SAGE
Salvia yunnanensis .... see DANSHEN
Salvinorin .... see DIVINER'S SAGE
Salvinorin A .... see DIVINER'S SAGE
Sambilata .... see ANDROGRAPHIS
Sambrani Chettu .... see BRAHMI
Sambuci Sambucus .... see ELDERBERRY
Sambucus .... see AMERICAN ELDER,
ELDERFLOWER
Sambucus canadensis .... see AMERICAN ELDER
Sambucus ebulus .... see DWARF ELDER
Sambucus Nigra .... see ELDERBERRY,
ELDERFLOWER
Samch'il .... see PANAX PSEUDOGINSENG
SAMe .... see SAMe
Samento .... see CAT'S CLAW
Samm Al Ferakh .... see ASHWAGANDHA
Sammy .... see SAMe
SAMPHIRE .... see SAMPHIRE
Sampier .... see SAMPHIRE
San Qi .... see PANAX PSEUDOGINSENG
San Qui .... see PANAX PSEUDOGINSENG
Sand Plantain .... see BLOND PSYLLIUM
Sand Sedge .... see GERMAN SARSAPARILLA
Sandalwood .... see WHITE SANDALWOOD wood
Sandalwood Padauk .... see RED SANDALWOOD
Sandberry .... see UVA URSI
Sanddorn .... see SEA BUCKTHORN
Sanderswood .... see WHITE SANDALWOOD oil
Sandriedgraswurzelstock
.... see GERMAN SARSAPARILLA
Sandwort .... see ARENARIA RUBRA
SANDY EVERLASTING ..... see SANDY EVERLASTING
Sang .... see GINSENG, AMERICAN,
GINSENG, PANAX
Sangre de Drago .... see SANGRE DE GRADO
Sangre de Dragon .... see SANGRE DE GRADO
SANGRE DE GRADO .... see SANGRE DE GRADO

Sangree Root .... see ARISTOLOCHIA
Sangrel .... see ARISTOLOCHIA
Sangue de Agua .... see SANGRE DE GRADO
Sangue de Drago .... see SANGRE DE GRADO
Sanguinaria .... see BLOODROOT
Sanguinaria Canadensis .... see BLOODROOT
Sanguinary .... see SHEPHERD'S PURSE,
                                                      YARROW
Sanguis Draconis .... see DRAGON'S BLOOD
Sanguisorba .... see GREATER BURNET
Sanguisorba officinalis .... see GREATER BURNET
SANICLE .... see SANICLE
Sanicula europaea .... see SANICLE
Saniculae herba .... see SANICLE
Sanshichi .... see PANAX PSEUDOGINSENG
Santa Maria .... see FEVERFEW
Santal Oil .... see WHITE SANDALWOOD oil
Santali Lignum Albi .... see WHITE SANDALWOOD wood
Santali lignum rubrum .... see RED SANDALWOOD
Santalum album .... see WHITE SANDALWOOD oil,
                                        WHITE SANDALWOOD wood
Santolina .... see LAVENDER COTTON
Santolina chamaecyparissias ..... see LAVENDER COTTON
Santonica .... see WORMSEED
Sapodilla .... see CHICLE
Sapodillbaum .... see CHICLE
Saponaria Officinalis .... see RED SOAPWORT
Saponariae rubrae radix .... see RED SOAPWORT
Sapota achras .... see CHICLE
Sapote .... see CHICLE
Sapotier .... see CHICLE
Sapotillier .... see CHICLE
Sappan .... see RED SANDALWOOD
Sarapin .... see PITCHER PLANT
Sardian Nut .... see EUROPEAN CHESTNUT
Sarothamnus scoparius .... see SCOTCH BROOM flower,
                                             SCOTCH BROOM herb
Sarothamnus vulgaris .... see SCOTCH BROOM flower,
                                             SCOTCH BROOM herb
Sarpagandha .... see INDIAN SNAKEROOT
Sarracenia purpurea .... see PITCHER PLANT
Sarsa .... see SARSAPARILLA
SARSAPARILLA .... see SARSAPARILLA
Sarsaparillae radix .... see SARSAPARILLA
Sarsaparillewurzel .... see SARSAPARILLA
Sasha Foster .... see CHANCA PIEDRA
SASSAFRAS .... see SASSAFRAS
Sassafras ablidum .... see SASSAFRAS
Sassafras officinale .... see SASSAFRAS
Sassafras varifolium .... see SASSAFRAS
Sassafrax .... see SASSAFRAS
Satan's Apple .... see EUROPEAN MANDRAKE
Sativari .... see ASPARAGUS
Satureja capitata .... see SPANISH ORIGANUM OIL
Satureja hortensis .... see SUMMER SAVORY
Satureja montana .... see WINTER SAVORY
Satureja obovata .... see WINTER SAVORY
Satyrion .... see SALEP
Sauerdorn .... see EUROPEAN BARBERRY
Sauerkirsche .... see SOUR CHERRY
Sauerkirschenbaum .... see SOUR CHERRY
Sauge .... see SAGE
Saussurea Lappa .... see COSTUS OIL, COSTUS root
Sauvignon Blanc .... see GRAPE fruit, skin

Savin .... see SAVIN TOPS
SAVIN TOPS .... see SAVIN TOPS
Savine .... see SAVIN TOPS
Savory .... see SUMMER SAVORY,
                                        WINTER SAVORY
SAW PALMETTO .... see SAW PALMETTO
Saw Palmetto Berry .... see SAW PALMETTO
Sawi .... see MARIJUANA
Saxifrage .... see PIMPINELLA above ground parts,
                                             PIMPINELLA root
Saxifrax .... see SASSAFRAS
Saynt Johannes Wort .... see ST. JOHN'S WORT
Scabiosa succisa .... see PREMORSE
Scabish .... see EVENING PRIMROSE OIL
Scabwort .... see ELECAMPANE
Scaldweed .... see DODDER
Scaley Dragon's Claw .... see CORAL ROOT
Scarlet Berry .... see BITTERSWEET NIGHTSHADE
Scarlet Monarda .... see OSWEGO TEA
SCARLET PIMPERNEL .... see SCARLET PIMPERNEL
Scarlet Sage .... see SAGE
Sceau D'Or .... see GOLDENSEAL
Sceitbezien .... see SEA BUCKTHORN
Scented Fern .... see TANSY
SCHISANDRA .... see SCHISANDRA
Schisandra Berry .... see SCHISANDRA
Schisandra chinensis .... see SCHISANDRA
Schisandra splenanthera .... see SCHISANDRA
Schisandrae .... see SCHISANDRA
Schizandra .... see SCHISANDRA
Schizandrae .... see SCHISANDRA
Schizophyllan (SPG) .... see BETA GLUCANS
Schmallblaettrige Kegelblumenwurzel .... see ECHINACEA
Schmallblaettriger Sonnenhut .... see ECHINACEA
Schollkraut
...... see GREATER CELANDINE dried above ground parts
Schwarze Walnuss .... see BLACK WALNUT
Schwarzkümmel .... see BLACK SEED
Schweintang .... see BLADDERWRACK
Scilla .... see SQUILL
Scilla indica .... see SQUILL
Scilla maritima .... see SQUILL
Sclerutin .... see RUTIN
Scoke .... see POKEWEED berry, POKEWEED root
Scolopendrium vulgare .... see HARTSTONGUE
Scoparium .... see SCOTCH BROOM herb
Scoparius .... see SCOTCH BROOM flower,
                                             SCOTCH BROOM herb
Scopola .... see SCOPOLIA
SCOPOLIA .... see SCOPOLIA
Scopolia carniolica .... see SCOPOLIA
Scopoliae Rhizoma .... see SCOPOLIA
Scotch Barley .... see BARLEY
Scotch Broom .... see SCOTCH BROOM flower,
                                             SCOTCH BROOM herb
SCOTCH BROOM flower ... see SCOTCH BROOM flower
SCOTCH BROOM herb .... see SCOTCH BROOM herb
Scotch Fir .... see PINE
Scotch Heather .... see HEATHER
Scotch Mercury .... see DIGITALIS
Scotch Pine .... see PINE
SCOTCH PINE NEEDLE ..... see SCOTCH PINE NEEDLE
Scotch Quelch .... see AGROPYRON,
                                             COUCH GRASS

SCOTCH THISTLE .... see SCOTCH THISTLE
Scouring Rush .... see HORSETAIL
Scraperoot .... see OREGON GRAPE
Scratchweed .... see CLIVERS
Scrophula Plant .... see FIGWORT
Scrophularia .... see FIGWORT
Scrophularia mailandica .... see FIGWORT
Scrophularia nodosa (Scrophylariaceae) ...... see FIGWORT
Scrubby Grass .... see SCURVY GRASS
Scubby Trefoil .... see WAFER ASH
SCULLCAP .... see SCULLCAP
Scurvy Grass .... see SCURVY GRASS,
                                                            WATERCRESS
Scurvy Root .... see ECHINACEA
Scute .... see BAIKAL SKULLCAP
Scutellaria baicalensis .... see BAIKAL SKULLCAP
Scutellaria lateriflora .... see SCULLCAP
Scutelluria .... see SCULLCAP
Se .... see SELENIUM
Sea Ash .... see SOUTHERN PRICKLY ASH
Sea Buckhorn .... see SEA BUCKTHORN
SEA BUCKTHORN .... see SEA BUCKTHORN
Sea Coral .... see CORAL
Sea Fennel .... see SAMPHIRE
Sea Girdles .... see LAMINARIA
Sea Grape .... see EPHEDRA
Sea Holly
.... see ERYNGO above ground parts, ERYNGO root
Sea Holme
.... see ERYNGO above ground parts, ERYNGO root
Sea Hulver
.... see ERYNGO above ground parts, ERYNGO root
Sea Onion .... see SQUILL
Sea Parsley .... see LOVAGE
Sea Sedge .... see GERMAN SARSAPARILLA
Sea Squill Bulb .... see SQUILL
Sea Wormwood .... see WORMSEED
Seabuckthorn .... see SEA BUCKTHORN
Seagirdle Thallus .... see LAMINARIA
Sealroot .... see SOLOMON'S SEAL
Sealwort .... see SOLOMON'S SEAL
Seawrack .... see BLADDERWRACK
Secale cereale .... see RYE GRASS
Secale cornutum .... see ERGOT
SECRETIN .... see SECRETIN
Sedum acre .... see COMMON STONECROP
Sedum rhodiola .... see ROSEROOT
Sedum rosea .... see ROSEROOT
See Bright .... see CLARY SAGE
Seed-Free Bean Pods .... see BEAN POD
Seed on the Leaf .... see CHANCA PIEDRA
Seedorn .... see SEA BUCKTHORN
Segg .... see ORRIS
Sehydrin .... see HYDRAZINE SULFATE
Selada-Air .... see WATERCRESS
Selagine .... see HUPERZINE A
Selenicereus grandiflorus .... see CEREUS
Selenite .... see SELENIUM
SELENIUM .... see SELENIUM
Selenium Dioxide .... see SELENIUM
Selenized Yeast .... see SELENIUM
Selenomethionine .... see SELENIUM
Self-Heal .... see SANICLE
SELF-HEAL .... see SELF-HEAL

Selleriefruchte .... see CELERY
Selleriesamen .... see CELERY
Semen Anisi .... see ANISE
Semen Cumini Pratensis .... see CARAWAY dried fruit, seed
Semences de Carvi .... see CARAWAY dried fruit, seed
Seminole Bead .... see PRECATORY BEAN
Sempervivum tectorum .... see HOUSELEEK
Sena Alejandrina .... see SENNA
Senaga Snakeroot .... see SENEGA
Séné d'Egypte .... see SENNA
Seneca .... see SENEGA
Seneca Snakeroot .... see SENEGA
Senecio aureus .... see GOLDEN RAGWORT
Senecio cineraria .... see DUSTY MILLER
Senecio Herb .... see ALPINE RAGWORT
Senecio jacoboea .... see TANSY RAGWORT
Senecio nemorensis .... see ALPINE RAGWORT
Senecio vulgaris .... see GROUNDSEL
SENEGA .... see SENEGA
Senega Snakeroot .... see SENEGA
Seneka .... see SENEGA
Seng .... see GINSENG, PANAX
Sengreen .... see HOUSELEEK
SENNA .... see SENNA
Senna Alexandrina .... see SENNA
Sennae folium .... see SENNA
Sennae fructus .... see SENNA
Sennae fructus acutifoliae .... see SENNA
Sennae fructus angustifolia .... see SENNA
Septfoil .... see TORMENTIL
Serenoa Repens .... see SAW PALMETTO
Serenoa Serrulata .... see SAW PALMETTO
Serpentaria .... see ARISTOLOCHIA,
                                                            MONEYWORT
Serpent's Tongue ..... see AMERICAN ADDER'S TONGUE,
                                        ENGLISH ADDER'S TONGUE
Serpyllum .... see WILD THYME
Serratula spicata .... see MARSH BLAZING STAR
Seso Vegetal .... see ACKEE
Sessile Oak .... see OAK bark
Seven Barks .... see HYDRANGEA
Seville Orange .... see BITTER ORANGE
Shaddock Oil .... see GRAPEFRUIT OIL
Shamrock .... see WOOD SORREL
Shangzhou Zhiqiao .... see BITTER ORANGE
Shanzha .... see HAWTHORN
SHARK CARTILAGE .... see SHARK CARTILAGE
Shark Cartilage Extract .... see SHARK CARTILAGE
Shark Cartilage Powder .... see SHARK CARTILAGE
Shark Liver .... see SHARK LIVER OIL
SHARK LIVER OIL .... see SHARK LIVER OIL
Shark Oil .... see SHARK LIVER OIL
Sharp-Lobe Hepatica .... see LIVERWORT
Shatter Stone .... see CHANCA PIEDRA
Shave Grass .... see HORSETAIL
Sheep Laurel .... see MOUNTAIN LAUREL
Sheep-Lice .... see HOUND'S TONGUE
Sheep Sorrel .... see YELLOW DOCK
Sheggs .... see ORRIS
Shelf Fungi .... see MAITAKE MUSHROOM
SHELLAC .... see SHELLAC
Shellflower .... see TURTLE HEAD
Shen Min .... see FO-TI
Shepherd's Barometer .... see SCARLET PIMPERNEL

Shepherd's Club .... see MULLEIN
Shepherd's Heart .... see SHEPHERD'S PURSE
Shepherd's Knapperty .... see TORMENTIL
Shepherd's Knot .... see TORMENTIL
Shepherd's Needle .... see SWEET CICELY
SHEPHERD'S PURSE .... see SHEPHERD'S PURSE
Shepherd's Purse Herb .... see SHEPHERD'S PURSE
Shepherd's Scrip .... see SHEPHERD'S PURSE
Shepherd's Sprout .... see SHEPHERD'S PURSE
Shepherd's Staff .... see MULLEIN
Shepherd's Thyme .... see WILD THYME
Shi Liu Gen Pi .... see POMEGRANATE
Shi Liu Pi .... see POMEGRANATE
Shield Fern .... see MALE FERN
Shigoka .... see GINSENG, SIBERIAN
Shih Yin Ch'en .... see YIN CHEN
Shitake .... see SHIITAKE MUSHROOM
SHIITAKE MUSHROOM ... see SHIITAKE MUSHROOM
Shitake .... see SHIITAKE MUSHROOM
Shoe .... see NERVE ROOT
Shore Cranberry .... see ALPINE CRANBERRY
Short Buchu .... see BUCHU
Sho-saiko-to .... see BUPLEURUM
Shoti .... see ZEDOARY
Shou Wu .... see FO-TI
Shouwu .... see FO-TI
Shovelweed .... see SHEPHERD'S PURSE
Shoyu .... see SOY
Shrubby Hare's-ear .... see BUPLEURUM
Shu-Wei Ts'ao .... see DANSHEN
Siberian Beaver .... see CASTOREUM
Siberian Ginseng .... see GINSENG, SIBERIAN
Sicilian Thyme .... see SPANISH ORIGANUM OIL
Sickle-leaf Hare's-ear .... see BUPLEURUM
Sicklewort .... see BUGLE, SELF-HEAL
Siclewort .... see SELF-HEAL
Sida Cordifolia .... see COUNTRY MALLOW
Side-Saddle Plant .... see PITCHER PLANT
Sigualuo .... see LUFFA
Silberdistelwurz .... see CARLINA
Silberweide .... see WILLOW BARK
Silerkraut .... see ALCHEMILLA
Silky Cornel .... see AMERICAN DOGWOOD
Silky Loofah .... see LUFFA
Silphium laciniatum .... see ROSINWEED
Silphium perfoliatum .... see CUP PLANT
Silver Birch .... see BIRCH
Silver in suspending agent .... see COLLOIDAL SILVER
Silver Leaf .... see QUEEN'S DELIGHT
SILVER LINDEN .... see SILVER LINDEN
Silver-Morning-Glory
.... see HAWAIIAN BABY WOODROSE
Silver Protein .... see COLLOIDAL SILVER
Silverweed .... see JEWELWEED,
POTENTILLA
Silybin .... see MILK THISTLE
Silybum .... see MILK THISTLE
Silybum marianum .... see MILK THISTLE
Silymarin .... see MILK THISTLE
SIMARUBA .... see SIMARUBA
Simaruba amara .... see SIMARUBA
Simmondsia chinensis .... see JOJOBA
Simpler's Joy .... see VERBENA
Simson .... see GROUNDSEL

Sinapis alba .... see WHITE MUSTARD
Sinapis albae semen .... see WHITE MUSTARD
Sine Semine .... see BEAN POD
Singer's Plant .... see HEDGE MUSTARD
Singletary Pea .... see LATHYRUS
Sinsemilla .... see MARIJUANA
Sisymbrium officinale ... see HEDGE MUSTARD
SITOSTANOL .... see SITOSTANOL
Sitosterin .... see BETA-SITOSTEROL
Sitosterol .... see BETA-SITOSTEROL
Sitosterolins .... see BETA-SITOSTEROL
Sitosterols .... see BETA-SITOSTEROL
Sium sisarum .... see SKIRRET
SJW .... see ST. JOHN'S WORT
Ska Maria .... see DIVINER'S SAGE
Ska Maria Pastora .... see DIVINER'S SAGE
Skewerwood .... see WAHOO
SKIRRET .... see SKIRRET
Skoke .... see POKEWEED berry,
POKEWEED root
Skullcap .... see BAIKAL SKULLCAP
SKULLCAP .... see SCULLCAP
SKUNK CABBAGE .... see SKUNK CABBAGE
Skunkweed .... see SKUNK CABBAGE
Slave Wood .... see SIMARUBA
Slipper Root .... see NERVE ROOT
Slipper Weed .... see JEWELWEED
SLIPPERY ELM .... see SLIPPERY ELM
Slippery Root .... see COMFREY
Sloe .... see BLACKTHORN berry
Sloe Berry .... see BLACKTHORN berry
Sloe Flower .... see BLACKTHORN flower
Slough-Heal .... see SELF-HEAL
Small Cranberry .... see CRANBERRY
Small Hemlock .... see FOOL'S PARSLEY
Small Nettle
.... see STINGING NETTLE above ground parts,
STINGING NETTLE root
Small Periwinkle .... see PERIWINKLE
Small Radish .... see RADISH
Small Spikenard .... see AMERICAN SPIKENARD
Smallage .... see CELERY, LOVAGE
Smallpox Plant .... see PITCHER PLANT
Smallwort .... see LESSER CELANDINE
SMARTWEED .... see SMARTWEED
Smell Fox .... see WOOD ANEMONE
Smellage .... see LOVAGE
Smilax .... see SARSAPARILLA
Smilax aristolochiaefolii .... see SARSAPARILLA
Smilax aristolochiifolia .... see SARSAPARILLA
Smilax febrifuga .... see SARSAPARILLA
Smilax medica .... see SARSAPARILLA
Smilax Officinalis .... see SARSAPARILLA
Smilax regelii .... see SARSAPARILLA
SMOKELESS TOBACCO ... see SMOKELESS TOBACCO
SMOOTH ALDER .... see SMOOTH ALDER
Smooth Hydrangea .... see HYDRANGEA
Smooth Lawsonia .... see HENNA
Smooth-Leaved Elm .... see ELM BARK
Smooth Loofah .... see LUFFA
Smut Rye .... see ERGOT
Snake Berry .... see BITTERSWEET NIGHTSHADE
Snake Butter .... see SHIITAKE MUSHROOM
Snake Leaf .... see AMERICAN ADDER'S TONGUE

Snake Lily .... see ORRIS
Snake Root .... see SENEGA
Snake Weed .... see WATER HEMLOCK
Snakeberry .... see WHITE COHOSH
Snakebite .... see BETH ROOT, BLOODROOT
Snakehead .... see TURTLE HEAD
Snakeroot .... see ARISTOLOCHIA,
                                                          ASARABACCA,
                                                  BITTER MILKWORT,
                                                          ECHINACEA,
                                                  WATER HEMLOCK
Snakeweed .... see ARISTOLOCHIA
                                          BISTORT, EUPHORBIA
Snap Bean .... see BEAN POD
Snapdragon .... see YELLOW TOADFLAX
Snapping Tobacco Wood .... see WITCH HAZEL
SNEEZEWORT .... see SNEEZEWORT
Snow Rose .... see RUSTY-LEAVED RHODODENDRON
Snowball Bush .... see CRAMP BARK
Snowdrop Tree .... see FRINGETREE
Snowflower .... see FRINGETREE
Snuff .... see SMOKELESS TOBACCO
Soap Tree .... see QUILLAIA
Soap Tree Bark .... see QUILLAIA
Soapbark .... see QUILLAIA
Soapweed .... see YUCCA
Soapwort .... see RED SOAPWORT,
                                              WHITE SOAPWORT
SOD .... see SUPEROXIDE DISMUTASE
Sodium 4-hydroxybutyrate
.... see GAMMA-HYDROXYBUTYRATE
Sodium Alginate .... see ALGIN
Sodium Ascorbate .... see VITAMIN C
Sodium Borate .... see BORON
Sodium Edetate .... see EDTA
Sodium gamma-hydroxybutyrate
.... see GAMMA-HYDROXYBUTYRATE
Sodium Gluconate .... see PANGAMIC ACID
Sodium Oxybate .... see GAMMA-HYDROXYBUTYRATE
Sodium Oxybutyrate
.... see GAMMA-HYDROXYBUTYRATE
Sodium Phosphate .... see PHOSPHATE SALTS
Sodium Pyruvate .... see PYRUVATE
Soja .... see SOY
Sojabohne .... see SOY
Solanum dulcamara ... see BITTERSWEET NIGHTSHADE
Solanum nigrum .... see BLACK NIGHTSHADE
Solanum tuberosum .... see POTATO
Soldiers .... see PURPLE LOOSESTRIFE
Soldier's Herb .... see BUCKHORN PLANTAIN
Soldier's Wound Wort .... see YARROW
Solidago canadensis (Canadian goldenrod)
.... see GOLDENROD
Solidago gigantea (Early goldenrod) ...... see GOLDENROD
Solidago serotina .... see GOLDENROD
Solidago virgaurea (European goldenrod)
.... see GOLDENROD
SOLOMON'S SEAL .... see SOLOMON'S SEAL
Solsequia .... see MARSH MARIGOLD
Soma .... see AGA
Somalien Myrrh .... see MYRRH
Sonnenhutwurzel .... see ECHINACEA
Sophora japonica .... see PAGODA TREE
Sophorin .... see RUTIN

Sophretin .... see QUERCETIN
Sorb Apple .... see MOUNTAIN ASH
Sorbi acupariae fructus .... see MOUNTAIN ASH
Sorbus aucuparia .... see MOUNTAIN ASH
Sorghum .... see BROOM CORN
Sorghum vulgare .... see BROOM CORN
Sorosi .... see BITTER MELON
Sorrel .... see SORREL, YELLOW DOCK
Sorrel Dock .... see SORREL
SOUR CHERRY .... see SOUR CHERRY
Sour Dock .... see SORREL, YELLOW DOCK
Sour Orange .... see BITTER ORANGE
Sour Trefoil .... see WOOD SORREL
Souring Rush .... see HORSETAIL
South African Star Grass .... see AFRICAN WILD POTATO
Southern Bayberry .... see BAYBERRY
Southern Black Haw .... see BLACK HAW
Southern Ginseng .... see JIAOGULAN
SOUTHERN PRICKLY ASH
.... see SOUTHERN PRICKLY ASH
Southern Schisandra .... see SCHISANDRA
Southern Wax Myrtle .... see BAYBERRY
Southernwood Root .... see CARLINA
Sow Berry .... see EUROPEAN BARBERRY
Sowbread .... see CYCLAMEN
SOY .... see SOYBEAN OIL
Soy .... see SOY
Soy Fiber .... see SOY
Soy Milk .... see SOY
Soy Phosphatidylserine .... see PHOSPHATIDYLSERINE
Soy Protein .... see SOY
Soy Protein Extract .... see SOY
Soy PS .... see PHOSPHATIDYLSERINE
Soya .... see SOY
Soybean .... see SOY, SOYBEAN OIL
Soybean Curd .... see SOY
Soybean Lecithin .... see LECITHIN
SOYBEAN OIL .... see SOYBEAN OIL
Soyca .... see SOYBEAN OIL
Soy-Protein .... see SOY
Soy-PS .... see PHOSPHATIDYLSERINE
SP-303 .... see SANGRE DE GRADO
Spadic .... see COCA
Spanish Bayonet .... see YUCCA
SPANISH BROOM .... see SPANISH BROOM
Spanish Chestnut .... see EUROPEAN CHESTNUT,
                                      HORSE CHESTNUT branch bark,
                                         HORSE CHESTNUT flower,
                                             HORSE CHESTNUT leaf
Spanish Jasmine .... see JASMINE
Spanish Lavender .... see LAVENDER
Spanish Licorice .... see LICORICE
Spanish Origanum .... see SPANISH ORIGANUM OIL
SPANISH ORIGANUM OIL
.... see SPANISH ORIGANUM OIL
Spanish Pimienta .... see ALLSPICE
Spanish Psyllium .... see BLACK PSYLLIUM
Spanish Saffron .... see SAFFRON
Spanish Sage .... see SAGE
Spanish Thyme .... see SPANISH ORIGANUM OIL,
                                            THYME flower, leaf,
                                                      THYME OIL
Spanish Vetchling .... see LATHYRUS
Spargelkraut .... see ASPARAGUS

Spargelwurzelstock .... see ASPARAGUS
Sparrow Grass .... see ASPARAGUS
Sparrow Tongue .... see KNOTWEED HERB
Spartium junceum .... see SPANISH BROOM
Spartium scoparium .... see SCOTCH BROOM flower,
            SCOTCH BROOM herb
Spathyema Foetida .... see SKUNK CABBAGE
SPEARMINT .... see SPEARMINT
Speckled Jewels .... see JEWELWEED
Speedwell .... see BROOKLIME, VERONICA
Spergularia rubra .... see ARENARIA RUBRA
Spiceberry .... see WINTERGREEN leaf,
            WINTERGREEN oil
Spigelia marilandica .... see PINK ROOT
Spignet .... see AMERICAN SPIKENARD
Spike Lavender .... see LAVENDER
Spiked .... see PURPLE LOOSESTRIFE
Spiked Loosestrife .... see PURPLE LOOSESTRIFE
Spikenard .... see AMERICAN SPIKENARD
SPINACH .... see SPINACH
Spinacia oleracea .... see SPINACH
Spinaciae folium .... see SPINACH
Spinatblatter .... see SPINACH
Spindle Tree .... see WAHOO
Spiny Dogfish Shark .... see SQUALAMINE
SPINY RESTHARROW .... see SPINY RESTHARROW
Spiraea ulmaria .... see MEADOWSWEET
Spiraeae flos .... see MEADOWSWEET
Spire Mint .... see SPEARMINT
Spireae herba .... see MEADOWSWEET
Spirit Plant .... see REISHI MUSHROOM
Spirits Of Turpentine .... see TURPENTINE OIL
Spirulina .... see BLUE-GREEN ALGAE
Spirulina maxima .... see BLUE-GREEN ALGAE
Spirulina platensis .... see BLUE-GREEN ALGAE
Spitzwegerichkraut .... see BUCKHORN PLANTAIN
Spleen .... see SPLEEN EXTRACT
Spleen Concentrate .... see SPLEEN EXTRACT
SPLEEN EXTRACT .... see SPLEEN EXTRACT
Spleen Factors .... see SPLEEN EXTRACT
Spleen Peptides .... see SPLEEN EXTRACT
Spleen Polypeptides .... see SPLEEN EXTRACT
Splenopentin .... see SPLEEN EXTRACT
Spogel .... see BLOND PSYLLIUM
Sponge Cucumber .... see LUFFA
Sponsa Solis .... see MARSH MARIGOLD
Spoon Laurel .... see MOUNTAIN LAUREL
Spoonwood .... see KAMALA
Spoonwort .... see SCURVY GRASS
Spotted Cowbane .... see WATER HEMLOCK
Spotted Elder .... see WITCH HAZEL
Spotted Hemlock .... see HEMLOCK,
            WATER HEMLOCK
Spotted Monarda .... see HORSEMINT
Spotted Parsley .... see WATER HEMLOCK
Spotted Thistle .... see BLESSED THISTLE
Spotted Touch-Me-Not .... see JEWELWEED
Spotted Wintergreen .... see PIPSISSEWA
Spring Grass .... see SWEET VERNAL GRASS
Spruce .... see FIR, HEMLOCK SPRUCE
Spruce Fir .... see FIR, HEMLOCK SPRUCE
Spumonto .... see KOMBUCHA TEA
Spurge Flax .... see MEZEREON
Spurge Laurel .... see MEZEREON

Spurge Olive .... see MEZEREON
Spurred Rye .... see ERGOT
SPV 30 .... see BOXWOOD
SQ-9453 .... see DMSO (DIMETHYLSULFOXIDE)
Sqaulus acanthias .... see SHARK LIVER OIL
SQUALAMINE .... see SQUALAMINE
Squalus acanthias .... see SHARK CARTILAGE
            SQUALAMINE
Squaw Balm .... see PENNYROYAL leaf,
            PENNYROYAL oil
Squaw Berry .... see SQUAWVINE
Squaw Root .... see BLUE COHOSH
Squaw Tea .... see MORMON TEA
Squaw Vine .... see SQUAWVINE
Squaw Weed .... see ALPINE RAGWORT,
            GOLDEN RAGWORT
Squawmint
    .... see PENNYROYAL leaf, PENNYROYAL oil
Squawroot .... see BLACK COHOSH
SQUAWVINE .... see SQUAWVINE
Squawweed
    .... see ALPINE RAGWORT, GOLDEN RAGWORT
SQUILL .... see SQUILL
Squirrel Corn .... see CORYDALIS,
            TURKEY CORN
SSG .... see BETA GLUCANS
ST-200 .... see ACETYL-L-CARNITINE
St. Anthony's Turnip .... see BULBOUS BUTTERCUP
St. Barbara's Hedge Mustard .... see HEDGE MUSTARD
St. Bartholemew's Tea .... see MATE
St. Benedict Thistle .... see BLESSED THISTLE
St. James' Weed .... see SHEPHERD'S PURSE
St. James Wort .... see TANSY RAGWORT
St. James's Tea .... see LABRADOR TEA
St. John's Bread .... see CAROB
St. John's Herb .... see HEMP AGRIMONY
St. John's Plant .... see MUGWORT
ST. JOHN'S WORT .... see ST. JOHN'S WORT
St. Josephwort .... see BASIL
St. Mary Thistle .... see MILK THISTLE
St. Mary's Seal .... see SOLOMON'S SEAL
Stabilized Liquid Oxygen .... see VITAMIN O
Stabilized Oxygen .... see VITAMIN O
Stabilized Rice Bran .... see RICE BRAN
Stachys officinalis .... see BETONY
Staff Vine .... see BITTERSWEET NIGHTSHADE
Stag Bush .... see BLACK HAW
Staggerweed .... see DELPHINIUM,
            LARKSPUR,
            TURKEY CORN
Staggerwort .... see TANSY RAGWORT
Stags Horn .... see CLUB MOSS
Stammerwort .... see TANSY RAGWORT
STAR ANISE .... see STAR ANISE
Star-Bu .... see SEA BUCKTHORN
Star Chickweed .... see CHICKWEED
Starbloom .... see PINK ROOT
Starchwort .... see ARUM
Starflower .... see BORAGE SEED OIL
Stargrass .... see ALETRIS
Starweed .... see CHICKWEED
Starwort .... see ALETRIS, FALSE UNICORN
Staunchweed .... see YARROW
Stave Oak .... see OAK bark

Stave Wood .... see SIMARUBA
STAVESACRE .... see STAVESACRE
Stay Plough .... see SPINY RESTHARROW
Stellaria .... see ALCHEMILLA
Stellaria media .... see CHICKWEED
Stemless Carlina Root .... see CARLINA
Stemless Gentian .... see GENTIAN
Sterculia Acuminata .... see COLA NUT
Sterculia Gum .... see KARAYA GUM
Sterculia tragacanth .... see KARAYA GUM
Sterculia urens .... see KARAYA GUM
Sterculia villosa .... see KARAYA GUM
Sterinol .... see BETA-SITOSTEROL
Sterolins .... see BETA-SITOSTEROL
Sterretjie .... see AFRICAN WILD POTATO
STEVIA .... see STEVIA
Stevia eupatorium .... see STEVIA
Stevia rebaudiana .... see STEVIA
Stick-a-Back .... see CLIVERS
Stickwort .... see AGRIMONY, WOOD SORREL
Stigma Maydis .... see CORN SILK
Stigmastanol .... see SITOSTANOL
Stillingia .... see QUEEN'S DELIGHT
Stillingia sylvatica .... see QUEEN'S DELIGHT
Stillingia treculeana .... see QUEEN'S DELIGHT
Stinging Nettle
    .... see STINGING NETTLE above ground parts
                        STINGING NETTLE root
STINGING NETTLE above ground parts
    .... see STINGING NETTLE above ground parts
STINGING NETTLE root .... see STINGING NETTLE root
Stingless Nettle ..... see WHITE DEAD NETTLE FLOWER
Stinking Arrach .... see ARRACH
Stinking Balm .... see PENNYROYAL leaf,
                        PENNYROYAL oil
Stinking Benjamin ....see BETH ROOT
Stinking Goosefoot .... see ARRACH
Stinking Motherwort .... see ARRACH
Stinking Nanny .... see TANSY RAGWORT
Stinking Nightshade .... see HENBANE
Stinking Prairie Bush ....see WAFER ASH
Stinking-Roger .... see TAGETES
Stinking Rose.................................. see GARLIC
Stinking Tommy .... see SPINY RESTHARROW
Stinking Willie .... see TANSY
Stinkweed .... see JIMSON WEED
Stinkwort .... see JIMSON WEED
Stizolobium pruriens .... see COWHAGE
Stone Breaker .... see CHANCA PIEDRA
Stone Oak .... see OAK bark
STONE ROOT .... see STONE ROOT
Stonebreaker .... see CHANCA PIEDRA
STORAX .... see STORAX
Storkbill ....see HERB ROBERT
Stractan .... see LARCH ARABINOGALACTAN
Strained Honey .... see HONEY
Stramonium .... see JIMSON WEED
Strangle Tare .... see DODDER
Straw .... see OAT STRAW
Strawberries .... see STRAWBERRY
STRAWBERRY .... see STRAWBERRY
Strawberry Bush .... see WAHOO
Strawberry Tomato .... see WINTER CHERRY
Strawberry Tree .... see WAHOO

String Bean .... see BEAN POD
String Of Sovereigns .... see MONEYWORT
Stringy Bark Tree .... see EUCALYPTUS dried leaf
Strong-Scented Lettuce .... see WILD LETTUCE
Strophanthi Grati Semen .... see STROPHANTHUS
Strophanthi Kombe Semen .... see STROPHANTHUS
STROPHANTHUS .... see STROPHANTHUS
Strophanthus gratus .... see STROPHANTHUS
Strophanthus kombe .... see STROPHANTHUS
Strophanthus Seeds .... see STROPHANTHUS
Strychni Semen .... see NUX VOMICA
Strychnos ignatii .... see IGNATIUS BEAN
Strychnos nux-vomica .... see NUX VOMICA
Strychnos Seed .... see NUX VOMICA
Stubwort .... see WOOD SORREL
Styrax .... see STORAX
Styrax benzoin .... see BENZOIN
Styrax paralleloneurus .... see BENZOIN
Subholz .... see LICORICE
Succory .... see CHICORY
Sudanese Tea .... see HIBISCUS
Sugar Maple .... see RED MAPLE
Sugar Pods .... see CAROB
Sugarbeet .... see BEET
Sulfated N-Carboxymethylchitosan .... see CHITOSAN
Sulfated O-Carboxymethylchitosan .... see CHITOSAN
Sulfated Saccharide .... see GLUCOSAMINE SULFATE
Sulfomucopolysaccharide .... see MESOGLYCAN
Sulfonyl Sulfur .... see MSM
Sulphinybismethanesee DMSO (DIMETHYLSULFOXIDE)
Sultanas .... see GRAPE fruit, skin
SUMA .... see SUMA
Sumaruba .... see SIMARUBA
Sumatra Benzoin .... see BENZOIN
SUMBUL .... see SUMBUL
SUMMER SAVORY .... see SUMMER SAVORY
Sumpfporst .... see MARSH TEA
Sun Drop .... see EVENING PRIMROSE OIL
Sun Rose .... see FROSTWORT
SUNDEW .... see SUNDEW
Sunflower .... see SUNFLOWER OIL
SUNFLOWER OIL .... see SUNFLOWER OIL
Sunflower Oils .... see SUNFLOWER OIL
Sunflower Seed Oil .... see SUNFLOWER OIL
Sunkfield .... see EUROPEAN FIVE-FINGER GRASS
Super Dioxide Dismutase
    .... see SUPEROXIDE DISMUTASE
SUPEROXIDE DISMUTASE
    .... see SUPEROXIDE DISMUTASE
Surelle .... see WOOD SORREL
Surgical Maggot .... see MAGGOTS
Surinam Quassia .... see QUASSIA
Surinam Wood ....see QUASSIA
Swallow-Wort .... see PLEURISY ROOT
Swamp Cabbage .... see SKUNK CABBAGE
Swamp Cedar.............................. see CEDAR leaf,
                        CEDAR LEAF OIL
Swamp Dogwood .... see AMERICAN DOGWOOD,
                        WAFER ASH
Swamp Laurel .... see MAGNOLIA bark
Swamp Maple .... see RED MAPLE
SWAMP MILKWEED .... see SWAMP MILKWEED
Swamp Root .... see YERBA MANSA
Swamp Sassafras .... see MAGNOLIA bark

INDEX

Swamp Silkweed .... see SWAMP MILKWEED
Swamp Tea .... see MARSH TEA
Sweating Plant .... see BONESET
Sweatroot .... see ABSCESS ROOT
Sweet Acacia .... see CASSIE ABSOLUTE
SWEET ALMOND .... see SWEET ALMOND
Sweet Almond Oil .... see SWEET ALMOND
SWEET ANNIE .... see SWEET ANNIE
Sweet Balm .... see LEMON BALM
Sweet Bark .... see CASCARILLA
Sweet Basil .... see BASIL
Sweet Bay .... see MAGNOLIA bark
SWEET BAY .... see SWEET BAY
Sweet Bracken .... see SWEET CICELY
Sweet Broom .... see BUTCHER'S BROOM
Sweet Bugle .... see BUGLEWEED
Sweet Cane .... see CALAMUS
Sweet Chamomile .... see ROMAN CHAMOMILE
Sweet Chervil .... see SWEET CICELY
Sweet Chestnut .... see EUROPEAN CHESTNUT
SWEET CICELY .... see SWEET CICELY
Sweet Cinnamon .... see CALAMUS
SWEET CLOVER .... see SWEET CLOVER
Sweet Cumin .... see ANISE
Sweet-Cus .... see SWEET CICELY
Sweet Dock .... see BISTORT
Sweet Elder .... see AMERICAN ELDER,
ELDERFLOWER
Sweet Elm .... see SLIPPERY ELM
Sweet False Chamomile .... see GERMAN CHAMOMILE
Sweet Fennel .... see FENNEL fruit, seed
Sweet-Fern .... see SWEET CICELY
Sweet Flag .... see BLUE FLAG, CALAMUS
SWEET GALE .... see SWEET GALE
Sweet Grass .... see CALAMUS
Sweet Gum .... see STORAX
Sweet-Humlock .... see SWEET CICELY
Sweet Leaf of Paraguay .... see STEVIA
Sweet Lucerne .... see SWEET CLOVER
Sweet Mandulin .... see HEMP AGRIMONY
Sweet Marjoram .... see MARJORAM
Sweet Mary .... see LEMON BALM
Sweet Melilot .... see SWEET CLOVER
Sweet Myrtle .... see CALAMUS
Sweet Oil .... see OLIVE OIL
SWEET ORANGE .... see SWEET ORANGE
Sweet Pea .... see LATHYRUS
Sweet Pepper .... see CAPSICUM
Sweet Root .... see CALAMUS, LICORICE
Sweet Rush .... see CALAMUS
Sweet Scented Cactus .... see CEREUS
Sweet Sedge .... see CALAMUS
Sweet Slumber .... see BLOODROOT
Sweet-Smelling Trefoil .... see HEMP AGRIMONY
SWEET SUMACH .... see SWEET SUMACH
Sweet Vernal .... see PHEASANT'S EYE
Sweet Vernal Grass .... see HAY FLOWER
SWEET VERNAL GRASS

.... see SWEET VERNAL GRASS
SWEET VIOLET .... see SWEET VIOLET
Sweet Violet Herb .... see SWEET VIOLET
Sweet Violet Root .... see SWEET VIOLET
Sweet Weed .... see MARSHMALLOW
Sweet Wood Bark .... see CASCARILLA

SWEET WOODRUFF .... see SWEET WOODRUFF
Sweet Wormwood .... see SWEET ANNIE
Sweethearts .... see CLIVERS
Sweetleaf .... see STEVIA
Sweets .... see SWEET CICELY
Swertia chirata .... see CHIRATA
Swine Snout .... see DANDELION above ground parts,
DANDELION entire plant
Swinebread .... see CYCLAMEN
Swine's Grass .... see KNOTWEED HERB
Swiss Mountain Pine .... see PINE
Swynel Grass .... see KNOTWEED HERB
Sycocarpus rusbyi .... see COCILLANA
Symphytum officinale .... see COMFREY
Symphytum Radix .... see COMFREY
Symplocarpus foetidus .... see SKUNK CABBAGE
Synkfoyle .... see EUROPEAN FIVE-FINGER GRASS
Syrian Tragacanth .... see TRAGACANTH
Syxygii cumini cortex .... see JAMBOLAN bark
Syxygii cumini semen .... see JAMBOLAN seed
Syzugium cumini .... see JAMBOLAN bark
Syzugium jambolana .... see JAMBOLAN bark
Syzygium aromaticum

.... see CLOVE dried flowerbud, leaf, stem
Syzygium aromaticum .... see CLOVE OIL
Syzygium cumini .... see JAMBOLAN seed
Syzygium cumini jambolana .... see JAMBOLAN seed
Tabasco Pepper .... see CAPSICUM
Tabebuia avellanedae .... see PAU D'ARCO
Tabebuia heptaphylla .... see PAU D'ARCO
Tabebuia impetiginosa .... see PAU D'ARCO
Tabernanthe iboga .... see IBOGA
Table Grapes .... see GRAPE fruit, skin
Tag Alder .... see SMOOTH ALDER
TAGETES .... see TAGETES
Tagetes Erecta .... see TAGETES
Tagetes glandulifera .... see TAGETES
Tagetes minuta .... see TAGETES
Tagetes patula .... see TAGETES
Taheebo .... see PAU D'ARCO
Taheebo Tea .... see PAU D'ARCO
Tahiti Vanilla .... see VANILLA
Tahitian Noni Juice .... see MORINDA
Tahitian Vanilla .... see VANILLA
Tailed Chubebs .... see CUBEBS
Tailed Pepper .... see CUBEBS
Takila .... see ANDROGRAPHIS
Talepetrako .... see GOTU KOLA
Tall Melilot .... see SWEET CLOVER
Tall Nasturtium .... see WATERCRESS
Tall Speedwell .... see BLACK ROOT
Tall Veronica .... see BLACK ROOT
Tallow Shrub .... see BAYBERRY
Tamalaka .... see CHANCA PIEDRA
TAMARIND .... see TAMARIND
Tamarindo .... see TAMARIND
Tamarindus indica .... see TAMARIND
Tame Withy .... see FIREWEED
Tamus .... see BRYONIA
Tamus communis .... see BLACK BRYONY
Tan Kue Bai Zhi .... see DONG QUAI
Tan Xiang .... see WHITE SANDALWOOD wood
Tanaceti parthenii .... see FEVERFEW
Tanacetum parthenium .... see FEVERFEW

Tanacetum vulgare .... see TANSY
Tang .... see BLADDERWRACK
Tang Kuei .... see DONG QUAI
Tangantangan Oil Plant .... see CASTOR OIL, CASTOR seed
Tanner's Bark .... see OAK bark
Tanner's Oak .... see OAK bark
TANNIC ACID .... see TANNIC ACID
Tan-Shen .... see DANSHEN
TANSY .... see TANSY
Tansy Flower .... see TANSY
Tansy Herb .... see TANSY
TANSY RAGWORT .... see TANSY RAGWORT
Tar Weed .... see GUMWEED
Taraxaci herba .... see DANDELION above ground parts
Taraxacum .... see DANDELION above ground parts, DANDELION entire plant

Taraxacum officinale
.... see DANDELION above ground parts, DANDELION entire plant

Taraxacum vulgare
.... see DANDELION above ground parts, DANDELION entire plant
Tare .... see TAUMELLOOLCH
Target-Leaved Hibiscus .... see AMBRETTE
TARRAGON .... see TARRAGON
Tart Cherry .... see SOUR CHERRY
Tartaric Acid .... see ALPHA HYDROXY ACIDS
Tarweed .... see YERBA SANTA
Tasmanian Blue Gum .... see EUCALYPTUS dried leaf
Taso-Ho-Hua .... see THUNDER GOD VINE
Taspine .... see SANGRE DE GRADO
Tatuaba .... see CATUABA
TAUMELLOOLCH .... see TAUMELLOOLCH
TAURINE .... see TAURINE
Tausendaugbram .... see YARROW
Taxus bacatta .... see YEW
Taxus brevifolia .... see YEW
TC-80 .... see IPRIFLAVONE
Tchaad .... see KHAT
T'Chai from the Sea .... see KOMBUCHA TEA
TCV-3b .... see VINPOCETINE
Tea .... see BLACK TEA, GREEN TEA
Tea Green .... see GREEN TEA
TEA TREE OIL .... see TEA TREE OIL
Teaberry .... see WINTERGREEN leaf, WINTERGREEN oil
Tea Green .... see GREEN TEA
Teamster's Tea .... see EPHEDRA, MORMON TEA
Teasel .... see BONESET, TEAZLE
TEAZLE .... see TEAZLE
Tecuitlatl .... see BLUE-GREEN ALGAE
Teinturière .... see POKEWEED berry, POKEWEED root
Tempeh .... see SOY
Temu Kuning .... see ZEDOARY
Temu Lawak .... see JAVANESE TURMERIC
Temu Lawas .... see JAVANESE TURMERIC
Temu Putih .... see ZEDOARY
Terebinthina Laricina .... see LARCH TURPENTINE
Terebinthina Veneta .... see LARCH TURPENTINE
Terebinthinae aetheroleum .... see TURPENTINE OIL
TERMINALIA .... see TERMINALIA
Terminalia Arjuna .... see TERMINALIA

Terminalia belerica .... see TERMINALIA
Terminalia bellirica .... see TERMINALIA
Terminalia chebula .... see TERMINALIA
Tetracosanol .... see POLICOSANOL
Tetracosanol (24-C) .... see OCTACOSANOL
Tetrahydro-2-Furanone
.... see GAMMA BUTYROLACTONE (GBL)
Tetramethylene glycol .... see BUTANEDIOL (BD)
Tetramethylene-1,4-diol .... see BUTANEDIOL (BD)
Tetratriacontanol .... see POLICOSANOL
Tetterberry .... see BRYONIA
Tetterwort .... see BLOODROOT, GREATER CELANDINE dried above ground parts
Teucrium chamaedrys .... see GERMANDER
Teucrium scordium .... see WATER GERMANDER
Teucrium scorodonia .... see WOOD SAGE
Tewon Lawa .... see JAVANESE TURMERIC
Texas Cedarwood
.... see CEDARWOOD bark, berry, leaf, seed, twig
Texas Snakeroot .... see ARISTOLOCHIA
Texturized Vegetable Protein .... see SOY
TFd .... see TRANSFER FACTOR
Thalictroc .... see HEDGE MUSTARD
The Roman Plant .... see SWEET CICELY
Thea bohea .... see BLACK TEA, GREEN TEA
Thea Sinesis .... see BLACK TEA, GREEN TEA
Thea viridis .... see BLACK TEA, GREEN TEA
Theobroma .... see COCOA
Theobroma cacao .... see COCOA
Thevetia peruviana .... see OLEANDER
Thiamin .... see THIAMINE (VITAMIN B1)
Thiamin Chloride .... see THIAMINE (VITAMIN B1)
Thiamin Hydrochloride ..... see THIAMINE (VITAMIN B1)
THIAMINE .... see THIAMINE (VITAMIN B1)
Thiamine (Vitamin B1) ...... see THIAMINE (VITAMIN B1)
Thiamine Chloride .... see THIAMINE (VITAMIN B1)
Thiamine Hydrochloride ... see THIAMINE (VITAMIN B1)
Thiaminium Chloride Hydrochloride
.... see THIAMINE (VITAMIN B1)
Thick-Leaved Pennywort .... see GOTU KOLA
Thimbleberry .... see BLACKBERRY leaf, BLACKBERRY root
Thioctacid .... see ALPHA-LIPOIC ACID
Thioctan .... see ALPHA-LIPOIC ACID
Thioctic Acid .... see ALPHA-LIPOIC ACID
Thomas Balsam .... see TOLU BALSAM
Thompson Seedless .... see GRAPE fruit, skin
Thormantle .... see TORMENTIL
Thorn-apple .... see JIMSON WEED
Thorny Bearer of Free Berries ... see GINSENG, SIBERIAN
Thorny Burr .... see BURDOCK
Thoroughwax .... see BUPLEURUM
Thoroughwort .... see BONESET, HEMP AGRIMONY
Thor's Beard .... see HOUSELEEK
Thousand-Leaf .... see YARROW
Three-Leafed Ivy .... see POISON IVY
Three-Leafed Nightshade .... see BETH ROOT
Three-Leaved Grass .... see WOOD SORREL
Three-Leaved Hop Tree .... see WAFER ASH
Three Seven .... see PANAX PSEUDOGINSENG
Threewingnut .... see THUNDER GOD VINE
Throat Root .... see WATER AVENS
Throatwort .... see DIGITALIS, FIGWORT

Throw-Wort .... see MOTHERWORT
Thuga .... see CEDAR leaf
Thuja .... see CEDAR leaf,
CEDAR LEAF OIL
Thuja occidentalis .... see CEDAR leaf,
CEDAR LEAF OIL
Thuja Oil .... see CEDAR LEAF OIL
Thuja orientalis .... see ORIENTAL ARBORVITAE
THUNDER GOD VINE .... see THUNDER GOD VINE
Thunder Plant .... see HOUSELEEK
Thyme .... see THYME flower, leaf
Thyme Aetheroleum .... see THYME OIL
THYME flower, leaf .... see THYME flower, leaf
Thyme-Leave Gratiola .... see BRAHMI
THYME OIL .... see THYME OIL
Thyme vulgaris .... see THYME OIL
Thymi herba .... see THYME flower, leaf
Thymomodulin .... see THYMUS EXTRACT
Thymosin .... see THYMUS EXTRACT
Thymostimulin .... see THYMUS EXTRACT
Thymus .... see THYMUS EXTRACT
Thymus Acid Lysate Derivative

.... see THYMUS EXTRACT
Thymus capitatus .... see SPANISH ORIGANUM OIL
Thymus Complex .... see THYMUS EXTRACT
Thymus Concentrate .... see THYMUS EXTRACT
Thymus-Derived Polypeptides .... see THYMUS EXTRACT
THYMUS EXTRACT .... see THYMUS EXTRACT
Thymus Factors .... see THYMUS EXTRACT
Thymus Polypeptides .... see THYMUS EXTRACT
Thymus serpyllum .... see WILD THYME
Thymus Substance .... see THYMUS EXTRACT
Thymus vulgaris .... see THYME flower, leaf
THYME OIL
Thymus zygis .... see THYME flower, leaf
THYME OIL
Tian-Hua-Fen .... see CHINESE CUCUMBER root
Tian Qi .... see PANAX PSEUDOGINSENG
Tiarella cordifolia .... see COOLWORT
Tickleweed .... see AMERICAN HELLEBORE
Tickweed .... see PENNYROYAL leaf,
PENNYROYAL oil
Tienchi Ginseng .... see GINSENG, AMERICAN
Tiglium .... see CROTON SEEDS
Tiglium Seeds .... see CROTON SEEDS
Tilia argentea .... see SILVER LINDEN
Tilia cordata .... see LINDEN CHARCOAL,
LINDEN dried flower,
LINDEN dried leaf,
LINDEN dried sapwood
Tilia platyphyllos .... see LINDEN CHARCOAL,
LINDEN dried flower,
LINDEN dried leaf,
LINDEN dried sapwood
Tilia tormentosa .... see SILVER LINDEN
Tiliae carbo .... see LINDEN CHARCOAL
Tiliae flos .... see LINDEN dried flower
Tiliae folium .... see LINDEN dried leaf
Tiliae lignum .... see LINDEN dried sapwood
Tiliae tormentosae flos .... see SILVER LINDEN
Tilki Uzumu .... see HERB PARIS
Timothy .... see HAY FLOWER
Tindved .... see SEA BUCKTHORN
Tinnevelly Senna .... see SENNA

Tipton Weed .... see ST. JOHN'S WORT
TIRATRICOL .... see TIRATRICOL
TMG .... see BETAINE ANHYDROUS
BETAINE HYDROCHLORIDE
Toadpipe .... see HORSETAIL,
YELLOW TOADFLAX
Tobacco ....see SMOKELESS TOBACCO
Tocopherol .... see VITAMIN E
Tocopheryl Acetate .... see VITAMIN E
Tocopheryl Acid Succinate .... see VITAMIN E
Tocopheryl Succinate .... see VITAMIN E
Tocotrienol .... see VITAMIN E
Tofu .... see SOY
Tohai .... see KHAT
Tohat .... see KHAT
Toliufera balsamum .... see TOLU BALSAM
Tolu .... see TOLU BALSAM
TOLU BALSAM .... see TOLU BALSAM
Toluiferum Balsamum .... see TOLU BALSAM
Tom Rong .... see GAMBOGE
TOMATO .... see TOMATO
To-Nezumimochi .... see GLOSSY PRIVET
Tonga .... see KAVA
Tonka .... see TONKA BEAN
TONKA BEAN .... see TONKA BEAN
Tonka Seed .... see TONKA BEAN
Tonquin Bean .... see TONKA BEAN
Tonquin Musk .... see MUSK
Toothache Bark .... see NORTHERN PRICKLY ASH
Toothache Tree .... see SOUTHERN PRICKLY ASH
Toothpick Ammi .... see KHELLA
Toothpick Plant .... see KHELLA
Torch Weed .... see MULLEIN
Torches .... see MULLEIN
TORMENTIL .... see TORMENTIL
Tormentilla .... see TORMENTIL
Tormentillae rhizoma .... see TORMENTIL
Toronja .... see GRAPEFRUIT
Torquin Bean .... see TONKA BEAN
Touch-Me-Not .... see GINSENG, SIBERIAN,
JEWELWEED
Toute Épice .... see BLACK SEED
Toxicodendron radicans .... see POISON IVY
Toywort .... see SHEPHERD'S PURSE
Trackleberry .... see BILBERRY dried ripe fruit,
BILBERRY leaf
TRAGACANTH .... see TRAGACANTH
Tragacanth Gum .... see TRAGACANTH
TRAILING ARBUTUS .... see TRAILING ARBUTUS
Trailing Mahonia .... see OREGON GRAPE
Trailing Swamp Cranberry .... see CRANBERRY
Trailing Tansy .... see POTENTILLA
Trametes versicolor .... see CORIOLUS MUSHROOM
Trans-10 .... see CONJUGATED LINOLEIC ACID
Trans-11 conjugated linoleic acid

.... see CONJUGATED LINOLEIC ACID
TRANSFER FACTOR .... see TRANSFER FACTOR
Trans-Resveratrol .... see RESVERATROL
TRAVELER'S JOY .... see TRAVELER'S JOY
Traveler's-Joy .... see WOODBINE
Travmulsion .... see SOYBEAN OIL
Tree Moss .... see OAK MOSS, USNEA
TREE OF HEAVEN .... see TREE OF HEAVEN
Tree of Life .... see CEDAR leaf,
CEDAR LEAF OIL

Tree's Dandruff .... see USNEA
Trefoil .... see LIVERWORT, RED CLOVER
Triac .... see TIRATRICOL
Triacontanol (30-C) .... see OCTACOSANOL
Triacylglycerol lipase .... see LIPASE
Tribule terrestre .... see PUNCTURE VINE
Tribulis .... see PUNCTURE VINE
Tribulis Terrestris .... see PUNCTURE VINE
Tricalcium Phosphate .... see CALCIUM
Tricholomopsis edodes .... see LENTINAN,
                                        SHIITAKE MUSHROOM
Trichosanthes .... see CHINESE CUCUMBER fruit,
                                CHINESE CUCUMBER root,
                                CHINESE CUCUMBER seed
Trichosanthes kirilowii ... see CHINESE CUCUMBER fruit,
                                CHINESE CUCUMBER root,
                                CHINESE CUCUMBER seed
Trifolium .... see RED CLOVER
Trifolium pratense .... see RED CLOVER
Trigonella .... see FENUGREEK
Trigonella foenum-graecum .... see FENUGREEK
triiodothyroacetic acid .... see TIRATRICOL
Trilisa odoratissima .... see DEERTONGUE
Trillium erectum .... see BETH ROOT
Trimethyl Glycine .... see BETAINE ANHYDROUS,
                                BETAINE HYDROCHLORIDE
Trimethylethanolamine .... see CHOLINE
Trimethylglycine .... see BETAINE ANHYDROUS,
                                BETAINE HYDROCHLORIDE
Trimethylglycine anhydrous
                .... see BETAINE ANHYDROUS
Trimethylglycine hydrochloride
                .... see BETAINE HYDROCHLORIDE
Tripsin .... see TRYPSIN
Tripterygium wilfordii .... see THUNDER GOD VINE
Trisodium ethylenediamine tetraacetic acid .... see EDTA
Triticum .... see AGROPYRON
Triticum aestrivum .... see WHEAT BRAN
Triticum repens .... see AGROPYRON,
                                        COUCH GRASS
Trivalent Chromium .... see CHROMIUM
Troène De Chine .... see GLOSSY PRIVET
Trollius europaeus .... see GLOBE FLOWER
Trompillo .... see COCILLANA
Tropaeolum majus .... see NASTURTIUM
True Angostura .... see ANGOSTURA
True Bay .... see SWEET BAY
True Chamomile .... see GERMAN CHAMOMILE
True Ivy .... see ENGLISH IVY
True Lavender .... see LAVENDER
True Saffron .... see SAFFRON
True Sage .... see SAGE
True Senna .... see SENNA
Trueno .... see GLOSSY PRIVET
Trumpet Bush .... see PAU D'ARCO
Trumpet Flower .... see GELSEMIUM
Trumpet Weed .... see GRAVEL ROOT
Truxillo Coca .... see COCA
TRYPSIN .... see TRYPSIN
Tryptophan .... see L-TRYPTOPHAN
Tschambucco .... see KOMBUCHA TEA
Tschut .... see KHAT
Tsubo-kusa .... see GOTU KOLA
Tsuga canadensis .... see PINUS BARK

Tsuru-kokemomo .... see CRANBERRY
Tu Si Zi .... see DODDER
Tu Sizi .... see DODDER
Tuber Root .... see PLEURISY ROOT
Tuckahoe .... see PORIA MUSHROOM
Tuftsin .... see SPLEEN EXTRACT
Tumeric .... see TURMERIC
Tuna Cardona .... see PRICKLY PEAR CACTUS
Tung .... see TUNG SEED
TUNG SEED .... see TUNG SEED
Tungchian .... see GOTU KOLA
Tun-Hoof .... see GROUND IVY
Turangi-Ghanda .... see ASHWAGANDHA
Turi Hutan .... see CHANCA PIEDRA
Turkey Claw .... see CORAL ROOT
Turkey Corn .... see CORYDALIS
TURKEY CORN .... see TURKEY CORN
Turkey Grass .... see VERBENA
Turkey Rhubarb .... see RHUBARB
Turkey Tail .... see CORIOLUS MUSHROOM
Turk's Cap .... see MARTAGON
TURMERIC .... see TURMERIC
Turmeric .... see ZEDOARY
Turmeric Root .... see GOLDENSEAL
                                        TURMERIC
Turnera aphrodisiaca .... see DAMIANA
Turnera diffusa .... see DAMIANA
Turnera microphylla .... see DAMIANA
Turnerae diffusae folium .... see DAMIANA
Turnerae diffusae herba .... see DAMIANA
Turnhoof .... see GROUND IVY
Turnip Radish .... see RADISH
Turpentine .... see TURPENTINE OIL
TURPENTINE OIL .... see TURPENTINE OIL
Turpentine Weed .... see CUP PLANT
TURTLE HEAD .... see TURTLE HEAD
Turtlebloom .... see TURTLE HEAD
Tussilage .... see COLTSFOOT
Tussilago Farfara .... see COLTSFOOT
Twinberry .... see SQUAWVINE
Twitchgrass .... see AGROPYRON,
                                        WHEATGRASS
Two-Eyed Berry .... see SQUAWVINE
Twopenny Grass .... see MONEYWORT
Tyosen-Azami .... see ARTICHOKE
Type II Collagen .... see CHICKEN COLLAGEN
Tyr .... see TYROSINE
TYROSINE .... see TYROSINE
Tyrosinum .... see TYROSINE
Tzu Tan-Ken .... see DANSHEN
Ubidecarenone .... see COENZYME Q-10
Ubiquinone .... see COENZYME Q-10
Ulmaria .... see MEADOWSWEET
Ulmus fulva .... see SLIPPERY ELM
Ulmus minor .... see ELM BARK
Ulmus rubra .... see SLIPPERY ELM
Umbellate Wintergreen .... see PIPSISSEWA
Umbrella Leaves .... see BUTTERBUR
Uña De Gato .... see CAT'S CLAW
Uncaria guianensis .... see CAT'S CLAW
Uncaria Tomentosa .... see CAT'S CLAW
Undi .... see LAURELWOOD
Unicorn Root .... see ALETRIS
Unsaturated Fatty Acid .... see OLIVE OIL

INDEX

Untouchable .... see GINSENG, SIBERIAN
Upas .... see COCILLANA
Upright Virgin's Bower .... see CLEMATIS
Upstart ....see AUTUMN CROCUS
Uragoga granatensis .... see IPECAC
Uragoga ipecacuanha .... see IPECAC
Urginea indica................................... see SQUILL
Urginea maritima .... see SQUILL
Urginea scilla .... see SQUILL
Urtica .... see STINGING NETTLE above ground parts,
                    STINGING NETTLE root
Urtica Dioica
.... see STINGING NETTLE above ground parts,
                    STINGING NETTLE root
Urtica Urens
.... see STINGING NETTLE above ground parts,
                    STINGING NETTLE root
Urticae herba et folium
.... see STINGING NETTLE above ground parts
Urticae Radix .... see STINGING NETTLE root
USNEA .... see USNEA
Usnea barbata .... see USNEA
Usnea florida .... see USNEA
Usnea hirta .... see USNEA
Usnea Lichen .... see USNEA
Usnea plicata .... see USNEA
Usnea species .... see USNEA
Ussuri .... see GINSENG, SIBERIAN
Ussurian Thorny Pepperbrush ... see GINSENG, SIBERIAN
Utricularia vulgaris .... see BLADDERWORT
Uva De Raposa .... see HERB PARIS
UVA URSI .... see UVA URSI
Uvae ursi folium .... see UVA URSI
UZARA .... see UZARA
Uzarae radix .... see UZARA
V .... see VANADIUM
V. fragrans..................................... see VANILLA
va. Capitata .... see CABBAGE
Vaccinium angustifolium .... see BLUEBERRY
Vaccinium ashei .... see BLUEBERRY
Vaccinium corymbosum .... see BLUEBERRY
Vaccinium hagerupii .... see CRANBERRY
Vaccinium macrocarpon .... see CRANBERRY
Vaccinium microcarpum .... see CRANBERRY
Vaccinium myrtillus........... see BILBERRY dried ripe fruit,
                    BILBERRY leaf
Vaccinium oxycoccos .... see CRANBERRY
Vaccinium pallidum .... see BLUEBERRY
Vaccinium palustre ....see CRANBERRY
Vaccinium uliginosum .... see BOG BILBERRY
Vaccinium vitis-idaea .... see ALPINE CRANBERRY
Valencia Orange............................ see SWEET ORANGE
VALERIAN .... see VALERIAN
Valeriana .... see VALERIAN
Valeriana edulis .... see VALERIAN
Valeriana jatamansii............................ see VALERIAN
Valeriana Officinalis .... see VALERIAN
Valeriana rhizome .... see VALERIAN
Valeriana sitchensis .... see VALERIAN
Valeriana wallichii .... see VALERIAN
Valerianae radix .... see VALERIAN
Valeriane .... see VALERIAN
Valine .... see BRANCHED-CHAIN AMINO ACIDS
Vanadate .... see VANADIUM

VANADIUM .... see VANADIUM
Vanadium Pentoxide .... see VANADIUM
Vanadyl .... see VANADIUM
Vanadyl Sulfate .... see VANADIUM
VANILLA .... see VANILLA
Vanilla Leaf .... see DEERTONGUE
Vanilla planifolia .... see VANILLA
Vanilla Plant .... see DEERTONGUE
Vanilla tahitensis .... see VANILLA
Vanilla Trilisa .... see DEERTONGUE
Vanillan .... see VANILLA
Vapor...................................... see FUMITORY
Varech .... see BLADDERWRACK
Varnish Tree .... see TREE OF HEAVEN,
                    TUNG SEED
Vegetable Antimony .... see BONESET
Vegetable Caterpillar .... see CORDYCEPS
Vegetable Gelatin............................... see AGAR
Vegetable Mercury .... see MANACA,
                    PODOPHYLLUM
Vegetable Pepsin .... see PAPAIN
Vegetable Sponge .... see LUFFA
Vegetable Sulfur .... see CLUB MOSS
Vegetable Tallow .... see BAYBERRY
Vegilecithin .... see LECITHIN
Vellorita ....see AUTUMN CROCUS
Velvet Antler .... see DEER VELVET
Velvet Bean .... see COWHAGE
Velvet Dock .... see ELECAMPANE
Velvet Flower............................... see AMARANTH
Velvet Leaf............................... see PAREIRA
Velvet of Young Deer Horn .... see DEER VELVET
Velvet Plant .... see MULLEIN
Velvetleaf................................... see ABUTA
Venastat .... see HORSE CHESTNUT seed
Venetian Turpentine .... see LARCH TURPENTINE
Venostasin Retard .... see HORSE CHESTNUT seed
Venostat .... see HORSE CHESTNUT seed
Venus' Basin .... see TEAZLE
Venus Hair .... see MAIDENHAIR FERN
Venus Shoe .... see NERVE ROOT
Veratro Verde .... see AMERICAN HELLEBORE
Veratrum album .... see WHITE HELLEBORE
Veratrum luteum .... see FALSE UNICORN
Veratrum viride .... see AMERICAN HELLEBORE
Verbasci flos .... see MULLEIN
Verbascum densiflorum .... see MULLEIN
Verbascum phlomides .... see MULLEIN
Verbascum thapiforme .... see MULLEIN
Verbascum thapsus .... see MULLEIN
VERBENA .... see VERBENA
Verbena citriodora .... see LEMON VERBENA
Verbena officinalis .... see VERBENA
Verbena triphylla .... see LEMON VERBENA
Verbenae herba .... see VERBENA
Vernis de Japon .... see TREE OF HEAVEN
VERONICA .... see VERONICA
Veronica beccabunga .... see BROOKLIME
Veronica Herb .... see VERONICA
Veronica officinalis .... see VERONICA
Veronica Virginica Root .... see BLACK ROOT
Veronicae herba .... see VERONICA
Veronicastrum Virginicum .... see BLACK ROOT
Verrucaria .... see MARSH MARIGOLD

Vervain .... see VERBENA
Vespula maculata (Hornet) .... see BEE VENOM
VETIVER .... see VETIVER
Vétiver .... see VETIVER
Vetivergras .... see VETIVER
Vetiveria zizanoides .... see VETIVER
Viable Antiseptic .... see MAGGOTS
Viburnum .... see BLACK HAW
Viburnum opulus .... see CRAMP BARK
Viburnum Prunifolium .... see BLACK HAW
Viburnum prunifolium ferrugineum .... see BLACK HAW
Viburnum rufidulum .... see BLACK HAW
Vinca Minor .... see PERIWINKLE
Vinca rosea .... see MADAGASCAR PERIWINKLE
Vincae minoris herba .... see PERIWINKLE
Vine Bower .... see WOODBINE
Vine of Mount Ida .... see ALPINE CRANBERRY
Vinettier .... see EUROPEAN BARBERRY
VINPOCETINE .... see VINPOCETINE
Viola .... see HEART'S EASE
Viola odorata .... see GARDEN VIOLET,
                                          SWEET VIOLET
Viola Tricolor .... see HEART'S EASE
Violae Odoratae Rhizoma .... see SWEET VIOLET
Violae Tricoloris Herba .... see HEART'S EASE
Violet .... see SWEET VIOLET
Violet Bloom .... see BITTERSWEET NIGHTSHADE
Violet Willow .... see WILLOW BARK
Virginia Cedarwood
             ...... see CEDARWOOD bark, berry, leaf, seed, twig
Virginia Creeper .... see AMERICAN IVY
Virginia Serpentary .... see ARISTOLOCHIA
Virginia Snakeroot .... see ARISTOLOCHIA
Virginia Water Horehound .... see BUGLEWEED
Virginian Poke .... see POKEWEED berry,
                                          POKEWEED root
Virginian Prune .... see WILD CHERRY
Virginian Strawberry .... see STRAWBERRY
Virgin's Bower .... see WOODBINE
Visci .... see EUROPEAN MISTLETOE
Visci albi folia .... see EUROPEAN MISTLETOE
Visci albi fructus .... see EUROPEAN MISTLETOE
Visci albi herba .... see EUROPEAN MISTLETOE
Visci albi stipites .... see EUROPEAN MISTLETOE
Viscum album .... see EUROPEAN MISTLETOE
Visnaga .... see KHELLA
Visnaga Fruit .... see KHELLA
Visnagae .... see KHELLA
Visnagafruchte .... see KHELLA
Visnagin .... see KHELLA
Vitacarn .... see L-CARNITINE
Vitadurin .... see VITAMIN B12
VITAMIN A .... see VITAMIN A
Vitamin A1 .... see VITAMIN A
Vitamin A2 .... see VITAMIN A
Vitamin B(t) .... see L-CARNITINE
Vitamin B(t) Acetate .... see ACETYL-L-CARNITINE
Vitamin B1 .... see THIAMINE (VITAMIN B1)
Vitamin B2 .... see RIBOFLAVIN (VITAMIN B2)
Vitamin B3
           .... see NIACIN AND NIACINAMIDE (VITAMIN B3)
Vitamin B5 ...... see PANTOTHENIC ACID (VITAMIN B5)
Vitamin B6 .... see PYRIDOXINE (VITAMIN B6)
Vitamin B8 .... see INOSITOL
Vitamin B9 .... see FOLIC ACID

Vitamin B10
           .... see PARA-AMINOBENZOIC ACID (PABA)
VITAMIN B12 .... see VITAMIN B12
Vitamin B15 .... see PANGAMIC ACID
Vitamin B17 .... see APRICOT
VITAMIN C (ASCORBIC ACID)
           .... see VITAMIN C (ASCORBIC ACID)
VITAMIN D .... see VITAMIN D
VITAMIN E .... see VITAMIN E
Vitamin G .... see RIBOFLAVIN (VITAMIN B2)
Vitamin H
        ...... see BIOTIN, PARA-AMINOBENZOIC ACID (PABA)
VITAMIN K .... see VITAMIN K
Vitamin K1: Methylphytyl Naphthoquinone
           .... see VITAMIN K
VITAMIN O .... see VITAMIN O
Vitamin PP
        .... see NIACIN AND NIACINAMIDE (VITAMIN B3)
Vitaminum A .... see VITAMIN A
Vitellin .... see LECITHIN
Vitex .... see CHASTEBERRY
Vitex Agnus Castus .... see CHASTEBERRY
Vitis coignetiae .... see GRAPE seed
Vitis pentaphylla .... see JIAOGULAN
Vitis vinifera .... see GRAPE fruit, skin,
                                          GRAPE leaf, GRAPE seed,
                                          WINE
Vizra Ufar .... see ANDROGRAPHIS
Vogelknoeterichkraut .... see KNOTWEED HERB
Vogelmistel .... see EUROPEAN MISTLETOE
Volatile Almond Oil .... see BITTER ALMOND
Vomit Wort .... see LOBELIA
Vysorel .... see EUROPEAN MISTLETOE
W Factor .... see BIOTIN
W-3 Fatty Acid
           .... see DHA (DOCOSAHEXAENOIC ACID),
                                          EPA (EICOSAPENTAENOIC ACID)
W-3 Fatty Acids .... see FISH OILS
Wacholderbeeren .... see JUNIPER
Wacholderteer .... see CADE OIL
WAFER ASH .... see WAFER ASH
WAHOO .... see WAHOO
Wake Robin .... see ARUM, BETH ROOT
Waldmeister .... see SWEET WOODRUFF
Walewort .... see DWARF ELDER
Wall Germander .... see GERMANDER
Wall Ginger .... see COMMON STONECROP
Wallflower .... see CANADIAN HEMP
WALLFLOWER .... see WALLFLOWER
Wallpepper .... see COMMON STONECROP
Wallstock-Gillofer .... see WALLFLOWER
Wallwort .... see COMFREY
Walnussblätter .... see ENGLISH WALNUT
Walnussfrüchtschalen .... see ENGLISH WALNUT
Walnut .... see ENGLISH WALNUT
Walnut Fruit .... see ENGLISH WALNUT
Walnut Hull .... see ENGLISH WALNUT
Walnut Leaf .... see ENGLISH WALNUT
Walpole Tea .... see NEW JERSEY TEA
Wandering Jenny .... see MONEYWORT
Wandering Tailor .... see MONEYWORT
Wang Sun .... see HERB PARIS
Warnera .... see GOLDENSEAL
Wartwort .... see CUDWEED

INDEX

Wasp Venom .... see BEE VENOM
Wasp .... see BEE VENOM
Wasserkresse .... see WATERCRESS
Wasser-Schierling .... see WATER HEMLOCK
Wasshanf .... see HEMP AGRIMONY
Wateorhiza palmata .... see COLOMBO
Water Agrimony .... see BURR MARIGOLD
WATER AVENS .... see WATER AVENS
Water Blobs .... see MARSH MARIGOLD
Water Bugle .... see BUGLEWEED
Water Cabbage .... see AMERICAN WHITE POND LILY
Water Chisch .... see WATER AVENS
Water-Cup .... see PITCHER PLANT
WATER DOCK .... see WATER DOCK
Water Dragon .... see MARSH MARIGOLD
Water Dropwort .... see WATER FENNEL
WATER FENNEL .... see WATER FENNEL
Water Flag .... see ORRIS
Water Flower .... see WATER AVENS
WATER GERMANDER .... see WATER GERMANDER
Water Gourd .... see LUFFA
WATER HEMLOCK .... see WATER HEMLOCK
Water Hoarhound .... see BUGLEWEED
Water-Holly .... see OREGON GRAPE
Water Horehound .... see BUGLEWEED
Water Lemon .... see PASSIONFLOWER
Water Lily .... see AMERICAN WHITE POND LILY
Water Maudlin .... see HEMP AGRIMONY
Water Mint .... see WILD MINT
Water Nymph .... see AMERICAN WHITE POND LILY
Water of Pimento .... see ALLSPICE
Water Pepper .... see SMARTWEED
Water Pimpernel .... see BROOKLIME
Water Pink .... see TRAILING ARBUTUS
WATER PLANTAIN .... see WATER PLANTAIN
Water Purslane .... see BROOKLIME
Water Shamrock .... see BOGBEAN
WATERCRESS .... see WATERCRESS
Waterhemp .... see HEMP AGRIMONY
Waterkres .... see WATERCRESS
Wax Bean .... see BEAN POD
Wax Cluster .... see WINTERGREEN leaf,
.... WINTERGREEN oil
Wax Dolls .... see FUMITORY
Wax Myrtle .... see BAYBERRY
Waxberry .... see BAYBERRY
Waxwork .... see AMERICAN BITTERSWEET
Waythorn .... see EUROPEAN BUCKTHORN
Weather Plant .... see PRECATORY BEAN
Weaver's Broom .... see SPANISH BROOM
Weed .... see MARIJUANA
Weeping Ash .... see ASH
Weibe Senfsamen .... see WHITE MUSTARD
Weidenrinde .... see WILLOW BARK
Weissdorn .... see HAWTHORN
Wermut .... see WORMWOOD above ground parts
Wermutkraut .... see WORMWOOD above ground parts
West Indian Cherry .... see ACEROLA
West Indian Dogwood .... see JAMAICAN DOGWOOD
West Indian Lemongrass .... see LEMONGRASS
Western Larch .... see LARCH ARABINOGALACTAN
Western Shisandra .... see SCHISANDRA
Western Yew .... see YEW
Westwood-Pear .... see PRICKLY PEAR CACTUS
Weyl Ash .... see GOUTWEED

WHEAT BRAN .... see WHEAT BRAN
Wheat Grass .... see WHEATGRASS
WHEATGRASS .... see WHEATGRASS
WHEY PROTEIN .... see WHEY PROTEIN
Whig Plant .... see ROMAN CHAMOMILE
White Archangel ... see WHITE DEAD NETTLE FLOWER
White Ash .... see ASH, GOUTWEED
White Baneberry .... see WHITE COHOSH
White Bay .... see MAGNOLIA bark
White Beeswax .... see BEESWAX
White Birch .... see BIRCH
White Bole .... see KAOLIN
White Bryony .... see BRYONIA
White Cedar .... see CEDAR leaf, CEDAR LEAF OIL
White Cinnamon .... see CANELLA
WHITE COHOSH .... see WHITE COHOSH
White Daisy .... see OX-EYE DAISY
WHITE DEAD NETTLE FLOWER
.... see WHITE DEAD NETTLE FLOWER
White Dragon Flower .... see ORRIS
White-Faced Hornet .... see BEE VENOM
White Fringe .... see FRINGETREE
White Gum .... see STORAX
WHITE HELLEBORE .... see WHITE HELLEBORE
WHITE HOREHOUND .... see WHITE HOREHOUND
White Laurel .... see MAGNOLIA bark
WHITE LILY .... see WHITE LILY
White Mulberry .... see BLACK MULBERRY
WHITE MUSTARD .... see WHITE MUSTARD
White Pepper
.... see BLACK PEPPER AND WHITE PEPPER
White Pond Lily .... see WHITE LILY
White Potato .... see POTATO
White Quebracho .... see QUEBRACHO
White Root .... see PLEURISY ROOT
White Rot .... see GOTU KOLA
White Sandalwood .... see WHITE SANDALWOOD oil,
.... WHITE SANDALWOOD wood
WHITE SANDALWOOD oil
.... see WHITE SANDALWOOD oil
WHITE SANDALWOOD wood
.... see WHITE SANDALWOOD wood
White Saunders .... see WHITE SANDALWOOD wood
White Saunders Oil .... see WHITE SANDALWOOD oil
WHITE SOAPWORT .... see WHITE SOAPWORT
White Sorrel .... see WOOD SORREL
White Spruce Oil .... see FIR NEEDLE OIL
White Squill .... see SQUILL
White Thyme Oil .... see THYME OIL
White Walnut .... see BUTTERNUT
White Wax .... see BEESWAX
White Waxtree .... see GLOSSY PRIVET
White Weed .... see OX-EYE DAISY
White Willow .... see WILLOW BARK
White Willow Bark .... see WILLOW BARK
White Wood .... see CANELLA
Whitehorn .... see HAWTHORN
Whitetube Stargrass .... see ALETRIS
Whole Adrenal Extract .... see ADRENAL EXTRACT
Whorlywort .... see BLACK ROOT
Whortleberry .... see BILBERRY dried ripe fruit,
.... BILBERRY leaf
Wickup .... see FIREWEED
Wicopy .... see FIREWEED
Wiesen-Feldkummel .... see CARAWAY dried fruit, seed

Wiesensauerampfer .... see SORREL
Wigandia californicum .... see YERBA SANTA
Wild Agrimony .... see POTENTILLA
Wild Angelica .... see ANGELICA root
Wild Balsam .... see JEWELWEED
Wild Bergamot .... see HORSEMINT
Wild Black Cherry .... see WILD CHERRY
Wild Boar Fruit .... see ROSE HIP
Wild Carrot .... see HEMLOCK,
                                                       WATER HEMLOCK
WILD CARROT .... see WILD CARROT
Wild Celandine .... see JEWELWEED
Wild Celery Root .... see OSHA
Wild Chamomile .... see GERMAN CHAMOMILE
WILD CHERRY .... see WILD CHERRY
Wild Chicory .... see CHICORY
Wild Cinnamon .... see CANELLA
Wild Clover .... see RED CLOVER
Wild Coleus .... see PERILLA
Wild Cotton .... see CANADIAN HEMP
Wild Crane's-Bill .... see HERB ROBERT
Wild Cucumber .... see BITTER MELON
Wild Cumin .... see CARAWAY OIL
Wild Curcuma .... see GOLDENSEAL
WILD DAISY .... see WILD DAISY
Wild Dill .... see WATER HEMLOCK
Wild Endive .... see DANDELION above ground parts
Wild Endive .... see DANDELION entire plant
Wild Fennel .... see FENNEL fruit, seed
Wild Garlic .... see BEAR'S GARLIC
Wild Gentian .... see GENTIAN
Wild Germander .... see GERMANDER
Wild Ginger .... see ASARABACCA
Wild Hops .... see BRYONIA
Wild Hydrangea .... see HYDRANGEA
Wild Ice Leaf .... see MULLEIN
WILD INDIGO .... see WILD INDIGO
Wild Iris .... see ORRIS
Wild Laburnum .... see SWEET CLOVER
Wild Lady's Slipper .... see JEWELWEED
Wild Lemon .... see PODOPHYLLUM
WILD LETTUCE .... see WILD LETTUCE
Wild Liquorice .... see SPINY RESTHARROW
Wild Mandrake .... see PODOPHYLLUM
Wild Marjoram .... see OREGANO
Wild Mexican Yam .... see WILD YAM
WILD MINT .... see WILD MINT
Wild Nard .... see ASARABACCA
Wild Nep .... see BRYONIA
Wild Oat Herb .... see OAT above ground parts
Wild Pansy .... see HEART'S EASE
Wild Parsnip .... see WATER HEMLOCK
Wild Passion Flower .... see PASSIONFLOWER
Wild Pea .... see LATHYRUS
Wild Pepper .... see GINSENG, SIBERIAN,
                                                       MEZEREON
Wild Pine .... see MORINDA
Wild Plum Flower .... see BLACKTHORN flower
WILD RADISH .... see WILD RADISH
Wild Red American Ginseng .... see CANAIGRE
Wild Red Desert Ginseng .... see CANAIGRE
Wild Rosemary .... see LABRADOR TEA
                                                       MARSH TEA
Wild Snowball .... see NEW JERSEY TEA
Wild Strawberry .... see STRAWBERRY

Wild Sunflower .... see ELECAMPANE
WILD THYME .... see WILD THYME
Wild Tobacco .... see LOBELIA
Wild Vanilla .... see DEERTONGUE
Wild Vine .... see BRYONIA
Wild Woodbine .... see AMERICAN IVY
Wild Woodvine .... see AMERICAN IVY
Wild Wormwood .... see MUGWORT
WILD YAM .... see WILD YAM
WILLARD WATER .... see WILLARD WATER
Williard's Water .... see WILLARD WATER
WILLOW BARK .... see WILLOW BARK
Willow Herb .... see FIREWEED
Willow Sage .... see PURPLE LOOSESTRIFE
Willowbark .... see WILLOW BARK
Willowherb .... see FIREWEED
Wind Flower .... see PULSATILLA,
                                                       WOOD ANEMONE
Wind Root .... see PLEURISY ROOT
WINE .... see WINE
Wine Grapes .... see GRAPE fruit, skin
Wineberry .... see BILBERRY dried ripe fruit,
                                                       BILBERRY leaf
Wingseed .... see WAFER ASH
Winter Bloom .... see WITCH HAZEL
Winter Cherry .... see ASHWAGANDHA,
                                                       WINTER CHERRY
Winter Clover .... see SQUAWVINE
Winter Marjoram .... see OREGANO
Winter Pink .... see TRAILING ARBUTUS
WINTER SAVORY .... see WINTER SAVORY
Wintera .... see WINTER'S BARK
Wintera Aromatica .... see WINTER'S BARK
Wintergreen .... see PERIWINKLE,
                                                       WINTERGREEN leaf,
                                                       WINTERGREEN oil
WINTERGREEN leaf .... see WINTERGREEN leaf
WINTERGREEN oil .... see WINTERGREEN oil
Winterlien .... see FLAXSEED
WINTER'S BARK .... see WINTER'S BARK
Winter's Cinnamon .... see WINTER'S BARK
Wintersweet .... see OREGANO
Wisconsin Ginseng .... see GINSENG, AMERICAN
Witch Grass .... see AGROPYRON
WITCH HAZEL .... see WITCH HAZEL
Witch Meal .... see CLUB MOSS
Witchazel .... see WITCH HAZEL
Witchen .... see MOUNTAIN ASH
Witches' Pouches .... see SHEPHERD'S PURSE
Witch's Bells .... see DIGITALIS
Withania .... see ASHWAGANDHA
Withania Somnifera .... see ASHWAGANDHA
Wogon .... see BAIKAL SKULLCAP
Wolfberry .... see LYCIUM
Wolfiporia Cocos .... see PORIA MUSHROOM
Wolf's Bane .... see ARNICA
Wolfs Claw .... see CLUB MOSS
Wolfsbane .... see ACONITE
Wolfstrapp .... see BUGLEWEED
Wolly Foxglove .... see DIGITALIS
Woman's Long Hair .... see USNEA
Wonder Bulb .... see AUTUMN CROCUS
Wonder Tree .... see CASTOR OIL, CASTOR seed
WOOD ANEMONE .... see WOOD ANEMONE
Wood Betony .... see BETONY

Wood Gum .... see LARCH ARABINOGALACTAN
Wood-Rose .... see HAWAIIAN BABY WOODROSE
WOOD SAGE .... see WOOD SAGE
Wood Sanicle .... see SANICLE
WOOD SORREL .... see WOOD SORREL
Wood Sour .... see WOOD SORREL
Wood Spider .... see DEVIL'S CLAW
Wood Strawberry .... see STRAWBERRY
Wood Sugar .... see LARCH ARABINOGALACTAN
Wood Vine .... see BRYONIA
Wood Waxen .... see DYER'S BROOM
Woodbind .... see ENGLISH IVY
Woodbine .... see GELSEMIUM,
HONEYSUCKLE
WOODBINE .... see WOODBINE
Woodruff .... see SWEET WOODRUFF
Woody .... see BITTERSWEET NIGHTSHADE
Woody Climber .... see AMERICAN IVY
Woody Nightshade .... see BITTERSWEET NIGHTSHADE
Woolen .... see MULLEIN
Woolly Morning Glory
.... see HAWAIIAN BABY WOODROSE
Woolly Parsnip .... see MASTERWORT
Woolly Thistle .... see SCOTCH THISTLE
Woolmat .... see HOUND'S TONGUE
Wordward .... see SWEET WOODRUFF
Worm Seed .... see WORMSEED
Wormgrass .... see PINK ROOT
WORMSEED .... see WORMSEED
Wormwood .... see WORMWOOD above ground parts,
WORMWOOD oil
WORMWOOD above ground parts
.... see WORMWOOD above ground parts
WORMWOOD oil .... see WORMWOOD oil
Wound Wort .... see YARROW
Woundwort .... see GOLDENROD, SELF-HEAL
WS 1442 .... see HAWTHORN
Wu-jia .... see GINSENG, SIBERIAN
Wu Jia Pi .... see GINSENG, SIBERIAN
Wu Wei Zi .... see SCHISANDRA
Wundkraut .... see ARNICA
Wurmkraut .... see WORMWOOD above ground parts
Wurzelstock .... see KAVA
Wuweizi .... see SCHISANDRA
Wymote .... see MARSHMALLOW
Xanthan .... see XANTHAN GUM
XANTHAN GUM .... see XANTHAN GUM
Xanthomonas campestris .... see XANTHAN GUM
Xanthophyll .... see LUTEIN
Xanthoxylum .... see NORTHERN PRICKLY ASH,
SOUTHERN PRICKLY ASH
Xian Ling Pi .... see EPIMEDIUM
Xianxao .... see JIAOGULAN
Xiwuweizi .... see SCHISANDRA
Xue Jie .... see DRAGON'S BLOOD
Xue Zhi Kang .... see RED YEAST
Xylit .... see XYLITOL
Xylite .... see XYLITOL
XYLITOL .... see XYLITOL
xylo-pentane-1,2,3,4,5-pentol .... see XYLITOL
Xysmalobium undulatum .... see UZARA
Yagona .... see KAVA
Yam .... see WILD YAM
YARROW .... see YARROW

Yavani .... see BISHOP'S WEED
Yaw Root .... see QUEEN'S DELIGHT
Yeast-Derived Beta Glucan .... see BETA GLUCANS
Yege .... see KUDZU
Yellow Astringent .... see EPHEDRA
Yellow Bark .... see CASCARA
Yellow Beeswax .... see BEESWAX
Yellow Beet .... see BEET
Yellow Broom .... see WILD INDIGO
Yellow Bugle .... see GROUND PINE
Yellow Chaste Weed .... see IMMORTELLE,
SANDY EVERLASTING
Yellow Cleavers .... see LADY'S BEDSTRAW
YELLOW DOCK .... see YELLOW DOCK
Yellow Flag .... see ORRIS
Yellow Galium .... see LADY'S BEDSTRAW
Yellow Gentian .... see GENTIAN
Yellow Ginseng .... see BLUE COHOSH
Yellow Hornet .... see BEE VENOM
Yellow Horse .... see EPHEDRA
Yellow Indian Paint .... see GOLDENSEAL
Yellow Indigo .... see WILD INDIGO
Yellow Iris .... see ORRIS
Yellow-Jacket Venom .... see BEE VENOM
Yellow Jasmine .... see GELSEMIUM
Yellow Jessamine Root .... see GELSEMIUM
YELLOW LUPIN .... see YELLOW LUPIN
Yellow Melilot .... see SWEET CLOVER
Yellow Oleander .... see OLEANDER
Yellow Paint .... see GOLDENSEAL
Yellow Pheasant's Eye .... see PHEASANT'S EYE
Yellow Puccoon .... see GOLDENSEAL
Yellow Rod .... see YELLOW TOADFLAX
Yellow Root .... see GOLDENSEAL
Yellow Sandalwood ..... see WHITE SANDALWOOD wood
Yellow Sandalwood Oil ... see WHITE SANDALWOOD oil
Yellow Saunders .... see WHITE SANDALWOOD wood
Yellow Saunders Oil .... see WHITE SANDALWOOD oil
Yellow Snakeleaf ..... see AMERICAN ADDER'S TONGUE
Yellow Snowdrop .... see AMERICAN ADDER'S TONGUE
Yellow Starwort .... see ELECAMPANE
Yellow Sweet Clover .... see SWEET CLOVER
YELLOW TOADFLAX .... see YELLOW TOADFLAX
Yellow Vine .... see THUNDER GOD VINE
Yellow Water Dropwort
.... see HEMLOCK WATER DROPWORT
Yellow Wax .... see BEESWAX
Yellow Willowherb .... see LOOSESTRIFE
Yellow Wood .... see NORTHERN PRICKLY ASH
Yellowdock .... see YELLOW DOCK
Yellowroot .... see GOLDTHREAD
Yellows .... see BUTTERCUP,
NERVE ROOT
Yellowweed .... see BUTTERCUP
Yemen Myrrh .... see MYRRH
Yerba buena .... see SPEARMINT
Yerba de Maria .... see DIVINER'S SAGE
Yerba Dulce .... see STEVIA
YERBA MANSA .... see YERBA MANSA
Yerba Manza .... see YERBA MANSA
Yerba Mate .... see MATE
Yerba Maté .... see MATE
YERBA SANTA .... see YERBA SANTA
YEW .... see YEW

YIN CHEN .... see YIN CHEN
Yin Ch'en .... see YIN CHEN
Yin Chen Hao .... see YIN CHEN
Yin Yang Huo .... see EPIMEDIUM
Yinhsing .... see GINKGO leaf (GINKGO leaf extract),
                                                GINKGO seed
Ylang Ylang .... see YLANG YLANG OIL
YLANG YLANG OIL .... see YLANG YLANG OIL
Yoghurt .... see YOGURT
YOGURT .... see YOGURT
YOHIMBE .... see YOHIMBE
Yohimbehe .... see YOHIMBE
Yohimbehe cortex .... see YOHIMBE
Youthwort .... see MASTERWORT, SUNDEW
YUCCA .... see YUCCA
Yucca aloifolia .... see YUCCA
Yucca arborescens .... see YUCCA
Yucca brevifolia .... see YUCCA
Yucca filamentosa .... see ADAM'S NEEDLE, YUCCA
Yucca glauca .... see YUCCA
Yucca mohavensis .... see YUCCA
Yucca schidigera .... see YUCCA
Yucca whipplei .... see YUCCA
Yuma .... see WILD YAM
Yun-Zhi (cloud mushroom)
     .... see CORIOLUS MUSHROOM
Zacate Violeta .... see VETIVER
Zaffer .... see SAFFLOWER
Zafran .... see SAFFLOWER
Zanthoxylum .... see NORTHERN PRICKLY ASH,
                                        SOUTHERN PRICKLY ASH
Zamericanum .... see NORTHERN PRICKLY ASH
Zanthoxylum clava-herculis
     .... see SOUTHERN PRICKLY ASH
Zanzibar Pepper .... see CAPSICUM
Zao .... see JUJUBE
Zapote .... see CHICLE
Zapotillo .... see CHICLE
Zea .... see CORN SILK
Zea mays .... see CORN SILK
Zeaxanthin .... see LUTEIN
Zedoaire .... see ZEDOARY
Zedoária .... see ZEDOARY
Zedoarie rhizoma .... see ZEDOARY
ZEDOARY .... see ZEDOARY
Zhi Qiao .... see BITTER ORANGE
Zi Shi .... see BITTER ORANGE
Zhi Tai .... see RED YEAST
Zhihe Shou Wu .... see FO-TI
Zhong Mahuang .... see EPHEDRA
Zi Shou Wu .... see FO-TI
Zibeth .... see CIVET
Zimbluten .... see CINNAMON flower
Zimbro .... see JUNIPER
ZINC .... see ZINC
Zinc Acetate .... see ZINC
Zinc Acexamate .... see ZINC
Zinc Aspartate .... see ZINC
Zinc Citrate .... see ZINC
Zinc Gluconate .... see ZINC
Zinc Methionine .... see ZINC
Zinc Monomethionine .... see ZINC
Zinc Oxide .... see ZINC
Zinc Picolinate .... see ZINC

Zinc Sulfate .... see ZINC
Zingiber Officinale .... see GINGER
Zingiberis rhizoma .... see GINGER
Zi Shou Wu .... see FO-TI
Zitwer .... see ZEDOARY
Zitwerwirtzelstock .... see ZEDOARY
Zizyphus .... see JUJUBE
Zn .... see ZINC
Zoom .... see GUARANA
Zyzyphus jujube .... see JUJUBE

INDEX

"*Tell the Editors...*"

This Database is constantly evolving. Our research and editorial team analyzes new studies every day and makes updates to the Web version of this Database every day. We view our work as similar to a clearing house of information on natural medicines. If you spot a statement that needs to be changed, or updated, you can use this form, or a copy of it, to communicate directly with the editors. Feel free to mail, email, or fax. *We appreciate your help!*

1. What part of the Database are you commenting about?

Page # _____   Section _____

2. What wording should be added?

Please be specific about exact wording that you propose adding. Use additional pages if needed.

_____

_____

_____

_____

3. What wording should be deleted?

Please tell us which words you think should be removed.

_____

_____

_____

4. What reference citations support this change?

Please give us specific reference citations. We base entries into this Database on reliable studies published in peer-reviewed professional literature. Please give us enough information so that we can find the reference.

_____

_____

5. How can we contact you?

Name _____

Address _____

Phone _____   Email _____

Please send this information to:

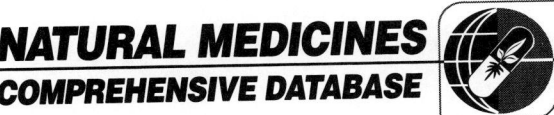

3120 W. March Lane
P.O. Box 8190, Stockton CA 95208
Phone: (209) 472-2244
Fax: (209) 472-2249
Email: Mail@NaturalDatabase.com
www.NaturalDatabase.com

"Tell the Editors..."

This Database is constantly evolving. Our research and editorial team analyzes new studies every day and makes updates to the Web version of this Database every day. We view our work as similar to a clearing house of information on natural medicines. If you spot a statement that needs to be changed, or updated, you can use this form, or a copy of it, to communicate directly with the editors. Feel free to mail, email, or fax. *We appreciate your help!*

1. What part of the Database are you commenting about?

Page # _____ Section _____

2. What wording should be added?

Please be specific about exact wording that you propose adding. Use additional pages if needed.

_____
_____
_____
_____

3. What wording should be deleted?

Please tell us which words you think should be removed.

_____
_____
_____

4. What reference citations support this change?

Please give us specific reference citations. We base entries into this Database on reliable studies published in peer-reviewed professional literature. Please give us enough information so that we can find the reference.

_____
_____

5. How can we contact you?

Name _____
Address _____
Phone _____ Email _____

Please send this information to:

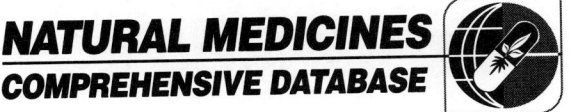

3120 W. March Lane
P.O. Box 8190, Stockton CA 95208
Phone: (209) 472-2244
Fax: (209) 472-2249
Email: Mail@NaturalDatabase.com
www.NaturalDatabase.com

PATIENT VERSION
available for licensure

There is a *Patient Version* of Natural Medicines Comprehensive Database for health care organizations to make available for their consumers and patients via the Web.

The *Patient Version* is huge and very patient-friendly. Most importantly it gives your patients highly reliable information.

Our editors update the *Patient Version* right along with the professional version. And the two versions go hand-in-hand.

The information in each is consistent. Medical professionals use the professional version of the Database and patients use the *Patient Version*.

Patients who use the *Patient Version* can find all the thousands upon thousands of product names just like in the professional version. Patients will be thrilled to see that they have the power to find info on thousands of products.

The information is written to make sense for consumers.

The *Patient Version* is for organizations who want their consumers to get the very best information. This is a powerful, comprehensive, useful resource.

We will be happy to provide interested organizations with a personalized demo site for you to explore, along with pricing information.

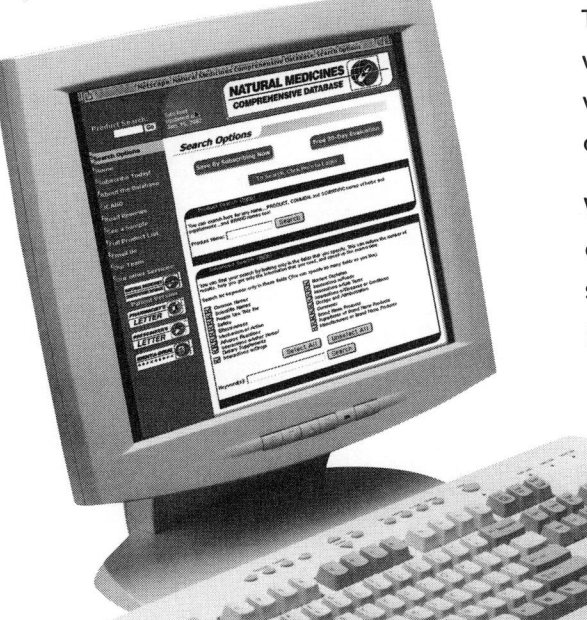

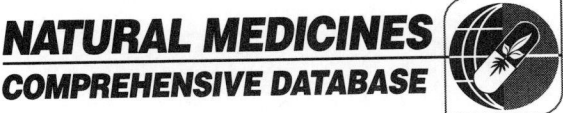

ORDER ADDITIONAL COPIES

☐ **New Order**

    ☐ Book .... $92 ($158 CAN)
    ☐ One year access to *www.NaturalDatabase.com* .... $92 per year ($158 CAN)
    ☐ Combination .... $132 ($198 CAN)
    (Book PLUS one year personal access to *www.NaturalDatabase.com*)

☐ **Extend existing subscription**

    ☐ Send me a new edition of the Book when it is published .... $92 ($158 CAN)
    ☐ Add one year to my access to *www.NaturalDatabase.com* .. $92 per year ($158 CAN)
    ☐ Combination .... $132 ($198 CAN)
    (Next edition of the Book PLUS one year access to *www.NaturalDatabase.com*)

☐ **I want Continuing Education credits. Send me the next two (2) CE booklets**
    Four (4) credits each booklet.

    If current subscriber, two (2) booklets are .... $19 ($32.60 CAN)
    If not current subscriber, two (2) booklets are .... $75 ($116.30 CAN)

    Please indicate your profession so we can send you the Booklets that are accredited for you
    ☐ Physician   ☐ Pharmacist   ☐ Nurse Practitioner
    ☐ Physician Assistant   ☐ Dietitian

    If you purchase Natural Medicines Comprehensive Database book, please add the following:

In California, add 7.75% sales tax .... $ _____
Shipping inside U.S. .... FREE
Shipping in Canada .... $19 CAN
Shipping outside of North America .... $18 US

                            TOTAL .... $ _____

Name _____ Degree _____ Member # *(optional)* _____

Address _____

City _____ State/Province _____ Zip Code _____

Phone _____ Email _____

☐ Bill my business or institution with this Purchase Order # _____

☐ Payment enclosed *(please make checks payable to Natural Database).*

☐ Charge my VISA, MasterCard, American Express, or Discover Card.

    Card No. _____ Exp. Date _____

Send or fax this order form to:

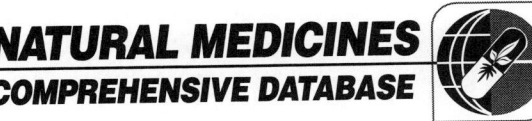

3120 W. March Lane
P.O. Box 8190, Stockton CA 95208
For fastest service call:
(209) 472-2244 fax (209) 472-2249
Email: Mail@NaturalDatabase.com
Order online: www.NaturalDatabase.com

GET *Continuing Education* CREDITS

Accredited for physicians, pharmacists, nurse practitioners, physician assistants and dietitians.

You can earn Continuing Education credits from this *Natural Medicines Comprehensive Database*. When you sign up for CE or CME, you get your first booklet right away, then a new booklet every six months. Each booklet gives you four (4) credits.

Please indicate your profession so we can send you the booklets that are accredited for you:

☐ Physician   ☐ Pharmacist   ☐ Nurse Practitioner

☐ Physician Assistant   ☐ Dietitian

Please select booklet(s) you would like to receive:

Booklet	Qty	Price †
☐ The next two (2) booklets in the series. A new CE booklet is released each Spring and Fall.		
☐ **#02002** – Natural Medicines in the Clinical Management of Osteoarthritis, Obesity, Chronic Fatigue Syndrome, and Eye Disorders.		
☐ **#01004** – Natural Medicines in the Clinical Management of Breast Cancer, HIV/AIDS, Anxiety, and Irritable Bowel Syndrome.		
☐ **#01002** – Natural Medicines in the Clinical Management of Colon Cancer Prevention, Premenstrual Syndrome, Congestive Heart Failure and Fibromyalgia.		
☐ **#00004** – Natural Medicines in the Clinical Management of Colds and Flu, Insomnia, Aging Skin and Urinary Tract Disorders.		
☐ **#00002** – Natural Medicines in the Clinical Management of Alzheimer's Disease, Diabetes and Men's Health.		
TOTALS:		$

† If you have a current version of *Natural Medicines Comprehensive Database* book or current access to the Web version, the price per booklet is **$9.50 ($16.30 CAN)**. If you DON'T have the Book or current access to the Web version, the price per booklet is **$37.50 ($58.15 CAN)**.

Name _____ Degree _____ Member # _____

Address _____

City _____ State/Province _____ Zip Code _____

Phone _____ Email _____

☐ Bill my business or institution with this Purchase Order # _____

☐ Payment enclosed *(please make checks payable to Natural Database).*

☐ Charge my VISA, MasterCard, American Express, or Discover Card.

     Card No. _____ Exp. Date _____

*PHYSICIANS: Prescriber's Letter is accredited by the Accreditation Council for Continuing Medical Education (ACCME) to provide continuing medical education for physicians. Prescriber's Letter designates each Booklet for up to 4 hours in category 1 credit towards the AMA Physician's Recognition Award. Each physician should claim only those hours of credit that he/she actually spent in the educational activity.
PHARMACISTS: Prescriber's Letter is accredited by the American Council on Pharmaceutical Education as a provider of continuing pharmaceutical education.
NURSE PRACTITIONERS: The individual Booklets in the series have been granted 4.0 pharmacology contact hours of continuing education by the American Academy of Nurse Practitioners.
PHYSICIAN ASSISTANTS: The American Academy of Physician Assistants accepts AMA category 1 CME credit for the Physician's Recognition Award from organizations accredited by the ACCME. Prescriber's Letter is accredited by ACCME.
DIETITIANS: Pharmacist's Letter/Prescriber's Letter is a Continuing Professional Education (CPE) Accredited Provider with the Commission on Dietetic Registration (CDR).

Send or fax this order form to:

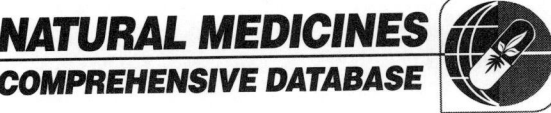

NATURAL MEDICINES
COMPREHENSIVE DATABASE

3120 W. March Lane
P.O. Box 8190, Stockton CA 95208
For fastest service call:
(209) 472-2244 fax (209) 472-2249
Email: Mail@NaturalDatabase.com
Order online: www.NaturalDatabase.com

GET *Continuing Education* CREDITS

Accredited for physicians, pharmacists, nurse practitioners, physician assistants and dietitians.

You can earn Continuing Education credits from this *Natural Medicines Comprehensive Database*. When you sign up for CE or CME, you get your first booklet right away, then a new booklet every six months. Each booklet gives you four (4) credits.

Please indicate your profession so we can send you the booklets that are accredited for you:

☐ Physician   ☐ Pharmacist   ☐ Nurse Practitioner

☐ Physician Assistant   ☐ Dietitian

Please select booklet(s) you would like to receive:

Booklet	Qty	Price †
☐ The next two (2) booklets in the series. A new CE booklet is released each Spring and Fall.		
☐ **#02002** – Natural Medicines in the Clinical Management of Osteoarthritis, Obesity, Chronic Fatigue Syndrome, and Eye Disorders.		
☐ **#01004** – Natural Medicines in the Clinical Management of Breast Cancer, HIV/AIDS, Anxiety, and Irritable Bowel Syndrome.		
☐ **#01002** – Natural Medicines in the Clinical Management of Colon Cancer Prevention, Premenstrual Syndrome, Congestive Heart Failure and Fibromyalgia.		
☐ **#00004** – Natural Medicines in the Clinical Management of Colds and Flu, Insomnia, Aging Skin and Urinary Tract Disorders.		
☐ **#00002** – Natural Medicines in the Clinical Management of Alzheimer's Disease, Diabetes and Men's Health.		
TOTALS:		$

† If you have a current version of *Natural Medicines Comprehensive Database* book or current access to the Web version, the price per booklet is **$9.50 ($16.30 CAN)**. If you DON'T have the Book or current access to the Web version, the price per booklet is **$37.50 ($58.15 CAN)**.

Name _____ Degree _____ Member # _____

Address _____

City _____ State/Province _____ Zip Code _____

Phone _____ Email _____

☐ Bill my business or institution with this Purchase Order # _____

☐ Payment enclosed *(please make checks payable to Natural Database).*

☐ Charge my VISA, MasterCard, American Express, or Discover Card.

Card No. _____ Exp. Date _____

*PHYSICIANS: Prescriber's Letter is accredited by the Accreditation Council for Continuing Medical Education (ACCME) to provide continuing medical education for physicians. Prescriber's Letter designates each Booklet for up to 4 hours in category 1 credit towards the AMA Physician's Recognition Award. Each physician should claim only those hours of credit that he/she actually spent in the educational activity.
PHARMACISTS: Pharmacist's Letter is accredited by the American Council on Pharmaceutical Education as a provider of continuing pharmaceutical education.
NURSE PRACTITIONERS: The individual Booklets in the series have been granted 4.0 pharmacology contact hours of continuing education by the American Academy of Nurse Practitioners.
PHYSICIAN ASSISTANTS: The American Academy of Physician Assistants accepts AMA category 1 CME credit for the Physician's Recognition Award from organizations accredited by the ACCME. Prescriber's Letter is accredited by ACCME.
DIETITIANS: Pharmacist's Letter/Prescriber's Letter is a Continuing Professional Education (CPE) Accredited Provider with the Commission on Dietetic Registration (CDR).

Send or fax this order form to:

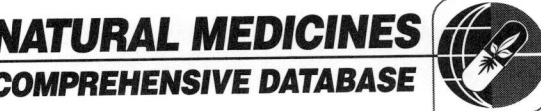

NATURAL MEDICINES
COMPREHENSIVE DATABASE

3120 W. March Lane
P.O. Box 8190, Stockton CA 95208
For fastest service call:
(209) 472-2244 fax (209) 472-2249
Email: Mail@NaturalDatabase.com
Order online: www.NaturalDatabase.com

SIGN UP FOR ACCESS TO
www.NaturalDatabase.com

This book version of *Natural Medicines Comprehensive Database* was current the day it was printed. But there is a huge amount of information coming out all the time, and we analyze the information and **update the Web version of the Database every day.** You can purchase access to this Database at *www.NaturalDatabase.com.*

NaturalDatabase.com gives you everything that is in this book version plus lots more. We are constantly adding **more brand name products.** The site also does **terrific searches** for you. You can have it search for interactions, uses, names, side effects, and many other criteria. You can even have the site help you **find products** or names for which you don't know the correct spelling. For each ingredient, you can click to see which brand name products contain it. For each monograph, you can click to see all the **references** used to compile the monograph, plus you can click on thousands of reference citations and read the **original journal abstract.** You can also post questions and comments, and **interact with the editors** and health professionals around the world.

You can also **get continuing education credits** fully accredited for pharmacists, MDs, DOs, PAs, NPs, and RDs.

A huge feature in *www.NaturalDatabase.com* is **Patient Education Handouts.** By using the Web site, you can click and print a Patient Education Handout for any product anytime you need. If you are part of a large organization, you can also arrange to have your name and logo included on these Patient Handout Sheets.

You can sign up for a complete access to *www.NaturalDatabase.com* as an **individual,** or get a **site license** for your organization.

☐   **YES,** please send me a personal access code so I can use *www.NaturalDatabase.com*

☐   Payment enclosed, $92 ($158 CAN) per year (payable to Natural Database).

☐   Please charge my VISA, MasterCard, American Express, or Discover Card.

    Card No. _____   Exp. Date _____

☐   Bill my business or institution with this Purchase Order # _____

☐   Contact me to arrange for a site license for my whole organization.

Name _____

Address _____

City _____   State/Province _____ Zip/Postal Code _____

Phone _____   Email _____

If you currently are a subscriber, please write **your member number:** _____

Send or fax this order form to:

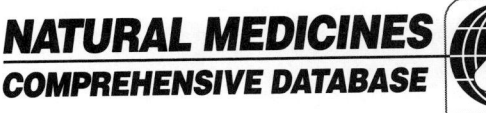

NATURAL MEDICINES
COMPREHENSIVE DATABASE

3120 W. March Lane
P.O. Box 8190, Stockton CA 95208
For fastest service call:
(209) 472-2244 fax (209) 472-2249
Email: Mail@NaturalDatabase.com
Order online: www.NaturalDatabase.com